# MEDICAL-SURGICAL NURSING

## Critical Thinking in Client Care

### THIRD EDITION

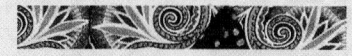

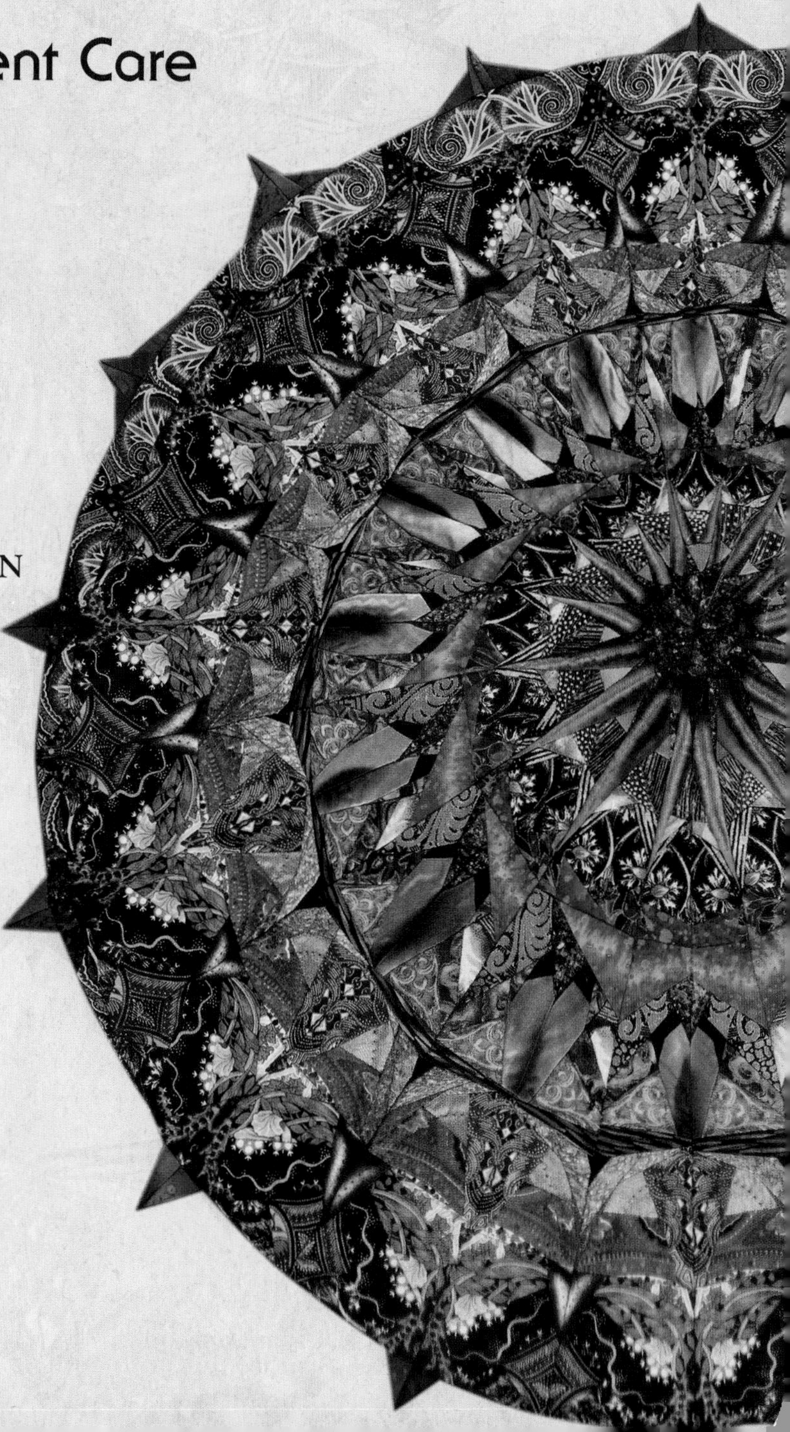

**PRISCILLA LEMONE**, RN, DSN
*Sinclair School of Nursing*
*University of Missouri—Columbia*
*Columbia, Missouri*

**KAREN BURKE**, RN, MS
*Clatsop Community College*
*Astoria, Oregon*

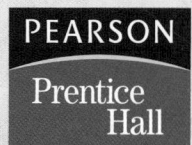

PEARSON

Prentice Hall

Upper Saddle River, New Jersey 07458

**Library of Congress Cataloging-in-Publication Data**

Medical-surgical nursing: critical thinking in client care/[edited by] Priscilla LeMone,
  Karen M. Burke.—3rd ed.
    p.; cm.
  Includes bibliographical references and index.
  ISBN 0-13-099075-2
  1. Nursing. 2. Surgical nursing. 3. Critical thinking. I. LeMone, Priscilla. II. Burke, Karen M.
  [DNLM: 1. Nursing Process. 2. Nursing Care. 3. Patient Care Planning. 4. Perioperative
  Nursing. WY 100 M4892 2004]
  RT41.M493 2004
  610.73'677—dc21                                                    2003043857

**Publisher:** Julie Levin Alexander
**Executive Assistant & Supervisor:** Regina Bruno
**Editor-in-Chief:** Maura Connor
**Senior Acquisitions Editor:** Nancy Anselment
**Development Editor:** Kim Wyatt
**Managing Development Editor:** Marilyn Meserve
**Editorial Assistant:** Malgorzata Jaros-White
**Managing Editor:** Patrick Walsh
**Production Liaison:** Cathy O'Connell
**Director of Manufacturing and Production:** Bruce Johnson
**Manufacturing Buyer:** Pat Brown
**Production Editor:** Amy Gehl, Carlisle Publishers Services
**Design Director:** Cheryl Asherman
**Senior Design Coordinator:** Maria Guglielmo Walsh
**Cover Designer:** Cheryl Asherman
**Interior Designer:** Janice Bielawa
**Senior Marketing Manager:** Nicole Benson
**Channel Marketing Manager:** Rachel Strober
**Marketing Coordinator:** Janet Ryerson
**Supplements Editor:** Sladjana Repic
**Media Editor:** John Jordan
**Media Production Manager:** Amy Peltier
**Media Project Manager:** Stephen Hartner
**Composition:** Carlisle, Inc.
**Printer/Binder:** RR Donnelley, Willard
**Cover Printer:** Phoenix Color Corp.

Cover and interior illustrations from Kaleidoscope XVIII: Chai by Paula Nadelstern,
as seen in *Kaleidoscope Artistry* by Cozy Baker.

**Notice:** Care has been taken to confirm the accuracy of information presented in this book. The authors, editors, and the publisher, however, cannot accept any responsibility for errors or omissions or for consequences from application of the information in this book and make no warranty, express or implied, with respect to its contents. The authors and publisher have exerted every effort to ensure that drug selections and dosages set forth in this text are in accord with current recommendations and practice at time of publication. However, in view of ongoing research, changes in government regulations, and the constant flow of information relating to drug therapy and drug reactions, the reader is urged to check the package inserts of all drugs for any change in indications of dosage and for added warnings and precautions. This is particularly important when the recommended agent is a new and/or infrequently employed drug.

Pearson Education LTD.
Pearson Education Australia PTY, Limited
Pearson Education Singapore, Pte. Ltd
Pearson Education North Asia Ltd
Pearson Education Canada, Ltd.

Pearson Educación de Mexico, S.A. de C.V.
Pearson Education—Japan
Pearson Education Malaysia, Pte. Ltd
Pearson Education, Upper Saddle River, NJ

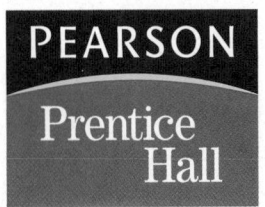

10 9 8 7 6 5 4 3 2
ISBN 0-13-099075-2

*I dedicate this book to the people I love.*
   *Priscilla LeMone*

*To my husband and best friend, Steve, who never waivers in his
love and support; our daughter, Kristin, who makes me unbelievably
proud and awestruck; and our son, Nathan, whose spirit, humor,
and incredible courage will always be with us.*
   *Karen Burke*

# DETAILED CONTENTS

## Unit 7
## Responses to Altered Urinary Elimination   693

**Chapter 25**
**Assessing Clients with Urinary System
    Disorders   694**

## Unit 9
## Responses to Altered Peripheral Tissue Perfusion 917

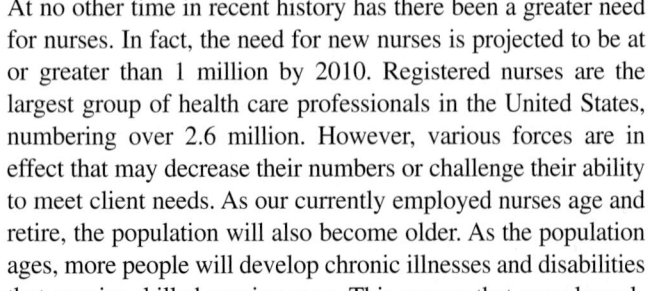

At no other time in recent history has there been a greater need for nurses. In fact, the need for new nurses is projected to be at or greater than 1 million by 2010. Registered nurses are the largest group of health care professionals in the United States, numbering over 2.6 million. However, various forces are in effect that may decrease their numbers or challenge their ability to meet client needs. As our currently employed nurses age and retire, the population will also become older. As the population ages, more people will develop chronic illnesses and disabilities that require skilled nursing care. This means that your knowledge and skills will be in demand to meet health care needs well into the future.

Students are expected to build on a knowledge foundation of basic sciences, social sciences, and fundamentals of nursing to synthesize and critically analyze new knowledge necessary to provide holistic care that addresses the individualized human responses to potential or actual alterations in health. The third edition of *Medical-Surgical Nursing: Critical Thinking in Client Care* has been completely revised to provide you with that knowledge and the skills needed to care for clients to promote health, facilitate recovery from illness and injury, and provide support when coping with disability or grieving.

The kaleidoscope cover image is a strong reflection of health care today. The meditative aspect of focusing on the images in the kaleidoscope calms and helps to integrate the mind, spirit, and body. As with nursing care, healing benefits are discovered through various complementary and alternative therapy methods. Nursing care, like the kaleidoscope, is the integration of mind-body-spirit.

## GOALS FOR THIS TEXTBOOK

Although the information has been totally updated, we continue to believe that students learn best within a nursing model of care with consistent organization and understandable text. From the first edition, we have held fast to our vision that this textbook will:

- Provide the most current information possible about the art and science of nursing.

- Provide clear explanations of the pathophysiologic processes of human illnesses and injury, integrating that information as a vital component of treatment and nursing care.

- Emphasize the nurse's role as an essential member of the health care team.

- Prioritize nursing diagnoses and interventions specific to altered responses to illness.

- Provide case studies for each major illness or injury so students can envision the client as a person requiring care.

- Foster critical thinking and decision-making skills in clinical practice.

## NEW TO THIS EDITION

The third edition of this textbook includes new content on cultural diversity that is integrated throughout the narrative as well as incorporated into the following feature boxes: Focus on Diversity, Nursing Care of the Older Adult, Meeting Individualized Needs, Nursing Research, and Multisystem Effects. Additionally, new content covers health promotion, gerontology, complementary and alternative therapies, genetics, and diseases specific to bioterrorism. The new health-promotion heads can be found in the nursing care section in every disorder chapter. Complementary and alternative therapies are integrated throughout the textbook where appropriate. Genetics as a risk factor or that increases incidence of a disease is included with the disorders, such as Huntington's chorea, Von Willebrand's disease, sickle cell disease, and hemophilia. Diseases are included if more prevalent as the result of inheritance (such as diabetes). Genetic counseling is included in nursing care as appropriate. Information about infections that may be caused by bioterrorism is included in Chapter 8. Based on reviewer feedback, two new chapters have been added: Chapter 12 concerns care of clients with substance abuse and Chapter 39 deals with care of clients with musculoskeletal disorders (two separate chapters in the previous edition). This combined chapter is more consistent and easier for students to follow.

## ORGANIZATION

The book has six major parts, organized by functional health patterns. Each part opens with a concept map illustrating the relationship of each functional health pattern to possible nursing diagnoses. The parts are then divided into units based on alterations in human structure and function. Each unit with a focus on altered health states opens with an assessment chapter that provides a review of normal anatomy and physiology, questions for a health history, and assessment techniques with possible abnormal findings. Students will find a detailed health history questionnaire, using functional health patterns as a guide, on the Companion Website. Also on the CD, students will find a comprehensive review of anatomy and physiology complete with animations, three-dimensional structures, and exercises. This draws upon the student's prerequisite knowledge, and serves to reinforce basic principles of anatomy and physiology as applied to physical assessment.

Following the assessment chapter in each unit, information about major conditions and diseases follows a consistent chapter format. Key components of the clinical chapters include the following:

***PATHOPHYSIOLOGY.*** The discussion of each major illness or condition begins with an overview of pathophysiology, followed by manifestations and complications. In the new edition, we have increased coverage of pathophysiology and highlighted it as a section within the disease. A new feature, Focus on Diversity, is included with some disorders to demonstrate, for example, how race, age, and gender affect differences in incidence, prevalence, and mortality.

*COLLABORATIVE CARE.* Collaborative care considers the treatment of the illness or condition by the health care team. Information in this section includes, as appropriate, diagnostic tests, medications, surgery and treatments, fluid management, dietary management, and complementary therapies.

*NURSING CARE.* Because the prevention of illness is a critical factor in health care today, this section begins with health-promotion information. A brief section on assessment provides a focused health history interview and physical examination guides, as well as information about assessment of the older adult. Nursing care is discussed within a context of priority nursing diagnoses and interventions, with rationales provided for each intervention. As care is increasingly provided in the home, nursing care is followed by a list of topics and resources for teaching about home care. Lastly, for each major disorder or condition, a narrative Nursing Care Plan is provided. Each plan begins with a brief case study, followed by the steps of the nursing process in action. Critical thinking questions specific to the care plan conclude this part, with a section called Evaluate Your Response that provides additional guidance for critical thinking. Suggested guidelines are found in Appendix C.

*CHAPTER REVIEW.* This new section at the end of each chapter concludes with five multiple-choice review questions, to reinforce comprehension of the chapter content. The student will also find the section entitled EXPLORE MediaLink, which encourages students to use the CD-ROM and the Companion Website to apply what they have learned from the textbook in case studies, to practice NCLEX questions, and to use additional resources such as animation tutorials and more.

## HALLMARK FEATURES

Thoughtful attention was given to existing features that students and faculty liked in the previous edition. We give them more emphasis in the new edition.

- **Manifestations** boxes reinforce understanding of the effects of illness or injury, and guide assessments and interventions.
- **Pathophysiology Illustrated** and **Multisystem Effects** features provide visual illustrations of the causes and consequences of pathophysiology.
- **Nursing Implications** boxes provide students with nursing implications that they need to be aware of when their client is undergoing a particular diagnostic test. These boxes address nursing care and client/family teaching.
- **Meeting Individualized Needs** boxes contain information specific to altered health, age, gender, race, and culture.

- **Procedure** boxes describe common or important procedures in detail.
- **Nursing Care of the Client** boxes describe nursing care for various medical or surgical procedures.

## NEW FEATURES

In addition to the hallmark features that have made this textbook so popular with students and faculty, we provide new items that help students learn the concepts in this textbook, apply them in clinical settings, and hone their clinical judgment skills. These include the following:

- **MediaLink,** at the beginning of each chapter, lists specific content, animations, anatomy and physiology review, NCLEX review questions, tools, and other interactive exercises that appear on the accompanying student CD-ROM and the Companion Website. Special MediaLink tabs appear throughout the chapter in the margins, encouraging the students to use the media supplements for specific activities, applications, and resources. The purpose of the MediaLink feature is to further enhance the student experience, build on knowledge gained from the textbook, prepare students for NCLEX, and foster critical thinking.
- **Medication Administration** boxes provide examples of drugs commonly prescribed for specific illnesses, followed by nursing responsibilities and client/family teaching. The medication boxes reflect the role of nurses, who administer medications.
- **Focus on Diversity** boxes list incidence, prevalence, etiology, and more for a particular disorder as effected by race or ethnicity.
- **Nursing Care of the Older Adult** boxes are found throughout the text, as well as in the assessment sections for disorders. As the population continues to age, this is critical information for nursing care in any setting, and provides guidelines for assessing and teaching in home care for the elderly.
- **Nursing Care Plans** throughout the text help students approach care from a nursing process perspective. The care plan is followed by critical thinking questions for students to apply their knowledge to a plan of care for a specific client. Suggested responses to the critical thinking questions can be found in Appendix C. Additional care plan activities can be found on the Companion Website at www.prenhall.com/lemone. These activities provide students with client scenarios so they can write comprehensive care plans and email them to instructors as homework assignments.
- **NANDA, NIC, and NOC** charts illustrate the most up-to-date information on nursing language, and demonstrate how these items are related for specific disorders.
- **Nursing Research: Evidence-Based Practice** boxes are included to show how nursing research is used to provide rationales for nursing care.
- **Practice Alerts** are integrated into nursing care purposefully to help students consider all aspects of nursing even

though they may be focusing on only one aspect of client needs.

- **End of Chapter Review Section** provides students with an opportunity to evaluate their comprehension of the chapter. The student-friendly section includes:

- **Test Yourself**—Review questions at the end of every chapter.

- **EXPLORE MediaLink**—at the end of every chapter, encourages students to use the CD-ROM and Companion Website to apply their knowledge of the chapter through additional case studies, practice NCLEX questions, A&P review, animation tutorials, and additional resources.

## COMPREHENSIVE TEACHING-LEARNING PACKAGE

### Clinical Handbook ISBN: 0-13-048397-4

Serves as a portable, quick reference to medical-surgical nursing. Organized alphabetizing provides a succinct review of common disorders and conditions, including pathophysiology, nursing diagnoses, interventions, client teaching, and home care. This handbook will allow students to bring the information they learn from class into any clinical setting.

### Study Guide ISBN: 0-13-113666-6

Provides anatomy and physiology review, study tips, review exercises, case studies, care plan activities, NCLEX review, and more. MediaLinks refer students to activities on the CD-ROM and Companion Website.

### Student CD-ROM

Packaged *free* with the textbook, the student CD-ROM provides an interactive study program that allows students to practice answering NCLEX-style questions with rationales for right and wrong answers. It also contains an audio glossary, animations, anatomy and physiology review, and a link to the Companion Website (an Internet connection is required).

### Companion Website

A *free* online study guide is designed to help students apply the concepts presented in the book. Each chapter-specific module features objectives, audio glossary, chapter summary for lecture notes, NCLEX review questions, case studies, care plan activities, MediaLink applications, WebLinks, and nursing tools, such as functional health pattern concept maps, assessment guides, and more.

## SUPPLEMENTS AND NEW MEDIA FOR INSTRUCTORS

### Instructor's Resource Manual ISBN: 0-13-143234-6

This manual contains a wealth of material to help faculty plan and manage the medical-surgical nursing course. It includes chapter overviews, detailed lecture suggestions and outlines, learning objectives, a complete test bank, answers to the textbook critical thinking exercises, teaching tips, and more for each chapter. The IRM also guides faculty how to assign and use the text-specific Companion Website, www.prenhall.com/lemone, and the free student CD-ROM that accompany the textbook.

### Instructor's Resource CD-ROM ISBN: 0-13-045581-4

This cross-platform CD-ROM provides illustrations in PowerPoint from the new third edition of this textbook for use in classroom lectures. It also contains an electronic test bank, answers to the textbook critical thinking exercises, and animations from the student CD-ROM. This supplement is available to faculty free upon adoption of the textbook.

### Companion Website Syllabus Manager

www.prenhall.com/lemone

Faculty adopting this textbook has *free* access to the online Syllabus Manager on the Companion Website, www.prenhall.com/lemone. Syllabus Manager offers a whole host of features that facilitate the students' use of the Companion Website, and allows faculty to post syllabi and course information online for students. For more information or a demonstration of Syllabus Manager, please contact a Prentice Hall sales representative.

### Online Course Management Systems

Also available are online companions for schools using course management systems. The online course management solutions feature interactive modules, electronic test bank, PowerPoint images, animations, assessment activities, and more. For more information about adopting an online course management system to accompany *Medical-Surgical Nursing,* please contact your Prentice Hall Health sales representative or go online to one of the following websites and select "courses."

WebCT: http://cms.prenhall.com/webct/index.html/

Blackboard: http://cms.prenhall.com/blackboard/index.html/

CourseCompass: http://cms.prenhall.com/coursecompass/

## Text Contributors

**Jane Bostick, PhD, RN**
Sinclair School of Nursing
University of Missouri-Columbia
　Columbia, MO

Chapter 12: Nursing Care of Clients
　with Problems of Substance Abuse

**Roxanne W. McDaniel, PhD, RN**
Sinclair School of Nursing
University of Missouri-Columbia
　Columbia, MO

Chapter 10: Nursing Care of Clients with
　Cancer

**Elaine Mohn-Brown, RN, EdD**
Chemeketa Community College
Salem, OR

Chapter 8: Nursing Care of Clients with
　Infection

Chapter 9: Nursing Care of Clients with
　Altered Immunity

Chapter 45: Nursing Care of Clients with
　Eye and Ear Disorders

**Margorie Whitman, RN, MSN, AOCN**
Sinclair School of Nursing
University of Missouri-Columbia
　Columbia, MO

Chapter 7: Nursing Care of Clients Having
　Surgery

## SUPPLEMENT AND MEDIA WRITERS

### Student CD-ROM

**Joseann DeWitt, RN, MSN, BC, CLNC**
Alcorn State University School of Nursing
Department of Baccalaureate Nursing
Natchez, MS

**Rebecca Gesler, RN, MSN**
Nursing Professor
Saint Catharine College
St. Catharine, KY

**Laurie Kaudewitz, RNC, BSN, MSN**
Assistant Professor
East Tennessee State University
Johnson City, TN

**Douglas Turner, PhD(C), RN, MSN, CNS, CRNA**
Lead Instructor
Forsyth Technical Community College
Winston-Salem, NC

**Linda White, PhD(C), MSN, CNS, RN**
Lead Instructor
Forsyth Technical Community College
Winston-Salem, NC

## Companion Website

**Joseann DeWitt, RN, MSN, BC, CLNC**
Alcorn State University School of Nursing
Department of Baccalaureate Nursing
Natches, MS

**Peggy Ellis, PhD, RNCS, ANP**
University of Missouri
Barnes College of Nursing
St. Louis, MO

**Lynne Bryant, PhD, RN, MSN**
Associate Professor, Nursing Technology
Broward Community College
Davie, FL

**Rebecca Gesler, RN, MSN**
Nursing Professor
Saint Catherine College
St. Catherine, KY

**Vincent Salyers, RN, EdD**
Associate Professor
Palomar College
San Marcos, CA
Adjunct Professor
University of Phoenix
San Diego, CA

## Study Guide

**Jacqueline B. Brinkman, RN, BSN, CPN**
College of the Redwoods
Eureka, CA

**Joseann DeWitt, RN, MSN, BC, CLNC**
Alcorn State University School of Nursing
Department of Baccalaureate Nursing
Natchez, MS

**Golden Tradewell, PhD, RN, MSN, MA**
Associate Professor
McNeese State University
College of Nursing
Lake Charles, LA

## Instructor's Resource Manual

**Joyce Hammer, RN, MSN**
Lourdes College
Sylvania, OH

**Edna Hull, RN, MSN, CPN**
Assistant Professor
Delgado Community College–Charity
　School of Nursing
New Orleans, LA

# REVIEWERS

**Marianne Adam, MSN, RN, CRNP**
Assistant Professor
Moravian College—St. Luke's School of
     Nursing
Bethlehem, PA

**Ellise D. Adams, CNM, MSN, CD, ICCE**
Nursing Faculty
Calhoun Community College
Decatur, AL

**Martha Baker, PhD, RN, CS, CCRN**
Associate Professor
Missouri Southern State College
Joplin, MO

**Claudia P. Barone, EdD, RN, LNC, CPC**
Clinical Assistant Professor, Dean for the
     Master's Program,
Chairperson Department of Nursing Practice
University of Arkansas for Medical Sciences
Little Rock, AR

**Gail Bolling, MS, RN, CCRN**
Associate Professor
Montgomery College
Takoma Park, MD

**Joanne Bonesteel, MS, RN**
Nursing Faculty
Excelsior College
Albany, NY

**Tara Brenner, MS, RN, CS**
Assistant Professor
SUNY Brockport
Brockport, NY

**Polly Cameron Haigler, PhD, RN**
Clinical Assistant Professor
University of South Carolina
Columbia, SC

**Candice Cherrington, PhD, RN**
Assistant Professor
Wright State University
Dayton, OH

**Betty Christeson, BSNE, MN, EdD**
Adjunct Faculty
Greenville Technical College
Greenville, SC

**Patty Clark, RN, MSN**
Associate Professor
Abraham Baldwin College
Tifton, GA

**Janet M. Clifton, MS**
Instructor
Danville Area Community College
Danville, IL

**Maureen Cochran, RN, PhD**
Nursing Faculty
Suffolk University
Boston, MA

**Ruth F. Craven, EdD, RN, BC, FAAN**
Professor and Associate Dean
University of Washington
Seattle, WA

**Janice A. Cullen, EdD, RN**
Associate Professor
University of South Carolina-Aiken
Aiken, SC

**Cynthia L. Dakin, RN, PHD**
Clinical Specialist
Northeastern University
Boston, MA

**Ann Denney, RN, MSN**
Assistant Professor
Thomas More College
Crestview Hills, KY

**Nancy Dentlinger, AS, BS, MS**
Assistant Director
Redlands Community College
El Reno, OK

**Susan DeSanto-Madeya, RN, DNSc**
Assistant Professor
Moravian College—St. Luke's School of
     Nursing
Bethlehem, PA

**Susan Dipert-Scott, RN, MS**
Adjunct Faculty
Wright State University
Dayton, OH

**Mary Jo Distel, MS**
Assistant Professor
Midwestern State University
Wichita Falls, TX

**Jean Forsha, MSN, RN**
Nursing Faculty
Westchester University
Westchester, PA

**Rebecca Gesler, RN, MSN**
Director
Saint Catherine College
St. Catherine, KY

**Paula Gilbert, BS, RN, ANP**
Nursing Instructor
Arnot Ogden Medical Center
Elmira, NY

**LaVerne Grant, MS, RN**
Assistant Professor
University of Mississippi Medical Center
Jackson, MS

**Corinne Grimes, RN, MSN, DNSc,
AOCN**
Assistant Professor
Texas Women's University
Dallas, TX

**Barbara F. Harrah, RN, MSN**
Assistant Professor
Kent State University
East Liverpool, OH

**Anne Helm, RN, BSN, MSN**
Associate Professor
Owens Community College
Toledo, OH

**Mary Ann Helm, MSN, MRE, RN**
Assistant Professor
Nursing Faculty
Tennessee State University
Nashville, TN

**Gayle Hofland, MSN, RN, BC**
Assistant Professor
Dickerson State University
Dickerson, MD

**Beverly K. Hogan, MSN, RN, CS**
Nursing Faculty
University of Alabama-Birmingham
Birmingham, AL

**Susan P. Holmes, MSN, CRNP**
Nursing Faculty
Auburn University
Auburn, AL

**Karen C. Johnson-Brennam, EdD,
RN, MSN**
Professor and Associate Director
San Francisco State University
San Francisco, CA

**Paula R. Klemm, DNSc, RN, OCN**
Associate Professor
University of Delaware
Newark, DE

**Wilma La Cava, RNC, MSN**
Assistant Professor
Riverside Community College
Riverside, CA

**Kristine M. Lecuyer, RN, MSN**
Adjunct Assistant Professor
Saint Louis University
St. Louis, MO

**Camille Little, MS, RN, CS**
Assistant Professor
Illinois State University
Normal, IL

**Karen Martin, RN, MS**
Assistant Professor
Pikeville College
Paintsville, KY

**Arlene McGrory, DNSc, RN**
Associate Professor
University of Massachusetts-Lowell
Lowell, MA

## PRISCILLA LEMONE, RN, DSN, FAAN

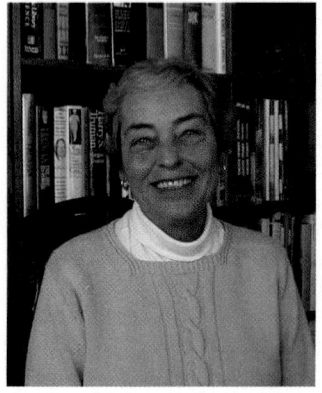

Priscilla LeMone has spent most of her career as a nurse educator, teaching medical-surgical nursing and pathophysiology at all levels from diploma to doctoral students. She has a diploma in nursing from Deaconess College of Nursing (St. Louis, Missouri), baccalaureate and master's degrees from Southeast Missouri State University, and a doctorate in nursing from the University of Alabama-Birmingham. She is currently an Associate Professor and Director of Undergraduate Studies, Sinclair School of Nursing, University of Missouri-Columbia.

Dr. LeMone has had numerous awards for scholarship and teaching during her over 30 years as a nurse educator. She is most honored for receiving the Kemper Fellowship for Teaching Excellence from the University of Missouri-Columbia, the Unique Contribution Award from the North American Nursing Diagnosis Association, and for being selected as a Fellow in the American Academy of Nursing.

She believes that her education gave her solid and everlasting roots in nursing. Her work with students has given her the wings that allow her love of nursing and teaching to continue through the years.

A widow, Dr. LeMone lives with her dog and shares time with her two children and her granddaughter. When she has time, she enjoys growing flowers and reading fiction.

## KAREN M. BURKE, RN, MS

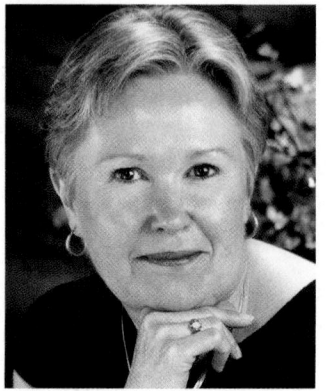

Karen Burke has practiced nursing in acute intensive and coronary care, in community-based settings, and in nursing education. As an educator, she has taught nursing skills, fundamentals, pathophysiology, and basic to advanced medical-surgical nursing. Ms. Burke has a diploma in nursing from Emanuel Hospital School of Nursing in Portland, Oregon, later completing baccalaureate studies at Oregon Health & Science University, and a master's degree at University of Portland.

Ms. Burke has been part of the nursing faculty at Clatsop Community College in Astoria, Oregon, since the inception of the Associate Degree Nursing program in 1983, most recently serving as Director of Health Occupations and Nursing. In this role, she is known as a leader and an innovator. She led the nursing faculty in developing an online program to deliver basic nursing education to a distant rural community. This program continues, serving as a model for other community college nursing programs to reach out to geographically isolated communities. Ms. Burke is actively involved in nursing education and developing strategies to address the nursing shortage in Oregon. She is a member of the Oregon Council of Associate Degree Nursing Programs (OCAP) and the Oregon Nursing Leadership Council (ONLC), currently serving as chair of the ONLC Education Committee. She is coauthor of several other texts: *Medical-Surgical Nursing Care,* with Priscilla LeMone and Elaine Mohn-Brown; *Fundamentals of Nursing: Concepts, Process, and Practice* (6th edition), with Barbara Kozier, Glenora Erb, and Audrey Berman; and a clinical handbook to accompany this text.

Ms. Burke sees herself as a nurse first, then a nurse educator and educational administrator. She strongly values the nursing profession and the importance of providing a solid education in the art and science of nursing for all students entering the profession.

When possible, Ms. Burke and her husband Steve spend time with their extended family and traveling. She enjoys a passion for quilting, and, when the weather allows, gardening.

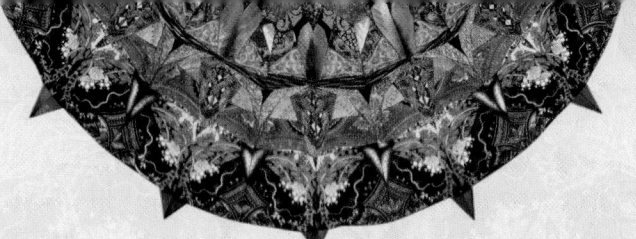

# Guide to
# MEDICAL-SURGICAL NURSING

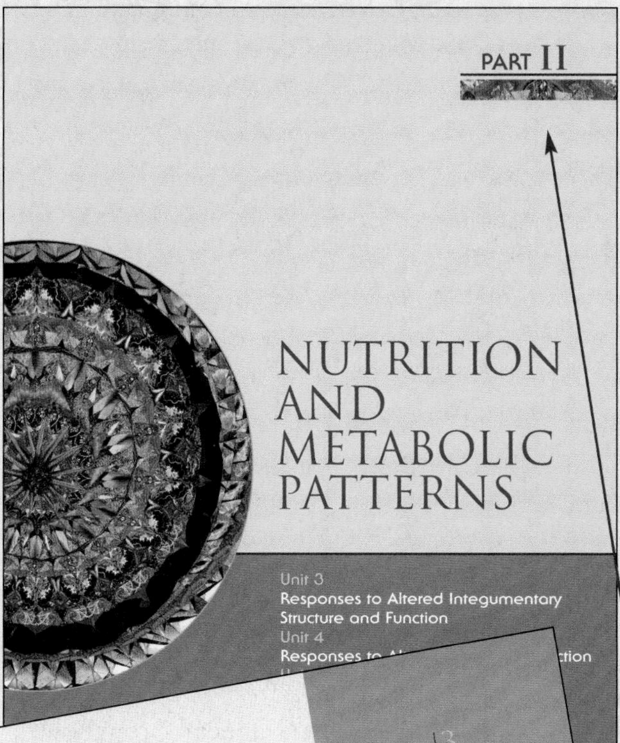

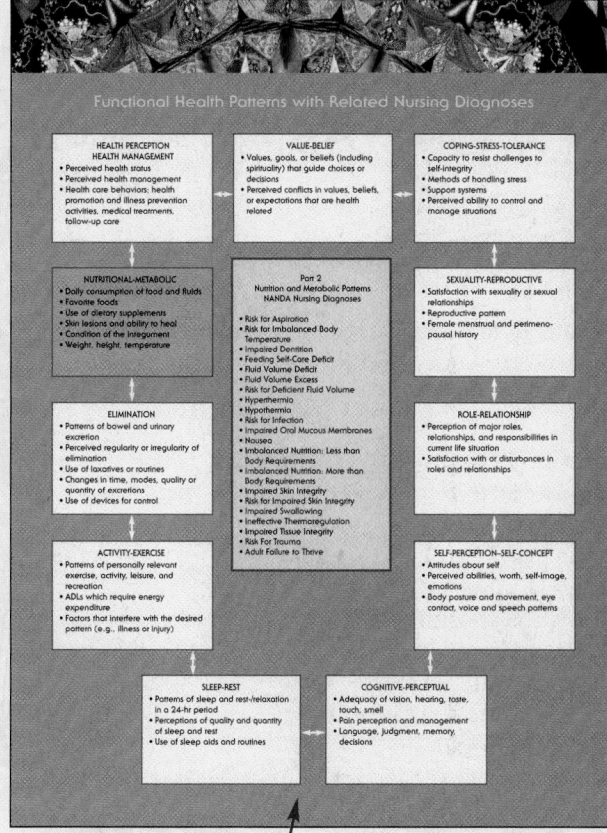

**PART II**

## NUTRITION AND METABOLIC PATTERNS

Unit 3
Responses to Altered Integumentary Structure and Function

Unit 4
Responses to A[...]ction

### Functional Health Patterns with Related Nursing Diagnoses

**HEALTH PERCEPTION HEALTH MANAGEMENT**
- Perceived health status
- Perceived health management
- Health care behaviors: health promotion and illness prevention activities, medical treatments, follow-up care

**VALUE-BELIEF**
- Values, goals, or beliefs (including spirituality) that guide choices or decisions
- Perceived conflicts in values, beliefs, or expectations that are health related

**COPING-STRESS-TOLERANCE**
- Capacity to resist challenges to self-integrity
- Methods of handling stress
- Support systems
- Perceived ability to control and manage situations

**NUTRITIONAL-METABOLIC**
- Daily consumption of food and fluids
- Favorite foods
- Use of dietary supplements
- Skin lesions and ability to heal
- Condition of the integument
- Weight, height, temperature

**Part 2 Nutrition and Metabolic Patterns NANDA Nursing Diagnoses**
- Risk for Aspiration
- Risk for Imbalanced Body Temperature
- Impaired Dentition
- Feeding Self-Care Deficit
- Fluid Volume Deficit
- Fluid Volume Excess
- Risk for Deficient Fluid Volume
- Hyperthermia
- Hypothermia
- Risk for Infection
- Impaired Oral Mucous Membranes
- Nausea
- Imbalanced Nutrition: Less than Body Requirements
- Imbalanced Nutrition: More than Body Requirements
- Impaired Skin Integrity
- Risk for Impaired Skin Integrity
- Impaired Swallowing
- Ineffective Thermoregulation
- Impaired Tissue Integrity
- Risk For Trauma
- Adult Failure to Thrive

**SEXUALITY-REPRODUCTIVE**
- Satisfaction with sexuality or sexual relationships
- Reproductive pattern
- Female menstrual and perimenopausal history

**ELIMINATION**
- Patterns of bowel and urinary excretion
- Perceived regularity or irregularity of elimination
- Use of laxatives or routines
- Changes in time, modes, quality or quantity of excretions
- Use of devices for control

**ROLE-RELATIONSHIP**
- Perception of major roles, relationships, and responsibilities in current life situation
- Satisfaction with or disturbances in roles and relationships

**ACTIVITY-EXERCISE**
- Patterns of personally relevant exercise, activity, leisure, and recreation
- ADLs which require energy expenditure
- Factors that interfere with the desired pattern (e.g., illness or injury)

**SELF-PERCEPTION-SELF-CONCEPT**
- Attitudes about self
- Perceived abilities, worth, self-image, emotions
- Body posture and movement, eye contact, voice and speech patterns

**SLEEP-REST**
- Patterns of sleep and rest-relaxation in a 24-hr period
- Perceptions of quality and quantity of sleep and rest
- Use of sleep aids and routines

**COGNITIVE-PERCEPTUAL**
- Adequacy of vision, hearing, taste, touch, smell
- Pain perception and management
- Language, judgment, memory, decisions

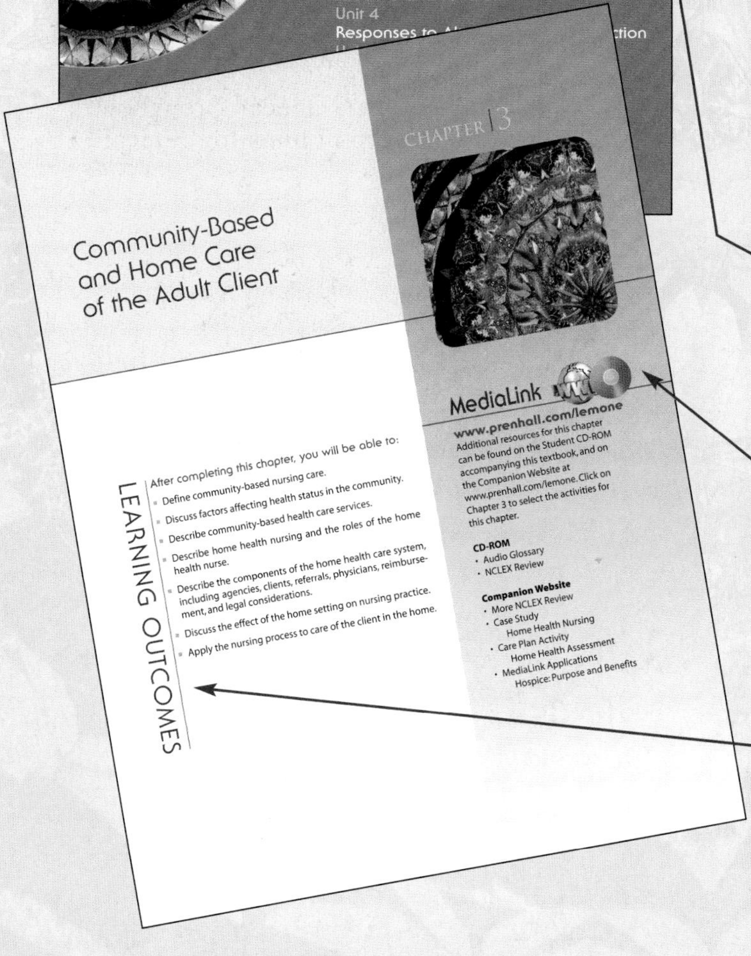

---

CHAPTER 3

## Community-Based and Home Care of the Adult Client

**MediaLink**

www.prenhall.com/lemone
Additional resources for this chapter can be found on the Student CD-ROM accompanying this textbook, and on the Companion Website at www.prenhall.com/lemone. Click on Chapter 3 to select the activities for this chapter.

**CD-ROM**
- Audio Glossary
- NCLEX Review

**Companion Website**
- More NCLEX Review
- Case Study
  Home Health Nursing
- Care Plan Activity
  Home Health Assessment
- MediaLink Applications
  Hospice: Purpose and Benefits

**LEARNING OUTCOMES**

After completing this chapter, you will be able to:
- Define community-based nursing care.
- Discuss factors affecting health status in the community.
- Describe community-based health care services.
- Describe home health nursing and the roles of the home health nurse.
- Describe the components of the home health care system, including agencies, clients, referrals, physicians, reimbursement, and legal considerations.
- Discuss the effect of the home setting on nursing practice.
- Apply the nursing process to care of the client in the home.

---

### Part Openers
Each Part Opener is followed by a Functional Health Pattern Concept Map. These concept maps relate nursing diagnoses to specific patterns covered in that part.

### MediaLink
introduces each chapter of the text and lists additional specific content, animations, NCLEX Review, tools, and other interactive exercises, which appear on the accompanying Student CD-ROM and the Companion Website.

### Learning Outcomes
appear at the start of each chapter, identifying important concepts students should know by the end of the chapter.

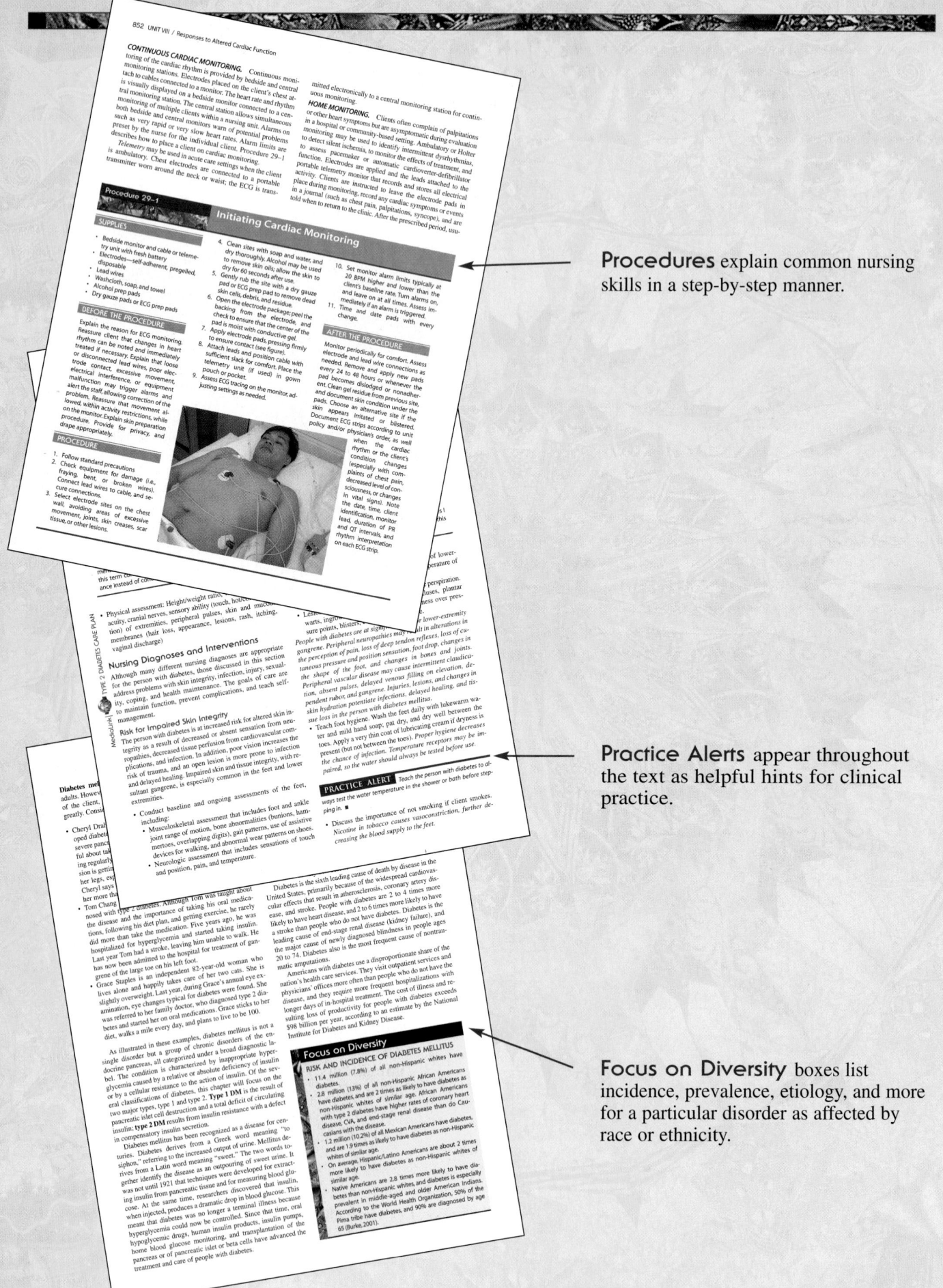

**Procedures** explain common nursing skills in a step-by-step manner.

**Practice Alerts** appear throughout the text as helpful hints for clinical practice.

**Focus on Diversity** boxes list incidence, prevalence, etiology, and more for a particular disorder as affected by race or ethnicity.

**Pathophysiology Illustrated** are three-dimensional illustrations that help students to visualize the pathophysiological process of a particular disorder. Additional animations can be found on the Student CD-ROM.

**Nursing Care Plan**
Throughout the text, nursing care plans help students approach care from a nursing process perspective. The care plan is followed by critical thinking questions for students to apply their knowledge to plan the care for a specific client. Suggested responses to the critical thinking questions can be found in Appendix C. Additional Care Plan activities can be found on the Companion Website.

**Multisystem Effects** are labeled illustrations that point out the effects a disorder has on various body systems.

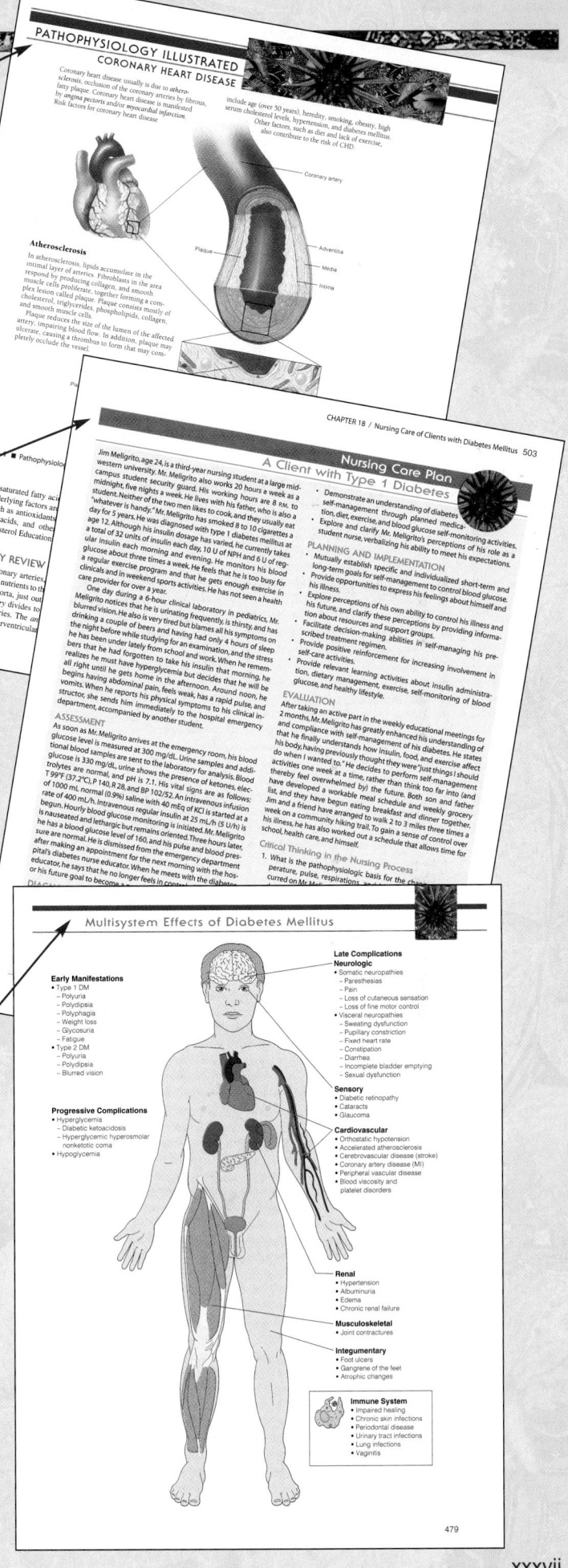

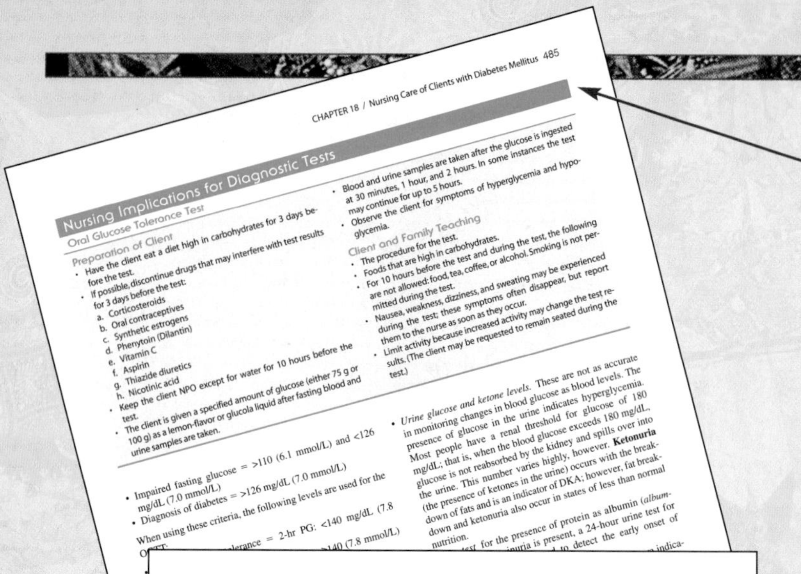
CHAPTER 18 / Nursing Care of Clients with Diabetes Mellitus 485

## Nursing Implications for Diagnostic Tests

### Oral Glucose Tolerance Test

#### Preparation of Client

- Have the client eat a diet high in carbohydrates for 3 days before the test.
- If possible, discontinue drugs that may interfere with test results for 3 days before the test:
  a. Corticosteroids
  b. Oral contraceptives
  c. Synthetic estrogens
  d. Phenytoin (Dilantin)
  e. Vitamin C
  f. Aspirin
  g. Thiazide diuretics
  h. Nicotinic acid
- Keep the client NPO except for water for 10 hours before the test.
- The client is given a specified amount of glucose (either 75 g or 100 g) as a lemon-flavor or glucola liquid after fasting blood and urine samples are taken.
- Blood and urine samples are taken after the glucose is ingested at 30 minutes, 1 hour, and 2 hours. In some instances the test may continue for up to 5 hours.
- Observe the client for symptoms of hyperglycemia and hypoglycemia.

#### Client and Family Teaching

- The procedure for the test.
- Foods that are high in carbohydrates.
- For 10 hours before the test and during the test, the following are not allowed: food, tea, coffee, or alcohol. Smoking is not permitted during the test.
- Nausea, weakness, dizziness, and sweating may be experienced during the test; these symptoms often disappear, but report them to the nurse as soon as they occur.
- Limit activity because increased activity may change the test results. (The client may be requested to remain seated during the test.)

- Impaired fasting glucose = >110 (6.1 mmol/L) and <126 mg/dL (7.0 mmol/L)
- Diagnosis of diabetes = >126 mg/dL (7.0 mmol/L)

When using these criteria, the following levels are used for the OGTT: ...

- *Urine glucose and ketone levels.* These are not as accurate in monitoring changes in blood glucose as blood levels. The presence of glucose in the urine indicates hyperglycemia. Most people have a renal threshold for glucose of 180 mg/dL; that is, when the blood glucose exceeds 180 mg/dL, glucose is not reabsorbed by the kidney and spills over into the urine. This number varies highly, however. **Ketonuria** (the presence of ketones in the urine) occurs with the breakdown of fats and is an indicator of DKA; however, fat breakdown and ketonuria also occur in states of less than normal nutrition.
- ... for the presence of protein as albumin (*albumin*...) ...

**Nursing Implications for Diagnostic Tests** provide students with information that they need to consider when clients undergo particular diagnostic tests.

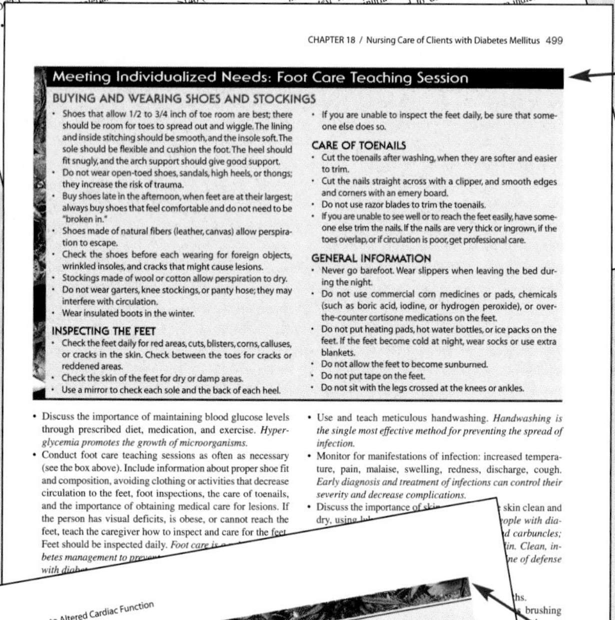
CHAPTER 18 / Nursing Care of Clients with Diabetes Mellitus 499

## Meeting Individualized Needs: Foot Care Teaching Session

**BUYING AND WEARING SHOES AND STOCKINGS**

- Shoes that allow 1/2 to 3/4 inch of toe room are best; there should be room for toes to spread out and wiggle. The lining and inside stitching should be smooth, and the insole soft. The sole should be flexible and cushion the foot. The heel should fit snugly, and the arch support should give good support.
- Do not wear open-toed shoes, sandals, high heels, or thongs; they increase the risk of trauma.
- Buy shoes late in the afternoon, when feet are at their largest; always buy shoes that feel comfortable and do not need to be "broken in."
- Shoes made of natural fibers (leather, canvas) allow perspiration to escape.
- Check the shoes before each wearing for foreign objects, wrinkled insoles, and cracks that might cause lesions.
- Stockings made of wool or cotton allow perspiration to dry.
- Do not wear garters, knee stockings, or panty hose; they may interfere with circulation.
- Wear insulated boots in the winter.

**INSPECTING THE FEET**

- Check the feet daily for red areas, cuts, blisters, corns, calluses, or cracks in the skin. Check between the toes for cracks or reddened areas.
- Check the skin of the feet for dry or damp areas.
- Use a mirror to check each sole and the back of each heel.
- If you are unable to inspect the feet daily, be sure that someone else does so.

**CARE OF TOENAILS**

- Cut the toenails after washing, when they are softer and easier to trim.
- Cut the nails straight across with a clipper, and smooth edges and corners with an emery board.
- Do not use razor blades to trim the toenails.
- If you are unable to see well or to reach the feet easily, have someone else trim the nails. If the nails are very thick or ingrown, if the toes overlap, or if circulation is poor, get professional care.

**GENERAL INFORMATION**

- Never go barefoot. Wear slippers when leaving the bed during the night.
- Do not use commercial corn medicines or pads, chemicals (such as boric acid, iodine, or hydrogen peroxide), or over-the-counter cortisone medications on the feet.
- Do not put heating pads, hot water bottles, or ice packs on the feet. If the feet become cold at night, wear socks or use extra blankets.
- Do not allow the feet to become sunburned.
- Do not put tape on the feet.
- Do not sit with the legs crossed at the knees or ankles.

- Discuss the importance of maintaining blood glucose levels through prescribed diet, medication, and exercise. *Hyperglycemia promotes the growth of microorganisms.*
- Conduct foot care teaching sessions as often as necessary (see the box above). Include information about proper shoe fit and composition, avoiding clothing or activities that decrease circulation to the feet, foot inspections, the care of toenails, and the importance of obtaining medical care for lesions. If the person has visual deficits, is obese, or cannot reach the feet, teach the caregiver how to inspect and care for the feet. Feet should be inspected daily. *Foot care is ... betes management to prevent ... with diab...*
- Use and teach meticulous handwashing. *Handwashing is the single most effective method for preventing the spread of infection.*
- Monitor for manifestations of infection: increased temperature, pain, malaise, swelling, redness, discharge, cough. *Early diagnosis and treatment of infections can control their severity and decrease complications.*
- Discuss the importance of ski... skin clean and dry, using ...

**Meeting Individualized Needs** focuses on the needs of specific populations, such as race, ethnicity, gender, and more.

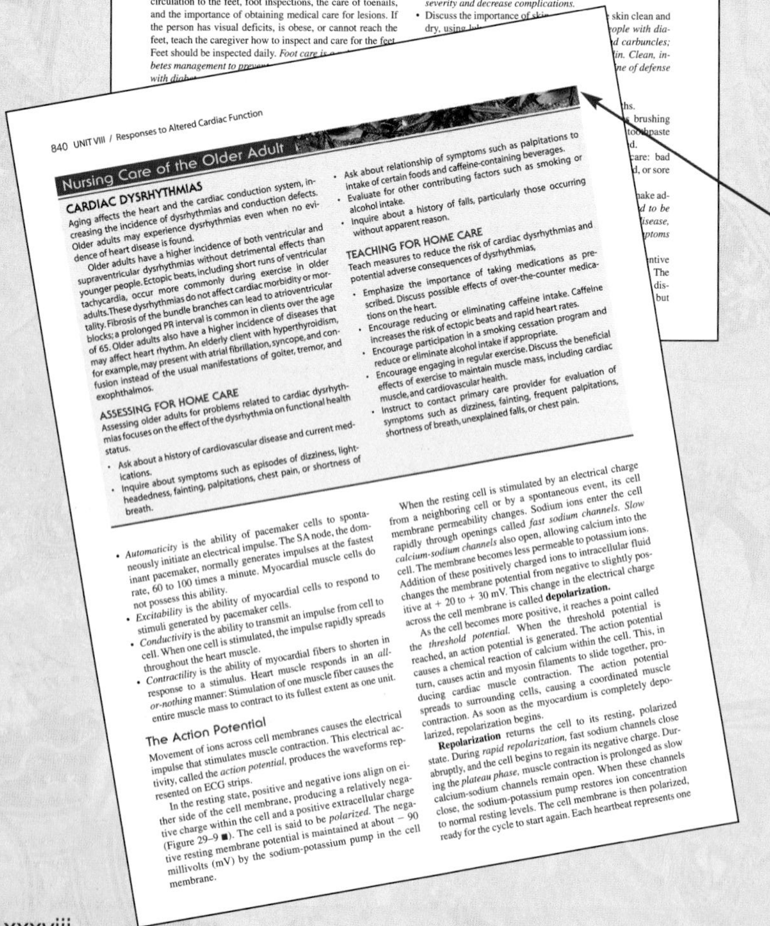
840 UNIT VIII / Responses to Altered Cardiac Function

## Nursing Care of the Older Adult

**CARDIAC DYSRHYTHMIAS**

Aging affects the heart and the cardiac conduction system, increasing the incidence of dysrhythmias and conduction defects. Older adults may experience dysrhythmias even when no evidence of heart disease is found.

Older adults have a higher incidence of both ventricular and supraventricular dysrhythmias without detrimental effects than younger people. Ectopic beats, including short runs of ventricular tachycardia, occur more commonly during exercise in older adults. These dysrhythmias do not affect cardiac morbidity or mortality. Fibrosis of the bundle branches can lead to atrioventricular blocks; a prolonged PR interval is common in clients over the age of 65. Older adults also have a higher incidence of diseases that may affect heart rhythm. An elderly client with hyperthyroidism, for example, may present with atrial fibrillation, syncope, and confusion instead of the usual manifestations of goiter, tremor, and exophthalmos.

**ASSESSING FOR HOME CARE**

Assessing older adults for problems related to cardiac dysrhythmias focuses on the effect of the dysrhythmia on functional health status.

- Ask about a history of cardiovascular disease and current medications.
- Inquire about symptoms such as episodes of dizziness, lightheadedness, fainting, palpitations, chest pain, or shortness of breath.
- Ask about relationship of symptoms such as palpitations to intake of certain foods and caffeine-containing beverages.
- Evaluate for other contributing factors such as smoking or alcohol intake.
- Inquire about a history of falls, particularly those occurring without apparent reason.

**TEACHING FOR HOME CARE**

Teach measures to reduce the risk of cardiac dysrhythmias and potential adverse consequences of dysrhythmias.

- Emphasize the importance of taking medications as prescribed. Discuss possible effects of over-the-counter medications on the heart.
- Encourage reducing or eliminating caffeine intake. Caffeine increases the risk of ectopic beats and rapid heart rates.
- Encourage participation in a smoking cessation program and reduce or eliminate alcohol intake if appropriate.
- Encourage engaging in regular exercise. Discuss the beneficial effects of exercise to maintain muscle mass, including cardiac muscle, and cardiovascular health.
- Instruct to contact primary care provider for evaluation of symptoms such as dizziness, fainting, frequent palpitations, shortness of breath, unexplained falls, or chest pain.

- *Automaticity* is the ability of pacemaker cells to spontaneously initiate an electrical impulse. The SA node, the dominant pacemaker, normally generates impulses at the fastest rate, 60 to 100 times a minute. Myocardial muscle cells do not possess this ability.
- *Excitability* is the ability of myocardial cells to respond to stimuli generated by pacemaker cells.
- *Conductivity* is the ability to transmit an impulse from cell to cell. When one cell is stimulated, the impulse rapidly spreads throughout the heart muscle.
- *Contractility* is the ability of myocardial fibers to shorten in response to a stimulus. Heart muscle responds in an *all-or-nothing* manner: Stimulation of one muscle fiber causes the entire muscle mass to contract to its fullest extent as one unit.

### The Action Potential

Movement of ions across cell membranes causes the electrical impulse that stimulates muscle contraction. This electrical activity, called the *action potential*, produces the waveforms represented on ECG strips.

In the resting state, positive and negative ions align on either side of the cell membrane, producing a relatively negative charge within the cell and a positive extracellular charge (Figure 29–9 ■). The cell is said to be *polarized*. The negative resting membrane potential is maintained at about − 90 millivolts (mV) by the sodium-potassium pump in the cell membrane.

When the resting cell is stimulated by an electrical charge from a neighboring cell or by a spontaneous event, its cell membrane permeability changes. Sodium ions enter the cell rapidly through openings called *fast sodium channels. Slow calcium-sodium channels* also open, allowing calcium into the cell. The membrane becomes less permeable to potassium ions. Addition of these positively charged ions to intracellular fluid changes the membrane potential from negative to slightly positive at + 20 to + 30 mV. This change in the electrical charge across the cell membrane is called **depolarization.**

As the cell becomes more positive, it reaches a point called the *threshold potential.* When the threshold potential is reached, an action potential is generated. The action potential causes a chemical reaction of calcium within the cell. This, in turn, causes actin and myosin filaments to slide together, producing cardiac muscle contraction. The action potential spreads to surrounding cells, causing a coordinated muscle contraction. As soon as the myocardium is completely depolarized, repolarization begins.

**Repolarization** returns the cell to its resting, polarized state. During *rapid repolarization,* fast sodium channels close abruptly, and the cell begins to regain its negative charge. During the *plateau phase,* muscle contraction is prolonged as slow calcium-sodium channels remain open. When these channels close, the sodium-potassium pump restores ion concentration to normal resting levels. The cell membrane is then polarized, ready for the cycle to start again. Each heartbeat represents one

**Nursing Care of the Older Adult** is found throughout the text, as well as in the assessment sections for disorders. As the population continues to age, this is critical information for nursing care in any setting, and provides guidelines for assessing and teaching in home care.

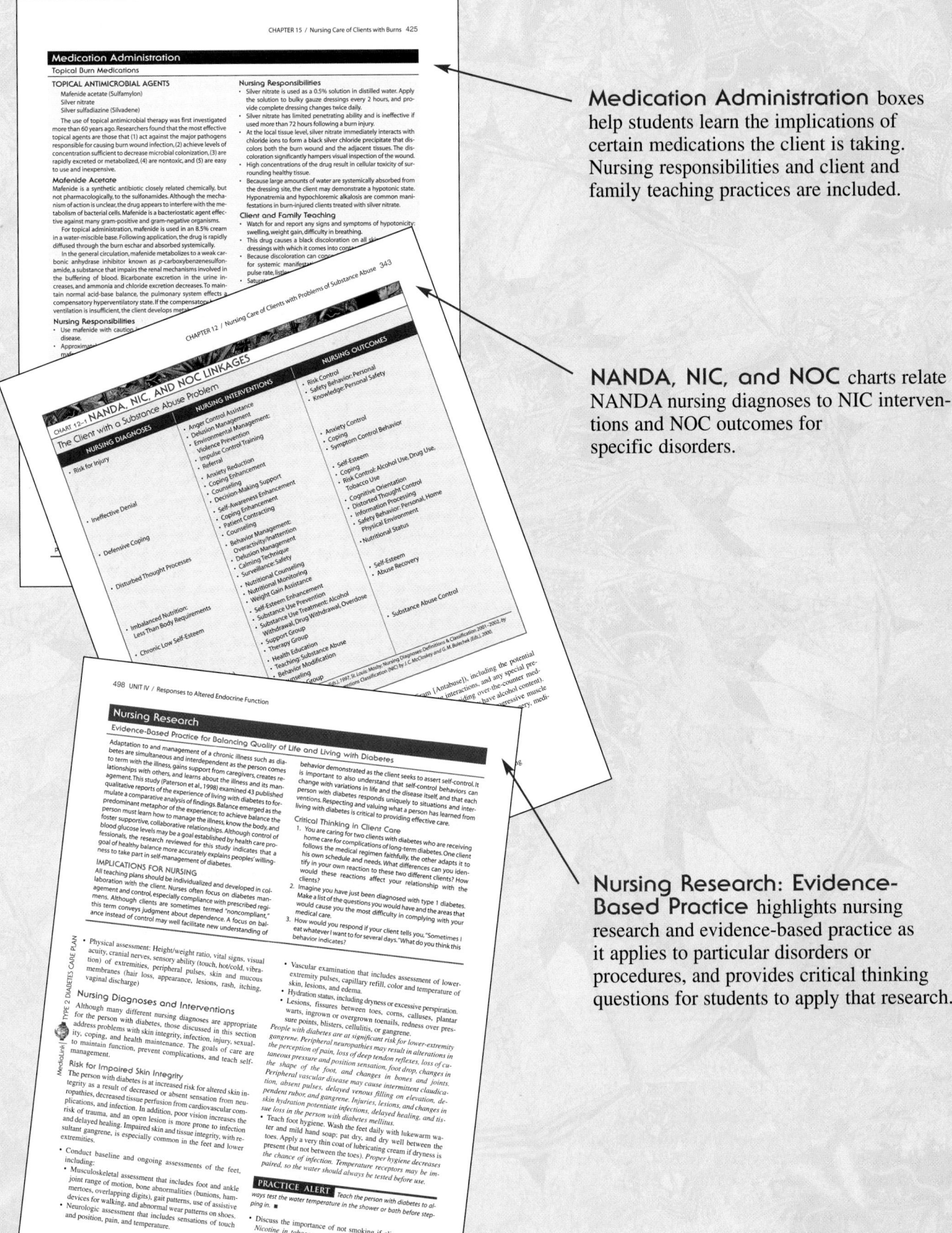

**Medication Administration** boxes help students learn the implications of certain medications the client is taking. Nursing responsibilities and client and family teaching practices are included.

**NANDA, NIC, and NOC** charts relate NANDA nursing diagnoses to NIC interventions and NOC outcomes for specific disorders.

**Nursing Research: Evidence-Based Practice** highlights nursing research and evidence-based practice as it applies to particular disorders or procedures, and provides critical thinking questions for students to apply that research.

**Nursing Care of the Client** describes nursing care for various medical or surgical procedures.

**EXPLORE MediaLink**

Found at the end of every chapter, EXPLORE MediaLink encourages students to use the CD-ROM and the Companion Website to apply what they have learned from the text in case studies, practice NCLEX questions, and use additional resources.

**Test Yourself** allows students to test their knowledge of the chapter.

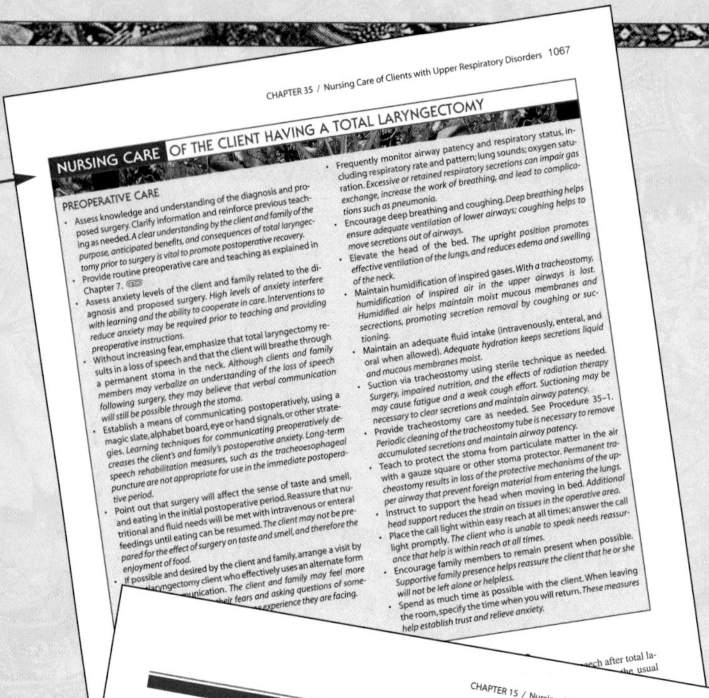
CHAPTER 35 / Nursing Care of Clients with Upper Respiratory Disorders 1067

NURSING CARE OF THE CLIENT HAVING A TOTAL LARYNGECTOMY

PREOPERATIVE CARE

- Assess knowledge and understanding of the diagnosis and proposed surgery. Clarify information and reinforce previous teaching as needed. *A clear understanding by the client and family of the purpose, anticipated benefits, and consequences of total laryngectomy prior to surgery is vital to promote postoperative recovery.*
- Provide routine preoperative care and teaching as explained in Chapter 7.
- Assess anxiety levels of the client and family related to the diagnosis and proposed surgery. *High levels of anxiety interfere with learning and the ability to cooperate in care. Interventions to reduce anxiety may be required prior to teaching and providing preoperative instructions.*
- Without increasing fear, emphasize that total laryngectomy results in a loss of speech and that the client will breathe through a permanent stoma in the neck. *Although clients and family members may verbalize an understanding of the loss of speech following surgery, they may believe that verbal communication will still be possible through the stoma.*
- Establish a means of communicating postoperatively, using a magic slate, alphabet board, eye or hand signals, or other strategies. *Learning techniques for communicating preoperatively decreases the client's and family's postoperative anxiety. Long-term speech rehabilitation measures, such as the tracheoesophageal puncture are not appropriate for use in the immediate postoperative period.*
- Point out that surgery will affect the sense of taste and smell, and eating in the initial postoperative period. Reassure that nutritional and fluid needs will be met with intravenous or enteral feedings until eating can be resumed. *The client may not be prepared for the effect of surgery on taste and smell, and therefore the enjoyment of food.*
- If possible and desired by the client and family, arrange a visit by a laryngectomy client who effectively uses an alternate form of communication. *The client and family may feel more ... their fears and asking questions of some... experience they are facing.*

- Frequently monitor airway patency and respiratory status, including respiratory rate and pattern; lung sounds; oxygen saturation. *Excessive or retained respiratory secretions can impair gas exchange, increase the work of breathing, and lead to complications such as pneumonia.*
- Encourage deep breathing and coughing. *Deep breathing helps ensure adequate ventilation of lower airways; coughing helps to move secretions out of airways.*
- Elevate the head of the bed. *The upright position promotes effective ventilation of the lungs, and reduces edema and swelling of the neck.*
- Maintain humidification of inspired gases. *With a tracheostomy, humidification of inspired air in the upper airways is lost. Humidified air helps maintain moist mucous membranes and secretions, promoting secretion removal by coughing or suctioning.*
- Maintain an adequate fluid intake (intravenously, enteral, and oral when allowed). *Adequate hydration keeps secretions liquid and mucous membranes moist.*
- Suction via tracheostomy using sterile technique as needed. *Surgery, impaired nutrition, and the effects of radiation therapy may cause fatigue and a weak cough effort. Suctioning may be necessary to clear secretions and maintain airway patency.*
- Provide tracheostomy care as needed. See Procedure 35–1. *Periodic cleaning of the tracheostomy tube is necessary to remove accumulated secretions and maintain airway patency.*
- Teach to protect the stoma from particulate matter in the air with a gauze square or other stoma protector. *Permanent tracheostomy results in loss of the protective mechanisms of the upper airway that prevent foreign material from entering the lungs.*
- Instruct to support the head when moving in bed. *Additional head support reduces the strain on tissues in the operative area.*
- Place the call light within easy reach at all times; answer the call light promptly. *The client who is unable to speak needs reassurance that help is within reach at all times.*
- Encourage family members to remain present when possible. *Supportive family presence helps reassure the client that he or she will not be left alone or helpless.*
- Spend as much time as possible with the client. When leaving the room, specify the time when you will return. *These measures help establish trust and relieve anxiety.*

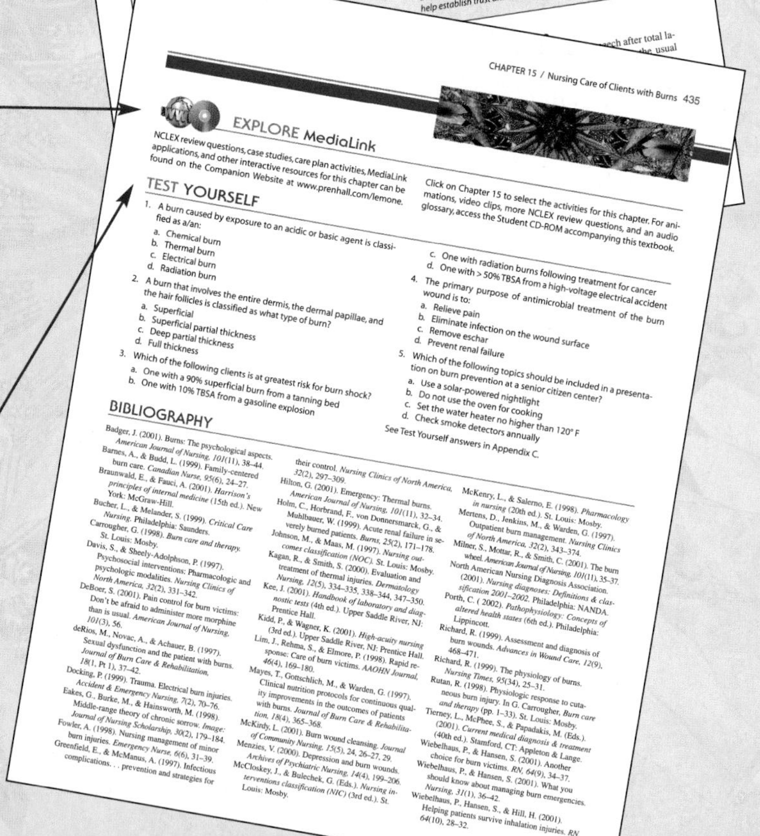
CHAPTER 15 / Nursing Care of Clients with Burns 435

EXPLORE MediaLink

NCLEX review questions, case studies, care plan activities, MediaLink applications, and other interactive resources for this chapter can be found on the Companion Website at www.prenhall.com/lemone.

Click on Chapter 15 to select the activities for this chapter. For animations, video clips, more NCLEX review questions, and an audio glossary, access the Student CD-ROM accompanying this textbook.

TEST YOURSELF

1. A burn caused by exposure to an acidic or basic agent is classified as a/an:
   a. Chemical burn
   b. Thermal burn
   c. Electrical burn
   d. Radiation burn
2. A burn that involves the entire dermis, the dermal papillae, and the hair follicles is classified as what type of burn?
   a. Superficial
   b. Superficial partial thickness
   c. Deep partial thickness
   d. Full thickness
3. Which of the following clients is at greatest risk for burn shock?
   a. One with a 90% superficial burn from a tanning bed
   b. One with 10% TBSA from a gasoline explosion
   c. One with radiation burns following treatment for cancer
   d. One with > 50% TBSA from a high-voltage electrical accident
4. The primary purpose of antimicrobial treatment of the burn wound is to:
   a. Relieve pain
   b. Eliminate infection on the wound surface
   c. Remove eschar
   d. Prevent renal failure
5. Which of the following topics should be included in a presentation on burn prevention at a senior citizen center?
   a. Use a solar-powered nightlight
   b. Do not use the oven for cooking
   c. Set the water heater no higher than 120° F
   d. Check smoke detectors annually

See Test Yourself answers in Appendix C.

BIBLIOGRAPHY


Badger, J. (2001). Burns: The psychological aspects. *American Journal of Nursing, 101*(11), 38–44.
Barnes, A., & Budd, L. (1999). Family-centered burn care. *Canadian Nurse, 95*(6), 24–27.
Braunwald, E., & Fauci, A. (2001). *Harrison's principles of internal medicine* (15th ed.). New York: McGraw-Hill.
Bucher, L., & Melander, S. (1999). *Critical Care Nursing.* Philadelphia: Saunders.
Carrougher, G. (1998). *Burn care and therapy.* St. Louis: Mosby.
Davis, S., & Sheely-Adolphson, P. (1997). Psychosocial interventions: Pharmacologic and psychologic modalities. *Nursing Clinics of North America, 32*(2), 331–342.
DeBoer, S. (2001). Pain control for burn victims: Don't be afraid to administer more morphine than is usual. *American Journal of Nursing, 101*(3), 56.
deRios, M., Novac, A., & Achauer, B. (1997). Sexual dysfunction and the patient with burns. *Journal of Burn Care & Rehabilitation, 18*(1, Pt 1), 37–42.
Docking, P. (1999). Trauma. Electrical burn injuries. *Accident & Emergency Nursing, 7*(2), 70–76.
Eakes, G., Burke, M., & Hainsworth, M. (1998). Middle-range theory of chronic sorrow. *Image: Journal of Nursing Scholarship, 30*(2), 179–184.
Fowler, A. (1998). Nursing management of minor burn injuries. *Emergency Nurse, 6*(6), 31–39.
Greenfield, E., & McManus, A. (1997). Infectious complications. . . prevention and strategies for their control. *Nursing Clinics of North America, 32*(2), 297–309.
Hilton, G. (2001). Emergency: Thermal burns. *American Journal of Nursing, 101*(11), 32–34.
Holm, C., Horbrand, F., von Donnersmarck, G., & Muhlbauer, W. (1999). Acute renal failure in severely burned patients. *Burns, 25*(2), 171–178.
Johnson, M., & Maas, M. (1997). *Nursing outcomes classification (NOC).* St. Louis: Mosby.
Kagan, R., & Smith, S. (2000). Evaluation and treatment of thermal injuries. *Dermatology Nursing, 12*(5), 334–335, 338–344, 347–350.
Kee, J. (2001). *Handbook of laboratory and diagnostic tests* (4th ed.). Upper Saddle River, NJ: Prentice Hall.
Kidd, P., & Wagner, K. (2001). *High-acuity nursing* (3rd ed.). Upper Saddle River, NJ: Prentice Hall.
Lim, J., Rehmar, S., & Elmore, P. (1998). Rapid response: Care of burn victims. *AAOHN Journal, 46*(4), 169–180.
Mayes, T., Gottschlich, M., & Warden, G. (1997). Clinical nutrition protocols for continuous quality improvements in the outcomes of patients with burns. *Journal of Burn Care & Rehabilitation, 18*(4), 365–368.
McKirdy, L. (2001). Burn wound cleansing. *Journal of Community Nursing, 15*(5), 24, 26–27, 29.
Menzies, V. (2000). Depression and burn wounds. *Archives of Psychiatric Nursing, 14*(4), 199–206.
McCloskey, J., & Bulechek, G. (Eds.). *Nursing interventions classification (NIC)* (3rd ed.). St. Louis: Mosby.
McKenry, L., & Salerno, E. (1998). *Pharmacology in nursing* (20th ed.). St. Louis: Mosby.
Mertens, D., Jenkins, M., & Warden, G. (1997). Outpatient burn management. *Nursing Clinics of North America, 32*(2), 343–374.
Milner, S., Mottar, R., & Smith, C. (2001). The burn wheel. *American Journal of Nursing, 101*(11), 35–37.
North American Nursing Diagnosis Association. (2001). *Nursing diagnoses: Definitions & classification 2001–2002.* Philadelphia: NANDA.
Porth, C. (2002). *Pathophysiology: Concepts of altered health states* (6th ed.). Philadelphia: Lippincott.
Richard, R. (1999). Assessment and diagnosis of burn wounds. *Advances in Wound Care, 12*(9), 468–471.
Richard, R. (1999). The physiology of burns. *Nursing Times, 95*(34), 25–31.
Rutan, R. (1998). Physiologic response to cutaneous burn injury. In G. Carrougher, *Burn care and therapy* (pp. 1–33). St. Louis: Mosby.
Tierney, L., McPhee, S., & Papadakis, M. (Eds.). (2001). *Current medical diagnosis & treatment* (40th ed.). Stamford, CT: Appleton & Lange.
Wiebelhaus, P., & Hansen, S. (2001). Another choice for burn victims. *RN, 64*(9), 34–37.
Wiebelhaus, P., & Hansen, S. (2001). What you should know about managing burn emergencies. *Nursing, 31*(1), 36–42.
Wiebelhaus, P., Hansen, S., & Hill, H. (2001). Helping patients survive inhalation injuries. *RN, 64*(10), 28–32.


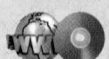

## ADDITIONAL MEDIA RESOURCES:

**Animation and Video Tutorials**—On the Student CD-ROM, the student will find animations illustrating difficult concepts or reinforcing content in the text.

**NCLEX Reviews**—Both the Student CD-ROM and the free Companion Website offer the student an abundance of NCLEX review questions for each chapter of the book. The questions provide comprehensive rationales, as well as identify how the questions correlate to the NCLEX test plan.

**Care Plan Activities**—Each clinical chapter on the Companion Website provides the student with a case scenario and asks the student to develop a care plan for the client. Students can e-mail these care plans to instructors as homework assignments.

**Case Studies**—For each clinical chapter on the Companion Website, the student can review a client scenario and answer critical thinking questions related to that client's care. Students can e-mail their responses to the case studies to instructors as homework assignments.

**MediaLink Applications**—Students are asked to go to websites to research the questions that are presented here.

# SPECIAL FEATURES

Focus on Diversity

 Meeting Individualized Needs

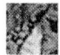

Procedures

 Multisystem Effects of ...

 Pathophysiology Illustrated

 Medication Administration

Manifestations of ...

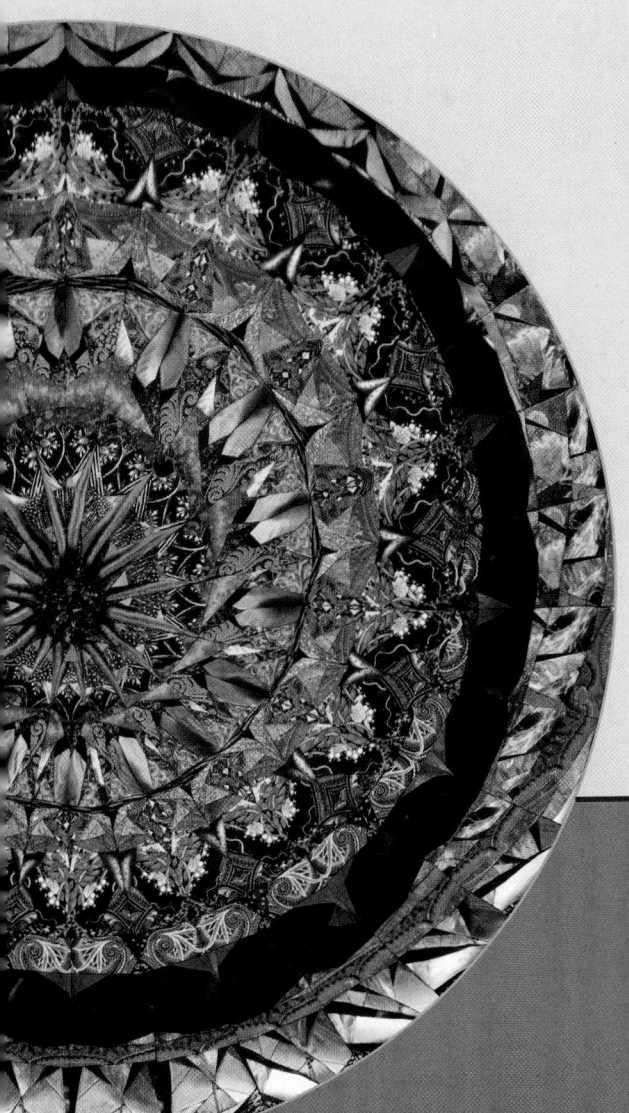

# MEDICAL-SURGICAL NURSING PRACTICE

Unit 1
**Dimensions of Medical-Surgical Nursing**

Unit 2
**Alterations in Patterns of Health**

# Functional Health Patterns with Related Nursing Diagnoses

### HEALTH PERCEPTION
### HEALTH MANAGEMENT
- Perceived health status
- Perceived health management
- Health care behaviors: health promotion and illness prevention activities, medical treatments, follow-up care

### VALUE-BELIEF
- Values, goals, or beliefs (including spirituality) that guide choices or decisions
- Perceived conflicts in values, beliefs, or expectations that are health related

### COPING-STRESS-TOLERANCE
- Capacity to resist challenges to self-integrity
- Methods of handling stress
- Support systems
- Perceived ability to control and manage situations

### NUTRITIONAL-METABOLIC
- Daily consumption of food and fluids
- Favorite foods
- Use of dietary supplements
- Skin lesions and ability to heal
- Condition of the integument
- Weight, height, temperature

### Part 1
### Medical-Surgical Nursing Practice
### NANDA Nursing Diagnoses
- Latex Allergy Response
- Caregiver Role Strain
- Chronic Sorrow
- Compromised Family Coping
- Death Anxiety
- Anxiety
- Decisional Conflict
- Disturbed Body Image
- Fatigue
- Fear
- Deficient Fluid Volume
- Excess Fluid Volume
- Ineffective Health Maintenance
- Health-Seeking Behaviors
- Risk for Infection
- Deficient Knowledge
- Nausea
- Acute Pain
- Chronic Pain
- Risk for Injury
- Powerlessness
- Disturbed Personal Identity
- Ineffective Protection
- Delayed Surgical Recovery
- Self-Care Deficit
- Low Self-Esteem
- Disturbed Sleep Pattern
- Ineffective Therapeutic Regimen Management
- Disturbed Thought Process
- Risk for Violence

### SEXUALITY-REPRODUCTIVE
- Satisfaction with sexuality or sexual relationships
- Reproductive pattern
- Female menstrual and perimeno-pausal history

### ELIMINATION
- Patterns of bowel and urinary excretion
- Perceived regularity or irregularity of elimination
- Use of laxatives or routines
- Changes in time, modes, quality or quantity of excretions
- Use of devices for control

### ROLE-RELATIONSHIP
- Perception of major roles, relationships, and responsibilities in current life situation
- Satisfaction with or disturbances in roles and relationships

### ACTIVITY-EXERCISE
- Patterns of personally relevant exercise, activity, leisure, and recreation
- ADLs which require energy expenditure
- Factors that interfere with the desired pattern (e.g., illness or injury)

### SELF-PERCEPTION–SELF-CONCEPT
- Attitudes about self
- Perceived abilities, worth, self-image, emotions
- Body posture and movement, eye contact, voice and speech patterns

### SLEEP-REST
- Patterns of sleep and rest-/relaxation in a 24-hr period
- Perceptions of quality and quantity of sleep and rest
- Use of sleep aids and routines

### COGNITIVE-PERCEPTUAL
- Adequacy of vision, hearing, taste, touch, smell
- Pain perception and management
- Language, judgment, memory, decisions

*Reprinted from Nursing Diagnosis: Process and Application, 3rd ed., by M. Gordon, pp. 80–96, Copyright © 1994, with permission from Elsevier Science.*

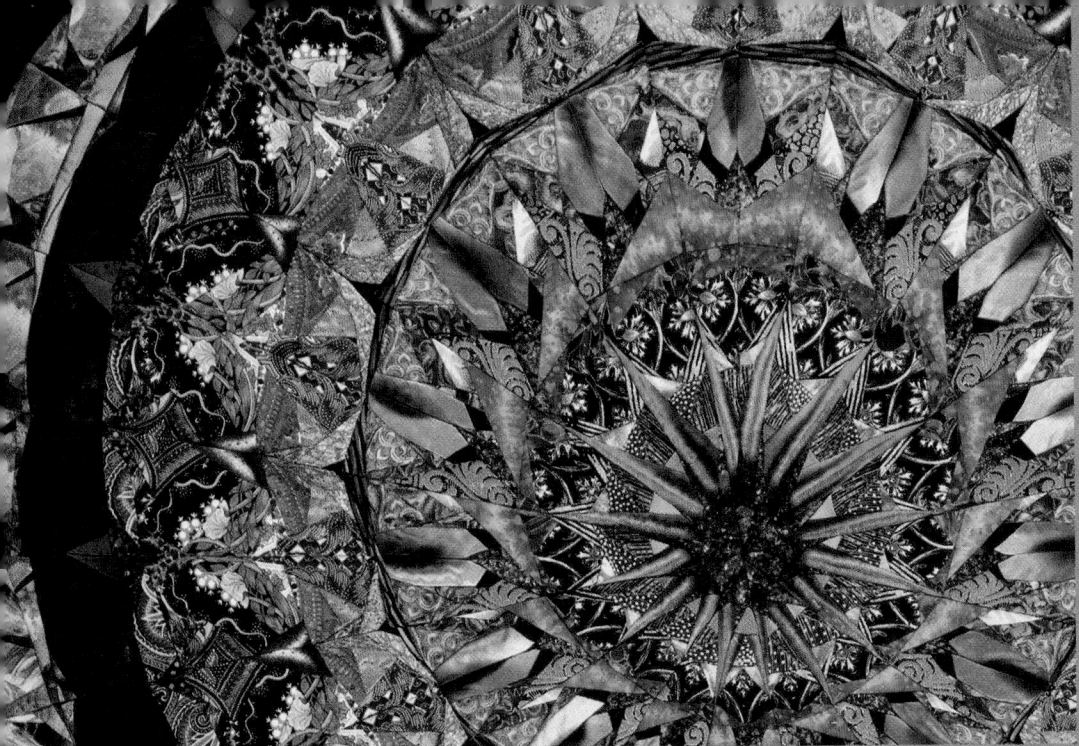

# DIMENSIONS OF MEDICAL-SURGICAL NURSING

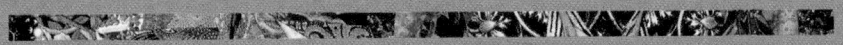

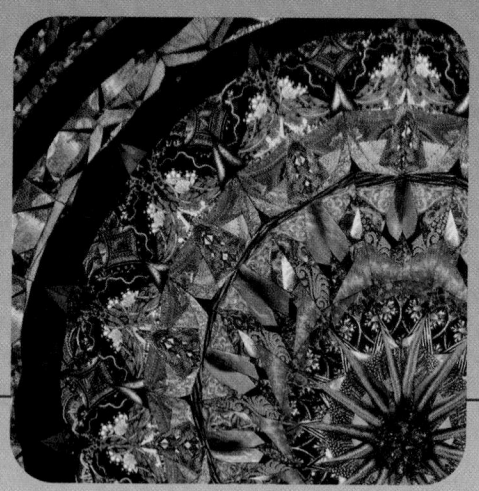

# The Medical-Surgical Nurse

## MediaLink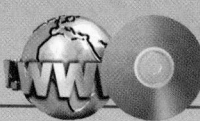

### www.prenhall.com/lemone

Additional resources for this chapter can be found on the Student CD-ROM accompanying this textbook, and on the Companion Website at www.prenhall.com/lemone. Click on Chapter 1 to select the activities for this chapter.

**CD-ROM**
• Audio Glossary
• NCLEX Review

**Companion Website**
• More NCLEX Review
• Case Study
  Advance Directive
• Care Plan Activity
  Nursing Process

## LEARNING OUTCOMES

After completing this chapter, you will be able to:

▪ Describe the activities and characteristics of the nurse as caregiver, educator, advocate, leader and manager, and researcher.

▪ Discuss the attitudes, mental habits, and skills necessary for critical thinking.

▪ Discuss the relationship between critical thinking and the nursing process in client care.

▪ Describe the importance of nursing codes and standards as guidelines for medical-surgical nursing care.

▪ Discuss the effect of legal and ethical dilemmas on nursing care.

▪ Discuss selected trends and issues in health care that affect medical-surgical nursing care.

**Medical-surgical nursing** is the health promotion, health care, and illness care of adults, based on knowledge derived from the arts and sciences and shaped by knowledge (the science) of nursing. Medical-surgical nursing focuses on the adult client's response to actual or potential alterations in health. In this textbook, discussions of those human responses are structured within the framework of functional health patterns, and nursing care is presented within the context of nursing diagnoses.

Medical-surgical nursing encompasses many interrelated components. The adult client—the person with whom and for whom nursing care is designed and implemented—ranges in age from the late teens to the early 100s. The human responses that nurses must consider when planning and implementing care result from changes in the structure and/or function of all body systems, as well as the interrelated effects of those changes on the psychosocial, cultural, spiritual, economic, and personal life of the client. The wide range of ages and the variety of health care needs specific to individual clients make medical-surgical nursing an ever-changing and challenging area of nursing practice.

## ROLES OF THE NURSE IN MEDICAL-SURGICAL NURSING PRACTICE

Health care today is a vast and complex system. It reflects changes in society, changes in the populations requiring nursing care, and a philosophical shift toward health promotion rather than illness care. Roles of the medical-surgical nurse have broadened and expanded in response to these changes. Medical-surgical nurses are not only caregivers but also educators, advocates, leaders and managers, and researchers. The nurse assumes these various roles to promote and maintain health, to prevent illness, and to facilitate coping with disability or death for the adult **client** (a person requiring health care services) in any setting.

### The Nurse as Caregiver

Nurses have always been caregivers. However, the activities carried out within the caregiver role have changed tremen-

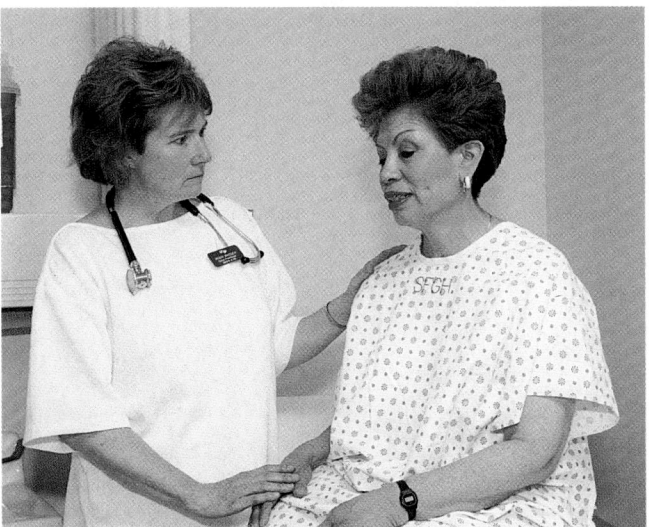

**Figure 1–1** ■ In the role of caregiver, the nurse provides comprehensive, individualized care to the adult client.

dously in the 21st century. From 1900 to the 1960s, the nurse was almost always female and was regarded primarily as the person who gave personal care and carried out physicians' orders. This dependent role has changed as a result of the increased education of nurses, research in and the development of nursing knowledge, and the recognition that nurses are autonomous and informed professionals.

The caregiver role for the nurse today is both independent and collaborative. Nurses independently make assessments and plan and implement client care based on nursing knowledge and skills (Figure 1–1 ■). Nurses also collaborate with other members of the health care team to implement and evaluate care.

As a caregiver, the nurse is a practitioner of nursing both as a science and as an art. Using **critical thinking** in the nursing process as the framework for care, the nurse provides interventions to meet not only the physical needs but also the psychosocial, cultural, spiritual, and environmental needs of clients and families. (Box 1–1 discusses culturally competent nursing care.) Considering all aspects of the client ensures a holistic approach to nursing. **Holistic nursing care** is based on a philosophical view that interacting wholes are greater than the sum of their parts. A holistic approach also emphasizes the uniqueness of the individual.

In providing comprehensive, individualized care, the nurse uses critical thinking skills to analyze and synthesize knowledge from the arts, the sciences, and nursing research and theory. The science (knowledge base) of nursing is translated into the art of nursing through caring. Caring is the means by which the nurse is connected with and concerned for the client (Benner & Wrubel, 1989). Thus, the nurse as caregiver is knowledgeable, skilled, empathic, and caring.

### The Nurse as Educator

The nurse's role as educator is becoming increasingly important for several reasons. Health care providers and consumers as well as local, state, and federal governments are placing greater emphasis on health promotion and illness prevention; hospital stays are becoming shorter; and the number of chronically ill in our society is increasing. All these factors make the educator role essential to maintaining the health and well-being of clients.

The framework for the role of educator is the teaching-learning process. Within this framework, the nurse assesses learning needs, plans and implements teaching methods to meet those needs, and evaluates the effectiveness of the teaching. To be an effective educator, the nurse must have effective interpersonal skills and be familiar with adult learning principles (Figure 1–2 ■).

A major component of the educator role today is discharge planning. **Discharge planning,** which begins on admission to a health care setting, is a systematic method of preparing the client and family for exit from the health care agency and for maintaining continuity of care after the client leaves the setting. Discharge planning also involves making referrals, identifying community and personal resources, and arranging for necessary equipment and supplies for home care.

## BOX 1–1 ■ Culturally Sensitive Nursing

The primary focus of nursing care is the client as the client relates to the environment and experiences events or situations related to health or illness. These experiences are given shape and personal meaning by culture—the socially inherited characteristics of a human group. These characteristics include the beliefs, practices, habits, likes, dislikes, customs, and rituals people learn from their families and pass on to their children. Cultural background is an essential component of a person's ethnic identity. A person's ethnic identity includes belonging to a social group within a culture and a social system and sharing a common religion, language, ancestry, and physical characteristics.

The health care system encompasses clients who are culturally diverse. This diversity includes differences in country of origin, health beliefs, sexual orientation, race, socioeconomic level, and age. Despite increasing diversity, nursing has been slow to address the need for culturally sensitive care. Many different factors account for this inattention, including ethnocentrism (people's belief that their own cultural group's beliefs and values are the only acceptable ones) and prejudice. The health care system is itself a culture, primarily, of white middle-class people, and it often serves as a barrier to culturally sensitive care.

The 1992 American Academy of Nursing Expert Panel on Culturally Competent Nursing Care identified several reasons why it has become increasingly important that nurses plan culturally sensitive care:

■ The demographic and ethnic composition of the population of the world in general, and the United States in particular, has changed markedly, and there is a lack of ethnic representation in health care professionals in the health care system. Information on and knowledge about values, beliefs, experiences, and health care needs of various populations is limited.

■ There is a growing awareness and acceptance of diversity and an increased willingness to maintain and support ethnic and cultural heritage.

■ People of color and immigrants are facing increasing unemployment, decreasing opportunity, and limited access to health care. These conditions may contribute to the establishment of new minorities, such as the homeless.

■ The international focus on providing health care for all people (within the context of inequity, barriers, and lack of access) may have raised the consciousness of health care professionals to some of the inequities inherent in health care systems in both developing countries and developed countries.

■ Nurses comprise the largest force in the delivery of health care and therefore have the potential to contribute to the changing inequities in and inaccessibility to health care.

■ Consumers are becoming increasingly aware of what is competent and sensitive health care.

This same panel of experts proposed general principles for nurses for becoming sensitive to cultural diversity and providing culturally sensitive care. For example:

■ Nurses must learn to appreciate intergroup and intragroup cultural diversity and commonalties in racial/ethnic minority populations.

■ Nurses must understand how social structure factors shape health behaviors and practices among members of racial/ethnic minorities.

■ Nurses must confront their own ethnocentrism and racism.

■ Nurses must begin rehearsing, practicing, and evaluating services provided to cross-cultural populations.

People of every culture have the right to have their cultural values known, respected, and addressed appropriately in nursing and other health care services (Leininger, 1991). To provide nursing care that is culturally sensitive, nurses must develop a sensitivity to personal fundamental values about health and illness; must accept the existence of differing values; and must be respectful of, interested in, and understanding of other cultures without being judgmental.

## The Nurse as Advocate

The client entering the health care system is often unprepared to make independent decisions. The nurse as client advocate actively promotes the client's rights to autonomy and free choice. The nurse as advocate speaks for the patient, mediates between the patient and other persons, and/or protects the patient's right to self-determination (Ellis & Hartley, 1998). The goals of the nurse as advocate are to:

• Assess the need for advocacy.
• Communicate with other health care team members.
• Provide client and family teaching.
• Assist and support client decision making.
• Serve as a change agent in the health care system.
• Participate in health policy formulation.

The nurse must practice advocacy based on the belief that clients have the right to choose treatment options, based on information about the results of accepting or rejecting the treatment, without coercion. The nurse must also accept and respect the decision of the client, even though it may differ from the decision the nurse would make.

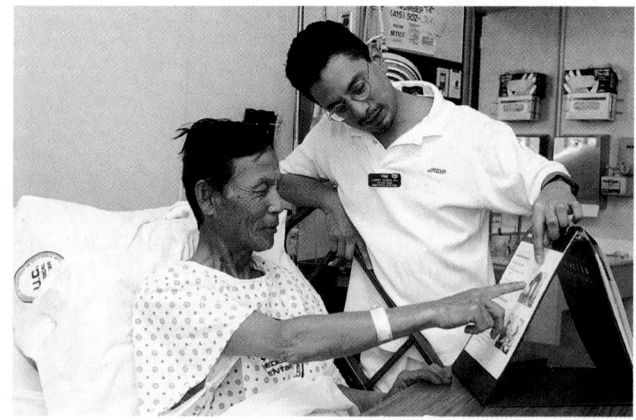

**Figure 1–2** ■ The nurse's role as educator is an essential component of care. As part of the discharge planning process, the nurse provides teaching for self-care at home.

## The Nurse as Leader and Manager

All nurses are leaders and managers. They practice leadership and they manage time, people, resources, and the environment in which they provide care. Nurses carry out these roles by directing, delegating, and coordinating nursing activities. Nurses also evaluate the quality of care provided.

### Models of Care Delivery

Nurses are leaders and managers of client care within a variety of models of care delivery. Examples are primary nursing, team nursing, and case management.

*PRIMARY NURSING.* **Primary nursing** allows the nurse to provide individualized direct care to a small number of clients during their entire inpatient stay. This model was developed to reduce the fragmentation of care experienced by the client and to facilitate family-centered continuity of care. In primary nursing, the nurse provides care; communicates with clients, families, and other health care providers; and carries out discharge planning.

*TEAM NURSING.* **Team nursing** is practiced by teams of variously educated health care providers. For example, a team may consist of a registered nurse, a licensed practical nurse, and two unlicensed assistive personnel. The registered nurse is the team leader. The team leader is responsible for making assignments and has overall responsibility for patient care by team members. All team members work together, each performing the activities for which he or she is best prepared.

*CASE MANAGEMENT.* **Case management** focuses on management of a caseload (group) of clients and the members of the health care team caring for those clients. The purpose of case management is to maximize positive outcomes and contain costs. The nurse who is case manager is usually a clinical specialist, and the caseload consists of clients with similar health care needs. As case manager, the nurse makes appropriate referrals to other health care providers and manages the quality of care provided, including accuracy, timeliness, and cost. The case manager also is in contact with clients after discharge, ensuring continuity of care and health maintenance.

### Delegation

**Delegation** is carried out when the nurse assigns appropriate and effective work activities to other members of the health care team. When the nurse delegates nursing care activities to another person, that person is authorized to act in the place of the nurse, while the nurse retains the accountability for the activities performed. Delegation skills are becoming increasingly important in health care as agencies restructure and implement cost containment measures. More categories of health care workers with often minimal nursing education and experience are being hired to assist the registered nurse as *nurse extenders*. Guidelines for delegation (Ellis & Hartley, 1998) include the following:

- Know the level of competence of each member of the health care team, the complexity of the task to be assigned, and the amount of time available to supervise the tasks.

- Know the level of nursing judgment and evaluation required for the task.
- Consider the potential harm and difficulty of performing the task.
- Know the state's nurse practice act and any practice limitations that may exist.
- Know the job descriptions for each category of worker.
- Assign the right job to the right person. Tasks that are routine and standard are the best to assign to others.
- Give clear and complete directions for assignments. Ask questions to be sure directions have been understood.
- Give the team member the authority to complete the task.
- Monitor the outcomes of the care provided and give constructive evaluation if necessary.

### Evaluating Outcomes of Nursing Care

*CRITICAL PATHWAYS.* A **critical pathway** is a health care plan designed to provide care with a multidisciplinary, managed action focus. Critical pathways, also called critical paths, are one model for this approach to health care. Such pathways are generally developed for specific diagnoses—usually high volume, high risk, and high cost case types—with the collaboration of members of the health care team. This client care management tool describes how resources will be used to achieve predetermined outcomes. It also establishes the sequence of multidisciplinary interventions, including education, discharge planning, consultations, medication administration, diagnostics, therapeutics, and treatments. Figure 1–3 ■ shows a sample critical pathway.

The goals of critical pathways are to:

- Achieve realistic, expected client and family outcomes.
- Promote professional and collaborative practice and care.
- Ensure continuity of care.
- Guarantee appropriate use of resources.
- Reduce costs and length of stay.
- Provide the framework for continuous improvement.

Critical pathways are often used in conjunction with case management models and/or quality improvement efforts. The overall goal is to design pathways that facilitate a reproducible standard of care for specific client populations and improve the quality and proficiency of that care.

The agency determines the process for developing a critical pathway. Information imperative to the development of any critical pathway includes literature reviews, chart reviews, expert opinion, and insurance reimbursements for the designated case type. A typical approach is to first identify high cost, high volume, and high risk case types for the agency. Next, a multidisciplinary team, including physicians, develops a consensus around the management of the case type and a critical pathway. The pathway is then piloted with a designated group of clients, and revisions are based on the number and types of variances. The goal is to develop a pathway that best meets the needs of clients in the particular practice setting.

When clients do not achieve expected outcomes, variances (deviations from the established plan) from the critical pathways are recorded and studied by the multidisciplinary team. In many agencies, critical pathways are designed so that

| | Date _____<br>Preoperative | Date _____<br>1st 24 hours following surgery |
|---|---|---|
| | Expected length of stay: less than 24 hours | |
| Daily outcomes | Client will<br>• Verbalize understanding of preoperative teaching, including turning, coughing, deep breathing, mobilization, and pain management.<br>• Demonstrate ability to cope. | Client will<br>• Be afebrile.<br>• Have a dry, clean dressing.<br>• Have nasal packing, splint/cast, and mustache dressing intact and in place.<br>• Manage pain with nonpharmacologic measures or oral medications.<br>• Be independent in self-care.<br>• Be fully ambulatory.<br>• Verbalize/demonstrate home care instructions.<br>• Tolerate usual diet.<br>• Demonstrate ability to cope with ongoing stressors. |
| Tests and treatments | CBC<br>Urinalysis<br>Baseline physical assessment with a focus on respiratory status<br>Anesthesia consultation | Vital signs and $O_2$ saturation, neurovascular assessment, dressing, edema, and wound drainage assessment q15min × 4, q30min × 4, q1h × 4, and then q4h if stable.<br>Assess for posterior nasal bleeding.<br>Assess lung sounds q4h and prn.<br>Assess voiding—if unable to void, try suggestive voiding techniques or catheterize q8h or prn if unable to void.<br>Cool compresses to nose, eyes, or face to reduce swelling and prevent excessive discoloration. |
| Knowledge deficit | Orient to room and surroundings.<br>Include family in teaching.<br>Provide simple, brief instructions.<br>Review preoperative preparation, including hospital and surgical routines.<br>Reinforce preoperative teaching regarding specific postoperative care: turning, coughing, deep breathing, mobilization, and pain management.<br>Assess understanding of teaching. | Reorient to room and postoperative routine.<br>Include family in teaching.<br>Review plan of care and importance of early mobilization, as well as any activity restrictions.<br>Complete discharge teaching regarding splint/cast care/dressing change, follow-up care, signs and symptoms to report, medications, and diet.<br>Instruct the client to avoid activities that might result in a blow or pressure on the nose and procedures to follow if bleeding occurs.<br>Instruct client to avoid the Valsalva's maneuver and to avoid aspirin and other nonsteroidal medications.<br>Assess understanding of teaching. |
| Psychosocial | Assess anxiety related to pending surgery.<br>Assess fears of the unknown and surgery.<br>Encourage verbalization of concerns.<br>Provide emotional support to client and family.<br>Provide information regarding surgery.<br>Minimize stimuli (e.g., noise, movement). | Assess level of anxiety.<br>Encourage verbalization of concerns.<br>Provide emotional support to client and family.<br>Provide information and ongoing support and encouragement. |
| Diet | NPO | Advance to clear liquids. If tolerated, advance to full liquids/soft diet following surgery. |
| Activity | OOB ad lib until premedicated for surgery. | Provide safety precautions.<br>Place in semi-Fowler's position.<br>Allow bathroom privileges with assistance on evening after surgery. Begin progressive ambulation to tolerance the morning following surgery until fully ambulatory. |
| Medications | NPO except ordered medications. | IM or PO analgesics.<br>Antibiotics if ordered.<br>IV fluids until adequate PO intake then intermittent IV.<br>Discontinue prior to discharge. |
| Transfer/ discharge plans | Assess discharge plans and support system. | Probable discharge within 24 hours of surgery.<br>Complete discharge home care teaching when client is fully awake and oriented and before discharge.<br>Provide a written copy of discharge instructions. |

**Figure 1—3** ■ Critical pathway for a client following a rhinoplasty.

interventions and variances can be easily documented. Most documentation systems require a checkoff when interventions are performed or variances occur.

In many agencies, critical pathways are replacing traditional nursing care plans. The advantages of critical pathways are that they are outcome driven and provide a time line to achieve specified goals. Additionally, critical pathways provide opportunities for health care workers to collaborate and establish dynamic plans of care that consider all of the clients' needs. Although initially developed for acute hospitalizations, critical pathways are now developed to manage clients in home health, outpatient, and long-term settings.

***QUALITY ASSURANCE.***   As a leader and manager, the nurse is responsible for the quality of client care through a process called **quality assurance.** It consists of the quality control activities that evaluate, monitor, or regulate the standard of services provided to the consumer. Clients are assured of quality care through professional and technical licensure of individual care providers; accreditation of hospitals (e.g., by the Joint Commission on Accreditation of Healthcare Organizations [JCAHO]); licensure of hospitals, pharmacies, and nursing homes; and certification in specialty areas.

Quality assurance methods also are used to evaluate client care. They commonly evaluate actual care against an established set of standards of care. Nurses and other health care providers make this evaluation by reviewing documentation, by conducting client surveys and nurse interviews, and/or by direct observation of nurse or client performance. The data are then used to identify differences between actual practice and established standards and to develop a plan of action to resolve the differences. The actions are then assessed through internal peer review or by an external medical review organization, called a utilization and quality control peer review organization (PRO), to determine whether they were effective in improving practice. These reviews have resulted in such health care changes as an increase in outpatient surgeries with a resultant decrease in the number of inpatient surgeries.

## The Nurse as Researcher

Nurses have always identified problems in client care. Although they have developed interventions to meet specific needs, the activities often have not been conducted within a scientific framework or communicated to other nurses through nursing literature. To develop the science of nursing, nursing knowledge must be established through clinical research and then published, so that the findings can be used by all nurses to provide evidence-based client care.

To be relevant, nursing research must have a goal to improve the care that nurses provide clients. This means that all nurses must consider the researcher role to be integral to nursing practice. Summaries of relevant nursing research are included in almost all the nursing care chapters of this textbook. After the summary and discussion of each study, a critical thinking section specifically related to the findings of the study encourages the student to apply the findings to the clinical setting.

## FRAMEWORK FOR PRACTICE: CRITICAL THINKING IN THE NURSING PROCESS

The **nursing process** is the series of critical thinking activities nurses use as they provide care to clients. These activities define a nursing model of care, differentiating nursing from other helping professions. The nursing process can be used in any setting. The purpose of care may be to promote wellness, maintain health, restore health, or facilitate coping with disability or death. Regardless of the purpose of care, the planned process of nursing allows for the inclusion of specific, individualized, and holistic activities.

## Critical Thinking

Critical thinking is, most basically, thinking about one's own thinking. It is self-directed thinking that is focused on what to believe or do in a specific situation. It involves attitudes and skills. Critical thinking occurs when the nurse uses knowledge to consider a client care situation and uses the nursing process to make judgments and decisions about what to do in that situation. As you practice critical thinking, you must consider:

- The purpose of the thinking (e.g., is it to collect more data or is it to report the data to someone else?).
- Your level of acquired knowledge.
- Prejudices that may influence thinking (e.g., believing that all people in poverty are dirty or that the aged are incapable of learning how to care for themselves, or letting emotions affect decision making).
- Information that is needed from other sources such as faculty members, a skilled clinical nurse, a textbook or journal article, or the policies of the health care agency.
- The ability to identify other possible options, evaluate the alternatives, and reach a conclusion.
- Personal values and beliefs.

Critical thinking takes practice so that it becomes an integral component of the nurse's attitudes and skills. Critical thinking exercises are included throughout this book to provide that practice.

### Attitudes and Mental Habits Necessary for Critical Thinking

Thinking critically involves more than just cognitive (knowledge) skills. It is strongly influenced by one's attitudes and mental habits. To think critically, you must focus your attention on your attitudes and how they affect your thinking. These attitudes and mental habits are:

- Being able to *think independently* so that you make clinical decisions based on sound thinking and judgment. This means, for example, you are not influenced by negative comments from other health care providers about a client.
- Being willing to listen to and be fair in your evaluation of others' ideas and beliefs by having *intellectual courage.* This involves listening carefully to other ideas and thoughts, and making a decision based on what you learn instead of how you feel.
- Having *intellectual empathy* by being able to put yourself in the place of another to better understand that other person.

For example, if you put yourself in the place of the person with severe pain, you are better able to understand why he or she is so upset when pain medications are late.

- Being fair-minded and considering all viewpoints before making a decision through an *intellectual sense of justice* and being *intellectually humble.* This means you consider the viewpoints of others that may be different from yours before reaching a conclusion. You also realize that you are constantly learning from others. You are not afraid to say, "I don't know the answer to that question, but I will find out and let you know."
- Being *disciplined* so that you do not stop at easy answers, but continue to consider alternatives.
- Being *creative* and *self-confident.* Nurses often need to consider different ways of providing care and constantly look for better, more cost-effective methods. Confidence in one's decisions is gained through critical thinking.

### Critical Thinking Skills

Critical thinking skills are the mental abilities that are used. Major critical thinking skills are as follows:

- *Divergent thinking* is having the ability to weigh the importance of information. This means that when you collect data from a client, you can sort out the data that are relevant for the care of your client from the data that are not relevant and explore alternatives to draw a conclusion. Abnormal data are usually considered relevant; normal data are helpful but may not change the care you provide.
- *Reasoning* is having the ability to discriminate between facts and guesses. By using known facts, problems are solved and decisions are made in a systematic, logical way. For example, when you take a pulse you must know the facts of normal pulse rate for a person of this age, types of medications the client is taking that may alter the pulse rate, and the emotional and physical state of the client. Based on these facts, you are able to decide if the pulse rate is normal or abnormal.
- *Clarifying* is defining terms and noting similarities and differences. For example, when caring for a client with chronic pain, you must know the definition of chronic pain and the similarities and differences between acute pain and chronic pain.
- *Reflection* occurs when you take time to think about something. It cannot take place in an emergency situation. As you reflect on your experiences in nursing, many of those experiences may in turn become alternatives when caring for a different client.

Critical thinking is an expected ability of all nurses. Using critical thinking to provide care that is structured by the nursing process allows the nurse to provide safe, effective, holistic, and individualized care. See Table 1–1.

## The Nursing Process

The five steps or phases in the nursing process are assessment, diagnosis, planning, implementation, and evaluation. These steps are interrelated and interdependent. The steps are most often used cyclically, as illustrated in Figure 1–4 ■ . The steps have been legitimized by the American Nurses Association (ANA) Standards of Practice, state nursing practice acts, and licensing examinations that are structured on a nursing model of care based on the nursing process.

This textbook assumes that the student already has a basic understanding of the nursing process and is now ready to expand and apply that knowledge to adult clients with medical-surgical health problems. The following discussion is intended to serve only as a review; for more information, consult books specifically focused on the use of the nursing process, and read the case studies in the nursing care chapters throughout this textbook.

### Assessment

Assessment is usually listed as the first step of the nursing process, but in actuality it is a critical element in each of the steps. It begins with the client's first encounter with the health care system and continues as long as the client requires care. During assessment, data (pieces of information) about health status are collected, validated, organized, clustered into patterns, and communicated either verbally or in written form. Assessment serves as the basis for deriving accurate nursing diagnoses, for planning and implementing both initial and ongoing individualized care, and for evaluating care.

The data that the nurse collects must be holistic; that is, the nurse must carefully consider all dimensions of an individual. The data collected are both objective and subjective. Information that the nurse perceives by the senses is **objective data;** it is seen, heard, touched, or smelled, and can be verified by another person (e.g., blood pressure, temperature, pulse, or the presence of infected drainage). Information that is perceived only by the person experiencing it (e.g., pain, dizziness, or anxiety) is **subjective data.**

Nurses assess clients in two ways: through an initial assessment and through focused assessments. The **initial assessment** of the client, conducted through a nursing history and physical assessment, is necessary to:

- Accumulate comprehensive data about health responses.
- Identify specific factors that contribute to these responses in a specific individual.
- Facilitate mutually established goals and outcomes of care. (Iyer, Taptich, & Bernocchi-Losey, 1994)

**Focused assessments** are ongoing and continuous, occurring whenever the nurse interacts with the client. They enable the nurse to evaluate nursing actions and make decisions about whether to continue or change interventions to meet outcomes. They also provide structure for documenting nursing care. In addition, focused assessments enable the nurse to identify responses to a disease process or treatment modality not present during the initial assessment, or to monitor the status of an actual or potential problem previously identified (Alfaro, 1998).

To make accurate and holistic assessments, nurses must have and use a wide variety of knowledge and skills. The ability to assess the physical status of the client is essential, as is the ability to use effective communication techniques. Nurses must be knowledgeable in pathophysiology and pharmacology and be able to identify abnormal laboratory and diagnostic test data. Finally, nurses must have a solid foundation of nursing knowledge and skill that will enable them to interpret assessment data and to use that interpretation as the basis for individualized care.

MediaLink   NURSING CARE PLAN

## TABLE 1-1 Using Critical Thinking in the Nursing Process

| Nursing Process Step | Critical Thinking Skills | Questions to Check Your Thinking |
|---|---|---|
| Assessment | Making reliable observations<br>Distinguishing relevant from irrelevant data<br>Distinguishing important from unimportant data<br>Validating data<br>Organizing data<br>Categorizing data according to a framework<br>Recognizing assumptions | What assumptions am I making about the patient?<br>Is my data correct and accurate?<br>How reliable are my sources?<br>What data is important? Relevant?<br>What biases do I have that might cause me to miss important information?<br>Am I listening carefully to get the patient's and family's perspective?<br>Do I have all the facts? What other data might I need? |
| Diagnosis | Finding patterns and relationships among cues<br>Identifying gaps in the data<br>Making inferences<br>Suspending judgment when lacking data<br>Making interdisciplinary connections<br>Stating the problem<br>Examining assumptions<br>Comparing patterns with norms<br>Identifying factors contributing to the problem | Do I know what is within normal limits for the data?<br>Do I have enough data to make a valid inference?<br>What biases might I have that could affect how I see the patient's problems?<br>Do I have enough data to make a nursing diagnosis or should I make a "possible" diagnosis?<br>What other problems might this data suggest other than the one that seems most obvious to me? |
| Planning | Forming valid generalizations<br>Transferring knowledge from one situation to another<br>Developing evaluative criteria<br>Hypothesizing<br>Making interdisciplinary connections<br>Prioritizing client problems<br>Generalizing principles from other sciences | Do I need help to plan interventions, or am I qualified to do it?<br>Did I remember to give high priority to the problems the patient and family identified as important?<br>What are the most important problems we need to solve?<br>What interventions worked in similar situations? Is this situation similar enough to merit using them with this patient?<br>Are there other plans that might be more agreeable to the patient, and therefore more likely to work?<br>Why do I expect these interventions to be effective? Based on what knowledge? |
| Implementation | Applying knowledge to perform interventions<br>Using interventions to test hypotheses | Has the patient's condition changed since the plan was made?<br>Have I overlooked any new developments?<br>What is the patient's initial response to the intervention?<br>Are there any safety issues I have overlooked? |
| Evaluation | Deciding whether hypotheses are correct<br>Making criterion-based evaluations | What are the patient reponses after the interventions?<br>Have I overlooked anything?<br>Does the data indicate that goals were met? Does the patient feel the goals were met?<br>Does the patient trust me enough to give honest answers?<br>Am I sure the problem is really resolved?<br>What might we have done that would have been more effective?<br>What nursing care is still needed, if any? |

*Note. From* Nursing Process and Critical Thinking *(3rd ed.) by J. M. Wilkinson, 2001. Reprinted by permission of Pearson Education, Inc., Upper Saddle River, NJ.*

## Diagnosis

The ANA defines nursing as "the diagnosis and treatment of human responses to actual or potential health problems" (1980, p. 9). The nurse labels each response with a **nursing diagnosis,** defined by the North American Nursing Diagnosis Association (NANDA) as "a clinical judgment about individual, family, or community responses to actual or potential health problems/life processes. Nursing diagnoses provide the basis for selection of nursing interventions to achieve outcomes for which the nurse is accountable" (NANDA, 2001,

p. 245). Nurses develop and implement a plan of care for actual responses; they also plan interventions to support health concerns and prevent illness concerns for potential human responses.

The nurse analyzes data collected during the assessment step to support appropriate nursing diagnoses. During analysis, the nurse clusters data into categories of information that can be used to identify actual or potential alterations in health. Data can be organized within a variety of frameworks and methods for identifying patterns of human behavior

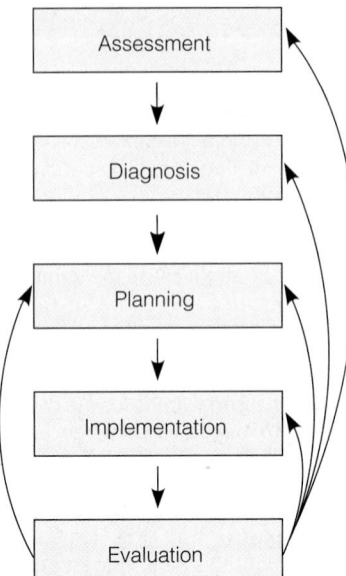

**Figure 1–4** ■ ■ Steps of the nursing process. Notice that the steps are interrelated and interdependent. For example, evaluation of the client might reveal the need for further assessment, additional nursing diagnoses, and/or a revision of the plan of care.

(Wilkinson, 2000). Methods commonly used are basic human needs (Maslow, 1970), body systems, human response patterns, and functional health patterns (Gordon, 1982). The broad organizational structure used to categorize information in this book is based on Gordon's (1994) functional health patterns, outlined in Box 1–2.

Making a diagnosis is a complex process that always involves uncertainty. Therefore, the nurse uses diagnostic reasoning to choose nursing diagnoses that best define the individual client's health problems. Diagnostic reasoning is a form of clinical judgment (Radwin, 1990) used to make decisions about which label (or diagnosis) best describes the patterns of data. Radwin's review of research about diagnostic reasoning

in nursing found that elements of the clinical judgment process include data gathering and validation, data categorization, intuition, and prior clinical experience.

Although there is no universal list of diagnoses used in nursing, the work of NANDA is widely accepted. The diagnoses are classified by a taxonomy; that is, they are grouped into classes and subclasses based on patterns and relationships. Work on both the nursing diagnoses and the taxonomy is ongoing. The NANDA system was accepted in 1988 by the ANA as the official system of diagnosis for the United States. Nursing diagnoses within the NANDA taxonomy are used in this book.

A diagnosis is written in two parts joined by the phrase "related to." The first part of the statement is the particular human response that has been identified from the analysis of data. It identifies what needs to change in a specific client as a result of nursing interventions, and it also identifies the client outcomes that measure the change. The part of the statement that follows the "related to" phrase identifies the physical, psychosocial, cultural, spiritual, and/or environmental factors (etiologies) that cause or contribute to the occurrence of the response.

Many nurses write nursing diagnoses using a method known as PES (Gordon, 1994). Diagnoses written with this method have three components:

1. The problem (P), which is the NANDA label.
2. The etiology (E) of the problem, which names the related factors and is indicated by the phrase "related to."
3. The signs and symptoms (S), which are the defining characteristics and are indicated by the phrase "as manifested by."

Examples of nursing diagnoses written with the PES method are as follows:

- *Anxiety* related to hospitalization as manifested by statements of nervousness and by crying
- *Bowel incontinence* related to loss of sphincter control as manifested by involuntary passage of stool

---

**BOX 1–2    ■ Functional Health Patterns**

1. *Health-perception–health-management pattern.* Describes client's perceived pattern of health and well-being and how health is managed.
2. *Nutritional-metabolic pattern.* Describes pattern of food and fluid consumption relative to metabolic need and pattern indicators of local nutrient supply.
3. *Elimination pattern.* Describes pattern of excretory function (bowel, bladder, and skin).
4. *Activity-exercise pattern.* Describes pattern of exercise, activity, leisure, and recreation.
5. *Cognitive-perceptual pattern.* Describes sensory-perceptual and cognitive patterns.
6. *Sleep-rest pattern.* Describes patterns of sleep, rest, and relaxation.

7. *Self-perception–self-concept pattern.* Describes self-concept pattern and perceptions of self (e.g., body comfort, body image, feeling state).
8. *Role-relationship pattern.* Describes patterns of role-engagements and relationships.
9. *Sexuality-reproductive pattern.* Describes client's patterns of satisfaction and dissatisfaction with sexuality; describes reproductive patterns.
10. *Coping–stress-tolerance pattern.* Describes general coping pattern and effectiveness of the pattern in terms of stress tolerance.
11. *Value-belief pattern.* Describes patterns of values, beliefs (including spiritual), or goals that guide choices or decisions.

*Note. Adapted from* Nursing Diagnosis: Process and Application *(3rd ed.) by M. Gordon, 1994, St. Louis: Mosby-Year Book.*

- *Fatigue* related to the side effects of chemotherapy as manifested by the inability to carry out normal daily routines and statements of overwhelming exhaustion

### Planning

During the **planning** step, the nurse develops a list of nursing interventions (actions) and client outcomes to promote healthy responses and to prevent, reverse, or decrease unhealthy responses. **Outcomes,** which are mutually established by the client and nurse, identify what the client will be able to do as a result of the nursing interventions. Both outcomes and nursing interventions are documented in a written plan of care that directs nursing activities and documentation and provides a tool for evaluation (Alfaro, 1998). The plan of care may be documented in a variety of formats.

Nurses plan interventions for two types of client problems: those that require nursing management, stated as nursing diagnoses; and those that require collaborative management, which may be referred to as collaborative or clinical problems. Nursing diagnoses provide the basis for selecting nurse-initiated interventions to achieve outcomes for which the nurse is accountable. Collaborative problems are pathophysiologic, treatment-related, personal, environmental, and maturational situations which nurses monitor for detection of onset or changes in status. Both physician-initiated and nurse-initiated interventions minimize the complications of collaborative problems (Carpenito, 1999).

Outcome criteria for nursing diagnoses are client centered, time specific, and measurable. They are classified into three domains: cognitive (knowing), affective (feeling), and psychomotor (doing). The nurse considers all three domains to ensure holistic care.

Outcome criteria for collaborative problems are nursing goals, usually written as statements that begin with "to detect and report early signs and symptoms of potential complications of . . . " and "to implement preventive and corrective nursing interventions ordered by . . . " (Alfaro, 1998). In many instances, these goals are not written as part of the plan of care. Preventive and corrective nursing interventions for collaborative problems may be ordered by the physician or by institutional policy, procedures, protocols, or standards.

The nursing interventions planned must be specific and individualized. If, for example, the nurse identifies that a client is at risk for fluid volume deficit, it is not enough that the nurse simply encourage the client to drink increased amounts of fluid. The nurse and the client together must identify those liquids the client prefers, the times that will be best for drinking them, and the amount of fluid (in ounces or milliliters); this information must be documented as a nursing order on the written care plan. Only then does care truly become a part of the plan of care.

### Implementation

The **implementation** step is the action or "doing" phase of the nursing process, during which the nurse carries out planned interventions. Ongoing assessment of the client before, during, and after the intervention is an essential component of implementation. Although the plan may be appropriate, many variables can modify or negate any planned intervention, making a change in the plan necessary. For example, the nurse would not be able to force fluids if the client were nauseated or vomiting.

When implementing the planned interventions, the nurse follows several important principles:

- Set daily priorities, based on initial assessments and on the client's condition as reported during the change of shift report and/or documented in the client's chart. Ensure that critical assessments (such as status of invasive lines, fluids infusing, or changes in health status during the preceding shift) take first priority.
- Be aware of the interrelated nature of nursing interventions. For example, while giving a bath the nurse can also assess physical and psychologic status, use therapeutic communication, teach the client, do range-of-motion exercises, and provide skin care.
- Determine the most appropriate interventions for each client, based on health status and illness treatment. Examples of appropriate interventions include:
  - Directly performing the activity for the client.
  - Assisting the client to perform the activity.
  - Supervising the client/family while they are performing the activity.
  - Teaching the client/family about health care.
  - Monitoring the client at risk for potential complications or problems.
- Use available resources to provide interventions that are realistic for the situation and practical in terms of equipment available, financial status of the client, and resources available (including staff, agency, family, and community resources).

Documenting interventions is the final component of implementation, and it is a legal requirement. There are many different ways of documenting care. The traditional narrative source-oriented and problem-oriented charting methods are used, as are newer methods such as focused charting, charting by exception, and computer-assisted documentation.

### Evaluation

The **evaluation** step allows the nurse to determine whether the plan was effective and either to continue the plan, to revise the plan, or to terminate the plan. The outcome criteria that were established during the planning step provide the basis for evaluation. Although evaluation is listed as the last part of the nursing process, it takes place continuously throughout client care.

To evaluate a plan, the nurse collects data from the client and reviews the chart. The nurse then compares the status of the client with the written outcomes. If the outcomes have been accomplished, the nurse may either continue or terminate the plan. If the outcomes have not been accomplished, the nurse must modify the nursing diagnoses, outcomes, or plan.

### Benefits of the Nursing Process

The nursing process benefits nurses who provide care, clients who receive care, and settings where care is provided. As nurses gain increasing autonomy in their practice, the use of the nursing process helps them identify their independent practice domain. The nursing process also provides a common reference system and a common terminology to serve as a base for improving

---

**BOX 1–3  ■ The International Council of Nurses Code for Nurses**

The fundamental responsibility of the nurse is fourfold: to promote health, to prevent illness, to restore health, and to alleviate suffering. The need for nursing is universal. Inherent in nursing is respect for life, dignity, and the rights of man. It is unrestricted by considerations of nationality, race, creed, color, age, sex, politics, or social status. Nurses render health services to the individual, the family, and the community and coordinate their services with those of related groups.

### NURSES AND PEOPLE

The nurse's primary responsibility is to those people who require nursing care. The nurse, in providing care, promotes an environment in which the values, customs, and spiritual beliefs of the individual are respected. The nurse holds in confidence personal information and uses judgment in sharing this information.

### NURSES AND PRACTICE

The nurse carries responsibility for nursing practice and for maintaining competence by continual learning. The nurse maintains the highest standards of nursing care possible within the reality of a specific situation. The nurse uses judgment in relation to individual competence when accepting and delegating responsibili-

ties. The nurse when acting in a professional capacity should at all times maintain standards of personal conduct that reflect credit upon the profession.

### NURSES AND SOCIETY

The nurse shares with other citizens the responsibility for initiating and supporting action to meet the health and social needs of the public.

### NURSES AND COWORKERS

The nurse sustains a cooperative relationship with coworkers in nursing and other fields. The nurse takes appropriate action to safeguard the individual when his or her care is endangered by a coworker or any other person.

### NURSES AND THE PROFESSION

The nurse plays the major role in determining and implementing desirable standards of nursing practice and nursing education. The nurse is active in developing a core of professional knowledge. The nurse, acting through the professional organization, participates in establishing and maintaining equitable social and economic working conditions in nursing.

Note. From ICN Code for Nurses: Ethical Concepts Applied to Nursing by International Council of Nurses, 1973, Geneva: Imprimeries Populaires. Copyright © 1973 by ICN. Reprinted by permission.

---

clinical practice through research. In addition, the nursing process can serve as a framework for the evaluation of quality care.

The nursing process also benefits the client receiving care and the agency or institution providing that care. The client receives planned, individualized interventions; participates in all steps of the process; and is assured continuity of care through the written care plan. The nursing process benefits the health care institution through better resource utilization, increased client satisfaction, and improved documentation of care.

### The Nursing Process in Clinical Practice

With experience, the nurse does not consciously stop and consider each step. Rather, using the process as a framework, the nurse provides care based on the client's specific, individualized needs. For example, when caring for a client who is hemorrhaging, the nurse uses all five steps simultaneously to meet critical, life-threatening needs. In contrast, when considering long-term needs for a client with a chronic illness or disability, the nurse makes in-depth assessments, mutually determines goals with the client, and provides documentation through a written plan of care that can be developed and revised as necessary by all nurses providing care. As a nurse becomes an expert practitioner, the nursing process becomes so much a part of the nurse that he or she may not even consciously consider it while providing care; the practice is the process (Benner, 1984).

## GUIDELINES FOR NURSING PRACTICE

Nursing practice is structured by codes of ethics and standards that guide nursing practice and protect the public. These guidelines are especially important because nurses encounter legal and ethical problems almost daily. A discussion of representative issues also is included.

## Codes for Nurses

An established code of ethics is one criterion that defines a profession. **Ethics** are principles of conduct. **Ethical behavior** is concerned with moral duty, values, obligations, and the distinction between right and wrong. Codes of ethics for nurses provide a frame of reference for "professionally valued and ideal nursing behaviors that are congruent with the principles expressed in the Code for Nurses" (Ketefian, 1987, p. 13).

The large number of ethical issues facing nurses in clinical practice makes the established codes for nurses critical to moral and ethical decision making. The codes also help to define the roles of nurses. The codes of ethics presented here were developed by and for members of the International Council of Nurses (ICN) and the ANA.

### The ICN Code

The ICN Code for Nurses (Box 1–3) helps guide nurses in setting priorities, making judgments, and taking action when they face ethical dilemmas in clinical practice.

### The ANA Code

The ANA Code for Nurses (Box 1–4) states principles of ethical concern, which guides the behavior of nurses and also defines nursing for the general public.

## Standards of Nursing Practice

A **standard** is a statement or criterion that can be used by a profession and by the general public to measure quality of practice. Established standards of nursing practice make each individual nurse accountable for practice. This means that each nurse providing care has the responsibility or obligation to account for his or her own behaviors within that role. Professional nursing

| BOX 1–4 | ■ The American Nurses Association Code of Ethics for Nurses |
|---|---|

- The nurse, in all professional relationships, practices with compassion and respect for the inherent dignity, worth, and uniqueness of every individual, unrestricted by considerations of social or economic status, personal attributes, or the nature of health problems.
- The nurse's primary commitment is to the patient, whether an individual, family, group, or community.
- The nurse promotes, advocates for, and strives to protect the health, safety, and rights of the patient.
- The nurse is responsible and accountable for individual nursing practice and determines the appropriate delegation of tasks consistent with the nurse's obligation to provide optimum patient care.
- The nurse owes the same duties to self as to others, including the responsibility to preserve integrity and safety, to maintain competence, and to continue personal and professional growth.

- The nurse participates in establishing, maintaining, and improving health care environments and conditions of employment conducive to the provision of quality health care and consistent with the values of the profession through individual and collective action.
- The nurse participates in the advancement of the profession through contributions in practice, education, administration, and knowledge development.
- The nurse collaborates with other health professionals and the public in promoting community, national, and international efforts to meet health needs.
- The profession of nursing, as represented by associations and their members, is responsible for articulating nursing values, for maintaining the integrity of the profession and its practice, and for shaping social policy.

*Note. Reprinted with permission from American Nurses Association, Code of Ethics for Nurses with Interpretive Statements, © 2001, American Nurses Publishing. American Nurses Foundation/American Nurses Association, Washington, DC.*

organizations develop and implement standards of practice to identify clearly the nurse's responsibilities to society.

The ANA standards of clinical nursing practice (1998) are outlined in Box 1–5. These standards allow objective evaluation of nursing licensure and certification, institutional accreditation, quality assurance, and public policy.

## LEGAL AND ETHICAL DILEMMAS AND ISSUES IN NURSING

A **dilemma** is a choice between two unpleasant, ethically troubling alternatives. Nurses who provide medical-surgical nursing care face dilemmas almost daily—so many that a complete discussion of them is impossible here. However, many com-

monly experienced dilemmas involve caring for the client with acquired immune deficiency syndrome (AIDS), client rights, and issues of dying and death. The nurse must use ethical and legal guidelines to make decisions about moral actions when providing care in these and in many other situations.

Nurses respect the right to confidentiality of client information found in the client's record or secured during interviews. (In most instances, state nursing practice acts legally require nurses to uphold this right.) Rights of the client as an individual, however, can result in dilemmas for the nurse in the clinical setting. For example, the right to privacy and confidentiality creates a dilemma when it conflicts with the nurse's right to information that may affect personal safety. The may happen when the nurse does not know a client's HIV status. The current

| BOX 1–5 | ■ The American Nurses Association Standards of Clinical Nursing Practice |
|---|---|

### STANDARDS OF CARE

Assessment: The nurse collects patient health data.

Diagnosis: The nurse analyzes the assessment data in determining diagnoses.

Outcome Identification: The nurse identifies expected outcomes individualized to the patient.

Planning: The nurse develops a plan of care that prescribes interventions to attain expected outcomes.

Implementation: The nurse implements the interventions identified in the plan of care.

Evaluation: The nurse evaluates the patient's progress toward attainment of outcomes.

### STANDARDS OF PROFESSIONAL PERFORMANCE

Quality of Care: The nurse systematically evaluates the quality and effectiveness of nursing practice.

Performance Appraisal: The nurse evaluates one's own nursing practice in relation to professional practice standards and relevant statues and regulations.

Education: The nurse acquires and maintains current knowledge and competency in nursing practice.

Collegiality: The nurse interacts with and contributes to the professional development of peers and other health care providers as colleagues.

Ethics: The nurse's decisions and actions on behalf of patients are determined in an ethical manner.

Collaboration: The nurse collaborates with the patient, family, and other health care providers in providing patient care.

Research: The nurse uses research findings in practice.

Resource Utilization: The nurse considers factors related to safety, effectiveness, and cost in planning and delivering patient care.

*Note. Reprinted with permission from American Nurses Association, Code of Ethics for Nurses with Interpretive Statements, © 2001, American Nurses Publishing. American Nurses Foundation/American Nurses Association, Washington, DC.*

law in most states mandates that HIV test results can be given to another person only if the client provides written consent for the release of that information. Many health care providers believe that this law violates their own right to personal safety and are actively working to change the law.

The right to refuse treatment (including surgery, medication, medical therapy, and nourishment) is another client right that raises nursing dilemmas. The nurse, as client advocate, must first establish that the client is competent. If the client is competent, the situation, the alternatives, and the potential harm from refusal must be carefully explained. By law, the client must establish an advance directive on admission to a health care agency stating the client's choice about preserving or prolonging life. An **advance directive,** or **living will,** is a document in which a client formally states preferences for health care in the event that he or she later becomes mentally incapacitated. The client also names a person who has durable power of attorney to serve as a substitute decision maker to implement the client's stated preferences. This document becomes a part of the client's hospital record and is honored even if the client becomes incompetent during the period of treatment. The dilemma arises when the client's preferences conflict with the law. For example, the client may indicate that there is to be no food or fluids given during end-of-life care. However, several states assert that artificial feeding is not a procedure that may be rejected under living will statutes. The nurse is faced with the dilemma of carrying out the client's wishes or following the law.

Questions about who lives, who dies, and who decides often arise in the health care setting. The issues surrounding dying and death have become increasingly pressing as advances in technology extend the lives of people with chronic debilitating illness and major trauma. These changes have altered concepts of living and dying, resulting in ethical conflicts regarding quality of life and death with dignity versus technologic methods of preserving life in any form.

Even if the client is competent and requests that no heroic measures be used to maintain life, many questions arise in nursing care. What constitutes an heroic measure? Should nursing interventions to provide comfort include administering narcotics at a level known to depress respirations? Should a feeding tube be placed in the client who is terminally ill? These and other questions are being debated not only within the health care system but also in the courts.

## TRENDS AND ISSUES IN MEDICAL-SURGICAL NURSING

Health care is a vast and complicated system, affected by, and reflecting changes in, society. The trends and issues facing medical-surgical nurses will shape both the philosophy and the provision of care in the 21st century. Following are some of the many trends and issues affecting nursing care today.

- The population over the age of 65 is increasing more rapidly than any other age group. Older adults have more chronic illnesses and recover less rapidly from acute illnesses than young and middle-aged adults. Treatment of illness requires a large number of hospital beds; the possibility exists that hospitals

will become intensive care settings for older adults. Older adults also require more long-term care, community services, and home care. As a result, nursing care will be increasingly geared toward meeting the needs of the older adult in health and illness. The older adult is discussed in Chapter 2.

- HIV infection is no longer ranked as a leading cause of death for all people in the United States. However, it still ranks as the fifth cause of death among 25 to 44 year olds, and is the leading cause of death for black men of this age. HIV infection is discussed in Chapter 9.

- Persons who are medically indigent—those without any type of public or private insurance and who cannot pay for health care out of pocket—put increasing demands on state and federal health care budgets. Many clients who are medically indigent either do not seek preventive and restorative health care interventions or receive them too late to avoid serious illness.

- The findings of the Human Genome Project may dramatically affect the way disease is diagnosed and treated. Scientists have identified at least 36 proteins that may be markers for ovarian, breast, and colon cancer; and may also indicate depression, bipolar disorder, and schizophrenia. Pharmaceutical companies are using data from the project in research to develop medications that may, for example, eliminate the beta amyloid tangles responsible for Alzheimer's disease.

- Health problems in the homeless population include both physical and mental alterations. People who are homeless are more prone to injuries and to acute illnesses such as respiratory infections, food poisoning, and skin infestations. Chronic problems affecting the homeless include high blood pressure, chronic respiratory problems (including tuberculosis), heart and peripheral vascular disorders, and malnutrition. Mental health problems that contribute significantly to physical alterations are schizophrenia, depression, and substance abuse. Most care is provided by community health nurses (Figure 1–5 ■).

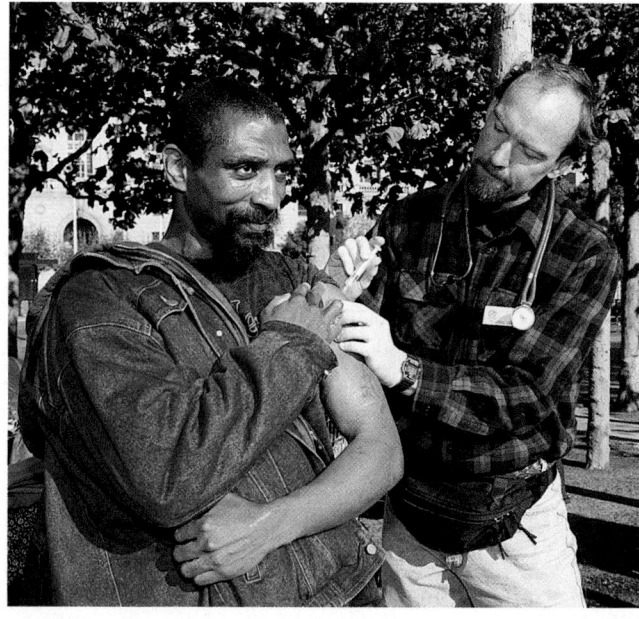

**Figure 1–5** ■ Care for the homeless is often provided by nurses working in the community setting.

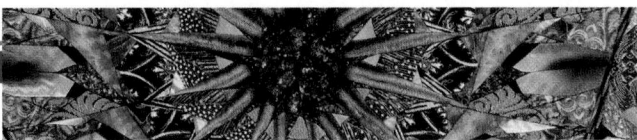

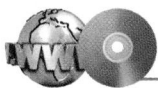 ## EXPLORE MediaLink

NCLEX review questions, case studies, care plan activities, MediaLink applications, and other interactive resources for this chapter can be found on the Companion Website at www.prenhall.com/lemone.

Click on Chapter 1 to select the activities for this chapter. For animations, video clips, more NCLEX review questions, and an audio glossary, access the Student CD-ROM accompanying this textbook.

## TEST YOURSELF

1. Which of the following is a collaborative nursing activity?
   a. Taking a health history on a newly admitted client
   b. Assessing changes in heart rate
   c. Teaching a client with diabetes how to give insulin
   d. Administering prescribed medications

2. What goal is a component of the nurse's role as advocate?
   a. Assisting and supporting client decision making
   b. Conducting research about the effects of exercise
   c. Delegating responsibilities for client care to others
   d. Performing range-of-motion exercises

3. A method of establishing a standard of care and evaluating outcomes of that standard involves:
   a. Writing a dress code policy for a health care agency
   b. Creating a critical pathway for a specific type of surgical client
   c. Establishing quality assurance regulations
   d. Implementing a new procedure to change dressings

4. Which one of the following statements is most true of assessment in the nursing process?
   a. Assessment is the first step in the nursing process
   b. Assessment is the last step in the nursing process
   c. Assessment is a component of all steps of the nursing process
   d. Assessment is rarely used as a step in the nursing process

5. A client tells you that he wants no treatment for his cancer. What must the nurse do first?
   a. Ask the client's family members if they agree
   b. Report the information to the legal department
   c. Establish that the client is competent
   d. Ignore the statement

See Test Yourself answers in Appendix C.

## BIBLIOGRAPHY

Alfaro, R. (1998). *Applying nursing diagnoses and nursing process: A step-by-step guide* (4th ed.). Philadelphia: Lippincott.

American Association of Retired Persons. (2002). *Profile of older Americans.* Washington, DC: Resource Services Group.

American Nurses Association. (1980). Nursing: A social policy statement. Kansas City, MO: ANA.

———. (1988). *Ethics in nursing: Position statement and guidelines.* Kansas City, MO: ANA.

———. (1991). *Nursing's agenda for health care reform.* Kansas City, MO: ANA.

———. (1995). *Nursing's social policy statement.* Washington, DC: American Nurses Publishing.

———. (1996). *Position statement on cultural diversity in nursing practice.* Washington, DC: ANA.

———. (1998). *Standards of clinical nursing practice.* Washington, DC: ANA.

———. (2001). *Code of ethics for nurses.* Washington, DC: ANA.

Anderson, C. A. (1999). Social change and its impact on nursing. *Nursing Outlook, 47*(2), 53–54.

Andrews, M., & Boyle, J. (1997). Competence in transcultural nursing care. *American Journal of Nursing, 97*(8), 16–20.

Benner, P. (1984). *From novice to expert: Excellence and power in clinical nursing practice.* Redwood City, CA: Addison-Wesley Nursing.

Benner, P., & Wrubel, J. (1989). *The primacy of caring: Stress and coping in clinical nursing practice.* Redwood City, CA: Addison-Wesley Nursing.

Carpenito, L. (1999). *Nursing care plans and documentation* (3rd ed.). Philadelphia: Lippincott.

———. (2000). *Nursing diagnoses: Application to clinical practice* (8th ed.). Philadelphia: Lippincott.

Centers for Disease Control, National Center for Health Statistics. (2002). *Deaths/mortality.* Hyattsville, MD: U.S. Department of Health and Human Services.

Chitty, K. (2001). *Professional nursing: Concepts & challenges* (3rd ed.). Philadelphia: Saunders.

Clemen-Stone, S., McGuire, S., & Eigsti, D. (1998). *Comprehensive community health nursing* (5th ed.). St. Louis: Mosby.

Ebert, J. (2000). Utilizing the nursing "team model" to enhance the role of case manager. *Nursing Case Management, 5*(5), 199–201.

Ellis, J., & Hartley, C. (1998). *Nursing in today's world: Challenges, issues, and trends* (6th ed.). Philadelphia: Lippincott.

Finkelman, A. W. (2001). *Managed care: A nursing perspective.* Upper Saddle River, NJ: Prentice Hall.

Flynn, L. (1997). The health practices of homeless women: A causal model. *Nursing Research, 46*(2), 72–77.

Gordon, M. (1982). *Nursing diagnosis: Process and application.* New York: McGraw-Hill.

———. (1987). *Nursing diagnosis: Process and application.* (2nd ed.) New York: McGraw-Hill.

———. (1994). *Nursing diagnosis: Process and application* (3rd ed.). St. Louis: Mosby.

Green, C. (2000). *Critical thinking in nursing: Case studies across the curriculum.* Upper Saddle River, NJ: Prentice Hall.

Hanshett, M., & OpNeal, J. (2001). Improving client education with the patient pathway. *Hospital Case Management, 9*(3), 39–42, 48.

International Council of Nurses. (1973). *ICN code for nurses: Ethical concept applied to nursing.* Geneva: Imprimeries Populaires.

Iyer, P., Taptich, B., & Bernocchi-Losey, D. (1994). *Nursing process and care planning* (2nd ed.). Philadelphia: Saunders.

Ketefian, S. (1987). Moral behavior in nursing. *Advances in Nursing Science, 9*(1), 10–19.

Klenner, S. (2000). Mapping out a clinical pathway. *RN, 63*(6), 33–36.

Leininger, M. (1991). Transcultural care principles, human rights, and ethical considerations. *Journal of Transcultural Nursing, 3*(1), 21–23.

Lipson, J., Dibble, S., & Minarik, P. (1996). *Culture & nursing care: A pocket guide.* San Francisco: UCSF Nursing Press.

Madigan, E. (2001). Home healthcare nurses can be leaders in evidence-based practice. *Home Healthcare Nurse, 19*(2), 120.

Maslow, A. (1970). *Motivation and personality.* New York: Harper & Row.

North American Nursing Diagnosis Association. (2001). *Nursing diagnoses: Definitions & classification 2001–2002.* Philadelphia: NANDA.

Radwin, L. (1990). Research on diagnostic reasoning in nursing. *Nursing Diagnosis, 1*(2), 70–77.

Roberts, S., & Cleary, V. (2000). Sustaining care delivery—team nursing with intensive care assistants. *Nursing in Critical Care, 5*(2), 68–71.

Rossi, P. (1999). *Case management in healthcare. A practical guide.* Philadelphia: Saunders.

Rosswurm, M. A., & Larrabee, J. H. (1999). A model for change to evidence-based practice.

*Image: Journal of Nursing Scholarship, 31*(4), 317–322.

Spector, R. (2000). *Cultural diversity in health and illness* (5th ed.). Norwalk, CT: Appleton & Lange.

Understanding differences can improve education: Examine own biases before teaching other cultures. (2001). *Patient Education Management, 8*(5), 57–58, 60.

Wilkinson, J. (2000). *Nursing process in action: A critical thinking approach.* Upper Saddle River, NJ: Prentice Hall.

# The Adult Client in Health and Illness

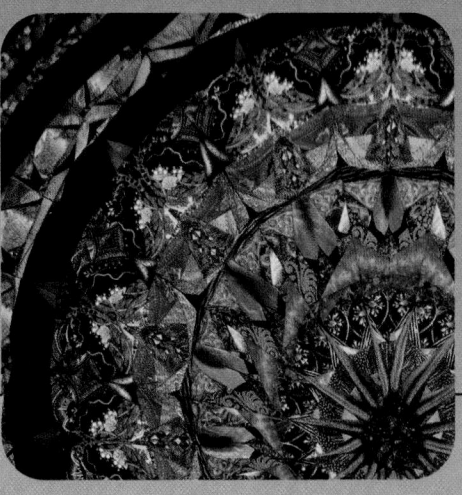

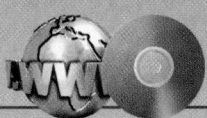

**MediaLink**

## www.prenhall.com/lemone

Additional resources for this chapter can be found on the Student CD-ROM accompanying this textbook, and on the Companion Website at www.prenhall.com/lemone. Click on Chapter 2 to select the activities for this chapter.

**CD-ROM**
- Audio Glossary
- NCLEX Review

**Companion Website**
- More NCLEX Review
- Case Study
  Developing Teaching Programs
- Care Plan Activity
  The Family and Chronic Illness
- MediaLink Application
  The Older Adult and Preventive Health

## LEARNING OUTCOMES

After completing this chapter, you will be able to:

- Compare and contrast the physical status, risks for alterations in health, assessment guidelines, and healthy behaviors of the young adult, middle adult, and older adult.

- Discuss the definitions, functions, and developmental stages and tasks of the family.

- Define health, incorporating the health-illness continuum and the concept of high-level wellness.

- Identify factors affecting health status.

- Discuss the nurse's role in health promotion.

- Describe the primary, secondary, and tertiary levels of illness prevention.

- Compare and contrast illness and disease.

- Describe illness behaviors and needs of the client with acute illness and chronic illness.

- Discuss the role of the nurse in providing care as a part of rehabilitation.

Gordon Hight, a 21-year-old college student, is admitted to the emergency room with multiple injuries and head trauma following a motorcycle accident. Mary Green, a 38-year-old homemaker, arrives at same-day surgery for biopsy of a tumor in her left breast. Sam Rosengarten, a 55-year-old attorney, is in the intensive care unit for treatment of a myocardial infarction. Margarite Schlefer, age 82, is receiving home health care following a fall that fractured her right hip. These examples demonstrate the striking variety among adult clients—the focus of care in medical-surgical nursing.

## THE ADULT CLIENT

The adult years commonly are divided into three stages: the young adult (age 18 to 40), the middle adult (age 40 to 65), and the older adult (over age 65). Although developmental markers are not as clearly delineated in the adult as in the infant or child, specific changes do occur with aging in intellectual, psychosocial, and spiritual development, as well as in physical structures and functions.

The developmental theories specific to the adult, with related stages and tasks, are listed in Table 2–1. Applying a vari-

### TABLE 2–1  Theories of Adult Development

| | Theorist | Age | Task |
|---|---|---|---|
| **Psychosocial Development** | Erikson | 18–25 | Identity versus role confusion<br>• Establishing an intimate relationship with another person<br>• Committing oneself to work and to relationships |
| | | 25–65 | Generativity versus stagnation<br>• Accepting one's own life as creative and productive<br>• Having concern for others |
| | | 65–death | Integrity versus despair<br>• Accepting worth of one's own life<br>• Accepting inevitability of death |
| **Spiritual Development** | Fowler | After 18<br><br>After 30 | • Having a high degree of self-consciousness<br>• Constructing one's own spiritual system<br>• Being aware of truth from a variety of viewpoints |
| | Westerhoff | Young adult | Searching Faith<br>• Acquiring a cognitive and an affective faith through questioning one's own faith |
| | | Middle–older adult | Owned Faith<br>• Putting faith into action and standing up for beliefs |
| **Moral Development** | Kohlberg | Adult | Post-Conventional Level<br>Social contract/legalistic orientation<br>• Defining morality in terms of personal principles<br>• Adhering to laws that protect the welfare and rights of others<br><br>Universal-Ethical Principles<br>• Internalizing universal moral principles<br>• Respecting others; believing that relationships are based on mutual trust |
| **Developmental Tasks** | Havighurst | 18–35 | • Selecting and learning to live with a mate<br>• Starting a family and rearing children<br>• Managing a home<br>• Starting an occupation<br>• Taking on civic responsibility<br>• Finding a congenial social group |
| | | 35–60 | • Achieving civic and social responsibility<br>• Establishing and maintaining an economic standard of living<br>• Assisting teenage children in becoming responsible and happy adults<br>• Developing leisure-time activities<br>• Relating to one's spouse as a person<br>• Accepting and adjusting to the physiologic changes of middle age<br>• Adjusting to aging parents |
| | | 60 and over | • Meeting civic and social obligations<br>• Establishing an affiliation with one's own age group<br>• Establishing satisfactory physical living arrangements<br>• Adjusting to decreasing physical strength, health, retirement, reduced income, death of spouse |

*Note. Adapted from Childhood and Society (2nd ed.) by E. Erickson, 1963, New York: Norton; Stages of Faith: The Psychology of Human Development and the Quest for Meaning by J. W. Fowler, 1981, New York: Harper & Row; Human Development and Education (3rd ed.) by R. J. Havighurst, 1972, New York: Longman; The Meaning and Measurement of Moral Development by L. Kohlberg, 1979, New York: Clark University; and Will Our Children Have Faith? by J. Westerhoff, 1976, New York: Seabury Press.*

ety of developmental theories is important to the holistic care of the adult client as nurses perform assessments, implement care, and provide teaching.

## THE YOUNG ADULT

From age 18 to 25, the healthy young adult is at the peak of physical development. All body systems are functioning at maximum efficiency. Then, during the 30s, some normal physiologic changes begin to occur. A comparison of physical status for young adults during their 20s and 30s is shown in Table 2–2.

### Risks for Alterations in Health

The young adult is at risk for alterations in health from accidents, sexually transmitted diseases, substance abuse, and physical or psychosocial stressors. These risk factors may be interrelated.

#### Accidents

Accidents are the leading cause of injury and death in people between ages 15 and 24 (Centers for Disease Control and Prevention [CDC], 1999b). Most injuries and fatalities occur as the result of motor vehicle accidents; but injuries and death also result from drowning, fire, guns, occupational accidents, and exposure to environmental hazards. Accidental injury or death is often associated with the use of alcohol or other chemical substances, or with psychologic stress.

#### Sexually Transmitted Diseases

Sexually transmitted diseases include genital herpes, chlamydia, gonorrhea, syphilis, and HIV/AIDS. The young adult who is sexually active with a variety of partners and who does not use condoms is at greatest risk for development of these diseases.

#### Substance Abuse

Substance abuse is a major cause for concern in the young adult population. Although alcohol abuse occurs at all ages, it is greater in the 20s than during any other decade of the life span. Alcohol contributes to motor vehicle accidents and physical violence, and it is damaging to the developing fetus in pregnant women. It can also cause liver disease and nutritional deficits.

Other substances that are commonly abused include nicotine, marijuana, amphetamines, cocaine, and crack. Smoking increases the risk of respiratory and cardiovascular diseases. Cocaine and crack can cause death from cardiovascular effects (increased heart rate and ventricular dysrhythmias), and can lead to addiction and health problems in the baby born to an addicted mother.

### Physical and Psychosocial Stressors

Physical stressors that increase the risk of illness include environmental pollutants and work-related risks (e.g., electrical hazards, mechanical injuries, or exposure to toxins or infectious agents). Other physical stressors include exposure to the sun, ingestion of chemical substances (e.g., caffeine, alcohol, nicotine), and pregnancy.

Many different and individualized psychosocial stressors may affect the young adult. Choices must be made about education, occupation, relationships, independence, and lifestyle. The young adult without adequate education or job skills may face unemployment, poverty, homelessness, and limited access to health care. Divorces in the United States are increasing. Three of every five marriages end in divorce, and this number is even higher among young adults (Edelman & Mandle, 2002). Divorce often results in loneliness, feelings of failure, financial difficulties, domestic violence, and child abuse. The inability of the young adult to cope with these stressors may result in suicide, which ranks next to accidents as a major cause of death in this age group. Although difficult to prove, it is believed that some accidental deaths, especially when associated with substance abuse, are actually suicides.

### Assessment Guidelines

The following guidelines are useful in assessing the achievement of significant developmental tasks in the young adult. Does the young adult:

- Feel independent from parents?
- Have a realistic self-concept?
- Like oneself and the direction in which life is going?
- Interact well with family?
- Cope with the stresses of constant change and growth?
- Have well-established bonds with significant others, such as marriage partners or close friends?
- Have a meaningful social life?

| TABLE 2–2 Physical Status and Changes in the Young Adult Years | | |
|---|---|---|
| **Assessment** | **Status During the 20s** | **Status During the 30s** |
| Skin | Smooth, even temperature | Wrinkles begin to appear |
| Hair | Slightly oily, shiny<br>Balding may begin | Graying may begin<br>Balding may begin |
| Vision | Snellen 20/20 | Some loss of visual acuity and accommodation |
| Musculoskeletal | Strong, coordinated | Some loss of strength and muscle mass |
| Cardiovascular | Maximum cardiac output<br>60–90 beats/min<br>Mean BP: 120/80 | Slight decline in cardiac output<br>60–90 beats/min<br>Mean BP: 120/80 |
| Respiratory | Rate: 12–20<br>Full vital capacity | Rate: 12–20<br>Decline in vital capacity |

- Have a career or occupation?
- Demonstrate emotional, social, and economic responsibility for own life?
- Have a set of values that guide behavior?
- Have a healthy lifestyle? (Kozier, Erb, Berman, & Burke, 2000)

Physical assessment of the young adult includes height and weight, blood pressure, and vision. During the health history, the nurse should ask specific questions about substance use, sexual activity and concerns, exercise, eating habits, menstrual history and patterns, coping mechanisms, any familial chronic illnesses, and family changes.

## Promoting Healthy Behaviors in the Young Adult

The nurse promotes health in the young adult by teaching the behaviors listed in Box 2–1. Health information for the young adult is primarily provided in community settings. Examples are as follows:

- Health-related courses and seminars at colleges and universities include information on the use of sports and exercise facilities, alcohol and drug abuse, smoking cessation, mental health, and sexual health.
- Workplace programs include blood pressure monitoring, exercise, smoking cessation, cafeteria nutrition guidelines, and stress-reduction activities.
- Community programs include media information, health fairs, support groups, and information about risk factors for disease and injury.

## THE MIDDLE ADULT

The middle adult, age 40 to 65, has physical status and function similar to that of the young adult. However, many changes take place between ages 40 and 65. Table 2–3 lists the physical changes that normally occur in the middle years.

## Risks for Alterations in Health

The middle adult is at risk for alterations in health from obesity, cardiovascular disease, cancer, substance abuse, and physical and psychosocial stressors. These factors may be interrelated.

### Obesity

The middle adult often has a problem maintaining a healthy weight. Weight gain in middle adulthood is usually the result of continuing to consume the same number of calories while decreasing physical activity and experiencing a decrease in basal metabolic rate. Obesity affects all the major organ systems of the body, increasing the risk of atherosclerosis, hypertension, elevated cholesterol and triglyceride levels, and diabetes. Obesity is also associated with heart disease, osteoarthritis, and gallbladder disease.

### Cardiovascular Disease

The major risk factors, especially for coronary artery disease, include age, male gender, physical inactivity, cigarette smoking, hypertension, elevated blood cholesterol levels, and diabetes. Other contributing factors include obesity, stress, and lack of exercise. The middle adult is at risk for disorders of peripheral vascular, cerebrovascular, and cardiovascular disease.

### Cancer

Cancer is the third leading cause of death in adults between ages 25 and 64 in the United States, with one-third of cases occurring between ages 35 and 64. Cancers of the breast, colon, lung, and reproductive system are common in the middle years. The middle adult is at risk for cancer as a result of increased length of exposure to environmental carcinogens, as well as alcohol and nicotine use.

### Substance Abuse

Although the middle adult may abuse a variety of substances, the most commonly abused are alcohol, nicotine, and prescription drugs. Excess alcohol use in the middle adult contributes

---

| BOX 2–1 ■ Healthy Behaviors in the Young Adult |
| --- |

- Choose foods from all food groups, and eat a variety of foods.
- Choose a diet low in fat (30% or less of total calories), saturated fat (less than 10% of calories), and cholesterol (less than 300 mg daily).
- Choose a diet that each day includes at least three servings of vegetables, two servings of fruits, and six servings of grains.
- Use sugar, salt, and sodium in moderation.
- For females, increase to or maintain 18 mg of iron daily in the diet, and 400 mg of folic acid per day through diet or supplements.
- Make exercise a regular part of life, carrying out activities that increase the heart rate to a set target, and maintain that rate for 30–60 minutes three or four times a week.
- Include exercise as part of any weight-reduction program.

- Have regular physical examinations, including assessment for cancer of the thyroid, ovaries, lymph nodes, and skin (every 3 years).
- Have a vision examination every 2–4 years.
- Have an annual dental checkup.
- For females between age 20 and 39 have a CBE[*] by a health care professional every 3 years.
- For females, have Pap tests as recommended by a physician: annually until three or more consecutive normal results, and then at physician's discretion.
- For males, have testicular and prostate examinations every 5 years.
- Conduct BSE[*] or testicular self-examination monthly.
- Maintain immunizations.

[*]CBE = clinical breast examination
BSE = breast self-examination

## TABLE 2–3   Physical Changes in the Middle Adult Years

| Assessment | Changes |
|---|---|
| Skin | • Decreased turgor, moisture, and subcutaneous fat result in wrinkles.<br>• Fat is deposited in the abdominal and hip areas. |
| Hair | • Loss of melanin in hair shaft causes graying.<br>• Hairline recedes in males. |
| Sensory | • Visual acuity for near vision decreases (presbyopia) during the 40s.<br>• Auditory acuity for high-frequency sounds decreases (presbycusis); more common in men.<br>• Sense of taste diminishes. |
| Musculoskeletal | • Skeletal muscle mass decreases by about age 60.<br>• Thinning of intervertebral discs results in loss of height (about 1 inch [2.5 cm]).<br>• Postmenopausal women may have loss of calcium and develop osteoporosis. |
| Cardiovascular | • Blood vessels lose elasticity.<br>• Systolic blood pressure may increase. |
| Respiratory | • Loss of vital capacity (about 1 L from age 20 to 60) occurs. |
| Gastrointestinal | • Large intestine gradually loses muscle tone; constipation may result.<br>• Gastric secretions are decreased. |
| Genitourinary | • Hormonal changes occur: menopause, women (↓ estrogen); andropause, men (↓ testosterone). |
| Endocrine | • Gradual decrease in glucose tolerance occurs. |

to an increased risk of liver cancer, cirrhosis, pancreatitis, hyperlipidemia, and anemia. Alcoholism also increases the risk of accidental injury or death and disrupts careers and relationships. Cigarette smoking increases the risk of cancer of the larynx, lung, mouth, pharynx, bladder, pancreas, esophagus, and kidney; of chronic obstructive pulmonary disorders; and of cardiovascular disorders.

### Physical and Psychosocial Stressors

The middle adult years are ones of change and transition, frequently resulting in stress. Both men and women must adapt to changes in physical appearance and function and accept their own mortality. Children may leave home or choose to remain at home longer than they are welcome. Parents are aging, with illness probable and death inevitable. The middle adult thus becomes part of what has been called "the sandwich generation," caught between the need to care for both children and aging parents. Both men and women may make career changes, and approaching retirement becomes a reality. Divorce in the middle years is a major emotional, social, and financial stressor.

### Assessment Guidelines

The following guidelines are useful in assessing the achievement of significant developmental tasks in the middle adult. Does the middle adult:

• Accept the aging body?
• Feel comfortable with and respect oneself?
• Enjoy some new freedom to be independent?
• Accept changes in family roles?
• Enjoy success and satisfaction from work and/or family roles?
• Interact well and share companionable activities with a partner?

• Expand or renew previous interests?
• Pursue charitable and altruistic activities?
• Consider plans for retirement?
• Have a meaningful philosophy of life?
• Follow preventive health care practices? (Kozier et al., 2000)

Physical assessment of the middle adult includes all body systems, including blood pressure, vision, and hearing. Monitoring for risks and onset of cancer symptoms is essential. During the health history, the nurse should ask specific questions about food intake and exercise habits, substance abuse, sexual concerns, changes in the reproductive system, and coping mechanisms.

### Promoting Healthy Behaviors in the Middle Adult

The nurse promotes health in the middle adult by teaching the behaviors listed in Box 2–2. Information about health for the middle adult may be provided in a variety of community settings, including outpatient clinics, occupational health clinics, and private practice. Examples are as follows:

• Specific programs emphasize accepting responsibility for one's own health. This type of teaching can be in a seminar or on a one-to-one basis, and includes information specific to a group of individuals with an identified need, such as smokers, women who have just entered the workforce, or men nearing retirement.
• The community and industries provide information about safety hazards in the home and workplace, as well as during leisure activities.
• Literature about community resources is available for health promotion, including programs offered at alcohol/drug abuse

| BOX 2–2 | ■ Healthy Behaviors in the Middle Adult |
| --- | --- |

- Choose foods from all food groups, and eat a variety of foods.
- Choose a diet low in fat (30% or less of total calories), saturated fat (less than 10% of calories), and cholesterol (less than 300 mg daily). Adjust daily calorie intake to maintain healthy weight.
- Choose a diet that each day includes at least three servings of vegetables, two servings of fruits, and six servings of grains.
- Use sugar, salt, and sodium in moderation.
- Increase calcium intake (in perimenopausal women) to 1200 mg daily.
- Consume high-fiber foods.
- Make exercise a part of life, carrying out regular exercise that is moderately strenuous, is consistent, and avoids overexertion; exercise for 30 minutes at least three times a week.
- Include exercise as part of any weight-reduction program.
- Have an annual vision examination.
- Have an annual dental checkup.

- Have a physical examination annually, including assessment for cancer of the thyroid, testes, prostate, mouth, ovaries, skin, colon, and lymph nodes.
- For females, have a mammogram every year from age 40 on. Have a CBE* annually.
- For females, have a Pap test as recommended for the young adult (see Box 2–1).
- Have an annual stool blood test; a digital rectal examination and a flexible sigmoidoscopy every 5 years; and a colonoscopy and digital rectal examination every 10 years or a double-contrast barium enema and a digital examination every 5–10 years.
- For males, have testicular and prostate examinations annually, including a PSA,* after age 50.
- Conduct BSE* or testicular self-examination every month. (The perimenopausal woman should set a specific date each month for the exam, as menstrual periods may be irregular or absent.)

*BSE = breast self-examination
CBE = clinical breast examination
PSA = prostate-specific antigen blood test

treatment centers, clinics and health centers, counseling services, crisis intervention centers, spouse abuse programs, and health education and promotion agencies (e.g., American Red Cross, American Cancer Society, American Heart Association, YWCA, YMCA).

## THE OLDER ADULT

The older adult period begins at age 65, but it can be further divided into three periods: the young-old (age 65 to 74), the middle-old (age 75 to 84), and the old-old (age 85 and over). With increasing age, a number of normal physiologic changes occur, as listed in Table 2–4.

The older adult population is increasing more rapidly than any other age group. In the last century, the number of adults in the United States living to age 65 or older increased from 4% in 1900 to 12.8% in 1999. There will be 70 million older adults by the year 2030, more than twice the number in 1999. The life expectancy in the United States is 73.6 years for men and 79.4 years for women (American Association of Retired Persons [AARP], 2001; CDC, 1999).

The increase in numbers of older adults has important implications for nursing. Clients needing health care in all settings will be older, requiring nursing interventions and teaching specifically designed to meet needs that differ from those of young and middle adults. Although **gerontologic nursing** (care of the older adult) is a nursing specialty area, it is also an integral component of medical-surgical nursing (Figure 2–1 ■).

## Risks for Alterations in Health

The older adult is at risk for alterations in health from a variety of causes. Approximately 40% of all older adults report having a limitation caused by a chronic illness, and more than 50% report having at least one disability (AARP, 2001). The most frequently occurring conditions in the older adult are arthritis, hypertension, hearing impairments, cardiovascular diseases, cataracts, sinusitis, orthopedic disorders, visual impairments, and diabetes. The leading causes of death are heart disease, cancer, and stroke.

Like the middle adult, the older adult is at risk for alterations in health from obesity, cardiovascular disease, and cancer. Other risk factors specific to this age group include injuries, pharmacologic effects, and physical and psychosocial stress.

### Injuries

Injuries in the older adult cause many different problems: illness, financial burdens, hospitalization, self-care deficits, loss of independence, and even death. The risk of injury is increased by normal physiologic changes that accompany aging, pathophysiologic alterations in health, environmental hazards, and lack of support systems. The three major causes of injury in the older adult are falls, fires, and motor vehicle accidents. Of these, falls with resultant hip fractures are the most significant in terms of long-term disability and death.

### Pharmacologic Effects

A number of risk factors predispose the older adult to experiencing drug toxicity. Age-related changes in tissue and organ structure and function alter the absorption of both oral and parenteral medications. Low nutritional levels and decreased liver function may alter drug metabolism. The aging kidney may not excrete drugs at the normal clearance rate. Self-administration of both prescribed and over-the-counter medications presents risks for error resulting from confusion, forgetfulness, or misreading the directions. In addition, the older adult may take several drugs at once, and it is difficult to know how drugs interact with each other (Weitzel, 2001).

### Physical and Psychosocial Stressors

The older adult is exposed to the same environmental hazards as the young and middle adult, but the accumulation of years of

MediaLink | OLDER ADULT RESOURCES

| TABLE 2–4 | Physical Changes in the Older Adult Years |
|---|---|
| **Assessment** | **Changes** |
| Skin | • Decreased turgor and sebaceous gland activity result in dry, wrinkled skin. Melanocytes cluster, causing "age spots" or "liver spots." |
| Hair and nails | • Scalp, axillary, and pubic hair thins; nose and ear hair thickens. Women may develop facial hair.<br>• Nails grow more slowly; may become thick and brittle. |
| Sensory | • Visual field narrows, and depth perception is distorted.<br>• Pupils are smaller, reducing night vision.<br>• Lenses yellow and become opaque, resulting in distortion of green, blue, and violet tones and increased sensitivity to glare.<br>• Production of tears decreases.<br>• Sense of smell decreases.<br>• Age-related hearing loss progresses, involving middle- and low-frequency sounds.<br>• Threshold for pain and touch increases.<br>• Alterations in proprioception (sense of physical position) may occur. |
| Musculoskeletal | • Loss of overall mass, strength, and movement of muscles occurs; tremors may occur.<br>• Loss of bone structure and deterioration of cartilage in joints results in increased risk of fractures and in limitation of range of motion. |
| Cardiovascular | • Systolic blood pressure rises.<br>• Cardiac output decreases.<br>• Peripheral resistance increases, and capillary walls thicken. |
| Respiratory | • Continued loss of vital capacity occurs as the lungs become less elastic and more rigid.<br>• Anteroposterior chest diameter increases; kyphosis.<br>• Although blood carbon dioxide levels remain relatively constant, blood oxygen levels decrease by 10% to 15%. |
| Gastrointestinal | • Production of saliva decreases, and decreased number of taste buds decrease accurate receptors for salt and sweet.<br>• Gag reflex is decreased, and stomach motility and emptying are reduced.<br>• Both large and small intestines have some atrophy, with decreased peristalsis.<br>• The liver decreases in weight and storage capacity; gallstones increase; pancreatic enzymes decrease. |
| Genitourinary | • Kidneys lose mass, and the glomerular filtration rate is reduced (by nearly 50% from young adulthood to old age).<br>• Bladder capacity decreases, and the micturition reflex is delayed. Urinary retention is more common.<br>• Women may have stress incontinence; men may have an enlarged prostate gland.<br>• Reproductive changes in men occur:<br>— Testosterone decreases.<br>— Sperm count decreases.<br>— Testes become smaller.<br>— Length of time to achieve an erection increases; erection is less full.<br>• Reproductive changes in women occur:<br>— Estrogen levels decrease.<br>— Breast tissue decreases.<br>— Vagina, uterus, ovaries, and urethra atrophy.<br>— Vaginal lubrication decreases.<br>— Vaginal secretions become alkaline. |
| Endocrine | • Pituitary gland loses weight and vascularity.<br>• Thyroid gland becomes more fibrous, and plasma $T_3$ decreases.<br>• Pancreas releases insulin more slowly; increased blood glucose levels are common.<br>• Adrenal glands produce less cortisol. |

exposure may now appear. For example, exposure to the sun in earlier years may be manifested by skin cancer, and the long-term effects of exposure to noise pollution can result in impaired hearing. The older adult (especially the older male) is at increased risk for respiratory disorders as a result of years of smoking, or from such pollutants as coal or asbestos dust. Living conditions and economic constraints may prevent the older adult from having necessary heating and cooling, contributing to thermal-related illness and even death. Elder abuse and neglect further increase the risk of injury or illness.

Psychosocial stressors for the older adult include the illness or death of a spouse, decreased or limited income, retirement, isolation from friends and family because of lack of transportation or distance, return to the home of a child, or relocation to

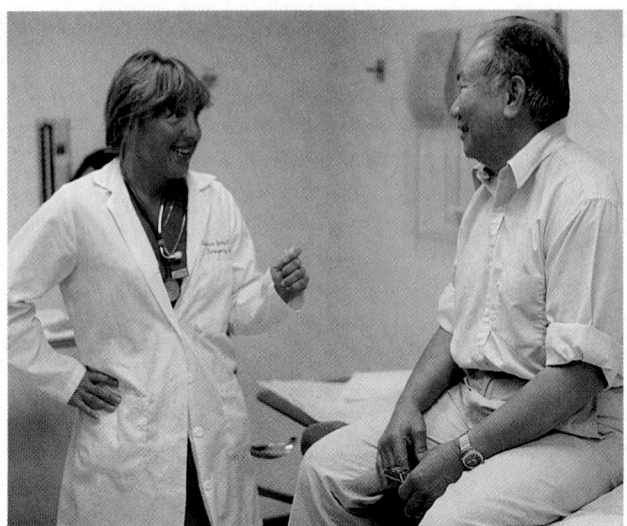

**Figure 2–1** ■ The older adult population is increasing more rapidly than any other age group, making gerontologic nursing an integral component of medical-surgical nursing practice.

a long-term health care facility. A further stressor may be role loss or reversal—for example, when the wife becomes the caretaker of her chronically ill husband.

## Assessment Guidelines

The following guidelines are useful in assessing the achievement of significant developmental tasks in the older adult. Does the older adult:

- Adjust to the physiologic changes related to aging?
- Manage retirement years in a satisfying manner?
- Have satisfactory living arrangements and income to meet changing needs?
- Participate in social and leisure activities?
- Have a social network of friends and support persons?
- View life as worthwhile?
- Have high self-esteem?
- Have the abilities to care for self or to secure appropriate help?
- Gain support from a value system or spiritual philosophy?
- Adapt lifestyle to diminishing energy and ability?
- Accept and adjust to the death of significant others? (Kozier et al., 2000)

Physical assessment of the older adult includes a careful examination of all body systems. During the health history, the nurse should ask specific questions about usual dietary patterns; elimination; exercise and rest; use of alcohol, nicotine, over-the-counter medications, and prescription drugs; sexual concerns; financial concerns; and support systems.

## Promoting Healthy Behaviors in the Older Adult

The nurse promotes health in the older adult by teaching the behaviors listed in Box 2–3. Older adults get the same benefits from health teaching as young adults and middle adults; they should never be viewed as being "too old" for healthy living

practices. However, nurses should structure teaching activities to meet age-related physiologic changes, such as using charts and literature with large print. Health education for the older adult is provided in hospitals, long-term care facilities, retirement centers, outpatient clinics, senior citizen centers, and other community settings. Examples are as follows:

- Educational seminars teach about accident prevention in the home, in automobiles, and when taking public transportation.
- Health screenings and information in health fairs can specifically aid the older adult.
- Community programs provide immunization for influenza and pneumonia.
- Literature is available about financial assistance for health care, crisis hot lines, community services and resources (as described earlier for the middle adult), transportation, and nutrition (such as the Meals-on-Wheels program).

## THE FAMILY OF THE ADULT CLIENT

Although some clients are totally alone in the world, most have one or more people who are significant in their lives. These significant others may be related or bonded to the client by birth, adoption, marriage, or friendship. Although not always meeting traditional definitions, people (or even pets) significant to the client are the client's family. The nurse includes the family as an integral component of care in all health care settings.

## Definitions and Functions of the Family

What is a **family?** The definitions of a family are changing as society changes. According to one definition, a family is a unit of people related by marriage, birth, or adoption (Duvall, 1977). An expanded definition states that "a family is composed of two or more people who are emotionally involved with each other and live in close geographical proximity" (Freidman, 1981, p. 8). In a global society, it may not be possible for family members to live in close proximity, but they do remain emotionally involved.

Although every family is unique, all families have certain structural and functional features in common. **Family structure** (family roles and relationships) and **family function** (interactions among family members and with the community) provide the following:

- *Interdependence.* The behaviors and level of development of individual family members constantly influence and are influenced by the behaviors and level of development of all other members of the family.
- *Maintaining boundaries.* The family creates boundaries that guide its members, providing a distinct and unique family culture. This culture, in turn, provides values.
- *Adapting to change.* The family changes as new members are added, current members leave, and the development of each member progresses.
- *Performing family tasks.* Essential tasks maintain the stability and continuity of the family. These tasks include physical maintenance of the home and the people in the home, the production and socialization of family members, and the maintenance of the psychologic well-being of members.

| BOX 2–3 | ■ Healthy Behaviors in the Older Adult |
|---|---|

- Choose foods from all food groups, and eat a variety of foods. Include some high-quality protein at each meal, such as low-fat milk and cheese, peanut butter, meat, fish, or poultry.
- Choose a diet low in fat (30% or less of total calories), saturated fat (less than 10% of calories), and cholesterol (less than 300 mg daily). Adjust daily caloric intake to balance energy expenditure and maintain healthy weight. A daily caloric intake of 1200 kcal is recommended, but it may vary according to body build and activity level.
- Choose a diet that each day includes at least three servings of vegetables, two servings of fruits, and six servings of grains. Increased amounts of high-fiber foods may be necessary; if so, fluid intake should also be increased.
- Use sugar, salt, and sodium in moderation.
- Increase calcium intake to at least 800 mg per day (1000–1500 mg per day may be recommended).
- Make exercise a part of life, following a regular program of moderate exercise, such as walking or swimming. Avoid overexertion.
- Have an annual vision examination.
- Have an annual dental checkup.
- Have an annual physical examination that includes urinalysis and assessment for cancer of the thyroid, testes, prostate, mouth, ovaries, skin, colon, and lymph nodes.
- For females, have a CBE* and a mammogram annually.
- For females, have Pap tests as recommended by health care provider.

- For males, have an annual testicular and prostate examination including a PSA.*
- Have a digital rectal examination and stool blood test annually. Have examinations as recommended for the middle adult (see Box 2–2).
- Conduct BSE* or testicular self-examination every month.
- Maintain immunizations for diphtheria and tetanus by having boosters every 10 years.
- Obtain annual immunizations against influenza, especially with a history of chronic cardiovascular or respiratory illness.
- Obtain pneumococcal pneumonia immunization.
- Practice the following to avoid injury:
  a. Have adequate lighting in all rooms of the house including stairs, basement, and bedrooms.
  b. Avoid sitting or standing rapidly; if dizziness occurs, remain in one position until dizziness is gone.
  c. Have handrails installed by the toilet and in the shower or bathtub.
  d. Do not use throw rugs.
  e. Install smoke alarms.
  f. Never step into a tub or shower without checking the temperature of the water.
  g. Always wear corrective lenses and/or hearing aids when driving.
  h. Do not drive a car after taking medications that cause drowsiness or dizziness.

*BSE = breast self-examination
CBE = clinical breast examination
PSA = prostate-specific antigen blood test

## Family Developmental Stages and Tasks

The family, like the individual, has developmental stages and tasks. Each stage brings change, requiring adaptation; each new stage also brings family-related risk factors for alterations in health. The nurse must consider the needs of the client both at a specific developmental stage and within a family with specific developmental tasks. Family developmental stages and developmental tasks are described next; related risk factors and health problems for each stage are listed in Table 2–5.

### Couple

Two people, living together with or without being married, are in a period of establishing themselves as a couple. The developmental tasks of the couple include adjusting to living together as a couple, establishing a mutually satisfying relationship, relating to kin, and deciding whether to have children.

### Family with Infants and Preschoolers

The family with infants or preschoolers must adjust to having and supporting the needs of more than two members. Other developmental tasks of the family at this stage are developing an attachment between parents and children, adjusting to the economic costs of having more members, coping with energy depletion and lack of privacy, and carrying out activities that enhance growth and development of the children.

### Family with School-Age Children

The family with school-age children has the developmental tasks of adjusting to the expanded world of children in school and encouraging educational achievement. A further task is promoting joint decision making between children and parents.

### Family with Adolescents and Young Adults

The developmental tasks of the family with adolescents and young adults focus on transition. While providing a supportive home base and maintaining open communications, parents must balance freedom with responsibility and release adult children as they seek independence.

### Family with Middle Adults

The family with middle adults (in which the parents are middle-aged and children are no longer at home) has the developmental tasks of maintaining ties with older and younger generations and planning for retirement. If the family consists of just the middle-aged couple, they have the developmental task of reestablishing the relationship and (if necessary) acquiring the role of grandparents.

### Family with Older Adults

The older adult family has the developmental tasks of adjusting to retirement, adjusting to aging, and coping with the loss of a spouse. If a spouse dies, further tasks include adjusting to living alone or closing the family home.

**TABLE 2–5   Family-Related Risk Factors for Alterations in Health**

| Stage | Risk Factors | Health Problems |
|---|---|---|
| Couple, or Family with Infants and Preschoolers | • Lack of knowledge about family planning, contraception, sexual and marital roles<br>• Inadequate prenatal care<br>• Altered nutrition: inadequate nutrition, overweight, underweight<br>• Smoking, alcohol/drug abuse<br>• First pregnancy before age 16 or after age 35<br>• Low socioeconomic status<br>• Lack of knowledge about child health and safety<br>• Rubella, syphilis, gonorrhea, AIDS | Premature pregnancy<br>Low-birth-weight infant<br>Birth defects<br>Injury to infant or child<br>Accidents |
| Family with School-Age Children | • Unsafe home environment<br>• Working parents with inappropriate or inadequate resources for child care<br>• Low socioeconomic status<br>• Child abuse or neglect<br>• Multiple, closely spaced children<br>• Repeated infections, accidents, and hospitalizations<br>• Unrecognized and unattended health problems<br>• Poor or inappropriate nutrition<br>• Toxic substances in the home<br>• Immature, dependent parents<br>• Generational pattern of using social agencies as a way of life | Behavior problems<br>Speech and vision problems<br>Learning disabilities<br>Communicable diseases<br>Physical abuse<br>Cancer<br>Developmental delay<br>Obesity, underweight |
| Family with Adolescents and Young Adults | • Family values of aggressiveness and competition<br>• Racial and ethnic family origin<br>• Socioeconomic factors contributing to peer relationships<br>• Lifestyle and behavior leading to chronic illness (substance abuse, inadequate diet)<br>• Lack of problem-solving skills<br>• Conflicts between parent and children | Violent death and injury<br>Alcohol/drug abuse<br>Unwanted pregnancy<br>Suicide<br>Sexually transmitted diseases<br>Domestic abuse |
| Family with Middle Adults | • High-cholesterol diet<br>• Overweight<br>• Hypertension<br>• Smoking, alcohol abuse<br>• Physical inactivity<br>• Genetic predisposition, heredity<br>• Personality patterns related to stress<br>• Habits: low-fiber and high-cholesterol diet; charcoal grilling<br>• Exposure to environment: sunlight, radiation, asbestos, water or air pollution<br>• Depression<br>• Gingivitis | Cardiovascular disease (coronary artery disease and cerebral vascular disease)<br>Cancer<br>Accidents<br>Suicide<br>Mental illness<br>Periodontal disease, loss of teeth |
| Family with Older Adults | • Age<br>• Depression<br>• Drug interactions<br>• Metabolic and endocrine disorders<br>• Chronic illness<br>• Death of spouse<br>• Reduced income<br>• Poor nutrition<br>• Lack of exercise<br>• Past environment and lifestyle | Impaired vision and hearing<br>Hypertension<br>Acute illness<br>Chronic illness<br>Infectious diseases (influenza, pneumonia)<br>Injuries from burns and falls<br>Depression<br>Alcohol abuse |

Note. Adapted from Healthy People: The Surgeon General's Report on Health Promotion and Disease Prevention, *Health and Human Services Pub. No. 79-55071, 1992, Washington, DC: US Government Printing Office, and* Healthy People 2001: National Health Promotion and Disease Prevention Objectives (Summary), *American Public Health Association, 2000, Washington, DC: US Government Printing Office.*

## HEALTH AND ILLNESS IN THE ADULT CLIENT
### Health

The World Health Organization (WHO) defines **health** as "a state of complete physical, mental, and social well-being, and not merely the absence of disease or infirmity" (WHO, 1974, p. 1). However, this definition does not take into account the various levels of health a person may experience, or that a person may be clinically described as ill and still define oneself as well. These additional factors, which greatly influence nursing care, include the health-illness continuum and high-level wellness.

### The Health-Illness Continuum and High-Level Wellness

The **health-illness continuum** represents health as a dynamic process, with high-level wellness at one extreme of the continuum and death at the opposite extreme (Figure 2–2 ■). Individuals place themselves at different locations on the continuum at specific points in time.

Dunn (1959) expanded the concept of a continuum of health and illness in his description of **high-level wellness.** Dunn conceptualized wellness as an active process influenced by the environment. He differentiated good health from wellness:

> Good health can exist as a relatively passive state of freedom from illness in which the individual is at peace with his environment. . . . Wellness is an integrated method of functioning, which is oriented toward maximizing the potential of which the individual is capable, within the environment where he is functioning. (1959, p. 4)

A variety of factors influence wellness, including self-concept, environment, culture, and spiritual values. Providing care based on a framework of wellness facilitates active involvement by both the nurse and the client in promoting, maintaining, or restoring health. It also supports the philosophy of holistic health care, in which all aspects of a person (physical, psychosocial, cultural, spiritual, and intellectual) are considered as essential components of individualized care.

### Factors Affecting Health

Many different factors affect a person's health or level of wellness. These factors often interact to promote health or to become risk factors for alterations in health. The factors affecting health are described next.

**GENETIC MAKEUP.**   Each person's genetic makeup influences health status throughout life. Genetic makeup affects personality, temperament, body structure, intellectual potential, and susceptibility to the development of hereditary alterations in health. Examples of chronic illnesses that are associated with genetic makeup include sickle cell disease, hemophilia, diabetes mellitus, and cancer.

**COGNITIVE ABILITIES AND EDUCATIONAL LEVEL.**   Although cognitive abilities are determined prior to adulthood, the level of cognitive development affects whether people view themselves as healthy or ill; cognitive levels also may affect health practices. Injuries to and illnesses affecting the brain may alter cognitive abilities. Educational level affects the ability to understand and follow guidelines for health. For example, if an individual is functionally illiterate, written information about healthy behaviors and health resources is worthless.

**RACE, ETHNICITY, AND CULTURAL BACKGROUND.**   Certain diseases occur at a higher rate of incidence in some races and ethnic groups than in others. For example, in the United States, hypertension is more common in African Americans, tuberculosis and diabetes mellitus are among the leading causes of illness in Native Americans, and eye disorders are more prevalent in Chinese Americans. The ethnic and cultural background of an individual also influences health values and behaviors, lifestyle, and illness behaviors. Every culture defines health and illness in a way that is unique; in addition, each culture has its own health beliefs and illness treatment practices.

**AGE, GENDER, AND DEVELOPMENTAL LEVEL.**   Age, gender, and developmental level are factors in health and illness. Cardiovascular disorders are uncommon in young adults, but the incidence increases after the age of 40. Myocardial infarctions are more common in men than women until women are past menopause. Some diseases occur only in one gender or the other (e.g., prostate cancer in men and cervical cancer in women). The older adult has increased incidence of chronic illness and increased potential for serious illness or death from infectious illnesses such as influenza and pneumonia.

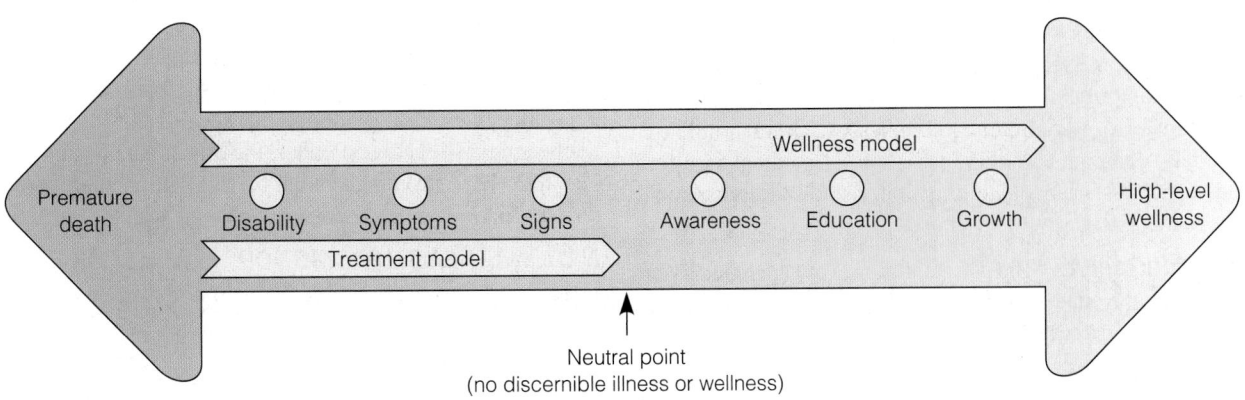

**Figure 2–2** ■ The health/illness continuum.

*From* Wellness Workbook *by J. W. Travis and R. S. Ryan, 1988, Berkeley, CA: Ten Speed Press. Used with permission.*

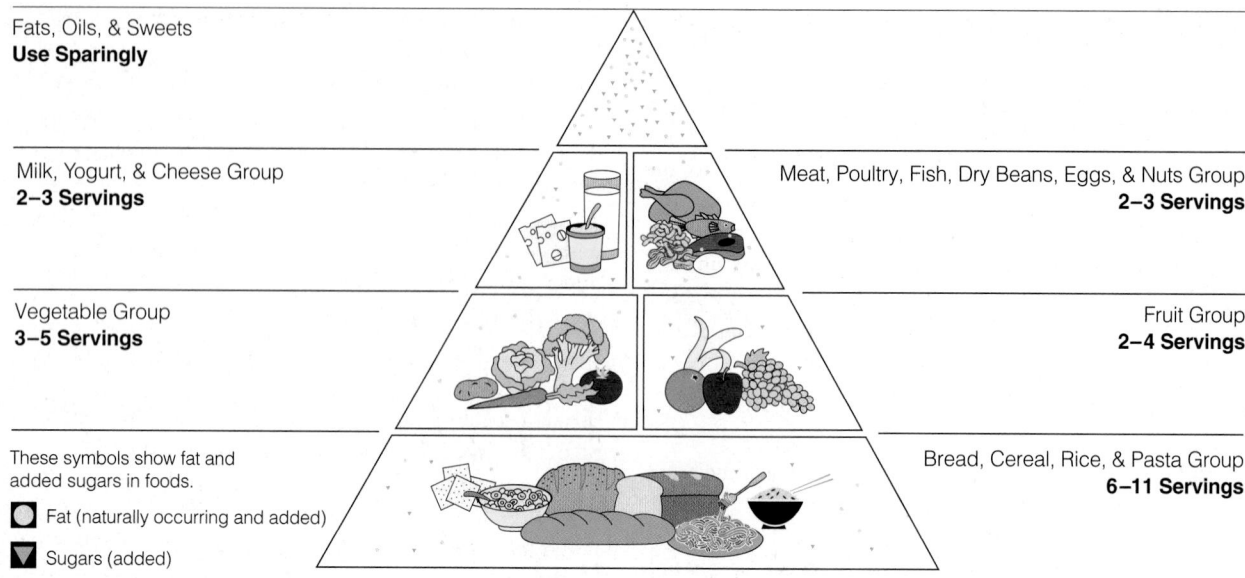

**Figure 2–3** ■ The food guide pyramid is designed to be used as a guide when buying foods and preparing meals.

*Source: U.S. Department of Agriculture and U.S. Department of Health and Human Services.*

**LIFESTYLE AND ENVIRONMENT.** The components of a person's lifestyle that affect health status include patterns of eating, use of chemical substances (alcohol, nicotine, caffeine, legal and illegal drugs), exercise and rest patterns, and coping methods. Examples of altered responses are the relationship of obesity to hypertension, cigarette smoking to chronic obstructive pulmonary disease, a sedentary lifestyle to heart disease, and a high-stress career to alcoholism. The environment has a major influence on health. Occupational exposure to toxic substances (such as asbestos and coal dust) increases the risk of pulmonary disorders. Air, water, and food pollution increase the risk of respiratory disorders, infectious diseases, and cancer. Environmental temperature variations can result in hypothermia or hyperthermia, especially in the older adult.

**SOCIOECONOMIC BACKGROUND.** Both lifestyle and environmental influences are affected by one's income level. The culture of poverty, which crosses all racial and ethnic boundaries, negatively influences health status. Living at or below the poverty level often results in crowded, unsanitary living conditions or homelessness. Housing often is overcrowded, lacks adequate heating or cooling, and is infested with insects and rats. Crowded living conditions increase the risk of transferring communicable diseases. Other problems include lack of infant and child care, lack of medical care for injuries or illness, inadequate nutrition, use of addictive substances, and violence.

**GEOGRAPHIC AREA.** The geographic area in which one lives influences health status. Such illnesses as malaria are more common in tropical areas of North America, whereas multiple sclerosis occurs with greater frequency in the northern United States and Canada. Other geographic influences are seen in the number of skin cancers in people living in sunny, hot areas and sinus infections in people living in areas of high humidity.

## Health Promotion and Maintenance

For many years, the emphasis in nursing was on care of the acutely ill client in the hospital setting. With changes in society and in health care, this emphasis is shifting toward preventive, community-based care. Although the focus of this textbook is not community health nursing, the importance of teaching health maintenance and providing continuity of care as a client moves among health care settings is an essential component of medical-surgical nursing.

**HEALTHY LIVING.** Practices that are known to promote health and wellness are:

- Eating three balanced meals a day and including foods according to the food guide pyramid (Figure 2–3 ■).
- Eating moderately to maintain a healthy weight.
- Exercising moderately, following a regular routine.
- Sleeping 7 to 8 hours each day.
- Limiting alcohol consumption to a moderate amount.
- Eliminating smoking.
- Keeping sun exposure to a minimum.

The nurse promotes health by teaching the activities that maintain wellness, by providing information about the characteristics and consequences of diseases when risk factors have been identified, and by supplying specific information about decreasing risk factors (Pender, Parsons, & Murdaugh, 2002). The nurse also promotes health by following healthy practices and serving as a role model.

**NATIONAL HEALTH PROMOTION.** The U.S. Department of Health and Human Services (2000) published national health objectives for the year 2010. Goals and leading health indicators are described in Box 2–4.

**ILLNESS PREVENTION.** Activities to prevent illness include any measures that limit the progression of an illness at any point of its course. Three levels of illness prevention have been

MediaLink | NATIONAL HEALTH GUIDELINES AND OBJECTIVES

| BOX 2–4 | ■ Goals and Leading Health Indicators: Healthy People 2010 |
|---|---|

Healthy People 2010 has two major goals: to increase the quality and years of healthy life and to eliminate health disparities.

The major goals are divided into 28 focus areas, with each area having a specific goal. For example, for cancer, the goal is to reduce the number of new cancer cases as well as the illness, disability, and death caused by cancer.

The leading indicators used to measure the expected goals are as follows:

- Physical activity
- Overweight and obesity
- Tobacco use
- Substance abuse
- Responsible sexual behavior
- Mental health
- Injury and violence
- Environmental quality
- Immunization
- Access to health care

*Note. Adapted from* Healthy People 2010 *by US Department of Health and Human Services, 2000, Washington, DC: USDHHS.*

defined (Leavell & Clark, 1965). Each level of prevention occurs at a distinct point in the development of a disease process and requires specific nursing interventions (Edelman & Mandle, 2002). The levels are as follows:

1. **Primary level of prevention** includes generalized health-promotion activities as well as specific actions that prevent or delay the occurrence of a disease. Following are examples of primary prevention activities:
   - Protecting oneself against environmental risks, such as air and water pollution
   - Eating nutritious foods
   - Protecting oneself against industrial hazards
   - Obeying seat belt and helmet laws
   - Obtaining sex counseling and practicing safe sex
   - Obtaining immunizations
   - Undergoing genetic screenings
   - Eliminating the use of alcohol and cigarettes
2. **Secondary level of prevention** involves activities that emphasize early diagnosis and treatment of an illness that is already present, to stop the pathologic process and enable the person to return to his or her former state of health as soon as possible. Following are examples of secondary prevention activities:
   - Having screenings for diseases such as hypertension, diabetes mellitus, and glaucoma
   - Obtaining physical examinations and diagnostic tests for cancer
   - Performing self-examination for breast and/or testicular cancer
   - Obtaining tuberculosis skin tests

   - Obtaining specific treatment of illness (e.g., the treatment of streptococcal infections of the throat will prevent secondary infections involving the heart and/or kidneys)
3. **Tertiary level of prevention** focuses on stopping the disease process and returning the affected individual to a useful place in society within the constraints of any disability. The activities primarily revolve around rehabilitation. Following are examples of tertiary prevention measures:
   - Obtaining medical or surgical treatment for an illness
   - Enrolling in specific rehabilitation programs for cardiovascular problems, head injuries, and strokes
   - Joining work training programs following illness or injury
   - Educating the public to employ rehabilitated people to the fullest possible extent

## Disease and Illness

*Disease* and *illness* are terms that are often used interchangeably, but in fact they have different meanings. In general, nursing is concerned with illness, whereas medicine is concerned with disease.

### Disease

**Disease** (literally meaning "without ease") is a medical term describing alterations in structure and function of the body or mind. Diseases may have mechanical, biologic, or normative causes. Mechanical causes of disease result in damage to the structure of the body and are the result of trauma or extremes of temperature. Biologic causes of disease affect body function and are the result of genetic defects, the effects of aging, infestation and infection, alterations in the immune system, and alterations in normal organ secretions. Normative causes are psychologic but involve a mind-body interaction, so that physical manifestations occur in response to the psychologic disturbance.

The cause of many diseases is still unknown. The following are generally accepted as common causes of disease:

- Genetic defects
- Developmental defects resulting from exposure to viruses, chemicals, or drugs that affect the developing fetus
- Biologic agents or toxins (including viruses, bacteria, rickettsia, fungi, protozoa, and helminths)
- Physical agents such as temperature extremes, radiation, and electricity
- Chemical agents such as alcohol, drugs, strong acids or bases, and heavy metals
- Generalized response of tissues to injury or irritation
- Alterations in the production of antibodies, resulting in allergies or hypersensitivities
- Faulty metabolic processes (e.g., a production of hormones or enzymes above or below normal)
- Continued, unabated stress

Diseases may be classified as acute or chronic, communicable, congenital, degenerative, functional, malignant, psychosomatic, idiopathic, or iatrogenic. These classifications are defined in Table 2–6. In all types of disease, alterations in structure or function cause signs and symptoms (**manifestations**) that

| TABLE 2-6 | Disease Classifications and Definitions |
|---|---|
| **Classification** | **Definition** |
| Acute | A disease that has a rapid onset, lasts a relatively short time, and is self-limiting |
| Chronic | A disease that has one or more of these characteristics: (1) is permanent, (2) leaves permanent disability, (3) causes nonreversible pathophysiology, (4) requires special training of the client for rehabilitation, (5) requires a long period of care |
| Communicable | A disease that can spread from one person to another |
| Congenital | A disease or disorder that exists at or before birth |
| Degenerative | A disease that results from deterioration or impairment of organs or tissues |
| Functional | A disease that affects function or performance but does not have manifestations of organic illness |
| Malignant | A disease that tends to become worse and cause death |
| Psychosomatic | A psychologic disease that is manifested by physiologic symptoms |
| Idiopathic | A disease that has an unknown cause |
| Iatrogenic | A disease that is caused by medical therapy |

prompt a person to seek treatment from a physician or traditional healer. Although both subjective symptoms and objective signs commonly appear with disease, objective signs often predominate. Examples include bleeding, vomiting, diarrhea, limitation of movement, swelling, visual disturbances, and changes in elimination. However, pain (a subjective symptom) is often the primary reason that prompts a person to seek health care.

## Illness

**Illness** is the response a person has to a disease. This response is highly individualized, as the person responds not only to his or her own perceptions of the disease but also to the perceptions of others. Illness integrates pathophysiologic alterations; psychologic effects of those alterations; effects on roles, relationships, and values; and cultural and spiritual beliefs. A person may have a disease and not categorize himself or herself as ill, or may validate feelings of illness through the comments of others ("You don't look as though you feel well today").

*ACUTE ILLNESS.* An **acute illness** occurs rapidly, lasts for a relatively short time, and is self-limiting. The condition responds to self-treatment or to medical-surgical intervention. Clients with uncomplicated acute illnesses usually have full recovery and return to normal pre-illness functioning.

**Illness behaviors** are the way people cope with the alterations in health and function caused by a disease. Illness behaviors are highly individualized and are influenced by age, gender, family values, economic status, culture, educational level, and mental status. Following is a sequence of illness behaviors (Suchman, 1972):

1. *Experiencing symptoms.* In the first stage of an acute illness, a person experiences one or more manifestations that serve as cues for an awareness that a change in normal health is occurring. The most significant manifestation is pain. Examples of other symptoms that signal an illness are bleeding, swelling, fever, or difficulty with breathing.

If the manifestations are mild or are familiar (such as symptoms of the common cold or influenza), the person usually uses over-the-counter medications or a traditional remedy for self-treatment. If the symptoms are relieved, no further action is taken; however, if the symptoms are severe or become worse, the person moves to the next stage.

2. *Assuming the sick role.* In the second stage of the sequence, the person assumes the sick role. This role assumption signals acceptance of the symptoms as proof that an illness is present. The person usually validates this belief with others and seeks support for the need to have professional treatment or to stay at home from school or work. Self-preoccupation is characteristic of this stage, and the person focuses on alterations in function resulting from the illness. If the illness is resolved, the person validates a return to health with others and resumes normal activities; however, if manifestations remain or increase in severity and others agree that no improvement has occurred, the person moves to the next stage by seeking medical care.

3. *Seeking medical care.* In our society, a physician or other health care provider most often provides validation of illness. People who believe themselves to be ill (and who are encouraged by others to contact a health care provider) make the medical contact for diagnosis, prognosis, and treatment of the illness. If the medical diagnosis is of an illness, the person moves to the next stage. If the medical diagnosis does not support illness, the client may return to normal functioning or may seek validation from a different health care provider.

4. *Assuming a dependent role.* The stage of assuming a dependent role begins when a person accepts the diagnosis and planned treatment of the illness. As the severity of the illness increases, so does the dependent role. It is during this stage that the person may enter the hospital for treatment and care. The responses of the person to care depend on many different variables: the severity of the illness, the

degree of anxiety or fear about the outcome, the loss of roles, the support systems available, individualized reactions to stress, and previous experiences with illness care.

5. *Achieving recovery and rehabilitation.* The final stage of an acute illness is recovery and rehabilitation. Institutional health care focuses on the acute care needs of the ill client, with recovery beginning in the hospital and completed at home. This focus makes client education and continuity of care a major goal for nursing. It has also contributed to the shift in settings for nursing care, with increasing numbers of nurses providing care in community settings and the home. The person now gives up the dependent role and resumes normal roles and responsibilities. As a result of education during treatment and care, the person may be at a higher level of wellness after recovery is complete. There is no set timetable for recovery from an illness. The degree of severity of the illness and the method of treatment both affect the length of time required, as does the person's compliance with treatment plans and motivation to return to normal health.

**CHRONIC ILLNESS.** **Chronic illness** is a term that encompasses many different lifelong pathologic and psychologic alterations in health. It is the leading health problem in the world today, and the number of people with chronic illnesses is estimated to triple by the year 2040. Current trends affecting an increased incidence of chronic illnesses include diseases of aging, diseases of lifestyle and behavior, and environmental factors.

Most descriptions of chronic illness are based on the definition by the National Commission on Chronic Illness, which states that a chronic illness is any impairment or deviation from normal functioning that has one or more of the following characteristics:

- It is permanent.
- It leaves permanent disability.
- It is caused by nonreversible pathologic alterations.
- It requires special training of the client for rehabilitation.
- It may require a long period of care.

Chronic illness is also characterized by impaired function in more than one body system; responses to this impaired function may occur in sensory perception, self-care abilities, mobility, cognition, and social skills. The demands on the individual and family as a result of these responses are often lifelong (Miller, 2000).

The intensity of a chronic illness and its related manifestations range from mild to severe, and the illness is usually characterized by periods of remission and exacerbation. During periods of **remission,** the person does not experience symptoms, even though the disease is still clinically present. During periods of **exacerbation,** the symptoms reappear. These periods of change in symptoms do not appear in all chronic diseases.

**Needs of the Chronically Ill Person.** Each person with a chronic illness has a unique set of responses and needs. The response of the person to the illness is influenced by the following factors:

- The point in the life cycle at which the onset of the illness occurs
- The type and degree of limitations imposed by the illness
- The visibility of impairment or disfigurement
- The pathophysiology causing the illness
- The relationship between the impairment and functioning in social roles
- Pain and fear

These factors are highly complex. They are interrelated within each person, resulting in individualized illness behaviors and needs. Because there are so many different chronic diseases and because the experience of each person with the illness is a composite of individualized responses, it is difficult to generalize about needs. However, almost all people with a chronic illness will need to:

- Live as normally as possible, despite the symptoms and treatment that make the person with a chronic illness feel alienated, lonely, and different from others without the illness.
- Learn to adapt activities of daily living and self-care activities.
- Grieve the loss of physical function and structure, income, status, roles, and dignity.
- Learn to live with chronic pain.
- Comply with a medical treatment plan.
- Maintain a positive self-concept and a sense of hope.
- Maintain a feeling of being in control.
- Confront the inevitability of death. (Miller, 2000; Pollock, 1986)

Some people with chronic illness successfully meet health-related needs, whereas others do not. Research indicates that adaptation is influenced by variables such as anger, depression, denial, self-concept, locus of control, hardiness, and disability. Nursing interventions for the person with a chronic illness focus on education to promote independent functioning, reduce health care costs, and improve well-being and quality of life.

**The Family of the Client with a Chronic Illness.** The client with a chronic illness may be hospitalized for diagnosis and treatment of acute exacerbations, but the care of the client is primarily provided at home. Chronic illness in a family member is a major stressor that may cause changes in family structure and function, as well as changes in performing family developmental tasks.

Many different factors affect family responses to chronic illness; family responses in turn affect the client's response to and perception of the illness. Factors influencing response to chronic illness include personal, social, and economic resources; the nature and course of the disease; and demands of the illness as perceived by family members.

Support for the family is essential. The following information should be considered when performing any family assessment and developing a client's plan of care:

- Cohesiveness and communication patterns within the family
- Family interactions that support self-care

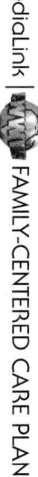

MediaLink  FAMILY-CENTERED CARE PLAN

- Number of friends and relatives available
- Family values and beliefs about health and illness
- Cultural and spiritual beliefs
- Developmental level of the client and family

It is important to remember that standardized teaching plans may not be effective. Rather, chronically ill clients and families should be given the freedom to choose appropriate literature, self-help or support groups, and interactions with others who have the same illness.

## REHABILITATION

**Rehabilitation** is the process of learning to live to one's maximum potential with a chronic impairment and its resultant functional disability. Rehabilitation nursing is based on a philosophy that each person has a unique set of strengths and abilities that can enable that person to live with dignity, self-worth, and independence. Nursing care to promote rehabilitation primarily focuses on clients with chronic illnesses or impairments.

The terms *impairment, disability,* and *handicap* are often used as synonyms, but they have different meanings. An **impairment** is a disturbance in structure or function resulting from physiologic or psychologic abnormalities. A **disability** is the degree of observable and measurable impairment. A **handicap** is the total adjustment to disability that limits functioning at a normal level (Stanhope & Lancaster, 1999). For example, following a motorcycle accident, Kim Rushin had damage to her left leg that resulted in an impairment in the ability to flex her knee. This resulted in a 50% disability of that leg and caused a handicap, because Kim was a school bus driver and could no longer operate the bus safely.

### A Team Approach to Care

Rehabilitation promotes reintegration into the client's family and community through a team approach. Many different aspects of the client's life are included in the plan of care, including physical function, mental health, interpersonal relationships, social interactions, and vocational status. This comprehensive consideration of the client requires the expertise of a team of health care providers.

The rehabilitation team usually meets weekly to discuss the achievement of client goals (Figure 2–4 ■). As a part of this comprehensive plan of care, the team assesses the client's level of function, develops an individualized plan of care, maintains ongoing evaluation of outcomes, and includes the family in the plan of care.

### Nursing in Rehabilitation

The nurse provides care for the chronically ill client of all ages and with many types of disability. The 20-year-old

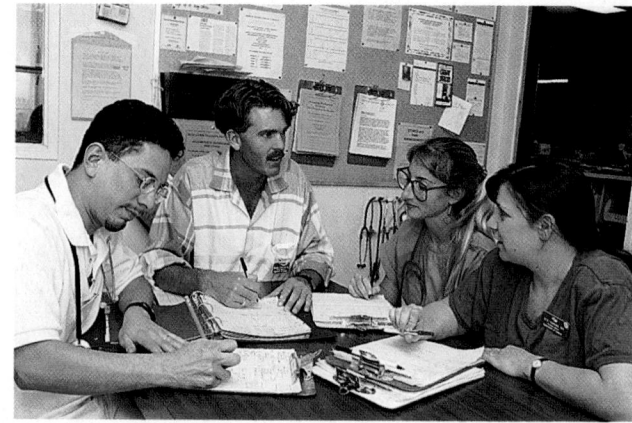

**Figure 2–4** ■ The rehabilitation team discusses the individualized plan of care and achievement of goals.

man with quadriplegia from a spinal cord injury has different needs than the 75-year-old woman who has had a stroke and is unable to move her left arm or speak. However, the plan of care developed for each of these clients considers common factors in assessing and planning individualized interventions.

Assessment of the client and family includes functional level and self-care abilities, educational needs, psychosocial needs, and the home environment. It is critical to determine the priorities of needs from the client and family perspective before establishing any plan of care. The nurse assesses the client's level of physical function, goals, concerns, stage of loss, home environment, and available resources.

Interventions to facilitate rehabilitation are revised to meet client and family needs as the client progresses toward reintegration. General areas of interventions include the following:

- Preventing complications
- Providing care as necessary and appropriate, with the goal of achieving a level of independence that is realistic for the client
- Implementing individualized teaching plans, with emphasis on care at home
- Making referrals to community agencies (for nursing care, special equipment or supplies, support groups, counseling, physical therapy, occupational therapy, respiratory therapy, vocational guidance, house cleaning, meals)

To ensure continuity of care during rehabilitation, the community health nurse is involved in the plan of care during the acute care stage. Continued education and support of the client and family are essential; the achievement of self-care and mobility does not guarantee independence in all areas of human functioning.

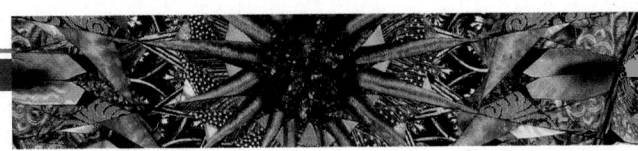

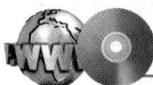 EXPLORE MediaLink

NCLEX review questions, case studies, care plan activities, MediaLink applications, and other interactive resources for this chapter can be found on the Companion Website at www.prenhall.com/lemone.

Click on Chapter 2 to select the activities for this chapter. For animations, video clips, more NCLEX review questions, and an audio glossary, access the Student CD-ROM accompanying this textbook.

## TEST YOURSELF

1. Which of the following physical stressors increases the risk for illness in the young adult?

    a. Sexually transmitted diseases
    b. Motor vehicle accidents
    c. Financial difficulties
    d. Exposure to environmental pollutants

2. Mr. Jones, age 50, is 20 pounds overweight, smokes, and rarely exercises. As a middle adult, these factors increase his risk for disorders of which body system?

    a. Cardiovascular
    b. Renal
    c. Gastrointestinal
    d. Nervous

3. You have been asked to present a health-related program at the local senior center. What would be an appropriate topic?

    a. The Hazards of Substance Abuse
    b. Accident Prevention in the Home
    c. Family Roles and Tasks
    d. Treating Acute Illness

4. Which of the following illustrates the primary level of prevention of illness?

    a. Health screenings for hypertension
    b. Stopping smoking
    c. Annual physical examination
    d. Rehabilitation programs

5. You call your instructor to say you have the "flu" and will not be in class. What level of illness behavior are you demonstrating?

    a. Experiencing symptoms
    b. Assuming the sick role
    c. Seeking medical care
    d. Assuming a dependent role

See Test Yourself answers in Appendix C.

## BIBLIOGRAPHY

Administration on Aging. (2002). *Profile of older Americans: 2002.* Bethesda, MD: National Aging Information Center, US Department of Health and Human Services.

American Association of Retired Persons. (2001). *Profile of older Americans: 2001.* Washington, DC: Resource Services Group.

American Cancer Society. (2002). *Summary of American Cancer Society recommendations for the early detection of cancer in asymptomatic people.* Atlanta, GA: American Cancer Society.

Artinian, N. (1994). Selecting a model to guide family assessment. *Dimensions in Critical Care Nursing, 14*(1), 4–12.

Burckhardt, C. (1987). Coping strategies of the chronically ill. *Nursing Clinics of North America, 22,* 543–550.

Centers for Disease Control and Prevention. (1999a). Births and deaths. *Monthly Vital Statistics Report, 47*(28). Washington, DC: US Department of Health and Human Services.

———. (1999b). *Deaths/mortality.* Washington, DC: National Center for Health Statistics.

Clemen-Stone, S., McGuire, S., & Eigsti, D. (1998). *Comprehensive community health nursing* (5th ed.). St. Louis: Mosby.

Crooks, E., & Clochesy, J. (2001, May). Special needs: Nurses can provide hope and quality care for the chronically, critically ill adult. *American Journal of Nursing* (Suppl.), 21–24, 48–50.

Dewar, A. L., & Lee, E. A. (2000). Bearing illness and injury. *Western Journal of Nursing Research, 22*(8), 912–926.

Duffy, B. (1997). Using a creative teaching process with adult patients. *Home Healthcare Nurse, 15*(2), 102–108.

Dunn, H. (1959). High-level wellness for man and society. *American Journal of Public Health, 49,* 786–972.

Duvall, E. (1977). *Marriage and family development.* Philadelphia: Lippincott.

Edelman, C., & Mandle, C. (2002). *Health promotion throughout the lifespan* (5th ed.). St. Louis: Mosby.

Eliopolous, C. (2000). *Gerontological nursing* (5th ed.). Philadelphia: Lippincott.

Erikson, E. (1963). *Childhood and society* (2nd ed.). New York: Norton.

Fowler, J. (1981). *Stages of faith: The psychology of human development and the quest for meaning.* New York: Harper & Row.

Fowler, S. (1997). Health promotion in chronically ill older adults. *Journal of Neuroscience Nursing, 29*(1), 39–43.

Freidman, M. (1981). *Family nursing: Theory and assessment.* New York: Appleton-Century-Crofts.

Grbich, C., Parker, D., & Maddocks, I. (2001). The emotions and coping strategies of caregivers of family members with a terminal cancer. *Journal of Palliative Care, 17*(1), 30–36.

Havighurst, R. (1972). *Human development and education* (3rd ed.). New York: Longman.

Kohlberg, L. (1979). *The meaning and measurement of moral development.* New York: Clark University.

Kozier, B., Erb, G., Berman, A., & Burke, K. (2000). *Fundamentals of nursing: Concepts, process and practice* (6th ed.). Upper Saddle River, NJ: Prentice Hall.

Leavell, H., & Clark, A. (1965). *Preventive medicine for doctors in the community.* New York: McGraw-Hill.

Lipson, J., Dibble, S., & Minarik, P. (1996). *Culture & nursing care: A pocket guide.* San Francisco: UCSF Nursing Press.

Lubkin, I. (1999). *Chronic illness: Impact and interventions* (4th ed.). Boston: Jones and Bartlett.

Lueckenotte, A. G. (2000). *Gerontologic nursing* (2nd ed.). St. Louis: Mosby.

Miller, C. (1998). *Nursing care of the older adult: Theory and practice* (3rd ed.). Philadelphia: Lippincott.

Miller, J. (2000). *Coping with chronic illness: Overcoming powerlessness* (3rd ed.). Philadelphia: F. A. Davis.

O'Neill, E. S., & Morrow, L. L. (2001). The symptom experience of women with chronic illness. *Journal of Advanced Nursing, 33*(2), 257–268.

Paterson, B. L. (2001). The shifting perspectives model of chronic illness. *Journal of Nursing Scholarship, 33*(1), 21–26.

Pender, N., Parsons, M., & Murdaugh, C. (2002). *Health promotion in nursing practice* (4th ed.). Upper Saddle River, NJ: Prentice Hall.

Pollock, S. (1986). Human responses to chronic illness: Physiologic and psychosocial adaptation. *Nursing Research, 35*(5), 90–95.

Stanhope, M., & Lancaster, J. (1999). *Community health nursing: Process and practice for promoting health* (5th ed.). St. Louis: Mosby.

Strauss, A., et al. (1984). *Chronic illness and the quality of life.* St. Louis: Mosby.

Suchman, E. (1972). Stages of illness and medical care. In E. Jaco (Ed.), *Patients, physicians and illness.* New York: Free Press.

Swanson, E., & Tripp-Reimer, T. (1997). *Chronic illness and the older adult.* New York: Springer.

US Census Department. (1999). *Statistical abstract of the United States.* Washington, DC: US Government Printing Office.

US Department of Health and Human Services. (2000). *Healthy people 2010.* Washington, DC: US Department of Health and Human Services.

_____. (1997). *Administration on aging: Aging into the 21st century.* Washington, DC: Department of Health and Human Services.

Weitzel, E. A. (2001). Risk for poisoning: Drug toxicity. In M. Maas, K. Buckwalter, M. Hardy, T. Tripp-Reimer, M. Titler, & J. Specht (Eds.), *Nursing care of older adults: Diagnoses, outcomes, & interventions* (pp. 34–46). St. Louis: Mosby.

Westerhoff, J. (1976). *Will our children have faith?* New York: Seabury Press.

Woods, N., Yates, B., & Primomo, J. (1989). Supporting families during chronic illness. *Image: Journal of Nursing Scholarship, 21*(1), 46–50.

World Health Organization. (1974). *Constitution of the World Health Organization: Chronicle of the World Health Organization.* Geneva: World Health Organization.

Wu, R. (1973). *Behavior and illness.* Englewood Cliffs, NJ: Prentice Hall.

# Community-Based and Home Care of the Adult Client

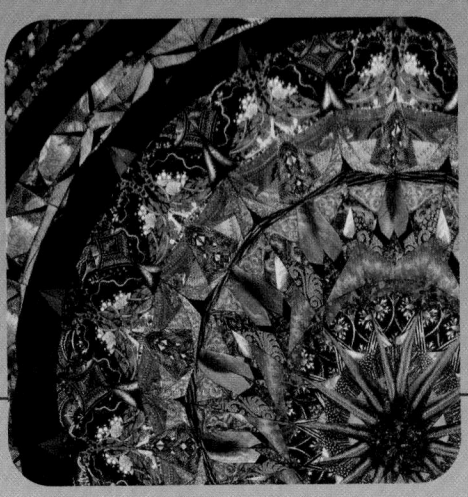

**MediaLink**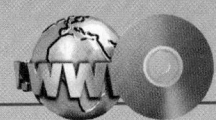

**www.prenhall.com/lemone**
Additional resources for this chapter
can be found on the Student CD-ROM
accompanying this textbook, and on
the Companion Website at
www.prenhall.com/lemone. Click on
Chapter 3 to select the activities for
this chapter.

**CD-ROM**
• Audio Glossary
• NCLEX Review

**Companion Website**
• More NCLEX Review
• Case Study
    Home Health Nursing
• Care Plan Activity
    Home Health Assessment
• MediaLink Application
    Hospice: Purpose and Benefits

## LEARNING OUTCOMES

After completing this chapter, you will be able to:

- Define community-based nursing care.

- Discuss factors affecting health status in the community.

- Describe community-based health care services.

- Describe home health nursing and the roles of the home health nurse.

- Describe the components of the home health care system, including agencies, clients, referrals, physicians, reimbursement, and legal considerations.

- Discuss the effect of the home setting on nursing practice.

- Apply the nursing process to care of the client in the home.

| BOX 3–1 | ■ Community-Based Nursing Care Settings |
| --- | --- |

- Hospitals
  - Inpatient care
  - Outpatient (ambulatory) surgery
  - Outpatient diagnostics and treatments
  - Cardiac rehabilitation
  - Support groups
  - Education groups
- County health departments
- Senior centers
- Long-term care
- Parish nursing
- Adult day care centers
- Homeless shelters
- Mobile vans

- Mental health centers
- Schools
- Crisis intervention centers
- Ambulatory surgery centers
- Alcohol/drug rehabilitation
- Health care provider offices
- Health care clinics
- Free clinics
- Urgent care centers
- Rural health centers
- Home care
- Hospice care
- Industry
- Jails and prisons

Hospitals have become primarily acute care providers with services focused on high-technology care for severely ill or injured people or for people having major surgery. Even those clients rarely remain in the hospital for long. They are moved as rapidly as possible to less acute care settings within the hospital and then to community-based care. Health care has become a managed care, community-based system. Although many nurses are still employed in hospitals, they are increasingly providing nursing care outside of the acute care, in-hospital setting.

## COMMUNITY-BASED NURSING CARE

A **community** may be a small neighborhood in a major urban city or a large area of rural residents. Communities are formed by the characteristics of people, area, social interaction, and common ties. Each community, however, is unique. People who live in a community may share a culture, history, or heritage. Although a community is where people live, have homes, raise families, and carry on daily activities, its members often cross community boundaries to work or to seek health care. Nurses who provide care within a community must know the composition and characteristics of the clients with whom they will work.

In contrast to *community health nursing,* which focuses on the health of the community, **community-based nursing** centers on individual and family health care needs. The nurse practicing community-based care provides direct services to individuals to manage acute or chronic health problems and to promote self-care. The care is provided in the local community, is culturally competent, and is family centered. The philosophy of community-based nursing directs nursing care for clients wherever they are, including where they live, work, play, worship, and go to school (Zotti, Brown, & Stotts, 1996).

Nurses provide community-based care in many different ways and locations, ranging from leading support groups in a hospital (for individuals and family members diagnosed with such illnesses as cancer or diabetes) to managing a freestanding clinic to

providing care at the client's home. Box 3–1 illustrates the varied settings within the community in which a nurse may provide care.

## FACTORS AFFECTING HEALTH IN THE COMMUNITY

Many factors affect health in a community. These factors include social support systems, the community health care structure, environmental factors, and economic resources.

### Social Support Systems

A person's social support system consists of the people who lend assistance to meet financial, personal, physical, or emotional needs. In most instances, family, friends, and neighbors provide the best social support within the community. To understand the community social structure, the nurse needs to know:

- The degree to which men and women are seen as equals and partners in health care.
- Available support for health care for the client and family, including neighbors, friends, their church, organizations, self-help groups, and professional providers.
- Cultural and ethnic background of the community.
- Level of neighborhood cooperation and communication.

### Community Health Care Structure

The health care structure of a community has a direct effect on the health of the people living and working within it. The size of the community often determines the type of services provided as well as the access to the services. For example, urban residents have various means of transportation to a variety of community health care providers, whereas rural residents must often travel long distances for any type of care. The financial base of the community is also important, often determining state and county funding of services.

Nurses who provide community-based care must know about public health services, the number and kind of health screenings offered, the location and specialty of health care professionals within the community, and the availability and accessibility of services and supplies. Other factors to consider include facilities (e.g., day care and long-term care), housing, and the number and kind of support agencies providing assistance (e.g., housing, shelter, and food).

## Environmental Factors

The environment within which a person lives and works may have both helpful and harmful effects on health. Air and water quality differs across communities. Air pollution may occur across a large area, or may be limited to the home. Within the home, pollution may occur from such sources as molds, pesticides, and fumes from new carpet. The water source also varies, with water supplies coming from rivers, lakes, reservoirs, or wells. No matter the source, chemical runoff or bacteria may contaminate water. It is critical to determine whether clients have a safe supply of running water.

Household and community safety and health resource accessibility are also important. Nurses must consider lighting, street and sidewalk or road upkeep and conditions, effects of ice and snow, condition of stairs and floors, and usefulness and availability of bathroom facilities. Physical barriers to accessing community resources include lack of transportation, distance to services, and location of services.

## Economic Resources

Economic resources encompass the financial and insurance coverages that provide the means to have health care within the community. As private medical insurance becomes more and more expensive, fewer citizens have it; and many U.S. citizens have no insurance at all. Most unskilled jobs do not provide health care benefits, resulting in a substantial percentage of what might be labeled "the working poor," those who have no financial assistance for illness care or health care screenings from an employer. Older adults on limited incomes often find their monthly income consumed by medicines and medical supplies.

Medicare and Medicaid are health assistance programs created by 1965 Social Security amendments. Medicare is a federal health insurance plan for acute care needs of the disabled and those over 65 years. This plan covers some services provided in hospitals, long-term facilities, and the home; however, many necessary health care components are not covered fully or at all, including prescribed and over-the-counter medications and adaptive equipment for safety, such as shower seats or raised toilet seats. Coverage for care at home continues only as long as skilled providers are needed, and the person is not considered homebound even if he or she needs a wheelchair and assistance from others to leave the home. Medicaid is a state-run health insurance program for people with limited incomes. Each state has different benefits and criteria for coverage.

## COMMUNITY-BASED HEALTH CARE SERVICES

Community-based health care services can take many forms. Some are discussed here, but a more detailed discussion of home health care is provided later in the chapter.

## Home Health Care

**Home health care** encompasses both health and social services provided to the chronically ill, disabled, or recovering person in his or her own home. Home care is usually provided when a person needs help that cannot be provided by a family member or friend. Among clients who benefit from home health care services are those who:

- Cannot live independently at home because of age, illness, or disability.
- Have chronic, debilitating illnesses such as congestive heart failure, heart disease, kidney disease, respiratory diseases, diabetes mellitus, or muscle-nerve disorders.
- Are terminally ill and want to die with comfort and dignity at home.
- Do not need in-patient hospital or nursing home care but require additional assistance.
- Need short-term help at home for postoperative care.

The services provided in the home may include professional nursing care, care provided by home health care aides, physical therapy, speech therapy, occupational therapy, medical social worker services, and nutritional services. Clients receiving home health care services are usually under the care of a physician, with the focus of care being treatment or rehabilitation. Registered nurses or licensed practical nurses provide nursing care based on physician orders. These nurses give direct care, supervise other health care providers, coordinate client care with the physician, advocate for the client and family, and teach family members and friends how to care for the client to assist the nurse as well as when professional services are no longer necessary.

**Hospice care** is a special component of home care, designed to provide medical, nursing, social, psychological, and spiritual care for terminally ill clients and their families. Hospice care relies on a philosophy of relieving pain and suffering and allowing the client to die with dignity in a comfortable environment. Licensed nurses, medical social workers, physicians, occupational and physical therapists, and volunteers provide care. Hospice care is discussed in Chapter 11. ♾

## Respite Care

**Respite care** provides short-term or intermittent home care, often using volunteers. These services exist primarily to give the family member or friend who is the primary caregiver some time away from care. Respite care does much to relieve the burden of full-time caregiving.

## Community Centers and Clinics

Community centers and clinics may be directed by physicians, advanced practice nurses in collaboration with physicians, or advanced practice nurses working independently (depending on state regulations). These health care settings may be located within a hospital, be part of a hospital but located in another area, or be independent of a hospital base. Health care centers and clinics provide a wide range of services and often meet the health needs of clients who are unable to access care elsewhere. This group includes the homeless, the poor, those with substance abuse problems, those with sexually transmitted diseases, and the victims of violent or abusive behavior.

## Day Care Programs

Day care programs, such as senior centers, are usually located where people gather for social, nutritional, and recreational purposes. These programs vary among communities. Meals may be provided at low cost.

## Parish Nursing and Block Nursing

Parish nursing and block nursing are nontraditional, community-based ways of providing health promotion and health restoration nursing interventions to specific groups of people. Both types of care meet the needs of people who are often underserved by the traditional health care system.

A nurse who practices **parish nursing** works with the pastor and staff of a faith community to promote health and healing through counseling, referrals, teaching, and assessment of health care needs. A parish nurse may be employed by a hospital and contracted by a church, be employed directly by a church, or work as a volunteer with the congregation of a church. The parish nurse helps bridge gaps between members of the church and the health care system.

**Block nursing** is nursing care provided to people who live on the same block as the nurse. Services are administered based on need rather than on eligibility for reimbursement. Other residents of the block often provide volunteer services to assist the nurse, with funding for care often coming from grants and demonstration projects.

## Meals-on-Wheels

Many communities have a food service, usually called Meals-on-Wheels, for older people who do not have assistance in the home for food preparation. A hot, nutritionally balanced meal is delivered once a day, usually at noon. Volunteers often deliver the meals, providing not only nutrition but also a friendly, caring visit each day.

## HOME HEALTH CARE

Home care is not easily defined. It is not simply illness care at home, nor is it the act of setting up a hospital room in someone's house. The National Association for Home Care (NAHC) 2000 defines **home care** as services for recovering, disabled, or chronically ill people who are in need of treatment or support to function effectively in the home environment. Home care is appropriate for adults and children in danger of abuse or neglect or for any person who needs either short-term or long-term assistance that cannot be provided by family members or friends.

The U.S. Department of Health and Human Services places home care along a continuum of health care. Home care is provided in the client's place of residence for the purpose of promoting, maintaining, or restoring health or of maximizing the level of independence while minimizing the effects of disability and illness, including terminal illness.

Home care is both professional and technical. Professional home care is provided by people who are practice driven, licensed, certified, and/or have special qualifications. Nurses, therapists, social workers, and home health aides are considered professional providers. Technical home care providers are business and product driven. Customer satisfaction, field service, reimbursement, and profits are their primary concerns. Durable medical equipment companies (businesses that deliver medical equipment to homes) are technical providers.

Many milestones marked the growth and development of home health care in the United States. The passage of Medicare in 1965, Medicaid in 1970, the addition of hospice benefits in 1973, and the introduction of diagnosis-related groups (DRGs) in 1983 dramatically affected home care. Medicare legislation entitled the nation's elderly to home care services, primarily skilled nursing and other curative or restorative therapies. This same benefit was extended to certain disabled younger Americans in 1973.

The introduction of DRGs to help control health care costs greatly increased home health care. DRGs are categories for reimbursement of inpatient services. The DRG system pays the same predetermined amount of money for the care of different persons with the same medical diagnosis. Many changes in the health care system have been attributed to the introduction of DRGs, including earlier discharge from hospitals and the increased need for home care services.

## Roles of the Home Health Nurse

The role expectations of the home health nurse are similar to those of the professional nurse in any setting. On behalf of clients in the home, the nurse serves as an advocate, a provider of direct care, an educator, and a coordinator of services (see Chapter 1).

### Advocate

As client advocate, the nurse explores, informs, supports, and affirms the choices of clients. Advocacy begins on the first visit, when the nurse discusses advanced directives, living wills, and durable power of attorney for health care. The home health agency's bill of rights also needs to be discussed. During the course of care, clients may need help negotiating the complex medical system (especially in regard to medical insurance), accessing community resources, recognizing and coping with required changes in lifestyle, and making informed decisions. When the family's desires differ from the client's, advocacy can be a challenge. If a conflict arises, the nurse must remain the client's primary advocate.

### Provider of Direct Care

Home health nurses usually are not involved in providing personal care for clients (bathing, changing linens, and so on). The family usually provides routine personal care, or the nurse may arrange for a home health aide. If a personal care need arises during the course of the skilled visit (e.g., if a client has an in-

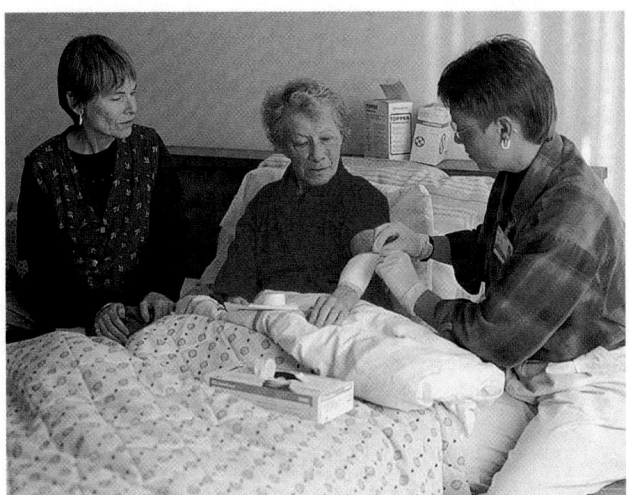

**Figure 3–1** ■ The home health nurse often provides client education. This nurse is teaching the client and a family member how to apply dressings.

continent episode), the nurse typically either bathes and changes the client or assists the caregiver to do so before moving on to the skilled activities planned for the visit.

As a provider of direct care, the nurse uses the nursing process to assess, diagnose, plan care, intervene, and evaluate client needs. During the course of this process, home health nurses frequently are involved in performing specific procedures and treatments such as physical assessments, care of intravenous lines, ostomy care, wound care, and pain management.

### Educator

Most of the home health nurse's time is spent teaching. Many nurses believe that their role as teacher is the crux of their nursing practice and that nurses in the home are always teaching (Figure 3–1 ■). For this reason, it is important that home health nurses develop expertise in the theory and principles of client education.

The greatest educational challenge may be motivating the client. Discovering what it takes to make the client want to learn and focusing the client on what is most important can tax the ingenuity of even the most dedicated nurse. Despite the work involved, nurses are rewarded by the knowledge that through their efforts, clients have learned to manage independently. Because the nurse's role as educator is becoming increasingly important, guidelines for home care are included in the discussion of each major disorder addressed in this textbook.

### Coordinator of Services

As coordinator of services, the home health nurse is the main contact with the client's physician and all other providers involved in the treatment plan. It is the responsibility of the registered nurse case coordinator (or clinical case manager) to report client changes, discuss responses, and develop and secure treatment plan revisions on an ongoing basis. This is accomplished both formally, through scheduled case and team conferences, and informally (often over the phone) with concerned providers. Documentation of all coordination activities is legally required.

## Standards for Nursing Practice in the Home

Home health nurses are responsible for adhering to the same codes and standards that guide all other nurses. These codes and standards, provided in Chapter 1, guide nursing practice and protect the public. In addition to these guidelines, other codes and statements give specific guidance on issues that affect care in the home. ⊕

### ANA Standards for Home Health Nursing Practice

The ANA Standards for Home Health Nursing Practice are used in conjunction with the ANA Standards of Community Health Nursing as a basis for the practice of nursing in the home. The standards address the nursing process, interdisciplinary collaboration, quality assurance, professional development, and research (see Box 3–2). The standards speak to two levels of practitioners (generalist, who is prepared on the baccalaureate level, and specialist, who is prepared on the graduate level) and outline what achievements are expected of the professional nurse in the home.

### NAHC Bill of Rights

Another source of guidance regarding home care is the NAHC Bill of Rights. Its use is a federal requirement for all home health agencies. Although they are permitted to make additions to the NAHC's original bill of rights, home health agencies are required by law to address the concepts in the NAHC Bill of Rights with all home health clients on the initial visit. Box 3–3 provides an example of a home health agency's bill of rights.

### ANA Position Statements

The ANA has published position statements addressing moral, ethical, and legal issues faced by home and community health nurses. Examples are as follows:

- *A Statement on the Scope of Home Health Nursing Practice*
- *Risk Versus Responsibility in Providing Nursing Care*
- *Cultural Diversity in Nursing Practice*
- *Foregoing Artificial Nutrition and Hydration*

## The Home Health Care System

Nurses who practice home care do so within a system that includes home health agencies, clients, referral sources, physicians, reimbursement sources, and legal considerations. The system is interactive and, like any other, functions best when its members communicate, cooperate, and collaborate with one another.

### Home Health Agencies

**Home health agencies** are either public or private organizations engaged in providing skilled nursing and other therapeutic services in the client's home. The several different types of

## BOX 3–2 ■ ANA Standards for Home Health Nursing Practice

**STANDARD I. ORGANIZATION OF HOME HEALTH SERVICES**

All home health services are planned, organized, and directed by a master's-prepared professional nurse with experience in community health and administration.

**STANDARD II. THEORY**

The nurse applies theoretical concepts as a basis for decisions in practice.

**STANDARD III. DATA COLLECTION**

The nurse continuously collects and records data that are comprehensive, accurate, and systematic.

**STANDARD IV. DIAGNOSIS**

The nurse uses health assessment data to determine nursing diagnoses.

**STANDARD V. PLANNING**

The nurse develops care plans that establish goals. The care plan is based on nursing diagnoses and incorporates therapeutic, preventive, and rehabilitative nursing actions.

**STANDARD VI. INTERVENTION**

The nurse, guided by the care plan, intervenes to provide comfort, to restore, improve, and promote health, to prevent complications and sequelae of illness, and to effect rehabilitation.

**STANDARD VII. EVALUATION**

The nurse continually evaluates the client's and family's responses to interventions in order to determine progress toward goal at-

tainment and to revise the database, nursing diagnoses, and plan of care.

**STANDARD VIII. CONTINUITY OF CARE**

The nurse is responsible for the client's appropriate and uninterrupted care along the health care continuum, and therefore uses discharge planning, case management, and coordination of community resources.

**STANDARD IX. INTERDISCIPLINARY COLLABORATION**

The nurse initiates and maintains a liaison relationship with all appropriate health care providers to assure that all efforts effectively complement one another.

**STANDARD X. PROFESSIONAL DEVELOPMENT**

The nurse assumes responsibility for professional development and contributes to the professional growth of others.

**STANDARD XI. RESEARCH**

The nurse participates in research activities that contribute to the profession's continuing development of knowledge of home care.

**STANDARD XII. ETHICS**

The nurse uses the code for nurses established by the American Nurses Association as a guide for ethical decision making in practice.

*Note. From* Standards for Home Health Nursing Practice *by American Nurses Association, 1986, Kansas City, MO: ANA.*

home health agencies differ only in the way their programs are organized and administered. All home health agencies are similar in that they must meet uniform standards for licensing, certification, and accreditation. Home health agencies include the following:

- *Official or public agencies.* State or local governments operate these agencies, which are financed primarily by tax funds. Most official agencies offer home care, health education, and disease-prevention programs in the community.
- *Voluntary or private not-for-profit agencies.* Donations, endowments, charities such as the United Way, and third-party (insurance company) reimbursement support these agencies. They are governed by a volunteer board of directors, which usually represents the community they serve.
- *Private, proprietary agencies.* Most of these agencies are for-profit organizations governed by either individual owners or national corporations. Although some participate in third-party reimbursement, others rely on clients paying their own bills (often called out-of-pocket expenses).
- *Institution-based agencies.* These agencies operate under a parent organization, such as a hospital. The home health

agency is governed by the sponsoring organization and the mission of both is similar. Often, the majority of home health referrals come from the parent organization.

Home health agency personnel typically include administrators, managers, professional providers, paraprofessionals, and business office staff. Depending on the agency and geographic location, professional providers may include registered nurses, practical nurses, nurse practitioners, enterostomal therapists, physical therapists, occupational therapists, speech therapists, respiratory therapists, social workers, a chaplain or pastoral minister, dietitians, and home health aides. It is not unusual for clients to require the services of several professionals simultaneously. No matter how many providers are in the home, the responsibility for case coordination (also called case management) remains with the registered nurse.

### Clients

The client in home health is the person receiving care and the person's family. The recognition that the family is also a client acknowledges the powerful influence that families exert on

| BOX 3-3 | ■ A Home Health Agency's Bill of Rights |
| --- | --- |

The agency acknowledges the client's rights and encourages the client and family to participate in their plan of care through informed decision making. In accordance with this belief, each client/family member will receive, prior to admission, the following bill of rights and responsibilities.

1. The client and the client's property will be treated with respect by the program's staff.
2. The client will receive care without regard to race, color, creed, age, sex, religion, national origin, or mental or physical handicap.
3. The client has the right to be free from mental and physical abuse.
4. The client's medical record and related information is maintained in a confidential manner by the program.
5. The client will receive a written statement of the program's objectives, scope of services, and grievance process prior to admission.
6. The client, family, or guardian has the right to file a complaint regarding the services provided by the program without fear of disruption of service, coercion, or discrimination.
7. The client will be advised of the following in advance of service:
   a. Description of services and proposed visit frequency
   b. Overview of the anticipated plan of care and its likely outcome
   c. Options that may be available
8. The client/family is encouraged to participate in the plan of care. The client will receive the necessary information concerning the client's condition and will be encouraged to participate in changes that may arise in care.
9. The program shall provide for the right of the client to refuse any portion of planned treatment to the extent permitted by law without relinquishing other portions of the treatment plan, except where medical contraindications exist. The client will be informed of the expected consequences of such action.
10. The client has a right to continuity of care:
    a. Services provided within a reasonable time frame
    b. A program that is capable of providing the level of care required by the client
    c. Timely referral to alternative services, as needed
    d. Information regarding impending discharge, continuing care requirements, and other services, as needed
11. The client will be informed of the extent to which payment will be expected for items or services to be furnished to clients by Medicare, Medicaid, and any other program that is funded partially or fully with federal funds. Upon admission, the client will be informed orally and in writing of any charges for items and services that the program expects will not be covered upon admission. The client will be informed of any change in this amount as soon as possible, but no later than within 25 days after the program is made aware of the change.
12. Upon request, the client may obtain:
    a. An itemized bill.
    b. The program's policy for uncompensated care.
    c. The program's policy for disclosure of the medical record.
    d. Identity of health care providers with which the program has contractual agreements, insofar as the client's care is concerned.
    e. The name of the responsible person supervising the client's care and how to contact this person during regular business hours.
13. The client has the right to obtain medical equipment and other health-related items from the company of the client's choice and assumes financial responsibility for such. The program's staff will assist in obtaining supplies and physician approvals as needed.
14. The client/family is responsible for:
    a. Giving the program accurate, necessary information.
    b. Being available and cooperative during scheduled visits.
    c. Assisting, as much as possible, in the plan of care.
    d. Alerting the staff to any problems as soon as possible.

*Note. Adapted from the Patient Bill of Rights and Responsibilities, Bon Secours Home Health Hospice Program, Baltimore, MD.*

health. A client's family is not limited to persons related by birth, adoption, or marriage. In the home, family members may include lovers, friends, colleagues, other significant people, and even animals that hold the potential of greatly affecting the health care environment.

Age and functional disability are the primary predictors of need for home care services. Information from a national survey conducted by the Agency for Health Care Policy and Research found that about half of all home care clients are over the age of 65 and that the number of home care services that clients need seems to increase with age (NAHC, 2000).

***PREPARING CLIENTS FOR CARE AT HOME.*** The old adage that discharge plans begin at admission makes more sense today than ever before. With shortened lengths of hospital stay, it is imperative for nurses to evaluate all clients for their ability to manage at home. Nurses preparing to send clients home must consider many of the questions outlined in the Meeting Individualized Needs Box on page 44.

***MEETING PRIORITY NEEDS.*** When preparing clients for discharge to home, the nurse focuses on safety and survival first. Even if health education is to continue with home care, a day or two may elapse before the nurse arrives, and clients must be able to manage by themselves until then. The nurse must not discharge clients without giving them the correct information and supplies to get them through the first few days at home. Additionally, clients should not be discharged without complete

## Meeting Individualized Needs

### THE CLIENT BEING DISCHARGED FROM ACUTE CARE TO HOME CARE

#### QUESTIONS FOR CONSIDERATION:

- Does the client need follow-up therapy, treatments, or additional education?
- What equipment, supplies, or information about community resources is necessary?
- What teaching materials can be sent home? Are they written at an acceptable reading level? Do they come in other languages?
- What cognitive abilities do the client and the caregiver seem to have? Are there any sensory deprivations that impede learning?

- Who will be the principal caregiver in the home? Is there one? Are all caregivers comfortable in doing what needs to be done? If not, what support do they need to become comfortable?
- Was the caregiver present during and included in instruction? How have the client and caregiver responded to health teaching thus far? Have they comprehended what has been taught? Was their stress level such that they could not listen?
- Has a devastating diagnosis and/or prognosis just been determined?
- Is high-technology intervention necessary?

---

information about their medications and the manifestations of complications they should report to their doctor. Finally, all clients should be able to at least minimally manage any necessary treatments. Management includes not only performing procedures safely but also knowing how to obtain necessary supplies in the community.

Clients need help understanding their situations, making health care decisions, and changing health behaviors. It is unrealistic, however, to believe that clients can be taught everything they need to know during today's shortened hospital stays. The nurse should therefore recommend a home health referral for anyone in need of follow-up teaching. Prioritized teaching is essential: Even under the best of circumstances, clients generally forget about one-third of what is said to them, and their recall of specific instructions and advice is less than 50%. Comprehensive information related to client and family teaching is included in most of the following chapters in this textbook. This can be used as a guide in planning teaching.

### Referrals

A referral source is a person recommending home health services and supplying the agency with details about the client's needs. The source may be a physician, nurse, social worker, therapist, or discharge planner. Families sometimes generate their own referrals, either by approaching one of the sources already mentioned or by calling a home health agency directly to make an inquiry. When the family seeks a referral and the agency believes that the client qualifies for services, usually the agency contacts the client's physician and requests a referral on the client's behalf.

The nurse may make a referral to either a home health agency, a hospice, or a community resource if the client seems to need formal follow-up beyond the present clinical setting. Hospital discharge planners, social workers, organizations for older adults, and local nonprofit agencies usually have a good command of the services and support groups available in their communities.

The nurse must talk to clients and their caregivers about concerns related to home management. It is not unusual for one family member to think that no additional help is necessary and for another to feel differently.

The nurse can facilitate an informal family meeting in which everyone shares concerns and can make inquiries about the family's insurance coverage for home health care. Suggesting services that families cannot afford only adds to the problem. For clients with limited means, the nurse can consult with staff in the institution who are most knowledgeable about funding. In every instance, it is important that the nurse avoid making assumptions: Well-educated and financially secure clients can be just as overwhelmed by illness as clients who are poor and less learned. Everyone is a referral candidate.

If the family believes that no help is necessary and the nurse believes otherwise, then the nurse may ask the family to consider an evaluation visit, explaining how the situation may look different once the client is home. If family members continue to refuse, the nurse can let them know that the door is never closed and give them contacts in the community that they can access independently should their needs change.

### Physicians

Home care cannot begin without a physician's order, nor can it proceed without a physician-approved treatment plan. This is a legal and reimbursement requirement. Only after a referral is made and an initial set of physician orders is obtained can a nursing assessment visit be scheduled to identify the client's needs. If the input of another provider, such as a physical therapist, is necessary to complete the initial assessment, then the nurse arranges for this visit.

At the nursing assessment visit, the nurse begins to formulate the plan of care. Box 3–4 lists Medicare's required data for the nursing plan of care. Once formulated, the nurse sends the plan of care back to the physician for review and approval. The physician's signature on the plan of care authorizes the home health agency's providers to continue with services and also

| BOX 3–4 | ■ Medicare's Required Data for the Plan of Care |
|---|---|

1. All pertinent diagnoses
2. A notation of the beneficiary's mental status
3. Types of services, supplies, and equipment ordered
4. Frequency of visits to be made
5. Client's prognosis
6. Client's rehabilitation potential
7. Client's functional limitations
8. Activities permitted
9. Client's nutritional requirements
10. Client's medications and treatments
11. Safety measures to protect against injuries
12. Discharge plans
13. Any other items the home health agency or physician wishes to include

*Note. From* Medicare Health Insurance Manual-11, *Section 204.2.*

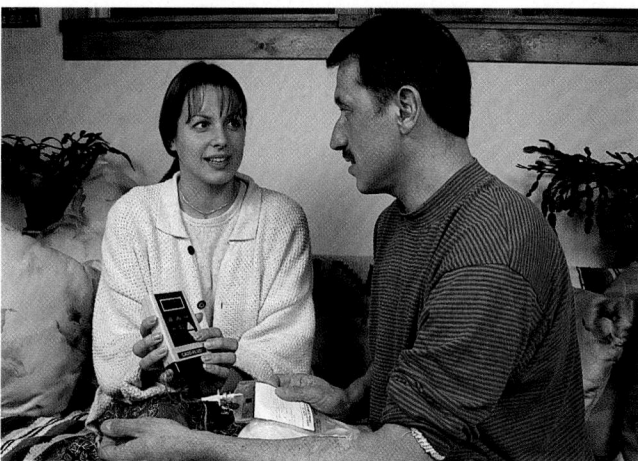

**Figure 3–2** ■ Demystifying high-technology home care equipment is a nursing challenge. This nurse demonstrates the use of a patient-controlled analgesia (PCA) pump used in management of chronic pain.

serves as a contract indicating agreement to participate in the care of the client on an ongoing basis. The plan is reviewed as necessary, but at least once every 60 days.

## Reimbursement for Services

A reimbursement source pays for home health services. Medicare is home care's largest single reimbursement source, although other sources exist (Medicaid, other public funding, private insurance, and public donation). The reimbursement source evaluates each treatment plan to determine if the goals and plans set forth by the professional providers match the needs assessed. Only interventions identified on the treatment plan are covered. Periodically the reimbursement source may ask for the home health provider's notes to substantiate what is being done in the home. This is one reason why accurate documentation is critical.

Medicare does not reimburse visits made to support general health maintenance, health promotion, or clients' emotional or socioeconomic needs. Both client and nurse must meet specific criteria to secure Medicare reimbursement. The client must meet all of the following criteria:

- The physician must decide that the client needs care at home and make a plan for home care.
- The client must need at least one of the following: intermittent (not full time) skilled nursing care, physical therapy, speech language pathology services, or occupational therapy.
- The client must be homebound. This means leaving the home is a major effort. When leaving the home, it must be infrequent, for a short time, to get medical care, or to attend religious services.
- The home health agency must be Medicare approved.

Medicare will reimburse only when the skilled provider performs at least one of the following tasks:

- Teaching about a new or acute situation.
- Assessing an acute process or a change in the client's condition.

- Performing a skilled procedure or a hands-on service requiring the professional skill, knowledge, ability, and judgment of a licensed nurse (Figure 3–2 ■).

The reimbursement guidelines present problems because they are not sensitive to the full scope of nursing practice. Many of the client and family needs that nurses encounter during home visits are complex and time consuming, reflecting both intense psychosocial and economic concerns. This situation presents a profound dilemma. How are nurses to reconcile spending time on issues for which their agency will receive no payment? How are they to meet agency home visit productivity standards when each home they enter requires more and more from them? How are they to document activities and interventions that are not considered "skilled"? There are no easy answers to these questions.

## Legal Considerations

The legal considerations in home health center around issues of privacy and confidentiality, the client's access to health information, the client's freedom from unreasonable restraint, witnessing of documents, informed consent, and matters of negligence and/or malpractice. Numerous sources suggest that nurses can best avoid lawsuits by familiarizing themselves with the standards of practice, providing care that is consistent with both the standards and their agency's policies, and documenting all care fully and accurately according to agency guidelines.

## Differences in Inpatient Care and Home Care

Nursing practice in the home is a unique experience that differs in many ways from nursing practice in a hospital setting. These differences include the following:

- *Nurses are invited into homes.* Nurses are guests and cannot assume entry, as they do in formal clinical settings. The environment belongs to the client, who retains control. Every nursing action must communicate respect for these boundaries. To negotiate both repeated entry and a share of power in the client's domain, the nurse must establish trust and rapport quickly. This is often difficult, because most home health nurses are with each client for only 1 hour a few times a week.

- *Home health nursing is solitary.* In the home, there are no colleagues present to consult, to assist, or to rely on for support. The home is a practice setting where nurses learn to trust their theoretical and intuitive knowledge and to be totally accountable.

- *The home is one of the richest symbols in Western culture.* The word *home* generates strong feelings of ownership, control, security, family history, independence, comfort, protection, and conflict. The family perceives a sharing of self when they consistently allow entry to a stranger. Because clients and nurses most often meet during periods of vulnerability and crisis, and because socializing is such an integral part of the home visit process, nurse providers are often perceived as friends or extended family members, blurring the boundaries of practice.

- *Intimacy and shared humanity are nurtured in the home.* During the course of establishing rapport and getting to know each other as people, the nurse-client relationship often becomes something more. Nurses and clients end up giving to each other and learning from each other. By connecting as human beings, they touch each other's spirits in profound ways (Carson, 1989). In home health, it is not unusual for nurses to realize suddenly not only that they do things to create a healing environment but also that their very presence has become the healing environment.

- *Family issues and relationships are more visible in the home.* Over time, as the nurse becomes a familiar presence and the family's behavior relaxes, the nurse can gain a clearer and more complete picture of family relationships, dynamics, lifestyle choices, and coping patterns. Multigenerational behavior patterns are more obvious, and working around them can become quite a feat.

- *Nurses play a variety of roles.* Although they focus on providing health care, home health nurses also understand that promoting the client's optimal wellness often necessitates interventions that are not treatment oriented. Nurses report that they find themselves functioning as social workers, friends, spiritual comforters, psychologists, financial counselors, and interpreters of medical information.

- *"Families of one" are a worrisome reality.* Today more older adults are living alone. Some may have current or potential caregivers nearby, whereas others, for any of various reasons, have no one. These people often require considerable nursing support to remain strong, independent, and resourceful. Caring for "families of one" can take a toll on even the strongest home health nurse. Some nurses have reported calling between visits, keeping in touch after discharge, and driving by on days off because they have such difficulty "letting go" their concerns about these clients.

- *Caregiver burden is not easily hidden in the home.* In more than 22 million American households, people are taking care of disabled relatives and friends (Health Care Financing Administration [HCFA], 1997). Many of these caregivers are themselves older adults. Health care planners visualize the home as a place where all kinds of medical services can occur but may give little thought to how people manage. Few ever ask whether families can cope with the level of care they are expected to assume. Caregiving has only recently been acknowledged as a complex activity, requiring adjustment in family living patterns, relationships, and finances. For some families, the crisis of caregiving is short lived, but for others it lasts for years. As a result, caregivers are at great risk for both physical and emotional illness. Because the success of home care heavily depends on the supports in place, addressing the needs of the support network is imperative.

- *Care in the home sometimes is inadequate.* Personal health habits, living conditions, resources, and support systems may leave much to be desired. It is not unusual for home health nurses to face unchanged dressings, undertreated infections, off-and-on self-medication, poor nutrition, filthy conditions, and unreliable caregivers. No matter how vigilant nurses may be, practice settings like these work against their best efforts. If the conditions cannot be changed, the nurse usually has two choices: to withdraw from the situation or to continue to practice within the environment.

## Practical Information from Home Health Nurses

A study (Stulginsky, 1993a, 1993b) of practicing home health nurses solicited knowledge about the art and science of home health nursing from their lived experience. The results have added a practical dimension to many of the interventions home health nurses typically implement during client care. The practical information gleaned from this research and from other home health experts follows.

### Establish Trust and Rapport

To establish trust and rapport in the client's home, nurses must try to find common ground and to let go of ethnocentric ("My culture's way is the best way") views. Nurses must be sure everything they say and do communicates an understanding that they are guests—offering suggestions in a way that acknowledges the client's right to say no, sensing and honoring "where people are in their situation," maintaining a respectful distance, and noticing and honoring family customs ("Gee, no one wears shoes in your house; I'll take mine off, too."). Nurses should try to negotiate their schedules around the family's needs; nursing should enhance family coping, not complicate it. Above all, nurses should validate clients' illness experiences, remembering that everyone needs someone who is willing to listen and say, "I hear what you are saying, and I think I have a sense of how you feel."

## Proceed Slowly

The nurse must enter the home with an awareness that the first contact is important. On the first nursing visit, the nurse can suggest to clients that they have someone else present "to help them listen." To avoid overwhelming clients with too much information, the nurse stresses the essential information and repeats it on subsequent visits. When making suggestions, the nurse offers clients the pluses and minuses of each alternative. Informed decisions are difficult to make if people are too overwhelmed to think of their options. The nurse speaks slowly, directly, and within the client's range of vision (the client may have to lip-read) and refrains from shouting at clients who are hearing-impaired. The nurse must allow time for families to process new information.

## Set Goals and Boundaries

The nurse explores clients' expectations of home care. In particular, the nurse explains the primary goal (to achieve self-care), defines nurse and client roles within this framework, and discusses limitations. The nurse may make statements such as, "No, a home health nurse is not the same as a private duty nurse" and "Home health nurses do not routinely do that, but today I will make an exception." It is important that the nurse stresses mutual accountability, choice, and negotiation as part of the process.

## Assess the Home Environment

The nurse surveys the overall home environment, using common sense, intuition, and imagination. Among the variables to note are sights, sounds, smells, dress, tone of voice, body language, and the use of touch; visiting patterns among family members; significant relationships; what is sacred and what is not; the appearance of the house, yard, sidewalk, and neighborhood; and the effect of illness on the family. The nurse asks questions and listens carefully to stories and offhand remarks.

## Set Priorities

It is important that nurses be flexible and realize they cannot tackle everything. Although it is necessary to enter the home with a plan in mind, nurses must be prepared to modify the plan according to conditions they encounter once inside. Safety, issues that are of concern to clients, and those problems that can most easily be solved should be addressed first. Alternatively, the nurse can focus on safety first, then short-term and long-term goals. If the priorities that are set are primarily the nurse's and not the client's, then they may not be met.

## Promote Learning

Instead of just teaching the client, the nurse tries actively to promote the client's ability to learn by, for example, identifying what is most important to the client and teaching that. Survival takes first priority; the nurse teaches the information people need to ensure their safety until the next visit. The nurse prioritizes material on a needs-to-know, wants-to-know, ought-to-know basis, assessing and responding to learner readiness.

Timing is important; people who are not ready to listen cannot be taught. In addition, the nurse must allow a sufficient amount of time to teach, ask clients how and when they learn best, use appropriate methods and materials when possible, and capitalize on clients' frustrations and desires to regain control of self-care. When possible, the nurse teaches while providing care.

The nurse can empower clients to learn by talking them through learning tasks, encouraging them to listen to their own bodies and to ask questions, and urging them to write thoughts and questions about their care and bring them to the next visit or doctor's appointment.

## Limit Distractions

Homes are full of events or circumstances that may divert attention from the job at hand. Such distractions as children, animals, noise, clutter, and mannerisms that are controlling, manipulative, or aggressive can try even the most experienced nurse. However, environmental and behavioral distractions can yield useful information about people, their relationships, and their values. For example, a dirty house could indicate a lack of interest in housekeeping, outright neglect and abuse, depression, or increased disability.

Distractions should be limited as much as possible. For example, the nurse might ask a client, "May I please turn off your television while we visit?" or "I would like to schedule my next visit for a time when the children are in school. Is that all right with you?" The nurse must be truthful about allergies, fear of a client's pet, or difficulty hearing in a particular room, but should not debate the priority of the visit over the distraction (such as a favorite television show). The nurse may not change the client's views and may also risk losing the client's trust and rapport. If all efforts at limiting distractions fail, the nurse should leave the home and return on another day: "I can see this is not going to work for us today. I will need to leave."

If any distraction originates with the nurse, such as fear of harm, reaction to the client's lifestyle, preoccupation with role or a feeling of being overwhelmed by the situation in the home, the nurse should seek out a colleague to discuss the problem. Often, another perspective helps when dealing with the issue.

## Put Safety First

Nurses must focus on safety and survival first, for themselves as well as their clients, in all that they do. When traveling in the community, the nurse takes such precautions as keeping car doors locked, having a cellular phone, keeping supplies out of sight, and staying inside the car in potentially dangerous situations. Colleagues, families, and community members can offer useful guidelines for maintaining safety and self-protection.

It is important to avoid overwhelming families with numerous health care providers in the home. Most people dislike having strangers in their home, no matter how helpful they may seem to be. The nurse can help families manage moments of crisis by staying as close as possible. If abuse is suspected, the nurse must notify authorities and/or remove clients from potentially dangerous situations.

| BOX 3-5 | ■ Home Safety Assessment Checklist |
| --- | --- |

**GENERAL HOUSEHOLD SAFETY**
1. Do stairwells and halls have good lighting?
2. Do staircases have handrails on both sides?
3. Are rugs securely tacked down?
4. Is the telephone readily accessible? Is the dial easy to read?
5. Are electrical cords in good condition and out of the way?
6. Is furniture sturdy?
7. Is the temperature of the home comfortable?
8. Are protective screens in front of fireplaces or heating devices?
9. Are smoke detectors present and working?

**BATHROOM**
1. Are grab bars present in the tub and/or shower? Around the toilet?
2. Are toilet seats high enough?
3. Are nonskid materials (rugs, mats) on the floor, tub/shower?
4. Are medications stored safely? Out of the reach of children?
5. Is the water temperature safe?
6. Are electrical outlets and appliances a safe distance from the tub?

**KITCHEN**
1. Are floors slippery? Are nonskid rugs used?
2. Is the stove in good working order?
3. Is the refrigerator in good working order? Clean?
4. Are electrical outlets overloaded with appliances?
5. Are sharp objects kept in a special container or safe area?
6. Is food storage adequate? Clean?
7. Are cleaning materials stored safely?

## Make Do

Nurses must learn to be resourceful and cost conscious with equipment, supplies, and services in the home. When needing to make do or improvise, they should do so in a low-key manner to avoid causing the family additional anxiety. The nurse must make every effort to convey the message that the situation is under control; after leaving the home, the nurse can react as necessary.

## Special Considerations in Home Care

### Ensuring Home Safety

Safety assessment in the home is a nursing responsibility and a legal requirement. Nurses cannot close their eyes to an unsafe environment. Upon entering the home and on a continuing basis, it is imperative that the nurse alert the family to unsafe and hazardous conditions, suggest remedies, and document in the clinical record the family's response to the nurse's suggestions. See Box 3–5 for a sample home safety assessment list. In particular, nurses must remain alert to:

- How clients handle stairs.
- How clients manage their own care if they are alone.
- The presence of a smoke detector in the home.
- The presence of bathroom safety equipment.
- Electrical hazards.
- Slippery throw rugs, clutter, or a furniture arrangement that may cause a fall.
- A supply of expired medications.
- Inappropriate clothing or shoes.
- Cooking habits that may precipitate a fire.
- An inadequate food supply.
- Poorly functioning utilities.
- Chipping paint.
- Signs of abusive behavior.

Nurses cannot go into homes and change the family's living space and lifestyle, but they can register their concern and re-act appropriately if the situation suggests that an injury is about to occur or if they suspect abuse or neglect. In the home and community setting, ignoring an unsafe environment is considered nursing negligence.

The disposal of toxic medications and sharp objects (such as needles used for injections) is also a safety issue in the home, especially if young children are present. Once again, it is imperative that the nurse address this with the client, demonstrate safe disposal, and provide the necessary equipment to accomplish that end. Documentation should address what information the nurse has covered, the family's response to the teaching, and assessment of the family's ongoing practice of safety precautions.

### Infection Control

Infection control in the home centers around protecting clients, caregivers, and the community from the spread of disease. Within the home, nurses may encounter clients with infectious or communicable diseases, clients who are immunocompromised, and/or clients having multiple access devices, drainage tubes, or draining wounds. The home presents a challenging environment in which to practice infection control for several reasons: Families typically are set in their own ways of doing things; caregivers often lack any formal education on the subject; the setting itself may not be conducive; and the facilities for even the most basic of aseptic practices (handwashing) may be lacking. Without a doubt, the single most important nursing intervention in controlling infection is health teaching. Clients and caregivers need to know the importance of effective handwashing, the use of gloves, the disposal of wastes and soiled dressings, the handling of linens, and the practice of standard precautions. Unfortunately, the imparting of important information does not always bring about a change in behavior. Trying to change a family's values frequently demands a great deal of ingenuity from the nurse.

## THE NURSING PROCESS IN HOME CARE

The nursing process used in home care is no different from that practiced in any other setting. The unique challenges of home care present themselves chiefly in the implementation step. Generally, the differences lie in assessing how the home's unique environment affects the need or problem and using outcome criteria and mutual participation to plan goals and interventions.

### Assessment

In home health care, nursing assessment and data collection center chiefly around the first home visit. This is not to say that nurses do not collect information on an ongoing basis, but because most agencies require the submission of a plan of care within 48 hours of the initial evaluation, the first visit carries tremendous weight. Under ideal circumstances, a preliminary review of background information initiates the assessment process; the reality in home health, however, is that few clients are referred with copies of either their medical records or their discharge summaries. If the client has received home health services in the past, records may be available, but often all the nurse has prior to initiating care is the referral form describing the present problem, some notations about past medical history, and a projection of the skilled interventions needed. Therefore, it falls to the nurse to try to obtain as complete a clinical picture as possible when meeting the client.

Assessment begins when the nurse calls the client to arrange a visit. This initial telephone call can yield much information to the nurse who pays close attention. For example:

- How alert, oriented, and stressed does the client (and/or family) seem to be?
- Does the client know the reason for the home health referral?
- How open to intervention do the client and family seem to be?
- Have they encountered any difficulties since discharge from the prior setting?
- Do they need any supplies on the first visit?

During the visit, much of the assessment process centers around collecting the information requested on the tools and forms contained in the agency's admission packet. These packets usually include a physical and psychosocial database; a medication sheet; forms for pain assessment, spiritual assessment, and financial assessment; and a family roster. It is extremely important that the data collected be as complete and accurate as possible and reflect subjective, objective, current, and historical information. Through interviewing, direct observation, and physical assessment, the nurse can achieve the goal of the initial visit, namely, to gain as clear and accurate a clinical picture of the client as possible.

### Diagnosis

After completing the initial assessment, the nurse identifies the real and/or potential client problems that emerge from the data. Nursing diagnoses describing the client's health problems and needs, based on data collection, must be part of the home health record both to organize care and to justify reimbursement.

In almost all home care situations, *deficient knowledge* is an appropriate nursing diagnosis. Nursing interventions for this diagnosis specific to a client with Alzheimer's disease and the client's family can be found in the Nursing Care of the Older Adult box on page 50.

### Planning

Planning in home health includes setting priorities, establishing goals, and deciding on intervention strategies designed to meet the needs of the client. The greatest level of success is achieved when clients feel an ownership of the suggested plan. For this reason, planned interventions and outcome criteria should be client centered, realistic, achievable, and mutually accepted. The nurse works with the client to:

- Identify significant issues and needs.
- Set mutually agreed-upon goals (outcome criteria).
- Make and initiate acceptable plans to meet the goals.

Outcome criteria should be verbally stated to clients and documented clearly and concisely, in timed, measurable, and observable terms. These measures help clients and care providers to better focus their work together and evaluate the effectiveness of care. In addition, outcome criteria provide the reimbursement source a measurable standard from which to judge the appropriateness of the plan of care.

### Implementation

The home health nurse implements most of the planned interventions, although some may be carried out by another agency provider, a paraprofessional introduced into the setting by the nurse case manager, or the client.

Nurses and clients reach an agreement about the implementation of care through a process called **contracting,** the negotiation of a cooperative working agreement between the nurse and client that is continuously renegotiated. Contracting is a concept used often in, but not exclusive to, many home and community health settings. Contracting can occur both formally and informally. It involves exploring a need, establishing goals, evaluating resources, developing a plan, assigning responsibilities, agreeing on a time frame, and, evaluating or terminating. Contracting requires the nurse to relinquish control as the expert and consider the client as an equal partner in the process.

Contracting is not appropriate with all clients. It is certainly inadvisable if the nurse-client relationship is to be no more than two visits or if the client has limited cognitive abilities. However, contracting is useful for clients who demonstrate a willingness to be active participants in their health care. It is empowering, can save time, and keeps the nursing goals directed and focused. Box 3–6 provides an example of verbal contracting.

MediaLink | HOME HEALTH CARE PLAN

## Nursing Care of the Older Adult

## HOME CARE BY FAMILY CAREGIVERS FOR THE OLDER ADULT WITH A DEMENTING DISORDER

### NURSING DIAGNOSIS

*Deficient knowledge* related to lack of information about Alzheimer's disease process and care

### OUTCOME CRITERIA

Short term: Adequate knowledge, as evidenced by family's stating of disease progression and treatment (expected within 1 week)

Long term: Adequate knowledge, as evidenced by family's following of the recommended interventions throughout illness course (within 1 month) or by discharge from home health

### INTERVENTIONS

- Alert the family to both environmental hazards and client habits that could threaten safety. (first visit)
- Provide the family with specific recommendations for keeping the client safe, for example, serving foods warm, not hot; allowing the client to eat with fingers; cutting food in small pieces; wearing an ID bracelet; discouraging daytime sleep. (first visit)
- Discuss the disease course (degenerative), the prognosis (incurable), typical issues of concern (promoting adequate nutrition, activity, rest, safety, and independence); supporting cognitive function; communication, socialization, and family caregiving; the supportive care available; and the ultimate need for long-term placement with disease progression. (first visit)
- Discuss local resources, including adult day care, support groups, and Alzheimer's Disease Association. Give family a list of these resources. (first visit)

- Include all family members or significant persons in teaching and planning care. (each visit)
- Prepare the family for typical types of Alzheimer's disease behaviors: forgetfulness, disorientation, agitation, screaming, crying, physical or verbal abuse, accusations of infidelity. (subsequent visits)
- Teach the family specific interventions for dealing with these behaviors: calm, unhurried manner, music, stroking, rocking, structuring the environment, distracting the client. (subsequent visits)
- Stress the importance of both exercise and recreation in terms of quality of life and decreasing nighttime restlessness. (subsequent visits)
- Reinforce the client's continued needs for socialization and intimacy. (subsequent visits)
- Suggest specific interventions for meeting socialization needs: limiting visitors to one or two at a time, pet therapy, use of the phone. (subsequent visits)
- Suggest useful interventions that are described in the literature and/or that are utilized in more formal Alzheimer's disease settings and may also be helpful in the home. (subsequent visits)
- Keep the environment safe for the client.
- Use reality orientation with client several times a day, and post clocks, calendars, and telephone numbers within easy sight of the client.
- Give client simple directions, using simple sentences and a quiet, monotone voice so as not to excite the client.
- Allow the use of the telephone, because calls will help orient the client.

## BOX 3-6   ■ Contracting

*Nurse:*  Mr. Ford, your mother is no longer safe alone in her home and requires help performing many of her activities of daily living. I can initiate home health aide services three times a week for 2 hours a day under Medicare, but she will need more assistance than that. Services beyond what Medicare provides must be contracted for by you on a private-pay basis.

*Mr. Ford:*  Can you arrange that for us?

*Nurse:*  I can give you a list of agencies here in the community that provide home health aide services, and I can recommend the ones that our clients have used successfully in the past, but the responsibility for choosing a service and negotiating hours and fees belongs to the family.

*Mr. Ford:*  I really don't know much about this. I'd really feel better if you did this for us.

*Nurse:*  Why don't the two of us discuss your mother's needs so that you'll have a clearer understanding of what type of help you

want to try to arrange. I can tell you about the local agencies we frequently refer our clients to, and I can give you suggestions about what questions to ask. We can also discuss the typical costs involved. This way, when you call to make inquiries, you'll be equipped with the right information.

*Mr. Ford:*  I still would rather you do this.

*Nurse:*  Mr. Ford, this is something the family must do. What I will do is teach whomever you hire what they will need to know about caring for your mother. Can we agree that by my next visit, you will have made some inquiries and will be ready to discuss what agency will best meet your family's situation?

*Mr. Ford:*  All right. I'll start making some calls. Give me 2 or 3 days.

*Nurse:*  Fine, then I'll plan for a longer visit Thursday so we can discuss what you find out.

## Evaluation

Evaluation in home health is both formative and summative. Formative evaluation is the systematic ongoing comparison of the plan of care with the goals actually being achieved from visit to visit. In summative evaluation, the nurse reviews the total plan of care and the client's progress toward goals to determine the client's eligibility for discharge.

Reimbursement guidelines may be helpful in driving the evaluation process. Because reimbursement sources require that all skilled services be justified, many home health agencies have designed their clinical notes to include areas for evaluation of the client's response to the visit's interventions and documentation of a plan of care for the next scheduled visit.

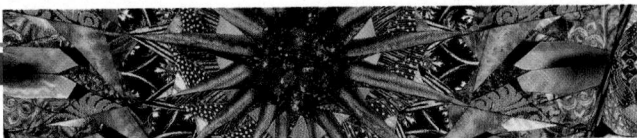

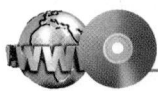

## EXPLORE MediaLink

NCLEX review questions, case studies, care plan activities, MediaLink applications, and other interactive resources for this chapter can be found on the Companion Website at www.prenhall.com/lemone.

Click on Chapter 3 to select the activities for this chapter. For animations, video clips, more NCLEX review questions, and an audio glossary, access the Student CD-ROM accompanying this textbook.

## TEST YOURSELF

1. What is the name given to nursing care provided by a faith community to promote health and healing?

   a. Respite care
   b. Parish nursing
   c. Block nursing
   d. Day care

2. While making the first home health visit, the nurse discusses advanced directives, living wills, and durable power of attorney for health care. These topics are part of which nursing role?

   a. Provider of direct care
   b. Coordinator of services
   c. Educator
   d. Advocate

3. Which of the following home health agency personnel is responsible for care coordination?

   a. Physician
   b. Social worker
   c. Registered nurse
   d. Home health aide

4. What agency is the largest single reimbursement source for home care?

   a. Medicare
   b. Medicaid
   c. Private insurance
   d. Self-pay

5. Nurses practicing in the home provide teaching for a variety of topics. Which of the following areas is essential to maintaining infection control?

   a. Fire and smoke detectors
   b. Handwashing
   c. Uncluttered floors and stairs
   d. Medications

See Test Yourself answers in Appendix C.

## BIBLIOGRAPHY

American Association of Retired People. (2000). Caregiving and long-term care. Available www.research.aarp.org

American Nurses Association. (1986). *Standards of home health nursing practice.* Kansas City, MO: Author.

_____. (2000). Reading room: Position statements. Available www.nursingworld.org

Boland, D., & Sims, S. (1996). Family care giving at home. *Image: Journal of Nursing Scholarship, 28*(1), 55–58.

Capone, L. (1997). Client challenge: Home care—a family affair. *Home Healthcare Nurse, 15*(1), 49–51.

Carson, V. (1989). *Spiritual dimensions of nursing practice.* Philadelphia: Saunders.

Chafey, K. (1996). "Caring" is not enough: Ethical paradigms for community-based care. *N & HC: Perspectives on Community, 17*(1), 10–15.

Clemen-Stone, S., McGuire, S., & Eigsti, D. (1998). *Comprehensive community health nursing* (5th ed.). St. Louis: Mosby.

Costello, M., & Todd-Magel, C. (1997). Bridging the gap: Hospital to home nutrition support. *MEDSURG Nursing, 6*(6), 328–337.

DeSavorgnani, A., & Haring, R. (1999). The impact of cultural issues on home care personnel and patients. *Caring, 18*(4), 22–27.

Grossman, D. (1996). Cultural dimensions in home health nursing. *American Journal of Nursing, 96*(7), 33–36.

Health Care Financing Administration. (1997). *Managed care in Medicare and Medicaid. Fact sheet.* Washington, DC: USDHHS.

_____ . (2001). *Medicare and home health care.* Washington, DC: USDHHS.

_____ . (2001). *Medicare & You 2001.* Washington, DC: USDHHS.

Jones, A., & Foster, N. (1997). Transitional care: Bridging the gap. *MEDSURG Nursing, 6*(1), 32–38.

National Association for Home Care. (2000). How to choose a home care provider. What are my rights as a patient? Available www.nahc.org

Paladichuk, A., & McNeal, G. (1997). Breaking down the walls: Critical care at home and on the road. *Critical Care Nurse, 17*(2), 94–99.

Rice, R. (2000). Home health care. Resources for home care nurses. *Geriatric Nursing, 21*(5), 276–279.

Roush, C., & Cox, J. (2000). The meaning of home. How it shapes the practice of home and hospice care. *Home Healthcare Nurse, 18*(6), 388–394.

Schoen, M., & Koenig, R. (1997). Home health care nursing: Past and present—part 1. *MEDSURG Nursing, 6*(4), 230–232.

Schumacher, K., Stewart, B., & Archbold, P. (1998). Conceptualization and measurement of doing family caregiving well. *Image: Journal of Nursing Scholarship, 30*(1), 63–69.

Shoultz, J., & Hatcher, P. (1997). Looking beyond primary care to primary health care: An approach to community-based action. *Nursing Outlook, 45*(1), 23–26.

Stulginsky, M. (1993a). Nurses' home health experience: Part I—The practice setting. *Nursing & Health Care, 14*(8), 402–407.

_____ . (1993b). Nurses' home health experience: Part II—The unique demands of home visits. *Nursing & Health Care, 14*(9), 476–485.

Swavely, D., Peter, D., & Stephens, D. (1999). Improving smooth sailing between hospital and home. *MEDSURG Nursing, 8*(5), 304–308.

Watson, J. (2000). Home health care. Reconsidering caring in the home. *Geriatric Nursing, 21*(6), 330–331.

Zotti, M., Brown, P., & Stotts, R. (1996). Community-based nursing versus community health nursing: What does it all mean? *Nursing Outlook, 44*(5), 211–217.

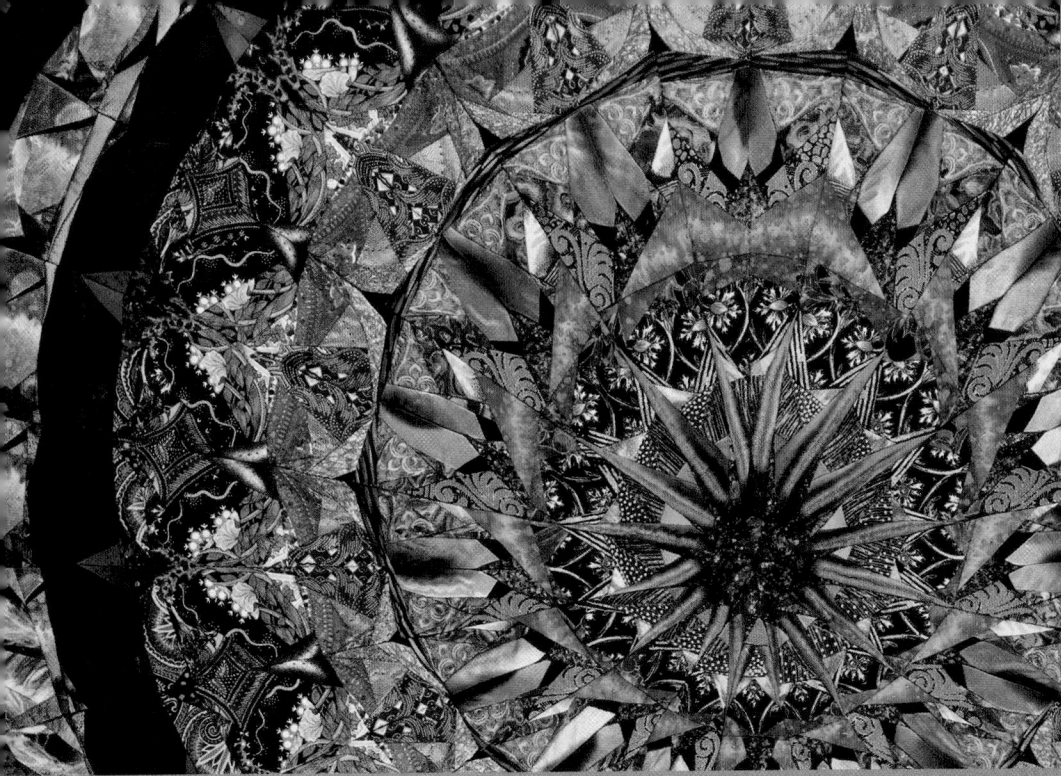

# ALTERATIONS IN PATTERNS OF HEALTH

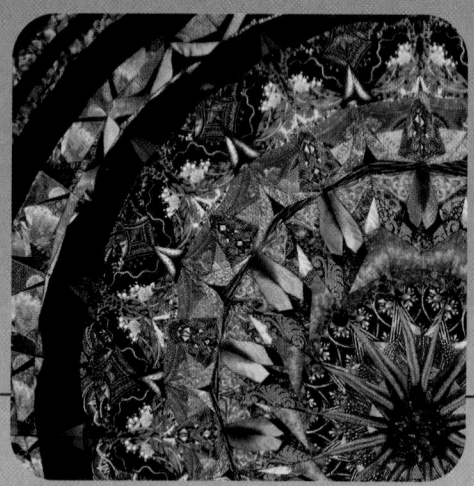

# Nursing Care of Clients in Pain

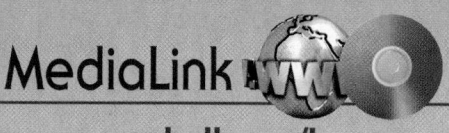

## MediaLink

**www.prenhall.com/lemone**
Additional resources for this chapter can be found on the Student CD-ROM accompanying this textbook, and on the Companion Website at www. prenhall.com/lemone. Click on Chapter 4 to select the activities for this chapter.

**CD-ROM**
• Audio Glossary
• NCLEX Review

*Animations*
• Components of a Reflex Arc
• Morphine

**Companion Website**
• More NCLEX Review
• Case Study
    Assessing the Client in Pain
• Care Plan Activity
    Nursing Care for the Client in Pain
• MediaLink Application
    Complementary Therapies

## LEARNING OUTCOMES

After completing this chapter, you will be able to:

▪ Describe the neurophysiology of pain.

▪ Compare and contrast definitions and characteristics of acute, chronic, central, phantom, and psychogenic pain.

▪ Discuss factors affecting individualized responses to pain.

▪ Clarify myths and misconceptions about pain.

▪ Discuss collaborative care for the client in pain, including medications, surgery, and transcutaneous electrical nerve stimulation, and complementary therapies.

▪ Use the nursing process as a framework for providing individualized nursing care for clients experiencing pain.

**Pain** is a subjective response to both physical and psychologic stressors. All people experience pain at some point during their lives. Although pain usually is experienced as uncomfortable and unwelcome, it also serves a protective role, warning of potentially health-threatening conditions. For this reason, pain is increasingly referred to as the *fifth* vital sign, with recommendations to assess pain with each vital sign assessment. The JCAHO (2000) has established pain standards that identify the relief of pain as a client right and requires health care facilities to implement specific procedures for, and provider education on, pain assessment and management.

Each individual pain event is a distinct and personal experience influenced by physiologic, psychologic, cognitive, sociocultural, and spiritual factors. Pain is the symptom most associated with describing oneself as ill, and it is the most common reason for seeking health care. Among the many definitions and descriptors of pain is the one most relevant: Pain is "whatever the person experiencing it says it is, and existing whenever the person says it does" (McCaffery, 1979, p. 11). This definition acknowledges the client as the only person who can accurately define and describe his or her own pain and serves as the basis for nursing assessment and care of clients in pain. It also supports the values and beliefs about pain necessary for holistic nursing care, including the following:

- Only the person affected can experience pain; that is, pain has a personal meaning.
- If the client says he or she has pain, the client is in pain. All pain is real.
- Pain has physical, emotional, cognitive, sociocultural, and spiritual dimensions.
- Pain affects the whole body, usually negatively.
- Pain may serve as both a response to and a warning of actual or potential trauma.

## THEORIES AND NEUROPHYSIOLOGY OF PAIN

One well-known theory, gate control, suggests that the interaction of two systems determines pain and its perception (Melzack & Wall, 1965, 1968). The first of these interrelated systems is the substantia gelatinosa in the dorsal horns of the spinal cord (Figure 4–1 ■). The substantia gelatinosa regulates impulses entering or leaving the spinal cord. The second system is an inhibitory system within the brainstem.

Small-diameter A-delta and C fibers in the spinal cord carry fast and slow pain impulses. In addition, large-diameter A-beta fibers carry impulses for tactile stimulation from the skin. In the substantia gelatinosa, these impulses encounter a "gate" that is thought to be opened and closed by the domination of either the large-diameter touch fibers or the small-diameter pain fibers. If impulses along the small-diameter pain fibers outnumber impulses along the large-diameter touch fibers, then the gate is open and pain impulses travel unimpeded to the brain. If impulses from the touch fibers predominate, then they will close the gate and the pain impulses will be turned away there. This explains why massaging a stubbed toe can reduce the intensity and duration of the pain.

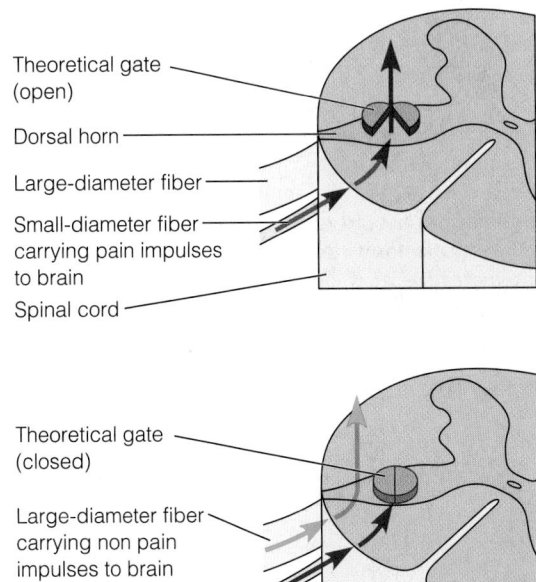

**Figure 4–1 ■** The spinal cord component of the gate control theory. Pain transmission by small-diameter fibers is blocked when large-diameter fibers carrying touch impulses dominate, closing the gate in the substantia gelatinosa.

The second system described by the gate control theory, the inhibitory system, is thought to be located in the brainstem. It is believed that cells in the midbrain, activated by a variety of stimuli such as opiates, psychologic factors, or even simply the presence of pain itself, signal receptors in the medulla. These receptors in turn stimulate nerve fibers in the spinal cord to block the transmission of impulses from pain fibers.

Ongoing research has demonstrated that the control and modulation of pain is much more complex than the description in the gate control theory, which served as a base for further research about pain-modulating systems. Tactile information is now known to be transmitted by both large-diameter and small-diameter fibers, and interactions between sensory neurons is known to occur at multiple levels of the central nervous system (Porth, 2002).

### Stimuli

Nerve receptors for pain are called *nociceptors* (Figure 4–2 ■). They are located at the ends of small afferent neurons and are woven throughout all the tissues of the body except the brain. Nociceptors are especially numerous in the skin and muscles. Pain occurs when biologic, mechanical, thermal, electrical, or chemical factors stimulate nociceptors (Table 4–1). The intensity and duration of the stimuli determine the sensation. Long-lasting, intense stimulation produces greater pain than brief, mild stimulation.

Nociceptors are stimulated either by direct damage to the cell or by the local release of biochemicals secondary to cell injury. *Bradykinin,* an amino acid, appears to be the most

**Figure 4–2** ■ *A,* Cutaneous nociceptors generate pain impulses that travel via A-delta and C fibers to the spinal cord's dorsal horn. *B,* Secondary neurons in dorsal horn pass impulses across spinal cord to anterior spinothalamic tract. *C,* Slow pain impulses ascend to the thalamus, while fast pain impulses ascend to the cerebral cortex. The reticular formation in the brainstem integrates the emotional, cognitive, and autonomic responses to pain.

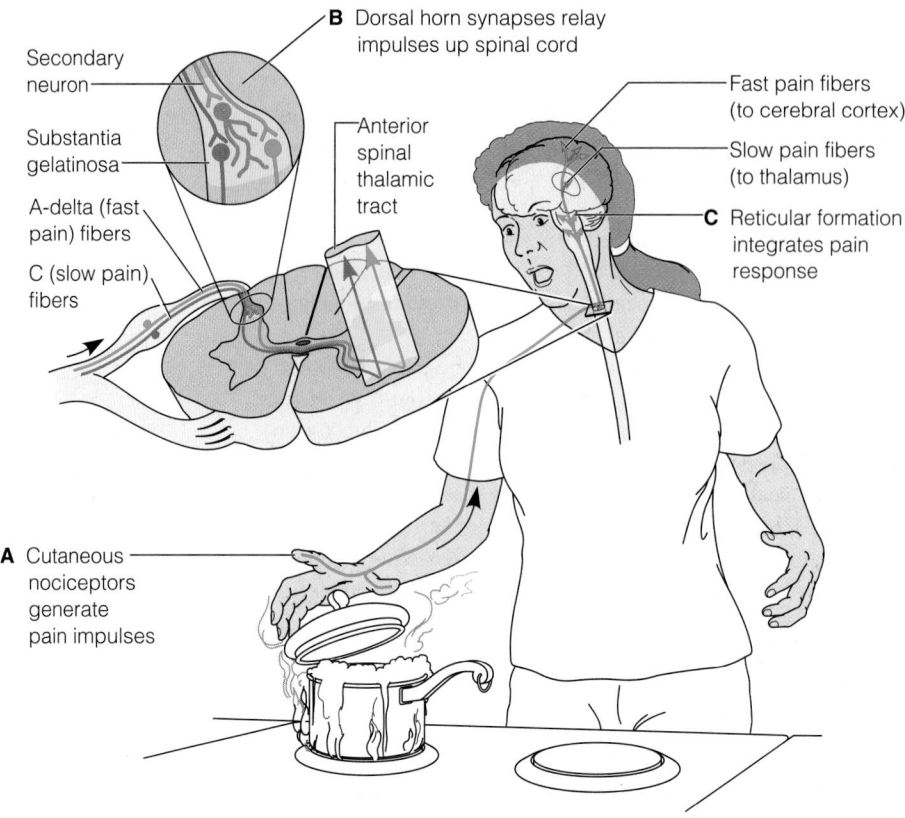

| TABLE 4–1 | Pain Stimuli |
|---|---|
| **Causative Factor** | **Example** |
| Microorganisms (e.g., bacteria, viruses) | Meningitis |
| Inflammation | Sore throat |
| Impaired blood flow | Angina |
| Invasive tumor | Colon cancer |
| Radiation | Radiation for cancer |
| Heat | Sunburn |
| Obstruction | Kidney stone |
| Spasm | Colon cramping |
| Compression | Carpal tunnel syndrome |
| Decreased movement | Pain after cast removal |
| Stretching or straining | Sprained ankle |
| Fractures | Fractured hip |
| Swelling | Arthritis |
| Deposits of foreign tissue | Endometriosis |
| Chemicals | Skin rash |
| Electricity | Electrical burn |
| Conflict, difficulty in life | Psychogenic pain |

abundant and potent pain-producing chemical; other biochemical sources of pain include prostaglandins, histamine, hydrogen ions, and potassium ions. These biochemicals are thought to bind to nociceptors in response to noxious stimuli, causing the nociceptors to initiate pain impulses.

## Pain Pathway

The neural pathway of pain illustrated in Figure 4–2 is summarized as follows:

1. Pain is perceived by the nociceptors in the periphery of the body (e.g., in the skin or viscera). Cutaneous pain is transmitted through small afferent A-delta and even smaller C nerve fibers to the spinal cord. A-delta fibers are myelinated and transmit impulses rapidly. They produce sharp, well-defined pain sensations, such as those that result from cuts, electric shocks, or the impact of a blow. A-delta fibers are associated with acute pain. C fibers are not myelinated and thus transmit pain impulses more slowly. The pain from deep body structures (such as muscles and viscera) is primarily transmitted by C fibers, producing diffuse burning or aching sensations. C fibers are associated with chronic pain. Both A-delta and C fibers are involved in most injuries. For example, if a person bangs the elbow, A-delta fibers transmit this pain stimulus within 0.1 second. The person feels this pain as a sharp, localized, smarting sensation. One or more seconds after the blow, the person experiences a duller, aching, diffuse sensation of pain impulses carried by the C fibers.

2. Secondary neurons transmit the impulses from the afferent neurons through the dorsal horn of the spinal cord, where they synapse in the substantia gelatinosa. The impulses then cross over to the anterior and lateral spinothalamic tracts.

3. The impulses ascend the anterior and lateral spinothalamic tracts and pass through the medulla and midbrain to the thalamus.

4. In the thalamus and cerebral cortex, the pain impulses are perceived, described, localized, and interpreted, and a response is formulated. A noxious impulse becomes pain when the sensation reaches conscious levels and is perceived and evaluated by the person experiencing the sensation.

Some pain impulses ascend along the paleospinothalamic tract in the medial section of the spinal cord. These impulses enter the reticular formation and the limbic systems, which integrate emotional and cognitive responses to pain. Interconnections in the autonomic nervous system may also cause an autonomic response to the pain. In addition, deep nociceptors often converge on the same spinal neuron, resulting in pain that is experienced in a part of the body other than its origin.

## Inhibitory Mechanisms

Efferent fibers run from the reticular formation and midbrain to the substantia gelatinosa in the dorsal horns of the spinal cord. Along these fibers, pain may be inhibited or modulated. The analgesia system is a group of midbrain neurons that transmits impulses to the pons and medulla, which in turn stimulate a pain inhibitory center in the dorsal horns of the spinal cord. The exact nature of this inhibitory mechanism is unknown.

The most clearly defined chemical inhibitory mechanism is fueled by *endorphins* (endogenous morphines), which are naturally occurring opioid peptides present in neurons in the brain, spinal cord, and gastrointestinal tract. Endorphins in the brain are released in response to afferent noxious stimuli, whereas endorphins in the spinal cord are released in response to efferent impulses. Endorphins work by binding with opiate receptors on the neurons to inhibit pain impulse transmission (Figure 4–3 ■).

## TYPES AND CHARACTERISTICS OF PAIN
## Acute Pain

**Acute pain** has a sudden onset, is usually temporary, and is localized. Pain that lasts for less than 6 months and has an identified cause is classified as acute pain. The sudden onset usually results from tissue injury from trauma, surgery, or inflammation. The pain is usually sharp and localized, although it may radiate. The three major types of acute pain are:

- **Somatic pain,** which arises from nerve receptors originating in the skin or close to the surface of the body. Somatic pain may be either sharp and well localized or dull and diffuse. It is often accompanied by nausea and vomiting.
- **Visceral pain,** which arises from body organs. Visceral pain is dull and poorly localized because of the low number of nociceptors. The viscera are sensitive to stretching, inflammation, and ischemia but relatively insensitive to cutting and

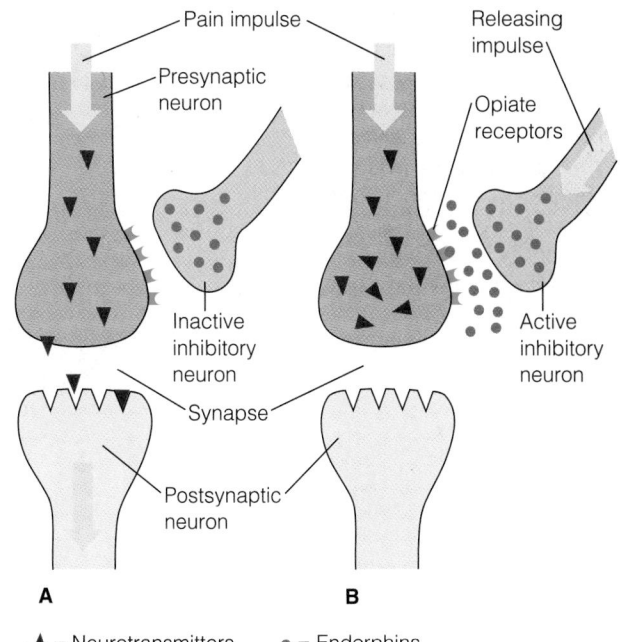

▲ = Neurotransmitters    ● = Endorphins

**Figure 4–3 ■** *A,* Pain impulse causes presynaptic neuron to release burst of neurotransmitters across synapse. These bind to postsynaptic neuron and propagate impulse. *B,* Inhibitory neuron releases endorphins, which bind to presynaptic opiate receptors. Neurotransmitter release is inhibited; pain impulse is interrupted.

temperature extremes. Visceral pain is associated with nausea and vomiting, hypotension, and restlessness. It often radiates or is referred.

- **Referred pain,** which is perceived in an area distant from the site of the stimuli. It commonly occurs with visceral pain, as visceral fibers synapse at the level of the spinal cord, close to fibers innervating other subcutaneous tissue areas of the body (Figure 4–4 ■). Pain in a spinal nerve may be felt over the skin in any body area innervated by sensory neurons that share that same spinal nerve route. Body areas defined by spinal nerve routes are called dermatomes (see Chapter 40). ⊚⊃

Acute pain warns of actual or potential injury to tissues. As a stressor, it initiates the fight-or-flight autonomic stress response. Characteristic physical responses include tachycardia, rapid and shallow respirations, increased blood pressure, dilated pupils, sweating, and pallor. The person experiencing the pain responds to this threat with anxiety and fear. This psychologic response may further increase the physical responses to acute pain.

## Chronic Pain

**Chronic pain** is prolonged pain, usually lasting longer than 6 months. It is not always associated with an identifiable cause and is often unresponsive to conventional medical treatment. Chronic pain is often described as dull, aching, and diffuse. Unlike acute pain, chronic pain has a much more complex and poorly understood purpose.

MediaLink | REFLEX ARC ANIMATION

**Figure 4–4** ■ Referred pain is the result of the convergence of sensory nerves from certain areas of the body before they enter the brain for interpretation. For example, a toothache may be felt in the ear, pain from inflammation of the diaphragm may be felt in the shoulder, and pain from ischemia of the heart muscle (angina) may be felt in the left arm.

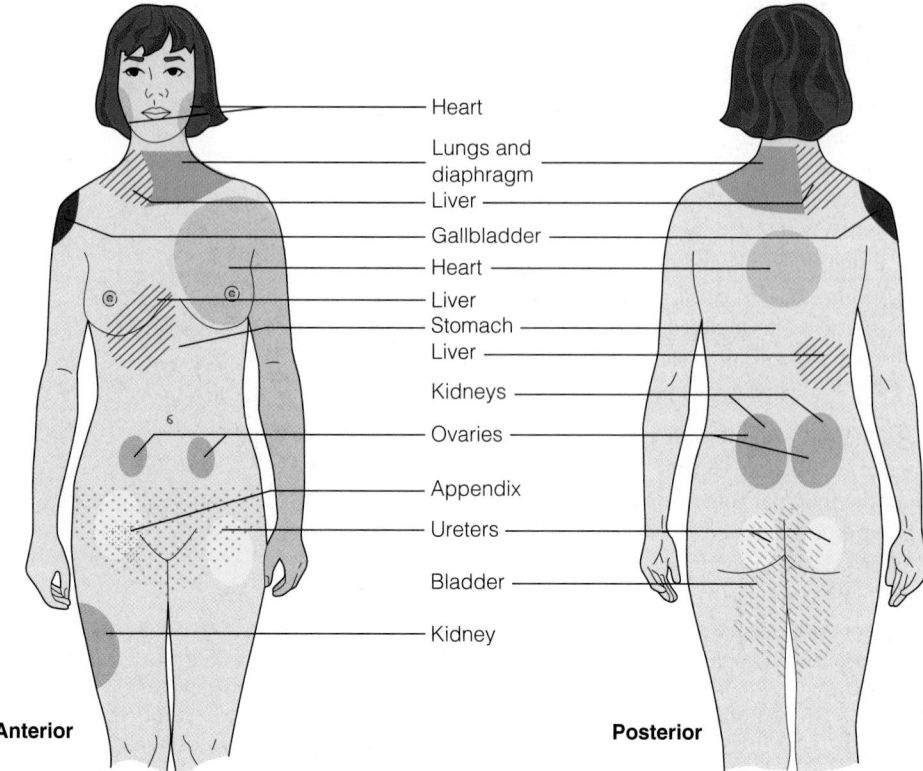

Heart
Lungs and diaphragm
Liver
Gallbladder
Heart
Liver
Stomach
Liver
Kidneys
Ovaries
Appendix
Ureters
Bladder
Kidney

**Anterior**                                      **Posterior**

Chronic pain can be subdivided into four categories:

- *Recurrent acute pain* is characterized by relatively well-defined episodes of pain interspersed with pain-free episodes. Examples of recurrent acute pain include migraine headaches and sickle cell crises.
- *Ongoing time-limited pain* is identified by a defined time period. Some examples are cancer pain, which ends with control of the disease or death, and burn pain, which ends with rehabilitation or death.
- *Chronic nonmalignant pain* is non-life-threatening pain that nevertheless persists beyond the expected time for healing. Chronic lower back pain falls into this category.
- *Chronic intractable nonmalignant pain syndrome* is similar to simple chronic nonmalignant pain, but is characterized by the person's inability to cope well with the pain and sometimes by physical, social, and/or psychologic disability resulting from the pain.

The client with chronic pain often is depressed, withdrawn, immobile, irritable, and/or controlling. Although chronic pain may range from mild to severe and may be continuous or intermittent, the unrelenting presence of the pain often results in the pain itself becoming the pathologic process requiring intervention. The most common chronic pain condition is lower back pain. Other common chronic pain conditions include the following (McCance & Huether, 2002):

- *Neuralgias* are painful conditions that result from damage to a peripheral nerve caused by infection or disease. Postherpetic neuralgia (following shingles) is an example.
- Reflex sympathetic *dystrophies* are characterized by continuous severe, burning pain. These conditions follow peripheral nerve damage and present the symptoms of pain, vasospasm, muscle wasting, and vasomotor changes (vasodilation followed by vasoconstriction).
- *Hyperesthesias* are conditions of oversensitivity to tactile and painful stimuli. Hyperesthesias result in diffuse pain that is usually increased by fatigue and emotional lability.
- Myofascial pain syndrome is a common condition marked by injury to or disease of muscle and fascial tissue. Pain results from muscle spasm, stiffness, and collection of lactic acid in the muscle. Fibromyalgia is an example.
- Cancer often produces chronic pain, usually due to factors associated with the advancing disease. These factors include a growing tumor that presses on nerves or other structures, stretching of viscera, obstruction of ducts, or metastasis to bones. The malignant tumor also may mechanically stimulate pain or the production of biochemicals that cause pain. Pain also may be associated with chemotherapy and radiation therapy.
- Chronic postoperative pain is rare but may occur following incisions in the chest wall, radical mastectomy, radical neck dissection, and surgical amputation.

## Central Pain

**Central pain** is related to a lesion in the brain that may spontaneously produce high-frequency bursts of impulses that are perceived as pain. A vascular lesion, tumor, trauma, or inflammation may cause central pain. Thalamic pain, one of the most common types, is severe, spontaneous, and often continuous. Hyperesthesia (an abnormal sensitivity to touch, pain, or other sensory stimuli) may occur on the side of the body opposite to the lesion in the thalamus. The perception of body position and movement may also be lost.

## Phantom Pain

**Phantom pain** is a syndrome that occurs following amputation of a body part. The client experiences pain in the missing body part even though he or she is completely mentally aware that it is gone. This pain may include itching, tingling, or pressure sensations, or it may be more severe, including burning or stabbing sensations. In some cases, the client may describe a sensation that an amputated limb is twisted or cramped. It is thought that this type of pain may be due to stimulation of the severed nerves at the site of the amputation. Treatment is complex and often unsuccessful.

## Psychogenic Pain

**Psychogenic pain** is experienced in the absence of any diagnosed physiologic cause or event. Typically psychogenic pain involves a long history of severe pain. It is thought that the client's emotional needs prompt the pain sensations. Psychogenic pain is real, and may in turn lead to physiologic changes, such as muscle tension, which may produce further pain. This condition may result from interpersonal conflicts, a need for support from others, or a desire to avoid a stressful or traumatic situation. Depression is often present.

## FACTORS AFFECTING RESPONSES TO PAIN

Physical response to pain involves specific and often predictable neurologic changes. In fact, everyone has the same pain threshold and perceives pain stimuli at the same stimulus intensity. For example, heat is perceived as painful at 44° to 46° C, the range at which it begins to damage tissue. What varies is the person's perception of and reaction to pain. The individualized response to pain is shaped by multiple and interacting factors including age, sociocultural influences, emotional state, past experiences with pain, source and meaning of the pain, and knowledge base.

When describing a person as being highly sensitive to pain, one is referring to the person's **pain tolerance,** which is the amount of pain a person can endure before outwardly responding to it. The ability to tolerate pain may be decreased by repeated episodes of pain, fatigue, anger, anxiety, and sleep deprivation. Medications, alcohol, hypnosis, warmth, distraction, and spiritual practices may increase pain tolerance.

## Age

Age influences a person's perception and expression of pain. The older adult with normal age-related changes in neurophysiology may have decreased perception of sensory stimuli and a higher pain tolerance. In addition, chronic disease processes more common in the older adult, such as peripheral vascular disease or diabetes, may interfere with normal nerve impulse transmission. Individuals in this age group may have atypical responses to pain: decreased perception of acute pain, heightened perceptions of chronic pain, and/or increased incidence of referred pain.

Often believing that pain is a part of growing older, the client may ignore pain or self-medicate with over-the-counter medications. As a result of these behaviors, the older adult is at increased risk of injury or serious illness. Table 4–2 lists age-related changes and their effects on pain.

## Sociocultural Influences

Each person's response to pain is strongly influenced by the family, community, and culture. Sociocultural influences affect the way in which a person tolerates pain, interprets the meaning of pain, and reacts verbally and nonverbally to the pain. For example, if the client's family believes that males should not cry and must tolerate pain stoically, then the male client often will appear withdrawn and refuse pain medication. If a family encourages open and intense emotional expression, then the client may cry freely and appear comfortable requesting pain medication.

Cultural standards also teach an individual how much pain to tolerate, what types of pain to report, to whom to report the pain, and what kind of treatment to seek. For example, clients of northern European ancestry may value "being a good patient," which may cause them to avoid "complaining" about their pain, whereas clients of Jewish ancestry may value seeking information about their pain, which may cause them to discuss their pain often and in detail. Note, however, that behaviors vary greatly within a culture and from generation to generation. The nurse should approach each client as an individual, observing the client carefully, taking the time to ask questions, and avoiding assumptions.

| TABLE 4–2 | Nursing Care of the Older Adult: Age-Related Changes and Their Effects on Pain | |
|---|---|---|
| **Factors Related to Aging** | **Effects** | **Outcomes** |
| Decreased blood flow | Ischemia, decreases in brain function | Client forgets to take medication |
| Changes in neurotransmitters related to sleep and mood | Decreased sleep resulting in vulnerability to pain | Greater risk of chronic pain, fatigue, increased withdrawal |
| Reduced levels of norepinephrine | Lowered transmission of pain | Less likely to notice an injury |
| Changes in sensory interpretation | Lowered pain sensation | Client may not take appropriate protective action |
| Decreased peripheral nerve conduction | Lowered response to pain | Not seeking appropriate care |
| Slowed reaction time | Slower avoidance response | Client receives more serious injury |
| Reduced movement | Increased risk for muscle wasting | May cause immobility |

The nurse also has a set of sociocultural values and beliefs about pain. If these values and beliefs differ from those of the client, the assessment and management of pain may be based on the values of the nurse rather than on the needs of the client. The nurse must be familiar with ethnic and cultural diversity in pain expression and management and respect cultural differences. It is particularly important to remember that pain behaviors are not an objective indicator of the amount of pain present for any individual client. Finally, most experts agree that cultural differences in the expression of, response to, and interpretation of the meaning of pain need further research.

## Emotional Status

Emotional status influences the pain perception. The sensation of pain may be blocked by intense concentration (e.g., during sports activities) or may be increased by anxiety or fear. Pain often is increased when it occurs in conjunction with other illnesses or physical discomforts such as nausea or vomiting. The presence or absence of support people or caregivers that genuinely care about pain management also may alter emotional status and the perception of pain.

Anxiety may increase the perception of pain, and pain in turn may cause anxiety. In addition, the muscle tension common with anxiety can create its own source of pain. This association explains why nonpharmacologic interventions such as relaxation or guided imagery are helpful in relieving or decreasing pain.

Fatigue, lack of sleep, and depression also are related to pain experiences. Pain interferes with a person's ability to fall asleep and stay asleep and thus induces fatigue. In turn, fatigue can lower pain tolerance. Depression is clearly linked to pain: Serotonin, a neurotransmitter, is involved in the modulation of pain in the central nervous system (CNS). In clinically depressed people, serotonin is decreased, leading to an increase in pain sensations. The reverse is also true: In the presence of pain, depression is common.

## Past Experiences with Pain

Previous experiences with pain are likely to influence the person's response to a current pain episode. If supportive adults responded to childhood experiences with pain appropriately, the adult usually will have a healthy attitude to pain. If, however, the person's pain was responded to with exaggerated emotions or neglectful indifference, that person's future responses to pain may be exaggerated or denied.

The responses of health care providers to the person in pain can influence the person's response during the next pain episode. If providers respond to pain with effective strategies and a caring attitude, the client will remain more comfortable during any subsequent pain episode, and anxiety will be avoided. If, however, the pain is not adequately relieved, or if the client feels that empathetic care was not given, anxiety about the next pain episode sets up the client for a more complex and therefore more painful event.

## Source and Meaning

The meaning associated with the pain influences the experience of pain. For example, the pain of labor to deliver a baby is experienced differently from the pain following removal of a major organ for cancer. Because pain is the major signal for health problems, it is strongly linked to all associated meanings of health problems, such as disability, loss of role, and death. For this reason, it is important to explain to clients the etiology and prognosis for the pain assessed.

If the client perceives the pain as deserved (e.g., "just punishment for sins"), then the client may actually feel relief that the "punishment" has commenced. If the client believes that the pain will relieve him or her from an unrewarding job, dangerous military service, or even stressful social obligations, there may similarly be a feeling of relief. In contrast, pain that is perceived as meaningless (e.g., chronic low back pain or the unrelieved pain of arthritis) can cause anxiety and depression.

## Knowledge

A lack of understanding of the source, outcome, and meaning of the pain can contribute negatively to the pain experience. It is important to assess the client's readiness to learn, use methods of teaching that are effective for the client and family, and evaluate learning carefully. Teaching must include the process of the pain, its predictable course (if possible), and the proposed plan of care. In addition, encourage clients to communicate preferences for pain relief. Learning how to let significant others know of the presence of pain and how to use their help can also promote effective pain management.

## MYTHS AND MISCONCEPTIONS ABOUT PAIN

Myths and misconceptions about pain and its management are common in both health care providers and clients. Following are some of the most common of these myths.

*Myth 1: Pain is a result, not a cause.* According to the traditional view, pain is only a symptom of a condition. However, it is now recognized that unrelieved or poorly relieved pain itself sets up further responses, such as immobility, anger, and anxiety; pain may also delay healing and rehabilitation.

*Myth 2: Chronic pain is really a masked form of depression.* Serotonin plays a chemical role in pain transmission and is also the major modulator of depression. Therefore, pain and depression are chemically related, not mutually exclusive. It is common to find them coexisting.

*Myth 3: Narcotic medication is too risky to be used in chronic pain.* This common misconception often deprives clients of the most effective source of pain relief. It is true that other methods should be tried first; if, however, they prove ineffective, narcotics should be considered as an appropriate alternative.

*Myth 4: It is best to wait until a client has pain before giving medication.* It is now widely accepted that anticipating pain has a noticeable effect on the amount of pain a client experiences. Offering pain relief before a pain event is well on its way can lessen the pain.

*Myth 5: Many clients lie about the existence or severity of their pain.* Very few clients lie about their pain.

*Myth 6: Postoperative pain is best treated with intramuscular injections.* The most commonly used postoperative pain relief for many years was meperidine (Demerol) given intramuscularly. However, meperidine has many adverse effects, such as irritating tissues and producing the CNS stimulant normeperidine. In addition, meperidine is short acting. Most contemporary experts do not recommend its use to manage postoperative pain.

# COLLABORATIVE CARE

Effective pain relief results from collaboration among health care providers. Pain clinics are centers staffed by a team of health care professionals who use a multidisciplinary approach to managing chronic pain. Therapies may include traditional pharmacologic agents as well as herbs, vitamins, and other dietary supplements; nutritional counseling; psychotherapy; biofeedback; hypnosis; acupuncture; massage; and other treatments. Hospices for dying clients also provide a multifaceted approach to pain management. Chapter 11 provides information about pain management during end-of-life care.

## Medications

Medication is the most common approach to pain management. Various drugs with many kinds of delivery systems are available. These drugs include nonnarcotic analgesics, nonsteroidal anti-inflammatory drugs (NSAIDs), narcotics, synthetic narcotics, antidepressants, and local anesthetic agents. In addition to administering prescribed medications, the nurse may act independently in choosing the dosage and timing. The nurse is also responsible for assessing the side effects of medications, evaluating a medication's effectiveness, and providing client teaching. The nurse's role in pain relief is client advocate and direct caregiver.

The World Health Organization "ladder of analgesia" effectively guides the use of medications (WHO, 1986/1990) (Figure 4–5 ■). NSAIDs and narcotic pain medications are used progressively until pain is relieved, reflecting the interactive nature of these two types of analgesics. Box 4–1 describes terms associated with pain medication.

### Nonnarcotic Analgesics
Nonnarcotic analgesics such as acetaminophen (Tylenol) produce analgesia and reduce fever. The exact mechanism of action is unknown. They are used to treat mild to moderate pain.

### NSAIDs
NSAIDs act on peripheral nerve endings and minimize pain by interfering with prostaglandin synthesis. Examples are aspirin, ibuprofen, and celecoxib (Celebrex). The NSAIDs have anti-inflammatory, analgesic, and antipyretic actions. NSAIDs are the treatment of choice for mild to moderate pain and continue to be effective when combined with narcotics for moderate to severe pain. Examples of NSAIDs and factors to consider when selecting an NSAID are provided in Table 4–3. Nursing implications for NSAIDs are found in the Medication Administration box on page 63.

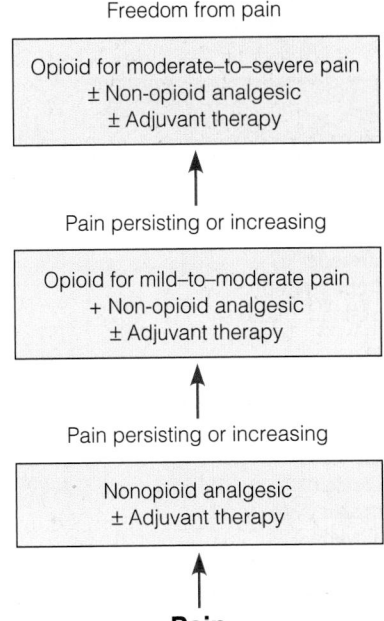

Figure 4–5 ■ The WHO analgesic ladder illustrates the process for selection of analgesic medications for pain management.

*From* Cancer Pain Relief and Palliative Care *by World Health Organization, 1990, (Technical Report Series, no. 804) Geneva: WHO. Reprinted by permission.*

| BOX 4–1 | ■ Terms Associated with Pain Medication |
| --- | --- |

- *Addiction:* The compulsive use of a substance despite negative consequences, such as health threats or legal problems.
- *Drug abuse:* The use of any chemical substance for other than a medical purpose.
- *Physical drug dependence:* A biologic need for a substance. If the substance is not supplied, physical withdrawal symptoms occur.
- *Psychologic drug dependence:* A psychologic need for a substance. If the substance is not supplied, psychologic withdrawal symptoms occur.
- *Drug tolerance:* The process by which the body requires a progressively greater amount of a drug to achieve the same results.
- *Equianalgesic:* Having the same pain-killing effect when administered to the same individual. Drug dosages are equianalgesic if they have the same effect as morphine sulfate 10 mg administered intramuscularly.
- *Pseudoaddiction:* Behavior involving drug seeking; a result of receiving inadequate pain relief.

### Narcotics (Opioids)
Narcotics, or opioids, are derivatives of the opium plant. These drugs (and their synthetic forms) are the pharmacologic treatment of choice for moderate to severe pain. Examples are morphine, codeine, and fentanyl (Durgesic, Actiq). Narcotic analgesics produce analgesia by binding to opioid receptors both within and outside the CNS. A summary of narcotic drugs, their

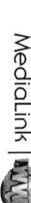

**TABLE 4-3  Factors to Consider When Selecting an NSAID**

| Chemical Class | Half Life (Hours) | Onset of Action (Hours) | Usual Dosing Interval (Times per Day) | Usual Daily Dose (Mg) |
|---|---|---|---|---|
| *Salicylates* | | | | |
| Acetylated | | | | |
|   Aspirin | 0.25 | 0.25–0.50 | 4–6 | 325–1000 |
|   Aspirin, buffered | | | | |
|   Aspirin, enteric coated | | | | |
|   Aspirin, sustained release | | | | |
| *Nonacetylated* | | | | |
|   Choline salicylate (Arthropan) | | 1–2 | 2–4 | 1200 |
|   Choline magnesium trisalicylate | | | | |
|     (Trilisate) | 2–19 | 2 | 2–4 | 1200 |
|   Diflunisal (Dolobid) | 8–12 | 2–3 | 2–3 | 250–500 |
|   Salsalate (Disalcid) | 2–19 | — | 2–3 | 325–3000 |
|   Magnesium salicylate | | | 3–4 | various |
|   Sodium salicylate | | | 4–6 | various |
| *Propionic Acids* | | | | |
|   Fenoprofen (Nalfon) | 2–3 | — | 3–4 | 300–600 |
|   Flurbiprofen (Ansaid) | 5.7 | — | 2–3 | 100 |
|   Ibuprofen (Motrin, others) | 2 | 0.5 | 3–4 | 300–800 |
|   Ketoprofen (Orudis) | 1.6–4 | — | 3–4 | 25–75 |
|   Ketoprofen SR (Oruvail) | | — | 1 | 200 |
|   Naproxen (Naprosyn) | 13 | 1 | 2 | 250–500 |
|   Naproxen sodium (Anaprox) | 13–15 | 1–2 | 2 | 250–500 |
|   Oxaprozin (Daypro) | 21–25 | 1–2 | 1–2 | 600 |
| *Acetic Acids* | | | | |
|   Diclofenac sodium (Voltaren) | 1.2–2 | 0.5 | 3 | 50 |
|   Etodolac (Lodine) | 6–7 | 0.5 | 3 | 200–400 |
|   Indomethacin (Indocin) | 4–6 | 0.5 | 2–4 | 25–50 |
|   Indomethacin SR (Indocin SR) | — | 2–4 | | 150 |
|   Ketoralac (Toradol) | 4–6 | 0.5–1 | 4–6 | 10–30 |
|   Sulindac (Clinoril, others) | 8 | — | 2 | 150–200 |
|   Tolmetin (Tolectin) | 5 | — | 3 | 400 |
| *Fenamates (Anthranilic Acids)* | | | | |
|   Meclofenamate (Meclomen) | 2–3 | — | 3–4 | 50 |
|   Mefenamic acid (Ponstel) | 2 | — | 4 | 250 |
| *Oxicams* | | | | |
|   Piroxican (Feldene) | 24 | 2–4 | 1–2 | 10–20 |
| *Nonacidic (Naphthylkanone)* | | | | |
|   Nabumetone (Relafon) | 22 | — | 1–2 | 500–1000 |
| *Pyrazolones* | | | | |
|   Phenylbutazone (Butazolidin) | 40–60 | 0.5–1 | 3–4 | 100–600 |

usual dosages, peak effect, and nursing implications is provided in Table 4–4.

A common myth among health care professionals is that using narcotics for pain treatment poses a real threat of addiction. Actually, when the medications are used as recommended, there is little to no risk of addiction. Rather, if pain is not adequately treated, the client may seek more and more narcotic relief, thus increasing the risk of tolerance. Nursing implications for narcotics are found in the Medication Administration box on page 65.

## Antidepressants

Antidepressants within the tricyclic and related chemical groups act on the production and retention of serotonin in the CNS, thus inhibiting pain sensation. They also promote normal sleeping patterns, further alleviating the suffering of the client in pain.

## Local Anesthetics

Drugs such as benzocaine and zylocaine are part of a large group of substances that block the initiation and transmission of nerve impulses in a local area, thus blocking pain as well. Local anesthetics can be delivered by a variety of methods. They are sometimes used to enable a client to begin moving and using a painful area to diminish long-term pain.

## Duration of Action

Each of the pharmacologic agents has a unique absorption and duration of action. The nurse caring for the client in pain must

# Medication Administration

## Nonsteroidal Anti-Inflammatory Drugs

Examples of NSAIDs are:

  aspirin (acetylsalicylic acid)
  fenoprofen calcium (Nalfon)
  ibuprofen (Motrin)
  rofecoxib (Vioxx)
  diflunisal (Dolobid)
  ketorolac tromethamine (Toradol)
  naproxen (Naprosyn)
  indomethacin (Indocin)
  celecoxib (Celebrex)

The NSAIDs have anti-inflammatory, analgesic, and antipyretic effects. It is believed that they inhibit the enzyme cyclooxygenase, thereby decreasing synthesis of prostaglandins. These drugs provide analgesic effects by reducing inflammation and by perhaps blocking the generation of noxious impulses.

### Nursing Responsibilities
- Do not administer aspirin with other NSAIDs.
- Assess and document if the client is taking a hypoglycemic agent or insulin; the NSAIDs may increase the hypoglycemic effect.
- Administer with meals, milk, or a full glass of water to decrease gastric irritation.
- Assess clients who are also taking anticoagulants for bleeding; the NSAIDs increase this risk.

### Client and Family Teaching
- Drugs may cause gastrointestinal bleeding (report nausea, vomiting of blood, dark stools), visual disturbances (report blurred or diminished vision), hearing problems, dizziness, skin rash, and renal problems (report weight gain or edema).
- Take medications with meals to decrease gastric irritation.
- Avoid drinking alcohol or taking any over-the-counter drug unless approved by the health care provider.
- The desired effects may not appear for 3–5 days, and the full effects may not appear for 2–4 weeks.
- Maintain regular health care appointments.

---

understand that no drug will have a totally predictable course of action, because each person absorbs, metabolizes, and excretes medications at different dosage levels. The only way to obtain reliable data about the effectiveness of the medication for the individual client is to assess how that client responds. Therefore, the best choice is to individualize the dosing schedule.

The two major descriptors of dosing schedules are *around the clock* (ATC) or *as necessary* (PRN). (The abbreviation PRN stands for *pro re nata,* Latin for "as circumstances may require.") An ATC administration is appropriate if the client experiences pain constantly and predictably during a 24-hour period. A PRN administration is appropriate for pain that is not predictable or constant. The PRN medication should be administered as soon as the pain begins.

Giving analgesics before the pain occurs or increases gives the client confidence in the certainty of pain relief and thereby avoids some of the untoward effects of pain. The benefits of a preventive approach can be summarized as follows:

- The client may spend less time in pain.
- Frequent analgesic administration may allow for smaller doses and less analgesic administration.
- Smaller doses will in turn mean fewer side effects.
- The client's fear and anxiety about the return of pain will decrease.
- The client will probably be more physically active and avoid the difficulties caused by immobility.

The side effects of a drug can become difficult to manage if the dosage is too high. The best formula for adequate dosage is a balance between effective pain relief and minimal side effects. Within prescribed limits, the nurse can choose the correct dose according to the client's response. It is also the role of the nurse to inform the physician if the prescribed dosage does not meet the client's needs.

## Routes of Administration

The route of administration significantly affects how much of the medication is needed to relieve pain. For example, oral doses of some narcotics must be up to 5 times greater than parenteral doses to achieve the same degree of pain relief. Different narcotics have different recommended dosages. Consulting an equianalgesic dosage chart helps ensure that dosages of different narcotics administered by different routes will have the same analgesic effect when administered to the same client. These charts are based on a comparison of an analgesic to 10 mg (IM) of morphine. Table 4–4 is an example of an equianalgesic chart.

**ORAL.** The simplest route for both client and nurse is the oral (PO) route. Special nursing care is still required, because some medications must be given with food, some are irritating to the gastrointestinal system, and some clients have trouble swallowing pills. Liquid and timed-release forms are available for special applications.

**RECTAL.** The rectal route is helpful for clients who are unable to swallow. Several of the opioid narcotics are available in this form. The rectal route is effective and simple, but the client and family may not accept it. To be effective, any rectal medication must be placed above the rectal sphincter.

**TRANSDERMAL.** The transdermal, or patch, form of medication is increasingly being used because it is simple, painless, and delivers a continuous level of medication (Figure 4–6 ■). Although expensive, transdermal medications are easy to store and apply. Additional short-acting medication is often needed for breakthrough pain.

To apply a medication transdermally, the nurse or client must clip any hair from the area, clean the site (which should be on the upper torso) with clear water, dry the cleansed area,

## TABLE 4-4  Equianalgesic Drug Chart

| Analgesic | Dosage (mg) | Peak (min) | Duration (h) | Nursing Considerations |
|---|---|---|---|---|
| Morphine sulfate | 10 IM<br>30–60 PO | 30–60 IM<br>60–120 PO | 4–5 IM<br>4–5 PO | PO dose is 3–6 times the IM dose. A lower dose may be appropriate for older clients with chronic pain. Contraindicated in clients with acute bronchial asthma or upper-airway obstruction. |
| Butorphanol tartrate (Stadol) | 2 IM<br>N/A PO | 30–60 IM | 3–4 IM | May cause withdrawal in clients physically dependent on narcotics. May cause hallucinations. Increases cardiac workload. Contraindicated in clients with myocardial infarction. |
| Codeine | 130 IM<br>200 PO | 30–60 IM<br>60–120 PO | 4 IM<br>4 PO | PO dose is about 1.5 times the IM dose. Often given synergistically with aspirin or acetaminophen for best effect. More toxic in high doses than morphine. Causes more nausea and vomiting than morphine and is constipating. |
| Hydromorphone HCl (Dilaudid) | 1.5 IM<br>7.5 PO | 15–30 IM<br>30 PO | 4 IM<br>4 PO | PO dose is 5 times IM dose. Shorter acting than morphine. May cause loss of appetite. Contraindicated in clients with increased intracranial pressure or status asthmaticus. |
| Levorphanol tartrate (Levo-Dromoran) | 2 IM<br>4 PO | 60 IM<br>90–120 PO | 4–5 IM<br>4–5 PO | Longer acting than morphine when given in repeated, regular doses. Accumulates, so analgesic effect may increase. SC recommended over IM route. Warn client drug has bitter taste. Contraindicated in clients with respiratory depression, asthma, alcoholism, or increased intracranial pressure. |
| Meperidine HCl (Demerol) | 75 IM<br>300 PO | 30–50 IM<br>60–90 PO | 2–4 IM<br>2–4 PO | Metabolized to normeperidine, a toxic CNS stimulant which may cause CNS hyperexcitability. Normeperidine's effects increased, not reversed, by naloxone. Use with caution in clients with renal disease. PO dose of 300 not recommended. |
| Methadone HCl (Dolophine) | 10 IM<br>20 PO | 60–120 IM<br>90–120 PO | 4–6 IM<br>4–6 PO | Initial PO dose is twice IM dose. Accumulates, so analgesic effect may increase. Warn client drug has bitter taste. Also used for heroin detoxification and temporary maintenance. Oral liquid form is legally required in maintenance programs. |
| Nalbuphine HCl (Nubain) | 10 IM<br>N/A PO | 30–60 IM | 3–6 IM | Longer acting and less likely to cause hypotension than morphine. Respiratory depression does not increase with increased dosages as compared to morphine. Similar to butorphanol, but does not increase cardiac workload. |
| Oxycodone HCl | N/A IM<br>30 PO | 60 PO | 3–6 PO | Now available as a single-entity product in tablet or liquid form. Also available in 5-mg dose in drugs such as Percodan and Percocet. Has faster onset and higher peak effect than most PO narcotics. |
| Oxymorphone HCl (Numorphan) | 1–1.5 IM<br>N/A PO | 30–60 IM | 3–6 IM | Also available as rectal suppository (10 mg equianalgesic), but more effective if given IM. |
| Pentazocine HCl | 60 IM<br>180 PO | 30–60 IM<br>30–90 PO | 3–4 IM<br>3–4 PO | PO dose is 3 times IM dose. May produce withdrawal in clients physically dependent on narcotics. May cause confusion, hallucinations, anxiety. Contraindicated in clients with head injury or increased intracranial pressure. Use with caution in clients with cardiac problems. |
| Propoxyphene HCl (Darvon) | N/A IM<br>500 PO | 120 PO | 4–6 PO | Available only in oral form in United States. Never give as much as 500 mg PO. PO dose of 65–130 mg recommended. Used for mild to moderate pain. May cause false decreases in urinary steroid excretion tests. Report suspected propoxyphene abuse; propoxyphene in excessive doses ranks second to barbiturates as a cause of drug-related deaths. |

*Note:* Morphine sulfate 10 mg IM is the analgesic dose to which all other IM and PO doses in this table are considered equianalgesic.

# Medication Administration

## Narcotic Analgesics

Examples of narcotic analgesics are:

> buprenorphine HCl (Buprenex)
> codeine
> hydromorphone HCl (Dilaudid)
> meperidine HCl (Demerol)
> morphine sulfate
> nalbuphine HCl (Nubain)
> oxymorphone HCl (Numorphan)
> pentazocine (Talwin)
> propoxyphene napsylate (Darvocet-N)

Narcotic analgesics are used to treat severe pain. The drugs in this category include opium, morphine, codeine, opium derivatives, and synthetic substances. Morphine and codeine are pure chemical substances isolated from opium. These drugs decrease the awareness of the sensation of pain by binding to opiate receptors in the brain and spinal cord. It is also believed that they diminish the transmission of pain impulses by altering cell membrane permeability to sodium and by affecting the release of neurotransmitters for efferent nerves sensitive to noxious stimuli. Narcotic analgesics affect the central nervous system; causing analgesia, euphoria, drowsiness, mental clouding, and lethargy. They also have various other effects: Depending on the drug used, the narcotics depress respirations, stimulate the vomiting center, depress the cough reflex, induce peripheral vasodilatation (resulting in hypotension), constrict the pupil, and decrease intestinal peristalsis. The narcotics are addictive, causing psychologic and physical dependence.

### Nursing Responsibilities

- Narcotics are regulated by federal law; the nurse must record the date, time, client name, type and amount of the drug used, and sign the entry in a narcotic inventory sheet. If the drug must be wasted after it is signed out, the act must be witnessed and the narcotic sheet signed by the nurse and the witness. Computerized narcotic documentation methods are also available.
- Keep a narcotic antagonist, such as naloxone, immediately available to treat respiratory depression.

- Assess allergies or adverse effects from narcotics previously experienced by the client.
- Meperidine (Demerol) is associated with CNS toxicity and thus involves significant patient risk. For any client who is receiving more than one dose, monitor for nervousness, restlessness, tremors, twitching, shakiness, myoclonic jerks, diaphoresis, changes in level of awareness, agitation, disorientation, confusion, delirium, hallucinations, violent shivering, and/or seizures. This toxicity can occur with any route of administration or any dosing regimen. This risk is increased with oral administration and in clients with decreased renal function (including normal changes with aging). Report these manifestations to the physician.
- Assess for any respiratory disease, such as asthma, that might increase the risk of respiratory depression.
- Assess the characteristics of the pain and the effectiveness of drugs that have been previously used to treat the pain.
- Take and record baseline vital signs before administering the drug.
- Administer the drugs, following established guidelines.
- Monitor vital signs, level of consciousness, pupillary response, nausea, bowel function, urinary function, and effectiveness of pain management.
- Teach noninvasive methods of pain management for use in conjunction with narcotic analgesics.
- Provide for client safety.

### Client and Family Teaching

- The use of narcotics to treat severe pain is unlikely to cause addiction.
- Do not drink alcohol.
- Do not take over-the-counter medications unless approved by the health care provider.
- Increase intake of fluids and fiber in the diet to prevent constipation.
- The drugs often cause dizziness, drowsiness, and impaired thinking; use caution when driving or making decisions.
- Report decreasing effectiveness or the appearance of side effects to the physician.

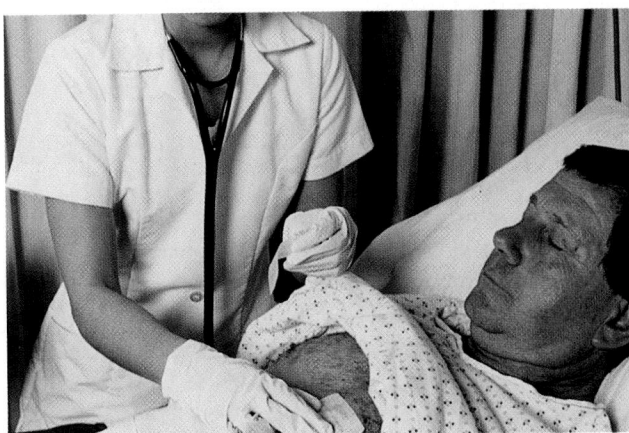

**Figure 4–6** ■ The transdermal patch administers medication in predictable doses.

apply the patch immediately upon opening the package, and ensure that the contact is complete, especially around the edges. The effectiveness of a patch lasts for a variable amount of time, and the next patch should be applied on a different site.

***INTRAMUSCULAR.*** Once the most popular route for pain medication administration, the intramuscular (IM) route is being reconsidered. Its disadvantages include uneven absorption from the muscle, discomfort on administration, and time consumed to prepare and administer the medication.

***INTRAVENOUS.*** The intravenous (IV) route provides the most rapid onset, usually ranging from 1 to 15 minutes. Medication can be given by drip, bolus, or **patient-controlled analgesia (PCA),** a pump with a control mechanism that affords the client self-management of pain (Figure 4–7 ■). Studies of PCA use for postoperative pain have shown that clients require less

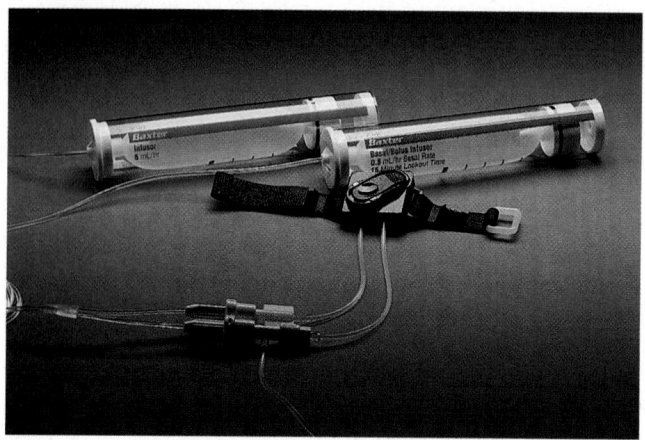

**Figure 4–7** ■ PCA units allow the client to self-manage severe pain. The units may be portable or mounted on intravenous poles.

*Courtesy of Baxter Healthcare Corporation.*

overall medication because of the even blood level of medication maintained, the feeling of control maintained by the client, and the absence of anxiety. Several drugs are available for this route. The disadvantages are the nursing care needed for any intravenous line, the potential for infection, and the cost of disposable supplies. The PCA method of administration requires careful client teaching.

***SUBCUTANEOUS.*** The subcutaneous (SC) route is accepted, but it is less commonly used than other methods. Its advantages and disadvantages are similar to those of the intravenous route.

***INTRASPINAL.*** The intraspinal route is invasive and requires more extensive nursing care. Nursing implications for clients receiving intraspinal analgesia can be found in box below.

***NERVE BLOCKS.*** In a nerve block, anesthetics, sometimes in combination with steroidal anti-inflammatory drugs, are injected by a physician or nurse anesthetist into or near a nerve,

# NURSING CARE | OF THE CLIENT RECEIVING INTRASPINAL ANALGESIA

Intraspinal analgesia is used to manage chronic and intractable cancer and severe postoperative pain. The intraspinal route may be either intrathecal (into the subarachnoid space) or epidural (into the epidural space). With the infusion of a narcotic into these spaces, there is a direct effect on the opiate receptors in the dorsal horn of the spinal cord; the narcotics are also absorbed systemically and affect the brain. This method provides complete pain relief but has some potentially dangerous side effects.

## PROCEDURE

The physician places a catheter into the epidural space. Tubing is attached to an infusion pump, and the prescribed medication is administered. A portable or implantable pump may be used for narcotic administration that lasts more than a few days.

## NURSING CARE

- Monitor vital signs every 15 minutes for the first 2–3 hours and every hour for the first 24 hours; the client is at risk for respiratory depression, which may not manifest itself for several hours.
- Ensure that naloxone, a narcotic antagonist, is immediately available to reverse respiratory depression.
- Monitor the effectiveness of the pain management.
- Monitor intake and output. Intraspinal narcotics may block the micturition reflex, causing urinary retention and necessitating the insertion of a Foley catheter.
- Use sterile technique to care for the catheter.

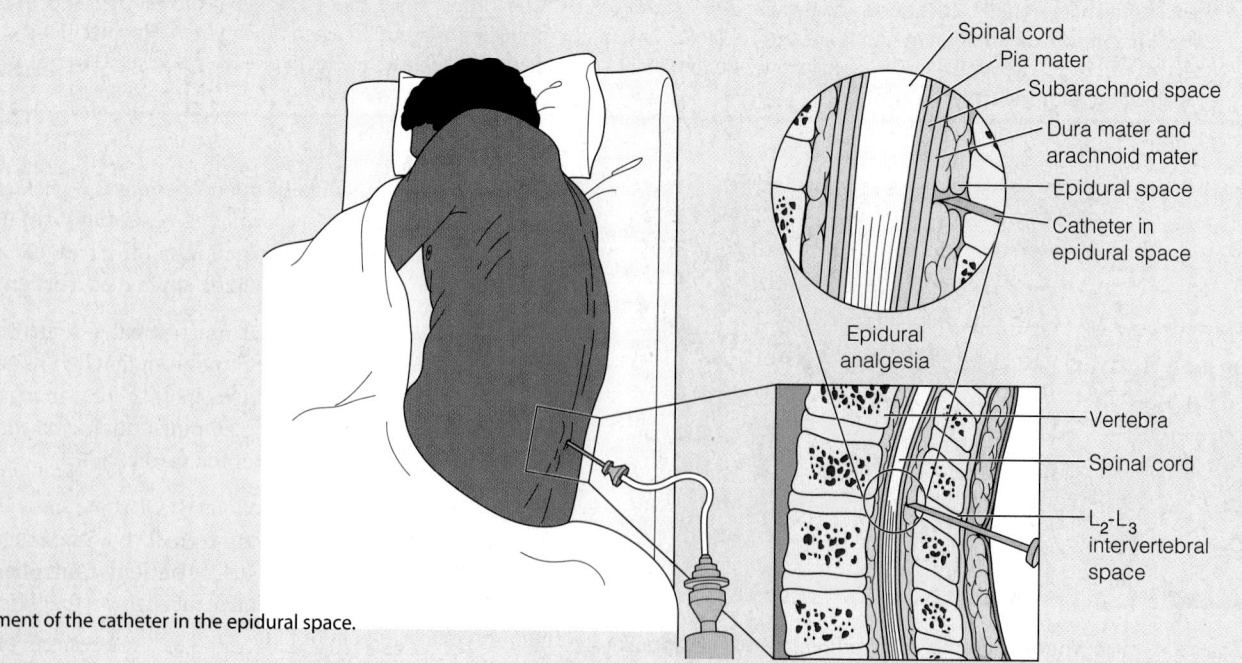

Placement of the catheter in the epidural space.

Spinal cord
Pia mater
Subarachnoid space
Dura mater and arachnoid mater
Epidural space
Catheter in epidural space
Epidural analgesia
Vertebra
Spinal cord
$L_2-L_3$ intervertebral space

usually in an area between the nociceptor and the dorsal root. The procedure may be performed to determine the precise location of the pain source: Pain relief indicates that the injection site is the site of the source of the pain.

Temporary (local) nerve blocks may give the client enough relief to (1) develop a more hopeful attitude that pain relief is possible, (2) allow local procedures to be performed without causing discomfort, or (3) exercise and move the affected part. Nerve blocks may also be performed to predict the results of neurosurgery. For long-term pain relief, a permanent neurolytic agent is used. Neurolytic blocks usually are reserved for terminally ill clients because of the risks of weakness, paralysis, and bowel and bladder dysfunction.

## Surgery

As a pain relief measure, surgery usually is performed only after all other methods have failed. Clients need thorough knowledge of the implications of the use of surgery for pain relief. For example, motor function loss is an unwelcome side effect of some surgeries. Surgical procedures used to relieve pain are shown in Figure 4–8 ■ and include cordotomy, neurectomy, sympathectomy, and rhizotomy.

### Cordotomy

A cordotomy is an incision into the anterolateral tracts of the spinal cord to interrupt the transmission of pain. Because it is difficult to isolate the nerves responsible for upper body pain, this surgery is most often performed for pain in the abdominal region and legs, including severe pain from terminal cancer. A percutaneous cordotomy produces lesions of the anterolateral surface of the spinal cord by means of a radio frequency current.

### Neurectomy

A neurectomy is the removal of a nerve. It is sometimes used for pain relief. A peripheral neurectomy is the severing of a nerve at any point distal to the spinal cord.

### Sympathectomy

The sympathetic nerves play an important role in producing and transmitting the sensation of pain. A sympathectomy involves destruction by injection or incision of the ganglia of sympathetic nerves, usually in the lumbar region or the cervicodorsal region at the base of the neck.

### Rhizotomy

Rhizotomy is surgical severing of the dorsal spinal roots. It is most often performed to relieve the pain of cancer of the head, neck, or lungs. A rhizotomy may be performed not only by surgically cutting the nerve fibers but also by injecting a chemical such as alcohol or phenol into the subarachnoid space or by using a radio frequency current to selectively destroy pain fibers.

## Transcutaneous Electrical Nerve Stimulation

A **transcutaneous electrical nerve stimulation (TENS)** unit consists of a low-voltage transmitter connected by wires to electrodes placed by the client as directed by the physical therapist (Figure 4–9 ■). The client experiences a gentle tapping or vibrating sensation over the electrodes. The client can adjust the voltage to achieve maximum pain relief.

The gate control theory clarifies how TENS works. It is believed that TENS electrodes stimulate the large-diameter A-beta touch fibers to close the gate in the substantia gelatinosa. It is also theorized that TENS stimulates endorphin release by inhibitory neurons.

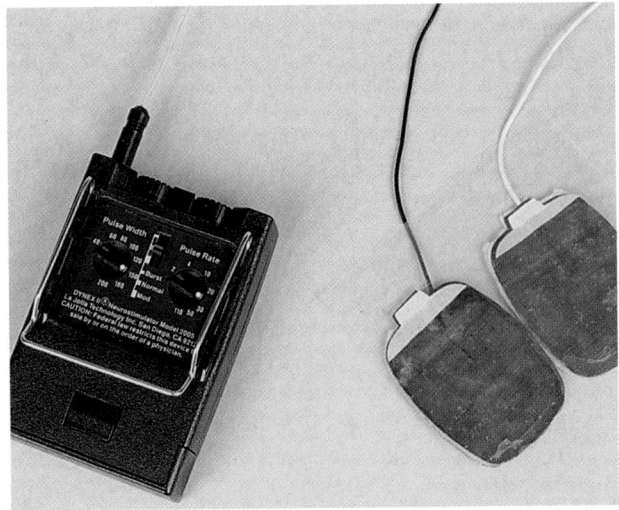

**Figure 4–9 ■** The TENS unit is believed to assist in pain management through the gate control theory. Electrodes that deliver low-voltage electrical stimuli are placed directly on the client over painful areas.

*Source: Rehabilicare, Inc./Complex Technologies.*

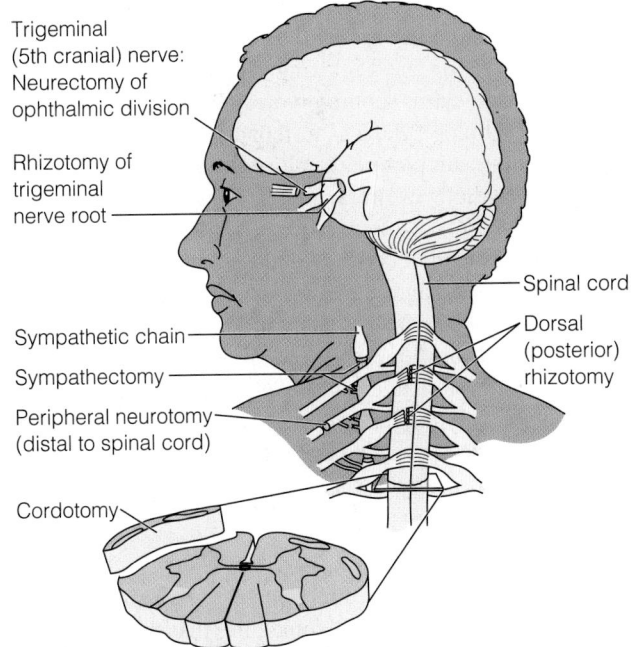

Trigeminal (5th cranial) nerve: Neurectomy of ophthalmic division

Rhizotomy of trigeminal nerve root

Sympathetic chain

Sympathectomy

Peripheral neurotomy (distal to spinal cord)

Cordotomy

Spinal cord

Dorsal (posterior) rhizotomy

**Figure 4–8 ■** Surgical procedures are used to treat severe pain that does not respond to other types of management.

A TENS unit is most commonly used to relieve chronic benign pain and acute postoperative pain. In either case, thorough client teaching is essential, including an explanation of manufacturer's directions, instructions on where to place the electrodes, and the importance of placing the electrodes on clean, unbroken skin. The client should assess the skin daily for signs of irritation.

TENS offers several advantages: avoidance of drug side effects, client control, and good interaction with other therapies. Disadvantages are its cost and the need for expert training for initiation.

## Complementary Therapies

### Acupuncture

Acupuncture is an ancient Chinese system involving the stimulation of certain specific points on the body to enhance the flow of vital energy (chi) along pathways called meridians. Acupuncture points can be stimulated by the insertion and withdrawing of needles; the application of heat, massage, laser, or electrical stimulation; or a combination of these methods. Only care providers with special training can use this method. Acupuncture is becoming a more widely accepted therapy, especially for the treatment of pain.

### Biofeedback

**Biofeedback** is an electronic method of measuring physiologic responses such as brain waves, muscle contraction, and skin temperature, and then "feeding" this information back to the client. Most biofeedback units consist of electrodes placed on the client's skin and an amplification unit that transforms data into visual cues, such as colored lights. The client thus learns to recognize stress-related responses and to replace them with relaxation responses. Eventually, the client learns to repeat independently those actions that produce the desired brain wave effect.

Relaxation helps the client avoid the anxiety that often accompanies and complicates pain. Additionally, biofeedback gives the client a measure of control over the response to pain.

### Hypnotism

Hypnosis is a trance state in which the mind becomes extremely suggestible. To achieve hypnosis, the client sits or lies down in a dimly lighted, quiet room. The therapist suggests that the client relax and fix attention on an object. The therapist then repeats in a calm, soothing voice simple phrases, such as instructions to relax and listen to the therapist's voice. The client gradually becomes more and more relaxed and falls into a trance in which the client is no longer aware of the physical environment and hears only the therapist's voice. During this state, the therapist may make suggestions to encourage pain relief. It is possible to achieve complete anesthesia or to modify pain in a variety of ways through hypnotism. For the technique to work, however, the client must be fully relaxed and must want to be hypnotized.

Advantages include client control and lack of side effects. Disadvantages include the need for a skilled practitioner; however, some clients can learn to hypnotize themselves to achieve pain relief.

### Relaxation

Relaxation involves learning activities that deeply relax the body and mind. Relaxation distracts the client, lessens the effects of stress from pain, increases pain tolerance, increases the effectiveness of other pain relief measures, and increases perception of pain control. In addition, by teaching the client relaxation techniques, the nurse acknowledges the client's pain and provides reassurance that the client will receive help in managing the pain (McCaffery & Beebe, 1999). Examples of relaxation activities are as follows:

- Diaphragmatic breathing can relax muscles, improve oxygen levels, and provide a feeling of release from tension. The use of diaphragmatic breathing is more effective when the client either lies down or sits comfortably, remains in a quiet environment, and keeps the eyelids closed. Inhaling and exhaling slowly and regularly is also helpful. The technique for diaphragmatic breathing is described and illustrated in Chapter 7.
- Progressive muscle relaxation may be used alone or in conjunction with deep breathing to help manage pain. The client should be taught to tighten one group of muscles (such as those of the face), hold the tension for a few seconds, and then relax the muscle group completely. The client should repeat these actions for all parts of the body. This method is also more effective when the client lies or sits comfortably, is in a quiet environment, and keeps the eyelids closed. Audiotapes are available to help the client with this relaxation process.
- Guided imagery, also called creative visualization, is the use of the imaginative power of the mind to create a scene or sensory experience that relaxes the muscles and moves the attention of the mind away from the pain experience. To use guided imagery, the client must be able to concentrate, use the imagination, and follow directions. The nurse can facilitate this technique by asking the client to describe places or situations that are most relaxing. The nurse then speaks to the client in a calm, soothing voice about them. The client usually must close the eyes to reduce visual stimulation so that the mind can picture the situation in as much detail as possible. Audiotapes are available to assist the client with guided imagery.
- Meditation is a process whereby the client empties the mind of all sensory data and, typically, concentrates on a single object, word, or idea. This activity produces a deeply relaxed state in which oxygen consumption decreases, muscles relax, and endorphins are produced. At its deepest level, the meditative state may resemble a trance. A variety of exercises can induce the meditative state, and all are relatively easy to learn. Many books and audiotapes are available commercially.

### Distraction

Distraction involves the redirection of the client's attention away from the pain and onto something that the client finds more pleasant. Examples of distracting activities are practicing focused breathing, listening to music, or doing some form of rhythmic activity to music. For example, the client using recorded music for distraction may sing along with the song, tap out the rhythm with the fingers or foot, clap to the music, conduct the music, or add harmony. Full participation in the music is key to pain relief.

Participating in an activity that promotes laughter, such as reading a joke book or viewing a comedy, has been found to be highly effective in pain relief. Laughing for 20 minutes or more is known to produce an increase in endorphins that may continue pain relief even after the client stops laughing.

### Cutaneous Stimulation

It is believed that stimulation of the skin is effective in relieving pain because it prompts closure of the gate in the substantia gelatinosa. Cutaneous stimulation may be accomplished by massage, vibration, application of heat and cold, and therapeutic touch (see Table 4–5).

## NURSING CARE

Nursing care of the client with pain presents perhaps more of a challenge than almost any other type of illness or injury. Regardless of the type of pain, the goal of nursing care is to assist the client to achieve optimal control of the pain.

### Assessment

A comprehensive approach to pain assessment is essential to ensure adequate and appropriate interventions. The assessment areas are client perceptions, physiologic responses, behavioral responses, and self-management of pain and the effectiveness of pain management strategies.

### Client Perceptions

The most reliable indicator of the presence and degree of pain is the client's own statement about the pain. The McGill Pain Questionnaire is a useful tool in assessing the client's subjective experience of the pain. It asks the client to locate the pain, to describe the quality of the pain, to indicate how the pain changes with time, and to rate the intensity of the pain (Figure 4–10 ■).

The client's perception of the pain can also be assessed by using the following PQRST technique.

- P = What precipitated (triggered, stimulated) the pain? Has anything relieved the pain? What is the pattern of the pain?
- Q = What are the quality and quantity of the pain? Is the pain sharp, stabbing, aching, burning, stinging, deep, crushing, viselike, gnawing?
- R = What is the region (location) of the pain? Does the pain radiate to other areas of the body?
- S = What is the severity of the pain?
- T = What is the timing of the pain? When does it begin, how long does it last, and how is it related to other events in the client's life?

The most common method to assess the severity of pain is a pain rating scale. Several scales are illustrated in Figure 4–11 ■.

---

### TABLE 4–5    Methods of Cutaneous Stimulation

| Method | Technique | Advantages | Disadvantages |
|---|---|---|---|
| Touch | Nurse places hands on client's body or less than 1 inch (about 2.5 cm) above client's body to realign energy. | May initiate gate closure. Communicates caring. | None. |
| Pressure | Nurse places hand firmly on or around the area where the client feels the pain. | May relieve pain, decrease bleeding, and prevent swelling. | Benefits are temporary—when pressure is lifted, pain returns. |
| Massage | Nurse gently or briskly stimulates client's subcutaneous tissues by kneading, pulling, or pressing with fingers, palms, or knuckles. | May initiate gate closure. Promotes relaxation and sedation. Minimal side effects. | Time consuming. |
| Vibration | Nurse uses an electrical or battery-operated vibrator to stimulate the client's subcutaneous tissues. | May initiate gate closure. Low risk of tissue damage. Less costly than TENS. | Expense of equipment. |
| Heat | Nurse applies a hot-water bottle, heating pad, or hot towels to client's body. A hot shower or hot bath may also be effective. A heat lamp or other heat-generating device may also be used. | May reduce muscle spasm and pain. Works best for localized pain. | Contraindicated if bleeding or swelling is present. |
| Cold | Nurse applies dry or moist cold packs, gel packs, towels, or bags of ice chips to the client's body. | May reduce muscle spasm and pain. Cold may slow the transmission of pain impulses, and is more effective than heat for pain relief. | Cannot be used on ischemic tissues. |

**Figure 4–10** ■ The McGill Pain Questionnaire.

*From* Pain Measurement and Assessment *by R. Melzack, 1983, New York: Raven. Reprinted by permission.*

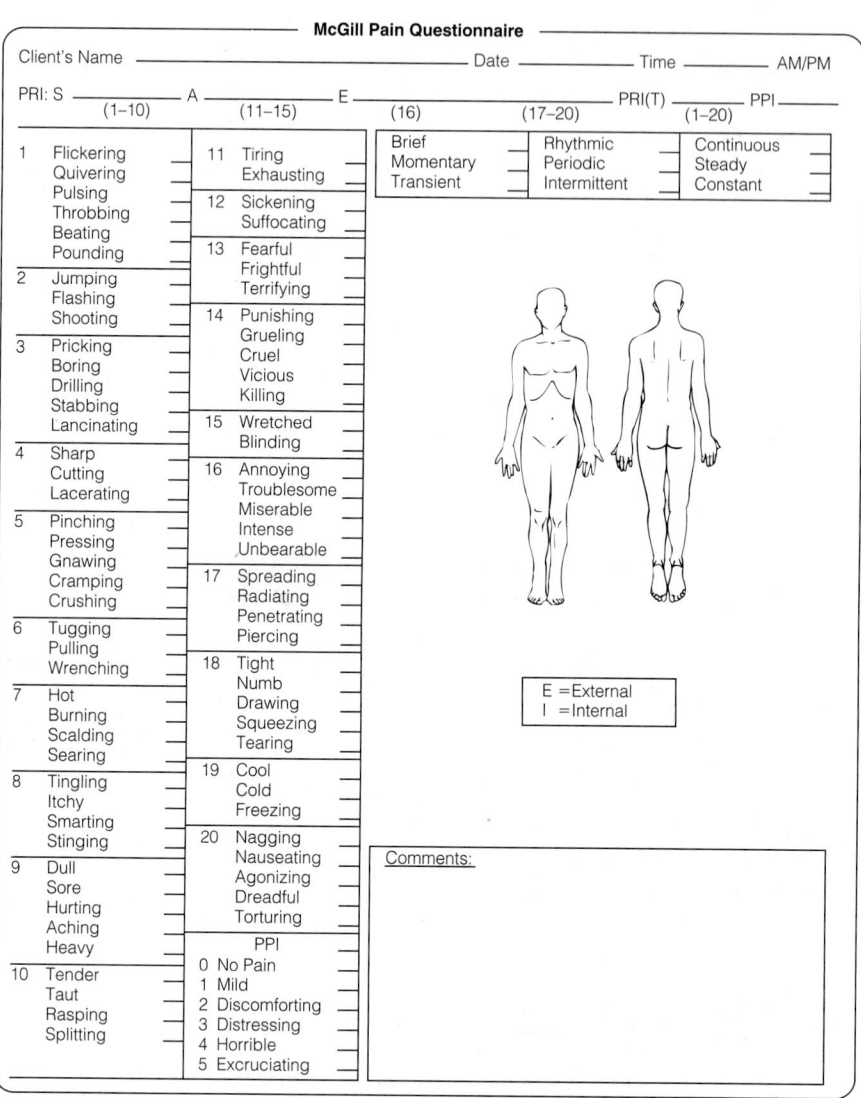

**Visual analog scale (VAS)**

No pain — Pain as bad as it could possibly be

**0–10 Numeric pain intensity scale**

0  1  2  3  4  5  6  7  8  9  10

No pain — Moderate pain — Worst possible pain

**Simple descriptive pain intensity scale**

No pain — Mild pain — Moderate pain — Severe pain — Very severe pain — Worst possible pain

**Figure 4–11** ■ Examples of commonly used pain scales.

For clients who do not understand English or numerals, a scale using colors (e.g., light blue for no pain through bright red for worst possible pain) or pictures may be helpful. The following nursing interventions will help the nurse use a pain rating scale to achieve optimal results.

- To ensure consistent communication, explain the specific pain rating scale being used. If a word descriptor scale is used, verify that the client can read the language being used. If a numerical scale is used, be sure the client can count to 10. If the client is not able to report pain because of communication difficulties, intubation, emotional disturbances, or cognitive impairments, follow these guidelines (Pasero & McCaffrey, 2000):
- Be sure the client is unable to report pain. Researchers have found that even residents in a nursing home who are cognitively impaired can validly self-report pain.
- Consider pathologic conditions and procedures that might cause pain and treat the client for pain.
- Look for indicators of pain, such as grimacing, restlessness, stillness, verbal or nonverbal vocalizations, and grasping an object.

- Ask a family member or caretaker about the client's pain to serve as a proxy pain rating.
- Discuss the definition of the word *pain* to ensure that the client and the provider are communicating on the same level. It is often helpful to use the client's own words when describing the pain.
- Explain that the report of pain is important for promoting recovery, not just for achieving temporary comfort.

### Physiologic Responses

Predictable physiologic changes occur in the presence of acute pain. These may include muscle tension; tachycardia; rapid, shallow respirations; increased blood pressure; dilated pupils; sweating; and pallor. Over time, however, the body adapts to the pain stimulus, and these physiologic changes may be extinguished in clients with chronic pain.

### Behavioral Responses

Some behaviors are so typical of people in pain that the behaviors are referred to as *pain behaviors.* They include bracing or guarding the painful part, taking medication, crying, moaning, grimacing, withdrawing from activity and socialization, becoming immobile, talking about pain, holding the painful area, breathing with increased effort, exhibiting a sad facial expression, and being restless.

Behavioral responses to pain may or may not coincide with the client's report of pain and are not reliable cues to the pain experience. For example, one client may rate pain at an 8 on a 1 to 10 scale while laughing or walking down the hall; another may deny pain completely while tachycardic, hypertensive, and grimacing. Discrepancies between the client's report of pain and behavioral responses may be the result of cultural factors, coping skills, fear, denial, or the utilization of relaxation or distraction techniques.

Clients may deny pain for a variety of reasons, including fear of injections, fear of drug/narcotic addiction, misinterpretation of terms (the client may not think that aching, soreness, or discomfort qualify as pain), or the misconception that health care providers know when clients experience pain. Some clients may deny pain as part of an attempt to deny that there is something wrong with them. Other clients, by contrast, may think that "as needed" medications will be given only if their pain rating is high. Clients may also use pain as a mechanism to gain attention from family and health care providers.

### Self-Management of Pain

The client's attempts to manage pain are useful additions to the assessment database. This information is individualized and client specific, including many factors such as culture, age, and client knowledge. Collect detailed descriptions of actions the client or significant others took, when and how these measures were applied, and how well they worked.

## Nursing Diagnoses and Interventions

The primary nursing diagnoses for clients in pain are acute pain and chronic pain. The interventions for these diagnoses are combined in this discussion.

### Acute Pain or Chronic Pain

- Assess the characteristics of the pain by asking the client to:
  - Point to the pain location or to mark the pain location on a figure drawing. *Pain location provides information about the etiology of the pain and the type of pain being experienced.*
  - Rate the intensity of the pain by using a pain scale (1 to 10, with 10 being the worst pain ever experienced), a visual analog scale (a scale on which pain is marked on a continuum from no pain to severe pain), or with word descriptors (such as the McGill Pain Questionnaire). Use the same scale with each assessment. *The intensity of pain is a subjective experience. The perception of the intensity of pain is affected by the client's degree of concentration or distraction, state of consciousness, and expectations. Some body tissues are more sensitive than others.*

> **PRACTICE ALERT** *Do not assume that the older client or the cognitively impaired client is not having pain or is unable to identify the intensity of pain.* ■

- Describe the quality of the pain, saying, for example, "Describe what your pain feels like." If necessary, provide word descriptors for the client to select. *Descriptive terms provide insight into the nature and perception of the pain. In addition, the location and type of pain (e.g., acute versus chronic) affect the quality.*
- Describe the pattern of the pain, including time of onset, duration, persistence, and times without pain. It is also important to ask if the pain is worse at regular times of the day and if it has any relationship to activity. *The pattern of pain provides clues about cause and location.*
- Describe any precipitating or relieving factors such as *sleep deficits, anxiety, temperature extremes, excessive noise, anxiety, fear, depression, and activity.*
- Describe the meaning of the pain, including its effects on lifestyle, self-concept, roles, and relationships. *Clients with acute pain may believe the pain is a normal response to injury or that it signals serious illness and death. Pain is a stressor that may affect the ability of the client to cope effectively. The client with chronic pain often has concerns about addiction to pain medication, costs, social interactions, sexual activities, and relationships with significant others.*
- Monitor manifestations of pain by taking vital signs; assessing skin temperature and moisture; observing pupils; observing facial expressions, position in bed, guarding of body parts; and noting restlessness. *Autonomic responses to pain may result in an increased blood pressure, tachycardia, rapid respirations, perspiration, and dilated pupils. Other responses to pain include grimacing, clenching the hands, muscle rigidity, guarding, restlessness, and nausea. The client with chronic pain may have an unexpressive, tired facial appearance.*

> **PRACTICE ALERT** *Consider pain the fifth vital sign and assess clients for pain every time you check temperature, pulse, respirations, and blood pressure.* ■

- Communicate belief in the client's pain by verbally acknowledging the presence of the pain, listening carefully to the description of pain, and acting to help the client manage the pain. *Because pain is a personal, subjective experience, the nurse must convey belief in the client's pain. By doing so, the nurse reduces anxiety and thereby lessens pain (see the Nursing Research box on this page for related research).*
- Provide optimal pain relief with prescribed analgesics, determining the preferred route of administration. Provide pain-relieving measures for severe pain on a regular around-the-clock basis or by self-administration (such as with a PCA pump). *The client is a part of the decision-making process and can exert some control over the situation by choosing the administration route. Analgesics are usually most effective when they are administered before pain occurs or becomes severe. Around-the-clock administration has been proven to provide better pain management for both acute and chronic pain.*
- Teach the client and family nonpharmacologic methods of pain management, such as relaxation, distraction, and cutaneous stimulation. *These techniques are especially useful when used in conjunction with pain medications and may also be useful in managing chronic pain.*
- Provide comfort measures, such as changing positions, back massage, oral care, skin care, and changing bed linens. *Basic comfort measures for personal cleanliness, skin care, and mobility promote physical and psychosocial well-being, lessening the perception of pain.*
- Provide client and family teaching and make referrals if necessary to assist with coping, financial resources, and home care. *The client (and family) with pain requires information about medications, noninvasive techniques for pain management, and sources of assistance with home-based care. The client with acute pain requires information about the expected course of pain resolution.*

## Using NANDA, NIC, and NOC

Chart 4–1 shows links between NANDA nursing diagnosis, NIC, and NOC when caring for the client in pain.

## Home Care

Teaching the client and family includes:

- Specific drugs to be taken, including the frequency, potential side effects, possible drug interactions, and any special precautions to be taken (such as taking with food or avoiding alcohol).
- How to take or administer the drugs (see Box 4–2).
- The importance of taking pain medications before the pain becomes severe.
- An explanation that the risk of addiction to pain medications is small when they are used for pain relief and management.
- The importance of scheduling periods of rest and sleep.

Suggest the following resources:

- Pain clinics
- Community support groups
- American Cancer Society
- American Pain Society

## Nursing Research

### Evidence-Based Practice for the Client Experiencing Pain

Pain is individualized to each person and to each painful experience. Nurses play a major role in assessing and managing pain, and must attend to the subjective quality of pain in order to successfully provide effective pain relief. The responses of the nurse to the client's expressions of pain may influence pain management, but limited research has explored this relationship. This study (Watt-Watson, Garkinel, Gallop, Stevens, & Streiner, 2000) was conducted to examine the relationship between nurses' empathic responses and their clients' pain intensity and analgesic administration after uncomplicated coronary artery bypass graft surgery. At the same time, the nurses' empathy and pain knowledge and beliefs were assessed.

The nurses were moderately empathic, and their responses did not significantly affect the clients' pain intensity or analgesia administered. The nurses showed a deficit of knowledge and misbeliefs about pain. It was postulated that the nurses may not have recognized the levels of pain intensity that occur with internal thoracic artery grafts. The researchers recommended having a better understanding of strategies to encourage clients to describe their pain experiences and to seek help. They also recommended that strategies are needed to encourage nurses to address the clients' pain experiences.

### IMPLICATIONS FOR NURSING

Findings from this study support other research that nurses (and other health care providers) are prone to undertreat pain. It is necessary for nurses to make greater efforts to understand the experiences of others. It is also necessary to make additional or more specific pain assessments; for example, although the clients' pain greatly increased with movement, this specific assessment was rarely conducted. Educational programs for nurses, related to pain, should include specific postoperative pain assessments, explore myths and misconceptions about pain medications, and clarify the individualized experiences of and responses to pain.

### Critical Thinking in Client Care

1. Reflect on your own experiences with pain. Will those experiences facilitate or hinder your assessments and interventions for clients in pain?
2. You are caring for a young man who has multiple injuries from a motorcycle accident. He tells you his pain is so bad that he "just wants to die." How would you respond?
3. You are caring for an 80-year-old man with diabetes who has had his left foot amputated for gangrene. He is restless and moaning. Another nurse tells you to give only one-half of the ordered dose of narcotics because "he is old and there is a danger of respiratory depression." What would you do?
4. Why do you think nurses tend to underestimate and undermedicate pain?

*Note. Adapted from* The Impact of Nurses' Empathic Responses on Patients' Pain Management in Acute Care *by J. Watt-Watson et al., 2000,* Nursing Research, 49(4), *pp. 191–200.*

## CHART 4–1 NANDA, NIC, AND NOC LINKAGES

### The Client Experiencing Pain

| NURSING DIAGNOSES | NURSING INTERVENTIONS | NURSING OUTCOMES |
|---|---|---|
| • Acute Pain<br>• Chronic Pain | • Pain Management<br>• Analgesic Administration<br>• Conscious Sedation<br>• PCA Assistance<br>• Cutaneous Stimulation<br>• Anxiety Reduction<br>• TENS<br>• Heat/Cold Application<br>• Accupressure<br>• Progressive Muscle Relaxation<br>• Environmental Management: Comfort | • Pain Control Behavior<br>• Pain: Disruptive Effects<br>• Pain Level |

*Note. Data from Nursing Outcomes Classification (NOC) by M. Johnson & M. Maas (Eds.), 1997, St. Louis: Mosby; Nursing Diagnoses: Definitions & Classification 2001–2002 by North American Nursing Diagnosis Association, 2001, Philadelphia: NANDA; Nursing Interventions Classification (NIC) by J.C. McCloskey & G. M. Bulechek (Eds.), 2000, St. Louis: Mosby. Reprinted by permission.*

## BOX 4–2 ■ Providing Long-Term Analgesia at Home

| Route | Drug | Nursing Implications |
|---|---|---|
| Oral | Oxycodone (OxyContin) | ■ Available in a timed-release formulation for 12-hour dosing and as fast-acting formulations (OxyIR, Oxyfast) for breakthrough pain. |
| Oral | Morphine (Kadian) | ■ Formulated of timed-release particles in a capsule. If client cannot swallow the capsule, it may be sprinkled over food or given by nasogastric or gastric tube. |
| Transdermal | Fentanyl (Duragesic) | ■ Absorbed slowly through the skin, allows 72-hour dose schedule. |
| Transdermal | Liocaine (Lidoderm) | ■ Effective for 12 hours for various neuropathic pains. Monitor clients also taking Class 1 antiarrhythmic drugs for increased effects. |
| Transmucosal | Fentanyl citrate (Actiq) | ■ A lozenge formulation used to treat breakthrough cancer pain in opioid-tolerant clients. |

## Nursing Care Plan
### A Client with Chronic Pain

Susan Akers, age 37, is currently being seen at an outpatient clinic for chronic nonmalignant pain. She works at a local paper factory. She has a 3-year history of neck and shoulder pain that usually is accompanied by headaches. She believes the pain is related to lifting objects at work, but it is now precipitated by activities of daily living. Susan is absent from work approximately three times a month and states that the absences are due to her pain and headaches. She has been seeking care in the local emergency department on the average of twice monthly for injections for pain. She does not regularly use medications but does take Darvocet-N 100 and Valium as needed (usually two to three times a day). Ms. Akers is divorced and has two children. She states that she has several friends in the area, but her parents and siblings live in another part of the United States.

### ASSESSMENT

During the nursing history, Susan rates her pain during an acute episode as a 7 on a 1 to 10 scale. She states that lifting objects and moving her hands and arms above shoulder level precipitates sharp pain. The pain never really goes away, but it does decrease with upper extremity rest. She says that when she lifts a lot at work, she has difficulty sleeping that night. She takes two Darvocet-N 100 tablets every 4 hours when the pain is severe, but does not get complete relief.

### DIAGNOSIS
• *Chronic pain* related to muscle inflammation

### EXPECTED OUTCOMES
• Return for follow-up visits with a journal of activities and pain experiences.
• After 3 to 5 days on regularly scheduled doses of pain medication, report a decrease in the level of pain from 7 to 3 or 4 on a 1 to 10 scale.
• Decrease number of absences from work.
• Modify activities at work and at home, especially when pain is intense.

*(continued on page 74)*

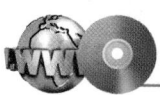

## Nursing Care Plan
## A Client with Chronic Pain *(continued)*

### PLANNING AND IMPLEMENTATION

- Encourage discussion of pain, and acknowledge belief in Susan's report of pain.
- Consult with a physician for a nonnarcotic analgesic with a minimum of side effects, and instruct in maintaining regular dosing schedules.
- For episodes of acute pain, take narcotic analgesics as soon as the pain begins and every 4 hours, while continuing the dosage of nonnarcotic analgesic.
- Teach one relaxation technique that is personally useful.
- Explore distraction techniques such as listening to music, watching comedies, or reading.
- Provide clinic phone number and instruct to call if pain is unrelieved with narcotic and nonnarcotic analgesics.

### EVALUATION

Susan returns for scheduled follow-up visits with a completed journal of her activities and associated pain. She reports that taking oral narcotic analgesics has relieved her pain and that within 3 weeks nonnarcotic analgesics brought her pain under control. She also reports that her supervisor has reassigned her to a position that requires no lifting. She now rates her pain at 2 or 3 on a 1 to 10 scale. She has missed only 1 day of work in the last 3 months and reports that her children and friends have helped with her household tasks when she has requested they do so.

### Critical Thinking in the Nursing Process

1. Describe three factors that support the statement, "Pain is a personal experience."
2. Susan asks you how often she should take her pain medications. You tell her to (a) take them on a regular basis or (b) wait until she experiences pain. Which action would you choose, and why?
3. Develop a care plan for Susan for the nursing diagnosis of *risk for constipation*. Why is this necessary?

See Evaluating Your Response in Appendix C.

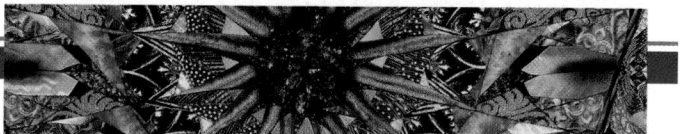

## EXPLORE MediaLink

NCLEX review questions, case studies, care plan activities, MediaLink applications, and other interactive resources for this chapter can be found on the Companion Website at www.prenhall.com/lemone.

Click on Chapter 4 to select the activities for this chapter. For animations, video clips, more NCLEX review questions, and an audio glossary, access the Student CD-ROM accompanying this textbook.

## TEST YOURSELF

1. Your neighbor has had lower back pain for 9 months. How would this pain be categorized?

   a. Acute pain
   b. Chronic pain
   c. Referred pain
   d. Somatic pain

2. Which of the following statements is a pain myth?

   a. "It is best to wait until a client has pain before giving medication."
   b. "Anxiety can cause pain; pain can cause anxiety."
   c. "Meperidine (Demerol) is no longer recommended for postoperative pain."
   d. "The rationale for use of a TENS unit is supported by the gate control theory."

3. You are taking a health history for a client who has taken an NSAID for several years. What would be an appropriate question to ask?

   a. "Do you understand what this drug could do to you?"

   b. "Have you ever vomited blood or had very dark stools?"
   c. "Do you know that you may become addicted to this drug?"
   d. "Have you noticed any problems with your breathing?"

4. You are replacing a transdermal pain medication. Where on the body would you place it?

   a. On one side of the buttocks
   b. Below the navel, midline on the abdomen
   c. On the anterior thigh
   d. On the upper torso

5. Which of the following statements would be most useful in determining the *quality* of a client's pain?

   a. "Tell me where you hurt."
   b. "Rate your pain on a scale of 0 to 10."
   c. "Describe what your pain feels like."
   d. "Tell me how this pain affects your sleep."

See Test Yourself answers in Appendix C.

# BIBLIOGRAPHY

Acello, B. (2000). Controlling pain. Facing fears about opioid addiction. *Nursing, 30*(5), 72.

Ackerman, C., & Turkoski, B. (2000). Using guided imagery to reduce pain and anxiety. *Home Healthcare Nurse, 18*(8), 524–530.

American Pain Society. 2001. *Pain: The fifth vital sign.* Available www.ampainsoc.org

American Pain Society Quality of Care Committee. (1995). Quality improvement guidelines for the treatment of acute pain and cancer pain. *Journal of the American Medical Association, 274*(23), 1874–1880.

Anonymous. (1997). The use of opioids for the treatment of chronic pain: A consensus statement from the American Academy of Pain Medicine and the American Pain Society. *Clinical Journal of Pain, 13*(1), 6–8.

Berkowitz, C. (1997). Epidural pain control—your job, too. *RN, 60*(8), 22–27.

Carpenito, L. (2000). *Nursing diagnosis: Application to clinical practice* (8th ed.). Philadelphia: Lippincott.

Coyne, M., Smith, J., Stein, D., Hieser, M., & Hoover, L. (1998). Describing pain management documentation. *MEDSURG Nursing, 7*(1), 45–51.

Dellasega, C., & Keiser, C. (1997). Pharmacologic approaches to chronic pain in the older adult. *American Journal of Primary Health Care, 22*(5), 20, 22–24, 26.

Joint Commission on Accreditation of Healthcare Organizations. (2000). *Joint Commission on Accreditation of Healthcare Organizations pain standards for 2001.* Available www.jcaho.org

Kodiath, M. (1997). Chronic pain: Contrasting two cultures. *Clinical Excellence for Nurse Practitioners, 1*(1), 59–61.

Lipson, J., Dibble, S., & Minarik, P. (1996). *Culture & nursing care: A pocket guide.* San Francisco: UCSF Nursing Press.

McCaffery, M. (1979). *Nursing management of the patient with pain.* Philadelphia: Lippincott.

McCaffery, M., & Beebe, A. (1999). *Pain: Clinical manual.* St. Louis: Mosby.

McCance, K., & Huether, S. (2002). *Pathophysiology: The biologic basic for disease in adults and children* (4th ed.). St. Louis: Mosby.

McKenry, L., & Salerno, E. (1998). *Pharmacology in nursing* (20th ed.). St. Louis: Mosby.

Melzack, R. (1975). The McGill Pain Questionnaire: Major properties and scoring methods. *Pain, 1,* 277.

Melzack, R., & Wall, P. (1965). Pain mechanisms: A new theory. *Science, 150,* 971–979.

_____ . (1968). Gate control theory of pain. In A. Soulairac, J. Cahn, & J. Carpentier (Eds.), *Pain: Proceedings of the International Association on Pain.* Baltimore: Williams & Wilkins.

Merboth, M. K., & Barnason, S. (2000). Managing pain: The fifth vital sign. *Nursing Clinics of North America, 35*(2), 375–383.

Pasero, C. (1999). Using agonist-antagonist opioids and antagonist drugs. *American Journal of Nursing, 99*(1), 20–21.

_____ . (2000). Oral patient-controlled analgesia. *American Journal of Nursing, 100*(3), 24.

Pasero, C., & McCaffrey, M. (1999). Opioids by the rectal route. *American Journal of Nursing, 99*(11), 20.

_____ . (2000). When patients can't report pain. *American Journal of Nursing, 100*(9), 22–23.

Porth, C. (2002). *Pathophysiology: Concepts of altered health states* (6th ed.). Philadelphia: Lippincott.

Seal, R. (1997). Choosing the right step on the analgesic ladder. *Community Nurse, 3*(2), 58–59.

U.S. Department of Health and Human Services. (1992). *Acute pain management: Operative or medical procedures and trauma* (AHCPR Publication No. 92-0032). Rockville, MD: Agency for Health Care Policy and Research, Public Health Service, USDHHS.

Victor, K. (2001). Properly assessing pain in the elderly. *RN, 64*(5), 45–49.

Waitman, J., & McCaffery, M. (2001). Meperidine—A liability. *American Journal of Nursing, 101*(1), 57–58.

Watt-Watson, J., Garfinkel, P., Gallop, R., Stevens, B., & Streiner, D. (2000). The impact of nurses' empathic responses on patients' pain management in acute care. *Nursing Research, 49*(4), 191–200.

Wilson, B. A., Shannon, M. T., & Stang, C. L. (2001). *Nursing drug guide 2001.* Upper Saddle River, NJ: Prentice Hall.

World Health Organization. (1986/1990). *Cancer pain relief.* Geneva: WHO.

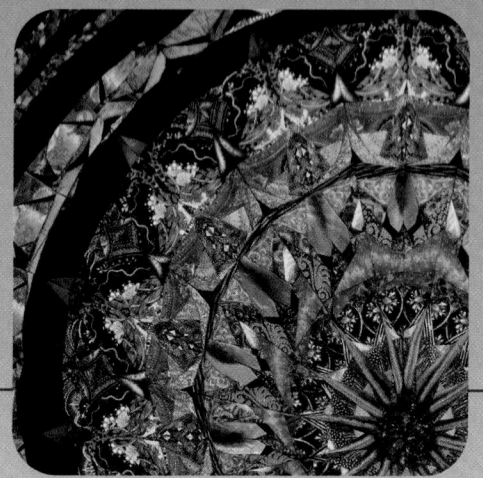

# CHAPTER 5

# Nursing Care of Clients with Altered Fluid, Electrolyte, or Acid-Base Balance

## MediaLink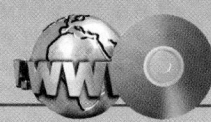

**www.prenhall.com/lemone**
Additional resources for this chapter can be found on the Student CD-ROM accompanying this textbook, and on the Companion Website at www.prenhall.com/lemone. Click on Chapter 5 to select the activities for this chapter.

**CD-ROM**
- Audio Glossary
- NCLEX Review

*Animations*
- Membrane Transport
- Acid-Base Balance
- Fluid Balance

**Companion Website**
- More NCLEX Review
- Case Study
    Hypernatremia
- Care Plan Activity
    Fluid Volume Deficit
    Hypocalcemia
- MediaLink Application
    Metabolic Acidosis and Type 1 Diabetes

## LEARNING OUTCOMES

After completing this chapter, you will be able to:

- Discuss the functions and regulatory mechanisms that maintain water and electrolyte balance in the body.

- Compare and contrast the causes, effects, and care of the client with fluid volume or electrolyte imbalance.

- Describe the pathophysiology and manifestations of imbalances of sodium, potassium, calcium, magnesium, and phosphorus.

- Discuss the causes and effects of acid-base imbalances.

- Identify laboratory and diagnostic tests used to diagnose and monitor treatment of fluid, electrolyte, and acid-base disorders.

- Recognize normal and abnormal values of electrolytes in the blood.

- Use arterial blood gas findings to identify the type of acid-base imbalance present in a client.

- Provide teaching about diet and medications used to treat or prevent electrolyte disorders.

- Use the nursing process as a framework to provide individualized nursing care to clients with fluid, electrolyte, and acid-base disorders.

Changes in the normal distribution and composition of body fluids often occur in response to illness and trauma. These changes affect fluid balance of the intracellular and extracellular compartments of the body, the concentration of electrolytes within fluid compartments, and the body's hydrogen ion concentration (pH). Normal physiologic processes depend on a relatively stable state in the internal environment of the body. The fluid volume, electrolyte composition, and pH of both intracellular and extracellular spaces must remain constant within a relatively narrow range to maintain health and life.

**Homeostasis** is the body's tendency to maintain a state of physiologic balance in the presence of constantly changing conditions. Homeostasis is necessary if the body is to function optimally at a cellular level and as a total organism. Homeostasis depends on multiple factors in both the external and internal environments, such as available oxygen in the air and nutrients in food, as well as normal body temperature, respiration, and digestive processes. The normal volume, composition, distribution, and pH of body fluids reflect a state of homeostasis.

The goal in managing fluid, electrolyte, and acid-base imbalances is to reestablish and maintain a normal balance. Nursing care includes assessing clients who are likely to develop imbalances, monitoring clients for early manifestations, and implementing collaborative and nursing interventions to prevent or correct imbalances. Effective nursing interventions require an understanding of the multiple processes that maintain fluid, electrolyte, and acid-base balance and an understanding of the causes and treatment of imbalances that occur.

Mechanisms that maintain normal fluid and electrolyte balance are discussed first, followed by sections on fluid imbalances and electrolyte imbalances. Discussion of normal acid-base balance precedes discussion of acid-base imbalances. Case studies related to selected fluid, electrolyte, and acid-base disorders are found throughout the chapter.

## OVERVIEW OF NORMAL FLUID AND ELECTROLYTE BALANCE

Fluid and electrolyte balance in the body involves regulatory mechanisms that maintain the composition, distribution, and movement of fluids and electrolytes. This section provides an overview of fluid and electrolyte balance in the body. It is followed by discussion of fluid volume and electrolyte balance disorders.

## Body Fluid Composition

Body fluid is composed of water and various dissolved substances (solutes).

### Water

Water is the primary component of body fluids. It functions in several ways to maintain normal cellular function. Water:

- Provides a medium for the transport and exchange of nutrients and other substances such as oxygen, carbon dioxide, and metabolic wastes to and from cells.
- Provides a medium for metabolic reactions within cells.
- Assists in regulating body temperature through the evaporation of perspiration.

- Provides form for body structure and acts as a shock absorber.
- Provides insulation.
- Acts as a lubricant.

Total body water constitutes about 60% of the total body weight, but this amount varies with age, gender, and the amount of body fat. Total body water decreases with aging; in people over age 65, body water may decrease to 45% to 50% of total body weight. Fat cells contain comparatively little water: In the person who is obese, the proportion of water to total body weight is less than in the person of average weight; in a person who is very thin, the proportion of water to total body weight is greater than in the person of average weight. Adult females have a greater ratio of fat to lean tissue mass than adult males; therefore, they have a lower percentage of body water content.

To maintain normal fluid balance, body water intake and output should be approximately equal. The average fluid intake and output usually is about 2500 mL over a 24-hour period. Table 5-1 shows the sources of fluid gain and loss.

### Electrolytes

Body fluids contain both water molecules and chemical compounds. These chemical compounds can either remain intact in solution or separate (dissociate) into discrete particles. **Electrolytes** are substances that dissociate in solution to form charged particles called ions. *Cations* are positively charged electrolytes; *anions* are negatively charged electrolytes. For example, sodium chloride (NaCl) in solution dissociates into a sodium ion, a cation carrying a positive charge ($Na^+$); and a chloride ion, an anion carrying a negative charge ($Cl^-$). Electrolytes may be *univalent,* with only one unit of electrical charge, such as sodium ($Na^+$) and chloride ($Cl^-$); or they may be *divalent,* carrying two units of electrical charge, such as magnesium ($Mg^{2+}$) and phosphate ($HPO_4^{2-}$).

Electrolytes have many functions. They:

- Assist in regulating water balance.
- Help regulate and maintain acid-base balance.
- Contribute to enzyme reactions.
- Are essential for neuromuscular activity.

The concentration of electrolytes in body fluids generally is measured in milliequivalents per liter of water (mEq/L).

| TABLE 5-1 Balanced Fluid Gain and Loss for an Adult | | |
|---|---|---|
| | **Source** | **Amount (mL)** |
| **Gain** | Fluids taken orally | 1200 |
| | Water in food | 1000 |
| | Water as by-product of food metabolism | 300 ↓ |
| | Total | 2500 |
| | | ↑ |
| **Loss** | Urine | 1500 |
| | Feces | 200 |
| | Perspiration | 300 |
| | Respiration | 500 |

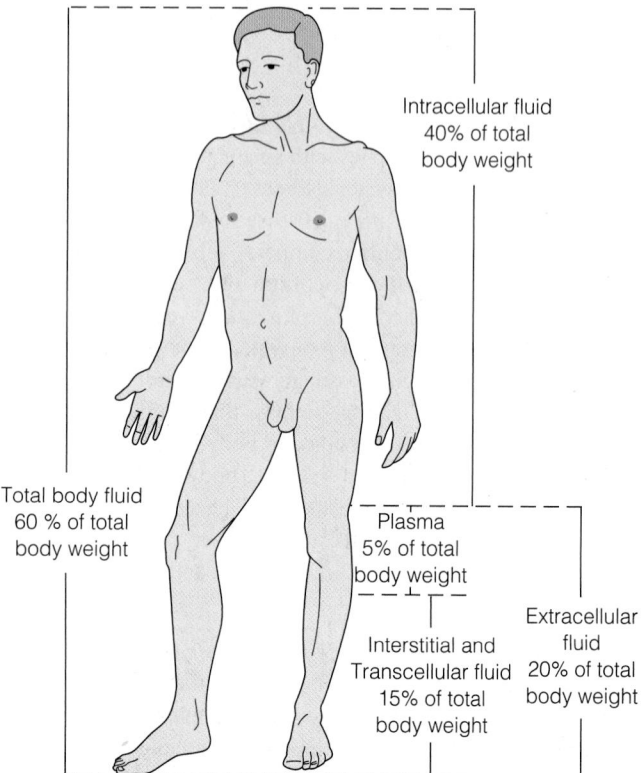

Intracellular fluid
40% of total
body weight

Total body fluid
60 % of total
body weight

Plasma
5% of total
body weight

Interstitial and
Transcellular fluid
15% of total
body weight

Extracellular
fluid
20% of total
body weight

**Figure 5–1** ■ The major fluid compartments of the body.

A milliequivalent is a measure of the chemical combining power of the ion. For example, 100 mEq of sodium ($Na^+$) can combine with 100 mEq of chloride ($Cl^-$) to form sodium chloride (NaCl). Sodium, potassium, and chloride usually are measured in milliequivalents. In some cases, the amount of an electrolyte in body fluid may be measured by weight in milligrams per 100 mL (1 deciliter [dL]) of water (mg/dL). Calcium, magnesium, and phosphorus often are measured by weight in milligrams per deciliter.

## Body Fluid Distribution

Body fluid is classified by its location inside or outside of cells. *Intracellular fluid (ICF)* is found within cells. It accounts for approximately 40% of total body weight (Figure 5–1 ■). ICF is essential for normal cell function, providing a medium for metabolic processes. *Extracellular fluid (ECF)* is located outside of cells. It accounts for approximately 20% of the total body weight. ECF is classified by location.

- Interstitial fluid is located in the spaces between most of the cells of the body. It accounts for approximately 15% of total body weight.
- Intravascular fluid, called plasma, is contained within the arteries, veins, and capillaries. It accounts for approximately 5% of total body weight.
- Transcellular fluid includes urine; digestive secretions; perspiration; and cerebrospinal, pleural, synovial, intraocular, gonadal, and pericardial fluids.

A trace amount of water is found in bone, cartilage, and other dense connective tissues; this water is not exchangeable with other body fluids.

ECF is the transport medium that carries oxygen and nutrients to and waste products from the cells. For example, plasma transports oxygen from the lungs and glucose from the digestive system to the tissues. These solutes diffuse through the capillary wall into the interstitial space, and from there across the cell membrane into the cells. Waste products of metabolism (e.g., carbon dioxide and hydrogen ion) diffuse from the intracellular space into the interstitial space, and from there into plasma via the capillary walls. Plasma then transports these waste products to the lungs and kidneys for elimination.

The concentration of various electrolytes in ICF and ECF differs significantly, as shown in Figure 5–2 ■. ICF contains high concentrations of potassium ($K^+$), magnesium ($Mg^{2+}$), and phosphate ($PO_4^{2-}$), as well as other solutes such as glucose and oxygen. Sodium ($Na^+$), chloride ($Cl^-$), and bicarbonate ($HCO_3^-$) are the principal extracellular electrolytes. The high sodium concentration in ECF is essential to regulating body fluid volume. The concentration of potassium in ECF is low. There is a minimal difference in electrolyte concentration between plasma and interstitial fluid. Normal values for electrolytes in plasma are shown in Table 5–2.

The body fluid compartments are separated by several types of membranes.

- Cell membranes separate interstitial fluid from intracellular fluid.
- Capillary membranes separate plasma from interstitial fluid.
- Epithelial membranes separate transcellular fluid from interstitial fluid and plasma. These membranes include the mucosa of the stomach, intestines, and gallbladder; the pleural, peritoneal, and synovial membranes; and the tubules of the kidney.

A cell membrane consists of layers of lipid and protein molecules. The layering of these molecules controls the passage of fluid and solutes between the cell and interstitial fluid. The cell membrane is selectively permeable; that is, it allows the passage of water, oxygen, carbon dioxide, and small water-soluble molecules, but bars proteins and other intracellular colloids.

The capillary membrane separating the plasma from the interstitial space is made of squamous epithelial cells. Pores in the membrane allow solute molecules (such as glucose and sodium), dissolved gases, and water to cross the membrane. Minute amounts of albumin and other proteins can also pass through the pores of a capillary membrane, but normally plasma proteins stay in the intravascular compartment.

### Body Fluid Movement

Four chemical and physiologic processes control the movement of fluid, electrolytes, and other molecules across membranes between the intracellular and interstitial space and the interstitial space and plasma. These processes are osmosis, diffusion, filtration, and active transport.

***OSMOSIS.*** The process by which water moves across a selectively permeable membrane from an area of lower solute concentration to an area of higher solute concentration is **osmosis** (Figure 5–3 ■). A *selectively permeable membrane* allows water molecules to cross but is relatively impermeable to dissolved substances (*solutes*). Osmosis continues until the solute

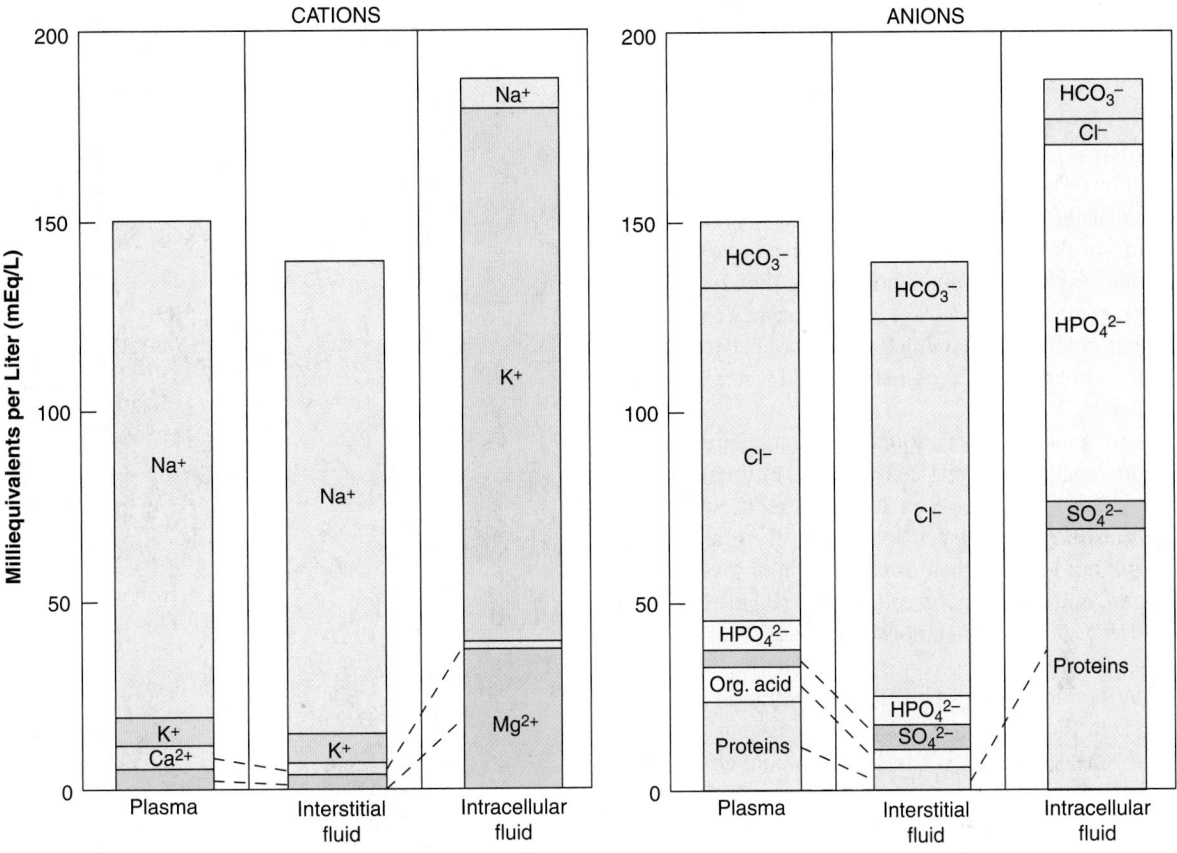

**Figure 5–2** ■ Electrolyte composition (cations and anions) of body fluid compartments.

*From* Fundamentals of Anatomy and Physiology 4e, *by Martini, Frederic. © Reprinted by permission of Pearson Education, Inc., Upper Saddle River, NJ.*

| TABLE 5-2 Normal Values for Electrolytes and Serum Osmolality | |
|---|---|
| **Serum Component** | **Values** |
| Electrolytes | |
| Sodium (Na$^+$) | 135–145 mEq/L |
| Chloride (Cl$^-$) | 98–106 mEq/L |
| Bicarbonate (HCO$_3$) | 22–26 mEq/L |
| Calcium (Ca$^{2+}$) (total) | 8.5–10 mg/dL |
| Potassium (K$^+$) | 3.5–5.0 mEq/L |
| Phosphate/inorganic phosphorus (PO$_4^{-2}$) | 1.7–2.6 mEq/L (2.5–4.5 mg/dL) |
| Magnesium (Mg$^{2+}$) | 1.6–2.6 mg/dL (1.3–2.1 mEq/L) |
| Serum osmolality | 275–295 mOsm/kg |

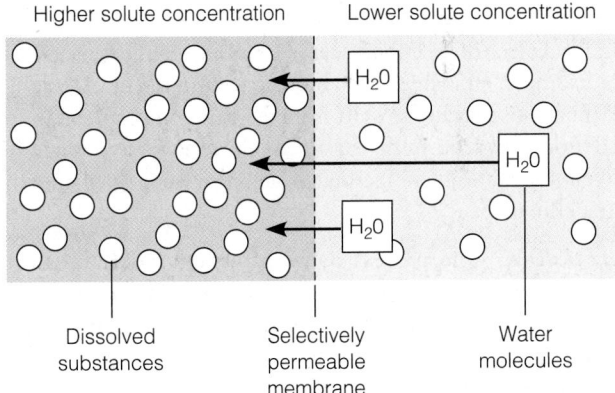

**Figure 5–3** ■ Osmosis. Water molecules move through a selectively permeable membrane from an area of low solute concentration to an area of high solute concentration.

concentration on both sides of the membrane is equal. For example, if pure water and a sodium chloride solution are separated by a selectively permeable membrane, then water molecules will move across the membrane to the sodium chloride solution. Osmosis is the primary process that controls body fluid movement between the ICF and ECF compartments.

**Osmolarity and Osmolality.**   The concentration of a solution may be expressed as the osmolarity or osmolality of the solution. *Osmolarity* refers to the amount of solutes per liter

of solution (by volume); it is reported in milliosmoles per liter (mOsm/L) in a solution. *Osmolality* refers to the number of solutes per kilogram of water (by weight); it is reported in milliosmoles per kilogram (mOsm/kg). Because osmotic activity in the body is regulated by the number of active particles (solutes) per kilogram of water, osmolality is used to describe the concentration of body fluids. The normal osmolality of both ICF and ECF ranges between 275 and 295 mOsm/kg. The osmolality of the extracellular fluid depends chiefly on sodium concentration. Serum osmolality may be estimated by doubling the serum sodium concentration (approximately 142 mEq/L).

**Osmotic Pressure and Tonicity.** The power of a solution to draw water across a membrane is known as the *osmotic pressure* of the solution. The composition of interstitial fluid and intravascular plasma is essentially the same except for a higher concentration of proteins in the plasma. These proteins (especially albumin) exert osmotic pressure, pulling fluid from the interstitial space into the intravascular compartment. This osmotic activity is important in maintaining fluid balance between the interstitial and intravascular spaces, helping hold water within the vascular system.

*Tonicity* refers to the effect a solution's osmotic pressure has on water movement across the cell membrane of cells within that solution. *Isotonic* solutions have the same concentration of solutes as plasma. Cells placed in an isotonic solution will neither shrink nor swell as there is no net gain or loss of water within the cell, and no change in cell volume (Figure 5–4 A ■). Normal saline (0.9% sodium chloride solution) is an example of an isotonic solution.

*Hypertonic* solutions have a greater concentration of solutes than plasma. In their presence, water is drawn out of a cell, causing it to shrink (Figure 5–4B). A 3% sodium chloride solution is hypertonic. *Hypotonic* solutions (such as 0.45% sodium chloride) have a lower solute concentration than plasma (Figure 5–4C). When red blood cells are placed in a hypotonic solution, water moves into the cells, causing them to swell and rupture (*hemolyze*).

The concepts of osmotic draw and tonicity are important in understanding the pathophysiologic changes that occur with fluid and electrolyte imbalances, as well as treatment measures. For example, an increased sodium concentration of extracellular fluid causes water to shift from the ICF compartment to the ECF compartment. In this case, administering a hypotonic intravenous solution will facilitate water movement back into the intracellular space.

*DIFFUSION.* The process by which solute molecules move from an area of high solute concentration to an area of low solute concentration to become evenly distributed is **diffusion** (Figure 5–5 ■). The two types of diffusion are simple and facilitated diffusion. *Simple diffusion* occurs by the random movement of particles through a solution. Water, carbon dioxide, oxygen, and solutes move between plasma and the interstitial space by simple diffusion through the capillary membrane. Water and solutes move into the cell by passing through protein channels or by dissolving in the lipid cell membrane. *Facilitated diffusion*, also called carrier-mediated diffusion, allows large water-soluble molecules, such as glucose and amino acids, to diffuse across cell membranes. Proteins embedded in the cell membrane function as *carriers*, helping large molecules cross the membrane.

The rate of diffusion is influenced by a number of factors, such as the concentration of solute and the availability of carrier proteins in the cell membrane. The effect of both simple and facilitated diffusion is to establish equal concentrations of the molecules on both sides of a membrane.

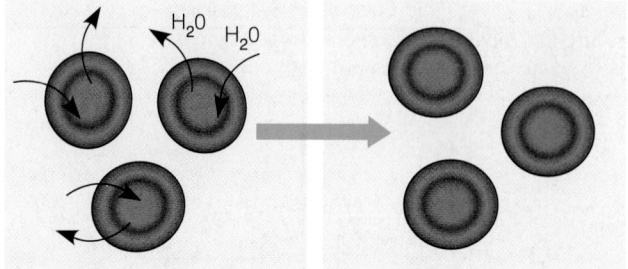

**A** Isotonic solution

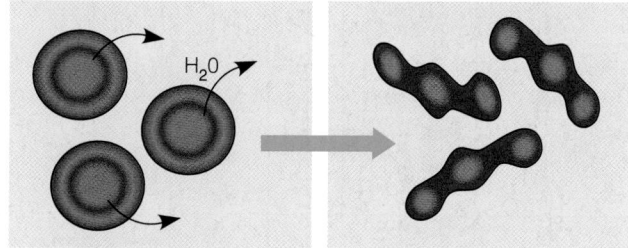

**B** Hypertonic solution

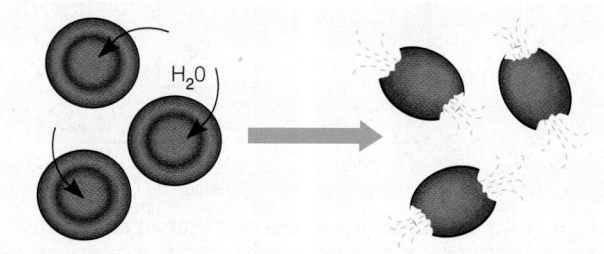

**C** Hypotonic solution

**Figure 5–4 ■** The effect of tonicity on red blood cells. *A,* In an isotonic solution, RBCs neither gain nor lose water. *B,* In a hypertonic solution, cells lose water and shrink in size. *C,* In a hypotonic solution, cells absorb water and may burst (hemolysis).

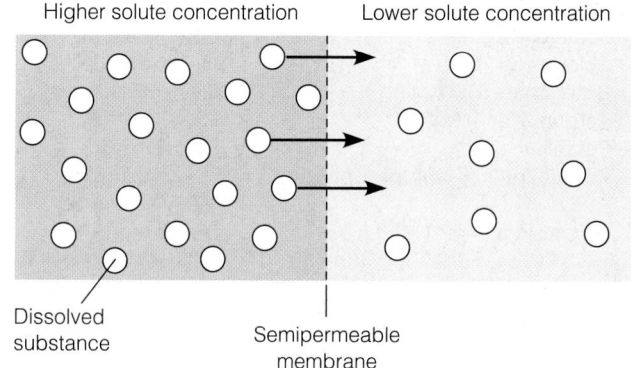

**Figure 5–5 ■** Diffusion. Solute molecules move through a semipermeable membrane from an area of high solute concentration to an area of low solute concentration.

*FILTRATION.* The process by which water and dissolved substances (solutes) move from an area of high hydrostatic pressure to an area of low hydrostatic pressure is **filtration**. This usually occurs across capillary membranes. *Hydrostatic pres-*

**Figure 5–6** ■ Fluid balance between the intravascular and interstitial spaces is maintained in the capillary beds by a balance of filtration at the arterial end and osmotic draw at the venous end.

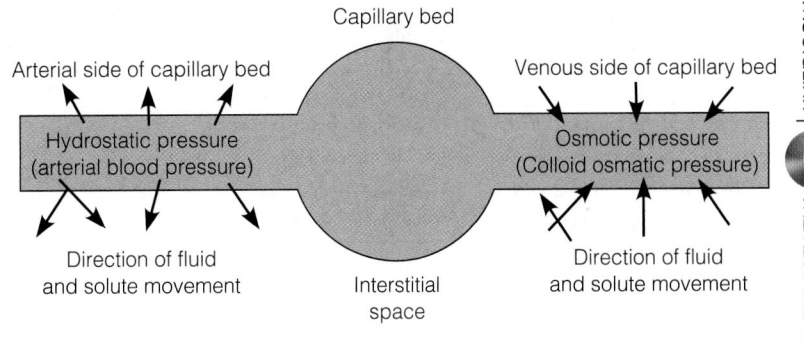

sure is created by the pumping action of the heart and gravity against the capillary wall. Filtration occurs in the glomerulus of the kidneys, as well as at the arterial end of capillaries.

A balance of hydrostatic (filtration) pressure and osmotic pressure regulates the movement of water between the intravascular and interstitial spaces in the capillary beds of the body. Hydrostatic pressure within the arterial end of the capillary pushes water into the interstitial space. Hydrostatic pressure within the interstitial space opposes this movement to some degree. At the venous end of the capillary, the osmotic force of plasma proteins draws fluid back into the capillary (Figure 5–6 ■).

***ACTIVE TRANSPORT.*** **Active transport** allows molecules to move across cell membranes and epithelial membranes against a concentration gradient. This movement requires energy (adenosine triphosphate, or ATP) and a carrier mechanism to maintain a higher concentration of a substance on one side of the membrane than on the other. The sodium-potassium pump is an important example of active transport (Figure 5–7 ■). High concentrations of potassium in intracellular fluids and of sodium in extracellular fluids are maintained because cells actively transport potassium from interstitial fluid (where the concentration of potassium is about 5 mEq/L) into intracellular fluid (where the potassium concentration is about 150 mEq/L).

## Body Fluid Regulation

Homeostasis requires several regulatory mechanisms and processes to maintain the balance between fluid intake and excretion. These include thirst, the kidneys, renin-angiotensin-aldosterone mechanism, antidiuretic hormone, and atrial natriuretic factor. These mechanisms affect the volume, distribution, and composition of body fluids.

## Thirst

Thirst is the primary regulator of water intake. Thirst plays an important role in maintaining fluid balance and preventing dehydration. The thirst center, located in the brain, is stimulated when the blood volume drops because of water losses or when serum osmolality (solute concentration) increases (Figure 5–8 ■).

The thirst mechanism is highly effective in regulating extracellular sodium levels. Increased sodium in ECF causes the serum osmolality to increase, stimulating the thirst center. Fluid intake in turn reduces the sodium concentration of ECF

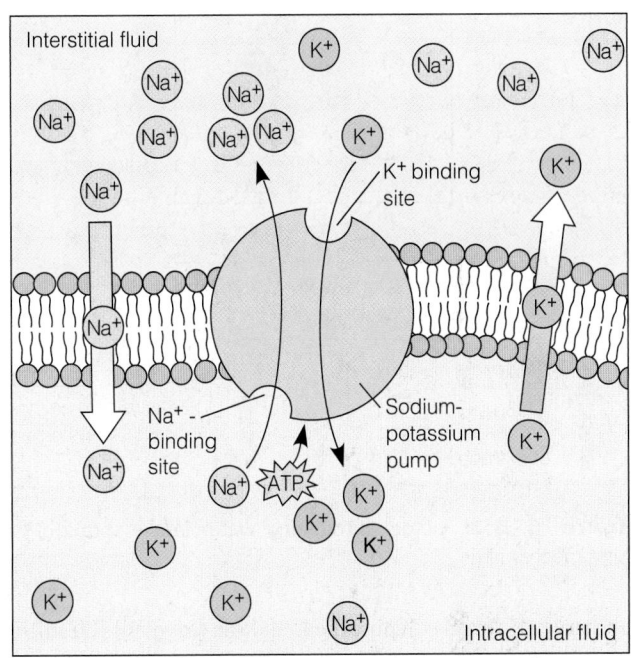

**Figure 5–7** ■ The sodium-potassium pump. Sodium and potassium ions are moved across the cell membranes against their concentration gradients. This active transport process is fueled by energy from adenosine triphosphate (ATP).

and lowers serum osmolality. Conversely, a drop in serum sodium and low serum osmolality inhibit the thirst center.

**PRACTICE ALERT** *The thirst mechanism declines with aging, making older adults more vulnerable to dehydration and hyperosmolality (high serum osmolality). Clients with an altered level of consciousness or who are unable to respond to thirst also are at risk.* ■

## Kidneys

The kidneys are primarily responsible for regulating fluid volume and electrolyte balance in the body. They regulate the volume and osmolality of body fluids by controlling the excretion of water and electrolytes. In adults, about 170 L of plasma are filtered through the glomeruli every day. By selectively reabsorbing water and electrolytes, the kidneys maintain the volume and osmolality of body fluids. About 99% of the

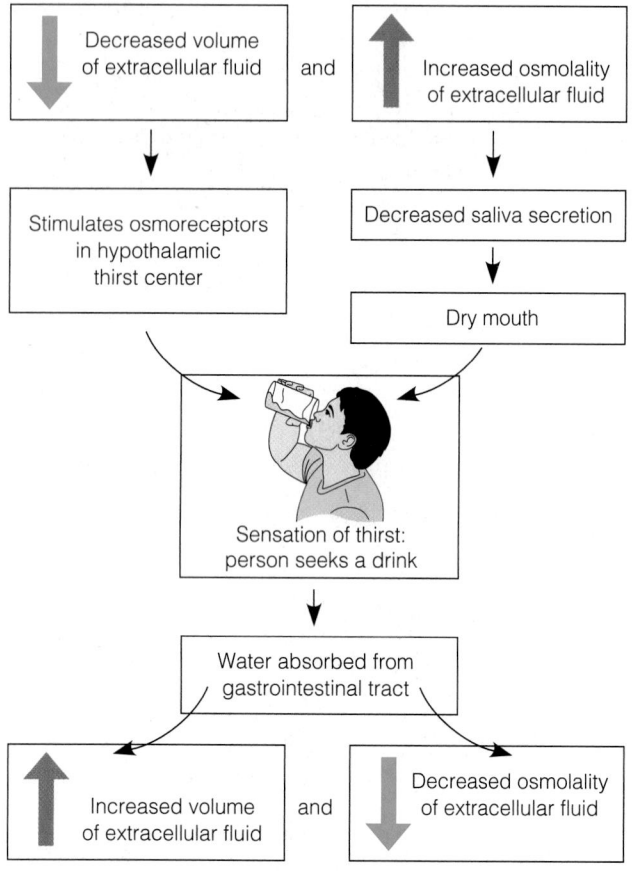

**Figure 5–8** ■ Factors stimulating water intake through the thirst mechanism.

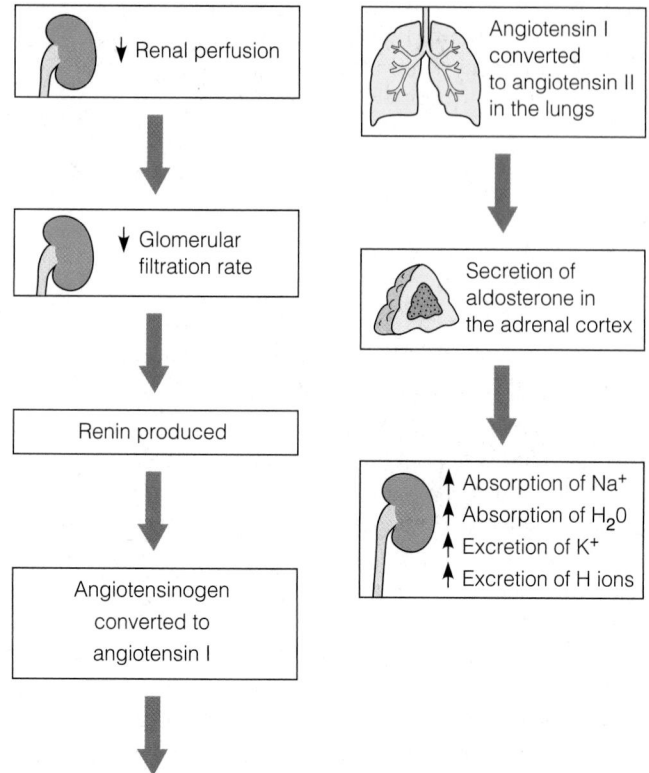

**Figure 5–9** ■ The renin-angiotensin-aldosterone system. Decreased blood volume and renal perfusion set off a chain of reactions leading to release of aldosterone from the adrenal cortex. Increased levels of aldosterone regulate serum K+ and Na+, blood pressure, and water balance through effects on the kidney tubules.

glomerular filtrate is reabsorbed, and only about 1500 mL of urine is produced over a 24-hour period.

## Renin-Angiotensin-Aldosterone System

The renin-angiotensin-aldosterone system works to maintain intravascular fluid balance and blood pressure. A fall in blood flow or blood pressure to the kidneys stimulates specialized receptors in the juxtaglomerular cells of the nephrons to produce *renin*, an enzyme. Renin converts angiotensinogen (a plasma protein) in the circulating blood into angiotensin I. Angiotensin I travels through the bloodstream to the lungs, where it is converted to angiotensin II by angiotensin-converting enzyme (ACE). Angiotensin II is a potent vasoconstrictor; it raises the blood pressure. It also stimulates the thirst mechanism to promote fluid intake and acts directly on the kidneys, causing them to retain sodium and water. Angiotensin II stimulates the adrenal cortex to release aldosterone. Aldosterone promotes sodium and water retention in the distal nephron of the kidney, restoring blood volume (Figure 5–9 ■).

## Antidiuretic Hormone

Antidiuretic hormone (ADH) regulates water excretion from the kidneys. Osmoreceptors in the hypothalamus respond to increases in serum osmolality and decreases in blood volume, stimulating ADH production and release. ADH acts on the distal tubules of the kidney, making them more permeable to water and thus increasing water reabsorption. With increased water reabsorption, urine

output falls, blood volume is restored, and serum osmolality drops as the water dilutes body fluids (Figure 5–10 ■).

Two disorders of ADH production illustrate this effect. First, diabetes insipidus is a condition characterized by a deficiency in ADH production. The lack of ADH causes the distal tubules and collecting ducts of the kidney to be impermeable to water, resulting in copious, very dilute urine output. ADH is not released in response to resulting serum hyperosmolality, but the thirst mechanism is stimulated and the client drinks additional fluids, maintaining high urine output. Second, in the syndrome of inappropriate ADH secretion (SIADH), excess ADH is released. Increased water reabsorption causes increased fluid volume and scant, concentrated urine output. These diseases of the pituitary gland are discussed in Chapter 17. ⊗

## Atrial Natriuretic Factor

**Atrial natriuretic factor (ANF)** is a hormone released by atrial muscle cells in response to distension from fluid overload. ANF affects several body systems, including the cardiovascular, renal, neural, gastrointestinal, and endocrine systems, but it primarily affects the renin-angiotensin-aldosterone system. ANF opposes this system by inhibiting renin secretion and blocking the secretion and sodium-retaining effects of aldosterone. As a result, ANF promotes sodium wasting and diuresis (increased urine output) and causes vasodilation.

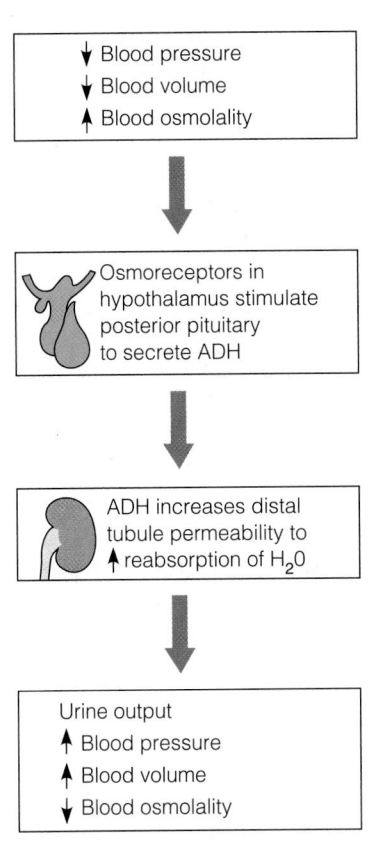

**Figure 5–10** ■ Antidiuretic hormone (ADH) release and effect. Increased serum osmolality or a fall in blood volume stimulates the release of ADH from the posterior pituitary. ADH increases the permeability of distal tubules, promoting water reabsorption.

FLUID VOLUME DEFICIT CARE PLAN

# FLUID AND ELECTROLYTE IMBALANCES

## THE CLIENT WITH FLUID VOLUME DEFICIT

**Fluid volume deficit (FVD)** is a decrease in intravascular, interstitial, and/or intracellular fluid in the body. Fluid volume deficits may be due to excessive fluid losses, insufficient fluid intake, or failure of regulatory mechanisms and fluid shifts within the body. Fluid volume deficit is a relatively common problem that may exist alone or in combination with other electrolyte or acid-base imbalances. The term **dehydration** refers to loss of water alone, even though it often is used interchangeably with fluid volume deficit.

## PATHOPHYSIOLOGY

The most common cause of fluid volume deficit is excessive loss of gastrointestinal fluids from vomiting, diarrhea, gastrointestinal suctioning, intestinal fistulas, and intestinal drainage. Other causes of fluid losses include:

- Excessive renal losses of water and sodium from diuretic therapy, renal disorders, or endocrine disorders.
- Water and sodium losses during sweating from excessive exercise or increased environmental temperature.
- Hemorrhage.
- Chronic abuse of laxatives and/or enemas.

Inadequate fluid intake may result from lack of access to fluids, inability to request or to swallow fluids, oral trauma, or altered thirst mechanisms. Older adults are at particular risk for fluid volume deficit (see Nursing Care of the Older Adult box on page 84).

Fluid volume deficit can develop slowly or rapidly, depending on the type of fluid loss. Loss of extracellular fluid volume can lead to **hypovolemia,** decreased circulating blood volume. Electrolytes often are lost along with fluid, resulting in an **isotonic fluid volume deficit.** When both water and electrolytes are lost, the serum sodium level remains normal, although levels of other electrolytes such as potassium may fall. Fluid is drawn into the vascular compartment from the interstitial spaces as the body attempts to maintain tissue perfusion. This eventually depletes fluid in the intracellular compartment as well.

Hypovolemia stimulates regulatory mechanisms to maintain circulation. The sympathetic nervous system is stimulated, as is the thirst mechanism. ADH and aldosterone are released, prompting sodium and water retention by the kidneys.

### Third Spacing

**Third spacing** is a shift of fluid from the vascular space into an area where it is not available to support normal physiologic processes. The trapped fluid represents a volume loss and is

## Nursing Care of the Older Adult

### FLUID VOLUME DEFICIT

The older adult is at risk for fluid volume deficit from a variety of factors. Physical changes include the following:

- The perception of thirst decreases with aging.
- As muscle tissue declines with aging, the amount of total body water decreases.
- Renal blood flow and glomerular filtration decline with aging, and the ability to concentrate urine decreases.
- Body temperature regulation is less effective with aging.

Functional changes of aging also affect fluid balance:

- Fear of incontinence can lead to self-limiting of fluid intake.

- Physical disabilities associated with age-related illnesses, such as arthritis or stroke, may limit access to fluids.
- Cognitive impairments can interfere with recognition of thirst and the ability to respond to it.

Older adults who have self-care deficits, or who are confused, depressed, tube fed, on bed rest, or taking medications (such as sedatives, tranquilizers, diuretics, and laxatives) are at greatest risk for fluid volume deficits. Older adults without air conditioning are at risk during extremely hot weather.

---

unavailable for normal physiologic processes. Fluid may be sequestered in the abdomen or bowel, or in such other actual or potential body spaces as the pleural or peritoneal space. Fluid may also become trapped within soft tissues following trauma or burns. Assessing the extent of fluid volume deficit resulting from third spacing is difficult. It may not be reflected by changes in weight or intake-and-output records, and it may not become apparent until after organ malfunction occurs (Metheny, 2000).

## MANIFESTATIONS

With a rapid fluid loss (such as hemorrhage or uncontrolled vomiting), manifestations of hypovolemia develop rapidly. When the loss of fluid occurs more gradually, the client's fluid volume may be very low before symptoms develop. The *Multisystem Effects of Fluid Volume Deficit* are illustrated on page 85.

Rapid weight loss is a good indicator of fluid volume deficit. Each liter of body fluid weighs about 1 kg (2.2 lb). Loss of interstitial fluid causes skin turgor to diminish. When pinched, the skin of a client with FVD remains elevated. Loss of skin elasticity with aging makes this assessment finding less accurate in older adults. Tongue turgor is not generally affected by age; therefore, assessing the size, dryness, and longitudinal furrows of the tongue may be a more accurate indicator of fluid volume deficit.

Postural or orthostatic hypotension is a sign of hypovolemia. A drop of more than 15 mmHg in systolic blood pressure when changing from a lying to standing position often indicates loss of intravascular volume. Venous pressure falls as well, causing flat neck veins, even when the client is recumbent. Loss of intravascular fluid causes the hematocrit to increase.

Compensatory mechanisms to conserve water and sodium and maintain circulation account for many of the manifestations of fluid volume deficit, such as tachycardia; pale, cool skin (vasoconstriction); and decreased urine output. The specific gravity of urine increases as water is reabsorbed in the tubules. Table 5–3 compares assessment findings for fluid deficit and fluid excess.

## COLLABORATIVE CARE

The primary goals of care related to fluid volume deficit are to prevent deficits in clients at risk and to correct deficits and their underlying causes. Depending on the acuity of the imbalance, treatment may include replacement of fluids and electrolytes by the intravenous, oral, or enteral route. When possible, the oral or enteral route is preferred for administering fluids. In acute situations, however, intravenous fluid administration is necessary.

### Diagnostic Tests

Laboratory and diagnostic tests may be ordered when fluid volume deficit is suspected. Such tests measure:

- *Serum electrolytes.* In an isotonic fluid deficit, sodium levels are within normal limits; when the loss is water only, sodium levels are high. Decreases in potassium are common.
- *Serum osmolality.* To help differentiate isotonic fluid loss from water loss. With water loss, osmolality is high; it may be within normal limits with an isotonic fluid loss.
- *Serum hemoglobin and hematocrit.* The hematocrit often is elevated due to loss of intravascular volume and hemoconcentration.
- *Urine specific gravity and osmolality.* As the kidneys conserve water, both the specific gravity and osmolality of urine increase.
- *Central venous pressure (CVP).* The CVP measures the mean pressure in the superior vena cava or right atrium, providing an accurate assessment of fluid volume status. The technique for measuring CVP is outlined in Box 5–1.

### Fluid Management

A fluid challenge may be done to evaluate fluid volume when urine output is low and cardiac or renal function is questionable. A fluid challenge helps prevent fluid volume overload resulting from intravenous fluid therapy when cardiac or renal function is compromised. Nursing responsibilities for a fluid challenge are as follows:

1. Obtain and document baseline vital signs, breath sounds, urine output, and mental status.

# Multisystem Effects of Fluid Volume Deficit (FVD)

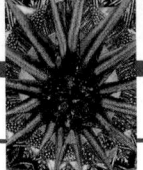

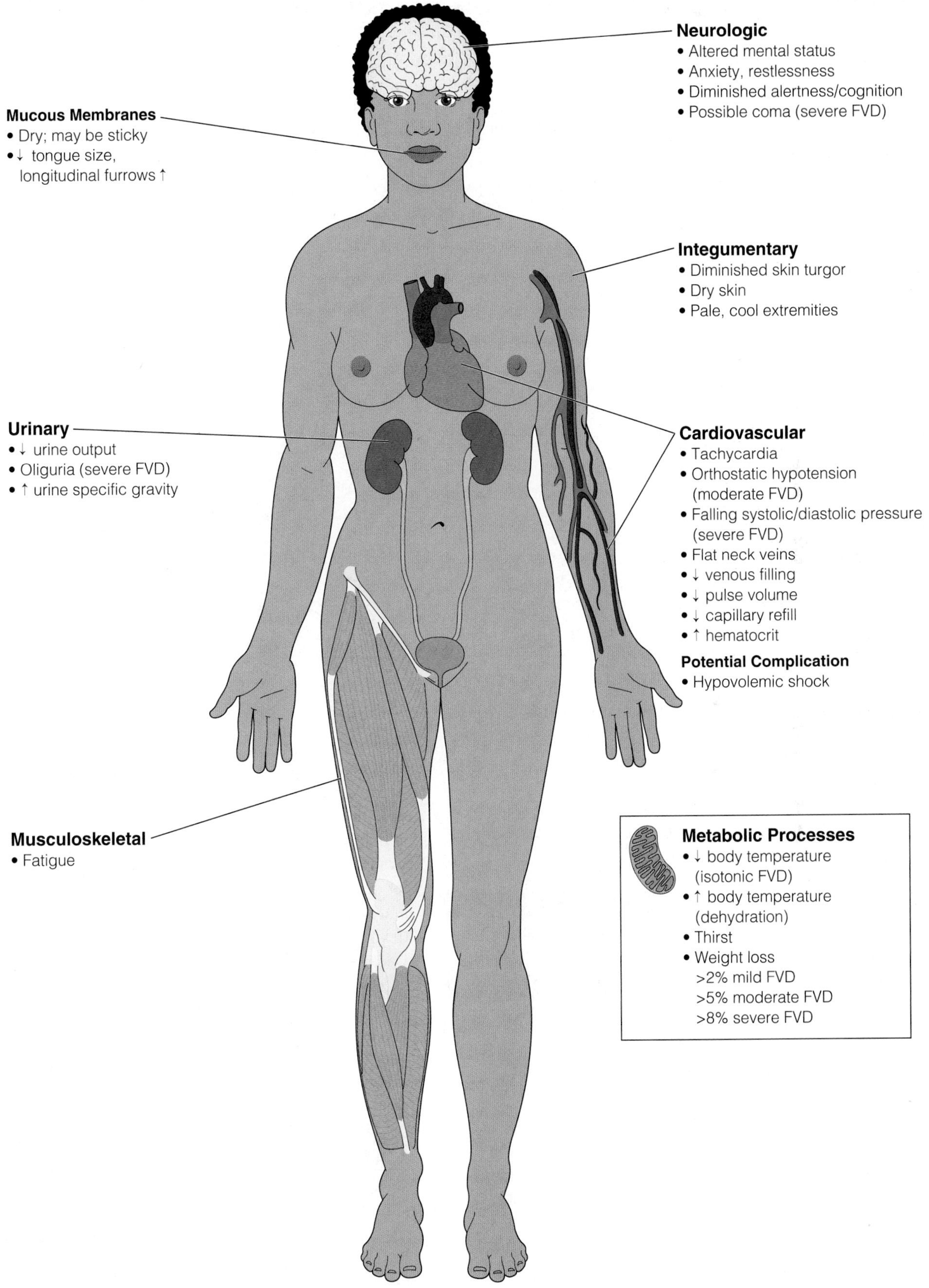

Neurologic
• Altered mental status
• Anxiety, restlessness
• Diminished alertness/cognition
• Possible coma (severe FVD)
Mucous Membranes
• Dry; may be sticky
• ↓ tongue size, longitudinal furrows ↑
Integumentary
• Diminished skin turgor
• Dry skin
• Pale, cool extremities
Urinary
• ↓ urine output
• Oliguria (severe FVD)
• ↑ urine specific gravity
Cardiovascular
• Tachycardia
• Orthostatic hypotension (moderate FVD)
• Falling systolic/diastolic pressure (severe FVD)
• Flat neck veins
• ↓ venous filling
• ↓ pulse volume
• ↓ capillary refill
• ↑ hematocrit
Potential Complication
• Hypovolemic shock
Musculoskeletal
• Fatigue
Metabolic Processes
• ↓ body temperature (isotonic FVD)
• ↑ body temperature (dehydration)
• Thirst
• Weight loss
>2% mild FVD
>5% moderate FVD
>8% severe FVD

## BOX 5–1  ■ Measuring Central Venous Pressure (CVP) with a Manometer

CVP is a hemodynamic monitoring method for evaluating fluid volume status. It measures mean right atrial pressure by means of a catheter. The CVP catheter is inserted by a physician, most often at the client's bedside, into the antecubital, internal jugular, or subclavian vein. Nursing responsibilities in measuring CVP are as follows:

1. Explain to the client and family what is being done.
2. Prior to the first measurement, take baseline vital signs, and measure the level of the right atrium on the client's thorax. This is usually at the fourth intercostal space on the lateral chest wall, midway between the anterior and posterior chest. This site is marked and used as the reference point for all measurements.
3. Place the bed in the same position for each reading, usually with the client supine and the head of the bed flat.
4. Use a carpenter's level to check the level of the measuring device to make sure the 0 on the manometer is level with the reference point on the client's chest (see figure).
5. Remove any air bubbles in the line.
6. Turn the stopcock on the manometer so that fluid flows into the manometer, filling it a few centimeters above the expected reading. Then turn the stopcock to open the line between the manometer and the client. The fluid level will fall and then reach a point at which it fluctuates with the client's respirations. This point is recorded as the CVP.
7. After the measurement is taken, turn the stopcock so that the fluid can again flow from the fluid source to the client.

### NORMAL VALUES

When CVP is measured by a manometer, normal values range from 2 to 8 cm water. A low CVP indicates inadequate venous return from fluid deficit and hypovolemia or due to peripheral vasodilation. A high CVP indicates fluid overload, cardiac problems that decrease cardiac contractility, or pulmonary disorders that increase pulmonary vascular resistance.

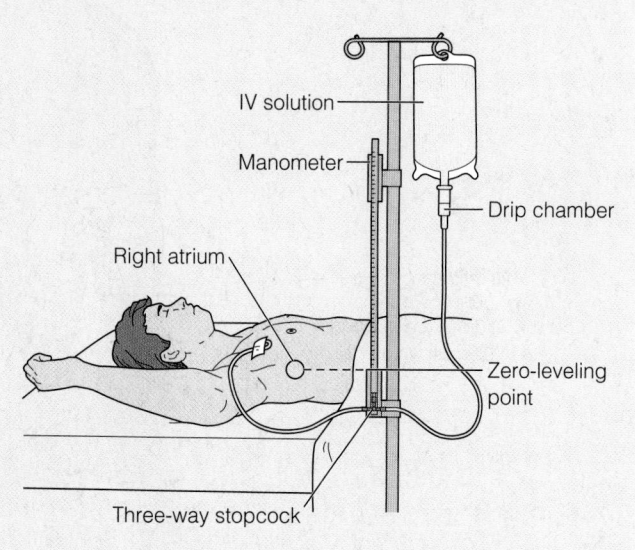

2. Administer (by IV infusion) an initial fluid volume of 200 to 300 mL over 5 to 10 minutes.
3. Reevaluate baseline data at the end of the 10-minute infusion period.
4. Administer additional fluid until a specified volume is infused or the desired hemodynamic parameters are achieved.

Intravenous fluids are often prescribed to correct FVD. Table 5–4 describes the types, tonicity, and uses of commonly administered intravenous fluids. Isotonic electrolyte solutions (0.9% NaCl or Ringer's solution) are used to expand plasma volume in hypotensive clients or to replace abnormal losses, which are usually isotonic in nature. Five percent dextrose in water (D5W) is given to provide water to treat total body water deficits. D5W is isotonic (similar in tonicity to the plasma) and thus does not provoke hemolysis of red blood cells. The dextrose is metabolized to carbon dioxide and water, leaving free water available for tissue needs.

Hypotonic saline solution (0.45% NaCl with or without added electrolytes) or hypotonic mixed electrolyte solutions are used as maintenance solutions. These solutions provide additional electrolytes such as potassium, a buffer (lactate or acetate) as needed, and water.

### NURSING CARE

Nurses are responsible for identifying clients at risk for fluid volume deficit, initiating and carrying out measures to prevent and treat fluid volume deficit, and monitoring the effects of therapy.

### Health Promotion

Health promotion activities focus on teaching clients to prevent fluid volume deficit. Discuss the importance of maintaining ad-

### TABLE 5–3  Comparison of Assessment Findings in Clients with Fluid Imbalance

| Assessment | Fluid Deficit | Fluid Excess |
|---|---|---|
| Blood pressure | Decreased systolic Postural hypotension | Increased |
| Heart rate | Increased | Increased |
| Pulse amplitude | Decreased | Increased |
| Respirations | Normal | Moist crackles Wheezes |
| Jugular vein | Flat | Distended |
| Edema | Rare | Dependent |
| Skin turgor | Loose, poor turgor | Taut |
| Output | Low, concentrated | May be low or normal |
| Urine specific gravity | High | Low |
| Weight | Loss | Gain |

TABLE 5-4  Commonly Administered Intravenous Fluids

| Fluid and Tonicity | Uses |
|---|---|
| **Dextrose in Water Solutions** | |
| 5% dextrose in water (D5W)<br>Isotonic | Replaces water losses<br>Provides free water necessary for cellular rehydration<br>Lowers serum sodium in hypernatremia |
| 10% dextrose in water (D10W)<br>Hypertonic | Provides free water<br>Provides nutrition (supplies 340 kcal/L) |
| 20% dextrose in water (D20W)<br>Hypertonic | Supplies 680 kcal/L<br>May cause diuresis |
| 50% dextrose in water (D50W)<br>Hypertonic | Supplies 1700 kcal/L<br>Used to correct hypoglycemia |
| **Saline Solutions** | |
| 0.45% sodium chloride<br>Hypotonic | Provides free water to replace hypotonic fluid losses<br>Maintains levels of plasma sodium and chloride |
| 0.9% sodium chloride<br>Isotonic | Expands intravascular volume<br>Replaces water lost from extracellular fluid<br>Used with blood transfusions<br>Replaces large sodium losses (as from burns) |
| 3% sodium chloride<br>Hypertonic | Corrects serious sodium depletion |
| **Combined Dextrose and Saline Solution** | |
| 5% dextrose & 0.45% sodium chloride<br>Isotonic | Provides free water<br>Provides sodium chloride<br>Maintenance fluid of choice if there are no electrolyte imbalances |
| **Multiple Electrolyte Solutions** | |
| Ringer's solution<br>Isotonic (electrolyte concentrations of sodium, potassium, chloride, and calcium are similar to plasma levels) | Expands the intracellular fluid<br>Replaces extracellular fluid losses |
| Lactated Ringer's solution<br>Isotonic (similar in composition of electrolytes to plasma but does not contain magnesium) | Replaces fluid losses from burns and the lower gastrointestinal tract<br>Fluid of choice for acute blood loss |

equate fluid intake, particularly when exercising and during hot weather. Advise clients to use commercial sports drinks to replace both water and electrolytes when exercising during warm weather. Instruct clients to maintain fluid intake when ill, particularly during periods of fever or when diarrhea is a problem.

Discuss the increased risk for fluid volume deficit with older adults (see p. 84) and provide information about prevention. Teach older adults (and their caretakers) that thirst decreases with aging and urge them to maintain a regular fluid intake of about 1500 mL per day, regardless of perception of thirst.

Carefully monitor clients at risk for abnormal fluid losses through routes such as vomiting, diarrhea, nasogastric suction, increased urine output, fever, or wounds. Monitor fluid intake in clients with decreased level of consciousness, disorientation, nausea and anorexia, and physical limitations.

## Assessment

Collect assessment data through the health history interview and physical examination.

- Health history: Risk factors such as medications, acute or chronic renal or endocrine disease; precipitating factors such

as hot weather, extensive exercise, lack of access to fluids, recent illness (especially if accompanied by fever, vomiting, and/or diarrhea); onset and duration of symptoms.
- Physical assessment: Weight; vital signs including orthostatic blood pressure and pulse; peripheral pulses and capillary refill; jugular neck vein distention; skin color, temperature, turgor; level of consciousness and mentation; urine output. See Box 5-2 for physical assessment changes in the older adult.

BOX 5-2    ■ Assessing Older Adults

**FLUID VOLUME DEFICIT**

With aging, the elasticity of skin decreases. As a result, turgor diminishes, even in the well-hydrated older adult. This makes skin turgor less reliable when assessing for fluid volume deficit. In addition, some older adults experience postural hypotension, even when well hydrated. Allow the older adult to stand quietly for a full minute before rechecking blood pressure and pulse when measuring orthostatic vital signs.

## Nursing Diagnoses and Interventions

The focus for nursing diagnoses and interventions for the client with fluid volume deficit is on managing the effects of the deficit and preventing complications.

### Deficient Fluid Volume

Clients with fluid volume deficit due to abnormal losses, inadequate intake, or impaired fluid regulation require close monitoring as well as immediate and ongoing fluid replacement.

- Assess intake and output accurately, monitoring fluid balance. In acute situations, hourly intake and output may be indicated. *Urine output should be 30 to 60 mL per hour (unless renal failure is present). Urine output of less than 30 mL per hour indicates inadequate renal perfusion and an increased risk for acute renal failure and inadequate tissue perfusion.*

**PRACTICE ALERT**   *Report a urine output of less than 30 mL per hour to the primary health care provider.* ■

- Assess vital signs, CVP, and peripheral pulse volume at least every 4 hours. *Hypotension, tachycardia, low CVP, and weak, easily obliterated peripheral pulses indicate hypovolemia.*
- Weigh daily under standard conditions (time of day, clothing, and scale). *In most instances (except third spacing), changes in weight accurately reflect fluid balance.* See the Nursing Research box on this page.
- Administer and monitor the intake of oral fluids as prescribed. Identify beverage preferences and provide these on a schedule. *Oral fluid replacement is preferred when the client is able to drink and retain fluids.*
- Administer intravenous fluids as prescribed using an electronic infusion pump. Monitor for indicators of fluid overload if rapid fluid replacement is ordered: dyspnea, tachypnea, tachycardia, increased CVP, jugular vein distension, and edema. *Rapid fluid replacement may lead to hypervolemia, resulting in pulmonary edema and cardiac failure, particularly in clients with compromised cardiac and renal function.*
- Monitor laboratory values: electrolytes, serum osmolality, BUN, and hematocrit. *Rehydration may lead to changes in serum electrolytes, osmolality, BUN, and hematocrit. In some cases, electrolyte replacement may be necessary during rehydration.*

### Ineffective Tissue Perfusion

A fluid volume deficit can lead to decreased perfusion of renal, cerebral, and peripheral tissues. Inadequate renal perfusion can lead to acute renal failure. Decreased cerebral perfusion leads to changes in mental status and cognitive function, causing restlessness, anxiety, agitation, excitability, confusion, vertigo, fainting, and weakness.

- Monitor for changes in level of consciousness and mental status. *Restlessness, anxiety, confusion, and agitation may indicate inadequate cerebral blood flow and circulatory collapse.*
- Monitor serum creatinine, BUN, and cardiac enzymes, reporting elevated levels to the physician. *Elevated levels may indicate impaired renal function or cardiac perfusion related to circulatory failure.*

### Nursing Research

**Evidence-Based Practice for Clients with Imbalanced Fluid Volume**

Nurses caring for clients with a fluid volume imbalance frequently monitor both 24-hour intake and output records and daily weights. These measurements require caregiver time, and may be providing redundant data. Nurse managers on three nursing units compared the results of continuous 48-hour intake and output records with daily weights for a total of 73 selected clients on their units. Their findings suggest that even when compliance with recording accurate intake and output is optimal, it is an unreliable measure of actual fluid balance (Wise, Mersch, Racioppi, Crosier, & Thompson, 2000).

#### IMPLICATIONS FOR NURSING

A significant shortage of licensed nurses is predicted for the early part of the 21st century. Tight nursing resources will require efficient nursing practice to maintain quality care. This study suggests that for the majority of clients (the exceptions being clients with kidney disease or who are on a fluid restriction), measuring accurate daily weights is a better indicator of fluid balance than intake and output records.

#### Critical Thinking

1. What factors can you identify that would affect the accuracy of intake and output records?
2. What measures can you and your institution take to ensure accurate daily weight measurements?
3. Compare intake and output records and daily weights for your assigned clients. Is the balance between intake and output accurately reflected by day-to-day weight changes? If not, what factors can you identify that might account for this discrepancy?

*Note. Adapted from "Evaluating the Reliability and Utility of Cumulative Intake and Output" by L.C. Wise et al., 2000,* Journal of Nursing Care Quality, 14(3), pp. 37–42.

- Turn at least every 2 hours.   Provide good skin care and monitor for evidence of skin or tissue breakdown. *Impaired circulation to peripheral tissues increases the risk of skin breakdown. Turn frequently to relieve pressure over bony prominences. Keep skin clean, dry, and moisturized to help maintain integrity.*

### Risk for Injury

The client with fluid volume deficit is at risk for injury because of dizziness and loss of balance resulting from decreased cerebral perfusion secondary to hypovolemia.

- Institute safety precautions, including keeping the bed in a low position, using side rails as needed, and slowly raising the client from supine to sitting or sitting to standing position.   *Using safety precautions and allowing time for the blood pressure to adjust to position changes reduce the risk of injury.*
- Teach client and family members how to reduce orthostatic hypotension:
  a. Move from one position to another in stages; for example, raise the head of the bed before sitting up, and sit for a few minutes before standing.

---

### CHART 5–1  NANDA, NIC, AND NOC LINKAGES

**The Client with Fluid Volume Deficit**

| NURSING DIAGNOSES | NURSING INTERVENTIONS | NURSING OUTCOMES |
|---|---|---|
| • Deficient Fluid Volume<br><br>• Decreased Cardiac Output | • Fluid Management<br>• Hypovolemia Management<br>• Circulatory Care | • Fluid Balance<br>• Hydration<br>• Circulatory Status<br>• Vital Signs Status |

*Note. Data from Nursing Outcomes Classification (NOC) by M. Johnson & M. Maas (Eds.), 1997, St. Louis: Mosby; Nursing Diagnoses: Definitions & Classification 2001–2002 by North American Nursing Diagnosis Association, 2001, Philadelphia: NANDA; Nursing Interventions Classification (NIC) by J.C. McCloskey & G. M. Bulechek (Eds.), 2000, St. Louis: Mosby. Reprinted by permission.*

---

  b. Avoid prolonged standing.

  c. Rest in a recliner rather than in bed during the day.

  d. Use assistive devices to pick up objects from the floor rather than stooping.

*Teaching measures to reduce orthostatic hypotension reduces the client's risk for injury. Prolonged bed rest increases skeletal muscle weakness and decreases venous tone, contributing to postural hypotension. Prolonged standing allows blood to pool in the legs, reducing venous return and cardiac output.*

## Using NANDA, NIC, and NOC

Chart 5–1 shows the links between NANDA nursing diagnoses, nursing interventions classification (NIC), and nursing outcomes classification (NOC) when caring for the client with fluid volume deficit.

## Home Care

Depending on the severity of the fluid volume deficit, the client may be managed in the home or residential facility, or may be admitted to an acute care facility. Assess the client's understanding of the cause of the deficit and the fluids necessary for providing replacement. Address the following topics when preparing the client and family for home care.

- The importance of maintaining adequate fluid intake (at least 1500 mL per day; more if extra fluid is being lost through perspiration, fever, or diarrhea)
- Manifestations of fluid imbalance, and how to monitor fluid balance
- How to prevent fluid deficit:
    Avoid exercising during extreme heat.
    Increase fluid intake during hot weather.
    If vomiting, take small frequent amounts of ice chips or clear liquids, such as weak tea, flat cola, or ginger ale.
    Reduce intake of coffee, tea, and alcohol, which increase urine output and can cause fluid loss.
- Replacement of fluids lost through diarrhea with fruit juices or bouillon, rather than large amounts of tap water
- Alternate sources of fluid (such as gelatin, frozen juices, or ice cream) for effective replacement of lost fluids

## THE CLIENT WITH FLUID VOLUME EXCESS

**Fluid volume excess** results when both water and sodium are retained in the body. Fluid volume excess may be caused by fluid overload (excess water and sodium intake) or by impairment of the mechanisms that maintain homeostasis. The excess fluid can lead to excess intravascular fluid (**hypervolemia**) and excess interstitial fluid (**edema**).

## PATHOPHYSIOLOGY

Fluid volume excess usually results from conditions that cause retention of both sodium and water. These conditions include heart failure, cirrhosis of the liver, renal failure, adrenal gland disorders, corticosteroid administration, and stress conditions causing the release of ADH and aldosterone. Other causes include an excessive intake of sodium-containing foods, drugs that cause sodium retention, and the administration of excess amounts of sodium-containing intravenous fluids (such as 0.9% NaCl or Ringer's solution). This iatrogenic cause of fluid volume excess primarily affects clients with impaired regulatory mechanisms.

In fluid volume excess, both water and sodium are gained together in about the same proportions as normally exists in extracellular fluid. The total body sodium content is increased, which in turn causes an increase in total body water. Because the increase in sodium and water is isotonic, the serum sodium and osmolality remain normal, and the excess fluid remains in the extracellular space.

## MANIFESTATIONS AND COMPLICATIONS

Excess extracellular fluid leads to hypervolemia and circulatory overload. Excess fluid in the interstitial space causes peripheral or generalized edema. The following manifestations of fluid volume excess relate to both the excess fluid and its effects on circulation.

- The increase in total body water causes weight gain (more than 5% of body weight) over a short period.
- Circulatory overload causes manifestations such as:
    - A full, bounding pulse.
    - Distended neck and peripheral veins.

- Increased central venous pressure (> 11–12 cm of water).
- Cough, **dyspnea** (labored or difficult breathing), **orthopnea** (difficulty breathing when supine).
- Moist crackles (rales) in the lungs; pulmonary edema (excess fluid in pulmonary interstitial spaces and alveoli) if severe.
- Increased urine output (**polyuria**).
- **Ascites** (excess fluid in the peritoneal cavity).
- Peripheral edema, or if severe, **anasarca** (severe, generalized edema).
- Dilution of plasma by excess fluid causes a decreased hematocrit and BUN.
- Possible cerebral edema (excess water in brain tissues) can lead to altered mental status and anxiety.

Heart failure is not only a potential cause of fluid volume excess, but it is also a potential complication of the condition if the heart is unable to increase its workload to handle the excess blood volume. Severe fluid overload and heart failure can lead to pulmonary edema, a medical emergency. See Chapter 30 ⊙⊃ for more information about heart failure and pulmonary edema.

## COLLABORATIVE CARE

Managing fluid volume excess focuses on prevention in clients at risk, treating its manifestations, and correcting the underlying cause. Management includes limiting sodium and water intake and administering diuretics.

## Diagnostic Tests

The following laboratory tests may be ordered.

- *Serum electrolytes* and *serum osmolality* are measured. Serum sodium and osmolality usually remain within normal limits.
- *Serum hematocrit* and *hemoglobin* often are decreased due to plasma dilution from excess extracellular fluid.

Additional tests of *renal* and *liver function* (such as serum creatinine, BUN, and liver enzymes) may be ordered to help determine the cause of fluid volume excess if it is unclear.

## Medications

Diuretics are commonly used to treat fluid volume excess. They inhibit sodium and water reabsorption, increasing urine output. The three major classes of diuretics, each of which acts on a different part of the kidney tubule, are as follows:

- Loop diuretics act in the ascending loop of Henle.
- Thiazide-type diuretics act on the distal convoluted tubule.
- Potassium-sparing diuretics affect the distal nephron.

The nursing implications for diuretics are outlined in the box below.

## Treatments

### Fluid Management

Fluid intake may be restricted in clients who have fluid volume excess. The amount of fluid allowed per day is prescribed by the primary care provider. All fluid intake must be calculated,

## Medication Administration

### Diuretics for Fluid Volume Excess

Diuretics increase urinary excretion of water and sodium. They are categorized into three major groups: loop diuretics, thiazide and thiazide-like diuretics, and potassium-sparing diuretics. Diuretics are used to enhance renal function and to treat vascular fluid overload and edema. Common side effects include orthostatic hypotension, dehydration, electrolyte imbalance, and possible hyperglycemia. Diuretics should be used with caution in the older adult. Examples of each major type follow.

### LOOP DIURETICS

Furosemide (Lasix)  Ethacrynic Acid (Edecrin)
Bumetanide (Bumex)  Torsemide (Demadex)

Loop diuretics inhibit sodium and chloride reabsorption in the ascending loop of Henle (see Chapter 25 for the anatomy of the kidneys). As a result, loop diuretics promote the excretion of sodium, chloride, potassium, and water.

### THIAZIDE AND THIAZIDELIKE DIURETICS

Bendroflumethiazide (Naturetin)  Polythiazide (Renese)
Chlorothiazide (Diuril)  Chlorthalidone (Hygroton)
Hydrochlorothiazide  Trichlormethiazide
(HydroDIURIL, Oretic)  (Naqua)
Metolazone (Zaroxolyn)  Indapamide (Lozol)

Thiazide and thiazidelike diuretics promote the excretion of sodium, chloride, potassium, and water by decreasing absorption in the distal tubule.

### POTASSIUM-SPARING DIURETICS

Spironolactone (Aldactone)
Amiloride HCl (Midamor)
Triamterene (Dyrenium)

Potassium-sparing diuretics promote excretion of sodium and water by inhibiting sodium-potassium exchange in the distal tubule.

### Client and Family Teaching

- The drug will increase the amount and frequency of urination.
- The drugs must be taken even when you feel well.
- Take the drugs in the morning and afternoon to avoid having to get up at night to urinate.
- Change position slowly to avoid dizziness.
- Report the following to your primary health care provider: dizziness; trouble breathing; or swelling of face, hands, or feet.
- Weigh yourself every day, and report sudden gains or losses.
- Avoid using the salt shaker when eating.
- If the drug increases potassium loss, eat foods high in potassium, such as orange juice and bananas.
- Do not use salt substitute if you are taking a potassium-sparing diuretic.

| BOX 5–3 | ■ Fluid Restriction Guidelines |
|---|---|

- Subtract requisite fluids (e.g., ordered IV fluids, fluid used to dilute IV medications) from total daily allowance.
- Divide remaining fluid allowance:
  - Day shift: 50% of total
  - Evening shift: 25% to 33% of total
  - Night shift: Remainder
- Explain the fluid restriction to the client and family members.
- Identify preferred fluids and intake pattern of client.
- Place allowed amounts of fluid in small glasses (gives perception of a full glass).
- Offer ice chips (when melted, ice chips are approximately half the frozen volume).
- Provide frequent mouth care.
- Provide sugarless chewing gum (if allowed) to reduce thirst sensation.

| BOX 5–4 | ■ Foods High in Sodium |
|---|---|

**HIGH IN ADDED SODIUM**

**Processed Meat and Fish**
- Bacon
- Luncheon meat and other cold cuts
- Sausage
- Smoked fish

**Selected Dairy Products**
- Buttermilk
- Cheeses
- Cottage cheese
- Ice cream

**Processed Grains**
- Graham crackers
- Most dry cereals

**Most Canned Goods**
- Meats
- Soups
- Vegetables

**Snack Foods**
- Salted popcorn
- Potato chips/pretzels
- Nuts
- Gelatin desserts

**Condiments and Food Additives**
- Barbecue sauce
- Catsup
- Chili sauce
- Meat tenderizers
- Worcestershire sauce
- Saccharin
- Pickles
- Soy sauce
- Salted margarine
- Salad dressings

**NATURALLY HIGH IN SODIUM**
- Brains
- Kidney
- Clams
- Crab
- Lobster
- Oysters
- Shrimp
- Dried fruit
- Spinach
- Carrots

including meals and that used to administer medications orally or intravenously. Box 5–3 provides guidelines for clients with a fluid restriction.

## Dietary Management

Because sodium retention is a primary cause of fluid volume excess, a sodium-restricted diet often is prescribed. Americans typically consume about 4 to 5 grams (g) of sodium every day; recommended sodium intake is 500 to 2400 mg per day. The primary dietary sources of sodium are the salt shaker, processed foods, and foods themselves (see Box 5–4).

A mild sodium restriction can be achieved by instructing the client and primary food preparer in the household to reduce the amount of salt in recipes by half, avoid using the salt shaker during meals, and avoid foods that contain high levels of sodium (either naturally or because of processing). In moderate and severely sodium-restricted diets, salt is avoided altogether, as are all foods containing significant amounts of sodium.

## NURSING CARE

Nursing care focuses on preventing fluid volume excess in clients at risk and on managing problems resulting from its effects.

## Health Promotion

Health promotion related to fluid volume excess focuses on teaching preventive measures to clients who are at risk (e.g., clients who have heart or kidney failure). Discuss the relationship between sodium intake and water retention. Provide guidelines for a low-sodium diet, and teach clients to carefully read food labels to identify "hidden" sodium, particularly in processed foods. Instruct clients at risk to weigh themselves on a regular basis, using the same scale, and to notify their primary care provider if they gain more than 5 lb in a week or less.

Carefully monitor clients receiving intravenous fluids for signs of hypervolemia. Reduce the flow rate and promptly report manifestations of fluid overload to the physician.

## Assessment

Collect assessment data through the health history interview and physical examination.

- Health history: Risk factors such as medications, heart failure, acute or chronic renal or endocrine disease; precipitating factors such as a recent illness, change in diet, or change in medications. Recent weight gain; complaints of persistent cough, shortness of breath, swelling of feet and ankles, or difficulty sleeping when lying down.
- Physical assessment: Weight; vital signs; peripheral pulses and capillary refill; jugular neck vein distention; edema; lung sounds (crackles or wheezes), dyspnea, cough, and sputum; urine output; mental status.

## Nursing Diagnoses and Interventions

Nursing diagnoses and interventions for the client with fluid volume excess focus on the multisystem effects of the fluid overload.

### Excess Fluid Volume

Nursing care for the client with fluid volume excess includes collaborative interventions such as administering diuretics and maintaining a fluid restriction, as well as monitoring the status and effects of the fluid volume excess. This is particularly critical in older clients because of the age-related decline in cardiac and renal compensatory responses.

- Assess vital signs, heart sounds, CVP, and volume of peripheral arteries. *Hypervolemia can cause hypertension, bounding peripheral pulses, a third heart sound ($S_3$) due to the volume of blood flow through the heart, and high CVP readings.*
- Assess for the presence and extent of edema, particularly in the lower extremities, the back, sacral, and periorbital areas. *Initially, edema affects the dependent portions of the body—the lower extremities of ambulatory clients and the sacrum in bedridden clients. Periorbital edema indicates more generalized edema.*

**PRACTICE ALERT** *Assess urine output hourly. Maintain accurate intake and output records. Note urine output less than 30 ml per hour or a positive fluid balance on 24-hour total intake and output calculations. Heart failure and inadequate renal perfusion may result in decreased urine output and fluid retention.* ∎

- Obtain daily weights at the same time of day, using approximately the same clothing and a balanced scale. *Daily weights are one of the most important gauges of fluid balance. Acute weight gain or loss represents fluid gain or loss. Weight gain of 2 kg is equivalent to 2 L of fluid gain.*
- Administer oral fluids cautiously, adhering to any prescribed fluid restriction. Discuss the restriction with the client and significant others, including the total volume allowed, the rationale, and the importance of reporting all fluid taken. *All sources of fluid intake, including ice chips, are recorded to avoid excess fluid intake.*
- Provide oral hygiene at least every 2 hours. *Oral hygiene contributes to client comfort and keeps mucous membranes intact; it also helps relieve thirst if fluids are restricted.*
- Teach client and significant others about the sodium-restricted diet, and emphasize the importance of checking before bringing foods to the client. *Excess sodium promotes water retention; a sodium-restricted diet is ordered to reduce water gain.*
- Administer prescribed diuretics as ordered, monitoring the client's response to therapy. *Loop or high-ceiling diuretics such as furosemide can lead to rapid fluid loss and signs of hypovolemia and electrolyte imbalance.*

## Risk for Impaired Skin Integrity

Tissue edema decreases oxygen and nutrient delivery to the skin and subcutaneous tissues, increasing the risk of injury.

- Frequently assess skin, particularly in pressure areas and over bony prominences. *Skin breakdown can progress rapidly when circulation is impaired.*
- Reposition the client at least every 2 hours. Provide skin care with each position change. *Frequent position changes minimize tissue pressure and promote blood flow to tissues.*
- Provide an eggcrate mattress or alternating pressure mattress, foot cradle, heel protectors, and other devices to reduce pressure on tissues. *These devices, which distribute pressure away from bony prominences, reduce the risk of skin breakdown.*

## Risk for Impaired Gas Exchange

With fluid volume excess, gas exchange may be impaired by edema of pulmonary interstitial tissues. Acute pulmonary edema is a serious and potentially life-threatening complication of pulmonary congestion.

- Auscultate lungs for presence or worsening of crackles and wheezes; auscultate heart for extra heart sounds. *Crackles and wheezes indicate pulmonary congestion and edema. A gallop rhythm ($S_3$) may indicate diastolic overloading of the ventricles secondary to fluid volume excess.*
- Place in Fowler's position if dyspnea or orthopnea is present. *Fowler's position improves lung expansion by decreasing the pressure of abdominal contents on the diaphragm.*
- Monitor oxygen saturation levels and **arterial blood gases (ABGs)** for evidence of impaired gas exchange ($SaO_2 <$ 92%–95%; $PaO_2 < 80$ mmHg). Administer oxygen as indicated. *Edema of interstitial lung tissues can interfere with gas exchange and delivery to body tissues. Supplemental oxygen promotes gas exchange across the alveolar-capillary membrane, improving tissue oxygenation.*

## Using NANDA, NIC, and NOC

Chart 5–2 shows links between NANDA nursing diagnoses, NIC, and NOC when caring for a client with fluid volume excess.

## CHART 5–2 NANDA, NIC, AND NOC LINKAGES

### The Client with Fluid Volume Excess

| NURSING DIAGNOSES | NURSING INTERVENTIONS | NURSING OUTCOMES |
| --- | --- | --- |
| • Excess Fluid Volume | • Fluid Management<br>• Fluid Monitoring | • Fluid Balance |
| • Impaired Gas Exchange | • Oxygen Therapy<br>• Respiratory Monitoring | • Respiratory Status: Gas Exchange |
| • Activity Intolerance | • Energy Management | • Activity Tolerance |

*Note. Data from Nursing Outcomes Classification (NOC) by M. Johnson & M. Maas (Eds.), 1997, St. Louis: Mosby; Nursing Diagnoses: Definitions & Classification 2001–2002 by North American Nursing Diagnosis Association, 2001, Philadelphia: NANDA; Nursing Interventions Classification (NIC) by J.C. McCloskey & G. M. Bulechek (Eds.), 2000, St. Louis: Mosby. Reprinted by permission.*

## Home Care

Teaching for home care focuses on managing the underlying cause of fluid volume excess and preventing future episodes of excess fluid volume. Address the following topics when preparing the client and family for home care.

- Signs and symptoms of excess fluid and when to contact the care provider
- Prescribed medications: when and how to take, intended and adverse effects, what to report to care provider
- Recommended or prescribed diet; ways to reduce sodium intake; how to read food labels for salt and sodium content; use of salt substitutes, if allowed. (See Box 5–5)
- If restricted, the amount and type of fluids to take each day; how to balance intake over 24 hours
- Monitoring weight; changes reported to care provider
- Ways to decrease dependent edema:
  a. Change position frequently.
  b. Avoid restrictive clothing.
  c. Avoid crossing the legs when sitting.
  d. Wear support stockings or hose.
  e. Elevate feet and legs when sitting.
- How to protect edematous skin from injury:
  a. Do not walk barefoot.
  b. Buy well-fitting shoes; shop in the afternoon when feet are more likely to be swollen.
- Using additional pillows or a recliner to sleep, to relieve orthopnea

### BOX 5–5 ■ Client Teaching

#### LOW-SODIUM DIET

- Reducing sodium intake will help the body excrete excess sodium and water.
- The body needs less than one-tenth of a teaspoon of salt per day.
- Approximately one-third of sodium intake comes from salt added to foods during cooking and at the table; one-fourth to one-third comes from processed foods; and the rest comes from food and water naturally high in sodium.
- Sodium compounds are used in foods as preservatives, leavening agents, and flavor enhancers.
- Many nonprescription drugs (such as analgesics, cough medicine, laxatives, and antacids) as well as toothpastes and mouthwashes contain high amounts of sodium.
- Low-sodium salt substitutes are not really sodium free and may contain half as much sodium as regular salt.
- Use salt substitutes sparingly; larger amounts often taste bitter instead of salty.
- The preference for salt will eventually diminish.
- Salt, monosodium glutamate, baking soda, and baking powder contain substantial amounts of sodium.
- Read labels.
- In place of salt or salt substitutes, use herbs, spices, lemon juice, vinegar, and wine as flavoring when cooking.

## Nursing Care Plan

### A Client with Fluid Volume Excess

Dorothy Rainwater is a 45-year-old Native American woman hospitalized with acute renal failure that developed as a result of acute glomerulonephritis. She is expected to recover, but she has very little urine output. Ms. Rainwater is a single mother of two teenage sons. Until her illness, she was active in caring for her family, her career as a high school principal, and community activities.

### ASSESSMENT

Mike Penning, Ms. Rainwater's nurse, notes that she is in the oliguric phase of acute renal failure, and that her urine output for the previous 24 hours is 250 mL; this low output has been constant for the past 8 days. She gained 1 lb (0.45 kg) in the past 24 hours. Laboratory test results from that morning are: sodium, 155 mEq/L (normal 135 to 145 mEq/L); potassium, 5.3 mEq/L (normal 3.5 to 5.0 mEq/L); calcium, 7.6 mg/dL (normal 8.0 to 10.5 mg/dL), and urine specific gravity 1.008 (normal 1.010 to 1.030). Ms. Rainwater's serum creatinine and blood urea nitrogen (BUN) are high; however, her ABGs are within normal limits.

In his assessment of Ms. Rainwater, Mike notes the following:

- BP 160/92; P 102, with obvious neck vein distention; R 28, with crackles and wheezes; head of bed elevated 30 degrees; T 98.6° F.
- Periorbital and sacral edema present; 3+ pitting bilateral pedal edema; skin cool, pale, and shiny.
- Alert, oriented; responds appropriately to questions.

- Client states she is thirsty, slightly nauseated, and extremely tired.

Ms. Rainwater is receiving intravenous furosemide and is on a 24-hour fluid restriction of 500 mL plus the previous day's urine output to manage her fluid volume excess.

### DIAGNOSES

- *Excess fluid volume* related to acute renal failure
- *Risk for impaired skin integrity* related to fluid retention and edema
- *Risk for impaired gas exchange* related to pulmonary congestion
- *Activity intolerance* related to fluid volume excess, fatigue, and weakness

### EXPECTED OUTCOMES

- Regain fluid balance, as evidenced by weight loss, decreasing edema, and normal vital signs.
- Experience decreased dyspnea.
- Maintain intact skin and mucous membranes.
- Increase activity levels as prescribed.

### PLANNING AND IMPLEMENTATION

- Weigh at 0600 and 1800 daily.

(continued on page 94)

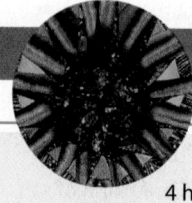

## Nursing Care Plan
### A Client with Fluid Volume Excess (continued)

- Assess vital signs and breath sounds every 4 hours.
- Measure intake and output every 4 hours.
- Obtain urine specific gravity every 8 hours.
- Restrict fluids as follows: 350 mL from 0700 to 1500; 300 mL from 1500 to 2300; 100 mL from 2300 to 0700. Prefers water or apple juice.
- Turn every 2 hours, following schedule posted at the head of bed. Inspect and provide skin care as needed; avoid vigorous massage of pressure areas.
- Provide oral care every 2 to 4 hours (can brush her own teeth, caution not to swallow water); use moistened applicators as desired.
- Elevate head of bed to 30 to 40 degrees; prefers to use own pillows.
- Assist to recliner chair at bedside for 20 minutes two or three times a day. Monitor ability to tolerate activity without increasing dyspnea or fatigue.

### EVALUATION

At the end of the shift, Mike evaluates the effectiveness of the plan of care and continues all diagnoses and interventions. Ms. Rainwater gained no weight, and her urinary output during his shift is 170 mL. Her urine specific gravity remains 1.008. Her vital signs are unchanged, but her crackles and wheezes have decreased slightly. Her skin and mucous membranes are intact. Ms. Rainwater tolerated the bedside chair without dyspnea or fatigue.

### Critical Thinking in the Nursing Process

1. What is the pathophysiologic basis for Ms. Rainwater's increased respiratory rate, blood pressure, and pulse?
2. Explain how elevating the head of the bed 30 degrees facilitates respirations.
3. Suppose Ms. Rainwater says, "I would really like to have all my fluids at once instead of spreading them out." How would you reply, and why?
4. Outline a plan for teaching Ms. Rainwater about diuretics.

See Evaluating Your Response in Appendix C.

# SODIUM IMBALANCE

Sodium is the most plentiful electrolyte in ECF, with normal serum sodium levels ranging from 135 to 145 mEq/L. Sodium is the primary regulator of the volume, osmolality, and distribution of ECF. It also is important to maintain neuromuscular activity. Because of the close interrelationship between sodium and water balance, disorders of fluid volume and sodium balance often occur together. Sodium imbalances affect the osmolality of ECF and water distribution between the fluid compartments. When sodium levels are low (**hyponatremia**), water is drawn into the cells of the body, causing them to swell. In contrast, high levels of sodium in ECF (**hypernatremia**) draw water out of body cells, causing them to shrink.

## OVERVIEW OF NORMAL SODIUM BALANCE

Most of the body's sodium comes from dietary intake. Although a sodium intake of 500 mg per day is usually sufficient to meet the body's needs, the average intake of sodium by adults in the United States is about 6 to 15 g per day (Porth, 2002). Other sources of sodium include prescription drugs and certain self-prescribed remedies. Sodium is primarily excreted by the kidneys. A small amount is excreted through the skin and the gastrointestinal tract.

The kidney is the primary regulator of sodium balance in the body. The kidney excretes or conserves sodium in response to changes in vascular volume. A fall in blood volume prompts several mechanisms that lead to sodium and water retention.

- The renin-angiotensin-aldosterone system (see Figure 5–9) is stimulated. Angiotensin II prompts the renal tubules to reabsorb sodium. It also causes vasoconstriction, slowing blood flow through the kidney and reducing glomerular filtration. This further reduces the amount of sodium excreted. Angiotensin II promotes the release of aldosterone from the adrenal cortex. In the presence of aldosterone, more sodium is reabsorbed in the cortical collecting tubules of the kidney, and more potassium is eliminated in the urine.
- Antidiuretic hormone (ADH) is released from the posterior pituitary (see Figure 5–10). ADH promotes sodium and water reabsorption in the distal tubules of the kidney, reducing urine output and expanding blood volume.

In contrast, when blood volume expands, sodium and water elimination by the kidneys increases.

- The **glomerular filtration rate** (the rate at which plasma is filtered through the glomeruli of the kidney) increases, allowing more water and sodium to be filtered and excreted.
- Atrial natriuretic peptide (ANP) is released by cells in the atria of the heart. ANP increases sodium excretion by the kidneys.
- ADH release from the pituitary gland is inhibited. In the absence of ADH, the distal tubule is relatively impermeable to water and sodium, allowing more to be excreted in the urine. Table 5–5 summarizes the causes and effects of sodium imbalances.

## THE CLIENT WITH HYPONATREMIA

Hyponatremia is a serum sodium level of less than 135 mEq/L. Hyponatremia usually results from a loss of sodium from the body, but it may also be caused by water gains that dilute ECF.

TABLE 5-5 Causes and Manifestations of Sodium Imbalances

| Imbalance | Possible Causes | Manifestations |
|---|---|---|
| **Hyponatremia**<br>Serum sodium <135 mEq/L<br><br>*Other Lab Values*<br>Serum osmolality<br> <280 mOsm/kg | • Excess sodium loss through kidneys, GI tract, or skin<br>• Water gains related to renal disease, heart failure, or cirrhosis of the liver<br>• Syndrome of inappropriate secretion of antidiuretic hormone (SIADH)<br>• Excessive hypotonic IV fluids | • Anorexia, nausea, vomiting, abdominal cramping, and diarrhea<br>• Headache<br>• Altered mental status<br>• Muscle cramps, weakness, and tremors<br>• Seizures and coma |
| **Hypernatremia**<br>Serum sodium >145 mEq/L<br><br>*Other Lab Values*<br>Serum osmolality<br> >295 mOsm/kg | • Altered thirst<br>• Inability to respond to thirst sensation or obtain water<br>• Profuse sweating<br>• Diarrhea<br>• Diabetes insipidus<br>• Oral electrolyte solutions or hyperosmolar tube-feeding formulas<br>• Excess IV fluids such as normal saline, 3% or 5% sodium chloride, or sodium bicarbonate | • Thirst<br>• Increased temperature<br>• Dry, sticky mucous membranes<br>• Restlessness<br>• Weakness<br>• Altered mental status<br>• Decreasing level of consciousness<br>• Muscle twitching<br>• Seizures |

## PATHOPHYSIOLOGY AND MANIFESTATIONS

Excess sodium loss can occur through the kidneys, gastrointestinal tract, or skin. Diuretic medications, kidney diseases, or adrenal insufficiency with impaired aldosterone and cortisol production can lead to excessive sodium excretion in urine. Vomiting, diarrhea, and gastrointestinal suction are common causes of excess sodium loss through the GI tract. Sodium may also be lost when gastrointestinal tubes are irrigated with water instead of saline, or when repeated tap water enemas are administered (Porth, 2002). Excessive sweating or loss of skin surface (as with an extensive burn) can also cause excessive sodium loss.

Water gains that can lead to hyponatremia may occur with:

• Systemic diseases such as heart failure, renal failure, or cirrhosis of the liver.
• Syndrome of inappropriate secretion of antidiuretic hormone (SIADH), in which water excretion is impaired.
• Excessive administration of hypotonic intravenous fluids.

Hyponatremia causes a drop in serum osmolality. Water shifts from ECF into the intracellular space, causing cells to swell and reducing the osmolality of intracellular fluid. Many of the manifestations of hyponatremia can be attributed to cellular edema and hypo-osmolality.

The manifestations of hyponatremia depend on the rapidity of onset, the severity, and the cause of the imbalance. If the condition develops slowly, manifestations are usually not experienced until the serum sodium levels reach 125 mEq/L. In addition, the manifestations of hyponatremia vary, depending on extracellular fluid volume. Early manifestations of hyponatremia include muscle cramps, weakness, and fatigue from its effects on muscle cells. Gastrointestinal function is affected, causing anorexia, nausea and vomiting, abdominal cramping, and diarrhea.

As sodium levels continue to decrease, the brain and nervous system are affected by cellular edema. Neurologic manifestations progress rapidly when the serum sodium level falls below 120 mEq/L, and include headache, depression, dulled sensorium, personality changes, irritability, lethargy, hyperreflexia, muscle twitching, and tremors. If serum sodium falls to very low levels, convulsions and coma are likely to occur.

When hyponatremia is associated with decreased ECF volume, the manifestations are those of hypovolemia. In hyponatremia associated with fluid volume excess, manifestations include those of hypervolemia.

## COLLABORATIVE CARE

Collaborative management of hyponatremia focuses on restoring normal blood volume and serum sodium levels.

### Diagnostic Tests

The following laboratory tests may be ordered.

• *Serum sodium* and *osmolality* are decreased in hyponatremia (serum sodium <135 mEq/L; serum osmolality <275 mOsm/kg).
• A *24-hour urine specimen* is obtained to evaluate sodium excretion. In conditions associated with normal or increased extracellular volume (such as SIADH), urinary sodium is increased; in conditions resulting from losses of isotonic fluids (e.g., sweating, diarrhea, vomiting, and third-space fluid accumulation), by contrast, urinary sodium is decreased.

### Medications

When both sodium and water have been lost (hyponatremia with hypovolemia), sodium-containing fluids are given to replace both water and sodium. These fluids may be given by mouth, nasogastric tube, or intravenously. Isotonic Ringer's solution or isotonic saline (0.9% NaCl) solution may be administered. Cautious administration of intravenous 3% or 5% NaCl solution may be necessary in clients who have very low plasma sodium levels (110 to 115 mEq/L).

Loop diuretics are administered to clients who have hyponatremia with normal or excess ECF volume. Loop diuretics promote an isotonic diuresis and fluid volume loss without hyponatremia (see p. 90). Thiazide diuretics are avoided because they cause a relatively greater sodium loss in relation to water loss.

In addition, drugs to treat the underlying cause of hyponatremia may be administered.

## Fluid and Dietary Management

If hyponatremia is mild, increasing the intake of foods high in sodium may restore normal sodium balance (see Box 5–4). Fluids often are restricted to help reduce ECF volume and correct hyponatremia (see Box 5–3).

# NURSING CARE

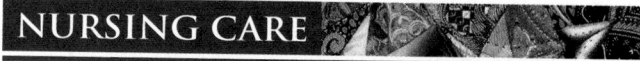

Nursing care of the client with hyponatremia focuses on identifying clients at risk and managing problems resulting from the systemic effects of the disorder.

## Health Promotion

People at risk for mild hyponatremia include those who participate in activities that increase fluid loss through excessive perspiration (diaphoresis) and then replace those losses by drinking large amounts of water. This includes athletes, people who do heavy labor in high environmental temperatures, and older adults living in non-air-conditioned settings during hot weather. Teach the following to clients who are at risk.

- Manifestations of mild hyponatremia, including nausea, abdominal cramps, and muscle weakness
- The importance of drinking liquids containing sodium and other electrolytes at frequent intervals when perspiring heavily, when environmental temperatures are high, and/or if watery diarrhea persists for several days

## Assessment

Assessment data related to hyponatremia include the following:

- Health history: Current manifestations, including nausea and vomiting, abdominal discomfort, muscle weakness, headache, other symptoms; duration of symptoms and any precipitating factors such as heavy perspiration, vomiting, or diarrhea; chronic diseases such as heart or renal failure, cirrhosis of the liver, or endocrine disorders; current medications.
- Physical assessment: Mental status and level of consciousness; vital signs including orthostatic vitals and peripheral pulses; presence of edema or weight gain.

## Nursing Diagnoses and Interventions

### Risk for Imbalanced Fluid Volume

Because of its role in maintaining fluid balance, sodium imbalances often are accompanied by water imbalances. In addition, treatment of hyponatremia can affect the client's fluid balance.

- Monitor intake and output, weigh daily, and calculate 24-hour fluid balance. *Fluid excess or deficit may occur with hyponatremia.*

**PRACTICE ALERT** *Carefully monitor clients receiving sodium-containing intravenous solutions for signs of hypervolemia (increased blood pressure and CVP, tachypnea, tachycardia, gallop rhythm, shortness of breath, crackles). Hypertonic saline solutions can lead to hypervolemia, particularly in clients with cardiovascular or renal disease.* ■

- Use an intravenous flow control device to administer hypertonic saline (3% and 5% NaCl) solutions; carefully monitor flow rate and response. *Hypertonic solutions can increase the risk of pulmonary and cerebral edema due to water retention. Careful monitoring is vital to prevent these complications and possible permanent damage.*
- If fluids are restricted, explain the reason for the restriction, the amount of fluid allowed, and how to calculate fluid intake. *Teaching increases the client's sense of control and compliance.*

For additional nursing interventions that may apply to the client with hyponatremia, review the discussions of fluid volume deficit and fluid volume excess.

### Risk for Decreased Intracranial Adaptive Capacity

The client with severe hyponatremia experiences fluid shifts that cause an increase in intracellular fluid volume. This can cause brain cells to swell, increasing pressure within the cranial vault.

- Monitor serum electrolytes and serum osmolality. Report abnormal results to the care provider. *As serum sodium levels fall, the manifestations and neurologic effects of hyponatremia become increasingly severe.*
- Assess for neurologic changes, such as lethargy, altered level of consciousness, confusion, and convulsions. Monitor mental status and orientation. Compare baseline data with continuing assessments. *Serum sodium levels of 115 to 120 mEq/L can cause headache, lethargy, and decreased responsiveness; sodium levels less than 110 to 115 mEq/L may cause seizures and coma.*
- Assess muscle strength and tone, and deep tendon reflexes. *Increasing muscle weakness and decreased deep tendon reflexes are manifestations of increasing hyponatremia.*

**PRACTICE ALERT** *Maintain a quiet environment, and institute seizure precautions in clients with severe hyponatremia. Severe hyponatremia can lead to seizures. A quiet environment reduces neurologic stimulation. Safety precautions, such as ensuring that side rails are up and having an airway readily available, reduce risk of injury from seizure.* ■

## Using NANDA, NIC, and NOC

Chart 5–3 shows links between NANDA nursing diagnoses, NIC, and NOC when caring for a client with a sodium imbalance.

## Home Care

Teaching for home care focuses on the underlying cause of the sodium deficit and often on prevention. Teach clients who have experienced hyponatremia and those who are at risk for developing hyponatremia about the following:

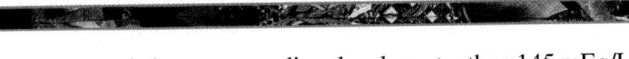

## CHART 5–3  NANDA, NIC, AND NOC LINKAGES

### The Client with a Sodium Imbalance

| NURSING DIAGNOSES | NURSING INTERVENTIONS | NURSING OUTCOMES |
|---|---|---|
| • Risk for Imbalanced Fluid Volume | • Electrolyte Management<br>• Fluid Monitoring | • Fluid Balance<br>• Electrolyte Balance |
| • Fatigue<br>• Risk for Injury | • Energy Management<br>• Environmental Management: Safety<br>• Fall Prevention | • Energy Conservation<br>• Risk Control<br>• Safety Status: Physical Injury |
| • Risk for Impaired Oral Mucous<br>  Membrane | • Oral Health Maintenance | • Tissue Integrity: Skin and Mucous<br>  Membranes |

*Note. Data from* Nursing Outcomes Classification (NOC) *by M. Johnson & M. Maas (Eds.), 1997, St. Louis: Mosby;* Nursing Diagnoses: Definitions & Classification 2001–2002 *by North American Nursing Diagnosis Association, 2001, Philadelphia: NANDA;* Nursing Interventions Classification (NIC) *by J.C. McCloskey & G. M. Bulechek (Eds.), 2000, St. Louis: Mosby. Reprinted by permission.*

- Manifestations of mild and more severe hyponatremia to report to the primary care provider
- The importance of regular serum electrolyte monitoring if taking a potent diuretic or on a low-sodium diet
- Types of foods and fluids to replace sodium orally if dietary sodium is not restricted

## THE CLIENT WITH HYPERNATREMIA

Hypernatremia is a serum sodium level greater than 145 mEq/L. It may develop when sodium is gained in excess of water, or when water is lost in excess of sodium. Either fluid volume deficit or fluid volume excess often accompany hypernatremia.

## PATHOPHYSIOLOGY AND MANIFESTATIONS

Two regulatory mechanisms protect the body from hypernatremia: (1) Excess sodium in ECF stimulates the release of ADH so more water is retained by the kidneys; and (2) the thirst mechanism is stimulated to increase the intake of water (Metheny, 2000). These two factors increase extracellular water, diluting the excess sodium and restoring normal levels. Because of the effectiveness of these mechanisms, hypernatremia almost never occurs in clients who have an intact thirst mechanism and access to water.

Water deprivation is a cause of hypernatremia in clients who are unable to respond to thirst due to altered mental status or physical disability. Excess water loss may occur with watery diarrhea or increased insensible losses (due to fever, hyperventilation, excessive perspiration, or massive burns). Unless water is adequately replaced, clients with diabetes insipidus also may develop hypernatremia. Excess sodium intake can result from ingestion of excess salt or hypertonic intravenous solutions. Clients who experience near-drowning in seawater are at risk for hypernatremia, as are clients with heatstroke.

Hypernatremia causes hyperosmolality of ECF. As a result, water is drawn out of cells, leading to cellular dehydration. The most serious effects of cellular dehydration are seen in the brain. As brain cells contract, neurologic manifestations develop. The brain itself shrinks, causing mechanical traction on cerebral vessels. These vessels may tear and bleed. Although the brain rapidly adapts to hyperosmolality to minimize the water loss, acute hypernatremia can cause widespread cerebral vascular bleeding (Metheny, 2000).

Thirst is the first manifestation of hypernatremia. If thirst is not relieved, the primary manifestations relate to altered neurologic function (see Table 5–5). Initial lethargy, weakness, and irritability can progress to seizures, coma, and death in severe hypernatremia. Both the severity of the sodium excess and the rapidity of its onset affect the manifestations of hypernatremia.

## COLLABORATIVE CARE

Treatment of hypernatremia depends on its cause. Hypernatremia is corrected slowly (over a 48-hour period) to avoid development of cerebral edema secondary to a shift of water into the brain cells.

### Diagnostic Tests

The following laboratory and diagnostic tests may be ordered.

- *Serum sodium levels* are greater than 145 mEq/L in hypernatremia.
- *Serum osmolality* is greater than 295 mOsm/kg in hypernatremia.
- The *water deprivation test* may be conducted to identify diabetes insipidus. Water and all other fluids are withheld for a specified period of time. During this time, urine specimens are obtained for osmolality and specific gravity. No change in these values supports the diagnosis of diabetes insipidus.

### Medications

The principal treatment for hypernatremia is oral or intravenous water replacement. Hypotonic intravenous fluids such as 5% dextrose in water or 0.45% NaCl solution may be administered to correct the water deficit. Diuretics may also be given to increase sodium excretion.

# NURSING CARE

## Health Promotion

Clients at risk for hypernatremia, as well as their care providers, need teaching to prevent this electrolyte disorder. Instruct caregivers of debilitated clients who are unable to perceive thirst or unable to respond to it to offer fluids at regular intervals. If the client is unable to maintain adequate fluid intake, contact the primary care provider about an alternate route for fluid intake (e.g., a feeding tube). Teach care providers the importance of providing adequate water for clients receiving tube feedings (many of which are hypertonic).

## Assessment

Assessment data related to hypernatremia include the following:

- Health history: Duration of symptoms and any precipitating factors such as water deprivation, increased water loss due to heavy perspiration, temperature or rapid breathing, diarrhea, excess salt intake, or diabetes insipidus; current medications; perception of thirst.
- Physical assessment: Vital signs including temperature; mucous membranes; altered mental status or level of consciousness; manifestations of fluid volume excess or fluid volume deficit.

## Nursing Diagnoses and Interventions

### Risk for Injury

Mental status and brain function may be affected by hypernatremia itself or by rapid correction of the condition that leads to cerebral edema. In either case, closely monitor the client and take precautions to reduce risk of injury.

- Monitor and maintain fluid replacement to within the prescribed limits. Monitor serum sodium levels and osmolality; report rapid changes to the care provider. *Rapid water replacement or rapid changes in serum sodium or osmolality can cause fluid shifts within the brain, increasing the risk of bleeding or cerebral edema.*
- Monitor neurologic function, including mental status, level of consciousness, and other manifestations such as headache, nausea, vomiting, elevated blood pressure, and decreased pulse rate. *Both hypernatremia and rapid correction of hypernatremia affect the brain and brain function. Careful monitoring is vital to detect changes in mental status that may indicate cerebral bleeding or edema.*
- Institute safety precautions as necessary: Keep the bed in its lowest position, side rails up and padded, and an airway at bedside. *Clients with sodium disorders are at risk for injury due to seizure activity and changes in mental status.*
- Keep clocks, calendars, and familiar objects at bedside. Orient to time, place, and circumstances as needed. Allow significant others to remain with the client as much as possible. *An unfamiliar environment and altered thought processes can further increase the client's risk for injury. Significant others provide a sense of security and reduce the client's anxiety.*

## Using NANDA, NIC, and NOC

Chart 5–3 shows links between NANDA nursing diagnoses, NIC, and NOC when caring for a client with a sodium imbalance.

## Home Care

When preparing the client who has experienced hypernatremia for home care, discuss the following topics.

- The importance of responding to thirst and consuming adequate fluids (If the client is dependent on a caregiver, stress the importance of regularly offering fluids to the caregiver.)
- If prescribed, guidelines for following a low-sodium diet (see Box 5–5)
- Use and effects (intended and unintended) of any prescribed diuretic or other medication
- The importance of following a schedule for regular monitoring of serum electrolyte levels and reporting manifestations of imbalance to care provider

# POTASSIUM IMBALANCE

Potassium, the primary intercellular cation, plays a vital role in cell metabolism, cardiac, and neuromuscular function. The normal serum (ECF) potassium level is 3.5 to 5.0 mEq/L.

## OVERVIEW OF NORMAL POTASSIUM BALANCE

Most potassium in the body is found within the cells (ICF), which have a concentration of 140 to 150 mEq/L. This significant difference in the potassium concentrations of ICF and ECF helps maintain the resting membrane potential of nerve and muscle cells; either a deficit or an excess of potassium can adversely affect neuromuscular and cardiac function. The higher intracellular potassium concentration is maintained by the sodium-potassium pump.

To maintain its balance, potassium must be replaced daily. Normally, potassium is supplied in food. Virtually all foods contain potassium, although some foods and fluids are richer sources of this element than others (see Box 5–6).

The kidneys eliminate potassium very efficiently; even when potassium intake is stopped, the kidneys continue to excrete it. Because the kidneys do not conserve potassium well, significant amounts may be lost through this route. However, because the kidneys are the principal organs involved in the elimination of potassium, renal failure can lead to potentially serious elevations of serum potassium.

Aldosterone helps regulate potassium elimination by the kidneys. An increased potassium concentration in ECF stimulates aldosterone production by the adrenal gland. The kidneys respond to aldosterone by increasing potassium excretion.

| BOX 5–6 ■ Foods High in Potassium |

**FRUITS**
- Apricots
- Avocados
- Bananas
- Cantaloupe
- Dates
- Oranges
- Raisins

**VEGETABLES AND VEGETABLE JUICES**
- Carrots
- Cauliflower
- Mushrooms
- Peas
- Potatoes
- Spinach
- Tomatoes
- V-8 Juice

**MEATS AND FISH**
- Beef
- Chicken
- Kidney
- Liver
- Lobster
- Pork loin
- Tuna
- Turkey
- Salmon

**MILK PRODUCTS**
- Buttermilk
- Chocolate milk
- Evaporated milk
- Low-fat yogurt
- Milk

Changes in aldosterone secretion can profoundly affect the serum potassium level.

Normally only small amounts of potassium are lost in the feces, but substantial amounts may be lost from the gastrointestinal tract with diarrhea or through drainage from an ileostomy (a permanent opening into the small bowel).

Potassium constantly shifts into and out of the cells. This movement between ICF and ECF can significantly affect the serum potassium level. For example, potassium shifts into or out of the cells in response to changes in hydrogen ion concentration (pH, discussed later in this chapter) as the body strives to maintain a stable acid-base balance. Table 5–6 summarizes potassium imbalances, their causes, and manifestations.

## THE CLIENT WITH HYPOKALEMIA

**Hypokalemia** is an abnormally low serum potassium (less than 3.5 mEq/L). It usually results from excess potassium loss, although hospitalized clients may be at risk for hypokalemia because of inadequate potassium intake.

### PATHOPHYSIOLOGY AND MANIFESTATIONS

Excess potassium may be lost through the kidneys or the gastrointestinal tract. These losses cause depletion of total potassium stores in the body.

- Excess potassium loss through the kidneys often is secondary to drugs such as potassium-wasting diuretics, corticosteroids, amphotericin B, and large doses of some antibiotics. Hyperaldosteronism, a condition in which the adrenal glands secrete excess aldosterone, also causes excess elimination of potassium through the kidneys. Glucosuria and osmotic diuresis (e.g., associated with diabetes mellitus) also cause potassium wasting through the kidneys (Metheny, 2000).
- Gastrointestinal losses of potassium result from severe vomiting, gastric suction, or loss of intestinal fluids through diarrhea or ileostomy drainage.

## TABLE 5–6 Causes and Manifestations of Potassium Imbalances

| Imbalance | Causes | Manifestations |
|---|---|---|
| **Hypokalemia**<br>Serum potassium <3.5 mEq/L | • Excess GI losses: vomiting, diarrhea, ileostomy drainage<br>• Renal losses: diuretics, hyperaldosteronism<br>• Inadequate intake<br>• Shift into cells: Alkalosis, rapid tissue repair | Cardiovascular<br>• Dysrhythmias<br>• ECG changes<br>Gastrointestinal<br>• Nausea and vomiting<br>• Anorexia<br>• Decreased bowel sounds<br>• Ileus<br>Musculoskeletal<br>• Muscle weakness<br>• Leg cramps |
| **Hyperkalemia**<br>Serum potassium >5.0 mEq/L | • Renal failure<br>• Potassium-sparing diuretics<br>• Adrenal insufficiency<br>• Excess potassium intake (e.g., excess potassium replacement)<br>• Aged blood<br>• Shift out of cells: Cell and tissue damage, acidosis | Cardiovascular<br>• Tall, peaked T waves, widened QRS<br>• Dysrhythmias<br>• Cardiac arrest<br>Gastrointestinal<br>• Nausea and vomiting<br>• Abdominal cramping<br>• Diarrhea<br>Neuromuscular<br>• Muscle weakness<br>• Paresthesias<br>• Flaccid paralysis |

Potassium intake may be inadequate in clients who are unable or unwilling to eat for prolonged periods. Hospitalized clients are at risk, especially those on extended parenteral fluid therapy with solutions that do not contain potassium. Clients with anorexia nervosa or alcoholism may develop hypokalemia due to both inadequate intake and loss of potassium through vomiting, diarrhea, or laxative or diuretic use.

A *relative* loss of potassium occurs when potassium shifts from ECF into the cells. This usually is due to loss of hydrogen ion and alkalosis, although it also may occur during periods of rapid tissue repair (e.g., following a burn or trauma), in the presence of excess insulin (insulin promotes potassium entry into skeletal muscle and liver cells), during acute stress, or because of hypothermia. In these instances, the total body stores of potassium remain adequate.

Hypokalemia affects the transmission of nerve impulses, interfering with the contractility of smooth, skeletal, and cardiac muscle, as well as the regulation and transmission of cardiac impulses.

- Characteristic electrocardiogram (ECG) changes of hypokalemia include flattened or inverted T waves, the development of U waves, and a depressed ST segment (Figure 5–11 ■). The most serious cardiac effect is an increased risk of atrial and ventricular **dysrhythmias** (abnormal rhythms). Hypokalemia increases the risk for digitalis toxicity in clients receiving this drug used to treat heart failure (see Chapter 30). ⊂⊃
- Hypokalemia affects both the resting membrane potential and intracellular enzymes in skeletal and smooth muscle cells. This causes skeletal muscle weakness and slowed peristalsis of the gastrointestinal tract. Muscles of the lower extremities are affected first, then the trunk and upper extremities.

Hypokalemia also can affect kidney function, particularly the ability to concentrate urine. Severe hypokalemia can lead to **rhabdomyolysis,** a condition in which muscle fibers disintegrate, releasing myoglobin to be excreted in the urine. The *Multisystem Effects of Hypokalemia* are summarized on page 101.

## COLLABORATIVE CARE

The management of hypokalemia focuses on prevention and treatment of a deficiency.

## Diagnostic Tests

The following laboratory and diagnostic tests may be ordered.

- *Serum potassium (K⁺)* is used to monitor potassium levels in clients who are at risk for or who are being treated for hypokalemia. A serum $K^+$ of 3.0 to 3.5 mEq/L is considered mild hypokalemia. Moderate hypokalemia is defined as a serum $K^+$ of 2.5 to 3.0 mEq/L, and severe hypokalemia as a serum $K^+$ of less than 2.5 mEq/L (Metheny, 2000).
- *Arterial blood gases (ABGs)* are measured to determine acid-base status. An increased pH (alkalosis) often is associated with hypokalemia.

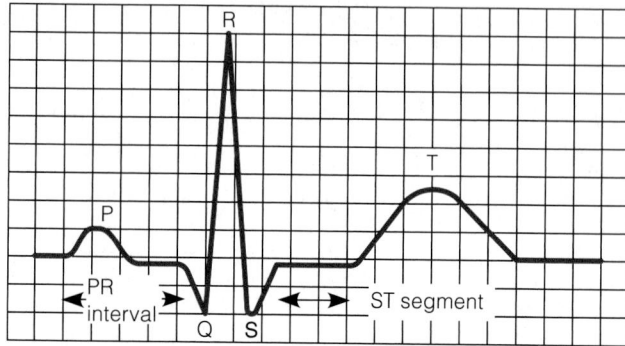

**A Normal ECG**

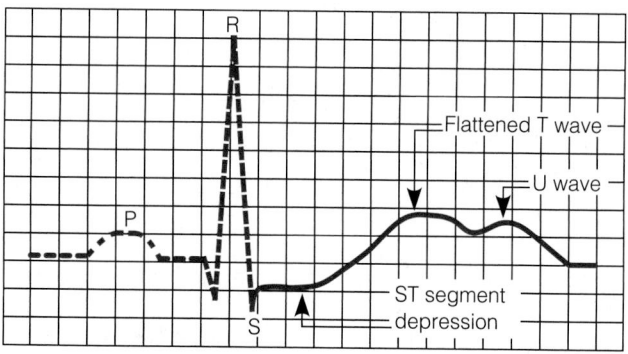

**B ECG in hypokalemia**

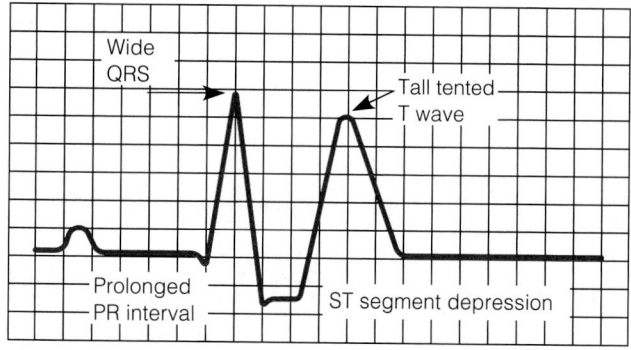

**C ECG in hyperkalemia**

**Figure 5–11** ■ The effects of changes in potassium levels on the electrocardiogram (ECG). *A,* Normal ECG; *B,* ECG in hypokalemia; *C,* ECG in hyperkalemia.

- *ECG recordings* are obtained to evaluate the effects of hypokalemia on the cardiac conduction system.

## Medications

Oral and/or parenteral potassium supplements are given to prevent and, as needed, treat hypokalemia. To prevent hypokalemia in the client taking nothing by mouth, 40 mEq of potassium chloride per day is added to intravenous fluids. The dose used to treat hypokalemia includes the daily maintenance requirement, replacement of ongoing losses (e.g., gastric suction), and additional potassium to correct the existing deficit.

# Multisystem Effects of Hypokalemia

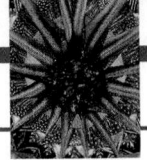

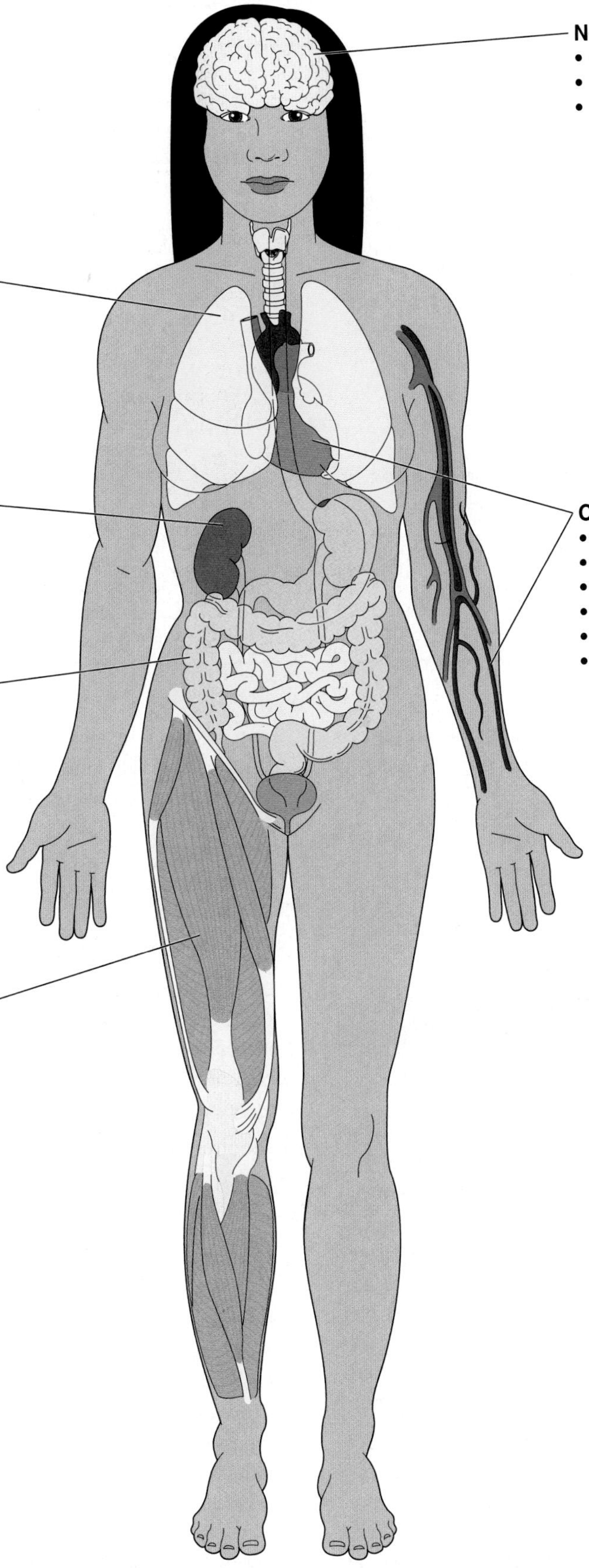
Neurologic
• Confusion
• Depression
• Lethargy
Respiratory
• Respiratory arrest (severe hypokalemia)
Urinary
• Dilute urine
• Polyuria
• Polydipsia
Cardiovascular
• Dysrhythmias
• Irregular pulse
• Postural hypotension
• ECG (conduction) abnormalities
• Increased risk of digitalis toxicity
• Cardiac arrest (severe hypokalemia)
Gastrointestinal
• Nausea and vomiting
• Anorexia
• Diarrhea
• Decreased bowel sounds
• Ileus
Musculoskeletal
• Fatigue
• Leg cramps
• Muscle weakness
• Poor muscle tone
• Paresthesias, paralysis

## Medication Administration

### Hypokalemia

**POTASSIUM SOURCES**
- Potassium acetate (Tri-K)
- Potassium bicarbonate (K + Care ET)
- Potassium citrate (K-Lyte)
- Potassium chloride (K-Lease, Micro-K 10, Apo-K)
- Potassium gluconate (Kaon Elixir, Royonate)

Potassium is rapidly absorbed from the gastrointestinal tract; potassium chloride is the agent of choice, because low chloride often accompanies low potassium. Potassium is used to prevent and/or treat hypokalemia (e.g., with parenteral nutrition and potassium-wasting diuretics, and prophylactically after major surgery).

**Nursing Responsibilities**
- When giving oral forms of potassium:
  a. Dilute or dissolve effervescent, soluable, or liquid potassium in fruit or vegetable juice or cold water.
  b. Chill to increase palatability.
  c. Give with food to minimize GI effects.
- When giving parenteral forms of potassium:
  a. Administer slowly
  b. *Do not* administer undiluted.

  c. Assess injection site frequently for signs of pain and inflammation.
  d. Use an infusion control device.
- Assess for abdominal pain, distention, gastrointestinal bleeding; if present, do not administer medication. Notify health care provider.
- Monitor fluid intake and output.
- Assess for manifestations of hyperkalemia: weakness, feeling of heaviness in legs, mental confusion, hypotension, cardiac arrhythmias, changes in ECG, increased serum potassium levels.

**Client and Family Teaching**
- Do not take potassium supplements if you are also taking a potassium-sparing diuretic.
- When parenteral potassium is discontinued, eat potassium-rich foods.
- Do not chew enteric-coated tablets or allow them to dissolve in the mouth; this may affect the potency and action of the medications.
- Take potassium supplements with meals.
- Do not use salt substitutes when taking potassium (most salt substitutes are potassium based).

---

Several days of therapy may be required. Commonly prescribed potassium supplements, their actions, and nursing implications are described in the box above.

## Dietary Management

A diet high in potassium-rich foods is recommended for clients at risk for developing hypokalemia or to supplement drug therapy (see Box 5–6).

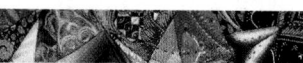

## NURSING CARE

## Health Promotion

When providing general health education, discuss using balanced electrolyte solutions (e.g., Pedialyte or sports drinks) to replace abnormal fluid losses (excess perspiration, vomiting, or severe diarrhea). Discuss the necessity of preventing hypokalemia with clients at risk. Provide diet teaching and refer clients with anorexia nervosa for counseling. Stress the potassium-losing effects of taking diuretics and using laxatives to enhance weight loss. Discuss the potassium-wasting effects of most diuretics with clients taking these drugs, and encourage a diet rich in high-potassium foods, as well as regular monitoring of serum potassium levels.

## Assessment

Assessment data related to hypokalemia include the following:

- Health history:  Current manifestations, including anorexia, nausea and vomiting, abdominal discomfort, muscle weakness or cramping, other symptoms; duration of symptoms and

any precipitating factors such as diuretic use, prolonged vomiting or diarrhea; chronic diseases such as diabetes, hyperaldosteronism, or Cushing's syndrome; current medications.
- Physical assessment:  Mental status; vital signs including orthostatic vitals, apical and peripheral pulses; bowel sounds, abdominal distension; muscle strength and tone.

## Nursing Diagnoses and Interventions

### Activity Intolerance

Muscle cramping and weakness are common early manifestations of hypokalemia. The lower extremities are usually affected initially. This muscle weakness can cause the client to fatigue easily, particularly with activity.

- Monitor skeletal muscle strength and tone, which are affected by moderate hypokalemia. *Increasing weakness, paresthesias, or paralysis of muscles or progression of affected muscles to include the upper extremities or trunk can indicate a further drop in serum potassium levels.*
- Monitor respiratory rate, depth, and effort; heart rate and rhythm; and blood pressure at rest and following activity. *Tachypnea, dyspnea, tachycardia, and/or a change in blood pressure may indicate decreasing ability to tolerate activities. Report changes to the care provider.*
- Assist with self-care activities as needed. *Increasing muscle weakness can lead to fatigue and affect the ability to meet self-care needs.*

### Decreased Cardiac Output

Hypokalemia affects the strength of cardiac contractions and can lead to dysrhythmias that further impair cardiac output.

Hypokalemia also alters the response to cardiac drugs, such as digitalis and the antidysrhythmics.

- Monitor serum potassium levels, particularly in clients at risk for hypokalemia (those with excess losses due to drug therapy, gastrointestinal losses, or who are unable to consume a normal diet). Report abnormal levels to the care provider. *Potassium must be replaced daily, as the body is unable to conserve it. Either lack of intake or abnormal losses of potassium in the urine or gastric fluids can lead to hypokalemia.*
- Monitor vital signs, including orthostatic vitals and peripheral pulses. *As cardiac output falls, the pulse becomes weak and thready. Orthostatic hypotension may be noted with decreased cardiac output.*

**PRACTICE ALERT** *Pace clients with severe hypokalemia on a cardiac monitor. Closely monitor cardiac rhythm and observe for characteristic ECG changes of hypokalemia (ST segment depression, flattened T waves, and U waves). Report rhythm changes and treat as indicated. Severe hypokalemia can cause life-threatening dysrhythmias.* ■

- Monitor clients taking digitalis for toxicity. Monitor response to antidysrhythmic drugs. *Hypokalemia potentiates digitalis effects and increases resistance to certain antidysrhythmics.*
- Dilute intravenous potassium and administer using an electronic infusion device. In general, potassium is given no faster than 10 to 20 mEq/hour. Closely monitor intravenous flow rate and response to potassium replacement. *Rapid potassium administration is dangerous and can lead to hyperkalemia and cardiac arrest.*

**PRACTICE ALERT** *Never administer undiluted potassium directly into the vein.* ■

### Risk for Imbalanced Fluid Volume

- Maintain accurate intake and output records. *Gastrointestinal fluid losses can lead to significant potassium losses.*

- Monitor bowel sounds and abdominal distention. *Hypokalemia affects smooth muscle function and can lead to slowed peristalsis and paralytic ileus.*

### Acute Pain

Discomfort is common when intravenous potassium chloride at a concentration of more than 40 mEq/L is given into a peripheral vein.

- When possible, administer intravenous KCl through a central line. *The rapid blood flow through central veins dilutes the KCl solution, decreasing discomfort.*
- Spread the total daily dose of KCl over 24 hours to minimize the concentration of intravenous solutions. *High concentrations of KCl are irritating to vein walls, particularly if inflammation is present.*
- Discuss with the physician using a small amount of lidocaine prior to or with the infusion. *Both a lidocaine bolus given at the infusion site and a small amount of lidocaine in the intravenous infusion have been shown to at least partially relieve discomfort associated with concentrated potassium solutions* (Metheny, 2000).

## Using NANDA, NIC, and NOC

Chart 5–4 shows links between NANDA nursing diagnoses, NIC, and NOC for clients with a potassium imbalance.

## Home Care

The focus in preparing the client with or at risk for hypokalemia is prevention. Discharge planning focuses on teaching self-care practices. Include the following topics when preparing the client and family for home care.

- Recommended diet, including a list of potassium-rich foods
- Prescribed medications and potassium supplements, their use, and desired and unintended effects
- Using salt substitutes (if recommended) to increase potassium intake; avoiding substitutes if taking a potassium supplement or potassium-sparing diuretic

---

## CHART 5–4  NANDA, NIC, AND NOC LINKAGES

### The Client with Potassium Imbalance

| NURSING DIAGNOSES | NURSING INTERVENTIONS | NURSING OUTCOMES |
|---|---|---|
| • Decreased Cardiac Output | • Cardiac Care<br>• Electrolyte Management: Hyperkalemia<br>• Electrolyte Management: Hypokalemia | • Cardiac Pump Effectiveness<br>• Vital Signs Status |
| • Activity Intolerance | • Energy Management | • Energy Conservation<br>• Activity Tolerance |
| • Risk for Ineffective Health Maintenance | • Health Education<br>• Risk Identification | • Health-Seeking Behavior |

*Note. Data from Nursing Outcomes Classification (NOC) by M. Johnson & M. Maas (Eds.), 1997, St. Louis: Mosby; Nursing Diagnoses: Definitions & Classification 2001–2002 by North American Nursing Diagnosis Association, 2001, Philadelphia: NANDA; Nursing Interventions Classification (NIC) by J.C. McCloskey & G. M. Bulechek (Eds.), 2000, St. Louis: Mosby. Reprinted by permission.*

- Manifestations of potassium imbalance (hypokalemia or hyperkalemia) to report to health care provider
- Recommendations for monitoring serum potassium levels
- If taking digitalis, manifestations of digitalis toxicity to report to health care provider
- Managing gastrointestinal disorders that cause potassium loss (vomiting, diarrhea, ileostomy drainage) to prevent hypokalemia

## THE CLIENT WITH HYPERKALEMIA

**Hyperkalemia** is an abnormally high serum potassium (greater than 5 mEq/L). Hyperkalemia can result from inadequate excretion of potassium, excessively high intake of potassium, or a shift of potassium from the intracellular to the ex-

tracellular space. *Pseudohyperkalemia* (an erroneously high serum potassium reading) can occur if the blood sample hemolyzes, releasing potassium from blood cells, before it is analyzed. Hyperkalemia affects neuromuscular and cardiac function.

## PATHOPHYSIOLOGY AND MANIFESTATIONS

Impaired renal excretion of potassium is a primary cause of hyperkalemia. Untreated renal failure, adrenal insufficiency (e.g., Addison's disease or inadequate aldosterone production), and medications (such as potassium-sparing diuretics, the antimicrobial drug trimethoprim, and some NSAIDs) impair potassium excretion by the kidneys.

In clients with normal renal excretion of potassium, excess oral potassium (e.g., by supplement or use of salt substitutes) rarely leads to hyperkalemia. Rapid intravenous administra-

## Nursing Care Plan
## A Client with Hypokalemia

Rose Ortiz is a 72-year-old widow who lives alone, although close to her daughter's home. Ms. Ortiz has mild heart failure and is being treated with digoxin (Lanoxin) 0.125 mg, furosemide (Lasix) 40 mg PO daily, and a mildly restricted sodium diet (2 g daily). For the last several weeks, Ms. Ortiz has complained that she feels weak and sometimes faint, light headed, and dizzy. Serum electrolyte tests ordered by her physician reveal a potassium level of 2.4 mEq/L. Potassium chloride solution (Kaochlor 10%, 20 mEq/15 mL) PO twice daily is prescribed, and Ms. Ortiz is referred to Nancy Walters, RN, for follow-up care.

### ASSESSMENT
Ms. Ortiz's health history reveals that she has rigidly adhered to her sodium-restricted diet and has been compliant in taking her prescribed medications, with the exception of occasionally taking an additional "water pill" when her ankles swell. She takes a laxative every evening to ensure a daily bowel movement. She states that she is reluctant to take the potassium chloride the doctor has ordered because her neighbor complains that his potassium supplement upsets his stomach. Physical assessment findings included T 98.4, P 70, R 20, and BP 138/84. Muscle strength in her upper extremities is normal and equal; lower extremity strength is weak but equal. Sensation is normal.

### DIAGNOSES
- *Risk for injury* related to muscle weakness
- *Risk for ineffective health maintenance* related to lack of knowledge about how diuretic therapy and laxative affect potassium levels

### EXPECTED OUTCOMES
- Maintain potassium level within normal limits (3.5 to 5.0 mEq/L).
- Regain normal muscle strength.
- Remain free of injury.
- Verbalize understanding of the effects of diuretic therapy and laxatives on potassium levels.

- Identify measures to avoid gastrointestinal irritation when taking oral potassium.
- Identify potassium-rich foods.

### PLANNING AND IMPLEMENTATION
- Explain need to use caution when ambulating, particularly when climbing or descending stairs.
- Discuss side effects of furosemide, and explain how taking additional tablets may have contributed to hypokalemia.
- Discuss alternative measures to prevent constipation without using laxatives on a regular basis (e.g., high-fiber diet, adequate fluid intake).
- Explain purpose of the prescribed potassium and its role in reversing muscle weakness.
- Teach to take potassium supplement after breakfast and supper, diluted in 4 oz of juice or water, and to sip it slowly over a 5- to 10-minute period. Advise to call if gastric irritation occurs.
- Discuss dietary sources of potassium; provide a list of potassium-rich foods.

### EVALUATION
On a follow-up visit 1 week later, Ms. Ortiz states that her muscle weakness, dizziness, and other symptoms have resolved. She is taking the prescribed drugs as directed and is using laxatives only two or three times a week. Ms. Ortiz reports that she has increased her intake of potassium-rich foods and fluids and of high-fiber foods. Her potassium level is within normal limits.

### Critical Thinking in the Nursing Process
1. What is the pathophysiologic basis for Rose's muscle weakness and dizziness?
2. How may the chronic overuse of laxatives contribute to hypokalemia?
3. Describe the interaction of digitalis, diuretics, and potassium.
4. Develop a plan of care for Ms. Ortiz for the nursing diagnosis *Constipation*.

See Evaluating Your Response in Appendix C.

tion of potassium or transfusion of aged blood can lead to hyperkalemia.

A shift of potassium ions from the intracellular space can occur in acidosis, with severe tissue trauma, during chemotherapy, and due to starvation. In acidosis, excess hydrogen ions enter the cells, causing potassium to shift into the extracellular space. The extent of this shift is greater with metabolic acidosis than with respiratory acidosis (see "Acid-Base Disorders" later in this chapter).

Hyperkalemia alters the cell membrane potential, affecting the heart, skeletal muscle function, and the gastrointestinal tract. The most harmful consequence of hyperkalemia is its effect on cardiac function. The cardiac conduction system is affected first, with slowing of the heart rate, possible heart blocks, and prolonged depolarization. ECG changes include peaked T waves, a prolonged PR interval, and widening of the QRS complex (see Figure 5–11). Ventricular dysrhythmias develop, and cardiac arrest may occur. Severe hyperkalemia decreases the strength of myocardial contractions.

Skeletal muscles become weak and paralysis may occur with very high serum potassium levels. Hyperkalemia causes smooth muscle hyperactivity, leading to gastrointestinal disturbances.

The seriousness of hyperkalemia is based on the serum potassium (K+) level and ECG changes.

- Mild hyperkalemia: serum K+ between 5 and 6.5 mEq/L; ECG changes limited to peaked T wave.
- Moderate hyperkalemia: serum K+ between 6.5 and 8 mEq/L; ECG changes limited to peaked T wave.
- Severe hyperkalemia: serum K+ greater than 8 mEq/L; ECG shows absent P waves and widened QRS pattern.

The manifestations of hyperkalemia result from its effects on the heart, skeletal, and smooth muscles. Early manifestations include diarrhea, colic (abdominal cramping), anxiety, paresthesias, irritability, and muscle tremors and twitching. As serum potassium levels increase, muscle weakness develops, progressing to flaccid paralysis. The lower extremities are affected first, progressing to the trunk and upper extremities.

## COLLABORATIVE CARE

The management of hyperkalemia focuses on returning the serum potassium level to normal by treating the underlying cause and avoiding additional potassium intake. The choice of therapy for existing hyperkalemia is based on the severity of the hyperkalemia.

### Diagnostic Tests

The following laboratory and diagnostic tests may be ordered.

- *Serum electrolytes* show a serum potassium level greater than 5.0 mEq/L. Low calcium and sodium levels may increase the effects of hyperkalemia; therefore, these electrolytes are usually measured as well.
- *ABGs* are measured to determine if acidosis is present.
- An *ECG* is obtained and *continuous ECG monitoring* is instituted to evaluate the effects of hyperkalemia on cardiac conduction and rhythm.

### Medications

Medications are administered to lower the serum potassium and to stabilize the conduction system of the heart. For moderate to severe hyperkalemia, calcium gluconate is given intravenously to counter the effects of hyperkalemia on the cardiac conduction system. While the effect of calcium gluconate lasts only for 1 hour, it allows time to initiate measures to lower serum potassium levels. To rapidly lower these levels, regular insulin and 50 g of glucose are administered. Insulin and glucose promote potassium uptake by the cells, shifting potassium out of ECF. In some cases, a $\beta_2$-agonist such as albuterol may be given by nebulizer to temporarily push potassium into the cells. Sodium bicarbonate may be given to treat acidosis. As the pH returns toward normal, hydrogen ions are released from the cells and potassium returns into the cells.

To remove potassium from the body, sodium polystyrene sulfonate (Kayexalate), a resin that binds potassium in the gastrointestinal tract, may be administered orally or rectally. If renal function is normal, diuretics such as furosemide are given to promote potassium excretion. Commonly prescribed drugs, their actions, and nursing implications are summarized on page 106.

### Dialysis

When renal function is severely limited, either peritoneal dialysis or hemodialysis may be implemented to remove excess potassium. These measures are invasive and typically used only when other measures are ineffective. See Chapter 27 for more information about dialysis.

## NURSING CARE

Nursing care focuses related to hyperkalemia include identifying clients at risk, preventing hyperkalemia, and addressing problems resulting from the systemic effects of hyperkalemia.

### Health Promotion

Clients at the greatest risk for developing hyperkalemia include those taking potassium supplements (prescribed or over-the-counter), using potassium-sparing diuretics or salt substitutes, and experiencing renal failure. Athletes participating in competition sports such as body building and using anabolic steroids, muscle-building compounds, or "energy drinks" also may be at risk for hyperkalemia.

Teach all clients to carefully read food and dietary supplement labels. Discuss the importance of taking prescribed potassium supplements as ordered, and not increasing the dose unless prescribed by the care provider. Advise clients taking a potassium supplement or potassium-sparing diuretic to avoid salt substitutes, which usually contain potassium. Discuss the importance of maintaining an adequate fluid intake (unless a fluid restriction has been prescribed) to maintain renal function to eliminate potassium from the body.

### Assessment

Assessment data related to hyperkalemia include the following:

- Health history:   Current manifestations, including numbness and tingling, nausea and vomiting, abdominal cramping, muscle weakness, palpitations; duration of symptoms and any precipitating factors such as use of salt substitutes, potassium supplements, or reduced urine output; chronic diseases such as renal failure or endocrine disorders; current medications.

- Physical assessment: Apical and peripheral pulses; bowel sounds; muscle strength in upper and lower extremities; ECG pattern.

## Nursing Diagnoses and Interventions

### Risk for Activity Intolerance

Both hypokalemia (low serum potassium levels) and hyperkalemia (high serum potassium levels) affect neuromuscular activity and the function of cardiac, smooth, and skeletal muscles. Hyperkalemia can cause muscle weakness and even paralysis.

- Monitor skeletal muscle strength and tone. *Increasing weakness, muscle paralysis, or progression of affected muscles to affect the upper extremities or trunk can indicate increasing serum potassium levels.*
- Monitor respiratory rate and depth. Regularly assess lung sounds. *Muscle weakness due to hyperkalemia can impair ventilation. In addition, medications such as sodium bicarbonate or sodium polystyrene sulfonate can cause fluid re-*

*tention and pulmonary edema in clients with preexisting cardiovascular disease.*

- Assist with self-care activities as needed. *Increasing muscle weakness can lead to fatigue and affect the ability to meet self-care needs.*

### Risk for Decreased Cardiac Output

Hyperkalemia affects depolarization of the atria and ventricles of the heart. Severe hyperkalemia can cause dysrhythmias with ventricular fibrillation and cardiac arrest. The cardiac effects of hyperkalemia are more pronounced when the serum potassium level rises rapidly. Low serum sodium and calcium levels, high serum magnesium levels, and acidosis contribute to the adverse effects of hyperkalemia on the heart muscle.

> **PRACTICE ALERT** *Monitor the ECG pattern for development of peaked, narrow T waves, prolongation of the PR interval, depression of the ST segment, widened QRS interval, and loss of the P wave. Notify the physician of changes. Progressive ECG changes from a peaked T wave to loss of the P wave and widening of the QRS complex indicate an increasing risk of dysrhythmias and cardiac arrest.* ■

## Medication Administration

### Hyperkalemia

#### DIURETICS

Potassium-wasting diuretics, such as furosemide (Lasix), may be used to enhance renal excretion of potassium.

##### Nursing Responsibilities
- Monitor serum electrolytes.
- Monitor and record weight at regular intervals under standard conditions (same time of day, balanced scale, same clothing).
- Monitor intake and output.

#### INSULIN, HYPERTONIC DEXTROSE, AND SODIUM BICARBONATE

Insulin, hypertonic dextrose (10% to 50%), and sodium bicarbonate are used in the emergency treatment of moderate to severe hyperkalemia. Insulin promotes the movement of potassium into the cell, and glucose prevents hypoglycemia. The onset of action of insulin and hypertonic dextrose occurs within 30 minutes and is effective for approximately 4 to 6 hours.

Sodium bicarbonate elevates the serum pH; potassium is moved into the cell in exchange for hydrogen ion. Sodium bicarbonate is particularly useful in the client with metabolic acidosis. Onset of effects occurs within 15 to 30 minutes and is effective for approximately 2 hours.

##### Nursing Responsibilities
- Administer intravenous insulin and dextrose over prescribed interval of time using an infusion pump.
- Administer sodium bicarbonate as prescribed. It may be administered as an intravenous bolus or added to a dextrose-in-water solution and given by infusion.
- In clients receiving sodium bicarbonate, monitor for sodium overload, particularly in clients with hypernatremia, heart failure, and renal failure.

- Monitor the ECG pattern closely.
- Monitor serum electrolytes ($K^+$, $Na^+$, $Ca^{2+}$, $Mg^{2+}$) frequently during treatment.

#### CALCIUM GLUCONATE AND CALCIUM CHLORIDE

Intravenous calcium gluconate or calcium chloride is used as a temporary emergency measure to counteract the toxic effects of potassium on myocardial conduction and function.

##### Nursing Responsibilities
- Closely monitor the ECG of the client receiving intravenous calcium, particularly for bradycardia.
- Calcium should be used cautiously in clients receiving digitalis, because calcium increases the cardiotonic effects of digitalis and may precipitate digitalis toxicity, leading to dysrhythmias.

#### SODIUM POLYSTYRENE SULFONATE (KAYEXALATE) AND SORBITOL

Sodium polystyrene sulfonate (Kayexalate) is used to treat moderate or severe hyperkalemia. Categorized as a cation exchange resin, Kayexalate exchanges sodium or calcium for potassium in the large intestine. Sorbitol is given with Kayexalate to promote bowel elimination. Kayexalate and sorbitol may be administered orally, through a nasogastric tube, or rectally as a retention enema. The usual dosage is 20 g three or four times a day with 20 mL of 70% sorbitol solution.

##### Nursing Responsibilities
- Because Kayexalate contains sodium, monitor clients with heart failure and edema closely for water retention.
- Monitor serum electrolytes ($K^+$, $Na^+$, $Ca^{2+}$, $Mg^{2+}$) frequently during therapy.
- Restrict sodium intake in clients who are unable to tolerate increased sodium load (e.g., those with CHF or hypertension).

- Closely monitor the response to intravenous calcium gluconate, particularly in clients taking digitalis. *Calcium increases the risk of digitalis toxicity.*

### Risk for Imbalanced Fluid Volume

Renal failure is a major cause of hyperkalemia. Clients with renal failure also are at risk for fluid retention and other electrolyte imbalances.

- Closely monitor serum potassium, BUN, and serum creatinine. Notify the physician if serum potassium level is greater than 5 mEq/L, or if serum creatinine and BUN levels are increasing. *Serum creatinine and BUN are the primary indicators of renal function. Levels of these substances rise rapidly in acute renal failure, more slowly in chronic renal failure* (see Chapter 27).
- Maintain accurate intake and output records. Report an imbalance of 24-hour totals and/or urine output less than 30 mL/hour. *Oliguria (scant urine) or anuria (no urine output) may indicate renal failure and an increased risk for hyperkalemia and fluid volume excess.*
- Monitor clients receiving sodium bicarbonate for fluid volume excess. *Increased sodium from injection of a hypertonic sodium bicarbonate solution can cause a shift of water into the extracellular space.*
- Monitor clients receiving cation exchange resins and sorbitol for fluid volume excess. *The resin exchanges potassium for sodium or calcium in the bowel. Excessive sodium and water retention may occur.*

### Using NANDA, NIC, and NOC

Chart 5–4 shows links between NANDA nursing diagnoses, NIC, and NOC when caring for a client with a potassium imbalance.

### Home Care

Preventing future episodes of hyperkalemia is the focus when preparing the client for home care. Include the family, a significant other, or a caregiver when teaching the following topics.

- Recommended diet and any restrictions including salt substitutes and foods high in potassium
- Medications to be avoided, including over-the-counter and fitness supplements
- Follow-up appointments for lab work and evaluation

## Nursing Care Plan
## A Client with Hyperkalemia

Montigue Longacre, a 51-year-old African American male, has end-stage renal failure. He arrives at the emergency clinic complaining of shortness of breath on exertion and extreme weakness.

### ASSESSMENT

Mr. Longacre tells the nurse, Janet Allen, RN, that he normally receives dialysis three times a week. He missed his last treatment, however, to attend his father's funeral. During the last several days, he has eaten a number of fresh oranges he received as a gift. Physical assessment findings include T 99.2, P 100, R 28, BP 168/96, 2+ pretibial edema, and a 6 lb (3.6 kg) weight gain since his last hemodialysis treatment 4 days ago. Laboratory and diagnostic tests show the following abnormal results.

- K+ 6.5 mEq/L (normal 3.5 to 5 mEq/L)
- BUN 118 mg/dL (normal 7 to 18 mg/dL)
- Creatinine 14 mg/dL (normal 0.7 to 1.3 mg/dL)
- HCO₃⁻ 17 mEq/L (normal 22 to 26 mEq/L)
- Peaked T wave noted on ECG

Mr. Longacre is placed on continuous ECG monitoring, and the physician prescribes hemodialysis. As an interim measure to lower the serum potassium, the physician prescribes D50W (25 g of dextrose), one ampule, to be administered intravenously with 10 units of regular insulin over 30 minutes.

### DIAGNOSIS

- *Activity intolerance* related to skeletal muscle weakness
- *Risk for decreased cardiac output* related to hyperkalemia
- *Risk for ineffective health maintenance* related to inadequate knowledge of recommended diet
- *Excess fluid volume* related to renal failure

### EXPECTED OUTCOMES

- Gradually resume usual physical activities.
- Maintain serum potassium level within normal range.

- Verbalize causes of hyperkalemia, the importance of hemodialysis treatments as scheduled, and the role of diet in preventing hyperkalemia.

### PLANNING AND IMPLEMENTATION

- Monitor intake and output.
- Monitor serum potassium and ECG closely during treatment.
- Teach causes of hyperkalemia and the relationship between hemodialysis and hyperkalemia.
- Discuss the importance of avoiding foods high in potassium to prevent or control hyperkalemia.

### EVALUATION

Following emergency treatment and hemodialysis, Mr. Longacre's ECG and serum potassium level have returned to normal. His muscle strength has returned to near normal, and he verbalizes an understanding of his prescribed hemodialysis regimen. Janet Allen provides verbal and written information about hyperkalemia, the importance of complying with the hemodialysis regimen, and the importance of limiting intake of dietary sources of potassium in renal failure. She also furnishes a list of foods high in potassium and cautions against using potassium-containing salt substitutes and nonprescription drugs.

### Critical Thinking in the Nursing Process

1. What information given by Mr. Longacre indicated that he might be experiencing hyperkalemia?
2. Why was continuous ECG monitoring instituted as an emergency measure?
3. What additional emergency measures might have been instituted if Mr. Longacre's serum potassium level was 8.5 mEq/L and his ECG showed changes in impulse conduction?
4. Develop a care plan for Mr. Longacre for the nursing diagnosis *anxiety*.

See Evaluating Your Response in Appendix C.

# CALCIUM IMBALANCE

Calcium is one of the most abundant ions in the body. The normal adult total serum calcium concentration is 8.5 to 10.0 mg/dL.

## OVERVIEW OF NORMAL CALCIUM BALANCE

Calcium is obtained from dietary sources, although only about 20% of the calcium ingested is absorbed into the blood. The remainder is excreted in feces. Extracellular calcium is excreted by the kidneys. Approximately 99% of the total calcium in the body is bound to phosphorus to form the minerals in bones and teeth. The remaining 1% is in extracellular fluid. About half of this extracellular calcium is ionized (free); it is this ionized calcium that is physiologically active. The remaining extracellular calcium is bound to protein or other ions.

Ionized calcium is essential to a number of processes:

- Stabilizing cell membranes
- Regulating muscle contraction and relaxation
- Maintaining cardiac function
- Blood clotting

Serum calcium levels are regulated by the interaction of three hormones: parathyroid hormone (PTH), calcitonin, and calcitriol (a metabolite of vitamin D). When serum calcium levels fall, the parathyroid glands secrete PTH, which mobilizes skeletal calcium stores, increases calcium absorption in the intestines, and promotes calcium reabsorption by the kidneys (Figure 5–12 ■). Calcitriol facilitates this process by stimulating calcium release from the bones, absorption in the intestines, and reabsorption by the kidneys. Calcitonin is secreted by the thyroid gland in response to high serum calcium levels. Its effect on serum calcium levels is the opposite of PTH: It inhibits the movement of calcium out of bone, reduces intestinal absorption of calcium, and promotes calcium excretion by the kidneys.

Serum calcium levels are also affected by acid-base balance. When hydrogen ion concentration falls and the pH rises (**alkalosis**), more calcium is bound to protein. While the total serum calcium remains unchanged, less calcium is available in the ionized, active form. Conversely, when hydrogen ion concentration increases and the pH falls (**acidosis**), calcium is released from protein, making more ionized calcium available. Table 5–7 summarizes the causes and manifestations of calcium imbalances.

## THE CLIENT WITH HYPOCALCEMIA

**Hypocalcemia** is a total serum calcium level of less than 8.5 mg/dL. Hypocalcemia can result from decreased total body calcium stores or low levels of extracellular calcium with normal amounts of calcium stored in bone. The systemic effects of hypocalcemia are caused by decreased levels of ionized calcium in extracellular fluid.

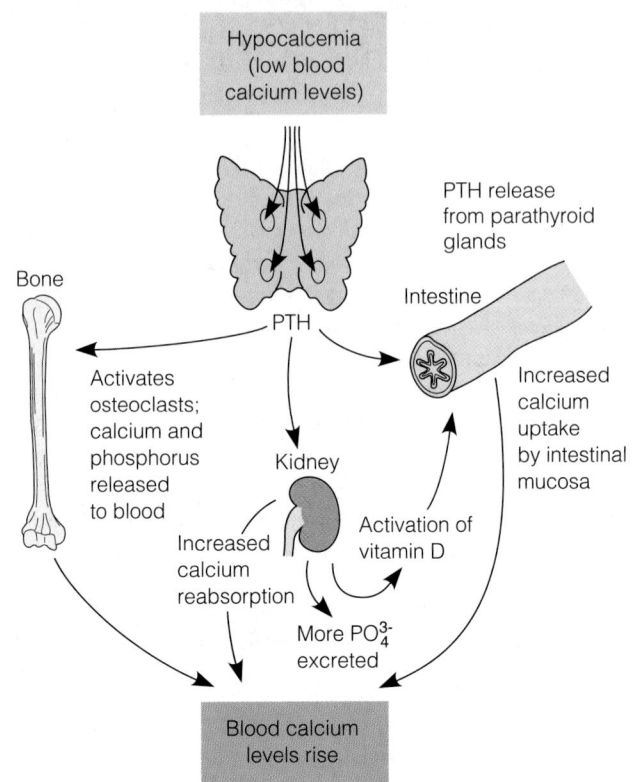

**Figure 5–12** ■ Low calcium levels (hypocalcemia) trigger the release of parathyroid hormone (PTH), increasing calcium ion levels through stimulation of bones, kidneys, and intestines.

## RISK FACTORS

Certain populations of people are at greater risk for hypocalcemia: people who have had a parathyroidectomy (removal of the parathyroid glands), older adults (especially women), people with lactose intolerance, and those with alcoholism. Older adults often consume less milk and milk products (good sources of calcium) and may have less exposure to the sun (a source of vitamin D). Older adults also may be less active, promoting calcium loss from bones. They are more likely to be taking drugs that interfere with calcium absorption or promote calcium excretion (e.g., furosemide). Older women are at particular risk after menopause because of reduced estrogen levels. Intolerance to lactose (found in milk and milk products) causes diarrhea and often limits the intake of milk and milk products, leading to possible calcium deficiency. Ethanol, or drinking alcohol, has a direct effect on calcium balance, reduces its intestinal absorption, and interferes with other processes involved in regulating serum calcium levels.

## PATHOPHYSIOLOGY

Common causes of hypocalcemia are hypoparathyroidism (see Chapter 17 ⊙ ) resulting from surgery (parathyroidectomy, thyroidectomy, radical neck dissection) and acute pancreatitis.

## TABLE 5-7 Causes and Manifestations of Calcium Imbalances

| Imbalance | Causes | Manifestations |
|---|---|---|
| **Hypocalcemia**<br>Serum calcium <4.3 mEq/L or 8.5 mg/dL | • Parathyroidectomy or neck surgery<br>• Acute pancreatitis<br>• Inadequate dietary intake<br>• Lack of sun exposure<br>• Lack of weight-bearing exercise<br>• Drugs: loop diuretics, calcitonin<br>• Hypomagnesemia, alcohol abuse | Neuromuscular<br>  • Tetany<br>    • Paresthesias<br>    • Muscle spasms<br>    • Positive Chvostek's sign<br>    • Positive Trousseau's sign<br>    • Laryngospasm<br>    • Seizures<br>  • Anxiety, confusion, psychoses<br>Cardiovascular<br>  • Decreased cardiac output<br>  • Hypotension<br>  • Dysrhythmias<br>Gastrointestinal<br>  • Abdominal cramping<br>  • Diarrhea |
| **Hypercalcemia**<br>Serum calcium >5.3 mEq/L or 10 mg/dL | • Hyperparathyroidism<br>• Some cancers<br>• Prolonged immobilization<br>• Paget's disease<br>• Excess milk or antacid intake<br>• Renal failure | Neuromuscular<br>  • Muscle weakness, fatigue<br>  • Decreased deep tendon reflexes<br>Behavioral<br>  • Personality changes<br>  • Altered mental status<br>  • Decreasing level of consciousness<br>Gastrointestinal<br>  • Abdominal pain<br>  • Constipation<br>  • Anorexia, nausea, vomiting<br>Cardiovascular<br>  • Dysrhythmias<br>  • Hypertension<br>Renal<br>  • Polyuria, thirst |

In the client who has undergone surgery, symptoms of hypocalcemia usually occur within the first 24 to 48 hours, but may be delayed.

**PRACTICE ALERT** *Carefully monitor clients who have undergone neck surgery for manifestations of hypocalcemia. Check serum calcium levels, and report changes to the care provider.* ■

Additional causes of hypocalcemia include other electrolyte imbalances (such as hypomagnesemia or hyperphosphatemia), alkalosis, malabsorption disorders that interfere with calcium absorption in the bowel, and inadequate vitamin D (due to lack of sun exposure or malabsorption). Massive transfusion of banked blood also can lead to hypocalcemia. Citrate is added to blood to prevent clotting and as a preservative. When blood is administered faster than the liver can metabolize the citrate, it can bind with calcium, temporarily removing ionized calcium from circulation. Many drugs increase the risk for hypocalcemia, including loop diuretics (such as furosemide), anticonvulsants (such as phenytoin and phenobarbital), phosphates (including phosphate enemas), and drugs that lower serum magnesium levels (such as cisplatin and gentamycin) (Metheny, 2000).

Hypocalcemia affects neuromuscular cell membranes, increasing neuromuscular irritability. The threshold of excitation of sensory nerve fibers is lowered as well, leading to paresthesias (altered sensation). The nervous system becomes more excitable, and muscle spasms develop. In the heart, this change in cell membranes can lead to dysrhythmias such as ventricular tachycardia and cardiac arrest. Hypocalcemia decreases the contractility of cardiac muscle fibers, leading to decreased cardiac output.

## MANIFESTATIONS AND COMPLICATIONS

The most serious manifestations of hypocalcemia are **tetany** (tonic muscular spasms) and convulsions. Numbness and tingling around the mouth (circumoral) and in the hands and feet develop. Muscle spasms of the face and extremities occur, and deep tendon reflexes become hyperactive. Chvostek's sign, contraction of the facial muscles produced by tapping the facial nerve in front of the ear (Figure 5–13A ■), and Trousseau's sign, carpal spasm induced by inflating a blood pressure cuff on the upper arm to above systolic blood pressure for 2 to 5 minutes (Figure 5–13B), indicate increased neuromuscular excitability in clients without obvious symptoms.

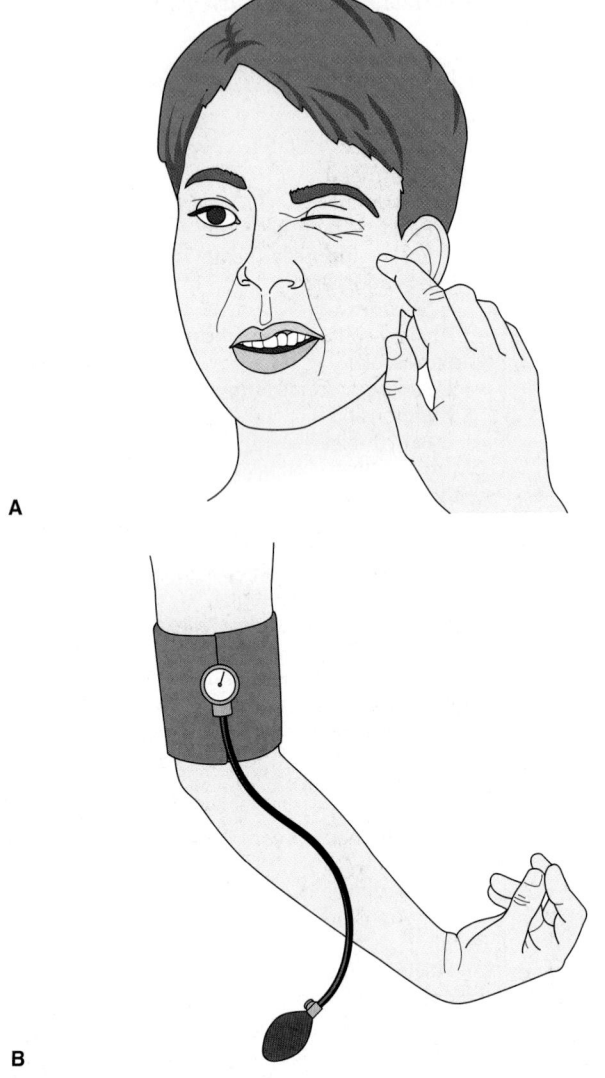

**A**

**B**

**Figure 5–13** ■ *A,* Positive Chvostek's sign. *B,* Positive Trousseau's sign.

Tetany can cause bronchial muscle spasms, simulating an asthma attack, and visceral muscle spasms, producing acute abdominal pain. Cardiovascular manifestations include hypotension, possible bradycardia (slow heart rate), and ventricular dysrhythmias.

Serious complications of hypocalcemia include airway obstruction and possible respiratory arrest from laryngospasm, ventricular dysrhythmias and cardiac arrest, heart failure, and convulsions.

## COLLABORATIVE CARE

Management of hypocalcemia is directed toward restoring normal calcium balance and correcting the underlying cause.

### Diagnostic Tests

The following laboratory and diagnostic tests may be ordered when hypocalcemia is known or suspected. Measurements include:

- *Total serum calcium* is the amount of ionized (active) calcium available usually is estimated. In critically ill clients, however, *ionized calcium* may be directly measured using ion-selective electrodes. Direct measurement of ionized calcium requires special handling of the blood specimen, including placing the specimen on ice and analyzing it immediately.
- *Serum albumin,* because the albumin level affects serum calcium results. When the albumin level is low (hypoalbuminemia), the amount of ionized calcium may remain normal even though the total calcium level is low.
- *Serum magnesium,* because hypocalcemia is often associated with hypomagnesemia (serum magnesium <1.6 mg/dL). In this case, normal magnesium levels must be restored to correct the hypocalcemia.
- *Serum phosphate* hyperphosphatemia (serum phosphate > 4.5 mg/dL) can lead to hypocalcemia because of the inverse relationship between phosphorus and calcium (as phosphate levels rise, calcium levels fall).
- *Parathyroid hormone (PTH),* to identify the possible diagnoses of hyperparathyroidism.
- An *ECG,* to evaluate the effects of hypocalcemia on the heart, such as a prolonged ST segment.

### Medications

Hypocalcemia is treated with oral or intravenous calcium. The client with severe hypocalcemia is treated with intravenous calcium to prevent life-threatening problems such as airway obstruction. The most common intravenous calcium preparations include calcium chloride and calcium gluconate. Although calcium chloride contains more elemental calcium than calcium gluconate, it also is more irritating to the veins and may cause venous sclerosis (hardening of the vein walls) if given into a peripheral vein. Intravenous calcium preparations can cause necrosis and sloughing of tissue if they extravasate into subcutaneous tissue. Rapid drug administration can lead to bradycardia and possible cardiac arrest due to overcorrection of hypocalcemia with resulting hypercalcemia. See page 111 for further information about calcium administration.

Oral calcium preparations (calcium carbonate, calcium gluconate, or calcium lactate) are used to treat chronic, asymptomatic hypocalcemia. Calcium supplements may be combined with vitamin D, or vitamin D may be given alone to increase gastrointestinal absorption of calcium.

### Dietary Management

A diet high in calcium-rich foods may be recommended for clients with chronic hypocalcemia or with low total body stores of calcium. Box 5–7 lists foods that are high in calcium.

## NURSING CARE

### Health Promotion

Because of the large stores of calcium in bones, most healthy adults have a very low risk of developing hypocalcemia. A deficit of total body calcium is often associated with aging,

## Medication Administration

### Calcium Salts

**CALCIUM SALTS**

Calcium carbonate (BioCal, Calsam, Caltrate, OsCal, Tums, others)
Calcium chloride
Calcium citrate (Citrical)
Calcium glubionate
Calcium gluceptate
Calcium gluconate (Calcinate)
Calcium lactate

Calcium salts are given to increase calcium levels when there is a deficit (a total body deficit or inadequate levels of extracellular calcium). Calcium is necessary to maintain bone structure and for multiple physiologic processes including neuromuscular and cardiac function as well as blood coagulation. In the presence of vitamin D, calcium is well absorbed from the gastrointestinal tract. Severe hypocalcemia is treated with intravenous calcium preparations.

#### Nursing Responsibilities

Oral calcium salts
- Administer 1 to 1.5 hours after meals and at bedtime.
- Give calcium tablets with a full glass of water.

Intravenous calcium salts
- Assess IV site for patency. Do not administer calcium if there is a risk of leakage into the tissues.
- May be given by slow IV push (dilute with sterile normal saline for injection prior to administering) or added to compatible parenteral fluids such as NS, lactated Ringer's solution, or $D_5W$.
- Administer into the largest available vein; use a central line if available.
- Do not administer with bicarbonate of phosphate.
- Continuously monitor ECG when administering IV calcium to clients taking digitalis due to increased risk of digitalis toxicity.
- Frequently monitor serum calcium levels and response to therapy.

#### Client and Family Teaching
- Take calcium tablets with a full glass of water 1 to 2 hours after meals. Do not take with food or milk. If possible, do not take within 1 to 2 hours of other medications.
- Maintain adequate vitamin D intake through diet or exposure to the sun to promote calcium absorption.
- Calcium carbonate can cause constipation. Eat a high-fiber diet and maintain a generous fluid intake to prevent constipation.

---

however, increasing the risk of osteoporosis, fractures, and disability. Women have a higher risk for developing osteoporosis than men due to lower bone density and hormonal influences. Teach women of all ages the importance of maintaining adequate calcium intake through diet and, as needed, calcium supplements. Stress the relationship between weight-bearing exercise and bone density, and encourage women to engage in a regular aerobic and weight-training exercise regime. Discuss hormone replacement therapy and its potential benefits during and after menopause. See Chapter 39 ⊕ for more information about osteoporosis.

### Assessment

Assessment data related to hypocalcemia include the following:

- Health history:   Current manifestations, including numbness and tingling around mouth and of hands and feet, abdominal pain, shortness of breath; acute or chronic diseases such as pancreatitis, liver or kidney disease; current medications.
- Physical assessment:   Muscle spasms; deep tendon reflexes; Chvostek's sign and Trousseau's sign; respiratory rate and

depth; vital signs and apical pulse; heart rate and rhythm; presence of convulsions.

### Nursing Diagnoses and Interventions

#### Risk for Injury

The client with hypocalcemia is at risk for injury from possible laryngospasm, cardiac dysrhythmias, or convulsions. In addition, too rapid administration of intravenous calcium or extravasation of the medication into subcutaneous tissues can lead to injury.

- Frequently monitor airway and respiratory status. Report changes such as respiratory **stridor** (a high-pitched, harsh inspiratory sound indicative of upper airway obstruction) or increased respiratory rate or effort to the physician. *These changes may indicate laryngeal spasm due to tetany.*

**PRACTICE ALERT**   *Laryngeal spasm is a respiratory emergency, requiring immediate intervention to maintain ventilation and gas exchange.* ■

- Monitor cardiovascular status including heart rate and rhythm, blood pressure, and peripheral pulses. *Hypocalcemia decreases myocardial contractility, causing reduced cardiac output and hypotension. It also can cause bradycardia or ventricular dysrhythmias. Cardiac arrest may occur in severe hypocalcemia.*
- Continuously monitor ECG in clients receiving intravenous calcium preparations, especially if the client also is taking digitalis. *Rapid administration of calcium salts can lead to hypercalcemia and cardiac dysrhythmias. Calcium administration increases the risk of digitalis toxicity and resultant dysrhythmias.*

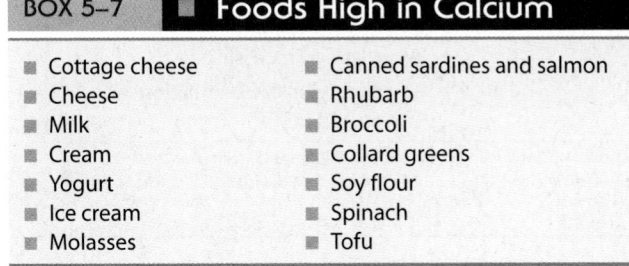

| BOX 5–7 | ■ Foods High in Calcium |
| --- | --- |
| ■ Cottage cheese | ■ Canned sardines and salmon |
| ■ Cheese | ■ Rhubarb |
| ■ Milk | ■ Broccoli |
| ■ Cream | ■ Collard greens |
| ■ Yogurt | ■ Soy flour |
| ■ Ice cream | ■ Spinach |
| ■ Molasses | ■ Tofu |

- Provide a quiet environment. Institute seizure precautions such as raising the side rails and keeping an airway at bedside. *A quiet environment reduces central nervous system stimuli and the risk of convulsions in the client with tetany.*

## Using NANDA, NIC, and NOC

Chart 5–5 shows links between NANDA nursing diagnoses, NIC, and NOC for the client with a calcium imbalance.

## Home Care

In preparing the client with hypocalcemia for discharge and home care, consider the circumstances leading to low serum calcium levels. Discuss risk factors for hypocalcemia specific to the client, and provide information about managing these risk factors to avoid future episodes of hypocalcemia. Teach about prescribed medications, including calcium supplements. Provide a list of foods high in calcium, as well as sources of vitamin D if recommended. Discuss symptoms to report to the care provider, and stress the importance of follow-up care as scheduled.

## THE CLIENT WITH HYPERCALCEMIA

**Hypercalcemia** is a serum calcium value greater than 10.0 mg/dL. Excess ionized calcium in ECF can have serious widespread effects.

## PATHOPHYSIOLOGY

Hypercalcemia usually results from increased resorption of calcium from the bones. The two most common causes of bone resorption are hyperparathyroidism and malignancies. In hyperparathyroidism, excess PTH is produced. This causes calcium to be released from bones, as well as increased calcium absorption in the intestines and retention of calcium by the kidneys. Hypercalcemia is a common complication of malignancies. It may develop as a result of bone destruction by the tu-

mor or due to hormonelike substances produced by the tumor itself. Prolonged immobility and lack of weight bearing also cause increased resorption of bone with calcium release into extracellular fluids. Self-limiting hypercalcemia also may follow successful kidney transplant.

Increased intestinal absorption of calcium also can lead to hypercalcemia. This may result from excess vitamin D, overuse of calcium-containing antacids, or excessive milk ingestion. Renal failure and some drugs such as thiazide diuretics and lithium can interfere with elimination of calcium by the kidneys, causing high serum calcium levels.

The effects of hypercalcemia largely depend on the degree of serum calcium elevation and the length of time over which it develops. In general, higher serum calcium levels are associated with more serious effects. Calcium has a stabilizing effect on the neuromuscular junction; hypercalcemia decreases neuromuscular excitability, leading to muscle weakness and depressed deep tendon reflexes. Gastrointestinal motility is reduced as well. In the heart, calcium exerts an effect similar to digitalis (see Chapter 30 ⊙ ), strengthening contractions and reducing the heart rate. Hypercalcemia affects the conduction system of the heart, leading to bradycardia and heart blocks. The ability of the kidneys to concentrate urine is impaired by hypercalcemia, causing excess sodium and water loss and increased thirst.

Extremely high serum calcium levels affect mental status. This is thought to be due to increased calcium in cerebrospinal fluid (CSF). Behavior differences range from personality changes to confusion, impaired memory, and acute psychoses.

## MANIFESTATIONS AND COMPLICATIONS

Manifestations of hypercalcemia relate to its effects on neuromuscular activity, the central nervous system, the cardiovascular system, and the kidneys. Decreased neuromuscular excitability causes muscle weakness and fatigue, as well as gastrointestinal manifestations such as anorexia, nausea, vom-

### CHART 5–5   NANDA, NIC, AND NOC LINKAGES

#### The Client with Calcium Imbalance

| NURSING DIAGNOSES | NURSING INTERVENTIONS | NURSING OUTCOMES |
|---|---|---|
| • Risk for Injury | • Seizure Precautions<br>• Environmental Management: Safety | • Risk Control<br>• Safety Status: Physical Injury |
| • Decreased Cardiac Output | • Cardiac Precautions<br>• Electrolyte Management: Hypocalcemia | • Cardiac Pump Effectiveness<br>• Vital Signs Status |
| • Disturbed Thought Processes | • Anxiety Reduction<br>• Delusion Management | • Cognitive Orientation<br>• Information Processing |
| • Risk for Ineffective Breathing Pattern | • Airway Management<br>• Respiratory Monitoring | • Respiratory Status: Ventilation<br>• Airway Patency |

*Note. Data from Nursing Outcomes Classification (NOC) by M. Johnson & M. Maas (Eds.), 1997, St. Louis: Mosby; Nursing Diagnoses: Definitions & Classification 2001–2002 by North American Nursing Diagnosis Association, 2001, Philadelphia: NANDA; Nursing Interventions Classification (NIC) by J.C. McCloskey & G. M. Bulechek (Eds.), 2000, St. Louis: Mosby. Reprinted by permission.*

iting, and constipation. CNS effects may include confusion, lethargy, behavior or personality changes, and coma. Cardiovascular effects include dysrhythmias, ECG changes, and possible hypertension. Hypercalcemia causes polyuria, and, as a result, increased thirst.

Complications of hypercalcemia can affect several different organ systems. Peptic ulcer disease may develop due to increased gastric acid secretion. Pancreatitis can occur as a result of calcium deposits in pancreatic ducts. Excess calcium can precipitate to form kidney stones. Hypercalcemic crisis, an acute increase in the serum calcium level, can lead to cardiac arrest.

## COLLABORATIVE CARE

The management of hypercalcemia focuses on correcting the underlying cause and reducing the serum calcium level. Treatment is particularly important in clients who have one or more of the following: serum calcium levels greater than 12 mg/dL, overt symptoms of hypercalcemia, compromised renal function, and an inability to maintain an adequate fluid intake.

### Diagnostic Tests

The laboratory and diagnostic tests that may be ordered and the resultant findings are as follows:

- *Serum electrolytes* show a total serum calcium greater than 10.0 mg/dL.
- *Serum PTH levels* are measured to identify or rule out hyperparathyroidism as the cause of hypercalcemia.
- *ECG* changes in hypercalcemia include a shortened QT interval, shortened and depressed ST segment, and widened T wave. Bradycardia or heart block may be identified on the ECG.

### Medications

Measures to promote calcium elimination by the kidneys and reduce calcium resorption from bone are used to treat hypercalcemia. In acute hypercalcemia, intravenous fluids are given (see "Fluid Management" that follows) with a loop diuretic such as furosemide to promote elimination of excess calcium. Calcitonin, which promotes the uptake of calcium into bones, also may be used to rapidly lower serum calcium levels.

A number of drugs that inhibit bone resorption are available. The bisphosphonates (pamidronate and etidronate) are commonly used to treat hypercalcemia associated with malignancies. These drugs also are used to prevent and treat osteoporosis. Their nursing implications for calcitonin and bisphosphonate drugs are presented in the boxes on pages 1226 and 1232. When a bisphosphonate drug is ineffective to correct hypercalcemia, mithramycin, a chemotherapeutic agent, may be used. Glucocorticoid drugs (see Chapter 17 ⟳) may be used in combination with other therapies to lower serum calcium levels by inhibiting intestinal calcium absorption and bone resorption.

Rapid reversal of hypercalcemia in emergency situations may be accomplished by intravenous administration of sodium phosphate or potassium phosphate. Calcium binds to phosphate, and serum calcium levels thereby decrease. Paradoxically, complications of this therapy can include fatal hypocalcemia resulting from binding of the ionized calcium and soft tissue calcifications.

Other drug therapies include the use of intravenous plicamycin (Mithracin) to inhibit bone resorption. Glucocorticoids (cortisone), which compete with vitamin D, and a low-calcium diet may be prescribed to decrease gastrointestinal absorption of calcium and to increase urinary calcium excretion. Also, calcitonin may be prescribed to decrease skeletal mobilization of calcium and phosphorus and to increase renal output of calcium and phosphorus.

### Fluid Management

Intravenous fluids, usually isotonic saline, are administered to clients with severe hypercalcemia to restore vascular volume and promote renal excretion of calcium. Isotonic saline is used because sodium excretion is accompanied by calcium excretion. Careful assessment of cardiovascular and renal function is done prior to fluid therapy; the client is carefully monitored for evidence of fluid overload during treatment.

## NURSING CARE

### Health Promotion

Identify and monitor clients at risk for hypercalcemia. Promote mobility in clients when possible. Ambulate hospitalized clients as soon as possible. In the home setting, discuss the benefits of weight-bearing activity with clients, families, and caregivers. Encourage a generous fluid intake of up to 3 to 4 quarts per day. Encourage clients at risk to limit their intake of milk and milk products, as well as calcium-containing antacids and supplements.

### Assessment

Assessment data related to hypercalcemia include the following:

- Health history: Current manifestations, including weakness or fatigue, abdominal discomfort, nausea or vomiting, increased urination and thirst; changes in memory or thinking; duration of symptoms and any risk factors such as excess intake of milk or calcium products, prolonged immobility, malignancy, renal failure, or endocrine disorders; current medications.
- Physical assessment: Mental status and level of consciousness; vital signs including apical pulse; bowel sounds; muscle strength of upper and lower extremities; deep tendon reflexes.

## PRACTICE ALERT *Remember, calcium has a stabilizing or sedative effect on neuromuscular transmission. Therefore:*

Hypo*calcemia* ➔ Increased *neuromuscular excitability, muscle twitching, spasms, and possible tetany*

Hyper*calcemia* ➔ Decreased *neuromuscular excitability, muscle weakness, and fatigue* ■

## Nursing Diagnoses and Interventions

### Risk for Injury

Clients with hypercalcemia are at risk for injury due to changes in mental status, the effects of hypercalcemia on muscle strength, and loss of calcium from bones.

- Institute safety precautions if confusion or other changes in mental status are noted. *Changes in mental status may impair judgment and the client's ability to maintain own safety.*

**PRACTICE ALERT** *Monitor cardiac rate and rhythm, treating and/or reporting dysrhythmias as indicated. Prepare for possible cardiac arrest; keep emergency resuscitation equipment readily available. Hypercalcemia can cause bradycardia, various heart blocks, and cardiac arrest. Immediate treatment may be necessary to preserve life.* ∎

- Observe for manifestations of digitalis toxicity, including vision changes, anorexia, and changes in heart rate and rhythm. Monitor serum digitalis levels. *Hypercalcemia increases the risk of digitalis toxicity.*
- Promote fluid intake (oral and/or intravenous) to keep the client well hydrated and maintain dilute urine. Encourage fluids such as prune or cranberry juice to help maintain acid urine. *Acidic, dilute urine reduces the risk of calcium salts precipitating out to form kidney stones.*
- If excess bone resorption has occurred, use caution when turning, positioning, transferring, or ambulating. *Bones that have lost excess calcium may fracture with minimal stress or trauma* (pathologic fractures).

### Risk for Excess Fluid Volume

Large amounts of isotonic intravenous fluid often are administered to help correct acute hypercalcemia, leading to a risk for hypervolemia. Clients with preexisting cardiac or renal disease are at particular risk.

- Closely monitor intake and output. *A loop diuretic such as furosemide may be necessary if urinary output does not keep up with fluid administration.*
- Frequently assess vital signs, respiratory status, and heart sounds. *Increasing pulse rate, dyspnea, adventitious lung sounds, and an $S_3$ on auscultation of the heart may indicate excess fluid volume and potential heart failure.*
- Place in semi-Fowler's to Fowler's position. *Elevating the head of the bed improves lung expansion and reduces the work of breathing.*
- Administer diuretics as ordered, monitoring response. *Loop diuretics may be ordered to help eliminate excess fluid and calcium.*

## Using NANDA, NIC, and NOC

Chart 5–5 shows links between NANDA nursing diagnoses, NIC, and NOC when caring for a client with a calcium imbalance.

## Home Care

Discuss the following topics when preparing the client for discharge.

- Avoid excess intake of calcium-rich foods and antacids.
- Use of prescribed drugs to prevent excess calcium resorption, their dose, use, and desired and possible adverse effects.
- Increase fluid intake to 3 to 4 quarts per day; increase the intake of acid ash foods (meats, fish, poultry, eggs, cranberries, plums, prunes); increase dietary fiber and fluid intake to prevent constipation.
- Maintain weight-bearing physical activity to prevent hypercalcemia.
- Early manifestations of hypercalcemia to report to care provider.
- Follow recommended schedule for monitoring serum electrolyte levels.

# MAGNESIUM IMBALANCE

Only about 1% of the magnesium in the body is in extracellular fluid; the rest is found within the cells and in bone. The normal serum concentration of magnesium ranges from 1.6 to 2.6 mg/dL (1.3 to 2.1 mEq/L).

## OVERVIEW OF NORMAL MAGNESIUM BALANCE

Magnesium is obtained through the diet (it is plentiful in green vegetables, grains, nuts, meats, and seafood) and excreted by the kidneys. Magnesium is vital to many intracellular processes, including enzyme reactions and synthesis of proteins and nucleic acids. Magnesium exerts a sedative effect on the neuromuscular junction, decreasing acetylcholine release. It is an essential ion for neuromuscular transmission and cardiovascular function. The physiologic effects of magnesium are affected by both potassium and calcium levels. Approximately 65% of extracellular magnesium is ionized; the re-

mainder is bound to protein. Table 5–8 summarizes common causes and manifestations of magnesium imbalances.

## THE CLIENT WITH HYPOMAGNESEMIA

**Hypomagnesemia** is a magnesium level of less than 1.6 mg/dL. It is a common problem, particularly in critically ill clients. Hypomagnesemia may be caused by deficient magnesium intake, excessive losses, or a shift between the intracellular and extracellular compartments.

## RISK FACTORS

Loss of gastrointestinal fluids, particularly from diarrhea, an ileostomy, or intestinal fistula is a major risk factor for hypomagnesemia. Disruption of nutrient absorption in the small intestine also increases the risk. Chronic alcoholism is the most

TABLE 5–8  Causes and Manifestations of Magnesium Imbalances

| Imbalance | Causes | Manifestations |
|---|---|---|
| **Hypomagnesemia**<br>Serum magnesium <1.6 mg/dL | • Chronic alcoholism<br>• GI losses: intestinal suction, diarrhea, ileostomy<br>• Impaired absorption<br>• Inadequate replacement<br>• Increased excretion: drugs, renal disease, osmotic diuresis | Neuromuscular<br>• Muscle weakness, tremors<br>• Tetany, seizures<br>Gastrointestinal<br>• Dysphagia<br>• Anorexia, nausea, vomiting, diarrhea<br>Cardiovascular<br>• Tachycardia<br>• Dysrhythmias<br>• Hypertension<br>CNS<br>• Mood and personality changes<br>• Paresthesias |
| **Hypermagnesemia**<br>Serum magnesium >2.1 mEq/L<br>or 2.6 mg/dL | • Renal insufficiency or failure<br>• Excess intake of antacids, laxatives<br>• Excess magnesium administration | Neuromuscular<br>• Muscle weakness<br>• Depressed deep tendon reflexes<br>Gastrointestinal<br>• Nausea and vomiting<br>Cardiovascular<br>• Hypotension<br>• Bradycardia<br>• Cardiac arrest<br>CNS<br>• Respiratory depression<br>• Coma |

common cause of deficient magnesium levels in the United States (Metheny, 2000). Multiple factors associated with alcoholism contribute to hypomagnesemia: deficient nutrient intake, increased gastrointestinal losses, impaired absorption, and increased renal excretion. Other risk factors for hypomagnesemia include:

• Protein-calorie malnutrition or starvation.
• Endocrine disorders including diabetic ketoacidosis.
• Drugs such as loop or thiazide diuretics, aminoglycoside antibiotics, amphotericin B, and cyclosporine.
• Rapid administration of citrated blood (banked blood).
• Kidney disease.

## PATHOPHYSIOLOGY

Magnesium deficiency usually occurs along with low serum potassium and calcium levels. The effects of hypomagnesemia relate not only to the magnesium deficiency but also to hypokalemia and hypocalcemia.

Hypomagnesemia causes increased neuromuscular excitability, with muscle weakness and tremors. The accompanying hypocalcemia contributes to this effect. In the central nervous system, this increased neural excitability can lead to seizures and changes in mental status.

Deficient intracellular magnesium in the myocardium increases the risk of cardiac dysrhythmias and sudden death. Hypokalemia increases this risk. Hypomagnesemia also increases the risk of digitalis toxicity. Chronic hypomagnesemia

may contribute to hypertension, probably due to increased vasoconstriction.

## MANIFESTATIONS AND COMPLICATIONS

Neuromuscular manifestations of hypomagnesemia include tremors, hyperreactive reflexes, positive Chvostek's and Trousseau's signs, tetany, paresthesias, and seizures. CNS effects include confusion, mood changes (apathy, depression, agitation), hallucinations, and possible psychoses.

An increased heart rate and ventricular dysrhythmias are common, especially when hypokalemia is present or the client is taking digitalis. Cardiac arrest and sudden death may occur. Gastrointestinal manifestations include nausea, vomiting, anorexia, diarrhea, and abdominal distention.

## COLLABORATIVE CARE

Hypomagnesemia is diagnosed by measuring serum electrolyte levels. The ECG shows a prolonged PR interval, widened QRS complex, and depression of the ST segment with T wave inversion.

Treatment is directed toward prevention and identification of an existing deficiency. Magnesium is added to intravenous total parenteral nutrition solutions to prevent hypomagnesemia.

In clients able to eat, a mild deficiency may be corrected by increasing the intake of foods rich in magnesium (see Box 5–8), or with oral magnesium supplements. Oral magnesium supplements may cause diarrhea, however, limiting their use.

| BOX 5–8 | ■ Foods High in Magnesium | |
|---|---|---|
| ■ Green, leafy vegetables | ■ Oranges | |
| ■ Seafood | ■ Grapefruit | |
| ■ Meat | ■ Chocolate | |
| ■ Wheat bran | ■ Molasses | |
| ■ Milk | ■ Coconut | |
| ■ Legumes | ■ Refined sugar | |
| ■ Bananas | | |

Clients with manifestations of hypomagnesemia are treated with parenteral magnesium sulfate. Treatment is continued for several days to restore intracellular magnesium levels. Magnesium may be given intravenously or by deep intramuscular injection. Renal function is evaluated prior to administration, and serum magnesium levels are monitored during treatment. The intravenous route is used for severe magnesium deficiency or if neurologic changes or cardiac dysrhythmias are present. See the box below for the nursing implications of parenteral magnesium sulfate.

## NURSING CARE

### Health Promotion

Discuss the importance of maintaining adequate magnesium intake through a well-balanced diet, particularly with clients at risk (people with alcoholism, malabsorption, or bowel surgery). Many hospitalized clients are at risk for hypomagnesemia due to protein-calorie malnutrition and other disorders. Monitor serum magnesium levels, reporting changes to the health care provider.

## Medication Administration

### Magnesium Sulfate

Magnesium sulfate is used to prevent or treat hypomagnesemia. It also is used as an anticonvulsant in severe eclampsia or preeclampsia. It may be given intravenously or by intramuscular injection.

### Nursing Responsibilities

- Assess serum magnesium levels and renal function tests (BUN and serum creatinine) prior to administering. Notify the care provider if magnesium levels are above normal limits or renal function is impaired.
- Frequently monitor neurologic status and deep tendon reflexes during therapy. Withhold magnesium and notify the care provider if deep tendon reflexes are hypoactive or absent.
- Monitor intake and output.
- Administer IM doses deep into the ventral or dorsal gluteal sites.
- Intravenous magnesium sulfate may be given by direct IV push or by continuous infusion.

### Client and Family Teaching

Explain purpose and duration of treatment. Discuss reason for frequent neurologic and reflex assessments.

### Assessment

In addition to asking questions related to risk factors for hypomagnesemia, use the guidelines for assessing clients with hypokalemia and hypocalcemia for subjective and objective assessment data.

### Nursing Diagnoses and Interventions

Nursing care for clients with hypomagnesemia focuses on careful monitoring of manifestations and responses to treatment, promoting safety, client and family teaching, and administering prescribed medications.

#### Risk for Injury

- Monitor serum electrolytes, including magnesium, potassium, and calcium. *Magnesium deficiency often is accompanied by deficiencies of potassium and calcium.*
- Monitor gastrointestinal function, including bowel sounds and abdominal distention. *Hypomagnesemia reduces gastrointestinal motility.*
- Initiate cardiac monitoring, reporting and treating (as indicated) ECG changes and dysrhythmias. In clients receiving digitalis, monitor for digitalis toxicity. *Low magnesium levels can precipitate ventricular dysrhythmias, including lethal dysrhythmias such as ventricular fibrillation.*
- Assess deep tendon reflexes frequently during intravenous magnesium infusions and prior to each intramuscular dose. *Depressed tendon reflexes indicate a high serum magnesium level.*
- Maintain a quiet, darkened environment. Institute seizure precautions. *Increased neuromuscular and CNS irritability can lead to seizures. A quiet, dark environment reduces stimuli.*

### Home Care

Prior to discharge, instruct the client to increase dietary intake of foods high in magnesium and provide information about magnesium supplements. In addition, if alcohol abuse has precipitated a magnesium deficit, discuss alcohol treatment options, including inpatient treatment and support groups such as Alcoholics Anonymous, Al-Anon, and/or Al-a-Teen.

## THE CLIENT WITH HYPERMAGNESEMIA

**Hypermagnesemia** is a serum magnesium level greater than 2.6 mg/dL. It is much less common than hypomagnesemia. Hypermagnesemia can develop in renal failure, particularly if magnesium is administered parenterally or orally (e.g., magnesium-containing antacids or laxatives). Older adults are at risk for hypermagnesemia as renal function declines with aging and they are more likely to use over-the-counter laxatives and other preparations that contain magnesium.

## PATHOPHYSIOLOGY AND MANIFESTATIONS

Elevated serum magnesium levels interfere with neuromuscular transmission and depress the central nervous system. Hypermagnesemia also affects the cardiovascular system, potentially causing hypotension, flushing, sweating, and bradydysrhythmias.

Predictable manifestations occur with increasing serum magnesium levels. With lower levels, nausea and vomiting, hypotension, facial flushing, sweating, and a feeling of warmth occur. As levels increase, signs of central nervous system depression appear (weakness, lethargy, drowsiness, weak or absent deep tendon reflexes). Marked elevations cause respiratory depression, coma, and compromised cardiac function (ECG changes, bradycardia, heart block, and cardiac arrest).

## COLLABORATIVE CARE

The management of hypermagnesemia focuses on identifying and treating the underlying cause. All medications or compounds containing magnesium (such as antacids, intravenous solutions, or enemas) are withheld. In the client with renal failure, hemodialysis or peritoneal dialysis is instituted to remove the excess magnesium.

Calcium gluconate is administered intravenously to reverse the neuromuscular and cardiac effects of hypermagnesemia. The client may require mechanical ventilation to support respiratory function, and a pacemaker to maintain adequate cardiac output.

## NURSING CARE

Nursing care includes instituting measures to prevent and identify hypermagnesemia in clients at risk, monitoring for critical effects of hypermagnesemia, and providing measures to ensure the client's safety. Consider the following nursing diagnoses for the client with hypermagnesemia.

- *Decreased cardiac output* related to altered myocardial conduction
- *Risk for ineffective breathing pattern* related to respiratory depression
- *Risk for injury* related to muscle weakness and altered level of consciousness
- *Risk for ineffective health maintenance* related to lack of knowledge about use of magnesium-containing supplements, antacids, laxatives, and enemas

### Home Care

Discharge teaching and planning focuses on instructions to avoid magnesium-containing medications, including antacids, mineral supplements, cathartics, and enemas (see Box 5–9).

| BOX 5–9 | ■ Medications Containing Magnesium |
|---|---|

| **Antacids** | **Laxatives** |
|---|---|
| ■ Gelusil | ■ Milk of Magnesia |
| ■ Maalox No. 1 | ■ Magnesium oxide |
| ■ Maalox Plus | ■ Haley's M-O |
| ■ Riopan | ■ Magnesium citrate |
| ■ Milk of Magnesia | ■ Epsom salts |
| ■ Mylanta | |
| ■ Di-Gel | |
| ■ Gaviscon | |

# PHOSPHATE IMBALANCE

Although most phosphate (85%) is found in bones, it is the primary intracellular anion. About 14% is in intracellular fluid, and the remainder (1%) is in extracellular fluid. The normal serum phosphate (or phosphorus) level in adults is 2.5 to 4.5 mg/dL. Phosphorus levels vary with age, gender, and diet.

## OVERVIEW OF NORMAL PHOSPHATE BALANCE

Phosphate is essential to intracellular processes such as the production of adenosine triphosphate (ATP), the fuel that supports muscle contraction, nerve cell transmission, and electrolyte transport. Phosphate is vital for red blood cell function and oxygen delivery to tissues; nervous system and muscle function; and the metabolism of fats, carbohydrates, and protein. It also assists in maintaining acid-base balance.

Phosphorus is ingested in the diet, absorbed in the jejunum, and primarily excreted by the kidneys. When phosphate intake is low, the kidneys conserve phosphorus, excreting less. An inverse relationship exists between phosphate and calcium levels: When one increases, the other decreases. Regulatory mechanisms for calcium levels (parathyroid hormone, calci-

tonin, and vitamin D) also influence phosphate levels. The causes and manifestations of phosphate imbalances are summarized in Table 5–9.

## THE CLIENT WITH HYPOPHOSPHATEMIA

**Hypophosphatemia** is a serum phosphorus of less than 2.5 mg/dL. Low serum phosphate levels may indicate a total body deficit of phosphate or a shift of phosphate into the intracellular space, the most common cause of hypophosphatemia. Decreased gastrointestinal absorption of phosphate or increased renal excretion of phosphate also can cause low phosphate levels. Hypophosphatemia often is *iatrogenic,* that is, related to treatment. Selected causes of hypophosphatemia include the following:

- *Refeeding* syndrome can develop when malnourished clients are started on enteral or total parenteral nutrition. Glucose in the formula or solution stimulates insulin release, which promotes the entry of glucose and phosphate into the cells, depleting extracellular phosphate levels.

**TABLE 5–9  Causes and Manifestations of Phosphate Imbalances**

| Imbalance | Causes | Manifestations |
|---|---|---|
| **Hypophosphatemia**<br>Serum phosphorus <2.5 mg/dL | • Shift of phosphorus into cells<br>• IV glucose administration<br>• Total parenteral nutrition without phosphorus<br>• Aluminum- or magnesium-based antacids<br>• Diuretic therapy<br>• Alcoholism | • Paresthesias<br>• Muscle weakness<br>• Muscle pain and tenderness<br>• Confusion, decreasing LOC<br>• Seizures<br>• Bone pain, osteomalacia<br>• Anorexia, dysphagia<br>• Decreased bowel sounds<br>• Possible acute respiratory failure |
| **Hyperphosphatemia**<br>Serum phosphate >4.5 mg/dL | • Renal failure<br>• Chemotherapy<br>• Muscle tissue trauma<br>• Sepsis<br>• Severe hypothermia<br>• Heat stroke | • Circumoral and peripheral paresthesias<br>• Muscle spasms<br>• Tetany<br>• Soft tissue calcification |

- Medications frequently contribute to hypophosphatemia, including intravenous glucose solutions, antacids (aluminum- or magnesium-based antacids bind with phosphate), anabolic steroids, and diuretics.
- Alcoholism affects both the intake and absorption of phosphate.
- Hyperventilation and respiratory alkalosis cause phosphate to shift out of extracellular fluids into the intracellular space.
- Other causes include diabetic ketoacidosis with excess phosphate loss in the urine, stress responses, and extensive burns.

## PATHOPHYSIOLOGY AND MANIFESTATIONS

Most effects of hypophosphatemia result from depletion of ATP and impaired oxygen delivery to the cells due to a deficiency of the red blood cell enzyme 2,3-DPG. Severe hypophosphatemia affects virtually every major organ system.

- Central nervous system: Reduced oxygen and ATP synthesis in the brain causes neurologic manifestations such as irritability, apprehension, weakness, paresthesias, lack of coordination, confusion, seizures, and coma.
- Hematologic: Oxygen delivery to the cells is reduced. Hemolytic anemia may develop due to lack of ATP in red blood cells.
- Musculoskeletal: Decreased ATP causes muscle weakness and release of creatinine phosphokinase (CPK, a muscle enzyme); acute rhabdomyolysis (muscle cell breakdown) can develop.
- Respiratory: Chest muscle weakness can interfere with effective ventilation, leading to respiratory failure.
- Cardiovascular: Hypophosphatemia decreases myocardial contractility; decreased oxygenation of the heart muscle can cause chest pain and dysrhythmias.
- Gastrointestinal: Anorexia can occur, as well as dysphagia (difficulty swallowing), nausea and vomiting, decreased bowel sounds, and possible ileus due to reduced gastrointestinal motility.

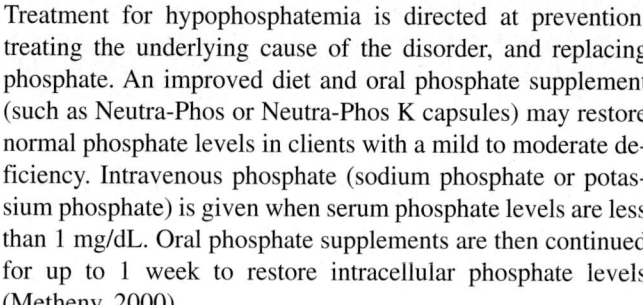

## COLLABORATIVE CARE

Treatment for hypophosphatemia is directed at prevention, treating the underlying cause of the disorder, and replacing phosphate. An improved diet and oral phosphate supplement (such as Neutra-Phos or Neutra-Phos K capsules) may restore normal phosphate levels in clients with a mild to moderate deficiency. Intravenous phosphate (sodium phosphate or potassium phosphate) is given when serum phosphate levels are less than 1 mg/dL. Oral phosphate supplements are then continued for up to 1 week to restore intracellular phosphate levels (Metheny, 2000).

## NURSING CARE

Nurses can be instrumental in identifying clients at risk for phosphate deficiency and preventing it from developing. Nurses should closely monitor serum electrolyte values in clients at risk, including those who are malnourished, receiving intravenous glucose solutions or total parenteral nutrition, or being treated with diuretic therapy or antacids that bind with phosphate. Nursing diagnoses that may be appropriate for the client with hypophosphatemia include:

- *Impaired physical mobility* related to muscle weakness and poor coordination
- *Ineffective breathing pattern* related to weakened muscles of respiration
- *Decreased cardiac output* related to reduced myocardial contractility
- *Risk for injury* related to muscle weakness and altered mental status

### Home Care

In preparing for discharge, teach the client and family about the causes and manifestations of hypophosphatemia. Discuss the importance of avoiding phosphorus-binding antacids, unless prescribed. Stress a well-balanced diet to maintain an adequate intake of phosphate.

## THE CLIENT WITH HYPERPHOSPHATEMIA

**Hyperphosphatemia** is a serum phosphate level greater than 4.5 mg/dL. As with other electrolyte imbalances, it may be the result of impaired phosphate excretion, excess intake, or a shift of phosphate from the intracellular space into extracellular fluids.

- Acute or chronic renal failure is the primary cause of impaired phosphate excretion.
- Rapid administration of phosphate-containing solutions can increase serum phosphate levels. This can include phosphate enemas. In addition, excess vitamin D increases phosphate absorption and can lead to hyperphosphatemia in clients with impaired renal function.
- A shift of phosphate from the intracellular to extracellular space can occur during chemotherapy, due to sepsis or hypothermia, or because of extensive trauma or heat stroke.
- Because phosphate levels are affected by serum calcium concentrations, disruption of the mechanisms that regulate calcium levels (e.g., hypoparathyroidism, hyperthyroidism, or vitamin D intoxication) can lead to hyperphosphatemia.

### PATHOPHYSIOLOGY AND MANIFESTATIONS

Excessive serum phosphate levels cause few specific symptoms. The effects of high serum phosphate levels on nerves and muscles (muscle cramps and pain, paresthesias, tingling around the mouth, muscle spasms, tetany) are more the result of hypocalcemia that develops secondary to an elevated serum phosphorus level. The phosphate in the serum combines with ionized calcium, and the ionized serum calcium level falls.

Calcification of soft tissues can occur with high phosphate levels. Phosphates bind with calcium to precipitate in soft tissues such as the kidneys and other organs. Soft tissue calcification can impair the function of affected organs.

## COLLABORATIVE CARE

Treatment of the underlying disorder often corrects hyperphosphatemia. When this is not feasible, phosphate-containing drugs are eliminated and intake of phosphate-rich foods such as organ meats and milk and milk products is restricted. Agents that bind with phosphate in the gastrointestinal tract (such as calcium-containing antacids) may be prescribed. If renal function is adequate, intravenous normal saline may be given to promote renal excretion of phosphate. Dialysis may be necessary to reduce phosphate levels in clients with renal failure.

## NURSING CARE

When providing nursing care for the client with hyperphosphatemia, monitor the client for laboratory data revealing an excess of phosphorus and a deficit of calcium, as well as the signs of hypocalcemia.

### Home Care

Discuss the risk of hyperphosphatemia related to using phosphate preparations as laxatives or enemas, particularly with clients who have other risk factors for the disorder. When preparing the client for discharge, teach about the use of phosphate-binding preparations as ordered and dietary phosphate restrictions.

# ACID-BASE DISORDERS

Homeostasis and optimal cellular function require maintenance of the hydrogen ion ($H^+$) concentration of body fluids within a relatively narrow range. Hydrogen ions determine the relative acidity of body fluids. **Acids** release hydrogen ions in solution; **bases** (or **alkalis**) accept hydrogen ions in solution. The hydrogen ion concentration of a solution is measured as its pH. The relationship between hydrogen ion concentration and pH is inverse; that is, as hydrogen ion concentration increases, the pH falls, and the solution becomes more acidic. As hydrogen ion concentration falls, the pH rises, and the solution becomes more alkaline or basic. The pH of body fluids is slightly basic, with the normal pH ranging from 7.35 to 7.45 (a pH of 7 is neutral).

## REGULATION OF ACID-BASE BALANCE

A number of mechanisms work together to maintain the pH of the body within this normal range. Metabolic processes in the body continuously produce acids, which fall into two categories: volatile acids and nonvolatile acids. **Volatile acids** can be eliminated from the body as a gas. Carbonic acid ($H_2CO_3$) is the only volatile acid produced in the body. It dissociates (separates) into carbon dioxide ($CO_2$) and water ($H_2O$); the carbon dioxide is then eliminated from the body through the lungs. All other acids produced in the body are *nonvolatile acids* that must be metabolized or excreted from the body in fluid. Lactic acid, hydrochloric acid, phosphoric acid, and sulfuric acid are examples of nonvolatile acids. Most acids and bases in the body are weak; that is, they neither release nor accept a significant amount of hydrogen ion.

Three systems work together in the body to maintain the pH despite continuous acid production: buffers, the respiratory system, and the renal system.

## Buffer Systems

**Buffers** are substances that prevent major changes in pH by removing or releasing hydrogen ions. When excess acid is present

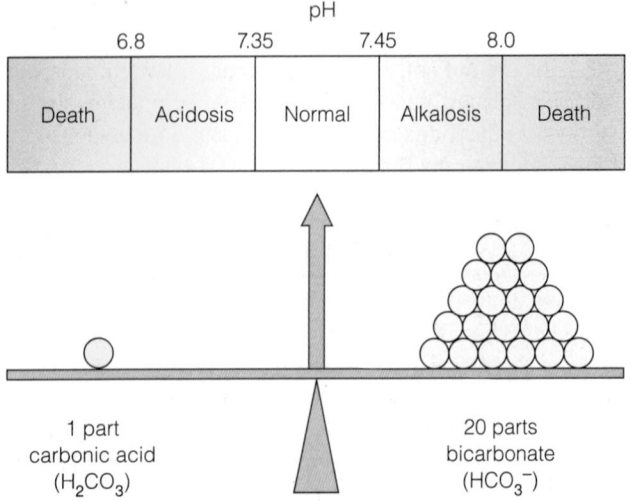

**Figure 5–14** ■ The normal ratio of bicarbonate to carbonic acid is 20:1. As long as this ratio is maintained, the pH remains within the normal range of 7.35 to 7.45.

in body fluid, buffers bind with hydrogen ions to minimize the change in pH. If body fluids become too basic or alkaline, buffers release hydrogen ions, restoring the pH. Although buffers act within a fraction of a second, their capacity to maintain pH is limited. The major buffer systems of the body are the bicarbonate-carbonic acid buffer system, phosphate buffer system, and protein buffers.

The bicarbonate-carbonic acid buffer system can be illustrated by the following equation:

$$CO_2 + H_2O \leftrightarrow H_2CO_3 \leftrightarrow H^+ + HCO_3^-$$

Bicarbonate ($HCO_3^-$) is a weak base; when an acid is added to the system, it combines with bicarbonate, and the pH changes only slightly. Carbonic acid ($H_2CO_3$) is a weak acid produced when carbon dioxide dissolves in water. If a base is added to the system, it combines with carbonic acid, and the pH remains within the normal range. Although the amounts of bicarbonate and carbonic acid in the body vary to a certain extent, as long as a ratio of 20 parts bicarbonate ($HCO_3^-$) to 1 part carbonic acid ($H_2CO_3$) is maintained, the pH remains within the 7.35 to 7.45 range (Figure 5–14 ■). The normal serum bicarbonate level is 24 mEq/L, and that of carbonic acid is 1.2 mEq/L. Thus, the ratio of bicarbonate to carbonic acid is 20:1. It is this ratio that maintains the pH within the normal range. Adding a strong acid to extracellular fluid depletes bicarbonate, changing the 20:1 ratio and causing the pH to drop below 7.35. This is known as acidosis. Addition of a strong base depletes carbonic acid as it combines with the base. The 20:1 ratio again is disrupted and the pH rises above 7.45, a condition known as alkalosis.

Intracellular and plasma proteins also serve as buffers. Plasma proteins contribute to buffering of extracellular fluids. Proteins in intracellular fluid provide extensive buffering for organic acids produced by cellular metabolism. In red blood cells, hemoglobin acts as a buffer for hydrogen ion when carbonic acid dissociates. Inorganic phosphates also serve as extracellular buffers, although their roles are not as important as the bicarbonate-carbonic acid buffer system. Phosphates are, however, important intracellular buffers, helping to maintain a stable pH.

## Respiratory System

The respiratory system (and the respiratory center of the brain) regulates carbonic acid in the body by eliminating or retaining carbon dioxide. Carbon dioxide is a potential acid; when combined with water, it forms carbonic acid (see previous equation). Acute increases in either carbon dioxide or hydrogen ions in the blood stimulate the respiratory center in the brain. As a result, both the rate and depth of respiration increase. The increased rate and depth of lung ventilation eliminates carbon dioxide from the body, and carbonic acid levels fall, bringing the pH to a more normal range. Although this compensation for increased hydrogen ion concentration occurs within minutes, it becomes less effective over time. Clients with chronic lung disease may have consistently high carbon dioxide levels in their blood.

Alkalosis, by contrast, depresses the respiratory center. Both the rate and depth of respiration decrease, and carbon dioxide is retained. The retained carbon dioxide then combines with water to restore carbonic acid levels and bring the pH back within the normal range.

## Renal System

The renal system is responsible for the long-term regulation of acid-base balance in the body. Excess nonvolatile acids produced during metabolism normally are eliminated by the kidneys. The kidneys also regulate bicarbonate levels in extracellular fluid by regenerating bicarbonate ions as well as reabsorbing them in the renal tubules. Although the kidneys respond more slowly to changes in pH (over hours to days), they can generate bicarbonate and selectively excrete or retain hydrogen ions as needed. In acidosis, when excess hydrogen ion is present and the pH falls, the kidneys excrete hydrogen ions and retain bicarbonate. In alkalosis, the kidneys retain hydrogen ions and excrete bicarbonate to restore acid-base balance.

## Assessment of Acid-Base Balance

Acid-base balance is evaluated primarily by measuring arterial blood gases.

**PRACTICE ALERT** *Arteries are high-pressure vessels in contrast to veins. Obtaining an arterial blood sample requires specialized training. It may be done by a registered nurse, respiratory therapist, or laboratory technician who has been trained in drawing ABGs. Apply firm pressure to the puncture site for 5 minutes after the needle is withdrawn to prevent bleeding into the surrounding tissues.* ■

Arterial blood is used because it reflects acid-base balance throughout the entire body better than venous blood. Arterial blood also provides information about the effectiveness of the lungs in oxygenating blood. The elements measured are pH, the $Paco_2$, the $Pao_2$, and bicarbonate level.

## TABLE 5–10  Normal Arterial Blood Gas Values

| Value | Normal Range | Significance |
|---|---|---|
| pH | 7.35 to 7.45 | Reflects hydrogen ion ($H^+$) concentration<br>• <7.35 = acidosis<br>• >7.45 = alkalosis |
| $Pa_{CO_2}$ | 35 to 45 mmHg | Partial pressure of carbon dioxide ($CO_2$) in arterial blood<br>• <35 mmHg = hypocapnia<br>• >45 mmHg = hypercapnia |
| $Pa_{O_2}$ | 80 to 100 mmHg | Partial pressure of oxygen ($O_2$) in arterial blood<br>• <80 mmHg = hypoxemia |
| $HCO_3^-$ | 22 to 26 mEq/L | Bicarbonate concentration in plasma |
| BE | −3 to +3 | Base excess; a measure of buffering capacity |

**PRACTICE ALERT**  *You will see the abbreviations $Pa_{CO_2}$ and $Pa_{O_2}$ used interchangeably with $P_{CO_2}$ and $P_{O_2}$. The P stands for partial pressure: the pressure exerted by the gas dissolved in the blood. The a indicates that the sample is arterial blood. Because these measurements rarely are done on venous blood, the a often is deleted from the abbreviation.* ■

The $Pa_{CO_2}$ measures the pressure exerted by dissolved carbon dioxide in the blood. The $Pa_{CO_2}$ reflects the respiratory component of acid-base regulation and balance. The $Pa_{CO_2}$ is regulated by the lungs. The normal value is 35 to 45 mmHg. A $Pa_{CO_2}$ of less than 35 mmHg is known as *hypocapnia;* a $Pa_{CO_2}$ greater than 45 mmHg is *hypercapnia.*

The $Pa_{O_2}$ is a measure of the pressure exerted by oxygen that is dissolved in the plasma. Only about 3% of oxygen in the blood is transported in solution; most is combined with hemoglobin. However, it is the dissolved oxygen that is available to the cells for metabolism. As dissolved oxygen diffuses out of plasma into the tissues, more is released from hemoglobin. The normal value for $Pa_{O_2}$ is 80 to 100 mmHg. A $Pa_{O_2}$ less than 80 mmHg is indicative of *hypoxemia.* The $Pa_{O_2}$ is valuable for evaluating respiratory function, but is not used as a primary measurement in determining acid-base status.

The **serum bicarbonate** ($HCO_3^-$) reflects the renal regulation of acid-base balance. It is often called the metabolic component of arterial blood gases. The normal $HCO_3^-$ value is 22 to 26 mEq/L.

The **base excess (BE)** is a calculated value also known as buffer base capacity. The measurement of base excess reflects the degree of acid-base imbalance by indicating the status of the body's total buffering capacity. It represents the amount of acid or base that must be added to a blood sample to achieve a pH of 7.4. This is essentially a measure of increased or decreased bicarbonate. The normal value for base excess for arterial blood is − 3.0 to + 3.0. Normal ABG values are summarized in Table 5–10.

ABGs are analyzed to identify acid-base disorders and their probable cause, to determine the extent of the imbalance, and to monitor treatment. When analyzing ABG results, it is important to use a systematic approach. First evaluate each individual measurement, then look at the interrelationships to determine the client's acid-base status (see Box 5–10).

## ACID-BASE IMBALANCE

Acid-base disorders fall into two major categories: acidosis and alkalosis. Acidosis occurs when the hydrogen ion concentration increases above normal (pH below 7.35). Alkalosis occurs when the hydrogen ion concentration falls below normal (pH above 7.45).

Acid-base imbalances are further classified as *metabolic* or *respiratory* disorders. In metabolic disorders, the primary change is in the concentration of bicarbonate. In **metabolic acidosis,** the amount of bicarbonate is decreased in relation to the amount of acid in the body (Figure 5–15A ■). It can develop as a result of abnormal bicarbonate losses or because of excess nonvolatile acids in the body. The pH falls below 7.35 and the bicarbonate concentration is less than 22 mEq/L. **Metabolic alkalosis,** by contrast, occurs when there is an excess of bicarbonate in relation to the amount of hydrogen ion (Figure 5–15B). The pH is above 7.45 and the bicarbonate concentration is greater than 26 mEq/L.

In respiratory disorders, the primary change is in the concentration of carbonic acid. **Respiratory acidosis** occurs when carbon dioxide is retained, increasing the amount of carbonic acid in the body (Figure 5–16A ■). As a result, the pH falls to less than 7.35, and the $Pa_{CO_2}$ is greater than 45 mmHg. When too much carbon dioxide is "blown off," carbonic acid levels fall and **respiratory alkalosis** develops (Figure 5–16B). The pH rises to above 7.45 and the $Pa_{CO_2}$ is less than 35 mmHg.

Acid-base disorders are further defined as *primary* (simple) and *mixed.* Primary disorders usually are due to one cause. For example, respiratory failure often causes respiratory acidosis due to retained carbon dioxide; renal failure usually causes metabolic acidosis due to retained hydrogen ion and impaired bicarbonate production. Table 5–11 summarizes primary acid-base imbalances with common causes

## BOX 5–10 ■ Interpreting Arterial Blood Gases

1. Look at the pH.
   - pH <7.35 = acidosis
   - pH >7.45 = alkalosis
2. Look at the $Paco_2$.
   - $Paco_2$ <35 mmHg = hypocapnia; more carbon dioxide is being exhaled than normal
   - $Paco_2$ >45 mmHg = hypercapnia; carbon dioxide is being retained
3. Evaluate the pH–$Paco_2$ relationship for a possible respiratory problem.
   - If the pH is <7.35 (acidosis) and the $Paco_2$ is >45 mmHg (hypercapnia), retained carbon dioxide is causing increased $H^+$ concentration and *respiratory acidosis*.
   - If the pH is >7.45 (alkalosis) and the $Paco_2$ is <35 mmHg (hypocapnia), low carbon dioxide levels and decreased $H^+$ concentration are causing *respiratory alkalosis*.
4. Look at the bicarbonate.
   - If the $HCO_3^-$ is <22 mEq/L, bicarbonate levels are lower than normal.
   - If the $HCO_3^-$ is >26 mEq/L, bicarbonate levels are higher than normal.
5. Evaluate the pH, $HCO_3^-$, and BE for a possible metabolic problem.
   - If the pH is <7.35 (acidosis), the $HCO_3^-$ is <22 mEq/L, and the BE is <−3 mEq/L, then low bicarbonate levels and high $H^+$ concentrations are causing *metabolic acidosis*.
   - If the pH is >7.45 (alkalosis), the $HCO_3^-$ is >26 mEq/L, and the BE is > + 3 mEq/L, then high bicarbonate levels are causing *metabolic alkalosis*.
6. Look for compensation.
   - *Renal compensation:*
     - In respiratory acidosis (pH < 7.35, $Paco_2$ > 45 mmHg), the kidneys retain $HCO_3^-$ to buffer the excess acid, so the $HCO_3^-$ is > 26 mEq/L.
     - In respiratory alkalosis (pH >7.45, $Paco_2$ <35 mmHg), the kidneys excrete $HO_3^-$ to minimize the alkalosis, so the $HCO_3^-$ is <22 mEq/L.
   - *Respiratory compensation*
     - In metabolic acidosis (pH <7.35, $HCO_3^-$ <22 mEq/L), the rate and depth of respirations increase, increasing carbon dioxide elimination, so the $Paco_2$ is <35 mmHg.
     - In metabolic alkalosis (pH >7.45, $HCO_3^-$ >26 mEq/L), respirations slow, carbon dioxide is retained, so the $Paco_2$ is >45 mmHg.
7. Evaluate oxygenation.
   - $Pao_2$ <80 mmHg = hypoxemia; possible hypoventilation
   - $Pao_2$ > mmHg = hyperventilation

of each. Mixed disorders occur from combinations of respiratory and metabolic disturbances. For example, a client in cardiac arrest develops a mixed respiratory and metabolic acidosis due to lack of ventilation (and retained $CO_2$) and hypoxia of body tissues that leads to anaerobic metabolism and acid by-products (excess nonvolatile acids).

## Compensation

With primary acid-base disorders, compensatory changes in the other part of the regulatory system occur to restore a normal pH and homeostasis. In metabolic acid-base disorders, the change in pH affects the rate and depth of respirations. This, in turn, affects carbon dioxide elimination and the $Paco_2$, helping restore the carbonic acid to bicarbonate ratio. The kidneys

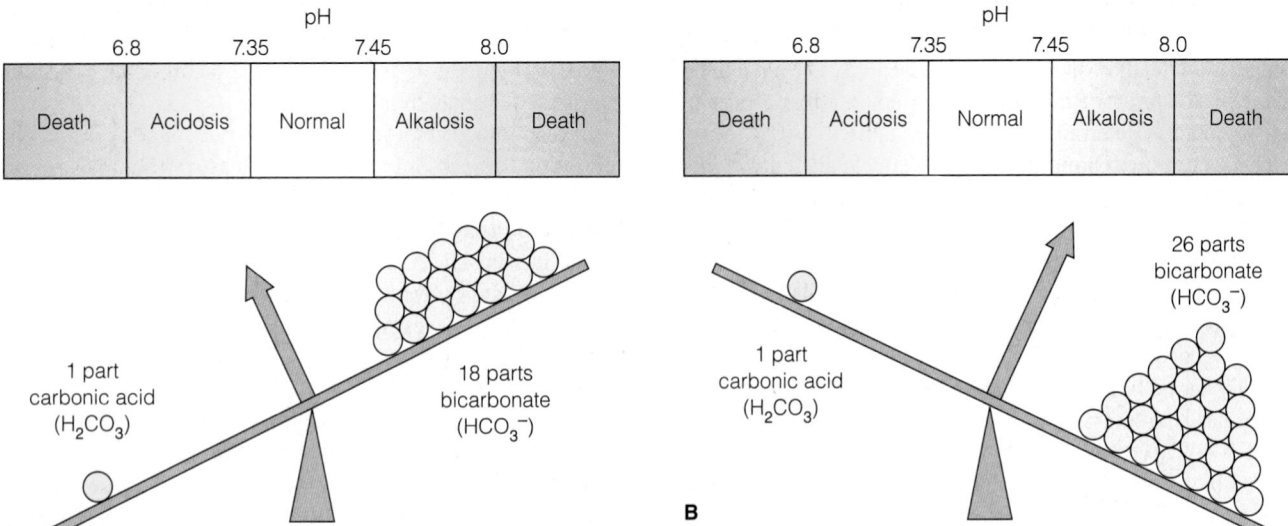

**Figure 5–15** ■ Metabolic acid-base imbalances. *A,* Metabolic acidosis. *B,* Metabolic alkalosis.

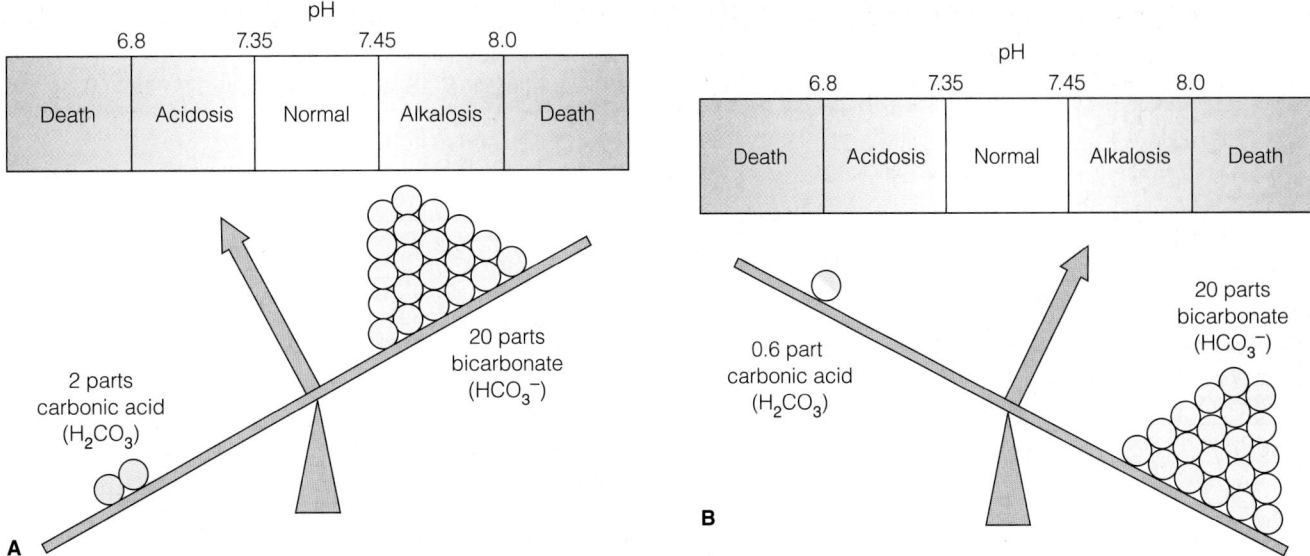

**Figure 5-16** ■ Respiratory acid-base imbalances. *A,* Respiratory acidosis. *B,* Respiratory alkalosis.

TABLE 5-11  Common Causes of Primary Acid-Base Imbalances

| Imbalance | Common Causes |
|---|---|
| Metabolic acidosis<br>pH < 7.35<br>$HCO_3^-$ <22 mEq/L | ↑ Acid production<br>• Lactic acidosis<br>• Ketoacidosis related to diabetes, starvation, or alcoholism<br>• Salicylate toxicity<br>↓ Acid excretion<br>• Renal failure<br>↑ Bicarbonate loss<br>• Diarrhea, ileostomy drainage, intestinal fistula<br>• Biliary or pancreatic fistulas<br>↑ Chloride<br>• Sodium chloride IV solutions<br>• Renal tubular acidosis<br>• Carbonic anhydrase inhibitors |
| Metabolic alkalosis<br>pH >7.45<br>$HCO_3^-$ >26 mEq/L | ↑ Acid loss or excretion<br>• Vomiting, gastric suction<br>• Hypokalemia<br>↑ Bicarbonate<br>• Alkali ingestion (bicarbonate of soda)<br>• Excess bicarbonate administration |
| Respiratory acidosis<br>pH <7.35<br>$Pa_{CO_2}$ >45 mmHg | Acute respiratory acidosis<br>• Acute respiratory conditions (pulmonary edema, pneumonia, acute asthma)<br>• Opiate overdose<br>• Foreign body aspiration<br>• Chest trauma<br>Chronic respiratory acidosis<br>• Chronic respiratory conditions (COPD, cystic fibrosis)<br>• Multiple sclerosis, other neuromuscular diseases<br>• Stroke |
| Respiratory alkalosis<br>pH >7.45<br>$Pa_{CO_2}$ <35 mmHg | • Anxiety-induced hyperventilation (e.g., anxiety)<br>• Fever<br>• Early salicylate intoxication<br>• Hyperventilation with mechanical ventilator |

TABLE 5-12 Compensation for Simple Acid-Base Imbalances

| Primary Disorder | Cause | Compensation | Effect on ABGs |
|---|---|---|---|
| Metabolic acidosis | Excess nonvolatile acids; bicarbonate deficiency | Rate and depth of respirations increase, eliminating additional $CO_2$ | ↓ pH<br>↓ $HCO_3^-$<br>↓ $Paco_2$ |
| Metabolic alkalosis | Bicarbonate excess | Rate and depth of respirations decrease, retaining $CO_2$ | ↑ pH<br>↑ $HCO_3^-$<br>↑ $Paco_2$ |
| Respiratory acidosis | Retained $CO_2$ and excess carbonic acid | Kidneys conserve bicarbonate to restore carbonic acid:bicarbonate ratio of 1:20 | ↓ pH<br>↑ $Paco_2$<br>↑ $HCO_3^-$ |
| Respiratory alkalosis | Loss of $CO_2$ and deficient carbonic acid | Kidneys excrete bicarbonate and conserve $H^+$ to restore carbonic acid:bicarbonate ratio | ↑ pH<br>↓ $Paco_2$<br>↓ $HCO_3^-$ |

compensate for simple respiratory imbalances. The change in pH affects both bicarbonate conservation and hydrogen ion elimination (see Table 5–12).

Compensatory changes in respirations occur within minutes of a change in pH. These changes, however, become less effective over time. The renal response takes longer to restore the pH, but is a more effective long-term mechanism. If the pH is restored to within normal limits, the disorder is said to be *fully compensated*. When these changes are reflected in ABG values but the pH remains outside normal limits, the disorder is said to be *partially compensated*.

## THE CLIENT WITH METABOLIC ACIDOSIS

Metabolic acidosis (bicarbonate deficit) is characterized by a low pH (< 7.35) and a low bicarbonate (< 22 mEq/L). It may be caused by excess acid or loss of bicarbonate from the body. When metabolic acidosis develops, the respiratory system attempts to return the pH to normal by increasing the rate and depth of respirations. Carbon dioxide elimination increases, and the $Paco_2$ falls (< 35 mmHg).

### RISK FACTORS

Metabolic acidosis rarely is a primary disorder; it usually develops during the course of another disease.

- *Acute lactic acidosis* usually results from tissue hypoxia due to shock or cardiac arrest.
- Clients with type 1 diabetes mellitus are at risk for developing *diabetic ketoacidosis* (see Chapter 18 ⊙ for more information about diabetes and its complications).
- *Acute or chronic renal failure* impairs the excretion of metabolic acids.
- Diarrhea, intestinal suction, or abdominal fistulas increase the risk for excess *bicarbonate loss*.

Other common causes of metabolic acidosis are listed in Table 5–11.

### PATHOPHYSIOLOGY

Three basic mechanisms that can cause metabolic acidosis are:

- Accumulation of metabolic acids.
- Excess loss of bicarbonate.
- An increase in chloride levels.

An accumulation of metabolic acids can result from excess acid production or impaired elimination of metabolic acids by the kidney. Lactic acidosis develops due to tissue hypoxia and a shift to anaerobic metabolism by the cells. Lactate and hydrogen ions are produced, which form lactic acid. Both oxygen and glucose are necessary for normal cell metabolism. When intracellular glucose is inadequate due to starvation or a lack of insulin to move it into cells, the body breaks down fatty tissue to meet its metabolic needs. In this process, fatty acids are released, which are converted to ketones; ketoacidosis develops. Aspirin (acetylsalicylic acid) breaks down into salicylic acid in the body. Substances such as aspirin, methanol (wood alcohol), and ethylene (contained in antifreeze and solvents) cause a toxic increase in body acids by either breaking down into acid products (salicylic acid) or stimulating metabolic acid production (Porth, 2002). Renal failure impairs the body's ability to excrete excess hydrogen ions and form bicarbonate.

Excess metabolic acids increase the hydrogen ion concentration of body fluids. The excess acid is buffered by bicarbonate, leading to what is known as a high **anion gap** acidosis (see Box 5–11).

The pancreas secretes bicarbonate-rich fluid into the small intestine. Intestinal suction, severe diarrhea, ileostomy drainage, or fistulas can lead to excess losses of bicarbonate. Hyperchloremic acidosis can develop when excess chloride solutions (such as NaCl or ammonium chloride) are infused, causing a rise in chloride concentrations. It also may be related to renal disease or administration of carbonic anhydrate inhibitor diuretics. The anion gap remains normal in metabolic acidosis due to bicarbonate loss or excess chloride.

## BOX 5-11   ■ Unraveling the Anion Gap

Calculation of the anion gap can help identify the underlying mechanism in metabolic acidosis if it is unclear.

The number of cations (positively charged ions) and anions (negatively charged ions) in ECF normally is equal (refer to Figure 5–2). Not all of these ions, however, are measured in laboratory testing (e.g., organic acids and proteins). The anion gap is calculated by subtracting the sum of two measured anions, chloride and bicarbonate, from the concentration of the major cation, sodium (see accompanying Figure 5–17 ■). The normal anion gap is 8 to 12 mEq/L.

Excess acids in ECF are buffered by bicarbonate, reducing serum bicarbonate levels and the total measured concentration of anions. This increases the anion gap (B in figure). When bicarbonate is lost from the body or chloride levels increase, however, the anion gap remains within normal limits (C in figure). This occurs because an increase or decrease in one of these negatively charged ions causes a corresponding change in the other to maintain balance (e.g., $\downarrow HCO_3^- \leftrightarrow \uparrow Cl^-$), and there is no change in the amount of unmeasured anions.

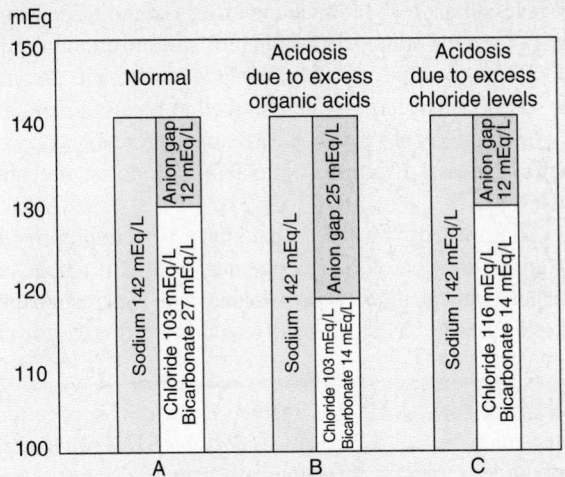

**Figure 5–17** ■ Illustration of the anion gap in metabolic acidosis. *A,* Normal anion gap. *B,* High anion gap caused by excess acids. *C,* Normal anion gap with hyperchloremia.

---

Acidosis depresses cell membrane excitability, affecting neuromuscular function. It also increases the amount of free calcium in ECF by interfering with protein binding. Severe acidosis (pH of 7.0 or less) depresses myocardial contractility, leading to a fall in cardiac output. If kidney function is normal, acid excretion and ammonia production increase to eliminate excess hydrogen ions.

Acid-base imbalances also affect electrolyte balance. In acidosis, potassium is retained as the kidney excretes excess hydrogen ion. Excess hydrogen ions also enter the cells, displacing potassium from the intracellular space to maintain the balance of cations and anions within the cells. The effect of both processes is to increase serum potassium levels. Also in acidosis, calcium is released from its bonds with plasma proteins, increasing the amount of ionized (free) calcium in the blood. Magnesium levels may fall in acidosis (Bullock & Henze, 2000).

## MANIFESTATIONS

Metabolic acidosis affects the function of many body systems. Its general manifestations include weakness and fatigue, headache, and general malaise. Gastrointestinal function is affected, causing anorexia, nausea, vomiting, and abdominal pain. The level of consciousness declines, leading to stupor and coma. Cardiac dysrhythmias develop, and cardiac arrest may occur. The skin is often warm and flushed. Skeletal problems may develop in chronic acidosis, as calcium and phosphate are released from the bones. Manifestations of compensatory mechanisms are seen. The respirations are deep and rapid, known as **Kussmaul's respirations.** The client may complain of shortness of breath or dyspnea. See the box on this page.

## COLLABORATIVE CARE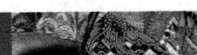

Management of metabolic acidosis focuses on treating the underlying cause of the disorder and correcting the acid-base imbalance.

### Diagnostic Tests

The following laboratory and diagnostic tests may be ordered.

- *ABGs* generally show a pH of less than 7.35 and a bicarbonate level of less than 22 mEq/L. A compensatory decrease in $Paco_2$ to less than 35 mmHg is usually present.
- *Serum electrolytes* demonstrate elevated serum potassium levels and possible low magnesium levels. The total calcium may remain unchanged, although more physiologically active ionized calcium is available. Sodium, chloride, and bicarbonate levels are used to calculate the anion gap.
- The *ECG* may show changes which reflect both the acidosis (particularly when severe) and the accompanying hyperkalemia.

## Manifestations of Metabolic Acidosis

- Anorexia
- Nausea and vomiting
- Abdominal pain
- Weakness
- Fatigue
- General malaise
- Decreasing levels of consciousness
- Dysrhythmias
- Bradycardia
- Warm, flushed skin
- Hyperventilation (Kussmaul's respirations)

## Medications

An alkalinizing solution such as bicarbonate may be given if the pH is less than 7.2 to reduce the effects of the acidosis on cardiac function. Sodium bicarbonate is the most commonly used alkalinizing solution; others include lactate, citrate, and acetate solutions (which are metabolized to bicarbonate). Alkalinizing solutions are given intravenously for severe acute metabolic acidosis. In chronic metabolic acidosis, the oral route is used.

The client treated with bicarbonate must be carefully monitored. Rapid correction of the acidosis may lead to metabolic alkalosis and hypokalemia. Hypernatremia and hyperosmolality may develop as well, leading to water retention and fluid overload.

**PRACTICE ALERT** *As metabolic acidosis is corrected, potassium shifts back into the intracellular space. This can lead to hypokalemia and cardiac dysrhythmias. Carefully monitor serum potassium levels during treatment.* ■

Treatment for diabetic ketoacidosis includes intravenous insulin and fluid replacement. Alcoholic ketoacidosis is treated with saline solutions and glucose. Treatment for lactic acidosis from decreased tissue perfusion (e.g., shock or cardiac arrest) focuses on correcting the underlying problem and improving tissue perfusion. Clients with chronic renal failure and mild or moderate metabolic acidosis may or may not require treatment, depending on the pH and bicarbonate levels. When metabolic acidosis is due to diarrhea, treatment includes correcting the underlying cause and providing fluid and electrolyte replacement.

## NURSING CARE

## Health Promotion

To promote health in clients at risk for metabolic acidosis, discuss management of their underlying disease process (e.g., type 1 diabetes or renal failure) to prevent complications such as diabetic ketoacidosis and metabolic acidosis. Because early manifestations of metabolic acidosis (e.g., fatigue, general malaise, anorexia, nausea, abdominal pain) resemble those of common viral disorders such as "the flu," stress the importance of promptly seeking treatment if these symptoms develop.

## Assessment

Assessment data related to metabolic acidosis include the following:

- Health history: Current manifestations, including anorexia, nausea, vomiting, abdominal discomfort, fatigue, lethargy, other symptoms; duration of symptoms and any precipitating factors such as diarrhea, ingestion of a toxin such as aspirin, methanol, or ethylene; chronic diseases such as diabetes or renal failure, cirrhosis of the liver, or endocrine disorders; current medications.

- Physical assessment: Mental status and level of consciousness; vital signs including respiratory rate and depth; apical and peripheral pulses; skin color and temperature; abdominal contour and distention; bowel sounds; urine output.

## Nursing Diagnoses and Interventions

### Decreased Cardiac Output

Metabolic acidosis affects cardiac output by decreasing myocardial contractility, slowing the heart rate, and increasing the risk for dysrhythmias. The accompanying hyperkalemia increases the risk for decreased cardiac output as well (see earlier discussion about hyperkalemia).

- Monitor vital signs, including peripheral pulses and capillary refill. *Hypotension, diminished pulse strength, and slowed capillary refill may indicate decreased cardiac output and impaired tissue perfusion. Poor tissue perfusion can increase the risk for lactic acidosis.*
- Monitor the ECG pattern for dysrhythmias and changes characteristic of hyperkalemia. Notify the physician of changes. *Progressive ECG changes such as widening of the QRS complex indicate an increasing risk of dysrhythmias and cardiac arrest. Dysrhythmias further decrease cardiac output, possibly intensifying the degree of acidosis.*
- Monitor laboratory values, including arterial blood gases, serum electrolytes, and renal function studies (serum creatinine and BUN). *Frequent monitoring of laboratory values allows evaluation of the effectiveness of treatment as well as early identification of potential problems.*

### Risk for Excess Fluid Volume

Administering bicarbonate to correct acidosis increases the risk for hypernatremia, hyperosmolality, and fluid volume excess.

- Monitor and maintain fluid replacement as ordered. Monitor serum sodium levels and osmolality. *Bicarbonate administration can cause hypernatremia and hyperosmolality, leading to water retention.*
- Monitor heart and lung sounds, CVP, and respiratory status. *Increasing dyspnea, adventitious lung sounds, a third heart sound ($S_3$) due to the volume of blood flow through the heart, and high CVP readings are indicative of hypervolemia and should be reported to the care provider.*
- Assess for edema, particularly in the back, sacral, and periorbital areas. *Initially, edema affects dependent tissues—the back and sacrum in clients who are bedridden. Periorbital edema indicates more generalized edema.*
- Assess urine output hourly. Maintain accurate intake and output records. Note urine output less than 30 mL/hour or a positive fluid balance on 24-hour total intake and output calculations. *Heart failure and inadequate renal perfusion may lead to decreased urine output.*
- Obtain daily weights using consistent conditions. *Daily weights are an accurate indicator of fluid balance.*
- Administer prescribed diuretics as ordered, monitoring the client's response to therapy. *Loop or high-ceiling diuretics such as furosemide can lead to further electrolyte imbal-*

## CHART 5–6  NANDA, NIC, AND NOC LINKAGES

### The Client with Metabolic Acidosis

| NURSING DIAGNOSES | NURSING INTERVENTIONS | NURSING OUTCOMES |
|---|---|---|
| • Decreased Cardiac Output | • Acid-Base Management<br>• Vital Signs Monitoring | • Cardiac Pump Effectiveness |
| • Risk for Excess Fluid Volume | • Electrolyte Management<br>• Fluid Management | • Electrolyte & Acid-Base Balance<br>• Vital Signs Status |
| • Risk for Injury | • Environmental Management: Safety | • Safety Status: Physical Injury |

*Note. Data from Nursing Outcomes Classification (NOC) by M. Johnson & M. Maas (Eds.), 1997, St. Louis: Mosby; Nursing Diagnoses: Definitions & Classification 2001–2002 by North American Nursing Diagnosis Association, 2001, Philadelphia: NANDA; Nursing Interventions Classification (NIC) by J.C. McCloskey & G. M. Bulechek (Eds.), 2000, St. Louis: Mosby. Reprinted by permission.*

*ances, especially hypokalemia. This is a significant risk as during correction of metabolic acidosis.*

### Risk for Injury

Mental status and brain function are affected by acidosis, increasing the risk for injury.

- Monitor neurologic function, including mental status, level of consciousness, and muscle strength. *As the pH falls, mental functioning declines, leading to confusion, stupor, and a decreasing level of consciousness.*
- Institute safety precautions as necessary; keep the bed in its lowest position, side rails raised. *These measures help protect the client from injury resulting from confusion or disorientation.*
- Keep clocks, calendars, and familiar objects at bedside. Orient to time, place, and circumstances as needed. Allow significant others to remain with the client as much as possible. *An unfamiliar environment and altered thought processes can further increase the risk for injury. Significant others provide a sense of security and reduce anxiety.*

Nursing care also includes measures to treat the underlying disorder, such as diabetic ketoacidosis. Refer to the chapters on diabetes (Chapter 18) and renal failure (Chapter 27) for specific interventions. ⏎

### Using NANDA, NIC, and NOC

Chart 5–6 shows links between potential NANDA nursing diagnoses, NIC, and NOC when caring for a client with metabolic acidosis.

### Home Care

Discharge planning and teaching focuses on the underlying cause of the imbalance. The client who has developed ketoacidosis as a result of diabetes mellitus, starvation, or alcoholism needs interventions and teaching to prevent future episodes of acidosis. Diet, medication management, and alcohol dependency treatment are vital teaching areas. When metabolic acidosis is related to renal failure, the client should be referred for management of the renal failure itself. Clients who have experienced diarrhea or excess ileostomy drainage leading to bicarbonate loss need information about appropriate diarrhea treatment strategies and when to call their primary care provider.

## THE CLIENT WITH METABOLIC ALKALOSIS

Metabolic alkalosis (bicarbonate excess) is characterized by a high pH (>7.45) and a high bicarbonate (>26 mEq/L). It may be caused by loss of acid or excess bicarbonate in the body. When metabolic alkalosis develops, the respiratory system attempts to return the pH to normal by slowing the respiratory rate. Carbon dioxide is retained, and the $Paco_2$ increases (>45 mmHg).

### RISK FACTORS

As is the case with other acid-base imbalances, metabolic alkalosis rarely occurs as a primary disorder. Risk factors include hospitalization, hypokalemia, and treatment with alkalinizing solutions (e.g., bicarbonate).

### PATHOPHYSIOLOGY

Hydrogen ions may be lost via gastric secretions, through the kidneys, or because of a shift of $H^+$ into the cells. Metabolic alkalosis due to loss of hydrogen ions usually occurs because of vomiting or gastric suction. Gastric secretions are highly acidic (pH 1 to 3). When these are lost through vomiting or gastric suction, the alkalinity of body fluids increases. This increased alkalinity results both from the loss of acid and selective retention of bicarbonate by the kidneys as chloride is depleted (chloride is the major anion in ECF; when it is lost, bicarbonate is retained as a replacement anion).

Increased renal excretion of hydrogen ions can be prompted by hypokalemia as the kidneys try to conserve potassium, excreting hydrogen ion instead. Hypokalemia contributes to metabolic alkalosis in another way as well. When potassium shifts out of cells to maintain extracellular potassium levels, hydrogen ions shift into the cells to maintain the balance between cations and anions within the cell.

## Manifestations of Metabolic Alkalosis

- Confusion
- Decreasing levels of consciousness
- Hyperreflexia
- Tetany
- Dysrhythmias
- Hypotension
- Seizures
- Respiratory failure

Excess bicarbonate usually occurs as a result of ingesting antacids that contain bicarbonate (such as soda bicarbonate or Alka-Seltzer) or overzealous administration of bicarbonate to treat metabolic acidosis. Common causes of metabolic alkalosis are summarized in Table 5–11.

In alkalosis, more calcium combines with serum proteins, reducing the amount of ionized (physiologically active) calcium in the blood. This accounts for many of the common manifestations of metabolic alkalosis. Alkalosis also affects potassium balance: Hypokalemia not only can cause metabolic alkalosis (see above), but it also can result from metabolic alkalosis. Hydrogen ions shift out of the intracellular space to help restore the pH, prompting more potassium to enter the cells and depleting ECF potassium. The high pH depresses the respiratory system as the body retains carbon dioxide to restore the carbonic acid to bicarbonate ratio.

## MANIFESTATIONS AND COMPLICATIONS

Manifestations of metabolic alkalosis occur as a result of decreased calcium ionization and are similar to those of hypocalcemia, including numbness and tingling around the mouth and of fingers and toes, dizziness, Trousseau's sign, and muscle spasm (see box above). As the respiratory system compensates for metabolic alkalosis, respirations are depressed and respiratory failure with hypoxemia and respiratory acidosis may develop.

## COLLABORATIVE CARE

The management of metabolic alkalosis focuses on diagnosing and correcting the underlying cause.

## Diagnostic Tests

The following laboratory and diagnostic tests may be ordered.

- *ABGs* show a pH greater than 7.45 and bicarbonate level greater than 26 mEq/L. With compensatory hypoventilation, carbon dioxide is retained, and the $Paco_2$ is greater than 45 mmHg.
- *Serum electrolytes* often demonstrate decreased serum potassium (< 3.5 mEq/L) and decreased chloride (< 95 mEq/L) levels. The serum bicarbonate level is high. Although the total serum calcium may be normal, the ionized fraction of calcium is low.
- *Urine pH* may be low (pH 1 to 3) if metabolic acidosis is caused by hypokalemia. The kidneys selectively retain potassium and excrete hydrogen ion to restore ECF potassium levels. Urinary chloride levels may be normal or greater than 250 mEq/24 hours.

- The *ECG pattern* shows changes similar to those seen with hypokalemia. These changes may be due to hypokalemia or to the alkalosis.

## Medications

Treatment of metabolic alkalosis includes restoring normal fluid volume and administering potassium chloride and sodium chloride solution. The potassium restores serum and intracellular potassium levels, allowing the kidneys to more effectively conserve hydrogen ions. Chloride promotes renal excretion of bicarbonate. Sodium chloride solutions restore fluid volume deficits that can contribute to metabolic alkalosis. In severe alkalosis, an acidifying solution such as dilute hydrochloric acid or ammonium chloride may be administered. In addition, drugs may be used to treat the underlying cause of the alkalosis.

## NURSING CARE

## Health Promotion

Health promotion activities focus on teaching clients the risks of using sodium bicarbonate as an antacid to relieve heartburn or gastric distress. Stress the availability of other effective antacid preparations and the need to seek medical evaluation for persistent gastric symptoms.

In the hospital setting, carefully monitor laboratory values for clients at risk for developing metabolic alkalosis, particularly clients undergoing continuous gastric suction.

## Assessment

Focused assessment data related to metabolic alkalosis include the following:

- Health history:   Current manifestations, such as numbness and tingling, muscle spasms, dizziness, other symptoms; duration of symptoms and any precipitating factors such as bicarbonate ingestion, vomiting, diuretic therapy, or endocrine disorders; current medications.
- Physical assessment:   Vital signs including apical pulse and rate and depth of respirations; muscle strength; deep tendon reflexes.

## Nursing Diagnoses and Interventions

### Risk for Impaired Gas Exchange

Respiratory compensation for metabolic alkalosis depresses the respiratory rate and reduces the depth of breathing to promote carbon dioxide retention. As a result, the client is at risk for impaired gas exchange, especially in the presence of underlying lung disease.

- Monitor respiratory rate, depth, and effort. Monitor oxygen saturation continuously, reporting an oxygen saturation level of less than 95% (or as ordered). *The depressed respiratory drive associated with metabolic alkalosis can lead to hypoxemia and impaired oxygenation of tissues. Oxygen saturation levels of less than 90% indicate significant oxygenation problems.*

- Assess skin color; note and report cyanosis around the mouth. *Central cyanosis, seen around the mouth and oral mucous membranes, indicates significant hypoxia.*
- Monitor mental status and level of consciousness. Report decreasing LOC or behavior changes such as restlessness, agitation, or confusion. *Changes in mental status or behavior may be early signs of hypoxia.*
- Place in semi-Fowler's or Fowler's position as tolerated. *Elevating the head of the bed facilitates alveolar ventilation and gas exchange.*
- Schedule nursing care activities to allow rest periods. *The client who is hypoxemic has limited energy reserves, necessitating frequent rest and limited activities.*
- Administer oxygen as ordered or necessary to maintain oxygen saturation levels. *Supplemental oxygen can help maintain blood and tissue oxygenation despite depressed respirations.*

### Deficient Fluid Volume

Clients with metabolic alkalosis often have an accompanying fluid volume deficit.

**PRACTICE ALERT** *Assess intake and output accurately, monitoring fluid balance. In acute situations, hourly intake and output may be indicated. Urine output less than 30 mL/hour indicates inadequate tissue perfusion, inadequate renal perfusion and an increased risk for acute renal failure.* ■

- Assess vital signs, CVP, and peripheral pulse volume at least every 4 hours. *Hypotension, tachycardia, low CVP, and weak, easily obliterated peripheral pulses indicate hypovolemia.*
- Weigh daily under standard conditions (time of day, clothing, and scale). *Rapid weight changes accurately reflect fluid balance.*
- Administer intravenous fluids as prescribed using an electronic infusion pump. Monitor for indicators of fluid overload if rapid fluid replacement is ordered: dyspnea, tachypnea, tachycardia, increased CVP, jugular vein distension, and edema. *Rapid fluid replacement may lead to hypervolemia, resulting in pulmonary edema and cardiac failure, particularly in clients with compromised cardiac and renal function.*

- Monitor serum electrolytes, osmolality, and ABG values. *Rehydration and administration of potassium chloride will affect both acid-base and fluid and electrolyte balance. Careful monitoring is important to identify changes.*

Nursing care also includes interdependent care measures to treat the underlying disorder, such as excessive vomiting or hypokalemia.

### Using NANDA, NIC, and NOC

Chart 5–7 shows links between potential NANDA nursing diagnoses, NIC, and NOC when caring for a client with metabolic alkalosis.

### Home Care

When preparing the client with metabolic alkalosis for discharge and home care, consider the cause of the alkalosis and any underlying factors. For example, provide teaching about the following:

- Using appropriate antacids for heartburn and gastric distress
- Using potassium supplements as ordered or eating high-potassium foods to avoid hypokalemia if taking a potassium-wasting diuretic or if aldosterone production is impaired
- Contacting the primary care provider if uncontrolled or extended vomiting develops

## THE CLIENT WITH RESPIRATORY ACIDOSIS

Respiratory acidosis is caused by an excess of dissolved carbon dioxide, or carbonic acid. It is characterized by a pH of less than 7.35 and a $PaCO_2$ greater than 45 mmHg. Respiratory acidosis may be either acute or chronic. In chronic respiratory acidosis, the bicarbonate is higher than 26 mEq/L as the kidneys compensate by retaining bicarbonate.

### RISK FACTORS

Acute or chronic lung disease (e.g., pneumonia or chronic obstructive pulmonary disease) is the primary risk factor for respiratory acidosis. Other conditions that depress or interfere with ventilation, such as excess narcotic analgesics, airway

---

### CHART 5–7 NANDA, NIC, AND NOC LINKAGES

#### The Client with Metabolic Alkalosis

| NURSING DIAGNOSES | NURSING INTERVENTIONS | NURSING OUTCOMES |
|---|---|---|
| • Risk for Impaired Gas Exchange | • Acid-Base Management<br>• Fluid Management | • Respiratory Status: Gas Exchange |
| • Deficient Fluid Volume | • Intravenous Therapy | • Electrolyte & Acid-Base Balance<br>• Fluid Balance |

*Note. Data from Nursing Outcomes Classification (NOC) by M. Johnson & M. Maas (Eds.), 1997, St. Louis: Mosby; Nursing Diagnoses: Definitions & Classification 2001–2002 by North American Nursing Diagnosis Association, 2001, Philadelphia: NANDA; Nursing Interventions Classification (NIC) by J.C. McCloskey & G. M. Bulechek (Eds.), 2000, St. Louis: Mosby. Reprinted by permission.*

obstruction, or neuromuscular disease, also are risk factors for respiratory acidosis. Selected causes of respiratory acidosis are listed in Table 5–11.

## PATHOPHYSIOLOGY

Both acute and chronic respiratory acidosis result from carbon dioxide retention caused by alveolar hypoventilation. Hypoxemia (low oxygen in the arterial blood) frequently accompanies respiratory acidosis.

## Acute Respiratory Acidosis

Acute respiratory acidosis occurs due to a sudden failure of ventilation. Chest trauma, aspiration of a foreign body, acute pneumonia, and overdoses of narcotic or sedative medications can lead to this condition. Because acute respiratory acidosis occurs with the sudden onset of hypoventilation—as, for example, with cardiac arrest—the $PaCO_2$ rises rapidly and the pH falls markedly. A pH of 7 or lower can occur within minutes (Metheny, 2000). The serum bicarbonate level initially is unchanged because the compensatory response of the kidneys occurs over hours to days.

Hypercapnia (increased carbon dioxide levels) affects neurologic function and the cardiovascular system. Carbon dioxide rapidly crosses the blood-brain barrier. Cerebral blood vessels dilate, and if the condition continues, intracranial pressure increases and papilledema (swelling and inflammation of the optic nerve where it enters the retina) develops (Porth, 2002). Peripheral vasodilation also occurs, and the pulse rate increases to maintain cardiac output.

## Chronic Respiratory Acidosis

Chronic respiratory acidosis is associated with chronic respiratory or neuromuscular conditions such as chronic obstructive pulmonary disease (COPD), asthma, cystic fibrosis, or multiple sclerosis. These conditions affect alveolar ventilation because of airway obstruction, structural changes in the lung, or limited chest wall expansion. Most clients with chronic respiratory acidosis have COPD with chronic bronchitis and emphysema. In chronic respiratory acidosis, the $PaCO_2$ increases over time and remains elevated. The kidneys retain bicarbonate, increasing bicarbonate levels, and the pH often remains close to the normal range.

The acute effects of hypercapnia may not develop because carbon dioxide levels rise gradually, allowing compensatory changes to occur. When carbon dioxide levels are chronically elevated, the respiratory center becomes less sensitive to the gas as a stimulant of the respiratory drive. The $PaO_2$ provides the primary stimulus for respirations. Clients with chronic respiratory acidosis are at risk for developing *carbon dioxide narcosis* with manifestations of acute respiratory acidosis, if the respiratory center is suppressed by administering excess supplemental oxygen.

**PRACTICE ALERT**   *Carefully monitor neurologic and respiratory status in clients with chronic respiratory acidosis who are receiving oxygen therapy. Immediately report decreasing level of consciousness or depressed respirations.* ■

## Manifestations of Respiratory Acidosis

**ACUTE RESPIRATORY ACIDOSIS**
- Headache
- Warm, flushed skin
- Blurred vision
- Irritability, altered mental status
- Decreasing level of consciousness
- Cardiac arrest

**CHRONIC RESPIRATORY ACIDOSIS**
- Weakness
- Dull headache
- Sleep disturbances with daytime sleepiness
- Impaired memory
- Personality changes

## MANIFESTATIONS

The manifestations of acute and chronic respiratory acidosis differ. In acute respiratory acidosis, the rapid rise in $PaCO_2$ levels causes manifestations of hypercapnia. Cerebral vasodilation causes manifestations such as headache, blurred vision, irritability, and mental cloudiness. If the condition continues, the level of consciousness progressively decreases. Rapid and dramatic changes in ABGs can lead to unconsciousness and ventricular fibrillation, a potentially lethal cardiac dysrhythmia. The skin of the client with acute respiratory acidosis may be warm and flushed, and the pulse rate is elevated.

The manifestations of chronic respiratory acidosis include weakness and a dull headache. Sleep disturbances, daytime sleepiness, impaired memory, and personality changes also may be manifestations of chronic respiratory acidosis (see the box above).

## COLLABORATIVE CARE

Clients with acute respiratory failure usually require treatment in the emergency department or intensive care unit. The focus is on restoring adequate ventilation and gas exchange. Hypoxemia often accompanies acute respiratory acidosis, so oxygen is administered as well. Supplemental oxygen is administered with caution to clients with chronic respiratory acidosis.

## Diagnostic Tests

The following laboratory and diagnostic tests may be ordered.

- *ABGs* show a pH of less than 7.35 and a $PaCO_2$ of more than 45 mmHg. In acute respiratory acidosis, the bicarbonate level is initially within normal range but increases to greater than 26 mEq/L if the condition persists. In chronic respiratory acidosis, both the $PaCO_2$ and the $HCO_3^-$ may be significantly elevated.
- *Serum electrolytes* may show hypochloremia (chloride level < 98 mEq/L) in chronic respiratory acidosis.
- *Pulmonary function tests* may be done to determine if chronic lung disease is the cause of the respiratory acidosis. These studies would not be done during the acute period, however.

## Medications

Bronchodilator drugs may be administered to open the airways and antibiotics prescribed to treat respiratory infections. If excess narcotics or anesthetic has caused acute respiratory acidosis, drugs to reverse their effects (such as naloxone) may be given.

## Respiratory Support

Treatment of respiratory acidosis, either acute or chronic, focuses on improving alveolar ventilation and gas exchange. Clients with severe respiratory acidosis and hypoxemia may require intubation and mechanical ventilation (see Chapter 36 for more information about these procedures). ⊖ The $PaCO_2$ level is lowered slowly to avoid complications such as cardiac dysrhythmias and decreased cerebral perfusion. In clients with chronic respiratory acidosis, oxygen is administered cautiously to avoid carbon dioxide narcosis.

Pulmonary hygiene measures, such as breathing treatments or percussion and drainage, may be instituted. Adequate hydration is important to promote removal of respiratory secretions.

# NURSING CARE

## Health Promotion

Health promotion activities related to respiratory acidosis focus on identifying, monitoring, and teaching clients at risk. Carefully monitor clients receiving anesthesia, narcotic analgesics, or sedatives for signs of respiratory depression. Monitor the response of clients with a history of chronic lung disease to oxygen therapy. Teach clients who have an identified risk for respiratory acidosis (such as people using narcotic analgesia for cancer pain and people with chronic lung disease) and their families about early manifestations of respiratory depression and acidosis, and instruct them to immediately contact their care provider if manifestations develop.

## Assessment

Assessment data related to respiratory acidosis include the following:
- Health history: Current manifestations, including headache, irritability or lethargy, difficulty thinking, blurred vision, and other symptoms; duration of symptoms and any precipitating factors such as drug use or respiratory infection; chronic diseases such as cystic fibrosis or COPD; current medications.
- Physical assessment: Mental status and level of consciousness; vital signs; skin color and temperature; rate and depth of respirations, pulmonary excursion, lung sounds; examination of optic fundus for possible papilledema.

## Nursing Diagnoses and Interventions

### Impaired Gas Exchange
- Frequently assess respiratory status, including rate, depth, effort, and oxygen saturation levels. *Decreasing respiratory rate and effort along with decreasing oxygen saturation levels may signal worsening respiratory failure and respiratory acidosis.*

**PRACTICE ALERT** *Frequently assess level of consciousness. A decline in level of consciousness may indicate increasing hypercapnia and the need for increasing ventilatory support (such as intubation and mechanical ventilation).* ■

- Promptly evaluate and report ABG results to the physician and respiratory therapist. *Rapid changes in carbon dioxide or oxygen levels may necessitate modification of the treatment plan to prevent complications of overcorrection of respiratory acidosis.*
- Place in semi-Fowler's to Fowler's position as tolerated. *Elevating the head of the bed promotes lung expansion and gas exchange.*
- Administer oxygen as ordered. Carefully monitor response. Reduce the oxygen flow rate or percentage and immediately report increasing somnolence. *Supplemental oxygen can suppress the respiratory drive in clients with chronic respiratory acidosis.*

### Ineffective Airway Clearance
- Frequently auscultate breath sounds (whether on or off a mechanical ventilator). *Increasing adventitious sounds or decreasing breath sounds (faint or absent) may indicate worsening airway clearance due to obstruction or fatigue.*
- Encourage the client with chronic respiratory acidosis to use pursed-lip breathing. *Pursed-lip breathing helps maintain open airways throughout exhalation, promoting carbon dioxide elimination.*
- Frequently reposition and encourage out of bed as tolerated. *Repositioning, sitting at the bedside, and ambulation promote airway clearance and lung expansion.*
- Encourage fluid intake of up to 3000 mL per day as tolerated or allowed. *Fluids help liquify secretions and hydrate respiratory mucous membranes, promoting airway clearance.*
- Administer medications such as inhaled bronchodilators as ordered. *Inhaled bronchodilators help relieve bronchial spasm, dilating airways.*
- Provide percussion, vibration, and postural drainage as ordered. *Pulmonary hygiene measures such as these help loosen respiratory secretions so they can be coughed out of airways.*

## Using NANDA, NIC, and NOC

Chart 5–8 shows links between NANDA nursing diagnoses, NIC, and NOC when caring for a client with respiratory acidosis.

## Home Care

Planning and teaching for home care focuses on the problem that caused the client to develop respiratory acidosis. The client who developed acute respiratory acidosis as a result of acute pneumonia or chest trauma may only require teaching to prevent future problems. If acute respiratory acidosis occurred secondarily to a narcotic overdose, determine if the drug was prescribed for pain or if it was an illicit street drug. Provide teaching to the client who requires narcotic medication on a continuing basis. Refer the client using illicit drugs to a substance abuse counselor, treatment center, or Narcotics Anonymous as appropriate.

## CHART 5–8  NANDA, NIC, AND NOC LINKAGES

### The Client with Respiratory Acidosis

| NURSING DIAGNOSES | NURSING INTERVENTIONS | NURSING OUTCOMES |
| --- | --- | --- |
| • Impaired Gas Exchange<br>• Ineffective Airway Clearance | • Acid-Base Management:<br>  Respiratory Acidosis<br>• Respiratory Monitoring<br>• Ventilation Assistance | • Electrolyte & Acid-Base Balance<br>• Respiratory Status: Gas Exchange<br>• Respiratory Status: Ventilation |

Note. Data from Nursing Outcomes Classification (NOC) by M. Johnson & M. Maas (Eds.), 1997, St. Louis: Mosby; Nursing Diagnoses: Definitions & Classification 2001–2002 by North American Nursing Diagnosis Association, 2001, Philadelphia: NANDA; Nursing Interventions Classification (NIC) by J.C. McCloskey & G. M. Bulechek (Eds.), 2000, St. Louis: Mosby. Reprinted by permission.

For clients with chronic lung disease, discuss ways to avoid future episodes of acute respiratory failure. Encourage the client to be immunized against pneumococcal pneumonia and influenza. Discuss ways to avoid acute respiratory infections and measures to take when respiratory status is further compromised.

## THE CLIENT WITH RESPIRATORY ALKALOSIS

Respiratory alkalosis is characterized by a pH greater than 7.45 and a $PaCO_2$ of less than 35 mmHg. It is always caused by hyperventilation leading to a carbon dioxide deficit.

## Nursing Care Plan
### A Client with Acute Respiratory Acidosis

Marlene Hitz, age 76, is eating lunch with her friends when she suddenly begins to choke and is unable to breathe. After several minutes of trying, an attendant at the senior center successfully dislodges some meat caught in Ms. Hitz's throat using the Heimlich maneuver. Ms. Hitz is taken by ambulance to the emergency department for follow-up because she was apneic for 3 to 4 minutes, her respirations are shallow, and she is disoriented.

### ASSESSMENT

Ms. Hitz is placed in an observation room. Oxygen is started at 4 L/min per nasal cannula. David Love, the nurse admitting Ms. Hitz, makes the following assessments: T 98.2, P 102, R 36 and shallow, BP 146/92. Skin is warm and dry. Alert but restless and not oriented to time or place; she responds slowly to questions. Stat ABGs are drawn, a chest X-ray is done, and D5 ½ NS is started intravenously at 50 mL/hr.

The chest X-ray shows no abnormality. ABG results are pH 7.38 (normal: 7.35 to 7.45), $PaCO_2$ 48 mmHg (normal: 35 to 45 mmHg), $PaO_2$ 92 mmHg (normal: 80 to 100 mmHg), and $HCO_3^-$ 24 mEq/L (normal: 22 to 26 mEq/L).

### DIAGNOSES

- *Impaired gas exchange* related to temporary airway obstruction
- *Anxiety* related to emergency hospital admission
- *Risk for injury* related to confusion

### EXPECTED OUTCOMES

- Regain normal gas exchange and ABG values.
- Be oriented to time, place, and person.

- Regain baseline mental status.
- Remain free of injury.

### PLANNING AND IMPLEMENTATION

- Monitor ABGs, to be redrawn in 2 hours.
- Monitor vital signs and respiratory status (including oxygen saturation) every 15 minutes for the first hour then every hour.
- Assess color of skin, nail beds, and oral mucous membranes every hour.
- Assess mental status and orientation every hour.
- Monitor anxiety level as evidenced by restlessness and agitation.
- Maintain a calm, quiet environment.
- Provide reorientation and explain all activities.
- Keep side rails in place, and place call bell within reach.

### EVALUATION

Ms. Hitz remains in the emergency department for 6 hours. Her ABGs are still abnormal, and David Love now notes the presence of respiratory crackles and wheezes. She is less anxious and responds appropriately when asked who and where she is. Because she has not regained normal gas exchange, Ms. Hitz is admitted to the hospital for continued observation and treatment.

### Critical Thinking in the Nursing Process

1. Describe the pathophysiologic process that leads to acute respiratory acidosis in Marlene Hitz.
2. Describe the effect of acidosis on mental function.
3. What teaching would you provide to Marlene Hitz to prevent future episodes of choking?

See Evaluating Your Response in Appendix C.

## RISK FACTORS

Anxiety with hyperventilation is the most common cause of respiratory alkalosis; therefore, anxiety disorders increase the risk for this acid-base imbalance. In the client who is critically ill, mechanical ventilation is a risk factor for respiratory alkalosis.

## PATHOPHYSIOLOGY

In acute respiratory alkalosis, the pH rises rapidly as the $Paco_2$ falls. Because the kidneys are unable to rapidly adapt to the change in pH, the bicarbonate level remains within normal limits. Anxiety-based hyperventilation is the most common cause of acute respiratory alkalosis. Other physiologic causes of hyperventilation include high fever, hypoxia, gram-negative bacteremia, and thyrotoxicosis. Early salicylate intoxication (aspirin overdose), encephalitis, and high progesterone levels in pregnancy directly stimulate the respiratory center, potentially leading to hyperventilation and respiratory alkalosis. Hyperventilation also can occur during anesthesia or mechanical ventilation if the rate and tidal volume (depth) of ventilations is excessive.

If hyperventilation continues, the kidneys compensate by eliminating bicarbonate to restore the bicarbonate to carbonic acid ratio. The bicarbonate level is lower than normal in chronic respiratory alkalosis, and the pH may be close to the normal range.

Alkalosis increases binding of extracellular calcium to albumin, reducing ionized calcium levels. As a result, neuromuscular excitability increases and manifestations similar to hypocalcemia develop. Low carbon dioxide levels in the blood cause vasoconstriction of cerebral vessels, increasing the neurologic manifestations of the disorder.

## MANIFESTATIONS

The manifestations of respiratory alkalosis include lightheadedness, a feeling of panic and difficulty concentrating, circumoral and distal extremity paresthesias, tremors, and positive Chvostek's and Trousseau's signs. The client also may experience tinnitus, a sensation of chest tightness, and palpitations (cardiac dysrhythmias). Seizures and loss of consciousness may occur. See the box below.

## COLLABORATIVE CARE

Management of respiratory alkalosis focuses on correcting the imbalance and treating the underlying cause.

### Manifestations of Respiratory Alkalosis

- Dizziness
- Numbness and tingling around mouth, of hands and feet
- Palpitations
- Dyspnea
- Chest tightness

- Anxiety/panic
- Tremors
- Tetany
- Seizures, loss of consciousness

## Diagnostic Tests

*ABGs* generally show a pH greater than 7.45 and a $Paco_2$ less than 35 mmHg. In chronic hyperventilation, there is a compensatory decrease in serum bicarbonate to less than 22 mEq/L and the pH may be near normal.

## Medications

A sedative or antianxiety agent may be necessary to relieve anxiety and restore a normal breathing pattern. Additional drugs to correct underlying problems other than anxiety-induced hyperventilation may be ordered.

## Respiratory Therapy

The usual treatment for anxiety-related respiratory alkalosis involves instructing the client to breathe more slowly and having the client breathe into a paper bag or rebreather mask. This allows rebreathing of exhaled carbon dioxide, increasing $Paco_2$ levels and reducing the pH. If excessive ventilation by a mechanical ventilator is the cause of respiratory alkalosis, ventilator settings are adjusted to reduce the respiratory rate and tidal volume as indicated. When hypoxia is the underlying cause of hyperventilation, oxygen is administered.

## NURSING CARE

### Health Promotion

Identify clients at risk in the hospital (e.g., clients on mechanical ventilation or who have a fever or infection), and monitor assessment data and ABGs to identify early manifestations of hyperventilation and respiratory alkalosis.

### Assessment, Diagnoses, and Interventions

#### Ineffective Breathing Pattern

The usual cause of hyperventilation and respiratory alkalosis is psychologic, although physiologic disorders also can lead to hyperventilation. It is important to not only address the hyperventilation, but also to identify the underlying cause.

- Assess respiratory rate, depth, and ease. Monitor vital signs (including temperature) and skin color. *Assessment data can help identify the underlying cause, such as a fever or hypoxia.*
- Obtain subjective assessment data such as circumstances leading up to the current situation, current health and recent illnesses or medication use, and current manifestations. *Subjective data provide cues to the cause and circumstances of the hyperventilation response.*
- Reassure the client that he or she is not experiencing a heart attack and that symptoms will resolve when breathing returns to normal. *Manifestations of hyperventilation and respiratory alkalosis such as dyspnea, chest tightness or pain, and palpitations can mimic those of a heart attack.*
- Instruct the client to maintain eye contact and breathe with you to slow the respiratory rate. *These measures help to make*

## CHART 5–9 NANDA, NIC, AND NOC LINKAGES

### The Client with Respiratory Alkalosis

| NURSING DIAGNOSES | NURSING INTERVENTIONS | NURSING OUTCOMES |
|---|---|---|
| • Ineffective Breathing Pattern<br>• Risk for Injury | • Acid-Base Management:<br>  Respiratory Alkalosis<br>• Anxiety Reduction | • Anxiety Control<br>• Respiratory Status: Gas Exchange |

*Note. Data from* Nursing Outcomes Classification (NOC) *by M. Johnson & M. Maas (Eds.), 1997, St. Louis: Mosby;* Nursing Diagnoses: Definitions & Classification 2001–2002 *by North American Nursing Diagnosis Association, 2001, Philadelphia: NANDA;* Nursing Interventions Classification (NIC) *by J.C. McCloskey & G. M. Bulechek (Eds.), 2000, St. Louis: Mosby. Reprinted by permission.*

the client aware of respirations and provide a sense of support and control (Ackley & Ladwig, 2002).
- Have the client breathe into a paper bag. *This allows the client to rebreathe exhaled carbon dioxide, increasing the Paco₂ and decreasing the pH.*
- Protect the client from injury. *If hyperventilation continues to the point at which the client loses consciousness, respirations will return to normal, as will acid-base balance.*
- If the client has experienced repeated episodes of hyperventilation or has a chronic anxiety disorder, refer for counseling. *Counseling can help the client develop alternative strategies for dealing with anxiety.*

## Using NANDA, NIC, and NOC

Chart 5–9 shows links between NANDA nursing diagnoses, NIC, and NOC when caring for a client with respiratory alkalosis.

## Home Care

Planning and teaching for home care is directed toward the underlying cause of hyperventilation. If anxiety precipitated the episode, discuss anxiety-management strategies with the client. Refer the client and family to a counselor if appropriate. Teach the client to identify a hyperventilation reaction, and how to breathe into a paper bag to manage it at home.

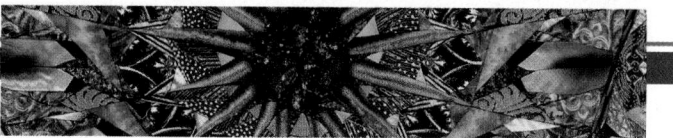

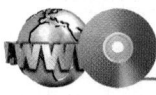 **EXPLORE MediaLink**

NCLEX review questions, case studies, care plan activities, MediaLink applications, and other interactive resources for this chapter can be found on the Companion Website at www.prenhall.com/lemone.

Click on Chapter 5 to select the activities for this chapter. For animations, video clips, more NCLEX review questions, and an audio glossary, access the Student CD-ROM accompanying this textbook.

## TEST YOURSELF

1. Isotonic intravenous fluids are recommended to restore intravascular fluid volume. Which solution would the nurse identify as an isotonic intravenous solution?
   a. Ringer's solution
   b. 10% dextrose in water
   c. 3% sodium chloride
   d. 0.45% sodium chloride

2. When assessing a client with fluid volume deficit, the nurse would expect to find:
   a. Increased pulse rate and blood pressure
   b. Dyspnea and respiratory crackles
   c. Headache and muscle cramps
   d. Orthostatic hypotension and flat neck veins

3. Laboratory results for a client show a serum potassium level of 2.2 mEq/L. Which of the following nursing actions is of highest priority for this client?
   a. Keep the client on bed rest
   b. Initiate cardiac monitoring
   c. Start oxygen at 2 L/min
   d. Initiate seizure precautions

4. The nurse evaluates teaching about calcium supplement therapy as effective when the client states that she will take her calcium tablets:
   a. All at one time in the morning
   b. With meals
   c. As needed for tremulousness
   d. With a full glass of water

5. Arterial blood gas results for a client show pH 7.21, $Pao_2$ 98 mmHg, $Paco_2$ 32 mmHg, and $HCO_3^-$ 17 mEq/L. The nurse correctly interprets these values as indicative of which of the following acid-base imbalances?

    a. Metabolic acidosis
    b. Metabolic alkalosis
    c. Respiratory acidosis
    d. Respiratory alkalosis

See Test Yourself answers in Appendix C.

# BIBLIOGRAPHY

Ackley, B. J., & Ladwig, G. B. (2002). *Nursing diagnosis handbook: A guide to planning care* (5th ed.). St. Louis: Mosby.

Braunwald, E., Fauci, A. S., Kasper, D. L., Hauser, S. L., Longo, D. L., & Jameson, J. L. (2001). *Harrison's principles of internal medicine* (15th ed.). New York: McGraw-Hill.

Bullock, B. A., & Henze, R. L. (2000). *Focus on pathophysiology.* Philadelphia: Lippincott.

Call-Schmidt, T. (2001). Interpreting lab results: A primer. *MEDSURG Nursing, 10*(4), 179–184.

Castiglione, V. (2000). Emergency. Hyperkalemia. *American Journal of Nursing, 100*(1), 55–56.

Cook, L. (1999). The value of lab values. *American Journal of Nursing, 99*(5), 66–69, 71, 73, 75.

Danner, K. (2000). Acid/base balance: Making sense of pH. *CIN PLUS* (On-line serial), *3*(1), 3.

Deglin, J. H., & Vallerand, A. H. (2001). *Davis's drug guide for nurses* (7th ed.). Philadelphia: F. A. Davis.

Edwards, S. (2001). Regulation of water, sodium and potassium: Implications for practice. *Nursing Standard, 15*(22), 36–44.

Gallo, J. J., Busby-Whitehead, J., Rabins, P. V., Silliman, R. A., & Murphy, J. B. (Eds.). (1999). *Reichel's care of the elderly: Clinical aspects of aging* (5th ed.). Philadelphia: Lippincott Williams & Wilkins.

Heater, D. W. (1999). If ADH goes out of balance: Diabetes insipidus. *RN, 62*(7), 42–46.

_____. (1999). If ADH goes out of balance: SIADH. *RN, 62*(7), 47–49.

Horne, C., & Derrico, D. (1999). Mastering ABGs. *American Journal of Nursing, 99*(8), 26–32.

Iggulden, H. (1999). Dehydration and electrolyte balance. *Nursing Standard, 13*(19), 48–56.

Incredibly easy! Understanding imbalances caused by GI fluid loss. (1999). *Nursing, 29*(8), 72.

Johnson, M., Bulechek, G., Dochterman, J. M., Maas, M., & Moorhead, S. (2001). *Nursing diagnoses, outcomes, & interventions: NANDA, NOC, and NIC linkages.* St. Louis: Mosby.

Kuhn, M. A. (1999). *Complementary therapies for health care providers.* Philadelphia: Lippincott.

Lehne, R. A. (2001). *Pharmacology for nursing care* (4th ed.). Philadelphia: Saunders.

Malarkey, L. M., & McMorrow, M. E. (2000). *Nurse's manual of laboratory tests and diagnostic procedures* (2nd ed.). Philadelphia: Saunders.

Meeker, M. H., & Rothrock, J. C. (1999). *Alexander's care of the patient in surgery* (11th ed.). St. Louis: Mosby.

Metheny, N. M. (2000). *Fluid and electrolyte balance: Nursing considerations* (4th ed.). Philadelphia: Lippincott.

Morrison, C. (2000). Helping patients maintain a healthy fluid balance. *Nursing Times,* (NTplus), *96*(31), 3–4.

Naxarko, L. (2000). How age affects fluid intake. *Nursing Times* (NTplus), *96*(31), 11–12.

North American Nursing Diagnosis Association. (2001). *NANDA nursing diagnoses: Definitions & classification 2001–2002.* Philadelphia: NANDA.

Porth, C. M. (2002). *Pathophysiology: Concepts of altered health states* (6th ed.). Philadelphia: Lippincott.

Powers, F. (1999). The role of chloride in acid-base balance. *Journal of Intravenous Nursing, 22*(5), 286–291.

Roper, M. (1996). Assessing orthostatic vital signs. *American Journal of Nursing, 96*(8), 43–46.

Rosenberger, K. (1998). Pharmacology update. Management of electrolyte abnormalities: Hypocalcemia, hypomagnesemia, and hypokalemia. *Journal of the American Academy of Nurse Practitioners, 10*(5), 209–217.

Sheehy, C. M., Perry, P. A., & Cromwell, S. L. (1999). Dehydration: Biological considerations, age-related changes, and risk factors in older adults. *Biological Research for Nuring, 1*(1), 30–37.

Shepherd, E. (2000). Fluids: A balancing act. *Nursing Times* (NTplus), *96*(31), 1.

Sheppard, M. (2001). Assessing fluid balance. *Nursing Times* (NTplus), *97*(6), XI–XII.

Shoulders-Odom, B. (2000). Using an algorithm to interpret arterial blood gases. *Dimensions of Critical Care Nursing, 19*(1), 36–41.

Springhouse. (1999). *Nurse's handbook of alternative & complementary therapies.* Springhouse, PA: Author.

Tasota, F. J., & Wesmiller, S. W. (1998). Balancing act: Keeping blood pH in equilibrium. *Nursing, 28*(12), 34–41.

Terpstra, T. L., & Terpstra, T. L. (2000). Syndrome of inappropriate antidiuretic hormone secretion: Recognition and management. *MEDSURG Nursing, 9*(2), 61–68.

Tierney, L. M., McPhee, S. J., & Papadakis, M. A. (2001). *Current medical diagnosis & treatment* (40th ed.). New York: Lange Medical Books/McGraw-Hill.

Wallace, L. S. (2000). Using color to simplify ABG interpretation. *MEDSURG Nursing, 9*(4), 205–208.

Whitney, E. N., & Rolfes, S. R. (2002). *Understanding nutrition* (9th ed.). Belmont, CA: Wadsworth.

Wilkinson, J. M. (2000). *Nursing diagnosis handbook with NIC interventions and NOC outcomes* (7th ed.). Upper Saddle River, NJ: Prentice Hall Health.

Wise, L. C., Mersch, J., Racioppi, J., Crosier, J., & Thompson, C. (2000). Evaluating the reliability and utility of cumulative intake and output. *Journal of Nursing Care Quality, 14*(3), 37–42.

Wong, F. W. (1999). A new approach to ABG interpretation. *American Journal of Nursing, 99*(8), 34–36.

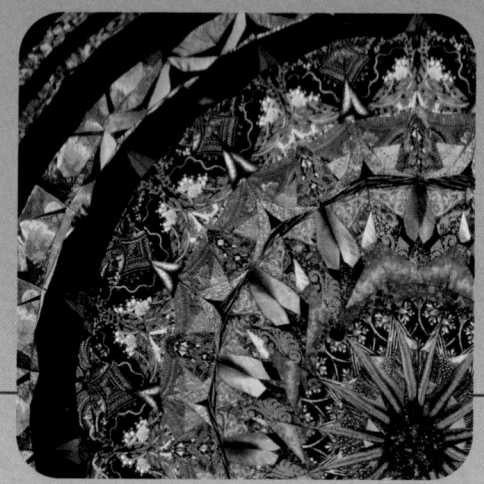

# CHAPTER 6

# Nursing Care of Clients Experiencing Trauma and Shock

## MediaLink

**www.prenhall.com/lemone**

Additional resources for this chapter can be found on the Student CD-ROM accompanying this textbook, and on the Companion Website at www.prenhall.com/lemone. Click on Chapter 6 to select the activities for this chapter.

**CD-ROM**
- Audio Glossary
- NCLEX Review

**Animation**
- Hypovolemic Shock

**Companion Website**
- More NCLEX Review
- Case Study
   A Client Experiencing Trauma
- MediaLink Applications
   Organ Donation
   Injury Prevention

## LEARNING OUTCOMES

After completing this chapter, you will be able to:

- Describe the components and types of trauma.

- Discuss causes, effects, and initial management of trauma.

- Discuss diagnostic tests used in assessing clients experiencing trauma and shock.

- Describe collaborative interventions for clients experiencing trauma and shock, including medications, blood transfusion, and intravenous fluids.

- Discuss organ donation and forensic implications of traumatic injury or death.

- Discuss cellular homeostasis and basic hemodynamics.

- Discuss the risk factors, etiologies, and pathophysiologies of hypovolemic shock, cardiogenic shock, obstructive shock, and distributive shock.

- Use the nursing process as a framework for providing individualized care to clients experiencing trauma and shock.

## THE CLIENT EXPERIENCING TRAUMA

Many different accidental or purposeful acts may cause trauma, including motor vehicle and farm machinery accidents, gunshot wounds, falls, violence toward others, or self-inflicted violence. The injuries, disabilities, and deaths resulting from these acts constitute a major health care challenge.

Trauma usually occurs suddenly, leaving the client and family with little time to prepare for its consequences. Nurses provide a vital link in both the physical and psychosocial care for the injured client and family. In caring for the client who has experienced trauma, nurses must consider not only the initial physical injury, but also its long-term consequences, including rehabilitation and the client's return to a previous way of life.

### COMPONENTS OF TRAUMA

Trauma results from an abnormal exchange of energy between a host and a mechanism in a predisposing environment. The *host* is the person or group at risk of injury. Multiple factors influence the host's potential for injury: age, sex, race, economic status, preexisting illnesses, and use of substances such as alcohol. Most trauma victims are young and unemployed, involved in substance abuse, likely to be reinjured within 5 years of their first injury, and at greater risk of dying young. Statistics show that trauma primarily afflicts males.

The *mechanism* is the source of the energy transmitted to the host. The energy exchanged can be mechanical, gravitational, thermal, electrical, physical, or chemical. Table 6–1 lists the most common mechanisms for each type of energy. Mechanical energy is the most common type of energy transferred to a host in trauma. The most common mechanical source of injury in all adult age groups is the motor vehicle.

Guns are another common mechanical source of injury. Trauma from gunshot wounds has steadily increased over the past 20 years and has become a major reason for emergency department and trauma center admissions, especially in large cities.

When describing a traumatic injury, *intention* is included as a component. Most gunshot and stab wounds are examples of intentional injuries. It is important to remember, however, that some gunshot wounds are unintentional, such as those that occur when children play with their parents' guns. Other common unintentional injuries result from motor vehicle crashes, falls, drowning, and fires.

The final component of trauma is the *environment.* For example, a road that has become slippery after a snowstorm is a physical environment that may contribute to an injury. Occupation is an important environmental factor to consider. Those in certain occupations face a high risk of trauma; examples include police officers, professional athletes, and racecar drivers. One's social environment also influences risk for injury. (See the box below for one example, domestic violence.)

| TABLE 6–1 | Common Mechanisms of Injury by Energy Source |
| --- | --- |
| **Energy Source** | **Common Mechanisms of Injury** |
| Mechanical | Motor vehicles<br>Firearms<br>Machines |
| Gravitational | Falls |
| Thermal | Heating appliances<br>Fire<br>Freezing temperatures |
| Electrical | Wires, sockets, and other electrical objects<br>Lightning |
| Physical | Fists, feet, and other body parts (as in physical assault)<br>Sharp objects, such as knives<br>Ultraviolet radiation<br>Ionizing radiation<br>Water (drowning)<br>Other submersion agents (e.g., grain)<br>Explosions |
| Chemical | Drugs<br>Poisons<br>Industrial chemicals |

### Meeting Individualized Needs

#### ASSESSING DOMESTIC VIOLENCE

Although domestic violence may involve either men or women, most victims are women. Domestic violence is the leading cause of injury to women, causing more injuries than muggings, stranger rapes, and car accidents combined. More than 4 million women are beaten by male partners every year. Health care is affected by this phenomenon, with women who were abused requiring 100,000 hospital days, 30,000 emergency room visits, and 40,000 trips to health care providers every year. These numbers mean that incorporating domestic violence awareness into nursing assessment is essential. The following guidelines (Speck & Whalley, 1996) are useful:

1. Include questions about domestic violence in a non-threatening way, such as with the question, "When you are arguing or fighting, does anyone ever get pushed or shoved?"
2. Use more specific open-ended questions once violence is disclosed, such as, "Tell me more" or "and then what happened?"
3. Evaluate the danger for the client by asking about the number and severity of past incidents, the use of alcohol and drugs, the presence of weapons in the home, and the desire of the couple to solve disputes in nonviolent ways.
4. Include in the physical assessment evidence of bruises, scars, or deformities, signs of neglect or malnutrition; presence of choke marks, wire marks, or cigarette burns.

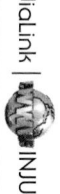

MediaLink | INJURY PREVENTION APPLICATION

## TYPES OF TRAUMA

Whether intentional or accidental, trauma causes injury to one or more parts of the body. **Minor trauma** causes injury to a single part or system of the body and is usually treated in the hospital or emergency department. A fracture of the clavicle, a small second-degree burn, and a cut requiring stitches are considered minor trauma. Major or multiple trauma involves serious single-system injury (such as the traumatic amputation of a leg) or multiple-system injuries. **Multiple trauma** (which is most often the result of a motor vehicle accident) requires immediate intervention specifically focused on ensuring survival. Clients who suffer multiple trauma receive immediate emergency care and often require long periods of intensive collaborative and nursing care.

Trauma also may be classified as either blunt or penetrating. **Blunt trauma** occurs when there is no communication from the damaged tissues to the outside environment. It is caused by a combination of forces including *deceleration* (a decrease in the speed of a moving object), *acceleration* (an increase in the speed of a moving object), *shearing* (forces occurring across a plane, with structures slipping across each other), *compression,* and *crushing.* Blunt forces often cause multiple injuries. Common blunt forces are motor vehicle accidents, falls, assaults, and sports activities. Blunt trauma often causes alterations in the anatomy and physiology of the head, spinal cord, bones, thorax, and abdomen.

**Penetrating trauma** occurs as the result of foreign objects set in motion. Penetration of tissues causes damage to body structures, most commonly the intestines, liver, spleen, and vascular system. Examples of penetrating trauma are gunshot or stab wounds and impalement.

Other types of trauma occur from inhalation, thermal changes, and blast forces. Inhalation of gases, smoke, and steam may injure the respiratory system. Thermal injuries are manifested as burns or freezing. Injuries from blasts (explosions) result from the velocity of air movement and the force of projectiles from the explosion. Blast injuries are more severe in water than in air (the blast wave travels farther and faster in water) and enclosed spaces. The trauma from blast injuries includes pulmonary edema and hemorrhage, damage to abdominal organs, burns, penetrating injuries, and ruptured tympanic membranes.

## EFFECTS OF TRAUMATIC INJURY

Death is a common result of serious traumatic injury, and may be immediate, early, or late. Immediate death happens at the scene from such injuries as a torn thoracic aorta or decapitation. Early death occurs within several hours of the injury from, for example, shock or delay in recognizing injuries. Late death generally occurs 1 or more days after the injury and results from complications or multiple organ failure.

Because of the serious consequences of trauma, it is important to rapidly identify the client's injuries and institute appropriate interventions quickly. Following are common effects of trauma and health care interventions at the scene of the accident or in the emergency department.

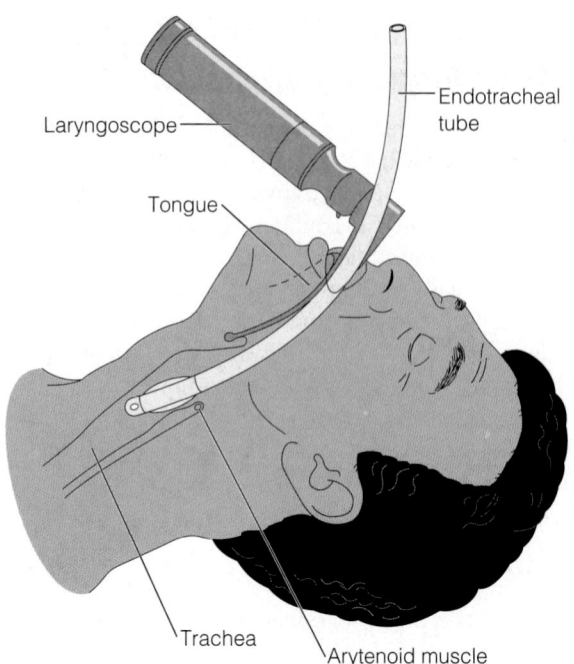

**Figure 6–1** ■ Placement of an oral endotracheal tube (ETT) for intubation. When the ETT is in place, air or oxygen can be blown into the external opening of the tube and enter the trachea.

### Airway Obstruction

The trauma client's airway may become obstructed by the presence of blood, teeth, the tongue, direct injury, or vomitus. After the client's cervical spine is immobilized (a procedure discussed later in this chapter), oxygen must be supplied. Airway interventions may include clearing the airway by suctioning, using airway adjuncts such as an oropharyngeal airway, or intubating with an oral endotracheal airway (Figure 6–1 ■). Intubation is the preferred method of airway management.

### Tension Pneumothorax

A **pneumothorax** results when air enters the pleural space due to blunt and penetrating injuries to the chest. When a one-way valve is created, most often by blunt trauma, air can enter the pleural space but not exit; thus, a **tension pneumothorax** may develop. Immediate needle thoracostomy (insertion of a large-bore needle into the appropriate thoracic space) and chest tube insertion are performed. Most often, the needle is inserted into the second intercostal space at the midclavicular line or a chest tube is placed into the fifth intercostal space at the midaxillary line (Figure 6–2 ■).

### Hemorrhage

When the client has suffered an injury that causes external hemorrhage, such as severing of an artery, the bleeding must be controlled immediately. This may be done by applying direct pressure over the wound and applying pressure over arterial pressure points (Figure 6–3 ■).

Internal hemorrhage may result from either blunt or penetrating traumatic injury. Discovering the cause and location of the injury, as well as the extent of related blood loss, are the most important concerns. Several potential spaces in the body

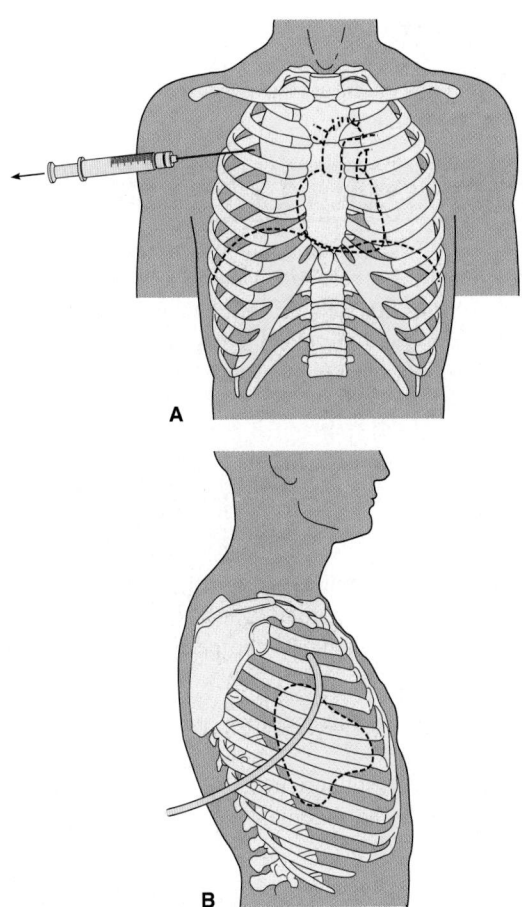

**Figure 6–2** ■ A needle thoracostomy may be used in the emergency treatment of a tension pneumothorax. *A,* A large-gauge needle is introduced, and air and fluid are aspirated. *B,* Alternatively, a chest tube may be inserted and connected to a chest drainage system.

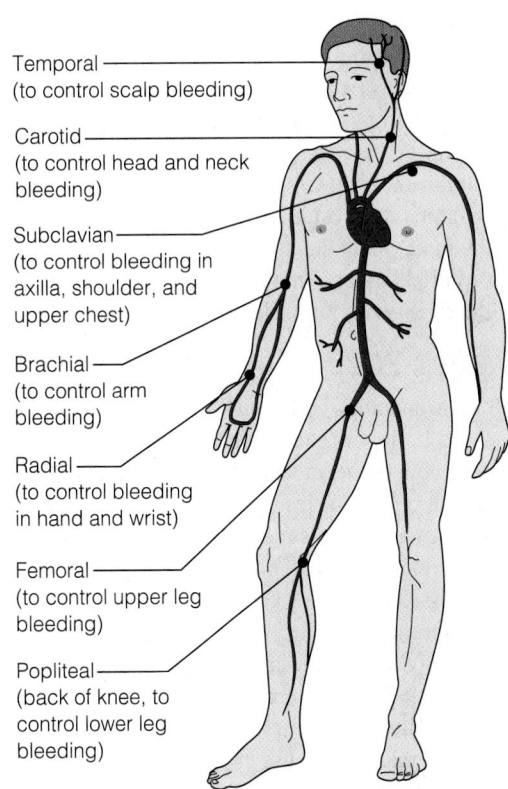

Temporal (to control scalp bleeding)

Carotid (to control head and neck bleeding)

Subclavian (to control bleeding in axilla, shoulder, and upper chest)

Brachial (to control arm bleeding)

Radial (to control bleeding in hand and wrist)

Femoral (to control upper leg bleeding)

Popliteal (back of knee, to control lower leg bleeding)

**Figure 6–3** ■ The major pressure points used for the control of bleeding.

can accommodate large amounts of blood that may accumulate (called *third spacing*) following injury. For example, bleeding into the pleural space may occur with chest trauma, and bleeding into the abdominal cavity may occur with abdominal trauma. A pelvic fracture may cause massive hemorrhage in the retroperitoneal region. Once the source of internal hemorrhage has been recognized, interventions are initiated, including operative control of bleeding and continual assessment of the client. Hemorrhage may result in hypovolemic shock (discussed later in the chapter).

## Integumentary Effects

Injuries to the integument generally are not as serious as other injuries, with the exception of burns (see Chapter 15). ⊂⊃ The primary organ involved in integumentary trauma is the skin; however, underlying structures may also be injured. Injuries may result from either blunt or penetrating sources. It is important to evaluate all injuries to the integument, because they may indicate a more serious injury such as an open fracture. Additionally, large wounds may contribute to significant blood loss.

Four specific injuries to the integument are contusions, abrasions, puncture wounds, and lacerations (Figure 6–4 ■).

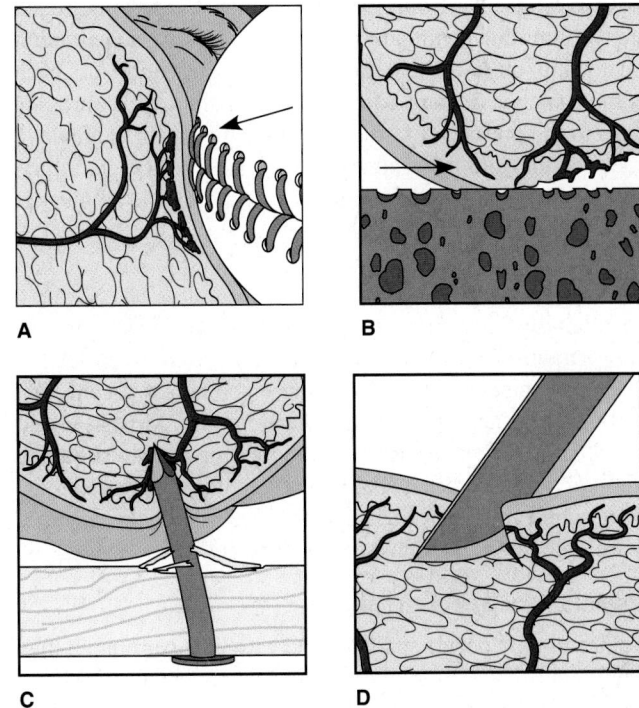

**Figure 6–4** ■ Traumatic injuries to the skin include: *A,* contusion; *B,* abrasion; *C,* puncture wound; and *D,* laceration.

**Contusions,** or superficial tissue injuries, result from blunt trauma that causes the breakage of small blood vessels and bleeding into the surrounding tissue. **Abrasions,** or partial-thickness denudations of an area of integument, generally result from falls or scrapes. **Puncture** wounds occur when a sharp or blunt object penetrates the integument. **Lacerations** are open wounds that result from sharp cutting or tearing. Injuries to the integument are at risk for contamination from dirt, debris, or foreign objects. Infection may cause further physical stress to the client with multiple injuries.

## Abdominal Effects

The abdomen contains both solid organs (liver, spleen, and pancreas) and hollow organs (stomach and intestines). Direct trauma to the abdomen can lacerate and compress the solid organs and cause burst injuries to the hollow organs. Blood vessels may be torn and organs may be displaced from their blood supply, producing life-threatening hemorrhage. Damage to the mesenteric vessels supplying the bowel can result in bowel ischemia and infarction. Injury to the stomach, pancreas, and small bowel may allow digestive enzymes to leak out into the abdominal cavity. Rupture of the large bowel results in escape of feces which causes peritonitis. Blunt or penetrating trauma to the abdomen may also cause rupture of the diaphragm with herniation of the abdominal organs into the thoracic cavity. The immediate threat following abdominal trauma is hemorrhage; the later threat is peritonitis.

## Musculoskeletal Effects

Musculoskeletal injuries may occur alone or with multiple injuries as the result of blunt or penetrating trauma. Musculoskeletal injuries usually are not considered a high priority in the care of the client with multiple injuries. Exceptions are the life- or limb-threatening musculoskeletal injury, such as a dislocated hip, pulseless extremity, or significant blood loss such as from a pelvic fracture. Musculoskeletal injuries may provide clues to the presence of other serious injuries; for example, a fractured clavicle may indicate an associated thoracic injury. Care of the client who has suffered a musculoskeletal injury is discussed in Chapter 38. ⌘

## Neurologic Effects

Head injuries are a common type of injury sustained as the result of trauma. Injuries to the spinal cord resulting in loss of neurologic function are devastating outcomes of trauma, but they are much less common than head injuries. Most head and spinal cord injuries result from blunt trauma and are sustained in motor vehicle crashes. Falls, sports injuries, and assault are other sources of neurologic injury. Care of the client with a neurologic injury is discussed in Chapters 41 and 42. ⌘

## Effects on the Family

Trauma usually occurs suddenly and with little warning. It may result in death or cause injury serious enough to alter both the client's and the family's lives. The suddenness and seriousness of the event are precipitating factors in the development of a psychologic crisis. Over the past decade, some emergency departments have instituted care plans that allow families to participate as active members of the resuscitation team. This type of care is not without controversy, but it should be considered when appropriate.

# COLLABORATIVE CARE

Collaborative care of the trauma client depends on a team approach. Providing trauma care with a team focus helps each team member know his or her role. Prompt delegation of tasks and responsibilities improves the client's chances for survival and decreases the morbidity that may result from traumatic injuries.

## Prehospital Care

The major functions of prehospital care include injury identification, critical interventions, and rapid transport.

### Injury Identification

Emergency care of the client experiencing trauma is based on rapid assessment to identify injuries and begin appropriate interventions. Injuries that indicate the need for trauma center care include:

- Penetrating injuries to the abdomen, pelvis, chest, neck, or head.
- Spinal cord injuries with deficit.
- Crushing injuries to the abdomen, chest, or head.
- Major burns.

Many methods help health care providers determine the seriousness of the client's injuries and the potential for survival. Scoring systems such as the Champion Revised Trauma Scoring System can be helpful (Table 6–2). A rapid

### TABLE 6-2 Champion Revised Trauma Scoring System

| Test | Score | Coded Value |
|---|---|---|
| Glasgow Coma Scale* | 13 to 15 | 4 |
| | 9 to 12 | 3 |
| | 6 to 8 | 2 |
| | 4 to 5 | 1 |
| | 3 | 0 |
| Systolic blood pressure | > 89 | 4 |
| | 76 to 89 | 3 |
| | 50 to 75 | 2 |
| | 1 to 49 | 1 |
| | 0 | 0 |
| Respiratory rate | 10 to 29 | 4 |
| | > 29 | 3 |
| | 6 to 9 | 2 |
| | 1 to 5 | 1 |
| | 0 | 0 |
| | Total score: | _____ |

The highest possible total score is 12. The lowest possible score is 0. The higher the total score, the greater the chance of survival.

*See Chapter 40 for instructions for using the Glasgow Coma Scale.*

Note. From "A Revision of the Trauma Score" by H. Champion et al., 1989, Journal of Trauma, 29(5): 624. Used with permission.

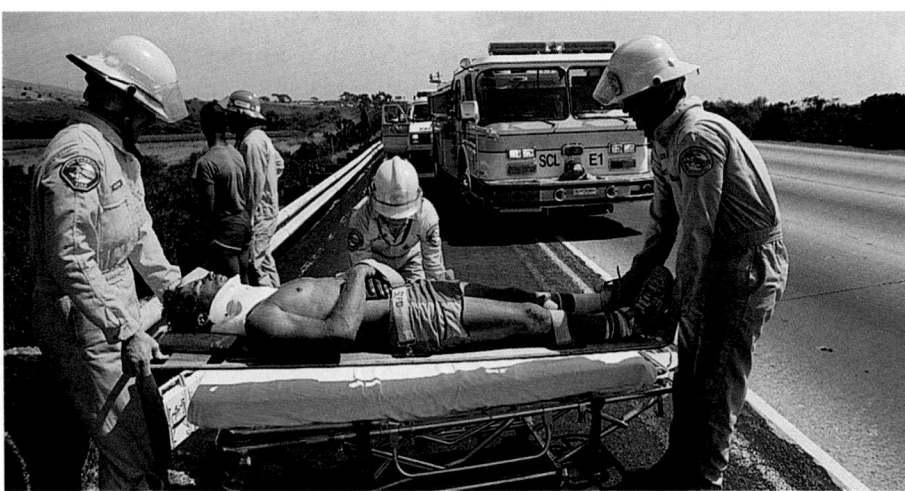

**Figure 6–5** ■ Immobilization of the cervical spine at the scene of the accident is essential to preventing further injury to the spinal cord. The combined use of a hard cervical collar, sandbags, and tape best restricts flexion, extension, rotation, and lateral bending of the neck.

*Source: Spencer Grant/Photo Researchers, Inc.*

but comprehensive trauma assessment, completed on the scene, includes:

- Airway and breathing assessments to determine if the airway is patent, maintainable, or nonmaintainable, and if ventilations are impeded, such as by rib fractures or a collapsed lung.
- Circulation assessment to palpate peripheral and central pulses; to assess capillary refill, skin color, and temperature; and to identify any external sources of bleeding.
- Level of consciousness and pupillary function.
- Any obvious injuries.

### Critical Interventions

As life-threatening problems are identified during the primary assessment, appropriate on-the-scene interventions must be performed immediately. These include providing life support, immobilizing the cervical spine, managing the airway, and treating hemorrhage and shock.

Immobilization of the client's cervical spine is a primary intervention. The client is placed on a spine board, and a cervical collar and a head immobilizer are applied (Figure 6–5 ■). The cervical spine may also be immobilized by logrolling the client onto a board, placing towel rolls or a head immobilizer along the sides of the client's head, and securing the client to the board. If the client was wearing a helmet at the time of injury, the helmet should remain on until the client arrives at the hospital, unless the client's airway is at risk. If necessary, health care personnel at the scene will remove the helmet by manipulating it over the client's nose and ears while holding the client's head and neck immobile; safe removal requires at least two people. Improper removal risks injury or additional injury to the spinal cord.

If the client's airway is patent, oxygen is administered. Ventilations may be assisted with a bag-valve-mask resuscitator until airway management is achieved. Active external bleeding is controlled by direct pressure. Measures to reverse shock (discussed later in the chapter) are initiated.

### Rapid Transport

Clients who have multiple injuries must be transported as soon as possible to a regional trauma center. The most common modes of rapid transport are ground ambulance and air ambulance, which includes helicopters specially staffed and equipped to care

for trauma victims. Figure 6–6 ■ shows a flight nurse assessing a client. Stable clients within access of a ground ambulance are best transported by ground. Unstable clients and those injured in the wilderness or other areas in which ground access is difficult may best be transported by air. When these transport systems are unavailable, the client is transported by any possible means.

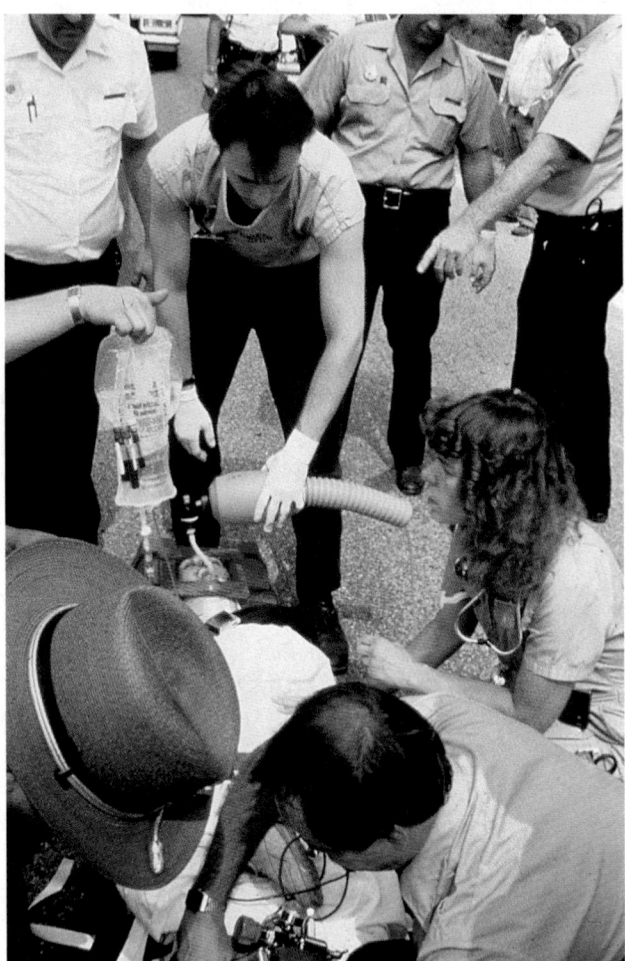

**Figure 6–6** ■ Flight nurses provide initial assessment, stabilization, and support for clients with trauma.

*Courtesy of University Air Care/University of Cincinnati Hospital.*

# Emergency Department Care

## Diagnostic Tests

The diagnostic tests ordered once the client reaches the hospital depend on the type of injury the client has sustained. Tests that may be ordered for victims of trauma include the following:

- *Blood type and crossmatch* involves typing the client's blood for ABO antigens and Rh factor, screening the blood for antibodies, and crossmatching the client's serum and donor red blood cells.
- *Blood alcohol level* measures the amount of alcohol in a client's blood. It has been found that between 20% and 50% of people who are injured may be intoxicated. Alcohol alters the client's level of consciousness and response to pain.
- *Urine drug screen* may also be ordered. Like alcohol, such drugs as cocaine alter the client's level of consciousness and overall response to the primary survey.
- *Pregnancy test* for any woman of childbearing age rules out the potential for pregnancy and fetal injury.
- *Diagnostic peritoneal lavage* determines the presence of blood in the peritoneal cavity, which may indicate abdominal injury. The test is generally done in the emergency department. A local anesthetic (such as lidocaine) is injected subcutaneously, and a small incision is made in the lower abdomen. A catheter is placed into the peritoneal cavity, and any free blood is aspirated. If 10 mL of blood is found, the client is taken to the operating room for exploratory surgery. If no free blood is aspirated, 1 L of a warm isotonic solution (Ringer's solution or normal saline) is rapidly infused into the peritoneal cavity and then allowed to drain by gravity. If the solution returns pink and is found to have a red blood cell count of 100,000 mm$^3$, a white blood cell count of > 500, or bile, food, or feces, the test is considered positive and the client is taken to the operating room for exploratory surgery.
- *Computerized tomography (CT) scans* can discover injuries to the brain, skull, spine, spinal cord, chest, and abdomen.
- *Magnetic resonance imaging (MRI) scans* can discover injuries to the brain and spinal cord.

## Medications

Medications used to treat the client who has experienced trauma depend on the type and severity of the injuries, as well as the degree of traumatic shock that is present. The following general categories of medications may be used. (Fluid administration and the drugs listed are covered later in the chapter in discussion of the collaborative care of the client in shock.)

- Blood components and crystalloids are administered intravenously in the initial treatment of traumatic shock to replace intravascular volume.
- Inotropic drugs (drugs that increase myocardial contractility) are given to increase cardiac output and improve tissue perfusion. These drugs, administered only after fluid volume restoration, include dopamine (Dopastat, Intropin), dobutamine (Dobutrex), and isoproterenol (Isuprel).
- Vasopressors may be administered in conjunction with fluid replacement to treat neurogenic, septic, or anaphylactic shock. Examples of vasopressors include dopamine, epinephrine, norepinephrine, and phenylephrine.
- Opioids, administered by bolus or continuous infusion, are used to treat pain as soon as possible. However, the effects of the pain medications may alter client responses to injury and mask potential injuries. If pain medications are administered, they must be carefully regulated, and the client must be closely monitored. If the client has penetrating and open wounds, tetanus immunization status must be determined. If the client is unable to remember when the last tetanus immunization was given or is unable to answer, tetanus prophylaxis is given.

## Blood Transfusions

Blood and blood components are initially produced in the body and then donated for use by another person through a **transfusion** (an infusion of blood or blood components). A client may be given whole blood, packed red blood cells (RBCs), platelets, plasma, albumin, clotting factors, prothrombin, or cryoprecipitate (Table 6–3). Blood and blood components increase the amount of hemoglobin available to carry oxygen to the cells, improve hemoglobin and hematocrit levels during active bleeding, increase intravascular volume, and replace deficient substances such as platelets and clotting factors.

Each person has one of four blood types: A, B, AB, or O. The blood group antigens A and B, present on RBC membranes, form the basis for the ABO blood categorization. The presence or absence of these inherited antigens determines one's blood type. People with blood type A have A antigens, those with type B have B antigens, those with type AB have both antigens, and those with neither antigen have blood type O (called a universal donor).

ABO antibodies develop in the serum of people whose RBCs lack the corresponding antigen; these antibodies are called anti-A and anti-B. The person with blood type B has A antibodies, the person with type A has B antibodies, the person with type O has both types of antibodies, and the person with blood type AB has no antibodies (called a universal recipient).

A third antigen on the RBC membrane is D. People who are Rh positive have the D antigen, whereas people who are Rh negative do not. These antigens and antibodies may cause ABO and Rh incompatibilities.

A transfusion of incompatible blood causes hemolysis (breakdown) of the RBCs and agglutination of erythrocytes. (Agglutination is the clumping of cells that results from their interaction with specific antibodies.) The ABO blood group names and compatibilities are listed in Table 6–4.

Before RBCs or whole blood can be administered, a series of procedures determine donor and recipient ABO types and Rh groups. These procedures, called a type and crossmatch, are performed by mixing the donor cells with the recipient's serum and watching for agglutination. If none occurs, the blood is considered compatible.

Despite meticulous procedures for matching blood types and antigens, blood transfusion reactions may still occur. The most common is a *febrile reaction*. Antibodies within the client

**TABLE 6-3    Types of Blood Components Used in Transfusion Therapy**

| Type | Use | Limitations |
|---|---|---|
| Whole blood | Replaces blood volume and oxygen-carrying capacity in hemorrhage and shock. Contains RBCs, plasma proteins, clotting factors, and plasma. | Contains few platelets or granulocytes; deficient in clotting factors V and VII. Greatest risks are for incompatibility or circulatory overload. |
| Red cells | Increase oxygen-carrying capacity in slow bleeding or in clients with anemia, with leukemia, or having surgery. | Has no viable platelets or granulocytes. Incompatibility may cause hemolytic reactions. |
| Platelets | Used to control or prevent bleeding in clients with platelet deficiencies. | If given for an extended period of time, antibodies may develop. Hypersensitivity reactions may occur. |
| Plasma | Expands blood volume; can be administered to any blood group or type. Contains all clotting factors and is used to restore those deficient in bleeding disorders. | May cause vascular overload, hypersensitivity reactions, or hemolytic reactions. |
| Albumin | Expands blood volume in shock and trauma. Used to treat clients in shock from trauma or infection and in surgery to replace blood volume and proteins. | Is not a substitute for whole blood. May cause hypersensitivity reactions. |
| Clotting factors | Factor VIII concentrate is used to treat clients with hemophilia A and von Willebrand's disease. Factor IX concentrate is used to treat clients with hemophilia B and other clotting factor deficiencies. | |
| Prothrombin complex | Contains prothrombin, clotting factors VII, IX, X, and part of XI. Used to treat clients with deficiencies of these factors. | |
| Cryoprecipitate | Contains factor VIII, factor XIII, von Willebrand's factor, and fibrinogen. Used to treat clients with clotting factor deficiencies. | May cause ABO incompatibilities. |

receiving the blood are directed against the donor's white blood cells, causing fever and chills. Febrile reactions typically begin during the first 15 minutes of the transfusion. Using leukocyte-poor blood avoids future febrile reactions.

*Hypersensitivity reactions* result when antibodies in the client's blood react against proteins, such as immunoglobulin A, in the donor blood. Hypersensitivity reactions may appear during or after the transfusion. The manifestations of hypersensitivity reaction include *urticaria* (the appearance of reddened wheals of various sizes on the skin) and itching.

*Hemolytic reactions,* the most dangerous transfusion reactions, usually result from an ABO incompatibility. Clumping RBCs block capillaries, decreasing blood flow to vital organs. In addition, macrophages engulf the clumped RBCs, releasing free hemoglobin into the circulating blood; the hemoglobin is then filtered by the kidneys and may block the renal tubules, causing renal failure. Hemolytic reactions usually begin after infusion of 100 to 200 mL of the incompatible blood. Manifestations of a hemolytic reaction include flushing of the face, a burning sensation along the vein, headache, urticaria, chills, fever, lumbar pain, abdominal pain, chest pain, nausea and vomiting, tachycardia, hypotension, and dyspnea. If any of these manifestations appear, the blood transfusion must be immediately discontinued.

Other risks to clients receiving blood include circulatory overload, electrolyte imbalances, and infectious diseases such as hepatitis or cytomegalovirus.

Clients who have experienced trauma of any severity have had substantial blood loss and are usually in hypovolemic shock. Blood replacement is the treatment of choice to restore

**TABLE 6-4    Blood Group Types and Compatibilities**

| Blood Group | RBC Agglutinogens | Serum Agglutinogens | Compatible Donor Blood Groups | Incompatible Donor Blood Groups |
|---|---|---|---|---|
| A | A | Anti-B | A, O | B, AB |
| B | B | Anti-A | B, O | A, AB |
| AB | A, B | None | A, B, AB, O | None |
| O | None | Anti-A, Anti-B | O | A, B, AB |

*Note: Group O is often called the universal donor, and group AB is called the universal recipient.*

# Medication Administration

## Blood Transfusion

The risk for and seriousness of blood transfusion reactions require that extreme caution be taken when blood is administered. Most fatal transfusion reactions are the result of human error. Although general guidelines are provided here, each institution has specific policies and procedures that must be followed. Prior to beginning the transfusion, the nurse must determine that typed and cross-matched blood is available and collect the needed equipment a Y-tubing blood administration set with a filter, a large-bore intravenous catheter, Usually 18 or 19 gauge, and normal saline solution. Only normal saline is used with a blood transfusion. Dextrose causes clumping of RBCs, and distilled water causes hemolysis.

### Nursing Responsibilities

- Assess for any previous reactions to blood.
- Explain the procedure to the client, and answer any questions.
- Prepare the intravenous equipment. Shut off one side of the Y tubing, and attach the other side to the saline solution. Flush the tubing and filter with the saline.
- If venous access is not already in place, insert the intravenous needle (following body substance precautions), and begin administering the saline.
- Using institutional procedure, obtain the blood from the blood bank or laboratory. Administer the blood immediately; if this is not possible, return it to the blood bank or laboratory.
- Check and document that the donor and recipient blood have been tested and are compatible. This usually involves two nurses, each verifying that:
  a. An order for blood has been written.
  b. Type and crossmatch have been done.
  c. The name of the client and the name on the blood bag are identical.

  d. The number assigned to the unit of blood is identical to the one on the requisition for the blood.
  e. Blood type and Rh factor are compatible.
  f. The blood has not exceeded its expiration date.
  g. The unit of blood is intact and has no bubbles or discoloration.
- Identify the client by reading the arm band and asking the client to tell you his or her name. Check the arm band against the unit of blood.
- Gently invert the blood bag several times to mix the plasma and RBCs.
- Take and record vital signs as a baseline.
- Attach the open side of the Y tubing to the blood unit, and begin the transfusion at a slow rate of about 2 mL per minute. (Some trauma clients may have blood infused at a rapid rate. If blood is infused rapidly, it may need to be warmed prior to administration to prevent hypothermia.) Stay with the client for at least the first 15 minutes of the transfusion, monitoring for manifestations of a reaction and taking the client's vital signs.
- Continue to monitor the client during the transfusion, assessing for manifestations of hypersensitivity or hemolytic reactions and taking and recording vital signs as directed by institutional policy.
- After the first 15 minutes, the rate of infusion is increased. If there is no danger of fluid volume overload, most clients can tolerate an infusion of a unit of blood (ranging from 250 to 500 mL, depending on the blood component administered) in 2 hours. The unit of blood should be administered in 3 to 4 hours; after this time, it has warmed and begins to deteriorate.

---

oxygen-carrying capacity. Clients in severe shock with active bleeding are given universal, type O red blood cells immediately. Clients with less severe injuries or bleeding may be stabilized with other types of fluids until type-specific or cross-matched blood is available.

Some emergency departments and trauma centers use auto-transfusion to provide blood for transfusions for the client with multiple injuries and/or severe shock. Autotransfusion is a method of blood administration in which special equipment collects and returns the client's own blood. The chest cavity is the typical source of blood to be autotransfused.

Nursing considerations for blood transfusion therapy are described in the Medication Administration box above.

## Emergency Surgery

Immediate surgical intervention is indicated when the client remains in shock despite resuscitation and there is no obvious external sign of blood loss. Abdominal and chest X-ray studies and a diagnostic peritoneal lavage or CT scan may be performed to help identify the potential source of the blood loss. It is important that the emergency or trauma nurse speak with the family as soon as possible and keep pthem informed about what is happening to their family member. Unfortunately, the need for

emergency surgery may not allow time for family members or significant others to see their loved one before transfer to the operating room.

## Organ Donation

The **Uniform Anatomical Gift Act** (1968, 1987) requires that people be informed about their options for organ donation. Under this act, consent for organ donation may be given not only by the donor but also by a spouse, adult children, parents, adult siblings, guardian, or any adult authorized to do so. The act also encourages people to carry donor cards.

The increased success of organ transplant has made it a more common and valuable method of prolonging and improving life; however, many people are still waiting for organs, and many people who may be suitable organ donors die each year from trauma. Organs and tissues that may be transplanted include bones, eyes, liver, lungs, skin, muscles and tendons, pancreas, kidneys, heart, and heart valves.

The organ donation process begins with identification of the potential organ donor. Most people are potential organ donors. Exceptions include those who:

- Currently abuse intravenous drugs.
- Have preexisting untreated infections, such as septicemia.

# Medication Administration

## Blood Transfusion (continued)

- Take the following actions if manifestations of a reaction occur:
  a. Stop the infusion of blood immediately, and notify the physician. Continue to infuse the saline.
  b. Take vital signs and assess manifestations.
  c. Compare the blood slip with the unit of blood to ensure that an identification error was not made.
  d. Save the blood bag and any remaining blood for return to the laboratory for further tests to determine the cause of the reaction.
  e. Follow institutional policy for collecting urine and venous blood samples.
  f. Continue to monitor the client and provide prescribed interventions to treat hypersensitivity or hemolytic manifestations.
- Do not add medications to blood infusions or tubing.
- When the blood is totally infused, use the saline to flush the tubing to ensure complete administration of the blood.
- Return the empty blood bag to the blood bank or laboratory.

### Client and Family Teaching

- The possible risks of blood transfusions include infectious diseases and acquired immune deficiency syndrome (AIDS). However, because of careful handling and storage of blood, bacterial contamination is rare. Although hepatitis may be transmitted by contaminated blood, new tests for hepatitis antibodies in the donor blood are reducing this risk. Many people are afraid of contracting AIDS from blood; however, donor screening and HIV-antibody testing of donor blood has virtually eliminated the transmission of HIV by blood transfusion.
- During the transfusion, immediately report any warm feelings, chills, itching, feelings of weakness or fainting, or difficulty breathing.
- Report any signs of a delayed transfusion reaction: chills, fever, cough, difficulty breathing, hives, itching, or changes in circulation. Report difficulty with breathing, and seek medical care immediately.

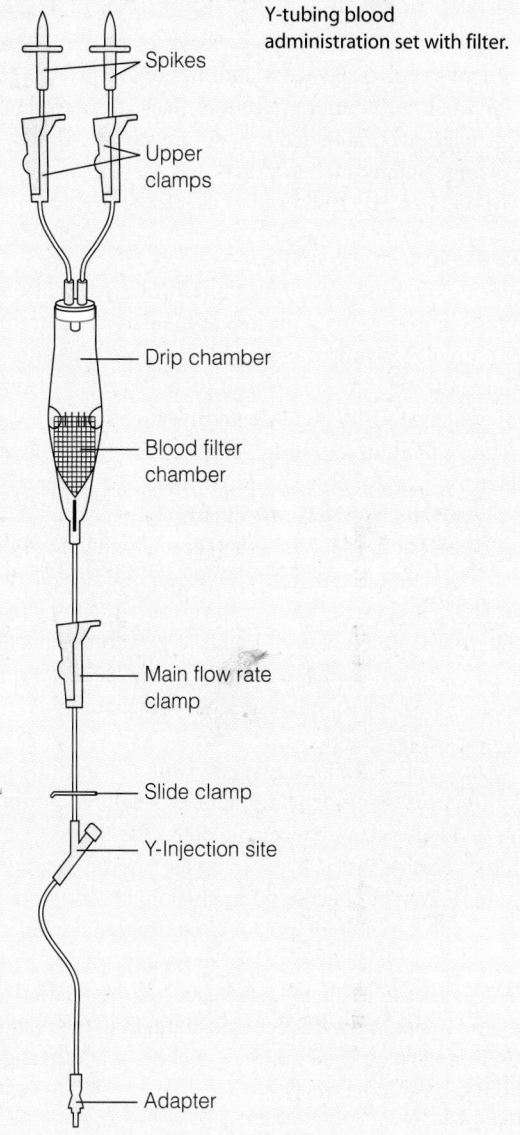

Y-tubing blood administration set with filter.

Spikes

Upper clamps

Drip chamber

Blood filter chamber

Main flow rate clamp

Slide clamp

Y-Injection site

Adapter

- Are HIV positive.
- Have any malignancy other than a primary brain tumor.
- Have active tuberculosis.

The family needs to be made aware of the client's prognosis and presented with the option of donating the client's organs. Both the family's and the client's feelings about organ donation must be explored. Even if the client carries an organ donation card, many institutions will not remove any organs without a signature from a family member or other authorized person. The nurse must always respect the family's concerns and feelings in this process. Some members of certain cultural groups may have religious constraints or issues of mistrust that may interfere with the donation process.

Before any organs can be removed, the client must be declared brain dead. Box 6–1 lists **brain death criteria.** Once

---

### BOX 6–1   ■ Brain Death Criteria

#### CLINICAL SIGNS

- Irreversible condition
- Apnea with a $PaCO_2$ greater than 60 mmHg
- No response to deep stimuli
- No spontaneous movement (some spinal cord reflexes may be present)
- No gag or corneal reflex
- No oculocephalic or oculovestibular reflex
- Absence of toxic or metabolic disorders

#### CONFIRMATORY TESTS

- Cerebral blood flow study
- Electroencephalogram

brain death has been confirmed, the family must also understand the diagnosis and be allowed time to accept the client's death.

When caring for an adult client who is brain dead and an organ donor, the nurse carries out the following:

- Maintain systolic blood pressure of 90 mmHg to keep the client's organs perfused until removal.
- Maintain urine output at more than 30 mL per hour. This is usually accomplished by administering fluids and/or inotropic agents such as dopamine.
- Maintain oxygen saturation at 90% or greater.

### Forensic Considerations

Injuries often happen under circumstances that require legal investigation. Many injuries, particularly penetrating trauma, may involve criminal activity. Therefore, the nurse must recognize the need to identify, store, and properly transfer potential evidence for medical-legal investigations.

Each item of clothing removed from the client must be placed in a breathable container, such as a paper bag, and documented appropriately. Bullets or knives should be labeled, with their source specified, and given to the proper authorities.

The client's hands may yield important evidence, such as powder burns on the skin or tissue or hair samples beneath the fingernails. In the case of death, it is recommended that paper bags be placed over the client's hands if the presence of evidence is suspected; otherwise, the evidence should be collected by nail clippings.

Look for entrance and exit wounds and document these findings with pictures, diagrams, or written descriptions. Once the evidence has been collected, identified, and properly stored, ensure that it is given to the appropriate authorities. A chain of custody needs to be maintained throughout the entire process. All evidence must be identified and labeled, and documentation procedures must chronicle where and in whose possession the evidence has been. For the chain of custody to remain intact, the evidence must remain in the continuous possession of identified people and be marked and sealed in tamper-proof containers.

## NURSING CARE

Nursing care of the client who has been injured begins with a primary assessment and the initiation of collaborative interventions for any life-threatening injuries. Nursing care is directed toward the client's specific responses to trauma.

### Health Promotion

Prevention efforts can reduce the incidence and severity of trauma. Areas of health promotion and trauma prevention interventions for individuals and communities include the following (Bucher & Melander, 1999):

- Motor vehicle safety: seatbelts, airbags, helmets, driving under the influence of alcohol or drugs, reckless driving, visual or cognitive deficits in the older adult
- Home safety: snow and ice removal, electrical wiring, falls, burns, drowning

- Farm safety: operating heavy equipment
- Work safety: operating work equipment, wearing safety equipment
- Relationships: domestic violence, child abuse, elder abuse, or neglect
- Communities: gun control, gangs, condition of streets, neighborhood safety

(In providing information about trauma prevention to members of the community, the nurse serves as a health care educator, political activist, and safety advocate.)

### Assessment

Assessment of the client experiencing trauma was discussed with collaborative care.

### Nursing Diagnoses and Interventions

The trauma client has many complex and interrelated actual or potential alterations in health. The nursing care in this section focuses on client and family problems with respirations, infection, immobility, and spirituality. Nursing interventions for decreased cardiac output and altered perfusion are discussed in the section of the chapter on nursing care of the client in shock.

#### Ineffective Airway Clearance

The client with multiple injuries is at great risk for developing airway obstruction and apnea. Facial injuries, loose teeth, blood, and vomitus increase the risk for aspiration and obstruction. Neurologic injuries and cerebral edema alter the client's respiratory drive and ability to keep the airway clear.

- Assess if airway is patent, maintainable, or nonmaintainable. Assess for manifestations of airway obstruction: stridor, tachypnea, bradypnea, cough, cyanosis, dyspnea, decreased or absent breath sounds, changes in oxygen levels, and changes in level of consciousness. *Assessing the airway and initiating interventions are the first steps in managing the client with multiple injuries.*
- Monitor oxygen saturation by applying a pulse oximeter. Adjust oxygen flow to maintain oxygen saturation from 94% to 100%. *Changes in oxygen saturation as measured by the pulse oximeter indicate the effectiveness of the client's airway.*
- Monitor level of consciousness. *An early sign of an ineffective airway is change in the client's behavior. If the client becomes restless, anxious, combative, or unresponsive, the effectiveness of the airway needs to be immediately evaluated and appropriate interventions initiated.*

#### Risk for Infection

Traumatic injuries are considered dirty wounds. Projectiles enter the body through dirty surfaces and clothing, carrying dirt and debris into the wound. Open fractures provide a portal for the entry of bacteria and dirt. Even with surgical intervention, the wounds often remain contaminated.

- Use careful handwashing practices. *Handwashing remains the single most important factor in preventing the spread of infection.*
- Use strict standard precautions and aseptic technique when caring for wounds. *Standard precautions are essential to protect the client and the nurse from infection.* In addition:

- Monitor wounds for odor, redness, heat, swelling, and copious or purulent drainage.
- Monitor hidden wounds, such as those under casts, by asking the client whether the pain has increased and observing for increased drainage and heat over the area of the wound.
- Ensure that cross-contamination between wounds does not occur. Collect drainage in ostomy bags if it is copious. *The skin is the first line of defense against infection. Wounds provide a portal of entry for organisms. Risk factors for wound infection include contamination, inadequate wound care, and the condition of the wound at the time of closure. Aseptic techniques used in applying and changing dressings reduce the entry of organisms.*
- Take and record vital signs, including temperature, every 2 to 4 hours. *Vital signs, particularly an elevated body temperature, indicate the presence of an infection.*
- Provide adequate fluids and nutrition. *Adequate fluids, calories, and protein are essential to wound healing.*
- Assess for manifestations of gas gangrene: fever, pain, and swelling in traumatized tissues; drainage with a foul odor. *Gas gangrene is usually caused by the organism* Clostridium perfringens. *This bacterium is found in the soil and can be introduced into the body during a traumatic injury. The organism grows in the tissues, causing necrosis; hydrogen and carbon dioxide are released, with resultant swelling of tissues. If the infection continues, tissues are progressively destroyed, and sepsis and death may result.*
- Assess status of tetanus immunization and administer tetanus toxoid or human toxin-antitoxin (TAT) as prescribed. *Tetanus is caused by an exotoxin produced by* Clostridium tetani, *usually introduced through an open wound. The organism is commonly found in the soil.*
- Use strict aseptic technique when inserting catheters, suctioning, administering parenteral medications, or performing any other invasive procedure. *Using aseptic technique during invasive procedures reduces the risk of entry of organisms.*

## Impaired Physical Mobility

The client with trauma injuries is often unable to change positions independently and is at risk for complications of the integumentary, cardiovascular, gastrointestinal, respiratory, musculoskeletal, and renal systems. Clients at greatest risk are those who have had multiple injuries, spinal cord injuries, peripheral nerve injuries, and traumatic amputations. Collaborate with the physical therapist and occupational therapist (if available) to determine the most effective types and schedule of exercises and assistive devices.

- If active bleeding or edema is not present, provide active or passive exercises to affected and unaffected extremities at least once every 8 hours. *Exercise improves muscle tone, maintains joint mobility, improves circulation, and prevents contractures.*
- Help the client turn, cough, and deep breathe and use the incentive spirometer at least every 2 hours. *Changing positions, coughing, deep breathing and incentive spirometry reduce the risk of integumentary and respiratory complications.*

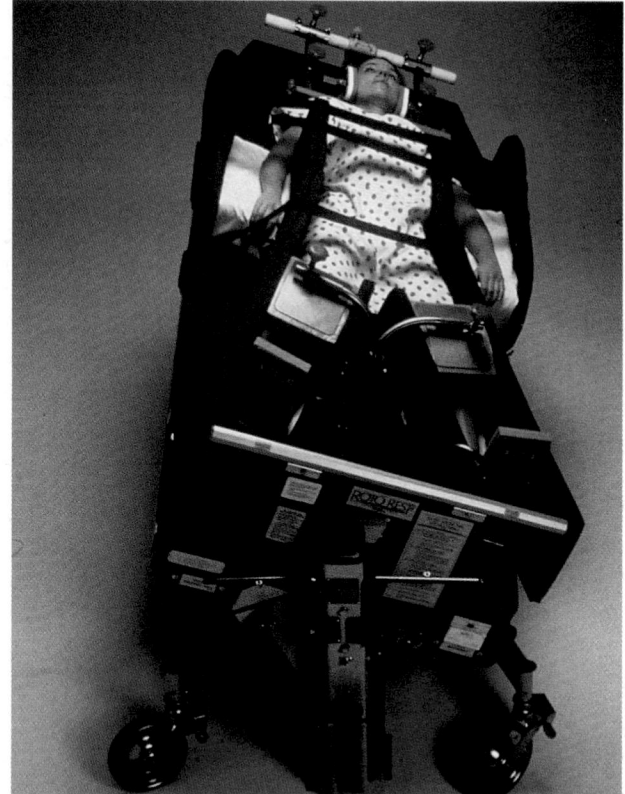

**Figure  6–7 ■** A kinetic continuous rotation bed provides a means of turning the client with multiple injuries to decrease the hazards of immobility.

*Courtesy of Kinetic Concepts, Inc.*

- If the client is unable to be moved and positioned, consider a specialty bed, such as the kinetic continuous rotation bed (Figure 6–7 ■). *The kinetic continuous rotation bed allows continuous turning of the client; the motion decreases pulmonary complications, venous stasis, postural hypotension, urinary stasis, muscle wasting, and bone demineralization.*
- Monitor the lower extremities each day for manifestations of deep vein thrombosis: heat, swelling, and pain. Measure and record the circumference of the thigh and calf each day. If antiemboli stockings are used, remove them for 1 hour during each shift and assess the skin. *Venous stasis results when surrounding muscles are unable to contract and help move the blood through the veins. Thrombus (clot) formation in deep veins is a major risk for pulmonary embolism.*

## Spiritual Distress

Trauma generally strikes without warning and carries potentially devastating consequences, including severe alterations in the lives of the victim and family, and death. The traumatic death of a loved one may be the most difficult event a family may ever experience. The decision to cease life support systems or to donate organs challenges the family's belief systems and psychologic stability. Nursing care of the family (or client) experiencing spiritual distress includes the following:

- Give the family information about the option to donate the client's organs. *The decision to donate organs needs to be*

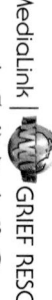

*based on information about the client's condition, prognosis, and criteria by which brain death is determined. It is important to convey to family members that organ donation is only an option and that they should not feel they are obligated to consent or are doing something wrong if they do not consent.*

- Encourage the family to ask questions and express their feelings about the traumatic event and/or organ donation. *Allowing families to express their feelings may help prevent long-term consequences such as guilt.*
- Refer the family for follow-up care. Long-term follow-up is important for the family facing the sudden death of a loved one. *Grieving is not an overnight process, and providing the family with resources that may be used in the future may help prevent future crises and dysfunction.* (For more information, see Chapter 11.) 🔗

### Risk for Posttrauma Syndrome

Posttrauma syndrome is an intense, sustained emotional response to a disastrous event. It is characterized by emotions that range from anger to fear and by flashbacks or psychic numbing. In the initial stage, the client may be calm or may express feelings of anger, disbelief, terror, and shock. In the long-term phase, which begins anywhere from a few days to several months after the event, the client often experiences flashbacks and nightmares of the traumatic event. The client may call on ineffective coping mechanisms, such as alcohol or drugs, and withdraw from relationships.

- Assess emotional responses while providing physical care. Observe for crying, sleep problems, suspiciousness, and fear during the initial phase of treatment. If the client is unconscious, encourage family members and friends to express their feelings. *These assessments provide valuable information about the client's ability to cope with the trauma.*

- Be available if the client wishes to talk about the trauma, and encourage expression of feelings. *The client may initially deny negative feelings; this denial is a coping mechanism in the initial phase of recovery.*
- Teach relaxation techniques, such as deep breathing, progressive muscle relaxation, or imagery (see Chapter 4). 🔗 *These techniques are often useful in coping when thoughts of the trauma recur.*
- Refer the client and family members for counseling, psychotherapy, or support groups as appropriate. *Continued therapy may be necessary in assisting the client and family to resolve the acute and long-term effects of trauma.*

## Using NANDA, NIC, and NOC

Chart 6–1 shows links between NANDA nursing diagnoses, NIC, and NOC when caring for the patient with multiple injuries.

## Home Care

Address the following topics to prepare the client and family for home care.

- The type of home environment to which the client will be returning, including any changes that will be required to let the client function in that environment
- Medications, dressings, wound care, equipment, and supplies
- Special diet, if needed
- Rehabilitation plan and its effect on the client's family
- Follow-up appointments with the physician or at the trauma clinic
- Emotional changes that the client may undergo as a result of the trauma
- Helpful resources:
  - Home health care
  - Community support groups
  - National Institute of Neurological Disorders and Stroke

---

**CHART 6–1  NANDA, NIC, AND NOC LINKAGES**

### The Client Experiencing Trauma

| NURSING DIAGNOSES | NURSING INTERVENTIONS | NURSING OUTCOMES |
|---|---|---|
| • Risk for Falls<br>• Risk for Injury | • Fall Prevention<br>• Surveillance: Safety | • Safety Behavior: Fall Prevention<br>• Safety Behavior: Personal<br>• Risk Control |
| • Posttrauma Syndrome | • Counseling | • Coping<br>• Grief Resolution |
| • Risk for Trauma | • Environmental Management: Safety<br>• Vehicle Safety Promotion | • Safety Status: Physical Injury |
| • Impaired Tissue Integrity | • Bleeding Reduction<br>• Blood Products Administration<br>• Fluid Management<br>• Hemorrhage Control<br>• Infection Protection | • Tissue Integrity: Skin and Mucous Membranes<br>• Wound Healing<br>• Fluid Balance<br>• Circulation Status<br>• Infection Control |

*Note. Data from Nursing Outcomes Classification (NOC) by M. Johnson & M. Maas (Eds.), 1997, St. Louis: Mosby; Nursing Diagnoses: Definitions & Classification 2001–2002 by North American Nursing Diagnosis Association, 2001, Philadelphia: NANDA; Nursing Interventions Classification (NIC) by J.C. McCloskey & G. M. Bulechek (Eds.), 2000, St. Louis: Mosby. Reprinted by permission.*

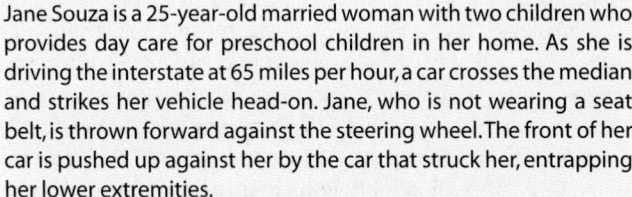

## Nursing Care Plan
## A Client with Multiple Injuries

Jane Souza is a 25-year-old married woman with two children who provides day care for preschool children in her home. As she is driving the interstate at 65 miles per hour, a car crosses the median and strikes her vehicle head-on. Jane, who is not wearing a seat belt, is thrown forward against the steering wheel. The front of her car is pushed up against her by the car that struck her, entrapping her lower extremities.

After extensive efforts to extricate her from the car, Jane is transported to the local trauma center. She is still conscious, is receiving high-flow oxygen by mask, and has one intravenous line in place. Her vital signs are a palpable systolic blood pressure of 80, a pulse rate of 120, and a respiratory rate of 36. On arrival, she states that she is having difficulty breathing.

### ASSESSMENT
- Airway: Maintainable with high-flow oxygen in place.
- Breathing: Respiratory rate of 36, multiple bruising and abrasions on right side of her chest, decreased breath sounds on the right side.
- Circulation: No palpable radial pulses; palpable brachial pulses. Monitor shows sinus tachycardia. No active external bleeding noted. Skin color pale, cool to the touch, and diaphoretic.
- Neurologic: Moved her fingers when asked; complains of difficulty breathing; denies that she is hurt. Pupils 4 mm, equal, and react to light. Has a broken right arm and an open fracture of the left ankle; because of these injuries, extremity movement is limited.

Because of Jane's respiratory distress, she is intubated and ventilated with 100% oxygen. Another intravenous line is inserted and O-negative blood administered.

### DIAGNOSES
- *Ineffective breathing pattern* related to multiple bruises and abrasions on the right side of the chest, and respiratory difficulty
- *Deficient fluid volume* related to acute internal blood loss (presumed because no active bleeding can be found)

- *Risk for injury* related to trauma resuscitation

### EXPECTED OUTCOMES
- Maintain adequate oxygenation.
- Maintain adequate circulating blood volume.

### PLANNING AND IMPLEMENTATION
- Monitor airway and assist in any needed airway management.
- Explain all procedures.
- Monitor the effects of fluid and blood administration, including any changes in blood pressure and pulse.
- Prepare for transfer to the operating room for emergency surgery.
- Keep family informed about her condition.

### EVALUATION
Jane is transferred to the operating room, where it is determined that she has a ruptured spleen and a serious pelvic fracture. Jane's treatment continues in the operating room.

### Critical Thinking in the Nursing Process
1. Is the nursing diagnosis deficient fluid volume appropriate for Jane Souza? Why or why not?
2. The assessment of a client who has experienced trauma is, in order: A = airway, B = breathing, and C = circulation. What is the rationale for this sequence?
3. Following surgery, Jane is moved to the surgical intensive care unit. She is very anxious and restless. What assessments would you make to identify the cause of her restlessness?
4. Infection is a common complication for the trauma client. Describe five risks for infection that are present from the time of injury to the time of hospital discharge.

See Evaluating Your Response in Appendix C.

## THE CLIENT EXPERIENCING SHOCK

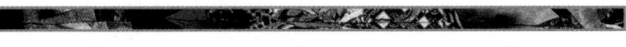

**Shock** is a clinical syndrome characterized by a systemic imbalance between oxygen supply and demand. This imbalance results in a state of inadequate blood flow to body organs and tissues, causing life-threatening cellular dysfunction.

### OVERVIEW OF CELLULAR HOMEOSTASIS AND HEMODYNAMICS

To maintain cellular metabolism, cells of all body organs and tissues require a regular and consistent supply of oxygen and the removal of metabolic wastes. This homeostatic regulation is maintained primarily by the cardiovascular system and depends on four physiologic components.

1. A cardiac output sufficient to meet bodily requirements

2. An uncompromised vascular system, in which the vessels have a diameter sufficient to allow unimpeded blood flow and have good tone (the ability to constrict or dilate to maintain normal pressure)
3. A volume of blood sufficient to fill the circulatory system, and a blood pressure adequate to maintain blood flow
4. Tissues that are able to extract and use the oxygen delivered through the capillaries

In a healthy person, these components function as a system to maintain tissue perfusion. During shock, however, one or more of these components are disrupted. An understanding of basic hemodynamics is necessary to understand the pathophysiology of shock.

- **Stroke volume (SV)** is the amount of blood pumped into the aorta with each contraction of the left ventricle.
- **Cardiac output (CO)** is the amount of blood pumped per minute into the aorta by the left ventricle. CO is determined

by multiplying the stroke volume (SV) by the heart rate (HR): CO = SV × HR.

- **Mean arterial pressure (MAP)** is the product of cardiac output and systemic vascular resistance (SVR): MAP = CO × SVR. When CO, SVR, or total blood volume rises, MAP and tissue perfusion increase. Conversely, when CO, SVR, or total blood volume falls, MAP and tissue perfusion decrease.
- The sympathetic nervous system maintains the smooth muscle surrounding the arteries and arterioles in a state of partial contraction called sympathetic tone. Increased sympathetic stimulation increases vasoconstriction and SVR; decreased sympathetic stimulation allows vasodilatation, which decreases SVR.

## PATHOPHYSIOLOGY

When one or more cardiovascular components do not function properly, the body's hemodynamic properties are altered. Consequently, tissue perfusion may be inadequate to sustain normal cellular metabolism. The result is the clinical syndrome known as shock. The manifestations of shock result from the body's attempts to maintain vital organs (heart and brain) and to preserve life following a drop in cellular perfusion. However, if the injury or condition triggering shock is severe enough or of long enough duration, then cellular hypoxia and cellular death occur.

Shock is triggered by a sustained drop in mean arterial pressure. This drop can occur after a decrease in cardiac output, a decrease in the circulating blood volume, or an increase in the size of the vascular bed due to peripheral vasodilatation. If intervention is timely and effective, the physiologic events that characterize shock may be stopped; if not, shock may lead to death.

### Stage I: Early, Reversible, and Compensatory Shock

The initial stage of shock begins when baroreceptors in the aortic arch and the carotid sinus detect a sustained drop in MAP of less than 10 mmHg from normal levels. The circulating blood volume may decrease (usually to less then 500 mL), but not enough to cause serious effects.

The body reacts to the decrease in arterial pressure as it would to any physical stressor. The cerebral integration center initiates the body's response systems, causing the sympathetic nervous system to increase the heart rate and the force of cardiac contraction, thus increasing cardiac output. Sympathetic stimulation also causes peripheral vasoconstriction, resulting in increased systemic vascular resistance and a rise in arterial pressure. The net result is that the perfusion of cells, tissues, and organs is maintained.

Symptoms are almost imperceptible during the early stage of shock. The pulse rate may be slightly elevated. If the injury is minor or of short duration, arterial pressure is usually maintained, and no further symptoms occur.

Compensatory shock begins after the MAP falls 10 to 15 mmHg below normal levels. The circulating blood volume is reduced by 25% to 35% (1000 mL or more), but compensatory mechanisms are able to maintain blood pressure and tissue perfusion to vital organs, thereby preventing cell damage.

- Stimulation of the sympathetic nervous system results in the release of epinephrine from the adrenal medulla and the release of norepinephrine from the adrenal medulla and the sympathetic fibers. Both hormones rapidly stimulate the alpha- and beta-adrenergic fibers. Stimulated alpha-adrenergic fibers cause vasoconstriction in the blood vessels supplying the skin and most of the abdominal viscera. Perfusion of these areas decreases. Stimulated beta-adrenergic fibers cause vasodilatation in vessels supplying the heart and skeletal muscles (beta one response), and increase the heart rate and force of cardiac contraction (beta two response). Further, blood vessels in the respiratory system dilate, and the respiratory rate increases (beta two response). Thus, stimulation of the sympathetic nervous system results in increased cardiac output and oxygenation of these tissues.
- The renin-angiotensin response occurs as the blood flow to the kidneys decreases. Renin released from the kidneys converts a plasma protein to angiotensin II, which causes vasoconstriction and stimulates the adrenal cortex to release aldosterone. Aldosterone causes the kidneys to reabsorb water and sodium and to lose potassium. The absorption of water maintains circulating blood volume while increased vasoconstriction increases SVR, maintaining central vascular volume and raising blood pressure.
- The hypothalamus releases adrenocorticotropic hormone (ACTH), causing the adrenal glands to secrete aldosterone. Aldosterone promotes the reabsorption of water and sodium by the kidneys, preserving blood volume and pressure.
- The posterior pituitary gland releases antidiuretic hormone (ADH), which increases renal reabsorption of water to increase intravascular volume. The combined effects of hormones released by the hypothalamus and posterior pituitary glands work to conserve central vascular volume.
- As MAP falls in the compensatory stage of shock, decreased capillary hydrostatic pressure causes a fluid shift from the interstitial space into the capillaries. The net gain of fluid raises the blood volume.

Working together, these compensatory mechanisms can maintain MAP for only a short period of time. During this period, the perfusion and oxygenation of the heart and brain are adequate. If effective treatment is provided, the process is arrested, and no permanent damage occurs. However, unless the underlying cause of shock is reversed, these compensatory mechanisms soon become harmful, and shock perpetuates shock.

### Stage II: Intermediate or Progressive Shock

The progressive stage of shock occurs after a sustained decrease in MAP of 20 mmHg or more below normal levels and a fluid loss of 35% to 50% (1800 to 2500 mL of fluid). Although the compensatory mechanisms in the previous state remain activated, they are no longer able to maintain MAP at a level sufficient to ensure perfusion of vital organs.

The vasoconstriction response that first helped sustain MAP eventually limits blood flow to the point that cells become oxygen deficient. To remain alive, the affected cells switch from aerobic to anaerobic metabolism. The lactic acid formed as a by-product of anaerobic metabolism contributes to an acidotic state at the cellular level. As a result, adenosine triphosphate (ATP), the source of cellular energy, is produced inefficiently. Lacking energy, the sodium-potassium pump fails. Potassium moves out of the cell, while sodium and water move inward. As this process continues, the cell swells, cell membrane integrity is lost, and cell organelles are damaged. Lysosomes within the cell spill out their digestive enzymes, which disintegrate any remaining organelles. Some enzymes spread to adjacent cells, where they erode and rupture cell membranes.

The acid by-products of anaerobic metabolism dilate the precapillary arterioles and constrict the postcapillary venules. This causes increased hydrostatic pressure within the capillary, and fluid shifts back into the interstitial space. The capillaries also become increasingly permeable, allowing serum proteins to shift from the vascular space into the interstitium. The buildup of plasma proteins increases the osmotic pressure in the interstitium, further accelerating the fluid shift out of the capillaries.

Throughout this period, the heart rate and vasoconstriction increase; however, perfusion of the skin, skeletal muscles, kidneys, and gastrointestinal organs is greatly diminished. Cells in the heart and brain become hypoxic while other body cells and tissues become ischemic and anoxic. A generalized state of acidosis and hyperkalemia ensues (see Chapter 5 ⊂⊃). Unless this stage of shock is treated rapidly, the client's chances of survival are poor.

## Stage III: Refractory or Irreversible Shock

If shock progresses to the irreversible stage, tissue anoxia becomes so generalized and cellular death so widespread that no treatment can reverse the damage. Even if MAP is temporarily restored, too much cellular damage has occurred to maintain life. Death of cells is followed by death of tissues, which results in death of organs. Death of vital organs contributes to subsequent death of the body.

## Effects of Shock on Body Systems

Whatever its causes, shock produces predictable effects on the body's organ systems. (See *Multisystem Effects of Shock* on page 152.)

### Cardiovascular System

The perfusion and oxygenation of the heart are adequate in the early stages of shock. As shock progresses, myocardial cells become hypoxic, and myocardial muscle function diminishes. Initially, the blood pressure may be normal or even slightly elevated (as a result of compensatory mechanisms) and the heart rate only slightly increased. Sympathetic stimulation increases the heart rate (a sinus tachycardia of 120 beats per minute is common) in an effort to increase cardiac output. As a result of vasoconstriction and decreased blood volume, the palpated pulse is rapid, weak, and thready; as shock progresses, peripheral pulses are usually nonpalpable.

Tachycardia reduces the time available for left ventricular filling and coronary artery perfusion, further reducing cardiac output. With progressive shock, altered acid-base balance, hypoxia, and hyperkalemia damage the heart's electrical systems

and contractility. Consequently, cardiac dysrhythmias may develop. Decreased blood volume with decreased venous return also decreases cardiac output, and blood pressure falls.

The blood pressure changes produced by shock are characterized by a progressive decrease in both systolic and diastolic pressures and a narrowing pulse pressure. Auscultation of blood pressure is often difficult or impossible and is an inaccurate reflection of blood pressure status. For this reason, hemodynamic monitoring is usually instituted to follow the client's cardiovascular status accurately.

### Respiratory System

During shock, oxygen delivery to cells may be impaired by a drop in circulating blood volume or, in the case of blood loss, by an insufficient number of red blood cells that carry oxygen. Although the respiratory rate increases because of compensatory mechanisms that promote oxygenation, the number of alveoli that are perfused decreases, and gas exchange is impaired. As a result, oxygen levels in the blood decrease, and carbon dioxide levels increase. As perfusion of the lungs diminishes, carbon dioxide is retained, and respiratory acidosis occurs.

A complication of decreased perfusion of the lungs is acute respiratory distress syndrome (ARDS), or "shock lung." The exact mechanism that produces ARDS is unknown, but some contributing factors have been identified. The pulmonary capillaries become increasingly permeable to proteins and water, resulting in noncardiogenic pulmonary edema. Production of surfactant (which controls surface tension within alveoli) is impaired, and the alveoli collapse or fill with fluid. This potentially lethal form of respiratory failure may result from any condition that causes hypoperfusion of the lungs, but it is more common in shock caused by hemorrhage, severe allergic responses, trauma, and infection. (ARDS is discussed further in Chapter 36.) ⊂⊃

### Gastrointestinal and Hepatic Systems

The gastrointestinal organs normally receive 25% of the cardiac output through the splanchnic circulation. Shock constricts the splanchnic arterioles and redirects arterial blood flow to the heart and brain. Consequently, gastrointestinal organs become ischemic and may be irreversibly damaged.

Gastric mucosa tends to ulcerate when it becomes ischemic. Lesions of the gastric and duodenal mucosa (called *stress ulcers*) can develop within hours of severe trauma, sepsis, or burns (Porth, 2002). Gastrointestinal ulcers may hemorrhage within 2 to 10 days following the original cause of shock. In addition, the permeability of damaged mucosa increases, allowing enteric bacteria or their toxins to enter the abdominal cavity and then progress to the circulation, resulting in sepsis.

Gastric and intestinal motility is impaired during shock, and paralytic ileus may result. If the episode of shock is prolonged, necrosis of the bowel may occur. In many cases, alterations in the structure and function of the gastrointestinal tract impair absorption of nutrients, such as protein and glucose.

Shock also alters the metabolic functions of the liver. Initially, *gluconeogenesis* (the process of forming glucose from noncarbohydrate sources) and *glycogenolysis* (the breakdown of glycogen into glucose) increase. This process allows blood glucose

# Multisystem Effects of Shock

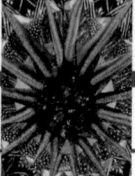

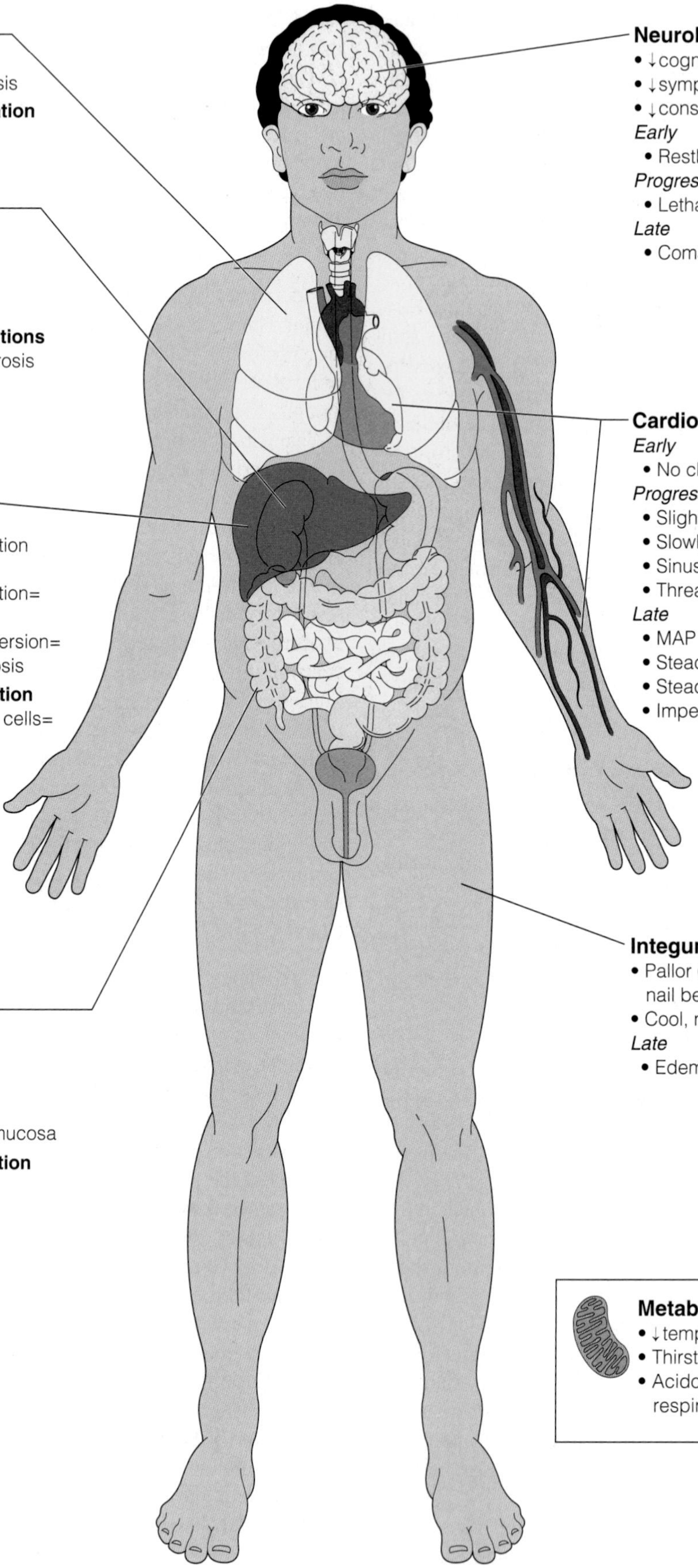

**Respiratory**
- ↑ respiratory rate
- Respiratory acidosis

**Potential Complication**
- ARDS

**Urinary**
- ↓ renal perfusion
- ↓GFR

*Late*
- Oliguria

**Potential Complications**
- Acute tubular necrosis
- Kidney failure

**Hepatic**

*Early*
- ↑ glucose production

*Progressive*
- ↓glucose production= hypoglycemia
- ↓lactic acid conversion= metabolic acidosis

**Potential Complication**
- Destroyed Kupffer cells= systemic bacterial infections

**Gastrointestinal**

*Early*
- ↓GI motility

*Late*
- Paralyticileus
- Ulceration of GI mucosa

**Potential Complication**
- Bowel necrosis

**Neurologic**
- ↓cognition
- ↓sympathetic activity
- ↓consciousness

*Early*
- Restlessness, apathy

*Progressive*
- Lethargy

*Late*
- Coma

**Cardiovascular**

*Early*
- No change

*Progressive*
- Slightly ↑BP
- Slowly rising HR
- Sinus tachycardia
- Thready pulse

*Late*
- MAP <60mmHg
- Steadily ↓BP
- Steadily ↓C/O
- Imperceptible pulses

**Integumentary**
- Pallor (skin, lips, oral mucosa, nail beds, conjunctiva)
- Cool, moist skin

*Late*
- Edema

**Metabolic Processes**
- ↓temperature
- Thirst
- Acidosis (metabolic and respiratory)

levels to increase as the body attempts to respond to the stressor; however, as shock progresses, liver functions are impaired, and hypoglycemia develops. Metabolism of fats and protein is impaired, and the liver can no longer effectively remove lactic acid, contributing to the development of metabolic acidosis.

The destruction of the liver's reticuloendothelial Kupffer cells (phagocytes that destroy bacteria) causes a further problem. Bacteria may proliferate within the circulatory system, causing overwhelming bacterial infection and toxicity.

### Neurologic System

The primary effects of shock on the neurologic system involve changes in mental status and orientation. Cerebral hypoxia produces altered levels of consciousness, beginning with apathy and lethargy and progressing to coma. A common early symptom of cerebral hypoxia is restlessness. Continued ischemia of brain cells eventually causes swelling, resulting in cerebral edema, neurotransmitter failure, and irreversible brain cell damage.

As cerebral ischemia worsens, the sympathetic activity and vasomotor centers are depressed. This leads to a loss of sympathetic tone, causing systemic vasodilatation and pooling of blood in the periphery. As a result, venous return and cardiac output further decrease.

### Renal System

Blood that normally perfuses the kidneys is shunted to the heart and brain during the progressive stage of shock, resulting in renal hypoperfusion. The drop in renal perfusion is reflected in a corresponding decrease in the glomerular filtration rate. Urine output is reduced, and the urine that is produced is highly concentrated. Oliguria of less than 20 mL per hour indicates progressive shock.

Healthy kidneys can tolerate a drop in perfusion for only about 20 minutes; thereafter, acute tubular necrosis develops (Porth, 2002). As tubular necrosis occurs, epithelial cells slough off and block the tubules, disrupting nephron function. The accumulating loss of functional nephrons eventually causes renal failure. Without normal renal function, metabolic waste products are retained in the plasma.

If treatment restores renal perfusion, the kidneys can regenerate the lost epithelial cells in the tubules, and renal function usually returns to normal. However, in the older or chronically ill client or in the client with sustained shock, loss of renal function may become permanent.

### Effects on Skin, Temperature, and Thirst

In most types of shock, blood vessels supplying the skin are vasoconstricted, and the sweat glands are activated. As a result, changes in skin color occur. The skin of Caucasian clients becomes pale. In people with darker skin (such as those of African, Hispanic, or Mediterranean descent), shock-related skin color changes may be assessed as paleness of the lips, oral mucous membranes, nail beds, and conjunctiva. The skin is usually cool and moist and, in the later stages of shock, often edematous.

The body temperature decreases as shock progresses, the result of a decrease in overall body metabolism. Some people in shock become thirsty, probably a response to decreased blood volume and increased serum osmolality (Porth, 2002).

## TYPES OF SHOCK

Shock is identified according to its underlying cause. All types of shock progress through the same stages and exert similar effects on body systems. Any differences are noted in the following discussion.

### Hypovolemic Shock

**Hypovolemic shock** is caused by a decrease in intravascular volume of 15% or more (Porth, 2002). In hypovolemic shock, the venous blood returning to the heart decreases, and ventricular filling drops. As a result, stroke volume, cardiac output, and blood pressure decrease. Hypovolemic shock is the most common type of shock, and it often occurs simultaneously with other types.

The decrease in circulating blood volume that triggers hypovolemic shock may result from:

- Loss of blood volume from hemorrhage (from surgery, trauma, gastrointestinal bleeding, blood coagulation disorders, ruptured esophageal varices).
- Loss of intravascular fluid from the skin due to injuries such as burns (see Chapter 15). 🔗
- Loss of blood volume from severe dehydration.
- Loss of body fluid from the gastrointestinal system due to persistent and severe vomiting or diarrhea, or continuous nasogastric suctioning.
- Renal losses of fluid due to the use of diuretics or to endocrine disorders such as diabetes insipidus.
- Conditions causing fluid shifts from the intravascular compartment to the interstitial space.
- Third spacing due to such disorders as liver diseases with ascites, pleural effusion, or intestinal obstruction.

Hypovolemic shock affects all body systems. Its effects vary depending on the client's age, general state of health, extent of injury or severity of illness, length of time before treatment is provided, and the rate of volume loss.

The manifestations of hypovolemic shock result directly from the decrease in circulating blood volume and the initiation of compensatory mechanisms (Figure 6–8 ■). The loss of circulating blood volume reduces cardiac output by decreasing venous return to the heart. As a result, blood pressure drops. The carotid and cardiac baroreceptors sense the decrease in blood pressure and communicate it to the vasomotor centers in the brainstem. The vasomotor centers then induce the sympathetic compensatory responses. If the fluid loss is less than 500 mL, activation of the sympathetic response is generally adequate to restore cardiac output and blood pressure to near normal, although the heart rate may remain elevated.

With a sustained loss of blood volume (1000 mL or more), the shock stage progresses. Heart rate and vasoconstriction increase, and blood flow to the skin, skeletal muscles, kidneys, and abdominal organs decreases. Several renal mechanisms and a decline in capillary pressure help conserve blood volume. Eventually, the amount of blood flowing to cells is too low to oxygenate them and sustain production of cellular energy. Anaerobic metabolism begins, producing an acidotic environment for cells. As a result, cells lose their physical integrity.

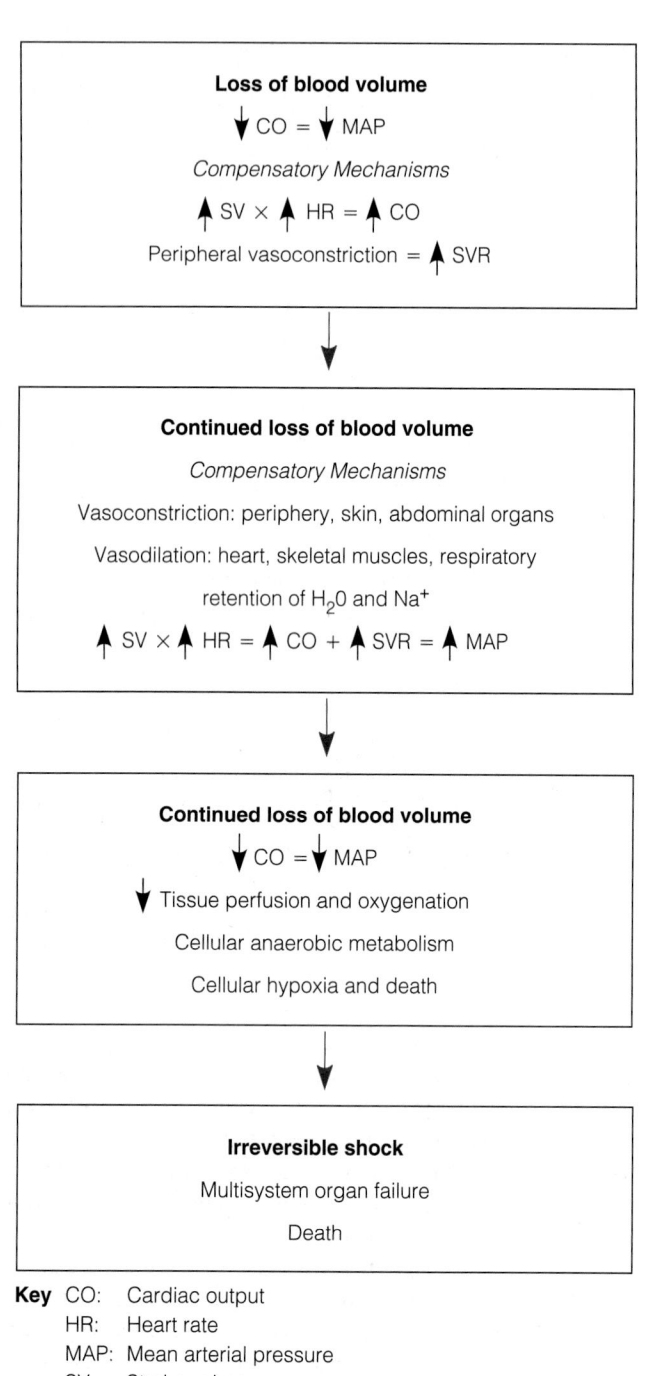

**Loss of blood volume**

$\downarrow$ CO = $\downarrow$ MAP

*Compensatory Mechanisms*

$\uparrow$ SV $\times$ $\uparrow$ HR = $\uparrow$ CO

Peripheral vasoconstriction = $\uparrow$ SVR

---

**Continued loss of blood volume**

*Compensatory Mechanisms*

Vasoconstriction: periphery, skin, abdominal organs

Vasodilation: heart, skeletal muscles, respiratory

retention of $H_2O$ and $Na^+$

$\uparrow$ SV $\times$ $\uparrow$ HR = $\uparrow$ CO + $\uparrow$ SVR = $\uparrow$ MAP

---

**Continued loss of blood volume**

$\downarrow$ CO = $\downarrow$ MAP

$\downarrow$ Tissue perfusion and oxygenation

Cellular anaerobic metabolism

Cellular hypoxia and death

---

**Irreversible shock**

Multisystem organ failure

Death

**Key**  CO:   Cardiac output
HR:   Heart rate
MAP:  Mean arterial pressure
SV:   Stroke volume
SVR:  Systemic vascular resistance

**Figure 6–8** ■ The stages of hypovolemic shock.

If untreated, shock causes multiple organ failure, and death results. Manifestations of various stages of hypovolemic shock are listed in Box 6–2.

## Cardiogenic Shock

**Cardiogenic shock** occurs when the heart's pumping ability is compromised to the point that it cannot maintain cardiac output and adequate tissue perfusion. Cardiac disorders are discussed in Chapters 29 and 30; this section focuses only on the effects of shock caused by these disorders. ⌾

---

**BOX 6–2** ■ **Assessment Findings in Clients in Hypovolemic Shock**

**INITIAL STAGE**
- Blood pressure: normal to slightly decreased
- Pulse: slightly increased from baseline
- Respirations: normal (baseline)
- Skin: cool, pale (in periphery), moist
- Mental status: alert and oriented
- Urine output: slight decrease
- Other: thirst, decreased capillary refill time

**COMPENSATORY AND PROGRESSIVE STAGES**
- Blood pressure: hypotension
- Pulse: rapid, thready
- Respirations: increased
- Skin: cool, pale (includes trunk); poor turgor with fluid loss, edematous with fluid shift
- Mental status: restless, anxious, confused, or agitated
- Urine output: oliguria (less than 30 mL/hour)
- Other: marked thirst, acidosis, hyperkalemia, decreased capillary refill time, decreased or absent peripheral pulses

**IRREVERSIBLE STAGE**
- Blood pressure: severe hypotension (often, systolic pressure is below 80 mmHg)
- Pulse: very rapid, weak
- Respirations: rapid, shallow; crackles and wheezes
- Skin: cool, pale, mottled with cyanosis
- Mental status: disoriented, lethargic, comatose
- Urine output: anuria
- Other: loss of reflexes, decreased or absent peripheral pulses

---

The loss of the pumping action of the heart may be caused by the following conditions.

- Myocardial infarction
- Cardiac tamponade
- Restrictive pericarditis
- Cardiac arrest
- Dysrhythmias, such as fibrillation or ventricular tachycardia
- Pathologic changes in the valves
- Cardiomyopathies from hypertension, alcohol, bacterial or viral infections, or ischemia
- Complications of cardiac surgery
- Electrolyte imbalances (especially changes in normal potassium and calcium levels)
- Drugs affecting cardiac muscle contractility
- Head injuries causing damage to the cardioregulatory center

Myocardial infarction is the most common cause of cardiogenic shock. Clients admitted to the hospital for treatment of myocardial infarction or cardiac surgery are at risk for cardiogenic shock. The severity and progression of shock are related to the amount of myocardial damage.

Whatever the cardiogenic cause, the decrease in cardiac output causes a decrease in MAP. Heart rate may increase in response to compensatory mechanisms. However, tachycardia increases myocardial oxygen consumption and decreases coronary perfusion. The myocardium becomes progressively de-

| BOX 6–3 | ■ Assessment Findings in Clients in Cardiogenic Shock |
|---|---|

- Blood pressure: hypotension
- Pulse: rapid, thready; distention of veins of hands and neck
- Respirations: increased, labored; crackles and wheezes; pulmonary edema
- Skin: pale, cyanotic, cold, moist
- Mental status: restless, anxious, lethargic progressing to comatose
- Urine output: oliguria to anuria
- Other: dependent edema; elevated CVP; elevated pulmonary capillary wedge pressure; arrhythmias

pleted of oxygen, causing further myocardial ischemia and necrosis. The typical sequence of shock is essentially unchanged in cardiogenic shock.

Cyanosis, however, is more common in cardiogenic shock, because stagnating blood increases extraction of oxygen from the hemoglobin at the capillary beds. As a result, the skin, lips, and nail beds may appear cyanotic. As cardiac failure (and cardiogenic shock) progresses, left ventricular end-diastolic pressure increases. The increase is transmitted to the pulmonary capillary bed, and pulmonary edema may occur. Retention of blood in the right side of the heart increases right atrial pressure, which leads to jugular venous distention as a result of backflow through the vena cava. Manifestations of cardiogenic shock are listed in Box 6–3.

## Obstructive Shock

**Obstructive shock** is caused by an obstruction in the heart or great vessels that either impedes venous return or prevents effective cardiac pumping action. The causes of obstructive shock are impaired diastolic filling (e.g., pericardial tamponade or pneumothorax), increased right ventricular afterload (e.g., pulmonary emboli), and increased left ventricular afterload (e.g., aortic stenosis, abdominal distention). The manifestations are the result of decreased cardiac output and blood pressure, with reduced tissue perfusion and cellular metabolism.

## Distributive Shock

**Distributive shock** (also called **vasogenic shock**) includes several types of shock that result from widespread vasodilatation and decreased peripheral resistance. As the blood volume does not change, relative hypovolemia results.

### Septic Shock

**Septic shock,** the leading cause of death for clients in intensive care units, is one part of a progressive syndrome called systemic inflammatory response syndrome (SIRS). This condition is most often the result of gram-negative bacterial infections (i.e., *Pseudomonas, E. coli, Klebsiella*), but may also follow gram-positive infections from *Staphyloccus* and *Streptococcus* bacteria. Gram-negative sepsis has greatly increased in the past 10 years, with a 60% mortality rate despite treatment. The pathophysiology of septic shock is complex and not completely understood.

Clients at risk for developing infections leading to septic shock include those who are hospitalized, have debilitating chronic illnesses, or have poor nutritional status. The risk is heightened after invasive procedures or surgery. Other clients at risk of septic shock include older adults and those who are immunocompromised. Portals of entry for infection that may lead to septic shock are as follows:

- Urinary system: catheterizations, suprapubic tubes, cystoscopy
- Respiratory system: suctioning, aspiration, tracheostomy, endotracheal tubes, respiratory therapy, mechanical ventilators
- Gastrointestinal system: peptic ulcers, ruptured appendix, peritonitis
- Integumentary system: surgical wounds, intravenous catheters, intra-arterial catheters, invasive monitoring, decubitus ulcers, burns, trauma
- Female reproductive system: elective surgical abortion, ascending infections from transmission of bacteria during the intrapartal and postpartal periods, tampon use, sexually transmitted diseases

Septic shock begins with *septicemia* (the presence of pathogens and their toxins in the blood). As pathogens are destroyed, their ruptured cell membranes allow endotoxins to leak into the plasma. The endotoxins disrupt the vascular system, coagulation mechanism, and immune system and trigger an immune and inflammatory response (see Chapter 8 ⊙⊃ for more information). For this reason, the initial effects of septic shock differ from those of hypovolemic and cardiogenic shock; cardiac output is high and systemic vascular resistance is low.

Endotoxins directly damage the endothelial lining of small blood vessels first; the small blood vessels of the kidneys and lungs are most susceptible. Cellular damage stimulates the release of vasoactive proteins and activates coagulation factor XII. The vasoactive proteins stimulate peripheral vasodilatation and increase capillary permeability; the activation of coagulation factors results in the production of multiple intravascular blood clots.

As a result of the increased capillary permeability and vasodilatation, fluid shifts from the intravascular space to the interstitial space. Hypovolemia results as fluid volume is lost from the circulating blood. Hypovolemia and intravascular coagulation alter oxygenation and cellular metabolism, leading to anaerobic metabolism, lactic acidosis, and cellular death.

Septic shock has an early phase and a late phase. In early septic shock (sometimes called the *warm* phase), vasodilatation results in weakness and warm, flushed skin, and the septicemia often causes high fever and chills. In late septic shock (sometimes called the *cold* phase), hypovolemia and activity of the compensatory mechanisms result in typical shock manifestations, including cold, moist skin; oliguria; and changes in mental status. Death may result from respiratory failure, cardiac failure, or renal failure. Manifestations of septic shock are listed in Box 6–4.

*Toxic shock syndrome* is an especially virulent form of septic shock, occurring most frequently in menstruating women who use tampons. It is thought that bacterial toxins diffuse

| BOX 6–4 | ■ Assessment Findings in Clients in Septic Shock |
| --- | --- |

**EARLY (WARM) SEPTIC SHOCK**
- Blood pressure: normal to hypotension
- Pulse: increased, thready
- Respirations: rapid and deep
- Skin: warm, flushed
- Mental status: alert, oriented, anxious
- Urine output: normal
- Other: increased body temperature; chills; weakness; nausea, vomiting, diarrhea; decreased CVP

**LATE (COLD) SEPTIC SHOCK**
- Blood pressure: hypotension
- Pulse: tachycardia, arrhythmias
- Respirations: rapid, shallow, dyspneic
- Skin: cool, pale, edematous
- Mental status: lethargic to comatose
- Urine output: oliguria to anuria
- Other: normal to decreased body temperature; decreased CVP

| BOX 6–5 | ■ Assessment Findings in Clients in Neurogenic Shock |
| --- | --- |

- Blood pressure: hypotension
- Pulse: slow and bounding
- Respirations: vary
- Skin: warm, dry
- Mental status: anxious, restless, lethargic progressing to comatose
- Urine output: oliguria to anuria
- Other: lowered body temperature

from the site of infection in the vagina into the circulation. The toxins then trigger a widespread inflammatory response and septic shock. The manifestations of toxic shock syndrome include extreme hypotension, hyperpyrexia, headache, myalgia, confusion, skin rash, vomiting, and diarrhea (Porth, 2002).

Disseminated intravascular coagulation (DIC), a generalized response to injury, is a potential risk in septic shock. This condition is characterized by simultaneous bleeding and clotting throughout the vasculature. Sepsis injures blood cells, causing platelet aggregation and decreased blood flow. As a result, blood clots form throughout the microcirculation. The clotting slows circulation further while stimulating excess fibrinolysis. As the body's stores of clotting factors are depleted, generalized bleeding begins. DIC is further discussed in Chapter 32. ⊝⊝

### Neurogenic Shock

**Neurogenic shock** is the result of an imbalance between parasympathetic and sympathetic stimulation of vascular smooth muscle. If parasympathetic overstimulation or sympathetic understimulation persists, sustained vasodilatation occurs, and blood pools in the venous and capillary beds.

Neurogenic shock causes dramatic reduction in systemic vascular resistance as the size of the vascular compartment increases. As systemic vascular resistance decreases, pressure in the blood vessels becomes too low to drive nutrients across capillary membranes, and cellular metabolism is impaired.

The following conditions can cause neurogenic shock by increasing parasympathetic stimulation or inhibiting sympathetic stimulation of the smooth muscle of blood vessels.

- Head injury
- Trauma to the spinal cord (spinal shock, a form of neurogenic shock, is described in Chapter 41) ⊝⊝
- Insulin reactions (which cause hypoglycemia, decreasing glucose to the medulla)
- Central nervous system depressant drugs (such as sedatives, barbiturates, or narcotics)

- Anesthesia (spinal and general)
- Severe pain
- Prolonged exposure to heat

Bradycardia occurs early, but tachycardia begins as compensatory mechanisms are initiated. Central venous pressure drops as veins dilate, venous return to the heart decreases, stroke volume decreases, and MAP falls. In early stages, the extremities are warm and pink (from the pooling of blood), but as shock progresses, the skin becomes pale and cool. Manifestations of neurogenic shock are listed in Box 6–5.

### Anaphylactic Shock

**Anaphylactic shock** is the result of a widespread hypersensitivity reaction (called *anaphylaxis*). The pathophysiology in this type of shock includes vasodilatation, pooling of blood in the periphery, and hypovolemia with altered cellular metabolism. These physiologic alterations occur when a sensitized person has contact with an *allergen* (a foreign substance to which an individual is hypersensitive). Many different allergens can cause anaphylactic shock, including medications, blood administration, latex, foods, snake venom, and insect stings.

Anaphylactic shock does not occur with the first exposure to an allergen. With the first exposure to a foreign substance (the *antigen*), the body produces specific immunoglobulin E (IgE) antibodies against this antigen. The person is thus sensitized to that specific antigen. With subsequent exposure, the antigen reacts with the already formed IgE antibodies, disrupting cellular integrity. In addition, large amounts of histamine and other vasoactive amines are released and distributed through the circulatory system. These substances cause increased capillary permeability and massive vasodilatation, resulting in profound hypotension and eventual vascular collapse.

Histamine also causes constriction of smooth muscles in the bladder, uterus, intestines, and bronchioles. Respiratory distress, bronchospasm, laryngospasm, and severe abdominal cramping result. Serotonin (a neurotransmitter with vasoconstrictive properties) is released, further affecting respiratory status by increasing capillary permeability in the lungs. As a result, plasma leaks into the alveoli, gas exchange is impaired, and pulmonary edema may occur.

Anaphylactic shock begins and progresses rapidly. Manifestations may begin within 20 minutes of contact with an antigen. Unless appropriate intervention is provided, death can occur within a matter of minutes. Because anaphylaxis is rapid and potentially lethal, people with known allergies should carry some form of

| BOX 6–6 | ■ Assessment Findings in Clients in Anaphylactic Shock |
|---|---|

- Blood pressure: hypotension
- Pulse: increased, dysrhythmias
- Respirations: dyspnea, stridor, wheezes, laryngospasm, bronchospasm, pulmonary edema
- Skin: warm, edematous (lips, eyelids, tongue, hands, feet, genitals)
- Mental status: restless, anxious, lethargic to comatose
- Urine output: oliguria to anuria
- Other: paresthesias; pruritus; abdominal cramps, vomiting, diarrhea

warning (such as a MedicAlert bracelet) informing others of their susceptibility. Health care providers should be extremely careful to assess and document allergies or previous drug reactions. Manifestations of anaphylactic shock are listed in Box 6–6.

## COLLABORATIVE CARE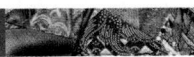

Medical care for the client in shock focuses on treating the underlying cause, increasing arterial oxygenation, and improving tissue perfusion. Depending on the cause and type of shock, interventions include emergency care measures, oxygen therapy, fluid replacement, and medications. Emergency care is often the first course of collaborative action taken to arrest shock, as discussed earlier in this chapter.

### Diagnostic Tests

The following diagnostic tests can help identify the type of shock and assess the client's physical status. Measurements include:

- *Blood hemoglobin* and *hematocrit.* Changes in hemoglobin and hematocrit concentrations usually occur in hypovolemic shock. These changes reflect the underlying etiology. In hypovolemic shock resulting from hemorrhage, the hemoglobin and hematocrit concentrations are lower than normal; in hypovolemic shock resulting from intravascular fluid loss, by contrast, the hemoglobin and hematocrit concentrations are higher than normal.
- *Arterial blood gases (ABGs),* to determine oxygen and carbon dioxide levels and pH. The effects of shock and of the body's compensatory mechanisms cause a decrease in pH (indicating acidosis), a decrease in the partial pressure of oxygen ($PaO_2$) and in total oxygen saturation, and an increase in the partial pressure of carbon dioxide ($PaCO_2$).
- *Serum electrolytes,* to monitor the severity and progression of shock. As shock progresses, glucose levels decrease, sodium levels decrease, and potassium levels increase.
- *Blood urea nitrogen (BUN), serum creatinine levels, urine specific gravity,* and *osmolality,* to check renal function. As perfusion of the kidneys is decreased and renal function is reduced, the BUN and creatinine levels increase as does urine specific gravity and osmolality.
- *Blood cultures,* to identify the causative organism in septic shock.

- *White blood cell count* and *differential,* in the client with septic or anaphylactic shock. The total WBC count is increased in septic shock. Elevated neutrophils indicate acute infection, increased monocytes indicate a bacterial infection, and increased eosinophils indicate an allergic response.
- *Serum cardiac enzymes,* which are elevated in cardiogenic shock: lactate dehydrogenase (LDH), creatine phosphokinase (CPK), and serum glutamic-oxaloacetic transaminase (SGOT).
- *Central venous catheter,* to aid in the differential diagnosis of shock and to provide information about the preload of the heart. A pulmonary artery catheter may be inserted to monitor cardiac dynamics, fluid balance, and the effects of vasoactive medications.

Other diagnostic tests may be ordered to determine the extent of injury or damage or to locate the site of internal hemorrhage. These tests might include X-ray studies, computerized tomography (CT) scans, magnetic resonance imaging (MRI), endoscopic examinations, and echocardiograms. Newer diagnostic methods for hypoperfusion include gastric tonometry and sublingual $PCO_2$. Gastric tonometry measures the partial pressure of carbon dioxide in the gastric lumen. The measurement of sublingual carbon dioxide correlates well with decreased MAP (Sole, Lamborn, & Hartshorn, 2001).

### Medications

When fluid replacement alone is not sufficient to reverse shock, vasoactive drugs (drugs causing vasoconstriction or vasodilatation) and inotropic drugs (drugs improving cardiac contractility) may be administered. When used to treat shock, these drugs increase venous return through vasoconstriction of peripheral vessels; they also improve the pumping ability of the heart by facilitating myocardial contractility and by dilating coronary arteries to increase perfusion of the myocardium.

Drugs used to treat shock are discussed in the Medication Administration box on page 158. Other drugs that may be administered to the client in shock include:

- Diuretics to increase urine output after fluid replacement has been initiated.
- Sodium bicarbonate to treat acidosis.
- Calcium to replace calcium lost as a result of blood transfusions.
- Antiarrhythmic agents to stabilize heart rhythm.
- Antibiotics to suppress organisms responsible for septic shock.
- A cardiotonic glycoside (such as digitalis) to treat cardiac failure.
- Steroids to treat anaphylactic shock.

### Oxygen Therapy

Establishing and maintaining a patent airway and ensuring adequate oxygenation are critical interventions in reversing shock. All clients in shock (even those with adequate respirations) should receive oxygen therapy (usually by mask or nasal cannula) to maintain the $PaO_2$ at greater than 80 mmHg during the first 4 to 6 hours of care. If the client's unassisted respiration cannot maintain $PaO_2$ at this level, ventilatory assistance may be necessary. Care of the client requiring ventilatory assistance is discussed in Chapter 36. ∞

# Medication Administration

## The Client in Shock

### ADRENERGICS (SYMPATHOMIMETICS)

Adrenergic drugs (also called sympathomimetics) mimic the fight-or-flight response of the sympathetic nervous system, selectively stimulating alpha-adrenergic and beta-adrenergic receptors. Many of these drugs have both vasopressor (vasoconstricting) effects and positive inotropic effects (Table 6–5). Stimulation of alpha-adrenergic receptors results in vasoconstriction and increased systemic blood pressure. Stimulation of beta-adrenergic receptors increases the force and rate of myocardial contraction.

The physiologic effect of these drugs includes improved perfusion and oxygenation of the heart, with increased stroke volume and heart rate, and increased cardiac output. Increased cardiac output in turn increases tissue perfusion and oxygenation. The major disadvantage is that increases in stroke volume and heart rate also increase the oxygen requirements of the myocardium. These drugs may be used in the early stages of shock, especially in types of shock characterized by vasodilation.

### Nursing Responsibilities

- Carefully monitor responses in the older adult, who may be especially sensitive to sympathomimetics and require lower doses.
- When administering these drugs by the subcutaneous route, carefully aspirate the injection site to avoid injecting the drug directly into a blood vessel.
- Use the intravenous route only with continuous infusion pumps. Carefully adjust the dose to accommodate the client's cardiovascular status (as ordered by the physician or by written protocol).
- Document lung sounds, vital signs, and hemodynamic parameters before starting the medication, and then according to institutional policy (usually every 5 to 15 minutes).
- Record and monitor urine output, report output of less than 30 mL per hour.
- Be aware that the sympathomimetics are incompatible with sodium bicarbonate or alkaline solutions.

**Table 6–5** Adrenergic Drugs Used to Treat Shock

| Action | Drug | Receptor |
|---|---|---|
| Vasoconstrictors | Norepinephrine (Levophed) | A |
| | Metaraminol (Aramine) | A |
| Inotropes | Dopamine (Inotropin)* | A, B¹ |
| | Dobutamine (Dobutrex) | B¹ |
| | Isoprotenernol (Isuprel) | B¹, B² |

*Receptors are dose dependent.

- When administering drugs that cause vasoconstriction, such as norepinephrine (Levophed) and metaraminol (Aramine), monitor the intravenous insertion site for infiltration. If infiltration does occur, stop the infusion and notify the physician immediately. (Infiltration may cause ischemia and necrosis of tissue.)

### Client Teaching

- Because these drugs mimic a physiologic reaction to stress, they may cause feelings of anxiety.
- Close monitoring to adjust the dose will be carried out by qualified nurses using written protocols.
- Report heart palpitations or chest pain immediately.

### VASODILATORS

Nitroglycerin (Tridil)
Nitroprusside (Nipride)

Drugs that cause vasodilation act directly on smooth muscle, affecting both arterioles and veins. Peripheral resistance, cardiac output, and pulmonary wedge pressure are all reduced as a result of the vasodilation. These effects decrease the oxygen need of the heart and decrease pulmonary congestion. Vasodilators are used primarily in the treatment of cardiogenic shock and may be combined with a sympathomimetic (e.g., dopamine).

### Nursing Responsibilities

- Protect these drugs from light by wrapping the intravenous bag in the package that is provided.
- Mix with D5W only.
- Infuse with an infusion pump, and use within 4 hours of reconstitution.
- Do not add other medications to the solution.
- Assess mental status, blood pressure, and pulse prior to initiating medication. Thereafter, assess blood pressure and pulse according to institutional policy (usually every 5 minutes initially, then every 15 minutes until stable, and then every hour).
- Monitor for confusion, dizziness, tachycardia, arrhythmias, hypotension, and adventitious breath sounds. Report these immediately if they occur, and slow infusion to a keep-open rate.
- Monitor for signs of thiocyanate poisoning (nausea, disorientation, muscle spasms, decreased or absent reflexes) if infusion lasts longer than 72 hours.
- Keep client in bed with side rails up.

### Client and Family Teaching

- It is important to stay in bed and change positions slowly to avoid dizziness.
- The blood pressure and pulse are taken frequently to adjust the dose of medication.
- Headache is a common side effect.

## Fluid Replacement

The most effective treatment for the client in hypovolemic shock is the administration of intravenous fluids or blood. Fluids also treat septic and neurogenic shock. However, the client with cardiogenic shock may require either fluid replacement or restriction, depending on pulmonary artery pressure.

Various fluids may be administered alone or in combination as part of fluid replacement therapy in treating shock. Whole blood or blood products increase the oxygen-carrying capacity of the blood and thus increase oxygenation of cells. Fluid replacements, such as crystalloid and colloid solutions, increase circulating blood volume and tissue perfusion. Fluid replacements are administered in massive amounts through two large-bore peripheral lines or through a central line.

### Crystalloid Solutions

Crystalloid solutions contain dextrose or electrolytes dissolved in water; they are either isotonic or hypotonic. Isotonic solutions include normal saline (0.9%), lactated Ringer's solution, and Ringer's solution. Hypotonic solutions include one-half normal saline (0.45%) and 5% dextrose in water (D5W).

All crystalloid solutions increase fluid volume in both the intravascular and the interstitial space. Of the total amount infused, only about 25% remains in the intravascular system; the remaining 75% moves into the interstitial space. Consequently, fluid volume is only minimally expanded and the potential for peripheral edema is increased when crystalloid solutions are used. However, Ringer's lactate (an electrolyte solution) and 0.9% saline are the fluids of choice in treating hypovolemic shock, especially in the emergency phase of care while blood is being typed and crossmatched. Large amounts of these solutions may be infused rapidly, increasing blood volume and tissue perfusion.

### Colloid Solutions

Colloid solutions contain substances (colloids) that should not diffuse through capillary walls. Hence, colloids tend to remain in the vascular system and increase the osmotic pressure of the serum, causing fluid to move into the vascular compartment from the interstitial space. As a result, plasma volume expands.

Colloid solutions used to treat shock include 5% albumin, 25% albumin, hetastarch, plasma protein fraction, and dextran.

Colloid products reduce platelet adhesiveness and have been associated with reductions in blood coagulation. Consequently, the client's prothrombin time (PT), INR, platelet count, and activated partial thromboplastin time (PTT) should be monitored when these solutions are administered. Normal values are as follows:

| | |
|---|---|
| PT | 10–15 seconds |
| INR | 1–1.2 seconds |
| Platelets | 150,000–400,000 |
| APTT | < 35 seconds |

See the box below for further information about colloid solutions and associated nursing responsibilities and client teaching.

### Blood and Blood Products

If hypovolemic shock is due to hemorrhage, the infusion of blood and blood products may be indicated. The goal of blood administration is to keep the hematocrit at 30% to 35% and the hemoglobin level between 12.5 and 14.5 g/100 mL. Available blood and blood products include fresh whole blood, stored whole blood, packed red blood cells, platelet concentrate, fresh-frozen plasma, and cryoprecipitate. Often, packed red blood cells are given to provide hemoglobin concentration and are supplemented with crystalloids to maintain an adequate circulatory volume (see discussion of blood administration earlier in the chapter).

## Medication Administration

### Colloid Solutions

#### COLLOID SOLUTIONS (PLASMA EXPANDERS)

Albumin 5% (Albuminar-5, Buminate 5%)
Albumin 25% (Albuminar-25, Buminate 25%)
Dextran 40 (Gentran 40)
Dextran 70 (Gentran 70, Macrodex)
Dextran 75 (Gentran 75)
Hetastarch (Hespan [HES])
Plasma protein fraction (Plasmanate, Plasma-Plex, Plasmatein, Protenate)

These solutions are blood volume expanders and are used to treat hypovolemic shock due to surgery, hemorrhage, burns, or other trauma. Albumin and plasma protein fraction are prepared from healthy blood donors. Dextran and hetastarch are synthetically prepared large molecules. The solutions promote circulatory volume and tissue perfusion by rapidly expanding plasma volume. Dextran solutions are infrequently used.

#### Nursing Responsibilities
- Before infusion begins, establish baseline of vital signs, lung sounds, heart sounds, and (if possible) CVP and pulmonary artery wedge pressure.
- Start administration of ordered intravenous fluids, using a large-gauge (18 or 19 gauge) infusion needle.
- Take and record vital signs as required by institutional policy (usually every 15 to 60 minutes) and client status.
- Take and record intake and output every 1 to 2 hours.

- Monitor for manifestations of congestive heart failure or pulmonary edema (dyspnea, cyanosis, cough, crackles, wheezes). If these manifestations appear, stop the fluids and notify the physician immediately.
- Monitor for bleeding from new sites; an increase in blood pressure may cause bleeding in severed vessels that did not bleed with decreased blood pressure.
- Monitor for manifestations of dehydration (dry lips; scant, dark-colored urine; loss of skin turgor). Increased intravenous fluids are usually ordered if the client becomes dehydrated.
- Monitor for manifestations of circulatory overload (jugular vein distention, increase in CVP, increase in pulmonary artery wedge pressure). If these manifestations occur, slow rate of infusion and notify physician.
- Monitor prothrombin time, partial thromboplastin time, and platelet counts.
- If administering dextran or plasma protein fraction, have epinephrine and antihistamines readily available for any manifestations of a hypersensitivity reaction (fever, chills, rash, headache, wheezing, flushing).
- Maintain client on bed rest with side rails elevated.

#### Client and Family Teaching
- The solutions are given to replace lost serum protein, which helps maintain the volume of blood.
- The vital signs are taken frequently to ensure the safety of the client.

# NURSING CARE

Nursing assessments and interventions to prevent shock are an essential part of the nursing care of every client. The primary nursing interventions to prevent shock are assessment and monitoring.

## Health Promotion and Assessment

Nursing assessments are critical in preventing shock. Identifying clients at risk and making focused assessments are essential. Although shock may occur at any age, physiologic changes with aging make the older adult a high-risk population (see the box below).

- *Hypovolemic shock:* Clients who have undergone surgery, have sustained multiple traumatic injuries, or have been seriously burned are most likely to develop hypovolemic shock. Monitoring fluid status is essential in preventing shock and includes daily assessments of weight, fluid intake by all routes, measurable fluid loss (e.g., urine, vomitus, wound drainage, gastric drainage, and chest tube drainage), and fluid loss that must be estimated, such as profuse perspiration and wound drainage. Assessments for the critically ill client are ongoing and include fluid balance, hemodynamic values, and vital signs.
- *Cardiogenic shock:* Clients with left anterior wall myocardial infarctions are at risk for developing cardiogenic shock. Nursing care to prevent the development of cardiogenic shock focuses on maintaining or improving myocardial oxygen supply by providing immediate pain relief, maintaining rest, and administering supplemental oxygen.
- *Neurogenic shock:* The risk of neurogenic shock is increased in clients who have spinal cord injuries and those who have received spinal anesthesia. Preventive nursing care includes maintaining immobility of clients with spinal cord trauma and elevating the head of the bed 15 to 20 degrees following spinal anesthesia. Elevations of more than 20 degrees, however, can potentiate headaches following spinal anesthesia and should be avoided.
- *Anaphylactic shock:* Prevent anaphylactic shock by collecting information about allergies and drug reactions during the health history. Note these allergies clearly on all documents and place a special armband on the client. Careful and frequent assessments during blood administration may prevent serious reactions to blood or blood products.

- *Septic shock:* Clients who are hospitalized, are debilitated, are chronically ill, or have undergone invasive procedures or tube insertions are at high risk for septic shock. Nursing care to prevent septic shock includes careful and consistent handwashing, the use of aseptic techniques for procedures (e.g., catheterizations, suctioning, changing dressings, starting and maintaining intravenous fluids or medications), and monitoring for local and systemic manifestations (e.g., white blood cell and differential counts) of infection.

## Nursing Diagnoses and Interventions

Nursing care for the client in shock focuses on assessing and monitoring overall tissue perfusion and on meeting psychosocial needs of the client and the family. This section discusses nursing diagnoses that are appropriate for the client with hypovolemic shock.

### Decreased Cardiac Output

Decreased cardiac output is the primary problem for the client in shock. Although much of the care related to this diagnosis is collaborative, many independent nursing interventions are critical to the care of the client in shock.

- *Assess and monitor cardiovascular function via the following:*
  - Blood pressure
  - Heart rate and rhythm
  - Pulse oximetry
  - Peripheral pulses
  - Hemodynamic monitoring of arterial pressures, pulmonary artery pressures, and central venous pressures (CVPs)

    *A baseline assessment is necessary to establish the stage of shock. If palpable peripheral pulses and audible (to auscultation) blood pressure are lost, inserting central arterial, venous, and pulmonary artery catheters is essential to establish progression of shock accurately and to evaluate the client's response to therapy.*
- Measure and record intake and output (total output and urinary output) hourly. *A decrease in circulating blood volume with hypotension and the effect of the compensatory mechanisms associated with shock can cause renal failure. Urinary output of less than 30 mL per hour in an acutely ill adult indicates reduced renal blood flow.*
- Monitor bowel sounds, abdominal distention, and abdominal pain. *Decreased splanchnic blood flow reduces bowel motility and peristalsis; paralytic ileus may result.*

## Nursing Care of the Older Adult

### VARIATIONS IN ASSESSMENT FINDINGS—SHOCK

- Cardiac changes may include a thickened left ventricular wall, decreased elasticity of the myocardium, and more rigid valves. These changes result in a decreased stroke volume and cardiac output, thus decreasing responses to shock in general and increasing the risk of cardiogenic shock.
- Decreased arterial wall elasticity and vasomotor tone reduce the older adult's ability to respond to a decrease in oxygenation.

- Decreased elasticity and turgor of the skin make assessments of skin turgor more difficult.
- Previous medication and blood administration increase the risk of anaphylactic shock.
- Decreased immune system response increases the risk of septic shock.

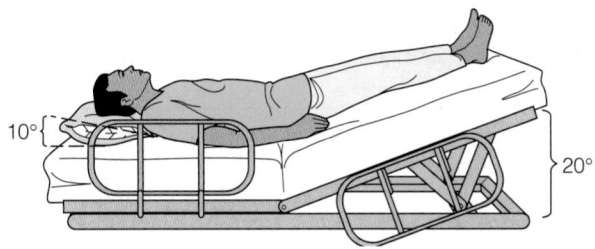

**Figure 6–9** ■ The client in shock should be positioned with the lower extremities elevated approximately 20 degrees (knees straight), trunk horizontal, and the head elevated about 10 degrees.

- Monitor for sudden sharp chest pain, dyspnea, cyanosis, anxiety, and restlessness. *Hemoconcentration and increased platelet aggregation may result in pulmonary emboli.*
- Maintain bed rest and provide (to the extent possible) a calm, quiet environment. Place in a supine position with the legs elevated to about 20 degrees, trunk flat, and head and shoulders elevated higher than the chest (Figure 6–9 ■). *Limiting activity and ensuring rest decreases the workload of the heart. The supine position with legs elevated increases venous return; however, this position should not be used for clients in cardiogenic shock. The Trendelenburg position is no longer recommended, because it causes the abdominal organs to press against the diaphragm (limiting respirations), decreases filling of the coronary arteries, and initiates aortic and carotid sinus reflexes.*

### Altered Tissue Perfusion

As shock progresses, diminished tissue perfusion causes ischemia and hypoxia of major organ systems. As shock worsens, blood flow and oxygenation of the lungs, heart, and brain are also impaired. Hypoxia and ischemia result from decreased tissue perfusion in the kidneys, brain, heart, lungs, gastrointestinal tract, and the periphery.

- Monitor skin color, temperature, turgor, and moisture. *Decreased tissue perfusion is evidenced by the skin's becoming pale, cool, and moist; as hemoglobin concentrations decrease, cyanosis occurs.*
- Monitor cardiopulmonary function by assessing/monitoring the following:
  - Blood pressure (by auscultation or by hemodynamic monitoring)
  - Rate and depth of respirations
  - Lung sounds
  - Pulse oximetry
  - Peripheral pulses (brachial, radial, dorsalis pedis, and posterior tibial); include presence, equality, rate, rhythm, and quality (If unable to palpate pulses, use a device such as a Doppler ultrasound flowmeter to assess peripheral arterial blood flow.)
  - Jugular vein distention
  - CVP measurements

*Baseline vital signs are necessary to determine trends in subsequent findings. As shock progresses, the blood pressure decreases, and the pulse becomes rapid, weak, and thready. As perfusion of the lungs decreases, crackles, wheezes, and dyspnea are commonly assessed. Capillary refill is prolonged, and peripheral pulses are weak or nonpalpable. Neck veins that cannot be seen when the client is in the supine position indicate decreased intravascular volume. CVP is an accurate means of determining fluid status in the client in shock; the findings will be low (5 to 15 cm of water is normal) in hypovolemic shock because of the decreased blood volume. (See Chapter 5 ∞ for a discussion of CVP.)*

- Monitor body temperature. *An elevated body temperature increases metabolic demands, depleting reserves of bodily energy. It also increases myocardial oxygen demand and may place the client with previous cardiac problems at even greater risk for hypoperfusion.*
- Monitor urinary output per Foley catheter hourly, using a urimeter. *Urine output is a reliable indicator of renal perfusion.*
- Assess mental status and level of consciousness. *The appropriateness of the client's behavior and responses reflects the adequacy of cerebral circulation. Restlessness and anxiety are common early in shock; in later stages, the client may become lethargic and progress to a comatose state. Altered levels of consciousness are the result of both cerebral hypoxia and the effects of acidosis on brain cells.*

### Anxiety

Many clients in hypovolemic shock have experienced some form of major trauma and may have life-threatening, multiple injuries. Following on-the-scene treatment, the client is usually admitted to the health care setting through the emergency department. Surgery may be required to treat injuries, followed by care in a critical care unit. Throughout this sequence of crisis events, treatment is invasive, and contact with family is minimal. Client and family responses to these situations of uncertainty, instability, and change include anxiety, fear, and powerlessness (see page 162). These responses are affected by age, developmental level, cultural and ethnic group, experience with illness and the health care system, and support systems.

- Assess the cause(s) of the anxiety, and manipulate the environment to provide periods of rest. *Reducing stimuli that cause anxiety is calming and facilitates rest, which is necessary in the client at risk for bleeding.*
- Administer prescribed pain medications on a regular basis. *Pain precipitates and/or aggravates anxiety.*
- Provide interventions to increase comfort and reduce restlessness:
  - Maintain a clean environment.
  - Provide skin and oral care.
  - Monitor the effectiveness of ventilation or oxygen therapy.
  - Eliminate all nonessential activities.
  - Remain with the client during procedures.
  - Speak slowly and calmly, using short sentences.
  - Use touch to provide support.

*Unfamiliar sounds, sights, and odors can increase anxiety. Damp skin or a dry mouth increases discomfort. Inadequate gas exchange with a decrease in oxygen or an increase in carbon dioxide in the blood may cause the client to experience a "feeling of doom." Activity increases the body's need*

## Nursing Research

### Evidence-Based Practice for Care of ICU Clients

The purpose of this study (Hupcey, 2000) was to describe the psychosocial needs of critically ill clients and behaviors of family members, friends, and ICU staff who helped or hindered meeting those needs. Data were collected by interviewing 45 adult clients who were in a medical or surgical ICU for a minimum of 3 days, and grounded theory methodology was used to analyze and conceptualize the experiences of the patients. A model of the psychosocial needs of this population was developed around the overarching need of all subjects in this study to feel safe. This core variable encompassed the four categories of identified needs: knowing, regaining control, hoping, and trusting.

- Knowing what was happening provided reassurance and helped the subjects "get through a terrible experience." Those who did not know or understand refused treatments, felt frightened, and even fought with staff.
- Regaining control emerged from an initial sense of total loss of control. Loss of control was frustrating and led to feelings of insecurity.
- Maintaining hope was essential to not giving up and survival. Sources of hope included family members, friends, staff, and religious beliefs.
- Trusting the ICU staff was essential to feel safe.

### IMPLICATIONS FOR NURSING

Nurses in the ICU can provide interventions to make clients feel safe. Nurses can incorporate family members as part of the team to provide support and can encourage the use of hospital or individual resources of spiritual strength. Hope can be assessed, and interventions designed to meet individualized needs. Control and independence can be fostered by having clients make decisions about such areas as control of lights and television. Based on the findings of this study, feeling safe is also fostered in ICU clients when nurses are technically competent and genuinely caring. In addition, nurses need to be aware that clients require frequent and repeated explanations and reorientations.

### Critical Thinking in Client Care

1. Make a list of the barriers to feeling safe for clients who are in the ICU. Consider the physical environment, the client's physical condition, and factors such as medications. Do you believe any of these barriers could be changed? If not, why not?
2. Consider the verbal and nonverbal methods of demonstrating genuine caring. Conversely, think about the verbal and nonverbal ways that health care providers may not demonstrate caring. If you were a nurse manager in an ICU unit, how could you encourage caring?
3. Considering the information from this study, what level of health care provider would you delegate to provide care for a 75-year-old woman who has had a stroke and is unable to verbally communicate? How would your decision differ if it were a 55-year-old woman who had suffered serious head trauma in an automobile crash (driving while intoxicated)?

---

*for oxygen. Listening and touch provide support in an environment in which the client often feels alone and abandoned. Severe anxiety interferes with the ability to understand others and to respond appropriately.*

- Provide support for the client and family:
  - Provide time, space, and privacy for family members.

- Allow family members access to the client when feasible.
- Encourage the expression of feelings and concerns. Provide anticipatory guidance to prepare for recovery or death and to support realistic hope.
- Acknowledge the beliefs, values, and expectations of the client and family.

---

### CHART 6–2  NANDA, NIC, AND NOC LINKAGES

## The Client Experiencing Shock

| NURSING DIAGNOSES | NURSING INTERVENTIONS | NURSING OUTCOMES |
|---|---|---|
| • Ineffective Tissue Perfusion | • Cardiac Care: Acute<br>• Shock Management<br>• Acid-Base Monitoring<br>• Fluid Management<br>• Hypovolemia Management<br>• Hemodynamic Regulation<br>• Vital Signs Monitoring | • Tissue Perfusion: Cardiac<br>• Electrolyte and Acid-Base Balance<br>• Fluid Balance<br>• Tissue Perfusion: Peripheral<br>• Vital Sign Status |
| • Decreased Cardiac Output | • Cardiac Care<br>• Hemodynamic Regulation | • Circulatory Pump Effectiveness<br>• Circulatory Status<br>• Tissue Perfusion: Abdominal Organs<br>• Tissue Perfusion: Peripheral<br>• Vital Signs Status |

*Note. Data from Nursing Outcomes Classification (NOC) by M. Johnson & M. Maas (Eds.), 1997, St. Louis: Mosby; Nursing Diagnoses: Definitions & Classification 2001–2002 by North American Nursing Diagnosis Association, 2001, Philadelphia: NANDA; Nursing Interventions Classification (NIC) by J.C. McCloskey & G. M. Bulechek (Eds.), 2000, St. Louis: Mosby. Reprinted by permission.*

*Allowing the family access to the client reduces anxiety and gives both the client and the family some feeling of control. If prognosis is poor, access and involvement allow the family to begin the grieving process. If recovery is expected, contact provides the client and family with a feeling of hope. Supporting the client and family facilitates concrete problem solving, promotes acceptance of the illness and its implications, and helps them begin to establish ways of managing the illness experience.*

- Provide information about the current setting to both the client and family; give the family information about available resources (such as pastoral care, social services, temporary housing, meals). *Knowing what to expect and how to control the environment to meet basic needs reduces anxiety.*

## Using NANDA, NIC, and NOC

Chart 6–2 shows links between NANDA nursing diagnoses, NIC, and NOC when caring for the client who is experiencing shock.

## Home Care

Home care for the client who has experienced shock is highly individualized, depending on the cause and the illness or injury that caused shock. Therefore, topics for consideration are not included in this section.

---

## Nursing Care Plan
## A Client with Septic Shock

Huang Mei Lan is a 43-year-old unmarried female who lives alone in a major West Coast city. Ms. Huang came to America 15 years ago from China and now speaks English well. Her family still lives in China. She worked in a neighborhood sewing shop until 3 years ago, when she was diagnosed with breast cancer. Her treatment included mastectomy of the affected breast and follow-up chemotherapy.

Last month, Ms. Huang experienced a recurrence of cancer in the lymph glands of the affected side. Surgery to remove the glands was performed and chemotherapy started. Ms. Huang has a central line, a urinary catheter, and a surgical incision. She is underweight, weak, and depressed. Although she has multiple physical problems, she never complains or asks for any kind of medication.

### ASSESSMENT

Ms. Huang's primary nurse, Robert O'Brien, enters her room early in the morning to make an initial assessment. He finds Ms. Huang huddled in the middle of the bed, shivering violently. Her vital signs are T 104° F, P 110, R 30, and BP 106/66. Her skin is hot, dry, and flushed with poor turgor. She is alert and oriented, but is restless and appears anxious. Ms. Huang states she is nauseated and suddenly begins vomiting and is incontinent of liquid stool. Laboratory data indicate leukocytosis, respiratory alkalosis, and reduced platelet count. Blood cultures, as well as cultures of Ms. Huang's sputum, urine, and wound drainage, are conducted. She is diagnosed as having septic shock.

Hetastarch is ordered per intravenous line, and intravenous broad-spectrum antibiotics are begun until the organism and its portal of entry can be determined. Despite treatment, Ms. Huang's condition worsens. Her blood pressure continues to drop, her skin becomes cool and cyanotic, and she begins to have periods of disorientation. She is transferred to the critical care unit. As she is being prepared for the transfer, she begins to cry and asks, "Am I going to die?"

### DIAGNOSES

- *Deficient fluid volume* related to vomiting, diarrhea, high fever, and shift of intravascular volume to interstitial spaces
- *Ineffective breathing pattern* related to rapid respirations and progression of septic shock
- *Ineffective tissue perfusion* related to progression of septic shock with decreased cardiac output, hypotension, and massive vasodilatation
- *Anxiety* related to feelings that illness is worsening and is potentially life threatening, and the transfer to the critical care unit

### EXPECTED OUTCOMES

- Maintain adequate circulating blood volume.
- Regain and maintain blood gas parameters within normal limits.
- Regain and maintain stable hemodynamic levels.
- Verbalize increased ability to cope with stressors.

### PLANNING AND IMPLEMENTATION

- Monitor neurologic status, including mental status and level of consciousness.
- Monitor cardiovascular status, including arterial blood pressure; rate, rhythm, and quality of pulses; central venous pressure; pulmonary artery pressure; and cardiac output.
- Monitor color and character of skin.
- Monitor results of arterial blood gases, blood counts, clotting times, and platelet counts.
- Monitor respiratory status, including respiratory rate, rhythm, and breath sounds.
- Monitor body temperature every 2 hours.
- Monitor urinary output hourly, reporting any output of less than 30 mL per hour.
- Explain procedures and provide comfort measures (oral care, skin care, turning, positioning).

### EVALUATION

Despite intensive nursing and medical care, Ms. Huang's condition remains critical. The interventions are continued.

### Critical Thinking in the Nursing Process

1. Vasopressors may be used in the treatment of septic shock. Explain the rationale for their use.
2. While monitoring Ms. Huang's arterial blood gases, the nurse notes that her $Pao_2$ is < 60 mmHg and her $PaCo_2$ is > 50. What do these findings indicate, and why have they occurred?
3. Ms. Huang has been given large amounts of colloids intravenously. Hemodynamic monitoring indicates a higher than normal CVP and pulmonary artery pressure. What do these findings indicate? What physical assessments would you make to confirm the changes?

See Evaluating Your Response in Appendix C.

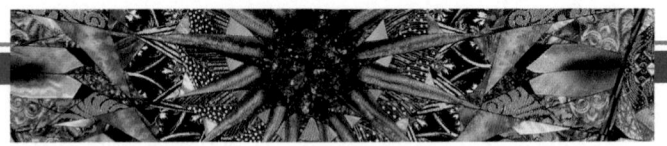

## EXPLORE MediaLink

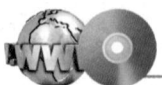

NCLEX review questions, case studies, care plan activities, MediaLink applications, and other interactive resources for this chapter can be found on the Companion Website at www.prenhall.com/lemone.

Click on Chapter 6 to select the activities for this chapter. For animations, video clips, more NCLEX review questions, and an audio glossary, access the Student CD-ROM accompanying this textbook.

## TEST YOURSELF

1. What is the most common mechanical source of injury in adults of all ages?

   a. Gunshot wounds
   b. Fire
   c. Drowning
   d. Motor vehicles

2. Severe facial injuries, such as those resulting from going through a windshield, increase the risk for all of the following. What would you assess first?

   a. Airway obstruction
   b. Hemorrhage
   c. Contusions
   d. Fractures

3. Which on-the-scene intervention would be a priority?

   a. Determine cause of injury
   b. Assess airway patency

   c. Assess peripheral capillary refill
   d. Palpate for internal hemorrhage

4. You are monitoring blood administration to a trauma victim in shock. Which of the following assessments indicate a dangerous transfusion reaction?

   a. Red raised areas (wheals) on the skin that itch
   b. An increase in body temperature by 3°
   c. Decreasing blood pressure and dyspnea
   d. Increasing blood pressure and pulse

5. What type of shock causes widespread vasodilatation and decreased peripheral resistance?

   a. Cardiogenic shock
   b. Septic shock
   c. Hypovolemic shock
   d. Obstructive shock

See Test Yourself answers in Appendix C.

## BIBLIOGRAPHY

A crash course in skin trauma. (1998). *Homecare Education Management, 3*(2), 24–25.

American College of Surgeons. Committee on Trauma. (1997). *Advanced trauma life support manual.* Chicago: ACS.

Asuncion, M., & Koushik, V. (2000). Shock states in the elderly40. *Clinical Geriatriacs, 8*(8), 40–42, 45–48.

Bucher, L., & Melander, S. (1999). *Critical care nursing.* Philadelphia: Saunders.

Carpenito, L. (2000). *Nursing diagnoses: Application to clinical practice* (8th ed.). Philadelphia: Lippincott.

Champion, H., Copes, W., Gann, D., Gennarelli, T., & Flanagan, M. (1989). A revision of the trauma score. *Journal of Trauma, 29*(5), 624.

Craven, A. (1998). Trauma. In C. Hudak, B. Gall, & P. Morton (Eds.), *Critical care nursing: A holistic approach* (7th ed.) (pp. 973–990). Philadelphia: Lippincott-Raven.

DeJong, M. (1997). Emergency! Cardiogenic shock. *American Journal of Nursing, 97*(6), 40–41.

Emergency Nurses Association. (1992). *Trauma resource document.* Park Ridge, IL: ENA.

Fitzpatrick, L., & Fitzpatrick, T. (1997). Blood transfusions: Keeping your patient safe. *Nursing 97, 27*(8), 34–42.

Hupcey, J. (2000). Feeling safe: The psychosocial needs of ICU patients. *Journal of Nursing Scholarship, 32*(4), 361–367.

Huston, C. (1996). Emergency! Hemolytic transfusion reaction. *American Journal of Nursing, 96*(3), 47.

Johnson, M., & Maas, M. (Eds.). (1997). *Nursing outcomes classification (NOC).* St. Louis: Mosby.

Jordan, K. S. (2000). Fluid resuscitation in acutely injured patients. *Journal of Intravenous Nursing, 23*(2), 81–87.

Labovich, T. (1997). Transfusion therapy: Nursing implications. *Clinical Journal of Oncology Nursing, 1*(3), 61–72.

Liepert, D., & Rosenthal, M. (2000). Management of cardiogenic, hypovolemic, and hyperdynamic shock. *Current Reviews for Perianesthesia Nurses, 22*(9), 1–3, 113, back cover.

Lisanti, P. (1996). Emergency! Anaphylaxis. *American Journal of Nursing, 96*(11), 51.

McCloskey, J. C., & Bulechek, G. M. (Eds.). (2000). *Nursing interventions classification (NIC).* St. Louis: Mosby.

McConnell, E. (1997). Safely administering a blood transfusion. *Nursing 97, 27*(6), 30.

McCracken, L. (2001). The forensic ABC's of trauma care. *Canadian Nurse, 97*(3), 30–33.

McKenny, L., & Salerno, E. (1998). *Pharmacology in nursing* (20th ed.). St. Louis: Mosby.

Mower-Wade, D., Bartley, M., & Chiari-Allwein, J. (2001). How to respond to shock. *Dimensions of Critical Care Nursing, 20*(2), 22–27.

North American Nursing Diagnosis Association. (2001). *Nursing diagnoses: Definitions & classification 2001–2002.* Philadelphia: NANDA.

Porth, C. (2002). *Pathophysiology: Concepts of altered health states* (6th ed.). Philadelphia: Lippincott.

Sole, M., Lamborn, M., & Hartshorn, J. (2001). *Introduction to critical care nursing* (3rd ed.). Philadelphia: Saunders.

Speck, P., & Whalley, A. (1996). Domestic violence: Role of the RN. *Tennessee Nurse, 59*(3), 27, 31.

Stamatos, C., Sorensen, P., & Tefler, K. (1996). Meeting the challenge of the older trauma patient. *American Journal of Nursing, 96*(5), 40–47.

Stoll, E. (2001). Sepsis and septic shock. *Clinical Journal of Oncology Nursing, 5*(2), 71–72.

Tierney, L., McPhee, S., & Papadakis, M. (Eds.). (2001). *Current diagnosis & treatment* (40th ed.). Stamford, CT: Appleton & Lange.

Waldsburger, W. J. (1999). Massive transfusion in trauma. *AACN Clinical Issues: Advanced Practice in Acute & Critical Care, 10*(1), 69–84.

Watts, D., Abrahams, E., MacMillan, C., Sanat, J., Silver, R., VanGorder, S., Waller, M., & York, D. (1998). Insult after injury: Pressure ulcers in trauma patients. *Orthopaedic Nursing, 17*(4), 84–91.

Wilson, B., Shannon, M., & Stang, C. (2001). *Nursing drug guide 2001.* Upper Saddle River, NJ: Prentice Hall.

# CHAPTER 7

# Nursing Care of Clients Having Surgery

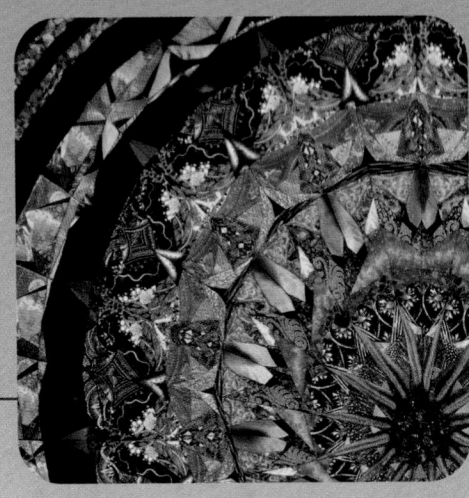

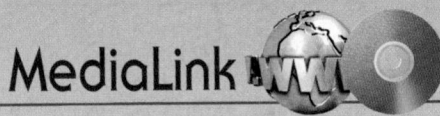

## www.prenhall.com/lemone

Additional resources for this chapter can be found on the Student CD-ROM accompanying this textbook, and on the Companion Website at www.prenhall.com/lemone. Click on Chapter 7 to select the activities for this chapter.

**CD-ROM**
- Audio Glossary
- NCLEX Review

**Companion Website**
- More NCLEX Review
- Case Study
    The Circulating Nurse
- Care Plan Activity
    Providing Postoperative Care
- MediaLink Application
    Anesthesia and Outpatient Surgery

## LEARNING OUTCOMES

After completing this chapter, you will be able to:

- Describe the various classifications of surgical procedures.

- Identify diagnostic tests used in the perioperative period.

- Describe nursing implications for medications prescribed for the surgical client.

- Provide appropriate nursing care for the client in the perioperative, intraoperative, and postoperative phases of surgery.

- Identify variations in perioperative care for the older adult.

- Describe principles of pain management specific to acute postoperative pain control.

- Discuss the differences and similarities between outpatient and inpatient surgery.

- Use the nursing process as a framework for providing individualized care for the client undergoing surgery.

TABLE 7-1 Classification of Surgical Procedures

|  | Classification | Function | Examples |
|---|---|---|---|
| **Purpose** | Diagnostic | Determine or confirm a diagnosis | Breast biopsy, bronchoscopy |
|  | Ablative | Remove diseased tissue, organ, or extremity | Appendectomy, amputation |
|  | Constructive | Build tissue/organs that are absent (congenital anomalies) | Repair of cleft palate |
|  | Reconstructive | Rebuild tissue/organ that has been damaged | Skin graft after a burn, total joint replacement |
|  | Palliative | Alleviate symptoms of a disease (not curative) | Bowel resection in client with terminal cancer |
|  | Transplant | Replace organs/tissue to restore function | Heart, lung, liver, kidney transplant |
| **Risk Factor** | Minor | Minimal physical assault with minimal risk | Removal of skin lesions, dilation and curettage (D&C), cataract extraction |
|  | Major | Extensive physical assault and/or serious risk | Transplant, total joint replacement, cholecystectomy, colostomy, nephrectomy |
| **Urgency** | Elective | Suggested, though no foreseen ill effects if postponed | Cosmetic surgery, cataract surgery, bunionectomy |
|  | Urgent | Necessary to be performed within 1 to 2 days | Heart bypass surgery, amputation resulting from gangrene, fractured hip |
|  | Emergency | Performed immediately | Obstetric emergencies, bowel obstruction, ruptured aneurysm, life-threatening trauma |

Surgery is an invasive medical procedure performed to diagnose or treat illness, injury, or deformity. Although surgery is a medical treatment, the nurse assumes an active role in caring for the client before, during, and after surgery. **Collaborative care** and **independent nursing care** together prevent complications and promote the surgical client's optimal recovery.

**Perioperative nursing** is a specialized area of practice. It incorporates the three phases of the surgical experience: preoperative, intraoperative, and postoperative. The **preoperative phase** begins when the decision for surgery is made and ends when the client is transferred to the operating room. The **intraoperative phase** begins with the client's entry into the operating room and ends with admittance to the postanesthesia care unit (PACU), or recovery room. The **postoperative phase** begins with the client's admittance to the PACU and ends with the client's complete recovery from the surgical intervention.

Surgical procedures can be classified according to purpose, risk factor, and urgency (Table 7–1). Based on this information, nursing care can be individualized to best meet client needs.

Although the perioperative nurse works in collaboration with other health care professionals to identify and meet the client's needs, the perioperative nurse has the primary responsibility and accountability for nursing care of the client undergoing surgery.

## SETTINGS FOR SURGERY

Surgical patients may be inpatients or outpatients. The complexity of the surgery and recovery and the expected disposition of the client following the surgery are the major differences. Sometimes outpatients, clients intending to be discharged home immediately, are admitted to the hospital. Cataract removal with or without lens implants, hernia repairs,

tubal ligations, vasectomies, dilation and curettage (D&C), hemorrhoidectomies, and biopsies are commonly performed outpatient surgeries.

Inpatient and outpatient surgeries are performed in the same operating suites in most hospitals. There are also **freestanding outpatient surgical facilities**, which are not physically or financially connected to a hospital. Surgeons may practice in both hospital and freestanding surgical facilities. The number of outpatient surgeries has rapidly grown in the past decade as part of the effort to contain the high costs of surgery. Moreover, increasingly complex surgeries on clients with complicated medical problems are now commonly performed on an outpatient basis. This increase in number of procedures and acuity level of the clients has presented a challenge to the perioperative nurse, the patient, and the family.

Outpatient surgery offers several advantages:

- Decreased cost to the client, hospital, and insuring agency
- Reduced risk of hospital-acquired infection
- Less interruption in the client's and family's routine
- Possible reduction in time lost from work and/or other responsibilities
- Less physiologic stress to the client and family

Outpatient surgery also presents some disadvantages:

- Less time for the nurse to establish rapport with client and family
- Less time for the nurse to assess, evaluate, and teach the client and family
- Lack of opportunity for the nurse to assess for the risk of postoperative complications that may occur after discharge

Many similarities exist between nursing care of the inpatient and outpatient surgical clients. Physical care is provided in much the same manner in the preoperative, intraoperative, and postoperative phases of surgery. The major differences lie in the degree of teaching and emotional support that must be provided for outpatient surgical clients and their families. In addition to the physiologic insult of surgery, the outpatient surgical client must cope with the additional stress of needing to learn a great deal of information in a short span of time. The nurse teaches the client and family in both the preoperative and postoperative periods to enable the client to perform self-care following discharge. More extensive teaching and emotional support is mandated as clients requiring more complex surgical procedures and experiencing more complicated health problems undergo outpatient surgery.

**PRACTICE ALERT** *Clients having outpatient surgery should wear or bring clothing that will be easy to put on after surgery and accommodate any dressings or appliances. Furthermore, despite being NPO, clients must bring any medications they regularly use (especially those prescribed by other providers), such as steroids, antibiotics, anticoagulants, antivirals, diuretics, oral contraceptives, hypotensives, cardiotonics, hypoglycemics, asthma medications, seizure medications, and analgesics. Clients should consult with the surgeon and anesthesiologist before taking these medications.* ■

Following outpatient surgery, the client is discharged after meeting the institution's criteria:

- Vital signs are stable.
- Client is able to stand and begin to walk without dizziness or nausea.
- Pain is controlled or alleviated.
- Client is able to urinate.
- Client is oriented.
- Client demonstrates understanding of postoperative instructions.

## LEGAL REQUIREMENTS

It is the responsibility of the surgeon who performs the procedure to obtain the client's consent for care. The surgeon should discuss the above information with the client and family in language they can understand. **Informed consent** (or an **operative permit**) is a legal document required for certain diagnostic procedures or therapeutic measures, including surgery. This legal document protects the client, nurse, physician, and health care facility. Informed consent includes the following information:

- Need for the procedure in relation to the diagnoses
- Description and purpose of the proposed procedure
- Possible benefits and potential risks
- Likelihood of a successful outcome
- Alternative treatments or procedures available
- Anticipated risks should the procedure not be performed
- Physician's advice as to what is needed
- Right to refuse treatment or withdraw consent

Ideally, the nurse should be present when the information is provided. Later, the nurse can discuss the information with the client and family, if necessary. If the client has questions or concerns that were not discussed or made clear, or if the nurse questions the client's understanding, the surgeon is responsible for supplying further information. If these situations arise, the nurse should contact the surgeon before having the client give informed consent. Following a thorough discussion of the informed consent, the nurse witnesses the client's signature on the informed consent form (Figure 7–1 ■ ). The nurse also signs the form, indicating that the correct person is signing the form and that the client was alert and aware of what was being signed.

## SURGICAL RISK FACTORS

Prior to planning and implementing care for the surgical client, the nurse must first assess the client's needs and the factors that may increase the risks associated with surgery. The type of surgical procedure directs the assessment and interventions planned by the nurse. However, a complete assessment is also necessary to identify *risk factors* and to determine the client's overall health status. Table 7–2 lists common risk factors for the client undergoing surgery, and the related nursing interventions and implications. For example, when a client is admitted for surgery on the right knee, it should be of concern to the nurse if this client has diabetes, smokes 1.5 packs of cigarettes per day, has numbness in the right foot, and takes insulin. This information should be incorporated into a care plan, using appropriate nursing diagnoses and interventions to meet all of the client's needs and assist the client toward full postoperative recovery.

Interpreting and responding to identified risk factors requires nursing judgment. It is important to bring information to the attention of the surgeons and anesthesiologists prior to surgery, so necessary modifications can be made for the patient.

**PRACTICE ALERT** *Remind diabetic clients that the stress of surgery increases rather than decreases blood sugar. Coordinate insulin injection and/or hypoglycemic medication with the client, surgeon, and anesthesiologist.* ■

## COLLABORATIVE CARE

The client undergoing surgery receives care from a number of health care providers. This collaborative approach focuses on placing the client in the best possible health status before, during, and after surgery.

### Diagnostic Tests

Diagnostic tests performed prior to surgery provide baseline data or detect problems that may place the client at additional risk during and after surgery. Because of the trend toward shortened hospital stays, many diagnostic studies and procedures are performed in a preadmission clinic within a week prior to elective surgery.

M.R. # _____

**Informed Consent to Operation, Administraton of Anesthetics,**
**and to the Rendering of Other Medical Services**

Saint
Francis
Medical
Center

**1.** I do hereby authorize and direct _____ M.D./D.O./D.D.S., my physician, and/or such associates or assistants of his choice, to perform the following operation or procedure:

_____

_____

upon _____ (patient's name). I understand that the above named physician and his associates or assistants are employed by me and will be occupied solely with performing such operation or procedure.

**2.** The nature of the operation or procedure has been explained to me and no warranty or guarantee has been made as to result or cure. I have been advised that additional surgical and/or medical procedures or treatment may be deemed necessary during the course of the operation or procedure consented hereto, and I fully consent to such additional procedures and treatment which, in the opinion of my physician, are deemed necessary or desirable for the well being of the patient. The possible risks and complications of the operation or procedure have been explained to me. The physician has explained to me the above medical terminology and I satisfactorily understand the type of operation/procedure.

**3.** I hereby authorize and direct the above named physician and/or his associates or assistants or those working under his direction to provide for _____ (patient's name) such additional services as he or they may deem reasonable and necessary, including, but not limited to, the administration and maintenance of anesthesia, blood or blood derivatives, and the performance of services involving pathology and radiology and I hereby consent thereto. The possible risks and complications of blood transfusions and the administration of anesthetics have also been explained to me.

**4.** I understand also that the persons in attendance at such operation or procedure for the purpose of administering anesthesia, and the radiologists in attendance at such operation or procedure for the purpose of performing radiological (x-ray) service are not the agents, servants or employees of St. Francis Medical Center nor of any physician, but are independent health care providers who are employed by me in the same way that my surgeon and physician are employed by me.

**5.** I hereby authorize the Medical Center pathologist or personnel to use their discretion in the disposal of any severed tissue or member.

**6.** I hereby grant permission for St. Francis Medical Center to obtain clinical photographs for educational purposes or for my patient record as deemed necessary by my physician.

**7.** *The exception to this consent:* (If none, write "none".) _____

_____ and I assume full responsibility for these exceptions.

_____     _____
PATIENT'S SIGNATURE                                                  DATE

*If the patient is a minor or incompetent or is unable to sign, the following must be completed:*

I hereby certify that I am the (relationship) _____ of the above named patient

who is unable to sign because _____ ,

and I am fully authorized to give the consent herein granted.

_____     _____
SIGNATURE                                                                  DATE

_____     _____
WITNESSED BY/date                                              WITNESSED BY/date

*If signed in the physician's office, the following MUST be completed by the Medical Center.*

_____     _____
REVIEWED BY (patient name) /date                     WITNESSED BY /date

**Figure 7–1** ■ Informed consent form.

TABLE 7–2    Nursing Implications for Surgical Risk Factors

| Factor | Associated Risk | Nursing Implications |
|---|---|---|
| Advanced age | Older adults have age-related changes that affect physiologic, cognitive, and psychosocial responses to the stress of surgery; decrease tolerance of general anesthesia and postoperative medications; and delay wound healing. | Selected nursing interventions are summarized in Table 7–6. |
| Obesity | The obese client is at increased risk for delayed wound healing, wound dehiscence, infection, pneumonia, atelectasis, thrombophlebitis, arrhythmias, and heart failure. | Promote weight reduction if time permits. Monitor closely for wound, pulmonary, and cardiovascular complications postoperatively. Encourage coughing, turning, and diaphragmatic breathing exercises and early ambulation. |
| Malnutrition | Reserves may not be sufficient to allow the body to respond satisfactorily to the physical assault of surgery; organ failure and shock may result. Increased metabolic demands may result in poor wound healing and infection. | With the physician and dietitian, promote weight gain by providing a well-balanced diet high in calories, protein, and vitamin C. Administer total parenteral nutrition intravenously, nutritional supplements, and tube feedings as prescribed. Daily weights and calorie counts also may be ordered. |
| Dehydration/ electrolyte imbalance | Depending on the degree of dehydration and/or type of electrolyte imbalance, cardiac dysrhythmia or heart failure may occur. Liver and renal failure may also result. | Administer intravenous fluids as ordered. Monitor I&O. Monitor client for evidence of electrolyte imbalance (see Chapter 5). 🔗 |
| Cardiovascular disorders | Presence of cardiovascular disease increases the risk of hemorrhage and shock, hypotension, thrombophlebitis, pulmonary embolism, stroke (especially in the older client), and fluid volume overload. | Diligently monitor vital signs, especially pulse rate, regularity, and rhythm, and general condition of the client. Closely monitor fluid intake (oral and parenteral) to prevent circulatory overload.<br><br>Assess skin color. Assess for chest pain, lung congestion, and peripheral edema. Observe for signs of hypoxia, and administer oxygen as ordered. Early postoperative ambulation and leg exercises reduce the risk of vascular problems, such as thrombophlebitis and pulmonary embolism. |
| Respiratory disorders | Respiratory complications such as bronchitis, atelectasis, and pneumonia are some of the most common and serious postoperative complications. Respiratory depression from general anesthesia and acid-base imbalance may also occur. Clients with pulmonary disease are more at risk for developing these complications. | Closely monitor respirations, pulse, and breath sounds. Also assess for hypoxia, dyspnea, lung congestion, and chest pain. Encourage coughing, turning, and diaphragmatic breathing exercises and early postoperative ambulation. Encourage the client to quit smoking or at least to reduce the number of cigarettes smoked. |
| Diabetes mellitus | Diabetes causes an increased risk for fluctuating blood glucose levels, which can lead to life-threatening hypoglycemia or ketoacidosis. Diabetes also increases the risk for cardiovascular disease, delayed wound healing, and wound infection. | Monitor the client closely for signs and symptoms of hypoglycemia and hyperglycemia. Monitor blood glucose levels every 4 hours or as ordered. Administer insulin as prescribed. Encourage intake of food at the designated meal and snack times. |
| Renal and liver dysfunction | The client with renal or liver dysfunction may poorly tolerate general anesthesia, have fluid/electrolyte and acid-base imbalances, decreased metabolism and excretion of drugs, increased risk for hemorrhage, and delayed wound healing. | Monitor for fluid volume overload, I&O, and response to medication. Evaluate closely for drug side effects and evidence of acidosis or alkalosis. |
| Alcoholism | The client may be malnourished and experience delirium tremens (acute withdrawal symptoms). More general anesthesia may be required. Hemorrhage and delayed wound healing can result from liver damage and poor nutritional status. | Monitor closely for signs of delirium tremens. Encourage well-balanced diet. Monitor for wound complications. Administer supplemental nutrients parenterally as ordered. |

(continued on page 170)

TABLE 7–2    Nursing Implications for Surgical Risk Factors (continued)

| Factor | Associated Risk | Nursing Implications |
|--------|-----------------|----------------------|
| Nicotine use | Cigarette smokers are at increased risk for respiratory complications such as pneumonia, atelectasis, and bronchitis because of increased mucous secretions and a decreased ability to expel them. | Ideally, the client should quit smoking. Be supportive of the client, and monitor closely for respiratory difficulties. Coughing, turning, and diaphragmatic breathing exercises with early ambulation are very important. Increase daily fluid intake to 2500–3000 mL (unless contraindicated) to help liquefy respiratory secretions to aid expectoration. |
| Adolescence | Diversity in age, and physical, cognitive, and psychological maturation makes preparation for surgery vary in content and inclusion of significant others. Increased need for control, privacy, and peer interaction poses special challenges in the acute care setting. | Adapt assessment and interventions to the development level of individual clients, involving them in preparation and care to the extent possible. Allow for regressive and independent behavior including rejection of adult support. |
| Medications | Anesthesia interaction with some medications can cause respiratory difficulties, hypotension, and circulatory collapse. Other medications can produce side effects that may increase surgical risk. | Inform the anesthesiologist of all prescribed or over-the-counter medications. |
| Anticoagulants (including aspirin) | May cause intraoperative and postoperative hemorrhage. | Monitor for bleeding. Assess PT/PTT values. |
| Diuretics (particularly thiazides) | May lead to fluid and electrolyte imbalances, producing altered cardiovascular response and respiratory depression. | Monitor I&O and electrolytes. Assess cardiovascular and respiratory status. |
| Antihypertensives (particularly phenothiazines) | Increase the hypotensive effects of anesthesia. | Closely monitor blood pressure. |
| Antidepressants (particularly monoamine oxidase inhibitors) | Increase the hypotensive effects of anesthesia. | Closely monitor blood pressure. |
| Antibiotics (particularly the "mycin" group) | May cause apnea and respiratory paralysis. | Monitor respirations. |
| Herbal supplements | Some may prolong the effects of anesthesia. Others may increase the risks of bleeding or raise blood pressure. | Inquire about the use of herbs or other dietary supplements. These should be discontinued at least 1 week before surgery. |

Complete blood counts, electrolyte studies, coagulation studies, and urinalysis are the most commonly performed preoperative laboratory tests. Table 7–3 discusses the significance and nursing implications of abnormal findings for these common tests. Additional diagnostic tests may be performed as the history and physical findings indicate. For example, if the client has a low hemoglobin and hematocrit, and significant blood loss during surgery is anticipated, then the surgeon may order a type and crossmatch of the client's blood for a possible transfusion.

In addition to laboratory tests, elderly clients or those with risk factors related to heart and lung function typically have a chest X-ray. This radiologic procedure provides baseline information about the size, shape, and condition of the heart and lungs. Pulmonary complications such as lung disease, tuberculosis, calcification, infiltration, or pneumonia may require that surgery be postponed to allow the client to

undergo further evaluation or treatment. If findings are abnormal and the surgery cannot be postponed, information from the chest X-ray study can be used to determine the safest form of anesthesia.

Another commonly performed preoperative diagnostic procedure is the electrocardiogram (ECG). This test is ordered routinely on clients undergoing general anesthesia when they are over 40 years of age or have cardiovascular disease. The ECG provides data for evaluation about either new or preexisting cardiac conditions. The client's surgery may be cancelled or postponed if a life-threatening cardiac condition is discovered.

In addition to the chest X-ray study and ECG, other diagnostic tests may be performed preoperatively to gather further assessment data. For example, for clients who have chronic obstructive pulmonary disease, pulmonary function studies often are performed to determine the extent of respiratory dysfunction. This information guides the anesthesiologist before

TABLE 7-3   Laboratory Tests for Perioperative Assessment

| Test | Significance of Increased Values | Significance of Decreased Values | Nursing Implications |
|---|---|---|---|
| Hemoglobin (Hgb) and hematocrit (Hct) | Dehydration, excessive fluid plasma loss, polycythemia vera | Fluid overload, excessive blood loss, anemia | Monitor oxygenation, intake and output (I&O), and vital signs; assess for bleeding. |
| White blood cell (WBC) count | Infectious/inflammatory processes, leukemia | Immune deficiencies | Monitor for signs of inflammation; monitor drainage, temperature, and pulse. Use strict universal precautions. |
| Platelet count | Malignancies, polycythemia vera | Clotting deficiency disorders, chemotherapy | If decreased, assess for bleeding at incision sites and drainage tubes, and assess for hematomas. |
| Carbon dioxide ($CO_2$) | Emphysema, chronic bronchitis, asthma, pneumonia, respiratory acidosis, vomiting, nasogastric suctioning | Metabolic acidosis, hyperventilation | Monitor respiratory status and arterial blood gases (ABGs). |
| Electrolytes Potassium ($K^+$) | Kidney dysfunction, dehydration, suctioning | Side effects of diuretics, vomiting, NG suctioning | Monitor $K^+$ level, cardiac and neurologic function, and preoperative diuretic therapy. |
| Sodium ($Na^+$) | Kidney dysfunction, normal saline-containing intravenous fluids | Side effects of diuretics, vomiting, NG suctioning | Monitor $Na^+$ level and I&O; assess for peripheral edema and effects of perioperative diuretic therapy. |
| Chloride ($Cl^-$) | Kidney dysfunction, dehydration, alkalosis | Side effects of diuretics, vomiting, NG suctioning | Monitor $Cl^-$ level and I&O; assess for peripheral edema and perioperative diuretic therapy. |
| Prothrombin time (protime, or PT) and partial thromboplastin time (PTT) | Defect in mechanism for blood clotting, anticoagulant therapy (aspirin, heparin, warfarin), side effect of other drugs affecting clotting time | Hypercoagulability of the blood may lead to thrombus formation in the veins | If clotting time is elevated, monitor PT/PTT values. Assess for bleeding at incision site and drainage tubes and for hematomas. If clotting time is decreased, monitor for thrombus formation (pulmonary emboli, thrombophlebitis), and evaluate PT and PTT values. |
| Urinalysis | Varied | Varied | Used to detect abnormal substances (e.g., protein, glucose, red blood cells, or bacteria) in the urine. Notify surgeon if abnormalities are detected. |

and during surgery in choosing the type of anesthetic to be used, and it guides the surgeon and nursing staff in the recovery phase.

## Medications

The client having surgery receives medications before, during, and after surgery to achieve specific therapeutic outcomes. Traditionally, all medication orders are cancelled when the client goes to surgery and must be rewritten by the physician when the client returns to the postsurgical care unit.

### Preoperative Medications

The surgical client usually is given preoperative medications 45 to 70 minutes before the scheduled surgery. Any delay in administration should be reported promptly to the surgical department. Preoperative medications may also be given in the surgical holding room to produce the desired effects.

A combination of preoperative drugs may be ordered to achieve the desired outcomes with minimal side effects. Such outcomes include sedation, reducing anxiety, inducing amnesia to minimize unpleasant surgical memories, increasing comfort during preoperative procedures, reducing gastric acidity and volume, increasing gastric emptying, decreasing nausea and

vomiting, and reducing the incidence of aspiration by drying oral and respiratory secretions. Table 7–4 outlines commonly prescribed preoperative medications.

### Intraoperative Medications

**Anesthesia** is used to produce unconsciousness, analgesia, reflex loss, and muscle relaxation during a surgical procedure. General anesthesia produces these effects, whereas regional anesthesia results in analgesia, reflex loss, and muscle relaxation but does not cause the client to lose consciousness. An anesthesiologist (physician) or certified registered nurse anesthetist (CRNA) administers the anesthetics during the intraoperative phase of surgery.

***GENERAL ANESTHESIA.*** **General anesthesia** is most commonly administered by inhalation and, to a lesser extent, by the intravenous route. It produces central nervous system depression. As a result, the client loses consciousness and does not perceive pain, skeletal muscles relax, and reflexes diminish.

Advantages to general anesthesia include rapid excretion of the anesthetic agent and prompt reversal of its effects when desired. Additionally, general anesthesia can be used with all age groups and any type of surgical procedure. It produces amnesia.

TABLE 7–4    Preoperative Medications

| Generic | Trade | Dose and Route | Action by Category | Nursing Implications |
|---|---|---|---|---|
| *Benzodiazepines*<br>Midazolam<br>Diazepam<br>Lorazepam | Versed<br>Valium<br>Ativan | 3–5 mg IM<br>5–2 mg PO<br>1–4 mg IM or IV | Decreases anxiety and produces sedation to some extent<br>Induces amnesia<br>May induce substantial amnesia | Monitor for respiratory depression, hypotension, drowsiness, and lack of coordination. |
| *Opioid Analgesics*<br>Morphine<br>Meperidine | Morphine<br>Demerol | 5–15 mg IM<br>50–150 mg IM | Decreases anxiety, provides analgesia, allows decreased anesthetics | Monitor for respiratory depression, nausea, vomiting, orthostatic hypotension, and pruritus. Smaller doses may be given to frail or older clients. |
| *Antacids*<br>Sodium citrate | Bicitra | 15–30 mL PO | Increases the pH and reduces volume of gastric fluid; used in clients with GERD and/or trauma | No significant factors in this setting |
| *$H_2$-Receptor Antagonists*<br>Cimetidine<br>Famotidine<br>Ranitidine | Tagamet<br>Pepcid<br>Zantac | 300 mg IV, IM, or PO<br>20 mg IV<br>50 mg IV, IM, or PO | Reduces gastric acid volume and concentration | Monitor for confusion and dizziness in older adults. |
| *Gastric Acid Pump Inhibitors*<br>Lansoprazole<br>Omeprazole | Prevacid<br>Prilosec | 15–60 mg PO<br>20–40 mg PO | Suppresses gastric acid secretion | Monitor for dizziness and headache, rash, or thirst. |
| *Antiemetics*<br>Metoclopramide<br>Droperidol | Reglan<br>Inapsine | 10 mg IV<br>10–15 mg PO<br>0.625–2.5 mg IM | Enhances gastric emptying<br>Tranquilizer | Monitor for sedation and extrapyramidal reaction (involuntary movement, muscle tone changes, and abnormal posture). |
| *Anticholinergics*<br>Atropine sulfate<br><br>Glycopyrrolate<br>Scopolamine | Atropine Sulfate<br>Robinul<br>Scopolamine | 0.4–0.6 mg IM or IV<br>0.1–0.3 IM mg or IV<br>0.4–0.6 mg IM or IV | Reduces oral and respiratory secretions to decrease risk of aspiration; decreases vomiting and laryngospasm | Monitor for confusion, restlessness, and tachycardia.<br>Prepare client to expect a dry mouth. |

Disadvantages of general anesthesia include risks associated with circulatory and respiratory depression. Clients with serious respiratory or circulatory diseases, such as emphysema or congestive heart failure, are at greater risk for complications.

The phases of general anesthesia are divided into three distinct categories: induction, maintenance, and emergence. During the induction phase, the client receives the anesthetic agent intravenously or by inhalation. During this phase, airway patency is achieved with endotracheal intubation. The next phase of general anesthesia is maintenance. During this period, the client is positioned, the skin is prepared, and surgery is performed. The anesthesiologist maintains the proper depth of anesthesia while constantly monitoring physiologic parameters such as heart rate, blood pressure, respiratory rate, temperature, and oxygen and carbon dioxide levels. The final phase of anesthesia is the client's emergence from this altered physiologic state. As the anesthetic agents are withdrawn or the effects reversed pharmacologically, the client begins to awaken. The endotracheal tube is removed (extubated) once the client is able to reestablish voluntary breathing. It is critical to ensure airway patency in this period, because extubation may cause bronchospasm or laryngospasm.

***REGIONAL ANESTHESIA.*** **Regional anesthesia** is a type of local anesthesia in which medication instilled around the nerves blocks transmission of nerve impulses in a particular area. Regional anesthesia produces analgesia, relaxation, and reduced reflexes. The client is awake and conscious during the surgical procedure but does not perceive pain. Regional anesthesia may be classified in several ways:

- Surface or topical anesthesia is applied to the skin or mucous membranes to block nerve impulses at that site. Skin wounds or burns are anesthetized using a cocaine solution, lidocaine (Xylocaine), or benzocaine.

- Local nerve infiltration is achieved by injecting lidocaine or tetracaine around a local nerve to depress nerve sensation over a limited area of the body. This technique may be used when a skin or muscle biopsy is obtained or when a small wound is sutured.
- Nerve blocks are accomplished by injecting an anesthetic agent at the nerve trunk to produce a lack of sensation over a specific area, such as an extremity.
- Epidural blocks are local anesthetic agents injected into the epidural space, outside the dura mater of the spinal cord. This type of intraspinal anesthesia can be used for surgeries of the abdomen and lower extremities.
- Spinal anesthesia is accomplished by injecting a local anesthetic agent into the subarachnoid space. Surgeries of the lower abdomen, perineum, and lower extremities are likely to use this type of regional anesthesia. Leakage of cerebrospinal fluid (CSF) from the needle insertion site may cause reduced CSF pressure and postoperative headaches. Bed rest, hydration, and pressure to the infusion site combat this common side effect.

***CONSCIOUS SEDATION.*** Conscious sedation is described in Box 7–1.

## Postoperative Medications

Management of acute postoperative pain by medication follows the principles outlined later in the chapter. For more information on pain management, see the nursing care section on managing acute postoperative pain, and see Chapter 4. ⌘

---

| BOX 7–1 | ■ Conscious Sedation |
|---|---|

An increased number of surgical and diagnostic procedures are being performed using **conscious sedation.** This type of anesthesia provides analgesia and amnesia, but the client remains conscious. The pharmacologic effects are produced by administering a combination of intravenous medications with opioids (such as morphine sulfate, meperidine hydrochloride [Demerol], and fentanyl [Sublimaze]) and sedatives (such as diazepam [Valium] and midazolam [Versed]). During conscious sedation the client is able to independently maintain an open airway. This allows the client to respond to verbal and physical stimulation.

Common adverse side effects include venous thrombosis, phlebitis, local irritation, confusion, drowsiness, hypotension, and apnea. Reversal agents (naloxone hydrochloride [Narcan] and flumazenil [Romazicon]) are used as needed to enhance the safety of conscious sedation.

The American Society of Perianesthesia Nurses (1995) and the Association of Operating Room Nurses (1993) include management and monitoring before, during, and after the procedure using conscious sedation. Included in the standards are knowledge of anatomy, physiology, and complications; physiologic monitoring; use of oxygen delivery devices and airway management; and understanding of legal ramifications of administering or monitoring clients receiving intravenous conscious sedation.

---

Established, severe pain is more difficult to treat than pain that is at its onset. Therefore, postoperative analgesics should be administered initially at regular intervals to maintain a therapeutic blood level. Administering analgesics as needed (prn) lowers this therapeutic level; delays in the medication administration further increase pain intensity. Therefore, prn administration of analgesics is not recommended in the first 36 to 48 hours postoperatively.

> **PRACTICE ALERT** *Nurses are responsible for assessing clients' pain level and administering pain medication. Work collaboratively with surgeons to schedule postoperative analgesics rather than rely on prn administration orders.* ■

Nonsteroidal anti-inflammatory drugs (NSAIDs) treat mild to moderate postoperative pain. This category of drugs should be given soon after surgery (orally, parenterally, or rectally) along with opioids unless contraindicated. Although NSAIDs may not be sufficient to control pain completely, they allow lower doses of opioid analgesics and, therefore, fewer side effects. NSAIDs can be given safely to older clients, but observe closely for side effects, particularly gastric and renal toxicity.

Opioid analgesics, such as morphine and meperidine (Demerol), are considered the foundation for managing moderate to severe postoperative pain. Opioid dosage requirements vary greatly from one client to another, so the dosage must be individually tailored. Later in the postoperative recovery period, opioid analgesics (oral or intramuscular) may be given prn. In this way, pain relief can be maintained, while the potential for drug side effects is decreased.

Contrary to the belief of many health care providers (including nurses), physical dependence and tolerance to opioid analgesics is uncommon in short-term postoperative use. Additionally, opioid analgesics, when used to treat acute pain, rarely lead to psychologic dependence and addiction.

Older clients tend to be more sensitive to the analgesic effects of opioids, experiencing a higher peak effect with a longer duration of pain control. The Nursing Research box on page 174 provides additional information.

> **PRACTICE ALERT** *Oral analgesia requires a significantly greater dose than parenteral for most analgesics. Teach clients who are being discharged, and their caregivers, the relative strength of oral analgesics. (Caution them to not rely on trade names to gauge effectiveness. Two Tylenol with codeine (30 mg) is equianalgesia to 10 mg parenteral morphine; however, oral Demerol 100 mg does not provide equianalgesia with 10 mg parenteral morphine.)* ■

## Surgery
### Members of the Surgical Team
Because of the complexity of the intraoperative environment, members of the surgical team must function as a coordinated unit. The surgeon, surgical assistant(s), anesthesiologist or *certified registered nurse anesthetist* (CRNA), *circulating* nurse, and *scrub*

## Nursing Research

### Evidence-Based Practice for Managing Postoperative Pain in Frail Older Women

As the population continues to age, increasing numbers of older adults are hospitalized for surgical procedures. Older adults, and especially those over age 75, are more likely to have a longer postoperative period of pain, find analgesics less helpful, and have more confusion. It is not known if pain perception in this population is decreased, if pain tolerance is different, or if pain relief is adequate. Zalon (1997) conducted a study to understand postoperative pain from the perspective of frail, older women after surgery. Analysis of data from 16 women revealed three themes: (1) the immediate reality of pain, (2) security, and (3) dealing with pain.

The women in the study found it difficult to put the pain experience into words, suggesting it was a unique and solitary experience. Feeling secure was manifested by seeking comfort and was influenced by trust. The comfort of nursing care was valued, and was facilitated by the nurses' demeanor, words, and actions. The women dealt with pain through endurance, asking for medication for intolerable pain. Other strategies for handling pain included using medication for sleep and lying still.

### Implications for Nursing

Findings from this study highlight the importance of assessing pain in postoperative older adults, and asking probing questions if nonverbal cues are different than verbal reports of pain. Establishing trust within the nurse-client relationship is critical to relieving pain. Teaching is necessary to dispel myths about addiction, and to allow clients control and independence so they ask for pain medications. Exploring with older clients their perception of pain, as well as the significance it has for recovery from illness, are necessary elements in providing adequate pain relief and restoring health.

### Critical Thinking in Client Care

1. What physiologic changes make pain management more difficult for an 80-year-old client following surgery than for a 30 year old?
2. Your older client says: "I deserved this pain, so I don't want to take anything to make it better." What would be your response and why?
3. A man of Native American descent, age 76, replies that "something doesn't feel right" when asked to rate his pain on a scale of 0 to 10. His pulse is increased and he is protective of his abdominal incision. What could you ask or do to accurately assess his pain?
4. If your grandfather was having surgery tomorrow, what would you like him to be taught about pain management?
5. An independent, 85-year-old woman has a PCA pump for analgesia following major surgery. She continuously presses the pump button, but continues to complain of severe pain. What do you do now?

nurse or operating room technician (Figure 7–2 ■) constitute the surgical team. Each member provides specialized skills and is essential to the successful outcome of the surgery. Risks to members of the surgical team from bloodborne pathogens or injury are minimized when the surgical team is well organized and prepared.

The surgeon is the physician performing the procedure. As head of the surgical team, the surgeon is responsible for all medical actions and judgments.

The surgical assistant works closely with the surgeon in performing the operation. The number of assistants varies according to the complexity of the procedure. The assistant may be another physician, a nurse, a physician assistant, or other trained personnel. The assistant performs such duties as exposing the operative site, retracting nearby tissue, sponging and/or suctioning the wound, ligating bleeding vessels, and suturing or helping suture the surgical wound.

The anesthesiologist or CRNA relieves the surgeon of the responsibility for the client's general well-being, thus allowing the surgeon to focus on the technical aspects of the procedure. The anesthesiologist or CRNA evaluates the client preoperatively, administers the anesthesia and other required medications, transfuses blood or other blood products, infuses intravenous fluids, continuously monitors the client's physiologic status, alerts the surgeon to developing problems and treats them as they arise, and supervises the client's recovery in the PACU.

The circulating nurse is a highly experienced registered nurse who coordinates and manages a wide range of activities before, during, and after the surgical procedure. For example,

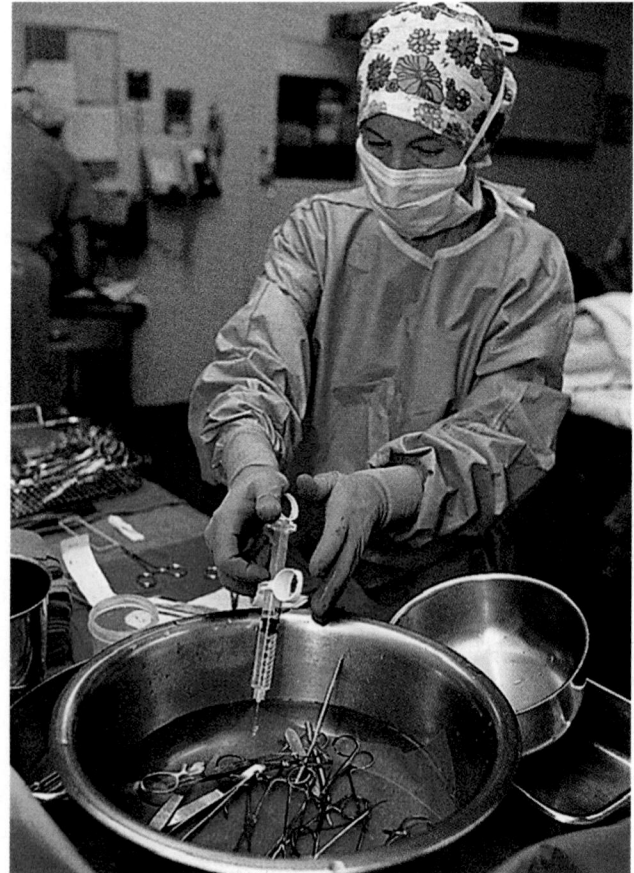

**Figure 7–2** ■ A scrub nurse in the operating room.

the circulating nurse oversees the physical aspects of the operating room itself, including the equipment. The circulating nurse also assists with transferring and positioning the client, prepares the client's skin, ensures that no break in aseptic technique occurs, and counts all sponges and instruments. The circulating nurse assists all other team members, including the anesthesiologist or CRNA. Thorough documentation in the surgical area is essential, and the circulating nurse is responsible for documenting intraoperative nursing activities, medications, blood administration, placement of drains and catheters, and length of the procedure. The circulating nurse also formulates a care plan based on physiologic and psychosocial assessments of the client. Finally, the circulating nurse is at all times an advocate for the safety and well-being of the client.

The role of the scrub nurse primarily involves technical skills, manual dexterity, and in-depth knowledge of the anatomic and mechanical aspects of a particular surgery. The scrub nurse handles sutures, instruments, and other equipment immediately adjacent to the sterile field. Although the title implies that the person who performs these duties is a nurse, the role of the scrub nurse may also be assumed by an operating room technician (ORT), depending on hospital policy and the complexity of the surgery.

The role of nurses in surgery continues to evolve to improve client care. In recent years, nurses have begun to specialize within the already specialized field of perioperative nursing. Specialty surgical teams have developed in response to the demands of increasingly complex technical surgeries. For example, a designated open heart surgical team may be responsible for all open heart cases and ordinarily not be involved with other procedures. The use of specialty surgical teams allows nurses to become highly skilled in a particular range of procedures.

### Surgical Attire

Strict dress codes are necessary in the surgical department to provide infection control within the operating room suites, reduce cross-contamination between the surgery department and other hospital units or departments, and promote both personnel and client health and safety. Based on research and recommendations by hospital infection control authorities, guidelines for attire differ among surgical facilities. Following institutional guidelines, all personnel in the surgical department must be in proper surgical attire. The design and composition of the surgical attire minimize bacterial shedding, thus reducing wound contamination. The area in the surgical department is divided into *unrestricted, semirestricted,* and *restricted* zones. The unrestricted zones permit access by those in hospital uniforms or street clothes. These areas may also allow limited access for communicating with operating room personnel.

The semirestricted zones require scrub attire, including a scrub suit, shoe covers, and a cap or hood (Figure 7–3 ■). Hallways, work areas, and storage areas are considered semirestricted.

Restricted zones are within operating rooms. Personnel wear masks, sterile gowns, and gloves in addition to appropriate scrub attire (Figure 7–3). The entire surgical attire is changed between procedures or when it becomes soiled or wet.

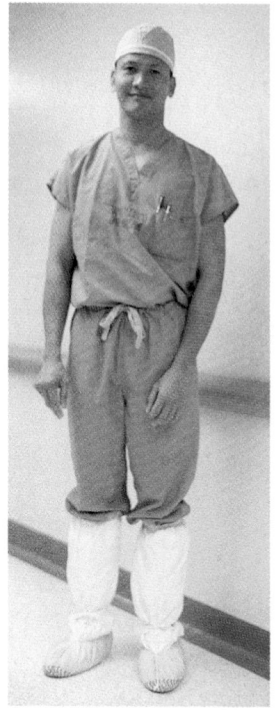 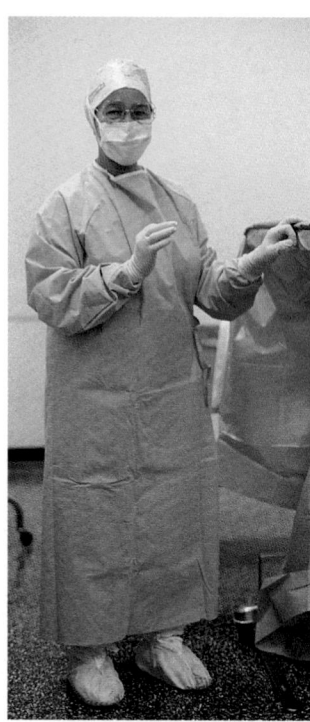

**Figure 7–3** ■ Surgical attire. *A,* Scrub attire includes scrub suit, shoe covers, and cap or hood to cover hair. *B,* Sterile attire includes scrub suit, shoe covers, and cap or hood, plus gown, gloves, and mask.

### The Surgical Scrub

The surgical scrub is performed to render hands and arms as clean as possible in preparation for a procedure. All personnel who participate directly in the procedure must perform a surgical scrub with a brush and antimicrobial soap. Skin cannot be rendered sterile, but it can be considered "surgically clean" following the scrub. The purposes of the surgical scrub are to:

- Remove dirt, skin oils, and transient microorganisms from hands and forearms.
- Increase client safety by reducing microorganisms on surgical personnel.
- Leave an antimicrobial residue on the skin to inhibit growth of microbes for several hours.

Following the 5- to 10-minute surgical scrub, hands and arms are dried with sterile towels.

### Preparing the Client

Although much preparation has taken place prior to the client's transfer to the surgical department, additional activities such as shaving and positioning may be performed. The skin preparation, which usually includes cleansing the area with a prescribed antimicrobial agent, already may have been performed either by the client or by nursing personnel before the transfer to the surgical department. Additional skin cleansing is performed in the surgical department to further decrease microorganisms on the skin and thereby reduce the possibility of wound infection.

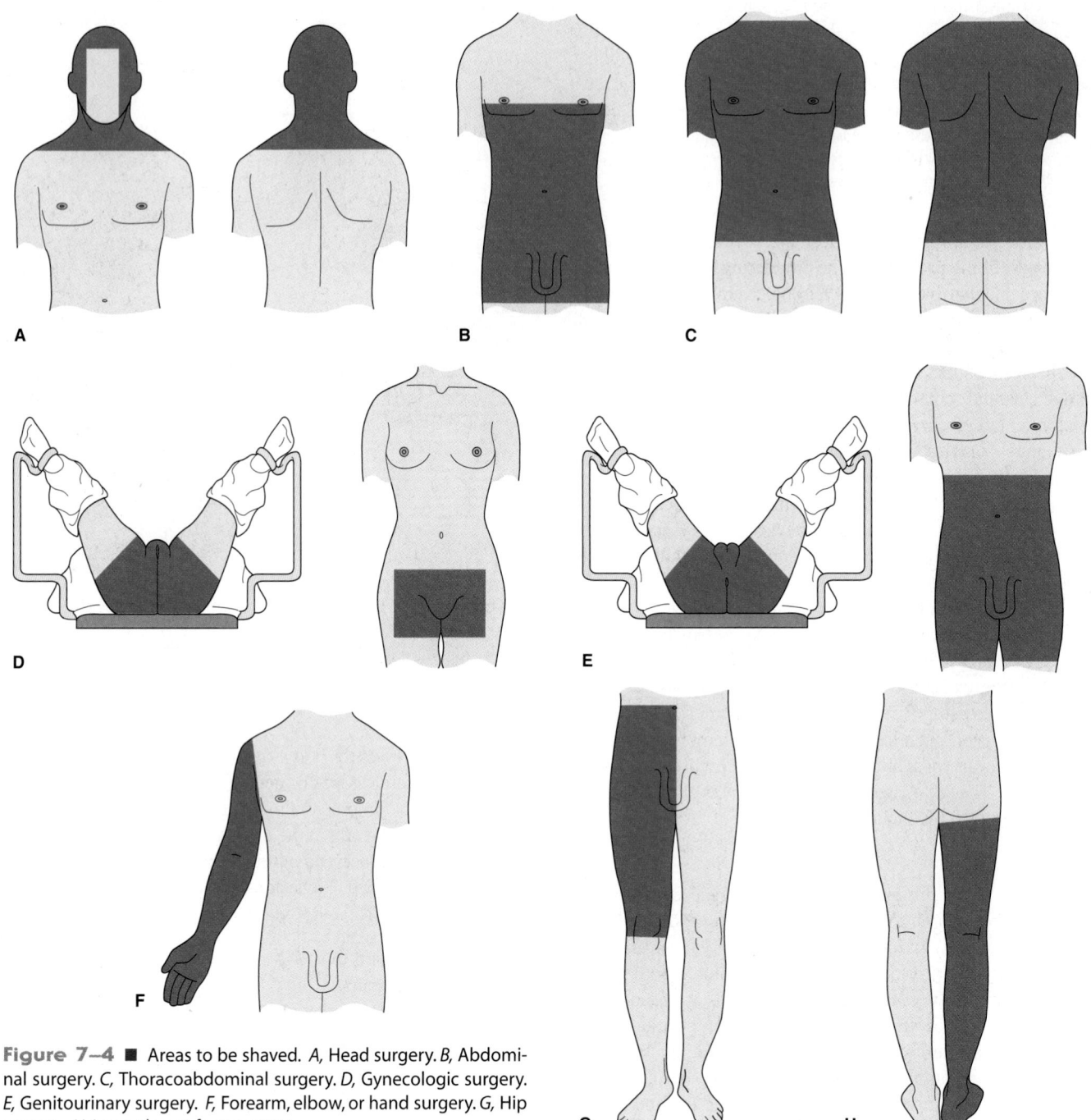

**Figure 7–4** ■ Areas to be shaved. *A*, Head surgery. *B*, Abdominal surgery. *C*, Thoracoabdominal surgery. *D*, Gynecologic surgery. *E*, Genitourinary surgery. *F*, Forearm, elbow, or hand surgery. *G*, Hip surgery. *H*, Lower leg or foot surgery.

The surgeon also may order the skin shaved in and around the proposed incision area (Figure 7–4 ■). Shaving may be completed preoperatively, but more often it is performed in the surgical department. The extent of shaving varies. Generally, the area shaved is wider than the planned incision because of the possibility of unexpected extension of the incision. Disposable, sterile supplies are used, in accordance with aseptic techniques. However, the benefit of shaving the incisional site has become controversial. Physical trauma to the shaved area can weaken the client's defense against organisms, thus increasing the chance of wound infection. An altered body image

also may result from the physiologic trauma of a surgical shave, particularly if the shave involves the head or groin area. Hospital policy and surgeon preference should be followed.

Preparing the client for surgery also includes **positioning** the client on the operating table. Table 7–5 shows frequently used positions and describes corresponding surgical procedures and possible adverse effects. Positioning exposes the operative site and gives access for anesthesia administration. Proper positioning is imperative to prevent injury to the client. Pressure, rubbing, and/or shearing forces can cause injury to the tissue over bony prominences. If positioning

TABLE 7–5    Common Surgical Positions

| Position and Use | Possible Adverse Effects and Nursing Interventions |
|---|---|
| (a) The *dorsal recumbent* (or *supine*) *position* is used for many abdominal surgeries (e.g., colostomy and herniorrhaphy) as well as for some thoracic surgeries (e.g., open heart surgery) and some surgeries on the extremities. 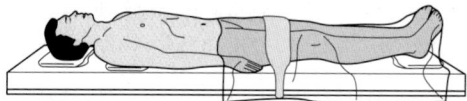 | This position may cause excessive pressure on posterior bony prominences, such as the back of the head, scapulae, sacrum, and heels. Pad these areas with soft materials. To avoid compression of blood vessels and sluggish circulation, ensure that the knees are not flexed. Use trochanter rolls or other padding to avoid internal or external rotation of the hips and shoulders. |
| (b) The *semisitting position* is used for surgeries on the thyroid and neck areas. 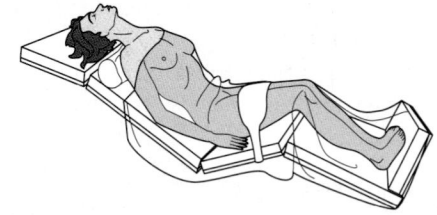 | This position can lead to postural hypotension and venous pooling in the legs. It may promote skin breakdown on the buttocks. Sciatic nerve injury is possible. Assess for hypotension. Ensure that knees are not sharply flexed. Use soft padding to prevent nerve compression. |
| (c) The *prone position* is used for spinal fusions and removal of hemorrhoids. 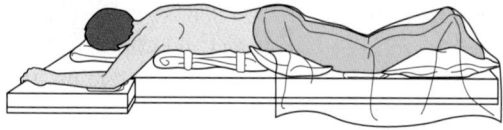 | This position causes pressure on the face, knees, thighs, anterior ankles, and toes. Pad bony prominences, and support the feet under the ankles. To promote optimum respiratory function, raise the client's chest and abdomen, and support with padding. Corneal abrasion could occur if the eyes are not closed or are insufficiently padded. |
| (d) The *lateral chest position* is used for some thoracic surgeries, as well as hip replacements. 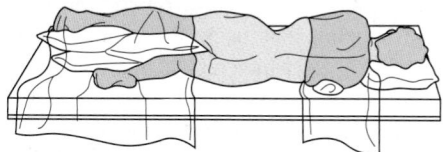 | This may cause excessive pressure on the bony prominences on the side on which the client is positioned. Ensure adequate padding and support, especially of the downside arm. The weight of the upper leg may cause peroneal nerve injury on the downside leg. Both legs must therefore be padded. |
| (e) The *lithotomy position* is used for gynecologic, perineal, or rectal surgeries. 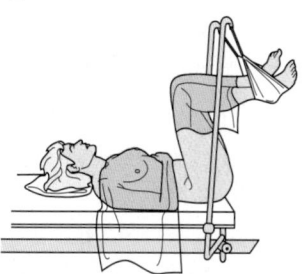 | This position causes an 18% decrease (from a standing position) in vital capacity of the lungs. Monitor respirations, and assess for hypoxia and dyspnea. The lithotomy position can lead to joint damage, peroneal nerve damage, and damage to peripheral blood vessels. To avoid injury, ensure adequate padding, and manipulate both legs into the stirrups simultaneously. |
| (f) The *jackknife position* is used for proctologic surgeries, such as removal of hemorrhoids, and for some spinal surgeries. 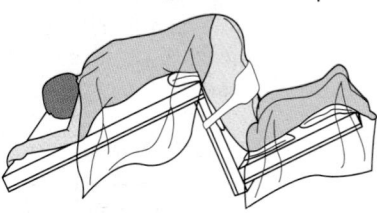 | This position causes a 12% decrease (from a standing position) in vital capacity of the lungs. Monitor respirations, and assess for hypoxia and dyspnea. In this position, the greatest pressure is felt at the bends in the table. Therefore, the client is supported with pads at the groin and knees, as well as at the ankles. Padding of the chest and knees helps prevent skin breakdown. Padding and proper positioning help prevent pressure on the ear, the neck, and the nerves of the upper arm. |

causes normal joint range of motion to be exceeded, injury to muscles and joints can occur. Improper positioning also can lead to sensory and motor dysfunction, resulting in nerve damage. Pressure on peripheral blood vessels can decrease venous return to the heart and negatively affect the client's blood pressure. Additionally, oxygenation of the blood can be decreased if the client is not properly positioned to promote lung expansion.

Because the anesthetized client cannot respond to discomfort, it is the surgical team's responsibility to position the client not only for the best surgical advantage but also for client safety and comfort. The circulating nurse refers to hospital policy, the surgeon's preference, and the client's history to ensure optimal positioning, and continuously assesses the client.

### Intraoperative Awareness

Prior to induction of anesthesia, the circulating nurse establishes rapport with the client to assess the client's psychologic status. This assessment is continued throughout the surgical procedure. After anesthetic medications have been given, the client may appear oblivious to the surroundings; however, studies have shown that the client's awareness during the intraoperative period may be greater than once believed. Intraoperative awareness is the client's subconscious awareness of what is being said and done during surgery. Although most clients do not consciously remember what happened or what was said, psychologic trauma can result. Because there is no reliable method of preventing this phenomenon, conversations during surgery should be professional.

**PRACTICE ALERT** *Do not say anything while the client is unconscious that would be inappropriate if the client were awake. Maintain a respectful, professional demeanor throughout the operative period.* ∎

### Special Considerations for the Older Adult

Because of cardiovascular and tissue changes that result from aging, surgeries longer than 2 hours place the older adult at increased risk for complications. The older adult is more prone to hypotension, hypothermia, and hypoxemia resulting from anesthesia and the cool temperature in the operating room.

Positioning may also cause complications in the older adult. Intraoperative positioning of arthritic joints can cause postoperative joint pain unrelated to the operative site. Also, the longer the surgery, the greater the chance of decubitus ulcer (pressure sore) formation. The older client is at increased risk for developing pressure sores because of decreased subcutaneous fat tissue and reduced peripheral circulation.

Finally, the older adult often has some degree of hearing and/or visual impairment. These impairments coupled with a strange environment can make the operating room a frightening, disorienting place. By effectively communicating with the client, the nurse can provide support and reassurance to minimize these factors. To decrease confusion and assist in communication, hearing aids and glasses should be used when appropriate and possible.

### Dietary Management

Wound healing after surgery depends on adequate nutritional intake. During the immediate postoperative phase, dietary intake is withheld until evidence of peristalsis is found and the client can tolerate liquids without nausea and vomiting. While intravenous fluids maintain hydration and electrolyte balance, they do not provide nutrition. Some clients believe that intravenous fluids are the same as intravenous "feeding," but this is a myth. Unless balanced nutrition through the gastrointestinal intake can be reestablished within 3 to 4 days, parenteral hyperalimentation is critical for homeostasis and wound healing.

- Protein and calories are needed for wound healing and recovery from surgery.
- Low-fat, high-fiber diets are important for chronic cardiovascular fitness, but are contraindicated in the wound healing phase following surgery.
- Failure to use the gastrointestinal tract for more than 4 or 5 days allows the intestinal mucosa to atrophy, putting the client at risk for infection.

Fluid administered through peripheral veins must be isotonic or only moderately hypertonic to prevent sclerosing the small peripheral veins. Solutions of 10% dextrose are tolerable peripherally for a short time but do not provide adequate calories for healing and maintenance. To provide adequate nutrition, central vein access must be established and solutions must be prepared with protein, carbohydrates, lipids, vitamins, and minerals. This is important for clients who have extended recovery periods without eating after surgery.

Parenteral nutrition has serious risks. Central vein access may cause infection and sepsis. Normal stimulation to the intestinal tract is lost when the parenteral approach is used alone. Using the gut is better than using the vein because it (1) prevents intestinal atrophy, which results in a very thin bowel wall poorly suited to absorb nutrients; (2) prevents bacteria and inert particles from translocating across the bowel lining into the bloodstream; (3) introduces fats and other large particles into the lymphatic circulation and stimulates the immune system; and (4) is safer and far less expensive than parenteral nutritional support (Hiemburger & Weinsier, 1997). Education and counseling to support adequate nutritional intake should be ongoing throughout the preoperative and postoperative period.

## NURSING CARE

The following section will discuss nursing care in each of the three phases of surgery. A case study at the end of the section follows one client through the postoperative experience, bringing this information together. Perioperative nursing diagnoses are provided in Box 7–2 to assist in identifying the needs of the surgical client. This is not an exhaustive list, but it can serve as a guide in identifying possible nursing diagnoses.

### Preoperative Nursing Care

The client's response to planned surgery varies greatly. When planning and implementing nursing care, consider individual

| BOX 7–2 | ■ Examples of Perioperative Nursing Diagnoses |
|---|---|

**Preoperative**
- Knowledge, Deficient
- Anxiety
- Fear
- Anticipatory Grieving
- Decisional Conflict
- Coping, Ineffective
- Sexuality Patterns, Ineffective
- Sleep Pattern, Disturbed
- Thought Processes, Disturbed
- Family Processes, Interrupted

**Intraoperative**
- Knowledge, Deficient
- Anxiety
- Fear
- Airway Clearance, Ineffective
- Aspiration, Risk for
- Decreased Cardiac Output
- Hypothermia
- Infection, Risk for
- Thought Processes, Disturbed
- Gas Exchange, Impaired
- Urinary Elimination, Impaired
- Fluid Volume, Deficient
- Fluid Volume, Excessive
- Verbal Communication, Impaired

**Postoperative**
- Knowledge, Deficient
- Pain
- Breathing Pattern, Ineffective
- Airway Clearance, Ineffective
- Skin Integrity, Impaired
- Nutrition Imbalanced: Less Than Body Requirements
- Sexuality Patterns, Ineffective
- Sleep Pattern, Disturbed
- Fatigue
- Urinary Retention
- Urinary Elimination, Impaired
- Adjustment, Impaired
- Body Image, Disturbed
- Physical Mobility, Impaired
- Activity Intolerance, Risk for
- Injury, Risk for
- Self-Care, Deficient
- Health Maintenance, Ineffective
- Diversional Activity, Deficient
- Social Isolation

psychologic and physical differences, the type of surgery, and the circumstances surrounding the need for surgery. A thorough nursing assessment is needed to determine the most appropriate care for each client undergoing surgery.

Before planning and implementing care for the surgical client, gather assessment information by taking a nursing history and performing a physical examination. Use this information to establish baseline data, identify physical needs, determine teaching needs and psychologic support for the client and family, and prioritize nursing care. The type of surgical procedure directs the assessment and intervention planned by the nurse.

**PRACTICE ALERT**  *Be sure to assess information about use of over-the-counter medications including herbal supplements. These drugs can interact with medications administered in the perioperative period.* ■

Surgery is a significant and stressful event. Regardless of the nature of the surgery (whether major or minor), the client and family will be anxious. The degree of anxiety they will feel is not necessarily proportional to the magnitude of the surgical procedure. For example, a client scheduled to have a biopsy to rule out cancer, which is considered minor surgery, may be more anxious than a client undergoing gallbladder removal, which is considered major surgery.

The nurse's ability to listen actively to both verbal and nonverbal messages is imperative to establishing a trusting relationship with the client and family. Therapeutic communication can help the client and family identify fears and concerns. The nurse can then plan nursing interventions and supportive care to reduce the client's anxiety level and assist the client to cope successfully with the stressors encountered during the perioperative period.

## Preoperative Client and Family Teaching

Client teaching is an essential nursing responsibility in the preoperative period. Client education and emotional support have a positive effect on the client's physical and psychologic well-being, both before and after surgery. In an analysis of 102 studies, surgical clients receiving client education and/or supportive interventions had less pain and anxiety, experienced fewer complications, were discharged sooner, were more satisfied with their care, and returned to normal activities sooner than clients who did not receive this type of care. These positive outcomes may be attributed in part to the sense of control the client gains through the nurse's teaching.

Client teaching should begin as soon as the client learns of the upcoming surgery. Teaching may begin as early as in the physician's office or at the time of preadmission testing. Although education continues during postoperative care, most teaching is done before surgery, because pain and the effects of anesthesia can greatly diminish the client's ability to learn.

The amount of information desired varies from client to client. Therefore, assess the client's need for and readiness to accept information. The teaching will be directed in part by the particular surgical procedure that is being performed. The information in Box 7–3 is relevant to most clients undergoing major surgery.

In addition to teaching the client and family about measures that will decrease the risk of complications, provide other preoperative information to prepare the client and family for surgery. This information should include the following:

- Diagnostic tests—reasons and preparations
- Arrival time if surgery is scheduled in early morning
- Preparations for the day of surgery after midnight prior to a morning surgery, skin preparation, indwelling catheter or bladder elimination, start of intravenous infusion, preoperative medication, handling of valuables (rings, watch, money)

## BOX 7–3 ■ Preoperative Client Teaching

### DIAPHRAGMATIC BREATHING EXERCISE

Diaphragmatic (abdominal) breathing exercises are taught to the client who is at risk for developing pulmonary complications, such as atelectasis or pneumonia. Risk factors for pulmonary complications include general anesthesia, abdominal or thoracic surgery, history of smoking, chronic lung disease, obesity, and advanced age.

In diaphragmatic breathing, the client inspires deeply while allowing the abdomen to expand outward. On expiration, the abdomen contracts inward as air from the lungs is expelled.

1. Explain to the client that the diaphragm is a muscle that makes up the floor of the abdominal cavity and assists in breathing. The purpose of diaphragmatic breathing is to promote lung expansion and ventilation and enhance blood oxygenation.
2. Position the client in a high or semi-Fowler's position (see figure below).
3. Ask the client to place the hands lightly on the abdomen.
4. Instruct the client to breathe in deeply through the nose, allowing the chest and abdomen to expand.
5. Have the client hold the breath for a count of 5.
6. Tell the client to exhale completely through pursed (puckered) lips, allowing the chest and abdomen to deflate.

7. Have the client repeat the exercise five times consecutively.

Encourage the client to perform diaphragmatic breathing exercises every 1 to 2 waking hours, depending on the client's needs and institutional protocol.

### COUGHING EXERCISE

Coughing exercises are also taught to the client who is at risk for developing pulmonary complications. The purpose of coughing is to loosen, mobilize, and remove pulmonary secretions. Splinting the incision decreases the physical and psychologic discomfort associated with coughing.

1. Assist the client in following steps 1 through 4 for diaphragmatic breathing.
2. Ask the client to splint the incision with interlocked hand or pillow (see figure below).
3. Tell the client to take three deep breaths and then cough forcefully.
4. Have the client repeat the exercise five times consecutively every 2 hours while awake, taking short rest periods between coughs, if necessary.

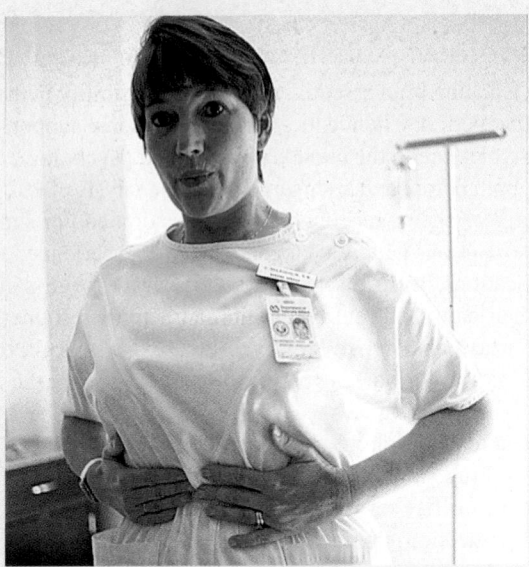

Diaphragmatic breathing exercise.

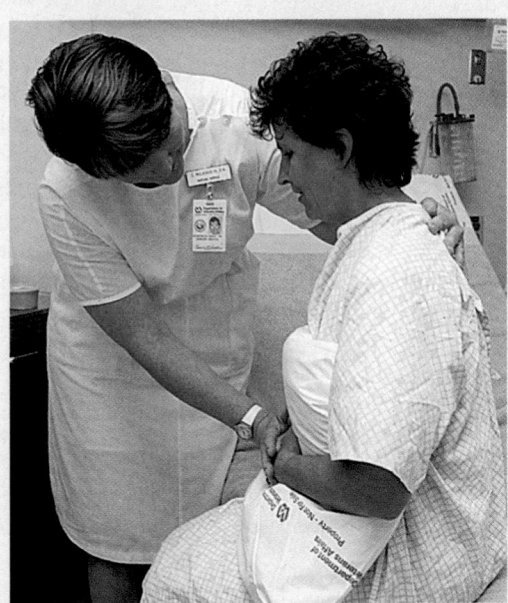

Splinting abdomen while coughing.

- Sedative/hypnotic medication to be taken the night before surgery to promote rest and sleep
- Counseling on whether to take significant medications the morning of surgery
- Informed consent
- Expected timetable for surgery and the recovery room
- Transfer to the surgery department
- Location of the surgical waiting room
- Transfer to recovery room
- Anticipated postoperative routine and devices or equipment (drains, tubes, equipment for IV infusions, oxygen or humidifying mask, dressings, splints, casts)
- Plans for postoperative pain control

**PRACTICE ALERT** *Researchers report that many patients experience unnecessarily long preoperative fasts.* ■

The American Society of Anesthesiologists guidelines for preoperative fasting in healthy patients undergoing elective procedures are available online at www.asahq.org/practice/npo/npoguide.html. Withdrawal from caffeine in beverages such as coffee or colas may cause headaches and irritability. Dehydration, hypovolemia, and hypoglycemia are other recognized side effects. Thirst, worry, and hunger are reported by patients to be related to fasting. Fasting does not ensure that the stomach will be empty or that the gastric contents will be less acidic.

## BOX 7–3  ■  Preoperative Client Teaching (continued)

### LEG, ANKLE, AND FOOT EXERCISES

Leg exercises are taught to the client who is at risk for developing thrombophlebitis (inflammation of a vein, which is associated with the formation of blood clots). Risk factors for developing thrombophlebitis include decreased mobility preoperatively and/or postoperatively; a history of difficulties with peripheral circulation; and cardiovascular, pelvic, or lower extremity surgeries.

The purpose of leg exercises is to promote venous blood return from the extremities. As the leg muscles contract and relax, blood is pumped back to the heart, promoting cardiac output and reducing venous stasis. These exercises also maintain muscle tone and range of motion, which facilitate early ambulation.

Teach the client to perform the following exercises while lying in bed:

1. Muscle pumping exercise: Contract and relax calf and thigh muscles at least 10 times consecutively.
2. Leg exercises:
   a. Bend the knee and raise it toward the chest (see figure below).
   b. Straighten out leg and hold for a few seconds before lowering the leg back to the bed.
   c. Repeat exercise five times consecutively prior to alternating to the other foot.
3. Ankle and foot exercises:
   a. Rotate both ankles by making complete circles, first to the right and then to the left (see figure below).
   b. Repeat five times and then relax.
   c. With feet together, point toes toward the head and then to the foot of the bed (see figure below).
   d. Repeat this pumping action 10 times, and then relax.

Encourage the client to perform leg, ankle, and foot exercises every 1 to 2 hours while awake, depending on the client's needs and ambulatory status, the physician's preference, and institutional protocol.

### TURNING IN BED

The client who is at risk for circulatory, respiratory, or gastrointestinal dysfunction following surgery is taught to turn in bed. Although this may be a simple task prior to surgery, after surgery (particularly after abdominal surgery) the client may find it a difficult procedure. To make the procedure more comfortable, the client may need to splint the incision by using the hand placed on a small pillow or blanket. Additionally, the client should be taught that analgesics can be given to ease postoperative discomfort involved with turning. Encourage the client to turn every 2 hours while awake.

1. Tell the client to grasp the side rail toward the direction to be turned, to rest the opposite foot on the mattress, and to bend the knee.
2. Instruct the client to roll over in one smooth motion by pulling on the side rail while pushing off with the bent knee.
3. Pillows may need to be positioned behind the client's back to help the client maintain a side-lying position. The older client may also need padding over pressure points between the knees and ankles to decrease the chance of decubitus ulcer formation from pressure.

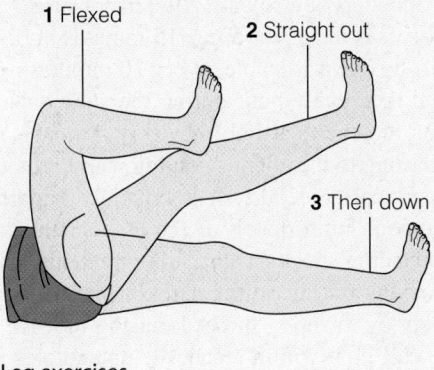

Leg exercises.

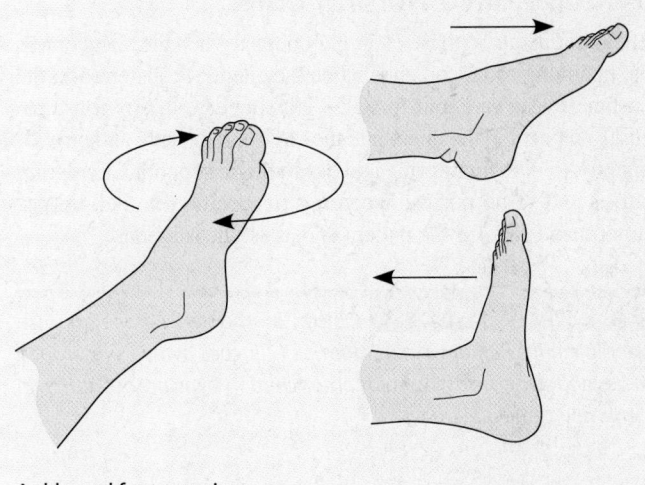

Ankle and foot exercises.

## Preoperative Client Preparation

A preoperative surgical checklist serves as an outline for finalizing preparation of the client for surgery in most institutions. Complete the checklist before the client is transported to surgery. Nursing responsibilities the day of surgery are as follows:

- Assist with bathing, grooming, and changing into operating room gown.
- Ensure that the client takes nothing by mouth (NPO). Provide additional teaching, and reinforce prior teaching.
- Remove nail polish, lipstick, and makeup to facilitate circulatory assessment during and after surgery.

- Ensure that identification, blood, and allergy bands are correct, legible, and secure.
- Remove hair pins and jewelry; a wedding ring may be worn if it is removed from the finger, covered with gauze, and then taped to the finger.
- Complete skin or bowel preparation as ordered.
- Insert an indwelling catheter, intravenous line, or nasogastric tube as ordered.
- Remove dentures, artificial eye, and contact lenses, and store them in a safe place.
- Leave a hearing aid in place if the client cannot hear without it, and notify the operating room nurse.

- Verify that the informed consent has been signed prior to administering preoperative medications.
- Verify that the client's height and weight are recorded in the chart (for dosage of anesthesia).
- Verify that all ordered diagnostic test reports are in the chart.
- Have the client empty the bladder immediately before the preoperative medication is administered (unless an in-dwelling catheter is in place).
- Administer preoperative medication as scheduled (refer to "Preoperative Medications" earlier in the chapter).
- Ensure the safety of the client once the medication has been given by placing the client on bed rest with raised side rails and by placing the call light within reach.
- Obtain and record vital signs.
- Provide ongoing supportive care to the client and the client's family.
- Document all preoperative care in the appropriate location, such as the preoperative surgical checklist, the medication record, or the narrative preoperative nursing notes.
- Verify with the surgical personnel the client's identity, and verify that all client information is documented appropriately.
- Help the surgical personnel transfer the client from the bed to the gurney.
- Prepare the client's room for postoperative care, including making the surgical bed and ensuring that the anticipated supplies and equipment are in the room.

## Intraoperative Nursing Care

The intraoperative phase of surgery begins when the client enters the operating room and ends when the client is transferred to the postanesthesia care unit (PACU). Nursing care in this phase focuses on keeping the client and the environment safe and providing physiologic monitoring and psychologic support. Circulating nurses and scrub nurses, according to specific role definitions, support and care for the patient and assist the surgeons.

**PRACTICE ALERT** *Objects on the sterile drape are considered sterile. Remain a minimum of 12 inches away from draped tables and sterile fields to avoid contamination if you are not attired in sterile gown and gloves.* ∎

## Postoperative Nursing Care
### Immediate Postoperative Care

Immediate postoperative care begins when the client has been transferred from the operating room to the PACU. The nurse monitors the client's vital signs and surgical site to determine the response to the surgical procedure and to detect significant changes. Assessing mental status and level of consciousness is another ongoing nursing responsibility, and the client may require repeated orientation to time, place, and person. Emotional support also is essential, because the client is in a vulnerable and dependent position. Assessing and evaluating hydration status by monitoring intake and output is crucial to detecting cardiovascular or renal complications. In addition, the PACU nurse assesses the client's pain level. Careful administration of analgesics provides comfort without compounding the potential side effects from the anesthesia.

### Care When the Client Is Stable

After being stabilized and awake, the client is transferred to his or her room. The PACU nurse communicates information about the client's condition and postoperative orders to the floor nurse prior to the client's arrival. This prepares the floor nurse for additional problems or needed equipment.

Immediate and continuing assessment is essential to detect and/or prevent complications. In documenting assessment findings, the nurse completes a flow record of the individual client's situation. Baseline data are obtained and compared with preoperative data. A postoperative head-to-toe assessment includes but may not be limited to the following:

- General appearance
- Vital signs
- Level of consciousness
- Emotional status
- Quantity of respirations
- Skin color and temperature
- Discomfort/pain
- Nausea/vomiting
- Type of intravenous fluids and flow rate
- Dressing site
- Drainage on the dressing and/or bed linen
- Urinary output (catheter or ability to urinate)
- Ability to move all extremities

The hospital policy or physician's orders dictate the frequency of follow-up assessments. After major surgery, the nurse generally assesses the client every 15 minutes during the first hour and, if the client is stable, every 30 minutes for the next 2 hours, and then every hour during the subsequent 4 hours. Assessments are then carried out every 4 hours, subject to change according to the client's condition and protocol for the particular surgical procedure. It is critically important to inform the surgeon immediately if the assessment reveals any signs of impending shock or other life-threatening changes.

After carrying out the initial assessment and ensuring the client's safety by lowering the bed, raising the side rails, and placing the call light within reach, the nurse notes the physician's postoperative orders. These orders guide the nurse in the care of the postoperative client. For example, the orders specify activity level, diet, medications for pain and nausea, antibiotics, continuation of preoperative medications, frequency of vital sign assessments, administration of intravenous fluids, and laboratory tests such as hemoglobin and potassium level. In most institutions, orders written prior to surgery must be reordered following surgery because the client's condition is presumed to have changed.

## Common Postoperative Complications

Several factors place the client at risk for postoperative complications. Nursing care before, during, and after surgery is aimed at preventing and/or minimizing the effects of these complications.

Preoperative care and teaching to decrease postoperative complications have been discussed. Let us now address postoperative cardiovascular, respiratory, and wound complications, and problems associated with elimination.

## Cardiovascular Complications

Common postoperative cardiovascular complications include shock, hemorrhage, deep venous thrombosis, and pulmonary embolism.

**SHOCK.** Shock is a life-threatening postoperative complication. It results from an insufficient blood flow to vital organs, an inability to use oxygen and nutrients, or the inability to rid tissues of waste material. Hypovolemic shock, the most common type in the postoperative client, results from a decrease in circulating fluid volume. Decreased fluid volume develops with blood or plasma loss or, less commonly, from severe prolonged vomiting or diarrhea. Symptoms vary according to the severity of the shock; the greater the loss of fluid volume, the more severe the symptoms. Chapter 6 ⬤⬤ provides a detailed discussion of nursing care of the client with various types of shock.

**HEMORRHAGE.** Hemorrhage is an excessive loss of blood. A concealed hemorrhage occurs internally from a blood vessel that is no longer sutured or cauterized or from a drainage tube that has eroded a blood vessel. An obvious hemorrhage occurs externally from a dislodged or ill-formed clot at the wound. Hemorrhage also may result from abnormalities in the blood's ability to clot; these abnormalities may result from a pathologic condition, or they may be a side effect of medications.

Hemorrhage from a venous source oozes out quickly and is dark red, whereas an arterial hemorrhage is characterized by bright red spurts of blood pulsating with each heartbeat. Whether the hemorrhage is from a venous or an arterial source, hypovolemic shock will occur if sufficient blood is lost from the circulation.

Common assessment with hemorrhage depends on the amount and rate of blood loss. Restlessness and anxiety are observed in the early stage of hemorrhage. Frank bleeding will be present if the hemorrhage is external. The client will have symptoms characteristic of shock.

Care of the client who is hemorrhaging centers around stopping the bleeding and replenishing the circulating blood volume. Nursing care includes providing care for shock and one or more of the following:

- Applying one or more sterile gauze pads and a snug pressure dressing to the area
- Applying pressure with gloved hands (may be necessary for severe external bleeding)
- Preparing client and family for emergency surgery (in severe situations when bleeding cannot be stopped)

**DEEP VEIN THROMBOSIS.** Deep venous thrombosis (DVT) is the formation of a thrombus (blood clot) in association with inflammation in deep veins. This complication most often occurs in the lower extremities of the postoperative client. It may result from the combination of several factors, including trauma during surgery, pressure applied under the knees, and sluggish blood flow during and after surgery. Clients particularly at risk for developing DVT include those who are over age 40 and who:

- Have undergone orthopedic surgery to lower extremities; urologic, gynecologic, or obstetric surgeries; or neurosurgery.
- Have varicose veins.
- Have a history of thrombophlebitis or pulmonary emboli.
- Are obese.
- Have an infection.
- Have a malignancy.

Common assessment findings reveal pain or cramping in the involved calf or thigh. Redness and edema of the entire extremity may occur along with a slightly elevated temperature. The client may have a positive Homans' sign (pain in the calf on dorsiflexion of the affected foot).

Nursing care of the client with DVT focuses on preventing a portion of the clot from dislodging and becoming an embolus (traveling blood clot) circulating to the heart, brain, or lungs; preventing other clots from forming; and supporting the client's own physiologic mechanism for dissolving clots. Nursing care includes the following measures:

- Administer anticoagulants and analgesics as prescribed. (NSAIDs are not usually given along with anticoagulants, because doing so increases the anticoagulant effects.)
- Monitor laboratory values for clotting times.
- Maintain bed rest and keep affected extremity at or above heart level.
- Apply thigh-high antiemboli stockings or devices to stimulate venous return.
- Ensure that the affected area is not rubbed or massaged.
- Apply heat as prescribed.
- Record bilateral calf or thigh circumferences every shift.
- Teach and support the client and family.
- Assess color and temperature of involved extremity every shift.

**PULMONARY EMBOLISM.** A pulmonary embolism is a dislodged blood clot or other substance that lodges in a pulmonary artery. For the postoperative client with DVT, the threat that a portion of the thrombus may dislodge from the vein wall and travel to the lung, heart, or brain is a constant concern. Early detection of this potentially life-threatening complication depends on the nurse's astute, continuing assessment of the postoperative client.

Common assessment findings of the client experiencing a pulmonary embolism include mild to moderate dyspnea, chest pain, diaphoresis, anxiety, restlessness, rapid respirations and pulse, dysrhythmias, cough, and cyanosis. The severity of the symptoms is determined by the degree of pulmonary vascular blockage. Sudden death can occur if a major pulmonary artery becomes completely blocked.

Stabilizing respiratory and cardiovascular functioning while preventing the formation of additional emboli is of utmost importance in the care of the client with a pulmonary embolism. Nursing care includes the following measures:

- Immediately notify the physician and nursing supervisor.
- Frequently assess and record general condition and vital signs.
- Maintain the client on bed rest, and keep the head of the bed elevated.
- Provide oxygen as ordered and monitor pulse oximetry.
- Administer prescribed intravenous fluids to maintain fluid balance while preventing fluid overload.
- Administer prescribed anticoagulants.
- Maintain comfort by administering analgesics and sedatives (use caution to prevent respiratory depression).
- Provide supportive measures for the client and family.

Refer to Chapter 36 for a detailed discussion of pulmonary embolism. ᏣᎠ

### Respiratory Complications

Common postoperative respiratory complications include pneumonia and atelectasis.

***PNEUMONIA.*** Pneumonia is an inflammation of lung tissue. Inflammation is caused either by a microbial infection or by a foreign substance in the lung, which leads to an infection. Numerous factors may be involved in the development of pneumonia, including aspiration infection, retained pulmonary secretions, failure to cough deeply, and impaired cough reflex and decreased mobility.

Common assessment findings of the client with pneumonia are as follows:

- High fever
- Rapid pulse and respirations
- Chills (may be present initially)
- Productive cough (may be present depending on the type of pneumonia)
- Dyspnea
- Chest pain
- Crackles and wheezes

Treating the pulmonary infection, supporting the client's respiratory efforts, promoting lung expansion, and preventing the organisms' spread are the goals in the care of the client with pneumonia. Nursing care includes the following measures:

- Obtain sputum specimens for culture and sensitivity testing.
- Position client with the head of the bed elevated.
- Encourage the client to turn, cough, and perform deep-breathing exercises at least every 2 hours.
- Assist with incentive spirometry, intermittent positive pressure breathing (IPPB), and/or nebulizer treatments as ordered.
- Ambulate client as condition permits and as prescribed.
- Administer oxygen as ordered.
- Assess vital signs, breath sounds, and general condition.
- Maintain hydration to help liquefy pulmonary secretions.
- Administer antibiotics, expectorants, antipyretics, and analgesics as ordered.
- Provide or assist with frequent oral hygiene.

- Prevent the spread of microorganisms by teaching proper disposal of tissues, covering mouth when coughing, and good handwashing technique.
- Provide supportive measures for the client and family.

Chapter 36 provides a detailed discussion of pneumonia. ᏣᎠ

***ATELECTASIS.*** Atelectasis is an incomplete expansion or collapse of lung tissue resulting in inadequate ventilation and retention of pulmonary secretions. Common assessment findings include dyspnea, diminished breath sounds over the affected area, anxiety, restlessness, crackles, and cyanosis.

Promoting lung expansion and systemic oxygenation of tissues is a goal in the care of the client with atelectasis. Nursing care includes:

- Positioning the client with the head of bed elevated.
- Administering oxygen as prescribed.
- Encouraging coughing, turning, and deep breathing every 2 hours.
- Ambulating the client as condition permits and as prescribed.
- Assisting with incentive spirometry or other pulmonary exercises, such as inflating a balloon, as ordered.
- Administering analgesics as prescribed.
- Promoting hydration.
- Providing supportive measures to the client and family.

### Wound Complications

Discussion of the complications associated with surgical wounds follows an overview of wound healing, wound drainage, and nursing care of wounds.

Wounds heal by either *primary, secondary,* or *tertiary intention* (Figure 7–5 ■). Healing by primary intention takes place when the wound is uncomplicated and clean and has sustained little tissue loss. The edges of the incision are well approximated (have come together well) with sutures or staples. This type of surgical incision heals quickly, and very little scarring is expected.

Secondary intention refers to the healing that occurs when the wound is large, gaping, and irregular. Tissue loss prevents wound edges from approximating; therefore, granulation fills in the wound. This type of wound takes longer to heal, is more prone to infection, and develops more scar tissue.

If enough time passes before a wound is sutured, healing by tertiary intention occurs. Infection is more likely to take place. Because the wound edges are not approximated, tissue is regenerated by the granulation process. Closure of the wound results in a wide scar.

From the time the surgical incision is made until the wound is completely healed, all wounds progress through four stages of healing. However, healing time varies according to many factors, such as age, nutritional status, general health, and the type and location of the wound. Figure 7–5 also provides a summary of the stages of wound healing.

Wound drainage (exudate) results from the inflammatory process in the first two stages of wound healing. The drainage is from the rich blood supply that surrounds the wound tissue and is composed of escaped fluid and cells. The drainage is described as serous, sanguineous, or purulent.

## Stages of Wound Healing

- *Stage I: from surgery through day 2.* Inflammatory process occurs to prepare the surrounding tissue for healing. Blood vessels constrict, and clotting occurs. Vasodilation follows, bringing more blood, white blood cells, and fibroplastin to the wound site. Epithelial cells begin to form and reestablish blood flow in the wound tissue. A mild temperature elevation is normal.
- *Stage II: day 3 through day 14 following surgery.* Fewer white blood cells are present. Collagen tissue forms in the wound tissue. Granulation tissue, red with a rich blood supply, is established.
- *Stage III: day 15 to week 6 following surgery.* Collagen fibers continue to strengthen the wound. As the blood supply decreases, the scar tissue appears pink and somewhat raised.
- *Stage IV: several months to a year following surgery.* As the wound tissue constricts, the scar becomes flat, smaller, and white.

**Primary intention**

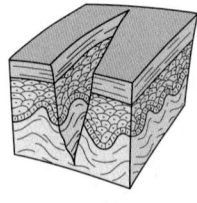 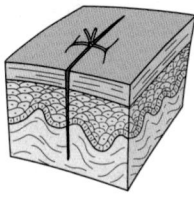 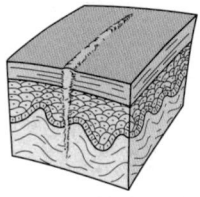

Clean incision          Early suture          "Hairline" scar

**Secondary intention**

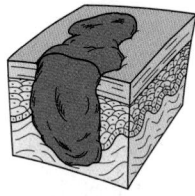 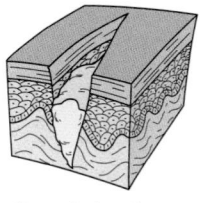 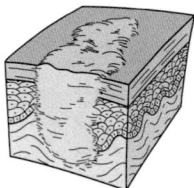

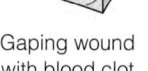

Gaping wound        Granulation tissue        Large scar
with blood clot        fills in wound

**Tertiary intention**

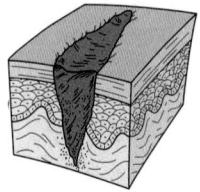 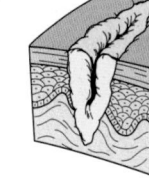 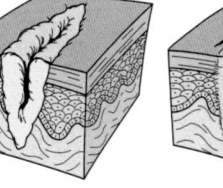

Contaminated wound     Granulation tissue     Closure with
                                              wide scar

**Figure 7–5** ■ Wound healing by primary, secondary, and tertiary intention.

- Serous drainage contains mostly the clear serous portion of the blood. The drainage appears clear or slightly yellow and is thin in consistency.
- Sanguineous drainage contains a combination of serum and red blood cells and has a thick, reddish appearance. This is the most common type of drainage from a noncomplicated surgical wound.
- Purulent drainage is composed of white blood cells, tissue debris, and bacteria. Purulent drainage is the result of infection and tends to be of a thicker consistency, with various colors specific to the type of organism. It also may have an unpleasant odor.

Box 7–4 describes and illustrates various types of wound drainage devices. These devices decrease pressure in the wound area by removing excess fluid, which promotes healing and decreases complications.

Nursing care of the postoperative client with a surgical wound focuses on preventing and monitoring for wound complications. The nurse assumes a leading role in supporting the wound healing process, providing emotional support to the client and teaching wound care to the client.

Common assessment findings of an infected wound include purulent, odorous discharge and redness, warmth, and edema around the edges of the incision. Additionally, the client may have a fever, chills, and increased respiratory and pulse rates. Nursing care includes the following measures:

- Maintain medical asepsis (e.g., by using a good handwashing technique).
- Follow Centers for Disease Control and Prevention (CDC) guidelines for wound care.
- Observe aseptic technique during dressing changes and handling of tubes and drains.
- Assess vital signs, especially temperature.
- Evaluate the characteristics of wound discharge (color, odor, and amount).
- Assess the condition of the incision (approximation of the edges, sutures, staples, or drains).
- Clean, irrigate, and pack the wound in the prescribed manner. Sterile normal saline is often prescribed; povidone-iodine (Betadine) is no longer recommended for wound care.
- Maintain the client's hydration and nutritional status.
- Culture the wound prior to beginning antibiotic therapy.
- Administer antibiotics and antipyretics as prescribed.
- Provide supportive measures to client and family.

**Dehiscence** is a separation in the layers of the incisional wound (Figure 7–6A ■). Treatment depends on the extent of wound disruption. If the dehiscence is extensive, the incision must be resutured in surgery. **Evisceration** is the protrusion of body organs from a wound dehiscence (Figure 7–6B). These serious complications may result from delayed wound healing or may occur immediately following surgery. They also may occur after forceful straining (coughing, sneezing, or vomiting). When dehiscence occurs, immediately cover the wound with a sterile dressing moistened with normal saline. Emergency surgery is performed to repair these conditions.

## BOX 7–4   ■   Wound Drainage Devices

A Penrose drain, used for passive wound drainage, promotes healing from the inside to the outside (see figure A below). The use of the drain decreases the chance of abscess formation. The safety pin in the Penrose drain prevents the exposed end from slipping down into the wound. Wound care focuses on cleaning around the drain with a prescribed solution, such as sterile normal saline, and replacing the precut gauze dressing as necessary to keep the surrounding skin dry and encourage further drainage. An absorbent dressing is placed over the drain and gauze (not shown).

Wound suction devices promote drainage of fluid from the incision site, decreasing pressure on healing tissues and reducing abscess formation. Shown are the Jackson-Pratt and Hemovac wound suction devices (see figures B and C below).

The frequency with which the nurse empties the device depends on the time elapsed since surgery, type of surgery, amount of drainage, and hospital policy. For example, immediately after surgery the nurse may empty the device every 15 to 60 minutes. With time, as drainage decreases, the device is emptied every 2 to 4 hours (per hospital policy). Amount, color, consistency, and odor of drainage are documented.

Usually, the nurse removes the drain on the second to fourth day after surgery (depending on hospital policy). Removal causes minor client discomfort. The drain site is cleaned, and a sterile dressing is applied.

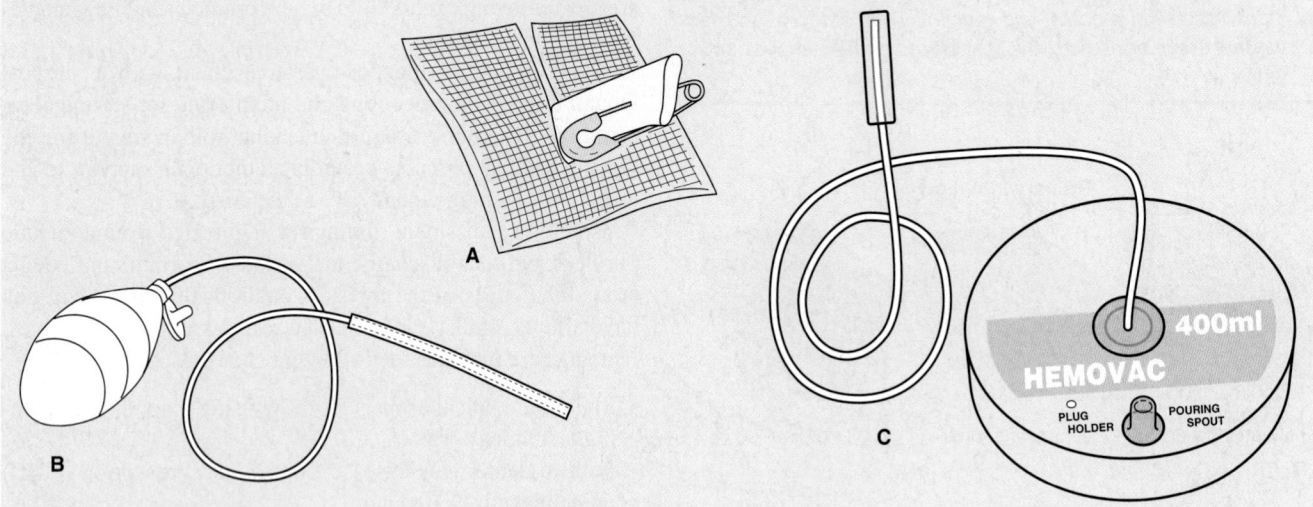

Wound drainage devices. A, Penrose passive wound drainage device. B, Jackson-Pratt wound suction device. C, Hemovac wound suction device.

Either the nurse or physician removes sutures or staples after the wound has healed sufficiently (usually 5 to 10 days after surgery). Removal is performed using medical aseptic technique. Additional support may be provided to the incision by applying strips of tape (or Steri-Strips) as directed by institutional policy or by the physician.

### Complications Associated with Elimination

Common postoperative complications associated with elimination include urinary retention and altered bowel elimination. The inability to urinate with urinary retention may occur postoperatively as a result of the recumbent position, effects of anesthesia and narcotics, inactivity, altered fluid balance, nervous tension, or surgical manipulation in the pelvic area. Nursing care centers around promoting normal urinary elimination and includes the following measures.

- Assess for bladder distention if the client has not voided within 7 to 8 hours after surgery or if the client is urinating small amounts frequently.
- Assess the amount of urine in the bladder with a portable ultrasound scanner. This noninvasive procedure decreases the potential for urinary tract infections and urethral trauma from repeated catheterizations.
- Monitor intake and output.

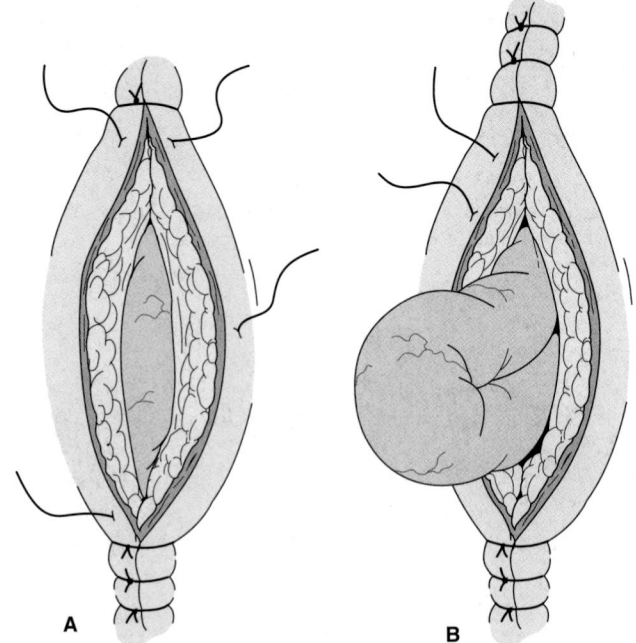

**Figure 7–6** ■ Wound complications. A, Dehiscence is a disruption in the incision resulting in a separation of the layers of the wound. B, Evisceration is a protrusion of a body organ through a surgical incision.

- Maintain intravenous infusion if fluids are prescribed.
- Increase daily oral fluid intake to 2500 to 3000 mL if the client's condition permits.
- Insert a straight or indwelling catheter if ordered.
- Promote normal urinary elimination by:
  a. Assisting and providing privacy when the client uses a bedpan.
  b. Helping the client use the bedside commode or walk to the bathroom.
  c. Assisting male clients to stand to void.
  d. Pouring a measured amount of warm water over the peritoneal area. (If urination occurs, subtract the amount of water from the total amount for an accurate output measurement.)

  Bowel elimination frequently is altered after abdominal or pelvic surgery and sometimes after other surgeries. Return to normal gastrointestinal function may be delayed by general anesthesia, narcotic analgesia, decreased mobility, or altered fluid and food intake during the perioperative period.

  Nursing care centers around the return of normal bowel function and includes the following measures.

- Assess for the return of normal peristalsis:
  a. Auscultate bowel sounds every 4 hours while the client is awake.
  b. Assess the abdomen for distention. (A distended abdomen with absent or high-pitched bowel sounds may indicate paralytic ileus.)
  c. Determine whether the client is passing flatus.
  d. Monitor for passage of stool, including amount and consistency.
- Encourage early ambulation within prescribed limits.
- Facilitate a daily fluid intake of 2500 to 3000 mL (unless contraindicated).
- Provide privacy when the client is using the bedpan, bedside commode, or bathroom.

If no bowel movement has occurred within 3 to 4 days after surgery, a suppository or an enema may be ordered.

## Special Considerations for Older Adults

Physiologic, cognitive, and psychosocial changes associated with the aging process place the older adult at increased risk for postoperative complications. These age-related changes with selected nursing interventions are summarized in Table 7–6. With an ever-increasing population of older adults, particularly the very old, the nurse must be aware of these normal changes and modify nursing care accordingly in an effort to provide safe, supportive care.

## TABLE 7–6    Nursing Interventions for Older Surgical Clients

| System | Age-Related Changes | Nursing Interventions |
|---|---|---|
| General appearance | Change in height, weight, and fat distribution | Assess physical parameters. Provide for warmth. Turn frequently. |
| Integument | Diminished integrity secondary to loss of subcutaneous fat and decreased oil production, elasticity, and hydration | Provide careful preoperative preparation to avoid trauma. Use other means to assess oxygenation and hydration, such as evaluation of mucous membranes, laboratory studies, and urine output. |
| Sensory-perceptual | Decline in vision and hearing ability; dryness of mouth | Compensate for sensory deficits: speak low, not loud; minimize noise in environment; provide adequate room light; stay within client's field of vision when speaking; encourage client to wear hearing aid to the operating room. Provide comfort measures when NPO. |
| Respiratory | Decreased efficiency of cough reflex and decreased aeration of lung fields | Teach and encourage coughing and diaphragmatic breathing exercises. Assess baseline parameters. Constantly monitor lung sounds and respiratory status. |
| Cardiovascular | Less efficient, decreased adaptation to stress | Monitor for hypotension and shock. Assess for thrombus formation, cardiac dysrhythmias, peripheral pulses, and edema. |
| Gastrointestinal | Decline in gastric motility | Encourage intake of adequate fluids, nutritious meals, soft diet. Assist with feeding; monitor bowel function. |
| Genitourinary | Decreased efficiency of kidney; loss of bladder control | Monitor I&O and electrolyte levels. Assess for drug side effects. Assist with voiding as needed. |
| Musculoskeletal | Stiffness of joints; decrease in strength; brittleness of bones | Carefully position on OR table. Move carefully and gently. Prevent pressure sores. |
| Cognitive-psychosocial | Decreased reaction time; stable intellectual ability stable; proneness to delirium and altered mental status while in hospital | Provide ample time for making decisions. Implement safety measures. Talk to client as adult, not as child. Orient frequently. |

*Note. Adapted from "Perioperative Nursing Care for the Elderly Surgical Patient" by C. Dellasea and C. Burgunder, 1991, Today's O.R. Nurse, 13(6): 12–17.*

## Managing Acute Postoperative Pain

Pain is expected after surgery. It is neither realistic nor practical to eliminate postoperative pain completely. Nevertheless, the client should receive substantial relief from and control of this discomfort. Controlling postoperative pain not only promotes comfort but also facilitates coughing, turning, deep-breathing exercises, earlier ambulation, and decreased length of hospitalization, resulting in fewer postoperative complications, and therefore reducing health care costs. Despite the apparent benefits of effective pain control, recent studies indicate that about 50% of postoperative clients do not receive adequate pain relief or control (Acute Pain Management Guideline Panel, 1992).

Managing acute postoperative pain is an important nursing role before, during, and after surgery. Successful pain manage- ment involves the cooperative efforts of the client, physician, and nurse. Preoperatively, the client should learn how much pain to anticipate and what methods are available to control pain. After discussing options with the client, health care providers must respect the client's personal preferences. The information that follows is based on *Acute Pain Management in Adults: Operative Procedures* (Acute Pain Management Guideline Panel, 1992).

Postoperative medications were discussed earlier in the chapter. Various nonpharmacologic approaches to pain management are used alone or in combination to control acute postoperative pain. Relaxation, distraction, and imagery techniques can decrease mild pain and anxiety. Massage and the application of heat or cold can also relieve postoperative pain. Transcutaneous electrical nerve stimulation (TENS) has been used

---

### CHART 7–1  NANDA, NIC, AND NOC LINKAGES

#### The Postoperative Client

| NURSING DIAGNOSES | NURSING INTERVENTIONS | NURSING OUTCOMES |
|---|---|---|
| • Acute Pain | • Analgesic Administration<br>• Pain Management<br>• Patient-Controlled Analgesia (PCA) Assistance<br>• Postanesthesia Care | • Pain Level<br>• Comfort Level<br>• Pain Control Behavior |
| • Risk for Infection | • Infection Protection<br>• Infection Control<br>• Cough Enhancement<br>• Nutrition Management<br>• Wound Care<br>• Incision Site Care<br>• Vital Signs Monitoring | • Risk Control<br>• Tissue Integrity: Skin<br>• Immobility Consequences: Physiological<br>• Nutritional Status |
| • Risk for Imbalanced Fluid Volume | • Electrolyte Management<br>• Fluid Management<br>• Fluid Monitoring<br>• Intravenous (IV) Therapy<br>• Vital Signs Monitoring | • Fluid Balance<br>• Hydration |
| • Nausea | • Nausea Management<br>• Vomiting Management<br>• Medication Administration<br>• Pain Management | • Nausea Level |
| • Ineffective Protection | • Surgical Precautions<br>• Postanesthesia Care<br>• Infection Control<br>• Wound Care<br>• Surveillance: Safety | • Infection Status<br>• Neurological Status: Consciousness<br>• Wound Healing<br>• Cognitive Orientation |
| • Delayed Surgical Recovery | • Exercise Management: Ambulation<br>• Incision Site Care<br>• Infection Control<br>• Nutrition Management<br>• Pain Management<br>• Urinary Elimination Management<br>• Sleep Enhancement<br>• Discharge Planning | • Immobility Consequences: Physiological<br>• Wound Healing<br>• Nutritional Status<br>• Comfort Level<br>• Urinary Elimination<br>• Sleep<br>• Knowledge: Diet, Health Resources, Infection Control, Medication, Prescribed Activity, Treatment Regimen |

*Note. Data from Nursing Outcomes Classification (NOC) by M. Johnson & M. Maas (Eds.), 1997, St. Louis: Mosby; Nursing Diagnoses: Definitions & Classification 2001–2002 by North American Nursing Diagnosis Association, 2001, Philadelphia: NANDA; Nursing Interventions Classification (NIC) by J.C. McCloskey & G. M. Bulechek (Eds.), 2000, St. Louis: Mosby. Reprinted by permission.*

successfully to decrease postoperative incisional pain. Other approaches include acupuncture, acupressure, and therapeutic touch. Additional information on pain management techniques is found in Chapter 4. ⬭

Opioid dosage requirements vary greatly from one client to another and by the route they are taken. Remember that oral doses of analgesics are not equal to parenteral doses. Oral doses need to be higher to provide equianalgesia. See Table 4–4 regarding equianalgesics.

The client's input and participation in assessing pain and pain relief is essential to a successful pain control regime. For example, the client can rate the pain on a scale of 0 to 10 (where 0 signifies no pain and 10 signifies unbearable pain). Assess and document pain at scheduled intervals to determine the degree of pain control, to observe for drug side effects, and to assess the need for changes in the dosage and/or frequency of medication administration.

## Using NANDA, NIC, and NOC

Chart 7–1 shows links between NANDA nursing diagnoses, NIC, and NOC when caring for the postoperative client.

## Home Care

Because the postoperative phase does not end until the client has recovered completely from the surgical intervention, the nurse plays a vital role as the client nears discharge. As the client prepares to recuperate at home, provide information and support to help the client successfully meet self-care demands. All aspects of teaching should be accompanied by written guidelines, directions, and information. This is particularly helpful when a large amount of unfamiliar, detailed information is presented. Because the hospital stay is often brief, make an organized, coordinated effort to educate the client and family. Teaching needs vary, but the most common needs include:

- How to perform wound care. Teaching is more effective if the nurse first demonstrates and explains the procedure for the client and family or other caregiver. The client and family should then participate in the care. To evaluate the effectiveness of the teaching, ask the client or caregiver to demonstrate the procedure in return. Ideally, teaching is carried out over several days, evaluated, and periodically reinforced.
- Signs and symptoms of a wound infection. The client should be able to determine what is normal and what should be reported to the physician.
- Method and the frequency of taking one's temperature.
- Limitations or restrictions that may be imposed on such activities as lifting, driving, bathing, sexual activity, and other physical activities.
- Control of pain. If analgesics are prescribed, instruct the client in the dosage, frequency, purpose, common side effects, and other side effects to report to the physician. Reinforce the use of relaxation, distraction, imagery, or other pain control techniques that the client has found useful in controlling postoperative pain.

## Nursing Care Plan
## A Client Having Surgery

Martha Overbeck is a 74-year-old widow of German descent who lives alone in a senior citizens' housing complex. She is active there, as well as in the Lutheran Church. She has been in good health and is independent, but she has become progressively less active as a result of arthritic pain and stiffness. Mrs. Overbeck has degenerative joint changes that have particularly affected her right hip. On the recommendation of her physician and following a discussion with her friends, Mrs. Overbeck has been admitted to the hospital for an elective right total hip replacement. Her surgery has been scheduled for 8:00 A.M. the following day.

Mrs. Eva Jackson, a close friend and neighbor, accompanies Mrs. Overbeck to the hospital. Mrs. Overbeck explains that her friend will help in her home and assist her with the wound care and prescribed exercises.

### ASSESSMENT

Gloria Nobis, RN, is assigned to Mrs. Overbeck's care on return to her room. Ms. Nobis performs a complete head-to-toe assessment and determines that Mrs. Overbeck is drowsy but oriented. Her skin is pale and slightly cool. Mrs. Overbeck states she is cold and requests additional covers. Ms. Nobis places a warmed cotton blanket next to Mrs. Overbeck's body, adds another blanket to her covers, and adjusts the room's thermostat to increase the room temperature. Mrs. Overbeck states that she is in no pain and would like to sleep. She has even, unlabored respirations and stable vital signs as compared to preoperative readings.

Mrs. Overbeck is NPO. An intravenous solution of dextrose and water is infusing at 100 mL/h per infusion pump. No redness or edema is noted at the infusion site. Ms. Nobis notes that the antibiotic ciprofloxacin hydrochloride (Cipro) is to be administered by mouth when the client is able to tolerate fluids. Mrs. Overbeck has a large gauze dressing over her right upper lateral thigh and hip with no indications of drainage from the wound. Tubing protrudes from the distal end of the dressing and is attached to a passive suctioning device (Hemovac). Ms. Nobis empties 50 mL of dark red drainage from the suctioning device and records the amount and characteristics on a flow record. Mrs. Overbeck has a Foley catheter in place with 250 mL of clear, light amber urine in the dependent gravity drainage bag.

When assessing Mrs. Overbeck's lower extremities, Ms. Nobis finds her feet slightly cool and pale with rapid capillary refill time bilaterally. Dorsalis pedis and posterior tibial pulses are strong and equal bilaterally. Ms. Nobis notes slight pitting edema in the right foot and ankle as compared with the left extremity. She also notes sensation and ability to move both feet and toes, without numbness or tingling (paresthesia).

Ms. Nobis records the above findings on a postoperative flowsheet. After ensuring that Mrs. Overbeck is safely positioned and can reach her call light, Ms. Nobis gives Mrs. Overbeck's friend, Mrs. Jackson, a progress report. They then go into Mrs. Overbeck's room.

(continued on page 190)

## Nursing Care Plan
### A Client Having Surgery (continued)

### DIAGNOSES

Ms. Nobis makes the following postoperative nursing diagnoses for Mrs. Overbeck.

- *Risk for infection* of right hip wound related to disruption of normal skin integrity by the surgical incision
- *Risk for injury* related to potential dislocation of right hip prosthesis secondary to total hip replacement
- *Pain* related to right hip incision and positioning of arthritic joints during surgery

### EXPECTED OUTCOMES

The expected outcomes established in the plan of care specify that Mrs. Overbeck will:

- Regain skin integrity of the right hip incision without experiencing signs or symptoms of infection.
- Demonstrate (along with Mrs. Jackson) proper aseptic technique while performing the dressing change.
- Verbalize signs and symptoms of infection to be reported to her physician.
- Describe measures to be taken to prevent dislocation of right hip prosthesis.
- Report control of pain at incision and in arthritic joints.
- Remain afebrile.

### PLANNING AND IMPLEMENTATION

Ms. Nobis develops a care plan that includes the following interventions to assist Mrs. Overbeck during her postoperative recovery.

- Use aseptic technique while changing dressing.
- Monitor temperature and pulse every 4 hours to assess for elevation.
- Assess wound every 8 hours for purulent drainage and odor. Assess edges of wound for approximation, edema, redness, or inflammation in excess of expected inflammatory response.
- Teach Mrs. Overbeck and Mrs. Jackson how to use aseptic technique while assessing the wound and performing the dressing change.
- Teach Mrs. Overbeck and Mrs. Jackson the signs and symptoms of infection and when to report findings to the physician.

- Review and discuss with Mrs. Overbeck the written materials on total hip replacement.
- Convey empathetic understanding of Mrs. Overbeck's incisional and arthritic joint pain.
- Medicate Mrs. Overbeck every 4 hours (or as ordered) to maintain a therapeutic analgesic blood level.

### EVALUATION

Throughout Mrs. Overbeck's hospitalization, Ms. Nobis works with Mrs. Overbeck and Mrs. Jackson to ensure that Mrs. Overbeck can care for herself after discharge from the hospital. Five days after her surgery, Mrs. Overbeck is discharged with a well-approximated incision with no indications of an infection. Prior to discharge, Ms. Nobis is confident that with Mrs. Jackson's help, Mrs. Overbeck can properly assess the incision. With minimal help, Mrs. Overbeck is able to replace the dressing using aseptic technique. She can cite the signs and symptoms of an infection, take her own oral temperature, and describe preventive measures to decrease the chances of dislocating her prosthetic hip. Because of her reduced mobility the past 5 days, Mrs. Overbeck says she can tell the arthritis in her "old bones" is "acting up." She reports less pain in her right hip than before the surgery. Mrs. Overbeck tells Ms. Nobis she will be back the following winter to have her left hip replaced.

### Critical Thinking in the Nursing Process

1. Describe risk factors for Mrs. Overbeck's safety; what changes in her home environment would you suggest to promote safety until she recovers more fully?
2. Why is Mrs. Overbeck placed on the antibiotic Cipro although she has no indications of an infection? What teaching would you do?
3. Mrs. Overbeck's clotting time is slightly elevated as a result of an ordered anticoagulant. Why would this medication be ordered? Consider the client's age and the area of surgery.
4. Mrs. Overbeck is 30 pounds above her ideal weight and has osteoarthritis. Develop a care plan for the nursing diagnosis *altered health maintenance* related to intake in excess of metabolic requirements.

See Evaluating Your Response in Appendix C.

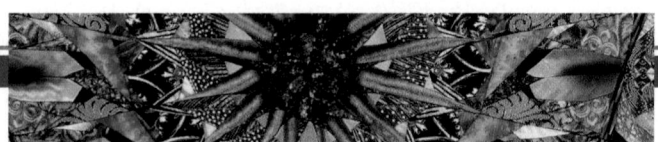

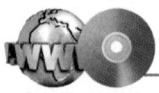

## EXPLORE MediaLink

NCLEX review questions, case studies, care plan activities, MediaLink applications, and other interactive resources for this chapter can be found on the Companion Website at www.prenhall.com/lemone.

Click on Chapter 7 to select the activities for this chapter. For animations, video clips, more NCLEX review questions, and an audio glossary, access the Student CD-ROM accompanying this textbook.

# TEST YOURSELF

1. The nurse's primary responsibility related to informed consent is:
   a. Defining the risks and benefits of the surgery
   b. Witnessing the client's signature on the consent form
   c. Explaining the right to refuse treatment or withdraw consent
   d. Advising the client and family about what is needed for the diagnosis

2. Obtaining a preoperative blood pressure measurement serves the following purpose:
   a. Fulfills a legal requirement
   b. Informs anesthesiologist so proper level of anesthesia can be given
   c. Prevents atelectasis
   d. Provides a baseline to compare postoperative blood pressure levels

3. Nonsteroidal anti-inflammatory drugs are given in the postoperative period to:
   a. Stimulate appetite
   b. Increase amnesia
   c. Potentiate analgesia
   d. Improve renal function

4. Discharge planning for a client with a total knee replacement will include dietary management guidelines. Specifically, the client will eat a diet:
   a. Low in cholesterol, high in fat
   b. High in protein, moderate in calories
   c. Low in fat, high in fiber
   d. Regular diet without dairy products

5. In the immediate postoperative period for knee surgery, assessment distal to the site includes:
   a. Urinary pH
   b. Rebound tenderness
   c. Chvostek's sign
   d. Neurovascular assessment

See Test Yourself answers in Appendix C.

# BIBLIOGRAPHY

Acute Pain Management Guideline Panel. (1992). *Acute pain management in adults: Operative procedures* (AHCPR Publication No. 92-0019). Rockville, MD: Agency for Health Care Policy and Research, Public Health Service, USDHHS.

American Society of Perianesthesia Nurses. (1995). *Standards of perianesthesia nursing practice*. Thorofare, NJ: ASPAN.

Arndt, K. (1999). Inadvertent hypothermia in the OR. *AORN Journal, 70,* 204–214.

Association of Operating Room Nurses. (1993). *AORN standards and recommended practices for perioperative nursing*. Denver, CO: AORN.

Bailes, B.K. (2000). Perioperative care of the elderly surgical patient. *AORN Journal, 72,* 186–207.

Brown, B., Riippa, M., & Shaneberger, K. (2001). Promoting patient safety through preoperative patient verification. *AORN Journal, 74*(5), 690–698.

Busen, N.H. (2001). Perioperative preparation of the adolescent surgical patient. *AORN Journal, 73,* 337–363.

Carpenito, L. (1997). *Nursing diagnosis: Application to clinical practice* (7th ed.). Philadelphia: Lippincott.

Crensha, J.T., & Winslow, E.H. (2002). Preoperative fasting: Old habits die hard. *American Journal of Nursing, 102*(5), 36–45.

Cuzzell, J. (1994). Back to basics: Test your wound assessment. *American Journal of Nursing, 94*(6), 34–35.

DeFazio-Quinn, D. (1997). Ambulatory surgery . . . an evolution. *Nursing Clinics of North America, 32*(2), 377–386.

Fairchild, S. (1996). *Perioperative nursing: Principles and practice* (2nd ed.). Boston: Little, Brown and Company.

Flanagan, M. (1997). *Wound management*. New York: Churchill Livingstone.

Heimberger, D.C., & Weinsier, R.L. (1997). *Handbook of clinical nutrition* (3rd ed.). St. Louis: Mosby.

Hollingsworth, H. (1995). Nurses' assessment and management of pain at wound dressing changes. *Journal of Wound Care, 4*(2), 77–83.

Ireland, D. (1997). Legal issues in ambulatory surgery. *Nursing Clinics of North America, 32*(2), 469–476.

Kee, J. (1995). Laboratory & diagnostic tests with nursing implications. Upper Saddle River, NJ: Prentice Hall.

Kreger, C. (2001). Getting to the root of pain: Spinal anesthesia and analgesia. *Nursing 2001, 31*(6), 37–42.

Lancaster, K. (1997). Patient teaching in ambulatory surgery. *Nursing Clinics of North America, 32*(2), 417–427.

McKenry, L., & Salerno, E. (1998). *Pharmacology in nursing* (20th ed.). St. Louis: Mosby.

Nash, P., & O'Malley, M. (1997). Streamlining the perioperative process. *Nursing Clinics of North America, 32*(1), 141–151.

New, S., & Gutierrez, L. (1997). Quality improvement in the ambulatory surgical setting. *Nursing Clinics of North America, 32*(2), 477–488.

Ozawa, S., Shander, A., & Ochani, T.D. (2001). A practical approach to achieving bloodless surgery. *AORN Journal, 74*(1), 34–47.

Pasero, C., & McCaffery, M. (1996). Managing postoperative pain in the elderly. *American Journal of Nursing, 96*(10), 38–45.

Pontieri-Lewis, V. (1997). The role of nutrition in wound healing. *MEDSURG Nursing, 6*(4), 187–190, 221.

Porth, C. (1998). *Pathophysiology: Concepts of altered health states* (5th ed.). Philadelphia: Lippincott.

Ruzicka, S. (1997). The impact of normal aging processes and chronic illness on perioperative care of the elderly. *Seminars in Perioperative Nursing, 6*(1), 3–13.

Schick, L. (1998). The postanesthesia patient. In C. Hudak, B. Gallo, & P. Morton (Eds.), *Critical care nursing: A holistic approach* (7th ed.) (pp. 137–150). Philadelphia: Lippincott.

Scott, E.M., Leaper, D.J., Clark, N., & Kelly, P.J. (2001). Effects of warming therapy on pressure ulcers—A randomized trial. *AORN Journal, 73*(5), 921–928.

Steelman, V., Bulechek, G., & McCloskey, J. (1994). Toward a standardized language to describe perioperative nursing. *AORN Journal, 60*(5), 786–795.

Stringer, B., Infante-Revard, C., & Hanley, J. (2001). Quantifying and reducing the risk of bloodborne pathogen exposure. *AORN Journal, 73,* 1135–1146.

Tappen, R.M., Muzic, J., & Kennedy, P. (2001). Preoperative assessment and discharge planning for older adults undergoing ambulatory surgery. *AORN Journal, 73,* 464–474.

Walton, J. (2001). Helping high-risk surgical patients beat the odds. *Nursing 2001, 31*(3), 54–59.

Whitman, M. (2000). The starving patient. *Clinical Journal of Oncology Nursing, 4*(3), 121–125.

Williams, G. (1997). Preoperative assessment and health history review. *Nursing Clinics of North America, 32*(2), 395–416.

Zalon, M. (1997). Pain in frail, elderly women after surgery. *Image: Journal of Nursing Scholarship, 29*(1), 21–26.

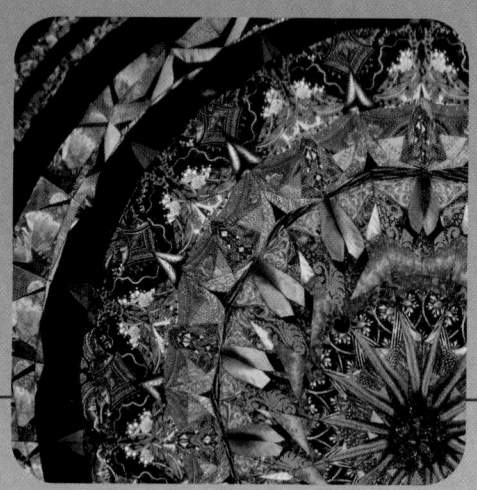

# CHAPTER 8

# Nursing Care of Clients with Infection

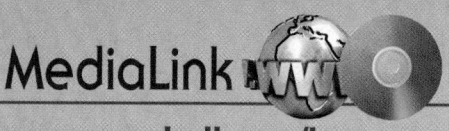

## MediaLink

**www.prenhall.com/lemone**
Additional resources for this chapter can be found on the Student CD-ROM accompanying this textbook, and on the Companion Website at www.prenhall.com/lemone. Click on Chapter 8 to select the activities for this chapter.

**CD-ROM**
- Audio Glossary
- NCLEX Review

**Animations**
- Inflammatory Response
- White Blood Cells
- Penicillin

**Companion Website**
- More NCLEX Review
- Case Study
  Bioterrorism Preparedness
- Care Plan Activity
  Postoperative Infection
- MediaLink Application
  Antibiotic-Resistant Organisms

## LEARNING OUTCOMES

After completing this chapter, you will be able to:

- Discuss the components and functions of the immune system and the immune response.

- Compare antibody-mediated and cell-mediated immune response.

- Describe the pathophysiology of wound healing, inflammation, and infection.

- Compare natural and acquired immunity and active and passive immunity.

- Identify factors responsible for nosocomial infections.

- Provide teaching for clients with inflammation or an infection and their families.

- Use the nursing process as a framework to provide individualized care to clients with inflammation and infection.

The human body is continually threatened by foreign substances, infectious agents, and abnormal cells. The immune system is the body's major defense mechanism against infectious organisms and abnormal or damaged cells. Recent years have seen the emergence of resistant microorganisms such as methicillin-resistant *Staphylococcus aureus* and altered strains of familiar diseases, such as multiple-drug-resistant tuberculosis. New diseases have also emerged, such as Lyme disease and human immunodeficiency virus (HIV).

A thorough knowledge of the immune system increases understanding of the local and systemic inflammatory response, resistance to infectious disease, and the importance of immunization. This foundation can help the nurse teach clients and families to follow recommended treatment regimens, to promote and maintain health, and to prevent disease. In addition, the nurse can prescribe appropriate rehabilitative measures, such as increased rest and attention to optimal nutrition.

## OVERVIEW OF THE IMMUNE SYSTEM

The immune system is a complex and intricate network of specialized cells, tissues, and organs. Cells of the immune system seek out and destroy damaged cells and foreign tissue, yet recognize and preserve host cells (Porth, 2002). The immune system performs the following functions:

- Defending and protecting the body from infection by bacteria, viruses, fungi, and parasites

- Removing and destroying damaged or dead cells
- Identifying and destroying malignant cells, thereby preventing their further development into tumors

The immune system is activated by minor injuries, such as small lacerations or bruises, or by major injuries, such as burns, surgeries, and systemic diseases (e.g., pneumonia). The response of the immune system may be nonspecific or specific. Nonspecific responses prevent or limit the entry of invaders into the body, thereby limiting the extent of tissue damage and reducing the workload of the immune system. **Inflammation** is a nonspecific response activated by both minor and major injuries. When the inflammatory process is unable to destroy invading organisms or toxins, a more specific response, called the immune response, is activated.

## Immune System Components

The immune system consists of molecules, cells, and organs that produce the immune response (Table 8–1). These components may be involved in the nonspecific inflammatory response, the specific immunologic response, or both.

### Leukocytes

**Leukocytes,** or white blood cells (WBCs), are the primary cells involved in both nonspecific and specific immune system responses. Like all blood cells, leukocytes derive from stem cells, the hemocytoblasts, in the bone marrow (Figure 8–1 ■). Unlike red blood cells (RBCs), which are confined to the circulation,

| TABLE 8–1 | Cells and Tissues of the Immune System | |
|---|---|---|
| **Component** | **Location** | **Function** |
| **Leukocytes** | | |
| Granulocytes | | |
| Neutrophils | Circulation | Phagocytosis and chemotaxis |
| Eosinophils | Circulation, respiratory tract, and gastrointestinal tract | Phagocytosis  Protection against parasites  Involved in allergic response |
| Basophils | Circulation | Release of chemotactic substances |
| Monocytes and macrophages | Circulation (monocytes) and body tissue, such as skin (histocytes), liver (Kupffer's cells), alveoli, spleen, tonsils, lymph nodes, bone marrow, brain | Trapping and phagocytizing of foreign substances and cellular debris  Secretion of interleukin-1 to stimulate lymphocyte growth |
| Lymphocytes | | |
| T cells  (mature in thymus gland) | Circulation, lymph system, tissues | Activation of T and B cells  Control of viral infections and destruction of cancer cells  Involved in hypersensitivity reactions and graft tissue rejection |
| B cells  (mature in bone marrow) | Circulation, spleen | Production of antibodies (immunoglobulins) to specific antigens |
| NK (natural killer) cells | Circulation | Cytotoxic; killing of tumor cells, fungi, viral-infected cells, and foreign tissue |
| **Lymphoid Tissues** | | |
| Primary or central lymphoid structures | Bone marrow and thymus gland | Production of immune cells; sites for cell maturation |
| Secondary or peripheral lymphoid structures | Lymph nodes, spleen, tonsils, intestinal lymphoid tissue, lymphoid tissue in other organs | Sites for activation of immune cells by antigens |

**Figure 8-1** ■ The development and differentiation of leukocytes from hemocytoblasts.

Hemocytoblasts (stem cells)

Myeloid stem cells

Lymphoid stem cells

Megakaryoblasts

Proerythroblasts

Myeloblasts

Monoblasts

Lymphoblasts

Thrombocytes (platelets)

Erythrocytes (RBCs)

Eosinophils   Neutrophils   Basophils   Monocytes   Lymphocytes

Granulocytes

(some become)

(some become)

Macrophages

Plasma cells

Leukocytes

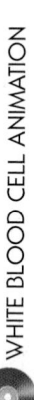

leukocytes use the circulation to transport themselves to the site of an inflammatory or immune response. As the mobile units of the immune system, leukocytes detect, attack, and destroy anything that is recognized as "foreign." They are able to move through tissue spaces, locating damaged tissue and infection by responding to chemicals released by other leukocytes and damaged tissue.

The normal number of circulating leukocytes is 4,500 to 10,000 cells per cubic millimeter (mm³) of blood (Kee, 2001). Many more leukocytes are marginated; that is, they adhere to vascular epithelial cells along the vessel walls, in other tissue spaces, or in the lymph system. In the presence of an attack such as an infection, additional WBCs are released from the bone marrow, leading to **leukocytosis,** a WBC count of greater than 10,000/mm³. As WBCs move out of the bone marrow into the blood, the bone marrow increases its production of additional leukocytes. A decrease in the number of circulating leukocytes, known as **leukopenia,** occurs when bone marrow activity is suppressed or when leukocyte destruction increases.

Leukocytes are divided into three major groups: granulocytes, monocytes, and lymphocytes. The granulocytes and monocytes derive from the myeloid stem cells of the bone marrow and are instrumental in the inflammatory response. Lymphocytes derive from the lymphoid stem cells of the bone marrow

and are the primary cells involved in the specific immune response. In laboratory tests, the WBC count indicates the total number of circulating leukocytes. The WBC differential identifies the portion of the total represented by each type of leukocyte.

**GRANULOCYTES.** Granulocytes constitute 60% to 80% of the total number of normal blood leukocytes. Their cytoplasm has a granular appearance, and their nuclei are distinctively multilobular (see Figure 8–1). Granulocytes have a short life span, measured in hours to days, compared to the life span of monocytes, which is measured in months to years. Granulocytes play a key role in protecting the body from harmful microorganisms during acute inflammation and infection. There are three types of granulocytes: neutrophils, eosinophils, and basophils.

*Neutrophils,* also called polymorphonuclear leukocytes (PMNs or polys), are the most plentiful of the granulocytes, constituting 55% to 70% of the total number of circulating leukocytes. Neutrophils are *phagocytic* cells, responsible for engulfing and destroying foreign agents, particularly bacteria and small particles. Neutrophils are the first phagocytic cells to arrive at the site of invasion, drawn by chemicals released by damaged tissue and invading organisms.

Neutrophils are produced in the bone marrow and released into the circulation when they mature. Segmented neutrophils (or segs) are mature forms, and usually account for about 55% of total leukocytes. *Bands* are immature neutrophils and usually comprise 5% of leukocytes. It takes about 10 days for a neutrophil to mature and be released into the circulation. Once released, neutrophils have a circulating half-life of 6 to 10 hours. They cannot replicate and must be replaced constantly to maintain adequate numbers in the circulation. They do not return to the bone marrow.

*Eosinophils* account for 1% to 4% of the total number of circulating leukocytes. They mature in the bone marrow in 3 to 6 days before being released into the circulation. Eosinophils have a circulating half-life of 30 minutes and a tissue half-life of 12 days. They too are phagocytic cells, but are less efficient at this process than neutrophils. Eosinophils are found in large numbers in the respiratory and gastrointestinal tracts, where they are thought to be responsible for protecting the body from parasitic worms, including tapeworms, flukes, pinworms, and hookworms. Eosinophils surround the parasite and release toxic enzymes from their cytoplasmic granules. The parasite, although too large to be phagocytized, is destroyed. Eosinophils are also involved in a hypersensitivity response, inactivating some of the inflammatory chemicals released during the inflammatory response.

*Basophils* constitute about 0.5% to 1% of the circulating leukocytes. These cells are not phagocytic. Granules within basophils contain proteins and chemicals such as heparin, histamine, bradykinin, serotonin, and a slow-reacting substance of anaphylaxis (leukotrienes). These substances are released into the bloodstream during an acute hypersensitivity reaction or stress response.

**MONOCYTES AND MACROPHAGES.** *Monocytes* are the largest of the leukocytes and constitute 2% to 3% of circulating leukocytes. After their release from the bone marrow, monocytes are mobile for 1 to 2 days. They then migrate to various tissues throughout the body, attaching themselves to the tissues, where they remain for months or even years until they are activated. Monocytes mature into **macrophages** after settling into the tissues. Once they have migrated and matured, macrophages are differentiated by the tissues in which they reside. *Histiocytes* are tissue macrophages in loose connective tissue, *Kupffer cells* are found in the liver, *alveolar macrophages* in the lungs, and *microglia* in the brain. Tissue macrophages are also found in the spleen, tonsils, lymph nodes, and bone marrow.

Monocytes and macrophages are actively phagocytic, with the capacity to phagocytize large foreign particles and cell debris. Once they are in the tissue, macrophages can multiply to encapsulate and trap foreign matter that cannot be phagocytized. Like neutrophils, macrophages are drawn to an inflamed area by chemicals released from damaged tissue, a process known as chemotaxis. Monocytes and macrophages are particularly important in the body's defense against chronic infections such as tuberculosis, viral infections, and certain intracellular parasitic infections.

**LYMPHOCYTES.** Small and nondescript cells, the **lymphocytes** account for 20% to 40% of circulating leukocytes. Lymphocytes are the principal effector and regulator cells of specific immune responses. Along with monocytes and macrophages, lymphocytes protect the body from microorganisms, foreign tissue, and cell mutations or alterations. Through a process known as immune surveillance, lymphocytes monitor the body for cancerous cells and eliminate or destroy them.

Like other leukocytes, lymphocytes derive from the stem cells in the bone marrow (Figure 8–2 ■). Lymphocytes have "homing" patterns: They constantly circulate, then return to concentrate in lymphoid tissues (the lymph nodes, spleen, thymus, tonsils, Peyer's patches in the submucosa of the distal ileum, and the appendix). On contact with an **antigen,** lymphocytes are activated and mature into either effector cells (e.g., plasma cells or cytotoxic cells), which are instrumental in destruction of the antigen, or memory cells. Memory cells stay inactive, sometimes for years, but activate immediately with subsequent exposure to the same antigen. They then proliferate rapidly, producing an intense immune response. Memory cells are responsible for providing acquired immunity.

Lymphocyte types are difficult to distinguish by appearance. They have distinct differences in how and where they mature, and in life cycle, surface characteristics, and function.

The three types of lymphocytes are **T lymphocytes (T cells), B lymphocytes (B cells),** and **natural killer cells (NK cells or null cells).** None of these cells acts independently. Their functions are closely interrelated.

T cells mature in the thymus gland, whereas B cells complete their maturation in the bone marrow. T cells and B cells are integral to the specific immune response and are discussed further in that section of this chapter.

NK cells are large, granular cells found in the spleen, lymph nodes, bone marrow, and blood. They constitute 15% of circulating lymphocytes. NK cells provide immune surveillance and resistance to infection, and they play an important role in the destruction of early malignant cells. Like B cells and T cells, NK cells are cytotoxic, but whereas T cells and B cells can attack only specific infected cells or malignant cells, NK cells can attack any target.

**ANTIGENS.** Substances that are recognized as foreign or "nonself" are called antigens; they provoke a specific immune response when introduced into the body. Typically, antigens are large protein molecules, although polysaccharides, polypeptides, and nucleic acids may also be antigenic. Many antigens are proteins found on the cell membrane or cell wall of microorganisms or tissues such as transplanted tissue or organs, incompatible blood cells, vaccines, pollen, egg white, and insect or snake venom.

Complete antigens, known as immunogens, have two characteristics:

- *Immunogenicity* is the ability to stimulate a specific immune response.
- *Specific reactivity* is the stimulation of specific immune system components.

The portion of an antigen that incites a specific immune response is called its antigenic determinant site (epitope). Complete antigens typically are large molecules with multiple antigenic sites; examples include proteins and certain polysaccharides. Small molecules (e.g., chemical toxins, drugs, and

**Figure 8–2** ■ The development and differentiation of lymphocytes from the lymphoid stem cell (lymphoblasts).

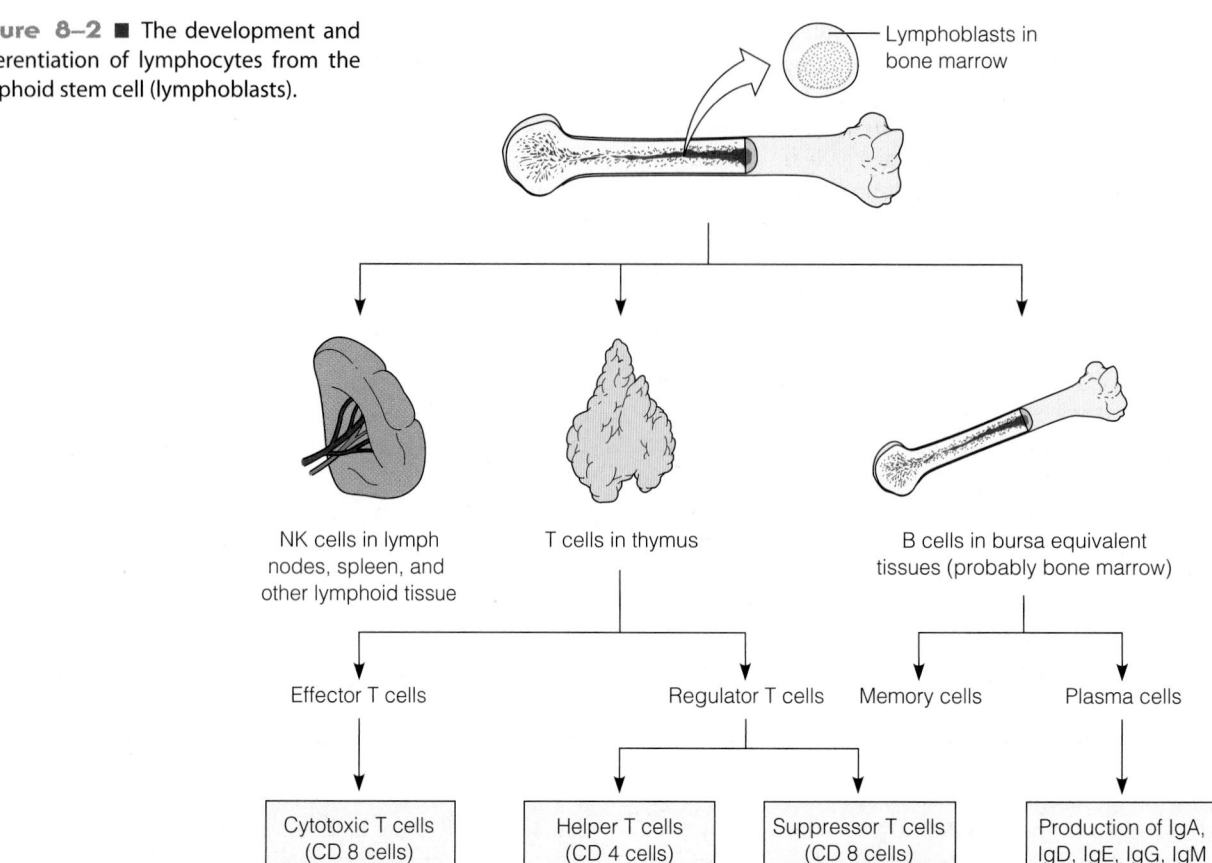

dust) that cannot evoke an antigenic response alone may link to proteins to function as complete antigens. These substances are known as haptans.

When an antigen is encountered in the body, a specific receptor on a lymphocyte "recognizes" it, and an immune response is generated. Two separate but overlapping immune responses may occur, depending on the antigen itself and the type of immune cell activated by contact with the antigen. Antigens such as bacteria, bacterial toxins, and free viruses usually activate B cells to produce **antibodies,** molecules that bind with the antigen and inactivate it. This is the **antibody-mediated (humoral) immune response.** Other antigens, such as viral-infected cells, cancer cells, and foreign tissue, activate T cells, which are the primary agents of the **cell-mediated (cellular) immune response.** In this immune response, the lymphocytes themselves inactivate the antigen, either directly or indirectly.

## Lymphoid System

The *lymphoid system* consists of the lymph nodes, spleen, thymus, tonsils, lymphoid tissue scattered in connective tissues and mucosa, and the bone marrow. The thymus and bone marrow, in which T cells and B cells mature, are considered central lymphoid organs. The spleen, lymph nodes, tonsils, and other peripheral lymphoid tissue are peripheral lymphoid organs (Figure 8–3 ■).

Lymph nodes, the most numerous elements of the lymphoid system, are small, round or bean-shaped encapsulated bodies that vary in size from 1 mm to 2 cm. Distributed throughout the

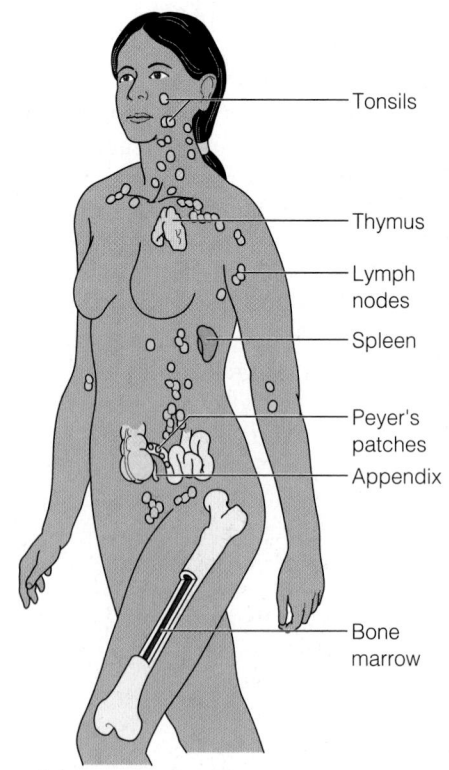

**Figure 8–3** ■ The lymphoid system: the central organs of the thymus and bone marrow, and the peripheral organs, including the spleen, tonsils, lymph nodes, and Peyer's patches.

body, lymph nodes generally occur in groups at the junction of the lymphatic vessels. They can be found in the neck, axillae, abdomen, and groin.

Lymph nodes have two functions: (1) to filter foreign products or antigens from the lymph, and (2) to house and support proliferation of lymphocytes and macrophages. Lymph, a clear, protein-containing fluid transported by lymph vessels, enters the node through afferent lymphatic vessels. Inside the node, the lymph flows through sinuses in the cortex of the lymph node where T and B lymphocytes and macrophages are abundant, then through sinuses of the medulla of the lymph node, which contains macrophages and plasma cells. The presence of a foreign antigen stimulates lymphocytes and macrophages to proliferate in the lymph nodes. Macrophages destroy the antigen by phagocytosis. Immune cells and lymph then leave the lymph node through efferent vessels. An abundant blood supply to the node also facilitates lymphocyte movement.

The *spleen* is the largest lymphoid organ in the body and the only lymphoid organ that can filter blood. The spleen is located in the upper left quadrant of the abdomen. The spleen has two kinds of tissue, white pulp and red pulp. White pulp is lymphoid tissue that serves as a site for lymphocyte proliferation and immune surveillance. B cells predominate in the white pulp. Blood filtration occurs in the red pulp. In blood-filled venous sinuses, phagocytic cells dispose of damaged or aged RBCs and platelets. Other debris and foreign matter, such as bacteria, viruses, and toxins, are also removed from the blood. The spleen also stores blood and the breakdown products of RBCs for future use. The spleen is not essential for life. If it is removed because of disease or trauma, the liver and the bone marrow assume its functions.

The *thymus gland* is located in the superior anterior mediastinal cavity beneath the sternum. It reaches its maximum size at puberty, then begins to atrophy slowly. By adulthood, it is difficult to differentiate from surrounding adipose tissue even though it remains active. In the elderly, the vast majority of thymus tissue has been replaced by adipose and fibrous connective tissue. During fetal life and childhood, the thymus serves as a site for the maturation and differentiation of thymic lymphoid cells, the T cells. Thymosin, an immunoregulatory hormone of the thymus, stimulates lymphopoiesis, the formation of lymphocytes or lymphoid tissue.

*Bone marrow* is soft organic tissue found in the hollow cavity of the long bones, particularly the femur and humerus, as well as the flat bones of the skull, sternum, ribs, and vertebrae. Bone marrow produces and stores hematopoietic stem cells, from which all cellular components of the blood are derived (see Figure 8–1).

Lymphoid tissues are also located at key sites of potential invasion by microorganisms: the submucosa of the genitourinary, respiratory, and gastrointestinal tracts and the skin. Plasma cells in these lymphoid tissues defend the body against bacterial invasion at areas exposed to the external environment. In general, these tissues are known as *mucosa-associated lymphoid tissue* (MALT). Diffuse collections of lymphocytes, plasma cells, and phagocytes are scattered throughout the respiratory tract, concentrating at bifurcations of the bronchi and bronchioles. Gastrointestinal lymphoid tissue occurs as both diffusely scattered MALT and in more clearly defined tissues, such as the appendix and Peyer's patches, which are lymph nodules located on the distal ileum near its junction with the colon. Tonsils and adenoids protect the body from inhaled or ingested foreign agents. Skin-associated lymphoid tissue contains lymphocytes and Langerhans cells in the epidermis, which transport antigens to regional lymph nodes for phagocytosis.

## Nonspecific Inflammatory Response

Barrier protection is the body's first line of defense against infection. The skin is the primary barrier. When intact, it prevents invasion by external organisms. When the skin is damaged or lost (e.g., as a result of injury, surgery, or burns), infection is much more likely. The membranes lining inner surfaces of the body are protected by a barrier of mucus, which traps microorganisms and other foreign substances. These can then be removed by other protective mechanisms, such as ciliary movement or the washing action of tears or urine. In addition, many body fluids contain bactericidal substances that provide barrier protection. These include acid in gastric fluid, zinc in prostatic fluid, and lysozyme in tears, nasal secretions, saliva, and sweat (Copstead & Banasik, 2000).

When these first-line defenses are breached, resulting tissue damage or foreign material entering the body induces a nonspecific immune response known as inflammation. Inflammation is an adaptive response to injury that brings fluid, dissolved substances, and blood cells into the interstitial tissues where the invasion or damage has occurred. The response is called nonspecific because the same events occur regardless of cause of the inflammatory process. Through the inflammatory reaction, the invader is neutralized and eliminated, destroyed tissue removed, and the process of healing and repair initiated.

There are three stages in the inflammatory response: (1) a vascular response characterized by vasodilation and increased permeability of blood vessels, (2) a cellular response and phagocytosis, and (3) tissue repair.

### Vascular Response

After tissue cells are damaged, local blood vessels briefly constrict. Vasodilation follows almost immediately as inflammatory mediators such as histamine and kinins are released from damaged tissue (see Box 8–1). Increased blood flow causes vasocongestion at the injury site with resultant redness and heat. The congestion also increases local hydrostatic pressure. This, along with increased vessel permeability that results from chemical mediators, moves fluid out of the capillaries and into the interstitial spaces of the tissue. The escaping fluid, called fluid exudate, contains large amounts of protein and causes local edema. Fluid exudate has three functions: (1) It provides protection to the injured tissue by bringing certain nutrients needed for tissue healing; (2) it dilutes bacterial toxins; and (3) it transports cells needed for phagocytosis. Mild tissue damage such as a blister produces a *serous* exudate of primarily plasma fluid and a few proteins. With moderate to severe tissue damage, fluid exudate is *sanguineous* or *hemorrhagic*, containing large amounts of RBCs. A mixture of RBCs and

## BOX 8–1 ■ Inflammatory Mediators

Many of the manifestations of inflammation are produced by *inflammatory mediators,* which are chemicals released as a result of immunologic processes or tissue injury or damage. These inflammatory mediators are broadly classified as follows:

■ Vasoactive substances produce smooth muscle constriction, postcapillary vasodilation, and increased capillary permeability.
■ Chemotactic factors attract leukocytes to the damaged tissue.
■ Plasma enzymes activate the clotting cascade, plasminogen system, and complement system.
■ Miscellaneous cell products (e.g., oxygen metabolites and lysosomal enzymes) damage surrounding tissue.

Many of the outward manifestations of inflammation result from vasoactive substances such as *histamine, serotonin,* and *leukotrienes* (formerly known as slow-reacting substance of anaphylaxis, or SRS-A). Stored in mast cells, basophils, and platelets, histamine is released when an injury occurs or with stimulation by the immune system. An important component of the early inflammatory response, histamine causes vasodilation and vascular permeability in the affected area. Histamine is also a key factor in

many hypersensitivity reactions. Serotonin is released from platelets and produces effects similar to those of histamine. The leukotrienes play a significant vasoactive role in the later stages of the inflammatory response.

*Prostaglandins* are chemotactic substances drawing leukocytes to the inflamed tissue. In addition, they play a vasoactive role and are pain and fever inducers. Aspirin and other nonsteroidal anti-inflammatory drugs (NSAIDs) as well as the glucocorticoids inhibit prostaglandin synthesis, thereby reducing fever, pain, and inflammation.

Plasma factors such as Hageman factor activate the clotting cascade, plasminogen system (involved in the lysis of clots), and complement system. With activation of the clotting cascade, bacteria and other foreign substances are trapped in the area of tissue damage. Fibrin, which has vasoactive by-products, is also released. (See Chapter 32 for a full description of the clotting process.) The complement system serves a chemotactic role and facilitates the phagocytic process.

Major chemical mediators of inflammation are summarized in Table 8–4.

---

serum is referred to as *serosanguineous* exudate. *Fibrinous* exudate forms a thick, sticky meshwork of fibrinogen, in effect "walling off" inflamed tissues and preventing the spread of infection (Porth, 2002). In more severe or acute inflammation, the fluid contains fibrin, RBCs, and dead and live bacteria. This type of exudate, called *purulent* exudate, has an odor and color characteristic of the bacteria present.

The vascular response localizes invading bacteria and keeps them from spreading. Increased capillary permeability enhances the release of clotting factors such as fibrinogen, which converts to fibrin threads, entrapping the bacteria and walling them off from contact with the rest of the body.

### Cellular Response

The cellular stage of the inflammatory process begins within less than an hour after the injury. This stage is marked by the margination and emigration of leukocytes into the damaged tissue, chemotaxis, and phagocytosis (Porth, 2002).

As serous fluid escapes the capillaries, the viscosity of blood in the area increases and its flow becomes more sluggish. Leukocytes marginate, moving to the edges of the blood vessels, and begin to adhere to the capillary endothelium. This process is known as pavementing. After margination and pavementing, leukocytes emigrate from the blood vessel into the tissue spaces (Figure 8–4 ■). Within hours, millions of leukocytes emigrate into the area of inflammation (Price & Wilson, 1997).

Once leukocytes have emigrated, they are drawn to the damaged or inflamed tissues by chemotactic signals. Infectious agents, damaged tissues, and activated plasma substances such as complement fractions provide chemotaxic signals that attract an army of neutrophils, monocytes, and macrophages to the injury site.

The number of neutrophils around the site increases to about 15,000/mm³ to 25,000/mm³, and they begin their role in

phagocytosis within a few hours. Monocytes become transient macrophages to augment the activity of the fixed macrophages; together they engulf dead cells, damaged tissue, nonfunctioning neutrophils, and invading bacteria.

### Phagocytosis

**Phagocytosis** is a process by which a foreign agent or target cell is engulfed, destroyed, and digested. Neutrophils and macrophages, known as *phagocytes,* are the primary cells involved in phagocytosis. Once attracted to the inflammatory site, phagocytes select and engulf foreign material.

The following factors or processes help phagocytes differentiate foreign tissue from normal cells.

- *Smooth surface.* Normal tissue has a smooth surface that is resistant to phagocytosis, whereas the rough surface of a foreign agent or target cell promotes phagocytosis.
- *Surface charge.* Healthy body cells present an electronegative surface charge that repels phagocytes. Cellular debris and foreign agents, by contrast, have an electropositive charge that attracts them.
- *Opsonization.* This immune system process coats the surface of bacteria or target cells with a substance (an opsonin) as in the complement system (see Box 8–2). Opsonization enables the phagocyte to bind tightly with the foreign tissue, facilitating phagocytosis (Figure 8–5A■).

Phagocytes engulf the foreign agent or target cell by projecting pseudopodia ("false feet") in all directions around it (Figure 8–5B). This produces a chamber called a *phagosome* containing the antigen, which is ingested into the cytoplasm (Figure 8–5C). Once the phagosome has been engulfed, lysosomes fuse with the phagosome, killing any live organism and releasing digestive enzymes which destroy the antigen (Figure 8–5D).

Phagocytes—in particular, neutrophils and macrophages—contain bactericidal agents that kill most of the bacteria they in-

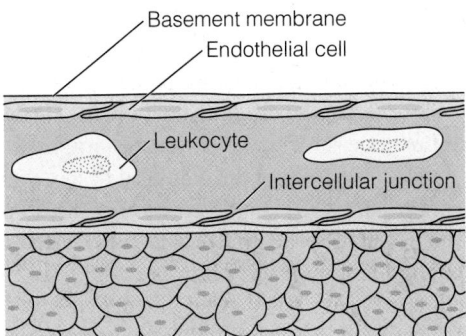

**A** Leukocytes in circulation

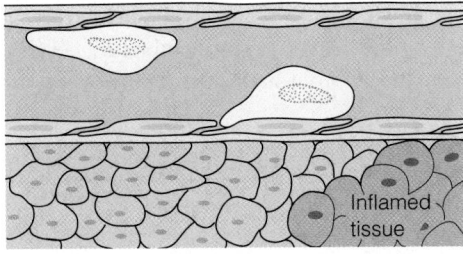

**B** Margination and pavementing

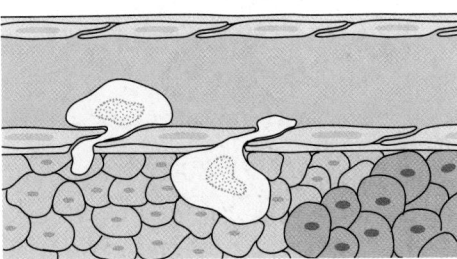

**C** Emigration

**Figure 8–4** ■ The process of leukocyte emigration at the site of inflammation. *A,* Normal blood flow with free movement of formed elements. *B,* As blood flow slows, leukocytes move toward the periphery of stream and begin to cling to capillary endothelium, a process known as margination and pavementing. *C,* Leukocytes emigrate from the vessel into inflamed tissues.

gest before the bacteria can multiply and destroy the phagocyte itself. The phagocyte kills bacteria in a number of ways; for example, it alters the intracellular pH and produces bactericidal agents. Oxidizing agents, such as superoxide, hydrogen peroxide, and hydroxyl ions, are bactericidal. Two lysosomal substances that kill bacteria are lysozyme and phagocytin.

Some antigens, such as the tubercle bacterium, have coats or secrete substances that are resistant to lysosomal and bactericidal agents. To destroy such antigens, lysosomes release digestive enzymes into the phagosome. The lysosomes of neutrophils and macrophages contain an abundance of proteolytic (protein-destroying) enzymes that digest bacteria and other foreign protein components. The macrophage's lysosomes also contain lipases (fat-splitting enzymes) capable of digesting the

**BOX 8–2   ■ The Complement System**

The *complement system* consists of approximately 20 complex plasma proteins that are activated by a tissue injury or antigen-antibody reaction. The complement system is involved in both nonspecific and specific immune responses. Its activation results in the production of effector molecules that are involved in the processes of inflammation, phagocytosis, and cell lysis or destruction (Porth, 1998; Roitt, 1994). Specifically, complement activation leads to

■ *Mediation of the inflammatory response.* When the complement system is activated, chemical mediators such as histamine are released from mast cells and basophils, leading to smooth muscle contraction, increased vascular permeability and edema, and the attraction of leukocytes.
■ *Opsonization (or coating) of antigen-antibody complexes to facilitate phagocytosis.*
■ *Alteration of the cell membrane or viral capsule.* When the cell surface is altered, lysis results. Bacteria and viruses are destroyed; certain normal cells, such as RBCs, platelets, and lymphocytes, that are damaged or old may also be destroyed through this process.

The complement system has two "arms," or pathways, of protein and enzyme reactions. The *classic pathway* is activated by antibody-containing immunoglobulins and other substances such as DNA and C-reactive protein. The *alternate pathway* is activated by tissue injury, polysaccharides, or enzymes. When either pathway is activated, the results are mediation of the inflammatory process, attraction of phagocytes, facilitation of phagocytosis, and lysis of microbes.

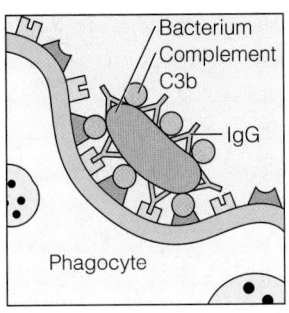

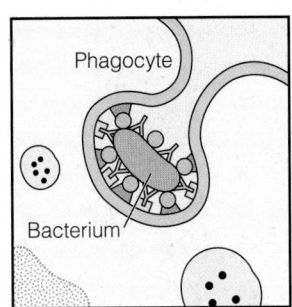

**A**

**B**

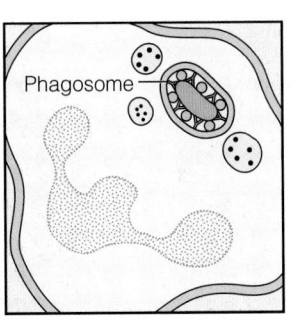

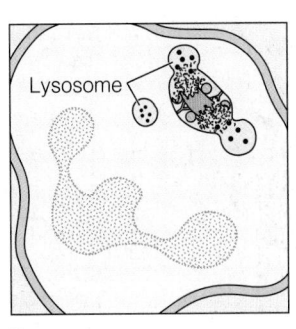

**C**

**D**

**Figure 8–5** ■ The process of phagocytosis. *A,* Opsonization coats the surface of the bacterium with IgG (an antibody) and complement. *B,* The bacterium is bound to and engulfed by the phagocyte. *C,* The phagosome is ingested into the cytoplasm of the phagocyte. *D,* Lysosomes fuse with the phagosome, releasing digestive enzymes and destroying the antigen.

thick lipid membranes of such bacteria as *Mycobacterium tuberculosis* and *Mycobacterium leprae.*

Once neutrophils have ingested toxic substances to their capacity, they in turn are killed. Neutrophils have the capacity to phagocytize 5 to 20 bacteria before they become inactive. Macrophages then digest the dead neutrophils. Monocytes or macrophages are capable of phagocytizing up to 100 bacteria. Because of their size, they can ingest larger particles than neutrophils can ingest, such as whole RBCs, necrotic tissue, cell fragments, malarial parasites, and dead neutrophils. Macrophages have the ability to extrude (release) the toxic substances and lysosomal enzymes within their phagosomes. As a result, they can continue to function for months and even years.

### Healing

*Inflammation* is the first phase of the healing process. During the inflammatory process, particulate matter, bacteria, damaged cells,

and inflammatory exudate are removed by phagocytosis. This process, called debridement, prepares the wound for healing.

The second phase of the healing process, known *as reconstruction,* may overlap the inflammatory phase. The ideal result of the healing process is *resolution,* the restoration of the original structure and function of the damaged tissue. Simple resolution occurs when there is no destruction of the normal tissue and the body is able to neutralize and remove the offending agent through the inflammatory process.

Resolution may also occur when the damaged tissue is capable of regeneration. The ability to regenerate, or replace lost parenchyma (functional tissue) with new, functional cells varies by tissue and cell type. *Labile cells* continue to regenerate throughout life. These cells are found in tissues where there is a daily turnover of cells—namely, bone marrow and the epithelial cells of the skin, mucous membranes, cervix, gastrointestinal tract, and genitourinary tract. *Stable cells* normally stop

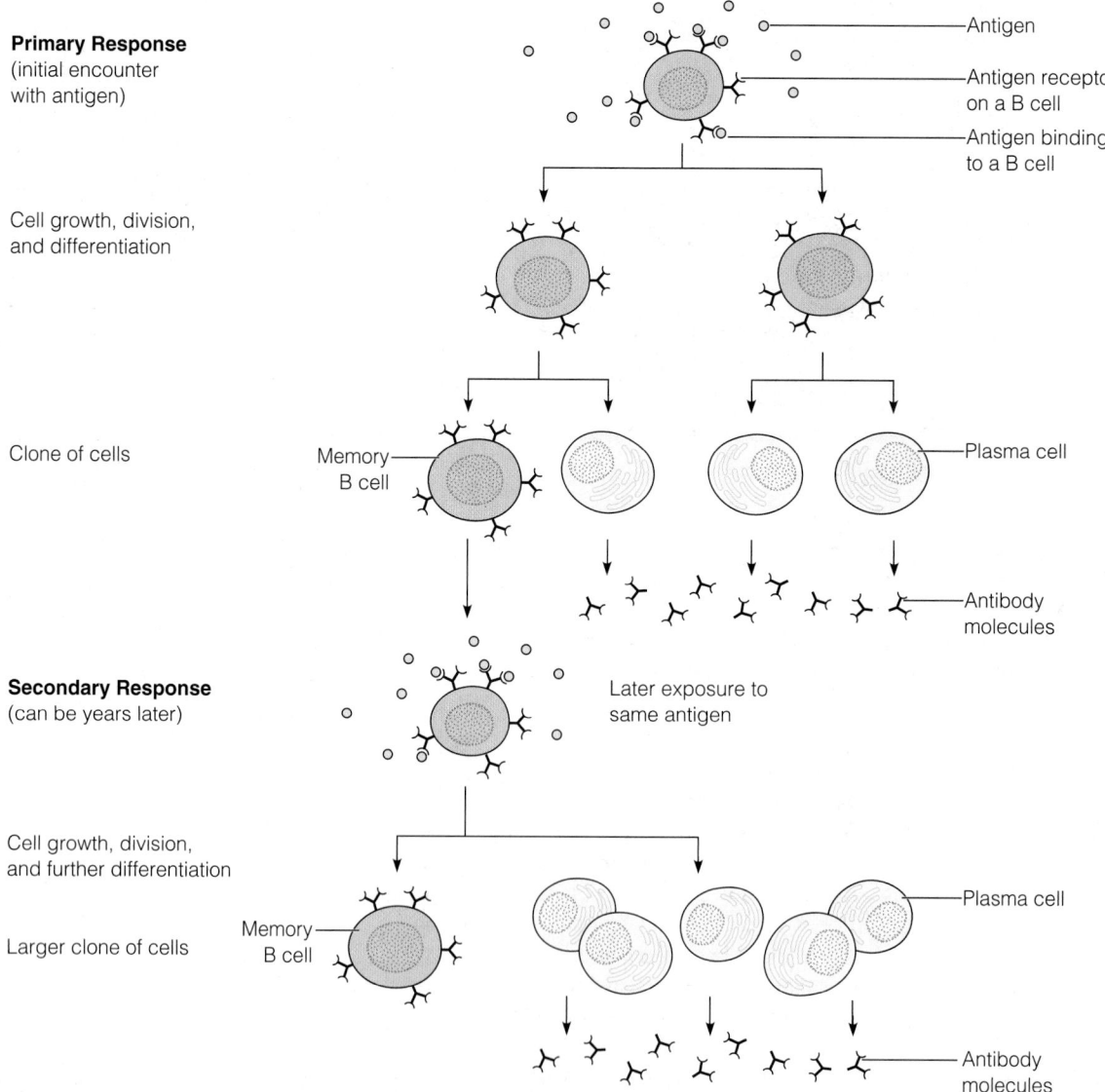

**Figure 8–6** ■ Antibody-mediated (humoral) immunity. On initial exposure to the antigen, B cells with appropriate receptor sites are activated to become plasma cells and produce antibodies or memory cells. This is known as the primary response. With subsequent exposures, memory cells respond rapidly with antibody production. This is known as the secondary response.

replicating when growth ceases, but are capable of regeneration when stimulated by an injury. Osteocytes (which are found in bone) and parenchymal cells of the kidneys, liver, and pancreas are stable cells. *Permanent* or *fixed cells* are unable to regenerate. When these cells are destroyed, they are replaced by fibrous scar tissue. Nerve cells, skeletal muscle cells, and cardiac muscle cells are fixed cells (Porth, 1998).

When regeneration and complete resolution is not possible, healing occurs by replacement of the destroyed tissue with collagen scar tissue. This process is known as *repair*. Although tissue that has undergone repair lacks the physiologic function of the destroyed tissue, the scar fills the lesion and provides tensile tissue strength. The healing process is discussed further in Chapter 7. ⌘

## Specific Immune Response

The introduction of antigens into the body causes a more specific reaction than the nonspecific inflammatory response. On the first exposure to an antigen, a change occurs in the host, resulting in a specific and rapid response following subsequent exposures. This specific response is known as the *immune response.*

The immune response to an antigen has the following distinctive properties:

- The immune response typically is directed against materials recognized as foreign (i.e., from outside the body) and is not usually directed against the self (i.e., cells or structures produced by the body). This property is known as self-recognition.
- The immune response is *specific*. It is initiated by and directed against particular antigens (such as a specific virus, bacterium, or transplanted tissue).
- Unlike a localized inflammatory response, the immune response is systemic. Immunity is generalized; it is not restricted to the initial site of infection or entry of foreign tissue.
- The immune response has memory. Repeated exposures to an antigen produce a more rapid response.

A client whose immune system is able to identify antigens and effectively destroy or remove them is said to be **immunocompetent.** Health problems may occur when the immune response is altered (see Chapter 9 for further discussion). ⌘

### Antibody-Mediated Immune Response

The antibody-mediated (humoral) immune response is produced by B lymphocytes (B cells). B cells are constantly replaced through cell division and proliferation in the bone marrow. It is believed that B cells mature in the bone marrow and then migrate to the spleen to await activation. They normally constitute 10% to 15% of circulating lymphocytes.

B cells are activated by contact with an antigen and by T cells (discussed in the next section). Each B cell has receptor sites for a specific antigen or antigens. When the antigen is encountered, the activated B cell proliferates and differentiates into antibody-producing plasma cells and memory cells (Figure 8–6 ■). Plasma cells are short-lived, lasting only about 1 day. While alive, however, they can produce thousands of antibody molecules per second. Memory cells retain antibody-producing information, allowing a rapid response if the antigen is again encountered.

An antibody is an **immunoglobulin (Ig)** molecule with the ability to bind to and inactivate a specific antigen. Immunoglobulins comprise the gamma globulin portion of the blood proteins. The immune system produces numerous antibodies, each active against a specific antigen. Antibodies fall into five classes of immunoglobulins: IgG, IgA, IgM, IgD, and IgE. Each has a slightly different structure and function. Their roles are summarized in Table 8–2.

### TABLE 8–2    Immunoglobulin Characteristics and Functions

| Class | Percentage of Total | Characteristics and Function |
|-------|---------------------|------------------------------|
| IgG | 75% | Most abundant Ig; also known as gamma globulin; found in blood, lymph, and intestines<br>Active against bacteria, bacterial toxins, and viruses<br>Activates complement<br>The only Ig to cross the placenta, providing immune protection to neonate |
| IgA | 10% to 15% | Found in saliva, tears, and bronchial, gastrointestinal, prostatic, and vaginal secretions, as well as blood and lymph<br>Provides local protection on exposed mucous membrane surfaces and potent antiviral activity by preventing binding of the virus to cells of the respiratory and gastrointestinal tracts<br>Levels decrease during stress |
| IgM | 5% to 10% | Found in blood and lymph<br>First antibody produced with primary immune response<br>High concentrations early in infection, decreases within about a week<br>Mediates cytotoxic response and activates complement |
| IgD | <1% | Found in blood, lymph, and surfaces of B cells<br>Exact function unknown; may be receptor-binding antigens to B-cell surface |
| IgE | <0.1% | Found on mast cells and basophils<br>Involved in release of chemical mediators responsible for immediate hypersensitivity (allergic and anaphylactic) response |

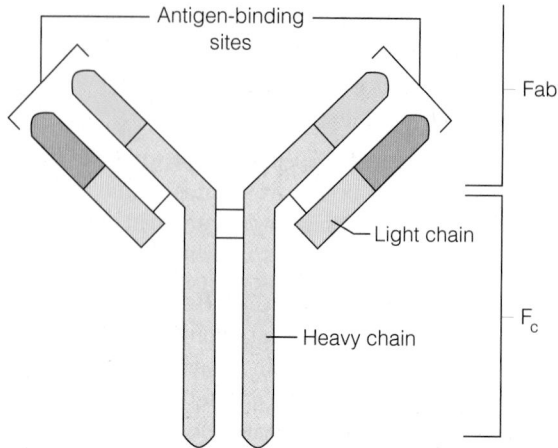

**Figure 8–7** ■ An antibody molecule. The Fab section is unique, providing an antigen-specific binding site. The F$_c$ section is common to each class of immunoglobulin (IgG, IgA, IgM, IgD, IgE).

Antibodies are Y-shaped molecules of two light and two heavy polypeptide chains (Figure 8–7 ■). The top portion of the Y, called the *Fab* or *antigen-binding fragment,* is chemically variable and specific to the antigen. The lower portion, the *F$_c$*, or *crystallized fragment,* is constant for its class of immunoglobulin and directs the biologic activity of the immunoglobulin (the manner in which it functions). For example, the lower portion of immunoglobulin molecules produced against hepatitis A and hepatitis B are the same (IgG), but the upper portion is different and specific to the virus.

The antibodies produced by B cells (see Figure 8–7) link with the antigen (Figure 8–8 ■) and inactivate it through one of the following processes.

- Promoting phagocytosis of the antigen by neutrophils
- Precipitation: combining with soluble antigens to form an insoluble complex or precipitate

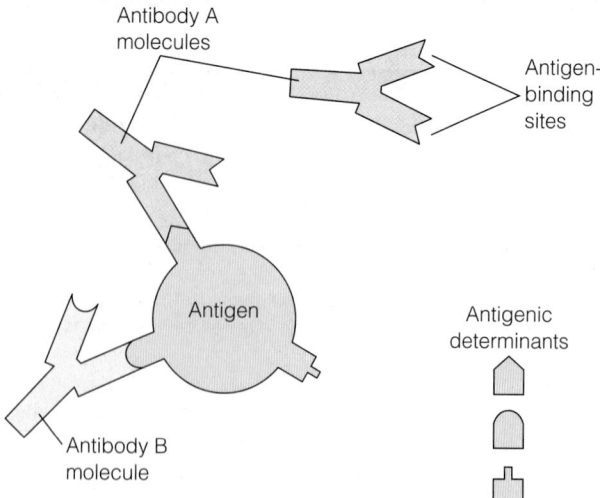

**Figure 8–8** ■ Antigen-antibody binding. The unique Fab site on the antibody binds with specific receptor sites on the antigen. As shown, more than one kind of antibody may be produced to an antigen.

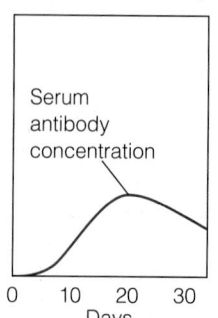
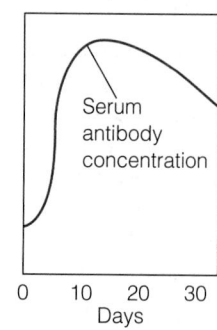

**Figure 8–9** ■ Antibody production in the primary and secondary responses of the antibody-mediated immune response. Note the more rapid and effective production following subsequent exposure.

- Neutralization: combining with a toxin to neutralize its effects; the antigen-antibody complex is then destroyed by the process of phagocytosis
- Lysis of the antigen cell membrane caused by combination with antibodies and complement
- Agglutination (clumping) of antigens to form a noninvasive aggregate
- Opsonization: coating of the antigen with antibodies and complement, making them more susceptible to phagocytosis

The complete antibody-mediated response occurs in two phases. With initial exposure to an antigen, the primary response develops. B cells are activated to proliferate and begin producing antibodies. There is a latency period of 3 to 6 days before antibodies become detectable in the blood. Levels then continue to rise, peaking at 10 to 14 days after the initial exposure. With many illnesses (e.g., chickenpox), this peak correlates with recovery.

Subsequent exposure to the same antigen elicits a secondary response. Memory cells (Figure 8–6) formed during the primary response stimulate the production of plasma cells, and an almost immediate rise in antibody levels occurs (Figure 8–9 ■). This rapid secondary response is the basis of acquired immunity and is instrumental in preventing disease. It is also the mechanism through which vaccines provide protection from disease.

## Cell-Mediated Immune Response

Many antigens cannot stimulate the antibody-mediated response or are "hidden" from it because they live inside the body's cells (viruses and mycobacteria are examples of such antigens). The immune response providing protection against these antigens is the cell-mediated immune response, also called *cellular immunity.* T lymphocytes (T cells) initiate this type of immune response.

Approximately 70% to 80% of circulating lymphocytes are T cells. T cells migrate to the thymus during fetal and early life, establishing the lifetime pool of cells. T cells have a life span measured in years, maintaining their numbers through proliferation, primarily in the lymph nodes.

T cells are much more complex than B cells. There are two major classes of T cells, *effector cells* and *regulator cells.* The main effector T cell is the *cytotoxic cell,* also called the *killer T cell.* Regulator T cells are further classified into two groups: *helper T cells* and *suppressor T cells.*

T cells are antigen specific; that is, each subset is activated by a particular antigen. The antigens that activate T cells must be presented on another cell surface, such as pieces of virus presented on the surface of an infected cell, or the histocompatibility locus antigen (HLA) on a cell of transplanted tissue. When activated, T cells divide and proliferate, forming antigen-specific clones (Figure 8–10 ■). (A clone is an exact copy of another cell.)

Cytotoxic T cells bind with cell surface antigens on virus-infected or foreign cells. Killer T cells destroy the antigen by combining with it and then either destroying its cell membrane or releasing cytotoxic substances into the cell. They are vital in the control of viral and bacterial infections.

Regulator T cells play a key role in controlling the immune response. The majority of regulator T cells are helper T cells. They stimulate the proliferation of other T cells, amplify the cytotoxic activity of killer T cells, and activate B cells to proliferate and differentiate. They interact directly with B cells to promote their multiplication and conversion into plasma cells capable of producing antibodies. The other regulatory T-cell group, suppressor T cells, provide negative feedback, making the immune response a self-limiting process.

On activation, both effector and regulator T cells synthesize and release lymphokines, a type of soluble protein. Lymphokines are a subgroup of nonspecific defense mechanisms known as **cytokines** (Box 8–3). Lymphokines secreted by cytotoxic and helper T cells are important in amplifying the im-

---

### BOX 8–3  ■ Cytokines

**Cytokines** are hormonelike polypeptides produced primarily by monocytes, macrophages, and T cells. Cytokines secreted by monocytes and macrophages may be called *monokines;* those secreted by T cells are known as *lymphokines.* Cytokines are also produced in small quantities in many different tissues throughout the body. Cytokines act as messengers of the immune system, facilitating communication between the cells to adjust or vary the inflammatory reaction or to initiate immune cell proliferation and differentiation. Cytokines are an essential component of an adequate immune response. The major cytokines and their functions are summarized in Table 8–3.

*Interferons* are a class of cytokine with broad antiviral effects. A number of different forms of interferon exist, broadly grouped as alpha, beta, and gamma interferons. Interferon is synthesized by cells infected with a virus and secreted into extracellular fluid. It then binds to specific receptors on uninfected neighboring cells, protecting them from infection. The spread of the virus is thus inhibited, and recovery from infection enhanced. It appears that interferons also moderate the activity of NK cells and may be involved in preventing the spread of abnormal malignant cells.

---

mune response and the nonspecific inflammatory response. They stimulate the following:

* B cells to become plasma cells and produce antibodies
* Macrophages to become activated macrophages (the most aggressive phagocyte)
* Proliferation of killer T cells

**Figure 8–10** ■ Cellular immune response. *A,* An infected cell, abnormal cell, or phagocyte presents antigen on its surface that binds with a receptor site on a killer T or a helper T cell. The killer T cell is activated to proliferate into memory cells or mature cytotoxic cells. *B,* The helper T cell is activated to augment the cytotoxic response and stimulate the antibody-mediated immune response.

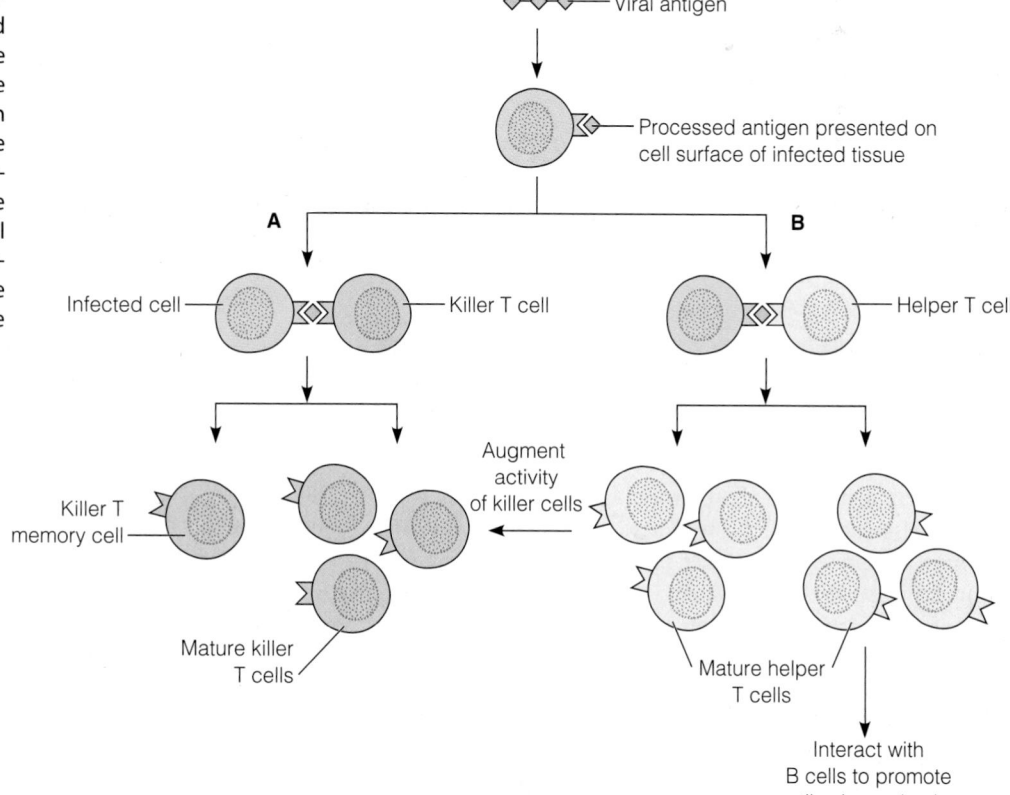

TABLE 8-3  Major Cytokines and Their Functions

| Cytokine | Where Produced | Primary Functions |
| --- | --- | --- |
| Interleukin-1 (IL-1) | Monocytes and macrophages; other cells | Activates T and B cells<br>Induces fever and tissue catabolism<br>Enhances NK activity<br>Attracts neutrophils, macrophages, and lymphocytes<br>Stimulates endothelial cell growth, collagen, and collagenases |
| Interleukin-2 (IL-2) | Helper T cells | Stimulates T and B cell proliferation<br>Activates killer T and NK cells |
| Interleukin-3 (IL-3) | T cells | Stimulates growth and differentiation of bone marrow stem cells |
| Interleukin-4 (IL-4) | Activated helper T cells | Stimulates proliferation of T and B cells<br>Increases IgE secretion by B cells |
| Interleukin-5 (IL-5) | T cells and activated mast cells | Promotes differentiation of B cells and eosinophils<br>Stimulates production of IgA |
| Gamma interferon | T and NK cells | Stimulates phagocytosis by neutrophils and macrocytes<br>Activates NK cells<br>Augments B cell proliferation, enhancing both cellular and humoral immune responses |
| Alpha and beta interferons | Virus-infected cells; macrophages | Activate macrophages and endothelial cells<br>Augment NK cell activity<br>Act at gene level to protect neighboring cells from invasion by intracellular parasites, such as viruses, rickettsia, malaria |
| Tumor necrosis factor (TNF) | Activated macrophages, T cells, and NK cells | Major chemical mediator of inflammatory response<br>Stimulates T-cell activation, antibody production, and accumulation of leukocytes at inflammatory site<br>Directly cytotoxic to some tumor cells<br>Induces fever |

Suppressor T cells release lymphokines, which inhibit the activity of other T cells and B cells.

Although T cells can be activated only by specific antigens, much of the resulting effect is nonspecific—in other words, an enhanced inflammatory response. Like the antibody-mediated response, the cell-mediated response has memory. Subsequent exposures to an antigen result in a more rapid and effective inflammatory response and more effective phagocytosis by macrophages. This memory provides the basis for skin testing. A client previously exposed to tuberculosis, for example, develops a more pronounced inflammatory response when minute amounts are injected under the skin.

# NORMAL IMMUNE RESPONSES

## THE CLIENT WITH TISSUE INFLAMMATION AND HEALING

As noted, inflammation is a nonspecific response to injury that serves to destroy, dilute, or contain the injurious agent or damaged tissue. Inflammation may be either acute or chronic. Acute inflammation is a short-term reaction of the body to all types of tissue damage. It is immediate and aimed at protecting the body and preventing further invasion or injury. Acute inflammation usually lasts less than 1 to 2 weeks. Once the injurious agent is removed, the inflammation subsides. Healing with tissue repair or scar formation occurs, and the body functions in normal or near-normal capacity.

Chronic inflammation is slower in onset and may not have an acute phase. Its clinical manifestations occur over months or years. It involves cell proliferation and is debilitating, with long-term adverse effects. There is increased cellular exudate, necrosis, fibrosis, and sometimes tissue scarring, resulting in severe tissue damage.

## PATHOPHYSIOLOGY OF TISSUE INFLAMMATION

The tissue damage that evokes an inflammatory response may be caused by specific or nonspecific agents. These agents may be *exogenous,* from outside the body, or *endogenous,* from within the body. Causes of inflammation include the following:

- Mechanical injuries, such as cuts or surgical incisions
- Physical damage, such as burns
- Chemical injury from toxins or poisons
- Microorganisms, such as bacteria, viruses, or fungi
- Extremes of heat or cold
- Immunologic responses, such as hypersensitivity reactions
- Ischemic damage or trauma, such as a stroke or myocardial infarction

| TABLE 8-4 | Major Chemical Mediators of Inflammation | |
|---|---|---|
| **Factor** | **Source** | **Effect** |
| Histamine | Mast cells, basophils, and platelets | Vasodilation and increased capillary permeability, producing tissue redness, warmth, and edema |
| Kinins (bradykinin and others) | Plasma protein factors | Histaminelike effects; chemotaxis and pain inducers |
| Prostaglandins | Metabolism of anachidonic acid from cell membranes | Histaminelike effects; chemotaxis, pain, and fever inducers |
| Leukotrienes | Anachidonic acid metabolism | Smooth muscle constriction (especially bronchoconstriction), increased vascular permeability, chemotaxis |

## Acute Inflammation

Regardless of the cause, location, or extent of the injury, the acute inflammatory response follows the previously outlined sequence of vascular response, cellular and phagocytic response, and healing.

Many of the manifestations of inflammation are produced by inflammatory mediators such as histamine and prostaglandins released when tissue is damaged (see Table 8–4 and Box 8–1 on inflammatory mediators).

The cardinal signs of inflammation include the following:

- Erythema (redness)
- Local heat caused by the increased blood flow to the injured area (hyperemia)
- Swelling due to accumulated fluid at the site
- Pain from tissue swelling and chemical irritation of nerve endings
- Loss of function caused by the swelling and pain

The degree of functional loss depends on the location and extent of the injury. With increased tissue damage, more fluid exudate is formed, resulting in more swelling, pain, and functional impairment. Pain may be immediate or delayed. Prostaglandins intensify and prolong the pain. Kinins cause irritation to the nerve endings and contribute to the pain sensation.

Dead neutrophils, necrotic tissue, and digested bacteria accumulate as a result of inflammation and phagocytosis, forming *pus.* It usually forms and remains until after the infection subsides. Pus may push itself to the surface of the body or become internalized. In the latter case, pus is gradually autolyzed (self-digested) by enzymes over a period of days. The end product is then absorbed by the body. On occasion, pus may remain after the infection is resolved. Pockets of pus, called abscesses, may need to be artificially drained with a procedure called *incision and drainage (I&D).* Ectopic calcifications are another possible result of residual collections of pus.

Systemic responses to inflammation include an increase in the size of lymph nodes due to the accumulation of bacteria, phagocytes, and destroyed lymph tissue. Enlarged lymph nodes are usually noted in the groin, axillae, and neck (Figure 8–11 ■). Fever, often precipitated by inflammatory mediators or bacterial toxins, inhibits the growth of many microorganisms and increases tissue repair functions. Loss of appetite and fatigue may occur in the effort to conserve energy during the inflammatory process. Leukocytosis occurs with increased WBC production to support inflammation and phagocytosis.

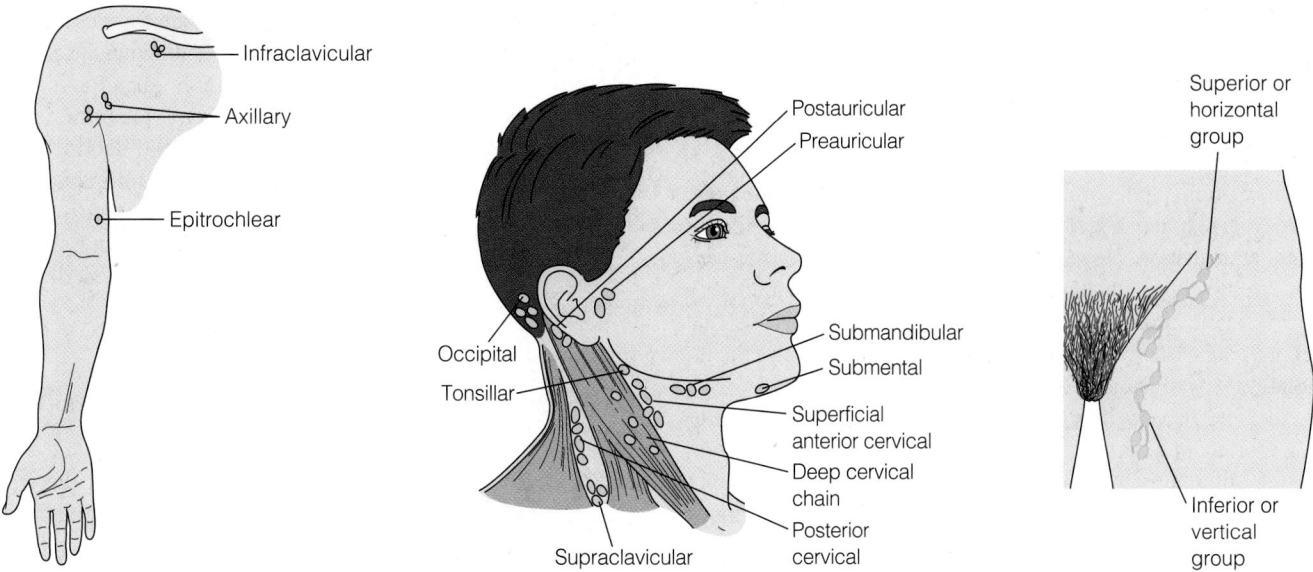

**Figure 8-11** ■ Lymph nodes that may be assessed by palpation.

## Manifestations of Inflammation

### LOCAL MANIFESTATIONS

- Erythema
- Warmth
- Pain
- Edema
- Functional impairment

### SYSTEMIC MANIFESTATIONS

- T >100.4°F (38°C) or <96.8°F (36°C)
- P >90/min
- R >20/min (tachypntea)
- WBC >12,000/mm³ or >10% bands

Local and systemic manifestations of inflammation are summarized in the box above.

## Chronic Inflammation

Whereas acute inflammation is a self-limiting process lasting less than 2 weeks, chronic inflammation tends to be self-perpetuating, lasting weeks to months or years. Chronic inflammation may develop when the acute inflammatory process has been ineffective in removing the offending agent. For example, mycobacteria have cell walls with high lipid and wax content, making them resistant to phagocytosis. Chronic inflammation and granuloma formation is common with *Mycobacterium tuberculosis* infection. Persistent irritation by chemicals, particulate matter, or physical irritants such as talc, asbestos, or silica may also result in chronic inflammation.

The chronic inflammatory process is characterized by a dense infiltration of the site by lymphocytes and macrophages. The macrophages mass or coalesce to form a multinucleated giant cell surrounded by lymphocytes, in a lesion called a *granuloma*. The granuloma is effective in walling off the offending agent, isolating it from the rest of the body; however, the infectious agent or offending irritant may not be destroyed and can survive within the granuloma for a long period of time. The granuloma formed in tuberculosis is called a tubercle. *Mycobacterium tuberculosis* may survive for many years within the tubercle, emerging when the client's immune system is no longer able to contain it.

## Complications

Inflammation and wound healing are highly metabolic processes that may be affected by a number of factors. Without adequate nutrition, blood supply, and oxygenation, tissues cannot effectively complete the process. Impaired inflammatory and immune processes can interfere with phagocytosis and preparation of the wound for healing. Infection prolongs the inflammatory process and delays healing.

Chronic diseases may also impair healing. Diabetes mellitus is a prominent example. With high blood glucose levels associated with poorly controlled diabetes, chemotaxic and phagocytic function is decreased. Collagen formation and tensile strength of the wound are also impaired. Small blood vessel disease is common in people with diabetes, a factor that further impairs the healing process.

### TABLE 8–5   Factors That May Impair Healing

| Factor | Effect |
|---|---|
| Malnutrition Protein deficit | Prolongs inflammation and impairs healing process |
| Carbohydrate and kilocalorie deficit | Impairs metabolic processes and promotes catabolism; proteins are used for energy rather than for healing |
| Fat deficit | Impairs cell membrane synthesis in tissue repair |
| Vitamin deficits Vitamin A | Limits epithelialization and capillary formation |
| B-Complex | Inhibits enzymatic reactions that contribute to wound healing |
| Vitamin C | Impairs collagen synthesis |
| Tissue hypoxia | Associated with an increased risk of infection and impaired healing, because oxygen is required to support cell function and collagen synthesis |
| Impaired blood supply | Inadequate delivery of oxygen and nutrients to healing tissues and removal of waste products |
| Impaired inflammatory and immune processes | Decreased phagocytosis and wound debridement; increased risk of infection; delayed healing |

Drug therapy, particularly corticosteroid medications, may suppress the immune and inflammatory responses, delaying healing (Porth, 2002). Other external factors, such as exposure to ionizing radiation and wound cleansing agents, can also affect healing. Table 8–5 summarizes major factors that affect the inflammatory process and wound healing.

## COLLABORATIVE CARE

Management of the client with inflamed tissue focuses on promoting healing. Care is generally supportive, allowing the client's own physiologic processes to remove foreign matter and damaged cells. Wound care may be minimal, involving only simple cleaning, or extensive, involving irrigations and debridement. The client is encouraged to rest, to increase fluid intake, and to eat a well-balanced, nutritious diet. Anti-inflammatory medications are administered only when the inflammatory process has become problematic. Antibiotics may also be prescribed to help eliminate infectious causes of inflammation.

## Diagnostic Tests

The following diagnostic tests may be ordered to identify the source and extent of inflammation.

- *WBC with differential* provides information about the type and extent of inflammatory response. The differential count (the percentage of the total WBC made up by each type of leukocyte) provides further clues about inflammatory processes (Table 8–6).

## TABLE 8-6  The White Blood Cell Count and Differential

| Cell Type and Normal Value | Increased | Decreased |
|---|---|---|
| Total WBCs:<br>4000 to 10,000 per mm³ | *Leukocytosis:* Infection or inflammation, leukemia, trauma or stress, tissue necrosis | *Leukopenia:* Bone marrow depression, overwhelming infection, viral infections, immunosuppression, autoimmune disease, dietary deficiency |
| Neutrophils<br>(segs, PMNs, or polys):<br>55% to 70% | *Neutrophilia:* Acute infection or stress response, myelocytic leukemia, inflammatory or metabolic disorders | *Neutropenia:* Bone marrow depression, overwhelming bacterial infection, viral infection, Addison's disease |
| Eosinophils (eos):<br>1% to 4% | *Eosinophilia:* Parasitic infections, hypersensitivity reactions, autoimmune disorders | *Eosinopenia:* Cushing's syndrome, autoimmune disorders, stress, certain drugs |
| Basophils (basos):<br>0.5% to 1% | *Basophilia:* Hypersensitivity responses, chronic myelogenous leukemia, chickenpox or smallpox, splenectomy, hypothyroidism | *Basopenia:* Acute stress or hypersensitivity reactions, hyperthyroidism |
| Monocytes (monos):<br>2% to 8% | *Monocytosis:* Chronic inflammatory disorders, tuberculosis, viral infections, leukemia, Hodgkin's disease, multiple myeloma | *Monocytopenia:* Bone marrow depression, corticosteroid therapy |
| Lymphocytes (lymphs):<br>20% to 40% | *Lymphocytosis:* Chronic bacterial infection, viral infections, lymphocytic leukemia | *Lymphocytopenia:* Bone marrow depression, immunodeficiency, leukemia, Cushing's syndrome, Hodgkin's disease, renal failure |

*Note. Data are from* Laboratory Tests and Diagnostic Procedures *(2nd ed.) by R. Chernecky and B. J. Berger, 1997, Philadelphia: W. B. Saunders; and* Mosby's Diagnostic and Laboratory Test Reference *(3rd ed.) by K. D. Pagana and T. J. Pagana, 1997, St. Louis: Mosby-Year Book.*

- *Erythrocyte sedimentation rate (ESR or sed rate)* is a nonspecific test to detect inflammation. The rate at which RBCs fall to the bottom of a vertical tube is an indicator of inflammation. An increased ESR may indicate acute or chronic inflammation, tuberculosis, autoimmune disorders, some malignancies, and nephritis. Decreased ESR is found in congestive heart failure, sickle cell anemia, and polycythemia vera.
- *C-reactive protein (CRP) test* is used to detect CRP. This abnormal glycoprotein is produced by the liver and is excreted into the bloodstream during the acute phase of an inflammatory process. The expected result of this test is negative for CRP. A positive result indicates an acute or chronic inflammatory process. It may also indicate the client's response to therapy, because it decreases when inflammation subsides (Kee, 2001).

In addition to the above diagnostic tests, cultures of the blood and other body fluids may be ordered to determine if infection is the cause of inflammation.

## Medications

Medications may be prescribed for the client with an inflammatory response to help alleviate distressing symptoms or destroy infectious agents.

Acetaminophen (Tylenol) may be administered to reduce the fever and pain associated with inflammation. Acetaminophen has no anti-inflammatory effect; it will not reduce the inflammatory process but will relieve associated symptoms. Acetaminophen decreases fever by acting directly on the hypothalamus heat-regulating center. It also works on the central nervous system to relieve pain sensations.

Antibiotics may be used either prophylactically to prevent infection from interfering with the healing process of damaged tissue, or therapeutically to treat the infection. If infection is present, the organism and its response or sensitivity to various antibiotics are used to guide therapy. Antibiotic therapy is presented in greater depth in the section of this chapter on infectious diseases.

Although inflammation is a beneficial process to prepare acutely injured tissue for healing, it can have damaging effects as well. When these effects are a concern or the manifestations of inflammation are deleterious to the client, anti-inflammatory medications may be prescribed. Anti-inflammatory medications fall into three broad groups: salicylates, such as aspirin; other nonsteroidal anti-inflammatory drugs (NSAIDs); and corticosteroids.

Aspirin (also called acetylsalicylic acid, or ASA) is an NSAID that has antipyretic, analgesic, and antiplatelet effects. Its beneficial effects are largely dose related. Low doses (as little as 81 mg per day) inhibit platelet aggregation and normal blood clotting. Higher doses (650 to 1000 mg 4 to 5 times per day) are required to accomplish its anti-inflammatory effects. However, 650 mg of aspirin is an effective analgesic and antipyretic dosage. To relieve pain, aspirin acts primarily on peripheral sensory nerves by inhibiting the synthesis of prostaglandins and kinins, which are chemical stimuli of sensory nerves. As an antipyretic, aspirin acts both centrally and peripherally. It inhibits the formation of pyrogenic substances that raise the hypothalamic thermostat. It also dilates peripheral blood vessels and promotes diaphoresis, increasing the dissipation of heat (Shannon, Wilson, & Stang, 2001).

In therapeutic doses, aspirin mediates the inflammatory process by inhibiting the synthesis of prostaglandins and acting on the mobility and activation of leukocytes. Inflammation is reduced, along with the swelling, redness, and impaired function that accompanies it.

The other NSAIDs have activity similar to that of aspirin. They inhibit prostaglandin synthesis, reducing the inflammatory and pain response. NSAIDs fall into the following classifications.

- *Salicylates,* which include aspirin and related compounds
- *Acetic acids,* including indomethacin (Indocin), ketorolac (Toradol), sulindac (Clinoril), and tolmetin (Tolectin)
- *Propionic acids,* including ibuprofen (Motrin and numerous nonprescription preparations), fenoprofen (Nalfon), and naproxen (Naprosyn)
- *Fenamates,* including meclofenamate (Meclomen)
- *Pyrazoles,* including phenylbutazone (Butazolidin)
- *Oxicams,* including piroxicam (Feldene)

Each group has a slightly different mode of action for prostaglandin inhibition. Clients may have varying degrees of relief with different NSAIDs; sometimes, several different agents must be tried before the most effective is identified. Side effects also differ to a certain extent; however, all have a potential cross-sensitivity with aspirin, all irritate the gastrointestinal tract, and all cause some degree of sodium and water retention. They also are more costly than aspirin, but they have a longer duration of action; therefore, fewer daily doses are required to achieve the desired effect. Indomethacin and phenylbutazone are the most toxic of the NSAIDs. Their use is limited to short-term therapy. (See Chapter 4 for further information on NSAIDs.)

For acute hypersensitivity reactions, such as reactions to poison oak, or for inflammation that cannot be managed by aspirin or NSAID therapy, corticosteroid therapy may be prescribed. The glucocorticoids are hormones produced by the adrenal cortex that have widespread effects on body metabolism and the immune response. Glucocorticoids inhibit inflammation and may be lifesaving in acute fulminating or chronic progressive inflammation. They do not cure disease; they are palliative to manage the inflammatory process.

When glucocorticoids are prescribed to manage inflammation, the following principles are used to guide therapy.

- The smallest possible effective dose is used.
- If a local-acting preparation such as a topical agent or intra-articular injection will be effective, it is prescribed.
- To minimize suppression of adrenal gland activity, an alternate-day dose schedule is used when possible.
- High-dose corticosteroid therapy is never stopped abruptly, but tapered, allowing the client's adrenal glands to resume normal function.

The incidence of potentially harmful side effects increases with higher doses and prolonged therapy.

The nursing implications of caring for a client receiving corticosteroid medications are discussed in Chapter 23. 🔗

## Nutrition

Healing depends on cell replication, protein synthesis, and the function of specific organs—the liver, heart, and lungs in particular. Weight loss and protein depletion are risk factors for poor healing and wound complications. Even a few days of severely impaired nutritional intake can noticeably affect healing.

The client with an inflammatory process or healing wound requires a well-balanced diet of sufficient kilocalories to meet the metabolic needs of the body (see Table 8–5). Inflammation often produces *catabolism,* a state in which body tissues are broken down. Healing, by contrast, is a process of *anabolism,* or building up. Without sufficient kilocalories and nutrients, catabolism may predominate, impairing healing.

Carbohydrates are important to meet energy demands, as well as to support leukocyte function. Adequate protein is necessary for tissue healing and the production of antibodies and WBCs. Lack of adequate protein increases the risk of infection. Complete protein sources, those that provide the essential amino acids, are preferred. Dietary fats are used in the synthesis of cell membranes.

Vitamins A, B-complex, C, and K are also important to the healing process. Vitamin A is necessary for capillary formation and epithelialization. B-complex vitamins promote wound healing, and vitamin C is necessary for collagen synthesis. Vitamin K provides a vital component for the synthesis of clotting factors in the liver.

Although it has been established that minerals contribute to the inflammatory and healing processes, less is known about required amounts. Zinc appears to be important for tissue growth, skin integrity, cell-mediated immunity, and other general immune mechanisms (Lutz & Przytulski, 2001).

## NURSING CARE

Acute inflammation may be self-limiting or extensive and require hospitalization. Nursing care includes teaching clients with acute and chronic inflammatory conditions self-management at home.

### Health Promotion

Health promotion activities to prevent inflammation focus on reducing the risk for accidents and exposure to harmful agents that can result in subsequent injury. It is important to educate the public about potential hazards in both the work and home environments. In addition, safety education guidelines such as not drinking and driving, wearing a protective helmet when riding a bicycle, and using a safety belt in the car are important areas for discussion. Because most injuries occur at home, it is also important to discuss ways to make the home safer.

### Assessment

The following data are collected through the health history and physical examination. Further focused assessments are described with nursing interventions in the next section.

- Health history: risk factors, nutrition, medication use (anti-inflammatory and corticosteroids), location, duration, and type (redness, heat, pain, swelling, and impaired function) of symptoms
- Physical assessment: movement of injured area, circulation, wounds, lymph nodes

## Nursing Diagnoses and Interventions

The nursing care needs of the client with an inflammatory process are related to the manifestations of inflammation (pain in particular) and altered tissue integrity. Priority nursing diagnoses include *pain, impaired tissue integrity,* and *risk for infection.*

### Pain

Along with redness, warmth, swelling, and impaired function, pain is one of the cardinal manifestations of inflammation. Depending on the cause, affected area, and degree of inflammation, pain may be acute and immobilizing or chronic and demoralizing. It is important to remember that pain is a subjective experience and that client responses to pain vary. (Refer to Chapter 4 for more information about pain and its management.) ⊖⊝

- Assess pain using a scale of 0 to 10, with 0 being no pain and 10 being the worst pain; note the character and location of the pain. *Because pain is subjective, the client provides the most accurate information regarding his or her pain experience.*
- Use physical and nonverbal cues to further assess the level of pain. *This intervention is especially important if the client is nonverbal or tends to underreport pain.*
- Administer anti-inflammatory medications as prescribed. *These medications help reduce the pain resulting from acute inflammation.*
- Administer analgesic medications as prescribed. *Although most analgesics do little to reduce inflammation, they provide additional pain relief by reducing the perception of pain.*
- Monitor effectiveness of interventions. *Results may call for modifications in the regimen.*
- Provide comfort measures, such as back rubs, position changes, or relaxation techniques. *These measures reduce muscle tension, relieve areas of pressure, and provide distraction.*
- Encourage activities such as reading, watching television, and taking part in social interactions. *Such activities provide distraction from the pain experience.*
- Encourage rest. *Strenuous activity or exercising an inflamed body part may increase discomfort and tissue damage.*
- Provide cold or heat as pain-relief measures, as ordered. *For an acute injury, cold reduces swelling and relieves pain; after the initial stage, heat increases blood flow to the affected tissue and relieves pain and swelling by promoting absorption of edema. Either heat or cold may be contraindicated with some inflammatory processes; for example, if the appendix is acutely inflamed, applying heat to the abdomen may prompt the appendix to rupture, increasing the risk of peritonitis. If unsure, check with the client's primary care provider.*

**PRACTICE ALERT** *Use heat or cold application cautiously in older clients who have fragile skin and are at risk for tissue injury.* ∎

- Elevate the inflamed area if possible. *Elevation promotes venous return and reduces swelling.*
- Teach about the appropriate use and expected effects of anti-inflammatory medications. *If the client's pain continues after the initial doses of anti-inflammatory medication, he or she may become discouraged and stop taking the medication before it becomes fully effective.*

### Impaired Tissue Integrity

The inflammatory response can either precipitate or result from an impairment in the integrity of skin, support, or other tissues. Whatever the cause of the tissue alteration, it is vital that the nurse consider this alteration in delivering care.

- Assess general health and nutritional status. *Poor general health or chronic diseases such as diabetes mellitus or renal failure interfere with the healing processes and increase the risk of infection.*
- Assess circulation to the affected area. *Adequate tissue perfusion and oxygenation are necessary for healing.*
- Monitor the skin and surrounding tissue for increased signs of inflammation. *Inflammation can spread to adjacent tissues leading to conditions such as cellulitis.*
- Provide protection and support for inflamed tissue. *This reduces discomfort and decreases the risk of further tissue damage.*
- Clean inflamed tissue gently; if possible, use water, normal saline, or nontoxic wound cleansers such as Comfeel (Coloplast Corporation) only. *Soap and harsh cleansers such as povidone-iodine (Betadine) and hydrogen peroxide can cause further drying and tissue damage. Granulation tissue in a healing wound is fragile and easily damaged.* (See Chapter 7 for further discussion of wound care.) ⊖⊝
- Keep the inflamed area dry, and expose it to air as much as possible. *This promotes healing and helps prevent infection.*
- Balance rest with the tolerable degree of mobility. *Rest decreases metabolic demands and allows for cell regeneration while mobility helps to promote oxygenation and perfusion of the tissues.*
- Provide supplemental oxygen as ordered. *Supplemental oxygen improves tissue oxygenation and reduces hypoxia.*
- Provide a well-balanced diet with adequate kilocalories to meet the body's metabolic and healing needs. If the client is allowed nothing by mouth (NPO), suggest parenteral or enteral nutrition. For the client who is unable to consume an adequate diet, consult with a dietitian for between-meal supplements, and/or multivitamin supplements. *Careful attention to diet and nutrient intake is important to provide the nutrients necessary for immune function and healing and to prevent catabolism.*

### Risk for Infection

The inflammatory response often indicates that body defense mechanisms have been set in motion to protect against invading microorganisms. Wounds, whether traumatic or surgical in nature, are typically contaminated, as attested to by subsequent wound infections. The client with a healing wound is at particular risk for infection.

- Assess the wound for specific signs of infection, including purulent drainage, odor, and poor healing. *The normal inflammatory response can indicate infection and, on occasion, mask its presence.*

- Monitor temperature, pulse, and respirations at least every 4 hours. *In response to the inflammatory process the temperature rises, usually in the range of 99°F (37.2°C) to 100.9°F (38.2°C). A temperature of 101.0°F (38.3°C) or above indicates infection. Fever is usually accompanied by increased heart and respiratory rates.*
- Culture purulent or odorous wound drainage. *Wound culture is used to determine the infectious organism and to direct antibiotic therapy.*
- Apply dry or moist heat to the affected area for no longer than 20 minutes several times a day. *Heat increases the circulation of blood to and from the inflamed tissue. Time is limited to prevent burns.*
- Provide fluid intake of 2500 mL per day. *Adequate hydration promotes blood flow and nutrient supply to the tissues as well as dilutes and removes waste products from the body.*
- Assure adequate nutrition. *Adequate nutrition enhances the function and production of T cells and B cells, which are important in the immune response.*
- Use good handwashing techniques. *Handwashing removes transient microorganisms and is the best mechanism to prevent the spread of infection to a susceptible person.*
- Wear sterile gloves when providing wound care. *Using sterile gloves helps prevent further contamination of the wound and the spread of infection to other clients.*

## Using NANDA, NIC, and NOC

Chart 8–1 shows links between NANDA, NIC, and NOC when caring for the client with inflammation.

## Home Care

Client and family teaching enhances understanding of the inflammatory process, its cause, and its management. Teaching is also important to prevent further compromise that could result in infection.

Instructions, verbal and written, should include the following:

- Increase fluid intake to 2500 mL (approximately 2.5 quarts) per day.
- Eat a well-balanced diet high in vitamins and minerals and with adequate protein and kilocalories for healing.
- Use good handwashing techniques, particularly when caring for wounds or inflamed tissue and after using the bathroom.
- Elevate the inflamed area to reduce swelling and pain.
- Apply heat or cold for no longer than 20 minutes at a time to reduce the risk of tissue damage from burns or frostbite.
- Take all medications as prescribed, notifying the physician if adverse effects or hypersensitivity responses are noted.
- Rest acutely inflamed tissue; do not engage in strenuous activity until the inflammation has subsided.

## THE CLIENT WITH NATURAL OR ACQUIRED IMMUNITY

**Immunity** refers to the protection of the body from disease. Immunity to disease may be either natural or acquired, active or passive (see Table 8–7).

---

### CHART 8–1 NANDA, NIC, AND NOC LINKAGES

#### The Client with Tissue Inflammation and Healing

| NURSING DIAGNOSES | NURSING INTERVENTIONS | NURSING OUTCOMES |
|---|---|---|
| • Activity Intolerance<br>• Imbalanced Nutrition: Less than Body Requirements | • Energy Management<br>• Fluid Monitoring<br>• Nutrition Monitoring | • Energy Conservation<br>• Self-Care: Activities of Daily Living<br>• Nutritional Status: Food & Fluid Intake |

*Note. Data from Nursing Outcomes Classification (NOC) by M. Johnson & M. Maas (Eds.), 1997, St. Louis: Mosby; Nursing Diagnoses: Definitions & Classification 2001–2002 by North American Nursing Diagnosis Association, 2001, Philadelphia: NANDA; Nursing Interventions Classification (NIC) by J.C. McCloskey & G. M. Bulechek (Eds.), 2000, St. Louis: Mosby. Reprinted by permission.*

---

### TABLE 8–7 Types of Acquired Immunity

| Type of Immunity | | How Developed | Examples |
|---|---|---|---|
| *Active Immunity* | Natural | Acquired by infection with an antigen, resulting in the production of antibodies | Chickenpox, hepatitis A |
| | Artificial | Acquired by immunization with an antigen, such as attenuated live virus vaccine | MMR, polio, DPT, hepatitis B vaccines |
| *Passive Immunity* | Natural | Acquired by transfer of maternal antibodies to the fetus or neonate via the placenta or breast milk | Neonate initially protected against MMR if mother immune |
| | Artificial | Acquired by administration of antibodies or antitoxins in immune globulin | Gamma globulin injection following hepatitis A exposure |

Immunity develops from the activation of the body's immune response. Depending on the antigen, antibody-mediated or cell-mediated responses are activated. The immune response typically involves components of both. In the immunocompetent client, these responses inactivate and remove the antigen, allowing recovery to occur or preventing the development of disease.

## PATHOPHYSIOLOGY

The processes of antibody-mediated and cell-mediated immunity result in the development of **acquired immunity** or **active immunity.** Active immunity occurs when the body produces antibodies or develops immune lymphocytes against specific antigens. Memory cells, which can produce an immediate immune response on reexposure to the antigen, provide long-term immunity.

Active immunity can be naturally acquired, resulting from contact with the disease-producing antigen and subsequent development of the disease. Naturally acquired immunity is common for diseases such as chickenpox and hepatitis A, making the risk of developing the disease a second time very low.

For many diseases, the potential consequences of a single disease episode on the individual and society make prevention desirable, especially for highly contagious diseases capable of causing epidemics. In these instances, immunization or vaccination is used to provide artificially acquired immunity. The purpose of vaccination is to establish adequate levels of antibody and/or memory cells to provide effective immunity (Roitt, 1994). Vaccination introduces the disease-producing antigen into the body in a manner that will stimulate the immune system to form antibodies and memory cells but will not produce disease. Vaccines may be made of killed organisms or of live organisms that have been attenuated or modified to reduce their disease-producing capability. Typhoid is an example of a killed organism vaccine; measles-mumps-rubella (MMR) vaccine, by contrast, is made from attenuated organisms. Many newer vaccines use subunits of the antigen; these are portions of the organism that have antigenic properties but are unable to produce disease.

**Passive immunity** provides temporary protection against disease-producing antigens. Passive immunity is provided by antibodies produced by other people or animals. These acquired antibodies are used up; they either combine with the antigen or are naturally degraded by the body, and their protection is gradually lost. Naturally acquired passive immunity is provided by the transfer of maternal antibodies via the placenta and breast milk to the infant. Rabies human immune globulin and hepatitis B immune globulin (HBIG) are examples of immunizations used to provide artificially acquired passive immunity. The types of active and passive immunity are summarized in Table 8–7.

## COLLABORATIVE CARE

Collaborative care focuses primarily on assessing the client's immune status and ensuring acquired immunity to prevent disease.

## Diagnostic Tests

A number of diagnostic tests can be performed to assess the client's immune status.

- *Serum protein* measures the total protein in the blood including albumin and globulins. Normal levels for the adult are 6 to 8 g/dL; albumin is approximately 60% (3.2 to 4.5 g/dL) of the total serum protein; and globulins are normally 2.3 to 3.4 g/dL. Total protein levels, albumin, and globulin are decreased in malnutrition and liver disease. Decreased globulin levels are noted with immunologic deficiencies.

- *Protein electrophoresis* analyzes protein content especially for albumin and gamma globulin and is used to assess immune function. Gamma globulins subjected to further electrophoresis separate into immunoglobulins: IgA, IgD, IgE, IgG, and IgM (see Table 8–3.) Analysis of specific levels of each provides clues about the immune status of the client. IgG levels are increased during acute infection. Decreased levels of IgG, IgA, and IgM are found in malignancies.

- *Antibody testing* is ordered to determine if a client has developed antibodies in response to an infection or immunization. Antibodies for hepatitis, HIV, rubella, toxoplasmosis, and *Treponema pallidum* (the organism causing syphilis) can be identified. An elevated titer level for hepatitis and rubella indicates immunity. For the other disorders and hepatitis, it may also be used to determine if the client has the disease.

- *Skin testing* can assess cell-mediated immunity. A known antigen such as streptokinase, tuberculin purified protein derivative (PPD), or candida is injected intradermally. The site is then observed for induration and erythema, which typically peaks at 24 to 48 hours. An induration of at least 10 mm in diameter is a positive reaction indicating previous exposure and sensitization to the antigen. (See Chapter 9 for further information on skin testing for hypersensitivity reactions.) ⊘ No reaction, or **anergy,** indicates depressed cell-mediated immunity.

## Immunizations

**Vaccines** are suspensions of whole or fractionated bacteria or viruses that have been treated to make them nonpathogenic. Vaccines are given to induce an immune response and subsequent immunity. Although vaccine development has been a major factor in improving public health, no vaccine is completely effective or entirely safe. Table 8–8 outlines the vaccines recommended for the adult client to maintain optimal health and immune status.

Adults born before 1956 are generally considered to be immune to measles, mumps, and rubella by prior infection. For persons born after 1956 whose immunologic status is unclear or who are at significant risk of exposure to these diseases (e.g., persons entering health care careers), reimmunization is recommended.

Tetanus and diphtheria toxoids are combined in a single immunization. The pediatric form of the vaccine is known as DT; the adult form is Td. The vaccine stimulates active immunity by inducing the production of antibodies and antitoxins. After

TABLE 8–8  Recommended Immunizations for Adults

| Vaccine | Type | Dose | Indications | Precautions and Nursing Implications |
|---|---|---|---|---|
| Measles / mumps / rubella (MMR) | Live virus | 0.5 mL SC | All adults born after 1956, particularly those who are at risk for infection, such as college students and military recruits. Measles and mumps vaccination particularly recommended for males without history of previous infection; rubella vaccination recommended for all seronegative females. | As a live virus vaccine, should not be administered to pregnant women or immunocompromised clients. Do not administer to clients with a history of anaphylactic reaction to egg protein or neomycin. |
| Tetanus and diphtheria toxoids (Td) | Inactivated toxins | 0.5 mL IM | Initial series of 3 injections (2 doses, 4 to 6 weeks apart; third dose 6 to 12 months after dose 2) if never immunized; booster every 10 years; following a major or contaminated wound if more than 5 years since last booster | Do not give in first trimester of pregnancy or to clients with a history of anaphylactic reaction to horse serum; administer deep IM in deltoid of dominant arm. |
| Hepatitis B (HB) | Inactive viral antigen | 1.0 mL IM | Series of 3 doses: initial and at 1 and 6 months. Recommended for anyone at risk for exposure and for postexposure prophylaxis | Use with caution in pregnant or lactating females, older clients, and clients with active infection; have epinephrine 1:1000 available on unit in case of anaphylaxis and laryngospasm. |
| Influenza | Inactivated virus or viral components | 0.5 mL IM | Yearly for all clients over age 65 and those at risk for complications, including debilitated clients and clients with chronic disease | Do not administer to acutely ill clients or clients with history of anaphylactic reaction to egg protein. |
| Pneumococcal | Bacterial polysaccharides | 0.5 mL IM or SC | One dose for clients over age 65 and those at risk for pneumococcal pneumonia, including clients with chronic lung disease or other chronic diseases | Do not administer to pregnant women. |

an initial series of three immunizations, an intramuscular (IM) booster injection of 0.5 mL is recommended every 10 years to maintain protection. Older clients, particularly those who never entered the workforce (e.g., older female adults), may have never received the initial series of DT vaccine.

Hepatitis B (HB) vaccine is given as a series of three or four immunizations to promote active immunity to hepatitis B. This vaccine is recommended for everyone at high risk for exposure through blood or other body fluids. It is mandated by the Occupational Health and Safety Administration (OSHA) for all health care workers at risk. Other high-risk populations include intravenous drug users, sexual partners of infected individuals, clients on hemodialysis, prison guards, and athletic coaches.

Influenza vaccine is recommended for persons at high risk for serious sequelae of influenza, including older adults, persons with lung disease or other chronic illness, and immunosuppressed individuals. The antigenic strain included in influenza vaccine varies each year according to the predicted predominant strains affecting the population. Yearly reimmunization is therefore required.

Pneumococcal vaccine is generally recommended for the same populations as influenza vaccine. A single dose of this vaccine confers lifetime immunity, although repeating immunization every 6 years may be considered for high-risk clients.

In addition to routine immunizations, people traveling outside the United States and Canada should receive vaccines against diseases that are endemic in certain regions of the world.

Other immunologic substances may be administered as indicated. Immune globulins provide passive immunity as protection against a known or potential exposure to an antigen. Standard immune globulin is given to household contacts of clients with hepatitis A and persons traveling to areas in which it is endemic. Hepatitis B immune globulin (HBIG) contains higher titers of antibody to hepatitis B virus and is used for persons exposed by blood or sexual contact. Following confirmed or suspected contact with a pathogen, selected vaccines may be administered to stimulate an immediate immune response (Table 8–9).

For most vaccines, a sensitivity test should be performed prior to administration to detect sensitivity to substances such as horse serum or eggs. The substance is injected intradermally; if after 20 minutes there is no evidence of a reaction, the selected vaccine can be administered.

Moderate to severe local reactions may occur following administration of an immunization. Common reactions include redness, swelling, tenderness, and muscle ache. Administering the vaccine in the dominant arm of the client helps minimize local reactions, because use and movement of the arm facilitates absorption of the solution. Applying heat to the site is

**TABLE 8–9  Preparations for Postexposure Prophylaxis**

| Disease | Preparation and Dose | Indications |
|---|---|---|
| Hepatitis A | Human immune globulin (IG), 0.02 mL/kg IM | Contacts in day care centers, households, custodial institutions; patrons of eating establishments known to have been exposed by infected food worker |
| Hepatitis B | Hepatitis B immune globulin (HBIG), 0.06 mL/kg IM | Possible percutaneous or sexual contact with blood or body fluids of an infected individual; usually given concurrently with hepatitis B vaccine |
| Varicella | Varicella-zoster immune globulin (VZIG), 12.5 units/kg; minimum dose 125 units, maximum 625 units | Susceptible adults exposed to varicella virus (e.g., chickenpox or shingles) |
| Tetanus | Tetanus immune globulin (TIG), 500 to 3000 units IM (part infiltrated around wound) | Clients with major or contaminated wounds who have no history of tetanus immunization or an unclear one that is not up-to-date; Td usually given as well |
| Rabies | Human rabies immune globulin (HRIG), 20 IU/kg, half IM, half infiltrated around wound | Persons with a significant exposure to a rabid or potentially rabid animal; followed with 5-dose course of rabies vaccine |
| Measles | Human immune globulin (IG), 0.25 mL/kg IM | Susceptible close contacts, especially people who are immunosuppressed; postpone immunization with measles vaccine until 3 months after IG |
| Rubella | Human immune globulin (IG), 0.55 mL/kg IM | Pregnant women exposed in first trimester when termination of pregnancy is not an option; does not ensure protection of fetus |

*Note. Table adapted from Harrison's Principles of Internal Medicine (14th ed.) by A. S. Fauci et al. (Eds.), 1998, New York: McGraw-Hill.*

also beneficial. Occasionally local ulcerations occur; when they do, warm, wet pack, or sterile wet-to-dry dressings may be prescribed.

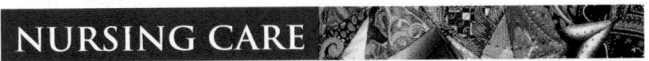

## NURSING CARE

Maintaining a population that is fully immunized against common, potentially epidemic, and devastating diseases is a major public health task for nursing. Nurses not only recommend and administer vaccines to individual clients and their families, but also plan and implement preventive care for whole communities.

Although this process may appear to be straightforward, multiple issues affect society's ability to immunize the entire population. For some people, for example, religious beliefs may preclude the use of immunizations to prevent disease. Also, people who are not citizens and the medically indigent population have difficulty accessing immunization services. Lack of immunization not only puts the individual at increased risk for infectious disease, but also increases the cost of medical services and the possibility of exposing immunocompromised people to disease.

### Health Promotion

In the public health setting, the nurse looks at the immunization needs and illness risk for an entire community. Communities include not only cities and localities but also groups of people, such as college populations and employees in a workplace. Public education needs may be met through presentations to groups of people, feature articles in newspapers and other local publications, advertising, radio presentations and public service announcements, and one-to-one discussion and teaching.

### Assessment

Collect the following data through the health history and physical examination. Further focused assessments are described with nursing interventions in the next section.

- Health history: age, medication use (corticosteroids and antibiotics) and blood transfusion, nutrition, allergies, infection, immunizations, autoimmune disorders, chronic diseases such as diabetes mellitus, cancer
- Physical assessment: skin lesions or rashes, breath sounds, respiratory rate

### Nursing Diagnoses and Interventions

Nursing care focuses on preventing injury from the immunization and educating the client.

#### Health-Seeking Behaviors: Immunization

For individual clients and their families, nurses promote immunocompetence by assessing immune status, recommending appropriate immunizations, and administering vaccines as ordered or indicated. Once a person reaches adulthood, routine immunizations often become a neglected part of health care.

- Determine knowledge level, understanding, attitudes, and religious beliefs about immunization. *This provides a basis for further education and determines if religious beliefs may contraindicate immunization.*
- Discuss the value and reasons for recommended immunizations. *Understanding promotes adherence.*

- Reinforce positive health-seeking behaviors. *This will help promote future health maintenance activities.*
- Using recommended immunization schedules, develop a plan to attain optimal immunization status. *Adherence with recommended schedules for immunization is important in preventing disease and disability.*
- Do not administer MMR or influenza vaccine if allergic to eggs or tetanus antitoxin if sensitive to horse serum. *Vaccines prepared from chicken or duck embryos are contraindicated in clients who are allergic to eggs. Tetanus antitoxin is prepared from horse serum. Both will cause a severe allergic reaction.*
- Withhold administration of active immunologic products in the presence of an upper respiratory infection (URI) or other infection. *Active immunizations can cause a greater inflammatory reaction in the presence of infections.*
- Do not administer oral polio vaccine (OPV), MMR, or any live virus vaccine to immunosuppressed clients or to clients who are in close household contact with an immunosuppressed person. *Live virus vaccines can cause disease in the immunosuppressed client. The virus may be transmitted from close household contacts during the initial postvaccination period.*
- Do not administer live attenuated virus vaccines and passive immunizations such as gamma globulin simultaneously. *Passive antibodies interfere with the response of the live attenuated virus.*
- Prior to administering prescribed vaccine, check expiration date and manufacturer's instructions. *Outdated vaccines cannot provide adequate immunization protection. Certain injection sites have better absorption than others.*
- Keep epinephrine 1:1000 readily available when administering immunizations. *Epinephrine causes vasoconstriction and reduces laryngospasm; in acute anaphylaxis, it can be lifesaving.*

**PRACTICE ALERT**  *Observe the client for 20 to 30 minutes following inoculation to monitor for possible adverse reactions.* ■

## Using NANDA, NIC, and NOC

Chart 8–2 shows links between NANDA, NIC, and NOC when caring for the client who is receiving an immunization.

## Home Care

Educating individual clients, families, and the public about the maintenance of immune status is a significant nursing responsibility. For individual clients and their families, instructions focus on the following areas.

- Appropriate immunizations and recommended schedules for initial vaccination and boosters
- How and where to obtain immunizations
- The need to observe the client for up to 30 minutes following a vaccine for possible adverse reactions
- Possible side effects and adverse effects of the immunization administered
- Self-care measures for side effects and postvaccination discomfort
- Responses to immunization that should be reported immediately to the primary care provider
- Maintenance of a permanent immunization record
- Beneficial resources:
  - County or public health departments
  - Centers for Disease Control and Prevention National Immunization Program
  - National Institute of Allergy and Infectious Diseases

## THE CLIENT WITH AN INFECTION

In an effort to find a suitable environment in which to grow and reproduce, microorganisms—including bacteria, viruses, fungi, and parasites—often invade the human body. In most cases, contact between humans and microorganisms is incidental and may even be beneficial to both organisms. Resident bacteria of the skin, mucous membranes, and gastrointestinal tract are an important part of the body's defense system. However, many microorganisms are virulent; that is, they have the ability to cause disease. **Pathogens** are virulent organisms rarely found in the absence of disease. Some microorganisms known as opportunistic pathogens rarely, if ever, cause harm to persons with intact immune systems, but are capable of producing infectious disease in the immunocompromised host (Porth, 2002).

Infectious disease has been pervasive throughout history. Modern medicine, antibiotic therapy, immunizations, and

## CHART 8–2  NANDA, NIC, AND NOC LINKAGES

### The Client with Acquired Immunity

| NURSING DIAGNOSIS | NURSING INTERVENTIONS | NURSING OUTCOMES |
|---|---|---|
| • Risk for Injury | • Health Screening<br>• Immunization/Vaccination Management<br>• Health Education<br>• Health Beliefs | • Immune Status<br>• Immunization Behaviors |

*Note. Data from Nursing Outcomes Classification (NOC) by M. Johnson & M. Maas (Eds.), 1997, St. Louis: Mosby; Nursing Diagnoses: Definitions & Classification 2001–2002 by North American Nursing Diagnosis Association, 2001, Philadelphia: NANDA; Nursing Interventions Classification (NIC) by J.C. McCloskey & G. M. Bulechek (Eds.), 2000, St. Louis: Mosby. Reprinted by permission.*

## Nursing Care Plan
## A Client with Acquired Immunity

Terry Adams is a 48-year-old executive who is planning a trip to central Africa. In preparation, he contacts his local health care provider to obtain the necessary immunizations. Jane Wong, the registered nurse in the clinic, obtains a nursing history on Mr. Adams.

### ASSESSMENT

Mr. Adams's history reveals that he has always been very healthy and active, apart from a mild case of asthma. As an adult, he has had little problem with his asthma, "except for those rare occasions on which I am dumb enough to smoke more than one cigarette!" He is divorced and is not currently in a continuing relationship. He has two grown daughters with whom his relationship is good. Since contracting hepatitis A several years ago, he drinks alcohol only rarely, and never more than one or two drinks at any one time. He confesses to little organized exercise but plays golf two or three times a week and states that he is such a hyperactive workaholic that he rarely sits for any length of time. Mr. Adams has not seen a physician since recovering from the hepatitis and is unsure when he last received any immunizations. He does know if he had all recommended childhood immunizations, but recalls getting both Salk and Sabin polio vaccines when they became available. His physical examination reveals an alert and healthy individual with no abnormalities noted. His vital signs are as follows: T 97.4°F, P 64, R 14, and BP 142/82.

The physician orders the following immunizations for Mr. Adams:

- Measles-mumps-rubella (MMR)
- Combined tetanus and diphtheria toxoids (Td)
- Yellow fever vaccine
- Typhoid vaccine
- Meningococcal meningitis vaccine

### DIAGNOSES

- *Health-seeking behaviors: immunization* related to impending international travel
- *Altered health maintenance* related to apparent lapse in immunization status

- *Risk for injury* related to adverse response to immunization

### EXPECTED OUTCOMES

- Obtain necessary immunizations.
- Verbalize a schedule for maintaining up-to-date immunization status.
- Experience no significant adverse effects from immunization.

### PLANNING AND IMPLEMENTATION

- Administer MMR, Td, and meningococcal meningitis vaccines prior to discharge from clinic.
- Observe closely for 30 minutes following immunization for potential adverse responses.
- Schedule return visit in 1 week for typhoid vaccine.
- Provide referral to a registered vaccination center for yellow fever vaccine and documentation of vaccination.
- Provide instructions for comfort measures to relieve local and systemic adverse effects of vaccines. Provide written instructions on manifestations that should be reported to the physician.
- Document immunizations on a permanent record at the clinic and for the client.

### EVALUATION

Terry Adams completes his prescribed immunizations without major adverse effects, although he does complain of fever, malaise, and general achiness for several days following the typhoid vaccination. His trip to Africa is successful, and he returns to the United States without contracting any infectious diseases.

### Critical Thinking in the Nursing Process

1. Explain why it is important for adults to continue receiving immunizations throughout their life span.
2. If a client says said to you, "I don't believe in immunizations. I hear they are dangerous," how would you respond?
3. When should a client contact the primary caregiver after receiving an immunization?

See Evaluating Your Responses in Appendix C.

---

other public health measures to protect food and water supplies have significantly reduced the prevalence of infectious diseases in many parts of the world. In spite of these advances, many infections, including malaria, typhoid, and tuberculosis, remain prevalent in developing nations. Sexually transmitted infections (STIs) rage through modern cities and industrialized populations. New varieties and strains of pathogens, such as human immunodeficiency virus (HIV), evolve to cause disease.

To a certain extent, modern medicine has contributed to the development of infectious diseases caused by antibiotic-resistant strains of microorganisms. Tuberculosis is on the rise in the United States, partially because organisms have become resistant to standard therapies. Clients receive immunosuppressive therapy following organ or tissue transplant or in the treatment of neoplasms, making them more susceptible to in-

fection. Metal and plastic prosthetic devices are implanted, providing potential sites for colonization by disease-producing organisms (Fauci et al., 1998). It has also become apparent that many diseases long considered unrelated to microorganisms may actually be infectious; for example, colonization of the gastric mucosa with *Helicobacter pylori* may be the predominant cause of peptic ulcer disease, and oncogenic viruses have the ability to transform normal cells into malignant cells.

## PATHOPHYSIOLOGY

**Infection** occurs when an organism is able to colonize and multiply within a host. The host can be any organism capable of supporting the nutritional and physical growth requirements of the microorganism—for example, humans. When the host experiences injury, pathologic changes, inflammation, or organ dysfunction in response to an infection or from intoxication

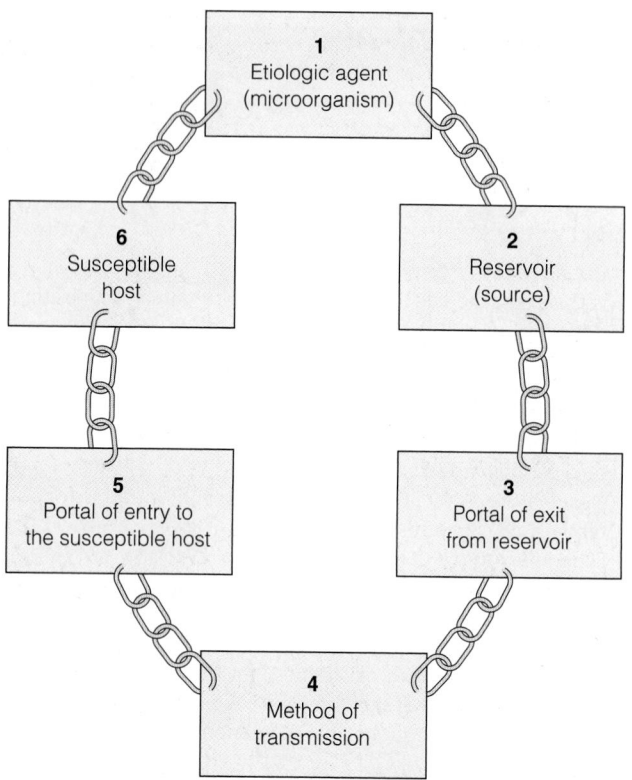

**Figure 8–12** ■ The chain of infection.

by cellular poisons produced by a pathogen, it is called an infectious disease.

For a microorganism to cause infection, it must have disease-causing potential (virulence), be transmitted from its reservoir, and gain entry into a susceptible host. This is known as the chain of infection (Figure 8–12 ■).

## Pathogens

Pathogens capable of infecting and causing disease in a susceptible host include bacteria, viruses, mycoplasma, rickettsia, chlamydia, fungi, and parasites such as protozoa, helminths (worms), and arthropods (Box 8–4). Each organism causes a different specific reaction in the host.

A number of different mechanisms have evolved in pathogens to facilitate their transmission and increase their ability to invade the host and cause disease. Factors influencing the transmission of an organism include its resistance to drying and to variations in environmental temperature. For example, spore-forming organisms are extremely resistant to drying.

Many microorganisms are capable of producing toxins or enzymes to facilitate their invasion of the host, increase their resistance to host defenses, and increase their ability to cause disease. Adhesion factors produced by or incorporated into the cell wall or membrane of the pathogen improve its ability to attach and colonize the host. Pathogens may also produce enzymes to enhance their spread to local tissues, chemicals to block specific

---

**BOX 8–4    ■   Pathogenic Organisms**

### BACTERIA

Bacteria are single-celled organisms capable of autonomous reproduction. Relatively small and simple organisms, they contain a single chromosome: A flexible cell membrane and rigid cell wall surrounds their cytoplasm, giving them a distinctive shape; some also have an extracellular capsule for additional protection. Bacteria have different characteristics and growth requirements: *aerobes* require oxygen for survival, whereas *anaerobes* cannot survive in the presence of oxygen; *gram-positive* bacteria stain purple when subjected to crystal violet stain, whereas *gram-negative* bacteria do not stain with crystal violet but turn red when subjected to safranin stain; the colonies formed by replicating bacteria differ from one another.

### VIRUSES

Viruses are obligate intracellular parasites that are incapable of reproducing outside of a living cell. Viruses consist of a protein coat around a core of either DNA or RNA. Some viruses are shed continuously from infected cell surfaces; others, after inserting their genetic material into that of the infected cell, remain latent until they are stimulated to replicate. Viruses may or may not cause lysis and death of the host cell during replication. Oncogenic viruses are able to transform normal cells into malignant cells.

### MYCOPLASMA

Although similar to bacteria, mycoplasma are smaller and have no cell wall, making them resistant to antibiotics that inhibit cell wall synthesis (e.g., penicillins).

### RICKETTSIA AND CHLAMYDIA

As obligate intracellular parasites with a rigid cell wall, rickettsia and *Chlamydia* have some features of both bacteria and viruses. Rather than depending on the host cell for reproduction, they use vitamins, nutrients, or products of metabolism (e.g., ATP) from the host. *Chlamydia* are transmitted by direct contact, whereas many rickettsiae infect the cells of arthropods (e.g., fleas, ticks, and lice) and are transmitted from these vectors to humans.

### FUNGI

Fungi are prevalent throughout the world, but few are capable of causing disease in humans. Most fungal infections are self-limited, affecting the skin and subcutaneous tissue. Some fungi, such as *Pneumocystis carinii,* can cause life-threatening opportunistic infections in the immunocompromised host.

### PARASITES

The term *parasite* is typically applied to members of the animal kingdom that infect and cause disease in other animals. Protozoa, helminths, and arthropods are considered parasites. Protozoa are single-celled organisms transmitted via direct or indirect contact or an arthropod vector. Helminths are wormlike parasites: roundworms, tapeworms, and flukes are examples. They gain entry into humans primarily through ingestion of fertilized eggs or penetration of larvae through the skin or mucous membranes. Arthropod parasites, such as scabies (mites), lice, and fleas, typically infest external body surfaces, causing localized tissue damage and inflammation. Transmission is by direct contact with the arthropod or its eggs.

*Note. Data summarized from* Pathophysiology: Concepts of Altered Health States *(6th ed.) by C. M. Porth, 2002, Philadelphia: Lippincott.*

immune processes or deplete neutrophils and macrophages, or extracellular capsules to discourage phagocytosis.

Pathogens are often capable of producing toxins that alter or destroy the normal function of host cells and promote colonization, proliferation, and invasion by the pathogen. Toxins often increase the disease-producing capability of the pathogen and, in some cases, are totally responsible for it; for example, cholera, tetanus, and botulism result from bacterial toxins, not from the direct effects of the infection. **Exotoxins** are soluble proteins secreted into surrounding tissue by the microorganism. Exotoxins are highly poisonous, causing cell death or dysfunction. **Endotoxins** are found in the cell wall of gram-negative bacteria and are released only when the cell is disrupted. Endotoxins have less specific effects than exotoxins, but they act as activators of many human regulatory systems, producing fever, inflammation, and potentially clotting, bleeding, or hypotension when released in large quantities.

## Reservoir and Transmission

The reservoir or source, where the pathogen lives and multiplies, may be either endogenous or exogenous. Organisms that reside on skin or mucosal surfaces of the host are endogenous. Exogenous sources can include other humans, animals, soil, water, intravenous fluid, or equipment. Infectious diseases are usually transmitted from human sources, that is, persons who have clinical disease or carriers with subclinical infection. Carriers harbor the pathogen without showing evidence of clinical disease. Pathogens exit human hosts via respiratory secretions, body fluids from the gastrointestinal and genitourinary tracts, skin or mucous membrane lesions, the placenta, and blood.

Organisms may be transmitted from the source to the susceptible host by direct or indirect contact, droplet or airborne transmission, or a vector. Direct contact includes person-to-person spread or contact with infected body fluids, as well as transmission from contaminated food or water. Indirect contact occurs when the infectious agent is contracted by use of inanimate objects, such as dirty eating utensils. Sneezing, talking, and coughing allow transmission by droplet contact when the host is within 2 to 3 feet of the source. Smaller respiratory particles that stay suspended in air and are carried via air currents allow airborne transmission. Vectors are insects and animals such as flies, mosquitoes, or rodents that act as intermediate hosts between the source and host. Microorganisms usually first colonize the portal of entry: nonintact skin, wounds, mucous membranes, and the respiratory, gastrointestinal, or genitourinary tracts.

## Host Factors

The susceptible host is the final link in the chain of infection. Exposure to pathogens does not automatically cause infection or infectious disease. The outcome of contact with a pathogenic microorganism is determined by the balance of microbial virulence and host resistance. Factors that can enable the host to resist infection include the following:

- Physical barriers, such as the skin and mucous membranes
- The hostile environment created by acid stomach secretions, urine, and vaginal secretions
- Antimicrobial factors in saliva, tears, and prostatic fluid
- Respiratory defenses, including humidification, filtration, the mucociliary escalator, cough reflex, and alveolar macrophages
- Specific and nonspecific immune responses to pathogenic invasion

## Stages of the Infectious Process

When infectious disease develops in the host, it typically follows a predictable course with stages based on the progression and intensity of manifestations.

The initial stage is the incubation period, during which the pathogen begins active replication but does not yet cause symptoms. Depending on the organism and host factors, the incubation period may last from hours, as with salmonella, to years, as with HIV infection.

The prodromal stage follows, during which symptoms first begin to appear. At this stage, symptoms are often nonspecific and include general malaise, fever, myalgias, headache, and fatigue.

Maximal impact of the infectious process is felt during the acute phase as the pathogen proliferates and disseminates rapidly. Toxic by-products of microorganism metabolism and cell lysis, along with the immune response, produce tissue damage and inflammation during this stage (Porth, 2002). Manifestations are more pronounced and specific to the infecting organism and site during the acute stage. Fever and chills may be significant during this phase. However, alcoholic clients and the very old may respond to severe infection by becoming hypothermic. The client is often tachycardic and tachypneic because of increased metabolic demands. Localized manifestations include redness, heat, swelling, pain, and impaired function. When the infectious disease affects an internal organ, manifestations are related to inflammatory changes in that organ and surrounding tissue. The client may experience tenderness to palpation over the site or show signs of impaired function, such as the hematuria and proteinuria characteristic of renal infections.

If the infectious process is prolonged, manifestations of the continuing immune response may become apparent. Catabolic and anorexic effects of the infection can lead to loss of body fat and muscle wasting. Immune complexes may be deposited at sites other than the primary infection, resulting in an inflammatory process. Glomerulonephritis (e.g., following strep throat) and vasculitis are possible results. Another possible consequence of prolonged infection and immune response is the triggering of an autoimmune disease process (discussed in Chapter 9), such as rheumatic cardiomyopathy or celiac disease. Juvenile-onset diabetes mellitus is thought to be the result of such a response (Fauci et al., 1998).

As the infection is contained and the pathogen eliminated, the convalescent stage of the disease occurs. During this stage, affected tissues are repaired and manifestations resolve. Resolution of the infection is total elimination of the pathogen from the body without residual manifestations. If a balance between organism and host factors occurs with neither predominating, chronic disease may develop or the organism may be driven into a protected site, such as an abscess. A carrier state develops when host defenses eliminate the infectious disease but the organism continues to multiply on mucosal sites (Fauci et al., 1998).

## Complications

Multiple and varied complications are associated with infectious diseases. They are typically specific to the infecting organism and the body system affected.

Acute invasion of the blood by certain microorganisms or their toxins can result in septicemia and septic shock. Whereas bacteremia, the presence of bacteria in the blood, may not have serious effects, septicemia refers to systemic disease associated with their presence or toxins. Septic shock indicates a state of hypotension and impaired organ perfusion resulting from sepsis. Unless treated aggressively, septic shock leads to diffuse cell and tissue injury, and potentially to organ failure. See Chapter 6 for an in-depth discussion of septic shock, other shock syndromes, and their management. ⌖

## Nosocomial Infections

**Nosocomial infections** are acquired in a health care setting, such as a hospital or nursing home. Currently, 5% of clients acquire a nosocomial infection while hospitalized, but this rate may rise to 10% in larger institutions (Wenzel and Edmond, 2001). Hospital-acquired infections add over 7.5 million hospital days, directly result in approximately 20,000 deaths, and contribute to 60,000 more deaths yearly in the United States (Fauci et al., 1998).

Clients entering hospitals are often the least able to mount immune defenses to infection. Immunologic responses may be compromised and normal defenses impaired in clients with, for example, cancer or chronic diseases, pressure ulcers, or organ transplants (Tierney et al., 2001). Nosocomial infections also occur when antibiotic therapy has altered natural defenses and impaired resistance to harmful microorganisms. Endogenous organisms outside their normal habitats (such as in *Escherichia coli* in the urinary tract) become a threat to the client. Other pharmacologic and therapeutic procedures such as chemotherapy, the use of corticosteroids, or radiation therapy also contribute to nosocomial infections. Gram-negative enteric bacteria and gram-positive *Staphylococcus aureus* are the most common bacteria responsible.

Invasive procedures and altered immune defenses are the main factors contributing to infection. Urinary catheterization is the number-one cause; cardiac catheterization, peripheral and central intravenous lines, respiratory care procedures, and surgical procedures are also closely linked to nosocomial infection (Box 8–5). Consequently, the urinary tract, surgical wounds, the respiratory tract, and invasive catheter sites on the skin are most often affected by hospital-acquired infection. The American Hospital Association (2001) reports that hospital-acquired pneumonia is the second most common nosocomial infection, and has the highest morbidity and mortality. Organisms causing the infection are often resistant to many drugs, not responding to antibiotics usually effective in treating infections acquired outside the hospital.

---

### BOX 8–5   ■ Nosocomial Infections

- Nosocomial infections typically manifest after 48 hours of hospitalization.
- Urinary tract infection is the most common type, accounting for about 45% of all nosocomial infections.
- Pneumonia accounts for 15% of all nosocomial infections related to endotracheal or nasogastric intubation.
- Surgical wounds account for 30% of all nosocomial infections.
- Bacteremia accounts for 7% of all nosocomial infections related to invasive devices (e.g., intravenous catheters, arterial lines).
- Antibiotic-associated diarrhea accounts for less than 3% of all nosocomial infections related to prophylactic antibiotic doses.

---

Prevention is the most important control measure for nosocomial infections. The pathogens causing these infections are transmitted primarily by contact with hospital personnel. **Effective hand washing is the single most important measure in infection control.** Although infections may also be transmitted by the airborne route, contaminated equipment, or from the environment, these are less significant causes. Invasive procedures and equipment should be used only when absolutely necessary; for example, it is not appropriate to insert an indwelling catheter when the only indication is incontinence. Peripheral intravenous equipment and sites must be changed regularly: intravenous bags and bottles every 24 hours, tubing every 24 to 72 hours, and sites every 2 to 3 days according to agency policy (Smith, Duell, & Martin, 2000).

## Antibiotic-Resistant Microorganisms

Antibiotic-resistant microorganisms are increasing at an alarming rate primarily due to prolonged or inappropriate use of antibiotic therapy. Although antibiotic therapy is expected to eradicate all targeted microorganisms, sometimes a few bacteria survive, leading to bacteria that reproduce with antibiotic resistance already encoded into their genetic makeup (Glover, 2000). Other bacteria produce enzymes that inactivate drugs, change drug binding sites, or alter their cell membrane to prevent drug absorption.

Some of the current resistant strains include:

- Methicillin-resistant *Staphylococcus aureus* (MRSA)
- Multidrug-resistant tuberculosis (MDR-TB)
- Penicillin-resistant *Streptococcus pneumoniae* (PRSP)
- Vancomycin-resistant *Enterococci* (VRE)
- Vancomycin intermediate-resistant *Staphylococcus aureus* (VISA)

**Methicillin-resistant *Staphylococcus aureus* (MRSA)** exists not only in hospitals but also is becoming more prevalent in nonhospital settings. MRSA colonizes in the nares and skin; health care personnel often transmit *S. aureus* unknowingly on their hands. Most *S. aureus* strains resist treatment by methicillin and other similar drugs, the treatment of choice for *S. aureus* infections. Vancomycin has been the only uniformly effective drug for MRSA; however, in 1997, a new form of

MediaLink | WWW BIOTERRORISM PREPAREDNESS CASE STUDY

*S. aureus* emerged with intermediate resistance to vancomycin, known as **vancomycin intermediate-resistant Staphylococcus aureus (VISA).** Clients with MRSA and VISA are isolated in a private room using contact precautions.

*Enterococci* are part of the normal flora of the gastrointestinal and female genital tracts. Frequent use of vancomycin caused *Enterococci* to develop resistance, leading to **vancomycin-resistant Enterococci (VRE).** Direct transmission occurs on the hands of health care personnel or contact with contaminated equipment. Stringent infection control measures are instituted; care is provided using contact precautions and clients are placed either alone or with other VRE-infected clients.

*Streptococcus pneumoniae,* the most common cause of community-acquired pneumonia, has developed into its resistant form, **penicillin-resistant Streptococcus pneumoniae (PRSP).** Unlike MRSA and VRE, PRSP is transmitted by droplets from the respiratory tract and requires transmission-based droplet precautions.

## Biological Threat Infections

Following the terrorist attacks on September 11, 2001, and the development of anthrax cases in the United States, concern has arisen about the possible use of biological weapons. The most likely pathogens to be used for this purpose include anthrax, smallpox, botulism, pneumonic plague, and viral hemorrhagic fevers.

*Anthrax* is an acute bacterial infection caused by *Bacillus anthracis,* a gram-positive, spore-producing organism that occurs in inhaled, cutaneous, and gastrointestinal forms. The spores are impervious to temperature and sunlight, and remain viable for years.

Inhalation anthrax carries the highest mortality rate because spores of 1 to 5 microns are easily inhaled and deposited in the alveoli (Coleman, 2001). The client initially exhibits influenzalike symptoms such as fever, nonproductive cough, headache, and malaise that advances to respiratory failure and hemodynamic collapse. Untreated clients die in 2 to 3 days. The characteristic lesion of cutaneous anthrax progresses from an itching papule to a painless, serosanguinous-filled vesicle that forms a black necrotic center. Clients who ingest the anthrax bacillus develop nausea, vomiting, severe abdominal pain, and bloody diarrhea. Diagnosis is confirmed by a positive blood culture, polymerase chain reaction, and serology. On confirmation of anthrax exposure, prophylaxis is initiated with oral ciprofloxacin (Cipro) or doxycycline (Doxylin) for 60 days; whereas people with confirmed systemic anthrax cases must receive anti-infectives intravenously.

In 1980, the World Health Organization certified that *smallpox* was eradicated. Routine smallpox vaccination was discontinued in 1972, leaving people under the age of 30 at risk for this disease if it reappears or is used as a weapon. Smallpox spreads by direct contact or by inhalation of respiratory droplets. Symptoms include a high fever, headache, and malaise, followed by a vesicular/pustular rash appearing simultaneously on the face and extremities. Once the pustules become scabs, people are highly contagious and should be placed in negative-pressure rooms. Anyone exposed to the client should be vaccinated and monitored closely. Vaccination within 2 to 3 days of exposure provides almost complete protection.

Health care providers should be alert to illness patterns that could indicate an unusual infectious disease outbreak. Indicators of a biological agent release include increased disease incidence among people in the same geographic area (e.g., people who attended the same event); the disease pattern is inconsistent with client age, such as chickenpox among adults; and a client presents with symptoms of a rare disease (Centers for Disease Control and Prevention [CDC], 2001). Presence of one or more of these indicators should be reported to public health authorities to determine the infectious disease source and to prevent further exposure.

## Infectious Process in Older Adults

Older adults, particularly those over the age of 75 years, are at greater risk of acquiring an infection. Although the incidence of septicemia in the United States is increasing in all age groups, the greatest increase is among people over the age of 65 years (Schlossberg, 2001). Physiologic changes of aging that put the elderly at an increased risk for infection include the following:

- Cardiovascular changes: decreased cardiac output, loss of capillaries, and decreased tissue perfusion delaying inflammatory response and healing
- Respiratory system changes: decreased mucociliary escalator, decreased elastic recoil, and a diminished cough reflex leading to decreased clearance of respiratory secretions
- Genitourinary changes: loss of muscle tone, reduced bladder contractility, altered bladder reflexes, and prostatic hypertrophy in men leading to reduced bladder capacity and incomplete emptying
- Gastrointestinal system changes: impaired swallow reflex, decreased gastric acidity, and delayed gastric emptying thus increasing the risk of aspiration
- Skin and subcutaneous tissue changes: thinning of skin, decreased cushioning, and decreased sensation leading to increased risk of injury and ulceration
- Immune changes: decreased phagocytosis, reduced inflammatory response, slowed or impaired healing processes leading to reduced immunity

In addition to the previous physiologic changes, other factors that may contribute to the older adult's increased risk for infectious disease are as follows:

- Decreased activity level related to musculoskeletal, neurologic, or balance problems
- Poor nutrition and an increased risk of dehydration (see the Nursing Research box on page 220)
- Chronic diseases, such as diabetes mellitus, cardiac disease, and renal disease
- Chronic medication use
- Lack of recent immunizations against preventable infectious diseases
- Altered mentation and dementias
- Hospitalization or residence in a long-term care facility
- Presence of invasive devices, such as indwelling urinary catheters and gastric tubes

## Nursing Research

### Evidence-Based Practice for Meeting Nutritional Needs in Older Adults

Inadequate nutrition decreases normal functioning of the immune system. Older adults with declining immunity and often poor dietary habits have an increased risk for developing infections. Family members who provide nutritional assistance to older clients are challenged to provide an adequate nutritional intake.

A pilot project conducted to determine what family caregivers know about older adults' nutritional needs, the judgments and decisions they make regarding the nutritional needs of their elderly family members, and their actions in providing appropriate food intake (Biggs & Freed, 2000). Family caregivers assume a key role in promoting the nutritional status of their elderly family members; yet they often provide such assistance with minimal knowledge of sound nutritional principles. For instance, they may supply smaller, low-calorie meals mistakenly believing that the elderly need less food regardless of their medical condition. However, when provided with appropriate nutrition information, family caregivers can make correct nutritional decisions and meet the dependent older person's needs.

#### IMPLICATIONS FOR NURSING

Nurses in community health settings assume an important role in assessing the nutritional status and potential risk factors of dependent elderly persons. Equally important is determining the nutritional knowledge base of both the elderly client and the family caregiver. Because caregiver assistance may range from buying groceries to feeding the older adult, the nurse must identify the caregiver's level of involvement.

Therefore, the nurse needs to include the family caregiver in all nutritional teaching sessions and evaluate the caregiver's level of understanding and adherence to the guidelines provided. If older clients are malnourished and have an infection, their risk for prolonged recovery increases. An increased balanced nutritional intake should improve immune system function, shorten recovery time, and reduce the risk of future infections.

#### Critical Thinking in Client Care

1. Develop strategies that a family caregiver can use to improve the nutritional intake of an elderly family member who has no interest in eating.
2. An 86-year-old woman is being discharged to her home following repair of a broken hip. Identify the nutritional factors you would assess before she is discharged.
3. Discuss how prescription and over-the-counter medications affect the nutritional needs of the older adult.
4. Discuss the interrelationship between malnutrition and immune system function.

In addition, the thymus gland atrophies and by age 50 to 60 years thymic hormone levels are undetectable. Although the exact relationship of these events to T-cell function is unclear, some T-cell populations decrease or decline in function as the person ages. The ability of T cells to proliferate following activation also declines with advancing age; in addition, a portion of T cells cannot be activated in the elderly (Hazzard, Bierman, Blass, Ettinger, & Halter, 1994). With these changes, cell-mediated immune function declines. The client has reduced resistance to antigens such as *Mycobacterium tuberculosis*, influenza and varicella-zoster viruses, malignant cells, and tissue grafts.

Immunoglobulin levels remain relatively stable, but primary and secondary antibody responses decline with aging. This diminished antibody production has clinical implications in that immunizations (single-dose and booster) may not produce the expected protective immune response.

The older adult is not only at increased risk for infection, but also may not exhibit the classic manifestations of inflammation and infection. Older adults are more likely to take nonsteroidal anti-inflammatory agents and corticosteroids that interfere with inflammation and healing. The cardinal signs of inflammation—redness, heat, and swelling—tend to be diminished or absent in older adults. The classic signs of infection—fever and chills—may be absent altogether because of age-related changes in the immune system, loss of central temperature control mechanisms, decreased muscle mass, and loss of shivering ability. The older adult may have only subtle signs of sepsis, including changes in mental status, disorientation, and tachypnea (Hazzard et al., 1994). Infectious diseases commonly seen in the elderly client are outlined on page 221.

## COLLABORATIVE CARE

The goals of care for the client with an infection are to identify the organ system affected by the infection, to identify the causative agent, and to achieve a cure by the least toxic, least expensive, and most effective means. Fortunately, most infectious diseases are self-limiting and will resolve with little or no medical care. However, medical treatment can be lifesaving in an overwhelming infection or immunocompromised host.

The body part or organ system affected by the infection is often obvious from the client's history and presenting signs and symptoms. Identifying the system allows the range of possible infecting organisms to be narrowed to those known to affect that system. The manner of presentation provides further cues as to the diagnosis. For example, pneumococcal pneumonia typically presents with an acute onset of chills, fever, and cough in a previously healthy adult, whereas the client with viral pneumonia relates a gradual onset of symptoms, with systemic manifestations such as muscle aches and headache often predominant. A history of recent activities also provides clues. Family members who all vomit and have diarrhea within 12 hours after a picnic probably do not have the flu.

Once the infecting agent has been identified, either positively or by probability, therapy can be specifically tailored to the client's needs. Viral infections often resolve without treatment other than supportive care, such as providing rest and fluids. Skin infections may respond to a topical agent, avoiding the potential adverse effects of one administered systemically.

## Nursing Care of the Older Adult

### INFECTION

Because immune function declines with aging, older adults are more susceptible to infections. In fact, infections are among the top 10 causes for hospitalization and 1 of the 5 leading causes of death among people over 65 years of age.

Age-related changes may obscure the presentation of infection in older adults. Rather than an elevated temperature to signal an infection, confusion and subtle changes in behavior such as restlessness may be observed. The white blood cell count may be slightly elevated.

In addition to monitoring for changes in the client's mental status or behavior, the nurse should collect data on the amount of fluids consumed, urinary output, activity levels, complaints of fatigue, and respiratory status. A thorough assessment is necessary to facilitate an early diagnosis and prompt treatment that will improve outcomes for the older adult. Delay in treating infection may prolong the client's immobility and reduce the ability to perform activities of daily living.

### URINARY TRACT INFECTIONS

Urinary tract infection (UTI) is not only the most common infection but also the leading cause of bacteremia and sepsis in older adults. Factors that contribute to UTI include poor hygiene, incomplete bladder emptying, inadequate fluid intake, and long-term indwelling catheters. In addition, chronic conditions and medications may contribute to retention, which can result in urinary tract infection.

### RESPIRATORY TRACT INFECTIONS

The leading causes of pneumonia in older adults include *Streptococcus pneumoniae, Hemophilus influenzae, Klebsiella pneumoniae, Staphylococcus aureus,* and pneumococci. As a result of physiological changes, the older adult with pneumonia may not present with cough or sputum production. Influenza A and B are prevalent in the aged; however, strain A accounts for greater illness severity and death (Eliopoulus, 2000). Both pneumonia and influenza cause high mortality rates in the older person.

Frail older adults, especially those with chronic respiratory conditions such as emphysema, are at risk for developing pneumonia as a complication of influenza. To prevent this complication, all persons over 65 should receive an annual immunization for influenza. In addition, pneumonia caused by pneumococcus bacteria can be deadly for older adults. Therefore, it is recommended that individuals over 65 also receive the pneumococcal immunization.

Tuberculosis has a relatively high incidence in older adults, especially those living in long-term care facilities. It often occurs as reactivation or secondary tuberculosis when the immune system can no longer contain the bacteria.

### OTHER INFECTIONS

Older adults have the highest incidence of gangrene of the appendix and gallbladder. Diverticulitis increases due to chronic constipation and changes in the intestinal wall. Postoperative wound infections and decubitus ulcers are also most prevalent in older adults.

### NOSOCOMIAL INFECTIONS

Nosocomial infections are more common in older adults. Nursing interventions should focus on prevention strategies such as (1) avoiding prolonged bed rest unless the medical condition contraindicates mobilization, (2) encouraging clients to take deep breaths, (3) providing adequate fluids, and (4) providing regular toileting schedules with good hygiene. The nurse must steadfastly adhere to principles of infection control.

### HOME CARE

To prevent infection, the older adult should be taught to:

- Eat a well-balanced diet.
- Drink adequate fluids.
- Get adequate rest.
- Obtain an annual influenza immunization.
- Use good handwashing techniques.

Older adults and families should be taught to seek medical attention if they:

- Develop a fever or other signs and symptoms of infection.
- Exhibit changes in mental status and/or behavior.
- Experience fatigue or changes in activity levels.

## Diagnostic Tests

To assess the client's response to infection, identify the infecting organism, and monitor the progress of therapy, the following diagnostic tests may be ordered.

- *WBC count* provides clues about the infecting organism and the body's immune response to it (see Table 8–6).
- *WBC differential* is also ordered (see Table 8–6). Neutrophilia, increased numbers of circulating neutrophils (or PMNs), is a common response with infection as the bone marrow responds to an increased need for phagocytes. Along with neutrophilia, a shift to the left is common in acute infection. This means that there are more immature neutrophils in circulation than normal (Figure 8–13 ■), indicating an appropriate bone marrow response.
- *Cultures of the wound, blood, or other infected body fluids* are used to identify probable microorganisms by their characteristics, such as shape, growth patterns, and Gram-staining qualities. After the organism is cultured, it is subjected to various antibiotics known to be effective against its particular strain to determine which antibiotic is likely to be most effective. This is known as sensitivity testing. Generally 24 to 48 hours are required to grow the organism, potentially delaying the institution of therapy. Because antibiotics (and possibly oxygen therapy) can alter the ability to culture an organism, specimens should be obtained before instituting therapy.
- *Serologic testing* provides an indirect means of identifying infecting agents by detecting antibodies to the suspected organism. When the antibody titer against a specific organism rises during the acute phase of an infectious disease and begins to fall during convalescence, the diagnosis is supported. Although it is not as accurate as culture, serology is particularly useful for organisms that cannot easily be cultured, such as hepatitis B or HIV (Porth, 2002).

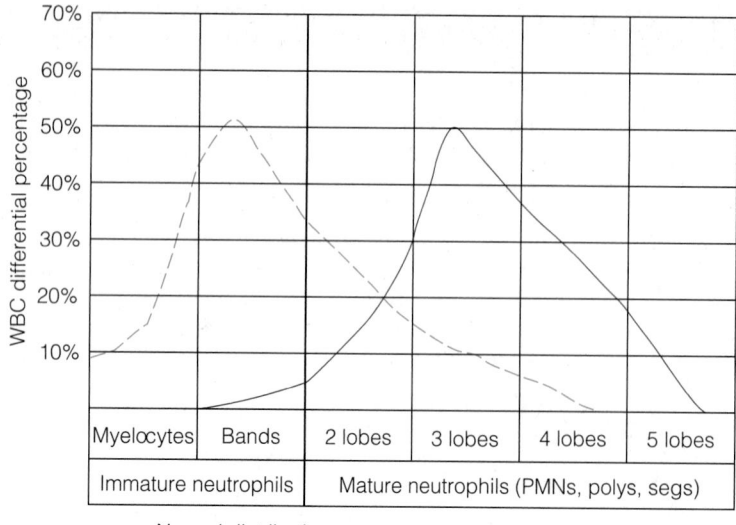

| Type of WBC | Normal differential | Shift to left |
|---|---|---|
| Myelocytes | 0% | Present |
| Band neutrophils (bands) | 3% to 5% | Increased |
| Segmented neutrophils (segs, polys, PMNs) | 50% to 65% | May be stable, increased, or decreased |

Figure 8–13 ■ Neutrophils by stage of maturity and normal distribution in the blood.

- *Direct antigen detection methods* are in the process of being developed. These tests use monoclonal antibodies, which are purified antibody forms, to detect antigens in specimens from the diseased host (Porth, 2002). See Box 8–6. These tests offer rapid and accurate identification of the offending microorganism.
- *Antibiotic peak and trough levels* monitor therapeutic blood levels of the prescribed medication(s). The therapeutic range, that is, the minimum and maximum blood levels at which the drug is effective, is known for a given drug. By measuring blood levels at the predicted peak (1 to 2 hours after oral administration, 1 hour after intramuscular administration, and 30 minutes after intravenous administration) and trough (lowest level, usually a few minutes before the next scheduled dose), health care personnel can determine that the client is maintaining a level within the therapeutic range at all times, ensuring maximal effect from the drug. It is also possible to determine whether the drug is reaching a toxic or harmful level during therapy, increasing the likelihood of adverse effects.
- *Radiologic examination of the chest, abdomen, or urinary system* may be ordered to detect organ abnormalities indicating an inflammatory response or tissue damage.
- *Lumbar puncture* is performed to obtain cerebrospinal fluid (CSF) for examination and culture if a central nervous system (CNS) infection, such as meningitis or encephalitis, is suspected.
- *Ultrasonic examination* is a noninvasive diagnostic test to evaluate organ function such as an echocardiogram or renal ultrasonography.

## Medications

Once the infecting organism and affected body system have been identified, specific therapy to cure the infectious disease can be instituted. The number of antimicrobial agents available makes choosing the appropriate one seem overwhelming. The

perfect anti-infective agent would destroy pathogens while preserving host cells, would be effective against many different organisms while not promoting the development of resistance, would distribute to necessary tissues, and would remain in the body for relatively long periods.

Because no currently available antimicrobial meets all the above criteria, physicians look for the agent that will be effective, has little toxicity, can be administered with relative convenience, and is cost-effective. Characteristics of both the host and the infecting organism are considered in making the selection. The following host factors are considered in choosing an antimicrobial agent.

- *History of hypersensitivity.* Previous hypersensitivity responses to an antimicrobial contraindicate the use of that agent or one of its class.
- *Age and childbearing status of the client.* Sulfonamides and tetracyclines as well as some less common agents are contraindicated for pregnant women due to their possible effects on the fetus.
- *Renal function.* Because most antimicrobials are excreted through the kidneys, renal function is important. Impaired renal function may contraindicate a specific drug, such as an aminoglycoside, because of its nephrotoxicity, or it may call for a reduced dosage.
- *Hepatic function.* Because hepatic function may alter the metabolism of a particular antimicrobial, the risk of toxicity increases. Again, certain drugs are avoided with impaired hepatic function; others may dictate a reduced dosage.
- *Site of the infection.* The infection site is critical in choosing both the antimicrobial to be used and the route by which it is administered. Antimicrobials can be applied topically or administered by oral, intramuscular, intravenous, interperitoneal, intrathecal, or intramedullary routes. Oral and intravenous routes are most commonly used.
- *Other host factors.* Chronic diseases or other medications in the treatment regimen are also considered.

## BOX 8-6 ■ Monoclonal Antibodies

Antigens typically have numerous antigenic determinant sites, each capable of stimulating a different subset of B cells. Each clone secretes a slightly different antibody from the others. The immunoglobulin produced as a result is therefore *polyclonal*, with multiple different antibodies. In 1975, researchers devised a technique for making a single clone of "immortal" B cells that could be maintained indefinitely in a laboratory and would produce a single antibody to a specific antigen (see figure below). This pure antibody, known as a *monoclonal* antibody, offers the following advantages:

- It can target specific antigens.
- It has a single, constant binding affinity for the antigen.
- It can be diluted to a specific titer or concentration, because it is not mixed with other antibodies.
- It can be purified to avoid adverse responses (McCance & Huether, 1998).

In addition to their use in providing passive protection from disease, multiple other uses are being identified for monoclonal antibodies, including the diagnosis and treatment of cancer, immunosuppression to prevent rejection of transplanted tissue or organs, immune response analysis, imaging techniques for diagnostic uses, and the early detection of viral infections (McCance & Huether, 1998, Roitt, 1994).

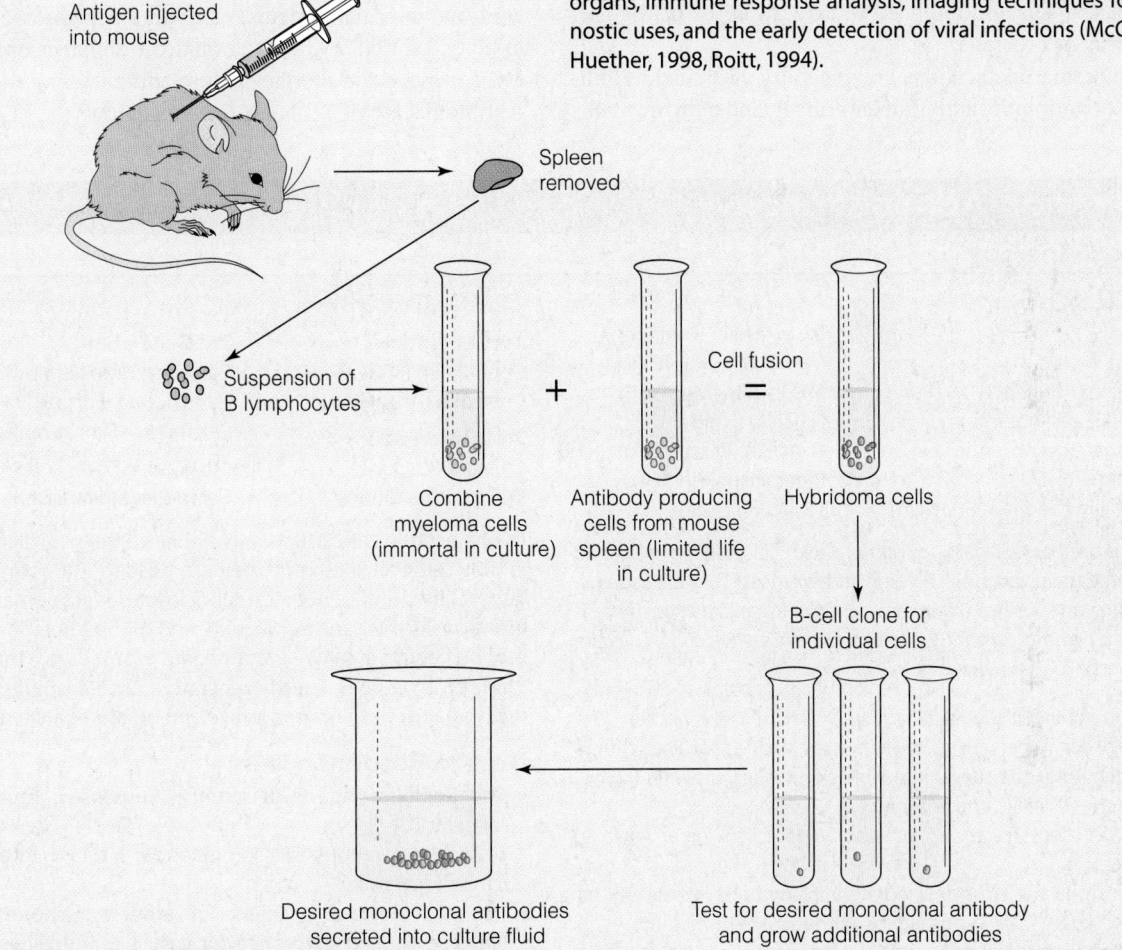

Antigen injected into mouse

Spleen removed

Suspension of B lymphocytes

Combine myeloma cells (immortal in culture)

+

Antibody producing cells from mouse spleen (limited life in culture)

Cell fusion

=

Hybridoma cells

B-cell clone for individual cells

Desired monoclonal antibodies secreted into culture fluid

Test for desired monoclonal antibody and grow additional antibodies

*Note. Figure adapted from* The World of the Cell *by W. Becker & D. Deane, 1986, Redwood City, CA: Benjamin Cummings;* Textbook of Diagnostic Microbiology *by C. R. Mahon & G. Manuselis Jr., 1995, Philadelphia: W.B. Saunders. Reprinted by permission.*

Antimicrobial preparations are broadly classified as bacteriostatic or bactericidal. **Bacteriostatic** agents inhibit the growth of the microorganism, leaving its destruction to the host's immune system. These agents are generally not indicated for the immunocompromised host. Tetracyclines, erythromycin, and chloramphenicol are bacteriostatic preparations. **Bactericidal** agents are capable of killing the organism without immune system intervention. These include the penicillins, cephalosporins, and aminoglycoside antibiotics.

The activity of antimicrobial agents on bacteria, fungi, and viruses falls under five basic mechanisms:

- Impairing cell wall synthesis, leading to lysis and cell destruction
- Inhibiting protein synthesis, causing impaired microbial function
- Altering cell membrane permeability, causing intracellular contents to leak
- Inhibiting the synthesis of nucleic acids
- Inhibiting cell metabolism and growth

Obviously, agents that work on the cell wall will not be effective against organisms that have no cell wall, such as mycoplasma and viruses. The antimicrobial's spectrum of activity is also considered in making a selection. Therapy is often initiated with a broad-spectrum antimicrobial until the specific organism is identified.

Finally, many microorganisms have the ability to develop resistance to an anti-infective agent; that is, the pathogen continues to live and grow in the presence of the anti-infective. Resistance develops as a result of a chance mutation by the pathogen, allowing a subpopulation of cells to survive. The chance of an organism's becoming resistant to an agent is partially related to the dose delivered. Resistance is less likely to occur when a lethal dose is administered; therefore, it is vital that clients understand the need to take all doses of the prescribed drug as ordered.

Antimicrobial medications are generally classified as antibacterial or antibiotic, antiviral, antifungal, and antiparasitic.

## Antibiotics

Medications used to treat bacterial infections are generally known as antibiotics. Their development and use began before World War II and has proliferated rapidly since. Most antibiotics are biologic substances, that is, substances produced by other microorganisms. Antibiotics fall into classes of drugs with related chemical structure and activity. Some are effective against only gram-positive bacteria, and others are effective against only gram-negative organisms. Newer broad-spectrum antibiotics have activity against a wide variety of bacteria, including both gram-positive and gram-negative forms. No antibiotic is totally safe. Hypersensitivity responses occur, and some drugs are toxic to organ systems, exhibiting hepatotoxicity, nephrotoxicity, ototoxicity, or bone marrow suppression. Therefore, always check for allergies before administering the first dose. Antibiotics are presented in the box below.

# Medication Administration

## Antibiotic Therapy

### PENICILLINS

| | |
|---|---|
| Penicillin G | Dicloxacillin (Dynapen) |
| Penicillin V | Methicillin (Staphcillin) |
| Amoxicillin (Amoxil) | Mezlocillin (Mezlin) |
| Amoxicillin and potassium clavulanate (Augmentin) | Nafcillin (Unipen) |
| | Oxacillin (Prostaphlin) |
| Ampicillin (Polycillin) | Piperacillin (Pipracil) |
| Carbenicillin (Geopen, Geocillin) | Ticarcillin (Ticar) |

Penicillins are bactericidal and interfere with cell wall synthesis and the enzymes involved in cell division and synthesis. They are more effective on gram-positive than gram-negative organisms. Resistance is now more common among *Streptococci* and *Staphylococci*. They are considered to be safe, effective, and of low toxicity.

### Nursing Responsibilities

- Monitor for hypersensitivity responses such as local erythema and itching at the site of injection, skin rashes, urticaria (hives), itching, fever, chills, and anaphylaxis.
- Observe clients receiving parenteral penicillin for at least 30 minutes.
- Discontinue the drug immediately if any hypersensitivity response occurs. Be prepared to administer antihistamines or corticosteroids for a mild reaction. Anaphylaxis is treated with epinephrine subcutaneously or intravenously and airway support.
- Do not administer penicillin to anyone with a history of a severe allergic reaction to any form of the drug; a cross-reactivity may occur in clients allergic to cephalosporin antibiotics.
- Assess for superinfection (vaginitis, stomatitis, or diarrhea) due to elimination of resident bacteria.
- Monitor for therapeutic response.

### Client and Family Teaching

- Notify the physician if you see white patches are noted on the oral mucosa or if vaginitis develops. An antifungal drug may be prescribed and the antibiotic continued.
- Consuming yogurt or buttermilk may prevent superinfection. Do not take these products within 1 hour of taking the drug.

### CEPHALOSPORINS

| **1st Generation** | **3rd Generation** |
|---|---|
| Cephalexin (Keflex) | Cefoperazone (Cefobid) |
| Cefazolin (Ancef) | Ceftazidime (Fortaz) |
| **2nd Generation** | Ceftriaxone (Rocephin) |
| Cefaclor (Ceclor) | **4th Generation** |
| Cefuroxime (Zinacef) | Cefepime (Moxapime) |

Cephalosporins are structurally similar to the penicillins and also inhibit cell wall synthesis. They are divided into four groups, or generations. First-generation cephalosporins act primarily against gram-positive organisms. Second- and third-generation drugs are more effective against gram-negative organisms than against gram-positive ones. Fourth-generation cephalosporins act effectively against both gram-positive and gram-negative organisms.

### Nursing Responsibilities

- Monitor for previous hypersensitivity response to cephalosporins or penicillins.
- Assess intravenous site for phlebitis; intramuscular site may cause local pain.
- Monitor laboratory results for adverse response, such as leukopenia and thrombocytopenia, nephrotoxicity (elevated BUN and serum creatinine), or hepatotoxicity (elevated bilirubin, LDH, ALT, AST, and alkaline phosphatase).
- Assess for signs of superinfections.

### Client and Family Teaching

- Take the medication on an empty stomach, 1 hour before or 2 hours after meals.
- Space doses of the medication relatively evenly throughout the day and evening hours.
- Increase consumption of buttermilk or yogurt to prevent intestinal superinfection.

### AMINOGLYCOSIDES

| | |
|---|---|
| Amikacin (Amikin) | Netilmicin (Netromycin) |
| Gentamicin (Garamycin) | Streptomycin (Stepolin) |
| Kanamycin (Kantrex) | Tobramycin (Nebcin) |

# Medication Administration

## Antibiotic Therapy (continued)

Aminoglycosides are bactericidal, interfering with protein synthesis in the pathogen. They are especially effective against gram-negative organisms. To provide a broader spectrum of activity, they are often combined with other antibiotics, especially penicillins. Aminoglycosides can be administered in multiple or single daily doses. They are ototoxic and nephrotoxic; the risk is highest for older adults, clients with preexisting renal disease, and persons receiving other ototoxic or nephrotoxic drugs.

### Nursing Responsibilities

- Assess renal function before and during aminoglycoside therapy. Monitor intake and output, daily weight, BUN, and serum creatinine.
- Assess for adverse effects on hearing such as loss of perception of high tones, tinnitus, and vertigo.
- Notify the physician if the client is receiving other nephrotoxic or ototoxic drugs such as furosemide (Lasix) and ethacrynic acid (Edecrin).
- Administer intravenous preparations separately from other drugs; flush tubing before and after administration.

### Client and Family Teaching

- Monitor for a sudden weight gain that may indicate adverse effects on the kidney and report it to the physician.

### FLUOROQUINOLONES

Ciprofloxacin (Cipro)                    Levofloxacin (Levaquin)
Gatifloxacin (Tequin)

Fluoroquinolones are bactericidal and especially active against gram-negative and some gram-positive organisms. They are used to manage infections of the respiratory, gastrointestinal, and genitourinary tracts.

### Nursing Responsibilities

- Increase fluid intake to 2000 to 3000 mL per day unless contraindicated to prevent crystalluria.
- Monitor laboratory results for hepatotoxicity (elevated ALT, AST).

### Client and Family Teaching

- Drink six to eight glasses of water per day.
- Avoid exposure to sunlight while taking these drugs.

### TETRACYCLINES

Tetracycline HCl                         Minocycline HCl (Minocin)
Doxycycline (Vibramycin)                 Oxytetracycline (Terramycin)

Tetracyclines are active against many gram-positive and gram-negative bacteria, such as Mycoplasma, Rickettsia, and Chlamydia. They are bacteriostatic, interfering with microbial protein synthesis. Tetracycline binds readily with metal and solid elements in the bowel, limiting its absorption when administered with food; the other preparations are highly soluble in lipids and can be administered with food.

### Nursing Responsibilities

- Schedule doses 1 hour before or 2 hours after meals. Do not give with milk or milk products or antacids.
- Monitor for signs of superinfection.
- If the client is taking an anticoagulant, monitor prothrombin time, and for signs of bleeding.

### Client and Family Teaching

Avoid excessive sun exposure to reduce the risk of photosensitivity reactions.

### MACROLIDES

Erythromycin (E-Mycin)                   Erythromycin salts (Ilosone,
Azithromycin (Zithromax)                 E.E.S., Erythrocin)

Macrolides are bacteriostatic and act effectively against gram-positive and gram-negative organisms. Erythromycin is used to treat streptococcal pharyngitis in clients who are allergic to penicillin. Azithromycin is ordered more frequently because the client takes the drug for 5 days, increasing client adherence.

### Nursing Responsibilities

- Administer erythromycin on an empty stomach or immediately before meals.
- Give the drug with a full glass of water. Do not administer with acidic fruit juice.

### Client and Family Teaching

- Gastric distress is a common side effect with erythromycin.

### SULFONAMIDES AND TRIMETHOPRIM

Sulfamethizole (Thiosulfil Forte)
Sulfamethoxazole (Gantanol; in combination with Trimethoprim, TMP-SMZ, Bactrim, Septra)
Sulfisoxazole (Gantrisin)

Sulfonamides are bacteriostatic. Trimethoprim is an antibiotic effective against most gram-positive and many gram-negative organisms. It is often combined with sulfamethoxazole to manage urinary tract infections, *Pneumocystis carinii* pneumonia (PCP), and otitis media. Skin rashes and pruritus are the most common hypersensitivity reactions. Severe reactions include exfoliative dermatitis and Stevens-Johnson syndrome. *(continued)*

### Nursing Responsibilities

- Assess for history of hypersensitivity to sulfonamides and related medications, such as thiazide diuretics and hypoglycemic preparations.
- Monitor intake and output. Maintain a fluid intake of at least 1500 mL per day.
- Assess for evidence of bleeding, easy bruising, or systemic infection, and monitor blood count for possible bone marrow depression.

### Client and Family Teaching

- Take medication on an empty stomach with a full glass of water. Maintain a fluid intake of at least 2 quarts per day.
- Protect the skin from excessive sun exposure with clothing and sunscreens to reduce the risk of photosensitivity.

### METRONIDAZOLE (FLAGYL)

Metronidazole is effective against anaerobic gram-negative bacteria and protozoan infections caused by amebiasis, giardiasis, and trichomoniasis. It is commonly used to prevent and treat infections following intestinal surgery.

(continued on page 226)

## Medication Administration

### Antibiotic Therapy (continued)

#### Nursing Responsibilities

- Monitor for central nervous system effects of dizziness, headache, ataxia, confusion, depression, and peripheral neuropathy.
- Administer with food to minimize gastric distress and metallic taste. Infuse intravenous metronidazole over 60 minutes.
- Discontinue the medication and notify the physician if neurologic reactions occur.
- Increase fluid intake to 2500 mL per day to minimize the risk of nephrotoxicity.

#### Client and Family Teaching

- This medication may turn urine reddish brown; caution client that this is expected and not harmful.
- Discontinue the drug and notify the physician if hypersensitivity reaction or adverse effects occur, such as changes in mentation or coordination, painful or frequent urination, painful or difficult intercourse, impotence.
- Do not drink alcohol while taking this medication; an Antabuse-type reaction (flushing, sweating, headache, vomiting, and abdominal cramps) may occur.
- Maintain a fluid intake of 2.5 to 3 quarts per day.
- When the drug is prescribed for Trichomonas infections, treatment of both partners is necessary.
- While taking metronidazole, use condoms to prevent cross-contamination during intercourse.

### Antivirals

Antiviral therapy is a relatively new phenomenon. Most antibiotics have little effect on viruses, because the virus has no cell wall and no cytoplasm, produces no enzymes, and sequesters itself in a host cell to reproduce. Antiviral agents must be very selective in differentiating normal cellular activity from viral activity. In addition, the immune function of the host is a vital component in fighting viral infections; antiviral therapy may be relatively ineffective in the severely immunocompromised host. Making a timely diagnosis to allow institution of antiviral therapy can be an additional problem, because viruses are less easily identified using laboratory techniques. Antiviral agents in common use are summarized in the box to the right. Antiretroviral agents used in the management of HIV and AIDS are presented in Chapter 9. ᴄᴐ

### Antifungals

Antifungal agents are available in both topical and systemic forms. They act by interfering with the cytoplasmic membrane of the fungus. Topical agents include preparations for cutaneous use to treat candidiasis, tineas, and ringworm. Vaginal preparations to treat vulvovaginal candidiasis are also available, as are several nonprescription topical and vaginal antifungal agents.

Amphotericin B (Fungizone) is a systemic antifungal agent for parenteral administration. It is used to treat severe, life-threatening fungal infections including histoplasmosis, blastomycosis, and candidiasis. Another systemic antifungal in current use is flucytosine (Ancobon). Unlike amphotericin B, flucytosine

can be administered orally. It is used to treat severe candidiasis infections such as candidae septicemia, endocarditis, pulmonary or urinary tract infections, and *Cryptococcus* meningitis.

Fluconazole (Diflucan) has the broadest use as an antifungal agent. It can be administered either orally or parenterally and is used to treat candidiasis infections as well as *Cryptococcus* meningitis. It is generally better tolerated than other systemic antifungal medications.

### Antiparasitics

Drugs used to treat parasitic infections are as varied as the organisms that cause them. Generally, agents classified as antiparasitic are both expensive and likely to be toxic. Quinine was one

## Medication Administration

### Antiviral Agents

#### AMANTADINE (SYMMETREL)

Amantadine is used to prevent and treat influenza A. It has been shown to be 55% to 80% or more effective in preventing the disease. When administered within 24 to 72 hours after the onset of symptoms, it reduces common manifestations of influenza. It is generally well tolerated; minimal central nervous system side effects, such as dizziness, anxiety, insomnia, and difficulty concentrating, may occur.

#### ACYCLOVIR (ZOVIRAX) AND GANCICLOVIR (CYTOVENE)

Acyclovir and ganciclovir are related compounds used primarily in the treatment of herpesviruses. Acyclovir is prescribed mainly in the treatment of genital herpes simplex infections. Although it does not kill the virus, acyclovir is effective in reducing the severity, duration, and frequency of recurrence of symptoms. Ganciclovir is indicated primarily in the treatment of cytomegalovirus infection. Although acyclovir is generally well tolerated with little toxicity, ganciclovir may profoundly suppress bone marrow function, and its use is therefore limited.

#### ZIDOVUDINE (AZT, RETROVIR)

Zidovudine inhibits replication of HIV, although it does not kill it. Zidovudine's use is limited to clients with symptomatic HIV infection or CD4 cell counts of less than 200/mm³. Zidovudine may be administered either orally or parenterally. Many clients are unable to tolerate recommended doses because of the drug's adverse effects, including nausea, anorexia, malaise, severe anemia, and granulocytopenia. Zidovudine is usually administered in combination with other antiretroviral medications.

#### VIDARABINE (VIRA-A)

Vidarabine inhibits viral DNA synthesis and is effective against many herpesvirus infections. Its primary use is in treatment of herpes simplex encephalitis.

#### INTERFERONS

Interferons are naturally produced cytokines whose use as antiviral agents is being explored. When administered intranasally, interferons have been shown to be effective in preventing rhinovirus upper respiratory infections. Other uses being explored include treatment of human papillomavirus (genital warts) and preventing or reducing Kaposi's sarcoma in clients with AIDS.

of the first antiparasitic drugs developed in the treatment of malaria. Quinine is highly toxic, but newer forms such as chloroquine (Aralen, Chlorocon) and hydroxychloroquine (Plaquenil) are widely used as antimalarial drugs. Metronidazole (e.g., Flagyl) is used to treat infections of protozoan parasites (see the Medication Administration box on pages 225–226).

## Isolation Techniques

Controlling the spread of infectious diseases in the hospital or long-term care setting is particularly important to preventing nosocomial infection. Handwashing remains the single most important factor in preventing the transmission of infections. Not all infectious diseases spread readily, necessitating special techniques or procedures. However, diseases such as chickenpox (varicella) and pulmonary tuberculosis are highly contagious and are spread by the airborne route, requiring special precautions to protect other hospitalized clients.

In determining the need for isolation precautions, health care personnel consider the usual reservoir or source of the microorganism, the mode of transmission, and susceptibility of hospital staff and other clients. For example, clients with *Pneumocystis carinii* pneumonia do not require isolation, because immunocompetent persons are not susceptible to this infection.

The Centers for Disease Control and Prevention (CDC) has published guidelines for isolation precautions to be used in health care facilities. These guidelines include both *standard precautions* and *category-specific isolation precautions*.

### Standard Precautions

*Standard Precautions*, published by the Hospital Infection Control Practices Advisory Committee of the Centers for Disease Control in 1996, provides guidelines for the handling of blood and other body fluids. These guidelines are used with all clients, regardless if they have a known infectious disease. The guidelines were developed in light of the realization that many clients with an infectious disease such as HIV or hepatitis B have no apparent symptoms, but can transmit the disease to others. Standard precautions are used by all health care workers who have direct contact with clients or with their body fluids or have indirect contact, such as by emptying trash, changing linens, or cleaning the room.

Standard precautions apply to the following:

- Blood
- All body fluids, secretions, and excretions, regardless if they contain visible blood
- Nonintact skin
- Mucous membranes

Barrier protection is used to prevent exposing skin and mucous membrane surfaces to blood and body fluids. Barrier protection involves using gloves for touching or handling body fluids, and adding other protection such as gowns, masks, and goggles if splashing or spraying is likely. Needles and other sharp objects are not recapped or bent, but disposed of in puncture-proof containers to prevent inadvertent percutaneous (needle-stick) exposure. Standard precautions are presented in Appendix A. 🔗

### Transmission-Based Precautions

In addition to handwashing and standard precautions, the nature and spread of some infectious diseases require that special techniques be used to protect uninfected clients and workers. The CDC identifies three types of transmission-based precautions: airborne, droplet, and contact precautions. Transmission-based precautions may be combined for diseases that have multiple routes of transmission. Indications for the use of transmission-based isolation precautions and the specific measures to be taken are outlined in Table 8–10.

## NURSING CARE

Nursing management related to infectious disease has two foci: (1) *prevention* and (2) *health promotion and maintenance*. Prevention focuses on assessing the client's risk for infection based on underlying conditions, immune response, and prophylactic measures such as immunizations.

### Health Promotion

Preventing infection requires education of not only health care personnel but also the general public. Part of an education program includes understanding the importance of immunizations, the guidelines for using antibiotics to prevent drug-resistant microorganisms, and the ways to prevent the spread of infection. Check immunization records for all family members and encourage them to keep immunizations up to date. Increase public awareness regarding appropriate antibiotic use. Guidelines for preventing the spread of infection to others include the following:

- Avoid crowds and contact with susceptible persons, especially those who are immunosuppressed (e.g., persons who have HIV infection, who are undergoing therapy for cancer, or who have had an organ transplant).
- Use disposable tissues to contain respiratory secretions when coughing or sneezing.
- Use appropriate food-handling precautions for diseases spread via the fecal-oral route, such as hepatitis A.
- Avoid contact with or sharing of body fluids. For example, do not share needles or razors; use a condom during sexual activity, or abstain; have each person clean their own blood spills or wounds if possible.

### Assessment

The following data are collected through the health history and physical examination. Further focused assessments are described with nursing interventions in the next section.

- Health history: age, medication use (antipyretics and anti-infectives), nutrition, exposure to infectious persons, immunizations, invasive procedures and therapies, chronic diseases such as diabetes mellitus, cancer
- Physical assessment: vital signs, body system(s) where infection is suspected, lymph node enlargement, and tenderness

### TABLE 8–10  Transmission-Based Precautions

| Category | Infectious Diseases | Purpose | Precautions |
|---|---|---|---|
| Airborne precautions | Pulmonary tuberculosis, chicken-pox (with contact precautions), measles, respiratory infections (pneumonia) | Reduce risk of airborne transmission of infectious agents. Airborne transmission occurs by dissemination of either airborne droplet nuclei or dust particles containing the infectious agent. | Private room with handwashing, toilet facilities, and special ventilation that does not allow air to circulate to general hospital ventilation; mask or special filter respirator for everyone entering room. |
| Droplet precautions | Meningitis, pertussis | Reduce risk of droplet transmission of infectious agents. Droplet transmission involves contact of conjunctivae of the eyes or mucous membranes of the nose or mouth with large-particle droplets generated during coughing, sneezing, talking, or procedures such as suctioning. | Private room with handwashing and toilet facilities; mask, eye protection, and/or face shields worn by everyone entering room. |
| Contact precautions | Acute diarrhea, chickenpox, (with airborne precautions), respiratory syncytial virus (RSV); skin, wound, or urinary tract infection with multidrug-resistant organisms; *Staphylococcus aureus* infections | Reduce risk of transmission by direct or indirect contact. Direct contact transmission involves skin-to-skin contact and physical transfer of organisms. It may occur between clients or during direct care activities such as bathing or turning clients. Indirect contact involves contact with a contaminated object. | Private room with handwashing and toilet facilities; gowns and protective apparel to provide barrier protection; disposable supplies or decontamination of all articles leaving room. |

## Nursing Diagnoses and Interventions

Clients with an infection may be managed in the hospital or at home. During the acute phase, nursing care includes administering prescribed antibiotics, implementing and maintaining aseptic technique and infection control measures, and encouraging a balance of rest and activity, good nutritional intake, and other general health measures to support immunologic function and healing. The key nursing diagnoses are *risk for infection, anxiety,* and *hyperthermia.*

### Risk for Infection

The spread of infection is a risk in any facility that houses many people. It is a particular risk in hospitals, where many clients have at least some degree of immunosuppression and many drug-resistant strains of pathogens are prevalent. It is vital that nurses use good handwashing techniques at all times, employ standard precautions with all clients, and use category-specific isolation techniques as indicated to prevent infectious spread to other clients, themselves, and their families.

- Admit clients with known or suspected infections to a private room. *This is important to minimize the risk to other clients.*
- Wash hands on entering and leaving the client's room, using a 10- to 15-second vigorous scrub with soap or antibacterial scrub solution. *A 10- to 15-second scrub removes transient microorganisms from the skin and helps prevent transmission of infection to or from the client.*
- Use standard precautions and personal protective devices to reduce the risk of transmission. *Gloves, gowns, and masks are to be worn whenever there is a risk of skin or mucous*

*membrane contamination by direct contact with infectious material, airborne spread of organisms, or droplet nuclei.*

- Explain the reasons for and importance of isolation procedures during hospitalization. *Clients with isolation precautions may feel neglected, dirty, or shunned. Explanation of reasons and procedures can enhance the client's and family's understanding and acceptance.*
- Place a mask on the client and/or cover all infectious lesions or wounds completely when transporting the client to other parts of the facility for diagnostic or treatment procedures. *These measures help minimize air contamination and the risk to visitors and personnel.*
- Collect a culture and sensitivity (C&S) specimen as ordered or indicated by purulent drainage, pyuria, or other manifestations of infection. *C&S is performed to determine the presence and type of infectious organisms as well as antibiotics most likely to be effective in eradicating it.*

**PRACTICE ALERT** *Collect the specimen before the first dose of antibiotics is administered to ensure adequate organisms for culture.* ■

- Administer prescribed anti-infective agents. *Anti-infectives are used to destroy the invading microorganism.*
- Inform all personnel having contact with the client of the diagnosis. *This is particularly important for a client with a disease requiring category-specific isolation so that personnel can take appropriate precautions.*

- Ensure that visitors don appropriate protective wear before they enter the client's room. *Protective wear reduces their risk of infection.*
- Use appropriate measures for disposing of contaminated tissues, dressings, or other material and for removing soiled linens and equipment from the client's room. *Check hospital policy or published guidelines for category-specific isolation.*
- Teach the importance of complying with prescribed treatment for the entire course of the regimen. *Because anti-infective agents kill only a portion of the pathogen population with each dose, completion of the entire course of therapy is necessary to reduce the risk of relapse and of creating drug-resistant organisms.*

### Anxiety

The client with an infectious disease may experience anxiety related to his or her manifestations, treatment measures, the prognosis, and expected outcome of the disease. The diagnosis of an infection can be traumatic, causing feelings of uneasiness, isolation, guilt (e.g., in regard to sexually transmitted diseases), apprehension, or depression.

- Assess level of anxiety. *The level of anxiety influences the client's response to and interpretation of the situation and degree of threat it poses.*
- Discuss the infection, treatments, prognosis, and outcomes. *Discussions help to allay fears and misconceptions.*
- Support and enhance the client's coping strategies. *A person uses intrapersonal and interpersonal mechanisms to reduce or relieve anxiety.*
- Include significant others in the plan of care. *Inclusion of the client and family members provides assurance and confidence, and promotes understanding of the unknown.*
- Explain isolation procedures, and answer any concerns. *Isolation may be necessary to prevent the spread of infection but can cause great anxiety for the client and family members.*
- Provide referrals as needed for continuing care, for example, to home health agencies, for dressing changes or periodic assessment. *Referrals are often necessary to provide ongoing interventions and maintain continuity of care.*

### Hyperthermia

Hyperthermia is an expected consequence of the infectious disease process. Fever may produce mild, short-term effects or, when prolonged, may cause serious life-threatening effects.

- *Monitor temperature especially during episodes of chills; note heart rate and rhythm. Chills indicate a rising temperature. Hyperthermia can cause dysrhythmias.*

**PRACTICE ALERT**   *Monitor temperature between 5 P.M. and 7 P.M. as the body's daily temperature cycle peaks at this point.* ■

- Administer prescribed antipyretic as indicated for elevated temperature. *Although antipyretics lower the temperature and enhance comfort for the client, this benefit must be weighed against the possible beneficial effect of an elevated temperature in the immune response. Fever increases the motility and activity of WBCs, stimulates the production of interferon, and activates T cells. In addition, temperatures above the normal range inhibit the growth of many microorganisms* (Porth, 2002).
- Promote body cooling through lowering room temperature. *Rapid cooling stimulates the hypothalamus to increase the body's temperature; this increases both shivering and metabolic rate.*

**PRACTICE ALERT**   *Use ice packs, cool/tepid baths, or hypothermia blanket with caution to prevent unnecessary shivering.* ■

- Monitor fluid loss; encourage increased fluid and electrolyte intake either orally or intravenously. *Hyperthermia causes fluid loss from evaporation and may result in dehydration and electrolyte imbalance.*
- If diaphoretic, bathe and provide dry clothing and bedding. *These measures increase client comfort and decrease further water evaporation.*
- Promote rest periods. *Rest increases energy reserve that is depleted by an increased metabolic, heart, and respiratory rate.*

### Using NANDA, NIC, and NOC

Chart 8–3 shows links between NANDA, NIC, and NOC when caring for the client with an infection.

---

## CHART 8–3  NANDA, NIC, AND NOC LINKAGES

### The Client with an Infection

| NURSING DIAGNOSES | NURSING INTERVENTIONS | NURSING OUTCOMES |
|---|---|---|
| • Risk for Deficient Fluid Volume<br>• Risk for Activity Intolerance<br>• Ineffective Health Maintenance | • Fluid Management<br>• Fluid Monitoring<br>• Energy Management<br>• Health Education<br>• Teaching Individual | • Fluid Balance<br>• Hydration<br>• Endurance<br>• Health-Promoting Behavior<br>• Health-Seeking Behavior |

*Note. Data from Nursing Outcomes Classification (NOC) by M. Johnson & M. Maas (Eds.), 1997, St. Louis: Mosby; Nursing Diagnoses: Definitions & Classification 2001–2002 by North American Nursing Diagnosis Association, 2001, Philadelphia: NANDA; Nursing Interventions Classification (NIC) by J.C. McCloskey & G. M. Bulechek (Eds.), 2000, St. Louis: Mosby. Reprinted by permission.*

## Home Care

Client and family teaching is directed toward helping the client recover from the infection or disease, preventing its spread to others, and preventing life-threatening complications. Instructions should include the following points.

- Use good handwashing techniques, particularly after touching infected wounds or lesions, coughing, sneezing, blowing the nose, or using the bathroom. Wash hands thoroughly before eating or performing any procedures such as dressing changes.
- Take all prescribed antibiotics as ordered even after symptoms have subsided. Notify your health care provider if:
  - Symptoms do not improve within 24 to 48 hours after antibiotic therapy is instituted.
  - Signs of antibiotic allergy (itching, rash, difficulty breathing) occur.
  - Adverse responses, such as gastrointestinal distress, interfere with completion of the prescription.
  - Signs of superinfection (vaginitis, oral candidiasis, or diarrhea) occur.
  - Manifestations of infection recur after completing prescribed antibiotic.
- Report redness, swelling, or drainage around wounds or persistent high fever.
- Increase fluid intake to at least 2500 mL (2.5 quarts) per day.
- In addition, suggest the following resources:
  - County or public health department
  - Centers for Disease Prevention and Control

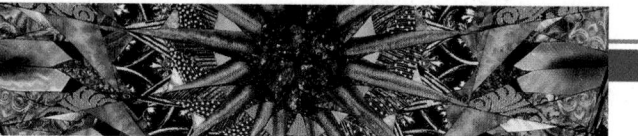

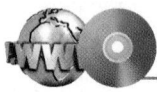 **EXPLORE MediaLink**

NCLEX review questions, case studies, care plan activities, MediaLink applications, and other interactive resources for this chapter can be found on the Companion Website at www.prenhall.com/lemone.

Click on Chapter 8 to select the activities for this chapter. For animations, video clips, more NCLEX review questions, and an audio glossary, access the Student CD-ROM accompanying this textbook.

## TEST YOURSELF

1. When a client receives gamma globulin following exposure to hepatitis A, the nurse expects the client to develop:
   a. Natural passive immunity
   b. Natural active immunity
   c. Acquired passive immunity
   d. Acquired active immunity

2. When performing a physical assessment of a client, the nurse should expect which of these findings related to a systemic infection?
   a. Erythema
   b. Enlarged lymph nodes
   c. Pain
   d. Decreased heart rate

3. Which one of the following medications is known to inhibit prostaglandin synthesis?
   a. Acetaminophen (Tylenol)
   b. Prednisone
   c. Penicillin
   d. Aspirin

4. The client with an acute infection shows a shift to the left on the WBC differential count. The nurse recognizes a shift to the left because of which laboratory finding?
   a. Increased band neutrophils
   b. Increased eosinophils
   c. Decreased leukocytes
   d. Decreased monocytes

5. A client is admitted with methicillin-resistant *Staphylococcus aureus* in a draining sacral wound. The client should be placed in which type of isolation precautions?
   a. Droplet precautions
   b. Contact precautions
   c. Airborne precautions
   d. Protective precautions

See Test Yourself answers in Appendix C.

# BIBLIOGRAPHY

Ackley, B. J., & Ladwig, G. B. (2002). *Nursing diagnosis handbook* (5th ed.). St. Louis: Mosby.

American Hospital Association. (2001). ATS: Hospital-acquired pneumonia remains a serious problem. Available http://www.ahanews.com

Andreoli, T., Bennett, J., Carpenter, C., & Plum, F. (Eds.). (1997). *Cecil essentials of medicine* (4th ed.). Philadelphia: Saunders.

Biggs, A. J., & Freed, P. E. (2000). Nutrition and older adults What do family caregivers know and do? *Journal of Gerontological Nursing, 26*(8), 6–14.

Bullock, B. L., & Henze, R. L. (2000). *Focus on pathophysiology*. Philadelphia: Lippincott.

Burggraf, V., & Weinstein, B. F. (2000). Don't miss this opportunity: Promote adult immunizations. *MEDSURG Nursing, 9*(6), 198–200.

Centers for Disease Control. (1996). Guidelines for isolation precautions in hospitals. *American Journal of Infection Control, 24* (1), 32–52.

_____ . (2000a). *Preventing emerging infectious diseases. A strategy for the 21st century.* Atlanta: CDC.

_____ . (2002). *Recommended adult immunization schedule, United States, 2002–2003.* Atlanta: CDC.

_____ . (2000b). *Vaccine-preventable adult diseases.* Atlanta: CDC.

_____ . (2001, October). Update: Investigation of anthrax associated with intentional exposure and interim public health guidelines. *MMWR, 50*(41), 889–897.

Coleman, E. A. (2001). Anthrax. *American Journal of Nursing, 101*(12), 48–52.

Copstead, L. C., & Banasik, J. L. (2000). *Pathophysiology, biological, and behavioral responses* (2nd ed.). Philadelphia: W.B. Saunders.

Eliopoulous, C. (2000). *Gerontological nursing* (5th ed.). Philadelphia: Lippincott.

Fauci, A., et al. (1998). *Harrison's principles of internal medicine* (14th ed.). New York: McGraw-Hill.

Fraser, D. (1997). Assessing the elderly for infections. *Journal of Gerontological Nursing, 23*(11), 5–10, 52–58.

Glover, T. L. (2000). How drug-resistant microorganisms affect nursing. *Orthopaedic Nursing, 19*(2), 19–27.

Gylys, K. H. (1999). Antimicrobial resistance. *Journal of Cardiovascular Nursing, 13*(2), 66–69.

Hazzard, W., Bierman, E., Blass, J., Ettinger, W., & Halter, J. (Eds.). (1994). *Principles of geriatric medicine and gerontology* (3rd ed.). New York: McGraw-Hill.

Inman, W. B. (2000). Pathogens invade 21st century. *Nursing 2000, 30*(8), 22–23.

Jackson, M. M., Rickman, L. S., & Pugliese, G. (1999). Pathogens, old and new: An update for cardiovascular nurses. *Journal of Cardiovascular Nursing, 13*(2), 1–22.

Johnson, M., Maas, M., & Moorhead, S. (2000). *Iowa outcomes project: Nursing outcomes classification (NOC)* (2nd ed.). St. Louis: Mosby.

Kee, J. (2001). *Handbook of laboratory & diagnostic tests with nursing implications* (4th ed.). Upper Saddle River, NJ: Prentice Hall.

Lueckenotte, A. G. (2000). *Gerontologic nursing* (2nd ed.). St. Louis: Mosby.

Lutz, C., & Przytulski, K. (2001). *Nutrition and diet therapy* (3rd ed.) Philadelphia: F.A. Davis.

Markis, A. T., Morgan, L., Gaber, D. J., Richter, A., & Rubino, J. R. (2000). Effect of comprehensive infection control program on the incidence of infections in long-term care facilities. *American Journal of Infection Control, 28*(1), 3–7.

McCance, K., & Huether, S. (1998). *Pathophysiology: The biologic basis for disease in adults and children.* St. Louis: Mosby.

McCloskey, J., & Bulechek, G. (2000). *Iowa intervention project: Nursing interventions classification (NIC)* (3rd ed.). St. Louis: Mosby.

Miller, J. M., Walton, J. C., & Tordicella, L. L. (1998). Recognizing and managing *Clostridium difficile*–associated diarrhea. *MEDSURG Nursing, 7*(6), 348–356.

Miller, N. C., & Rudoy, R. C. (2000). Vancomycin intermediate-resistant *Staphylococcus aureus* (VISA). *Orthopaedic Nursing, 19*(6), 45–50.

National Institute of Allergy and Infectious Diseases. (2000). *Antimicrobial resistance.* Bethesda: National Institutes of Health.

Porth, C. (2002). *Pathophysiology: Concepts of altered health states* (6th ed.). Philadelphia: Lippincott.

Price, S., & Wilson, L. (2003). *Pathophysiology: Clinical concepts of disease processes* (6th ed.). St. Louis: Mosby.

Reece, S. M. (1999). The emerging threat of antimicrobial resistance: Strategies for change. *The Nurse Practitioner, 24*(11), 70, 73, 77–80, 85–86.

Roitt, I. (1994). *Essential immunology* (8th ed.). London: Blackwell.

Rowsey, P. J. (1997a). Pathophysiology of fever. Part 1: The role of cytokines. *Dimensions of Critical Care Nursing, 16*(4), 202–207.

_____ . (1997b). Pathophysiology of fever. Part 2: Relooking at cooling interventions. *Dimensions of Critical Care Nursing, 16*(5), 251–256.

Sandhu, S. K., & Mossad, S. B. (2001). Influenza in the older adult. *Geriatrics, 56*(1), 43–44, 47–48, 51.

Schlossberg, D. (2001). *Current therapy of infectious disease* (2nd ed.). St. Louis: Mosby.

Shannon, M., Wilson, B., & Stang, C. (2001). *Nursing drug guide 2001.* Upper Saddle River, NJ: Prentice Hall.

Sheff, B. (1998). VRE & MRSA: Putting bad bugs out of business. *Nursing 98, 28*(3), 40–45.

_____ . (1999). Minimizing the threat of *C. difficile. Nursing 99, 29*(2), 33–39.

Silverblatt, F. J., Tibert, C., Mikolich, D., Blazek-D'Arezzo, J., Alves, J., Tack, M., & Agatiello, P. (2000). Preventing the spread of vancomycin-resistant enterococci in a long-term care facility. *Journal of the American Geriatrics Society, 48*(10), 1211–1214.

Smith, S. F., Duell, D. J., & Martin, B. C. (2000). *Clinical nursing skills* (5th ed.). Upper Saddle River: Prentice Hall.

Tenover, F. C., & McGownan, J. E. (1997). Antimicrobial resistance. *Infectious Disease Clinics of North America, 11*(4), 813–928.

Tierney, L., McPhee, S., & Papadakis, M. (Eds). (2001). *Current medical diagnosis & treatment* (40th ed.). Stamford, CT: Appleton & Lange.

Wenzel, R. P., & Edmond, M. B. (2001). The impact of hospital-acquired bloodstream infections. *Emerging Infectious Diseases, 7*(2), 174–177.

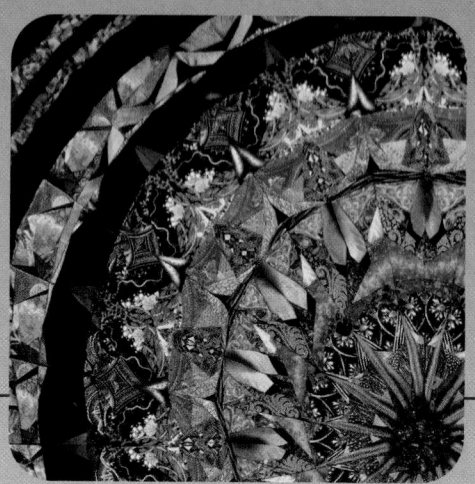

# CHAPTER 9

# Nursing Care of Clients with Altered Immunity

## MediaLink

**www.prenhall.com/lemone**

Additional resources for this chapter can be found on the Student CD-ROM accompanying this textbook, and on the Companion Website at www. prenhall.com/lemone. Click on Chapter 9 to select the activities for this chapter.

**CD-ROM**
- Audio Glossary
- NCLEX Review

*Animations*
- Histamine
- T-Cell Destruction of HIV

**Companion Website**
- More NCLEX Review
- Case Study
  HIV Prevention
- Care Plan Activity
  A Clients with AIDS
- MediaLink Application
  At Risk for HIV/AIDS

## LEARNING OUTCOMES

After completing this chapter, you will be able to:

- Review normal anatomy and physiology of the immune system and the immune response (see Chapter 8).
- Describe the four types of hypersensitivity reactions.
- Discuss the pathophysiology of autoimmune disorders and tissue transplant rejection.
- Discuss the characteristics of immunodeficiencies.
- Identify laboratory and diagnostic tests used to diagnose and monitor immune response.
- Describe pharmacologic and other collaborative therapies used in treating clients with altered immunity.
- Provide teaching for clients with altered immune responses and their families.
- Correlate the pathophysiological alterations with the manifestations of HIV/AIDS infection.
- Use the nursing process as a framework to provide individualized care to clients with altered immune responses.

Recent years have seen the emergence of new diseases affecting the immune system. These diseases include human immunodeficiency virus (HIV) infection and altered strains of familiar diseases such as multidrug-resistant tuberculosis. At the same time, understanding of the components of the immune system and specific immune responses is increasing. It is therefore vital that today's nurses understand the foundations of the immune system and the immune response.

## OVERVIEW OF THE IMMUNE SYSTEM

The immune system functions to protect the body from invasion by foreign antigens, to identify and destroy potentially harmful cells, and to remove cellular debris. This realm is accomplished by the lymphoid organs and specifically designed lymphocytes through the processes of antibody-mediated immune response and cell-mediated immune response.

The effectiveness of the immune system depends on its ability to differentiate normal host tissue from abnormal or foreign tissue. Body cells, tissues, and fluids have unique antigenic properties recognized by the immune system as "self." External agents, such as microorganisms, cells and tissues from other humans or animals, and some inorganic substances, have antigenic properties recognized by the immune system as "nonself."

Each body cell displays specific cell surface characteristics, or markers, that are unique to each person. These are known as human leukocyte antigens (HLA). A person's HLA characteristics are coded within a large cluster of genes known as the major histocompatibility complex (MHC) located on chromosome 6. Recall that chromosomes are paired; each person inherits one member of the pair from each parent. A chromosome pair contains multiple genes, each carrying instructions for production of one polypeptide chain. The number of genes in the MHC results in a multitude of HLA combinations. As a result, the possibility of two people having the same HLA type is extremely remote. Identical twins may be the exception, and some siblings have very similar HLA patterns. In tissue grafting and organ transplants, matching the HLA type as closely as possible tends to decrease rejection.

Immunocompetent clients have an immune system that identifies antigens and effectively destroys or removes them. When the immune system functions improperly, the result may be an overreaction or deficiency resulting in health problems. Overreaction of the immune system leads to hypersensitivity disorders, such as allergies. When the immune system loses the ability to recognize self, autoimmune disorders may ensue (see Table 9–1). Immunodeficiency diseases or malignancies can develop when the immune system is incompetent or unable to respond effectively, as is the case with acquired immunodeficiency disorder. These alterations in immunity are discussed later in this chapter.

As discussed previously in Chapter 8, the *antibody-mediated immune response* is accomplished by B lymphocytes (B cells) that are further divided into memory cells and plasma cells. They are activated by contact with an antigen and by T cells. B cells produce antibodies, also known as immunoglobulins

(see Table 8–2), and serve to inactivate an invading antigen. One immunoglobulin in particular, IgM, forms natural antibodies, such as those for ABO blood group antigens, and is an important component of the immune system complexes seen in autoimmune disorders. Memory cells "remember" an antigen and when exposed to it a second time, immediately initiate the immune response. This action provides the foundation of acquired immunity.

In contrast, *cell-mediated immunity* acts at the cellular level by attacking antigens directly and by activating B cells. T lymphocytes comprise the cell-mediated immune response and are subdivided into effector cells and regulator cells. The cytotoxic cell or killer T cell is the primary effector cell. Regulator T cells are divided into two subsets known as helper T cells and suppressor T cells.

Proteins on the surface of the T cell help define its function and also provide a marker that can be used to identify the cell class. These proteins are known as the cluster of differentiation antigen or *CD antigen*. The two primary CD proteins are CD4 and CD8. Both cytotoxic and suppressor T cells carry the CD8 antigen. Helper T cells have the CD4 antigen and are often called CD4 cells. CD4 cells are the most numerous of the T lymphocytes, making up 70% of the circulating population.

Helper T cells initiate the immune response, whereas suppressor T cells limit it. Helper T cells accomplish their role by promoting growth of additional T cells, by stimulating proliferation of B cells, and by activating killer T cells. It is believed that suppressor T cells are important in preventing autoimmune disorders. Proper immune system function depends on the correct balance between helper and suppressor T cells.

In addition to destroying viruses and bacteria, cytotoxic T lymphocytes also attack malignant cells. They also are responsible for the rejection of transplanted organs and grafted tissues.

## CHANGES IN IMMUNE FUNCTION IN THE OLDER ADULT

Immune function declines with aging, although many of the mechanisms leading to this decline are not clear. External factors, such as nutritional status and the effects of chemical exposure, ultraviolet radiation, and environmental pollution, affect the older adult's immune status. Internal factors affect it as well, including genetics, the function of the neurologic and endocrine systems, chronic and prior illnesses, and individual anatomic and physiologic variations. These myriad influences make it difficult to determine the effect of aging on the immune system. In some older individuals, the immune system is as effective as that of younger persons.

Whereas the antibody response to foreign antigens is diminished, autoantibodies (antibodies that react to the client's own tissues) are more common in older persons. The presence of autoantibodies suggests impaired regulation of the immune system, but it is not associated with an increased incidence of autoimmune disorders (discussed later in this chapter). There is also reduced or delayed hypersensitivity response.

## ASSESSMENT OF ALTERED IMMUNE SYSTEM FUNCTION

Unlike body systems that are composed of a few closely related organs, the immune system is diverse and scattered. Optimal immune function depends on intact skin and mucous membrane barriers, adequate blood cell production and differentiation, a functional system of lymphatics and the spleen, and the ability to differentiate foreign tissue and pathogens from normal body tissue and flora. Because of this diversity of organs and function, assessment of the immune system is often integrated throughout the history and physical examination.

### Health History

Prior to interviewing the client, review the biographic data, including age, sex, race, and ethnic background. This information can provide valuable clues about possible immunologic disorders. For example, many autoimmune disorders are more prevalent in women than in men. Family history is also important, because there is a genetic component in the etiology of many disorders affecting the immune system.

Many interview questions related to the immune system and disorders that affect it are of a sensitive nature. Be sure to provide for privacy prior to the interview. If family members are present, request that they leave as well. Establish a trusting relationship with the client prior to asking the most sensitive questions (e.g., those related to the use of illicit drugs or sexual activity).

### Physical Assessment

The techniques of inspection and palpation are especially important in assessing a client's immune system.

- *Assess the general appearance.* Note whether the client's stated and apparent age coincide. Evident fatigue or weakness may indicate acute or chronic illness or immunodeficiency. Assess height, weight, and body type for apparent weight loss or wasting. Observe ease of movement and note any evident stiffness or difficulty moving. Check vital signs. An elevated temperature may indicate an infection or inflammatory response.
- *Assess skin color, temperature, and moisture.* Pale or jaundiced skin may indicate a hemolytic reaction. Pallor may also indicate bone marrow suppression with accompanying immunodeficiency. Inspect the skin for evidence of rashes or lesions, such as petechiae, numerous bruises, purple or blue patches or lesions indicative of Kaposi's sarcoma, and wounds that are infected, inflamed, or unhealed. Note the location and distribution of any rashes or lesions.
- *Inspect the mucous membranes of the nose and mouth for color and condition.* Pale, boggy (edematous) nasal mucosa is often associated with chronic allergies. Note petechiae, white patches, or lacy white plaques in the oral mucosa; they may indicate hemolysis or immunodeficiency.
- *Inspect and palpate the cervical lymph nodes for evidence of lymphadenopathy (swelling) or tenderness.* Palpate the nodes of the axillae and groin as well (see Figure 8–11).
- *Assess the musculoskeletal system by inspecting and palpating the joints for redness, swelling, tenderness, or deformity.* Such changes may indicate an autoimmune disorder such as rheumatoid arthritis or systemic lupus erythematosus (SLE). Check joint range of motion as well, including that of the spine.

## ALTERED IMMUNE RESPONSES

Considering the complexity of the immune system, it is not surprising that abnormal or harmful responses occur. Altered immune system responses include those characterized by hyperresponsiveness of the immune system and those characterized by an impaired immune response. Allergies, autoimmune disorders, and reactions to organ or tissue transplants are all examples of hyperresponsive immune function. AIDS and other immunodeficiency disorders result from impairment of the immune system.

### THE CLIENT WITH A HYPERSENSITIVITY REACTION

**Hypersensitivity** is an altered immune response to an antigen that results in harm to the client. When the antigen is environmental or exogenous, it is called an **allergy,** and the antigen is referred to as an *allergen.* The tissue response to a hypersensitivity reaction may be simply irritating or bothersome, causing a runny nose or itchy eyes, or it may be life threatening, leading to blood cell hemolysis or laryngospasm.

Hypersensitivity reactions are primarily classified by the type of immune response that occurs on contact with the allergen. They may also be classified as immediate or delayed hypersensitivity responses. Anaphylaxis and transfusion reactions are examples of immediate hypersensitivity reactions; contact dermatitis is a typical delayed response. Allergies are sometimes referred to by the affected organ system (e.g., allergic rhinitis) or the allergen involved, as in hay fever. Classification by immunologic response is the most accurate and preferred means of studying allergies (Tierney, McPhee, & Papadakis, 2001).

### PATHOPHYSIOLOGY

In a hypersensitivity reaction, an antigen-antibody or antigen-lymphocyte interaction causes a response that is damaging to body tissues. Antigen-antibody responses characterize types I, II, and III, also known as immediate hypersensitivity responses. Type IV hypersensitivity is an antigen-lymphocyte reaction, resulting in a delayed hypersensitivity response.

## Type I IgE-Mediated Hypersensitivity

Common hypersensitivity reactions, such as allergic asthma, allergic rhinitis (hay fever), allergic conjunctivitis, hives, and anaphylactic shock, are typical of type I or IgE-mediated hypersensitivity. This type of hypersensitivity response is triggered when an allergen interacts with IgE bound to mast cells and basophils. The antigen-antibody complex prompts release of histamine and other chemical mediators, complement, acetylcholine, kinins, and chemotactic factors (Figure 9–1 ■).

When a potent allergen such as bee or wasp venom or a drug is injected, resulting in widespread antibody-antigen reaction and response to these chemical mediators, a systemic response such as anaphylaxis, urticaria, or angioedema results.

Anaphylaxis is an acute systemic type I response that occurs in highly sensitive persons following injection of a specific antigen. Substances known to trigger anaphylaxis are summarized in Box 9–1. Anaphylaxis rarely follows oral ingestion, although this is possible. The reaction begins within minutes of exposure to the allergen and may be almost instantaneous. The release of histamine and other mediators causes vasodilation and increased capillary permeability, smooth muscle contraction, and bronchial constriction. These chemical mediators

MediaLink | HISTAMINE ANIMATION

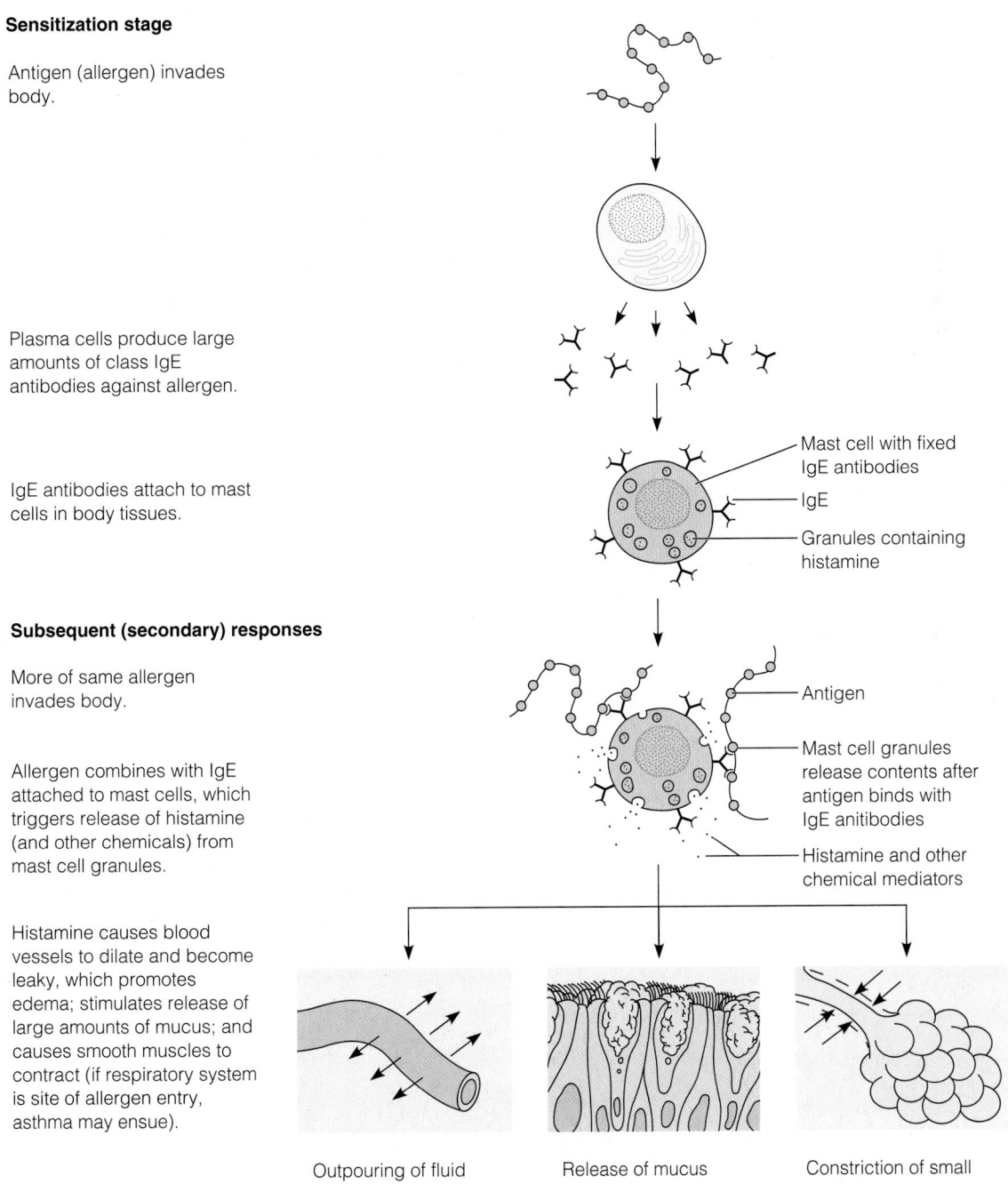

**Sensitization stage**

Antigen (allergen) invades body.

Plasma cells produce large amounts of class IgE antibodies against allergen.

IgE antibodies attach to mast cells in body tissues.

**Subsequent (secondary) responses**

More of same allergen invades body.

Allergen combines with IgE attached to mast cells, which triggers release of histamine (and other chemicals) from mast cell granules.

Histamine causes blood vessels to dilate and become leaky, which promotes edema; stimulates release of large amounts of mucus; and causes smooth muscles to contract (if respiratory system is site of allergen entry, asthma may ensue).

Mast cell with fixed IgE antibodies

IgE

Granules containing histamine

Antigen

Mast cell granules release contents after antigen binds with IgE anitbodies

Histamine and other chemical mediators

Outpouring of fluid from capillaries

Release of mucus

Constriction of small respiratory passages (bronchioles)

**Figure 9–1** ■ Type I IgE-mediated hypersensitivity response.

cause the client to experience the typical manifestations of anaphylaxis. Initially, a sense of foreboding or uneasiness, lightheadedness, and itching palms and scalp may be noted. Hives may develop, along with angioedema (localized tissue swelling) of the eyelids, lips, tongue, hands, feet, and genitals. Swelling can also affect the uvula and larynx, impairing breathing. This is further complicated by the bronchial constriction. The client exhibits air hunger, stridor and wheezing, and a barking cough. These respiratory effects can be lethal if the reaction is severe and intervention is not immediately available. Vasodilation and fluid loss from the vascular system can lead to impaired tissue perfusion and hypotension, a condition known as anaphylactic shock.

Fortunately, localized responses are more common manifestations of type I hypersensitivity. These are typically atopic responses; that is, they have a strong genetic predisposition. Atopic reactions are the result of localized, rather than systemic, IgE-mediated responses to an allergen. They are prompted by contact of the allergen with cell-bound IgE in the bronchial tree, nasal mucosa, and conjunctival tissues. Chemical mediators are released locally, producing symptoms such as asthma, allergic rhinitis (hay fever), conjunctivitis, or atopic dermatitis. Allergens commonly associated with atopic reactions of this type include pollens, fungal spores, house dust mites, animal dander, and feathers (Porth, 2002). Food allergens can also cause localized responses such as diarrhea or vomiting. If the gastrointestinal mucosa is altered by a local

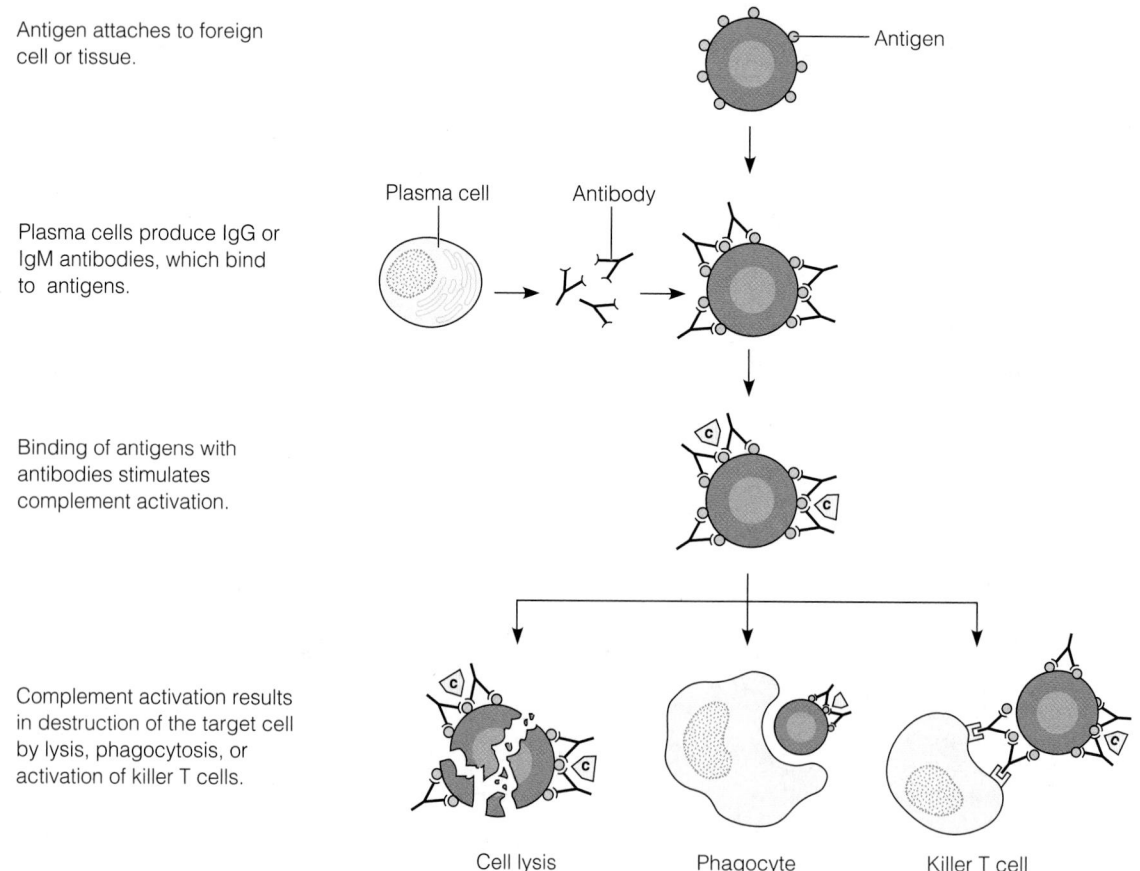

Antigen attaches to foreign cell or tissue.

Antigen

Plasma cells produce IgG or IgM antibodies, which bind to antigens.

Plasma cell

Antibody

Binding of antigens with antibodies stimulates complement activation.

Complement activation results in destruction of the target cell by lysis, phagocytosis, or activation of killer T cells.

Cell lysis

Phagocyte

Killer T cell

**Figure 9–2** ■ Type II cytotoxic hypersensitivity response.

allergic response, then the allergen may be absorbed, leading to a systemic reaction. Urticaria (hives) is the most common systemic response to food allergies.

## Type II Cytotoxic Hypersensitivity

A hemolytic transfusion reaction to blood of an incompatible type is characteristic of a type II or cytotoxic hypersensitivity reaction. IgG or IgM type antibodies are formed to a cell-bound antigen such as the ABO or Rh antigen. When these antibodies bind with the antigen, the complement cascade is activated, resulting in destruction of the target cell (Figure 9–2 ■).

Type II reactions may be stimulated by an exogenous antigen, such as foreign tissue or cells, or a drug reaction, in which the drug forms an antigenic complex on the surface of a blood cell, stimulating the production of antibodies. The affected cell is then destroyed in the resulting antigen-antibody reaction; for example, hemolytic anemia is sometimes associated with the administration of chlorpromazine (Thorazine). Withdrawal of the drug stops the reaction and cell destruction (Roitt, 1994).

Endogenous antigens can also stimulate a type II reaction, resulting in an autoimmune disorder such as Goodpasture's syndrome, in which antigens are formed to specific tissues in the lungs and kidneys. Hashimoto's thyroiditis and autoimmune hemolytic anemia are additional examples of autoimmune type II reactions.

## Type III Immune Complex–Mediated Hypersensitivity

Type III hypersensitivity reactions result from the formation of IgG or IgM antibody-antigen immune complexes in the circulation. When these complexes are deposited in vessel walls and extravascular tissues, complement is activated and chemical mediators of inflammation such as histamine are released. Chemotactic factors attract neutrophils to the site of inflammation. When neutrophils attempt to phagocytize the immune complexes, lysosomal enzymes are released, increasing tissue damage (Figure 9–3 ■).

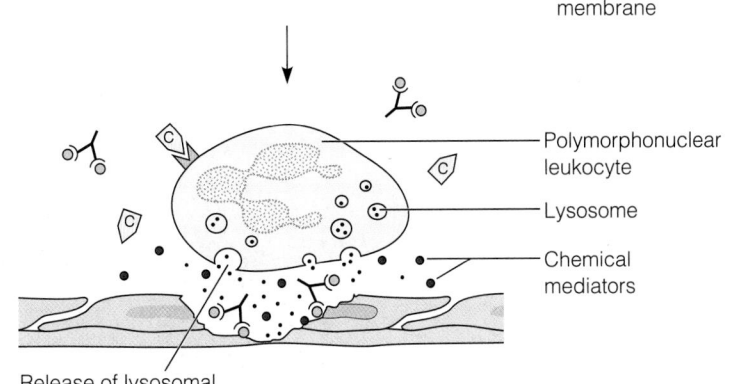

Antigens invade body and bind to antibodies in circulation. Antigen-antibody complexes are formed.

Antigen-antibody complexes are deposited in the basement membrane of vessel walls and other body tissues, activating complement.

Complement activation leads to release of inflammatory chemical mediators. Infiltration of polymorphonuclear leukocytes (PMNs) is followed by release of lysozymes. Tissue damage may be extensive.

Antigen

Antibody

Antigen-antibody complex

Basement membrane

Polymorphonuclear leukocyte

Lysosome

Chemical mediators

Release of lysosomal granules

**Figure 9–3** ■ Type III immune complex–mediated hypersensitivity response.

Either systemic or local responses may be seen with type III reactions. For example, serum sickness is a systemic response, so named because it was first identified after administration of foreign serum (e.g., horse antitetanus toxin). Although foreign serums are no longer administered, serum sickness occurs in response to some drugs, such as penicillin and sulfonamides. Immune complexes are deposited in walls of small blood vessels, the kidneys, and joints. Manifestations of serum sickness include fever, urticaria or rash, arthralgias, myalgias, and lymphadenopathy.

Localized responses may occur at a number of different sites. As immune complexes accumulate in the glomerular basement membrane of the kidneys—for example, following a streptococcal infection or with systemic lupus erythematosus—glomerulonephritis develops. When an antigen such as dust from moldy hay is inhaled, an acute alveolar inflammatory response can occur. This condition can develop in agricultural workers.

## Type IV Delayed Hypersensitivity

Type IV reactions differ from other hypersensitivity responses in two ways. First, these reactions are cell mediated rather than antibody mediated, involving T cells of the immune system. Second, type IV reactions are delayed rather than immediate, developing 24 to 48 hours after exposure to the antigen. Type IV hypersensitivity responses result from an exaggerated interaction between an antigen and normal cell-mediated mechanisms. This exaggerated interaction results in the release of soluble inflammatory and immune mediators (from the lysozymes within the macrophages) and recruitment of killer T cells, causing local tissue destruction (Figure 9–4 ■).

Contact dermatitis is a classic example of a type IV reaction. Intense redness, itching, and thickening affect the skin in the area exposed to the antigen. Fragile vesicles are often present as well. Many antigens can provoke this response; poison ivy is a prime perpetrator. In the health care setting, an allergic response to latex can also produce contact dermatitis. An estimated 8% to 12% of health care workers are allergic to latex (National Institute of Occupational Safety and Health [NIOSH], 1997). Other examples of cell-mediated responses include a positive tuberculin test and graft rejection episodes.

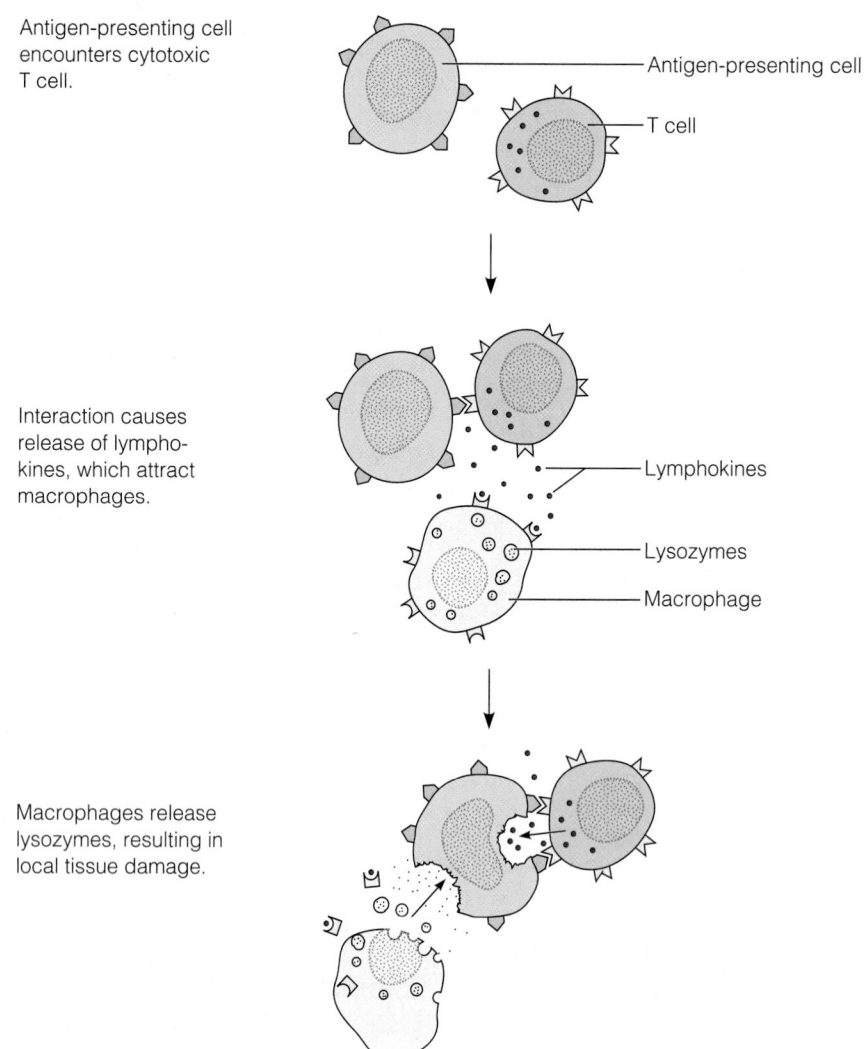

Antigen-presenting cell encounters cytotoxic T cell.

Antigen-presenting cell

T cell

Interaction causes release of lympho-kines, which attract macrophages.

Lymphokines

Lysozymes

Macrophage

Macrophages release lysozymes, resulting in local tissue damage.

**Figure 9–4** ■ Type IV delayed hypersensitivity response.

## COLLABORATIVE CARE

The focus of care for clients with allergic responses is on the following:

- Minimize exposure to the allergen.
- Prevent a hypersensitivity response.
- Provide prompt, effective interventions for allergic responses when they occur.

Identifying allergens for the individual to reduce the likelihood of exposure is a key aspect of management. A complete history of the client's allergies is obtained, including medications, foods, animals, plants, and other materials. The type of hypersensitivity response is documented, as is its onset, manifestations, and usual treatment.

When a documented or suspected hypersensitivity reaction occurs, the allergen (e.g., intravenous medication or transfusion) is withdrawn immediately. With a type I hypersensitivity response, managing the client's airway takes highest priority, followed by maintaining cardiac output. Type II hypersensitivity responses may necessitate aggressive management of bleeding or renal failure. Type III (immune complex) reaction is treated by removing the offending antigen and interrupting the inflammatory response.

With a hypersensitivity response, supportive care is important to relieve discomfort. This often involves the administration of selected antihistamine or anti-inflammatory medications. Other therapies, such as plasmapheresis, may be prescribed in selected instances.

## Diagnostic Tests

To identify possible allergens or hypersensitivity reactions, the following laboratory tests may be ordered.

- *WBC count with differential* can detect high levels of circulating eosinophils. Normally, eosinophils constitute a very small percentage (1% to 4%) of the total WBCs. Eosinophilia, however, is often present in clients with type I hypersensitivities.
- *Radioallergosorbent test (RAST)* measures the amount of IgE directed toward specific allergens. Test results are compared with control values and used to identify hypersensitivities. RAST poses no risk for an anaphylactic reaction. It is particularly useful in detecting allergies to some occupational chemicals and toxic allergens (Tierney et al., 2001).
- *Blood type and crossmatch* are ordered prior to any anticipated transfusions. The client's ABO blood group and Rh status are determined. Two major antigens, designated A and B, may be present on RBCs. Clients with the A antigen are designated as blood type A; those with blood type B have the B antigen. When neither antigen is found on the RBCs, the person is identified as type O. A third major RBC antigen is the Rh antigen. Persons with this antigen are called Rh positive; those without are Rh negative. Because a blood transfusion is actually a transplant of living tissue, antigen matching is vital to prevent significant hypersensitivity reactions. Once blood type is determined, a sample of the client's blood is mixed with a sample of matching donor blood and observed for antigen-antibody reactions in the crossmatch portion of this test. Although this procedure greatly reduces the risk of a hemolytic transfusion reaction (type II hypersensitivity), it does not totally eliminate it.
- *Indirect Coombs' test* detects the presence of circulating antibodies (other than ABO antibodies) against RBCs. The client's serum is mixed with the donor's RBCs. If the client's serum contains antibodies to an RBC antigen, agglutination (clumping together) will occur. This is called a positive response. The normal value is negative, or no agglutination. This test is also part of the crossmatch of a blood type and crossmatch.
- *Direct Coombs' test* detects antibodies on the client's RBCs that damage and destroy the cells. This is used following a suspected transfusion reaction to detect antibodies coating the transfused RBCs. It can also identify hemolytic anemia when the cause is unknown. In the direct Coombs' test, the client's RBCs are mixed with Coombs' serum, which contains antibodies to IgG and several complement components. Agglutination will occur if the client's RBCs are coated with antibodies, resulting in a positive test. As with the indirect Coombs' test, the normal test result is negative.
- *Immune complex assays* may be performed to detect the presence of circulating immune complexes in suspected type III hypersensitivity responses. The assays are particularly useful in diagnosing suspected autoimmune disorders. Nonspecific assays of IgG-, IgM-, and IgA-containing immune complexes, which do not detect specific antibodies, as well as specific antibody assays may be done. The normal result is a test negative for circulating immune complexes. A negative test does not, however, rule out an immune complex hypersensitivity response. In some cases, a negative result may indicate that the disease process has reached a later stage, in which complexes are no longer circulating but have initiated extensive tissue damage, such as glomerulonephritis (Braunwald et al., 2001).
- *Complement assay* is also useful in detecting immune complex disorders. In these disorders, complement is, in effect, used up by the development of antigen-antibody complexes. Decreased levels are seen on examination. Both total complement level and amounts of individual components of the complement cascade can be determined.

Skin tests are also used to determine causes of hypersensitivity reactions. These tests are used to identify specific allergens to which a person may be sensitive. Allergens for testing are selected according to the client's history. Test solutions made from extracts of inhaled, ingested, or injected materials, such as pollens, mites, venoms, or some drugs, are used for the prick test and intradermal testing. Epicutaneous testing (prick testing) is generally done first to avoid a systemic reaction; it is followed by intradermal testing of allergens with a negative response to prick testing (Tierney et al., 2001).

- *Prick (epicutaneous or puncture) test:* A drop of diluted allergenic extract is placed on the skin, and the skin is then pricked or punctured through the drop. With a positive test,

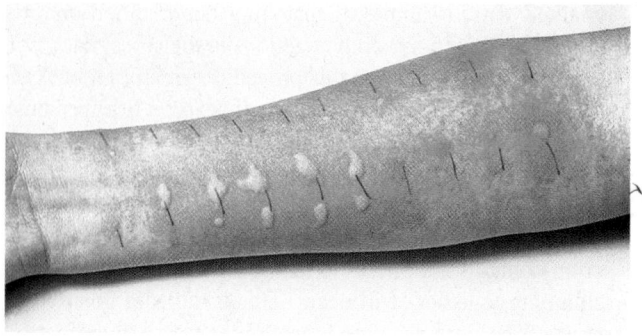

**Figure 9–5** ■ Skin testing on the forearm showing induration and erythema typical of a positive response to an antigen.

*Source: Southern Illinois University/Photo Researchers, Inc.*

a localized pruritic wheal and erythema occurs. The response is maximal at 15 to 20 minutes.

- *Intradermal:* A small amount (just enough to create a wheal) of allergen extract at a 1:500 or 1:1000 dilution is injected on the forearm or intrascapular area. If several allergens are being tested, injections are spaced 0.25 to 0.5 inches apart. As control measures, plain diluent (negative control) and histamine (positive control) are also injected. If there is no response to a particular allergen at 15 to 20 minutes, the test is negative. The appearance of a wheal and erythema, with a wheal diameter at least 5 mm greater than that produced by the control, indicates a positive response (Figure 9–5 ■).
- *Patch:* A 1-inch patch impregnated with the allergen (e.g., perfume, cosmetics, detergents, or clothing fibers) is applied to the skin for 48 hours. Absence of a response indicates a negative test result. Positive responses are graded from mild (erythema in the exposed area) to severe (erythema, papules, vesicles, or ulceration).
- *Food allergy testing* is done when a food allergy is suspected but the source or implicated food item has not been clearly identified. Food allergy symptoms are typically demonstrated within hours of eating. Initially, the client is asked to keep a diary of foods consumed and allergic responses for a week. An elimination diet is then prescribed. The diet excludes most common food allergens and all suspected foods for 1 week. Any foods that may contain allergens in combination, such as breads, are also eliminated. If symptoms do not improve, a different variation of the elimination diet is prescribed. If symptoms are relieved, foods are reintroduced to the diet one at a time until symptoms recur, indicating allergy to that food.

## Medications

When it is impossible to avoid the offending allergen and allergic manifestations are severe or disrupt the client's activities of daily living (ADLs), pharmacologic intervention is prescribed. *Immunotherapy,* also called hyposensitization or desensitization, consists of injecting an extract of the allergen(s) in gradually increasing doses. Immunotherapy is used primarily for allergic rhinitis or asthma related to inhaled allergens. It has also been shown to be effective in preventing anaphylactic responses to insect venom. With weekly or biweekly subcutaneous injections of the allergen, the client develops IgG antibodies to the allergen that appear to block effectively the allergic IgE-mediated response. Once a therapy plateau is reached, injections are continued indefinitely either monthly or bimonthly.

Antihistamines are the major class of drugs used in treating the symptoms of hypersensitivity responses, type I in particular. They are also useful to some extent in relieving manifestations (such as urticaria) of some type II and type III reactions.

Antihistamines block H1-histamine receptors, acting as a competitive antagonist to histamine, but they do not affect the production or release of histamine. The prototype antihistamine is diphenhydramine (Benadryl). It and other antihistamines alleviate the systemic effects of histamine such as urticaria and angioedema. They are also useful in relieving allergic rhinitis, although they are not effective in all clients. Antihistamines are available in both prescription and nonprescription preparations. The preferred route of administration is oral, although diphenhydramine and others can be given parenterally, particularly when immediate action is needed, as in anaphylaxis. They also dry respiratory secretions through an anticholinergic effect. Their use is limited by their side effects, especially drowsiness and dry mouth. Antihistamines are not effective in relieving asthmatic responses to allergens and may actually worsen symptoms by their drying effect on respiratory secretions.

Antihistamines are often combined with a sympathomimetic agent such as pseudoephedrine to improve their decongestant activity and counteract their sedative effect. Antihistamines are discussed further in Chapter 35. ☒

The immediate treatment for anaphylaxis is parenteral epinephrine, an adrenergic agonist (sympathomimetic) drug that has both vasoconstricting and bronchodilating effects. These qualities, combined with its rapid action, make epinephrine ideal for treating an anaphylactic reaction. For mild reactions with wheezing, pruritus, urticaria, and angioedema, a subcutaneous injection of 0.3 to 0.5 mL of 1:1000 epinephrine is generally sufficient. For clients with an injected toxin such as a bee sting, an additional amount equivalent to one-half the above may be injected directly into the site of the sting and a tourniquet applied above it to prevent further systemic absorption. Intravenous epinephrine using a 1:100,000 concentration may be used in the client with a more severe anaphylactic reaction.

Clients who have experienced an anaphylactic reaction to insect venom or other potentially unavoidable allergen should carry a kit (commonly called a bee sting kit) for immediate treatment of future exposures. This kit typically includes a prefilled syringe of epinephrine and an epinephrine nebulizer, allowing prompt self-treatment.

Cromolyn sodium (Intal, Nasalcrom) is a drug used to treat allergic rhinitis and asthma. Cromolyn sodium acts by stabilizing the mast cell membrane, thus preventing chemical mediator release (Shannon, Wilson, & Stang, 2001). Because it is effective only when applied directly to involved tissue, it is delivered by inhaler or nasal spray. It has few side effects and a wide margin of safety, making it a good choice for clients in whom it is effective (Tierney et al., 2001).

Glucocorticoids (corticosteroids) are used in both systemic and topical forms for many types of hypersensitivity responses. Their anti-inflammatory effects, rather than their immunosuppressive effects, are of most benefit. A short course of corticosteroid therapy is often used for severe asthma, allergic contact dermatitis, and some immune-complex disorders (Tierney et al., 2001). Corticosteroids in topical forms or delivered by inhaler may be used for longer periods of time with few side effects; however, systemic absorption can occur.

## Other Therapies

Other treatments used for hypersensitivity responses are generally dictated by the severity of the response and the organ system affected. Airway management takes highest priority for the client with an acute anaphylactic reaction. Insertion of an endotracheal tube or emergency tracheostomy may be required to maintain airway patency with severe laryngospasm. Because anaphylaxis places the person at risk for vasomotor collapse and significant hypotension, it is necessary to insert an intravenous line and initiate fluid resuscitation with an isotonic solution such as Ringer's lactate.

*Plasmapheresis,* removal of harmful components in the plasma, may be used to treat immune complex responses such as glomerulonephritis and Goodpasture's syndrome. Plasma and the glomerular-damaging antibody-antigen complexes are removed by passing the client's blood through a blood cell separator. The RBCs are then returned to the client along with an equal amount of albumin or human plasma. This procedure is usually done in a series rather than as a one-time treatment. It is not without risk, and informed consent is required. Potential complications of plasmapheresis include those associated with intravenous catheters, shifts in fluid balance, and alteration of blood clotting.

## NURSING CARE

Nursing care related to hypersensitivity reactions is primarily directed toward prevention, early identification, and providing prompt, effective treatment.

## Health Promotion

Health promotion activities include helping clients to identify possible allergens that prompt a hypersensitivity response and discussing possible strategies to avoid these allergens. Anyone with severe food allergies may need assistance from a dietitian to discuss necessary dietary changes and ways to continue meeting nutrient needs. It is important that persons with hypersensitivities inform health care personnel of all allergens. People who experience anaphylactic reactions should wear a bracelet or tag at all times to identify the substance(s) that provokes this response.

## Assessment

Collect the following data through the health history and physical examination. Further focused assessments are described with nursing interventions in the next section.

- Health history: risk factors, hypersensitivities (medications, household dust, bee stings, etc.), reaction (rash, hives, difficulty breathing), type of treatment for hypersensitivity reactions; allergy skin testing; asthma, hay fever, or dermatitis
- Physical assessment: mucous membranes of nose and mouth, skin for lesions or rashes, eyes (tearing and redness), respiratory rate, and adventitious breath sounds

## Nursing Diagnoses and Interventions

Priority nursing diagnoses will vary according to the type of hypersensitivity reaction experienced by the client. Because nurses are most likely to become involved with a client experiencing a type I or type II response, this section focuses on diagnoses for these clients. Airway, breathing, and circulation (the ABCs) are of greatest importance for the client with an anaphylactic reaction. When a hemolytic reaction to an incompatible blood transfusion occurs, the client is at risk for injury.

### Ineffective Airway Clearance

In anaphylactic reactions, the airway may be obstructed due to facial angioedema, bronchospasm, or laryngeal edema. Establishing and maintaining a patent airway is of highest priority.

- Administer oxygen per nasal cannula at a rate of 2 to 4 L/min. *This increases the alveolar oxygen and its availability to cells of the body.*

**PRACTICE ALERT**   *Placing in Fowler's to high-Fowler's position allows optimal lung expansion and ease of breathing.* ∎

- Assess respiratory rate and pattern, level of consciousness and anxiety, nasal flaring, use of accessory muscles of respiration, chest wall movement, audible stridor; palpate for respiratory excursion; auscultate lung sounds and any adventitious sounds, such as wheezes. *Extreme anxiety or agitation, nasal flaring, stridor, and diminished lung sounds indicate air hunger and possible airway obstruction, necessitating immediate intervention.*
- Insert a nasopharyngeal or oropharyngeal airway, and arrange for immediate intubation as indicated. *Assuring an adequate airway is vital to preserve life.*
- Administer subcutaneous epinephrine 1:1000, 0.3 to 0.5 mL as prescribed. This may be repeated in 20 to 30 minutes if necessary. Administer parenteral diphenhydramine (deep intramuscular or intravenous) as prescribed. *Epinephrine is a potent vasoconstrictor and bronchodilator, counteracting the effects of histamine. Diphenhydramine is an antihistamine that blocks histamine receptors and its effect. These medications can be effective in rapidly reversing manifestations of anaphylaxis.*
- Provide calm reassurance. *Hypoxemia and air hunger are terrifying for the client. Anxiety can impair the client's ability to cooperate with treatment and increase the respiratory rate, making breathing less effective.*

### Decreased Cardiac Output

Peripheral vasodilation and increased capillary permeability from the release of histamine can significantly impair cardiac output. When it falls to the degree that tissue perfusion becomes impaired and hypoxia results, a state of anaphylactic shock exists.

- Monitor vital signs frequently, noting fall in blood pressure, decreasing pulse pressure, tachycardia, and tachypnea. *These vital sign changes may indicate shock.*
- Assess skin color, temperature, capillary refill, edema, and other indicators of peripheral perfusion. *As cardiac output falls, peripheral vessels constrict and tissue perfusion is impaired.*
- Monitor level of consciousness. *A change in level of consciousness (lethargy, apprehension, or agitation) is often the first indicator of decreased cardiac output.*
- Insert one or more large-bore (18-gauge or larger) intravenous catheters. *It is important to insert intravenous catheters as soon as possible to provide sites for rapid fluid replacement.*
- Administer warmed intravenous solutions of lactated Ringer's or normal saline, as prescribed. *These isotonic solutions help maintain intravascular volume. Warmed solutions are used to prevent hypothermia from the rapid administration of large amounts of fluid at room temperature (about 70°F, or 21.1°C).*
- Insert an indwelling catheter, and monitor urinary output frequently. *As the cardiac output drops, the glomerular filtration rate (GFR) falls. With an output of less than 30 mL per hour, the client is at risk for acute renal failure from ischemia.*
- Place a tourniquet above the site of an injected venom (such as a bee sting), and infiltrate the site with epinephrine as prescribed. *Use of a tourniquet and the vasoconstriction resulting from epinephrine infiltration reduce further absorption of the allergen.*
- Once breathing is established, place the client flat with the legs elevated. *This position enhances perfusion of the central organs, such as the brain, heart, and kidneys.*

**PRACTICE ALERT** *Aggressive fluid therapy may lead to hypervolemia and pulmonary edema; assess for shortness of breath and crackles in the lungs. ∎*

### Risk for Injury

As noted, the potential for hypersensitivity responses is high in clients subjected to medical treatments. Because a blood transfusion is a transplant of living tissue, the risk for adverse immunologic response and injury is particularly significant.

- Obtain and record a thorough history of previous blood transfusions and any reactions experienced, *no matter how mild.* Alert the physician if previous transfusion reactions have occurred. *The client who has received prior blood transfusions is at increased risk for a hypersensitivity reaction, because antibody production may have been stimulated by prior exposure to antigens.*
- Check for a signed informed consent to administer blood or blood products. *It is important to obtain informed consent for this invasive and risky procedure.*
- Using two licensed health care professionals, double-check the type, Rh factor, crossmatch, and expiration date for all

blood and blood components received from the blood bank with the client's data. *This is an important safety measure to reduce the risk of a hemolytic transfusion reaction due to incompatible blood types.*

**PRACTICE ALERT** *Begin a blood transfusion within 30 minutes of its delivery from the blood bank to reduce bacterial contamination. ∎*

- Take and record vital signs within 15 minutes prior to initiating the blood infusion. *This provides a baseline for evaluating any changes related to the blood transfusion.*
- Infuse blood into a site separate from any other intravenous infusion. Use at least an 18-gauge catheter for the infusion. *This reduces the risk of damage to the blood cells due to incompatibility with other intravenous solutions or physical trauma. When blood is administered with dextrose solutions (e.g., D5W, D5NS), blood cell hemolysis and aggregation occurs; administration with lactated Ringer's can cause agglutination of cells.*
- Administer 50 mL of blood during the first 15 minutes of the transfusion. *Reactions generally occur within the first 15 minutes.*
- During transfusion, monitor for complaints of back or chest pain, an increase in the temperature of more than 1.8°F, chills, tachycardia, tachypnea, wheezing, hypotension, hives, rashes, or cyanosis. *These signs may indicate an adverse reaction to the blood transfusion.*
- Stop the blood transfusion immediately if a reaction occurs, no matter how mild, keeping the intravenous line open with normal saline. Notify the physician and the blood bank.
- If a reaction is suspected, send the blood and administration set to the laboratory with a freshly drawn blood sample and urine specimen from the client. *These will be used to identify the cause of the reaction as well as its effect on the client.*
- If no adverse reaction occurs, administer the transfusion over 2 to 4 hours. *This time frame is important to limit the risk of bacterial growth.*

## Using NANDA, NIC, and NOC

Chart 9–1 shows links between NANDA, NIC, and NOC when caring for the client with hypersensitivities.

## Home Care

The vast majority of hypersensitivity responses are appropriately treated by the client and/or family members with little or no medical intervention. Teaching, therefore, is a vital component of care. If the client is at risk for anaphylaxis, involving the family in teaching is essential because the response may occur with such rapidity that the client will be unable to provide self-care.

Include the following points in teaching the client and family about managing hypersensitivities.

- When and how to use an anaphylaxis kit containing epinephrine and antihistamines in injectable, inhaler, and oral forms
- When to seek medical attention

## CHART 9–1 NANDA, NIC, AND NOC LINKAGES

### The Client with a Hypersensitivity Reaction

| NURSING DIAGNOSES | NURSING INTERVENTIONS | NURSING OUTCOMES |
| --- | --- | --- |
| • Ineffective Health Maintenance<br><br>• Risk for Latex Allergy Response | • Health Education<br>• Teaching: Individual<br>• Allergy Management<br>• Latex Precautions | • Health-Promoting Behavior<br>• Health-Seeking Behavior<br>• Immune Hypersensitivity Control<br>• Risk Detection |

*Note. Data from Nursing Outcomes Classification (NOC) by M. Johnson & M. Maas (Eds.), 1997, St. Louis: Mosby; Nursing Diagnoses: Definitions & Classification 2001–2002 by North American Nursing Diagnosis Association, 2001, Philadelphia: NANDA; Nursing Interventions Classification (NIC) by J.C. McCloskey & G. M. Bulechek (Eds.), 2000, St. Louis: Mosby. Reprinted by permission.*

- Use and adverse reactions of prescription and nonprescription antihistamines and decongestants
- Advantages of autologous blood transfusion if future surgery is scheduled
- Preventing an immune complex reaction such as glomerulonephritis
- Skin care to prevent contact dermatitis, including:
    Expose affected areas to air and sun as much as possible.
    Avoid direct contact with people who have an infection.
    Wear cool, light, nonrestrictive clothing of natural fibers, such as cotton, to avoid irritating affected areas.
    Avoid exposure to extremes of heat or cold.
    Use bath oils or plain water instead of soaps and detergents.
    Take tub baths in cool to lukewarm water rather than showers.
    To decrease pruritus, maintain a cool environment and avoid exercising.
    Trim fingernails to reduce the risk of skin damage.
- Helpful resources:
    - ALERT, Inc., Allergy to Latex Education and Resource Team
    - Food Allergy Network

## THE CLIENT WITH AN AUTOIMMUNE DISORDER

Maintaining optimal health and preventing disease depend not only on the immune system's ability to recognize and destroy foreign tissues and other antigens, but also on the immune system's ability to recognize self. When this self-recognition is impaired and immune defenses are directed against normal host tissue, the result is an **autoimmune disorder.**

Autoimmune disorders can affect any tissue in the body. Some are tissue or organ specific, affecting particular tissue or a particular organ. Hashimoto's thyroiditis is an example of an organ-specific autoimmune disorder. Circulating antibodies are formed to certain thyroid components, resulting ultimately in destruction of the gland. In other disorders, autoantibodies are formed that are not tissue specific, but tend to accumulate and cause an inflammatory response in certain tissue, for example, the renal glomerulus or the hepatic small bile ductules.

Autoimmune disorders may also be systemic, with neither antibodies nor the resulting inflammatory lesions confined to any one organ. Rheumatologic disorders, such as rheumatoid arthritis and systemic lupus erythematosus (SLE), are characteristic of systemic autoimmune disorders (Roitt, 1994). A list of selected autoimmune disorders is included in Table 9–1.

## PATHOPHYSIOLOGY

The mechanism that causes the immune system to recognize host tissue as a foreign antigen is not clear. The following factors are under study as possible contributors to the development of autoimmune disorders.

- The release of previously "hidden" antigens into the circulation, such as DNA or other components of the cell nucleus, which elicits an immune response
- Chemical, physical, or biologic changes in host tissue that cause self-antigens to stimulate the production of autoantibodies
- The introduction of an antigen, such as a bacteria or virus, whose antigenic properties closely resemble those of host tissue, resulting in the production of antibodies which target not only the foreign antigen but also normal tissue
- A defect in normal cellular immune function that allows B cells to produce autoantibodies unchecked
- Initiation of the autoimmune response by very slow-growing mycobacteria

Although the exact mechanism producing autoimmunity is unclear, several characteristics of autoimmune diseases are known. It is apparent that genetics plays a role, because a higher incidence is seen in family members of people with autoimmune disorders. Autoimmune disorders are far more prevalent in females than in males. The disorders tend to overlap, so that the client with one autoimmune disorder may develop another or some manifestations of another. The onset of an autoimmune disorder is frequently associated with an abnormal stressor, either physical or psychologic. Autoimmune disorders are frequently progressive relapsing-remissing disorders characterized by periods of exacerbation and remission.

Specific autoimmune disorders are discussed in the sections of this textbook related to the affected organ systems or functional disruption.

## TABLE 9–1  Selected Autoimmune Disorders

| More organ specific ⟶ Less organ specific ⟶ Non–organ specific | | |
|---|---|---|
| More organ specific | Hashimoto's thyroiditis | A chronic progressive inflammatory disease of the thyroid with lymphocyte infiltration and gradual destruction of the gland. See Chapter 17. |
| | Primary myxedema | Thyroid deficiency resulting from destruction of the thyroid gland due to an autoimmune process, often Hashimoto's thyroiditis. See Chapter 17. |
| | Thyrotoxicosis | Hyperthyroidism resulting from thyroid-stimulating immunoglobulins that stimulate activity of the gland. See Chapter 17. |
| | Pernicious anemia | Anemia resulting from absence of intrinsic factor associated with loss of parietal cells; most clients have antibodies to parietal cells. See Chapter 32. |
| | Addison's disease | Atrophy and hypofunction of the adrenal cortex, probably autoimmune in origin. See Chapter 17. |
| | Myasthenia gravis | A disease characterized by episodic muscle weakness caused by antibodies to the acetylcholine receptor of the neuromuscular junction. See Chapter 43. |
| | Insulin-dependent diabetes mellitus | Impaired insulin secretion, often the result of islet cell destruction by antibodies directed at the cell surface or cytoplasm. See Chapter 18. |
| | Goodpasture's syndrome | A type II hypersensitivity disorder with pulmonary hemorrhage and progressive glomerulonephritis characterized by circulating antiglomerular basement membrane antibodies. See Chapter 27. |
| | Multiple sclerosis | A probable autoimmune process resulting in disseminated patches of demyelination in the brain and spinal cord and varied neurologic manifestations. See Chapter 43. |
| | Idiopathic thrombocytopenic purpura | A chronic disorder characterized by petechiae, purpura, mucosal bleeding, and antibodies against platelets. See Chapter 32. |
| | Primary biliary cirrhosis | Inflammation and fibrosis of the bile ducts, probably of autoimmune origin. See Chapter 22. |
| | Active chronic hepatitis | A serious liver disease often resulting in hepatic failure and/or cirrhosis; may be autoimmune with infiltration by T cells and plasma cells. See Chapter 22. |
| Less organ specific | Ulcerative colitis | A chronic inflammatory disease of colon mucosa, possibly of autoimmune origin. See Chapter 21. |
| | Sjogren's syndrome | A systemic inflammatory disorder characterized by dryness of the mouth, eye, and other mucous membranes with lymphocyte infiltration of affected tissues. See Chapter 39. |
| | Rheumatoid arthritis | A chronic syndrome with inflammation of peripheral joints and generalized manifestations, characterized by infiltration of synovium by lymphocytes and plasma cells. See Chapter 39. |
| | Scleroderma | Diffuse fibrosis, degenerative changes, and vascular abnormalities of skin, joint structures, and internal organs; probably of autoimmune origin. See Chapter 39. |
| Non–organ specific | Systemic lupus erythematosus | An inflammatory connective tissue disorder characterized the presence of antinuclear antibodies. See Chapter 39. |

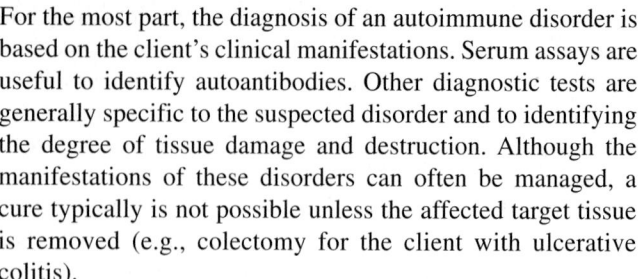

## COLLABORATIVE CARE

For the most part, the diagnosis of an autoimmune disorder is based on the client's clinical manifestations. Serum assays are useful to identify autoantibodies. Other diagnostic tests are generally specific to the suspected disorder and to identifying the degree of tissue damage and destruction. Although the manifestations of these disorders can often be managed, a cure typically is not possible unless the affected target tissue is removed (e.g., colectomy for the client with ulcerative colitis).

### Diagnostic Tests

Serologic assays are used to identify and measure antibodies directed toward host tissue antigens or normal cellular components. Many detectable autoantibodies are not specific to a single autoimmune disorder and are used to establish the au-

toimmune process rather than the specific disorder. Although healthy people often have low levels of autoantibodies, levels are much higher in clients affected by an autoimmune disorder. The following serologic assays may be ordered.

- *Antinuclear antibody (ANA)* detects antibodies produced to DNA and other nuclear material. These antibodies can cause tissue damage characteristic of autoimmune disorders, such as SLE. The client's serum is combined with nuclear material and tagged antihuman antibody to detect ANA-antihuman antibody complexes. A negative, or normal, result is a titer <1:20. When complexes are detected at higher titer levels (>1:20), the test is positive for ANA. This test is not specific for SLE, because high levels of ANA may be present in rheumatoid arthritis and cirrhosis of the liver; nevertheless, 95% of clients with SLE have a positive ANA titer.
- *Lupus erythematosus (LE) cell test* is also used to detect SLE and monitor its treatment. Neutrophils that contain

large masses of phagocytized DNA from the nuclei of PMNs are called LE cells. Like the ANA, the LE cell prep is non-specific for SLE. A positive result may also be seen in rheumatoid arthritis or with medications such as isoniazid, penicillin, phenytoin, procainamide, streptomycin, or sulfonamide drugs.

- *Rheumatoid factor (RF)* is an immunoglobulin present in the serum of approximately 80% of clients with rheumatoid arthritis. Low titer levels (<1:20) may be present in the elderly. An RF titer 1:80 or higher indicates rheumatoid arthritis. A titer between 1:20 and 1:80 could indicate SLE, scleroderma, or liver cirrhosis (Kee, 1999).
- *Complement assay* may also be useful in identifying autoimmune disorders. In these disorders, complement may be consumed in the development of antigen-antibody complexes. Decreased levels are seen on examination. Both total complement level and amounts of individual components of the complement cascade can be determined.

## Medications

Various approaches are used in the treatment of autoimmune disorders. Anti-inflammatory medications such as aspirin, NSAIDs, and corticosteroids may be prescribed to reduce the inflammatory response and minimize tissue damage. (Refer to Chapter 4 for additional detail on these drugs.) When these agents are not effective or well tolerated by the client, slow-acting anti-inflammatory medications may be prescribed. Slow-acting or antirheumatic drugs include such medications as gold salts, hydroxychloroquine (Plaquenil), and penicillamine. Their use is further detailed in Chapter 39. Cytotoxic drugs may be used in combination with plasmapheresis in treating many autoimmune disorders. Cytotoxic drugs are discussed in further detail in the next section of this chapter. ∞

## NURSING CARE

Nursing care measures for the client with an autoimmune disorder are individualized and tailored to needs dictated by manifestations of the disorder. Nurses often will be involved with the client in an outpatient setting such as an office or home, evaluating the client's response to therapy and self-care management.

Consider the following nursing diagnoses in planning care for the client with an autoimmune disorder.

- *Activity intolerance* related to inflammatory effects of autoimmune disorder
- *Ineffective coping* related to chronic disease process
- *Interrupted family processes* related to lack of understanding about autoimmune disorder and its effects
- *Ineffective protection* related to disordered immune function
- *Risk for ineffective therapeutic regimen management* related to lack of understanding

## Home Care

Because many autoimmune disorders are chronic, teaching the client and family about the disorder and its management is a key nursing care component. The client may be taking drugs with multiple side effects or long-term effects, necessitating effective teaching. Clients with autoimmune disorders often do not appear to be ill, making it difficult for friends and families to understand their care needs. The chronicity of these disorders also puts the client at high risk for unproven remedies and quackery. Provide psychologic support, listening, and teaching. In addition, suggest resources such as local support groups and the American Autoimmune Related Diseases Association.

## THE CLIENT WITH A TISSUE TRANSPLANT

Since the first kidney transplant performed from one identical twin to the other in 1954, organ and tissue transplantation has become an increasingly popular and viable treatment option. The transplantation of avascular tissues, such as skin, cornea, bone, and heart valves, is considered routine, with little need for tissue matching and immunosuppression. Transplants of organs (e.g., the kidney, heart, heart and lung, liver, and bone marrow) are increasingly common and are no longer considered experimental or extraordinary procedures. Common organ transplants are outlined in Table 9–2.

Transplant success is closely tied to obtaining an organ with tissue antigens as close to those of the recipient as possible. As noted earlier in this chapter, every body cell has cell surface antigens known as human leukocyte antigens that are unique to the individual. Although identical twins may have the same HLA type, the chance is reduced to 1 in 4 for siblings, and less than 1 in several thousand for unrelated individuals (Tierney et al., 2001). Matching the HLA type of the donor and recipient as closely as possible decreases the potential for rejection of the transplanted organ or tissue but does not eliminate it.

## PATHOPHYSIOLOGY

An **autograft,** a transplant of the client's own tissue, is the most successful type of tissue transplant. Skin grafts are the most common examples of autografts. Increasingly, autologous bone marrow transplants and blood transfusions are being used to reduce immunologic responses. When the donor and recipient are identical twins, the term **isograft** is used. Because of the high likelihood of an HLA match, the success of these grafts is good and rejection episodes are mild. Few people, however, have an identical twin to provide tissue for donation; and when the need is for an organ such as the heart, liver, or lungs, a living-donor transplantation is not possible. Most often, organ and tissue transplants are **allografts,** which are grafts between members of the same species but who have different genotypes and HLA. Allografts may come from living donors; examples are bone marrow, blood, and a kidney. Most often, however, organs for transplantation are obtained from a cadaver. Donors are typically people who meet the criteria for brain death; are less than 65 years old; and are free of systemic disease, malignancy, or infection, including HIV, hepatitis B, or hepatitis C. The organ is removed immediately

## TABLE 9–2   Organ Transplants

| Organ | Graft Type | Indications for Transplant | Success Rate |
|---|---|---|---|
| Kidney | Allograft; may be isograft | End-stage renal disease | 80% to 90% at 1 year |
| Heart | Allograft | End-stage cardiac disease refractory to medical management | 74% at 5 years |
| Lung | Allograft | Pulmonary hypertension, cystic fibrosis, pulmonary fibrosis, chronic obstructive pulmonary disease | 70% at 1 year for combined heart-lung; 60% for single lung |
| Liver | Allograft | Severe liver dysfunction due to chronic active hepatitis, primary biliary cirrhosis, sclerosing cholangitis | 70% to 90% 1-year survival |
| Bone marrow | Autograft or allograft | Leukemia, aplastic anemia, congenital immunologic defects | 40% to 75% at 1 year |
| Skin | Autograft, allograft, or xenograft | Severe burns, plastic surgery | >95% at 5 years |
| Cornea | Allograft | Corneal ulceration and opacification | >95% at 5 years |
| Pancreas | Allograft | Pancreatic insufficiency, diabetes | 65% at 1 year |

Note. Summarized from Current Medical Diagnosis and Treatment (40th ed.) by L. M. Tierney, S. J. McPhee, and M. A. Papadakis, 2001, New York: Lange Medical Books / McGraw-Hill.

before or after cardiac arrest and preserved until it is transplanted into the waiting recipient. Finally, **xenograft** is a transplant from an animal species to a human. These transplants are the least successful but may be used in selected instances, such as the use of pig skin as a temporary covering for a massive burn.

Tissue typing is used to determine the **histocompatibility,** the ability of cells and tissues to survive transplantation without immunologic interference by the recipient. Tissue typing is performed in an attempt to match the donor and recipient as closely as possible for HLA type and blood type (ABO, Rh) and to identify preformed antibodies to the donor's HLA.

Both antibody-mediated and cell-mediated immune responses are involved in the complex process of transplant rejection. Host macrophages process donor antigen, presenting it to T and B lymphocytes. Activated lymphocytes produce both antibody- and cell-mediated effects. Killer T cells bind with cells of the transplanted organ, resulting in cell lysis.

Helper T cells stimulate the multiplication and differentiation of B cells, and antibodies are produced to graft endothelium. Complement activation or antibody-dependent cell-mediated cytotoxicity leads to transplant cell destruction. Rejection typically begins after the first 24 hours of the transplant, although it may present immediately. Rejection episodes are characterized as hyperacute, acute, or chronic, as summarized in Table 9–3.

*Hyperacute tissue rejection* occurs immediately to 2 to 3 days after the transplant of new tissue. Hyperacute rejection is due to preformed antibodies and sensitized T cells to antigens in the donor organ. Hyperacute rejection is most likely to occur in clients who have had a previous organ or tissue transplant, such as a blood transfusion. Hyperacute rejection may be evident even before the transplant procedure is completed. The grafted organ initially appears pink and healthy, but soon becomes soft and cyanotic as blood flow is impaired. Organ function deteriorates rapidly, and symptoms of organ failure develop.

## TABLE 9–3   Transplant Rejection Episodes

| Type | Cause | Presentation | Treatment |
|---|---|---|---|
| Hyperacute | Preexisting antibodies to donor ABO or HLA antigens | Occurs within minutes to hours or days of the transplant<br>Rapid deterioration of organ function | The transplant usually cannot be saved; prevent with crossmatch, and use antimetabolites or anti-inflammatory drugs before surgery. |
| Acute | Primarily a cell-mediated immune response to HLA antigens; antibody-mediated response may also contribute | Occurs within days to months after the transplant<br>Signs of inflammation and impaired organ function | Increase immunosuppression using steroids, cyclosporine, monoclonal antibodies, or antilymphocyte globulins. |
| Chronic | Probably antibody-mediated response; may also involve inflammatory damage to vessel endothelium | Occurs 4 months to years after the transplant<br>Gradual deterioration of organ function | None; loss of graft will occur, requiring retransplant. |

*Acute tissue rejection* is the most common and treatable type of rejection episode. It occurs between 4 days and 3 months after the transplant. Acute rejection is mediated primarily by the cellular immune response, resulting in transplant cell destruction. The client experiencing acute rejection demonstrates manifestations of the inflammatory process, with fever, redness, swelling, and tenderness over the graft site. Signs of impaired function of the transplanted organ may be noted (e.g., elevated BUN and creatinine, liver enzyme and bilirubin elevations, or elevated cardiac enzymes and signs of cardiac failure).

*Chronic tissue rejection* occurs from 4 months to years after transplant of new tissue. Chronic rejection is most likely the result of antibody-mediated immune responses. Antibodies and complement are deposited in transplant vessel walls, causing narrowing and decreased function of the organ due to ischemia. The gradual deterioration of transplanted organ function is seen with chronic tissue rejection.

*Graft-versus-host disease (GVHD)* is a frequent and potentially fatal complication of bone marrow transplant. When there is no close match between donor and recipient HLA, immunocompetent cells in the grafted tissue recognize host tissue as foreign and mount a cell-mediated immune response. If the host is immunocompromised, as is often the case when a bone marrow transplant is performed, host cells are unable to destroy the graft and instead become the targets of destruction. Of clients with very closely matched bone marrow, 30% to 60% nevertheless develop GVHD. Acute GVHD occurs within the first 100 days following a transplant and primarily affects the skin, liver, and gastrointestinal tract. The client develops a maculopapular pruritic rash beginning on the palms of the hands and soles of the feet. The rash may spread to involve the entire body and lead to desquamation. Gastrointestinal manifestations include abdominal pain, nausea, and bloody diarrhea. GVHD that lasts longer than 100 days is said to be chronic. If it is limited to the skin and liver, the prognosis is good. If multiple organs are involved, the prognosis is poor (Porth, 2002; Roitt, 1994).

## COLLABORATIVE CARE

Pretransplant care and posttransplant care are directed toward reducing the risk that transplanted tissue will be rejected or result in GVHD. Diagnostic studies are directed first at identifying a suitable donor, then at monitoring the immune response to the transplant. Immunosuppressive therapy with medications is a vital part of posttransplant care. Indeed, the development of effective immunosuppressive drugs is responsible for the success of organ transplants using allografts.

### Diagnostic Tests

The following diagnostic tests may be ordered prior to organ or tissue transplantation.

- *Blood type and Rh factor* of both the donor and recipient are determined. Although there is some question about the benefit of histocompatibility testing prior to transplant of a cadaver organ, there is no question about the need for ABO blood group compatibility.

- *Crossmatching* of the client's serum against the donor's lymphocytes is performed to identify any preformed antibodies against antigens on donor tissues. If present, these antibodies would likely result in an immediate or hyperacute graft rejection with probable loss of the transplant.

- *HLA histocompatibility testing* identifyies donors with an HLA type close to that of the recipient. It is used primarily to identify living donors for bone marrow and kidney transplant. Because of GVHD, histocompatibility tests to identify an identical or very close HLA match are particularly important in bone marrow transplant. HLA tests are performed using lymphocytes from a blood sample. The sample should not be obtained within 72 hours of a blood transfusion, because this will interfere with results.

- *Mixed lymphocyte culture (MLC) assay tests* also are used to determine histocompatibility between the donor and the recipient. This test identifies whether mononuclear cells of the recipient will react against the potential donor's leukocyte antigens. The disadvantage of this test is that results cannot be obtained until 7 to 10 days later (Chernecky & Berger, 1997). Factors that could interfere with the results of this test include use of oral contraceptives, a radioisotope scan within 1 week prior to the test, and chemotherapy.

- *Ultrasonography* or *magnetic resonance imaging (MRI)* of the transplanted organ may be performed to evaluate its size, perfusion, and function.

- *Tissue biopsies* of the transplanted organ are performed routinely to assess for evidence of tissue rejection.

### Medications

Prior to transplantation, several antibiotic and antiviral drugs may be prescribed, including the following:

- Trimethoprim-sulfamethoxazole (Septra, Bactrim), which decreases the incidence of gram-negative bacterial infections
- Acyclovir (Zovirax), which prevents the development of herpes simplex virus (HSV) pneumonia in bone marrow transplant recipients
- Ganciclovir (Cytovene), which prevents the development of cytomegalovirus (CMV) pneumonia with bone marrow transplant recipients

The mainstays of drug therapy for clients following a tissue or organ transplant are immunosuppressive agents. Varying regimens of these drugs are used, depending on the transplanted tissue and the medical center; however, a combination of corticosteroids and cyclosporine is common for maintenance therapy. Antilymphocyte therapy and the use of monoclonal antibodies are increasingly common in the immediate posttransplant period and for treating steroid-resistant rejection episodes.

Corticosteroids, primarily prednisone (Deltasone, others) and methylprednisolone (Solu-Medrol, others) were among the first medications used to prevent transplant rejection, and they remain important agents today. Although the exact anti-inflammatory and immunosuppressive activity of corticosteroids is unknown, they are known to suppress production of interleukin 1 and 2, decrease monocyte migration, and suppress proliferative and cytotoxic T-cell activity. Although they are very effective, large doses of corticosteroids used posttransplant are associated with significant adverse effects. Wound healing is impaired, and the metabolism of fats, proteins, and carbohydrates is altered. Fat distribution changes, producing a cushingoid appearance with moon facies, increased truncal fat, and "buffalo hump." Fluid retention and hypertension are potential problems, as are osteoporosis, gastrointestinal bleeding, and emotional disturbances.

Azathioprine (Imuran) has been in use as an immunosuppressant for more than 25 years and continues to be a component of many regimens. Azathioprine inhibits both cell-mediated and antibody-mediated immunity, although its activity is more specific for T cells than B cells. Because it is rapidly metabolized by the liver, azathioprine can be given to clients with impaired renal function but may not be effective in clients with impaired hepatic function. Bone marrow suppression is the most common adverse effect of this drug, necessitating frequent evaluation of the CBC. Hepatotoxicity, pancreatitis, and increased risk of neoplasm are also associated with azathioprine administration. Nursing responsibilities related to azathioprine are included in the box below. Clients who cannot tolerate azathioprine may receive a newer immunosuppressant, mycophenolate mofetil (CellCept). Primarily, it is prescribed following renal and cardiac transplants.

# Medication Administration

## Immunosuppressive Agents

### CYTOTOXIC AGENTS
- Azathioprine (Imuran)
- Cyclophosphamide (Cytoxan)
- Mycophenolate (CellCept)
- Cyclosporine (Sandimmune, Neoral)

Certain drugs that are identified as cytotoxic or antineoplastic agents are effective as immunosuppressive agents. They act by decreasing the proliferation of cells within the immune system and are widely used to prevent rejection following a tissue or organ transplant. They are usually administered concurrently with corticosteroid therapy, allowing lower doses of both preparations and resulting in fewer side effects.

#### Nursing Responsibilities
- Monitor blood count, with particular attention to the WBC and platelet counts. Notify the physician if WBCs fall below 4000 or platelets below 75,000.
- Monitor renal and liver function studies, including creatinine, BUN, creatinine clearance, and liver enzymes. Report abnormal levels to the physician.
- Administer the drug as ordered. Administer oral preparations with food to minimize gastrointestinal effects. Antacids may be ordered.
- Increase fluids to maintain good hydration and urinary output.
- Monitor intake and output.
- Monitor for signs of abnormal bleeding bleeding gums, bruising, petechiae, joint pain, hematuria, and black or tarry stools.
- Use meticulous handwashing and other appropriate measures to protect the client from infection. Assess for signs of infection.
- Pulmonary fibrosis is a potential adverse effect of cyclophosphamides. Therefore, monitor respiratory function using pulmonary function studies and clinical signs of dyspnea or cough.

#### Client and Family Teaching
- Avoid large crowds and situations where exposure to infection is probable.
- Report signs of infection, such as chills, fever, sore throat, fatigue, or malaise, to the physician.
- Use contraceptive measures to prevent pregnancy while on immunosuppressive therapy; these drugs are teratogenic.
- Avoid the use of aspirin or ibuprofen while taking these drugs. Report any signs of bleeding to the physician.

- With cyclophosphamide, amenorrhea may occur. The menses will resume after the drug is discontinued.
- If taking cyclophosphamide, report difficulty breathing or cough to the physician.

### MONOCLONAL ANTIBODY
Muromonab-CD3 or OKT3 (Orthoclone)

This monoclonal antibody against T cells is formed by immunizing a mouse with an antigen to produce a specific antibody. Lymphocytes producing the antibody, OKT3, are cloned, and the antibody is harvested. When injected into humans, OKT3 binds with a surface antigen on T cells, removing them from circulation and inactivating those bound to allograft cells. Due to the high incidence of adverse effects, the first two doses of OKT3 are administered by a physician and the client closely observed for 2 hours following each dose.

#### Nursing Responsibilities
- Be sure a chest X-ray has been performed within 24 hours preceding initiation of OKT3 therapy and that no congestion is present. The risk of anaphylaxis is greater in the client with fluid overload.
- Premedicate as ordered with hydrocortisone, acetaminophen, and diphenhydramine to reduce potential adverse effects.
- Position a crash cart or code cart with emergency medications in the client's room or in close proximity to it.
- After each of the first two doses, monitor vital signs every 15 minutes for 2 hours, then every 30 minutes for 2 hours.
- After the first two doses, administer a 2.5- to 10-mg dose by intravenous push over 1 to 2 minutes.
- Observe closely for potential adverse effects, including chills and fever; tachycardia; headache and tremor; hypertension or hypotension; nausea, vomiting, and diarrhea; chest pain, dyspnea, and wheezing.
- OKT3 can also cause anaphylaxis; observe for evidence of urticaria, angioedema, laryngeal edema, wheezing, or other signs of anaphylactic reaction.
- Monitor CBC for evidence of leukopenia or pancytopenia.
- Assess for infection. Remember that typical signs of infection, including symptoms such as fever and inflammation, may be masked or reduced by immunosuppressive therapy.

## Risk for Impaired Tissue Integrity: Allograft

As noted, the risk for transplant rejection is highest in the initial postoperative period, but it is never completely eliminated for the client who has had an allograft. The client who has had a bone marrow transplant has the additional risk of developing GVHD, which can affect the integrity of skin, mucous membranes, and other organs.

- Administer immunosuppressive therapy as prescribed. *Suppression of the immune response is necessary to reduce the risk of graft destruction by normal immune responses and to preserve its function.*
- Assess for evidence of graft rejection, including tenderness, erythema, and swelling over the site; sudden weight gain, edema, and hypertension; chills and fever; malaise; and an increased WBC count and sedimentation rate. Report any changes immediately. *Early identification of rejection allows adjustment of medication regimens and, possibly, preservation of the graft.*
- Monitor results of laboratory studies for function of the transplanted organ. *With a functional graft, results (e.g., renal or liver function studies) will improve; a functional decline may be an early indicator of rejection.*
- Assess for and report signs of GVHD immediately, including maculopapular rash, erythema of the skin and possible desquamation, hair loss, abdominal cramping and diarrhea, jaundice with elevated bilirubin and liver enzymes (AST, ALT). *GVHD is a potentially lethal complication in the immunosuppressed client and necessitates immediate intervention.*
- Stress the importance of maintaining immunosuppressive therapy and reporting signs of graft rejection promptly to the physician. *Continued immunosuppression and prompt treatment of rejection are vital to preserving graft function.*

## Anxiety

The client who undergoes an organ or tissue transplantation often faces the unwelcome choices of death from organ failure or receiving an organ that his or her body will likely attempt to reject. In most cases, the client understands that to receive this transplant, someone else must die and be willing to give up an organ. When the transplant comes from a living donor (bone marrow or kidney), the client may worry not only about himself or herself, but also about the condition of the donor. Fear of rejection and guilt may be even greater in this instance.

- Assess level of anxiety by noting such cues as expressions of apprehension, fear, or inadequacy; facial expression, tension, or shakiness; difficulty focusing; helplessness; poor eye contact; and restlessness. *Clients may have difficulty identifying or verbalizing feelings of fear and anxiety. Nonverbal cues are often useful in recognizing states of anxiety.*
- Provide opportunities to express feelings. Use opening statements such as, "Facing an organ transplant must be very stressful." Listen attentively. *Encouragement and active listening allow the client to express feelings of anxiety or fear.*
- Arrange tasks to allow as much time with the client as possible. When leaving, tell the client when you will return. *Time spent with the client facilitates the development of trust.*
- Provide clear, concise directions. *Highly anxious clients have difficulty focusing and retaining information.*
- Encourage involvement in care but do not request unnecessary decisions. *The client needs to feel a sense of control but may become irritated if asked to make decisions unrelated to the situation.*
- Encourage family members to remain with the client as much as possible. *This can help reduce the client's anxiety.*
- Encourage the use of coping behaviors that have been effective for the client in the past. *Coping mechanisms and behaviors help lower anxiety to a more acceptable level.*
- Reduce or eliminate environmental stressors to the extent possible. *This gives the client a better sense of control.*
- Assist with stress-reduction and relaxation techniques, such as guided imagery, meditation, and muscle relaxation. *These techniques help the client gain control over physical responses to anxiety.*
- Arrange for a counselor or mental health specialist to work with the client. *Counseling can help the client identify and deal with his or her feelings.*

## Using NANDA, NIC, and NOC Linkages

Chart 9–2 shows links between NANDA, NIC, and NOC when caring for a client posttransplant.

---

## CHART 9–2 NANDA, NIC, AND NOC LINKAGES

### The Client with a Tissue Transplant

| NURSING DIAGNOSES | NURSING INTERVENTIONS | NURSING OUTCOMES |
|---|---|---|
| • Ineffective Protection | • Infection Protection | • Immune Status<br>• Infection Status |
| • Disturbed Body Image | • Body Image Enhancement | • Self-Esteem<br>• Psychosocial Adjustment: Life Change |
| • Anxiety | • Anxiety Reduction | • Anxiety Control<br>• Coping |
| • Ineffective Health Maintenance | • Health Education<br>• Teaching: Individual | • Health-Promoting Behavior<br>• Health-Seeking Behavior |

*Note. Data from Nursing Outcomes Classification (NOC) by M. Johnson & M. Maas (Eds.), 1997, St. Louis: Mosby; Nursing Diagnoses: Definitions & Classification 2001–2002 by North American Nursing Diagnosis Association, 2001, Philadelphia: NANDA; Nursing Interventions Classification (NIC) by J.C. McCloskey & G. M. Bulechek (Eds.), 2000, St. Louis: Mosby. Reprinted by permission.*

## Home Care

Teaching of the client and family regarding an organ or tissue transplant begins well before the transplant and continues throughout hospitalization and follow-up treatment.

Initial teaching focuses on the options, risks, and potential benefits of the transplant itself. Include the procedure by which the organ is selected and obtained, as well as the procedure by which it is transplanted into the client. If a living related donor is an option, discuss the risks and benefits for both the client and the donor. Outline the posttransplant treatment regimen, including any lifestyle changes that may be necessary.

Following the transplant, provide verbal and written instructions, including the following:

- Manifestations of transplant rejection and the importance of notifying the physician
- Immunosuppressive drug regimen and side effects
- Wound care
- Avoiding exposure to infectious diseases, particularly respiratory infections, and wearing a mask when going outside
- Meticulous personal hygiene, handwashing technique, and frequent mouth care
- Wearing a medical alert bracelet or tag
- Follow-up visits to the physician or clinic
- Helpful resources:
  - American Council on Transplantation
  - Local and state support groups related to specific organ transplant, such as the National Kidney Foundation

# IMPAIRED IMMUNE RESPONSES

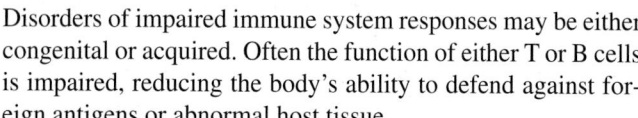

Disorders of impaired immune system responses may be either congenital or acquired. Often the function of either T or B cells is impaired, reducing the body's ability to defend against foreign antigens or abnormal host tissue.

No matter what the cause, clients with immunodeficiency disorders demonstrate an unusual susceptibility to infection. When the antibody-mediated response is primarily affected, the client is at particular risk for severe and chronic bacterial infections. These clients also do not develop long-lasting immunity to such diseases as chickenpox and are prone to recurrent cases. Clients with a defect of cell-mediated immunity tend to develop disseminated viral infections such as herpes simplex and CMV. Candidiasis and other fungal infections are also common. Because T cells are involved with activating antibody-mediated immune responses as well, overwhelming bacterial infections may occur. Immunodeficiency in its most severe form occurs when both antibody-mediated and cell-mediated responses are impaired. Clients with combined immunodeficiency are susceptible to all varieties of infectious organisms, including those not normally considered to be pathogens.

Most immunodeficiency diseases are genetically determined and rare. They affect children more than adults. The noted exception is AIDS, an infectious disease caused by a virus.

## THE CLIENT WITH HIV INFECTION

In 1981, five cases of *Pneumocystis carinii* pneumonia (PCP) and 26 cases of a rare cancer, Kaposi's sarcoma, were diagnosed in young, previously healthy homosexual males in Los Angeles and New York City. The term **acquired immunodeficiency syndrome (AIDS)** was ascribed to this new phenomenon to describe the immune system deficits associated with these opportunistic disorders. Prior to this time, both PCP and Kaposi's had been seen only in elderly, debilitated, or severely immunodeficient people. Other groups at risk for AIDS were soon identified: injection drug users, persons with hemophilia, recipients of blood transfusions, and immigrants from Haiti.

Research to identify the cause of this apparently new disease progressed feverishly, and in 1983, a common antibody was identified in clients with AIDS. The **human immunodeficiency virus (HIV)** was isolated in 1984. It then became apparent that AIDS was the final, fatal stage of HIV infection.

> It began, like so many epidemics, with a few isolated cases, a whisper that caught the ear of only a few in medical research. Today, that whisper has become a roar heard around the world. AIDS—acquired immunodeficiency syndrome—is now the epidemic of our generation, invading our lives in ways we never imagined—testing our scientific knowledge, probing our private values, and sapping our strength. AIDS no longer attracts our attention—it commands it. (Novello, 1993)

### INCIDENCE AND PREVALENCE

As of December 2000, the CDC estimated that 800,000 to 900,000 persons in the United States were infected with HIV, with AIDS as the fifth leading cause of death among adults age 25 to 44. As many as one-third of those infected are unaware of their HIV infection. By the end of June 2000, a cumulative total of 753,907 cases of AIDS had been reported. By 1999, death rates among people with AIDS had decreased (Bihari, Levin, Malebranche, & Valdez, 2000), the result of a slowing of the epidemic and improved treatments.

Among men with new HIV infection, 60% were men who have sex with men, 25% were those injecting drugs, and 15% were people having heterosexual contact (primarily with injecting drug users). The majority (75%) of women were infected through heterosexual contact, with the remaining 25% through injection drug use. Among risk groups, the most rapid increases are noted in young gay and bisexual men, women, and inner-city intravenous drug users, especially African Americans and Hispanics (Bihari et al., 2000). In the United States, the reported rate of adult/adolescent AIDS cases (per 100,000 population) reported was 84.2 among African Americans, 34.6 among Hispanics, 11.3 among American Indians/Alaska Natives, 9.0 among whites, and 4.3 among Asians/Pacific Islanders (National Institute of Allergy and Infectious Diseases [NIAID], 2001). The rapid increase of AIDS cases among women is of special concern; those numbers increased from 7% of cases in 1985 to 23% of newly reported cases in 2000 (NIAID, 2000).

In addition, AIDS in the adult over age 50 accounts for 10% of all reported cases in the United States. Declining immune system function in older adults significantly increases their risk for contracting HIV/AIDS, along with the belief that they cannot be affected by it. Just as younger persons with HIV/AIDS contract the diseases primarily through sexual intercourse, so does the elderly population. Because older adults are beyond childbearing years, they often fail to use condoms when engaging in sexual activity. Manifestations may be overlooked by health care professionals, leading to a delayed diagnosis and increased severity of the disease.

There are an estimated 36.2 million people infected with AIDS worldwide, with virtually every country in the world reporting cases of AIDS (Joint United Nations Programme on HIV/AIDS [UNAIDS], 2000). The highest incidence is found in sub-Saharan Africa, South and Southeast Asia, the United States, western Europe, South America, and Canada. Approximately 70% of all people infected with HIV or who have AIDS live in sub-Saharan Africa, and another 16% live in South and Southeast Asia, especially in Thailand and India. The most common mode of transmission is heterosexual intercourse. The cofactors of general health status, the presence of genital ulcers, and the number of sexual partners correlate with incidence (Tierney et al., 2001).

HIV is a retrovirus transmitted by direct contact with infected blood and body fluids. Significant concentrations of the virus are present in blood, semen, vaginal and cervical secretions, and cerebrospinal fluid (CSF) of infected individuals. It is also found in breast milk and saliva. Sexual contact is the primary mode of transmission. HIV is also transmitted through contact with infected blood via needle sharing during injection drug use or by transfusion. Approximately 15% to 30% of infants born to HIV-positive mothers are infected perinatally.

The risk factors for HIV infection are behavioral. Among adults in the United States, 60% of reported cases are in men who have sex with other men, including homosexuals, bisexuals, and such groups as prison populations. Unprotected anal intercourse is the major route of transmission in this group. Injection drug use is the second leading risk factor, accounting for approximately 25% of cases. Sharing of needles and other drug paraphernalia is the primary route of transmission in this group. Heterosexual intercourse with an infected drug user and exchanging sex for drugs are major risk factors for women. Hemophiliacs who require large amounts of intravenous clotting factors and people infected through blood transfusion account for a small number of cases, approximately 2% to 3%.

Among the general population of the United States, the prevalence of HIV infection is very low. Less than 0.04% of people voluntarily donating blood (a process that generally excludes people with high-risk behavior) are found to be HIV positive. HIV is not transmitted by casual contact, nor is there any evidence of its transmission by vectors such as mosquitoes. Blood donation also poses no risk of contracting HIV to the donor, because only new sterile equipment is used. A small but real occupational risk exists for health care workers. Percutaneous exposure to infected blood or body fluids through a needle-stick injury or nonintact skin is the primary route of transmission. Documented evidence indicates that parenteral exposure poses a 0.3% risk of becoming HIV positive (Carrico, 2001). Mucosal exposures, such as splashing in the eyes or mouth, pose a much smaller risk.

## PATHOPHYSIOLOGY AND MANIFESTATIONS

HIV is a retrovirus, meaning it carries its genetic information in RNA. On entry into the body, the virus infects cells which have the CD4 antigen. Once inside the cell, the virus sheds its protein coat and uses an enzyme called *reverse transcriptase* to convert the RNA to DNA (Figure 9–6 ■). This viral DNA is then integrated into host cell DNA and duplicated during normal processes of cell division. Within the cell, the virus may remain latent or become activated to produce new RNA and to form virions. The virus then buds from the cell surface, disrupting its cell membrane and leading to destruction of the host cell.

Although the virus may remain inactive in infected cells for years, antibodies are produced to its proteins, a process known as **seroconversion.** These antibodies are usually detectable 6 weeks to 6 months after the initial infection. Helper T or CD4 cells are the primary cells infected by HIV. It also infects macrophages and certain cells of the CNS. Helper T cells play a vital role in normal immune system function, recognizing foreign antigens and infected cells and activating antibody-producing B cells. They also direct cell-mediated immune activity and influence the phagocytic activity of monocytes and macrophages. The loss of these helper T cells leads to the immunodeficiencies seen with HIV infection (Porth, 2002). Figure 9–7 ■ illustrates the typical course of HIV infection.

Pathologic changes are also noted in the CNS of many infected individuals. Although the mechanism of neurologic dysfunction is unclear, neurologic manifestations of HIV infection may be seen in clients who have no apparent immune deficiency (Porth, 2002; Tierney et al., 2001). The clinical manifestations of HIV infection range from no symptoms to severe immunodeficiency with multiple opportunistic infections and cancers (see the Manifestations box on page 255). It appears that the majority of clients develop an acute mononucleosis-type illness within days to weeks after contracting the virus. Typical manifestations include fever, sore throat, arthralgias and myalgias, headache, rash, and lymphadenopathy. The client may also experience nausea, vomiting, and abdominal cramping. The client often attributes this initial manifestation of HIV infection to a common viral illness such as influenza, upper respiratory infection, or stomach virus.

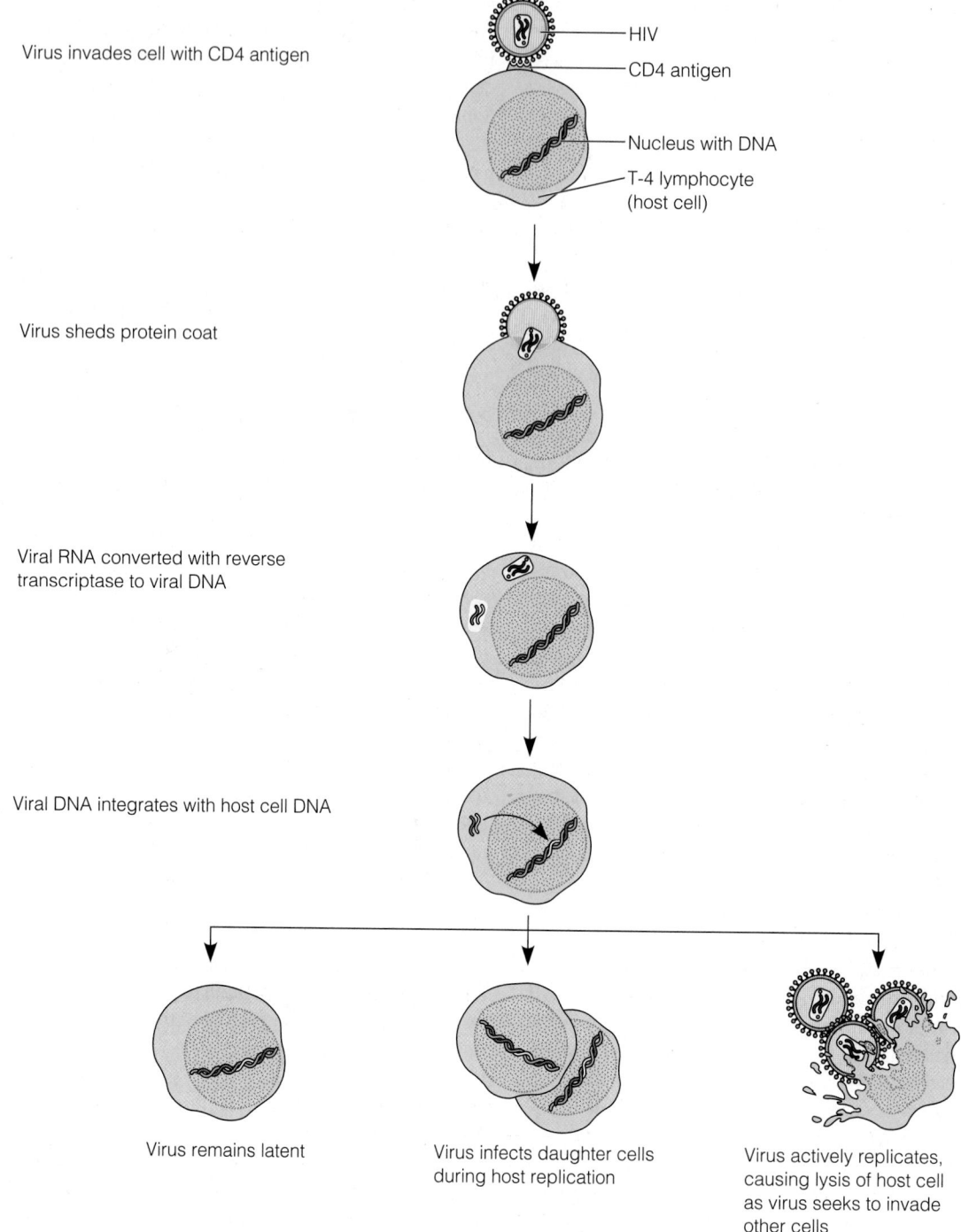

Virus invades cell with CD4 antigen

HIV
CD4 antigen
Nucleus with DNA
T-4 lymphocyte (host cell)

Virus sheds protein coat

Viral RNA converted with reverse transcriptase to viral DNA

Viral DNA integrates with host cell DNA

Virus remains latent

Virus infects daughter cells during host replication

Virus actively replicates, causing lysis of host cell as virus seeks to invade other cells

**Figure 9–6 ■** How HIV infects and destroys CD4 cells.

Following this acute illness, clients enter a long-lasting asymptomatic period. Although the virus is present and can be transmitted to others, the infected host has few or no symptoms. Clearly, the majority of HIV-infected persons are in this stage of the disease. The length of the asymptomatic period varies widely, but its mean length is estimated to be 8 to 10 years.

Some clients with few other symptoms develop persistent generalized lymphadenopathy. This is defined as enlargement of two or more lymph nodes outside the inguinal chain with no other illness or condition to account for the lymphadenopathy.

The move from asymptomatic disease or persistent lymphadenopathy to AIDS is often not clearly defined. The client may complain of general malaise, fever, fatigue, night sweats, and involuntary weight loss. Persistent skin dryness and rash may be a problem. Diarrhea is common, as are oral lesions such as hairy leukoplakia, candidiasis, and gingival inflammation and ulceration.

With the development of significant constitutional disease, neurologic manifestations, or opportunistic infections or cancers, the client has manifestations that are characteristic of

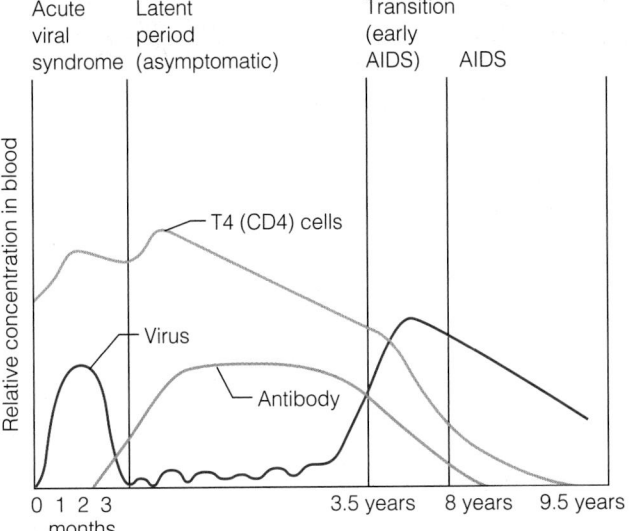

**Figure 9–7 ■** The progression of HIV infection. Acute illness develops shortly after the virus is contracted, corresponding with a rapid rise in viral levels. Antibodies are formed and remain present throughout the course of infection. Late in the disease, viral activation results in a marked increase in virus while CD4 (T4) cells diminish as they are destroyed with viral replication. Antibody levels gradually decrease as immune function is impaired.

AIDS and a very poor prognosis. HIV infection and AIDS may be classified by using the CDC's matrix classification system. Under this system, HIV disease is determined by the presence of clinical symptoms (clinical categories A, B, and C) and by T4 cell counts (categories 1, 2, and 3) (see Box 9–2).

When clinical manifestations develop, the outcome varies. With improvements in therapy, many clients are living longer after being diagnosed with AIDS. For example, in San Francisco, mean survival after a first bout with PCP is 18 to 24 months. The time of survival has increased from about 12 months at the start of the epidemic; however, survival after diagnosis of HIV-related lymphomas still averages less than 8 months.

## AIDS Dementia Complex and Neurologic Effects

Neurologic manifestations of HIV are common, affecting 40% to 60% of clients with AIDS. They result from both the direct effects of the virus on the nervous system and opportunistic infections.

AIDS dementia complex is the most common cause of mental status changes for clients with HIV infection. This dementia results from a direct effect of the virus on the brain and affects cognitive, motor, and behavioral functioning. Fluctuating memory loss, confusion, difficulty concentrating, lethargy, and diminished motor speed are typical manifestations of AIDS dementia complex. Clients become apathetic, losing interest in work and social and recreational activities. As the complex progresses, the client develops severe dementia with motor disturbances such as ataxia, tremor, spasticity, incontinence, and paraplegia (Porth, 2002; Braunwald et al., 2001).

## Manifestations of HIV Infection and AIDS

I. Acute Retroviral Syndrome (ARS) or Primary HIV Infection
 • Fever
 • Sore throat
 • Arthralgias and myalgias
 • Headache
 • Rash
 • Nausea, vomiting, and abdominal cramping
II. Asymptomatic Infection
 • None; converts to seropositive status
III. Persistent Generalized Lymphadenopathy
 • Enlargement of two or more extrainguinal sites for more than 3 months
IV. Other Acute Disease Symptoms
 • General malaise, fatigue
 • Low grade fever
 • Night sweats
 • Involuntary weight loss
 • Skin dryness, or rashes
V. Other Diseases and AIDS
 A. *AIDS Dementia Complex*
 B. *Secondary Infectious Diseases*
  • *Pneumocystis carinii* pneumonia
  • *Mycobacterium* tuberculosis
  • *Mycobacterium avium* complex
  • Candidiasis
  • Cryptosporidiosis
  • Cryptococcosis
  • Toxoplasmosis
  • Herpes simplex or herpes zoster
  • Cytomegalovirus
 C. *Secondary Cancers*
  • Kaposi's sarcoma
  • Non-Hodgkin's lymphoma
  • Cervical dysplasia and cervical cancer
 D. *Other Conditions*
  • Pelvic inflammatory disease
  • Human papillomavirus

Infections and lesions common with AIDS may also affect the CNS. Toxoplasmosis and non-Hodgkin's lymphoma are space-occupying lesions that may cause headache, altered mental status, and neurologic deficits. Cryptococcal meningitis and CMV infection also are common in people with AIDS.

Peripheral nervous system manifestations are also common in HIV-infected clients. Sensory neuropathies with manifestations of numbness, tingling, and pain in the lower extremities affect about 30% of clients with AIDS. A Guillain-Barré type of inflammatory demyelinating polyneuropathy can also occur, resulting in progressive weakness and paralysis.

## Opportunistic Infections

Opportunistic infections are the most common manifestations of AIDS, often occurring simultaneously. The risk of opportunistic infections is predictable by the T4 or CD4 cell count. The normal CD4 cell count is greater than 1000/mm³. When the CD4 count falls to less than 500/mm³, manifestations of

| BOX 9–2 | ■ Classification System for HIV Infection and Expanded AIDS Surveillance Case Definition for Adolescents and Adults |
|---|---|

| | Diagnostic Categories | | Clinical Categories | |
|---|---|---|---|---|
| CD4 + T-cell Categories | A Asymptomatic, Acute (Primary) HIV or PGL | | B Symptomatic, Not (A) or (C) Conditions | C AIDS-Indicator Conditions |
| (1) ≥500/mm$^3$ | A1 | | B1 | C1 |
| (2) 200–499/mm$^3$ | A2 | | B2 | C2 |
| (3) <200/mm$^3$ | A3 | | B3 | C3 |

As of January 1, 1993, people with AIDS-indicator conditions (clinical category C) and those in categories A3 or B3 were considered to have AIDS.

## CLINICAL CATEGORY A

One or more of the following conditions in an adolescent or adult with documented HIV infection and without conditions in categories B and C:

- Asymptomatic HIV infection
- Persistent generalized lymphadenopathy
- Acute HIV infection with accompanying illness or history of acute HIV infection

## CLINICAL CATEGORY B

Examples of conditions but are not limited to:

- Candidiasis, oral (thrush), or vulvovaginal (persistent, frequent, or poorly responsive to therapy)
- Cervical dysplasia / cervical carcinoma in situ
- Constitutional symptoms, such as fever (38.5°C) or diarrhea exceeding 1 month duration
- Hairy leukoplakia
- Herpes zoster involving at least two distinct episodes
- Pelvic inflammatory disease
- Peripheral neuropathy

## CLINICAL CATEGORY C

- Candidiasis of bronchi, trachea, or lungs; esophagus
- Coccidioidomycosis
- Cryptococcosis
- Cryptosporidiosis with persistant diarrhea
- Cytomegalovirus infection (other than of liver, spleen, or lymph nodes)
- CMV retinitis
- HIV encephalopathy
- Herpes simplex: chronic ulcers or bronchitis, pneumonitis, or esophagitis
- *Mycobacterium avium* complex or disseminated
- *Mycobacterium* tuberculosis
- *Pneumocystis carinii* pneumonia
- Progressive multifocal leukoencephalopathy
- *Salmonella* septicemia
- Toxoplasmosis of the brain
- Kaposi's sarcoma
- Cervical cancer, invasive
- Lymphoma
- HIV wasting syndrome

Note. Adapted from "Revised Classification System for HIV Infection and Expanded Case Definition for AIDS Among Adolescents and Adults," 1993, MMWR, CDC Recommendations and Reports, 41 (RR 17), pp. 1–19.

immunodeficiency are seen. With a count of less than 200/mm$^3$, opportunistic infections and cancers are likely.

## Pneumocystis Carinii Pneumonia

*Pneumocystis carinii* pneumonia (PCP) is the most common opportunistic infection affecting clients with AIDS. Approximately 75% to 80% of clients develop PCP at some point in their disease (Tierney et al., 2001). It tends to be recurrent, and is the cause of death in about 20% of clients with AIDS. PCP is caused by a common environmental fungus that is not pathogenic in clients with intact immune systems.

Unlike many pneumonias, the manifestations of PCP are nonspecific and may progress insidiously. Clients often present with fever, cough, shortness of breath, tachypnea, and tachycardia. Complaints of mild chest pain and sputum may also be present. Breath sounds may initially be normal. With severe disease, the client may present with cyanosis and significant respiratory distress.

## Tuberculosis

An estimated 4% of clients with AIDS develop tuberculosis, contributing significantly to the rise in incidence of this disease in the United States. In some clients, active tuberculosis results from reactivation of a prior infection. In other clients, it is a new, primary disease facilitated by impaired immune function. Rapid progression, diffuse pulmonary infiltrates, and disseminated disease occur more commonly in clients with AIDS. Multidrug-resistant strains of tuberculosis present a significant problem (Tierney et al., 2001).

Clients with pulmonary tuberculosis present with a cough productive of purulent sputum, fever, fatigue, weight loss, and lymphadenopathy. Disseminated disease affects the bone marrow, bone, joints, liver, spleen, CSF, skin, kidneys, gastrointestinal tract, lymph nodes, brain, and other sites.

## Candidiasis

*Candida albicans* infection is a common opportunistic infection in clients with AIDS. It is usually manifested as oral thrush or esophagitis. In women, vaginal candidiasis is frequent and often recurrent. Oral thrush presents as white, friable plaques on the buccal mucosa or tongue and, in the HIV-infected client, is often the first indication of progression to AIDS. Clients with esophagitis have difficulty swallowing and substernal pain or burning which increases with swallowing.

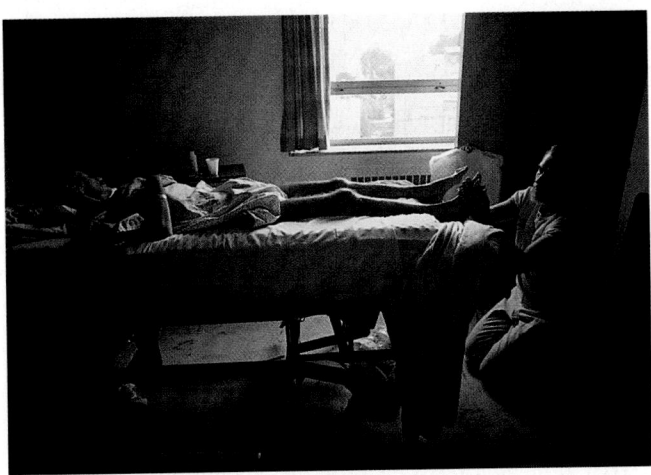

**Figure 9–8** ■ Wasting syndrome in a client with AIDS.

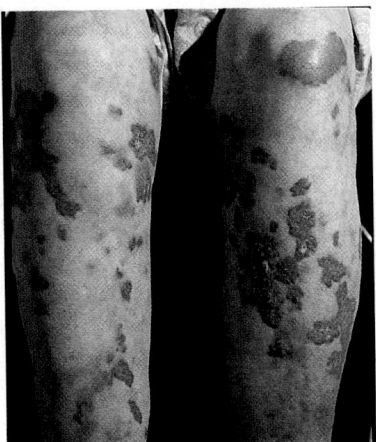

**Figure 9–9** ■ Kaposi's sarcoma lesions.

*Source: Zeva Oelbaum/Peter Arnold, Inc.*

## Mycobacterium Avium Complex

*Mycobacterium avium* complex (MAC) affects up to 25% of clients with AIDS, typically occurring late in the course of the disease when CD4 cell counts are less than 50/mm$^3$. MAC is more common in women than men. MAC is caused by organisms commonly found in food, water, and soil. It is a major cause of "wasting syndrome" in persons with AIDS (Figure 9–8 ■). Manifestations of MAC include chills and fever, weakness, night sweats, abdominal pain and diarrhea, and weight loss. Nearly every organ can be infected, and most people with MAC develop disseminated disease.

## Other Infections

Herpes virus infections are common in clients with AIDS and may be severe. CMV can affect the retina, the gastrointestinal tract, or lungs. Disseminated herpes simplex or herpes zoster may occur, although severe mucocutaneous manifestations are more common.

Parasitic infections with *Toxoplasma gondii* and *Cryptococcus neoformans* commonly affect the CNS. Toxoplasmosis occurs as encephalitis or an intracerebral mass lesion. Changes in mental status, focal neurologic signs, and seizures may result. *Cryptococcus* infection may present as either meningitis or disseminated disease, primarily affecting the lungs. *Cryptosporidium,* a protozoon affecting the gastrointestinal tract, is an important cause of prolonged diarrhea in AIDS clients. Bacterial salmonella infections are also a relatively common cause of diarrhea.

Women with AIDS have a high incidence of pelvic inflammatory disease (PID). Although the pathogens appear to be the same as those in PID affecting non-HIV-infected women, the disease is more severe. Inpatient treatment with intravenous antibiotics is often necessary.

## Secondary Cancers

As cell-mediated immune function declines, the risk of malignancy increases. The CDC classification of AIDS currently includes four cancers: Kaposi's sarcoma, non-Hodgkin's lymphoma, primary lymphoma of the brain, and invasive cervical carcinoma.

## Kaposi's Sarcoma

**Kaposi's sarcoma (KS)** is often the presenting symptom of AIDS. It remains the most common cancer associated with the disease. KS affects homosexual males with AIDS predominantly, occurring much less commonly in injection drug users and heterosexuals. At this time, the reason for the discrepancy is unknown.

A tumor of the endothelial cells lining small blood vessels, KS presents as vascular macules, papules, or violet lesions affecting the skin and viscera (Figure 9–9 ■). The face is a common site for skin lesions, especially the tip of the nose and pinnae of the ears. Common sites for visceral disease include the gastrointestinal tract, lungs, and lymphatic system.

The lesions of KS are usually painless initially, but may become painful as the disease progresses. Internally, the tumors may obstruct organ function or cause bleeding. When the lungs are involved, gas exchange may be severely impaired, resulting in pulmonary hemorrhage. This disease may progress slowly or rapidly. KS is an indicator of late-stage HIV disease, with an average survival time of 18 months after diagnosis.

## Lymphomas

Lymphomas are malignancies of the lymphoid tissue, including lymphocytes, lymph nodes, and the lymphoid organs such as the spleen and bone marrow. In AIDS, two lymphomas are common, non-Hodgkin's lymphoma and primary lymphoma of the brain. Hodgkin's disease also occurs 5 times more frequently in clients with HIV infection. The CNS is the usual site for these lymphomas, although they may be found in the bone marrow, gastrointestinal tract, liver, skin, and mucous membranes. They are aggressive tumors, growing and spreading rapidly. Headache and changes in mental status are common early symptoms of lymphomas affecting the CNS.

## Cervical Cancer

Of women with HIV infection, 40% have cervical dysplasia. Cervical cancer develops frequently and tends to be aggressive. Women with concurrent HIV infection and cervical cancer usually die of the cervical cancer, not AIDS. Because of this, it is recommended that women with HIV infection have Papanicolaou

(Pap) smears every 6 months and aggressive treatment of cervical dysplasia with colposcopic examination and cone biopsy.

## COLLABORATIVE CARE

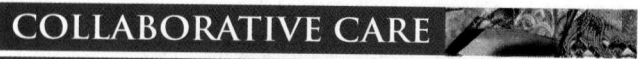

Although multiple research studies to identify a cure for HIV infection and AIDS are underway, no cure is currently available. This fact, plus the apparent universally fatal nature of the disease, make prevention a vital strategy in HIV care. New treatments are under investigation (see Box 9–3 below).

The goals of care for the client with HIV disease are as follows:

- Early identification of the infection
- Promoting health-maintenance activities to prolong the asymptomatic period as long as possible
- Prevention of opportunistic infections
- Treatment of disease complications, such as cancers
- Providing emotional and psychosocial support

### Diagnostic Tests

Diagnostic testing is used to screen and identify the infection, as well as to monitor the client's disease and immune status. The following diagnostic tests may be ordered.

- *Enzyme-linked immunosorbent assay (ELISA)* is the most widely used screening test for HIV infection. The ELISA test was developed in 1985 to screen blood donors. ELISA tests for HIV antibodies; it does not detect the virus. Therefore, a client may have a negative ELISA test early in the course of infection, before detectable antibodies have developed. The test has a 99.5% or higher sensitivity when performed at least 12 weeks after infection. This means that more than 99.5% of tests performed on blood containing HIV antibodies will show a positive result. False positives can occur; therefore, an initial positive result is always tested repeatedly and confirmed using a different method of antibody detection, usually the Western blot.

- *Western blot antibody testing* is more reliable but more time consuming and more expensive than ELISA. When combined with ELISA, however, a specificity of greater than 99.9% is achieved. Specificity is a measure of the probability that a negative test result indicates that no antibodies are present. In this test, the client's serum is mixed with HIV proteins to detect reaction. If antibodies to HIV are present, a detectable antigen-antibody response will occur.

- *HIV viral load tests* measure the amount of actively replicating HIV. Levels correlate with disease progression and response to antiretroviral medications. Levels greater than 5000 to 10,000 copies/mL indicate the need for treatment.

- *CBC* is performed to detect anemia, leukopenia, and thrombocytopenia, which are often present in HIV infection. Lymphopenia (or low levels of lymphocytes) is especially common in this disease.

- *CD4 cell count* is the most widely used test to monitor the progress of the disease and guide therapy. The CD4 cell count correlates so closely with the immunodeficiency disorders seen in AIDS. AIDS is now defined not only by the presence of opportunistic infections and other diseases indicative of immunodeficiency, but also by HIV-seropositive status and a CD4 count of less than 200/mm$^3$ or a percentage of CD4 lymphocytes of less than 14%. CD4 counts are recommended every 3 to 6 months for all people with HIV disease.

---

**BOX 9–3 ■ Investigational Immune-Based Treatment for HIV**

HIV infection progressively alters the function of and destroys CD4+ lymphocytes. CD4+ cells are essential to the function of the immune system, including the body's ability to respond to infections. These cells initiate, direct, and regulate immune responses and may also directly attack infected cells. They also are a source of cytokines, the chemical messengers of the immune system. Destruction of CD4+ cells by HIV devastates the immune system, facilitating the development of fatal infections and neoplasms in the infected person. Immune-based treatments indirectly affect the HIV by improving the function of the immune system through actions that inhibit cytokines, replenish cytokines, or restore immune function. These treatments, used alone or in combination with antiretroviral drugs, are being investigated for use in the treatment of HIV.

### INHIBITING CYTOKINES

Tumor necrosis factor alpha (TNF-alpha) is a cytokine secreted by activated monocytes and macrophages in response to infection, infestation, or tumor growth. It causes a proliferation of B cells and T cells. However, high levels of this cytokine may actually facilitate the development of disease by blocking the normal inflammatory response. It is believed that blocking the effect of TNF-alpha can suppress HIV production, although caution must be used.

### REPLENISHING CYTOKINES

Some cytokines (interleukin-2 [IL-2], interleukin-12 [IL-12], and interferon alpha [IFN-alpha]) may be helpful in treating HIV by stimulating the production of killer cells as well as increasing the function of lymphocytes. The interferons are part of the body's first line of defense against viruses. All of these agents have toxic side effects, requiring careful nursing assessment and care.

### RESTORING IMMUNE SYSTEM FUNCTION

HIV infection not only destroys CD4+ cells, but also eventually destroys the lymphoid organs, such as bone marrow and the thymus gland. Lymphocytes, including the CD4+ cells, are derived from stem cells in bone marrow and mature in the thymus. Two investigational treatments to restore the immune system are bone marrow transplant and thymus transplant. Bone marrow transplants have been used to correct other types of immune disorders (such as leukemia or lymphoma) but have yet to be effective in persons with HIV. A few thymus transplants have been done in HIV-infected persons, but have provided only temporary benefits.

In addition to these widely used tests, several other diagnostic tests may be performed:

- *Blood culture for HIV* provides the most specific diagnosis but is an expensive and cumbersome test that is not widely available in the United States.
- *Immune-complex-dissociated p24 assay* is a test for p24 (HIV) antigen in the blood. This antigen indicates active reproduction of HIV and tends to be positive prior to seroconversion and with advanced disease. It is most useful in monitoring disease progress and the antiviral activity of medications (Tierney et al., 2001).

Other diagnostic tests are used primarily to detect secondary cancers and opportunistic infections in the client with HIV. Tests ordered are both general and specific to the client's manifestations and may include the following:

- *Tuberculin skin testing* to detect possible tuberculosis infection
- *Magnetic resonance imaging (MRI)* of the brain to identify lymphomas
- *Specific cultures and serology examinations for opportunistic infections* such as PCP, toxoplasmosis, and others
- *Pap smears* every 6 months for early detection of cervical cancer in women

## Medications

Pharmacologic management of the client with HIV disease has two primary foci: (1) *to suppress the infection itself,* decreasing symptoms and prolonging life, and (2) *to treat opportunistic infections and malignancies.* Effectiveness of treatment is monitored by viral load and CD4 cell counts; positive results are indicated by a reduction in viral load along with preserving the CD4 count above 500 mm$^3$.

Three classes of drugs used in antiretroviral treatment include nucleoside reverse transcriptase inhibitors (NRTIs), nonnucleoside reverse transcriptase inhibitors (NNRTIs), and protease inhibitors. The new treatment protocol, highly active antiretroviral therapy (HAART), combines three or four antiretroviral drugs to reduce the incidence of drug resistance. However, when clients with AIDS at earlier stages or at lower risk of rapid progression are treated, combination therapies may burden them with complicated and expensive medication schedules and increase the potential of developing drug toxicities and drug resistance (Tierney et al., 2001). Clients beginning the HAART protocol must understand the benefits, risks, costs, and affects on daily life. HAART medications are expensive, costing more than $15,000 per year, and this does not include medications to prevent or treat opportunistic infections or cancer. Medications are scheduled for specific times throughout the day; therefore, leading a normal life becomes a challenge. In addition, all HAART medications cause major adverse reactions. Adherence to the treatment regimen is less than perfect, as with most chronic diseases, but in this case, the outcome could be fatal.

### Nucleoside Reverse Transcriptase Inhibitors

The NRTIs (also called nucleoside analogs) inhibit the action of viral reverse transcriptase, a retroviral enzyme that catalyzes the substrates for conversion and copying of viral RNA to DNA sequences. This enzyme is necessary for viral integration into cellular DNA and replication. The nucleoside analogs act as a chemical decoy for building blocks of the formation of the DNA copy, preventing the RNA from being copied into DNA. Each drug substitutes for a particular nucleoside base at different points on the chain. Medication administration guidelines for this group of drugs are discussed in the box below.

## Medication Administration

### Antiretroviral Nucleoside Analogs

#### ZIDOVUDINE (AZT, RETROVIR, ZDT)

Zidovudine is the first antiretroviral agent developed to treat HIV infection. It interferes with reverse transcriptase, thus inhibiting replication of the virus. Zidovudine is used for clients with CD4 cell counts of less than 500/μL. The usual dose is 500 to 600 mg per day in divided doses. It is administered orally.

#### Nursing Responsibilities

- Assess for possible contraindications to therapy including allergic response or a CD4 count of greater than 500/mm$^3$.
- Administer by mouth, instructing the client to swallow capsules whole.
- Assess for adverse effects. Nausea and headache are common. They may be self-limiting, decreasing with time, or significant and continuing, necessitating a change of therapy. Other adverse effects include insomnia, malaise, and confusion.
- Assess CBC and differential. Notify the physician of significant changes.

#### Client and Family Teaching

- Zidovudine will not cure HIV infection but slows its progress and reduces significant symptoms.
- Take the drug as prescribed every 4 to 6 hours to maintain an effective blood level.
- Take the drug at least ½ hour before or 1 hour after meals if tolerated.
- With this and all antiretroviral drugs, it is important to emphasize that the client is still infective and can pass the infection to others. Use safer sex practices and other measures to prevent transmission to partners. Do not donate blood.
- Notify the physician if signs of an infection or adverse response to zidovudine develop: sore throat, swollen lymph glands, fever; unusual fatigue or weakness; easy bruising, bleeding gums, or an injury that will not heal; persistent or intractable nausea; muscle pain or wasting.
- Continue all scheduled follow-up visits and laboratory studies to monitor for drug toxicity.

*(continued on page 260)*

## Medication Administration

### Antiretroviral Nucleoside Analogs (continued)

- Check with the physician before taking any prescription or over-the-counter drug containing aspirin or other NSAID.

### DIDANOSINE (DDI, VIDEX)

As with zidovudine, didanosine does not kill HIV but inhibits its replication within the cells. Its activity is similar to that of zidovudine. Didanosine has been shown to increase CD4 cell counts and lower p24 antigen levels (Tierney et al., 2001). Didanosine is used alone for clients who are intolerant or resistant to zidovudine. It is also being used with zidovudine in combination therapy regimens. Didanosine does not cause the anemia associated with zidovudine, but it may cause granulocytopenia. Didanosine is also associated with an increased risk of pancreatitis, peripheral neuritis, and dry mouth.

### Nursing Responsibilities

- Assess for possible contraindications to didanosine therapy, including previous episodes of pancreatitis and impaired renal or liver function.
- Administer as directed. Tablets are to be chewed thoroughly or dissolved in 1 ounce of water at room temperature. The powder form is dissolved in water prior to administration.
- Administer with caution to clients taking vincristine, rifampin, pentamidine, ethambutol, or metronidazole; the action of both drugs may be affected by concurrent administration. Intravenous pentamidine and trimethoprim-sulfamethoxazole taken concurrently may increase the risk of acute and fatal pancreatitis.
- Didanosine interferes with the absorption of ketoconazole and dapsone. Doses of these drugs should be scheduled at least 2 hours apart from didanosine doses.
- Evaluate for therapeutic response and possible adverse effects. Notify the physician if manifestations of peripheral neuropathy, diarrhea, depression, or other adverse effects develop.
- Stop the drug and notify the physician immediately if the client develops manifestations of pancreatitis or hepatic failure, including nausea and vomiting, severe abdominal pain, elevated bilirubin, or elevated serum enzymes (e.g., amylase, AST, ALT).

### Client and Family Teaching

- Take the drug as directed. The prescribed two-tablet dose must always be taken to get the required amount of antacid to prevent the drug from being destroyed by stomach acid.
- Take on an empty stomach, at least 1 hour before or 2 hours after meals.
- Do not use alcohol while taking didanosine; alcohol may increase the risk of pancreatitis.

- Stop the drug and call the doctor immediately if nausea, vomiting, abdominal pain, or diarrhea develops. These may indicate pancreatitis.
- Call the doctor if extremity pain, weakness, numbness, or tingling occurs. These side effects usually disappear when didanosine is discontinued.
- Other side effects to report to the physician include unusual bleeding or bruising, fatigue, weakness, fever, or persistent sore throat.

### ZALCITABINE (DDC, HIVID)

Another inhibitor of retroviral replication, zalcitabine is generally used in combination therapy regimens with zidovudine. It may also be used alone in clients who have become resistant to zidovudine. Unlike zidovudine and didanosine, zalcitabine is not toxic to the bone marrow, is inexpensive, and easy to administer (Tierney et al., 2001). It is, however, associated with severe peripheral neuropathy and an increased risk of pancreatitis. Other adverse effects include stomatitis, rash, fever, and arthritis.

### Nursing Responsibilities

- Assess for possible contraindications to zalcitabine: history of pancreatitis or evidence of impaired hepatic function.
- Check with the physician prior to administering the drug concurrently with vincristine, rifampin, intravenous pentamidine, ethambutol, pyrimethamine, dapsone, acyclovir, or metronidazole.
- Administer as prescribed, generally every 8 hours.
- Evaluate for desired effect of increased CD4 counts and lower blood levels of p24 antigen.
- Notify the physician if the client develops evidence of pancreatitis, impaired hepatic function, or painful peripheral neuropathy.

### Client and Family Teaching

- Take the medication on an empty stomach, 1 hour before or 2 hours after meals.
- Check with the physican before taking any other prescription or over-the-counter medication.
- Do not consume alcohol while taking this medication; alcohol increases the risk of pancreatitis.
- Notify the physician immediately if symptoms of peripheral neuropathy (see above section on didanosine) or pancreatitis develops.
- Report to the physician signs of infection or changes in condition.

---

- Zidovudine (Retrovir, AZT) was the first antiretroviral agent approved for use with HIV infection. It remains in widespread use and has been shown to decrease symptoms and prolong the lives of clients with AIDS. Zidovudine is often given to clients with a CD4 cell count of less than 500 because of evidence that it slows the progression to severe disease (Tierney et al., 2001). Zidovudine may also be used prophylactically following a documented parenteral exposure to HIV. AZT is used in combination with ddI, ddC, or 3TC.

- Didanosine (ddI, Videx) also inhibits reverse transcriptase and viral replication. It is used in combination therapy with AZT.
- Zalcitabine (ddC, Hivid) is also a retroviral inhibitor that interferes with the reproduction of HIV. It provides a valuable combination agent with AZT.
- Stavudine (d4T, Zerit) is a retroviral inhibitor that has been shown to increase CD4 cell counts and decrease serum p24 antigen levels. Current use is for clients who are intolerant of AZT.

- Lamivudine (3-TC, Epivir) is used for low CD4 cell counts or symptomatic disease as a first-line treatment in combination with AZT.
- Abacavir (Ziagen) is a potent inhibitor of reverse transcriptase; however, it may cause serious hypersensitivity reactions.
- Zidovudine plus lamivudine (Combivir) is the first combination drug and currently decreases HIV zidovudine-resistant strains.

## Protease Inhibitors

Protease is a viral enzyme necessary for the formation of specific viral protein needs for viral assembly and maturation. Protease inhibitors bond chemically with protease to block the function of the enzyme and result in the production of immature, noninfectious viral particles. When combined with other antiviral drugs, these chemicals increase the chance of eliminating the virus by interfering with different stages of its life cycle. However, viral resistance occurs rather quickly.

- Saquinavir (Invirase) is used in combination with nucleoside analogs to treat progression of the disease.
- Ritonavir (Norvir) is used in combination with nucleoside analogs to treat progression of the disease.
- Indinavir (Crixivan) is used in combination with nucleoside analogs to treat progression of the disease.

- Nelfinavir (Viracept) is used in cases of failure of or intolerance to other protease inhibitors.
- Amprenavir (Agenerase) is the newest protease inhibitor.
- Lopinavir/Ritonavir (Kaletra) is the first combination of protease inhibitors active against some HIV strains resistant to other protease inhibitors.

## Nonnucleoside Reverse Transcriptase Inhibitors

Nevirapine (Viramune), Delavirdine (Rescriptor), and Efavirenz (Sustiva) are NNRTIs that may be used in combination with nucleoside analogs and protease inhibitors. However, one limitation to NNRTIs is the high incidence of cross-resistance to NRTIs. Some studies have shown that Nevirapine and Efavirenz may significantly reduce serum levels of the protease inhibitors. Optimal combinations of these agents have not been established.

Other agents may also be administered in combination with antiretroviral therapy. Interferons, which are naturally occurring lymphokines, have been used alone and in combination. Alpha-interferon may be used to treat KS and in combination with zidovudine to slow disease progression. Gamma-interferon is also used.

A number of pharmacologic agents are used to prevent and treat opportunistic infections and malignancies in the client with HIV. These agents are outlined in Table 9–4.

**TABLE 9–4   Pharmacologic Treatment of Common Opportunistic Infections and Malignancies in HIV Disease**

| Condition | Treatment | Potential Adverse Effects |
|---|---|---|
| **Infections** | | |
| *Pneumocystis carinii* pneumonia | Trimethoprim/sulfamethoxazole<br>Pentamidine | Rash, neutropenia, anemia, thrombocytopenia, Stevens-Johnson syndrome<br>Hypotension, altered blood glucose levels, hypocalcemia, anemia and leukopenia, liver and renal toxicity, pancreatitis |
| Tuberculosis | Combination drug therapy using isoniazid, rifampin, ethambutol, pyrazinamide, or streptomycin | Multiple; see Chapter 36 |
| Candidiasis<br>  Oral thrush | Clotrimazole troches<br>Nystatin suspension | Few toxic responses noted for either medication |
|   Esophagitis or recurrent vaginitis | Ketoconazole<br>Fluconazole<br>Amphotericin B | Hepatitis, adrenal insufficiency<br>Hepatitis<br>Bone marrow toxicity, acute renal or hepatic failure; nausea, vomiting; chills, fever, headache |
| *Mycobacterium avium* complex | Combination therapy using<br>• Clarithromycin, plus<br>• Clofazimine<br>• Ethambutol<br>• Rifampin<br>• Ciprofloxacin<br>• Amikacin | <br>• Hepatitis, nausea, diarrhea<br>• Diarrhea, nausea, vomiting; skin discoloration, pruritus, rash<br>• Thrombocytopenia, hepatitis, optic neuritis<br>• Bone marrow depression, renal failure, hepatitis<br>• Nausea, rash<br>• Bone marrow depression, renal failure, ototoxicity, hepatitis |
| Cytomegalovirus | Ganciclovir<br>Foscarnet | Bone marrow depression, fever<br>Renal failure, electrolyte imbalances, seizures |
| Herpes simplex or herpes zoster | Acyclovir | Nausea, vomiting, diarrhea; CNS effects; renal failure |
| Toxoplasmosis | Pyrimethamine, plus<br>Sulfadiazine or clindamycin and folinic acid | Bone marrow depression, rash; respiratory failure; nausea, vomiting, abdominal pain; hematuria |
| **Malignancies**<br>Kaposi's sarcoma | Intralesional vinblastine | Inflammation and pain at injection site |
| Lymphoma | Combination chemotherapy | Nausea, vomiting; bone marrow toxicity; alopecia |

Many clients at some point require an implanted venous access device, such as a Groshong catheter, to facilitate blood sampling, intravenous medication administration, transfusions, and parenteral nutrition. See Chapter 10 for nursing care of the client with an intravenous access device implant. ⊝⊃

It is recommended that all HIV-infected clients receive pneumococcal, influenza, hepatitis B, and *Haemophilus influenzae b* vaccines. Persons with a positive PPD and negative chest X-ray are given prophylactic isoniazid (INH). When the client's CD4 cell count falls to less than 200, prophylactic treatment for PCP is begun, usually with trimethoprim-sulfamethoxazole. Clients with a CD4 count of less than 100 are started on prophylactic treatment for MAC.

## NURSING CARE

The client with HIV and AIDS has many care needs, including both physical and psychosocial support (see the Nursing Research box below). Because there is as yet no cure or effective treatment for HIV disease, many of these needs fall within the realm of nursing to promote knowledge and understanding, self-care, comfort, and quality of life. As with many diseases that have an ultimately fatal outcome, the course of HIV infection may well be affected by the client's social support systems, control, perceived self-efficacy in management, and coping mechanisms.

As the epidemic spreads, nurses are providing care for increasing numbers of clients with HIV infection. These clients are not only in special care settings, but also on general units, maternal-child units, hospice, and home settings. As clients with HIV disease live longer, nurses will increasingly encounter clients in whom HIV disease is a secondary diagnosis, with another primary diagnosis, for example, heart disease, diabetes mellitus, or an operative procedure.

## Prevention

To date, no safe immunization to protect against HIV infection has been developed. Education, counseling, and behavior modification are the primary tools for AIDS prevention. The benefit of education and behavior modification is evident in the homosexual male population. The incidence of new HIV infections in this population has declined dramatically in high-prevalence cities such as San Francisco. Nurses play a vital role in providing education about this epidemic and infection prevention for individuals and communities.

All sexually active individuals need to know how HIV is spread. Following are the only *totally* safe sex practices:

- No sex
- Long-term mutually monogamous sexual relations between two uninfected people
- Mutual masturbation without direct contact

Clients who do engage in sexual activity need to know and practice safer sex (see Box 9–4). Reducing the number of sexual partners—for example, by entering into and remaining in a long-term mutually monogamous relationship with an unin-

## Nursing Research

### Evidence-Based Practice and Nurses' Willingness to Care for People with AIDS

As reported by the Centers for Disease Control, the number of deaths from AIDS has declined. This is believed to be the result of both the slowing of the epidemic and of improved treatment, which has lengthened the life span of people with AIDS. However, as treatment continues to improve survival, a key challenge will be the increasing number of people living with HIV and AIDS—and the additional resources needed for services, treatment, and care.

Several studies have found that some professional nurses and students are resistant to caring for clients with AIDS. The willingness to provide care for clients with this illness involves moral choices about one's own mortality (death anxiety), spirituality, and social support. Sherman (1996) conducted a descriptive study to examine relationships among these choices and nurses' willingness to care for clients with AIDS. In a survey of 220 registered nurses employed in eight hospitals in the New York Metropolitan area, she found that willingness to care for AIDS patients was positively correlated with spirituality and perceived social support and negatively correlated with death anxiety. It is suggested that nurses' willingness to care for people with AIDS may be related not only to nurses' personal values and beliefs (expressed in spirituality) but also to their professional identity and role expectations.

#### Implications for Nursing
Standards of professional nursing clearly state that nurses will care for people with AIDS. To increase nurses' willingness to do so, students need to be better socialized into their roles and respon-

sibilities. Discussions within the classroom and clinical settings provide a safe means of bringing fears into the open and sharing experiences, one means of increasing self-awareness and developing a spiritual frame of reference. Student groups can thus serve as support groups, improving communications, decreasing isolation and anxiety, and improving self-esteem and morale. Within the work setting, perceived support from colleagues and administrators as well as increased contact with people with AIDS are important factors in making caring a rewarding and positive experience.

#### Critical Thinking in Client Care
1. This study was of registered nurses. What differences do you think might have been found if the study had been of student nurses in their first clinical course?
2. Carefully consider each of the following clients with AIDS and write a brief paragraph about how you would feel if you were assigned to care for them:
   a. A heterosexual female, age 25
   b. A homosexual male, age 35
   c. A newborn baby girl
   d. A 40-year-old single mother of three teenagers
   e. A 30-year-old homeless drug user
   f. A 17-year-old male with hemophilia, infected by blood transfusions

| BOX 9–4 | ■ Guidelines for Safer Sex |
| --- | --- |

- Practice mutual monogamy; if you are not in a mutually monogamous relationship, limit the number of sexual partners.
- Do not engage in unprotected sex, especially if HIV status of partner is unknown (remember that a person may be infected and infective for up to 6 months before converting to seropositive status).
- When entering into a new monogamous relationship, both partners should undergo HIV testing initially. If both are negative, practice abstinence or safer sex for 6 months, followed by retesting. If results still indicate that both partners are negative, sexual activity can probably be considered safe.
- Use latex condoms for oral, vaginal, or anal intercourse; avoid natural or animal skin condoms, which allow passage of HIV.
- For vaginal or anal sex, lubricate the condom with the spermicidal agent nonoxynol-9 for additional protection.
- Do not use an oil-based lubricant such as petroleum jelly, which can result in condom damage; water-based lubricants are acceptable.
- Women should carry and use a female condom.

- Remember that use of other means of birth control, such as oral contraceptives, provide no protection against HIV; barrier protection with a condom is necessary.
- Engage in safer sexual practices that are less damaging to sensitive tissues (e.g., mutual masturbation, avoiding anal or oral sex).
- Do not use drugs or alcohol.
- Do not share needles, razors, toothbrushes, sexual toys, or other items that may be contaminated with blood or body fluids.
- If HIV positive:
  a. Do not engage in unprotected sexual activity.
  b. Inform all current and former sexual partners of HIV status.
  c. Inform all health care personnel—primary care providers, physicians and dentists in particular—of HIV status.
  d. Do not donate blood, plasma, blood products, sperm, organs, or tissue.
  e. If female, do not become pregnant.

fected partner—reduces the risk. Clients should not engage in unprotected sex, especially if the HIV status of the partner is unknown. Latex condoms have been shown to reduce the risk of transmitting HIV. Their effectiveness is improved when nonoxynol-9, a spermicide, is used for lubrication; however, it may cause genital ulcers which can facilitate HIV transmission. To be effective, condoms must be used with every sexual encounter involving vaginal, oral, or anal intercourse. They also need to be applied and removed properly. A female condom is also available for use.

The most difficult group of high-risk people to reach and educate has been injection drug users. People in this group should never share needles, syringes, or other drug paraphernalia. Many cities have initiated needle-exchange programs, providing a sterile needle and syringe in exchange for a used one. A fresh solution of household bleach and water in a 1:10 ratio is effective to clean "works" when sterile supplies are not available. It is important to also teach people in this population about safer sex practices, because most heterosexual HIV transmission occurs between injection drug users and their partners.

Screening of voluntary blood donors and donated blood supplies has reduced the risk of transmission by transfusion to 1 in 100,000. Because current blood-screening methods use antibody testing, receiving donated blood continues to carry a small risk. Clients in the *window period* between contraction of the virus and the development of detectable antibodies are able to transmit the virus to others, even though they do not yet test positive for HIV. This window period usually lasts from 6 weeks to 6 months; rarely, it lasts up to 1 year. When possible, encourage clients to use autologous transfusion, donating their own blood prior to an anticipated surgery. Seeking donations from family members is not encouraged for several reasons. Family members may have engaged in high-risk behaviors but lie about their risk because of embarrass-

ment or fear of discovery. Furthermore, the family member may have a different blood type or have other contraindications to donating.

Encourage HIV-positive clients to abstain from donating blood, organs, or sperm. They should understand tactics to avoid exchange of body fluids by not sharing needles or other drug paraphernalia, not sharing razors, and not obtaining a tattoo. Stress the importance of informing all medical personnel providing direct care (especially anyone performing a dental, surgical, or obstetric procedure) about the diagnosis.

Health care workers can prevent most exposures to HIV by using standard precautions (refer to Appendix and see Figure 9–10 ■). Testing to determine HIV status remains voluntary and relies on the use of antibody-screening methods. It is therefore impossible to identify every client who is HIV positive. With standard precautions, all clients are treated alike, eliminating the need to know the client's HIV status. All high-risk body fluids are treated as if they are infectious, and barrier precautions are used to prevent skin, mucous membrane, or percutaneous exposure to them. Counseling and testing are provided to health care workers with a documented needle-stick exposure. Some clinicians and facilities recommend prophylactic AZT therapy after needle-stick or splash exposure; however, it must be initiated immediately, and its effectiveness has yet to be established.

## Assessment

Collect the following data through health history and physical examination. Further focused assessments are described with nursing interventions below.

- Health history: risk factors (transfusion, unprotected sex, needle exposure), infections (sexually transmitted diseases, hepatitis, TB), medications, recreational drug use, foreign travel, pets

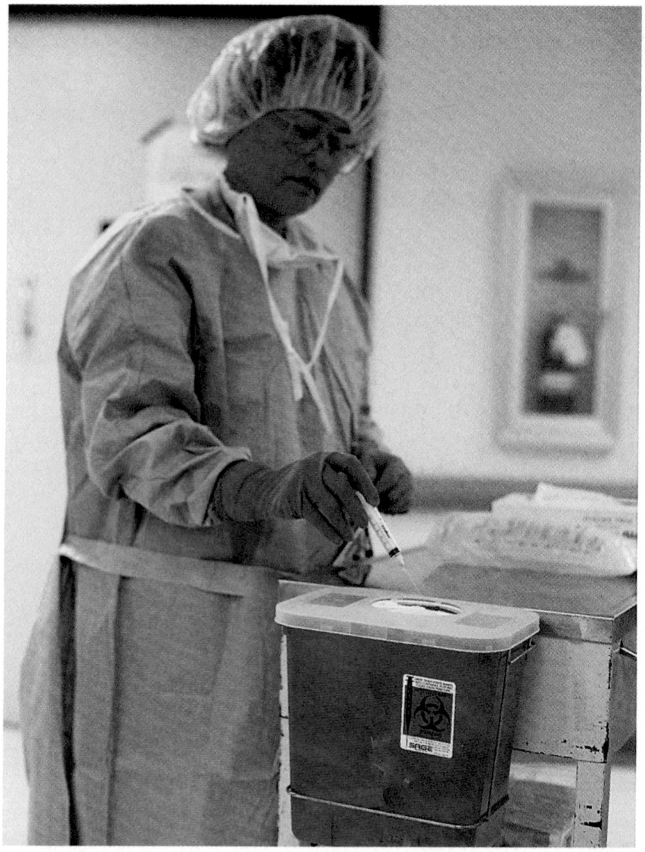

**Figure 9–10** ■ This nurse is disposing of a needle and syringe in a special container, a necessary practice to avoid the transmission of HIV through needle sticks with contaminated needles.

- Physical assessment: height, weight, nutrition, skin and mucous membranes, vision, lymph nodes, breath sounds, abdominal tenderness, motor strength, coordination, cranial nerves, gait, deep tendon reflexes, genitourinary examination, mental status

## Nursing Diagnoses and Interventions

Nursing care needs for the client with HIV infection change over the course of the disease. Preventive health care measures, health maintenance activities, education, and support of coping mechanisms are important in the early stages of the disease. Counseling the client with a new diagnosis of HIV infection is vital. HIV infection and AIDS continue to carry a social stigma that may interfere with the client's usual support systems and coping mechanisms. As the disease progresses and the client experiences more physical symptoms, direct care needs become more important while the need for psychosocial support continues. Acute exacerbation of opportunistic infections may necessitate hospitalization, but typically the client is managed at home.

### Ineffective Coping

On receiving the test results indicating HIV seropositive status, the person with HIV infection is faced with multiple issues rarely affecting other clients. First and foremost, HIV is a disease for which there is no known cure and which is, at this time,

thought to be almost universally fatal. Social support systems, family relationships, and the ability to obtain and retain useful work and health insurance may be disrupted by the disease. The client may experience guilt about his or her lifestyle and how the disease was contracted. As the disease progresses, social isolation, fatigue, body image changes, medication side effects, and multiple other issues affect the client's abilities to cope.

- Assess social support network and usual methods of coping. *This will help both the nurse and the client identify people and mechanisms that can help the client cope more effectively with the disease.*
- If possible, assign a primary nurse, whether the setting is home health, hospice, or acute care. *This helps promote the development of a therapeutic and trusting relationship and provides for continuity of care.*
- Plan for consistent, uninterrupted time with the client. *Time and a consistent presence encourage the client to express feelings and work through issues related to HIV infection.*
- Interact at every opportunity outside of providing specific nursing care treatments. *This purposeful interaction communicates caring and acceptance without fear of HIV disease.*
- Support the client's social network. *Nontraditional families may offer more support than the traditional family. This in turn may necessitate a liberal interpretation of the term* family *if unit policy is* immediate family only.
- Promote interaction between the client, significant others, and family. *Hospitalization and manifestations of HIV disease may bring about isolation from others and decrease the client's ability to cope.*
- Encourage involvement in making care decisions. *This gives the client a greater sense of self-worth and control over the situation, increasing coping abilities.*
- Set and maintain limits on manipulative and other destructive behaviors. *The client who is unable to limit inappropriate behaviors needs the external control established by setting limits.*
- Assist to accept responsibility for actions without blaming others. *Effective coping cannot occur without accepting responsibility for one's actions.*
- Support positive coping behaviors, decisions, actions, and achievements. *As self-esteem is enhanced, coping improves.*

### Impaired Skin Integrity

Dryness, malnutrition, immobility from fatigue, and skin lesions on pressure sites contribute to impaired integrity of the skin for the client with HIV disease. Maintaining skin integrity is important because of the progressive and debilitating nature of the disease. It is also a consideration both as the first line of defense against infection in an immunosuppressed client and as a site for secondary manifestations such as KS and herpes.

- Monitor the skin frequently for lesions and areas of breakdown. *Early identification of impaired skin integrity allows prompt intervention.*
- Monitor lesions for signs of infection or impaired healing. *Infection or poor tissue perfusion not only impairs healing but may lead to further skin breakdown.*

- Turn at least every 2 hours, more frequently if necessary. *Turning decreases unrelieved pressure on bony prominences and improves circulation to the tissues.*
- Use pressure-relieving devices, such as pressure and egg crate mattresses, or sheep skin pads for elbows and heels. *These devices provide prophylactic relief of pressure.*
- Keep skin clean and dry using mild, nondrying soaps or oils for cleansing. *Night sweats and diarrhea, if present, can cause breakdown and damage to the skin. Frequent cleansing with nondrying products discourages bacterial growth, thus reducing the risk of infection.*

**PRACTICE ALERT**  *Applying protective creams to reddened areas in the rectal area protects skin from the caustic effects of diarrhea.* ■

- Massage around but not over affected pressure sites to increase circulation to the surrounding tissue. *Massaging over the affected area can cause skin breakdown.*
- If blisters are noted, leave intact, and dress with a hydrocolloid (Duoderm) dressing. *Blisters provide natural sterile coverings for damaged tissue, improving healing and preventing bacterial invasion.*
- Caution against scratching. If confused, trim fingernails and use mitts or soft restraints to prevent scratching. Check for circulation of hands and fingers frequently if mitts or restraints are used. *Scratching and skin damage allow bacteria to be introduced into lesions, increasing the risk of infection. Tight or restrictive restraints or mitts may compromise circulation.*
- Avoid the use of heat or occlusive dressings. *Heat can further dry and damage the skin; occlusive dressings may impair circulation and lead to ulceration.*
- Prevent skin shearing by using a turnsheet and adequate personnel when repositioning. *Shearing causes tissue trauma that can lead to decubitus ulcers.*
- Encourage ambulation if possible; if the client is confined to bed, encourage active or passive range-of-motion exercises. *Activity increases circulation, decreases pressure and skin breakdown, and helps maintain muscle tone.*
- Monitor nutritional intake and albumin levels. *Maintenance of optimal nutrition decreases the risk of tissue breakdown and improves resistance to infection.*

### Imbalanced Nutrition: Less Than Body Requirements

Many factors associated with HIV disease, including manifestations of the disease itself, put the client at risk for altered nutrition and weight loss. Nausea and anorexia may be manifestations of the disease or the result of antiretroviral therapy. Chronic diarrhea is a common manifestation of constitutional HIV disease. Wasting syndrome is also common. It is manifested by involuntary weight loss of greater than 10% to 15% of baseline weight, severe diarrhea, fever, and chronic fatigue and weakness. The exact cause of wasting syndrome is unclear, but the diarrhea and fatigue contribute, as does the increased metabolic rate associated with fever. Oral and esophageal candidiasis and KS of the gastrointestinal tract may cause painful

swallowing, making eating difficult and thereby contributing to anorexia. Poor nutritional status in the client with HIV can ultimately result in altered comfort, a change in body image, muscle wasting, increased risk of infection, and higher mortality and morbidity.

- Assess nutritional status, including weight; body mass; caloric intake; and laboratory studies, such as total protein and albumin levels, hemoglobin, and hematocrit. *These factors provide a baseline to determine the effectiveness of interventions.*
- Identify possible causes of altered nutrition. *Identification of causes provides direction for planned interventions.*
- Administer prescribed medications for candidiasis and other manifestations as ordered. *Eliminating this opportunistic infection improves comfort and facilitates food intake. Topical viscous anesthetic can help reduce pain and improve oral intake.*
- Administer antidiarrheal medications after stools and antiemetics prior to meals. Provide antipyretics as needed to control fever. *Reducing diarrhea will improve nutrient absorption; preprandial medication with an antiemetic reduces nausea and improves food intake. Reduction of fever lowers the body's metabolic demands.*

**PRACTICE ALERT**  *High-fiber foods can increase intestinal motility and the incidence of diarrhea.* ■

- Provide a diet high in protein and kilocalories. *A high-protein, high-kilocalorie diet provides the necessary nutrients to meet metabolic and tissue healing needs.*
- Offer soft foods and serve small portions. *Soft foods are easily digested. Small portions are more appealing to the anorectic or nauseated client.*
- Involve in meal planning and encourage significant others to bring favorite foods from home. *The client is more likely to consume adequate amounts of preferred foods. Allowing food choices enhances the client's sense of control.*
- Assist with eating as needed. *Fatigue and weakness can prevent the client from eating an adequate amount of food.*
- Provide supplementary vitamins and enteral feedings, such as Ensure. *This improves nutritional status and caloric intake.*
- Provide or assist with frequent oral hygiene. *Oral hygiene improves comfort and appetite, and reduces the risk of mucosal lesions.*
- Administer appetite stimulants, such as megestrol (Megace) and dronabinol (Marinol) as ordered. *Both drugs may increase appetite and promote weight gain.*

### Ineffective Sexuality Patterns

The diagnosis of HIV infection can significantly alter the client's expressions of sexuality. Guilt over the diagnosis may interfere with libido. The client may be angry with a significant other or partner if that person was the probable source of infection. The client may fear spreading the disease to others via sexual relations. As the disease progresses, its manifestations can affect body image and self-esteem, impairing sexuality. Other symptoms, such as nausea, fatigue, and weakness, may also interfere with libido and sexual satisfaction.

- Examine your feelings about sexuality, your role in dealing with a client's sexuality, the client's lifestyle, and sexual preferences. *To deal effectively with the client's concerns, it is vital that the nurse be comfortable with his or her own feelings of sexuality and be able to accept the client's lifestyle. Referring the client to another nurse or counselor may be necessary.*
- Establish a trusting, therapeutic relationship through the use of time, active listening, caring, and self-disclosure. Maintain a nonthreatening, nonjudgmental attitude toward the client. *Sexuality is a private issue that will be uncomfortable or impossible for the nurse and client to discuss without a mutually trusting relationship.*
- Provide factual information about HIV infection and its effects. *This helps the client separate fears and myths from reality.*
- Discuss safer sex practices, including hugging, cuddling, nonsexual contact, the use of latex condoms and spermicidal lubricant, and mutual masturbation. *Alternative forms of sexual activity and expressing affection can allow the client and significant other to remain close throughout the course of the disease.*
- Encourage discussion of fears and concerns with significant other. *Open communication helps them to deal with issues related to sexuality.*
- For the client without a significant other, stress the need to continue to meet people and develop social relationships while practicing safer sex. *The risk of isolation is high in the client with HIV infection, and relationships with others help the client to cope with the disease.*
- Refer the client and significant other to local support groups for people and partners of people with HIV. *Support groups provide a social and support network of people facing the same issues.*

## Using NANDA, NIC, and NOC

Chart 9–3 shows links between NANDA, NIC, and NOC when caring for the client with AIDS.

## Home Care

Teaching needs for both the client and significant other are extensive. The primary need is information about the disease, its spread, and its expected course. The client and family need current factual information to plan realistically and to combat myths, misperceptions, and prejudices. At the same time, it is important to include information about current research and progress in treating the disease to maintain a sense of hopefulness.

The following topics should be discussed with the client and family to prepare for home care.

- Guidelines for safer sex practices
- Nutrition, rest and exercise, stress reduction, lifestyle changes, and maintaining a positive outlook
- Infection prevention and transmission including handwashing and wearing gloves when handling client's secretions or excretions
- Importance of regular medical follow-up and monitoring of immune status
- Signs and symptoms of opportunistic infections and malignancies, as well as other symptoms that should be reported
- Medications and adverse effects
- Use and care of implanted venous access devices, total parenteral nutrition, intravenous pumps and continuous medication delivery systems, and intravenous or aerosolized medications
- Cessation of smoking, alcohol, and recreational or illicit drug use
- Home health services
- Hospice and respite care services
- Community resources, such as support groups, social agencies, and counselors
- Helpful resources:
  - CDC National AIDS Hotline
  - Gay Men's Health Crisis Network
  - National Association of People with AIDS
  - National Organization for HIV over Fifty

*MediaLink | AIDS/HIV RESOURCES*

### CHART 9–3 NANDA, NIC, AND NOC LINKAGES

#### The Client with HIV Infection

| NURSING DIAGNOSES | NURSING INTERVENTIONS | NURSING OUTCOMES |
|---|---|---|
| • Disturbed Body Image | • Body Image Enhancement | • Self-Esteem |
| • Caregiver Role Strain | • Caregiver Support | • Caregiver Emotional Health |
| | | • Caregiver Performance: Direct Care |
| • Diarrhea | • Diarrhea Management | • Electrolyte and Acid-Base Balance |
| | | • Fluid Balance |
| • Fatigue | • Energy Management | • Endurance |
| | | • Nutritional Status: Energy |
| • Ineffective Airway Clearance | • Airway Management | • Respiratory Status: Gas Exchange |
| • Risk for Disturbed Thought Processes | • Dementia Management | • Cognitive Orientation |

*Note. Data from Nursing Outcomes Classification (NOC) by M. Johnson & M. Maas (Eds.), 1997, St. Louis: Mosby; Nursing Diagnoses: Definitions & Classification 2001–2002 by North American Nursing Diagnosis Association, 2001, Philadelphia: NANDA; Nursing Interventions Classification (NIC) by J.C. McCloskey & G. M. Bulechek (Eds.), 2000, St. Louis: Mosby. Reprinted by permission.*

## Nursing Care Plan
## A Client with HIV Infection

Sara Lu is a 26-year-old elementary school teacher who lives with her parents and two younger sisters. Ms. Lu is very close to her parents and sisters; they share everything with each other. During the required physical for admission to graduate school, Ms. Lu tells her physician that lately she has felt fatigued. She also states that she has had a persistent sore throat, intermittent bouts of diarrhea, and mild shortness of breath for about a month. She takes no routine medications other than a daily multivitamin and an occasional acetaminophen tablet for a headache. She is active in a drama club in her community, and she jogs 3 miles three to four times a week. She is engaged to be married; her wedding date is 6 months away. Her fiancé is the only person with whom she has had sexual relations. Her sexual activity has been unprotected. Ms. Lu has a history of open heart surgery 7 years ago to correct a congenital valve defect. She has been physically healthy since that time, until about a month or two ago. The physician orders a mononucleosis test, enzyme-linked immunosorbent assay (ELISA), Western blot analysis, CD4 T-cell count, a p24 antigen test, and an erythrocyte sedimentation rate (ESR). She has been asked to return in 1 week for follow-up.

### ASSESSMENT

On Ms. Lu's follow-up visit, Carole Kee, RN, obtains her nursing history. Ms. Lu continues to have flulike symptoms but has improved somewhat. She states that she just has not been as active as usual and is worried about her health. Her appetite has decreased because of soreness in her mouth, and she has noted some whitish patches on her tongue and cheeks.

A chest X-ray film reveals no abnormality. The results of her laboratory tests are as follows:

- ELISA: positive for antibodies against HIV
- Western blot analysis: positive for antibodies against HIV
- p24 antigen test: positive for circulating HIV antigens
- ESR: increased to 25 mm/h (normal for women is 15 to 20 mm/h; normal for men is 10 to 15 mm/h)
- CD4 T-cell count: 599/mm$^3$ (normal range is 600 to 1200 mm$^3$)

Ms. Lu's physical examination reveals that she has enlarged lymph nodes in her neck and white patches on her oral mucosa. Her skin is warm to the touch. Her vital signs are as follows: T 99.9°F (37.7°C), P 84, R 20, and BP 120/78.

Ms. Lu is told of the results of her laboratory tests and the medical diagnosis of HIV infection. Ms. Lu is obviously distressed and wants to know how this happened, its meaning, whether she has infected her loved ones, and whether she will get better.

### DIAGNOSIS

- *Imbalanced nutrition: Less than body requirements* related to soreness in mouth
- *Risk for deficient fluid volume* related to decreased fluid intake and diarrhea
- *Risk for infection* related to altered immune protection
- *Anxiety* related to diagnosis and fear
- *Deficient knowledge* about the HIV disease process

### EXPECTED OUTCOMES

- Maintain adequate nutrition for optimal body and cellular function.

- Consume at least 2500 mL of fluid per day.
- Remain free of infections and their complications.
- Verbalize anxiety and use appropriate coping mechanisms.
- Verbalize and demonstrate knowledge of HIV disease.
- Verbalize measures to prevent HIV transmission to others, including safer sex practices.

### PLANNING AND IMPLEMENTATION

- Monitor daily weight and intake and output.
- Monitor dietary habits and serum albumin levels.
- Teach Ms. Lu the importance of consuming a nutritionally balanced diet and maintaining adequate fluid intake.
- Suggest strategies for coping with anorexia and nausea.
- Provide dietary consultation referral.
- Encourage oral care before and after meals.
- Assess bowel sounds and monitor elimination pattern.
- Administer antiemetic and antimotility medications as ordered.
- Monitor for signs of dehydration, such as poor skin turgor, oliguria, and orthostatic hypotension.
- Increase fluid to 2500 mL daily.
- Use strict aseptic technique for all invasive procedures.
- Teach Ms. Lu to avoid exposure to infection and people with known illnesses.
- Administer antiretroviral medications and antibiotics as prescribed, and monitor response.
- Encourage maintenance of regular physical exercise.
- Provide opportunities for Ms. Lu to verbalize her feelings.
- Avoid false reassurances.
- Provide appropriate and adequate information about HIV/AIDS.
- Teach safer sex practices and other measures to prevent HIV transmission.
- Teach anxiety-controlling techniques, such as deep breathing and meditation.

### EVALUATION

Ms. Lu is eager to learn about her illness and wants her family to come with her for further explanation. She states that she is sure her fiancé will be available as well. Ms. Lu is taking home antifungal medication, diet plans, and a schedule for increased exercise. She will return in 1 week for counseling and in 1 month for a follow-up physical.

### Critical Thinking in the Nursing Process

1. How does age effect the body's response to fighting HIV? What other factors affect the risk of HIV infection and its progression?
2. Are the laboratory results for Ms. Lu a true indication that she is HIV positive? What additional tests might be ordered?
3. What is the most likely source of Ms. Lu's infection? What measures are used to reduce this risk, and how did she contract HIV? What is another possible source of Ms. Lu's HIV infection?
4. Ms. Lu says that her fiancé would like to have a child. How will you counsel her regarding pregnancy and childbearing?

See Evaluating Your Response in Appendix C.

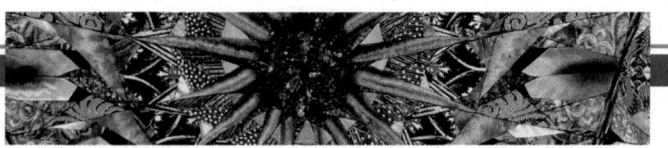

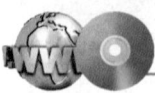 ## EXPLORE MediaLink

NCLEX review questions, case studies, care plan activities, MediaLink applications, and other interactive resources for this chapter can be found on the Companion Website at www.prenhall.com/lemone.

Click on Chapter 9 to select the activities for this chapter. For animations, video clips, more NCLEX review questions, and an audio glossary, access the Student CD-ROM accompanying this textbook.

## TEST YOURSELF

1. Which one of the following conditions is caused by a type I IgE-mediated hypersensitivity reaction?

   a. Autoimmune hemolytic anemia
   b. Systemic lupus erythematosus
   c. Graft rejection
   d. Anaphylaxis

2. A client received a liver transplant 1 day ago. If the client were to develop an acute transplant rejection episode, when should the nurse expect to see the manifestations?

   a. Approximately 4 days to 3 months later
   b. Approximately 2 days later
   c. Within the first 24 hours
   d. Within the first 8 hours

3. The nurse notes a cough, shortness of breath, and tachypnea in a client with AIDS. Which opportunistic infection is probably causing these manifestations?

   a. *Toxoplasma gondii*
   b. *Cytomegalovirus*
   c. *Pneumocystis carinii*
   d. *Cryptococcus neoformans*

4. Which of the following explanations should the nurse give to a client who has tested positive for HIV?

   a. "You have been diagnosed with AIDS."
   b. "At this point, AIDS is not active in your blood."
   c. "This means that you will not develop AIDS in the future."
   d. "Antibodies to the AIDS virus are present in the blood."

5. Clients taking zidovudine (Retrovir) should be monitored for which of the following adverse reactions?

   a. Cardiotoxicity
   b. Leukopenia
   c. Nephrotoxicity
   d. Polycythemia

See Test Yourself answers in Appendix C.

## BIBLIOGRAPHY

Abramowicz, M. (Ed.). (2000). *Drugs for HIV infection.* New Rochelle, NY: The Medical Letter, Inc.

Abrams, A. C. (2001). *Clinical drug therapy: Rationales for practice* (6th ed.). Philadelphia: Lippincott.

Ackley, B. J., & Ladwig, G. B. (2002). *Nursing diagnosis handbook* (5th ed.). St. Louis: Mosby.

American Nurses Association. (1997). *Position statement: Needle exchange and HIV.* Washington, DC: ANA.

Bihari, B., Levin, S., Malebranche, D., & Valdez, H. (2000). Caring for diverse populations: Identifying HIV infection. *Patient Care, 34*(9), 55–56, 58, 60–62, 65–66, 68, 73, 76–77.

Braunwald, E., Fauci, A. S., Kasper, D. L., Hauser, S. L., Longo, D. L., & Jameson, J. L. (2001). *Harrison's Principles of internal medicine* (15th ed.). New York: McGraw-Hill.

Bullock, B. A., & Henze, R. L. (2000). *Focus on pathophysiology.* Philadelphia: Lippincott.

Carrico, R.M. (2001). What to do if you're exposed to a bloodborne pathogen. *Home Health-care Nurse, 19*(6), 362–368.

Centers for Disease Control. (1992). 1993 Revised classification system for HIV infection and expanded case definition for AIDS among adolescents and adults. *MMWR, CDC Recommendations and Reports, 41*(RR-17), 1–19.

_____ . (1996). Update: Provisional public health recommendations for chemoprophylaxis after occupational exposure to HIV. *MMWR, 45,* 468–472.

Cheng, C., & Umland, E.M. (2001). A practical update on antiretroviral therapy. *Patient Care, 35*(10), 99–106.

Chernecky, R., & Berger, B. (1997). *Laboratory tests and diagnostic procedures* (2nd ed.). Philadelphia: Saunders.

Cournoyer, S. (1997). How much do you know about the opportunistic diseases of AIDS? *Nursing97, 27*(6), 1–2, 4, 6.

Early HIV Infection Guideline Panel. (1994). *Evaluation and management of early HIV infection: Clinical practice guidelines* (AHCPR Publication No. 94-0572). Rockville, MD: AHCPR Public Health Service, USDHHS.

Esch, J.F., & Frank, S.V. (2001). HIV drug resistance and nursing practice. *American Journal of Nursing, 101*(6), 30–36.

Fryback, P., & Reinert, B. (1997). Alternative therapies and control for health in cancer and AIDS. *Clinical Nurse Specialist, 11*(2), 64–69.

Joint United Nations Programme on HIV/AIDS. (2000). Men make a difference. Press kit: world AIDS day. HIV/AIDS in Africa. Available http://www.unaids.org/wac/2000/wad00/files/FS_Africa.htm

Kee, J. (1999). *Laboratory & diagnostic tests with nursing implications* (5th ed.). Upper Saddle River, NJ: Prentice Hall.

Kirton, C.A., Ferri, R.S., & Eleftherakis, V. (1999). Primary care and case management of persons with HIV/AIDS. *Nursing Clinics of North America, 34*(1), 71–94.

Johnson, M., Maas, M., & Moorhead, S. (2000). *Iowa outcomes project: Nursing outcomes classification (NOC)* (2nd ed.). Upper Saddle River, NJ: Prentice Hall.

Lueckenotte, A.G. (2000). *Gerontologic nursing* (2nd ed.). St. Louis: Mosby.

Lutz, C., & Przytulski, K. (2001). *Nutrition and diet therapy* (3rd ed.). Philadelphia: F.A. Davis.

Lyon, D.E., & Munro, C. (2001). Disease severity and symptoms of depression in black Americans infected with HIV. *Applied Nursing Research, 14*(1), 3–10.

McCloskey, J.C., & Bulechek, G. M. (2000). *Iowa interventions project: Nursing interventions classifications (NIC)* (3rd ed.). Upper Saddle River, NJ: Prentice Hall.

Muehlbauer, P., & White, R. (1998). Are you prepared for interleukin-2? *RN, 61*(2), 34, 36–38.

National Institute of Allergy and Infectious Diseases. (2000). *HIV infection in women.* Bethesda, MD: National Institutes of Health.

_____ . (2001). HIV/AIDS statistics (fact sheet). Available, http://www.niaid.nih.gov/factsheets/aidstat.htm

National Institute of Occupational Safety and Health. (1997). *Preventing allergic reactions to natural rubber latex in the workplace.* Washington, DC: USDHHS.

Novello, A. (1993, June). *Surgeon General's report to the American public on HIV infection and AIDS—extracts.* Rockville, MD: CDC National AIDS Clearinghouse.

Panel on Clinical Practices for Treatment of HIV Infection. (2000). Guidelines for the use of antiretroviral agents in HIV-infected adults and adolescents. Available http://www.hivatis.org

Porche, D.J. (1999). State of the art: Antiretroviral and prophylactic treatments in HIV/AIDS. *Nursing Clinics of North America, 34*(1), 95–112.

Porth, C. (2002). *Pathophysiology: Concepts of altered health states* (6th ed.). Philadelphia: Lippincott.

Roitt, I. (1994). *Essential immunology* (8th ed.). London: Blackwell.

Shannon, M.T., Wilson, B.A., & Stang, C.L. (2001). *Nursing drug guide 2001.* Upper Saddle River, NJ: Prentice Hall.

Sherman, D. (1996). Nurses' willingness to care for AIDS patients and spirituality, social support, and death anxiety. *Image: Journal of Nursing Scholarship, 28*(3), 205–213.

Sowell, R.L., Moneyham, L., & Aranda-Naranjo, B. (1999). The care of women with AIDS. *Nursing Clinics of North America, 34*(1), 179–199.

Swenson, M.R. (2000). Autoimmunity and immunotherapy. *Journal of Intravenous Nursing, 23*(5S), S8–S13.

Szirony, T.A. (1999). Infection with HIV in the elderly population. *Journal of Gerontological Nursing, 25*(10), 25–31.

Thurlow, K.L. (2001). Latex allergies: Management and clinical responsibilities. *Home Healthcare Nurse, 19*(6), 369–376.

Tierney, L., McPhee, S., & Papadakis, M. (Eds). (2001). *Current medical diagnosis & treatment* (40th ed.). New York: Lange Medical Books/McGrawHill.

Trzcianowska, H., & Mortensen, E. (2001). HIV and AIDS: Separating fact from fiction. *American Journal of Nursing, 101*(6), 53, 55, 57, 59.

Ungvarski, P. (1996). Waging war on HIV wasting. *RN, 59*(2), 26–32.

_____ . (2001). The past 20 years of AIDS. *American Journal of Nursing, 101*(6), 26–29.

Valdez, M.R. (2001). A metaphor for HIV-positive Mexican and Puerto Rican women. *Western Journal of Nursing Research, 23*(5), 517–535.

Williams, A.B. (2001). Adherence to HIV regimens: 10 vital lessons. *American Journal of Nursing, 101*(6), 37–44.

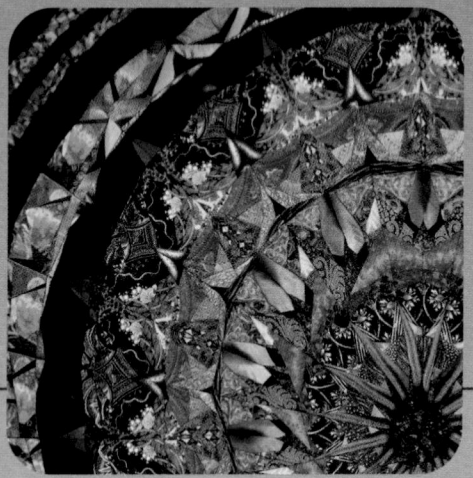

# CHAPTER 10

# Nursing Care of Clients with Cancer

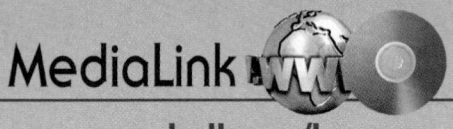

## MediaLink

**www.prenhall.com/lemone**

Additional resources for this chapter can be found on the Student CD-ROM accompanying this textbook, and on the Companion Website at www.prenhall.com/lemone. Click on Chapter 10 to select the activities for this chapter.

**CD-ROM**
- Audio Glossary
- NCLEX Review

**Companion Website**
- More NCLEX Review
- Case Study
   Pain Management
- Care Plan Activity
   Weight Loss and Chemotherapy
- MediaLink Application
   Terminal Cancer Support Groups

## LEARNING OUTCOMES

After completing this chapter, you will be able to:

- Define cancer and differentiate benign from malignant neoplasms.

- Discuss the theories of carcinogenesis, known carcinogens, and risk factors for cancer.

- Compare the mechanisms and characteristics of normal cells with those of malignant cells.

- Describe the effects of cancer on the body.

- Describe the laboratory and diagnostic tests used to diagnose cancer.

- Discuss the role of chemotherapy in cancer treatment.

- Discuss the use of surgery, radiation therapy, and biotherapy in the treatment of cancer.

- Describe the nursing interventions required for selected oncologic emergencies.

- Provide teaching to the client and family experiencing cancer.

- Use the nursing process as a framework for providing individualized care to the client with cancer.

Cancer is a family of complex diseases with manifestations that vary according to the body system affected and the type of tumor cells involved. This disease can affect people of any age, gender, ethnicity, or geographic region. Although the incidence and mortality rates of cancer have continued to decline since 1990, it remains one of the most feared diseases. The fear engendered by even the suggestion of a cancer diagnosis often brings forth feelings of dread and helplessness.

This chapter looks at the general pathogenesis, pathophysiology, and etiology of cancer; identifies current diagnostic and treatment modalities; and discusses nursing care appropriate for most clients with cancer. Discussions of cancers that affect specific body systems (e.g., leukemia, lung cancer) can be found in corresponding body system chapters in the text.

Cancer results when normal cells mutate into abnormal, deviant cells that then perpetuate within the body. Cancer can affect any body tissue. Providing cancer care is a potentially complex process, reflecting cancer's many different types and manifestations.

Nursing focuses on cancer not as one disease, but as many diseases. The nurse recognizes that cancer is a disruptive process that affects the whole person and that person's significant others. Nursing interventions reflect the fact that cancer is a chronic disease that has acute episodes, that the client is often treated in the home, and that the client is usually treated with a combination of therapeutic modalities. Equally important, the nurse recognizes that caring for the client with cancer involves prevention, detection, rehabilitation, long-term follow-up, and terminal care (Oncology Nursing Society [ONS], 1997).

**Oncology** is the study of cancer. The term is derived from the Greek word *oncoma* ("bulk"). Oncologists specialize in caring for clients with cancer; they may be medical doctors, surgeons, radiologists, immunologists, or researchers. Another significant member of the oncology team is the oncology nurse, who has received specialized training in such cancer treatment modalities as chemotherapy. Oncology nurses also have special skills in assisting the client and family with the psychosocial issues associated with cancer and terminal illness. Often the client with cancer has the benefit of a team of physicians, nurses, and other health care professionals who collaborate to provide the most effective treatment.

## INCIDENCE AND PREVALENCE

Only heart disease has a higher mortality rate than cancer. Despite continuing research, the rates of death from some forms of cancer continue to rise. Statistics from the American Cancer Society (ACS) show that approximately 25% of all deaths were attributable to cancer in the year 2001. It was estimated that 1.28 million new cases of cancer would occur in that year, with a projected death rate of 555,500 (ACS, 2002).

In 1994, prostate cancer surpassed lung and colon cancer for the position of highest incidence. Despite remaining the most frequently occurring cancer in men (189,000 new cases in 2002), the incidence of prostate cancer has begun to decline, due to the effects of prostate-specific antigen screening that allowed for diagnosis of cases earlier. Breast cancer is the most frequently occurring cancer in women, with an incidence of 203,500 in 2002. Lung and bronchial cancer (169,400 cases in 2002) and colorectal cancer (148,300 cases in 2002) rank second and third for both men and women. One of the most rapidly increasing cancers is melanoma (53,600 new cases in 2002) which has increased an average of 3% per year since 1981. The mortality rates for different cancers vary. In 2002, lung cancer is predicted to have the highest mortality rate with 154,900 estimated deaths, followed by colorectal (56,600), breast (40,000), and prostate cancer (30,2500). Information about the most recent cancer cases and mortality rates are available on the World Wide Web at www.cancer.org. The number of new cancer cases and cancer deaths is declining in the United States, and the 5-year survival rate for individual cancers continues to improve. Still, the gains are not equal for men and women nor for European Americans versus African Americans. The 5-year survival rate for all cancers is 62%, but African Americans are 33% more likely to die of cancer than whites (ACS, 2002). For example, although breast cancer occurs more commonly in white women than in black women, the survival rate is 86% for white women compared to only 71% for African Americans. Similar disparities are seen in survival rates for colorectal, prostate, and endometrial cancers in these ethnic groups. For information about diversity and cancer risk and incidence see the Focus on Diversity box below.

Cancer is a disease associated with aging; 80% of cancer diagnoses occur after age 55. The mortality rate for adults over 65 with cancer is 70%. These data are significant for health care as our elderly population increases.

## RISK FACTORS

Risk factors make an individual or a population vulnerable to a specific disease or other unhealthy outcome. Risk factors can be divided into those that are controllable and those that are not controllable. Knowledge and assessment of risk factors are especially important in counseling clients and families about measures to prevent cancer.

### Focus on Diversity

#### RISK AND INCIDENCE OF CANCER

- The incidence and mortality rates for all types of cancer are 35% to 39% lower in Hispanics.
- The incidence of cervical, stomach, and liver cancer is almost twice as high in Hispanics.
- Blacks are more likely to develop cancer than any other ethnic or racial group in the United States.
- Blacks have the highest incidence and mortality for colorectal and lung cancers.
- Breast cancer occurrence is about 13% lower in black women than in white women, but the mortality rate is approximately 28% higher.
- Black men are at least 50% more likely to develop prostate cancer than men of any other ethnic or racial group.
- Cancer incidence and mortality are lower in American Indian men and women than in any other ethnic or racial group.

## Heredity

It is estimated that 5% to 10% of cancers may have a hereditary component. The familial pattern of some breast and colon cancers has been well documented. Lung, ovarian, and prostate cancers have also shown some familial relationships. The Human Genome Project has identified new cancer-linked genes (Futreal et al., 2001). For most cancers, research has yet to distinguish true genetic transfer from environmental causes. So although further research is needed to identify cancers that are due to the inheritance of defective genes, familial predisposition to malignancies should be counted among risk factors so that people at risk can reduce behaviors that promote cancer. For example, a client with a family history of lung cancer should be counseled to avoid smoking, to avoid areas where smoking is allowed, and to avoid working in an occupation that may expose the client to inhaled carcinogens.

## Age

Approximately 70% of all cancers occur in people over age 65. A number of factors are associated with this increased risk in older adults. One possible factor is that at least five cycles of genetic mutations seem necessary to cause permanent damage to the afflicted cells. In addition, long-term exposure to high doses of promotional agents is usually necessary to allow the cancer to take hold. Evidence indicates that the immune response alters with aging; its actions become more generalized and less spe-

cific. Another problem is that free radicals (molecules resulting from the body's metabolic and oxidative processes) tend to accumulate in the cells over time, causing damage and mutation.

Hormonal changes that occur with aging can be associated with cancer. Postmenopausal women receiving exogenous estrogen have an increased risk for breast and uterine cancers. Older men are at risk for prostate cancer, possibly due to breakdown of testosterone into carcinogenic forms. See the box below for a discussion about older adults and cancer.

Severe and/or cumulative losses also are implicated in promoting cancer. These losses, which are common to older adults, include the death of a spouse or friends, loss of position and status in society, and a decline in physical abilities (Selye, 1984). These repeated stressors are related to changes in the immune system that may lead to the development of cancer.

## Gender

Gender is a risk factor for certain types of cancer, rather than for acquiring cancer in general. For example, thyroid cancer occurs more commonly among females, whereas bladder cancer is seen more often among male clients. Chapters 47 and 48 provide more information on gender-specific cancers. ∞

## Poverty

The poor are at higher risk for cancer than the population in general. Inadequate access to health care, especially preventive

---

# Meeting Individualized Needs

## OLDER ADULTS WITH CANCER

Nurses need to be aware of how cancer and cancer treatments affect older adults. Cancer is the second leading cause of death in people over age 65. The incidence of cancer increases with advancing age, probably as a result of the accumulated exposure to carcinogens and to age-related declines in the action of the immune system. The most commonly seen cancers in older women are colorectal, breast, lung, pancreatic, and ovarian. In older men, lung, colorectal, prostate, pancreatic, and gastric cancers occur most frequently.

The importance of screening and early detection of cancer does not diminish with age. Unfortunately, many older adults do not receive adequate cancer screening. Because the older adult is closer to the end of life, some health care providers may believe that cancer screening is not as important as it is for the younger client. This attitude may result in delayed diagnosis and treatment.

Older adults may not participate in screening programs or seek treatment for cancer due to fear, depression, cognitive impairments, poor access to health care, or financial constraints. Some older adults (and health care providers) mistake cancer symptoms for normal age-related changes. Believing that little can be done, they do not seek health care for their symptoms. Fear of the cancer diagnosis also keeps older adults from seeking appropriate health care. When they do seek treatment, chronic conditions frequently seen in older adults may make the diagnosis of cancer more difficult by masking or confounding the usual symptoms associated with cancer.

Older adults are at greater risk for side effects associated with cancer treatment because of age-related physiologic changes and chronic conditions associated with aging. This is particularly true for the side effects of chemotherapeutic agents. Older adults have increased incidence of cardiotoxicity and toxicity of the central nervous system when undergoing chemotherapy than younger adults. The side effects of chemotherapy can contribute to fatigue and cause problems related to immobility and functional decline. Alterations in the function of the immune system are also more frequent in older adults, which increases their risk for developing infection.

The problems associated with chemotherapy do not rule out its use, but the nurse must be aware of potential problems and monitor the client closely for the development of side effects. The nurse must consider how the aging process will alter the response to the disease and treatment plan when planning care for older adults.

### Client and Family Teaching
- Discuss the warning signs of cancer.
- Stress the importance of seeking health care if any of the warning signs develop.
- Get an annual physical examination.
- For women, learn how to perform a breast self-exam and perform the exam every month.
- For men, undergo prostate-specific antigen (PSA) screening for prostate cancer.

screening and counseling, may be a major factor. Although other factors that may be involved, such as diet and stress, usually come under the category of controllable risks, these risks are frequently uncontrollable in this population.

## Stress

Continuous unmanaged stress that keeps hormones such as epinephrine and cortisol at high levels can result in systematic "fatigue" and impaired immunologic surveillance. When the body attempts to adapt to physiologic and psychologic stressors, it goes through a series of stages called the general adaptation syndrome (GAS) (Selye, 1984). First, the "alarm reaction" occurs, in which adrenal hormones increase, allowing the body to cope with the stressor. Eventually, the body reaches the "stage of resistance," in which the stress hormones are significantly reduced, indicating that adaptation has occurred. If the physiologic adaptation is supported by appropriate coping strategies, the stressor is considered managed and body systems return to the prealarm functioning. However, if adaptation continues and the stress hormones remain elevated, the "stage of exhaustion" sets in. This stage will maintain life, but at great expense to body systems, resulting in general wear-and-tear and depression of the immune system (Selye, 1984).

The literature mentions a type C, or "cancer personality," describing people who have unhealthy coping behaviors for life stressors. Type C people are identified as those who tend to others' needs to the exclusion of their own and who rarely ask for help or support, even in personal crises. These people tend to be emotionally, and sometimes even physically, isolated and have a great deal of buried, unexpressed anger. It is thought that this kind of behavior pattern harms the immune system over time, promoting vulnerability to cancer. Depression is also considered a major risk factor, especially depression that is chronic or related to multiple or major losses. It is thought that depression and hopelessness tend to shut down the energizing chemicals in the body and depress immune responses (Kaye, Morton, Bowcutt, & Maupin, 2000).

## Diet

Some foods are considered genotoxic, such as the nitrosamines and nitrosindoles found in preserved meats and pickled, salted foods. Migrant workers have been found to have a high incidence of esophageal and gastric cancers related to their excessive consumption of these items. Other foods, such as high-fat, low-fiber foods—the mainstay of many American diets—promote colon, breast, and sex hormone–dependent tumors. When fish and meat are excessively fried or broiled, potent carcinogenic compounds can form that may cause tumors in the mammary glands, colon, liver, pancreas, and bladder. Also, repeatedly using fat to fry foods at high temperatures produces high levels of polycyclic hydrocarbons, which increase cancer risk considerably. Although many people profess to have changed their dietary habits, one only has to observe the large number of people who still lunch on cheeseburgers and french fries (and who teach their children to do the same) to realize that much more educational and motivational work is needed in this area. Other food-related substances believed to increase cancer risk include sodium saccharine, red food dyes, and both regular and decaffeinated coffee.

## Occupation

Occupational risk might be considered to be either controllable or uncontrollable. For many people, both education and ability limit their choice of occupation; during times of high unemployment, moreover, changing one's occupation because it poses risk factors may not be a viable option. Federal standards are designed to protect workers from hazardous substances, but many believe that these standards are not strict enough and that inspections are not frequent enough to prevent violations.

Specific risks vary according to the occupation. For example, outdoor workers such as farmers and construction workers are exposed to solar radiation; health care workers such as X-ray technicians and biomedical researchers are exposed to ionizing radiation and carcinogenic substances; and exposure to asbestos is a problem for people who work in old buildings with asbestos insulation in the walls. Table 10–1 correlates known carcinogens and occupations.

### TABLE 10–1   Chemical Carcinogens and Relationship to Occupation

| Chemical Agent | Action | Occupation Affected |
|---|---|---|
| Polycyclic hydrocarbons (smoke, soot, tobacco, smoked foods) Benzopyrene | Genotoxic | Miners, coal/gas workers, chimney sweeps, migrant workers, workers in offices where smoking is allowed in closed areas |
| Arsenic | Genotoxic | Pesticide manufacturers, mining |
| Vinyl chloride polymers | Promotional | Plastics workers Artists |
| Methylaminobenzine | Genotoxic | Fabric workers Rubber and glue workers |
| Asbestos | Promotional | Construction workers, workers in old, run-down buildings with asbestos insulation, insulation makers |
| Wood and leather dust | Promotional | Woodworkers, carpenters, leather toolers |
| Chemotherapy drugs | Genotoxic | Drug manufacturers, pharmacists, nurses |

## Infection

Because a number of viruses have been linked to some cancers, avoiding those specific infections will decrease risk. Although some infections may be unavoidable (Epstein-Barr, for example), others, such as genital herpes and papillomavirus-induced genital warts, can often be avoided by following safe sex practices (e.g., the use of condoms).

## Tobacco Use

Lung cancer is considered highly preventable because of its relationship to smoking. The genotoxic carcinogenic substances in tobacco are considered weak; therefore, stopping smoking can reverse the damage it causes. However, many other substances in tobacco are highly promotional, so that the larger the dose and longer the use, the higher the risk for developing cancer. Research has shown a significantly lower lung cancer death risk for former smokers compared to current smokers. Smokers who quit before middle age avoid more than 90% of the risk of lung cancer that can be attributed to tobacco (Peto et al., 2000).

Tobacco is also related to other forms of cancer. Smokers face an increased risk for oropharyngeal, esophageal, laryngeal, gastric, pancreatic, and bladder cancers. Pipe and cigar smokers are especially susceptible to oropharyngeal and laryngeal cancers. Oral and esophageal cancers are more common among those who chew tobacco or use snuff. Smokers who have a genetic decrease in alpha-1 antitripsin (an enzyme that protects lung tissue) that results in emphysema face an even higher cancer risk than smokers without this defect.

Additional research has documented the deleterious effects of secondhand tobacco smoke (Williams & Sandler, 2001). Tobacco-specific nitrosamines were recovered in the urine of children living with smokers. It is now accepted that nonsmokers exposed to tobacco smoke over long periods of time, whether in the workplace or the home, have an increased risk for lung or bladder cancers.

## Alcohol Use

Alcohol promotes cancer by modifying the metabolism of carcinogens in the liver and esophagus, thus increasing the effectiveness of the carcinogens in some tissues. People who both smoke and drink a considerable amount of alcohol daily have an increased risk for oral, esophageal, and laryngeal cancers.

## Recreational Drug Use

Recreational drug use often promotes an unhealthy lifestyle that increases general cancer risk; for example, drug users often do not maintain adequate nutrition. Furthermore, recreational drugs are implicated as promoters because of their suppressive effect on the immune system. Although it has not been directly implicated in cancer development, marijuana has been demonstrated to cause chromosomal damage that may over time also result in cancer-causing DNA damage and genetic mutations. Marijuana smoke is also much more injurious to lung tissue than tobacco smoke.

## Obesity

Excessive body fat has been linked to an increased risk of hormone-dependent cancers. Because sex hormones are synthesized from fat, obese people often have excessive amounts of the hormones that feed hormone-dependent malignancies of the breast, bowel, ovary, endometrium, and prostate.

## Sun Exposure

As the protective ozone layer thins, more of the sun's damaging ultraviolet radiation reaches the earth. As a consequence, the rate of skin cancers has increased. Sun-related skin cancers are now considered to be a problem for all people, regardless of skin color, but people of Northern European extraction with very fair skin, blue or green eyes, and light-colored hair are most vulnerable. Elderly people with decreased pigment are also more at risk, even those with darker skin.

Figure 10–1 ■ summarizes the interaction of factors that promote cancer.

## PATHOPHYSIOLOGY

Cancer is a complex disease with hundreds of agents that can contribute to its pathogenesis. Advances in research have greatly increased the understanding of how cancer develops. It is now known that the development of cancer is a process in which normal cells are changed and acquire malignant properties. Before a discussion of the various theories of the causes of cancer, it is useful to review how normal cells divide and adapt to changing conditions.

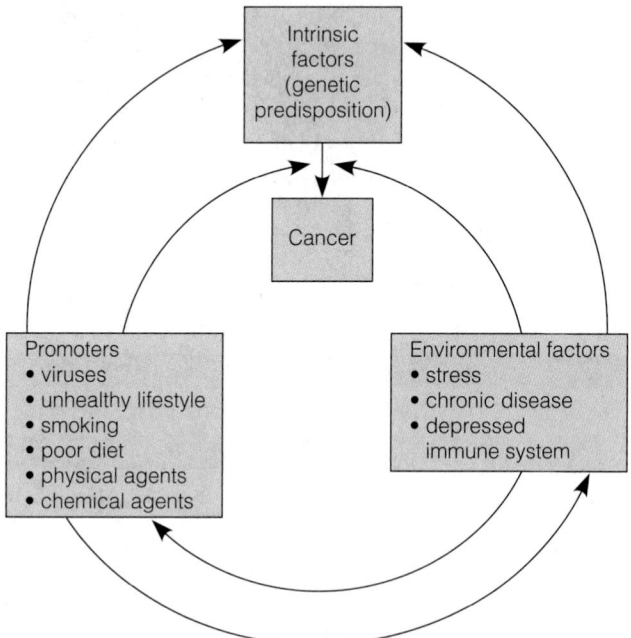

**Figure 10–1** ■ Interaction of factors that promote cancer. Most people have immune systems that are competent enough to resist the establishment of cancer from an initiated cell. Cancer takes hold when a number of promotional factors occur together and over enough time to weaken immune resistance. Like factors are grouped together for ease of presentation but may occur in any combination.

- Orders production of enzymes.
- Instructs cells to produce specific chemicals.
- Instructs cells to develop specific structures.
- Determines individual traits and characteristics.
- Controls other DNA by telling a cell to "switch on" and use some portion of the genetic information stored in it.

## Normal Cell Growth

Mature normal cells are uniform in size and have nuclei that are characteristic of the tissue to which the cells belong. Within the nucleus of normal cells, chromosomes containing deoxyribonucleic acid (DNA) molecules carry the genetic information that controls the synthesis of polypeptides (proteins). Genes are subunits of chromosomes and consist of portions of DNA that specify the production of particular sets of proteins. Thus, genes control the development of specific traits. The genetic code in the DNA of every gene is translated into protein structures that determine the type, maturity, and function of a cell. Any change or disruption in a gene can result in an inaccurate "blueprint" that can produce an aberrant cell, which may then become cancerous. Box 10–1 lists some of the functions of DNA.

## The Cell Cycle

Two coordinated events are responsible for cellular reproduction. Reproduction occurs as the result of replication of cellular DNA and mitosis, when the cell divides into two daughter cells with identical DNA.

The cell cycle consists of four phases. In the gap 1 or $G_1$ phase, the cell enlarges and synthesizes proteins to prepare for DNA replication. During this phase the cell prepares to replicate and enter into the synthesis phase. During the synthesis (S) phase, DNA is replicated and the chromosomes in the cell are duplicated. During the next phase, gap 2 ($G_2$), the cell prepares itself for mitosis. Finally, with all preparation complete, the cell begins mitosis (M). This phase culminates in the division of the parent cell into two exact copies called daughter cells, each having identical genetic material. The cells then immediately enter $G_1$ where they begin the cell cycle again, or divert into a resting phase called $G_0$. The cell cycle is controlled by cyclins, which combine with and activate enzymes called cyclin-dependent kinases (CDKs). Some cyclins cause a "braking" action and prevent the cycle from proceeding (Dunlop & Campbell, 2000). Checkpoints in the cell cycle ensure that it proceeds in the correct order.

A malfunction of any of these regulators of cell growth and division can result in the rapid proliferation of immature cells. In some cases, these cells are considered cancerous (malignant). Knowledge of cell cycle events is used in the development of chemotherapeutic drugs, which are designed to disrupt the cancer cells during different stages of their cell cycle. These drugs and their use are discussed later in the chapter.

## Differentiation

**Differentiation** is a normal process occurring over many cell cycles that allows cells to specialize in certain tasks. For example, some epithelial cells lining the lungs develop into tall columnar cells with cilia. These columnar cells sweep potentially dangerous debris out of the lungs. When adverse conditions occur in body tissues during differentiation, protective adaptations can produce alterations in cells. Some of these alterations are helpful, but in other cases the cells mutate beyond usefulness and become liabilities (Porth, 1998). Following are potentially unproductive cellular alterations occurring during cell differentiation.

- **Hyperplasia** is an increase in the number or density of normal cells. Hyperplasia occurs in response to stress, increased metabolic demands, or elevated levels of hormones. Examples include the hyperplasia of myocardial cells in response to a prolonged increase in the body's demand for oxygen, and hyperplasia of uterine cells in response to rising levels of estrogen during pregnancy. Hyperplastic cells are under normal DNA control.
- **Metaplasia** is a change in the normal pattern of differentiation such that dividing cells differentiate into cell types not normally found in that location in the body. The metaplastic cell is normal for its particular type, but it is not in its normal location. Some metaplastic cells are less functional than the cells they replace. Metaplasia is a protective response to adverse conditions. Metaplastic cells are under normal DNA control and are reversible when the stressor or other disruptive condition ceases.
- **Dysplasia** represents a loss of DNA control over differentiation occurring in response to adverse conditions. Dysplastic cells show abnormal variation in size, shape, and appearance and a disturbance in their usual arrangement. Examples of dysplasia include changes in the cervix in response to continued irritation, such as from the human papillomavirus (HPV), or leukoplakia on oral mucous membranes in response to chronic irritation from smoking.
- **Anaplasia** is the regression of a cell to an immature or undifferentiated cell type. Anaplastic cell division is no longer under DNA control. Anaplasia usually occurs when a damaging or transforming event takes place inside the dividing, still undifferentiated cell, leading to loss of useful function. Anaplasia may occur in response to overwhelmingly destructive conditions inside the cell or in surrounding tissue (Porth, 2002).

Although hyperplasia, metaplasia, and dysplasia often reverse after the irritating factor is eliminated, they can lead to malignancy under certain conditions. This is especially true of dysplasia, which represents a loss of DNA control. Anaplasia is not reversible, but the degree of anaplasia determines the potential risk for cancer.

## Etiology

Intensive research efforts during the past several decades have led to an increased understanding of how cancer develops. The Human Genome Project, begun in 1990, has provided critical information about the development of cancer. Continuing research will provide information that will be key in the detection and prevention of cancer.

Cancer research has brought new options for cancer treatment and improved clients' overall survival rate. Almost daily, people hear of research studies indicating that certain foods, habits, or environmental factors may cause cancer. Although much of this is true and is inspiring a welcome preventive focus to health care, it is not true that one can determine the specific factors that cause cancer in any individual. Although taking responsibility for one's own health is a positive step, the emphasis on prevention may have a negative result if clients feel so guilty and blameworthy that they fail to seek out early and appropriate health care. Also, clients who feel that their bodies have failed them may become depressed, and such feelings can impair the functioning of an already stressed immune system.

Factors that cause cancer are both external (chemicals, radiation, and viruses) and internal (hormones, immune conditions, and inherited mutations). Causal factors may act together or in sequence to initiate or promote carcinogenesis. Ten or more years often pass between exposures or mutations and detectable cancer.

## Theories of Carcinogenesis

### Cellular Mutation

The theory of cellular mutation suggests that carcinogens cause mutations in cellular DNA. It is believed that the carcinogenic process has three stages: initiation, promotion, and progression. The initiation stage involves permanent damage in the cellular DNA as a result of exposure to a carcinogen (e.g., radiation, chemicals) that was not repaired or had a defective repair. Promotion may last for years and includes conditions, such as smoking or alcohol use, that act repeatedly on the already affected cells. In the progression stage further inherited changes acquired during the cell replication develop into a cancer.

### Oncogenes

**Oncogenes** are genes that promote cell proliferation and are capable of triggering cancerous characteristics. Oncogenes can be classified according to their overall function. Several oncogenes and their relationship to human cancers have been identified. For example, BRCA-1 and BRCA-2 are associated with breast cancer (Surbone, 2001).

A decrease in the body's immune surveillance may allow the expression of oncogenes; this can occur during times of stress or in response to certain carcinogens. For example, clients with AIDS, who have a decreased number of helper T lymphocytes, have a much higher than normal incidence of certain cancers, including non-Hodgkin's lymphoma and Kaposi's sarcoma (Donahue, Wernz, & Cooper, 2000).

### Tumor Suppressor Genes

Tumor suppressor genes normally suppress oncogenes. They can become inactive by deletion or mutation. Inherited cancers have been associated with tumor suppressor genes. An example is p53, a suppressor gene that has been associated with sarcoma and cancer of the breast and brain.

Central to these theories are two important concepts about the etiology of cancer. First, damaged DNA, whether inherited or from external sources, sets up the necessary initial step for cancer to occur. Second, impairment of the human immune system, from whatever cause, lessens its ability to destroy abnormal cells.

## Known Carcinogens

A number of agents are known to cause cancer, or at least are strongly linked to certain kinds of cancers. These known carcinogens include viruses, drugs, hormones, and chemical and physical agents.

**Carcinogens** can be categorized in two groups: Genotoxic carcinogens directly alter DNA and cause mutations, and promoter substances cause other adverse biologic effects, such as cytotoxicity, hormonal imbalances, altered immunity, or chronic tissue damage. Promoter substances do not cause cancer in the absence of previous cell damage (initiation) and often require high-level and long-term contact with the altered cells (see Table 10–1).

Note also that although everyone comes into contact with a vast number of substances that are considered carcinogenic, not everyone develops cancer. Other factors, such as genetic predisposition, impairment of the immune response, and repeated exposure to the carcinogen, are necessary for a cancer to develop.

### Viruses

Several viruses have been associated with the development of cancer. They damage cells and induce hyperplastic cell growth. Viral infection may play a role in cell mutation that can progress to malignant cells. Most people are able to suppress this progression (Spitalnick & diSant'Agnese, 2001). Box 10–2 identifies these viruses and the cancers with which they are associated.

---

**BOX 10–2 ■ Cancers Associated with Different Viruses**

**HERPES SIMPLEX VIRUS TYPES I AND II (HSV-1 AND HSV-2)**
- Carcinoma of the lip
- Cervical carcinoma
- Kaposi's sarcoma

**HUMAN CYTOMEGALOVIRUS (HCMV)**
- Kaposi's sarcoma
- Prostate cancer

**EPSTEIN-BARR VIRUS (EBV)**
- Burkitt's lymphoma

**HUMAN HERPESVIRUS-6 (HHV-6)**
- Lymphoma

**HEPATITIS B VIRUS (HBV)**
- Primary hepatocellular cancer

**PAPILLOMAVIRUS**
- Malignant melanoma
- Cervical, penile, and laryngeal cancers

**HUMAN T-LYMPHOTROPIC VIRUSES (HTLV)**
- Adult T-cell leukemia and lymphoma
- T-cell variant of hairy-cell leukemia
- Kaposi's sarcoma

In addition, viruses play a significant role in weakening immunologic defenses against neoplasms. For example, HIV, which infects helper T lymphocytes and monocytes, impairs the person's protection against certain cancers such as lymphoma and Kaposi's sarcoma.

Other viruses have also been associated with human malignancies. Hepatitis B virus (HBV) integrates its DNA with liver cell DNA and is believed to cause primary hepatocellular carcinoma. Papillomaviruses cause plantar, common, and flat warts, which are benign and usually regress spontaneously; however, they also cause genital warts and laryngeal papillomas, which are associated with malignant melanoma and cervical, penile, and laryngeal cancers. Retroviruses have been found to cause cancer in animals. Adult T-cell leukemia is the only human cancer known to be associated with a retrovirus (Hill, 2001).

Vaccines to prevent virus-induced cancers are being investigated. Preliminary results of the use of vaccines to treat malignancies, such as melanoma, have been encouraging (Berd, 2001).

### Drugs and Hormones

Certain drugs can be either genotoxic or promotional. For example, chemotherapeutic drugs used to disrupt the cell cycle of malignant cells can be genotoxic for normal cells. They can also be promotional: By drastically reducing the number of leukocytes, they impair immune function. Examples of these chemotherapeutic drugs include busulfan, chlorambucil, and cycloposphamide. Some recreational drugs also are implicated as carcinogens. These include the genotoxic betel nut chewed by many Pacific Islanders and the immunosuppressant promoters heroin and cocaine.

Hormones are also potential genotoxic carcinogens or promoters. Gonadotropic hormones often mediate cancers of the reproductive organs. Estrogen, both natural and synthetic, and diethylstilbestrol (DES) have been linked to cervical, endometrial, and breast cancers. Estrogen-containing contraceptive pills have been implicated in breast cancer, but they also have been shown to decrease the risk of ovarian cancer. Investigators have not reached a final conclusion about the cancer risk posed by contraceptives. Newer research suggests that alterations in the molecular structure of testosterone in older men may promote the development of prostate cancer. Also, glucocorticosteroids (cortisone) and anabolic steroids may act as promoters by altering the immune response or endocrine balance (Chapman & Goodman, 2000; Held-Warmkessel, 2000; Rubin, Williams, Okunieff, Rosenblatt, & Sitzmann, 2001).

### Chemical Agents

Many chemicals have been demonstrated to be both genotoxic and promotional. Because many of these substances are encountered in the workplace, they constitute occupational hazards, which will be discussed more thoroughly. Examples of industrial and environmental carcinogens include polycyclic hydrocarbons, found in soot; benzopyrene, found in cigarette smoke; and arsenic, found in pesticides. These chemicals have some genotoxic action; some alter DNA replication. Other industrial and environmental chemicals are considered promotional agents. These include wood and leather dust, polymer esters (used in plastics and paints), carbon tetrachloride, asbestos, and phenol.

Natural substances in the body may also be carcinogenic or promotional. For example, end products of metabolism that are produced in excess amounts or are ineffectively eliminated, such as bile acids from a high-fat diet, may promote cancer.

Some foods contain carcinogens added during preparation or preservation. Examples include the sugar substitute sodium saccharine and nitrosamines and nitrosindoles, which are found in pickled, salted foods. In some cases, food contaminants produce carcinogenic chemicals. The Aspergillus fungi produce aflatoxin, a highly potent carcinogen. These organisms grow on improperly stored vegetable products, such as grains and peanuts.

Polycyclic aromatic hydrocarbons, nitrosamines, phenols, and other chemicals in tobacco act as either carcinogens or promoters of cancer (see Table 10–1).

### Physical Agents

It has been well documented that excessive exposure to radiation causes increased rates of cancer by damaging the DNA in cells, by activating other oncogenetic factors, or by suppressing antitumor activity (protein inhibitors). Both solar radiation from ultraviolet rays and ionizing radiation from industrial or medical sources are carcinogenic. This fact has implications for workers exposed to these agents and for the population in general. Radon, a naturally formed radioactive gas found in the basements of many homes, is also a known carcinogen. People who have lived in areas where nuclear weapons have been tested or whose groundwater has been polluted by nuclear wastes are at risk for developing cancers. The effects of high-dose radiation exposure and subsequent cancer development have been demonstrated in the survivors of the atomic bomb at Nagasaki and Hiroshima and workers exposed to radiation during the cleanup of nuclear disasters such as Chernobyl.

## Types of Neoplasms

A **neoplasm** is a mass of new tissue (a collection of cells) that grows independently of its surrounding structures and has no physiologic purpose. The term *neoplasm* is often used interchangeably with *tumor*, from the Latin word meaning "swelling." Neoplasms are said to be autonomous because of the following:

- They grow at a rate uncoordinated with the needs of the body.
- They function independently of usual homeostatic controls.
- They share some of the properties of the parent cells but with altered size and shape.
- They do not benefit the host and in some cases are actively harmful.

Neoplasms are not completely autonomous, however, because they require a blood supply with nutrients and oxygen to sustain their growth. Neoplasms typically are classified as benign or malignant on the basis of their potential to damage the body and on their growth characteristics.

## Benign Neoplasms

Benign neoplasms are localized growths. They form a solid mass, have well-defined borders, and frequently are encapsulated. Benign neoplasms tend to respond to the body's homeostatic controls. Thus, they often stop growing when they reach the boundaries of another tissue (a process called contact inhibition). They grow slowly and often remain stable in size. Because they are usually encapsulated, benign neoplasms often are easily removed and tend not to recur.

Although typically harmless, benign neoplasms nevertheless can be destructive if they crowd surrounding tissue and obstruct the function of organs. For example, a benign meningioma (from the meninges of the brain and spinal cord) can cause severely increased intracranial pressure (ICP), which progressively impairs the person's cerebral function. Unless the meningioma can be successfully removed, the steadily rising ICP will eventually lead to coma and death.

## Malignant Neoplasms

In contrast to benign neoplasms, malignant neoplasms grow aggressively and do not respond to the body's homeostatic controls. Malignant neoplasms are not cohesive, and present with an irregular shape. Instead of slowly crowding other tissues aside, malignant neoplasms cut through surrounding tissues, causing bleeding, inflammation, and necrosis (tissue death) as they grow. This invasive quality of malignant neoplasms is reflected in the word origin of *cancer,* from the Greek *karkinos,* meaning "crab." Health care professionals are referring to a malignant neoplasm when they use the term *cancer.*

Malignant cells from the primary tumor may travel through the blood or lymph to invade other tissues and organs of the body and form a secondary tumor called a metastasis. This term also refers to the process by which such spreading of malignant neoplasms—perhaps their most destructive trait—occurs. Malignant neoplasms can recur after surgical removal of the primary and secondary tumors and after other treatments. Table 10–2 compares benign and malignant neoplasms.

Malignant neoplasms vary in their degree of differentiation from the parent tissue. Highly differentiated cancer cells try to mimic the specialized function of the parent tissue, but undifferentiated cancers, consisting of immature cells, have almost no resemblance to the parent tissue and so perform no useful function. To make matters worse, undifferentiated cancers rob the body of its energy and nutrition as they grow. Undifferentiated anaplastic cells have little structural or functional relationship to the parent cells and are the basis of many malignant neoplasms. The degree of differentiation of anaplastic cells is a consideration in the classification and staging of neoplasms, discussed later in this chapter.

## Characteristics of Malignant Cells

Malignant neoplasms may be identified by the following predictable cellular characteristics.

- *Loss of regulation of the rate of mitosis.* This results in rapid cell division and growth of the neoplasm.
- *Loss of specialization and differentiation.* Malignant cells do not perform typical cellular functions. Many produce hormones and enzymes similar to those of the parent tissue, but usually in excessive amounts, possibly revealing their presence.
- *Loss of contact inhibition.* Malignant cells do not respect other cellular boundaries. They easily invade and destroy other tissues.
- *Progressive acquisition of a cancerous phenotype.* Cellular mutation seems to be a sequential process involving successive generations of cells, each generation becoming more deviant than the previous one. Additionally, malignant cells seem to be "immortal"; that is, they do not stop growing and die, as do normal cells, which have a genetically determined life span.
- *Irreversibility.* The transformation into a malignant cell is irreversible. Rarely does a malignant neoplasm revert to a benign state.
- *Altered cell structure.* Cytologic examination of malignant cells reveals distinct differences in the cell nucleus and cytoplasm as well as an overall cell shape that differs from that of normal cells of the particular tissue type.
- *Simplified metabolic activities.* The work of malignant cells is simpler than that of normal cells; they show an increased synthesis of substances needed for cell division, and they have no need to create proteins for the specialized functions of the tissues they invade.
- *Transplantability.* Malignant cells often break away from the primary tissue site and travel to other locations in the body, where they establish new growths.
- *Ability to promote their own survival.* Malignant cells may create ectopic sites to produce the hormones they need for their growth. By their very presence and their ability to initiate vascular permeability, malignant cells promote the development of nonneoplastic stroma, a connective tissue framework consisting of collagen and other components, which then supports the neoplasm. They may also create their own blood supply. Through a process called angiogenesis, tumor cells secrete a polypeptide angiogenic growth factor that stimulates blood vessels from surrounding normal tissue to grow into the tumor. Finally, malignant cells divert nutrition from the host to meet their own needs, by diffusion when the tumor is less than 1 mm and thereafter by means of the newly formed blood vessels. If unchecked, malignant cells eventually destroy their host.

| TABLE 10–2 | Comparison of Benign and Malignant Neoplasms |
|---|---|
| **Benign** | **Malignant** |
| Local | Invasive |
| Cohesive | Noncohesive |
| Well-defined borders | Does not stop at tissue border |
| Pushes other tissues out of the way | Invades and destroys surrounding tissues |
| Slow growth | Rapid growth |
| Encapsulated | Metastasizes to distant sites |
| Easily removed | Not always easy to remove |
| Does not recur | Can recur |

The characteristics of malignant cells are summarized in Box 10–3.

## Tumor Invasion and Metastasis

The ability of cancer cells to invade adjacent tissues and travel to distant organs is considered their most ominous characteristic. This quality makes treatment a considerable challenge (Hawkins, 2001).

### Invasion

Aggressive tumors possess several qualities that facilitate invasion (Figure 10–2 ■):

- *Ability to cause pressure atrophy.* The pressure of a growing tumor can cause atrophy and necrosis of adjacent tissues. The malignancy then moves into the vacated space.
- *Ability to disrupt the basement membrane of normal cells.* Many cancer cells can bind to elements of the basement membrane and secrete enzymes that degrade that physical barrier, thus facilitating their movement into normal tissues, lymph, and blood circulation.
- *Motility.* Because malignant cells are less tightly bound to each other than normal cells (reduced adhesiveness), they easily separate from the neoplasm and move into surrounding body fluids and tissues.
- *Response to chemical signals from adjacent tissues.* Chemotaxis (the movement of cells in response to a chemical stimulus) calls the tumor cells into the normal tissues, possibly as a result of the degrading of the basement membranes of the normal cells. This breakdown of normal cellular membranes releases the chemical stimulus physiologically designed to draw normal phagocytic cells to clean up the debris. (See Chapter 8 on the inflammatory response for more information on chemotaxis. ◯◯ ) Malignant cells are also known to respond chemotactically to the end product of cellular metabolism. Some cancer cells even produce a substance called autocrine motility factor, which calls other malignant cells to a normal tissue. The first invading cells produce this substance, which then actively draws other malignant cells from the primary tumor into the invaded normal tissue.

### Metastasis

The factors that favor invasion also contribute to the process of metastasis. **Metastasis** can occur by means of one or more mechanisms including embolism in the blood or lymph or spread by way of body cavities.

A blood- or lymph-borne metastasis allows a new tumor to be established in a distant organ. Figure 10–3 ■ shows metastasis through the bloodstream. A tumor's ability to metastasize in this manner requires the following steps:

1. Intravasation of malignant cells through blood or lymphatic vessel walls and into the circulation

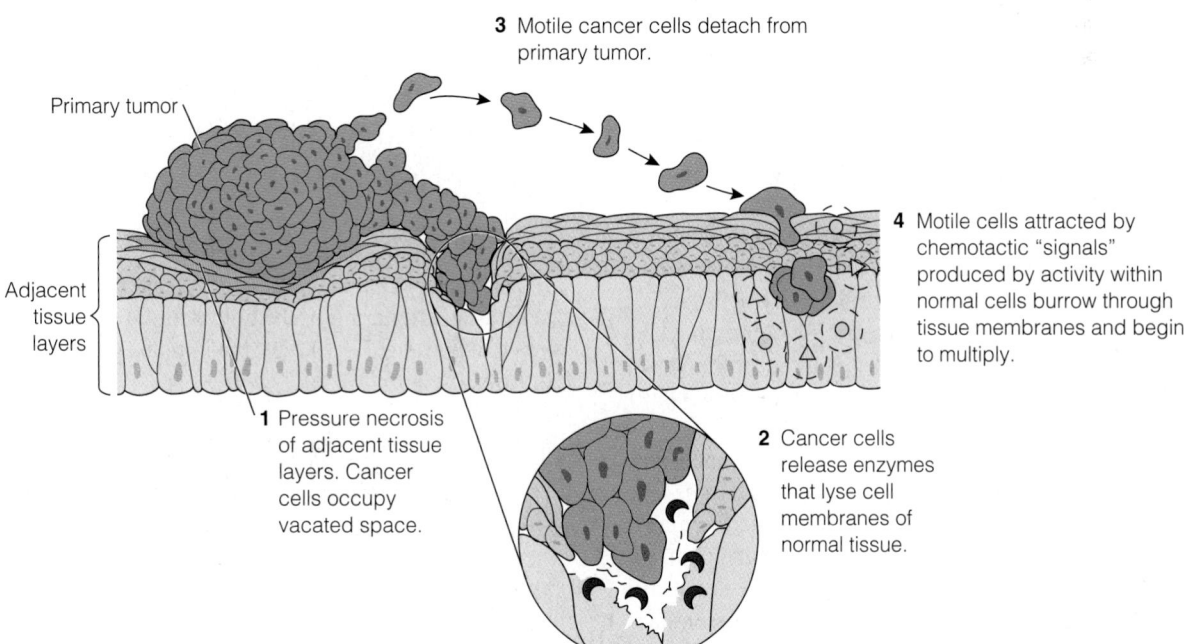

**3** Motile cancer cells detach from primary tumor.

Primary tumor

Adjacent tissue layers

**1** Pressure necrosis of adjacent tissue layers. Cancer cells occupy vacated space.

**2** Cancer cells release enzymes that lyse cell membranes of normal tissue.

**4** Motile cells attracted by chemotactic "signals" produced by activity within normal cells burrow through tissue membranes and begin to multiply.

**Figure 10–2** ■ How cancer cells invade normal tissue.

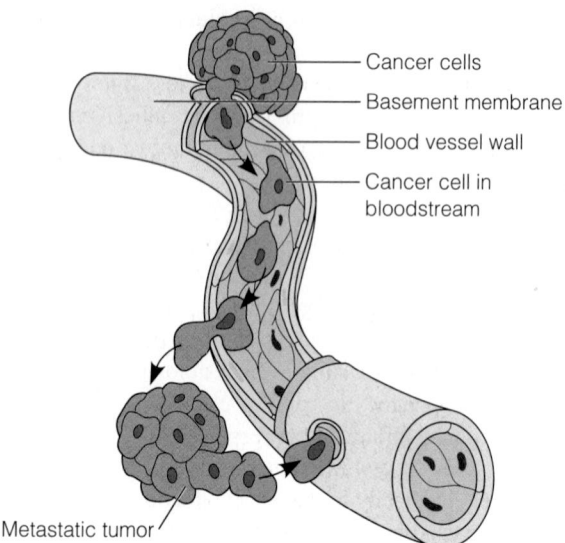

**Figure 10–3** ■ Metastasis through the bloodstream. Cancer cells secrete enzymes and a motility factor that disrupt the basement membrane in the blood vessel. In this way, the cancer cells gain access into the circulation. Once in the blood, only about 1 cell in 1000 escapes immune detection, but that can be enough. Undetected cells move out of the blood, again secreting enzymes and cutting through the vessel wall into new tissue. The tissue selected for establishing a new tumor may be downstream from the original tumor, or a chemical attraction may cause the malignant cells to target a specific site. Once in the new site, the malignant cells multiply and establish a metastatic tumor.

2. Survival of the malignant cells in the blood (To survive, the cells must escape the notice of the body's immune surveillance; only about 1 in 1000 cells does so.)
3. Extravasation from the circulation and implantation in a new tissue

The tumor cells tend to clump together, forming an embolus, and continue growing until their size prevents further travel in the vessel or lymph channel. The growing neoplastic mass then uses its invasive abilities (secreting enzymes and motility factor) to move into the nearest organ.

About 60% of metastatic lesions tend to occur in a schema reflecting the pattern of blood or lymph circulation. However, it has been demonstrated that some malignant cells defy a bloodborne pattern and actually target specific organs to which they prefer to metastasize. For example, lung cancer frequently metastasizes to the adrenal glands and breast cancer frequently metastasizes to bone.

Malignant cells that gain access to the lymph channels may travel to a preferred organ and then move into it the same way they emigrate through blood vessels. Alternatively, the malignant cells may become trapped in the lymph node and continue to grow. Eventually, the malignant cells replace the node's tissues. At this point, emboli from the cancerous node disseminate to other nodes, creating a cascade reaction. The malignant cascade causes widespread transfer of the tumor to uncharacteristic sites.

| TABLE 10–3 | Various Cancers and Sites of or Metastases |
|---|---|
| **Primary Tumor** | **Common Metastatic Sites** |
| Bronchogenic (lung) | Spinal cord, brain, liver, bone |
| Breast | Regional lymph nodes, vertebrae, brain, liver, lung, bone |
| Colon | Liver, lung, brain, ovary, bone |
| Prostate | Bladder, bone (especially vertebrae), liver |
| Malignant melanoma | Lung, liver, spleen, regional lymph nodes, brain |

A malignant tumor may break through the walls of the organ in which it is primarily housed, shedding cells into the nearby body cavity. The cells then are free to establish new tumors in a distant area of that cavity. For example, malignant cells from a colon cancer may be seeded into the peritoneal cavity, establishing a new tumor in the mesenteric epithelium.

Metastatic lesions are differentiated from primary neoplasms by cell morphology: Metastatic cells do not resemble the tissue in which they reside. The most common sites of metastasis are the lymph nodes, liver, lungs, bones, and brain. Table 10–3 lists different cancers and common sites of metastasis.

For metastasis to occur, the cancerous cells must avoid detection by the immune system. Thus, impairment of the immune system is a major factor in the establishment of metastatic lesions. Cells may escape detection in several different ways:

- Aggressive cancer cells may compile a large mass (greater than 1 cm) so rapidly that the immune system is unable to overcome the tumor before it takes hold in a new tissue.
- For tumor cells to be recognized as foreign by the immune system, they must display on their surface a special antigen called tumor-associated antigen (TAA). TAA marks tumor cells for destruction by the lymphocytes. Some oncogenic viruses depress the expression of TAA on infected cells. Also, some tumors in advanced stages of growth no longer display TAA. Thus, such tumor cells escape detection as they travel through the blood or lymph.
- If the person's immune response is weakened or altered, then a metastatic tumor may take hold with little opposition. Factors that may weaken or alter the immune response are listed in Box 10–4.

| BOX 10–4 | ■ Factors That May Weaken or Alter the Immune Response |
|---|---|

- Accumulated stress
- Depression
- Increased age
- Pregnancy
- Chronic disease
- Chemotherapy treatment for the primary cancer

An estimated 50% to 60% of all cancers have already metastasized by the time the primary tumor is identified. This may account for the current 50% death rate and certainly supports the need for client education to facilitate early diagnosis. The time it takes for metastasis to occur is extremely variable and often difficult to predict. Some cancers, such as basal cell carcinomas, do not metastasize. The aggressiveness and location of the tumor, and the state of the person's immune system, determine whether and how rapidly metastasis takes place.

## Physiologic and Psychologic Effects of Cancer

Much of the nursing care for clients with cancer is related to the generalized effects of cancer on the body and the side effects of the treatments used to remove or destroy the cancer. Although pathophysiologic effects of the cancer vary with the type and location of the cancer, the following effects usually are observed.

### Disruption of Function

Physiologic functioning can be upset by obstruction or pressure. For example, a large tumor in the bowel can stop intestinal motility, resulting in a bowel obstruction. Prostatic tumors can obstruct the bladder neck or urethra, resulting in urine retention. Intracranial pressure can be dangerously increased by a glioma.

Obstruction or pressure can cause anoxia and necrosis of surrounding tissues, which in turn cause a loss of function of the involved organ or tissue. For example, a kidney tumor may progress to renal failure. Pressure against the superior vena cava from an adjacent lung tumor or tumor-infiltrated lymph nodes can interrupt the blood flow to the heart.

In the liver, either a primary hepatocellular cancer or metastatic lesion can have several significant effects:

- In liver parenchymal tissue, it impairs the multiple life-sustaining functions of the liver, such as carbohydrate metabolism, synthesis of plasma proteins, detoxification, and immunologic functions. These functional impairments result in severe nutritional, hormonal, hematologic, and immunologic problems. (See Chapter 19 for a more complete discussion of liver functions and effects of disruption. )
- Because more than 1 L of blood per minute passes through the liver via the portal vein, obstruction to this flow by a tumor can cause portal hypertension. This results in backup of fluid and increased pressure in the splanchnic circulation. The end result is ascites (third-spaced fluid in the peritoneal cavity) and varices (friable, overdistended blood vessels) of the esophageal, gastric, mesenteric, and hemorrhoidal vessels.

### Hematologic Alterations

Hematologic alterations can impair the normal function of blood cells. For example, in leukemia, a malignant proliferative disease of the hematopoietic (blood cell–producing) system, the immature leukocytes cannot perform the normal protective phagocytic functions and immunity is compromised. Additionally, the excessive numbers of immature leukocytes in the bone marrow diminish erythrocyte and thrombocyte (platelet) production, resulting in secondary anemia and clotting disorders (Scigliano, Vlachos, Najfeld, & Shank, 2001).

Other examples of hematologic alteration include the following:

- Gastrointestinal tumors disrupt the absorption of vitamin $B_{12}$ and iron.
- Growing tumors need purines and folate and have a unique ability to accumulate and store these substances. Thus, the tumor deprives the bone marrow of these substances, which are needed for erythropoiesis (red blood cell production).
- Renal cell carcinoma produces its own erythropoietin hormone, which causes an excessively large number of red blood cells to be produced and dumped into the bloodstream. The resulting polycythemia causes viscous blood, which impairs circulation, plugs small capillaries, and promotes thrombus formation.

### Infection

If the tumor invades and connects two incompatible organs, such as the bowel and bladder, and thus creates a fistula, infection becomes a serious problem. As they destroy viable tissue and thus their source of nutrition, tumors may become necrotic and septicemia may result. Some tumors are less efficient in creating capillaries; as a consequence, the center of the tumor may become necrotic and infected. When a tumor grows near the surface of the body, it may erode through to the surface, thus breaking down the natural defenses of intact skin and mucous membranes and providing a site for the entry of microorganisms. Any malignant involvement of the organs or tissues of immunity—such as the liver, bone marrow, Peyer's patches in the small intestine, spleen, or lymph nodes—can seriously impair the immune response, allowing infections to develop in vulnerable tissues.

### Hemorrhage

Tumor erosion through blood vessels can cause extensive bleeding, giving rise to severe anemia. Hemorrhage can be serious enough to cause life-threatening hypovolemic shock.

### Anorexia-Cachexia Syndrome

A characteristic feature of cancer is the wasted appearance of its victims, called **cachexia.** In many cases, unexplained rapid weight loss is the first symptom that brings the client to a health care provider. This can be due to a variety of problems associated with cancer, such as pain, infection, depression, or the side effects of chemotherapy and radiation. Usually, however, the emaciation, malnutrition, and loss of energy are attributed to the anorexia-cachexia syndrome.

This syndrome is specific to cancer because of the effect of cancer cells on the host's metabolism. The neoplastic cells divert nutrition to their own use while causing changes that reduce the client's appetite. Early in the disease, glucose metabolism is altered, causing an increase in serum glucose levels. Through the process of negative feedback, anorexia (loss of appetite) results. In addition, the tumor secretes substances that decrease appetite by altering taste and smell and producing early satiety. Pain, infection, and depression also contribute to anorexia. Some types of cancers cause specific food aversions, such as to red meat, coffee, or chocolate.

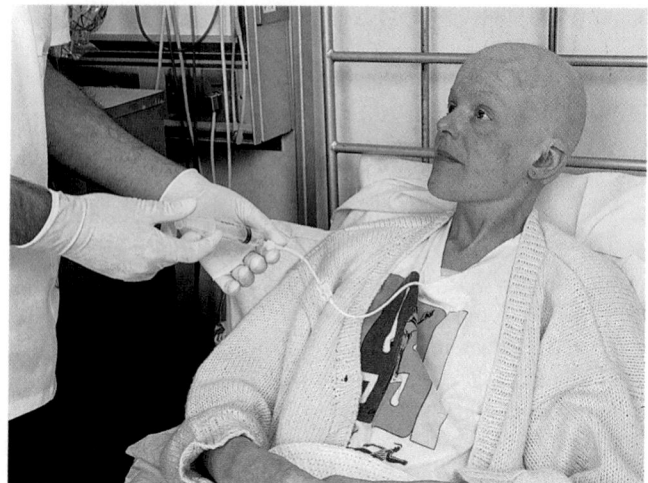

**Figure 10–4** ■ Cachexic person. Cancer robs its host of nutrients and increases body catabolism of fat and muscle to meet its metabolic needs.

*Source: Simon Fraser/SPL/Photo Researchers, Inc.*

| TABLE 10–4 | Laboratory Indicators of Ectopic Functioning |
|---|---|
| **Hormone** | **Specific Laboratory Test** |
| Antidiuretic hormone (ADH) | Serum and urine osmolality |
| Adrenocorticotropic hormone (ACTH) | Plasma ACTH<br>ACTH suppression test<br>ACTH stimulation test<br>Urine catecholamines |
| Calcitonin | Serum calcitonin |
| Insulin | Serum glucose<br>Glucose tolerance test |
| Parathyroid hormone (PTH) | Serum PTH<br>Serum calcium |
| Thyroxine | Serum thyroid-stimulating hormone (TSH), $T_3$, $T_4$ |

Avaricious cancer cells support their growth through widespread catabolism of the body's tissue and muscle proteins. This catabolism, coupled with inadequate nutrient intake, results in the typical cachexia. Normally, a starvation state reduces the body's basal metabolic rate. However, in many people with cancer, the metabolic rate is increased, probably because of the hyperactive metabolic and reproductive activities of the malignant cells. One theory suggests that cytokinins the body produces in response to the tumor are responsible for both early satiety and cachexia. One specific cytokine, called tumor necrosis factor-alpha or cachectin, is believed to enhance the increased metabolic consumption of nutrients. Cancers of the gastrointestinal system further promote anorexia-cachexia by decreasing absorption and use of nutrients; the side effects of some treatment modalities enhance this effect. Figure 10–4 ■ shows the characteristic appearance of a cachexic person.

### Paraneoplastic Syndromes

Paraneoplastic syndromes are indirect effects of cancer. They may be early warning signs of cancer or indicate complications or return of a malignancy. The most frequently occurring paraneoplastic syndromes are endocrine, occurring when cancers set up ectopic sites of hormone production (Haapoja, 2000). Table 10–4 lists laboratory indicators of ectopic funtioning. These ectopic sites produce excessive amounts of the hormone, which harm the host. Consider the following examples.

- Breast, ovarian, and renal cancers may set up ectopic parathyroid hormone sites, causing severe hypercalcemia.
- Oat cell and other lung cancers may produce ectopic secretions of insulin (causing hypoglycemia), parathyroid hormone (PTH), antidiuretic hormone (ADH, which causes excessive fluid retention, hypertension, and peripheral edema), and adrenocorticotropic hormone (ACTH). See Chapter 20 for the description of the multiple problems caused by excessive secretions of cortisone. ⧉

Other paraneoplastic syndromes include hematological abnormalities such as anemia, thrombocytopenia, and coagulation abnormalities; nephrotic syndrome; cutaneous syndromes; and neurological syndromes, such as distant tumors that produce increased intracranial pressure (Haapoja, 2000).

### Pain

Pain is ranked as one of the most serious concerns of clients, families, and oncology health care professionals. Because pain management for people with cancer has a reputation for being ineffective, the anticipation of pain may engender fear in even the most stoic people. Most persons fear pain and suffering even more than possible death, although pain management strategies have improved tremendously. The findings from a 10-year study of over 2000 patients in a palliative care program are encouraging. Following the World Health Organization Guidelines for cancer pain relief, 88% of patients reported good to satisfactory pain relief (Zech, Grond, Lynch, Hertel, & Lehmann, 1995). Research on pain with its devastating statistics has led to great improvement in the pain management strategies.

***TYPES OF CANCER PAIN.*** Cancer pain can be divided into two main categories, acute and chronic, with subgroupings. These classifications serve to indicate appropriate therapeutic approaches. Acute pain has a well-defined pattern of onset, exhibits common signs and symptoms, and is often identified with hyperactivity of the autonomic system. Chronic pain, which lasts more than 6 months, frequently lacks the objective manifestations of acute pain, primarily because the autonomic nervous system adapts to this chronic stress. Unfortunately, chronic pain often results in personality changes, alterations in functional abilities, and lifestyle disruptions that can seriously affect compliance with treatment and the quality of life.

Most cancer clients who cite acute pain as the primary symptom that led to the diagnosis tend to associate pain with the introduction to their disease. If these clients experience pain during the illness or after therapy, they often perceive the pain as introducing another cancer or as a recurrence of the original cancer. Other clients report experiencing pain as a component of cancer therapy. These clients often are able to endure the pain in anticipation of a successful outcome of treatment.

Chronic pain may be related to treatment or may indicate progression of the disease. Identifying the pain as treatment related rather than tumor related is extremely important because it has a definite effect on the client's psychologic outlook. For the client whose pain is due to the advancement of the disease, psychologic factors play an even more important role. Hopelessness and fear of impending death intensify physiologic pain and contribute to overall suffering (which goes well beyond just physical pain).

Three other categories used to classify clients with cancer pain are worth mentioning: clients with preexisting pain, those with a history of drug abuse, and dying clients with cancer-related pain. The first two groups may have altered perceptions of pain and may not have the anticipated response to pain medication. For the dying client, pain is strongly associated with both the client's and family's confrontation of issues of hopelessness and death. Confronting these issues can intensify the perception of pain (see Chapter 4). ⨮

### CAUSES OF CANCER PAIN.
Direct tumor involvement is the primary cause of the pain experienced by people with cancer. This includes metastatic bone disease, nerve compression, and involvement of visceral organs. The pain from tumor involvement is believed to be mechanical, resulting from stretching of tissues and compression. Chemicals from ischemia or tumor metabolites and toxins that activate and sensitize nociceptors and mechanoreceptors are also responsible for tumor pain. See Chapter 4 for a more complete discussion of the mechanics of pain.

Side effects or toxic effects of cancer therapies (e.g., surgery, radiation, and chemotherapy) may also cause cancer pain. These are usually the result of traumatized tissue; one example of this is the oropharyngeal ulcerations that occur with some types of chemotherapy. However, these therapies may also be used to manage pain, such as radiation to decrease pain associated with bone metastasis.

### Physical Stress
When the immune system discovers a neoplasm, it tries to destroy it using the resources of the body. The body mounts an all-out assault on the foreign invader, calling on many resources:

- Chemical mediators
- Hormones and enzymes
- Blood cells
- Antibodies
- Proteins
- Inflammatory and immune responses

These protective responses also mobilize fluid, electrolytes, and nutritional systems. This massive effort requires tremendous energy. See Chapters 5 and 19 for specific information on these systems. ⨮ If the neoplasm is small enough (i.e., microscopic), the immune system can destroy it, and a tumor will never manifest. A neoplasm of 1 cm is large enough to overwhelm most immune systems; however, the body will continue

to try to fight it until it reaches the stage of exhaustion and is no longer capable (Selye, 1984). Thus, many clients with cancer present with fatigue, weight loss, anemia, dehydration, and altered blood chemistries (e.g., decreases in electrolytes).

### Psychologic Stress
People confronted with the diagnosis of cancer exhibit a variety of psychologic and emotional responses. Some people see cancer as a death sentence and experience overwhelming grief, often giving up. Others may feel guilt, considering the cancer a punishment for past behaviors, such as smoking, unhealthy eating habits, or for delaying diagnosis or treatment. The person may experience anger, especially if the person believes that he or she had been practicing a healthful lifestyle; beneath that anger may reside feelings of powerlessness. Fear is common: fear of the outcome of the illness, fear of the

MediaLink | PAIN MANAGEMENT CASE STUDY

---

**BOX 10–5 ■ Physiologic and Psychosocial Effects of Cancer**

- Disruption of function (due to obstruction or pressure)
- Hematologic alterations
  a. Decreased leukocytes, erythrocytes, and thrombocytes
  b. Altered erythropoiesis
- Infections
  a. Fistula between noncompatible organs
  b. Necrosis of tumor center
  c. Malignant involvement of organs of immunity
- Hemorrhage (caused by erosion of neoplasm through blood vessels or surface of skin)
- Anorexia-cachexia syndrome
  a. Hyperglycemia
  b. Catabolism of tissue and muscle proteins
  c. Altered taste and smell
- Creation of ectopic sites of hormones
  a. PTH            c. ADH
  b. Insulin         d. ACTH
- Paraneoplastic syndromes
  a. Deep-vein thrombosis
  b. Peripheral nerve problems
  c. Increased intracranial pressure
  d. Anorexia-cachexia syndrome
  e. Nephritic syndrome
- Pain
  a. Acute and chronic
  b. Caused by direct tumor involvement or side effects of therapy
- Physical stress
  a. Increased general adaptation syndrome activity
  b. Increased immunologic activity
  c. Increased inflammatory response activity
  d. Nutritional, fluid, and electrolyte alterations
- Psychologic stress
  a. Grief           e. Fear
  b. Hopelessness    f. Isolation
  c. Guilt           g. Body image concerns
  d. Anger           h. Sexual dysfunction

*Note. Manifestations depend on the type and location of the cancer.*

effects of treatment, fear of pain, fear of death. Some people feel isolated because of the stigma of cancer and old beliefs of contagion. Body image concerns and sexual dysfunction may be present but often unexpressed, especially if the cancer is of the breast or sexual organs or causes visible body changes. Box 10–5 summarizes the physiologic and psychosocial effects of cancer.

# COLLABORATIVE CARE

Collaborative care begins with a variety of specialized laboratory and diagnostic tests. Once cancer is diagnosed, the initial focus is on medical treatment. The goals of treatment are:

- Eliminating the tumor or malignant cells.
- Preventing metastasis.
- Reducing cellular growth and the tumor burden.
- Promoting functional abilities and providing pain relief to those whose disease has not responded to treatment.

## Laboratory and Diagnostic Tests

### Diagnosis

Several procedures are used to diagnose cancer. X-ray imaging, computed tomography, ultrasonography, and magnetic resonance imaging can locate abnormal tissues or tumors. However, only microscopic histologic examination of the tissue reveals the type of cell and its structural difference from the parent tissue. Tissue samples are acquired through biopsy, shedded cells (e.g., Papanicolaou smear), or collections of secretions (e.g., sputum). Lymph nodes are also biopsied to determine whether metastasis has begun. Simple screening procedures can be used to pick up substances secreted by the tumor, such as the prostatic-specific antigen (PSA) blood test now being used to identify early prostatic cancers. Increases in enzymes or hormones released by normal tissues when they are damaged can also contribute to the diagnosis. Increased alkaline phosphatase noted in bone metastases and osteosarcoma is one example of an enzyme increase associated with cancer. Recent research has identified tumor markers; they are used for early diagnosis, tracking response to therapy, and for devising immunologic treatments.

Some investigators studying chemical mediators of the immune system have noted that there seems to be communication between the chemical mediators and the emotional centers of the brain. A person who states, "I feel I have cancer," should be listened to, and the complaint investigated thoroughly.

### Classification

To help standardize diagnosis and treatment protocols, an elaborate identification system has been developed. This consists of naming the tumor (classification) and describing its aggressiveness (grading) and spread within or beyond the tissue of origin (staging).

Tumors are classified and named by the tissue or cell of origin. Tumor nomenclature often incorporates the Latin stem identifying the tissue from which the tumor arises. For example, a carcinoma arises from epithelial tissue; adjectives are added to further specify the location. A glandular malignancy arising from epithelial tissue is classified as an adenocarcinoma. A tumor arising from supportive tissues is called a sarcoma; the specific type of tissue is added as a prefix. For example, a cancer of fibrous connective tissue is called fibrosarcoma, and a smooth muscle cancer is a leiomyosarcoma. A tumor from seminal or germ tissue is called a seminoma. Table 10–5 compares the nomenclature of benign and malignant neoplasms.

Other names for tumors incorporate the name of the discoverer of that particular cancer, such as Burkitt's lymphoma or Hodgkin's disease. Hematopoietic malignancies (also known as "liquid tumors") are usually named by the type of immature blood cell that predominates. An example is myelocytic leukemia, named for the immature form of the granulocyte that is predominant in this malignancy.

### Grading and Staging

Grading evaluates the amount of differentiation (level of functional maturity) of the cell and estimates the rate of growth based on the mitotic rate. Cells which are the most differentiated—that is, most like the parent tissue and therefore the least malignant—are classified as grade 1 and are associated with a better prognosis. Grade 4 is reserved for the least differentiated and most aggressively malignant cells. Because of the differences inherent in tumor appearance and biologic behavior, grading criteria may vary with different locations and types of tumors.

Staging is used to classify solid tumors and refers to the relative size of the tumor and extent of the disease. The TNM classification system is an internationally agreed upon staging system: The T stands for the relative tumor size, depth of invasion, and surface spread; N indicates the presence and extent of lymph node involvement; and M denotes the presence or absence of distant metastases. Table 10–6 shows the basic outline of the TNM system; however, there are other systems used to differentiate types and locations of tumors (e.g., melanomas, cervical cancer, Hodgkin's disease).

### Cytologic Examination

For the malignant tissues to be identified by name, grade, and stage, they must first be subjected to histologic and cytologic examination by light or electron microscope. Specimens are collected by three basic methods:

1. *Exfoliation from an epithelial surface.* Examples include scraping cells from the cervix (Pap smear) or bronchial washings.
2. *Aspiration of fluid from body cavities or blood.* Examples include white blood cells for evaluation of hematopoietic cancers, pleural fluid, and cerebral spinal fluid.
3. *Needle aspiration of solid tumors.* This could include the breast, lung, or prostate.

Cytologic examination is also carried out on specimens from biopsied tissues or tumors and on collected body secretions, such as sputum or urine.

### TABLE 10-5  Nomenclature for Benign and Malignant Neoplasms

| | Tissue of Origin | Benign | Malignant |
|---|---|---|---|
| Ectoderm/Endoderm | Epithelium | Papilloma | Carcinoma |
| | Gland | Adenoma | Adenocarcinoma |
| | Liver cells | Hepatocellular adenoma | Hepatocellular carcinoma |
| | Neuroglia | Glioma | Glioma |
| | Melanocytes | Melanoma | Malignant melanoma |
| | Basal cells | | Basal cell carcinoma |
| | Germ cells | Tetroma | Seminoma |
| Mesoderm | Connective tissue | | |
| | Adipose tissue | Lipoma | Liposarcoma |
| | Fibrous tissue | Fibroma | Fibrosarcoma |
| | Bone tissue | Osteoma | Osteosarcoma |
| | Cartilage | Chondroma | Chondrosarcoma |
| | Muscle | | |
| | Smooth muscle | Leiomyoma | Leiomyosarcoma |
| | Striated muscle | Rhabdomyoma | Rhabdomyosarcoma |
| | Neural tissue | | |
| | Nerve cells | Ganglioneuroma | Neuroblastoma |
| | Endothelial tissues | | |
| | Blood vessels | Hemangioma | Angiosarcoma |
| | | | Kaposi's sarcoma |
| | Meninges | Meningioma | Malignant meningioma |
| Hematopoietic Tissues | Granulocytes | Granulocytosis | Leukemia |
| | Plasma cells | | Multiple myeloma |
| | Lymphocytes | | Lymphomas |

After collection, specimens are spread on a glass slide, fixed, and stained if necessary. The morphologic features of the cells are examined, with special attention to the nucleus and cytoplasm. Other special pathologic procedures can be carried out on the specimen, but they must be ordered ahead of time if special preparations of the specimen are necessary.

Several special diagnostic cytologic procedures, such as cytogenetics, are proving useful in diagnosing and monitoring client response to treatment.

### TABLE 10-6  TNM Staging Classification System

| | Stage | Manifestations |
|---|---|---|
| Tumor | $T_0$ | No evidence of primary tumor. |
| | $T_{IS}$ | Tumor in situ. |
| | $T_1, T_2, T_3, T_4$ | Ascending degrees of tumor size and involvement. |
| Nodes | $N_0$ | No abnormal regional nodes. |
| | $N_{1a}, N_{2a}$ | Regional nodes—no metastasis. |
| | $N_{1b}, N_{2b}, N_{3b}$ | Regional lymph nodes— metastasis suspected. |
| | $N_x$ | Regional nodes cannot be assessed clinically. |
| Metastasis | $M_0$ | No evidence of distant metastasis. |
| | $M_1, M_2, M_3$ | Ascending degrees of metastatic involvement of the host including distant nodes. |

## Tumor Markers

A tumor marker is a protein molecule detectable in serum or other body fluids. This marker is used as a biochemical indicator of the presence of a malignancy. Small amounts of tumor marker proteins are found in normal body tissues or benign tumors and are not specific for malignancy. However, high levels are suspicious and mandate follow-up diagnostic studies. Tumor marker tests are in the developmental and investigational phase and are most useful for monitoring the client's response to therapy and for detecting residual disease. However, one marker, prostatic-specific antigen (PSA) has received a great deal of media attention as a detector of prostate cancer. As a result, many health care practitioners recommend screening for it in men over 40, much as Pap smears and mammograms are recommended for women.

Tumor markers fall into two general categories: those derived from the tumor itself and those associated with host (immune) response to the tumor. Examples of tumor markers include the following:

- *Antigens.* These are present in fetal tissue but normally are suppressed after birth. Thus, their presence in large amounts may reflect an anaplastic process in tumor cells. Alpha-fetoprotein (AFP) and carcinoembryonic antigen (CEA) are oncofetal antigens.
- *Hormones.* Hormones are, of course, present in considerable amounts in human blood and tissues, but very high levels not related to other conditions may signify the presence

## TABLE 10-7  Tumor-Derived Markers Associated with Specific Neoplasms

| | Tumor Marker | Associated Neoplasm |
|---|---|---|
| Oncofetal Antigens | Carcinoembryonic antigen (CEA)<br>Alpha-fetoprotein (AFP) | Adenocarcinomas of colon, lung, breast, ovary, stomach, pancreas<br>Hepatocellular carcinoma, gonadal germ cell tumors (seminoma) |
| Hormones | Human chorionic gonadotropin (HCG)<br>Calcitonin<br>Catecholamines/metabolites | Gonadal germ cell tumors<br>Medullary cancer of thyroid<br>Pheochromocytoma |
| Isoenzymes | Prostatic acid phosphatase (PAP)<br>Neuron-specific enolase | Adenocarcinoma of prostate<br>Small-cell lung carcinoma, neuroblastoma |
| Specific Proteins | Prostate-specific antigen (PSA)<br>Immunoglobin<br>CA 125<br>CA 19-9<br>CA 15-3 | Adenocarcinoma of prostate<br>Multiple myeloma<br>Epithelial ovarian cancer<br>Adenocarcinoma of pancreas, colon<br>Breast cancer |

Note. Adapted from "The Pathologic Evaluation of Neoplastic Disease" by J. D. Pfeifer and M. R. Wick, in American Cancer Society Textbook of Clinical Oncology (pp. 75–95) by A. I. Holleb, D. J. Fink, and G. P. Murphy, Eds., 1995, Atlanta: American Cancer Society.

of a hormone-secreting malignancy. Some common hormones seen as tumor markers include human chorionic gonadotropin (HCG), antidiuretic hormone (ADH), parathyroid hormone (PTH), calcitonin, and catecholamines.

- *Proteins.* These narrow down the type of tissue that may be malignant, although they can also be increased in hyperplastic disorders. Examples of tissue-specific proteins include serum immunoglobin and beta-2 microglobulin.
- *Enzymes.* Rapid, excessive growth of a tissue may cause some of the enzymes and isoenzymes normally present in that particular tissue to spill into the bloodstream. Elevated levels can point to either hyperplasia of the tissue or cancer. Prostatic acid phosphatase (PAP) and neuron-specific enolase (NSE) are examples. Table 10–7 compares selected tumor-derived markers with their presence in neoplasms and other conditions.

### Oncologic Imaging

Because physical assessment usually cannot detect cancer until the tumor has reached a size that poses a major risk for metastasis, radiologic examination is extremely important in early diagnosis. This diagnostic process may involve routine X-ray imaging (usually for screening only), computed tomography, magnetic resonance imaging, ultrasonography, nuclear imaging, angiography, positron emission tomography, and tagged antibodies.

**X-RAY IMAGING.** Considered the least expensive and least invasive diagnostic procedure, film screen imaging (standard X-ray imaging) is the method of choice for screening such body areas as the breast (mammography), lung, and bone to identify changes in tissue density that may indicate malignancies. X-ray studies are limited in that they do not easily distinguish among calcifications, benign cystic growths, and true malignancies. However, as a screening tool, X-ray imaging can usually reas-

sure the client if findings are negative or encourage follow-up studies if findings are suspicious. X-ray imaging is still the method of choice for lung cancer. Unfortunately, it does not usually reveal tumors until they have reached about 1 cm in size, which is late in their development.

**COMPUTED TOMOGRAPHY.** Computed tomography (CT) has vastly advanced the effectiveness of traditional X-ray methods. By applying computers and mathematics to diagnostic imaging, CT allows the visualization of cross sections of the anatomy. Because CT scans reveal subtle differences in tissue densities, they provide much greater accuracy in tumor diagnosis. This procedure, although more expensive than X-ray imaging, is useful in the screening for some cancers such as renal cell and most gastrointestinal tumors. CT scans are especially useful to evaluate possible lymph node involvement.

**MAGNETIC RESONANCE IMAGING.** Like CT, magnetic resonance imaging (MRI) involves computerized mathematical technology. The patient is placed within a strong magnetic field, pulsed radio waves are directed at the patient, and transmitted signals based on tissue characteristics are analyzed by a computer. Related diagnostic imaging procedures—positron emission tomography (PET) and single photon emission computed tomography (SPECT)—create visible images by measuring electrical impulses from different body structures. Although MRI is relatively expensive, it is the diagnostic tool of choice for both screening and follow-up of cranial and head and neck tumors.

Some clients become claustrophobic during the MRI procedure because they must be placed inside the diagnostic imaging machine, an experience that has been likened to being encased in a small tube. In addition, some machines make loud thumping sounds that can be frightening if the client is not informed beforehand that this is normal.

**ULTRASONOGRAPHY.** Ultrasonography is relatively safe and noninvasive. It measures sound waves as they bounce off various body structures, giving an image of normal anatomy as well as revealing abnormalities that indicate tumors. Ultrasonography has been adapted for diagnosing some specific tumors. For example, transrectal ultrasonography has provided excellent imaging of early prostate cancers and is used to guide needle biopsy. Ultrasound imaging is also more useful for detecting masses in the denser breast tissue of young women.

**NUCLEAR IMAGING.** Nuclear imaging involves the use of a special scintillation scanner in conjunction with the ingestion or injection of specific radioactive isotopes. This is an invasive but usually safe diagnostic method for identifying tumors in various body tissues. For the client with a newly diagnosed cancer, the procedure is often used to check for possible bone or other organ metastases. This evaluation helps the health care provider determine appropriate treatment.

The principle underlying the technology is that certain isotopes have an affinity for specific tissues; for example, radioactive iodine (I 131) has an affinity for the thyroid gland. Malignancies in these tissues sequester an abnormally large amount of the isotope, which then can be traced and measured by the scintillation scanner. This procedure is considered safe because the amount of isotope used is small enough not to damage normal cells.

The procedure is usually minimally distressing for clients. Drinking the isotope solution is not pleasant but is tolerable; some anxious clients may have difficulty lying still during the scan. Antianxiety medication may help. Some clients may experience nausea from drinking the isotope and require antiemetic drugs to complete the procedure. Client preparation may include allowing nothing by mouth or clear fluids only after midnight.

**ANGIOGRAPHY.** An expensive and invasive procedure, angiography is used infrequently for tumor diagnosis. Angiography is performed when the precise location of the tumor cannot be identified or there is a need to visualize the tumor's extent prior to surgery. The procedure involves injecting a radiopaque dye into a major blood vessel proximal to the organ or tissue to be examined. The movement of the dye through the vasculature of the organ or tissue is then traced by means of fluoroscopy or serial X-ray films. In some cases, small catheters are threaded through the vein under fluoroscopy to ensure the specific placement of the dye. Blockage to the flow of the dye indicates the tumor's location. Dye may also be used to identify blood vessels supplying a tumor, allowing the surgeon to know where to safely ligate vessels. Angiography requires preparation similar to that for minor surgery. This includes ensuring that the client takes in only fluids on the day of the examination, performing skin preparation at the insertion site, and administering sedative drugs prior to the procedure. Clients should be informed that injection of the dye used to enhance imaging may cause a hot, flushing sensation or nausea and vomiting. Although angiography is usually done on an outpatient basis, the client will be kept in a short-stay unit for several hours and monitored for such complications as bleeding at the catheter insertion site.

### Direct Visualization

Direct visualization procedures are invasive but do not require the use of radiography. Examples include the following:

- Sigmoidoscopy (viewing the sigmoid colon with a fiberoptic flexible sigmoidoscope)
- Cystoscopy (viewing the urethra and bladder)
- Endoscopy (viewing the upper gastrointestinal tract)
- Bronchoscopy (inspecting the tracheobronchial tree)

These methods allow the visual identification of the organs within the limits of the scope and usually permit biopsy of suspicious lesions or masses. Flexible fiberoptic scopes may be more useful, because they allow deeper penetration than do traditional scopes. These procedures all require some client preparation, cause moderate to considerable discomfort, and may require sedation or even anesthesia, as in the case of bronchoscopy. Some procedures, such as sigmoidoscopy and cystoscopy, may be performed in the physician's office and therefore cost less, making them more accessible screening procedures.

Client preparation includes a thorough bowel cleansing prior to the sigmoidoscopy and cystoscopy; the client may ingest only liquids the morning of the procedure. Because anesthesia may be required, clients undergoing bronchoscopy and endoscopy may be instructed to have nothing by mouth from midnight until the procedure. These procedures are discussed in greater detail in later chapters of this textbook. A more radical method of direct visualization for suspected malignancies is exploratory surgery with biopsy. The client undergoes the usual preoperative preparation (see Chapter 7 ⊂⊃ ) for the type of surgery anticipated. When the tumor is exposed, a sample of tissue (biopsy) is sent to the pathology laboratory for a "frozen-section" histologic examination. This can be done rapidly while the client remains on the operating table under anesthesia. If the initial report is negative, the benign mass is usually removed to prevent further symptoms. If the report is positive for cancer, the tumor and, often, adjacent lymph nodes are resected, along with any other suspicious tissue. The tumor, nodes, and any other specimens are sent to the pathology laboratory for more in-depth analysis. The client then receives the usual postoperative care.

### Laboratory Tests

Most laboratory tests of blood, urine, and other body fluids are used to rule out nutritional disorders and other noncancerous conditions that may be causing the client's symptoms. For example, a complete blood count (CBC) helps screen for such problems as anemia, infection, and impaired immunity. Blood chemistries can point out nutritional disturbances and electrolyte imbalances. However, in conjunction with other diagnostic studies, some laboratory tests can be quite useful either in screening for other pathologic conditions or for validating the cancer diagnosis (Kee, 2002). These

TABLE 10–8    Laboratory Tests Used for Cancer Diagnosis*

| Test | Reference Value | Abnormality Indicated |
|---|---|---|
| Acid phosphatase (ACP) | 0.0 to 0.8 U/L | Elevated in prostate, breast, and bone cancer and in multiple myeloma |
| Adrenocorticotropic hormone (ACTH) | 8 to 80 pg/mL | Decreased in adrenal cancer<br>Elevated in pituitary cancer or with tumor that secretes ACTH (bronchiogenic cancer) |
| Alanine aminotransferase (ALT) | 5 to 35 U/mL (Frankel) | Moderate elevation in liver cancer |
| Albumin | 3.5 to 5.0 g/dL | Decreased in malnutrition, metastatic liver cancer |
| Alkaline phosphatase (ALP) | 20 to 90 U/L | Elevated in cancer of liver, bone, breast, and prostate, in leukemia, and in multiple myeloma |
| Alpha fetoprotein (AFP) | Male and nonpregnant female: <15 ng/mL | Elevated in germ cell tumors (e.g., seminoma), testicular cancer |
| Aspartate aminotransferase (AST) | 5 to 40 U/mL (Frankel) | Elevated in liver cancer |
| Bilirubin | Total: 0.1 to 1.2 mg/dL<br>Direct: 0.0 to 0.3 mg/dL | Elevated in liver and gallbladder cancer |
| Bleeding time | Ivy method: 3 to 7 minutes | Prolonged in leukemia and metastatic liver cancer |
| Blood urea nitrogen (BUN) | 5 to 25 mg/dL | Decreased in malnutrition; increased in renal cancer |
| Calcitonin | Male: <40 pg/mL<br>Female: <20 pg/mL | Elevated to >500 pg/mL in thyroid medullary cancer, breast cancer, and lung cancer |
| Calcium (Ca) | 4.5 to 5.5 mEq/L<br>9.0 to 11.0 mg/dL | Elevated in bone cancer and ectopic parathyroid hormone production (paraplastic syndrome) |
| Carcinoembryonic antigen (CEA) | 2.5 ng/mL in nonsmokers<br>5 ng/mL in smokers; >12 ng/mL neoplasms | Elevated with GI cancers, lung, breast, bladder, kidney, cervical, leukemias<br>Used to evaluate effectiveness of cancer treatment |
| Chloride (Cl) | 95 to 105 mEq/L | Decreased in vomiting, diarrhea, syndrome of inappropriate antidiuretic hormone (SIADH) |
| C-reactive protein | >1:2 titer is positive | Elevated in metastatic cancer and Burkitt's lymphoma |
| Creatinine | 0.5 to 1.5 mg/dL | Decreased in malnutrition; elevated in most cancers |
| Dexamethasone suppression test | >50% reduction in plasma cortisol | Nonsuppression in adrenal cancer and ACTH-producing tumors, severe stress |
| Estradiol-Serum | Female: 20 to 300 pg/mL<br>Menopausal female: <20 pg/mL<br>Male: 15 to 50 pg/mL | Elevated in estrogen-producing tumors and testicular tumors |
| Fibrinogen | 200 to 400 mg/dL | Decreased in leukemia and as a side effect of chemotherapy |
| Gamma glutamyltransferase (GGT) | Male: 10 to 80 IU/L<br>Female: 5 to 25 IU/L | Elevated in cancer of liver, pancreas, prostate, breast, kidney, lung, and brain |
| Fasting blood sugar | 70 to 110 mg/dL | Decreased in malnutrition, cancer of stomach, liver, and lung |
| Haptoglobin | 20 to 240 mg/dL | Elevated in Hodgkin's disease and cancer of lung, large intestine, stomach, breast, and liver |
| Hematocrit (Hct) | Male: 40% to 54%<br>Female: 36% to 46% | Decreased in anemia, leukemia, Hodgkin's disease, lymphosarcoma, multiple myeloma, and malnutrition and as a side effect of chemotherapy |
| Hemoglobin (Hgb) | Male: 13.5 to 18 g/dL<br>Female: 12 to 16 g/dL<br>1:3 ratio of Hgb:Hct | Decreased in anemia, many cancers, Hodgkin's disease, leukemia, and malnutrition and as a side effect of chemotherapy |
| Human chorionic gonadotropin (HCG) | Nonpregnant female <0.01 IU/L | Elevated in choriocarcinoma |
| Insulin | 5 to 25 µU/mL | Elevated in insulinoma (islet cell tumor) and insulin-secreting cancers (e.g., lung cancer) |
| Lactic dehydrogenase (LDH) | 100 to 190 IU/L | Elevated in liver, brain, kidney, muscle cancers, acute leukemia, anemia |

*All values refer to serum values unless otherwise indicated. Values are approximate; check the reference standards specified by your own agency's laboratory.

**TABLE 10-8    Laboratory Tests Used for Cancer Diagnosis\* (continued)**

| Test | Reference Value | Abnormality Indicated |
|---|---|---|
| Occult blood | Negative | Positive in gastric and colon cancers |
| Serum osmolality | 280 to 300 mOsm/kg $H_2O$ | Decreased in SIADH |
| Urine osmolality | 50 to 1200 mOsm/kg $H_2O$ | Increased in SIADH |
| Parathyroid hormone (PTH) | 400 to 900 pg/mL | Increased in PTH-secreting tumors |
| Platelet (thrombocyte) count | 150,000/mm³ to 400,000/mm³ | Decreased in bone, gastric, and brain cancer, in leukemia, and as a side effect of chemotherapy |
| Potassium (K) | 3.5 to 5.0 mEq/L | Decreased in vomiting and diarrhea and in malnutrition |
| Prostate-specific antigen (PSA) | 0 to 4 ng/mL | Elevated from 10 to 120+ in prostate cancer |
| Total protein | 6.0 to 8.0 g/dL | Decreased in malnutrition, gastrointestinal cancer, Hodgkin's disease; elevated in vomiting, diarrhea, multiple myeloma |
| Red blood cells (RBCs) | Male: 4.6 to 6.0 million/mm³ Female: 4.0 to 5.0 million/mm³ | Decreased in anemia, leukemia, infection, multiple myeloma |
| Sodium (Na) | 135 to 145 mEq/L | Decreased in SIADH, vomiting; elevated in dehydration |
| Uric acid | Male: 3.5 to 8.0 mg/dL Female: 2.8 to 6.8 mg/dL | Increased in leukemia, metastatic cancer, multiple myeloma, Burkitt's lymphoma, after vigorous chemotherapy |
| White blood cells (WBC) Total leukocytes | 4,500/mm³ to 10,000/mm³ | Elevated in acute infection, leukemias, tissue necrosis; decreased as a side effect of chemotherapy |
| Neutrophils | 50% to 70% | Elevated in bacterial infection Hodgkin's disease; decreased in leukemia and malnutrition and as a side effect of chemotherapy |
| Eosinophils | 1% to 3% | Elevated in cancer of bone, ovary, testes, and brain |
| Basophils | 0.4% to 1.0% | Elevated in leukemia and healing stage of infection |
| Monocytes | 4% to 6% | Elevated in infection, monocytic leukemia and cancer; decreased in lymphocytic leukemia and as a side effect of chemotherapy |
| Lymphocytes | 25% to 35% | Elevated in lymphocytic leukemia, Hodgkin's disease, multiple myeloma, viral infections, and chronic infections; decreased in malnutrition, cancer, and other leukemias and as a side effect of chemotherapy |

tests include evaluating levels of enzymes such as alanine aminotransferase (ALT), aspartate aminotransferase (AST), and lactic dehydrogenase (LDH) for liver metastases. Special protein tumor markers such as PSA for prostate cancer and CEA for colon cancer are also used. Table 10–8 identifies some useful laboratory tests, their normal values, and their possible indications.

## Psychologic Support During Diagnosis

Preparing for and awaiting the results of diagnostic tests can create extreme anxiety. Many clients compare the experience to that of a prisoner awaiting trial and sentencing: After they know what the "sentence" is, then they can prepare for the future. In addition to coping with the possibility of a life-threatening disease, or at least a life-altering one, clients often also face the prospect of uncomfortable, even painful, diagnostic procedures. They have important decisions to make that depend on the outcome of those tests. Many unspoken questions may exist, including the following:

- Do I have cancer?
- If so, what kind, and how serious?
- Has it spread?
- Will I survive?
- What kind of treatment is needed?
- How will this affect my lifestyle?
- How will this affect family members and friends?

Denial or intellectualization serve some clients well, but others display signs of anxiety and stress as they attempt to cope with this perceived menace. The nurse can provide valuable support during this very difficult stage by helping clients become actively involved in managing their life and disease. Talk with clients as soon as they enter the health care system, asking what they know already about what is going to happen and soliciting questions from them. Taking this approach and encouraging clients to share what knowledge and experience they have allows them to maintain control. From there, the nurse can provide the information needed.

It is essential that clients thoroughly understand the preparation required for their tests, especially if they will be preparing at home. They also need to be informed of any unusual effects that may occur as a result of the procedure, such as nausea from radioactive dye. If possible, a phone call the evening before to verify the client's understanding of the procedure and to answer questions can be helpful and supportive.

As clients begin to feel more comfortable with the nurse, they may express concerns, fears, and other emotions. The nurse should actively listen and be supportive, but avoid giving advice and false reassurance, providing appropriate information when needed. For clients who are not ready to discuss concerns or for those who appear angry, being nonjudgmental and providing nonverbal support may facilitate more open communication. An atmosphere of calmness, warmth, caring, and respect can ease the tension and often unspoken terror of this initial period.

Support of and communication with the client's significant others is extremely important. Often they try to be strong for the client but have many fears and emotional concerns that they do not feel comfortable expressing. The nurse needs to be available to the family while the client is undergoing diagnostic procedures. Allowing them to talk without the need to edit for the client's benefit can help them manage their own difficulties in coping with their loved one's potential cancer diagnosis.

## Chemotherapy

The goals of cancer treatment are aimed at cure, control, or palliation of symptoms. These goals may overlap. Cancer may be treated through chemotherapy, surgery, radiation therapy, or biotherapy. **Chemotherapy** involves the use of cytotoxic medications to cure some cancers, such as leukemias, lymphomas, and some solid tumors; to decrease tumor size, adjunctive to surgery or radiation therapy; or to prevent or treat suspected metastases. Chemotherapy may also be used in conjunction with biotherapy. All chemotherapy has side effects or toxic effects. The type and severity depend upon the drugs used.

Chemotherapy disrupts the cell cycle in various phases by interrupting cell metabolism and replication. It also works by interfering with the ability of the malignant cell to synthesize vital enzymes and chemicals. Phase-specific drugs work during only some phases of the cell cycle; non-phase-specific drugs work through the entire cell cycle. Figure 10–5 ■ lists some of the drugs useful in each phase of the cell cycle.

Most chemical treatment involves combinations of drugs in specific protocols given over varying periods of time. For example, one protocol for adult acute lymphocytic leukemia (ALL) uses the acronym DVPA: daunorubicin given on days 1 through 3; vincristine given on days 1, 8, 15, and 22; prednisone given on days 1 through 28, and asparaginase given on days 17 through 28. The treatment regimen is given in cycles with rest periods allowed, especially if toxic effects such as liver dysfunction or severe neutropenia occur. The treatment is continued until the disease goes into remission. If the disease progresses, the particular protocol is abandoned and a new one may be tried.

Researchers have examined the possibility of basing chemotherapy administration on the body's circadian rhythms. Some drugs work better if they follow the normal cyclic fluctuations of body hormones during the night, whereas others are more effective when given during daytime hours. Chemotherapy administration that follows circadian rhythms appears to be

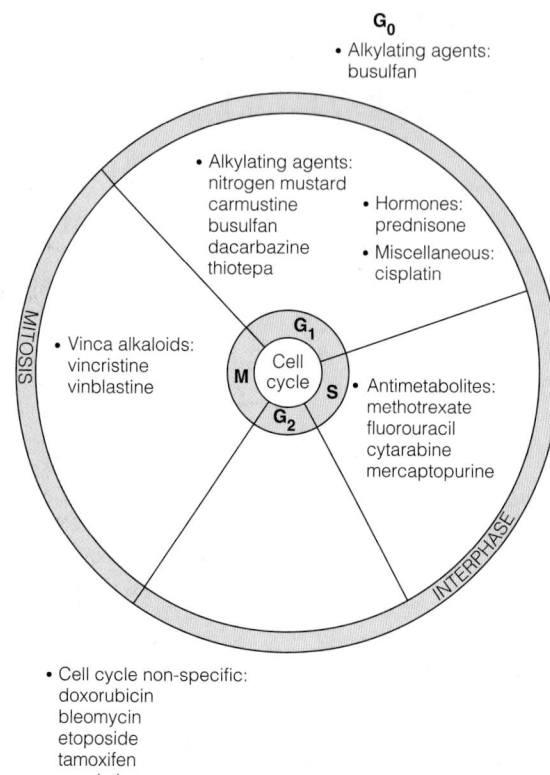

**Figure 10–5** ■ Chemotherapeutic drugs useful in each phase of the cell cycle. Based on their chemical makeup and biologic activity, different drugs used for cancer treatment act in specific phases and subphases of the cell cycle. Some drugs, called non-phase-specific drugs, are generalized and act throughout the cycle. Chemotherapy often involves combinations of drugs designed to attack the cancer cells at many different times in the cycle and thus to enhance effectiveness.

more effective and causes fewer side effects with some types of cancer. A study of people with advanced colon cancer who were treated in this cyclic fashion (circadian rhythmic delivery, or CRD) demonstrated a 51% shrinkage in their tumors, compared with a shrinkage of only 28% in people who received chemotherapy in a steady dosage over 24 hours. In addition, the frequency and severity of side effects was decreased in the CRD group (Misset & Levi, 1995).

The cell-kill hypothesis explains why several courses of chemotherapy are necessary. A 1 cm tumor contains about $10^9$ (10 billion) total cells, most of which are viable. During each cell cycle, the chemotherapy kills a fixed percentage of cells, always leaving some behind. With each reduction, the tumor burden of cells decreases until the number of viable, clonogenic cells (i.e., those that are able to clone daughter cells) becomes small enough to allow the body's immune system to finish the job. For this reason, oncologists usually give the maximum amount of chemotherapy tolerated by the client. High-dose chemotherapy (HDCT) remains controversial (Weiss et al., 2000). In a randomized study of 525 women with high-risk early breast cancer, individually tailored chemotherapy was compared with standard chemotherapy followed by HDCT. Women in the tailored chemotherapy group had significantly improved relapse-free survival and fewer severe side effects compared to women in the HDCT group (Bergh et al., 2000). Another study examined outcomes of women with metastatic breast cancer who were eligible for HDCT, but who were treated with standard-dose chemotherapy. The findings that progression-free survival and overall survival were higher for the HDCT group could be due in part to selection of subjects with better prognoses. The researchers concluded that the findings emphasize the importance of completing ongoing studies with randomized comparison groups (Rahman et al., 1997).

### Classes of Chemotherapy Drugs

Chemotherapeutic agents fall basically into six major classes: alkylating agents, antimetabolites, antitumor antibiotics, mitotic inhibitors, hormones and hormone antagonists, and miscellaneous agents.

***ALKYLATING AGENTS.*** Alkylating agents are non-phase specific and basically act on preformed nucleic acids by creating defects in tumor DNA. They cause cross linking of DNA strands, which can permanently interfere with replication and transcription.

Alkylating agents work with both proliferating and nonproliferating cells (those in $G_0$ phase). Their toxicity relates to their ability to kill slowly cycling stem cells and manifests in delayed, prolonged, or permanent bone marrow failure. Toxicity can also cause a mutagenic effect on bone marrow stem cells, culminating in a treatment-resistant form of acute myelogenous leukemia. Because of the alkylating agents' effect on stem cells, they also cause irreversible infertility. Other common adverse effects include nephrotoxicity and hemorrhagic cystitis.

The several subclasses of alkylating agents include nitrogen mustard (mechlorethamine), nitrosoureas (carmustine), alkyl sulfonates (busulfan), triazines (dacarbazine), ethylenimines (thiotepa), and cisplatin. Cisplatin is an alkylating agent containing platinum and chlorine atoms. It is most active in the $G_1$ subphase, but it is also non-phase specific. Cisplatin binds to DNA and acts much like alkylating agents by forming intrastrand DNA cross links (gluing strands of DNA together so that they cannot separate). Its major toxic effect is reversible renal tubular necrosis. Cisplatin may be used alone or in combination with other chemotherapeutic drugs for testicular and ovarian cancers.

***ANTIMETABOLITES.*** Antimetabolites, a group of somewhat diverse drugs, are phase specific, working best in the S phase and having little effect in $G_0$. They interfere with nucleic acid synthesis by either displacing normal metabolites at the regulatory site of a key enzyme or by substituting for a metabolite that is incorporated into DNA or RNA molecules.

Toxic effects usually do not occur until very high levels of the drug are administered. Toxicity is also more likely when the drugs accumulate in third-spaced fluid, such as pleural fluid (a characteristic that also makes them useful in treating malignant pleural effusions). Because the drug diffuses out slowly from the third-spaced fluid, exposure of the tissue to the drug is prolonged. Most toxic effects relate to rapidly

proliferating cells, such as cells in the gastrointestinal tract, hair, and skin and WBCs. Signs and symptoms include the following:

- Nausea and vomiting
- Stomatitis
- Diarrhea
- Alopecia
- Leukopenia

Some of the drugs can also cause liver and pulmonary toxicity.

The different types of antimetabolites include folic acid analogues (methotrexate), pyrimidine analogues (5-fluorouracil), cytosine arabinoside (ARA-C), and purine analogues (6-mercaptopurine).

***ANTITUMOR ANTIBIOTICS.*** Antitumor antibiotics are originally derived from natural sources that are generally too toxic to be used as antibacterial agents. They are non-phase specific and act in several ways: They disrupt DNA replication and RNA transcription; create free radicals, which generate breaks in DNA and other forms of damage; and interfere with DNA repair. In addition, these drugs bind to cells and kill them, probably by damaging the cell membrane. Their main toxic effect is damage to the cardiac muscle. This limits the amount and duration of treatment. Examples of these antibiotics include actinomycin D, doxorubicin, bleomycin, mitomycin-C, and mithramycin.

***MITOTIC INHIBITORS.*** Mitotic inhibitors are drugs that act to prevent cell division during the M phase. Mitotic inhibitors include the plant alkaloids and taxoids. Plant alkaloids consist of medications extracted from plant sources: Vinca alkaloids (e.g., vincristine and vinblastine) and etoposide (also called VP-16). The Vinca alkaloids are phase specific, acting during mitosis. They bind to a specific protein in tumor cells that promotes chromosome migration during mitosis and serves as a conduit for neurotransmitter transport along axons. The toxicity of these drugs is characterized by depression of deep-tendon reflexes, paresthesias (pain and altered sensation), motor weakness, cranial nerve disruptions, and paralytic ileus. Etoposide acts in all phases of the cell cycle, causing breaks in DNA and metaphase arrest. Although etoposide may cause bone marrow suppression and nausea and vomiting, the most common toxic effect is hypotension resulting from too rapid intravenous administration.

The taxoids act during the $G_2$ phase to inhibit cell division. Paclitaxel is used for the treatment of Kaposi's sarcoma and metastatic breast and ovarian cancer. Taxotere is used for breast cancer. Toxicities associated with these drugs include alopecia, bone marrow depression, and severe hypersensitivity reactions (e.g., hypotension, dyspnea, and urticaria).

***HORMONES AND HORMONE ANTAGONISTS.*** The main hormones used in cancer therapy are the corticosteroids (e.g., prednisone), which are phase specific ($G_1$). These act by binding to specific intracellular receptors, repressing transcription of mRNA and thereby altering cellular function and growth. Corticosteroids have multiple side effects such as impaired healing, hyperglycemia, hypertension, osteoporosis, and hirsutism.

Hormone antagonists work with hormone-binding tumors, usually those of the breast, prostate, and endometrium. They block the hormone's receptor site on the tumor and prevent it from receiving normal hormonal growth stimulation. These drugs do not cure, but do cause regression of the tumor in about 40% of breast and endometrial tumors and 80% of prostate tumors. Tamoxifen competes with estradiol receptors in breast tumors. Raloxifene blocks estrogen in the breast. Diethylstilbestrol competes with hormone receptors in endometrial and prostate tumors. Antiandrogen (flutamide) and luteinizing hormone–releasing hormone (LHRH) block testosterone synthesis in prostate cancers. The main side effects of these drugs are alterations of the secondary sexual characteristics.

**MISCELLANEOUS AGENTS.** Several miscellaneous agents act at different phases in the cell cycle. L-asparaginase and hydroxyurea are examples of miscellaneous agents.

## Effects of Chemotherapeutic Drugs

As described, the side effects and toxic effects of chemotherapy vary with the drug used and the length of treatment. Because most of these drugs act on fast-growing cells, the side effects are manifestations of damage to normal rapidly dividing somatic cells. The side effects of hormones express the action of the hormone used or suppression of the normal hormone, such as the masculinizing effects of male hormones administered for ovarian cancers.

Tissues usually affected by cytotoxic drugs include the following:

- Mucous membranes of the mouth, tongue, esophagus, stomach, intestine, and rectum. This may result in anorexia, loss of taste, aversion to food, erythema and painful ulcerations in any portion of the gastrointestinal tract, nausea, vomiting, and diarrhea.
- Hair cells, resulting in alopecia.
- Bone marrow depression affecting most blood cells (e.g., granulocytes, lymphocytes, thrombocytes, and erythrocytes). This results in an impaired ability to respond to infection, a diminished ability to clot blood, and severe anemia.
- Organs, such as heart, lungs, bladder, kidneys. This kind of damage is related to specific agents, such as cardiac toxicity with doxorubicin or pneumonitis with bleomycin.
- Reproductive organs, resulting in impaired reproductive ability or altered fetal development.

Table 10–9 gives the classifications of chemotherapeutic drugs, common examples, target malignancies, adverse effects and side effects, and nursing implications. Consult current pharmacology textbooks for additional drugs and for new combination therapies as they are developed.

| TABLE 10–9 | Classifications of Chemotherapeutic Drugs | | | |
|---|---|---|---|---|
| **Drug Classification** | **Common Drugs** | **Target Malignancies** | **Adverse Effects or Side Effects** | **Nursing Implications** |
| Alkylating agents | Mechlorethamine (Mustargen) | Hodgkin's disease Lymphosarcoma Lung cancer Chronic leukemia | Nausea and vomiting Leukopenia Thrombocytopenia Hyperuricemia | Maintain good hydration. Alkalinize urine. Administer antiemetics prior to chemotherapy. Monitor WBC, uric acid. Assess for infection. |
| | Busulfan (Myleran) | Chronic myelogenous leukemia | Leukopenia Thrombocytopenia Renal failure Pulmonary fibrosis | Monitor WBCs, BUN. Maintain adequate fluid intake. Assess for infection. Assess lungs for fibrotic (coarse, loud) rales. |
| | Cyclophosphamide (Cytoxan) | Lymphomas Multiple myeloma Leukemias Adenocarcinoma of lung and breast | Hemorrhagic cystitis Renal failure Alopecia Stomatitis Liver dysfunction | Encourage daily fluid intake of 2 to 3 L during treatment. Monitor WBCs, BUN, liver enzymes. Teach ways to manage hair loss. |
| Antimetabolites | Methotrexate | Acute lymphoblastic leukemia Osteosarcoma Gestational trophoblastic carcinoma | Oral and gastrointestinal ulcerations Anorexia and nausea Leukopenia Thrombocytopenia Pancytopenia | Monitor CBC, WBC differential, BUN, uric acid, creatinine. Assess oral mucous membranes; treat ulcers prn. Assess for infection, bleeding. |

TABLE 10–9  Classifications of Chemotherapeutic Drugs (continued)

| Drug Classification | Common Drugs | Target Malignancies | Adverse Effects or Side Effects | Nursing Implications |
|---|---|---|---|---|
| | 5-Fluorouracil (5-FU) | Colon carcinoma<br>Rectal carcinoma<br>Breast carcinoma<br>Gastric carcinoma<br>Pancreatic cancer | Stomatitis<br>Alopecia<br>Nausea and vomiting<br>Gastritis<br>Enteritis<br>Diarrhea<br>Anemia<br>Leukopenia<br>Thrombocytopenia | Monitor CBC with differential, BUN, uric acid.<br>Administer antiemetics prn.<br>Assess for bleeding; check stool occult blood.<br>Evaluate hydration and nutrition status.<br>Teach oral care for stomatitis.<br>Assess for infection.<br>Teach care for hair loss. |
| Antitumor antibiotics | Doxorubicin (Adriamycin) | Acute lymphoblastic leukemia (ALL)<br>Acute myeloblastic leukemia<br>Neuroblastoma<br>Wilms' tumor<br>Breast, ovarian, thyroid, lung cancer | Stomatitis<br>Alopecia<br>Nausea and vomiting<br>Gastritis<br>Enteritis<br>Diarrhea<br>Anemia<br>Leukopenia<br>Thrombocytopenia<br>Cardiac toxicity | Monitor ECG; assess for arrythmias, gallops, and congestive heart failure (CHF).<br>Monitor CBC with differential, BUN, uric acid.<br>Administer antiemetics prn.<br>Assess for bleeding; check stool for occult blood.<br>Evaluate hydration and nutrition status.<br>Teach oral care for stomatitis.<br>Assess for infection.<br>Teach care for hair loss. |
| | Bleomycin (Blenoxane) | Squamous cell carcinoma<br>Lymphosarcoma<br>Reticulum cell sarcoma<br>Testicular carcinoma<br>Hodgkin's disease | Mucocutaneous ulcerations<br>Alopecia<br>Nausea and vomiting<br>Chills and fever<br>Pneumonitis and pulmonary fibrosis | Check for fever 3 to 6 hours after administration.<br>Have chest X-ray films taken every 2 to 3 weeks.<br>Assess respiratory status, and check for coarse rales.<br>Evaluate hydration and nutrition status.<br>Teach oral care for stomatitis.<br>Assess for infection.<br>Teach care for hair loss. |
| Plant alkaloids | Vincristine (Oncovin) | Combination therapy for acute leukemia, Hodgkin's and non-Hodgkin's lymphomas, rhabdomyosarcoma, neuroblastoma, Wilm's tumor | Areflexia<br>Muscle weakness<br>Peripheral neuritis<br>Constipation<br>Paralytic ileus<br>Mild bone marrow Depression | Assess neuromuscular function.<br>Monitor CBC with differential.<br>Evaluate gastrointestinal function.<br>Manage constipation. |
| | Vinblastine (Velban) | Combination therapy for Hodgkin's disease, lymphocytic and histocytic lymphoma.<br>Kaposi's sarcoma, advanced testicular carcinoma, unresponsive breast cancer | Areflexia<br>Alopecia<br>Nausea and vomiting<br>Bone marrow depression | Assess neuromuscular function.<br>Monitor CBC with differential.<br>Administer antiemetics prn.<br>Teach ways to manage hair loss. |

(continued on page 294)

TABLE 10–9    Classifications of Chemotherapeutic Drugs (continued)

| Drug Classification | Common Drugs | Target Malignancies | Adverse Effects or Side Effects | Nursing Implications |
|---|---|---|---|---|
| Plant alkaloids *continued* | Etoposide, also called VP-16 (VePesid) | Nonresponsive testicular tumors<br>Small-cell lung cancer | Alopecia<br>Hypotension with rapid infusion | Hydrate adequately before administration.<br>Administer for 60 minutes.<br>Monitor vital signs every 15 minutes during administration and every 2 to 4 hours thereafter.<br>Teach ways to manage hair loss. |
| | Prednisone | Combination therapy for many tumors<br>Leukemia<br>Lymphoma | Fluid retention<br>Hypertension<br>Steroid diabetes<br>Emotional lability<br>Silent bleeding ulcers<br>Increased risk for infection | Monitor vital signs.<br>Administer diuretics prn.<br>Check blood glucose regularly.<br>Evaluate mental status.<br>Administer oral medications with food.<br>Administer hydrogen ion antagonist drugs (antacids) as ordered.<br>Monitor WBC with differential.<br>Check for signs of systemic infection. |
| | Diethylstilbestrol (DES) | Advanced breast and prostrate cancers | Fluid retention<br>Feminization<br>Uterine bleeding | Monitor vital signs.<br>Administer diuretics prn as ordered.<br>Explain reason for feminization to men, bleeding to women.<br>Monitor for excessive bleeding. |
| | Tamoxifen (Nolvadex) | Breast cancer | Hot flashes<br>Nausea and vomiting | Teach ways to manage hot flashes.<br>Explain reason for hot flashes.<br>Administer antiemetics as ordered. |
| Miscellaneous drugs | Cisplatin (CDDP) (Platinol) | Combination and single therapy for metastatic testicular and ovarian cancers, advanced bladder cancer, head and neck tumors, non-small-cell lung carcinoma, osteogenic sarcoma, neuroblastoma | Bone marrow depression: leukopenia and thrombocytopenia<br>Renal tubular damage<br>Deafness | Monitor WBC with differential and platelets, BUN, creatinine, uric acid.<br>Watch for bleeding.<br>Monitor for signs of infection.<br>Evaluate hearing; check for tinnitus.<br>Ensure that client is well hydrated before drug is administered.<br>Encourage 2 to 3 L of fluid intake daily. |

## Preparation and Administration

Many states and individual hospitals require that personnel be trained and certified to administer chemotherapy. Pharmacists in large hospitals and independent home care agencies usually prepare chemotherapeutic drugs for parenteral administration under specific safety guidelines established by the federal government or the Oncology Nursing Society. In some agencies, nurses both prepare and administer these drugs. Because of the potential carcinogenic effects, it is usually recommended that the health care professional wear gloves, a mask, and gown while preparing and administering the drug and disposing of equipment. The nurse must use care when handling excretory products of clients undergoing chemotherapy and teach clients to dispose of their own body fluids safely. Oral medications pose a lesser risk of exposure, but a risk nonetheless, primarily through excretion in the urine.

Chemotherapeutic drugs can be administered orally, such as cyclophosphamide (Cytoxan) and chlorambucil (Leukeran). Other drugs, such as hormones or hormone-blocking agents, may also be given intramuscularly. However, many drugs require intravenous infusion or direct injection into intraperitoneal or intrapleural body cavities. Intravenous preparations can be given through large peripheral veins, but the risk of extravasation or irritation to the vein may preclude this method for long-term therapy. Many clients now receive vascular access devices (VADs), especially if their treatment requires several cycles over weeks or months. VADs are also useful for adjunctive parenteral nutrition in the client who needs continuous intravenous infusions to manage pain or frequent blood drawing to monitor blood counts. Different types of VADs are available:

- Catheters that are inserted nonsurgically by threading them through a large peripheral vein into the vena cava. Called peripherally inserted central catheters (PICCs), they have multiple lumens that facilitate blood drawing. Placement is usually monitored by fluoroscopy.
- Catheters tunneled under the skin on the chest into a major vein, such as the subclavian vein. Hickman or Groshong catheters may be used.
- Surgically implanted ports, which are placed under the skin with a connected catheter inserted into a major vein. These are

accessed by means of a special needle with a 90-degree angle inserted through the skin directly into the rubber dome of the port, which has a hard plastic back to prevent tissue damage.

Figure 10–6 ■ shows examples of different catheters and vascular access ports.

Risk of infection, catheter obstruction, and extravasation are the main problems associated with VADs. Nurses therefore must teach clients and family members to observe for redness, swelling, pain, or exudate at the insertion site, which may indicate infection; to observe for swelling of the neck or skin near the VAD for extravasation and infiltration; and to flush catheters and provide site care (cleaning and dressing changes) on a regular basis. During each encounter with the client, the nurse always inspects the site; observes for infection, infiltration, and catheter occlusion; and provides site care when necessary.

## Management of Clients Receiving Chemotherapy

In addition to providing the above nursing interventions, nurses help identify and manage toxic effects or side effects of the drugs and provide psychosocial support. Careful assessment and monitoring of the client's signs and symptoms, including appropriate laboratory tests, alert the nurse to the onset of toxicity. Nausea and vomiting, diarrhea, inflammation and ulceration of oral mucous membranes, hair loss, skin changes, anorexia, and fatigue require specific medical and nursing

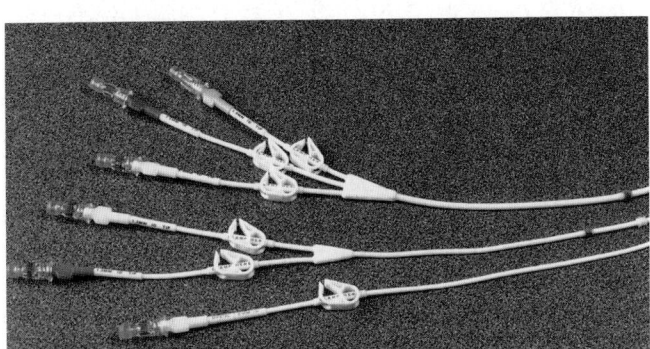

**A**

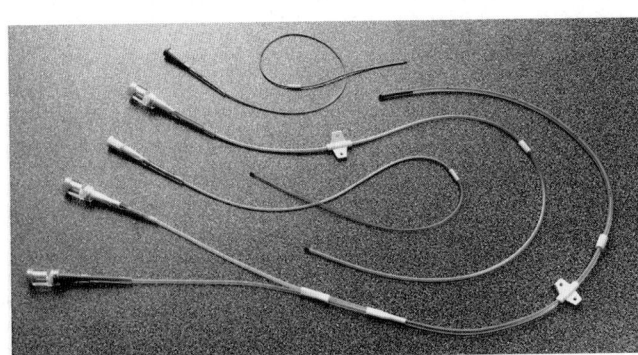

**B**

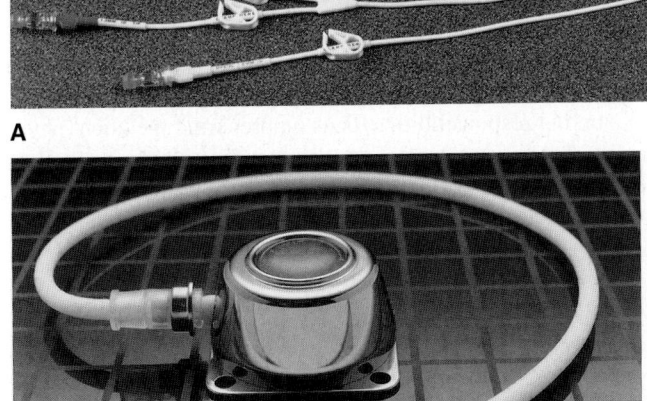

**C**

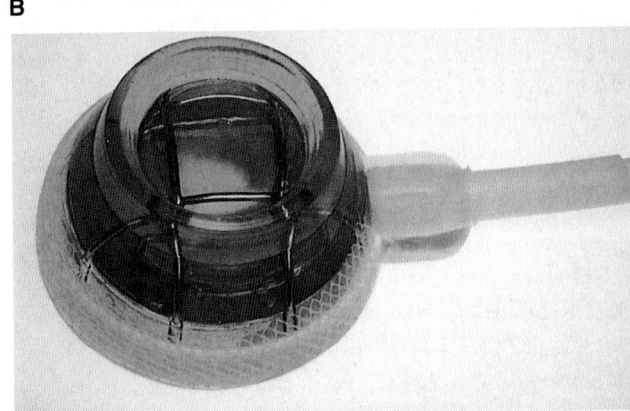

**D**

**Figure 10–6** ■ Vascular access devices. *A,* Single-, double-, and triple-lumen catheters; *B,* single- and double-lumen Groshong catheters; *C,* Port-a-Cath Access System; *D,* Norport-SP, a side-entrance port.

*Photos A, B: Courtesy of Bard Access Systems, Salt Lake City, UT; Photo C, S/MS Deltec, Inc., St. Paul, MN; Photo D, Norfolk Medical, Skokie, Il.*

actions. These actions are discussed later in this chapter under the appropriate nursing diagnoses. Indicators of organ toxicities, such as nephrotoxicity, neurotoxicity, or cardiac toxicity, must be reported immediately to the physician. Another aspect of managing clients undergoing chemotherapy is to teach them how to care for access sites and to dispose of used equipment and excretions safely. Nurses also teach clients to increase fluid intake to flush out the drugs; to get extra rest, which can both assist therapy and help the client avoid other illnesses; to identify major complications of their particular drug protocol; to know when to call the physician or emergency medical services; and, if their WBC count is low, to limit their exposure to other people, especially those with infections or children.

During chemotherapy, a number of psychologic issues that can cause moderate to severe emotional distress may arise. The need to plan activities around chemotherapy treatments and their side effects can impair the client's ability to work, manage a household or care for family members, function sexually, or participate in social and recreational activities. Weight loss and alopecia may prompt feelings of powerlessness and depression. The nurse can assist by carefully evaluating symptoms, providing specific interventions as indicated, and allowing clients opportunities to express their fears, concerns, and feelings. Clients should be encouraged to participate in their care and maintain control over their life as much as possible (McDaniel & Rhodes, 1998). Specific interventions will be discussed later in the chapter under the appropriate nursing diagnoses. Table 10–9 includes nursing implications for specific adverse effects of common chemotherapy drugs.

## Surgery

Surgical resection is used for diagnosis and staging of more than 90% of all cancers and for primary treatment of more than 60% of cancers. When possible, the tumor is removed in its entirety. This sometimes necessitates mutilation of the body and the creation of new structures to assume function of the lost structures. For example, removal of the distal sigmoid colon and rectum requires a new means of bowel elimination, so the remaining healthy segment of the bowel is brought out through a created opening (stoma) in the abdominal wall, resulting in a permanent colostomy (see Chapter 24). In like manner, when the bladder is removed, the ureters are transplanted into a created pouch just under the abdominal wall. This serves as a continent ileostomy, a substitute reservoir for urine (see Chapter 26). Surgery can also destroy sensitive nerve plexes, resulting in alteration or loss of normal functioning; for example, prostate surgery may result in incontinence and impotence. ⊂⊃

Not all surgery results in such radical changes in functioning. The following surgeries can eliminate cancer successfully with less distressing results.

- Removing a nonessential portion of the organ or tissue containing the tumor, such as in situ small bowel tumors
- Removing an organ whose function can be replaced chemically, such as the thyroid
- Resecting one of a pair of organs when the unaffected organ can take over the function of the missing one, such as a lung

Although the removal of any major body part has physiologic and psychologic consequences, the alternative—terminal disease—is usually less desirable.

If the tumor is in a nonresectable location or deeply invasive with metastases, surgery may be only a palliative measure to allow the involved organs to function as long as possible, to relieve pain, or to bypass an obstruction. Surgery may also be done to reduce the bulk of the tumor in advanced disease, both at primary and metastatic sites. Decreasing the tumor size enhances the ability to control the remaining disease through other modalities. Surgery is often used in conjunction with other treatments to effect a cure. For example, in cases when extensive removal of tissue is contraindicated (e.g., in surgical removal of a brain tumor), radiation may be used prior to surgery in an attempt to shrink the tumor before it is removed.

Surgical intervention may also be used for reconstruction and rehabilitation. One example is the construction of transabdominal mycocutaneous (TRAM) flaps in conjunction with or following modified radical mastectomy (see Chapter 48). For surgical interventions for cancers affecting specific body systems, refer to later chapters. ⊂⊃

Surgical oncologists are working with researchers to identify premalignant disease earlier in high-risk populations and to conduct studies on ways to reverse oncogenic cell activity. Surgeons also work with molecular biologists using sophisticated techniques to develop monoclonal antibodies. Laser technology is being explored for use in different types of cancer surgery because it minimizes blood loss, reduces deformity, increases the accuracy of tissue resection, and enhances healing. Lasers are currently being used to treat radical prostectomy in order to preserve urinary continence and sexual functioning. Another collaborative strategy under development is intraoperative radiation therapy, in which radiosensitive, nondiseased organs that may be damaged by radiation therapy are moved away from the radiation field and shielded. Radiation is then administered while the patient is on the operating table. This technique allows more penetrating radiation to be directed to the malignant tumor with less trauma to normal, vulnerable tissues or organs.

Nursing responsibilities focus on preparing the client physically and psychologically for the specific surgery, as well as teaching routine postoperative care in which the client is expected to participate. For example, the nurse teaches the client about respiratory care and the use of the incentive spirometer to improve postoperative ventilation, early ambulation to prevent circulatory problems, and how the client will receive fluids and nutrition (intravenously or orally, depending on the type of surgery). In addition, the nurse explains the specific surgical procedure and any anticipated alterations to the client's body, especially those that require major lifestyle adjustments, such as a colostomy. Before surgery, the nurse should give the client the opportunity to ask questions and to discuss concerns and fears. In some cases, the client may want to discuss alternative treatment options. In the latter case, the nurse should avoid trying to persuade the client to accept any one option; rather, the nurse should contact the oncologist and the surgeon and set up a conference for the client before surgery.

## Radiation Therapy

Still the treatment of choice for some tumors or by some oncologists, radiation may be used to kill the tumor, to reduce its size, to decrease pain, or to relieve obstruction. Lymph nodes and adjacent tissues are irradiated when beginning metastasis is suspected. Radiation therapy consists of delivering ionizing radiations of gamma and X-rays in one of two ways:

- **Teletherapy.** Also called external radiation, teletherapy involves delivery of radiation from a source at some distance from the client. A relatively uniform dosage is delivered to the tumor.
- **Brachytherapy.** In brachytherapy, the radioactive material is placed directly into or adjacent to the tumor, a technique that delivers a high dose to the tumor and a lower dose to the normal tissues. This allows delivery of high doses of radiation to the tumor while sparing adjacent tissue. Brachytherapy is also referred to as internal, interstitial, or intracavitary radiation.

For many common neoplasms, a combination of these two therapies is used.

Lethal injury to DNA is believed to be the primary mechanism by which radiation kills cells, especially cells in faster growing tumors and tissues. As a result, when given over time, radiation can destroy not only rapidly multiplying cancer cells but also rapidly dividing normal cells, such as those of the skin and mucous membranes. A malignant tumor is considered cured when there are no surviving tumor stem cells. The goal of radiation therapy is to achieve maximum tumor control with a minimum of damage to normal tissue.

Implanted or ingested radiation can be dangerous for those living with, taking care of, or treating the client. Caregivers must use protection by, for example, shielding themselves from the source of radiation, limiting the time of exposure to the client, increasing the distance from the client, and using specific safety procedures for handling secretions. Box 10–6 identifies safety principles to be followed by those caring for clients undergoing internal radiation.

Tumors have differing sensitivities to radiation. Tumors that have the greatest number of rapidly proliferating cancer cells usually exhibit the best early response to radiation. The decision to use radiation rather than other modalities is based on balancing the probability of controlling the tumor against the probability of causing complications, such as tissue damage. The decision is usually made by risk-benefit analysis. Planning for radiation therapy includes assessing the disease site, tumor size, and histologic findings. Treatment schedules vary based on these factors (Neal & Hoskin, 1997). Box 10–7 lists the degree of radiosensitivity for selected cancers.

The client receiving external radiation may experience skin changes such as blanching, erythema, desquamation, sloughing, or hemorrhage. Ulcerations of mucous membranes may cause severe pain; in addition, oral secretions can decrease, making the client more vulnerable to infection and dental caries. Gastrointestinal effects include nausea and vomiting, diarrhea, or bleeding. Lungs may develop interstitial exudate, a condition called radiation pneumonia. Occasionally, external

---

### BOX 10–6 ■ Safety Principles for Radiation

These recommendations apply to caregivers working with clients receiving internal radiation (brachytherapy).

- Maintain the greatest possible distance from the source of radiation.
- Spend the minimum amount of time close to the radiation source.
- Shield yourself from the radiation with lead gloves and aprons when possible.
- If pregnant, avoid contact with radiation sources.
- If you work routinely near radiation, wear a monitoring device to measure whole-body exposure.
- Avoid direct exposure with radioisotope containers; for example, do not touch the container.
- Keep clients with implanted radioisotopes in a private room with private bath and as far away from other hospitalized persons as possible.
- Dispose of body fluids of clients with unsealed implanted radioisotopes with special care and in specially marked containers.
- Handle bed linen and clothing with care and according to agency protocol.
- Use long-handled forceps to place any dislodged implants into a lead container.
- Consult with the radiation therapy department for any questions or problems in caring for clients with radioactive implants.

---

radiation therapy may cause fistulas or necrosis of adjacent tissues. Implanted radioactive materials can lead to similar problems; moreover, the excretory products of these clients are usually considered dangerous and need special disposal. See the Nursing Care box on page 298 for nursing implications for clients receiving radiation therapy.

---

### BOX 10–7 ■ Degree of Radiosensitivity for Selected Cancers

#### VERY RADIOSENSITIVE
- Neuroblastoma
- Lymphomas
- Chronic leukemia

#### MODERATELY RADIOSENSITIVE
- Bronchogenic carcinoma
- Esophageal carcinoma
- Squamous cell carcinoma
- Prostate carcinoma
- Cervical carcinoma
- Testicular carcinoma

#### NONRADIOSENSITIVE
- Many adenocarcinomas
- Fibrosarcoma
- Osteogenic carcinoma

# NURSING CARE OF THE CLIENT RECEIVING RADIATION THERAPY

## NURSING RESPONSIBILITIES FOR EITHER EXTERNAL OR INTERNAL RADIATION THERAPY

- Carefully assess and manage any complications, usually in collaboration with the radiation oncologist.
- Assist in documenting the results of the therapy; for example, clients receiving radiation for metastases to the spine will show improved neurologic functioning as tumor size diminishes.
- Provide emotional support, relief of physical and psychologic discomfort, and opportunities to talk about fears and concerns. For some clients, radiation therapy is a last chance for cure or even just for relief of physical discomfort.

## EXTERNAL RADIATION

Prior to the start of treatments, the treatment area will be specifically located by the radiation oncologist and marked with colored semipermanent ink or tatoos. Treatment is usually given 5 days per week for 15 to 30 minutes per day over 2 to 7 weeks.

### Nursing Responsibilities

- Monitor for adverse effects: skin changes, such as blanching, erythema, desquamation, sloughing, or hemorrhage; ulcerations of mucous membranes; nausea and vomiting, diarrhea, or gastrointestinal bleeding.
- Assess lungs for rales, which may indicate interstitial exudate. Observe for any dyspnea or changes in respiratory pattern.
- Identify and record any medications that the client will be taking during the radiation treatment.
- Monitor white blood cell counts and platelet counts for significant decreases.

### Client and Family Teaching

- Wash the skin that is marked as the radiation site only with plain water, no soap; do not apply deodorant, lotions, medications, perfume, or talcum powder to the site during the treatment period. Take care not to wash off the treatment marks.
- Do not rub, scratch, or scrub treated skin areas. If necessary, use only an electric razor to shave the treated area.
- Apply neither heat nor cold (e.g., heating pad or ice pack) to the treatment site.
- Inspect the skin for damage or serious changes, and report these to the radiologist or physician.

- Wear loose, soft clothing over the treated area.
- Protect skin from sun exposure during treatment and for at least 1 year after radiation therapy is discontinued. Cover skin with protective clothing during treatment; once radiation is discontinued, use sun-blocking agents with a sun protection factor (SPF) of at least 15.
- External radiation poses no risk to other people for radiation exposure, even with intimate physical contact.
- Be sure to get plenty of rest and eat a balanced diet.

## INTERNAL RADIATION

The radiation source, called an implant, is placed into the affected tissue or body cavity and is sealed in tubes, containers, wires, seeds, capsules, or needles. An implant may be temporary or permanent. Internal radiation may also be ingested or injected as a solution into the bloodstream or a body cavity or be introduced into the tumor through a catheter. The radioactive substance may transmit rays outside the body or be excreted in body fluids.

### Nursing Responsibilities

- Place the client in a private room.
- Limit visits to 10 to 30 minutes, and have visitors sit at least 6 feet from the client.
- Monitor for side effects such as burning sensations, excessive perspiration, chills and fever, nausea and vomiting, or diarrhea.
- Assess for fistulas or necrosis of adjacent tissues.

### Client and Family Teaching

- While a temporary implant is in place, stay in bed and rest quietly to avoid dislodging the implant.
- For outpatient treatments, avoid close contact with others until treatment has been discontinued.
- If the radiologist indicates the need for such measures, dispose of excretory materials in special containers or in a toilet not used by others.
- Carry out daily activities as able; get extra rest if feeling fatigued.
- Eat a balanced diet; frequent, small meals often are better tolerated.
- Contact the nurse or physician for any concerns or questions after discharge.

## Biotherapy

**Biotherapy** modifies the biologic processes that result in malignant cells, primarily through enhancing the person's own immune responses. The development of this therapy was based on the immune surveillance hypothesis. Although it has been established that a competent immune system is the body's most important defense against any disease, the role that various immune cells play in combating different types of malignancies continues to be investigated. Currently, biotherapy is used for both hematological malignancies, such as lymphoma and hairy cell leukemia, and solid tumors, such as renal cancer and melanoma.

Tumor immunology has the following applications: detection screening in high-risk groups, differential diagnosis and classification of tumor cells, monitoring the course of the disease with early detection of recurrence, and active therapies to halt or limit the disease. The theory underlying tumor immunology is that most tumor cells have a structural appearance recognizable by the immune cells. Tumor-associated antigens (TAAs) exist on tumor cells but not on normal cells. TAAs elicit an immune response that, in a person with a competent immune system, destroys or inhibits tumor growth. Thus, TAAs can be isolated from serum and used for both diagnosis and various treatment modalities. The prostate-specific antigen (PSA) is one such TAA currently in successful diagnostic use.

Tumor cells are often in a stage of arrested development (i.e., in the differentiation stage) for the cell type they represent; thus, they express antigens characteristic of that particular stage of development. The immaturity of the cells provides the physician with information about the relative aggressiveness of the cancer.

Another aspect of immunotherapy is the development of monoclonal antibodies that enhance the immune system's ability to fight the cancer. Monoclonal antibodies are developed by inoculating an animal with the tumor antigen and recovering the specific antibodies produced. The antibodies are then given to the person with that cancer to assist in the destruction of the tumor. Monoclonal antibodies are also recreated, or cloned, in the genetic laboratory by recombining DNA to produce the specific antibody. Techniques involving recombinant DNA have been used to combine these antibodies with toxins and drugs that are then delivered selectively to the tumor sites.

A number of cytokines (normal growth-regulating molecules) with antitumor activity have been synthesized. Alpha interferon, bacillus Calmette-Guérin (BCG, which has been used for many years as an inoculation against tuberculosis), and interleukin-2 (IL-2) have shown some therapeutic benefit in eliciting increased immune responses. Combination strategies have also helped stimulate the function of macrophages.

A most promising discovery has been the recently identified natural killer (NK) cells. These cells are like large granular lymphocytes, but have a cell surface phenotype different from that of T lymphocytes or macrophages. They have demonstrated a spontaneous cytotoxic effect on some types of cancer cells. They also provide a strong resistance to metastasis and secrete cytokines. When augmented by biologic response modifiers such as IL-2, they show increased tumor destructive activity (Battiato & Wheeler, 2000).

The use of hematopoietic growth factors (HGF) has been one of the most successful in biotherapy. HGF, such as granu-locyte colony-stimulating factor (G-CSF) and erythropoietin, offset the suppression of granulocytes and erythrocytes that results from chemotherapy (Battiato & Wheeler, 2000).

As promising as these biotherapies are, they are accompanied by serious side effects and toxicities. IL-2 can cause acute alterations in renal, cardiac, liver, gastrointestinal, and mental functioning. Alpha interferon causes mental slowing, confusion, and lethargy and, when used in combination with 5-fluorouracil or IL-2, severe flulike symptoms—chills and fever of 103° to 106°F (39.4° to 41.1°C), nausea, vomiting, diarrhea, anorexia, severe fatigue, and stomatitis—may result. The toxic effects are probably exaggerations of the normal systemic effects that these substances cause when fighting infection. For example, IL-2 is known to raise body temperature substantially in an attempt to create a hostile environment for foreign invaders.

The box below discusses nursing implications for clients receiving immunotherapy. For nursing care of specific problems, refer to the appropriate nursing diagnoses later in this chapter.

## Photodynamic Therapy

Photodynamic therapy is a method of treating certain kinds of superficial tumors. It is known by several different names: phototherapy, photoradiation, and photochemotherapy. Clients suffering from tumors growing on the surface of the bladder, peritoneal cavity, chest wall, pleura, bronchus, or head and neck are candidates for this treatment. The client is given an intravenous dose of a photosensitizing compound, Photofrin, which is selectively retained in higher concentrations in malignant tissue. This drug is activated by a laser treatment that is started 3 days after the drug injection and administered for 3 days. The drug interacts with oxygen molecules in the tissue to produce a cytotoxic oxygen molecule called singlet oxygen.

---

## NURSING CARE OF CLIENTS RECEIVING IMMUNOTHERAPY

Immunotherapy can consist of various substances used alone, such as interleukin-2, or combination biotherapy, such as alpha interferon with 5-fluorouracil. The nurse's role is to enhance the client's quality of life.

### Nursing Responsibilities

- Monitor for side effects: Alpha interferon may cause mental slowing, confusion, and lethargy; combination therapy of 5-fluorouracil or interleukin-2 and alpha interferon may cause severe flulike symptoms, with chills and fever of 103° to 106°F (39.4° to 41.1°C), nausea, vomiting, diarrhea, anorexia, severe fatigue, and stomatitis; erythropoietin may cause acute hypertension.
- Monitor enzymes and other appropriate biochemical indicators for acute alterations in renal, cardiac, liver, or gastrointestinal functioning, which can be side effects of interleukin-2.
- Evaluate response to therapy by conducting a thorough evaluation of clients' symptoms.
- Assess clients' coping behaviors and teach new strategies as needed.

- Manage fatigue and depression.
- Encourage self-care and participation in decision making.
- Provide close supervision for clients with altered mental functioning, either by caretakers or frequent nursing visits to the client's home.
- If client is unable to manage alone, teach medication administration and care of equipment to caregivers.

### Client and Family Teaching

- Minimize symptoms by managing fever and flulike symptoms: increase fluid intake, take analgesic and antipyretic medications, and maintain bed rest until symptoms abate.
- Seek help for serious problems not managed by usual means, such as dehydration from diarrhea.
- Use correct techniques for providing subcutaneous injections.
- Identify how to work and care for ambulatory pumps when medication is administered through an intercatheter or vascular access device.

At the time of the first intravenous injection, clients are observed for adverse hypersensitivity reactions, such as nausea, chills, and hives. Systemic or long-term toxicities are rare. The main side effects are local skin reactions and temporary photosensitivity, transiently elevated liver enzymes, and inflammatory responses of the tissues being treated, such as peritoneal or pleural tissues. This treatment has been used successfully with early-stage lung cancer with response rates as high as 90% (Bruce, 2001).

The major nursing responsibilities associated with photodynamic therapy are to address the client and family's anxiety about undergoing a relatively new treatment procedure and to educate them in managing side effects. The drug remains in the subcutaneous tissues for 4 to 6 weeks after injection. Any direct or indirect exposure to the sun activates the drug, resulting in a chemical sunburn. Clients are taught to protect themselves from sunlight (even on cloudy days) by covering themselves from head to toe in opaque clothing, including a wide-brimmed hat, gloves, shoes and stockings, and sunglasses with 100% ultraviolet block. Long-term care of treated skin includes moisturizing lotions and protection from trauma or irritation.

## Bone Marrow and Peripheral Blood Stem Cell Transplantations

Bone marrow transplantation (BMT) is an accepted treatment to stimulate a nonfunctioning marrow or to replace marrow. BMT is given as an intravenous infusion of bone marrow cells from donor to client. Most commonly used in leukemias, this therapy is being expanded to include treatment of other cancers including melanoma and testicular cancer. Chapter 32 provides an in-depth discussion of this procedure. ⊂⊃ Peripheral blood stem cell transplantation (PBSCT) is the process of removing circulating stem cells from the peripheral blood through apheresis and returning these cells to the patient after dose-intensive chemotherapy. PBSCT has fewer side effects, shorter hospitalization, and decreased cost compared to BMT.

## Pain Management

Pain management is an important component of oncology care and is considered a crucial part of the collaborative treatment plan. It is estimated that 20% to 50% of clients with early-stage cancer and up to 95% of clients with advanced cancer experience pain that requires analgesia (Cady, 2001). There are three main categories of pain syndromes in clients with cancer, and the category influences the type of treatment.

- *Pain associated with direct tumor involvement.* The most common causes are metastatases to bone, nerve compression or infiltration, and involvement of hollow visceral organs.
- *Pain associated with treatment.* This may include postsurgical incisional or wound pain; peripheral neuropathy, ulceration of mucous membranes, and pain from herpes zoster outbreaks secondary to chemotherapy; and pain in nerve plexes, muscles, and peripheral nerves from radiation therapy.
- *Pain from a cause not related to either the cancer or therapy,* such as diabetic neuropathy.

The goal of pain therapy is to provide relief that allows clients to function as they wish and, in the case of terminally ill clients, to die relatively free of pain. Drug therapy with opioid and nonopioid analgesics as well as adjuvant medications (those that enhance the effect of the analgesic) is the basis of most physician-guided pain management. Other therapies include injection of anesthetic drugs into spinal cord or specific nerve plexes, surgical severing of nerves, radiation to reduce tumor size and pressure, and behavioral approaches. Pharmacologic pain management follows these steps:

1. Conduct careful initial and ongoing assessment of the pain.
2. Evaluate the client's functional goals.
3. Establish a plan with combinations of nonnarcotic drugs (such as aspirin or ibuprofen) with adjuvants (such as corticosteroids or antidepressants).
4. Evaluate the degree of pain relief.
5. Progress to stronger drugs as needed, from mild narcotics such as oxycodone (Percodan) or propoxyphene (Darvon) to strong narcotics such as morphine or hydromorphone (Dilaudid), and monitor side effects.
6. Continue to try combinations and escalate dosages until maximal pain relief balanced with client's need to function is achieved.

Medication usually is administered by the oral route as long as this route continues to be effective. Medication is given on a regular time schedule (e.g., every 4 hours) with additional medication prescribed to cover breakthrough pain. When the oral route alone becomes inadequate, the primary narcotic can be administered intramuscularly, subcutaneously, or rectally on an intermittent schedule or continuously by transdermal patches or intravenously by a continuous drip, usually controlled by an infusion pump. Some newer pumps are portable, deliver medication continuously, and allow clients to control their breakthrough pain with a limited number of boluses. When narcotic doses are increased gradually, there is no limit to the amount the client can receive, as long as adverse reactions can be managed. Clients have received up to 4800 mg daily (200 mg per hour) of morphine sulfate with up to six 200- to 400-mg breakthrough doses daily without major ill effects and with good pain control. The body develops tolerance to the sedative after a short period, and most clients are able to tolerate the level of medication needed to control the pain. Other side effects, such as constipation, nausea and vomiting, and itching, can be managed through the usual means and are discussed under the appropriate nursing diagnoses. If the client has persistent untoward side effects that do not respond to treatment, or if the client does not get adequate relief from the narcotic, different narcotics and combinations are tried. Morphine sulfate and transdermal fentanyl are the most commonly used drugs for relief of cancer pain (Ferrell & McCaffery, 1997).

Clients receiving high-dose narcotics should not have the medication abruptly stopped, because withdrawal symptoms will occur. If the drug needs to be stopped, it must be tapered gradually. For more information on pain management, and on alternative therapies in particular, see Chapter 4. ⊂⊃

## NURSING CARE

Nurses face a major challenge in educating clients about preventive measures and lifestyle changes to reduce the risk of cancer. At the same time, clients with cancer must be reassured that they are not responsible for having acquired cancer.

Once a cancer diagnosis is established, nurses help clients recover and support them during the rehabilitation phase. In cases of terminal cancer, nurses provide comfort and facilitate positive growth for the client and significant others.

### Health Promotion

Early detection and treatment are considered the most important factors influencing the prognosis of those afflicted with cancer. However, many people do not seek early diagnosis and treatment because of denial, fear and anxiety, stigma, or the absence of specific early signs such as pain or weight loss (which usually are late signs). For this reason, screening procedures such as mammograms, PSA, occult blood stool tests, and sigmoidoscopy may be lifesaving.

The American Cancer Society (ACS) promotes early detection through public education using the CAUTION model (see Box 10–8). This model encourages people to seek medical attention when they discover signs and symptoms characteristic of cancer. For people without symptoms, the ACS recommends a cancer checkup every 3 years for those ages 20 to 39 and yearly for those over 40. If a person is at special risk due to heredity, environment, occupation, or lifestyle, special tests or more frequent examinations may be necessary. A routine cancer checkup should include counseling to improve health behaviors and physical examination with related tests of the breast, uterus, cervix, colon, rectum, testes, prostate, skin, thyroid, and lymph nodes. Box 10–9 lists the tests recommended for a cancer checkup. Nurses have a special role in public education and should encourage all with whom they come into contact to schedule their cancer checkup. Nurses must be familiar with the ACS guidelines so that they can advise clients, their families, and significant others.

### Assessment

#### Focused Interview

During this initial phase of the nursing process, collect the following significant data about the client.

---

**BOX 10–8  ■  American Cancer Society CAUTION Model**

**C**hange in bowel or bladder habits
**A** sore that does not heal
**U**nusual bleeding or discharge
**T**hickening or lump in breast or elsewhere
**I**ndigestion or difficulty in swallowing
**O**bvious change in wart or mole
**N**agging cough or hoarseness

If you have a warning signal, see your doctor!

*Note. From the American Cancer Society.*

---

**BOX 10–9  ■  American Cancer Society Recommendations for Cancer Checkups**

**BREAST CANCER**
- Routine monthly breast self-examination starting at age 20
- Breast examination by a health care professional every 3 years from age 20 to 39 and yearly thereafter
- Screening mammography every year from age 40

**COLON AND RECTUM CANCER—FOR PEOPLE AT AVERAGE RISK**
- Fecal occult blood test every year beginning at age 50
- Flexible sigmoidoscopy every 5 years with digital rectal exam
- Colonoscopy double-contrast barium enema every 10 years with digital rectal exam

**CERVIX OR UTERINE CANCER**
- Yearly pelvic examination and Pap test for sexually active girls and any women over 18; less often for women with three consecutive negative results
- An endometrial tissue sample at menopause for high-risk women with repeated samples at physician's discretion

**PROSTATE CANCER**
- Digital rectal exam yearly beginning at age 50 (higher risk begin at age 40)
- Prostate-specific antigen (PSA) test yearly beginning at age 50 (begin at age 45 for African American men and men with first-degree relative)

*Note. From the American Cancer Society.*

---

- History of the client's disease, including the signs and symptoms that led the client to seek health care
- Other concurrent diseases, such as diabetes
- Current physical or psychologic problems resulting from the cancer, such as pain or depression
- Understanding of the treatment plan
- Expectations of the treatment plan
- Functional limitations due to illness or treatment (see Box 10–10)
- Effect of the disease on current lifestyle
- Reliable support systems or caretakers for the client
- Coping strategies and how well they are working

**INTERVIEW QUESTIONS.**  The following are appropriate questions to ask the client during the initial interview and at subsequent assessments.

- "What brought you in to see the doctor?" Asking this question allows clients to tell their story in their own way, which may elicit more information than asking specific questions. The answer should elicit not only data about the signs and symptoms but also fears or concerns. If the cancer was discovered during a routine physical examination or checkup, the client may have some difficulty accepting the disease, especially if there were no symptoms. For clients who offer insufficient information in response to this open-ended question, more specific questions may be necessary, such as "Did you have pain or any specific physical problems that caused you to seek health care?"

## BOX 10–10 ■ Two Scales of Functional Status for Cancer Clients

### KARNOFSKY SCALE: CRITERIA OF PERFORMANCE STATUS (PS)

100  Normal; no complaints; no evidence of disease.
90  Able to carry on normal activity; minor signs or symptoms of disease.
80  Able to carry on normal activity with effort; some signs or symptoms of disease.
70  Cares for self; unable to carry on normal activity or to do active work.
60  Requires occasional assistance but is able to care for most of own needs.
50  Requires considerable assistance and frequent medical care.
40  Disabled; requires special care and assistance.
30  Severely disabled; hospitalization indicated, although death not imminent.
20  Very sick; hospitalization necessary; active supportive treatment necessary.
10  Moribund; fatal processes progressing rapidly.
0  Dead.

### EASTERN COOPERATIVE ONCOLOGY GROUP SCALE (ECOG)

0  Fully active, able to carry on all predisease activities without restriction. (Karnofsky 90 to 100)
1  Restricted in physically strenuous activity, but ambulatory and able to carry out work of a light or sedentary nature, for example, light housework or office work. (Karnofsky 70 to 80)
2  Ambulatory and capable of all self-care, but unable to carry out work activities. Up and about more than 50% of waking hours. (Karnofsky 50 to 60)
3  Capable of only limited self-care, confined to bed or chair 50% or more of waking hours. (Karnofsky 30 to 40)
4  Completely disabled, cannot carry out any self-care, totally confined to bed or chair. (Karnofsky 10 to 20)

*Note. "Nitrogen Mustards in the Palliative Treatment of Carcinoma" by D. A. Karnofsky, L. Craver, & J. Burchenal, 1948. Cancer 1, pp. 634–656. Copyright © American Cancer Society. Reprinted by permission of Wiley-CISS, Inc. a subsidiary of John Wiley & Sons.*

• "Do you have any other medical conditions or problems that are troubling you at this time?" It may be necessary to ask about specific diseases to help the client focus. For example, "Do you have high blood pressure?" or "Are you having any problems with your lungs?" Information gained from these questions can help you anticipate problems and formulate potential nursing diagnoses related to other diseases that may interact with the cancer.

• "What kinds of physical problems are you having at this time? Do you have pain? Are you nauseated? Have you lost a great deal of weight? Are you so tired you have difficulty carrying on your daily activities? Are you feeling blue or discouraged because of your illness?" For each positive response, ask follow-up questions to narrow down or define the exact nature of the problem. Again, these data help identify what nursing diagnoses should be included in the care plan.

• "What options has your physician suggested for treating your cancer?" The answer will indicate clients' knowledge about their treatment and, possibly, their communication with the physician. Often, under the stress of a cancer diagnosis, clients do not hear or understand what the doctor is saying and are afraid to ask questions. Lack of knowledge indicates a need to collaborate with the physician to explain the information to the client so that the client can absorb and understand it. If the client has a good understanding of the treatment plan, discussing how he or she feels about it can be useful in exposing fears, concerns, and emotional responses.

• "What do you expect to happen as a result of this treatment?" The answer may reveal unrealistic expectations or lack of understanding of consequences of the treatment.

• "What effect is the disease and/or treatment having on your ability to carry on with your usual daily activities?" Additional questions may also be needed to pinpoint the types of limitations. The response to this question should provide information on the client's functional status such as those shown in Box 10–10. This information can also be used to identify the need to collaborate with professionals from other disciplines. For example, if the client is the sole financial support of the family and is unable to work, a social worker may be able to help with resources; if the client is extremely weak, referral to a physical therapist may help with energy conservation strategies and strengthening exercises.

• "Who is available to help you at home and run errands for you? Who can provide transportation for you to get to your appointments or treatments? Who can you rely on to be a good listener when you're sad or just to be a comfortable companion? Is there someone you would like to make health care decisions for you if there is a time that you are unable to make them for yourself?" It often seems that the person with cancer is the one who takes care of everyone else; asking for help may be difficult for this person. This information can identify how much support and help the client has access to. The last question introduces the concept of advanced directives and durable power of attorney regarding health care (see Chapter 11). ⊂⊃

• "How do you manage your stress or your feelings of discomfort? What helps you feel better? Do you think these measures work well for you?" The responses to these questions provide information about the client's coping strategies and may identify maladaptive strategies such as alcohol or drug use. Lack of appropriate coping methods can interfere with the client's response to treatment and decrease overall quality of life.

Other assessment questions may be useful at different stages of the client's illness. For example, if the client is not expected to survive the cancer, it is important to ask whether the client has made decisions about last wishes (e.g., for a funeral and burial), whether these have been discussed with significant others, and whether the client has made out a will.

### Physical Assessment

As soon as the client is admitted to the health care service or agency, conduct a complete physical assessment to establish a

TABLE 10–10   Signs of Nutritional Status

| System | Good Nutrition | Poor Nutrition |
|---|---|---|
| General | Alert, energetic, good endurance, psychologically stable | Withdrawn, apathetic, easily fatigued, irritable |
| | Weight within range for height, age, body size | Over- or underweight |
| Integumentary | Skin glowing, good turgor, smooth, free of lesions | Skin dull, pasty, scaly-dry, bruises, multiple lesions |
| | Hair shiny, lustrous, minimal loss | Hair brittle, dull, falls out easily |
| Head, eyes, ears, nose, and throat | Eyes bright, clear, no fatigue circles | Eyes dull, conjunctiva pale, discoloration under eyes |
| | Oral mucous membranes pink-red and moist | Oral mucous membranes pale |
| | Gums pink, firm | Gums red, spongy, and bleed easily |
| | Tongue pink, moderately smooth, no swelling | Tongue bright to dark red, swollen |
| Abdomen | Abdomen flat, firm | Abdomen flaccid or distended (ascites) |
| Musculoskeletal | Firm, well-developed muscles | Flaccid muscles, wasted appearance |
| | Good posture | Stooped posture |
| | No skeletal changes | Skeletal malformations |
| Neurologic | Good attention span, good concentration, astute thought processes | Inattentive, easily distracted, impaired thought processes |
| | Good reflexes | Paresthesias, reflexes diminished or hyperactive |

baseline against which to evaluate later changes. It is especially important to document the nutritional status of the client using anthropomorphic measurements (i.e., frame size, height, weight, body fat, and muscle mass), and to evaluate laboratory results and note any specific signs and symptoms. Table 10–10 compares the manifestations of good nutrition with those of malnutrition.

It is also important to assess the client's hydration status, especially if the client is not taking oral food and fluids well or is having bouts of vomiting. Box 10–11 lists specific assessments for hydration status. Other recommended assessments are discussed under the specific nursing diagnoses that follow. They can also be found in other chapters that address specific body systems affected by the cancer.

## Nursing Diagnoses and Interventions

Nursing goals focus on supporting the whole person and managing specific problems such as pain, poor nutrition, dehydration, fatigue, adverse emotional responses, altered individual and family coping, and the side effects of medical treatment. Nursing also focuses on improving the quality of life by promoting rehabilitation for survivors of cancer and helping those who succumb to the disease maintain their dignity in the dying process. Because cancer affects the whole family, nursing care

BOX 10–11  ■  **Factors to Consider in Assessing Hydration Status**

- Intake and output
- Rapid weight changes
- Skin turgor and moisture
- Venous filling
- Vital sign changes
- Tongue furrows and moisture
- Eyeball softness
- Lung sounds
- Laboratory values

includes everyone involved with the client from the onset of diagnosis through the entire disease and treatment process and the ultimate outcome. Many diagnoses are pertinent to clients with cancer; this section addresses only the most common diagnoses. Diagnoses specific to individual diseases can be found in their respective chapters.

### Anxiety

Early in the disease continuum, for example, during diagnosis and treatment, threats to or changes in health status, physical comfort, role functioning, or even socioeconomic status can cause anxiety. Later, anxiety may result from the anticipation of pain, disfigurement, or the threat of death. In particular, clients whose coping skills have been poor in the past (e.g., in managing anger) may find themselves at a loss to manage this current crisis. The client may manifest overt signs of anxiety: trembling, restlessness, irritability, hyperactivity, stimulation of the sympathetic nervous system (increased blood pressure, pulse, respiration, excessive perspiration, pallor), withdrawal, worried facial expressions, and poor eye contact. The client may report insomnia and feelings of tension and apprehension, or express concerns regarding perceived changes brought about by the disease and fear of future events.

- Carefully assess the client's level of anxiety (moderate anxiety, severe anxiety, or panic) and the reality of the threats represented in the client's current situation. The level of anxiety and the reality of the perceived threat influence the type of intervention that is appropriate for the client. *A client in panic may need medical intervention with appropriate medications, whereas those with moderate or severe anxiety are often managed by the nurse through counseling and teaching new coping skills.*
- Establish a therapeutic relationship by conveying warmth and empathy and listening nonjudgmentally. *A client who feels safe in the relationship with the nurse more easily expresses feelings and thoughts. The client will be able to trust*

*the nurse and perhaps be willing to try new behaviors as suggested. The amount of time this relationship may take to develop depends on the client's current emotional and mental state and the stage of the disease process.*

- Encourage the client to acknowledge and express feelings, no matter how inappropriate they may seem to the client. *Just by expressing their feelings, clients often can significantly diminish anxiety. Expressing feelings also allows the client to direct energy toward healing and thus has a positive therapeutic effect. Moreover, by acknowledging feelings, especially those the client considers unacceptable, the client can lay a groundwork for new coping behaviors.*

- Review the coping strategies the client has used in the past and build on past successful behaviors, introducing new strategies as appropriate. Explain why inappropriate strategies, such as repressing anger or turning to alcohol, are not helpful. *The client will be more willing to make changes that build on what has already worked in the past. The client will also be more willing to reject inappropriate strategies if he or she is given a persuasive reason why they have not had the desired effect in managing previous crises.*

- Identify resources in the community, such as crisis hotlines and support groups, that can help the client manage anxiety-producing situations. *The client may not have support systems available, or the client's significant others may be having their own difficulties in dealing with the cancer diagnosis. Programs such as "I Can Cope," sponsored by the American Cancer Society in most communities, provide education, counseling, and support in a group setting with other cancer clients.*

- Provide specific information for the client about the disease, its treatment, and what may be expected, especially for those clients with obvious misinformation. *Knowing what is to come gives the client a sense of control and enables the client to make decisions. Also, knowing that every effort will be made to keep the client as free of pain as possible can do a great deal to relieve anxiety.*

- Provide a safe, calm, and quiet environment for the client in panic. Remain with the client and administer antianxiety medications as ordered. *Staying with the client and displaying calmness and confidence can protect the client from injury and prevent further panic. If the panic does not subside with the nurse's presence and support, referral to the physician for medication management may be necessary.*

- Use crisis intervention theory to promote growth in the client and significant others, regardless of the outcome of the disease. *During a major crisis, people can, with assistance, transform the experience from one that causes defeat and despair to one that enhances personal and spiritual growth.* If you are not skilled in this area, a referral to an appropriate mental health professional may be helpful to the client and family.

## Disturbed Body Image

Cancer and cancer treatments frequently result in major physiologic and psychologic body image changes. See the box on this page for manifestations of cancer. Loss of a body part (e.g., amputation, prostatectomy, or mastectomy), skin changes and hair loss from chemotherapy or radiation therapy, or creation

### Manifestations of Cancer

- Hair loss
- Depression
- Fever
- Bleeding gums
- Oropharyngeal ulcerations
- Stomatitis
- Anorexia
- Nausea and vomiting
- Diarrhea
- Emaciation
- General weakness
- Flaccid muscles
- Stooped posture
- Pallor
- Excessive bruising
- Radiation burns
- Visible tumor (abdomen)
- Odor of decay
- Hypotension

of unnatural openings on the body for elimination (e.g., colostomy or ileostomy) may have a major effect on the person's self-image. The gaunt, wasted appearance of the cachexic client or draining, malodorous lesions that result when cancer breaks through the skin are other significant etiologies of body image disturbance. This may also give rise to fear of rejection, which plays a major role in sexual dysfunction. In addition to all of the other afflictions the cancer brings about, the client may undergo major changes in appearance and function. The client may exhibit a visible physical alteration of some portion of the body, verbalize negative feelings about the body and/or fear of rejection by others, refuse to look at the affected site, and depersonalize the body change or lost part (e.g., by calling the colostomy "that thing").

- Discuss the meaning of the loss or change with the client. *Doing so helps the nurse discover the best approach for this particular client and involves the client more actively in interventions. A small, seemingly trivial loss may have a big impact, especially when viewed in light of the other changes that are occurring in the client's life. Likewise, a major loss may not be as important as the nurse might imagine. To ensure more appropriate and individualized care, evaluate each situation in terms of the reactions of the specific client.*

- Observe and evaluate interaction with significant others. *People who are important to the client may unintentionally reinforce negative feelings about body image; on the other hand, the client may perceive rejection where none exists.*

- Allow denial, but do not participate in the denial; for example, if a client does not want to look at the wound, the nurse may say, "I am going to change the dressing to your breast incision now." *During the initial stage of shock at the loss of a body part, denial is a protective mechanism and should not be challenged, nor should it be promoted. A matter-of-fact approach and an empathetic attitude will go far to facilitate the eventual acceptance of the change.*

- Assist the client and significant others to cope with the changes in appearance:
  a. Provide a supportive environment.
  b. Encourage the client and significant others to express feelings about the situation.
  c. Give matter-of-fact responses to questions and concerns.
  d. Identify new coping strategies to resolve feelings.

e. Enlist family and friends in reaffirming the client's worth. *A supportive, safe environment in which feelings are respected and new coping strategies can be tried promotes acceptance, as does reaffirming that the client's worth is not diminished by any physical changes.*

- Teach the client or significant others to participate in the care of the afflicted body area. Provide support and validation of their efforts. *Active involvement in providing care, such as changing a dressing or emptying a colostomy bag, empowers the client and/or significant others. This intimate involvement also desensitizes feelings about disfigurement and promotes acceptance. Involving significant others reduces the risk of their rejecting the client and can promote closeness. Positive reinforcement from the nurse encourages them to continue these behaviors.*

- Teach strategies for minimizing physical changes, such as providing skin care during radiation therapy and dressing to enhance appearance and minimize change in the body part. *Early intervention can limit the negative side effects of treatment and actually promote recovery. Involving the client provides an additional way for the client to be in control of a difficult situation.*

- Teach ways to reduce the alopecia that results from chemotherapy and to enhance appearance until the hair grows back:
  a. Discuss the pattern and timing of hair loss. *This allows the client to cope with changes and incorporate them into daily activities.*
  b. Encourage wearing cheerful, brightly colored head coverings; assist in color coordinating them with usual clothing. *Attractive head coverings protect the bald head while allowing the client to feel stylish and well dressed.*
  c. Refer to a good wig shop before hair loss is experienced. *Hair color and texture can be matched to minimize obvious changes in appearance.*
  d. Refer to support programs such as "Look Good . . . Feel Better," which is sponsored by the American Cancer Society and the Cosmetic, Toilet, and Fragrance Association Foundation. *A support group can diminish feelings of isolation and provide practical tips for managing problems. For a list of community resources available to clients with cancer, refer to a local phone book.*
  e. Reassure that hair will grow back after chemotherapy is discontinued, but also inform that the color and texture of the new hair may be different. Hair loss has been identified as the most distressing symptom by many clients (Ferrell, 2000; Williams, Wood, & Cunningham-Warburton, 1999). *Interventions to reduce that loss can have a significant impact on body image concerns. Moreover, knowing what to expect may decrease anxiety and distress.*

### Anticipatory Grieving

Anticipatory grieving is a response to loss that has not yet occurred. Overall, only 50% of people with cancer fully recover, and certain types of cancer have a much higher death rate; thus, the client with cancer is often confronted with facing death and making preparations for it. This can be a healthy response that allows the client and family to work through the dying process and achieve growth in the final stage of life. Perceived changes in body image and lifestyle also can prompt anticipatory grieving. The client or significant others may show sorrow, anger, depression, or withdrawal, expressing distress at the potential loss or verbalizing concern about unfinished life business.

- Use the therapeutic communication skills of active listening, silence, and nonverbal support to provide an open environment for the client and significant others to discuss their feelings realistically and to express anger or other negative feelings appropriately. *This helps the client and family to get in touch with feelings and confront the possibility of the loss or death.*

- Answer questions about illness and prognosis honestly, but always encourage hope. *This allows for realistic appraisal of the situation and planning, and it also helps combat feelings of hopelessness and depression.*

- Encourage the dying client to make funeral and burial plans ahead of time and to be sure the will is in order. Make sure the necessary phone numbers can be easily located. *This gives a sense of control and relieves family members of these concerns at a time when the client is most in need of their support and when they themselves are extremely stressed.*

- Encourage the client to continue taking part in activities he or she enjoys, including maintaining employment as long as possible. *This gives a sense of continuity of life even in the face of severe losses.*

### Risk for Infection

Malnutrition, impaired skin and mucous membrane integrity, tumor necrosis, and suppression of the white blood cells from chemotherapy or radiation may contribute to the risk for infection. Anorexia, as well as the disease itself, deprives the body of nutrients needed for healing, while impaired integrity of skin and mucous membranes (a result of chemotherapy and/or radiation therapy) compromise the first lines of defense against microbial invasion. Cells in the center of large or not very vascular tumors may die from malnutrition, eventually eroding through tissues to increase the risk of sepsis. Bone marrow depression resulting from the effects of certain types of cancers and from chemotherapy undermine the body's ability to respond to infection. The client may exhibit the classic signs of infection: lassitude, fever, anorexia, pain in the affected area, and physical evidence of infection, such as a purulent, draining lesion or wound. If the bone marrow is compromised, the usual signs and symptoms of infection may be absent or reduced.

- Monitor vital signs. *Fever and sympathetic nervous system responses, such as increased pulse and respiration, are usual early signs of infection. However, severely immunosuppressed clients may be unable to mount a fever; therefore, the absence of fever cannot rule out infection.*

- Monitor white blood cell counts frequently, especially if the client is receiving chemotherapy known to cause bone marrow suppression. *This allows the nurse to notify the physician at the first sign of diminishing white blood cell counts so that corrective action can be taken.*

- Teach the client to avoid crowds, small children, and people with infections when white blood cell count is at nadir (lowest point during chemotherapy) and to practice scrupulous personal hygiene. *During periods of leukopenia, the client may lose immunity to his or her own natural flora. Careful attention to hygiene reduces the risk of infection. Crowds, which promote contact with a greater variety of infectious agents, and friends with minor infections can be very dangerous for the immunosuppressed. Small children should be avoided because they often have microbes to which most people are usually immune but which the client may not be able to resist.*
- Protect skin and mucous membranes from injury. Teach appropriate skin care measures, such as good hygiene, use of a moisturizing lotion to prevent dryness and cracking, frequent changes of position for the bed-bound, and immediate attention to skin breaks or lesions. *Ensuring intact skin strengthens the first line of defense against infection.*
- Encourage the client to consume a diet high in protein, minerals, and vitamins, especially vitamin C. *Improving nutrition decreases the risk of infection. Vitamin C has been shown to help prevent certain types of infection, such as colds.*

### Risk for Injury

In addition to infection, cancer can pose a risk for injury from, for example, obstruction by a large tumor or one located in a limited body space (e.g., in the brain, bowel, or bronchial airways). If the cancer is one that creates ectopic sites of hormones, elevated levels of hormones that are not under the control of the pituitary gland can injure the client in a variety of ways. Signs of obstruction depend on the organ involved: Bowel obstruction presents with pain, distention, and cessation of bowel activities; obstruction in the brain gives signs of increased intracranial pressure or personality/behavioral change; bronchial obstruction manifests as respiratory distress, cyanosis, and altered arterial blood gases. Ectopic production of parathyroid hormone manifests as high serum calcium levels as well as signs of hypercalcemia; ectopic production of antidiuretic hormone causes fluid retention and manifests as hypertension and peripheral and pulmonary edema.

- Assess frequently for signs and symptoms indicating problems with organ obstruction. *Early detection of major problems allows the nurse to seek medical help before the problem evolves into a physiologic crisis.*
- Teach to differentiate minor problems from those of a serious nature. Encourage the client to consult with the nurse or physician if in doubt or to call 911 if the client becomes very ill. Box 10–12 provides guidelines to help clients identify serious problems. *Having guidelines for when to call the doctor provides an anxiety-reducing safety net for the client and family and promotes early detection of complications.*
- Monitor laboratory values that may indicate the presence of ectopic functioning and report abnormal findings to physicians immediately. (See Table 10–4 for laboratory indicators of ectopic functions.) *Early detection promotes early medical intervention and prevents serious consequences from the ectopic secretion.* Refer to Chapters 5, 17, and 18 for

---

### BOX 10–12 ■ When to Call for Help

Instruct the client or family member to call the nurse or physician if any of the following signs or symptoms occur:

- Oral temperature greater than 101.5°F (38.6°C)
- Severe headache; significant increase in pain at usual site, especially if the pain is not relieved by the medication regimen; or severe pain at a new site
- Difficulty breathing
- New bleeding from any site, such as rectal or vaginal bleeding
- Confusion, irritability, or restlessness
- Withdrawal, greatly decreased activity level, or frequent crying
- Verbalizations of deep sadness or a desire to end life
- Changes in body functioning, such as the inability to void or severe diarrhea or constipation
- Changes in eating patterns, such as refusal to eat, extreme hunger, or a significant increase in nausea and vomiting
- Appearance of edema in the extremities or significant increase in edema already present

Instruct the client or family member to call 911 if the client

- Is having much difficulty breathing or if the lips or face has a bluish tinge.
- Becomes unconscious or has a convulsion.
- Exhibits unmanageable behavior, such as being physically abusive, hurting self, or engaging in uncontrollable activity.

---

specific signs and symptoms of electrolyte imbalances and endocrine disorders. ∞

### Imbalanced Nutrition: Less Than Body Requirements

The anorexia-cachexia syndrome (described earlier in this chapter) is a common cause of malnutrition in cancer clients. Metabolism increases in response to increased cancer cell production while the cancer's parasitic activity reduces the nutrients available to the body. Loss of appetite, food aversion, nausea and vomiting, and painful oral lesions from chemotherapy or radiation may contribute to impaired nutrition. Tumors of the gastrointestinal tract that affect absorption also contribute to the problem. Manifestations include wasted appearance, considerable weight loss over a relatively short period of time, anthropometric measurements below 85% of standard for fat and muscle tissue, decreases in serum proteins, and negative responses to antigen testing.

- Assess current eating patterns, including usual likes and dislikes, and identify factors that impair food intake. *This allows for a more individualized plan based on needs and preferences.*
- Evaluate degree of malnutrition:
  a. Check laboratory values for total serum protein, serum albumin and globins, total lymphocyte count, serum transferrin, hemoglobin, and hematocrit. *These values represent the laboratory values that are most likely to decrease with malnutrition.*
  b. Calculate nitrogen balance and creatinine-height index. Calculate skeletal muscle mass, and compare findings to

normal ranges. *Urinary creatinine is an index of lean body mass and decreases in malnutrition. Lean muscle mass is catabolized for energy in clients with cancer.*

c. Take anthropometric measurements and compare them to standards: height, weight, elbow breadth, arm circumference, triceps skinfold thickness, and arm muscle mass. *This estimates the degree of wasting; findings below 85% of standard are considered malnutrition.*

- Teach the principles of maintaining good nutrition by using the food guide pyramid and adapting the diet to medical restrictions and current preferences. *This tailors the food plan to the client's needs and thereby promotes compliance.*
- Manage problems that interfere with eating:
  a. Encourage eating whatever is appealing and consider adding nutritional supplements such as Ensure or Isocal to diet. *It is better to eat something even if it is not nutritionally balanced.*
  b. Eat small, frequent meals. *These are more easily digested and absorbed and usually better tolerated by the client with anorexia.*
  c. Encourage to try icy cold foods (such as ice cream) or those that are more highly seasoned if food has no taste. *Chemotherapy and radiation therapy may harm taste buds and prevent distinguishing the taste of foods. Strong seasonings and coldness make food more enjoyable to the client with diminished taste.* However, spicy foods are not recommended for patients with stomatitis.
  d. Encourage cold and bland semisoft and liquid foods with painful oropharyngeal ulcers; use a nonalcohol anesthetic mouthwash prior to eating. *These foods are less irritating to sensitive mucous membranes; deadening the pain can make chewing and swallowing easier.*
  e. Manage nausea and vomiting by administering antiemetic drugs (around-the-clock medication may be an effective preventive measure). Encourage client to eat small, frequent, low-fat meals with dry foods such as crackers and toast, to avoid liquids with meals, and to sit upright for an hour after meals. Remove emesis basins, and encourage oral hygiene before eating. *Dry, low-fat foods are more readily tolerated when nauseated. Removing vomiting cues, such as odor and supplies associated with vomiting, can reduce nausea.*
- Teach to supplement meals with nutritional supplements such as Ensure Plus or Isocal and to take multivitamin and mineral tablets with meals. Suggest increasing calories by adding ice cream or frozen yogurt to the liquid supplement or commercial protein-carbohydrate powders to milk or fruit juice. *Because the food intake is usually less than that needed to maintain or gain weight, these supplements can add calories in a manner often tolerated.*
- Teach to keep a food diary to document daily intake. *If the client can see how little is being consumed, he or she may eat more. A food diary also helps the nurse keep a calorie count and alert the physician if more drastic nutritional measures, such as a feeding tool or parenteral nutrition, need to be instituted.*
- Teach to administer parenteral nutrition via a central line or other VAD. Teach safety measures and care of the VAD, and explain how the pump delivering the solution works. Provide an emergency phone number for help with administration problems. (See Chapter 20 for safety guidelines for administering parenteral nutrition.) ⬭ *The client with chronic or terminal cancer requiring parenteral nutrition is usually managed at home, so information on how to manage the entire process may be needed.*

## Impaired Tissue Integrity

The most common impairment of tissue integrity occurs in the oral-pharyngeal-esophageal mucous membranes. It is secondary to the effects of some chemotherapeutic drugs and radiation treatment to the head and neck. The oral-pharyngeal-esophageal tissues are lined with cells with a high mitotic turnover rate and are therefore vulnerable to many chemotherapeutic drugs. Leukemias, bone marrow transplants, and herpes viral infections are other etiologic factors in the disruption of oral-pharyngeal-esophageal tissue. Manifestations of this problem may include the following:

- Small ulcers occur on the tongue and mucous membranes in the mouth and throat.
- Herpes simplex type I lesions or vesicles evolve into ulcerations.
- Fungal infections, such as thrush (due to Candida infections), are manifested by a white, yellow, or tan coating with dry, red, fissured tissue underneath.
- Red, swollen, friable gums bleed with minimal or no trauma.
- **Xerostomia** is excessive dryness of the mucous membranes (due to chemotherapy or radiation).

Manage such problems with the following interventions.

- Carefully assess and evaluate the type of tissue impairment present. Identify possible sources, such as chemotherapy or radiation therapy to head and neck. *This allows the nurse to implement corrective measures appropriate to the type of problem.*
- Implement and teach measures for preventing oropharyngeal infection:
  a. Observe for systemic signs of infection. Be suspicious of any fever that has no apparent cause. *This facilitates early identification of an infection before it spreads.*
  b. Encourage cleaning teeth gently and using a nonalcohol mouthwash several times a day. This can be done after waking up in the morning, after any oral intake, and before bedtime. Soak dentures nightly in hydrogen peroxide and floss gently with waxed floss after meals and bedtime; this measure may be contraindicated for people with leukemia or thrombocytopenia. *Disrupted mucous membranes allow the normal oral bacterial flora into the systemic circulation, which can result in sepsis in the immunocompromised person. Reducing the oral flora by frequent hygiene decreases the risk of infection.*
  c. Culture any oral lesions, and report the problem to the physician. Herpes lesions may not follow a typical pattern in immunosuppressed clients. *Identifying the cause of the infection, whether viral, fungal, or bacterial, allows the physician to prescribe the appropriate treatment.*

- Implement and teach measures for reducing trauma to delicate tissues:
  a. Counteract dry mouth (xerostomia) with lubricating and moisturizing agents, such as Gatoraid, sugarless gum, and Blistex. *This protects mucous membranes from infection and trauma.*
  b. Avoid putting sharp instruments in the mouth. Use smooth plastic spoons and forks for eating, especially with a bleeding disorder. Dental work should be done by dental oncologists.
  c. Brush teeth with a very soft toothbrush and obtain a new toothbrush monthly. If gums are friable and bleeding, clean teeth with a soft cloth or toothpaste over finger. Chlorhexidine mouthwash (Peridex) may be used. *This protects gums from trauma and decreases risk of hemorrhage.*
- Administer specific medications as ordered to control infection and/or pain:
  a. Acyclovir is often used to treat viral infections.
  b. Systemic antibiotics are used to treat bacterial infections.
  c. Nystatin or clotrimazole solution for "swish and swallow" or lozenges that dissolve slowly in the mouth are used for fungal infections.
  d. Use viscous xylocaine or various combination mouthwashes before meals and as needed. These agents reduce pain and inflammation. See Box 10–13 for the ingredients of combination mouthwashes. *Knowing the contents of each mouthwash can prevent hypersensitivity reactions (e.g., to lidocaine) and assist in client teaching.*

## Nursing Interventions for Oncologic Emergencies

In caring for clients with cancer, nurses may encounter a number of emergency situations in which their role may be pivotal to the client's survival. Most of these emergencies require astute observations, accurate judgments, and rapid action once the problem has been identified. A brief description of the more common oncologic emergencies with nursing interventions follows. In all cases, immediate notification of the physician or emergency team is the first step.

## Pericardial Effusions and Neoplastic Cardiac Tamponade

Malignant pericardial effusion is an accumulation of excess fluid in the pericardial sac that compresses the heart, restricts heart movement, and results in a cardiac tamponade. The signs of cardiac tamponade are caused by compression of the heart leading to decreased cardiac output and impaired cardiac function. Signs include hypotension, tachycardia, tachypnea, dyspnea, cyanosis, increased central venous pressure, anxiety, restlessness, and impaired consciousness.

Interventions include the following:

- Start oxygen and alert respiratory therapy for other respiratory support as needed.
- Insert an intravenous catheter if one is not already in place.
- Monitor vital signs and initiate hemodynamic monitoring.
- Prepare vasopressor drugs.
- Bring emergency to bedside.
- Set up for and assist physician with a pericardial tap (pericardiocentesis).
- Reassure the client.

## Superior Vena Cava Syndrome

The superior vena cava can be compressed by mediastinal tumors or adjacent thoracic tumors. The most common cause is small-cell or squamous-cell lung cancers. Occasionally the problem is caused by thrombus around a central venous catheter that then plugs up the vena cava, resulting in obstruction and backup of the blood flowing into the superior vena cava.

Obstruction of the venous system causes increased venous pressure, venous stasis, and engorgement of veins that are drained by the superior vena cava. Signs and symptoms may develop slowly; facial, periorbital, and arm edema are early signs. As the problem progresses, respiratory distress, dyspnea, cyanosis, tachypnea, and altered consciousness and neurologic deficits may occur. Figure 10–7 ■ illustrates the superior venal cava syndrome.

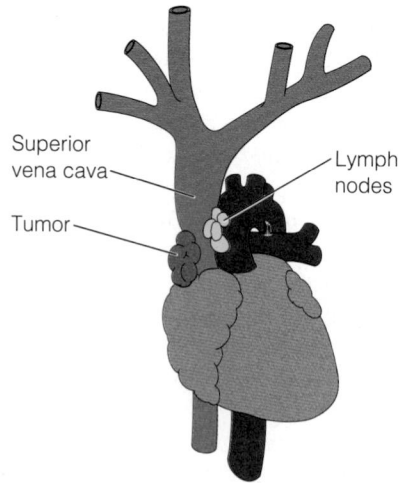

**Figure 10–7** ■ The superior vena cava syndrome. The enlargement of a tumor adjacent to the superior vena cava (usually in the lung or mediastinum) compresses that major blood vessel, which leads into the right atrium of the heart. As a result, blood backs up into the venous system behind the obstruction, diminishing blood flow into the heart.

| BOX 10–13 ■ | Combination Mouthwashes for Oropharyngeal Pain Control |
| --- | --- |

| *Kaiser Mouthwash* | *Xyloxylin Suspension* |
| --- | --- |
| ■ Nystatin | ■ Benylin syrup |
| ■ Hydrocortisone | ■ Lidocaine |
| ■ Tetracycline | ■ Maalox suspension |
| *Stanford Mouthwash* | *Stomafate Suspension* |
| ■ Nystatin | ■ Sucralfate |
| ■ Tetracycline | ■ Sterile water |
| ■ Lidocaine | ■ Benylin syrup |
| ■ Hydrocortisone | ■ Maalox suspension |

Emergency measures include the following:

- Provide respiratory support with oxygen, and prepare for tracheostomy.
- Monitor vital signs.
- Administer corticosteroids (e.g., dexamethasone) to reduce edema.
- If the disorder is due to a clot, administer antifibrinolytic or anticoagulant drugs.
- Provide a safe environment, including seizure precautions.

After the emergency is managed, the client often receives radiation or chemotherapy to reduce the tumor size.

### Sepsis and Septic Shock

Tumor necrosis, immune deficiency, antineoplastic therapy, malnutrition, and comorbid conditions can lead to the development of sepsis. Bacteria gain entrance to the blood, grow rapidly, and produce septicemia. Because malignant tumors are more likely to use anaerobic metabolic pathways, the bacteria of tumor sepsis are usually gram negative and damage the body through a combination of bacterial endotoxins and an uncontrolled immune reaction. Gram-negative sepsis progresses to systemic shock and eventually results in multisystem failure. Signs and symptoms appear in two phases. The first phase is characterized by vasodilation with vascular dehydration, high fever, peripheral edema, hypotension, tachycardia, tachypnea, hot flushed skin with creeping mottling beginning in the lower extremities, and anxiety or restlessness. Without treatment, the shock progresses to the second phase which shows the more classic signs of shock: hypotension, rapid thready pulse, respiratory distress, cyanosis, subnormal temperature, cold clammy skin, decreased urinary output, and altered mentation. Identifying the problem while the client is still in the hyperdynamic state is crucial to the client's survival. See Chapter 6 for further discussion of septic shock. ⌾

### Spinal Cord Compression

Spinal cord compression is most commonly associated with pressure from expanding tumors of the breast, lung, or prostate; lymphoma; or metastatic disease. Spinal cord compression constitutes an emergency because of the potential for irreversible paraplegia. Back pain is the initial symptom in 95% of the cases of spinal cord compression. This may progress to leg pain, numbness, paresthesias, and coldness. Later, bowel and bladder dysfunction occur and, finally, neurologic dysfunction progressing from weakness to paralysis. Treatment often consists of radiation or surgical decompression, but early detection is essential. See Chapter 41 for further discussion of spinal cord compression. ⌾

### Obstructive Uropathy

Clients with intraabdominal, retroperitoneal, or pelvic malignancies, such as prostate, cervical, or bladder cancers, may experience obstruction of the bladder neck or the ureters. Bladder neck obstruction usually manifests as urinary retention, flank pain, hematuria, or persistent urinary tract infections, but ureteral obstruction is not often evident until the client is in renal failure. See Chapters 26 and 47 for further discussion of obstructive uropathy.

### Hypercalcemia

Hypercalcemia in clients with cancer results from the excessive ectopic production of parathyroid hormone and is most commonly associated with cancers of the breast, lung, esophagus, thyroid, head, and neck and with multiple myeloma. Bone metastases may also cause hypercalcemia. When the rate of calcium mobilization from the bone exceeds the renal threshold for excretion, serum calcium levels can become dangerously elevated. Clients with hypercalcemia often present with nonspecific symptoms of fatigue, anorexia, nausea, polyuria, and constipation. Neurologic symptoms include muscle weakness, lethargy, apathy, and diminished reflexes. Without treatment, hypercalcemia progresses to alterations in mental status, psychotic behavior, cardiac arrythmias, seizures, coma, and death (see Chapter 5). ⌾

### Hyperuricemia

Hyperuricemia usually is a complication of rapid necrosis of tumor cells after vigorous chemotherapy for lymphomas and leukemias. Hyperuricemia may be related to increased uric acid production or to the tumor lysis syndrome associated with Burkitt's lymphoma. Uric acid crystals are deposited in the urinary tract, causing renal failure and uremia. Clients with hyperuricemia manifest with nausea, vomiting, lethargy, and oliguria.

### Syndrome of Inappropriate Antidiuretic Hormone Secretion

Occurring in only about 2% of cancer clients, syndrome of inappropriate antidiuretic hormone secretion (SIADH) is related to an ectopic secretion of antidiuretic hormone (ADH) that is usually associated with small-cell lung carcinoma, but also occasionally with prostate and adrenal cancers. The kidney secretes an excessive amount of sodium and conserves a disproportionate amount of free water, causing profound hyponatremia. Signs and symptoms include anorexia, nausea, muscle aches, and subtle neurologic symptoms that can progress to lethargy, confusion, seizures, and coma from cerebral edema (see Chapter 42). ⌾

## Using NANDA, NIC, and NOC

Chart 10–1 shows links between NANDA, NIC, and NOC when caring for the client with cancer.

## Client and Family Teaching
### Prevention

The ACS makes specific recommendations for cancer prevention in addition to the screening measures discussed earlier in this chapter. Based on these recommendations, nurses teach clients and families to decrease risk factors by:

- Avoiding tobacco and excessive alcohol use.
- Avoiding situations where secondhand smoke is abundant.
- Eating a low-fat, high-fiber diet.
- Consuming ample amounts of antioxidant foods, such as those containing beta carotene (a vitamin A precursor), vitamins E and C, and omega-3 oils.

## CHART 10–1 NANDA, NIC, AND NOC LINKAGES

### The Client with Cancer

| NURSING DIAGNOSES | NURSING INTERVENTIONS | NURSING OUTCOMES |
|---|---|---|
| • Chronic Pain | • Analgesia Administration<br>• Anxiety Reduction<br>• Pain Management | • Pain Level<br>• Symptom Severity |
| • Fatigue<br>• Imbalanced Nutrition:<br>  Less than Body Requirements<br>• Fear | • Energy Management<br>• Nutrition Management<br>• Nutritional Therapy<br>• Anxiety Reduction<br>• Emotional Support<br>• Spiritual Support<br>• Support Group | • Energy Conservation<br>• Nutritional Status (Nutrient Intake, Body Mass, Energy)<br>• Anxiety Control<br>• Coping |

*Note. Data from Nursing Outcomes Classification (NOC) by M. Johnson & M. Maas (Eds.), 1997, St. Louis: Mosby; Nursing Diagnoses: Definitions & Classification 2001–2002, by North American Nursing Diagnosis Association, 2001, Philadelphia: NANDA; Nursing Interventions Classification (NIC) by J. C. McCloskey and G. M. Bulechek (Eds.), 2000, St. Louis: Mosby. Reprinted by permission.*

### BOX 10–14 ■ American Cancer Society Dietary Guidelines to Prevent Cancer

- ■ Avoid obesity.
- ■ Cut down on total fat intake.
- ■ Include a variety of vegetables and fruits in the daily diet.
- ■ Eat more high-fiber foods, such as whole-grain cereals, vegetables, and fruits.
- ■ Limit consumption of alcoholic beverages, if you drink at all.
- ■ Limit consumption of salt-cured, smoked, and nitrate-cured foods.

*Note. From the American Cancer Society.*

- Avoiding foods with carcinogenic additives, dyes, or chemicals used in processing. Box 10–14 lists the ACS dietary guidelines.
- Taking certain medications and hormones, such as estrogen or tamoxifen, only under close medical supervision.
- Limiting exposure to radiation, including sun exposure.
- Using extreme caution if employed in an industry that uses carcinogenic chemicals or airborne particles (smoke). Seek new employment if at risk for related cancers.
- Protecting self from viral diseases known to cause cancer.
- Improving immunity by maintaining a healthy lifestyle and managing stress.

In addition, encourage people to report to the public health department any known leaking of chemicals or radioactive materials into the water or air and any noted increase in the incidence of cancer, especially of one specific type, in their communities.

### Rehabilitation and Survival

Rehabilitation from cancer not only involves regaining strength, recovering from surgery or chemotherapy, and learning to live with an altered body part or appliance, but also entails recovering from associated psychologic and emotional turmoil.

Rehabilitation centers provide physical therapy, occupational therapy, speech therapy, job retraining, and an opportunity to recuperate before resuming full responsibilities. In addition, many clients go home to convalesce and receive in-home support in the form of nursing supervision, direct care, and teaching. Hygiene and home maintenance can be provided by a certified home health aide. Physical and occupational therapists provide muscle strengthening and mobility training (especially with prostheses), and home safety teaching.

Psychologic rehabilitation of cancer survivors addresses quality of life issues. Three "seasons of cancer survival" have been described (Mullan, 1985). The first starts with diagnosis but is dominated by treatment. The second stage is one of extended survival, which occurs when treatment ends and the watchful waiting period begins. This period is characterized by fear of recurrence. Permanent survival is said to begin when the survival period has gone on long enough that the risk of recurrence is small. In this period, the client has to deal with secondary problems related to health and social issues resulting from the cancer experience. Employment may be a problem, health insurance may be cancelled, and life insurance may be difficult to get. Relationships may have suffered from the strain of the illness on significant others and the essential self-focusing required for recovery. However, both the client and significant others may have undergone a personal and spiritual growth that ushers in a new and enriching period of their lives.

New self-help groups are emerging in many communities to support others through their "seasons of survival." Many cancer survivors speak to groups about assisting other cancer survivors. Clients and families need to be informed about the many resources available through community agencies as well as the survivor support groups.

### Home Care

Before the client is discharged, teach both the client and significant others or caregivers to manage the client at home. Discuss problems that may result from the type of cancer and the treatment received, and provide information on how to manage these problems and when to call the physician.

- Teach wound care to the client with an open wound or draining lesion, and provide a referral to a home health nurse to monitor progress.
- Explain special diets clearly, or refer the client to a dietitian before discharge.
- Carefully review the physician's instructions with the client and family, making sure they understand medications to be taken, any other treatments, and when to see the doctor for follow-up care.
- Provide or order equipment and supplies needed for home care, especially any specialized bed or equipment to aid mobility and ensure safety in the home.
- For the client who will need complex care, such as parenteral nutrition, provide a referral to a home health nurse before discharge.

Because the hospital stay is often short, the client and family will benefit from follow-up phone calls at home for several days. People do not learn well under the stress of going home; give the client and family a number to call if they have concerns or questions.

## Hospice Care

More and more cancer clients with terminal disease are electing to die at home. This decision has been made easier by the increased availability of hospice programs. When a client and family or significant others elect hospice care, they are usually precluding additional hospitalizations other than those re-quired to manage reversible problems. Hospice clients also refuse resuscitation measures (CPR and other extraordinary measures).

Hospice care involves a multidisciplinary team and is designed to give the client comfort and to assist in a peaceful death with support to caretakers. The team usually consists of a nurse case manager, a physician, an anesthesiologist or pharmacist, an infusion therapist, a social worker, a physical therapist, a home health aide, and volunteers.

Many hospice services are connected with an inpatient respite care unit, where the client can receive 24-hour care for up to several weeks. This source provides the necessary care to the client if a family member becomes ill or needs to be relieved temporarily of the tremendous burden of caring for a dying loved one. Veterans Administration medical centers are very good models for these programs.

Studies of families that have participated in hospice services have found that family members were very positive about the experience (Teno et al., 2001). The aspects of hospice they most appreciated were the 24-hour accessibility and availability of the health team and the quality of communication from all team members. Family members emphasized that "the nurses listened, answered questions honestly, and prepared us for changes in the patient's condition." Team members were rated as very professional, but more relaxed and friendly than hospital staff; they talked with the family and displayed accepting, nonjudgmental attitudes. Team members were also seen as well informed, knowledgeable, and competent with excellent problem-solving skills. Chapter 11 provides more information on hospice care. ඏ

## Nursing Care Plan
### A Client with Cancer

James Casey, age 72, is of Northern European heritage. He has been receiving medical care for chronic obstructive pulmonary disease, chronic bronchitis, status postmyocardial infarction, and type I diabetes mellitus for over 15 years. He reports that he lost his wife from lung cancer 5 years ago and still "misses her terribly." He describes his bad habits as smoking two packs of cigarettes a day for 52 years (104 packs/year), one to two six-packs of beer a week, one "bourbon and water" a night, and "a lot of sugar-free junk food, like french fries." He assures the nurse that he quit smoking 2 years ago, when he could no longer walk a block without considerable shortness of breath, and just quit drinking alcohol a few weeks ago at his physician's insistence. About a year ago, he had a basal-cell carcinoma removed from his right ear. Six months ago, cancerous tumors were discovered in his bladder, and he underwent two 6-week chemotherapy courses of bladder instillations of BCG. His latest report indicates that the tumors have grown back and no further chemotherapy would be useful. The urologist had considered surgery but believed that Mr. Casey's other medical problems would compromise his chances of survival. Mr. Casey decides to let the disease run its course and to be managed at home through hospice care. Because he lives alone in a modest home, he asks his daughter, Mary, and her family to move in with him to provide care and support during his final months. The daughter accepts, saying she is glad to be able to spend this time with her father; she has been informed of the physical and emotional stress this will entail.

### ASSESSMENT

Glynis Jackson, RN, the hospice nurse assigned as case manager for James Casey, completes a health history and physical examination during her first two visits in his home, 1 day apart. She gathers this information over 2 days to conserve his strength and allow more time for Mr. Casey and his daughter to talk about their concerns.

During the physical assessment, Glynis notes that Mr. Casey is pale with pink mucous membranes, thin with a wasted appearance and a strained, worried facial expression. He complains of severe back pain no longer adequately relieved by Percodan and Vicodin alternating every 2 to 4 hours. His blood pressure is 90/50, right arm in the reclining position with no significant orthostatic change; his apical pulse is 102, regular and strong; respiratory rate 24 and unlabored; breath sounds are clear but diminshed in the bases; oral temperature is 96.8°F.

(continued on page 312)

## Nursing Care Plan
### A Client with Cancer (continued)

A tunnelled Groshong catheter as a VAD is present in the right anterior chest. There is no drainage, redness, or swelling at the site. The catheter was placed last week when the client was being evaluated at the anesthesiologist's office for pain management, but no medication is running via the VAD. Mary reports that his urinary output is adequate. Approximately 200 mL of yellow, cloudy, nonmalodorous urine is present in the urinal at the bedside from his last voiding.

Mr. Casey states that he spends most of his time either in bed or sitting up in a chair in his room. He reports that he has no energy any more and is unable to walk to the bathroom unassisted, dress himself, or take care of his own personal hygiene. Glynis rates Mr. Casey's functional level at ECOG level 4: capable of only limited self-care, confined to bed or chair 50% or more of waking hours (Karnofsky 10 to 20). He tells the nurse that his daughter "is working day and night to help me and is looking awfully tired."

Many reports that Mr. Casey is eating very poorly: He usually eats a small bowl of oatmeal with milk for breakfast and vegetable soup and crackers for lunch, but he tells her that he is too tired for dinner and wants only fruit juice. Mr. Casey tells the nurse that he has no appetite and eats just to please Mary. He does drink at least three to four glasses of water a day plus juice. His fingerstick blood sugars remain within normal range.

His current weight is 120 pounds at 67 inches tall, down from 180 pounds a year ago. He has lost about 30 pounds over the last 2 months.

Available laboratory values from his visit with the doctor show the following:

Total protein: 4.1 g/dL (normal range: 6.0 to 8.0 g/dL)
Albumin: 2.2 g/dL (normal range: 3.5 to 5.0 g/dL)
Hemoglobin: 10.2 g/dL (normal range: 13.5 to 18.0 g/dL)
Hematocrit: 30.5% (normal range: 40.0% to 54.0%)
BUN: 30 mg/dL (normal range: 5 to 25 mg/dL slightly higher in older people)
Creatinine: 2.2 mg/dL (normal range: 0.5 to 1.5 mg/dL)

### DIAGNOSIS

- *Imbalanced nutrition: Less than body requirements* related to anorexia and fatigue
- *Risk for caregiver role strain* related to severity of her father's illness and lack of help from other family members
- *Chronic pain* related to progression of disease process
- *Impaired physical mobility* related to pain, fatigue, and beginning neuromuscular impairment
- *Risk for impaired skin integrity* related to impaired physical mobility and malnourished state

### EXPECTED OUTCOMES

- Increase oral intake and show improvement in serum protein values.
- Daughter will be able to maintain supportive caretaking activities as long as Mr. Casey needs them.
- Minimal pain for the rest of his life.
- Able to continue his current activity level.
- Maintain intact skin.

### PLANNING AND IMPLEMENTATION

- Ask about favorite foods, and ask Mary to offer a small portion of one of these foods each day.
- Encourage drinking up to four cans of liquid nutritional supplement with fiber a day, sipping them throughout the day.
- Talk with the physician about prescribing a medication to help stimulate the appetite.
- Plan to have a home health aide come to the home, give him a shower or bed bath daily, and assist his daughter with some of the household chores.
- Talk with Mary about having her adult son and daughter relieve her of the housework and stay with Mr. Casey so that she can get out of the house occasionally. Offer to talk with them if she is uncomfortable doing so.
- Request a volunteer to spend up to 4 hours a day, twice a week with Mr. Casey so that Mary can attend to outside activities and chores.
- Talk with the anesthesiologist, and work out a pain control program, using the VAD and a CADD-PCA infusion pump with a continuous morphine infusion.
- Call the infusion therapist to set up the equipment and supplies (including the medication) for the morphine infusion.
- Teach how to use the pump and about the side effects of the morphine infusion, including those that require a call to the nurse for assistance. Teach which untoward effects should be reported.
- Request a physical therapy consultation to evaluate current level of functioning and determine how to maintain current level.
- Instruct Mary to allow ample rest periods for James between activities.
- Order a hospital bed with electronic controls to be delivered to the house.
- Order a special foam pad for bed and chair and a bedside commode from the medical supply house.
- Instruct Mary and the home health aide to inspect skin daily, give good skin care with emollient lotion after bathing, and report any beginning lesions immediately to the nurse.

### EVALUATION

James Casey did increase his oral intake a little, sometimes eating the special treats his daughter prepared and drinking one or two cans of liquid nutritional supplement a day. However, his weight did not increase; it stayed at about 120 pounds until his death 2 weeks later. His daughter was very grateful for the extra help from the home health aide and the volunteer, though she could not bring herself to ask her son and daughter for help and did not want the nurse to do so. She did become more rested and reported that "Dad and I had some wonderful 3:00 A.M. talks when he couldn't sleep."

Mr. Casey was started on 20 mg of morphine per hour with boluses of 10 mg 4 times a day, for breakthrough pain. This medication relieved his pain quite well; after 2 days he was alert enough most of the time to carry on a normal conversation and still walk to the bathroom with help up until 2 days before he died.

## Nursing Care Plan

### A Client with Cancer *(continued)*

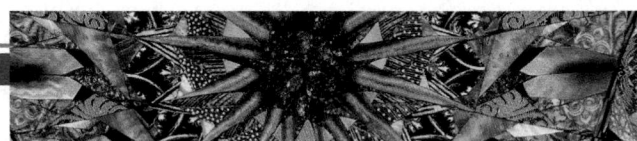

The hospital bed simplified Mr. Casey's care and made it much easier for him to rest comfortably and change position. His skin remained intact and in good condition.

Mary reported that Mr. Casey died peacefully in his sleep, about 2 weeks after care was started. She said spending the last weeks of his life together was a healing experience for both of them.

### Critical Thinking in the Nursing Process

1. What other tests could be done to evaluate James Casey's nutritional status?
2. Mr. Casey had severe back pain. What were the possible pathophysiologic reasons for his pain?

3. One of the specified interventions was to consult the physician regarding medication to increase Mr. Casey's appetite. What medications might fulfill that function? What side effects might they have that would contraindicate these medications for him?
4. If Mr. Casey had developed signs and symptoms of sepsis, what manifestations would you expect to see? As the nurse making the home visits, what would be your nursing actions, and in what order of priority?

See Evaluating Your Response in Appendix C.

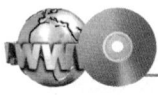

## EXPLORE MediaLink

NCLEX review questions, case studies, care plan activities, MediaLink applications, and other interactive resources for this chapter can be found on the Companion Website at www.prenhall.com/lemone.

Click on Chapter 10 to select the activities for this chapter. For animations, video clips, more NCLEX review questions, and an audio glossary, access the Student CD-ROM accompanying this textbook.

## TEST YOURSELF

1. Mr. Lawrence has a history of colon cancer. Cells from the colon tumor have traveled to his liver. This process is called:

    a. Carcinogenesis
    b. Dysplasia
    c. Metastasis
    d. Mutation

2. A client diagnosed with lung cancer reports he is having difficulty sleeping and often feels tense. The most appropriate initial nursing intervention would be to:

    a. Encourage the client to express his feelings about the cancer diagnosis
    b. Document the client's report of difficulty sleeping and tenseness in the chart
    c. Obtain an order for medication for sleep from the physician
    d. Offer an antianxiety drug such as Ativan (Lorazepam)

3. Mr. Roberts is receiving external radiation for treatment of lung cancer. Client education for care of the skin in the marked area includes:

    a. Apply antibacterial ointment daily
    b. Avoid contact with others

    c. Avoid rubbing or scratching treated skin areas
    d. Cleanse the skin with mild soap and water

4. Ms. Smith complains of nausea and vomiting following her daily chemotherapy treatment. The *most* appropriate nursing intervention would be to:

    a. Keep Ms. Smith NPO until her daily chemotherapy is completed
    b. Provide antiemetic medication 30 to 40 minutes prior to each treatment
    c. Provide clear liquids until the chemotherapy is completed
    d. Schedule chemotherapy administration for bedtime

5. Mrs. Smith experiences bone marrow depression as a result of chemotherapy. Which of the following would the nurse expect to find?

    a. Alopecia
    b. Nausea and vomiting
    c. Platelet count 50,000
    d. Temperature 102°F

See Test Yourself answers in Appendix C.

# BIBLIOGRAPHY

American Cancer Society. (2002). *Cancer facts and figures—2002*. Atlanta: Author.

Battiato, L. A., & Wheeler, V. S. (2000). Biotherapy. In C. H. Yarbro, M. H. Frogge, M. Goodman, & S. L. Groenwald (Eds.), *Cancer nursing: Principles and practice* (5th ed.) (pp. 543–579). Boston: Jones and Bartlett.

Berd, D. (2001). Autologous, hapten-modified vaccine as a treatment for human cancers. *Vaccine, 19*, 2565–2570.

Bergh, J., Wiklund, T., Erikstein, B., Lidbrink, E., Lindman, H., Malmström, P., et al. (2000). Tailored fluorouracil, epirubicin, and cyclophosphamide compared with marrow-supported high-dose chemotherapy as adjuvant treatment for high-risk breast cancer: A randomised trial. *Lancet, 356*, 1384–1391.

Bruce, S. (2001). Photodynamic therapy: Another option in cancer care. *Clinical Journal of Oncology Nursing, 5*, 95–99.

Cady, J. (2001). Understanding opioid tolerance in cancer pain. *Oncology Nursing Forum, 28*, 1561–1568.

Chapman, D., & Goodman, M. (2000). Breast cancer. In C. H. Yarbro, M. H. Frogge, M. Goodman, & S. L. Groenwald (Eds.), *Cancer nursing: Principles and practice* (5th ed.) (pp. 994–1047). Boston: Jones and Bartlett.

Donahue, B. R., Wernz, J. C., & Cooper, J. S. (2000). HIV-associated malignancies. In J. D. Roseblatt, P. Okunieff, & J. V. Sitzmann (Eds.), *Clinical oncology: A multidisciplinary approach for physicians and students* (8th ed.) (pp. 199–207). Philadelphia: W.B. Saunders.

Dunlop R. J., & Campbell C. W. (2000). Cytokines and advanced cancer. *Journal of Pain & Symptom Management, 20*(3), 214–232.

Ferrell, B. (2000). Article captures the essence and meaning of alopecia. *Oncology Nursing Forum, 27*, 17.

Ferrell, B., & McCaffery, M. (1997). Nurses' knowledge about equianalgesia and opioid dosing. *Cancer Nursing, 20*, 201–212.

Foltz, A. (2000). Nutritional disturbances. In C. H. Yarbro, M. H. Frogge, M. Goodman, & S. L. Groenwald (Eds.), *Cancer nursing: Principles and practice* (5th ed.) (pp. 754–775). Boston: Jones and Bartlett.

Futreal, P. A., Kasprzyk, A., Birney, E., Mullikin, J. C., Wooster, R., & Stratton, M. R. (2001). Cancer and genomics. *Nature, 409*(6822), 850–852.

Haapoja, I. (2000). Paraneoplastic syndromes. In C. H. Yarbro, M. H. Frogge, M. Goodman, & S. L. Groenwald (Eds.), *Cancer nursing: Principles and practice* (5th ed.) (pp. 792–812). Boston: Jones and Bartlett.

Hawkins, R. (2001). Mastering the intricate maze of metastasis. *Oncology Nursing Forum, 28*(6), 959–965.

Held-Warmkessel, J. (2000). Prostate cancer. In C. H. Yarbro, M. H. Frogge, M. Goodman, & S. L. Groenwald (Eds.), *Cancer nursing: Principles and practice* (5th ed.) (pp. 1427–1451). Boston: Jones and Bartlett.

Hill, R. P. (2001). The biology of cancer. In P. Rubin (Ed.), *Clinical oncology: A multidisciplinary approach for physicians and students* (pp. 32–45). Philadelphia: W. B. Saunders.

Holland, J. (2001). New treatment modalities in radiation therapy. *Journal of Intravenous Nursing, 24*, 95–101.

Karnofsky, D., Abelmann, W., Craver, L., & Burchenal, J. (1948). The use of nitrogen mustard in the palliative treatment of carcinoma. *Cancer, 1,* 634–656.

Kaye, J., Morton, J., Bowcutt, M., & Maupin, D. (2000). Stress, depression, and psychoneuroimmunology. *Journal of Neuroscience Nursing, 32,* 93–100.

LeFever Kee, J. (2002). *Laboratory and diagnostic tests with nursing implications* (6th ed.) Upper Saddle River, NJ: Prentice Hall.

McDaniel, R., & Rhodes, V. (1998). Development of a sensory information videotape for women receiving chemotherapy for breast cancer. *Cancer Nursing, 21,* 143–148.

Misset, J., & Levi, F. (1995). Chronomodulated chemotherapy combining 5-fluorouracil, folinic acid, and oxaliplatin in advanced colorectal cancer: An overview of seven years of experience (Meeting abstract). *Cancer Investigation, 13*(Suppl 1), 49–50.

Mullan, F. (1985). Seasons of survival: Reflections of a physician with cancer. *New England Journal of Medicine, 313,* 270–273.

Neal, A., & Hoskin, P. (1997). *Clinical oncology: Basic principles and practice* (2nd ed.). New York: Oxford University Press.

Oncology Nursing Society Board of Directors. (1997). Oncology Nursing Society position paper on quality cancer care. *Oncology Nursing Forum, 24,* 951–953.

Pace, J. C. (2000). AIDS-related malignancies. In C. H. Yarbro, M. H. Frogge, M. Goodman, & S. L. Groenwald (Eds.), *Cancer nursing: Principles and practice* (5th ed.) (pp. 933–949). Boston: Jones and Bartlett.

Peto, R., Darby, S., Deo, H., Silcocks, P., Whitley, E., & Doll, R. (2000). Smoking, smoking cessation, and lung cancer in the UK since 1950: Combination of national statistics with two case-control studies. *BMJ, 321*(7257), 323–329.

Porth, C. (2002). *Pathophysiology: Concepts of altered health states* (6th ed.). Philadelphia: Lippincott.

Rahman, Z., Frye, D., Buzdar, A., Smith, T., Asmar, L., Champlin, R., & Hortobagyi, G. (1997). Impact of selection process on response rate and long-term survival of potential high-dose chemotherapy candidates treated with standard-dose doxorubicin-containing chemotherapy in patients with metastatic breast cancer. *Journal of Clinical Oncology, 15,* 3171–3177.

Rosenthal, D. (1998). Changing trends. *A Cancer Journal for Clinicians, 48*(1), 3–4.

Rubin, P., Williams, J. P., Okunieff, P., Rosenblatt, J. D., & Sitzmann, J. V. (2001). Statement of the clinical oncologic problem. In P. Rubin (Ed.). *Clinical oncology: A multidisciplinary approach for physicians and students* (pp. 1–31). Philadelphia: W. B. Saunders.

Scigliano, E., Vlachos, A., Najfeld, V., & Shank, B. (2001). The leukemias. In P. Rubin (Ed.), *Clinical oncology: A multidisciplinary approach for physicians and students* (pp. 565–614). Philadelphia: W. B. Saunders.

Selye, H. (1984). *The stress of life* (rev. 2nd ed.). New York: McGraw-Hill.

Spitalnick, P. F., & diSant' Angnese, P. A. (2001). The pathology of cancer. In P. Rubin (Ed.), *Clinical oncology: A multidisciplinary approach for physicians and students* (pp. 47–61). Philadelphia: W. B. Saunders.

Surbone, A. (2001). Ethical implications of genetic testing for breast cancer susceptibility. *Critical Reviews in Oncology-Hematology, 40*(2), 149–157.

Teno, J. M., Clarridge, B., Casey, V., Edgman-Levitan, S., & Fowler, J. (2001). Validation of toolkit after-death bereaved family member interview. *Journal of Pain & Symptom Management, 22,* 752–758.

Weiss, R. B., Rifkin, R.M., Stewart, F. M., Theriault, R. L., Williams, L. A., Herman, A. A., & Beveridge, R. A. (2000). High dose chemotherapy for high-risk primary breast cancer: An on-site review of the Bezwoda study. *Lancet, 355,* 999–1003.

Williams, J., Wood, C., & Cunningham-Warburton, P. (1999). A narrative study of chemotherapy-induced alopecia. *Oncology Nursing Forum, 26,* 1463–1468.

Williams, M. D., & Sandler, A. B. (2001). The epidemiology of lung cancer. *Cancer Treatment & Research, 105,* 31–52.

Yarbro, J. (2000). Carcongenesis. In C. H. Yarbro, M. H. Frogge, M. Goodman, & S. L. Groenwald (Eds.), *Cancer nursing: Principles and practice* (5th ed.) (pp. 48–57). Boston: Jones and Bartlett.

Zech, D., Grond, S., Lynch, J., Hertel, D., & Lehmann, K. (1995). Validation of World Health Organization Guidelines for cancer pain relief: A 10-year prospective study. *Pain, 63,* 65–76.

(Zenapax), are a combination of mouse and human antibodies and cause fewer side effects.

Polyclonal antilymphocyte antibodies are also used as adjunctive immunosuppressant therapy. These are administered as antilymphocyte globulin (ALG) or antithymocyte globulin (ATG). These globulins contain antibodies against both T and B cells, as well as other mononuclear leukocytes. When administered, they deplete circulating lymphocytes, platelets, and granulocytes.

## NURSING CARE

The client who has an organ or tissue transplant has both immediate and long-term nursing care needs. Both the client and the family must be considered in providing nursing care.

### Health Promotion

Part of health promotion activities focus on preventing the need for a tissue transplant. It is important to increase public awareness regarding unhealthy lifestyle behaviors, such as excessive alcohol consumption and illegal drug use, and their relationship to organ failure. Clients with chronic diseases like diabetes mellitus and hypertension must understand that inadequate management of these disorders could lead to end-stage renal disease. Other risk factors may simply relate to a person's heredity; understanding how heredity could affect future health might influence their lifestyle choices.

### Assessment

Assessment data collected following a tissue transplant focus on identifying potential rejection episodes. Further focused assessments are described with nursing interventions in the next section.

### Nursing Diagnoses and Interventions

Because of the continuing risk of transplant rejection and the need for immunosuppression, *ineffective protection* and *risk for impaired tissue integrity* are priority nursing care foci. The client's underlying disease process, the transplant, and the continuing need for immunosuppressive drug therapy also have emotional and psychologic consequences. Many nursing diagnoses, such as *powerlessness* or *ineffective coping,* may be appropriate. The diagnosis *anxiety* related to potential transplant rejection is considered in this section.

#### Ineffective Protection

Altered protection is a problem for the transplant client at all stages. Before the transplant occurs, failure of the affected organ may put the client at risk for infection and other multisystemic problems. Incisions and invasive perioperative procedures impair skin and mucous membrane protection from infectious organisms and other antigens. Immunosuppressive drugs given postoperatively to prevent graft rejection disarm the immune response to a certain extent, increasing the risk of infections and neoplastic growths.

- Wash hands on entering room and before providing direct care. *Handwashing removes transient organisms from the skin, reducing the risk of transmission to the client.*

**PRACTICE ALERT** *Use strict aseptic technique in changing dressings and caring for invasive catheters such as intravenous lines and indwelling urinary catheters to protect against external and resident host microorganisms.* ■

- Assess frequently for signs and symptoms of infection. Monitor the temperature and vital signs every 4 hours. Assess for evidence of inflammation, abnormal wound drainage, changes in urine or other body secretions, complaints of pain, or behavior changes that may indicate infection. Culture abnormal wound drainage. *The client on immunosuppressive therapy is more susceptible to infection, and usual signs and symptoms may not be evident. Both the temperature and inflammatory response can be suppressed by therapy. Prompt identification and intervention for infection is important in the immunosuppressed client.*
- Monitor laboratory values, including CBC and tests of organ function; report changes to the physician. *An elevation in the WBC count with increased numbers of immature cells (bands) or a decline in function of the transplanted organ (e.g., a rising BUN and creatinine in the renal transplant client) may be early indications of infection or transplant failure.*
- Initiate reverse or protective isolation procedures as indicated by the client's immune status. *These procedures further protect the severely immunocompromised client from infection.*
- Instruct ill family members and visitors to avoid contact with the client. *A "minor" upper respiratory infection can be a significant illness in the immunocompromised host.*
- Help ensure adequate nutrient intake, offering supplementary feedings as indicated or maintaining parenteral nutrition if necessary. *Adequate nutrition is important for healing and immune system function.*
- Change intravenous bags and tubing at least every 24 hours, and change peripheral intravenous sites every 48 to 72 hours, unless contraindicated. Remove invasive catheters and lines as soon as they are no longer necessary. *Changing lines and sites is important to reduce bacterial contamination. Fewer invasive lines provide fewer sites for bacterial invasion of the body.*
- Emphasize the importance of washing hands thoroughly after using the bathroom and before eating. *This reduces the risk of infection with endogenous organisms.*
- Provide good mouth care. *Good mouth care reduces the population of oral microorganisms and helps maintain an intact mucous membrane lining.*
- Monitor for potential adverse effects of medications:
    Thrombocytopenia and possible bleeding
    Fluid retention with edema and possible hypertension
    Loss of bone density, osteoporosis, and possible pathologic fractures
    Renal or hepatic toxicity
    Cardiac effects, particularly in the presence of fluid retention and hypervolemia
  *Medications used to maintain immunosuppression and preserve the allograft have many potential adverse effects that can alter normal protective and homeostatic mechanisms.*

Cyclosporine has contributed significantly to the success of organ transplantation since its introduction in the 1970s. Cyclosporine inhibits T-cell function and the normal cell-mediated immune response. The incidence of cyclosporine toxicity and side effects is related to blood levels, so blood levels are monitored closely. Cyclosporine is both nephrotoxic and hepatotoxic, especially at high doses. Observable toxic effects include hypertension and CNS symptoms such as flushing or tingling of the extremities, confusion, visual disturbances, and seizures or coma.

Muromonab-CD3, also known as OKT3 or Orthoclone, is the first monoclonal antibody produced for therapeutic use in humans. As a monoclonal antibody, OKT3 is specific to T cells, blocking their generation and function. It binds with a surface antigen on T cells, inactivating and removing them from circulation. It also blocks killer T cells attached to the graft. Because of significant side effects, the use of OKT3 is limited primarily to treatment of steroid-resistant rejection. Two newer monoclonal antibodies, basiliximab (Simulect) and daclizumab

# Medication Administration

## Immunosuppressive Agents (continued)

### Client and Family Teaching
- Teach about the drug and its purpose.
- Discuss potential adverse and side effects, and emphasize the need to report symptoms promptly.
- Inform the client that adverse effects are most likely to occur following the first two doses, necessitating close observation at that time. Reassure the client that this is standard protocol for this medication.

### ANTILYMPHOCYTE GLOBULINS
- Antithymocyte globulin or ATG (ATGAM)
- Antilymphocyte globulin or ALG

These globulins containing antilymphocyte antibodies are produced by immunizing horses (the main source), rabbits, or sheep with human lymphocytes to stimulate production of antibodies (see figure at right). Serum from the animal is then recovered, and the active IgG fraction is isolated, purified, and administered parenterally to the client. It binds with periheral lymphocytes and mononuclear cells, removing them from circulation.

ATG or ALG is used both to induce immunosuppression immediately following a transplant and to treat steroid-resistant rejection episodes. As with monoclonal antibody, multiple side effects are associated with ATG or ALG.

### Nursing Responsibilities
- Perform a skin test for sensitivity to horse serum prior to initial dose. Report any positive reaction to the physician and hold administration until desensitization therapy has been completed.
- Premedicate as ordered with acetaminophen and diphenhydramine prior to each dose. Steroids may also be administered before the initial dose. Have epinephrine and hydrocortisone injections available at the bedside in case of anaphylactic reaction.
- Administer by intravenous infusion into a central line over 4 to 6 hours.
- Monitor vital signs hourly while medication is infusing.
- Assess for adverse effects, including chills and fever, erythema, and pruritus. Notify the physician, these may be treated symptomatically.
- Monitor CBC daily, notify the physician if WBC falls to less than 3000/mm$^3$ or platelet count to less than 100,000/mm$^3$. The medication may be stopped or reduced.
- Assess renal function studies to monitor for serum sickness. Report complaints of joint pain.
- Monitor for signs of infection, and report any signs promptly.

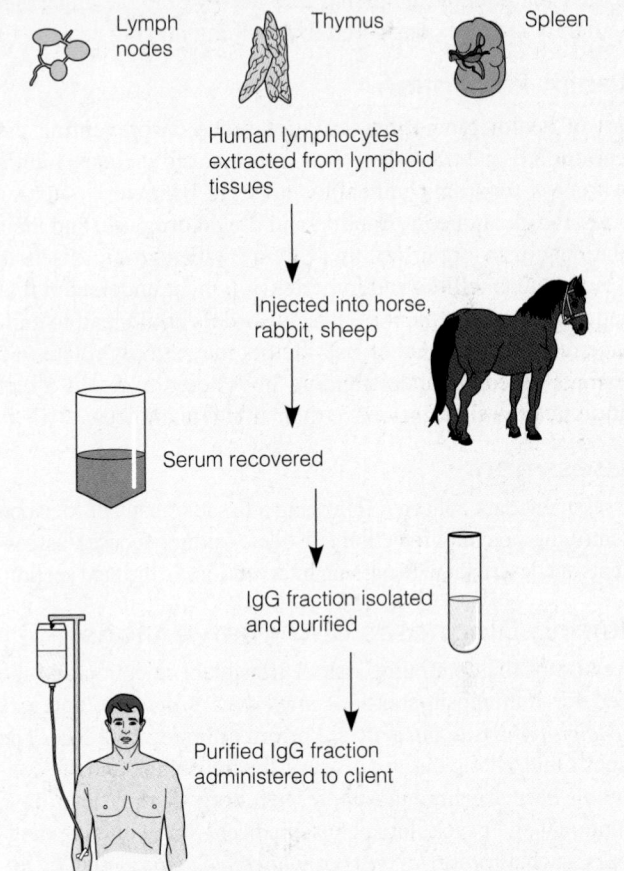

Lymph nodes    Thymus    Spleen

Human lymphocytes extracted from lymphoid tissues

Injected into horse, rabbit, sheep

Serum recovered

IgG fraction isolated and purified

Purified IgG fraction administered to client

A horse is inoculated with washed human lymphocytes, stimulating the production of immunoglobulin with polyclonal antilymphocyte antibodies. These are then extracted from horse serum, purified, and administered intravenously to the client.

### Client and Family Teaching
- Explain the need for special precautions and close monitoring while this drug is being administered.
- Instruct the client to report any adverse effects, including malaise or joint pain, promptly.
- Ask the client to report any evidence of easy bruising, bleeding gums, or black stools.
- Teach family members about the importance of not exposing the client to persons with infectious diseases.

# CHAPTER 11

# Nursing Care of Clients Experiencing Loss, Grief, and Death

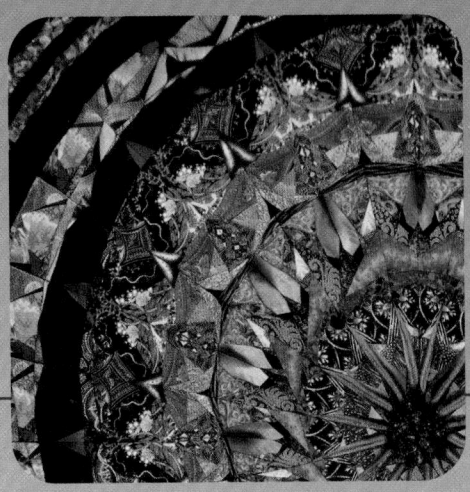

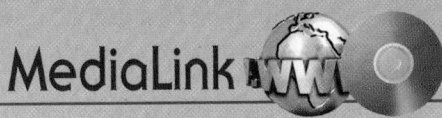

## LEARNING OUTCOMES

After completing this chapter, you will be able to:

- Describe theories of loss and grief.

- Discuss factors affecting responses to loss.

- Begin to assess own feelings and values related to loss, grief, and death.

- Discuss legal and ethical issues in end-of-life care.

- Describe the philosophy and activities of hospice.

- Identify physiological changes in the dying client.

- Provide nursing interventions to promote a comfortable death.

- Use the nursing process as a framework for providing individualized care for clients and families experiencing loss, grief, or death.

## www.prenhall.com/lemone

Additional resources for this chapter can be found on the Student CD-ROM accompanying this textbook, and on the Companion Website at www.prenhall.com/lemone. Click on Chapter 11 to select the activities for this chapter.

**CD-ROM**
- Audio Glossary
- NCLEX Review

**Companion Website**
- More NCLEX Review
- Case Study
    Dysfunctional Grieving
- Care Plan Activity
    Anticipatory Grieving
- MediaLink Application
    Grief and Unexpected Death

## BOX 11–1  ■ Types of Losses

- Death
- Health
- Body part
- Social status
- Lifestyle
- Marital relationship (i.e., through divorce)
- Reproductive function
- Sexual function

**Loss** may be defined as an actual or potential situation in which a valued object, person, body part, or emotion that was formerly present is lost or changed and can no longer be seen, felt, heard, known, or experienced. A loss may be temporary or permanent, complete or partial, objectively verifiable or perceived, physical or symbolic. Only the person who experiences the loss can determine the meaning of the loss. Although the order of importance varies with the person, people most commonly fear the losses listed in Box 11–1.

Loss always results in change. The stress associated with the loss may be the precipitating factor leading to physiologic or psychologic change in the person or family. The effective or ineffective resolution of feelings surrounding the loss determines the person's ability to deal with the resulting changes.

**Grief** is the emotional response to loss and its accompanying changes. Grief as a response to loss is an inevitable dimension of the human experience. The loss of a job, a role (e.g., the loss of the role of spouse, as occurs in divorce), a goal, body integrity, a loved one, or the impending loss of one's own life may trigger grief. Loss is also integral to death. Although death is the ultimate loss, losses that occur in any phase of the life cycle may produce grief responses as intensely painful as those observed in the death experience.

Grieving may be thought of as the internal process the person uses to work through the response to loss. *Bereavement,* a form of depression accompanied by anxiety, is a common reaction to the loss of a loved one. *Mourning* describes the actions or expressions of the bereaved, including the symbols, clothing, and ceremonies that make up the outward manifestations of grief. Both grieving and mourning are healthy responses to loss because they ultimately lead the person to invest energy in new relationships and to develop positive self-regard.

**Death** is defined in many ways. One commonly used definition of death is an irreversible cessation of circulatory and respiratory functions or irreversible cessation of all functions of the entire brain, including the brainstem. With the current life-support systems available, the most often used criterion for determining death is whole-brain death (permanent irreversible cessation of the functioning of all areas of the brain). The criteria for whole-brain death are listed in Chapter 6. ⊙⊃

Although death is an inevitable part of life, it is often an immensely difficult loss for the person who is dying and for his or her loved ones. Death may be accidental (such as from trauma) or the end of a long and painful struggle with a terminal illness such as cancer or AIDS. It may also be purposeful, if a person commits suicide.

## THEORIES OF LOSS, GRIEF, AND DYING

Medical-surgical nurses often care for clients exhibiting responses typical of various stages of the grieving process. Highly individual in quality and duration, the grief process may range from discomforting to debilitating, and it may last a day or a lifetime, depending on what the loss means to the person experiencing it. Although each person experiences loss in a different manner, knowledge of some of the major theories of loss, grief, and dying can give the nurse a framework for holistic care of the client and family anticipating or experiencing a loss. Table 11–1 summarizes these theories.

### Freud: Psychoanalytic Theory

Freud (1917, 1957) wrote about grief and mourning as reactions to loss. Freud described the process of mourning as one in which the person gradually withdraws attachment from the lost object or person. He observed that with normal grieving, this

### TABLE 11–1  Summary of Theories of Loss

| Theorist | Dynamics |
|---|---|
| Freud | Grief and mourning are reactions to loss. Grieving is the inner labor of mourning a loss. Inability to grieve a loss results in depression. |
| Bowlby | The successful grieving process initiated by a loss or separation during childhood ends with feelings of emancipation from the lost person or object. |
| Engel | After the person perceives and evaluates the loss, the person adapts to it. Shock and disbelief, developing awareness, and restitution occur during the first year following the loss; in the months following, the person puts the lost relationship into perspective. |
| Lindemann | A sequence of responses is experienced following a catastrophic event; defined concepts of anticipatory grieving and morbid grief reactions. |
| Caplan | Periods of psychologic crisis are precipitated by hazardous circumstances; successful resolution of grief involves feelings of hope and engaging in activities of ordinary living. |
| Kübler-Ross | There are five stages defining the response to loss: denial, anger, bargaining, depression, and acceptance. Stages are not necessarily sequential. |
| Carter | Identified the quality of grief's changing character, the need to hold on to that which was good in the loved one's lost existence, expectations of how to react to the experience, and the ways in which personal history affects the quality and meaning of the loss. |

withdrawal of attachment is followed by a readiness to make new attachments. In comparing melancholia (prolonged gloominess, depression) with the "normal" emotions of grief, and its expression in mourning, Freud observed that the "work of mourning" is a nonpathologic condition that reaches a state of completion after a period of inner labor.

## Bowlby: Protest, Despair, and Detachment

Bowlby (1973, 1980) believed that the grieving process initiated by a loss or separation from a loved object or person successfully ends when the grieving person experiences feelings of emancipation from the lost object or person. He divided the grieving process into three phases and identified behaviors characteristic of each phase.

- *Protest.* The protest phase is marked by a lack of acceptance of the loss. All energy is directed toward protesting the loss. The person experiences feelings of anger toward self and others, and feelings of ambivalence toward the lost object or person. Crying and angry behaviors characterize this phase.
- *Despair.* The person's behavior becomes disorganized. Despair mounts as efforts to deny the loss compete with acceptance of permanent loss. Crying and sadness, coupled with a desire for the lost object or person to return, result in disorganized thoughts as the client recognizes the reality of the loss.
- *Detachment.* As the person realizes the permanence of the loss and gradually relinquishes attachment to the lost object, a reinvestment of energy occurs. Both the positive and negative aspects of the relationship are remembered. Expressions of hopefulness and readiness to move forward are characteristic of this phase.

## Engel: Acute Grief, Restitution, and Long-Term Grief

Engel (1964) related the grief process to other methods of coping with stress: After the person perceives and evaluates the loss (the stressful event), the person adapts to it. Engel's recognition of the impact of cognitive factors on the grieving process was an important contribution to our understanding of grieving.

Engel described three main stages in the grief process: an acute stage, a restitution stage, and a long-term stage. The acute stage occurs in two phases. The first phase, shock and disbelief, begins immediately after the person receives the news of the loss. The initial response may be denial, which may help the person to cope with the overwhelming pain. Alternatively, the grieving person in this phase may appear to accept the loss, making statements such as, "It was for the best," while repressing his or her feelings. This phase of shock and disbelief normally lasts only a few hours; however, it may continue for 1 or 2 days.

As the shock and disbelief begin to fade, the second phase, developing awareness, follows. The finality of the loss becomes a reality, and pain, anguish, anger, guilt, and blame surface. The person feels a need to make someone responsible for the loss. "If only" and "why" frequently punctuate the expressed or inner dialogue of the bereaved. Crying is common. "It is during this time that the greatest degree of anguish or despair, within the limits imposed by cultural patterns, is experienced or expressed" (Engel, 1964, p. 93). Culturally patterned behaviors, such as maintaining a stoic pose in public or weeping openly, characterize this phase.

The acute stage is followed by a stage of restitution, in which the mourning is institutionalized. Friends and family gather to support the grieving person through rituals dictated by the culture. As time passes, the mourner continues to feel a painful void and is preoccupied with thoughts of the loss. The mourner may join a support group or seek other social support for coping with the loss.

After the restitution stage, which lasts at least a year, the mourner begins to come to terms with the loss. In this long-term stage, interest in people and activities is renewed. The person puts the lost relationship in perspective as he or she begins to form new relationships. Engel observed that this period might last another 1 to 2 years.

## Lindemann: Categories of Symptoms

Lindemann (1944) interviewed people who had lost a loved one during the course of medical treatment, disaster victims, and relatives of members of the armed forces who had died. Lindemann's research led him to describe normal grief, anticipatory grieving, and morbid grief reactions. He described symptoms characteristic of normal grief into categories of somatic (physical symptoms without an organic cause) distress, preoccupation with the image of the deceased, feelings of guilt, hostile reactions, and loss of patterns of conduct

**Anticipatory grieving** was defined as a cluster of predictable responses to an anticipated loss. These responses include the range of feelings experienced by the person or family preoccupied with an anticipated loss. The term *morbid grief reaction* described delayed and dysfunctional reactions to loss; a variety of debilitating health problems were seen in people who displayed excessive or delayed responses to loss.

## Caplan: Stress and Loss

Caplan's (1990) theory of stress and its relationship to loss is useful in understanding the grief process. He expanded the focus of the grief process to include not only bereavement but also other episodes of stress that people experience, such as may result from surgery or childbirth. Caplan described these periods as "psychological crises precipitated by hazardous circumstances that lead to a temporary upset in the normal homeostatic balance of forces that characterizes transactions between an individual and his environment" (p. 28). He believed these "hazardous circumstances" lead to psychologic disequilibrium in some people because their coping skills are inadequate in helping them gain mastery over their predicament.

Caplan described three factors that influence the person's ability to deal with a loss. He believed these factors might cause distress for a year or more following the loss.

- The psychic pain of the broken bond and the agony of coming to terms with the loss
- Living without the assets and guidance of the lost person or resource
- The reduced cognitive and problem-solving effectiveness associated with the distressing emotional arousal

Caplan described the process of building new attachments to replace those that have been lost. This process involves two elements: a feeling of hope and the assumption of regular activity as a form of participating in ordinary living.

## Kübler-Ross: Stages of Coping with Loss

Kübler-Ross's (1969, 1978) research on death and dying provided a framework for gaining insight about the stages of coping with an impending or actual loss. According to Kübler-Ross, not all people dealing with a loss go through these stages, and those who do may not experience the stages in the sequence described. In identifying the stages of death and dying, Kübler-Ross (1978) repeatedly stressed the danger of prematurely labeling a "stage" and emphasized that her goal was to describe her observations of how people come to terms with situations of loss.

Some or all of the following reactions may occur during the grieving process and may reappear as the person experiences the loss:

- *Denial.* A person may react with shock and disbelief after receiving word of an actual or potential loss. After receiving a terminal diagnosis, notification of a death, or other serious loss, people may make such statements as "This can't be happening to me" or "This can't be true." This initial stage of denial serves as a buffer in helping the person or family mobilize defenses to cope with the situation.
- *Anger.* In the anger stage, the person resists the loss. The anger is often directed toward family and health care providers.
- *Bargaining.* The bargaining stage serves as an attempt to postpone the reality of the loss. The person makes a secret bargain with God, expressing a willingness to do anything to postpone the loss or change the prognosis. This is the individual's plea for an extension of life or the chance to "make everything right" with a dying family member or friend.
- *Depression.* The person enters a stage of depression as the full impact of the actual or perceived loss is realized. The person prepares for the impending loss by working through the struggle of separation. While grieving over "what cannot be," the person may either talk freely about the loss or withdraw from others.
- *Acceptance.* The person begins to come to terms with the loss and resumes activities with an air of hopefulness for the future. Some dying people reach a stage of acceptance in which they may appear to be almost devoid of emotion. The struggle is past, and the emotional pain is gone.

## Carter: Themes of Bereavement

Carter (1989) focused on identifying themes of bereavement expressed by grieving persons. She identified themes disclosed by people who had experienced the death of a loved one as:

- Grief's changing character, including "waves" of intense pain that may be triggered years after the death by a photograph of the loved one, a favorite song, a fragrance, or anything that calls the loved one to mind.
- Holding, an individual process of preserving the fact and the meaning of the loved one's existence.

- Expectations, both social and personal, regarding how the bereaved should react to the experience.
- The critical importance of personal history in affecting the quality and meaning of individual bereavement.

## FACTORS AFFECTING RESPONSES TO LOSS

A variety of factors affect a person's responses to loss. These include age, social support, families, spirituality, and rituals of mourning.

### Age

The understanding of and reaction to loss is influenced by the age of the person experiencing the loss. In general, as people experience life transitions, their ability to understand and accept the losses associated with the transitions increases. From the age of 3 years, the development of the concept of death as a loss proceeds rapidly. Table 11–2 outlines the development of the concept of death throughout the life span.

| TABLE 11–2 | Development of the Concept of Death |
| --- | --- |
| **Age** | **Beliefs/Attitudes about Death** |
| 3 | Fears separation; lacks comprehension of permanent separation. |
| 3 to 5 | Believes death is like sleeping and is reversible. Expresses curiosity about what happens to the body. |
| 6 to 10 | Understands finality of death. Views own death as avoidable. Associates death with violence. Believes wishes can be responsible for death. |
| 11 to 12 | Reflects views of death expressed by parents. Expresses interest in afterlife as an understanding of mortality develops. Recognizes death as irreversible and inevitable. |
| 13 to 21 | Usually has a religious and philosophic view of death but seldom thinks about it. Views own death as distant or a challenge, acting out defiance through reckless behavior. Previously held developmental awareness of death may still be present. |
| 22 to 45 | Does not think about death unless confronted with it. Emotionally distances self from death. Attitude toward death influenced by religious and cultural beliefs. |
| 46 to 65 | Experiences the death of parents or friends. Accepts own mortality. Experiences waves of death anxiety. Puts life in order to prepare for death and decrease anxiety. |
| 66 and older | Fears lingering, incapacitating illness. Views death as inevitable but from a philosophical viewpoint: that is, as freedom from pain and illness or as a spiritual reunion with deceased friends and loved ones. |

## Social Support

Grieving is painful and lonely. One's social support system is important because of its potentially positive influence on the successful resolution of grief. Some losses may lead to social isolation, placing clients at high risk for dysfunctional grief reactions. For example, survivors of people with AIDS often report feeling excluded by the deceased person's family and by health care providers. Characteristic factors that can interfere with successful grieving include the following:

- Perceived inability to share the loss
- Lack of social recognition of the loss
- Ambivalent relationships prior to the loss
- Traumatic circumstances of the loss

A move, a divorce, or even the death of a pet can cause a person to feel extremely isolated, yet the person experiencing these types of loss does not ordinarily receive the same social support offered to the person mourning the death of a loved one. A woman having an abortion or giving up a child for adoption seldom receives the same social support as the mother of a child who died at birth. It is therefore especially important that the nurse does not place a value on the client's loss when assessing the need for support.

The painful nature of grief can cause the client to withdraw from a previously established social support system, thereby increasing the feelings of loneliness caused by the loss. A recently widowed woman, for example, may refuse invitations involving married couples with whom she had socialized while her husband was alive. The client's needs for social interaction remain similar to those established before the loss.

## Families

A well-functioning family usually rallies after the initial shock and disbelief and provides support for each other during all phases of the grieving process. After a loss, the functional family is able to shift roles, levels of responsibility, and ways of communicating.

The family may have negative as well as positive effects. For example, the dying client may request that someone the family perceives as an outsider be near, and the family may respond with anger to the perceived "intrusion." Similarly, certain family members may express hurt feelings or anger if the client is unresponsive to other family members. Well-meaning family members also may try to shield the client from the pain of grieving. It is rare for the family and the client to experience anger, denial, and acceptance in unison. While one member is in denial, another may be angry because "not enough is being done."

## Spirituality

Spirituality is at the core of human existence, integrating and transcending the physical, emotional, intellectual, and social dimensions (Reed, 1996). The principles, values, personal philosophy, and meaning of life by which the client has pursued goals and self-actualization, however, may be called into question when the client responds to an actual or perceived loss. Because of a fear of intruding on the personal spiritual beliefs and practices of the client, the nurse often feels at a loss in implementing interventions that would be helpful to the client responding to a loss.

## Rituals of Mourning

Through the participation in religious ceremonies such as baptism, confirmation, and Bat or Bar Mitzvah, people joyously celebrate progression to a new stage of life and loss of a former way of being. The funeral ceremony serves many of the same purposes in meeting the needs of the bereaved as people gather to share loss. Through the ceremony, people symbolically express triumph over death and deny the fear of death. Culture is the primary factor that dictates the rituals of mourning. See the Focus on Diversity box on page 320 for examples of values and rituals for death in selected cultures.

## NURSES' SELF-ASSESSMENT

Nurses care for clients and families at various stages of the grief process and may feel that crisis situations are not the time for self-reflection. However, because the nurse's conscious or unconscious reactions to the client's responses to the loss will influence the outcome of any interventions, nurses need to take time to analyze their own feelings and values related to loss and the expression of grief. The nurse can promote self-awareness by reflecting on the following questions.

- What are my personal feelings about how grief should be expressed?
- Am I making judgments about the meaning of this loss to the client?
- Are unresolved losses in my own life preventing me from relating therapeutically to the client?

## END-OF-LIFE CONSIDERATIONS

Nurses care for the dying client in intensive care units, emergency rooms, hospital units, long-term care facilities, and the home. Regardless of the setting, the client's wishes about death should be respected. The Dying Person's Bill of Rights states that each person has "the right to be cared for by caring, sensitive, knowledgeable people who will attempt to understand my needs and will be able to gain some satisfaction in helping me face my death" (Barbus, 1975).

## Legal and Ethical Issues

Issues such as those involved in advance directives and living wills, euthanasia, and quality of life are especially important to nurses in upholding the specific care requests of their clients.

### Advance Directives and Living Wills

**Advance directives** are legal documents that allow a person to plan for health care and/or financial affairs in the event of incapacity. A **durable power of attorney for health care** (or health care proxy) is a legal document written by a competent (mentally healthy) adult that gives another competent adult the

## Focus on Diversity

### CULTURAL ASPECTS OF DYING AND DEATH

| Culture/Ethnicity | Nursing Interventions |
|---|---|
| American Indian | Some tribes prefer not to openly discuss terminal prognosis and DNR decisions, as negative thoughts may make inevitable loss occur sooner. Suggest a family meeting to discuss care and end-of-life issues. If the family feels comfortable, all members of the family and close friends may remain 24 hours a day (eating, joking, singing). Mourning is done in private, away from the dying person. After death, the family may hug, touch, sing, and stay close to the deceased. |
| Black/African American | Suggest that the family have a family meeting or talk with a minister or family elder. Client may decide to have older family member disclose a poor prognosis. Care for the dying family member is often done at home until death is imminent. |
| Chinese American | Ensure the head of the family is present when terminal illness is discussed. The client may not want to discuss approaching death. Special amulets or cloths may be brought from home. Family members may prefer to bathe the body after death. |
| Iranian | Information about a terminal illness should be presented by a trusted member of the health care team to the family, and never to the client when he or she is alone. Most Iranians believe in *tagdir* (will of God) in life and death as a predestined journey. When death occurs, notify the head of the family first. DNR decisions are often made by the family. The family may want to bathe the body. |
| Mexican American | Based on the belief that worry may make health worse, the family may want to protect the client from seriousness of illness. The information is often handled by an older daughter or son. Extended family members are obligated to pay respects to the sick and dying, although pregnant women do not care for dying persons or attend funerals. May prefer the client die at home. Prayers, amulets, and rosary beads are used, and the priest should be notified. Death is seen as an important spiritual event. The family may bathe the body and spend time with the body. |
| Vietnamese | Consult head of family before telling client about a terminal illness. Entire family will make DNR decision, often with assistance from a priest or monk. Clients often prefer to die at home. Family should have extra time with the body, and may cry loudly and uncontrollably. Spiritual/religious rites are often conducted in the room. |

*Note. Adapted from* Culture & Nursing Care: A Pocket Guide *by J.G. Lipson, S. L. Dibble, & P. A. Minarik (Eds.), 1996, San Francisco: UCSF Nursing Press.*

right to make health care decisions on his or her behalf if he or she cannot. The legal authority is limited to decisions about health care.

A **living will** is a legal document that formally expresses a person's wishes regarding life-sustaining treatment in the event of terminal illness or permanent unconsciousness (Figure 11–1 ■). It is not a type of durable power of attorney and usually does not designate a substitute decision maker. It is the responsibility of the nurse as client advocate to request and record the client's preference for care and include it in the plan of care. The nurse's documentation helps communicate these preferences to the other members of the health care team.

All facilities that receive Medicare and Medicaid funds are required to provide all clients with written information and counseling about advance directives and the institution's policies governing them (see the Nursing Research box on page 322). The specific terms of this requirement are found in the Patient Self-Determination Act (PSDA). A copy of the signed advance directive must be kept in the client's medical record, but clients do not have to sign it in order to be treated. Nurses are the ones in close contact with clients, so they are often left with unresolved feelings about the moral, ethical, and legal aspects of their actions. Although advance directives do not ease the pain of seeing clients die, they do help nurses provide clients with the care that the clients have chosen.

### Do-Not-Resuscitate Orders

A **do-not-resuscitate (DNR, or "no-code") order** is written by the physician for the client who is near death. This order is usually based on the wishes of the client and family that no cardiopulmonary resuscitation be performed for respiratory or cardiac arrest. A **comfort measures only order** indicates that

**Directive**

I,_____ recognize that the best health care is based on a partnership of trust and communication with my physician. My physician and I will make health care decisions together as long as I am of sound mind and able to make my wishes known. If there comes a time that I am unable to make medical decisions about myself because of illness or injury, I direct that the following treatment preferences be honored:

If, in the judgment of my physician, I am suffering with a terminal condition from which I am expected to die within six months, even with available life-sustaining treatment provided in accordance with prevailing standards of medical care:

_____ I request that all treatment other than those needed to keep me comfortable be discontinued or withheld and my physician allow me to die as gently as possible; OR

_____ I request that I be kept alive in this terminal condition using available life-sustaining treatment. (This Selection Does Not Apply To Hospice Care)

If, in the judgment of my physician, I am suffering with an irreversible condition so that I cannot care for myself or make decisions for myself and am expected to die without life-sustaining treatment provided in accordance with prevailing standards of care:

_____ I request that all treatment other than those needed to keep me comfortable be discontinued or withheld and my physician allow me to die as gently as possible; OR

_____ I request that I be kept alive in this irreversible condition using available life-sustaining treatment. (This Section Does Not Apply to Hospice Care)

Addition request:

_____

_____

After signing this directive, if my representative or I elect hospice care, I understand and agree that only those treatments needed to keep me comfortable would be provided and I would not be given available life-sustaining treatment.

If I do not have a Medical Power of Attorney, and I am unable to make my wishes known, I designate the following person(s) to make treatment decisions with my physician compatible with my personal values:

1. _____
      (name of person)

2. _____
      (name of second person)

SIGNED _____ DATE _____
                (your name)               (date)

City, County, State of Residence

_____ , _____ , _____
      (city)              (county)             (state)

WITNESS #1: _____

WITNESS #2: _____

Excerpted. *Texas Directive to Physicians and Family or Surrogates.* Courtesy of Partnership for Caring Inc., Washington, DC 800-989-9455

**Figure 11–1** ■ Sample living will. For more information and a complete document, contact Concern for Dying or the Society for the Right to Die.

Excerpted. *Texas Directive to Physicians and Family or Surrogates.* Courtesy of Partnership for Caring, Inc., 1620 Eye Street, NW, Suite 2002, Washington, DC.

## Nursing Research

### Evidence-Based Practice for Advance Directives

In accordance with the Patient Self-Determination Act (PSDA), passed in 1990, all health care institutions that receive any government funding are required to have written policies and procedures concerning the formulation and execution of advance directives. The PSDA requires institutions to ask clients upon admission whether they have an advance directive already prepared and then to provide them with information regarding advance directives, including any applicable state laws and the institution's policies. Public education is a major responsibility defined in the PSDA.

Although advance directives have been mandated for a decade, a noticeably small percentage of patients have completed them. One study (Ott & Hardie, 1997) suggested that a client's inability to understand advance directives may explain why this is true. It is known that many people read below the level of their completed education and that older adult clients often read at a 4th- to 8th-grade level. Teaching-learning guidelines recommend that written materials given to clients not be above the 6th-grade reading level, but studies have shown the mean client readability level for health-related materials to range from grades 11.2 to 17.5. The purpose of this study was to assess the readability of 10 advance directive documents from various sources. The estimated readability for all documents was at levels much more difficult than recommended reading levels. Based on these findings, the authors advised that any document used to document client decisions about future treatment decisions be readable by clients. Poor readability prevents understanding and adversely affects choices about advance directives.

### IMPLICATIONS FOR NURSING

The American Nurses Association (1992) has stated that nurses have a responsibility to ensure that clients have the knowledge necessary to make informed decisions about treatment. There is a need for documents and supporting materials designed for clients with low reading levels. The following suggestions may help.

1. Use a readability formula as a screening device to determine whether documents are written at appropriate reading levels.
2. Increase collaboration and documentation of communications about treatment decisions among all health care providers and clients.
3. Provide client education about advance directives in community-based settings if at all possible, so that decisions are made before a client is seriously ill.
4. Encourage consumer and advocacy groups to develop documents and other supporting materials that have good readability.
5. Evaluate client education materials used in client education and print the readability level on each document. Use larger print for older adults.
6. Include considerations about cultural, ethnic, religious, and illness-related variables in all printed materials.

### Critical Thinking in Client Care

1. Which factors may influence clients to prepare an advance directive?
2. What members of the health care team should be included in a discussion about end-of-life decisions?
3. What are the responsibilities of the hospital to ensure that clients receive accurate and compassionate information regarding advance directives?

---

no further life-sustaining interventions are necessary and that the goal of care is a comfortable, dignified death. Confusing or conflicting DNR orders create dilemmas, because nurses are involved in resuscitation and either begin CPR or ensure that unwanted attempts do not occur. The ANA has made specific recommendations related to a DNR order (see Box 11–2).

The ANA further recommends that guidelines and policies be developed to help resolve conflicts between clients and their families, between clients and health care professionals, and among health care professionals.

### Euthanasia

**Euthanasia** (from the Greek for painless, easy, gentle, or good death) is now commonly used to signify a killing prompted by some humanitarian motive. There are many arguments for and against euthanasia, and nurses have often found themselves at the center of the debate. As a result, nurses have pushed for the development of appropriate guidelines and procedures for DNR orders. When no such orders exist, the nurse faces a dilemma. Certainly, there are situations in which the nurse's role is clear. For example, it is considered malpractice to participate in "slow codes" (in which the nurse does not hurry to alert the emergency team when a terminally ill client who does not have a DNR order stops breathing).

The natural death laws seek to preserve the notion of voluntary versus involuntary euthanasia. In *voluntary euthanasia,* the competent adult client and a physician, nurse, or adult friend or relative make the decision to terminate life. *Involuntary euthanasia* ("mercy killing") is performed without the client's consent. Because care settings offer many complex and technologic interventions, it is not likely that the ethical aspects of euthanasia will soon be resolved. However, advance directives do give clients a much more active role in decisions about their own care.

### Hospice

**Hospice** is a model of care (rather than a place of care) for clients and their families when faced with a limited life expectancy. Hospice care is initiated for clients as they near the end of life, emphasizing quality rather than quantity of life. Emotional, spiritual, and practical support is provided based on the wishes of the client and the needs of the family. Hospice regards dying as a normal part of life and provides support for a dignified and peaceful death.

## BOX 11-2 ■ The ANA Position on Nursing Care and Do-Not-Resuscitate Decisions

■ The choices and values of the competent patient should always be given highest priority, even when these wishes conflict with those of health care providers and families.

■ In the case of the incompetent or never competent patient, any existing advance directives or the decisions of surrogate decision makers acting in the patient's best interest should be determinative.

■ The DNR decision should always be a subject of explicit discussion among the patient, the family, any designated surrogate decision maker acting in the patient's best interest, and the health care team. The decision should include consideration of the efficacy and desirability of CPR, a balancing of benefits and burdens to patients, and therapeutic goals.

■ DNR orders must be clearly documented, reviewed, and updated periodically to reflect changes in the patient's condition.

■ Nurses have a responsibility to educate patients and their families about various forms of advance directives such as living wills and durable power of attorney.

■ If it is the nurse's personal belief that his or her moral integrity is compromised by professional responsibility to carry out a particular DNR order, the nurse should transfer the responsibility for the patient's care to another nurse.

*Note. From Task Force on the Nurse's Role in End of Life Decisions by ANA Board of Directors, 1992, new position statement.*

The American hospice movement was originally led by volunteers (many of whom were nurses) who wanted to make life better for those who were dying. These devoted volunteers promoted the dignity of patients during their death and decreased their institutionalization. In 1986, Congress passed the Medicare Hospice Benefit and also gave states the option of including hospice services in their Medicaid programs. Since then, patients dying of cancer or any other terminal illness may receive hospice care in the comfort of their homes with their families.

Hospice care usually begins when the patient has 6 months or less to live and ends with the family 1 year after the death. Nurses providing hospice care work with an interdisciplinary team of other health professionals such as social workers, pastoral counselors, home health aides, and volunteers to provide comprehensive palliative care. The hospice nurse must combine all of the skills of the home care nurse with the ability to provide daily emotional support to dying patients and their families. Hospice nurses are especially skilled in pain and symptom management. Their focus is on improving quality of life and preserving dignity for the patient in death.

## End-of-Life Care

End-of-life nursing care that ensures a peaceful death was mandated by the International Council of Nurses' (1997) and further supported by the American Association of Colleges of Nursing (AACN) (1999). The principles of hospice care are basic to end-of-life care: that people live until the moment they die; that care until death may be offered by a variety of health care professionals; and that such care is coordinated, is sensitive to diversity, offered around the clock, and incorporates the physical, psychological, social, and spiritual concerns of the patient and the patient's family. Following are selected competencies necessary for nurses to provide high-quality end-of-life care as defined by the AACN (1999).

• Promote the provision of comfort care to the dying as an active, desirable, and important skill, and an integral component of nursing care (Figure 11–2 ■).

• Communicate effectively and compassionately with the patient, family, and health care team members about end-of-life issues.

• Recognize one's own attitudes, feelings, values, and expectations about death and the individual, cultural, and spiritual diversity existing in those beliefs and customs.

• Demonstrate respect for the patient's views and wishes during end-of-life care.

• Use scientifically based standardized tools to assess symptoms (e.g., pain, dyspnea, constipation, anxiety, fatigue, nausea/vomiting, and altered cognition) experienced by patients at the end of life.

• Use data from symptom assessment to plan and intervene in symptom management using state-of-the-art traditional and complementary approaches.

• Assist the patient, family, colleagues, and one's self to cope with suffering, grief, loss, and bereavement in end-of-life care.

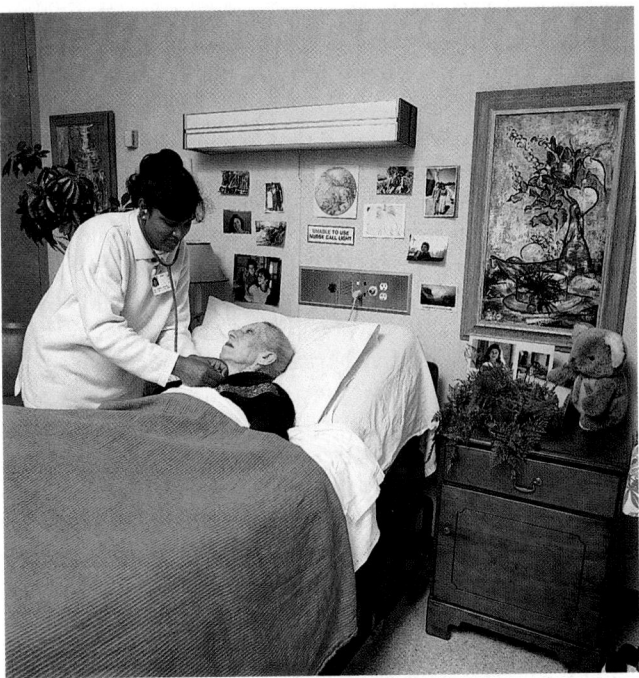

**Figure 11–2** ■ The nurse helps the client visualize the hospital room as a safe, comfortable place to die by surrounding the client with familiar articles brought from the client's home.

## Manifestations of Impending Death

- Difficulty talking or swallowing
- Nausea, flatus, abdominal distention
- Urinary and/or bowel incontinence, constipation
- Decreased sensation, taste, and smell
- Weak, slow, and/or irregular pulse
- Decreasing blood pressure
- Decreased, irregular, or Cheyne-Stokes respirations
- Changes in level of consciousness
- Restlessness, agitation
- Coolness, mottling, and cyanosis of the extremities

## Physiological Changes in the Dying Client

Death may occur rapidly or slowly. Physiological changes are a part of the dying process. These changes result in any or all of the manifestations listed in the box above as death nears.

- *Weakness and fatigue.* Weakness and fatigue cause discomfort, especially in joints, and contribute to an increased risk for pressure ulcers.
- *Anorexia and decreased food intake.* Although anorexia and a decrease in food intake are normal in the dying client, the family often views this as "giving up." Anorexia may be a protective mechanism; the breakdown of body fats results in ketosis, which leads to a sense of well-being and helps decrease pain. Parenteral or enteral feedings do not improve symptoms or prolong life and may actually cause discomfort. As weakness and difficulty swallowing progress, the gag reflex is decreased and clients are at increased risk for aspiration if oral foods are given.
- *Fluid and electrolyte imbalances.* Decreased oral fluid intake is normal at the end of life and does not cause distress. Parenteral fluids are sometimes given to decrease delirium, but they may cause increased edema, breathlessness, cough, and respiratory secretions. If the client has edema or *ascites* (a collection of fluid in the abdominal cavity), excess body water is present so dehydration is not a problem.
- *Hypotension and renal failure.* As cardiac output decreases, so does intravascular blood volume. As a result, renal perfusion decreases and the kidneys cease to function. Urinary output is scanty. The client will have tachycardia, hypotension, cool extremities, and cyanosis with skin mottling.
- *Neurologic dysfunction.* Neurologic dysfunction results from any or all of the following: decreased cerebral perfusion, hypoxemia, metabolic acidosis, sepsis, an accumulation of toxins from liver and renal failure, the effects of medications, and disease-related factors. These changes may result in decreased level of consciousness or agitated delirium. Clients with terminal delirium may be confused, restless, or agitated. Moaning, groaning, and grimacing often accompany the agitation and are often misinterpreted as pain. Level of consciousness often decreases to the point where the client cannot be aroused. Although decreased consciousness and agitation are both normal states at the end of life, they are very distressing to the client's family. A client near death often has altered cerebral function, so the nurse must

## BOX 11-3 ■ Providing Comfort for the Client Nearing Death

- Maintain clean skin and bed linens.
- Use a draw sheet to turn the client as often as possible so the client is comfortable.
- Position the client to promote comfort and protect bony areas with padding. Reposition the client and raise the head of the bed if fluids accumulate in the upper airways and back of the throat.
- Use bed pads or insert a Foley catheter (if ordered) for urinary incontinence.
- Use gentle massage to improve circulation and shift edema.
- Provide small, frequent sips of fluids, ice chips, or popsicles.
- Provide oral care, using a soft moist brush or glycerin swab.
- Clean secretions from the eyes and nose.
- Administer ordered pain medications as needed to maintain comfort.
- Administer oxygen as prescribed to relieve dyspnea.

stand near the bedside and speak clearly. Hearing is thought to be the last sense a dying client loses; the nurse should never whisper or engage in conversation with the family as if the client were not there.

- *Respiratory changes.* Respiratory changes are normal at this time. The client may have dyspnea, apnea, or Cheyne-Stokes respirations, and may use accessory muscles to breathe. Fluids accumulated in the lungs and oropharynx may lead to what is sometimes called "the death rattle." Oxygen may not relieve these manifestations.
- *Bowel and/or bladder incontinence.* Loss of sphincter control may lead to incontinence of feces or urine.
- *Pain.* A common problem for clients at the end of life, pain is what people often say they fear the most. It is of utmost importance to keep the client comfortable through general comfort measures (see Box 11–3) and by administering ordered medications for pain and anxiety.

**PRACTICE ALERT** *There is no maximum allowable dose for opioids such as morphine sulfate; the dose should be increased to whatever is necessary to relieve pain (Tierney, McPhee, & Papadakis, 2001).* ■

## Support for the Client and Family

As the client's condition deteriorates, the nurse's knowledge of the client and family guides the care provided. It may be necessary to provide opportunities for clients to express personal preferences about where they want to die and about funeral and burial arrangements. If the family feels that this is morbid, the nurse explains that it helps clients to keep a sense of control as they approach death.

The client needs the opportunity to say goodbye to others. The nurse encourages and supports the client and family as they terminate relationships as a necessary part of the grief process. The nurse acknowledges that termination is painful and, if the client or family desires, stays with them during this

## Manifestations of Death

- Absence of respirations, pulse, and heartbeat
- Fixed and dilated pupils; eyes may stay open
- Release of stool and urine
- Waxen color (pallor) as blood settles to dependent areas
- Body temperature drops
- Lack of reflexes
- Flat encephalogram

time. Family members are often afraid to be present at the moment of death, yet dying alone is the greatest fear expressed by clients.

## DEATH

The manifestations listed in the box above are seen after death occurs, and are the basis for pronouncing death. They appear gradually and not in any special order. Pronouncement of death is legally required by a physician or other health care provider to confirm death. The time of death, with any related data, is documented in the client's chart.

The nurse may also fear being present at the moment of the client's death. In fact, Kübler-Ross (1969) noted that the nurse's fear of death frequently interferes with the ability to provide support for the dying client and family. Thoughts such as, "Please, God, don't let him die on my shift," are common, and they express the nurse's emotional turmoil in dealing with the task. Nurses who have worked through their own feelings about death and dying are more at ease in assisting the dying client toward a peaceful death.

After the death, the family is encouraged to acknowledge the pain of loss. The nurse's presence and support as the bereaved express their sorrow, anger, or guilt can help them resolve their grief. It is important for the bereaved not to suppress the pain of grieving with drugs. By accepting variations in the expression of grief, the nurse supports the family's grief reactions and helps prevent dysfunctional grieving. Dysfunctional grieving is an extended and unsuccessful resolution of grief.

Resolution of grief begins with acceptance of the loss. The nurse can encourage this acceptance by maintaining open, honest dialogue and by providing the family with the opportunity to view, touch, hold, and kiss the person's body (Carpenito, 2000). As family members realize the finality of the death, they are often comforted by the presence of the nurse who cared for the client during the final days.

## Postmortem Care

The nurse documents the time of death (required for the death certificate and all official records), notifies the physician, and assists the family (if needed) in choice of a funeral home. If the client dies at home, death must be pronounced before the body is removed. In some states and in some situations, nurses can pronounce death; for specifics, consult state practice acts, laws, and agency policy. All jewelry is removed and given to the family unless they ask that it be left on. The body is kept in place until the family is ready and gives permission. If an au-

topsy is required or requested, the body must be left undisturbed (e.g., do not remove any tubes) for transportation to the medical examiner.

Documentation of the death is completed by sending a completed death certificate to the funeral home (for a death in the home), or by completing the required paperwork and sending the body to the morgue or funeral home (for a death in the hospital or long-term care setting).

## Nurses' Grief

The nurse who has developed a close relationship with the client who has died may experience strong feelings of grief. Sharing grief with the family after the death of a loved one helps both the nurse and family to cope with their feelings about the loss. Taking time to grieve after the death of a client provides a release that can help prevent "blunting" of feelings, a problem often experienced by nurses who care for clients who are terminally ill.

**PRACTICE ALERT**   *Crying with families (at one time considered unprofessional) is now recognized as simply an expression of empathy and caring.* ■

Nurses working with critically or terminally ill clients should be aware that witnessing a client's death and the family's grief may reactivate feelings about some unresolved grief in their own lives. In these cases, nurses may need to reflect on their responses to their own losses. Also, nurses who work with dying clients need support from peers and other professionals to work through the often overwhelming feelings that result from dealing with death, grief, and loss (Figure 11–3 ■).

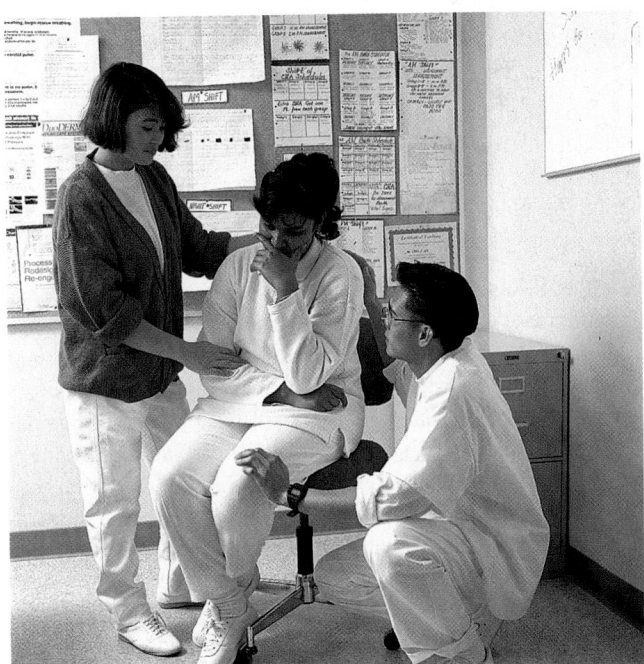

**Figure 11–3** ■ Nurses who work with dying clients need support from their colleagues to work through their often overwhelming feelings of grief.

## COLLABORATIVE CARE

Interventions for loss and grief may be planned and implemented by any or all members of the health care team. Nurses and social workers provide interventions to help clients or families adapt to a loss. They also make referrals to mental health professionals (grief counselors, social services), support groups, chaplains, or legal or financial assistance agencies.

Grieving clients frequently enter the health care system with significant somatic symptoms. In some cases, the symptoms of grief and loss are overlooked until the client reaches a crisis state requiring psychiatric medical intervention. Collaborative care by the physician and the nurse early in the normal grieving process can help the client achieve an early and effective resolution of grief and avoid physical or psychiatric health problems.

## NURSING CARE

Nurses practicing in all types of settings care for clients who are in various stages of the grieving process. Grief is highly individual. The grief process may range from uncomfortable to debilitating, and it may last for a day or a lifetime, depending on what the loss means to the person experiencing it.

### Health Promotion

In planning and implementing nursing care for the client experiencing a loss, the nurse considers the individual responses, which may vary greatly. In an era of short acute care stays for clients, nurses may feel that an elaborate grief assessment is impossible or, at the least, impractical. But research and clinical experience suggest that clients who delay the grieving process after a loss are prone to have health problems that may last a lifetime.

### Assessment

Knowledge of the expected physical reactions to loss provides the nurse with a basis for identifying reactions requiring further assessment. To assess the extent of somatic distress, the nurse observes for changes in sensory processes and asks questions about the client's sleeping and eating patterns, activities of daily living, general health status, and pain.

### Physical Assessment

Clients may experience one or more predictable somatic symptoms as they become aware of a loss. Gastrointestinal symptoms occur frequently. They may include indigestion, nausea or vomiting, anorexia, weight gain or loss, constipation, or diarrhea. The shock and disbelief that accompany a loss may cause shortness of breath, a choking sensation, hyperventilation, or loss of strength. Some clients also report insomnia, preoccupation with sleep, fatigue, and decreased or increased activity level.

Crying and sadness are observed during normal grief states. Crying may make the client feel exhausted and interfere with carrying out activities of daily living. However, a person who is unable to cry may have difficulty completing the mourning process. If the client does not express feelings of grief, somatic symptoms may increase.

It is imperative that the client's concerns about pain be assessed, especially if the client has cancer or another painful illness. Knowledge of pain theories and pain assessment can help the nurse assess the need for pain medication (see Chapter 4). ⌾⌾ During the last stages of dying, the client usually becomes very weak, and sensations and reflexes decrease; these changes call for careful assessment of the client's physical needs.

Reactions to loss are not always obvious. For example, in clients who experience an illness following a serious loss, assessment may reveal somatic complaints related to the grief state as well as the illness. When a person who has been healthy begins to develop patterns of increased illness, the nurse should be aware that this may signal dysfunctional grieving. This is especially common in the loss and grieving associated with a change in body image. In addition to making a physical assessment, assess the client's perception of the alteration in body image. The loss of a body part, weight gain or loss, and scars from surgery or trauma can be difficult for the client to accept. Some clients may grieve hair loss that accompanies chemotherapy used in cancer treatment.

### Spiritual Assessment

Because spiritual beliefs and practices greatly influence people's reaction to loss, it is important to explore them with the client when assessing a loss. The spiritually healthy client has inner resources that help work through the grief process. Faith, prayer, trust in God or a superior being, perception of a purpose in life, or belief in immortality are examples of the inner resources that may sustain the client during an actual or perceived loss (Reed, 1996).

Assessing the client's spiritual life and its significance to the client and family helps identify spiritual support systems. Some nurses are uncomfortable with assessing the client's spiritual needs; the following questions may be helpful.

- What are the spiritual aspects of the client's philosophy about life? Death?
- Are the values and beliefs about life and death congruent with those of people who are important to the client?
- Which spiritual resources and rituals have significance for the client?

Belief systems that are incompatible with those of family members can be an additional source of stress for clients dealing with a loss. The anger and resentment often observed among families faced with decisions concerning dying members may be avoided if the nurse assesses the potential impact of differing beliefs.

Clients coping with a loss often perceive that it is a punishment from God for their wrongdoing or for their failure to remain faithful to their religious practices. Therefore, it is important to assess the level of guilt the client or family expresses. Assessing the client's comments regarding feelings of responsibility for the loss helps determine whether these feelings are an expected phase of grieving or indicate dysfunctional grieving.

Clients who had not considered themselves religious before the actual or perceived loss often turn to religion to seek comfort or to cope with feelings of despair, helplessness, hopelessness, or guilt. They may utter anguished statements such as "Why, God?" or "Please help me, God." The nurse continues to assess the client's verbalization of such feelings to determine the best interventions to help the client cope with the loss.

## Psychosocial Assessment

When working through the grief process, clients can be overwhelmed by the fears associated with the loss and the changes it will produce. The client responding to an actual or perceived loss commonly expresses anxiety (fear of the unknown). An extreme level of anxiety can threaten the client's well-being. Assessment includes helping clients openly acknowledge their fears. Some clients may fear the feelings they experience while proceeding through the grief process more than the loss itself. The most common fear expressed by clients facing a loss is that of losing self-control.

Focusing on the meaning of the loss to the client is more important than attempting to place the client in a sequence or phase of grief. The degree of caring and sensitivity shown when asking questions about the meaning of the loss influences the amount of information the client will be willing to reveal. Asking such questions as, "Why do you feel this way?" or "What does this loss mean to you?" is less helpful than making a statement such as, "This must be difficult for you." The latter more effectively conveys a genuine interest in hearing how the client feels about the loss.

Awareness of the altered sensorium observed during the stage of shock and disbelief provides parameters for assessment. The nurse may note in the client feelings of numbness, unreality, emotional distance, intense preoccupation with the lost object, helplessness, loneliness, and disorganization. As awareness of the loss begins to develop, preoccupation with the lost person or object may increase, and self-accusation and ambivalence toward the lost person or object may follow.

## Nursing Diagnoses and Interventions

A variety of nursing diagnoses may be appropriate for the client experiencing loss and grief, as well as for the client who is nearing death. Nurses practicing medical-surgical nursing will most often provide interventions for anticipatory grieving, chronic sorrow, and death anxiety.

### Anticipatory Grieving

Anticipatory grieving is a combination of intellectual and emotional responses and behaviors by which people adjust their self-concept in the face of a potential loss. Anticipatory grieving may be a response to one's own future death; to potential loss of body parts or functions; to potential loss of a significant person, animal, or possession; or to potential loss of a social role. Nursing interventions are designed to assist with grief resolution.

- Assess for factors causing or contributing to the grief. Ask about support systems, how many losses have occurred, relationship with the lost person, significance of the body part, and previous experiences with loss and grief. *Grief and mourning occur when a person experiences any type of loss.*
- Use open-ended questions to encourage the person to share concerns and the possible effect on the family. *Grief resolution cannot occur until the client acknowledges the loss.*

- Promote a trusting nurse-client relationship: Allow enough time for communications; speak clearly, simply, and concisely; listen; be honest in responses to questions; do not give unrealistic hope; offer support; and demonstrate respect for the person's age, culture, religion, race, and values. *An effective nurse-client relationship begins with acceptance of the client's feelings, attitudes, and values related to the loss. If the client is ready to talk, listening and being present are the most appropriate interventions.*
- Ask about strengths and weakness in coping with the anticipated loss. *Current responses are influenced by past experiences with loss, illness, and death. Socioeconomic and cultural background, as well as cultural and spiritual beliefs and values, affect a person's ability to adapt to loss.*
- Teach the client and family the stages of grief. *This helps them to be aware of their emotions in each stage and reassures them that their reactions are normal.*
- Provide time for decision making. *In periods of stress, people may need extra time to make informed decisions.*
- Provide information about appropriate resources, including support from family, friends, and support groups, community resources, and legal/financial aides. *Support from others decreases feelings of loneliness and isolation and facilitates grief work.*

### Chronic Sorrow

Chronic sorrow is a cyclical, recurring, and potentially progressive pattern of pervasive sadness experienced in response to continual loss, throughout the trajectory of an illness or disability. It is triggered by situations that bring to mind the person's losses, disappointments, or fears. It may be experienced by a client, parent or caregiver, or person with chronic illness or disability.

- Explain the difference between chronic sorrow and chronic grieving. *Grieving is time-limited and ends in adaptation to the loss. Chronic sorrow may vary in intensity, but it persists as long as the person with the disability or chronic sorrow condition lives.*
- Encourage verbalization of feelings about the loss, and about the personal relevance of the changes to hopes for the future. *Expressing feelings is normal and necessary to decrease the emotional pain.*
- Help identify triggers that intensify the sorrow, such as birthdays, anniversaries, and holidays. *When triggers have been identified, role-playing may make the events less painful.*
- Refer to appropriate community support groups. *Participating in support groups with others experiencing grief is helpful in coping with loss.*
- Encourage use of personal, family, significant other, and spiritual support systems *to facilitate coping with loss.*

### Death Anxiety

Death anxiety is worry or fear related to death or dying. It may be present in clients who have an acute life-threatening illness, who have a terminal illness, who have experienced the death of a family member or friend, or who have experienced multiple deaths in the same family.

- Explore the client's knowledge of the situation. For example, ask, "What has your doctor told you about your condition?" *This informs you of the client's knowledge base about the condition and about his or her ability to make informed decisions.*
- Ask the client to identify specific fears about death. *This provides data about any unrealistic expectations or misperceptions.*
- Determine the client's perceptions of strengths and weakness in coping with death. *Identifying past strengths can help the client cope with loss, illness, and death.*
- Ask the client to identify needed help. *This determines whether available resources are adequate.*
- Encourage independence and control in decisions about treatment and care. *This promotes self-esteem, decreases feelings of powerlessness, and allows the client to retain dignity in dying.*
- Facilitate access to culturally appropriate spiritual rituals and practices. *This provides spiritual comfort.*
- Explain advance directives and assist with them if necessary. *Advance directives help ensure that the client's wishes for end-of-life care are carried out.*
- Encourage life review and reminiscence. *Life review is self-affirming.*
- Encourage activities such as listening to music, aromatherapy, massage, or relaxation exercises. *These activities decrease anxiety.*
- Suggest keeping a journal or leaving a written legacy. *A written document provides continuing support to others after death.*

## Using NANDA, NIC, and NOC

Chart 11–1 shows linkages between NANDA, NIC, and NOC when caring for the client experiencing loss, grief, and death.

## Home Care

In addition to teaching clients and families to carry out the physical skills that are necessary to the client's care, nurses also provide information on identifying signs of deterioration and additional sources of support. General guidelines for teaching clients and families about grief include those suggested in the box below. In addition, suggest the following resources:

- Hospice
- Support groups
- Home health care agencies
- Public health departments

---

### Meeting Individualized Needs

#### TEACHING FOR CLIENTS EXPERIENCING A LOSS

- Encourage both children and adults to discuss expected or impending loss and to express feelings.
- Teach problem-solving skills: Define what the possible changes and problems are related to the predicted loss, develop potential strategies for dealing with problems, list pros and cons of each strategy, and decide which strategies might be most useful to try first to solve potential problems associated with loss.
- Teach individuals and families how to support a person who is dealing with an impending loss.
- Explain what to expect with a loss: sadness, fear, rejection, anger, guilt, loneliness.
- Teach signs of grief resolution:
  - No longer living in the past, becoming future oriented
  - Breaking ties with the lost object or person (Acute stage often shows signs of resolving in 6 to 12 months.)
  - The possibility of having painful "waves" of grief years after the loss, especially on the anniversary of the loss and in response to "triggers" such as pictures, events, songs, or memories

---

### CHART 11–1  NANDA, NIC, AND NOC LINKAGES

#### The Client Experiencing Loss

| NURSING DIAGNOSES | NURSING INTERVENTIONS | NURSING OUTCOMES |
|---|---|---|
| • Anticipatory Grieving | • Grief Work Facilitation<br>• Emotional Support<br>• Family Support<br>• Hope Instillation | • Grief Resolution<br>• Coping |
| • Dysfunctional Grieving | • Coping Enhancement<br>• Counseling<br>• Emotional Support<br>• Spiritual Support | • Coping<br>• Self-Esteem |
| • Death Anxiety | • Dying Care<br>• Spiritual Support<br>• Forgiveness Facilitation<br>• Simple Guided Imagery<br>• Medication Management | • Dignified Dying<br>• Spiritual Well-Being<br>• Acceptance: Health Status<br>• Quality of Life<br>• Knowledge: Medication |

*Note. Data from* Nursing Outcomes Classification (NOC) *by M. Johnson & M. Maas (Eds.), 1997, St. Louis: Mosby;* Nursing Diagnoses: Definitions & Classification 2001–2002, *by North American Nursing Diagnosis Association, 2001, Philadelphia: NANDA;* Nursing Interventions Classification (NIC) *by J. C. McCloskey and G. M. Bulechek (Eds.), 2000,  St. Louis: Mosby. Reprinted by permission.*

## Nursing Care Plan
## A Client Experiencing Loss and Grief

Pearl Rogers is a 79-year-old African American woman who is admitted to the Methodist Home Nursing Center. Mrs. Rogers lived with her husband of 58 years until his death 9 months ago. She had one son who died in an auto accident 2 years ago, and she has one daughter who lives nearby. After her husband's death, Mrs. Rogers lived with her daughter until her admission to the nursing center. Mrs. Rogers has become increasingly agitated and helpless, complaining constantly of pain. Her daughter states that Mrs. Rogers is chronically constipated, has difficulty sleeping, and has stopped engaging in all social activities, including weekly church services. She cries frequently. Extensive medical testing prior to her admission to the nursing center revealed Mrs. Rogers has arthritis but no other pathologic disorder.

### ASSESSMENT

On admission to the nursing center, Mrs. Rogers says, "I'm a sick woman, and no one will listen to me! I can't walk, I'm so weak. My head hurts, and I'm always sick at my stomach. I haven't had a bowel movement in a week, and I never sleep more than 3 hours a night." Physical assessment finding include swollen knees and ankles, with limited mobility of the lower extremities.

### DIAGNOSES

- *Dysfunctional grieving* related to stress of husband's death
- *Sleep pattern disturbance* related to grieving
- *Constipation* related to inactivity

### EXPECTED OUTCOMES

- Engage in normal grief work: Work through grief process, discuss reality of losses, use nondestructive coping mechanisms, and discuss positive and negative aspects of the loss.
- Experience adequate and restful sleep: Fall asleep 20 to 30 minutes after retiring and awaken feeling rested after 7 to 8 hours of sleep.
- Have a bowel movement with soft formed stools at least every other day.

### PLANNING AND IMPLEMENTATION

- Promote trust: Show empathy and caring, demonstrate respect for her culture and values, offer support and reassurance, be honest, engage in active listening.

- Assist in labeling her feelings: anger, fear, loneliness, guilt, isolation.
- Explore previous losses and the ways in which the client has coped.
- Encourage review of her relationship with her dead husband.
- Reinforce expressions of behaviors associated with normal grieving.
- Encourage participation in usual spiritual practices.
- Encourage participation in a grief group that meets at the facility.
- Consult with the physical and recreational therapist to help the nursing staff provide afternoon activities.
- Provide measures that assist in bowel evacuation: Encourage exercise as tolerated, including walks and rocking in a rocking chair. Offer foods that stimulate bowel movements. Offer privacy: Close the door, ensuring that the emergency call bell is within reach, and do not interrupt.
- Administer a mild laxative and/or stool softener, if necessary, but discontinue as soon as possible.

### EVALUATION

After 4 weeks at the nursing center, Mrs. Rogers states, "I don't feel any better, but I know I have to accept my situation." Although Mrs. Rogers states that she doesn't feel better, she is walking the length of the hall, sleeping better, and having regular bowel movements. Mrs. Rogers is also less withdrawn and has openly discussed her feelings related to her husband's death, including her anger at the loss of her son and her husband less than 2 years apart. She has attended the grief group once and has attended chapel services on Sunday for the past 2 weeks. Her daughter visits her each Saturday and takes her in a wheelchair to the shopping mall.

### Critical Thinking in the Nursing Process

1. What common physical manifestations of grief did Mrs. Rogers experience?
2. How might Mrs. Rogers's daughter be more involved in developing and implementing her mother's plan of care?
3. Suppose Mrs. Rogers says that she does not want any help, that she just wants to be left alone to die. How would you respond?

See Evaluating Your Response in Appendix C.

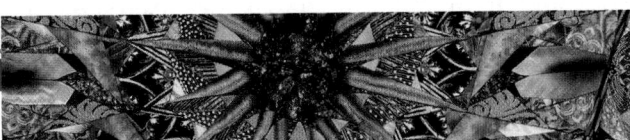

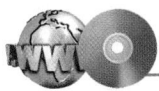

## EXPLORE MediaLink

NCLEX Review questions, case studies, care plan activities, MediaLink applications, and other interactive resources for this chapter can be found on the Companion Website at www.prenhall.com/lemone.

Click on Chapter 11 to select the activities for this chapter. For animations, video clips, more NCLEX review questions, and an audio glossary, access the Student CD-ROM accompanying this textbook.

# TEST YOURSELF

1. Which of the following statements *best* describes loss?
   a. It is determined by one's cultural values
   b. It is largely dependent on support of family and friends
   c. It can be determined only by the person who experiences it
   d. It is the same as grief and mourning

2. Kübler-Ross believed that one usually first responds to a situation of loss with:
   a. Anger
   b. Bargaining
   c. Depression
   d. Denial

3. What document expresses a person's wishes for life-sustaining treatment in the event of terminal illness or permanent unconsciousness?
   a. Durable power of attorney for health care
   b. Living will
   c. Physician's no-code order
   d. Patient Self-Determination Act

4. Which of the senses is believed to be the last one lost as a person nears death?
   a. Hearing
   b. Vision
   c. Touch
   d. Smell

5. Which of the following statements best describes the treatment of pain at the end of life?
   a. As client nears death, no pain is perceived and no medications are necessary
   b. It is important to withhold pain medications if the client has respiratory changes
   c. There is no maximum allowable dose for opioids during end-of-life care
   d. Nurses should not administer opioids to the dying client

See Test Yourself answers in Appendix C.

# BIBLIOGRAPHY

American Association of Colleges of Nursing. (1999). *Peaceful death: Recommended competencies and curricular guidelines for end-of-life nursing care.* Washington, DC: AACN.

American Nurses Association. (1992). *Position statement on nursing and the Patient Self-Determination Act.* Kansas City: ANA.

_____. (1992). *Report from the task force on the nurse's role in end of life decisions.* Kansas City: ANA.

Barbus, A. J. (1975). The dying person's bill of rights. *The American Journal of Nursing, 75* (1), 99.

Bowlby, J. (1973). Attachment and loss, *Separation, anxiety, and anger* (Vol. 2). New York: Basic Books.

_____. (1980). Attachment and loss, *Loss, sadness, and depression* (Vol. 3). New York: Basic Books.

Caplan, G. (1990). Loss, stress, and mental health. *Community Mental Health Journal, 26*(1), 27–48.

Carpenito, L. (2000). *Nursing diagnoses: Application to clinical practice* (8th ed.). Philadelphia: Lippincott.

Carter, S. (1989). Themes of grief. *Nursing Research, 36*(6), 354–358.

Collins, D. (2001). Grief and loss experienced by patients with Alzheimer's disease and their caregivers. *Geriaction, 19*(1), 17–20.

Duffield, P. (1998). Advance directives in primary care. *American Journal of Nursing, 61*(4), 16CCC–16DDD.

Durham, E., & Weiss, L. (1997). How patients die. *American Journal of Nursing, 97*(12), 41–46.

Engel, G. (1964). Grief and grieving. *American Journal of Nursing, 64,* 93.

Freud, S. (1917/1957). Mourning and melancholia. In J. Strachey & A. Tyson (Eds.), *The complete psychological works of Sigmund Freud* (Vol. 14). London: Hogarth Press.

Goetschius, S. (1997). Families and end-of-life care: How do we meet their needs? *Journal of Gerontological Nursing, 23*(3), 43–49.

International Council of Nurses. (1997). *Basic principles of nursing care.* Washington, DC: American Nurses Publishing.

Johnson, M., & Maas, M. (Eds.). (1997). *Nursing outcomes classification (NOC).* St. Louis: Mosby.

Kaunonen, M., Tarkka, M., Paunonen, M., & Laippala, P. (1999). Grief and social support after the death of a spouse. *Journal of Advanced Nursing, 30*(6), 1304–1311.

Kübler-Ross, E. (1969). *On death and dying.* New York: Macmillan.

_____. (1978). *To live until we say goodbye.* Englewood Cliffs, NJ: Prentice Hall.

Libson, J., Dibble, S., & Minarik, P. (1996). *Culture & nursing care: A pocket guide.* San Francisco: UCSF Nursing Press.

Lindemann, E. (1944). Symptomatology and management of acute grief . *American Journal of Psychiatry, 32,* 141.

Matzo, P. L., & Sherman, D. W. (Eds.). (2001). *Palliative care nursing: Quality care to the end of life.* New York: Springer.

McCloskey, J.C., & Bulechek, G. M. (Eds.). (2000). *Nursing interventions classification (NIC)* (3rd ed.). St. Louis: Mosby.

McCorkle, R., Robinson, L., Nuamah, I., Lev, E., & Benoliel, J. (1998). The effects of home nursing care for patients during terminal illness on the bereaved's psychological distress. *Nursing Research, 47*(1), 2–10.

Ott, B., & Hardie, T. (1997). Readability of advance directive documents. *Image: Journal of Nursing Scholarship, 29*(1), 53–57.

Perrin, K. (1997). Giving voice to the wishes of elders for end-of-life care. *Journal of Gerontological Nursing, 23*(3), 18–27.

Poor, B., & Poirrier, G. (2001). *End of life nursing care.* Boston: Jones & Bartlett.

Reed, P. G. (1996). Transcendence: Formulating nursing perspectives. *Nursing Science Quarterly, 9*(1), 2–4.

Rushton, C., & Scanlon, C. (1998). A road map for navigating end-of-life care. *MEDSURG Nursing, 7*(1), 57–59.

Tierney, L. M., McPhee, S. J., & Papadakis, M. A. (2001). *Current medical diagnosis & treatment* (40th ed.). New York: McGraw Hill.

Tipton, K. (1997). How to discuss death with patients and families. *Nursing97, 27*(32), 10–12.

Ufema, J. (2000). Terminal illness: Compassion and raspberry tea. *Nursing, 30*(12), 66–67.

# CHAPTER 12

# Nursing Care of Clients with Problems of Substance Abuse

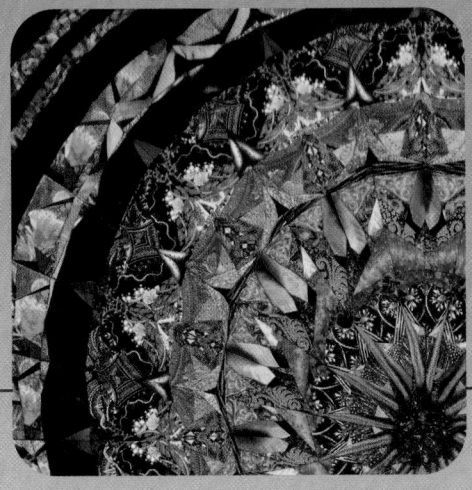

## LEARNING OUTCOMES

After completing this chapter, you will be able to:

- Discuss risk factors associated with substance abuse.

- Describe common characteristics of substance abusers.

- Identify major addictive substances.

- Explain the effects of addictive substances on physiological, cognitive, psychological, and social well-being.

- Discuss collaborative care for the client with substance abuse problems, including diagnostic tests, emergency care for overdose, and treatment of withdrawal.

- Use the nursing process as a framework for providing individualized nursing care for clients experiencing problems with substance abuse.

## MediaLink

**www.prenhall.com/lemone**
Additional resources for this chapter can be found on the Student CD-ROM accompanying this textbook, and on the Companion Website at www.prenhall.com/lemone. Click on Chapter 12 to select the activities for this chapter.

**CD-ROM**
- Audio Glossary
- NCLEX Review

*Animation*
- Cocaine

**Companion Website**
- More NCLEX Review
- Case Study
  Alcohol Abuse
- Care Plan Activity
  Alcohol Withdrawal
- MediaLink Application
  Support in Recovery

**Substance abuse** refers to the use of any chemical in a fashion inconsistent with medical or culturally defined social norms despite physical, psychological, or social adverse effects. Anxiety and depressive disorders frequently occur with substance abuse and more than 90% of people who commit suicide have a depressive or substance abuse disorder (National Institute of Mental Health [NIMH], 2001).

In a recent report of the surgeon general, 6% of the adult U.S. population are estimated to have an addictive disorder and 3% have both mental and addictive disorders (U.S. Department of Health and Human Services [USDHHS], 1999). Consequently, 9% of the population (15.4 million) have a substance abuse disorder. The costs of addictive disorders are exceedingly high. Direct costs of all mental health services in the United States totaled $69 billion with nearly 20% ($12.6 billion) spent on substance abuse treatment (USDHHS, 1999).

Alcohol is the most commonly used and abused substance in the United States. One of every 10 persons in America is alleged to be alcoholic (American Psychiatric Association [APA], 2000a). Two thirds of the nation's adult population consume alcohol regularly. When used in moderation, alcohol can have positive physiological effects by decreasing coronary artery disease and protecting against stroke; however, when consumed in excess, alcohol can severely diminish one's ability to function and will ultimately lead to life-threatening conditions.

The *Diagnostic and Statistical Manual of Mental Disorders,* fourth edition, text revision (DSM-IV-TR) (APA, 2000b) includes a classification scheme for distinguishing between substance abuse and substance dependence. **Substance dependence** refers to a severe condition occurring when the use of the chemical substance is no longer under an individual's control for at least 3 months. Continued use of the substance usually persists despite adverse effects on the person's physical condition, psychological health, and interpersonal relationships. The DSM-IV-TR criteria deals with the behavioral aspects and the maladaptive patterns of substance use, emphasizing the physical symptoms of **tolerance** and **withdrawal.** Tolerance is a cumulative state in which a particular dose of the chemical elicits a smaller response than before. With increased tolerance, the individual needs higher and higher doses to obtain the desired effect. When a person is physically addicted to the drug and stops taking it, **withdrawal symptoms** can occur within hours. Withdrawal is an uncomfortable state lasting several days, manifested by tremors, diaphoresis, anxiety, high blood pressure, tachycardia, and possibly convulsions. An overview of the DSM-IV-TR diagnostic criteria for substance abuse and substance dependence is shown in Box 12–1.

## RISK FACTORS

Various risk factors help explain why one person becomes addicted while another does not. Biological, psychological, and sociocultural factors shed light on how a person may abuse or become dependent on a substance.

- *Biological factors* include an apparent hereditary factor, especially with alcohol. Studies have shown that children of alcoholic parents are more likely to develop alcoholism than children of nonalcoholic parents (Kutlenios, 1998). This is primarily true with male relatives. One type of alcoholism seen mostly in the sons of alcoholic fathers is thought to be connected with an early onset, inability to abstain, and an antisocial personality (Stuart & Laraia, 2001). Another type of alcoholism may be more environmentally influenced and is linked with onset after the age of 25, inability to stop after one drink, and a passive-dependent personality (Stuart & Laraia, 2001). More recent studies have demonstrated that alcohol and drug use has specific effects

---

**BOX 12–1  ■ Substance Abuse versus Substance Dependence**

| **Substance Abuse** | **Substance Dependence** |
|---|---|
| Maladaptive pattern of substance use leading to clinically significant impairment or distress, manifested by **one or more** of the following within a 12-month period: | Maladaptive pattern of substance use leading to clinically significant impairment or distress, manifested by **three or more** of the following within a 12-month period: |
| 1. Failure to fulfill major role obligations at work, school, and home. | 1. Presence of tolerance to the drug. |
| 2. Involvement in physically hazardous situations while impaired (driving while intoxicated, operating a machine, exacerbation of physical symptoms such as ulcers). | 2. Presence of withdrawal symptoms. |
| 3. Recurrent legal or interpersonal problems. | 3. Substance is taken in larger amounts or for longer periods than is intended. |
| 4. Continued use despite recurrent social and interpersonal problems. | 4. Unsuccessful or persistent desire to cut down or control substance use. |
| | 5. More time spent in getting, taking, and recovering from the substance. May withdraw from family or friends and spend more time using substance in private. |
| | 6. Decline in or absence of important social, occupational, or recreational activities. |
| | 7. Continued use of substance despite knowledge of adverse effects. |

Note. Adapted from *Diagnostic and Statistical Manual of Mental Disorders (4th ed., text rev.) (DSM-IV-TR)* by American Psychiatric Association, 2000, Washington, DC: APA.

on selected biochemicals in the brain. Alcohol and other CNS depressants, such as benzodiazepines and barbiturates, act on gamma-aminobutyric acid (GABA). This may be why additive and cross-tolerance effects occur when alcohol and other CNS depressants are used in combination (Varcarolis, 2002).

- *Psychological factors* attempt to explain substance abuse through a combination of psychoanalytic, behavioral, and family system theories. Psychoanalytic theorists view substance abuse as a fixation at the oral stage of development, while behavioral theorists see addiction as a learned, maladaptive behavior. Family system theory focuses on the pattern of family relationships throughout several generations. No addictive personality type has been identified; however, several common factors seem to exist among alcoholics and drug users. Many substance abusers have experienced sexual or physical abuse in their childhood and as a result have low self-esteem and difficulty expressing emotions. A link also exists between substance abuse and psychiatric disorders such as depression, anxiety, and antisocial and dependent personalities. The habit of using a substance becomes a form of self-medication to cope with day-to-day problems, and over time develops into an addiction.

- *Sociocultural factors* often influence individuals' decisions as to when, what, and how they use substances. Many Asian people do not drink alcohol because of an uncomfortable physiological response characterized by flushing and tachycardia. About half of the Asian population have a deficiency of aldehyde dehydrogenase, the chemical that breaks down alcohol acetaldehyde (APA, 2000b). A buildup of acetaldehyde causes toxic symptoms and therefore keeps the prevalence rate of alcoholism lower in Asians. Europeans, on the other hand, have higher alcoholism rates. Religious background may also correlate with the likelihood that a person will abuse alcohol. Among major religions, people of Jewish faith have the lowest rate of alcoholism while Roman Catholics have the highest rate. Many people have a desire for social acceptance and initiate drug use to "fit in" with a peer group. Others may suffer from social anxiety and need drugs or alcohol to feel less inhibited while interacting with others.

Many factors place a person at risk for substance use, abuse, and dependence. No single cause can explain why one individual develops a pattern of drug use and another person does not. Thorough assessment of these factors is necessary to understand the whole person and plan appropriate interventions.

## CHARACTERISTICS OF ABUSERS

As mentioned, no addictive personality type exists; however, many abusers have several characteristics in common. There is a tendency for drug users to indulge in impulsive, risk-taking behaviors. Abusers often have a low tolerance for frustration and pain. The human tendency to seek pleasure and avoid stress and pain is partially responsible for substance abuse. The reinforcing properties of drugs can create a pleasurable experience and reduce the intensity of unpleasant experiences. Often, drug users are rebellious against social norms and engage in antisocial behaviors such as stealing, promiscuity, driving while intoxicated, and violence against others.

There is also a tendency toward anxiety, anger, and low self-esteem in substance abusers. Although there is no greater prevalence of psychiatric illness in substance abusers than in the general population, dual diagnosis is often present. **Dual diagnosis,** or **dual disorder,** refers to the coexistence of substance abuse or dependence and a psychiatric disorder in one individual. One disorder can be an indication of another, such as the relationship with alcoholism and depression. A depressed person may use self-medication in the form of alcohol to treat the depression, or the alcoholic person may become depressed. One recent study described the prevalence and characteristics of co-occurring serious mental illness (SMI) and substance abuse or dependence (Virgo et al., 2001). Most dual diagnoses in adult mental health patients were (1) alcohol and/or cannabis abuse with psychoses and heroin and/or (2) alcohol abuse or dependence with depression. Compared with other SMI patients, those who were dually diagnosed were younger, more often male, in less stable accommodation, more likely to be unemployed, and more likely to have more than one psychiatric diagnosis and personality disorder. They also tended to have more crises and pose greater risk to themselves and others (Virgo et al., 2001). Box 12–2 lists terminology associated with substance abuse.

## ADDICTIVE SUBSTANCES AND THEIR EFFECTS
### Nicotine

**Nicotine** enters the system via the lungs (cigarettes and cigars) and oral mucous membranes (smokeless tobacco as well as smoking). In low doses, nicotine stimulates nicotinic receptors in the brain to release norepinephrine and epinephrine, causing vasoconstriction. As a result, the heart rate accelerates and the force of ventricular contractions increases. Gastrointestinal (GI) effects include an increase in gastric acid secretion, tone and motility of GI smooth muscle, and promotion of vomiting. Nicotine acts on the central nervous system (CNS) as a stimulant, increasing respiration and arousal. Nicotine also activates the pleasure system in the mesolimbic system (Lehne, 2001). Moderate doses of nicotine can cause tremors. With high doses, such as acute poisoning from insecticides, convulsions and death can occur.

Tolerance can develop to nausea and dizziness, but not to the cardiovascular effects. Nicotine dependence results from chronic use with withdrawal seen as craving, nervousness, restlessness, irritability, impatience, increased hostility, insomnia, impaired concentration, increased appetite, and weight gain. Gradual reduction in nicotine use seems to prolong suffering. Chronic toxicity from smoking has been well established in the form of vascular diseases; chronic lung disease; and cancers of the larynx, esophagus, oral cavity, lung, bladder, and pancreas (Lehne, 2001). In addition, secondhand effects from smoking have been demonstrated, especially to fetuses during pregnancy. Smoking during pregnancy leads to increased risks for infants such as low birth weight, spontaneous abortions, perinatal mortality, and sudden infant death.

## BOX 12–2 ■ Terminology Associated with Substance Abuse

| Term | Definition |
| --- | --- |
| Abstinence | Voluntarily going without drugs |
| Addiction | A disease process characterized by the continued use of a specific chemical substance despite physical, psychological, or social harm (used interchangeably with substance dependence) |
| Codependence | A cluster of maladaptive behaviors exhibited by significant others of a substance abusing individual that serves to enable and protect the abuse at the expense of living a full and satisfying life |
| Cross dependence | Ability of one drug to support physical dependence on another drug |
| Cross-tolerance | Tolerance to one drug confers tolerance to another |
| Delirium tremens | A medical emergency usually occurring 3 to 5 days following alcohol withdrawal and lasting 2 to 3 days. Characterized by paranoia, disorientation, delusions, visual hallucinations, elevated vital signs, vomiting, diarrhea, and diaphoresis |
| Detoxification | The process of helping an addicted individual safely through withdrawal |
| Dual diagnosis | The coexistence of substance abuse/dependence and a psychiatric disorder in one individual (used interchangeably with dual disorder) |
| Dual disorder | Concurrent diagnosis of a substance use disorder and a psychiatric disorder. One disorder can precede and cause the other, such as the relationship between alcoholism and depression. |
| Korsakoff's psychosis | Secondary dementia caused by thiamine ($B_1$) deficiency that may be associated with chronic alcoholism; characterized by progressive cognitive deterioration, confabulation, peripheral neuropathy, and myopathy |
| Physical dependence | A state in which withdrawal syndrome will occur if drug use is discontinued |
| Polysubstance abuse | The simultaneous use of many substances |
| Psychologic dependence | An intensive subjective need for a particular psychoactive drug |
| Substance abuse | Continued use of a chemical substance in a fashion inconsistent with medical or social norms, for at least 1 month, despite related problems |
| Substance dependence | A severe condition occurring when the use of the chemical substance is no longer under control, for at least 3 months; continued use persists despite adverse effects (used interchangeably with addiction) |
| Tolerance | State in which a particular dose elicits a smaller response than it formerly did. With increased tolerance the individual needs higher and higher doses to obtain the desired response. |
| Wernicke's encephalopathy | Caused by thiamine ($B_1$) deficiency, characterized by nystagmus, ptosis, ataxia, confusion, coma, and possible death. Thiamine deficiency is common in chronic alcoholism. |
| Withdrawal syndrome | Constellation of signs and symptoms that occurs in physically dependent individuals when they discontinue drug use |

## Cannabis

**Cannabis sativa** is the source of marijuana. Use of cannabis is on the rise in the United States, with 10% of children age 12 to 17 using marijuana (Lehne, 2001). One recent study revealed that lifetime use of marijuana in a sample of 918 adolescents aged 12 to 21 years was 59%, while 18.4% reported frequent weekly use (Siqueira, Diab, Bodian, & Rolnitzky, 2001). Contributing factors to marijuana use in this population were negative life events, anger, and less parental support. The greatest psychoactive substances are in the flowering tops of the cannabis plant. Marijuana (also know as grass, weed, pot, dope, joint, and reefer) and hashish are the most common derivatives. The psychoactive component of marijuana is an oily chemical known as delta-9-tetrahydrocannabinol (THC). THC activates specific cannabinoid receptors in the brain. Recent evidence suggests that marijuana may act like opioids and cocaine in producing a pleasurable sensation, probably by causing release of endogenous opioids and then dopamine (Lehne, 2001).

Physiologic effects of cannabis are dose related and can cause an increase in heart rate and bronchodilation in short-term use, but airway constriction with chronic use leading to bronchitis, sinusitis, asthma, and possibly cancer. The reproductive system is also affected by marijuana; it causes decreased spermatogenesis and testosterone levels in males and decreased levels of follicle-stimulating, luteinizing, and prolactin hormones in females. Birth defects may also be associated with cannabis use. Subjective effects of marijuana include euphoria, sedation, and hallucinations. In addition, chronic use of marijuana can result in amotivational behaviors such as apathy, dullness, poor grooming, reduced interest in achievement, and disinterest. At extremely high doses, tolerance and physical dependence result.

## Alcohol

**Alcohol** acts as a CNS depressant and enhances the action of gamma aminobutyric acid (GABA). Chronic use of alcohol can cause severe neurologic and psychiatric disorders. Severe damage to the liver occurs with chronic alcohol abuse, and can progress from fatty liver to other liver diseases such as hepatitis or cirrhosis. Chronic alcoholism is the major cause of fatal cirrhosis. Alcohol causes damaging effects to many other systems; its effects include myocardial disease, erosive gastritis, acute and chronic pancreatitis, sexual dysfunction, and an increased risk of breast cancer.

Malnutrition is another serious complication of chronic alcoholism, especially thiamine ($B_1$) deficiency that can result in neurological impairments. Thiamine depletion is thought to cause the Wernicke-Korsakoff syndrome observed in chronic alcoholics (Stuart & Laraia, 2001). Severe cognitive impairment is a principal feature of **Wernicke's encephalopathy** and **Korsakoff's psychosis.** Although alcohol is a CNS depressant, it actually disrupts sleep, thus altering the sleep cycle, decreasing the quality of sleep, intensifying obstructive sleep apnea, and reducing total sleeping time. Heavy drinkers have a higher mortality rate and many fatalities occur from alcohol-related accidents. Blood alcohol levels (BALs) are highly predictive of CNS effects. Euphoria, reduced inhibitions, impaired judgment, and increased confidence are seen at 0.05% (Vacarolis, 2002). The legal level of intoxication in most states is 0.10%. Toxic levels in excess of 0.5% can cause coma, respiratory depression, peripheral collapse, and death (Vacarolis, 2002). Chronic consumption of alcohol produces tolerance and creates cross-tolerance to general anesthetics, barbiturates, benzodiazepines, and other CNS depressants. If alcohol is withdrawn abruptly, withdrawal symptoms such as tachycardia, hypertension, diaphoresis, nausea, vomiting, tremors, sleeplessness, irritability, **delirium tremens (DT),** seizures, and convulsions result.

## CNS Depressants

**Central nervous system depressants** including barbiturates, benzodiazepines, paraldehyde, meprobamate, and chloral hydrate are also subject to abuse. Cross dependence exists among all CNS depressants and cross-tolerance can develop to alcohol and general anesthetics. Chronic users of barbiturates require progressively higher doses to achieve subjective effects as tolerance develops, but they develop little tolerance to respiratory depression. The depressant effects related to barbiturates are dose dependent and range from mild sedation to sleep to coma to death. With larger doses over time and a combination of alcohol and barbiturates, the risk of death increases greatly. Benzodiazepines alone are safer than barbiturates, because an overdose of oral benzodiazepines rarely results in death.

## Psychostimulants

**Psychostimulants** such as cocaine and amphetamines have a high potential for abuse. Euphoria is the main subjective effect associated with cocaine and amphetamines, leading to addiction. Cocaine base (freebase, cocaine, or "crack") is heat stable and is usually smoked (freebasing). Cocaine hydrochloride (HCl) is diluted or cut before sale and the pure form ("rocks") is administered intranasally (snorted) or in-

jected intravenously. "Skin popping" is a method many substance abusers are using to administer drugs, perhaps leading to the formation of abscesses under the skin. The use of crack cocaine reached epidemic proportions especially in teens (who have a high risk of lethal overdose) in 1985, but has declined in use over the past few years (Lehne, 2001). Mild overdose of cocaine produces agitation, dizziness, tremor, and blurred vision. Severe overdose produces anxiety, hyperpyrexia, convulsions, ventricular dysrhythmias, severe hypertension, and hemorrhagic stroke with possible angina or myocardial infarction (MI). The use of cocaine during pregnancy is especially problematic, because the drug crosses the placenta and enters the fetal bloodstream. Spontaneous abortion, premature delivery, retardation of intrauterine growth, congenital abnormalities, and fetal addiction can result. Long-term intranasal use of cocaine can cause atrophy of the nasal mucosa, necrosis and perforation of the nasal septum, and lung damage.

Amphetamine use is on the rise in the United States and poses a severe health risk to society. Between 1993 and 1999, amphetamine treatment admission rates increased by 250% or more in 14 states and 100% to 249% in another 10 states (USDHHS, 2001). Dextroamphetamine, methamphetamine, and amphetamine can be taken orally or intravenously. Methamphetamine is the primary form of amphetamine seen in the United States, comprising 94% of all amphetamine treatment admissions in 1999 (USDHHS, 2001). A form of dextroamphetamine ("ice" or "crystal meth") can be smoked. Amphetamines cause arousal and an elevation of mood with a sense of increased strength, mental capacity, self-confidence, and a decreased need for food and sleep. A psychotic state with hallucinations and paranoia are common with long-term use, requiring treatment similar to other psychotic disorders. The cardiovascular effects of amphetamines are comparable to those of cocaine, including vasoconstriction, tachycardia, hypertension, angina, and dysrhythmias. Tolerance to mood elevation, appetite suppression, and cardiovascular effects develops with amphetamines; however, dependence is more psychological than physical. Withdrawal from amphetamines produces dysphoria and craving with fatigue, prolonged sleep, excessive eating, and depression.

## Opiates

**Opiates** such as morphine and heroin have been abused for many centuries and are major drugs of abuse. The urban poor constitute the majority of abusers, although opiates are used and abused by people of all socioeconomic status. A small percentage of individuals are originally exposed to opiates in the context of pain management; however, most people use opiates under social or illicit circumstances. Heroin is usually the opiate of choice, except among health care workers, who usually select meperidine (Demerol). Health care professionals have a higher risk for opiate abuse than other professionals due to the high accessibility of opiates in their line of work. If colleagues are showing signs of a substance abuse problem, information about impaired nurse programs is available through state boards of nursing to help individual nurses.

Heroin is usually administered intravenously and induces a "rush" or "kick" that lasts less than a minute, followed by a sense of euphoria for an extended period. Tolerance develops to the euphoria, respiratory depression, and nausea but not to constipation and miosis. Physical dependence occurs with long-term use of opiates. Initial withdrawal symptoms such as drug craving, lacrimation, rhinorrhea, yawning, and diaphoresis usually take 10 days to run their course, with the second phase of opiate withdrawal lasting for months with insomnia, irritability, fatigue, and potential GI hyperactivity and premature ejaculation as problems.

## Hallucinogens

**Hallucinogens** are also called psychedelics or psychotomimetics and include d-lysergic acid diethylamide (LSD), mescaline, dimethyltryptamine (DMT), and psilocin. Psychedelics bring on the same types of thoughts, perceptions, and feelings that occur in dreams. LSD was first used to simulate psychosis. It affects serotonin receptors at multiple sites in the brain and spinal cord. LSD is usually taken orally but can be injected or smoked. The individual's response to a "trip," the experience of being high on LSD, cannot be predicted and psychological effects and "flashbacks" are common. Ecstasy (3,4-methylenediosy-methamphetamine or MDMA) had high use in the 1980s as a popular recreational "rave" drug and has reappeared in recent years as a date or rape drug. Current research has revealed that women might be more susceptible to the neurotoxic effects on serotonin neurons when using MDMA (Reneman et al., 2001). Serotonin imbalance is thought to affect impulse control and may be responsible for uninhibited sexual responses in women who have been given the drug without their knowledge. Phencyclidine (PCP, also called angel dust and peace pill) was formerly an anesthetic similar to ketamine used for animals but caused emergence delirium in humans. Other hallucinogens are similar to LSD but with different potency and time course of action.

## Inhalants

**Inhalants** are categorized into three types: anesthetics, volatile nitrites, and organic solvents. Nitrous oxide (laughing gas) and ether are the most abused anesthetics. Amyl nitrite, butyl nitrite, and isobutyl nitrite are volatile nitrites used especially by homosexual males to induce venodilation and anal sphincter relaxation. Amyl nitrite is manufactured for medical use, but butyl and isobutyl nitrites are sold for recreational use. Other names for butyl and isobutyl nitrites are climax, rush, and locker room. Street names for amyl nitrite are "poppers" or "snappers." (See Table 12–1.) Brain damage or sudden death can occur from the first, tenth, or hundredth time an individual uses an inhalant, resulting in "sudden sniffing death." This danger makes the use of inhalants more hazardous than some other substances.

Organic solvents are ingested in three different methods: bagging, huffing, or sniffing. *Bagging* involves pouring the solvent in a plastic bag and inhaling the vapor. *Huffing* refers to pouring the solvent on a rag and inhaling. *Sniffing* refers to inhaling the solvent directly from the container. Common organic solvents are toluene, gasoline, lighter fluid, paint thinner, nail polish remover, benzene, acetone, chloroform, and model airplane glue. The effects from inhaling organic solvents are similar to alcohol, with prolonged use leading to multiple toxicity. There are no antidotes for these inhalants; therefore, management of toxicity is supportive.

### TABLE 12–1 Common Street Names for Abused Substances

| Substance | Street Name |
|-----------|-------------|
| Alcohol | Booze, brew, spirits, juice |
| Amphetamines | Bennies, crystal, crystal meth, diet pills, dolls, eye-openers, ice, lid poppers, pep pills, purple hearts, speed, uppers |
| Barbiturates | Barbs, beans, black beauties, blue angels, candy, downers, goof balls, nebbies, reds, sleepers, yellow jackets, yellows |
| Cocaine | Bernice, bernies, big C, blow, charlie, coke, dust, girl, heaven, jay, lady, nose candy, nose powder, snow, sugar, white lady Crack: conan, freebase, rock, toke, white cloud, white tornado |
| Heroin | H, horse, harry, boy, scag, shit, smack, stuff, white junk, white stuff |
| Marijuana | Acapulco gold, aunt mary, broccoli, dope, grass, grunt, hay, hemp, herb, J, joint, joy stick, killer weed, maryjane, pot ragweed, reefer, smoke, weed |
| Hallucinogens | Acid, big D, blotter, blue heaven, cap D, deeda, flash, L, mellow yellows, microdots, paper acid, sugar, ticket, yello, Ecstasy |

## COLLABORATIVE CARE

Effective treatment of substance abuse and dependence results from the collaborative efforts of an interdisciplinary team specializing in the treatment of psychiatric and substance abuse disorders. Therapies may include detoxification, aversion therapy to maintain abstinence, group and/or individual psychotherapy, psychotropic medications, cognitive-behavioral strategies, family counseling, and self-help groups. Clients suffering from substance abuse can be treated in either inpatient or outpatient settings. A substance overdose is a life-threatening condition that requires emergency hospitalization to stabilize the client medically before implementing any of the above interventions. Several diagnostic tests can provide valuable information about the patients physical condition and set the course for treatment.

### Diagnostic Tests

The body fluids most often tested for drug content are blood and urine. A urine drug screen (UDS) and/or blood alcohol level (BAL) are useful biological measures for assessment purposes. The length of time that drugs can be found in blood and urine varies according to dosage and metabolic properties of the drug. All traces of the drug may disappear within 24 hours or may still be detectable 30 days later. Knowledge of the

BAL is helpful in ascertaining the level of intoxication, the level of tolerance, and whether the person accurately reported recent drinking. At 0.10% (after 5 to 6 drinks in 1 to 2 hours), voluntary motor action becomes clumsy and reaction time is impaired. The degree of impairment varies with gender, weight, and food ingestion. Small women who drink alcohol on an empty stomach will experience intoxication more rapidly than large males who have eaten a full meal. At 0.20% (after 10 to 12 drinks in 2 to 4 hours), function of the motor area in the brain is depressed, causing staggering and ataxia (Vacarolis, 2002). A level above 0.10% without associated behavioral symptoms indicates the presence of tolerance. A BAL greater than 0.10% is considered legal intoxication in most states. High tolerance is a sign of physical dependence. Assessing for withdrawal symptoms is important when the BAL is high. Medications given for treatment of withdrawal from alcohol are usually not started until the BAL is below a set norm (usually below 0.10%) unless withdrawal symptoms become severe. BAL may be repeated several times, several hours apart, to determine the body's metabolism of alcohol and when it is safe to give the patient medication to minimize the withdrawal symptoms.

## Emergency Care for Overdose

The care of a patient who has overdosed on any substance is a serious medical emergency. Respiratory depression may require mechanical ventilation. The patient may become severely sedated and difficult to arouse. Every effort must be made to keep the patient awake; however, stupor and coma may often result. A seizure is another serious complication that requires emergency treatment. If the overdose was intentional, the patient must be constantly monitored for further signs of suicidal ideation. Never leave an actively suicidal patient alone. Signs of overdose and withdrawal from major substances are summarized in Table 12–2 along with their recommended treatments.

## Treatment of Withdrawal

All CNS depressants, including alcohol, benzodiazepines, and barbiturates, have a potentially dangerous progression of

### TABLE 12–2  Signs and Treatment of Overdose and Withdrawal

| Drug | Overdose | | Withdrawal | |
| | Signs | Treatment | Signs | Treatment |
|---|---|---|---|---|
| **CNS Depressants:** Alcohol Barbiturates Benzodiazepines | Cardiovascular or respiratory depression or arrest (mostly with barbiturates) Coma Shock Convulsions Death | *If awake:* Keep awake Induce vomiting Activated charcoal to absorb drug VS q 15 minutes *Coma:* Clear airway, intubate IV fluids Gastric lavage Seizure precautions Possible hemo or peritoneal dialysis Frequent VS Assess for shock and cardiac arrest | Nausea and vomiting Tachycardia Diaphoresis Anxiety or agitation Tremors Marked insomnia Grand mal seizures Delirium (after 5–15 years of heavy use) | Carefully titrated detoxification with similar drug NOTE: Abrupt withdrawal can lead to death. |
| **Stimulants:** Cocaine-crack Amphetamines | Respiratory distress Ataxia Hyperpyrexia Convulsions Coma Stroke Myocardial infarction (MI) Death | Antipsychotics Management for: 1. Hyperpyrexia 2. Convulsions 3. Respiratory distress 4. Cardiovascular shock 5. Acidify urine (ammonium Cl for amphetamine) | Fatigue Depression Agitation Apathy Anxiety Sleepiness Disorientation Lethargy Craving | Antidepressants (desipramine) Dopamine agonist Bromocriptine |
| **Opiates:** Heroin Meperidine Morphine Methadone | Pupil dilation due to anoxia Respiratory depression-arrest Coma Shock Convulsions Death | Narcotic antagonist, (Narcan) quickly reverses CNS depression | Yawning, insomnia Irritability Rhinorrhea Panic Diaphoresis Cramps Nausea and vomiting Muscle aches Chills and fever Lacrimation Diarrhea | Methadone tapering Clonidine-naltrexone detoxification Buprenorphine substitution |

*(continued on page 338)*

## TABLE 12-2 Signs and Treatment of Overdose and Withdrawal (continued)

| Drug | Overdose | | Withdrawal | |
|------|----------|------------|------------|-----------|
| | Signs | Treatment | Signs | Treatment |
| **Hallucinogens:**<br>Lysergic acid<br>diethylamide<br>(LSD) | LSD:<br>Psychosis<br>Brain damage<br>Death | Low stimuli with minimal light,<br>sound, activity<br>Have one person "talk down<br>client," reassure<br>Speak slowly and clearly<br>Diazepam or chloral hydrate for<br>anxiety | No pattern of<br>withdrawal | |
| Phencyclidine<br>piperidine<br>(PCP) | Possible hypertensive<br>crisis<br>Respiratory arrest<br>Hyperthermia<br>Seizures | Acidify urine to help excrete drug<br>(cranberry juice, ascorbic acid); in<br>acute stage: ammonium chloride<br>Minimal stimulis<br>Do NOT attempt to talk down,<br>speak slowly in low voice<br>Diazepam or Haldol | | |
| **Inhalants:**<br>Volatile<br>Solvents such as<br>butane, paint thinner,<br>airplane glue, or<br>nail polish remover | Intoxication:<br>1. Excitation<br>2. Drowsiness<br>3. Disinhibition<br>4. Staggering<br>5. Lightheadedness<br>6. Agitation<br>Side Effects:<br>1. Damage to nervous<br>system<br>2. Death | Support affected systems | No pattern of<br>withdrawal | |
| Nitrates<br><br>Anesthetics such<br>as nitrous oxide | Enhance sexual pleasure<br><br>Giggling, laughter<br>Euphoria | Neurological symptoms may<br>respond to vitamin $B_{12}$ and folate<br>Chronic users may experience<br>polyneuropathy and myelopathy | | |

## BOX 12-3 ■ Drugs Used in the Treatment of Substance Withdrawal/Abuse

| Drug | Dose | Purpose |
|------|------|---------|
| **Benzodiazepines** | | |
| 1. Clordiazepoxide (Librium) | 15–100 mg | Diminishes anxiety and has anticonvulsant qualities to |
| 2. Diazepam (Valium) | 4–40 mg | provide safe withdrawal. May be ordered q4h or prn to |
| 3. Oxazepam (Serax) | 30–120 mg | manage adverse effects from withdrawal, then dose is |
| 4. Lorazepam (Ativan) | 2–6 mg | tapered to zero. |
| **Vitamins** | | |
| 1. Thiamine (Vitamin $B_1$) | 100 mg/day | Prevents Wernicke's encephalopathy |
| 2. Folic acid | 1 mg/day | Corrects vitamin deficiency caused by heavy long-term alcohol |
| 3. Multivitamins | I tab/cap daily | abuse |
| **Anticonvulsants** | | |
| 1. Phenobarbital | 30–320 mg | For seizure control and sedation |
| 2. Magnesium sulfate | 1 g q6h | Reduces postwithdrawal seizures |
| **Abstinence medications** | | |
| 1. Disulfiram (Antabuse) | 250 mg/day | Prevents breakdown of alcohol |
| 2. Naltrexone (ReVia) | 50 mg/day | Diminishes cravings for alcohol and opioids |
| 3. Methadone | 40 mg/day | Blocks craving for heroin |
| **Antidepressants** | | |
| 1. Fluoxetine (Prozac) | 20–80 mg/day | Enhances and stabilizes mood and diminishes anxiety |
| 2. Sertraline (Zoloft) | 50–200 mg/day | |

withdrawal. Alcohol and the entire class of CNS depressants share the same withdrawal syndrome. Early signs of withdrawal appear within a few hours following cessation of the drug, peak after 24 to 48 hours, and then rapidly disappear unless the withdrawal progresses to delirium tremens. Severe withdrawal or delirium tremens is a medical emergency that usually occurs 2 to 5 days following alcohol withdrawal and persists 2 to 3 days. The symptoms of severe withdrawal include disorientation, paranoid delusions, visual hallucinations, and marked withdrawal symptoms. Seizures may also occur, requiring the use of emergency equipment. Treatment of severe withdrawal during detoxification is mostly symptomatic through acetaminophen, vitamins, and medications to minimize discomfort. Withdrawal symptoms from opiates and stimulants can be very unpleasant but are generally not life threatening. The patient experiencing an acute phase of cocaine withdrawal may become suicidal. Common drugs used in the treatment of substance abuse and withdrawal are presented in Box 12–3.

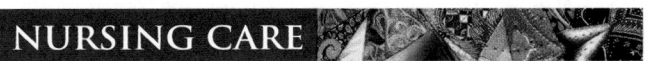

## NURSING CARE

### Health Promotion

Nursing care of the client with substance abuse or dependence is challenging and requires a nonjudgmental atmosphere promoting trust and respect. Health promotion efforts are aimed at preventing drug use among children and adolescents and reducing the risks among adults. Adolescence is the most common phase for the first experience with drugs (Stuart & Laraia, 2001), therefore teenagers are a vulnerable population, often succumbing to peer pressure. Healthy lifestyles, parental support, stress management, good nutrition, and information about ways to steer clear of peer pressure are important topics for the nurse to provide in school programs.

Nurses should provide adults with information on healthy coping mechanisms, relaxation, and stress reduction techniques to decrease the risks of substance abuse. Nurses have a responsibility to educate their clients about the physiological effects of substances on the body as well as ways to manage stress and anxiety. Nurses must encourage and support periods of abstinence while assisting clients to make major changes in lifestyles, habits, relationships, and coping methods. See the box below for nursing research about older clients with substance abuse problems.

### Assessment

A comprehensive approach to the assessment of substance use is essential to ensure adequate and appropriate intervention. Three important areas to be assessed are a history of the client's past substance use, medical and psychiatric history, and the presence of psychosocial concerns. Ask questions in a nonthreatening, matter-of-fact manner, phrased as to not imply wrongdoing (Henderson-Martin, 2000). For instance, a nonthreatening question such as, "How much alcohol do you drink?" is preferable to the judgmental question, "You don't drink too much alcohol, do you?" Open-ended questions that

## Nursing Research

### Evidence-Based Practice for the Older Client with a Substance Abuse Problem

People of any age can have substance abuse problems, but the consequences in older adults can be more critical. Falls and accidents can rob older adults of their independence, and substance abuse increases the risk of falls by affecting alertness, judgment, coordination, and reaction time. In addition, older adults are more likely than younger people to use prescription or over-the-counter medicines, which can be harmful when mixed with alcohol and/or illicit drugs. Alcohol and drug abuse also can make some medical problems hard to diagnose, for example, by dulling a pain sensation that might warn of a heart attack.

The purpose of this study (Blixen, McDougall, & Suen, 1997) was to examine the prevalence and correlates of dual diagnosis in older adults and compare the findings with studies of younger clients. The leading psychiatric diagnosis for hospitalized elders was depression. Over one-third (37.6%) had a substance abuse disorder in addition to a psychiatric disorder. Almost three-fourths (71%) of this dual diagnosis group abused alcohol and 29% abused both alcohol and other substances. Because affective disorders in conjunction with alcohol abuse are the most frequently found disorders in completed suicides, the authors' findings have important relevance for routinely using screening tools for both substance abuse and mental disorders in this population.

#### IMPLICATIONS FOR NURSING

Findings from this study support other research that substance abuse in older adults is likely to increase over subsequent decades as baby boomers reach retirement age. Estimates of alcohol abuse in the older adult population range from 4% to 20% in the community-dwelling elderly and approximately 25% among hospitalized older adults (Adams & Cox, 1995; Adams & Kinney, 1995; Beresford, Blow, & Brower, 1990).

Unfortunately, a substance abuse problem in an older adult can be difficult to detect because many of the symptoms of abuse (e.g., insomnia, depression, loss of memory, anxiety, musculoskeletal pain) may be confused with conditions commonly seen in older patients. Health care professionals frequently fail to recognize and address the misuse and abuse of alcohol and drugs in the elderly (Ondus, Hujer, Mann, & Mion, 1999).

#### Critical Thinking in Client Care

1. You are caring for an 85-year-old man who tells you that since his wife died 6 months ago, he only feels like drinking to dull the pain of her loss. How would you respond?

2. Why do you think nurses and other health care professionals often fail to recognize and address substance abuse problems in the older adult?

3. You are caring for an older adult who denies that alcohol has become a serious problem, even though this is the third hospitalization for this client in 6 months due to accidents, falls, and blackouts. What would you do?

| BOX 12–4 | ■ Examples of Open-Ended Questions for Assessment |
|---|---|

- On average, how many days per week do you drink alcohol or use drugs?
- On a typical day when you use drugs or alcohol, how many hits or drinks do you have?
- What is the greatest number of drinks you've had at any one time during the past month?
- What drug(s) did you take before coming to the hospital or clinic?
- How long have you been using the substances?
- How often and how much do you usually use?
- What kinds of problems has substance use caused for you, your family, friends, finances, and health?

elicit more than a simple yes or no answer help to determine the direction of future counseling. Examples of open-ended questions are provided in Box 12–4. Use therapeutic communication techniques to establish trust prior to the assessment process.

### History of Past Substance Use

A thorough history of the client's past substance use is important to ascertain the possibility of tolerance, physical dependence, or withdrawal syndrome. The following questions are helpful in eliciting a pattern of substance use behavior.

- How many substances has the client used simultaneously (**polysubstance abuse** or simultaneous use of many substances) in the past?
- How often, how much, and when did the client first use the substance(s)?
- Is there a history of blackouts, delirium, or seizures?
- Is there a history of withdrawal syndrome, overdoses, and complications from previous substance use?
- Has the client ever been treated in an alcohol or drug abuse clinic?
- Has the client ever been arrested for driving under the influence (DUI) or charged with any criminal offense while using drugs or alcohol?
- Is there a family history of drug or alcohol use?

### Medical and Psychiatric History

The client's medical history is another important area for assessment and should include the existence of any concomitant physical or mental condition (e.g., HIV, hepatitis, cirrhosis, esophageal varices, pancreatitis, gastritis, Wernicke-Korsakoff syndrome, depression, schizophrenia, anxiety, or personality disorder). Ask about prescribed and over-the-counter medications as well as any allergies or sensitivity to drugs. A brief overview of the client's current mental status is also significant.

- Is there a history of abuse (physical or sexual) or family violence?
- Has the client ever tried to commit suicide?
- Is the client currently having suicidal or homicidal ideation?

### Psychosocial Issues

Information about the client's level of stress and other psychosocial concerns can help in the assessment of substance use problems.

- Has the client's substance use affected his or her ability to hold a job?
- Has the client's substance use affected relationships with spouse, family, friends, or coworkers?
- How does the client usually cope with stress?
- Does the client have a support system that helps in time of need?
- How does the client spend his or her leisure time?

### Assessment Tools

Several screening tools such as the Michigan Alcohol Screening Test (MAST) (Pokorny, Miller, & Kaplan, 1972), Drug Abuse Screening Test (DAST) (Skinner, 1982), and the CAGE questionnaire (Ewing, 1984) may help the nurse determine the degree of severity of substance abuse or dependence (see Figure 12–1 ■). These screening tools provide a nonjudgmental, brief, and easy method to ascertain patterns of substance abuse behaviors.

- *Michigan Alcohol Screening Test (MAST) Brief Version* is a 10-question, dichotomous, self-administered questionnaire that takes 10 to 15 minutes to complete. An answer of yes to 3 or more questions indicates a potentially dangerous pattern of alcohol abuse.
- *CAGE questionnaire* is more useful when the client may not recognize he or she has an alcohol problem or is uncomfortable acknowledging it. This questionnaire is designed to be a self-report of drinking behavior or may be administered by a professional. One affirmative response indicates the need for further discussion and follow-up. Two or more yes answers signify a problem with alcohol that may require treatment.

  Have you ever felt you should *cut* down on your drinking?
  Have people *annoyed* you by criticizing your drinking?
  Have you ever felt bad or *guilty* about your drinking?
  Have you ever had a drink first thing in the morning (an "*eye-opener*") to steady your nerves or to get rid of a hangover?

- *Drug Abuse Screening Test (DAST)* is a yes/no self-administered questionnaire that is useful in identifying people who are possibly addicted to drugs other than alcohol. A positive response to one or more questions suggests significant drug abuse problems and warrants further evaluation. Because the tools can be incorrect if the client is not answering truthfully, all clients who are screened positive for drug addiction should be evaluated according to diagnostic criteria.

## Nursing Diagnoses and Interventions

The primary nursing diagnoses and interventions for clients with substance abuse problems are listed below. Implications for nursing care in acute and home care settings are combined in this discussion.

### Risk for Injury

- Assess client's level of disorientation to determine specific risks to safety. *Knowledge of the client's level of cognitive functioning is essential to the development of an appropriate plan of care.*

- Obtain a drug history as well as urine and blood samples for laboratory analysis of substance content. *Subjective history is often not accurate and knowledge regarding substance use is important for accurate assessment.*
- Place client in a quiet, private room to decrease excessive stimuli, but do not leave client alone if excessive hyperactivity or suicidal ideation is present. *Excessive stimuli increase client's agitation.*
- Frequently orient client to reality and the environment, ensuring that potentially harmful objects are stored outside the client's access. *Client may harm self or others if disoriented and confused.*
- Monitor vital signs every 15 minutes until stable and assess for signs of intoxication or withdrawal. *The most reliable information about withdrawal symptoms are vital signs; they provide information about the need for medication during detoxification.*

## Ineffective Denial

- Be genuine, honest, and respectful of client. Keep all promises and convey an attitude of acceptance of the client. *The development of a nonjudgmental, therapeutic nurse-client relationship is essential to gain the client's trust.*
- Identify maladaptive behaviors or situations that have occurred in client's life and discuss how the use of substances may have been a contributing factor. *The first step in combating denial is for the client to recognize the relationship between substance use and personal problems.*
- Do not accept the use of defense mechanisms such as rationalization or projection as the client attempts to blame others or make excuses for his or her behavior. Use confrontation with caring to avoid placing client on the defensive. *Confrontation interferes with the client's ability to use denial.*
- Encourage client participation in therapeutic group activities such as dual diagnosis or Alcoholics Anonymous (AA)

---

### Scoring Yes to 3 or more indicates alcoholism

1. Do you feel you are a normal drinker?
2. Do friends or relatives think you are a normal drinker?
3. Have you ever attended a meeting of Alcoholics Anonymous?
4. Have you ever gotten in trouble at work because of drinking?
5. Have you ever lost friends or girlfriends/boyfriends because of drinking?
6. Have you ever neglected your obligations, your family, or your work for 2 or more days in a row because of your drinking?
7. Have you ever had delirium tremens (DTs), severe shaking, or heard voices or seen things that were not there after heavy drinking?
8. Have you ever gone to anyone for help about your drinking?
9. Have you ever been in a hospital because of your drinking?
10. Have you ever been arrested for drunken driving or other drunken behavior?

**The following questions concern information about your involvement with drugs *not including alcoholic beverages* during the past 12 months.**

**In the statements, "drug abuse" refers to (1) the use of prescribed or OTC drugs in excess of the directions and (2) any nonmedical use of drugs. The various classes of drugs may include cannabis, solvents, antianxiety drugs, sedative-hypnotics, cocaine, stimulants, hallucinogens, and narcotics. Remember that the questions *do not include alcoholic beverages.***

| | | |
|---|---|---|
| Have you used drugs other than those required for medical purposes? | Yes ___ | No ___ |
| Do you abuse more than one drug at a time? | Yes ___ | No ___ |
| Are you always able to stop using drugs when you want to? | Yes ___ | No ___ |
| Have you had "blackouts" or "flashbacks" as a result of drug use? | Yes ___ | No ___ |
| Do you ever feel bad about your drug abuse? | Yes ___ | No ___ |
| Does your spouse (or parents) ever complain about your involvement with drugs? | Yes ___ | No ___ |
| Have you neglected your family because of your use of drugs? | Yes ___ | No ___ |
| Have you engaged in illegal activities in order to obtain drugs? | Yes ___ | No ___ |
| Have you ever experienced withdrawal symptoms (felt sick) when you stopped taking drugs? | Yes ___ | No ___ |
| Have you had medical problems as a result of your drug use (e.g., memory loss, hepatitis, convulsions, bleeding, etc.)? | Yes ___ | No ___ |
| Scoring: one positive response warrants further evaluation | Yes ___ | No ___ |

**Figure 12–1** ■ Screening tools for alcohol and drug abuse.

*From "The Brief MAST: A Shortened Version of the Michigan Alcohol Screening Test" by A. D. Porkorny, B. A. Miller, and H. B. Kaplan, 1972, American Journal of Psychiatry, 129, pp. 342–345. Copyright 1972 by the American Psychiatric Association; and Drug Abuse Screening Test (DAST) (p. 363) by H. A. Skinner, 1982, Langford Lance, England: Elsevier Science Ltd. Copyright 1982. Both reprinted by permission.*

meetings with other people who are experiencing or have experienced similar problems. *Peer feedback is often more accepted than feedback from authority figures.*

## Ineffective Individual Coping

- Establish trusting relationship. *Trust is essential to the nurse-client relationship.*
- Set limits on manipulative behavior and maintain consistency in responses. *Client is unable to set own limits and must begin to accept responsibility without being manipulative.*
- Encourage client to verbalize feelings, fears, or anxieties. Use attentive listening and validate client's feelings with observations or statements that acknowledge feelings. *Verbalization of feelings helps client to develop insight into behaviors and long-standing problems.*
- Explore methods of dealing with stressful situations other than resorting to substance use. Provide encouragement for changing to a healthier lifestyle. Teach healthy coping mechanisms (e.g., physical exercise, progressive muscle relaxation, deep breathing exercises, meditation, and imagery). *Client needs knowledge about how to adapt to stress without resorting to drug use.*

## Imbalanced Nutrition: Less Than Body Requirements

- Administer vitamins and dietary supplements as ordered by physician. *Vitamin $B_1$ is necessary to prevent complications from chronic alcoholism such as Wernicke's syndrome.*
- Monitor lab work (e.g., total albumin, complete blood count, urinalysis, electrolytes, and liver enzymes) and report significant changes to physician. *Objective laboratory tests provide necessary information to determine the extent of malnourishment.*
- Collaborate with dietitian to determine number of calories needed to provide adequate nutrition and realistic weight gain. Document intake, output, and calorie count. Weigh daily if condition warrants. *Weight loss or gain is important assessment information so that an appropriate plan of care can be developed.*
- Teach the importance of adequate nutrition by explaining the food guide pyramid and relating the physical effects of malnutrition on body systems. *Client may have inadequate knowledge of proper nutritional habits.*

## Low Self-Esteem

- Spend time with client and convey an attitude of acceptance. Encourage client to accept responsibility for own behaviors and feelings. *An attitude of acceptance enhances self-worth.*
- Encourage client to focus on strengths and accomplishments rather than weaknesses and failures. *Minimize attention to negative ruminations.*
- Encourage participation in therapeutic group activities. Offer recognition and positive feedback for actual achievements. *Success and recognition increase self-esteem.*
- Teach assertiveness techniques and effective communication techniques such as the use of "I feel" rather than "You make me feel" statements. *Previous patterns of communication may have been aggressive and accusatory, causing barriers to interpersonal relationships.*

## Deficient Knowledge

- Assess client's level of knowledge and readiness to learn the effects of drugs and alcohol on the body. *Baseline assessment is required to develop appropriate teaching material.*
- Develop teaching plan that includes measurable objectives. Include significant others, if possible. *Lifestyle changes often affect all family members.*
- Begin with simple concepts and progress to more complex issues. Use interactive teaching strategies and written materials appropriate to the client's educational level. Include information on physiological effects of substances, the propensity for physical and psychological dependence, and the risks to a fetus if the client is pregnant. *Active participation and handouts enhance retention of important concepts.*

## Disturbed Sensory Perceptions

- Observe for withdrawal symptoms. Monitor vital signs. Provide adequate nutrition and hydration. Place on seizure precautions. *These actions provide supportive physical care during detoxification.*
- Assess level of orientation frequently. Orient and reassure client of safety in presence of hallucinations, delusions, or illusions. *Client may be frightened.*
- Explain all interventions before approaching client. Avoid loud noises and talk softly to client. Decrease external stimuli by dimming lights. *Excessive stimuli increase agitation.*
- Administer prn medications according to detoxification schedule. *Benzodiazepines help to minimize the discomfort of withdrawal symptoms.*

## Disturbed Thought Processes

- Give positive reinforcement when thinking and behavior are appropriate or when client recognizes that delusions are not based in reality. *Drugs and alcohol can interfere with client's perception of reality.*
- Use simple, step-by-step instructions and face-to-face interaction when communicating with client. *Client may be confused or disoriented.*
- Express reasonable doubt if client relays suspicious or paranoid beliefs. Reinforce accurate perception of people or situations. *It is important to communicate that you do not share that false belief as reality.*
- Do not argue with delusions or hallucinations. Convey acceptance that the client believes a situation to be true, but that the nurse does not see or hear what is not there. *Arguing with the client or denying the belief serves no useful purpose, because delusions are not eliminated.*
- Talk to client about real events and real people. Respond to feelings and reassure client that he or she is safe from harm. *Discussions that focus on the delusions may aggravate the condition. Verbalization of feelings in a nonthreatening environment may help the client develop insight.*

## Using NANDA, NIC, and NOC

Chart 12–1 shows links between NANDA, NIC, and NOC when caring for the client with a substance abuse problem.

## CHART 12–1   NANDA, NIC, AND NOC LINKAGES

### The Client with a Substance Abuse Problem

| NURSING DIAGNOSES | NURSING INTERVENTIONS | NURSING OUTCOMES |
|---|---|---|
| • Risk for Injury | • Anger Control Assistance<br>• Delusion Management<br>• Environmental Management: Violence Prevention<br>• Impulse Control Training<br>• Referral | • Risk Control<br>• Safety Behavior: Personal<br>• Knowledge: Personal Safety |
| • Ineffective Denial | • Anxiety Reduction<br>• Coping Enhancement<br>• Counseling<br>• Decision-Making Support | • Anxiety Control<br>• Coping<br>• Symptom Control Behavior |
| • Defensive Coping | • Self-Awareness Enhancement<br>• Coping Enhancement<br>• Patient Contracting<br>• Counseling | • Self-Esteem<br>• Coping<br>• Risk Control: Alcohol Use, Drug Use, Tobacco Use |
| • Disturbed Thought Processes | • Behavior Management: Overactivity/Inattention<br>• Delusion Management<br>• Calming Technique<br>• Surveillance: Safety | • Cognitive Orientation<br>• Distorted Thought Control<br>• Information Processing<br>• Safety Behavior: Personal, Home Physical Environment |
| • Imbalanced Nutrition: Less Than Body Requirements | • Nutritional Counseling<br>• Nutritional Monitoring<br>• Weight Gain Assistance | • Nutritional Status |
| • Chronic Low Self-Esteem | • Self-Esteem Enhancement<br>• Substance Use Prevention<br>• Substance Use Treatment: Alcohol Withdrawal, Drug Withdrawal, Overdose<br>• Support Group<br>• Therapy Group | • Self-Esteem<br>• Abuse Recovery |
| • Deficient Knowledge (Specify) | • Health Education<br>• Teaching: Substance Abuse<br>• Behavior Modification<br>• Counseling<br>• Support Group | • Substance Abuse Control |

Note. *Data from Nursing Outcomes Classification (NOC) by M. Johnson & M. Maas (Eds.), 1997, St. Louis: Mosby; Nursing Diagnoses: Definitions & Classification 2001–2002, by North American Nursing Diagnosis Association, 2001, Philadelphia: NANDA; Nursing Interventions Classification (NIC) by J. C. McCloskey and G. M. Bulechek (Eds.), 2000, St. Louis: Mosby. Reprinted by permission.*

## Home Care

Teaching the client and family includes:

- The negative effects of substance abuse including physical and psychological complications of substance abuse.
- The signs of relapse and the importance of after care programs and self-help groups to prevent relapse. An acronym that can assist the client in recognizing behaviors that lead to relapse is HALT: **h**ungry, **a**ngry, **l**onely, and **t**ired. Stress the importance of adequate sleep and nutrition, healthy recreation activities, and a caring support system in managing stressful situations.
- Information about specific medications that help to reduce the craving for alcohol (naltrexone [ReVia]) and maintain abstinence (disulfiram [Antabuse]), including the potential side effects, possible drug interactions, and any special precautions to be taken (e.g., avoiding over-the-counter medications such as cough syrup that may have alcohol content).
- Stress management techniques such as progressive muscle relaxation, abdominal breathing techniques, imagery, meditation, and effective coping skills.

In addition, suggest the following resources:

- Self-help groups
- Employee assistance programs
- Individual, group, and/or family counseling
- Community rehabilitation programs
- National Alliance for the Mentally Ill

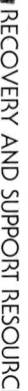

MediaLink | RECOVERY AND SUPPORT RESOURCES

# Nursing Care Plan
## A Client Experiencing Withdrawal from Alcohol

George Russell, age 58, fell at home and broke his arm. His wife took him to the ER and an open reduction internal fixation (ORIF) of his right wrist was performed under general anesthetic in the operating room. He was admitted to the postoperative unit for observation following surgery because he required large amounts of anesthesia during the procedure.

Mr. Russell has a ruddy complexion and looks older than his stated age. He discloses that he was laid off from his factory job 2 years ago and has been working odd jobs until last week when he was hired by a local assembly plant. His father was a recovering alcoholic and his 30-year-old son has been treated for alcohol abuse in the past. Mr. Russell states that he knows alcoholism runs in the family, but he feels that he has his drinking under control. However, he cannot remember the events that led up to his fall and how he might have broken his arm.

### ASSESSMENT

During the nursing assessment, Mr. Russell is hesitant to provide information and refuses to make eye contact. Prior to his operation, a BAL was drawn because the ER nurse detected alcohol on his breath. His BAL was 0.42 % which is 4 times the legal limit for intoxication in many states. His vital signs are within the upper limits of normal, but he is confused and disoriented with slurred speech and a slight tremor of the hands. He is 6 feet tall and weighs 140 pounds. His total albumin is 3.5 mg and he has elevated liver enzymes. His wife states that he rarely eats the meals she prepares because he is usually drinking and has no appetite for food.

### DIAGNOSIS

- *Ineffective individual coping* related to possible hereditary factor and personal vulnerability

### EXPECTED OUTCOMES

- Client will express his true feelings associated with using alcohol as a method of coping with stressful situations.
- Client will identify three adaptive coping mechanisms he can use as alternatives to alcohol in response to stress.

- Client will verbalize the negative effects of alcohol and agree to seek professional help with his drinking.

### PLANNING AND IMPLEMENTATION

- Establish trusting relationship with client and spend time with him discussing his feelings, fears, and anxieties.
- Consult with a physician regarding a schedule for medications during detoxification and observe for signs of withdrawal syndrome.
- Explain the effects of alcohol abuse on the body and emphasize that prognosis is closely associated with abstinence.
- Teach a relaxation technique that is useful in the client's opinion.
- Provide information about self-help groups and, if receptive, a list of meeting times and phone numbers.

### EVALUATION

Mr. Russell was discharged from the postoperative unit without complications. He successfully underwent detoxification and contacted the Employee Assistance Program (EAP) at his new place of employment. He was on medical leave while his arm completely healed and now attends Alcoholics Anonymous meetings 5 days a week. He reports that he enjoys taking long walks with his wife in the warm weather and that his appetite has returned. He has gained 10 pounds in the past 6 weeks and feels physically better than he has in many years.

### Critical Thinking in the Nursing Process

1. Explain why it would be important to include questions about Mr. Russell's medication history and his use of other medications during the initial nursing assessment.
2. Mr. Russell asks you to explain the risks of taking disulfiram (Antabuse). What should you tell him?
3. Develop a care plan for Mr. Russell for the nursing diagnosis of *Alteration in nutrition: Less than body requirements.* Why is this necessary?

See Evaluating Your Response in Appendix C.

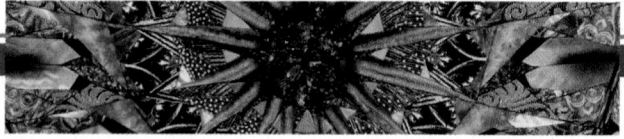

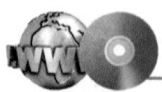

## EXPLORE MediaLink

NCLEX review questions, case studies, care plan activities, MediaLink applications, and other interactive resources for this chapter can be found on the Companion Website at www.prenhall.com/lemone.

Click on Chapter 12 to select the activities for this chapter. For animations, video clips, more NCLEX review questions, and an audio glossary, access the Student CD-ROM accompanying this textbook.

## TEST YOURSELF

1. What is the minimum level of alcohol in the blood for an individual to be considered intoxicated in most states?

   a. 0.05%
   b. 0.10%
   c. 0.50%
   d. 1.00%

2. Which of the following questions is *most* appropriate when interviewing the client who is suspected of alcohol abuse problems?

   a. "Typically, how many days per week do you drink alcoholic beverages?"
   b. "Have you been drinking lately?"
   c. "You don't drink much alcohol, do you?"
   d. "Has your drinking caused a lot of problems between you and your spouse?"

3. What is the rationale behind ordering thiamine (vitamin $B_1$) for a person with a history of chronic alcoholism?

   a. To prevent acute pancreatitis
   b. To prevent cirrhosis of the liver
   c. To prevent hepatic encephalopathy
   d. To prevent Wernicke's encephalopathy

4. Which of the following substances present the highest medical danger during withdrawal?

   a. CNS stimulants and amphetamines
   b. Opiates and marijuana
   c. Alcohol and CNS depressants
   d. Amphetamines and hallucinogens

5. What is the rationale for prescribing naltrexone (Trexan, ReVia) for a person who suffers from substance abuse?

   a. To decrease the discomfort of withdrawal symptoms
   b. To decrease the pleasant, reinforcing effects of the drug
   c. To inhibit impulsive drinking
   d. To block the signs and symptoms of opioid withdrawal

See Test Yourself answers in Appendix C.

## BIBLIOGRAPHY

Adams, W. L., & Cox, N. S. (1995). Epidemiology of problem drinking among elderly people. *International Journal of the Addictions, 30*, 1693–1716.

Adams, W. L., & Kinney, J. (1995). *The clinical manual of substance abuse.* St. Louis: Mosby.

American Psychiatric Association. (2000a). *Practice guidelines for the treatment of psychiatric disorders compendium 2000.* Washington, DC: APA.

_____ (2000b). *Diagnostic and statistical manual of mental disorders* (4th ed., text revision) (DSM-IV-TR). Washington, DC: APA.

Beresford, T. P., Blow, F. C., & Brower, K. J. (1990). Alcoholism in the elderly. *Comprehensive Therapeutics, 16*, 38–43.

Blixen, C. E., McDougall, G. J., & Suen, L. J. (1997). Dual diagnosis in elders discharged from a psychiatric hospital. *International Journal of Geriatric Psychiatry, 12*(3), 307–313.

Ewing, J. A. (1984). Detecting alcoholism: The CAGE questionnaire. *Journal of the American Medical Association, 252*(14), 1905–1907.

Henderson-Martin, B. (2000). No more surprises: Screening patients for alcohol abuse. *American Journal of Nursing, 100*(9), 26–32.

Johnson, M., & Maas, M. (Eds.). (1997). *Nursing outcomes classification (NOC).* St. Louis: Mosby.

Kutlenios, R.M. (1998). Genetics and alcoholism—implications for advance practice psychiatric/mental health nursing. *Archives of Psychiatric Nursing, 12*(3), 154.

Lehne, R. A. (2001). *Pharmacology for nursing care.* Philadelphia: W.B. Saunders.

McCloskey, J. C., & Bulechek, G. M. (Eds.). (2000). *Nursing interventions classification (NIC).* St. Louis: Mosby.

National Institute of Mental Health. (2001). *Mental disorders in America.* NIH Publication No. 01-4584. Bethesda, MD: NIMH. Available. http://www.nimh.nih.gov/publicat/numbers.cfm (accessed on 4/11/02).

North American Nursing Diagnosis Association. (2001). *Nursing diagnoses: Definitions & classification 2001–2002.* Philadelphia: NANDA.

Ondus, K. A., Hujer, M. E., Mann, A. E., & Mion, L. C. (1999). Substance abuse and the hospitalized elderly. *Orthopaedic Nursing, 18*(4), 27–36.

Pokorny, A. D., Miller, B. A., & Kaplan, H. B. (1972). The brief MAST: A shortened version of the Michigan Alcohol Screening Test. *American Journal of Psychiatry, 129*: 342–345.

Reneman, L., Booij, J., de Bruin, K., Reitsma, J. B., de Wolff, F. A., Gunning, W. B., den Heeten, G. J., & van den Brink, W. (2001). Effects of dose, sex, and long-term abstention from use on toxic effects of MDMA (ecstasy) on brain serotonin neurons. *Lancet, 358*(9296), 1864–1869.

Siqueira, L., Diab, M., Bodian, C., & Rolnitzky, L. (2001). The relationship of stress and coping methods to adolescent use. *Substance Abuse, 22*(3), 157–166.

Skinner, H. A. (1982). *Drug Abuse Screening Test (DAST)* (p. 363). Langford Lance, England: Elsevier Science Ltd.

Stuart, G. W., & Laraia, M. T. (2001). *Stuart & Sundeen's principles and practice of psychiatric nursing* (7th ed.). St. Louis: Mosby.

U.S. Department of Health and Human Services. (1999). *Mental health: A report of the surgeon general—Executive summary.* Rockville, MD: USDHHS, Substance Abuse and Mental Health Services Administration, Center for Mental Health Services, National Institutes of Health, National Institute of Mental Health. Available http://www.surgeongeneral.gov/Library/MentalHealth (accessed on 4/11/02).

_____ (2001). *The DASIS Report: Amphetamine treatment admission increase: 1993–1999.* Rockville, MD: USDHHS, Substance Abuse and Mental Health Services Administration, Center for Mental Health Services, National Institutes of Health, National Institute of Mental Health. Available http://www.samhsa.gov/oas/facts/speed.cfm (accessed on 4/23/02).

Varcarolis, E. (2002). *Foundations of psychiatric mental health nursing: A clinical approach* (4th ed). Philadelphia: W.B. Saunders.

Virgo, N., Bennett, G., Higgins, D., Bennett, L., & Thomas, P. (2001). The prevalence and characteristics of co-occurring serious mental illness (SMI) and substance abuse or dependence in the patients of Adult Mental Health and Addictions Services in eastern Dorset. *Journal of Mental Health, 10*(2), 175–188.

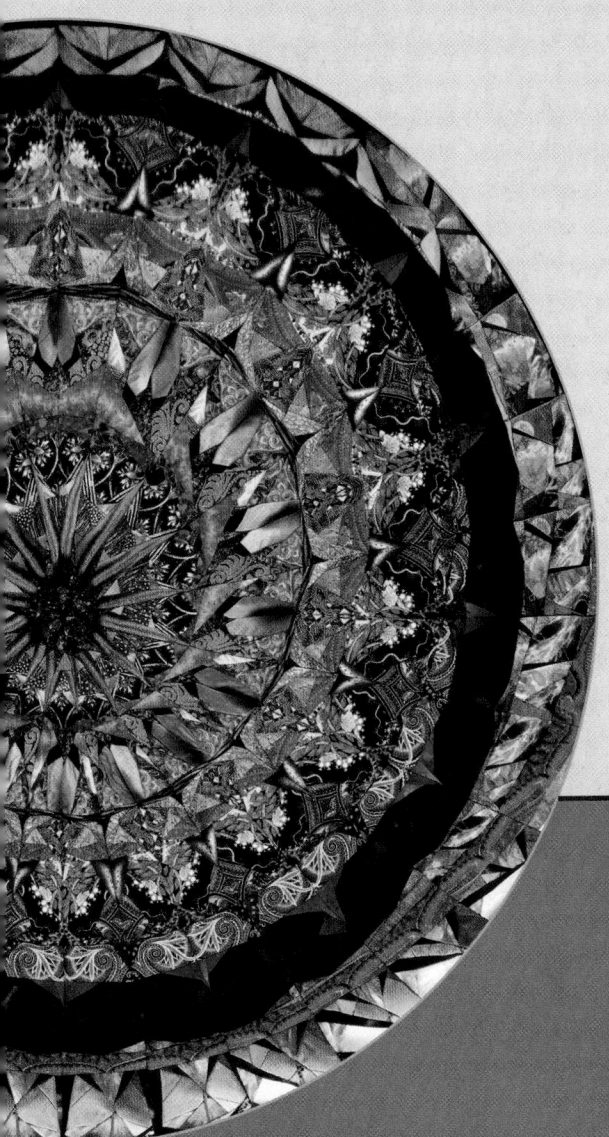

# NUTRITION AND METABOLIC PATTERNS

# Functional Health Patterns with Related Nursing Diagnoses

## HEALTH PERCEPTION HEALTH MANAGEMENT
- Perceived health status
- Perceived health management
- Health care behaviors: health promotion and illness prevention activities, medical treatments, follow-up care

## VALUE-BELIEF
- Values, goals, or beliefs (including spirituality) that guide choices or decisions
- Perceived conflicts in values, beliefs, or expectations that are health related

## COPING-STRESS-TOLERANCE
- Capacity to resist challenges to self-integrity
- Methods of handling stress
- Support systems
- Perceived ability to control and manage situations

## NUTRITIONAL-METABOLIC
- Daily consumption of food and fluids
- Favorite foods
- Use of dietary supplements
- Skin lesions and ability to heal
- Condition of the integument
- Weight, height, temperature

## Part 2
### Nutrition and Metabolic Patterns
### NANDA Nursing Diagnoses
- Risk for Aspiration
- Risk for Imbalanced Body Temperature
- Impaired Dentition
- Feeding Self-Care Deficit
- Fluid Volume Deficit
- Fluid Volume Excess
- Risk for Deficient Fluid Volume
- Hyperthermia
- Hypothermia
- Risk for Infection
- Impaired Oral Mucous Membranes
- Nausea
- Imbalanced Nutrition: Less than Body Requirements
- Imbalanced Nutrition: More than Body Requirements
- Impaired Skin Integrity
- Risk for Impaired Skin Integrity
- Impaired Swallowing
- Ineffective Thermoregulation
- Impaired Tissue Integrity
- Risk For Trauma
- Adult Failure to Thrive

## SEXUALITY-REPRODUCTIVE
- Satisfaction with sexuality or sexual relationships
- Reproductive pattern
- Female menstrual and perimeno-pausal history

## ELIMINATION
- Patterns of bowel and urinary excretion
- Perceived regularity or irregularity of elimination
- Use of laxatives or routines
- Changes in time, modes, quality or quantity of excretions
- Use of devices for control

## ROLE-RELATIONSHIP
- Perception of major roles, relationships, and responsibilities in current life situation
- Satisfaction with or disturbances in roles and relationships

## ACTIVITY-EXERCISE
- Patterns of personally relevant exercise, activity, leisure, and recreation
- ADLs which require energy expenditure
- Factors that interfere with the desired pattern (e.g., illness or injury)

## SELF-PERCEPTION–SELF-CONCEPT
- Attitudes about self
- Perceived abilities, worth, self-image, emotions
- Body posture and movement, eye contact, voice and speech patterns

## SLEEP-REST
- Patterns of sleep and rest-/relaxation in a 24-hr period
- Perceptions of quality and quantity of sleep and rest
- Use of sleep aids and routines

## COGNITIVE-PERCEPTUAL
- Adequacy of vision, hearing, taste, touch, smell
- Pain perception and management
- Language, judgment, memory, decisions

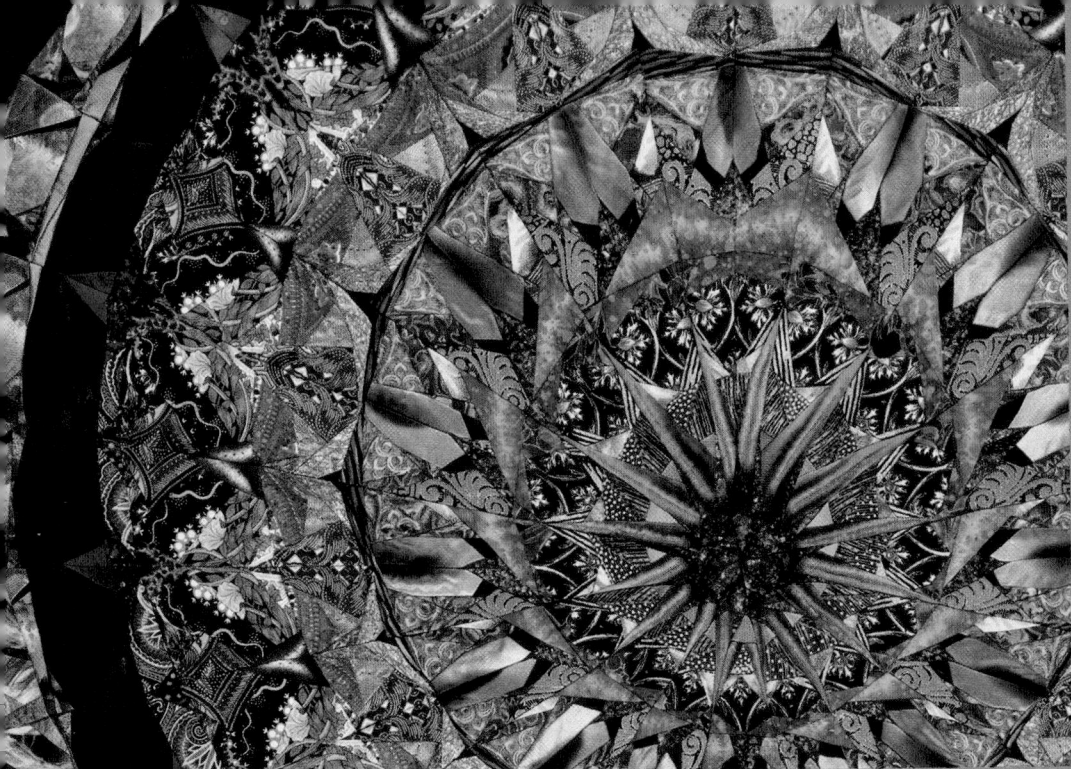

# RESPONSES TO ALTERED INTEGUMENTARY STRUCTURE AND FUNCTION

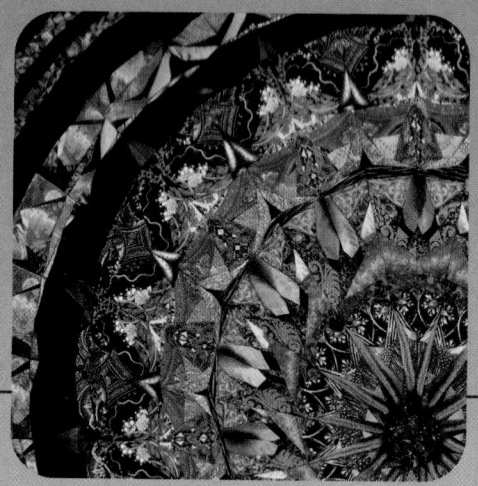

# Assessing Clients with Integumentary Disorders

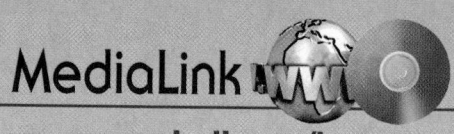

**MediaLink**

## www.prenhall.com/lemone

Additional resources for this chapter can be found on the Student CD-ROM accompanying this textbook, and on the Companion Website at www.prenhall.com/lemone. Click on Chapter 13 to select the activities for this chapter.

**CD-ROM**
- Audio Glossary
- NCLEX Review

*Animation*
- Integumentary Repair

**Companion Website**
- More NCLEX Review
- Functional Health Pattern Assessment
- Case Study
    Assessing a Rash

## LEARNING OUTCOMES

After completing this chapter, you will be able to:

- Review the anatomy and physiology of the skin, hair, and nails.

- Discuss factors that influence skin color.

- Identify specific topics for consideration during a health history interview of the client with problems involving the skin, hair, and nails.

- Describe techniques for assessing the skin, hair, and nails.

- Describe normal variations in assessment findings for the client with dark skin.

- Identify abnormal findings that may indicate impairment of the integumentary system.

The skin, the hair, and the nails make up the integumentary system. The skin provides an external covering for the body, separating the body's organs and tissues from the external environment. It is the largest organ of the body and has many functions, summarized in Table 13–1.

In addition, the integumentary system:

- Protects the body from injury from the external environment.
- Provides a barrier to the loss of body fluids and electrolytes.
- Maintains the integrity of the body surface through wound repair.
- Serves as a sense organ for touch, pressure, pain, and temperature.
- Provides a film over the body through the action of glandular secretions, which protects the body from bacterial and fungal invasion.
- Dissipates body heat through the evaporation of sweat.
- Participates in the production of vitamin D.
- Serves as an indicator of emotions and health or illness through color changes.

## REVIEW OF ANATOMY AND PHYSIOLOGY
## The Skin

The **skin** has a total surface area of 15 to 20 square feet and weighs about 9 pounds. It has been estimated that each square inch of skin contains 15 feet of blood vessels, 4 yards of nerves, 650 sweat glands, 100 oil glands, 1500 sensory receptors, and over 3 million cells that are constantly dying and being replaced. The skin is composed of two regions: the epidermis and the dermis (Figure 13–1 ■).

### The Epidermis
The **epidermis,** which is the surface or outermost part of the skin, consists of epithelial cells. The epidermis has either four or five layers, depending on its location; there are five layers over the palms of the hands and the soles of the feet, and four layers over the rest of the body.

The stratum basale is the deepest layer of the epidermis. It contains melanocytes, cells that produce the pigment melanin, and keratinocytes, which produce keratin. **Melanin** forms a protective shield to protect the keratinocytes and the nerve endings in the dermis from the damaging effects of ultraviolet light. Melanocyte activity probably accounts for the difference in skin color in humans. **Keratin** is a fibrous, water-repellent protein that gives the epidermis its tough, protective quality. As keratinocytes mature, they move upward through the epidermal layers, eventually becoming dead cells at the surface of the skin. Millions of these cells are worn off by abrasion each day, but millions are simultaneously produced in the stratum basale. The next layer of the epidermis is the stratum spinosum. Several cells thick, this layer contains abundant Langerhans cells that arise from the bone marrow and migrate to the epidermis. Mitosis occurs at this layer, although not as abundantly as in the stratum basale.

The stratum granulosum is only two to three cells thick, and also contains Langerhans cells. The cells of the stratum granulosum contain a glycolipid that slows water loss across the epidermis. *Keratinization,* a thickening of the cells' plasma membranes, begins in the stratum granulosum. The stratum lucidum is present only in areas of thick skin. It is made up of flattened, dead keratinocytes.

The outermost layer of the epidermis, the stratum corneum, is also the thickest, making up about 75% of the epidermis's total thickness. It consists of about 20 to 30 sheets of dead cells filled with keratin fragments arranged in "shingles" that flake off as dry skin.

### The Dermis
The **dermis** is the second, deeper layer of skin. Made of a flexible connective tissue, this layer is richly supplied with blood cells, nerve fibers, and lymphatic vessels. Most of the hair follicles, sebaceous glands, and sweat glands are located in the dermis. The dermis consists of a papillary and a reticular layer. The papillary layer contains ridges that indent the overlying epidermis. It also contains capillaries and receptors for pain and touch. The deeper, reticular layer contains blood vessels, sweat and sebaceous glands, deep pressure receptors, and dense bundles of collagen fibers. The regions between these

### TABLE 13–1 Functions of the Skin and Its Appendages

| Structure | Functions |
|---|---|
| Epidermis | Protects tissues from physical, chemical, and biologic damage. <br> Prevents water loss and serves as a water-repellent layer. <br> Stores melanin, which protects tissues from harmful effects of the ultraviolet radiation in sunlight. <br> Converts cholesterol molecules to vitamin D when exposed to sunlight. <br> Contains phagocytes, which prevent bacteria from penetrating the skin. |
| Dermis | Regulates body temperature by dilating and constricting capillaries. <br> Transmits messages via nerve endings to the central nervous system. |
| Sebaceous (oil) glands | Secrete sebum, which lubricates skin and hair and plays a role in killing bacteria. |
| Eccrine sweat glands | Regulate body heat by excretion of perspiration. |
| Apocrine sweat glands | Unknown. |
| Hair | Cushions the scalp. Eyelashes and cilia protect the body from foreign particles. Provides insulation in cold weather. |
| Nails | Protect the fingers and toes, aid in grasping, and allow for various other activities, such as scratching the skin, picking up small items, peeling an orange, and so on. |

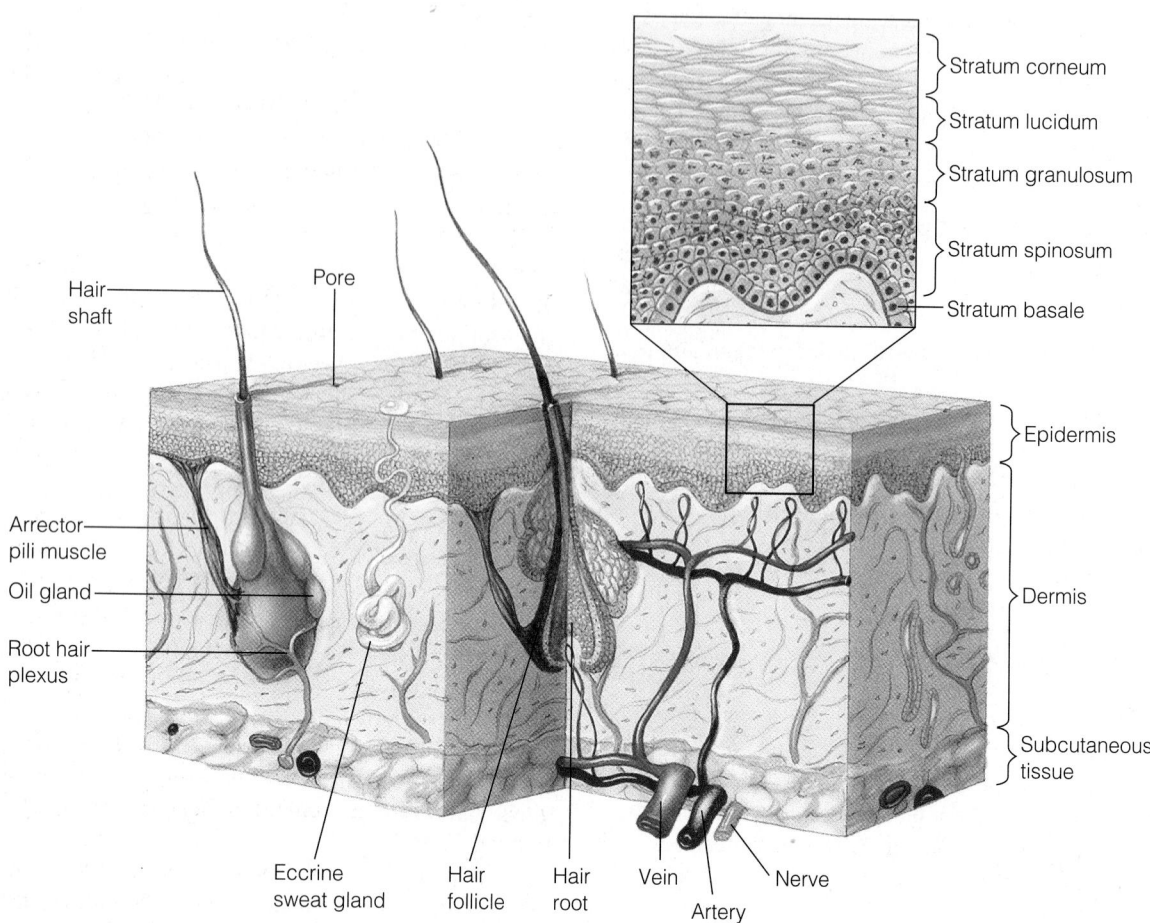

Stratum corneum
Stratum lucidum
Stratum granulosum
Stratum spinosum
Stratum basale

Epidermis
Dermis
Subcutaneous tissue

Hair shaft
Pore
Arrector pili muscle
Oil gland
Root hair plexus
Eccrine sweat gland
Hair follicle
Hair root
Vein
Artery
Nerve

**Figure 13–1** ■ Anatomy of the skin.

bundles form lines of cleavage in the skin. Surgical incisions parallel to these lines of cleavage heal more easily and with less scarring than incisions or traumatic wounds across cleavage lines.

## Superficial Fascia

Underlying the skin is a layer of subcutaneous tissue called the **superficial fascia.** It consists primarily of adipose (fat) tissue, and helps the skin adhere to underlying structures.

## Skin Color

The color of the skin is the result of varying levels of pigmentation. Melanin, a yellow-to-brown pigment, is darker and is produced in greater amounts in persons with dark skin color than in those with light skin. Exposure to the sun causes a buildup of melanin and a darkening or tanning of the skin in people with light skin. Carotene, a yellow-to-orange pigment, is found most in areas of the body where the stratum corneum is thickest, such as the palms of the hands. Carotene is more abundant in the skins of persons of Asian ancestry and, together with melanin, accounts for their golden skin tone. The epidermis in Caucasian skin has very little melanin and is almost transparent. Thus, the color of the hemoglobin found in red blood cells circulating through the dermis shows through, lending Caucasians a pinkish skin tone.

Skin color is influenced also by emotions and illnesses. **Erythema,** a reddening of the skin, may occur with embarrassment (blushing), fever, hypertension, or inflammation. It may also result from a drug reaction, sunburn, acne rosacea, or other factors. A bluish discoloration of the skin and mucous membranes, called **cyanosis,** results from poor oxygenation of hemoglobin. **Pallor,** or paleness of skin, may occur with shock, fear, or anger or in anemia and hypoxia. **Jaundice** is a yellow-to-orange color visible in the skin and mucous membranes; it is most often the result of a hepatic disorder.

## Glands of the Skin

The skin contains sebaceous (oil) glands, sweat (sudoriferous) glands, and ceruminous glands. Each of these glands has a different function (see Table 13–1).

**Sebaceous glands** are found all over the body except on the palms and soles. These glands secrete an oily substance called sebum, which usually is ducted into a hair follicle. Sebum softens and lubricates the skin and hair and also decreases water loss from the skin in low humidity. Sebum also protects the body from infection by killing bacteria. The secretion of sebum is stimulated by hormones, especially androgens. If a sebaceous gland becomes blocked, a pimple or whitehead appears on the surface of the skin; as the material oxidizes and dries, it forms a blackhead. Acne vulgaris is an inflammation of the sebaceous glands.

There are two types of sweat glands: eccrine and apocrine. **Eccrine sweat glands** are more numerous on the forehead, palms, and soles. The gland itself is located in the dermis; the duct to the skin rises through the epidermis to open in a pore at the surface. **Sweat,** the secretion of the eccrine glands, is composed mostly of water but also contains sodium, antibodies, small amounts of metabolic wastes, lactic acid, and vitamin C. The production of sweat is regulated by the sympathetic nervous system and serves to maintain normal body temperature. Sweating also occurs in response to emotions. Most **apocrine sweat glands** are located in the axillary, anal, and genital areas. The secretions from apocrine glands are similar to those of

sweat glands, but they also contain fatty acids and proteins. Their function is unknown.

Ceruminous glands are modified apocrine sweat glands. Located in the skin of the external ear canal, they secrete yellow-brown waxy cerumen. This substance provides a sticky trap for foreign materials.

## The Hair

**Hair** is distributed all over the body, except the lips, nipples, parts of the external genitals, the palms of the hands, and the soles of the feet. Hair is produced by a hair bulb, and its root is enclosed in a hair follicle (Figure 13–2 ■). The exposed part, called the shaft, consists mainly of dead cells. Hair follicles extend into the dermis and in some places, such as the scalp, below the dermis. Many factors, including nutrition and hormones, influence hair growth.

Hair in various parts of the body has protective functions: The eyebrows and eyelashes protect the eyes; hair in the nose helps keep foreign materials out of the upper respiratory tract; and hair on the head protects the scalp from heat loss and sunlight. Table 13–1 summarizes the various functions of the hair.

## The Nails

A **nail** is a modified scalelike epidermal structure. Like hair, nails consist mainly of dead cells. They arise from the stratum germinativum of the epidermis. The body of the nail rests on the nail bed (Figure 13–3 ■). The nail matrix is the active, growing part of the nail. The proximal visible end of the nail has a white crescent, called a lunula. The sides of the nail are overlapped by skin, called nail folds. The proximal nail fold is thickened and is called the eponychium or cuticle. Nails form a protective coating over the dorsum of each digit on the fingers and toes.

## ASSESSING THE INTEGUMENTARY SYSTEM

The function of the integumentary system (skin, glands, hair, and nails) is assessed by both a health assessment interview to

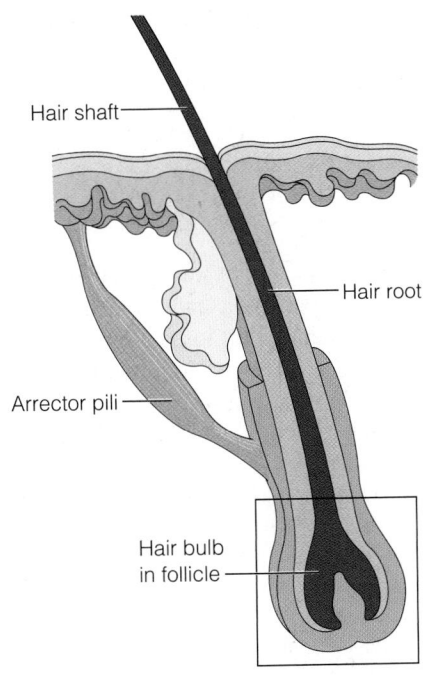

**Figure 13–2 ■** Anatomy of a hair follicle.

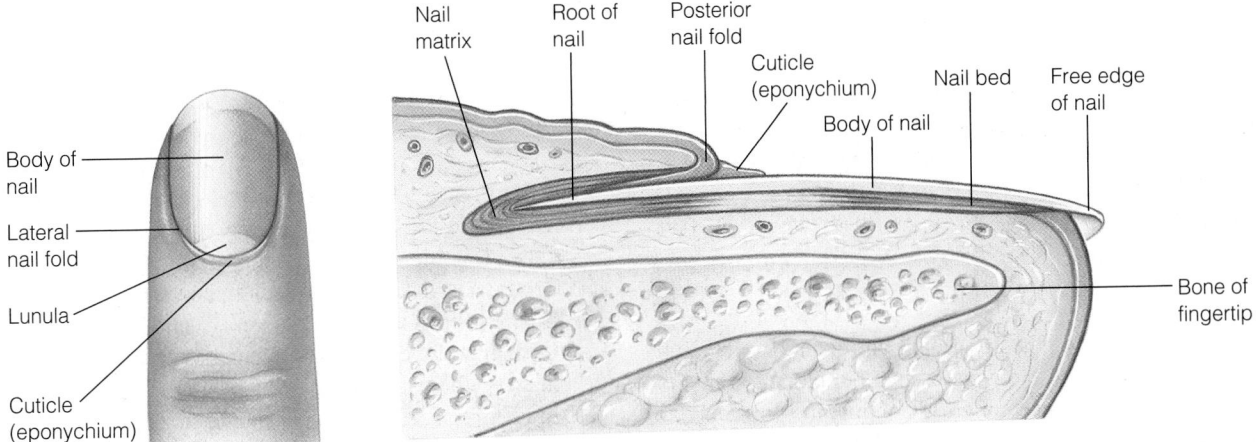

**Figure 13–3 ■** Anatomy of a nail.

collect subjective data and a physical assessment to collect objective data.

## The Health Assessment Interview

This section provides guidelines for collecting subjective data through a health assessment interview specific to the skin and its appendages. A health assessment interview to determine problems with the integumentary system may be conducted as part of a health screening or total health assessment, or it may focus on a chief complaint (such as itching or a rash). If the client has a skin problem, analyze its onset, characteristics and course, severity, precipitating and relieving factors, and any associated symptoms, noting the timing and circumstances. For example, ask the client:

- What type of itching have you experienced?
- When did you first notice a change in this mole?
- Did you change to any different kinds of shampoo or other hair products just before you started to lose your hair?

Ask about any change in health, rashes, itching, color changes, dryness or oiliness, growth of or changes in warts or moles, and the presence of lesions. Precipitating causes, such as medications, the use of new soaps, skin-care agents, cosmetics, pets, travel, stress, or dietary changes, must also be explored. In assessing hair problems, ask about any thinning or baldness, excessive hair loss, change in distribution of hair, use of hair-care products, diet, and dieting. When assessing nail problems, ask about nail splitting or breakage, discoloration, infection, diet, and exposure to chemicals.

The client's medical history is important. Questions focus on previous problems, allergies, and lesions. Skin problems may be manifestations of other disorders, such as cardiovascular disease, endocrine disorders, hepatic disease, and hematologic disorders. Occupational and social history may provide cues to skin problems; ask the client about travel, exposure to toxic substances at work, use of alcohol, and responses to stress.

Assess the presence of risk factors for skin cancer carefully. These include male gender; age over 50; family history of skin cancer; extended exposure to sunlight; tendency to sunburn; history of sunburn or other skin trauma; light-colored hair or eyes; residence in high altitudes or near the equator; and exposure to radiation, X-rays, coal, tar, or petroleum products.

Also explore the risk factors for malignant melanoma. These include a large number of moles, the presence of atypical moles, a family history of melanoma, prior melanoma, repeated severe sunburns, ease of freckling and sunburning, or inability to tan.

Interview questions categorized by functional health patterns can be found on the Companion Website.

## Physical Assessment

Physical assessment of the skin, hair, and nails may be performed either as part of a total assessment or alone for clients with known or suspected problems. Conduct the physical examination of the skin, hair, and nails by inspection and palpation. Assess the skin for color, presence of lesions (observable changes from normal skin structure), temperature, texture, moisture, turgor, and presence of edema. Characteristics of lesions to note include location and distribution, color, pattern, edges, size, elevation, and type of exudate (if present). Examine the hair for color, texture, quality, and scalp lesions. Determine the shape, color, contour, and condition of the nails.

The equipment necessary for assessment of the skin includes a ruler (to measure lesions), a flashlight (to illuminate lesions), and disposable rubber gloves to protect the examiner. Prior to the examination, collect all necessary equipment and explain techniques to the client to decrease anxiety.

The examination should be conducted in a warm, private room. The client removes all clothing and puts on a gown or drape. The areas to be examined should be fully exposed, but protect the client's modesty by keeping other areas covered. The client may be standing, sitting, or lying down at various times of the examination.

## Integumentary Assessments with Abnormal Findings (✓)

- **Inspect skin color.**
  - ✓ Pallor and/or cyanosis are seen with exposure to cold and with decreased perfusion and oxygenation. In cyanotic dark-skinned clients, skin loses glow and appears ashen. Cyanosis may be more visible in the mucous membranes and nail beds of these clients.
  - ✓ In dark-skinned clients, jaundice may be most apparent in the sclera of the eyes.
  - ✓ Redness, swelling, and pain are seen with various rashes, inflammations, infections, and burns. First-degree burns cause areas of painful erythema and swelling. Red, painful blisters appear in second-degree burns, whereas white or blackened areas are common in third-degree burns.
  - ✓ **Vitiligo,** an abnormal loss of melanin in patches, typically occurs over the face, hands, or groin. Vitiligo is thought to be an autoimmune disorder.
- **Inspect the skin for lesions.** Primary, secondary, and vascular lesions are described and shown in Tables 13–2 through 13–4.
  - ✓ Pearly edged nodules with a central ulcer are seen in basal cell carcinoma.
  - ✓ Scaly, red, fast-growing papules are seen in squamous cell carcinoma.
  - ✓ Dark, asymmetric, multicolored patches (sometimes moles) with irregular edges appear in malignant melanoma.
  - ✓ Circular lesions are usually present in ringworm and in tinea versicolor.
  - ✓ Grouped vesicles may be seen in contact dermatitis.
  - ✓ Linear lesions appear in poison ivy and herpes zoster.
  - ✓ **Urticaria** (hives) appears as patches of pale, itchy wheals in an erythematous area.
  - ✓ In psoriasis, scaly red patches appear on the scalp, knees, back, and genitals.

✓ In herpes zoster, vesicles appear along sensory nerve paths, turn into pustules, and then crust over.

✓ Bruises are raised bluish or yellowish vascular lesions. Multiple bruises in various stages of healing suggest abuse.

- **Palpate skin temperature.**

✓ Skin is warm and red in inflammation and is generally warm with elevated body temperature.

✓ Decreased blood flow decreases the skin temperature; this may be generalized, as in shock, or localized, as in arteriosclerosis.

- **Palpate skin texture.**

✓ Changes in the texture of the skin may indicate irritation or trauma.

✓ The skin is soft and smooth in hyperthyroidism and coarse in hypothyroidism.

- **Palpate skin moisture.**

✓ Dry skin often is present in the elderly and clients with hypothyroidism.

✓ Oily skin is common in adolescents and young adults. Oily skin may be a normal finding, or it may accompany a skin disorder such as acne vulgaris.

✓ Excessive perspiration may be associated with shock, fever, increased activity, or anxiety.

- **Palpate skin turgor.**

✓ Pinch the client's skin gently over the collarbone. Tenting, in which the skin remains pinched for a few moments before resuming its normal position, is common in elderly clients who are thin (Figure 13–4 ■).

✓ Skin turgor is decreased in dehydration. It is increased in edema and scleroderma.

## TABLE 13–2  Primary Skin Lesions

| | | | |
|---|---|---|---|
| **Macule, Patch** 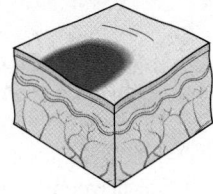 | Flat, nonpalpable change in skin color. Macules are smaller than 1 cm, with a circumscribed border, and patches are larger than 1 cm and may have an irregular border. **Examples** Macules: freckles, measles, and petechiae. Patches: Mongolian spots, port-wine stains, vitiligo, and chloasma. | **Vesicle, Bulla** 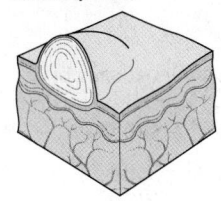 | Elevated, fluid-filled, round or oval shaped, palpable mass with thin, translucent walls and circumscribed borders. Vesicles are smaller than 0.5 cm; bullae are larger than 0.5 cm. **Examples** Vesicles: herpes simplex/zoster, early chickenpox, poison ivy, and small burn blisters. Bullae: contact dermatitis, friction blisters, and large burn blisters. |
| **Papule, Plaque** 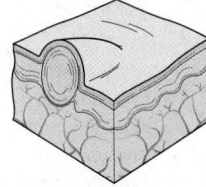 | Elevated, solid, palpable mass with circumscribed border. Papules are smaller than 0.5 cm; plaques are groups of papules that form lesions larger than 0.5 cm. **Examples** Papules: elevated moles, warts, and lichen planus. Plaques: psoriasis, actinic keratosis, and also lichen planus. | **Wheal** 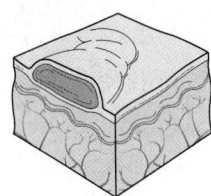 | Elevated, often reddish area with irregular border caused by diffuse fluid in tissues rather than free fluid in a cavity, as in vesicles. Size varies. **Examples** Insect bites and hives (extensive wheals). |
| **Nodule, Tumor** 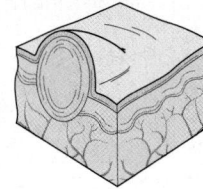 | Elevated, solid, hard or soft palpable mass extending deeper into the dermis than a papule. Nodules have circumscribed borders and are 0.5 to 2 cm; tumors may have irregular borders and are larger than 2 cm. **Examples** Nodules: small lipoma, squamous cell carcinoma, fibroma, and intradermal nevi. Tumors: large lipoma, carcinoma, and hemangioma. | **Pustule** 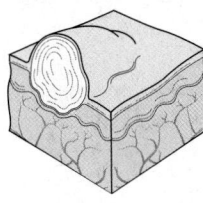 | Elevated, pus-filled vesicle or bulla with circumscribed border. Size varies. **Examples** Acne, impetigo, and carbuncles (large boils). |
| | | **Cyst** 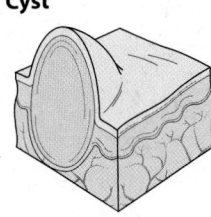 | Elevated, encapsulated, fluid-filled or semisolid mass originating in the subcutaneous tissue or dermis, usually 1 cm or larger. **Examples** Varieties include sebaceous cysts and epidermoid cysts. |

## TABLE 13–3  Secondary Skin Lesions

**Atrophy**

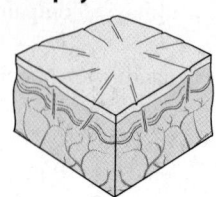

A translucent, dry, paperlike, sometimes wrinkled skin surface resulting from thinning or wasting of the skin due to loss of collagen and elastin.

**Examples**  Striae, aged skin.

**Erosion**

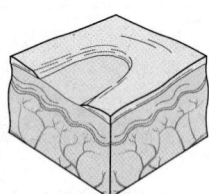

Wearing away of the superficial epidermis causing a moist, shallow depression. Because erosions do not extend into the dermis, they heal without scarring.

**Examples**  Scratch marks, ruptured vesicles.

**Lichenification**

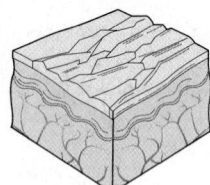

Rough, thickened, hardened area of epidermis resulting from chronic irritation such as scratching or rubbing.

**Example**  Chronic dermatitis.

**Scales**

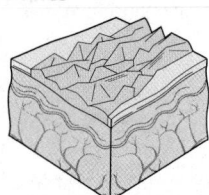

Shedding flakes of greasy, keratinized skin tissue. Color may be white, gray, or silver. Texture may vary from fine to thick.

**Examples**  Dry skin, dandruff, psoriasis, and eczema.

**Crust**

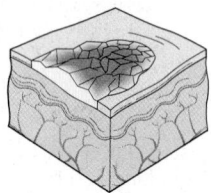

Dry blood, serum, or pus left on the skin surface when vesicles or pustules burst. Can be red-brown, orange, or yellow. Large crusts that adhere to the skin surface are called scabs.

**Examples**  Eczema, impetigo, herpes, or scabs following abrasion.

**Ulcer**

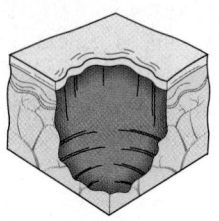

Deep, irregularly shaped area of skin loss extending into the dermis or subcutaneous tissue. May bleed. May leave scar.

**Examples**  Decubitus ulcers (pressure sores), stasis ulcers, chancres.

**Fissure**

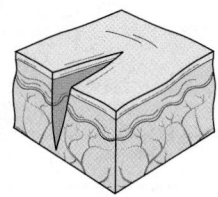

Linear crack with sharp edges, extending into the dermis.

**Examples**  Cracks at the corners of the mouth or in the hands, athlete's foot.

**Scar**

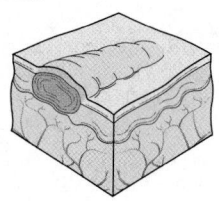

Flat, irregular area of connective tissue left after a lesion or wound has healed. New scars may be red or purple; older scars may be silvery or white.

**Examples**  Healed surgical wound or injury, healed acne.

**Keloid**

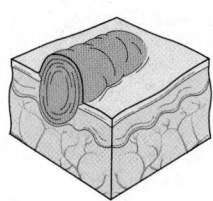

Elevated, irregular, darkened area of excess scar tissue caused by excessive collagen formation during healing. Extends beyond the site of the original injury. Higher incidence in people of African descent.

**Examples**  Keloid from ear piercing or surgery.

TABLE 13–4   Vascular Skin Lesions

**Port-Wine Stain**

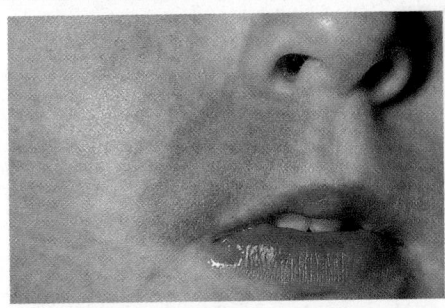

*Source: Photo Researchers, Inc.*

Flat, irregularly shaped lesion ranging in color from pale red to deep purple-red. Color deepens with exertion, emotional response, or exposure to extremes of temperature. It is present at birth and typically does not fade.

**Cause** A large, flat mass of blood vessels on the skin surface.

**Localization/Distribution** Most commonly appears on the face and head but may occur elsewhere.

**Strawberry Mark**

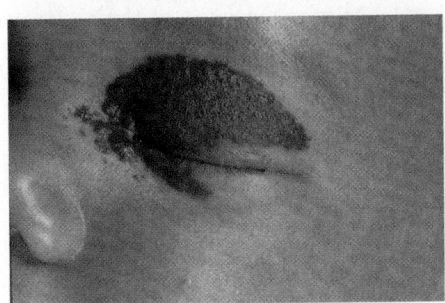

*Source: NMSB/Custom Medical Stock Photo.*

A bright red, raised lesion about 2 to 10 cm in diameter. It does not blanch with pressure. It is usually present at birth or within a few months of birth. Typically, it disappears by age 3. The lesion pictured here is located on the upper and lower lid of the left eye.

**Cause** A cluster of immature capillaries.

**Localization/Distribution** Can appear on any part of the body.

**Spider Angioma**

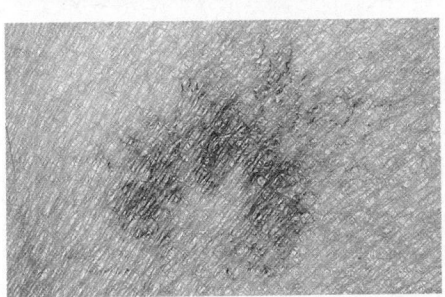

*Source: Photo Researchers, Inc.*

A flat, bright red dot with tiny radiating blood vessels ranging in size from a pinpoint to 2 cm. It blanches with pressure.

**Cause** A type of telangiectasis (vascular dilatation) caused by elevated estrogen levels, pregnancy, estrogen therapy, vitamin B deficiency, or liver disease, or may not be pathological.

**Localization/Distribution** Most commonly appear on the upper half of the body.

**Venous Star**

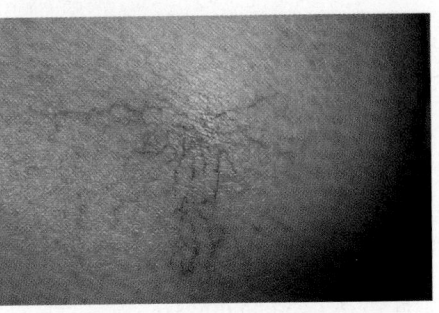

*Source: Medichrome.*

A flat blue lesion with radiating, cascading, or linear veins extending from the center. It ranges in size from 3 to 25 cm.

**Cause** A type of telangiectasis (vascular dilatation) caused by increased intravenous pressure in superficial veins.

**Localization/Distribution** Most commonly appear on the anterior chest and the lower legs near varicose veins.

**Petechiae**

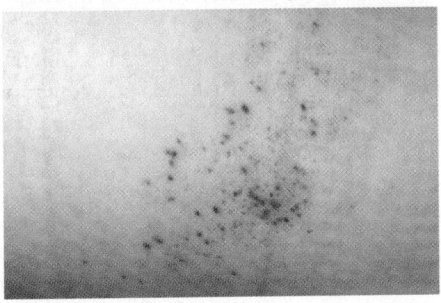

*Source: Custom Medical Stock.*

Flat red or purple rounded "freckles" approximately 1 to 3 mm in diameter. Difficult to detect in dark skin. Do not blanch.

**Cause** Minute hemorrhages resulting from fragile capillaries, petechiae are caused by septicemias, liver disease, or vitamin C or K deficiency. They may also be caused by anticoagulant therapy.

**Localization/Distribution** Most commonly appear on the dependent surfaces of the body (e.g., back, buttocks). In the client with dark skin, look for them in the oral mucosa and conjunctivae.

*(continued on page 358)*

## TABLE 13-4  Vascular Skin Lesions (continued)

**Purpura**

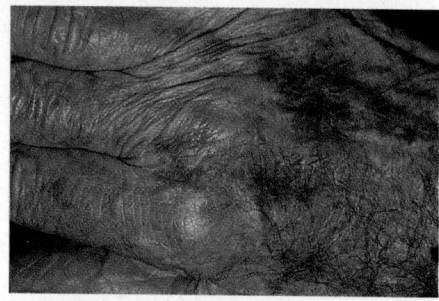

Flat, reddish blue, irregularly shaped extensive patches of varying size.

**Cause**  Bleeding disorders, scurvy, and capillary fragility in the older adult (senile purpura).

**Localization/Distribution**  May appear anywhere on the body, but are most noticeable on the legs, arms, and backs of hands.

**Ecchymosis**

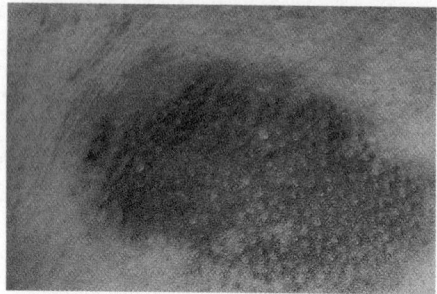

Source: DeGrazia/Custom Medical Stock Photo.

A flat, irregularly shaped lesion of varying size with no pulsation. Does not blanch with pressure. In light skin, it begins as bluish purple mark that changes to greenish yellow. In brown skin, it varies from blue to deep purple. In black skin, it appears as a darkened area.

**Cause**  Release of blood from superficial vessels into surrounding tissue due to trauma, hemophilia, liver disease, or deficiency of vitamin C or K.

**Localization/Distribution**  Occurs anywhere on the body at the site of trauma or pressure.

**Hematoma**

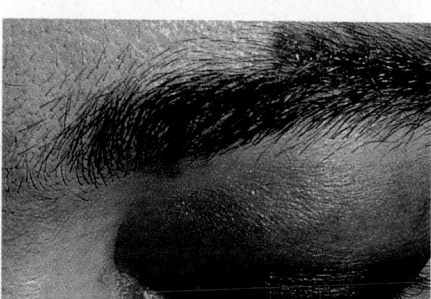

Source: Science Photo/Custom Medical Stock.

A raised, irregularly shaped lesion similar to an ecchymosis except that it elevates the skin and looks like a swelling.

**Cause**  A leakage of blood into the skin and subcutaneous tissue as a result of trauma or surgical incision.

**Localization/Distribution**  May occur anywhere on the body at the site of trauma, pressure, or surgical incision.

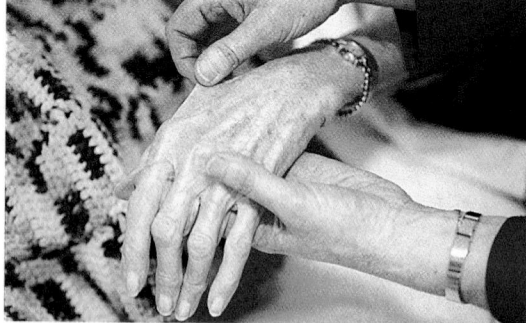

**Figure 13-4** ■ Tenting in an elderly client.

- **Assess for edema.**
  ✓ Assess **edema** (accumulation of fluid in the body's tissues) by depressing the client's skin over the ankle (Figure 13-5 ■). Record findings as follows:

1+ Slight pitting, no obvious distortion
2+ Deeper pit, no obvious distortion
3+ Pit is obvious; extremities are swollen
4+ Pit remains with obvious distortion

✓ Edema is common in cardiovascular disorders, renal failure, and cirrhosis of the liver. It also may be a side effect of certain drugs.

- **Inspect distribution and quality of hair.**
  ✓ A deviation in the normal hair distribution in the male or female genital area may indicate an endocrine disorder. **Hirsutism** (increased growth of coarse hair, usually on the face and trunk) is seen in Cushing's syndrome, acromegaly, and ovarian dysfunction. **Alopecia** (hair loss) may be related to changes in hormones, chemical or drug treatment, or radiation. In adult males whose hair loss follows the normal male pattern, the cause is usually genetic.

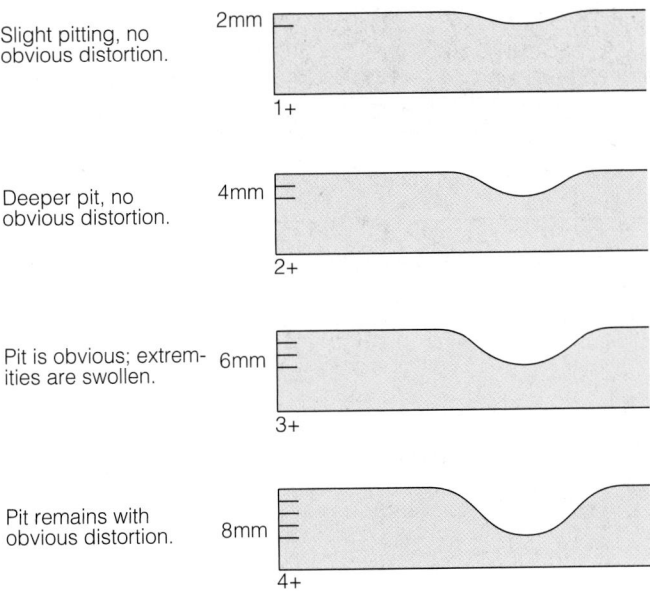

Slight pitting, no obvious distortion.   2mm   1+

Deeper pit, no obvious distortion.   4mm   2+

Pit is obvious; extremities are swollen.   6mm   3+

Pit remains with obvious distortion.   8mm   4+

**Figure 13–5** ■ Degrees of pitting in edema.

- **Palpate hair texture.**
  - ✓ Some systemic diseases change the texture of the hair. For instance, hypothyroidism causes the hair to coarsen, whereas hyperthyroidism causes the hair to become fine.
- **Inspect the scalp for lesions.**
  - ✓ Mild dandruff is normal, but excessive, greasy flakes indicate seborrhea requiring treatment.
  - ✓ Hair loss, pustules, and scales appear on the scalp in tinea capitis (scalp ringworm).
  - ✓ Red, swollen pustules appear around infected hair follicles and are called furuncles.
  - ✓ Head lice may be seen as oval nits (eggs) adhering to the base of the hair shaft. Head lice are usually accompanied by itching.
- **Inspect nail curvature.**
  - ✓ Clubbing (Figure 13–6 ■), in which the angle of the nail base is greater than 180 degrees, is seen in respiratory disorders, cardiovascular disorders, cirrhosis of the liver, colitis, and thyroid disease. The nail becomes thick, hard, shiny, and curved at the free end.
- **Inspect the surface of the nails.**
  - ✓ The nail folds become inflamed and swollen and the nail loosens in paronychia, an infection of the nails.
  - ✓ Inflammation and transverse rippling of the nail is associated with chronic paronychia and/or eczema.

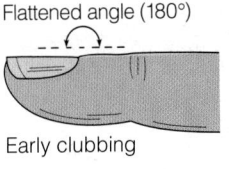

Flattened angle (180°)

Early clubbing

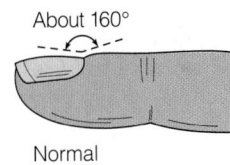

About 160°

Normal

**Figure 13–6** ■ Assessing clubbing of the nails.

- ✓ The nail plate may separate from the nail bed in trauma, psoriasis, and Pseudomonas and Candida infections. This separation is called oncolysis.
- ✓ Nail grooves may be caused by inflammation, by planus, or by nail biting.
- ✓ Nail pitting may be seen with psoriasis.
- ✓ A transverse groove (Beau's line) may be seen in trachoma and/or acute diseases.
- ✓ Thin spoon-shaped nails (Figure 13–7 ■) may be seen in anemia.
- **Inspect nail color.**
  - ✓ The sudden appearance of a pigmented band may indicate melanoma. However, pigmented bands are normally found in over 90% of African Americans.
  - ✓ Yellowish nails are seen in psoriasis and fungal infections.
  - ✓ Dark nails occur with trauma, Candida infections, and hyperbilirubinemia.
  - ✓ Blackish-green nails are apparent in injury and in Pseudomonas infection.
  - ✓ Red splinter longitudinal hemorrhages may be seen in injury and/or psoriasis.
- **Inspect nail thickness.**
  - ✓ Trauma to the nails usually causes thickening. Other causes of thick nails include psoriasis, fungal infections, and decreased peripheral vascular blood supply.
  - ✓ Thinning of the nails is seen in nutritional deficiencies.

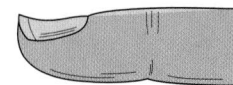

**Figure 13–7** ■ Spoon-shaped nails.

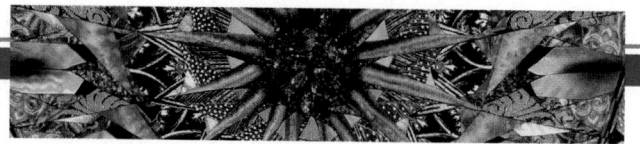

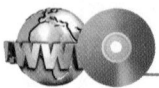

## EXPLORE MediaLink

NCLEX review questions, case studies, care plan activities, MediaLink applications, and other interactive resources for this chapter can be found on the Companion Website at www.prenhall.com/lemone.

Click on Chapter 13 to select the activities for this chapter. For animations, video clips, more NCLEX review questions, and an audio glossary, access the Student CD-ROM accompanying this textbook.

## TEST YOURSELF

1. Which layer of the skin contains most of the hair follicles, sebaceous glands, and sweat glands?

   a. Epidermis
   b. Dermis
   c. Stratum basale
   d. Stratum spinosum

2. What pigment is responsible for skin tanning?

   a. Carotene
   b. Red blood cells
   c. Melanin
   d. Sebum

3. You are assessing the skin of an elderly client for dehydration. What finding would indicate this condition?

   a. Decreased turgor
   b. Increased moisture
   c. Presence of lesions
   d. Pallor

4. What part of the body would you palpate to assess edema?

   a. The scalp
   b. The fingers
   c. The clavicle
   d. The ankle

5. You note that your client with chronic dermatitis has rough, thickened areas of skin. You document these areas as:

   a. Ulcers
   b. Papules
   c. Atrophy
   d. Lichenification

See Test Yourself answers in Appendix C.

## BIBLIOGRAPHY

Andresen, G. (1998). Assessing the older patient. *RN, 61*(3), 46–56.

Lawton, S. (2001). Assessing the patient with a skin condition. *Journal of Tissue Viability, 11*(3), 113–115.

McConnell, E. (1996). Assessing pruritus. *Nursing 96, 26*(12), 32.

Rupp, J., & Kaplan, D. (1999). Scratching the surface of pruritic disorders. *Consultant, 39*(11), 3161–3164, 3167.

Talbot, L., & Curtis, L. (1996). The challenge of assessing skin indicators in people of color. *Home Healthcare Nurse, 14*(3), 167–173.

Weber, J., & Kelley, J. ( 2002). *Health assessment in nursing* (2nd ed). Philadelphia: Lippincott-Raven.

Wilson, S., & Giddens, J. (2001). *Health assessment for nursing practice* (2nd ed.). St. Louis: Mosby.

Young, T. (1997). Skin assessment and usual presentations. *Community Nurse, 3*(5), 33–36.

# CHAPTER 14

# Nursing Care of Clients with Integumentary Disorders

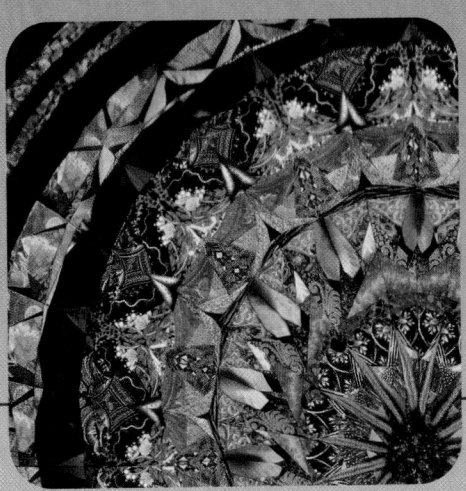

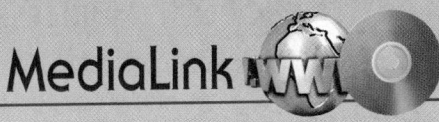

## MediaLink

### www.prenhall.com/lemone

Additional resources for this chapter can be found on the Student CD-ROM accompanying this textbook, and on the Companion Website at www. prenhall.com/lemone. Click on Chapter 14 to select the activities for this chapter.

**CD-ROM**
- Audio Glossary
- NCLEX Review

**Companion Website**
- More NCLEX Review
- Case Study
    Lesions and Pruritis
- Care Plan Activity
    Pressure Ulcers

## LEARNING OUTCOMES

After completing this chapter, you will be able to:

- Apply knowledge of normal anatomy, physiology, and assessments of the integument when providing nursing care for clients with disorders of the skin, hair, and nails (see Chapter 13).

- Describe the manifestations and nursing care of common skin problems and lesions.

- Compare and contrast the pathophysiology and collaborative care of clients with infections and infestations of the skin.

- Discuss the etiology, pathophysiology, and collaborative care of inflammatory disorders of the skin.

- Describe the pathophysiology and collaborative care of clients with malignant skin neoplasms.

- Explain the risk factors for, pathophysiology of, and nursing interventions to prevent and care for pressure ulcers.

- Discuss surgical options for excision of neoplasms, reconstruction of facial or body structures, and cosmetic procedures.

- Explain the pathophysiology of selected disorders of the hair and nails.

- Discuss nursing implications for pharmacologic agents used to treat disorders of the integument.

- Provide teaching appropriate for prevention and self-care of disorders of the integumentary system.

- Use the nursing process as a framework for providing individualized care to clients with disorders of the integument.

The skin and its accessory structures (the integumentary system) enclose the body, providing protection by serving as a barrier between the internal and external environments. The skin contains receptors for touch and sensation, helps regulate body temperature, and maintains fluid and electrolyte balance. The skin also provides cues to racial and ethnic background, and plays a major role in determining self-concept, roles, and relationships.

There are many disorders of the integument. The client with minor or benign disorders is usually treated in a health care provider's office or outpatient setting; but the client with disorders that involve large areas of the body, are chronic, or are malignant may require inpatient care. This chapter discusses disorders of the skin, hair, and nails; Chapter 15 discusses the client with burns. Primary and secondary skin lesions are described and illustrated in Tables 13–2 and 13–3. These terms are used throughout this and the next chapter.

# COMMON SKIN PROBLEMS AND LESIONS

The disorders discussed in this section of the chapter are those experienced by a large number of people. Although they are considered minor health problems in terms of health care, they may cause major problems for the person experiencing a high level of discomfort and/or chronicity.

## THE CLIENT WITH COMMON SKIN PROBLEMS AND LESIONS

### PRURITUS

**Pruritus** is a subjective itching sensation producing an urge to scratch. Pruritus may occur in a small, circumscribed area, or it may involve a widespread area; it may or may not be associated with a rash. Pruritus is believed to result from either stimulation of itch receptors in the skin or as a response to the stimulation of skin receptors for pain and touch. The CNS interprets these stimuli as an itch through central summation (Porth, 2002).

Almost anything in the internal or external environment can cause pruritus. Insects, animals, plants, fabrics, metals, medications, allergies, and even emotional distress are among the most common causes. Pruritus also may occur as a secondary manifestation of systemic disorders, such as certain types of cancer, diabetes mellitus, hepatic disease, and renal failure. Although the exact physiology is unknown, it is known that heat and prostaglandins trigger pruritus and that histamine and morphine increase it.

The pathophysiologic response of pruritus to stimulation or irritation follows a similar pathway, regardless of cause. The irritating agent stimulates receptors in the junction between the epidermis and dermis, and may also trigger the release of histamine and other chemical mediators that either further stimulate or mediate the itch response. The response of the person experiencing the itch is to scratch or rub the affected area. This may irritate the skin and cause further inflammation, which in turn sets off a cycle of increasingly intense itching and scratching, called the *itch-scratch-itch cycle.*

Secondary effects of pruritus include skin excoriation, erythema (redness of the skin), wheals, changes in pigmentation, and infections. Persistent pruritus may interrupt sleep patterns, because the itching sensation is often more intense at night. Long-term pruritus may be debilitating and increases the risk of infection as excoriation occurs.

Management of pruritus focuses on identifying and eliminating the cause and providing medications to relieve the itch. Antihistamines may relieve pruritus in some clients. Tranquilizers provide sedation, which may in turn relieve the emotional stress associated with pruritus; however, eliminating the stressors produces a more successful result. Systemic antibiotics are used to treat the infection resulting from the scratching and excoriation. Topical medications that contain corticosteroids are often used to relieve the pruritus and inflammation. Topical medications may also be administered through therapeutic baths or soaks with agents that relieve pruritus, such as cornstarch and baking soda or coal tar concentrates. Creams containing a topical anesthetic or antibiotic may also be used. Therapeutic baths are discussed in the Medication Administration box on page 363. Table 14–1 lists examples of topical agents used to treat skin disorders.

| TABLE 14–1 | Medications Used to Treat Skin Disorders | |
| --- | --- | --- |
| **Type** | **Use** | **Examples** |
| Creams | Moisturize the skin | Aquacare Curel Nutraderm |
| Ointments | Lubricate the skin Retard water loss | Aquaphor Vaseline |
| Lotions | Moisturize the skin Lubricate the skin | Alpha-Keri Dermassage Lubriderm |
| Anesthetics | Relieve itching | Xylocaine |
| Antibiotics | Treat infection | Bacitracin Polysporin Gentamicin Silvadene |
| Corticosteroids | Suppress inflammation Relieve itching | Dexamethasone Hydrocortisone Clocortolone Desonide |

## Medication Administration

### Therapeutic Baths

#### AGENTS USED IN THERAPEUTIC BATHS

Saline or tap water

Antibacterial agents: Potassium permanganate, acetic acid, hexachlorophene

Colloid substances: Oatmeal (Aveeno), cornstarch, sodium bicarbonate

Coal tar derivatives: Balnetar, Zetar, Polytar

Potassium permanganate

Emollients: Alpha-Keri, Lubath, mineral oil

Therapeutic baths have a variety of uses in treating skin disorders. Depending on the agent used, therapeutic baths soothe the skin, lower the skin bacteria count, clean and hydrate the skin, loosen scales, and relieve itching.

#### Nursing Responsibilities

- Ensure that the bath water is at a comfortable temperature that is neither too hot nor too cool (usually 110° to 115°F [45° to 46°C]).
- Fill the tub one-third to one-half full.

- Mix the agent well with the water.
- Assist the client into and out of the tub to prevent falls.
- Dry the client by blotting with the towel.

#### Client and Family Teaching

- Use a bath mat in the tub, the medications may cause the tub to become slippery.
- Keep the bathroom warm but adequately ventilated.
- Follow directions carefully for the amount of medication to use in the bath.
- Fill the bath one-third to one-half full of water that is at a comfortable temperature.
- Stay in the bath for 20 to 30 minutes, and immerse the areas to be treated.
- Do not get the bathwater in your eyes.
- Dry by blotting (not rubbing) with the towel.
- If the medications cause staining, use old towels or linens.
- If the itching is not relieved or the skin becomes excessively dry, call your health care provider.

## DRY SKIN (XEROSIS)

Dry skin, also called **xerosis**, is most often a problem in the older adult (Figure 14–1 ■). Xerosis commonly results, especially in the older adult, from a decrease in the activity of sebaceous and sweat glands, which reduces the skin's lubrication and moisture retention. However, dry skin may occur at any age from exposure to environmental heat and low humidity, sunlight, excessive bathing, and a decreased intake of liquids.

Two types of severe dry skin are xeroderma and ichthyosis. **Xeroderma** is a chronic skin condition characterized by dry, rough skin. **Ichthyosis** is an inherited dermatological condition in which the skin is dry, fissured, and hyperkeratotic; the surface of the skin has the appearance of fish scales.

The primary manifestation of dry skin is pruritus. Other manifestations include visible flaking of surface skin and an observable pattern of fine lines over the area. If the skin has been excessively dry and pruritic for a long period, the client may have secondary skin lesions and *lichenification* (thickening).

### NURSING CARE

Nursing care focuses on teaching the client and family how to reduce the dry skin and relieve the pruritus:

- Wash clothing in a mild detergent and rinse twice; do not use fabric softeners.
- Avoid using perfumes and lotions containing alcohol.
- Apply skin lubricants after a bath to help retain moisture.
- Soaps and hot water are drying. Clean the skin with tepid water and either a mild soap or cleansing creams. If soap is used, rinse it off carefully.
- It is not necessary to take a bath every day.
- If bath oils are used, add them to the bath water at the end of the bath (the moist skin is more likely to retain the oil). Use care not to slip in the tub.
- Use a humidifier to humidify the air.
- Apply creams and lotions when the skin is slightly damp after bathing.
- Increase fluid intake.
- Keep nails trimmed short, wear loose clothing, and keep the environment cool.
- A brief application of pressure or cold may relieve pruritus.
- Cotton gloves may be worn at night if scratching during sleep causes skin excoriation.
- Distraction or relaxation techniques may prove helpful.

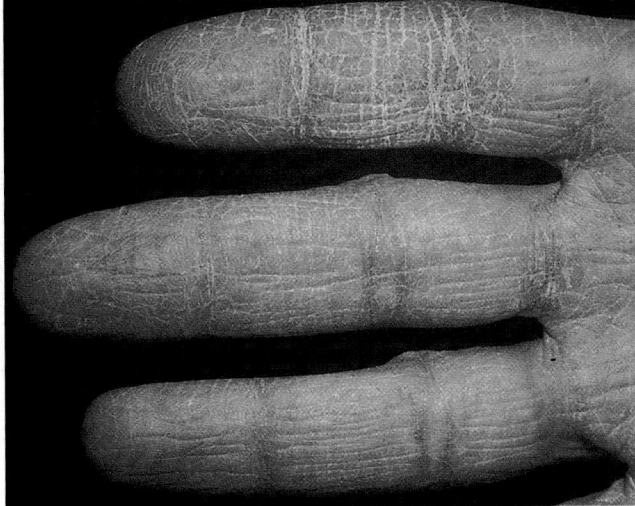

**Figure 14–1** ■ Severe xerosis, or dry skin, produces dry, rough skin with visible flaking of the skin surface.

*Source: Camera M. D. Studios. Carroll H. Weiss, Director. 8290 N. W. 26th Place. Sunrise, FL 33322.*

MediaLink | LESIONS AND PRURITIS CASE STUDY

## BENIGN SKIN LESIONS

The skin is subject to many different types and kinds of benign skin lesions, including cysts, keloids, nevi, angiomas, skin tags, and keratoses. Although these benign lesions are often considered more of a nuisance than an illness, they do require monitoring for an increase in size that interferes with the skin's appearance or function.

### Cysts

**Cysts of the skin** are benign closed sacs in or under the skin surface that are lined with epithelium and contain fluid or a semisolid material. Epidermal inclusion cysts and pilar cysts are the most common types.

Epidermal inclusion cysts may occur anywhere on the body but are most often found on the head and trunk. Although they are painless, they may grow so large that they become irritated by contact with clothing (e.g., if located on the back of the neck) or cause obstruction (e.g., if located on the nose). The cysts contain a semisolid material mainly of keratin. Pilar cysts are found on the scalp and originate from sebaceous glands. They are also painless. Both types of cysts rarely require treatment unless they become large and bothersome.

### Keloids

**Keloids** are elevated, irregularly shaped, progressively enlarging scars. They arise from excessive amounts of collagen in the stratum corneum during scar formation in connective tissue repair. These lesions are more common in young adults and appear within 1 year of the initial trauma.

This abnormal response most often occurs in people of African and Asian descent who sustain burns of the skin, although, even seemingly minor trauma can result in keloid formation. There is a familial tendency to develop keloids. Other risk factors for keloid formation include excessive tension on a wound and poor alignment of skin edges following accidental or intentional skin trauma. Certain skin surfaces are also more likely to develop keloids: the chin, ears, shoulders, back, and lower legs.

The excessive scar formation is associated with increased metabolic activity of fibroplasts and increased type III collagen. The principal cells of the keloids are myofibroblasts, which have characteristics of both fibroblasts and smooth muscle cells. The swollen appearance of the keloids is the result of an excess of extracellular material.

The keloids first appear as red, firm, rubbery plaques that persist for several months after the initial trauma (Figure 14–2 ■). Uncontrolled overgrowth over time causes the keloids to extend beyond the original scar. Eventually, the keloid becomes smooth and hyperpigmented.

### Nevi

**Nevi,** more commonly called *moles,* are flat or raised macules or papules with rounded, well-defined borders (Figure 14–3 ■). Nevi arise from melanocytes during early childhood, with the cells initially accumulating at the junction of the dermis and epidermis. Over time, the cluster of cells moves into the dermis, and the lesion becomes visible. Almost all adults have nevi.

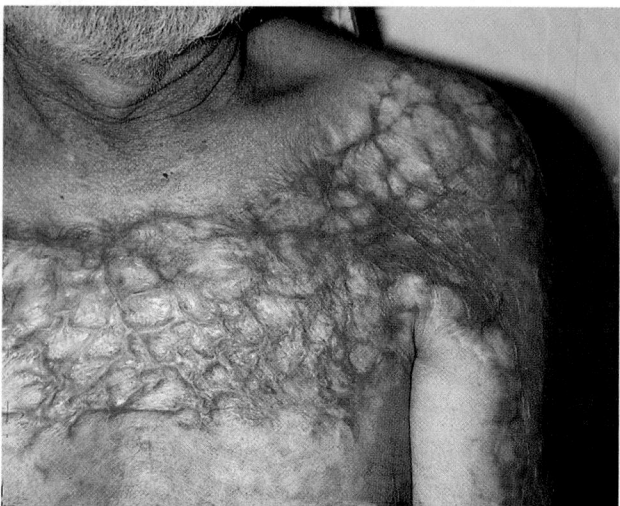

**Figure 14–2 ■** Keloids form from the deposit of excessive amounts of collagen during scar formation.

*Source: Camera M. D. Studios. Carroll H. Weiss, Director. 8290 N. W. 26th Place. Sunrise, FL 33322.*

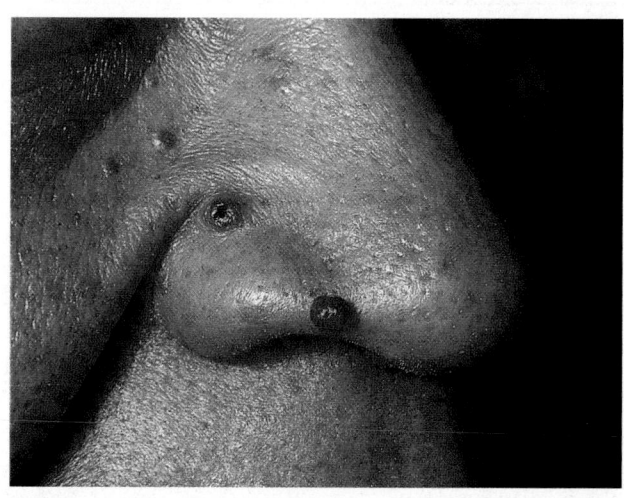

**Figure 14–3 ■** Nevi, more commonly called moles, arise from melanocytes and are common in all adults.

*Source: Camera M. D. Studios. Carroll H. Weiss, Director. 8290 N. W. 26th Place. Sunrise, FL 33322.*

Nevi range from flesh colored to black and occasionally contain hair. They can occur on any skin surface of the body and may arise as single lesions or in groups. Some pigmented nevi can transform into malignant lesions. Although the average adult has about 20 nevi, only 4 people out of 100,000 develop a malignant melanoma (Porth, 2002). However, it is important to monitor nevi for changes in size, thickness, color, bleeding, or itching. If any of these changes occur, the person should seek immediate professional assessment.

### Angiomas

**Angiomas,** also called **hemangiomas,** are benign vascular tumors. They appear in the adult in different forms:

- Nevus flammeus (port-wine stain) is a congenital vascular lesion that involves the capillaries. The lesions tend to occur on the upper body or face as macular patches that range from light red to dark purple. These lesions are present at birth and grow proportionally with the child into adulthood.

- Cherry angiomas are small, rounded papules that may occur at any age, but they most commonly arise in the 40s and gradually increase in number. The lesions range in color from bright red to purple. These lesions are often found on the trunk.
- Spider angiomas are dilated superficial arteries. They are common in pregnant women and in clients with hepatic disease. Spider angiomas occur most often on the face, neck, and upper chest. The lesions are usually small, bright red papules with radiating lines.
- Telangiectases are single dilated capillaries or terminal arteries that appear often on the cheeks and nose. These lesions are most common in older adults and result from photoaged skin. The lesions look like broken veins.
- Venous lakes are small, flat, blue blood vessels. They are seen on the exposed skin of the older adult: the ears, lips, and backs of the hands.

## Skin Tags

**Skin tags** are soft papules on a pedicle. They can be as small as a pinhead or as large as a pea and are most often found on the front or side of the neck and in the axillae, as well as in areas where clothing (such as underwear) rubs the skin. These lesions have normal skin color and texture.

## Seborrheic Keratoses

A **keratosis** is any skin condition in which there is a benign overgrowth and thickening of the cornified epithelium. These lesions most often appear in adults after age 50. *Seborrheic keratoses* are lesions that appear as superficial flat, smooth, or warty-surfaced growths, 5 to 20 mm in diameter, most often on the face and trunk. The lesions may be tan, waxy yellow, dark brown, or flesh colored, and they often appear greasy. These lesions are most often seen in the older adult and do not appear to be related to damage from sun exposure.

## COLLABORATIVE CARE

Most benign skin lesions do not require treatment, although excision or laser surgery may sometimes be necessary. Cysts may enlarge, skin tags may become irritated and bleed, nevi may change in appearance, or any of the lesions may cause discomfort with appearance.

## THE CLIENT WITH PSORIASIS

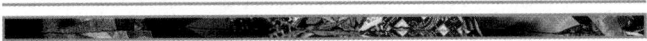

**Psoriasis** is a chronic skin disorder characterized by raised, reddened, round circumscribed plaques covered by silvery white scales (Figure 14–4 ■). The size of these lesions varies. The lesions may appear anywhere on the body; but they are most commonly found on the scalp, extensor surfaces of the arms and legs, elbows, knees, sacrum, and around the nails.

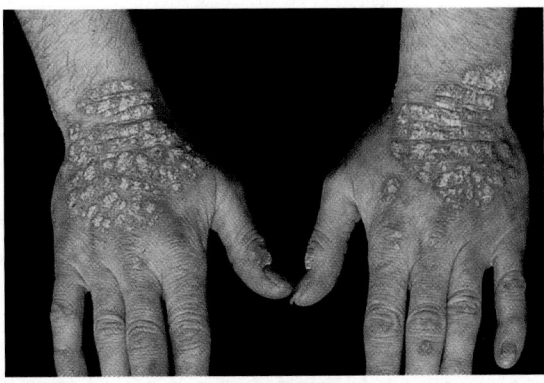

**Figure 14–4** ■ The characteristic lesions of psoriasis are raised, red, round plaques covered with thick, silvery scales.

*Source: NMSB/Custom Medical Stock Photo.*

The characteristic lesions in psoriasis are well-demarcated regions of erythematous plaques that shed thick gray flakes. As with any chronic illness, the skin manifestations may occur and disappear throughout life, with no discernible pattern to the recurrence.

## PATHOPHYSIOLOGY

Psoriasis affects about 1% of the U.S. population. The incidence is lower in warm, sunny climates. Onset usually occurs in the 20s, but it may occur at any age. Psoriasis occurs more often in Caucasians, but men and women are affected equally.

Sunlight, stress, seasonal changes, hormone fluctuations, steroid withdrawal, and certain drugs (such as alcohol, corticosteroids, lithium, and chloroquine) appear to exacerbate the disorder. About one-third of clients have a family history of psoriasis. Trauma to the skin from such events as surgery, sunburn, or excoriation is also a common precipitating factor; lesions that result from trauma are called Koebner's reaction (Porth, 2002).

Normally, the keratinocyte (an epidermal cell making up 95% of the epidermis) migrates from the basal cell to the stratum corneum (the outer skin layer) in about 14 days and is sloughed off 14 days later. Psoriatic skin cells, by contrast, have a shorter cycle of growth, completing the journey to the stratum corneum in only 4 to 7 days, a condition called *hyperkeratosis*. These immature cells produce an abnormal keratin that forms thick, flaky scales at the surface of the skin. The increased cell metabolism stimulates increased vascularity, which contributes to the erythema of the lesions.

*Psoriasis vulgaris* is the most common form of psoriasis. The lesions can be found anywhere on the skin but most commonly involve the skin over the elbows, knees, and scalp. Initially, the lesions are papules that form into well-defined erythematous plaques with thick, silvery scales. The plaques in darker-skinned persons may appear purple.

Permanent remission of psoriasis is rare. The prognosis depends on the type, extent, and severity of the initial attack. The age of onset is also a factor; early-onset disease is usually more severe.

## MANIFESTATIONS AND COMPLICATIONS

Pruritus is common over the psoriatic lesions. If the lesions are located in an intertriginous zone, such as between the toes, under the breasts, or in the perianal region, the psoriatic scales may soften, allowing painful fissures to form. When psoriasis affects the nails, pitting and a yellow or brown discoloration results. The nail may separate from the nail bed, thicken, and crumble. The involved nails, which are more often fingernails than toenails, are at high risk for infection.

## COLLABORATIVE CARE

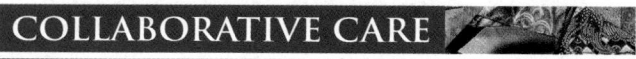

Treatment is based on the type of psoriasis, the extent and location of the lesions, the age of the client, and the degree of disfigurement or disability.

### Diagnostic Tests

- *Skin biopsy* may be done if the client presents with atypical manifestations, or to differentiate psoriasis from other inflammatory or infectious skin disorders.
- *Ultrasonography* may be performed to measure skin thickness; results reveal typical psoriatic changes in the stratum corneum and dermal inflammation.

### Medications

A variety of medications and treatments may be prescribed, including topical medications and photochemotherapy. Although there is no cure, treatment decreases the severity and pain of the lesions.

Topical medications are administered to decrease inflammation, prolong the maturity time of keratinocytes, and increase remission time. Corticosteroids, tar preparations, anthralin, and the retinoids are typically used. Box 14–1 outlines general guidelines for teaching clients to apply topical medications.

Topical corticosteroids decrease inflammation, suppress mitotic activity of psoriatic cells, and delay the movement of keratinocytes to the surface of the skin (thus giving them time to

mature and decreasing hyperkeratinosis). Tazarotene gel, a topical retinoid, is useful in treating clients with mild to moderate cases. The most effective topical corticosteroids are potent preparations that are well absorbed through the skin and are used under an occlusive dressing. Corticosteroids may also be taken systemically or injected directly into the lesions.

Tar preparations (such as Estar, Psorigel, and Fototar) suppress mitotic activity and are also anti-inflammatory. Their exact mechanism of action is unknown, but they are effective in removing scales and increasing remission time. Preparations made of coal tar are messy, cause staining, and have an unpleasant odor, but they are an effective form of treatment.

Topical anthralin (dithranol) inhibits the mitotic activity of epidermal cells and is effective in some cases of chronic, localized psoriasis that do not respond to other topical agents. The medication is applied to the plaque patches at bedtime and left in place for 8 to 12 hours. Clients should be tested for sensitivity to the drug before use, and it should not be applied to inflamed or open areas of skin.

Calcipotriene (Dovonex) has been shown to be effective and safe in both the short-term and long-term treatment of psoriasis. It inhibits cell proliferation in the epidermis and facilitates cell differentiation. Although a derivative of topical vitamin D, calcipotriene does not seem to affect bone or calcium metabolism.

### Treatments

#### Photochemotherapy

Photochemotherapy is the preferred treatment modality for severe psoriasis (Porth, 2002). A light-activated form of the drug methoxsalen is used. This drug is an antimetabolite that inhibits DNA synthesis and thereby prevents cell mitosis, decreasing hyperkeratosis. Exposure to ultraviolet-A (UVA) rays activates methoxsalen; it is administered orally, and the client is exposed to UVA 2 hours later. Treatments are administered 2 to 3 times a week; usually 10 to 20 total treatments are given over 1 to 2 months. The eyes are covered by dark glasses during the treatment. Treatment causes tanning, and direct sunlight must be avoided for

---

**BOX 14–1    ■  General Guidelines for Applying Topical Medications**

Each time a medication is applied, the skin surface must be clean and dry. Remove the medication from the previous application: Remove creams by washing the skin with tap water; remove ointments by washing the skin first with mineral oil and then with a mild soap and water.

- To apply gels, creams, and pastes: Squeeze about 1/2 to 1 inch of the gel or cream into the palm of the hand. Rub the hands together until they are covered. Apply gels and creams to the affected areas with long strokes until the skin is thinly covered. Differences from these general guidelines follow:
  - a. Corticosteroids are usually applied two to three times a day in small amounts and rubbed directly onto the lesions. Apply the medication after a bath and cover with an occlusive dressing.

- b. Apply medications containing tar in the direction of hair growth. Do not apply these medications to the face, to the genitals, or in skinfolds. If the tar is water based or oil based, it will stain clothing.
  - c. Wear gloves when applying anthralin stains.
- To apply lotions: Shake the bottle of lotion well. Pour a small amount into the palm of the hand, and pat the medication onto the skin. If the lotion is thin, apply it with a gauze pad.
- To apply sprays: Hold the container about 6 inches from the skin, and apply the medication in a short spray.
- To apply medicated shampoo: Rinse out medication from the previous application. Apply the shampoo, massage into the hair and over the scalp carefully, and allow it to remain for the prescribed time. Rinse.
- To apply pastes: Use enough paste on an applicator (such as a wooden tongue depressor) to cover the lesion thinly.

8 to 12 hours thereafter. If the client exhibits erythema, the treatments are stopped until the redness and swelling resolve.

Photochemotherapy has had a high success rate in achieving remission of psoriasis, but it can accelerate aging of exposed skin, induce cataract development, alter immune function, and increase the risk of melanoma.

### Ultraviolet Light Therapy

Ultraviolet-B (UVB) light is often used to treat psoriasis. UVB light decreases the growth rate of epidermal cells, thereby decreasing hyperkeratosis. Mercury vapor lights or fluorescent UV tubes provide the UVB light; the latter are often arranged in a cabinet so the client can stand and expose psoriatic lesions more easily. These units may be purchased or constructed to be used in the client's home.

The light therapy is administered in gradually increasing exposure times, until the client experiences a mild erythema, like a mild sunburn. Treatments are given daily and are measured in seconds of exposure. The eyes are shielded during the treatment. The erythema response occurs in about 8 hours. Careful assessment is necessary to prevent more severe burning, which could exacerbate the psoriasis. In clients with extensive psoriasis, UVB treatments may be combined with tar preparations, which increase the photosensitivity of the skin.

## NURSING CARE

The client with psoriasis requires nursing care to meet physical and psychologic responses to the illness. The nursing interventions discussed in this section focus on common problems of the client with psoriasis: risk for impaired skin integrity and body image disturbance.

## Nursing Diagnoses and Interventions

### Impaired Skin Integrity

Psoriatic lesions range from several scales to large, open areas. Typical psoriatic skin lesions increase the risk of infection, which can further compromise healing. In addition, certain treatments (e.g., the use of UVA or retinoids) may cause erythema or peeling of the skin, further altering skin integrity.

- Demonstrate methods to reduce injury to the skin when taking therapeutic baths or treatments:
  - Use warm, not hot, water.
  - Gently rub lesions with a soft washcloth, using a circular motion.
  - Dry the skin with a soft towel, using a blotting or patting motion.
  - Keep the skin lubricated at all times.

*Hot water and dry skin increase pruritus, further stimulating the itch-scratch-itch cycle. Dry skin also worsens psoriasis. Washing or drying the skin with rough linens or pressure may excoriate the skin over the psoriatic lesions.*

- Demonstrate application of topical medications:
  - Apply the medication as prescribed in a thin layer, using hands (gloved, if appropriate), wooden tongue depressors, or a gauze pad.
  - Avoid getting medications in the eyes, on mucous membranes, or in skinfolds.
  - Apply a covering (occlusive dressing) over the medicated areas as prescribed, especially when using corticosteroids. Usually, the covering is applied for only 12 hours, often during the evening and night hours. Choose some type of plastic wrap that covers the area well.

*Applying a thin layer of medication more frequently is often more effective than applying a single thick layer of medication. The medications used to treat psoriasis may irritate the eyes and mucous membranes; when applied in skinfolds, they may also cause maceration (skin breakdown due to prolonged exposure to moisture). Topical corticosteroids are often covered with occlusive dressing to increase absorption and thus facilitate treatment. However, constant occlusion may increase the effects of the medications to undesired levels and also increases the risk for infections.*

- Teach manifestations of infection and how to contact the health care provider if these occur: elevated temperature, increased swelling, redness, pain, increase in drainage, and any change in the color of the drainage. *The client with skin lesions is at high risk for infection, as the skin is the body's first line of defense.*
- Teach manifestations of the complications of treatment: excoriation, increased erythema, increased peeling, and blister formation. *The medications or treatments may damage cells through chemical burns or excessive exposure to ultraviolet light. Times and methods of treatment need to be adjusted if these manifestations occur.*

### Disturbed Body Image

The obvious skin lesions that accompany psoriasis often cause clients to isolate themselves from social contacts, withdraw from normal roles and responsibilities, and feel helpless or powerless.

- Establish a trusting relationship by expressing acceptance of the client, both verbally and nonverbally. For example, touch the client during social communications, demonstrating that the lesions are not contagious or offensive. *One's body image is affected not only by self-perception but also by the responses of others. Nonjudgmental acceptance helps the client adapt to the change in body image. By touching the client during interactions, the nurse demonstrates that acceptance.*
- Encourage to verbalize feelings about self-perception in view of the chronic nature of psoriasis and to ask questions about the disease and treatment. *The client adapts to a changed body image through a process of recognition, acceptance, and resolution. Each person responds individually to disfigurement and loss.*
- Promote social interaction through family involvement in care, and referral to support groups of people with psoriasis or other chronic skin conditions. *Acceptance by others is critical to acceptance of self. Psoriasis treatment is lifelong, time consuming, and often unappealing. By becoming involved in care, the family communicates acceptance. Sharing experiences with others who have the same health problem is a source of strength in adjusting to a visible, chronic illness.*

## Home Care

Client and family teaching focuses on treatments and skin care needs. The following topics should be addressed:

- The chronic nature of the disease, factors that may precipitate an exacerbation, and methods to reduce stress
- Interventions for pruritus and dry skin, and specific care for psoriasis:
  - Expose the skin to sunlight, but avoid sunburn.
- Avoid trauma to the skin (e.g., do not scrub off scales, and use only an electric razor).
- Avoid exposure to contagious illnesses such as influenza and colds.
- Discuss current medications with the health care provider. Certain drugs (such as indomethacin (Indocin), lithium, and beta-adrenergic blocking agents) are known to precipitate exacerbations of psoriasis.
- In addition, suggest the National Psoriasis Foundation as a resource.

# INFECTIONS AND INFESTATIONS OF THE SKIN

The skin's resistance to infections and infestations is provided by protective mechanisms, including skin flora, sebum, and the immune response. Although the skin is normally resistant to infections and infestations, these disorders may occur as a result of a break in the skin surface, a virulent agent, and/or decreased resistance due to a compromised immune system. This section discusses skin disorders resulting from bacterial infections, fungal infections, parasitic infestations, and viral infections.

## THE CLIENT WITH A BACTERIAL INFECTION OF THE SKIN

A number of bacteria normally inhabit the skin and do not cause an infection. However, when a break in the skin allows invasion by pathogenic bacteria, an infection, called a **pyoderma,** may occur. The most common bacterial infections are caused by gram-positive *Staphylococcus aureus* and beta-hemolytic streptococci.

Bacterial infections of the skin may be primary or secondary. Primary infections are caused by a single pathogen and arise from normal skin; secondary infections develop in traumatized or diseased skin.

Most bacterial infections are treated by a primary care provider, and the client remains at home for care. If the infection becomes more serious, however, inpatient care is required. In addition, nosocomial infections of wounds or open lesions in hospitalized clients are often the result of bacterial infections, especially by methicillin-resistant *Staphylococcus aureus (MRSA).*

## PATHOPHYSIOLOGY

Bacterial infections of the skin arise from the hair follicle, where bacteria can accumulate and grow and cause a localized infection. However, the bacteria also can invade deeper tissues and cause a systemic infection, a potentially life-threatening disorder. Various types of bacterial infections involve the skin, including folliculitis, furuncles, carbuncles, cellulitis, erysipelas, and impetigo.

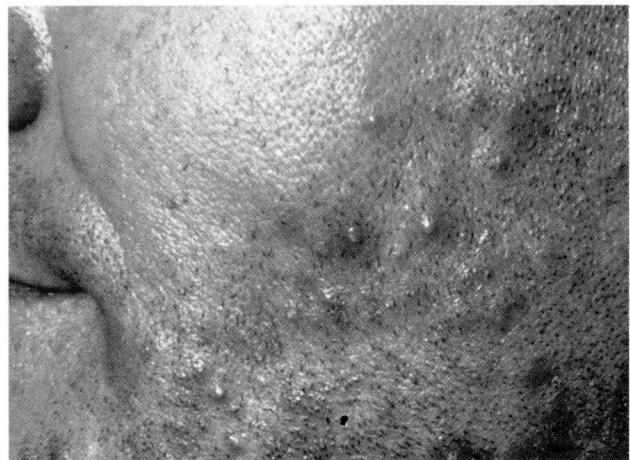

**Figure 14–5 ■** The lesions of folliculitis are pustules surrounded by areas of erythema.

## Folliculitis

**Folliculitis** is a bacterial infection of the hair follicle, most commonly caused by *Staphylococcus aureus*. The infection begins at the follicle opening and extends down into the follicle. The bacteria release enzymes and chemical agents that cause an inflammation. The lesions appear as pustules surrounded by an area of erythema on the surface of the skin (Figure 14–5 ■). Folliculitis is found most often on the scalp and extremities. It is also often seen on the face of bearded men (called sycosis barbae), on the legs of women who shave, and on the eyelids (called a *stye*). Although folliculitis may appear without any apparent cause, contributing factors include poor hygiene, poor nutrition, prolonged skin moisture, and trauma to the skin.

## Furuncles

**Furuncles,** often called boils, are also inflammations of the hair follicle. They often begin as folliculitis, but the infection spreads down the hair shaft, through the wall of the follicle, and into the dermis. The causative organism is commonly *Staphylococcus aureus*. A furuncle is initially a deep, firm, red, painful nodule from 1 to 5 cm in diameter (Figure 14–6 ■). After a few

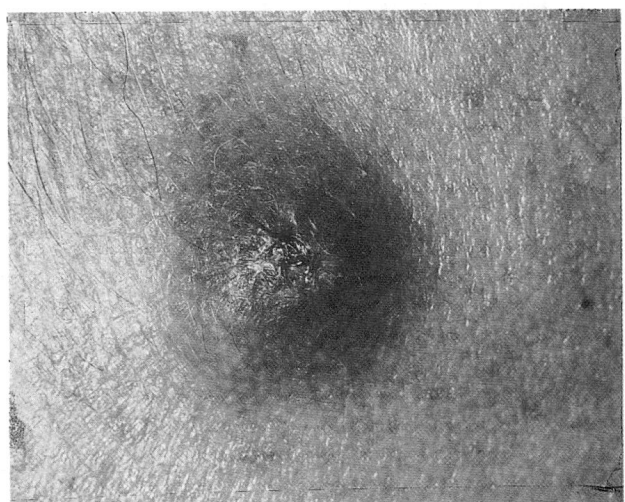

**Figure 14–6** ■ A furuncle (or boil) is a deep, firm, red, painful nodule.

*Source: Camera M.D. Studios. Carroll H. Weiss, Director. 8290 N.W. 26th Place. Sunrise, FL 33322.*

days, the nodule changes into a large, tender cystic nodule. The cysts may drain substantial amounts of purulent drainage.

One or more furuncles may occur on any part of the body that has hair. Contributing factors include poor hygiene, trauma to the skin, areas of excessive moisture (including perspiration), and systemic diseases such as diabetes mellitus and hematologic malignancies.

## Carbuncles

A **carbuncle** is a group of infected hair follicles. The lesion begins as a firm mass located in the subcutaneous tissue and the lower dermis. This mass becomes swollen and painful and has multiple openings to the skin surface. Carbuncles are most frequently found on the back of the neck, the upper back, and the lateral thighs. In addition to the local manifestations, the client may experience chills, fever, and malaise. The contributing factors for carbuncles are the same as for furuncles. Both infections are more common in hot, humid climates.

## Cellulitis

**Cellulitis** is a localized infection of the dermis and subcutaneous tissue. Cellulitis can occur following a wound or skin ulcer or as an extension of furuncles or carbuncles. The infection spreads as a result of a substance produced by the causative organism, called spreading factor (hyaluronidase). This factor breaks down the fibrin network and other barriers that normally localize the infection. The area of cellulitis is red, swollen, and painful (Figure 14–7 ■). In some cases, vesicles may form over the area of cellulitis. The client may also experience fever, chills, malaise, headache, and swollen lymph glands.

## Erysipelas

**Erysipelas** is an infection of the skin most often caused by group A streptococci. Chills, fever, and malaise are prodromal symptoms, occurring from 4 hours to 20 days before the skin lesion appears. The initial infection appears as firm red spots

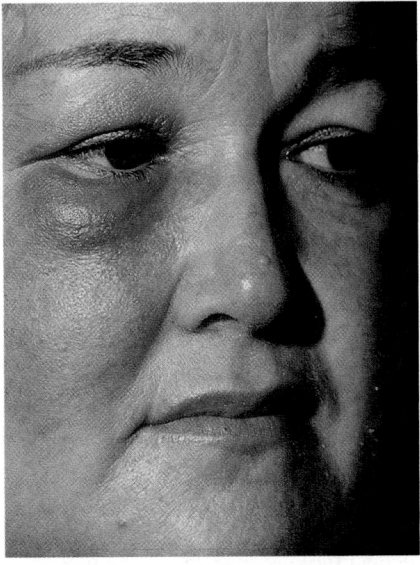

**Figure 14–7** ■ Cellulitis is a bacterial infection localized in the dermis and subcutaneous tissue. The involved area is red, swollen, and painful.

*Source: Camera M.D. Studios. Carroll H. Weiss, Director. 8290 N.W. 26th Place. Sunrise, FL 33322.*

that enlarge and join to form a circumscribed, bright red, raised, hot lesion. Vesicles may form over the surface of the erysipelas lesion. The area usually is painful, itches, and burns. Erysipelas most commonly appears on the face, ears, and lower legs.

## Impetigo

**Impetigo** is an infection of the skin caused by either *Staphylococcus aureus* or beta-hemolytic streptococci. Impetigo typically begins with a vesicle or pustule. This lesion ruptures, leaving an open area that discharges a honey-colored serous liquid that hardens into a crust (Figure 14–8 ■). Within

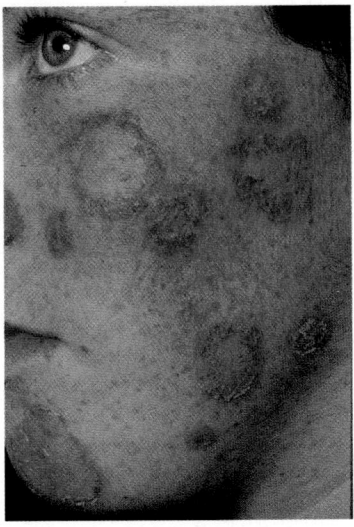

**Figure 14–8** ■ Impetigo is characterized by red, macular lesions as well as broken, crusted vesicles.

*Source: NMSB/Custom Medical Stock Photography.*

hours, more vesicles form. The pruritus that accompanies the eruptions causes scratching and excoriation, which spreads the infection. This disease occasionally occurs in adults but is much more common in children.

## COLLABORATIVE CARE

The diagnosis of a bacterial infection of the skin is made by assessing the appearance of the lesion and by identifying the causative organism. Antibiotics specific to the organism are used in treatment.

### Diagnostic Tests

- Culture and sensitivity of the drainage from the lesion may be ordered to identify the organism and to target the most effective antibiotics.
- If the infection is systemic, a blood culture may be ordered to identify a causative organism.
- People who experience repeated bacterial skin infections, or who provide care for others who exhibit infections, may have a culture taken from the external nares to determine whether they are carriers of bacteria (e.g., MSRA) and are reinfecting themselves or others.

### Medications

The primary treatment for bacterial infections of the skin is an antibiotic specific to the organism. The antibiotic is usually taken orally, and may also be applied topically. Multiple furuncles and carbuncles may be treated with cloxacillin (a penicillinase-resistant penicillin); the cephalosporins also are often effective.

## NURSING CARE

Nursing care focuses on preventing the spread of infection and restoring normal skin integrity. Most clients provide self-care at home, but the incidence of secondary bacterial infections in the inpatient population is great enough to warrant their inclusion in planning and implementing care. Nursing interventions for inpatient and long-term care clients include the following:

- Practice good handwashing and teach its importance. Careful handwashing is one of the most effective methods to reduce the spread of infection both in and out of the hospital setting. Health care providers must wash their hands with soap and water before and after client care and between each client contact. All clients, family members, and visitors (both in the home and hospital setting) should be taught the importance of handwashing, but it is even more important for the client with a bacterial infection.
- Assess the client for any increase in infection, which may be manifested systemically by fever, tachycardia, chills, and malaise. Local manifestations of the spread of the infection include an increase in erythema, the size of the lesion, and drainage. This assessment is especially important for older, debilitated, or immunosuppressed clients, and for those who have large or dirty wounds.

- Place the client on isolation precautions to limit the spread of the organisms to other patients. All health care providers and visitors follow the procedures and protocols of the institution exactly to prevent cross-contamination.
- Cover draining lesions with a sterile dressing, and handle soiled dressings or linens according to standard precautions. When changing dressings, always wear disposable rubber gloves and masks.

### Home Care

Client and family teaching focuses on facilitating tissue healing and eliminating the infection. Address the following topics:

- The importance of maintaining good nutrition
- The importance of maintaining cleanliness through careful handwashing and proper handling and disposal of dressings
- Preventing the spread of infection in the home by not sharing linens and towels and washing clothing and linens in hot water
- The importance of not squeezing or trying to open a bacterial lesion
- Avoiding the plucking of nasal hair or picking the nose
- The importance of taking the full course of prescribed antibiotics on a regular schedule until the prescribed supply is finished
- Bathing daily with an antibacterial soap (The client can gently wash off crusts during the bath. Warm compresses may be applied to the lesions two to three times a day to increase comfort and decrease swelling.)

## THE CLIENT WITH A FUNGAL INFECTION

Fungi are free-living plantlike organisms that live in the soil, on animals, and on humans. The fungi that cause superficial skin infections are called **dermatophytes.** In humans, the dermatophytes live on keratin in the stratum corneum, hair, and nails. Fungal disorders are also called *mycoses.*

### PATHOPHYSIOLOGY

#### Dermatophytoses (Tinea)

Superficial fungal infections of the skin are called **dermatophytoses** or, more commonly, *ringworm*. Fungal infections occur when a susceptible host comes in contact with the organism. The organism may be transmitted by direct contact with animals or other infected persons or by inanimate objects such as combs, pillowcases, towels, and hats. The most important factor in the development of the infection is moisture; the onset and spread of the fungal infection is greatest in areas where moisture content is high, such as within skinfolds, between the toes, and in the mouth. Other factors that increase the risk of a fungal infection include the use of broad-spectrum antibiotics that kill off normal flora and allow the fungi to grow, the presence of diabetes mellitus, immunodeficiencies, nutritional deficiencies, pregnancy, increasing age, and iron deficiency. Fungal infections of the skin are more common in

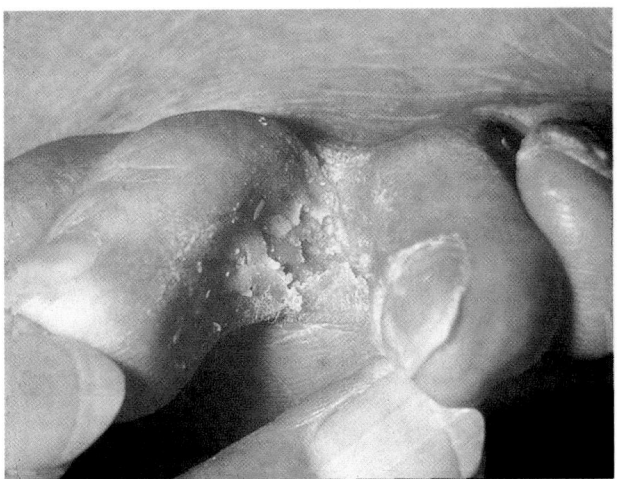

**Figure 14–9** ■ Tinea pedis (athlete's foot) is a fungal infection that often occurs between the toes.

*Source: Camera M. D. Studios. Carroll H. Weiss, Director. 8290 N. W. 26th Place. Sunrise, FL 33322.*

warm, humid climates. The dermatophyte infections are named by the body part affected, as follows:

- **Tinea pedis** is a fungal infection of the soles of the feet, the space between the toes, and/or the toenail (Figure 14–9 ■). More often called *athlete's foot,* this is the most common tinea infection. The lesions vary from mild scaliness to painful fissures with drainage, and they are usually accompanied by pruritus and a foul odor. The infection is often chronic, reappearing in hot weather, when perspiring feet are encased in shoes.
- **Tinea capitis** is a fungal infection of the scalp. The primary lesions are gray, round, bald spots, often accompanied by erythema and crusting (Figure 14–10 ■). The hair loss is usually temporary. Tinea capitis is seen more often in children than in adults.

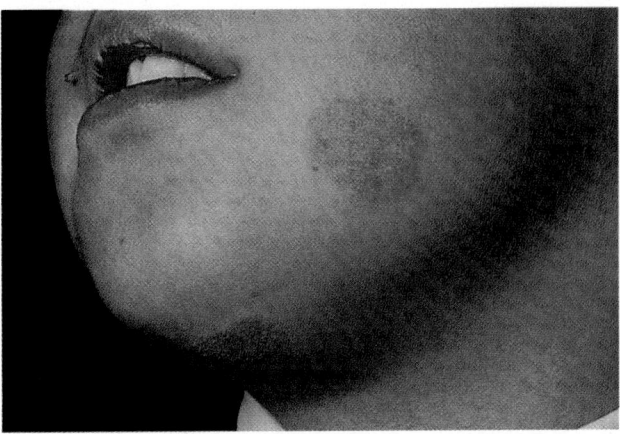

**Figure 14–11** ■ Tinea corporis commonly causes large, circular lesions with raised red borders.

*Source: Custom Medical Stock, Inc.*

- **Tinea corporis** is a fungal infection of the body. It can be caused by several different fungi, and the lesions vary according to the causative organism. The most common lesions are large circular patches with raised red borders of vesicles, papules, or pustules (Figure 14–11 ■). Pruritus and erythema are also present.
- **Tinea versicolor** is a fungal infection of the upper chest, back, and sometimes the arms. The lesions are yellow, pink, or brown sheets of scaling skin. The patches do not have pigment and do not tan when exposed to ultraviolet light.
- **Tinea cruris** is a fungal infection of the groin that may extend to the inner thighs and buttocks (Figure 14–12 ■). Often called "jock itch," it is often associated with tinea pedis

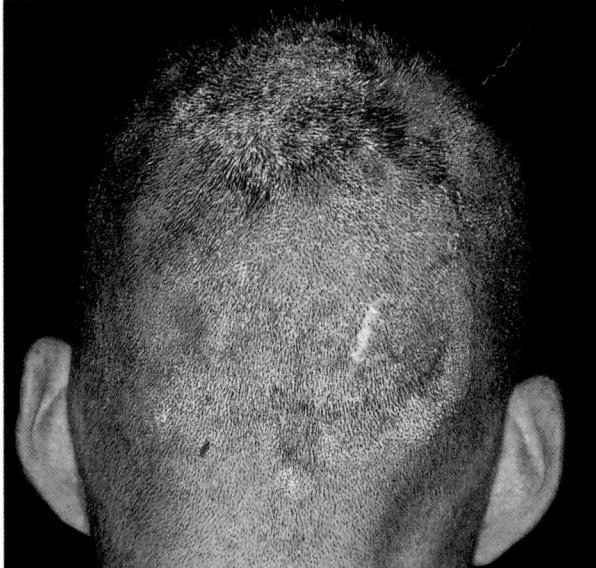

**Figure 14–10** ■ Tinea capitis is a fungal infection of the scalp that causes erythema, crusting, and hair loss.

*Source: Camera M. D. Studios. Carroll H. Weiss, Director. 8290 N. W. 26th Place. Sunrise, FL 33322.*

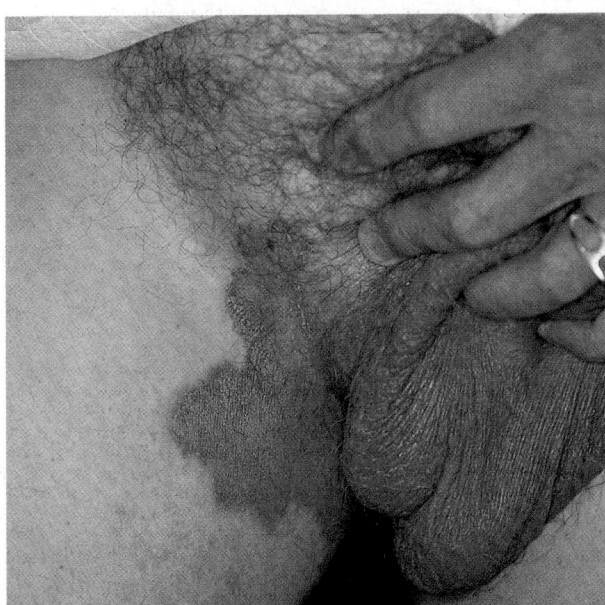

**Figure 14–12** ■ Tinea cruris (jock itch) is a fungal infection of the groin and inner thighs.

*Source: Camera M. D. Studios. Carroll H. Weiss, Director. 8290 N. W. 26th Place. Sunrise, FL 33322.*

and is more common in people who are physically active, are obese, and/or wear tight underclothing.

## Candidiasis

**Candidiasis** infections are caused by *Candida albicans,* a yeastlike fungus. This fungus is normally found on mucous membranes, on the skin, in the vagina, and in the gastrointestinal tract. The fungus becomes a pathogen when the following factors encourage its growth:

- A local environment of moisture, warmth, or altered skin integrity
- The administration of systemic antibiotics
- Pregnancy
- The use of birth control pills
- Poor nutrition
- The presence of diabetes mellitus, Cushing's disease, or other chronic debilitating illnesses
- Immunosuppression
- Some malignancies of the blood

Candidiasis affects the outer layers of the skin and mucous membranes of the mouth, vagina, uncircumcised penis, nails, and deep skinfolds. The first sign of infection is a pustule that extends under the stratum corneum. The pustule has an inflamed base and often burns and itches. As the infection spreads, the accumulation of inflammatory cells and shedding of surface cells produce a white to yellow curdlike substance that covers the infected area (Figure 14–13 ■). Satellite lesions (maculopapular areas found outside the clearly demarcated border of the original infection) are characteristic of candidiasis. The appearance of the infection differs by location, as summarized in Table 14–2.

| TABLE 14–2 | Characteristics of Candidiasis Infections by Location |
|---|---|
| **Location** | **Characteristics** |
| Skinfolds (under breasts, in groin, axillae, anus, umbilicus, and between toes or fingers) | Erythematous lesions that are either dry or moist. The lesions have clear borders, and satellite lesions are present. |
| Nails | Nail bed is red, swollen, and painful. |
| Mouth (thrush) | Mucous membranes are red and may be swollen; surface is covered with white, creamy material. Eroded areas may be present over the tongue and the oral cavity. |
| Penis (balanitis) (glans and shaft) | The penis is covered with small, red, clearly demarcated lesions that are painful and itch. The lesions may be covered with a white plaque. |
| Vagina | Red mucous membranes contain brighter red, demarcated, oozing lesions. The cervix may be covered with white plaque. A white, cheesy, foul-smelling vaginal discharge is present, accompanied by itching and burning. The vaginal and labial membranes may be swollen; the infection may extend to the anus and groin. |

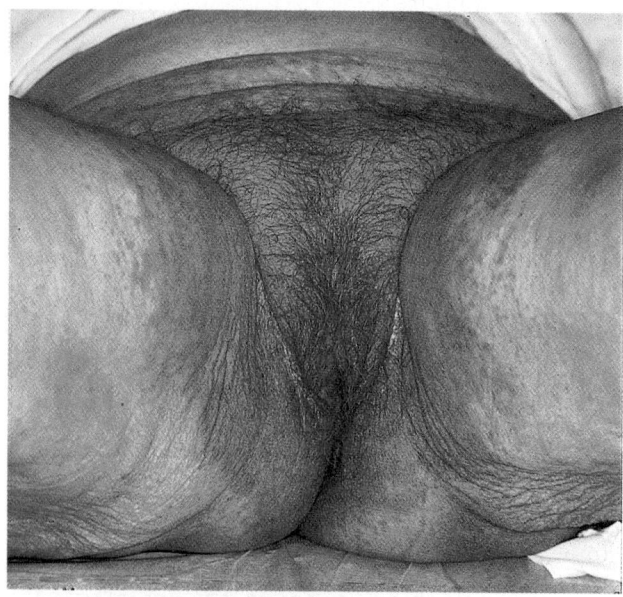

**Figure 14–13** ■ *Candida albicans,* a fungus, causes a skin infection characterized by erythema, pustules, and a typical white substance covering the area.

*Source: Camera M.D. Studios. Carroll H. Weiss, Director. 8290 N.W. 26th Place. Sunrise, FL 33322.*

## COLLABORATIVE CARE

Fungal infections are primarily diagnosed in outpatient settings and treated at home, but may also occur in hospitalized clients. The treatment is the same, regardless of the setting.

### Diagnostic Tests

Diagnostic tests are conducted to determine the causative fungi and may include:

- Cultures of skin scrapings, nail scrapings, or hairs.
- Microscopic examination of scrapings from the lesions. The scrapings are prepared in a solution of 10% potassium hydroxide (KOH) to reveal more clearly the spores and filaments (hyphae) of each fungus.
- Observation of the skin under ultraviolet light (called a Wood's lamp). The fungal spores fluoresce blue-green.

### Medications

Fungal infections of the skin are treated by topical or systemic antifungal medications. Nursing implications for the antifungal medications are described in the Medication Administration box on page 373.

## Medication Administration

### Treating Fungus Infections

#### ANTIFUNGAL AGENTS

Examples:

| | |
|---|---|
| Butenafine (Mentax) | Undecylenic acid (Desenex) |
| Clotrimazole (Mycelex) | Ketoconazole (Nizoral) |
| Nystatin (Mycostatin, Nilstat) | Fluconazole (Diflucan) |
| Econazole (Spectazole) | Amphotericin B (Fungizone) |
| Oxiconazole (Oxistat) | Griseofulvin (Fulvicin) |
| Miconazole (Monistat) | |

Antifungal medications are prepared in a variety of forms, depending on the specific drug: powders, creams, shampoos, suspensions, troches, vaginal suppositories, and oral tablets. Some drugs interfere with the permeability of the fungal cell membrane; others interfere with DNA synthesis. Most of these medications are fungistatic but in large doses they may be fungicidal.

#### Nursing Responsibilities

- When taking the health history, ask about known hypersensitivity reactions to these agents; document carefully.
- Assess for side effects: skin rash, local irritation, gastrointestinal symptoms (if given PO), and mental status.
- Administer ketoconazole with food to minimize gastrointestinal irritation.
- Shake suspensions well before administration, and ask the client to swish them around the mouth before swallowing.
- Tell the client to allow oral tablets to dissolve in the mouth.

#### Client and Family Teaching

- Therapy usually continues over a long period of time, but regular use of medications for the recommended period is necessary. Do not miss doses, and complete the full treatment.
- For griseofulvin: Take with meals or foods high in fat (such as ice cream) to avoid stomach upset and help with absorption. Avoid alcohol (which may cause rapid pulse and flushing) and exposure to sunlight (this drug causes increased sensitivity).
- For nystatin: Dissolve lozenges completely in the mouth. Hold suspensions in the mouth and swish throughout the mouth as long as possible before swallowing. Insert intravaginal medication high in the vagina. Continue with intravaginal applications throughout the menses.
- For antifungal shampoo: Use two times a week for 4 weeks, allowing at least 3 days between each shampoo. Wet hair, apply shampoo to produce lather, leave in place for 1 minute, then rinse. Apply shampoo a second time, lather, leave in place for 3 minutes, then rinse thoroughly.
- For topical application: Rub well into the affected areas, but do not get the medication in your eyes.
- For vaginal candidiasis infections: During therapy, refrain from sexual intercourse or advise partner to use a condom.
- Your sexual partner will need to be treated at the same time so that you do not pass the infection back and forth to each other.

---

- Tinea capitis is treated by shampooing the hair two to three times a week, applying a topical antifungal to inactivate organisms on the hair, and taking griseofulvin (Fulvicin), an antifungal agent, orally.
- Tinea pedis is treated by soaking the feet in Burrow's solution, potassium permanganate solution, or saline solution to remove crusts and scales. Topical antifungals are applied to the infected areas for several weeks.
- Mild cases of tinea cruris are treated with topical medications for 3 to 4 weeks. More severe cases may require oral griseofulvin.

Candidiasis infections are treated, depending on the location, with oral medication or with powder or vaginal suppositories. Nystatin (Mycostatin) is an antibiotic effective in controlling the infection. Fluconazole (Diflucan), an oral antifungal agent, is also effective.

## NURSING CARE

Many people treat themselves with over-the-counter antifungal medications. It is recommended, however, that the person be professionally diagnosed the first time the infection occurs. If symptoms reappear, self-treatment is usually satisfactory. The interventions discussed for nursing care of the client with a bacterial infection are also appropriate for the client with a fungal infection. Teaching topics specific to fungal infections are as follows:

- Fungal diseases are contagious. Do not share linens or personal items with others.
- Use a clean towel and washcloth each day.
- Carefully dry all skinfolds, including those under the breasts, under the arms, and between the toes.
- Wear clean cotton underclothing each day.
- Fungi grow in moist environments, such as on sweaty feet. To prevent further infections:
  - Do not wear the same pair of shoes every day.
  - Wear socks that permit moisture to wick away from the skin surface.
  - Do not wear rubber- or plastic-soled shoes.
  - Use talcum powder or an over-the-counter antifungal powder twice a day.
- For vaginal *Candida albicans* infection:
  - Avoid tight clothing, such as jeans and pantyhose.
  - Wear cotton or cotton-crotch underwear.
  - Bathe more frequently, and dry the genital area well.
  - Have your sexual partner treated at the same time to avoid passing the infection back and forth to each other.

**PRACTICE ALERT** *Recommend the client have a blood glucose test for repeated infections, as they may indicate diabetes mellitus.* ∎

## THE CLIENT WITH A PARASITIC INFESTATION

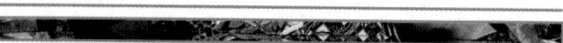

Infestations of the skin by parasites are more common in developing countries but may occur in any geographic area of the world. They affect people of all social classes but are associated with crowded or unsanitary living conditions.

## PATHOPHYSIOLOGY

Two of the more common parasitic infestations of the skin are caused by lice and mites. These parasites do not normally live on the skin, but infest the skin through contact with an infested person or contact with clothing, linens, or objects infested with the parasites.

### Pediculosis

Pediculosis is an infestation with lice. Lice are parasites that live on the blood of an animal or human host. The louse is a 2- to 4-mm oval organism with a stylet that pierces the skin; an anticoagulant in its saliva prevents host blood from clotting while it eats. The female louse lays its eggs (small pearl-gray or brown eggs, called nits) on hair shafts. The louse within the egg hatches, reaches the adult reproductive stage, and dies in 30 to 50 days (Porth, 2002).

There are three types of human pediculosis:

- **Pediculosis corporis** is an infestation with body lice. This type of infestation is more common in people who do not have access to facilities for bathing or washing clothes, such as the homeless. The lice live in clothing fibers and are transmitted primarily by contact with infested clothing and bed linens. The skin lesions occur at the site of a louse bite; macules appear initially, followed by wheals and papules. Pruritus is common, and scratching often results in linear excoriations. Secondary infections cause hyperpigmentation and scarring. The lesions are most often seen on the shoulders, trunk, and buttocks.
- **Pediculosis pubis** is an infestation with pubic lice (often called crabs). This infestation is spread through sexual activity with someone already infested or by contact with infested clothing or linens. The lice are found in the pubic region and occasionally spread to the axillae or men's beards. The lice cause skin irritation and intense itching.
- **Pediculosis capitis** is an infestation with head lice. This infestation primarily affects Caucasians and is more common in female children. The lice are most often found behind the ears and at the nape of the neck but may also spread to other hairy areas of the body: the eyebrows, pubic area, or beard. The lice are transmitted by contact with an infected person. Manifestations of head lice include pruritus, scratching, and erythema of the scalp. If untreated, the hair appears matted and crusted with a foul-smelling substance.

### Scabies

**Scabies** is a parasitic infestation caused by a mite (Sarcoptes scabiei). The pregnant female mite burrows into the skin and lays two to three eggs each day for about a month. The eggs hatch in 3 to 5 days, and the larvae migrate to the surface of the skin but burrow into the skin for food or protection. The larvae develop, and the cycle repeats. Scabies infestation affects people of all socioeconomic classes. Formerly it was seen most often in times of war or famine, but it has become more common as a result of international travel and sexual activity. The infestation is found in webs between the fingers, the inner surfaces of the wrist and elbow, the axillae, the female nipple, the penis, the belt line, and the gluteal crease. The lesions are a small redbrown burrow, about 2 mm in length, sometimes covered with vesicles, which appears as a rash. Pruritus in response to the mite or its feces is common, especially at night, and excoriations may develop. The excoriations predispose the person to secondary bacterial infections.

## COLLABORATIVE CARE

Parasitic infestations are diagnosed by identifying the organism and are treated with medications that kill the lice or mites.

### Diagnostic Tests

- When a client exhibits manifestations of pediculosis, the hair shaft and the clothing are examined to identify the lice or the nits. Microscopic examination of the parasite provides a positive diagnosis.
- Scabies is diagnosed by skin scrapings and microscopic examination for the mites or their feces.

### Medications

Lice are eradicated with agents that kill the parasite. Infestations of the body and pubic area are treated with topical medications that contain gamma benzene hexachloride, malathion (Prioderm lotion), or permethrin (NIX).

Infestations of the head are treated with shampoos containing lindane, such as Kwell. The shampoo is applied to dry hair and massaged in. A small amount of water is added to produce a lather, and the head is scrubbed for 4 minutes, then rinsed. The treatment may need to be repeated in a week to kill newly hatched lice. A fine-toothed comb can be used to comb the dead nits off the hair shaft. Infestations of the eyebrows are treated by applying a thick covering of petroleum jelly for several days.

Scabies may be eradicated by a single treatment of lindane lotion or Kwell applied to the entire skin surface for 12 hours.

The associated itching is treated with systemic or topical medications, including corticosteroids. Secondary bacterial infections are treated with the appropriate antibiotic.

## NURSING CARE

Nursing care for clients with a parasite infestation most often focuses on teaching to prevent infestation or to eradicate an existing infestation. For a hospitalized client with pediculosis, isolation procedures are instituted until the client no longer has the infestation.

Client and family teaching is necessary to facilitate treatment at home, to prevent the spread of the infestation, and to dispel the myth that lice infest only people with poor hygiene or in dirty living conditions. Specific information includes the following:

- Wash clothing and linens in soap and hot water, or have them dry cleaned.
- Ironing the clothes kills any lice eggs.
- Personal care items, such as combs or brushes, may be boiled to kill the parasites.
- All family members and sexual partners must also be treated.
- Avoid using the combs, brushes, or hats of others.
- Lice and mites may infest anyone.

## THE CLIENT WITH A VIRAL INFECTION OF THE SKIN

Viruses are pathogens that consist of an RNA or DNA core surrounded by a protein coat. They depend on live cells for reproduction and so are classified as intracellular pathogens. The viruses that cause skin lesions invade the keratinocyte, reproduce, and either increase cellular growth or cause cellular death.

An increase in the incidence of viral skin disorders has been attributed to a variety of causes. Some commonly used drugs, such as birth control medications and corticosteroids, are known to have immunosuppressive properties that allow the viruses to multiply. Other drugs, such as antibiotics, kill off normal skin bacteria that would otherwise serve as defense against viral infections.

### PATHOPHYSIOLOGY

Viral infections cause many different kinds of skin disorders, including warts, herpes simplex infections, and herpes zoster infections.

### Warts

**Warts,** or *verrucae,* are lesions of the skin caused by the human papillomavirus (HPV). Over 60 types of HPVs are found on the human skin and mucous membranes (Porth, 2002). Warts may be found on nongenital skin or genital skin and mucous membranes. Nongenital warts are benign lesions; genital warts may be precancerous. Warts are transmitted through skin contact. Wart lesions may be flat, fusiform (tapered at both ends), or round, but most are round and raised and have a rough, gray surface. There are many different types of warts; location and appearance of the warts depend on the causative virus. Those most common are as follows:

- A common wart (*verruca vulgaris*) may appear anywhere on the skin and mucous membranes of the body; most commonly appear on the fingers. Common warts grow above the skin surface and may be dome-shaped with ragged borders (Figure 14–14 ■).
- *Plantar warts* occur at pressure points on the soles of the feet. The pressure of shoes and walking prevents these warts

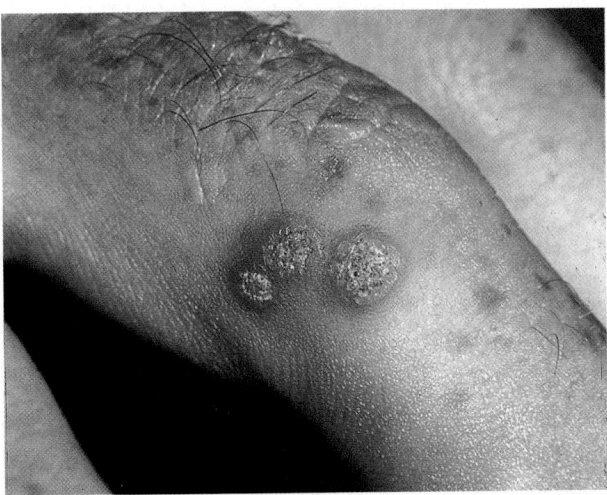

**Figure 14–14 ■** The common wart is a lesion of the skin caused by a virus. It commonly appears as a raised, dome-shaped lesion.

Source: Camera M. D. Studios. Carroll H. Weiss, Director. 8290 N. W. 26th Place. Sunrise, FL 33322.

from growing outward, so they tend to extend deeper beneath the skin surface than do common warts. Plantar warts are often painful.
- A flat wart (*verruca plana*) is a small flat lesion, usually seen on the forehead or dorsum of the hand.
- *Condylomata acuminata,* also called venereal warts, occur in moist areas, along the glans of the penis, in the anal region, and on the vulva. They are usually cauliflowerlike in appearance and have a pink or purple color.

Warts resolve spontaneously when immunity to the virus develops. This response may take up to 5 years.

### Herpes Simplex

**Herpes simplex** (also called a **fever blister** or **cold sore**) virus infections of the skin and mucous membranes are caused by two types of herpesvirus: HSV I and HSV II. Most infections above the waist are caused by HSV I, with herpes simplex lesions most often found on the lips, face, and mouth. (Genital herpes infections, which result from either HSV I or HSV II, are classified as sexually transmitted diseases and are discussed in Chapter 49.) ⊂⊃ The virus may be transmitted by physical contact, oral sex, or kissing.

The infection begins with a burning or tingling sensation, followed by the development of erythema, vesicle formation, and pain (Figure 14–15 ■). The vesicles progress through pustules, ulcers, and crusting until healing occurs in 10 to 14 days.

The initial infection is often severe and accompanied by systemic manifestations, such as fever and sore throat; recurrences are more localized and less severe. The virus lives in nerve ganglia and may cause recurrent lesions in response to sunlight, menstruation, injury, or stress. Oral acyclovir may be used prophylactically to prevent reoccurrences and to treat recurrent outbreaks.

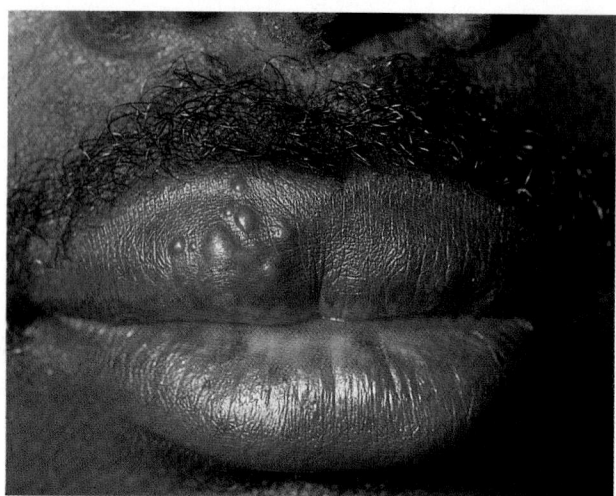

**Figure 14–15** ■ Herpes simplex is a viral infection of the skin and mucous membranes. This client has lesions in the early stage, with erythema and vesicles.

*Source: Camera M. D. Studios. Carroll H. Weiss, Director. 8290 N. W. 26th Place. Sunrise, FL 33322.*

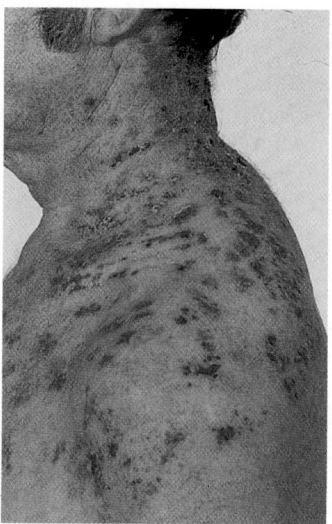

**Figure 14–16** ■ Herpes zoster is a viral infection of a dermatome section of the skin. The typical lesions are painful vesicles lying along the path of the nerve.

*Source: Custom Medical Stock, Inc.*

## Herpes Zoster

**Herpes zoster,** also called **shingles,** is a viral infection of a dermatome section of the skin caused by varicella zoster (the herpesvirus that also causes chickenpox). The infection is believed to result from reactivation of a varicella virus remaining in the sensory dorsal ganglia after a childhood infection of chickenpox. When reactivated, the virus travels from the ganglia to the corresponding skin dermatome area.

Herpes zoster affects an estimated 10% to 20% of the population, most often adults over the age of 50. Clients with Hodgkin's disease, certain types of leukemia, and lymphomas are more susceptible to an outbreak of the disease. Herpes zoster is more prevalent in immunocompromised people, such as those with HIV infections, those receiving radiation therapy or chemotherapy, and those who have had major organ transplants. The appearance of the lesions in people with HIV infections may be one of the first manifestations of immune compromise.

### MANIFESTATIONS AND COMPLICATIONS

Herpes zoster lesions are vesicles with an erythematous base. The vesicles appear on the skin area supplied by the neurons of a single or associated group of dorsal root ganglia (although they may occur beyond this area in immunosuppressed people). The lesions usually appear unilaterally on the face, trunk, and thorax (Figure 14–16 ■). New lesions continue to erupt for 3 to 5 days, then crust and dry. Recovery occurs in 2 to 3 weeks. The client often experiences severe pain for up to 48 hours before and during eruption of the lesions. The pain may continue after the lesions have disappeared. The older adult is especially sensitive to the pain and often experiences more severe outbreaks of herpes zoster lesions.

Complications of herpes zoster include postherpetic neuralgia (a sharp, spasmodic pain along the course of one or more

nerves) and visual loss. The neuralgia, described as burning or stabbing, results from inflammation of the root ganglia. This complication is more common in clients over the age of 55 (Tierney, McPhee, & Papadakis, 2001). Permanent loss of vision may follow occurrence of lesions that arise from the ophthalmic division of the trigeminal nerve. The disease may disseminate in immunocompromised clients, causing lesions beyond the dermatome, visceral lesions, and encephalitis. This serious complication may cause death.

## COLLABORATIVE CARE

The treatment for viral skin infections focuses on stopping viral replication and treating client responses, such as itching and pain.

### Diagnostic Tests

Although diagnosis is usually based on manifestations and appearance of the lesions, laboratory tests may be necessary to differentiate herpes zoster from impetigo, contact dermatitis, and herpes simplex. The laboratory tests include the following:

- A Tzanck smear identifies the herpes virus, but it does not distinguish herpes zoster from herpes simplex. This is a microscopic examination of cells from the base of the lesion.
- Cultures of fluid from the vesicles and antibody tests are used to make the differential diagnosis of herpesvirus types.
- Immunofluorescent methods can identify varicella in skin cells.

### Medications

Most viral skin disorders are treated with antiviral medications, and other types of medications are used to relieve pruritus and pain in clients with herpes zoster.

- *Warts.* Depending on their size, location, and any associated discomfort, warts may be treated with medications, cryotherapy, or electrodesiccation and curettage. A common method of wart removal is acid therapy, using a colloidal solution of 16% salicylic acid and 16% lactic acid. The solution is applied to the wart every 12 to 24 hours; the wart disappears in 2 to 3 weeks. Other methods of eradicating warts are cryosurgery, freezing with liquid nitrogen, and electrodesiccation of the wart with an electric current followed by excision of the dead tissue. Venereal warts are further described in Chapter 49. ⬤

- *Herpes simplex.* Herpes simplex lesions are treated with acyclovir (Zovirax), an antifungal agent. Acyclovir shortens the time of symptoms and speeds healing. Other antiviral mediations are discussed with herpes zoster.

- *Herpes zoster.* Antiviral drugs are used to treat herpes zoster infections. Acyclovir (Zovirax) interferes with viral synthesis and replication. Although it does not cure herpes infections, it does decrease the severity of the illness and also decreases pain. It may be administered topically, orally, or parenterally. It is more effective if administration begins within the first 1 to 2 days after the first vesicles appear. Acyclovir has little effect on postherpetic neuralgia. Famciclovir (Famvir) may have an advantage over acyclovir as it is more intracellularly stable in infected cells, inhibits DNA synthesis in infected cells, and has longer-lasting antiviral activity. Valacyclovir (Valtrex) is an antiviral agent that is hydrolyzed to acyclovir in the intestinal wall or liver, resulting in a higher plasma level that acyclovir when both are taken orally. Another antiviral drug that may be prescribed is vidarabine (Ara-A, Vira-A). This drug is given either by intravenous infusion or as an ophthalmic ointment.

Narcotic and nonnarcotic analgesics are prescribed for pain management, and antihistamines may be administered for relief of pruritus. Clients with eye involvement are treated with topical steroid ophthalmic ointments and mydriatics. Antivirals may sometimes be administered.

## NURSING CARE

This section discusses care of the client with herpes zoster, focusing on the nursing diagnoses of acute pain, sleep pattern disturbance, and risk for infection.

## Nursing Diagnoses and Interventions

### Acute Pain

The client with herpes zoster often experiences severe pain over the entire dermatome supplied by the affected nerve root. The pain is described as burning, tearing, or stabbing. The client may avoid movement and does not want clothing or bed linens to touch the affected area.

- Monitor the location, duration, and intensity of the pain. *Each person experiences and expresses pain in his or her own manner. Pain tolerance is also individual. Accurate as-*sessment of the client's perception and tolerance of pain is essential in facilitating pain management.

- Explain the rationale for taking prescribed medications on a regular schedule. *Delaying or withholding medications may allow the pain to reach an intensity at which the medication is less effective in promoting relief.*

- Teach measures to relieve pruritus:
  - Take prescribed antipruritic medications.
  - Apply calamine lotion or wet compresses, if prescribed.
  - Keep the room temperature cool.
  - Use a bed cradle to keep sheets off affected areas of the body.

*Pruritus is a common problem for clients with herpes zoster; scratching may excoriate the skin and increase the risk for secondary infections. Pruritus may intensify the experience of pain. Lotions and cool, wet compresses are effective in decreasing the itch-scratch-itch cycle. Warmth and touch intensify pruritus.*

- Encourage the use of distraction (such as music) or a specific relaxation technique (such as progressive muscle relaxation or deep breathing). *Noninvasive methods to relieve pain not only help the client manage the pain experience but also increase the effectiveness of pain medications.*

### Disturbed Sleep Pattern

The pain and pruritus of herpes zoster interferes with normal sleep patterns. Those responses often are more intense at night, probably as a result of decreased distraction.

- Use appropriate measures to relieve pain and pruritus (as described above). *Pain and pruritus interfere with normal sleep. Analgesics and noninvasive methods of relief may be necessary before the client prepares for sleep.*

- Maintain a cool environment and avoid heavy bed covering. *Heat and touch intensify pruritus. Pruritus stimulates scratching, which awakens the client. The client may then perceive the pain more acutely. A cycle is established that interferes with sleep.*

### Risk for Infection

Clients with herpes zoster have impaired skin integrity and pruritus with scratching and possible excoriation; moreover, they may be immunocompromised. All of these factors contribute to a high risk for secondary bacterial infection. In addition, the client is contagious to others who did not have chickenpox as children.

- Teach client the manifestations of infection:
  - Increased temperature
  - Increased redness, formation of pustules, and/or purulent drainage
  - Monitoring white blood cell count
  - Assessing for lymph gland enlargement

*Secondary bacterial infections may occur in any client with impaired skin integrity; if the client is immunocompromised, the risk is even greater. Fever, changes in lesions or drainage, an increased white blood cell count, and lymph gland enlargement are manifestations of an infection.*

- Teach interventions to decrease the itch-scratch-itch cycle, thereby decreasing the possibility of excoriation (see discussion about nursing care of clients with pruritus and psoriasis, earlier in this chapter). *Excoriation from scratching provides an avenue for bacterial invasion.*
- Institute infection control procedures for clients who are hospitalized:
  - Maintain strict isolation for immunocompromised clients.
  - Wear gloves and gown if contact with lesions is likely.
  - Instruct pregnant women to avoid exposure until lesions have crusted over.

*Isolation procedures are instituted for the immunocompromised client to prevent client infection. Wear gloves and gown to prevent spreading the infection to self or others.*

**PRACTICE ALERT** *Pregnant women must avoid exposure because the herpesvirus can cross the placental barrier.* ■

## Using NANDA, NIC, and NOC

Chart 14-1 shows links between NANDA, NIC, and NOC when caring for the client with herpes zoster.

## Home Care

Because most clients with viral infections provide self-care at home, the nurse focuses on teaching the client and family how to provide the necessary care. With herpes zoster increasing in incidence in clients who are older or have a serious chronic illness, it may also be necessary to make a referral to a community health provider for continued support. Provide the following information and instructions:

- The diseases are usually self-limiting and heal completely. Second occurrences of herpes zoster are rare.
- Do not have social contact with children or pregnant women until crusts have formed over the blistered areas with herpes zoster, as the disease is contagious to people who have not had chickenpox.
- Use pain medications regularly.
- Follow suggestions to help reduce itching, scratching, and pain: Use medications as prescribed, wear lightweight cotton clothing, keep room temperatures cool, wear cotton gloves at night if scratching is a problem, and practice relaxation and distraction activities.
- Report any increase in pain, fever, chills, drainage that smells bad and has pus, or a spread in the blisters to your health care provider.

## CHART 14–1 NANDA, NIC, AND NOC LINKAGES

### The Client with Herpes Zoster

| NURSING DIAGNOSES | NURSING INTERVENTIONS | NURSING OUTCOMES |
|---|---|---|
| • Impaired Skin Integrity | • Skin Surveillance<br>• Medication Administration<br>• Infection Control | • Tissue Integrity: Skin and Mucous Membranes |
| • Disturbed Sleep Pattern | • Sleep Enhancement<br>• Pain Management | • Pain Level<br>• Pain Control Behavior |
| • Acute Pain | • Analgesia Administration<br>• Environmental Management: Comfort | • Pain Level<br>• Symptom Severity |

*Note. Data from Nursing Outcomes Classification (NOC) by M. Johnson & M. Maas (Eds.), 1997, St. Louis: Mosby; Nursing Diagnoses: Definitions & Classification 2001–2002 by North American Nursing Diagnosis Association, 2001, Philadelphia: NANDA; Nursing Interventions Classification (NIC) by J.C. McCloskey & G. M. Bulechek (Eds.), 2000, St. Louis: Mosby. Reprinted by permission.*

# INFLAMMATORY DISORDERS OF THE SKIN

Inflammatory skin disorders are rarely associated with systemic manifestations. The inflammatory skin disorders discussed in this section include dermatitis, acne, pemphigus, lichen planus, and toxic epidermal necrolysis.

## THE CLIENT WITH DERMATITIS

**Dermatitis** is an inflammation of the skin characterized by erythema and pain or pruritus. Dermatitis may be acute or chronic.

## PATHOPHYSIOLOGY

In dermatitis, various exogenous and endogenous agents cause an inflammatory response of the skin. Different types of skin eruptions occur, often specific to the causative allergen, infection, or disease. The initial skin responses to these agents or illnesses include erythema, formation of vesicles and scales, and pruritus (Figure 14–17 ■). Subsequently, irritation from scratching promotes edema, a serous discharge, and crusting. Long-term irritation in chronic dermatitis causes the

## Nursing Care Plan
## A Client with Herpes Zoster

Jesus Rivera is a 34-year-old migrant farm worker who currently lives in temporary housing in a rural area of the southwestern United States. His family includes his wife, Marta, who is 3 months' pregnant, and two children, ages 3 and 5. He takes his wife to a medical clinic staffed by volunteer nurses, physicians, and students from a nearby university for a prenatal checkup. The clinic is open only on Saturday and provides care on a sliding fee scale or for free if the family is unable to pay. While Mrs. Rivera is being examined, Mr. Rivera asks the nurse to have someone look at some very painful blisters on his chest that developed about a week ago. He is afraid that exposure to pesticides has caused the sores.

### ASSESSMENT

Mr. Rivera speaks Spanish and is able to communicate only slightly in English. The initial assessment of Mr. Rivera is performed by Anita Mendez, a student nurse fluent in Spanish. Mr. Rivera's history reveals problems with lower back pain but no significant past medical illnesses. He is not aware of any allergies and cannot remember having had chickenpox as a child. Two years ago, both children were sick and had blisters on their bodies, and a friend told them it was chickenpox. Mrs. Rivera thinks she had chickenpox as a child.

Because Mr. Rivera has not had any medical care for several years, baseline laboratory tests are ordered to screen for any other illnesses; the complete blood count (CBC), blood chemistry, and urinalysis are all within normal limits.

Mr. Rivera says that he did not feel well for several days before the blisters appeared, having experienced chills and general achiness. He had not taken his temperature because the family does not own a thermometer. Current vital signs are as follows: T 99°F (37.2°C), p 74, R 22, and BP 148/88.

Physical examination of the trunk reveals a bandlike pattern of lesions across the left thorax. Some of the lesions are vesicles filled with serous fluid; others are darker in color and are oozing a light yellow drainage. The skin around the lesions is red and inflamed. Mr. Rivera complains of a severe, burning pain with itching across his chest. He is diagnosed with herpes zoster.

### DIAGNOSIS

- *Risk for infection* related to open oozing areas on the left thorax
- *Acute pain* related to the presence of lesions and pruritus
- *Deficient knowledge* of the cause of the skin disorder and recommended treatment
- *Anxiety* related to need to work in areas of pesticide application
- *Altered health maintenance* related to limited access to health care, transitory work conditions, and cultural and language barriers

### EXPECTED OUTCOMES

- Skin lesions will heal without evidence of a secondary infection.
- Limit exposure (as much as possible) to his wife and children and to persons with debilitating illnesses to prevent the spread of the virus.
- Obtain relief of pain and pruritus with the proper use of medications.
- Verbalize an understanding of the disease process and participate in the treatment plan.

- Obtain follow-up care.
- Make an appointment for a referral for information about occupational hazards.

### PLANNING AND IMPLEMENTATION

- Provide verbal and written instructions (in Spanish) for self-care:
  - Wear a clean cotton undershirt each day.
  - Trim the fingernails short, and keep the hands clean.
  - Wash the hands each time the area is touched.
  - Wash any soiled clothes or linens in hot water and soap.
  - Do not allow other family members to use your towels.
  - Take medications as prescribed for itching and pain.
  - Take the medicine for your sores every 4 hours, even during nighttime hours, for 7 days.
  - As much as possible, do not touch your wife and children until the sores are covered with scabs. Do not have sex with your wife while you have these sores.
- Teach how to take care of skin lesions:
  - Wear the rubber gloves every time you do this treatment.
  - Wash the sores and the skin around them very gently with a soft washcloth and a mild soap.
  - Using your fingers, carefully rub the cream on the sores. Do this once every morning after breakfast and once every evening after supper.
  - Wash your hands carefully before and after each treatment.
- Make a follow-up appointment for the next week.
- Provide Mr. Rivera with the name and phone number of the Occupational Safety and Health Administration (OSHA) and recommend he call for an appointment to discuss his concerns about pesticides.

### EVALUATION

Mrs. Rivera explains how she has taken care of her husband, and Mr. Rivera is careful to describe how he has followed the nurse's instructions. The skin lesions are dry and crusty, with no new blister formation. Mr. Rivera says he has not called OSHA and is not sure that he will, but he thanks Miss Mendez for the phone number. The nurses make an appointment in 1 month for a prenatal checkup for Mrs. Rivera and for follow-up of Mr. Rivera's herpes zoster. Mr. Rivera promises to return if they are still living close enough to keep the appointment.

### Critical Thinking in the Nursing Process

1. Identify barriers to care present in this case study. How may nursing interventions promote health care delivery to disadvantaged populations?
2. Although most cases of herpes zoster are self-limiting, what further assessments and interventions might have been indicated had the lesions shown little improvement over time and/or the pain remained severe?
3. If Mr. Rivera is advised not to work until his lesions heal, the family may face economic and sociocultural hardships. Develop a plan of care for Mr. Rivera for the nursing diagnosis *Ineffective role performance.*

See Evaluating Your Response in Appendix C.

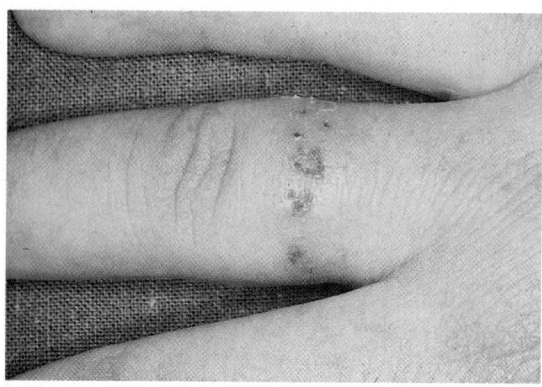

**Figure 14–17** ■ Inflammation of the skin, or dermatitis, may be a response to allergens, infections, or chemicals. This client has contact dermatitis resulting from the metal salts in jewelry.

*Source: Biophoto Associates/Photo Researchers, Inc.*

skin to become thickened and leathery (a condition called *lichenification*) and darker in color.

## Contact Dermatitis

**Contact dermatitis** is a type of dermatitis caused by a hypersensitivity response or chemical irritation. The major sources known to cause contact dermatitis are dyes, perfumes, poison plants (ivy, oak, sumac), chemicals, and metals (Box 14–2). A contact dermatitis common in the health care field is latex (glove) dermatitis.

Allergic contact dermatitis is a cell-mediated or delayed hypersensitivity to a wide variety of allergens. Sensitizing antigens include microorganisms, plants, chemicals, drugs, metals, or foreign proteins. On initial contact with the skin, the allergen binds to a carrier protein, forming a sensitizing antigen. The antigen is processed and carried to the T cells, which in turn become sensitized to the antigen. The first exposure is the sensitizing contact; skin manifestations occur with subsequent exposures. These manifestations include erythema, swelling, and pruritic

vesicles in the area of allergen contact. For example, a person hypersensitive to metal may have lesions under a ring or watch.

Irritant contact dermatitis is an inflammation of the skin from irritants; it is not a hypersensitivity response. Common sources of irritant contact dermatitis include chemicals (such as acids), soaps, and detergents. The skin lesions are similar to those seen in allergic contact dermatitis.

## Atopic Dermatitis

**Atopic dermatitis** is an inflammatory skin disorder that is also called **eczema.** The exact cause is unknown, but related factors include depressed cell-mediated immunity, elevated IgE levels, and increased histamine sensitivity. The disorder is seen more often in children, but chronic forms persist throughout life.

Clients with atopic dermatitis have a family history of hypersensitivity reactions, such as dry skin, eczema, asthma, and allergic rhinitis. Although up to one-third of clients with atopic dermatitis also have food allergies, a positive correlation has not been found.

The dermatitis results when mast cells, T lymphocytes, monocytes, and other inflammatory cells are activated and release histamine, lymphokines, and other inflammatory mediators. The immune response interacts with the allergen to create a chronic inflammatory condition. In the adult form of atopic dermatitis, characteristic lesions include chronic lichenification, erythema, and scaling, the result of pruritus and scratching. The lesions are usually found on the hands, feet, or flexor surfaces of the arms and legs (Figure 14–18 ■). Scratching and excoriation increase the risk of secondary infections, as well as invasion of the skin by viruses such as herpes simplex.

## Seborrheic Dermatitis

**Seborrheic dermatitis** is a chronic inflammatory disorder of the skin that involves the scalp, eyebrows, eyelids, ear canals, nasolabial folds, axillae, and trunk. The cause is unknown. This disorder is seen in all ages, from the very young (called "cradle cap") to the very old. Clients taking methyldopa (Aldomet) for hypertension occasionally develop this disorder, and it is a component of Parkinson's disease. Seborrheic dermatitis is also frequently seen in clients with AIDS.

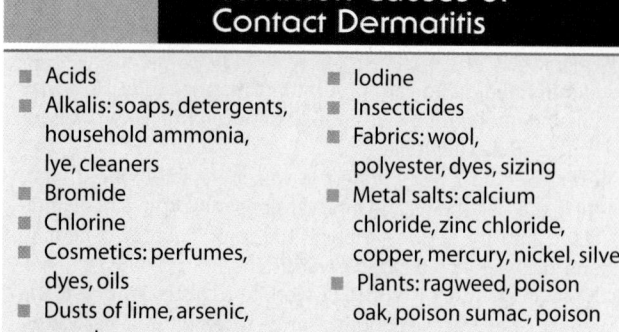

| BOX 14–2 | ■ Common Causes of Contact Dermatitis |
| --- | --- |

- Acids
- Alkalis: soaps, detergents, household ammonia, lye, cleaners
- Bromide
- Chlorine
- Cosmetics: perfumes, dyes, oils
- Dusts of lime, arsenic, wood
- Hydrocarbons: crude petroleum, lubricating oil, mineral oil, paraffin, asphalt, tar
- Iodine
- Insecticides
- Fabrics: wool, polyester, dyes, sizing
- Metal salts: calcium chloride, zinc chloride, copper, mercury, nickel, silver
- Plants: ragweed, poison oak, poison sumac, poison ivy, pine
- Coloring agents
- Rubber products
- Soot

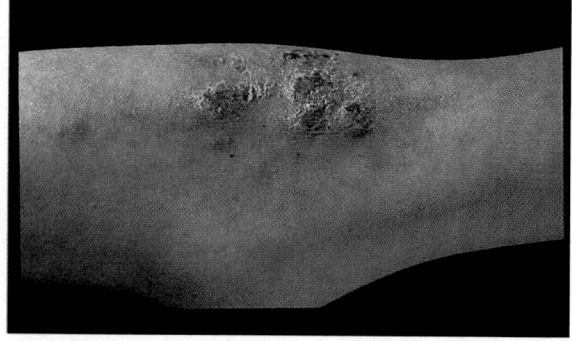

**Figure 14–18** ■ Atopic dermatitis, or eczema, causes pruritus, resulting in lichenification, erythema, and scaling.

*Source: NMSB/Custom Medical Stock Photo.*

The lesions are yellow or white plaques with scales and crusts. The scales are often yellow or orange and have a greasy appearance. Mild pruritus is also present. Diffuse dandruff with erythema of the scalp often accompanies the skin lesions.

## Exfoliative Dermatitis

**Exfoliative dermatitis** is an inflammatory skin disorder characterized by excessive peeling or shedding of skin. The cause is unknown in about half of all cases, but a preexisting skin disorder (such as psoriasis, atopic dermatitis, contact dermatitis, or seborrheic dermatitis) is found in about 40% of the cases (Tierney et al., 2001). Exfoliative dermatitis is also associated with leukemia and lymphoma.

Both systemic and localized manifestations may appear. Systemic manifestations include weakness, malaise, fever, chills, and weight loss. Scaling, erythema, and pruritus may be localized or involve the entire body (Figure 14–19 ■). In addition to peeling of skin, the client may lose the hair and nails.

Generalized exfoliative dermatitis may cause debility and dehydration. The impairment of skin integrity increases the risk for local and systemic infections.

## COLLABORATIVE CARE

The client with dermatitis is treated primarily with topical medications and therapeutic baths. If the dermatitis is due to hypersensitivity to an allergen, the client avoids exposure to environmental irritants and suspected foods. The client also discontinues as many medications as possible to determine whether the dermatitis is the result of a drug allergy.

### Diagnostic Tests

The diagnosis is often based on the manifestations of the disorder. Diagnostic tests may include the following:

- Scratch tests and intradermal tests are conducted to identify a specific allergen.
- Serum studies may find elevated eosinophil and IgE levels in atopic dermatitis.
- Skin biopsy may reveal specific changes in inflammatory dermatitis.

### Medications

The medications used depend on the cause of the dermatitis and the severity of the manifestations. Minor cases are treated with antipruritic medications, whereas more severe cases are treated with oral antihistamines, oral and/or topical corticosteroids, and wet dressings. Topical anti-infectives may be prescribed if necessary.

## NURSING CARE

Nursing care of the client with dermatitis focuses primarily on providing information for self-care at home. The client is responsible for managing skin problems and requires education and support. Address the following topics:

- Medications and treatments do not cure the disease; they only relieve the symptoms.
- Dry skin increases pruritus, which stimulates scratching. Scratching may in turn cause excoriation, and excoriation increases the risk of infection.
- It may be necessary to change the diet or environment to avoid contact with allergens.
- When using steroid preparations, apply only a thin layer to slightly damp skin (e.g., after taking a bath).
- If occlusive dressings are necessary, a plastic suit may be used.
- When using oral corticosteroids, never abruptly stop taking the medication. Rather, follow instructions to taper the dosage gradually.
- Antihistamines cause drowsiness. When using these medications, avoid alcohol and use caution when driving or working around machinery.

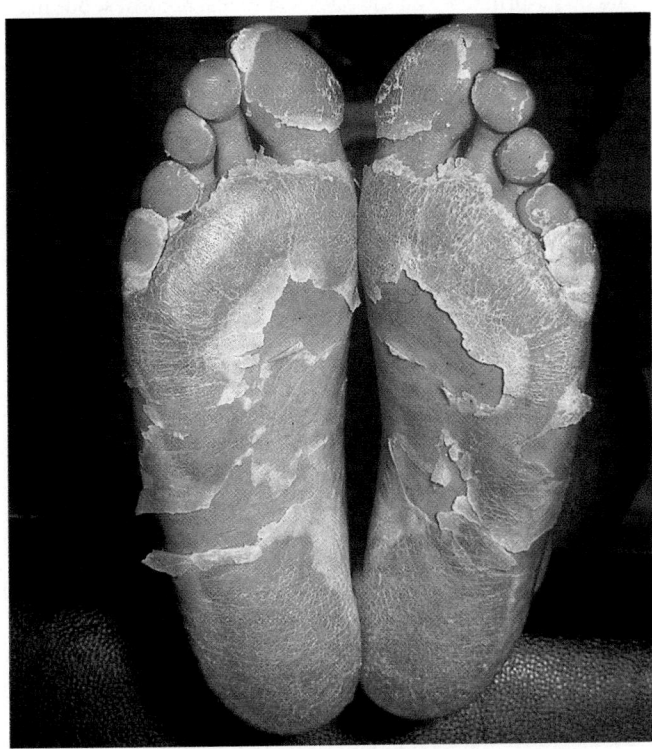

**Figure 14–19** ■ Exfoliative dermatitis is an inflammatory skin disorder causing excessive skin peeling.

*Source: Camera M. D. Studios. Carroll H. Weiss, Director. 8290 N. W. 26th Place. Sunrise, FL 33322.*

## THE CLIENT WITH ACNE

**Acne** is a disorder of the pilosebaceous (hair and sebaceous gland) structure, which opens to the skin surface through a pore. The sebaceous glands, which empty directly into the hair follicle, produce sebum, a lipid substance. Sebaceous glands are present over the entire skin surface except the soles of the feet and the palms of the hands, but the largest glands are on the face, scalp, and scrotum. Sebum production is a response to direct hormonal stimulation by testicular androgens in men and adrenal and ovarian androgens in women.

## PATHOPHYSIOLOGY

Acne may be noninflammatory or inflammatory. Noninflammatory acne lesions are primarily *comedones,* more commonly called pimples, whiteheads, and blackheads. Whiteheads are pale, slightly elevated papules categorized as closed comedones (Figure 14–20A ■). Blackheads are plugs of material that accumulate in the sebaceous glands. They are categorized as open comedones. The color is the result of the movement of melanin into the plug from surrounding epidermal cells. Inflammatory acne lesions include comedones, erythematous pustules, and cysts (Figure 14–20B). Inflammation close to the skin surface results in pustules; deeper inflammation results in cysts. The inflammation is believed to result from irritation from fatty acid constituents of the sebum and from substances produced by *Propionibacterium acnes* bacteria, both of which escape into the dermis when the follicular wall of closed comedones ruptures.

Several forms of acne occur at different periods of the life span. The most common are acne vulgaris, acne rosacea, and acne conglobata.

### Acne Vulgaris

Acne vulgaris is the form of acne common in adolescents and young to middle adults. Although the lesions may persist longer in women, the incidence is greater in men. The actual cause of acne vulgaris is unknown. Possible causes include androgenic influence on the sebaceous glands, increased sebum production, and proliferation of the organism *Propionibacterium acnes.* Many factors once thought to cause acne vulgaris, including high-fat diets, chocolate, infections, and cosmetics, have been disproved (Porth, 2002).

Mild cases may involve only a few scattered comedones, but severe cases are manifested by multiple lesions of all types. Most acne vulgaris lesions form on the face and neck, but they also occur on the back, chest, and shoulders. The lesions are usually mildly painful and may itch. The complications of acne vulgaris, especially in severe cases, are formation of cysts, pigment changes in persons with dark skin, severe scarring, and lowered self-concept from the obvious skin eruptions.

### Acne Rosacea

Acne rosacea is a chronic type of facial acne that occurs more often in middle and older adults. The cause is unknown. The lesions of acne rosacea begin with erythema over the cheeks and nose. Other skin lesions may or may not appear. Over years of time, the skin color changes to dark red, and the pores over the area become enlarged (Figure 14–21 ■). The soft tissue of the nose may exhibit *rhinophyma,* an irregular bullous thickening that can be treated with plastic surgery.

### Acne Conglobata

Acne conglobata is also a chronic type of acne of unknown cause that begins in middle adulthood. This type causes serious skin lesions: Comedones, papules, pustules, nodules, cysts, and scars occur primarily on the back, buttocks, and chest but may occur on other body surfaces. The comedones have multiple openings and a discharge that ranges from serous to purulent with a foul odor.

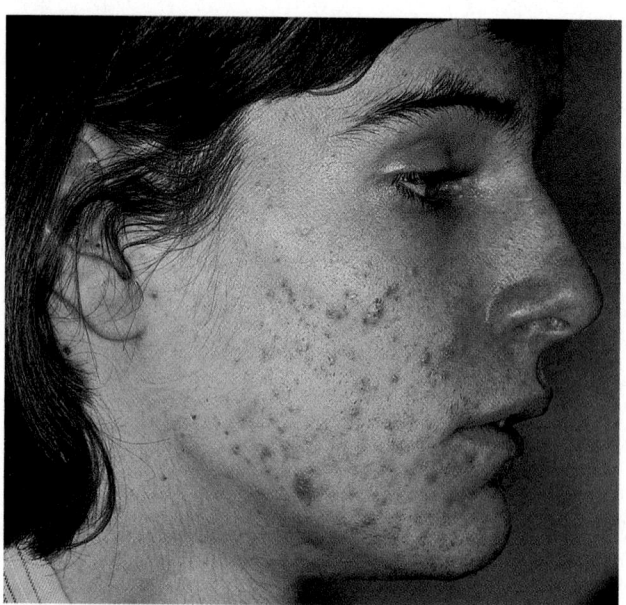 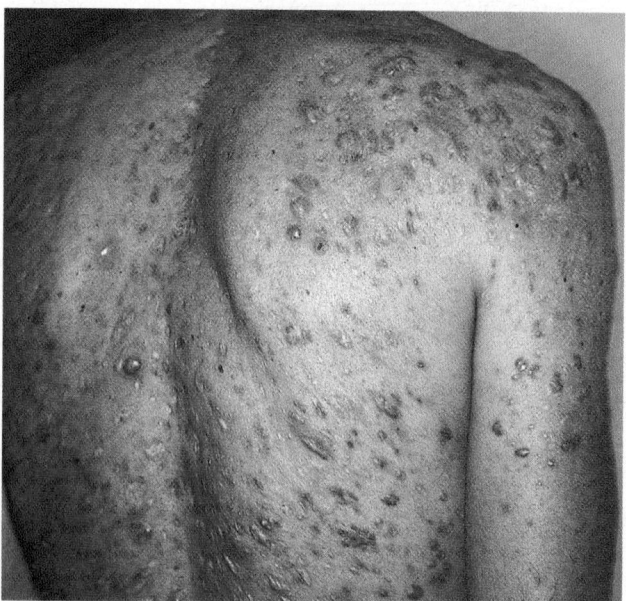

**Figure 14–20** ■ Acne is a disorder of the hair and sebaceous skin structures. *A,* In noninflammatory forms of acne, the characteristic lesions are comedones (pimples). *B,* Inflammatory acne lesions include comedones, erythematous pustules, and cysts. These lesions often leave scars when they heal.

*Source: Camera M.D. Studios. Carroll H. Weiss, Director, 8290 N.W. 26th Place, Sunrise, FL 33322.*

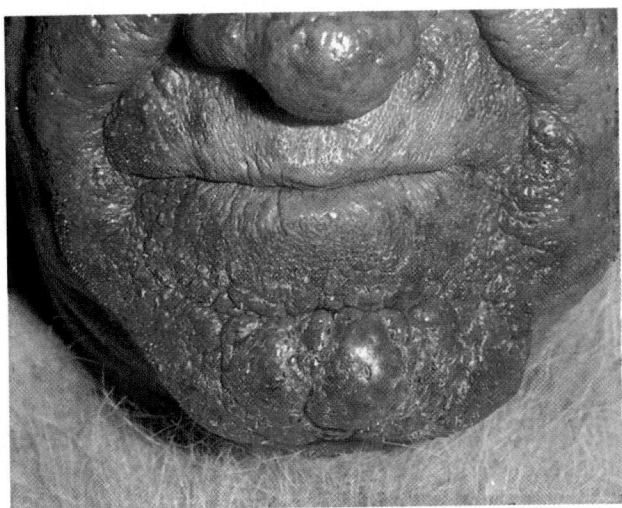

**Figure 14–21** ■ Acne rosacea is more common in the middle to older adult. It causes changes in skin color, enlarged pores, and in some cases thickening of the soft tissues of the nose.

*Source: Camera M. D. Studios. Carroll H. Weiss, Director. 8290 N. W. 26th Place. Sunrise, FL 33322.*

## COLLABORATIVE CARE

The management of acne is similar, regardless of type. Because acne vulgaris is most common, the discussions of collaborative and nursing care focus on that type.

Treatment is primarily by medications and continues for several weeks. Treatment is based on the type and severity of the lesions.

### Diagnostic Tests

The disease is diagnosed by the typical location and appearance of lesions. If the client has pustules, a culture of the drainage is performed to differentiate viral or bacterial dermatitis from acne.

### Medications

The treatment of acne is tailored to the individual and is based on the severity of the lesions. For acne with comedones, tretinoin (retinoic acid, Retin-A) or benzoyl peroxide preparations are prescribed. Azelaic acid (Azelex) may also be used. The administration of these vitamin A analogues is discussed in the Medication Administration box on this page. Benzoyl peroxide preparations are found in over-the-counter medications such as Fostex, Acne-Dome, Desquam-X, Benzagel, Clear By Design, and Xerac BP. These products are keratolytic and loosen the comedones.

Mild forms of papular inflammatory acne are treated with topical clindamycin (Cleocin T), a bacteriostatic agent that decreases the amount of fatty acids on the skin surface. This medication may be combined with tretinoin therapy.

Moderate forms of papular inflammatory acne are treated with oral or topical antibiotics, such as tetracycline, erythromycin, and minocycline. These antiacne antibiotics are admin-

istered for 3 to 4 months; if the client's skin is clear, the dose is lowered gradually to a maintenance dose that will maintain clear skin.

Severe forms of papular inflammatory acne are treated with isotretinoin (Accutane). This drug is effective, but has serious side effects. Isotretinoin, with nursing responsibilities, is discussed below.

## Medication Administration

### Acne Medications

#### ANTIACNE RETINOIDS
Tretinoin (Retin-A)        Isotretinoin (Accutane)

Tretinoin is a vitamin A derivative classified as an acne agent. This topical agent acts as an irritant to decrease cohesiveness of follicular epithelial cells, thereby decreasing comedone formation while increasing the extrusion of comedones from the skin surface.

Isotretinoin is a vitamin A analogue classified as an acne product. It reduces the size of sebaceous glands, inhibits sebaceous gland differentiation to decrease sebum production, and alters sebum lipid composition.

#### Nursing Responsibilities
- Administer tretinoin with caution to pregnant women, the effects of absorption on the developing fetus are not clearly defined.
- Isotretinoin is absolutely contraindicated for pregnant women or for women who want to become pregnant. The medication poses a high risk of major deformities in the infant if pregnancy occurs during use, even use that continues only for short periods.
- Do not administer to clients with eczema or to those who are hypersensitive to the sun.

#### Client and Family Teaching
*Tretinoin*
- Use the cream in a test area twice at night to test for sensitivity; if no reaction occurs, increase applications gradually to the prescribed frequency.
- A pea-sized amount of the cream is enough to cover the entire face.
- Apply the cream to clean, dry skin.
- Do not apply the cream to the eyes, mouth, angles of the nose, or mucous membranes.
- Wash your face no more than two to three times a day, using a mild soap. Do not use skin preparations (such as aftershave lotion or perfumes) that contain alcohol, menthol, spice, or lime, they may irritate your skin.
- The medication may cause a temporary stinging or warm sensation but should not cause pain.
- The skin where you apply the cream will be mildly red and may peel; if you experience a more severe reaction, consult your health care provider.
- The medication may cause increased sensitivity to sunlight, use sunscreens and wear protective clothing when outdoors.
- Your acne may become worse during the first 2 weeks of treatment; this is an expected response.

*(continued on page 384)*

## Medication Administration

### Acne Medications (continued)

*Isotretinoin*

- Take the pills with food.
- Your acne may become worse during the initial period of treatment; this is an expected response.
- The medication causes dryness of the eyes, so you may have trouble wearing contact lenses during and after treatment.
- Do not take vitamin A supplements; they will increase the effects of the medication.
- Avoid prolonged exposure to sunlight; use sunscreen and protective clothing when in the sun.
- Notify the physician at once if you have abdominal pain, severe diarrhea, rectal bleeding, headache, nausea or vomiting, or visual disturbances.
- Do not drink alcohol while taking this medication (it causes an increase in triglycerides).
- Night vision may become worse; use caution when driving at night.
- Do not donate blood while or for 1 month after taking this medication.
- (*For female clients*) You must use two reliable forms of contraception simultaneously for at least 1 month before, during, and at least 1 month after therapy with this medication. The medication may cause deformities in a baby conceived at this time.

## Treatments

### Dermabrasion and Laser

Dermabrasion of inactive acne lesions can improve the client's appearance, especially if the scars are flat. (Dermabrasion is discussed in greater detail later in this chapter.) Laser excision of deep scars may also be used.

## NURSING CARE

Nursing care is individualized to the client's developmental needs and is conducted primarily through teaching in clinics or the home setting. Regardless of the client's age or gender, it is important to remember that almost all clients with acne are embarrassed by and self-conscious of their appearance. Prior to teaching, establish rapport with the client and clarify beliefs; for example, the client may believe the lesions result from poor hygiene, masturbation, use of cosmetics, eating the wrong types of foods, or lack of sexual activity. It is critical to teach the client about the causes of and factors involved in acne prior to teaching self-care.

## Home Care

The teaching plan for the client with acne includes general guidelines for skin care and health as well as specific guidelines for care of the acne lesions. The following topics should be addressed:

- Wash the skin with a mild soap and water at least twice a day to remove accumulated oils.
- Shampoo the hair often enough to prevent oiliness.

- Eat a regular, well-balanced diet. Foods do not cause or increase acne.
- Expose the skin to sunlight, but avoid sunburn.
- Get regular exercise and sleep.
- Try to avoid putting your hands on your face.
- Do not squeeze a pimple. Squeezing forces the material of the pimple deeper into the skin and usually causes the pimple to become larger and infected.
- The treatment for acne lasts months, in some cases for the rest of one's life. It is very important to take the medications each day for the prescribed length of time.

## THE CLIENT WITH PEMPHIGUS VULGARIS

**Pemphigus vulgaris** is a chronic disorder of the skin and oral mucous membranes characterized by vesicle (blister) formation. The disease is caused by autoantibodies that cause *acantholysis* (the separation of epidermal cells from one another). The disorder is associated with IgG antibodies and HLA-A10 antigen. If untreated, the disease is usually fatal within 5 years (Tierney et al., 2001). However, better methods of diagnosis and treatment have improved the prognosis.

The disease occurs in middle and older adults of all races and ethnic backgrounds. The disorder has been associated with other autoimmune disorders and with the administration of certain drugs, such as penicillamine and captopril.

### MANIFESTATIONS

The blisters that form in pemphigus vulgaris usually appear first in the mouth and scalp and then spread in crops or waves to involve large areas of the body, including the face, back, chest, umbilicus, and groin. Blisters in the mouth ulcerate. The blisters form in the epidermis and cause the epidermal cells to separate above the basal layer. These blisters rupture, leaving denuded skin, crusting, and oozing of fluid with a musty odor (Figure 14–22 ■). The lesions are painful. Pressure on a blister

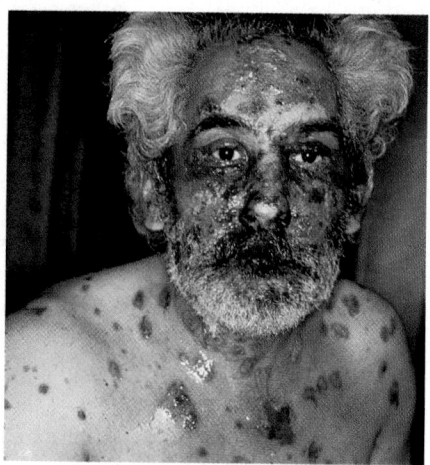

**Figure 14–22** ■ Pemphigus vulgaris is a chronic skin disorder characterized by vesicles that ooze fluid and form crusts.

causes it to spread to adjacent skin (Nikolsky's sign). The loss of fluid from the blisters may result in fluid and electrolyte imbalances. Secondary bacterial infections are a serious risk and a major cause of death.

## COLLABORATIVE CARE

The goals of treatment are to control the severity of the disease, to prevent infection and loss of fluids, and to promote healing. Clients who experience severe attacks or secondary infections are usually hospitalized. Although the disease cannot be cured, the manifestations can be controlled.

### Diagnostic Tests

Pemphigus vulgaris is diagnosed by clinical manifestations and laboratory and diagnostic tests. These tests may include the following:

- Immunofluorescence microscopy is done to identify the presence of IgG antibodies in the epidermis and serum.
- Skin biopsy may be performed to determine the presence of acantholysis.

### Medications

Early lesions are treated with highly potent topical corticosteroids. As the disease becomes more severe, systemic corticosteroids or immunosuppressive agents (such as azathioprine or methotrexate) are prescribed. Secondary infections are treated with topical and/or systemic antibiotics.

### Treatments

Plasmapheresis is occasionally used to treat pemphigus. In this procedure, the plasma is selectively removed from whole blood and reinfused into the client. This decreases the serum level of antibodies for a period of time. Plasmapheresis with related nursing care is discussed in Chapter 43. ⬤⬤

## NURSING CARE

The hospitalized client with pemphigus requires careful assessment of skin lesions and monitoring for manifestations of infection. Provide skin care through bathing and applying dressings to denuded areas, using aseptic technique to prevent infection. The client may be placed on reverse isolation as a protective measure. Monitor the client's hydration status to prevent fluid volume deficit and incorporate pain medications and noninvasive pain management techniques in the plan of care. Oral lesions often make eating difficult; the client requires meticulous oral hygiene and nonirritating foods. The client often is depressed and fearful; establishing a therapeutic relationship is essential, and referrals for counseling may be necessary.

### Home Care

Teaching the client and family how to provide care at home also involves skin care, oral care, diet, pain management, and prevention of infection. In addition, the nurse teaches the client and family how to take prescribed medications. A referral to a home health agency or local health department may be necessary.

## THE CLIENT WITH LICHEN PLANUS

**Lichen planus** is an inflammatory disorder of the mucous membranes and skin. It has no known cause but has been associated with exposure to drugs or to film processing chemicals. The disease affects adults from 30 to 70 years of age.

The lesions first appear as violet papules, 2 to 10 mm in size, commonly occurring on the wrists, ankles, lower legs, and genitals (Figure 14–23 ■). The lesions are intensely pruritic. Over time, persistent lesions thicken and become dark red, forming hypertrophic lichen planus. Lesions on the oral mucous membranes appear as white lacey rings; lesions may also appear on the mucous membranes of the vaginal area and the penis. The nails become thin and may shed.

Lichen planus lesions are self-limiting but last for an average of 12 to 18 months. The disorder is diagnosed by clinical manifestations. Corticosteroids are used to control the inflammation, and antihistamines are used to control the pruritus. Lesions recur in about 20% of cases.

## THE CLIENT WITH TOXIC EPIDERMAL NECROLYSIS

**Toxic epidermal necrolysis (TEN)** is a rare, life-threatening disease in which the epidermis peels off the dermis in sheets, leaving large areas of denuded skin. Conjunctivitis and mucositis of the mouth, upper airway, esophagus, and sometimes the genitourinary tract are often associated with TEN. The client

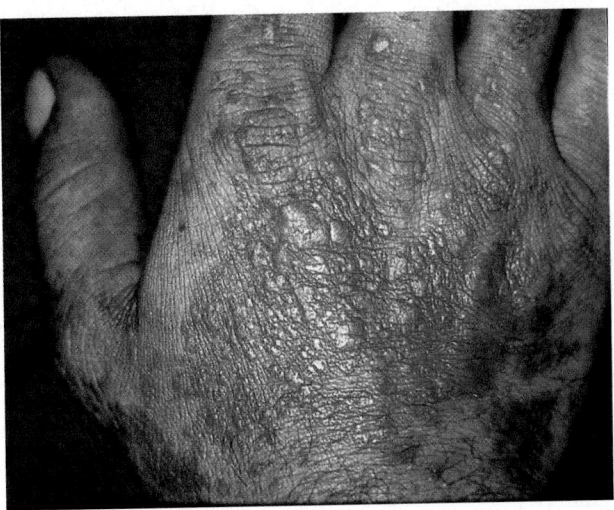

**Figure 14–23 ■** These violet lesions are typical of lichen planus, a benign inflammatory disease of the skin and mucous membranes.

*Source: Camera M. D. Studios. Carroll H. Weiss, Director. 8290 N. W. 26th Place. Sunrise, FL 33322.*

usually requires critical care, often in a burn center. The incidence of TEN has not been documented, but it is seen more often in men and in people of African descent. The mortality rate ranges from 25% to 100% but is decreasing because of current methods of care. The cause of death is almost always sepsis.

Most cases result from a drug reaction, and others are associated with a serious concomitant illness, such as cancer or AIDS. In other cases, the disease has no known cause. Drugs that have been associated with TEN are the sulfonamides, barbiturates, NSAIDs, phenytoin, allopurinol, and penicillin.

The pathophysiologic process in TEN is not completely understood, but the triggering mechanism is believed to be a hypersensitivity or immune response. TEN begins with a painful, localized erythema of the face and extremities, accompanied by fever, chills, muscle aches, and generalized malaise. A macular rash develops, followed by the formation of large, flaccid blisters over the body surface during the next 24 to 96 hours. The skin begins to slough, leaving the dermal surface exposed. Even in areas without blistering, the skin may peel off in layers. The skin sloughing continues over several days and can expose 95% or more of the dermal surface (Figure 14–24 ■). Other manifestations include conjunctivitis, pharyngitis, stomatitis, and enlargement of lymph glands. Urethral slough is common, causing such painful voiding that the client voluntarily retains urine. The client is often disoriented, may be nearly comatose, and is seriously ill.

The loss of skin leads to fluid and electrolyte imbalances and secondary infections, as well as systemic effects on all other body systems. These complications may cause death. However, if the complications can be prevented, healing by epidermal regeneration occurs in about a month. The long-term

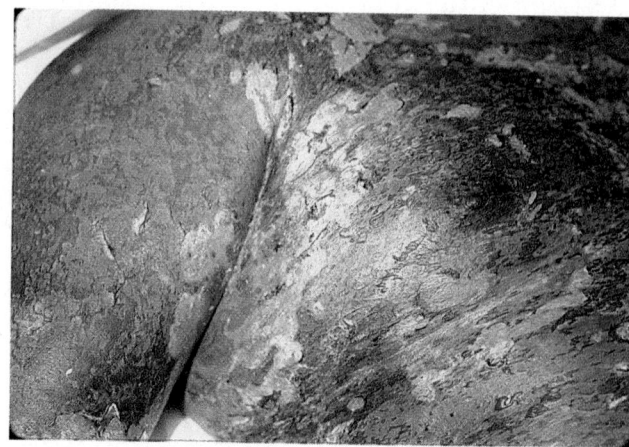

**Figure 14–24 ■** Toxic epidermal necrolysis (TEN) is a life-threatening skin disease characterized by the sloughing of large skin surfaces.

*Source: Camera M. D. Studios. Carroll H. Weiss, Director. 8290 N. W. 26th Place. Sunrise, FL 33322.*

complications of TEN include blindness, lacrimal duct occlusion, scarring and contractures, loss of nails, esophageal strictures, and glomerulonephritis.

The client is hospitalized and requires rapid diagnosis and treatment. Any medication in use by the client is stopped immediately. Collaborative care involves fluid replacement, correction of electrolyte imbalances, prevention or management of infection, and pain control. The collaborative and nursing care are essentially the same as for the client with burns, discussed in Chapter 15.

# MALIGNANT SKIN DISORDERS

The skin is a common site for malignant lesions. Many of these lesions are found on skin surfaces that have undergone long-term exposure to the sun or the environment. Malignant skin tumors are the most common of all cancers.

## ACTINIC KERATOSIS

**Actinic keratosis,** also called senile or solar keratosis, is an epidermal skin lesion directly related to chronic sun exposure and photodamage. The prevalence is highest in people with light-colored skin; these lesions are rare in people with dark skin. Actinic keratosis may progress to squamous cell carcinoma. Fewer than 1% of early lesions become malignant, but many of those that persist progress to malignancy (Porth, 2002). Because of this tendency, the lesions are classified as premalignant.

The lesions are erythematous rough macules a few millimeters in diameter. They are often shiny but may be scaly; if the scales are removed, the underlying skin bleeds. They occur in multiple patches, primarily on the face, dorsa of the hands, the forearms, and sometimes on the upper trunk (Figure 14–25 ■).

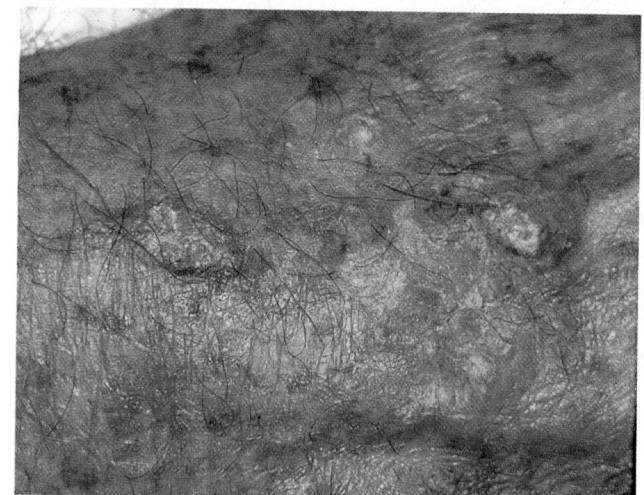

**Figure 14–25 ■** The effects of long-term sun exposure are illustrated in this epidermal skin lesion, called actinic keratosis.

*Source: Camera M. D. Studios. Carroll H. Weiss, Director. 8290 N. W. 26th Place. Sunrise, FL 33322.*

Enlargement or ulceration of the lesions suggests transformation to malignancy.

# THE CLIENT WITH NONMELANOMA SKIN CANCER

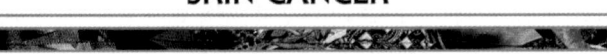

The skin, despite its ability to protect the internal body from external damage, is a fragile organ and is subject to damage from ultraviolet radiation and chemicals. Over time, this damage results in alterations in cellular structure and function, and malignancies of the skin occur. The nonmelanoma skin cancers are basal cell cancer and squamous cell cancer.

## INCIDENCE

Nonmelanoma skin cancer is the most common malignant neoplasm found in fair-skinned Americans. The American Cancer Society estimates that more than 1 million new cases of nonmelanoma skin cancer occur in the United States each year. Of that number 95% to 99% can be cured if detected and treated early. Men develop nonmelanoma skin cancer more often than do women, probably because of occupational exposures. Although nonmelanoma skin cancer may occur at any age, the incidence increases with each decade of life. Adults between the ages of 30 and 60 have the majority of these cancers.

## PATHOPHYSIOLOGY AND MANIFESTATIONS

The two nonmelanoma skin cancers, basal cell cancer and squamous cell cancer, arise from epithelial tissue but have different pathophysiology, classifications, and manifestations.

### Basal Cell Carcinoma

**Basal cell carcinoma** is an epithelial tumor believed to originate either from the basal layer of the epidermis or from cells in the surrounding dermal structures. These tumors are characterized by an impaired ability of the basal cells of the epidermis to mature into keratinocytes, with mitotic division beyond the basal layer. This results in a bulky neoplasm that grows by direct extension and destroys surrounding tissue, including healthy skin, nerves, blood vessels, lymphatic tissue, cartilage, and bone. Basal cell cancer is the most common but least aggressive type of skin cancer, rarely metastasizing.

Basal cell cancer is classified into different types: nodular, superficial, pigmented, morpheaform, and keratotic. These types are described below and are summarized in Table 14–3.

- Nodular basal cell cancer, the most common type of basal cell cancer, most often appears on the face, neck, and head. The tumor is made up of masses of cells that resemble epidermal basal cells and grow in a bulky, nodular form from lack of keratinization. In early stages, the tumor is a papule that looks like a smooth pimple. It is often pruritic and continues to grow at a steady rate, doubling in size every 6 to 12 months. As the tumor grows, the epidermis thins, but it remains intact. The skin over the tumor is shiny, and either pearly white, pink, or

| TABLE 14–3 | Types and Characteristics of Basal Cell Cancers | |
|---|---|---|
| **Type** | **Common Location** | **Manifestation** |
| Nodular | Face, neck, head | Small, firm papule; pearly, white, pink, or flesh colored; telangiectasis; enlarges; may ulcerate. |
| Superficial | Trunk, extremities | Papules or plaque that is flat, erythematous, or scaling; pink color; well-defined borders; may have shallow erosions and surface crusting. |
| Pigmented | Head, neck, face | Dark brown, blue, or black color; border is shiny and well defined. |
| Morpheaform | Head, neck | Looks like a flat scar; ivory or flesh colored. |
| Keratotic | Ear | Small, firm papule; pearly, white, pink, or flesh colored; may ulcerate. |

skin colored. Telangiectasis may be visible over the area of the tumor. As the tumor continues to increase in size, the center or periphery may ulcerate, and the tumor develops well-circumscribed borders. It bleeds easily from mild injury.

- Superficial basal cell cancer, found most often on the trunk and extremities, is the second most common type of basal cell cancer. This tumor is a proliferating tissue that attaches to the undersurface of the epithelium. The tumor is a flat papule or plaque, often erythematous, with well-defined borders. The tumor may ulcerate and be covered with crusts or shallow erosions (Figure 14–26 ■).

- Pigmented basal cell cancer, found on the head, neck, and face, is less common. This tumor concentrates melanin pigment in the center of the basal cancer cells, giving it a dark brown, blue, or black appearance. The border of the tumor is shiny and well defined.

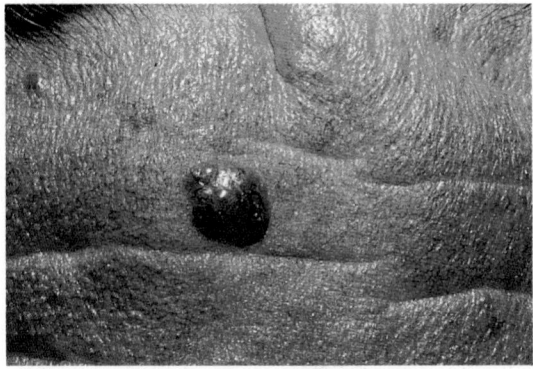

**Figure 14–26** ■ A superficial basal cell cancer often is erythematous, has well-defined borders, and ulcerations.

*Source: From American Academy of Dermatology. Reprinted with permission. All rights reserved.*

- Morpheaform basal cell cancer, the rarest form of basal cell cancer, usually develops on the head and neck. The tumor forms fingerlike projections that extend in any direction along dermal tissue planes. The tumor resembles a flat ivory or flesh-colored scar. This form is more likely to extend into and destroy adjacent tissue, especially muscle, nerve, and bone. It is often more difficult to diagnose because of its appearance.
- Keratotic basal cell cancer (basosquamous) is found on the preauricular and postauricular groove. It contains both basal cells and squamoid-appearing cells that keratinize. Its appearance is much like that of nodular basal cell cancer. This type of basal cell cancer tends to recur locally and also is the type most likely to metastasize.

Basal cell cancers tend to recur. Tumors greater than 2 cm in diameter have a high recurrence rate. Predisposing factors for metastasis are the size of the tumor and the client's resistance to treatment with surgery or chemotherapy. Even though they rarely metastasize, untreated basal cell cancers invade surrounding tissue and may destroy body parts, such as the nose or eyelid.

## Squamous Cell Cancer

**Squamous cell cancer** is a malignant tumor of the squamous epithelium of the skin or mucous membranes. It occurs most often on areas of skin exposed to ultraviolet rays and weather, such as the forehead, helix of the ear, top of the nose, lower lip, and back of the hands. Squamous cell cancer may also arise on skin that has been burned or has chronic inflammation. This is a much more aggressive cancer than basal cell cancer, with a faster growth rate and a much greater potential for metastasis if untreated.

The tumors arise when the keratinizing cells of the squamous epithelium proliferate, producing a growth that eventually fills the epidermis and invades the dermal tissue planes. Keratinization of some cells is present, and the formation of keratin "pearls" is common. The keratin formation diminishes as the tumor grows. As the tumor grows, the tumor cells increase in number and rate of mitosis, forming odd shapes.

Squamous cell cancer begins as a small, firm red nodule. The tumor may be crusted with keratin products. As it grows, it may ulcerate, bleed, and become painful. As the tumor extends into the surrounding tissue and becomes a nodule, the area around the nodule becomes indurated (hardened) (Figure 14–27 ■).

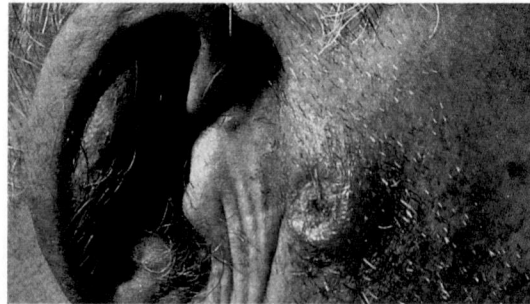

**Figure 14–27** ■ As a squamous cell cancer grows, it tends to invade surrounding tissue. It also ulcerates, may bleed, and is painful.

Recurrent squamous cell cancer can be invasive, increasing the risk of metastasis. Invasive squamous cell cancer may arise from preexisting skin lesions, such as scars and actinic keratosis, and extend into the dermis (called intraepidermal squamous cell cancer). This form appears as a slightly raised erythematous plaque with well-defined borders. Metastasis occurs most often via the lymphatics. The degree of risk for metastasis depends on the size and depth of penetration of the tumor.

## RISK FACTORS

There are multiple etiologic factors involved in the development of nonmelanoma skin cancer, including environmental factors and host factors.

### Environmental Factors

The environmental factors implicated in the nonmelanoma skin cancers are ultraviolet radiation, pollutants, chemicals, ionizing radiation, viruses, and physical trauma.

Ultraviolet radiation (UVR) from the sun is believed to be the cause of most nonmelanoma skin cancers. Sunlight contains both short-length rays (UVB) and long-length rays (UVA). UVB rays are absorbed by the top layer of skin and cause sunburn. UVA rays penetrate deeper into the skin layers, causing tissue damage. Both types of rays are believed to cause DNA alterations and also suppress T-cell and B-cell immunity. The amount of ultraviolet radiation reaching the earth is increasing, most likely from depletion of the ozone layer surrounding the planet. The U.S. Environmental Protection Agency predicts that for every 1% decrease in the ozone layer, a corresponding 1% to 3% increase in nonmelanoma skin cancer per year will occur.

Geographic, environmental, and lifestyle factors affect the amount of exposure to the sun and the risk for nonmelanoma skin cancer. People who live in latitudes close to the equator and those who live at higher altitudes receive greater ultraviolet radiation exposure. The amount of clothing worn, the time of day, and amount of time in the sun also determine the amount of exposure. Exposure to ultraviolet radiation in tanning booths has also been implicated in the development of nonmelanoma skin cancer.

Certain chemicals have long been associated with nonmelanoma skin cancer. Polycyclic aromatic hydrocarbons, found in mixtures of coal, tar, asphalt, soot, and mineral oils, have been linked with skin cancers. Psoralens, used in conjunction with UVA for treatment of psoriasis and cutaneous T-cell lymphoma, increase the risk of squamous cell cancer.

Other factors associated with nonmelanoma skin cancer are the use of ionizing radiation, viruses, and physical trauma. X-ray therapy for tinea capitis and the use of radium to treat other malignancies are risk factors. Human papillomavirus is implicated in the development of squamous cell cancer, as is damage to the skin from burns.

### Host Factors

Certain host factors increase the risk of nonmelanoma skin cancer. These include skin pigmentation as well as the presence of premalignant lesions.

Skin pigmentation is an important factor in the development of nonmelanoma skin cancer. The amount of melanin pigment produced by the melanocytes determines a person's skin color. The more melanin, the more the skin is protected from the damage produced by ultraviolet rays. Thus, African Americans, Asian Americans, and people of Mediterranean descent have a much lower incidence of nonmelanoma skin cancer than do people who have fair complexions and tend to freckle or sunburn easily, such as people of Irish, Scandinavian, or English ancestry.

Although most people have numerous pigmented lesions on their body, almost all of these are normal. However, a major risk factor in the development of nonmelanoma skin cancer is a change in an existing lesion or the presence of a premalignant lesion, such as actinic keratosis. Organ transplant recipients who undergo immunosuppression to prevent rejection are also at risk for the development of squamous cell cancer.

## COLLABORATIVE CARE

Treatment of nonmelanoma skin cancer focuses on removal of all malignant tissue using such methods as surgery, curettage and electrodesiccation, cryotherapy, or radiotherapy. These modalities offer a greater than 90% cure rate. After the malignant tissue is removed, the client should have regular examinations for recurrence.

## Diagnostic Tests

Nonmelanoma cancer is diagnosed by microscopic examination of tissue biopsied from the tumor. The biopsy is usually done as an office procedure under local anesthesia. The types of biopsy commonly conducted follow:

- Shave biopsy, in which the lesion is shaved with a scalpel to the level of the mid-dermis
- Punch biopsy, in which a circular punch removes a section of tissue in a "cookie cutter" fashion to a level of the reticular dermis or subcutaneous tissue
- Incisional biopsy, in which a part of the tumor is removed with a scalpel
- Excisional biopsy, in which the entire tumor is removed and analyzed

## Treatments

### Surgical Excision

Both basal cell and squamous cell cancers are excised surgically. The surgery may be minor or major, depending on the size and location of the tumor. Surgery for small tumors is most often performed in the outpatient surgery department or in the surgeon's office. Surgical excision allows rapid healing and yields good cosmetic results, but as does any surgery, carries the risk of infection.

The goal of surgical excision is to remove the tumor completely, so some surrounding tissue is excised along with the tumor. If the tumor is on the face, the incision is made along normal wrinkle or anatomic lines so that the scars will be less obvious. The incision is closed in layers to leave the smallest possible scar. A pressure dressing is usually applied over the incision to provide support.

If a large tumor is removed, a skin graft or skin flap may be performed to cover the excised area. If grafting is necessary, the client is hospitalized.

### Mohs' ChemoSurgery Technique

In Mohs' chemosurgery technique, thin layers of the tumor are horizontally shaved off. A frozen section of the tissue is stained at each level to determine tumor margins. This method is the most accurate in assessing the extent of nonmelanoma skin cancer and the method that conserves the most normal tissue. It is often used in areas such as the nose, the nasolabial fold, the medial canthus, and the ear.

### Curettage and Electrodesiccation

Curettage and electrodesiccation are used to treat basal cell cancers that are less than 2 cm in diameter, are superficial, or recur because of poor margin control. It may also be used for primary squamous cell cancers that are less than 1 cm in diameter and have distinct borders. This type of treatment is most successful for tumors on anatomic sites over a fixed underlying surface, such as the ear, chest, and temple.

Abnormal tissue is scraped away (curettage) within 1 to 2 mm of the margin and then a low-voltage electrode is used to abrade the tumor base (electrodesiccation). Tumor tissue is much softer and more friable than normal tissue. Therefore, curettage and electrodesiccation is not used for lesions where the dermis is thin (such as the eyelid) or where the tumor extends into the subcutaneous tissue.

Curettage and electrodesiccation provide good cosmetic results and preserve normal tissue. However, healing time is longer, and it is difficult to ensure that all tumor margins have been removed.

Instead of a low-voltage electrode, some physicians use a carbon dioxide laser to vaporize the tumor. When used in conjunction with curettage, this treatment is effective on superficial basal cell cancers. Carbon dioxide vaporization results in minimal thermal injury to adjacent cells, less pain, and quicker healing.

### Radiation Therapy

Radiation is most often used for lesions that are inoperable because of their location (such as tumors on the corner of the nose, the eyelid, the canthus, and the lip) or size (between 1 cm and 8 cm). Radiotherapy is also used for clients who are older and of poor surgical risk. Radiation is painless and can be used to treat areas surrounding the tumor if necessary. However, the treatment is given over 3 to 4 weeks in a clinical facility, does not allow control of tumor margins, and may itself cause skin cancer.

## NURSING CARE

The increasing number of people with skin cancer requires that nurses be involved in prevention and early detection, as well as provide nursing interventions. Nurses have the opportunity to teach preventive behaviors in all settings, including the hospital, home, community, school, and clinic.

Nursing care for the client with nonmelanoma skin cancer depends on the treatment employed. Surgical excision is the most common form of treatment; nursing care depends on the extent of the procedure. However, regardless of the type of treatment, the client will have impaired skin integrity, an increased risk for infection, and anxiety about the future following a diagnosis of cancer. Interventions with rationale for the client with any type of skin cancer are discussed in the section on malignant melanoma.

## Health Promotion

It is well known that cumulative sun exposure positively correlates with nonmelanoma skin cancers. Many skin cancers can be prevented by limiting exposure to risk factors. Primary prevention behaviors recommended by the American Cancer Society and the Skin Cancer Foundation follow:

- Minimize exposure to the sun between the hours of 10 A.M. and 3 P.M., when ultraviolet rays are the strongest.
- Cover up with a wide-brimmed hat, sunglasses, long-sleeved shirt, and long pants made of tightly woven material when you are in the sun.
- Use a waterproof or water-resistant sunscreen with an SPF of 15 or more before every exposure to the sun. Apply sunscreen not only on sunny days but also on cloudy days, when ultraviolet rays can penetrate 70% to 80% of the cloud cover. Reapply the sunscreen before the protection time is up. See Box 14–3 for information about sunscreens.
- Use sunscreen and protective clothing when you are on or near sand, snow, concrete, or water, which can reflect more than half of the ultraviolet rays onto the skin.
- Avoid tanning booths; UVA radiation emitted by tanning booths damages the deep skin layers.

Nurses also provide client and family education for early detection of nonmelanoma skin cancer. Numerous brochures describing the types of skin cancers, photographs of lesions, and prevention behaviors are available from the American Cancer Society, health education and support agencies, and pharmaceutical companies that manufacture sunscreen. Most of this literature is free.

The client or family at risk for or diagnosed with a skin cancer must be taught how to conduct a self-examination of the skin as well as the importance of conducting the examination on the same day of each month. Family members can help with areas that are hard to examine, such as the ears, scalp, and back.

## Home Care

Teach the client and family specific measures for self-care following surgery, including information about:

- How and when to change dressings.
- The use of aseptic technique and careful handwashing when caring for the wound.
- Symptoms to report (such as bleeding, fever, or signs of wound infection), and how to protect the operative site against trauma and irritations.

---

**BOX 14–3 ■ Sunscreen Information**

### TYPES OF SUNSCREEN
**Chemical**
Chemical sunscreens absorb ultraviolet light and act as a radiation filter. Examples follow:

- p-aminobenzoic acid (PABA)
- Benzophenones
- Anthranilates
- Salicylates

**Physical**
Physical sunscreens reflect and scatter ultraviolet light. Examples follow:

- Zinc oxide
- Titanium dioxide
- Magnesium silicate
- Ferric chloride
- Kaolin
- Ichthyol

### ADVERSE REACTIONS ASSOCIATED WITH SUNSCREENS
Adverse reactions associated with sunscreens include contact and photocontact dermatitis. People with previous hypersensitivity reactions to benzocaine, procaine, sulfonamides, or paraphenylenediamine may develop hypersensitivity responses to PABA. People who are also taking systemic thiazide diuretics or sulfonamides may develop eczematous dermatitis.

### SUNSCREEN RATINGS
In the United States, the Food and Drug Administration (FDA) rates commercial sunscreens according to their "sun protection factor," or SPF. The SPF value is the ratio of the time required to produce minimal skin redness through a sunscreen product with the time required to produce the same degree of redness without the sunscreen. A person who can tolerate 1/2 hour of sun without a sunscreen should be able to tolerate 3 hours of sun when a sunscreen of SPF 6 is applied to the skin. SPF values of sunscreens range from 2 to 50.

---

# THE CLIENT WITH MALIGNANT MELANOMA

**Malignant melanoma** arises from melanocytes. This serious skin cancer is increasing in incidence each year. At the current rate, it is predicted that 1 in 58 males and 1 in 82 females in the United States will develop melanoma in his or her lifetime (American Cancer Society, 2002).

## INCIDENCE

This disease is over 10 times more common in fair-skinned people than in dark-skinned people. As with the nonmelanoma skin cancers, an increase in the incidence of malignant melanoma is believed to be related to the thinning ozone layer and increased exposure to ultraviolet rays. The incidence is highest in Caucasian upper-middle-class professionals who work indoors (Porth, 2002). This group of people often had severe sunburn with blistering during childhood and tend to vacation in areas of intense sun exposure. Malignant melanoma is also more common in people who live in sunny climates, burn easily, and patronize tanning parlors. However, malignant melanoma may arise from already present lesions or from skin normally covered with clothing.

## PATHOPHYSIOLOGY AND MANIFESTATIONS

Melanocytes are located at or near the basal layer (the deepest epidermal layer). These cells produce melanin, the dark skin pigment. Melanin is made in granules and transferred to keratinocytes, where it accumulates on the superficial side of each keratinocyte and forms a shield of pigment over the nucleus as protection against ultraviolet rays. Malignant melanomas can develop wherever there is pigment, but about one-third of them originate in existing nevi.

Almost all malignant melanomas are more than 6 mm in diameter, are asymmetric, and initially develop within the epidermis over a long period. While they are still confined to the epidermis, the lesions (called *malignant melanoma in situ*) are flat and relatively benign. However, when they penetrate the dermis, they mingle with blood and lymph vessels and are capable of metastasizing. At this latter stage, the tumors develop a raised or nodular appearance and often have smaller nodules, called satellite lesions, around the periphery.

The prognosis for survival for people diagnosed with malignant melanoma is determined by several variables, including tumor thickness, ulceration, metastasis, site, age, and gender. Younger clients and women have a somewhat better chance of survival. Tumors on the hands, feet, and scalp have a poorer prognosis; tumors of the feet and scalp are less visible and may not be diagnosed until they grow into the dermis.

### Precursor Lesions

The three specific precursor lesions for the development of malignant melanoma are congenital nevi, dysplastic nevi, and lentigo maligna. A precursor lesion is also called a premalignant lesion, a name that indicates that the lesion's risk of becoming malignant is greater than normal.

### Congenital Nevi

Congenital nevi are present at birth. Some lesions are small; others are large enough to cover an entire body area. Their color can range from brown to black. They are often slightly raised, with an irregular surface and a fairly regular border.

### Dysplastic Nevi

Dysplastic nevi are also called atypical moles. Although dysplastic nevi are not present at birth, they appear as normal nevi during childhood and become dysplastic (having abnormal development) after puberty. A client with classic dysplastic nevi has more than 100 nevi, at least one of which is larger than 8 mm in diameter, and at least one has the characteristics of malignant melanoma (asymmetry, irregular border, color variegation, and a diameter greater than 6 mm). A familial tendency to dysplastic nevi increases the risk for the development of malignant melanoma. However, it is not known whether people with dysplastic nevi and no family history of melanoma face a higher risk of melanoma.

Dysplastic nevi most often appear on the face, trunk, and arms but also are seen on the scalp, female breast, groin, and buttocks. The pigmentation of the nevi is irregular, with mixtures of tan, brown, black, red, and pink. An area of lighter pigmentation is surrounded by a papular area of deeper pigmentation (described as a "fried egg appearance"). The borders of the nevi are irregular.

### Lentigo Maligna

Lentigo maligna, also called Hutchinson's freckle, is a tan or black patch on the skin that looks like a freckle. It grows slowly, becoming mottled, dark, thick, and nodular. It is usually seen on one side of the face of an older adult who has had a large amount of sun exposure.

### Classification

Malignant melanomas are classified into different types. The major types are superficial spreading melanoma, lentigo maligna melanoma, nodular melanoma, and acral lentiginous melanoma. Each of these tumors is characterized by a radial and/or vertical growth phase. During the initial radial phase, which may last from 1 to 25 years (depending on the type), the melanoma grows parallel to the skin surface. During this phase, the tumor rarely metastasizes and is often curable by surgical excision. However, during the vertical growth phase, atypical melanocytes rapidly penetrate into the dermis and subcutaneous tissue, greatly increasing the risk for metastasis and death.

### Superficial Spreading Melanoma

Superficial spreading melanoma is the most common type, comprising about 70% of all melanomas (Porth, 2002). The lesions are usually flat and scaly or crusty and are about 2 cm in diameter. They often arise from a preexisting nevus. This type of melanoma is found on the trunk and back of men and on the legs of women. Superficial spreading melanomas occur more often in women than in men. The median age of occurrence is the 50s.

The radial growth phase lasts from 1 to 5 or more years. When the lesion enters the vertical growth phase, it grows rapidly, and its color changes from a mixture of tan, brown, and black to a characteristic red, white, and blue. The lesion also develops irregular borders and often has raised nodules and ulcerations (Figure 14–28 ■).

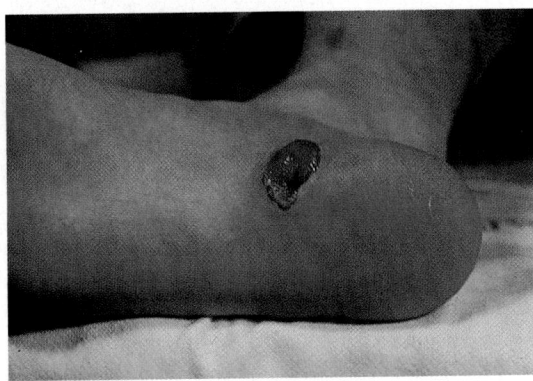

**Figure 14–28 ■** Malignant melanoma is a serious skin cancer that arises from melanocytes.

*Source: L. Solomon/Custom Medical Stock Photography.*

### Lentigo Maligna Melanoma

Lentigo maligna melanoma often arises from the precursor lesion, lentigo maligna. The lesions are large and tan with different shades of brown. This type of melanoma makes up 4% to 10% of malignant melanomas and is the least serious form (Porth, 2002). It occurs on skin that has had long-term sun exposure, such as the face, neck, and sometimes the dorsal surface of the hands and lower extremities. Lentigo maligna melanoma affects women more than men. It is typically diagnosed in people in their 60s and 70s.

Lentigo maligna melanoma is characterized by a proliferation of atypical melanocytes parallel to the basal layer of the epidermis. The radial growth phase may last from 10 to 25 years, with the lesion growing to as large as 10 cm. The lesion becomes malignant as soon as the melanocytes invade the dermis. In the vertical growth phase, raised nodules may appear on the surface of the lesion. The lesion tends to acquire a freckled or mottled appearance.

### Nodular Melanoma

Nodular melanoma lesions are raised, dome-shaped blueblack or red nodules on areas of the head, neck, and trunk that may or may not have been exposed to the sun. The lesions may look like a blood blister, or they may ulcerate and bleed. The lesions arise from unaffected skin rather than from a preexisting lesion. This type makes up 15% to 30% of malignant melanomas and is often diagnosed in people in their 50s (Porth, 2002).

Nodular melanoma has only a vertical growth phase, but it grows aggressively during that phase. However, the absence of a radial growth phase makes this type more difficult to diagnose before it metastasizes.

### Acral Lentiginous Melanoma

Acral lentiginous melanoma, also called mucocutaneous melanoma, is less common in people with fair skin and more common in people with dark skin. The lesions progress from tan, brown, or black flat lesions to elevated nodules and are about 3 cm in diameter. The radial phase lasts from 2 to 5 years. They are found on the palms of the hands, soles of the feet, the mucous membranes, and the nailbeds. Acral lentiginous melanoma affects both men and women equally and is most often diagnosed in people in their 50s and 60s.

## COLLABORATIVE CARE

The management of the client with malignant melanoma begins with identification, diagnosis, and tumor staging. If treatable, the tumor is removed through surgical excision. Malignant melanoma is also treated with chemotherapy, immunotherapy, and radiation therapy. Other therapies used with success include biological therapies with interleukin-2 and interferon and therapeutic vaccines containing melanoma antigens.

### Identification

Malignant melanoma is most often found on the trunk of men and on the lower extremities of women. Nevertheless, it is important for the client to have a complete physical examination and total skin assessment. In addition to a visual examination of all skin surfaces, palpation of regional lymph nodes, the liver, and the spleen is essential to assess for metastasis when a melanoma is suspected or found.

A change in the color or size of a nevus is reported in 70% of people diagnosed with a malignant melanoma. The ABCD rule is used to assess suspicious lesions:

A = asymmetry (one half of the nevus does not match the other half)
B = border irregularity (edges are ragged, blurred, or notched)
C = color variation or dark black color
D = diameter greater than 6 mm (size of a pencil eraser)

### Diagnostic Tests

In addition to biopsy of any suspicious lesion, diagnostic tests are conducted to determine whether the tumor has metastasized. Because malignant melanoma may metastasize to any organ or tissue of the body, a variety of tests may be conducted.

- Epiluminescence microscopy helps identify lesions that require a biopsy.
- Biopsy of the lesion is the only definitive method of diagnosing a malignant melanoma. An excisional biopsy is the diagnostic procedure of choice because this allows the most complete histologic evaluation and microstaging.
- Prior to excision, lymphoscintigraphy may be performed to detect microscopic metastasis.
- If the client has manifestations indicating possible metastasis, diagnostic tests specific to the suspected site include liver function tests and CT scan of the liver, a complete blood count, serum blood chemistry profile, chest X-ray, bone scan, and CT scan or MRI of the brain.

### Microstaging

The term *microstaging* describes the assessment of the level of invasion of a malignant melanoma and the maximum tumor thickness. In the Clark system of microstaging, the vertical growth of the lesion is measured from the epidermis to the subcutaneous tissue to determine the level of invasion (Figure 14–29 ■). However, variations in individual skin thicknesses

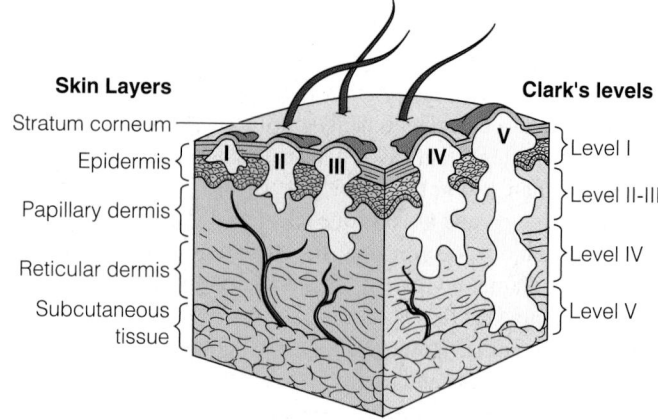

**Figure 14–29 ■** Clark's levels for staging measure the invasion of a melanoma from the epidermis to the subcutaneous tissue.

and different anatomic sites can affect the accuracy of the measurement. In the Breslow system, an adaptation of the Clark system of assessment, the vertical thickness is measured from the granular level of the epidermis to the deepest level of tumor invasion. This determination is important, because as the thickness of the melanoma increases, survival rate decreases.

After the thickness and depth of the tumor are determined, a clinical stage is assigned. The traditional three-stage system is still used, although it does not include tumor thickness. The American Joint Committee on Cancer has adopted a four-stage system that includes tumor thickness, level of invasion, lymph node involvement, and evidence of metastasis.

## Treatments

Surgical excision is the preferred treatment for malignant melanoma. Other methods are chemotherapy, immunotherapy, and radiation therapy.

### Surgery

If a biopsy identifies the lesion as a melanoma, a wide excision is performed that includes the full thickness of the skin and subcutaneous tissue. Because the risk of local recurrence for thin melanomas (those less than 0.76 mm) is quite low, margins of 0.5 to 1.0 cm of normal skin are excised around the tumor. Thick tumors require a 1- to 3-cm margin excision because they are at risk for local recurrence or satellite lesions.

Regional lymph nodes are the most common sites for metastasis of malignant melanoma. Standard surgical treatment for clinically suspicious lymph node involvement includes excision of the primary lesions as well as surgical dissection of the involved lymph nodes. Elective lymph node dissection (ELND) in the treatment of localized malignant melanoma remains controversial. Advocates of ELND believe that the procedure benefits clients with intermediate-thickness tumors because approximately 20% of people whose lymph nodes were clinically negative at diagnosis show some metastasis on removal of the nodes. Those opposed to ELND believe the risks associated with the procedure are too high for the 80% of people who have no evidence of metastasis after removal of the nodes.

Surgery also is indicated for palliative management of isolated metastasis. Removal of metastatic tumors in the brain, liver, lung, gastrointestinal tract, or subcutaneous tissue may relieve symptoms and prolong life.

### Immunotherapy

Immunotherapy is a relatively new treatment modality for malignant melanoma. The role of the immunologic response initially was recognized because of the numerous spontaneous remissions seen in clients with melanoma—a higher occurrence than with any other adult tumor. In addition, researchers have recently identified tumor-specific antigen-antibodies in clients with melanoma. This also has stimulated an interest in immunotherapeutic interventions for the treatment of malignant melanoma.

Agents such as interferons, interleukins, monoclonal antibodies, bacille Calmette-Guérin (BCG), levamisole, transfer factors, and tumor vaccines have shown activity in melanoma, with varying response rates. The effectiveness of these agents, used either alone, in combination with chemotherapy, or in combination with each other, is under investigation. The use of immunotherapy in the treatment of melanoma is still new and requires further investigation.

### Radiation Therapy

Melanoma responds to higher dose radiation, especially if the tumor is small. Response rates to radiation therapy depend on the site of the tumor, the thickness of the tumor, the type of melanoma, and the client's general health, but may range from 0% to 71%. Radiation frequently is used for palliation of symptoms resulting from metastasis to the brain, bone, lymph nodes, gastrointestinal tract, skin, or subcutaneous tissue. Liver and lung metastases are not treated with radiation therapy because a loss of organ function may result.

## NURSING CARE

The nurse has the opportunity to assess the skin of clients requiring care for many different health problems and may be the first person to identify suspicious lesions. Wide excision and the high risk of metastasis from malignant melanoma usually requires inpatient surgical treatment, with the nurse providing care and teaching.

## Health Promotion

The most important aspect of preventing malignant melanoma is a health history and skin assessment. The American Cancer Society recommends that people between the ages of 20 and 40 see a skin specialist every 3 years and those over 40 have annual skin checkups. People with actinic keratoses should also have their skin checked regularly for any signs of change. Clients at risk (those with precancerous lesions and with personal risk factors) should conduct a monthly skin self-examination (e.g., the first day of each month). Using a mirror to examine lesions on the back of the body and extremities, the client looks for a change in:

- Color, especially any lesion that becomes darker or variegated in shades of tan, brown, black, red, white, or blue.
- Size, especially any lesion that becomes larger or spreads out.
- Shape, especially any lesion that protrudes more from the skin or begins to have an irregular outline.
- Appearance of a lesion, especially bleeding, drainage, oozing, ulceration, crusting, scaliness, or development of a mushrooming outward growth.
- Consistency, especially any lesion that becomes softer or is more easily irritated.
- Skin around a lesion, such as redness, swelling, or leaking of color from a lesion into the surrounding skin.
- Sensation, such as itching or pain.

## Assessment

Skin assessment is discussed in Chapter 13. Specific health history questions and assessments for skin cancer are outlined in Box 14–4.

## BOX 14–4 ■ Nursing Assessment for Skin Cancer

### INTERVIEW QUESTIONS

■ Have any members of your family ever been treated for skin cancer?

■ Have you had a skin cancer removed from any part of your body?

■ Have you noticed any change in the size, shape, or color of a mole, wart, birthmark, or scar?

■ Do you have any moles, warts, birthmarks, or scars that itch, are painful, have crusting, or bleed?

■ In what parts of the country or world have you lived?

■ Have you ever been badly sunburned?

■ Do you visit tanning salons?

■ Are you exposed to any hazardous chemicals in your job?

■ Have you been taught how to examine your skin? If so, how do you do this examination? How often?

### Physical Assessment

1. Ask the client to remove all clothing and put on an examination gown. Ensure good light; natural, bright light is best for inspection of lesions. The client may sit, stand, or lie down.
2. Inspect and palpate the skin. Stretching the skin tightly during assessment facilitates assessment of nodular and scaly lesions and lesions in the dermis. Assess for:
   a. Obvious lesions
   b. Visible swellings
   c. Alterations in normal contour and borders of nevi
   d. Enlarged lymph glands
   e. Skin or mucosal discolorations
   f. Areas of ulceration, scaling, crusting, or erosion
3. The order of assessment follows:
   a. Head and neck: entire scalp, eyelids, external ear, auditory canals, external surface of the nose, internal surface of the nose, the oral cavity, facial skin, the facial glands (parotid, submaxillary, sublingual)
   b. Thyroid and neck, including lymph glands
   c. Chest and abdomen, with special attention under pendulous breasts, in skinfolds, and in areas covered with hair
   d. Back and buttocks, with special attention to the area between the buttocks
   e. Extremities, with special attention to the axillae, nail beds, webs between the fingers and toes, and soles of the feet
   f. External genitals, with special attention to skinfolds, mucous membranes, and areas covered with hair
4. Measure and record a description of all skin lesions on an anatomic chart. Take photographs (if possible) of any suspicious lesion, and include them in the client's record for future reference.

## Nursing Diagnoses and Interventions

Although many different nursing diagnoses may be appropriate for the client with a malignant melanoma, the most common responses are impaired skin integrity, hopelessness, and anxiety.

### Impaired Skin Integrity

Impaired skin integrity is a common problem for the client with malignant melanoma. These cancers not only destroy skin layers but also invade body structures. Certain types of tumors may ulcerate prior to diagnosis, and treatment typically involves some type of surgical biopsy and excision. Any open lesion or incision increases the risk for secondary infection.

• Monitor for manifestations of infection: fever, tachycardia, malaise, incisional erythema, swelling, pain, or drainage that increases or becomes purulent. *Intact skin is the first line of defense against infection; impaired skin integrity increases the risk for infection. If infection is present, the client may have both systemic and local manifestations.*

• Keep the incision line clean and dry by changing dressings as necessary. *Moisture increases the risk of infection.*

• Follow principles of medical and surgical asepsis when caring for client's incision. Teach family members and visitors the importance of careful hand washing. Maintain standard precautions if drainage is present. Careful hand washing is essential in preventing the spread of infection. *Aseptic techniques are necessary when caring for any surgical incision to prevent infection.*

• Encourage and maintain adequate caloric and protein intake in the diet. Suggest a consultation with the dietitian if client does not want to eat. *Adequate kcalories and protein are necessary for proper healing. The client with cancer has increased metabolic needs; if these needs are not met, nutritional problems that impair healing may result.*

### Hopelessness

Hopelessness is often described in the literature as a response to the diagnosis of cancer. It is an emotional state in which a person feels that there is no possibility that life will improve. Clients who experience hopelessness are often withdrawn, passive, and apathetic.

The diagnosis of malignant melanoma threatens the quality and quantity of life as the client faces the possibility or reality of metastasis; the possibility that the cancer may recur and cause death; and alterations in self-concept, roles, and relationships. Inspiring hope in clients during this health crisis is a legitimate nursing action.

• Provide an environment that encourages the client to identify and express feelings, concerns, and goals:
  • Use active listening, ask open-ended questions, and reflect on the client's statements.
  • Acknowledge and respect the client's feelings of apathy and/or anger as expressions of distress.
  • Convey an empathetic understanding of the client's fears and concerns.
  • Provide opportunities for the client to express positive emotions: hope, faith, a sense of purpose, and the will to live.

- Explore the client's perceptions, and modify or clarify them if necessary by providing information and correcting misconceptions.
- Encourage the client to identify support systems and sources of strength and coping in the past.

*Verbalizing feelings, concerns, and goals allows others to validate or correct them, promotes a therapeutic nurse-client relationship, and fosters feelings of self-worth. Expressing positive emotions and calling on support systems and sources of strength that were effective in coping with past crises help the person resolve the crisis and develop hope.*

- Encourage the client to participate actively in self-care as well as in mutual decision making and goal setting. *Meeting self-care needs and making decisions about care increase personal confidence in one's capacity for coping.*
- Encourage the client to focus not only on the present but also on the future: Review past occasions for hope, discuss the client's personal meaning of hope, establish and evaluate short-term goals with the client and family, and encourage them to express hope for the future. *The nurse mobilizes the client's resources to strengthen motivation, hope, and the will to live.*

## Anxiety

Anxiety is aroused by a perceived threat; its intensity depends on the severity of the present situation and the client's ability to handle the threat. Anxiety is one of the most common psychosocial responses in clients with cancer. Anxiety increases at the time of diagnosis and remains a constant emotion throughout the course of treatment, regardless of treatment type or setting. Interventions center on helping the client recognize the manifestations of anxiety, determining whether the client wishes to do anything about the anxiety, and facilitating coping strategies (McCloskey & Bulechek, 2000).

- Provide reassurance and comfort:
  - Set aside time to sit quietly with the client.
  - Speak slowly and calmly.
  - Convey empathetic understanding by touch and supporting present coping mechanisms, such as crying and talking.
  - Do not make demands or expect the client to make decisions.

*Coping behaviors differ from situation to situation and from person to person. Anxiety at moderate to severe levels narrows perceptions and the ability to function.*

- Decrease sensory stimuli by using short, simple sentences; focusing on the here and now; and providing concise information. *Higher levels of anxiety result in a focus on the present, inability to concentrate, and difficulty in understanding verbal communications.*
- Provide interventions that decrease anxiety levels and increase coping:
  - Provide accurate information about the illness, treatment, and expected length of recovery.
  - Encourage discussion of expected physical changes and ways to minimize disfigurement through cosmetics and clothing.
  - Include family members in teaching sessions.
  - Provide the client with strategies for participating in the recovery process.

*Although the prognosis and treatment of melanoma depend on various factors, the prognosis of complete cure is decreased with metastasis. Surgical incisions include excision with wide margins, which may cause disfigurement. Active participation in care give the client some control over the future and is often an effective means of coping with anxiety.*

## Using NANDA, NIC, and NOC

Chart 14–2 shows links between NANDA, NIC, and NOC when caring for the client with malignant melanoma.

### CHART 14–2  NANDA, NIC, AND NOC LINKAGES

#### The Client with Malignant Melanoma

| NURSING DIAGNOSES | NURSING INTERVENTIONS | NURSING OUTCOMES |
|---|---|---|
| • Impaired Skin Integrity | • Skin Surveillance<br>• Medication Administration<br>• Infection Control | • Tissue Integrity:<br>  Skin and Mucous Membranes |
| • Impaired Tissue Integrity | • Incision Site Care<br>• Infection Protection<br>• Wound Care | • Wound Healing<br>• Tissue Integrity: Skin and Mucous Membranes |
| • Risk for Infection | • Infection Control<br>• Wound Care | • Risk Control |
| • Hopelessness | • Hope Instillation<br>• Sleep Enhancement<br>• Spiritual Support | • Hope<br>• Sleep<br>• Spiritual Well-Being |

*Note. Data from Nursing Outcomes Classification (NOC) by M. Johnson & M. Maas (Eds.), 1997, St. Louis: Mosby; Nursing Diagnoses: Definitions & Classification 2001–2002 by North American Nursing Diagnosis Association, 2001, Philadelphia: NANDA; Nursing Interventions Classification (NIC) by J.C. McCloskey & G. M. Bulechek (Eds.), 2000, St. Louis: Mosby. Reprinted by permission.*

## Home Care

Teaching the client and family experiencing the diagnosis and treatment of malignant melanoma involves self-care and ongoing self-monitoring. Education for the client and family is specific to the type of treatment. In addition to wound care, clients who have had a lymph node dissection need instructions in how to protect the extremity from bleeding, trauma, and infection. In addition, address the following topics.

- Clients should schedule regular medical checkups every 3 months for the first 2 years, every 6 months for the next 5 years, and yearly thereafter.
- Emphasize that proper self-care combined with regular medical care can help the client lead a fairly normal life.
- If assistance for home care is necessary, provide referrals to a community health agency or a home care agency. In addition, refer the client to a local cancer support group if the client believes this will be helpful.

## Nursing Care Plan
## A Client with Malignant Melanoma

Geoff Sanders, age 69, is retired from the postal service. He has always been an avid participant in outdoor sports: When he was younger he played baseball and tennis, and for the last 10 years he has played golf at least twice a week. He now lives in Connecticut, but as a younger man he lived in Florida for almost 15 years. Mr. Sanders has a variety of warts and moles and rarely pays attention to them. However, after taking a shower one day he noticed that a mole on his left lower leg looked bigger and darker. Mr. Sanders had just seen a public announcement on television about the dangers of changes in moles, and he immediately called his primary HMO physician for an appointment at the dermatology clinic.

### ASSESSMENT

On arriving at the clinic, Mr. Sanders is interviewed and examined by Tom Hall, a clinical nurse specialist. Following the assessment, Tom documents the following information.

Mr. Sanders has a family history of skin cancer; his father had several squamous cell cancers removed from his face. He has numerous nevi on his body; the one causing concern is located on the medial anterior left leg, 2 inches below the patella. Mr. Sanders states that the mole has been present for years but that he noticed just yesterday that it has become larger and darker. On further questioning, he states that the mole itches sometimes but has never hurt or bled. Mr. Sanders lived in Florida for 15 years and now experiences a sunburn early each summer before he tans. The sunburn involves the lower legs because Mr. Sanders wears shorts during his twice-weekly golf game.

A complete skin assessment reveals various freckles, warts, and nevi. With the exception of the nevus that prompted Mr. Sanders to come to the clinic, all lesions appear normal. The nevus in question is raised, 3 cm in diameter, with irregular borders and a nodular surface. It is variegated in color, with various shades of brown. The skin surrounding the nevus is slightly erythematous. Inguinal lymph nodes are not enlarged or painful. Tom Hall takes a photograph of the lesion with Mr. Sanders's permission.

Following the assessment, Mr. Sanders discusses the lesion with a surgeon, who recommends excision. They discuss the possibility of skin cancer and the importance of early detection and treatment. Mr. Sanders is scheduled for a biopsy of the nevus under a local anesthetic the following morning. Following the biopsy, histologic examination reveals lentigo maligna melanoma. Staging of the tumor reveals that it is a melanoma in situ, with no metastasis to regional lymph nodes. Mr. Sanders undergoes a wide excision of the lesion the following afternoon.

### DIAGNOSIS

- *Impaired skin integrity* related to excision of melanoma from the left lower leg
- *Risk for infection* related to surgical wound on left lower leg
- *Acute pain* related to wide excision of melanoma on left lower leg
- *Anxiety* related to diagnosis of skin cancer

### EXPECTED OUTCOMES

- Demonstrate complete healing of the incision without manifestations of infection.
- Verbalize relief of pain by the time the incision is healed.
- Verbalize fears and concerns about his diagnosis.

### PLANNING AND IMPLEMENTATION

- Make the first dressing change, but ensure that Mr. Sanders can safely change the dressing himself prior to discharge the day after surgery.
- On discharge, provide adequate dressings and tape for the first home dressing change; include in discharge instructions necessary information about where to buy supplies and how many dressing supplies will be needed.
- Review and provide written instructions for prescribed systemic antibiotic and pain medication.
- Provide written instructions for dressing change, manifestations of infection, and phone number of clinic; stress importance of calling if any abnormal symptoms occur.
- Teach how to protect the incision from bumps and to protect the site from irritants.
- Discuss diagnosis, positive outlook for treatment of melanoma in situ, and the client's concerns.
- Stress importance of lifelong regular health care evaluations to identify any recurrence or metastasis.

### EVALUATION

Mr. Sanders returned to the dermatology clinic 1 week after his surgical incision. His incision is well approximated and shows no signs of infection. He is taking his antibiotic 4 times a day as prescribed and reports that his need for pain medications is decreasing. During his clinic visit the following week, Tom Hall removes the sutures and assesses the wound as healed. Mr. Sanders completed his antibiotics and no longer requires pain medications. He says he is still "scared to death" about having cancer, but he has decided to join a local cancer support group. He also says he had gotten a list of skin safety rules from the American Cancer

(continued on page 397)

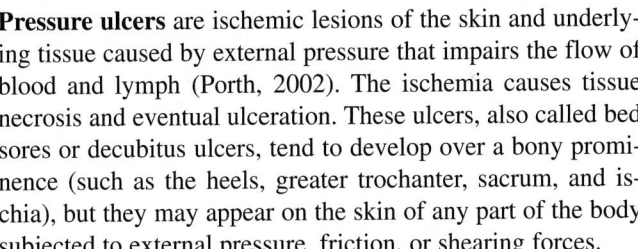

## Nursing Care Plan

### A Client with Malignant Melanoma *(continued)*

Society and will be sure to cover up and use sunscreens when he plays golf. Mr. Sanders makes an appointment for follow-up care in 3 months.

#### Critical Thinking in the Nursing Process

1. Consider reasons why people who notice a change in a skin lesion put off seeking health care. What can nurses do to effect change?
2. Design a teaching plan for young adults for preventing skin cancers.

3. What would you say to Mr. Sanders if he called the clinic and said that the antibiotics were making him sick and he didn't think he needed them anyway?
4. Design a nursing care plan for Mr. Sanders for the diagnosis *Powerlessness.*

See Evaluating Your Response in Appendix C.

# SKIN TRAUMA

Trauma to the skin can be unintentional or intentional (as in the case of surgery). Chemicals, radiation, pressure, or thermal changes cause skin trauma. This section discusses pressure ulcers and frostbite, as well as intentional trauma from cutaneous and plastic surgery or treatment. Thermal injury, or burns, is discussed in Chapter 15.

## THE CLIENT WITH A PRESSURE ULCER

**Pressure ulcers** are ischemic lesions of the skin and underlying tissue caused by external pressure that impairs the flow of blood and lymph (Porth, 2002). The ischemia causes tissue necrosis and eventual ulceration. These ulcers, also called bed sores or decubitus ulcers, tend to develop over a bony prominence (such as the heels, greater trochanter, sacrum, and ischia), but they may appear on the skin of any part of the body subjected to external pressure, friction, or shearing forces.

### INCIDENCE

The incidence of pressure ulcers in hospitals, long-term care facilities, and home settings is high enough to warrant concern for health care providers. The incidence in hospitals has been reported as ranging from 3.5% to 29%, whereas the incidence in long-term care facilities is reported to be around 23%. Little research has been done to determine the extent of the problem in the home setting. However, with increasing numbers of clients (and especially older adult clients) being cared for in the home, it is probable that the incidence is great enough to warrant plans of care to prevent their occurrence.

### PATHOPHYSIOLOGY

Pressure ulcers develop from external pressure that compresses blood vessels or from friction and shearing forces that tear and injure vessels. Both types of pressure cause traumatic injury and initiate the process of pressure ulcer development.

External pressure that is greater than capillary pressure and arteriolar pressure interrupts blood flow in capillary beds. When pressure is applied to skin over a bony prominence for 2 hours, tissue ischemia and hypoxia from external pressure cause irreversible tissue damage. For example, when the body is in the supine position, the body's weight applies pressure to the sacrum. The same amount of pressure causes more damage when it is applied to a small area than when it is distributed over a large surface.

Shearing forces result when one tissue layer slides over another. The stretching and bending of blood vessels cause injury and thrombosis. Clients in hospital beds are subject to shearing forces when the head of the bed is elevated and the torso slides down toward the foot of the bed. Pulling the client up in bed also subjects the client to shearing forces. (For this reason, always lift clients up in bed). In both cases, friction and moisture cause the skin and superficial fascia to remain fixed to the bed sheet, while the deep fascia and bony skeleton slides in the direction of body movement.

When a person lies or sits in one position for an extended length of time without moving, pressure on the tissue between a bony prominence and the external surface of the body distorts capillaries and interferes with normal blood flow. If the pressure is relieved, blood flow to the area increases, and a brief period of reactive hyperemia occurs without permanent damage. However, if the pressure continues, platelets aggregate in the endothelial cells surrounding the capillaries and form microthrombi. These microthrombi impede blood flow, resulting in ischemia and hypoxia of tissues. Eventually, the cells and tissues of the immediate area of pressure and of the surrounding area die and become necrotic.

Alterations in the involved tissue depend on the depth of the injury. Injury to superficial layers of skin results in blister formation, whereas injury to deeper structures causes the pressure ulcer area to appear dark reddish-blue. As the tissues die, the ulcer becomes an open wound that may be deep enough to expose the bone. The necrotic tissue elicits an inflammatory

## BOX 14–5   ■ Pressure Ulcer Staging

**STAGE I**

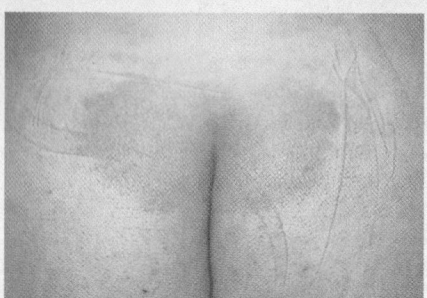

Nonblanchable erythema of intact skin; the heralding lesion of skin ulceration. Identification of stage I pressure ulcers may be difficult in clients with darkly pigmented skin. *Note:* Reactive hyperemia can normally be expected to be present for one-half to three-fourths as long as the pressure occluded blood flow to the area. This should not be confused with stage I pressure ulcer.

**STAGE II**

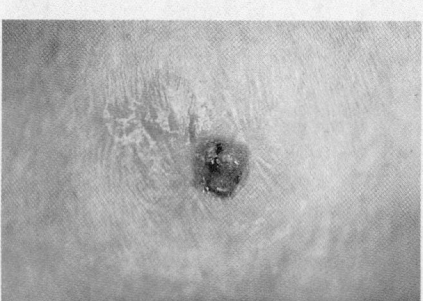

Partial-thickness skin loss involving epidermis and/or dermis. The ulcer is superficial and presents clinically as an abrasion, blister, or shallow crater.

**STAGE III**

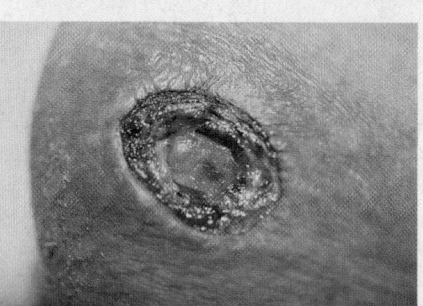

Full-thickness skin loss involving damage or necrosis of subcutaneous tissue that may extend down to, but not through, underlying fascia. The ulcer presents clinically as a deep crater with or without undermining of adjacent tissue.

**STAGE IV**

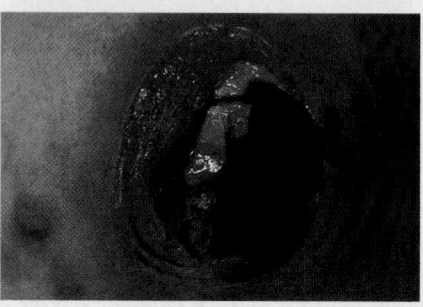

Full-thickness skin loss with extensive destruction, tissue necrosis, or damage to muscle, bone, or supporting structures (for example, tendon or joint capsule). Sinus tracts may also be associated with stage IV ulcers.

*Note:* When eschar is present, accurate staging of the pressure ulcer is not possible until the eschar has sloughed or the wound has been debrided.

*Note. Text is from* Pressure Ulcers in Adults: Prediction and Prevention *by the Agency for Health Care Policy and Research, 1992, Rockville, MD: U.S. Department of Health and Human Services. Photos courtesy of Karen Lou Kennedy, RN, FPN.*

response, and the client experiences increases in temperature, pain, and white blood cell count. Secondary bacterial invasion is common. Enzymes from bacteria and macrophages dissolve necrotic tissue, resulting in a foul-smelling drainage.

Pressure ulcers are graded or staged to classify the degree of damage. The stages are listed in Box 14–5.

## RISK FACTORS

Although a pressure ulcer may develop in an adult of any age who has an impairment in mobility, those most at risk are older adults with limited mobility (see page 399), people with quadriplegia, and clients in the critical care setting (Porth, 2002).

Other clients prone to develop pressure ulcers are those with fractures of large bones (e.g., hip or femur) or who have undergone orthopedic surgery or sustained spinal cord injury. In addition to deficits in mobility and activity, incontinence and nutritional deficit also increase the risk of pressure ulcer development. Clients with chronic illnesses, such as renal failure and anemia, and those with edema or infection are also at increased risk.

Because of age-related skin changes, the older adult is at increased risk for the development of pressure ulcers. The skin of the older adult has a thicker epidermis, a thinner dermis with decreased vascularity, decreased sebaceous gland activity, and

## Meeting Individualized Needs

### PRESSURE ULCER PREVENTION IN OLDER ADULTS

Older adults are at a greater risk for developing pressure ulcers because of age-related changes in the integumentary system. Cell renewal slows, resulting in skin that has decreased elasticity. The margin between the epidermis and the dermis separates more easily, making the skin more prone to tearing. In addition, thinning subcutaneous tissue provides less cushioning over bony prominences. Water content decreases, and the skin becomes drier. These changes increase the older adult's susceptibility to skin trauma and prolong wound healing.

Chronic conditions associated with immobility and self-care deficit place older adults at risk of developing pressure ulcers. For example, bowel or bladder incontinence can produce regions of wet skin that are prone to infections and breakdown. Furthermore, sensory-perceptual alterations and impaired cognitive functioning may reduce the frequency in which the older adult shifts position when sitting or lying in bed. Finally, undernutrition, which is often seen in older adults, heightens the risk for developing pressure ulcers.

To prevent pressure ulcers, the skin of older adults should be kept clean, dry, and well hydrated. Moisturizers are recommended to keep the skin free of excessive dryness. Older adults should be taught to avoid bumping into furniture and to wear long skirts or pants to help protect the lower extremities from trauma.

When hospitalized, older adults should have a validated risk assessment for pressure ulcers completed on admission and as often as the tool suggests. A daily systematic skin inspection with particular attention to bony prominences should be completed.

Once pressure ulcers develop in older adults, the treatment is the same as for younger clients. However, there are additional steps that may need to be taken. Because local perfusion to tissues is compromised, steps should be taken to prevent under or over hydration. It is essential that optimal nutritional status be maintained. Also, keep in mind that it may take a longer time for the pressure ulcer to heal.

decreased strength and elasticity. As a result, the more fragile and less nourished dermal layer is more prone to shear and friction problems. In addition, the skin of the older adult responds more slowly to inflammation, and wounds heal more slowly; when pressure ulcers occur, they are more difficult to reverse.

## COLLABORATIVE CARE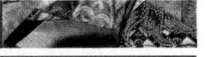

For the client at risk for pressure ulcers, the goal is prevention. Existing ulcers require collaborative treatment to promote healing and restore skin integrity.

Diagnostic tests are conducted to determine the presence of a secondary infection and to differentiate the cause of the ulcer.

If the ulcer is deep or appears infected, drainage or biopsied tissue is cultured to determine the causative organism.

Topical and systemic antibiotics specific to the infectious organism eradicate any infection present. Additionally, a variety of topical products promote healing. Examples are listed in Table 14–4.

Surgical debridement may be necessary if the pressure ulcer is deep; if subcutaneous tissues are involved; or if an eschar (a scab or dry crust that forms over skin damaged by burns, infections, or excoriations) has formed over the ulcer, preventing healing by granulation. Large wounds may require skin grafting for complete closure.

### TABLE 14–4  Products Used to Treat Pressure Ulcers

| Stage | Product | Purpose |
|---|---|---|
| I | Skin Prep | Toughens intact skin and preserves skin integrity. |
| | Granulex | Prevents skin breakdown, increases blood supply, adds moisture, contains trypsin to aid in removal of necrotic tissue. |
| | Hydrocolloid dressing (e.g., DuoDerm) | Prevents skin breakdown and promotes healing without the formation of a crust over the ulcer. Is permeable to air and water vapor; prevents the growth of anaerobic organisms. |
| | Transparent dressing (e.g., Tegaderm) | Prevents skin breakdown; prevents entrance of moisture and bacteria but allows oxygen and moisture vapor permeability. |
| II | Transparent dressing | Enhances healing (see above). |
| | Hydrocolloid dressing | Enhances healing (see above). Note: If infection is present, these types of dressings are contraindicated. A sterile dressing should be applied instead. |
| III | Wet-to-dry gauze dressing with sterile normal saline | Allows necrotic material to soften and adhere to the gauze, so that the wound is debrided. |
| | Hydrocolloid dressing | Enhances healing (see above). |
| | Proteolytic enzymes (such as Elase) | Proteolytic enzymes serve as a debriding agent in inflamed and infected lesions. |
| IV | Wet-to-dry gauze dressing with sterile normal saline | Enhances healing (see above). Note: Transparent or hydrocolloid dressings or skin barriers are contraindicated. |
| | Vacuum-assisted closure (V.A.C.) | Creates a negative pressure to help reduce edema, increase blood supply and oxygenation, and decrease bacterial colonization. Also helps promote moist wound healing and the formation of granulation tissue. |

## Nursing Research

### Evidence-Based Practice for Preventing Pressure Ulcers in Acute Care and Home Care Settings

Chronic wounds treated in the United States are a growing and costly health care problem. It is estimated that 5.6 million chronic wounds are treated each year, and that the cost for pressure ulcers alone is $1.3 billion. One way to decrease the human and economic cost is to prevent pressure ulcers from forming in the first place. Pieper et al. (1997a, 1997b) have studied this problem extensively, examining the presence of pressure ulcer methods for at-risk clients (those with more medical diagnoses and longer hospitalizations) as compared to not-at-risk clients in hospital, acute rehabilitation, and home settings. Findings from these studies were that at-risk clients were more likely to have the head of the bed in a low position, a pressure-reducing bed surface, a positioning wedge, incontinence cleanser and ointment, heel protection, a trapeze, and a posted turning schedule. At-risk clients were also more likely to have a prevention care plan and documentation of prevention methods. It is important to implement these preventive methods as soon as possible, as ulcers develop quickly.

#### IMPLICATIONS FOR NURSING

The design and implementation of a pressure ulcer care plan is essential for any person who is at risk, including the older adult, those with disorders limiting mobility, and those with debilitating or multiple illnesses. Nursing care is critical to the prevention of this problem. As documented in these studies, the percentage of clients placed on a pressure ulcer–prevention program was low for those considered both at-risk and not-at-risk. Health care providers and institutions must continue to explore this critical area affecting client outcomes.

#### Critical Thinking in Client Care

1. Describe the differences and similarities in a pressure ulcer–prevention plan of care you would develop for two clients: a 76-year-old man in a nursing home who has had a stroke that paralyzed the left side of his body, and a 36-year-old man with spinal cord damage from a motorcycle accident who cannot walk and lives at home.
2. Consider the activities necessary to prevent pressure ulcers. If you were managing a client's care, what would you do about the following:
   a. What level of health care provider would you assign to care for the client?
   b. How much time in an 8-hour period would be needed for nursing care?
   c. What would you teach family caregivers about providing activities at home?

## NURSING CARE

The client with one or more pressure ulcers not only has impaired skin integrity but also is at increased risk for infection, pain, and decreased mobility. Pressure ulcers also prolong treatment for other conditions, increase health care costs, and diminish the client's quality of life (see the box above).

## Nursing Diagnoses and Interventions

The following interventions and rationales are adapted from the clinical guidelines developed by the Agency for Health Care Policy and Research (1992, 1994) in identifying adults at risk and treating those with stage I pressure ulcers.

### Risk for Impaired Skin Integrity

- Identify at-risk individuals needing prevention and the specific factors placing them at risk.
- Assess bed- and chair-bound clients, as well as those who are unable to reposition themselves, for additional risk factors: immobility, incontinence, nutritional factors (such as inadequate dietary intake and impaired nutritional status), and altered level of consciousness.
- Assess clients on admission to acute care and rehabilitation hospitals, nursing homes, home care programs, and other health care facilities.
- Use a systematic risk assessment by using a validated risk assessment tool (such as the Braden scale).
- Document all assessments of risk.

*Individuals at risk for pressure ulcers must be identified so that risk factors can be reduced through intervention. The primary risk factors for pressure ulcers are immobility and limited activity; therefore, assess clients who cannot reposition themselves or whose activity is limited to bed or chair. Validated tools ensure systematic evaluation of individual risk factors. The client requires periodic reassessment for pressure ulcers. Accurate and complete documentation of all risk assessments ensures continuity of care and may be used as a foundation for the skin care plan.*

- Conduct a systematic skin inspection at least once a day, paying particular attention to the bony prominences. Systematic, comprehensive, and routine skin care may decrease pressure ulcer incidence (although the exact role is unknown. Inspect the following to assess a pressure ulcer:
  - Location of any lesion or ulcer
  - Estimation of the stage
  - Dimensions of the ulcer: length, width, depth
  - Presence of any abnormal pathways in the wound
    - Sinus tract: a cavity or channel underneath the wound
    - Tunneling: a passageway or opening that may be visible at skin level, but with most of the tunnel under the surface of the skin
    - Undermining: areas of tissue destruction underneath intact skin along wound margins
  - Visible necrotic tissue (Slough is necrotic tissue that is in the process of separating from viable tissue.)
  - Presence of an exudate
  - Presence or absence of granulation tissue

*Skin inspection provides data the nurse uses in designing interventions to reduce risk and in evaluating outcomes of those interventions.*

- Clean the skin at the time of soiling and at routine intervals, as frequently as the client's need or preference dictates. Avoid hot water, use a mild cleansing agent, and clean the skin gently, applying as little force and friction as possible. *Metabolic wastes and environmental contaminants accumulate on the skin; these potentially irritating substances should be removed frequently. Feces and urine cause chemical irritation and should be removed as soon as possible. Hot water may cause skin injury. Mild cleansing agents are less likely to remove the skin's natural barrier.*

- Minimize environmental factors leading to skin drying, such as low humidity and exposure to cold. Treat dry skin with moisturizers. *Well-hydrated skin resists mechanical trauma. Hydration decreases as the ambient air temperature decreases, especially when the air humidity is low. Poorly hydrated skin is less pliable, and severe dryness is associated with fissuring and cracking of the stratum corneum. Moisturizers reduce dry skin.*

- Avoid massage over bony prominences. *Although massage has been practiced for years, evidence now suggests that massage over bony prominences may lead to deep tissue trauma in clients at risk for or with beginning skin manifestations of a pressure ulcer.*

- Minimize skin exposure to moisture due to incontinence, perspiration, or wound drainage. When these sources of moisture cannot be controlled, use underpads or briefs made of materials that absorb moisture and present a quick-drying surface to the skin. Change underpads and briefs frequently. Do not place plastic directly against the skin. *Moisture from incontinence, perspiration, or wound drainage may contain factors that irritate the skin; moisture alone can increase the susceptibility of the skin to injury.*

- To minimize skin injury due to friction and shearing forces, use proper positioning, transferring, and turning techniques. Lubricants (such as cornstarch or creams), protective films (such as transparent dressings and skin sealants), protective dressings (such as hydrocolloids), and protective padding may also reduce friction injuries. *Shear injury occurs when skin remains stationary and the underlying tissue shifts. This shift diminishes the blood supply to the skin and results in ischemia and tissue damage. Proper positioning, however, can eliminate most shear injuries. Friction injuries to the skin occur when it moves across a coarse surface, such as bed linens. Most friction injuries can be avoided by using appropriate techniques to move clients so that their skin is never dragged across the linens. Any agent that eliminates contact or decreases the friction between the skin and the linens reduces the potential for injury.*

- Assess factors involved in inadequate dietary intake of protein or kilocalories. Offer nutritional supplements, and support the client during mealtimes. If dietary intake remains inadequate, consult with a dietitian about other dietary interventions. *The role nutrition plays in the development of (and to a lesser degree, the healing of) pressure ulcers is not understood, but poor dietary intake of kilocalories, protein, and iron has been associated with the development of pressure ulcers.*

- Maintain the client's current level of activity, mobility, and range of motion. *Frequent turning, repositioning, and movement are essential in reducing the risk of pressure ulcers.*

- For the client on bed rest or who is immobile, provide interventions against the adverse effects of external mechanical forces of pressure, friction, and shear:
  - Reposition all at-risk clients at least every 2 hours, using a written schedule for systematic turning and repositioning.
  - For clients on bed rest, use positioning devices, such as pillows or foam wedges, to protect bony prominences.

- For completely immobile clients, use devices to totally relieve pressure on the heels (the most common method is to raise the heels off the bed). Do not use donut-type devices.

- Avoid placing clients in the side-lying position directly on the trochanter.

- Maintain the head of the bed at the lowest degree of elevation consistent with the client's medical condition and other restrictions. Limit the amount of time the head of the bed is elevated.

- Use assistive devices, such as a trapeze or bed linen, to move clients in bed who cannot assist during transfers and position changes.

- Place any at-risk client on a pressure-reducing device, such as foam, static air, alternating air, gel, or water mattress.

*Data indicate that the more spontaneous movements that bedridden, older adult clients make, the lower the incidence of pressure ulcers. Studies reveal that fewer pressure ulcers develop in at-risk clients who are turned every 2 to 3 hours. Proper positioning can reduce pressure on bony prominences. It is difficult to redistribute pressure under heels; suspending the heels is the best method. Donut cushions are more likely to cause than to prevent pressure ulcers. Shearing forces are exerted on the body when the head of the bed is elevated. Lifting (rather than dragging) is less likely to cause injury from friction. Pressure-reducing devices and beds can decrease the incidence of pressure ulcers.*

- For chair-bound clients, use pressure-reducing devices. Consider postural alignment, distribution of weight, balance and stability, and pressure relief when positioning these clients. Avoid uninterrupted sitting in a chair or wheelchair. Reposition the client every hour. Teach clients who can do so to shift their weight every 15 minutes. Use a written plan for positioning, movement, and the use of positioning devices. Do not use donut devices. *Prolonged, uninterrupted mechanical pressure results in tissue breakdown. The client's weight should be shifted at least every hour.*

## Home Care

Client and family teaching for care of a pressure ulcer also focuses on prevention and includes much of the same information presented in the preceding section. Because many clients with pressure ulcers are older or have other serious illnesses, a caregiver may require teaching on such topics as the following:

- Definition and description of pressure ulcers
- Common locations of pressure ulcers
- Risk factors for the development of pressure ulcers
- Skin care
- Ways to avoid injury
- Diet

Depending on the stage of the pressure ulcer, the nurse teaches the client or caregiver how to care for ulcers that are already present: how to change wet-to-dry dressings, apply skin barriers, and avoid injury and infection. Referrals to a home health agency or community health department can help the family through the lengthy healing process.

## THE CLIENT WITH FROSTBITE

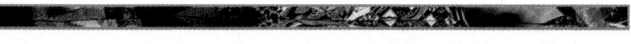

**Frostbite** is an injury of the skin from freezing. If the exposure to freezing temperatures is limited, only the skin and subcutaneous tissues become involved. However, as exposure increases, deeper structures freeze. The skin freezes when the temperature drops to 14° to 24.8°F (210° to 24°C). Frostbite is most common on exposed or peripheral areas of the body, such as the nose, ears, feet, and hands.

As human tissues freeze, ice crystals form and increase intracellular sodium content. Small blood vessels initially vasoconstrict but then vasodilate and become more permeable, causing cellular and tissue swelling. With continued exposure, vasoconstriction and increased viscosity of the blood cause infarction and necrosis of the affected tissue.

Superficial frostbite causes numbness, itching, and prickling. The skin appears cyanotic, reddened, or white. Deeper frostbite causes stiffness and paresthesias. As the skin and tissues thaw, the skin becomes white or yellow and loses its elasticity. The client experiences burning pain. Edema, blisters, necrosis, and gangrene may appear.

Rapid thawing may significantly decrease tissue necrosis. General guidelines for rewarming areas of frostbite follow:

- If you are outdoors, treat superficial frostbite by applying firm pressure with a warm hand or by placing frostbitten hands in the axillae. If the feet are frostbitten, remove wet footwear, dry the feet, and put on dry footwear. Do not rub the areas with snow.
- In the hospital, rapidly rewarm affected areas in circulating warm water, 104° to 105°F (40° to 40.5°C) for 20 to 30 minutes. Do not rub or massage the areas.

Following rewarming, the client is kept on bed rest with the affected parts elevated. Pain medications and anti-inflammatory agents are administered. Blisters are debrided. Whirlpool therapy may be used to clean the skin and debride necrotic tissue. Recovery from frostbite is usually complete if the involved area has not become necrotic. Necrotic tissue may require amputation.

## THE CLIENT UNDERGOING CUTANEOUS AND PLASTIC SURGERY

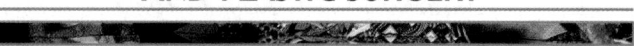

Although many skin disorders are so small and benign that no treatment is necessary, others require some type of surgery of the skin to remove the lesion. Other surgeries and treatments for skin lesions and deformities are used to restore function and change appearance. This section discusses both cutaneous and plastic surgery, as well as other types of treatment modalities used in the care of the client with a skin disorder.

## CUTANEOUS SURGERY AND PROCEDURES

The basic types of cutaneous surgery described here are excision, electrosurgery, cryosurgery, curettage, and laser surgery. Two nonsurgical procedures, chemical destruction and sclerotherapy, are also discussed. Most of these procedures are performed in the office or outpatient clinic.

### Fusiform Excision

**Fusiform excision** is the removal of a full thickness of the epidermis and dermis, usually with a thin layer of subcutaneous tissue. It is used to remove tissue for biopsies and for complete removal of benign and malignant lesions of the skin. Most fusiform excisions have a length-to-width ratio of 3 to 1.

Excision of small, superficial lesions is performed under a local anesthetic, and care is taken to place the incision in a way that will provide good cosmetic results. The incision line is usually closed with sutures, and the wound is covered with a dry dressing, an occlusive dressing, or a hydrocolloid dressing.

### Electrosurgery

**Electrosurgery** involves the destruction or removal of tissue with high-frequency alternating current. A variety of surgical procedures may be performed, including *electrodesiccation* (which produces superficial skin destruction), *electrocoagulation* (which produces deeper tissue destruction), and *electrosection* (which can cut through skin and tissue). Electrodesiccation is used to remove benign surface lesions, such as skin tags, keratoses, warts, and angiomas. It is also used to produce hemostasis for capillary bleeding. Electrocoagulation is used to remove telangiectases, warts, and superficial nonmelanoma skin cancers. Electrosection is used to make incisions, excise tissue, and perform biopsies.

### Cryosurgery

**Cryosurgery** is the destruction of tissue by cold or freezing with agents such as fluorocarbon sprays, carbon dioxide snow, nitrous oxide, and liquid nitrogen. Cryosurgery is used to treat many skin lesions (e.g., keratoses, lentigo maligna, venous lakes, nevi, keloids, and Kaposi's sarcoma). The freezing agents are applied topically to the lesion.

The effects of freezing depend on the degree of freeze. Light freezing causes damage to the epidermis with blistering or crusting that heals without scarring. Deeper freezes, used to treat malignant cells, cause edema, necrosis, and tissue slough. The effects of cryosurgery may not be obvious until 24 hours following the treatment. Postoperatively, infection is prevented by applying a topical antibiotic and keeping the treated areas clean. Healing occurs in 2 to 3 weeks.

## Curettage

**Curettage** is the removal of lesions with a curette (a semisharp cutting instrument). The design of the curette allows it to cut through soft or weak tissue, but not through normal tissue. It is used primarily to remove benign and malignant superficial epidermal lesions. Benign lesions removed by curettage include keratoses, nevi, and angiomas. Nonmelanoma skin lesions are removed by curettage if they are small, well-defined, primary tumors. Curettage is also used to remove specimens of tissue for biopsy.

Following curettage, the wound may be treated with electrodesiccation to destroy any remaining malignant cells and to provide hemostasis. These wounds are not closed; rather, they are left open to heal by second intention. Topical antibiotic ointments and dressings may be used in the postoperative period.

## Laser Surgery

Laser surgery is used to treat clients with a wide variety of skin disorders, including port-wine stains, telangiectases, and venous lakes. A laser is an intense light that produces a thermal injury on contact with tissue. The injury causes coagulation, vaporization, excision, and ablation (removal of a growth). Argon, pulsed dye, carbon dioxide, and Nd: YAG lasers are used in cutaneous and plastic surgery. A local anesthetic may be used, although pulsed dye laser causes minimal pain and rarely requires anesthesia.

The response differs by type of laser. Following treatment with the argon laser, the lesion appears from white to black in color, a blister forms, and the skin may peel. The area weeps, and an eschar forms; in 10 to 14 days, the eschar separates, revealing an underlying red area. The redness fades over a period of up to 1 year. However, pulsed dye laser does not result in blistering or weeping; only rarely does it result in eschar.

## Chemical Destruction

Chemical destruction is the application of a specific chemical to produce destruction of skin lesions. Chemical destruction is used to treat both benign and premalignant lesions. The chemical is applied to the lesion or is used to cause peeling. After application, the treated area forms a thin crust that sloughs off in about a week.

## Sclerotherapy

**Sclerotherapy** is the removal of benign skin lesions with a sclerosing agent that causes inflammation with fibrosis of tissue. Agents that cause therapeutic sclerosis include aethoxysklerol (Sclerodex) and hypertonic sodium chloride. This type of treatment is used for telangiectases and superficial spider veins of the lower extremities. The solution is injected into the affected veins, causing a reaction that closes the lumen of the vein.

## PLASTIC SURGERY

**Plastic surgery** is the alteration, replacement, or restoration of visible portions of the body, performed to correct a structural or cosmetic defect. The word *plastic* comes from the Greek word *plastikos,* which means "able to be molded."

Many skin disorders discussed in this chapter cause changes in appearance. For example, acne may leave deep pitting scars, nevi and keloids are often disfiguring, and skin cancers may require wide excision and skin grafting. These scars, lesions, and wounds often cause embarrassment and alterations in body image. In addition, the removal of lesions may leave unsightly scars or areas of obviously missing tissue.

**Cosmetic surgery,** also called **aesthetic surgery,** is one of two fields within plastic surgery. Cosmetic surgery enhances the attractiveness of normal features. The other field, **reconstructive surgery,** uses similar techniques; however, its purpose is to improve the function or appearance of parts of the body damaged by trauma, disease, or birth defects. Reconstructive surgeries comprise approximately 60% of all plastic surgeries performed in the United States.

Many of the plastic surgeries permanently alter body image. To provide the client with a preview of what surgery will accomplish, some surgeons integrate computer imaging into preoperative teaching. The computer projects a photograph of the targeted area onto a monitor and uses graphics to demonstrate how the size and or shape of the body part or area will change as a result of the surgery.

## Skin Grafts and Flaps

Skin grafts and flaps are used to restore function while also maintaining an acceptable appearance. Both of these procedures involve the movement of skin from one part of the body to another part.

A **skin graft** is a surgical method of detaching skin from a donor site and placing it in a recipient site, where it develops a new blood supply from the base of the wound. Skin grafting is an effective way to cover wounds which have a good blood supply, which are not infected, and in which bleeding can be controlled.

Skin grafts may be either split thickness or full thickness (Figure 14–30 ■). A *split-thickness graft* contains epidermis and only a portion of dermis of the donor site. Split-thickness grafts range in thickness from 0.010 inch to greater than 0.015 inch. A common donor site for a skin graft is the anterior thigh. Skin is removed in sheets from the donor site with a dermatome. Donor sites of split-thickness grafts heal by reepithelialization. A meshed graft is a type of split-thickness graft that is rolled under a special cutting machine to form a mesh pattern with perforations. The perforations allow drainage of serum and blood from under the graft. After healing, however, the skin has a rough appearance. A *full-thickness graft* contains both epidermis and dermis. These layers contain the greatest number of skin elements (sweat glands, sebaceous glands, or

**Figure 14–30** ■ Skin depth of split-thickness and full-thickness grafts.

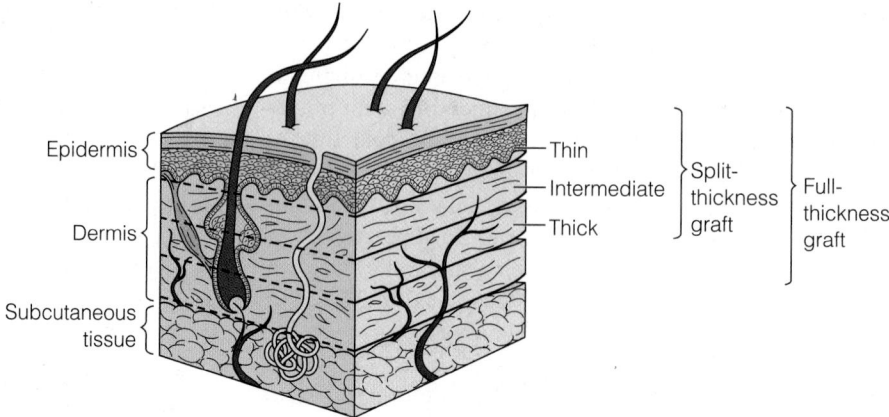

hair follicles) and are best able to withstand trauma. Areas of thin skin are the best donor sites for full-thickness skin grafts. The donor site must be surgically closed and will scar.

Other types of grafts are composite grafts and cultured epithelial grafts. Composite grafts are free grafts and are usually used on the face. They contain skin, subcutaneous tissue, cartilage, or other tissue. Cultured epithelial grafts are made from epithelial cells cultured in vivo, coalesced into sheets, and then used to cover full-thickness wounds. They are used primarily to treat burns.

A **flap** is a piece of tissue whose free end is moved from a donor site to a recipient site while maintaining a continuous blood supply through its connection at the base or pedicle. Flaps carry their own blood supply and are therefore used to cover recipient sites that have a poor blood supply or have sustained a major tissue loss. They are often used for reconstruction or closure of large wounds. Microsurgical techniques, with anastomosis of small blood vessels and nerves, allow reconstruction with free flaps (in which the flap is completely removed from its donor site and moved to the recipient site).

## Chemical Peeling

**Chemical peeling** is the application of a chemical to produce a controlled and predictable injury that alters the anatomy of the epidermis and superficial dermis. The result is skin that appears firmer, smoother, and less wrinkled. This form of cosmetic surgery is more useful in people who have fair, thin skin with fine wrinkling.

Chemical agents used for peeling include phenol, trichloroacetic acid (TCA), and alpha-hydroxy acids (AHA). Phenol, a keratocoagulant, penetrates the epidermis and dermis; regeneration of the epithelium produces the desired results. After treatment, the entire surface of the face except the eyelids is covered with adhesive tape for 1 to 2 days. The adhesive is then removed, and the treated area forms a crust that heals in about a week. TCA has been used for years to obtain the desired effect. A light peel causes mild erythema followed by peeling (as from a mild sunburn) in 3 to 5 days. AHA are organic acids used to produce light to moderate peeling to remove acne, fine lines, seborrheic keratosis, warts, and mild scarring. Both TCA and AHA treatments may be repeated weekly. One complica-

tion of chemical peeling is bleaching of the skin (due to removal of melanocytes).

## Liposuction

**Liposuction** is a method of changing the contours of the body by aspirating fat from the subcutaneous layer of tissue. This treatment is used to remove excess fat from the buttocks, flanks, abdomen, thighs, upper arms, knees, ankles, and chin. It is not a cure for obesity and should not be used as a substitute for weight loss. The procedure is usually done for younger clients because their skin is more elastic. Liposuction may be performed on either an outpatient or inpatient basis.

To aspirate the fat, a small incision is made close to the area, and a suction cannula or curette is inserted and attached to a suction apparatus. The high vacuum pressure caused by the suction machine causes fat cells to emulsify, and they are aspirated out of the body. Following removal of the fat, a pressure dressing is applied to help the skin conform to the new tissue size.

## Dermabrasion

Dermabrasion is a method of removing facial scars, severe acne, and pigment from unwanted tattoos. The area is sprayed with a chemical to cause light freezing and is then abraded with sandpaper or a revolving wire brush to remove the epidermis and a portion of the dermis.

## Facial Reconstructive Surgery

Many different reconstructive surgeries may be performed to correct deformities or improve cosmetic appearance. Those discussed here are rhinoplasty, blepharoplasty, and rhytidectomy (face-lift).

- A *rhinoplasty* is conducted to improve the appearance of the external nose. The nasal skeleton is reshaped, and the overlying skin and subcutaneous tissue are allowed to redrape over the new framework. A submucous resection of the nasal septum is often done at the same time; this surgery resects a segment of the septal cartilage to improve the nasal airway and also to alter the appearance of the nose. This surgery is done through incisions within the nose, so no visible scars remain after healing.

- A *blepharoplasty* is a cosmetic surgery in which loose skin and protruding periorbital fat is removed from the upper and lower eyelids. With aging, the eyelid skin sags, allowing the periorbital fat to bulge; the skin of the upper eyelid can be so lax that it partially obstructs vision. The procedure is performed under local anesthesia, and excess skin and fat are excised. The incision is made in the normal eyelid lines so that scars are not visible after healing.

- A *rhytidectomy,* or face-lift, is a cosmetic surgery done to improve appearance by removing excess skin (and sometimes fat) from the face and neck. As one ages, the skin of the face and neck tends to become loose and wrinkled. The procedure is usually performed with local anesthesia. To perform the surgery, bilateral incisions are made from the scalp at the temple, in front of the ear in the natural skin line, around the ear lobe, and to the occipital scalp. The skin is then elevated, fat is removed or suctioned, and excess skin is excised. The incision lines are sutured, and a pressure dressing is applied.

## NURSING CARE

Nursing care for the client having cutaneous or plastic surgery is highly individualized. It depends on the type of surgery or procedure performed, the type of deficit treated, the reason for the surgery or procedure, the expected results of the treatment, and the response of the client to the lesion or surgery. Although some surgeries, such as skin grafts and flaps, require in-hospital care, many of the surgeries are carried out in the primary care setting, and the client provides self-care at home following or between treatments.

## Nursing Diagnoses and Interventions

Although a variety of nursing diagnoses may be appropriate for the client having cutaneous or plastic surgery or procedures, the most common are *Impaired skin integrity, Acute pain,* and *Disturbed body image.*

### Impaired Skin Integrity

The client having surgery of the skin has impaired skin integrity. Skin grafts and flaps are performed to repair large wounds, and it is necessary to inflict further wounds to collect the graft or flap from a donor site. Excisions and various cosmetic surgeries cause wounds. Skin is traumatized by freezing, chemicals, abrasion, sclerosing agents, electrical currents, and lasers. Although all of these treatment modalities are conducted to remove lesions, improve function, or improve appearance, they first impair the integrity of the skin. These impairments increase the risk for infection, which would further impair the skin integrity and may negate the benefits of surgery.

Nurses provide preoperative care and teaching, intraoperative assistance, and postoperative care and teaching; in each case, care and teaching are specific to the type of surgical treatment and the individual client. In all cases, the nurse provides appropriate preoperative interventions to prepare the client physically and emotionally for surgery and the postoperative period. The following interventions are appropriate for the client having inpatient skin grafts or flaps.

- Monitor incisions and graft, and flap donor and recipient sites, for manifestations of infection and necrosis:
  - Take and record vital signs every 4 hours.
  - Monitor all wounds for changes in color, consistency, amount, and odor of drainage every 4 to 8 hours.
  - Monitor wounds for increased swelling, redness, and pain every 4 to 8 hours.
  - Monitor and document assessment of graft every 4 hours.
  - Monitor and document temperature, turgor, color, dermal bleeding, and capillary refill of flaps every 4 hours.

*When bacterial infection is present, the inflammatory phase of wound healing is prolonged, retarding healing. Increased body temperature and tachycardia are manifestations of infection. The drainage in wounds that become infected is often increased in amount, purulent, thicker, and has a musty or foul odor. Tissue response to infection includes edema, increased erythema, and pain. Grafts and flaps that do not have adequate blood supply will appear black instead of the normal pink-red color.*

- Provide care for the donor site:
  - Position the client to minimize pressure on the donor site.
  - Use a bed cradle to keep linens off the area.
  - If the donor site is left open and a heat lamp is to be applied to the area, place the lamp no closer than 2 feet from the wound.
  - Avoid moving the body part containing the donor site, if possible.
  - If the donor site is on the posterior portion of the body, place the client on a special bed (such as a low-pressure or fluidized bed) to decrease pressure and allow air circulation around the donor site.

*Minimizing trauma from pressure and movement facilitates healing of the donor site. Leaving the site open to the air and providing heat increase healing. Special beds minimize ischemia and allow donor sites on the posterior side of the body to dry.*

- Encourage a diet high in protein, ascorbic acid, vitamins, and minerals. *An adequate protein intake is necessary to supply amino acids for tissue repair. Vitamin C is necessary for collagen formation and wound strength. Vitamins and minerals contribute to the healing process.*
- Change dressings as prescribed, or if the frequency is not indicated, as necessary. Determine which dressings are not to be removed during the healing process and which are to be changed, and whether the wound is to be kept dry or moist.
  - Use aseptic technique and follow standard precautions when changing dressings.
  - Remove old dressings carefully and gently.
  - Choose the appropriate dressing materials.

*Donor sites may be covered with an adherent gauze dressing that is allowed to dry and remains adherent through the healing process. Aseptic techniques prevent secondary bacterial infections. Standard precautions protect the nurse from HIV infection. Unless care is taken, the removal of adherent old dressings may damage the wound by traumatizing granulation tissue or wound edges. The use of semipermeable transparent dressings provides an environment that optimizes wound healing by promoting collagen synthesis and the formation of granulation tissue; it also increases cell migration and epithelial resurfacing and prevents the formation of scabs, crusts, and eschar.*

### Acute Pain

The client having a graft or flap has two wounds; in fact, the donor site may be more painful than the recipient site. Cutaneous surgeries, dermabrasions, and chemical treatments result in blistering, swelling, and loss of epidermal tissue. The client having facial reconstructive surgery has edema.

- Administer pain medications on a regular basis, following guidelines for controlling pain in clients having operative procedures (see Chapter 4). ⊖⊃ *Established, severe pain is difficult to control and has negative physical and psychological consequences.*
- Use alternative pain relief measures as appropriate and prescribed, such as ice bags or cold compresses. *Cold reduces swelling, acts as a local anesthetic, and decreases pain.*
- Teach the client noninvasive methods of pain relief, such as deep breathing, relaxation, and guided imagery. *Noninvasive methods of pain relief increase the effectiveness of pain medications and also allow the client some control and self-management of pain.*

### Disturbed Body Image

Cosmetic surgery is performed for a variety of reasons in adult clients of all ages. Changes in appearance, especially in a society that values youth and beauty, affect one's self-perception. Lesions or scars, especially of the face, may decrease self-esteem and cause a person to avoid social interactions and relationships. With aging, the skin becomes looser and wrinkles appear; this can be a source of anxiety and despair, especially to the woman who has always prided herself on her youthful appearance. Most clients cite one reason for having plastic surgery: to "feel better about myself."

- Provide preoperative teaching:
  - Explain that bruising and swelling will be present and that it will be several weeks before these responses to surgery disappear.
  - Explain that it may take a year for healing to complete and the final results to appear.

*Expectations differ; many people expect immediate results. Knowledge of postoperative responses is necessary for the client to adapt to change. The client may need to make arrangements to take time off from work during the initial healing stage.*

- Provide time for the client to verbalize feelings and concerns. Be empathetic, and listen nonjudgmentally. *Such nurse-client interaction facilitates acceptance of changes in body image.*
- Refer to a consultant who can provide information on the use of cosmetics and apparel to enhance personal appearance. *Knowledgeable use of cosmetics and clothing can make scars much less noticeable. If the client feels better about appearance, body image is improved.*

### Home Care

The nurse teaches the client and family to provide self-care at home after inpatient and outpatient cutaneous and plastic surgery and procedures. The nurse asks about the client's expectations and stresses that final results will not be seen for several months, providing written instructions about the following topics.

- Wound care, including application of topical medications and dressing changes. If the client is to return to the office or clinic for removal of tape or pressure dressings, or for dressing changes in the first weeks after surgery, an appointment is made. For some procedures, the wound is left open to the air.
- Manifestations of wound infection, such as increased temperature, malaise, changes in the appearance of the wound, or changes in drainage. If any of these manifestations occur, the client should notify the health care provider immediately.
- Specific care for the type of surgery or procedure, such as type of oral care, avoiding blowing the nose, or limiting talking.
- Limitations on physical activity, especially lifting or straining.
- When to resume bathing or showering, shampooing the hair, and using cosmetics.
- The need to avoid picking at crusts or scabs. If the healing wound itches, the client should contact the health care provider for a topical medication.
- Use of a 15 (or higher) SPF sunblock when the client is outdoors. This may be prescribed for several months or for the rest of the client's life.

# HAIR AND NAIL DISORDERS

## THE CLIENT WITH A DISORDER OF THE HAIR

Although hair disorders are not serious threats to health, they may cause embarrassment and a negative body image. Changes in hair growth and pattern occur secondary to other illnesses and treatment for illness and also as a part of the aging process.

The hair grows at various rates. The male beard grows the most rapidly, followed by the hair of the scalp, axillae,

thighs, and eyebrows. Normally, an adult's hair grows at a rate of 10 to 12 mm per month; however, the growth rate is influenced by both the person's state of health and the environment (hair grows faster in hot climates, more slowly in cold climates).

Racial characteristics and gender influence the amount and type of hair. Caucasians have more facial and body hair than do Asians. People of Mongolian or Native American descent have straight hair, those of African descent have wavy to curly hair, and Caucasians have straight to curly hair. In addition, male hair growth characteristics (such as facial hair and hair on the lower extremities) are normal in certain women of some races and families. Women do not normally become bald.

## PATHOPHYSIOLOGY

Hair color, growth, and pattern vary from person to person, and they are determined largely by genetic inheritance. However, changes do occur. For example, in some instances, hair loss recurs in successive generations of males in a family; in other cases, hair loss may be the result of chemotherapy. Excessive facial hair may be a response to certain endocrine disorders or to the loss of estrogen after menopause. These changes may seem minor, but they may create psychosocial problems for the person experiencing the changes.

### Hirsutism

**Hirsutism,** also called hypertrichosis, is the appearance of excessive hair in normal and abnormal areas of the body in women. Hirsutism most often occurs in a male distribution (that is, on the upper lip, chin, abdomen, and chest) in women. The excess hair is primarily the result of an increase in androgen levels (especially testosterone) which may be due to any of the following:

- Familial predisposition (considered normal)
- Polycystic ovary syndrome
- Ovarian, adrenal, or pituitary tumors
- Cushing's syndrome
- Central nervous system disorders
- Medications, such as minoxidil, cyclosporine, phenytoin, certain progestins, and anabolic steroids

The manifestations of hirsutism include increased male pattern hair growth, acne, and menstrual irregularities. If the androgen excess is great, defeminization (a decrease in breast size and loss of normal adipose tissue) and virilization (frontal balding, increased muscle mass, deepening of the voice, and enlargement of the clitoris) may occur. Virilization indicates the presence of an androgen-producing tumor (Tierney et al., 2001).

### Alopecia

**Alopecia** is loss of hair, or baldness (Figure 14–31 ■). Alopecia may result from scarring, various systemic diseases, or genetic predisposition. Scarring from trauma, radiation, and severe bacterial, fungal, or viral infections causes permanent and irreversible hair loss over the scarred area. Systemic diseases that may cause alopecia include systemic lupus erythematosus, thyroid disorders, and pituitary insufficiency. The hair loss from these disorders may be reversible. Hair loss from androgenic causes may also occur in the postmenopausal woman. Alopecia may be drug induced and is a side effect of a variety of medications (see Box 14–6).

Types of alopecia follow:

- Male pattern baldness is the most common cause of alopecia in men and is genetically predetermined. The hair loss begins at the temples, with recession of the hairline and baldness of the crown.

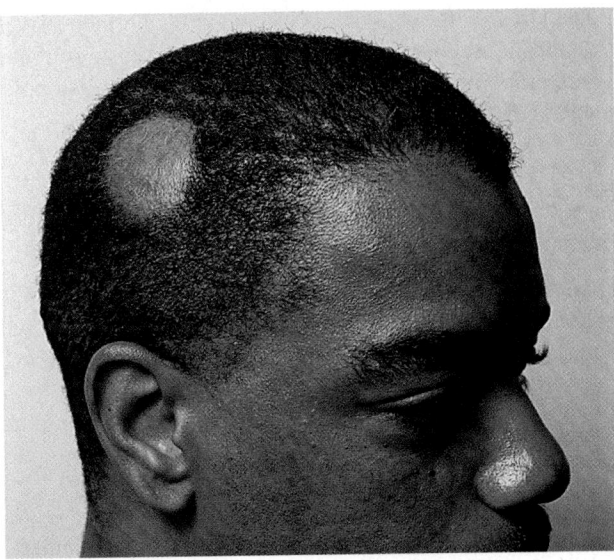

**Figure 14–31 ■** Alopecia, or baldness, may be the result of scarring, disease, or genetic predisposition.

| BOX 14–6 | ■ Medications Causing Alopecia |
|---|---|
| ■ Thallium | ■ Allopurinol |
| ■ Retinoids | ■ Propranolol |
| ■ Anticoagulants | ■ Indomethacin |
| ■ Antimitotic agents | ■ Amphetamines |
| ■ Antithyroid drugs | ■ Salicylates |
| ■ Oral contraceptives | ■ Levodopa |
| ■ Trimethadione | ■ Gentamicin |
| ■ Excessive use of vitamin A | ■ Chemotherapy |

- Female pattern alopecia begins in women in their 20s and 30s, with progressive thinning and loss of hair over the central part of the scalp. Unlike men, women do not lose hair from the frontal hairline. Many of these women have elevated adrenal androgens.
- Alopecia areata is characterized by round or oval bald patches on the scalp as well as on other hairy parts of the body. The cause is unknown. This type of alopecia is usually self-limiting and reverses without treatment, although it often recurs.
- Alopecia totalis is the loss of all hair on the scalp. This rare condition is irreversible.
- Alopecia universalis is the total loss of hair on all parts of the body.

## COLLABORATIVE CARE

Alopecia is diagnosed by assessing the appearance of the hair and hair loss and by assessing the client for other systemic diseases and the use of medications that may cause hair loss. Various treatments are used to restore hair.

The client with hirsutism is examined for hormone levels and indications of other systemic illnesses. Hirsutism is treated by addressing the underlying systemic disorder and stopping medications that may be causing the problem.

## Diagnostic Tests

The following diagnostic tests may be ordered for the client with hirsutism.

- Serum testosterone levels are measured; levels above 200 ng/dL indicate the need for further diagnostic work, including a pelvic examination and tests of ovarian function in women.
- Adrenal CT scan may be performed to assess for an adrenal tumor.

## Medications

Hirsutism is treated with medications specific to the underlying cause. Oral contraceptives containing estrogen decrease ovarian androgen production and decrease free testosterone levels. Dexamethasone (Decadron) may be prescribed for people with high cortisol levels. Ketoconazole (Nizoral) inhibits androgen production. Antiandrogenic medications cause congenital abnormalities in male infants and are therefore given only to nonpregnant women, who are cautioned to avoid pregnancy while taking the medications.

Male pattern baldness has been successfully treated with topical minoxidil (Loniten) or Rogaine, a commercial product that contains minoxidil. These drugs, which are vasodilators, stimulate vertex hair growth, probably by stimulating the epithelium of the hair follicle. These agents have been most successful in clients who have a recent onset of alopecia or are less than 50 years old. About 40% of clients treated two times a day for a year will have moderate to dense regrowth of hair at the temples (Tierney et al., 2001).

## Surgery

Surgical movement of tissue containing hair is used to restore hair or reduce the size of areas of alopecia. These surgical procedures include punch grafting, scalp reduction, and flaps.

- Punch grafting of small hair plugs taken from the back or sides of the scalp is an effective means of replacing hair to areas of alopecia. This procedure is done on an outpatient office or clinic every 1 to 2 months.
- Scalp reduction is done by excising a portion of the affected scalp. In some cases, a tissue expander (such as a silicone balloon) is first implanted under the scalp to enlarge the hair-bearing scalp so that larger areas of alopecia can be removed.
- Flaps from hair-bearing areas of the scalp can be surgically transplanted from adjacent areas into areas of alopecia. This procedure may be done in stages.

## NURSING CARE

The client with either hirsutism or alopecia is often self-conscious about appearance and tries a variety of over-the-counter treatments before seeking medical care. Nursing care

for the client with hair disorders focuses on teaching the client self-care and providing support during long-term care. Women with hirsutism are taught to use various means of removing unwanted hair, such as shaving, applying depilatories, waxing, or undergoing electrolysis. Women with mild hirsutism may bleach facial hair to make it less obvious. Clients with alopecia may wear hair pieces or wigs.

## THE CLIENT WITH A DISORDER OF THE NAILS

Nail disorders may be due to systemic diseases, trauma, allergies, or irritants. They may also be congenital or genetic. Nails may be discolored, multicolored, malformed, infected, or separated from underlying tissue.

## PATHOPHYSIOLOGY

The nail disorders discussed here are separation of the nail, infection, and ingrown toenails.

- **Onycholysis** is the separation of the distal nail plate from the nail bed. It occurs most often in the fingernails. This disorder may result from many different factors, including excessive or prolonged exposure to water, soaps, detergent, alkalies, and industrial keratolytic agents; Candida infections; nail hardeners; and thyroid disorders. Prolonged application of false fingernails may also cause this disorder.
- A **paronychia** is an infection of the cuticle of the fingernails or toenails (Figure 14–32 ■). The disorder often follows a minor trauma and secondary infection with staphylococci, streptococci, or Candida. The acute form begins with a painful inflammation that may progress to an abscess. The chronic form is seen most often in people who have frequent exposure to water. In the chronic form, the skin around the nail is painful, edematous, and infected. The nail plate may become ridged and discolored.
- An **onychomycosis** is a fungal or dermatophyte infection of the nail plate. The nail plate elevates and becomes yellow or white. Psoriasis infections of the nail plate cause the nails to pit.

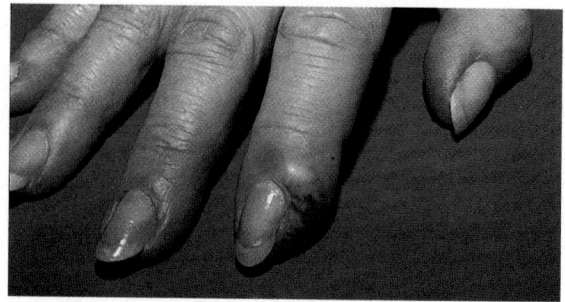

**Figure 14–32** ■ A paronychia is an infection of the cuticle of the fingernails or toenails.

Source: Leonard Morse, Medical Images, Inc.

- An ingrown toenail (*unguis incarnatus*) results when the edge of the nail plate grows into the soft tissue of the toe. Pain and infection may occur. The infection, if untreated, may spread to the bone. This disorder is especially dangerous for the person with diabetes mellitus or peripheral vascular disease.

## COLLABORATIVE CARE

The treatment of disorders of the nail vary from pharmacologic treatment to surgical removal. Infections of the nails are treated, depending on the causative agent, with antifungal or antibiotic medications. If the causative agent is a fungus or chronic dermatologic disorder, treatment is difficult and may not be effective. Persistently painful and/or infected nails are in some cases surgically removed.

## NURSING CARE

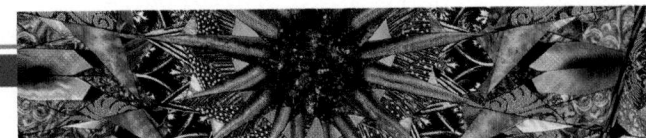

Nursing care of the client with a disorder of the nail focuses on teaching self-care. Clients with nail disorders that are caused by frequent exposure to water are taught to protect the hands or feet by wearing rubber gloves or boots and to keep the nails as clean and dry as possible. Clients with ingrown toenails are cautioned not to cut into the lateral nail bed, but rather to soak the nail twice a day and insert a piece of cotton or gauze under the softened nail until the nail has grown out enough to trim.

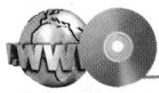

## EXPLORE MediaLink

NCLEX review questions, case studies, care plan activities, MediaLink applications, and other interactive resources for this chapter can be found on the Companion Website at www.prenhall.com/lemone.

Click on Chapter 14 to select the activities for this chapter. For animations, video clips, more NCLEX review questions, and an audio glossary, access the Student CD-ROM accompanying this textbook.

## TEST YOURSELF

1. Your elderly client has severe xerosis. What topic should be included in your teaching plan?

   a. Take a hot bath every day
   b. Use fabric softeners when laundering clothing
   c. Apply skin lotions after a bath
   d. Maintain a warm environment

2. Which of the following clients is at risk for the development of a candidiasis infection?

   a. An older adult with pruritus
   b. A young woman who is pregnant
   c. An older man with a premalignant skin condition
   d. A young man with multiple nevi

3. What question should be included in a health history of a client with a linear pattern of painful vesicles over the left thorax?

   a. Do you remember being sunburned as a child?
   b. Are you a regular patron of tanning booths?
   c. Have you ever been diagnosed with acne?
   d. Did you have chickenpox when you were young?

4. Of the following, which is most significant to the development of a malignant melanoma?

   a. A change in the color or size of a nevus
   b. Sexual contact with a person who has a herpes virus infection
   c. Inadequate knowledge about infection prevention
   d. A dietary intake of high-calorie foods

5. The rationale for lifting, rather than pulling, a client up in bed is that:

   a. Lifting a client allows a brief period of increased capillary circulation
   b. Lifting a client prevents tissue injury from shearing forces
   c. Pulling a client up in bed decreases tissue ischemia and hypoxia
   d. Pulling a client up in bed promotes capillary blood flow

See Test Yourself answers in Appendix C.

# BIBLIOGRAPHY

Agency for Health Care Policy and Research. (1992). *Pressure ulcers in adults: Prediction and prevention*. Rockville, MD: USDHHS.

———. (1994). *Treatment of pressure ulcers*. Rockville, MD: USDHHS.

American Cancer Society. (2002). *Cancer facts and figures 2002*. Atlanta: American Cancer Society.

American Melanoma Foundation/National Cancer Institute. (2001). Skin cancer treatment. Available http://cancernet.nci.nih.gov

Appling, S. (1997). Promoting healthy skin. *MEDSURG Nursing, 6*(6), 377–378.

Bielan, B. (1997a). What's your assessment . . . papular urticaria. *Dermatology Nursing, 9*(3), 191, 201.

———. (1997b). What's your assessment . . . tinea pedis. *Dermatology Nursing, 9*(2), 105, 117.

Bjorgen, S. (1998). Clinical snapshot: Herpes zoster. *American Journal of Nursing, 98* (2 Continuing Care Extra), 46–47.

Blawat, D., & Banks, P. (1997). Comforting touch: Using topical skin preparations. *Nursing 97, 27*(5), 46–48.

Center for Disease Control. (2001). Cancer prevention and control. Available www.cdc.gov/cancer/nscpep/skin

Boston, M. (1997). Acne: Avoiding permanent damage. *Community Nurse, 3*(4), 15–16.

Davis, P. (1998). Pain from herpes zoster and postherapetic neuralgia. *American Journal of Nursing, 98*(2 Continuing Care Extra), 18, 20.

Hardy, M. (1996). What can you do about your patient's dry skin? *Journal of Gerontological Nursing, 22*(5), 10–18, 52–53.

Johnson, M., & Maas, M. (1997). *Iowa outcome project: Nursing outcomes classification (NOC)*. St. Louis: Mosby.

Landow, K. (1998). Hand dermatitis: The perennial scourge. *Postgraduate Medicine, 103*(1), 141–142, 145–148, 151–152.

Lapka, D. (2000). Oncology today. New horizons: Skin cancer. *RN, 63*(7), 32–40.

Lebwohl, M. (1997). Understanding psoriasis. *Women's Health Digest, 3*(3), 159–164.

Leshaw, S. (1998). Itching in active patients: Causes and cures. *Physician & Sportsmedicine, 26*(1), 47–50.

Marghoob, A. (1997). Basal and squamous cell carcinomas. *Postgraduate Medicine, 102*(2), 139–142.

McCloskey, J., & Bulechek, G. (Eds.). (2000). *Iowa intervention project: Nursing interventions classification (NIC)* (3rd ed.). St. Louis: Mosby.

McKay, S. (2000). Why we need to worry about warts. *RN, 63*(9), 68–74.

Metules, T. (2000). Tips for nurses who wash too much. *RN, 63*(3), 34–37.

North American Nursing Diagnosis Association. (2001) *Nursing diagnoses: Definitions & classification 2001–2002*. Philadelphia: NANDA.

Penzer, R., & Finch, M. (2001). Promoting healthy skin in older people. *Nursing Standard, 15*(34), 46–52.

Pieper, B., & Weiland, M. (1997a). Pressure ulcer prevention within 72 hours of admission in a rehabilitation setting. *Ostomy Wound Management, 43*(8), 14–16, 18, 20.

Pieper, B., Sugrue, M., Weiland, M., Sprague, K., & Heimann, C. (1997b). Presence of ulcer prevention methods used among patients considered at-risk versus those considered not-at-risk. *Journal of WOCN, 24*(4), 191–199.

Porth, C. (2002). *Pathophysiology: Concepts of altered health states* (6th ed.). Philadelphia: Lippincott.

Reifsnider, E. (1997). Common adult infectious skin conditions. *Nursing Practitioner: American Journal of Primary Health Care, 22*(11), 17–18, 20, 23–24.

Rigel, D., & Carucci, J. (2000). Malignant melanoma: Prevention, early detection, and treatment in the 21st century. *CA: A Cancer Journal for Clinicians, 50*(4), 209–213.

Russell, J. (2000). Topical therapy for acne. *American Family Physician, 61*(2), 357–366.

Sarver-Steffensen, J. (1999). When MRSA reaches into long-term care. *RN, 62*(3), 39–41.

Tierney, L., McPhee, S., & Papadakis, M. (Eds.). (2001). *Current medical diagnosis & treatment* (40th ed.). Stamford, CT: Appleton & Lange.

Wilson, B., Shannon, M., & Stang, C. (2001). *Nursing drug guide 2001*. Upper Saddle River, NJ: Prentice Hall.

Yarbo, C., Frogge, M, Goodman, M., & Groenwald, S. (Eds.) (2001). *Cancer nursing: Principles and practice*. (5th ed.). Sudbury, MA: Jones & Bartlett.

# CHAPTER 15

# Nursing Care of Clients with Burns

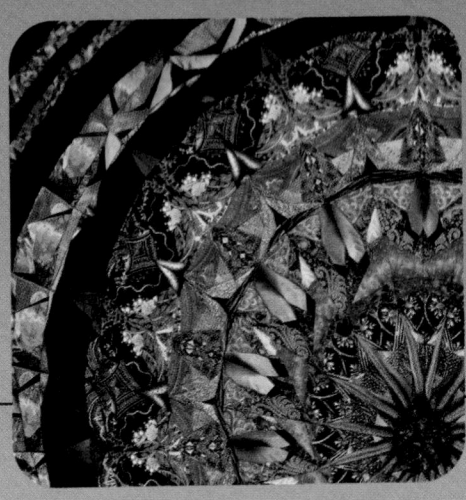

## MediaLink

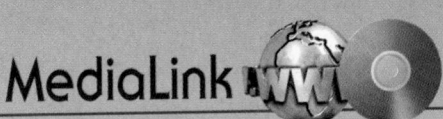

**www.prenhall.com/lemone**
Additional resources for this chapter can be found on the Student CD-ROM accompanying this textbook, and on the Companion Website at www. prenhall.com/lemone. Click on Chapter 15 to select the activities for this chapter.

**CD-ROM**
- Audio Glossary
- NCLEX Review

**Companion Website**
- More NCLEX Review
- Case Study
    Full-Thickness Burns
- Care Plan Activity
    Inhalation Injury
- MediaLink Application
    Teaching Plan: Fire Prevention

## LEARNING OUTCOMES

After completing this chapter, you will be able to:

- Apply knowledge of normal integumentary anatomy, physiology, and assessments when providing nursing care for clients with burns (see Chapter 13).

- Discuss types and causative agents of burns.

- Explain burn classification by depth and extent of injury.

- Describe the stages of burn wound healing.

- Explain the pathophysiology, collaborative care, and nursing care for the client with a minor burn.

- Discuss the systemic pathophysiologic effects of a major burn.

- Identify the collaborative care necessary during the emergent/resuscitative stage, the acute stage, and the rehabilitative stage of a major burn.

- Discuss the nursing implications of medications administered to the client with a major burn.

- Discuss the nursing implications for burn wound management.

- Use the nursing process as a framework for providing individualized care to clients with a burn.

A **burn** is an injury resulting from exposure to heat, chemicals, radiation, or electric current. A transfer of energy from a source of heat to the human body initiates a sequence of physiologic events that in the most severe cases leads to irreversible tissue destruction. Burns range in severity from a minor loss of small segments of the outermost layer of the skin to a complex injury involving all body systems. Treatments vary from simple application of a topical antiseptic agent in an outpatient clinic to an invasive, multisystem, interdisciplinary health team approach in the aseptic environment of a burn center.

It is estimated that more than 2 million burn injuries occur each year in the United States, and, of those, about 70,000 require hospitalization (Braunwald & Fauci, 2001). The home is the most common site for fire-related burns. Home fires cause 73% of all fire-related deaths, with about 12 people dying in home fires each day. Factors associated with deaths from burns are age (especially children and older adults), careless smoking, alcohol or drug intoxication, and physical and mental disabilities. Occupation is also a factor, with electricians and chemical workers among those at greatest risk (Rutan, 1998).

## TYPES OF BURN INJURY

The four types of burn injury are thermal, chemical, electrical, and radiation. Although all four types can lead to generalized tissue damage and multisystem involvement, the causative agents and priority treatment measures are unique to each (Table 15–1).

## Thermal Burns

Thermal burns result from exposure to dry heat (flames) or moist heat (steam and hot liquids). They are the most common burn injuries and occur most often in children and older adults. Direct exposure to the source of heat causes cellular destruction that can result in charring of vascular, bony, muscle, and nervous tissue.

## Chemical Burns

Chemical burns are caused by direct skin contact with either acid or alkaline agents. More than 25,000 products found in the home or workplace can cause chemical burns. The chemical destroys tissue protein, leading to necrosis. Burns caused by alkalis (such as lye) are more difficult to neutralize than are burns caused by acids. They also tend to have deeper penetration with a correspondingly more severe burn than from acid. Organic compound burns, such as by petroleum distillates, cause cutaneous damage through fat solvent action and may also cause renal and liver failure if absorbed.

Chemical agents are further classified according to the manner by which they structurally alter proteins. Oxidizing agents, such as household bleach, alter protein configuration through the chemical process of reduction. Corrosives, such as lye, cause extensive protein denaturation. Protoplasmic poisons, such as organic compounds, form salts with proteins, inhibiting calcium and other ions needed for cell viability. The severity of the chemical burn is related to the type of agent, the concentration of the agent, the mechanism of action, the duration of contact, and the amount of body surface area exposed. Box 15–1 lists household cleaning agents that may cause burns.

## Electrical Burns

The severity of electrical burns depends on the type and duration of current, and amount of voltage. It is particularly difficult to assess the extent of the electrical burn injury, because the destructive processes initiated by the electrical insult are concealed and may persist for weeks beyond the time of the incident. It is difficult to assess the depth and extent of the burn, as electricity follows the path of least resistance, which in the human body tends to lie along muscles, bone, blood vessels, and nerves. Necrosis of the tissue results from impaired blood flow, secondary to blood coagulation at the site of the electrical injury. More than 90% of electrical burn wounds of the extremities that develop gangrene result in amputation.

Alternating current, as is found in conventional households, produces repeated electrical surges that lead to tetanic muscle contractions. Such sustained muscle contractions inhibit respiratory efforts for the duration of contact and result in respiratory arrest. The contractions also cause the person to clamp

**TABLE 15–1  Types, Causative Agents, and Priority Treatment Measures for Burns**

| Type | Causative Agent | Priority Treatment |
|------|-----------------|--------------------|
| Thermal | Open flame | Extinguish flame (stop, drop, and roll). |
| | Steam | Flush with cool water. |
| | Hot liquids (water, grease, tar, metal) | Consult fire department. |
| Chemical | Acids | Neutralize or dilute chemical. |
| | Strong alkalis | Remove clothing. |
| | | Consult Poison Control Center. |
| Electrical | Direct current | Disconnect source of current. |
| | Alternating current | Initiate CPR if necessary. |
| | Lightning | Move to area of safety. |
| | | Consult electrical experts. |
| Radiation | Solar (ultraviolet) | Shield the skin appropriately. |
| | X-rays | Limit time of exposure. |
| | Radioactive agents | Move the client away from the radiation source. |
| | | Consult a radiation expert. |

**BOX 15–1  ■ Household Cleaning Agents That May Cause Burns**

- Drain cleaners
- Lye
- Industrial-strength ammonia
- Household ammonia
- Oven cleaners
- Toilet bowl cleaners
- Dishwasher detergents
- Bleach

down on the power source (such as an electrical cord) and thus may increase the duration of contact with the source. Direct current, as in injury from a lightning bolt, exposes the body to very high voltage for an instantaneous period of time. High voltage (lightning) injury usually results in entry and exit wounds. The flash-over effect, a phenomenon unique to lightning injury, actually saves the client from death. It is seen in those instances in which the current travels over the moist surface of the skin rather than through deeper structures.

## Radiation Burns

Radiation burns are usually associated with sunburn or radiation treatment for cancer. These kinds of burns tend to be superficial, involving only the outermost layers of the epidermis. All functions of the skin remain intact. Symptoms are limited to mild systemic reactions: headache, chills, local discomfort, nausea, and vomiting. More extensive exposure to radiation or radioactive substances, as in nuclear power accidents, leads to the same degree of tissue damage and multisystem involvement associated with other types of burns.

## FACTORS AFFECTING BURN CLASSIFICATION

Tissue damage following a burn is determined primarily by two factors: depth of the burn (the layers of underlying tissue affected) and the extent of the burn (the percentage of body surface area involved).

## Depth of the Burn

The depth of burn of injury is determined by the elements of the skin that have been damaged or destroyed. Burn depth results from a combination of the temperature of the burning agent and the length of contact. Burns are classified as either superficial, partial thickness, or full thickness. Characteristics of

burns are described below, summarized in Table 15–2, and illustrated in Figure 15–1 ■.

### Superficial Burns

A **superficial burn** (often called a first-degree burn) involves only the epidermal layer of the skin. This type of burn most often results from damage from sunburn, ultraviolet light, minor flash injury (from a sudden ignition or explosion), or mild radiation burn associated with cancer treatment. Because the skin remains intact, this degree of burn is not calculated into the estimates of burn injury. The skin color ranges from pink to bright red, and there may be slight edema over the burned area. Superficial burns involving large body surface areas may be manifested by chills, headache, nausea, and vomiting. The injury usually heals in 3 to 6 days, with dryness and peeling of the outer layer of skin. There is no scar formation. Superficial burns are treated with mild analgesics and the application of water-soluble lotions. Extensive superficial burns, especially in older adults, may require intravenous fluid treatment.

### Partial-Thickness Burns

**Partial-thickness burns** (often called second-degree burns) may be subdivided into superficial partial-thickness and deep dermal partial-thickness burns. The classification depends on the depth of the burn.

A *superficial partial-thickness burn* involves the entire dermis and the papillae of the dermis. Causes may include such injuries as a brief exposure to flash flame or dilute chemical agents, or contact with a hot surface. This burn is often bright red, but has a moist, glistening appearance with blister formation (Figure 15–2 ■). The burned area will blanch on pressure, and touch and pain sensation remain intact. Pain in response to temperature and air is usually severe. These injuries heal within 21 days with minimal or no scarring, but pigment changes are common. Analgesics are administered, and if large blistered areas are disrupted, skin substitutes may be used.

## TABLE 15–2 Characteristics of Burns by Depth

| Characteristic | Superficial | Split Thickness | Full Thickness |
|---|---|---|---|
| Skin layers lost | Epidermis | Epidermis and dermis | Epidermis, dermis, and underlying tissues |
| Skin appearance over burn | Red to gray; may have local edema | Fluid-filled blisters; bright pink, may appear waxy white with deep partial-thickness burns | Waxy white; dry, leathery, charred |
| Skin function | Present | Absent | Absent |
| Pain sensation | Present | Present | Absent |
| Manifestations at the burn site | Pain; local edema | Severe pain; edema; weeping of fluid | Little pain; edema |
| Treatment | Regular cleaning Topical agent of choice | Regular cleaning Topical agent of choice May require skin grafting | Regular cleaning Topical agent of choice Skin substitutes Excision of eschar Skin grafting |
| Scarring | None | May occur in deep burns | Of grafted area |
| Time to heal | 3 to 6 days | 14 to >21 days | Requires skin grafting to heal |

**Figure 15-1** ■ Burn injury classification according to the depth of the burn.

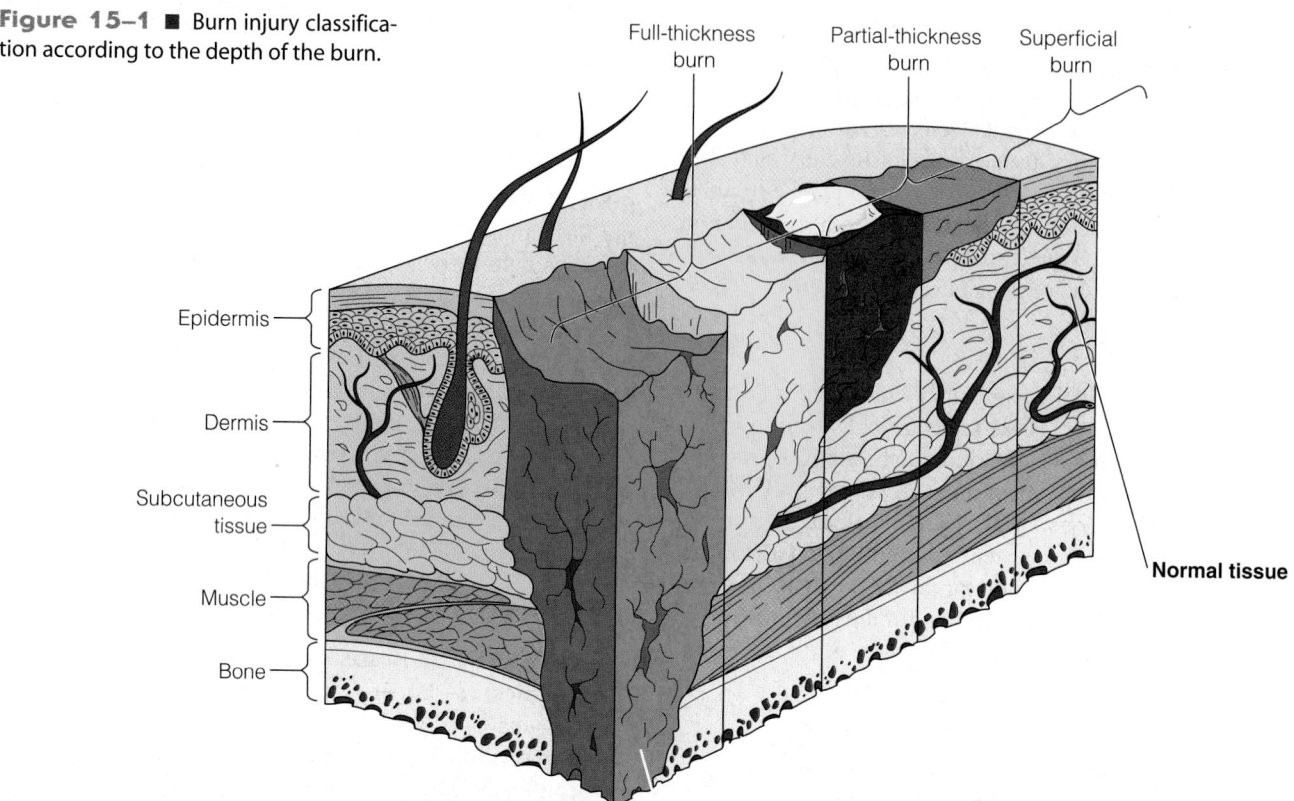

A *deep partial-thickness burn* also involves the entire dermis, but extends further into the dermis than a superficial partial-thickness burn. Hair follicles, sebaceous glands, and epidermal sweat glands remain intact (Porth, 2002). Hot liquids or solids, flash flame, direct flame, intense radiant energy, or chemical agents may cause this level of burn wound. The surface of the burn wound appears pale and waxy and may be moist or dry. Large, easily ruptured blisters may be present, or the blisters may look like flat, dry tissue paper. Capillary refill is decreased, and sensation to deep pressure is present. The burn wound is less painful than a superficial partial-thickness burn, but areas of pain and areas of decreased sensation may be present. Deep partial-thickness burn wounds often require more

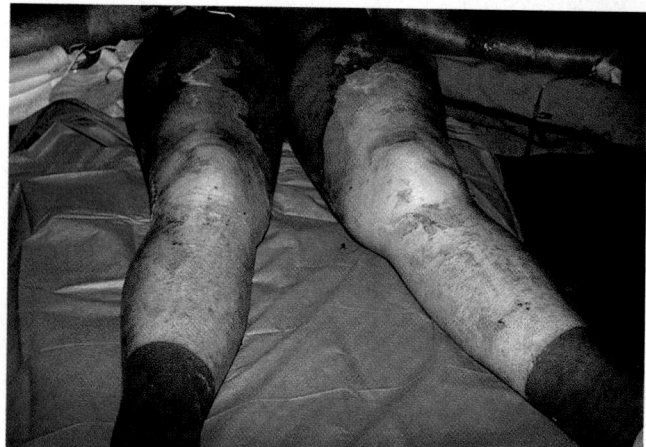

**Figure 15-2** ■ Partial-thickness burn injury.

*Courtesy of Dr. William Dominic, Valley Medical Center.*

than 21 days for healing and may convert to a full-thickness injury as necrosis extends the depth of the wound. Contractures are possible, as are hypertrophic scarring and functional impairment. Excision and grafting may be necessary to decrease scarring and loss of function.

### Full-Thickness Burns

A **full-thickness burn** (often called a third-degree burn) involves all layers of the skin, including the epidermis, the dermis, and the epidermal appendages (Figure 15-3 ■). The burn wound may extend into the subcutaneous fat, connective tissue, muscle, and bone. Full-thickness burns are caused by prolonged contact with flames, steam, chemicals, or high-voltage electric current.

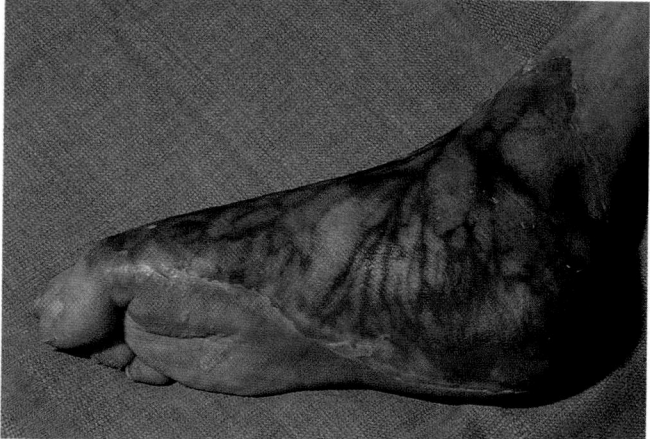

**Figure 15-3** ■ Full-thickness burn injury.

*Courtesy of Dr. William Dominic, Valley Medical Center.*

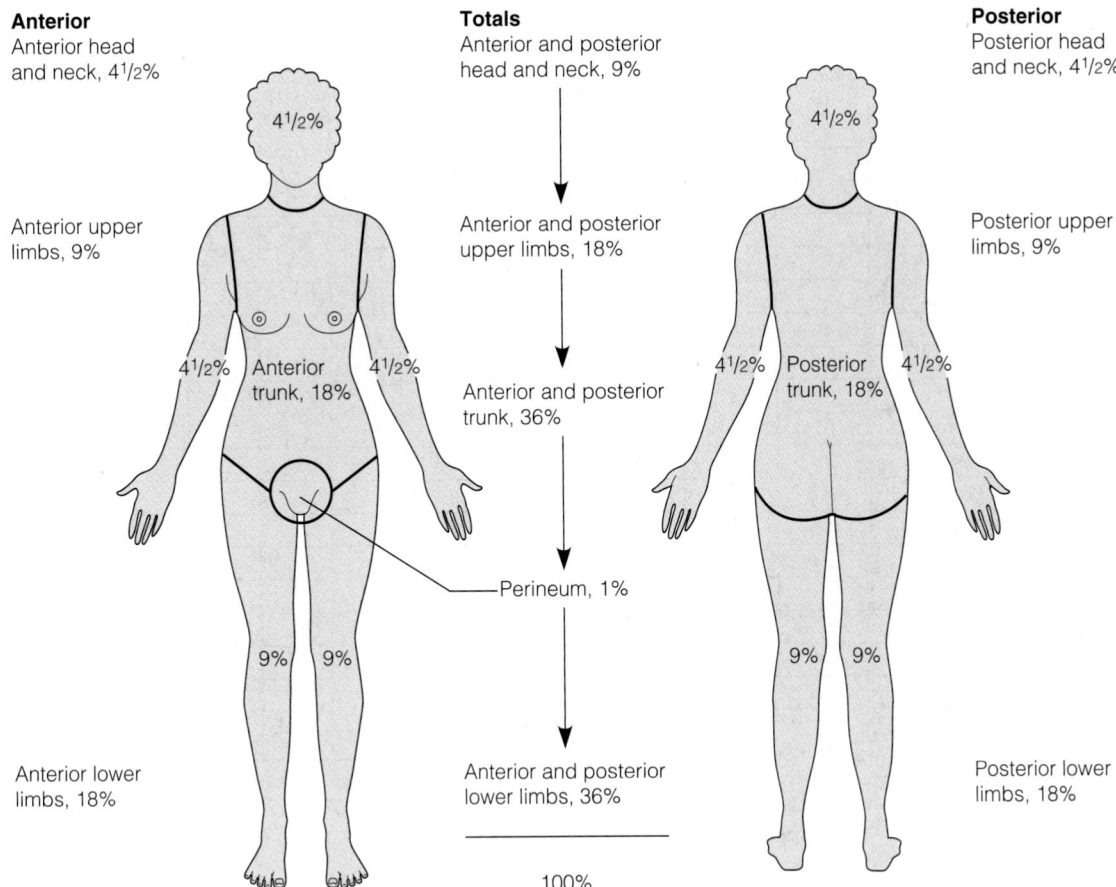

**Figure 15–4** ■ The "rule of nines" is a method of quickly estimating the percentage of TBSA affected by a burn injury. Although useful in emergency care situations, the rule of nines is not accurate for estimating TBSA for adults who are short, obese, or very thin.

Depending on the cause of injury, the burn wound may appear pale, waxy, yellow, brown, mottled, charred, or nonblanching red. The wound surface is dry, leathery, and firm to the touch. Thrombosed blood vessels may be visible under the surface of the wound. There is no sensation of pain or light touch, as pain and touch receptors have been destroyed. Full-thickness burns require skin grafting to heal.

## Extent of the Burn

The extent of the burn injury is expressed as a percentage of the total body surface area (TBSA). There are several methods used for determining the extent of injury. The "rule of nines" is a rapid method of estimation used during the prehospital and emergency care phases. In this method, the body is divided into five surface areas—head, trunk, arms, legs, and perineum—and percentages that equal or total a sum of nines are assigned to each body area (Figure 15–4 ■). For example, a client with burns of the face, anterior right arm, and anterior trunk has burn injury involving 27% of the total body surface area (in this example, face = 4.5%, arm = 4.5%, and trunk = 18% to total 27%). Only partial- and full-thickness burns are included in the estimation.

On the client's admission to the hospital, critical care area, or burn center, more accurate methods for estimating the extent of injury are employed. For example, the Lund and Browder

method (Figure 15–5 ■) determines surface area measurements for each body part according to the age of the client.

A recognized system for describing a burn injury, developed by the American Burn Association, uses both the extent and depth of burn to classify burns as minor, moderate, or major (Table 15–3).

## BURN WOUND HEALING

Burns heal in the same processes as do other wounds, but the wound healing phases occur more slowly and last longer. The healing process involves four phases: hemostasis, inflammation, proliferation, and remodeling. The following physiologic events occur (Carrougher, 1998):

- *Hemostasis.* Immediately following the injury, platelets coming in contact with the damaged tissue aggregate and degranulate (releasing growth factors). Fibrin is deposited, trapping further platelets, and a thrombus is formed. The thrombus, combined with local vasoconstriction, leads to hemostasis which walls off the wound from the systemic circulation.
- *Inflammation.* Local vasodilation and an increase in capillary permeability follows hemostasis. Neutrophils infiltrate the wound and peak in about 24 hours, and then monocytes predominate. The monocytes are converted into macrophages, which consume pathogens and dead tissue, and also

| Area | Age (years) | | | | | % 1° | % 2° | % 3° | % Total |
|------|------|------|------|------|------|------|------|------|------|
| | 0–1 | 1–4 | 5–9 | 10–15 | Adult | | | | |
| Head | 19 | 17 | 13 | 10 | 7 | | | | |
| Neck | 2 | 2 | 2 | 2 | 2 | | | | |
| Ant. trunk | 13 | 13 | 13 | 13 | 13 | | | | |
| Post. trunk | 13 | 13 | 13 | 13 | 13 | | | | |
| R. buttock | $2\frac{1}{2}$ | $2\frac{1}{2}$ | $2\frac{1}{2}$ | $2\frac{1}{2}$ | $2\frac{1}{2}$ | | | | |
| L. buttock | $2\frac{1}{2}$ | $2\frac{1}{2}$ | $2\frac{1}{2}$ | $2\frac{1}{2}$ | $2\frac{1}{2}$ | | | | |
| Genitalia | 1 | 1 | 1 | 1 | 1 | | | | |
| R.U. arm | 4 | 4 | 4 | 4 | 4 | | | | |
| L.U. arm | 4 | 4 | 4 | 4 | 4 | | | | |
| R.L. arm | 3 | 3 | 3 | 3 | 3 | | | | |
| L.L. arm | 3 | 3 | 3 | 3 | 3 | | | | |
| R. hand | $2\frac{1}{2}$ | $2\frac{1}{2}$ | $2\frac{1}{2}$ | $2\frac{1}{2}$ | $2\frac{1}{2}$ | | | | |
| L. hand | $2\frac{1}{2}$ | $2\frac{1}{2}$ | $2\frac{1}{2}$ | $2\frac{1}{2}$ | $2\frac{1}{2}$ | | | | |
| R. thigh | $5\frac{1}{2}$ | $6\frac{1}{2}$ | $8\frac{1}{2}$ | $8\frac{1}{2}$ | $9\frac{1}{2}$ | | | | |
| L. thigh | $5\frac{1}{2}$ | $6\frac{1}{2}$ | $8\frac{1}{2}$ | $8\frac{1}{2}$ | $9\frac{1}{2}$ | | | | |
| R. leg | 5 | 5 | $5\frac{1}{2}$ | 6 | 7 | | | | |
| L. leg | 5 | 5 | $5\frac{1}{2}$ | 6 | 7 | | | | |
| R. foot | $3\frac{1}{2}$ | $3\frac{1}{2}$ | $3\frac{1}{2}$ | $3\frac{1}{2}$ | $3\frac{1}{2}$ | | | | |
| L. foot | $3\frac{1}{2}$ | $3\frac{1}{2}$ | $3\frac{1}{2}$ | $3\frac{1}{2}$ | $3\frac{1}{2}$ | | | | |
| | | | | | Total | | | | |

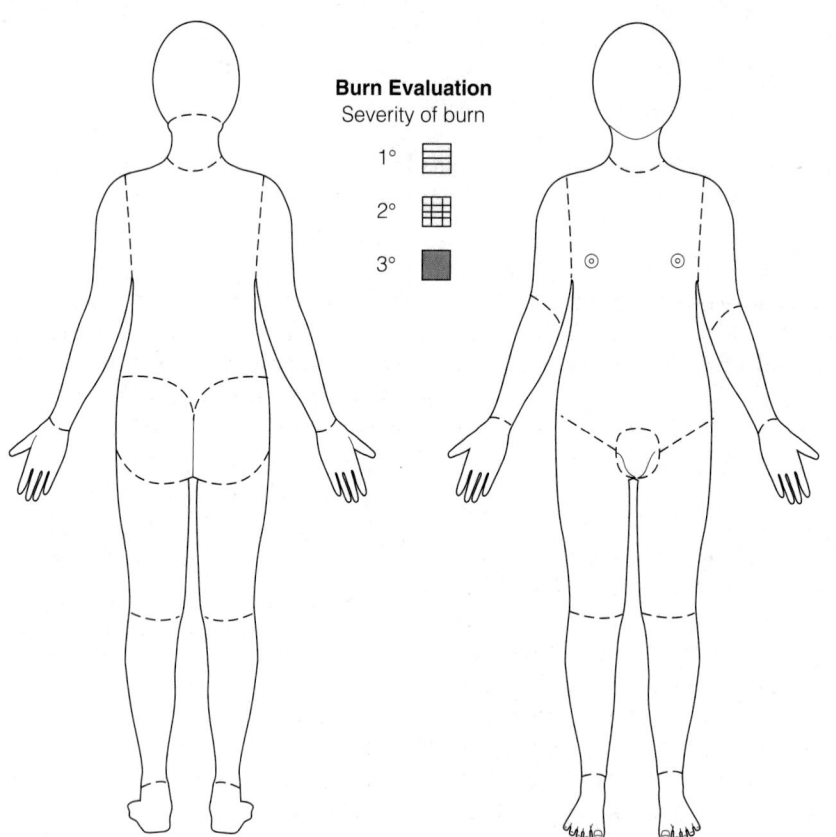

**Burn Evaluation**
Severity of burn

1°
2°
3°

**Figure 15–5** ■ The Lund and Browder burn assessment chart. This method of estimating TBSA affected by a burn injury is more accurate than the "rule of nines" because it accounts for changes in body surface area across the life span.

TABLE 15-3 American Burn Association Classification of Burn Injury

| Minor Burn Injury | Moderate Burn Injury | Major Burn Injury |
|---|---|---|
| Excludes electrical injury, inhalation injury, complicated injuries (such as multiple trauma), and all clients who are considered to be at high risk (such as older adults and those with chronic illnesses)<br><br>Second-degree burns of less than 15% of the total body surface area in adults<br><br>Third-degree burns of less than 2% of the total body surface area not involving special care areas (eyes, ears, face, hands, feet, perineum) | Excludes electrical injury, inhalation injury, complicated injuries (such as multiple trauma), and all clients who are considered to be at high risk (such as older adults and those with chronic illnesses)<br><br>Second-degree burns of 15% to 25% of the total body surface area in adults<br><br>Third-degree burns of less than 10% of the total body surface area not involving special care areas (eyes, ears, face, hands, feet, perineum) | Includes all burns of the hands, face, eyes, ears, feet, and perineum; all electrical injuries, inhalation injuries, multiple trauma injuries, and all clients who are considered to be at high risk<br><br>Second-degree burns of greater than 25% of the total body surface area in adults<br><br>All third-degree burns of 10% or greater of the total body surface area |

*Note. Burn injuries described in this table (except minor burns) should be treated in a specialized burn center. These criteria have been established by the American Burn Association.*

secrete various growth factors. These growth factors stimulate the proliferation of fibroblasts and a deposit of a provisional wound matrix.

- *Proliferation.* Within 3 to 4 days postburn, fibroblasts are the major cell within the wound. Their number peaks at about 14 days after the injury. Granulation tissue begins to form, with complete reepithelialization occurring during this stage. Epithelial cells cover the wound as each cell stretches across the wound surface to join with other epithelial cell sheets or the other side of the wound. The proliferation phase lasts until complete reepithelialization occurs, by epithelial cell migration, surgical intervention, or a combination of the two.

- *Remodeling.* This phase may last for years. Collagen fibers, laid down during the proliferative phase, are reorganized into more compact areas. Scars contract and fade in color. In normal healing following a minor burn injury, the newly formed skin closely resembles its neighboring tissue. However, when a burn injury extends into the dermal layer of skin, two types of excessive scar may develop. A **hypertrophic scar** is an overgrowth of dermal tissue that remains within the boundaries of the wound. A **keloid** is a scar that extends beyond the boundaries of the original wound. People with dark skin are at greater risk for hypertrophic scars and keloids.

## THE CLIENT WITH A MINOR BURN

Minor burn injuries consist of superficial burns that are not extensive, superficial split-thickness burns that involve less than 15% of TBSA, and full-thickness burns that involve less than 2% of TBSA, excluding the special care areas (eyes, ears, face, hands, feet, perineum, and joints). Minor burn injuries are not associated with immunosuppression, hypermetabolism, or increased susceptibility to infection.

A minor burn injury is usually treated in an outpatient facility. The goal of therapy is to promote wound healing, eliminate discomfort, maintain mobility, and prevent infection.

## PATHOPHYSIOLOGY

### Sunburn

Sunburns result from exposure to ultraviolet light. Such injuries, which tend to be superficial, are more commonly seen in clients with lighter skin. Because the skin remains intact, the manifestations in most cases are mild and are limited to pain, nausea, vomiting, skin redness, chills, and headache. Treatment is performed on an outpatient basis and generally consists of applying mild lotions, increasing liquid intake, administering mild analgesics, and maintaining warmth. Older adults should be monitored for evidence of dehydration. Proper use of sunscreen and limiting sun exposure to the less hazardous hours of the day (before 10 A.M. and after 3 P.M.) can prevent sunburn.

### Scald Burn

Minor scald burns result from exposure to moist heat and involve superficial and superficial split-thickness burns of less than 15% of TBSA. The goals of therapy are to prevent wound contamination and to promote healing. The nurse teaches the client to apply antibiotic solutions and light dressings and to maintain adequate nutritional intake. Mild analgesics may be ordered to help the client carry out activities of daily living. Tetanus toxoid is administered as appropriate.

## COLLABORATIVE CARE

In the outpatient facility, the wound may be washed with mild soap and water. Tar and asphalt can be removed with mineral oil, petroleum ointments, or Medisol (a citrus and petroleum distillate with hydrocarbon structure). Tetanus toxoid booster is recommended for all clients whose immunization histories are in doubt. Although controversy regarding the care of blisters remains, blisters may be managed in one of three ways: left intact, evacuated, or debrided. Follow-up care for the minor burn injury includes twice daily wound cleansing with application of bland ointment, range-of-motion exercises to affected joints, and weekly clinic appointments until the wound heals completely.

## NURSING CARE

Although the nurse seldom treats the minor burn in the acute care environment, the burn treatment methods used in the outpatient setting follow the same standard approaches to care. General nursing measures include taking the history, estimating the extent and depth of the injury, cleansing the wound, applying topical agents, dressing the wound, controlling pain, and establishing follow-up care.

### Home Care

The nurse should address the following topics to facilitate self-care at home of minor burns.

- How to identify and report manifestations of impaired wound healing:
  - Change in healthy appearance of the wound (altered skin integrity, swelling, blister formation, erythema)
  - Signs of infection (fever, purulent drainage, foul odor)
- Wound care:
  - Daily cleansing with mild soap and water
  - Using sterile technique to change dressings
  - Correct application of ordered topical agents
- Pain management:
  - Use mild analgesics as ordered
  - Use alternative pain management therapies

## THE CLIENT WITH A MAJOR BURN

A major burn involves serious injury to the underlying layers of skin and covers a large body surface area. The American Burn Association defines a major burn as one that involves:

- >25% TBSA in adults less than 40 years of age
- >20% TBSA in adults more than 40 years of age

- >10% TBSA full-thickness burn
- Injuries to the face, eyes, ears, hands, feet, or perineum
- High-voltage electrical injuries
- All burn injuries with inhalation injury or major trauma

## PATHOPHYSIOLOGY

The pathophysiologic changes that result from major burn injuries involve all body systems. Extensive loss of skin (the body's protective barrier) can result in massive infection, fluid and electrolyte imbalances, and hypothermia. Often the person inhales the products of combustion, thus compromising respiratory function. Cardiac dysrhythmias and circulatory failure are common manifestations of serious burn injuries. A profound catabolic state dramatically increases caloric expenditure and nutritional deficiencies. An alteration in gastrointestinal motility predisposes the client to developing paralytic ileus, and hyperacidity leads to gastric and duodenal ulcerations. Dehydration slows glomerular filtration rates and renal clearance of toxic wastes and may lead to acute tubular necrosis and renal failure. Overall body metabolism may be profoundly altered. Systemic responses to burns are shown in Figure 15–6 ■ and discussed in the following sections.

### Integumentary System

Heat transfer to skin is a complex phenomenon. If the microcirculation of the skin remains intact during burning, it cools and protects the deeper portions of the skin and cools the outer surface once the heat source is removed. With extensive burn injury, the integrity of the microcirculation is lost, and the burning process continues even after the heat source is removed.

Burns have a characteristic skin surface appearance that resembles a bull's-eye, with the most severe burn located centrally and the lesser burns located along the peripheral wound edges. Depending on their intensity, burns consist of one, two, or three concentric three-dimensional zones closely corresponding on the skin surface to the depth of the burn.

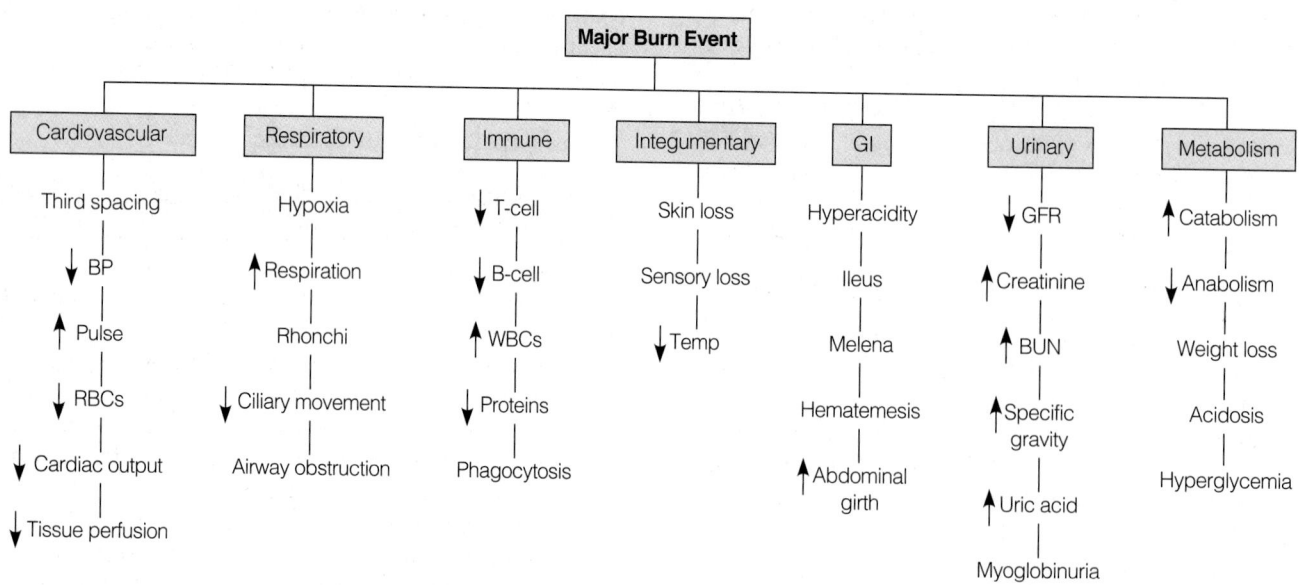

**Figure 15–6** ■ Effects of a severe burn on major body systems and metabolism.

- The outer zone of hyperemia blanches on pressure and heals in 2 to 7 days postburn.
- The medial zone of stasis is initially moist, red, and blistered and blanches on pressure. It becomes pale and necrotic on days 3 to 7 postburn.
- The inner zone of coagulation immediately appears leathery and coagulated. It merges with the necrotic zone of stasis in 3 to 7 days postburn.

The overall thickness of the dermis and epidermis varies considerably from one area of the body to another. Similar temperatures produce different depths of injury to different body parts. For example, in the adult, skin covering the medial aspect of the forearm is thinner and more easily damaged than the skin covering the back of the same person. Skin dissipates heat maximally in areas of greatest vascularization. When heat absorption exceeds the rate of dissipation, cellular temperatures rise, and skin tissue is destroyed.

The burn injury results in the formation of necrotic skin and subcutaneous tissue. During the acute stage of the injury, a hard crust (**eschar**) forms, which covers the wound and harbors necrotic tissue. The eschar is characteristically leathery and rigid. Removal of the eschar facilitates healing.

## Cardiovascular System

The effects of a major burn are manifested in all components of the vascular system, and include hypovolemic shock (burn shock), cardiac dysrrhythmias (such as ventricular fibrillation), cardiac arrest, and vascular compromise.

### Hypovolemic Shock (Burn Shock)

Within minutes of the burn injury, a cascade of cellular events is initiated, and a massive amount of fluid shifts from the intracellular and intravascular compartments into the interstitium. This shift is a type of hypovolemic shock called **burn shock,** and it continues until capillary integrity is restored, usually within 24 to 36 hours of the injury. Although the pathophysiologic mechanisms of postburn vascular changes and fluid volume shifts are not clearly understood, three processes occur early in the postburn phase in clients with ≥ 40% TBSA:

- Increase in microvascular permeability at the burn wound site
- Generalized impairment of cell wall function, resulting in intracellular edema
- Increase in osmotic pressure of the burned tissue, leading to extensive fluid accumulation

During burn shock, the shifting of fluid is the direct result of a loss of cell wall integrity at the site of injury and in the capillary bed. Fluid leaks from the capillaries into interstitial compartments located at the burn wound site and throughout the body, resulting in a decrease in fluid volume within the intravascular space. Plasma proteins and sodium escape into the interstitium, enhancing edema formation. Blood pressure falls as cardiac output diminishes.

Vasoconstriction results as the vascular system attempts to compensate for fluid loss. Abnormal platelet aggregation and white blood cell (WBC) accumulation result in ischemia in the deeper tissue below the burn, leading to eventual thrombosis.

Red blood cells (RBCs) and WBCs remain in the circulation, producing an elevation in erythrocyte and leukocyte counts secondary to hemoconcentration.

The leakage of fluid into the interstitium compromises the lymphatic system, resulting in intravascular hypovolemia and edema at the burn wound site. Edematous body surfaces impair peripheral circulation and result in necrosis of the underlying tissue. During burn shock, potassium ions leave the intracellular compartment, predisposing the client to developing cardiac dysrhythmias. The process of burn shock continues until capillary integrity is restored, usually within 24 hours of the injury.

Burn shock reverses when fluid is reabsorbed from the interstitium into the intravascular compartment. The blood pressure rises as cardiac output increases, and urinary output improves. Diuresis continues from several days to 2 weeks postburn. During this phase, the extra cardiac workload may predispose the older client, or the client with cardiovascular disease, to fluid volume overload.

### Cardiac Rhythm Alterations

Burns of more than 40% TBSA cause significant myocardial dysfunction, with a decrease in myocardial contractibility and cardiac output. These changes, which occur prior to a decrease in plasma volume, are believed to be due to the release of substances and oxygen-free radicals from the burn wound and from ischemic myocardial cells. Electrical burns often result in cardiac dysrhythmias or cardiac arrest caused by heat damage to the myocardium or electrical interference with cardiac electrical activity.

### Peripheral Vascular Compromise

Direct heat damage to extremities, especially if circumferential burns are present, results in damage to blood vessels. Circulation to extremities may be further impaired by edema and by peripheral vasoconstriction that occurs during burn shock. In addition, **compartment syndrome** (in which the tissue pressure within a muscle compartment exceeds microvascular pressure, interrupting cellular perfusion) may result from circumferential burns and edema.

### Respiratory System

Pulmonary damage may result from either direct inhalation injury or as part of the systemic response to the injury. Inhalation injury is a frequent and often lethal complication of burns. The injury may range from mild respiratory inflammation to massive pulmonary failure. Exposure to heat, asphyxiants, and smoke initiates the pathophysiologic process associated with inhalation injury.

Inflammation occurs at localized sites within the airway and is manifested as hyperemia. As a result, cells are destroyed and the bronchial cilia are rendered inactive. Because the mucociliary transport mechanism no longer functions, the client may develop bronchial congestion and infection.

Interstitial pulmonary edema develops secondary to the escape of fluid from the pulmonary vasculature into the interstitial compartment of the lung tissue. Surfactant is inactivated, resulting in atelectasis and alveolar collapse. Sloughing of the damaged and dead lung tissue occasionally produces debris that may lead to complete airway obstruction.

Upper airway (above the level of the glottis) thermal injury results from the inhalation of heated air or chemicals dissolved in water. Physical findings include the presence of soot, charring, edema, blisters, and ulcerations along the mucosal lining of the oropharynx and larynx. The resulting edema in the airway peaks within the first 24 to 48 hours of injury. Lower airway thermal injury is a rare occurrence. Because the lower airway is protected by laryngeal reflexes, thermal injury below the vocal cords is seldom seen. However, when it does occur, it is typically associated with the inhalation of steam or explosive gases or the aspiration of hot liquids.

Smoke poisoning results when toxic gases and particulate matter, the products of incomplete combustion, deposit directly onto the pulmonary mucosa. The composition of the products of combustion depends on the combustible material, the rate at which the temperature increases, and the amount of ambient oxygen present. Irritant gases and particulate matter have a direct cytotoxic effect. The degree of injury is determined by their solubility in water, duration of exposure, and the size of the particulate or aerosol droplet.

Carbon monoxide, a common asphyxiant, is a colorless, tasteless, odorless gas that has a 200 times greater affinity for hemoglobin than does oxygen. It displaces oxygen to bind with hemoglobin, forming carboxyhemoglobin. As a result, the decrease in arterial oxyhemoglobin produces tissue hypoxia. Carbon monoxide impairs both oxygen delivery and cellular oxygen use. The clinical manifestations of carbon monoxide poisoning range from mild visual impairment to coma and death (Table 15–4).

## Gastrointestinal System

Dysfunction of the gastrointestinal system is directly related to the size of the burn wound. Clients with ≥20% TBSA experience decreased peristalsis with resultant gastric distention and increased risk of aspiration. A decrease in or absence of bowel sounds is a manifestation of paralytic ileus (adynamic bowel) secondary to burn trauma. The resulting cessation of intestinal motility leads to gastric distention, nausea, vomiting, and hematemesis.

| TABLE 15–4 | Manifestations of Carbon Monoxide Poisoning |
|---|---|
| **Level of Carbon Monoxide** | **Manifestations** |
| 10% to 20% | Headache, dizziness, nausea, abdominal pain |
| 21% to 40% | Headache, nausea, drowsiness, dizziness, irritability, confusion, stupor, hypotension, bradycardia, skin color ranging from pale to dark red |
| 41% to 60% | Convulsion, coma, hypotension, tachycardia |
| >60% | Death |

Stress ulcers (**Curling's ulcers**) are acute ulcerations of the stomach or duodenum that form following the burn injury. Abdominal pain, acidic gastric pH levels, hematemesis, and melana in the stool may indicate a gastric ulcer.

In addition, ischemia of the intestine from splanchnic vasoconstriction increases the intestinal mucosal permeability. As a result, normal intestinal bacteria move from the lumen of the bowel to extraluminal sites, a process called *bacterial translocation*. This process is believed to be one of the mechanisms causing systemic sepsis and multiple organ dysfunction syndrome.

## Urinary System

During the early stages of the burn injury, renal blood flow and glomerular filtration rates are greatly reduced from the decreased intravascular blood volume and the release of antidiuretic hormone (ADH) by the posterior pituitary. Urine output decreases, and serum creatinine and blood urea nitrogen increase.

Dark brown concentrated urine may indicate myoglobinuria, the result of the release of large amounts of dead or damaged erythrocytes after a major burn injury. When large amounts of these pigments are released, the liver cannot keep pace with conjugation and the pigments pass through the glomeruli. The pigments can occlude the renal tubules and cause renal failure, especially when dehydration, acidosis, or shock is also present.

## Immune System

The function of the immune system is to protect the human body from invasion by foreign microorganisms. The capillary leak that occurs in the early stages of the burn injury continues throughout the burn shock phase and impairs the active components of both the cell-mediated and humoral immune systems.

The humoral immune system relies on B cells to produce antibodies or immunoglobulins (see Chapter 9). ⏳ In the burn client, the serum levels of all immunoglobulins are significantly diminished. Serum protein levels remain persistently low throughout the clinical course until wound closure is effected. A marked decrease in T-cell counts results in a reduction of cytotoxic activity and suppression of the cell-mediated immune system.

The compromise in the humoral and cell-mediated immune systems constitutes a state of acquired immunodeficiency, which places the burn client at risk for infection. The period of vulnerability is transient and may last from 1 to 4 weeks following the onset of the burn injury. During this time frame, opportunistic infections can be fatal despite aggressive antimicrobial therapy.

## Metabolism

Two distinct phases characterize the body's metabolic response to the burn injury. The ebb phase, occurring during the first 3 days of the injury, is manifested by decreased oxygen consumption, fluid imbalance, shock, and inadequate circulating volume. These responses protect the body from the initial impact of the injury.

A second phase, the flow phase, occurs when adequate burn resuscitation has been accomplished. This phase is characterized by increases in cellular activity and protein catabolism, lipolysis, and gluconeogenesis. The basal metabolic rate (BMR) significantly increases, reaching twice the normal rate. Body weight and heat drop dramatically. Total energy expenditure may exceed 100% of normal BMR. Hypermetabolism persists until after wound closure has been accomplished and may reappear if complications occur.

## COLLABORATIVE CARE

The burn team is composed of an interdisciplinary group of health care professionals, who together plan the care and treatment of the burn-injured client during the acute and rehabilitative stages. The burn team consists of the nurse, physician, physical therapist, dietitian, social worker, and burn technician. The team members meet regularly to discuss client progress and to determine collaboratively the most effective regimen of care and psychosocial support.

## Stages of Collaborative Care

The clinical course of treatment for the burn client is divided into three stages: the emergent/resuscitative stage, the acute stage, and the rehabilitative stage. Although these stages are useful predictors of the clinical needs of the burn client, it is important to recognize that the process of burn injury is dynamic and that, in many cases, the clinical stage may not be clearly delineated. Assessment and management of the burn-injured client are ongoing processes determined by the clinical picture; they last throughout the course of treatment. Figure 15–7 ■ shows the burn client's progression through the health care system during each clinical stage of burn care.

During each stage, different groups of nurses, physicians, and allied health care specialists collaborate to manage the client's recovery.

## The Emergent/Resuscitative Stage

The emergent/resuscitative stage lasts from the onset of injury through successful fluid resuscitation. During this stage, health care workers estimate the extent of burn injury, institute first-aid measures, and implement fluid resuscitation therapies. The client is assessed for shock and evidence of respiratory distress. If indicated, intravenous lines are inserted, and the client may be prophylactically intubated. During this stage, health care workers determine whether the client is to be transported to a burn center for the complex intervention strategies of the professional, interdisciplinary burn team.

Although many burn injuries are treated in local tertiary care facilities, the American Burn Association has developed guidelines for determining whether the client should be transported to a burn center for interdisciplinary approaches to treatment and rehabilitation. Adult clients who should be treated at burn centers include those with:

- Second- or third-degree burns >10% TBSA and older than 50 years of age.
- Second- or third-degree burns >20% TBSA in adults to the age of 50.
- Third-degree burns >5% TBSA in adults of any age.
- Burns involving the hands, feet, face, eyes, ears, or perineum.
- Electrical (including lightning), chemical, and inhalation injuries.
- Circumferential burns of the extremities and/or chest.

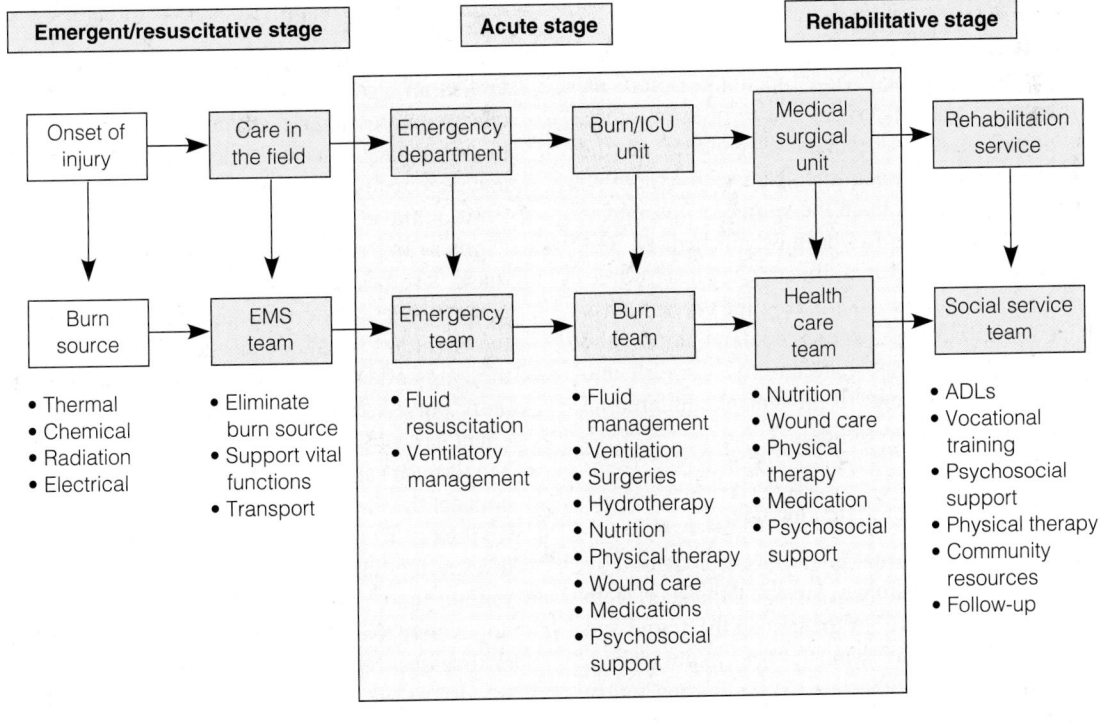

**Figure 15–7** ■ The client's progression through the health care system during the emergent, acute, and rehabilitative stages of burn injury.

- Any burn associated with extenuating problems, preexisting illness, fractures, or other trauma.

## Acute Stage

The acute stage begins with the start of diuresis and ends with closure of the burn wound (either by natural healing or by using skin grafts). During this stage, wound care management, nutritional therapies, and measures to control infectious processes are initiated. Hydrotherapy and excision and grafting of full-thickness wounds are performed as soon as possible after injury. Enteral and parenteral nutritional interventions are started early in the treatment plan to address caloric needs resulting from extensive energy expenditure. Measures to combat infection are implemented during this stage, including the administration of topical and systemic antimicrobial agents. Pain management constitutes a significant segment of the nursing care plan throughout the clinical course of the burn-injured client. The administration of narcotic pharmaceutical agents must precede all invasive procedures to maximize client comfort and to reduce the anxieties associated with wound debridement and intensive physical therapy.

## Rehabilitative Stage

The rehabilitative stage begins with wound closure and ends when the client returns to the highest level of health restoration, which may take years. During this stage, the primary focus is the biopsychosocial adjustment of the client, specifically the prevention of contractures and scars and the client's successful resumption of work, family, and social roles through physical, vocational, occupational, and psychosocial rehabilitation. The client is taught to perform range-of-motion exercises to enhance mobility and to support injured joints.

# Prehospital Client Management

Treatment at the injury scene includes measures to limit the severity of the burn and support vital functions. Before attempting to remove the client from the source of burn injury, rescuers must ensure their own safety. Depending on the causative agent, rescuers may need to consult with experts to determine the best way to eliminate the source of the injury. Once the safety of the rescuers has been established, all prehospital interventions are aimed at eliminating the heat source, stabilizing the client's condition, identifying the type of burn, preventing heat loss, reducing wound contamination, and preparing for emergency transport. Restrictive jewelry and clothing is removed at the scene to prevent circumferential constriction of the torso and extremities.

## Stop the Burning Process

Emergency measures, by type of injury, include:

**THERMAL BURNS.**  If the thermal injury has been caused by dry heat, smother inflamed clothing or lavage with water. Help the person "stop, drop, and roll" to extinguish the flame and limit the extent of burn. Once the flame has been extinguished, cover the body to prevent hypothermia. If the thermal injury has been caused by moist heat, lavage the area with cool water. Ice is not used for cooling as it causes vasoconstriction and may result in further injury.

**CHEMICAL BURNS.**  For chemical burns, immediately remove the clothing and use a hose or shower to lavage the involved area thoroughly for a minimum of 20 minutes. Many chemicals are in powder form and as much dry chemical needs to be removed as possible before flushing the surface with water. Unusual chemicals may require consultation with the poison control center about appropriate treatment. Protective clothing should be worn during this process to protect the rescuer from chemical exposure.

**ELECTRICAL BURNS.**  Electrical injuries pose serious potential harm to both rescuer and burn victim. Ensure that the source of electrical current has been disconnected, or move the person to safety and away from the energy source using a nonconductive device such as a broomstick. If the person is unresponsive, assess for the presence of cardiac and respiratory function. If indicated, begin cardiopulmonary resuscitation (CPR). A spinal cord injury may be present secondary to the forceful contraction of the muscles of the neck and back during exposure to the current. If possible, place the person in a cervical collar and transport on a spinal board.

**RADIATION BURNS.**  Radiation injuries are usually minor and involve only the epidermal layer of skin. Treatment focuses on helping normal body mechanisms promote wound healing. For severe radiation burns, such as those that result from industrial radiation accidents, trained personnel may need to render the area safe for entry prior to rescue. All interventions are aimed at shielding, establishing distance, and limiting the time of exposure to the radioactive source.

## Support Vital Function

The initial assessment of the client's respiratory and hemodynamic status begins with an evaluation of the client's airway, breathing, and circulation (the ABCs of care).

- If the client has no pulse and is not breathing, begin CPR. Establish an airway, and start mouth-to-mouth breathing and chest compressions. Continue CPR until spontaneous cardiopulmonary function returns or until the emergency management team takes over.
- Position the client with the head elevated at greater than 30 degrees, and administer 100% humidified oxygen by face mask. Use nasotracheal suction as necessary to maintain a patent airway. Endotracheal intubation may be necessary if the client has facial edema and inhalation injury. Auscultate the lungs often onsite to monitor respiratory status. Continuous pulse oximetry provides ongoing assessment of the client's oxygen saturation levels.
- Monitor for cardiac dysrrhythmias or arrest. When available, connect the client to a cardiac monitor and observe for dysrhythmias. Elevate burned extremities above the level of the heart to facilitate circulation.
- Initiate fluid replacement therapy for burn wounds that involve more than 20% of the total body surface area. Continuously assess heart and lung sounds and observe level of consciousness, cardiac rate and rhythm, blood pressure, and urine output.
- Cover the client to maintain body temperature and to prevent further wound contamination and tissue damage.

## Emergency and Acute Care

Prehospital personnel report to the emergency department staff all findings and medical interventions that occurred at the scene of the injury. The nurse obtains a history of the injury, estimates the depth and extent of the burn, begins fluid resuscitation, and maintains ventilation according to protocol.

### Fluid Resuscitation

**Fluid resuscitation** is the administration of intravenous fluids to restore the circulating blood volume during the acute period of increasing capillary permeability. To counteract the effects of burn shock, fluid resuscitation guidelines are used to replace the extensive fluid and electrolyte losses associated with major burn injuries. Fluid replacement is necessary in all burn wounds that involve ≥20% TBSA.

Crystalloid fluids are administered through two large-bore (14 to 16 gauge) catheters, preferably inserted through unburned skin. Warmed Ringer's lactate solution is the intravenous fluid most widely used during the first 24 hours after burn injury, as it most closely approximates the body's extracellular fluid composition. Several formulas may be used to replace fluid loss. Two commonly used formulas are as follows:

- Parkland formula, in which lactated Ringer's solution is administered 4 mL × kg × % TBSA burn.
- Modified Brooke formula, in which lactated Ringer's solution is administered 2 mL × kg × % TBSA burn.

These formulas specify the volume of fluid to be infused in the first 24 hours after the injury, with 50% of the fluid to be infused during the first 8 hours, followed by the remaining 50% over the next 16 hours (25% per 8 hours). Over the second 24 hours, fluids for clients with larger burns (such as more than 30% TBSA) are changed to a crystalloid solution of 5% dextrose in water titrated to maintain urine output (Bucher & Melander, 1999).

Hourly urine output is often used as the indicator of effective fluid resuscitation, with 30 to 50 cc for an adult considered adequate. (With electrical burns, a urine output of 75 to 100 cc should be maintained). Another valuable indicator is heart rate; if fluid resuscitation is adequate, the rate should be less than 120 beats per minute or in the upper limits of normal for age. A higher rate may indicate a need for additional fluid (Bucher & Melander, 1999).

During the fluid resuscitation stage, the client may require invasive hemodynamic monitoring (see Chapter 29). ⊙⊙ A pulmonary artery catheter can be used to monitor cardiac output, cardiac index, and pulmonary artery wedge pressures. All measurements must be maintained within normal limits to effect adequate fluid resuscitation.

### Respiratory Management

Upon the client's admission to the emergency department, several baseline assessments of respiratory status must be obtained: chest X-ray study, ABGs, vital signs, and carboxyhemoglobin levels. Intubation is indicated for all clients with burns of the chest, face, or neck. The primary treatment plan is oriented toward preventing atelectasis and maintaining alveolar oxygen exchange. The following interventions should be initiated.

- Maintain the head of the bed at 30 degrees or greater to maximize the client's ventilatory efforts. Turn the client side to side every 2 hours to prevent hypostatic pneumonia.
- To keep airway passages clear, suction the client frequently, encourage the client to use incentive spirometry hourly, and help the client perform coughing and deep-breathing exercises every 2 hours.
- In the face of impending airway obstruction, the client will require intubation. Nasotracheal tube placement is the preferred route because it seems to be better tolerated and can be more effectively secured. If the client has suffered nasolabial burns, however, the orotracheal route is preferred. Nasotracheal and orotracheal intubation is reserved for short-term ventilatory management. For long-term ventilatory management (i.e., greater than 3 weeks), a tracheostomy is performed.
- Humidification of either room air or oxygen helps prevent the drying of tracheal secretions. Ambient air or oxygen flow is based on ABG results. The client may be placed on a face mask, steam collar, T-piece, mechanical ventilation with PEEP, pressure support ventilation, or high-frequency jet ventilation. The goal of all therapies is to maintain adequate tissue oxygenation with the least amount of inspired oxygen flow necessary.
- Medications to dilate constricted bronchial passages are administered intravenously and as inhalants to control bronchospasms and wheezing. Mucolytic agents liquefy tenacious sputum and aid in expectoration.
- An arterial line is placed in the client with major burn injury for continuous assessment of ABGs. Pulmonary artery pressure catheters may be inserted to measure pulmonary vascular resistance (PVR), pulmonary artery pressure (PAP), pulmonary capillary wedge pressure (PCWP), and mixed venous oxygen saturation ($SVO_2$). The PVR and PAP rise in the presence of hypoxia. The $SVO_2$ is the average percentage of hemoglobin bound with oxygen in the venous blood and reflects overall tissue utilization of oxygen. Pulse oximetry monitors arterial oxygen saturation levels.
- Pain medications are administered if the client is not in shock.

After stabilization in the emergency department, the client is transferred to the critical care unit or a specialized burn center (a facility that has a burn physician as director of a specialized nursing unit with dedicated burn beds). In both settings, continuous monitoring of diagnostic tests, administration of medications, pain control, wound management, and nutrition support therapies constitute the initial plan of care.

## Diagnostic Tests

The following diagnostic tests are used to evaluate the client's progress and to modify intervention strategies.

- *Urinalysis* indicates the adequacy of renal perfusion and the client's nutritional status. In catabolic states, nitrogen is excreted in large amounts into the urine. Nitrogen loss is measured through 24-hour urine collections for total nitrogen, urea nitrogen, and amino acid nitrogen. *Myoglobinuria,* which manifests as a dark brown, wine-colored urine, signals the development of acute tubular necrosis. Loss of plasma protein and dehydration lead to proteinuria and elevated urine specific gravity. Glycosuria is a transient development following major burn injury; it indicates a need to adjust the nutritional program.

- The *complete blood count* is monitored regularly. Hematocrit is elevated secondary to hemoconcentration and fluid shifts from the intravascular compartment. Hemoglobin is decreased secondary to hemolysis. White blood cells are elevated if infection is present.
- *Serum electrolytes* are monitored regularly. Sodium levels are decreased secondary to massive fluid shifts into the interstitium. Potassium levels initially are elevated during burn shock, as a result of cell lysis and fluid shifts into the extracellular space. Potassium levels decrease after burn shock resolves, as fluid shifts back to intracellular and intravascular compartments.
- *Renal function* test results are closely monitored. Blood urea nitrogen (BUN) is elevated secondary to dehydration. Creatinine is elevated in the presence of renal insufficiency.
- *Total protein, albumin, transferrin, prealbumin, retinol binding protein, alpha 1-acid glycoprotein, and C-reactive protein* indicate protein synthesis and nutritional status. Because of the fluid shifts that occur during the early stages of the burn injury, they are more useful markers during the rehabilitative phase of care.
- *Creatine phosphokinase (CPK)* is elevated following an electrical burn, secondary to extensive muscle damage.
- *Blood glucose* is transiently elevated after major burn injury.
- *Serial ABGs* indicate the presence of hypoxia and acid-base disturbances and indicate client responses to changes in oxygen therapies. The burn-injured client may demonstrate elevated or lowered pH, decreased $Pco_2$, decreased $Po_2$, and low-normal bicarbonate levels.
- *Pulse oximetry* allows continuous assessment of oxygen saturation levels. The burn-injured client may have saturation levels below 95%.
- *Serial chest X-ray* studies document changes within the first 24 to 48 hours that may reflect the presence of atelectasis, pulmonary edema, or acute respiratory disease (ARD).
- *Serial electrocardiograms (EKGs)* are necessary to monitor the development of dysrhythmias, especially those associated with hypokalemic and hyperkalemic states.

## Medications

### Pain Control

Burns often cause excruciating pain. In the early stages of care, intravenously administered narcotics such as morphine, meperidine, or fentanyl are the best means of managing pain. Morphine is the drug of choice. Once the client has been stabilized, it is appropriate to administer narcotics prior to initiating hydrotherapy or intensive exercising routines. The oral, subcutaneous, or intramuscular route of administration should be avoided until hemodynamic stability and unimpaired tissue perfusion returns.

As the client enters the rehabilitative stage of care, alternative therapies for pain control may be added to the plan of care.

Distraction, self-hypnosis, guided imagery, and relaxation techniques are helpful adjuncts in managing pain and coping with loss. Patient-controlled analgesia (PCA) enhances the client's ability to cope with pain. See Chapter 4 for a discussion of strategies for managing pain. ⊝

### Antimicrobial Agents

Systemic infection is a leading cause of death in major burn patients. Gram-positive organisms such as Staphylococcus and Streptococcus colonize the burn surface during the first week postburn; gram-negative enteric organisms become more common with longer periods of hospitalization. To eliminate infection on the surface of the burn wound, topical antimicrobial therapy is used, depending on protocol. Of the many antimicrobial agents available, the three most widely used are mafenide acetate (Sulfamylon) cream, sulfadiazine (Silvadene) cream, and silver nitrate 0.5% soaks. All three are broad-spectrum antibiotics. The choice of topical antibiotic is based on the extent of the burn wound, the presence of identified bacterial organisms, whether an open (exposing the wound to the air) or closed (using bulky dressings) method of treatment is used, and client response.

The increasing trend is toward prophylactic antibiotic administration in burn clients (Tierney, McPhee, & Papadakis, 2001). Systemic antimicrobial therapy is indicated in the immediate preoperative and postoperative period associated with excision and autografting. Postoperatively, the therapy is discontinued as soon as the client's hemodynamic status returns to normal, usually within the first 24 hours. In the long-term treatment of identified infectious processes, drug administration is limited to the least amount of time required to eradicate the infection. See the box on the following page for nursing implications for topical antimicrobial therapy for the burn client.

### Tetanus Prophylaxis

If the client's immunization status is in doubt, tetanus toxoid is administered intramuscularly early in the acute phase of care to prevent *Clostridium tetani* infection.

### Preventing Gastric Hyperacidity

Hyperacidity must be controlled to prevent Curling's ulcer. A nasogastric tube is placed during the emergent phase of care, and gastric aspirant is obtained hourly. The gastric pH should be assessed and maintained at levels above 5. To control gastric acid secretion during the acute phase of care, histamine $H_2$ blockers (e.g., famotidine [Pepcid] and ranitidine [Zantac]) can be administered intravenously, either intermittently or as continuous infusions. As soon as bowel sounds become audible, the client is placed on an antacid regimen.

## Treatments

### Surgery

Three surgical interventions are commonly employed to manage the burn wound: surgical debridement, escharotomy, and autografting.

***ESCHAROTOMY.*** When the burn eschar forms circumferentially around the torso or extremities, it acts as a tourniquet, impairing circulation. Left unchecked, the affected body part becomes gangrenous.

# Medication Administration
## Topical Burn Medications

## TOPICAL ANTIMICROBIAL AGENTS
Mafenide acetate (Sulfamylon)
Silver nitrate
Silver sulfadiazine (Silvadene)

The use of topical antimicrobial therapy was first investigated more than 60 years ago. Researchers found that the most effective topical agents are those that (1) act against the major pathogens responsible for causing burn wound infection, (2) achieve levels of concentration sufficient to decrease microbial colonization, (3) are rapidly excreted or metabolized, (4) are nontoxic, and (5) are easy to use and inexpensive.

### Mafenide Acetate
Mafenide is a synthetic antibiotic closely related chemically, but not pharmacologically, to the sulfonamides. Although the mechanism of action is unclear, the drug appears to interfere with the metabolism of bacterial cells. Mafenide is a bacteriostatic agent effective against many gram-positive and gram-negative organisms.

For topical administration, mafenide is used in an 8.5% cream in a water-miscible base. Following application, the drug is rapidly diffused through the burn eschar and absorbed systemically.

In the general circulation, mafenide metabolizes to a weak carbonic anhydrase inhibitor known as *p*-carboxybenzenesulfonamide, a substance that impairs the renal mechanisms involved in the buffering of blood. Bicarbonate excretion in the urine increases, and ammonia and chloride excretion decreases. To maintain normal acid-base balance, the pulmonary system effects a compensatory hyperventilatory state. If the compensatory hyperventilation is insufficient, the client develops metabolic acidosis.

### Nursing Responsibilities
- Use mafenide with caution in clients with renal or pulmonary disease.
- Approximately 3% to 5% of clients develop a hypersensitivity to mafenide, resulting in a maculopapular rash on the unburned areas. Assess the client for the following:

| | |
|---|---|
| Pruritus | Urticaria |
| Facial edema | Blisters |
| Swelling | Eosinophilia |

  If hypersensitivity reactions occur, discontinue the drug and administer antihistamines.
- Monitor the client for superinfection within the burn eschar, in the subeschar tissue, or in viable tissue adjacent to the wound.

### Client and Family Teaching
- Expect pain or a burning sensation following drug application. Take appropriate measures to control pain before applying the drug.
- Apply the drug to clean, debrided burn wounds once or twice daily. Continue applications until healing is apparent.
- If any signs of allergy develop, discontinue the drug and notify the physician.
- Report any sudden and prolonged increases in respiratory rate.

### Silver Nitrate
Silver nitrate is a bacteriostatic agent that inhibits a wide variety of gram-positive and gram-negative organisms. Its antimicrobial effect is due to the actions of silver ions, which markedly alter the microbial cell wall and membrane. Additionally, the drug denatures bacterial protein, thereby inactivating and precipitating the microbes.

### Nursing Responsibilities
- Silver nitrate is used as a 0.5% solution in distilled water. Apply the solution to bulky gauze dressings every 2 hours, and provide complete dressing changes twice daily.
- Silver nitrate has limited penetrating ability and is ineffective if used more than 72 hours following a burn injury.
- At the local tissue level, silver nitrate immediately interacts with chloride ions to form a black silver chloride precipitate that discolors both the burn wound and the adjacent tissues. The discoloration significantly hampers visual inspection of the wound.
- High concentrations of the drug result in cellular toxicity of surrounding healthy tissue.
- Because large amounts of water are systemically absorbed from the dressing site, the client may demonstrate a hypotonic state. Hyponatremia and hypochloremic alkalosis are common manifestations in burn-injured clients treated with silver nitrate.

### Client and Family Teaching
- Watch for and report any signs and symptoms of hypotonicity: swelling, weight gain, difficulty in breathing.
- This drug causes a black discoloration on all skin surfaces and dressings with which it comes into contact.
- Because discoloration can conceal evidence of infection, watch for systemic manifestations of infection fever, malaise, rapid pulse rate, listlessness.
- Saturate the wound dressings every 2 hours with a 0.5% aqueous solution of the drug. Change the dressings completely twice daily.

### Silver Sulfadiazine
Silver sulfadiazine, a sulfonamide, is the most commonly used topical agent. The drug acts on the cell membrane and cell wall of susceptible bacteria and binds to cellular DNA. The drug is bactericidal and effective against a wide variety of gram-negative and gram-positive organisms.

### Nursing Responsibilities
- Many clients develop a marked leukopenia in response to this drug, which tends to improve spontaneously over the course of therapy. This finding does not contraindicate use of the drug.
- Hypersensitivity to silver sulfadiazine has been reported in a small number of cases. If the client develops hypersensitivity, administer antihistamine, and change the topical agent.
- If sulfa crystals form in the urine, keep the client well hydrated.
- Treatment with this drug can cause systemic uptake of propylene glycol, which results in an elevated serum osmolality and high urine specific gravity in the client who is not dehydrated. These findings tend to create confusion during the fluid resuscitative stage of care. Whenever the serum osmolality and urine specific gravity fail to correlate with a clinical picture that reflects fluid volume overload (elevated CVP/PCWP, rhonichi/wheezing, edema), suspect systemic propylene glycol uptake.

### Client and Family Teaching
- Apply the drug to clean, debrided wounds once or twice daily, completely covering the burn wound at all times.
- Continue applying the drug until healing is apparent.
- If any signs of allergy develop, discontinue the drug and notify the physician.
- Watch for evidence of concentrated urine, and notify the physician.
- If not contraindicated, drink large amounts of fluids to prevent sulfa crystals from forming in the urine.

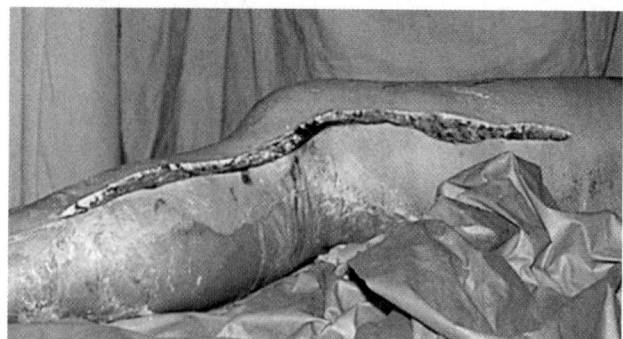

**Figure 15–8** ■ Escharotomy. The surgical procedure consists of removing the eschar formed on the skin and underlying tissue following severe burns. The procedure is particularly helpful in restoring circulation to the extremities of clients when scar tissue forms a tight, constrictive band around the circumference of a limb.

*Courtesy of Dr. William Dominic, Valley Medical Center.*

To prevent circumferential constriction of the torso or extremity, an **escharotomy** is performed by the physician with a scalpel or by electrocautery (Figure 15–8 ■). A sterile surgical incision is made longitudinally along the extremity or the trunk to release taut skin and allow for expansion caused by edema formation. In the first 24 hours following the procedure, the incision should be gently packed with fine mesh gauze. After 24 hours, the site may be treated with a direct application of a topical antimicrobial agent. See the box below for nursing implications for care of the client undergoing escharotomy.

**SURGICAL DEBRIDEMENT.** **Surgical debridement** refers to the process of excising the wound to the level of fascia (fascial excision) or sequentially removing thin slices of the burn wound to the level of viable tissue (sequential excision). Because **fascial excision**, or **fasciectomy**, sacrifices potentially viable fat and lymphatic tissue, its use is reserved for clients with extensive or full-thickness burns. The most common technique is electrocautery with cutting and coagulating current capabilities. Sequential excision is performed with the use of a dermatome. Shallow burns and some of moderate depth bleed briskly after one slice. If bleeding does not occur, the procedure is repeated until a viable bed of dermis or subcutaneous fat is reached. Following surgical debridement, the client is returned to the burn unit.

**AUTOGRAFTING.** A procedure performed in the surgical suite, **autografting** is used to effect permanent skin coverage. Early burn wound excision and skin grafting decreases the hospital stay and enhances rehabilitation. Skin is removed from healthy tissue (donor site) of the burn-injured client and applied to the burn wound (Figures 15–9 ■ and 15–10 ■). (Skin grafts and flaps are discussed in Chapter 14.) After the autograft is applied, the grafted area is immobilized. The site is assessed daily for evidence of adherence. The client resumes range-of-motion exercises 5 days postgraft. As the wound heals, the client may complain of itching, which can be treated with mild lotions.

Cultured epithelial autografting is a technique in which skin cells are removed from unburned sites on the client's body, then minced and placed in a culture medium for growth. Over a 5- to 7-day period, the cells expand 50 to 70 times the size of the initial biopsies. The cells are again separated out and placed in

---

## Nursing Implications for Circumferential Wound Management:

### Escharotomy

When a burn wound totally encircles an extremity, the torso, or the neck, the client is at risk for impaired tissue perfusion of the involved area. To prevent arterial occlusion, a circumferential burn wound may need to be excised. An escharotomy is a lengthwise incision made by the physician along the circumferential burn wound to release tension and permit unobstructed arterial blood flow. The nurse continuously assesses the involved area and notifies the physician of the need to perform this emergent procedure, which is done at the bedside. Because only the dead burn wound tissue is excised, the client experiences very little pain.

#### Nursing Responsibilities
- For circumferential burn wounds of the extremity, assess the extremity for absence of blood flow:
  a. Using a Doppler ultrasound stethoscope, check hourly for the presence of a pulse.
  b. Assess the extremity hourly for warmth, color, sensation, and capillary refill.
  c. Observe for evidence of numbness or tingling.
- For circumferential burn wounds of the torso, assess for evidence of respiratory distress:
  a. Obtain ABGs as needed.

  b. Auscultate lung sounds hourly.
  c. Observe for evidence of cyanosis, tachypnea, anxiety, or restlessness.
- For circumferential burn wounds of the neck, assess for evidence of respiratory distress. Prepare the client for prophylactic intubation.
- Monitor for excessive blood loss, and transfuse the client if indicated.
- Dress the open wound (escharotomy) with topical antimicrobial agents as ordered.

#### Client Teaching
- Teach the client the importance of reporting any evidence of impaired circulation: numbness, tingling, blue color to the extremity, absence of sensation.
- Assure the client that the procedure will not be painful and will provide immediate relief.
- Teach the client the importance of protecting the open wound (escharotomy) from infection.
- Explain the rationale supporting prophylactic intubation for burn wounds involving the head and neck.
- Provide assurance that all blood loss will be replaced and that bleeding at the site will be controlled.

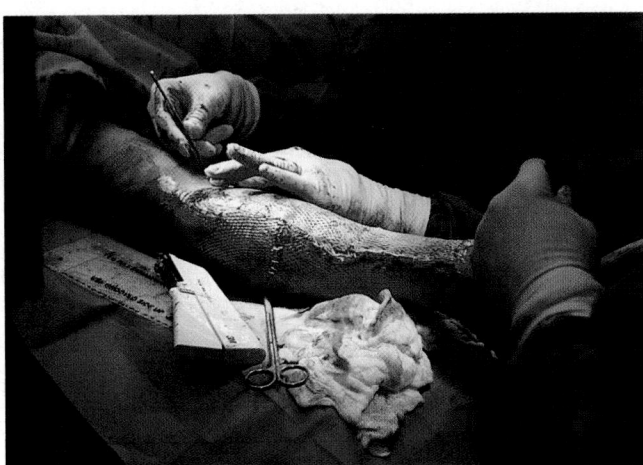

**Figure 15–9** ■ Skin grafting procedure.

*Courtesy of Dr. William Dominic, Valley Medical Center.*

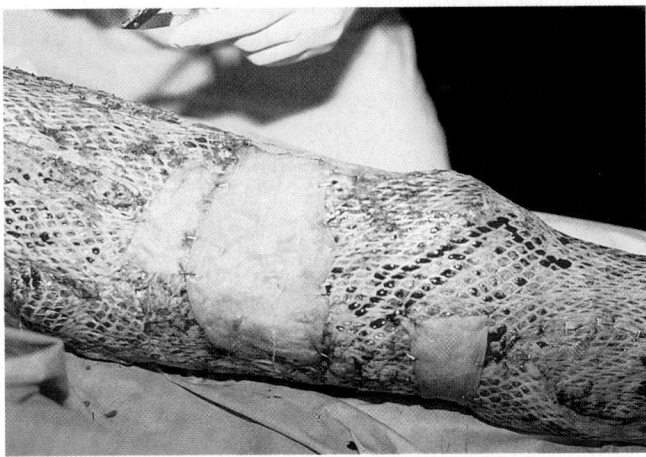

**Figure 15–10** ■ Skin graft for burn injury (autograft).

*Courtesy of Dr. William Dominic, Valley Medical Center.*

a new culture medium for continued growth. With this technique, enough skin can be grown over a period of 3 to 4 weeks to cover an entire human body. The cells are prepared in sheets and attached to petroleum jelly gauze backing, which is applied to the burn wound site. Problems with infection and lack of attachment have occurred.

## Biologic and Biosynthetic Dressings

The terms *biologic dressing* and *biosynthetic dressing* refer to any temporary material that rapidly adheres to the wound bed, promotes healing, and/or prepares the burn wound for permanent autograft coverage. Ideally, these kinds of dressings should be easy to apply and remove, inexpensive, nonantigenic, elastic, able to reduce pain, able to serve as a bacterial barrier, and able to enhance the natural healing process. The dressings are applied to the burn wound as soon as possible. Covering the wound eliminates the loss of water through evaporation, reduces infection, and promotes wound healing. Biologic and biosynthetic dressings that are currently in use include homograft (allograft), heterograft (xenograft), amnionic membranes, and synthetic materials.

**Homograft,** or **allograft,** is human skin that has been harvested from cadavers. It is stored in skin banks located throughout the nation. The development of methods to achieve prolonged storage of frozen, viable skin has increased the use of this dressing; however, its short supply and expense still pose problems. It is manufactured as strips cut to the pattern of the burn and applied using sterile technique. Under normal circumstances, a homograft is rejected within 14 to 21 days following application.

**Heterograft,** or **xenograft,** is skin obtained from an animal, usually a pig. Although fresh porcine heterograft is available to some centers, frozen heterograft is much more commonly used. Once applied, heterograft appears to undergo early softening and lysis from enzymatic action from the wound. As a result, frequent changes of the heterograft dressing are necessary. Because of the high infection rates associated with this dressing, silver-nitrate-treated porcine heterograft has been developed to retard microbial growth.

The multiple problems associated with the use of biologic dressings have driven the development of synthetic materials. One such material is Biobrane, a composite material consisting of nylon mesh bonded to silicone that has proved successful in the temporary coverage of second- and third-degree burns. Whereas Biobrane adheres well to moderately clean wounds, it cannot adhere to or lower bacterial counts in grossly contaminated wounds. Biobrane dressing is supplied in various sizes, cut to fit the wound site, and secured with tape or Steri-Strips. It spontaneously separates from the wound when the underlying tissue heals. Hydrocolloid dressings are another type of biosynthetic material. They are occlusive wafers of gumlike materials that provide a water-resistant outer layer for coverage of the donor site. They protect healing tissue from excessive drying, liquefy necrotic tissue, and absorb wound drainage.

If dermal thickness is lost in deep partial-thickness or full-thickness burns, several products can serve as a dermal replacement. Integra is a synthetic dermal substitute and Alloderm is human cadaver allograft dermis that is nonimmunogenic. These products are placed in the wound, and split-thickness autografts are then placed over the dermal replacement. These products are used to provide temporary wound coverage, reduce pain, and facilitate healing.

The most recent temporary skin substitute is TransCyte. This bioengineered substance is derived from human fibroblast cells grown within mesh. As the cells grow, they secrete human dermal collagen, matrix proteins, and growth factors. The product is produced, extensively tested for any infectious agents, and then frozen. It is used for temporary covering for surgically debrided full-thickness and deep partial-thickness burn wounds, and is an alternative to silver sulfadiazine and cadaver skin. TransCyte forms a transparent, protective barrier over the wound surface and is typically applied only once. The best results have been obtained when it was applied within 24 hours of injury.

## Wound Management

The outcomes of care for the client with a major burn depends on the prevention and treatment of infection through daily topical wound care, wound monitoring, and wound excision and closure. The goals of wound management are as follows (Bucher & Melander, 1999):

- Remove nonviable tissue.
- Control microbial colonization.
- Promote reepithelialization.
- Achieve wound coverage as early as possible.

***DEBRIDING THE WOUND.*** Burned tissue releases chemical mediators that stimulate phagocytosis in an attempt to digest debris left by decaying necrotic tissue. Necrotic tissue that remains despite phagocytic action retards healing and prolongs inflammation. **Debridement** is the process of removing all loose tissue, wound debris, and eschar (dead tissue) from the wound. Three methods of debridement are employed: mechanical, enzymatic, and surgical (surgical debridement was previously discussed).

A nurse may perform mechanical debridement by applying and removing gauze dressings (wet-to-dry or wet-to-moist), hydrotherapy, irrigation, or scissors and tweezers. During hydrotherapy (in an immersion tank, a shower, or on a spray table) the burn injury may be gently washed with a mild soap or wound cleaner solution to remove dead skin and separate eschar. The solution is then rinsed off with warm saline or tap water. Body hair (except for eyebrows) should be shaved within the burn and to within 2.5 cm of the wound edges. Blistered skin is grasped with a dry gauze and gently removed. The edges of blisters or eschar are trimmed with blunt scissors. The wound is then covered with a topical antimicrobial agent.

Enzymatic debridement involves the use of a topical agent to dissolve and remove necrotic tissue. An enzyme (such as sutilains, collagenase [Santyl], or fibrinolysis-deoxyribonuclease [Elase]) is applied in a thin layer directly to the wound and covered with one layer of fine mesh gauze. A topical antimicrobial agent is then applied and covered with a bulky wet dressing; the wound is immobilized with expandable mesh gauze.

***DRESSING THE WOUND.*** Once the wound has been cleaned and debrided, it may be dressed using one of two methods. In the open method, the burn wound remains open to air, covered only by a topical antimicrobial agent. This method allows the wound to be easily assessed. Topical agents must be frequently reapplied because they tend to rub off onto the bedding.

In the closed method, a topical antimicrobial agent is applied to the wound site, which is covered with gauze or a nonadherent dressing and then gently wrapped with a gauze roll bandage (Figure 15–11 ■). With the closed method, burn wounds are usually dressed twice daily and as needed. Dressings are applied circumferentially in a distal-to-proximal manner. All fingers and toes are wrapped separately.

***POSITIONING, SPLINTS, AND EXERCISE.*** During therapy, the client must be maintained in positions that prevent **contractures** from forming. Because flexion is the natural resting position of joints and extremities, early physical therapy may include maintaining antideformity positions. Splints immobi-

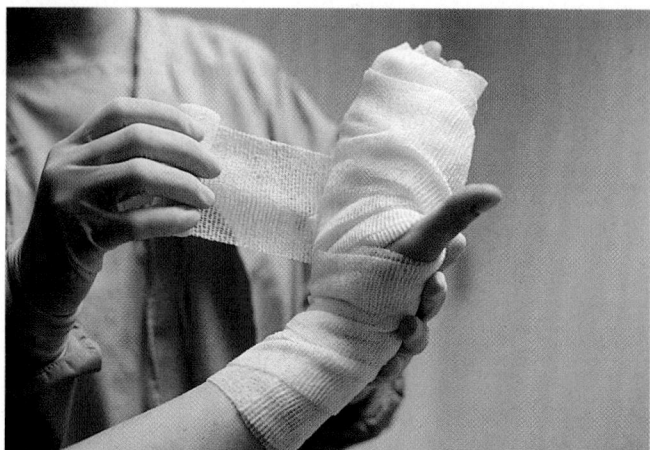

**Figure 15–11** ■ Closed method of dressing a burn.
*Courtesy of Dr. William Dominic, Valley Medical Center.*

lize body parts and prevent contractures of the joints. They are applied and removed according to schedules established by the physical therapist.

Early in the acute phase of care, the physical therapist prescribes active and passive ROM exercises, which are performed every 2 hours at the bedside, most often by physical therapy. Early ambulation is also part of the plan of care once the client's condition becomes stable.

***SUPPORT GARMENTS.*** Applying uniform pressure can prevent or reduce hypertrophic scarring. Tubular support bandages are applied 5 to 7 days postgraft to maintain a tension ranging from 10 to 20 mmHg to control scarring. The client wears custom-made elastic pressure garments for 6 months to a year postgraft.

## Nutritional Support

The client with a major burn is in a hypermetabolic and catabolic state. The resting energy expenditure after severe burn injury can increase by as much as 100% above normal levels, depending on the extent of catabolism and the client's physical activity, size, age, and gender. This increase is believed due to heat loss from the burn wound, an increase in beta-adrenergic activity, pain, and infection. As a result, total caloric needs may be as great as 4000 to 6000 kcal per day.

Traditional dietary management based on oral intake seldom meets the kcal requirements necessary to reverse negative nitrogen balance and begin the healing process. Enteral feedings with a nasointestinal feeding tube are therefore instituted within 24 to 48 hours of the burn injury to offset hypermetabolism, improve nitrogen balance, and decrease length of hospital stay. A nasointestinal feeding tube is placed under fluoroscopy, with the tip extending past the pylorus to prevent reflux and aspiration.

Although enteral feeding is the preferred nutritional therapy, it is contraindicated in Curling's ulcer, bowel obstruction, feeding intolerance, pancreatitis, or septic ileus. When the enteral route cannot be used, a central venous catheter is inserted via the subclavian or jugular vein for the administration of total parenteral nutrition (TPN).

TABLE 15-5 Interventions in Various Stages of Burn Injury

| Stage of Burn Injury | Onset | End Point | Interventions |
| --- | --- | --- | --- |
| Emergent/Resuscitative | Occurrence of burn injury | Successful fluid resuscitation | Remove client from heat source. Initiate first aid. Assess extent of burn injury. Prevent hypothermia. Assess for shock. Determine need for intubation. Determine need for intravenous therapy. Follow protocol for fluid resuscitation. Obtain history. Transport to tertiary care facility. |
| Acute | Diuresis | Wound closure | Begin hydrotherapy. Determine need for excision of burn wound. Control spread of infection. Institute wound care. Start nutrition support. Graft burn wound. Initiate physical therapy. Manage pain. |
| Rehabilitative | Wound closure | Return to highest level of health restoration | Prevent scar formation. Continue physical therapy. Address psychosocial, cultural, and spiritual needs. Consider occupational therapy. Consider vocational training. Assess home maintenance management. |

## NURSING CARE

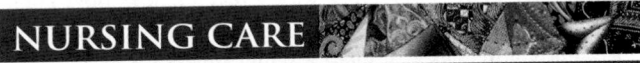

The client with a major burn has complex, multisystem needs. Table 15–5 lists overall nursing interventions for the emergent, acute, and rehabilitative stages of burn injury.

### Health Promotion

Although treatments have improved significantly over the last several decades, there is no cure for burns. Prevention remains the primary goal. With the public's increasing attention to health promotion and disease prevention, the nursing profession currently is well positioned to collaborate with other disciplines to develop initiatives to reduce the number of burn injuries. For example, as client advocates, nurses can alert political leaders to the need to pass legislation aimed at reducing the incidence of burns. Appropriate legislative themes might center on safety in the workplace (e.g., requirements for smoke alarms and sprinkler systems), on the highways (e.g., regulations regarding the transportation of flammable liquids), and in the home (e.g., requirements for safety devices for water heaters and wood-burning stoves, and for self-extinguishing cigarettes). As educators, nurses can develop teaching plans for families and communities to heighten awareness of the problem. As researchers, nurses can investigate conditions leading to burn injury and suggest methods to reduce its prevalence. Working together with health care policymakers and community leaders, nurses can join the effort to lower the number of annual burn cases.

### Assessment

Nursing assessment is continuous from the initial contact with the client with a burn injury. This section describes the secondary survey, conducted when the client arrives at the emergency department. Once there, the staff must act quickly to obtain the client's history of the burn injury, including the time of injury, causative agents, early treatment, medical history, and client's age and body weight. In most cases, the client is awake and oriented and able to relate the information during the emergent phase of care. Because changes in sensorium will become evident within the first few hours following a major burn injury, the nurse obtains as much information as is possible immediately on the client's arrival.

- *Time of injury.* In many cases, the client is admitted to the emergency department an hour or more after the injury occurred. The time of the burn injury must be documented as precisely as possible at the scene, because all fluid resuscitation calculations are based on the time of the burn injury, not on the client's time of arrival at the ER.
- *Cause of the injury.* Because the type of burn injury determines which nursing measures take priority, identify the specific causative agent to establish the appropriate plan of care.
- *First-aid treatment.* Prior to the arrival of medical personnel, the client or family may have applied home remedies to treat the burn wound. It is important for the nurse to ascertain and document the nature of all home treatment interventions, including the application of neutralizing agents, liquids, and immobilizing devices used to splint associated injuries.

## Meeting Individualized Needs

### BURNS IN THE OLDER ADULT

Older adults are at greater risk for burns of all degrees of severity, with burns and fires being a major cause of death. Most burns are accidental, the result of slower reaction times, decreased mobility, visual deficits, a decreased sense of smell, forgetfulness, and impaired sensation. Many older adults are burned by stoves, hot water, hot food, irons, cookware, and heating pads. Older adults with cognitive impairments or dementias may start fires by leaving foods cooking unattended. The most common burns in this age group are the result of catching clothing on fire and scalding from tap water that is too hot.

The care of the older adult with burns often presents unique challenges. They may delay seeking treatment, thus increasing the risk of infection. Their care is often complicated by the presence of other chronic illnesses. They may live alone, and have no one to care for them during rehabilitation. Even small burns have the potential to become lethal in older adults.

Burn prevention topics for older adults are as follows:

- Have a relative or neighbor routinely check for the odor of gas.
- Check the smoke detector battery once a month.
- Wear close-fitting clothing when cooking.
- Use a cooking timer with a loud alarm.
- Never lay anything over a heating device.
- Set the temperature of the hot water heater no higher than 120°F.
- Install antiscald devices in bathroom plumbing.

---

- *Past medical history.* Clients with histories of respiratory, cardiac, renal, metabolic, neurologic, gastrointestinal, or skin diseases; alcohol abuse; or altered immune states require more intense observation. Known allergies are obtained.
- *Age.* Older adults tend to require more supportive care (see the box above).
- *Medications.* Drugs, either prescribed or recreational, taken by the client prior to the burn injury may further complicate the treatment regimen. Drugs that affect any of the major body systems or cause mood alterations will need to be factored into the treatment plan. As part of the early assessment, obtain and document blood levels of therapeutic pharmaceutical agents and mood-altering substances.
- *Body weight.* During the acute and rehabilitative phases of the burn injury, the client will lose as much as 20% of preburn weight. This fact will have significant implications for all clients, especially for those who are underweight or cachectic at the time of the injury.

### Nursing Diagnoses and Interventions

A major burn affects virtually every body system, as well as social, cultural, economic, psychological, and spiritual well-being. Immediate treatment in an intensive care setting is followed by years of rehabilitation and a lifetime of change in what was possible for an individual before the injury. Many nursing diagnoses are appropriate for the client with a major burn injury; those described here are *Altered skin integrity, Deficient fluid volume, Acute pain, Risk for infection, Impaired physical mobility, Imbalanced nutrition: Less than body requirements,* and *Powerlessness.*

### Impaired Skin Integrity

The burn injury significantly impairs skin integrity. The severity of wounds varies according to the depth and extent of the burn. General treatment measures are designed to restore normal skin function as quickly as possible. Nursing care focuses on assessing and cleansing the wound and controlling infection.

- Estimate the extent and depth of the burn wound and recalculate extent of unhealed burns weekly. *The severity of the*

*burn injury is the basis for determining which type of interventions are appropriate. Reassessment on a regular basis is necessary to monitor the healing process.*
- Provide daily wound care (including debridement method, dressing method, and medication administration) as prescribed, *to remove dead tissue, control infection, and promote reepithelialization as soon as possible.*
- Provide special skin care to sensitive body areas:
  - Clean burns involving the eyes with normal saline or sterile water, *to prevent corneal and conjunctival drying and adherence.* If contracture of the eyelid develops, apply drops or ointment to the eye, *to prevent corneal abrasion.*
  - Gently wipe burns of the lips with saline-soaked pads. Apply an antibiotic ointment as prescribed. Assess the mouth frequently, and perform mouth care routinely. If an oral endotracheal tube is in place, reposition it often, *to prevent pressure ulcer formation.*
  - Gently debride burns of the nose, and apply mafenide acetate (Sulfamylon) cream. Position nasogastric and nasotracheal tubes, *to prevent excessive pressure.*
  - Apply mafenide acetate (Sulfamylon) cream to burns of the ear. Gently debride and thoroughly clean the wound with a water spray. Do not cover ears with dressings. Do not use pillows; to reduce pressure to the area, use a foam doughnut instead. *Burns of the ears are prone to infection; special positioning devices are necessary to decrease pressure ulcer formation.*

### Deficient Fluid Volume

Fluid resuscitation rates are adjusted periodically throughout the emergent stage of care. The nurse should be particularly aware of several situations that may warrant the administration of fluids at rates in excess of the calculations needed to maintain adequate urine output: initial underestimation of the burn size, sequestration of fluid into the lung tissue in inhalation injury, electrical injury (which tends to cause more extensive damage than is immediately visible), full-thickness burns, and inordinately delayed starts of fluid resuscitation.

- Assess blood pressure and heart rate frequently. *Vital signs rapidly deteriorate when fluid resuscitation is inadequate.*

- Monitor hemodynamic status, including CVP and PCWP. *Inadequate fluid resuscitation is manifested by a drop in the central venous pressure and pulmonary capillary wedge pressure.*
- Follow prescribed protocols for intravenous fluid resuscitation. *Therapy for burn shock is aimed at supporting the client through the period of hypovolemic instability.*
- Monitor intake and output hourly. *Report urine outputs of less than 50 mL/h. Intake and output measurements indicate the adequacy of fluid resuscitation, and should range from 30 to 50 mL per hour in an adult.*
- Weigh daily. *Body weight is used to calculate fluid requirements.*
- Test all stools and emesis for the presence of blood. *Occult blood in emesis or stool indicates gastrointestinal bleeding.*
- Maintain a warm environment. *Hypothermia leads to shivering and further loss of body fluid through increased energy expenditure and catabolism.*
- Monitor for fluid volume overload. *Older clients and those with underlying cardiac disease may demonstrate symptoms of congestive heart failure during the fluid resuscitation stage.*

**PRACTICE ALERT**  *Manifestations of fluid overload include weight gain in a short time; an intake that exceeds output; an increase in blood pressure and CVP; jugular vein distention; dyspnea, orthopnea, crackles; and restlessness.* ■

### Acute Pain

The client experiences excruciating pain with extensive superficial and all partial-thickness burns. Intense pain is also experienced during wound care and physical therapy. In addition, increased levels of anxiety about treatments and outcomes may further increase the perception of pain.

- Measure the client's level of pain, using a consistent measurement tool. *Pain tolerance is the duration and intensity of pain that the client is able to endure. Pain tolerance differs from one client to the next and may vary in the same client in different situations.*
- Medicate before painful procedures and determine when PCA is appropriate. *The inability to manage pain results in feelings of despair and frustration.*
- Administer intravenous narcotic analgesics as prescribed. *Nurses' fear of precipitating addiction often makes them reluctant to administer narcotics. During the acute stage of burn injury, however, invasive procedures and exposed neurosensory nerve endings dictate the need for narcotic pharmaceutical agents.*

**PRACTICE ALERT**  *Narcotics are never administered orally, subcutaneously, or intramuscularly in the acute stage of a burn.* ■

- Explain all procedures and expected levels of discomfort. *Clients who are prepared for painful procedures and know beforehand the actual sensations they will feel experience less stress.*

- Use methods of nonnarcotic pain control in combination with medications for pain. *Noninvasive pain relief measures (e.g., relaxation, massage, distraction) can enhance the therapeutic effects of pain relief medications.*
- Allow the client to verbalize the pain experience. *Each person experiences and expresses pain in his or her own manner, using various sociocultural adaptation techniques.*

### Risk for Infection

From the onset of the burn injury, loss of the body's natural barrier to the external environment increases the risk of infection. Nursing interventions focus on controlling infectious processes. Monitor the results of diagnostic tests, maintain nutritional therapies, and apply antimicrobial agents to monitor and prevent the spread of infection, a major complication of the burn injury.

- Monitor daily for manifestations of wound infection. Remove topical medications and wound exudate and examine the entire wound. *Early manifestations of wound infection include swelling and inflammation in intact skin surrounding the wound; a change in the color, odor, or amount of exudate; increased pain; and loss of previously healed skin grafts.*

**PRACTICE ALERT**  *An increased body temperature, without other manifestations of infection, is not indicative of infection in clients with large burn wounds (in which the hypermetabolic response resets the core temperature to a higher level).* ■

- Monitor for positive blood cultures, *which indicate bacteremia.*
- Monitor for hyperermia, cough, chest pain, wheezing, rhonchi, decreased oxygen saturation, and purulent sputum, *which are manifestations of pneumonia.*
- Monitor for the presence of bacteria in the urine, fever, urgency, frequency, dysuria and superpubic pain, *which are manifestations of urinary tract infections.*

**PRACTICE ALERT**  *If the client has an indwelling catheter, assess the urine for cloudiness and a foul odor, and obtain a urine culture and sensitivity at least weekly.* ■

- Obtain daily WBC counts. *Leukocyte counts are indicators of immune system function, and increase in the presence of infection.*
- Determine tetanus immunization status. *Burn clients are at risk for anaerobic infection caused by* Clostridium tetani.
- Maintain high kcal intake. *Nutritional support provides the nutrients needed to maintain the body's defense mechanisms.*
- Maintain an aseptic environment, using standard precautions (including gloving, gowning, and sterile procedures). *Strict isolation technique deters the development of nosocomial infection.*
- Culture all wounds and body secretions per protocol. *Culture and sensitivity reports identify the presence of infectious microbes and indicate appropriate antimicrobial therapies.*
- Administer prescribed antimicrobial medications, *to decrease invasive wound infections.*

## Impaired Physical Mobility

As the burn wound heals and new skin tissue forms, the involved area tends to shrink. Contractures form at the site and significantly limit mobility, especially when a joint is involved. Physical therapy is important, beginning in the early stages of treatment. The nurse institutes ambulation and planned exercise regimens as soon as the client's condition stabilizes.

- Perform active or passive ROM exercises to all joints every 2 hours. Ambulate when stable. *Regular exercise prevents further loss of motion, restores movement, and improves functional status.*
- Apply splints as prescribed. Maintain antideformity positions, and reposition the client hourly. *Splinting and positioning retard the formation of contractures.*

**PRACTICE ALERT** *Assess all clients, but especially the older adult, for indications of pressure ulcer formation under a splint.* ■

- Maintain limbs in functional alignment, *to preserve joint mobility.*

- Anticipate the need for analgesia. *Administering analgesics promotes the client's comfort during exercising sessions.*

## Imbalanced Nutrition: Less Than Body Requirements

The burn injury initiates a complex series of events that have a profound effect on the body's use of nutrients and expenditure of energy. Daily kcal requirements are determined by the nutritionist, and as soon as possible, enteral feedings are initiated. Duodenal tubes are placed to enhance intestinal absorption and retard gastric reflux. Parenteral nutrition is reserved for instances in which enteral feedings are contraindicated. Nursing measures focus on assessing feeding tolerance and use of nutrients.

- Maintain nasogastric/nasointestinal tube placement. *Correct tube placement ensures appropriate absorption of nutrients and prevents aspiration.*
- Maintain enteral/parenteral nutritional support as prescribed. Observe and report any evidence of feeding intolerance: diarrhea, vomiting, excessive gastric residue, abdominal distention, absent bowel sounds, and constipation. *The dietitian, in collaboration with the physician, selects and individualizes the feeding formula according to the client's daily en-*

---

# Nursing Research

## Evidence-Based Practice for the Client with a Major Burn

The personal losses resulting from burns include changes in body image and self-concept, altered functional ability, inability to provide self-care, changes in roles and relationships, threats to employment and income, and fear of death. In the initial stage of burn treatment the client gives up most, if not all, control over all aspects of life.

In an investigation of chronic sorrow (Eakes et al., 1998), sorrow is presented as a normal response to an abnormal situation within a model of chronic sorrow. Chronic sorrow is defined as cyclical, with periodic recurrences as long as the disparity created by the loss exists. Characterized as pervasive, permanent, periodic, and potentially progressive in nature, the periodic return of grief is experienced by both individuals and caregivers. Chronic sorrow may be precipitated by a loss without a predictable end such as a chronic health problem or by a circumscribed loss such as the loss of a loved one. Chronic sorrow is most often triggered in individuals with chronic health problems when the individual experiences disparity with accepted social, developmental, or personal norms; and when treatment such as hospitalization brings the ongoing disparity into focus.

Individuals draw on a variety of strategies to cope with the periodic grief associated with chronic sorrow. Positive coping skills include taking part in personal interest and activities, seeking information, living one day at a time, talking with others in the same or similar situation, talking with someone close, and relying on religious or personal beliefs and practices for comfort.

### IMPLICATIONS FOR NURSING

It is important that nurses provide interventions for chronic sorrow based on a personal belief that chronic sorrow is normal and

does occur. Being aware of the situations that trigger grief allows the nurse to provide anticipatory guidance drawn from the client's personal coping strategies. Simply asking "what helps?" is often a good way to assess coping strategies. Specific nursing interventions have been identified as being helpful in reducing the emotional pain of grief in clients with chronic health conditions. These interventions are taking time to listen, being empathic, offering support and reassurance, recognizing and focusing on feelings, and appreciating the uniqueness of each client and family. Interventions helpful to caregivers are empathic presence and providing accurate situation-specific information and helpful tips for dealing with the caregiver role.

### Critical Thinking in Client Care

1. Support groups are available for clients and care-givers with many different situations of loss. Would you recommend a support group for a young adult with major burns? Why or why not?
2. Why do you think chronic sorrow in a client with severely disfiguring burns differs from that in a client whose child died at the age of 3?
3. Develop a plan for facilitating positive coping strategies for the following clients:
   a. A 22-year-old woman with full-thickness thermal burns over half the face and the skull, with loss of an ear.
   b. A 76-year-old man with deep split-thickness burns of the right hand (he is right-handed) from a hot-water heater explosion.
   c. A 35-year-old single mother of three school-age children, struck by lightning, with burns ranging from superficial to full thickness.

*ergy expenditure requirements and feeding tolerance. Failure to maintain rates of infusion predisposes the client to continued catabolism and negative nitrogen balance.*

- Weigh the client daily. *Anthropometric measurements indicate the adequacy of nutritional support therapies.*
- Obtain daily laboratory values for protein, iron, CBC, glucose, and albumin. *Decreased serum values indicate inadequate nutritional intake.*

### Powerlessness

Usually, the client with a major burn injury endures a lengthy hospital stay involving many treatments and care protocols that are beyond his or her control. During the early stages, much of the care regimen involves excruciating pain. Further, the foreign environment of the burn unit makes it difficult for the client to relate to the immediate surroundings. For example, the need to control infection in the burn unit requires hospital personnel and family members to don sterile clothing prior to coming to the client's bedside. Family members and nursing personnel appear radically different when they are masked and gowned, and their odd appearance can add to the burn-injured client's sense of alienation.

- Allow the client as much control over the surroundings and daily routine as possible. For example, allow the client to choose times of dressing changes. *Powerlessness derives from the belief that one is unable to influence the outcome of a situation.*
- Keep needed items within reach, such as call bell, urinal, water pitcher, and tissues, *to reinforce the client's feelings of control.*
- Allow the client to express feelings. *The nurse can help the client cope by therapeutically listening, displaying a caring presence, clarifying misconceptions, and providing positive feedback* (see the Nursing Research box on previous page).
- Set short-term, realistic goals (e.g., set a goal for the client to ambulate from bedside to chair twice daily). *Small incremental gains are easier to achieve and allow for frequent positive reinforcement.*

### Using NANDA, NIC, and NOC

Chart 15–1 shows links between NANDA, NIC, and NOC when caring for the client with a major burn.

## CHART 15–1  NANDA, NIC, AND NOC LINKAGES

### The Client with a Major Burn

| NURSING DIAGNOSES | NURSING INTERVENTIONS | NURSING OUTCOMES |
|---|---|---|
| • Impaired Skin Integrity | • Skin Surveillance<br>• Circulatory Precautions<br>• Wound Care<br>• Medication Administration: Skin<br>• Skin Care: Topical Treatments<br>• Positioning<br>• Splinting<br>• Exercise Therapy: Stretching<br>• Exercise Therapy: Joint Mobility<br>• Infection Protection | • Tissue Integrity: Skin<br>• Wound Healing<br>• Risk Control |
| • Deficient Fluid Volume | • Electrolyte Management Balance<br>• Fluid Management<br>• Fluid Monitoring<br>• Hypovolemia Management<br>• Intravenous Therapy<br>• Shock Management: Volume<br>• Vital Signs Monitoring | • Electrolyte<br>• Fluid Balance |
| • Anxiety | • Anxiety Reduction<br>• Coping Enhancement | • Anxiety Control<br>• Coping |
| • Disturbed Body Image | • Body Image Enhancement<br>• Active Listening<br>• Coping Enhancement<br>• Emotional Support<br>• Grief Work Facilitation<br>• Pain Management<br>• Support Group | • Body Image<br>• Grief Resolution |

*Note. Data from Nursing Outcomes Classification (NOC) by M. Johnson & M. Maas (Eds.), 1997, St. Louis: Mosby; Nursing Diagnoses: Definitions & Classification 2001–2002 by North American Nursing Diagnosis Association, 2001, Philadelphia: NANDA; Nursing Interventions Classification (NIC) by J.C. McCloskey & G. M. Bulechek (Eds.), 2000, St. Louis: Mosby. Reprinted by permission.*

## Home Care

Client and family teaching is an important component of all phases of burn care. As treatment progresses, the nurse encourages family members to assume more responsibility in providing care. From admission to discharge, the nurse teaches the client and family to assess all findings, implement therapies, and evaluate progress. The following topics should be addressed in preparing the client and family for home care.

- The long-term goals of rehabilitation care: to prevent soft tissue deformity, protect skin grafts, maintain physiologic function, manage scars, and return the client to an optimal level of independence
- Avoiding exposure to people with colds or infections and following aseptic technique meticulously when caring for the wound
- The need for progressive physical activity
- How to apply splints, pressure support garments, and other assistive devices
- Dietary requirements with required kcal
- Alternative pain control therapies, such as guided imagery, relaxation techniques, and diversional activities
- Care of the graft and donor sites
- Referral for occupational therapy, social service, clergy, and/or psychiatric services as appropriate
- Helpful resources:
  - American Burn Association
  - International Society for Burn Injuries
  - American Academy of Facial Plastic and Reconstructive Surgery
  - The Phoenix Society for Burn Survivors, Inc.

## Nursing Care Plan
## The Client with a Major Burn

Craig Howard, a 39-year-old truck driver, is admitted to the hospital following an accident in which the cab of his truck caught on fire. He was freed from the truck by a passing motorist, who stayed with him until the rescue team arrived and transported him to a local ED. Mr. Howard's wife, Mary, and twin daughters, Jessica and Jane, age 10, have been notified.

### ASSESSMENT

On his admission to the ED, Mr. Howard is diagnosed with deep split-thickness and full-thickness burns of the anterior chest, arms, and hands. A quick assessment based on the rule of nines estimates the extent of his burn injury at 36% of TBSA. His vital signs are as follows: T 96.2°F (35.6°C), P 140, R 40, and BP 98/60. In the field, the paramedics had inserted a large-bore central line into Mr. Howard's right subclavian vein and started the rapid infusion of lactated Ringer's solution. Mr. Howard is receiving 40% humidified oxygen via face mask. Initial ABGs are: pH 7.49, $Po_2$ 60 mmHg, $Pco_2$ 32 mmHg, and bicarbonate 22 mEq/L. Lung sounds indicate inspiratory and expiratory wheezing, and a persistent cough reveals sooty sputum production. A Foley catheter is inserted and initially drains a moderate amount of dark, concentrated urine. A nasogastric tube is connected to low-intermittent suction. Mr. Howard is alert and oriented and complains of severe pain associated with the burn injuries. The burn unit is notified, and Mr. Howard is transferred there.

### DIAGNOSIS

- *Risk for ineffective airway clearance,* related to increasing lung congestion secondary to smoke inhalation
- *Deficient fluid volume,* related to abnormal fluid loss secondary to burn injury
- *Risk for ineffective tissue perfusion,* related to peripheral constriction secondary to circumferential burn wounds of the arms

### EXPECTED OUTCOMES

- Demonstrate a patent airway, as evidenced by clear breath sounds; absence of cyanosis; and vital signs, chest X-ray findings, and ABGs within normal limits.
- Demonstrate adequate fluid volume and electrolyte balance, as evidenced by urine output, vital signs, mental status, and laboratory findings within normal limits.
- Demonstrate adequate tissue perfusion, as evidenced by palpable pulses, warm extremities, normal capillary refill, and absence of paresthesia.

### PLANNING AND IMPLEMENTATION

- Prepare for prophylactic nasotracheal intubation to maintain airway patency.
- Initiate fluid resuscitation therapy using the Parkland/Baxter formula to calculate intravenous fluid rate for the first 24 hours postburn.
- Assist the physician to perform escharotomies of both upper extremities.

### EVALUATION

The nurse anesthetist inserted a nasotracheal tube and connected Mr. Howard to a T-piece delivering 40% oxygen. Vigorous respiratory toileting has significantly improved his ABGs. Bronchodilators have been parenterally administered and mucolytic agents added to his respiratory treatments. His tracheal secretions have begun to show evidence of clearing. Hourly urine outputs indicate adequate fluid resuscitation. Urine output has been maintained at 50 mL/h, and color and concentration have improved. CVP readings have been maintained at 6 cm $H_2O$, and blood pressure has increased to 100/64. The pulse rate has decreased to 100.

To improve tissue perfusion of both arms, the physician has performed bilateral escharotomies and the wounds are dressed, using sterile procedure. The extremities have demonstrated improved circulation.

### Critical Thinking in the Nursing Process

1. Explain the rationale for the immediate insertion of a Foley catheter and nasogastric tube.
2. An escharotomy was performed on both arms. Why was this procedure necessary in Mr. Howard's case?
3. What is the rationale supporting the intravenous administration of narcotics to control Mr. Howard's pain?
4. Explain the sequence of events that led to a fluid and electrolyte shift during the first 24 to 48 hours after Mr. Howard sustained his injury.

See Evaluating Your Response in Appendix C.

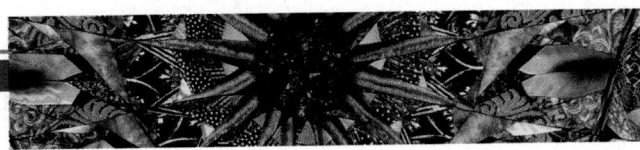

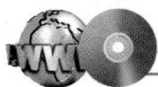 ## EXPLORE MediaLink

NCLEX review questions, case studies, care plan activities, MediaLink applications, and other interactive resources for this chapter can be found on the Companion Website at www.prenhall.com/lemone.

Click on Chapter 15 to select the activities for this chapter. For animations, video clips, more NCLEX review questions, and an audio glossary, access the Student CD-ROM accompanying this textbook.

## TEST YOURSELF

1. A burn caused by exposure to an acidic or basic agent is classified as a/an:
   a. Chemical burn
   b. Thermal burn
   c. Electrical burn
   d. Radiation burn

2. A burn that involves the entire dermis, the dermal papillae, and the hair follicles is classified as what type of burn?
   a. Superficial
   b. Superficial partial thickness
   c. Deep partial thickness
   d. Full thickness

3. Which of the following clients is at greatest risk for burn shock?
   a. One with a 90% superficial burn from a tanning bed
   b. One with 10% TBSA from a gasoline explosion
   c. One with radiation burns following treatment for cancer
   d. One with > 50% TBSA from a high-voltage electrical accident

4. The primary purpose of antimicrobial treatment of the burn wound is to:
   a. Relieve pain
   b. Eliminate infection on the wound surface
   c. Remove eschar
   d. Prevent renal failure

5. Which of the following topics should be included in a presentation on burn prevention at a senior citizen center?
   a. Use a solar-powered nightlight
   b. Do not use the oven for cooking
   c. Set the water heater no higher than 120° F
   d. Check smoke detectors annually

See Test Yourself answers in Appendix C.

## BIBLIOGRAPHY

Badger, J. (2001). Burns: The psychological aspects. *American Journal of Nursing, 101*(11), 38–44.

Barnes, A., & Budd, L. (1999). Family-centered burn care. *Canadian Nurse, 95*(6), 24–27.

Braunwald, E., & Fauci, A. (2001). *Harrison's principles of internal medicine* (15th ed.). New York: McGraw-Hill.

Bucher, L., & Melander, S. (1999). *Critical Care Nursing.* Philadelphia: Saunders.

Carrougher, G. (1998). *Burn care and therapy.* St. Louis: Mosby.

Davis, S., & Sheely-Adolphson, P. (1997). Psychosocial interventions: Pharmacologic and psychologic modalities. *Nursing Clinics of North America, 32*(2), 331–342.

DeBoer, S. (2001). Pain control for burn victims: Don't be afraid to administer more morphine than is usual. *American Journal of Nursing, 101*(3), 56.

deRios, M., Novac, A., & Achauer, B. (1997). Sexual dysfunction and the patient with burns. *Journal of Burn Care & Rehabilitation, 18*(1, Pt 1), 37–42.

Docking, P. (1999). Trauma. Electrical burn injuries. *Accident & Emergency Nursing, 7*(2), 70–76.

Eakes, G., Burke, M., & Hainsworth, M. (1998). Middle-range theory of chronic sorrow. *Image: Journal of Nursing Scholarship, 30*(2), 179–184.

Fowler, A. (1998). Nursing management of minor burn injuries. *Emergency Nurse, 6*(6), 31–39.

Greenfield, E., & McManus, A. (1997). Infectious complications. . . prevention and strategies for their control. *Nursing Clinics of North America, 32*(2), 297–309.

Hilton, G. (2001). Emergency: Thermal burns. *American Journal of Nursing, 101*(11), 32–34.

Holm, C., Horbrand, F., von Donnersmarck, G., & Muhlbauer, W. (1999). Acute renal failure in severely burned patients. *Burns, 25*(2), 171–178.

Johnson, M., & Maas, M. (1997). *Nursing outcomes classification (NOC).* St. Louis: Mosby.

Kagan, R., & Smith, S. (2000). Evaluation and treatment of thermal injuries. *Dermatology Nursing, 12*(5), 334–335, 338–344, 347–350.

Kee, J. (2001). *Handbook of laboratory and diagnostic tests* (4th ed.). Upper Saddle River, NJ: Prentice Hall.

Kidd, P., & Wagner, K. (2001). *High-acuity nursing* (3rd ed.). Upper Saddle River, NJ: Prentice Hall.

Lim, J., Rehma, S., & Elmore, P. (1998). Rapid response: Care of burn victims. *AAOHN Journal, 46*(4), 169–180.

Mayes, T., Gottschlich, M., & Warden, G. (1997). Clinical nutrition protocols for continuous quality improvements in the outcomes of patients with burns. *Journal of Burn Care & Rehabilitation, 18*(4), 365–368.

McKirdy, L. (2001). Burn wound cleansing. *Journal of Community Nursing, 15*(5), 24, 26–27, 29.

Menzies, V. (2000). Depression and burn wounds. *Archives of Psychiatric Nursing, 14*(4), 199–206.

McCloskey, J., & Bulechek, G. (Eds.). *Nursing interventions classification (NIC)* (3rd ed.). St. Louis: Mosby.

McKenry, L., & Salerno, E. (1998). *Pharmacology in nursing* (20th ed.). St. Louis: Mosby.

Mertens, D., Jenkins, M., & Warden, G. (1997). Outpatient burn management. *Nursing Clinics of North America, 32*(2), 343–374.

Milner, S., Mottar, R., & Smith, C. (2001). The burn wheel. *American Journal of Nursing, 101*(11), 35–37.

North American Nursing Diagnosis Association. (2001). *Nursing diagnoses: Definitions & classification 2001–2002.* Philadelphia: NANDA.

Porth, C. ( 2002). *Pathophysiology: Concepts of altered health states* (6th ed.). Philadelphia: Lippincott.

Richard, R. (1999). Assessment and diagnosis of burn wounds. *Advances in Wound Care, 12*(9), 468–471.

Richard, R. (1999). The physiology of burns. *Nursing Times, 95*(34), 25–31.

Rutan, R. (1998). Physiologic response to cutaneous burn injury. In G. Carrougher, *Burn care and therapy* (pp. 1–33). St. Louis: Mosby.

Tierney, L., McPhee, S., & Papadakis, M. (Eds.). (2001). *Current medical diagnosis & treatment* (40th ed.). Stamford, CT: Appleton & Lange.

Wiebelhaus, P., & Hansen, S. (2001). Another choice for burn victims. *RN, 64*(9), 34–37.

Wiebelhaus, P., & Hansen, S. (2001). What you should know about managing burn emergencies. *Nursing, 31*(1), 36–42.

Wiebelhaus, P., Hansen, S., & Hill, H. (2001). Helping patients survive inhalation injuries. *RN, 64*(10), 28–32.

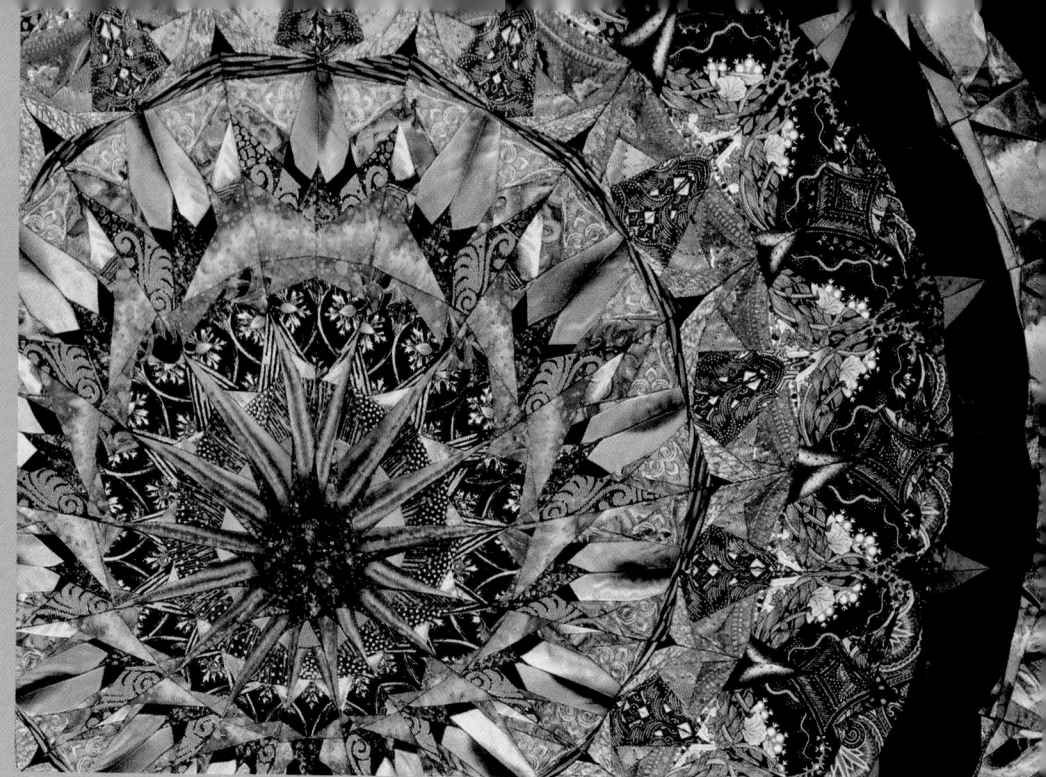

UNIT 4

# RESPONSES TO ALTERED ENDOCRINE FUNCTION

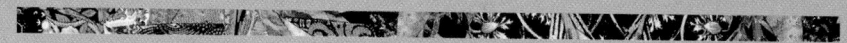

# Assessing Clients with Endocrine Disorders

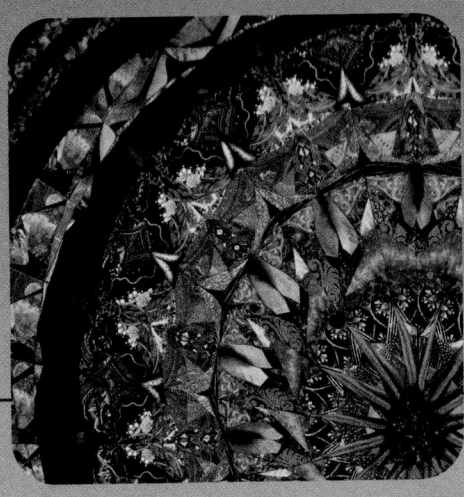

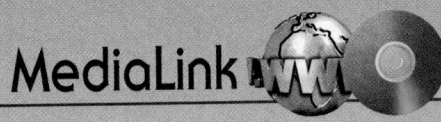

**www.prenhall.com/lemone**
Additional resources for this chapter can be found on the Student CD-ROM accompanying this textbook, and on the Companion Website at www. prenhall.com/lemone. Click on Chapter 16 to select the activities for this chapter.

**CD-ROM**
- Audio Glossary
- NCLEX Review

*Animation*
- Endocrine System

**Companion Website**
- More NCLEX Review
- Functional Health Pattern Assessment
- Case Study
  Endocrine Assessment
- MediaLink Application
  Endocrine Hormones

## LEARNING OUTCOMES

After completing this chapter, you will be able to:

- Review the anatomy and physiology of the endocrine glands.

- Explain the functions of the hormones secreted by the endocrine glands.

- Identify specific topics to consider during a health history interview of the client with health problems involving endocrine function.

- Describe techniques for physical assessment of endocrine structure and function.

- Identify abnormal findings that may indicate malfunction of the endocrine system.

The endocrine system is an essential regulator of the body's internal environment. Through hormones secreted by its glands, the endocrine system regulates such varied functions as growth, reproduction, metabolism, fluid and electrolyte balance, and gender differentiation. It also helps the body adapt to constant alterations in the internal and external environment.

## REVIEW OF ANATOMY AND PHYSIOLOGY

The major endocrine organs are the pituitary gland, thyroid gland, parathyroid glands, adrenal glands, pancreas, and gonads (reproductive glands). The locations of these glands are illustrated in Figure 16–1 ■. Table 16–1 summarizes the role of the endocrine organs and their hormones. Specific information about the gonads is found in Chapters 46 through 49. ◯◯

### Pituitary Gland

The pituitary gland (or *hypophysis*) is located in the skull beneath the hypothalamus of the brain. It often is called the "master gland" because its hormones regulate many body functions. The pituitary gland has two parts: the anterior pituitary (or *adenohypophysis*) and the posterior pituitary (or *neurohypophysis*). The anterior pituitary is glandular tissue, whereas the posterior pituitary is actually an extension of the hypothalamus.

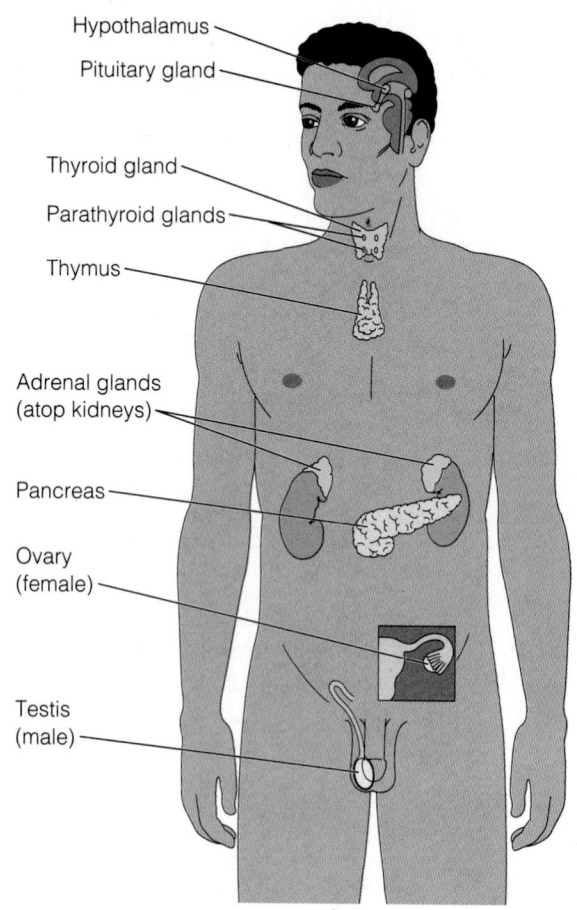

Hypothalamus
Pituitary gland
Thyroid gland
Parathyroid glands
Thymus
Adrenal glands (atop kidneys)
Pancreas
Ovary (female)
Testis (male)

**Figure 16–1** ■ Location of the major endocrine glands.

### Anterior Pituitary

The *anterior pituitary* has several types of endocrine cells and secretes at least six major hormones (Figure 16–2 ■).

- Somatotropic cells secrete growth hormone (GH) also called *somatotropin*. GH stimulates growth of the body by signaling cells to increase protein production and by stimulating the epiphyseal plates of the long bones.
- Lactotropic cells secrete prolactin (PRL). Prolactin stimulates the production of breast milk.
- Thyrotropic cells secrete thyroid-stimulating hormone (TSH). TSH stimulates the synthesis and release of thyroid hormones from the thyroid gland.
- Corticotropic cells secrete adrenocorticotropic hormone (ACTH). ACTH stimulates release of hormones, especially the *glucocorticoids,* from the adrenal cortex.
- Gonadotropic cells secrete the gonadotropin hormones, follicle-stimulating hormone (FSH), and luteinizing hormone (LH). These hormones stimulate the ovaries and testes (the gonads). In women, FSH stimulates the development of ovarian follicles and induces the secretion of estrogenic female sex hormones. In men, FSH is involved in the development and maturation of sperm. In women, increasing levels of LH work together with FSH to lead to ovulation and the formation of the corpus luteum from an ovarian follicle. In men, LH is called interstitial cell–stimulating hormone (ICSH). This hormone stimulates the interstitial cells of the testes to produce male sex hormones.

### Posterior Pituitary

The *posterior pituitary* is made of nervous tissue. Its primary function is to store and release two hormones produced in the hypothalamus:

- Antidiuretic hormone (ADH), also called *vasopressin,* inhibits urine production by causing the renal tubules to reabsorb water from the urine and return it to the circulating blood.
- Oxytocin induces contraction of the smooth muscles in the reproductive organs. In women, oxytocin stimulates the myometrium of the uterus to contract during labor. It also induces milk ejection from the breasts.

### Thyroid Gland

The thyroid gland is anterior to the upper part of the trachea and just inferior to the larynx. This butterfly-shaped gland has two lobes connected by a structure called the *isthmus.*

The glandular tissue consists of follicles filled with a jelly-like colloid substance called thyroglobin, a glycoprotein-iodine complex. Cells within the follicles secrete thyroid hormone (TH), a general name for two similar hormones: *thyroxine* ($T_4$) and *triiodothyronine* ($T_3$). The primary role of thyroid hormones is to increase metabolism; they are also responsible for growth and development in children. TH secretion is initiated by the release of TSH by the pituitary gland and is dependent on an adequate supply of iodine.

The thyroid gland also secretes calcitonin, a hormone that decreases excessive levels of calcium in the blood by slowing the calcium-releasing activity of bone cells.

TABLE 16-1  Organs, Hormones, Functions, and Feedback Mechanisms of the Endocrine System

| Endocrine Organ | Hormone Secreted | Target Organ and Feedback Mechanism |
| --- | --- | --- |
| Thyroid gland | Thyroid hormone (TH): thyroxine ($T_4$) is the major hormone secreted by the thyroid gland. It is converted to triiodothyronine ($T_3$) at the target tissues. | Maintains metabolic rate and growth and development of all tissues. $T_3$ and $T_4$ are secreted in response to thyroid-stimulating hormone (TSH). |
| | Calcitonin | Maintains serum calcium levels by decreasing bone resorption and decreasing resorption of calcium in the kidneys whenever levels of plasma calcium are elevated. |
| Parathyroid gland | Parathyroid hormone (PTH) | Maintains serum calcium levels by stimulating bone resorption and formation and by stimulating kidney resorption of calcium in response to falling levels of plasma calcium. |
| Adrenal cortex | Mineralocorticoids (e.g., aldosterone) | Promote kidney tubule reabsorption of sodium and water and excretion of potassium in response to elevated levels of potassium and low levels of sodium, thereby increasing blood pressure and blood volume. |
| | Glucocorticoids (e.g., cortisol) | Help regulate metabolism of carbohydrates, fats, and proteins. Activate anti-inflammatory responses to stressors. Low cortisol levels stimulate hypothalamic secretion of corticotropin-releasing hormone (CRH), which stimulates the anterior pituitary gland to release ACTH, which in turn stimulates the adrenal cortex to secrete cortisol. |
| | Gonadocorticoids (androgens and small amounts of estrogen and progesterone) | The quantity of sex hormones produced here is small, and the mechanism is not well understood. |
| Adrenal medulla | Catecholamines (epinephrine and norepinephrine) | Stimulate the heart, constrict blood vessels, inhibit visceral muscles, dilate bronchioles, increase respiration and metabolism, promote hyperglycemia. Secreted in response to physical or psychologic stress. |
| Anterior pituitary (adenohypophysis) | Growth hormone (GH) | Promotes growth of body tissues by enhancing protein synthesis and promoting use of fat for energy and thus conserving glucose. Release is stimulated by growth hormone releasing hormone (GHRH) in response to low GH levels, hypoglycemia, increased amino acids, low fatty acids, and stress. |

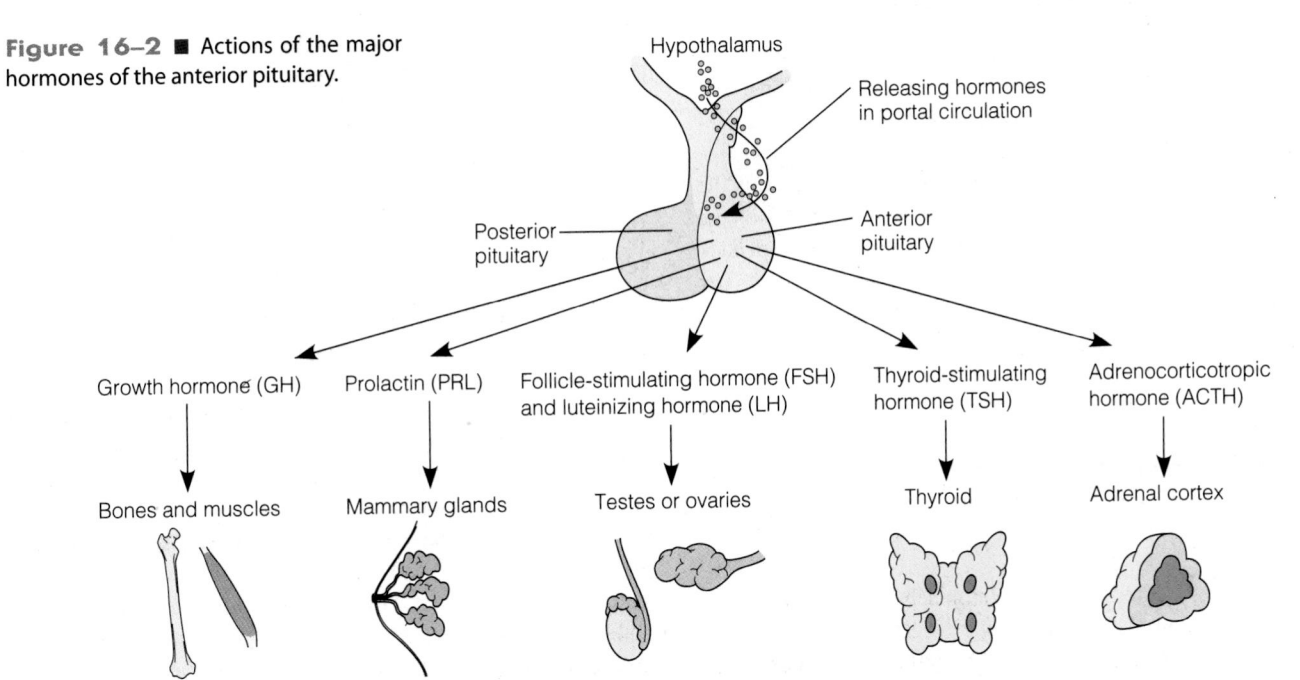

**Figure 16-2** ■ Actions of the major hormones of the anterior pituitary.

## Parathyroid Glands

The parathyroid glands (usually four to six) are embedded on the posterior surface of the lobes of the thyroid gland. They secrete parathyroid hormone (PTH), or *parathormone*. When calcium levels in the plasma fall, PTH secretion increases. PTH also controls phosphate metabolism. It acts primarily by increasing renal excretion of phosphate in the urine, by decreasing the excretion of calcium, and by increasing bone reabsorption to cause the release of calcium from bones. Normal levels of vitamin D are necessary for PTH to exert these effects on bone and kidneys.

## Adrenal Glands

The two adrenal glands are pyramid-shaped organs that sit on top of the kidneys. Each gland consists of two parts, which are distinct organs: an inner medulla and an outer cortex.

### Adrenal Medulla

The adrenal medulla produces two hormones (also called catecholamines): epinephrine (also called *adrenaline*) and norepinephrine (or *noradrenaline*.) These hormones are similar to substances released by the sympathetic nervous system and thus are not essential to life. Epinephrine increases blood glucose levels and stimulates the release of ACTH from the pituitary; ACTH in turn stimulates the adrenal cortex to release glucocorticoids. Epinephrine also increases the rate and force of cardiac contractions; constricts blood vessels in the skin, mucous membranes, and kidneys; and dilates blood vessels in the skeletal muscles, coronary arteries, and pulmonary arteries.

Norepinephrine increases both heart rate and the force of cardiac contractions. It also vasoconstricts blood vessels throughout the body.

### Adrenal Cortex

The adrenal cortex secretes several hormones, all corticosteroids. They are classified into two groups: mineralocorticoids and glucocorticoids. These hormones are essential to life. The release of the mineralocorticoids is controlled primarily by an enzyme called renin. When a decrease in blood pressure or sodium is detected, specialized kidney cells release renin to act on a substance called angiotensinogen, manufactured by the liver. Angiotensinogen is modified by renin and other enzymes to become angiotensin, which stimulates the release of aldosterone from the adrenal cortex. Aldosterone prompts the distal tubules of the kidneys to release increased amounts of water and sodium back into the circulating blood to increase volume and pressure. The glucocorticoids include cortisol and cortisone. These hormones affect carbohydrate metabolism by regulating glucose use in body tissues, mobilizing fatty acids from fatty tissue, and shifting the source of energy for muscle cells from glucose to fatty acids. Glucocorticoids are released in times of stress. An excess of glucocorticoids in the body depresses the inflammatory response and inhibits the effectiveness of the immune system.

## Pancreas

The pancreas, located behind the stomach between the spleen and the duodenum, is both an endocrine gland (producing hormones) and an exocrine gland (producing digestive enzymes).

The endocrine cells of the pancreas produce hormones that regulate carbohydrate metabolism. They are clustered in bodies called pancreatic islets (or islets of Langerhans) scattered throughout the gland. Pancreatic islets have at least four different cell types:

- Alpha cells produce glucagon, which decreases glucose oxidation and promotes an increase in the blood glucose level by signaling the liver to release glucose from glycogen stores.
- Beta cells produce insulin, which facilitates the uptake and use of glucose by cells and prevents an excessive breakdown of glycogen in the liver and muscle. In this way, insulin decreases blood glucose levels. Insulin also facilitates lipid formation, inhibits the breakdown and mobilization of stored fat, and helps amino acids move into cells to promote protein synthesis. In general, the actions of glucagon and insulin oppose one another, helping to maintain a stable blood glucose level.
- Delta cells secrete somatostatin, which inhibits the secretion of glucagon and insulin by the alpha and beta cells.
- F cells secrete pancreatic polypeptide, which is believed to inhibit the exocrine activity of the pancreas.

## Gonads

The gonads are the testes in men and the ovaries in women. These organs are the primary source of steroid sex hormones in the body. The hormones of the gonads are important in regulating body growth and promoting the onset of puberty.

In men, androgens (primarily testosterone) produced by the testes maintain reproductive functioning and secondary sex characteristics. Androgens also promote the production of sperm. In women, the ovaries secrete estrogens and progesterone to maintain reproductive functioning and secondary sex characteristics. Progesterone also promotes the growth of the lining of the uterus to prepare for implantation of a fertilized ovum.

The structure and functions of the gonads are discussed in Chapter 46.

## AN OVERVIEW OF HORMONES

Hormones are chemical messengers secreted by the endocrine organs and transported throughout the body, where they exert their action on specific cells called target cells. Hormones do not cause reactions directly but rather regulate tissue responses. They may produce either generalized or local effects.

Hormones are transported from endocrine gland cells to target cells in the body in one of four ways:

- Endocrine glands release most hormones, including TH, insulin, and others, into the bloodstream. Some require a protein carrier.
- Neurons release some hormones, such as epinephrine, into the bloodstream. This is called the neuroendocrine route.
- The hypothalamus releases its hormones directly to target cells in the posterior pituitary by nerve cell extension.
- With the paracrine method, released messengers diffuse through the interstitial fluid. This method of transport involves a number of hormonal peptides that are released throughout various organs and cells and act locally. An example is endorphins, which act to relieve pain.

Hormones act by binding to specific receptor sites located on the surfaces of the target cells. These receptors recognize a specific hormone and translate the message into a cellular response. The receptor sites are structured so that they respond only to a specific hormone; in other words, receptors in the thyroid gland are responsive to TSH but not to LH.

Hormone levels are controlled by the pituitary gland and by feedback mechanisms. Although most feedback mechanisms are negative, a few are positive. Negative feedback is controlled much as the thermostat in a house regulates temperature. Sensors in the endocrine system detect changes in hormone levels and adjust hormone secretion to maintain normal body levels. When the sensors detect a decrease in hormone levels, they begin actions to cause an increase in hormone levels; when hormone levels rise above normal, the sensors cause a decrease in hormone production and release. For example, when the hypothalamus or anterior pituitary gland senses increased blood levels of TH, it releases hormones causing a reduction in the secretion of TSH, which in turn prompts a decrease in the output of TH by the thyroid gland.

With positive feedback mechanisms, increasing levels of one hormone cause another gland to release a hormone. For example, the increased production of estradiol (a female ovarian hormone) during the follicular stage of the menstrual cycle in turn stimulates increased FSH production by the anterior pituitary gland. Estradiol levels continue to increase until the ovarian follicle disappears, eliminating the source of the stimulation for FSH, which then decreases. Stimuli for hormone release may also be classified as hormonal, humoral, or neural (Figure 16–3 ■). In hormonal release, hypothalamic hormones stimulate the anterior pituitary to release hormones. Fluctuations in the serum level of these hormones in turn prompt other endocrine glands to release hormones. In humoral release, fluctuations in the serum levels of certain ions and nutrients stimulate specific endocrine glands to release hormones to bring these levels back to normal. In neural release, nerve fibers stimulate the release of hormones.

## ASSESSING ENDOCRINE FUNCTION

Function of the endocrine glands is assessed both by a health assessment interview to collect subjective data and a physical assessment to collect objective data. Hormones affect all body tissues and organs, and manifestations of dysfunction are often nonspecific, making assessment of endocrine function often more difficult than assessment of other body systems.

### Health Assessment Interview

A health assessment interview to determine problems with the endocrine system may be part of a health screening or total health assessment, or it may focus on a chief complaint (such as increased urination or changes in energy levels). If the client has a problem with endocrine function, the nurse analyzes its onset, characteristics and course, severity, precipitating and relieving factors, and any associated symptoms, noting the timing and circumstances. For example, the nurse may ask the client:

- Describe the swelling you noticed in the front of your neck. When did it begin? Have you noticed any changes in your energy level?
- When did you first notice that your hands and feet were getting larger?
- Have you noticed that your appetite has increased even though you have lost weight?

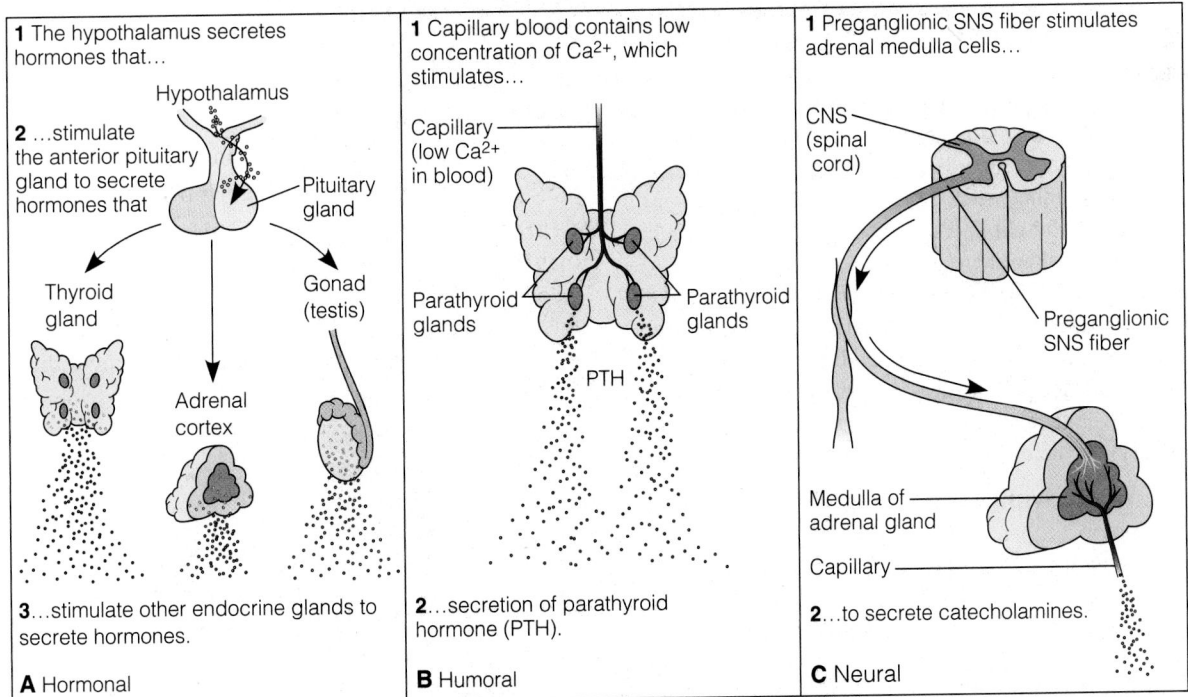

**Figure 16–3** ■ Examples of three mechanisms of hormone release: *A*, hormonal; *B*, humoral; *C*, neural.

The health history includes information about the client's medical history, family history, and social and personal history. Ask the client about any changes in normal growth and development as well as in height and weight. Changes in the size of extremities can often be detected by asking whether the client has had to have rings enlarged or to buy increasingly larger gloves and shoes. Enlargement of the neck may be identified by asking whether the client has difficulty finding shirts or blouses with a collar that fits. Also explore changes including difficulty swallowing; increased or decreased thirst, appetite, and/or urination; visual changes; sleep disturbances; altered patterns of hair distribution (such as increased facial hair in women); changes in menstruation; changes in memory or ability to concentrate; and changes in hair and skin texture. Ask the client about any blow to the head, as well as previous hospitalizations, chemotherapy, radiation (especially to the neck), and the use of medications (especially hormones or steroids).

Because many endocrine disorders have a familial tendency, ask the client about a family history of such diseases as diabetes mellitus, diabetes insipidus, thyroid disorders, hypertension, tumors, autoimmune disorders, and obesity. Ask women about problems with pregnancy, menstruation, and/or menopause.

The nurse also asks about the client's occupational and social history. Include questions about the client's satisfaction with occupation, personal relationships, and lifestyle. Other areas of assessment include the client's usual means of coping; use of alcohol, smoking, or drugs; diet; exercise patterns; and sleep patterns. Although the client may not recognize changes in behavior, family members may be able to provide important information.

## Physical Assessment

Physical assessment of the endocrine system may be performed as part of a total health assessment, or it may be a focused assessment of clients with known or suspected problems with endocrine function.

The only endocrine organ that can be palpated is the thyroid gland; however, other assessments that provide information about endocrine problems include inspection of the skin, hair and nails, facial appearance, reflexes, and musculoskeletal system. Measurement of height and weight as well as vital signs also provides clues to altered endocrine system function.

The client may sit during the examination. A reflex hammer is used to test deep-tendon reflexes. Prior to the examination, the nurse collects the necessary equipment and explains the techniques to the client to decrease anxiety. Additional techniques for assessing hypocalcemic tetany, a complication of endocrine disorders or surgery, are included in the examination sequence.

### Skin Assessments with Abnormal Findings
- Inspect skin color.
  - ✓ Hyperpigmentation may be seen in clients with Addison's disease or Cushing's syndrome.
  - ✓ Hypopigmentation may be seen in diabetes mellitus, hyperthyroidism, or hypothyroidism.
  - ✓ A yellowish cast to the skin might indicate hypothyroidism.
  - ✓ Purple striae over the abdomen and bruising may be present in the client with Cushing's syndrome.

- Palpate the skin, assessing texture, moisture, and the presence of lesions.
  - ✓ Rough, dry skin is often seen in clients with hypothyroidism, whereas smooth and flushed skin can be a sign of hyperthyroidism.
  - ✓ Lesions on the lower extremities might indicate diabetes mellitus.

### Nails and Hair Assessment with Abnormal Findings
- Assess texture and condition of nails and hair.
  - ✓ Increased pigmentation of the nails is often seen in clients with Addison's disease.
  - ✓ Dry, thick, brittle nails and hair may be apparent in hypothyroidism; thin, brittle nails and thin, soft hair may be apparent in hyperthyroidism.
  - ✓ Hirsutism (excessive facial, chest, or abdominal hair) may be seen in Cushing's syndrome.

### Facial Assessments with Abnormal Findings
- Inspect the symmetry and form of the face.
- Inspect position of eyes.
  - ✓ Variations of form and structure may indicate growth abnormalities such as acromegaly.

### Thyroid Gland Assessment with Abnormal Findings
- Palpate the thyroid gland for size and consistency.
  - ✓ Stand behind the client, and place your fingers on either side of the trachea below the thyroid cartilage (Figure 16–4 ■). Ask the client to tilt the head to the right. Now ask the client to swallow. As the client swallows, displace the left lobe while palpating the right lobe. Repeat to palpate the left lobe.
  - ✓ Exophthalmos (protruding eyes) may be seen in hyperthyroidism.
  - ✓ The thyroid may be enlarged in clients with Graves' disease or a goiter.
  - ✓ Multiple nodules may be seen in metabolic disorders, whereas the presence of only one nodule may indicate a cyst or a benign or malignant tumor.
  - ✓ One enlarged nodule suggests malignancy.

### Motor Function Assessment with Abnormal Findings
- Assess the deep-tendon reflexes. See Chapter 40 for guidelines on assessment. ∞
  - ✓ Increased reflexes may be seen in hyperthyroidism; decreased reflexes may be seen in hypothyroidism.

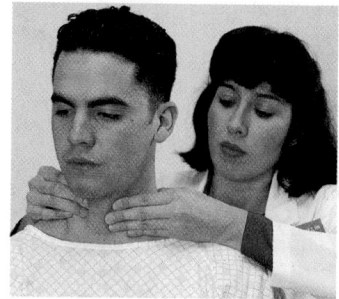

**Figure 16–4** ■ Palpating the thyroid gland from behind the client.

## Sensory Function Assessment with Abnormal Findings

- Test the client's sensitivity to pain, temperature, vibration, light touch, and stereognosis (the ability to identify an object merely by touch). Compare symmetric areas on both sides of the body, and compare the distal to the proximal regions of the extremities.

  Ask the client to close his or her eyes.
  - To test pain, use the blunt and sharp ends of a new safety pin. Discard the pin after use.
  - To test temperature, use cups or other containers of cold and hot water.
  - To test vibration, use a tuning fork over one of the client's finger or toe joints.
  - To test light touch, use a cotton wisp.
  - To test stereognosis, place in the client's hand a simple, familiar object, such as a rubber band, cotton ball, or button. Ask the client to identify the object.

✓ Peripheral neuropathy and paresthesias (altered sensations) may occur in diabetes, hypothyroidism, or acromegaly.

## Musculoskeletal Assessment with Abnormal Findings

- Inspect the size and proportions of the client's body structure.
  - ✓ Extremely short stature may indicate dwarfism, which is caused by insufficient growth hormone.
  - ✓ Extremely large bones may indicate acromegaly, which is caused by excessive growth hormone.

## Assessing for Hypocalcemic Tetany

- Assess for **Trousseau's sign:** Inflate pressure cuff above antecubital space to occlude blood supply to the arm.
  - ✓ Decreased calcium levels cause the client's hand and fingers to contract (*carpal spasm*).
- Assess for **Chvostek's sign:** Tap your finger in front of the client's ear at the angle of the jaw.
  - ✓ Decreased calcium levels cause the client's lateral facial muscles to contract.

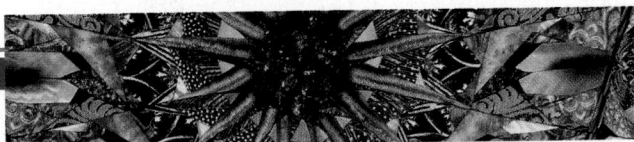

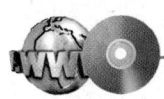

## EXPLORE MediaLink

NCLEX review questions, case studies, care plan activities, MediaLink applications, and other interactive resources for this chapter can be found on the Companion Website at www.prenhall.com/lemone.

Click on Chapter 16 to select the activities for this chapter. For animations, video clips, more NCLEX review questions, and an audio glossary, access the Student CD-ROM accompanying this textbook.

## TEST YOURSELF

1. Antidiuretic hormone (ADH) is produced by which endocrine gland?
   a. Pancreas
   b. Adrenals
   c. Thyroid
   d. Pituitary
2. Excessive amounts of glucocorticoids, produced by the adrenal cortex, result in what pathophysiologic health problem?
   a. Inhibited immune response
   b. Increased response to glucagon
   c. Delayed onset of puberty
   d. Decreased metabolic rate
3. When conducting a health history focused on the endocrine system, which of the following questions should be included?
   a. "When did you first notice the pain in your abdomen?"
   b. "Do your children have problems with urination?"
   c. "Are your menstrual periods regular?"
   d. "How did you get this scar on your leg?"
4. What assessments are made when palpating the thyroid gland?
   a. Edema and movement
   b. Size and consistency
   c. Character and texture
   d. Pain and pulse rate
5. Decreased calcium levels can be assessed with Chvostek's sign. To conduct this assessment, the nurse:
   a. Inflates a blood pressure cuff above the antecubital space
   b. Taps the finger in front of the client's ear
   c. Depresses the skin over the shin
   d. Pinches a fold of skin over the sternum

See Test Yourself answers in Appendix C.

## BIBLIOGRAPHY

Andresen, G. (1998). Assessing the older patient. *RN, 61*(3), 46–56.

Loriaux, T. (1996). Endocrine assessment: Red flags for those on the front line. *Nursing Clinics of North America, 31*(4), 695–713.

Rusterholtz, A. (1996). Interpretation of diagnostic laboratory tests in selected endocrine disorders. *Nursing Clinics of North America, 31*(4), 715–724.

Watson, R. (2001). Assessing endocrine system function in older people. *Nursing Older People, 12*(9), 27–28.

Weber, J., & Kelley, J. (2002). *Health assessment in nursing* (2nd ed.). Philadelphia: Lippincott-Raven.

Wilson, S., & Giddens, J. (2001). *Health assessment for nursing practice.* St. Louis: Mosby.

Winger, J., & Hornick, T. (1996). Age-associated changes in the endocrine system. *Nursing Clinics of North America, 31*(4), 827–844.

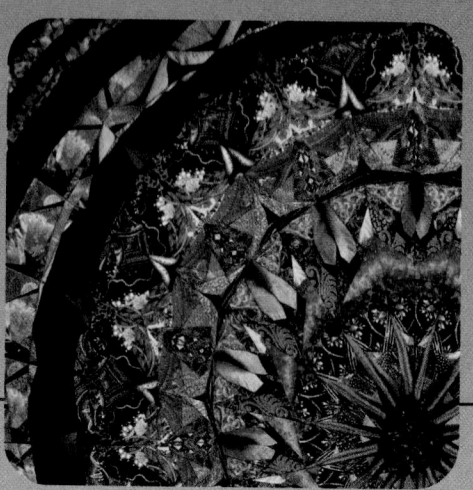

# CHAPTER 17

# Nursing Care of Clients with Endocrine Disorders

## MediaLink

**www.prenhall.com/lemone**

Additional resources for this chapter can be found on the Student CD-ROM accompanying this textbook, and on the Companion Website at www.prenhall.com/lemone. Click on Chapter 17 to select the activities for this chapter.

**CD-ROM**
- Audio Glossary
- NCLEX Review

**Companion Website**
- More NCLEX Review
- Case Study
  Hyperthyroidism
- Care Plan Activity
  Cushing's Syndrome
- MediaLink Application
  Exophthalmos

## LEARNING OUTCOMES

After completing this chapter, you will be able to:

- Apply knowledge of normal anatomy, physiology, and assessments of the thyroid, parathyroid, adrenal, and pituitary glands when providing nursing care for clients with endocrine disorders (see Chapter 16).

- Identify diagnostic tests used to diagnose disorders of the thyroid, parathyroid, adrenal, and pituitary glands.

- Compare and contrast the manifestations of disorders that result from hyperfunction and hypofunction of the thyroid, parathyroid, adrenal, and pituitary glands.

- Explain the nursing implications for medications prescribed to treat disorders of the thyroid and adrenal glands.

- Provide appropriate nursing care for the client before and after a subtotal thyroidectomy and an adrenalectomy.

- Use the nursing process as a framework for providing individualized care to clients with disorders of the thyroid, parathyroid, adrenal, and pituitary glands.

The thyroid, parathyroid, adrenal, and pituitary glands are part of the endocrine system. Disorders of the structure and function of these glands alter normal hormone levels and the way body tissues use those hormones. When hormone production increases or decreases, people experience alterations in health.

Clients with disorders of the glands discussed in this chapter require nursing care for multiple problems. They often face exhausting diagnostic tests, changes in physical appearance and emotional responses, and permanent alterations in lifestyle. Nursing care is directed toward meeting physiologic needs, providing education, and ensuring psychologic support for the client and family. A holistic approach to the complex needs of clients with these endocrine disorders is an essential component of nursing care.

## DISORDERS OF THE THYROID GLAND

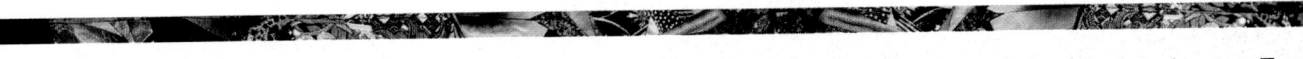

Altered thyroid hormone (TH) production or use affects all major organ systems. In the adult, TH changes primarily affect metabolism, cardiovascular function, gastrointestinal function, and neuromuscular function. Thyroid disorders—both hyperthyroidism and hypothyroidism—are among the most common endocrine disorders.

## THE CLIENT WITH HYPERTHYROIDISM

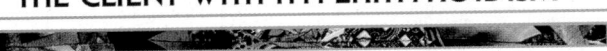

**Hyperthyroidism** (also called **thyrotoxicosis**) is a disorder caused by excessive delivery of TH to the peripheral tissues. Because the primary effect of TH is to increase metabolism and protein synthesis, hyperthyroidism affects all major organ systems of the body. The increase in metabolic rate and the alterations in cardiac output, peripheral blood flow, oxygen consumption, and body temperature are similar to those found in increased sympathetic nervous system activity (Porth, 2002).

The effects of hyperthyroidism are the result of increased circulating levels of TH. This hormonal excess increases the metabolic rate and heightens the sympathetic nervous system's physiologic response to stimulation. The sensitizing effect of abnormally elevated TH levels increases the cardiac rate and stroke volume. As a result, cardiac output and peripheral blood flow increase. Elevated TH levels also increase carbohydrate, protein, and lipid metabolism. Lipids are depleted, and glucose tolerance decreases. Protein degradation increases, resulting in a negative nitrogen balance. Over time, the hypermetabolic effects of excess TH result in caloric and nutritional deficiencies.

## PATHOPHYSIOLOGY AND MANIFESTATIONS

Hyperthyroidism results from many different factors, including autoimmune reactions (as in Graves' disease), excess secretion of thyroid-stimulating hormone (TSH) by the pituitary gland, thyroiditis, neoplasms (such as toxic multinodular goiter), and an excessive intake of thyroid medications. The most common etiologies of hyperthyroidism are Graves' disease and toxic multinodular goiter.

The client with hyperthyroidism typically has an increased appetite, yet loses weight and may have hypermotile bowels and diarrhea. Additional manifestations related to hypermetabolism include heat intolerance and increased sweating. The client's hair is fine, and the skin is smooth and warm. Emotional lability is common. The *Multisystem Effects of Hyperthyroidism* are shown on page 446.

### Graves' Disease

**Graves' disease,** the most common cause of hyperthyroidism, is an autoimmune disorder. The serum of more than 90% of clients with Graves' disease contains TSH-R (stim) Ab, an antibody directed against the TSH receptor site in the thyroid follicles (Tierney et al., 2001). When this antibody binds to the TSH receptors, it stimulates hormone synthesis and secretion. The cause is unknown, but there is a hereditary link. Other factors associated with Graves' disease include an immune response against a viral antigen, a defect of the lymphocyte T helper cells, and the presence of other autoimmune disorders (such as myasthenia gravis and pernicious anemia) (Porth, 2002).

Graves' disease is seen 5 times more often in women than in men and occurs most frequently between the ages of 20 and 40. It is seen worldwide, with the incidence often correlated with the amount of iodine in the diet. Increased iodine intake (such as from radiocontrast dyes used in diagnostic tests or from ingestion of kelp tablets) has been associated with an increased frequency of hyperthyroidism.

Clients with Graves' disease have an enlarged thyroid gland (**goiter**) and manifestations of hyperthyroidism (as illustrated in Table 17–1). The hypertrophy of the gland can result from excess TSH stimulation (when the amount of circulating TH is deficient), growth-stimulating immunoglobulins, or substances that inhibit TH synthesis. A goiter may be present in hyperthyroidism or hypothyroidism.

| TABLE 17–1 Laboratory Findings in Hyperthyroidism | | |
|---|---|---|
| **Test** | **Normal Values** | **Findings** |
| Serum TA | Negative to 1:20 | Increased |
| Serum TSH (Sensitive assay) | >1.0 mµ/L | Decreased in primary hyperthyroidism |
| Serum T₄ | 5 to 12 mµ/dL | Increased |
| Serum T₃ | 80 to 200 ng/dL | Increased |
| T₃ uptake (T₃RU) | 25 to 35 relative percentage | Increased |
| Thyroid suppression | | Increased RAI uptake and T₄ levels |

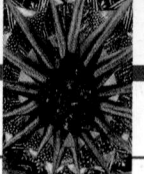

# Multisystem Effects of Hyperthyroidism

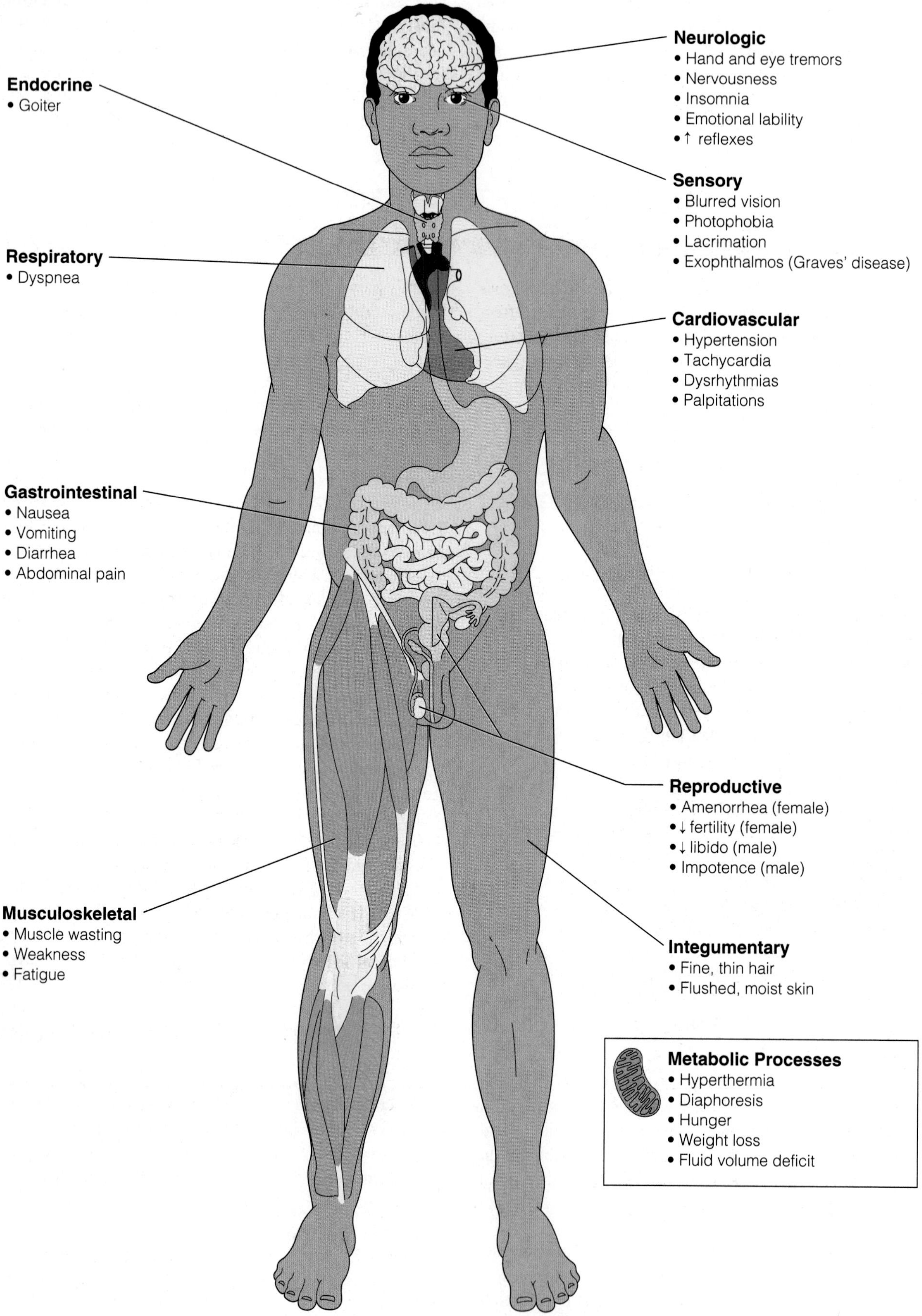

**Endocrine**
• Goiter

**Respiratory**
• Dyspnea

**Gastrointestinal**
• Nausea
• Vomiting
• Diarrhea
• Abdominal pain

**Musculoskeletal**
• Muscle wasting
• Weakness
• Fatigue

**Neurologic**
• Hand and eye tremors
• Nervousness
• Insomnia
• Emotional lability
• ↑ reflexes

**Sensory**
• Blurred vision
• Photophobia
• Lacrimation
• Exophthalmos (Graves' disease)

**Cardiovascular**
• Hypertension
• Tachycardia
• Dysrhythmias
• Palpitations

**Reproductive**
• Amenorrhea (female)
• ↓ fertility (female)
• ↓ libido (male)
• Impotence (male)

**Integumentary**
• Fine, thin hair
• Flushed, moist skin

**Metabolic Processes**
• Hyperthermia
• Diaphoresis
• Hunger
• Weight loss
• Fluid volume deficit

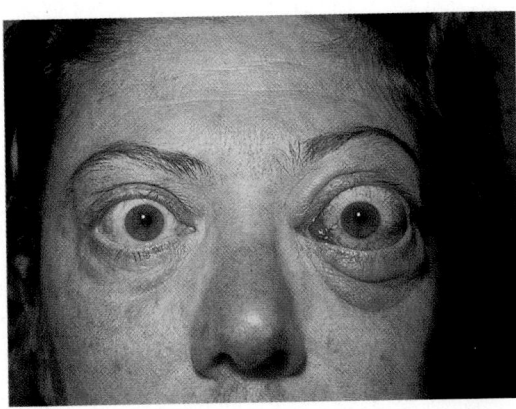

**Figure 17–1** ■ Exophthalmos in a client with Graves' disease. The disease causes edema of fat deposits behind the eyes and inflammation of the extraocular muscles. The accumulating pressure forces the eyes outward from their orbits.

*Source: University of Illinois, Custom Medical Stock Photo, Inc.*

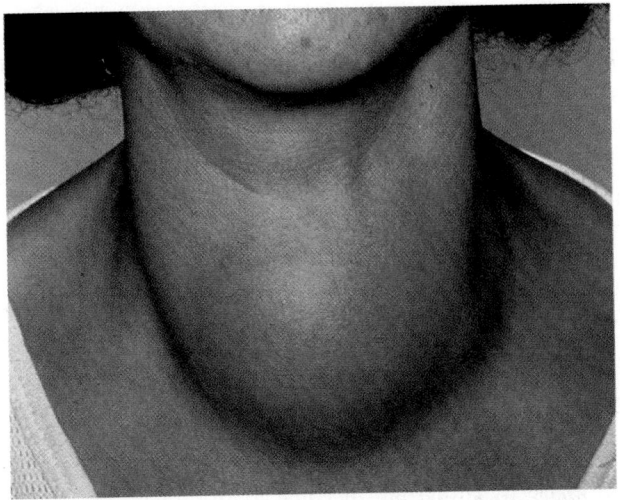

**Figure 17–2** ■ Toxic multinodular goiter. The formation and growth of numerous nodules in the thyroid gland cause the characteristic massive enlargement of the neck.

*Source: Custom Medical Stock Photo, Inc.*

**Proptosis** (forward displacement) of the eye occurs in about one-third of cases (Porth, 2002). The forward protrusion of the eyeballs (also called **exophthalmos**) results from an accumulation of fat deposits and inflammation by-products in the retro-orbital tissues. Often the sclera is visible above the iris. The upper lids are often retracted, and the person has a characteristic unblinking stare (Figure 17–1 ■). Proptosis is usually bilateral, but it may involve only one eye. The client may experience blurred vision, diplopia, eye pain, lacrimation, and photophobia. The inability to close the eyelids completely over the protruding eyeballs increases the risk of corneal dryness, irritation, infection, and ulceration. The treatment of Graves' disease does not reverse these changes in the eyes.

Other manifestations include fatigue, difficulty sleeping, hand tremors, and changes in menstruation ranging from decreased flow to amenorrhea. Older clients may present with atrial fibrillation, angina, or congestive heart failure.

### Toxic Multinodular Goiter

**Toxic multinodular goiter** (Figure 17–2 ■) is characterized by small, discrete, independently functioning nodules in the thyroid gland tissue that secrete excessive amounts of TH. It is not known how these nodules grow or become independent, but a genetic mutation of follicle cells is suspected. Elevated TH levels result in manifestations of hyperthyroidism; however, they are slower to develop and differ somewhat from those of Graves' disease. The client with this type of hyperthyroidism is usually a woman in her 60s or 70s who has had a goiter for a number of years.

### Excess TSH Stimulation

Overproduction of TSH by the pituitary usually stimulates the thyroid gland to produce excess TH. The elevation in TSH secretion often results from a pituitary adenoma. This secondary form of hyperthyroidism is rare.

### Thyroiditis

**Thyroiditis** (inflammation of the thyroid gland) is most often the result of a viral infection of the thyroid gland. The symptoms of thyroiditis are those of acute inflammation and the effects of increased TH. Thyroiditis is an acute disorder that may become chronic, resulting in a hypothyroid state as repeated infections destroy gland tissue. See the discussion of Hashimoto's thyroiditis later in this chapter.

### Thyroid Crisis

**Thyroid crisis** (also called **thyroid storm**) is an extreme state of hyperthyroidism that is rare today because of improved diagnosis and treatment methods (Porth, 2002). When it does occur, those affected are usually people with untreated hyperthyroidism (most often Graves' disease) and people with hyperthyroidism who have experienced a stressor, such as an infection, trauma, untreated diabetic ketoacidosis, or manipulation of the thyroid gland during surgery. Thyroid crisis is a life-threatening condition.

The rapid increase in metabolic rate that results from the excessive TH causes the manifestations of thyroid crisis. The manifestations include hyperthermia, with body temperatures ranging from 102°F (39°C) to 106°F (41°C); tachycardia; systolic hypertension; and gastrointestinal symptoms (abdominal pain, vomiting, diarrhea). Agitation, restlessness, and tremors are common, progressing to confusion, psychosis, delirium, and seizures. The mortality rate is high. Rapid treatment of thyroid crisis is essential to preserve life. Treatment includes relieving respiratory distress, stabilizing cardiovascular function, and reducing TH synthesis and secretion.

## COLLABORATIVE CARE

Treatment of hyperthyroidism focuses on reducing the production of TH by the thyroid gland, thus establishing a **euthyroid** (normal thyroid) state, and preventing or treating complications. Depending on the client's age and physical status, either medications, radioactive iodine therapy, or surgery may be used.

## Diagnostic Tests

Hyperthyroidism is diagnosed according to the manifestations of the specific disorders causing excessive TH, and by diagnostic test results. Elevated levels of TH (both $T_3$ and $T_4$) and increased radioactive iodine (RAI) uptake are diagnostic criteria of hyperthyroidism. Laboratory findings in hyperthyroidism are shown in Table 17–1.

The following diagnostic tests may be ordered:

- *TA test.* Serum thyroid antibodies (TA) are measured to determine whether a thyroid autoimmune disease is causing the client's symptoms. TA is elevated in Graves' disease.
- *TSH test (sensitive assay).* Serum TSH levels are measured and compared with thyroxine ($T_4$) levels to differentiate pituitary from thyroid dysfunction. The best indicator of primary hyperthyroidism (such as in Graves' disease) is suppression of TSH below 0.1 µg/mL. When the sensitive TSH is not suppressed, the hyperthyroidism is caused by a TSH-secreting pituitary tumor.
- *$T_4$ test.* Serum thyroxine ($T_4$) levels are measured to determine TH concentration and to test thyroid gland function. $T_4$ levels are elevated in hyperthyroidism and in acute thyroiditis.
- *$T_3$ test.* Serum triiodothyronine ($T_3$) is measured by radioimmunoassay ($T_3$RIA), which measures bound and free forms of this hormone. This test is effective for the diagnosis of hyperthyroidism. $T_3$ levels may also be elevated in thyroiditis.
- *$T_3$ uptake test.* $T_3$ uptake ($T_3$RU) is measured by an in vitro test in which the client's blood is mixed with radioactive $T_3$; the results are elevated in hyperthyroidism.

- *RAI uptake test.* A radioactive iodine (RAI) uptake test (thyroid scan) measures the absorption of $^{131}I$ or $^{123}I$ by the thyroid gland. A calculated dose of radioactive iodine is given orally or intravenously, and the thyroid is then scanned (often after 24 hours). The distribution of radioactivity in the gland is recorded (increased uptake of radioactive iodine is seen in Graves' disease). In addition, the scan reveals the size and shape of the gland.
- *Thyroid suppression test.* RAI and $T_4$ levels are measured first. The client then takes TH for 7 to 10 days, after which the tests are repeated. Failure of hormone therapy to suppress RAI and $T_4$ indicates hyperthyroidism.

## Medications

Hyperthyroidism is treated by administering antithyroid medications that reduce TH production. Because these drugs do not affect the release or activity of hormone that is already formed, therapeutic effects may not be seen for several weeks. Some commonly prescribed drugs, their actions, and nursing implications are shown in the Medication Administration box below.

## Radioactive Iodine Therapy

Because the thyroid gland takes up iodine in any form, radioactive iodine ($^{131}I$) concentrates in the thyroid gland and damages or destroys thyroid cells so that they produce less TH. Radioactive iodine is given orally. Results typically occur in 6 to 8 weeks. In most instances, the client is not hospitalized during treatment and does not require radiation precautions. This type of therapy is contraindicated in pregnant women

## Medication Administration

### Hyperthyroidism

#### IODINE SOURCES

Potassium iodide (SSKI, Thyro-Block)
Potassium iodide (Pima)

Large doses of iodine inhibit TH synthesis and release. Iodine also makes the hyperplastic thyroid less vascular prior to surgery and hastens the ability of other antithyroid drugs to reduce natural hormone output.

#### Nursing Responsibilities

- Assess for hypersensitivity to iodine before giving medication; for example, ask client about allergies to shellfish.
- Dilute liquid iodine sources in water or orange juice to disguise bitter taste.
- Monitor for increased bleeding tendencies if the client is also taking anticoagulants; iodine increases their effect.

#### Client and Family Teaching

- The maximum effect of iodine in large doses usually occurs in 1 to 2 weeks.
- Long-term iodine therapy is not effective in controlling hyperthyroidism.

#### ANTITHYROID DRUGS

Methimazole (Tapazole)
Propylthiouracil (PTU, Propyl-Thracil)

Antithyroid drugs inhibit TH production. They do not affect already formed hormones; thus, several weeks may elapse before the client experiences therapeutic effects.

#### Nursing Responsibilities

- Monitor for side effects: pruritus, rash, elevated temperature, (for iodides) swelling of the eyelids, anorexia, loss of taste, changes in menstruation.
- Administer drugs at the same time each day to maintain stable blood levels.
- Monitor for symptoms of hypothyroidism: fatigue, weight gain.

#### Client and Family Teaching

- Watch for unusual bleeding, nausea, loss of taste, or epigastric pain. Report any such symptoms to the physician.
- If you are also taking anticoagulants, report any signs of bleeding.
- If you are taking lithium, be aware of symptoms of hypothyroidism.
- It may take up to 12 weeks before you experience the full effects of the drugs. Take the medication regularly and exactly as prescribed.

because radioactive iodine crosses the placenta and can have negative effects on the developing fetal thyroid gland. Because the amount of gland destroyed is not readily controllable, the client may become hypothyroid and require lifelong TH replacement.

## Surgery

Some hyperthyroid clients have such enlarged thyroid glands that pressure on the esophagus or trachea causes breathing or swallowing problems. In these cases, removal of all or part of the gland is indicated. A *subtotal thyroidectomy* is usually performed. This procedure leaves enough of the gland in place to produce an adequate amount of TH. A total **thyroidectomy** is performed to treat cancer of the thyroid; the client then requires lifelong hormone replacement.

Before surgery, the client should be in as nearly a euthyroid state as possible. The client may be given antithyroid drugs to reduce hormone levels and iodine preparations to decrease the vascularity and size of the gland (which also reduces the risk of hemorrhage during and after surgery). Nursing care of the client having a subtotal thyroidectomy is discussed in the box below.

## NURSING CARE

### Health Promotion

Although hyperthyroidism is not preventable, it is important to teach clients the importance of regular health care provider visits and medication intake.

### Assessment

The following data are collected through the health history and physical examination (see Chapter 16). ⊝ Further focused assessments are described with nursing interventions.

- *Health history:* other diseases, family history of thyroid disease, when symptoms began, severity of symptoms, intake of thyroid medications, menstrual history, changes in weight, bowel elimination
- *Physical assessment:* muscle strength, tremors, vital signs, cardiovascular and peripheral vascular systems, integument, size of thyroid, presence of bruit over thyroid, eyes and vision

## NURSING CARE OF THE CLIENT HAVING A SUBTOTAL THYROIDECTOMY

### PREOPERATIVE CARE

- Administer ordered antithyroid medications and iodine preparations, and monitor their effects. *Antithyroid drugs are given before surgery to promote a euthyroid state. Iodine preparations are given to the client before surgery to decrease vascularity of the gland, thereby decreasing the risk of hemorrhage.*
- Teach the client to support the neck by placing both hands behind the neck when sitting up in bed, while moving about, and while coughing. *Placing the hands behind the neck provides support for the suture line.*
- Answer questions, and allow time for the client to verbalize concerns. *Because the incision is made at the base of the throat, clients (especially women) are often concerned about their appearance after surgery. Explain that the scar will eventually be only a thin line and that jewelry or scarves may be used to cover the scar.*

### POSTOPERATIVE CARE

- Provide comfort measures: Administer analgesic pain medications as ordered, and monitor their effectiveness; place the client in a semi-Fowler's position after recovery from anesthesia; support head and neck with pillows. *Analgesic medications reduce the perception of pain and reduce physical stress during the postoperative period. Positioning the client in a semi-Fowler's position and supporting the head and neck decrease strain on the suture line.*
- Perform focused assessments to monitor for complications:
  a. *Hemorrhage.* Assess dressing (if present) and the area under the client's neck and shoulders for drainage. Monitor blood pressure and pulse for symptoms of hypovolemic shock. Assess tightness of dressing (if present). *The vascularity of the gland increases the risk of hemorrhage. The location of the incision and the position of the client may cause the drainage to run back and under the client. The danger of hemorrhage is greatest in the first 12 to 24 hours after surgery.*
  b. *Respiratory distress.* Assess respiratory rate, rhythm, depth, and effort. Maintain humidification as ordered. Assist the client with coughing and deep breathing. Have suction equipment, oxygen, and a tracheostomy set available for immediate use. *Respiratory distress may result from hemorrhage and edema, which may compress the trachea; from tetany and laryngeal spasms resulting from decreased hormones due to removal or damage to the parathyroid glands; and from damage to the laryngeal nerve, causing spasms of the vocal cords. Equipment must be immediately available if the client experiences respiratory distress that requires interventions and treatment.*
  c. *Laryngeal nerve damage.* Assess for the ability to speak aloud, noting quality and tone of voice. *The location of the laryngeal nerve increases the risk of damage during thyroid surgery. Although hoarseness may be due to edema or the endotracheal tube used during surgery and will subside, permanent hoarseness or loss of vocal volume is a potential danger.*
  d. *Tetany.* Assess for signs of calcium deficiency, including tingling of toes, fingers, and lips; muscular twitches; positive Chvostek's and Trousseau's signs; and decreased serum calcium levels. Keep calcium gluconate or calcium chloride available for immediate intravenous use, if necessary. *The parathyroid glands are located in and near the thyroid gland; surgery of the thyroid gland may injure or remove parathyroid glands, resulting in hypocalcemia and tetany. Tetany may occur in 1 to 7 days after thyroidectomy.*

## Nursing Diagnoses and Interventions

In planning and implementing nursing care for the client with hyperthyroidism, the nurse considers the client's responses to the systemic effects of the disorder. Although each client may have different needs, nursing diagnoses discussed in this section focus on the most common problems: cardiovascular problems, visual deficits, altered nutrition, and body image disturbance.

### Risk for Decreased Cardiac Output

The client with hyperthyroidism is at risk for alterations in cardiac output. Excess TH directly affects the heart, resulting in increased rate and stroke volume. Increases in the metabolic demands and oxygen requirements of peripheral tissues increase the demands on the heart, and systolic hypertension, angina, arrhythmias, or cardiac failure may occur. The client often has palpitations and shortness of breath and is easily fatigued. The risk of complications is greater in clients with pre-existing cardiovascular disorders.

- Monitor blood pressure, pulse rate and rhythm, respiratory rate, and breath sounds. Assess for peripheral edema, jugular vein distention, and increased activity intolerance. *Increased TH increases cardiac rate, stroke volume, and tissue demand for oxygen, causing stress on the heart. This may result in hypertension, arrhythmias, tachycardia, and congestive heart failure.*
- Suggest keeping the environment as cool and free of distraction as possible. Decrease stress by explaining interventions and teaching relaxation procedures. *A physically comfortable and psychologically calm environment can reduce stimuli and stressors. Stress increases circulating catecholamines, which further increase cardiac workload.*
- Encourage the client to balance activity with rest periods. *Rest periods decrease energy expenditure and tissue requirements for oxygen, decreasing demands on the heart by decreasing cardiac workload.*

### Disturbed Sensory Perception: Visual

Visual changes that occur in clients with hyperthyroidism include difficulty in focusing, diplopia (double vision), or visual loss. If the client is unable to close the eyelids because of exophthalmos, the risk of corneal dryness with resultant infection or injury increases. Visual deficits may also result from pressure on the optic nerve from retro-orbital edema and the shortening of eye muscles. Although treatment of hyperthyroidism may stop the progression of eye changes, not all symptoms are reversible.

- Monitor visual acuity, photophobia, integrity of the cornea, and lid closure. *The cornea is at risk for dryness, injury, conjunctivitis, and corneal infections. Injury and infection of the cornea can result in further loss of visual acuity.*
- Teach measures for protecting the eye from injury and maintaining visual acuity:
  - Use tinted glasses or shields as protection.
  - Use artificial tears to moisten the eyes.
  - Use cool, moist compresses to relieve irritation.
  - Promptly report any pain or changes in vision.

**PRACTICE ALERT** *Teach the client to cover or tape the eyelids shut at night if they do not close and to sleep with the head of the bed elevated.* ■

*The measures outlined decrease the risk of injury, provide comfort, decrease periorbital edema that can further compromise vision, and ensure immediate care for problems, thereby minimizing the risk of further visual loss.*

### Imbalanced Nutrition: Less Than Body Requirements

The hypermetabolic state that occurs in hyperthyroidism causes gastrointestinal hypermotility, with nausea, vomiting, diarrhea, and abdominal pain. Although the client may have an increased appetite and eat more than usual, weight loss continues.

- Ask the client to weigh daily (at the same time each day), and keep a record of results. *The inability to meet metabolic demands results in loss of body weight. Regular monitoring detects continued weight loss.*
- In collaboration with a dietitian, teach the client the need for a diet high in carbohydrates and protein and including between-meal snacks. Six small meals a day may be more desirable than three large meals. Caloric intake may need to be increased to 4000 kcal per day if weight loss exceeds 10% to 17% for height and frame. *Increased nutrients as part of a well-balanced diet are necessary to meet metabolic demands. Clients are often better able to increase food intake by eating frequent, small meals. A 1-lb weight gain requires approximately 3500 extra kcal.*
- Monitor nutritional status through results of laboratory data. Serum albumin, transferrin, and total lymphocyte counts are commonly lower than normal in nutritional deficits. *A negative nitrogen balance signifies a catabolic state in which protein is lost and metabolic demands are not being met.*

### Disturbed Body Image

Physical changes common in hyperthyroidism include exophthalmos, goiter, tremors, hair loss, increased perspiration, loss of strength, fatigue (see the Nursing Research box on page 451), weight loss, and changes in reproductive and sexual function (amenorrhea in women, impotence in men, and increased libido in both men and women). In addition, the client often has mood changes and insomnia and is constantly nervous and anxious. There may even be periods of psychosis. These changes are frightening not only for the client but also for family members.

- Establish a trusting relationship; encourage the client to verbalize feelings about self and to ask questions about the illness and treatment. Provide reliable information, and clarify misconceptions. *Establishing trust facilitates open sharing of feelings and perceptions.*

MediaLink | ENDOCRINE DISORDER RESOURCES

## Nursing Research

### Evidence-Based Practice for Fatigue

This analysis of fatigue (Tiesinga et al., 1996) was conducted to document how it is defined in the literature, and to distinguish dimensions and identify indicators. As defined in this analysis, fatigue is a nonspecific manifestation, often related to different chronic illnesses and their treatments. Fatigue has physical, psychological, and social dimensions.

### IMPLICATIONS FOR NURSING

Although nurses both experience fatigue and assess fatigue in clients, little research has been conducted to clearly define and interpret the experience of fatigue. This is important, as the experience of fatigue may well be very different in the client with hyperthyroidism than in the client with fatigue-related radiation treatments. Continued research and the development of accurate assessment tools will increase the knowledge base necessary to holistic, individualized clinical practice.

### Critical Thinking in Client Care

1. What specific pathophysiologic processes in clients with hyperthyroidism or hypothyroidism increase the risk of fatigue?
2. What defining characteristics of the nursing diagnosis *Fatigue* would make implementation of a teaching plan more difficult? How could you adapt your teaching to ensure client and family knowledge?
3. How could fatigue interfere with following a therapeutic regimen that is prescribed? Could fatigue be a major factor when the client is said to be noncompliant? Why or why not?

## Home Care

Clients with hyperthyroidism primarily provide self-care at home. Teaching is individualized to meet the client's needs. Address the following topics:

- The client taking oral medications must understand the need for lifelong treatment.
- The client who has a thyroidectomy requires information about postoperative wound care.
- The client having radioactive iodine therapy needs to know the symptoms of hypothyroidism.
- Depending on the age of the client and the support systems available, referral to community health care agencies may be necessary.
- In addition, suggest the following resources:
  - American Thyroid Association
  - Thyroid Foundation of Canada
  - Endocrine Society

## Nursing Care Plan
### A Client with Graves' Disease

Mrs. Juanita Manuel is a 33-year-old mother of four small children. She is a second-year student at the local community college, within one semester of completing the requirements for an associate degree in child care. For the past 3 months, Juanita has been constantly hungry and has eaten more than usual, but she has still lost 15 lb (6.8 kg). She has repeated bouts of diarrhea and often feels nauseated. Her hands shake, she can feel her heart beating rapidly, and she finds herself laughing or crying for no apparent reason.

Mrs. Manuel makes an appointment with her family physician. The nurse at the office completes a health history and physical assessment. When asked how she has been feeling, Mrs. Manuel replies, "Well, I don't know what's wrong with me—but I keep losing weight and I cry at the drop of a hat. I am also just so hot all the time, and I've never had that problem before. I hope I find out what's wrong and it's nothing serious."

### ASSESSMENT

The health history indicates that although her appetite has increased, Mrs. Manuel has lost 15 lb (6.8 kg). She states that she has had diarrhea, nausea, palpitations, heat intolerance, and mood changes. Physical assessment findings include the following: T 101°F (38.3°C), P 110, R 24, and BP 162/86. Her skin is moist and warm, her hair thin and fine. She has visible tremors in her hands. Her eyeballs protrude, and she is unable to close her eyelids completely. Her thyroid is enlarged and palpable. Diagnostic tests reveal the following abnormal results: $T_3$, 350 g/dL (normal range: 80 to 200 ng/dL), $T_4$, 15.1 mg/dL (normal range: 5 to 12 mg/dL). A thyroid scan demonstrates an enlarged thyroid with increased iodine uptake. After the medical diagnosis of Graves' disease is made, Mrs. Manuel is started on the antithyroid medication propylthiouracil, 150 mg orally every 8 hours.

### DIAGNOSIS

- *Risk for imbalanced nutrition: Less than body requirements,* related to weight loss of 15 lb (6.8 kg), with present weight 10% less than normal for height
- *Diarrhea,* related to increased peristalsis as evidenced by 8 to 10 liquid stools per day
- *Risk for disturbed sensory perception: Visual,* related to an inability to close the eyelids completely
- *Anxiety,* related to a lack of knowledge about disease process

### EXPECTED OUTCOMES

- Gain at least 1 lb (0.45 kg) every 2 weeks.
- Regain normal bowel elimination patterns.
- Maintain normal vision (with no evidence of corneal damage) and verbalize measures to protect her eyes.
- Verbalize medical treatment and self-care needs.
- Verbalize a decrease in anxiety.

*(continued on page 452)*

## Nursing Care Plan

### A Client with Graves' Disease (continued)

#### PLANNING AND IMPLEMENTATION

- Request that she keep a record of daily weight.
- Discuss adopting a high-kcalorie diet. Identify food likes and dislikes, as well as foods that increase diarrhea, before instituting a plan to increase food intake.
- Request that she keep a stool chart, noting the time, type, and precipitating factors for diarrhea stools. Teach comfort measures for irritated anal area (clean washcloth and soap, nonirritating ointment).
- Teach how to apply eye drops (artificial tears).
- Explain the need to elevate the head of the bed to 45 degrees at night, and tape eye shields over eyes before sleep.
- Teach about Graves' disease, the medication's effects and side effects, and the need for continued medical care.

#### EVALUATION

By her next office visit, Mrs. Manuel has gained 1 lb (0.45 kg) and has discussed her dietary needs with the nurse and her husband.

She is having diarrhea less often. She has safely applied the eye drops and states that she uses the eye shields and elevates the head of her bed at night. The office nurse reviewed the written and verbal information about Graves' disease and the medication prescribed. Mrs. Manuel verbalizes her understanding, stating, "I'll always take my medicine—I never want to feel like that again!" She also says that she feels much less anxious now that she understands what has happened.

#### Critical Thinking in the Nursing Process

1. What is the pathophysiologic basis for Mrs. Manuel's abnormal vital signs?
2. What is the rationale for having the client with exophthalmos elevate the head of the bed at night?
3. Outline a teaching plan that could be given to clients for home care following a subtotal thyroidectomy.

See Evaluating Your Response in Appendix C.

## THE CLIENT WITH HYPOTHYROIDISM

**Hypothyroidism** is a disorder that results when the thyroid gland produces an insufficient amount of TH. Because a decrease in TH levels decreases metabolic rate and heat production, hypothyroidism affects all body systems (see the *Multisystem Effects of Hypothyroidism* on page 453). Hypothyroidism is more common in women between ages 30 and 60; the incidence rises after age 50. However, the disorder can occur at any stage of life. Careful evaluation of symptoms is important in the older adult because manifestations of hypothyroidism are often thought to be the result of aging instead of a pathologic process.

The hypothyroid state in adults is sometimes called **myxedema.** The term reflects the characteristic accumulation of nonpitting edema in the connective tissues throughout the body. The edema is the result of water retention in mucoprotein (hydrophilic proteoglycans) deposits in the interstitial spaces. The face of a client with myxedema appears puffy, and the tongue is enlarged (Porth, 2002).

## PATHOPHYSIOLOGY AND MANIFESTATIONS

Hypothyroidism may be either primary or secondary. Primary hypothyroidism (which is more common) may be caused by congenital defects in the gland, loss of thyroid tissue following treatment for hyperthyroidism with surgery or radiation, antithyroid medications, thyroiditis, or endemic iodine deficiency. The cardiac drug, amiodarone (Cordarone), which contains 75 mg of iodine per 200 mg tablet, is increasingly being implicated in causing thyroid problems (Porth, 2002). Secondary hypothyroidism may result from pituitary TSH deficiency or peripheral resistance to thyroid

hormones. Hypothyroidism has a slow onset, with manifestations occurring over months or even years. With treatment, the mental and physical symptoms rapidly reverse in clients of all ages.

When TH production decreases, the thyroid gland enlarges in a compensatory attempt to produce more hormone. The goiter that results is usually a simple or nontoxic form. People living in certain areas of the world where the soil is deficient in iodine, the substance necessary for TH synthesis and secretion, are more prone to become hypothyroid and develop simple goiter. (Iodine deficiency is discussed below.)

Hypothyroid clients characteristically have the manifestations of goiter, fluid retention and edema, decreased appetite, weight gain, constipation, dry skin, dyspnea, pallor, hoarseness, and muscle stiffness. Many clients have a decreased sense of taste and smell, menstrual disorders, anemias, and cardiac enlargement. The pulse is typically slow. Deficient amounts of TH cause abnormalities in lipid metabolism, with elevated serum cholesterol and triglyceride levels. As a result, the client is at increased risk for atherosclerosis and cardiac disorders. Decreased renal blood flow and glomerular filtration rate reduces the kidney's ability to excrete water, which may cause hyponatremia. Sleep apnea is more common in clients with hypothyroidism. Factors that result in decreased TH (in addition to those described) include iodine deficiency and Hashimoto's thyroiditis. A severe state of hypothyroidism is called *myxedema coma.*

### Iodine Deficiency

Iodine is necessary for TH synthesis and secretion. Iodine deficiency may result from certain goitrogenic drugs (which block TH synthesis); lithium carbonate, used to treat bipolar mental disorders; and antithyroid drugs. Goitrogenic compounds in foods such as turnips, rutabagas, and soybeans may

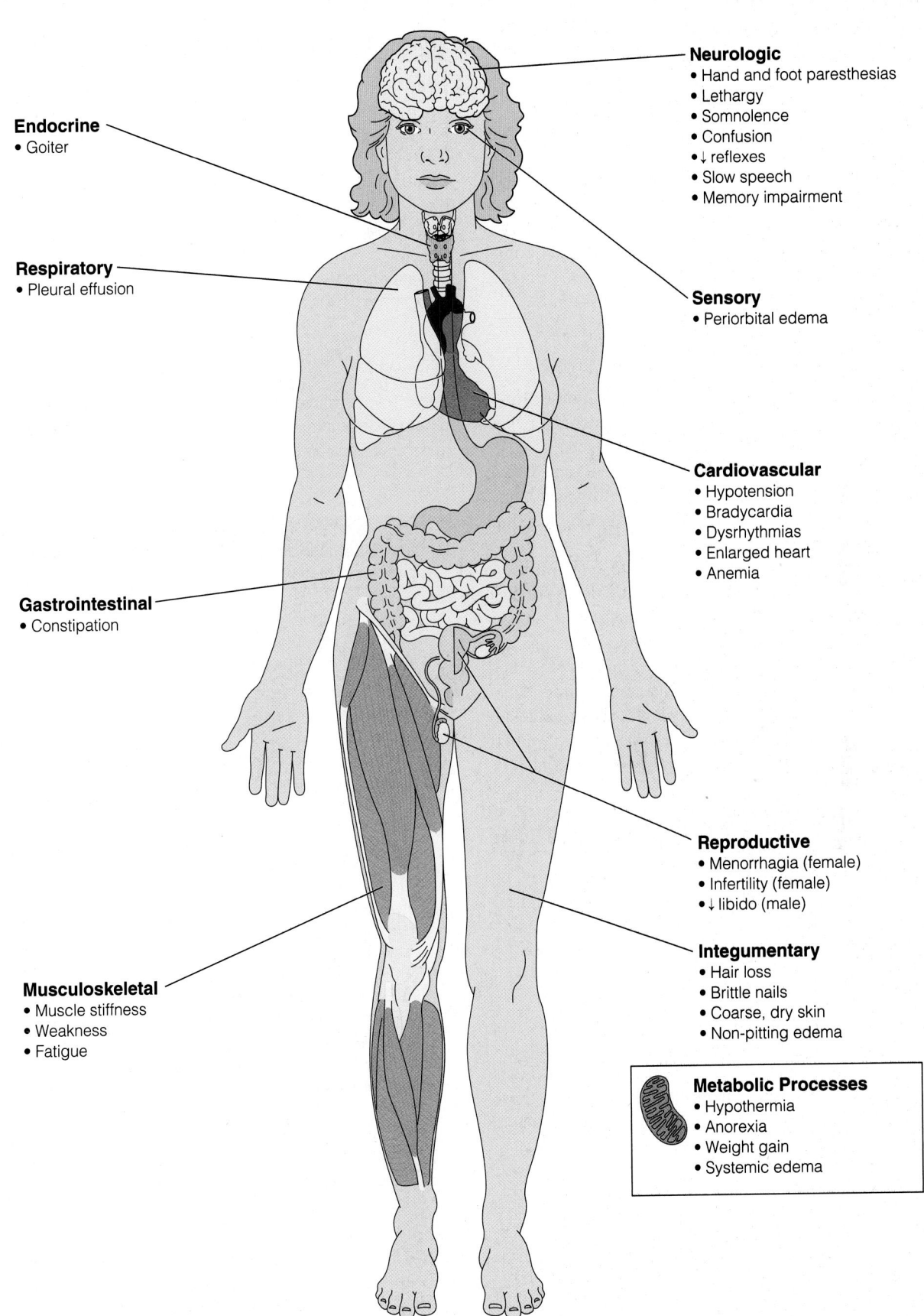

**Neurologic**
- Hand and foot paresthesias
- Lethargy
- Somnolence
- Confusion
- ↓ reflexes
- Slow speech
- Memory impairment

**Endocrine**
- Goiter

**Respiratory**
- Pleural effusion

**Sensory**
- Periorbital edema

**Cardiovascular**
- Hypotension
- Bradycardia
- Dysrhythmias
- Enlarged heart
- Anemia

**Gastrointestinal**
- Constipation

**Reproductive**
- Menorrhagia (female)
- Infertility (female)
- ↓ libido (male)

**Integumentary**
- Hair loss
- Brittle nails
- Coarse, dry skin
- Non-pitting edema

**Musculoskeletal**
- Muscle stiffness
- Weakness
- Fatigue

**Metabolic Processes**
- Hypothermia
- Anorexia
- Weight gain
- Systemic edema

also block TH synthesis if consumed in sufficient quantities. In areas of the world where the soil is deficient in iodine, dietary intake of iodine may be inadequate. However, the use of iodized salt has reduced this risk in the United States.

## Hashimoto's Thyroiditis

**Hashimoto's thyroiditis** is the most common cause of primary hypothyroidism. In this autoimmune disorder, antibodies develop that destroy thyroid tissue. Functional thyroid tissue is replaced with fibrous tissue, and TH levels decrease. In addition, decreasing levels of TH in the early stages of the disease prompt the gland to enlarge to compensate, causing a goiter. However, as the disease progresses, the thyroid gland becomes smaller. This disorder is more common in women and has a familial link.

## Myxedema Coma

**Myxedema coma** is a life-threatening complication of long-standing, untreated hypothyroidism. It is characterized by severe metabolic disorders (hyponatremia, hypoglycemia, lactic acidosis), hypothermia, cardiovascular collapse, and coma. Myxedema coma, although rare, most commonly occurs during the winter months in older women with long-standing chronic hypothyroidism (Porth, 2002).

Myxedema coma may be precipitated by trauma, infection, failure to take thyroid replacement medications, the use of central nervous system depressants, and exposure to cold temperatures (Porth, 2002). The treatment of myxedema coma addresses the precipitating factors and manifestations and involves maintaining a patent airway; maintaining fluid, electrolyte, and acid-base balance; maintaining cardiovascular status; increasing body temperature; and increasing TH levels. If untreated, the mortality rate is high (Tierney et al., 2001).

## COLLABORATIVE CARE

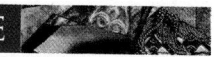

The treatment of the client with hypothyroidism focuses on diagnosis, prevention or treatment of complications, and replacement of the deficient TH. With early and continued treatment, both appearance and mental function return to normal.

### Diagnostic Tests

Hypothyroidism is diagnosed by the manifestations and by a decrease in TH, especially $T_4$. TSH concentration often is increased, because the negative hormonal feedback from TH is lost. The same laboratory and diagnostic tests used to diagnose hyperthyroidism are also used to diagnose hypothyroidism, with opposite results in most cases (see Table 17–2).

### Medications

Hypothyroidism is treated with medications that replace TH. Levothyroxine (thyroxine, $T_4$) is the treatment of choice (Tierney et al., 2001). Medications commonly used to treat hypothyroidism and their nursing implications are shown in the box on this page.

### TABLE 17-2 Laboratory Findings in Hypothyroidism

| Test | Normal Values | Findings |
| --- | --- | --- |
| Serum TA | None to 1:20 | Normal |
| Serum TSH | >1.0 mµ/L | Increased in primary hypothyroidism |
| Serum $T_4$ | 5 to 12 µg/dL | Decreased |
| Serum $T_3$ | 80 to 200 ng/dL | Decreased |
| $T_3$ uptake ($T_3$RU) | 25 to 35 relative percentage | Decreased |
| Thyroid suppression | | No change in RAI uptake or $T_4$ levels |

## Surgery

If the hypothyroid client has a goiter large enough to cause respiratory difficulties or dysphagia, a subtotal thyroidectomy may be performed (see page 449).

## Medication Administration

### Hypothyroidism

#### THYROID PREPARATIONS

Levothyroxine sodium ($T_4$) (Levoxyl, Levothroid, Synthroid)
Liothyronine sodium ($T_3$) (Cytomel)
Liotrix ($T_3 - T_4$) (Euthroid, Thyrolar)

Thyroid preparations increase blood levels of TH, thus raising the client's metabolic rate. As a result, cardiac output, oxygen consumption, and body temperature increase. The dosage depends on the drug chosen and the client's degree of thyroid dysfunction, sensitivity to TH, age, body size, and health. The older adult may require lower doses.

#### Nursing Responsibilities
- Give 1 hour before meals or 2 hours after meals for best absorption.
- Thyroid preparations potentiate the effect of anticoagulant drugs. If the client is also receiving an anticoagulant, monitor for bruising, bleeding gums, and blood in the urine.
- Thyroid medications potentiate the effect of digitalis. If the client is also receiving a digitalis preparation, monitor for signs of digitalis toxicity.
- Monitor for symptoms of coronary insufficiency: chest pain, dyspnea, tachycardia.
- If the client has insulin-dependent diabetes, monitor the effects of insulin. The effect of the insulin may change as thyroid function increases.
- During dose adjustment, take pulse before administering drug. Report pulse >100.

#### Client and Family Teaching
- Do not substitute brands of drugs or use generic equivalents without the physician's approval.
- The medications must be taken for the rest of one's life.

## Medication Administration

### Hypothyroidism (continued)

- Report symptoms of excess thyroid hormone to the physician: excess weight loss, palpitations, leg cramps, nervousness, or insomnia.
- If you have diabetes and use insulin, monitor blood glucose levels closely; the thyroid medications may alter the amount of insulin required.
- Thyroid preparations increase the risk of iodine toxicity. Do not use iodized salt or over-the-counter drugs containing iodine.
- If you are also taking an anticoagulant, report any signs of bleeding.
- Report any changes in menstrual periods.
- Take the thyroid preparation each morning to decrease the possibility of insomnia.
- Closely monitor blood pressure and pulse (older clients).
- Avoid excessive intake of foods that are known to inhibit TH utilization such as turnips, cabbage, carrots, spinach, and peaches.

## NURSING CARE

### Health Promotion

One of the most critical factors in preventing hypothyroidism is education of the public about the necessity of an adequate dietary intake of iodine. The use of iodized salt meets the requirements for hormone production. It is important to teach clients the importance of regular health care provider visits and medication intake.

### Assessment

Collect the following data through the health history and physical examination (see Chapter 16). ⌘ Further focused assessments are described with nursing interventions below. When assessing the older client, be aware of normal changes with aging, outlined in the box below.

- Health history: pituitary diseases, when symptoms began, severity of symptoms, treatment of hyperthyroidism with medications or radioactive iodine, thyroid surgery, treatment of head or neck cancer with radiation, diet, use of iodized salt, bowel elimination, respiratory difficulties

- Physical assessment: muscle strength, deep tendon reflexes, vital signs, cardiovascular and peripheral vascular systems, integument, thyroid gland, weight

### Nursing Diagnoses and Interventions

In planning and implementing care for clients with hypothyroidism, the nurse takes into account that the disorder affects all organ systems. Although many nursing diagnoses might be valid, this section focuses on client problems with cardiovascular function, elimination, and skin integrity.

### Decreased Cardiac Output

A TH deficit causes a reduction in heart rate and stroke volume, resulting in decreased cardiac output. There may also be an accumulation of fluid in the pericardial sac (from the edema characteristic of hypothyroidism), and coronary artery disease may be present, further compromising cardiac function.

- Monitor blood pressure, rate and rhythm of apical and peripheral pulses, respiratory rate, and breath sounds. *Hypotension indicates decreasing peripheral blood. Fluid in the pericardial sac restricts cardiac function. Monopolysaccharide deposits in the respiratory system decrease vital capacity and cause hypoventilation.*
- Suggest the client avoid chilling; increase room temperature, use additional bed covers, and avoid drafts. *Chilling increases metabolic rate and puts increased stress on the heart.*
- Explain the need to alternate activity with rest periods. Ask the client to report any breathing difficulties, chest pain, heart palpitations, or dizziness. *Activity increases demands on the heart and should be balanced with rest. Symptoms of cardiac stress include dyspnea, chest pain, palpitations, and dizziness.*

### Constipation

The hypothyroid client is likely to have a reduced appetite and decreased food intake, a diminished activity level because of muscle aches and weakness, and reduced peristalsis to the point that fecal impactions may occur.

- Encourage a fluid intake of up to 2000 mL per day. Discuss preferred liquids and the best times of day to drink fluids. If kcal intake is restricted, ensure that liquids have no kcal or are low in kcal. *Sufficient fluid intake is necessary to promote proper stool consistency.*

## Nursing Care of the Older Adult

### VARIATIONS IN ASSESSMENT FINDINGS—HYPOTHYROIDISM

#### NORMAL CHANGES WITH AGING

- The thyroid gland undergoes some degree of atrophy, fibrosis, and nodularity.
- Hair growth decreases.
- Nails are often thick, brittle, and yellow.
- Facial skin sags, and bones become more prominent.
- Deep tendon reflexes decrease.
- Response to questions may be slower.

- Discuss ways to maintain a high-fiber diet. *Diets high in fiber and fluid produce soft stools. Fiber that is not digested absorbs water, which adds bulk to the stool and assists in the movement of fecal material through the intestines.*

**PRACTICE ALERT** *High-fiber foods include beans, potatoes, fruits, breads, cereal, crackers, popcorn, and rice.* ■

- Encourage activity as tolerated. *Activity influences bowel elimination by improving muscle tone and stimulating peristalsis.*

### Risk for Impaired Skin Integrity

The client with hypothyroidism is at risk for impaired skin integrity related to the accumulation of fluid in the interstitial spaces and to dry, rough skin. Decreased peripheral circulation, decreased activity levels, and slow wound healing further increase the risk. These interventions are outlined for the older client who is hospitalized for surgery or severe hypothyroidism.

- Monitor skin surfaces for redness or lesions, especially if the client's activity is greatly reduced. Use a pressure ulcer risk assessment scale to identify clients at risk. *Hypothyroidism causes dry, rough, edematous skin conditions that increase the risk of skin breakdown.*
- Provide or teach the immobile client measures to promote optimal circulation:
  - Use a turning schedule if the client is on bed rest, or teach the client to change position every 2 hours.

**PRACTICE ALERT** *Lift the client up in bed to prevent tissue damage from shearing forces.* ■

- Limit the time for sitting in one position; shift weight or lift the body using arm rests every 20 to 30 minutes.
- Use pillows, pads, or sheepskin or foam cushions for bed and/or chair.
- Teach and implement a schedule of range-of-motion exercises.

*Prolonged pressure, especially in clients with edema and circulatory impairment, can occlude capillaries and cause hypoxic tissue damage.*

- Provide or teach the client measures to maintain skin integrity:
  - Take baths only as necessary; use warm (not hot) water.
  - Use gentle motions when washing and drying skin.
  - Use alcohol-free skin oils and lotions.

*Dry skin and edema increase the risk of skin breakdown. Hot water, rough massage, and alcohol-based preparations may increase skin dryness, further impairing the body's ability to maintain skin integrity.*

### Using NANDA, NIC, and NOC

Chart 17–1 shows links between NANDA, NIC, and NOC when caring for the client with hypothyroidism.

### Home Care

Clients with hypothyroidism require lifelong care, primarily at home. Address the following topics.

- The need to take medications for the rest of one's life
- The need for periodic dosage reassessments
- If the client is older or does not have support system, helpful community resources
- Additional resources:
  - American Thyroid Association
  - Thyroid Foundation of Canada
  - Endocrine Society

---

**CHART 17–1  NANDA, NIC, AND NOC LINKAGES**

### The Client with Hypothyroidism

| NURSING DIAGNOSES | NURSING INTERVENTIONS | NURSING OUTCOMES |
|---|---|---|
| • Risk for Constipation | • Bowel Management<br>• Constipation Management<br>• Fluid Management | • Bowel Elimination<br>• Hydration |
| • Excess Fluid Volume | • Fluid Management<br>• Electrolyte Management<br>• Vital Sign Monitoring | • Fluid Balance<br>• Electrolyte Balance |
| • Activity Intolerance | • Energy Management | • Energy Conservation<br>• Self-Care: Activities of Daily Living |
| • Altered Thought Processes | • Environmental Management: Safety | • Safety Behavior: Personal |

*Note. Data from Nursing Outcomes Classification (NOC) by M. Johnson & M. Maas (Eds.), 1997, St. Louis: Mosby; Nursing Diagnoses: Definitions & Classification 2001–2002 by North American Nursing Diagnosis Association, 2001, Philadelphia: NANDA; Nursing Interventions Classification (NIC) by J.C. McCloskey & G. M. Bulechek (Eds.), 2000, St. Louis: Mosby. Reprinted by permission.*

## Nursing Care Plan
### A Client with Hypothyroidism

Jane Lee is a 60-year-old retired nurse living with her husband and daughter on a farm that has been in the family for four generations. Mrs. Lee has gained 10 lb (4.5 kg) in the past few months, even though she is rarely hungry and eats much less than normal. She is always tired and weak—so tired that she has not even been able to help with the chores on the farm or do housework. She is concerned about her appearance and the way she sounds when she talks. Her face is puffy, and her tongue always feels thick. Mr. Lee convinces his wife to make an appointment at a health center in a nearby town.

### ASSESSMENT

Brian Henning, RN, completes the health assessment for Mrs. Lee at the health center. He finds that she now weighs 150 lb (68 kg), an increase of 10 lb (4.5 kg) over her weight at her last visit 6 months earlier. Mrs. Lee states that she always feels cold, tired, and weak. She also states that she is constipated, has difficulty remembering things, and looks different. Physical assessment findings include a palpable and bilaterally enlarged thyroid; dry, yellowish skin; nonpitting edema of the face and lower legs; and slow, slurred speech. Diagnostic tests revealed the following abnormal findings: $T_3$, 56 ng/dL (normal range: 80 to 200 ng/dL); $T_4$, 3.1 (normal range: 5 to 12 mg/dL); TSH increased. The medical diagnosis of hypothyroidism is made, and Mrs. Lee is started on levothyroxine 0.05 mg daily.

### DIAGNOSIS

- *Constipation,* related to decreased peristalsis, as evidenced by hard, formed stools every 4 days
- *Impaired verbal communication,* related to changes in speech patterns and enlarged tongue
- *Low self-esteem,* related to changes in physical appearance and activity intolerance

### EXPECTED OUTCOMES

- Regain normal bowel elimination patterns, having a soft, formed stool at least every other day.

- Experience improvement in verbal communication.
- Regain positive self-esteem as medication reduces physical changes and fatigue.

### PLANNING AND IMPLEMENTATION

- Teach to increase fluids, bulk, and fiber in the diet to help regain a normal bowel elimination pattern of a soft, formed stool every other day.
- Take medication as prescribed and do not expect immediate reversal of symptoms affecting speech.
- Plan activities around rest periods. Encourage husband and daughter to help with housecleaning and cooking.

### EVALUATION

On return to the health center 2 months later, Mrs. Lee reports that she is no longer constipated but that she is continuing to drink six glasses of water and eating oatmeal every day. She no longer feels cold, is regaining her normal energy, and even feels well enough to plant her garden. Her speech is clear and easy to understand. As she leaves the examining room, Mrs. Lee says, "It's hard to believe that I have changed so much—now I look and feel like the 'old' me!"

### Critical Thinking in the Nursing Process

1. What physical changes that normally occur with aging are similar to the manifestations of hypothyroidism?
2. Describe the factors that put Mrs. Lee's safety at risk. What alterations in her home environment would you suggest to promote safety until the prescribed medication takes effect?
3. The client taking oral thyroid medications may become hyperthyroid. List the manifestations you would include in a teaching plan to signal this condition.

See Evaluating Your Response in Appendix C.

## THE CLIENT WITH CANCER OF THE THYROID

Thyroid cancer is relatively rare, with an estimated rate of 23,000 new cases annually. Thyroid cancer accounts for approximately 1300 cancer deaths a year (American Cancer Society, 2002). The most consistent risk factor is exposure to ionizing radiation to the head and neck during childhood. For example, many adults in their 50s and 60s received X-ray treatments for colds and sinus infections during childhood.

Of the several types of thyroid cancer, the most common types are listed here.

- Papillary thyroid carcinoma is the most common thyroid malignancy. It is usually detected as a single nodule, but may arise from a multinodular goiter. The average age of diagnosis is 42, with 70% of cases occurring in women. Risks for

the development of this form are exposure to external X-ray treatments to the head or neck as a child, childhood exposure to radioactive isotopes of iodine in nuclear fallout, and a family history. Papillary thyroid carcinoma is the least aggressive type, but does metastasize to the local and regional lymph nodes and lungs.

- Follicular thyroid cancer is the second most common thyroid malignancy. The average age of diagnosis is 50, with 72% of cases occurring in women. This form is more aggressive, with metastasis commonly found in neck lymph nodes, bone, and lungs.

Thyroid cancer is manifested by a palpable, firm nontender nodule in the thyroid. If undetected, the tumor may grow and impinge on the esophagus or trachea, causing difficulty in swallowing or breathing. Most people with thyroid cancer do not have elevated thyroid hormone levels. The diagnosis is made by measuring thyroid hormones, performing thyroid scans, and by fine-needle biopsy of the nodule. The usual treatment is subtotal or total thyroidectomy. TSH suppression therapy with levothyroxine may be conducted prior to surgery. Radioactive iodine therapy ($^{131}$I) and chemotherapy are additional therapeutic options. The 5-year survival rate, if the tumor has not metastasized, is 95% (American Cancer Society, 2002). Nursing care for the client with cancer is discussed in Chapter 10.

# DISORDERS OF THE PARATHYROID GLANDS

Disorders of the parathyroid glands, hyperparathyroidism and hypoparathyroidism, are not as common as those of the thyroid gland. Hypercalcemia and hypocalcemia (the primary results of alterations in parathyroid function) are discussed in Chapter 5.

## THE CLIENT WITH HYPERPARATHYROIDISM

**Hyperparathyroidism** results from an increase in the secretion of parathyroid hormone (PTH), which regulates normal serum levels of calcium. The increase in PTH affects the kidneys and bones, resulting in the following pathophysiologic changes:

- Increased resorption of calcium and excretion of phosphate by the kidneys, which increases the risk of hypercalcemia and hypophosphatemia
- Increased bicarbonate excretion and decreased acid excretion by the kidneys, which increases the risk of metabolic acidosis and hypokalemia
- Increased release of calcium and phosphorus by bones, with resultant bone decalcification
- Deposits of calcium in soft tissues and the formation of renal calculi

## PATHOPHYSIOLOGY AND MANIFESTATIONS

Hyperparathyroidism occurs more often in older adults and is 3 times more common in women. The disorder itself is not common. The three types of hyperparathyroidism are as follows:

- Primary hyperparathyroidism occurs when there is hyperplasia or an adenoma in one of the parathyroid glands. These disorders interrupt the normal regulatory mechanism between serum calcium levels and PTH secretion and increase the absorption of calcium through the gastrointestinal tract.
- Secondary hyperparathyroidism is a compensatory response by the parathyroid glands to chronic hypocalcemia. It is characterized by an increased secretion of PTH.
- Tertiary hyperparathyroidism results from hyperplasia of the parathyroid glands and a loss of response to serum calcium levels. This disorder is most often seen in clients with chronic renal failure.

Many clients with hyperparathyroidism are asymptomatic. When symptoms occur, they are related to hypercalcemia and various musculoskeletal, renal, and gastrointestinal manifestations. Bone reabsorption results in pathologic fractures, while

## Manifestations of Hyperparathyroidism

**Musculoskeletal System**
- Bone pain (back, joints, shins)
- Pathologic fractures (women)
- Muscle weakness
- Muscle atrophy

**Renal Effects**
- Renal calculi
- Polyuria
- Polydipsia

**Gastrointestinal System**
- Abdominal pain
- Peptic ulcers
- Pancreatitis
- Nausea
- Constipation

**Cardiovascular System**
- Arrhythmias
- Hypertension

**Central Nervous System**
- Paresthesias
- Depression
- Psychosis

**Metabolic Effects**
- Acidosis
- Weight loss

elevated calcium levels alter neural and muscular activity, leading to muscle weakness and atrophy. Proximal renal tubule function is altered, and metabolic acidosis, renal calculi formation, and polyuria occur.

Manifestations of the effect of hypercalcemia on the gastrointestinal tract include abdominal pain, constipation, anorexia, and peptic ulcer formation. Hypercalcemia also affects the cardiovascular system, causing arrhythmias, hypertension, and increased sensitivity to cardiotonic glycosides (e.g., digitalis preparations). The manifestations of hyperparathyroidism are summarized in the box above.

## COLLABORATIVE CARE

Hyperparathyroidism is diagnosed by excluding all other possible causes of hypercalcemia; by at least a 6-month history of symptoms; by laboratory analysis of levels of calcium, phosphorus, magnesium, bicarbonate, and chloride; and by bone X-ray studies and scans (Tierney et al., 2002).

Treatment of hyperparathyroidism focuses on decreasing the elevated serum calcium levels. Clients with mild hypercalcemia are urged to drink fluids and keep active. They should avoid immobilization, thiazide diuretics, large doses of vitamins A and D, antacids containing calcium, and calcium supplements. Severe hypercalcemia requires hospitalization and intensive treatment with intravenous saline. Medications to inhibit bone reabsorption and reduce hypercalcemia, such as pamidronate (Aredia) and alendronate (Fosamax), are administered.

Surgical removal of the parathyroid glands affected by hyperplasia or adenoma treats primary hyperparathyroidism. The preoperative and postoperative nursing care of the client having surgery of the parathyroids is essentially the same as that for the client having a thyroidectomy (see page 449).

## NURSING CARE

Nursing care of the client with hypercalcemia is discussed in Chapter 5.

## THE CLIENT WITH HYPOPARATHYROIDISM

**Hypoparathyroidism** results from abnormally low PTH levels. The most common cause is damage to or removal of the parathyroid glands during thyroidectomy. The lack of circulating PTH causes hypocalcemia and an elevated blood phosphate level.

### PATHOPHYSIOLOGY AND MANIFESTATIONS

Reduced levels of PTH result in impaired renal tubular regulation of calcium and phosphate. In addition, decreased activation of vitamin D results in decreased absorption of calcium by the intestines. The low calcium levels cause changes in neuromuscular activity, affecting peripheral motor and sensory nerves. Hypocalcemia lowers the threshold for nerve and muscle excitability; a slight stimulus anywhere along a nerve or muscle fiber initiates an impulse.

The neuromuscular manifestations that result include numbness and tingling around the mouth and in the fingertips, muscle spasms of the hands and feet, convulsions, and laryngeal spasms. Tetany, a continuous spasm of muscles, is the primary symptom of hypocalcemia. In severe cases of tetany, death may occur. Assessments for **tetany** include Chvostek's sign and

| Manifestations of Hypoparathyroidism | |
| --- | --- |
| **Musculoskeletal System** | |
| • Muscle spasms | • Carpopedal spasms |
| • Facial grimacing | • Tetany or convulsions |
| **Integumentary System** | |
| • Brittle nails | • Dry, scaly skin |
| • Hair loss | |
| **Gastrointestinal System** | |
| • Abdominal cramps | • Malabsorption |
| **Cardiovascular System** | |
| • Arrhythmias | |
| **Central Nervous System** | |
| • Paresthesias (lips, hands, feet) | • Hyperactive reflexes |
| • Mood disorders (irritability, depression, anxiety) | • Psychosis |
| | • Increased intracranial pressure |

Trousseau's sign (see Chapter 16). The manifestations of hypoparathyroidism are summarized in the box above.

## COLLABORATIVE CARE

Hypoparathyroidism is diagnosed by low serum calcium levels and high phosphorus levels in the absence of renal failure, an absorption disorder, or a nutritional disorder.

Treatment of hypoparathyroidism focuses on increasing calcium levels. Intravenous calcium gluconate is given immediately to reduce tetany. Long-term therapy includes supplemental calcium, increased dietary calcium, and vitamin D therapy.

## NURSING CARE

Nursing care for the client with hypocalcemia is discussed in Chapter 5.

# DISORDERS OF THE ADRENAL GLANDS

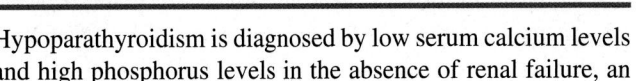

Disorders of the adrenal cortex or adrenal medulla result in changes in the production of adrenocorticotropic hormone (ACTH). Hormones of the adrenal cortex are essential to life. They maintain homeostasis in response to stressors. Disorders of the adrenal cortex result in complex physical, psychologic, and metabolic alterations that are potentially life threatening. Hormones of the adrenal medulla are not essential to life, because the sympathetic nervous system produces similar body responses. The disorders that occur are hyperfunction and hypofunction of the adrenal cortex and hyperfunction of the adrenal medulla.

## THE CLIENT WITH HYPERCORTISOLISM (CUSHING'S SYNDROME)

**Cushing's syndrome** is a chronic disorder in which hyperfunction of the adrenal cortex produces excessive amounts of circulating cortisol or ACTH. Cushing's syndrome is more common in women, with the average age of onset between 30 and 50 years (Figure 17–3 ■). However, the disorder may occur at any age, especially as the result of pharmacologic therapy. People who take steroids for long periods of time (e.g., for

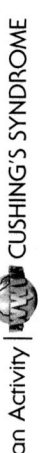

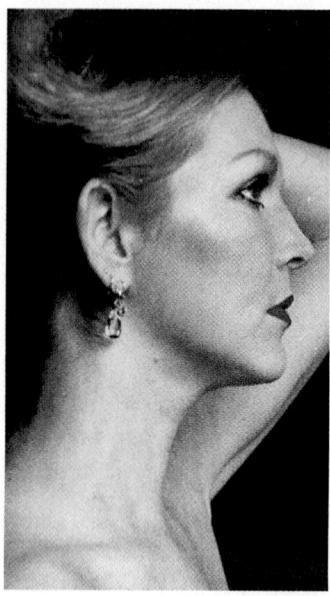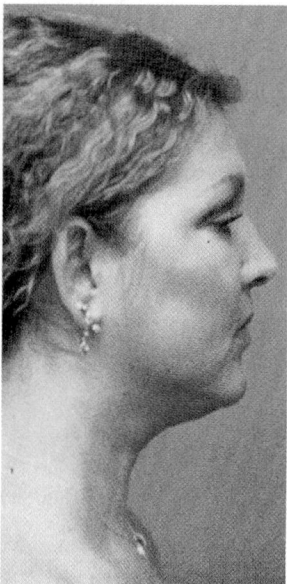

**Figure 17–3** ■ A woman before and after developing Cushing's syndrome. In the photo at right, notice the swollen facial features.

*Courtesy of Dr. Charles Wilson, University of California, San Francisco.*

the treatment of arthritis, after an organ transplant, or as an adjunct to chemotherapy) are at increased risk for developing the disorder.

## PATHOPHYSIOLOGY

Cushing's syndrome may be the result of various causes. The most common etiologies of the disorder are (Porth, 2002):

- The pituitary form, with ACTH hypersecretion by a tumor of the pituitary (called *Cushing's disease*). This is most commonly caused by a small pituitary adenoma, with persistent but disorderly and random overproduction of ACTH.
- The ectopic form, caused by ACTH-secreting tumors (such as small-cell lung cancer). In this form, the ACTH is also random and episodic, but greater than in Cushing's disease.
- The adrenal form, resulting from excessive cortisol secretion by a benign or malignant adrenal tumor. The excess secretion suppresses pituitary ACTH production, resulting in atrophy of the uninvolved adrenal cortex.
- Iatrogenic Cushing's syndrome, resulting from long-term therapy with potent pharmacologic glucocorticoid preparations.

## MANIFESTATIONS

The manifestations of Cushing's syndrome result from the ACTH or cortisol excess, and manifest as exaggerated cortisol actions. Obesity and a redistribution of body fat result in fat deposits in the abdominal region (central obesity), fat pads under the clavicle, a "buffalo hump" over the upper back, and a round "moon" face. Changes in protein metabolism cause muscle weakness and wasting, especially in the extremities. Glucocorticoid excess inhibits fibroblasts, resulting in loss of collagen and connective tissue. Thinning of skin, abdominal

striae (reddish purple "stretch marks"), easy bruising, poor wound healing, and frequent skin infections result. Glucose metabolism is altered in the majority of clients, and diabetes mellitus may occur. Electrolyte imbalances also occur with the increased hormone levels. Changes in calcium absorption result in osteoporosis, compression fractures of the vertebrae, fractures of the ribs, and renal calculi. Hypokalemia and hypertension occur as potassium is lost and sodium is retained. Inhibited immune responses increase the risk of infection, and increased gastric acid secretion increases the risk of peptic ulcers. Emotional changes range from depression to psychosis. In women, increasing androgen levels cause hirsutism (excessive facial hair in particular), acne, and menstrual irregularities. The manifestations and effects of Cushing's syndrome are grouped by body system in the box below.

The complications of untreated Cushing's syndrome include electrolyte imbalances (hyperglycemia, hypernatremia, and hypokalemia), hypertension, and emotional disturbances. Increased susceptibility to infections is also a factor. Compression fractures from osteoporosis and aseptic necrosis of the femoral head may result in serious disability. If the client undergoes a bilateral adrenalectomy as a treatment for Cushing's syndrome, an acute deficit of cortisol (addisonian crisis) may result.

## COLLABORATIVE CARE

The treatment of Cushing's syndrome includes medications, radiation therapy, or surgery, depending on the etiologic origin of the disorder.

### Manifestations of Cushing's Syndrome

**Musculoskeletal System**
- Weakness
- Muscle wasting
- Osteoporosis

**Integumentary System**
- Thin, easily bruised skin
- Skin infections
- Poor wound healing
- Eccymosis
- Purple striae (around thighs, breasts, abdomen)
- Hirsutism

**Central Nervous System**
- Emotional lability
- Psychoses

**Gastrointestinal System**
- Peptic ulcers

**Cardiovascular System**
- Hypertension

**Renal Effects**
- Renal calculi
- Polyuria
- Polydipsia
- Glycosuria

**Metabolic Effects**
- Hypokalemia
- Hypernatremia
- Truncal obesity

**Reproductive System**
- Oligomenorrhea or amenorrhea
- Impotence
- Decreased libido

## TABLE 17–3 Laboratory Findings in Cushing's Syndrome

| | Test | Normal Values | Findings |
|---|---|---|---|
| Serum | Cortisol | 8 a.m. to 10 a.m.: 5 to 23 µg/dL 4 p.m. to 6 p.m.: 3 to 13 µg/dL | Increased |
| | Blood urea nitrogen (BUN) | 5 to 25 mg/dL | Normal |
| | Sodium | 135 to 145 mEq/L | Increased |
| | Potassium | 3.5 to 5.0 mEq/L | Decreased |
| | Glucose (serum) | 70 to 100 mg/dL | Increased |
| Urine | 17-KS | Male: 5 to 25 mg/24h Female: 5 to 15 mg/24h >65: 4 to 8 mg/24h | Increased |

## Diagnostic Tests

Cushing's syndrome is diagnosed through a variety of diagnostic tests. Findings are shown in Table17–3.

- *Plasma cortisol levels* are measured. If Cushing's disease is present, test results show a loss of the normal diurnal variations of higher levels in the morning and lower levels in the afternoon.
- *Plasma ACTH levels* are measured to determine the etiology of the syndrome. Normally, plasma ACTH levels are highest from 7 A.M. to 10 A.M. and lowest from 7 P.M. to 10 P.M. In secondary Cushing's syndrome, ACTH is elevated; in primary Cushing's syndrome, ACTH is decreased.
- *24-hour urine tests* (*17-ketosteroids* and *17-hydroxycorticosteroids*) are conducted to measure free cortisol and androgens; these hormones are increased in Cushing's syndrome.

- *Serum potassium, calcium, and glucose levels* are measured to identify electrolyte imbalances.
- *ACTH suppression test* may be conducted to identify the cause of the disorder. A synthetic cortisol (dexamethasone) is given to suppress the production of ACTH, and plasma cortisol levels are measured. If an extremely high dose of cortisol is necessary to suppress ACTH, the primary disorder is adrenal cortex hyperplasia. If ACTH is not suppressed with the synthetic cortisol, an adrenal tumor is suspected.

## Medications

Cushing's syndrome that results from a pituitary tumor is treated by medications as an adjunct to surgery or radiation. Medications are also used for clients with inoperable pituitary or adrenal malignancies. Although the drugs control symptoms, they do not effect a cure. Examples of some commonly prescribed drugs follow:

- Mitotane directly suppresses activity of the adrenal cortex and decreases peripheral metabolism of corticosteroids. It is used to treat metastatic adrenal cancer.
- Metyrapone or ketoconazole (or both) inhibit cortisol synthesis by the adrenal cortex and may be administered to clients with ectopic ACTH-secreting tumors that cannot be surgically removed.
- Somatostatis analog (octreotide) suppresses ACTH secretion in some clients.

## Surgery

When Cushing's syndrome is caused by an adrenal cortex tumor, an adrenalectomy may be performed to remove the tumor. Only one adrenal gland is usually involved; however, if an ACTH-producing ectopic tumor is involved, a bilateral adrenalectomy is performed. Lifelong hormone replacement is necessary if both adrenal glands are removed. Nursing care of the client having an adrenalectomy is discussed below.

# NURSING CARE OF THE CLIENT HAVING AN ADRENALECTOMY

## PREOPERATIVE CARE

- Request a dietary consultation to discuss with the client about a diet high in vitamins and proteins. If hypokalemia exists, include foods high in potassium. *Glucocorticoid excess increases catabolism. Vitamins and proteins are necessary for tissue repair and wound healing following surgery.*
- Use careful medical and surgical asepsis when providing care and treatments. *Cortisol excess increases the risk of infection.*
- Monitor the results of laboratory tests of electrolytes and glucose levels. *Electrolyte and glucose imbalances are corrected before the client has surgery.*
- Teach the client to turn, cough, and perform deep-breathing exercises. *Although they are important for all surgical clients, these activities are even more important for the client who is at risk for infection. Having the client practice and demonstrate the activities increases postoperative compliance.*

## POSTOPERATIVE CARE

- Take and record vital signs, measure intake and output, and monitor electrolytes on a frequent schedule, especially during the first 48 hours after surgery. *Removal of an adrenal gland, especially a bilateral adrenalectomy, results in adrenal insufficiency. Addisonian crisis and hypovolemic shock may occur. Cortisol is often given on the day of surgery and in the postoperative period to replace inadequate hormone levels. Intravenous fluids are also administered.*
- Assess body temperature, WBC levels, and wound drainage. Change dressings using sterile technique. *Impaired wound healing increases the risk of infection in clients with adrenal disorders. Use aseptic technique to decrease this risk.*

Surgical removal of the pituitary gland (hypophysectomy) is indicated when Cushing's syndrome is the result of a pituitary disorder. The gland is removed either by a transphenoidal route or by a craniotomy. Nursing care for the client having cranial surgery is discussed in Chapter 42. ⚭

# NURSING CARE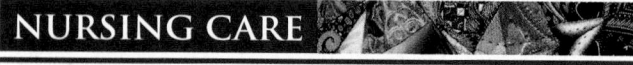

## Health Promotion

Stress the risk of developing Cushing's syndrome for clients taking long-term steroids. The risk of abruptly discontinuing the medications is an essential component of teaching.

## Assessment

Collect the following data through the health history and physical examination (see Chapter 16). Further focused assessments are described with nursing interventions below.

- Health history: history of pituitary, adrenal, pancreatic, or pulmonary tumor; frequent infections; gastrointestinal bleeding; stress fractures; pain, changes in weight distribution; change in height; fatigue; weakness; change in appearance; bruising; skin infections; menstrual history; sexual function
- Physical assessment: vital signs, behavior, appearance, fat distribution, face, skin, hair quantity and distribution, muscle size and strength, gait

## Nursing Diagnoses and Interventions

The nurse caring for the client with Cushing's syndrome must take a holistic approach to plan and implement interventions for a wide variety of responses, including problems related to fluid and electrolyte balance, injury, infection, and body image. For additional information about clients with alterations in fluid and electrolyte balance, see Chapter 5. ⚭

### Fluid Volume Excess

The excess cortisol secretion associated with Cushing's syndrome results in sodium and water reabsorption, causing fluid volume excess. The client will have weight gain, edema, and hypertension.

- Ask the client to weigh at the same time each day, and maintain a record of results. *Body weight is an accurate indicator of fluid status. One liter of fluid retention corresponds to about 2 lb (0.9 kg) of body weight.*
- Monitor blood pressure, rate and rhythm of pulse, respiratory rate, and breath sounds. Assess for peripheral edema and jugular vein distention. *Extracellular fluid volume excess resulting from sodium and water retention is manifested by hypertension and a bounding, rapid pulse. There may also be crackles and wheezes, dependent edema, and venous distention.*
- Teach the client and family the reasons for restricting fluid and the importance of limiting fluids if ordered. *Restricting fluid can help decrease the risk of fluid volume excess. Involving the client and family in the plan of care and teaching the rationale for interventions helps achieve goals.*

### Risk for Injury

The client with Cushing's syndrome is at risk for injury from several causes. Excess cortisol causes increased absorption of calcium and demineralization of bones, resulting in risk of pathologic fractures. Muscle weakness and fatigue are common, increasing the potential for accidental falls.

- Teach the client and family to maintain a safe environment:
  - Keep unnecessary clutter and equipment out of the way and off the floor.
  - Ensure adequate lighting, especially at night.
  - Encourage the use of assistive devices for ambulation or to ask for help if needed.
  - If the client wears corrective lenses, be sure they are available and clean.
  - Encourage the use of nonskid slippers or shoes.
  - Monitor for signs of fatigue (increased pulse and respirations); plan rest periods.

*A well-lighted environment free of clutter decreases the risk of falls and injury. Sensory and motor deficits increase the risk of falls; corrective lenses, assistive devices, and nonslip footwear can decrease this risk. Rest relieves fatigue. To reduce energy expenditure, include alternating periods of rest and activity in daily schedules.*

### Risk for Infection

Elevated cortisol levels impair the immune response and put the client with Cushing's syndrome at increased risk for infection. Increased cortisol also affects protein synthesis, causing delayed wound healing, and inhibits collagen formation, which results in epidermal atrophy, further inhibiting resistance to infection. In addition, impaired blood flow to edematous tissue results in altered cellular nutrition, which increases the potential for infection. The following interventions are outlined for the client with Cushing's syndrome who is hospitalized.

- Place in a private room, and limit visitors. *The client must avoid exposure to environmental infection.*
- Monitor vital signs and verbalizations of subjective manifestations (e.g., the client's response to, "How do you feel?") every 4 hours. *Increased body temperature and pulse are systemic indicators of infection; however, because Cushing's syndrome impairs the normal inflammatory response, the usual indicators of inflammation may not be present.*

**PRACTICE ALERT**   *A generalized feeling of malaise may be the primary manifestation of infection.* ■

- Use principles of medical and sterile asepsis when caring for the client, conducting procedures, or providing wound care. *Impaired skin and tissues make aseptic techniques even more necessary to decrease the risk of infection. Intact skin is the first line of defense against infection; if invasive procedures are performed or a wound is present, this defense is lost.*

- If wounds are present, assess the color, odor, and consistency of wound drainage, and look for increased pain in and around the wound. *Cortisol excess delays wound healing and closure.*
- Teach the importance of increasing intake of protein and vitamins C and A. *Protein, vitamin C, and vitamin A are necessary to collagen formation; collagen helps support and repair body tissues.*

### Disturbed Body Image

The client with Cushing's syndrome has obvious physical changes in appearance. The abnormal fat distribution, moon face, buffalo hump, striae, acne, and facial hair (in women) all contribute to disruptions in the way clients with this disorder perceive themselves.

- Encourage clients to express feelings and to ask questions about the disorder and its treatment. *The loss of one's normal body image may prompt feelings of hopelessness, powerlessness, anger, and depression. Understanding the disease and adapting to changes from that disease are the first steps in regaining control of one's own body.*
- Discuss strengths and previous coping strategies. Enlist the support of family or significant others in reaffirming the client's worth. *Disturbances in body image are often accompanied by low self-esteem. Self-esteem derives from one's perception of competence and from appraisals of others.*
- Discuss signs of progress in controlling symptoms; for example, decreased facial edema or increased activity tolerance. *Many physical changes from cortisol excess disappear with treatment. Clearly communicate this fact, because the client may believe changes are permanent.*

### Using NANDA, NIC and NOC

Chart 17–2 shows links between NANDA, NIC, and NOC when caring for the client with Cushing's syndrome.

### Home Care

The client with Cushing's syndrome requires education about self-care at home specific to the type of treatment given. Address the following topics:

- Safety measures to prevent falls if fatigue, weakness, and osteoporosis are present
- Taking medications as prescribed, with information about side effects. Clients often require medications for the rest of their lives, and dosage changes are highly likely.
- Having regular health assessments
- Wearing a medical ID indicating the client has Cushing's syndrome
- Helping the older client with referrals to social services or community health services because of the complexity of the treatment and care required
- Providing helpful resources:
  - American Association of Clinical Endocrinologists
  - Endocrine Society

## THE CLIENT WITH CHRONIC ADRENOCORTICAL INSUFFICIENCY (ADDISON'S DISEASE)

**Addison's disease** is a disorder resulting from destruction or dysfunction of the adrenal cortex. The result is chronic deficiency of cortisol, aldosterone, and adrenal androgens, accompanied by skin pigmentation. It can occur at any age, although it is more common in adults under the age of 60. Like many endocrine disorders, Addison's disease is more common in women.

### CHART 17–2  NANDA, NIC, AND NOC LINKAGES

#### The Client with Cushing's Syndrome

| NURSING DIAGNOSES | NURSING INTERVENTIONS | NURSING OUTCOMES |
|---|---|---|
| • Risk for Infection | • Infection Protection<br>• Environmental Management<br>• Skin Surveillance<br>• Wound Care | • Risk Control<br>• Risk Detection |
| • Impaired Skin Integrity | • Infection Control<br>• Skin Surveillance | • Tissue Integrity: Skin |
| • Risk for Injury | • Fall Prevention<br>• Teaching: Disease Process<br>• Home Maintenance Assistance | • Safety Behavior: Fall Prevention<br>• Safety Behavior: Home Physical Environment |
| • Disturbed Body Image | • Body Image Enhancement | • Body Image |

*Note. Data from* Nursing Outcomes Classification (NOC) *by M. Johnson & M. Maas (Eds.), 1997, St. Louis: Mosby;* Nursing Diagnoses: Definitions & Classification 2001–2002 *by North American Nursing Diagnosis Association, 2001, Philadelphia: NANDA;* Nursing Interventions Classification (NIC) *by J.C. McCloskey & G. M. Bulechek (Eds.), 2000, St. Louis: Mosby. Reprinted by permission.*

## Nursing Care Plan
## A Client with Cushing's Syndrome

Sara Domico is a 30-year-old lawyer living in a major metropolitan area. She has never been married, and she shares her life with her cat, Beau, and her parents, who live nearby. Her physician recently diagnosed Ms. Domico as having Cushing's syndrome and admits her to the hospital for surgery for an adrenal cortex tumor (adrenalectomy). She has been having increased muscle weakness, so much so that she has difficulty climbing the one flight of stairs to her apartment. She has also had difficulty sleeping, irregular menstrual periods, and hypertension. Ms. Domico is especially concerned about her protruding abdomen, round face, development of facial hair, and the numerous bruises that have appeared on her skin.

### ASSESSMENT

When Ms. Domico arrives at the hospital the morning of surgery, she is admitted by her case manager, Ann Sprengel, RN, CNS. Ann completes a physical assessment that includes abnormal findings of thin lower extremities, an enlarged abdomen, purple striae over the abdomen and buttocks, a round face, and obvious facial hair. Her blood pressure is 160/96. Ms. Domico tells Ann that she is always tired and that sometimes it "just wears me out to walk from the bedroom to the kitchen." Diagnostic tests conducted prior to admission reveal the following abnormal findings (all except cortisol levels are corrected before surgery).

Glucose: 186 mg/dL (normal range: 70 to 110 mg/dL)
Sodium: 152 mEq/L (normal range: 135 to 145 mEq/L)
Potassium: 3.2 mEq/L (normal range: 3.5 to 5.0 mEq/L)
Calcium: 4.3 mEq/L (normal range: 4.5 to 5.5 mEq/L)
Cortisol: 35 mg/dL (normal for A.M.: 5 to 23 mg/dL)

### DIAGNOSIS

- *Fluid volume excess,* related to sodium retention causing edema and hypertension
- *Risk for injury,* related to generalized fatigue and weakness
- *Risk for infection,* related to impaired immune response and edema
- *Body image disturbance,* related to physical changes secondary to Cushing's syndrome

### EXPECTED OUTCOMES

- Regain a normal body fluid balance.

- Remain free of injury.
- Remain free of infection.
- Verbalize understanding of the physical effects of the disease process and realistic expectations of desired changes in appearance.

### PLANNING AND IMPLEMENTATION

- Weigh each morning, using the same scale.
- Maintain an accurate record of intake and output.
- Ensure adequate lighting in the room, and wear glasses and shoes when getting out of bed.
- Develop a written schedule of rest and activity periods.
- If agreeable, provide a private room, and restrict visitors to parents at this time.
- Use strict medical and surgical asepsis when providing care.
- Provide time for discussion of the disease and treatment; encourage verbalization of feelings and identify successful coping mechanisms used in the past.
- Encourage turning, coughing, and deep breathing and/or incentive spirometry every 2–4 hours.

### EVALUATION

Ms. Domico states that she is "ready to have surgery and start feeling better." She has not fallen or injured herself, and she has remained free of infection. Although edema is still present, she has lost 8 lb (3.6 kg), and her blood pressure is decreased. Ms. Domico has openly discussed her concerns about the way she looks and feels; she understands that symptoms will improve following surgery. She has strong religious beliefs and family support, both of which provide strength and help her cope with the effects of the disorder and the need for any further treatment.

### Critical Thinking in the Nursing Process

1. When Ms. Domico was admitted to the hospital, several of her test results were abnormal. Describe the pathophysiologic reason for those results.
2. List the assessments that nurses can make to determine body fluid balance.
3. Develop a plan of care for this client for the nursing diagnosis *Fatigue.*

See Evaluating Your Response in Appendix C.

## PATHOPHYSIOLOGY

There are many possible causes of Addison's disease. The etiologies include:

- Autoimmune destruction of the adrenals. This is the most common cause, accounting for about 80% of spontaneous cases (Tierney et al., 2001). It may occur alone, or as part of a polyglandular autoimmune syndrome (PGA). Type 2 PGA is seen in adults, often associated with autoimmune thyroid disease (usually hypothyroidism), type 1 diabetes, primary ovarian or testicular failure, and pernicious anemia.
- Clients who are taking anticoagulants, have major trauma, or are having open heart surgery. Such clients may have bilateral adrenal hemorrhage.

- Adrenoleukodystrophy, an X-linked disorder characterized by an accumulation of very long chain fatty acids in the adrenal cortex, testes, brain, and spinal cord.
- ACTH deficit, resulting from pituitary tumors, pituitary surgery or irradiation, and the use of exogenous steroids.
- Clients who are abruptly withdrawn from long-term, high-dose steroid therapy. Other clients at risk are those with tuberculosis or acquired immune deficiency syndrome (AIDS); the pathogens responsible for either disease can infiltrate and destroy adrenal tissue.

Adrenocortical destruction initially causes a decrease in adrenal glucocorticoid reserve. Basal glucocorticoid secretion is normal, but does not increase in response to stress and surgery. Trauma or infection can precipitate an adrenal crisis. As the destruction of the adrenal cortex continues, even basal secretion of glucocorticoids and mineralocorticoids is deficient. Decreasing plasma cortisol reduces the feedback inhibition of pituitary ACTH and plasma ACTH rises.

Secondary adrenocortical insufficiency occurs when large doses of glucocorticoids are given for their anti-inflammatory and immunosuppressive effects to treat diseases such as arthritis and asthma. Treatment that extends for longer than 4 to 5 weeks suppresses ACTH and cortisol secretion. If the steroid medications are suddenly discontinued, the hypothalamus and pituitary cannot respond normally to the reduced level of circulating glucocorticoids. The client may develop manifestations of chronic adrenocortical insufficiency or, if subjected to stress, adrenal crisis (Tierney et al., 2001).

## MANIFESTATIONS

The onset of Addison's disease is slow; the client experiences symptoms after about 90% of the function of the gland is lost. The primary manifestations are the result of elevated ACTH levels and decreased aldosterone and cortisol (see the box below.) Aldosterone deficiency affects the ability of the distal tubules of the nephron to conserve sodium. Sodium is lost, potassium is retained, extracellular fluid is depleted, and the blood volume is decreased. Postural hypotension and syncope are common, and hypovolemic shock may occur. Hyponatremia causes dizziness, confusion, and neuromuscular irritability. Hyperkalemia causes cardiac arrhythmias.

Cortisol insufficiency also causes decreased hepatic glyconeogenesis with hypoglycemia. The client tolerates stress poorly and experiences lethargy, weakness, anorexia, nausea, vomiting, and diarrhea. The increased ACTH levels stimulate hyperpigmentation in about 98% of clients with Addison's disease (Porth, 2002). In Caucasian clients, the skin looks deeply suntanned or bronzed in both exposed and unexposed areas.

## Manifestations of Addison's Disease

**Integumentary System**
- Delayed wound healing
- Hyperpigmentation

**Cardiovascular System**
- Postural hypotension
- Arrhythmias
- Tachycardia

**Central Nervous System**
- Lethargy
- Tremors
- Emotional lability
- Confusion

**Musculoskeletal System**
- Weakness
- Muscle wasting
- Joint pain
- Muscle pain

**Gastrointestinal System**
- Anorexia
- Nausea and vomiting
- Diarrhea

**Reproductive System**
- Menstrual changes

**Metabolic Effects**
- Hyperkalemia
- Hyponatremia
- Hypoglycemia

## ADDISONIAN CRISIS

**Addisonian crisis** is a life-threatening response to acute adrenal insufficiency. This response can occur in any person with Addison's disease; however, it is most commonly precipitated by major stressors, especially if the disease is poorly controlled. Addisonian crisis may also occur in clients who are abruptly withdrawn from glucocorticoid medications or who have hemorrhage into the adrenal glands from either septicemia or anticoagulant therapy.

The client with addisonian crisis may have any of the manifestations of Addison's disease, but the primary symptoms are a high fever, weakness, abdominal pain, severe hypotension, circulatory collapse, shock, and coma. Treatment of the crisis is rapid intravenous replacement of fluids and glucocorticoids. Fluid balance is usually restored in 4 to 6 hours.

## COLLABORATIVE CARE

The client with Addison's disease requires early diagnosis and treatment. Medical treatment includes cortisol replacement therapy.

### Diagnostic Tests

Addison's disease is diagnosed through findings of decreased levels of cortisol, aldosterone, and urinary 17-ketosteroids. Dehydration may result in increased hematocrit and blood urea nitrogen (BUN). Blood glucose levels are decreased, and potassium is increased. A list of laboratory findings in Addison's disease is shown in Table 17–4. The following diagnostic tests are used:

- *Serum cortisol levels,* which are decreased in adrenal insufficiency
- *Blood glucose levels,* which are decreased in adrenal insufficiency
- *Serum sodium levels,* which are decreased in adrenal insufficiency

| TABLE 17–4 Laboratory Findings in Addison's Disease | | | |
|---|---|---|---|
| | **Test** | **Normal Values** | **Findings** |
| *Serum* | Cortisol | 8 a.m. to 10 a.m.: 5 to 23 µg/dL 4 p.m. to 6 p.m.: 3 to 13 µg/dL | Decreased |
| | Blood urea nitrogen (BUN) | 5 to 25 mg/dL | Increased |
| | Sodium | 135 to 145 mEq/L | Decreased |
| | Potassium | 3.5 to 5.0 mEq/L | Increased |
| | Glucose (serum) | 70 to 100 mg/dL | Decreased |
| *Urine* | 17-KS | Male: 5 to 25 mg/24h Female: 5 to 15 mg/24h >65: 4 to 8 mg/24h | Low/Absent |

- *Serum potassium levels,* which are increased in adrenal insufficiency
- *Blood urea nitrogen (BUN) levels,* which are increased in adrenal insufficiency
- *Urinary 17-hydroxycorticoids* and *17-ketosteroids (17-KS) levels,* which are decreased in adrenal insufficiency
- *Plasma ACTH levels,* which are increased in primary adrenal insufficiency but decreased in secondary adrenal insufficiency
- Possibly *ACTH stimulation test.* (Cortisol levels rise with pituitary deficiency but do not rise in primary adrenal insufficiency.)
- *CT scans* of the head, which identify any intracranial lesion impinging on the pituitary gland

## Medications

The primary medical treatment of Addison's disease is replacement of corticosteroids and mineralocorticoids, accompanied by increased sodium in the diet. Hydrocortisone is given orally to replace cortisol; fludrocortisone (Florinef) is given orally to replace mineralocorticoids. Nursing implications in cortisol replacement are given in the box below.

# NURSING CARE

## Health Promotion

Health promotion interventions for the client with or at risk for Addison's disease focus on careful assessments during anticoagulant therapy, open heart surgery, and trauma treatment. If the disease is present, teaching to prevent or treat an addisonian crisis is essential.

## Assessment

Collect the following data through the health history and physical examination (see Chapter 16). Further focused assessments are described with nursing interventions below.

- Health history: weight loss, changes in skin color, nausea and vomiting, anorexia, diarrhea, abdominal pain, weakness, amenorrhea, changes in sexual desire, confusion, intolerance of stress
- Physical assessment: height and weight, vital signs, skin, hair quality and distribution, muscle size and strength

# Medication Administration

### Addison's Disease

#### CORTISOL REPLACEMENTS

Cortisone (Cortone, Cortogen)
Hydrocortisone (Cortisol, Hydrocortone, Cortef)
Prednisone (Meticorten, Deltasone, Orasone)
Fludrocortisone acetate (Florinef, F-Cortef)
Dexamethasone (Decadron, Hexadrol, Dexasone)
Prednisolone (Meticortelone)
Methylprednisolone (Medrol, Solu-Medrol)

Adrenocorticosteroids are used for replacement therapy in acute and chronic adrenal insufficiency. These drugs have anti-inflammatory and immunosuppressant effects. They also facilitate coping with stress.

Because corticosteroids are immunosuppressants, their use is contraindicated when an infection is suspected because they mask the signs of infection. Corticosteroids are also contraindicated in many other disorders, including peptic ulcer, Cushing's syndrome, cardiac disease, hyperthyroidism, hypothyroidism, and tuberculosis.

When these drugs are administered in small doses for replacement therapy, side effects are uncommon. Large doses or prolonged therapy may cause a Cushing-like syndrome, with atrophy of the adrenal cortex. Older clients, especially postmenopausal women, are more prone to develop hypertension and osteoporosis when undergoing glucocorticoid therapy. These drugs are used with caution in children and the older adult and are not usually administered to pregnant women.

#### Nursing Responsibilities
- Establish baseline data, including mental status, neurologic function, vital signs, and weight.
- Identify medications that might interact with corticosteroids: antidiabetic agents, cardiac glycosides, oral contraceptives, anticoagulants.

- Document and report increased blood pressure, edema or weight gain, bleeding or bruising, weakness, or manifestations of Cushing's syndrome.
- Administer oral forms of the drug with food to minimize its ulcerogenic effect.
- Monitor electrolyte levels for increased sodium and decreased potassium.

#### Client and Family Teaching
- Take medications with food or milk, and report any gastric distress or dark stools.
- Most people need to take the medications for the rest of their lives.
- Consume a diet that is high in potassium, low in sodium, and high in protein.
- Weigh yourself each day at the same time, and report any consistent weight gain, which indicates fluid retention.
- Use safety measures in the home to prevent falls and injuries.
- Corticosteroids may impair the effectiveness of oral contraceptives.
- Take the medication regularly and continuously. *Abruptly discontinuing the medication is dangerous.*
- Obtain a MedicAlert bracelet.
- Monitor for increased stressors (infection, dental work, personal crisis) and increase the dose as indicated by the physician.
- Anticoagulant drugs or insulin may decrease the effectiveness of corticosteroids.
- Report the following to the physician: dizziness on sitting or standing, nausea and vomiting, pain, thirst, feelings of anxiety, malaise, infections.

## Nursing Diagnoses and Interventions

The client with Addison's disease requires nursing care for a wide variety of responses to the decrease in cortisol levels. Nursing diagnoses discussed in this section are directed toward problems with fluid and electrolyte balance and compliance with lifelong self-care.

### Deficient Fluid Volume

Fluid volume deficit in the client with Addison's disease results from loss of water and sodium, as well as from vomiting and diarrhea. Extracellular fluid volume deficit, decreased cardiac output, hypotension, and hypovolemic shock may occur, especially in crisis situations. Interventions for this diagnosis are outlined for the client who is hospitalized.

- Monitor intake and output, and assess for signs of dehydration: dry mucous membranes; thirst; poor skin turgor; sunken eyeballs; scanty, dark urine; increased urine specific gravity; weight loss; and increased hemoconcentration (increased hematocrit and BUN). *Glucocorticoid and mineralocorticoid depletion causes fluid volume deficit. Fluid volume deficit may reach crisis levels if undetected, causing altered tissue perfusion and hypovolemic shock.*
- Monitor cardiovascular status: Take and record vital signs, assess character of pulses, monitor potassium levels and ECGs. *Fluid volume deficit may lead to hypotension and a rapid, weak, or thready pulse. As aldosterone levels fall, renal excretion of potassium decreases, increasing blood levels of potassium.*

**PRACTICE ALERT** *Hyperkalemia causes changes in cardiac muscle function, which are reflected in ECG changes.* ■

- Weigh the client daily at the same time and in the same clothing. *Dehydration is manifested by weight loss.*
- Encourage an oral fluid intake of 3000 mL per day and an increased salt intake. *Cortisol deficiency increases fluid loss, leading to extracellular fluid volume depletion. Oral fluid replacement is necessary to balance this loss. An increase in dietary sodium can decrease the hyponatremia characteristic of adrenal insufficiency.*
- Teach to sit and stand slowly, and provide assistance as necessary. *Extracellular fluid volume deficit causes orthostatic hypotension, dizziness, and possible loss of consciousness. These manifestations increase the risk of injury from falls.*

### Risk for Ineffective Therapeutic Regimen Management

Clients with Addison's disease must learn to provide lifelong self-care that involves varied components: medications, diet, and recognizing and responding to responses to stress. Changes in lifestyle are difficult to maintain permanently.

- Teach the effects of illness and treatment. Discuss client and family concerns. *Lack of knowledge about the illness, as well as the possibility of complications from disregarding or altering the treatment, can negatively affect compliance.*

- Include the following in the teaching plan:
  - Self-administration of steroids
  - The importance of carrying at all times an emergency kit containing parenteral cortisone and a syringe/needle
  - Wearing a MedicAlert bracelet that says "Adrenal insufficiency—takes hydrocortisone"
  - Increasing oral fluid intake
  - Maintaining a diet high in sodium and low in potassium
  - The necessity of altering the medication dose when experiencing emotional or physical stressors
  - The importance of continuing health care
    *One of the most important components of caring for the client with Addison's disease is teaching both the client and family to provide care. The length of treatment and the side effects of medications can discourage compliance.*

## Home Care

The client with Addison's disease provides self-care at home. One of the most important components of caring for the client with Addison's disease is teaching both the client and family to provide care. Family stability, an awareness of the serious nature of the disease, and the effectiveness of treatment all promote compliance. The length of treatment and the side effects of medications, however, can discourage compliance. In addition to the information in the teaching topics included with nursing diagnoses and interventions, include the following topics:

- The importance of continuing health care
- Referral to social worker, if appropriate
- Referral to community agencies for continued education and support
- Helpful resources:
  - National Institute of Diabetes and Digestive and Kidney Diseases (Addison's disease)
  - Endocrine Society
  - American Association of Clinical Endocrinologists

# THE CLIENT WITH PHEOCHROMOCYTOMA

**Pheochromocytomas** are tumors of chromaffin tissues in the adrenal medulla. These tumors, which are usually benign, produce catecholamines (epinephrine or norepinephrine) that stimulate the sympathetic nervous system. Although many organs are affected, the most dangerous effects are peripheral vasoconstriction and increased cardiac rate and contractility with resultant paroxysmal hypertension. Systolic blood pressure may rise to 200 to 300 mmHg, the diastolic to 150 to 175 mmHg. Attacks are often precipitated by physical, emotional, or environmental stimuli. This condition is life threatening.

A pheochromocytoma is diagnosed by increased catecholamine levels in the blood or urine, by X-ray studies, and by surgical exploration. Surgical removal of the tumor(s) by adrenalectomy is the treatment of choice.

## Nursing Care Plan
## A Client with Addison's Disease

A 51-year-old unemployed salesman, Mr. Don Sardoff, is brought to the emergency room by his wife, Ellen, at 8 A.M. Mrs. Sardoff tells the emergency room nurse that her husband has not been feeling well for the last week, but that when he got up this morning, he was so weak he couldn't dress himself and didn't know where he was. Mrs. Sardoff also tells the nurse that her husband has been taking a cortisone drug for treatment of his rheumatoid arthritis for the past 2 years, but notes, "We didn't have the money to buy it this month."

### ASSESSMENT

On admission to the emergency room, Mr. Sardoff is dehydrated, with dry oral mucous membranes and tongue, poor skin turgor, and sunken eyeballs. His blood pressure is 94/44, and his pulse is rapid and thready. He is weak, dizzy, and disoriented about time and place. Diagnostic tests reveal the following abnormal findings at 8:30 A.M.:

- EKG: widening QRS complex and increased PR interval
- Sodium: 129 mEq/L (normal range: 135 to 145 mEq/L)
- Glucose: 54 mg/dL (normal range: 70 to 110 mg/dL)
- Potassium: 5.3 mEq/L (normal range: 3.5 to 5 mEq/L)
- Cortisol: 2 mg/dL (normal for A.M.: 5 to 23 mg/dL)

The medical orders for Mr. Sardoff include intravenous administration of 5% dextrose in normal saline ($D_5NS$) at 250 mL/h and hydrocortisone (Solu-Cortef) 200 mg. After the fluids and medication are initiated, Mr. Sardoff is moved to an in-hospital medical bed.

### DIAGNOSIS

- *Deficient fluid volume*, related to hypovolemia secondary to adrenal insufficiency
- *Ineffective tissue perfusion: Peripheral*, related to fluid volume deficit
- *Anxiety*, related to lack of knowledge about the effects and treatment of adrenal insufficiency

### EXPECTED OUTCOMES

- Regain normal fluid balance.

- Regain normal peripheral perfusion with blood pressure within normal range.
- Verbalize knowledge of the causes and effects of adrenal insufficiency.

### PLANNING AND IMPLEMENTATION

- Monitor intake and output closely.
- Take and record weight at the same time daily.
- Monitor blood pressure, pulses, and skin turgor every 2 hours until stable, then 4 times a day.
- Monitor electrolytes, and report abnormal results.
- Discuss a diet that is high in sodium, low in potassium, and has an increased fluid intake (3000 mL per day). Discuss the types of fluids desired and the best times for intake of increased fluids.
- Assist during activity to prevent falls.
- Provide verbal and written instructions, and encourage verbal feedback about the causes and effects of the disease, the effects of medications, the effects of not taking long-term cortisone drugs, the diet, and self-care at home.

### EVALUATION

Following treatment for acute adrenal insufficiency, Mr. Sardoff is no longer dehydrated, and his blood pressure has returned to his normal reading of 132/88. He is alert and oriented, and anxious to learn to care for himself at home. After dietary instructions and teaching for self-care that included his wife, Mr. Sardoff verbalizes an understanding of his illness and the need to take his medication carefully and accurately. A referral is made to a social worker for assistance with costs of medications.

### Critical Thinking in the Nursing Process

1. Adrenal insufficiency is often diagnosed only when the client becomes seriously ill in response to a stressor. Explain why this statement is or is not true.
2. Describe the physical assessments that are found in the severely dehydrated client.
3. Outline a teaching plan for Mr. Sardoff with foods for a high-sodium, low-potassium diet.

See Evaluating Your Response in Appendix C.

# DISORDERS OF THE PITUITARY GLAND

The pituitary gland produces hormones that affect multiple body systems through regulation of endocrine function. Target tissues include the thyroid, adrenal cortex, ovary, uterus, mammary glands, testes, and kidneys. Disorders result from an excess or deficiency of one or more of the pituitary hormones due to a pathologic condition within the gland itself or to hypothalamic dysfunction.

Although disorders of the pituitary cause diverse and serious problems, they are not as common as disorders of other endocrine glands. Hyperpituitarism and hypopituitarism are discussed in this section.

## THE CLIENT WITH DISORDERS OF THE ANTERIOR PITUITARY GLAND

Hyperfunction of the anterior pituitary gland, characterized by excess production and secretion of one or more trophic hormones, is usually the result of a pituitary tumor or pituitary hyperplasia. The most common cause of hyperpituitarism is a benign adenoma. The manifestations result from an excess of growth hormone (GH), prolactin (PRL), or ACTH.

Hypofunction of the anterior pituitary gland results in a deficiency of one or more of the gland's hormones. Conditions causing hypopituitarism include pituitary tumors, surgical removal of the pituitary gland, radiation, and pituitary infarction, infection, or trauma.

## PATHOPHYSIOLOGY AND MANIFESTATIONS

Growth hormone (also called somatotropin) is produced by cells in the anterior pituitary throughout life. GH is necessary for growth and also contributes to metabolic regulation. GH stimulates all aspects of cartilage growth, and one of its major effects is to stimulate the growth of the epiphyseal cartilage plates of long bones. In addition, other body tissues respond to the metabolic effect of GH with increases in bone width and the growth of visceral and endocrine organs, skeletal and cardiac muscle, skin, and connective tissue. Gigantism and acromegaly (discussed below) result from overstimulation. Growth retardation and short stature result from deficient production of GH.

Hypersecretion of PRL affects reproductive and sexual function. Women may have irregular or absent menses, difficulty in becoming pregnant, and decreased libido. Men may be impotent and have decreased libido. PRL deficiency in postpartal women causes a failure to lactate. An excess secretion of ACTH overstimulates the adrenal cortex, which in turn increases secretion of adrenal hormones. The result is Cushing's syndrome. A deficit of TSH causes hypothyroidism.

## Gigantism

**Gigantism** occurs when GH hypersecretion begins before puberty and the closure of the epiphyseal plates. The person becomes abnormally tall, often exceeding 7 ft (213 cm) in height, but body proportions are relatively normal. Most often the result of a tumor, the condition is rare today as a result of improved diagnosis and treatment.

## Acromegaly

**Acromegaly,** which literally means "enlarged extremities," occurs when sustained GH hypersecretion begins during adulthood, most commonly because of pituitary tumors. As a result of constant stimulation, bone and connective tissue continue to grow. The forehead enlarges, the maxilla lengthens, the tongue enlarges, and the voice deepens (Figure 17–4 ■). Overgrowth of bone and soft tissue in the hands and feet causes clients to buy increasingly larger rings, gloves, and shoes.

Other manifestations include peripheral nerve damage from entrapment of nerves, headache, hypertension, congestive heart failure, seizures, and visual disturbances. Impaired glucose tolerance and diabetes may also occur.

## COLLABORATIVE CARE

Acromegaly is treated by surgical removal or irradiation of the pituitary tumor. A transphenoidal or transfrontal surgical procedure is most commonly used (see Chapter 42).

## NURSING CARE

Clients with anterior pituitary disorders require interventions to help in coping with physical and emotional changes, as well as to prevent complications involving other organs and functions of the endocrine system. Nursing care for the client having cranial surgery is discussed in Chapter 42.

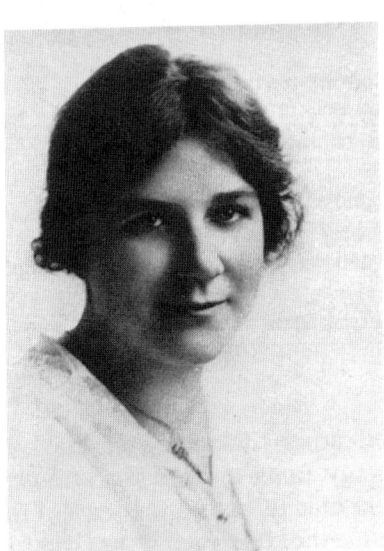 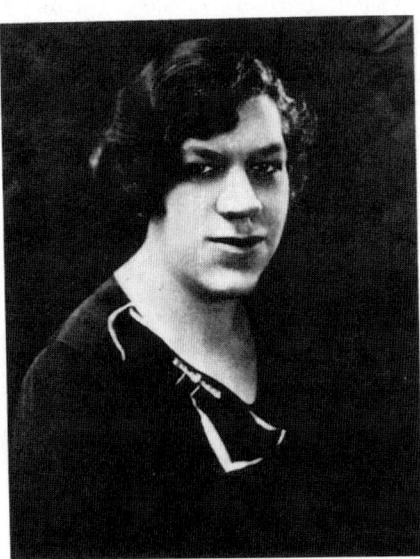 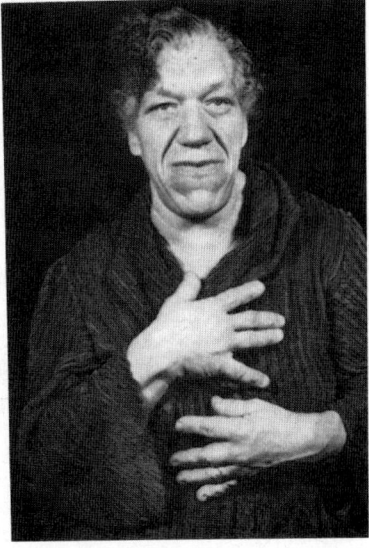

**Figure 17–4** ■ Manifestations of acromegaly. Progressive alterations in facial appearance include enlargement of the cheekbones and jaw along with thickening of soft-tissue structures such as the nose, lips, cheeks and the flesh above the brows.

*Courtesy of Clinical Pathological Conference, American Journal of Medicine.*

## THE CLIENT WITH DISORDERS OF THE POSTERIOR PITUITARY GLAND

Disorders of the posterior pituitary are related primarily to excessive or deficient antidiuretic hormone (ADH) secretion. The disorders discussed here are the syndrome of inappropriate ADH secretion and diabetes insipidus.

## PATHOPHYSIOLOGY AND MANIFESTATIONS

Antidiuretic hormone is secreted in response to serum osmolality, which is monitored by osmoreceptors in the hypothalamus. When a condition of hyperosmolality occurs, ADH secretion increases, and renal water is reabsorbed. Hypo-osmolality causes the suppression of ADH, and renal water excretion increases.

### Syndrome of Inappropriate ADH Secretion

The **syndrome of inappropriate ADH secretion (SIADH)** is characterized by high levels of ADH in the absence of serum hypo-osmolality. This disorder is most often caused by the ectopic production of ADH by malignant tumors (e.g., oat cell carcinoma of the lung, pancreatic carcinoma, leukemia, and Hodgkin's disease). A transient form may follow a head injury, pituitary surgery, or the use of medications such as barbiturates, anesthetics, or diuretics.

Manifestations of SIADH occur as a result of water retention, hyponatremia, and serum hypo-osmolality. Blood volume expands, but the plasma is diluted. Aldosterone is suppressed; as a result, renal excretion of sodium increases. Water moves from the hypotonic plasma and the interstitial spaces into the cells.

Manifestations of SIADH (see Chapter 5 ) are usually nonspecific but are related to hyponatremia and water intoxication. Brain cells swell, causing neurologic symptoms: headache, changes in level of consciousness, muscle twitches, and seizures. Usually no edema is present, because water is distributed between the intracellular and extracellular spaces.

### Diabetes Insipidus

**Diabetes insipidus** is the result of ADH insufficiency. The two types are as follows:

- *Neurogenic diabetes insipidus* can either result from a disruption of the hypothalamus and pituitary gland (as from trauma, irradiation, or cranial surgery) or be idiopathic.
- *Nephrogenic diabetes insipidus* is a disorder in which the renal tubules are not sensitive to ADH. This may be familial in origin or the result of renal failure.

Diabetes insipidus may result from brain tumors or infections, pituitary surgery, cerebral vascular accidents, and renal and organ failure. It is also a complication of closed-head trauma with increased intracranial pressure.

A deficit of ADH causes excretion of large amounts of dilute urine (*polyuria*), in some instances as much as 12 L per day. The client has extreme thirst and drinks large volumes of water (*polydipsia*). If unable to replace the water loss, the client becomes dehydrated and hypernatremic. Even though hyperosmolality is present, the urine is dilute and has a low specific gravity.

If this disorder is caused by cerebral injury, symptoms commonly appear 3 to 6 days after the initial injury and last for 7 to 10 days. If the increased intracranial pressure is relieved, symptoms of diabetes insipidus usually disappear. However, diabetes insipidus may also be a chronic illness requiring lifelong treatment and care.

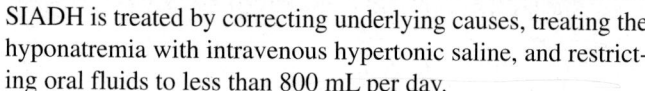

## COLLABORATIVE CARE

SIADH is treated by correcting underlying causes, treating the hyponatremia with intravenous hypertonic saline, and restricting oral fluids to less than 800 mL per day.

Diabetes insipidus is also treated by correcting underlying causes, if possible. Other medical interventions include administering intravenous hypotonic fluids, increasing oral fluids, and replacing ADH hormone. Desmopressin acetate, administered intranasally, orally, or parenterally, is the treatment of choice (Tierney et al., 2001).

## NURSING CARE

Nursing care for the client with SIADH and diabetes insipidus focuses on client problems with fluid and electrolyte balance, as discussed in Chapter 5.

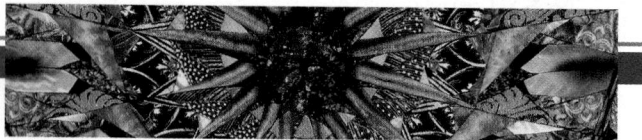

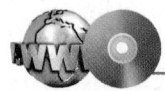

## EXPLORE MediaLink

NCLEX review questions, case studies, care plan activities, MediaLink applications, and other interactive resources for this chapter can be found on the Companion Website at www.prenhall.com/lemone.

Click on Chapter 17 to select the activities for this chapter. For animations, video clips, more NCLEX review questions, and an audio glossary, access the Student CD-ROM accompanying this textbook.

# TEST YOURSELF

1. Graves' disease, the most common cause of hyperthyroidism, is categorized as what type of disorder?

   a. Immune
   b. Infectious
   c. Allergic
   d. Genetic

2. What principle supports the treatment of hyperthyroidism with radioactive iodine?

   a. Radioactive iodine reduces the vascularity of the thyroid gland
   b. Doses of radioactive iodine are too small to be hazardous to other body parts
   c. The thyroid gland takes up iodine in any form
   d. Irradiation of the thyroid gland decreases the risk of hypothyroidism

3. You assess a client with newly diagnosed hypothyroidism as having an enlarged thyroid gland (goiter). What physiologic process causes this enlargement?

   a. An excess of TH stimulates thyroid follicles
   b. An increased dietary iodine intake
   c. A compensatory effort to produce more TH
   d. Tissue hypertrophy in response to increased TH

4. Mrs. Jonah has taken cortisone for her rheumatoid arthritis for several years. What endocrine disorder is she most at risk for developing?

   a. Hyperthyroidism
   b. Hypothyroidism
   c. Acromegaly
   d. Cushing's syndrome

5. Which statement illustrates that the client with Addison's disease understands your teaching?

   a. "I will be sure to stop taking my medications when I have an infection."
   b. "I have purchased an emergency kit and keep it with me all the time."
   c. "I know I should never alter my dose of medications."
   d. "I wonder why I look suntanned all the time."

See Test Yourself answers in Appendix C.

# BIBLIOGRAPHY

American Cancer Society. (2002). *Cancer facts & figures.* New York: American Cancer Society.

Burton, M. (1997). Emergency! Pheochromocytoma. *American Journal of Nursing, 97*(11), 57.

Clayton, L., & Dilley, K. (1998). Cushing's syndrome. *American Journal of Nursing, 98*(7), 40–41.

Cooper, D. S. (Ed.). (2001). *Medical management of thyroid disease.* New York: Marcel Dekker, Inc.

Gumowski, J., & Loughran, M. (1996). Disease of the adrenal gland. *Nursing Clinics of North America, 31*(4), 747–768.

Johnson, M., & Maas, M. (Eds.). (1997). *Nursing outcomes classification (NOC).* St. Louis: Mosby.

Kee, J. (2001). *Handbook of laboratory and diagnostic tests with nursing implications* (4th ed.). Upper Saddle River, NJ: Prentice Hall.

McCloskey, J., & Bulechek, G. (Eds.). (2000). *Iowa intervention project: Nursing interventions classification (NIC)* (3rd ed.). St. Louis: Mosby.

McKenry, L., & Salerno, E. (1998). *Pharmacology in nursing* (20th ed.). St. Louis: Mosby.

McPhee, S., Lingappa, V., Ganong, W., & Lange, J. (2000). *Pathophysiology of disease: An introduction to clinical medicine.* New York: Appleton & Lange.

Mead, M. (2000). Thyroid function tests. *Practice Nurse, 19*(6), 283.

New guidelines for detecting thyroid dysfunction. (2000). *Consultant, 40*(9), 1676.

North American Nursing Diagnosis Association. (2001). *Nursing diagnoses: Definitions & classification 2001–2002.* Philadelphia: NANDA.

O'Donnell, M. (1997). Emergency! Addisonian crisis. *American Journal of Nursing, 97*(3), 41.

Porth, C. (2002). *Pathophysiology: Concepts of altered health states* (6th ed.). Philadelphia: Lippincott.

Romeo, J. (1996). Hyperfunction and hypofunction of the anterior pituitary. *Nursing Clinics of North America, 31*(4), 769–778.

Sabol, V. (2001). Addisonian crisis: This life-threatening condition may be triggered by a variety of stressors. *American Journal of Nursing, 101*(7, Advanced Practice Extra), 24AAA, 24CCC–DDD.

Sache, D. (2001). Acromegaly. *American Journal of Nursing, 101*(11), 69, 71, 73–75, 77.

Schilling, J. (1997). Hyperthyroidism: Diagnosis and management of Graves' disease. *Nurse Practitioner, 22*(6), 72, 74–75, 78.

Shannon, M., Wilson, B., & Stang, C. (2002). *Health professional's drug guide 2002.* Upper Saddle River, NJ: Prentice Hall.

Sheppard, M. (2001). Assessing fluid balance. *Nursing Times, 97*(6 Ntplus), XI–XII.

Terpstra, T., & Terpstra, T. L. (2000). Syndrome of inappropriate antidiuretic hormone secretion: Recognition and management. *MEDSURG Nursing, 9*(2), 61–70.

Thyroid disorders and women's health. (2000). *National women's health report, 22*(5), 1–2, 4–6.

Tierney, L., McPhee, S., & Papadakis, M. (Eds.). (2001). *Current medical diagnosis & treatment* (40th ed.). Stamford, CT: Appleton & Lange.

Tiesinga, L., Dassen, T., & Halfens, R. (1996). Fatigue: A summary of the definitions, dimensions, and indicators. *Nursing Diagnosis, 7*(2), 51–62.

Trotto, N. (1999). Hypothyroidism, hyperthyroidism, hyperparathyroidism. *Patient Care, 33*(14), 186–188, 191, 195–200.

Wartofsky, L. (1998). Q & A. . . Thyroid tests and food. *New Choices: Living Even Better After 50, 38*(1), 79.

Yarbro, C., Frogge, M., Goodman, M., & Broenwald, S. (2001). *Cancer nursing: Principles and practice.* Sudbury, MA: Jones and Bartlett.

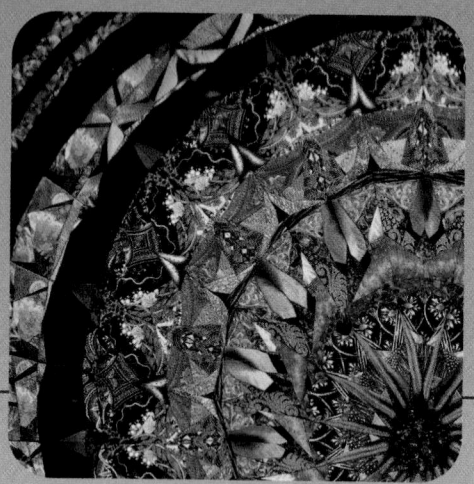

# CHAPTER 18

# Nursing Care of Clients with Diabetes Mellitus

## LEARNING OUTCOMES

After completing this chapter, you will be able to:

- Apply knowledge of normal endocrine anatomy, physiology, and assessments when providing nursing care for clients with diabetes mellitus (see Chapter 16).

- Describe the prevalence and incidence of diabetes mellitus.

- Explain the pathophysiology, risk factors, manifestations, and complications of type 1 and type 2 diabetes mellitus.

- Compare and contrast the manifestations and collaborative care of hypoglycemia, diabetic ketoacidosis (DKA), and hyperosmolar hyperglycemic state (HHS).

- Identify the diagnostic tests used for screening, diagnosis, and monitoring of diabetes mellitus.

- Discuss the nursing implications for insulin and oral hypoglycemic agents used to treat clients with diabetes mellitus.

- Provide accurate information to clients with diabetes mellitus to facilitate self-management of medications, diet planning, exercise, and self-assessment, including foot care.

- Use the nursing process as a framework for providing individualized care to clients with diabetes mellitus.

Diabetes mellitus (DM) is a common chronic disease of adults. However, depending on the type of diabetes and the age of the client, both client needs and nursing care may vary greatly. Consider the following examples.

- Cheryl Draheim is a 45-year-old schoolteacher. She developed diabetes at age 34 after an automobile accident caused severe pancreatic injuries. Cheryl has always been very careful about taking her insulin, following her diet, and exercising regularly. However, she is beginning to notice that her vision is getting worse and that she is having increasing pain in her legs, especially after standing for long periods of time. Cheryl says that sometimes she believes the disease controls her more than she controls it.
- Tom Chang is 53 years old. Early in his 40s, Tom was diagnosed with type 2 diabetes. Although Tom was taught about the disease and the importance of taking his oral medications, following his diet plan, and getting exercise, he rarely did more than take the medication. Five years ago, he was hospitalized for hyperglycemia and started taking insulin. Last year Tom had a stroke, leaving him unable to walk. He has now been admitted to the hospital for treatment of gangrene of the large toe on his left foot.
- Grace Staples is an independent 82-year-old woman who lives alone and happily takes care of her two cats. She is slightly overweight. Last year, during Grace's annual eye examination, eye changes typical for diabetes were found. She was referred to her family doctor, who diagnosed type 2 diabetes and started her on oral medications. Grace sticks to her diet, walks a mile every day, and plans to live to be 100.

As illustrated in these examples, diabetes mellitus is not a single disorder but a group of chronic disorders of the endocrine pancreas, all categorized under a broad diagnostic label. The condition is characterized by inappropriate hyperglycemia caused by a relative or absolute deficiency of insulin or by a cellular resistance to the action of insulin. Of the several classifications of diabetes, this chapter will focus on the two major types, type 1 and type 2. **Type 1 DM** is the result of pancreatic islet cell destruction and a total deficit of circulating insulin; **type 2 DM** results from insulin resistance with a defect in compensatory insulin secretion.

Diabetes mellitus has been recognized as a disease for centuries. Diabetes derives from a Greek word meaning "to siphon," referring to the increased output of urine. Mellitus derives from a Latin word meaning "sweet." The two words together identify the disease as an outpouring of sweet urine. It was not until 1921 that techniques were developed for extracting insulin from pancreatic tissue and for measuring blood glucose. At the same time, researchers discovered that insulin, when injected, produces a dramatic drop in blood glucose. This meant that diabetes was no longer a terminal illness because hyperglycemia could now be controlled. Since that time, oral hypoglycemic drugs, human insulin products, insulin pumps, home blood glucose monitoring, and transplantation of the pancreas or of pancreatic islet or beta cells have advanced the treatment and care of people with diabetes.

Clients with DM face lifelong changes in lifestyle and health status. Nursing care is provided in many settings for the diagnosis and care of the disease and treatment of complications. A major role of the nurse is that of educator in both hospital and community settings.

## INCIDENCE AND PREVALENCE

Approximately 1 million new cases of DM are diagnosed each year in the United States. This chronic illness affects an estimated 17 million people; of that number, 11.1 million have been diagnosed and an estimated 5.9 million are undiagnosed (National Institutes of Health [NIH], 2002, 1999). There is an increased prevalence of diabetes (especially type 2 diabetes) among older adults and in minority populations. See the Focus on Diversity box below.

Diabetes is the sixth leading cause of death by disease in the United States, primarily because of the widespread cardiovascular effects that result in atherosclerosis, coronary artery disease, and stroke. People with diabetes are 2 to 4 times more likely to have heart disease, and 2 to 6 times more likely to have a stroke than people who do not have diabetes. Diabetes is the leading cause of end-stage renal disease (kidney failure), and the major cause of newly diagnosed blindness in people ages 20 to 74. Diabetes also is the most frequent cause of nontraumatic amputations.

Americans with diabetes use a disproportionate share of the nation's health care services. They visit outpatient services and physicians' offices more often than people who do not have the disease, and they require more frequent hospitalizations with longer days of in-hospital treatment. The cost of illness and resulting loss of productivity for people with diabetes exceeds $98 billion per year, according to an estimate by the National Institute for Diabetes and Kidney Disease.

### Focus on Diversity

#### RISK AND INCIDENCE OF DIABETES MELLITUS

- 11.4 million (7.8%) of all non-Hispanic whites have diabetes.
- 2.8 million (13%) of all non-Hispanic African Americans have diabetes, and are 2 times as likely to have diabetes as non-Hispanic whites of similar age. African Americans with type 2 diabetes have higher rates of coronary heart disease, CVA, and end-stage renal disease than do Caucasians with the disease.
- 1.2 million (10.2%) of all Mexican Americans have diabetes, and are 1.9 times as likely to have diabetes as non-Hispanic whites of similar age.
- On average, Hispanic/Latino Americans are about 2 times more likely to have diabetes as non-Hispanic whites of similar age.
- Native Americans are 2.8 times more likely to have diabetes than non-Hispanic whites, and diabetes is especially prevalent in middle-aged and older American Indians. According to the World Health Organization, 50% of the Pima tribe have diabetes, and 90% are diagnosed by age 65 (Burke, 2001).

## PATHOPHYSIOLOGY

### Overview of Endocrine Pancreatic Hormones and Glucose Homeostasis

#### Hormones

The endocrine pancreas produces hormones necessary for the metabolism and cellular utilization of carbohydrates, proteins, and fats. The cells that produce these hormones are clustered in groups of cells called the islets of Langerhans. These islets have three different types of cells:

- Alpha cells produce the hormone *glucagon,* which stimulates the breakdown of glycogen in the liver, the formation of carbohydrates in the liver, and the breakdown of lipids in both the liver and adipose tissue. The primary function of glucagon is to decrease glucose oxidation and to increase blood glucose levels. Through *glycogenolysis* (the breakdown of liver glycogen) and *gluconeogenesis* (the formation of glucose from fats and proteins), glucagon prevents blood glucose from decreasing below a certain level when the body is fasting or in between meals. The action of glucagon is initiated in most people when blood glucose falls below about 70 mg/dL.
- Beta cells secrete the hormone *insulin,* which facilitates the movement of glucose across cell membranes into cells, decreasing blood glucose levels. Insulin prevents the excessive breakdown of glycogen in the liver and in muscle, facilitates lipid formation while inhibiting the breakdown of stored fats, and helps move amino acids into cells for protein synthesis. After secretion by the beta cells, insulin enters the portal circulation, travels directly to the liver, and is then released into the general circulation. Circulating insulin is rapidly bound to receptor sites on peripheral tissues (especially muscle and fat cells) or is destroyed by the liver or kidneys. Insulin release is regulated by blood glucose; it increases when blood glucose levels increase, and it decreases when blood glucose levels decrease. When a person eats food, insulin levels begin to rise in minutes, peak in 30 to 60 minutes, and return to baseline in 2 to 3 hours.
- Delta cells produce *somatostatin,* which is believed to be a neurotransmitter that inhibits the production of both glucagon and insulin.

#### Blood Glucose Homeostasis

All body tissues and organs require a constant supply of glucose; however, not all tissues require insulin for glucose uptake. The brain, liver, intestines, and renal tubules do not require insulin to transfer glucose into their cells. Skeletal muscle, cardiac muscle, and adipose tissue do require insulin for glucose movement into the cells.

Normal blood glucose is maintained in healthy people primarily through the actions of insulin and glucagon. Increased blood glucose levels, amino acids, and fatty acids stimulate pancreatic beta cells to produce insulin. As cells of cardiac muscle, skeletal muscle, and adipose tissue take up glucose, plasma levels of nutrients decrease, suppressing the stimulus to produce insulin. If blood glucose falls, glucagon is released to raise glucose levels. Epinephrine, growth hormone, thyroxine, and glucocorticoids (often referred to as glucose counter-regulatory hormones) also stimulate an increase in glucose in times of hypoglycemia, stress, growth, or increased metabolic demand. The regulation of blood glucose levels by insulin and glucagon is illustrated in Figure 18–1 ■.

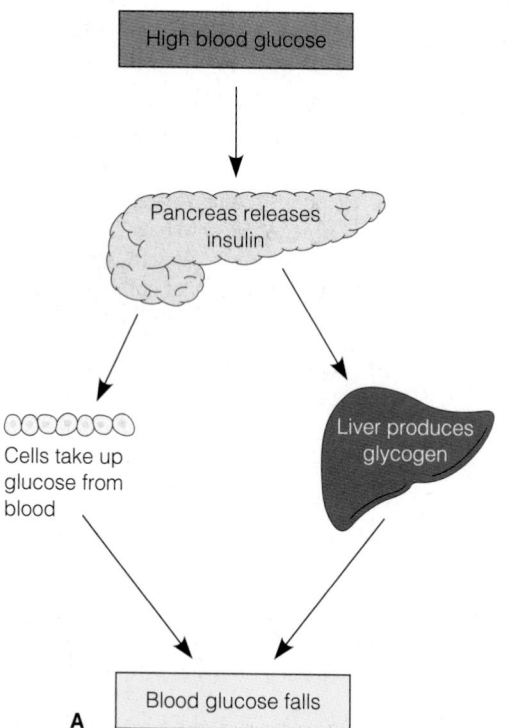

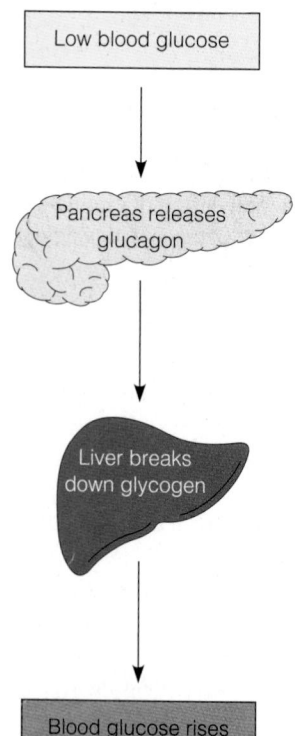

**Figure 18–1 ■** Regulation (homeostasis) of blood glucose levels by insulin and glucagon. *A,* High blood glucose is lowered by insulin release. *B,* Low blood glucose is raised by glucagon release.

## Pathophysiology of Diabetes

DM is a group of metabolic diseases characterized by hyperglycemia resulting from defects in the secretion of insulin, the action of insulin, or both. There are four major types of DM. Type I diabetes (5% to 10% of diagnosed cases) was formerly called juvenile-onset diabetes or insulin-dependent diabetes mellitus (IDDM). Type 2 diabetes (90% to 95% of diagnosed cases) was formerly labeled non-insulin-dependent diabetes mellitus (NIDDM) or adult-onset diabetes. The other major types are gestational diabetes (2% to 5% of all pregnancies) and other specific types of diabetes (1% to 2% of diagnosed cases). The classification and characteristics of the four types are described in Table 18–1.

## Type 1 Diabetes

Type 1 diabetes most often occurs in childhood and adolescence, but it may occur at any age, even in the 80s and 90s. This disorder is characterized by **hyperglycemia** (elevated blood glucose levels), a breakdown of body fats and proteins, and the development of **ketosis** (an accumulation of ketone bodies produced during the oxidation of fatty acids). Type 1 DM is the result of the destruction of the beta cells of the islets of Langerhans in the pancreas. When beta cells are destroyed, insulin is no longer produced. Although type 1 DM may be classified as either an autoimmune or idiopathic disorder, 90% of the cases are immune mediated. The disorder begins with insulinitis, a chronic inflammatory process that occurs in response to the

### TABLE 18–1   Classification and Characteristics of Diabetes

| | Classification | Characteristics |
|---|---|---|
| **I. Type 1 diabetes** | A. Immune-mediated | Beta cells are destroyed, usually leading to absolute insulin deficiency. Markers to the immune destruction of the beta cells include islet cell autoantibodies (ICAs) and insulin autoantibodies (IAAs). The rate of beta cell destruction is variable, usually more rapid in infants and children and slower in adults. Destruction of the beta cells has genetic predispositions and is also related to environmental factors as yet undefined. |
| | B. Idiopathic | Has no known etiologic causes. Most clients are of African or Asian descent. Is strongly inherited. Need for insulin may be intermittent. |
| **II. Type 2 diabetes** | | May range from predominantly insulin resistance with relative insulin deficiency to a predominantly secretory defect with insulin resistance. There is no immune destruction of beta cells. Initially, and in some cases for the entire life, insulin is not necessary. Most people with this form are obese, or have an increased amount of abdominal fat. Risks for development include increasing age, obesity, and a sedentary lifestyle. Occurs more frequently in women who have had gestational diabetes, and in people with lipid disorders or hypertension. There is a strong genetic predisposition. |
| **III. Other specific types** | A. Genetic defects of beta cell | Hyperglycemia occurs at an early age (usually before age 25). This type is referred to as maturity-onset diabetes of the young (MODY). |
| | B. Genetic defects in insulin action | Are genetically determined. Dysfunctions may range from hyperinsulinemia to severe diabetes. |
| | C. Diseases of the exocrine pancreas | Acquired processes causing diabetes include pancreatitis, trauma, infection, pancreatectomy, and pancreatic cancer. Severe forms of cystic fibrosis and hemochromatosis may also damage beta cells and impair insulin secretion. |
| | D. Endocrine disorders | Excess amount of hormones (e.g., growth hormone, cortisol, glucagon, and epinephrine) impair insulin secretion, resulting in diabetes in people with Cushing's syndrome, acromegaly, and pheochromocytoma. |
| | E. Drug or chemical induced | Many drugs impair insulin secretion, precipitating diabetes in people with predisposing insulin resistance. Examples are nicotinic acid, glucocorticoids, thyroid hormone, thiazides, and dilantin. |
| | F. Infections | Certain viruses may cause beta cell destruction, including congenital measles, cytomegalovirus, adenovirus, and mumps. |
| **IV. Gestational diabetes mellitus (GDM)** | | Any degree of glucose intolerance with onset or first recognition during pregnancy. |

autoimmune destruction of islet cells. This process slowly destroys beta cell production of insulin, with the onset of hyperglycemia occurring when 80% to 90% of beta cell function is lost. This process usually occurs over a long preclinical period. It is believed that both alpha-cell and beta-cell functions are abnormal, with a lack of insulin and a relative excess of glucagon resulting in hyperglycemia.

***RISK FACTORS.*** Genetic predisposition plays a role in the development of type 1 DM. Although the risk in the general population ranges from 1 in 400 to 1 in 1000, the child of a person with diabetes has a 1 in 20 to 1 in 50 risk. Genetic markers that determine immune responses—specifically, DR3 and DR4 antigens on chromosome 6 of the human leukocyte antigen (HLA) system—have been found in 95% of people diagnosed with type 1 DM. (HLAs are cell surface proteins, controlled by genes on chromosome 6.) Although the presence of these markers does not guarantee that the person will develop type 1 DM, they do indicate increased susceptibility (Haire-Joshu, 1996).

Environmental factors are believed to trigger the development of type 1 DM. The trigger can be a viral infection (mumps, rubella, or coxsackievirus B4) or a chemical toxin, such as those found in smoked and cured meats. As a result of exposure to the virus or chemical, an abnormal autoimmune response occurs in which antibodies respond to normal islet beta cells as though they were foreign substances, destroying them. The manifestations of type 1 DM appear when approximately 90% of the beta cells are destroyed. However, manifestations may appear at any time during the loss of beta cells if an acute illness or stress increases the demand for insulin beyond the reserves of the damaged cells. The actual cause and exact sequence are not completely understood, but research continues to identify the genetic markers of this disorder and to investigate ways of altering the immune response to prevent or cure type 1 DM.

***MANIFESTATIONS.*** The manifestations of type 1 DM are the result of a lack of insulin to transport glucose across the cell membrane into the cells (Figure 18–2 ■). Glucose molecules accumulate in the circulating blood, resulting in **hyperglycemia.** Hyperglycemia causes serum hyperosmolality, drawing water from the intracellular spaces into the general circulation. The increased blood volume increases renal blood flow, and the hyperglycemia acts as an osmotic diuretic. The resulting osmotic diuresis increases urine output. This condition is called **polyuria.** When the blood glucose level exceeds the renal threshold for glucose—usually about 180 mg/dL—glucose is excreted in the urine, a condition called **glucosuria.** The decrease in intracellular volume and the increased urinary output cause dehydration. The mouth becomes dry and thirst sensors are activated, causing the person to drink increased amounts of fluid (**polydipsia**).

Because glucose cannot enter the cell without insulin, energy production decreases. This decrease in energy stimulates hunger, and the person eats more food (**polyphagia**). Despite increased food intake, the person loses weight as the body loses water and breaks down proteins and fats in an attempt to restore

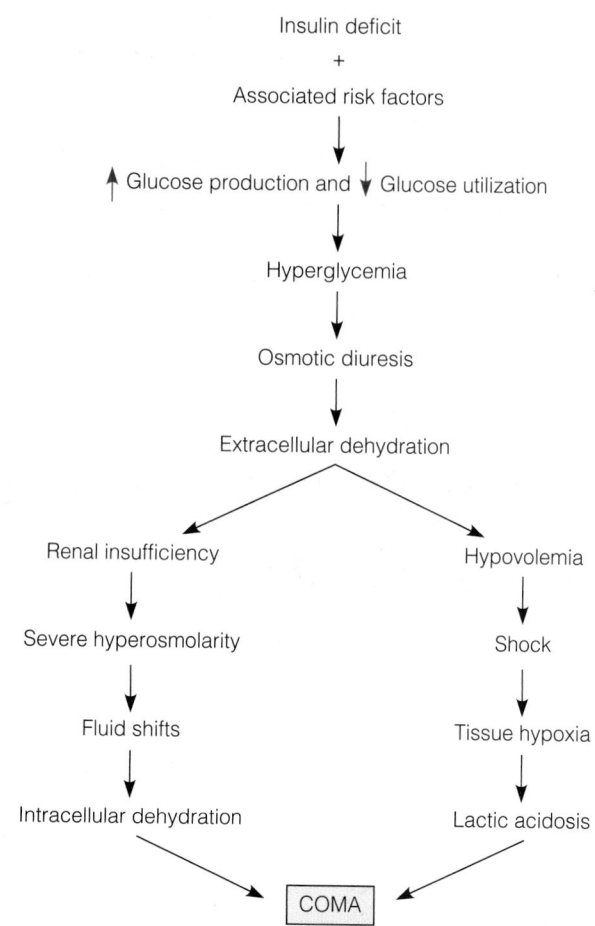

**Figure 18–2** ■ Pathophysiologic results of type 1 DM.

energy sources. Malaise and fatigue accompany the decrease in energy. Blurred vision is also common, resulting from osmotic effects that cause swelling of the lenses of the eyes.

Thus, the classic manifestations are polyuria, polydipsia, and polyphagia, accompanied by weight loss, malaise, and fatigue. Depending on the degree of insulin lack, the manifestations vary from slight to severe. People with type 1 DM require an exogenous source of insulin to maintain life.

***DIABETIC KETOACIDOSIS.*** As the pathophysiology of untreated type 1 DM continues, the insulin deficit causes fat stores to break down, resulting in continued hyperglycemia and mobilization of fatty acids with a subsequent ketosis (see Figure 18–2). **Diabetic ketoacidosis (DKA)** develops when there is an absolute deficiency of insulin and an increase in the insulin counterregulatory hormones. Glucose production by the liver increases, peripheral glucose use decreases, fat mobilization increases, and ketogenesis (ketone formation) is stimulated. Increased glucagon levels activate the gluconeogenic and ketogenic pathways in the liver. In the presence of insulin deficiency, hepatic overproduction of beta-hydroxybutyrate and acetoacetic acids (ketone bodies) causes increased ketone concentrations and an increased release of free fatty acids. As a result of a loss of bicarbonate (which occurs when the ketone is formed), bicarbonate buffering does not occur, and a metabolic acidosis occurs, called DKA. Depression of the central nervous system (CNS) from the accumulation of ketones and the resulting acidosis may cause coma and death if left untreated.

DKA also may occur in a person with diagnosed diabetes when energy requirements increase during physical or emotional stress. Stress states initiate the release of gluconeogenic hormones, resulting in the formation of carbohydrates from protein or fat. The person who is sick, has an infection, or who decreases or omits insulin doses is at a greatly increased risk for developing DKA.

DKA involves four metabolic problems:

- Hyperosmolarity from hyperglycemia and dehydration
- Metabolic acidosis from an accumulation of ketoacids
- Extracellular volume depletion from osmotic diuresis
- Electrolyte imbalances (such as loss of potassium and sodium) from osmotic diuresis

Manifestations of DKA result from severe dehydration and acidosis. These manifestations are summarized in the box below. Laboratory findings include the following:

- Blood glucose levels higher than 250 mg/dL
- Plasma pH less than 7.3
- Plasma bicarbonate less than 15 mEq/L
- Presence of serum ketones
- Presence of urine ketones and glucose
- Abnormal levels of serum sodium, potassium, and chloride

## Type 2 Diabetes

Type 2 DM is a condition of fasting hyperglycemia that occurs despite the availability of endogenous insulin (Porth, 2002). Type 2 DM can occur at any age, but it is usually seen in middle-age and older people. Heredity plays a role in its transmission. Although the exact cause of type 2 DM is unknown, several theories have been suggested. These theories include limited beta-cell response to hyperglycemia, peripheral insulin resistance, and insulin-receptor or postreceptor abnormalities. Whatever the cause, there is sufficient insulin production to prevent the breakdown of fats with resultant ketosis; thus, type 2 DM is characterized as a nonketotic form of diabetes. However, the amount of insulin available is not sufficient to lower blood glucose levels through the uptake of glucose by muscle and fat cells.

A major factor in the development of type 2 DM is cellular resistance to the effect of insulin. This resistance is increased by obesity, inactivity, illnesses, medications, and increasing age. In obesity, insulin has a decreased ability to influence glucose metabolism and uptake by the liver, skeletal muscles, and adipose tissue. Although the exact reason for this is not clear, it is known that weight loss may improve the mechanism responsible for insulin receptor-binding or postreceptor activity (McCance & Huether, 2002).

***RISK FACTORS.*** The major risk factors for type 2 DM are:

- History of diabetes in parents or siblings. Although there is no identified HLA linkage, the children of a person with type 2 DM have a 15% chance of developing type 2 DM and a 30% risk of developing a glucose intolerance (the inability to metabolize carbohydrate normally).
- Obesity, defined as being at least 20% over desired body weight or having a body mass index (BMI) of at least 27 kg/m$^2$. Obesity, especially of the upper body, decreases the number of available insulin receptor sites in cells of skeletal muscles and adipose tissues, a process called *peripheral insulin resistance*. In addition, obesity impairs the ability of the beta cells to release insulin in response to increasing glucose levels.
- Physical inactivity.
- Race/ethnicity (see Box 18–1).
- In women, a history of gestational DM, polycystic ovary syndrome, or delivering a baby weighing more than 9 lb.
- Hypertension (≥130/85 in adults), HDL cholesterol of ≥35 mg/dL and/or a triglyceride level of ≥250 mg/dL.

***MANIFESTATIONS.*** The person with type 2 DM experiences a slow onset of manifestations and is often unaware of the disease until seeking health care for some other problem. The hyperglycemia in type 2 is usually not as severe as in type 1, but similar symptoms occur, especially polyuria and polydipsia. Polyphagia is not often seen, and weight loss is uncommon. Other manifestations are also the result of hyperglycemia: blurred vision, fatigue, paresthesias, and skin infections. If available insulin decreases, especially in times of physical or emotional stress, the person with type 2 DM may develop DKA, but this occurrence is uncommon.

***HYPEROSMOLAR HYPERGLYCEMIC STATE.*** The metabolic problem called **hyperosmolar hyperglycemic state (HHS)** occurs in people who have type 2 DM. HHS is characterized by a plasma osmolarity of 340 mOsm/L or greater (the normal range is 280 to 300 mOsm/L), greatly elevated blood glucose levels (over 600 mg/dL and often 1000 to 2000 mg/dL), and altered levels of consciousness. HHS is a serious, life-threatening medical emergency and has a higher mortality rate than DKA. Mortality is high not only because the metabolic changes are serious but also because people with diabetes are usually older

## Manifestations of Diabetic Ketoacidosis (DKA)

**Dehydration (from hyperglycemia)**
- Thirst
- Warm, dry skin with poor turgor
- Soft eyeballs
- Dry mucous membranes
- Weakness
- Malaise
- Rapid, weak pulse
- Hypotension

**Metabolic Acidosis (from ketosis)**
- Nausea and vomiting
- Ketone (fruity, alcohol-like) breath odor
- Lethargy
- Coma

**Other Manifestations**
- Abdominal pain (cause unknown)
- Kussmaul's respirations (increased rate and depth of respirations, with a longer expiration; a compensatory response to prevent a further decrease in pH)

## BOX 18–1 ■ Factors Associated with Hyperosmolar Hyperglycemic State (HHS)

**Therapeutic Agents**
- Glucocorticoids
- Diuretics
- Beta-adrenergic blocking agents
- Immunosuppressants
- Chlorpromazine
- Diazoxide

**Acute Illness**
- Infection
- Gangrene
- Urinary infection
- Burns
- Gastrointestinal bleeding
- Myocardial infarction
- Pancreatitis
- Stroke

**Therapeutic Procedures**
- Peritoneal dialysis
- Hemodialysis
- Hyperosmolar alimentation (oral or parenteral)
- Surgery

**Chronic Illness**
- Renal disease
- Cardiac disease
- Hypertension
- Previous stroke
- Alcoholism

and have other medical problems that either cause or are caused by HHS. The precipitating factors associated with HHS include infection, therapeutic agents, therapeutic procedures, acute illness, and chronic illness (Box 18–1). The most common precipitating factor is infection. The manifestations of this disorder may be slow to appear, with onset ranging from 24 hours to 2 weeks. The manifestations are initiated by hyperglycemia, which causes increased urine output. With increased output, plasma volume decreases and glomerular filtration rate (GFR) drops. As a result, glucose is retained and water is lost. Glucose and sodium accumulate in the blood and increase serum osmolarity.

Serum hyperosmolarity results in severe dehydration, reducing intracellular water in all tissues, including the brain. The person has dry skin and mucous membranes, extreme thirst, and altered levels of consciousness (progressing from lethargy to coma). Neurologic deficits may include hyperthermia, motor and sensory impairment, positive Babinski's sign, and seizures. Treatment is directed toward correcting fluid and electrolyte imbalances, lowering blood glucose levels with insulin, and treating underlying conditions.

## COMPLICATIONS OF DIABETES

The person with DM, regardless of type, is at increased risk for complications involving many different body systems. Alterations in blood glucose levels, alterations in the cardiovascular system, neuropathies, an increased susceptibility to infection, and periodontal disease are common. In addition, the interaction of several complications can cause problems of the feet. The *Multisystem Effects of Diabetes Mellitus* illustration on the next page shows the progression from cardinal signs to acute and late complications for the client with diabetes. A discussion of each of these complications follows; related collaborative care and nursing care are discussed later in the chapter.

## Alterations in Blood Glucose Levels

The following discussion provides additional information about hyperglycemia and hypoglycemia. Table 18–2 compares DKA, HHS, and hypoglycemia.

### Hyperglycemia

The major problems resulting from hyperglycemia in the person with diabetes are DKA and HHS. Two other problems are the dawn phenomenon and the Somogyi phenomenon.

The **dawn phenomenon** is a rise in blood glucose between 4 A.M. and 8 A.M. that is not a response to hypoglycemia. This condition occurs in people with both type 1 and type 2 DM. The exact cause is unknown but is believed to be related to nocturnal increases in growth hormone, which decreases peripheral uptake of glucose. The **Somogyi phenomena** is a combination of hypoglycemia during the night with a rebound morning rise in blood glucose to hyperglycemic levels. The hyperglycemia stimulates the counterregulatory hormones, which stimulate gluconeogenesis and glycogenolysis and also inhibit peripheral glucose use. This may cause insulin resistance for 12 to 48 hours (McCance & Huether, 2002).

### Hypoglycemia

**Hypoglycemia** (low blood glucose levels) is common in people with type 1 DM and occasionally occurs in people with type 2 DM who are treated with oral hypoglycemic agents. This condition is often called insulin shock, **insulin reaction,** or "the lows" in clients with type 1 DM. Hypoglycemia results primarily from a mismatch between insulin intake (e.g., an error in insulin dose), physical activity, and carbohydrate availability (e.g., omitting a meal). The intake of alcohol and drugs such as chloramphenicol (Chloromycetin), coumadin, monoamine oxidase (MAO) inhibitors, probenecid (Benemid), salicylates, and sulfonamides can also cause hypoglycemia.

The manifestations of hypoglycemia (see below) result from a compensatory autonomic nervous system (ANS) response and from impaired cerebral function due to a decrease in glucose available for use by the brain. The manifestations vary, particularly in older adults. The onset is sudden, and blood

## Manifestations of Hypoglycemia

**Manifestations Caused by Responses of the Autonomic Nervous System**
- Hunger
- Nausea
- Anxiety
- Pale, cool skin
- Sweating
- Shakiness
- Irritability
- Rapid pulse
- Hypotension

**Manifestations Caused by Impaired Cerebral Function**
- Strange or unusual feelings
- Headache
- Difficulty in thinking
- Inability to concentrate
- Change in emotional behavior
- Slurred speech
- Blurred vision
- Decreasing levels of consciousness
- Seizures
- Coma

# Multisystem Effects of Diabetes Mellitus

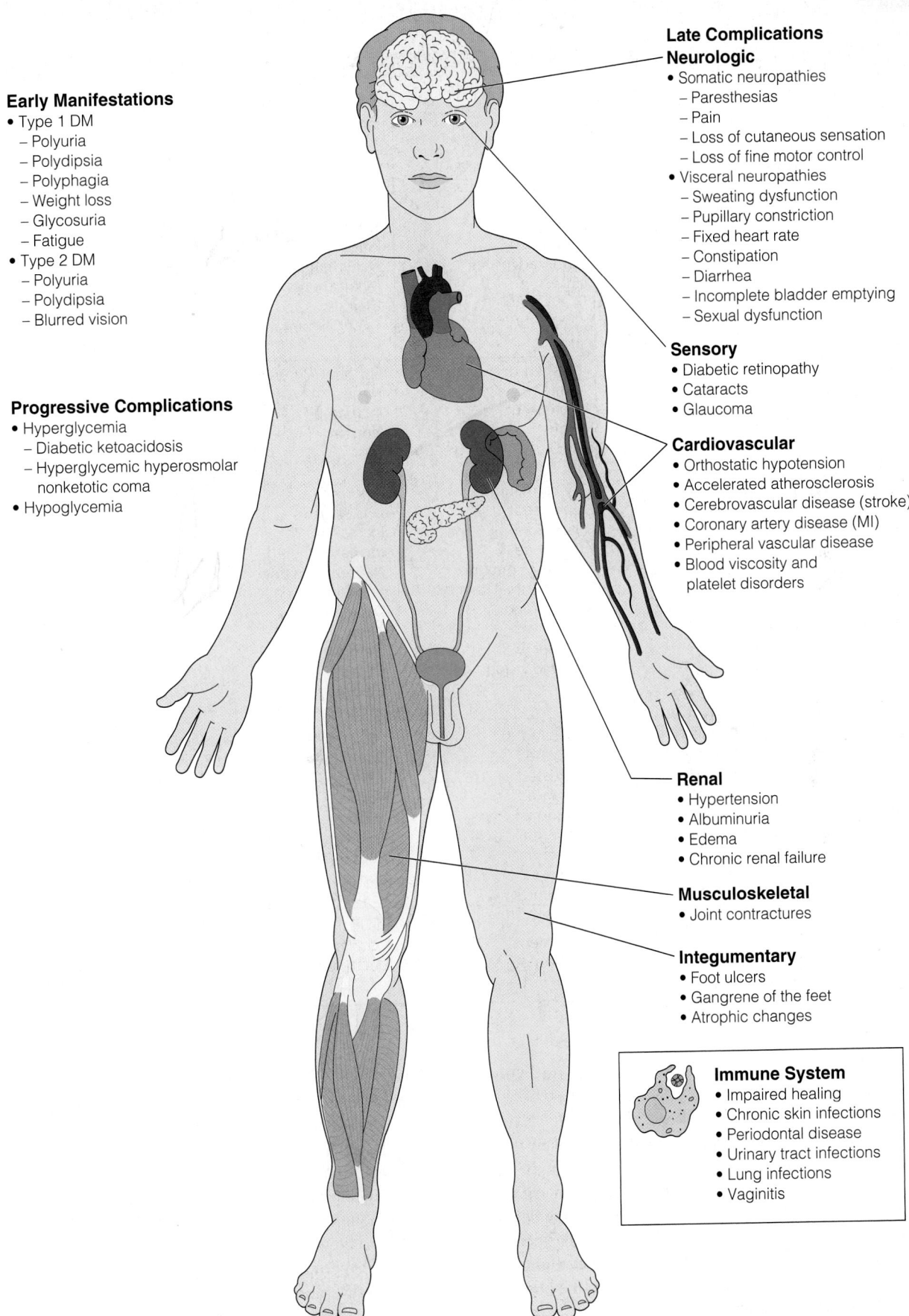

**Early Manifestations**
- Type 1 DM
  - Polyuria
  - Polydipsia
  - Polyphagia
  - Weight loss
  - Glycosuria
  - Fatigue
- Type 2 DM
  - Polyuria
  - Polydipsia
  - Blurred vision

**Progressive Complications**
- Hyperglycemia
  - Diabetic ketoacidosis
  - Hyperglycemic hyperosmolar nonketotic coma
- Hypoglycemia

**Late Complications**

**Neurologic**
- Somatic neuropathies
  - Paresthesias
  - Pain
  - Loss of cutaneous sensation
  - Loss of fine motor control
- Visceral neuropathies
  - Sweating dysfunction
  - Pupillary constriction
  - Fixed heart rate
  - Constipation
  - Diarrhea
  - Incomplete bladder emptying
  - Sexual dysfunction

**Sensory**
- Diabetic retinopathy
- Cataracts
- Glaucoma

**Cardiovascular**
- Orthostatic hypotension
- Accelerated atherosclerosis
- Cerebrovascular disease (stroke)
- Coronary artery disease (MI)
- Peripheral vascular disease
- Blood viscosity and platelet disorders

**Renal**
- Hypertension
- Albuminuria
- Edema
- Chronic renal failure

**Musculoskeletal**
- Joint contractures

**Integumentary**
- Foot ulcers
- Gangrene of the feet
- Atrophic changes

**Immune System**
- Impaired healing
- Chronic skin infections
- Periodontal disease
- Urinary tract infections
- Lung infections
- Vaginitis

TABLE 18-2    DKA, HHS, and Hypoglycemia Compared

| | | DKA | HHS | Hypoglycemia |
|---|---|---|---|---|
| **Diabetes Type** <br> **Onset** <br> **Cause** | | Primary Type 1 <br> Slow <br> ↓ Insulin <br> <br> Infection | Type 2 <br> Slow <br> ↓ Insulin <br> <br> Older age | Both <br> Rapid <br> ↑ Insulin <br> Omitted meal/snack <br> Error in insulin dose |
| **Risk Factors** | | Surgery <br> Trauma <br> Illness <br> Omitted insulin <br> Stress | Surgery <br> Trauma <br> Illness <br> Dehydration <br> Medications <br> Dialysis <br> Hyperalimentation | Surgery <br> Trauma <br> Illness <br> Exercise <br> Medications <br> Lipodystrophy <br> Renal failure <br> Alcohol intake |
| **Assessments** | Skin <br> Perspiration <br> Thirst <br> Breath <br> Vital signs <br><br><br><br> Mental status <br> Thirst <br> Fluid intake <br> Gastrointestinal effects <br><br> Level of consciousness <br> Energy level <br> Other | Flushed; dry; warm <br> None <br> Increased <br> Fruity <br> BP ↓ <br> P ↑ <br> R Kussmaul's <br> Confused <br> Increased <br> Increased <br> Nausea/vomiting; <br>  abdominal pain <br> Decreasing <br> Weak <br> Weight loss <br> Blurred vision | Flushed; dry; warm <br> None <br> Increased <br> Normal <br> BP ↓ <br> P ↑ <br> R normal <br> Lethargic <br> Increased <br> Increased <br> Nausea/vomiting; <br>  abdominal pain <br> Decreasing <br> Weak <br> Weight loss <br> Malaise <br> Extreme thirst <br> Seizures | Pallor; moist; cool <br> Profuse <br> Normal <br> Normal <br> BP ↓ <br> P ↑ <br> R normal <br> Anxious; restless <br> Normal <br> Normal <br> Hunger <br><br> Decreasing <br> Fatigue <br> Headache <br> Altered vision <br> Mood changes <br> Seizures |
| **Laboratory** <br> **Findings** | Blood glucose <br> Plasma ketones <br> Urine glucose <br> Urine ketones <br> Serum potassium <br> Serum sodium <br> Serum chloride <br> Plasma pH <br> Osmolality | >300 mg/dL <br> Increased <br> Increased <br> Increased <br> Abnormal <br> Abnormal <br> Abnormal <br> <7.3 <br> >340 mOsm/L | >600 mg/dL <br> Normal <br> Increased <br> Normal <br> Abnormal <br> Abnormal <br> Abnormal <br> Normal <br> >340 mOsm/L | <50 mg/dL <br> Normal <br> Normal <br> Normal <br> Normal <br> Normal <br> Normal <br> Normal <br> Normal |
| **Treatment** | | Insulin <br> Treatment <br> Intravenous fluids <br> Electrolytes | Insulin <br> Intravenous fluids <br> Electrolytes | Glucagon <br> Rapid-acting carbohydrate <br> Intravenous solution of 50% <br>  glucose |

glucose is usually less than 45 to 60 mg/dL. Severe hypoglycemia may cause death.

People who have type 1 DM for 4 or 5 years fail to secrete glucagon in response to a decrease in blood glucose. They then depend on epinephrine to serve as a counterregulatory response to hypoglycemia. However, this compensatory response can become absent or blunted. The person then develops a syndrome called *hypoglycemia unawareness*. The person does not experience symptoms of hypoglycemia, even though it is present. Because treatment is not initiated in the absence of symptoms, the person is likely to have episodes of severe hypoglycemia.

## Alterations in the Cardiovascular System

The macrocirculation (large blood vessels) in people with diabetes undergoes changes due to atherosclerosis; abnormalities in platelets, red blood cells, and clotting factors; and changes in arterial walls. It has been established that atherosclerosis has an increased incidence and earlier age of onset in people with diabetes (although the reason is unknown). Other risk factors that contribute to the development of macrovascular disease of diabetes are hypertension, hyperlipidemia, cigarette smoking, and obesity. Alterations in the vascular system increase the risk of the long-term complications of coronary artery disease, cerebral vascular disease, and peripheral vascular disease.

Alterations in the microcirculation in the person with diabetes involve structural defects in the basement membrane of smaller blood vessels and capillaries. (The basement membrane is the structure that supports and serves as the boundary around the space occupied by epithelial cells.) These defects cause the capillary basement membrane to thicken, eventually resulting in decreased tissue perfusion. Changes in basement membranes are believed to be due to one or more of the following: the presence of increased amounts of sorbitol (a substance formed as an intermediate step in the conversion of glucose to fructose), the formation of abnormal glycoproteins, or problems in the release of oxygen from hemoglobin (Porth, 2002). The effects of alterations in the microcirculation affect all body tissues but are seen primarily in the eyes and the kidneys.

### Coronary Artery Disease

Coronary artery disease is a major risk factor in the development of myocardial infarction in people with diabetes, especially in the middle to older adult with type 2 DM. Coronary artery disease is the most common cause of death in people with diabetes, accounting for 40% to 60% of all cases of mortality (Haire-Joshu, 1996). People with diabetes who have myocardial infarction are more prone to develop congestive heart failure as a complication of the infarction and are also less likely to survive in the period immediately following the infarction. (Myocardial infarction is fully discussed in Chapter 29.) ⊖⊃

### Hypertension

Hypertension (blood pressure ≥140/90 mmHg) is a common complication of DM. It affects 20% to 60% of all people with diabetes, and is a major risk factor for cardiovascular disease and microvascular complications such as retinopathy and nephropathy. Hypertension may be reduced by weight loss, exercise, and decreasing sodium intake and alcohol consumption. If these methods are not effective, treatment with antihypertensive medications is necessary.

### Stroke (Cerebrovascular Accident)

People with diabetes, especially older adults with type 2 DM, are 2 to 6 times more likely to have a stroke. Although the exact relationship between diabetes and cerebral vascular disease is unknown, hypertension (a risk factor for stroke) is a common health problem in those who have diabetes. In addition, atherosclerosis of the cerebral vessels develops at an earlier age and is more extensive in people with diabetes (Porth, 1998).

The manifestations of impaired cerebral circulation (see Chapter 41 ⊖⊃ ) are often similar to those of hypoglycemia or HHS: blurred vision, slurred speech, weakness, and dizziness. People with these manifestations have potentially life-threatening health problems and require constant medical attention.

### Peripheral Vascular Disease

Peripheral vascular disease of the lower extremities accompanies both types of DM, but the incidence is greater in people with type 2 DM. Atherosclerosis of vessels in the legs of people with diabetes begins at an earlier age, advances more rap-

idly, and is equally common in both men and women. Impaired peripheral vascular circulation leads to peripheral vascular insufficiency with intermittent claudication (pain) in the lower legs and ulcerations of the feet. Occlusion and thrombosis of large vessels and small arteries and arterioles, as well as alterations in neurologic function and infection, result in gangrene (necrosis, or the death of tissue). Gangrene from diabetes is the most common cause of nontraumatic amputations of the lower leg. In people with diabetes, dry gangrene is most common, manifested by cold, dry, shriveled, and black tissues of the toes and feet. The gangrene usually begins in the toes and moves proximally into the foot.

### Diabetic Retinopathy

**Diabetic retinopathy** is the name for the changes in the retina that occur in the person with diabetes. The retinal capillary structure undergoes alterations in blood flow, leading to retinal ischemia and a breakdown in the blood-retinal barrier. Diabetic retinopathy is the leading cause of blindness in people between ages 25 and 74. Retinopathy has three stages:

- *Stage I:* Nonproliferative retinopathy. Dilated veins, microaneurysms, edema of the macula, and the presence of exudates characterize this stage.
- *Stage II:* Preproliferative retinopathy. Retinal ischemia causes infarcts of the nerve fiber layer, with characteristic "cotton wool" patches on the retina. Shunts form between occluded and patent vessels.
- *Stage III:* Proliferative retinopathy. As fibrous tissue and new vessels form in the retina or optic disc, traction on the vitreous humor may cause hemorrhage or retinal detachment.

After 20 years of diabetes, almost all clients with type 1 DM and more than 60% of clients with type 2 DM will have some degree of retinopathy (American Diabetes Association [ADA], 2002). If exudate, edema, hemorrhage, or ischemia occurs near the fovea, the person experiences visual impairment at any stage. In addition, the person with diabetes is at increased risk for developing cataracts (opacity of the lens) as a result of increased glucose levels within the lens itself. Screening for retinopathy is important, as laser photocoagulation surgery has proven beneficial in preventing loss of vision.

### Diabetic Nephropathy

**Diabetic nephropathy** is a disease of the kidneys characterized by the presence of albumin in the urine, hypertension, edema, and progressive renal insufficiency. This disorder is the most common cause of renal failure requiring dialysis or transplantation in the United States. Nephropathy occurs in 20% to 40% of people with diabetes (ADA, 2002).

Despite research, the exact pathologic origin of diabetic nephropathy is unknown; it has been established, however, that thickening of the basement membrane of the glomeruli eventually impairs renal function. It is suggested that an increased intracellular concentration of glucose supports the formation of abnormal glycoproteins in the basement membrane. The accumulation of these large proteins stimulates glomerulosclerosis (fibrosis of the glomerular tissue). Glomerulosclerosis severely impairs the filtering function of the glomerulus, and protein is lost in the urine. *Kimmelstiel-Wilson syndrome* is a type of glomerulosclerosis found only in people with diabetes. In advanced nephropathy, tubular atrophy occurs, and end-stage renal disease results. (Renal failure is discussed in Chapter 27.) 🔗

The first indication of nephropathy is **microalbuminuria,** a low but abnormal level of albumin in the urine. Without specific interventions, people with type 1 DM with sustained microalbuminuria will develop overt nephropathy, accompanied by hypertension, over a period of 10 to 15 years. People with type 2 DM often have microalbuminuria and overt nephropathy shortly after diagnosis, because the diabetes has often been present but undiagnosed for many years. Because the hypertension accelerates the progress of diabetic nephropathy, aggressive antihypertensive management should be instituted. Management includes control of hypertension with ACE inhibitors such as captopril (Capoten), weight loss, reduced salt intake, and exercise.

## Alterations in the Peripheral and Autonomic Nervous Systems

Peripheral and visceral neuropathies are disorders of the peripheral nerves and the autonomic nervous system. In people with diabetes, these disorders are often called **diabetic neuropathies.** The etiology of diabetic neuropathies involves (1) a thickening of the walls of the blood vessels that supply nerves, causing a decrease in nutrients; (2) demyelinization of the Schwann cells that surround and insulate nerves, slowing nerve conduction; and (3) the formation and accumulation of sorbitol within the Schwann cells, impairing nerve conduction. The manifestations depend on the locations of the lesions.

### Peripheral Neuropathies

The peripheral neuropathies (also called *somatic neuropathies*) include polyneuropathies and mononeuropathies. *Polyneuropathies,* the most common type of neuropathy associated with diabetes, are bilateral sensory disorders. The manifestations appear first in the toes and feet and progress upward. The fingers and hands may also be involved, but usually only in later stages of diabetes. The manifestations of polyneuropathy depend on the nerve fibers involved.

The person with polyneuropathy commonly has distal paresthesias (a subjective feeling of a change in sensation, such as numbness or tingling); pain described as aching, burning, or shooting; and feelings of cold feet. Other manifestations may include impaired sensations of pain, temperature, light touch, two-point discrimination, and vibration. There is no specific treatment for polyneuropathy.

*Mononeuropathies* are isolated peripheral neuropathies that affect a single nerve. Depending on the nerve involved, manifestations may include the following:

- Palsy of the third cranial (oculomotor) nerve, with headache, eye pain, and an inability to move the eye up, down, or medially
- Radiculopathy, with pain over a dermatome and loss of cutaneous sensation, most often located in the chest

- Diabetic femoral neuropathy, with motor and sensory deficits (pain, weakness, areflexia) in the anterior thigh and medial calf
- Entrapment or compression of the medial nerve at the wrist, resulting in carpal tunnel syndrome with pain and weakness of the hand; the ulnar nerve at the elbow, with weakness and loss of sensation over the palmar surface of the fourth and fifth fingers; and the peroneal nerve at the head of the fibula, with foot drop.

### Visceral Neuropathies

The visceral neuropathies (also called *autonomic neuropathies*) cause various manifestations, depending on the area of the ANS involved. These neuropathies may include the following:

- Sweating dysfunction, with an absence of sweating (*anhydrosis*) on the hands and feet and increased sweating on the face or trunk
- Abnormal pupillary function, most commonly seen as constricted pupils that dilate slowly in the dark
- Cardiovascular dysfunction, resulting in such abnormalities as a fixed cardiac rate that does not change with exercise, postural hypotension, and a failure to increase cardiac output or vascular tone with exercise
- Gastrointestinal dysfunction, with changes in upper gastrointestinal motility (*gastroparesis*) resulting in dysphagia, anorexia, heartburn, nausea, and vomiting and altered blood glucose control. Constipation is one of the most common gastrointestinal symptoms associated with diabetes, possibly a result of hypomotility of the bowel. Diabetic diarrhea is not as common, but it does occur and is often associated with fecal incontinence during sleep due to a defect in internal sphincter function.
- Genitourinary dysfunction, resulting in changes in bladder function and sexual function. Bladder function changes include an inability to empty the bladder completely, loss of sensation of bladder fullness, and an increased risk of urinary tract infections. Sexual dysfunctions in men include ejaculatory changes and impotence. Sexual dysfunctions in women include changes in arousal patterns, vaginal lubrication, and orgasm. Alterations in sexual function in people with diabetes are the result of both neurologic and vascular changes.

## Increased Susceptibility to Infection

The person with diabetes has an increased risk of developing infections. The exact relationship between infection and diabetes is not clear, but many dysfunctions that result from diabetic complications predispose the person to develop an infection. Vascular and neurologic impairments, hyperglycemia, and altered neutrophil function are believed to be responsible (Porth, 2002).

The person with diabetes may have sensory deficits resulting in inattention to trauma, and vascular deficits that decrease circulation to the injured area; as a result, the normal inflammatory response is diminished and healing is slowed. Nephrosclerosis and inadequate bladder emptying with retention of urine predispose the person with diabetes to pyelonephritis and urinary tract infections. Bacterial and fungal infections of the skin, nails, and mucous membranes are common. Tuberculosis is more prevalent in people with diabetes than in the general population.

## Periodontal Disease

Although periodontal disease does not occur more often in people with diabetes, it does progress more rapidly, especially if the diabetes is poorly controlled. It is believed to be caused by microangiopathy, with changes in vascularization of the gums. As a result, gingivitis (inflammation of the gums) and periodontitis (inflammation of the bone underlying the gums) occur.

## Complications Involving the Feet

The high incidence of both amputations and problems with the feet in people with diabetes is the result of angiopathy, neuropathy, and infection. People with diabetes are at high risk for amputation of a lower extremity, with increased risk in those who have had DM for more than 10 years, are male, have poor glucose control, or have cardiovascular, retinal, or renal complications.

Vascular changes in the lower extremities of the person with diabetes result in arteriosclerosis. Diabetes-induced arteriosclerosis tends to occur at an earlier age, occurs equally in men and women, is usually bilateral, and progresses more rapidly. The blood vessels most often affected are located below the knee. Blockages form in the large, medium, and small arteries of the lower legs and feet. Multiple occlusions with decreased blood flow result in the manifestations of peripheral vascular disease (see the box below). Peripheral vascular disease is discussed in Chapter 33. 

Diabetic neuropathy of the foot produces multiple problems. Because the sense of touch and perception of pain is absent, the person with diabetes may have some type of foot trauma without being aware of it. The person thus is at increased risk for trauma to tissues of the feet, leading to ulcer development. Infections commonly occur in traumatized or ulcerated tissue (see Figure 18–3 ■).

Despite the many potential sources of foot trauma in the person with diabetes, the most common are cracks and fissures caused by dry skin or infections such as athlete's foot, blisters caused by improperly fitting shoes, pressure from stockings or

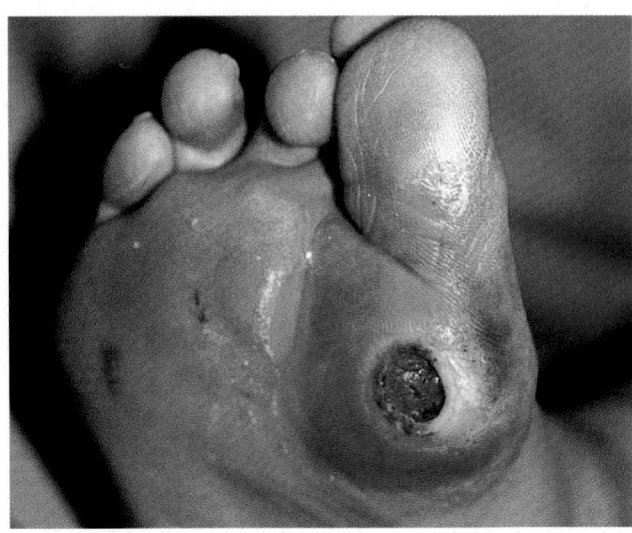

**Figure 18–3 ■** Ulceration following trauma in the foot of the person with diabetes.

*Source: Harry Przekop, Medichrome/The Stock Shop, Inc.*

shoes, ingrown toenails, and direct trauma (cuts, bruises, or burns). It is important to remember that the person with diabetic neuropathy who has lost the perception of pain may not be aware that these injuries have occurred. In addition, when a part of the body loses sensation, the person tends to dissociate from or ignore the part, so that an injury may go unattended for days or weeks. The injury may even be forgotten entirely.

Foot lesions usually begin as a superficial skin ulcer. In time, the ulcer extends deeper into muscles and bone, leading to abscess or osteomyelitis. Gangrene can develop on one or more toes; if untreated, the whole foot eventually becomes gangrenous. (Care of the feet, an essential part of client and family education, is discussed later in the chapter.)

## DIABETES IN THE OLDER ADULT

Although the older adult may have either type 1 or type 2 DM, most have type 2. The National Institute of Diabetes and Kidney Disease estimates that nearly 11% of the U.S. population between the ages of 65 and 74 have diabetes. The prevalence of diabetes becomes greater with age, increasing from 8.2% with diagnosed diabetes in those age 20 years or older to 18.4% for those equal to or older than age 65 (ADA, 2002). It is predicted that the number of older adults with diabetes will continue to increase, because the incidence of the disease increases with age and because the number of people over 65 is increasing.

Although most older adults with diabetes have type 2 DM, the improved survival rates for people with diabetes have resulted in an increased number of older adults with type 1. The picture is complicated by the fact that blood glucose levels increase with age, beginning in the 50s. For this reason, it is more difficult to diagnose diabetes in the older adult; conversely, the older adult may be mistakenly diagnosed with the disease simply for exhibiting essentially normal age-related changes in glucose. The relationship between normal increases in glucose levels and the presence of diabetes is not yet understood.

## Manifestations of Peripheral Vascular Disease

- Loss of hair on lower leg, feet, and toes
- Atrophic skin changes: shininess and thinning
- Cold feet
- Feet and ankles darker than leg
- Dependent rubor, blanching on elevation
- Thick toenails
- Diminished or absent pulses
- Nocturnal pain
- Pain at rest, relieved by standing or walking
- Intermittent claudication
- Patchy areas of gangrene on feet and toes

## TABLE 18–3 Implications for Nursing Care of the Older Adult with Diabetes

| Health Problem/Complication | Implications for Nursing Care |
|---|---|
| Urinary incontinence | Polyuria, a classic manifestation of diabetes, often is ignored. This problem also often leads to social isolation. |
| Decreased thirst | Polydipsia, a classic manifestation of diabetes, often is ignored. This further increases the risk of dehydration and electrolyte imbalances. |
| Decreased hunger and weight loss | Polyphagia, a classic manifestation of diabetes, often is ignored. The aging process, medications, depression, or lack of socialization may decrease hunger. Weight loss may be gradual and go unnoticed. |
| Fatigue | Fatigue is a common symptom of diabetes but may be blamed on increased age. |
| Hypoglycemia | The older adult may have either very mild manifestations or none at all. As a result, hypoglycemia is often ignored until it causes serious effects. |
| Peripheral neuropathy | Manifestations may be thought to be due to arthritis, and over-the-counter drugs often are used to self-medicate. The risk of falls increases, as does the risk of gangrene and amputation. |
| Peripheral vascular disease | May go undetected if the person does not get enough exercise to cause claudication. May also impair abilities to climb stairs and walk. |
| Diabetic retinopathy | May be undetected if the person has cataracts. Diabetic clients also have an increased incidence of cataracts and glaucoma. Deficits in vision threaten independence, mobility, and social interactions. |
| Hypertension | Treatment with diuretics may further impair glucose tolerance and result in electrolyte imbalances. |
| Arthritis | Older adults may believe the pain from arthritis to be more important than the diabetes management. Also, depression from chronic pain as well as inactivity and loss of appetite may interfere with diabetes self-care. |
| Parkinson's disease | The tremors and rigidity of this disease make self-care involving fine and gross motor skills difficult or impossible. |
| Medications | Older adults commonly take more than one type of medication and are at increased risk for problems relating to drug interactions. |

*Note. Adapted from "Diabetes Mellitus and the Older Adult" by M. M. Funnell and J. H. Merritt, pp. 755–830, in D. Haire-Joshu (Ed.), Management of Diabetes Mellitus: Perspectives of Care Across the Lifespan (2nd ed.) 1996, St. Louis: Mosby.*

The older adult with diabetes has multiple, complex health care problems and needs. The normal physiologic changes of aging may mask manifestations of the onset of diabetes and may also increase the potential for complications. Table 18–3 presents common problems in the older adult that make the diagnosis and management of diabetes more difficult. The older adult with diabetes also has a longer recovery period after surgery or serious illness, often requiring insulin to maintain blood glucose levels.

## COLLABORATIVE CARE

The results of a 10-year Diabetes Control and Complications Trial (DCCT), sponsored by the National Institutes of Health (NIH), have significant implications for the management of type 1 DM. People in the study who kept their blood glucose levels close to normal by frequent monitoring, several daily insulin injections, and lifestyle changes that included exercise and a healthier diet reduced by 60% their risk for the development and progression of complications involving the eyes, the kidneys, and the nervous system. Treatment of the client with diabetes focuses on maintaining blood glucose at levels as nearly normal as possible through medications, dietary management, and exercise. Treatment of the acute complications of diabetes (hypoglycemia, DKA, and HHS) is also included in this section.

## Diagnostic Tests

Diagnostic tests are conducted for screening purposes to diagnose diabetes, and ongoing laboratory tests are conducted to evaluate the effectiveness of diabetic management. Definitions of normal blood glucose levels vary in clinical practice, depending on the laboratory that performs the assay.

### Diagnostic Screening

Three diagnostic tests may be used to diagnose DM, and each must be confirmed, on a subsequent day, with one of the three tests. The diagnostic criteria recommended by the ADA (2002) are:

1. Symptoms of diabetes plus causal plasma glucose (PG) concentration >200 mg/dL (11.1 mmol/L). Causal is defined as any time of day without regard to time since last meal.
2. Fasting plasma glucose (FPG) >126 mg/dL (7.0 mmol/L). Fasting is defined as no caloric intake for 8 hours.
3. Two-hour PG >200 mg/dL (11.1 mmol/L) during an oral glucose tolerance test (OGTT). The test should be performed with a glucose load containing the equivalent of 75 anhydrous glucose dissolved in water (see the Nursing Implications box on the next page).

When using these criteria, the following levels are used for the FPG:

- Normal fasting glucose = 110 mg/dL (6.1 mmol/L)

## Nursing Implications for Diagnostic Tests

### Oral Glucose Tolerance Test

#### Preparation of Client

- Have the client eat a diet high in carbohydrates for 3 days before the test.
- If possible, discontinue drugs that may interfere with test results for 3 days before the test:
  a. Corticosteroids
  b. Oral contraceptives
  c. Synthetic estrogens
  d. Phenytoin (Dilantin)
  e. Vitamin C
  f. Aspirin
  g. Thiazide diuretics
  h. Nicotinic acid
- Keep the client NPO except for water for 10 hours before the test.
- The client is given a specified amount of glucose (either 75 g or 100 g) as a lemon-flavor or glucola liquid after fasting blood and urine samples are taken.

- Blood and urine samples are taken after the glucose is ingested at 30 minutes, 1 hour, and 2 hours. In some instances the test may continue for up to 5 hours.
- Observe the client for symptoms of hyperglycemia and hypoglycemia.

#### Client and Family Teaching

- The procedure for the test.
- Foods that are high in carbohydrates.
- For 10 hours before the test and during the test, the following are not allowed: food, tea, coffee, or alcohol. Smoking is not permitted during the test.
- Nausea, weakness, dizziness, and sweating may be experienced during the test; these symptoms often disappear, but report them to the nurse as soon as they occur.
- Limit activity because increased activity may change the test results. (The client may be requested to remain seated during the test.)

---

- Impaired fasting glucose = >110 (6.1 mmol/L) and <126 mg/dL (7.0 mmol/L)
- Diagnosis of diabetes = >126 mg/dL (7.0 mmol/L)

When using these criteria, the following levels are used for the OGTT:

- Normal glucose tolerance = 2-hr PG: <140 mg/dL (7.8 mmol/L)
- Impaired glucose tolerance = 2-hr PG: ≥140 (7.8 mmol/L) and <200 mg/dL (11.1 mmol/L)
- Diagnosis of diabetes = 2-hr PG: ≥200 mg/dL (11.1 mmol/L)

Note that although either method may be used to diagnose diabetes, in a clinical setting the FPG is the recommended screening test for nonpregnant adults (ADA, 2002).

### Diagnostic Tests to Monitor Diabetes Management

The following diagnostic tests may be used to monitor diabetes management.

- *Fasting blood glucose (FBG).* This test is often ordered, especially if the client is experiencing symptoms of hypoglycemia or hyperglycemia. In most people, the normal range is 70 to 110 mg/dL.
- *Glycosylated hemoglobin (c) (A1C).* This test determines the average blood glucose level over approximately the previous 2 to 3 months. When glucose is elevated or control of glucose is erratic, glucose attaches to the hemoglobin molecule and remains attached for the life of the hemoglobin, which is about 120 days. The normal level depends on the type of assay done, but values above 7% to 9% are considered elevated. The ADA recommends that A1C be performed at the initial assessment, and then at regular intervals, individualized to the medical regimen used.

- *Urine glucose and ketone levels.* These are not as accurate in monitoring changes in blood glucose as blood levels. The presence of glucose in the urine indicates hyperglycemia. Most people have a renal threshold for glucose of 180 mg/dL; that is, when the blood glucose exceeds 180 mg/dL, glucose is not reabsorbed by the kidney and spills over into the urine. This number varies highly, however. **Ketonuria** (the presence of ketones in the urine) occurs with the breakdown of fats and is an indicator of DKA; however, fat breakdown and ketonuria also occur in states of less than normal nutrition.
- *Urine test* for the presence of protein as albumin (*albuminuria*). If albuminuria is present, a 24-hour urine test for creatinine clearance is used to detect the early onset of nephropathy.
- *Serum cholesterol and triglyceride levels.* These are indicators of atherosclerosis and an increased risk of cardiovascular impairments. The ADA (2002) recommends treatment goals to lower LDL cholesterol to <100 mg/dL, raise HDL cholesterol to >45 mg/dL, and lower triglycerides to <150 mg/dL.
- *Serum electrolytes.* Levels are measured in clients who have DKA or HHS to determine imbalances.

### Monitoring Blood Glucose

People with diabetes must monitor their condition daily by testing glucose levels. Two types of tests are available. The first type, long used prior to the development of devices to directly measure blood glucose, is urine testing for glucose and ketones. Urine testing is less commonly used today. The second type, direct measurement of blood glucose, is widely used in all types of health care settings and in the home.

### Urine Testing for Ketones and Glucose

Urine testing for glucose and ketones was at one time the only available method for evaluating the management of diabetes.

## Procedure 18–1 — Testing Urine for Ketones and Glucose

### TO TEST THE URINE FOR KETONES

1. Ask the client to void, discard the urine, and drink a full glass of water.
2. Thirty minutes later, collect a urine sample.
3. For Acidtest tablets: Place the tablet on a white paper towel, place 1 drop of urine on the tablet, and wait 30 seconds. If the tablet turns any shade from lavender to deep purple, the test is positive for ketones.

4. For Ketostix: Dip the reagent stick into the urine sample. Wait 15 seconds, and compare the color of the pad at the end of the stick to an accompanying color chart. Purple is indicative of ketones.

### TO TEST THE URINE FOR GLUCOSE

1. Follow the same procedure to collect a urine sample.

2. Dip the reagent stick into the urine sample, and wait the time indicated. Compare the color of the pad on the end of the reagent stick with an accompanying color chart. The glucose is expressed as a percentage (for example, 0.5%, 1%, 2%). Remember that normally no glucose is found in the urine, so the presence of glucose is an abnormal manifestation indicating hyperglycemia.

---

An inexpensive and noninvasive test, it has unpredictable results and cannot be used to detect or measure hypoglycemia. Urine testing is recommended to monitor hyperglycemia and ketoacidosis in people with type 1 DM who have unexplained hyperglycemia during illness or pregnancy. Urine testing may also be used by people who choose not to self-monitor blood glucose by other methods. (See Procedure 18–1.)

### Self-Monitoring of Blood Glucose

Self-monitoring of blood glucose (SMBG) allows the person with diabetes to monitor and achieve metabolic control and decrease the danger of hypoglycemia. The ADA recommends that all clients with diabetes must be taught some method of monitoring glycemic control. The timing of SMBG is highly individualized, depending on the person's diagnosis, general disease control, and physical state. SMBG is recommended three or more times a day for clients with type 1 DM. Clients with type 2 DM should be sufficient to help them reach glucose goals. When adding or modifying therapy, clients with both types of DM should test more often than usual. SMBG is also useful when the person is ill or pregnant, or has symptoms of hypoglycemia or hyperglycemia.

The ADA annually publishes a comprehensive list of currently available blood glucose monitoring machines and strips with approximate prices in *Diabetes Forecast*. Most medical insurance policies cover the cost of these machines.

Following is the equipment needed for SMBG.

- Some type of lancet device to perform a finger-stick for obtaining a drop of blood (such as an Autolet, Penlet, or Soft Touch)
- Chemically impregnated test strips that change color when they come into contact with glucose or that can be read by machine (e.g., Glucostix and Chemstrip bG). The strip may also be read by comparing its color with a color chart on the side of the container or on an insert (Figure 18–4 ■).
- A blood glucose monitor (e.g., the Glucometer, the AccuChek, or the One Touch) if the most accurate measurement is desired or recommended. The manufacturer's instructions must be followed carefully. If the timing of the blood on the

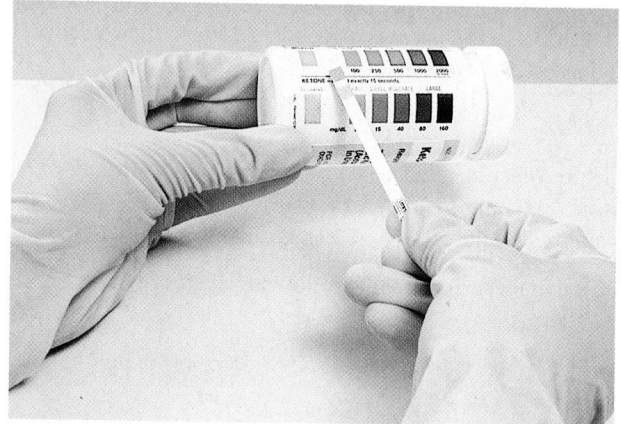

**Figure 18–4** ■ Determination of blood glucose levels by visual reading. The color of the strip is compared with the color chart on the side of the container.

strip is not exact, the test will not be accurate. In addition, the machine must be cleaned according to the manufacturer's directions to ensure accuracy. Monitors that use no-wipe technology improve the accuracy of glucose measurement. Other monitors are computerized and/or include a memory of previous glucose readings to show a pattern of control.

Factors that may alter blood glucose results when testing with a monitor (Passaniza, 2001) are as follows:

- Increased triglyceride levels, which can interfere with the way light is reflected in light reflectance monitors, such as the AccuChek
- Insufficient amounts of blood on the testing strip, outdated strips, and exposure of the strips to air and humidity
- Both increased and decreased hematocrits, with blood glucose values varying as much as 30% for every 10% change in hematocrit
- High altitudes, which cause a decrease in blood oxygen
- High doses of acetaminophen (Tylenol), ascorbic acid (vitamin C), ibuprofen (Motrin, Advil), salicylates (Aspirin), and tetracycline.

## Medications

The pharmacologic treatment for diabetes mellitus depends on the type of diabetes. People with type 1 must have insulin; those with type 2 are usually able to control glucose levels with an oral hypoglycemic medication, but they may require insulin if control is inadequate.

### Insulin

The person with type 1 DM requires a lifelong exogenous source of the insulin hormone to maintain life. Insulin is not a cure for diabetes; rather, it is a means of controlling hyperglycemia. Insulin is also necessary in other situations, such as:

- People with diabetes who are unable to control glucose levels with oral antidiabetic drugs and/or diet. Approximately 40% of people with type 2 diabetes require insulin (NIH, 2002).
- People with diabetes who are experiencing physical stress (such as an infection or surgery) or who are taking corticosteroids.
- Women with gestational diabetes who are unable to control glucose with diet.
- People with DKA or HHS.
- People who are receiving high-calorie tube feedings or parenteral nutrition.

**SOURCES OF INSULIN.** Preparations of insulin are derived from animal (pork pancreas) or synthesized in the laboratory from either an alteration of pork insulin or recombinant DNA technology, using strains of *E. coli* to form a biosynthetic human insulin. Insulin analogs have been developed by modifying the amino acid sequence of the insulin molecule. Although different types are prescribed on an individualized basis, it is standard practice to prescribe human insulin.

**INSULIN PREPARATIONS.** Insulins are available in rapid-acting, short-acting, intermediate-acting, and long-acting preparations. The trade names and times of onset, peak, and duration of action are listed in Table 18–4.

Insulin lispro (Humalog) is a human insulin analog that is derived from genetically altered *E. coli* that includes the gene for insulin lispro. It is classified as a rapid-acting or ultra-short-acting insulin. Compared to regular insulin, insulin lispro has a more rapid onset (<15 minutes), an earlier peak of glucose lowering (30 to 60 minutes), and a shorter duration of activity (3 to 4 hours). This means that lispro should be administered 15 minutes before a meal, rather than 30 to 60 minutes before as recommended for regular insulin. Clients with type 1 DM usually also require concurrent use of a longer-acting insulin product. Lispro is much less likely than regular insulin to cause tissue changes and may lower the risk of nocturnal hypoglycemia in clients with type 1 DM.

Regular insulin is unmodified crystalline insulin, classified as a short-actin insulin. Regular insulin is clear in appearance and can be given by the intravenous route; the other types are suspensions and could be harmful if given by this route. Regular insulin is also used to treat DKA, to initiate treatment for newly diagnosed type 1 DM, and in combination with intermediate-acting insulins to provide better glucose control.

The onset and peak and duration of action of insulin can be changed by adding zinc, acetate buffers, and protamine. Zinc is added to make lente insulin, and zinc and protamine are added to NPH insulin to prolong their action, and they are classified as intermediate- or long-acting insulins. These preparations appear cloudy when properly mixed prior to injection. Protamine and zinc are foreign substances and may cause hypersensitivity reactions.

Insulin glargine (Lantus) is a 24-hour long-acting rDNA human insulin analog that is given subcutaneously once a day at bedtime to treat clients with both type 1 and type 2 diabetes. It has a relatively constant effect (meaning it does not have a peak time of effect). It may be used in combination with intermediate-acting or long-acting insulins.

**CONCENTRATIONS OF INSULIN.** Insulin is dispensed as 100 U/mL (U-100) and 500 U/mL (U-500) in the United States. U-100 is the standard insulin concentration used. U-500 insulin

| TABLE 18–4 | Insulin Preparations | | | |
|---|---|---|---|---|
| **Preparation** | **Name** | **Onset (h)** | **Peak (h)** | **Duration (h)** |
| Rapid acting | Lispro | 0.25 | 1–1.5 | 3–4 |
| Short acting | Regular<br>Regular Humulin (R)<br>Regular Iletin II<br>Velosulin | 0.5–1.0 | 2–3 | 4–6 |
| Intermediate acting | Lente Humulin (L)<br>Lente Iletin II<br>NPH Humulin (N)<br>NPH Iletin II<br>NPH | 2 | 6–8 | 12–16 |
| Long acting | Ultralente (U)<br>Lantus | 2<br>(onset and peak not defined) | 16–20 | 24+<br>24 |
| Combinations | Humulin 50/50<br>Humulin 70/30<br>Novolin 70/30 | 0.5<br>0.5<br>0.5 | 3<br>4–8<br>4–8 | 22–24<br>24<br>24 |

is only used in rare cases of insulin resistance when clients require very large doses. U-500 and the insulin analog lispro are the only insulins that require a prescription.

***INSULIN ADMINISTRATION.***   Nursing implications for administering insulin are outlined in the Medication Administration box below and further discussion follows in the chapter. The considerations for administering insulin include routes of administration, syringe and needle selection, preparing the injection, sites of injection, mixing insulins, and insulin regimens.

### Routes of Administration.
All insulins are given parenterally, although current research is investigating the development of a nasal spray and an oral preparation of insulin. Only regular insulin is given by both subcutaneous and intravenous routes; all others are given only subcutaneously. If the intravenous route is not available, regular insulin may also be administered intramuscularly in an emergency situation.

### Continuous Subcutaneous Insulin Infusion.
Regular insulin is also used in continuous subcutaneous insulin infusion (CSII) devices, often called *insulin pumps* (e.g., Minimed and Disetronic pumps). CSII devices have a small pump that holds a syringe of insulin, connected to a subcutaneous needle by tubing. The pump is about the size of a pager and can be worn on a belt or tucked into a pocket. The needle is placed in the skin, usually in the abdomen. This device delivers a constant amount of programmed insulin throughout each 24-hour period. It also can be used to deliver a bolus of insulin manually (e.g., before meals).

# Medication Administration

## Insulin

### Nursing Responsibilities
- Discard vials of insulin that have been open for several weeks or whose expiration date has passed.
- Refrigerate extra insulin vials not currently in use, but do not freeze them.
- Store insulin in a cool place, and avoid exposure to temperature extremes or sunlight.
- Store compatible mixtures of insulin for no longer than 1 month at room temperature or 3 months at 36° to 46°F (2° to 8°C).
- Discard any vials with discoloration, clumping, granules, or solid deposits on the sides.
- If breakfast is delayed, also delay the administration of rapid-acting insulin.
- Monitor and maintain a record of blood glucose readings 30 minutes before each meal and bedtime (or as prescribed).
- Monitor food intake, and notify the physician if food is not being consumed.
- Monitor electrolytes (especially potassium), blood urea nitrogen (BUN) levels, and creatinine.
- Observe injection sites for manifestations of hypersensitivity, lipodystrophy, and lipoatrophy.
- If symptoms of hypoglycemia occur, confirm by testing blood glucose level, and administer an oral source of a fast-acting carbohydrate, such as juice, milk, or crackers. Hypoglycemic symptoms may vary but commonly include feelings of shakiness, hunger, and/or nervousness accompanied by sweating, tachycardia, or palpitations.
- If symptoms of hyperglycemia occur, confirm by testing blood glucose level, and notify the physician.

### Client and Family Teaching
- The manifestations of diabetes mellitus.
- Self-administration of insulin, with a return demonstration.
  a. Wash hands carefully.
  b. Have a vial of insulin, the insulin syringe with needle, and alcohol pads ready to use.
  c. Remove the cover from the needle.
  d. Fill the syringe with an amount of air equal to the number of units of insulin, and insert the needle into the vial.
  e. Push air into the vial, invert the vial, and withdraw the prescribed units of insulin.
  f. Replace the cover over the needle.
  g. Wipe the selected site with alcohol. The injection is less likely to be painful if the alcohol is allowed to dry.
  h. Pinch up a fold of skin, and insert the needle into the tissue at the recommended angle.
  i. Insert the insulin.
  j. Withdraw the needle; if desired, apply firm pressure to the site for a few seconds.
  k. Recap the needle. Many people with diabetes reuse disposable syringes with attached needles without adverse effects. The primary reason for discarding after several uses is that the needle becomes dull and makes the injection painful.
- Follow instructions for mixing insulins (refer to the box on page 490).
- Always keep an extra vial of insulin available.
- Always have a vial of regular insulin available for emergencies.
- Be aware of the signs of hypersensitivity responses, hypoglycemia, and hyperglycemia.
- Keep candy or a sugar source available at all times to treat hypoglycemia, if it occurs.
- Vision may be blurred during the first 6 to 8 weeks of insulin therapy; this is the result of fluid changes in the eye and should clear up in 8 weeks.
- Avoid alcoholic beverages, which may cause hypoglycemia.
- Follow these guidelines for sick days:
  a. Never omit insulin.
  b. Always monitor blood glucose and/or urine ketones at least every 2 to 4 hours.
  c. Always drink plenty of fluids, try to drink at least one glass of water or other calorie-free, caffeine-free liquid each hour.
  d. Get as much rest as possible.
  e. Contact the physician if there is persistent fever, vomiting, shortness of breath, severe pain in the abdomen, dehydration, loss of vision, chest pain, persistent diarrhea, blood glucose levels above 250, or ketones in the urine.
- Establish a plan for rotating injection sites, and observe closely for changes in tissues such as hardness, dimpling, or sunken areas.

Programming the amount of insulin to be delivered is determined by frequent blood glucose monitoring. Several different pumps are available, and each has rechargeable batteries, a syringe, a programmable computer, and a motor and drive mechanism. The rapid-acting insulin analog lispro is an appropriate insulin for insulin pumps, and short-acting regular insulin may also be used. Lispro is not approved for use in pregnancy (Tierney et al., 2001).

Many people with diabetes believe the pump allows more normal regulation of blood glucose and provides greater lifestyle flexibility. Pumps are as safe as multiple-injection therapy when recommended procedures are followed. A potential complication is an undetected interruption in insulin delivery, which may result in a rapid onset of DKA. The needle site must be kept clean and changed on a regular basis (usually every 2 to 3 days) to prevent inflammation and infection. Although the client who chooses an insulin pump has more to learn, many are very satisfied with having more normal glucose control.

**Syringe and Needle Selection.**    Insulin is administered in sterile, single-use, disposable insulin syringes, calibrated in units per milliliter. This means that in U-100 insulin, there are 100 U of insulin in 1 mL. Syringes for administering U-100 insulin can be purchased in either 0.3 mL (30 U), 0.5 mL (50 U), or 1.0 mL (100 U) size. The advantage of the 0.3 mL and 0.5 mL sizes is that the distance between unit markings is greater, making it easier to measure the dose accurately.

Most insulin syringes are manufactured with the needle permanently attached in a 25 to 27 gauge, 0.5 inch size. If this type of syringe is not available, an insulin syringe and a 25 gauge, 0.5 inch, or 0.75 inch needle should be used.

Other special injection products are available for people with physical handicaps. These products include automatic injectors and jet spray injectors. Prefilled syringes are useful for people who are visually impaired or traveling. Prefilled syringes are stable for up to 30 days if stored in the refrigerator.

**Preparing the Injection.**    The vial of insulin in use may be kept at room temperature for up to 4 weeks. Stored vials should be kept in the refrigerator and brought to room temperature prior to administration.

Regular insulin does not require mixing. If the solution is cloudy or discolored, the vial should be discarded. The other types of insulin must be mixed to disperse the particles evenly throughout the solution. Mix the vial by gently rolling it between the hands; vigorous shaking causes bubble formation and frothing, which makes the dose inaccurate. It is critical that no air bubbles remain in the prepared dose, because even a small bubble can displace several units of insulin.

**Sites of Injection.**    Although in theory any area of the body with subcutaneous tissue may be used for injections of insulin, certain sites are recommended (Figure 18–5 ■). The rate of absorption and peak of action of insulin differs according to the site. The site that allows the most rapid absorption is the abdomen, followed by the deltoid muscle, then the thigh, and then the hip. Because of the rapid absorption, the abdomen is the

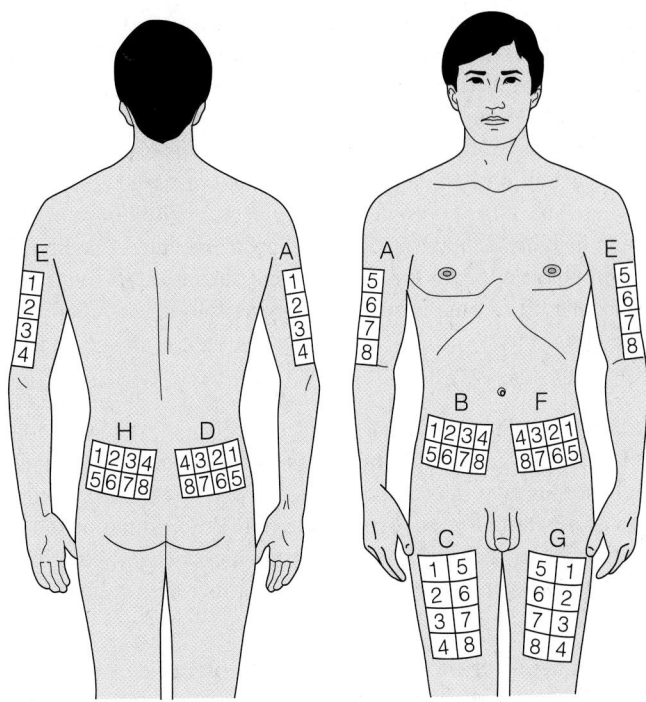

**Figure 18–5 ■** Sites of insulin injection.

recommended site. See Box 18–2 on techniques to minimize painful injections.

When administering insulin, gently pinch a fold of skin and inject the needle at a 90-degree angle. If the person is very thin, a 45-degree angle may be required to avoid injecting into muscle. Routine aspiration to check for blood is not necessary. Do not massage the site after administering the injection, because this may interfere with absorption; pressure, however, may be applied for about 1 minute. Rotation of injection sites is recommended for clients using pork insulin; rotation within sites is recommended for those using human or purified pork insulin. The distance between injections should be about 1 inch (avoiding the area within a 2-inch radius around the umbilicus). Insulin should not be injected into an area to be exercised (such as the thigh before a vigorous walk) or to which heat will be applied; exercise or heat may increase the rate of absorption and cause a more rapid onset and peak of action.

| BOX 18–2 | ■ Techniques to Minimize Painful Injections |
|---|---|

■ Inject insulin that is at room temperature.
■ Make sure no air bubbles remain in the syringe before the injection.
■ Wait until alcohol on the skin completely dries before the injection.
■ Relax muscles in the injection area.
■ Penetrate the skin with the needle quickly.
■ Don't change the direction of the needle during insertion or withdrawal.
■ Don't reuse dull needles.

*Note: Adapted from "Insulin Administration" by the American Diabetes Association, 1998, Diabetes Care, 21 (Supplement 1), 572–575.*

**Lipodystrophy.** Lipodystrophy (hypertrophy of subcutaneous tissue) or **lipoatrophy** (atrophy of subcutaneous tissue) may result if the same injection sites are used repeatedly, especially with pork and beef insulins. The tissues become hardened and have an orange-peel appearance. The use of refrigerated insulin may trigger the development of tissue atrophy or hypertrophy. These problems rarely occur with the use of human insulins. Lipodystrophy and lipoatrophy alter insulin absorption, delaying its onset or retaining the insulin in the tissue for a period of time instead of allowing it to be absorbed into the body. Lipodystrophy usually resolves if the area is unused for a minimum of 6 months.

**Mixing Insulins.** When a person with diabetes requires more than one type of insulin, mixing is recommended to avoid administering two injections per dose. Two different concentrations are administered, because a single dose of intermediate-acting or long-acting insulin rarely provides adequate control of blood glucose levels. The procedure for mixing insulins is described in Box 18–3. Following are some general guidelines.

- Commercially mixed insulins are recommended if the insulin ratio is appropriate for the requirements of the client.
- Regular insulin may be mixed with all other types of insulin; it may be injected immediately after mixing or stored for future use.
- NPH insulin and PZI insulin may be mixed only with regular insulin.

- Lente insulin preparations may be mixed with each other; mixing with regular insulin or with PZI and NPH insulin is not recommended.
- Do not mix human and animal insulins.
- Always withdraw regular insulin first to avoid contaminating the regular insulin with intermediate-acting insulin.

**Insulin Regimens.** The appropriate insulin dosage is individualized by achieving a balance among insulin, diet, and exercise. For most people with diabetes, the timing of insulin action requires two or more injections each day, often a mixture of rapid-acting and intermediate-acting insulins. Timing of the injections depends on blood glucose levels, food consumption, exercise, and types of insulin used. The objective is to avoid daytime hypoglycemia while achieving adequate blood glucose control overnight. Typical insulin regimens are discussed in Table 18–5.

**Hypersensitivity Responses.** When injected, insulin may cause local and systemic hypersensitivity responses. Manifestations of local reactions are a hardening and reddening of the area that develops over several hours. Local reactions result from a contaminant in the insulin and are more likely to occur when less purified insulin products are used.

Systemic reactions occur rapidly and are characterized by widespread red, intensely pruritic welts. Respiratory difficulty may occur if the respiratory system is involved. Systemic responses are due to an allergy to the insulin itself and are most

---

**BOX 18–3   ■   Mixing Insulins: 10 Units of Regular and 20 Units of NPH**

1. Wash hands.
2. Inspect regular insulin for clarity.
3. Gently rotate NPH insulin to mix well.
4. Wipe off the top of both vials with an alcohol pad.
5. Draw 20 U of air into the syringe, and inject air into the NPH vial (Figure A). Withdraw needle.
6. Draw 10 U of air into the syringe, and inject air into the regular vial (Figure B).
7. Invert the vial, and withdraw 10 U of regular insulin (Figure C). Withdraw the needle.
8. Insert the needle into the NPH vial, and carefully withdraw 20 U of NPH insulin (Figure D).
9. Administer the insulin.
10. Wash hands, and properly dispose of the syringe.

A   Injecting air into the NPH vial.

B   Injecting air into the regular insulin vial.

C   Withdrawing regular insulin.

D   Withdrawing NPH insulin.

## TABLE 18-5   Insulin Regimens

| Regimen | Insulin Type* | General Information |
|---|---|---|
| One injection per day | NPH or NPH/R before breakfast | One injection is used to cover all meals (see figure at left). This is a simple regimen, but it is often difficult to control FBG levels, and afternoon hypoglycemia may result from increases in NPH. |
| Two injections per day | NPH or NPH/R before breakfast and dinner | This regimen is the least complex of those aiming to mimic normal pancreatic function; the person must have a fairly rigid schedule of food intake and exercise. |
| Three or four injections per day | R before each meal; NPH at dinner or bedtime | This regimen more closely mimics normal pancreatic function; it allows greater choice in mealtimes and exercise (see figure at left). However, each prandial dose of R must be determined by blood glucose tests. |

*Insulin types are abbreviated as follows: NPH = intermediate acting, R = regular, rapid acting.*

common with beef insulin. The client can be desensitized by administering small doses of purified pork or human insulin, followed by progressively larger doses.

### Oral Hypoglycemic Agents

Oral hypoglycemic agents are used to treat people with type 2 DM. Nursing implications for this category of drugs are discussed in the Medication Administration box on page 492.

### Aspirin Therapy

People with diabetes are up to 4 times more likely to die from cardiovascular disease. It is recommended that a once daily dose of 75 to 325 mg of enteric-coated aspirin be given to re-

duce atherosclerosis in clients with vascular disease or increased cardiovascular risk factors. Aspirin therapy is contraindicated for clients with aspirin allergy, bleeding tendency, recent gastrointestinal bleeding, or active liver disease.

### Diet Therapy

The management of diabetes requires a careful balance between the intake of nutrients, the expenditure of energy, and the dose and timing of insulin or oral antidiabetic agents. Although everyone has the same need for basic nutrition, the person with diabetes must eat a more structured diet to prevent hyperglycemia. The goals for dietary management for adults with

# Medication Administration

## Oral Hypoglycemic Agents

### SULFONYLUREAS

Glimepiride (Amaryl)
Glipizide (Glucotrol, Glucotrol XL)
Glyburide (Diaβeta, Micronase)
Tolazamide (Tolinase)
Tolbutamide (Orinase)

These drugs are used primarily to treat mild, nonketotic type 2 DM in people who are not obese. Glyburide, glipizide, and glimepiride are 100 to 200 times more potent than tolbutamide. These clients cannot control the symptoms by diet alone, but they do not require insulin. The drugs act by stimulating the pancreatic cells to secrete more insulin and by increasing the sensitivity of peripheral tissues to insulin. The most common side effect is hypoglycemia.

### MEGLITINIDES

Repaglinide (Prandin)

This drug lowers blood glucose levels by stimulating release of insulin from the pancreatic islet cells.

### BIGUANIDES

Metformin (Glucophage)

Metformin reduces both the FBG and the degree of postprandial hyperglycemia in clients with type 2 DM. It primarily decreases the overproduction of glucose by the liver, and may also make insulin more effective in peripheral tissues. It is used as an adjunct to diet, especially in clients who are obese or not responding to the sufonylureas.

### ALPHA-GLUCOSIDE INHIBITORS

Acarbose (Precose)
Miglitol (Glyset)

These drugs work locally in the small intestine to slow carbohydrate digestion and delay glucose absorption. As a result, postprandial glucose and glycosylated hemoglobin are better controlled, reducing the risk of long-term complications.

### THIAZOLIDINEDIONES

Rosiglitazone (Avandia)
Pioglitazone (Actos)

This class of drugs acts by sensitizing peripheral tissue to insulin. Both drugs can be used alone or in combination with sulfonylureas, metformin, and insulin.

### D-PHENYLALANINE (AMINO ACID) DERIVATIVE

Netaglinide (Starlix)

This is the first in a new class of oral medications for treatment of type 2 diabetes. It stimulates rapid and short insulin secretion from the pancreatic beta cells to decrease spikes in glucose following meals and also reduces the overall blood glucose level.

### Nursing Responsibilities

- Assess clients taking oral hypoglycemic agents closely for the first 7 days to determine therapeutic response.
- Administer the drug with food.
- Teach the client the importance of maintaining a prescribed diet and exercise program.
- Monitor for hypoglycemia if the client is also taking nonsteroidal anti-inflammatory agents (NSAIDs), sulfonamide antibiotics, ranitidine, cimetidine, or beta blockers; these drugs intensify the action of sulfonylureas.
- Monitor for hyperglycemia if the client is also taking calcium channel blockers, oral contraceptives, glucocorticoids, phenothiazines, or thiazide diuretics; these drugs decrease the hypoglycemic responses to sulfonylureas.
- Do not administer these drugs to pregnant or lactating women.
- Assess for side effects: nausea, heartburn, diarrhea, dizziness, fever, headache, jaundice, skin rash, urticaria, photophobia, thrombocytopenia, leukopenia, or anemia.
- If the client is to have a thyroid test, determine whether the drug has been taken; sulfonylureas interfere with the uptake of radioactive iodine.
- Monitor for hypoglycemia with concurrent administration of an oral antidiabetic agent and insulin.
- Temporarily hold metformin for 2 days prior to injection of any radiocontrast agent to avoid potential lactic acidosis if renal failure occurs.
- Closely monitor liver function tests with administration of rosiglitazone and pioglitazone.

### Client and Family Teaching

- Maintain prescribed diet and exercise regimen.
- You may need insulin if you have surgery, trauma, fever, or infection.
- Follow instructions to monitor blood glucose.
- Report illness or side effects to the health care provider.
- Undergo periodic laboratory evaluations as prescribed by your health care provider.
- Avoid alcohol intake, which may cause a reaction involving flushing, palpitations, and nausea.
- The medication interferes with the effectiveness of oral contraceptives; other birth control measures may be required.
- Mild symptoms of hyperglycemia may appear if a different agent is begun.
- Take medications as prescribed; for example, once a day at the same time each day. If you are taking acarbose, take the pill with the first bite of food at breakfast, lunch, and dinner.

---

diabetes, based on guidelines established by the ADA (2002), are as follows:

- Maintain as near normal blood glucose levels as possible by balancing food intake with insulin or oral glucose.
- Achieve optimal serum lipid levels.
- Provide adequate calories to maintain or attain reasonable weights, and to recover from catabolic illness.

- Prevent and treat the acute complications of insulin-treated DM, short-term illnesses, and exercise-related problems; or the long-term complications of diabetes.
- Improve overall health through optimal nutrition, using Dietary Guidelines for Americans and the food guide pyramid (see Chapter 2).

## Carbohydrates

The ADA recommends that carbohydrates should be individualized to the client's needs, with the combination of carbohydrates and monosaturated fats constituting 60% to 70% of the daily diet. Carbohydrates contain 4 kcal per gram. This group of nutrients consists of plant foods (grains, fruits, vegetables), milk, and some dairy products. Carbohydrates can be divided into simple sugars and complex carbohydrates. Despite a long-held belief, research does not support that sugars are more rapidly digested and therefore aggravate hyperglycemia. Fruits and milk have a lower glycemic response than most starches, and the glycemic response of sucrose is similar to that of bread, rice, and potatoes (ADA, 2002)

The use of sucrose as part of the total carbohydrate content in the diet does not impair blood glucose control in people with diabetes. Sucrose and sucrose-containing foods must be substituted for other carbohydrates gram for gram. Dietary fructose (from fruits and vegetables or from fructose-sweetened foods) produces a smaller rise in plasma glucose than sucrose and most starches, so it may offer an advantage as a sweetening agent. However, large amounts of fructose have potentially adverse effects on serum cholesterol and LDL cholesterol, so amounts used should be controlled.

## Protein

The recommended daily protein intake is 15% to 20% of total daily kcal intake. Protein has 4 kcal per gram. Sources of protein should be low in fat, low in saturated fat, and low in cholesterol. Although this amount of protein is much less than that which most people normally consume, it is recommended to help prevent or delay renal complications. To help the client accept the decrease in the amount of protein, the nurse may suggest a less severe restriction at diagnosis with a gradual decrease to take place over a period of years.

## Fats

Dietary fats should be low in saturated fat and cholesterol. Saturated fats should be no higher than 10% of the total kcal allowed per day, with dietary cholesterol less than 300 mg per day. Fat has 9 kcal per gram. Sources of the different types of fat include:

- *Saturated fat.* Sources are animal meats (meat and butter fats, lard, bacon), cocoa butter, coconut oil, palm oil, and hydrogenated oils.
- *Polyunsaturated fat.* Sources are oils of corn, safflower, sunflower, soybean, sesame seed, and cottonseed.
- *Monosaturated fat.* Sources are peanut oil, olive oil, and canola oil.

Limiting fat and cholesterol intake may help prevent or delay the onset of atherosclerosis, a common complication of diabetes.

## Fiber

Dietary fiber may be helpful in treating or preventing constipation and other gastrointestinal disorders, including colon cancer. It also helps provide a feeling of fullness, and large amounts of soluble fiber may be beneficial to serum lipids. Soluble fiber is found in dried beans, oats, barley, and in some vegetables and fruits (e.g., peas, corn, zucchini, cauliflower, broccoli, prunes, pears, apples, bananas, oranges). Insoluble fiber, which is found in wheat, corn, and in some vegetables and fruits (e.g., carrots, brussels sprouts, eggplant, green beans, pears, apples, strawberries), does facilitate intestinal motility and give a feeling of fullness.

The ideal level of fiber has not been determined, but an intake of 20 to 35 g per day is recommended. An increase in fiber may cause nausea, diarrhea or constipation, and increased flatulence, especially if the person does not also increase fluid intake. Fiber in the diet should therefore be increased gradually.

## Sodium

Although the body requires sodium, most people consume much more than is needed each day, especially in processed foods. The recommended daily intake is 1000 mg of sodium per 1000 kcal, not to exceed 3000 mg. The primary concern with sodium is its association with hypertension, a common health problem in people with diabetes. It is suggested that table salt (which is 40% sodium) and processed foods high in sodium be avoided in the diabetes meal plan.

## Sweeteners

The diet plan for people with diabetes restricts the amount of refined sugars. As a result, many people use noncaloric sweeteners and foods or drinks made with noncaloric sweeteners. Commercially produced nonnutritive sweeteners are approved for use by the Food and Drug Administration (FDA). Although questions have been raised about the safety of these substances in laboratory animal studies, they are considered safe for use by humans. Included in this category of sweeteners are saccharin (Sweet & Low), aspartame (Nutrasweet, Equal), and acesulfame potassium (Sunnette). The nonnutritive sweeteners have negligent amounts of or no kilocalories and produce very little or no changes in blood glucose levels.

People with diabetes also use nutritive sweeteners, including fructose, sorbitol, and xylitol. The kcal content of these substances is similar to that of table sugar (sucrose), but they cause less elevation in blood glucose. They are often included in foods labeled as "sugar free." Sorbitol may cause flatulence and diarrhea.

Researchers are continuing to study the safety and effectiveness of the sweeteners. In addition, the FDA recommends that the food industry label products with the amount of each ingredient in milligrams per serving and the number of servings per container. When teaching clients about diet, the nurse should include information about the kilocalorie content of sweeteners and the meaning of such words as sugar free and dietetic on labels.

## Alcohol

Although drinking alcoholic beverages is not encouraged, neither is it totally prohibited for the client with diabetes. Alcohol consumption may potentiate the hypoglycemic effects of insulin and oral agents. The ADA recommends that men with diabetes consume no more than two drinks and women with diabetes no more than one drink per day. In the following list are guidelines for people who include alcohol in their diet plan.

- The signs of intoxication and hypoglycemia are similar; thus, the person with type 1 DM is at increased risk for an insulin reaction.
- Two oral hypoglycemic agents (chlorpropamide and tolbutamide) may interact with the alcohol, causing headache, flushing, and nausea.
- Liqueurs, sweet wines, wine coolers, and sweet mixes contain large amounts of carbohydrate.
- Light beer is the recommended alcoholic drink.
- Alcohol should be consumed with meals and added to the daily food intake. In most instances, the alcohol is substituted for fat in calculating the diet; a drink with 1.5 oz of alcohol is the equivalent of two fat exchanges (90 kcal). (Food exchanges are discussed below.)

## Meal Planning

Several different systems for meal planning are available to the person with diabetes. These systems include a consistent-carbohydrate diabetes meal plan, exchange lists, point systems, food groups, and calorie counting. No matter what system is used, however, it must take into account the person's individualized eating habits, diet history, food values, and special needs. Altering foods and meal patterns are often one of the most difficult parts of diabetes management; careful consideration of individualized preferences enhances compliance with the diet. Although the ADA recommends that a registered dietitian provide the nutrition prescription, nurses must know what is prescribed and be able to reinforce teaching and answer questions.

### THE CONSISTENT-CARBOHYDRATE DIABETES MEAL PLAN.

The consistent-carbohydrate diabetes meal plan, which is replacing the traditional exchange list plan, focuses on carbohydrate content. The client eats a similar amount of carbohydrates at each meal or snack each day, based on an individual diet prescription and the food guide pyramid. Carbohydrates in a meal have the most effect on postprandial (after meals) blood glucose levels. They also determine, to a greater extent than do proteins and fats, insulin requirements before meals. Clients should be taught to count carbohydrates so they can administer 1 unit of regular insulin or insulin lispro for each 10 or 15 g of carbohydrate eaten at a meal. This method provides a better connection between food, medications, and exercise.

### THE EXCHANGE LISTS.

The exchange list diet is based on the person's ideal (or reasonable) weight, activity level, age, and occupation. These factors determine the total kilocalories that the person may consume each day. After the calories have been determined, the proportions of carbohydrates, proteins, and fats are calculated, using guidelines established by the American Diabetes Association and the American Dietetic Association.

The distribution of foods throughout the day is based on exchange lists. The name and quantity of food that make up one exchange (or serving) are listed; standard household measurements are used. One food portion on the list can be substituted ("exchanged") for another with very little difference in calories or amount of carbohydrates, proteins, and fats. The meal plan prescribes how many exchanges are allowed for each food group per meal and snacks.

### DIET PLAN FOR TYPE 1 DIABETES.

Diet and insulin prescription must be integrated for optimal energy metabolism and the prevention of hyperglycemia or hypoglycemia. The goals of the diet plan are to achieve optimal glucose and lipid levels, improve overall health, and maintain reasonable body weight. To meet these goals, the following strategies must be implemented.

- Glucose regulation requires correlating eating patterns with insulin onset and peak of action.
- Meals, snacks, and insulin regimens should be based on the person's lifestyle.
- Meal planning depends on the specific insulin regimen prescribed.
- Snacks are an important consideration in relation to the amount and timing of exercise.
- The diet plan must consider the availability of foods, based on occupational, financial, religious, and ethnic constraints.
- Self-monitoring of blood glucose levels helps the client make adjustments for planned and unplanned changes in routines.

### DIET PLAN FOR TYPE 2 DIABETES.

The goals of the diet plan are to improve blood glucose levels, improve overall health, prevent or delay complications, and attain or maintain reasonable body weight. Because the majority of these clients are overweight, weight loss is important and facilitates achieving the other goals.

There are no specific guidelines for the type 2 diet, but in addition to decreasing kilocalories, it is recommended that the client consume three meals of equal size, evenly spaced approximately 4 to 5 hours apart, with one or two snacks. The person with type 2 DM should also decrease fat intake. If the exchange list is difficult to use, calorie counting or designing the diet by grams of fat may be more useful.

## Sick-Day Management

When the person with diabetes is sick or has surgery, blood glucose levels increase, even though food intake decreases. The person often mistakenly alters or omits the insulin dose, causing further problems. The guidelines for dietary management during illness focus on preventing dehydration and providing nutrition for promoting recovery. In general, sick-day management includes the following:

- Monitoring blood glucose at least four times a day throughout an illness
- Testing urine for ketones if blood glucose is greater than 240 mg/dL
- Continuing to take the usual insulin dose or oral hypoglycemic agent
- Sipping 8 to 12 oz of fluid each hour
- Substituting easily digested liquids or soft foods if solid foods are not tolerated (The substituted liquids and foods should be carbohydrate equivalents, for example, 1/2 cup sweetened gelatin, 1/2 cup fruit juice, one Popsicle, 1/4 cup sherbet, and 1/2 cup regular soft drink.)
- Calling the health care provider if the client is unable to eat for more than 24 hours or if vomiting and diarrhea last for more than 6 hours.

## Diet Plan for the Older Adult

The majority of older adults have type 2 DM and should follow the general guidelines for that diet plan. However, special considerations for the older adult are important if the diet plan is to be followed, including:

- Dietary likes and dislikes
- Who prepares the meals
- Age-related changes in taste perception
- Dental health
- Transportation to buy foods
- Available income

Other factors to consider in planning the diet for the older adult include the age-related decline in kcal requirements, decline in physical activity due to age and/or chronic illnesses, and the onset or progression of other chronic illnesses. The older adult who is overweight should reduce kcal intake to ensure weight loss, but at the same time, careful monitoring for malnutrition is necessary. It is possible for the older adult to revert to normal glucose tolerance if ideal body weight is regained.

## Exercise

The third component of diabetes management is a regular exercise program. The benefits of exercise are the same for everyone, with or without diabetes: improved physical fitness, improved emotional state, weight control, and improved work capacity. In people with diabetes, exercise increases the uptake of glucose by muscle cells, potentially reducing the need for insulin. Exercise also decreases cholesterol and triglycerides, reducing the risk of cardiovascular disorders. People with diabetes should consult their primary health care provider before beginning or changing an exercise program. The ability to maintain an exercise program is affected by many different factors, including fatigue and glucose levels. It is as important to assess the person's usual lifestyle before establishing an exercise program as it is before planning a diet. Factors to consider include the client's usual exercise habits, living environment, and community programs. The exercise that the person enjoys most is probably the one that he or she will continue throughout life.

All people with diabetes should follow the recommendations of the ADA when exercising: Use proper footwear, inspect the feet daily and after exercise, avoid exercise in extreme heat or cold, and avoid exercise during periods of poor glucose control. The ADA further recommends that people over age 35 have an exercise-stress electrocardiogram prior to beginning an exercise program.

### Type 1 Diabetes

In the person with type 1 DM, glycemic responses to exercise vary according to the type, intensity, and duration of the exercise. Other factors that influence responses include the timing of exercise in relation to meals and insulin injections, and the time of day of the activity. Unless these factors are integrated into the exercise program, the person with type 1 DM has an increased risk of hypoglycemia and hyperglycemia. Following are general guidelines for an exercise program.

- People who have frequent hyperglycemia or hypoglycemia should avoid prolonged exercise until glucose control improves.
- The risk of exercise-induced hypoglycemia is lowest before breakfast, when free-insulin levels tend to be lower than they are before meals later in the day or at bedtime.
- Low-impact aerobic exercises are encouraged.
- Exercise should be moderate and regular; brief, intense exercise tends to cause mild hyperglycemia, and prolonged exercise can lead to hypoglycemia.
- Exercising at a peak insulin action time may lead to hypoglycemia.
- Self-monitoring of blood glucose levels is essential both before and after exercise.
- Food intake may need to be increased to compensate for the activity.
- Fluid intake, especially water, is essential.

Young adults may continue participating in sports with some modifications in diet and insulin dosage. Athletes should begin training slowly, extend activity over a prolonged period, take a carbohydrate source (such as a drink consisting of 5% to 10% carbohydrate) after about 1 hour of exercise, and monitor blood glucose levels for possible adjustments. In addition, a snack should be available after the activity is completed. It may be necessary to omit the usual regular insulin dose prior to an athletic event; even if the athlete is hyperglycemic at the beginning of the event, blood glucose levels will fall to normal after the first 60 to 90 minutes of exercise.

### Type 2 Diabetes

An exercise program for the person with type 2 DM is especially important. The benefits of regular exercise include weight loss in those who are overweight, improved glycemic control, increased well-being, socialization with others, and a reduction of cardiovascular risk factors. A combination of diet, exercise, and weight loss often decreases the need for oral hypoglycemic agents. This decrease is due to an increased sensitivity to insulin, increased kcal expenditure, and increased self-esteem. Regular exercise may prevent type 2 DM in high-risk individuals (ADA, 2002).

Following are general guidelines for an exercise program.

- Before beginning the program, have a medical screening for previously undiagnosed hypertension, neuropathy, retinopathy, nephropathy, and cardiac ischemia.
- Begin the program with mild exercises, and gradually increase intensity and duration.
- Self-monitor blood glucose before and after exercise.
- Exercise at least three times a week or every other day, for at least 20 to 30 minutes.
- Include muscle-strengthening and low-impact aerobic exercises in the program.

## Treatments

### Surgery

Surgical management of diabetes involves replacing or transplanting the pancreas, pancreatic cells, or beta cells. Although it is still in the investigative stage, many researchers believe that transplantation of the tail of the pancreas is the most promising technique for achieving long-term disease control. Islet cell transplantation has had moderate success, and research is continuing. Other research is being conducted in the use of an internally implanted artificial pancreas, or closed-loop artificial beta cell.

Surgery is a stressor that often alters self-management and glycemic control in people with diabetes. In response to stress, levels of catecholamines, cortisol, glucagon, and growth hormones increase, as does insulin resistance. Hyperglycemia occurs, and protein stores are decreased. In addition, diet and activity patterns change, and medication types and dosages vary. As a result, surgical clients who have diabetes are at increased risk for postoperative infection, delayed wound healing, fluid and electrolyte imbalances, hypoglycemia, and DKA.

Preoperatively, all clients should be in the best possible metabolic state. Screening for complications and regular blood glucose monitoring are part of preoperative preparation. Oral hypoglycemic agents may be withheld for 1 or 2 days before surgery, and regular insulin is often administered to the client with type 2 DM during the perioperative period. The client with type 1 DM follows a carefully prescribed insulin regimen individualized to specific needs.

The insulin regimen in the preoperative, intraoperative, and immediate postoperative periods is individualized and may involve any of the following:

- No intermediate- or long-acting insulin is given the day of surgery; regular insulin is given with intravenous glucose.
- Half of the usual intermediate- or long-acting insulin is given before surgery and the remaining half is given in the recovery room.
- The total daily dose of insulin is divided into four equal doses of regular insulin, and one dose is administered subcutaneously every 6 hours. An intravenous solution of 5% dextrose in 0.45% normal saline is administered for fluid replacement, and blood glucose monitoring precedes each insulin dose (Guthrie & Guthrie, 1997).

The surgical procedure should be scheduled for as early as possible in the morning to minimize the length of fasting. If there is no food intake after surgery, intravenous dextrose should be administered, accompanied by subcutaneous regular insulin every 6 hours. The dose can be adjusted to blood glucose levels. Although kcal intake is decreased postoperatively, stress can increase insulin requirements. Glucose control is also affected postoperatively by nausea and vomiting, anorexia, and gastrointestinal suction.

During the postoperative period, the client with type 2 DM may continue to require insulin or may resume oral medications, depending on glucose control. The client with type 1 DM may require reduced insulin as healing progresses and stress diminishes. Regular blood glucose monitoring is essential, as are assessments for hypoglycemia.

## Treatment of Hypoglycemia

***MILD HYPOGLYCEMIA.*** When mild hypoglycemia occurs, immediate treatment is necessary. People experiencing hypoglycemia should take about 15 g of a rapid-acting sugar. This amount of sugar is found, for example, in three glucose tablets, 1/2 cup of fruit juice or regular soda, 8 oz of skim milk, five Life Savers candies, three large marshmallows, or 3 tsp of sugar or honey. Sugar should not be added to fruit juice. Adding sugar to the fruit sugar already in the juice could cause a rapid rise in blood glucose, with persistent hyperglycemia.

If the manifestations continue, the 15/15 rule should be followed: Wait 15 minutes, monitor blood glucose, and, if it is low, eat another 15 g of carbohydrate. This procedure can be repeated until blood glucose levels return to normal (Haire-Joshu, 1996). People with diabetes should have some source of carbohydrate readily available at all times so that hypoglycemic symptoms can be quickly reversed. If hypoglycemia occurs more than two or three times a week, the diabetes management plan should be adjusted.

***SEVERE HYPOGLYCEMIA.*** People with diabetes who have severe hypoglycemia are often hospitalized. The criteria for hospitalization are one or more of the following:

- Blood glucose is less than 50 mg/dL, and the prompt treatment of hypoglycemia has not resulted in recovery of sensorium.
- The client has coma, seizures, or altered behavior.
- The hypoglycemia has been treated, but a responsible adult cannot be with the client for the following 12 hours.
- The hypoglycemia was caused by a sulfonylurea drug.

If the client is conscious and alert, 10 to 15 g of an oral carbohydrate may be given. If the client has altered levels of consciousness, parenteral glucose or glucagon is administered.

Glucose is administered intravenously as a 25% to 50% solution, usually at a rate of 10 mL over 1 minute by intravenous push, followed by intravenous infusion of 5% dextrose in water (D5W) at 5 to 10 g/h (Haire-Joshu, 1996). This is the most rapid method of increasing blood glucose levels.

Glucagon is an antihypoglycemic agent that raises blood glucose by promoting the conversion of hepatic glycogen to glucose. It is used in severe insulin-induced hypoglycemia and may be given in the recommended dose of 1 mg by the subcutaneous, intramuscular, or intravenous route. Glucagon has a short period of action; an oral (if the client is conscious) or intravenous carbohydrate should be administered following the glucagon to prevent a recurrence of hypoglycemia. If the client has been unconscious, glucagon may cause vomiting when consciousness returns.

## Treatment of DKA

DKA requires immediate medical attention. Admission to the hospital is appropriate when the person has a blood glucose of greater than 250 mg/dL, a decreasing pH, and ketones in the urine. If the client is alert and conscious, fluids may be replaced orally. However, alterations in levels of consciousness, vomiting, and acidosis are common, necessitating intravenous fluid replacement. The initial fluid replacement may be accomplished by administering 0.9% saline solution at a rate of 500 to 1000 mL/h. After 2 to 3 hours (or when blood pressure is returning to normal), the administration of 0.45% saline at

## Medication Administration

### Intravenous Insulin

#### General Guidelines

- Regular insulin may be given undiluted directly into the vein or through a Y-tube or three-way stopcock.
- Insulin is usually diluted in 0.9% saline or 0.45% saline solution for infusion.
- The glass or plastic infusion container and plastic tubing may reduce insulin potency by at least 20% and possibly by up to 80% before the insulin reaches the venous system.

#### Nursing Responsibilities

- Monitor blood glucose levels hourly.

- Infuse the insulin solution separately from the hydration solution.
- Flush the intravenous tubing with 50 mL of insulin mixed with normal saline solution to saturate binding sites on the tubing before administering the insulin to the client; this step increases the amount of insulin delivered over the first few hours.
- Do not discontinue the intravenous infusion until subcutaneous administration of insulin is resumed.
- Monitor for manifestations of hypoglycemia.
- Ensure that glucagon is readily available as an antidote for insulin overdose.

---

200 to 500 mL/h may continue for several more hours. When the blood glucose levels reach 250 mg/dL, dextrose is added to prevent rapid decreases in glucose; hypoglycemia could result in fatal cerebral edema.

Regular insulin is used in the management of DKA and may be given by various routes, depending on the severity of the condition. Mild ketosis may be treated with subcutaneous insulin, whereas severe ketosis requires intravenous insulin infusion. Nursing responsibilities for the client receiving intravenous insulin are described in the Medication Administration box above.

The electrolyte imbalance of primary concern is depletion of body stores of potassium. Initially, serum potassium levels may be normal, but they decrease during treatment. In DKA (and from rehydration), the body loses potassium from increased urinary output, acidosis, catabolic state, and vomiting or diarrhea. Potassium replacement is begun early in the course of treatment, usually by adding potassium to the rehydration fluids. Replacement is essential for preventing cardiac dysrhythmias secondary to hypokalemia. Cardiac rhythms and potassium levels must be monitored every 2 to 4 hours.

### Treatment of HHS

HHS is a serious, life-threatening metabolic condition. The client admitted to the intensive care unit for treatment typically manifests blood glucose levels over 700 mg/dL, increased serum osmolarity, and altered levels of consciousness or seizures. Treatment is similar to that of DKA: correcting fluid and electrolyte imbalances and providing insulin to lower hyperglycemia. In general, treatment modalities include the following:

- Establishing and maintaining adequate ventilation
- Correcting shock with adequate intravenous fluids
- Instituting nasogastric suction if comatose to prevent aspiration
- Maintaining fluid volume with intravenous isotonic or colloid solutions
- Administering potassium intravenously to replace losses
- Administering insulin to reduce blood glucose, usually discontinuing administration when blood glucose levels reach 250 mg/dL (Because ketosis is not present, there is no need to continue insulin, as with DKA.)

## NURSING CARE

The responses of the person with diabetes to the illness are often complex and individual, involving multiple body systems. Assessments, planning, and implementation differ for the person with newly diagnosed diabetes, the person with long-term diabetes, and the person with acute complications of diabetes. The plan of care and content of teaching also differ according to the type of diabetes, the person's age and culture, and the person's intellectual, psychological, and social resources. However, nursing care often focuses on teaching the client to manage the illness. The Nursing Research box on the following page describes a study of quality of life in people with diabetes.

### Health Promotion

Health promotion activities primarily focus on preventing the complications of diabetes. The prevention of the disease has not been determined, although it is recommended that all people should prevent or decrease excess weight, follow a sensible and well-balanced diet, and maintain a regular physical exercise program. Blood glucose screening at 3-year intervals beginning at age 45 is recommended for those in the high-risk groups. These same activities, when combined with medications and self-monitoring, are also beneficial in reducing the onset of complications.

### Assessment

The following data are collected through the health history and physical examination (see Chapter 16). ⊙⊙ Further focused assessments are described with nursing interventions below. When assessing the older client, be aware of normal aging changes in all body systems that may alter interpretation of findings.

- Health history: Family history of diabetes; history of hypertension or other cardiovascular problems; history of any change in vision (e.g. blurring) or speech, dizziness, numbness or tingling in hands or feet; pain when walking; frequent voiding; change in weight, appetite, infections, and healing; problems with gastrointestinal function or urination; or altered sexual function

## Nursing Research

### Evidence-Based Practice for Balancing Quality of Life and Living with Diabetes

Adaptation to and management of a chronic illness such as diabetes are simultaneous and interdependent as the person comes to term with the illness, gains support from caregivers, creates relationships with others, and learns about the illness and its management. This study (Paterson et al., 1998) examined 43 published qualitative reports of the experience of living with diabetes to formulate a comparative analysis of findings. Balance emerged as the predominant metaphor of the experience; to achieve balance the person must learn how to manage the illness, know the body, and foster supportive, collaborative relationships. Although control of blood glucose levels may be a goal established by health care professionals, the research reviewed for this study indicates that a goal of healthy balance more accurately explains peoples' willingness to take part in self-management of diabetes.

#### IMPLICATIONS FOR NURSING

All teaching plans should be individualized and developed in collaboration with the client. Nurses often focus on diabetes management and control, especially compliance with prescribed regimens. Although clients are sometimes termed "noncompliant," this term conveys judgment about dependence. A focus on balance instead of control may well facilitate new understanding of

behavior demonstrated as the client seeks to assert self-control. It is important to also understand that self-control behaviors can change with variations in life and the disease itself, and that each person with diabetes responds uniquely to situations and interventions. Respecting and valuing what a person has learned from living with diabetes is critical to providing effective care.

#### Critical Thinking in Client Care

1. You are caring for two clients with diabetes who are receiving home care for complications of long-term diabetes. One client follows the medical regimen faithfully, the other adapts it to his own schedule and needs. What differences can you identify in your own reaction to these two different clients? How would these reactions affect your relationship with the clients?
2. Imagine you have just been diagnosed with type 1 diabetes. Make a list of the questions you would have and the areas that would cause you the most difficulty in complying with your medical care.
3. How would you respond if your client tells you, "Sometimes I eat whatever I want to for several days." What do you think this behavior indicates?

---

MediaLink | TYPE 2 DIABETES CARE PLAN

- Physical assessment: Height/weight ratio, vital signs, visual acuity, cranial nerves, sensory ability (touch, hot/cold, vibration) of extremities, peripheral pulses, skin and mucous membranes (hair loss, appearance, lesions, rash, itching, vaginal discharge)

## Nursing Diagnoses and Interventions

Although many different nursing diagnoses are appropriate for the person with diabetes, those discussed in this section address problems with skin integrity, infection, injury, sexuality, coping, and health maintenance. The goals of care are to maintain function, prevent complications, and teach self-management.

### Risk for Impaired Skin Integrity

The person with diabetes is at increased risk for altered skin integrity as a result of decreased or absent sensation from neuropathies, decreased tissue perfusion from cardiovascular complications, and infection. In addition, poor vision increases the risk of trauma, and an open lesion is more prone to infection and delayed healing. Impaired skin and tissue integrity, with resultant gangrene, is especially common in the feet and lower extremities.

- Conduct baseline and ongoing assessments of the feet, including:
  - Musculoskeletal assessment that includes foot and ankle joint range of motion, bone abnormalities (bunions, hammertoes, overlapping digits), gait patterns, use of assistive devices for walking, and abnormal wear patterns on shoes.
  - Neurologic assessment that includes sensations of touch and position, pain, and temperature.

- Vascular examination that includes assessment of lower-extremity pulses, capillary refill, color and temperature of skin, lesions, and edema.
- Hydration status, including dryness or excessive perspiration.
- Lesions, fissures between toes, corns, calluses, plantar warts, ingrown or overgrown toenails, redness over pressure points, blisters, cellulitis, or gangrene.

*People with diabetes are at significant risk for lower-extremity gangrene. Peripheral neuropathies may result in alterations in the perception of pain, loss of deep tendon reflexes, loss of cutaneous pressure and position sensation, foot drop, changes in the shape of the foot, and changes in bones and joints. Peripheral vascular disease may cause intermittent claudication, absent pulses, delayed venous filling on elevation, dependent rubor, and gangrene. Injuries, lesions, and changes in skin hydration potentiate infections, delayed healing, and tissue loss in the person with diabetes mellitus.*

- Teach foot hygiene. Wash the feet daily with lukewarm water and mild hand soap; pat dry, and dry well between the toes. Apply a very thin coat of lubricating cream if dryness is present (but not between the toes). *Proper hygiene decreases the chance of infection. Temperature receptors may be impaired, so the water should always be tested before use.*

**PRACTICE ALERT** *Teach the person with diabetes to always test the water temperature in the shower or bath before stepping in.* ■

- Discuss the importance of not smoking if client smokes. *Nicotine in tobacco causes vasoconstriction, further decreasing the blood supply to the feet.*

## Meeting Individualized Needs: Foot Care Teaching Session

### BUYING AND WEARING SHOES AND STOCKINGS

- Shoes that allow 1/2 to 3/4 inch of toe room are best; there should be room for toes to spread out and wiggle. The lining and inside stitching should be smooth, and the insole soft. The sole should be flexible and cushion the foot. The heel should fit snugly, and the arch support should give good support.
- Do not wear open-toed shoes, sandals, high heels, or thongs; they increase the risk of trauma.
- Buy shoes late in the afternoon, when feet are at their largest; always buy shoes that feel comfortable and do not need to be "broken in."
- Shoes made of natural fibers (leather, canvas) allow perspiration to escape.
- Check the shoes before each wearing for foreign objects, wrinkled insoles, and cracks that might cause lesions.
- Stockings made of wool or cotton allow perspiration to dry.
- Do not wear garters, knee stockings, or panty hose; they may interfere with circulation.
- Wear insulated boots in the winter.

### INSPECTING THE FEET

- Check the feet daily for red areas, cuts, blisters, corns, calluses, or cracks in the skin. Check between the toes for cracks or reddened areas.
- Check the skin of the feet for dry or damp areas.
- Use a mirror to check each sole and the back of each heel.
- If you are unable to inspect the feet daily, be sure that someone else does so.

### CARE OF TOENAILS

- Cut the toenails after washing, when they are softer and easier to trim.
- Cut the nails straight across with a clipper, and smooth edges and corners with an emery board.
- Do not use razor blades to trim the toenails.
- If you are unable to see well or to reach the feet easily, have someone else trim the nails. If the nails are very thick or ingrown, if the toes overlap, or if circulation is poor, get professional care.

### GENERAL INFORMATION

- Never go barefoot. Wear slippers when leaving the bed during the night.
- Do not use commercial corn medicines or pads, chemicals (such as boric acid, iodine, or hydrogen peroxide), or over-the-counter cortisone medications on the feet.
- Do not put heating pads, hot water bottles, or ice packs on the feet. If the feet become cold at night, wear socks or use extra blankets.
- Do not allow the feet to become sunburned.
- Do not put tape on the feet.
- Do not sit with the legs crossed at the knees or ankles.

---

- Discuss the importance of maintaining blood glucose levels through prescribed diet, medication, and exercise. *Hyperglycemia promotes the growth of microorganisms.*
- Conduct foot care teaching sessions as often as necessary (see the box above). Include information about proper shoe fit and composition, avoiding clothing or activities that decrease circulation to the feet, foot inspections, the care of toenails, and the importance of obtaining medical care for lesions. If the person has visual deficits, is obese, or cannot reach the feet, teach the caregiver how to inspect and care for the feet. Feet should be inspected daily. *Foot care is a priority in diabetes management to prevent serious problems. Many people with diabetes are unaware of lesions or injury until infection and compromised circulation are far advanced. The hows and whys of each component must be included in teaching. A variety of methods may be used, including demonstration, return demonstration, audiovisual aids, and written lists. If the person is wearing shoes and socks, ask him or her to remove them to practice foot care effectively.*

**PRACTICE ALERT**   *Suggest the use of a hand mirror to check the bottom of the feet and the back of the heel.* ■

### Risk for Infection

The person with diabetes is at increased risk for infection. The risk of infection is believed to be due to vascular insufficiency that limits the inflammatory response, neurologic abnormalities that limit the awareness of trauma, and a predisposition to bacterial and fungal infections.

- Use and teach meticulous handwashing. *Handwashing is the single most effective method for preventing the spread of infection.*
- Monitor for manifestations of infection: increased temperature, pain, malaise, swelling, redness, discharge, cough. *Early diagnosis and treatment of infections can control their severity and decrease complications.*
- Discuss the importance of skin care. Keep the skin clean and dry, using lukewarm water and mild soap. *People with diabetes are more prone to develop furuncles and carbuncles; the infection often increases the need for insulin. Clean, intact skin and mucous membranes are the first line of defense against infection.*
- Teach dental health measures:
  - Obtain a dental examination every 4 to 6 months.
  - Maintain careful oral hygiene, which includes brushing the teeth with a soft toothbrush and fluoridated toothpaste at least twice a day and flossing as recommended.
  - Be aware of the symptoms requiring dental care: bad breath; unpleasant taste in the mouth; bleeding, red, or sore gums; and tooth pain.
  - If dental surgery is necessary, monitor for need to make adjustments in insulin. *All people with diabetes need to be taught proper oral hygiene, the risk of periodontal disease, and the importance of obtaining dental care for symptoms of oral or dental problems.*
- Teach women with diabetes the symptoms and preventive measures for vaginitis caused by *Candida albicans*. The symptoms are an odorless, white or yellow cheeselike discharge and itching. Sexual transmission is unlikely, but

*discomfort may cause the client to avoid sexual activity. Diabetes is a predisposing factor for Candida albicans vaginitis, the most common form of vaginitis. Poor personal hygiene and wearing clothing that keeps the vaginal area warm and moist increase the risk of vaginitis. The infection may spread to the urinary tract, resulting in urinary tract infections; preventing and treating vaginitis decrease this risk.*

**PRACTICE ALERT** *Teach women with DM to take preventive measures by maintaining good personal hygiene, wiping front to back after voiding, wearing cotton underwear, avoiding tight jeans and nylon pantyhose, and avoiding douching.* ■

### Risk for Injury

The person with diabetes is at risk for injury from multiple factors. Neuropathies may alter sensation, gait, and muscle control. Cataracts or retinopathy may cause visual deficits. Hyperglycemia often causes osmotic changes in the lenses of the eye, resulting in blurred vision. In addition, changes in blood glucose alter levels of consciousness and may cause seizures. The impaired mobility, sensory deficits, and neurologic effects of complications of diabetes increase the risk of accidents, burns, falls, and trauma.

- Assess for the presence of contributing or causative factors that increase the risk of injury: blurred vision, cataracts, decreased adaptation to dark, decreased tactile sensitivity, hypoglycemia, hyperglycemia, hypovolemia, joint immobility, unstable gait. *A knowledge base is necessary to develop an individualized plan of care. The risk of injury increases with the number of factors identified.*
- Reduce environmental hazards in the health care facility, and teach the client about safety in the home and in the community.

#### IN THE HEALTH CARE FACILITY
- Orient the client to new surroundings on admission.
- Keep the bed at the lowest level.
- Keep the floors free of objects.
- Use a night light.
- Check the temperature of the bath or shower water before the client uses it.
- Instruct the client to wear shoes or slippers when out of bed.
- Monitor blood glucose levels regularly.
- Monitor for side effects of prescribed medications, such as dizziness or drowsiness.

#### IN THE HOME AND COMMUNITY
- Use a night light, preferably one with a soft, nonglare bulb.
- Turn the head away when switching on a bright light.
- Avoid directly looking into headlights when driving at night.
- Test the temperature of the bath or shower water before use.
- Conduct a daily foot inspection.
- Wear shoes and slippers with nonskid soles.
- Do not use throw rugs.
- Install hand grips in the tub and shower and next to the toilet.
- Wear a seat belt when driving or riding in a car.

*Strange environments and the presence of hazardous environmental factors increase the risk of falls or other accidents. Glare is often responsible for falls in people with visual deficits. The nurse can reduce factors that increase the risk of injury by implementing care and teaching safe practices during the activities of daily life.*

- Monitor for and teach the client and family to recognize and seek care for the manifestations of DKA in the client with type 1 DM: hyperglycemia, thirst, headaches, nausea and vomiting, increased urine output, ketonuria, dehydration, and decreasing level of consciousness. *Blood glucose levels increase if the insulin need is unmet or insufficiently met; the cellular use of fats for fuel results in ketosis. Osmotic diuresis increases urinary output, resulting in thirst and dehydration.*
- Monitor for and teach the client and family to recognize and seek care for the manifestations of HHS in the client with type 2 DM: extreme hyperglycemia, increased urinary output, thirst, dehydration, hypotension, seizures, and decreasing level of consciousness. *HHS is a life-threatening condition requiring recognition and treatment.*

**PRACTICE ALERT** *Make frequent assessments to monitor for symptoms of HHS in the older adult who has had major surgery.* ■

- Monitor for and teach the client and family to recognize and treat the manifestations of hypoglycemia: low blood glucose, anxiety, headache, uncoordinated movements, sweating, rapid pulse, drowsiness, and visual changes. Teach client and family to carry some form of rapid-acting sugar source at all times. *Severe hypoglycemia causes a decrease in the level of consciousness. The decrease in blood glucose most often results from too much insulin, too little food, or too much exercise.*
- Recommend that the client wear a MedicAlert bracelet or necklace identifying self as a person with diabetes. *In case of sudden, severe illness or accident, a MedicAlert bracelet can allow immediate medical attention for diabetes to be instituted.*

### Sexual Dysfunction

Sexuality is a complex and inseparable part of every person. It involves not only physical sexual activities but also a person's self-perception as male or female, roles and relationships, and attractiveness and desirability. Changes in sexual function and in sexuality have been identified in both men and women with diabetes.

Alterations in erectile ability occur in approximately 50% of all men with diabetes. The incidence of impotence increases with the duration of the diabetes and is often associated with peripheral neuropathy. Libido is usually unaffected, even when impotence is present.

Women with diabetes also have alterations in sexual function, although the reason is less clear. The problems reported by women involve decreased desire and decreased vaginal lubrication. Women with diabetes are also at increased risk for vaginitis and may avoid sexual intercourse in order to avoid pain.

- Include a sexual history as a part of the initial and ongoing assessment of the client with diabetes. A specific history form may be used that addresses sexual development, personal and family values, current sexual practices and concerns, and changes desired. Ask a nonthreatening, open-ended question to elicit information, such as, "Tell me about your experience with sexual function since you have been diagnosed with diabetes." *Obtaining accurate information to assess the sexual health of a client is necessary before counseling can begin or referrals can be made.*

**PRACTICE ALERT** *Sexual function is a private matter, and clients rarely share concerns unless the nurse initiates the discussion.* ■

- Provide information about the actual and potential physical effects of diabetes on sexual function. Include the effect of poor control of blood glucose on sexual function as part of any teaching plan. *Clients benefit from basic information about male and female anatomy and the sexual response cycle, and how diabetes can affect this part of the body. Changes in blood glucose levels not only may cause changes in desire and physical response but also may alter sexual responses as a result of depression, anxiety, and fatigue.*
- Provide counseling or make referrals as appropriate. The nurse is responsible for knowing about sexuality and sexual health throughout the life span and provides information based on knowledge of the effects of illness and treatment on sexual function. For example, men who are impotent may regain the ability to have sexual intercourse through penile implants, suction apparatus, the use of sildenafil citrate (Viagra), or injections of medications (such as yohimbine, an alpha-2 adrenergic blocker) that increase vascular blood flow into the corpus of the penis. Women with decreased vaginal lubrication can decrease painful intercourse by using vaginal lubricants (such as K-Y Jelly) or estrogen creams. *The nurse may make specific suggestions to facilitate positive sexual functioning, referring the client to the appropriate health care provider as necessary for intensive therapy.*

### Ineffective Coping

Coping is the process of responding to internal or environmental stressors or potential stressors. When coping responses are ineffective, the stressors exceed the individual's available resources for responding. The person diagnosed with diabetes is faced with lifelong changes in many parts of his or her life. Diet, exercise habits, and medications must be integrated into the person's lifestyle and be carefully controlled. Daily injections may be a reality. Fear of potential complications and of negative effects on the future is common.

If the person is unable to cope successfully with these changes, emotional stress can interfere with glycemic control. In addition, unsuccessful coping often results in noncompliance with prescribed treatment modalities, further impairing glycemic control and increasing the potential for acute and chronic complications.

- Assess the client's psychosocial resources, including emotional resources, support resources, lifestyle, and communication skills. *Chronic illness affects all dimensions of a person's life, as well as the lives of family members and significant others. A comprehensive assessment of strengths and weaknesses is the first step in developing an individualized plan of care to facilitate coping.*
- Explore with the client and family the effects (actual and perceived) of the diagnosis and treatment of diabetes on finances, occupation, energy levels, and relationships. *Common frustrations associated with diabetes are the disease itself, the treatment modalities, and the health care system. Effective coping involves maintaining a healthy self-concept and satisfying relationships, emotional balance, and handling emotional stress.*
- Teach constructive problem-solving techniques. *Problem-focused behaviors include setting attainable and realistic goals, learning about all aspects of the problem, learning new procedures or skills that increase self-esteem, and reaching out to others for support.*
- Provide information about support groups and resources, such as suppliers of products, journals, books, and cookbooks for people with diabetes. *Sharing with others who have similar problems provides opportunities for mutual support and problem solving. Using available resources improves the ability to cope.*

## Using NANDA, NIC, and NOC

Chart 18–1 shows links between NANDA, NIC, and NOC when caring for the client with diabetes.

## Home Care

Teaching the client and family to self-manage diabetes is a nursing responsibility. Even if a formal teaching plan is developed and implemented by advanced practice nurses, all nurses must be able to reinforce knowledge and answer questions. Teaching is necessary for both the person who is newly diagnosed and for the person who has had diabetes for years. In fact, the latter may need almost as much teaching as the newly diagnosed person (Guthrie & Guthrie, 1997).

The American Diabetes Association recommends that teaching be carried out on three levels. The first level focuses on survival skills, with the person learning basic knowledge and skills to be able to provide diabetes management for the first week or two while he or she adjusts to the idea of having the disease. The second level focuses on home management, emphasizing self-reliance and independence in the daily management of diabetes. The third level aims at improving lifestyle and educating clients to individualize self-management of the illness.

For the hospitalized client with diabetes, teaching should begin on admission. Prior to designing the teaching plan, the nurse makes an initial assessment of the client's and family's knowledge and learning needs, outlining past diabetes management practices and identifying physical, emotional, and sociocultural needs. Educational level, preferred learning methods and style, life experiences, and support systems are also assessed.

It is important that the nurse and client mutually establish goals based on the assessment data. It is equally important that

## CHART 18–1   NANDA, NIC, AND NOC LINKAGES

### The Client with Diabetes

| NURSING DIAGNOSES | NURSING INTERVENTIONS | NURSING OUTCOMES |
|---|---|---|
| • Ineffective Therapeutic Regimen Management | • Hyperglycemia Management | • Knowledge: Treatment Regimen |
| | • Nutritional Counseling | • Nutritional Status: Food and Fluid Intake |
| • Imbalanced Nutrition: More than Body Requirements | • Weight Management | • Knowledge: Diet |
| • Fatigue | • Energy Management | • Energy Conservation |
| • Risk for Peripheral Neurovascular Dysfunction | • Peripheral Sensation | • Circulation Status |
| | • Circulatory Care: Arterial Insufficiency | • Neurological Status |
| • Powerlessness | • Self-Esteem Enhancement | • Health Beliefs: Perceived Control |
| • Altered Protection | • Infection Control | • Infection Status |

Note. Data from Nursing Outcomes Classification (NOC) by M. Johnson & M. Maas (Eds.), 1997, St. Louis: Mosby; Nursing Diagnoses: Definitions & Classification 2001–2002 by North American Nursing Diagnosis Association, 2001, Philadelphia: NANDA; Nursing Interventions Classification (NIC) by J.C. McCloskey & G. M. Bulechek (Eds.), 2000, St. Louis: Mosby. Reprinted by permission.

family members understand that the responsibility for daily management lies with the client and that the primary role of the family is supportive. The client is the person with the disease, and it is the client who each day must take medications or inject insulin, test blood or urine, calculate and balance foods, exercise, adjust medications, inspect the body for injury, and determine whether and when medical assistance is needed. However, family members require the same knowledge so that they can provide emotional support as well as physical care if necessary.

The following should be included in teaching the client and family about care at home.

- Information about normal metabolism, diabetes mellitus, and how diabetes changes metabolism
- Diet plan: how diet helps keep blood glucose in normal range; number of kcal required and why; amount of carbohydrates, meats, and fats allowed and why; and how to calculate the diet, integrating personal food preferences
- Exercise: how it helps lower blood glucose; the importance of a regular program; types of exercise; integrating personal exercise preferences; how to handle increased activity
- Self-monitoring of blood glucose: how to perform the tests accurately, how to care for equipment, what to do for high or low blood glucose
- Medications:
  - Insulin: type, dosage, mixing instructions (if necessary), times of onset and peak actions, how to get and care for equipment, how to give injections, where to give injections
  - Oral agents: type, dosage, side effects, interaction with other drugs
- Manifestations of acute complications of hypoglycemia and hyperglycemia; what to do when they occur
- Hygiene: skin care, dental care, foot care
- Sick days: what to do about food, fluids, and medications
- Helpful resources:
  - The American Diabetes Association
  - The American Dietetic Association

- National Diabetes Information Clearinghouse
- Department of Veterans Affairs
- Indian Health Service
- National Council of La Raza

Teaching may have to be adapted to the special needs of the older adult. Because 40% of all people with diabetes are over the age of 65, considering the special needs of this population is essential. Uncontrolled diabetes in the older adult increases the potential for functional loss, social disengagement, and increased morbidity and mortality. Education for self-care allows the older adult to be more actively involved in his or her diabetes management and decreases the potential for acute and long-term complications from the disease. Considerations for teaching the older adult with diabetes include the following:

- Changes in diet may be difficult to implement for many reasons. Favorite foods are difficult to give up. Balanced meals at regular intervals may not have been part of the client's lifestyle. Purchasing, storing, and preparing foods may be a problem. Dentures may not fit well. Changes in taste sensation often cause the client to increase the use of salt and sugar.
- Exercise of any type may not have been part of the activities of daily living. Exercise must be individualized for any physical limitations imposed by other chronic illnesses, such as arthritis, Parkinson's disease, chronic respiratory diseases, and/or cardiovascular diseases.
- The diagnosis of a chronic illness threatens independence and self-worth. After years of taking care of self, the older adult with diabetes may now have to depend on others for help in meeting self-care needs. This in turn often leads to withdrawal from social interactions with others.
- Money to purchase medications and supplies often must be taken out of a fixed income.
- Visual deficits make insulin administration difficult or impossible. Visual deficits also interfere with blood glucose monitoring, food preparation, exercises, and foot care.

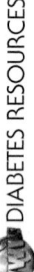

MediaLink | DIABETES RESOURCES

## Nursing Care Plan
## A Client with Type 1 Diabetes

Jim Meligrito, age 24, is a third-year nursing student at a large mid-western university. Mr. Meligrito also works 20 hours a week as a campus student security guard. His working hours are 8 P.M. to midnight, five nights a week. He lives with his father, who is also a student. Neither of the two men likes to cook, and they usually eat "whatever is handy." Mr. Meligrito has smoked 8 to 10 cigarettes a day for 5 years. He was diagnosed with type 1 diabetes mellitus at age 12. Although his insulin dosage has varied, he currently takes a total of 32 units of insulin each day, 10 U of NPH and 6 U of regular insulin each morning and evening. He monitors his blood glucose about three times a week. He feels that he is too busy for a regular exercise program and that he gets enough exercise in clinicals and in weekend sports activities. He has not seen a health care provider for over a year.

One day during a 6-hour clinical laboratory in pediatrics, Mr. Meligrito notices that he is urinating frequently, is thirsty, and has blurred vision. He also is very tired but blames all his symptoms on drinking a couple of beers and having had only 4 hours of sleep the night before while studying for an examination, and the stress he has been under lately from school and work. When he remembers that he had forgotten to take his insulin that morning, he realizes he must have hyperglycemia but decides that he will be all right until he gets home in the afternoon. Around noon, he begins having abdominal pain, feels weak, has a rapid pulse, and vomits. When he reports his physical symptoms to his clinical instructor, she sends him immediately to the hospital emergency department, accompanied by another student.

### ASSESSMENT

As soon as Mr. Meligrito arrives at the emergency room, his blood glucose level is measured at 300 mg/dL. Urine samples and additional blood samples are sent to the laboratory for analysis. Blood glucose is 330 mg/dL, urine shows the presence of ketones, electrolytes are normal, and pH is 7.1. His vital signs are as follows: T 99°F (37.2°C), P 140, R 28, and BP 102/52. An intravenous infusion of 1000 mL normal (0.9%) saline with 40 mEq of KCl is started at a rate of 400 mL/h. Intravenous regular insulin at 25 mL/h (5 U/h) is begun. Hourly blood glucose monitoring is initiated. Mr. Meligrito is nauseated and lethargic but remains oriented. Three hours later, he has a blood glucose level of 160, and his pulse and blood pressure are normal. He is dismissed from the emergency department after making an appointment for the next morning with the hospital's diabetes nurse educator. When he meets with the diabetes educator, he says that he no longer feels in control of the diabetes or his future goal to become a nurse anesthetist.

### DIAGNOSIS

- *Powerlessness* related to a perceived lack of control of diabetes due to present demands on time
- *Deficient knowledge* of self-management of diabetes
- *Risk for ineffective role performance* related to uncertainty about capacity to achieve desired role as registered nurse

### EXPECTED OUTCOMES

- Identify those aspects of diabetes that can be controlled and participate in making decisions about self-managing care.

- Demonstrate an understanding of diabetes self-management through planned medication, diet, exercise, and blood glucose self-monitoring activities.
- Explore and clarify Mr. Meligrito's perceptions of his role as a student nurse, verbalizing his ability to meet his expectations.

### PLANNING AND IMPLEMENTATION

- Mutually establish specific and individualized short-term and long-term goals for self-management to control blood glucose.
- Provide opportunities to express his feelings about himself and his illness.
- Explore perceptions of his own ability to control his illness and his future, and clarify these perceptions by providing information about resources and support groups.
- Facilitate decision-making abilities in self-managing his prescribed treatment regimen.
- Provide positive reinforcement for increasing involvement in self-care activities.
- Provide relevant learning activities about insulin administration, dietary management, exercise, self-monitoring of blood glucose, and healthy lifestyle.

### EVALUATION

After taking an active part in the weekly educational meetings for 2 months, Mr. Meligrito has greatly enhanced his understanding of and compliance with self-management of his diabetes. He states that he finally understands how insulin, food, and exercise affect his body, having previously thought they were "just things I should do when I wanted to." He decides to perform self-management activities one week at a time, rather than think too far into (and thereby feel overwhelmed by) the future. Both son and father have developed a workable meal schedule and weekly grocery list, and they have begun eating breakfast and dinner together. Jim and a friend have arranged to walk 2 to 3 miles three times a week on a community hiking trail. To gain a sense of control over his illness, he has also worked out a schedule that allows time for school, health care, and himself.

### Critical Thinking in the Nursing Process

1. What is the pathophysiologic basis for the changes in temperature, pulse, respirations, and blood pressure that occurred on Mr. Meligrito's admission to the hospital emergency department?
2. How can smoking and poor self-management of diabetes increase the risk of long-term complications?
3. Is powerlessness a common response to a chronic illness? Why or why not?
4. Consider that you are teaching Mr. Meligrito and another client, Mr. McDaniel (age 75, newly diagnosed with type 2 DM). What components of your teaching plan would be the same and what components would be different?

See Evaluating Your Response in Appendix C.

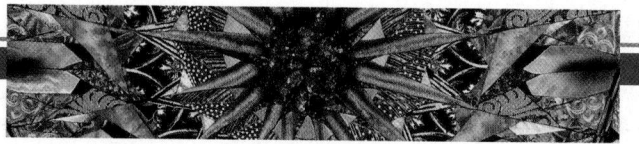

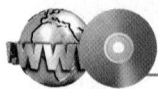 ## EXPLORE MediaLink

NCLEX review questions, case studies, care plan activities, MediaLink applications, and other interactive resources for this chapter can be found on the Companion Website at www.prenhall.com/lemone.

Click on Chapter 18 to select the activities for this chapter. For animations, video clips, more NCLEX review questions, and an audio glossary, access the Student CD-ROM accompanying this textbook.

## TEST YOURSELF

1. Increased susceptibility to the development of type 1 diabetes is indicated by which of the following:
   a. Genetic markers that determine immune response
   b. Persistent obesity throughout the adolescent years
   c. Delivery of a baby that weighs less than 6 lb
   d. Excessive amounts of plasma glucagon

2. Diabetic ketoacidosis is the result of which pathologic process?
   a. An excess amount of insulin drives all glucose into the cells
   b. A decreased amount of glucagon causes low protein levels
   c. A deficit of insulin causes fat stores to be used as an energy source
   d. An increase occurs in the breakdown of glucose molecules with hypoglycemia

3. Which of the following clients would be most at risk for the development of type 2 DM?
   a. Young adult who is a professional basketball player
   b. Middle-age man who maintains normal weight

   c. Middle-age woman who is the sole caretaker of her parents
   d. Woman over age 70 who is overweight and sedentary

4. You note that your assigned client has a nursing diagnosis of *Peripheral neurovascular dysfunction* involving both feet. Which of the following assessments would support this diagnosis?
   a. Normal sensation to touch
   b. Loss of normal reflexes
   c. States "I can't feel my feet anymore."
   d. States "I have been having chest pain."

5. Which of the following statements would indicate your client understands teaching about foot care at home?
   a. "I will walk barefooted as long as I am in the house."
   b. "I always buy my shoes as soon as the stores open."
   c. "I will check my feet for cuts and bruises every night."
   d. "If I get a blister, I just put alcohol on it and let it go."

See Test Yourself answers in Appendix C.

## BIBLIOGRAPHY

American Diabetes Association. (2002). *Clinical practice recommendations 2002, 25* (Supplement 1).

Batts, M., Gary, T., Huss, K., Hill, M., Bone, L., & Brancatt, F. (2001). Patient priorities and needs for diabetes care among urban African American adults. *Diabetes Educator, 27*(3), 405–412.

Bohannon, N. (1998). Treatment of vulvovaginal candidiasis in patients with diabetes. *Diabetes Care, 21*(3), 451–456.

Bulpitt, C., Palmer, A., Battersby, C., & Fletcher, A. (1998). Association of symptoms of type 2 diabetic patients with severity of disease, obesity, and blood pressure. *Diabetes Care, 21*(1), 111–115.

Burke, D. (2001). Diabetes education for the Native American Population. *Diabetes Educator, 27*(2), 181–189.

Cameron, B. (2002). Making diabetes management routine. *American Journal of Nursing, 102*(2), 26–33.

Carter, J., Gilliland, S., Perez, G., Levin, S., Broussand, B., Valdez, L., Cunningham-Sabo, L., & Davis, S. (1997). Tool chest. Native American

Diabetes Project: Designing culturally relevant education materials. *Diabetes Educator, 23*(2), 133–134.

Fishman, T., Freedline, A., & Town, L. (1997). Helping diabetic patients treat their feet right. *Nursing97, 27*(6), 10–12.

Goldberg, J. M. (2001). Nutrition and exercise. *RN, 64*(7), 34–39.

Guthrie, D., & Guthrie, R. (1997). *Nursing management of diabetes mellitus* (4th ed.). New York: Springer.

Haire-Joshu, D. (Ed.) (1996). *Management of diabetes mellitus: Perspectives of care across the life span* (2nd ed.). St. Louis: Mosby.

Hanna, K., & Guthrie, D. (2001). Health-compromising behavior and diabetes mismanagement among adolescents and young adults. *Diabetes Educator, 27*(2), 223–230.

Hernandez, D. (1998). Microvascular complications of diabetes: Nursing assessment and intervention. *American Journal of Nursing, 98*(6), 26–31.

Johnson, M., & Maas, M. (Eds.) (1997). *Nursing outcomes classification (NOC)*. St. Louis: Mosby.

Kee, J. (1999). *Laboratory & diagnostic tests with nursing implications* (5th ed.). East Norwalk, CT: Appleton & Lange.

Lipton, R., Losy, L., Giachello, A., Mendez, J., & Girotti, M. (1998). Attitudes and issues in treating Latino patients with type 2 diabetes. *Diabetes Educator, 24*(1), 67–71.

Lupo, M. (1997). An overview of foot disease associated with diabetes mellitus. *MEDSURG Nursing, 6*(4), 225–229.

McCance, K., & Huether, S. (2002). *Pathophysiology: The biologic basis for disease in adults and children.* (4th ed.). St. Louis: Mosby.

McCloskey, J. C., & Bulechek, G. M. (Eds.). (2000). *Nursing interventions classification (NIC).* St. Louis: Mosby.

McKenry, L., & Salerno, E. (1998). *Pharmacology in nursing* (20th ed.). St. Louis: Mosby.

National Institutes of Health. (2002). *Diabetes statistics in the United States.* NIH Publication No. 99–3892. Washington, DC: NIH.

North American Nursing Diagnosis Association. (2001). *Nursing diagnoses: Definitions & Classification 2001–2002.* Philadelphia: NANDA.

Passanza, C. (2001). Diabetes update: Monitor options. *RN, 64*(6), 36–43.

Paterson, B., Thorne, S., & Dewis, M. (1998). Adapting to and managing diabetes. *Image: Journal of Nursing Scholarship, 30*(1), 57–62.

Porth, C. (2002). *Pathophysiology: Concepts of altered health states* (6th ed.). Philadelphia: Lippincott.

Robertson, C. (1998). When your patient is on an insulin pump. *RN, 61*(3), 30–33.

Shannon, M., Wilson, B., & Stang, C. (2002). *Health professional's drug guide 2002.* Upper Saddle River, NJ: Prentice Hall.

Stanley, K. (1998). Assessing the nutritional needs of the geriatric patient with diabetes. *Diabetes Educator, 24*(1), 29–30, 35–36, 38.

Strowig, S. (2001). Insulin therapy. *RN, 64*(9), 38–44.

Sullivan, E., & Joseph, D. (1998). Struggling with behavior changes: A special case for clients with diabetes. *Diabetes Educator, 24*(1), 72–77.

Tierney, L., McPhee, S., & Papadakis, M. (Eds.). (2001). *Current medical diagnosis & treatment* (40th ed.). Stamford, CT: Appleton & Lange.

Tkacs, N. (2002). Hypoglycemia unawarenesss. *American Journal of Nursing, 102*(2), 34–41.

Whittemore, R. (2000). Strategies to facilitate lifestyle change associated with diabetes mellitus. *Journal of Nursing Scholarship, 32*(3), 225–232.

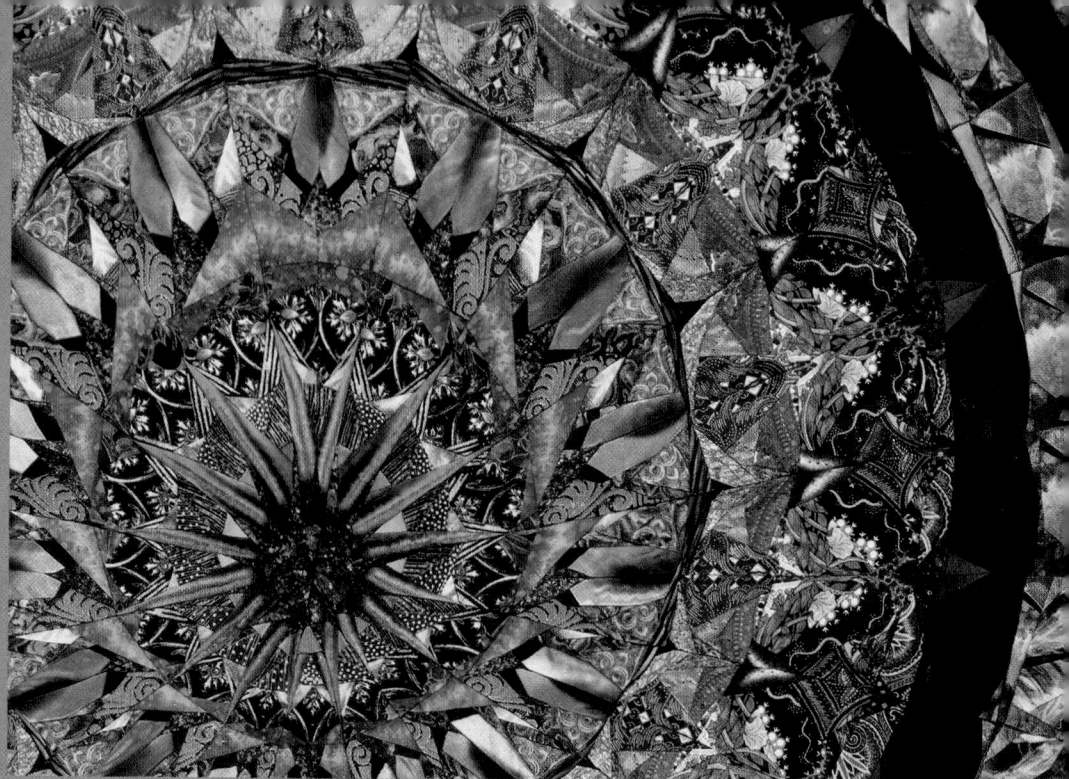

UNIT 5

# RESPONSES TO ALTERED NUTRITION

# CHAPTER 19

# Assessing Clients with Nutritional and Gastrointestinal Disorders

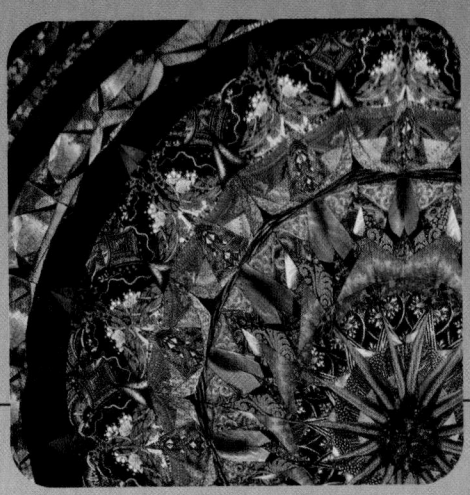

## LEARNING OUTCOMES

After completing this chapter, you will be able to:

- Review the anatomy and physiology of the gastrointestinal system.

- Describe the processes of carbohydrate, fat, and protein metabolism.

- Describe the sources of nutrients and vitamins and their functions in the human body.

- Identify specific topics to consider during a health history assessment interview of the client with nutritional and gastrointestinal disorders.

- Describe physical assessment techniques used to evaluate nutritional and gastrointestinal status.

- Identify abnormal findings that may indicate impairment in gastrointestinal function.

## MediaLink

**www.prenhall.com/lemone**
Additional resources for this chapter can be found on the Student CD-ROM accompanying this textbook, and on the Companion Website at www. prenhall.com/lemone. Click on Chapter 19 to select the activities for this chapter.

### CD-ROM
- Audio Glossary
- NCLEX Review

### *Animations*
- Digestive System
- Carbohydrates
- Lipids
- Proteins

### Companion Website
- More NCLEX Review
- Functional Health Pattern Assessment
- Case Study
  Weight Loss

**Nutrition** is the process by which the body ingests, absorbs, transports, uses, and eliminates food. The digestive organs responsible for these processes are the gastrointestinal tract (also called the alimentary canal) and the accessory digestive organs. The gastrointestinal tract consists of the mouth, pharynx, esophagus, stomach, small intestine, and large intestine. The accessory digestive organs include the liver, gallbladder, and pancreas (Figure 19–1 ■). This chapter discusses the assessment of these organs except the large intestine. Assessment of the large intestine, which is primarily responsible for elimination, is discussed in Chapter 23. ⊘⊘

## REVIEW OF ANATOMY AND PHYSIOLOGY

The gastrointestinal (GI) tract is a continuous hollow tube, extending from the mouth to the anus. Once foods are ingested into the mouth, they are subjected to a variety of processes that move them and break them down into end products that can be absorbed from the lumen of the small intestine into the blood or lymph. These digestive processes are as follows:

- Ingestion of food
- Movement of food and wastes
- Secretion of mucus, water, and enzymes
- Mechanical digestion of food
- Chemical digestion of food
- Absorption of digested food

## The Mouth

The mouth, also called the oral or buccal cavity, is lined with mucous membranes and is enclosed by the lips, cheeks, palate, and tongue (Figure 19–2 ■).

The lips and cheeks are skeletal muscle covered externally by skin. Their function is to keep food in the mouth during chewing. The palate consists of two regions: the hard palate and the soft palate. The hard palate covers bone and provides a hard surface against which the tongue forces food. The soft palate is primarily muscle; it ends at the back of the mouth as a fold called the uvula. When food is swallowed, the soft palate rises as a reflex to close off the oropharynx.

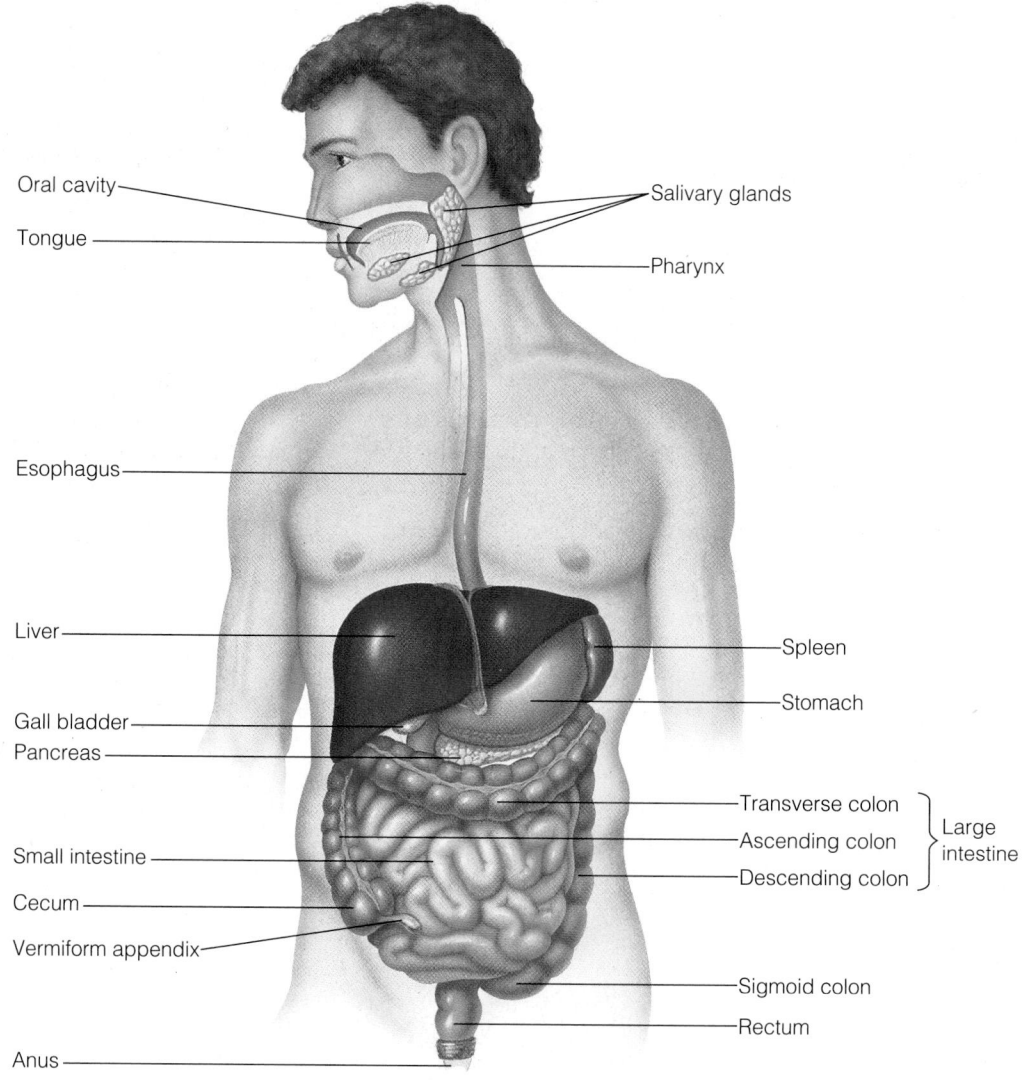

Oral cavity
Tongue
Salivary glands
Pharynx
Esophagus
Liver
Spleen
Stomach
Gall bladder
Pancreas
Transverse colon
Ascending colon
Descending colon
Large intestine
Small intestine
Cecum
Vermiform appendix
Sigmoid colon
Rectum
Anus

**Figure 19–1** ■ Organs of the gastrointestinal tract and accessory digestive organs.

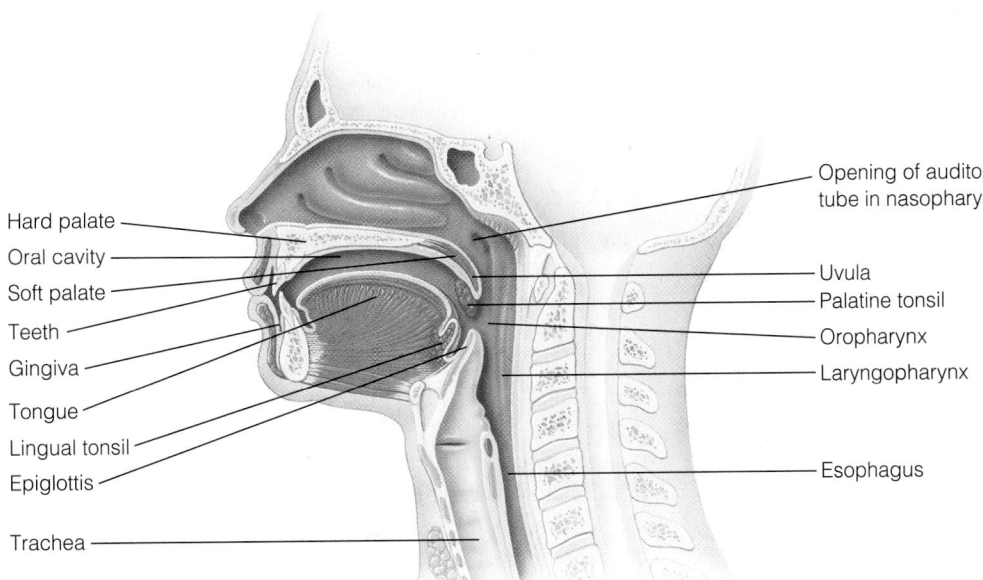

**Figure 19–2** ■ Structures of the mouth, the pharynx, and the esophagus.

The tongue, composed of skeletal muscle and connective tissue, is located in the floor of the mouth. It contains mucous and serous glands, taste buds, and papillae. The tongue mixes food with saliva during chewing, forms the food into a mass (called a bolus), and initiates swallowing. Some papillae provide surface roughness to facilitate licking and moving food; other papillae house the taste buds.

Saliva moistens food so it can be made into a bolus, dissolves food chemicals so they can be tasted, and provides enzymes (such as amylase) that begin the chemical breakdown of starches. Saliva is produced by salivary glands, most of which lie superior or inferior to the mouth and drain into it. The salivary glands include the parotid, the submaxillary, and the sublingual glands.

The teeth chew (masticate) and grind food to break it down into smaller parts. As the food is masticated, it is mixed with saliva. Adults have 32 permanent teeth. The teeth are embedded in the gingiva (gums), with the crown of each tooth visible above the gingiva.

## The Pharynx

The pharynx consists of the oropharynx and the laryngopharynx (see Figure 19–2). Both structures provide passageways for food, fluids, and air. The pharynx is skeletal muscles and is lined with mucous membranes. The skeletal muscles move food to the esophagus via the pharynx through **peristalsis** (alternating waves of contraction and relaxation of involuntary muscle). The mucosa of the pharynx contains mucus-producing glands that provide fluid to facilitate the passage of the bolus of food as it is swallowed.

## The Esophagus

The esophagus, a muscular tube about 10 inches (25 cm) long, serves as a passageway for food from the pharynx to the stomach (see Figures 19–1 and 19–2). The epiglottis, a flap of cartilage over the top of the larynx, keeps food out of the larynx during swallowing. The esophagus descends through the tho-

rax and diaphragm, entering the stomach at the cardiac orifice. The gastroesophageal sphincter surrounds this opening. This sphincter, along with the diaphragm, keeps the orifice closed when food is not being swallowed.

For most of its length, the esophagus is lined with stratified squamous epithelium; simple columnar epithelium lines the esophagus where it joins the stomach. The mucosa and submucosa of the esophagus lie in longitudinal folds when the esophagus is empty.

## The Stomach

The stomach, located high on the left side of the abdominal cavity, is connected to the esophagus at the upper end and to the small intestine at the lower end (Figure 19–3 ■). Normally about 10 inches (25 cm) long, the stomach is a distensible organ that can expand to hold up to 4 L of food and fluid. The

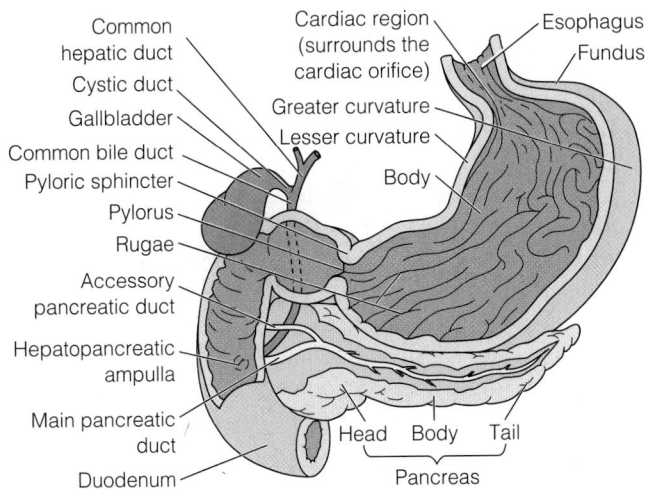

**Figure 19–3** ■ The internal anatomic structures of the stomach, including the pancreatic, cystic, and hepatic ducts; the pancreas; and the gallbladder.

concave surface of the stomach is called the lesser curvature; the convex surface is called the greater curvature. The stomach may be divided into regions extending from the distal end of the esophagus to the opening into the small intestine. These regions are the cardiac region, fundus, body, and pylorus (see Figure 19–3). The pyloric sphincter controls emptying of the stomach into the duodenal portion of the small intestine. The stomach is a storage reservoir for food, continues the mechanical breakdown of food, begins the process of protein digestion, and mixes the food with gastric juices into a thick fluid called **chyme.**

The stomach is lined with columnar epithelial, mucus-producing cells. Millions of openings in the lining lead to gastric glands that can produce 4 to 5 L of gastric juice each day. The gastric glands contain a variety of secretory cells, including the following:

- Mucous cells produce alkaline mucus that clings to the lining of the stomach and protects it from gastric juice.
- Zymogenic cells produce pepsinogen (an inactive form of pepsin, a protein-digesting enzyme).
- Parietal cells secrete hydrochloric acid and intrinsic factor. Hydrochloric acid activates and increases the activity of protein-digesting cells and also is bactericidal. Intrinsic factor is necessary for the absorption of vitamin $B_{12}$ in the small intestine.
- Enteroendocrine cells secrete gastrin, histamine, endorphins, serotonin, and somatostatin. These hormones or hormone-like substances diffuse into the blood. Gastrin is important in regulating secretion and motility of the stomach.

The secretion of gastric juice is under both neural and endocrine control. Stimulation of the parasympathetic vagus nerve increases secretory activity; in contrast, stimulation of sympathetic nerves decreases secretions. The three phases of secretory activity are the cephalic phase, the gastric phase, and the intestinal phase.

- The cephalic phase prepares for digestion and is triggered by the sight, odor, taste, or thought of food. During this initial phase, motor impulses are transmitted via the vagus nerve to the stomach.
- The gastric phase begins when food enters the stomach. Stomach distention (stimulating stretch receptors) and chemical stimuli from partially digested proteins initiate this phase. Gastrin-secreting cells produce gastrin, which in turn stimulates the gastric glands (especially the parietal cells) to produce more gastric juice. Histamine also stimulates hydrochloric acid secretion.
- The intestinal phase is initiated when partially digested food begins to enter the small intestine, stimulating mucous cells of the intestine to release a hormone that promotes continued gastric secretion.

Mechanical digestion in the stomach is accomplished by peristaltic movements that churn and mix the food with the gastric juices to form chyme. Gastric motility is enhanced or retarded by the same factors that affect secretion, namely, distention and the effect of gastrin. After a person eats a normal, well-balanced meal, the stomach empties completely in approximately 4 to 6 hours. Gastric emptying depends on the volume, chemical composition, and osmotic pressure of the gastric contents. The stomach empties large volumes of content more rapidly, while gastric emptying is slowed by solids and fats.

## The Small Intestine

The small intestine begins at the pyloric sphincter and ends at the ileocecal junction at the entrance of the large intestine (see Figure 19–1). The small intestine is about 20 ft (6 m) long but only about 1 inch (2.5 cm) in diameter. This long tube hangs in coils in the abdominal cavity, suspended by the mesentery and surrounded by the large intestine. The small intestine has three regions: the duodenum, the jejunum, and the ileum. The duodenum begins at the pyloric sphincter and extends around the head of the pancreas for about 10 inches (25 cm). Both pancreatic enzymes and bile from the liver enter the small intestine at the duodenum. The jejunum, the middle region of the small intestine, extends for about 8 ft (2.4 m). The ileum, the terminal end of the small intestine, is approximately 12 ft (3.6 m) long and meets the large intestine at the ileocecal valve.

Food is chemically digested, and most of it absorbed, as it moves through the small intestine. Circular folds (deep folds of the mucosa and submucosa layers), villi (fingerlike projections of the mucosa cells), and microvilli (tiny projections of the mucosa cells) increase the surface area of the small intestine to enhance absorption of food. Although up to 10 L of food, liquids, and secretions enter the GI tract each day, less than 1 L reaches the large intestine.

Enzymes in the small intestine break down carbohydrates, proteins, lipids, and nucleic acids. Pancreatic amylase acts on starches, converting them to maltose, dextrins, and oligosaccharides; the intestinal enzymes dextrinase, glucoamylase, maltase, sucrase, and lactase further break down these products into monosaccharides. Pancreatic enzymes (trypsin and chymotrypsin) and intestinal enzymes continue to break down proteins into peptides. Pancreatic lipases digest lipids in the small intestine. Triglycerides enter as fat globules and are coated by bile salts and emulsified. Nucleic acids are hydrolyzed by pancreatic enzymes and then broken apart by intestinal enzymes. Both pancreatic enzymes and bile are excreted into the duodenum in response to the secretion of secretin and cholecystokinin, hormones produced by the intestinal mucosa cells when chyme enters the small intestine.

Nutrients are absorbed through the mucosa of the intestinal villi into the blood or lymph by active transport, facilitated transport, and passive diffusion. Almost all food products and water, as well as vitamins and most electrolytes, are absorbed in the small intestine, leaving only indigestible fibers, some water, and bacteria to enter the large intestine.

## The Accessory Digestive Organs
### The Liver and Gallbladder

The liver is the largest gland in the body, weighing about 3 lb (1.4 kg) in the average-size adult. It is located in the right side of the abdomen, inferior to the diaphragm and anterior to the stomach (see Figure 19–1). The liver has four lobes: right, left, caudate, and quadrate. A mesenteric ligament separates the right and left lobes and suspends the liver from the diaphragm and anterior abdominal wall. The liver is encased in a fibro-elastic capsule.

Liver tissue consists of units called lobules, which are composed of plates of hepatocytes (liver cells). A branch of the hepatic artery, a branch of the hepatic portal vein, and a bile duct communicate with each lobule. Sinusoids, blood-filled spaces within the lobules, are lined with Kupffer cells. These phagocytic cells remove debris from the blood.

The liver performs the following digestive and metabolic functions.

- Secretes bile
- Stores fat-soluble vitamins (A, D, E, and K)
- Metabolizes bilirubin
- Stores blood and releases blood into the general circulation during hemorrhage
- Synthesizes plasma proteins to maintain plasma oncotic pressure
- Synthesizes prothrombin, fibrinogen, and factors I, II, VII, IX, and X, which are necessary for blood clotting
- Synthesizes fats from carbohydrates and proteins to be either used for energy or stored as adipose tissue
- Synthesizes phospholipids and cholesterol necessary for the production of bile salts, steroid hormones, and plasma membranes
- Converts amino acids to carbohydrates through deamination
- Releases glucose during times of hypoglycemia
- Takes up glucose during times of hyperglycemia and stores it as glycogen or converts it to fat
- Alters chemicals, foreign molecules, and hormones to make them less toxic
- Stores iron as ferritin, which is released as needed for the production of red blood cells

Bile production is the liver's primary digestive function. **Bile** is a greenish, watery solution containing bile salts, cholesterol, bilirubin, electrolytes, water, and phospholipids. These substances are necessary to emulsify and promote the absorption of fats. Liver cells make from 700 to 1200 mL of bile daily. When bile is not needed for digestion, the sphincter of Oddi (located at the point at which bile enters the duodenum) is closed, and the bile backs up the cystic duct into the gallbladder for storage.

Bile is concentrated and stored in the gallbladder, a small sac cupped in the inferior surface of the liver. When food containing fats enters the duodenum, hormones stimulate the gallbladder to secrete bile into the cystic duct. The cystic duct joins the hepatic duct to form the common bile duct, from which bile enters into the duodenum (see Figure 19–3).

### The Pancreas

The pancreas, a gland located between the stomach and small intestine, is the primary enzyme-producing organ of the digestive system. It is a triangular gland extending across the abdomen, with its tail next to the spleen and its head next to the duodenum (see Figure 19–3). The body and tail of the pancreas are retroperitoneal, lying behind the greater curvature of the stomach. The pancreas is actually two organs in one, having both exocrine and endocrine structures and functions. The exocrine portion of the pancreas, through secretory units called acini, secretes alkaline pancreatic juice containing many different enzymes. The acini, clusters of secretory cells surrounding ducts, drain into the pancreatic duct. The pancreatic duct joins with the common bile duct just before it enters the duodenum (so that pancreatic juice and bile from the liver enter the small intestine together). The pancreas also has endocrine functions (see Chapter 16).

The pancreas produces from 1 to 1.5 L of pancreatic juice daily. Pancreatic juice is clear and has high bicarbonate content. This alkaline fluid neutralizes the acidic chyme as it enters the duodenum, optimizing the pH for intestinal and pancreatic enzyme activity. The secretion of pancreatic juice is controlled by the vagus nerve and the intestinal hormones secretin and cholecystokinin. Pancreatic juice contains enzymes that aid in the digestion of all categories of foods: lipase promotes fat breakdown and absorption; amylase completes starch digestion; and trypsin, chymotrypsin, and carboxypeptidase are responsible for half of all protein digestion. Nucleases break down nucleic acids.

## METABOLISM

After nutrients (carbohydrates, fats, and proteins) are ingested, digested, absorbed, and transported across cell membranes, they must be metabolized to produce and provide energy to maintain life. **Metabolism** is the complex of biochemical reactions occurring in the body's cells. Metabolic processes are either catabolic or anabolic. Catabolism involves the breakdown of complex structures into simpler forms, for example, the breakdown of carbohydrates to produce adenosine triphosphate (ATP), an energy molecule that fuels cellular activity. In the process of anabolism, simpler molecules combine to build more complex structures, for example, amino acids bond to form proteins.

The biochemical reactions of metabolism produce water, carbon dioxide, and ATP (Figure 19–4 ■). The energy value of foods is measured in kilocalories (kcal). A kilocalorie is defined as the amount of heat energy needed to raise the temperature of 1 kilogram (kg) of water 1 degree centigrade.

## NUTRIENTS

Nutrients are substances found in food and are used by the body to promote growth, maintenance, and repair. The categories of nutrients are carbohydrates, proteins, fats, vitamins, minerals, and water.

## Carbohydrates

The primary sources of carbohydrates (which include sugars and starches) are plant foods. Monosaccharides and disaccharides come from milk, sugar cane, sugar beets, honey, and fruits. Polysaccharide starch is found in grains, legumes, and root vegetables. Following ingestion, digestion, and metabolism, carbohydrates are converted primarily to glucose, the

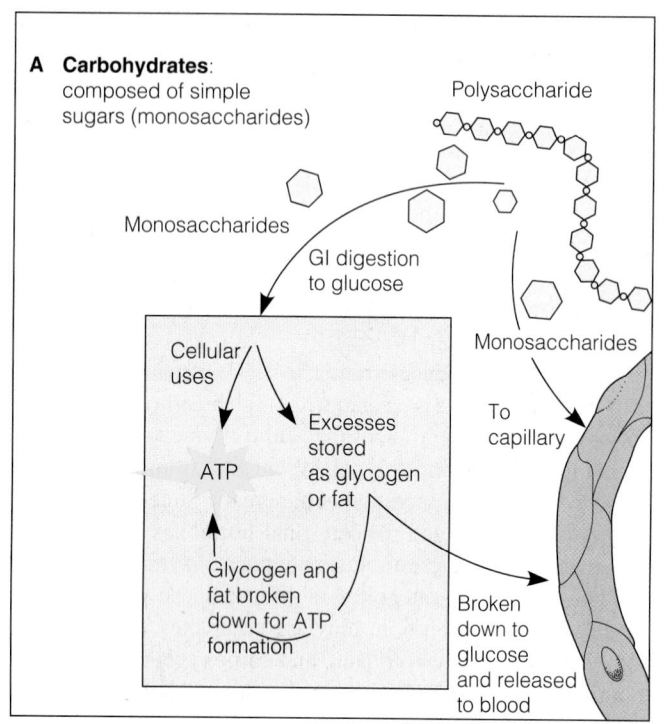

**A Carbohydrates:** composed of simple sugars (monosaccharides)

Polysaccharide

Monosaccharides

GI digestion to glucose

Cellular uses

ATP

Excesses stored as glycogen or fat

Glycogen and fat broken down for ATP formation

Monosaccharides

To capillary

Broken down to glucose and released to blood

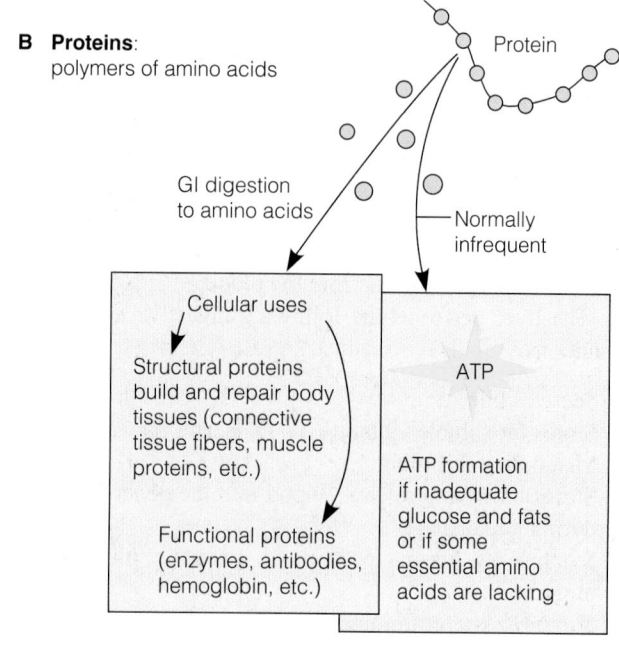

**B Proteins:** polymers of amino acids

Protein

GI digestion to amino acids

Normally infrequent

Cellular uses

Structural proteins build and repair body tissues (connective tissue fibers, muscle proteins, etc.)

Functional proteins (enzymes, antibodies, hemoglobin, etc.)

ATP

ATP formation if inadequate glucose and fats or if some essential amino acids are lacking

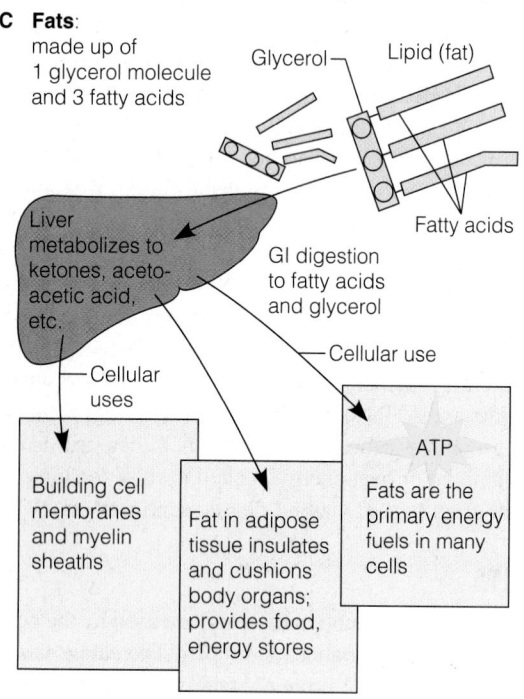

**C Fats:** made up of 1 glycerol molecule and 3 fatty acids

Glycerol

Lipid (fat)

Fatty acids

Liver metabolizes to ketones, aceto-acetic acid, etc.

GI digestion to fatty acids and glycerol

Cellular use

Cellular uses

Building cell membranes and myelin sheaths

Fat in adipose tissue insulates and cushions body organs; provides food, energy stores

ATP

Fats are the primary energy fuels in many cells

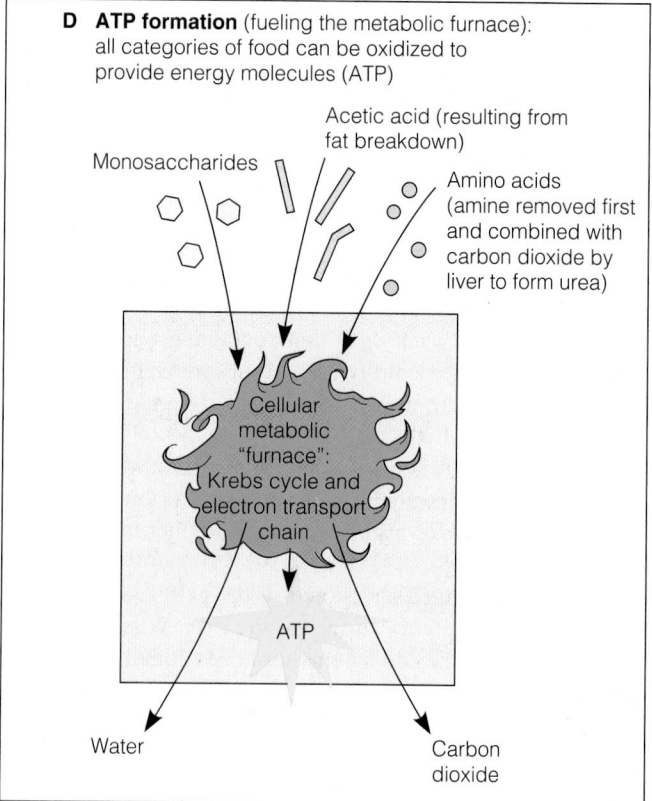

**D ATP formation** (fueling the metabolic furnace): all categories of food can be oxidized to provide energy molecules (ATP)

Acetic acid (resulting from fat breakdown)

Monosaccharides

Amino acids (amine removed first and combined with carbon dioxide by liver to form urea)

Cellular metabolic "furnace": Krebs cycle and electron transport chain

ATP

Water

Carbon dioxide

**Figure 19–4** ■ A schematic overview of nutrient use by body cells, including *A.* carbohydrates; *B.* proteins; *C,* fats; and *D,* ATP formation.

molecule body cells use to make ATP. Glucose is carefully regulated to maintain cellular functions. Excess glucose in the healthy person is converted to glycogen or fat. Glycogen is stored in the liver and muscles; fat is stored as adipose tissue. Carbohydrate use by the body is shown in Figure 19–4A.

Regardless of source, all carbohydrates supply 4 kcal per gram. The minimum necessary daily carbohydrate intake is unknown, but the recommended daily intake is 125 to 175 g, most of which should be complex carbohydrates (such as milk, potatoes, and whole grains). Excess intake of carbohydrates over time can result in obesity, dental caries, and elevated plasma triglycerides. Over extended periods of time, carbohydrate deficiencies lead to tissue wasting from protein breakdown and metabolic acidosis from an excess of ketones as a by-product of fat breakdown.

## Proteins

Proteins are classified as either complete or incomplete. Complete proteins are found in animal products such as eggs, milk, milk products, and meat. They contain the greatest amount of amino acids and meet the body's amino acid requirements for tissue growth and maintenance. Incomplete proteins are found in legumes, nuts, grains, cereals, and vegetables. These sources are low in or lack one or more of the amino acids essential for building complete proteins.

The body uses proteins to build many different structures, including skin keratin, the collagen and elastin in connective tissues, and muscles. They also are used to make enzymes, hemoglobin, plasma proteins, and some hormones. Protein use by the body is shown in Figure 19–4B.

Proteins provide 4 kcal per gram. The recommended daily intake of protein is 56 g for men and 45 g for women. Healthy people with adequate caloric intake have an equal rate of protein synthesis and protein breakdown and loss, reflected as nitrogen balance. If the breakdown and loss of proteins exceeds intake, a negative nitrogen balance results. This may be due to starvation, altered physical states (e.g., from injury or illness), and altered emotional states (such as depression or anxiety). A positive nitrogen balance, which results when protein intake exceeds breakdown, is normal during growth, tissue repair, and pregnancy. Anabolic steroids affect the rate of protein; for example, the adrenal corticosteroids are released in times of stress to increase protein breakdown and conversion of amino acids to glucose. Excessive intake of proteins may lead to obesity, whereas deficits cause weight loss and tissue wasting, edema, and anemia.

## Fats (Lipids)

Fats, or lipids, include phospholipids; steroids, such as cholesterol; and neutral fats, more commonly known as triglycerides. Neutral fats are the most abundant fats in the diet. They may be either saturated or unsaturated. Saturated fats are found in animal products (milk and meats) and in some plant products (such as coconut). Unsaturated fats are found in seeds, nuts, and most vegetable oils. Sources of cholesterol include meats, milk products, and egg yolks. Fat use by the body is shown in Figure 19–4C.

Fats are a necessary part of the structure and function of the body. For example:

- Phospholipids are a part of all cell membranes.
- Triglycerides are the major energy source for hepatocytes and skeletal muscle cells.
- Adipose tissue serves as a protection around body organs, as a layer of insulation under the skin, and as a concentrated source of fuel for cellular energy.
- Dietary fats facilitate absorption of fat-soluble vitamins.
- Linoleic acid, an essential fatty acid, helps form prostaglandins, regulatory molecules that assist in smooth muscle contraction, maintenance of blood pressure, and control of inflammatory responses.
- Cholesterol is the essential component of bile salts, steroid hormones, and vitamin D. Fats supply 9 kcal per gram. The recommended intake of fats is 30% or less of the total daily caloric intake. Saturated fats should account for no more than 10% of the total daily caloric intake, and cholesterol intake should not exceed 250 mg per day. When a person consumes more than the body requires, the excess is stored as adipose tissue, increasing the risk of obesity and heart disease. A deficit of fats may cause excessive weight loss and skin lesions.

## Vitamins

Vitamins are organic compounds that facilitate the body's use of carbohydrates, proteins, and fats. All of the vitamins except vitamins D and K must be ingested in foods or taken as supplements. Vitamin D is made by ultraviolet irradiation of cholesterol molecules in the skin, and vitamin K is synthesized by bacteria in the intestine. Vitamins are categorized as either fat soluble or water soluble. The fat-soluble vitamins (A, D, E, and K) bind to ingested fats and are absorbed as the fats are absorbed. Water-soluble vitamins (the B complex and C) are absorbed with water in the GI tract (however, vitamin $B_{12}$ must become attached to intrinsic factor to be absorbed). Fat-soluble vitamins are stored in the body, and excesses may cause toxicity; water-soluble vitamins in excess of body requirements are excreted in the urine. The recommended amounts of vitamins, previously labeled recommended daily allowances (RDAs), are now labeled by the National Academy of Sciences as dietary reference intakes (DRIs) per day. DRIs are provided for each vitamin in the following discussion.

### Fat-soluble vitamins:

- Vitamin A (retinol) is found in fish liver oils, egg yolk, liver, fortified milk, and margarine. Vitamin A is necessary to vision, skin and mucous membrane integrity, normal reproductive function, and cell membrane structure. The DRI is 1000 µg for men and 800 µg for women.
- Vitamin D is formed by the action of sunlight on cholesterol in the skin. Vitamin D is necessary for blood calcium homeostasis, which in turn is essential to normal blood clotting, bone formation, and neuromuscular function. The DRI is 7.5 µg.
- Vitamin E is found in vegetable oils, margarine, whole grains, and dark green leafy vegetables. Vitamin E is believed to be

an antioxidant; that is, it helps prevent the oxidation of vitamins A and C in the intestine and decreases the oxidation of unsaturated fatty acids to facilitate cell membrane integrity. The DRI is 15 mg.

- Vitamin K is synthesized by coliform bacteria in the large intestine and is found in green leafy vegetables, cabbage, cauliflower, and pork. Vitamin K is essential for the formation of clotting proteins in the liver. The DRI is 2 g.

**Water-soluble vitamins:**

- Vitamin $B_1$ (thiamin) is found in lean meats, liver, eggs, green leafy vegetables, legumes, and whole grains. This B vitamin is an essential coenzyme for carbohydrate catabolism and use. It is essential for the healthy functioning of the nerves, muscles, and heart. The DRI is 1.5 mg for men and 1.1 mg for women.
- Vitamin $B_2$ (riboflavin) is found in liver, egg whites, whole grains, meat, poultry, and fish; a major source is milk. This B vitamin is involved in the catabolism and use of carbohydrates, fats, and proteins, and the use of other B vitamins. It is also important in the production of adrenal hormones. The DRI is 1.7 mg for men and 1.3 mg for women.
- Vitamin $B_6$ (pyridoxine) is found in meat, poultry, fish, potatoes, tomatoes, sweet potatoes, and spinach. This B vitamin is necessary for amino acid metabolism, formation of antibodies, and formation of hemoglobin. The DRI is 2.2 mg for men and 2 mg for women.
- Vitamin $B_{12}$ (cyanocobalamin) is found in liver, meat, poultry, fish, dairy foods (except butter), and eggs. Vitamin $B_{12}$ is not found in any plant foods, however. It is essential for the production of nucleic acids and of red blood cells in the bone marrow. It also plays an important role in the use of folic acid and carbohydrates and in the healthy functioning of the nervous system. The DRI is 3 µg.
- Vitamin C (ascorbic acid) is found in citrus fruits, fresh potatoes, tomatoes, and green leafy vegetables. Vitamin C acts as an antioxidant and a vasoconstrictor. It also serves in the formation of connective tissue, in the conversion of cholesterol to bile salts, in iron absorption and use, and in the conversion of folic acid to its active form. The DRI is 90 mg for men and 75 mg for women.
- Niacin (nicotinamide) is found in meat, poultry, fish, liver, peanuts, and green leafy vegetables. Niacin plays an important role in the metabolism of carbohydrates and fats and inhibits cholesterol synthesis. It is important for the health of the integumentary, nervous, and digestive systems, and assists in the manufacture of reproductive hormones. The DRI is 19 mg for men and 14 mg for women.
- Biotin is found in liver, egg yolk, nuts, and legumes. Biotin is essential for the catabolism of fatty acids and carbohydrates. It also helps dispose of the waste products of protein catabolism. The DRI is 100 to 200 mg.
- Pantothenic acid is found in meats, whole grains, egg yolk, liver, yeast, and legumes. Pantothenic acid assists in the synthesis of steroids and the heme of hemoglobin. It is essential for the metabolism of carbohydrates and fats and for the manufacture of reproductive hormones. The DRI is 10 mg.

- Folic acid (folacin) is found in liver, dark green vegetables, lean beef, eggs, veal, and whole grains. Folic acid is also synthesized by bacteria in the intestine. Folic acid is the basis of a coenzyme necessary to the manufacture of nucleic acids and is therefore essential for the formation of red blood cells, growth and development, and the health of the nervous system. The RDA is 0.4 mg. (DRI not available.)

## Minerals

Minerals work with other nutrients to maintain the structure and function of the body. An adequate supply of calcium, phosphorus, potassium, sulfur, sodium, chloride, and magnesium—as well as other trace elements such as iron, iodine, copper, and zinc—is necessary to health. Most minerals in the body are found in body fluids or are bound to organic compounds. The best sources of minerals are vegetables, legumes, milk, and some meats. Dietary sources for minerals are discussed in Chapter 5. The recommended daily intake for each is as follows: ⊂⊃

- Calcium: 1000 mg, although after menopause, women who do not take estrogen supplements should increase their uptake to 1200 mg.
- Phosphorus: 700 mg
- Iron: 15 mg
- Zinc: 12 mg
- Iodine: 150 µg
- Fluoride: 3.1 mg
- Selenium: 55 µg
- Potassium: 2 g

## ASSESSING NUTRITIONAL STATUS AND THE GASTROINTESTINAL SYSTEM

The nurse conducts both a health assessment interview (to collect subjective data) and a physical assessment (to collect objective data) to assess the client's nutritional status and gastrointestinal function. Physical assessment of the integumentary system, nervous system, musculoskeletal system, cardiovascular system, and respiratory system may also reflect the client's nutritional status. Table 19–1 summarizes abnormal nutritional assessment findings related to these body systems.

## The Health Assessment Interview

This section provides guidelines for collecting subjective data through a health assessment interview specific to nutritional status, the gastrointestinal system, and the accessory digestive organs.

A health assessment interview to determine problems with nutrition and digestion may be conducted during a health screening, may focus on a chief complaint (such as nausea or unexplained weight loss), or may be part of a total health assessment. If the client has a health problem involving nutrition and digestion, analyze its onset, characteristics and course, severity, precipitating and relieving factors, and any associated symptoms, noting the timing and circumstances. For example, ask the client:

- Have you had any episodes of indigestion, nausea, vomiting, diarrhea, or constipation? If so, describe the appearance of what was vomited or the stools and anything that makes

| TABLE 19-1 | Assessment Findings Due to Malnutrition |
|---|---|
| **Body System** | **Assessment Findings** |
| Nails | Soft and spoon-shaped in iron deficiency. Splinter hemorrhages in vitamin C deficiency. |
| Hair | Dry, dull, and scarce in zinc, protein, and linoleic acid deficiencies. |
| Skin | Flaky and dry in vitamin A, vitamin B, and/or linoleic acid deficiency. Cracks and/or hyperpigmentation in niacin deficiency. Bruising in vitamin C or vitamin K deficiency. |
| Eyes | Eyes become dry and soft with decrease in vitamin A. Conjunctiva is pale with a decrease in iron, and red with a decrease in riboflavin. |
| Nervous system | Reflexes are decreased and client may have peripheral neuropathies with thiamine deficiency. Client may be irritable and/or disoriented with thiamine deficiency. |
| Musculoskeletal system | Muscle wasting is seen with deficits in protein, carbohydrate, and fat metabolism. Calf pain occurs with thiamine deficiency; joint pain may occur with vitamin C deficiency. |
| Cardiovascular system | Heart size and rate may increase with thiamine deficiency. Diastolic blood pressure may be increased with a high intake of fat. Lowered cardiac output and decreased blood pressure may occur with caloric deficiencies over a long time period. |
| Respiratory system | Excessive fat can restrict respirations, and excessive fluids can impair gas exchange. |
| Gastrointestinal system | Cheilosis (sores at corner of mouth) seen in vitamin B-complex deficiencies, especially riboflavin. Stomatitis and spongy, bleeding gums may also be seen in malnutrition. |

these problems better or worse. How long have you had these problems?

- What is your usual dietary intake pattern during a 24-hour period?
- Describe what you believe to be a "healthy" diet.

When collecting information about the client's current health status, ask about any changes in weight, appetite, and the ability to taste, chew, or swallow. What is the client's perception of the role of nutrition in maintaining health? Who buys and prepares the food? What medications (prescribed, over-the-counter, or vitamins) is the client currently taking? Does the client take any vitamins, herbal supplements, or other "health-food" items? Does the client consume alcohol (how much and type)? If the client has experienced nausea or vomiting, ask whether the vomitus contains bright red blood, dark (old) blood, bile, or fecal material. If the client is very thin or verbalizes concerns about body size incongruent with the ratio

of height to weight, ask whether the client induces vomiting or uses laxatives to control weight. Ask whether the client has appliances such as braces, bridges, or dentures, and what self-care measures are used for such appliances, as well as oral hygiene practices and frequency of dental visits.

Ask the client to describe any heartburn, indigestion, abdominal discomfort, or pain. Explore the location of the pain, the type of pain, the time it occurs, foods that aggravate or relieve it, and how it is relieved. Abdominal pain is often referred to other sites (see Chapter 4). ∞ For example, a client with a liver disorder may experience pain over the right shoulder (Kehr's sign). Epigastric (middle upper abdominal) pain is experienced in cases of acute gastritis, obstruction of the small intestine, and acute pancreatitis. Pain in the right upper quadrant is associated with cholecystitis. Pain in the left upper quadrant may be related to a gastric ulcer.

The health history should include questions about any prior surgeries or trauma of the gastrointestinal tract. Explore the past history of any medical condition that may affect the client's ingestion, digestion, and/or metabolism (for example, Crohn's disease, diabetes mellitus, irritable bowel syndrome, peptic ulcers, or pancreatitis). Other areas significant to assessment of nutritional status and the gastrointestinal system are food allergies (especially to milk, which is evidenced as lactose intolerance with abdominal cramping, excessive flatus, and loose stools) and a family history that may provide clues to increased risk for health problems.

Other questions and leading statements, categorized by functional health patterns, can be found on the Companion Website.

## Physical Assessment

Physical assessment of gastrointestinal and nutritional status may be performed as part of a total health assessment, in combination with assessment of the urinary and reproductive systems (problems which may cause clinical manifestations similar to those of the gastrointestinal system), or alone for clients with known or suspected health problems. The techniques of inspection, auscultation, percussion, and palpation are used. Palpation is the last method used in assessing the abdomen, because pressure on the abdominal wall and contents may interfere with bowel sounds and cause pain, ending the examination.

Collect objective data by obtaining **anthropometric measurements** (height, weight, triceps skinfolds, and midarm circumference) and by examining the mouth and abdomen. The equipment necessary for the assessment are a stethoscope, a scale, a tape measure, and skinfold calipers. Prior to the examination, collect all necessary equipment and explain techniques to the client to decrease anxiety. The client may be seated during assessment of the mouth, but is supine during the abdominal assessment.

The quadrants of the abdomen, with related internal structures, are illustrated in Figure 19–5 ■.

## Anthropometric Assessment with Abnormal Findings

- Weigh the client and compare the client's actual weight to ideal body weight (IBW) (Table 19–2).

MediaLink | FUNCTIONAL HEALTH PATTERN ASSESSMENT

**Figure  19–5** ■ The four quadrants of the abdomen, with anatomic location of organs within each quadrant.

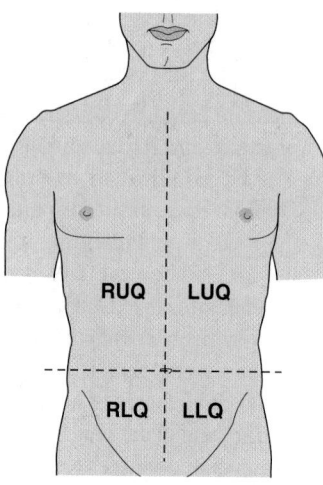

**Midline**
Aorta
Bladder
Uterus

○ = Umbilicus

**Right Upper Quadrant**
Liver and gallbladder
Pylorus
Duodenum
Head of pancreas
Right adrenal gland
Portion of right kidney
Hepatic flexure of colon
Portions of ascending and
    transverse colon

**Left Upper Quadrant**
Left lobe of liver
Spleen
Stomach
Body of pancreas
Left adrenal gland
Portion of left kidney
Splenic flexure of colon
Portions of transverse and
    descending colon

**Right Lower Quadrant**
Lower pole of right kidney
Cecum and appendix
Portion of ascending colon
Bladder (if distended)
Right ovary and salpinx
Right spermatic cord
Right ureter

**Left Lower Quadrant**
Lower pole of left kidney
Sigmoid colon
Portion of descending colon
Bladder (if distended)
Left ovary and salpinx
Uterus (if enlarged)
Left spermatic cord
Left ureter

TABLE 19–2  Example of a Height and Weight Table

| | Height | | Weight* | | |
|---|---|---|---|---|---|
| | Feet | Inches | Small Frame | Medium Frame | Large Frame |
| **Men** (ages 25–29) | 5 | 2 | 128–134 | 131–134 | 138–150 |
| | 5 | 3 | 130–136 | 133–143 | 140–153 |
| | 5 | 4 | 132–138 | 135–145 | 142–156 |
| | 5 | 5 | 134–140 | 137–148 | 144–160 |
| | 5 | 6 | 136–142 | 139–151 | 146–164 |
| | 5 | 7 | 138–145 | 142–154 | 149–168 |
| | 5 | 8 | 140–148 | 145–157 | 152–172 |
| | 5 | 9 | 142–151 | 148–160 | 155–176 |
| | 5 | 10 | 144–154 | 151–163 | 158–180 |
| | 5 | 11 | 146–157 | 154–166 | 161–184 |
| | 6 | 0 | 149–160 | 157–170 | 164–188 |
| | 6 | 1 | 152–164 | 160–174 | 168–192 |
| | 6 | 2 | 155–168 | 164–178 | 172–197 |
| | 6 | 3 | 158–172 | 167–182 | 176–202 |
| | 6 | 4 | 162–176 | 171–187 | 181–207 |
| **Women** (ages 25–29) | 4 | 10 | 102–111 | 109–121 | 118–131 |
| | 4 | 11 | 103–113 | 111–123 | 120–134 |
| | 5 | 0 | 104–115 | 113–126 | 122–137 |
| | 5 | 1 | 106–118 | 115–129 | 125–140 |
| | 5 | 2 | 108–121 | 118–132 | 128–143 |
| | 5 | 3 | 111–124 | 121–135 | 131–147 |
| | 5 | 4 | 114–127 | 124–138 | 134–151 |
| | 5 | 5 | 117–130 | 127–141 | 137–155 |
| | 5 | 6 | 120–133 | 130–144 | 140–159 |
| | 5 | 7 | 123–136 | 133–147 | 143–163 |
| | 5 | 8 | 126–139 | 136–150 | 146–167 |
| | 5 | 9 | 129–142 | 139–153 | 149–170 |
| | 5 | 10 | 132–145 | 142–156 | 152–173 |
| | 5 | 11 | 135–148 | 145–159 | 155–176 |
| | 6 | 0 | 138–151 | 148–162 | 158–179 |

*Weight in pounds. Men: allow 5 lb of clothing. Women: allow 3 lb of clothing.*

*Note.* Courtesy of Metropolitan Life Insurance Company, 1983.

| TABLE 19-3 | Indications of Nutritional Status by Body Weight | |
|---|---|---|
| %IBW | %UBW | Nutritional Status |
| >120 | —— | Obese |
| 110–120 | —— | Overweight |
| 80–90 | 85–95 | Mildly undernourished |
| 70–79 | 75–84 | Moderately undernourished |
| <70 | <75 | Severely undernourished |

| TABLE 19-4 | Values for Anthropometric Measurements | |
|---|---|---|
| | Standard Value | |
| Measurement | Male | Female |
| Triceps skinfold thickness | 12.5 mm | 16.5 mm |
| Midarm circumference | 29.3 cm | 28.5 cm |
| Midarm muscle circumference | 25.3 cm | 23.2 cm |

- A weight 10% to 20% less than ideal body weight indicates malnutrition.
- A weight 10% above ideal body weight is considered overweight.
- A weight 20% above ideal body weight is considered obese.
- Calculate the client's percentage of ideal body weight (%IBW).
  - Use the formula in Table 19–3 to determine the presence of obesity and/or malnutrition based on percentage of ideal body weight.
- Calculate the client's percentage of usual body weight (%UBW) to determine weight change, using this formula:

$$\frac{\text{current weight}}{\text{usual weight}} \times 100$$

  - Using %IBW may result in overlooking malnutrition in a very obese client. Refer to Table 19–3 to determine nutritional status based on %UBW.
- Measure triceps skinfold thickness (TSF).
  - Find the midpoint between the client's olecranon and acromion processes.
  - Grasp the skin and fat, and pull it away from the muscle. Apply skinfold calipers for 3 seconds, and record reading (Figure 19–6 ■).
  - Repeat three times, and average the three readings.
  - Compare the client's reading to the standard values shown in Table 19–4.
  - Triceps readings are 10% or more below standards in malnutrition and 10% or more above standards in obesity or overnutrition.
- Measure midarm circumference (MAC).
  - Find the midpoint between the client's olecranon and acromion processes.
  - Wind tape measure around arm (Figure 19–7 ■). Compare the client's reading to the standard values shown in Table 19–4.
- MAC decreases with malnutrition and increases with obesity.
- Calculate midarm muscle circumference (MAMC).
  - Use the client's triceps skinfold measurement and midarm circumference readings to calculate the client's MAMC, using: MAMC = MAC − (0.314 × TSF).
  - Compare the result to the standard values shown in Table 19–4.
- In mild malnutrition, the MAMC is 90% of the standard; in moderate malnutrition, 60% to 90%. In severe malnutrition (muscle wasting), the MAMC is less than 60% of the standard.

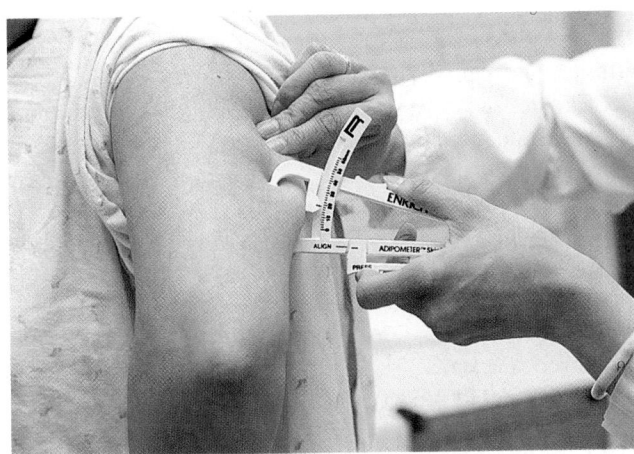

**Figure 19–6 ■** Measuring triceps skinfold thickness with calipers.

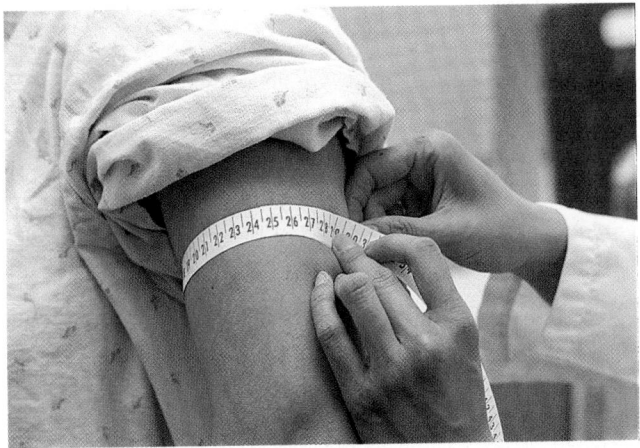

**Figure 19–7 ■** Measuring midarm circumference with a tape measure.

## Oral Assessment with Abnormal Findings

Note: Wear gloves!

- Inspect and palpate the lips.
  - ✓ *Cheilosis* (painful lesions at corners of mouth) is seen with riboflavin and/or niacin deficiency.
  - ✓ Cold sores or clear vesicles with a red base are seen in herpes simplex I.

- Inspect and palpate the tongue.
  - ✓ Atrophic smooth glossitis is characterized by a bright red tongue. It is seen in $B_{12}$, folic acid, and iron deficiencies.
  - ✓ Vertical fissures are seen in dehydration.
  - ✓ A black, hairy tongue may be seen following antibiotic therapy.
- Inspect and palpate the buccal mucosa.
  - ✓ *Leukoplakia* (small white patches) may be a sign of a premalignant condition.
  - ✓ A reddened, dry, swollen mucosa may be seen in stomatitis.
  - ✓ *Candidiases* (white cheesy patches that bleed when scraped) may be seen in immune-suppressed clients receiving antibiotics or chemotherapy and in terminally ill clients.
- Inspect and palpate the teeth.
  - ✓ Cavities and excessive plaque are seen with poor nutrition and/or poor oral hygiene.
- Inspect and palpate the gums.
  - ✓ Swollen, red gums that bleed easily (*gingivitis*) are seen in periodontal disease, vitamin C deficiencies, or with hormonal changes.
- Inspect the throat and tonsils.
  - ✓ In acute infections, tonsils are red and swollen and may have white spots.
- Note the client's breath.
  - ✓ Sweet, fruity breath is noted in diabetic ketoacidosis.
  - ✓ Acetone breath may be a sign of uremia.
  - ✓ Foul breath may result from liver disease, respiratory infections, and poor oral hygiene.

## Abdominal Assessment with Abnormal Findings

Box 19–1 provides guidelines for abdominal assessment.

- Inspect abdominal contour, skin integrity, venous pattern, and aortic pulsation.
  - ✓ Generalized abdominal distention may be seen in gas retention or obesity.
  - ✓ Lower abdominal distention is seen in bladder distention, pregnancy, or ovarian mass.
  - ✓ General distention and an everted umbilicus is seen with ascites and/or tumors.
  - ✓ A scaphoid (sunken) abdomen is seen in malnutrition or when fat is replaced with muscle.
  - ✓ *Striae* (whitish-silver stretch marks) are seen in obesity and during or after pregnancy.
  - ✓ Spider angiomas may be seen in liver disease.
  - ✓ Dilated veins are prominent in cirrhosis of the liver, ascites, portal hypertension, or venocaval obstruction.
  - ✓ Pulsation is increased in aortic aneurysm.
- Auscultate all four quadrants of the abdomen with the diaphragm of the stethoscope (Figure 19–8 ■). Begin in the lower right quadrant, where bowel sounds are almost always present. Normal bowel sounds (gurgling or clicking) occur every 5 to 15 seconds. Listen for at least 5 minutes in each of the four quadrants to confirm the absence of bowel sounds.
  - ✓ *Borborygmus* (hyperactive high-pitched, tinkling, rushing, or growling bowel sounds) is heard in diarrhea or at the onset of bowel obstruction.
  - ✓ Bowel sounds may be absent later in bowel obstruction, with an inflamed peritoneum, and/or following surgery of the abdomen.
- Auscultate the abdomen for vascular sounds with the bell of the stethoscope (Figure 19–9 ■).
  - ✓ *Bruits* (blowing sound due to restriction of blood flow through vessels) may be heard over constricted arteries. A bruit over the liver may be heard in hepatic carcinoma.

---

**BOX 19–1 ■ Guidelines for Assessing the Abdomen**

Ask the client to empty the bladder before beginning the examination. Assist the client to the dorsal recumbent (supine) position, with a small pillow under the head, a pillow under the knees (if desired), and the arms at the sides of the body. Warm the stethoscope before applying it to the client's skin. Ask the client to point to areas that are painful, and explain that those areas will be examined last. Expose the abdomen from below the breasts to the pubic symphysis, and drape the client's thoracic and genital areas. When you document your findings, specify the location by abdominal quadrant.

General guidelines for abdominal assessment are as follows:

1. Inspect the abdomen under a good light source that is shining across the abdomen. Sit at the right side of the client, and note symmetry, distention, masses, visible peristalsis, and respiratory movements. If masses are detected, ask the client to take a deep breath, which decreases the size of the abdominal cavity and makes any abnormality more visible.
2. Auscultate each quadrant of the abdomen, using the diaphragm of the stethoscope. Listen for bowel sounds, arterial bruits, venous hums, and friction rubs.
3. Percuss several areas within each quadrant of the abdomen, using a systematic path. (For example, always begin in the lower left quadrant, then proceed to the lower right quadrant, upper right quadrant, and upper left quadrant, respectively). The predominant percussion tones for the entire abdomen are tympany and dullness. Tympany is present over gas-filled intestines. Dullness is present over the liver, the spleen, an enlarged kidney, or a full stomach. Percuss for fluid, gaseous distention, and masses.
4. Palpate each quadrant of the abdomen for shape, position, mobility, size, consistency, and tenderness of the major abdominal organs. Begin this part of the assessment with light palpation, and increase the depth of palpation to elicit tenderness or better identify organ size and shape. Deep palpation should be conducted only by nurses with considerable experience. Remember to palpate areas of indicated tenderness last and to use gentle pressure. Palpation may be difficult or impossible if the client exhibits muscle guarding from pain or is ticklish. The gallbladder and the spleen are normally not palpable.

✓ A venous hum (continuous medium-pitched sound) may be heard over a cirrhotic liver.

✓ Friction rubs (rough grating sounds) may be heard over an inflamed liver or spleen.

• Percuss the abdomen in all four quadrants (Figure 19–10 ■). Normally, tympany is heard over the stomach and gas-filled bowels.

✓ Dullness is heard when the bowel is displaced with fluid or tumors or filled with a fecal mass.

• Percuss the liver (see Box 19–2 for guidelines for liver percussion and palpation; see Figure 19–11 ■ for landmarks).

✓ In cirrhosis and/or hepatitis, the liver is greater than 6 to 10 cm in the MCL and greater than 4 to 8 cm in the midsternal line (MSL).

• Percuss the spleen for dullness posterior to the midaxilliary line at the level of the 6th to 11th rib (Figure 19–12 ■).

✓ A large area of dullness that extends to the left anterior axcillary line on inspiration is associated with an enlarged

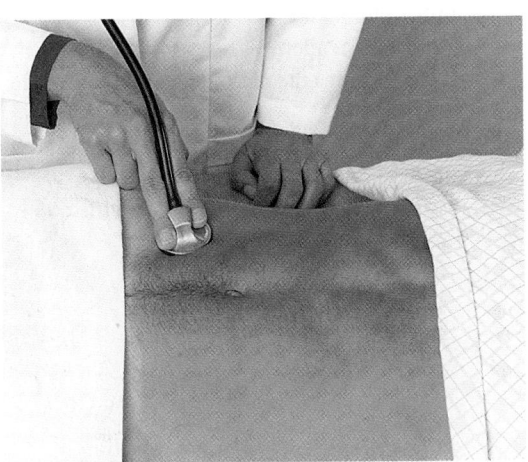

Figure 19–8 ■ Auscultating the abdomen with the diaphragm of the stethoscope.

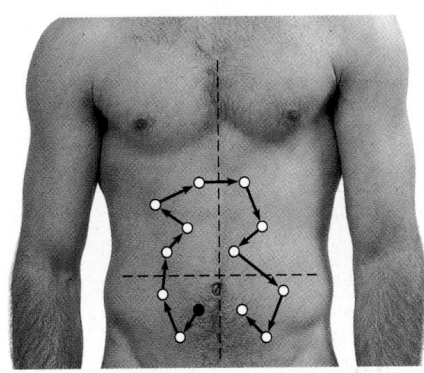

Figure 19–10 ■ Location of sites for systematic percussion of all four quadrants.

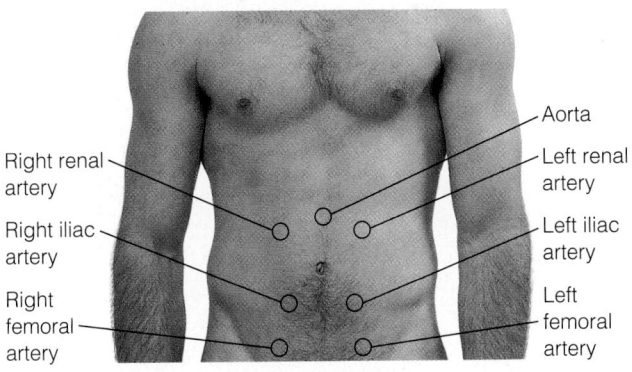

Right renal artery

Right iliac artery

Right femoral artery

Aorta

Left renal artery

Left iliac artery

Left femoral artery

Figure 19–9 ■ Location of placement of the stethoscope for auscultation of arteries of the abdomen.

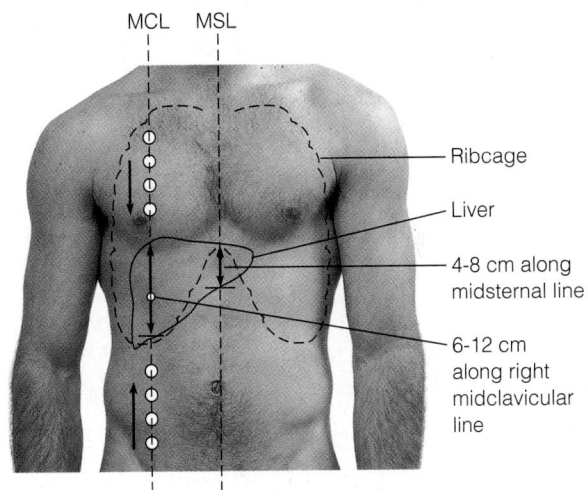

MCL    MSL

Ribcage

Liver

4-8 cm along midsternal line

6-12 cm along right midclavicular line

Figure 19–11 ■ Anatomic location of the liver, with the midclavicular line (MCL) and midsternal line (MSL) superimposed. The normal liver span is 6 to 12 cm.

## BOX 19–2  ■  Guidelines for Percussing and Palpating the Liver

The size of the liver may be determined by percussion and palpation, as follows:

1. Percuss in the midclavicular line (MCL), beginning below the umbilicus (see Figure 19–11). Begin to percuss over a region of typmpany, and move upward. The first dull percussion tone occurs at the lower border of the liver. Determine the upper liver border by beginning percussion over an area of lung resonance (in the MCL) and percussing downward to the first dull tone, usually at the 5th to 7th interspace. Mark each of these loca-

tions, and measure the distance from one mark to the other to determine liver size. The normal liver size is 6 to 12 cm in the MCL; however, men have larger livers than women.

2. Conduct bimanual palpation of the liver by placing your left hand under the client at the level of the 11th to 12th ribs and applying upward pressure. Place your right hand below the costal margin, ask the client to take a deep breath, and palpate for the liver border. The liver is not normally palpable in a healthy adult, although it may be in very thin people.

spleen and may be related to in trauma, infection, or mononucleosis.

- Percuss for shifting dullness (Figure 19–13 ■).
  ✓ In a client with ascites, the level of dullness increases when the client turns to the side.
- Palpate the abdomen in all four quadrants.
  - Use a circular motion to move the abdominal wall over underlying structures (Figure 19–14 ■). Feel for masses and note any tenderness or pain the client may have during this part of the exam. Palpate lightly at first (0.5 to 0.75 inch), then deeply (1.5 to 2 inches) with caution.
  - Never use deep palpation in a client who has had a pulsatile abdominal mass, renal transplant polycystic kidneys, or is at risk for hemorrhage.

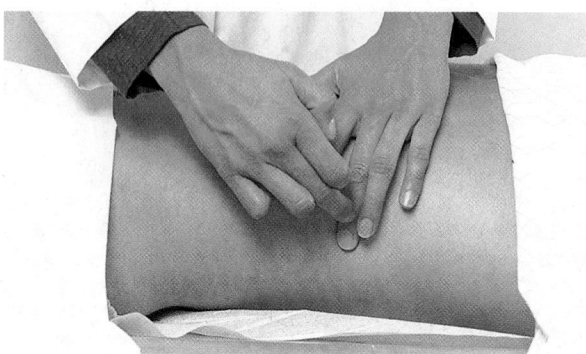

**Figure 19–12 ■** Percussing the spleen.

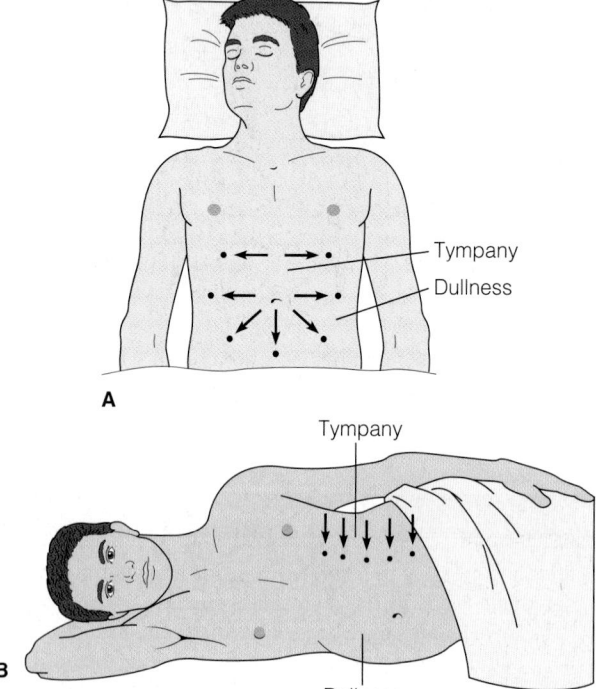

**Figure 19–13 ■** Percussing for shifting dullness in ascites. *A,* Common percussion tones when the client is lying supine; *B,* changes in percussion tones (shfiting dullness) when the client turns to the side.

- ✓ In cases of peritoneal inflammation, palpation causes abdominal pain and involuntary muscle spasms.
- ✓ Abnormal masses include aortic aneurysms, neoplastic tumors of the colon or uterus, and a distended bladder or distended bowel due to obstruction.
- ✓ A rigid, boardlike abdomen may be palpated when the client has a perforated duodenal ulcer.
- ✓ If a mass is palpated, ask the client to raise head and shoulders. A mass in the abdomen may become more prominent with this maneuver, as will a ventral abdominal wall hernia. If the mass is no longer palpable, it is deeper in the abdomen.
- Palpate for rebound tenderness.
  ✓ Press the fingers into the abdomen slowly and release the pressure quickly.
    ✓ In peritoneal inflammation, pain occurs when the fingers are withdrawn.
    ✓ Right upper quadrant pain occurs with acute cholecystitis.

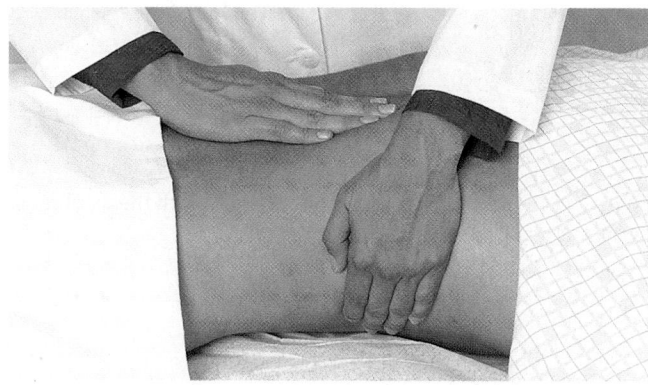

A

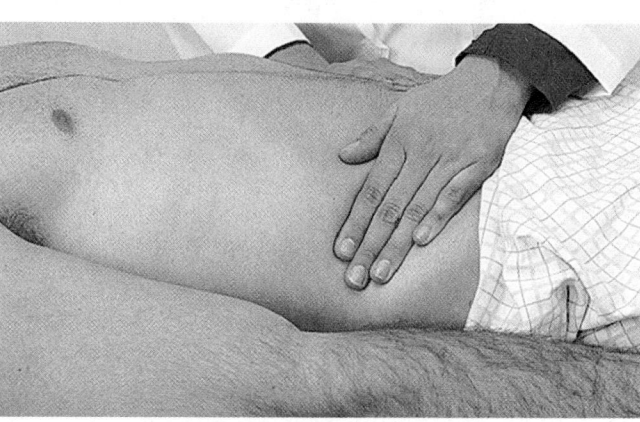

B

**Figure 19–14 ■** Light to moderate palpation of the abdomen. *A,* in light palpation, the examiner, keeping the fingers approximated, gently depresses the abdominal wall about 1 cm to assess for large masses, slight tenderness, and muscle guarding. *B,* The examiner performs moderate palpation by using the palm or the side of the hand to depress the abdominal wall to a slightly greater depth than in light palpation. This technique is useful for assessing abdominal organs that move with respiration (such as the liver and the spleen).

✓ Upper middle abdominal pain occurs with acute pancreatitis.

✓ Right lower quadrant pain occurs with acute appendicitis.

✓ Left lower quadrant pain is seen in acute diverticulitis.

- Palpate the liver (Figure 19–15 ■).

  ✓ An enlarged liver with a smooth, tender edge may indicate hepatitis or venous congestion.

  ✓ An enlarged, nontender liver may be felt in malignant condition.

  ✓ Note whether the client guards the abdomen or reports any sharp pain, especially on inspiration.

  ✓ The client with inflammation of the gallbladder feels sharp pain on inspiration and stops inspiring. This is called Murphy's sign.

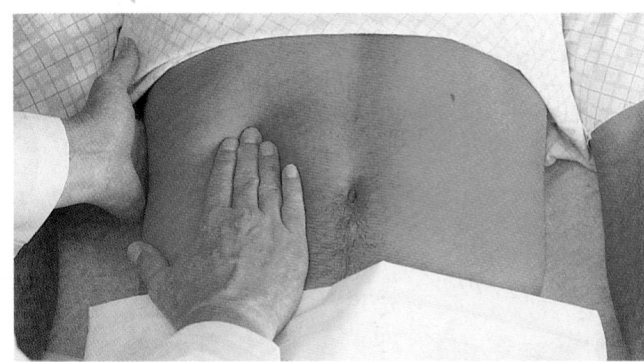

**Figure 19–15** ■ Palpating the liver with the bimanual method.

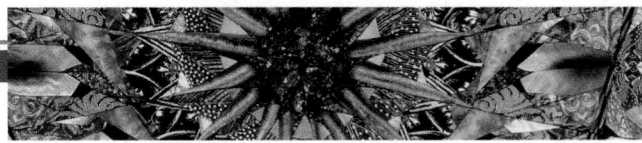

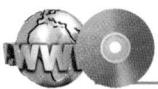

## EXPLORE MediaLink

NCLEX review questions, case studies, care plan activities, MediaLink applications, and other interactive resources for this chapter can be found on the Companion Website at www.prenhall.com/lemone.

Click on Chapter 19 to select the activities for this chapter. For animations, video clips, more NCLEX review questions, and an audio glossary, access the Student CD-ROM accompanying this textbook.

## TEST YOURSELF

1. What is the digestive function of the liver?

   a. To secrete bile
   b. To release glucose
   c. To synthesize plasma proteins
   d. To store iron as ferritin

2. The breakdown of carbohydrates to produce ATP is an example of:

   a. Metabolism
   b. Anabolism
   c. Catabolism
   d. Lipidism

3. During a health history for nutritional problems, it is important to ask the client to describe:

   a. The type, amount, and character of pain experienced
   b. The odor and color of urine

   c. The ability to put joints through full range-of-motion
   d. The usual food and fluid intake for a 24-hour period

4. In which quadrant of the abdomen would you palpate to assess the liver?

   a. Right upper
   b. Right lower
   c. Left upper
   d. Left lower

5. Clients with ascites are assessed for changes in what type of percussion sounds?

   a. Inaudible bowel sounds
   b. Resonance
   c. Alternating amplitude
   d. Shifting dullness

See Test Yourself answers in Appendix C.

## BIBLIOGRAPHY

Curl, P., & Warren, J. (1997). Nutritional screening for the elderly: A CNS role. *Clinical Nurse Specialist, 11*(4), 153–158.

Evans-Stoner, N. (1997). Nutrition assessment: A practical approach. *Nursing Clinics of North America, 32*(4), 637–650.

Kirton, C. (1996). Assessing for ascites. *Nursing 96, 26*(4), 53.

Langan, J. (1998). Abdominal assessment in the home: From A to Zzz. *Home Healthcare Nurse, 16*(1), 50–58.

O'Hanlon-Nichols, T. (1998). Basic assessment series: The gastrointestinal system. *American Journal of Nursing, 98*(4), 48–53.

Watson, J., Miller, J., & Tordecilla, L. (2001). Elder oral assessment and care. *MEDSURG Nursing, 10*(1), 37–44.

Watson, R. (2000a). Assessing the gastrointestinal tract in older people: The lower GI tract. *Nursing Older People, 13*(1), 27–28.

_____ . (2000b). Assessing the gastrointestinal tract in older people: The upper GI tract. *Nursing Older People, 12*(10), 27–28.

Weber, J., & Kelley, J. (2002). *Health assessment in nursing* (2nd ed). Philadelphia: Lippincott-Raven.

Wood, S. (1998). Nutrition assessment. *Nursing Times, 94*(29), insert 2p.

Wright, J. (1997). Seven abdominal assessment signs every emergency nurse should know. *Journal of Emergency Nursing, 23*(5), 446–450.

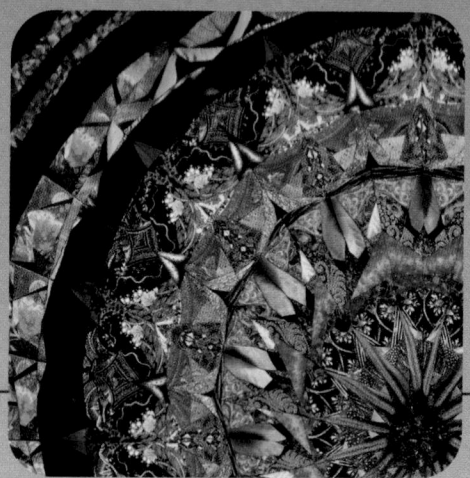

# CHAPTER 20

# Nursing Care of Clients with Nutritional Disorders

## LEARNING OUTCOMES

After completing this chapter, you will be able to:

- Compare and contrast the pathophysiology and manifestations of nutritional disorders.

- Identify diagnostic tests used to find nutritional disorders.

- Discuss nursing implications for collaborative care for clients with nutritional disorders.

- Provide appropriate nursing care for a client receiving enteral or parenteral nutrition.

- Use appropriate techniques to assess clients with nutritional disorders (see Chapter 19).

- Use the nursing process as a framework for providing individualized nursing care for clients with nutritional disorders.

Obesity and malnutrition, the major nutritional disorders in the world today, affect many systems and organs. They often cause serious health problems, such as hypertension, heart disease, fluid and electrolyte imbalances, disability, and even death.

Clients with nutritional disorders require complex, skilled nursing care. Developmental, sociocultural, psychologic, and physiologic factors may play a role in these disorders: A holistic approach to nursing care is vital. Nursing care focuses on identifying causes, meeting nutritional and physiologic needs, providing client education, and meeting the psychologic needs of clients and families.

## THE CLIENT WITH OBESITY

**Obesity,** an excess of adipose tissue, is one of the most prevalent, preventable health problems in the United States. While obesity is often defined by weight, it is more accurately defined by amount of body fat, or adipose tissue. Adipose tissue is created when energy consumption exceeds energy expenditure. Obesity has serious physiologic and psychologic consequences, and is associated with increased morbidity and mortality. Health-related problems associated with obesity are listed in Box 20–1.

### INCIDENCE AND PREVALENCE

Up to one-third of the population in the United States is obese. The incidence of obesity is higher in women, African Americans, and economically disadvantaged people of all races (Braunwald et al., 2001; Tierney et al., 2001). Of particular concern is the increasing incidence of obesity in children and young adults.

### OVERVIEW OF NORMAL PHYSIOLOGY

All body activities require energy, including activities of daily living, as well as those necessary to maintain cell and tissue function. Nutrients in food (or enteral or parenteral feedings)

| BOX 20–1 | ■ Health-Related Problems in Obesity |
|---|---|

- Arthritis
- Atherosclerosis
- Cancers of the breast, uterus, prostate, and colon
- Cholecystitis and cholelithiasis
- Heart failure
- Diabetes mellitus, type 2
- Hiatal hernia
- Postoperative complications
- Hypertension
- Low back pain
- Muscle strains and sprains
- Stress incontinence
- Thrombophlebitis
- Varicosities

provide this energy and the building blocks for growth and tissue repair. The body stores excess nutrients and energy (measured as kilocalories) to meet the body's needs when required nutrients are unavailable. This ability to store and release energy is important to maintaining body function.

Energy is primarily stored as fat in adipose tissue. Although mature fat cells (adipocytes) do not multiply, the immature cells in adipose tissue can multiply, particularly when exposed to estrogen during puberty, in late adolescence, during breastfeeding, and in middle-aged adults who are overweight. Fat cells store excess energy as **triglycerides,** formed from dietary fats and carbohydrates. The body breaks down the triglycerides in fat cells when needed to provide energy (Porth, 2002).

### PATHOPHYSIOLOGY

Obesity occurs when excess calories are stored as fat. It can result from excess energy intake, decreased energy expenditure, or a combination of both.

Appetite, which affects food intake, is regulated by the central nervous system and by emotional factors. The hunger center in the hypothalamus stimulates appetite in response to stimuli such as hypoglycemia. As nutrient levels rise, the satiety center (also in the hypothalamus) sends the message to stop eating. Gastrointestinal filling and hormonal factors also signal *satiety* (a sensation of fullness). Appetite may have little relationship to hunger: People may eat to relieve depression or anxiety.

Several hormones are involved in regulating obesity, including thyroid hormone, insulin, and leptin (a peptide produced by fatty tissue that suppresses appetite and increases energy expenditure). Some studies suggest that leptin resistance is a cause of obesity. Insulin is associated with body fat distribution (Bullock & Henze, 2000). The two major types of body fat distribution are upper body and lower body obesity.

**Upper body obesity** (also called central obesity) is identified by a waist/hip ratio of greater than 1 in men or 0.8 in women. People with upper body obesity tend to have more intra-abdominal fat and higher levels of circulating free fatty acids (Porth, 2002). As a result, upper body obesity is associated with a greater risk of complications such as hypertension, abnormal blood lipid levels, heart disease, stroke, and elevated insulin levels. Men tend to have more intra-abdominal fat than women, although women develop a central fat distribution pattern after menopause.

**Lower body obesity** (also known as peripheral obesity), in which the waist/hip ratio is less than 0.8, is more commonly seen in women. The risk for hyperinsulinemia, abnormal lipids, and heart disease is lower in people with lower body obesity than in those with upper body obesity. Lower body obesity may be more difficult to treat, however.

### Risk Factors

Many factors contribute to obesity, including genetic, physiologic, psychologic, environmental, and sociocultural factors. There is a strong link between heredity and obesity. A person with one obese parent has a 40% chance of becoming obese;

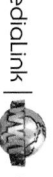

one with two obese parents, an 80% chance. Researchers have reported a strong correlation between the weight of adopted children and their biologic parents.

Physical inactivity is probably the most important factor contributing to obesity. Inactive people may consume fewer calories than active people and continue to gain weight due to lack of energy expenditure.

Environmental influences, such as an abundant and readily accessible food supply, fast-food restaurants, advertising, and vending machines, contribute to increased food intake. Socio-cultural influences that contribute to obesity include overeating at family meals, rewarding behavior with food, religious and family gatherings that promote food intake, and sedentary lifestyles.

Psychologic factors, such as low self-esteem, also play a role in obesity. Low self-esteem may precipitate unhealthy eating behaviors, and the resulting weight gain in turn may diminish self-image even further. A person may overeat as a result of anxiety, depression, guilt, or boredom or as a means of getting attention. Some experts characterize overeating as a food addiction and as a coping mechanism for stressful life events.

## Complications of Obesity

As obesity increases, adverse consequences of obesity increase. Individuals with **morbid obesity** (those whose weight is more than 100% over ideal body weight) have a risk of dying that is 12 times that of people who are not obese (Braunwald et al., 2001). Obesity increases the risk of insulin resistance and type 2 diabetes. It affects reproductive function in both men and women. Androgen (male sex hormone) levels are reduced in obese men; menstrual irregularities and polycystic ovarian syndrome (PCOS) are more common in obese women. Obesity is a significant risk factor for cardiovascular disease, including hypertension, coronary heart disease, and heart failure. Other health-related problems associated with obesity are listed in Box 20–1.

## COLLABORATIVE CARE

Because obesity has many contributing factors, its treatment is far more complex than just reducing the amount of food consumed. Treatment is an ongoing process requiring a number of strategies. Most experts recommend an individualized program of exercise, diet, and behavior modification designed to meet the client's specific needs.

---

**BOX 20–2 ■ Calculating Body Mass Index (BMI)**

BMI = weight (kg)/height$^2$ (m$^2$)
Normal = BMI 18.5–24.9 kg/m$^2$
Overweight = BMI 25–29.9 kg/m$^2$
Obese = BMI > 30 kg/m$^2$
Morbidly obese = BMI > 40 kg/m$^2$

---

## Diagnostic Tests

Although body weight may be used to identify obesity, measures of body fat are more accurate. Males at ideal body weight have 10% to 20% body fat, whereas females at ideal body weight have 20% to 30% body fat.

- *Body mass index (BMI)* is used to identify excess adipose tissue. BMI is calculated by dividing the weight (in kilograms) by the height in meters squared (m$^2$). See Box 20–2.
- *Anthropometry,* skinfold or fatfold measurements, uses calipers to measure skinfold thickness at various sites on the body (see Chapter 19).
- *Underwater weighing (hydrodensitometry)* is considered the most accurate way to determine body fat. This technique involves submerging the whole body and then measuring the amount of displaced water.
- *Bioelectrical impedance* uses a low-energy electrical impulse to determine the percentage of body fat by measuring the electrical resistance of the body.

Other diagnostic tests may be done to help identify a physiologic cause of obesity, as well as complications of obesity.

- A *thyroid profile,* including a T$_3$, T$_4$, and TSH, is done to rule out thyroid disease (see Chapter 16). ☞
- *Serum glucose* is measured to identify coexisting diabetes mellitus.
- *Serum cholesterol* is measured to assess for elevated levels.
- A *lipid profile* is ordered; high-density lipoprotein (HDL) levels are reduced in obese clients, whereas low-density lipoprotein (LDL) levels are elevated.
- An *electrocardiogram (ECG)* is performed to detect effects of obesity on the heart, such as rate or rhythm disruptions, myocardial infarction, or heart enlargement.

## Treatments

Treatment of obesity focuses on changing both eating and exercise habits. A pound of body fat is equivalent to 3500 kcal. To lose 1 pound, therefore, a person must reduce daily caloric intake by 250 kcal for 14 days or increase activity enough to burn the equivalent kcal.

### Exercise

Exercise is a critical element in weight loss and maintenance. Physical activity increases energy consumption and promotes weight loss while preserving lean body mass. Physical activity improves physical fitness, decreases appetite, promotes self-esteem, and increases the basal metabolic rate. An exercise or activity program should reflect the client's physical condition, interest, lifestyle, and abilities. Evaluation by a health care practitioner is important before beginning an exercise program. The practitioner instructs the client to increase the duration and intensity of activity and to stop exercising and report symptoms if chest pain or shortness of breath occurs. An aerobic exercise program of 30 minutes of exercise 3 to 5 days a week promotes weight loss while reducing adipose tissue, increasing lean body mass, and promoting long-term weight control.

## BOX 20–3 ■ Behavioral Change Strategies for the Obese Client

### CONTROLLING THE ENVIRONMENT
- Purchase low-calorie foods.
- Shop from a prepared list and on a full stomach.
- Keep all foods in the kitchen.
- Store all foods in the refrigerator or in the cabinets in opaque containers.
- Prepare exact portions of food to eliminate leftovers.
- Eat all foods in the same place, avoiding the kitchen.
- Avoid eating when watching television or reading.
- Reduce frequency of eating out at restaurants, parties, and picnics.

### CONTROLLING PHYSIOLOGIC RESPONSES TO FOOD
- Eat slowly by taking small bites, allowing 20 minutes for a meal.
- Eat a salad or drink a hot beverage before a meal.
- Chew each bite thoroughly and slowly.
- Put eating utensils or food down between bites.
- Concentrate on the eating process, savor the food.
- Stop eating with the first feelings of fullness.

### CONTROLLING PSYCHOLOGIC RESPONSES TO FOOD
- Appreciate the aesthetic experience of eating.
- Use attractive dinnerware, and prepare a formal setting for eating.
- Use small plates and cups to make servings of food look larger.
- Concentrate on conversations and socialization during the meal.
- Use nonfood rewards for meeting a goal.
- Acknowledge small successes and improvements in all behavior.
- Substitute other activities for eating (e.g., reading, exercise, hobbies).

## Dietary Management

The diet should be low in kilocalories and fat and contain adequate nutrients, minerals, and fiber. The client should eat regular meals with small servings. A gradual, slow weight loss of no more than 1 to 2 pounds per week is recommended. For most people, this means a diet of 1000 to 1500 kcal per day. Fewer than 1200 kcal each day may lead to loss of lean tissue and nutritional deficiencies. The recommended diet generally is low in fat and high in dietary fiber. Excessive calorie restrictions can lead to failure to follow the prescribed diet, feelings of guilt, and overeating. "Yo-yo" dieting (repeated cycles of weight loss and gain) may lead to a metabolic deficiency that makes subsequent weight loss efforts increasingly difficult. Therefore, it is critical that dieters take any weight loss effort seriously and include plans for long-term maintenance. The best approach is to modify dietary intake without severe restrictions, eating a well-balanced, low-fat diet and developing improved eating habits.

**Very low calorie diets (VLCD)** are generally reserved for clients who are more than 35% overweight. This type of program offers a protein-sparing modified fast (400 to 800 kcal/day or less) under close medical supervision. In a typical program, the client observes a 12-week fast, ingesting only a liquid protein supplement. This initial fast is followed by a 12-week refeeding program with nutrition and behavior modification counseling. The client generally experiences a dramatic and rapid weight loss while maintaining lean body mass. This type of program is indicated for short-term use only and requires very close medical supervision.

## Behavior Modification

Behavior modification is a critical component of successful weight management. Strategies such as keeping food records, eliminating cues that precipitate eating, and changing the act of eating are often helpful.

Recording food intake, amount, location of eating, and situations that induce eating often help the dieter gain self-control. These strategies are often most effective when used in combination with other behavior modification approaches.

Researchers have found that most overweight people are stimulated to eat by external cues, such as the proximity to food and the time of day. In contrast, hunger and satiety are the cues that regulate eating in adults of normal weight. Strategies to control food cues include keeping food out of view, eliminating snack foods, and eating only in designated areas. See Box 20–3 for a list of behavior modification strategies.

Other behavior modification approaches focus on helping clients examine factors that affect eating behaviors. Examining lifestyle, personality, and environment helps the client understand eating behaviors and their consequences. The goal is to empower the person who is stimulated to eat to choose activities that are not related to food.

Social support and group programs such as Weight Watchers, Overeaters Anonymous, and Take Off Pounds Sensibly (TOPS) promote weight loss success through peer support. Most organized programs require participants to pay a fee, which may improve compliance.

## Medications

Many prescription and over-the-counter drugs have been used to help people lose weight. When used in combination with diet and exercise, drugs can help promote weight loss. Their long-term efficacy, however, is questionable. In addition, tolerance, addiction, and side effects may occur. These products are usually recommended only as an adjunct to therapy and only when traditional therapies have been unsuccessful.

Amphetamines (which have a high potential for abuse) and nonamphetamine appetite suppressants (such as phenteramine) may be used for a short time to promote weight loss. Sibutramine (Meridia) is an appetite suppressant that acts on the CNS. Sibutramine also may increase the metabolic rate, promoting weight loss. It has the additional benefit of lowering

## Medication Administration
### Drugs to Treat Obesity

**APPETITE SUPPRESSANT**

- Sibutramine (Meridia)

Sibutramine reduces hunger and increases sensations of satiety by inhibiting the uptake of seroatonin, norepinephrine, and dopamine. It is used to treat obesity in clients with a BMI of >30 kg/m² and obese clients who have risk factors such as diabetes or hypertension.

#### Nursing Responsibilities

- Assess for contraindications to this drug, such as pregnancy or lactation, use of other appetite suppressants, impaired liver or kidney function, history of coronary heart disease, or alcohol abuse.
- Regularly monitor blood pressure and heart rate during treatment. Increases may indicate need to reduce dose or discontinue treatment.

#### Client and Family Teaching

- Take as directed; do not exceed recommended dose. Do not take if you may be pregnant or are nursing.
- You may experience difficulty sleeping, nervousness, or palpitations while taking this drug.
- Increase your fluid intake to reduce possible side effects of dry mouth and constipation.

- This drug does not replace diet and exercise for weight loss; continue to follow your prescribed regimen.

**LIPASE INHIBITOR**

- Orlistat (Xenical)

Orlistat inhibits lipases necessary for the breakdown and absorption of fat, thus decreasing the absorption of dietary fat. Its action is primarily local, within the GI tract, with few systemic effects.

#### Nursing Responsibilities

- Administer with meals or up to 1 hour following a meal.
- Provide a fat-soluble vitamin supplement (A, D, E, and K) daily. Separate administration time from orlistat by at least 2 hours.

#### Client and Family Teaching

- Take as directed; do not increase dose. You may skip a dose if you do not consume a meal.
- Use in conjunction with a low-calorie, low-fat diet.
- Common gastrointestinal side effects include oily or fatty stools, flatulence, oily discharge, or frequent stools with difficulty controlling defecation. These side effects may diminish with time or increase if a meal high in fat is consumed.
- Notify your health care provider if you become pregnant while taking this medication.

---

cholesterol and triglyceride levels. Orlistat (Xenical) has a different mechanism of action: It inhibits fat absorption from the GI tract, leading to weight loss. It has the added benefit of lowering blood glucose and cholesterol. See the box above for the nursing implications of these drugs.

Over-the-counter products such as phenylpropanolamine, benzocaine, and bulk-forming agents are commonly used in weight management efforts. Phenylpropanolamine (Acutrim, Dexatrim) is an adrenergic agent that suppresses appetite. This product is contraindicated in clients with hypertension, coronary heart disease, diabetes mellitus, and thyroid disease. Methylcellulose and other bulk-forming products may decrease appetite by producing a sensation of fullness. Clients taking these products may experience flatulence or diarrhea and may need to increase fluid intake.

## Surgery

Surgical treatment of obesity generally is limited to morbidly obese clients (BMI of over 40 kg/m² or 100% over ideal body weight). In addition, clients must be able to tolerate surgery and be free of addiction to alcohol or other drugs. A thorough psychologic evaluation is done before surgery.

The most common surgical procedures used in the United States to treat obesity are the vertical banded gastroplasty and Roux-en-Y gastric bypass (Figure 20–1 ■). These procedures reduce stomach capacity. Although the risk for postoperative complications is high, the mortality rate for these procedures is low. Possible postoperative complications include anasto-

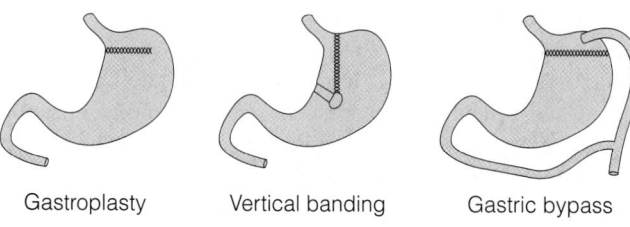

Gastroplasty     Vertical banding     Gastric bypass

**Figure 20–1 ■** Surgical procedures to treat obesity.

mosis leak with peritonitis, abdominal wall hernia, wound infections, deep vein thrombosis, nutritional deficiencies, and gastrointestinal symptoms (Tierney et al., 2001). Clients may lose as much as half their initial body weight following surgery.

## Maintaining Weight Loss

Losing weight and maintaining that loss are two separate but related issues. Most experts agree that the majority of dieters regain lost weight within a 2-year period. The potential risks associated with regaining weight make maintenance a critical issue. Clients are encouraged to continue exercise, self-monitoring, and treatment support. Long-term weight loss and maintenance mean a lifelong commitment to significant lifestyle changes, including food and eating habits, activity and exercise routines, and behavior modification.

## NURSING CARE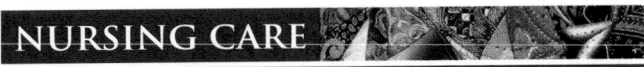

### Health Promotion

Maintaining a healthy weight throughout the life span begins in childhood. Obese children and teenagers become obese adults. Promote healthy eating, including a diet rich in whole grains, fruits, and vegetables and low in fat. Encourage all children and adults to maintain an active lifestyle, engaging in at least 30 minutes of aerobic activity daily. Encourage parents to limit time children spend watching television, using the computer, and playing video games. Discuss the effect of smoking and excess alcohol use on nutrition and activity.

Adults commonly gain about 20 pounds between early and middle adulthood. Encourage clients to reduce the amount of calories consumed as energy needs change.

### Assessment

Collect the following data through the health history and physical examination (see Chapter 19).

- Health history: risk factors; current and usual weight; recent weight gains or losses; perception of weight and effect on health; usual diet and food intake; exercise/activity patterns; prior weight-loss efforts; current medications; coexisting disorders such as cardiovascular disease and diabetes
- Physical examination: vital signs; weight and height; skin-fold measurements; waist/hip ratio; BMI

### Nursing Diagnoses and Interventions

Nursing care for overweight and obese clients is community based and holistic, focusing on both physiologic and psychologic responses to weight and appearance.

#### Imbalanced Nutrition: More Than Body Requirements

Although many factors contribute to obesity, it always involves an imbalance of kcal consumption to energy expenditure.

- Encourage the client to identify the factors that contribute to excess food intake. *Identification of cues to eating helps the client eliminate or reduce these cues.*
- Establish realistic weight-loss goals and exercise/activity objectives. *Small, reasonable goals, such as loss of 1 to 2 pounds per week, increase the likelihood of success.*
- Assess the client's knowledge and discuss well-balanced diet plans. Provide necessary teaching about diet. *Knowledge empowers the client to participate and make appropriate diet choices.*
- Discuss behavior modification strategies, such as self-monitoring and environmental management. *Behavior modification, diet, and exercise are critical to promoting successful, long-term weight loss.*

#### Activity Intolerance

Obese clients may experience excess fatigue, tachycardia, and shortness of breath with activity due to the physiologic effects of excess weight as well as a sedentary lifestyle. A medical evaluation may be needed before beginning an exercise program.

- Assess current activity level and tolerance of that activity. Assess vital signs. *This provides baseline information to plan an activity program and assess response to that activity.*
- After medical clearance, plan with the client a program of regular, gradually increasing exercise. Consider a consultation with an exercise physiologist. *An individualized exercise program promotes activities within the client's physical capabilities.*

#### Ineffective Therapeutic Regimen Management

Most overweight or obese clients experience some difficulty integrating all the components of a weight-loss program into a daily routine. For a weight loss and maintenance program to be successful, the overweight client must modify dietary intake in a world of daily temptations. There may be many obstacles to exercise, including a busy schedule, activity intolerance, impaired physical mobility, lack of equipment, and the embarrassment of being fat.

- Discuss ability and willingness to incorporate changes into daily patterns of diet, exercise, and lifestyle. *This provides data from which to set realistic goals with the client.*
- Help the client identify behavior modification strategies and support systems for weight loss and maintenance. *Weight loss and maintenance are most successful if the client establishes lifestyle patterns that promote interest and motivation and thus exercise and diet management. Family and social support is critical to successful adherence to the therapeutic regime.*
- Have the client establish strategies for dealing with "stress" eating or interruptions in the therapeutic regime. *A sense of failure associated with overeating or lack of exercise can lead to further overeating. Identifying positive strategies to deal with these situations promotes self-acceptance and limits self-punishment through overeating.*

#### Chronic Low Self-Esteem

Although many obese clients may have accepted their weight and body appearance on some level, most overweight and obese individuals verbalize the experience of "fat prejudice" in their family, workplace, or community. Obese clients may experience ridicule, prejudice, and health problems attributed to being "fat." These experiences, coupled with day-to-day problems such as finding attractive clothing or a chair large enough to sit on can affect self-esteem. Many clients report that "fat" jokes or comments contribute to a sense of negative self-worth.

- Encourage the client to verbalize the experience of being overweight, and validate the client's experience. *This provides baseline data to use in developing individualized interventions to addresses self-esteem issues.*
- Set small goals with the client and offer positive feedback and encouragement. *Small goals provide more opportunities for success. Positive feedback and encouragement provide a comfortable environment in which to develop self-esteem.*
- Refer for counseling as appropriate. *Many clients benefit from counseling for issues related to self-esteem.*

## CHART 20–1  NANDA, NIC, AND NOC LINKAGES

### The Obese Client

| NURSING DIAGNOSES | NURSING INTERVENTIONS | NURSING OUTCOMES |
| --- | --- | --- |
| • Imbalanced Nutrition: More than Body Requirements | • Nutrition Management<br>• Weight Reduction Assistance<br>• Behavior Modification | • Nutritional Status<br>• Nutrient Intake<br>• Weight Control |
| • Disturbed Body Image | • Body Image Enhancement | • Body Image |
| • Chronic Low Self-Esteem | • Self-Esteem Enhancement | • Self-Esteem |

*Note. Data from* Nursing Outcomes Classification (NOC) *by M. Johnson & M. Maas (Eds.), 1997, St. Louis: Mosby;* Nursing Diagnoses: Definitions & Classification 2001–2002 *by North American Nursing Diagnosis Association, 2001, Philadelphia: NANDA;* Nursing Interventions Classification (NIC) *by J.C. McCloskey & G. M. Bulechek (Eds.), 2000, St. Louis: Mosby. Reprinted by permission.*

## Using NANDA, NIC, and NOC

Chart 20–1 shows links between NANDA nursing diagnoses, NIC, and NOC for obese clients.

## Home Care

Weight reduction usually occurs in community-based settings. Weight loss and maintenance requires a long-term commitment

## Nursing Care Plan
### A Client with Obesity

Sam Elliott, age 57, has gained 30 pounds since his retirement 2 years ago. The most active thing he does each day is "puttering around" and "walking to the end of the driveway to get the mail." His diet includes juice, oatmeal, muffin, and coffee with cream for breakfast; donuts and coffee with friends midmorning; a bologna-and-cheese sandwich with chips and a root beer for lunch; and cheese, crackers, and wine before a dinner of meat, potatoes, vegetables, and dessert. He tells the nurse, "I have never had to diet. I just don't know how to get this weight off."

### ASSESSMENT

Mr. Elliott is 5′ 8″ (173 cm) tall and weighs 201 lb (91.2 kg). His BMI is 30.1 kg/m². His cholesterol is 240 mg/dL (normal 150 to 200 mg/dL) with an HDL of 37 mg/dL (normal male value > 45 mg/dL) and an LDL of 180 mg/dL (normal <130 mg/dL). His BP is 138/90. His fasting blood glucose is normal at 103 mg/dL. His ECG shows normal sinus rhythm. He reports fatigue and shortness of breath with activity. His health care provider has advised a weight loss of 30 pounds and a regular exercise program.

### DIAGNOSES

- *Imbalanced nutrition: More than body requirements* related to food intake in excess of energy expenditure
- *Risk for ineffective therapeutic regimen management* related to knowledge deficit
- *Activity intolerance* related to sedentary lifestyle

### EXPECTED OUTCOMES

- Lose 1 pound each week.
- Walk 30 minutes 5 days each week.
- Verbalize an understanding of the relationship between weight loss, weight control, and exercise.
- Identify behavior modification strategies to avoid overeating.
- Identify support systems for behavior modification.

### PLANNING AND IMPLEMENTATION

- Assess weight and blood pressure once or twice each week.
- Discuss current eating habits and strategies to reduce fat and calorie intake.
- Discuss cues that promote eating. Identify strategies to eliminate or reduce eating cues.
- Teach to keep a food diary to examine and change eating habits.
- Discuss the role of regular exercise in weight loss and weight control. Instruct to maintain an exercise record to track the intensity and duration of activity.
- Discuss lifestyle and behavior modification strategies to promote successful weight loss and control.

### EVALUATION

Two weeks after changing his diet and beginning to exercise, Mr. Elliott has lost 2 pounds. He has maintained a food diary. He has identified boredom as a cue to eating. In light of that fact, he has started volunteering at the local hospital, where he is working with children. He is walking for 30 minutes 5 days a week. He plans to increase his activity periods to 45 minutes. He verbalizes commitment to a lifelong plan of exercising and eating a low-fat diet. His BP has ranged from 132/76 to 136/84. He plans to have the employee health nurse at the hospital check his weight and BP each week and to join Weight Watchers for ongoing support.

### Critical Thinking in the Nursing Process

1. What are some possible pathophysiologic bases for Mr. Elliott's abnormal cholesterol, HDL, and LDL levels?
2. Develop a teaching plan for a group of overweight men and women.
3. Identify potential barriers to losing weight and strategies to reduce or eliminate these barriers.

See Evaluating Your Response in Appendix C.

by the client, family, and support systems. Address the following topics with the client and family.

- Lifestyle changes are more effective than diets. Fad diets promote rapid weight loss but often are not nutritionally sound or may be difficult to maintain for a lifetime.
- All household members should consume a diet that is nutritionally sound, low in fat, and high in fiber.
- Establish realistic weight loss goals and a system of nonfood rewards for achieving each goal.
- Identify an "exercise buddy" or support system to promote continued physical activity.
- Expect occasional failures. Resume prescribed diet and exercise routine as soon as possible; the goal is long-term weight management.
- Community resources such as Weight Watchers, TOPS, or health care–based programs provide information, strategies, and support for successful weight management.

## THE CLIENT WITH MALNUTRITION

**Malnutrition** results from inadequate intake of nutrients. There may be a lack of major nutrients (calories, carbohydrates, proteins, and fats) or micronutrients such as vitamins and minerals. Malnutrition may be caused by inadequate nutrient intake, impaired absorption and use of nutrients, or increased metabolic needs.

## INCIDENCE AND PREVALENCE

Malnutrition is a widespread cause of disease and mortality throughout the world. It is endemic in regions affected by famine. Groups at risk for malnutrition in the United States include the young, poor, elderly, homeless, low-income women, and ethnic minorities. Even when food is plentiful, clients may be undernourished because of poor food choices.

More than half of all hospitalized clients are malnourished (Braunwald et al., 2001). Malnutrition may be present on admission or develop as a result of surgery or serious illness. See Box 20–4 for conditions commonly associated with malnutrition.

## PATHOPHYSIOLOGY

Carbohydrates and fats in the diet are the body's primary energy source. Approximately 15% to 25% of the body is fat, the

| BOX 20–4 ■ Conditions Associated with Malnutrition |
| --- |

| | |
| --- | --- |
| ■ Acute respiratory failure | ■ Gastrointestinal disorders |
| ■ Aging | ■ Neurologic disorders |
| ■ AIDS | ■ Renal disease |
| ■ Alcoholism | ■ Short bowel syndrome |
| ■ Burns | ■ Surgery |
| ■ COPD | ■ Trauma |
| ■ Eating disorders | |

body's energy reservoir. The remainder (muscles, bones, other body tissues and organs) is lean body mass, metabolically active tissue. Proteins in the diet primarily are used to maintain this tissue. Glycogen and proteins in this lean body mass also act as energy stores.

When dietary intake does not meet the body's energy needs, the body uses glycogen, body proteins, and lipids (fats) to support metabolism. In **starvation** (inadequate dietary intake), glycogen initially is used to provide energy. After the first 24 hours of starvation, gluconeogenesis (formation of glucose from proteins) is the major source of energy. As starvation continues, the body breaks down fats into free fatty acids and ketones, which provide energy for the brain. The size of all body compartments is reduced as body fats and muscle proteins are used to meet energy needs. As lean body mass is reduced, metabolically active tissue is lost, and energy expenditure decreases.

The stress of acute illness or trauma produces a different response. The acute stress response produces a state of hypermetabolism and **catabolism** (cell and tissue breakdown). This hypermetabolic state increases energy expenditure and nutrient needs. Lean body mass is broken down to meet these needs. If untreated, up to half of the body's protein stores can be used within 3 weeks.

Many hospitalized clients are malnourished (starved) on admission. Surgery or illness promote a stress response, resulting in **protein-calorie malnutrition (PCM)**. In PCM, both protein and calories are deficient. Chronic protein deficiency with adequate calories to meet energy needs is called **kwashiorkor.** When both proteins and calories are insufficient to meet the body's needs, PCM is known as **marasmus.**

### Risk Factors

Risk factors for malnutrition include the following:

- Age—older adults are at greater risk for malnutrition due to a variety of factors (see the Meeting Individualized Needs box on page 530)
- Poverty, homelessness, inadequate food storage and preparation facilities
- Functional health problems that limit mobility or vision
- Oral or gastrointestinal problems that affect food intake, digestion, and absorption
- Chronic pain or chronic diseases such as pulmonary, cardiovascular, renal, or endocrine disorders
- Medications or treatments that affect appetite
- Acute problems such as infection, surgery, or trauma

### Manifestations and Complications

The manifestations of malnutrition may vary among clients. Weight loss is the most apparent manifestation of malnutrition. The malnourished client may have a body weight of less than 90% of ideal. Body mass also is reduced (see Box 20–2), as is skinfold thickness. Other manifestations include a wasted appearance, dry and brittle hair, and pale mucous membranes. Peripheral or abdominal edema may be present. Manifestations of specific nutritional deficiencies may be present (Table 20–1). See page 531 for the *Multisystem Effects of Malnutrition.*

## Meeting Individualized Needs

### NUTRITION FOR THE OLDER ADULT

Older adults are at greater risk for malnutrition. Age-related changes that contribute to this problem include changes in taste and smell, a higher incidence of gastrointestinal disease, poor oral health, loss of teeth or ill-fitting dentures, anorexia caused by medications, and functional limitations that impair the ability to shop and cook. Psychosocial issues also contribute to the problem. Older adults living on fixed incomes, many at the poverty level, may not be able to afford well-balanced meals. Loss of appetite is a problem commonly seen with depression. Social isolation and loneliness contribute to the problem. Eating is a social event, and older adults who eat alone may not eat as well as those who share meals with companions, and may consume too few, or too many, calories.

Conduct a thorough assessment to determine nutritional status. Assess psychological factors that influence eating habits, such as loneliness, isolation, and depression. Note the client's general appearance and obtain a diet history, including infor-

mation about foods and nutrients the client consumes, and recent weight loss or gain. Review laboratory values, including complete blood count, total protein, and albumin.

### Teaching for Home Care

To maintain nutritional status, the older client should be advised to:

- Eat a well-balanced diet.
- Eat fresh fruits and vegetables.
- Shop wisely to get the most value for the money.
- Avoid processed foods.
- Avoid foods high in fat.
- Drink adequate fluids.
- Exercise regularly.
- Contact local agencies for the availability of congregate meals (e.g., at local senior centers) or home-delivered meals (e.g., Meals-on-Wheels).

---

Subcutaneous fat and muscle proteins are broken down in PCM, impairing mobility and increasing the risk for skin and tissue breakdown (pressure ulcers). Protein synthesis is inhibited and wound healing delayed. Serum albumin levels fall, leading to abdominal edema, diarrhea, and impaired nutrient absorption. Immune function is impaired, increasing the risk of infection. Cardiac output falls, and the risk for postural hypotension increases.

| TABLE 20–1 | Manifestations of Specific Nutrient Deficiencies |
| --- | --- |
| **Deficiency** | **Assessment Data** |
| Calorie | Weight Loss<br>Weakness, listlessness<br>Loss of subcutaneous fat<br>Muscle wasting |
| Protein | Thin or sparse hair<br>Flaking skin<br>Hepatomegaly |
| Vitamin A | Night blindness<br>Altered taste and smell<br>Dry, scaling, rough skin |
| Thiamine | Confusion, apathy<br>Cardiomegaly, dyspnea<br>Muscle cramping and wasting<br>Paresthesia, neuropathy<br>Ataxia |
| Riboflavin | Cheilosis, stomatitis<br>Neuropathy, glossitis |
| Vitamin C | Swollen, bleeding gums<br>Delayed wound healing<br>Weakness, depression<br>Easy bruising |
| Iron | Smooth tongue<br>Listlessness, fatigue<br>Dyspnea |

## COLLABORATIVE CARE

The goal of treatment for the malnourished client is to restore ideal body weight while replacing and restoring depleted nutrients and minerals. The client's age, severity of malnutrition, and coexisting health problems help determine interventions. Treatment may include oral supplementation, tube feedings, or total parenteral nutrition (TPN).

### Diagnostic Tests

As with obesity, the standard measurements to assess for malnutrition include height, weight, calculation of BMI, and skinfold measurements. A BMI of less than 18 to 20 kg/m² may indicate malnutrition. The following laboratory studies also may be ordered.

- *Serum albumin* is reduced in PCM, and may be below 3.0 mg/dL.
- The *total lymphocyte count* is evaluated by multiplying the WBC by the percentage of lymphocytes. The total lymphocyte count is reduced in PCM.
- *Serum electrolytes* are measured. Potassium levels are low in severe malnutrition.

The following specialized procedures to evaluate the extent of malnutrition may be ordered.

- *Bioelectric impedance analysis* measures body fat and total body water. Differences in the conductivity of a weak current (measured between the hands and feet) allow calculation of body fat and water (current flows more slowly through fat tissue than through water).
- *Total daily energy expenditure* (which includes resting energy expenditure, energy needed for digestion, plus physical activity needs) may be measured to help determine the client's calorie intake needs.

# Multisystem Effects of Malnutrition

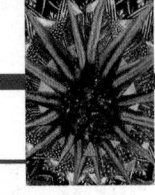

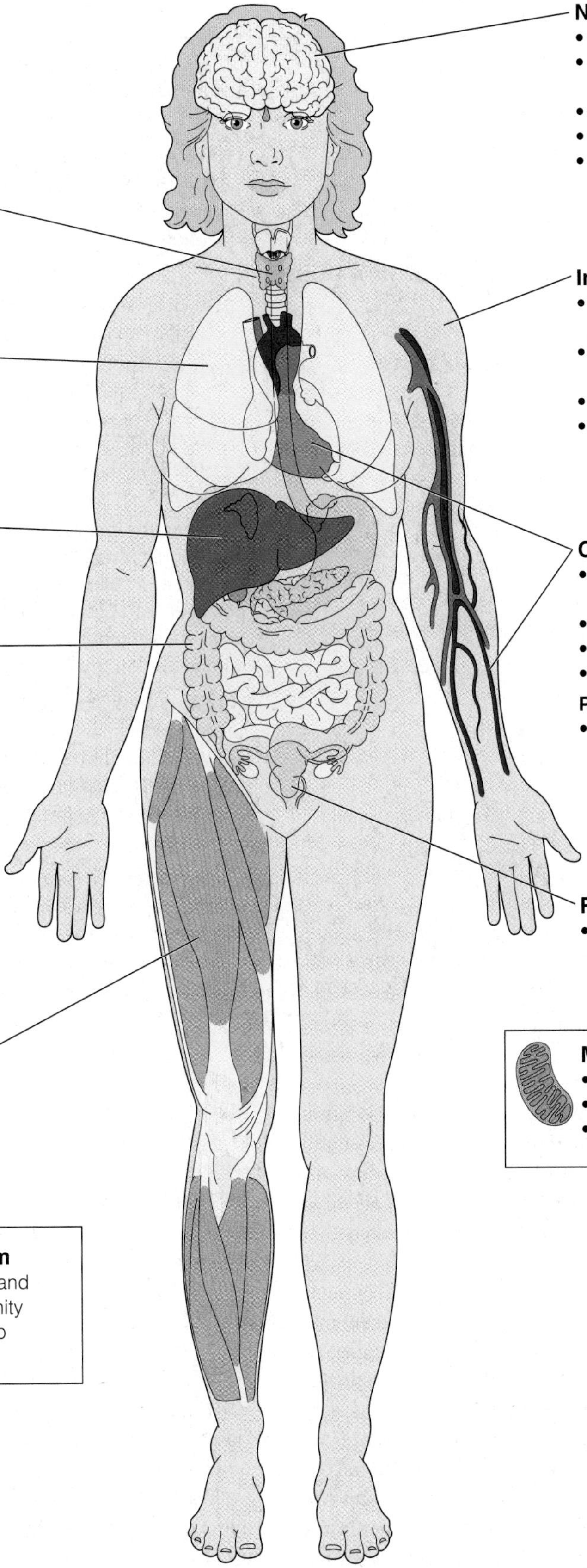

Neurologic
• ↓ Cognition
• ↓ Consciousness (drowsiness, lethargy)
• Tremors
• Paresthesias
• Impaired coordination
Endocrine
• ↓ Thyroid hormones
• ↓ Testosterone (male)
• ↓ Estrogen (female)
Integumentary
• Hair: brittle, dull, dry, loss of color
• Nails: fragile, brittle, spoon-shaped
• Petechiae
• Poor wound healing
Respiratory
• ↓ Respiratory rate
• ↓ Vital capacity
Hepatic
• Hepatomegaly
• ↓ Bile synthesis
Cardiovascular
• Dysrythmias and conduction disturbances
• ↓ HR
• ↓ BP
• Enlarged heart
Potential Complication
• Heart failure
Gastrointestinal
Oral/esophageal:
• Cheilosis
• Glossitis
• Gingivitis
Stomach/intestines:
• Ascites
• Constipation
• Intestinal atrophy
• Steatorrhea
• ↓ Gastric and pancreatic secretions
Potential Complication
• Malabsorption syndrome
Reproductive
• Amenorrhea
Metabolic Processes
• ↓Weight
• ↓Core body temperature
• Edema
Musculoskeletal
• Muscle wasting
• Tenderness
• Impaired strength
Immune System
• ↓ Cell-mediated and humoral immunity
• ↑ Susceptibility to infections

# Medication Administration

## Vitamin & Mineral Supplements

### FAT-SOLUBLE VITAMINS

Vitamin A
Vitamin D
Vitamin E
Vitamin K

The fat-soluble vitamins are absorbed in the gastrointestinal tract. Vitamins A and D are stored in the liver.

All fat-soluble vitamins may become toxic if taken in excess amounts.

### Nursing Responsibilities

- Monitor for manifestations of vitamin excess as well as for adverse effects from vitamin administration.
- Monitor carefully for hypersensitivity reactions during the parenteral administration. Have emergency equipment available.
- Administer vitamin A with food.
- Do not administer vitamin K intravenously.

### Client and Family Teaching

- Teach the importance of eating a well-balanced diet. If indicated, provide lists of foods high in specific vitamins.
- Caution that excessive intake of these vitamins may lead to vitamin toxicity.

### WATER-SOLUBLE VITAMINS

Vitamin C (ascorbic acid)
Vitamin B complex:
Thiamine ($B_1$)
Riboflavin ($B_2$)
Niacin (Nicotinic acid)
Pyridoxine hydrochloride ($B_6$)
Pantothenic acid
Biotin

These vitamins are used to prevent or treat deficiency problems. If the diet is deficient in one vitamin, it is usually deficient in other vitamins as well; therefore, multivitamin preparations are often administered. Most of these vitamins are well absorbed from the gastrointestinal tract.

### Nursing Responsibilities

- Monitor for responses to replacement therapy.
- Monitor for hypersensitivity reactions from parenteral administration. Have emergency equipment available.

### Client and Family Teaching

- Do not exceed the recommended daily allowances for the specific vitamin.

### MINERALS

| | | |
|---|---|---|
| Sodium | Copper | Manganese |
| Potassium | Fluoride | Chromium |
| Magnesium | Iodine | Selenium |
| Calcium | Zinc | |

Minerals are inorganic chemicals that are vital to a variety of physiologic functions. Also called trace elements, these minerals are part of a balanced diet. Recommended daily allowances have not been established for all mineral substances. The dosage of prescribed minerals depends on the specific deficiency, route of administration, and the client's general health.

### Nursing Responsibilities

- Monitor for manifestations of mineral imbalance.
- Prior to administration dilute oral mineral preparations.
- Prior to the administration of iodine, assess for history of hypersensitivity to iodine or seafood; if hypersensitive notify the physician.

### Client and Family Teaching

- Encourage the client to avoid exceeding the known recommended daily allowances of the mineral.
- Instruct the client to take minerals other than fluoride and zinc with or after meals.

## Medications

Malnourished clients generally require supplemental vitamins and minerals to restore these essential micronutrients. A multivitamin and mineral supplement may be given, or therapy may be tailored to correct specific deficiencies. See the box above for nursing implications of vitamin and mineral supplements.

## Fluid and Dietary Management

Fluids and nutrients are carefully reintroduced in severely malnourished clients. First, fluid and electrolyte imbalances are corrected, with particular attention paid to restoring normal potassium, magnesium, and calcium levels, as well as acid-base balance. Once fluid and electrolyte imbalances are corrected, protein and calories are gradually reintroduced into the diet. Vitamin and mineral supplements are provided along with refeeding. Fat and lactose are reintroduced into the diet last.

Gradual refeeding is necessary to prevent electrolyte imbalances from developing as potassium, magnesium, phosphorus, and glucose move into the cells. Heart failure may occur due to depressed cardiac function. Abnormalities in gastrointestinal function can lead to malabsorption and diarrhea with refeeding (Tierney et al., 2001). Commercially available nutritional supplements (such as Carnation Instant Breakfast, Ensure, and Sustacal) may supplement protein and calorie intake. Administering 2 ounces of nutritional supplement with each medication given (unless the medication must be given on an empty stomach) may be an effective way to increase clients' calorie and protein intake (Bender et al., 2000).

## Enteral Nutrition

**Enteral nutrition,** or tube feeding, may be used to meet calorie and protein requirements in clients unable to consume adequate food. Indications for tube feedings include difficulty swallowing, unresponsiveness, oral or neck surgery or trauma, anorexia, or serious illness. Tube feedings may provide part or all of a client's nutritional needs.

Tube feedings are usually administered through a soft, small-caliber nasogastric or nasoduodenal tube with a weighted

## Nursing Research

### Evidence-Based Practice for Determining Feeding Tube Placement

The auscultatory method of determining the location for feeding tubes on initial placement and prior to initiating feeding is commonly recommended in nursing textbooks and is frequently used. The premise is that injecting a small amount of air into the tube will produce a distinctive sound if the tube is correctly located, presumably in the stomach. Sounds produced by tubes located in the esophagus, intestines, and respiratory tract are presumed to be different enough to alert the nurse to the improper location. However, based on a series of studies (Metheny et al., 1998), the auscultory method for determining placement is not reliable. This is especially true for small-bore feeding tubes. Testing the pH level of aspirates from newly inserted feeding tubes and of tubes from clients receiving intermittent feedings can help distinguish gastric from respiratory and intestinal placement. Based on the pH of a large number of samples of aspirates from feeding tubes, a pH between 0 and 4 suggests gastric placement and a pH of 7 or greater indicates respiratory placement. As the tube advances through the stomach into the intestine, pH levels increase and the color of the aspirate changes. If placement in the small intestine is required, a confirmatory X-ray should be taken. These researchers recommend that the pH method be used rather than the auscultory method and that protocols be updated to reflect current information.

### IMPLICATIONS FOR NURSING

With the advent of small-bore nasogastric and nasointestinal feeding tubes and the increasing use of gastrostomy and jejunostomy feeding tubes, more and more clients are receiving enteral feedings. Nurses need to use alternative methods to auscultation to determine correct initial and continued placement of these tubes. Aspiration of contents and pH testing is more effective for determining tube placement.

### Critical Thinking in Client Care

1. This study investigated differences in auscultatory sounds through small-lumen feeding tubes. Would the sound be more noticeably different with the larger bore tubes used for gastric lavage and drainage?
2. What other methods for determining tube placement are recommended in fundamentals and skills texts?
3. Compare the normal pH of aspirates obtained from the respiratory tract, esophagus, stomach, duodenum, and jejunum.
4. Develop a teaching plan for the client being discharged with a gastrostomy or jejunostomy feeding tube.

---

mercury tip. They also can be administered through a gastrostomy or jejunostomy tube. Small-bore feeding tubes are easily displaced; appropriate tube placement should be periodically checked by aspirating the tube and checking the pH of aspirated contents. A pH of <4 indicates placement in the stomach; pH >6 indicates the tube is in the jejunum. See the Nursing Research box above.

Most tube feeding formulas provide 1 kcal/mL with approximately 14% of the calories from protein, 60% from carbohydrates, and 25% to 30% from fat. Administering 1500 mL per day provides the recommended daily intake of all vitamins and minerals. Formulas that provide more calories per mL, more grams of protein, added fiber, or lower fat also are available. Commercial products provide instructions for initiating therapy. Some formulas are initially diluted to half strength for the first day of therapy. If tolerated, the formula is given at three-fourths strength on the second day and at full strength thereafter. Some formulas are started with smaller volumes of full-strength formula with a gradual increase in volume. Formulas may be administered as a bolus feeding or as a continuous- drip feeding regulated by a feeding pump.

Aspiration and diarrhea are the most common complications of enteral feedings. Continuous infusion of the formula reduces the risk of aspiration. The risk also is reduced by placing the feeding tube in the jejunum rather than the stomach. To avoid aspiration, the nurse elevates head of the bed at least 30 degrees during feeding and for at least 1 hour after feeding. Formulas that contain fiber can reduce the incidence of diarrhea. Fluid and electrolyte status is monitored carefully, and additional water is administered as needed.

## Parenteral Nutrition

**Total parenteral nutrition (TPN),** also known as *hyperalimentation,* is the intravenous administration of carbohydrates (high concentrations of dextrose), protein (amino acids), electrolytes, vitamins, minerals, and fat emulsions. These solutions usually are administered through a central vein, such as the subclavian vein (Figure 20–2 ■).

TPN is initiated when a client's nutritional requirements cannot be met through diet, enteral feedings, or peripheral vein infusions. Clients who have undergone major surgery or trauma or are seriously undernourished are often candidates for TPN. TPN is used for both short- and long-term management of nutritional deficiencies, and many clients are discharged to home with TPN and monitored by home health nurses.

To begin therapy, the physician inserts the central venous catheter under aseptic conditions. The location of the catheter tip is confirmed by X-ray. A triple-lumen catheter is most commonly used. This type of catheter permits administration of medications, intralipids, or blood through other lumens. Parenteral nutrition solutions are mixed using sterile technique under a laminar-flow-air hood. A commonly used solution includes 500 mL of 50% dextrose, 500 mL of an 8.5% amino acid solution, electrolytes, minerals, and vitamins. The sterility of the solution is maintained, and no medication, other than intralipids, is added to the solution or to the lumen through which the TPN is being administered. Most hospitals have specific policies and procedures for changing the tubing and the dressing at the insertion site as well as for hanging new containers. TPN solutions are always administered with an infusion pump to ensure the correct rate of infusion.

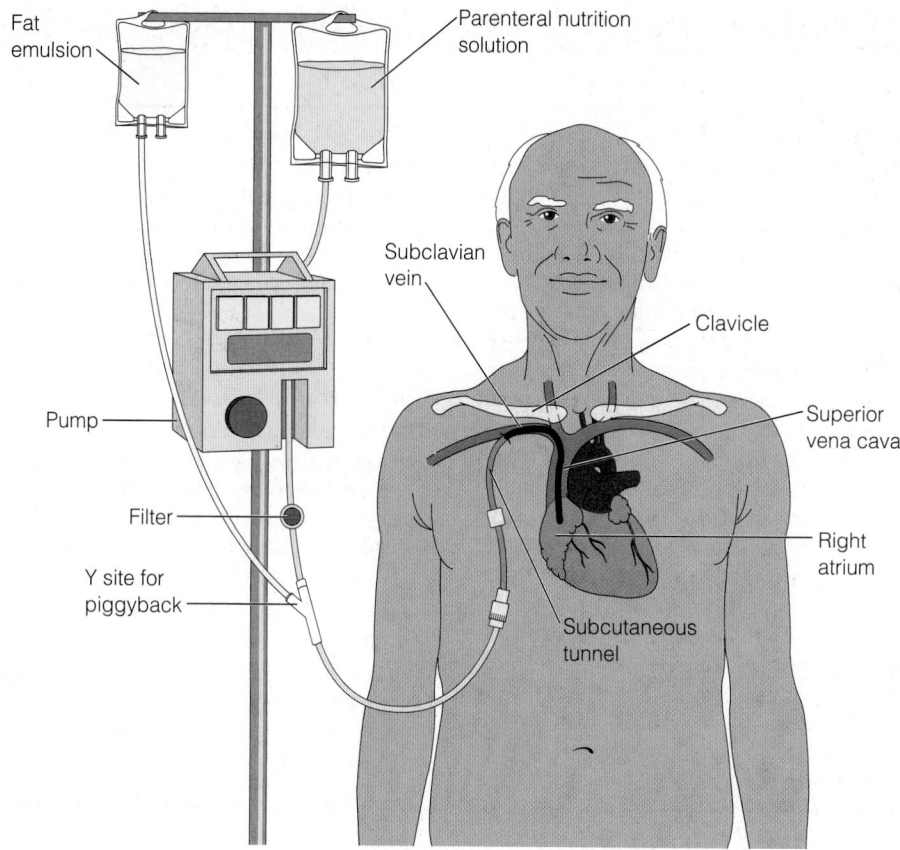

**Figure 20–2** ■ Total parenteral nutrition through a catheter in the right subclavian vein.

The client receiving parenteral nutrition is at risk for mechanical, metabolic, and infectious complications. Pneumothorax, hemothorax, brachial plexus injury, and improper position are possible complications of central venous catheter insertion. Once in place, the catheter may dislodge, leak, or break and become an embolus. Clots also may form within or around the catheter.

Fluid overload is a risk with parenteral nutrition, particularly in older adults. The high-glucose formulas can lead to osmotic diuresis or shifts of electrolytes, potassium and phosphorus in particular, into the cells. Blood glucose and serum electrolyte levels are carefully monitored during treatment. Long-term use of parenteral nutrition can lead to gallstone formation and liver disease.

Disruption of the skin barrier and administration of a solution high in glucose presents a risk for infection in clients receiving TPN. The temperature and other manifestations of infection are carefully monitored. Meticulous sterile technique is used for site and catheter care and bag and tubing changes.

## NURSING CARE

### Health Promotion

Aggressive nursing assessment and interventions can help prevent malnutrition associated with hospitalization or long-term care. In hospitalized clients, carefully monitor food intake.

When the client is placed on NPO status for surgery or tests, ask the care provider to restore diet orders as soon as possible. If allowed, encourage family members to provide favorite foods to promote intake. In long-term care settings, promote socialization during meals. Assess food likes and dislikes for clients, and provide foods they are likely to eat.

### Assessment

Collect nutritional assessment data on admission and periodically (once or twice a week) during long-term institutionalization.

- Health history: usual daily dietary pattern (type and amount of foods consumed); usual weight and recent changes; appetite and food tolerance; specific food likes and dislikes; difficulty swallowing; problems such as anorexia, nausea, diarrhea, or constipation; history of surgery and/or chronic diseases (e.g., chronic lung disease) and medications
- Physical examination: height, weight, skinfold thickness, BMI; vital signs; general appearance, muscle wasting, mobility; skin and mucous membranes; bowel sounds; laboratory studies

### Nursing Diagnoses and Interventions

The complex effects of malnutrition on multiple body systems place the client at high risk for a number of other problems. This section addresses problems with nutrition, infections, fluid volume, and skin integrity.

## Imbalanced Nutrition: Less Than Body Requirements

The nurse plays a critical role in the ongoing assessment of the malnourished client, while collaborating with the multidisciplinary team to provide nutritional therapies.

- If the client is able to eat, provide an environment and nursing measures that encourage eating. Eliminate foul odors, provide oral hygiene before and after meals, make meals appetizing, and offer frequent, small meals including preferred foods. Consult with the nutrition support team to provide adequate protein, calories, minerals, and vitamins. *Oral hygiene and a pleasant environment make food more appetizing. Small, frequent meals are generally more appealing and less overwhelming to a client with anorexia. Many clients require complicated nutritional therapy such as enteral or parenteral therapy to meet nutritional needs.*
- Provide a rest period before and after meals. *Eating requires energy, and the malnourished client may have decreased physical strength and energy.*
- Assess knowledge and provide appropriate teaching. *Lack of knowledge often contributes to undernutrition. Education empowers the client to make healthy choices.*

## Risk for Infection

Malnourished clients have a much higher risk for infection than well-nourished people. Malnutrition affects many components of the immune system, including the skin, mucous membranes, and lymph tissue and cells.

- Monitor temperature and assess for manifestations of infection every 4 hours. *Although the baseline temperature may be subnormal in malnourished clients, any elevation from baseline may indicate infection. Manifestations of infection may include chills, malaise, erythema, and leukocytosis. Early detection of infection may prevent complications.*
- Maintain medical asepsis when providing care and surgical asepsis when carrying out procedures. *Handwashing is the best strategy to prevent the spread of pathogens. Sterile technique is required for procedures such as inserting central lines and changing dressings.*

- Teach the signs and symptoms of infection, good handwashing technique, and factors that increase the risk for infection. *Knowledge empowers the client to participate in self-care, thus reducing exposure to infectious pathogens.*

## Risk for Deficient Fluid Volume

The client with malnutrition may also have a fluid volume deficit. Difficulty swallowing food and fluids or administration of hyperosmolar nutritional solutions may lead to dehydration or electrolyte disturbances.

- Monitor oral mucous membranes, urine specific gravity, level of consciousness, and laboratory findings every 4 to 8 hours. *Dry mucous membranes, increased urine specific gravity, decreased level of consciousness, and electrolyte imbalances may indicate dehydration.*
- Weigh daily and monitor intake and output. *Daily weights and intake and output measurements help monitor fluid balance.*
- If allowed, offer fluids frequently in small amounts, considering the client's preferences. *Frequent, small amounts of fluids are better tolerated and promote adequate intake.*

## Risk for Impaired Skin Integrity

Skin integrity depends on adequate nutrition. Loss of subcutaneous tissue and muscle increase the risk of pressure ulcers. In addition, healing is impaired in malnourished clients.

- Assess skin every 4 hours. *Baseline and ongoing assessments allow prompt identification of early manifestations of skin breakdown.*
- Turn and position at least every 2 hours. Encourage passive and active range-of-motion exercises. *These measures reduce pressure and promote oxygenation of cells.*
- Keep skin dry and clean, and minimize shearing forces. Keep linens smooth, clean, and dry. Provide therapeutic beds, mattresses, or pads. *These nursing measures promote comfort and reduce the risk of skin breakdown.*

## Using NANDA, NIC, and NOC

Chart 20–2 shows links between NANDA nursing diagnoses, NIC, and NOC for the client with malnutrition.

MediaLink | MALNUTRITION CARE PLAN

---

### CHART 20–2 NANDA, NIC, AND NOC

#### The Malnourished Client

| NURSING DIAGNOSES | NURSING INTERVENTIONS | NURSING OUTCOMES |
|---|---|---|
| • Imbalanced Nutrition: Less than Body Requirements<br>• Adult Failure to Thrive<br>• Ineffective Protection<br>• Ineffective Therapeutic Regimen Management | • Fluid Monitoring<br>• Weight Gain Assistance<br>• Nutrition Therapy<br>• Infection Protection<br>• Teaching: Procedure/Treatment | • Nutritional Status: Nutrient Intake<br>• Nutritional Status<br>• Immune Status<br>• Knowledge: Treatment Regimen |

*Note. Data from Nursing Outcomes Classification (NOC) by M. Johnson & M. Maas (Eds.), 1997, St. Louis: Mosby; Nursing Diagnoses: Definitions & Classification 2001–2002 by North American Nursing Diagnosis Association, 2001, Philadelphia: NANDA; Nursing Interventions Classification (NIC) by J.C. McCloskey & G. M. Bulechek (Eds.), 2000, St. Louis: Mosby. Reprinted by permission.*

## Nursing Care Plan
## A Client with Malnutrition

Rose Chow is an 88-year-old widow who lives alone. She typically rises early and has a cup of tea before spending her morning puttering in her garden. She consumes her main meal of the day at lunch, which usually includes rice and some vegetables. For dinner, she generally eats a bowl of rice with "whatever seems to be in the refrigerator." She admits to little interest in cooking or eating since her husband died 10 years ago and her group of friends has been "dying off, too."

### ASSESSMENT

Mrs. Chow weighs 95 lb (43.1 kg) and is 5'3" (160 cm) tall, for a BMI of 16.8. She reports weighing 118 lb (53.5 kg) 5 years ago. Her triceps skinfold thickness measurement is 11 mm (normal values for a female: >13 mm). Her skin is pale, and she appears thin and wasted. Her temperature is 97°F (36.1°C). Diagnostic test results include serum albumin 2.9 g/dL (normal 3.4 to 4.8 g/dL) and serum cholesterol 130 mg/dL (normal 150 to 200 mg/dL). A diagnosis of protein-calorie malnutrition is made, and a 1500-calorie per day diet is recommended.

### DIAGNOSES

- *Imbalanced nutrition: Less than body requirements* related to lack of knowledge and inadequate food intake
- *Risk for infection* related to protein-calorie malnutrition
- *Impaired social interaction* related to widowhood and reduced social support group

### EXPECTED OUTCOMES

- Gain at least 1 pound per week.
- Verbalize understanding of nutritional requirements and identify strategies to incorporate requirements into daily diet after discharge.
- Remain infection free, evidenced by normal vital signs.

- Identify strategies to increase social interaction, such as participating in senior citizens' lunches at local senior center.

### PLANNING AND IMPLEMENTATION

- Weigh weekly at a consistent time of day.
- Refer to dietitian for evaluation of nutritional needs.
- Teach about nutritional requirements, and plan an eating program that includes high-calorie, high-protein foods and supplements and reflects her food preferences. Encourage small, frequent meals.
- Encourage to keep a food intake diary.
- Teach strategies to reduce risks for infection.
- Provide information about communal meals available to seniors in the community, and help Mrs. Chow develop a plan to participate.

### EVALUATION

One month later, Mrs. Chow has gained 3 pounds and reports feeling "more energetic." A friend is helping her shop to ensure that she purchases foods to maintain her protein, calorie, and nutrient intake. She has begun attending senior lunches twice a week, and is enjoying "being around people again." Although she still doesn't enjoy cooking like she used to, she is using prepared foods and supplements to maintain her nutrient intake.

### Critical Thinking in the Nursing Process

1. What is the physiologic basis for Mrs. Chow's low albumin and cholesterol levels?
2. Mrs. Chow asks, "Can I get better by just taking more vitamins?" How will you respond?
3. Design a teaching plan for a Hispanic client with protein-calorie malnutrition.

See Evaluating Your Response in Appendix C.

## Home Care

Clients with malnutrition may be cared for at home or in the hospital with diet, enteral, or parenteral therapy. Each year, it is more common to see clients managing tube feeding or TPN at home. Teaching for the client and family includes the following topics.

- Diet recommendations and use of nutritional supplements
- Where to obtain recommended foods and nutritional supplements
- If continuing enteral or parenteral nutrition, how to (1) prepare and/or handle solutions, (2) add them to either the feeding tube or central line, (3) manage infusion pumps, (4) care for the feeding tube or central catheter, (5) recognize and manage problems and complications, and (6) how and when to notify the health care provider of problems.

## THE CLIENT WITH AN EATING DISORDER

Eating disorders are characterized by severely disturbed eating behavior and weight management. Eating disorders are more common in affluent societies where food is plentiful. Women are much more commonly affected than men. **Anorexia nervosa** is characterized by a body weight less than 85% of expected for age and height, and an intense fear of gaining weight. Anorexia nervosa affects about 0.5% to 1% of women in the United States. **Bulimia nervosa,** which affects 1% to 3% of women in the United States, is characterized by recurring episodes of binge eating followed by purge behaviors such as self-induced vomiting, use of laxatives or diuretics, fasting, or excessive exercise.

## ANOREXIA NERVOSA

Anorexia nervosa typically begins during adolescence. Clients with anorexia nervosa have a distorted body image and irrational fear of gaining weight. They maintain weight loss by restricted calorie intake, often accompanied by excessive exercise. Some clients may exhibit binge–purge behavior. A number of risk factors, both biologic and psychosocial, have been identified for anorexia nervosa. Abnormal levels of neurotransmitters and other hormones may play a role. Women who develop anorexia nervosa tend to be obsessive

TABLE 20-2   Manifestations and Complications of Anorexia Nervosa and Bulimia Nervosa

| Disorder | Manifestations | Complications |
|---|---|---|
| Anorexia nervosa | • Weight < 85% of normal, muscle wasting<br>• Fear of weight gain, refusal to eat<br>• Disturbed body image, excessive exercise<br>• Amenorrhea<br>• Skin and hair changes<br>• Hypotension, bradycardia<br>• Hypothermia<br>• Constipation<br>• Insomnia | • Electrolyte and acid-base disturbances<br>• Reduced cardiac muscle mass, low cardiac output, dysrhythmias<br>• Anemia<br>• Hypoglycemia, elevated serum uric acid levels<br>• Osteoporosis<br>• Enlarged salivary glands<br>• Delayed gastric emptying<br>• Abnormal liver function |
| Bulimia nervosa | • Weight often normal; may be slightly overweight<br>• Binge–purge behavior<br>• Oligomenorrhea or amenorrhea<br>• Lacerations of palate; callous on fingers or dorsum of hand | • Enlarged salivary glands<br>• Stomatitis, loss of dental enamel<br>• Fluid, electrolyte, and acid-base imbalances<br>• Dysrhythmias<br>• Esophageal tears, stomach rupture |

and perfectionistic. Family, social, or occupational (e.g., a career in modeling or ballet) pressures to maintain low body weight also contribute.

The manifestations and complications of anorexia nervosa are listed in Table 20–2. Clients who engage in binge–purge behavior have a higher risk for complications.

## BULIMIA NERVOSA

Bulimia nervosa develops in late adolescence or early adulthood, often following a diet. The client with bulimia typically reports binge eating followed by purging 5 to 10 times per week (Braunwald et al., 2001). Foods consumed during a binge often are high calorie, high fat, and sweet. After binge eating, the client induces vomiting (usually by stimulating the gag reflex), or may take excessive quantities of laxatives or diuretics. In contrast to anorexia, the client's weight often is normal. Fluid and electrolyte balance, in contrast, may be severely disrupted by loss of fluid and gastrointestinal secretions. The complications of bulimia nervosa (Table 20–2) primarily result from the purging behavior.

## COLLABORATIVE CARE

Eating disorders, anorexia nervosa in particular, are difficult to effectively treat. Because of the intense fear of weight gain and the distorted body image of clients with anorexia, they strongly resist increasing food intake. A combination of nutritional, behavioral, and psychologic treatment is necessary.

Clients with anorexia nervosa may require hospitalization, particularly if their weight is less than 75% of normal. Refeeding is gradually introduced to avoid complications such as heart failure. Meals must be supervised and a firm but empathetic attitude conveyed about the importance of adequate food intake. Psychologic treatment focuses on providing emotional support during weight gain and helping the client base their

self-esteem on factors other than weight (e.g., personal relationships, satisfaction with achieving occupational goals) (Braunwald et al., 2001).

An antidepressant drug such as fluoxetine (Prozac) may benefit the client with bulimia nervosa. Cognitive behavioral therapy also is used to treat bulimia, focusing on excessive concerns about weight, persistent dieting, and binge–purge behaviors.

## NURSING CARE

Nurses can be instrumental in identifying clients with anorexia nervosa or bulimia nervosa and referring them for treatment. It is particularly important to identify these disorders early to prevent adverse effects on growth and increase the success of treatment.

The nurse is an integral part of the eating disorders treatment team. Although *Imbalanced nutrition: Less than body requirements* is a primary nursing diagnosis for clients with anorexia or bulimia, the following nursing diagnoses also should be considered.

- *Ineffective sexuality patterns*
- *Chronic low self-esteem*
- *Disturbed body image*
- *Ineffective family therapeutic regimen management*

When planning and implementing care, consider the following nursing activities.

- Regularly monitor weight, using standard conditions. *Weight gain or loss provides information about the effectiveness of care, as well as the client's risk for complications.*
- Monitor food intake during meals, recording percentage of meal and snack consumed. Maintain close observation for at least one hour following meals; do not allow client alone in bathroom. *Observing the client during and after meals helps*

*prevent disposal of food and purging behavior after eating. Recording actual food intake allows accurate calculation of calorie intake.*

- Serve balanced meals, including all nutrient groups. Increase serving size gradually. *The client may find "normal" food servings overwheming, reducing the desire to eat. Calorie intake is initially limited to prevent complications associated with refeeding, then gradually increased.*
- Serve frequent, small feedings of cold or room temperature foods. *Cool foods reduce sensations of early satiety, promoting greater food intake at a meal or snack.*
- Administer a multivitamin and mineral supplement to replace losses.

Clients with anorexia nervosa or bulimia nervosa require extended treatment of the disorder. Involvement of the family and social support persons is vital to success. Encourage family members to participate in teaching and diet counseling sessions. Discuss the value of family therapy to address issues that have contributed to the disorder. Emphasize the need to provide consistent messages of support for healthy eating habits. Discuss using rewards for food and calorie intake rather than weight gain. Provide referrals to a dietitian, nutritional support team, counseling, and support groups for people with eating disorders.

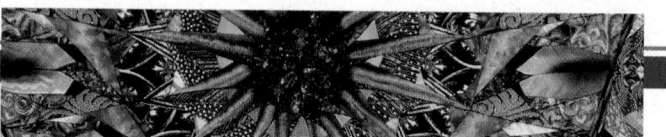

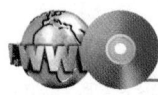 EXPLORE MediaLink

NCLEX review questions, case studies, care plan activities, MediaLink applications, and other interactive resources for this chapter can be found on the Companion Website at www.prenhall.com/lemone.

Click on Chapter 20 to select the activities for this chapter. For animations, video clips, more NCLEX review questions, and an audio glossary, access the Student CD-ROM accompanying this textbook.

## TEST YOURSELF

1. Of the following noted in a client's history, which does the nurse identify as the greatest risk factor for obesity?

   a. Adopted at 2 months of age
   b. Usual diet includes "fast food" lunches twice a week
   c. Does not engage in regular activity
   d. Allergic to chocolate and strawberries

2. A client on a reduced calorie diet asks the nurse what she can do to lose weight faster, because most weeks she loses no more than 0.5 lb. "At this rate, it will take me years to get to my goal!" The most appropriate response by the nurse would be:

   a. "Let's reevaluate your long-term goal. Perhaps it was set too low for you."
   b. "A pound of body fat equals 3500 calories. Let's reevaluate your diet and exercise plan for calorie intake and expenditure."
   c. "Perhaps we should look into a diet supplement since you are unable to stick with your prescribed diet plan."
   d. "You sound frustrated. Would you like to take some time off from your diet and exercise plan?"

3. An expected finding in a client admitted with a diagnosis of protein-calorie malnutrition would be:

   a. Recent 5 lb weight loss
   b. Increased skinfold thickness measurements
   c. Hyperactive bowel sounds
   d. Anxiety and agitation

4. Before administering an intermittent enteral feeding, the nurse confirms placement of the small bore feeding tube in the stomach by:

   a. Instilling water and listening for the gastric gurgle
   b. Withdrawing the tube slightly, then reinserting it
   c. Aspirating gastric contents and check for a pH of <4
   d. Obtaining a flat-plate X-ray of the stomach

5. The nurse identifies which of the following as a realistic goal for a client with anorexia nervosa?

   a. Will consume 100% of a 2500 calorie diet
   b. Will gain 2 pounds per week
   c. Will rest alone in room following meals
   d. Will participate in family counseling

See Test Yourself answers in Appendix C.

# BIBLIOGRAPHY

Ackley, B. J., & Ladwig, G. B. (2002). *Nursing diagnosis handbook: A guide to planning care* (5th ed.). St. Louis: Mosby.

Ainley, H. (2001). Analysis. . . managing obesity. *Practice Nurse, 22*(3), 14–15.

Bender, S., Pusateri, M., Cook, A., Ferguson, M., & Hall, J. C. (2000). Malnutrition: Role of the TwoCal® HN med pass program. *MEDSURG Nursing, 9*(6), 284–295.

Braunwald, E., Fauci, A. S., Kasper, D. L., Hauser, S. L., Longo, D. L., & Jameson, J. L. (2001). *Harrison's principles of internal medicine* (15th ed.). New York: McGraw-Hill.

Bullock, B. A., & Henze, R. L. (2000). *Focus on pathophysiology*. Philadelphia: Lippincott.

Cammons, A. R., & Hackshaw, H.S. (2000). Are we starving our patients? *American Journal of Nursing, 100*(5), 43–46.

Crogan, N. L., Shultz, J. A., & Massey, L. K. (2001). Nutrition knowledge of nurses in long-term care facilties. *Journal of Continuing Education in Nursing, 32*(4), 171–176.

Deglin, J. H., & Vallerand, A. H. (2001). *Davis's drug guide for nurses* (7th ed.). Philadelphia: F.A. Davis.

Devlin, M. (2000). The nutritional needs of the older person. *Professional Nurse, 16*(3), 951–955.

Dudek, S. G. (2000). Malnutrition in hospitals: Who's assessing what patients eat? *American Journal of Nursing, 100*(4), 36–42.

Ferguson, M., Cook, A, Bender, S., Rimmasch, H., & Voss, A. (2001). Diagnosing and treating involuntary weight loss. *MEDSURG Nursing, 10*(4), 165–175.

Gallo, J. J., Busby-Whitehead, J., Rabins, P. V., Silliman, R. A., & Murphy, J. B. (Eds.). (1999). *Reichel's care of the elderly: Clinical aspects of aging* (5th ed.). Philadelphia: Lippincott Williams & Wilkins.

Green, S., & O'Kane, M. (2001). Obesity. *Practice Nurse, 22*(3), 20, 22, 24.

Jeffrey, S. (2001). The role of the nurse in obesity management. *Journal of Community Nursing, 15*(3), 20, 22, 26.

Johnson, M., Bulechek, G., Dochterman, J. M., Maas, M., & Moorhead, S. (2001). *Nursing diagnoses, outcomes, & interventions*. St. Louis: Mosby.

Ledsham, J., & Gough, A. (2000). Screening and monitoring patients for malnutrition. *Professional Nurse, 15*(11), 695–698.

Lehne, R. A. (2001). *Pharmacology for nursing care* (4th ed.). Philadelphia: Saunders.

Malarkey, L.M., & McMorrow, M.E. (2000). *Nurse's manual of laboratory tests and diagnostic procedures* (2nd ed.). Philadelphia: Saunders.

Meeker, M. H., & Rothrock, J. C. (1999). *Alexander's care of the patient in surgery* (11th ed.). St. Louis: Mosby.

Metheny, N. A., & Titler, M. G. (2001). Assessing placement of feeding tubes. *American Journal of Nursing, 101*(5), 36–45.

Metheny, N., Wehrle, M., Wiersema, L., & Clark, J. (1998). pH, color, and feeding tubes. *RN, 61*(1), 25–27.

North American Nursing Diagnosis Association. (2001). *NANDA nursing diagnoses: Definitions & classification 2001–2002*. Philadelphia: NANDA.

Nutrition. Clinical guidelines to manage malnutrition in nursing homes. (2001). *Geriatric Nursing, 22*(1), 46.

Orbanic, S. (2001). Understanding bulimia. *American Journal of Nursing, 101*(3), 35–41.

Porth, C. M. (2002). *Pathophysiology: Concepts of altered health states* (5th ed.). Philadelphia: Lippincott.

Robinson, F. (2001). Analysis . . . management of excess weight in primary care. *Practice Nurse, 21*(5), 16, 19.

Saunders, C. S. (2001). Diet and nutrition in your practice. Intervening in the obesity epidemic. *Patient Care for the Nurse Practitioner, 4*(3), 12–14, 16, 18+.

Tierney, L. M., McPhee, S. J., & Papadakis, M. A. (2001). *Current medical diagnosis & treatment* (40th ed.). New York: Lange Medical Books/McGraw-Hill.

Vender, S., Pusateri, M., Cook, A., Ferguson, M., & Hall, J.C. (2000). Malnutrition: Role of the TwoCal® med pass program. *MEDSURG Nursing, 9*(6), 284–295.

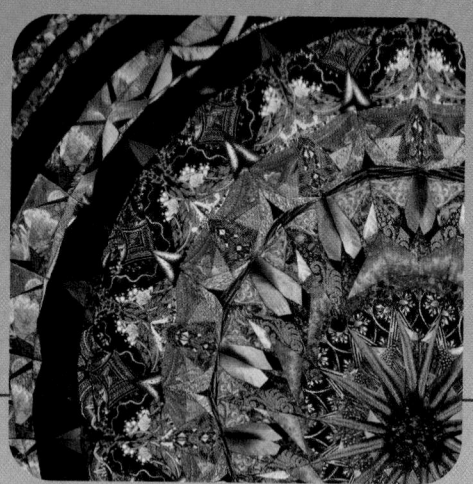

# CHAPTER 21

# Nursing Care of Clients with Upper Gastrointestinal Disorders

## MediaLink

**www.prenhall.com/lemone**
Additional resources for this chapter can be found on the Student CD-ROM accompanying this textbook, and on the Companion Website at www.prenhall.com/lemone. Click on Chapter 21 to select the activities for this chapter.

**CD-ROM**
• Audio Glossary
• NCLEX Review

*Animations*
• Mouth and Throat
• Ranitidine

**Companion Website**
• More NCLEX Review
• Case Study
    Peptic Ulcer Disease
• Care Plan Activity
    Peptic Ulcer Disease and Pain
• MediaLink Application
    Oral Cancer

## LEARNING OUTCOMES

After completing this chapter, you will be able to:

■ Describe the pathophysiology of common disorders of the mouth, esophagus, and stomach.

■ Relate the manifestations of upper gastrointestinal disorders to the pathophysiologic processes.

■ List diagnostic tests used to identify disorders of the upper gastrointestinal tract.

■ Discuss the nursing implications for collaborative care measures used to treat clients with upper gastrointestinal disorders.

■ Use knowledge of normal anatomy and physiology and assessments to provide nursing care for clients with upper gastrointestinal disorders (see Chapter 19).

■ Use the nursing process to assess needs, plan, and implement individualized care for the client with an upper gastrointestinal disorder.

The upper gastrointestinal tract includes the mouth, esophagus, stomach, and proximal small intestine. Food and fluids, ingested through the mouth, move through the esophagus to the stomach. The stomach and upper intestinal tract (duodenum and jejunum) are responsible for the majority of food digestion. When an acute or chronic disease process interferes with the function of this portion of the gastrointestinal (GI) tract, nutritional status can be affected and the client may experience symptoms that interfere with lifestyle.

Nurses provide both acute care for the hospitalized client and teaching about the skills and knowledge needed to manage these conditions at home.

# DISORDERS OF THE MOUTH

Inflammations, infections, and neoplastic lesions of the mouth affect food ingestion and nutrition. Oral lesions may have a variety of causes, including infection, mechanical trauma, irritants such as alcohol, and hypersensitivity. Appropriate treatment of the disorder, any underlying factors, and associated symptoms is essential.

## THE CLIENT WITH STOMATITIS

**Stomatitis,** inflammation of the oral mucosa, is a common disorder of the mouth. It may be caused by viral (herpes simplex) or fungal (Candida albicans) infections, mechanical trauma (e.g., cheek biting), and irritants such as tobacco or chemotherapeutic agents.

## PATHOPHYSIOLOGY

The oral mucosa, which lines the oral cavity, is a relatively thin, fragile layer of stratified squamous epithelial cells. The blood supply to the oral mucosa is rich. Frequent exposure to the environment, a rich blood supply, and the oral mucosa's delicate nature increase the risk of infection or inflammation, reaction to toxins, and trauma.

The clinical manifestations of stomatitis vary according to its cause. Table 21–1 outlines common causes of stomatitis with their manifestations and treatment. Chemotherapy or chemical irritation may result in generalized redness, swelling, and ulcerations.

## COLLABORATIVE CARE

Stomatitis is diagnosed by direct physical examination and, if indicated, cultures, smears, and evaluation for systemic illness. Treatment addresses both the underlying cause and any coexisting illnesses. An undiagnosed oral lesion present for more than 1 week and that does not respond to therapy must be evaluated for malignancy.

Direct smears and cultures of lesions may be obtained to identify causative organisms. If systemic illness is suspected, a variety of diagnostic tests may be ordered to identify the underlying cause.

General treatment measures include using a topical anesthetic, such as 2% viscous lidocaine, as an oral rinse. This

| TABLE 21–1 | Manifestations and Treatment of Common Stomatitis Conditions | | |
|---|---|---|---|
| **Type** | **Cause** | **Manifestations** | **Complications** |
| Cold sore, fever blister | Herpes simplex virus | • Initial burning at site<br>• Clustered vesicular lesions on lip or oral mucosa | • Self-limiting<br>• Acyclovir to shorten course |
| Aphthous ulcer (canker sore, ulcerative stomatitis) | Unknown, may be type of herpes virus | • Well-circumscribed, shallow erosions with white or yellow center encircled by red ring<br>• Less than 1 cm in diameter<br>• Painful | • Topical steroid ointment<br>• Amlexanox oral paste (Aphthasol)<br>• Oral prednisone |
| Candidiasis (thrush) | *Candida albicans* | • Creamy white, curdlike patches<br>• Red, erythematous mucosa | • Fluconazole (Diflucan)<br>• Ketoconazole (Nizoral)<br>• Clotrimazole troches<br>• Nystatin vaginal troches (dissolved orally) or mouth rinse |
| Necrotizing ulcerative gingivitis (trench mouth, Vincent's infection) | Infection with spirochetes and bacilli or systemic infection | • Acute gingival inflammation and necrosis<br>• Bleeding, halitosis<br>• Fever<br>• Cervical lymphadenopathy | • Correct any underlying disorders<br>• Warm, half-strength peroxide mouthwashes<br>• Oral penicillin |

solution is not swallowed to avoid impairment of the swallowing mechanism. Orabase, a protective paste, may be applied to oral ulcers to promote comfort. Triamcinolone acetonide may be mixed in Orabase to reduce inflammation and promote healing. Sodium bicarbonate mouthwashes may provide relief and promote cleansing, whereas alcohol-based mouthwashes may cause pain and burning.

Fungal infections often are treated with a nystatin oral suspension; clients "swish and swallow" the solution. Clotrimazole lozenges also treat oral fungal infections. If the infection does not resolve, oral antifungal medications such as fluconazole or ketoconazole may be used. Antifungals are usually continued for at least 3 days after symptoms disappear.

Herpetic lesions may be treated with topical or oral acyclovir. Acyclovir ointment provides comfort and lubrication while limiting the spread of the virus. Acyclovir capsules reduce the severity of symptoms and the duration of the lesions.

Bacterial infections are treated with antibiotics based on cultures and smears. Oral penicillin is the treatment of choice if the client is not allergic and the cultured bacteria is sensitive. Nursing implications for selected drugs used to treat stomatitis are outlined below.

## NURSING CARE

Nursing care for the client with stomatitis focuses not only on the oral inflammation, but also on any underlying systemic diseases and the effects of the condition on the client's comfort and nutrition.

## Nursing Diagnoses and Interventions

### Impaired Oral Mucous Membrane

Stomatitis disrupts the integrity of the oral mucous membrane. Regardless of cause, the pain and symptoms of stomatitis must be relieved to promote comfort as well as food and fluid intake.

- Assess and document oral mucous membranes and the character of any lesions every 4 to 8 hours. *Baseline and ongoing assessment data provide the basis for evaluation.*
- Assist with thorough mouth care after meals, at bedtime, and every 2 to 4 hours while awake. If unable to tolerate a toothbrush, offer sponge or gauze toothettes. Avoid using alcohol-based mouthwashes. *Mouth care promotes hygiene, comfort, and healing. Alcohol-based mouthwashes may be irritating to mucous membranes, causing pain and further tissue damage.*
- Assess knowledge and teach about condition, mouth care, and treatments. Instruct to avoid alcohol, tobacco, and spicy or irritating foods. *Knowledge promotes client participation in the plan of care and compliance. Alcohol, tobacco, and hot, spicy rough foods may injure the inflamed mucous membranes.*

### Imbalanced Nutrition: Less Than Body Requirements

Oral lesions and pain may limit oral intake, which may in turn lead to nutritional deficits. Anorexia and general malaise may also contribute to decreased intake.

- Assess food intake as well as the client's ability to chew and swallow. Weigh daily. Provide appropriate assistive de-

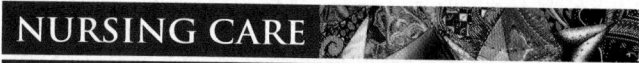

## Medication Administration

### Drugs Used to Treat Stomatitis

#### TOPICAL ORAL ANESTHETICS

| | |
|---|---|
| Orajel | Anbesol |
| Viscous lidocaine | Triamcinolone acetonide |

These drugs reduce the pain associated with mucous membrane lesions or stomatitis. They provide temporary relief of pain. Any oral lesion that persists longer than 1 week should be evaluated by an oral surgeon.

##### Nursing Responsibilities
- Instruct the client to seek medical attention for any oral lesion that does not heal within 1 week.
- Monitor for local hypersensitivity reactions, and discontinue use if they occur.

##### Client and Family Teaching
- Apply every 1 to 2 hours as needed.
- Perform oral hygiene after meals and at bedtime.

#### TOPICAL ANTIFUNGAL AGENTS

| | |
|---|---|
| Clotrimazole | Nystatin |

These products help in the topical treatment of candidiasis. Their effects are primarily local rather than systemic.

##### Nursing Responsibilities
- Instruct the client to dissolve lozenges in the mouth.

- Instruct the client to rinse mouth with oral suspension for at least 2 minutes and expectorate or swallow as directed.
- These drugs are contraindicated in pregnancy.

##### Client and Family Teaching
- Take medication as prescribed.
- Do not eat or drink 30 minutes after medication.
- Contact physician if symptoms worsen.
- Perform good oral hygiene after meals and at bedtime; remove dentures at bedtime.

#### ANTIVIRAL AGENT

Acyclovir (Zovirax)

Acyclovir is useful in the treatment of oral herpes simplex virus. It helps reduce the severity and frequency of infections. It interferes with the DNA synthesis of herpes simplex virus.

##### Nursing Responsibilities
- Start therapy with acyclovir as soon as herpetic lesions are noted.
- Administer with food or on an empty stomach.

##### Client and Family Teaching
- The virus remains latent and can recur during stressful events, fever, trauma, sunlight exposure, and treatment with immunosuppressive drugs.
- Take the medication as ordered, and contact the physician if symptoms worsen.

vices such as straws or feeding syringes. *Adequate nutrition is essential for healing. Daily weights allow monitoring of the adequacy of food intake. Assistive devices may allow food intake while avoiding irritation of ulcerations or lesions.*

- Encourage a high-calorie, high-protein diet considerate of food preferences. Offer soft, lukewarm, or cool foods or liquids such as eggnogs, milk shakes, nutritional supplements, popsicles, and puddings frequently in small amounts. Obtain nutritional consultation. *Oral intake may be limited, and enriched foods and liquids enhance nutrition. A nutritional consultation can help ensure an adequate diet and assist in meeting nutritional needs.*

## Home Care

Clients with stomatitis generally provide self-care. Include the following topics in teaching for home care.

- Managing any underlying health conditions and ongoing treatments such as chemotherapy
- The recommended diet and oral hygiene regime
- Nutritional supplements to help meet nutritional requirements
- Prescribed medication, its route, side effects, frequency of administration, and signs and symptoms to report
- The importance of completing the full course of antibiotic, antiviral, or antifungal treatment
- Manifestations to report and the importance of follow-up care

## THE CLIENT WITH ORAL CANCER

Oral cancer, malignancy of the oral mucosa, may develop on the lips, tongue, floor of the mouth, or other oral tissues. It is uncommon, accounting for only 5% of all cancers. It has, however, a high rate of morbidity and mortality. The incidence of this type of head and neck cancer is twice as high in men as in women, and it is seen more often in men over 40. The stage of an oral cancer determines the prognosis, treatment, and degree of disability. The primary risk factors for oral cancer are smoking, drinking alcohol, and chewing tobacco. Marijuana use, occupational exposures to chemicals, and viruses such as human papilloma virus (HPV) also may contribute to the risk for oral cancer.

## PATHOPHYSIOLOGY AND MANIFESTATIONS

Oral cancer is usually a squamous cell carcinoma. Most early cancers of the mouth, lips, tongue, or pharynx present as inflamed areas with irregular, ill-defined borders. More advanced cancers appear as deep ulcers that are fixed to deeper tissues. Early lesions involve the mucosa or submucosa, whereas more advanced tumors may involve the tongue, oropharynx, mandible, or maxilla.

The earliest symptom of oral cancer is a painless oral ulceration or lesion (Figure 21–1 ■). Later symptoms vary and may include difficulty speaking, swallowing, or chewing; swollen lymph nodes; and blood-tinged sputum. See the box above for

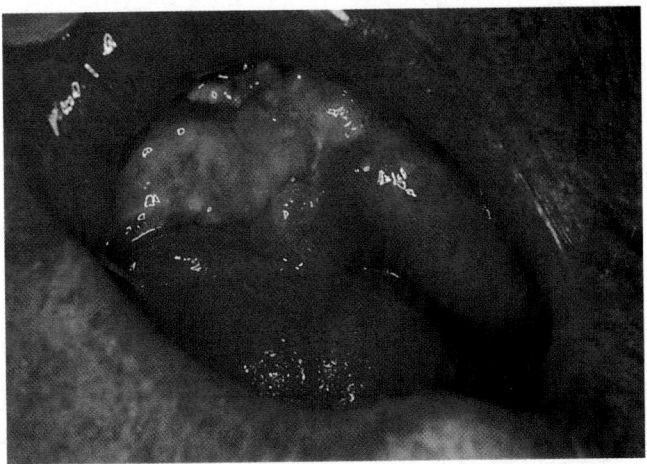

**Figure 21–1** ■ Oral cancer.

*Source: Biophoto Associates/Photo Researchers, Inc.*

### Manifestations of Oral Cancer

- White patches (leukoplakia)
- Red patches (erythroplakia)
- Ulcers
- Masses
- Pigmented areas (brownish or black)
- Fissures
- Asymmetry of the head, face, jaws, or neck

other manifestations of oral cancer. Any oral lesion that does not heal or respond to treatment within 1 to 2 weeks should be evaluated for malignancy.

## COLLABORATIVE CARE

The first component of treatment is eliminating any causative factors such as chewing tobacco, smoking, or drinking alcohol. Tumor staging then determines therapy. A biopsy of the oral lesion allows direct visualization of cells to determine the presence or absence of cancerous cells. Staging may require additional diagnostic studies such as CT scans or an MRI.

Radiation and chemotherapy may be considered based on age, tumor stage, general condition, and preferences. Radiation therapy may be used preoperatively to "shrink" the tumor or postoperatively to limit the risks of metastasis. Chemotherapy may be indicated depending on the stage of the tumor. See Chapter 10 for more information about radiation and chemotherapy to treat cancer.

Following the biopsy and staging of the tumor, surgery is generally indicated, although an advanced or extensive tumor may be considered unresectable. If the tumor involves surrounding tissues, the cosmetic effects of surgery are important considerations. The goal of surgery is removal of the lesion and potentially cancerous surrounding tissue or lymph nodes. Advanced carcinomas may require extensive excision or a *radical neck dissection,* a potentially disfiguring procedure in which the lymph nodes and muscles of the neck are removed. A tracheostomy is performed at the time of surgery. The tracheostomy may be temporary, but often is permanent. See Chapter 35 ⟨∞⟩ for more information about caring for a client following radical neck dissection and a tracheostomy

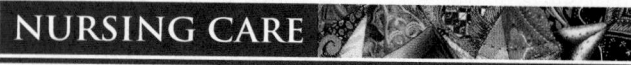

## NURSING CARE

### Health Promotion

Reducing or eliminating tobacco use (smoking and smokeless tobacco) and excess alcohol consumption can significantly reduce the incidence of oral cancer. Teach children and adolescents about the dangers of using tobacco and alcohol. Emphasize the relationship between smokeless tobacco and oral cancer. Discuss strategies to deal with peer pressure to use tobacco and alcohol.

### Assessment

Early precancerous oral lesions are very treatable. Unfortunately, these lesions usually are painless, so diagnosis and treatment often is delayed. Assess the oral cavity of all clients, particularly those with risk factors for oral cancer.

- Health history: complaints of oral lesions that fail to heal; use (current or past) of tobacco products or excess alcohol
- Physical examination: Inspect and palpate lips and oral mucosa (including tongue and floor of mouth under the tongue) for tumors or lesions. Lesions may appear as velvety red or white patches that do not scrape off, or as ulcers or areas of necrosis.

### Nursing Diagnoses and Interventions

The mouth allows food ingestion, and the lips are integral to verbal and nonverbal expression. The head, mouth, and lips are important to self-perception and body image. Nursing diagnoses discussed in this section consider such problems as airway clearance, nutrition, communication, and body image.

### Risk for Ineffective Airway Clearance

The location and the extent of an oral cancer and its excision may compromise the airway. Swelling of adjacent tissues, increased oral secretions, or difficulty swallowing may contribute to respiratory distress. If extensive surgery is performed, a tracheostomy usually is performed to maintain airway patency.

**PRACTICE ALERT** *In the initial postoperative period, assess airway patency and respiratory status at least hourly. A patent airway is vital to maintain respirations and oxygenation of tissues. Frequent assessment allows early identification of possible airway compromise.* ∎

- Unless contraindicated, place in Fowler's position, supporting arms. Assist the client to turn, cough, and deep

breathe at least every 2 to 4 hours. *Fowler's position promotes lung expansion. Turning, coughing, and deep breathing help maintain a patent airway by preventing pooling of secretions.*
- Maintain adequate hydration (2000 to 3000 mL per day unless contraindicated) and humidity of inspired air. *Adequate hydration helps thin and loosen secretions.*

### Imbalanced Nutrition: Less Than Body Requirements

Surgery affects oral food and fluid intake. Enteral feedings or total parenteral nutrition may be required. A gastrostomy tube usually is inserted during surgery to maintain nutrition. If an oral diet is permitted, anorexia or pain may affect intake.

- Weigh daily. Assess oral intake for adequacy of protein, calories, and nutrients. *Daily weights and nutritional assessments provide information about the adequacy of diet.*
- Offer soft, bland foods with supplements as indicated. Provide small, frequent feedings, making mealtimes pleasant. *Soft, bland foods may be better tolerated following oral surgery. Large meals may be overwhelming; small, frequent meals promote food and nutrient intake.*
- Provide enteral feedings per gastrostomy tube as ordered. Elevate the head of the bed 30 to 40 degrees. *Enteral feedings maintain nutritional status in the client who is unable to consume foods orally. Elevating the head of the bed reduces the risk of regurgitation and aspiration of gastric contents.*
- Assess for gastric residual volume per facility protocol for the type of feeding (intermittent or continuous). See the Nursing Research box page 545. Notify the physician of volumes greater than 200 mL or 50% of previous feeding if feeding is intermittent. *Excess residual volume may increase the risk for aspiration.*
- Consider a nutritional consultation to assess diet and plan appropriate supplements. *A registered dietitian can calculate energy requirements and develop an individualized diet plan to meet nutritional requirements.*

### Impaired Verbal Communication

Oral surgery can interfere with communication. Effective communication is vital to postoperative recovery and prevention of complications.

- Before surgery, establish and practice a communication plan such as using a magic slate or flash cards. *Practicing communication techniques reduces fear and anxiety while promoting communication.*
- Provide ample time for communication efforts and do not answer for the client. Be alert for nonverbal communications. Use yes/no questions and simple phrases. *Providing adequate time allows the client opportunity to express ideas and thoughts. Nonverbal communication provides cues regarding comfort or other needs. Simple yes/no questions are easily answered nonverbally.*
- If indicated, refer to or consult with a speech therapist. *A speech therapist can help promote or restore effective communication.*

## Nursing Research

### Evidence-Based Practice for Clients with Enteral Feeding Tubes

Practices and protocols for assessing gastric residual volume in clients with nasogastric or gastrostomy feeding tubes are inconsistent. Researchers have come to varying conclusions about the amount of gastric residual volume that is safe and does not increase gastric distention and the risk for aspiration. In one study, while more than 30% of the clients had residual volumes greater than 150 mL, only 4% had evidence of formula in their airways. In an extensive review of the literature regarding measurement of gastric residual volume, Edwards and Metheny (2000) also found that nursing practice often was inconsistent with hospital protocols.

### IMPLICATIONS FOR NURSING

Gastric motility slows following surgery or trauma, in diabetes, sepsis, or electrolyte imbalance, and with medications such as narcotic analgesics. Excessive gastric distention appears to increase the risk for aspiration of gastric contents. However, when enteral feedings are withheld unnecessarily, the nutritional status of the client is at risk. Impaired nutrition affects healing and recovery.

The authors suggest a protocol for enteral infusions that includes: (1) checking residual volume every 4 hours; (2) assessing the client and contacting the physician if the residual volume is greater than 200 mL or 50% of the previous bolus feeding; and (3) withholding the feeding only when directed to do so by the physician (Edwards & Metheny, 2000).

### Critical Thinking in Client Care

1. What factors might influence the accuracy of residual volume measurements? What measures can be taken to obtain accurate measurements?
2. What would be the effect of withholding one bolus feeding of 240 mL of a standard enteral formula? If this is repeated daily for a week, what is the cumulative effect?
3. One reason frequently cited for avoiding checking residual volume is the risk of plugging the feeding tube. Identify measures to prevent this potential problem.

---

**PRACTICE ALERT** *Provide an emergency call system and respond promptly. Make all staff aware that the client cannot respond over an intercom system by posting an alert on the intercom. Nonverbal clients rely on an emergency call system to summon help. Answering promptly reduces fear and anxiety and maintains safety.* ■

### Disturbed Body Image

Radical surgery of the head or neck seriously affects body image. An altered speech pattern and any disfigurement affect the ability to feel attractive or effective in work or social roles. Clients may defer lifesaving surgery to postpone disfiguring interventions or therapies.

- Assess coping style, self-perception, and responses to altered appearance or function. *This information can be used to identify appropriate interventions and care.*
- Encourage verbalization of feelings regarding perceived and actual changes. *Nonjudgmental acceptance of feelings and fears helps establish trust.*
- Provide emotional support, encourage self-care, and provide decision-making opportunities. *Self-care promotes self-acceptance and independence. Giving choices empowers the client to participate in care.*

### Using NANDA, NIC, and NOC

Chart 21–1 shows links between NANDA nursing diagnoses, NIC, and NOC when caring for the client with oral cancer.

---

## CHART 21–1  NANDA, NIC, AND NOC LINKAGES

### The Client with Oral Cancer

| NURSING DIAGNOSES | NURSING INTERVENTIONS | NURSING OUTCOMES |
|---|---|---|
| • Impaired Oral Mucous Membrane | • Oral Health Restoration | • Oral Health<br>• Self-Care: Oral Hygiene |
| • Acute Pain | • Pain Management<br>• Patient-Controlled Analgesia (PCA) Assistance | • Comfort Level<br>• Pain Control |
| • Risk for Imbalanced Nutrition: Less Than Body Requirements | • Nutrition Management<br>• Fluid Monitoring<br>• Swallowing, Therapy | • Nutritional Status<br>• Nutritional Status: Food and Fluid Intake |

*Note. Data from Nursing Outcomes Classification (NOC) by M. Johnson & M. Maas (Eds.), 1997, St. Louis: Mosby; Nursing Diagnoses: Definitions & Classification 2001–2002 by North American Nursing Diagnosis Association, 2001, Philadelphia: NANDA; Nursing Interventions Classification (NIC) by J.C. McCloskey & G. M. Bulechek (Eds.), 2000, St. Louis: Mosby. Reprinted by permission.*

## Home Care

Discharge planning for the client with oral cancer depends on the type of treatment planned and surgery performed. Depending on the client's age, condition, and availability of support systems, referral to community health care agencies may be an essential component of care. Visits from home care nurses can assist in meeting health care needs.

Discuss the following topics with the client and family members or care providers:

- Diagnosis and prescribed care
- Monitoring for new lesions or recurrences
- Diet, nutrition, and activity
- Pain management
- Airway management, care of incision, and signs and symptoms to report

## Nursing Care Plan
## A Client with Oral Cancer

Juan Chavez, a married 44-year-old farmer, has two adult children. He and his wife raise and sell fruits and vegetables. Two months ago, Mr. Chavez developed a sore on his tongue that would not heal. Mr. Chavez tells his admission nurse, Sara Bucklin, "The doctor says he will have to remove part of my tongue," and anxiously asks, "Will I ever look the same? How will I be able to talk?"

### ASSESSMENT

Mr. Chavez's admission history reveals that he has been healthy, but has smoked two packs of cigarettes a day for over 20 years, and usually drinks two to four beers per day. He admits to being anxious and fearful of surgery and its outcomes. He says he quit smoking and drinking 2 weeks ago. The biopsy report is positive for squamous cell carcinoma of the tongue. Mr. Chavez has no enlarged cervical nodes and says he has no bloody sputum or saliva, difficulty swallowing, chewing, or talking. His weight is in the normal range for his height. A wide excision of the oral lesion is planned.

### DIAGNOSES

- *Risk for ineffective airway clearance* related to oral surgery
- *Risk for imbalanced nutrition: Less than body requirements* related to oral surgery
- *Impaired verbal communication* related to excision of a portion of the tongue
- *Disturbed body image* related to surgical excision of the tongue

### EXPECTED OUTCOMES

- Maintain a patent airway and remain free of respiratory distress.
- Maintain a stable weight and level of hydration.
- Effectively communicate with staff and family using a magic slate and flash cards.
- Communicate an increased ability to accept changes in body image.

### PLANNING AND IMPLEMENTATION

- Assess airway patency and respiratory status every hour until stable.

- Maintain semi-Fowler's position, supporting arms. Encourage to turn, cough, and deep breathe every 2 to 4 hours.
- Teach the importance of activity, turning, coughing, and deep breathing.
- Monitor daily weights.
- Consult with dietitian to assess calorie needs and plan appropriate enteral feeding. Assess response to enteral feedings.
- Demonstrate and allow to practice using magic slate and flash cards prior to surgery.
- Allow adequate time for communication efforts.
- Keep emergency call system in reach at all times and answer light promptly. Alert all staff of inability to respond verbally.
- Encourage expression of feelings regarding perceived and actual changes.
- Provide emotional support, encourage self-care and participation in decision making.

### EVALUATION

At the time of discharge, Mr. Chavez has maintained his weight and has started on oral liquids, including supplements and enriched liquids. His airway has remained clear, and he is effectively coughing and deep breathing. He has used the magic slate to communicate throughout his hospital stay. He is regaining use of his tongue, and can speak a few words. Although initially distressed, he is communicating an increased ability to cope with loss of part of his tongue. He and his wife say they understand his discharge instructions, including diet, activity, follow-up care, and signs and symptoms to report.

### Critical Thinking in the Nursing Process

1. What measures can you, as a nurse, implement to reduce the incidence of oral cancer?
2. Plan a health education program for young athletes who chew tobacco.
3. Mr. Chavez's wife calls you 2 weeks after discharge. She tells you that he refuses to try to talk and is relying on his magic slate to communicate. How will you respond?

See Evaluating Your Response in Appendix C.

# DISORDERS OF THE ESOPHAGUS

The esophagus plays an essential role in the ingestion of food and liquids. Disorders of the esophagus can be inflammatory, mechanical, or cancerous. Because of its location and neighboring organs, the symptoms of esophageal disorders may mimic those of a variety of other illnesses.

## THE CLIENT WITH GASTROESOPHAGEAL REFLUX DISEASE

**Gastroesophageal reflux** is the backward flowing of gastric contents into the esophagus. When this occurs, the client experiences heartburn. Many people with gastroesophageal reflux have few symptoms, while others develop inflammatory esophagitis as a result of exposure to gastric juices.

**Gastroesophageal reflux disease (GERD)** is a common gastrointestinal disorder that affects 15% to 20% of adults. As many as 10% of people experience daily symptoms such as heartburn and indigestion (Braunwald et al., 2001; Mattonen, 2001; Tierney et al., 2001).

### PATHOPHYSIOLOGY

Normally, the lower esophageal sphincter remains closed except during swallowing. Reflux (backflow) of gastric contents into the esophagus is prevented by pressure differences between the stomach and the lower esophagus. The diaphragm, the lower esophageal sphincter, and the location of the gastroesophageal junction below the diaphragm help maintain this pressure difference (Figure 21–2 ■).

Gastroesophageal reflux may result from transient relaxation of the lower esophageal sphincter, an incompetent lower esophageal sphincter, and/or increased pressure within the stomach (Figure 21–3 ■). Factors contributing to gastroesophageal reflux include increased gastric volume (e.g., after meals), positioning that allows gastric contents to remain close to the gastroesophageal junction (e.g., bending over, lying down), and increased gastric pressure (e.g., obesity or wearing tight clothing). A hiatal hernia may contribute to GERD.

Gastric juices contain acid, pepsin, and bile, which are corrosive substances. Esophageal peristalsis and bicarbonate in salivary secretions normally clear and neutralize gastric juices in the esophagus. During sleep, however, and in clients with impaired esophageal peristalsis or salivation, the esophageal mucosa is damaged by gastric juices, causing an inflammatory response. With prolonged exposure, esophagitis develops. Superficial ulcers develop, and the mucosa becomes red, friable (easily torn), and may bleed. If untreated, scarring and esophageal stricture may develop.

### MANIFESTATIONS AND COMPLICATIONS

GERD causes heartburn, usually after meals, with bending over, or when reclining. Regurgitation of sour material into the mouth, or difficulty and pain with swallowing may develop. Other manifestations may include atypical chest pain, sore throat, and hoarseness. See the Manifestations box on page 548. Aspiration of gastric contents can cause hoarseness or respiratory symptoms.

Complications include esophageal strictures and Barrett's esophagus. Strictures can lead to dysphagia. Barrett's esophagus

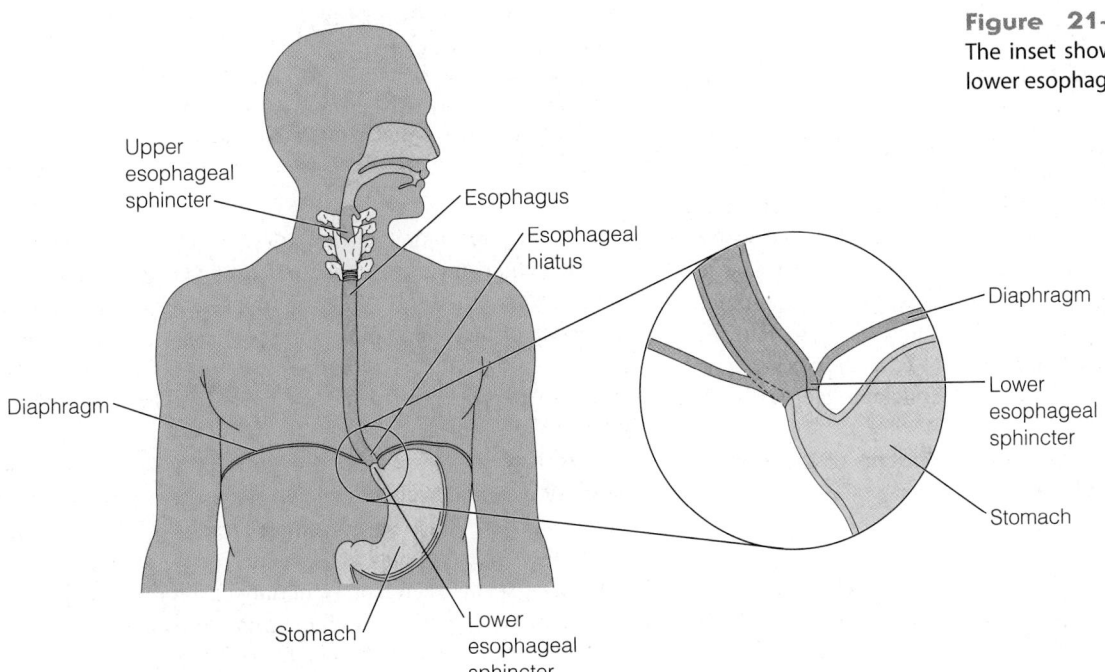

**Figure 21–2 ■** The esophagus. The inset shows a closer view of the lower esophageal sphincter.

Upper esophageal sphincter

Esophagus

Esophageal hiatus

Diaphragm

Diaphragm

Lower esophageal sphincter

Stomach

Stomach

Lower esophageal sphincter

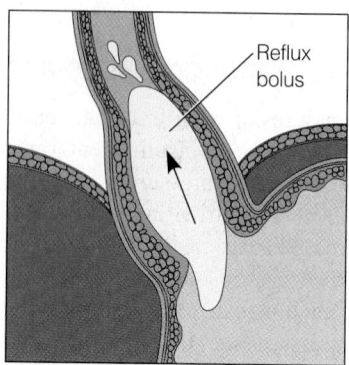

Transient lower esophageal sphincter relaxation

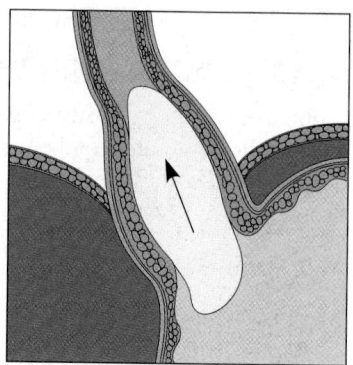

Incompetent lower esophageal sphincter

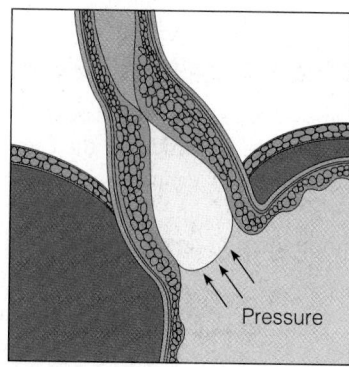

Increased intragastric pressure

**Figure 21–3** ■ Mechanisms of gastroesophageal reflux.

## Manifestations of GERD

- Heartburn
- Regurgitation
- Pain after eating
- Dysphagia
- Chest pain
- Belching

is characterized by changes in the cells lining the esophagus and an increased risk of developing esophageal cancer (Porth, 2002).

## COLLABORATIVE CARE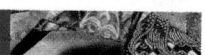

Often the diagnosis of GERD is made by the history of symptoms and predisposing factors. Collaborative care focuses on lifestyle changes, diet modification, and for more severe cases, drug therapy. Surgery is reserved for clients who develop serious complications.

### Diagnostic Tests

Diagnostic tests that may be ordered for clients with manifestations of GERD include:

- *Barium swallow* to evaluate the esophagus, stomach, and upper small intestine.
- *Upper endoscopy* to permit direct visualization of the esophagus. Tissue may be obtained for biopsy to establish the diagnosis and rule out malignancy. See the accompanying box for nursing care of the client undergoing an upper endoscopy.
- *24-hour ambulatory pH monitoring* may be performed to establish the diagnosis of GERD. For this test, a small tube with a pH electrode is inserted through the nose into the esophagus. The electrode is attached to a small box worn on the belt which records the data. The data are later analyzed by computer.
- *Esophageal manometry* measures pressures of the esophageal sphincters and esophageal peristalsis.

### Medications

Antacids, such as Mylanta or Maalox, relieve mild or moderate symptoms by neutralizing stomach acid. Gaviscon, which forms a floating barrier between the gastric contents and the esophageal mucosa when the client is upright, may also be used.

## Nursing Implications for Diagnostic Tests: Upper Endoscopy

### Client Preparation

- Schedule at least 2 days after barium swallow or upper gastrointestinal series.
- Ensure the informed consent is signed prior to premedication.
- Encourage questions, and provide answers and support.
- Withhold food and fluids for 6 to 8 hours before the procedure.
- Remove dentures and eyewear. Provide mouth care.

### Client and Family Teaching

- Do not eat or drink anything for 6 to 8 hours before the procedure.
- The procedure is somewhat uncomfortable but requires only 20 to 30 minutes to complete.
- A local anesthetic will be used in your throat and you will be given a sedative during the procedure.
- After the procedure, you will be allowed to eat and drink as soon as your gag reflex returns and you are able to swallow.
- You may experience mild bloating, belching, or flatulence following the procedure.
- Contact your physician immediately if you develop any of the following: difficulty swallowing; epigastric, substernal or shoulder pain; vomiting blood or black tarry stools; or fever.

Histamine$_2$-receptor (H$_2$-receptor) blockers reduce gastric acid production and are effective in treating GERD symptoms. When treating GERD, H$_2$-receptor blockers are usually given twice a day or more frequently for a prolonged period of time. Cimetidine, ranitidine, famotidine, and nizatidine are all approved by the FDA for the treatment of GERD and are available over the counter.

Omeprazole (Prilosec), lansoprazole (Prevacid), pantoprazole (Protonix), and rabeprazole (Aciphex) are proton-pump inhibitors (PPIs) that reduce gastric secretions. PPIs promote healing of erosive esophagitis as well as relieve symptoms. An 8-week course of treatment is initially prescribed, although some clients may require 3 to 6 months of therapy.

A promotility agent, such as metoclopramide (Reglan), may be ordered to enhance esophageal clearance and gastric emptying. Metoclopramide is used to treat clients with regurgitation, symptoms of indigestion, and nighttime symptoms. However, it is not recommended for long-time use. See the Medication Administration box below for the nursing implications of drugs used to treat GERD.

## Dietary and Lifestyle Management

GERD is a chronic condition. Dietary and lifestyle changes are important to reduce symptoms and long-term effects of the disorder. Acidic foods such as tomato products, citrus fruits, spicy foods, and coffee are eliminated from the diet. Fatty foods, chocolate, peppermint, and alcohol relax the lower esophageal

# Medication Administration

## Drugs Used to Treat GERD, Gastritis, and Peptic Ulcer Disease

### ANTACIDS

| | | | |
|---|---|---|---|
| Maalox | Gaviscon | Gelusil | Tums |
| Mylanta | Aludrox | Riopan | Amphojel |

Antacids buffer or neutralize gastric acid, usually acting locally. Antacids are used in GERD, gastritis, and peptic ulcer disease to relieve pain and prevent further damage to esophageal and gastric mucosa.

#### Nursing Responsibilities

- Antacids interfere with the absorption of many drugs given orally; separate administration times by at least 2 hours.
- Monitor for constipation or diarrhea resulting from antacid therapy. Notify the physician should either develop; a different antacid may be ordered.
- Although most antacids have little systemic effect, electrolyte imbalances can develop. Monitor serum electrolytes, particularly sodium, calcium, and magnesium levels.

#### Client and Family Teaching

- Take your antacid frequently as prescribed, 1 to 3 hours after meals and at bedtime. To be effective, the antacid must be in your stomach.
- Avoid taking an antacid for approximately 2 hours before and 1 hour after taking another medication.
- Shake suspensions well prior to administration.
- Chew tablets thoroughly, and follow with 4 to 6 ounces of water.
- Report worsening symptoms, diarrhea, or constipation to your primary care provider.
- Continue taking the antacid for the duration prescribed. While pain and discomfort often are relieved soon after treatment begins, healing takes 6 to 8 weeks.

### H$_2$-RECEPTOR BLOCKERS

| | |
|---|---|
| Cimetidine (Tagamet) | Ranitidine (Zantac) |
| Famotidine (Pepcid) | Nizatidine (Axid) |

H$_2$-receptor blockers reduce acidity of gastric juices by blocking the ability of histamine to stimulate acid secretion by the gastric parietal cells. As a result, both the volume and concentration of hydrochloric acid in gastric juice is reduced. H$_2$-receptor blockers are given orally or intravenously. Both prescription and over-the-counter preparations are available.

#### Nursing Responsibilities

- To ensure absorption, do not give an antacid within 1 hour before or after giving an H$_2$-receptor blocker.
- When administered intravenously, do not mix with other drugs. Administer in 20 to 100 mL of solution over 15 to 30

minutes. Rapid intravenous injection as a bolus may cause dysrhythmias and hypotension.
- Monitor for interaction with such drugs as oral anticoagulants, beta blockers, benzodiazepines, tricyclic antidepressants, and others. H$_2$-receptor blockers may inhibit the metabolism of other drugs, increasing the risk of toxicity.

#### Client and Family Teaching

- Take the drug as directed, even if pain and gastric discomfort are relieved early in the course of therapy.
- Take at bedtime if once-a-day dosing is ordered. If spaced through the day, take before meals. Avoid taking antacids for 1 hour before and 1 hour after taking this drug.
- To promote healing, avoid cigarette smoking (which increases gastric acid secretion) and gastric mucosal irritants such as alcohol, aspirin, and NSAIDs.
- Long-term use of these drugs can lead to gynecomastia (breast enlargement) and impotence in men and breast tenderness in women. Discontinuing the drug will reverse these effects.
- Report possible adverse effects such as diarrhea, confusion, rash, fatigue, malaise, or bruising to your care provider.

### PROTON-PUMP INHIBITORS

Lansoprazole (Prevacid)
Omeprazole (Prilosec)
Pantoprazole (Protonix)
Rabeprazole (Aciphex)

Proton-pump inhibitors (PPIs) are the drugs of choice for severe GERD. PPIs inhibit the hydrogen-potassium-ATP pump, reducing gastric acid secretion. Initially, the PPI may be given twice a day, with the dose reduced to once daily (at bedtime) after 8 weeks.

#### Nursing Responsibilities

- Administer before breakfast and at bedtime if ordered twice a day; at bedtime if once a day.
- Do not crush tablets.
- Monitor liver function tests for possible abnormal values, including increased AST, ALT, alkaline phosphatase, and bilirubin levels.

#### Client and Family Teaching

- Take the drug as ordered for the full course of therapy, even if symptoms are relieved.
- Do not crush, break, or chew tablets.
- Avoid cigarette smoking, alcohol, aspirin, and NSAIDs while taking this drug as these substances may interfere with healing.
- Report black tarry stools, diarrhea, or abdominal pain to your primary care provider.

(continued on page 550)

## Medication Administration

### Drugs Used to Treat GERD, Gastritis, and Peptic Ulcer Disease (continued)

#### ANTI-ULCER AGENT

Sucralfate (Carafate)

Sucralfate reacts with gastric acid to form a thick paste which adheres to damaged gastric mucosal tissue. It protects gastric mucosa and promotes healing through this local action.

#### Nursing Responsibilities

- Administer on an empty stomach, 1 hour before meals and at bedtime.
- Do not crush tablets.
- Separate administration time from antacids by at least 30 minutes.

#### Client and Family Teaching

- Take as directed, even after symptoms have been relieved.
- Do not crush or chew tablets; shake suspension well.
- Increase your intake of fluids and dietary fiber to prevent constipation.

#### PROMOTILITY AGENT

Metoclopramide (Reglan)

By acting on the central nervous system, metoclopramide stimulates upper gastrointestinal motility and gastric emptying. As a result, nausea, vomiting, and symptoms of GERD are reduced.

#### Nursing Implications

- Do not administer this drug to clients with possible gastrointestinal obstruction or bleeding, or a history of seizure disorders, pheochromocytoma, or Parkinson's disease.
- Monitor for extrapyramidal side effects (e.g., difficulty speaking or swallowing, loss of balance, gait disruptions, twitching or twisting movements, weakness of arms or legs) or manifestations of tardive dyskinesia (uncontrolled rhythmic facial movement, lip-smacking, tongue rolling). Report immediately.
- Give oral doses 30 minutes before meals and at bedtime.
- May be given by direct intravenous push over 1 to 2 minutes, or diluted by slow infusion over 15 to 30 minutes.

#### Client and Family Teaching

- Take this drug as directed. If you miss a dose, take as soon as you remember unless it is close to time for the next dose.
- Do not drive or engage in other activities that require alertness if this drug makes you drowsy.
- Avoid using alcohol or other CNS depressants while you are taking this drug.
- Immediately contact your health care provider if you develop involuntary movements of your eyes, face, or limbs.

---

sphincter or delay gastric emptying, so should be avoided. The client is advised to maintain ideal body weight, eat smaller meals, refrain from eating for 3 hours before bedtime, and stay upright for 2 hours after meals. Elevating the head of the bed on 6- to 8-inch blocks often is beneficial. Stopping smoking is a necessary lifestyle change. Avoiding tight clothing and avoiding bending may help to relieve symptoms.

## Surgery

Surgery may be used for clients who do not respond to pharmacologic and lifestyle management. Antireflux surgeries increase pressure in the lower esophagus, inhibiting gastric content reflux. Laparoscopic procedures for GERD include tightening the lower esophageal sphincter with an endoscopic suturing system or burning spots on the muscle surrounding the lower esophageal sphincter to create scar tissue (Mattonen, 2001). An open surgical procedure known as Nissen fundoplication also may be done (Figure 21–4 ■).

## NURSING CARE

### Assessment

Assessment data related to GERD include the following:

- Health history: manifestations such as frequent heartburn; intolerance of foods that are acidic, spicy, or fatty; regurgitation of acidic gastric juice; increased symptoms when bending over, lying down, or wearing tight clothing; difficulty swallowing
- Physical assessment: Epigastric tenderness

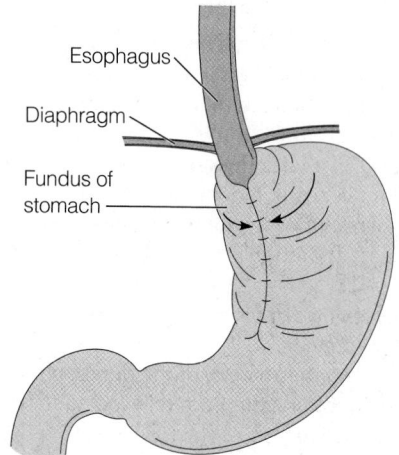

Esophagus

Diaphragm

Fundus of stomach

**Figure 21–4** ■ Nissen fundoplication. The fundus of the stomach is wrapped around the lower esophagus and the edges are sutured together.

## Nursing Diagnoses and Interventions

### Pain

The epigastric pain associated with GERD can be severe, interfering with rest and causing anxiety.

- Provide small, frequent meals. Restrict intake of fat, acidic foods, coffee, and alcohol. *Limiting the size of meals reduces pressure in the stomach, reducing esophageal reflux. Fatty, acidic foods, coffee, and alcohol increase gastric acidity and interfere with gastric emptying, increasing the incidence of gastroesophageal reflux.*

## CHART 21–2 NANDA, NIC, AND NOC LINKAGES

### The Client with GERD

| NURSING DIAGNOSES | NURSING INTERVENTIONS | NURSING OUTCOMES |
|---|---|---|
| • Pain: Heartburn | • Behavior Modification | • Pain: Disruptive Effects |
| • Imbalanced Nutrition: Less Than Body Requirements | • Nutrition Management | • Nutritional Status: Food and Fluid Intake |
| | • Nutrition Monitoring | |
| • Ineffective Health Maintenance | • Teaching: Individual | • Knowledge: Treatment Regimen |

*Note. Data from* Nursing Outcomes Classification (NOC) *by M. Johnson & M. Maas (Eds.), 1997, St. Louis: Mosby;* Nursing Diagnoses: Definitions & Classification 2001–2002 *by North American Nursing Diagnosis Association, 2001, Philadelphia: NANDA;* Nursing Interventions Classification (NIC) *by J.C. McCloskey & G. M. Bulechek (Eds.), 2000, St. Louis: Mosby. Reprinted by permission.*

• Instruct to stop smoking. Refer to a smoking cessation clinic or program as needed. *Cigarette smoking increases gastric acidity and interferes with healing of damaged mucosa.*

• Administer antacids, H$_2$-receptor blockers, and proton-pump inhibitors as ordered. Instruct client to continue therapy as prescribed, even after symptoms have been relieved. *These drugs neutralize or reduce gastric acid secretion, relieving symptoms and promoting healing.*

• Discuss the long-term nature of GERD and its management. *Lifestyle changes need to be continued after healing and symptom relief to manage the long-term effects of GERD.*

### Using NANDA, NIC, and NOC

Chart 21–2 shows links between NANDA nursing diagnoses, NIC, and NOC for clients with GERD.

### Home Care

GERD is a lifelong condition best managed by the client. Teach the client and family about continuing management strategies, including dietary changes, remaining upright after meals, and avoiding eating for at least 3 hours before bedtime. Suggest elevating the head of the bed on 6- to 8-inch wooden blocks placed under the legs. Discuss the need for continued gastric acid reduction using antacids, H$_2$-receptor blockers, or proton-pump inhibitors. All are effective to reduce the acidity of gastric juices. Antacids, the most cost-effective measure, require frequent doses to neutralize gastric acid. H$_2$-receptor blockers, also available over the counter, are a cost-effective management strategy that require only twice-a-day dosing.

## THE CLIENT WITH HIATAL HERNIA

A **hiatal hernia** occurs when part of the stomach protrudes through the esophageal hiatus of the diaphragm into the thoracic cavity. While hiatal hernia is thought to be a common problem, most affected individuals are asymptomatic. The incidence of hiatal hernia increases with age.

In a *sliding hiatal hernia*, the gastroesophageal junction and the fundus of the stomach slide upward through the esophageal hiatus (Figure 21–5A). Several factors may contribute to a sliding hiatal hernia, including weakened gastroesophageal-diaphragmatic anchors, shortening of the esophagus, or increased intra-abdominal pressure. Small sliding hiatal hernias produce few symptoms.

In a *paraesophageal hiatal hernia,* the junction between the esophagus and stomach remains in its normal position below the diaphragm while a part of the stomach herniates through the esophageal hiatus (Figure 21–5B). A paraesophageal hernia can become incarcerated (constricted) and strangulate, impairing blood flow to the herniated tissue. Clients with

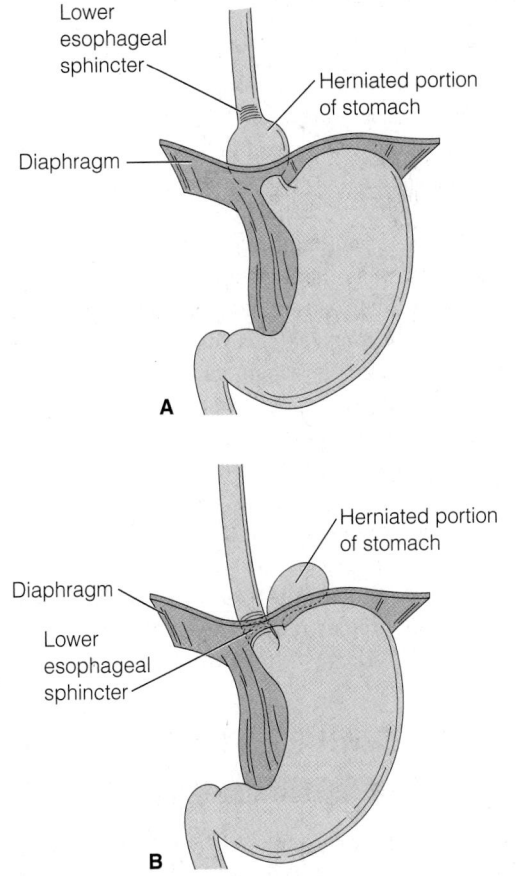

**Figure 21–5** ■ Hiatal hernias. *A,* Sliding hiatal hernia. *B,* Paraesophageal hiatal hernia.

## Manifestations of Hiatal Hernia

- Reflux, heartburn
- Substernal chest pain
- Occult bleeding
- Feeling of fullness
- Dysphagia
- Belching, indigestion

paraesophageal hernia may develop gastritis, or chronic or acute gastrointestinal bleeding. The manifestations of hiatal hernias are listed in the box above.

A barium swallow or an upper endoscopy may be done to diagnose hiatal hernia. Many clients with hiatal hernia require no treatment. If symptoms are present, treatment measures such as those for clients with GERD may be ordered. If medical management is ineffective or the hernia becomes incarcerated, surgery may be required. The most common surgical procedure is the Nissen fundoplication (see Figure 21–4). This surgery prevents the gastroesophageal junction from slipping into the thoracic cavity.

Nursing care for the client with a hiatal hernia is similar to that for the client with GERD. If surgery is performed, nursing care is similar to that for clients undergoing gastric or thoracic surgery (see Chapter 7). 

## THE CLIENT WITH IMPAIRED ESOPHAGEAL MOTILITY

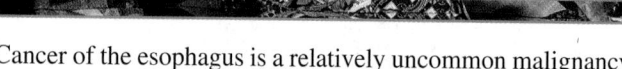

Disorders of esophageal motility can cause dysphagia or chest pain. **Achalasia**, a disorder of unknown etiology, is characterized by impaired peristalsis of the smooth muscle of the esophagus and impaired relaxation of the lower esophageal sphincter. The client experiences gradually increasing dysphagia with both solid foods and liquids. Fullness in the chest during meals, chest pain, and nighttime cough are additional manifestations. Other clients may experience **diffuse esophageal spasm** that causes nonperistaltic contraction of esophageal smooth muscle. This disorder causes chest pain and/or dysphagia. The chest pain can be severe, and usually occurs at rest.

Treatment of achalasia may include endoscopically guided injection of botulinum toxin into the lower esophageal sphincter or balloon dilation of the LES. Botulinum toxin injection lowers LES pressure, but may need to be repeated every 6 to 9 months. Balloon dilation tears muscle fibers in the LES, reducing its pressure (Figure 21–6 ■). A laparoscopic myotomy (incision into the circular muscle layer of the LES) also reduces pressure and relieves symptoms.

## THE CLIENT WITH ESOPHAGEAL CANCER

Cancer of the esophagus is a relatively uncommon malignancy in the United States. It does, however, have a high mortality rate, primarily because symptoms often are not recognized until late in the course of the disease.

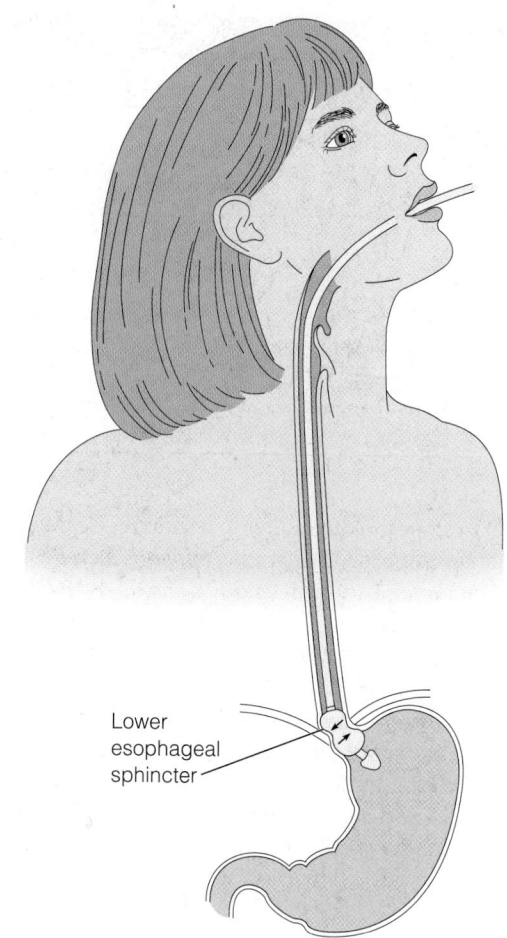

**Figure 21–6 ■** Balloon dilation of the lower esophageal sphincter.

Lower esophageal sphincter

## PATHOPHYSIOLOGY AND MANIFESTATIONS

Squamous cell carcinoma is the most common type of esophageal cancer. It usually affects the middle or distal portion of the esophagus. Squamous cell cancer is much more common in blacks than in whites. Cigarette smoking and chronic alcohol use are strong risk factors for squamous cell esophageal tumors.

Adenocarcinoma, nearly as common as squamous cell, is more common in whites. It usually develops in the distal portion of the esophagus. Adenocarcinoma is commonly associated with Barrett's esophagus, a possible complication of chronic GERD and achalasia.

The most common symptom of esophageal carcinoma is progressive dysphagia. Other manifestations are listed in the box below. The cancer often is advanced and incurable by the time the disease is diagnosed.

## Manifestations of Esophageal Cancer

- Dysphagia
- Weight loss
- Regurgitation
- Chest pain
- Anemia
- GERD-like symptoms
- Anorexia
- Persistent cough

## COLLABORATIVE CARE

Controlling dysphagia and maintaining nutritional status is an essential goal of therapy for clients with esophageal cancer, regardless of the stage of the disease. Treatment may involve surgery, radiation therapy, and/or chemotherapy.

### Diagnostic Tests

Diagnostic and staging procedures for esophageal cancer may include esophagography, bronchoscopy, and scans to detect metastasis. The following diagnostic tests may be done.

- *Barium swallow* to identify irregular mucosal patterns or narrowing of the lumen, which suggest esophageal cancer.
- *Esophagoscopy* to allow direct visualization of the tumor and obtain tissue for biopsy.
- *Chest X-ray, CT scans,* or *MRI* to identify possible tumor metastases to other organs or tissues.
- *Complete blood count (CBC)* may indicate anemia due to chronic blood loss. *Serum albumin levels* may be low due to malnutrition, and *liver function tests (ALT, alkaline phosphatase, AST,* and *bilirubin)* are elevated if liver metastases are present.

### Treatments

The treatment of esophageal cancer depends on the stage of the disease, as well as factors such as the client's condition and preference.

Clients with early, "curable" esophageal cancer may be treated with surgery alone. Surgery involves resection of the affected portion of the esophagus, and possible anastamosis of the stomach to the remaining esophagus. Mediastinal lymph nodes may be resected at the time of surgery. Other approaches to early esophageal cancer include combined radiation and chemotherapy, or a combination of radiation therapy and chemotherapy prior to surgical resection of the tumor. Complications associated with radiation therapy to the esophagus include perforation, hemorrhage, and strictures. When the tumor has spread locally or to distant sites, palliative therapy relieves dysphagia and pain (Tierney et al., 2001). Palliative therapy may include surgical resection, radiation therapy, or local treatments such as wire stents or laser therapy to keep the esophagus patent.

## NURSING CARE

### Health Promotion

Health promotion measures to reduce the risk for and incidence of esophageal cancer include educating people (especially young people) about the dangers of cigarette smoking and excess alcohol use. Refer to smoking cessation and alcohol treatment programs as indicated.

### Assessment

Early diagnosis and treatment of esophageal cancer can make a difference in the client's prognosis. Collect the following assessment data related to esophageal cancer.

- Health history: current symptoms such as chest pain, dysphagia, odynophagia (pain with swallowing), coughing or hoarseness; duration of symptoms; recent weight loss; smoking history; current and past patterns of alcohol consumption
- Physical examination: weight; general health status; skin color; supraclavicular and cervical lymph nodes for lymphadenopathy

### Nursing Diagnoses and Interventions

#### Imbalanced Nutrition: Less Than Body Requirements

The client diagnosed with esophageal cancer may already suffer from some degree of malnutrition because of difficulty and pain with swallowing. Enteral nutrition via nasogastric feeding tube or gastrostomy tube or parenteral nutrition maintain nutritional status after surgery or if the tumor is inoperable and obstruction occurs. See Chapter 20 for nursing interventions related to enteral and parenteral feedings.

#### Risk for Ineffective Airway Clearance

After surgery for esophageal cancer, the client is at high risk for aspiration and difficulty maintaining a patent airway due to disruption of the esophagus and incision into the thoracic cavity.

- Assess mental and respiratory status (including rate, depth, breath sounds, and oxygen saturation levels) every hour during the initial postoperative period. *Altered mental status increases the risk for aspiration. An increased respiratory rate, dyspnea, diminished breath sounds, or decreased oxygen saturation levels may indicate impaired airway clearance or possible aspiration pneumonia.*
- Encourage coughing and deep breathing every 2 to 4 hours and as needed. *These activities help mobilize respiratory secretions.*
- Verify enteral tube feeding placement by checking the pH of gastric aspirate (see Chapter 20). Stop enteral feedings if feelings of fullness or nausea occur. Suction gastrointestinal contents as needed, positioning the client on the side. *Overdistention of the stomach or delayed gastric emptying may result in regurgitation of stomach contents. Nausea or a feeling of fullness may indicate stomach overdistention. Suctioning and positioning limit the risk of aspiration.*

#### Anticipatory Grieving

Upon a diagnosis of cancer, the client and family may experience a grief reaction. The pessimistic prognosis associated with esophageal cancer and the disruptions in relationships may result in an intense sense of loss. Chapter 11 discusses care of client experiencing grief and loss.

### Using NANDA, NIC, and NOC

Chart 21–3 shows links between NANDA nursing diagnoses, NIC, and NOC for clients with esophageal cancer.

The Client with Esophageal Cancer

| NURSING DIAGNOSES | NURSING INTERVENTIONS | NURSING OUTCOMES |
|---|---|---|
| • Impaired Swallowing | • Aspiration Precautions<br>• Positioning | • Aspiration Control<br>• Swallowing Status |
| • Imbalanced Nutrition: Less Than Body Requirements | • Fluid Monitoring<br>• Nutrition Management | • Nutritional Status: Food and Fluid Intake |
| • Fear | • Anxiety Reduction | • Anxiety Control |

Note. Data from Nursing Outcomes Classification (NOC) by M. Johnson & M. Maas (Eds.), 1997, St. Louis: Mosby; Nursing Diagnoses: Definitions & Classification 2001–2002 by North American Nursing Diagnosis Association, 2001, Philadelphia: NANDA; Nursing Interventions Classification (NIC) by J.C. McCloskey & G. M. Bulechek (Eds.), 2000, St. Louis: Mosby. Reprinted by permission.

## Home Care

Most care for clients with esophageal cancer is provided in community-based and home settings. Include the following topics in client and family teaching for home care:

• Planned treatment options including the risks, benefits, and potential adverse effects of each

• Wound and follow-up care following surgery
• How to prepare, implement, and care for tube feedings or home parenteral nutrition

Based on the client's needs and prognosis, referral to a home health agency and/or hospice may be appropriate.

# DISORDERS OF THE STOMACH AND DUODENUM

The stomach and upper small intestine (duodenum and jejunum) are responsible for the majority of food digestion. The major disorders that affect digestion are gastritis, peptic ulcer disease, and cancer of the stomach. Nursing roles in managing these disorders include both acute care for the hospitalized client and teaching to give the client the skills and knowledge to manage these conditions at home.

## OVERVIEW OF NORMAL PHYSIOLOGY

Normally, the stomach is protected from the digestive substances it secretes—namely hydrochloric acid and pepsin—by the **gastric mucosal barrier** (Figure 21–7 ■). The gastric mucosal barrier includes:

• An impermeable hydrophobic lipid layer that covers gastric epithelial cells. This lipid layer prevents diffusion of water-soluble molecules, but substances such as aspirin and alcohol can diffuse through it.
• Bicarbonate ions secreted in response to hydrochloric acid secretion by the parietal cells of the stomach. When bicarbonate ($HCO_3^-$) secretion is equal to hydrogen ion ($H^+$) secretion, the gastric mucosa remains intact. Prostaglandins, chemical messengers involved in the inflammatory response, support bicarbonate production and blood flow to the gastric mucosa.
• Mucus gel that protects the surface of the stomach lining from the damaging effects of pepsin and traps bicarbonate to neutralize hydrochloric acid. This gel also acts as a lubricant, preventing mechanical damage to the stomach lining from its contents.

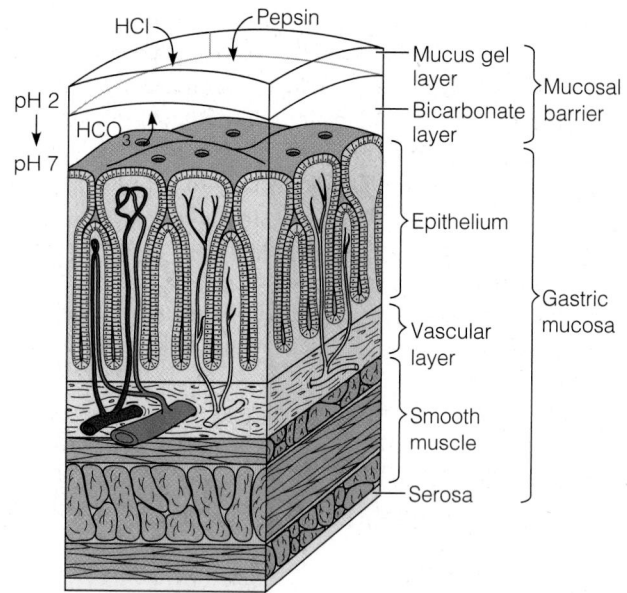

**Figure 21–7 ■** The gastric mucosa and mucosal barrier. The mucus gel and bicarbonate of the mucosal barrier protect the gastric mucosa (the epithelial, vascular, and smooth muscle layers) from damage by digestive substances such as hydrochloric acid and pepsin.

When an acute or chronic irritant disrupts the mucosal barrier, or when disease alters the processes that maintain the barrier, the gastric mucosa becomes irritated and inflamed. Lipid-soluble substances such as aspirin and alcohol penetrate the gastric mucosal barrier, leading to irritation and possible inflammation. Bile acids also break down the lipids in the mucosal barrier, increasing the potential for irritation (Porth, 2002). In addition, aspirin and other nonsteroidal anti-inflammatory drugs (NSAIDs) inhibit prostaglandins. Aspirin and NSAIDs also alter the nature of gastric mucus, affecting its protective function.

## THE CLIENT WITH GASTRITIS

**Gastritis,** inflammation of the stomach lining, results from irritation of the gastric mucosa. Gastritis is common, and may be caused by a variety of factors. The most common form of gastritis, **acute gastritis,** is generally a benign, self-limiting disorder associated with the ingestion of gastric irritants such as aspirin, alcohol, caffeine, or foods contaminated with certain bacteria. Manifestations of acute gastritis may range from asymptomatic to mild heartburn to severe gastric distress, vomiting, and bleeding with **hematemesis** (vomiting blood).

**Chronic gastritis** is a separate group of disorders characterized by progressive and irreversible changes in the gastric mucosa (Porth, 2002). Chronic gastritis is more common in the elderly, chronic alcoholics, and cigarette smokers. When symptoms of chronic gastritis occur, they are often vague, ranging from a feeling of heaviness in the epigastric region after meals to gnawing, burning, ulcerlike epigastric pain unrelieved by antacids.

## PATHOPHYSIOLOGY
### Acute Gastritis

Acute gastritis is characterized by disruption of the mucosal barrier by a local irritant. This disruption allows hydrochloric acid and pepsin to come into contact with the gastric tissue, resulting in irritation, inflammation, and superficial erosions. The gastric mucosa rapidly regenerates, generally making acute gastritis a self-limiting disorder, with resolution and healing occurring within several days.

The ingestion of aspirin or other NSAIDS, corticosteroids, alcohol, and caffeine is commonly associated with the development of acute gastritis. Accidental or purposeful ingestion of a corrosive alkali (such as ammonia, lye, Lysol, and other cleaning agents) or acid leads to severe inflammation and possible necrosis of the stomach. Gastric perforation, hemorrhage, and peritonitis are possible results. Iatrogenic causes of acute gastritis include radiation therapy and administration of certain chemotherapeutic agents.

### Erosive Gastritis

A severe form of acute gastritis, **erosive** or **stress-induced gastritis,** occurs as a complication of other life-threatening conditions such as shock, severe trauma, major surgery, sepsis, burns, or head injury. When these erosions follow a major burn, they are called **Curling's ulcers,** after Thomas Curling, a British physician, who first described them in 1842. When stress ulcers occur following head injury or central nervous system surgery, they are referred to as **Cushing's ulcers,** after Harvey Cushing, a U.S. surgeon.

The primary mechanisms leading to erosive gastritis appear to be ischemia of the gastric mucosa resulting from sympathetic vasoconstriction, and tissue injury due to gastric acid. As a result, multiple superficial erosions of the gastric mucosa develop. Maintaining the gastric pH at greater than 3.5 and inhibiting gastric acid secretion with medications help prevent erosive gastritis.

### Manifestations

The client with acute gastritis may have mild symptoms such as **anorexia** (loss of appetite), or mild epigastric discomfort relieved by belching or defecating. More severe manifestations include abdominal pain, nausea, and vomiting. Gastric bleeding may occur, with hematemesis or **melena** (black, tarry stool that contains blood). Erosive gastritis is not typically associated with pain. The initial symptom often is painless gastric bleeding occurring 2 or more days after the initial stressor. Bleeding typically is minimal, but can be massive. Corrosive gastritis can cause severe bleeding, signs of shock, and an *acute abdomen* (severely painful, rigid, boardlike abdomen) if perforation occurs. See the Manifestations box below.

### Chronic Gastritis

Unrelated to acute gastritis, chronic gastritis is a progressive disorder that begins with superficial inflammation and gradually leads to atrophy of gastric tissues. The initial stage is characterized by superficial changes in the gastric mucosa and a decrease in mucus. As the disease evolves, glands of the gastric mucosa are disrupted and destroyed. The inflammatory process involves deep portions of the mucosa, which thins and atrophies. There appear to be at least two different forms of chronic gastritis, classified as type A and type B.

*Type A gastritis,* the less common form of chronic gastritis, usually affects people of Northern European heritage. This

## Manifestations of Acute and Chronic Gastritis

### ACUTE GASTRITIS

| **Gastrointestinal** | **Systemic** |
|---|---|
| • Anorexia | • Possible shock |
| • Nausea and vomiting | |
| • Hematemesis | |
| • Melena | |
| • Abdominal pain | |

### CHRONIC GASTRITIS

| **Gastrointestinal** | **Systemic** |
|---|---|
| • Vague discomfort after eating; may be asymptomatic | • Anemia |
| | • Fatigue |

type of gastritis is thought to have an autoimmune component. In type A or autoimmune gastritis, the body produces antibodies to parietal cells and to intrinsic factor. These antibodies destroy gastric mucosal cells, resulting in tissue atrophy and the loss of hydrochloric acid and pepsin secretion. Because intrinsic factor is required for the absorption of vitamin $B_{12}$, this immune response also results in pernicious anemia. For further discussion of pernicious anemia, see Chapter 32. ⊙⊙

*Type B gastritis* is the more common form of chronic gastritis. Its incidence increases with age, reaching nearly 100% in people over the age of 70. Type B gastritis is caused by chronic infection of the gastric mucosa by *Helicobacter pylori* (*H. pylori*), a gram-negative spiral bacterium. *H. pylori* infection causes inflammation of the gastric mucosa, with infiltration by neutrophils and lymphocytes. The outermost layer of gastric mucosa thins and atrophies, providing a less effective barrier against the autodigestive properties of hydrochloric acid and pepsin.

Infection with *H. pylori* also is associated with an increased risk for peptic ulcer disease. *H. pylori* infection significantly increases the risk of developing gastric cancer. See the sections that follow for more information about these disorders.

### Manifestations

Chronic gastritis is often asymptomatic until atrophy is sufficiently advanced to interfere with digestion and gastric emptying. The client may complain of vague gastric distress, epigastric heaviness after meals, or ulcerlike symptoms. These symptoms typically are not relieved by antacids. In addition, the client may experience fatigue and other symptoms of anemia. If intrinsic factor is lacking, paresthesias and other neurologic manifestations of vitamin $B_{12}$ deficiency may be present. See the Manifestations box on previous page.

## COLLABORATIVE CARE

Acute gastritis is usually diagnosed by the history and clinical presentation. In contrast, the vague symptoms of chronic gastritis may require more extensive diagnostic testing.

Clients with acute and chronic gastritis are generally managed in community settings. The client requires acute care only when nausea and vomiting are severe enough to interfere with normal fluid and electrolyte balance and nutritional status. If hemorrhage results, surgical intervention may be required.

### Diagnostic Tests

Diagnostic tests that may be ordered for the client with gastritis include the following:

- *Gastric analysis* to assess hydrochloric acid secretion. A nasogastric tube is passed into the stomach, and pentagastrin is injected subcutaneously to stimulate gastric secretion of hydrochloric acid. Secretion may be decreased in clients with chronic gastritis.

- *Hemoglobin, hematocrit,* and *red blood cell indices* are evaluated for evidence of anemia. The client with gastritis may develop pernicious anemia because of parietal cell destruction, or iron-deficiency anemia because of chronic blood loss.
- *Serum vitamin $B_{12}$ levels* are measured to evaluate for possible pernicious anemia. Normal values for vitamin $B_{12}$ are 200 to 1000 pg/mL, with lower levels seen in older adults.
- *Upper endoscopy* may be done to inspect the gastric mucosa for changes, identify areas of bleeding, and obtain tissue for biopsy. Bleeding sites may be treated with electro- or laser coagulation or injected with a sclerosing agent during the procedure. See the Nursing Implications box on page 548 for client preparation and teaching related to an upper endoscopy.

### Medications

Drugs such as a proton-pump inhibitor (PPI), histamine$_2$ (H$_2$)-receptor blocker, or sucralfate may be ordered to prevent or treat acute stress gastritis. PPIs and H$_2$-receptor blockers reduce the amount or effects of hydrochloric acid on the gastric mucosa. Lansoprazole (Prevacid) and omeprazole (Prilosec) are examples of PPIs. H$_2$-receptor blockers include cimetidine (Tagamet), ranitidine (Zantac), famotidine (Pepcid), and nizatidine (Axid). These drugs also are available in nonprescription strength. Sucralfate (Carafate) works locally to prevent the damaging effects of acid and pepsin on gastric tissue. It does not neutralize or reduce acid secretion. Nursing implications for drugs commonly used in managing gastritis are included in the Medication Administration box on pages 549–550.

The client with type B chronic gastritis may be treated to eradicate the *H. pylori* infection. This generally involves combination therapy consisting of two antibiotics (such as metronidazole and clarithromycin or tetracycline) and a PPI. In some cases, eradication of the infection is not warranted, and the client is treated symptomatically.

### Treatments

In acute gastritis, gastrointestinal tract rest is provided by 6 to 12 hours of NPO status, then slow reintroduction of clear liquids (broth, tea, gelatin, carbonated beverages), followed by ingestion of heavier liquids (cream soups, puddings, milk) and finally a gradual reintroduction of solid food.

If nausea and vomiting threaten fluid and electrolyte balance, intravenous fluids and electrolytes are ordered.

#### Gastric Lavage

Acute gastritis resulting from ingestion of a poisonous or corrosive substance (acid or strong alkali), is treated with immediate dilution and removal of the substance. Vomiting is not induced because it might further damage the esophagus and possibly the trachea; instead, **gastric lavage,** washing out of the stomach contents, is performed. See Procedure 21–1.

## Procedure 21–1 — Gastric Lavage

When it is important to remove or dilute gastric contents rapidly, gastric lavage, irrigation or washing out of the stomach, may be indicated. In acute poisoning or ingestion of a caustic substance, a large-bore 30- to 36- French nasogastric tube is inserted, and lavage performed. When gastric hemorrhage occurs, lavage may be used to remove blood from the GI tract. Because the GI tract is not sterile, clean technique is appropriate for use, although the solution used will generally be sterile.

- Obtain baseline assessment, including vital signs, abdominal inspection, girth, and bowel sounds. *It is important to have assessment data documented prior to instituting the procedure for comparison.*
- Explain the procedure, answering questions and clarifying perceptions. Instruct to report any pain, difficulty breathing, or other problems during the procedure. *A client who is able to understand and cooperate with the procedure will tolerate lavage better. The client may be aware of symptoms of complications such as perforation or tube displacement before they are evident to the nurse.*
- Place in semi-Fowler's or Fowler's position. If unable to tolerate elevation of the head of the bed because of hypotension, place in left side-lying position. *Elevating of the head of the bed or side-lying position will minimize the risk of aspiration.*
- Insert a nasogastric tube if one is not already in place. Verify tube placement by aspirating gastric contents and test pH of aspirate. *Proper placement is vital to prevent aspiration or overdistention of the small bowel with irrigating solution.*

### CLOSED SYSTEM IRRIGATION

- Wearing clean gloves, connect bag or bottle of normal saline irrigating solution to nasogastric tube using a Y connector. Attach drainage or suction tube to other arm of connector (Figure 21–8 ■). Empty the stomach, clamp drain tube or turn off suction, and allow 50 to 200 mL of solution to run into stomach by gravity. Stop solution and allow to drain or suction out. Repeat until ordered amount has been used or desired results are obtained, for example, no further clots and solution returns clear or light pink. Measure the amount of drainage, subtracting the amount of irrigant instilled, to obtain gastric output. *The closed system minimizes the risk of contact with body fluids for the nurse. Measuring gastric output is important in monitoring fluid balance.*

### INTERMITTENT OPEN SYSTEM

- Wearing clean gloves and other personal protective equipment as necessary (gown and face protection), empty the stomach using suction or a 50-mL catheter-tip syringe. Measure and discard the aspirate. Using the syringe, draw up approximately 50 mL of irrigation solution, and instill it using gentle pressure. Aspirate the nasogastric tube, and discard the solution into a measuring container. Continue this procedure until the desired amount of irrigant or desired results have been obtained. *Manual irrigation with a catheter-tip syringe may be more effective in removing clots from the stomach and nasogastric tube.*
- Continue to monitor vital signs (including temperature), tolerance of the procedure, and other assessment data. *The client may be unstable and require continuous reevaluation Gastric lavage may cause hypothermia; therefore, monitor temperature and indications of hypothermia, such as lethargy and changes in cardiac rate and rhythm.*
- If the aspirate has not cleared to light pink or pink-tinged after 20 to 30 minutes of lavage or if the client is unable to tolerate the procedure, notify the physician. *Medical or surgical intervention may be necessary to stop hemorrhage in some instances.*
- On completion of lavage, provide mouth and nares care. Continue to monitor vital signs, abdominal status, and other assessment data.
- Document the procedure, including the amount and type of irrigant used, gastric output character and amount, and the client's condition and tolerance of the procedure.

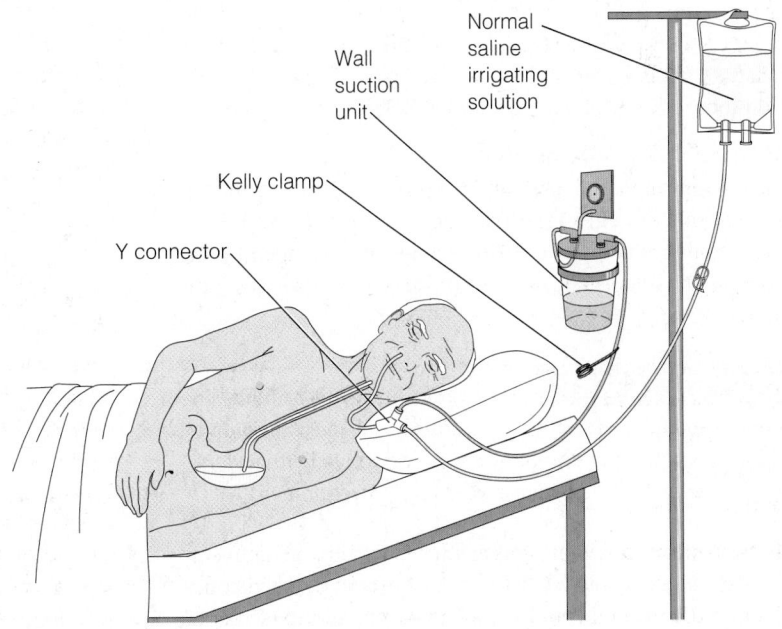

**Figure 21–8** ■ The client with a closed system gastric lavage.

## NURSING CARE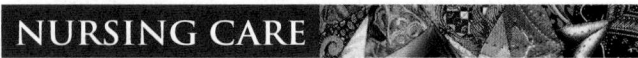

### Health Promotion

Teach all clients and community members about measures to prevent acute gastritis. Food contaminated with bacteria is a significant cause of acute gastritis. Discuss food safety measures such as fully cooking meats and egg products, and promptly refrigerating foods after cooking to avoid bacterial growth. Stress that food contaminated with potential pathogens often looks, smells, and tastes good, making it difficult to identify. Teach clients to abstain from eating or drinking anything during an acute episode of vomiting, then reintroduce clear liquids gradually once vomiting has stopped (2 to 4 hours after the last episode of vomiting). Suggest using liquids such as Pedialyte or sport drinks to replace lost electrolytes and fluid. Instruct clients to avoid milk and milk products until they easily tolerate clear liquids and solid foods such as dry toast or saltine crackers.

### Assessment

Assessment data to collect for clients with acute or chronic gastritis include the following:

- Health history: current symptoms and their duration; relieving and aggravating factors; history of ingestion of toxins, contaminated food, alcohol, aspirin, or NSAIDs; other medications
- Physical examination: vital signs including orthostatic vitals if indicated; peripheral pulses; general appearance; abdominal assessment including appearance, bowel sounds, and tenderness

### Nursing Diagnoses and Interventions

In planning and implementing nursing care for the client with acute or chronic gastritis, consider both the direct effects of the disorder on the gastrointestinal system and nutritional status as well as its effects on lifestyle and psychosocial integrity. This section focuses on problems of fluid balance and nutrition.

#### Deficient Fluid Volume

Nausea, vomiting, and abdominal distress are the primary manifestations of acute gastritis. The risk for fluid and electrolyte imbalance is high because of inadequate intake of food and fluids, and abnormal losses of fluids and electrolytes with vomiting.

**PRACTICE ALERT** *Tachycardia, tachypnea, and hypotension, especially orthostatic hypotension, may indicate fluid volume deficit. Electrolyte or acid-base imbalances resulting from vomiting may cause cardiac dysrhythmias or changes in respirations.* ■

- Monitor and record vital signs at least every 2 hours until stable, then every 4 hours. Check for orthostatic hypotension.
- Weigh daily. Monitor and record intake and output; record urine output every 1 to 4 hours as indicated. *Daily weights are an accurate indicator of fluid volume. Urine output of less than 30 mL per hour indicates decreased cardiac output and a need for prompt fluid replacement.*

- Monitor skin turgor, color, and condition and status of oral mucous membranes frequently. Provide skin and mouth care frequently. *Skin turgor and mucous membrane assessments indicate hydration status. Good skin and mouth care are necessary to maintain skin and mucous membrane integrity.*
- Monitor laboratory values for electrolytes and acid-base balance. Report significant changes or deviations from normal. *Electrolytes are lost through vomiting, increasing the risk of electrolyte and acid-base imbalances. These imbalances, in turn, affect multiple body systems.*
- Administer oral or parenteral fluids as ordered. *Oral fluids may be withheld until vomiting has ceased, then gradually reintroduced. Intravenous fluids restore or maintain hydration until adequate oral intake is resumed.*
- Administer antiemetic and other drugs as ordered to relieve vomiting and facilitate oral feeding. Encourage fluids as soon as feasible. *The oral route is preferred for fluid and nutrient intake; medications may be used to allow earlier resumption of feeding.*

**PRACTICE ALERT** *Ensure safety: Place call light within reach, put up the side rails, instruct to avoid getting up without assistance. Orthostatic hypotension may lead to syncope and to falls if the client attempts to get up without assistance.* ■

#### Imbalanced Nutrition: Less Than Body Requirements

Manifestations of chronic gastritis may lead to reduced food intake and malnutrition. The client often associates these unpleasant sensations with eating, and may gradually reduce food intake. Associated anorexia also contributes to poor food intake.

- Monitor and record food and fluid intake and any abnormal losses (such as vomiting). *Careful monitoring can help in developing a dietary plan to meet the caloric needs of the client.*
- Monitor weight and laboratory studies such as serum albumin, hemoglobin, and red blood cell indices. *Weights and laboratory values provide data regarding nutritional status and the effectiveness of interventions.*
- Arrange for dietary consultation to determine caloric and nutrient needs and develop a dietary plan. Consider food preferences and tolerances in menu planning. *A diet high in protein, vitamins, and minerals may be prescribed to meet nutritional needs of the client with chronic gastritis. In addition, specific food intolerances may need to be considered. Planning to include preferred foods in the diet helps ensure consumption of the prescribed diet.*
- Provide nutritional supplements between meals or frequent small feedings as needed. *Many clients with chronic gastritis tolerate small, frequent feedings better than three large meals per day.*
- Maintain tube feedings or parenteral nutrition as ordered. Refer to Chapter 20 for further information on enteral and parenteral feedings.

## CHART 21-4  NANDA, NIC, AND NOC LINKAGES

### The Client with Gastritis or Peptic Ulcer Disease

| NURSING DIAGNOSES | NURSING INTERVENTIONS | NURSING OUTCOMES |
|---|---|---|
| • Pain | • Medication Management | • Comfort Level |
| • Nausea | • Nausea Management | • Nutritional Status: Food and Fluid Intake |
| • Risk for Deficient Fluid Volume | • Fluid/Electrolyte Management | • Hydration |
| • Ineffective Health Maintenance | • Teaching: Disease Process | • Knowledge: Treatment Regimen |
| • Fatigue | • Energy Management | • Nutritional Status: Energy |

*Note. Data from Nursing Outcomes Classification (NOC) by M. Johnson & M. Maas (Eds.), 1997, St. Louis: Mosby; Nursing Diagnoses: Definitions & Classification 2001–2002 by North American Nursing Diagnosis Association, 2001, Philadelphia: NANDA; Nursing Interventions Classification (NIC) by J.C. McCloskey & G. M. Bulechek (Eds.), 2000, St. Louis: Mosby. Reprinted by permission.*

## Using NANDA, NIC, and NOC

Chart 21–4 shows links between NANDA nursing diagnoses, NIC, and NOC when caring for a client with gastritis.

## Home Care

Because acute or chronic gastritis is usually managed in community-based settings, teaching is vital. For the client with acute gastritis, teaching focuses on managing acute symptoms, reintroducing fluids and solid foods, indicators of possible complications (e.g., continued vomiting, signs of fluid and electrolyte imbalance), and preventing future episodes.

Provide the following information for clients with chronic gastritis.

- Maintaining optimal nutrition
- Helpful dietary modifications
- Using prescribed medications
- Avoiding known gastric irritants, such as aspirin, alcohol, and cigarette smoking

Referral to smoking-cessation classes or programs to treat alcohol abuse may be necessary.

## THE CLIENT WITH PEPTIC ULCER DISEASE

**Peptic ulcer disease (PUD),** a break in the mucous lining of the gastrointestinal tract where it comes in contact with gastric juice, is a chronic health problem. PUD affects approximately 10% of the population or 4 million people in the United States every year (Braunwald et al., 2001; Tierney et al., 2001).

Peptic ulcers occur in any area of the gastrointestinal tract exposed to acid-pepsin secretions, including the esophagus, stomach, or duodenum. **Duodenal ulcers** are the most common. They usually develop between the ages of 30 and 55, and are more common in men than women. **Gastric ulcers** more often affect older clients, between the ages of 55 and 70. Ulcers are more common in people who smoke and who are chronic users of NSAIDs. Alcohol and dietary intake do not seem to cause PUD, and the role of stress is uncertain. Although the incidence of PUD has dramatically decreased, the incidence of

### BOX 21-1  ■ Risk Factors for Peptic Ulcer Disease

- ■ *H. pylori* infection
  - ■ Low socioeconomic status
  - ■ Crowded, unsanitary living conditions
  - ■ Unclean food or water
- ■ Use of NSAIDs
  - ■ Advanced age
  - ■ History of ulcer
  - ■ Concurrent use of other drugs such as glucocorticoids or other NSAIDs
- ■ Cigarette smoking
- ■ Family history of PUD
- ■ Possible risk factors: psychological stress; alcohol and/or caffeine consumption

gastric ulcers is increasing, believed due to the widespread use of NSAIDs (Tierney et al., 2001).

## Risk Factors

Chronic *H. pylori* infection and use of aspirin and NSAIDs are the major risk factors for PUD. Contributing risk factors are listed in Box 21–1. Overall, an estimated one in six clients infected with *H. pylori* develop PUD. Of the NSAIDs, aspirin is the most ulcerogenic. A strong familial pattern suggests a genetic factor in the development of PUD. Cigarette smoking is a significant risk factor, doubling the risk of PUD. Cigarette smoking inhibits the secretion of bicarbonate by the pancreas and possibly causes more rapid transit of gastric acid into the duodenum.

## PATHOPHYSIOLOGY

The innermost layer of the stomach wall, the gastric mucosa, consists of columnar epithelial cells, supported by a middle layer of blood vessels and glands, and a thin outer layer of smooth muscle. The mucosal barrier of the stomach, a thin coating of mucous gel and bicarbonate, protects the gastric mucosa. The mucosal barrier is maintained by bicarbonate secreted by the epithelial cells, by mucus gel production stimulated by prostaglandins, and by an adequate blood supply to the mucosa (see the overview of normal physiology on page 554).

An **ulcer,** or break in the gastrointestinal mucosa, develops when the mucosal barrier is unable to protect the mucosa from damage by hydrochloric acid and pepsin, the gastric digestive juices.

*H. pylori* infection, found in about 70% of people who have PUD, is unique in colonizing the stomach. It is spread person to person (oral–oral or fecal–oral), and contributes to ulcer formation in several ways. The bacteria produce enzymes that reduce the efficacy of mucus gel in protecting the gastric mucosa. In addition, the host's inflammatory response to *H. pylori* contributes to gastric epithelial cell damage without producing immunity to the infection. Although the gastric mucosa is the usual site for *H. pylori* infection, this infection also contributes to duodenal ulcers. This is possibly related to increased gastric acid production associated with *H. pylori* infection.

NSAIDs contribute to PUD through both systemic and topical mechanisms. Prostaglandins are necessary for maintaining the gastric mucosal barrier. NSAIDs interrupt prostaglandin synthesis by disrupting the action of the enzyme cyclooxygenase (COX). The two forms of this enzyme are COX-1 and COX-2. The COX-1 enzyme is necessary to maintain the integrity of the gastric mucosa, but the anti-inflammatory effects of NSAIDs are due to their ability to inhibit the COX-2 enzyme. The COX-2 selective NSAIDs are less damaging to the gastric mucosa because they have less effect on the COX-1 enzyme. In addition to their systemic effect, aspirin and many NSAIDs cross the lipid membranes of gastric epithelial cells, damaging the cells themselves.

The ulcers of PUD may affect the esophagus, stomach, or duodenum. They may be superficial or deep, affecting all layers of the mucosa (Figure 21–9 ■). Duodenal ulcers, the most common, usually develop in the proximal portion of the duodenum,

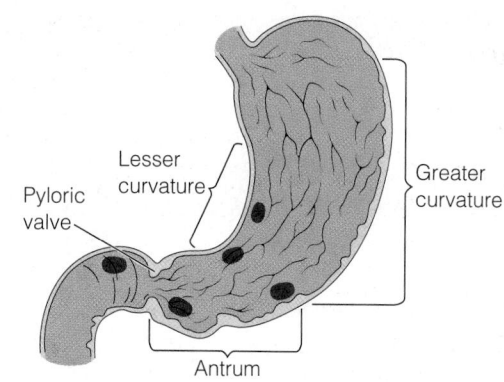

**Figure 21–10** ■ Common sites affected by peptic ulcer disease.

close to the pyloris (Figure 21–10 ■). They are sharply demarcated and usually less than 1 cm in diameter (Figure 21–11 ■). Gastric ulcers often are found on the lesser curvature and the area immediately proximal to the pylorus. Gastric ulcers are associated with an increased incidence of gastric cancer.

Peptic ulcer disease may be chronic, with spontaneous remissions and exacerbations. Exacerbations of the disease may be associated with trauma, infection, or other physical or psychologic stressors.

## MANIFESTATIONS

Pain is the classic symptom of peptic ulcer disease. The pain is typically described as gnawing, burning, aching, or hungerlike and is experienced in the epigastric region, sometimes radiating to the back. The pain occurs when the stomach is empty (2 to 3 hours after meals and in the middle of the night) and is relieved by eating with a classic "pain-food-relief" pattern. The client may complain of heartburn or regurgitation and may vomit.

The presentation of peptic ulcer disease in the older adult is often less clear, with vague and poorly localized discomfort, perhaps chest pain or dysphagia, weight loss, or anemia. In the older adult, a complication of PUD such as upper GI hemorrhage or perforation of the stomach or duodenum may be the presenting symptom.

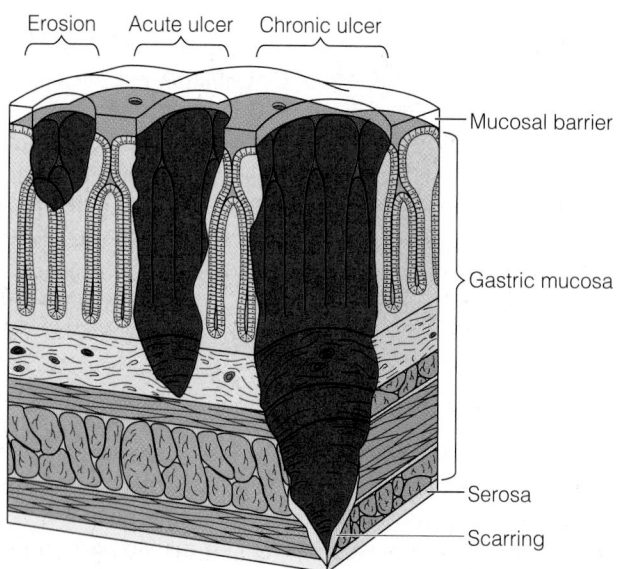

**Figure 21–9** ■ Erosion and ulcerations of the upper gastrointestinal tract.

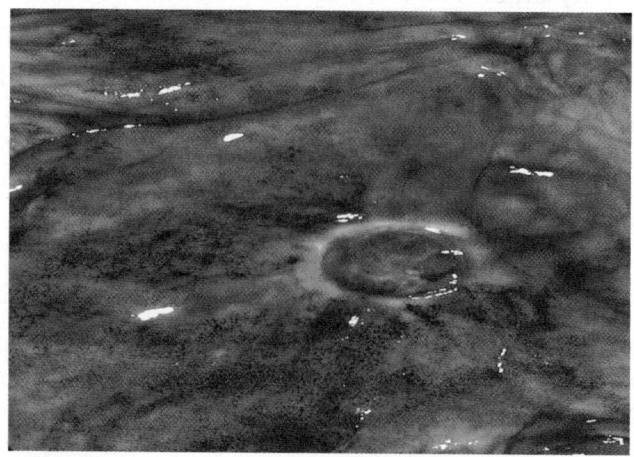

**Figure 21–11** ■ A superficial peptic ulcer.

*Source: SPL/Photo Researchers, Inc.*

## Manifestations of PUD Complications

### HEMORRHAGE
- Occult or obvious blood in the stool
- Hematemesis
- Fatigue
- Weakness, dizziness
- Orthostatic hypotension
- Hypovolemic shock

### OBSTRUCTION
- Sensations of epigastric fullness
- Nausea and vomiting
- Electrolyte imbalances
- Metabolic alkalosis

### PERFORATION
- Severe upper abdominal pain, radiating to the shoulder
- Rigid, boardlike abdomen
- Absence of bowel sounds
- Diaphoresis
- Tachycardia
- Rapid, shallow respirations
- Fever

## Complications

The complications associated with peptic ulcers include hemorrhage, obstruction, and perforation. See the box above for the manifestations of these complications.

Among people with PUD, 10% to 20% experience **hemorrhage** as a result of ulceration and erosion into the blood vessels of the gastric mucosa. In the older adult, bleeding is the most frequent complication. When small blood vessels erode, blood loss may be slow and insidious, with occult blood in the stool the only initial sign. If bleeding continues, the client becomes anemic and experiences symptoms of weakness, fatigue, dizziness, and orthostatic hypotension. Erosion into a larger vessel can lead to sudden and severe bleeding with hematemesis, melena, or **hematochezia** (blood in the stool), and signs of hypovolemic shock.

**Gastric outlet obstruction** may result from edema surrounding the ulcer, smooth muscle spasm, or scar tissue. Generally, obstruction is a gradual rather than an acute process. Symptoms include a feeling of epigastric fullness, accentuated ulcer symptoms, and nausea. If the obstruction becomes complete, vomiting occurs. Hydrochloric acid, sodium, and potassium are lost in vomitus, potentially leading to fluid and electrolyte imbalance and metabolic alkalosis.

The most lethal complication of PUD is **perforation** of the ulcer through the mucosal wall. When perforation occurs, gastric or duodenal contents enter the peritoneum, causing an inflammatory process and peritonitis. Chemical peritonitis from the hydrochloric acid, pepsin, bile, and pancreatic fluid is immediate; bacterial peritonitis follows within 6 to 12 hours from gastric contaminants entering the normally sterile peritoneal cavity. When an ulcer perforates, the client has immediate, severe upper abdominal pain, radiating throughout the abdomen and possibly to the shoulder. The abdomen becomes rigid and boardlike, with absent bowel sounds. Signs of shock may be present, including diaphoresis, tachycardia, and rapid, shallow respirations. Classic symptoms of perforation may not be present in an older adult. The older adult may instead present with mental confusion and other nonspecific symptoms. This atypical presentation can lead to delays in diagnosis and treatment, increasing the associated mortality rate.

## Zollinger-Ellison Syndrome

**Zollinger-Ellison syndrome** is peptic ulcer disease caused by a gastrinoma, or gastrin-secreting tumor of the pancreas, stomach, or intestines. Gastrinomas may be benign, although 50% to 70% are malignant tumors. Gastrin is a hormone that stimulates the secretion of pepsin and hydrochloric acid. The increased gastrin levels associated with these tumors result in hypersecretion of gastric acid, which in turn causes mucosal ulceration.

The peptic ulcers of Zollinger-Ellison syndrome may affect any portion of the stomach or duodenum, as well as the esophagus or jejunum. Characteristic ulcerlike pain is common. The high levels of hydrochloric acid entering the duodenum may also cause diarrhea and **steatorrhea** (excess fat in the feces), from impaired fat digestion and absorption. Complications of bleeding and perforation are often seen with Zollinger-Ellison syndrome. Fluid and electrolyte imbalances may also result from persistent diarrhea with resultant losses of potassium and sodium in particular.

## COLLABORATIVE CARE

Treatment for PUD focuses on eradicating *H. pylori* infection and treating or preventing ulcers related to use of NSAIDs.

## Diagnostic Tests

- *Upper GI series* using barium as a contrast medium can detect 80% to 90% of peptic ulcers. It commonly is the diagnostic procedure chosen first; it is less costly and less invasive than gastroscopy. Small or very superficial ulcers may be missed, however.
- *Gastroscopy* allows visualization of the esophageal, gastric, and duodenal mucosa and direct inspection of ulcers. Tissue also can be obtained for biopsy. Nursing care of the client undergoing a gastroscopy is outlined in the box on page 548.
- Biopsy specimens obtained during a gastroscopy can be tested for the presence of *H. pylori* using several different methods. In the *biopsy urease test,* the specimen is put into a gel containing urea. If *H. pylori* is present, the urease that it produces changes the color of the gel, often within minutes. Biopsy specimen cells also can be microscopically examined or cultured for evidence of *H. pylori*.
- Noninvasive methods of detecting *H. pylori* infection include *serologic testing* (to detect IgG antibodies through ELISA) and the *urea breath test.* In this test, radiolabeled urea is given orally. The urease produced by *H. pylori* bacteria converts the urea to ammonia and radiolabeled carbon dioxide, which can then be measured as the client exhales. This test also can be used to evaluate the effectiveness of treatment to eradicate *H. pylori*.

- If Zollinger-Ellison syndrome is suspected, *gastric analysis* may be performed to evaluate gastric acid secretion. Stomach contents are aspirated through a nasogastric tube and analyzed. In Zollinger-Ellison syndrome, gastric acid levels are very high.

## Medications

The medications used to treat PUD include agents to eradicate *H. pylori,* drugs to decrease gastric acid content, and agents that protect the mucosa. Nursing responsibilities related to selected drugs to treat GERD, gastritis, and PUD are found in the Medication Administration box on pages 549–550.

Eradication of *H. pylori* is often difficult. Combination therapies that use two antibiotics with either bismuth or proton-pump inhibitors (e.g., a combination of omeprazole, metronidazole, and clarithromycin or bismuth subsalicylate, tetracycline, and metronidazole) are necessary. With complete eradication of *H. pylori,* reinfection rates are less than 0.5% per year.

In clients who have NSAID-induced ulcers, the NSAID in use should be discontinued if at all possible. If this is not possible, twice-daily PPIs enable ulcer healing.

Medications that decrease gastric acid content include proton-pump inhibitors and the $H_2$-receptor antagonists.

- Proton pump inhibitors bind the acid-secreting enzyme ($H^+$, $K^+$ ATPase) that functions as the proton pump, disabling it for up to 24 hours. These drugs are very effective, resulting in over 90% ulcer healing after 4 weeks. Compared to the $H_2$-receptor blockers, the proton-pump inhibitors provide faster pain relief and more rapid ulcer healing.
- Histamine$_2$-receptor blockers inhibit histamine binding to the receptors on the gastric parietal cells to reduce acid secretion. These drugs are very well tolerated and have few serious side effects; however, drug interactions can occur. These drugs must be continued for 8 weeks or longer for ulcer healing.

Agents that protect the mucosa include sucralfate, bismuth, antacids, and prostaglandin analogs.

- Sucralfate binds to proteins in the ulcer base, forming a protective barrier against acid, bile, and pepsin. Sucralfate also stimulates the secretion of mucus, bicarbonate, and prostaglandin.
- Bismuth compounds (Pepto-Bismol) stimulate mucosal bicarbonate and prostaglandin production to promote ulcer healing. In addition, bismuth has an antibacterial action against *H. pylori.* There are very few side effects, other than a harmless darkening of stools.
- Prostaglandin analogs (misoprostol) promote ulcer healing by stimulating mucus and bicarbonate secretions and by inhibiting acid secretion. Although not as effective as the other drugs discussed, misoprostol is used to prevent NSAID-induced ulcers.
- Antacids stimulate gastric mucosal defenses, thereby aiding in ulcer healing. They provide rapid relief of ulcer symptoms, and are often used as needed to supplement other antiulcer medications. Antacids are inexpensive, but clients often have difficulty with a regular regimen because the drugs must be taken frequently and may cause either constipation (from the aluminum-type antacids) or diarrhea (from the magnesium-based antacids). Antacids also interfere with the absorption of iron, digoxin, some antibiotics, and other drugs.

## Treatments

### Dietary Management

In addition to pharmacologic treatment, clients are encouraged to maintain good nutrition, consuming balanced meals at regular intervals. It is important to teach clients that bland or restrictive diets are no longer necessary. Mild alcohol intake is not harmful. Smoking should be discouraged, as it slows the rate of healing and increases the frequency of relapses.

### Surgery

The identification of *H. pylori* as a cause of PUD and the availability of drugs to treat the infection and heal peptic ulcers has all but eliminated surgery as a treatment option for peptic ulcer disease. Older clients, however, may have undergone gastric resection surgery for PUD, and may have long-term complications related to the surgery. See the section on gastric cancer for more information about gastric surgery and its potential complications.

### Treatment of Complications

The client hospitalized with a complication of PUD such as bleeding, gastrointestinal obstruction, or perforation and peritonitis requires additional interventions to restore homeostasis.

In hemorrhage associated with PUD, initial interventions focus on restoring and maintaining circulation. Normal saline, lactated Ringer's, or other balanced electrolyte solutions are administered intravenously to restore intravascular volume if signs of shock (tachycardia, hypotension, pallor, low urine output, and anxiety) are present. Whole blood or packed red blood cells may be administered to restore hemoglobin and hematocrit levels.

Gastroscopy with direct injection of a clotting or sclerosing agent into the bleeding vessel may be performed. Laser photocoagulation, using light energy, or electrocoagulation, which uses electric current to generate heat, can also be done via gastroscopy to seal bleeding vessels.

The client is kept NPO until bleeding is controlled. Antacids are administered hourly via the nasogastric tube to protect the bleeding ulcer from gastric acid and to prevent acid reflux. $H_2$-receptor blockers such as cimetidine, ranitidine, and famotidine are administered intravenously until the client can resume oral intake. Surgery may be necessary if medical measures are ineffective in controlling bleeding. Older adults who experience bleeding as a complication of PUD are more likely to rebleed or require surgery to control the hemorrhage. See page 568 for nursing care of the client having gastric surgery.

Repeated inflammation, healing, scarring, edema, and muscle spasm can lead to gastric outlet (pyloric) obstruction. Initial treatment includes gastric decompression with nasogastric suction and administration of intravenous normal saline and potassium chloride to correct fluid and electrolyte imbalance. $H_2$-receptor blockers are given intravenously as well. Balloon dilation of the gastric outlet may be done via upper endoscopy. If these measures are unsuccessful in relieving obstruction, surgery may be required.

Gastric or duodenal perforation resulting in contamination of the peritoneum with gastrointestinal contents often requires immediate intervention to restore homeostasis and minimize peritonitis. Intravenous fluids maintain fluid and electrolyte balance. Nasogastric suction removes gastric contents and minimizes peritoneal contamination. Placing the client in Fowler's or semi-Fowler's position allows peritoneal contaminants to pool in the pelvis. Intravenous antibiotics aggressively treat bacterial infection from intestinal flora. Laparoscopic surgery or an open laparotomy may close the perforation.

## NURSING CARE

### Health Promotion

Although it is difficult to predict which clients will develop peptic ulcer disease, promote health by advising clients to avoid risk factors such as excessive aspirin or NSAID use and cigarette smoking. In addition, encourage clients to seek treatment for manifestations of gastroesophageal reflux disease (GERD) or chronic gastritis, both of which also are associated with *H. pylori* infection.

### Assessment

Collect the following subjective and objective data when assessing the client with peptic ulcer disease.

- Health history: complaints of epigastric or left upper quadrant pain, heartburn, or discomfort; its character, severity, timing and relationship to eating, measures used for relief; nausea or vomiting, presence of bright blood or "coffee-ground" appearing material in vomitus; current medications including use of aspirin or other NSAIDs; cigarette smoking and use of alcohol or other drugs
- Physical examination: general appearance including height and weight relationship; vital signs including orthostatic measurements; abdominal examination including shape and contour, bowel sounds, and tenderness to palpation; presence of obvious or occult blood in vomitus and stool

### Nursing Diagnoses and Interventions

#### Pain

The pain of peptic ulcer disease is often predictable and preventable. Pain is typically experienced 2 to 4 hours after eating, as high levels of gastric acid and pepsin irritate the exposed mucosa. Measures to neutralize the acid, minimize its production, or protect the mucosa often relieve this pain, minimizing the need for analgesics.

- Assess pain, including location, type, severity, frequency, and duration, and its relationship to food intake or other contributing factors.

**PRACTICE ALERT** *Avoid making assumptions about pain. Acute pain may indicate a complication, such as perforation (often heralded by sudden, severe epigastric pain and a rigid, boardlike abdomen) or it may be totally unrelated to PUD (e.g., angina, gallbladder disease, or pancreatitis).* ■

- Administer proton-pump inhibitors, H₂-receptor antagonists, antacids, or mucosal protective agents as ordered. Monitor for effectiveness and side effects or adverse reactions. *The pain associated with PUD is generally caused by the effect of gastric juices on exposed mucosal tissue. These medications reduce pain and promote healing by reducing acid production, neutralizing acid, or providing a barrier for the damaged mucosa.*
- Teach relaxation, stress-reduction, and lifestyle management techniques. Refer for stress management counseling or classes as indicated. *Although there is no clear relationship between stress and PUD, measures to relieve stress and promote physical and emotional rest help reduce the perception of pain and may reduce ulcer genesis.*

#### Sleep Pattern Disturbance

Nighttime ulcer pain, which typically occurs between 1:00 and 3:00 A.M., may disrupt the sleep cycle and result in inadequate rest. Anticipation of pain may lead to insomnia or other sleep disruptions.

- Stress the importance of taking medications as prescribed. *The bedtime dose of proton-pump inhibitor or H₂-receptor blocker minimizes hydrochloric acid production during the night, reducing nighttime pain.*
- Instruct to limit food intake after the evening meal, eliminating any bedtime snack. *Eating before bed can stimulate the production of gastric acid and pepsin, increasing the likelihood of nighttime pain.*
- Encourage use of relaxation techniques and comfort measures such as soft music as needed to promote sleep. *Once the pain associated with PUD has been controlled, these measures help reduce anxiety and reestablish a normal sleep pattern.*

#### Imbalanced Nutrition: Less Than Body Requirements

In an attempt to avoid discomfort, the client with peptic ulcer disease may gradually reduce food intake, sometimes jeopardizing nutritional status. Anorexia and early satiety are additional problems associated with PUD.

- Assess current diet, including pattern of food intake, eating schedule, and foods that precipitate pain or are being avoided in anticipation of pain. *The client may not realize the extent of self-imposed dietary limitations, especially if symptoms have persisted for an extended time. Assessment increases awareness and also helps identify the adequacy of nutrient intake.*
- Refer to a dietitian for meal planning to minimize PUD symptoms and meet nutritional needs. Consider normal eating patterns and preferences in meal planning. *Although no specific diet is recommended for PUD, clients should avoid foods that increase pain. Six small meals per day often help increase food tolerance and decrease postprandial discomfort.*
- Monitor for complaints of anorexia, fullness, nausea, and vomiting. Adjust dietary intake or medication schedule as indicated. *PUD and resultant scarring can lead to impaired gastric emptying, necessitating a treatment change.*

MediaLink | PEPTIC ULCER DISEASE CARE PLAN

*Advise the client to report increasing or persistent symptoms of anorexia, nausea and vomiting, or fullness to the care provider.* ∎

- Monitor laboratory values for indications of anemia or other nutritional deficits. Monitor for therapeutic and side effects of treatment measures such as oral iron replacement. Instruct the client taking oral iron replacement to avoid using an antacid within 1 to 2 hours of taking the iron preparation. *Anemia can result from poor nutrient absorption or chronic blood loss in clients with PUD. Oral iron supplements may cause GI distress, nausea, and vomiting; if these side effects are intolerable, notify the physician for a possible change of therapy. Antacids bind with oral iron preparations, blocking absorption.*

## Deficient Fluid Volume

Erosion of a blood vessel with resultant hemorrhage is a significant risk for the client with peptic ulcer disease. Acute bleeding can lead to hypovolemia and fluid volume deficit, which can lead to a decrease in cardiac output and impaired tissue perfusion.

*Monitor and record blood pressure and apical pulse every 15 to 30 minutes until stable; monitor central venous pressure or pulmonary artery pressure as indicated. Insert a Foley catheter and monitor urinary output hourly. Weigh daily. Continuous monitoring of cardiac output parameters is essential in clients with an acute hemorrhage to identify possible shock and intervene at an early stage.* ∎

- Monitor stools and gastric drainage for overt and occult blood. Assess gastric drainage (vomitus or from a nasogastric tube) to estimate the amount and rapidity of hemorrhage. *Drainage is bright red with possible clots in acute hemorrhage; dark red or the color of coffee grounds when blood has been in the stomach for a period of time. Hematochezia (stool containing red blood and clots) is present in acute hemorrhage; melena (black, tarry stool) is an indicator of less acute bleeding. When small vessels are disrupted, bleeding may be slow and not overtly evident. With chronic or slow gastrointestinal bleeding, the risk of a fluid volume deficit is minimal; anemia and activity intolerance are more likely.*
- Maintain intravenous therapy with fluid volume and electrolyte replacement solutions; administer whole blood or packed cells as ordered. *Both fluids and electrolytes are lost through vomiting, nasogastric drainage, and diarrhea in an episode of acute bleeding. To prevent shock, it is essential to maintain a blood volume and cardiac output sufficient to perfuse body tissues. Whole blood and packed cells replace both blood volume and red blood cells, providing additional oxygen-carrying capacity to meet cell needs.*
- Insert a nasogastric tube and maintain its position and patency; if ordered, irrigate with sterile normal saline until returns are clear. Initially, measure and record gastric output every hour (be sure to subtract the volume of irrigant), then every 4 to 8 hours. *Nasogastric suction removes blood from*

*the gastrointestinal tract, preventing vomiting and possible aspiration. Irrigation with sterile saline solution at room temperature has a vasoconstrictive effect, slowing active bleeding. Water is not used as an irrigant to avoid water intoxication. Sterile solution is used because of the possibility of perforation. Gastric output is replaced milliliter for milliliter with a balanced electrolyte solution to maintain homeostasis.*

- Monitor hemoglobin and hematocrit, serum electrolytes, BUN, and creatinine values. Report abnormal findings. *Hemoglobin and hematocrit are lower than normal with acute or chronic GI bleeding. In acute hemorrhage, initial results may be within normal range because both cells and plasma are lost. Loss of fluids and electrolytes with gastric drainage and diarrhea will alter normal levels. Digestion and absorption of blood in the GI tract may result in elevated BUN and creatinine levels.*
- Assess abdomen, including bowel sounds, distention, girth, and tenderness every 4 hours and record findings. *Borborygmi or hyperactive bowel sounds with abdominal tenderness are common with acute GI bleeding. Increased distention, increasing abdominal girth, absent bowel sounds, or extreme tenderness with a rigid, boardlike abdomen may indicate perforation.*
- Maintain bed rest with the head of the bed elevated. Ensure safety. *Loss of blood volume may cause orthostatic hypotension with resultant syncope or dizziness upon standing.*

## Using NANDA, NIC, and NOC

Chart 21–4 shows links between NANDA nursing diagnoses, NIC, and NOC when caring for a client with peptic ulcer disease (see page 559).

## Home Care

Peptic ulcer disease is managed in home and community-based settings; only its complications typically require treatment in an acute care setting. Provide the following information when preparing the client for home care.

- Prescribed medication regimen, including desired and potential adverse effects
- Importance of continuing therapy even when symptoms are relieved
- Relationship between peptic ulcers and factors such as NSAID use and smoking. If indicated, refer to a smoking-cessation clinic or program.
- Importance of avoiding aspirin and other NSAIDs; stress the necessity of reading the labels of over-the-counter medications for possible aspirin content
- Manifestations of complications that should be reported to the care provider, including increased abdominal pain or distention, vomiting, black or tarry stools, lightheadedness, or fainting
- Stress and lifestyle management techniques that may help prevent exacerbation. Refer to resources for stress management, such as classes, counseling, and formal or informal groups.

## Nursing Care Plan
### A Client with Peptic Ulcer Disease

Sean O'Donnell is a 47-year-old police officer who lives and works in a metropolitan area. Mr. O'Donnell has had "heartburn" and abdominal discomfort for years, but thought it went along with his job. Last year, after becoming weak, lightheaded, and short of breath, he was found to be anemic and was diagnosed as having a duodenal ulcer. He took omeprazole (Prilosec) and ferrous sulfate for 3 months before stopping both, saying he had "never felt better in his life." Mr. O'Donnell has now been admitted to the hospital with active upper GI bleeding.

### ASSESSMENT
Rachel Clark is Mr. O'Donnell's admitting nurse and case manager. On initial assessment, Mr. O'Donnell is alert and oriented, though very apprehensive about his condition. Skin pale and cool; BP 136/78, P 98; abdomen distended and tender with hyperactive bowel sounds; 200 mL bright red blood obtained on nasogastric tube insertion. Hemoglobin 8.2 g/dL and hematocrit 23% on admission. Mr. O'Donnell is taken to the endoscopy lab where his bleeding is controlled using laser photocoagulation. On his return to the nursing unit, he receives two units of packed red blood cells and intravenous fluids to restore blood volume. A 5-day course of high-dose oral omeprazole (40 mg bid) is ordered to prevent re-bleeding, and Mr. O'Donnell is allowed to begin a clear liquid diet 24 hours after his endoscopy. Tissue biopsy obtained during endoscopy confirms the presence of H. pylori infection.

### DIAGNOSES
- *Deficient fluid volume* related to acute bleeding duodenal ulcer
- *Risk for injury* related to acute blood loss
- *Fear* related to threat to well-being
- *Ineffective therapeutic regimen management* related to lack of knowledge regarding PUD and its treatment

### EXPECTED OUTCOMES
- Maintains normal blood pressure, pulse, and urine output (>30 mL/hr).
- Remains free of injury.
- Seeks information to reduce fear.
- Identifies and uses coping strategies to manage fear.
- Describes prescribed therapeutic regimen.
- Verbalizes ability to manage prescribed regimen.

### PLANNING AND IMPLEMENTATION
- Place call light within reach and encourage to ask for help when getting up or ambulating. Remind to rise slowly from lying to sitting and sitting to standing.
- Discuss situation and provide information about all procedures and treatments.
- Reassure about the effectiveness of treatment in reducing the risk for further bleeding.
- Discuss current and planned treatment measures; stress the importance of completing the prescribed treatment to reduce the risk of further ulcer development.
- Encourage to avoid using aspirin or NSAIDs in the future; suggest alternative medications such as acetaminophen.
- Discuss stress reduction techniques and refer for stress reduction counseling or workshops as indicated.

### EVALUATION
Mr. O'Donnell is discharged 48 hours after admission. He has had no further evidence of bleeding, and has resumed a regular diet. His hemoglobin and hematocrit remain low, and he has a prescription for ferrous sulfate. He will complete the prescribed high-dose omeprazole regimen at home, then begin treatment with omeprazole, amoxicillin, and clarithromycin (Biaxin) to eradicate the H. pylori infection detected during endoscopy. After 2 weeks of this regimen, he will continue taking omeprazole at bedtime for 4 to 8 weeks. He verbalizes a good understanding of his treatment and the importance of completing the entire regimen. Mr. O'Donnell expresses concern about his ability to "keep his cool on the inside" when under stress. Ms. Clark, his case manager, gives him the names of several resources to help with stress management in case he wants help.

### Critical Thinking in the Nursing Process
1. How does *H. pylori* infection contribute to the development of peptic ulcers?
2. Describe the physiologic responses to fear and anxiety. Why is it important to alleviate fear and its physical consequences in clients with PUD?
3. What suggestions can you make to help Mr. O'Donnell manage his complex treatment regimen over the next 3 months?
4. Develop a teaching plan that includes stress reduction techniques Mr. O'Donnell can use while performing his duties as a police officer.

See Evaluating Your Response in Appendix C.

## THE CLIENT WITH CANCER OF THE STOMACH

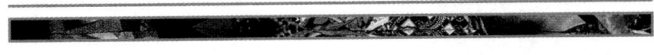

Worldwide, cancer of the stomach is the most common cancer (other than skin cancer); but it is less common in the United States, with an estimated 21,500 new cases annually. The incidence of gastric cancer is highest in Hispanics, African Americans, and Asian Americans, with men affected twice as often as women. Older adults are more likely to develop gastric cancer: The mean age at time of diagnosis is 63. People in lower socioeconomic groups are more often affected by gastric cancer.

### Risk Factors

*H. pylori* infection is a major risk factor for cancer of the distal portion of the stomach; from 35% to 89% of cases can be attributed to this infection. Other risk factors are a genetic predisposition, chronic gastritis, pernicious anemia, gastric polyps, and carcinogenic factors in the diet (such as smoked foods and nitrates). Achlorhydria, a lack of hydrochloric acid in the stomach, is a known risk factor. The risk for gastric cancer also is increased in people who have had a partial gastric resection.

## PATHOPHYSIOLOGY

Adenocarcinoma, which involves the mucus-producing cells of the stomach, is the most common form of gastric cancer. These carcinomas may arise anywhere on the mucosal surface of the stomach but are most frequently found in the distal portion. Half of all gastric cancers occur in the antrum or pyloric region (Porth, 2002). Gastric cancer begins as a localized lesion (in situ), then progresses to involve the mucosa or submucosa (early gastric carcinoma). Lesions may spread by direct extension to tissues surrounding the stomach, the liver in particular. The lesion may ulcerate or appear as a polypoid (polyplike) mass (Figure 21–12 ■). Lymph node involvement and metastasis occur early due to the rich blood and lymphatic supply to the stomach. Metastatic lesions are often found in the liver, lungs, ovaries, and peritoneum.

## MANIFESTATIONS

Few symptoms are associated with gastric cancer. Unfortunately, the disease is often quite advanced and metastases are usually present at the time of diagnosis. Early symptoms are vague, including feelings of early satiety, anorexia, indigestion, and possibly vomiting. The client may experience ulcerlike pain unrelieved by antacids, typically occurring after meals. As the disease progresses, weight loss occurs, and the client may be **cachectic** (in very poor health and malnourished) at the time of diagnosis. An abdominal mass may be palpable, and occult blood may be present in the stool, indicating gastrointestinal bleeding.

## COLLABORATIVE CARE

### Diagnostic Tests

Anemia detected by a CBC often is the first indication of gastric cancer. An upper GI X-ray with barium swallow is useful to identify lesions, and ultrasound or other radiologic techniques may identify a mass. Upper endoscopy with visualization and biopsy of the lesion provides the definitive diagnosis.

### Surgery

When gastric cancer is identified prior to the development of metastasis, surgical removal of part or all of the stomach and regional lymph nodes is the treatment of choice. **Partial gastrectomy** involves removal of a portion of the stomach, usually the distal half to two-thirds. In partial gastrectomy, the surgeon constructs an anastamosis from the remainder of the stomach directly to the duodenum or to the proximal jejunum. The **gastroduodenostomy,** or **Billroth I,** and the **gastrojejunostomy,** or **Billroth II,** are commonly used partial gastrectomy procedures (Figure 21–13 ■ A and B).

**Early Gastric Cancer**

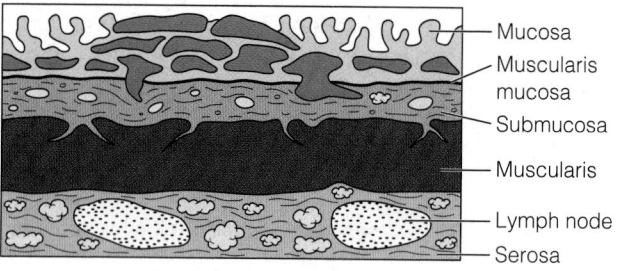

- Mucosa
- Muscularis mucosa
- Submucosa
- Muscularis
- Lymph node
- Serosa

**Polypoid Carcinoma**

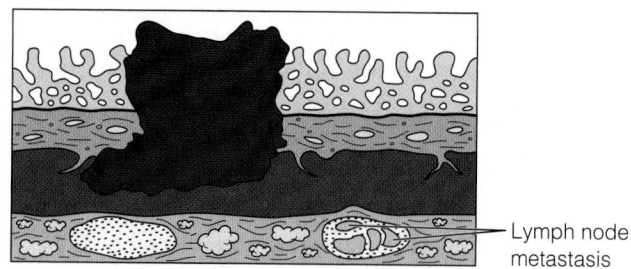

- Lymph node metastasis

**Ulcerating Carcinoma**

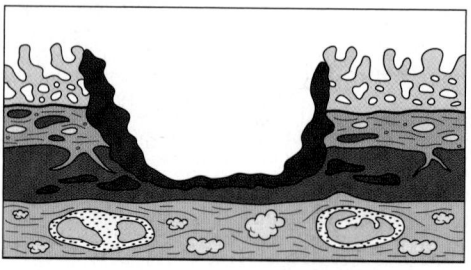

**Figure 21–12** ■ The spread and forms (polypoid and ulcerating) of gastric cancer.

A **total gastrectomy,** removal of the entire stomach, may be done for diffuse cancer that is spread throughout the gastric mucosa but limited to the stomach. In a total gastrectomy, the surgeon constructs an anastamosis from the esophagus to the duodenum or jejunum. Total gastrectomy with **esophagojejunostomy** is illustrated in Figure 21–13C.

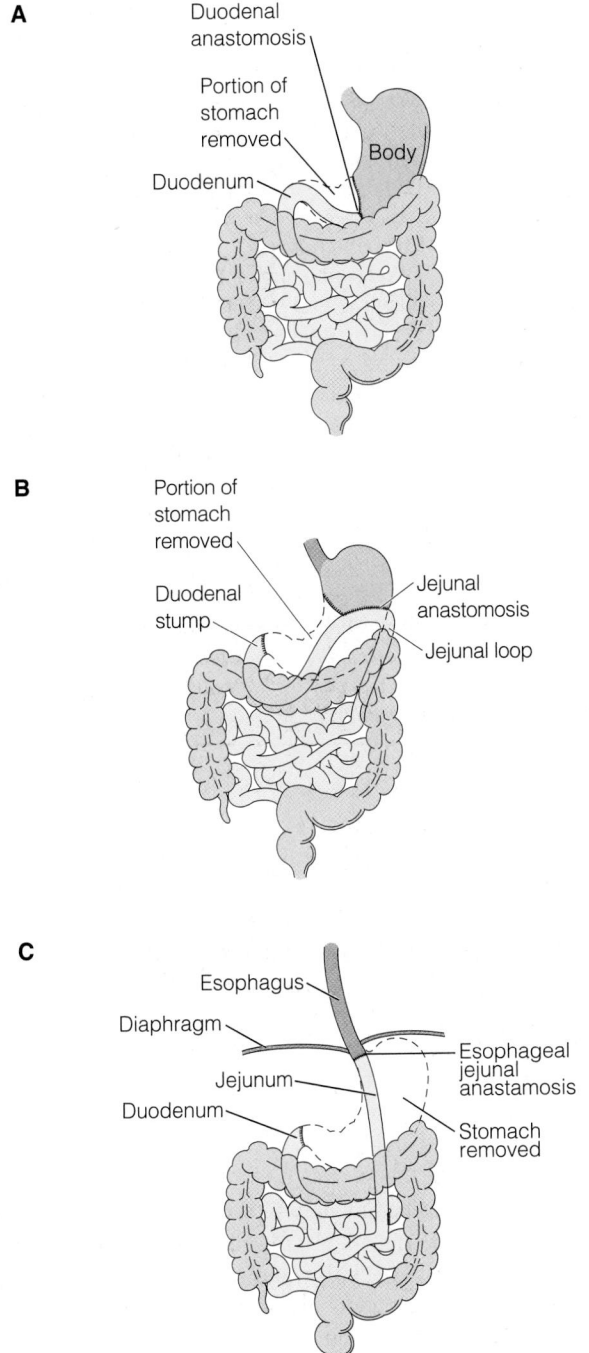

**Figure 21–13** ■ Partial and total gastrectomy procedures. *A,* Partial gastrectomy with anastomosis to the duodenum. *B,* Partial gastrectomy with anastomosis to the jejunum. *C,* Total gastrectomy with anastomosis of the esophagus to the jejunum.

Nursing care of the client who has undergone gastric surgery is outlined in the box on page 568.

## Complications

Several long-term complications may develop following gastrectomy procedures. **Dumping syndrome** is the most common problem. It may follow a partial gastrectomy with duodenal or jejunal anastamosis. When the pylorus has been resected or bypassed, a hypertonic, undigested food bolus may rapidly enter the duodenum or jejunum. Water is pulled into the lumen of the intestine by the hyperosmolar character of the chyme, resulting in decreased blood volume and intestinal dilation. Peristalsis is stimulated, and intestinal motility is increased.

Early symptoms of dumping syndrome occur within 5 to 30 minutes after eating. These symptoms result from intestinal dilation, peristaltic stimulation, and hypovolemia caused by undigested food in the proximal small intestine. Manifestations include nausea with possible vomiting, epigastric pain with cramping and borborygmi (loud, hyperactive bowel sounds), and diarrhea. Systemic symptoms from the hypovolemia and reflex sympathetic stimulation include tachycardia, orthostatic hypotension, dizziness, flushing, and diaphoresis.

The entry of hyperosmolar chyme into the jejunum also causes a rapid rise in the blood glucose. This stimulates the release of an excessive amount of insulin, leading to hypoglycemic symptoms 2 to 3 hours after the meal. The pathogenesis and clinical manifestations of dumping syndrome are represented in Figure 21–14 ■. Dumping syndrome is typically self-limiting,

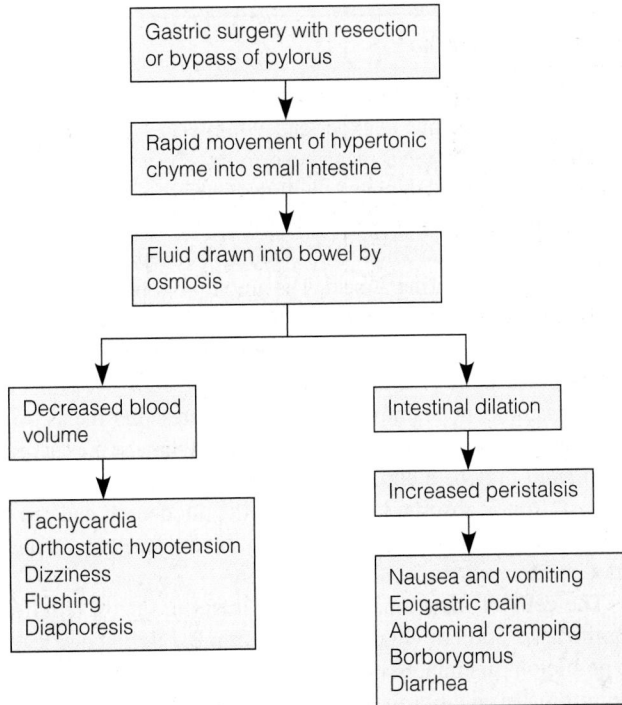

**Figure 21–14** ■ The pathogenesis and manifestations of dumping syndrome.

# NURSING CARE OF THE CLIENT HAVING GASTRIC SURGERY

## PREOPERATIVE NURSING CARE

- See Chapter 7 for routine preoperative care and teaching. ⊂⊃
- Insert a nasogastric tube if ordered preoperatively. *Although it is often inserted in the surgical suite just prior to surgery, the nasogastric tube may be placed preoperatively to remove secretions and empty stomach contents.*

## POSTOPERATIVE NURSING CARE

- Provide routine care for the surgical client as outlined in Chapter 7.
- Assess position and patency of nasogastric tube, connecting it to low suction. Gently irrigate with sterile normal saline if tube becomes clogged. *The nasogastric tube will be placed in surgery to avoid disruption of the gastric suture lines and should be well secured. If repositioning or tube replacement is needed, notify the surgeon. Patency must be maintained to keep the stomach decompressed, reducing pressure on sutures.*
- Assess color, amount, and odor of gastric drainage, noting any changes in these parameters or the presence of clots or bright bleeding. *Initial drainage is bright red. It becomes dark, then clear or greenish-yellow over the first 2 to 3 days. A change in the color, amount, or odor may indicate a complication such as hemorrhage, intestinal obstruction, or infection.*
- Maintain intravenous fluids while nasogastric suction is in place. *The client on nasogastric suction is not only unable to take oral food and fluids but also is losing electrolyte-rich fluid through the nasogastric tube. If replacement fluid and electrolytes are not maintained, the client is at risk for dehydration imbalances of sodium, potassium, and chloride; and metabolic alkalosis.*

- Provide antiulcer and antibiotic therapy as ordered. *These medications may be ordered for the postoperative client, depending on the procedure performed. Antibiotic therapy is a common preventive measure for infection that may result from contamination of the abdominal cavity with gastric contents.*
- Monitor bowel sounds and abdominal distention. *Bowel sounds indicate resumption of peristalsis. Increasing distention may indicate third-spacing, obstruction or infection.*
- Resume oral food and fluids as ordered. Initial feedings are clear liquids, progressing to full liquids and then frequent small feedings of regular foods. Monitor bowel sounds and for abdominal distention frequently during this period. *Oral feedings are reintroduced slowly to minimize trauma to the suture lines by possible gastric distension.*
- Encourage ambulation. *Ambulation stimulates peristalsis.*
- Begin discharge planning and teaching. Consult with a dietitian for diet instructions and menu planning; reinforce teaching. Teach the client about potential postoperative complications, such as abdominal abscess, dumping syndrome, postprandial hypoglycemia, or pernicious anemia. Also, teach the client to recognize signs and symptoms and preventive measures. *The client's gastric capacity is reduced after partial gastrectomy, necessitating a corresponding reduction in meal size. Changes in gastric emptying and reduction in gastric secretions may change the client's tolerance for many foods, requiring slow reintroduction of these foods. Dumping syndrome, postprandial hypoglycemia, and pernicious anemia are possible long-term complications of partial gastrectomy. For most clients, dietary modifications can control both dumping syndrome and postprandial hypoglycemia.*

---

lasting 6 to 12 months after surgery; however, a small percentage of people continue to experience long-term symptoms.

Dumping syndrome is managed primarily by a dietary pattern that delays gastric emptying and allows smaller boluses of undigested food to enter the intestine. Meals should be small and more frequent. Liquids and solids are taken at separate times instead of together during a meal. The amount of proteins and fats in the diet is increased, because they exit the stomach more slowly than carbohydrates. Carbohydrates, especially simple sugars, are reduced. The client is instructed to rest in a recumbent or semirecumbent position for 30 to 60 minutes after meals. Anticholinergics, sedatives, and antispasmodics may be prescribed.

*Anemia* may be a chronic problem after a major gastric resection. Iron is absorbed primarily in the duodenum and proximal jejunum; rapid gastric emptying or a gastrojejunostomy may interfere with adequate absorption.

The cells of the stomach produce intrinsic factor, required for the absorption of vitamin $B_{12}$. Vitamin $B_{12}$ deficiency leads to pernicious anemia. Because of hepatic stores of vitamin $B_{12}$, symptoms of anemia may not be seen for 1 to 2 years after surgery. Vitamin $B_{12}$ levels are routinely monitored following extensive gastric resections.

Other nutritional problems seen following surgery include folic acid deficiency and decreased absorption of calcium and vitamin D. Poor absorption of nutrients, combined with the inability to eat large meals, puts the client at risk for weight loss in addition to the more specific nutrient deficiencies. Nearly 50% of clients who have gastric surgery experience significant weight loss, primarily because of insufficient calorie intake. Factors contributing to insufficient intake of calories include early satiety (feeling of fullness), decreased stomach size, and altered emptying patterns.

## Other Therapies

Radiation or chemotherapy may be used to eliminate any lymphatic or metastatic spread. For the client with more advanced disease, treatment is palliative and may include surgery and chemotherapy. These clients may require a gastrostomy or jejunostomy feeding tube (Figure 21–15 ■).

See the box on page 569 for nursing care of the client with a gastrostomy or jejunostomy tube.

Because gastric cancer is generally advanced by the time of diagnosis, the prognosis is poor. The 5-year survival rate of all clients treated for gastric carcinoma is 10%.

# NURSING CARE OF THE CLIENT WITH A GASTROSTOMY OR JEJUNOSTOMY TUBE

Clients who have had extensive gastric surgery or who require long-term enteral feedings to maintain nutrition may have a gastrostomy or jejunostomy tube inserted.

## PROCEDURE

Gastrostomy tubes are surgically placed in the stomach, with the stoma in the epigastric region of the abdomen (see Figure 21–15). Jejunostomy tubes are placed in the proximal jejunum. Immediately following the procedure, the tube may be connected to low suction or plugged. If the client has been receiving tube feedings, these may be reinitiated shortly after tube placement.

## NURSING CARE

- Assess tube placement by aspirating stomach contents and checking the pH of aspirate to determine gastric or intestinal placement. A pH of 5 or less indicates gastric placement; the pH is generally 7 or higher with intestinal placement. *Recent studies show auscultation to be ineffective in determining feeding tube placement. Measuring the pH of aspirate from the tube is more reliable as a means of determining tube placement.*
- Inspect the skin surrounding the insertion site for healing, redness, swelling, and the presence of any drainage. If drainage is present, note the color, amount, consistency, and odor. *Changes in the insertion site, drainage, or lack of healing may indicate an infection.*
- Assess the abdomen for distention, bowel sounds, and tenderness *to evaluate functioning of the gastrointestinal tract.*
- Until the stoma is well healed, use sterile technique for dressing changes and site care. Clean technique is appropriate for use once healing is complete. *Sterile technique reduces the risk of wound contamination by pathogens that can lead to infec-*

*tion. Once healing has occurred, clean technique is acceptable because the gastrointestinal tract is not a sterile body cavity.*
- Wearing clean gloves, remove old dressing. Cleanse the site with saline or soap and water, and rinse as appropriate. A well-healed stoma may be cleansed in the shower with the tube clamped or plugged. Pat dry with 4X4 gauze pads, and allow to air dry. Apply Stomadhesive, karaya, or other protective agents around tube as needed to protect the skin. *Gastric acid and other wound drainage is irritating to the skin. Meticulous care is important to maintain the integrity of the skin surrounding the stoma.*
- Redress the wound using a stoma dressing or folded 4X4 gauze pads. *Do not cut gauze pads, because threads may enter the wound, causing irritation and increasing the risk of inflammation.*
- Irrigate the tube with 30 to 50 mL of water, and clean the tube inside and out as indicated or ordered. Soft gastric tubes may require cleaning of the inner lumen with a special brush to maintain patency. *Tube feeding formulas may coat the inside of the gastrostomy tube and eventually cause it to become occluded. Regular irrigation with water and brushing as indicated maintain tube patency.*
- Provide mouth care or remind the client to do so. *When feedings are not being taken orally, the usual stimulus to do mouth care is lost. In addition, salivary fluids may not be as abundant, and oral mucous membranes may become dry and cracked.*
- If indicated, teach the client and family how to care for the tube and feedings. Refer to a home health agency or visiting nurse for support and reinforcement of learning. *Gastrostomy tubes are often in place long term. When the client and family are able to assume care, independence and self-image are enhanced.*

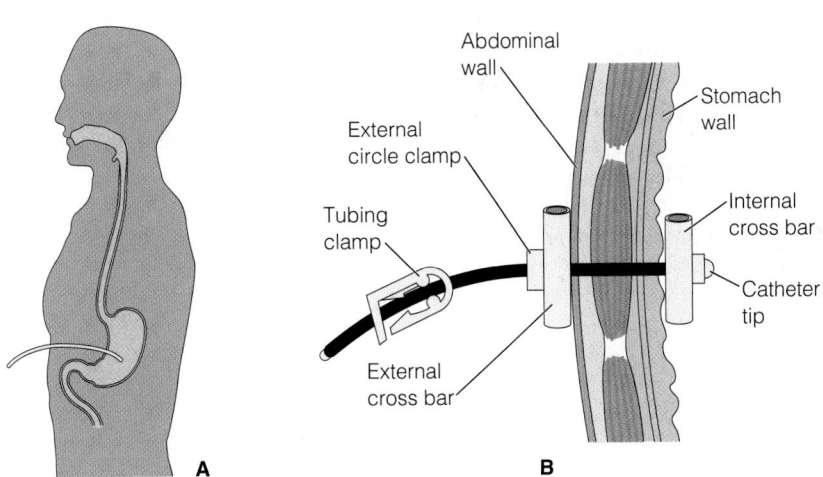

**Figure 21–15** ■ Gastrostomy. *A,* Gastrostomy tube placement. *B,* The tube is fixed against both the abdomen and stomach walls by cross bars.

## NURSING CARE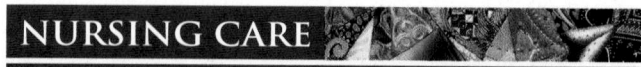

### Health Promotion

Although the exact causes of gastric cancer are unknown, contributing factors such as *H. pylori* infection and consumption of foods preserved with nitrates have been identified. To reduce their risk of developing gastric cancer, encourage clients with known *H. pylori* infection to complete the prescribed course of treatment and verify that it has eradicated the infection. With all clients, discuss the relationship between gastric cancer and consumption of foods preserved with nitrates (such as bacon and other processed meats), and encourage limited consumption of these products.

### Assessment

Assessment data related to gastric cancer include the following:

- Health history: manifestations such as anorexia, early satiety, indigestion, or vomiting; epigastric pain after meals; recent unintentional weight loss
- Physical assessment: general appearance, weight for height; abdominal distention or a palpable upper abdominal mass; occult blood in stool or vomitus

### Nursing Diagnoses and Interventions

#### Imbalanced Nutrition: Less Than Body Requirements

The client with gastric cancer may be malnourished because of anorexia, early satiety, and increased metabolic needs related to the tumor. Extensive gastric resection also makes it difficult to consume an adequate diet. Malnourishment, in turn, impairs healing and the client's ability to tolerate cancer treatment.

- Consult with dietitian for a complete nutrition assessment and diet planning. *The client is at risk for protein-calorie malnutrition, which impairs the ability to heal and recover from extensive surgery.*
- Weigh daily. Monitor laboratory values such as hemoglobin, hematocrit, and serum albumin levels. *Daily weights are a valuable measurement of both fluid and nutritional status. Laboratory values provide further evidence of nutritional status.*
- Provide preferred foods; have family prepare meals when possible. Provide supplemental feedings between meals. *Small, frequent feedings and preferred foods encourage intake of nutrients.*

**PRACTICE ALERT** *Assess ability to consume adequate nutrients. Nausea and feelings of early satiety may impair nutrient consumption, indicating a need to institute enteral or parenteral feedings.* ∎

- Arrange for visitors to be present during meals. *Eating is a social function as well as a physiologic one. Companionship often improves food intake.*
- Administer pain and antiemetic medications as needed before meals. *Pain and nausea suppress the appetite; relief promotes food intake.*

#### Anticipatory Grieving

- Encourage family members to spend as much time as possible with the client. *The family may feel helpless and ineffectual. Supporting family members' presence can encourage this vital interaction.*
- Do not negate denial if present. *Denial is a coping mechanism that protects the client from hopelessness.*
- Allow clients to talk openly if desired about their condition and the prognosis. *Acceptance of the client's fears helps reduce anxiety and promote coping behaviors.*
- Actively listen to the client's and family's expressions of grieving. Avoid interrupting or offering meaningless words of consolation. *Being present and active listening are often the most effective interventions for the grieving client.*

### Home Care

Although the client with gastric cancer may be hospitalized for surgery, most care is provided in the home and community-based settings such as hospice care. When preparing the client and family for home care, discuss the following topics.

- Care of incision and feeding tube (if present) or central venous line
- Maintaining nutrition and preventing complications of surgery such as dumping syndrome
- Pain management

Provide referrals to home care agencies, hospice, and cancer support groups as appropriate. Provide information about services available through the local chapter of the American Cancer Society.

## Nursing Care Plan
## A Client with Gastric Cancer

George Harvey is a 61-year-old estate attorney who lives with his wife, Harriet. For the last 3 months, Mr. Harvey has had increasing anorexia and difficulty eating. He has lost 10 pounds. His physician has diagnosed gastric cancer, and Mr. Harvey is admitted for a partial gastrectomy and gastrojejunostomy. The oncologist has recommended postoperative chemotherapy and radiation. Mr. Harvey reports that the doctor told him "that will give me the best chance for cure."

### ASSESSMENT

On admission before surgery, Mr. Harvey tells his nurse, Lauren Walsh, that he has eaten very little in the past few weeks. He asks, "What will happen to my wife if something happens to me? I'm afraid this cancer will get me." Mr. Harvey weighs 147 lb (67 kg) and is 72 inches (183 cm) tall. He is pale and thin; his vital signs are BP 148/86, P 92, R 18, and T 97.8° F PO. A firm mass is palpable in the left epigastric region. The rest of his physical assessment data are within normal limits. Mr. Harvey's hemoglobin is 12.8 g/dL, hematocrit is 39%, and serum albumin level is 3.2 g/dL, indicating that he is mildly malnourished. All other preoperative laboratory and diagnostic studies are within normal limits.

### DIAGNOSES

- *Imbalanced nutrition: Less than body requirements* related to anorexia and difficulty eating
- *Acute pain* related to surgical incision and manipulation of abdominal organs
- *Risk for ineffective airway clearance* related to upper abdominal surgery
- *Anticipatory grieving* related to recent diagnosis of cancer

### EXPECTED OUTCOMES

- Maintain present weight during hospitalization.
- Resume a high-calorie, high-protein diet by time of discharge.
- Verbalize effective pain management, maintaining a reported pain level of 3 or less on a scale of 1 to 10.
- Maintain a patent airway and clear breath sounds.
- Verbalize feelings regarding diagnosis and participate in decision making.

### PLANNING AND IMPLEMENTATION

- Weigh daily.
- Maintain nasogastric tube placement, patency, and suction as ordered.

- Maintain intravenous fluids and total parenteral nutrition as ordered until oral food intake is resumed.
- Arrange for diet teaching, including strategies to prevent dumping syndrome, before discharge.
- Maintain patient-controlled analgesia (PCA) until able to take oral analgesics.
- Assess respiratory status including rate, depth, and breath sounds every hour initially, then every 4 hours.
- Assist to cough, deep breathe, and use inspirometer every 2 to 4 hours and as needed. Splint abdomen during coughing.
- Encourage verbalization of feelings about diagnosis and perceived losses.
- Encourage participation in decision making.

### EVALUATION

Mr. Harvey's weight remained stable through his hospitalization. On discharge he is taking a high-protein, high-calorie diet in six small feedings per day. He and his wife have reviewed his diet with the dietitian and are planning on using some dietary supplements at home to meet protein needs. He verbalizes an understanding of measures to prevent dumping syndrome, including separating his intake of solid foods and liquids. Mr. Harvey is using oral analgesics in the morning and at bedtime to control his pain. He and his wife have begun to discuss the meaning of his diagnosis. Mrs. Harvey tells the discharge nurse, "We are going to a support group called 'Coping with Cancer' when George is stronger."

### Critical Thinking in the Nursing Process

1. What is the rationale for maintaining nasogastric suction after gastrojejunostomy?
2. Develop a preoperative teaching plan for a client undergoing an partial gastrectomy.
3. Mr. Harvey calls you just before the initial dose of chemotherapy and says, "Everyone tells me that chemotherapy will cause vomiting, and I don't think I can take being sick again." How would you respond?
4. Design interventions to ensure adequate nutrition for people with advanced gastric cancer.

See Evaluating Your Response in Appendix C.

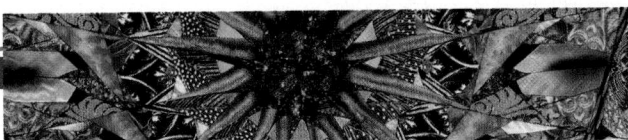

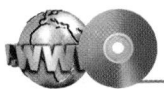

## EXPLORE MediaLink

# TEST YOURSELF

1. The nurse assessing for oral cancer risk factors in a client with a persistent sore on his tongue asks about:

    a. Consumption of highly spiced foods
    b. Thumb sucking or pacifier use as a child
    c. Regular use of dental floss
    d. Tobacco use in any form

2. The nurse teaching a client with gastroesophageal reflux disease includes which of the following instructions?

    a. This is a benign disease requiring no treatment
    b. Elevate the head of the bed on 6- to 8-inch blocks
    c. Take antacids or H$_2$-receptor blockers only when symptoms are severe
    d. Surgery frequently is required to relieve manifestations of the disease

3. The nurse evaluates his teaching of a client with acute stress gastritis as effective when the client states that she will:

    a. Avoid using aspirin or NSAIDs for routine pain relief
    b. Consume only bland foods
    c. Return for yearly upper endoscopy exams
    d. Fully cook all meats, poultry, and egg products

4. The nurse identifies which of the following nursing diagnoses as highest priority for the client admitted with peptic ulcer disease and possible perforation:

    a. *Acute pain*
    b. *Ineffective health maintenance*
    c. *Nausea*
    d. *Impaired tissue integrity: Gastrointestinal*

5. Following a partial gastrectomy for gastric cancer, a client complains of nausea, abdominal pain and cramping, and diarrhea after eating. Recognizing manifestations of dumping syndrome, the nurse recommends:

    a. Fasting for a period of 6 to 12 hours before meals
    b. Decreasing the protein content of meals
    c. Frequent small meals that contain solid foods or liquids, but not both
    d. A diet rich in carbohydrates to maintain blood glucose levels

See Test Yourself answers in Appendix C.

# BIBLIOGRAPHY

Ackley, B.J., & Ladwig, G. B. (2002). *Nursing diagnosis handbook: A guide to planning care* (5th ed.). St. Louis: Mosby.

Ahya, S. N., Flood, K., & Paranjothi, S. (Eds.). (2001). *The Washington manual of medical therapeutics* (30th ed.). Philadelphia: Lippincott Williams & Wilkins.

Braunwald, E., Fauci, A. S., Kasper, D. L., Hauser, S. L., Longo, D. L., & Jameson, J. L. (2001). *Harrison's principles of internal medicine* (15th ed.). New York: McGraw-Hill.

Brooks-Brunn, J. A. (2000). Esophageal cancer: An overview. *MEDSURG Nursing, 9*(5), 248–254.

Bullock, B. A., & Henze, R. L. (2000). *Focus on pathophysiology.* Philadelphia: Lippincott.

Chait, M. M. (2000). The many complications of gastroesophageal reflux disease. *Home Health Care Consultant, 7*(1), 25–27.

Edwards, S. J., & Metheny, N. A. (2000). Measurement of gastric residual volume: State of the science. *MEDSURG Nursing, 9*(3), 125–128.

Gallo, J. J., Busby-Whitehead, J., Rabins, P. V., Silliman, R. A., & Murphy, J. B. (Eds.). (1999). *Reichel's care of the elderly: Clinical aspects of aging* (5th ed.). Philadelphia: Lippincott Williams & Wilkins.

Galvin, T. J. (2001). Dysphagia: Going down and staying down. *American Journal of Nursing, 101*(1), 37–42.

Johnson, M., Bulechek, G., Dochterman, J. M., Maas, M., & Moorhead, S. (2001). *Nursing diagnoses, outcomes, & interventions.* St. Louis: Mosby.

Malarkey, L. M., & McMorrow, M. E. (2000). *Nurse's manual of laboratory tests and diagnostic procedures* (2nd ed.). Philadelphia: Saunders.

Mattonen, M. C. (2001). Managing heartburn in adults. *MEDSURG Nursing, 10*(5), 269–276.

McManus, T. J. (2000). *Helicobacter pylori.* An emerging infectious disease. *Nurse Practitioner, 25*(8), 40, 43–44, 47–48+

Meeker, M. H., & Rothrock, J. C. (1999). *Alexander's care of the patient in surgery* (11th ed.). St. Louis: Mosby.

Metheny, N. A., & Titler, M. G. (2001). Assessing placement of feeding tubes. *American Journal of Nursing, 101*(5), 36–45.

North American Nursing Diagnosis Association. (2001). *NANDA Nursing diagnoses: Definitions & classification 2001–2002.* Philadelphia: NANDA.

Porth, C. M. (2002). *Pathophysiology: Concepts of altered health states* (6th ed.). Philadelphia: Lippincott.

Resto, M. A. (2000). Hospital extra. Gastroesophageal reflux disease. *American Journal of Nursing, 100*(9), 24D, 24F, 24H.

Terrado, M., Russell, C., & Bowman, J. B. (2001). Dysphagia: An overview. *MEDSURG Nursing, 10*(5), 233–248.

Tierney, L. M., McPhee, S. J., & Papadakis, M. A. (2001). *Current medical diagnosis & treatment* (40th ed.). New York: Lange Medical Books/McGraw-Hill.

Walton, J. C., Miller, J., & Tordecilla, L. (2001). Elder oral assessment and care. *MEDSURG Nursing, 10*(1), 37–44.

Wilkinson, J. M. (2000). *Nursing diagnosis handbook with NIC interventions and NOC outcomes* (7th ed.). Upper Saddle River, NJ: Prentice Hall Health.

# CHAPTER 22

# Nursing Care of Clients with Gallbladder, Liver, and Pancreatic Disorders

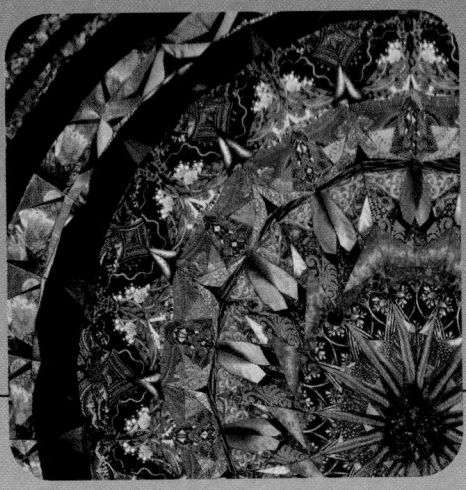

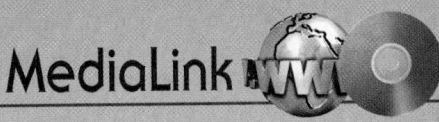

## www.prenhall.com/lemone

Additional resources for this chapter can be found on the Student CD-ROM accompanying this textbook, and on the Companion Website at www.prenhall.com/lemone. Click on Chapter 22 to select the activities for this chapter.

**CD-ROM**
- Audio Glossary
- NCLEX Review

**Animation**
- Cirrhosis

**Companion Website**
- More NCLEX Review
- Case Study
  Hepatitis B
- Care Plan Activity
  Hepatitis A
- MediaLink Application
  Treatment of Liver Cancer

## LEARNING OUTCOMES

After completing this chapter, you will be able to:

- Describe the pathophysiology of commonly occurring disorders of the gallbladder, liver, and exocrine pancreas.

- Relate knowledge of normal anatomy and physiology to the manifestations and effects of biliary, hepatic, and pancreatic disorders.

- Discuss diagnostic tests, including client preparation, used to identify biliary, hepatic, and pancreatic disorders.

- Discuss nursing implications for dietary and pharmacologic interventions used for clients with these disorders.

- Provide appropriate nursing care for the client who has surgery of the gallbladder, liver, or pancreas.

- Relate changes in normal assessment data to the pathophysiology and manifestations of gallbladder, liver, and exocrine pancreatic disorders.

- Use the nursing process to plan and provide individualized care for clients with disorders of the gallbladder, liver, or exocrine pancreas.

Gallbladder, liver, and exocrine pancreatic disorders may occur as primary disorders, or develop secondarily to other disease processes. One organ's functioning frequently affects that of another. Duct inflammation or obstruction, and changes in the multiple functions of these organs, can cause significant health effects.

Clients with a gallbladder, liver, or pancreatic disorder may experience pain, multiple metabolic and nutritional disturbances, and altered body image. Nursing care addresses physiologic and psychosocial needs of the client and family.

# GALLBLADDER DISORDERS

Altered bile flow through the hepatic, cystic, or common bile duct is a common problem. It often leads to inflammation and other complications. Gallstones are the most common cause of obstructed flow. Tumors and abscesses also can obstruct bile flow.

## THE CLIENT WITH CHOLELITHIASIS AND CHOLECYSTITIS

**Cholelithiasis** is the formation of stones (*calculi*) within the gallbladder or biliary duct system. Cholelithiasis is a common problem in the United States, affecting more than 10% of men and 20% of women by age 65 (Tierney et al., 2001).

### PHYSIOLOGY REVIEW

Normally, bile is formed by the liver and stored in the gallbladder. Bile contains bile salts, bilirubin, water, electrolytes, cholesterol, fatty acids, and lecithin. In the gallbladder, some of the water and electrolytes are absorbed, further concentrating the bile. Food entering the intestine stimulates the gallbladder to contract and release bile through the common bile duct and sphincter of Oddi into the intestine. The bile salts in bile increase the solubility and absorption of dietary fats.

### PATHOPHYSIOLOGY AND MANIFESTATIONS

#### Cholelithiasis

Gallstones form when several factors interact: abnormal bile composition, biliary stasis, and inflammation of the gallbladder. Most gallstones (80%) consist primarily of cholesterol; the rest contain a mixture of bile components. Excess cholesterol in bile is associated with obesity, a high-calorie, high-cholesterol diet, and drugs that lower serum cholesterol levels. When bile is supersaturated with cholesterol, it can precipitate out to form stones. Biliary stasis, or slowed emptying of the gallbladder, contributes to cholelithiasis. Stones do not form when the gallbladder empties completely in response to hormonal stimulation. Slowed or incomplete emptying allows cholesterol to concentrate and increases the risk of stone formation. Finally, inflammation of the gallbladder allows excess water and bile salt reabsoprtion, increasing the risk for lithiasis. Box 22–1 lists the risk factors for cholelithiasis.

**PRACTICE ALERT** *Certain very low-calorie diets are associated with a high risk of cholelithiasis. Increased cholesterol concentration in the bile and decreased gallbladder contractions associated with fasting increase the risk of gallstone formation.* ■

**BOX 22–1** ■ **Risk Factors for Cholelithiasis**

- Age
- Family history of gallstones
- Race or ethnicity: Native American (either Northern or Southern hemisphere); Northern European heritage
- Obesity, hyperlipidemia
- Rapid weight loss
- Female gender; use of oral contraceptives
- Biliary stasis: pregnancy, fasting, prolonged parenteral nutrition
- Diseases or conditions: cirrhosis; ileal disease or resection; sickle cell anemia; glucose intolerance

Most gallstones are formed in the gallbladder. They then may migrate into the ducts (Figure 22–1 ■), leading to *cholangitis* (duct inflammation). Although some people with cholelithiasis are asymptomatic, many develop manifestations. Early manifestations of gallstones may be vague: epigastric fullness or mild gastric distress after eating a large or fatty meal. Stones that obstruct the cystic duct or common bile duct lead to distention and increased pressure behind the stone. This causes **biliary colic,** a severe, steady pain in the epigastric region or right upper quadrant of the abdomen.

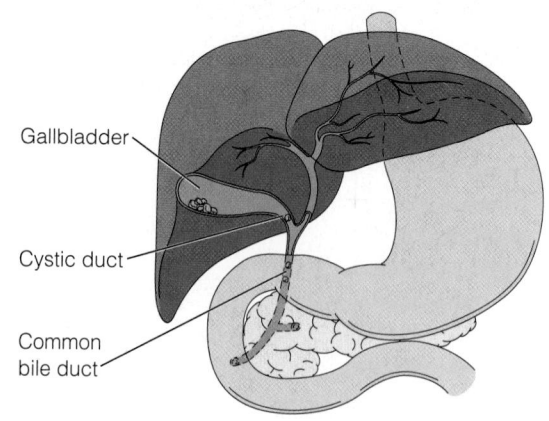

Gallbladder

Cystic duct

Common bile duct

**Figure 22–1** ■ Common locations of gallstones.

The pain may radiate to the back, right scapula, or shoulder. The pain often begins suddenly following a meal, and may last as long as 5 hours. It often is accompanied by nausea and vomiting.

Obstruction of the common bile duct may cause bile reflux into the liver, leading to jaundice, pain, and possible liver damage. If the common duct is obstructed, pancreatitis (discussed later in this chapter) is a potential complication.

## Cholecystitis

**Cholecystitis** is inflammation of the gallbladder. *Acute cholecystitis* usually follows obstruction of the cystic duct by a stone. The obstruction increases pressure within the gallbladder, leading to ischemia of the gallbladder wall and mucosa. Chemical and bacterial inflammation often follow. The ischemia can lead to necrosis and perforation of the gallbladder wall.

Acute cholecystitis usually begins with an attack of biliary colic. The pain involves the entire right upper quadrant (RUQ), and may radiate to the back, right scapula, or shoulder. Movement or deep breathing may aggravate the pain. The pain usually lasts longer than biliary colic, continuing for 12 to 18 hours. Anorexia, nausea, and vomiting are common. Fever often is present, and may be accompanied by chills. The RUQ is tender to palpation.

*Chronic cholecystitis* may result from repeated bouts of acute cholecystitis or from persistent irritation of the gallbladder wall by stones. Bacteria may be present in the bile as well. Chronic cholecystitis often is asymptomatic.

Complications of cholecystitis include *empyema*, a collection of infected fluid within the gallbladder; gangrene and perforation with resulting peritonitis or abscess formation; formation of a fistula into an adjacent organ (such as the duodenum, colon, or stomach); or obstruction of the small intestine by a large gallstone (*gallstone ilius*). Table 22–1 compares the manifestations and complications of acute cholelithiasis with those of cholecystitis.

## COLLABORATIVE CARE

Treatment of the client with cholelithiasis or cholecystitis depends of the acuity of the condition and the client's overall health status. When gallstones are present but asymptomatic and the client has a low risk for complications, conservative treatment is indicated. However, when the client experiences frequent symptoms, has acute cholecystitis, or has very large stones, the gallbladder and stones are usually surgically removed.

### Diagnostic Tests

Diagnostic tests are ordered to identify the presence and location of stones, identify possible complications, and help differentiate gallbladder disease from other disorders.

- *Serum bilirubin* is measured. Elevated direct (conjugated) bilirubin may indicate obstructed bile flow in the biliary duct system (see Box 22–2).
- *Complete blood count (CBC)* may indicate infection and inflammation if the WBC is elevated.
- *Serum amylase* and *lipase* are measured to identify possible pancreatitis related to common duct obstruction.
- *Abdominal X-ray* (flat plate of the abdomen) may show gallstones with a high calcium content.
- *Ultrasonography of the gallbladder* is a noninvasive exam that can accurately diagnose cholelithiasis. It also can be used to assess emptying of the gallbladder.
- *Oral cholecystogram* is performed using a dye administered orally to assess the gallbladder's ability to concentrate and excrete bile.
- *Gallbladder scans* use an intravenous radioactive solution that is rapidly extracted from the blood and excreted into the biliary tree to diagnose cystic duct obstruction and acute or chronic cholecystitis.

### Medications

Clients who refuse surgery or for whom surgery is inappropriate may be treated with a drug to dissolve the gallstones.

---

### TABLE 22–1   Manifestations and Complications of Cholelithiasis and Cholecystitis

| Manifestations | Cholelithiasis | Cholecystitis |
|---|---|---|
| Pain | • Abrupt onset<br>• Severe, steady<br>• Localized to epigastrium and RUQ of abdomen<br>• May radiate to back, right scapula, and shoulder<br>• Lasts 30 minutes to 5 hours | • Abrupt onset<br>• Severe, steady<br>• Generalized in RUQ of abdomen<br>• May radiate to back, right scapula, and shoulder<br>• Lasts 12 to 18 hours<br>• Aggravated by movement, breathing |
| Associated symptoms | • Nausea, vomiting | • Anorexia, nausea, vomiting<br>• RUQ tenderness and guarding<br>• Chills and fever |
| Complications | • Cholecystitis<br>• Common bile duct obstruction with possible jaundice and liver damage<br>• Common duct obstruction with pancreatitis | • Gangrene and perforation with peritonitis<br>• Chronic cholecystitis<br>• Empyema<br>• Fistula formation<br>• Gallstone ilius |

## BOX 22–2 ■ Sorting Out Total, Direct, and Indirect Bilirubin Levels

When serum bilirubin levels are drawn, the results usually are reported as the total bilirubin, direct bilirubin, and indirect bilirubin levels. Most bilirubin is formed from hemoglobin, as aging or abnormal RBCs are removed from circulation and destroyed. It is then bound to protein and transported to the liver. This protein-bound bilirubin is called *indirect* or *unconjugated* bilirubin. Once in the liver, bilirubin is separated from the protein and converted to a soluble form, *direct* or *conjugated* bilirubin. Conjugated bilirubin is then excreted in the bile.

■ **Total** (serum) **bilirubin,** the total bilirubin in the blood, includes both indirect and direct forms. In adults, the normal total bilirubin is 0.3 to 1.2 mg/dL or SI 5 to 21 µmol/L. Total bilirubin levels increase when more is being produced (e.g., RBC hemolysis), or when its metabolism or excretion are impaired (e.g., liver disease or biliary obstruction).

■ **Direct** (conjugated) **bilirubin** levels, normally 0 to 0.2 mg/dL or SI <3.4 µmo/L in adults, rise when its excretion is impaired by obstruction within the liver (e.g., in cirrhosis, hepatitis, exposure to hepatotoxins) or in the biliary system.

■ **Indirect** (unconjugated) **bilirubin** levels, normally <1.1 mg/dL or SI <19 µmol/L in adults, rise in RBC hemolysis (e.g., sickle cell disease or transfusion reaction).

Ursodiol (Actigall) and chenodiol (Chenix) reduce the cholesterol content of gallstones, leading to their gradual dissolution. These drugs are most effective in treating stones with high cholesterol content. They are less effective in treating radiopaque stones with high calcium salt content. Ursodiol is generally well tolerated with few side effects, while chenodiol has a high incidence of diarrhea at therapeutic doses. It also is hepatotoxic, so periodic liver function studies are required during therapy.

The primary disadvantages of pharmacologic treatment for gallstones include its cost, long duration (2 years or more), and the high incidence of recurrent stone formation when treatment is discontinued. If infection is suspected, antibiotics may be ordered to cure the infection and reduce associated inflammation and edema. Clients with pruritus (itching) due to severe obstructive jaundice and an accumulation of bile salts on the skin may be given cholestyramine (Questran). This drug binds with bile salts to promote their excretion in the feces. A narcotic analgesic such as morphine may be required for pain relief during an acute attack of cholecystitis.

## Treatments

### Surgery

**Laparoscopic cholecystectomy** (removal of the gallbladder) is the treatment of choice for symptomatic cholelithiasis or cholecystitis. This minimally invasive procedure has a low risk of complications and generally requires a hospital stay of less than 24 hours. Not all clients are candidates for laparoscopic cholecystectomy, and there is a risk that a laparoscopic cholecystectomy may be converted to a *laparotomy* (surgical opening into the abdomen) during the procedure. See the box below for nursing care for a client having laparoscopic cholecystectomy.

When stones are lodged within the ducts, a **cholecystectomy** with common bile duct exploration may be done. A T-tube (Figure 22–2 ■) is inserted to maintain patency of the duct and promote bile passage while the edema decreases. Excess bile is collected in a drainage bag secured below the surgical site. If it is suspected that a stone has been retained following surgery, a postoperative cholangiogram via the T-tube or direct visualization of the duct with an endoscope may be performed. See the box on page 577 for nursing care for a client with a T-tube.

Some clients who are poor surgical risks and for whom laparoscopic cholecystectomy is inappropriate may have either a *cholecystostomy* to drain the gallbladder, or a *choledochostomy* to remove stones and position a T-tube in the common bile duct.

### Dietary Management

Food intake may be eliminated during an acute attack of cholecystitis, and a nasogastric tube inserted to relieve nausea and vomiting. Dietary fat intake may be limited, especially if the

## NURSING CARE OF THE CLIENT WITH LAPAROSCOPIC CHOLECYSTECTOMY

### BEFORE SURGERY

• Provide routine preoperative care as ordered (see Chapter 7).
• Reinforce teaching about the procedure and postoperative expectations, including pain management, deep breathing, and mobilization. *Preoperative teaching reduces anxiety and promotes rapid postoperative recovery.*

### AFTER SURGERY

• Provide routine postoperative recovery care as outlined in Chapter 7.
• Assist to chair at bedside as allowed. *Early mobilization promotes lung ventilation and circulation, reducing the potential for postoperative complications.*

• Advance oral intake from ice chips to regular diet as tolerated. *Oral intake can be rapidly resumed due to minimal disruption of the gastrointestinal tract during surgery.*
• Provide and reinforce teaching: pain management, incision care, activity level, postoperative follow-up appointments. *With early discharge, the client and family assume responsibility for the majority of postoperative care. A clear understanding of this care and expected needs reduces anxiety and the risk of postoperative complications.*
• Initiate follow-up contact 24 to 48 hours after discharge to evaluate adequacy of pain control, incision management, and discharge understanding. *Contact following discharge provides an opportunity to evaluate care and reinforce teaching.*

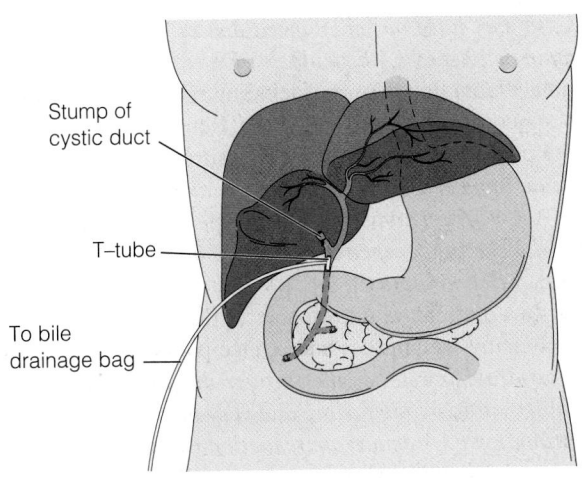

**Figure 22–2** ■ T-tube placement in the common bile duct. Bile fluid flows with gravity into a drainage collection device below the level of the common bile duct.

Stump of cystic duct

T–tube

To bile drainage bag

client is obese. If bile flow is obstructed, fat-soluble vitamins (A, D, E, and K) and bile salts may need to be administered.

## Other Therapies

In some cases, shock wave lithotripsy may be used with drug therapy to dissolve large gallstones. In *extracorporeal shock wave lithotripsy (ESWL)*, ultrasound is used to align the stones with the source of shock waves and the computerized lithotripter. Positioning is of prime importance throughout the procedure, which usually takes an hour. Mild sedation may be given during the procedure. Postprocedure nursing care includes monitoring for biliary colic that may result from the gallbladder contracting to remove stone fragments, nausea, and transient hematuria. *Percutaneous cholecystostomy*, ultrasound-guided drainage of the gallbladder, may be done in high-risk clients to postpone or even eliminate the need for surgery.

## Complementary Therapies

The herb goldenseal has been used in treating cholecystitis. One of the active ingredients in goldenseal, berberine, stimu-lates secretion of bile and bilirubin. It also inhibits the growth of many common pathogens, including those known to infect the gallbladder. A study of the effectiveness of berberine in clients with cholecystitis demonstrated relief of all symptoms. Goldenseal can stimulate the uterus, so it is contraindicated for use during pregnancy. It also should not be used by nursing mothers.

## NURSING CARE

### Health Promotion

While most risk factors for cholelithiasis cannot be controlled or modified, several can. Modifiable risk factors include obesity, hyperlipidemia, extreme low-calorie diets, and diets high in cholesterol. Encourage clients who are obese to increase their activity level and follow a low-carbohydrate, low-fat, low-cholesterol diet to promote weight loss and reduce their risk for developing gallstones. Discuss the dangers of "yo-yo" dieting, with cycles of weight loss followed by weight gain, and of extremely low calorie diets. Encourage clients with high serum cholesterol levels to discuss using cholesterol-lowering drugs with their primary care provider.

### Assessment

Assessment data related to cholelithiasis and cholecystitis include the following:

- Health history: current manifestations, including RUQ pain, its character and relationship to meals, duration, and radiation, nausea and vomiting or other symptoms; duration of symptoms; risk factors or previous history of symptoms; chronic diseases such as diabetes, cirrhosis, or inflammatory bowel disease; current diet; use of oral contraceptives or possibility of pregnancy
- Physical assessment: current weight; color of skin and sclera; abdominal assessment including light palpation for tenderness; color of urine and stool

## NURSING CARE   OF THE CLIENT WITH A T-TUBE

- Ensure that the T-tube is properly connected to a sterile container; keep the tube below the level of the surgical wound. *This position promotes the flow of bile and prevents backflow or seepage of caustic bile onto the skin. The tube itself decreases biliary tree pressure.*
- Monitor drainage from the T-tube for color and consistency; record as output. Normally, the tube may drain up to 500 mL in the first 24 hours after surgery; drainage decreases to less than 200 mL in 2 to 3 days, and is minimal thereafter. Drainage may be blood tinged initially, changing to green-brown. Report excessive drainage immediately (after 48 hours, drainage greater than 500 mL is considered excessive). *Stones or edema and inflammation can obstruct ducts below the tube, requiring treatment.*

- Place in Fowler's position. *This promotes gravity drainage of bile.*
- Assess skin for bile leakage during dressing changes. *Bile irritates the skin: it may be necessary to apply skin protection with karaya or another barrier product.*
- Teach client how to manage the tube when turning, ambulating, and performing activities of daily living. *Direct pulling or traction on the tube must be avoided.*
- If indicated, teach care of the T-tube, how to clamp it, and signs of infection. *Clients may be discharged home with the tube in place. Reporting early signs of infection facilitates prompt treatment.*

## Nursing Diagnoses and Interventions

Priority nursing diagnoses for the client with cholelithiasis or cholecystitis often include pain related to biliary colic or surgery, imbalanced nutrition related to the effects of altered bile flow and to nausea and anorexia, and risk for infection related to potential rupture of an acutely inflamed gallbladder. Nursing interventions for the client who has undergone a laparoscopic or open cholecystectomy are similar to those for other clients having abdominal surgery. See Chapter 7. ⊂⊃

### Pain

The pain associated with cholelithiasis can be severe. Sometimes a combination of interventions is indicated.

- Discuss the relationship between fat intake and the pain. Teach ways to reduce fat intake (see Box 22–3). *Fat entering the duodenum initiates gallbladder contractions, causing pain when gallstones are present in the ducts.*
- Withhold oral food and fluids during episodes of acute pain. Insert nasogastric tube and connect to low suction if ordered. *Emptying the stomach reduces the amount of chyme entering the duodenum and the stimulus for gallbladder contractions, thus reducing pain.*
- For severe pain, administer meperidine or other narcotic analgesia as ordered. *Recent research indicates that morphine is no more likely to cause spasms of the sphincter of Oddi than meperidine.*
- Place in Fowler's position. *Fowler's position decreases pressure on the inflamed gallbladder.*
- Monitor vital signs, including temperature, at least every 4 hours. *Bacterial infection often is present in acute cholecystitis, and may cause an elevated temperature and respiratory rate.*

### Imbalanced Nutrition: Less Than Body Requirements

The client with severe gallbladder disease may develop nutritional imbalances related to anorexia, pain and nausea following meals, and impaired bile flow that alters absorption of fat and fat-soluble vitamins (A, D, E, K) from the gut.

- Assess nutritional status, including diet history, height and weight, and skinfold measurements (see Chapters 19 and 20). ⊂⊃ *Even though often obese, clients with gallbladder*

| BOX 22–3 | ■ Examples of High-Fat Foods |
| --- | --- |

- Whole-milk products (e.g., cream, ice cream, cheese)
- Doughnuts, deep-fried
- Avocados
- Sausage, bacon, hot dogs
- Gravies with fat, cream
- Most nuts (e.g., pecans, cashews)
- Corn chips and potato chips
- Butter and cooking oils
- Fried foods (e.g., cheeseburgers, hamburgers, french fries)
- Peanut butter
- Chocolate candies

*disease may have an imbalanced diet or may have specific vitamin deficiencies, particularly of the fat-soluble vitamins.*

- Evaluate laboratory results, including serum bilirubin, albumin, glucose, and cholesterol levels. Report abnormal results to the primary care provider. *Elevated serum bilirubin may indicate impaired bilirubin excretion due to obstructed bile flow. A low serum albumin may indicate poor nutritional status. Glucose intolerance and hypercholesterolemia are risk factors for cholelithiasis.*
- Refer to a dietitian or nutritionist for diet counseling to promote healthy weight loss and reduce pain episodes. *A low-carbohydrate, low-fat, higher-protein diet reduces symptoms of cholecystitis. While fasting and very-low-calorie diets are contraindicated, a moderate reduction in calorie intake and increased activity levels promote weight loss.*
- Administer vitamin supplements as ordered. *Clients who do not absorb fat well due to obstructed bile flow may require supplements of the fat-soluble vitamins.*

### Risk for Infection

An acutely inflamed gallbladder may become necrotic and rupture, releasing its contents into the abdominal cavity. While the resulting infection often remains localized, peritonitis can result from chemical irritation and bacterial contamination of the peritoneal cavity.

**PRACTICE ALERT** *Rupture of an acutely inflamed gallbladder may be heralded by abrupt but transient pain relief as contents are released from the distended gallbladder into the abdomen. Promptly report this change to the physician.* ■

Following open cholecystectomy (*laparotomy*), the risk for pulmonary infection is significant due to the high abdominal incision.

- Monitor vital signs including temperature every 4 hours. Promptly report vital sign changes or temperature elevation. *Tachycardia, increased respiratory rate, or an elevated temperature may indicate an infectious process.*
- Assess abdomen every 4 hours and as indicated (e.g., when pain level changes abruptly). *Increasing abdominal tenderness or a rigid, boardlike abdomen may indicate rupture of the gallbladder with peritonitis.*
- Assist to cough and deep breathe or use incentive spirometer every 1 to 2 hours while awake. Splint abdominal incision with a blanket or pillow during coughing. *The high abdominal incision of an open cholecystectomy interferes with effective coughing and deep breathing, increasing the risk of atelectasis and respiratory infections such as pneumonia.*
- Place in Fowler's position and encourage ambulation as allowed. *Fowler's position and ambulating promote lung expansion and airway clearance, reducing the risk of respiratory infections.*
- Administer antibiotics as ordered. *Antibiotics may be given preoperatively to reduce the risk of infection from infected gallbladder contents, and may be continued postoperatively to prevent infection.*

## CHART 22–1  LINKAGES BETWEEN NANDA, NIC, AND NOC

### The Client with Gallbladder Disease

| NURSING DIAGNOSES | NURSING INTERVENTIONS | NURSING OUTCOMES |
|---|---|---|
| • Pain | • Pain Management<br>• Patient-Controlled Analgesia Assistance | • Pain Control |
| • Imbalanced Nutrition: Less Than Body Requirements<br>• Ineffective Health Maintenance | • Fluid Monitoring<br>• Nutrition Management<br>• Nutrition Monitoring<br>• Teaching: Procedure /Treatment<br>• Decision-Making Support | • Nutritional Status: Food and Fluid Intake<br><br>• Knowledge: Treatment Regimen<br>• Participation: Health Care Decisions |

*Data from Nursing Outcomes Classification (NOC) by M. Johnson & M. Maas (Eds.), 1997, St. Louis: Mosby; Nursing Diagnoses: Definitions & Classification 2001–2002 by North American Nursing Diagnosis Association, 2001, Philadelphia: NANDA; Nursing Interventions Classification (NIC) by J.C. McCloskey & G. M. Bulechek (Eds.), 2000, St. Louis: Mosby. Reprinted by permission.*

## Using NANDA, NIC, and NOC

Chart 22–1 shows links between NANDA nursing diagnoses, NIC, and NOC when caring for a client with cholelithiasis or cholecystitis.

## Home Care

Teaching varies, depending on the choice of treatment options for cholelithiasis and cholecystitis. If surgery is not an option, teach about medications that dissolve stones, their use and adverse effects (diarrhea is a common side effect), and maintaining a low-fat, low-carbohydate diet if indicated. Include an explanation about the role of bile and the function of the gallbladder in terms that the client and family can understand.

Provide appropriate preoperative teaching for the planned procedure. Discuss the possibility of open cholecystectomy even when a laparoscopic procedure is planned. Teach postoperative self-care measures to manage pain and prevent complications. If the client will be discharged with a T-tube, provide instructions about its care (see the Nursing Care box on page 577). Discuss manifestations of complications to report to the physician. Stress the importance of follow-up appointments.

Following cholecystectomy, a low-fat diet may be initially recommended. Refer the client and food preparer to a dietitian to review low-fat foods. Higher fat foods may be gradually added to the diet as tolerated.

## Nursing Care Plan
## A Client with Cholelithiasis

Joyce Red Wing is a 44-year-old married mother of three children. A member of the Chickasaw tribe, she is active in tribal activities and works part time as a cook at a community kitchen. Recently Mrs. Red Wing has noticed a dull pain in her upper abdomen that gets worse after eating fatty foods; nausea and sometimes vomiting accompany the pain. She had a similar pain after the birth of her last child. She is diagnosed with cholelithiasis, and is admitted for a laparoscopic cholecystecomy.

### ASSESSMENT

David Corbin, RN, takes Mrs. Red Wing's admission history. It includes intolerance to fatty foods and intermittent "stabbing" abdominal pain that radiates to her back. Her usual diet includes tacos or fried bread and biscuits with gravy for breakfast. She reports "not wanting to eat much of anything lately." She states she has never had surgery before and hopes "everything goes well." Physical assessment includes T 100° F (37.7° C), P 88, R 20, and BP 130/84. She has had a recent 5 lb weight loss, currently weighing 130 lb (59 kg). She is 63 inches (160 cm) tall. Abdominal examination elicits tenderness in the right upper abdominal quadrant.

She has no jaundice, chills, or evidence of complications.

### DIAGNOSES

- *Imbalanced nutrition: Less than body requirements* related to anorexia and recent weight loss
- *Pain* related to inflamed gallbladder and surgical incisions
- *Risk for infection* related to potential bacterial contamination of abdominal cavity
- *Anxiety* related to lack of information about perioperative experience

### EXPECTED OUTCOMES

- Maintain present weight within 5 lb (2.3 kg) over the next 3 weeks.
- Resume regular diet, decreasing intake of foods high in fat.
- Verbalize adequate pain control after surgery and with activity resumption.
- Remain free of infection.
- Verbalize a decrease in anxiety before surgery.

(continued on page 580)

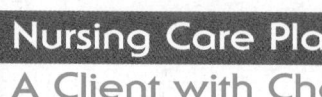

## Nursing Care Plan
## A Client with Cholelithiasis *(continued)*

### PLANNING AND IMPLEMENTATION

- Teach about the gallbladder and the function of bile.
- Discuss pre- and postoperative care, including self-care following discharge.
- Promote mobility as soon as allowed after surgery.
- Teach home care of stab wounds and recognition of signs of infection.
- Review specific high-fat foods to avoid and ways to maintain her weight.
- Provide analgesia as needed postoperatively. Teach appropriate analgesic use after discharge.

### EVALUATION

Mrs. Red Wing is discharged the morning after her surgery. She is afebrile, has no signs of infection, and is able to appropriately care for her stab wounds. She identifies signs of infection and

talks about ways to reduce her fat intake while keeping her weight stable. She verbalizes understanding of initial activity restrictions and resumption of normal activities. Mrs. Red Wing states, "It wasn't as bad as I thought it would be at first." She has an appointment to see her surgeon in 1 week.

### Critical Thinking in the Nursing Process

1. What is the rationale for a low-fat diet with cholelithiasis? Discuss nutritional practices as they relate to the medical problem and Mrs. Red Wing's culture.
2. How would your discharge teaching for Mrs. Red Wing differ if she had had an open cholecystectomy instead of a laparoscopic cholecystectomy?
3. Design a nursing care plan for Mrs. Red Wing for the nursing diagnosis: *Fatigue.*

See Evaluating Your Response in Appendix C.

## THE CLIENT WITH CANCER OF THE GALLBLADDER

Gallbladder cancer is rare, primarily affecting people over age 65. Women are more likely to develop the disorder. Manifestations of gallbladder cancer include intense pain and a palpable mass in the RUQ of the abdomen. Jaundice and weight loss are common. Gallbladder cancers spread by direct

extension to the liver, and metastasize via the blood and lymph system.

At the time of diagnosis, the cancer usually is too advanced to treat surgically. Ninety-five percent of clients with primary cancer of the gallbladder die within 1 year. Radical and extensive surgical interventions may be performed, but the prognosis is poor regardless of treatment (Tierney et al., 2001). Nursing care is palliative, focusing on maintaining comfort and independence to the extent possible.

# LIVER DISORDERS

The liver is a complex organ with multiple metabolic and regulatory functions. Optimal liver function is essential to health. Because of the significant amount of blood in the liver at all times, it is exposed to the effects of pathogens, drugs, toxins, and possibly malignant cells. As a result, liver cells may become inflamed or damaged, or cancerous tumors may develop.

## THE CLIENT WITH HEPATITIS

**Hepatitis** is inflammation of the liver. It is usually caused by a virus, although it may result from exposure to alcohol, drugs and toxins, or other pathogens. Hepatitis may be acute or chronic in nature. Cirrhosis, discussed in the next section, is a potential consequence of severe hepatocellular damage.

### PATHOPHYSIOLOGY AND MANIFESTATIONS

The essential functions of the liver are multiple. One of its primary functions is the metabolism and elimination of bilirubin.

Bilirubin is a breakdown product of hemoglobin, released when RBCs are broken down and destroyed. This insoluble form of bilirubin (unconjugated bilirubin) is metabolized by the liver into a soluble form (conjugated bilirubin), which is then eliminated in bile. The liver also metabolizes carbohydrates, proteins, and fats. Most drugs are metabolized in the liver, and substances such as alcohol and many toxins are detoxified. These metabolic functions and bile elimination are disrupted by the inflammation of hepatitis. See Chapter 19 for more information about the liver. ∞

## Viral Hepatitis

At least five viruses are known to cause hepatitis: hepatitis A virus (HAV), hepatitis B virus (HBV), hepatitis C virus (HCV), the hepatitis B-associated delta virus (HDV), and hepatitis E virus (HEV). These viruses differ from one another in mode of transmission, incubation period, the severity and type of liver damage they cause, and their ability to become chronic or develop a carrier (asymptomatic) state. Table 22–2 identifies unique features of the primary hepatitis viruses. Two additional

**TABLE 22–2  Comparison of Types of Viral Hepatitis**

| Virus | Hepatitis A (HAV) | Hepatitis B (HBV) | Hepatitis C (HCV) | Hepatitis D (HDV) | Hepatitis E (HEV) |
|---|---|---|---|---|---|
| Mode of transmission | Fecal–oral | Blood & body fluids; perinatal | Blood & body fluids | Blood & body fluids; perinatal | Fecal–oral |
| Incubation (in weeks) | 2–6 | 6–24 | 5–12 | 3–13 | 3–6 |
| Onset | Abrupt | Slow | Slow | Abrupt | Abrupt |
| Carrier state | No | Yes | Yes | Yes | Yes |
| Possible complications | Rare | Chronic hepatitis Cirrhosis Liver cancer | Chronic hepatitis Cirrhosis Liver cancer | Chronic hepatitis Cirrhosis Fulminant hepatitis | May be severe in pregnant women |
| Laboratory findings | Anti-HAV antibodies present | Positive HBsAg (HBV surface antigen); anti-HBV antibodies present | Anti-HCV antibodies present | Positive HDVAg (delta antigen) early; anti-HDV antibodies later | Anti-HEV antibodies present |

viruses, hepatitis F and hepatitis G, have recently been identified. Their characteristics are yet to be defined.

Hepatitis viruses replicate in the liver, damaging liver cells (hepatocytes). The viruses provoke an immune response that causes inflammation and necrosis of hepatocytes as well. Although the extent of damage and the immune response vary among the different hepatitis viruses, the disease itself usually follows a predictable pattern.

No manifestations are present during the incubation period after exposure to the virus. The *prodromal* or *preicteric* (before jaundice) *phase* may begin abruptly or insidiously, with general malaise, anorexia, fatigue, and muscle and body aches. These manifestations often are mistaken for the flu. Nausea, vomiting, diarrhea, or constipation may develop, as well as mild RUQ abdominal pain. Chills and fever may be present.

The *icteric* (jaundiced) *phase* usually begins 5 to 10 days after the onset of symptoms. It is heralded by jaundice of the sclera, skin, and mucous membranes. Inflammation of the liver and bile ducts prevents bilirubin from being excreted into the small intestine. As a result, the serum bilirubin levels are elevated, causing yellowing of the skin and mucous membranes. Pruritus may develop due to deposition of bile salts on the skin. The stools are light brown or clay colored because bile pigment is not excreted through the normal fecal pathway. Instead, the pigment is excreted by the kidneys, causing the urine to turn brown.

During the icteric phase, the initial prodromal manifestations usually diminish even though the serum bilirubin increases. The appetite increases, and the temperature returns to normal. When uncomplicated, spontaneous recovery usually begins within 2 weeks of the onset of jaundice.

The *convalescent phase* follows jaundice and lasts several weeks. During this time, manifestations gradually improve: Serum enzymes decrease, liver pain decreases, and gastrointestinal symptoms and weakness subside. See the box on this page for the manifestations of each phase of hepatitis.

### Hepatitis A

Hepatitis A, or *infectious hepatitis*, often occurs in either sporadic attacks or mild epidemics. It is transmitted by the fecal–oral route via contaminated food, water, shellfish, and direct contact with an infected person. The virus is in the stool of infected persons up to 2 weeks before symptoms develop. Although hepatitis A usually has an abrupt onset, it is typically a benign and self-limited disease with few long-term consequences. Symptoms last up to 2 months.

### Hepatitis B

Hepatitis B can cause acute hepatitis, chronic hepatitis, fulminant hepatitis, or a carrier state. This virus is spread through contact with infected blood and body fluids. Health care workers are at risk through exposure to blood and needle-stick injuries. Other high-risk groups for hepatitis B include injection drug users, people with multiple sex partners, men who have sex with other men, and people frequently exposed to blood products (such as people on hemodialysis). Hepatitis B is a major risk factor for primary liver cancer.

## Manifestations of Acute Hepatitis

### PREICTERIC PHASE
- "Flulike" symptoms: malaise, fatigue, fever
- Gastrointestinal: anorexia, nausea, vomiting, diarrhea, constipation
- Muscle aches, polyarthritis
- Mild right upper abdominal pain and tenderness

### ICTERIC PHASE
- Jaundice
- Pruritus
- Clay-colored stools
- Brown urine
- Decrease in preicteric phase symptoms (e.g., appetite improves; no fever)

### POSTICTERIC/CONVALESCENT PHASE
- Serum bilirubin and enzymes return to normal levels
- Energy level increases
- Pain subsides
- Gastrointestinal: minimal to absent

MediaLink | HEPATITIS B CASE STUDY

In hepatitis B, liver cells are damaged by the immune response to this antigen. Damage may affect only portions or the majority of the liver. The liver shows evidence of injury and scarring, regeneration, and proliferation of inflammatory cells (Bullock & Henze, 2000).

### Hepatitis C

Hepatitis C, formerly known as non-A, non-B hepatitis, is the primary worldwide cause of chronic hepatitis, cirrhosis, and liver cancer (Porth, 2002). It is transmitted through infected blood and body fluids. Injection drug use is the primary risk factor for HCV infection. The initial manifestations of this type of hepatitis often are mild and nonspecific. The disease often is recognized long after exposure occurred, when secondary effects of the disease (such as chronic hepatitis or cirrhosis) develop.

### Hepatitis Delta

Hepatitis delta (HDV) only causes infection in people who also are infected with hepatitis B. It can cause acute or chronic infection, and can increase the severity of HBV infection (Porth, 2002). It is transmitted in the same manner as HBV.

### Hepatitis E

Hepatitis E is rare in the United States. It is transmitted by fecal contamination of water supplies in developing areas such as southeast Asia, parts of Africa, and Central America. It primarily affects young adults. It can cause fulminant, fatal hepatitis in pregnant women.

## Chronic Hepatitis

**Chronic hepatitis** is chronic infection of the liver. While it may cause few symptoms, it is the primary cause of liver damage leading to cirrhosis, liver cancer, and liver transplantation. Three of the known hepatitis viruses cause chronic hepatitis: HBV, HCV, and HDV. Manifestations of chronic hepatitis include malaise, fatigue, and hepatomegaly. Occasional icteric (jaundiced) periods may occur. Liver enzymes, particularly serum aminotransferase levels, typically are elevated.

## Fulminant Hepatitis

**Fulminant hepatitis** is a rapidly progressive disease, with liver failure developing within 2 to 3 weeks after the onset of symptoms. Although uncommon, it is usually related to HBV with concurrent HDV infection.

## Toxic Hepatitis

Many substances, including alcohol, certain drugs, and other toxins, can directly damage liver cells. Alcoholic hepatitis can result from chronic alcohol abuse or from an acute toxic reaction to alcohol. Alcoholic hepatitis causes necrosis of hepatocytes and inflammation of the liver parenchyma (functional tissue). Unless alcohol intake is avoided, progression to cirrhosis is common.

Other potential hepatotoxins include acetaminophen, benzene, carbon tetrachloride, halothane, chloroform, and poisonous mushrooms. These substances directly damage liver cells, leading to necrosis. The degree of damage often depends on age and the extent of exposure (dose) to the hepatoxin. Acetaminophen is a common cause of hepatocellular damage.

## Hepatobiliary Hepatitis

Hepatobiliary hepatitis is due to cholestasis, the interruption of the normal flow of bile. Cholestasis may result from obstruction of the hepatic duct with stones or inflammation secondary to cholelithiasis. Other agents, such as oral contraceptives and allopurinol (a drug used to lower uric acid levels), also can cause cholestasis. When bile flow is disrupted, the liver parenchyma may become inflamed. Reestablishing bile flow by removing the stone or other causative agent is the treatment for hepatobiliary hepatitis.

## COLLABORATIVE CARE

Management of hepatitis focuses on determining its cause, providing appropriate treatment and support, and teaching strategies to prevent further liver damage. Effective management begins with thorough assessment of diagnostic and laboratory data.

### Diagnostic Tests

Liver function tests, such as blood levels of bilirubin and enzymes commonly released when liver cells are damaged, are obtained. These include the following:

- *Alanine aminotransferase (ALT)* is an enzyme contained within each liver cell. When liver cells are damaged, it is released into the blood. Levels may exceed 1000 IU/L or more in acute hepatitis.
- *Aspartate aminotransferase (AST)* is an enzyme found predominantly in heart and liver cells. AST levels rise when liver cells are damaged; with severe damage, blood levels may be 20 to 100 times normal values (Malarkey & McMorrow, 2000).
- *Alkaline phosphatase (ALP)* is an enzyme present in liver cells and bone. Serum ALP levels often are elevated in hepatitis.
- *Gamma-glutamyltransferase (GGT)* is an enzyme present in cell membranes. Its blood levels rise in hepatitis and obstructive biliary disease, and remain elevated until function is restored.
- *Lactic dehydrogenase (LDH),* an enzyme present in many body tissues, is a nonspecific indicator of tissue damage. Its isoenzyme, LDH5, is a specific indicator of liver damage.
- *Serum bilirubin* levels, including *conjugated* and *unconjugated,* are elevated in viral hepatitis due to impaired bilirubin metabolism and obstruction of the hepatobiliary ducts by inflammation and edema. The bilirubin level decreases as inflammation and edema subside.
- Laboratory tests for viral antigens and their specific antibodies may be done to identify the infecting virus and its state of activity. These tests are summarized in Table 22–2.
- A *liver biopsy* may be done to detect and evaluate chronic hepatitis. (Nursing implications for this test are outlined in the box on page 590.)

## Medications

### Prevention

Hepatitis A and hepatitis B are preventable diseases. Vaccines are available, as are preparations to prevent the disease following known or suspected exposure.

***VACCINES.*** Hepatitis A vaccine provides long-term protection against HAV infection. It is an inactivated whole virus vaccine available in pediatric and adult formulations. Although more than 95% of adults achieve immunity after one dose of the vaccine, two doses are recommended for full protection. See Table 22–3.

Three doses of hepatitis B vaccine provide immunity to HBV infection in 90% of healthy adults. Hepatitis B vaccine is a recombinant vaccine. Vaccines produced by different manufacturers may be used interchangeably, although their dosages differ. Older adults are less likely to achieve immunity than younger adults. Clients on hemodialysis and people who are immunocompromised may need larger or more doses of the vaccine to achieve adequate protection. Serologic testing for immunity is recommended on completion of the series for people in these high-risk groups.

***POSTEXPOSURE PROPHYLAXIS.*** Postexposure prophylaxis may be recommended for household or sexual contacts of peo-ple with HAV or HBV and other people who are known to have been exposed to these viruses. It is not necessary if the exposed person has been vaccinated and is known to be immune.

Hepatitis A prophylaxis is provided by a single dose of immune globulin (IG) given within 2 weeks after exposure. IG is recommended for all people with household or sexual contact with a person known to be infected with hepatitis A. See Table 22–3 for further recommendations.

Hepatitis B postexposure prophylaxis is indicated for people exposed to the hepatitis B virus. Hepatitis B immune globulin (HBIG) is given to provide for short-term immunity. HBV vaccine may be given concurrently. Candidates for postexposure prophylaxis include those with known or suspected percutaneous or permucosal contact with infected blood, sexual partners of clients with acute HBV or who are HBV carriers, and household contacts of clients with acute HBV infection (Atkinson, et al, 2000).

### Treatment

In most cases of acute viral hepatitis, pharmacologic treatment of the infection is not indicated. Acute hepatitis C may be treated with interferon alpha, an antiviral agent, to reduce the risk of chronic hepatitis C.

Interferon alpha is used to treat both chronic hepatitis B and chronic hepatitis C. Interferon alpha interferes with viral replication, reducing the viral load. It is given by intramuscular or

---

### TABLE 22–3    CDC Recommendations for Hepatitis Prevention in Adults

| Disease/Strategy | Immunization | Adverse Reactions | Population Recommendations |
|---|---|---|---|
| **Hepatitis A** Prevention | Hepatitis A vaccine (Havrix; VAQTA), 2 doses (initial dose with booster in 6–12 months) IM into deltoid muscle | Pain at injection site | • Children >2 yr<br>• International travelers<br>• Homosexual men<br>• Drug users<br>• Persons with clotting-factor disorders, chronic liver disease, hepatitis C<br>• Persons with occupational risk |
| Postexposure prophylaxis | Standard immune globulin IM into large muscle mass within 2 weeks of exposure | Rare; risk of anaphylaxis in people with IgA deficiency | • Close contacts of people with known hepatitis A<br>• People potentially exposed to hepatitis A at child care center or restaurant with infected food handler |
| **Hepatitis B** Prevention | Recombinant hepatitis B vaccine (Recombivax HB; Engerix-B), 3 doses (initial dose followed by doses at 4 weeks and 5 months later) given IM into deltoid muscle | Pain at injection site; fatigue, headache | • Infants and adolescents<br>• Adults with increased risk of HBV<br>• Homosexual males; heterosexuals with multiple sexual partners<br>• Injection drug users<br>• Long-term male prisoners<br>• People on hemodialysis<br>• Health care workers |
| Postexposure prophylaxis | Hepatitis B immune globulin (HBIG) given IM into large muscle mass within 24 hr to 7 days of exposure, second dose 28 to 30 days after exposure; concurrent initiation of hepatitis B vaccine series | Infrequent; muscle stiffness, pain | • Infants born to women with HBV infection<br>• Percutaneous or permucosal exposure to HBV when unvaccinated or antibody response is negative or unknown |

*Note.* From *Epidemiology and Prevention of Vaccine-Preventable Diseases* (6th ed.) by Centers for Disease Control and Prevention (CDC), January 2000, Atlanta: Department of Health and Human Services.

subcutaneous injection. Virtually all clients treated with interferon alpha develop a flulike syndrome with fever, fatigue, muscle aches, headache, and chills. Acetaminophen helps alleviate some of these adverse effects. Depression also is a common adverse effect of this drug.

An alternate drug for treating chronic hepatitis B is lamivudine (Epivir HBV), an antiviral drug that can reduce liver inflammation and fibrosis. Although it has minimal side effects, clients may become resistant to the beneficial effects of lamivudine.

The treatment of choice for chronic hepatitis C is combination therapy of interferon alpha with ribavirin (Rebetol), an oral antiviral drug. This combination therapy improves the response rate over either drug used alone. Ribavirin has two major adverse effects: hemolytic anemia and birth defects. Blood counts are obtained before and during treatment to detect early signs of hemolytic anemia. Because of the risk for birth defects, this drug is contraindicated for use during pregnancy, and two reliable methods of birth control must be used by women taking the drug and female sexual partners of men taking the drug.

### Treatments

Treatment of acute hepatitis also includes as-needed bed rest, adequate nutrition as tolerated, and avoidance of strenuous activity, alcohol, and agents that are toxic to the liver. In most cases, clinical recovery takes 3 to 16 weeks.

#### Complementary Therapies

Milk thistle, with its active ingredient silymarin, has been used by herbalists to treat liver disease for over 2000 years. Clinical studies have demonstrated that treatment with silymarin promotes recovery and reduces complications in clients with viral hepatitis. It also is beneficial for clients who have liver damage due to toxins, cirrhosis, and alcoholic liver disease. Silymarin's beneficial effects are attributed to its ability to promote liver cell growth, block toxins from entering and damaging liver cells, and reduce liver inflammation. It also is a powerful antioxidant.

Herbalists also may use licorice root to treat hepatitis. It has both antiviral and anti-inflammatory effects. Long-term use of licorice root, however, can lead to hypertension and affect fluid and electrolyte balance.

Herbal preparations also may be used to relieve the adverse effects of interferon alpha. Ginger can help relieve nausea, and St. John's wort is used for the depression associated with interferon alpha.

## NURSING CARE

### Health Promotion

Nurses play an instrumental role in preventing the spread of hepatitis. Stress the importance of hygiene measures such as handwashing after toileting and before all food handling. Discuss the dangers of injection drug use, and, with drug users, of sharing needles or other equipment. Encourage all sexually ac-

tive clients to use safer sexual practices such as abstinence, mutual monogamy, and barrier protection (such as male or female condoms).

Discuss recommendations for hepatitis A and hepatitis B vaccine with people in high or moderate risk groups for these infections. Encourage all people with known or probable exposure to HAV or HBV to obtain postexposure prophylaxis.

### Assessment

Collect assessment data related to hepatitis, such as the following:

- Health history: current manifestations, including anorexia, nausea, vomiting, abdominal discomfort, changes in bowel elimination or color of stools; muscle or joint pain, fatigue; changes in color of skin or sclera; duration of symptoms; known exposure to hepatitis; high-risk behaviors such as injection drug use or multiple sexual partners; previous history of liver disorders; current medications, prescription and over the counter
- Physical assessment: vital signs including temperature; color of sclera and mucous membranes; skin color and condition; abdominal contour and tenderness; color of stool and urine

### Nursing Diagnoses and Interventions

Clients with acute or chronic hepatitis usually are treated in community settings; rarely is hospitalization required. Nursing care focuses on preventing spread of the infection to others and promoting the client's comfort and ability to provide self-care.

#### Risk for Infection (Transmission)

An important goal when caring for clients with acute viral hepatitis is preventing spread of the infection.

- Use standard precautions. Practice meticulous handwashing. *The hepatitis viruses are spread by direct contact with feces or blood and body fluids. Standard precautions and good handwashing protect both health care workers and other clients from exposure to the virus.*
- For clients with HAV or HEV, use standard precautions and contact isolation if fecal incontinence is present. *The fecal–oral route is the primary mode of transmission of these viruses. Other hepatitis viruses are transmitted through blood and other body fluids.*
- Encourage prophylactic treatment of all members of household and intimate sexual contacts. *Prophylactic treatment of people in close contact with the client decreases their risk of contacting the disease, or if already infected, the severity of the disease.*

**PRACTICE ALERT**   *If the client diagnosed with hepatitis A is employed as a food handler or child care worker, contact the local health department to report possible exposure of patrons. Maintain confidentiality. Prophylactic treatment of people who have possibly been exposed to the virus can prevent a local epidemic of the disease.* ■

## Fatigue

Fatigue, and possible weakness, is common in acute hepatitis. Although bed rest is rarely indicated, adequate rest periods and limitation of activities may be necessary. Many clients with acute hepatitis may be unable to resume normal activity levels for 4 or more weeks.

- Encourage planned rest periods throughout the day. *Adequate rest is necessary for optimal immune function.*
- Assist to identify essential activities and those that can be deferred or delegated to others. *Identifying essential and nonessential activities promotes the client's sense of control.*
- Suggest using level of fatigue to determine activity level, with gradual resumption of activities as fatigue and sense of well-being improves. *Fatigue associated with activity is an indicator of appropriate and inappropriate activity levels. As recovery progresses, increasing activity levels are tolerated with less fatigue.*

## Imbalanced Nutrition:
## Less Than Body Requirements

Adequate nutrition is important for immune function and healing in clients with acute or chronic hepatitis.

- Help plan a diet of appealing foods that provides a high kilocaloric intake of approximately 16 carbohydrate kilocalories per kilogram of ideal body weight. *Sufficient energy is required for healing; adequate carbohydrate intake can spare protein.*
- Encourage planning food intake according to symptoms of the disease. Discuss eating smaller meals and using between-meal snacks to maintain nutrient and calorie intake. *Clients with acute hepatitis often are more anorexic and nauseated in the afternoon and evening; planning the majority of calorie intake in the morning helps maintain adequate intake. Limiting fat intake and the size of meals may reduce the incidence of nausea.*
- Instruct to avoid alcohol intake and diet drinks. *Alcohol avoidance is vital to prevent further liver damage and pro-mote healing. Diet drinks (e.g. diet sodas or juice drinks) provide few calories when an increased calorie intake is needed for healing.*
- Encourage use of nutritional supplements such as Ensure or Instant Breakfast drinks to maintain calorie and nutrient intake. *Nutritional supplement drinks are an additional source of concentrated calories and nutrients.*

## Disturbed Body Image

Jaundice and associated rashes and itching can affect the client's body image. Nursing measures to prevent skin breakdown and address body image are discussed in the following section on cirrhosis.

## Using NANDA, NIC, and NOC

Chart 22–2 shows links between NANDA nursing diagnoses, NIC, and NOC when caring for a client with hepatitis.

## Home Care

Provide discharge teaching to clients and their families for home care. Include the following topics.

- Recommended prophylactic treatment
- Infection control measures such as frequent handwashing, not sharing eating utensils, avoiding food handling or preparation activities by the client with hepatitis A; abstaining from sexual relations during acute infection and using barrier protection if a carrier or for chronic infection
- Managing fatigue and limited activity
- Promoting nutrient intake
- Avoiding hepatic toxins such as alcohol, acetaminophen, and selected other drugs; encourage to alert all care providers to presence of infection
- Recommended follow-up

If chronic hepatitis B or C is being treated with medications, teach how to administer the drug, its dosing schedule, precautions, and management of adverse effects. Stress the importance of keeping follow-up appointments, including recommended laboratory testing.

MediaLink | HEPATITIS A CARE PLAN

### CHART 22–2 LINKAGES BETWEEN NANDA, NIC, AND NOC

#### The Client with Hepatitis

| NURSING DIAGNOSES | NURSING INTERVENTIONS | NURSING OUTCOMES |
|---|---|---|
| • Fatigue | • Energy Management | • Energy Conservation |
| • Imbalanced Nutrition: Less Than Body Requirements | • Nutrition Management | • Nutritional Status: Nutrient Intake |
| • Ineffective Health Maintenance | • Self-Responsibility Facilitation | • Self-Direction of Care |
| | • Teaching: Disease Process | • Treatment Behavior: Illness or Injury |
| • Social Isolation | • Family Involvement Promotion | • Social Support |
| | • Social System Enhancement | |

*Data from Nursing Outcomes Classification (NOC) by M. Johnson & M. Maas (Eds.), 1997, St. Louis: Mosby; Nursing Diagnoses: Definitions & Classification 2001–2002 by North American Nursing Diagnosis Association, 2001, Philadelphia: NANDA; Nursing Interventions Classification (NIC) by J.C. McCloskey & G. M. Bulechek (Eds.), 2000, St. Louis: Mosby. Reprinted by permission.*

# THE CLIENT WITH CIRRHOSIS

**Cirrhosis** is the end stage of chronic liver disease. It is a progressive, irreversible disorder, eventually leading to liver failure. Cirrhosis is the tenth leading cause of death in the United States (Tierney et al, 2001). **Alcoholic** or **Laënnec's cirrhosis** is the most common type of cirrhosis in North America and many parts of Europe and South America (Braunwald et al., 2001). Cirrhosis also may result from chronic hepatitis B or C; prolonged obstruction of the biliary (bile drainage) system; long-term, severe right heart failure; and other uncommon liver disorders.

## PHYSIOLOGY REVIEW

The portal venous system is the primary source of blood flow to the liver. This venous system drains blood from the abdominal organs.

The essential functions of the liver include the metabolism of proteins, carbohydrates, and fats. It also is responsible for the metabolism of steroid hormones and most drugs. It synthesizes blood proteins, albumin and clotting factors in particular. The liver detoxifies alcohol and other toxic substances. Ammonia, a toxic by-product of protein metabolism, is converted to urea in the liver for elimination by the kidneys. The liver produces bile, an essential substance for absorbing fats and eliminating bilirubin from the body. Minerals and fat-soluble vitamins are stored in the liver, as is glycogen (stored carbohydrate for energy reserves). The Kupffer cells that line the sinusoids phagocytize foreign cells and damaged blood cells. See Chapter 19 for more information about the liver.

## PATHOPHYSIOLOGY

In cirrhosis, functional liver tissue is gradually destroyed and replaced by fibrous scar tissue. As hepatocytes and liver lobules are destroyed, the metabolic functions of the liver are lost. Structurally abnormal nodules encircled by connective tissue form. This fibrous connective tissue forms constrictive bands that disrupt blood and bile flow within liver lobules. Blood no longer flows freely through the liver to the inferior vena cava. This restricted blood flow leads to portal hypertension, increased pressure in the portal venous system.

## Alcoholic Cirrhosis

Alcoholic or Laënnec's cirrhosis is the end result of alcoholic liver disease. Alcohol causes metabolic changes in the liver: triglyceride and fatty acid synthesis increases, and the formation and release of lipoproteins decrease, leading to fatty infiltration of hepatocytes (fatty liver). At this stage, abstinence from alcohol can allow the liver to heal. With continued alcohol abuse, the disease progresses. Inflammatory cells infiltrate the liver (alcoholic hepatitis), causing necrosis, fibrosis, and destruction of functional liver tissue. In the final stage of alcoholic cirrhosis, regenerative nodules form, and the liver shrinks and develops a nodular appearance (Bullock & Henze, 2000). Malnutrition commonly accompanies alcoholic cirrhosis.

## Biliary Cirrhosis

When bile flow is obstructed within the liver or in the biliary system, retained bile damages and destroys liver cells close to the interlobular bile ducts. This leads to inflammation, fibrosis, and formation of regenerative nodules.

## Posthepatic Cirrhosis

Advanced progressive liver disease resulting from chronic hepatitis B or C or from an unknown cause is known as posthepatic or postnecrotic cirrhosis. Chronic viral hepatitis appears to be the leading cause of posthepatic cirrhosis in the United States (Braunwald et al., 2001). The liver is shrunken and nodular, with extensive liver cell loss and fibrosis.

## MANIFESTATIONS AND COMPLICATIONS

Early in the course of cirrhosis, few manifestations may be present. The liver usually is enlarged and may be tender. A dull, aching pain in the RUQ may be present. Other early signs include weight loss, weakness, and anorexia. Bowel function is disrupted with diarrhea or constipation (Porth, 2002).

As the disease progresses, manifestations related to liver cell failure and portal hypertension develop. Impaired metabolism causes such manifestations as bleeding, ascites, gynecomastia (breast enlargement) in men and infertility in women, jaundice, and neurologic changes. Portal hypertension accounts from such manifestations as ascites, peripheral edema, anemia, and low WBC and platelet counts. See *Multisystem Effects of Cirrhosis* on page 587.

## Portal Hypertension

**Portal hypertension,** elevated pressure in the portal venous system, causes blood to be rerouted to adjoining lower pressure vessels. This *shunting* of blood involves collateral vessels. Affected veins, which become engorged and congested, are located in the esophagus, rectum, and abdomen. Portal hypertension increases the hydrostatic pressure in vessels of the portal system. Increased hydrostatic pressure in the capillaries pushes fluid out, contributing to ascites formation.

## Splenomegaly

The spleen enlarges (**splenomegaly**) as portal hypertension causes blood to be shunted into the splenic vein. Splenomegaly increases the rate at which red and white blood cells and platelets are removed from circulation and destroyed. This increased blood cell destruction leads to anemia, leukopenia, and thrombocytopenia (Porth, 2002).

## Ascites

**Ascites** is the accumulation of plasma-rich fluid in the abdominal cavity. Although portal hypertension is the primary cause of ascites, decreased serum proteins and increased aldosterone also contribute to the fluid accumulation. *Hypoalbuminemia,* low serum albumin, decreases the colloidal osmotic pressure of plasma. This pressure normally holds fluid in the intravascular compartment; when plasma colloidal osmotic pressure decreases, fluid escapes into extravascular compartments.

# Multisystem Effects of Cirrhosis

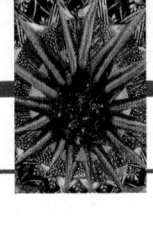

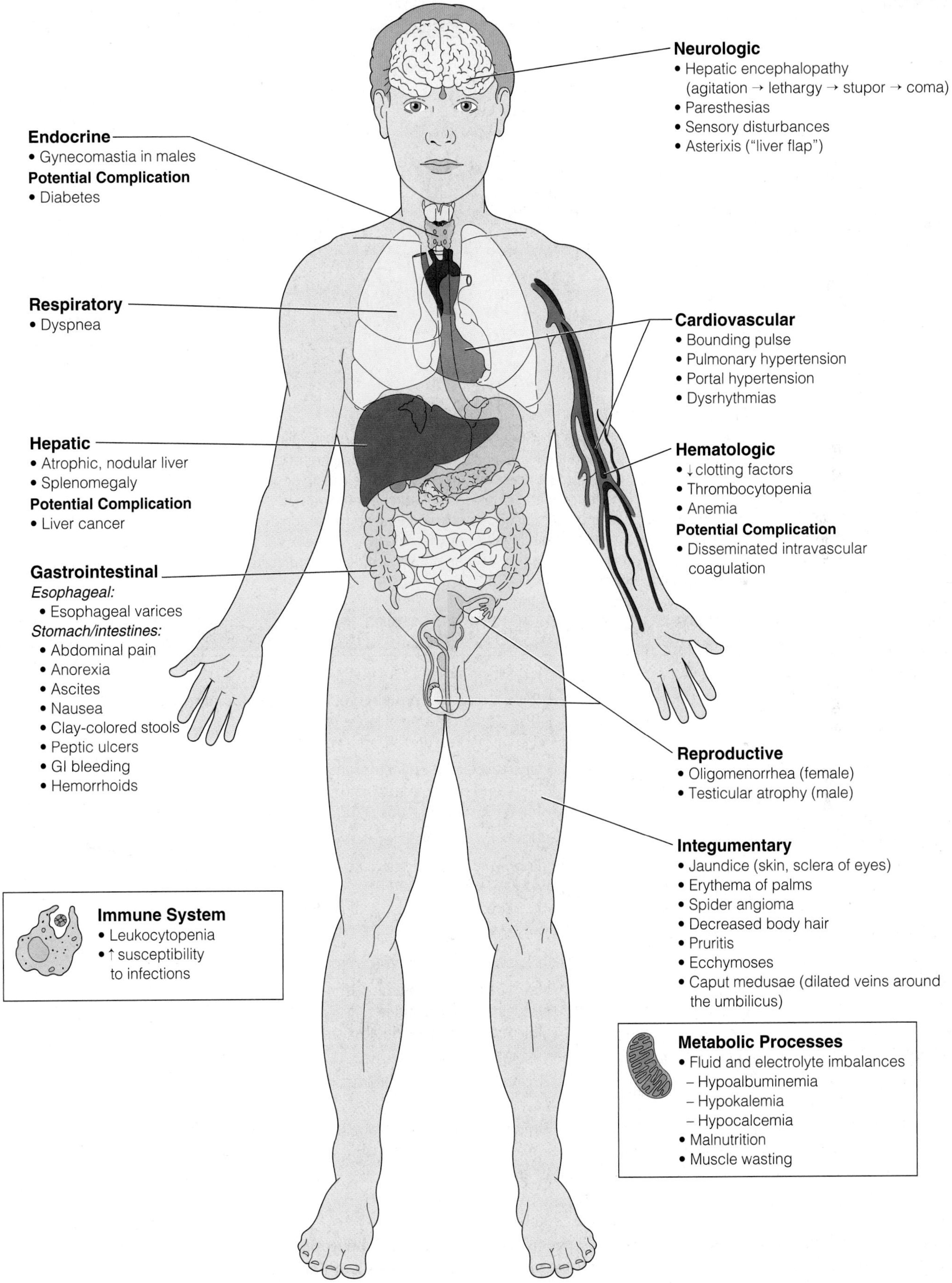
Neurologic
• Hepatic encephalopathy (agitation → lethargy → stupor → coma)
• Paresthesias
• Sensory disturbances
• Asterixis ("liver flap")
Endocrine
• Gynecomastia in males
Potential Complication
• Diabetes
Respiratory
• Dyspnea
Cardiovascular
• Bounding pulse
• Pulmonary hypertension
• Portal hypertension
• Dysrhythmias
Hepatic
• Atrophic, nodular liver
• Splenomegaly
Potential Complication
• Liver cancer
Hematologic
• ↓ clotting factors
• Thrombocytopenia
• Anemia
Potential Complication
• Disseminated intravascular coagulation
Gastrointestinal
Esophageal:
• Esophageal varices
Stomach/intestines:
• Abdominal pain
• Anorexia
• Ascites
• Nausea
• Clay-colored stools
• Peptic ulcers
• GI bleeding
• Hemorrhoids
Reproductive
• Oligomenorrhea (female)
• Testicular atrophy (male)
Integumentary
• Jaundice (skin, sclera of eyes)
• Erythema of palms
• Spider angioma
• Decreased body hair
• Pruritis
• Ecchymoses
• Caput medusae (dilated veins around the umbilicus)
Immune System
• Leukocytopenia
• ↑ susceptibility to infections
Metabolic Processes
• Fluid and electrolyte imbalances
– Hypoalbuminemia
– Hypokalemia
– Hypocalcemia
• Malnutrition
• Muscle wasting

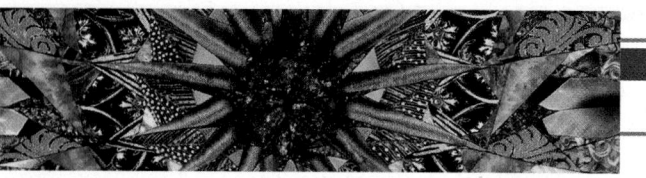

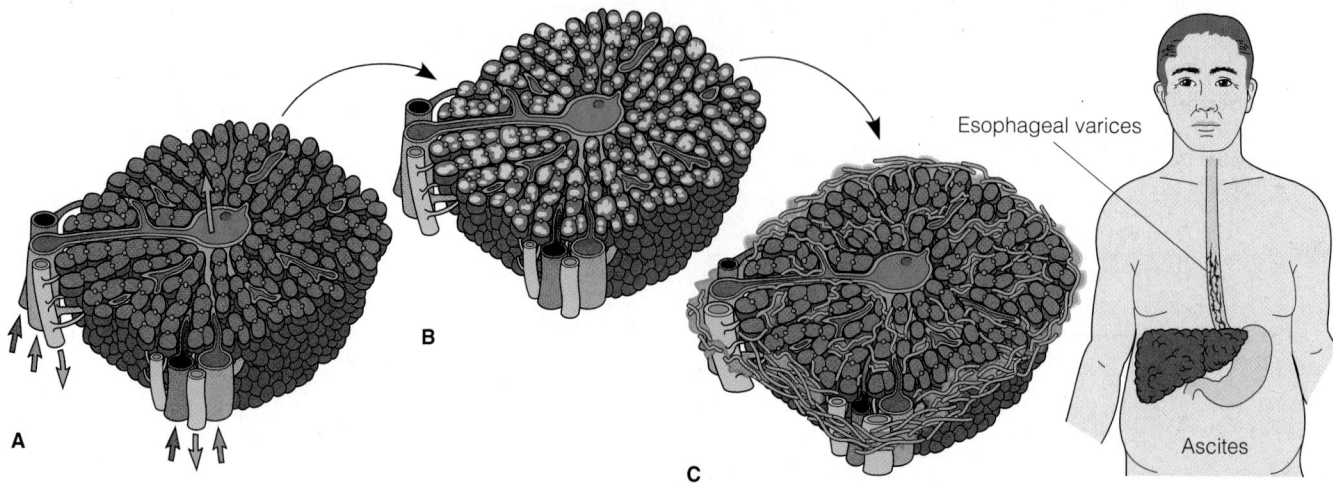

*A.* The portal vein (draining the capillary beds of the gut) provides 75% of the liver's blood supply; the hepatic artery provides the remainder. Venous and arterial blood mixes as it flows through the sinusoids and into the central hepatic vein, and from there into the inferior vena cava. *B.* Long-standing liver cell necrosis (from chronic infection, toxins such as alcohol, or obstructed bile flow) eventually overwhelms the liver's regenerative capacity, leading to fibrosis and scarring. Isolated hepatocytes continue to regenerate, forming nodules amongst the fibrous scar tissue. *C.* These nodules and scar tissue restrict blood flow through the liver, increasing pressure and congestion in the portal venous system. Blood is diverted into lower pressure collateral vessels, which become engorged, forming visible surface veins, hemorrhoids, and esophageal varices. Esophageal varices push the mucosa into its lumen, increasing the risk for trauma and bleeding due to food roughage or gastric reflux.

## Manifestations of Cirrhosis with Underlying Cause

| MANIFESTATION | UNDERLYING PATHOPHYSIOLOGY |
|---|---|
| Edema, ascites | • Impaired plasma protein synthesis (hypoalbuminemia)<br>• Disrupted hormone balance and fluid retention<br>• Increased pressure in portal venous system |
| Bleeding, bruising | • Decreased clotting factor synthesis<br>• Increased platelet destruction by enlarged spleen<br>• Impaired vitamin K absorption and storage |
| Esophageal varices, hemorrhoids | • Increased pressure in portal venous system with collateral vessel development |
| Gastritis, anorexia, diarrhea | • Engorged veins in gastrointestinal system<br>• Alcohol ingestion<br>• Impaired bile synthesis and fat absorption |
| Abdominal wall vein distention (caput medusae) | • Portal hypertension |
| Jaundice | • Impaired bilirubin metabolism and excretion |
| Malnutrition, muscle wasting | • Impaired nutrient metabolism<br>• Impaired fat absorption<br>• Impaired hormone metabolism |
| Anemia, leukopenia, increased risk for infection | • Bleeding<br>• Increased blood cell destruction by spleen |
| Asterixis, encephalopathy | • Accumulated metabolic toxins<br>• Impaired ammonia metabolism and excretion |
| Gynecomastia, infertility, impotence | • Altered sex hormone metabolism |

*Hyperaldosteronism,* an increase in aldosterone, causes sodium and water retention, contributing to ascites and generalized edema. See the box above for selected manifestations of cirrhosis and their underlying pathophysiology.

## Esophageal Varices

**Esophageal varices** are enlarged, thin-walled veins that form in the submucosa of the esophagus. See the *Pathophysiology Illustration* feature above. These collateral vessels form when blood

| BOX 22–4 | ■ Factors Precipitating Hepatic Encephalopathy |
| --- | --- |

- High serum ammonia level
- Constipation
- Blood transfusions
- Gastrointestinal bleeding
- Medications: sedatives, tranquilizers, narcotic analgesics, anesthetics
- Hypoxia
- High-protein diet
- Severe infection
- Surgery

is shunted from the portal system due to portal hypertension. The thin-walled varices may rupture, causing massive hemorrhage; even eating high-roughage foods can precipitate bleeding. Thrombocytopenia, platelet deficiency, and impaired production of clotting factors by the liver contribute to the risk for hemorrhage.

## Hepatic Encephalopathy

**Hepatic encephalopathy** results from accumulation of neurotoxins in the blood. Ammonia, a by-product of protein metabolism, contributes to hepatic encephalopathy. Ammonium ion is produced as proteins and amino acids are broken down by bacteria in the intestinal tract. Normally, the ammonia produced is then converted by the liver to urea before entering the general circulation. As functional liver tissue is destroyed, ammonia can no longer be converted to urea, and it accumulates in the blood. Other nervous system depressants, such as narcotics and tranquilizers, can contribute to hepatic encephalopathy. Box 22–4 lists selected precipitating factors for hepatic encephalopathy. *Asterixis* (liver flap), a flapping tremor of the hands when the arms are extended, is an early sign. Changes in personality and mentation develop; agitation, restlessness, impaired judgment, and slurred speech also are early manifestations of hepatic encephalopathy. As it progresses, confusion, disorientation, and incoherence develop. Deep coma is the final stage of hepatic encephalopathy.

## Hepatorenal Syndrome

Although the cause is unclear, renal failure with azotemia (excess nitrogenous waste products in the blood), sodium retention, oliguria, and hypotension may develop in clients with advanced cirrhosis and ascites. The syndrome may be precipitated by gastrointestinal bleeding, aggressive diuretic therapy, or by an unknown cause (Braunwald et al., 2001).

## COLLABORATIVE CARE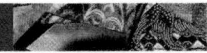

Care for the client with cirrhosis is holistic, addressing physiologic, psychosocial, and spiritual needs. The importance of including the family in the plan of care cannot be overemphasized, particularly if alcohol abuse is identified as the cause. Treatment includes medications to help regulate protein metabolism, maintenance of fluid and electrolyte balance, and supportive therapies, including treatment of underlying problems, such as malnutrition, anemia, bleeding, encephalopathy, renal failure, and infections.

## Diagnostic Tests

Studies to confirm the diagnosis of cirrhosis and identify its cause and effects are performed. Diagnostic tests may include the following:

- *Liver function studies* include *ALT, AST, alkaline phosphatase,* and *gamma-glutamyl transferase (GGT).* All may be elevated in cirrhosis, but usually not as severely as in acute hepatitis. Elevations in these enzymes may not correlate well with the extent of liver damage in cirrhosis.
- *CBC with platelets* is done. A low RBC count, hemoglobin, and hematocrit demonstrate anemia related to bone marrow suppression, increased RBC destruction, bleeding, and deficiencies of folic acid and vitamin $B_{12}$. Platelets are low, related to increased destruction by the spleen. Leukopenia (low WBC count) also relates to splenomegaly.
- *Coagulation studies* show a prolonged prothrombin time due to impaired production of coagulation proteins and lack of vitamin K.
- *Serum electrolytes* are measured. Hyponatremia is common, due to hemodilution. Hypokalemia, hypophosphatemia, and hypomagnesemia also are frequently seen, related to malnutrition and altered renal excretion of these electrolytes.
- *Bilirubin* levels are usually elevated in severe cirrhosis, including both direct (conjugated) and indirect (unconjugated) bilirubin.
- *Serum albumin* levels show hypoalbuminemia due to impaired liver production.
- *Serum ammonia* levels are elevated, as the liver fails to effectively convert ammonia to urea for renal excretion.
- *Serum glucose* and *cholesterol* levels frequently are abnormal in clients with cirrhosis.
- *Abdominal ultrasound* is performed to evaluate liver size, detect ascites, and identify liver nodules. Ultrasound may be used in conjunction with *doppler studies* to evaluate blood flow through the liver and spleen (Tierney et al., 2001).
- *Esophagascopy* (upper endoscopy) may be done to determine the presence of esophageal varices.
- *Liver biopsy* is not always necessary to diagnose cirrhosis, but may be done to distinguish cirrhosis from other forms of liver disease. See the box on page 590 for nursing implications for a client having a liver biopsy. Figure 22–3 ■ shows the site and position for liver biopsy. Biopsy may be deferred if the bleeding time is prolonged (such as a prothrombin time [PT] greater than 3 seconds over the control).

## Medications

Medications are used to treat the complications and effects of cirrhosis; they do not reverse or slow the process of cirrhosis itself. Known hepatotoxic drugs and alcohol are avoided, as are drugs metabolized by the liver (e.g., barbiturates, sedatives, hypnotics, and acetaminophen). Several groups of drugs are commonly prescribed. See the Medication Administration box on page 591 for nursing responsibilities and client teaching for commonly used drugs in clients with cirrhosis.

- Diuretics reduce fluid retention and ascites. Spironolactone (Aldactone) is frequently the drug of first choice because it

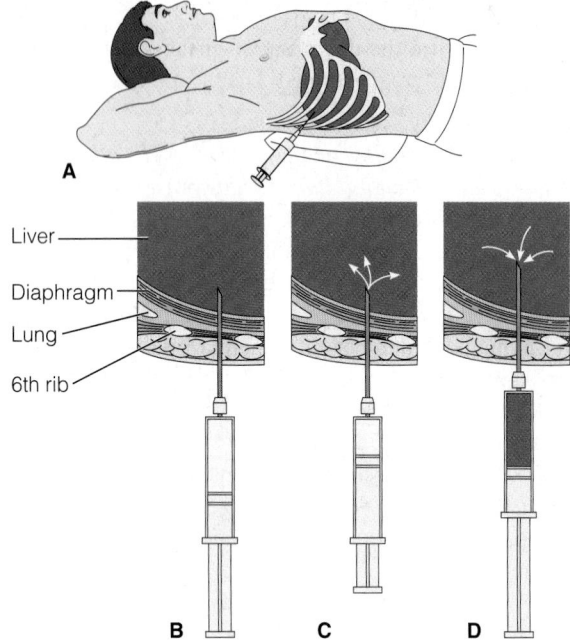

Liver

Diaphragm

Lung

6th rib

A

B          C          D

**Figure 22–3 ■** Liver biopsy. *A,* The client exhales completely, then holds his or her breath. This brings the liver and diaphragm to their highest position. *B,* The biopsy needle is inserted into the liver. *C,* Approximately 1 mL of saline is injected to clear the needle of blood and tissue. *D,* The needle is advanced, and a tissue sample is aspirated. Pressure is applied to the site immediately after the needle is withdrawn. The specimen is sent to the laboratory for analysis.

addresses one of the causes of ascites—increased aldosterone levels. If additional diuresis is necessary, a loop diuretic such as furosemide (Lasix) may be added to the regimen.

- Medications to reduce the nitrogenous load and lower serum ammonia levels are added when manifestations of hepatic encephalopathy develop. Two commonly administered medications are lactulose and neomycin. Both exert their effects locally, in the bowel. Lactulose reduces the number of ammonia-forming organisms in the bowel and increases the acidity of colon contents, converting ammonia into ammonium ion. Ammonium ion is not absorbable, and is excreted in the feces. Neomycin sulfate is a locally acting antibiotic that also reduces the number of ammonia-forming bacteria in the bowel.
- The beta-blocker nadolol (Corgard) may be given together with isosorbide mononitrate (Ismo, Imdur, Monoket) to prevent rebleeding of esophageal varices. This drug combination also lowers hepatic venous pressure.
- Ferrous sulfate and folic acid are given as indicated to treat anemia. Vitamin K may be ordered to reduce the risk of bleeding. When bleeding is acute, packed red blood cells, fresh frozen plasma, or platelets may be administered to restore blood components and promote hemostasis.
- Antacids are prescribed as indicated. A drug regimen to treat *H. pylori* infection may also be effective (see Chapter 21).
- Oxazepam (Serax), a benzodiazepine antianxiety/sedative drug, is not metabolized by the liver, and may be used to treat acute agitation.

## Nursing Implications for Diagnostic Tests
### Liver Biopsy

#### Preparation of Client
- Review chart for signed consent form.
- Withhold food and fluids per policy, usually 4 to 6 hours preprocedure.
- Assess and record baseline vital signs.
- Review prothrombin time (PT) and platelet count; administer vitamin K as ordered.
- Instruct to empty bladder immediately before the biopsy.
- Place in supine position on far right side of bed; turn head to left and extend right arm above head to improve access to the biopsy site.

#### Client and Family Teaching
- Discuss preparation for the biopsy and expected sensations during the procedure.
- Hold your breath following expiration during needle insertion to keep diaphragm and liver high and stabilized in the abdominal cavity.
- Obtaining the tissue sample usually requires only 10 to 15 seconds; there may be some pain or discomfort during this time.
- Direct pressure is applied to the site immediately after the needle is removed; you will be placed on your right side to maintain site pressure.
- You may develop pain in the right shoulder as the anesthetic loses effect.
- You will be monitored for bleeding after the procedure.
- Food and fluids are withheld for 2 hours after the biopsy; you then can resume your usual diet.
- Avoid coughing, lifting, or straining for 1 to 2 weeks.

## Treatments

Treatment of cirrhosis is supportive, directed at slowing the progression to liver failure and reducing complications.

### Dietary and Fluid Management
Dietary support is an essential part of care for the client with cirrhosis. Dietary needs change as hepatic function fluctuates.

- Sodium intake is restricted to under 2 g/day, and fluids are restricted as necessary to reduce ascites and generalized edema. Fluids are often limited to 1500 mL/day. Fluid needs are calculated based on response to diuretic therapy, urine output, and serum electrolyte values.
- Unless serum ammonia levels are high, a palatable diet with adequate calories and 75 to 100 g of protein per day is recommended. If hepatic encephalopathy is present, protein is restricted to 60 to 80 g/day (Tierney et al., 2001). When encephalopathy resolves and serum ammonia levels stabilize, protein intake is allowed as tolerated. The diet is high is calories and includes moderate fat intake to promote healing. Parenteral nutrition is used as needed to maintain nutritional status when food intake is limited.
- Vitamin and mineral supplements are ordered based on laboratory values. Deficiencies in the B-complex vitamins, particularly thiamin, folate, and B$_{12}$, and the fat-soluble vita-

## Medication Administration

### The Client with Cirrhosis

#### DIURETICS

Spironolactone (Aldactone)          Furosemide (Lasix)

Spironolactone is a potassium-sparing diuretic that competes with aldosterone. It reduces ascites by increasing renal excretion of fluid and decreasing aldosterone levels. Furosemide is a loop diuretic that promotes the excretion of potassium. Drugs may be given in combination if serum potassium level permits.

#### Nursing Responsibilities

- Monitor ECG, serum potassium, BUN, creatinine levels, and hydration status.
- Weigh daily.
- Carefully monitor intake and output.
- Monitor for signs of hyperkalemia if taking spironolactone alone: bradycardia; widening QRS, spiking T waves, or ST segment depression on ECG, diarrhea; and muscle twitching.
- Assess for hyponatremia: confusion, lethargy, apprehension.

#### Client and Family Teaching

- Maintain diet and fluid restrictions as prescribed.
- Report increases in weight or edema.
- Immediately report signs of hyponatremia, hyperkalemia, or hypokalemia (see Chapter 5).
- Expect increased urinary output; take medications in morning hours to avoid nocturia.

#### LAXATIVES

Lactulose (Cephulac, Chronulac)

Lactulose is a disaccharide laxative that is not absorbed by the gastrointestinal tract. It reduces the number of ammonia producing bacteria and lowers the pH in the colon. The lower pH (increased acidity) converts ammonia to ammonium ion, a nonabsorbable form that is excreted in the feces. Lactulose also pulls water into the bowel lumen, increasing the number of daily stools.

#### Nursing Responsibilities

- Assess bowel sounds and abdominal girth.
- Maintain accurate stool chart.
- Adjust dose to achieve two to three soft stools per day.
- Monitor electrolytes and hydration.

#### Client and Family Teaching

- Drink adequate fluids.
- Report diarrhea; if present, decrease dose.
- This drug may cause nausea. Continue taking the drug; taking it with crackers or a soft drink may reduce nausea.

#### ANTI-INFECTIVE AGENTS

Neomycin sulfate (Neo Tabs)

Neomycin sulfate is a nonsystemic aminoglycoside antibiotic that reduces intestinal bacteria and decreases ammonia production in the bowel lumen. The drug may be administered as an oral or rectal preparation.

#### Nursing Responsibilities

- Monitor hearing, renal, and neurologic functions. Drug is ototoxic, nephrotoxic, and neurotoxic.
- Prior to administration, check for previous hypersensitivity reaction.
- Monitor intake and output.
- Monitor BUN and creatinine levels.
- If the client is taking digitalis, monitor levels; oral neomycin interferes with its absorption.

#### Client and Family Teaching

- Report dizziness, tinnitus (ringing in ears), hearing loss, headaches, tremors, or vision changes immediately.
- Keep follow-up appointments.
- Maintain fluids, avoid dehydration. (Teach signs of dehydration.)

---

mins A, D, and E are common. These vitamins may need to be administered in a water-soluble form. Clients with alcohol-induced cirrhosis are at high risk for magnesium deficiency, which needs to be replaced.

### Complication Management

**Paracentesis,** aspiration of fluid from the peritoneal cavity, may be a diagnostic or a therapeutic procedure. It may be done therapeutically to relieve severe ascites that does not respond to diuretic therapy. The goal of paracentesis is to relieve respiratory distress caused by excess fluid in the abdomen. Ascites fluid may be withdrawn in moderate amounts of 500 mL to 1 L daily to reduce the risk of fluid and electrolyte imbalances. Large-volume paracentesis, withdrawal of 4 to 6 L of fluid at one time, may be used. Albumin is often administered intravenously during large volume paracentesis to maintain intravascular volume as the pressure of the ascites fluid in the abdomen is relieved. Nursing implications for the client undergoing paracentesis are listed in the box on page 592. Figure 22–4 ■ shows insertion sites and client positioning during paracentesis.

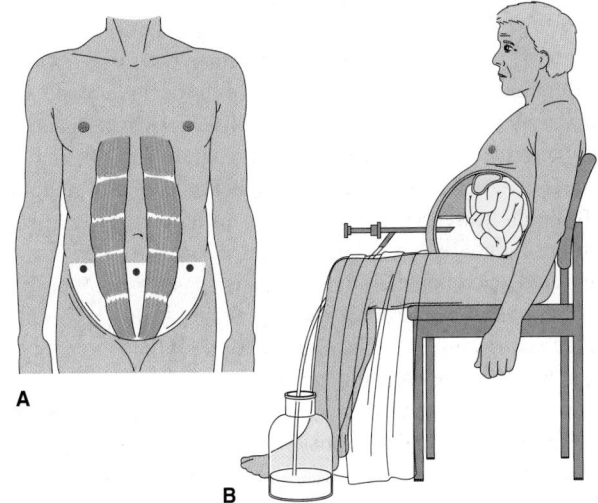

**Figure 22–4** ■ Sites and position for paracentesis. *A,* Potential sites of needle or trocar insertion to avoid abdominal organ damage. *B,* The client sits comfortably; in this position, the intestines float back and away from the insertion site.

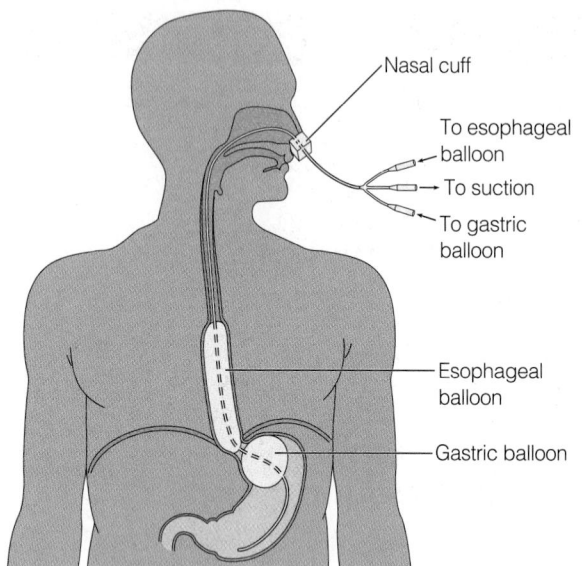

**Figure 22–5** ■ Triple-lumen nasogastric tube (Sengstaken-Blakemore) used to control bleeding esophageal varices.

Bleeding esophageal varices are life threatening and require intensive care management. Restoration of hemodynamic stability is the first priority. A central line is inserted and central venous and pulmonary artery pressures are monitored (see Chapter 30). ⏤ Blood is given to restore blood volume, and fresh frozen plasma may be administered to restore clotting factors. Somatostatin or octreotide, drugs that constrict blood vessels in the gut, are given intravenously to reduce blood flow in the portal venous system. Vasopressin, a drug that produces generalized vasoconstriction, also may be used.

When the blood pressure and cardiac output have stabilized, upper endoscopy is performed to evaluate and treat the varices. A large nasogastric tube is inserted prior to endoscopy, and **gastric lavage** (irrigation of the stomach with large quantities of normal saline) is performed to improve visualization. During endoscopy, the varices may be banded or sclerosed to reduce the risk of recurrent bleeding. In *banding (variceal ligation),* small rubber bands are placed on varices to occlude blood flow. *Endoscopic sclerosis* involves injecting a sclerosing agent directly into the varices to induce inflammation and clotting. See Chapter 21 ⏤ for the nursing implications of endoscopy.

**Balloon tamponade** of bleeding varices may be used if bleeding cannot be controlled through vasoconstriction or if endoscopy is unavailable. A multiple-lumen nasogastric tube (such as a Sengstaken-Blakemore tube or a Minnesota tube) is inserted, and the gastric and esophageal balloons are inflated to apply direct pressure on the bleeding varices (Figure 22–5 ■). Tension is applied to the tube to further compress the varices. Balloon tamponade carries a number of risks, including aspiration, airway obstruction, and tissue ischemia and necrosis. An endotracheal tube is inserted prior to nasogastric intubation to support the airway and reduce the risk of aspiration. This short-term measure is used only until more definitive treatment can be done.

**Transjugular intrahepatic portosystemic shunt (TIPS)** is used to relieve portal hypertension and its complications of

esophageal varices and ascites. A channel is created through the liver tissue using a needle inserted transcutaneously (Figure 22–6 ■). An expandable metal stent is inserted into this channel, to allow blood to flow directly from the portal vein into the hepatic vein, bypassing the cirrhotic liver. The shunt relieves pressure in esophageal varices and allows better control of fluid retention with diuretic therapy. Stenosis and occlusion of the shunt are frequent complications. TIPS also increases the risk of developing hepatic encephalopathy (due to decreased perfusion of the liver and impaired ammonia metabolism) and may reduce long-term survival. It generally is used as a short-term measure until liver transplant is performed.

### Surgery

**Liver transplantation** is indicated for some clients with irreversible, progressive cirrhosis. A decline in functional status, increasing bilirubin levels, falling albumin levels, and increasing problems with complications that respond poorly to treatment are indications for liver transplantation. Malignancy, active alcohol or drug abuse, and poor surgical risk are contraindications for the surgery. See the box on the next page for nursing care of the client having a liver transplant.

## NURSING CARE

### Health Promotion

For most clients, high-risk behaviors are the risk factors for cirrhosis. With all clients (including children and young adults), stress the relationship between alcohol and drug abuse and liver disorders. While many clients tolerate alcohol use in

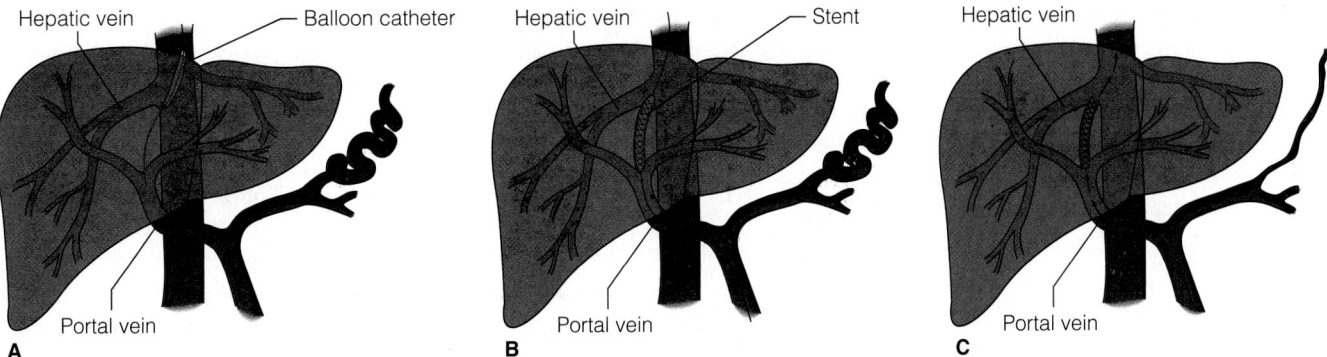

**Figure 22–6** ■ Transjugular intrahepatic portosystemic shunt (TIPS). *A,* Guided by angiography, a balloon catheter inserted via the jugular vein is advanced to the hepatic veins and through the substance of the liver to create a portacaval (portal vein-to-vena cava) channel. *B,* A metal stent is positioned into the channel, and expanded by inflating the balloon. *C,* The stent remains in place after the catheter is removed, creating a shunt for blood to flow directly from the portal vein into the hepatic vein.

## NURSING CARE OF THE CLIENT UNDERGOING LIVER TRANSPLANTATION

### PREOPERATIVE CARE

- Obtain a complete nursing history and physical examination. *A complete preoperative nursing assessment provides baseline data for comparison after surgery.*
- Provide routine preoperative care as ordered (see Chapter 7). *Preoperative care is similar to that provided for other clients undergoing major surgery.*
- Discuss preoperative and postoperative expectations with the client and family. Introduce to the intensive care unit, and discuss anticipated drainage tubes and supportive measures in the immediate postoperative period. Provide information about visiting policies and family accommodations (if available). *Preoperative teaching helps relieve anxiety in the client and family members. Clients return from surgery to an intensive care or specialized care unit. Restrictions on the number of visitors and the time they may spend with the client are common.*
- Once a donor liver is located, check for evidence of infection; if no infection is present, begin preoperative antibiotics as ordered. *An acute or chronic infection may contraindicate liver transplantation as drugs given postoperatively to suppress rejection of the transplanted organ also impair the ability to fight infection.*

### POSTOPERATIVE CARE

- Provide routine postoperative care as outlined in Chapter 7.
- Maintain airway and ventilatory support until awake and alert. *Until the new liver clears the anesthesia, the client requires measures to support respirations and ventilation.*
- Monitor temperature and implement rewarming measures (such as warming blankets, heating lamps, and head covers) as indicated. *The client often is hypothermic after liver transplant, necessitating careful rewarming while maintaining hemodynamic stability.*
- Frequently monitor hemodynamic pressures, including arterial blood pressure, central venous pressure, and pulmonary artery pressures. *Postoperative fluid volume status may be difficult to determine without careful pressure measurements. The rate and type of fluids administered are determined by hemodynamic status.*

- Monitor urine output hourly; maintain careful intake and output records. Weigh daily. *Urine output and weight provide additional information about fluid volume status. In addition, renal function may be altered after liver transplant; acute renal failure is a significant risk. See Chapter 27 for more information about acute renal failure and its management.*
- Monitor for signs of active bleeding, including excess drainage, increasing abdominal girth, bloody nasogastric drainage, black tarry stools, tachypnea, tachycardia, diminished peripheral pulses, or pallor. Report immediately. *Altered coagulation in the early postoperative period increases the risk for bleeding. Blood products to replace volume and clotting factors may be necessary.*
- Monitor serum electrolytes and laboratory values related to blood coagulation, liver function, and renal function. Report abnormal results or significant changes immediately. *Electrolyte imbalances are common postoperatively. Altered liver or renal function tests may indicate rejection of the transplanted liver or acute renal failure. Other early signs of transplant rejection include fever, a drop in bile output, or a change in bile color and viscosity (Urden, Stacy, & Lough, 2002).*
- Monitor neurologic status. *With good function of the transplanted organ, mental status should clear within days of the transplant.*
- Provide discharge teaching:
  a. Teach how to reduce risk of infection, and signs of infection to report.
  b. Instruct to recognize and report signs of organ rejection.
  c. Discuss all medications, including their purpose, schedule, adverse effects, and potential long-term effects. Stress the importance of complying with all prescribed medications and postoperative precautions for the remainder of the client's life.
  d. Discuss possible changes in body image and psychologic responses to receiving a transplanted organ. Refer to a counselor or support group as indicated.
  e. Refer for home health services for continued assessment and teaching.
  f. Stress importance of continued follow-up with transplant team and primary care provider.

moderation with no adverse effects on the liver, excess alcohol use is the leading cause of cirrhosis. Injection drug use also is a significant risk factor, increasing the risk for contracting blood-borne hepatitis (B, C, or D). These types of viral hepatitis can lead to chronic hepatitis and, ultimately, to cirrhosis. Discuss abstinence or safer sex practices as another measure to prevent viral hepatitis and potential liver damage.

## Assessment

Assessment data related to cirrhosis includes the following:

- Health history: current manifestations, including abdominal pain or discomfort, recent weight loss, weakness, and anorexia; altered bowel elimination; excess bleeding or bruising; abdominal distension; jaundice, pruritus; altered libido or impotence; duration of symptoms; history of liver or gallbladder disease; pattern and extent of alcohol or injection drug use; use of other prescription and nonprescription drugs.
- Physical assessment: vital signs; mental status; color and condition of skin and mucous membranes; peripheral pulses and presence of peripheral edema; abdominal assessment including appearance, shape and contour, bowel sounds, abdominal girth, percussion for liver borders, and palpation for tenderness and liver size.

## Nursing Diagnoses and Interventions

Nursing care of the client with cirrhosis presents many challenges because liver function affects all body systems. The nurse is responsible for coordinating care among care providers. Many nursing diagnoses may apply. The diagnoses discussed in this section focus on problems with fluid and electrolyte balance, altered thought processes, risk for bleeding, skin integrity, and nutrition.

### Excess Fluid Volume

Cirrhosis affects water and salt regulation due to portal hypertension, hypoalbuminemia, and hyperaldosteronism. Signs of fluid volume overload and portal hypertension may develop: ascites, peripheral edema, internal hemorrhoids and varices, and prominent abdominal wall veins. Careful monitoring is necessary, as treatment measures can lead to further fluid and electrolyte imbalances.

- Weigh daily. Assess for jugular vein distention, measure abdominal girth daily, and check for peripheral edema. Monitor intake and output. *Careful assessment is important to detect fluid shifts.*
- Assess urine specific gravity. *Specific gravity measures the concentration of urine, an indicator of hydration.*

**PRACTICE ALERT** *Monitor the client with cirrhosis for signs of impaired renal function, such as oliguria, a fixed specific gravity of about 1.012, central edema (around the eyes and of the face), and increasing serum creatinine and BUN levels. Such signs may indicate hepatorenal syndrome or acute renal failure from another cause.* ■

- Provide a low-sodium diet (500 to 2000 mg/day) and restrict fluids as ordered. *Excess sodium leads to water retention, and can increase fluid volume, ascites, and portal hypertension.*

### Disturbed Thought Processes

Accumulated nitrogenous waste products and other metabolites affect mental status and thought processes. Effects of hepatic encephalopathy can range from mild confusion to agitation to coma.

- Assess neurologic status, including level of consciousness and mental status. Observe for signs of early encephalopathy: changes in handwriting, speech, and asterixis. *Early identification of evidence of encephalopathy allows prompt intervention—subtle changes in neurologic functioning are important!*

**PRACTICE ALERT** *Closely monitor clients who have experienced gastrointestinal bleeding for signs of hepatic encephalopathy. Blood in the intestinal tract is digested as a protein, increasing serum ammonia levels and the risk for hepatic encephalopathy.* ■

- Avoid factors that may precipitate hepatic encephalopathy. Avoid hepatotoxic medications and CNS depressant drugs. *Cautious use of medications and close monitoring can eliminate iatrogenic causes of encephalopathy.*
- If possible, plan for consistent nursing care assignments. *Consistent care providers facilitate early identification of subtle neurologic changes indicative of hepatic encephalopathy.*
- Provide low-protein diet as prescribed; teach the family the importance of maintaining diet restrictions. *Nitrogenous by-products from dietary protein increase serum ammonia levels.*
- Administer medications or enemas as ordered to reduce nitrogenous products. Monitor bowel function and provide measures to promote regular elimination and prevent constipation. *Oral or rectally administered (per enema) medications are ordered to reduce intestinal bacteria and the ammonia they produce. Regular bowel elimination promotes protein and ammonia elimination in the feces.*
- Orient to surroundings, person, and place; provide simple explanations and reassurance. *Modification of verbal interactions to level of understanding and mental status may reduce anxiety and agitation.*

### Ineffective Protection

Impaired coagulation, esophageal varices, and possible acute gastritis place the client with cirrhosis at significant risk for hemorrhage. Clotting is altered by vitamin K deficiency, impaired manufacture of coagulation factors II, VII, IX, and X, and increased platelet destruction due to splenomegaly.

- Monitor vital signs; report tachycardia or hypotension. *Increased pulse and decreasing blood pressure may indicate hypovolemia due to hemorrhage.*
- Institute bleeding precautions (see Box 22–5). *Preventive measures can decrease the risk for active bleeding.*
- Monitor coagulation studies and platelet count. Report abnormal results. *Coagulation studies help determine the risk for bleeding and the need for treatment.*
- Carefully monitor the client who has had bleeding esophageal varices for evidence of rebleeding: hematemasis,

## BOX 22–5 ■ Bleeding Precautions

- Prevent constipation.
- Avoid rectal temperatures or enemas.
- Avoid injections; if needed, use small-gauge needle and apply gentle pressure.
- Monitor platelet count, PT, and PTT.
- Assess for ecchymotic areas and areas of purpura.
- Apply pressure to bleeding sites. After venipuncture, apply direct pressure for at least 5 minutes.
- Use only a soft toothbrush.
- Avoid blowing nose.
- Assess oral cavity for bleeding gums.

hematochezia (bright blood in the stool) or tarry stools, signs of hypovolemia or shock. *Rebleeding is common following variceal hemorrhage, especially within the first week.*

**PRACTICE ALERT** *Carefully monitor the respiratory status of the client with a Sengstaken-Blakemore or Minnesota tube. Displacement of the tube can obstruct the airway unless an endotracheal tube is in place. The esophageal balloon prevents the client from swallowing oral secretions, increasing the risk for aspiration. Keep the head of the bed elevated to 45 degrees to reduce the risk of aspiration and promote gas exchange.* ■

### Impaired Skin Integrity

Severe jaundice with bile salt deposits on the skin may cause pruritus. Scratching related to the pruritus damages the skin and impairs its integrity. Malnutrition, particularly protein deficiency, and edema also increase the risk for tissue breakdown and impaired skin integrity.

- Use warm water rather than hot water when bathing. *Hot water increases pruritus.*
- Use measures to prevent dry skin: Apply an emollient or lubricant as needed to keep skin moist, avoid soap or preparations with alcohol, and do not rub the skin. *Dry skin contributes to pruritus.*

- If indicated, apply mittens to the hands to prevent scratching. *Clients with encephalopathy may not understand the need to refrain from scratching.*
- Institute measures to prevent skin and tissue breakdown: Turn at least every 2 hours, use an alternating pressure mattress, and frequently assess skin condition. *Frequent position changes relieve pressure and promote circulation and tissue oxygenation.*
- Administer prescribed antihistamine (to relieve pruritus) cautiously. *Decreased liver function increases the risk for altered drug responses.*

### Imbalanced Nutrition: Less than Body Requirements

The client with cirrhosis is at risk for malnutrition for a number of reasons: possible chronic alcohol use, anorexia, impaired vitamin and mineral absorption, and impaired protein metabolism. In addition, salt and protein restrictions may make the diet less palatable and appealing to the client.

- Weigh daily. Instruct to weigh at least weekly at home. *Weight is a good indicator of both nutritional status and fluid balance. Short-term weight fluctuations tend to reflect fluid balance, while longer-term changes in weight are more reflective of nutritional status.*
- Provide small meals with between meal snacks. *A small meal is more appealing for an anorexic client. Between-meal snacks help maintain adequate calorie and nutrient intake.*
- Unless protein is restricted due to impending hepatic encephalopathy, promote protein and nutrient intake by providing nutritional supplements such as Ensure or Instant Breakfast. *The sodium and protein content of all meals and snacks must be calculated when maintaining restrictions of these nutrients.*
- Arrange for consultation with a dietitian for diet planning while hospitalized and at home. *The dietitian can provide detailed instructions, sample menus, and suggestions for improving the palatability of the diet and promoting intake.*

### Using NANDA, NIC, and NOC

Chart 22–3 shows links between NANDA nursing diagnoses, NIC, and NOC for the client with cirrhosis.

## CHART 22–3 LINKAGES BETWEEN NANDA, NIC, AND NOC

### The Client with Cirrhosis

| NURSING DIAGNOSES | NURSING INTERVENTIONS | NURSING OUTCOMES |
|---|---|---|
| • Disturbed Thought Processes | • Reality Orientation<br>• Environmental Management: Safety | • Cognitive Orientation<br>• Neurological Status: Consciousness |
| • Fatigue | • Energy Management | • Energy Conservation |
| • Ineffective Health Maintenance | • Self-Responsibility Facilitation | • Health-Promoting Behavior |
| • Ineffective Protection | • Bleeding Precautions | • Coagulation Status |
| • Risk for Impaired Skin Integrity | • Skin Surveillance | • Tissue Integrity: Skin and Mucous Membranes |

*Data from Nursing Outcomes Classification (NOC) by M. Johnson & M. Maas (Eds.), 1997, St. Louis: Mosby; Nursing Diagnoses: Definitions & Classification 2001–2002 by North American Nursing Diagnosis Association, 2001, Philadelphia: NANDA; Nursing Interventions Classification (NIC) by J.C. McCloskey & G. M. Bulechek (Eds.), 2000, St. Louis: Mosby. Reprinted by permission.*

## Nursing Care Plan
## A Client with Alcoholic Cirrhosis

Richard Wright is a 48-year-old divorced father of two teenagers. Mr. Wright has been admitted to the community hospital with ascites and malnutrition. He has had three previous hospital stays for cirrhosis, the most recent 6 months ago.

### ASSESSMENT

Mr. Wright is lethargic but responds appropriately to verbal stimuli. He complains of "spitting up blood the past week or so" and says, "I'm just not hungry." He has lost 20 lb (9 kg) since his previous admission. He is jaundiced and has petechiae and ecchymoses on his arms and legs. Liz Mowdi, Mr. Wright's nurse, notes pitting pretibial edema. Abdominal assessment reveals a tight, protuberant abdomen with caput medusae. The liver margin is not palpable; the spleen is enlarged. Vital signs are T 100°F (37.7°C), P 110, R 24, and BP 110/70.

Abnormal laboratory results include WBC 3700/mm$^3$ (normal 4300 to 10,800/mm$^3$); RBC 4.0 million/mm$^3$ (normal 4.6 to 5.9 million/mm$^3$); platelets 75,000/mm$^3$ (normal 150,000 to 350,000/mm$^3$); serum ammonia 105 μm/dL (normal 35 to 65 μm/dL); total bilirubin 4.9 μg/dL (normal 0.1 to 1.0 μg/dL); and serum sodium 150 mEq/L (normal 135 to 145 mEq/L). Potassium, hemoglobin, hematocrit, total protein, and albumin levels are markedly decreased. Hepatic enzymes are elevated. Blood urea nitrogen and creatinine levels are marginally elevated. Oxygen saturation (O$_2$ sat) is 88% (normal range: 96% to 100%) per pulse oximetry.

Endoscopy shows bleeding from gastric ulcer, and the diagnosis of alcoholic cirrhosis with gastritis is made. Mr. Wright is started on Aldactone, 25 mg PO q8h; Riopan, 30 mL 2 hr p.c. and hs; lactulose, 30 mL q h until onset of diarrhea, then 15 mL t.i.d.; and low-protein, 800 mg sodium diet; fluid restriction of 1500 mL/day.

### DIAGNOSES

- *Impaired gas exchange* related to pressure of ascites fluid on the diaphragm as manifested by tachypnea and decreased oxygen saturation
- *Excess fluid volume* related to electrolyte imbalance and hypoalbuminemia as manifested by ascites and peripheral edema
- *Imbalanced nutrition: less than body requirements* related to anorexia and possible alcohol abuse manifested by weight loss and low serum protein levels
- *Disturbed thought processes* related to effects of high ammonia levels as manifested by lethargy
- *Ineffective protection* related to impaired platelet formation and malnutrition

### EXPECTED OUTCOMES

- Respiratory rate and O$_2$ sats will be within normal limits.
- Abdominal girth will decrease by 1 to 2 cm per day; peripheral edema will decrease.
- Will gain 1 lb (0.45 kg) per week without evidence of increased fluid retention. Serum albumin levels will return to normal range.
- Will be alert and oriented; serum ammonia levels are within normal range.
- Will demonstrate no further evidence of active bleeding.
- Will verbalize willingness to join a community support group.

### PLANNING AND IMPLEMENTATION

- Weigh daily.
- Provide high-calorie, low-salt, low-protein diet with between-meal snacks.
- Maintain stool chart.
- Assign same nurses to care as much as possible to facilitate evaluation of mental status. Promptly report changes in status or laboratory values.
- Measure abdominal girth every 8 hr, marking level of measurement.
- Institute bleeding precautions.
- Elevate head of bed; assist to chair with legs elevated t.i.d. as tolerated.
- Include significant others in care and teaching; refer to community agencies for discharge follow-up.

### EVALUATION

A week after admission, Mr. Wright's ascites has decreased and no further active bleeding is noted. His serum protein levels have increased, and his laboratory values are improving. No further bruising is noted during hospitalization. Although he shows a 5 lb weight loss as excess water is eliminated, he is consuming 100% of his diet. His serum ammonia levels have returned to normal. On discharge, O$_2$ sat is 96%; respirations are 18. Lactulose will be continued on discharge.

Ms. Mowdi provides both written and verbal information about the medication and cirrhosis, including measures to prevent complications. Mr. Wright and his children express interest in Alcoholics Anonymous and Al Anon and are referred to those agencies. Prior to discharge, follow-up appointments are made with a psychiatric social worker and a primary caregiver.

### Critical Thinking in the Nursing Process

1. Describe the relationship between portal hypertension, liver dysfunction, and ascites.
2. Outline a 1-day menu for a low-protein, low-sodium high-calorie diet.
3. What is the pathophysiologic basis for hepatic encephalopathy? What are the nursing responsibilities related to lactulose and neomycin?
4. Design a nursing care plan for Mr. Wright for the diagnosis *Ineffective coping*.

See Evaluating Your Response in Appendix C.

## Home Care

Cirrhosis is a chronic, progressive disease. As such, the client and family assume major roles in managing the disease and its manifestations and in preventing complications. Teaching topics for home care include:

- The absolute necessity of avoiding alcohol and other hepatotoxic drugs. Suggest in-patient or community-based alcohol treatment programs and Alcoholics Anonymous as indicated.
- Diet and fluid intake restrictions and recommendations. Include suggestions to promote nutritional intake and increase the flavor of food when sodium is restricted.
- Prescribed medications; their timing, intended and adverse effects, and manifestations to report to the primary care provider.
- Bleeding precautions (see Box 22–5).
- Manifestations of potential complications to be reported to the primary care provider. Stress the importance of promptly reporting evidence of gastrointestinal bleeding for prompt intervention for potential hemorrhage.
- Skin care techniques to reduce pruritus and the risk of damage.
- Ways to manage fatigue and conserve energy.

Provide referrals for home health services, dietary consultation, social services, and counseling as needed by the client and family. Suggest local support groups where available. If appropriate, suggest hospice services for the client with end-stage liver disease.

## THE CLIENT WITH CANCER OF THE LIVER

Primary liver cancer is uncommon in the United States, accounting for only 0.5% to 2% of all cancers (Porth, 2002). It is, however, a common malignancy worldwide. Hepatocellular carcinoma is common in parts of Asia and Africa, where the incidence is as high as 500 cases per 100,000 people. This higher incidence is linked to chronic hepatitis B or C infection. The incidence of primary liver cancer is higher in men than it is in women. It typically develops in the fifth or sixth decade of life (Braunwald et al., 2001). The prognosis for primary liver cancer is poor, in part because the disease often is advanced at the time of diagnosis. Metastasis to the liver from primary tumors of the lung, breast, and gastrointestinal tract are relatively common.

## PATHOPHYSIOLOGY

About 80% to 90% of primary hepatic cancers arise from the liver's parenchymal cells (hepatocellular carcinoma); the remainder form in the bile ducts (cholangiocarcinoma). Regardless of the origin, the progress of the disease is similar. Several etiologic factors have been identified (Box 22–6). Most primary liver cancer in the United States is related to alcoholic cirrhosis, HBV, or HCV.

The underlying pathophysiology of primary liver cancer is damage to hepatocellular DNA. This damage may be caused by integration of HBV or HCV into the DNA or by repeated cycles of cell necrosis and regeneration that facilitate DNA mutations. HBV and aflatoxins damage a specific tumor sup-

### BOX 22–6 ■ Suspected Causes of Primary Liver Cancer

- Chronic hepatitis C infection
- Chronic hepatitis B infection
- Cirrhosis, regardless of type
- Chronic aflatoxin (a toxin produced by *Aspergillus* molds) exposure
- Arsenic-contaminated water
- Carcinogens in food
- Possible hormonal factors (e.g., long-term use of androgens)

pressor gene, p53. Tumors may be limited to one specific area, may occur as nodules throughout the liver, or may develop as surface infiltrates. The tumor interferes with normal hepatic function, leading to biliary obstruction and jaundice, portal hypertension, and metabolic disruptions (hypoalbuminemia, hypoglycemia, and bleeding disorders). It also may secrete bile products and produce hormones (paraneoplastic syndrome) that may lead to polycythemia, hypoglycemia, and hypercalcemia (Bullock & Henze, 2000). Tumors usually grow rapidly and metastasize early.

## MANIFESTATIONS

Initial manifestations of liver cancer develop insidiously and often are masked by the presence of cirrhosis or chronic hepatitis. Weakness, anorexia, weight loss, fatigue, and malaise are common early manifestations. Abdominal pain and a palpable mass in the right upper quadrant are common presenting symptoms. See the box below for manifestations of primary liver cancer. Ascites and jaundice may be present at diagnosis. Signs of liver failure with portal hypertension, splenomegaly, and altered metabolism develop as the tumor progresses. Most clients die within 6 months of the diagnosis (Porth, 2002).

## COLLABORATIVE CARE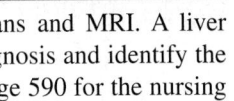

Liver tumors are identified by CT scans and MRI. A liver biopsy may be done to confirm the diagnosis and identify the tumor type or origin. See the box on page 590 for the nursing implications of liver biopsy. Serum αfetoprotein (AFP) levels, normally low in nonpregnant adults, rise in most clients with hepatocellular cancer.

### Manifestations of Primary Liver Cancer

- Malaise
- Anorexia
- Lethargy
- Weight loss
- Fever of unknown origin
- Feeling of abdominal fullness
- Painful right upper quadrant mass
- Manifestations of liver failure

Small, localized tumors may be surgically resected, offering the only viable chance for cure. Most tumors, however, have spread extensively or have distant metastasis at the time of diagnosis, so this is frequently not an option. Liver transplantation may be done; however, the tumor may recur in the transplanted organ.

Radiation therapy is used to shrink the tumor, decreasing pressure on surrounding organs and reducing pain. Chemotherapy may be used as primary treatment or adjunctive therapy. Direct continuous hepatic arterial infusion with an implanted pump has shown promise in prolonging survival rates. See Chapter 10 for nursing care for clients receiving radiation therapy or chemotherapy. ⚭

## NURSING CARE

Encourage clients with risk factors for primary liver cancer to avoid alcohol and other substances that may further damage the liver. Urge them to discuss regular screening for liver tumors (such as serum AFP levels) with their primary care physician.

Both the client and the family need extensive nursing support. Controlling pain is a priority. Because of the poor prognosis, early referral for hospice services may be appropriate.

Nursing diagnoses, interventions, and teaching for the client with liver cancer are similar to those for clients with cirrhosis.

## THE CLIENT WITH LIVER TRAUMA

Blunt or penetrating trauma to the abdomen can damage the liver. Liver trauma is frequently seen in combination with injuries to other abdominal organs. Motor vehicle crashes, stab or gunshot wounds, and iatrogenic sources such as liver biopsy are among the causes of these injuries.

## PATHOPHYSIOLOGY

Liver trauma generally causes bleeding due to the vascularity of the organ. Liver injury may cause a surface hematoma, hematoma within the liver parenchyma, laceration of liver tissue, or disruption of vessels leading to or from the liver. Severe bleeding can rapidly disrupt hemodynamic stability and lead to shock.

### PRACTICE ALERT
*Bleeding due to liver trauma may not be immediately apparent. Instruct the client with apparent or potential liver trauma to immediately report light-headedness, rapid heart rate, shortness of breath, thirst, or increasing abdominal pain.* ∎

## COLLABORATIVE CARE

*Diagnostic peritoneal lavage* is often used along with CT scan to diagnose liver trauma. The procedure is performed by making a small abdominal incision into the peritoneum (after the bladder has been emptied), and inserting a small catheter into the peritoneal cavity. If blood is immediately detected, the client is taken directly to surgery for abdominal exploration. If frank bleeding is not apparent, a liter of isotonic fluid is instilled into the abdomen, then drained and sent for laboratory analysis.

Intravenous fluids, fresh frozen plasma, platelets, and other clotting factors are administered to restore blood volume and promote hemostasis. Hemodynamic status is closely monitored; continued instability may indicate a need for surgical intervention to control hemorrhage. Postoperative nursing care focuses on preventing pulmonary complications, such as atelectasis, and detecting and preventing infection.

## NURSING CARE

Nursing care of the client with liver trauma focuses on fluid management and other supportive care related to shock. Keeping family members informed is an important aspect of care, especially during the period of client instability. Diagnoses include the following:

- *Deficient fluid volume* related to hemorrhage
- *Risk for infection* related to wound or abdominal contamination
- *Ineffective protection* related to impaired coagulation

## THE CLIENT WITH LIVER ABSCESS

Liver abscesses usually are bacterial or amebic (protozoal) in origin. Bacterial abscesses may follow trauma or surgical procedures, including biopsy. Multiple or single abscesses occur most commonly in the right lobe. Amebic abscesses most frequently occur following infestation of the liver by *Entamoeba histolytica*. Amebic infestation is associated with poor hygiene, unsafe sexual practices, or travel in areas where drinking water is contaminated.

## PATHOPHYSIOLOGY

Following bacterial or amebic invasion of the liver, healthy tissue is destroyed, leaving an area of necrosis, inflammatory exudate, and blood. This damaged region becomes walled off from the healthy liver tissue. Pyogenic (bacterial) liver abscess may be caused by cholangitis, or distant or intra-abdominal infections, such as peritonitis or diverticulitis. *Escherichia coli* is the most frequently identified causative organism. The onset of pyogenic abscess is usually sudden, causing acute symptoms such as fever, malaise, vomiting, hyperbilirubinemia, and pain in the right upper abdomen.

The infection pathway for amebic hepatic abscesses usually is the portal venous circulation from the right colon. Generally, the onset of amebic abscess is insidious.

## COLLABORATIVE CARE

Hepatic abscess is diagnosed through biopsy, hepatic aspirate, blood and fecal cultures, and CT scan and ultrasound studies. Therapy is based on identifying the causative organism through laboratory cultures. Pyogenic abscesses are treated with antibiotics to which the causitive organism is sensitive.

Pharmacologic agents used for amebic hepatic abscess are the same as those used for intestinal amebic infestation (see Chapter 24); combination therapy is commonly used. Two commonly used drugs for treating amebic liver abscesses are metronidazole (Flagyl) and iodoquinol (Diquinol). Both medications can cause gastrointestinal symptoms. Bone marrow suppression is a risk with metronidazole.

If the abscess does not respond to antibiotic therapy, percutaneous aspiration or surgical drainage may be done. In these procedures, a *percutaneous closed-catheter drain* is placed in the abscess to promote drainage of purulent material.

## NURSING CARE

A major aspect of nursing care is prevention; teaching clients to avoid contaminated water and foods is especially important. Nursing interventions include teaching hikers to treat water and food handlers to wash hands thoroughly.

Clients who have a liver abscess require supportive care to prevent dehydration from the accompanying fever, nausea, vomiting, and anorexia. Careful monitoring of fluid and electrolyte status is indicated, as are comfort measures for abdominal pain. Possible nursing diagnoses include the following:

- *Risk for deficient fluid volume,* related to effects of prolonged fever and vomiting
- *Deficient knowledge* about transmission of amebic abscess
- *Activity intolerance,* related to pain and weakness

# EXOCRINE PANCREAS DISORDERS

The pancreas is both an exocrine and an endocrine gland. It is made up of two basic cell types, each having different functions. The exocrine cells produce enzymes that empty through ducts into the small intestine, whereas the endocrine cells produce hormones that enter the bloodstream directly. Disorders of the exocrine pancreas affect the secretion and glandular control of digestive enzymes, whereas disorders of the endocrine pancreas affect the production of hormones necessary for normal carbohydrate, protein, and fat metabolism. Disorders of the exocrine pancreas are discussed in this section of the chapter; diabetes mellitus, a disorder of the endocrine pancreas, is discussed in Chapter 18. ○○

## THE CLIENT WITH PANCREATITIS

**Pancreatitis,** or inflammation of the pancreas, is characterized by release of pancreatic enzymes into the tissue of the pancreas itself, leading to hemorrhage and necrosis. Pancreatitis may be either acute or chronic. About 5000 new cases of acute pancreatitis are diagnosed every year in the United States. It is a serious disease, with a mortality rate of approximately 10% (Braunwald et al., 2001). Alcoholism and gallstones are the primary risk factors for acute pancreatitis.

The incidence of chronic pancreatitis is less clear, because many people with chronic pancreatitis do not have classic manifestations of the disease. Clients with pancreatitis may have long-term effects of the disease, with chronic changes in enzyme and hormone production.

## PHYSIOLOGY REVIEW

Knowledge of the normal structure and functions of the exocrine pancreas is important to understand how inflammation affects it and the client. The exocrine pancreas consists of lobules of acinar cells. The acinar cells secrete digestive enzymes and fluids (pancreatic juices) into ducts that empty into the main pancreatic duct (the duct of Wirsung). The pancreatic duct joins the common bile duct and empties into the duodenum through the ampulla of Vater (in some people the main pancreatic duct empties directly into the duodenum). The epithelial lining of the pancreatic ducts secretes water and bicarbonate to modify the composition of the pancreatic secretions. Pancreatic enzymes are secreted primarily in an inactive form and are activated in the intestine, a modification that prevents digestion of pancreatic tissue by its own enzymes (Porth, 2002). The pancreatic enzymes, with related functions, are as follows:

- Proteolytic enzymes, including trypsin, chymotrypsin, carboxypolypeptidase, ribonuclease, and deoxyribonuclease, which break down dietary proteins
- Pancreatic amylase, which breaks down starch
- Lipase, which breaks down fats into glycerol and fatty acids

## PATHOPHYSIOLOGY

### Acute Pancreatitis

Acute pancreatitis is an inflammatory disorder that involves self-destruction of the pancreas by its own enzymes through autodigestion. The milder form of acute pancreatitis, *interstitial edematous pancreatitis,* leads to inflammation and edema of pancreatic tissue. It often is self-limiting. The more severe form, *necrotizing pancreatitis,* is characterized by inflammation, hemorrhage, and ultimately necrosis of pancreatic tissue. Acute pancreatitis is more common in middle adults; its incidence is higher in men than in women. Acute pancreatitis is usually associated with gallstones in women and with alcoholism in men. Some clients recover completely, others experience recurring attacks, and still others develop chronic pancreatitis. The mortality and symptoms depend on the severity and type of pancreatitis: With mild pancreatic edema, mortality is low (6%); with severe necrotic pancreatitis, the mortality rate is high (23%) (Porth, 2002).

Although the exact cause of pancreatitis is not known, the following factors may activate pancreatic enzymes within the pancreas, leading to autodigestion, inflammation, edema, and/or necrosis.

- Gallstones may obstruct the pancreatic duct or cause bile reflux, activating pancreatic enzymes in the pancreatic duct system.
- Alcohol causes duodenal edema, and may increase pressure and spasm in the sphincter of Oddi, obstructing pancreatic outflow. It also stimulates pancreatic enzyme production, thus raising pressure within the pancreas.

Other factors associated with acute pancreatitis include tissue ischemia or anoxia, trauma or surgery, pancreatic tumors, third-trimester pregnancy, infectious agents (viral, bacterial, or parasitic), elevated calcium levels, and hyperlipidemia. Some medications have been linked with this disorder, including thiazide diuretics, estrogen, steroids, salicylates, and nonsteroidal anti-inflammatory drugs (NSAIDs). Regardless of the precipitating factor, the pathophysiologic process begins with the release of activated pancreatic enzymes into pancreatic tissue. Activated proteolytic enzymes, trypsin in particular, digest pancreatic tissue and activate other enzymes such as phospholipase A, which digests cell membrane phospholipids, and elastase, which digests the elastic tissue of blood vessel walls. This leads to proteolysis, edema, vascular damage and hemorrhage, and necrosis of parenchymal cells. Cellular damage and necrosis releases activated enzymes and vasoactive substances that produce vasodilation, increase vascular permeability, and cause edema. A large volume of fluid may shift from circulating blood into the retroperitoneal space, the peripancreatic spaces, and the abdominal cavity.

## Manifestations

Acute pancreatitis develops suddenly, with an abrupt onset of continuous severe epigastric and abdominal pain. This pain commonly radiates to the back and is relieved somewhat by sitting up and leaning forward. The pain often is initiated by a fatty meal or excessive alcohol intake.

Other manifestations include nausea and vomiting; abdominal distention and rigidity; decreased bowel sounds; tachycardia; hypotension; elevated temperature; and cold, clammy skin. Within 24 hours, mild jaundice may appear. Retroperitoneal bleeding may occur 3 to 6 days after the onset of acute pancreatitis; signs of bleeding include bruising in the flanks (Turner's sign) or around the umbilicus (Cullen's sign). See the Manifestations box on this page.

## Complications

Systemic complications of acute pancreatitis include intravascular volume depletion with acute tubular necrosis and renal failure (see Chapter 27 ⊙⊃ for more information about acute renal failure), and acute respiratory distress syndrome (ARDS). Acute renal failure usually develops within 24 hours after the

### Manifestations of Acute and Chronic Pancreatitis

**ACUTE PANCREATITIS**
- Abrupt onset of severe epigastric and LUQ pain, may radiate to back
- Nausea, vomiting; fever
- Decreased bowel sounds; abdominal distention and rigidity
- Tachycardia, hypotension; cold, clammy skin
- Possible jaundice
- Positive Turner's sign (flank ecchymosis) or Cullen's sign (periumbilical ecchymosis)

**CHRONIC PANCREATITIS**
- Recurrent epigastric and LUQ pain, radiates to back
- Anorexia, nausea and vomiting, weight loss
- Flatulence, constipation
- Steatorrhea

onset of acute pancreatitis. Manifestations of ARDS may be seen 3 to 7 days after its onset, particularly in clients who have experienced severe volume depletion. See Chapter 36 for more information about ARDS.

Localized complications include pancreatic necrosis, abscess, pseudocysts, and pancreatic ascites. Pancreatic necrosis causes an inflammatory mass which may be infected. It may lead to shock and multiple organ failure. A pancreatic abscess may form late in the course of the disease (6 or more weeks after its onset), causing an epigastric mass and tenderness (Tierney et al., 2001). Pancreatic pseudocysts, encapsulated collections of fluid, may develop both within the pancreas itself and in the abdominal cavity. They may impinge on other structures, or may rupture, causing generalized peritonitis. Rupture of a pseudocyst or of the pancreatic duct can lead to pancreatic ascites. Pancreatic ascites is recognized by gradually increasing abdominal girth and persistent elevation of the serum amylase level without abdominal pain.

## Chronic Pancreatitis

Chronic pancreatitis is characterized by gradual destruction of functional pancreatic tissue. In contrast to acute pancreatitis, which may completely resolve with no long-term effects, chronic pancreatitis is an irreversible process that eventually leads to pancreatic insufficiency. Alcoholism is the primary risk factor for chronic pancreatitis in the United States. Malnutrition is a major worldwide risk factor. About 10% to 20% of chronic pancreatitis is idiopathic, with no identified cause. A genetic mutation on a gene associated with cystic fibrosis may play a role in these cases. Children or young adults with cystic fibrosis may develop chronic pancreatitis as well.

In chronic pancreatitis related to alcoholism, pancreatic secretions have an increased concentration of insoluble proteins. These proteins calcify, forming plugs that block pancreatic ducts and the flow of pancreatic juices. This blockage leads to inflammation and fibrosis of pancreatic tissue. In other cases, a stricture or stone may block pancreatic outflow, causing chronic obstructive pancreatitis. In chronic pancreatitis, recurrent episodes of inflammation eventually lead to fibrotic changes in the parenchyma of the pancreas, with loss of exocrine function. This leads to malabsorption from pancreatic insufficiency. If endocrine function is disrupted as well, clinical diabetes mellitus may develop.

## Manifestations and Complications

Chronic pancreatitis typically causes recurrent episodes of epigastric and left upper abdominal pain that radiates to the back. This pain may last for days to weeks. As the disease progresses, the interval between episodes of pain becomes shorter. Other manifestations include anorexia, nausea and vomiting, weight loss, flatulence, constipation, and **steatorrhea** (fatty, frothy, foul-smelling stools caused by a decrease in pancreatic enzyme secretion). See page 600.

Complications of chronic pancreatitis include malabsorption, malnutrition, and possible peptic ulcer disease. Pancreatic pseudocyst or abscess may form, or stricture of the common bile duct may develop. Diabetes mellitus may develop, and there is an increased risk for pancreatic cancer. Narcotic addiction related to frequent, severe pain episodes is common.

## COLLABORATIVE CARE

Acute pancreatitis often is a mild, self-limiting disease. Treatment focuses on reducing pancreatic secretions and providing supportive care. Treatment to eliminate the causative factor is begun after the acute inflammatory process resolves. Severe necrotizing pancreatitis may require intensive care management. Treatment for chronic pancreatitis often focuses on managing pain and treating malabsorption and malnutrition.

## Diagnostic Tests

The laboratory tests that may be ordered when pancreatitis is suspected are summarized in Table 22–4. Diagnostic studies include the following:

- *Ultrasonography* can identify gallstones, a pancreatic mass, or pseudocyst.
- *Computed tomography (CT) scan* may be ordered to identify pancreatic enlargement, fluid collections in or around the pancreas, and perfusion deficits in areas of necrosis.
- *Endoscopic retrograde cholangiopancreatography (ERCP)* may be performed to diagnose chronic pancreatitis and to differentiate inflammation and fibrosis from carcinoma.
- *Endoscopic ultrasonography* can detect changes indicative of chronic pancreatitis in the pancreatic duct and parenchyma.
- *Percutaneous fine-needle aspiration biopsy* may be performed to differentiate chronic pancreatitis from cancer of the pancreas; the cells that are aspirated are examined for malignancy.

## Medications

The treatment of acute pancreatitis is largely supportive. Narcotic analgesics such as morphine sulfate are used to control pain. Antibiotics often are prescribed to prevent or treat infection.

Clients with chronic pancreatitis also require analgesics, but are closely monitored to prevent drug dependence. Narcotics are avoided when possible. Pancreatic enzyme supplements are given to reduce steatorrhea (see the Medication Administration box on page 602). $H_2$ blockers such as cimetidine (Tagamet) and ranitidine (Zantac), and proton-pump inhibitors such as omeprazole (Prilosec) may be given to neutralize or decrease gastric secretions. Octreotide (Sandostatin), a synthetic hormone, suppresses pancreatic enzyme secretion and may be used to relieve pain in chronic pancreatitis.

## Fluid and Dietary Management

Oral food and fluids are withheld during acute episodes of pancreatitis to reduce pancreatic secretions and promote rest of the organ. A nasogastric tube may be inserted and connected to suction. Intravenous fluids are administered to maintain vascular volume, and total parenteral nutrition (TPN) is initiated. Oral food and fluids are begun once the serum amylase levels

| TABLE 22–4 | Laboratory Tests in Exocrine Pancreatic Disorders | |
|---|---|---|
| **Test** | **Normal Value** | **Significance** |
| Serum amylase | 25 to 125 U/L | Rises within 2 to 12 hours of onset of acute pancreatitis to 2 to 3 times normal. Returns to normal in 3 to 4 days. |
| Serum lipase | <200 U/L | Levels rise in acute pancreatitis; remains elevated for 7 to 14 days. |
| Serum trypsinogen | <80 µg/L | Elevated in acute pancreatitis; may be decreased in chronic pancreatitis. |
| Urine amylase | 4 to 37 U/L/2h | Urine amylase levels rise in acute pancreatitis. |
| Serum glucose | 70 to 110 mg/dL | May be transient elevation in acute pancreatitis. |
| Serum bilirubin | 0.1 to 1.0 mg/dL | Compression of the common duct may increase bilirubin levels in acute pancreatitis. |
| Serum alkaline phosphatase | 30 to 95 U/L | Compression of the common duct may increase levels in acute pancreatitis. |
| Serum calcium | 8.9 to 10.3 mg/dL or 4.5 to 5.5 mEq/L | Hypocalcemia develops in up to 25% of clients with acute pancreatitis. |
| White blood cells | 4500/mm³ to 10,000/mm³ | Leukocytosis indicates inflammation and is usually present in acute pancreatitis. |

## Medication Administration

### The Client with Chronic Pancreatitis

**PANCREATIC ENZYME REPLACEMENT**

Pancrelipase (Lipancreatin)

Pancrelipase enhances the digestion of starches and fats in the gastrointestinal tract by supplying an exogenous source of the enzymes protease, amylase, and lipase. The drug promotes nutrition and decreases the number of bowel movements.

**Nursing Responsibilities**
- Assess for allergy to pork protein.
- Monitor frequency and consistency of stools.
- Weigh every other day. Record weights.

- Give with meals; if not enteric coated, $H_2$ antagonists or antacids may be given concurrently to prevent destruction of the enzymes by hydrochloric acid.
- Monitor for side effects: rash, hives, respiratory difficulty, hematuria, hyperuricemia, or joint pain.

**Client and Family Teaching**
- Take with meals or snacks.
- If medicine is enteric coated, do not crush, chew, or mix with alkaline foods (e.g., milk, ice cream)
- Be sure to follow prescribed diet.

---

have returned to normal, bowel sounds are present, and pain disappears. A low-fat diet is ordered, and alcohol intake is strictly prohibited.

### Surgery

If the pancreatitis is the result of a gallstone lodged in the sphincter of Oddi, an *endoscopic transduodenal sphincterotomy* may be performed to remove the stone. When cholelithiasis is identified as a causative factor, a cholecystectomy is performed once the acute pancreatitis has resolved. Surgical procedures to promote drainage of pancreatic enzymes into the duodenum or resection of all or part of the pancreas may be done to provide pain relief in clients with chronic pancreatitis. Large pancreatic pseudocysts may be drained endoscopically or surgically.

### Complementary Therapies

Several complementary therapies may be used in conjunction with traditional treatments for clients with acute or chronic pancreatitis. Fasting or use of low-salt, low-fat vegetarian diets may reduce episodes of recurrent pain. Qigong, a system of gentle exercise, meditation, and controlled breathing, is believed to balance the flow of qi (a vital life force) through the body. Qigong lowers the metabolic rate, and may reduce the stimulation of pancreatic enzyme secretion. Magnetic field therapy also may be employed for clients with pancreatitis. All complementary therapies should be prescribed by a trained and competent practitioner.

## NURSING CARE

### Health Promotion

Teach clients who abuse alcohol about the risk for developing pancreatitis. Advise abstinence to reduce this risk, and refer to an alcohol treatment program or Alcoholics Anonymous.

### Assessment

Assessment data related to acute or chronic pancreatitis include the following:

- Health history: current manifestations; abdominal pain (location, nature, onset and duration, identified precipitating

factors); anorexia, nausea or vomiting; flatulence, diarrhea, constipation, or stool changes; recent weight loss; history of previous episodes or gallstones; alcohol use (extent and duration); current medications
- Physical assessment: vital signs including orthostatic vitals and peripheral pulses; temperature; skin temperature and color, presence of any flank or periumbilical ecchymoses; abdominal assessment including bowel sounds, presence of distention, tenderness, or guarding

### Nursing Diagnoses and Interventions

Nursing care for the client with acute pancreatitis focuses on managing pain, nutrition, and maintaining fluid balance.

### Pain

Obstruction of pancreatic ducts and inflammation, edema, and swelling of the pancreas caused by pancreatic autodigestion cause severe epigastric, left upper abdominal, or midscapular back pain. The pain often is accompanied by nausea and vomiting, abdominal tenderness, and muscle guarding.

- Using a standard pain scale (see Chapter 4 ⊂⊃ ), assess pain, including location, radiation, duration, and character. Note nonverbal cues of pain: restlessness or remaining rigidly still; tense facial features; clenched fists; rapid, shallow respirations; tachycardia; and diaphoresis. Administer analgesics on a regular schedule. *Pain assessment before and after analgesic administration measures its effectiveness. Administering analgesics on a regular schedule prevents pain from becoming established, severe, and difficult to control. Unrelieved pain has negative consequences; for example, pain, anxiety, and restlessness may increase pancreatic enzyme secretion.*

**PRACTICE ALERT** *Regularly assess respiratory status (at least every 4 to 8 hours), including respiratory rate, depth, and pattern; breath sounds; oxygen saturation and arterial blood gas results. Report tachypnea, adventitious or absent breath sounds, oxygen saturation levels below 92%, $PaO_2$ <70 mmHg or $PacO_2$ >45 mmHg. Severe abdominal pain causes shallow respirations and hypoventilation, and suppresses cough effectiveness, which can lead to pooling of secretions, atelectasis, and pneumonia.* ■

- Maintain nothing by mouth (NPO) status and nasogastric tube patency as ordered. *Gastric secretions stimulate hormones that stimulate pancreatic secretion, aggravating pain. Eliminating oral intake and maintaining gastric suction reduces gastric secretions. Nasogastric suction also decreases nausea, vomiting, and intestinal distention.*
- Maintain bed rest in a calm, quiet environment. Encourage use of nonpharmacologic pain management techniques such as meditation and guided imagery. *Decreasing physical movement and mental stimulation decreases metabolic rate, gastrointestinal secretion, pancreatic secretions, and resulting pain. Adjunctive pain relief measures enhance the effectiveness of analgesics (see Chapter 4).*
- Assist to a comfortable position, such as a side-lying position with knees flexed and head elevated 45 degrees. *Sitting up, leaning forward, or lying in a fetal position tend to decrease pain caused by stretching of the peritoneum by edema and swelling.*
- Remind family and visitors to avoid bringing food into the client's room. *The sight or smell of food may stimulate secretory activity of the pancreas through the cephalic phase of digestion.*

## Imbalanced Nutrition:
## Less Than Body Requirements

The effects of pancreatitis and its treatment may result in malnutrition. Inflammation increases metabolic demand and frequently causes nausea, vomiting, and diarrhea. At a time of increased metabolic demand, NPO status and gastric suction further decrease available nutrients. In the client with chronic pancreatitis, loss of digestive enzymes affects the digestion and use of nutrients.

- Monitor laboratory values: serum albumin, serum transferrin, hemoglobin, and hematocrit. *Serum albumin, serum transferrin (which transports iron in the blood), hemoglobin, and hematocrit levels are decreased in malnutrition. Decreased pancreatic enzymes affect protein catabolism and absorption; decreased transferrin affects iron absorption and transport, thereby decreasing hematocrit and hemoglobin levels.*
- Weigh daily or every other day. *Short-term weight changes (over hours to days) accurately reflect fluid balance, whereas weight changes over days to weeks reflect nutritional status.*
- Maintain stool chart; note frequency, color, odor, and consistency of stools. *Protein and fat metabolism are impaired in pancreatitis; undigested fats are excreted in the stool. Steatorrhea indicates impaired digestion and, possibly, an increase in the severity of pancreatitis.*
- Monitor bowel sounds. *The return of bowel sounds indicates return of peristalsis; nasogastric suction usually is discontinued within 24 to 48 hours thereafter.*
- Administer prescribed intravenous fluids and/or TPN. *Intravenous fluids are given to maintain hydration. TPN is used to provide fluids, electrolytes, and kilocalories when fasting is prolonged (more than 2 to 3 days).*
- Provide oral and nasal care every 1 to 2 hours. *Fasting and nasogastric suction increase the risk for mucous membrane irritation and breakdown.*

- When oral intake resumes, offer small, frequent feedings. Provide oral hygiene before and after meals. *Oral hygiene decreases oral microorganisms that can cause foul odor and taste, decreasing appetite. Small, frequent feedings reduce pancreatic enzyme secretion and are more easily digested and absorbed.*

## Risk for Deficient Fluid Volume

Acute pancreatitis can lead to a fluid shift from the intravascular space into the abdominal cavity (third spacing). Third spacing of fluid may cause hypovolemic shock, affecting cardiovascular function, respiratory function, renal function, and mental status.

- Assess cardiovascular status every 4 hours or as indicated, including vital signs, cardiac rhythm, hemodynamic parameters (central venous and pulmonary artery pressures); peripheral pulses and capillary refill; skin color, temperature, moisture, and turgor. *These measurements are indicative of fluid volume status and are used to monitor response to treatment. Stable values are as follows: heart rate less than 100; blood pressure within 10 mmHg of baseline; central venous pressure 0 to 8 mmHg; pulmonary wedge pressure 8 to 12 mmHg; cardiac output approximately 5 L/min; and skin warm, dry, with good turgor and color. (See Chapter 6 for a full discussion of hypovolemic shock.)*
- Monitor renal function. Obtain hourly urine output; report if less than 30 mL per hour. Weigh daily. *Urine output of less than 30 mL per hour indicates decreased renal perfusion or acute renal failure, a major complication of acute pancreatitis. Weight changes are an effective indicator of fluid volume status.*
- Monitor neurologic function, including mental status, level of consciousness, and behavior. *Hypotension and hypoxemia may decrease cerebral perfusion, causing changes in mental status, decreased level of consciousness, and changes in behavior. In addition, alcohol withdrawal is a risk in the client with acute pancreatitis.*

## Using NANDA, NIC, and NOC

Chart 22–4 shows links between NANDA nursing diagnoses, NIC, and NOC for the client with acute or chronic pancreatitis.

## Home Care

The client with pancreatitis is often acutely ill and, along with family members, needs information about both hospital procedures and self-care at home following discharge. During the acute stage, keep explanations brief and simple.

Prior to discharge, teach the client and family about the disease and how to prevent further attacks of inflammation. Include the following topics as appropriate.

- Alcohol can cause stones to form, blocking pancreatic ducts and the outflow of pancreatic juice. Continued alcohol intake is likely to cause further inflammation and destruction of the pancreas. Avoid alcohol entirely.
- Smoking and stress stimulate the pancreas and should be avoided.

## CHART 22–4  LINKAGES BETWEEN NANDA, NIC, AND NOC

### The Client with Pancreatitis

| NURSING DIAGNOSES | NURSING INTERVENTIONS | NURSING OUTCOMES |
|---|---|---|
| • Pain | • Pain Management | • Pain Control |
| • Deficient Fluid Volume | • Fluid Management | • Fluid Balance |
| | • Hypovolemia Management | |
| • Imbalanced Nutrition: Less than Body Requirements | • Nutrition Management | • Nutritional Status: Food and Fluid Intake |
| • Ineffective Breathing Pattern | • Respiratory Monitoring | • Respiratory Status: Ventilation |

*Data from Nursing Outcomes Classification (NOC) by M. Johnson & M. Maas (Eds.), 1997, St. Louis: Mosby; Nursing Diagnoses: Definitions & Classification 2001–2002 by North American Nursing Diagnosis Association, 2001, Philadelphia: NANDA; Nursing Interventions Classification (NIC) by J.C. McCloskey & G. M. Bulechek (Eds.), 2000, St. Louis: Mosby. Reprinted by permission.*

- If pancreatic function has been severely impaired, discuss appropriate use of pancreatic enzymes, including timing, dose, potential side effects, and monitoring of effectiveness.
- A low-fat diet is recommended. Provide a list of high-fat foods to avoid. Crash dieting and binge eating also should be avoided as they may sometimes precipitate attacks. Spicy foods, coffee, tea, or colas, and gas-forming foods, stimulate gastric and pancreatic secretions and may precipitate pain. Avoid them if this occurs.
- Report symptoms of infection (fever of 102°F (38.8°C) or more, pain, rapid pulse, malaise) as a pancreatic abscess may develop after initial recovery.

Refer to a dietitian or nutritionist for diet teaching as needed. If appropriate, refer to community agencies, such as Alcoholics Anonymous, or to an alcohol treatment program. Provide referrals to community or home health agencies as needed for continued monitoring and teaching at home.

## Nursing Care Plan

### A Client with Acute Pancreatitis

Rose Schliefer is a 59-year-old wife, mother of three, and grandmother of four. She has been hospitalized for the past 6 weeks for acute hemorrhagic pancreatitis and pseudocyst. The pancreatitis was caused by gallstones. Mrs. Schliefer spent 3 weeks in intensive care, and then underwent surgery to remove the gallstones and to insert drains into the pseudocyst. Prior to discharge, she had progressed to a soft, high-carbohydrate, low-fat diet; had all drains removed; and was able to walk in the hall. Mrs. Schliefer was referred to a community health agency in her home town for continued follow-up.

### ASSESSMENT

Lee Quinn, the community health nurse, assesses Mrs. Schliefer at home after discharge. Mrs. Schliefer is thin and appears anxious and tired. She states that she lost 30 lb (13.6 kg) in the hospital and now weighs only 102 lb (46 kg). She is 66 inches (168 cm) tall. Her vital signs are within normal limits. Mrs. Schliefer has a well-healed upper abdominal scar and two round wounds (from drains) on each side of her abdomen. The wounds are closed but still have scabs. Her skin is cool and dry, and turgor is poor. She is alert and oriented and responds appropriately to questions. Blood glucose levels are normal. Mrs. Schliefer states that her main problems are lack of energy and lack of appetite for the low-fat diet that has been ordered. Mrs. Schliefer's husband and daughters express concern about their ability to provide care. Although they have been taught all about the disease and how to provide care, they still are not sure they know exactly what should be done now that Mrs. Schliefer is at home.

### DIAGNOSES

- *Fatigue* related to decreased metabolic energy production
- *Imbalanced nutrition: Less than body requirements* related to prolonged hospitalization, dietary restrictions, and impaired digestion
- *Bathing/hygiene self-care deficit* (Level II: requires help of another person, supervision, and teaching) related to decreased strength and endurance
- *Risk for caregiver role strain* related to inexperience with caregiving tasks

### EXPECTED OUTCOMES

- Set priorities for daily and weekly activities, and incorporate a rest period into daily activity.
- Gain 3 to 4 lb.
- Bathe and maintain personal hygiene without assistance.
- Family members will verbalize comfort with providing necessary care.

### PLANNING AND IMPLEMENTATION

- Explain causes of fatigue. Review effects of pancreatitis, surgery, and acute illness on energy levels.
- Develop activity goals, incorporating small, incremental steps toward achieving goal. Mrs. Schliefer indicates that she wants to cook a meal for the whole family. To reach this goal, she will:

## Nursing Care Plan

### A Client with Acute Pancreatitis (continued)

a. Schedule the meal when her energy level is highest.

b. List actions necessary to prepare the meal and delegate difficult tasks to family members.

c. Ask daughters to reorganize the kitchen to avoid unnecessary steps.

d. Plan the meal no sooner than the third week after being home.

- Instruct to:

a. Rest in bed each day from 1:00 P.M. to 3:00 P.M.

b. Eat six small meals a day with family members or friends.

c. Sit and rest quietly for 15 minutes before eating.

- Discuss dietary restrictions and how to adapt them to usual diet.

- Advice to use shower chair and develop self-care goals for bathing and hygiene in small steps. Add self-care tasks gradually as tolerated.

- Discuss division of responsibilities for physical care, home maintenance, and medical care with family members.

- Encourage family discussion of concerns about future; acknowledge family strengths.

### EVALUATION

One month after discharge, Mrs. Schliefer and her family have established new routines based on her energy levels. Mrs. Schliefer now fixes lunch because she feels best during midday. She and her husband share this time together without interruption. Mrs. Schliefer still rests during the day but can now provide self-care. She has gained only 2 lb, but states that she is getting used to the new diet and that "things are even starting to taste good without butter." She also says that sitting quietly before meals is helpful and that she prefers eating six small meals a day. Mr. and Mrs. Schliefer and their daughters agree that their initial worries about Mrs. Schliefer's care have been resolved; now they all know what they must do, and the future looks much brighter.

### Critical Thinking in the Nursing Process

1. Your client with acute pancreatitis is also an alcoholic. Describe assessments that indicate the beginnings of withdrawal.

2. Discuss the pathophysiologic basis of hypovolemic shock in acute necrotic pancreatitis.

3. Outline a teaching plan that includes specific foods to omit and to include in a high-carbohydrate, low-protein, low-fat diet.

4. Develop a plan of care for the nursing diagnosis, *Impaired home maintenance management.*

See Evaluating Your Response in Appendix C.

## THE CLIENT WITH PANCREATIC CANCER

Cancer of the pancreas accounts for approximately 2% of all cancers. It is, however, one of the most lethal cancers: More than 98% of people with pancreatic cancer die. An estimated 30,300 new cases occurred in the United States in 2002, with approximately 29,700 deaths from cancer of the pancreas (American Cancer Society, 2002). The incidence of pancreatic cancer increases after age 50. The incidence is slightly higher in women than men, and is higher in blacks than in whites. Most cancers of the pancreas occur in the exocrine pancreas, are adenocarcinomas, and cause death within 1 to 3 years after diagnosis.

The major risk factor for cancer of the pancreas is smoking; the incidence is twice as high in smokers as in nonsmokers. Other risk factors are exposure to industrial chemicals or environmental toxins, high-fat diet, chronic pancreatitis, and diabetes mellitus.

Cancer of the pancreas has a slow onset, with manifestations of anorexia, nausea, weight loss, flatulence, and dull epigastric pain. The pain increases in severity as the tumor grows. Other manifestations depend on the location of the tumor. Cancer of the head of the pancreas, which is the most common site, often obstructs bile flow through the common bile duct and the ampulla of Vater, resulting in jaundice, clay-colored stools, dark urine, and pruritus. Cancer of the body of the pancreas presses on the celiac ganglion, causing pain that increases when the person eats or lies supine. Cancer of the tail of the pancreas often causes no symptoms until it has metastasized. Other late manifestations include a palpable abdominal mass and ascites. Because the manifestations are nonspecific, up to 85% of clients with cancer of the pancreas do not seek health care until the cancer becomes too far advanced for a cure.

Early cancers of the head of the pancreas may be resectable. A pancreatoduodenectomy (commonly called Whipple's procedure) is performed to remove the head of the pancreas, the entire duodenum, the distal third of the stomach, a portion of the jejunum, and the lower half of the common bile duct. The common bile duct is then sutured to the end of the jejunum, and the remaining pancreas and stomach are sutured to the side of the jejunum (Figure 22–7 ■). Radiation and chemotherapy are often used in addition to surgery.

Postoperative nursing care of the client undergoing Whipple's procedure is outlined on page 606. Immediate postoperative care is often provided in the intensive care unit.

The client with pancreatic cancer has multiple problems requiring nursing care. Chapter 10 ∞ provides a discussion of care of the client with cancer; the nursing diagnoses and interventions discussed for the client with pancreatitis are also appropriate for the client with pancreatic cancer.

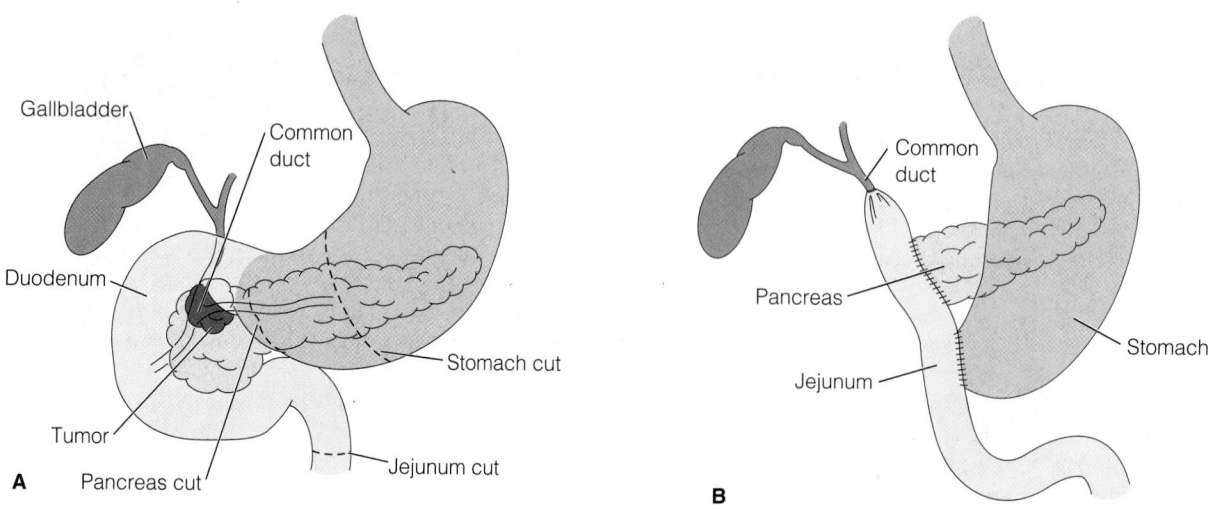

**Figure 22–7** ■ Pancreatoduodenectomy (Whipple's procedure): *A,* areas of resection; *B,* appearance following resection.

## NURSING CARE   OF THE CLIENT UNDERGOING WHIPPLE'S PROCEDURE

### PREOPERATIVE CARE

- Provide routine preoperative nursing care as outlined in Chapter 7. ⊝⊅
- Clarify teaching and learning as needed. Provide psychologic support for client and family. *The client and family faced with a diagnosis of pancreatic cancer may require reinforcement of teaching as anxiety, fear, and possible denial can interfere with learning.*

### POSTOPERATIVE CARE

- Provide postoperative care as outlined in Chapter 7.
- Maintain in semi-Fowler's position. *Semi-Fowler's position facilitates lung expansion and reduces stress on the anastomosis and suture line.*
- Maintain low gastrointestinal suction. If drainage is not adequate, obtain an order to irrigate, using minimal pressure. Do not reposition nasogastric tube. *Pressure within the operative area from retained secretions increases intraluminal pressure and places stress on the suture line. Forceful irrigations and repositioning of the nasogastric tube may disrupt the suture line.*
- Maintain pain control using analgesics as prescribed (PCA, infusion, or given on a regular basis). Assess effectiveness of pain management. *Doses higher than normal may be required if narcotic analgesics have been used prior to surgery to manage pain.*

*Increased pain may indicate complications such as disruption of suture line, leakage from anastomosis, or peritonitis. Adequate pain*

*management increases resistance to stress, facilitates healing and increases the ability to cough, deep breathe, and change position.*

- Assist with coughing, deep breathing, and changing position every 1 to 2 hours. Splint incision during coughing and deep breathing. *The location of the incision makes coughing and deep breathing more painful. The prolonged surgical procedure, anesthesia, location of incision, and immobility increase the risk of retained secretions, atelectasis, and pneumonia. Changing position facilitates drainage of secretions; effective coughing and deep breathing remove secretions and open distal alveoli.*
- Monitor for complications:
  a. Take vital signs every 2 to 4 hours or as indicated; immediately report changes (such as elevated temperature; hypotension; weak, thready pulse; increased or difficult respirations).
  b. Assess skin color, temperature, moisture, and turgor.
  c. Measure urinary output, gastrointestinal output, and drainage from any other tubes; monitor amount and type of would drainage.
  d. Assess level of consciousness.
  e. Monitor results of laboratory tests, especially arterial blood gases, hemoglobin, and hematocrit.

*The major complications following Whipple's procedure are hemorrhage, hypovolemic shock, and hepatorenal failure. The assessments listed provide information about the client's status and alert the nurse to abnormal findings that signal the onset of these complications.*

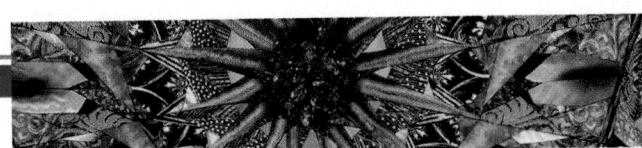

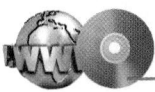

## EXPLORE MediaLink

NCLEX review questions, case studies, care plan activities, MediaLink applications, and other interactive resources for this chapter can be found on the Companion Website at www.prenhall.com/lemone.

Click on Chapter 22 to select the activities for this chapter. For animations, video clips, more NCLEX review questions, and an audio glossary, access the Student CD-ROM accompanying this textbook.

## TEST YOURSELF

1. When assessing the client admitted for a laparoscopic cholecystectomy, the nurse would expect to find:
   a. History of intermittent episodes of right upper quadrant pain
   b. Significant jaundice of the sclera and skin
   c. Complaints of recurrent heartburn and acid reflux
   d. Ascites and peripheral edema

2. During an outbreak of hepatitis A traced to a food handler at a local restaurant, the nurse teaches staff at the restaurant that the most cost-effective means of protecting customers from further outbreaks is to:
   a. Insist that all food handlers be immunized against hepatitis A
   b. Test all new employees for hepatitis A antigen
   c. Wash hands thoroughly before handling food and after using the bathroom
   d. Use gloves for handling food if any cuts or scrapes are on hands

3. The nurse would evaluate teaching as effective when a client with chronic hepatitis C states which of the following?
   a. "I will reduce my alcohol intake and use only acetaminophen for pain relief."
   b. "I understand that I must return to the doctor every year for a follow-up liver biopsy."
   c. "Even though no treatment is available for this disease, I plan to live a long life."
   d. "I will avoid donating blood and will use barrier protection during sex."

4. A client hospitalized with cirrhosis, ascites, and mild hepatic encephalopathy suddenly vomits 200 mL of bright red blood. Which of the following should the nurse do first?
   a. Insert a nasogastric tube
   b. Place in Fowler's position
   c. Contact the physician
   d. Check stool for occult blood

5. A 54-year-old woman admitted with acute pancreatitis says, "I don't understand how I got this disease. I thought alcoholics got pancreatitis—I never drink." Which of the following is the most appropriate response by the nurse?
   a. "Was there a time in your life that you did drink heavily?"
   b. "It also is prevalent in smokers; do you smoke cigarettes?"
   c. "Gallstones also are a risk factor. We'll evaluate for them."
   d. "Intravenous drug use is a risk factor. Do you use drugs by injection?"

See Test Yourself answers in Appendix C.

## BIBLIOGRAPHY

Ackley, B.J., & Ladwig, G. B. (2002). *Nursing diagnosis handbook: A guide to planning care* (5th ed.). St. Louis: Mosby.

American Cancer Society. (2002). *Cancer facts and figures 2002.* Atlanta: Author.

Atkinson, W., Wolfe, C., Humiston, S., & Nelson, R. (Eds.). (2000). *Epidemiology and prevention of vaccine-preventable diseases* (6th ed.). Atlanta: Centers for Disease Control.

Bockhold, K. M. (2000). Who's afraid of hepatitis C? *American Journal of Nursing, 100*(5), 26–31.

Braunwald, E., Fauci, A. S., Kasper, D. L., Hauser, S. L., Longo, D. L., & Jameson, J. L. (2001). *Harrison's principles of internal medicine* (15th ed.). New York: McGraw-Hill.

Bullock, B. A., & Henze, R. L. (2000). *Focus on pathophysiology.* Philadelphia: Lippincott.

Cole, L. (2001). Acute pancreatitis. *Nursing, 31*(12), 58–63.

Deglin, J. H., & Vallerand, A. H. (2001). *Davis's drug guide for nurses* (7th ed.). Philadelphia: F.A. Davis.

Dill, B., Dill, J. E., Berkhouse, L., & Palmer, S. T. (1999). Endoscopic ultrasound for chronic abdominal pain and gallbladder disease. *Gastroenterology Nursing, 22*(5), 209–212.

Dougherty, A. S., & Dreher, H. M. (2001). Hepatitis C: Current treatment strategies for an emerging epidemic. *MEDSURG Nursing, 10*(1), 9–13.

Farrar, J. A. (2001). Emergency! Acute cholecystitis. *American Journal of Nursing, 101*(1), 35–36.

Fontaine, K. L. (2000). *Healing practices: Alternative therapies for nursing.* Upper Saddle River, NJ: Prentice Hall Health.

Hession, M. C. (1998). Factors influencing successful discharge after outpatient laparoscopic sholecystectomy. *Journal of Perianesthesia Nursing, 13*(1), 11–15.

Johnson, M., Bulechek, G., Dochterman, J. M., Maas, M., & Moorhead, S. (2001). *Nursing diagnoses, outcomes, & interventions.* St. Louis: Mosby.

Johnson, M., Maas, M., & Moorhead, S. (Eds.). (2000). *Nursing outcomes classification (NOC)* (2nd ed.). St. Louis: Mosby.

Klainberg, M. (1999). Primary biliary cirrhosis. *American Journal of Nursing, 99*(12), 38–39.

Kuhn, M. A. (1999). *Complementary therapies for health care providers.* Philadelphia: Lippincott.

Lehne, R. A. (2001). *Pharmacology for nursing care* (4th ed.). Philadelphia: Saunders.

Malarkey, L.M., & McMorrow, M.E. (2000). *Nurse's manual of laboratory tests and diagnostic procedures* (2nd ed.). Philadelphia: Saunders.

Marx, J. F. (1998). Understanding the varieties of viral hepatitis. *Nursing, 28*(7), 43–49.

McCloskey, J. C., & Bulechek, G. M. (Eds.). (2000). *Nursing interventions classification (NIC)* (3rd ed.). St. Louis: Mosby.

Meeker, M. H., & Rothrock, J. C. (1999). *Alexander's care of the patient in surgery* (11th ed.). St. Louis: Mosby.

North American Nursing Diagnosis Association. (2001). *NANDA nursing diagnoses: Definitions & classification 2001–2002.* Philadelphia: NANDA.

Porth, C. M. (2002). *Pathophysiology: Concepts of altered health states* (6th ed.). Philadelphia: Lippincott.

Savage, R. B., Hussey, M. J., & Hurie, M. B. (2000). A successful approach to immunizing men who have sex with men against hepatitis B. *Public Health Nursing, 17*(3), 202–206.

Shovein, J. T., Damazo, R. J., & Hyams, I. (2000). Hepatitis A: How benign is it? *American Journal of Nursing, 100*(3), 43–47.

Springhouse. (1999). *Nurse's handbook of alternative & complementary therapies.* Springhouse, PA: Author.

Thorn, K. (1999). Hepatitis C: The lurking dragon. *Case Manager, 10*(4), 55–62.

Tierney, L. M., McPhee, S. J., & Papadakis, M. A. (2001). *Current medical diagnosis & treatment* (40th ed.). New York: Lange Medical Books/McGraw-Hill.

Urden, L. D., Stacy, K. M., & Lough, M. E. (2002). *Thelan's critical care nursing: Diagnosis and management* (4th ed.). St. Louis: Mosby

Wilkinson, J. M. (2000). *Nursing diagnosis handbook with NIC interventions and NOC outcomes* (7th ed.). Upper Saddle River, NJ: Prentice Hall Health.

Williamson, L. (1998). Self-destruction in the pancreas. *Nursing Times, 94*(29), 57–59.

Wrobleski, D. M., Barth, M. M., & Oyen, L. J. (1999). Necrotizing pancreatitis: Pathophysiology, diagnosis, and acute care management. *AACN Clinical Issues, 10*(4), 464–477.

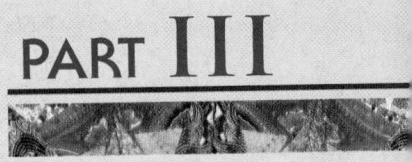

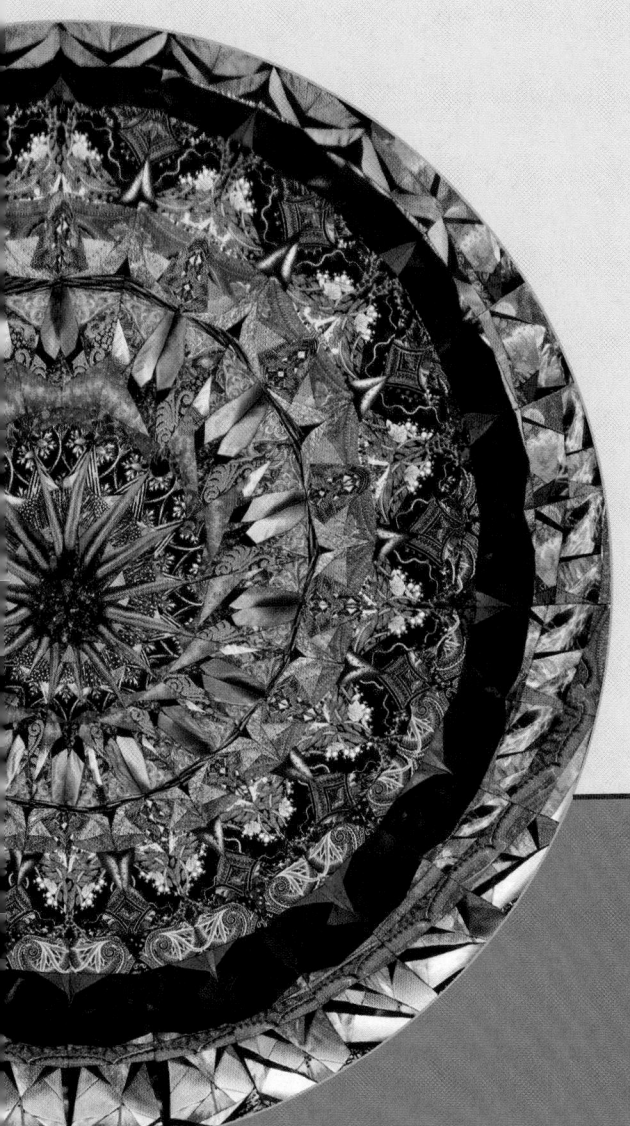

# ELIMINATION PATTERNS

Unit 6
**Responses to Altered Bowel Elimination**

Unit 7
**Responses to Altered Urinary Elimination**

# Functional Health Patterns with Related Nursing Diagnoses

## HEALTH PERCEPTION HEALTH MANAGEMENT
- Perceived health status
- Perceived health management
- Health care behaviors: health promotion and illness prevention activities, medical treatments, follow-up care

## VALUE-BELIEF
- Values, goals, or beliefs (including spirituality) that guide choices or decisions
- Perceived conflicts in values, beliefs, or expectations that are health related

## COPING-STRESS-TOLERANCE
- Capacity to resist challenges to self-integrity
- Methods of handling stress
- Support systems
- Perceived ability to control and manage situations

## NUTRITIONAL-METABOLIC
- Daily consumption of food and fluids
- Favorite foods
- Use of dietary supplements
- Skin lesions and ability to heal
- Condition of the integument
- Weight, height, temperature

## Part 3
### Elimination Patterns
### NANDA Nursing Diagnoses
- Bowel Incontinence
- Constipation
- Perceived Constipation
- Risk for Constipation
- Diarrhea
- Impaired Urinary Elimination
- Functional Urinary Incontinence
- Reflex Urinary Incontinence
- Stress Urinary Incontinence
- Total Urinary Incontinence
- Urge Urinary Incontinence
- Risk for Urge Urinary Incontinence
- Urinary Retention
- Self-Care Deficit: Toileting

## SEXUALITY-REPRODUCTIVE
- Satisfaction with sexuality or sexual relationships
- Reproductive pattern
- Female menstrual and perimenopausal history

## ELIMINATION
- Patterns of bowel and urinary excretion
- Perceived regularity or irregularity of elimination
- Use of laxatives or routines
- Changes in time, modes, quality or quantity of excretions
- Use of devices for control

## ROLE-RELATIONSHIP
- Perception of major roles, relationships, and responsibilities in current life situation
- Satisfaction with or disturbances in roles and relationships

## ACTIVITY-EXERCISE
- Patterns of personally relevant exercise, activity, leisure, and recreation
- ADLs which require energy expenditure
- Factors that interfere with the desired pattern (e.g., illness or injury)

## SELF-PERCEPTION–SELF-CONCEPT
- Attitudes about self
- Perceived abilities, worth, self-image, emotions
- Body posture and movement, eye contact, voice and speech patterns

## SLEEP-REST
- Patterns of sleep and rest/relaxation in a 24-hr period
- Perceptions of quality and quantity of sleep and rest
- Use of sleep aids and routines

## COGNITIVE-PERCEPTUAL
- Adequacy of vision, hearing, taste, touch, smell
- Pain perception and management
- Language, judgment, memory, decisions

*Reprinted from Nursing Diagnosis: Process and Application, 3rd ed., by M. Gordon, pp. 80–96, Copyright © 1994, with permission from Elsevier Science.*

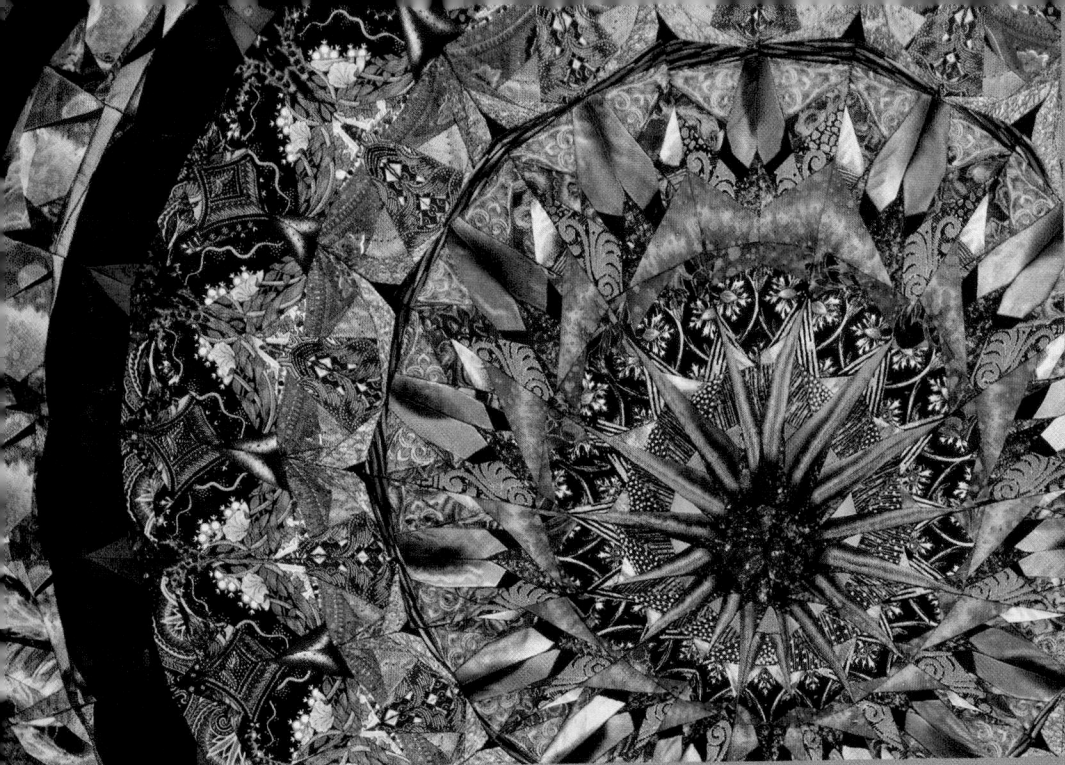

# RESPONSES TO ALTERED BOWEL ELIMINATION

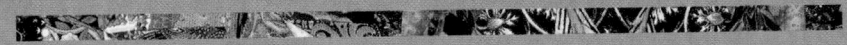

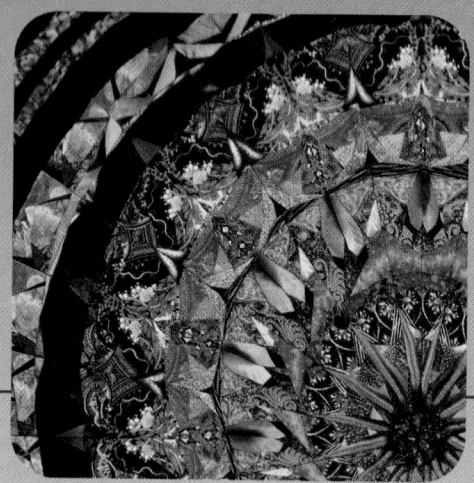

# Assessing Clients with Bowel Elimination Disorders

## MediaLink

**www.prenhall.com/lemone**

Additional resources for this chapter can be found on the Student CD-ROM accompanying this textbook, and on the Companion Website at www.prenhall.com/lemone. Click on Chapter 23 to select the activities for this chapter.

**CD-ROM**
- Audio Glossary
- NCLEX Review

**Companion Website**
- More NCLEX Review
- Functional Health Pattern Assessment
- Case Study
  Irritable Bowel Syndrome

## LEARNING OUTCOMES

After completing this chapter, you will be able to:

- Review the anatomy and physiology of the small and large intestines.

- Explain the physiologic processes involved in bowel elimination.

- Identify specific topics for consideration during a health history interview of the client with problems of bowel elimination.

- Describe physical assessment techniques of bowel function.

- Identify manifestations of impairment of bowel function.

After foods are eaten and broken down into usable elements, nutrients are absorbed and indigestible materials are eliminated. Bowel elimination is the end process in digestion. This chapter describes the structure and function of the large intestine, including the rectosigmoid region and the anus, as well as the assessment of bowel function. The anatomy and physiology of the small intestine are discussed more fully in Chapter 19; ⊖⊖ the information in this chapter is provided as a base for understanding health problems from altered bowel function. In addition, this chapter discusses the function of the small intestine in the absorption of digested end products. Malabsorption (impaired absorption of nutrients) is discussed fully in Chapter 24. ⊖⊖

## REVIEW OF ANATOMY AND PHYSIOLOGY
### The Small Intestine

The small intestine begins at the pyloric sphincter and ends at the ileocecal junction at the entrance of the large intestine. The small intestine is about 20 feet (6 m) long, but only about 1 inch (2.5 cm) in diameter. This long tube hangs in coils in the abdominal cavity, suspended by the mesentery and surrounded by the large intestine.

The small intestine has three regions: the duodenum, the jejunum, and the ileum. The duodenum begins at the pyloric sphincter and extends around the head of the pancreas for about 10 inches (25 cm). Both pancreatic enzymes and bile from the liver enter the small intestine at the duodenum. The jejunum is the middle region of the small intestine. It extends for about 8 feet (2.4 m). The ileum, the terminal end of the small intestine, is approximately 12 feet (3.6 m) long and meets the large intestine at the ileocecal valve.

Food is chemically digested and mostly absorbed as it moves through the small intestine. Circular folds (deep folds of the mucosa and submucosa layers), villi (fingerlike projections of the mucosa cells), and microvilli (tiny projections of the mucosa cells) all increase the surface area of the small intestine to enhance absorption of food. Although up to 10 L of food, liquids, and secretions enter the gastrointestinal tract each day, most is digested and absorbed in the small intestine; less than 1 L reaches the large intestine.

Enzymes in the small intestine break down carbohydrates, proteins, lipids, and nucleic acids.

- Pancreatic amylase acts on starches, converting them to maltose, dextrins, and oligosaccharides; the intestinal enzymes dextrinase, glucoamylase, maltase, sucrase, and lactase further break down these products into monosaccharides.
- Proteins are broken down into peptides by the pancreatic enzymes trypsin and chymotrypsin and by intestinal enzymes. Pancreatic enzymes (trypsin and chymotrypsin) and intestinal enzymes continue to break down proteins into peptides
- Pancreatic lipases break down lipids in the small intestine.
- Triglycerides enter as fat globules, and are then coated by bile salts and emulsified.
- Nucleic acids are hydrolyzed by pancreatic enzymes, then broken apart by intestinal enzymes.

Both pancreatic enzymes and bile are excreted into the duodenum in response to the secretion of secretin and cholecystokinin, hormones produced by the intestinal mucosa cells when chyme enters the small intestine.

Nutrients are absorbed through the mucosa of the intestinal villi into the blood or lymph by active transport, facilitated transport, and passive diffusion. Almost all food products and water, as well as vitamins and most electrolytes, are absorbed in the small intestine, leaving only indigestible fibers, some water, and bacteria to enter the large intestine.

### The Large Intestine

The large intestine, or colon, begins at the ileocecal valve and terminates at the anus (Figure 23–1 ■). It is about 5 feet (1.5 m) long. The large intestine frames the small intestine on three sides and includes the cecum, the appendix, the colon, the rectum, and the anal canal.

The first section of the large intestine is the cecum. The appendix is attached to its surface as an extension. The appendix, a twisted structure in which bacteria can accumulate, may become inflamed.

The colon is divided into ascending, transverse, and descending segments. The ascending colon extends along the right side of the abdomen to the hepatic flexure, where it makes a right-angle turn. The next segment, called the transverse colon, crosses the abdomen to the splenic flexure. At this juncture, the descending colon descends down the left side of the abdomen and ends at the S-shaped sigmoid colon. The sigmoid colon terminates at the rectum.

The rectum is a mucosa-lined tube approximately 12 cm in length (Figure 23–2 ■). The rectum has three transverse folds (*valves of Houston*) that retain feces yet allow flatus to be passed through the anus. The rectum ends at the anal canal, which terminates at the anus.

The anus, a hairless, dark-skinned area, is the end of the digestive tract. It has both an internal involuntary sphincter and an external voluntary sphincter. The sphincters are usually open only during defecation. The anorectal junction separates the rectum from the anal canal and may be the site of internal hemorrhoids (clusters of dilated veins in swollen anal tissue).

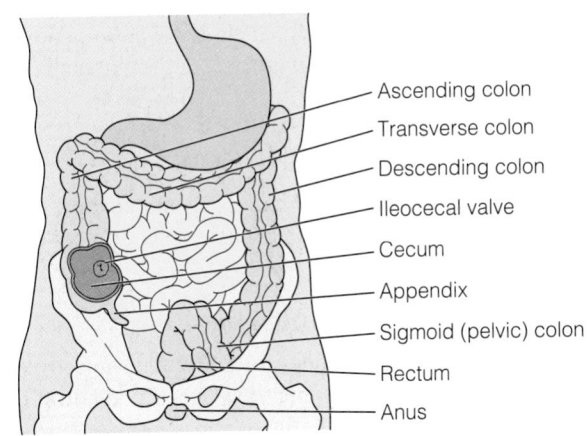

Figure 23–1 ■ Anatomy of the large intestine.

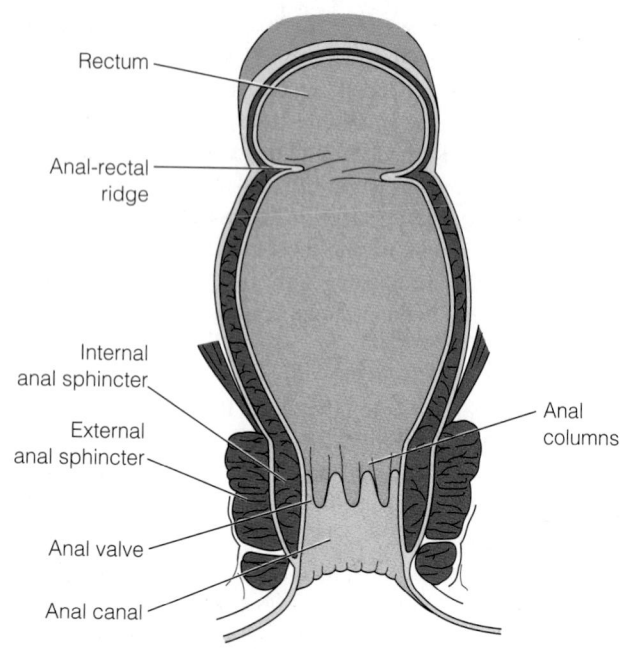

**Figure 23–2** ■ Structure of the rectum and anus.

The major function of the large intestine is to eliminate indigestible food residue from the body. The large intestine absorbs water, salts, and vitamins formed by the food residue and bacteria. The semiliquid chyme that passes through the ileocecal valve is formed into feces as it moves through the large intestine. Feces are moved along the intestine by peristalsis, waves of alternating contraction and relaxation. Goblet cells lining the large intestine secrete mucus that facilitates the lubrication and passage of feces.

The defecation reflex is initiated when feces enter the rectum and stretch the rectal wall. This spinal cord reflex causes the walls of the sigmoid colon to contract and the anal sphincters to relax. This reflex can be suppressed by voluntary control of the external sphincter. Closing the glottis and contracting the diaphragm and abdominal muscles to increase intra-abdominal pressure facilitates expulsion of feces; this movement is called *Valsalva's maneuver.* Prolonged suppression of defecation can result in a weakened reflex that may in turn lead to *constipation* (infrequent and often uncomfortable passage of hard, dry stool). Frequent bouts of constipation may lead to external hemorrhoids at the area of the external hemorrhoidal plexus.

## ASSESSING BOWEL FUNCTION

The nurse conducts both a health assessment interview (to collect subjective data) and a physical assessment (to collect objective data).

### Health Assessment Interview

This section provides guidelines for collecting subjective data through a health assessment interview specific to bowel function. Problems with bowel elimination may be assessed as part of a health screening, may focus on a chief complaint (such as abdominal pain or change in bowel patterns), or may be part of

a total health assessment. The assessment of bowel sounds is a common part of routine assessments.

Clients may feel embarrassed and hesitant to provide information about bowel elimination patterns. To promote effective rapport, remain nonjudgmental and ask for less personal information first.

If the client has a health problem involving bowel function, analyze its onset, characteristics and course, severity, precipitating and relieving factors, and any associated symptoms, noting the timing and circumstances. For example, ask the client:

* Can you describe the type of cramping and abdominal pain you are experiencing?
* Have you ever had bleeding from your rectum?
* Have you noticed increased constipation since your surgery?

Begin the interview by inquiring about any medical conditions that may influence the client's bowel elimination pattern, such as a stroke or spinal cord impairment, inflammatory gastrointestinal diseases, endocrine disorders, and allergies. Note any recent travel to other countries. Information about the client's psychosocial history is also important. Assess the client's lifestyle for any patterns of psychologic stress and/or depression, which may alter bowel elimination patterns. Depression may be associated with constipation, whereas *diarrhea* (frequent passage of loose, watery stools) may occur in situations of high stress and anxiety. Explore the client's activities of daily living, including exercise, sleep-rest patterns, and dietary and fluid intake. Changes in activities of daily living can influence bowel elimination patterns.

Determine whether the client has had any lower abdominal pain or rectal pain, which may be associated with a distended colon filled with gas or fluid. Crampy, colicky pains occur with diarrhea and/or constipation. Sudden onset of lower abdominal cramping occurs in obstruction of the colon. Left lower abdominal pain is associated with diverticulitis. Rectal pain may occur with stool retention and/or hemorrhoids.

Ask the client to describe the frequency and character of the stools. Ask about any history of diarrhea, constipation, or bleeding from the rectum, and collect information about the use of laxatives, suppositories, or enemas. Anticholinergic drugs, antihistamines, tranquilizers, or narcotics may cause constipation.

If the client has an **ostomy** (surgical opening into the bowel), ask about skin care problems, consistency of stool, foods that cause problems, the number of times that the client empties the appliance bag each day, and irrigation habits. Finally, explore the client's feelings about the appliance.

To obtain information about the client's nutritional status, ask about changes in weight, appetite, food preferences, food intolerances, special diets, and any cultural or ethnic influences on dietary intake. Ask whether the client is experiencing nausea and vomiting; if so, determine any relation to food intake, and ask the client to describe character of the emesis. In addition, ask about indigestion, the use of antacids or other over-the-counter medications, herbal preparations, and episodes of diarrhea and its character.

Explore any family history of colon cancer, colitis, gallbladder disease, or malabsorption syndromes, such as lactose intolerance and celiac sprue. Assess the client's risk factors for cancer, including age greater than 50; family member with colon cancer; history of endometrial, ovarian, or breast cancer; and previous diagnoses of colon inflammation, polyps, or cancer.

Other questions and leading statements, categorized by functional health patterns, can be found on the Companion Website.

## Physical Assessment

The function of the bowels is assessed through a rectal examination, an anal examination, and examination of the client's stool. A complete assessment also includes inspection of the abdomen and auscultation of bowel sounds. Guidelines for abdominal assessment and assessment of bowel sounds are outlined in Chapter 19. ⊖⊃

Physical assessment of the abdomen may be performed as part of a total health assessment, in combination with assessment of the urinary and reproductive systems (problems which may cause clinical manifestations similar to those of the gastrointestinal system), or alone for clients with known or suspected health problems. The techniques of inspection, auscultation, percussion, and palpation are used. Palpation is the last method used in assessing the abdomen, because pressure on the abdominal wall and contents may interfere with bowel sounds and cause pain, ending the examination.

Necessary equipment includes water-soluble lubricant, material for testing the stool, and disposable gloves for the examiner. Ask the client to empty the bladder before the examination and lie in the supine position. Have the client turn to the left lateral (Sims') position for the rectal examination. The older client or the client with limited mobility may need assistance in assuming this position.

Explain what will happen during the examination, and encourage the client to take deep, regular breaths to increase relaxation. Explain that during the examination, it may feel as though the client is about to have a bowel movement and that sometimes flatus (gas) is passed. Assure the client that this is normal. Ensure that the examination area is private and the client is draped properly to prevent unnecessary exposure.

### Abdominal Assessment with Abnormal Findings (✓)

- Inspect the abdomen.
  - ✓ Retention of flatus (gas) or stool may cause generalized abdominal distention.
  - ✓ Malnutrition causes a scaphoid (concave) abdomen.
- Auscultate the four quadrants of the abdomen with the diaphragm of the stethoscope. Begin in the lower right quadrant, where bowel sounds are almost always present. Normal bowel sounds (gurgling or clicking) occur every 5 to 15 seconds. Listen for at least 5 minutes in each of the four quadrants to confirm the absence of bowel sounds.
  - ✓ High-pitched, tinkling, rushing, or growling bowel sounds may be heard in the client who has diarrhea or who is experiencing the onset of a bowel obstruction.
  - ✓ Bowel sounds may be absent in later stages of a bowel obstruction or after surgery of the abdominal organs.

### Perianal Assessment with Abnormal Findings (✓)

- Inspect the perianal area. Wearing gloves, spread the client's buttocks apart. Observe the area, and ask client to bear down as if they were trying to have a bowel movement.
  - ✓ Swollen, painful, longitudinal breaks in the anal area may appear in clients with anal fissures. (These are caused by the passing of large, hard stools, or by diarrhea.)
  - ✓ Dilated anal veins appear with hemorrhoids.
  - ✓ A red mass may appear with prolapsed internal hemorrhoids.
  - ✓ Doughnut-shaped red tissue at the anal area may appear with a prolapsed rectum.
- Palpate the anus and rectum. Lubricate the gloved index finger and ask the client to bear down. Touch the tip of your finger to the client's anal opening. Flex the index finger, and slowly insert it into the anus, pointing the finger towards the umbilicus (Figure 23–3 ■). Rotate the finger in both directions to palpate any lesions or masses. (The prostate or cervix may also be examined at this time. See Chapter 46.) ⊖⊃
  - ✓ Movable, soft masses may be polyps.
  - ✓ Hard, firm, irregular embedded masses may indicate carcinoma.

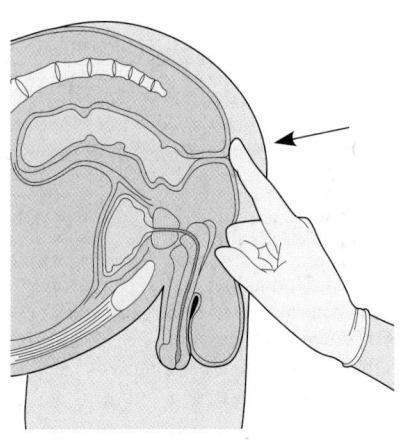

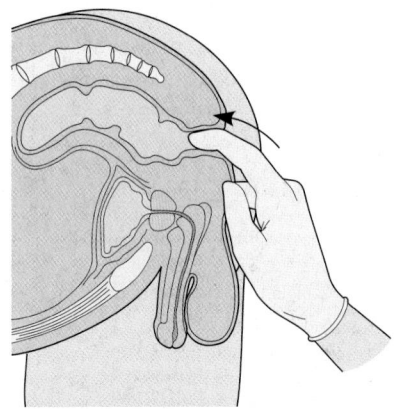

**Figure 23–3** ■ Digital examination of the anus and rectum.

## BOX 23-1 ■ Assessing Stool Characteristics

Inspect feces for color, odor, and consistency after the rectal exam or after defecation. Both hands are gloved.

### COLOR

■ Blood *on* the stool results from bleeding from the sigmoid colon, anus, or rectum. Blood *within* the stool indicates bleeding from the colon due to ulcerative colitis, diverticulosis, or tumors. Black, tarry stools, called **melena,** occur with upper gastrointestinal bleeding. Oral iron may turn stools black and mask melena.

■ Grayish or whitish stools can result from biliary tract obstruction due to lack of bile in stool.

■ Greasy, frothy, yellow stools, called **steatorrhea,** may appear with fat malabsorption.

### ODOR

■ Distinct, foul odors may be noted with stools containing blood or extra fat or in cases of colon cancer.

### CONSISTENCY

■ Hard stools or long, flat stools may result from a spastic colon or bowel obstruction due to a tumor or hemorrhoids. Hard stools may also result from ingestion of oral iron.

■ Mucousy, slimy feces may indicate inflammation and occur in irritable bowel syndrome.

■ Watery, diarrhea stools appear with malabsorption problems, irritable bowel syndrome, emotional or psychologic stress, ingestion of spoiled foods, or lactose intolerance.

## Fecal Assessment with Abnormal Findings (✓)

• Inspect the client's feces. After palpating the rectum, withdraw your finger gently. Inspect any feces on the glove. Note color and/or presence of blood. Also use gloved fingers to note consistency.

  ✓ See Box 23–1 for information about stool characteristics.

• Test the feces for occult blood. Use a commercial testing kit.

✓ A positive occult blood test requires further testing for colon cancer or gastrointestinal bleeding due to peptic ulcers, ulcerative colitis, or diverticulosis.

• Note the odor of the feces.

  ✓ Distinctly foul odors may be noted with stools containing blood or extra fat or in cases of colon cancer.

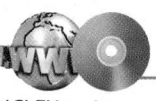

## EXPLORE MediaLink

NCLEX review questions, case studies, care plan activities, MediaLink applications, and other interactive resources for this chapter can be found on the Companion Website at www.prenhall.com/lemone.

Click on Chapter 23 to select the activities for this chapter. For animations, video clips, more NCLEX review questions, and an audio glossary, access the Student CD-ROM accompanying this textbook.

## TEST YOURSELF

1. What is the major function of the large intestine?
   a. To produce hormones necessary to digest food
   b. To break down lipids, proteins, and carbohydrates
   c. To secrete bile into the small intestine
   d. To eliminate undigested food residue

2. The appendix is attached to the surface of what segment of the large intestine?
   a. Cecum            c. Transverse colon
   b. Ascending colon  d. Rectum

3. Which of the following questions or statements would be appropriate for the client with an ostomy?

   a. "Have you had any bleeding from your hemorrhoids?"
   b. "Has your appetite changed lately?"
   c. "Tell me about your family."
   d. "Describe the consistency of your stools."

4. What assessment technique is used to assess bowel sounds?
   a. Inspection       c. Percussion
   b. Palpation        d. Auscultation

5. What term is used to describe black, tarry stools?
   a. Occult blood     c. Melena
   b. Hematemesis      d. Steatorrhea

See Test Yourself answers in Appendix C.

## BIBLIOGRAPHY

Dammel, T. (1997). Fecal occult-blood testing: Looking for hidden danger. *Nursing97, 27*(7), 44–45.

Goff, K. (1997). Assessment of the gastrointestinal tract. *Support Line, 19*(2), 3–7.

Hall, G., Karstens, M., Rakel, B., Swanson, E., & Davidson, A. (1995). Managing constipation using a research-based protocol. *MEDSURG Nursing, 4*(1), 11–18.

Kirton, C. (1997). Assessing bowel sounds. *Nursing97, 27*(3), 64.

Langan, J. (1998). Abdominal assessment in the home: From A to Zzz. *Home Healthcare Nurse, 16*(1), 50–58.

Lyneham, J. (2001). Physical examination (abdomen, thorax and lungs): A review. *Australian Journal of Advanced Nursing, 18*(3), 31.

Watson, R. (2001). Assessing the gastrointestinal tract in older people. 2: The lower GI tract. *Nursing Older People, 13*(1), 27–28.

Weber, J., & Kelley, J. (2002). *Health assessment in nursing* (2nd ed.). Philadelphia: Lippincott.

Wilson, S., & Giddens, J. (2001). *Health assessment for nursing practice* (2nd ed.). St. Louis: Mosby.

Wright, J. (1997). Seven abdominal assessment signs every emergency nurse should know. *Journal of Emergency Nursing, 23*(5), 446–450.

# CHAPTER 24

# Nursing Care of Clients with Bowel Disorders

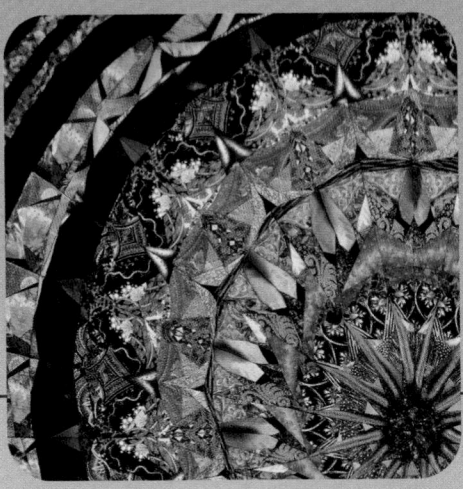

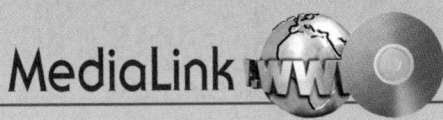

## MediaLink

**www.prenhall.com/lemone**
Additional resources for this chapter can be found on the Student CD-ROM accompanying this textbook, and on the Companion Website at www.prenhall.com/lemone. Click on Chapter 24 to select the activities for this chapter.

**CD-ROM**
- Audio Glossary
- NCLEX Review

**Companion Website**
- More NCLEX Review
- Case Study
    Irritable Bowel Syndrome
- Care Plan Activity
    Irritable Bowel Syndrome
- MediaLink Application
    Crohn's Disease

## LEARNING OUTCOMES

After completing this chapter, you will be able to:

- Relate the effects and manifestations of bowel disorders to normal physiology and assessment findings (Chapter 23).

- Discuss the pathophysiology, manifestations, and management of bowel absorption and elimination disorders.

- List diagnostic tests used to identify disorders of the small and large bowel.

- Discuss the nursing implications of medications used in managing bowel absorption and elimination disorders.

- Discuss care of clients with a colostomy or ileostomy.

- Provide appropriate nursing care for the client before and after intestinal surgery.

- Provide appropriate teaching for clients with bowel absorption and elimination disorders and their families.

- Use the nursing process as a framework for providing individualized care to clients with disorders of bowel absorption and elimination.

Disorders of intestinal absorption and bowel elimination can affect health, comfort, and well-being. Bowel function can be affected by inflammations, infections, tumors, obstructions, or changes in structure.

Clients with intestinal disorders often face extensive diagnostic testing, surgery, and permanent changes in physical appearance and lifestyle. Nursing care is directed toward meeting the client's physiologic needs, providing emotional support, and educating the client to adapt to changes in lifestyle.

# DISORDERS OF INTESTINAL MOTILITY

Few body functions respond as readily to internal and external influences as the process of defecation. Factors affecting the gastrointestinal (GI) tract directly, such as food intake and bacterial population, affect the number and consistency of stools. Indirect factors, such as psychologic stress or voluntary postponement of defecation, also affect elimination.

In modern society, "normal" bowel elimination patterns vary widely. For some clients, two to three stools per day is the usual pattern. Others may normally have as few as three stools per week. It is important to evaluate each client's elimination pattern against his or her own normal pattern.

## THE CLIENT WITH DIARRHEA

**Diarrhea** is an increase in the frequency, volume, and fluid content of the stool. In diarrhea, the water content of feces is increased, usually due to either malabsorption or water secretion in the bowel. It is a symptom rather than a primary disorder.

Diarrhea may be acute or chronic. Acute diarrhea, which usually lasts less than a week, is usually due to an infectious agent. Chronic diarrhea (diarrhea that persists longer than 3 to 4 weeks) may be caused by inflammatory bowel disorders, malabsorption, or even endocrine disorders.

### PATHOPHYSIOLOGY

About 1500 mL of digested material enters the large intestine daily. Most of the water and some of the solutes are reabsorbed in the bowel, leaving only about 200 mL of feces to be eliminated.

Large volume diarrhea, characterized by both increased numbers and volume of stools, is caused by increased water content of the stool. This increased water content may result from either osmotic or secretory processes. Water may be pulled into the bowel lumen by osmosis when the feces contains osmotically active molecules. Some stool softeners and laxatives work on this principle. When the lactose in milk is not broken down and absorbed, the lactose molecules exert an osmotic draw, causing diarrhea. The diarrhea associated with cholera and *Escherichia coli* infection is caused by increased water secretion in the small and large intestines. Unabsorbed dietary fat, some cathartics and other drugs, and other factors can cause secretory diarrhea.

Small volume diarrhea, characterized by frequent small stools, is usually caused by inflammation or disease of the colon. Diseases that affect the intestinal mucosa, such as inflammatory bowel disease, cause an exudative diarrhea. The mucosal inflammation causes plasma, serum proteins, blood, and mucus to accumulate in the bowel, increasing fecal bulk and fluidity. An increased rate of propulsion within the bowel can also decrease the amount of water normally absorbed from the chyme, leading to diarrhea. For this reason, laxatives that increase bowel motility and bowel resection or bypass can lead to diarrhea.

## MANIFESTATIONS AND COMPLICATIONS

The manifestations of diarrhea depend on its cause, duration, and severity, as well as the area of bowel affected and the client's general health. Diarrhea can present as several large, watery stools daily, or very frequent small stools that contain blood, mucus, or exudate.

Diarrhea can have devastating effects. Water and electrolytes are lost in diarrheal stool. This can lead to dehydration, particularly in the very young, the older adult, or the debilitated client unable to respond to thirst. With severe diarrhea, vascular collapse and hypovolemic shock may occur. Potassium and magnesium are lost, potentially leading to hypokalemia and hypomagnesemia. The loss of bicarbonate in the stool can lead to metabolic acidosis. See Chapter 5 ⊂⊃ for further discussion of the effects of these imbalances.

## COLLABORATIVE CARE

Management of diarrhea focuses on identifying and treating the underlying cause. In addition, the diarrhea itself may need to be treated to promote comfort and to prevent complications. The history (including the onset and associated circumstances of the diarrhea) and physical examination often provide enough information to identify its cause.

### Diagnostic Tests

The following laboratory and diagnostic tests may be ordered to help identify the cause of diarrhea.

- *Stool specimen* is obtained for gross and microscopic examination. Gross examination includes volume and water content, and the presence of any blood, pus, mucus, or excess fat. Microscopic examination evaluates the presence of WBCs, unabsorbed fat, and parasites. WBCs in the stool may indicate a bacterial infection or mucosal ulceration. Because parasites, ova, or larvae may not be continuously present in stool, a series of three specimens, spaced 2 to 3 days apart, is obtained when parasitic infection is suspected.

- *Stool culture* is ordered when an enteric pathogen is suspected (e.g., for persistent or bloody diarrhea accompanied by fever and/or recent travel out of the country).
- *Serum electrolytes, serum osmolality,* and *arterial blood gases* may be ordered to assess for adverse effects of diarrhea. Increased serum osmolality indicates water loss and dehydration. Other potential imbalances include hypokalemia, hypomagnesemia, and metabolic acidosis as a result of diarrhea. The serum sodium may be increased or decreased, depending on the type of diarrhea.
- *Sigmoidoscopy* allows direct examination of the bowel mucosa. Stool may also be obtained during sigmoidoscopy for microscopic examination. The preparation and teaching for a client undergoing sigmoidoscopy is in the box below.
- *Tissue biopsy* may be performed to identify chronic inflammatory processes, infection, and other causes of diarrhea. For biopsy, a small section of tissue (which may include the mucosal and muscle layers) is removed and examined for gross microscopic and histologic (cell character) changes.

## Nursing Implications for Diagnostic Tests

### Sigmoidoscopy

#### Client Preparation

- Ensure the presence of a signed informed consent form.
- Generally, clear liquid or a light diet is ordered for the evening before the procedure.
- Instruct to take a laxative.
- Administer an enema or rectal suppository before the procedure as ordered.

#### Client and Family Teaching

*Before Procedure*

- The procedure takes approximately 15 minutes.
- A mild sedative or tranquilizer may be given during the procedure.
- You may be positioned on your left side or in the knee-chest position.
- The scope will be inserted through the anus into the sigmoid colon.
- Feces may be suctioned.
- A biopsy may be taken. Polyps may be removed.
- Taking deep breaths when you feel discomfort may help you relax.

*After Procedure*

- Sit up slowly to avoid dizziness or lightheadedness.
- You may pass large amounts of flatus if air was instilled into the bowel.
- Report any abdominal pain, fever, chills, or rectal bleeding.
- If a polyp is removed, avoid heavy lifting for 7 days, and avoid high-fiber foods for 1 to 2 days.

## Medications

Antidiarrheal medications are used sparingly or not at all until the cause of diarrhea has been identified. In diarrhea associated with botulism or bacillary dysentery, giving an antidiarrheal agent can worsen or prolong the disease by slowing elimination of the toxin from the bowel. Once the underlying cause for diarrhea has been established, specific medications may be ordered to treat the underlying cause. Antibiotics are used with caution because they alter the normal bacterial population of the bowel and may actually worsen diarrhea. A balanced electrolyte solution may be required to replace fluid losses. Intravenous or oral potassium preparations may also be prescribed.

Opium and some of its derivatives, anticholinergics, absorbants, and demulcents are commonly used as antidiarrheal preparations. Specific preparations, their method of action, and the nursing implications for these medications are outlined in the box below and on the following page.

## Medication Administration

### Antidiarrheal Preparations

#### ABSORBANTS AND PROTECTANTS

Kaolin and pectin (Kaopectate, Donnagel-MB), Charcoal
Bismuth subsalicylate (Pepto-Bismol)

Absorbant preparations act locally in the intestines to bind substances that can cause diarrhea. Absorbants are safe and are generally available over the counter. Their efficacy has not been proved, although bismuth subsalicylate has been shown to be somewhat effective in preventing and managing traveler's diarrhea, usually related to contaminated water supplies. Bismuth salts also have a protective and antimicrobial effect.

#### Nursing Responsibilities

- Assess for contraindications to antidiarrheal therapy, such as some infections or chronic inflammatory bowel disease, including ulcerative colitis.
- If fever is present, check with physician before giving the medication.
- Administer these medications at least 1 hour before or 2 hours after other oral medications; they may interfere with the absorption of other drugs.
- Observe the client's response to the medication. Constipation is a potential problem.

#### Client and Family Teaching

- Take the recommended dosage at the onset of diarrhea and after each loose stool.
- Do not take any of these preparations for more than 48 hours. If diarrhea persists, notify the physician.
- Do not give antidiarrheal medications to debilitated older clients without physician supervision.
- Chew bismuth subsalicylate tablets, rather than swallowing them whole, for maximal effectiveness. This medication may cause harmless darkening of the tongue and stool.
- If you are allergic to aspirin, use bismuth subsalicylate with caution; as a general rule, avoid taking aspirin while taking bismuth subsalicylate.

*(continued on page 620)*

# Medication Administration

## Antidiarrheal Preparations (continued)

### OPIUM AND OPIUM DERIVATIVES

Camphorated tincture of opium (Paregoric)
Tincture of opium (laudanum, opium tincture)
Difenoxin (Motofen)
Diphenoxylate (Lomotil, Lotrol, others)
Loperamide hydrochloride (Imodium)

Opium and its derivatives act on the central nervous system (CNS) to decrease the motility of the ileum and colon, slowing transit time and promoting more water absorption. They also decrease the sensation of a full rectum and increase anal sphincter tone. Paregoric and tincture of opium have a greater potential for abuse and are prescription drugs subject to controls under the federal Controlled Substance Act of 1970. Difenoxin, diphenoxylate, and loperamide are derivatives of opium with few analgesic, euphoric, or abuse-promoting effects and are in more common use today.

### Nursing Responsibilities

- Assess for contraindications to antidiarrheal or narcotic medications prior to giving these drugs.
- Administer paregoric undiluted with water.
- Do not administer difenoxin and diphenoxylate to clients receiving monoamine oxidase inhibitors (MAOI); hypertensive crises may occur.
- Observe closely for increased effects of other CNS depressants, such as alcohol, narcotic analgesics, or barbiturate sedatives.
- Observe for abdominal distention; toxic megacolon may occur if these drugs are given to the client with ulcerative colitis.

### Client and Family Teaching

- Take the medication as recommended at the onset of diarrhea and after each loose stool.

- These drugs may be habit forming, use for no more than 48 hours.
- Avoid using alcohol and over-the-counter cold preparations while taking these drugs.
- These preparations may cause drowsiness, avoid driving or operating machinery while taking them.

### ANTICHOLINERGICS

Atropine
Belladonna alkaloids (Donnagel, Donnatal)

Anticholinergic medications reduce bowel spasticity and acid secretion in the stomach. They are used to treat diarrhea that is associated with peptic ulcer disease and irritable bowel syndrome. These are nonspecific drugs; their systemic effects are their major drawback.

### Nursing Responsibilities

- Assess for contraindications to atropine and other anticholinergic medications: glaucoma, prostatic hypertrophy, and gastrointestinal or genitourinary obstruction.
- Observe for side effects, such as eye pain, impaired urination, or constipation.

### Client and Family Teaching

- Take only as directed, stop the drug and notify the physician if you develop eye pain, impaired urination, constipation.
- Do not operate machinery while taking this medication; drowsiness may occur.
- Hard candies help relieve oral dryness associated with these preparations.

## Dietary Management

Fluid replacement is of primary importance in managing the client with diarrhea. If the client is able to tolerate oral fluids (i.e., if the client is not experiencing nausea and vomiting), an oral glucose/balanced electrolyte solution provides the best fluid replacement. Commercial preparations such as Gatorade and other sports drinks are available, as are pediatric solutions (e.g., Pedialyte), which can be used for adults as well as children. A solution of 5 mL (1 teaspoon) each of table salt and baking soda and 4 teaspoons (20 mL) of granulated sugar added with desired flavoring (such as lemon extract or juice) to 1 quart (1 L) of water can be made at home to replace water and electrolytes.

Solid food is withheld in the first 24 hours of acute diarrhea to rest the bowel. After that time, frequent, small, soft feedings can be added. Milk and milk products are added last, because the lactose they contain frequently aggravates the diarrhea. Raw fruits and vegetables, fried foods, bran, whole-grain cereals, condiments, spices, coffee, and alcoholic beverages are avoided during the recovery period.

Clients with chronic diarrhea may benefit by eliminating specific foods from the diet (see the Meeting Individual Needs box on page 621). Foods and nonfood substances that may aggravate diarrhea are outlined in Table 24–1. The diet should be high in calories and nutritional value. Vitamin supplements

### TABLE 24-1   Foods That May Aggravate Chronic Diarrhea

| Foods | Reason |
|---|---|
| Milk, ice cream, yogurt, soft cheeses, cottage cheese | Contain lactose; not tolerated by clients with lactase deficiency who cannot digest lactose. |
| Apple juice, pear juice, grapes, honey, dates, nuts, figs, fruit-flavored soft drinks | Contain fructose; when consumed in large quantities, fructose may not be totally absorbed, causing an osmotic draw of fluid into the bowel. |
| Table sugar | Contains sucrose; not tolerated by clients with sucrase deficiency. |
| Apple juice, pear juice, sugarless gums and mints | May contain sorbitol or mannitol, sugars that are not absorbed and can cause osmotic draw. |
| Antacids | Magnesium-containing antacids decrease bowel transit time and contain poorly absorbed salts that can exert an osmotic draw. |
| Coffee, tea, cola drinks, over-the-counter analgesics | Contain caffeine, which can decrease bowel transit time. |

## Meeting Individualized Needs

### LACTOSE INTOLERANCE

The enzyme lactase is necessary to digest and absorb lactose, or "milk sugar," a disaccharide found in milk. Lactase deficiency is common in adults; only about 30% of people worldwide are able to efficiently digest and absorb lactose throughout their lives. Lactose intolerance is common in Native North Americans and Southeast Asians. Scandinavians and other northern Europeans have the lowest incidence of lactose intolerance (Whitney & Rolfes, 2002).

may be necessary, particularly the fat-soluble vitamins (A, D, E, and K). Clients with severe chronic diarrhea may require parenteral nutrition (see Chapter 20 ⬭ ).

## Complementary Therapies

Herbal or homeopathic therapies may be used to help relieve diarrhea. Herbal treatments may include a strong tea of black pepper, chamomile, coriander, rosemary, sandalwood, or thyme. Homeopathic practitioners may use podophyllum tablets to treat diarrhea (Fontaine, 2000). Refer the client to a qualified practitioner for more information about using complementary therapies to treat diarrhea.

## NURSING CARE

### Health Promotion

Teach all clients about the importance of handwashing as a measure to prevent the spread of infectious diseases, including those that cause diarrhea. Teach safe food handling techniques to prevent bacterial contamination, and discuss measures to ensure safe drinking water. For clients planning to travel outside the United States or to wilderness areas, teach measures to purify water for drinking and cooking.

### Assessment

The nursing assessment can help identify the cause of the client's diarrhea, as well as early signs of complications. Collect the following assessment data.

- Health history: duration and extent of diarrhea; associated symptoms; dietary intake; recent travel out of the country or to wilderness areas; previous history of diarrhea; chronic diseases; prescription and nonprescription medications
- Physical examination: vital signs (including orthostatic vitals); peripheral pulses; skin temperature, moisture, turgor; color and moisture of mucous membranes; abdominal contour and girth; bowel sounds; stool for obvious or occult blood, pus, mucus, or steatorrhea (bulky, foul-smelling stool)

### Nursing Diagnoses and Interventions

Nursing care of the client with diarrhea focuses on identifying the cause, relieving the symptoms, preventing complications, and preventing the potential spread of infection to others.

### Diarrhea

Nursing interventions for diarrhea focus helping the client recover a normal elimination pattern without adverse consequences.

- Monitor and record the frequency and characteristics of bowel movements *to provide a measure of the effectiveness of treatment.*
- Measure abdominal girth and auscultate bowel sounds every 8 hours as indicated. *Loud, rushing bowel sounds (borborygmi) indicates increased peristalsis, and may be heard in clients with acute diarrhea. Diminished or absent bowel sounds may indicate a complication of treatment, such as constipation or toxic megacolon.*
- Use standard precautions, including gloves and handwashing. *Standard precautions help prevent the spread of infection to others.*
- Provide ready access to bathroom, commode, or bedpan. *The client may have little warning of the need to defecate. Easily accessed toileting facilities reduce the risk for soiling or injury.*
- Administer antidiarrheal medications as prescribed, *to promote comfort and prevent excess fluid loss.*
- Limit food intake if the diarrhea is acute, reintroducing solid foods slowly, in small amounts, *to allow the bowel to rest and mucosa to heal in acute diarrhea states.*

### Risk for Deficient Fluid Volume

The increased water content of diarrheal stool places the client at risk for fluid deficit.

- Record intake and output; weigh daily; assess skin turgor, mucous membranes, and urine specific gravity every 8 hours. *These assessments help monitor fluid volume status.*

**PRACTICE ALERT** *Assess skin turgor over the sternum in the older adult. Loss of subcutaneous fat associated with aging makes skin turgor assessment on the arms less reliable.* ∎

- Monitor vital signs, including orthostatic blood pressures. *Orthostatic hypotension is identified by a drop in BP of more than 10 mmHg and pulse increase of 10 BPM when changing from a lying to a sitting position or from a sitting to a standing position. It is an indicator of fluid volume deficit.*

**PRACTICE ALERT** *Institute safety precautions such as providing assistance when ambulating for the client with orthostatic hypotension. The fall in blood pressure with position changes can cause lightheadedness and syncope.* ∎

- Provide fluid and electrolyte replacement solutions as indicated. Ensure ready access to fluids; assist the debilitated client with fluid intake. Notify the care provider if the client is unable to tolerate oral fluids. *Oral fluids are encouraged as tolerated to prevent dehydration. Intravenous fluids are necessary if oral fluids are not tolerated. An intake of 3000 mL per day or more is often needed to replace fluid losses.*

## Risk for Impaired Skin Integrity

Decreased extracellular fluid volume and the irritating effects of diarrheal stool increase the risk for skin breakdown.

- Assist with cleaning the perianal area as needed. Use warm water, a gentle cleanser, and soft cloths. *Cleansing removes irritating substances in the stool. Gentle cleansing helps maintain integrity of dehydrated skin.*
- Apply protective ointment to the perianal area. *Moisture-barrier ointments or creams protect the skin from excoriation and help prevent tissue breakdown.*

## Using NANDA, NIC, and NOC

Chart 24–1 shows links between NANDA nursing diagnoses, NIC, and NOC for the client with diarrhea.

## Home Care

Acute and chronic diarrhea generally are managed by the client in the home. Teach the client and family members about the following subjects.

- Causes of diarrhea (as directed by the diagnosis)
- Importance of handwashing and hygiene measures
- Importance of maintaining adequate fluid intake to replace lost water and electrolytes
- Use of a balanced electrolyte solution such as Gatorade or a similar product (purchased or home prepared) for fluid replacement
- Recommendations to limit food intake during acute diarrhea, and resume gradually with small feedings of foods that have a constipating effect: applesauce, bananas, crackers, rice, potatoes
- To avoid foods high in fiber, milk products, and caffeine
- Ways to maintain nutrition if chronic diarrhea is a problem: frequent small meals, nutritional supplements, vitamin supplements
- Precautions and limitations of antidiarrheal preparations
- Importance of seeking medical intervention if diarrhea continues or recurs

# THE CLIENT WITH CONSTIPATION

**Constipation** is defined as the infrequent (two or fewer bowel movements weekly) or difficult passage of stools. Constipation affects older adults more frequently than younger people. Recent studies indicate that approximately 20% to 35% of people over age 65 report recurrent constipation and laxative use. Although fecal transit in the large intestine slows with aging, the increased incidence of constipation is thought to relate more to impaired general health status, increased medication use, and decreased physical activity in the older adult.

## PATHOPHYSIOLOGY AND MANIFESTATIONS

Constipation may be a primary problem or a symptom of another disease or condition. Acute constipation, a definite change in the bowel elimination pattern, often is caused by an organic process. A change in bowel patterns that persists or becomes more frequent or severe may be due to a tumor or other partial bowel obstruction. With chronic constipation, functional causes that impair storage, transport, and evacuation mechanisms impede the normal passage of stools. Common causes of constipation are listed in Table 24–2.

Psychogenic factors are the most frequent causes of chronic constipation. These factors include postponing defecation when the urge is felt, and the perception of satisfaction with defecation. Clients often abuse the use of laxatives and enemas to stimulate a bowel movement when constipation is perceived. Overuse of these measures can lead to real intestinal problems that worsen the condition. For example, *cathartic colon,* impaired colonic motility and changes in bowel structure, mimics ulcerative colitis in that the normal pouchlike or saccular appearance of the colon is lost. *Melanosis coli* is a brownish-black discoloration of the colon mucosa. Both conditions may be caused by long-term laxative use.

With significant constipation or long-term dependence on laxatives or enemas, **fecal impaction** may develop. Impaction

---

## CHART 24–1  LINKS BETWEEN NANDA, NIC, AND NOC

### The Client with Altered Bowel Motility

| NURSING DIAGNOSES | NURSING INTERVENTIONS | NURSING OUTCOMES |
|---|---|---|
| • Diarrhea | • Diarrhea Management<br>• Fluid / Electrolyte Management | • Bowel Elimination<br>• Electrolyte and Acid-Base Balance<br>• Fluid Balance |
| • Constipation | • Bowel Management<br>• Constipation / Impaction Management | • Bowel Elimination<br>• Symptom Control |
| • Bowel Incontinence | • Bowel Incontinence Care<br>• Bowel Training<br>• Perineal Care | • Bowel Continence<br>• Tissue Integrity: Skin and Mucous Membranes |

*Note. Data from Nursing Outcomes Classification (NOC) by M. Johnson & M. Maas (Eds.), 1997, St. Louis: Mosby; Nursing Diagnoses: Definitions & Classification 2001–2002 by North American Nursing Diagnosis Association, 2001, Philadelphia: NANDA; Nursing Interventions Classification (NIC) by J.C. McCloskey & G. M. Bulechek (Eds.), 2000, St. Louis: Mosby. Reprinted by permission.*

| TABLE 24–2 | Selected Causes of Constipation |
|---|---|
| **Factor** | **Related Cause** |
| Activity | Lack of exercise; bed rest |
| Dietary | Highly refined, low-fiber foods; inadequate fluid intake |
| Drugs | Antacids containing aluminum or calcium salts; narcotic analgesics; anticholinergics; many antidepressants, tranquilizers, and sedatives; antihypertensives, such as ganglionic blockers, calcium-channel blockers, beta-adrenergic blockers, and diuretics; iron salts |
| Large bowel | Diverticular disease, inflammatory disease, tumor, obstruction; changes in rectal or anal structure or function |
| Psychogenic | Voluntary suppression of urge; perceived need to defecate on schedule; depression |
| Systemic | Advanced age; pregnancy; neurologic conditions (trauma, multiple sclerosis, tumors, cerebrovascular accident, Parkinsonism); endocrine and metabolic disorders (hypothyroidism, hypercalcemia, uremia, porphyria) |
| Other | Chronic laxative or enema use |

may also occur following barium administration for radiologic exam. The impaction is felt as a rock-hard or puttylike mass of feces in the rectum. Abdominal cramping and a full sensation in the rectal area may be manifestations of impaction. Watery mucus or liquid stool may be passed around the impaction, causing the client to complain of diarrhea.

## COLLABORATIVE CARE

Initial evaluation of constipation is based on the history and physical examination. The abdomen may appear somewhat distended, and bowel sounds may be reduced. If an impaction is present, digital examination of the rectum reveals a palpable hard or puttylike fecal mass.

Simple or chronic constipation is treated with education (a daily bowel movement is not necessary for health), and modification of diet and exercise routines. If the problem is acute or does not resolve, further diagnostic examination may be ordered.

## Diagnostic Tests

- *Serum electrolytes* and *thyroid function tests* may be done to identify metabolic and endocrine problems that may contribute to constipation.
- *Barium enema* may be ordered to evaluate bowel structure and to identify tumors or diverticular disease. Barium is instilled into the large intestine and X-rays are taken. Nursing care for the client undergoing a barium enema is described in the following box.

## Nursing Implications for Diagnostic Tests

### Barium Enema

#### Client Preparation
Ensure presence of a signed informed consent for the procedure.

- Provide or instruct to follow a clear liquid diet for 24 hours prior to the test. All food and fluids may be withheld for 8 hours prior to the test.
- Administer or instruct to use laxatives, enemas, or suppositories as ordered the evening prior to the procedure. Additional bowel preparation may be ordered for the morning just prior to the procedure.

#### Client and Family Teaching

*Before Procedure*
- The procedure takes approximately 1 hour.
- The barium will be instilled through a lubricated tube inserted into your rectum. You will experience a sensation of fullness, and may feel the need to defecate.
- You will be positioned on the left side, on your back, and prone during this procedure.
- A fluoroscope will be used to follow the progress of the barium, and X-rays will be taken.
- You will expel the barium in the bathroom.

*After Procedure*
- Following the procedure, a laxative will be given.
- The stools may be white for the next 1 to 2 days.

- *Sigmoidoscopy* or *colonoscopy* may also be used to evaluate constipation, particularly when the problem is acute and a tumor or obstruction is suspected. A flexible endoscope is used to inspect bowel mucosa and structure. Suspicious lesions may be biopsied at the time of the scope. See the box on page 624 for nursing care for the client having a colonoscopy.

## Medications

Laxative and cathartic preparations to promote stool evacuation were among the earliest drugs. Milder preparations are generally known as laxatives; cathartics have a stronger effect. Most laxatives are appropriate only for short-term use. Cathartics and enemas interfere with normal bowel reflexes and should not be used for simple constipation. Laxatives should never be given if a bowel obstruction or impaction is suspected, nor to people with abdominal pain of undetermined origin (Tierney et al., 2001). When the bowel is obstructed, laxatives or cathartics may cause serious mechanical damage and perforate the bowel.

The only laxatives that are appropriate and safe for long-term use are bulking agents, such as psyllium seed, calcium polycarbophil, and methylcellulose. These agents act by increasing the bulk of the feces and drawing water into the bowel to soften it. Commonly prescribed laxatives and cathartics are discussed in the Medication Administration box on page 624.

## Nursing Implications for Diagnostic Tests

### Colonoscopy

#### Client Preparation

- Ensure presence of a signed informed consent for the procedure.
- A liquid diet may be prescribed for 2 days prior to the procedure, and the client is usually NPO for 8 hours just before the procedure.
- Administer or instruct the client in bowel preparation procedures such as taking citrate of magnesia or polyethylene glycol the evening before.
- Sedation is usually given during the procedure.

#### Client and Family Teaching

*Before Procedure*

- Explain dietary restrictions and their purpose.

- The procedure takes 30 minutes to 1 hour.
- The scope is inserted through the anus and advanced to the cecum.
- A biopsy may be taken, and polyps may be removed.
- Discomfort is minimal.
- Arrange for transportation as you may not be allowed to drive for 24 hours after the procedure.

*After Procedure*

- You may have increased flatus as air is instilled into the bowel during the procedure.
- Report any abdominal pain, chills, fever, rectal bleeding, or mucopurulent discharge.
- If a polyp has been removed, avoid heavy lifting for 7 days, and avoid high-fiber food for 1 to 2 days.

## Medication Administration

### Laxatives and Cathartics

#### BULK-FORMING AGENTS

> Bran
> Calcium polycarbophil (Fibercon)
> Methylcellulose (Citrucel)
> Psyllium hydrophilic mucilloid (Metamucil, Effer-Syllium)

Bulk-forming agents are the only safe laxatives for long-term use. They contain vegetable fiber, which is not digested or absorbed in the gut. This natural fiber creates bulk and draws water into the intestine, softening the stool mass.

##### Nursing Responsibilities

- Mix the agent with a full glass of cool liquid just prior to administering.
- Do not administer to clients with possible stool impaction or bowel obstruction.

##### Client and Family Teaching

- Drink at least 6 to 8 full glasses of nonalcoholic fluid per day. Adequate hydration is necessary to produce the drugs laxative effect.
- These agents may be mixed with water, milk, or fruit juice.
- Take the drug in the morning or with meals. To reduce the risk of impaction, do not take at bedtime.
- Because of the increased risk of impaction, check with the physician before increasing dietary fiber while you are taking these agents.

#### WETTING AGENTS

> Docusate (Colace, Surfak, Doxidan, others)

Wetting agents reduce stool surface tension and form an emulsion of fat and water, softening the stool. They are used primarily to prevent straining and reduce the discomfort of expelling hard stools.

##### Nursing Responsibilities

- Administer with ample fluids to promote softening effect.
- Wetting agents may alter the absorption of other drugs. Do not administer within 1 hour of other oral medications.

- Do not attempt to crush or open caplets; a liquid form is available for clients who cannot swallow pills or capsules.

##### Client and Family Teaching

- Do not use for more than 1 week or less unless specifically recommended by the physician.
- Take the medication in the morning or evening, but avoid taking it with other medications.
- Adequate fluid is necessary to obtain the beneficial effect of the drug. Drink 6 to 8 glasses of nonalcoholic fluid per day.

#### OSMOTIC AND SALINE LAXATIVES/CATHARTICS

> Lactulose (Rhodialose)
> Sorbitol
> Magnesium hydroxide (Milk of Magnesia)
> Magnesium citrate
> Polyethylene glycol (Klean-Prep)

Laxatives in this group contain poorly absorbed salts or carbohydrates that remain in the bowel, increasing osmotic pressure and drawing water into the intestine. Stool volume increases, consistency decreases, and peristalsis is stimulated. Many of these agents also have an irritant effect on the bowel, further stimulating peristalsis. They are used to stimulate rapid or complete bowel evacuation to relieve constipation and to prepare the bowel for diagnostic and surgical procedures. They should be limited to acute, short-term use; chronic use may suppress normal bowel reflexes.

##### Nursing Responsibilities

- Assess for possible contraindications to osmotic or saline laxatives, including bowel ulceration or obstruction, dehydration, electrolyte imbalances, heart failure (which may be aggravated by the sodium content), or renal failure.
- Administer with a full glass of liquid, preferably in the morning to avoid sleep disturbance.
- Monitor fluid and electrolyte status: skin turgor, mucous membranes, intake and output; daily weight, and laboratory studies, such as hemoglobin and hematocrit levels, serum osmolality and electrolytes, and urine specific gravity.

# Medication Administration

## Laxatives and Cathartics (continued)

### Client and Family Teaching

- Do not use these agents on a routine basis to treat or prevent constipation.
- Chill the solution to increase its palatability.
- Expect some abdominal cramping.
- Use only as directed. Increase fluid intake to at least 6 to 8 glasses of nonalcoholic fluid.
- Notify the physician if adverse effects occur, including abdominal pain, bloody stool, excessive skin or mucous membrane dryness, rapid weight loss, dizziness, or other unusual symptoms.
- These agents work in 3 to 6 hours; take them in the morning or early evening to avoid sleep disturbance.

### IRRITANT OR STIMULANT LAXATIVES

> Bisacodyl (Dulcolax, Bisco-Lax, Carter's Liver Pills, Codylax, others)
> Phenolphthalein (Evac-U-Gen, Evac-U-Lax, Feen-A-Mint, Phenolax, others)
> Cascara sagrada
> Senna (Senna laxative, Fletcher's Castoria)
> Castor oil

Stimulant laxatives work by stimulating the motility and secretion of intestinal mucosa. Their use results in watery stool, often accompanied by abdominal cramping and pain. They are used to relieve constipation, although they should not be used as the initial treatment. Stimulant laxatives are also used for preparing the bowel for diagnostic testing.

### Nursing Responsibilities

- Assess for potential contraindications to these laxatives, including abdominal pain and cramping, nausea and vomiting, anal or rectal fissures.
- Administer on an empty stomach to minimize the effects of food on its dissolution and absorption.
- Do not crush enteric-coated bisacodyl tablets or administer with alkaline products. This may hasten their dissolution in the stomach, leading to gastric distress.

### Client and Family Teaching

- Discourage the use of this type of laxative, even in over-the-counter preparations, for the initial or continuing relief of constipation.
- Do not use the laxative for more than 1 week; chronic use can be habit forming and may suppress normal bowel reflexes.

- These laxatives are excreted in breast milk and should not be used by lactating women.
- Phenolphthalein-containing products may discolor the urine pink or red. Report possible hypersensitivity manifestations, such as difficulty breathing, dizziness or lightheadedness, or skin rashes, to the primary care provider, and stop taking the medication.

### LUBRICANTS

> Mineral oil

Mineral oil is the only lubricant laxative available. It acts by forming an oily coat on the fecal mass, preventing the reabsorption of water, and resulting in softer stool. Problems associated with the use of mineral oil as a laxative include reduced absorption of the fat-soluble vitamins A, D, E, and K; possible damage to the liver and spleen due to systemic absorption, and potential pneumonitis from aspiration of oil droplets into the lungs.

### Nursing Responsibilities

- Assess for possible contraindications to use of mineral oil, including advanced age, preexisting lung disease, and hemorrhoids or other rectal lesions.
- Do not give mineral oil concurrently with wetting agents or stool softeners, because these increase the potential for systemic absorption and increase the effects of the mineral oil.
- Administer mineral oil in the evening before bedtime to reduce the effect on the absorption of fat-soluble vitamins and minimize the risk of aspiration.
- Assess for manifestations of vitamin deficiency. Monitor the client taking oral anticoagulants for evidence of increased bleeding, such as bleeding gums, easy bruising, or melena.

### Client and Family Teaching

- Long-term use of mineral oil is not recommended because of its risks and adverse effects.
- Do not use mineral oil if hemorrhoids or rectal lesions are present, leakage of the oil through the anal sphincter may cause itching and interfere with healing.
- Suck on a lemon or orange slice after taking oral mineral oil to reduce the oily aftertaste.

## Dietary Management

Foods that have a high fiber content are recommended. Vegetable fiber is largely indigestible and unabsorbable, so it increases stool bulk. Fiber also helps draw water into the fecal mass, softening the stool and making defecation easier. Raw fruits and vegetables are good sources of dietary fiber, as is cereal bran. Use 2 to 3 teaspoons of unprocessed bran with meals (sprinkled on fruit or cereal) or up to 1/4 cup daily to supply adequate fiber.

Fluids are also important to maintain bowel motility and soft stools. The client should drink 6 to 8 glasses of fluid per day.

In older adults, constipation may be due to inadquate food intake. Carefully evaluate diet history and usual daily intake.

## Enemas

Significant or chronic constipation or a fecal impaction may require the administration of an enema. As a general rule, enemas should be used only in acute situations and only on a short-term basis. They may also be ordered to prepare the bowel for diagnostic testing or examination. The following types of enemas may be prescribed.

- A saline enema using 500 to 2000 mL of warmed physiologic saline solution is the least irritating to the bowel.

- Tap-water enemas use 500 to 1000 mL of water to soften feces and irritate the bowel mucosa, stimulating peristalsis and evacuation.
- Soap-suds enemas consist of a tap-water solution to which soap is added as a further irritant.
- Phosphate enemas (e.g., Fleet) use a hypertonic saline solution to draw fluid into the bowel and irritate the mucosa, leading to evacuation.
- Oil retention enemas instill mineral or vegetable oil into the bowel to soften the fecal mass. The instilled oil is retained overnight or for several hours before evacuation.

The repeated use of enemas can lead not only to impaired bowel function, but also to fluid and electrolyte imbalances. Tap-water and phosphate enemas are particularly likely to cause these problems. In acute conditions with risk of bowel obstruction, perforation, ulceration, or other problem, enemas should not be administered until their safe use can be established.

## NURSING CARE

### Health Promotion

Education can prevent constipation. Teach clients the importance of maintaining a diet high in natural fiber. Foods such as fresh fruits, vegetables, whole-grain products, and bran provide natural fiber. Encourage reducing consumption of meats and refined foods, which are low in fiber and can be constipating. Emphasize the need to maintain a high fluid intake every day, particularly during hot weather and exercise. Discuss the relationship between exercise and bowel regularity. Encourage clients to engage in some form of exercise, such as walking daily.

Discuss normal bowel habits, and explain that a daily bowel movement is not the norm for all people. Encourage clients to respond to the urge to defecate when it occurs. Suggest setting aside a time, usually following a meal, for elimination.

### Assessment

To assess the client with real or perceived constipation, collect the following data.

- Health history: usual and current pattern of defecation, including time of day, amount, and stool consistency; usual diet, fluid intake, and activity pattern; possible contributing factors such as narcotic analgesics, activity limitations, painful hemorrhoids, perianal surgery; chronic diseases such as endocrine or neurologic disorders; prescribed and nonprescription medications
- Physical examination: abdominal girth and shape, bowel sounds, tenderness, and percussion tone; digital exam of the rectum if impaction is suspected.

For discussion of constipation in the older adult see the box on this page.

### Nursing Diagnoses and Interventions

Nursing interventions for the client with constipation focus chiefly on education.

### Meeting Individualized Needs

#### THE OLDER ADULT

Constipation and perceived constipation are common problems in older adults. While constipation is not a normal consequence of aging, factors such as slowed peristalsis, lowered activity levels, reduced food and fluid intake, and decreased sensory perception contribute to the higher incidence of constipation seen in the elderly. Chronic diseases such as diabetes, mobility problems, and medications also increase the risk of constipation in older adults.

Cultural influences and advertising lead many older adults to believe that a daily bowel movement is important for health. This belief contributes to an increased incidence of perceived constipation in the elderly. Because of this perception, the older adult may come to rely on laxatives, suppositories, or enemas to facilitate regular bowel movements. These external aids to defecation can further impair the ability to maintain "normal" bowel habits: a movement of soft stool every 2 to 3 days.

### Constipation

Whether real or perceived, constipation is disruptive to the client's activities of daily living (ADLs) and life satisfaction.

- Monitor pattern of defecation and stool consistency. *This information helps establish the client's usual pattern of defecation and differentiate between actual and perceived constipation.*
- Provide additional fluids to maintain an intake of at least 2500 mL per day. *A generous fluid intake helps maintain soft stool consistency and promote intestinal motility.*
- Encourage drinking a glass of warm water before breakfast. Provide time and privacy following breakfast for bowel elimination. *This helps develop a pattern of natural elimination; the warm water provides mild stimulation of bowel peristalsis.*
- Consult with the dietitian to provide a diet high in natural fiber unless contraindicated. Provide foods such as natural bran, prunes, or prune juice. *Natural fiber adds bulk to the stool and has a mild stimulant effect.*
- Encourage activities such as ambulation or chair exercises (range of motion, stretching, wheelchair lifts, etc.) as tolerated. *Activity stimulates peristalsis and strengthens abdominal muscles, facilitating elimination.*
- If indicated, consult with primary care provider about the use of bulk laxatives, stool softeners, or other laxatives as needed. *Laxatives may be necessary to relieve acute constipation. Clients with long-term activity or diet restrictions or impaired abdominal muscle strength may need a bulk-forming laxative to maintain normal elimination patterns and prevent constipation.*

### Using NANDA, NIC, and NOC

See Chart 24–1 on page 622 for links between NANDA nursing diagnoses, NIC, and NOC for the client with constipation.

## Home Care

Include the following topics when teaching for home care measures to prevent and treat constipation.

- Increasing dietary fiber intake by including fresh fruits and vegetables, whole grains, high-fiber breakfast cereals, and unprocessed bran in the diet (Bran can be sprinkled on cereals, mixed into bread or muffin recipes, or mixed with fruit juice to increase its palatability.)
- Maintaining fluid intake of 6 to 8 glasses of water per day (unless contraindicated)
- Suggestions for remaining physically active to promote bowel function and maintain muscle tone
- Responding to the urge to defecate when perceived
- Appropriate use of laxatives:
  - Do not use laxatives, suppositories, or enemas on a regular basis.
  - Bulk-forming agents provide insoluble fiber, and are safe for long-term use; it is important to drink at least 6 to 8 glasses of water daily when using these (or any) laxatives.
  - Other laxatives such as milk of magnesia, docusate (Colase, DSS, others), bisacodyl (Dulcolax, others), cascara, or castor oil should be used only occasionally to relieve constipation.
- The need to report any change in bowel habits such as new or persistent constipation or diarrhea, abdominal pain, black or bloody stools, nausea or anorexia, weakness, or unexplained weight loss to the primary care provider.

## THE CLIENT WITH IRRITABLE BOWEL SYNDROME

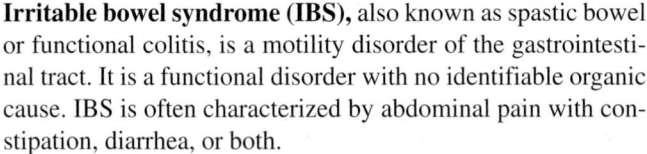

**Irritable bowel syndrome (IBS),** also known as spastic bowel or functional colitis, is a motility disorder of the gastrointestinal tract. It is a functional disorder with no identifiable organic cause. IBS is often characterized by abdominal pain with constipation, diarrhea, or both.

Irritable bowel syndrome is common, affecting up to 20% of people in Western civilization. It usually affects young people, although may also be prevalent in older adults. Women are affected 2 to 3 times more frequently than men (Braunwald et al., 2001).

## PATHOPHYSIOLOGY

In IBS, it appears that central nervous system (CNS) regulation of the motor and sensory functions of the bowel are altered. Clients with IBS often experience increased motor reactivity of the small bowel and colon in response to stimuli such as food intake, hormonal influences, and physiologic or psychologic stress. Sensory responses from the gut also are exaggerated in response to the movement of chime through the bowel (Braunwald et al., 2001). Hypersecretion of colonic mucus is a common feature of the syndrome.

### Manifestations of Irritable Bowel Syndrome

- Abdominal pain
  - May be relieved by defecation
  - May be intermittent and colicky or dull and continuous
- Altered bowel elimination
  - Constipation
  - Diarrhea
  - Mucous stools
- Abdominal bloating and flatulence
- Abdominal tenderness, especially over sigmoid colon
- Possible nausea, vomiting

A lower visceral pain threshold is often found in clients with IBS. Clients may complain of pain, bloating, and distention when intestinal gas levels are normal.

Psychologic factors such as depression or anxiety have been linked to IBS; however, they have not been identified as causes of the disorder. Clients with underlying psychologic factors may be more likely to seek medical attention for symptoms, but normal psychologic profiles are noted in clients with the disorder who do not seek medical attention (Tierney et al., 2001). Recent research does indicate a correlation between emotional, physical, and sexual abuse and IBS. Again, however, causation could not be established.

## MANIFESTATIONS

Irritable bowel syndrome is characterized by abdominal pain that often is relieved by defecation and a change in bowel habits (see the box above). The pain may be either colicky, occurring in spasms, or dull and continuous. Altered patterns of defecation may include:

- A change in frequency
- Abnormal stool form (hard or lumpy, loose or watery)
- Altered stool passage (straining, urgency, or a sensation of incomplete evacuation)
- Passage of mucus

The client may also complain of abdominal bloating and excess gas. Other manifestations include nausea, vomiting, and anorexia; fatigue, headache, depression, or anxiety. The abdomen is often tender to palpation, particularly over the sigmoid colon.

## COLLABORATIVE CARE

Irritable bowel syndrome is diagnosed based on the presence of abdominal pain or discomfort that has two of the following three characteristics: (1) relieved by defecation; (2) associated with a change in frequency of elimination; (3) associated with a change in stool form (Tierney et al., 2001). Management is directed toward relieving manifestations and reducing or eliminating precipitating factors. Stress reduction measures, exercises, or counseling may benefit the client.

## Diagnostic Tests

The primary purpose of diagnostic testing is to rule out other causes of abdominal pain and altered fecal elimination.

- *Stool* may be examined for *occult blood, ova and parasites,* and *culture.* A stool smear for WBCs may also be done; an elevated WBC count may indicate an inflammatory or infectious process.
- *Complete blood count (CBC) with differential* and *erythrocyte sedimentation rate (ESR)* are evaluated. Anemia may indicate blood loss and a possible tumor, polyps, or other organic problem. An elevated WBC may indicate bacterial infection, and an elevated ESR is seen with many inflammatory processes.
- *Sigmoidoscopy* or *colonoscopy* may be ordered to visually examine bowel mucosa, measure intraluminal pressures, and biopsy suspicious lesions. In IBS, the bowel appears normal, with increased mucus, marked spasm, and possible hyperemia (increased redness), but no suspicious lesions. Intraluminal pressures are often increased. The procedure itself may stimulate manifestations of the syndrome. Nursing care related to these procedures is found in the Nursing Implications boxes on pages 619 and 624.
- *Small bowel series (upper GI series with small bowel follow-through)* and *barium enema* may be ordered. For the small bowel series, an oral barium preparation is administered, and the small intestine is examined under fluoroscopy. With IBS, the entire GI tract may show increased motility. The box below outlines nursing care of the client undergoing a small bowel series. Nursing care of the client having a barium enema is described in the Nursing Implications box on page 623.

## Medications

Although not curative, medications may be prescribed to manage the symptoms of IBS. Bulk-forming laxatives (such as bran, methylcellulose, or psyllium) may help reduce bowel spasm and normalize the number and form of bowel movements. An anticholinergic drug such as dicyclomine (Antispas, Bentyl, others) or hyoscyamine (Anaspaz, others) may be ordered to inhibit bowel motility by interfering with parasympathetic stimulation of the gastrointestinal tract. It relieves postprandial abdominal pain when given 30 to 60 minutes before meals. In clients with diarrhea, loperamide (Imodium) or diphenoxylate (Lomotil) may be used prophylactically to prevent diarrhea in selected situations.

New drugs that affect GI motility by altering serotonin receptors in the GI tract are being researched. The initial approved drug, alosetron, was later withdrawn from the market due to severe complications associated with its use.

Antidepressant drugs, including tricyclics and selective serotonin reuptake inhibitors (SSRIs), may help relieve abdominal pain associated with IBS. While the anticholinergic side effects of the tricyclics (such as desipramine [Norpramin] and imipramine [Tofranil]) may help decrease diarrhea, they have more adverse effects than SSRIs such as sertraline (Zoloft) and fluoxetine (Prozac).

## Dietary Management

Many clients with IBS benefit from additional dietary fiber. Adding bran to meals provides added bulk and water content to the stool, reducing the incidence of both loose diarrheal stools and hard, constipated stools. Other dietary changes are specific to individual triggers for IBS symptoms. Some clients may benefit from limiting lactose, fructose, or sorbitol intake (see Table 24–1). When excess gas and flatulence is a problem, reducing the intake of gas-forming foods, such as beans, cabbage, apple and grape juices, nuts, and raisins, may be helpful. Caffeinated drinks, such as coffee, tea, and soft drinks, act as gastrointestinal stimulants; limiting intake of these fluids may also prove beneficial.

## Complementary Therapies

Herbal preparations may provide some benefit for clients with IBS. Herbs with an antispasmotic effect, such as anise, chamomile, peppermint, and sage, may be used to reduce the manifestations of IBS. Refer the client to a certified herbologist or naturopathic physician for treatment.

## Nursing Implications for Diagnostic Tests

### Small Bowel Series

#### Client Preparation

- Ensure the presence of a signed informed consent for the procedure.
- A low-residue diet may be ordered for 48 hours preceding the examination, and a tap-water enema or cathartic may be given the evening before.
- Instruct to withhold all food for 8 hours and water for 4 hours before the examination.
- Withhold medications affecting bowel motility for 24 hours prior to examination if possible (unless prescribed as part of the preparation procedure).

#### Client and Family Teaching

- Although the test is not uncomfortable, it requires several hours to complete. Bring reading material, paperwork, or crafts along to occupy time.
- For a small bowel exam, the barium may be administered orally, or instilled through a weighted tube inserted into the small bowel, or endoscopically.
- Increase intake of fluids for at least 24 hours after the procedure to facilitate evacuation of the barium. A laxative or cathartic may be prescribed.
- Stool will be chalky white for up to 72 hours after the exam. Normal stool color will return on complete evacuation of barium.

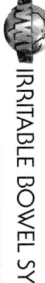

## NURSING CARE

Clients with irritable bowel syndrome rarely require acute care for IBS as a primary problem. However, nurses frequently interact with these clients in clinics and other outpatient settings.

### Assessment

Careful assessment is important to help identify the effects of IBS on the client. Collect the following assessment data.

- Health history: current symptoms, their onset and duration; current treatment measures; effect of symptoms on lifestyle; careful exploration of history of emotional, physical, or sexual abuse
- Physical examination: apparent general state of health; abdominal shape and contour, bowel sounds, tenderness

### Nursing Diagnoses and Interventions

The primary nursing responsibility is education; providing referrals and counseling are additional nursing responsibilities to clients who have irritable bowel syndrome.

The following nursing diagnoses may be appropriate for clients with IBS.

- *Constipation* related to altered gastrointestinal motility
- *Diarrhea* related to altered gastrointestinal motility and excess mucous secretion
- *Anxiety* related to situational stress
- *Ineffective coping* related to effects of disorder on lifestyle

Refer to the previous sections on diarrhea and constipation for selected nursing interventions.

### Home Care

Include the following topics in teaching for the client with irritable bowel syndrome.

- The nature of the disorder and the reality of the client's symptoms
- The relationship between irritable bowel syndrome and stress, anxiety, and depression
- Stress- and anxiety-reduction techniques, such as meditation, visualization, exercise, "time out," and progressive relaxation
- Dietary influences that may contribute to IBS and suggested dietary changes, such as additional fiber and water intake
- The use and role of prescribed medications, their adverse effects, and when to contact the physician
- The importance of routine follow-up appointments and of notifying the primary care provider if manifestations change (such as blood in the stool, significant constipation or diarrhea, increasing abdominal pain, or weight loss)

Refer the client to a counselor or other mental health professional for assistance in dealing with psychologic factors.

## THE CLIENT WITH FECAL INCONTINENCE

**Fecal incontinence,** the loss of voluntary control of defecation, occurs less frequently than urinary incontinence but is no less distressing to the client. Multiple factors contribute to fecal in-

---

### BOX 24–1   ■ Selected Causes of Fecal Incontinence

**Neurologic Causes**
- Spinal cord injury or disease
- Head injury, stroke, or brain tumor
- Degenerative neurologic disease, such as multiple sclerosis, amyotrophic lateral sclerosis (ALS), dementia
- Diabetic neuropathy

**Local Trauma**
- Obstetric tears
- Anorectal injury
- Anorectal surgery with sphincter damage

**Inflammatory Processes**
- Infection
- Radiation

**Other Physiologic Causes**
- Diarrhea
- Stool impaction
- Pelvic floor relaxation or loss of sphincter tone
- Tumors

**Psychologic Causes**
- Depression
- Confusion and disorientation

---

continence, including both physiologic and psychologic conditions (Box 24-1). Bowel incontinence is usually considered a manifestation of a disorder rather than a disorder unto itself. Clients often do not reveal fecal incontinence in discussing health concerns. Little information is available about its incidence and prevalence. Because many of the etiologic factors are more prevalent in the older adult, older clients are more often affected.

### PHYSIOLOGY REVIEW

To understand the pathophysiology of fecal incontinence, it is necessary to understand the normal mechanisms of defecation. The rectum is normally empty. When it is distended by feces entering from the sigmoid colon, the defecation reflex is stimulated. This reflex causes involuntary relaxation of the internal sphincter and stimulates the urge to defecate. When the external sphincter, which is under both voluntary and autonomic (involuntary) control, relaxes, defecation occurs. Adults normally can override the defecation reflex by voluntary contraction of the external sphincter and pelvic floor muscles. The wall of the rectum gradually relaxes, and the urge to defecate subsides.

### PATHOPHYSIOLOGY

The most common causes of fecal incontinence are those that interfere with either sensory or motor control of the rectum and anal sphincters. If the external sphincter is paralyzed as a result of spinal cord injury or disease, defecation occurs automatically when the internal sphincter relaxes with the defecation reflex. If sphincter muscles have been damaged or excessive pelvic floor relaxation has occurred, it may not be possible to override the defecation reflex with voluntary control.

Age-related changes in anal sphincter tone and response to rectal distention increase the risk for fecal incontinence in older adults. Resting and maximal anal sphincter pressures are decreased, particularly in older women. In addition, less rectal distension is needed to produce sustained relaxation of the anal sphincter in older females.

## COLLABORATIVE CARE

The diagnosis of fecal incontinence is based on the client's history. Physical examination of the pelvic floor and anus is performed to evaluate muscle tone and rule out a fecal impaction. Impaired sphincter muscle may be palpable on digital exam. *Anorectal manometry* or a rectal motility test may be used to evaluate the functional ability of the sphincter muscles. A small, flexible balloon catheter is introduced into the rectum, and pressures are measured in the rectum and internal and external sphincters. Normally, rectal dilation causes the internal sphincter to relax and the external sphincter to contract. *Sigmoidoscopy* also may be used to examine the rectum and anal canal.

Management of fecal incontinence is directed toward the identified cause. Medications to relieve diarrhea or constipation may be prescribed. A high-fiber diet, ample fluids, and regular exercise are helpful for many clients. Exercises to improve sphincter and pelvic floor muscle tone (Kegel exercises) may be of long-term benefit. See Chapter 26 ⟨∞⟩ for more information about Kegel exercises.

A bowel training program to establish a regular pattern of elimination often is effective. The client is taught to establish a regular time of day for elimination, usually 15 to 30 minutes after breakfast. A stimulant, such as a cup of coffee, a rectal suppository, or even a phosphate enema, may be given to prompt defecation. Clients with neurologic incontinence may learn to stimulate the anal canal digitally to initiate defecation.

Dietary changes may be useful in managing fecal incontinence. If incontinence occurs only when stools are loose or liquid, increasing dietary fiber or using a bulking agent to increase stool bulk and solidity may be effective (Bliss et al., 2001). When incontinence of solid stool occurs, a low-residue diet of foods that are easily digested and absorbed may be prescribed to reduce the frequency of defecation. Clients also may benefit from using loperimide before meals and prophylactically before running errands or leaving the house. (Tierney et al., 2001). Biofeedback therapy may be used for mentally alert clients with intact sphincter muscles but low muscle tone. With motivation and reinforcement, clients achieve improved sphincter control in response to a stimulus.

When damage to the sphincter or rectal prolapse (protrusion of rectal mucous membrane through the anus) is the cause of fecal incontinence, surgical repair is the treatment of choice. Surgery may also be indicated when conservative measures have not been effective. Permanent colostomy, the creation of an opening from the large bowel on the abdominal wall, is a last-choice option for some clients, but it can control fecal output when other measures fail.

## NURSING CARE

### Assessment

- Health history: extent, onset, and duration of incontinence; identified contributing factors; history of spinal cord or anorectal injury or surgery; chronic diseases such as diabetes, multiple sclerosis, or other neurologic disorders
- Physical examination: mental status; general health; examination of perineal tissues, digital rectal examination

### Nursing Diagnoses and Interventions
#### Bowel Incontinence

Nurses are often responsible for instituting bowel training programs and other measures to manage fecal incontinence.

- Teach caregivers to place the client on a toilet or commode and provide for privacy at a certain time of day. *Placing the client in a normal position to defecate at a consistent time of day stimulates the defecation reflex and helps reestablish a pattern of stool evacuation.*
- If necessary, insert a glycerine or bisacodyl (Dulcolax) suppository 15 to 20 minutes before positioning on the toilet or commode. *This helps to stimulate evacuation. Once a regular elimination pattern is established, it may be possible to discontinue suppository use.*
- Maintain a caring, nonjudgmental manner in providing care. *This promotes a feeling of acceptance when the client may feel unacceptable.*

### PRACTICE ALERT
*Provide room odor control with deodorizer tablets, sprays, or other devices. Controlling odor is important to preserve the client's self-esteem.* ∎

### Risk for Impaired Skin Integrity

Good skin care is vital for the client with fecal incontinence. Stool contains enzymes and other irritating substances that promote skin breakdown when they are not promptly removed. This can lead to pressure ulcers, particularly when a neurologic disorder (such as spinal cord injury, dementia, or stroke) impairs mobility.

- Clean the skin thoroughly with mild soap and water after each bowel movement. *Toilet tissue may be more irritating to the skin and less effective in removing fecal material.*
- Apply a skin barrier cream or ointment after each bowel movement. *These help protect the skin from irritating substances in the feces.*
- If incontinence pads or briefs are used, check frequently for soiling and change when feces is noted. *Although these help protect bedding and clothing from soilage, they can contribute to skin breakdown if they are not checked and changed frequently.*

### Using NANDA, NIC, and NOC

Chart 24–1 on page 622 shows links between NANDA nursing diagnoses, NIC, and NOC for the client with fecal incontinence.

## Nursing Research

### Evidence-Based Practice for Fecal Incontinence

Fecal incontinence is a distressing problem, particularly for clients residing in a community setting. In a prospective study, researchers at the University of Minnesota, Minneapolis, evaluated the effects of fiber supplementation on a group of community-living adults who were incontinent of loose or liquid stools.

Study participants recorded their dietary intake and stool characteristics and collected their stool for 8 days before addition of a fiber supplement. Participants were then randomly assigned to take psyllium, gum arabic, or placebo while continuing their usual diet. They again collected their stool and recorded dietary intake and stool characteristics for the final 8 days of the supplementation period.

On conclusion of the study period, the proportion of incontinent stools in subjects in both the psyllium and gum arabic groups was less than half that of the control group. Stool consistency also improved in the two groups taking fiber supplements.

#### IMPLICATIONS FOR NURSING

Fiber supplements are readily available in pharmacies and grocery stores as bulk-forming laxatives. These supplements have few contraindications and few adverse effects (other than a potential increase in flatus) when taken as directed with ample fluid. Nurses should feel comfortable recommending them for clients who have fecal incontinence associated with loose or liquid stool consistency.

#### Critical Thinking in Client Care

1. Why is fecal incontinence more frequently associated with loose or liquid stools than with soft, formed stools?
2. How do bulk-forming laxatives work to prevent constipation and reduce the frequency of liquid or loose stools?
3. What teaching will you provide for the client taking a bulk-forming laxative?

Note. From "Supplementation with dietary fiber improves fecal incontinence" by D. Bliss, H. Jung, K. Savik, A. Lowry, M. LeMoine, L. Jensen, C. Werner, & K. Schaffer (2001), Nursing Research, 50(4), 203–213.

## Home Care

Managing fecal incontinence is a challenging problem for the client and family caregivers. For the client with intact cognition, it can be psychologically devastating. The client may become socially isolated from fear of odor or clothing soilage. Self-esteem may suffer from a sense of lost control over body functions and the inability to provide self-care. It is important to stress that incontinence is never normal (i.e., aging alone is not a cause of incontinence) and often is treatable. Encourage the client to seek medical evaluation of the problem.

Topics of instruction for the client and family include:

- Recommended dietary measures such as consuming a high-fiber diet and ample fluids to maintain soft, formed stool, or a low-residue diet to reduce the number of stools
- Suggestions for regular exercise to stimulate bowel peristalsis and regular evacuation
- Use of bulk-forming laxatives, such as psyllium seed (Metamucil) to provide stool bulk and reduce the number of small, liquid stools. See the box above for research supporting the use of psyllium or gum arabic to reduce incontinent episodes.
- Prescribed medications (such as loperamide to reduce the number of stools), their appropriate use, and management of adverse effects (such as constipation)
- Bowel training program instructions, including techniques for digital anal stimulation, inserting suppositories, or administering enemas as recommended
  - For digital anal simulation, teach to insert a lubricated gloved finger through the anal sphincter into the rectum 1.5 to 2 inches while seated on the toilet or commode, then use a circular side-to-side movement to gently stretch the rectal wall until the internal sphincter relaxes.
- The importance of good skin care, particularly if neurologic impairment is present
- The potential benefits and associated risks of biofeedback and surgical treatment, if recommended

Provide referrals for home care or community health services as indicated.

# ACUTE INFLAMMATORY AND INFECTIOUS DISORDERS

The GI tract is particularly vulnerable to inflammation and infection because of its continual exposure to the external environment. Although most pathogens affecting the GI tract are ingested in food or water, infection also may be spread by direct contact, possibly by the respiratory route. Pathogens may also be transmitted sexually through anal intercourse.

Acute disease of the GI tract may be caused by the pathogen itself or by a bacterial or other toxin. Acute inflammatory disorders such as appendicitis and peritonitis result from contamination of damaged or normally sterile tissue by the client's own endogenous or resident bacteria.

## THE CLIENT WITH APPENDICITIS

**Appendicitis,** inflammation of the vermiform appendix, is a common cause of acute abdominal pain. It is the most common reason for emergency abdominal surgery in the United States

(Tierney et al., 2001). Appendicitis can occur at any age, but is more common in adolescents and young adults and slightly more common in males than females.

## PATHOPHYSIOLOGY

The appendix is a tubelike pouch attached to the cecum just below the ileocecal valve. It is usually located in the right iliac region, at an area designated as McBurney's point (Figure 24–1 ■). The function of the appendix is not fully understood, although it regularly fills with and empties digested food.

Obstruction of the proximal lumen of the appendix is apparent in most acutely inflamed appendices. The obstruction is often caused by a **fecalith,** or hard mass of feces. Other obstructive causes include a calculus or stone, a foreign body, inflammation, a tumor, parasites (e.g., pinworms), or edema of lymphoid tissue. Following obstruction, the appendix becomes distended with fluid secreted by its mucosa. Pressure within the lumen of the appendix increases, impairing its blood supply and leading to inflammation, edema, ulceration, and infection. Purulent exudate forms, further distending the appendix. Within 24 to 36 hours, tissue necrosis and gangrene result, leading to perforation if treatment is not initiated. Perforation results in bacterial peritonitis, which may remain localized.

Appendicitis can be classified as simple, gangrenous, or perforated, depending on the stage of the process. In *simple appendicitis,* the appendix is inflamed but intact. When areas of tissue necrosis and microscopic perforations are present in the appendix, the disorder is called *gangrenous appendicitis.* A *perforated appendix* shows evidence of gross perforation and contamination of the peritoneal cavity.

## MANIFESTATIONS AND COMPLICATIONS

Continuous mild generalized or upper abdominal pain is the initial characteristic symptom of acute appendicitis. Over the next 4 hours, the pain intensifies and localizes in the right lower quadrant of the abdomen. It is aggravated by moving, walking,

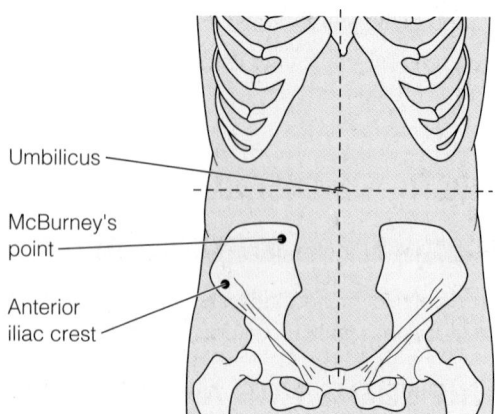

**Figure 24–1** ■ McBurney's point, located midway between the umbilicus and the anterior iliac crest in the right lower quadrant. It is the usual site for localized pain and rebound tenderness due to appendicitis.

or coughing. On palpation, localized and rebound tenderness are noted at McBurney's point. **Rebound tenderness** is demonstrated by relief of pain with direct palpation of McBurney's point followed by pain on release of pressure. Extension or internal rotation of the right hip increases the pain. In addition to pain, a low-grade temperature, anorexia, nausea, and vomiting are often present.

Pain and local tenderness may be less acute in older adults, delaying the diagnosis (Tierney et al., 2001). This can present a significant problem; the course of acute appendicitis in older adults is more virulent and complications develop sooner. Pregnant women may develop right lower quadrant, periumbilical, or right subcostal (under the rib cage) pain due to displacement of the appendix by the distended uterus (Tierney et al., 2001).

Perforation, peritonitis, and abscess are possible complications of acute appendicitis. Perforation is manifested by increased pain and a high fever. It can lead to a small, localized abscess, local peritonitis, or significant generalized peritonitis. (Peritonitis is discussed in the next section of this chapter.)

A less common disorder is chronic appendicitis, characterized by chronic abdominal pain and recurrent acute attacks at intervals of several months or more. Other conditions, such as inflammatory bowel disease and renal disorders, often cause symptoms attributed to chronic appendicitis.

## COLLABORATIVE CARE

Because the acutely inflamed appendix can perforate within 24 hours, rapid diagnosis and treatment are important. Because of this urgency and the low incidence of surgical complications, diagnostic testing and preoperative treatment are limited. The client is admitted to the hospital, and intravenous fluids are initiated. Oral food and fluids are withheld until a diagnosis is confirmed. Once the diagnosis is established, an appendectomy is performed.

### Diagnostic Tests

Laboratory tests are used to help confirm the diagnosis and rule out other possible causes for the symptoms. The following tests may be ordered.

- *WBC count with differential* is obtained. With appendicitis, the total white count is elevated ($10,000/mm^3$ to $20,000/mm^3$), with an increased number of immature WBCs.
- *Urinalysis* is performed to rule out a urinary tract infection or other urologic cause of the client's symptoms.
- *Abdominal X-rays* are taken with the client in the flat and upright positions. A fecalith or calculus may be noted in the right lower quadrant, or a localized ileus may be noted.
- *Abdominal ultrasound* is the most effective test for diagnosing acute appendicitis. In this noninvasive test, high-frequency sound waves are reflected back to a Doppler device to create a computer-generated image. The test requires fewer than 30 minutes to complete. Ultrasound examination has reduced the incidence of exploratory surgery and is particularly useful with clients with atypical symptoms, such as older adults.

- *Pelvic examination* is generally performed on female clients of childbearing age to rule out a gynecologic disorder, tubal pregnancy, or pelvic inflammatory disease (PID).
- *Intravenous pyelogram (IVP)* may be used to differentiate appendicitis from possible urinary tract disease.

## Medications

Prior to surgery, intravenous fluids are given to restore or maintain vascular volume and prevent electrolyte imbalance. Antibiotic therapy with a third-generation cephalosporin effective against many gram-negative bacteria, such as cefoperazone (Cefobid), cefotaxime (Claforan), ceftazidime (Fortaz), or ceftriaxone (Rocephin), is initiated prior to surgery. The antibiotic is repeated during surgery and continued for at least 48 hours postoperatively. The nursing implications for cephalosporin antibiotics are discussed in Chapter 8. ⊂⊃ Note that antibiotic therapy alone is not generally used to treat acute appendicitis.

## Surgery

The treatment of choice for acute appendicitis is an **appendectomy,** surgical removal of the appendix. Either a laparoscopic approach (insertion of an endoscope to view abdominal contents) or laparotomy (surgical opening of the abdomen) may be used for appendectomy. Laparoscopic appendectomy requires a very small incision through which the laparoscope is inserted. This procedure has several advantages: (1) direct visualization of the appendix allows definitive diagnosis without laparotomy; (2) postoperative hospitalization is short; (3) postoperative complications are infrequent; and (4) recovery and resumption of normal activities is rapid.

An open appendectomy is performed by laparotomy. A small transverse incision is made at McBurney's point; the appendix is isolated and ligated (tied off) to prevent contamination of the site with bowel contents, and then removed (Figure 24–2 ■). Laparotomy generally is used when the appendix has ruptured. It allows removal of contaminants from the peritoneal cavity by irrigation with sterile normal saline. Occasionally the wound may be left unsutured for periodic irrigation. Recovery is generally uneventful. Refer to Chapter 7 ⊂⊃ for further discussion of preoperative and postoperative nursing care.

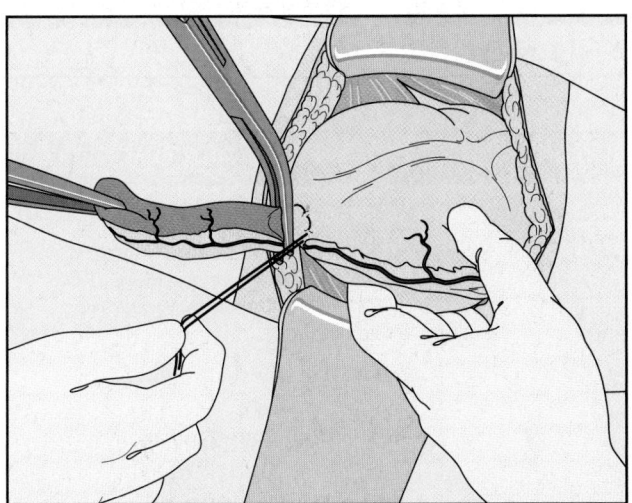

**Figure 24–2 ■** Appendectomy. The appendix and cecum are brought through the incision to the surface of the abdomen. The base of the appendix is clamped and ligated; the appendix is then removed.

## NURSING CARE

### Assessment

Because appendicitis can rapidly progress from inflammation to perforation, prompt assessment is vital. Obtain the following assessment data.

- Health history: current manifestations, including onset, duration, progression, and aggravating or relieving factors; most recent food or fluid intake; known medication or other allergies; current medications; history of chronic diseases
- Physical examination: vital signs including temperature; apparent general health; abdominal shape and contour, bowel sounds, tenderness to light palpation

### Nursing Diagnoses and Interventions

Preoperative nursing care is directed toward preparing the client physically and psychologically for emergency surgery. Limited time is available for preoperative teaching.

> **PRACTICE ALERT**  *Keep the client with suspected appendicitis NPO, and do not administer laxatives or enemas, which may cause perforation of the appendix. No heat should be applied to the abdomen; this may increase circulation to the appendix and also cause perforation.* ■

### Risk for Infection

Preventing complications during the preoperative and postoperative periods is a primary nursing care goal. Perforation and peritonitis are the most likely preoperative complications; postoperative complications include wound infection, abscess, and possible peritonitis.

> **PRACTICE ALERT**  *Assess abdominal status frequently, including distention, bowel sounds, and tenderness. Increasing generalized pain, a rigid, boardlike abdomen, and abdominal distention may indicate developing peritonitis.* ■

- Monitor vital signs, including temperature. *Tachycardia and rapid shallow respirations may indicate perforation of the appendix with resulting peritonitis. Fever may develop as well, and the blood pressure may fall if sepsis is present.*
- Maintain intravenous infusion until oral intake is adequate. *Intravenous fluids are given to maintain vascular volume and to provide a route for antibiotic administration.*
- Assess wound, abdominal girth, and postoperative pain. *Swelling of the wound, increased abdominal girth, or an increase in pain may indicate infection or peritonitis.*

## Pain

The client with appendicitis experiences pain before and after surgery. Analgesia is limited until the diagnosis is established. Postoperative pain is controlled by narcotic or nonnarcotic analgesics.

- Assess pain, including its character, location, severity, and duration. Report any unexpected changes in the nature of pain. *Both preoperatively and postoperatively, the client's pain provides important clues about the diagnosis and possible complications such as rupture of the appendix or peritonitis.*

**PRACTICE ALERT** *Sudden relief of preoperative pain may signal rupture of the distended and edematous appendix.* ■

- Administer analgesics as ordered. *Preoperatively, pain medication can be given after a diagnosis is established. Postoperatively, provide analgesics to maintain comfort and enhance mobility.*
- Assess effectiveness of medication 30 minutes after administration. Report unrelieved pain. *Pain unrelieved by prescribed analgesic may indicate a complication or the need for further assessment. For example, continued abdominal discomfort and distention may indicate excess intestinal gas which may be better relieved by ambulation.*

## Using NANDA, NIC, and NOC

Chart 24–2 shows links between NANDA nursing diagnoses, NIC, and NOC for the client with appendicitis or peritonitis.

## Home Care

Preoperative teaching may be limited by pain and the emergent nature of surgery. Explain why food and fluids are not permitted during this time. If time allows, teach postoperative turning, coughing, deep breathing, and pain management.

With uncomplicated appendectomy, the client often is discharged either the day of surgery or the day following surgery. Postoperative teaching includes:

- Wound or incision care, including handwashing and dressing change procedures as indicated.
- Instructions to report fever, increased abdominal pain, swelling, redness, drainage, bleeding, or warmth of the operative site to the physician.
- Activity limitations (e.g., lifting, driving), if any.
- Returning to work.

Provide a referral for community health or home health care nursing services as indicated, for example, if the client has preexisting illness or difficulty performing activities of daily living and self-care.

## THE CLIENT WITH PERITONITIS

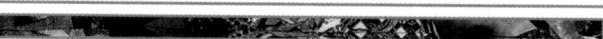

**Peritonitis,** inflammation of the peritoneum, is a serious complication of many acute abdominal disorders. It is usually caused by enteric bacteria entering the peritoneal cavity through a perforated ulcer, ruptured appendix, perforated diverticulum (discussed later in this chapter), necrotic bowel, or during abdominal surgery. Pelvic inflammatory disease, gallbladder rupture, or abdominal trauma also can lead to peritonitis.

### PHYSIOLOGY REVIEW

The peritoneum is a double-layered serous membrane lining the walls (parietal peritoneum) and organs (visceral peritoneum) of the abdominal cavity. There is a potential space

---

### CHART 24–2  LINKS BETWEEN NANDA, NIC, AND NOC

#### The Client with Appendicitis or Peritonitis

| NURSING DIAGNOSES | NURSING INTERVENTIONS | NURSING OUTCOMES |
|---|---|---|
| • Acute Pain | • Analgesic Administration<br>• Patient-Controlled Analgesia (PCA) Assistance | • Comfort Level<br>• Pain Control |
| • Deficient Fluid Volume | • Fluid Management<br>• Hypovolemia Management | • Electrolyte and Acid-Base Balance<br>• Fluid Balance |
| • Imbalanced Nutrition: Less Than Body Requirements | • Nutrition Monitoring | • Nutritional Status |
| • Ineffective Breathing Pattern | • Positioning<br>• Respiratory Monitoring | • Respiratory Status: Ventilation |
| • Risk for Infection | • Incision Site Care<br>• Wound Care | • Wound Healing: Primary Intention<br>• Wound Healing: Secondary Intention |

*Note: Data from Nursing Outcomes Classification (NOC) by M. Johnson & M. Maas (Eds.), 1997, St. Louis: Mosby; Nursing Diagnoses: Definitions & Classification 2001–2002 by North American Nursing Diagnosis Association, 2001, Philadelphia: NANDA; Nursing Interventions Classification (NIC) by J.C. McCloskey & G. M. Bulechek (Eds.), 2000, St. Louis: Mosby. Reprinted by permission.*

## Nursing Care Plan

## A Client with Acute Appendicitis

Jamie Lynn is a 19-year-old college student majoring in physical therapy. Ms. Lynn arrives at the emergency department at 1:00 A.M. complaining of general lower abdominal pain that had started the previous evening. By midnight, the pain was more localized over the right lower quadrant. She also reports nausea and vomiting.

### ASSESSMENT

Sue Grady, RN, completes the admission assessment in the emergency department. Ms. Lynn is complaining of nausea and severe abdominal pain, stating, "Walking makes my stomach hurt worse." Physical assessment findings include: T 100.2°F (37.8°C), P 84, R 16, and BP 110/70; skin warm to touch; abdomen flat and guarded, with marked tenderness in right lower quadrant. Ms. Lynn's complete blood count shows WBC 14,000/mm³; neutrophils 81.1%; lymphocytes 12.5%. The diagnosis of acute appendicitis is made, and Ms. Lynn is transferred to surgery for a laparoscopic appendectomy.

### DIAGNOSIS

- *Impaired skin integrity* related to surgical incisions
- *Pain* related to surgical intervention
- *Anxiety* related to situational crisis

### EXPECTED OUTCOMES

- Incisions will heal without infection or complications.
- Will verbalize adequate pain relief.
- Will verbalize decreased anxiety.
- Returns to preoperative activities.

### PLANNING AND IMPLEMENTATION

- Assess pain using a pain scale; provide analgesics as needed.
- Teach pain management following discharge.
- Teach abdominal splinting during coughing, turning, or ambulating as needed.
- Teach home care of incisions.
- Discuss activity limitations as ordered.
- Instruct to report fever or warmth, redness, or drainage from the incisions.

### EVALUATION

On discharge the following evening, Ms. Lynn is fully ambulatory. Her appetite has returned, and she is tolerating food and fluids well. Her temperature is normal. The nurse provides Ms. Lynn with written and verbal information on postoperative care following an appendectomy.

### Critical Thinking in the Nursing Process

1. What is the pathophysiologic basis for Ms. Lynn's elevated WBC?
2. How would Ms. Lynn's postoperative care and teaching differ if she had undergone a laparotomy instead of a laparoscopic appendectomy?
3. Outline a teaching plan to give to clients for home care following an appendectomy.
4. Develop a care plan for Ms. Lynn for the nursing diagnosis, *Anxiety* related to a situational crisis.

See Evaluating Your Response in Appendix C.

---

between the parietal and visceral layers of the peritoneum that contains a small amount of serous fluid. This space, the peritoneal cavity, normally is sterile.

## PATHOPHYSIOLOGY

Peritonitis results from contamination of the normally sterile peritoneal cavity by infection or a chemical irritant. Chemical peritonitis often precedes bacterial peritonitis. Perforation of a peptic ulcer or rupture of the gallbladder releases gastric juices (hydrochloric acid and pepsin) or bile into the peritoneal cavity, causing an acute inflammatory response.

Bacterial peritonitis usually is caused by infection by *Escherichia coli*, *Klebsiella*, *Proteus*, or *Pseudomonas* bacteria, which normally inhabit the bowel. Inflammatory and immune defense mechanisms are activated when bacteria enter the peritoneal space. These defenses can effectively eliminate small numbers of bacteria, but may be overwhelmed by massive or continued contamination. When this occurs, mast cells release histamine and other vasoactive substances, causing local vasodilation and increased capillary permeability. Polymorphonuclear leukocytes (PMNs, a type of WBC) infiltrate the peritoneum to phagocytize bacteria and foreign matter. Fibrinogen-rich plasma exudate promotes bacterial destruc-

tion and forms fibrin clots to seal off and segregate the bacteria. This process helps limit and localize the infection, allowing host defenses to eradicate it. Continued contamination, however, leads to generalized inflammation of the peritoneal cavity. The inflammatory process causes fluid to shift into the peritoneal space (third spacing). Circulating blood volume is depleted, leading to hypovolemia. *Septicemia*, systemic disease caused by pathogens or their toxins in the blood, may follow.

## MANIFESTATIONS

Manifestations of peritonitis depend on the severity and extent of the infection, as well as the age and general health of the client. Both local and systemic manifestations are present (see the box on page 636). The client often presents with evidence of an *acute abdomen*, an abrupt onset of diffuse, severe abdominal pain. The pain may localize and intensify near the area of infection. Movement may intensify the pain. The entire abdomen is tender, with guarding or rigidity of abdominal muscles. The acute abdomen is often described as boardlike. Rebound tenderness may be present over the area of inflammation. Peritoneal inflammation inhibits peristalsis, resulting in a paralytic ileus. (Paralytic ileus is discussed in a

## Manifestations of Peritonitis

**Abdominal Manifestations**
- Diffuse or localized pain
- Tenderness with rebound
- Boardlike rigidity
- Diminished or absent bowel sounds
- Distention
- Anorexia, nausea, and vomiting

**Systemic Manifestations**
- Fever
- Malaise
- Tachycardia
- Tachypnea
- Restlessness
- Confusion or disorientation
- Oliguria

later section of this chapter.) Bowel sounds are markedly diminished or absent, and progressive abdominal distention is noted. Pooling of GI secretions may cause nausea and vomiting. Systemic manifestations of peritonitis include fever, malaise, tachycardia and tachypnea, restlessness, and possible disorientation. The client may be oliguric and show signs of dehydration and shock.

The older, chronically debilitated, or immunosuppressed client may present with few of the classic signs of peritonitis. Increased confusion and restlessness, decreased urinary output, and vague abdominal complaints may be the only manifestations present. These clients are at increased risk for delayed diagnosis, contributing to a higher mortality rate.

### Complications

Complications of peritonitis may be life threatening. Abscess formation is common. The very defense mechanisms designed to isolate and localize the infection can protect it from immune responses and systemic antibiotics. Fibrous adhesions in the abdominal cavity are a late complication and may lead to subsequent obstruction.

Without prompt and effective treatment, septicemia and septic shock can develop. Fluid loss into the abdominal cavity may also lead to hypovolemic shock. These potentially lethal complications require immediate, aggressive intervention to prevent multiple organ failure and death. Shock and its management are discussed in Chapter 6. ⌘

The overall mortality rate associated with peritonitis is about 40%. Clients with other medical conditions, older clients, and those with greater bacterial contamination have a higher risk of dying. Young people with perforated ulcers or appendicitis, those with less extensive bacterial contamination, and those who receive early surgical intervention have mortality rates of less than 10%.

## COLLABORATIVE CARE

Care of the client with peritonitis focuses on establishing the diagnosis and identifying and treating its cause as well as the peritonitis. Preventing complications is an important aspect of care.

### Diagnostic Tests

Diagnostic testing is done to establish the diagnosis of peritonitis, rule out other disorders, and help identify the cause. The following tests may be ordered.

- *WBC count* is elevated to approximately 20,000/mm$^3$ in peritonitis. Increased numbers of immature blood cells are present as the bone marrow releases them in response to the infection.
- *Blood cultures* are ordered to identify the possible presence of bacteria in the blood (*bacteremia*). Bacteremia often precedes *septicemia,* a potential complication of peritonitis.
- *Liver* and *renal function studies* and *serum electrolytes* may be ordered to evaluate the systemic effects of peritonitis and help guide treatment.
- *Abdominal X-rays* (supine and standing) are obtained to detect intestinal distention, air-fluid levels (indicative of ileus or bowel obstruction), and free air under the diaphragm (indicative of GI perforation).
- *Paracentesis* is performed to obtain peritoneal fluid for analysis (see Chapter 22). ⌘ In peritonitis, the fluid contains increased protein and WBCs. Bacteria may be present. Amylase in the fluid may indicate acute pancreatitis. Peritoneal fluid analysis helps establish the diagnosis and underlying cause of acute peritonitis.

### Medications

Until the infecting organism has been identified, a broad-spectrum antibiotic effective against organisms commonly implicated in peritonitis is prescribed. Once culture results have been obtained, antibiotic therapy is modified to the specific organism(s) responsible. Cephalosporin antibiotics are often prescribed if gram-negative enteric bacteria are suspected. Other antibiotics that may be ordered include ampicillin (Omnipen, Polycillin, others), metronidazole (Flagyl, others), clindamycin (Cleocin), or an aminoglycoside antibiotic such as gentamycin (Garamycin) or amikacin (Amikin). Nursing implications for antibiotic therapy are discussed in Chapter 8. ⌘

In addition to antibiotic therapy, analgesics are usually ordered to promote comfort.

### Surgery

If the cause of peritonitis is a perforation, gangrenous bowel, or inflamed appendix, a laparotomy is done to close the perforation or remove the damaged and inflamed tissue. If an abscess is present, it also may be surgically drained or removed.

*Peritoneal lavage,* washing of the peritoneal cavity with copious amounts of warm isotonic fluid, may be done during surgery. This procedure dilutes residual bacteria and removes gross contaminants, blood, and fibrin clots. In rare instances, peritoneal lavage may be continued for several days following surgery. The solution is infused into the upper portion of the peritoneal cavity and removed via drains in the pelvic cul-de-sac. Careful attention to fluid and electrolyte status and strict aseptic technique are necessary.

Clients who have had laparotomy for peritonitis often return from surgery with either Penrose or closed drain systems such as a Jackson-Pratt drain. In some cases, the incision may be left unsutured. With severe and long-standing peritonitis, the abdomen may be closed temporarily with polypropylene mesh containing a nylon zipper or Velcro to allow repeated exploration of the abdomen and drainage of infectious sites.

## Treatments

Intravenous fluids and electrolyte replacements are administered to maintain vascular volume and fluid and electrolyte balance. Parenteral nutrition is given until adequate oral intake resumes. The client is placed on bed rest in Fowler's position to help localize the infection and promote lung ventilation. Oxygen is often ordered to facilitate cellular metabolism and healing.

## Intestinal Decompression

The inflammatory process of peritonitis often draws large amounts of fluid into the abdominal cavity and the bowel. In addition, peristaltic activity of the bowel is slowed or halted by the inflammation, causing **paralytic ileus** (or *ileus*), impaired propulsion or forward movement of bowel contents. Intestinal decompression is used to relieve abdominal distention, facilitate closure, and minimize postoperative respiratory problems. A nasogastric or long intestinal tube is inserted and connected to continuous drainage (Figure 24–3 ■). If prolonged intestinal decompression is anticipated, a jejunostomy may be performed for comfort. Suction is maintained until peristalsis resumes, bowel sounds are present, and the client is passing flatus. Food and fluids are withheld until intestinal motility has returned and suction is discontinued.

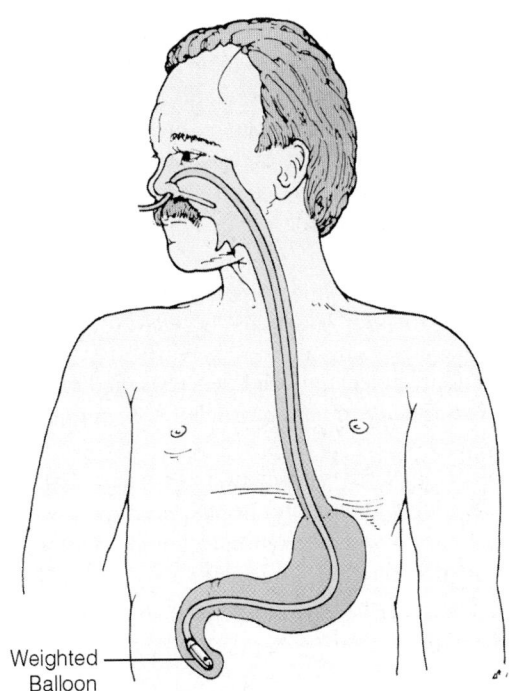

Weighted
Balloon

**Figure 24–3 ■** The weighted tip or inflated balloon at the end of an intestinal tube is drawn into the intestine by gravity and peristalsis.

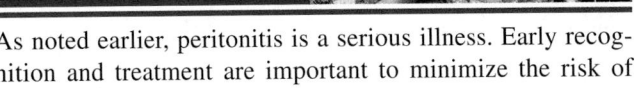

# NURSING CARE

As noted earlier, peritonitis is a serious illness. Early recognition and treatment are important to minimize the risk of complications.

## Assessment

- Health history: complaints of pain, its onset, character, severity, location, aggravating and relieving factors; associated symptoms such as anorexia, nausea, vomiting; current and previous history of peptic ulcer disease, gallbladder disease, other related conditions; chronic diseases; current medications
- Physical examination: vital signs including temperature; level of consciousness; skin color, temperature, warmth, capillary refill and turgor; abdominal shape, contour, bowel sounds, tenderness, and guarding

## Nursing Diagnoses and Interventions

Clients with peritonitis require intensive nursing and medical care to prevent complications and recover fully. Nursing care priorities include pain; altered fluid balance; altered protection due to infection, drains, and possibly repeated surgeries; and anxiety.

### Pain

Abdominal distention and acute inflammation contribute to the pain associated with peritonitis. Surgery further disrupts abdominal muscles and other tissues, causing pain. Effective pain management promotes immune function, healing, mobility, and recovery.

- Assess pain, including its location, severity (using a standard pain scale), and type. Monitor analgesic effectiveness. Report changes to the primary care provider.

> **PRACTICE ALERT** *Unrelieved pain or a change in the location, severity, or type of pain may indicate spread of infection, abscess formation, or other complications of peritonitis.* ■

- Place in Fowler's or semi-Fowler's position with the knees and feet elevated. *This position reduces stress on abdominal structures and facilitates respirations, promoting comfort.*
- Administer analgesics as ordered on a routine basis or using patient-controlled analgesia (PCA). *Routine analgesic administration maintains a therapeutic blood level and helps maintain comfort, facilitating healing and movement.*
- Teach and assist with adjunctive pain management techniques such as meditation, visualization, massage, and progressive relaxation. *Adjunctive measures augment analgesics and help promote a sense of control over pain.*

### Deficient Fluid Volume

In peritonitis, significant amounts of fluid are drawn into the abdominal cavity and bowel, reducing vascular volume and cardiac output. This fluid also may be lost from the body by intestinal suction or through drains placed in the abdomen during surgery. An unsutured incision causes additional significant fluid loss.

- Maintain accurate intake and output records. Measure urine output every 1 to 2 hours; report output of less than 30 mL/hr. Measure gastrointestinal output at least every 4 hours. *Intake and output records provide valuable information about fluid volume status.*

**PRACTICE ALERT** *Urine output of less than 30 mL/hr may indicate hypovolemia, decreased cardiac output, and impaired tissue perfusion.* ■

- Monitor vital signs and hemodynamic parameters such as central venous pressure, cardiac output, and pulmonary artery pressures every hour or as indicated. *These measurements provide important information about fluid and vascular volumes as well as cardiovascular status.*
- Weigh daily. *Weight is an accurate indicator of fluid status. Rapid weight gains or losses reflect changes in fluid volume.*
- Assess skin turgor, color, temperature, and mucous membranes at least every 8 hours. *Warm, dry skin with poor turgor and dry, shiny mucous membranes indicates dehydration.*
- Measure or estimate fluid losses through abdominal drains and on dressings. *Significant amounts of exudative fluid may be lost.*
- Monitor laboratory values, including hemoglobin and hematocrit, urine specific gravity, serum osmolality and electrolytes, and ABGs. Report changes to the physician. *Laboratory results provide information about fluid and electrolyte status and acid-base balance.*
- Administer intravenous fluids and electrolytes as ordered. Gastrointestinal drainage may be replaced milliliter for milliliter with a balanced electrolyte solution. *Intravenous fluids are necessary to meet daily fluid intake needs, as well as replace continuing losses of water and electrolytes.*
- Provide good skin care and frequent oral hygiene. *Fluid deficit increases the risk of skin breakdown and ulceration of mucous membranes.*

### Ineffective Protection

Repeated surgeries, an unsutured incision, and the presence of drains interrupt skin integrity and the body's first line of defense against microorganisms. In addition, immune defenses are stressed by the infection and potential malnutrition. As a result, the risk for impaired healing and further infection is increased.

- Monitor temperature, pulse rate, and for localized signs of infection such as redness and swelling around incisions and drain sites, increased or purulent drainage, and cloudy or malodorous urine. *Impaired defenses increase the risk for extension of the infection or unrelated infections.*
- Obtain cultures of purulent drainage from any site. *Early identification of any additional infection allows timely intervention.*
- Monitor WBC and differential, serum protein, and albumin. *An increased WBC with a higher percentage of immature*

cells present in the blood is an indicator of infection and normal immune response. Serum albumin and protein levels are indicators of nutritional status as well as immune function.

- Practice meticulous handwashing and use standard precautions at all times. *Handwashing reduces transient bacteria on the skin and remains the most important method of controlling infection. Standard precautions reduce the risk of spreading infection to or from the client.*
- Use strict aseptic technique for dressing changes, wound care, and irrigations. *Disruption of the protective barrier of the skin increases the risk of contamination and further infection.*
- Maintain fluid balance and nutritional status through enteral or parenteral feedings, as indicated. *Adequate nutrition and fluid balance are necessary for optimal immune system function.*

**PRACTICE ALERT** *An acute infection such as peritonitis causes a stress response with excess energy expenditure and loss of body proteins and cell mass. Glycogen stores are rapidly depleted, and body proteins are used to meet energy needs. Withholding food further complicates this process, leading to rapid development of protein-calorie malnutrition (PCM). PCM impairs the immune response and slows healing.* ■

### Anxiety

The severity and potential threat to life associated with peritonitis present a situational crisis for the client and family. Anxiety is a common response.

- Assess the client's and family's anxiety level and present coping skills. *Interventions need to be tailored to the needs and strengths of the client and family.*
- Present a calm, reassuring manner. Encourage expression of concerns; listen carefully, and acknowledge their validity. *This helps establish trust.*
- Maintain consistent caregiver assignments. *Consistency of nursing care and care providers helps reduce anxiety. Complex wound care and irrigation procedures are best performed by people who are very familiar with prescribed techniques.*
- Explain all treatments, procedures, tests, and examinations. *An increased understanding of what is being done can reduce anxiety.*
- Reinforce and clarify information as needed. *This improves understanding and promotes acceptance.*
- Teach and assist with relaxation techniques such as meditation, visualization, and progressive relaxation. *These measures promote positive coping skills and reduce physical manifestations of anxiety.*

### Using NANDA, NIC, and NOC

Linkages between NANDA nursing diagnoses, NIC, and NOC for the client with peritonitis are illustrated in Chart 24–2.

## Home Care

Teaching for the client with peritonitis is vital during hospitalization and prior to discharge. Provide brief but complete explanations of procedures, examinations, and expected sensations throughout hospitalization to reduce anxiety and improve cooperation.

Teaching for home care includes the following topics:

- Wound care procedures, including dressing changes or irrigations. Provide verbal and written instructions, and allow opportunities to practice and demonstrate the procedure prior to discharge.
- Where to obtain necessary supplies.
- Prescribed medications, including name and purpose of the drug, potential adverse effects, and their management.
- Manifestations of further infection (redness, heat, swelling, purulent drainage, chills, and fever) and potential complications to be reported to the care provider.
- Prescribed activity restrictions.
- Instructions for a high-calorie, high-protein diet for healing and optimal immune function.

Provide a referral to home health services for assessment, wound care, and further teaching, as needed.

## THE CLIENT WITH GASTROENTERITIS

**Gastroenteritis,** or enteritis, is an inflammation of the stomach and small intestine. Enteritis may be caused by bacteria, viruses, parasites, or toxins. Upper GI symptoms such as anorexia, nausea, and vomiting are common. Diarrhea of varying intensity and abdominal discomfort are nearly universal features of gastroenteritis.

The infectious organism usually enters the body in contaminated water or food. For this reason, gastroenteritis often is called "food poisoning." Viruses commonly cause acute diarrheal illness. Diarrhea due to rotaviruses or the Norwalk virus occurs year-round in both adults and children. These illnesses are generally mild and self-limited, but can have severe consequences in the very young, the very old, or in people with impaired immune function.

## PATHOPHYSIOLOGY

Bacterial or viral infection of the GI tract produces inflammation, tissue damage, and manifestations by two primary mechanisms.

- *The production of exotoxins.* A number of bacteria produce and excrete an exotoxin that enters the surrounding environment (intestinal lumen), causing damage and inflammation. Exotoxins in the GI tract are often referred to as *enterotoxins.* They impair intestinal absorption and can cause secretion of significant amounts of electrolytes and water into the bowel, resulting in diarrhea and fluid loss. Common bacterial enterotoxins include those produced by *Staphylococcus, Clostridium perfringens, Clostridium botulinum,* some strains of *Escherichia coli,* and *Vibrio cholerae.*
- *Invasion and ulceration of the mucosa.* Other bacteria, including some *Shigella, Salmonella,* and *Escherichia coli* species, damage tissue more directly. They invade the intestinal mucosa of the small bowel or colon, producing microscopic ulceration, bleeding, fluid exudate, and water and electrolyte secretion.

In some cases, the mechanism of injury is unclear. It may be a combination of direct and toxic damage. The Norwalk virus damages the mucosa of the jejunum, with fluid and electrolyte secretion.

## MANIFESTATIONS AND COMPLICATIONS

Although the manifestations of bacterial and viral enteritis vary according to the organism involved, several features are common (see the box below). Anorexia, nausea, and vomiting are caused by distension of the upper GI tract by unabsorbed chyme and excess water. Bowel distention, along with irritation of the bowel mucosa and gas production due to fermentation of undigested food, also lead to abdominal pain and cramping. *Borborygmi,* excessively loud and hyperactive bowel sounds, are another result. The abdomen is often distended and tender.

Diarrhea is usually predominant with enteritis. Fluid is secreted into the bowel lumen, and the unabsorbed chyme and electrolytes create an osmotic draw of fluid into the bowel. Motility is stimulated, and stools become watery and frequent. Loss of fluids and electrolytes through diarrhea can lead to the most serious manifestations of enteritis. Fluid volume can be rapidly depleted, leading to dehydration and hypovolemia. Orthostatic hypotension may be noted initially, along with an elevated temperature. If fluid loss continues, hypovolemic shock may develop.

Electrolyte and acid-base imbalances may result from gastroenteritis. Extensive vomiting can lead to metabolic alkalosis due to the loss of hydrochloric acid from the stomach. When diarrhea predominates, metabolic acidosis is more likely. Potassium is lost in either case, leading to hypokalemia. Hyponatremia may develop if fluids are replaced with pure water. Headache, cardiac irregularities, changes in respiratory rate

## Manifestations of Gastroenteritis

**Gastrointestinal Effects**
- Anorexia, nausea, and vomiting
- Abdominal pain and cramping
- Borborygmi
- Diarrhea

**General Effects**
- Malaise, weakness, and muscle aches
- Headache
- Dry skin and mucous membranes
- Poor skin turgor
- Orthostatic hypotension, tachycardia
- Fever

and pattern, malaise and weakness, muscle aching, and signs of neuromuscular irritability are the possible manifestations of these disturbances in homeostasis.

Several gastrointestinal infections produce specific effects that are discussed below and summarized in Table 24–3.

## Traveler's Diarrhea

People traveling to another country frequently develop diarrhea within 2 to 10 days, particularly when there is a significant difference in climate, sanitation standards, or food and drink. Strains of enterotoxin-producing *E. coli*, shigella species, and *Camylobacter* are the most frequent causes of traveler's diarrhea (Tierney et al., 2001). Other bacteria and viruses also may cause traveler's diarrhea.

Up to 10 or more loose stools per day and abdominal cramping are common manifestations. Nausea and vomiting are less frequent; fever is rare. Symptoms usually resolve within 2 to 5 days. Complications are rare.

| TABLE 24–3 Selected Bacterial Infections of the Bowel | | | | |
|---|---|---|---|---|
| **Disease and Organism** | **Incubation** | **Pathogenesis** | **Manifestations** | **Management** |
| Traveler's diarrhea: *Escherichia coli* | 24 to 72 hours | Enterotoxin causes hypersecretion of the small intestine. | Abrupt onset of diarrhea; vomiting rare | Prophylactic bismuth subsalicylate; anti-diarrheals such as loperamide or diphen-oxylate; 3- to 5-day course of norfloxacin, ciprofloxacin, or trimethoprim-sulfamethoxazole |
| Staphylococcal food poisoning | 2 to 8 hours | Enterotoxin impairs intestinal absorption and affects vomiting centers in the brain. | Severe nausea and vomiting; abdominal cramping and diarrhea; headache and fever | Fluid and electrolyte replacement as needed |
| Botulism: *Clostridium botulinum* | 1.5 to 8 days | Absorbed enterotoxin produces neuro-muscular blockade and progressive paralysis. | Diplopia, pupils fixed and dilated; dry mouth, dysphagia; progressive cephalocaudal weakness and paralysis; GI symptoms minimal; respiratory failure possible complication | Gastric lavage to remove toxin from gut; administration of botulinus antitoxin; respiratory, fluid, and nutritional support |
| Cholera: *Vibrio cholerae* | 1 to 3 days | Enterotoxin affects entire small intestine, causing secretion of water and electrolytes into bowel lumen. | Severe diarrhea with "rice water stool," grey, cloudy, odorless, with no blood or pus; vomiting; thirst, oliguria, muscle cramps, weakness; dehydration and vascular collapse | Oral or intravenous rehydration; possible antimicrobial therapy with ampicillin, tetra-cycline, trimethoprim-sulfamethoxazole, others |
| Hemorrhagic colitis: *E. coli* | 1 to 3 days | Enterotoxin causes direct mucosal damage in large intestine; also toxic to vascular endothelial cells. | Severe abdominal cramping, watery diarrhea that becomes grossly bloody; fever; possible complica-tions: hemolytic uremic syndrome and thrombotic thrombocytopenic purpura | Supportive care with fluid replacement and bland diet; may require dialysis or plasma-pheresis for complications |
| Salmonellosis: *Salmonella* | 8 to 48 hours | Superficial infection of the GI tract without invasion or production of toxins. | Diarrhea with abdominal cramping, nausea, and vomiting; low-grade fever, chills, weakness | Treatment of symptoms; trimethoprim-sulfamethoxazole, ampicillin, or ciproflox-acin for severe illness |
| Shigellosis (bacillary dysentery): *Shigella* | 1 to 4 days | Local tissue invasion, primarily involving large intestine and distal ileum; endotoxin causes fluid and electrolyte secretion into bowel lumen. | Watery diarrhea with severe abdominal cramping and tenesmus; lethargy | Fluid and electrolyte replacement; correction of acidosis; antibiotic therapy with trimethoprim-sulfamethoxazole, ciprofloxacin, or ampicillin |

## Staphylococcal Food Poisoning

Certain foods provide an excellent medium for staphylococcal growth when contaminated and left at room temperature. Examples include meats and fish, dairy products (e.g., custards), and bakery products (e.g., cream-filled pastries). The organism itself does not affect the bowel; the toxin it produces, however, impairs intestinal absorption and acts on receptors in the gut, stimulating the medullary center to produce vomiting.

The onset of staphylococcal food poisoning is abrupt, occurring within 2 to 8 hours after consuming the contaminated food. Nausea and vomiting are severe. Manifestations typically last 3 to 6 hours, and include abdominal cramping, diarrhea, headache, and fever. Complications such as fluid and electrolyte imbalances are rare, but may develop in older adults and people with underlying chronic disease processes.

## Botulism

**Botulism** is a severe, life-threatening form of food poisoning caused by *Clostridium botulinum*. These spore-forming anaerobic bacteria grow in improperly preserved foods, such as home-canned vegetables, smoked meats, and vacuum-packed fish. The spores are highly resistant to heat; a temperature of 248°F for 30 minutes is required to kill the bacteria. The bacterial toxin, however, is easily destroyed by temperatures as low as 176°F.

The bacterial toxin is absorbed into the bloodstream from the intestines. It blocks release of acetylcholine, a neurotransmitter, from nerve endings, causing bilateral and symmetric neurologic symptoms. Cranial nerves are often affected first, followed by descending weakness or paralysis. Diplopia (double vision) and loss of accommodation are common initial symptoms, often accompanied by dry mouth and dysphagia. Nausea, vomiting, and abdominal cramps may occur. Diarrhea is rare with botulism. As neuromuscular paralysis progresses, respiratory muscles become progressively weaker. Respiratory muscle paralysis may lead to death unless ventilatory support is provided. Sensation is not impaired, and the client remains mentally alert.

## Cholera

**Cholera** is an acute diarrheal illness caused by strains of *Vibrio cholerae*. It is endemic in parts of Asia, the Middle East, and Africa. Epidemics occur periodically. Cholera is spread by the fecal–oral route through contaminated water or food. The organism produces an enterotoxin, enzymes, and other substances that affect the entire small intestine. Water and electrolytes are secreted into the bowel lumen in response to the toxin. The enzymes and other substances produced by the bacteria may affect mucous protection of bowel endothelium.

Cholera ranges in severity from very mild, with few or no symptoms, to acute and fulminant. Its onset is typically abrupt, with severe, frequent, watery diarrhea. Up to 1 L of stool may be passed in an hour, rapidly producing depleting fluid volume. Stool is often described as "rice water stool" and characteristically gray and cloudy, with no fecal odor, blood, or pus. Vomiting may accompany the diarrhea. Other manifestations relate to the loss of fluid and electrolytes: thirst, oliguria, muscle cramps, weakness, and significant signs of dehydration. Metabolic acidosis and hypokalemia develop. If untreated, circulatory collapse and acute renal failure may occur.

Recovery from cholera usually occurs spontaneously within 3 to 6 days. With prompt and adequate fluid replacement, mortality is less than 1%.

## Escherichia coli Hemorrhagic Colitis

Most pathologic forms of *E. coli* bacteria cause little more than common traveler's diarrhea. Some strains, such as serotype 0157:H7, produce a potent enterotoxin in the large intestine after being ingested. This toxin damages bowel mucosa and the endothelial cells of blood vessels in the GI tract. If absorbed, the toxin can damage other blood vessels as well, such as those of the kidney.

Cattle provide the reservoir for *E. coli* 0157:H7. It is usually spread through undercooked beef (hamburger in particular) and unpasteurized milk or apple juice. It may also be spread by direct contact via the fecal–oral route. The onset of hemorrhagic colitis is abrupt, with severe abdominal cramping and watery diarrhea that becomes grossly bloody within 24 hours. Fever may be present.

Hemolytic uremic syndrome and thrombotic thrombocytopenic purpura are significant complications of *E. coli* hemorrhagic colitis, affecting about 5% of people with the disease. Children and older adults have the highest risk for developing complications.

## Salmonellosis

**Salmonellosis** is food poisoning caused by ingesting raw or improperly cooked meat, poultry, eggs, and dairy products contaminated with *Salmonella* bacteria. These bacteria cause superficial infection of the GI tract, rarely invading further. They do not produce a toxin.

Symptoms develop 8 to 48 hours after ingesting the bacteria. Diarrhea may be violent with abdominal cramping, nausea, and vomiting. A low-grade fever, chills, and weakness may accompany GI manifestations. The disease usually is self-limited, resolving within 3 to 5 days, although bacteremia may develop.

## Shigellosis (Bacillary Dysentery)

**Shigellosis** (or bacillary dysentery) occurs worldwide, accounting for up to 5% to 10% of diarrheal illness in some regions. It may be endemic or occur in epidemics. Humans are the reservoir for *Shigella* organisms, which are spread directly via the fecal–oral route or indirectly through contaminated food, fomites (such as inanimate objects), and vectors (such as fleas). The incubation period for shigellosis is 1 to 4 days.

*Shigella* organisms infect the lower intestine, and sometimes the distal ilium. They invade the tissue, causing inflammation, and they produce an enterotoxin. The result is watery diarrhea containing blood, mucus, and inflammatory exudate. The onset of diarrhea is abrupt, with severe abdominal cramping, and *tenesmus,* a sensation of urgent and continuing need to defecate. Lethargy is common; rarely, neurologic symptoms occur.

In adults, shigellosis is usually mild and self-limiting. Older adults and debilitated clients are at risk for volume depletion and electrolyte imbalances. Secondary infection is another potential complication, as is acute blood loss from mucosal ulcerations.

# COLLABORATIVE CARE

The goals of care for gastroenteritis are to manage the symptoms, prevent complications, identify the cause of the infection, and prevent its spread. The history and manifestations provide valuable cues about the cause. Diagnostic testing is used to identify the pathogen and evaluate its effects. In most cases, treatment is supportive, directed toward relieving symptoms, restoring fluid and electrolyte balance, and maintaining function.

## Diagnostic Tests

If symptoms are severe or do not resolve within about 48 hours, laboratory testing is used to identify the causative organism and to assess fluid, electrolyte, and acid-base balance.

- *Stool specimen for culture, ova and parasites, and fecal leukocytes.* Stool culture usually reveals the infective organism, but may require up to 6 weeks for some bacteria, making it impractical. In infections such as botulism, the toxin itself may be isolated in the stool. Contamination of the stool by urine or treatment with antibiotics, bismuth subsalicylate (Pepto-Bismol), or mineral oil may interfere with pathogen growth, altering stool culture results. Use a clean bedpan or collection device to obtain the stool specimen, and instruct the client to avoid mixing the stool with urine or toilet tissue.

- *Gram stain of vomitus* may reveal staphylococci in staphylococcal food poisoning.
- *Serum toxin levels* may be ordered, particularly if botulism is suspected.
- *Serum osmolality and electrolytes,* and *arterial blood gases* assess fluid, electrolyte, and acid-base balance. Common imbalances associated with enteritis and diarrhea are outlined in Table 24–4.

A *sigmoidoscopy* may be done to differentiate inflammatory bowel disease from infectious processes. It does not replace stool cultures, because the lesions associated with some infectious processes are indistinguishable from those of ulcerative colitis. Nursing care of the client undergoing a sigmoidoscopy is included in the Nursing Implications box on page 619.

## Medications

Acute enteritis usually resolves spontaneously, and no drug treatment is required. If the client is severely ill and symptoms are prolonged, medications may be prescribed.

Antibiotic therapy may used to treat cholera, salmonellosis, or shigellosis. Trimethoprim-sulfamethoxazole (Septra, Bactrim), ciprofloxacin (Cipro), ampicillin (Ampicin, Omnipen, Polycillin-N, others), or another antibiotic may be prescribed. Stool culture is obtained prior to starting antibiotics, but treatment may begin before culture results are available. A presumptive diagnosis based on history and presenting symptoms guides the choice of antibiotic.

An antidiarrheal drug may be prescribed to promote comfort and reduce fluid loss. Nursing measures related to antidiarrheal medications are outlined in the Nursing Implications box on page 619. It is vital to remember that antidiarrheal

## TABLE 24–4   Laboratory Values Associated with Enteritis and Diarrhea

| Test | Normal Value | Change with Significant Diarrhea |
|---|---|---|
| Serum osmolality | 275 to 295 mOsm/kg | Increased; levels above 320 mOsm/kg indicate significant dehydration |
| Serum potassium | 3.5 to 5.0 mEq/L | Decreased due to loss through stool and vomitus; levels below 2.5 mEq/L are critical |
| Serum sodium | 136 to 148 mEq/L | Decreased due to loss through stool and vomitus; may be significant when fluid losses are replaced with pure water; levels below 120 mEq/L may be critical |
| Serum chloride | 96 to 106 mEq/L | Increased when sodium loss is greater than chloride loss; decreased with severe diarrhea and with vomiting; possible critical values are below 80 mEq/L or above 115 mEq/L |
| Blood gases | | |
| • pH | Arterial: 7.35 to 7.45 | Decreased in metabolic acidosis, a possible result of severe diarrhea; increased in metabolic alkalosis, a possible result of severe vomiting and chloride loss; values below 7.25 or above 7.55 are critical |
| • $P_{CO_2}$ | Arterial: 35 to 45 mmHg | Typically decreased in metabolic acidosis as the body attempts to eliminate excess acid by "blowing off" $CO_2$; increased with metabolic alkalosis as the body retains $CO_2$ in an attempt to normalize pH |
| • Bicarbonate | 22 to 26 mEq/L | Decreased in metabolic acidosis; increased in metabolic alkalosis |
| Hematocrit | Males: 40% to 50% Females: 37% to 47% | Increased with dehydration and hypovolemia as a result of concentration of blood cells |
| Urine specific gravity | 1.010 to 1.025 | Increased with dehydration and hypovolemia as kidneys attempt to conserve fluid |

agents are not used to treat botulism. In fact, cathartics may be ordered to promote removal of the toxin from the bowel.

Botulism antitoxin is administered as soon as possible if botulism is suspected. The antitoxin may be given prophylactically, when ingestion of the bacteria or toxin is suspected. If the antitoxin is given more than 72 hours after symptom onset it may not be effective. The antitoxin neutralizes circulating toxin. It does not displace toxin bound to nerve endings, so existing paralysis continues when it is given. Botulism antitoxin is made from horse serum, so it can provoke an anaphylactic response and serum sickness (see Chapter 9). ⬡ Sensitivity testing and progressive desensitization is recommended prior to administering the antitoxin. This may not always be possible because of symptom progression. Keep epinephrine at the bedside to treat potential anaphylaxis.

## Treatments

Replacing lost fluids and electrolytes is vital when vomiting and/or diarrhea are severe or prolonged. In many cases of enteritis, fluid and electrolyte replacement are all that is required until the infection resolves.

Oral rehydration is preferred for replacing physiologic fluids. An oral glucose-electrolyte solution is often well tolerated in sips, even when vomiting is present. Commercial preparations such as Gatorade, All-Sport, and Pedialyte are available. A solution of 5 mL (1 teaspoon) table salt, 5 mL baking soda, 20 mL (4 teaspoons) granulated sugar, and flavoring (such as lemon extract or juice) to 1 L (1 quart) of water also is effective.

Intravenous rehydration may be necessary with severe diarrhea and fluid loss. In some cases, a combination of oral and intravenous fluids may be used to replace lost fluids and maintain vascular volume. Balanced electrolyte solutions, such as glucose in normal saline, Ringer's solution, and others, are used. Lactated Ringer's solution or another alkalinizing solution may be ordered if metabolic acidosis is present.

*Gastric lavage and catharsis*—in effect, "washing out" the stomach and intestines—may be done to remove unabsorbed toxin from the GI tract if botulism is suspected. The client with botulism is closely observed for signs of respiratory distress. Respiratory support with endotracheal intubation or tracheostomy and mechanical ventilation may be required (see Chapter 36).

*Plasmapheresis* (plasma exchange therapy) may be performed to remove circulating toxins for botulism or hemorrhagic colitis caused by *E. coli*. In plasmapheresis, harmful components in plasma are removed by withdrawing blood, separating the plasma from the blood cells, and returning the cells with an equal amount of albumin or human plasma to the client. This procedure is usually done in a series, rather than as a single treatment. Informed consent is required for plasmapheresis. Potential complications include those associated with intravenous catheters, shifts in fluid balance, and altered blood clotting.

Acute tubular necrosis and renal failure associated with hemorrhagic colitis may necessitate dialysis to remove wastes and prevent severe fluid and electrolyte imbalances and metabolic acidosis. Although acute renal failure often resolves spontaneously and renal function resumes, dialysis can be lifesaving. Either hemodialysis or peritoneal dialysis may be used, generally as a temporary measure. Nursing care related to acute renal failure and dialysis is discussed in Chapter 27. ⬡

## NURSING CARE

Few clients with acute enteritis require hospitalization. Most are treated in outpatient and community settings. Assessment, education, and support of self-care measures are major nursing responsibilities.

### Health Promotion

Nurses play a significant role in preventing enteritis as educators, community health providers, and advocates for environmental safety.

Teach the importance of proper food handling and maintaining appropriate temperatures. Adequate cooking of meat products is vital to prevent disorders such as staphylococcal food poisoning, *E. coli* hemorrhagic colitis, and salmonellosis. Emphasize the importance of not consuming raw meat products, and cooking hamburger in particular to the point that no redness is noted in the meat. The highly pathogenic *E. coli* serotype 0157:H7 is present in the gut of infected animals. Meats from the animal may be contaminated with bowel contents. The organism is readily destroyed by heat, so cuts of meat such as steaks or roasts are less likely to cause infection, since the organism is on the outside of the meat. However, the process of grinding hamburger allows *E. coli* to be mixed throughout the meat. Thorough cooking destroys the organism. This pathogen (and others) may also be spread through unpasteurized milk. Discuss the dangers of consuming milk that has not been pasteurized and encourage clients to avoid it.

Dairy products, eggs, and egg products left at room temperature provide a good growth medium for bacteria. Discuss the importance of prompt refrigeration of meats and these products to minimize this risk.

Nonacidic canned foods, such as vegetables, mushrooms, meats, and fish, are potential sources of botulism toxin. The high temperatures required to destroy the bacteria and its spores are achieved only by pressure canning with appropriate pressures and duration. Emphasize the importance of following directions precisely when home-canning foods. Advise boiling home-canned foods for 10 to 15 minutes to destroy any potential toxin. Any food that is discolored or comes from a can or jar that has been damaged or does not have a tight seal should be destroyed without tasting or touching. Food contaminated with botulism may have no unusual odor or color. If the seal is questionable, discard the food.

Many gastrointestinal infections are spread through contaminated water. Encourage travelers to consume only bottled water unless local water supplies are clearly safe. Water purification tablets are available for hikers and campers, and may also be used when traveling abroad.

## Assessment

- Health history: onset, duration, and severity of symptoms; recent activities such as attending a picnic or potluck, international travel, or camping; other affected members of the household; measures taken to relieve symptoms or replace fluids
- Physical examination: vital signs including temperature and orthostatic vitals; skin color, temperature, moisture, and turgor; peripheral pulses and capillary refill; abdominal shape, contour, bowel sounds, tenderness

## Nursing Diagnoses and Interventions

Diarrhea and fluid volume deficit are priority nursing diagnoses. See the earlier section of this chapter on diarrhea for specific nursing interventions related to these diagnoses.

Other nursing diagnoses that may be appropriate for the client with acute enteritis are as follows:

- *Risk for aspiration* related to impaired swallow reflex (botulism)
- *Nausea* related to effects of infection or toxins on GI tract and vomiting center of the brain
- *Impaired home maintenance* related to lack of knowledge about safe food preparation and storage practices
- *Impaired spontaneous ventilation* related to respiratory muscle paralysis (botulism)
- *Impaired urinary elimination* related to effects of enterotoxin on renal function (*E. coli* hemorrhagic colitis)

## Home Care

Discuss the following topics when preparing the client for home care.

- The importance of good handwashing, particularly before handling food and after each bowel movement
- The need to wash clothing and linens contaminated with feces separately in hot water and detergent
- Oral solutions to replace lost fluids and electrolytes
- Appropriate use of antidiarrheal medications if recommended
- Symptoms of complications to report to the health care-provider

# THE CLIENT WITH A PROTOZOAL BOWEL INFECTION

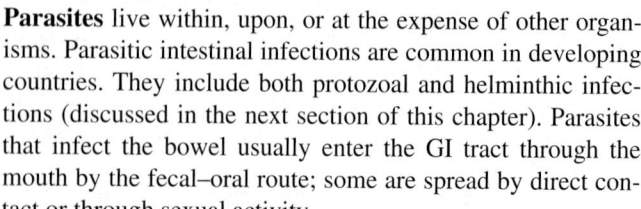

**Parasites** live within, upon, or at the expense of other organisms. Parasitic intestinal infections are common in developing countries. They include both protozoal and helminthic infections (discussed in the next section of this chapter). Parasites that infect the bowel usually enter the GI tract through the mouth by the fecal–oral route; some are spread by direct contact or through sexual activity.

Of the protozoal bowel infections, only giardiasis is common in the United States. Amebiasis is found chiefly in the tropics and where sanitation is poor. Cryptosporidiosis, a form of coccidiosis, is an important worldwide cause of sporadic mild diarrhea, traveler's diarrhea, and severe diarrhea in people who are immunocompromised.

## PATHOPHYSIOLOGY AND MANIFESTATIONS

The most common protozoal infections of the bowel are discussed below and summarized in Table 24–5.

### Giardiasis

*Giardiasis* is a protozoal infection of the upper small intestine caused by *Giardia lamblia*. It is the most common intestinal protozoal pathogen in the United States, affecting children more often than adults. Humans are the reservoir for *Giardia*. It is spread by the fecal–oral route, usually in contaminated food or water. It is also spread by direct contact.

When the cyst form of the organism is ingested, trophozoites emerge in the duodenum and jejunum, attaching themselves to the intestinal mucosa. This leads to superficial invasion, inflammation, and destruction of the mucosa of the small intestine.

Giardiasis may be asymptomatic, although manifestations may develop suddenly or insidiously. Diarrhea is common. It is usually mild, with one or several large, loose stools per day. Diarrhea may be severe, however, with frequent, copious, frothy, malodorous, and greasy stools. Other manifestations include weight loss and weakness; anorexia, nausea, and vomiting; epigastric pain, abdominal cramping and distention, flatulence, and belching. Malabsorption may develop (discussed later in this chapter).

### Amebiasis

*Amebiasis* (amebic dysentery) causes 40,000 to 100,000 deaths annually throughout the world. In the United States it tends to be mild and often asymptomatic.

Amebiasis is caused by the protozoon *Entamoeba histolytica*. Several strains of the protozoon have been identified. Tropical strains tend to be more virulent and pathogenic than those found in temperate climates. Humans are the host for this parasite. It usually is transmitted through food or water contaminated by feces and by person-to-person contact. The parasite enters the intestines, where it may live without causing disease. It may invade the intestinal wall to cause ulceration and inflammation. The cecum, appendix, ascending colon, sigmoid colon, and rectum are most often affected. Ulcers may spread to cause hemorrhage, edema, and mucosal sloughing. The infection may spread via the blood to the liver, lungs, or brain.

Amebiasis is usually asymptomatic. Mild manifestations include abdominal cramps, flatulence, and intermittent diarrhea containing blood and mucus. Severe manifestations of amebic dysentery include frequent watery stools containing blood, mucus, and necrotic tissue; colic, tenesmus, and abdominal tenderness; nausea and vomiting; and fever. The liver may be enlarged and tender to palpation.

Complications are rare, but may include appendicitis, bowel perforation with peritonitis, and fulminating colitis.

### Cryptosporidiosis (Coccidiosis)

*Cryptosporidiosis* causes sporadic mild diarrhea and traveler's diarrhea in all age groups. In people with impaired immune function, such as those with human immunodeficiency virus (HIV) disease, it causes severe diarrhea, malabsorption, and significant weight loss.

## TABLE 24–5    Common Protozoal Infections of the Bowel

| Disease and Organism | Incubation | Pathogenesis | Manifestations | Management |
|---|---|---|---|---|
| Giardiasis: *Giardia lamblia* | 1 to 3 weeks or more | Trophozoite attaches to mucosa in duodenum and jejunum, causing superficial invasion, inflammation, and tissue destruction. | Diarrhea, mild or severe, daily or intermittent; anorexia, nausea, vomiting; epigastric pain, cramping, distension; flatulence and belching; may be asymptomatic | Metronidazole, quinacrine, furazolidone |
| Amebiasis: *Entamoeba histolytica* | 2 to 4 weeks | Organisms may reside in large intestine without causing disease or can invade colon wall, causing ulceration; may be carried via blood to liver to produce abscess. | Usually asymptomatic; diarrhea may be mild, with few semiformed mucus-containing stools per day, or severe, with 10 to 20 blood-streaked liquid stools per day; abdominal cramps and flatulence; colic, tenesmus, vomiting, tenderness; fatigue, weight loss; prostration and toxicity | Metronidazole and diloxanide furoate or iodoquinol; chloroquine for hepatic abscess |
| Cryptosporidiosis: *Cryptosporidium* | 2 to 10 days | Organisms attach to epithelial surface of small bowel (jejunum), causing villous atrophy and mild inflammatory changes; may secrete enterotoxin. | In immunocompetent clients: Asymptomatic to profuse, watery diarrhea of sudden onset, abdominal cramping; malaise, fever; anorexia, nausea, vomiting. In immunodeficient clients: Profuse watery diarrhea with loss of up to 15 to 20 L per day; severe malabsorption, electrolyte imbalance; weight loss; lymphadenopathy | Self-limiting in immuno-competent clients. For immunodeficient clients: spiramycin, zidovudine (AZT), paromomycin (Humatin), octreotide, eflornithine; fluid and electrolyte replacement; paren-teral nutrition as needed |

This organism is transmitted by the fecal–oral route. Contaminated water is a frequent source of infection. The organism attaches to bowel epithelium, causing surface damage and inflammation. It does not invade the tissues, but secretes an enterotoxin that causes characteristic watery diarrhea. The disease is self-limited in people with competent immune systems. Watery diarrhea may be accompanied by low-grade fever, nausea, vomiting, abdominal cramps, and general malaise.

Immunocompromised clients develop profuse watery diarrhea with significant fluid and electrolyte losses and severe malabsorption. Lymphadenopathy also may develop.

## COLLABORATIVE CARE

Collaborative care includes identifying the causative organism and pharmacologic treatment. Diagnostic testing may include:

- *Stool examination for ova and parasites.* Many protozoa are shed intermittently rather than continuously. Stools are collected sequentially (e.g., every other day for a total of three specimens). Freshly collected stool is examined microscopically to identify protozoa, trophozoites (their immature forms), or their cysts. A laxative may be given prior to the specimen collection to increase protozoal shedding.
- *Indirect hemagglutination assay (IHA),* a blood test to detect antibodies to specific protozoa. This test may not differentiate current from previous infection.

- *Sigmoidoscopy,* to examine bowel mucosa and collect a stool or exudate specimen for examination. In this case, no bowel preparation is performed before the sigmoidoscopy.
- *Duodenal string test (Entero-Test), duodenal aspiration, or duodenal biopsy* when giardiasis is suspected. Duodenal aspirate is stained and examined microscopically for the protozoa. Small bowel biopsy can identify *Cryptosporidium* infection.

Pharmacologic treatment includes both local and systemic antiparasitic drugs, such as iodoquinol (Amebaquine), paromomycin (Humatin), and metronidazole (Flagyl), furazolidone (Furoxone), or albendazole (Albenza). Treatment is usually provided on an outpatient basis. Severe amebic dysentery may require hospitalization for intravenous fluid and electrolyte replacements. Nursing care related to common antiprotozoal drugs is outlined in the box on page 646.

## NURSING CARE

Nurses need to teach the public how parasitic diseases are transmitted and how to avoid spreading the infection. Prevention of amebiasis and giardiasis involves:

- Provision of safe water supplies.
- Appropriate disposal of human feces.
- Safe food storage, handling, and preparation.

# Medication Administration

## Antiprotozoal Agents

### LOCAL (GASTROINTESTINAL) AGENTS

Iodoquinol (Yodoxin, Amebaquine)
Paromomycin (Humatin)

These drugs exert a local amebicidal effect in the intestines and are poorly absorbed when administered orally. Local agents have the advantage of provoking fewer side effects than systemically active agents.

#### Nursing Responsibilities

- Assess for potential contraindications:
  a. Hypersensitivity to the drug or drug class.
  b. Iodoquinol: malnutrition, thyroid disorders; hepatic or renal impairment, optic neuropathy, or hypersensitivity to iodine.
  c. Paromomycin: ulcerative bowel lesions; hypersensitivity to aminoglycoside antibiotics, impaired renal function, intestinal obstruction.
- Observe for adverse effects: anorexia, nausea, vomiting, abdominal cramping, diarrhea, and increased flatulence; report skin rash, visual disturbances, or changes in blood work to primary care provider.

#### Client and Family Teaching

- Take as prescribed for the full course of therapy.
- Take with food to reduce gastrointestinal effects.
- Keep follow-up appointments as recommended to evaluate the effects of treatment.
- Report adverse effects to the physician.
  a. Any change in vision
  b. Numbness, tingling or pain in extremities
  c. Chills, fever, skin rash or boils
  d. A change in urination or character of urine
  e. Diminished hearing or tinnitus
  f. Weight loss, diarrhea, fatty stools
  g. Candidiasis of the mouth or vagina
- Practice good handwashing, particularly after using the toilet, to prevent spreading the disease to others.

### SYSTEMIC AGENTS

Metronidazole (Flagyl, Satric, Metzol, others)
Furazolidone (Furoxone), Albendazole (Albenza)

Clients with symptomatic protozoal infections are generally treated with a systemic antiprotozoal agent. Metronidazole is the most widely used of these antiprotozoal agents and is the drug of choice for treating amebiasis. Furazolidone, available as an elixir, often is used to treat children.

### Nursing Responsibilities

- Assess for possible contraindications to therapy:
  a. Hypersensitivity to the prescribed agent or related drugs.
  b. Liver dysfunction or blood dyscrasias
  c. Concurrent use of alcohol or an MAOI
  d. Pregnancy
- Administer as ordered.
  a. Metronidazole may be given orally after meals or as a continuous or intermittent intravenous infusion.
  b. Administer furazolidone and albendazole orally with meals to minimize gastric distress.
- Observe for possible adverse effects; notify the physician if significant. Gastrointestinal effects are common.
  a. Peripheral neuropathy and CNS effects may occur with metronidazole.
  b. Blood dyscrasias may develop with furazolidone or albendazole; monitor CBC and report abnormal results.
  c. Furazolidone can cause hypoglycemia; carefully monitor blood glucose in diabetic clients.
  d. Report abnormal liver function test results.
- Monitor the character and number of stools; obtain specimens as ordered to evaluate the effectiveness of therapy.

### Client and Family Teaching

- Take the drug as prescribed for the full duration of the prescription.
- Taking oral preparations after meals helps minimize gastrointestinal side effects. Notify the physician if nausea and vomiting continue.
- Do not use alcohol while taking these drugs. An Antabuse-type response with severe headache, flushing, and vomiting may occur.
- Report adverse effects to the physician, including dizziness and other nervous system changes, sore throats, fatigue, bruising, or infection.
- Candidiasis of the mouth or vagina may occur with metronidazole therapy. Report symptoms to the physician.
- A harmless change in urine color to deep yellow (quinacrine) or rust or brown (metronidazole or chloroquine) may occur while taking these drugs.
- If you are diabetic taking furazolidone, carefully monitor blood glucose levels as hypoglycemia may develop.
- Practice good handwashing, particularly after using the toilet, to prevent transmitting the protozoa to others.

- Adequate handwashing after defecating and before handling food.

Instruct people living in high-risk areas (tropical climates, areas with untreated water supplies) to boil, filter, or treat water supplies with iodine to eliminate protozoal contamination. Instruct them to avoid foods that cannot be peeled or cooked. Teach the manifestations of protozoal infections and where to obtain treatment.

Nursing assessment, diagnoses, and interventions for the client with a protozoal GI infection are similar to those indicated for clients with bacterial or viral infections. *Diarrhea* and *Risk for deficient fluid volume* are priority nursing diagnoses. See previous sections of this chapter for specific nursing interventions related to these diagnoses.

Emphasize the importance of keeping toilet areas clean and maintaining good personal hygiene. Advise the client to avoid rectal contact during sexual activity. Other household members should also have stool specimens examined for parasites. No drug is safe or effective to prevent protozoal infections of the bowel.

## THE CLIENT WITH A HELMINTHIC DISORDER

*Helminths* are parasitic worms, capable of causing infectious diseases in humans. Helminths are subclassified as round worms (nematodes), flukes (trematodes), or tapeworms (cestodes).

## PATHOPHYSIOLOGY AND MANIFESTATIONS

Although all helminths can infect humans, the definitive host and intermediate hosts vary with each organism. In nearly all instances of helminthic disorders, the organism enters the body through the gastrointestinal tract in contaminated and inadequately cooked foods. Some of these organisms remain in the intestinal tract; others migrate to infect the liver, lungs, or other structures. Few helminths are common in the United States; Table 24–6 summarizes the most common helminths and their effects.

### TABLE 24–6   Selected Helminthic Diseases

| | Infection | Host | Area | Pathogenesis | Manifestations |
|---|---|---|---|---|---|
| **Nematode Infections** | Ascariasis | Humans | Worldwide, cosmopolitan; warm, moist climates | Eggs are ingested in fecally contaminated food and drink; motile larvae migrate to lungs and back to small intestine, where they mature to produce more eggs. | Pulmonary: Low-grade fever, cough, blood-tinged sputum, wheezing, dyspnea, substernal chest pain. GI: Ulcerlike epigastric pain, vomiting, abdominal distention |
| | Enterobiasis (Pinworm infection) | Humans | Worldwide, cosmopolitan | Infect cecum; eggs deposit on perianal skin, organisms may be transmitted to others or reinfect host by oral ingestion. | Nocturnal perianal and perineal pruritus; insomnia, irritability, restlessness |
| | Hookworm disease | Humans | Tropics and subtropics | Larvae enter through skin or by ingestion and migrate to lungs, up bronchial tree, and down esophagus to mature in upper small bowel, where they attach and suck blood. | Skin: Pruritic dermatitis at site of entry  Pulmonary: Dry cough, wheezing, blood-tinged sputum  GI: Anorexia, diarrhea, abdominal pain  Systemic: Anemia, pallor, cardiac insufficiency |
| | Trichinosis | Pigs; dogs, cats, rats, many wild animals | Temperate areas where pork is consumed | Larvae are ingested in undercooked meat; adult female burrows into mucosa of small intestine to produce larvae that disseminate via blood and lymphatic system to body tissues and become encysted in striated muscle. | GI: Diarrhea, abdominal cramps, malaise  Muscle: Fever; muscle pain, tenderness, edema, and spasm  Systemic: Periorbital and facial edema, sweating; photophobia and conjunctivitis; manifestations of inflammation in tissues invaded by larvae |
| **Cestode Infections** | Fasciolopsiasis (intestinal fluke)  Tapeworm | Humans; other mammals and fish | Worldwide | Organism is ingested by eating uncooked fish or meat containing embryo cysts, by fecal contamination, or by swallowing infected intermediate hosts, such as arthropods, fleas, or lice; head (scolex) of adult worm attaches in upper small intestine, and eggs form in individual segments. | Large tapeworms: Often asymptomatic; infection may cause mild nausea, diarrhea, abdominal pain; anemia, thrombocytopenia, and mild leukopenia  Small tapeworms: May be asymptomatic; diarrhea, abdominal pain, anorexia, vomiting, weight loss, and irritability |

## COLLABORATIVE CARE

The primary means of diagnosing helminthic disorders is examination of the stool for ova and parasites. Enterobiasis is diagnosed by the presence of the parasite's eggs on the perianal skin or on cellulose tape placed over the anus. A CBC may also be ordered. Anemia may be present, particularly with hookworm disease. *Eosinophilia* (an increased percentage of eosinophils in the blood) is common in helminthic disorders. With trichinosis, serum muscle enzymes such as the creatinine kinase (CK) and aspartate aminotransferase (AST) are typically elevated. Serologic testing for antibodies to the worm may also be performed. Blood, duodenal washings, and cerebrospinal fluid (CSF) may be examined for the presence of the trichinosis larvae. Inflamed muscle may be biopsied.

Helminthic infections often are treated with a single oral dose or 3-day course of pyrantel pamoate (Antiminth) or mebendazole (Vermox). Doses may need to be repeated every 2 weeks for clients with heavy infections. These drugs are generally safe, requiring few precautions. Giving the drug after meals minimizes gastrointestinal side effects. Treatment is followed by a stool culture at 2 weeks to evaluate effectiveness. If necessary, an additional course of the drug is prescribed. Other members of the household are generally also treated.

Most clients with trichinosis recover spontaneously without long-term effects. The intestinal phase of the disease is treated with albendazole, taken twice daily for as long as 60 days, or a 13-day course of mebendazole. Hospitalization may be required during the muscle invasion phase of the disease if the infection is severe. Corticosteroids may be used to reduce the inflammation and manage the symptoms.

## NURSING CARE

Many helminthic disorders are acquired by consuming food that has been fecally contaminated or contains larvae of the organism. Emphasize the importance of not fertilizing food or grain crops with fecal material, particularly human feces. Teach clients to cook all meats and fish adequately to destroy possible larvae. In general, pickled or salt-preserved meats and fish are no safer than raw. Smoking, another means of preserving fish and meat, may not achieve temperatures high enough to destroy the organisms. Vegetables grown in soil that may be contaminated with eggs or larvae should be peeled or cooked prior to eating.

Emphasize the importance of safe water supplies. Encourage people traveling to areas in which water supplies are questionable to drink only bottled water or carry purification tablets. Work with clients who have private water systems to protect water from fecal contamination by either humans or animals.

Because many clients with these disorders are asymptomatic, nurses need to be alert for histories that indicate risk and subtle manifestations of the disorder.

Use standard precautions to minimize the risk of spreading these infections to other clients. Wear gloves and gowns as necessary to prevent fecal contamination of hands and uniforms. On rare occasions, parasites may be present in the sputum or vomitus, so handle these secretions with care also. Disinfect toilets, toilet seats, and commodes after use. To the client, emphasize the importance of washing hands after using the toilet and before handling food to prevent reinfection.

The client with a helminthic disorder may feel dirty or be ashamed of the disease. Emphasize the prevalence of these disorders, and assure the client that infection can occur despite good health practices when the eggs or larva of the organism are prevalent.

Discuss measures to prevent spread of the disease in the household. Emphasize the importance of hygiene measures including changing bedding, daily cleaning of toilets with disinfectant, and, of course, handwashing.

# CHRONIC INFLAMMATORY BOWEL DISEASE

## THE CLIENT WITH INFLAMMATORY BOWEL DISEASE

Chronic inflammatory bowel disease (IBD) includes two separate but closely related conditions: ulcerative colitis and Crohn's disease. These conditions have a number of similarities. The etiology of both illnesses is unknown, but both have a geographic distribution and a genetic component. IBD occurs more frequently in the United States and northern European nations than it does in southern Europe and countries in the Southern Hemisphere. IBD is 2 to 4 times more prevalent in Jewish populations of the United States and Europe than it is in non-Jewish Caucasians, African Americans, Hispanics, and Asians (Braunwald et al., 2001). It tends to run in families. Other studies suggest that factors such as an infectious agents and altered immune responses play a role in the development of IBD. Autoimmunity is thought to play a role (see Chapter 9). Lifestyle factors (such as smoking) may also affect its development.

The peak incidence of IBD is in young adults between the ages of 15 and 35 years. A second peak occurs between age 60 and 80 (Braunwald et al., 2001). IBD is a chronic and recurrent disease process. Responses to physiologic or psychologic stresses do not cause IBD, but often play a role in exacerbations of the disease.

Despite the similarities, ulcerative colitis and Crohn's disease have distinct differences. Ulcerative colitis primarily affects the large bowel in a continuous pattern, progressing distally to proximally. In Crohn's disease, a patchy pattern of

| TABLE 24-7 | | Characteristics of Ulcerative Colitis and Crohn's Disease | |
|---|---|---|---|
| | **Characteristic** | **Ulcerative Colitis** | **Crohn's Disease** |
| **Clinical** | Gender | Equal | Equal |
| | Age at onset | 15 to 35 years; secondary peak between 50 and 70 years | 10 to 30 years |
| | Course of disease | Typically chronic and intermittent | Slowly progressive, relapsing |
| | Diarrhea | 5 to 30 stools per day with blood and mucus | Common, usually less severe than colitis, with no obvious blood or mucus in stool |
| | Abdominal pain | Cramping in left lower quadrant; relieved by defecation | Cramping or steady right lower quadrant or periumbilical pain; tenderness and mass noted in right lower quadrant |
| | Nutritional deficit | Common; involves anemia, hypoalbuminemia, and weight loss | Common and significant: involves anemia, weight loss, and multiple vitamin and mineral deficits |
| | Constitutional manifestations | Fever rare; may have associated arthritic, skin, or other organ involvement, such as erythema nodosum or uveitis | Fever, malaise, fatigue; may have some associated conditions plus urinary complications |
| **Pathologic** | Depth of involvement | Mucosa and submucosa | Transmural (entire bowel wall) |
| | Portion of bowel involved | Typically rectum and sigmoid colon; may extend to involve entire large bowel | Any portion of GI tract; terminal ileum and ascending colon involvement predominates |
| | Distribution | Continuous from rectum | Patchy; skip lesions |
| | Appearance of mucosa | Granular, dull, hyperemic, friable; disease uniform in affected bowel; pseudopolyps may be seen | Cobblestone appearance, with areas of normal tissue surrounded by ulceration and fissures |
| **Complications** | Acute | Toxic megacolon, perforation, massive hemorrhage | Obstruction, fistulization, abscess formation, malabsorption |
| | Long-term | Colorectal cancer | Colon cancer |

involvement is seen, affecting primarily the small intestine. Ulcerative colitis shows mainly mucosal involvement; in Crohn's disease, the submucosal layers of the bowel are affected. A comparison of ulcerative colitis and Crohn's disease is found in Table 24–7. *Multisystem Effects of Inflammatory Bowel Disease* are illustrated on page 650.

## ULCERATIVE COLITIS

**Ulcerative colitis** is a chronic inflammatory bowel disorder that affects the mucosa and submucosa of the colon and rectum. Its annual incidence in the United States is about 11 per 100,000 people (Braunwald et al., 2001).

*Chronic intermittent colitis* (recurrent ulcerative colitis) is the most common form of the disease. Its onset is insidious, with attacks that last 1 to 3 months occurring at intervals of months to years. Typically, only the distal colon is affected, with few systemic manifestations of the disease. Approximately 15% of people with ulcerative colitis develop *fulminant colitis,* with involvement of the entire colon, severe bloody diarrhea, acute abdominal pain, and fever. Clients with fulminant disease are at high risk for complications.

## Physiology Review

The wall of the colon has three layers: the mucosa, the submucosa, and the muscularis externa. The mucosal layer contains an abundance of goblet cells and glands which secrete lubricating mucus to facilitate the movement of feces. The colon wall forms a series of pouches, or *haustra.* These pouches allow the colon to expand and contract. Feces moves through the colon by both peristaltic waves and by segmentation movements that mix the contents of adjacent haustra. As feces moves, water and other substances such as bile salts are reabsorbed.

## Pathophysiology

The inflammatory process of ulcerative colitis begins at the rectosigmoid area of the anal canal and progresses proximally. In most clients, the disease is confined to the rectum and sigmoid colon. It may progress to involve the entire colon, stopping at the ileocecal junction.

Ulcerative colitis begins with inflammation at the base of the crypts of Lieberkühn in the distal large intestine and rectum. Microscopic, pinpoint mucosal hemorrhages occur, and crypt abscesses develop (Figure 24–4 ■). These abscesses penetrate the superficial submucosa and spread laterally, leading to necrosis and sloughing of bowel mucosa. Further tissue damage is caused by inflammatory exudates and the release of inflammatory mediators, such as prostaglandins and other cytokines (see Chapter 8 ⊂⊃ for further discussion of the inflammatory process). The mucosa is red and edematous due to vascular congestion, friable (easily broken), and ulcerated. It bleeds easily,

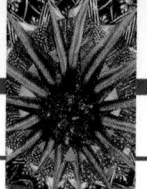

# Multisystem Effects of Inflammatory Bowel Disease

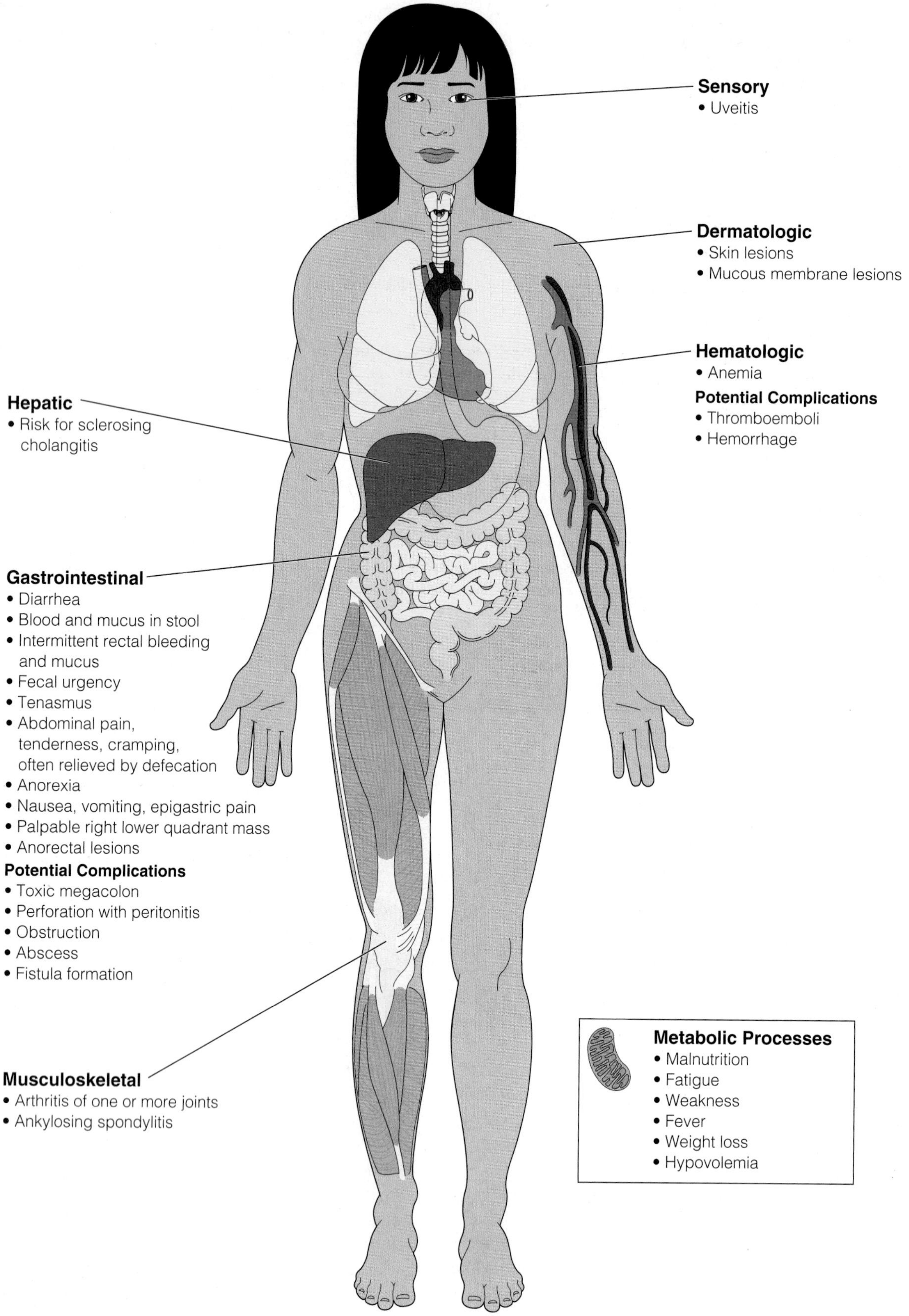

**Sensory**
- Uveitis

**Dermatologic**
- Skin lesions
- Mucous membrane lesions

**Hematologic**
- Anemia

**Potential Complications**
- Thromboemboli
- Hemorrhage

**Hepatic**
- Risk for sclerosing cholangitis

**Gastrointestinal**
- Diarrhea
- Blood and mucus in stool
- Intermittent rectal bleeding and mucus
- Fecal urgency
- Tenasmus
- Abdominal pain, tenderness, cramping, often relieved by defecation
- Anorexia
- Nausea, vomiting, epigastric pain
- Palpable right lower quadrant mass
- Anorectal lesions

**Potential Complications**
- Toxic megacolon
- Perforation with peritonitis
- Obstruction
- Abscess
- Fistula formation

**Musculoskeletal**
- Arthritis of one or more joints
- Ankylosing spondylitis

**Metabolic Processes**
- Malnutrition
- Fatigue
- Weakness
- Fever
- Weight loss
- Hypovolemia

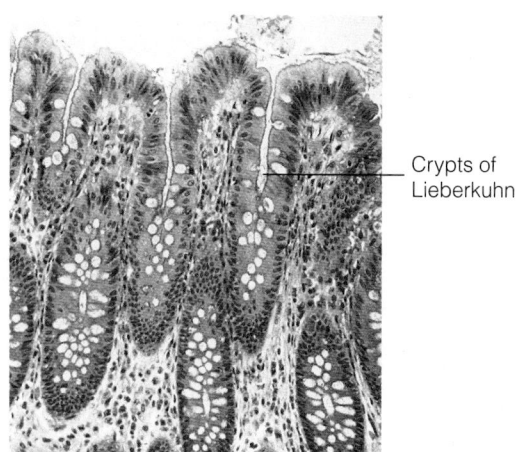

**Figure 24–4** ■ Photomicrograph of the mucosa of the large intestine showing the entrances to the crypts of Lieberkühn. The crypts are the focal points for ulcerative colitis.

Crypts of Lieberkuhn

*Source: Photo Researchers, Inc.*

and hemorrhage is common. Edema creates a granular appearance. Pseudopolyps, tonguelike projections of bowel mucosa into the lumen, may develop as the epithelial lining of the bowel regenerates. Chronic inflammation leads to atrophy, narrowing, and shortening of the colon, with loss of its normal haustra.

## MANIFESTATIONS

Diarrhea is the predominant symptom of ulcerative colitis. Stools contain both blood and mucus. Nocturnal diarrhea may occur. Mild ulcerative colitis is characterized by fewer than five stools per day, intermittent rectal bleeding and mucus, and few constitutional symptoms. Severe ulcerative colitis can lead to more than 6 to 10 bloody stools per day, extensive colon involvement, anemia, hypovolemia, and malnutrition. Rectal inflammation causes fecal urgency and tenesmus. Left lower quadrant cramping relieved by defecation is common. Other systemic manifestations include fatigue, anorexia, and weakness.

Clients with severe disease also may have systemic manifestations such as arthritis involving one or several joints, skin and mucous membrane lesions, or *uveitis* (inflammation of the uvea, the vascular layer of the eye, which may also involve the sclera and cornea). Some clients develop thromboemboli, with blood vessel obstruction due to clots carried from the site of their formation. Sclerosing cholangitis (inflammation and scarring of the bile ducts) may occur (Tierney et al., 2001).

## Complications

Acute complications of ulcerative colitis include hemorrhage, toxic megacolon, and colon perforation. Massive hemorrhage may occur with severe attacks of the disease. **Toxic megacolon,** a condition characterized by acute motor paralysis and dilation of the colon to greater than 6 cm, may affect part or all of the colon. The transverse segment of the bowel is most often affected. Toxic megacolon may be triggered by electrolyte imbalances or narcotic administration (Braunwald et al., 2001). Manifestations of toxic megacolon include fever, tachycardia,

hypotension, dehydration, abdominal tenderness and cramping, and a change in the number of stools per day. Perforation is rare, but the risk of this dangerous complication is increased with toxic megacolon. Perforation leads to peritonitis, and has a mortality rate of about 15% (Braunwald et al., 2001).

The risk for colorectal cancer is increased in clients with ulcerative colitis. When the entire colon is involved by ulcerative colitis, the risk is 20 to 30 times greater than for the general public (Porth, 2002). Beginning 8 to 10 years after the diagnosis, yearly colonoscopies with biopsy to detect masses or cell dysplasia are recommended for clients who have extensive ulcerative colitis (Tierney et al., 2001).

## CROHN'S DISEASE

Like ulcerative colitis, **Crohn's disease,** also known as regional enteritis, is a chronic, relapsing inflammatory disorder affecting the gastrointestinal tract. The overall incidence of Crohn's disease in the United States is approximately 7 per 100,000 people (Braunwald et al., 2001).

Crohn's disease can affect any portion of the GI tract from the mouth to the anus, but usually affects the terminal ileum and ascending colon. Only the small bowel is involved in about 30% to 40% of clients with Crohn's disease. The disease is limited to the colon only in 15% to 20% of those affected. Both the small and large intestine are involved in the majority (Braunwald et al., 2001).

## Pathophysiology

Crohn's disease typically begins as a small inflammatory *aphthoid lesion* (shallow ulcers with a white base and elevated margin, similar to a canker sore) of the mucosa and submucosa of the bowel. These initial lesions may regress, or the inflammatory process can progress to involve all layers of the intestinal wall. Deeper ulcerations, granulomatous lesions, and fissures (knifelike clefts that extend deeply into the bowel wall) develop. The inflammatory process involves the entire bowel wall (transmural).

The lumen of the affected bowel assumes a "cobblestone appearance" as fissures and ulcers surround islands of intact mucosa over edematous submucosa. The inflammatory lesions of Crohn's disease are not continuous; rather, they often occur as "skip" lesions with intervening areas of normal-appearing bowel. Some evidence suggests that despite its normal appearance, the entire bowel is affected by this disorder.

As the disease progresses, fibrotic changes in the bowel wall cause it to thicken and lose flexibility, taking on an appearance that has been likened to a rubber hose. The inflammation, edema, and fibrosis can lead to local obstruction, abscess development, and the formation of fistulas between loops of bowel or bowel and other organs (Figure 24–5 ■). Fistulas between loops of bowel are known as enteroenteric fistulas; those that occur between bowel and bladder are known as enterovesical fistulas; and fistulas that occur between bowel and skin are known as enterocutaneous fistulas. Perineal fistulas are relatively common, originating in the ileum.

Depending on the severity and extent of the disease, malabsorption and malnutrition may develop as the ulcers prevent

**Figure 24–5** ■ The progression of Crohn's disease.

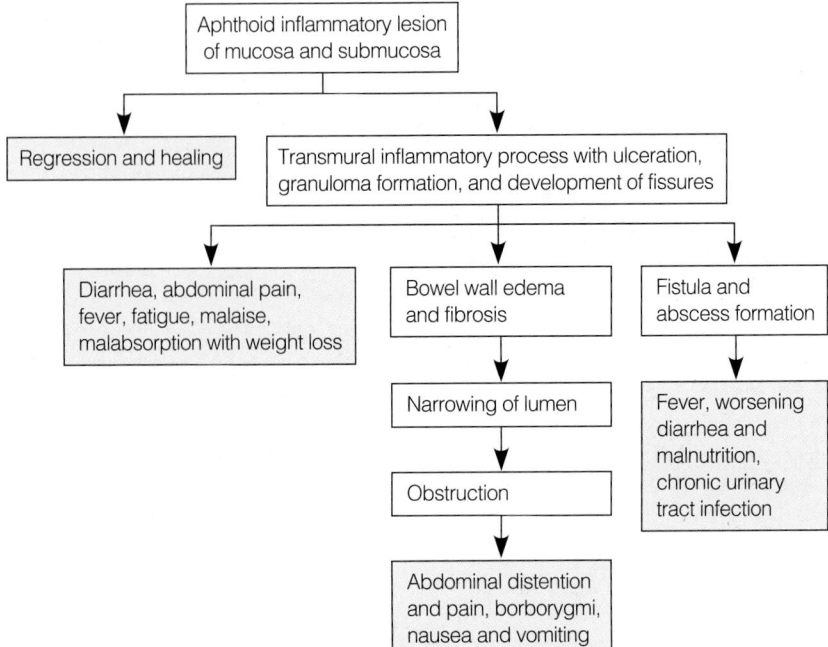

absorption of nutrients. When the jejunum and ileum are affected, the absorption of multiple nutrients may be impaired, including carbohydrates, proteins, fats, vitamins, and folate. Disease in the terminal ileum can lead to vitamin $B_{12}$ malabsorption and bile salt reabsorption. The ulcerations can also lead to protein loss and chronic, slow blood loss with consequent anemia.

## MANIFESTATIONS

Because the GI system involvement in Crohn's disease can be so diverse, manifestations may vary among clients. The majority of people with Crohn's disease experience continuous or episodic diarrhea. Stools are liquid or semiformed and typically do not contain blood, although blood may be passed if the colon is involved. Abdominal pain and tenderness is also common. The pain may be located in the right lower quadrant and relieved by defecation. A palpable right lower quadrant mass is often present. Systemic manifestations such as fever, fatigue, malaise, weight loss, and anemia are common. Anorectal lesions such as fissures, ulcers, fistulas, and abscesses also are common and may occur years before intestinal disease is apparent. If the stomach and duodenum are involved, nausea, vomiting, and epigastric pain may occur.

### Complications

Certain complications of Crohn's disease (e.g., intestinal obstruction, abscess, and fistula) are so common that they are considered part of the disease process. For many clients, the disease initially presents with one of these complications. Intestinal obstruction is a common complication caused by repeated inflammation and scarring of the bowel that leads to fibrosis and stricture. Obstruction of the bowel lumen causes abdominal distention, cramping pain, and borborygmi. Nausea and vomiting may occur.

Fistulas may be asymptomatic, particularly if they occur between loops of small bowel. When fistulization causes an abscess, chills and fever, a tender abdominal mass, and leukocy-

tosis develop. A fistula between the small bowel and colon may exacerbate diarrhea, weight loss, and malnutrition. When the bladder is involved, recurrent urinary tract infections occur.

Perforation of the bowel is uncommon, but can lead to generalized peritonitis. Massive hemorrhage also is an uncommon complication of Crohn's disease. Long-standing Crohn's disease increases the risk of cancer of the small intestine or colon by 5 to 6 times. This cancer risk, however, is significantly lower than the risk associated with ulcerative colitis.

## COLLABORATIVE CARE

Collaborative care for inflammatory bowel disease begins by establishing the diagnosis and the extent and severity of the disease. Treatment is supportive, including medications and dietary measures to decrease inflammation, promote intestinal rest and healing, and reduce intestinal motility. Many clients with IBD require surgery at some point to manage the disease or its complications.

### Diagnostic Tests

Diagnostic testing is used to establish the diagnosis of IBD, assess the extent of the disease, and evaluate the effects of the disorder.

- *Sigmoidoscopy* or *colonoscopy* is performed to inspect the bowel mucosa for characteristic changes of IBD: edema, inflammation, mucus and pus, mucosal ulcers or abscesses, and either a continuous or segmental pattern of involvement. Biopsy of bowel mucosa may differentiate ulcerative colitis or Crohn's disease from cancer and other inflammatory bowel disorders. There is a small risk of bowel perforation during these exams, particularly if the disease is severe. Nursing implications for these diagnostic tests are listed in the boxes on pages 619 and 624.

- *Radiologic examination* of the entire gastrointestinal tract includes an upper GI series with small bowel follow-through and a barium enema. These studies can show the characteristic small and large bowel changes of IBD, such as ulcerations, strictures, fistulas, shortening and loss of colon haustra, or complications such as a dilated colon in toxic megacolon. Nursing implications for the client having a barium enema are listed in the box on page 623; see the box on page 628 for nursing implications for a small bowel series.
- *Stool examination* for blood and mucus and *stool cultures* are done to rule out infectious causes of bowel inflammation and diarrhea.
- *CBC with hemoglobin* and *hematocrit* shows anemia from chronic inflammation, blood loss, and malnutrition; and leukocytosis due to inflammation and possible abscess formation. The sedimentation rate is typically elevated during periods of acute inflammation.
- *Serum albumin* may be decreased because of malabsorption, malnutrition, protein loss through intestinal lesions, and chronic inflammation.
- *Folic acid* and *serum levels* of most vitamins, including A, B complex, C, and the fat-soluble vitamins, often are decreased due to malabsorption.

- *Liver function tests* may show elevated liver enzymes (such as ALT, alkaline phosphatase, AST, GGTP, and LDH) and bilirubin levels if sclerosing cholangitis is present.

## Medications

The ultimate goal of care is to terminate acute attacks as quickly as possible and reduce the incidence of relapse. Drug therapy plays a key role in achieving this goal. Locally acting and systemic anti-inflammatory drugs are the primary medications used to manage mild to moderate IBD. Drugs to suppress the immune response may be used to treat clients with severe disease.

Sulfasalazine (Azulfidine) is a sulfonamide antibiotic that is poorly absorbed from the gastrointestinal tract and acts topically on the colonic mucosa to inhibit the inflammatory process. The active anti-inflammatory ingredient in sulfasalazine, 5-aminosalicylic acid, also is available in preparations that do not contain sulfa, such as olsalazine and mesalamine. They have the advantage of causing fewer adverse effects than sulfasalazine. Specific preparations, their method of action, and nursing implications for these medications are outlined in the box below and on the following page.

---

## Medication Administration

### Inflammatory Bowel Disease

#### SULFASALAZINE (AZULFIDINE)
Sulfasalazine is an anti-inflammatory drug used for its local effect on the intestinal mucosa in inflammatory bowel disease. The active part of the drug is 5-aminosalicylic acid, which inhibits prostaglandin production in the bowel. Prostaglandin is an important mediator of the inflammatory process; blocking its production reduces inflammation.

#### Nursing Responsibilities
- Assess for contraindications, including pregnancy or a history of hypersensitivity to sulfonamides or salicylates.
- Assess baseline values for renal function tests (serum creatinine, BUN, urinalysis), liver function tests, and CBC.
- Administer as ordered. Suppositories or retention enemas may be administered at bedtime. Administer oral forms with a full glass of water.
- Have resuscitation equipment available; anaphylactic responses may occur.
- Evaluate for therapeutic response, including reduced number of stools, reduced mucus and blood, and improved stool consistency.
- Monitor for possible adverse responses:
  a. Skin rash, dermatitis, urticaria, or pruritus
  b. Evidence of blood dyscrasias, such as bleeding, easy bruising, fever
  c. Leukopenia, thrombocytopenia, hemolytic anemia, or angranulocytosis
  d. Changes in urinary output or renal function studies
  e. Evidence of hepatitis or myocarditis

#### Client and Family Teaching
- Take oral preparations after meals to decrease gastric distress.

- Drink at least 2 quarts of fluid per day to reduce the risk of kidney damage.
- Use sunscreen to prevent burns; this drug increases sensitivity to sun.
- Do not take aspirin, vitamin C, or any other over-the-counter medications containing aspirin or vitamin C without consulting your doctor.
- This medication may interfere with the effectiveness of oral contraceptives; use alternative methods of contraception.
- Notify your doctor if you develop skin rash or hives, sore throat or mouth, bleeding gums, joint pain, easy bruising, or fever.

#### MESALAMINE (ASACOL ROWASA) AND OLSALAZINE (DIPENTUM)
Mesalamine and olsalazine contain the same active ingredient, 5-aminosalicylic acid, as sulfasalazine, but cause fewer adverse effects. Their mechanism of action is the same as that of sulfasalazine. These drugs are available as suppositories, suspension for enema, or oral tablets.

#### Nursing Responsibilities
- Assess for possible contraindications such as pregnancy, lactation, or hypersensitivity to these drugs or aspirin.
- Administer as ordered. If more than one dose per day is ordered, space doses evenly over the 24-hour period.
- Evaluate for desired effects (as for sulfasalazine) and potential adverse effects.
  a. Nausea, diarrhea, abdominal cramps, or flatulence
  b. CNS effects including headache, dizziness, insomnia, weakness, or fatigue
  c. Rash or itching
  d. Flulike symptoms, general malaise

*(continued on page 654)*

## Medication Administration
### Inflammatory Bowel Disease (continued)

#### Client and Family Teaching
- Teach the recommended method of administration, including how to insert rectal suppositories or administer a retention enema.
- Shake suspension forms well prior to using.
- Diarrhea is the most common side effect of these drugs. Notify your doctor if adverse effects occur.

#### CORTICOSTEROIDS

| | |
|---|---|
| Methylprednisolone (Medrol, Solu-Medrol) | Prednisolone (Delta-Cortel) |
| | Prednisone |

Glucocorticoids are hormones produced by the adrenal cortex. These hormones are necessary for the stress response. Cortisol, the main glucocorticoid, has potent anti-inflammatory effects. Corticosteroids are used to treat acute episodes of IBD. Because of their multiple and significant side effects, they are not used to maintain remission.

#### Nursing Responsibilities
- Assess for conditions that may be adversely affected by corticosteroid drugs: peptic ulcer disease, glaucoma or cataracts, diabetes, or psychiatric disorders.
- Obtain baseline vital signs and weight; monitor both routinely during therapy. Hypertension and weight gain may result from salt and water retention.
- Monitor for edema.
- Administer as ordered. For daily or alternate-day dosing, administer in the morning, when physiologic glucocorticoid levels are highest, to reduce adrenal cortisone suppression.
- Administer oral preparations with food to decrease gastrointestinal side effects. Antacids or histamine $H_2$-receptor blocking agents, such as cimetidine (Tagamet), may be prescribed during corticosteroid therapy.

- Monitor for desired effects reduced diarrhea, less blood and mucus in the stool, and less abdominal cramping.
- Monitor for adverse effects:
  a. Increased susceptibility to infection and masking of early signs of infection
  b. Hyperglycemia
  c. Hypokalemia, as manifested by muscle weakness, nausea, vomiting, and cardiac rhythm disturbances
  d. Edema, hypertension, and signs of heart failure
  e. Peptic ulcer formation and possible gastrointestinal hemorrhage (abdominal pain, black or tarry stools, and signs of bleeding)
  f. Changes in mental status, including depression, euphoria, aggression, and behavioral changes
  g. With long-term use, Cushingoid effects, such as abnormal fat deposits in the face (moon faces) and trunk (buffalo hump), muscle wasting and thin extremities, thinning of the skin, and osteoporosis

#### Client and Family Teaching
- Take as prescribed; do not change the dose or time of day. Do not stop the medication abruptly. The dose will be tapered down gradually when the drug is discontinued.
- Notify the physician if adverse or Cushingoid effects occur.
- Take with food or at mealtimes to decrease the gastrointestinal effects.
- Monitor weight. If a gain of more than 5 pounds is noted notify the physician.
- Moderate salt intake and avoid foods and snacks high in sodium, such as processed meats and potato chips. Increase intake of foods high in potassium, such as fruits, vegetables, and lean meats.
- Carry a card or wear a bracelet or tag at all times identifying corticosteroid use.

---

For acute exacerbations of IBD, corticosteroids are given to reduce inflammation and induce remission. For ulcerative colitis, the drug may be administered by enema for its local effect and to minimize systemic effects. Hydrocortisone can be administered by enema. Intravenous corticosteroids may be required to treat severe disease; oral preparations are used for less severe manifestations and long-term therapy. Many clients are unable to withdraw from steroid therapy without experiencing relapse and may need chronic low-dose therapy.

Mercaptopurine (6-MP, Purinethol) and other immunosuppressive agents such as azathioprine (Imuran) and cyclosporine (Sandimmune) may be used to treat clients who have not responded to other treatments or who require chronic steroid therapy. These drugs may allow withdrawal from corticosteroids, maintain remission, and facilitate healing. Long-term therapy may be required to produce a beneficial effect. For more information about immunosuppressive drugs, see Chapter 9. ↩

Newer treatments for IBD employ other immune response modifiers, such as monoclonal antibodies to suppress tumor necrosis factor (TNF, an inflammatory mediator substance),

and natural anti-inflammatory cyctokines such as interleukins (Braunwald et al., 2001).

Although antibiotic therapy generally is not indicated in IBD, metronidazole (Flagyl) has active anti-inflammatory effects. It may be prescribed to help prevent remission after ileal resection in Crohn's disease. See the Medication Administration box on page 646 for the nursing implications for metronidazole. Ciprofloxacin (Cipro) is an alternative to metronidazole.

Antidiarrheal agents, such as loperamide and diphenoxylate, may be given to slow gastrointestinal motility and reduce diarrhea. These drugs are safe for clients with mild, chronic symptoms, but they are not given during acute attacks because they may precipitate toxic dilation of the colon.

### Dietary Management

Antigens in the diet may stimulate the immune response in the bowel, exacerbating IBD. As a result, dietary management for inflammatory bowel disease is individualized. Some clients benefit from eliminating all milk and milk products from the diet. Increased dietary fiber may help reduce diarrhea and relieve rectal symptoms, but is contraindicated for clients with intestinal strictures caused by repeated inflammation and scarring.

All food is withheld to promote bowel rest during an acute exacerbation of Crohn's disease. Nutritional status is maintained using enteral or total parenteral nutrition (TPN). See Chapter 20 for more information about enteral feedings and TPN. TPN carries a higher risk of complications than does enteral nutrition. An elemental diet such as Ensure, which contains all essential nutrients in a residue-free formula, may be prescribed. Enteral diets provide essential nutrients to the small intestine to support cell growth, but are not always palatable.

## Surgery

Surgical interventions for IBD differ, depending on the primary disease process and the portion of the bowel affected. Generally, surgery is performed only when necessitated by complications of the disease or failure of conservative treatment measures.

Bowel obstruction is the leading indication for surgery in Crohn's disease. Other complications that may require surgical intervention include perforation, internal or external fistula, abscess, and perianal complications. Resection of the affected portion of bowel with an end-to-end anastomosis to preserve as much bowel as possible is the usual treatment. The disease process tends to recur in other areas following removal of affected bowel segments. There is an increased risk of fistula formation following surgery. Bowel strictures may be treated with a strictureplasty. In this procedure, longitudinal incisions are made in the narrowed segment to relieve the stricture while preserving bowel.

Clients with extensive chronic ulcerative colitis may require a **total colectomy** (surgical removal of the colon) to treat the disease itself, for complications such as toxic megacolon, perforation, or hemorrhage, or as a prophylactic measure due to the high colon cancer risk associated with extensive ulcerative colitis. The surgical procedure of choice for extensive ulcerative colitis is a *total colectomy with an ileal pouch-anal anastomosis (IPAA)*. In this procedure, the entire colon and rectum are removed; a pouch is formed from the terminal ileum; and the pouch is brought into the pelvis and anastomosed to the anal canal (Figure 24–6 ■). A temporary or loop ileostomy (described below) is generally performed at the same time and is maintained for 2 to 3 months to allow the anal anastomosis to heal. When the healing is complete, the ileostomy is closed, and the client has 6 to 8 daily bowel movements through the anus.

Advanced age, obesity, or other factors may preclude an IPAA. For these clients, a permanent ileostomy or continent ileostomy may be created.

An intestinal **ostomy** is a surgically created opening between the intestine and the abdominal wall which allows the passage of fecal material. The surface opening is called a **stoma** (Figure 24–7 ■).

The precise name of the ostomy depends on the location of the stoma. An **ileostomy** is an ostomy made in the ileum of the small intestine. In an ileostomy, the colon, rectum, and anus are usually completely removed (*total proctocolectomy with permanent ileostomy*). The anal canal is closed, and the end of the terminal ileum is brought to the body surface through the right abdominal wall to form the stoma. A temporary or *loop ileostomy* may be formed to eliminate feces and allow tissue healing for 2 to 3 months following an IPAA. A loop of ileum is

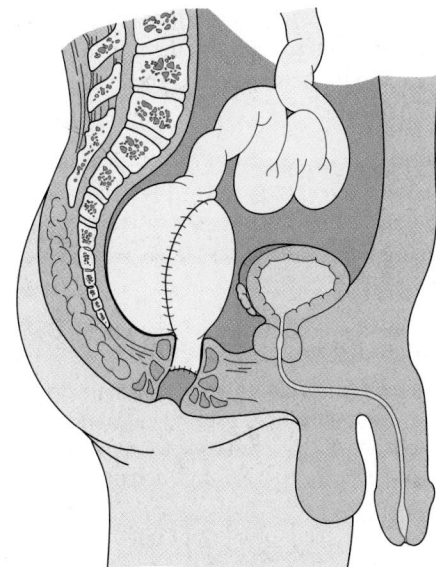

**Figure 24–6** ■ Ileal pouch-anal anastomosis.

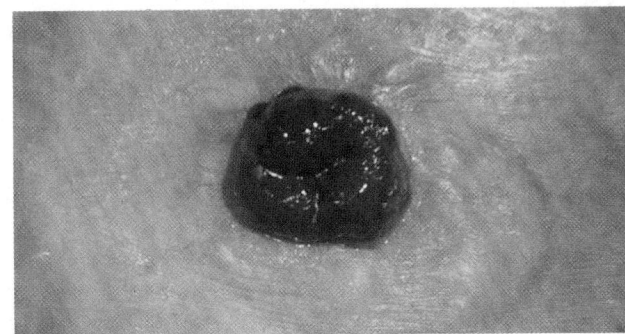

**Figure 24–7** ■ A healthy-appearing stoma.

*Courtesy of Carol Williams, RN, BS, UC Davis Medical Center.*

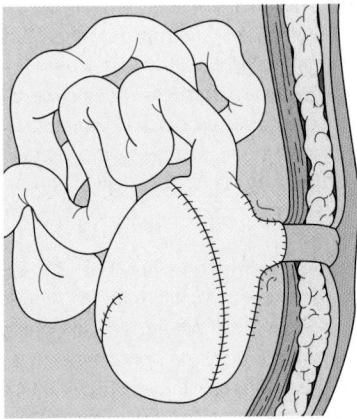

**Figure 24–8** ■ Continent (Kock's) ileostomy.

brought to the body surface to form a stoma and allow stool drainage into an external pouch. When the ileostomy is no longer necessary, a second surgery is performed to close the stoma and repair the bowel, restoring fecal elimination through the anus.

In a *continent* (or *Kock's) ileostomy,* (Figure 24–8 ■) an intra-abdominal reservoir is constructed and a nipple valve formed (the ileum folded back on itself) from the terminal ileum, before it is brought to the surface of the abdominal wall. Stool collects in the internal pouch; the nipple valve prevents it from leaking through the stoma. A catheter is inserted into the pouch to drain the stool.

Nursing care of the client with an ileostomy is outlined below and on the following page. Procedure 24–1 on page 658 describes how to apply one- and two-piece drainable ostomy pouches.

## NURSING CARE    OF THE CLIENT HAVING AN ILEOSTOMY

### PREOPERATIVE CARE

- Provide routine preoperative care and teaching as outlined in Chapter 7. ∞
- Refer to an enterostomal therapist for marking and teaching about the stoma location, ostomy care, and options for ostomy appliances. *It is important to begin teaching prior to surgery to facilitate learning and acceptance of the ostomy postoperatively.*
- Discuss the availability of a local United Ostomy Association chapter, and provide a referral as necessary or desired. *Local chapters often have members with ostomies who are willing to provide both preoperative and postoperative teaching, listening, and support.*
- Provide preoperative bowel preparation as ordered. *Cathartics, enemas, and preoperative antibiotics are often ordered to reduce the risk of abdominal contamination and infection after surgery.*

### POSTOPERATIVE CARE

- Provide routine postoperative care and teaching as outlined in Chapter 7.
- Apply an ostomy pouch over the stoma. (See Procedure 24–1.) *Stool from an ileostomy is expressed continuously or irregularly, and it is liquid in nature; continuous use of a pouch to collect the drainage is therefore necessary.*
- Assess frequently for bleeding, stoma viability, and function. In the early postoperative period, small amounts of blood in the pouch are expected. A healthy stoma appears pink or red and moist as a result of mucus production (Figure 24–7). It should protrude approximately 2 cm from the abdominal wall. *Frequent assessment is particularly important in the initial postoperative period to ensure stoma health and monitor for possible complications. A dusky, brown, black, or white stoma indicates circulatory compromise. Other possible stoma complications include retraction (indentation or loss of the external portion of the stoma) or prolapse (outward telescoping of the stoma, that is, an abnormally long stoma).*
- As the stoma starts to function, empty the pouch, explaining the procedure to the client. Initial drainage is dark green, viscid, and usually odorless. Drainage gradually thickens and becomes yellow-brown. Empty the pouch when it is one-third full. Measure drainage, and include it as output on intake and output records. Rinse the pouch and reapply the clamp. *Emptying the pouch when it is no more than one-third full helps prevent the skin seal from breaking as a result of the weight of the pouch. Because of the potential for excess fluid loss through ileostomy drainage, it is important to include it as fluid output.*
- Assess the peristomal skin. Skin around the stoma should remain clean and pink and free of irritation, rashes, inflammation, or excoriation. *Skin complications may arise from appliance irritation or hypersensitivity, excoriation from a leaking appliance, or Candida albicans, a yeast infection.*

- Protect peristomal skin from enzymes and bile salts in the ileostomy effluent. Using a skin barrier on the pouch is essential. Change the pouch if leakage occurs or if the client complains of burning or itching skin. *Enzymes and bile salts normally reabsorbed in the large intestine are irritating to the skin. Excoriation of skin surrounding the stoma impairs the first line of defense against microorganisms and can interfere with the ability to achieve a tight skin seal and prevent pouch leakage.*
- Report the following abnormal assessment findings to the physician:
  a. Allergic or contact dermatitis. *A rash may result from contact with fecal drainage or indicate sensitivity to pouch, paste, tape, or sealant.*
  b. Purulent ulcerated areas surrounding the stoma. *Disruption of the protective barrier of the skin allows bacterial entry.*
  c. A red, bumpy, itchy rash or white-coated area. *This is a manifestation of* Candida albicans, *a yeast infection.*
  d. Bulging around the stoma. *This finding may indicate herniation, caused by loops of intestine protruding through the abdominal wall.*
- Apply protective ointments to the perirectal area of clients with newly functioning ileoanal reservoirs and anastomoses. *This helps protect the skin from the initial stools. As stools thicken and become fewer per day, the client experiences less perirectal irritation.*

### CLIENT AND FAMILY TEACHING

- While caring for the ostomy, explain procedures to the client. *Teaching is immediate and ongoing to facilitate acceptance of the ostomy and self-care.*
- Teach to manage the pouch clamp, to empty, rinse, and perform pouch changes. *Self-care is vital to independence and self-esteem.*
- Instruct now to use an electric razor to shave the peristomal hair if necessary. *An electric razor prevents accidental cutting of the stoma with a razor blade.*
- Teach to check the stoma and peristomal skin with each pouch change. *Ongoing assessment is important for optimal health and function of the stoma and surrounding skin. Stripping of tape or excessively frequent pouch removal may cause mechanical trauma to peristomal skin. Chronic skin irritation by ileostomy effluent may lead to* pseudoveracous lesions, *or wartlike nodules.*
- Instruct to report abnormal appearance of the stoma or surrounding skin (as noted previously and below) to the physician:
  a. Narrowing of the stoma lumen. *This indicates stenosis and may interfere with fecal elimination.*
  b. Lacerations or cuts in the stoma. *The stoma contains no nerves, so trauma may occur without pain.*
  c. Separation of the stoma from the abdominal surface. *This potential complication may require surgical repair.*

(continued on page 657)

# NURSING CARE OF THE CLIENT HAVING AN ILEOSTOMY (continued)

- Emphasize the importance of adequate fluid and salt intake; the risk for dehydration and hyponatremia is increased particularly during hot weather, when fluid is lost through perspiration as well as ileostomy drainage. Water intake should be sufficient to maintain pale urine and an output of at least 1 quart per day. When exercising in hot weather, the client should consume extra water and salt. High-potassium foods, such as bananas and oranges, may also be recommended. *Loss of the reabsorptive surface of the large bowel increases the amount of water and sodium loss in the stool. If the ileostomy is high (more proximal in the ileum), additional potassium losses may also occur.*
- Discuss signs and symptoms of fluid and electrolyte imbalances:
  a. Extreme thirst
  b. Dry skin and oral mucous membrane
  c. Decreased urine output
  d. Weakness, fatigue
  e. Muscle cramps
  f. Abdominal cramps, nausea, vomiting
  g. Shortness of breath
  h. Orthostatic hypotension (feeling faint when suddenly changing positions)
- Discuss dietary concerns. A low-residue diet is recommended initially (see Table 24–8). Foods that may cause excessive odor or gas are typically avoided as well. *Because food blockage is a potential problem, high-fiber foods are limited, and foods that may cause blockage, such as popcorn, corn, nuts, cucumbers, cel-* *ery, fresh tomatoes, figs, strawberries, blackberries, and caraway seeds are avoided. Symptoms of food blockage include abdominal cramping, swelling of the stoma, and absence of ileostomy output for over 4 to 6 hours.*
- Teach self-care measures to relieve food blockage:
  a. Take a warm shower or tub bath. *This can help relax the abdominal muscles.*
  b. Assume a knee-chest position. *The knee-chest position reduces intra-abdominal pressure.*
  c. Drink warm fluids or grape juice if not vomiting. *This provides a mild cathartic effect.*
  d. Massage peristomal area. *Massage may stimulate peristalsis and fecal elimination.*
  e. Remove pouch if the stoma is swollen, and apply a pouch with a larger opening. *If the stoma swells, the pouch may create a mechanical obstruction to output.*
- Notify the physician or enterostomal therapy nurse if:
  a. The above measures fail to relieve the obstruction.
  b. Signs of a partial obstruction persist including high-volume odorous fluid output, abdominal cramps, nausea, and vomiting.
  c. There is no ileostomy output for 4 to 6 hours.
  d. Signs of fluid and electrolyte imbalance occur, such as weakness, dizziness, lightheadedness, or headache.

*Should self-care measures not succeed in breaking up a blockage,* ileostomy lavage, as *described in Procedure 24–2 may be required.*

## TABLE 24–8    Low-Residue Diet

| Food Group | Allowed | Avoid |
|---|---|---|
| Beverages | Coffee, teas, juices, carbonated beverages; milk limited to 2 cups per day | Alcohol, prune juice |
| Breads and cereals | Products made from refined flours (white bread, crackers) or finely milled grains (e.g., corn flakes, crisp rice cereal, puffed wheat) | Whole-grain breads, rolls, or cereal; breads or rolls with seeds, nuts, or bran |
| Desserts | Gelatins, tapioca, plain custards, or puddings; angel-food or sponge cake; ice cream or frozen desserts without fruit or nuts | Any desserts containing dried fruits, nuts, seeds, or coconut; rich pastries, pies |
| Fruits | Fruit juices and strained fruits; cooked or canned apples, apricots, cherries, peaches, pears; bananas | All other raw or cooked fruits |
| Meats and other protein sources | Roasted, baked, or broiled tender or ground beef, veal, pork, lamb, poultry, or fish; smooth peanut butter; cottage, cream, American, or mild chedder cheeses in small amounts | Tough or spiced meats and those prepared by frying; highly flavored cheeses; nuts |
| Potatoes, rice, and pasta | Peeled potatoes; white rice; most pasta products | Potato skins, potato chips, or fried potatoes; brown rice; whole-grain pasta products |
| Sweets | Sugar, honey, jelly, hard candy and gumdrops, plain chocolates | Jam, marmalade; candy made with seeds, nuts, coconut |
| Vegetables | Vegetable juices and strained vegetables; cooked or canned vegetables | Raw or whole cooked vegetables |
| Other | Salt, ground seasonings; cream sauce and plain gravy | Chili sauce, horseradish; popcorn, seeds of any kind; whole spices, olives, vinegar |

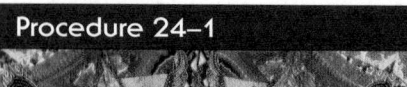

## Procedure 24–1

# Changing a One- or Two-Piece Drainable Ostomy Pouch

### SUPPLIES

- One- or two-piece pouch
- Skin barrier paste
- Skin prep
- Clamp
- Pouch deodorant
- Measuring guide
- Adhesive remover
- Skin cleanser
- Washcloths
- Plastic bag

Explain the procedure and provide for privacy Follow standard precautions.

### PROCEDURE

1. Remove soiled pouch (and the flange if a two-piece pouch) by gently pulling on the pouch or flange and pushing on skin. Use adhesive remover to remove skin barrier paste.
2. Empty pouch, discarding it and the flange (if applicable) in a plastic bag. Save the tail closure clamp. The pouch from a two-piece system may be cleaned out and reused.

3. Cleanse skin and stoma with warm water and skin cleanser or mild soap. Rinse skin and stoma, and pat dry.
4. Note stoma color and peristomal skin condition.
5. If necessary, clip or shave peristomal hair.
6. Use measuring guide or previous pattern to check size of stoma (Figure 24–9A ■).
   a. Presized pouch: check to verify that size is correct.
   b. Cut-to-fit pouch or flange: Trace the correct size of the stoma onto the back of the flange, and cut the opening to match the pattern. The opening should be no more than 1/8 inch larger than stoma.

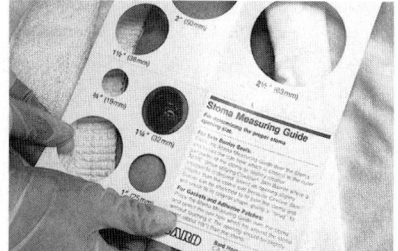

7. Apply skin prep to skin covered by a wafer, pouch, or tape. Allow to dry.
8. Remove backings from pouch or flange.
9. Apply a bead of skin barrier paste around the stoma base or around the opening of the pouch or flange. Allow the paste to air-dry for 1 to 2 minutes.
10. Center the pouch or flange over the stoma, and press to adhere (Figure 24–9B ■).
11. For a two-piece pouch, snap the pouch onto skin barrier flange.
12. Place deodorizing tablets or a few drops of liquid pouch deodorizer (in some cases, antiseptic mouthwash may be used) in the pouch. Apply the clamp.
13. "Picture frame" the pouch with tape to provide extra security.

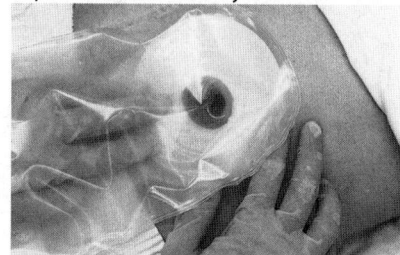

**Figure 24–9** ■ *A,* A guide for measuring the stoma. *B,* Applying the disposable pouch.

## Procedure 24–2

# Ileostomy Lavage

### SUPPLIES

- Disposable irrigation sleeve
- 60 mL catheter-tipped syringe
- #14 Fr. catheter
- Water-soluble lubricant
- Normal saline for irrigation
- Bedpan
- Clean ostomy pouch

Explain the procedure and provide for privacy. Follow standard precautions.

### PROCEDURE

1. Remove the pouch. Apply disposable irrigation sleeve.

2. Clamp the bottom of the sleeve, or place it into the bedpan.
3. Gently examine stoma digitally to break up any mass proximal to stoma and determine direction of the bowel.
4. Lubricate catheter, and insert into stoma until blockage is reached. If the catheter does not reach the blockage after 8 to 10 cm, notify the physician. This may indicate a more proximal obstruction.
5. Instill 30 to 50 mL normal saline.
6. Remove catheter. Allow stoma to drain.
7. Repeat the procedure until the mass is removed.

8. When the blockage is removed, remove the irrigation sleeve.
9. Clean peristomal skin.
10. Apply pouch and clamp.

### POSTPROCEDURE

1. Document the procedure, amount of solution used, consistency of results, and the client's tolerance of the procedure.

2. Discuss dietary concerns to help determine cause of blockage.

## Complementary Therapies

The chronic nature of inflammatory bowel disease and adverse effects of many prescribed treatments lead many clients with IBD to seek or use complementary therapies. Chiropractic care, megavitamin therapy, dietary supplements, and herbal medi-cine have been reported as common complementary therapies for IBD (Heuschkel et al., 2002; Verhoef et al., 2002). A study by Langmead et al (2002) concluded that herbal remedies such as slippery elm, fenugreek, devil's claw, Mexican yam, ter-mentil and wei tong ning have antioxidant effects and may provide an effect similar to that of 5-aminosalicylic acid preparations. Many complementary therapies for IBD may interact with prescribed medications; instruct the client to discuss all potential therapies with the primary care provider.

## NURSING CARE

### Health Promotion

Although inflammatory bowel disease cannot, at this time, be predicted or prevented, effective management may help the client avoid complications of the disease. Stress the importance of complying with the prescribed treatment regimen and promptly reporting manifestations of exacerbations to the physician.

### Assessment

Assessment data related to inflammatory bowel disease includes the following subjective and objective data.

- Health history: current manifestations, including onset, duration, severity (number of stools per day, presence of blood or mucus in stool, abdominal pain or cramping, tenesmus); usual diet, ability to maintain weight and nutrition, food intolerances; associated manifestations such as arthralgias, fatigue, malaise; current medications; previous treatment and diagnostic tests
- Physical examination: general appearance; weight; vital signs including orthostatic vitals and temperature; abdominal assessment including shape, contour, bowel sounds, palpation for tenderness and masses, presence of stoma or scars

### Nursing Diagnoses and Interventions

When planning nursing care for the client with inflammatory bowel disease, it is vital to consider the chronic, recurrent nature of the disorder. Teaching is a major aspect of care. Diarrhea and disturbed body image are significant nursing care problems for the client with IBD. With severe disease, impaired nutrition must be considered a priority problem as well.

### Diarrhea

During an acute exacerbation of IBD, diarrhea can be frequent and painful. The frequency of defecation and associated abdominal pain and cramping may interfere with ADLs and increase the risk for fluid volume deficit and impaired skin integrity.

- Record the frequency, amount, and color of stools using a stool chart. Measure and record liquid stool as output. *The severity of diarrhea is an indicator of the severity of the disease and helps determine the need for fluid replacement.*

**PRACTICE ALERT** *Observe stools for obvious blood and test for occult blood as indicated. Report grossly bloody stools or hematochezia, which may indicate hemorrhage and necessitate emergency surgery.* ■

- Assess vital signs every 4 hours. *Tachycardia, tachypnea, and fever may be indicators of fluid volume deficit.*

- Weigh daily and record. *Rapid weight loss (over days to a week) usually indicates fluid loss, whereas weight loss over weeks to months may indicate malnutrition.*
- Assess for other indications of fluid deficit: warm, dry skin, poor skin turgor, dry shiny mucous membranes, weakness, lethargy, complaints of thirst. *The extent of fluid loss may not be readily evident with diarrhea, particularly if the client uses the bathroom without assistance. Systemic manifestations of fluid volume deficit may be the first indicators of the problem.*
- Maintain bowel rest by keeping NPO or limiting oral intake to elemental feedings as indicated. *Bowel rest during an acute exacerbation of IBD promotes healing and reduces diarrhea and other symptoms.*
- Administer prescribed anti-inflammatory and antidiarrheal medications as indicated. *Anti-inflammatory medications reduce the extent of bowel inflammation and diarrhea. Unless contraindicated, antidiarrheal medications help reduce fluid loss and increase comfort.*

**PRACTICE ALERT** *When giving antidiarrheal medications to a client with ulcerative colitis, closely observe for manifestations of toxic megacolon: fever, tachycardia, hypotension, dehydration, abdominal pain and cramping, and an abrupt relief of diarrhea.* ■

- Maintain fluid intake by mouth or intravenously as indicated. *The client with IBD requires fluid to replace ongoing losses, as well as fluid to meet the usual daily needs of the body. If an elemental diet or total parenteral nutrition is prescribed, additional fluids may be required to meet fluid intake needs.*
- Provide good skin care. *Fluid deficit and tissue dehydration increase the risk for skin excoriations or breakdown.*
- Assess perianal area for irritation or denuded skin from the diarrhea. Use gentle cleansing agents, such as Periwash or Tucks, or cottonballs saturated with witch hazel. Apply a protective cream, such as zinc oxide–based preparations, to protect skin from the irritating effects of diarrheal stool. *Digestive enzymes in the stool are very corrosive, increasing the risk of skin breakdown where exposed to diarrheal stool.*

### Disturbed Body Image

The client with IBD may experience frustration at not being able to control, or even predict, fecal elimination, particularly when the disease is severe. Diarrhea can interfere with the ability to complete tasks, maintain employment or engage in social activities, and even meet basic needs such as eating, sleeping, and sexual activity. Body image can suffer as a result. Treatment of IBD, be it total colectomy with ileal pouch-anal anastomosis, ileostomy, or chronic corticosteroid therapy, also can affect the view of self.

- Accept feelings and perception of self. *Negating or denying the reality of the client's perception impairs trust.*
- Encourage discussion of physical changes and their consequences as they relate to self-concept. *This demonstrates acceptance and provides an opportunity to express the impact of the disease and its treatment on the client's life.*

- Encourage discussion about concerns regarding the effect of the disease or treatment on close personal relationships. *This demonstrates understanding and provides an opportunity for the client to express feelings about the impact of the disease on relationships and significant others.*
- Encourage the client to make choices and decisions regarding care. *This increases the client's sense of control over the disease and his or her future.*
- Discuss possible treatment options and their effects openly and honestly. *Open discussion allows more informed decisions.*
- Involve the client in care, teaching and demonstrating as needed. *This encourages and facilitates independence and decision making.*
- Provide care in an accepting, nonjudgmental manner. *Acceptance of the client despite potential embarrassment about odors or diarrhea enhances self-esteem.*
- Arrange for interaction with other clients or groups of people with IBD or ostomies. *The client may feel that no one who has not experienced a similar problem can understand his or her feelings.*
- Teach coping strategies (odor control, dietary modifications, and so on), and support their use. *This facilitates healthy adaptation to the disease.*

## Imbalanced Nutrition:
## Less Than Body Requirements

Crohn's disease can significantly alter the bowel's ability to absorb nutrients. In both forms of IBD, blood and protein-rich fluid may be lost in diarrheal stools. With malabsorption and continuing nutrient losses, multiple nutrient deficits can develop, affecting growth and development, healing, muscle mass, bone density, and electrolyte balances.

- Monitor laboratory results, including hemoglobin and hematocrit, serum electrolytes, and total serum protein and albumin levels. *These studies provide an indicator of nutritional status.*
- Provide the prescribed diet: high-kcal, high-protein, low-fat diet with restricted milk and milk products if lactose intolerance is present. *Calories and protein are important to replace lost nutrients. Fat restriction helps reduce diarrhea and nutrient loss, particularly when significant portions of the terminal ileum have been resected.*
- Provide parenteral nutrition as necessary if the client is unable to absorb enteral nutrients. *Parenteral nutrition can help reverse nutritional deficits and promote weight gain and healing in the client with acute symptoms.*
- Arrange for dietary consultation. Consider food preferences as allowed. *Providing preferred foods in the prescribed diet increases intake and supports nutritional status.*
- Provide or administer elemental enteral nutrition and supplements as ordered. *Elemental enteral nutritional supplements support healing while providing for bowel rest. They can replace losses and improve nutritional status more rapidly than diet alone.*
- Include family members, the primary food preparer in particular, in teaching and dietary discussions. *Families can reinforce teaching and help the client maintain required restrictions or kcal intake.*

## Using NANDA, NIC, and NOC

Chart 24–3 shows links between NANDA nursing diagnoses, NIC, and NOC when caring for the client with inflammatory bowel disease.

## Home Care

Inflammatory bowel disease is a chronic condition for which the client needs to provide daily self-management. For this rea-

---

## CHART 24–3 LINKS BETWEEN NANDA, NIC, AND NOC

### The Client with Inflammatory Bowel Disease

| NURSING DIAGNOSES | NURSING INTERVENTIONS | NURSING OUTCOMES |
|---|---|---|
| • Acute Pain | • Medication Management | • Comfort Level |
| • Deficient Fluid Volume | • Fluid Monitoring | • Fluid Balance |
| | • Fluid/Electrolyte Management | • Hydration |
| • Diarrhea | • Diarrhea Management | • Symptom Severity |
| • Imbalanced Nutrition: Less Than Body Requirements | • Nutrition Management | • Nutritional Status |
| | • Weight Gain Assistance | |
| • Risk for Impaired Skin Integrity | • Skin Surveillance | • Tissue Integrity: Skin and Mucous Membranes |
| • Ineffective Coping | • Coping Enhancement | • Coping |
| | • Decision-Making Support | • Decision Making |
| | • Emotional Support | • Social Support |
| | • Family Involvement Promotion | |

*Note: Data from Nursing Outcomes Classification (NOC) by M. Johnson & M. Maas (Eds.), 1997, St. Louis: Mosby; Nursing Diagnoses: Definitions & Classification 2001–2002 by North American Nursing Diagnosis Association, 2001, Philadelphia: NANDA; Nursing Interventions Classification (NIC) by J.C. McCloskey & G. M. Bulechek (Eds.), 2000, St. Louis: Mosby. Reprinted by permission.*

son, teaching is a vital component of care. Teach the client and family about the following topics.

- The type of inflammatory bowel disease affecting the client, including the disease process, short- and long-term effects, the relationship of stress to disease exacerbations, and the manifestations of complications
- Prescribed medications, including drug names, desired effects, schedules for tapering the doses if ordered (as with corticosteroids), and possible side effects or adverse reactions and their management
- The recommended diet and the rationale for any specific restrictions
- Use of nutritional supplements such as Ensure to maintain weight and nutritional status
- Indicators of malabsorption and impaired nutrition; recommendations for self-care and when to seek medical intervention
- If discharged with a central catheter and home parenteral nutrition, written and verbal instructions on catheter care, troubleshooting, and TPN administration (Have the client and a family member demonstrate catheter care and TPN maintenance.)
- The importance of maintaining a fluid intake of at least 2 to 3 quarts per day, increasing fluid intake during warm weather, exercise or strenuous work, and when fever is present
- The increased risk for colorectal cancer and importance of regular bowel exams
- Risks and benefits of various treatment options

If surgery is planned or has been done, include the following topics in home care instructions.

- Ileal pouch-anal anastomosis or ileostomy care as indicated
- Where to obtain ostomy supplies
- Use of nonprescription drugs, such as enteric-coated and timed-release capsules that may not be adequately absorbed before elimination through the ileostomy
- Community and national ostomy support groups (see Box 24–2)

Provide referrals to a dietary consultant or nutritionist, a community health care agency, home care services, and home intravenous care services as indicated. See the Nursing Care Plan on page 662.

---

**BOX 24–2 ■ Resources for Home Care**

Local and national resource groups that may be helpful for the client with an ostomy:

- Canadian Foundation for Ileitis and Colitis
  21 St. Clair Avenue E., Suite 301
  Toronto, Ontario M4T 1L9
  CANADA
  416-920-5035
- Crohn's and Colitis Foundation of America
  386 Park Avenue S.
  New York, NY 10016-8804
  800-932-2423
  www.ccfa.org
- United Ostomy Association, Inc.
  36 Executive Park, Suite 120
  Irvine, CA 92714
  800-826-0826
  www.uoa.org

*MediaLink | OSTOMY RESOURCES*

---

# MALABSORPTION SYNDROMES

**Malabsorption** is a condition in which the intestinal mucosa ineffectively absorbs nutrients—including carbohydrates, proteins, fats, water, electrolytes, minerals, and vitamins—resulting in their excretion in the stool. Multiple different bowel disorders can lead to malabsorption.

Diseases of the small intestine often cause malabsorption. Other medical and/or surgical conditions can result in malabsorption if they affect digestion or the intestinal mucosa. Primary diseases of the small bowel mucosa, such as sprue, Crohn's disease, and acute infections, can lead to malabsorption. It may also result from *maldigestion,* inadequate preparation of chyme for absorption. For example, major gastric resections, pancreatic disorders with impaired pancreatic enzyme secretion, and biliary disorders that affect bile secretion can impair digestion and absorption of chyme. Selected causes of impaired absorption and digestion are listed in Table 24–9.

Regardless of the cause, malabsorption causes common manifestations resulting from impaired absorption of chyme

**TABLE 24–9  Selected Causes of Malabsorption**

| Cause | Related Factors or Conditions |
|---|---|
| Impaired absorption | Sprue<br>Short bowel syndrome<br>Acute enteritis and other bowel infections or infestations<br>AIDS-related opportunistic infections and Kaposi's sarcoma<br>Celiac disease<br>Crohn's disease<br>Intestinal ischemia or infarction<br>Scleroderma |
| Impaired digestion | Lactose intolerance<br>Gastrectomy<br>Chronic pancreatitis, cancer of the pancreas<br>Cystic fibrosis<br>Biliary obstruction<br>Cirrhosis, hepatitis, or liver failure<br>Zollinger-Ellison syndrome |

## Nursing Care Plan
## A Client with Ulcerative Colitis

Cortez Lewis is a 42-year-old real estate agent and mother of three school-age children. She has had ulcerative colitis for 18 years and has been treated with prednisone and sulfasalazine. Over the past 4 months she has been having abdominal pain and cramping and frequent bloody diarrhea stools. During the same period, she has lost 20 lb (9 kg), and has had difficulty maintaining her career. She recently developed several lesions of the lower leg identified as erythema nodosum. A recent colonoscopy revealed extensive involvement of the entire colon. On admission, Mrs. Lewis states, "I'm tired of fighting this disease. I am a prisoner in my home because of the diarrhea." She is admitted for a total proctocolectomy and ileal pouch-anal anastomosis.

### ASSESSMENT

Janet Wheeler, RN, completes the admission assessment. Mrs. Lewis now weighs 115 lb (52.2 kg). She complains of abdominal cramping, pain, and frequent bloody diarrhea stools. Several reddened lesions are noted on her lower legs. Physical assessment findings include T 98° F (36.6° C), P 72, R 20, and BP 104/72. Skin cool and pale. Abnormal laboratory findings include hemoglobin 7.3 g/dL (normal 11.7 to 15.7 g/dL); hematocrit 23.3% (normal 35% to 47%); WBC 15,580/mm³ (normal 3500 to 11,000/mm³); platelet count 995,000/mm³ (normal 150,000 to 450,000/mm³); serum protein 4.6 g/dL (normal 6 to 8 g/dL); serum albumin 2.4 g/dL (normal 3.5 to 5 g/dL). Preparation for surgery is begun.

### DIAGNOSIS

- *Imbalanced nutrition: Less than body requirements* related to impaired absorption
- *Diarrhea* related to inflammation of bowel
- *Risk for deficient fluid volume* related to abnormal fluid loss
- *Risk for impaired tissue integrity* related to drainage from temporary ileostomy
- *Pain* related to surgical intervention
- *Risk for sexual dysfunction* related to temporary ileostomy

### EXPECTED OUTCOMES

- Resume prescribed diet within 5 days after surgery.
- Demonstrate normal fecal elimination through the temporary ileostomy.
- Maintain adequate fluid balance.

- Demonstrate appropriate ostomy care prior to discharge.
- Report a tolerable level of discomfort.
- Verbalize feelings about sexuality and acknowledge importance of discussing sexual issues with husband.

### PLANNING AND IMPLEMENTATION

- Discuss dietary modifications related to nutritional status and presence of ileostomy. Provide referral to dietitian for diet planning and teaching.
- Teach importance of maintaining a high fluid intake and manifestations of dehydration.
- Teach to empty and change ostomy pouch of choice.
- Teach stoma and peristomal skin assessment with each pouch change.
- Teach food blockage management.
- Refer to local United Ostomy Association.
- Provide list of local medical suppliers for ostomy appliances.

### EVALUATION

On discharge, Mrs. Lewis is caring for her ileostomy, demonstrating her ability to empty, rinse, and change the pouch. The ET nurse has provided written and verbal instructions on ileostomy care. Mrs. Lewis verbalizes her understanding of the recommended diet and the need to limit high-fiber food intake and avoid enteric-coated and timed-release medications. The ET nurse has discussed sexual aspects of having an ileostomy and has given Mrs. Lewis a booklet, "Sex and the Female Ostomate," available through the United Ostomy Association. Mrs. Lewis is looking forward to the planned surgery to close the temporary ileostomy.

### Critical Thinking in the Nursing Process

1. Why is the client with an ileostomy at risk for dehydration? How can Mrs. Lewis monitor her fluid status at home?
2. Why were Mrs. Lewis's hemoglobin and hematocrit low on admission? If her hemoglobin had been low but her hematocrit normal on admission, what might be the explanation?
3. Outline a teaching plan that could be given to clients for home care of an ileostomy.
4. Develop a care plan for Mrs. Lewis for the nursing diagnosis, *Risk for impaired skin integrity*.

See Evaluating Your Response in Appendix C.

---

and the nutrients it contains (Table 24–10). Predominant GI manifestations include anorexia; abdominal bloating; diarrhea with loose, bulky, foul-smelling stools; and steatorrhea (fatty stools). Weight loss, weakness, general malaise, muscle cramps, bone pain, abnormal bleeding, and anemia are common systemic manifestations of malabsorption. These manifestations result from malnutrition and fluid loss due to poor absorption.

Three common malabsorption disorders in adults are sprue, lactose intolerance, and short bowel syndrome.

## THE CLIENT WITH SPRUE

**Sprue** is a chronic primary disorder of the small intestine in which the absorption of nutrients, particularly fats, is impaired. The severity of the disease depends on the extent of mucosal involvement in the intestine and the duration of the disease. Two major forms of sprue are celiac disease (celiac sprue) and tropical sprue.

## TABLE 24-10 Local and Systemic Manifestations of Malabsorption

| Category | Manifestation | Cause |
|---|---|---|
| Local (GI) | Diarrhea | Impaired absorption of fluid and electrolytes, leading to excess water in the stool |
| | Abdominal distention | Gas formation from fermentation of undigested carbohydrates |
| | Steatorrhea | Impaired fat absorption leading to excess fat in feces |
| Systemic | Weight loss | Carbohydrate, protein, and fat deficit |
| | Weakness and malaise | Kcal deficit, anemia, fluid, and electrolyte losses |
| | Anemia | Vitamin $B_{12}$, folic acid, and iron deficits |
| | Bone pain | Calcium and vitamin D deficits |
| | Muscle cramps, paresthesias | Protein wasting, vitamin $B_{12}$ and electrolyte deficits |
| | Easy bruising and bleeding | Vitamin K deficit |
| | Glossitis, cheilosis | Iron, folic acid, and vitamin $B_{12}$ deficits |

## PHYSIOLOGY REVIEW

Most absorption of nutrients occurs in the small intestine. The mucosa of the small intestine is arranged in microscopic folds, which in turn contain even smaller fingerlike projections called *villi*. The cells of the villi are covered with microscopic hairs, *microvilli,* projecting from the cell membrane. The folds, villi, and microvilli of the intestinal mucosa provide a huge surface area for nutrient absorption. Cells of the intestines are specialized to absorb different nutrients. Readily digested nutrients are absorbed in the proximal intestine; others are absorbed more distally in the intestines. Nutrients are absorbed by the processes of simple diffusion (water and small lipids), facilitated diffusion (water soluble vitamins), and active transport (glucose and amino acids). Once absorbed into the cells of the villi, nutrients enter the blood or lymph for systemic distribution.

## PATHOPHYSIOLOGY AND MANIFESTATIONS

Sprue is characterized by flattening of the intestinal mucosa with a loss of villi and microvilli. With the loss of villi, intestinal absorptive surface is lost, and digestive enzyme production, including disaccharidase and particularly lactase, is reduced.

## Celiac Sprue

**Celiac sprue,** also known as *celiac disease* or *nontropical sprue,* is a chronic malabsorption disorder characterized by sensitivity to the gliadin fraction of gluten, a cereal protein. Gluten is found in wheat, rye, barley, and oats. It is also used as a filler in many prepared foods and in medications. The cause

of celiac sprue is unknown; however, genetic, environmental, and immune factors are known to play a role in its development. Caucasians of European descent are most commonly affected (Braunwald et al., 2001). Manifestations of celiac sprue often develop in childhood, but may develop at any age.

In celiac sprue, it appears that the intestinal mucosa is damaged by an immunologic response. Gliadin acts as an antigen (a substance that induces the formation of antibodies that interact specifically with it), prompting the formation of antibodies and immune complexes. These complexes may deposit in the intestinal mucosa, prompting an inflammatory response and loss of villi. Gluten also may directly damage the villi, causing cell loss, inflammation, and edema. The villi shorten and atrophy, resulting in loss of intestinal folds and absorptive surface.

Manifestations of celiac sprue may develop at any age. Local manifestations include abdominal bloating and cramps, diarrhea, and steatorrhea. Systemic manifestations result from the effects of malabsorption and resulting deficiencies. Anemia is common. Clients with celiac disease are often small in stature, and may have delayed maturity. Other signs of nutrient deficiencies include tetany, vitamin deficiencies, muscle wasting, and even rickets (impaired bone development). When gluten is removed from the diet, the manifestations resolve.

Gastrointestinal malignancies and intestinal lymphoma are potential complications of celiac sprue. Other complications include intestinal ulceration and development of refractory sprue, or disease that no longer responds to a gluten-free diet.

## Tropical Sprue

*Tropical sprue* is a chronic disease of unknown cause, although bacterial infection or toxins are thought to contribute. Tropical sprue occurs chiefly in the Caribbean, south India, and southeast Asia. Its onset may be abrupt or insidious. The pathophysiologic changes in bowel mucosa closely resemble those of celiac sprue, although gluten intake has no effect on this condition.

Manifestations of tropical sprue include sore tongue, diarrhea, and weight loss. Initially, diarrhea may be explosive and watery; as the disease progresses, stools become fewer in number and more solid with obvious steatorrhea. Folic acid deficiency is common. Vitamin $B_{12}$ and iron deficiencies may occur, resulting in glossitis; stomatitis; dry, rough skin; and anemia.

## COLLABORATIVE CARE

With any malabsorptive disorder, the initial focus of management is to identify the cause. Once this has been determined, specific therapy can be prescribed.

## Diagnostic Tests

Laboratory and diagnostic testing are used to make the differential diagnosis for various causes of malabsorption syndromes and to determine the severity of nutrient deficiencies.

- *Fecal fat* is measured to document the presence of steatorrhea. All stool is collected over a 72-hour period. The client is placed on a high-fat (100 g/day) diet for 3 days prior to and during the collection period. No alcohol is to be consumed for 24 hours prior to and during the collection period. The expected result is less than 7 g of fat per 24 hours (Malarkey & McMorrow, 2000). The fat content of stool is increased in many malabsorptive disorders, including celiac and tropical sprue.

- *Serologic testing* for IgA endomysial antibodies, and IgG and IgA antigliadin antibodies is used to diagnose celiac sprue and evaluate compliance with the prescribed gluten-free diet.
- *Serum levels of protein, albumin, cholesterol, electrolytes,* and *iron* may be ordered to evaluate for nutrient deficiencies. The *hemoglobin, hematocrit,* and *RBC indices* are used to evaluate anemia. *Prothrombin time* is increased in vitamin K deficiency.
- *Enteroscopy* uses an extra-long fiberoptic endoscope to visualize and biopsy the upper small intestine. This procedure permits direct examination of intestinal mucosa and collection of a tissue specimen for biopsy. This invasive procedure involves risks, such as perforation, bleeding, and aspiration of gastric contents, but provides valuable diagnostic information about malabsorptive syndromes. Nursing care of the client undergoing an enteroscopy is outlined in Chapter 21.
- *Upper GI series with small bowel follow-through* may be done to evaluate the structures of the upper GI tract. With sprue, the typical "feathery" pattern of barium in the small bowel is lost, and the barium may precipitate and clump. Nursing care of the client undergoing an upper gastrointestinal series with small bowel follow-through is in the Nursing Implications box on page 628.

## Medications

Clients with severe nutritional deficits may require vitamin and mineral supplements, as well as iron and folic acid to correct anemia. Vitamin K may be administered parenterally if the prothrombin time is prolonged. In clients whose disease fails to respond to dietary management, corticosteroids may be ordered to suppress the inflammatory response.

Tropical sprue is treated with a combination of folic acid and tetracycline. This regimen is continued for 1 to 2 months. Nutrient deficiencies are treated as for celiac sprue.

## Dietary Management

The client with celiac sprue is placed on a gluten-free diet. This treatment is generally successful, as long as the client avoids gluten totally. Gluten is so widely used in prepared foods that this may be no easy task. Consultation with a dietitian and detailed dietary instructions are necessary. Clients need to become aware of hidden sources of gluten and to analyze dietary labels. Common sources of gluten and foods to be avoided are indicated in Table 24–11.

The prescribed diet is also high in calories and protein to correct nutrient deficits. Fat content is restricted to minimize steatorrhea. Initially, the diet usually is restricted in lactose as well to compensate for the loss of lactase-containing microvilli. Foods containing lactose may be reintroduced once remission has occurred (Tierney et al., 2001).

## NURSING CARE

Nursing care for the client with sprue focuses on the effects of the disorder on health and nutrition, as well as the client's ability to manage the disease.

### Assessment

- Health history: onset, duration, and severity of symptoms; number and character of stools; history of travel to the Caribbean or southeast Asia; previous teaching related to disorder; current treatment and diet
- Physical examination: vital signs; abdominal shape, contour, bowel sounds; manifestations of malnutrition (e.g., anemia, small stature, muscle wasting, signs of other nutrient deficiencies)

| TABLE 24–11    Dietary Sources of Gluten | | |
|---|---|---|
| **Food Group** | **Contain Gluten** | **May Contain Gluten** |
| Cereals, grains, and grain products | Bread, crackers, cereal, and pasta containing wheat, rye, or barley grain or flour | Seasoned rice and potato mixes |
| Beverages | Malt, Postum, Ovaltine, beers, and ales | Commercial chocolate milk, cocoa, and other beverage mixes, such as instant tea mix, dietary supplements |
| Desserts | Cakes, cookies, and pastries made with wheat, rye, or barley flour | Commercial ice cream and sherbet |
| Meats and other protein sources | | Meat loaf, cold cuts and prepared meats, breaded meats; cheese products; soy protein meat substitutes; commercial egg products |
| Fruits and vegetables | | Commercial seasoned vegetable mixes or vegetables with sauce; canned baked beans; commercial pie fillings |
| Miscellaneous | | Commercial salad dressings and mayonnaise; ketchup and prepared mustard; gravy, white sauce; nondairy creamer; syrups; commercial pickles |

## Nursing Diagnoses and Interventions

Diarrhea and malnutrition are significant problems for the client with sprue and the priority foci for nursing intervention.

### Diarrhea

Steatorrhea and diarrhea typically occur with sprue because fat, water, and other nutrients are poorly absorbed, remaining in the bowel to be eliminated in the stool. Diarrhea can interfere with lifestyle, ADLs, skin integrity, and fluid and electrolyte balance.

- Assess and document the frequency and nature of stools. *Bowel elimination reflects the severity of the disease and efficacy of treatment. With effective treatment, stools become less frequent and more normal in color and appearance.*
- Weigh daily, monitor intake and output, and assess skin turgor and mucous membranes for indications of fluid balance. *Diarrhea increases the risk for hypovolemia and dehydration resulting from excess fluid loss in the stool.*
- Assess and document perianal skin condition. *Frequent defecation can irritate skin and mucous membranes, increasing the risk of breakdown.*
- Promote a liberal fluid intake. *Oral fluids help replace fluid lost through diarrheal stool.*

### Imbalanced Nutrition: Less than Body Requirements

Celiac sprue is a chronic condition. With continuing malabsorption, multiple nutrient deficits may occur, resulting in impaired growth and development, impaired healing, muscle wasting, bone disease, and electrolyte imbalances.

- Maintain accurate dietary intake records. *Assessment of dietary intake provides information about compliance with the prescribed diet as well as the adequacy of nutrient intake.*
- Monitor laboratory results, including hemoglobin and hematocrit, serum electrolytes, total serum protein, and albumin levels. *These studies provide information about nutritional status.*

- Arrange for dietary consultation. Provide for food preferences as allowed. *An individualized diet developed to address the client's food preferences as well as nutrient needs will promote appetite and food intake.*
- Provide the prescribed high-kcal, high-protein, low-fat, gluten-free diet for the client with celiac sprue. Restrict lactose (dairy product) intake as indicated. *Calories and protein are important to replace lost nutrients. Fat restriction helps reduce diarrhea and nutrient loss. Lactose may be restricted during initial treatment, then slowly reintroduced into the diet as the gut heals and its normal structure is restored.*
- Provide parenteral nutrition as ordered if the client is unable to absorb enteral nutrients. *Parenteral nutrition can help reverse nutritional deficits and promote weight gain when symptoms are acute.*
- Administer ordered nutritional supplements. *Nutritional supplements often are necessary to replace losses and restore nutrient levels to normal more rapidly than diet alone can achieve.*
- Include family members, the primary food preparer in particular, in teaching and dietary discussions. *Families can reinforce teaching and help the client maintain required restrictions or kcal intake.*

## Using NANDA, NIC, and NOC

Chart 24–4 shows links between NANDA nursing diagnoses, NIC, and NOC for the client with sprue and other malabsorption disorders.

## Home Care

Although tropical sprue can be treated with antibiotic and folic acid therapy, the client with celiac sprue has a chronic condition that requires continuing dietary management.

Provide a detailed list of foods that contain gluten and need to be eliminated from the diet, as well as foods that are allowed. Teach the client and family how to identify gluten-containing commercial products by reading labels and lists of ingredients. Encourage purchasing and using a gluten-free cookbook.

---

### CHART 24–4 LINKS BETWEEN NANDA, NIC, AND NOC

#### The Client with Malabsorption Syndrome

| NURSING DIAGNOSES | NURSING INTERVENTIONS | NURSING OUTCOMES |
|---|---|---|
| • Imbalanced Nutrition: Less Than Body Requirements | • Nutrition Management<br>• Weight Gain Assistance | • Nutritional Status |
| • Diarrhea | • Diarrhea Management<br>• Fluid Management | • Bowel Elimination<br>• Symptom Severity<br>• Hydration |
| • Deficient Knowledge | • Teaching: Prescribed Diet<br>• Teaching: Disease Process | • Knowledge: Diet<br>• Knowledge: Disease Process |

*Note: Data from Nursing Outcomes Classification (NOC) by M. Johnson & M. Maas (Eds.), 1997, St. Louis: Mosby; Nursing Diagnoses: Definitions & Classification 2001–2002 by North American Nursing Diagnosis Association, 2001, Philadelphia: NANDA; Nursing Interventions Classification (NIC) by J.C. McCloskey & G. M. Bulechek (Eds.), 2000, St. Louis: Mosby. Reprinted by permission.*

If corticosteroids have been prescribed, stress the importance of taking the medication as ordered. Emphasize the need to avoid stopping the medication abruptly and to notify all caregivers that a corticosteroid is part of the client's medication regimen. Instruct to frequently monitor weight. A weight gain of 5 lb (2.3 kg) or more in less than a week usually reflects fluid gain, a possible adverse effect of corticosteroids. Other potential effects include decreased resistance to infection, an impaired inflammatory response, and changes in the metabolism of carbohydrates, proteins, and fats.

## THE CLIENT WITH LACTASE DEFICIENCY

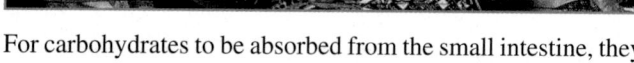

For carbohydrates to be absorbed from the small intestine, they first must be broken down into simple sugars, or monosaccharides. Lactose is the primary carbohydrate in milk and milk products. It is a disaccharide, requiring the enzyme lactase for digestion and absorption. Lactase deficiency can lead to *lactose intolerance* and symptoms of malabsorption.

Lactase deficiency affects up to 90% of Asians and Native Americans and 70% of African Americans. It also is common among Jewish Americans and Hispanics. Less than 25% of Caucasians are affected (Tierney et al., 2001). Lactase deficiency usually is genetic in origin, but also occurs secondarily to celiac sprue, Crohn's disease, and other disorders affecting the mucosa of the small intestine.

Many people with lactase deficiency are asymptomatic. Small to moderate amounts of milk (one to two 8-ounce glasses) of milk may be well tolerated. Symptoms of lactose intolerance include lower abdominal cramping, pain, and diarrhea following milk ingestion. Undigested lactose ferments in the intestine, forming gases that contribute to bloating and flatus. Lactic and fatty acids produced by this fermentation irritate the bowel, leading to increased motility and abdominal cramping. The undigested lactose draws water into the intestine, which contributes to increased motility and diarrhea. The diarrhea associated with lactose intolerance may be explosive.

## COLLABORATIVE CARE

The diagnosis of lactose intolerance usually is based on the history of intolerance to milk and milk products, and a trial of a lactose-free diet. If symptoms resolve when lactose intake is eliminated, the diagnosis of lactose intolerance is confirmed.

The *lactose breath test* is a noninvasive test that may be used to diagnose lactose intolerance. Expired hydrogen gas ($H_2$) is measured following oral administration of 50 g of lactose. If lactose is digested and absorbed normally, then little change occurs in the amount of exhaled $H_2$ from fasting to postlactose administration. With lactose intolerance, exhaled $H_2$ increases following lactose administration as the sugar ferments in the bowel.

For the *lactose tolerance test,* 100 g of lactose solution is orally administered, followed by measurement of blood glu-

cose levels at intervals of 30, 60, and 120 minutes. If lactose is digested and absorbed normally, the blood glucose rises more than 20 mg/dL. The expected blood glucose elevation does not occur in lactose intolerance.

A lactose-free or reduced lactose diet relieves the manifestations of the disorder. Some clients require total elimination of milk and milk products from the diet. Many can tolerate limited amounts of lactose. Milk pretreated with lactase is readily available. Nonprescription lactase enzyme preparations are available to improve milk tolerance. Yogurt containing bacterial lactases may be well tolerated. Calcium supplementation is often recommended, particularly for women on a reduced-lactose or lactose-free diet.

## NURSING CARE

Nursing care for the client with lactose intolerance focuses on providing education and support. Discuss sources of lactose: Milk, ice cream, and cottage cheese are high in lactose; aged cheese and yogurt contain much smaller amounts. Potential hidden sources of lactose include sherbets, desserts made from milk and milk chocolate, sauces and gravies, and cream soups. Suggest a trial of lactase-treated milk or lactase enzyme supplements. Emphasize the importance of obtaining nutrients contained in dairy products from other sources. Proteins may be obtained from meats, eggs, legumes, and grains. Other sources of calcium include sardines, oysters, and salmon, as well as plant sources such as beans, cauliflower, rhubarb, and green leafy vegetables.

## THE CLIENT WITH SHORT BOWEL SYNDROME

Resection of significant portions of the small intestine may result in a condition known as short bowel syndrome. The severity of the disorder depends on the total amount of bowel resected, as well as the portions of bowel removed. Removal of the proximal portions, including the duodenum, jejunum, and proximal ileum, and distal portion of the ileum are associated with more severe malabsorption and symptoms than resection of midportions of the ileum (Braunwald et al., 2001).

Small bowel may be resected due to tumors, infarction of bowel mucosa, incarcerated hernias, Crohn's disease, trauma, and enteropathy resulting from radiation therapy.

Resection of the small intestine affects the absorption of water, nutrients, vitamins, and minerals. Transit time of ingested foods and fluids is reduced, and digestive processes are impaired. The bowel undergoes an adaptive process in which the remaining villi enlarge and lengthen to increase absorptive surface following resection. For many clients, absorption and bowel function returns to preoperative or near-normal levels. Others have continued significant impairment of digestion and absorption, leading to nutrient deficiencies, weight loss, and diarrhea.

## COLLABORATIVE CARE

Laboratory and diagnostic studies are used to evaluate nutrient deficiencies. Total serum proteins and albumin are reduced, as are serum levels of folate, iron, vitamins, minerals, and electrolytes. Anemia and a prolonged prothrombin time (indicative of vitamin K deficiency) may develop.

Management of short bowel syndrome focuses on alleviating symptoms. Clients often simply require frequent, small, high-kcal, high-protein feedings. Multivitamin and mineral supplementation is also frequently necessary. Antidiarrheal medications are used to reduce bowel motility, allowing a greater amount of time for nutrient absorption. Some clients are affected by gastric hypersecretion following bowel resection. For these clients, a proton-pump inhibitor such as omeprazole (Prilosec) may be ordered. Clients with severe manifestations of short bowel syndrome may require total parenteral nutrition.

## NURSING CARE

Nursing care for the client with short bowel syndrome focuses on the problems of potential fluid volume deficit, malnutrition, and diarrhea.

Fluid losses are generally greatest in the initial periods following surgery, warranting the closest attention at that time. Frequent assessment of vital signs, intake and output, daily weights, skin turgor, and condition of mucous membranes is vital. It is important to remember that the risk also is high when other abnormal fluid losses occur through, for example, fever, increased respiratory rate, draining wounds, or excess perspiration.

Document nutritional status, including weight, anthropometric measurements, laboratory values, and kcal intake. Provide nutritional supplementation with enteral feedings as needed. Maintain central lines and total parenteral nutrition, using aseptic technique.

For diarrhea, document the number and character of stools. Administer antidiarrheal medications as ordered. If the client is lactose intolerant, limit intake of milk and milk products. Provide good skin care of the perianal region to prevent breakdown from frequent bowel movements. Refer to the discussion of nursing care for the client with sprue for other measures for altered nutrition and diarrhea.

The client and family affected by this condition require extensive education. Because there is no way to cure or replace the lost bowel at this time, the client must manage the disorder on a day-to-day basis. Provide instructions about the recommended diet and medication regimen. Emphasize the importance of maintaining an adequate fluid intake, particularly in hot weather or during strenuous exercise. Teach the client to monitor his or her weight frequently and report changes. Include teaching about possible manifestations of dehydration and nutrient deficiencies that should be reported to the physician. Referring the client to a dietitian or counselor can help the person cope with what may be a lifelong problem.

# NEOPLASTIC DISORDERS

Cancer remains the second leading cause of death in the United States, preceded only by heart disease. Although cancer may affect any portion of the digestive tract, the large intestine and rectum are the most common sites. Malignant neoplasms of the lower bowel are the second leading cause of death from cancer (after lung cancer), making this a significant health care concern.

## THE CLIENT WITH POLYPS

A **polyp** is a mass of tissue that arises from the bowel wall and protrudes into the lumen. Polyps may develop in any portion of the bowel, but they occur most often in the sigmoid colon and rectum. They vary considerably in size and may be single or multiple. It is estimated that approximately 30% of people over the age of 50 have polyps. Although most polyps are benign, some have the potential to become malignant.

### PATHOPHYSIOLOGY AND MANIFESTATIONS

Polyps are identified by their structure and tissue type. Most polyps are adenomas, benign epithelial tumors that are considered premalignant lesions. Less than 1% of polyps become malignant; however, virtually all colorectal cancers arise from adenomatous polyps (Braunwald et al., 2001; Porth, 2002).

Adenomatous polyps represent disruption of the normal process of cell proliferation to replace epithelial cells lining the intestine. Cells are constantly being reproduced to replace those shed as feces moves through the colon. Disruption of the normal process of cell division and maturation can lead to formation of a polyp composed of tightly packed epithelial cells. The cells may appear grossly normal or show signs of dysplasia. Polyps may develop as tubular, villous, or tubulovillous adenomas.

*Tubular adenomas* (also called *pedunculated* polyps) are more common, accounting for about 65% of benign polyps of the large intestine (Porth, 2002). A tubular adenoma is a globe-like structure attached to the intestinal wall by a thin, stalk-like stem (Figure 24–10 ■). The incidence of this type of polyp increases with age, although it occurs in all age groups and in both sexes. Most are small, 1 cm or less in diameter, although they may be as large as 4 to 5 cm. The malignant potential of these polyps seems to be related to their size. One percent of those under 1 cm in diameter are cancerous, whereas 35% of adenomas larger than 2 cm are cancerous (Porth, 2002).

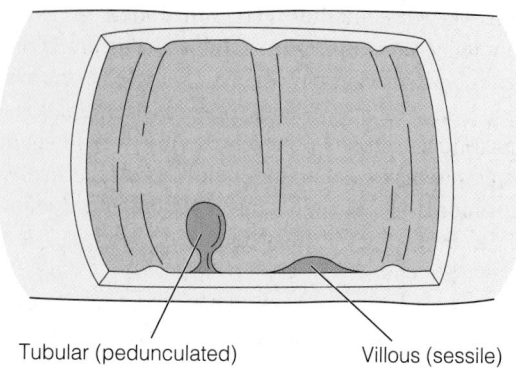

Tubular (pedunculated)          Villous (sessile)

**Figure 24–10** ■ Tubular (or pedumculated) and villous (or sessile) polyps.

*Villous adenomas* (also called *sessile* polyps) have a broad base and an elevated, cauliflower-like surface. They typically develop in the rectosigmoid colon. This type of polyp is often larger than tubular adenomas, usually more than 5 cm. Villous adenomas are less common, accounting for about 10% of colon polyps. They have a higher malignant potential than tubular adenomas, estimated at 25% to 40%. Some adenomatous polyps contain both tubular epithelium and villi and are known as *tubulovillous adenomas*.

Familial polyposis is an uncommon autosomal dominant genetic disorder characterized by hundreds of adenomatous polyps throughout the entire large intestine. Both pedunculated and sessile polyps are seen, usually developing after puberty. Unless treated, the risk of malignancy is almost 100% by age 40 (Braunwald et al., 2001).

Most polyps are asymptomatic, found coincidentally during routine examination or diagnostic testing. Intermittent painless rectal bleeding, bright or dark red, is the most common presenting complaint. A large polyp may cause abdominal cramping, pain, or manifestations of obstruction. Diarrhea and mucous discharge may be associated with a large villous adenoma.

## COLLABORATIVE CARE

The diagnosis of intestinal polyps is generally based on diagnostic studies such as sigmoidoscopy or colonoscopy. A rectal polyp may be palpable on digital examination, but further studies are necessary to determine its size and type, the extent of colon involvement, and to assess for malignancy.

- *Colonoscopy* provides the most reliable diagnosis of polyps, allowing visual inspection of the large intestine, biopsy of masses or lesions, and polypectomy. Nursing care of the client undergoing a colonoscopy is outlined in the Nursing Implications box on page 624.

Once identified, polyps are generally removed because of the risk of malignancy. Pedunculated polyps and small villous lesions may be removed during colonoscopy using an electrocautery snare or hot biopsy forceps passed through the scope. This relatively safe procedure has less than a 2% risk of complications such as perforation or hemorrhage. Large villous adenomas are completely excised and examined histologically for evidence of malignancy. In some cases, the colon segment containing the polyp is resected; a total colectomy with ileorectal anastomosis may be performed for multiple polyps in different anatomic parts of the colon.

Treatment following polypectomy depends on histologic examination of the excised tissue. Because polyps tend to recur, follow-up colonoscopy is recommended in 3 years and then every 5 years if no further polyps are detected. When the polyp is found to be malignant, follow-up care is determined by the tissue type and degree of invasion. See the next section of this chapter.

## NURSING CARE

### Health Promotion

The incidence of intestinal polyps increases with age. They affect men and women equally. It is believed that an adenomatous polyp requires more than 5 years of growth to become significant in size and malignant potential (Braunwald et al., 2001). Advise all clients to have a screening colonoscopy at age 50 and every 5 years thereafter for early detection of polyps.

### Assessment

Polyps are a "silent" disease, with few or no symptoms.

- Health history: rectal bleeding; personal or family history of intestinal polyps or colorectal cancer

### Nursing Diagnoses and Interventions

Nursing care for the client with polyps focuses on education and assisting the client through diagnostic testing and polyp removal. Before and after colonoscopy and polypectomy, provide direct care and teaching about the procedure, expected sensations during the procedure, and anticipated postoperative care. Cathartics are prescribed prior to colonoscopy; cleansing enemas also may be ordered. Observe for evidence of fluid and electrolyte imbalance during preoperative preparation. If enemas are ordered, use normal saline (not tap water) to reduce the risk of electrolyte imbalances. Following polypectomy, observe closely for possible complications such as hemorrhage.

The following nursing diagnoses may be appropriate for the client with polyps.

- *Risk for noncompliance* with recommended screening and follow-up, related to lack of understanding
- *Impaired tissue integrity* related to removal of polyps from bowel
- *Risk for deficient fluid volume* related to bowel preparation

### Home Care

Include the following topics when teaching for home care.

- The significance of polyps and their relationship to colorectal cancer
- The importance of keeping follow-up appointments and undergoing repeat colonoscopy as ordered: at 3 years following polypectomy, then every 5 years unless additional polyps are found; every 6 months for clients with familial polyposis

• Symptoms to report to the physician, such as diarrhea, pain, rectal bleeding, lightheadedness, or other indications of possible blood loss

Discuss the high risk for colorectal cancer with clients with familial polyposis and their families. Include its genetic transmission: Offspring have a 50% risk of inheriting the disorder. Referral to an enterostomal therapist for discussion about colectomy with ileoanal reservoir may help the client with decisions about treatment options.

## THE CLIENT WITH COLORECTAL CANCER

Colorectal cancer, malignancy of the colon or rectum, is the third most common cancer diagnosed in the United States. In the United States, about 148,300 new cases of colorectal cancer were diagnosed in 2002, and over 56,000 people died from this disease (American Cancer Society [ACS], 2002). Earlier diagnosis and improved treatment have improved the survival rate for colorectal cancer. Its incidence, which is nearly equal among men and women, is declining in the United States. Colorectal cancer occurs most frequently after age 50. The incidence continues to rise with increasing age. With early diagnosis and treatment, the 5-year survival rate for colorectal cancer is 90%; however, less than half of colorectal cancers are diagnosed at this early stage. The 5-year survival rate drops to 65% when it has spread locally at the time of diagnosis, and 8% when distant sites are involved (ACS, 2002).

Although the specific cause of colorectal cancer is unknown, a number of risk factors have been identified (Box 24–3). Genetic factors are strongly linked to the risk for colorectal cancer. Up to 25% of people who develop colorectal cancer have a family history of the disease (Braunwald et al., 2001). Persons with familial adenomatous polyposis inevitably will develop colon cancer unless the colon is removed (Tierney et al., 2001). Hereditary nonpolyposis colorectal cancer (also known as Lynch syndrome) is an autosomal dominant disorder that significantly increases the risk for developing colorectal and other cancers. Tumors associated with Lynch syndrome often affect the ascending colon, and tend to occur at an earlier age (Braunwald et al., 2001). Inflammatory bowel disease (ulcerative colitis and Crohn's disease) also increases the risk of colorectal cancer.

Diet plays a role in the development of colorectal cancer. The disease is prevalent in economically prosperous countries where people consume diets high in calories, meat proteins, and fats. This dietary pattern, common in the United States, is thought to increase the population of anaerobic bacteria in the gut. These anaerobes convert bile acids into carcinogens (Braunwald et al., 2001). Diets high in fruits and vegetables, folic acid, and calcium appear to reduce the risk of colorectal cancer. Cereal fiber, once thought to reduce colorectal cancer risk, does not now appear to play a role either way in its development. Other factors that may reduce the risk of colorectal cancer include use of aspirin and other NSAIDs and hormone replacement therapy in post menopausal women (Tierney et al., 2001).

## PATHOPHYSIOLOGY

Nearly all colorectal malignancies are adenocarcinomas that begin as adenomatous polyps. Most tumors develop in the rectum and sigmoid colon, although any portion of the colon may be affected (Figure 24–11 ■). The tumor typically grows undetected, producing few symptoms. By the time symptoms occur, the disease may have spread into deeper layers of the bowel tissue and adjacent organs. Colorectal cancer spreads by direct extension to involve the entire bowel circumference, the submucosa, and outer bowel wall layers. Neighboring structures such as the liver, greater curvature of the stomach, duodenum, small intestine, pancreas, spleen, genitourinary tract, and abdominal wall also may be involved by direct extension. Metastasis to regional lymph nodes is the most common form of tumor spread. This is not always an orderly process; distal nodes may contain cancer cells while regional nodes remain normal. Cancerous cells from the primary tumor may also spread by way of the lymphatic system or circulatory system to secondary sites such as the liver, lungs, brain, bones, and kidneys. "Seeding" of the tumor to other areas of the peritoneal cavity can occur when the tumor extends through the serosa or during surgical resection.

| BOX 24–3 | ■ Risk Factors for Colorectal Cancer |
| --- | --- |

- Age over 50 years
- Polyps of the colon and/or rectum
- Family history of colorectal cancer
- Inflammatory bowel disease
- Exposure to radiation
- Diet: high animal fat and kcal intake

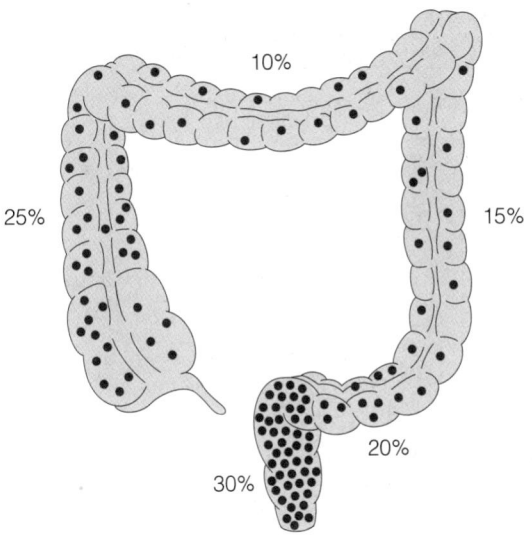

**Figure 24–11** ■ The distribution and frequency of cancer of the colon and rectum.

## MANIFESTATIONS AND COMPLICATIONS

As noted earlier, bowel cancer often produces no symptoms until it is advanced. Because it grows slowly, 5 to 15 years of growth may occur before symptoms develop. The manifestations depend on its location, type and extent, and complications. Bleeding is often the initial manifestation that prompts clients to seek medical care. Other common early symptoms include a change in bowel habits, either diarrhea or constipation. Pain, anorexia, and weight loss are characteristic in advanced disease. A palpable abdominal or rectal mass may be present. Occasionally the client presents with anemia from occult bleeding.

The primary complications associated with colorectal cancer: (1) bowel obstruction due to narrowing of the bowel lumen by the lesion; (2) perforation of the bowel wall by the tumor, allowing contamination of the peritoneal cavity by bowel contents; and (3) direct extension of the tumor to involve adjacent organs.

Most recurrences of colorectal cancer after tumor removal occur within the first 4 years. The size of the primary tumor does not necessarily relate to long-term survival. The number of involved lymph nodes, penetration of the tumor through the bowel wall, and tumor adherence to adjacent organs are better predictors of the prognosis for the disease (Braunwald et al., 2001).

## COLLABORATIVE CARE

The focus of collaborative care for colorectal cancer is early detection and intervention. Colorectal cancer is always treated by surgical resection, with chemotherapy and radiation therapy used as adjuncts.

### Screening

The American Cancer Society recommends annual digital rectal examination beginning at age 40, with annual fecal occult blood testing beginning at age 50. Because colorectal tumors bleed intermittently, several fecal occult blood specimens typically are collected over a period of several days. Debate exists regarding recommendations for periodic (every 3 to 5 years) flexible sigmoidoscopy or colonoscopy for everyone over age 50.

### Diagnostic Tests

- *CBC* is ordered to detect anemia resulting from chronic blood loss and tumor growth.
- *Fecal occult blood* (by guaiac or hemoccult testing) is ordered to detect blood in the feces, because nearly all colorectal cancers bleed intermittently.
- *Carcinoembryonic antigen (CEA)* is a tumor marker that can be detected in the blood of clients with colorectal cancer. CEA levels are used to estimate prognosis, monitor treatment, and detect cancer recurrence. Because this test is not specific for colorectal cancer and does not always detect early-stage cancer, it is not used as a screening measure (Malarkey & McMorrow, 2000).
- *Sigmoidoscopy* or *colonoscopy* is the primary diagnostic test used to detect and visualize tumors. It also allows tissue collection for biopsy. While flexible sigmoidoscopy can detect 50% to 65% of colorectal cancers, many clinicians recommend colonoscopy, endoscopic examination of the entire colon. Tumors typically appear as raised, red, centrally ulcerated, bleeding lesions. (See the boxes on pages 619 and 624 for nursing implications for these tests.)
- *Chest X-ray* is obtained to detect tumor metastasis to the lung.
- *Computed tomography (CT) scan, magnetic resonance imaging (MRI),* or *ultrasonic examination* may be used to assess tumor depth and involvement of other organs by direct extension or metastasis.
- *Tissue biopsy* is obtained at the time of endoscopy to confirm cancerous tissue and evaluate cell differentiation (see Chapter 10). Current staging methods primarily use the TNM system, as outlined in Table 24–12.

---

**TABLE 24–12    The TNM Classification for Colorectal Cancer**

| Stage | Primary Tumor (T) | Regional Lymph Nodes (N) | Distant Metastasis (M) |
|-------|-------------------|--------------------------|------------------------|
|  | TX—Primary tumor cannot be assessed<br>TO—No evidence of primary tumor | NX—Regional lymph node cannot be assessed | MX—Presence of distant metastasis cannot be assessed |
| Stage 0 | Tis—Carcinoma in situ | NO—No regional lymph node metastasis | MO—No distant metastasis |
| Stage I | T1—Tumor invades submucosa<br>T2—Tumor invades muscularis propria |  |  |
| Stage II | T3—Tumor invades through muscularis propria into subserosa or into non-peritonealized pericolic or perirectal tissues<br>T4—Tumor perforates visceral peritoneum or directly invades other organs or structures |  |  |
| Stage III | Any T | N1—Metastasis in 1 to 3 pericolic or perirectal lymph nodes<br>N2—Metastasis in 4 or more pericolic or perirectal lymph nodes<br>N3—Metastasis in any lymph node along course of a major named vascular trunk |  |
| Stage IV | Any T | Any N | M1—Distant metastasis |

## Surgery

Surgical resection of the tumor, adjacent colon, and regional lymph nodes is the treatment of choice for colorectal cancer. Options for surgical treatment vary from destruction of the tumor by laser photocoagulation performed during endoscopy to abdominoperineal resection with permanent colostomy. When possible, the anal sphincter is preserved and colostomy avoided.

*Laser photocoagulation* uses a very small, intense beam of light to generate heat in tissues toward which it is directed. The heat generated by the laser beam can be used to destroy small tumors. It is also used for palliative surgery of advanced tumors to remove obstruction. Laser photocoagulation can be performed endoscopically and is useful for clients who cannot tolerate major surgery.

Other surgical treatment options for small, localized tumors include local excision and fulguration. These procedures also may be performed during endoscopy, eliminating the need for abdominal surgery. Local excision may be used to remove a disk of rectum containing the tumor in clients with a small, well-differentiated, mobile polypoid lesion. *Fulguration* or electrocoagulation is used to reduce the size of some large tumors for clients who are poor surgical risks. This procedure requires general anesthesia and may need to be repeated at intervals.

Most clients with colorectal cancer undergo surgical resection of the colon with anastomosis of remaining bowel as a curative procedure. The distribution of regional lymph nodes determines the extent of resection as these may contain metastatic lesions. Most tumors of the ascending, transverse, descending, and sigmoid colon can be resected.

Tumors of the rectum usually are treated with an abdominoperineal resection in which the sigmoid colon, rectum, and anus are removed through both abdominal and perineal incisions. A permanent sigmoid colostomy is performed to provide for elimination of feces. Nursing care of the client having bowel surgery is outlined in the box below.

## NURSING CARE OF THE CLIENT HAVING BOWEL SURGERY

### PREOPERATIVE NURSING CARE

- Provide routine preoperative care for the surgical client as outlined in Chapter 7. ⊝⊃
- Arrange for consultation with enterostomal therapy (ET) specialist if appropriate. *The ET nurse is trained to identify and mark an appropriate stoma location, taking into consideration the level of ostomy, skinfolds, and the client's clothing preferences. Initial ostomy care teaching also is provided by the ET nurse during the preoperative visit.*
- Insert a nasogastric tube if ordered. *Although it is often inserted in the surgical suite just prior to surgery, the nasogastric tube may be placed preoperatively to remove secretions and empty stomach contents.*
- Perform bowel preparation procedures as ordered. *Oral and parenteral antibiotics as well as cathartics and enemas may be prescribed preoperatively to clean the bowel and reduce the risk of peritoneal contamination by bowel contents during surgery.*

### POSTOPERATIVE NURSING CARE

- Provide routine care for the surgical client (Chapter 7).
- Monitor bowel sounds and degree of abdominal distention. *Surgical manipulation of the bowel disrupts peristalsis, resulting in an initial ileus. Bowel sounds and the passage of flatus indicate a return of peristalsis.*
- Assess the position and patency of the nasogastric tube, connecting it to low suction. If the tube becomes clogged, gently irrigate with sterile normal saline. *A nasogastric or gastrostomy tube is used postoperatively to provide gastrointestinal decompression and facilitate healing of the anastomosis. Ensuring its patency is important for comfort and healing.*
- Assess color, amount, and odor of drainage from surgical drains and the colostomy (if present), noting any changes or the presence of clots or bright bleeding. *Initial drainage may be bright red and then become dark and finally clear or greenish yellow over the first 2 to 3 days. A change in the color, amount or odor of the drainage may indicate a complication such as hemorrhage, intestinal obstruction, or infection.*
- Alert all personnel caring for the client with an abdominoperineal resection to avoid rectal temperatures, suppositories, or other rectal procedures. *These procedures could disrupt the anal suture line, causing bleeding, infection, or impaired healing.*
- Maintain intravenous fluids while nasogastric suction is in place. *The client on nasogastric suction is unable to take oral food and fluids and, moreover, is losing electrolyte-rich fluid through the nasogastric tube. If replacement fluid and electrolytes are not maintained, the client is at risk for dehydration; sodium, potassium, and chloride imbalance; and metabolic alkalosis.*
- Provide antacids, histamine$_2$-receptor antagonists, and antibiotic therapy as ordered. *The above medications may be ordered for the postoperative client, depending on the procedure performed. Antibiotic therapy is a common measure to prevent infection resulting from contamination of the abdominal cavity with gastric contents.*
- Resume oral food and fluids as ordered. Initial feedings may be clear liquids, progressing to full liquids, and then frequent small feedings of regular foods. Monitor bowel sounds and monitor for abdominal distention frequently during this period. *Oral feedings are reintroduced slowly to minimize abdominal distention and trauma to the suture lines.*
- Begin discharge planning and teaching. Consult with a dietitian for instructions and menu planning; reinforce teaching. Teach about potential postoperative complications, such as abdominal abscess, or bowel obstruction, their signs and symptoms, and preventive measures.

## Colostomies

Surgical resection of the bowel may be accompanied by a colostomy for diversion of fecal contents. A **colostomy** is an ostomy made in the colon. It may be created if the bowel is obstructed by the tumor, as a temporary measure to promote healing of anastomoses, or as a permanent means of fecal evacuation when the distal colon and rectum are removed. Colostomies take the name of the portion of the colon from which they are formed: ascending colostomy, transverse colostomy, descending colostomy, and sigmoid colostomy (Figure 24–12 ■).

A *sigmoid colostomy* is the most common permanent colostomy performed, particularly for cancer of the rectum. It is usually created during an abdominoperineal resection. This procedure involves the removal of the sigmoid colon, rectum, and anus through abdominal and perineal incisions. The anal canal is closed, and a stoma formed from the proximal sigmoid colon. The stoma usually is located on the lower left quadrant of the abdomen.

When a *double-barrel colostomy* is performed, two separate stomas are created (Figure 24–13 ■). The distal colon is not removed, but bypassed. The proximal stoma, which is functional, diverts feces to the abdominal wall. The distal stoma, also called the mucus fistula, expels mucus from the distal colon. It may be pouched or dressed with a 4 × 4 gauge dressing. A double-barrel colostomy may be created for cases of trauma, tumor, or inflammation, and it may be temporary or permanent.

An emergency procedure used to relieve an intestinal obstruction or perforation is called a *transverse loop colostomy*. During this procedure, a loop of the transverse colon is brought out from the abdominal wall and suspended over a plastic rod or bridge, which prevents the loop from slipping back into the abdominal cavity. The loop stoma may be opened at the time of surgery or a few days later at the client's bedside. The bridge may be removed in 1 to 2 weeks. Transverse loop colostomies are typically temporary.

In a *Hartmann procedure,* a common temporary colostomy procedure, the distal portion of the colon is left in place and is oversewn for closure. A temporary colostomy may be done to

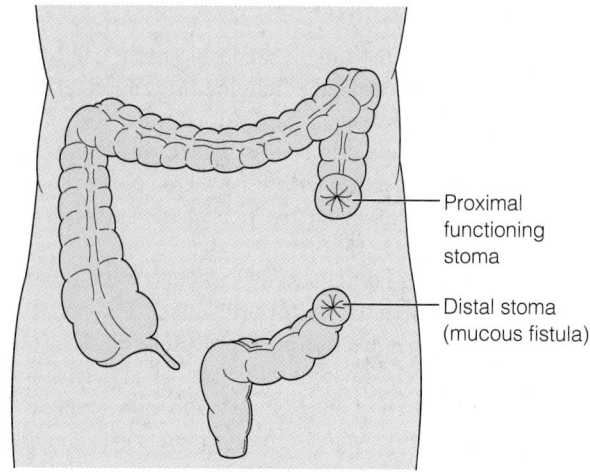

**Figure 24–13 ■** A double-barrel colostomy. The proximal stoma is the functioning stoma; the distal stoma expels mucus from the distal colon.

allow bowel rest or healing, such as following tumor resection or inflammation of the bowel. It also may be created following traumatic injury to the colon, such as a gunshot wound. Anastomosis of the severed portions of the colon is delayed because bacterial colonization of the colon would prevent proper healing of the anastomosis. About 3 to 6 months following a temporary colostomy, the colostomy is closed and the colon is reconnected. Clients with temporary colostomies require the same care as clients with permanent colostomies. See the Nursing Care box on page 673.

## Radiation Therapy

While radiation therapy is not used as a primary treatment for colon cancer, it is used along with surgical resection for treating rectal tumors. Small rectal cancers may be treated with intracavitary, external, or implantation radiation. Rectal cancer has a high rate of regional recurrence following complete surgical resection, particularly when the tumor has invaded tissues outside the bowel wall or regional lymph nodes. Pre- or postoperative radiation therapy reduces the recurrence of pelvic tumors, although the effect of radiation therapy on long-term survival is less clear. Radiation therapy also is used preoperatively to shrink large rectal tumors enough to permit surgical removal of the tumor (Braunwald et al., 2001).

## Chemotherapy

Chemotherapeutic agents, such as intravenous fluorouracil (5-FU) and folinic acid (leucovorin), are also used postoperatively as adjunctive therapy for colorectal cancer. When combined with radiation therapy, chemotherapy reduces the rate of tumor recurrence and prolongs survival for clients with stage II and stage III rectal tumors. The benefit for colon cancers is less clear, but chemotherapy may be used to reduce its spread to the liver and prevent recurrence. Irinotecan (CPT-11) or oxaliplatin also may be used in chemotherapy regimens for colorectal cancer. Further discussion about chemotherapy and nursing implications is included in Chapter 10. ↩

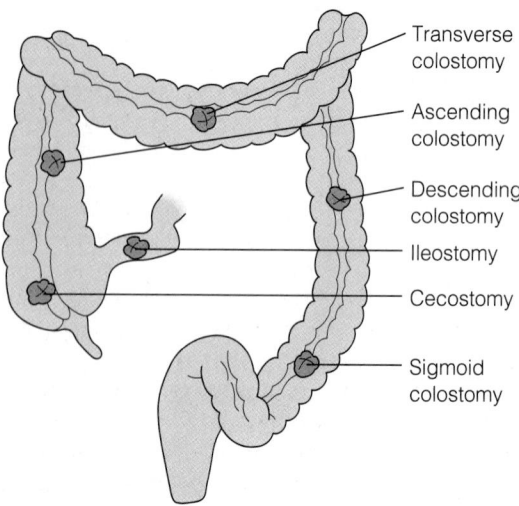

Transverse colostomy
Ascending colostomy
Descending colostomy
Ileostomy
Cecostomy
Sigmoid colostomy

**Figure 24–12 ■** Various ostomy levels and sites.

Proximal functioning stoma
Distal stoma (mucous fistula)

## NURSING CARE OF THE CLIENT WITH A COLOSTOMY

- Assess the location of the stoma and the type of colostomy performed. *Stoma location is an indicator of the section of bowel in which it is located and a predictor of the type of fecal drainage to expect.*
- Assess stoma appearance and surrounding skin condition frequently (see the box page 656). *Assessment of stoma and skin condition is particularly important in the early postoperative period, when complications are most likely to occur and most treatable.*
- Position a collection bag or drainable pouch over the stoma. *Initial drainage may contain more mucus and serosanguineous fluid than fecal material. As the bowel starts to resume function, drainage becomes fecal in nature. The consistency of drainage depends on the stoma location in the bowel.*
- If ordered, irrigate the colostomy, instilling water into the colon similar to an enema procedure. *The water stimulates the colon to empty.*
- When a colostomy irrigation is ordered for a client with a double-barrel or loop colostomy, irrigate the proximal stoma. Digital assessment of the bowel direction from the stoma can assist in determining which is the proximal stoma. *The distal bowel carries no fecal contents and does not need irrigation. It may be irrigated for cleansing just prior to reanastomosis.*
- Empty a drainable pouch or replace the colostomy bag as needed or when it is no more than one-third full. *If the pouch is allowed to overfill, its weight may impair the seal and cause leakage.*
- Provide stomal and skin care for the client with a colostomy as for the client with an ileostomy (see the box on page 656). *Good skin and stoma care is important to maintain skin integrity and function as the first line of defense against infection.*
- Use caulking agents, such as Stomahesive or karaya paste, and a skin barrier wafer as needed to maintain a secure ostomy pouch. This may be particularly important for the client with a loop colostomy. *The main challenge for a client with a transverse loop colostomy is to maintain a secure ostomy pouch over the plastic bridge.*
- A small needle hole high on the colostomy pouch will allow flatus to escape. This hole may be closed with a Band-Aid and opened only while the client is in the bathroom for odor control. *Ostomy bags may "balloon" out, disrupting the skin seal, if excess gas collects.*

### CLIENT AND FAMILY TEACHING

- Prior to discharge, provide written, verbal, and psychomotor instruction on colostomy care, pouch management, skin care, and irrigation for the client. *Whether the colostomy is temporary or permanent, the client will be responsible for its manage-*ment. *Good understanding of procedures and care enhances the ability to provide self-care, as well as self-esteem and control.*
- Allow ample time for the client (and family, if necessary) to practice changing the pouch, either on the client or a model. *Practice of psychomotor skills improves learning and confidence.*
- If an abdominoperineal resection has been performed, emphasize the importance of using no rectal suppositories, rectal temperatures, or enemas. Suggest that the client carry medical identification or a MedicAlert tag or bracelet. *These measures are important to prevent trauma to the tissues when the rectum has been removed.*
- The diet for a client with a colostomy is individualized and may require no alteration from that consumed preoperatively. Dietary teaching should, however, include information on foods that cause stool odor and gas and foods that thicken and loosen stools. Foods that cause these effects on ostomy output are listed below.

#### Foods That Increase Stool Odor

- Asparagus
- Beans
- Cabbage
- Eggs
- Fish
- Garlic
- Onions
- Some spices

#### Foods That Increase Intestinal Gas

- Beer
- Broccoli
- Brussels sprouts
- Cabbage
- Carbonated drinks
- Cauliflower
- Corn
- Cucumbers
- Dairy products
- Dried beans
- Peas
- Radishes
- Spinach

#### Foods That Thicken Stools

- Applesauce
- Bananas
- Bread
- Cheese
- Yogurt
- Pasta
- Pretzels
- Rice
- Tapioca
- Creamy peanut butter

#### Foods That Loosen Stools

- Chocolate
- Dried beans
- Fried foods
- Greasy foods
- Highly spiced foods
- Leafy green vegetables
- Raw fruits and juices
- Raw vegetables

#### Foods That Color Stools

- Beets
- Red gelatin

## NURSING CARE

### Health Promotion

Primary prevention of colorectal cancer is a significant nursing care issue. Teach clients about dietary recommendations provided by the American Cancer Society for the prevention of colorectal cancer. These recommendations include decreasing the amount of fat, refined sugar, and red meats in the diet while increasing intake of dietary fiber. Foods that contain high amounts of fiber include raw fruits and vegetables, legumes, and whole-grain products.

Stress the importance of regular health examinations, including digital rectal exams. Discuss recommendations for regular hemoccult testing of stool after age 40. Include the importance of seeking medical treatment if blood is noted in or on the stool. Teach clients the warning signs for cancer, including those specific to bowel cancer, such as a change in bowel habits.

## Assessment

- Health history: usual bowel patterns and any recent changes; weight loss, fatigue, decreased activity tolerance; presence of blood in the stool; pain with defecation, abdominal discomfort, perineal pain; usual diet; family history of colon cancer, other specific risk factors such as inflammatory bowel disease or colon polyps
- Physical examination: general appearance; weight; abdominal shape, contour; bowel sounds, abdominal tenderness; stool hemoccult or guaiac.

## Nursing Diagnoses and Interventions

In planning and implementing care, consider both physical care needs and emotional response to the diagnosis. Because colorectal cancer is often advanced at the time of diagnosis, the prognosis, even with treatment, may be poor. Denial and anger are common. Extensive abdominal surgery and potentially a colostomy may be necessary, and the effects of chemotherapy and radiation therapy can leave the client fatigued and discouraged.

**PRACTICE ALERT** *If an abdominoperineal resection has been performed, alert all care personnel to avoid rectal temperatures, suppositories, or other procedures that could damage sutures.* ■

Nursing care includes providing emotional support, teaching, and direct care before and after diagnostic procedures and surgery and during adjunctive treatments. Priority nursing diagnoses include *Pain, Imbalanced nutrition,* and *Anticipatory grieving. Risk for sexual dysfunction* should be considered as a priority diagnosis if a colostomy has been created.

### Pain

The client with colorectal cancer may experience pain related to preparatory procedures, diagnostic examinations, and surgery. Following an abdominoperineal resection, "phantom" rectal pain related to severing nerves during the wide excision of the rectum may develop. Finally, the primary tumor itself and, potentially, metastatic tumors may impinge on nerves and other organs, causing pain. In the early postoperative period, an epidural infusion or patient-controlled analgesia (PCA) often is used to manage pain. PCA, routine administration of ordered analgesics, or a continuous analgesia delivery (CAD) system also may be used for pain management when the tumor is far enough advanced to preclude surgical resection. See Chapter 4 for more information on caring for clients with pain. ⚭

- Assess frequently for adequate pain relief. Use subjective and objective information, including the location, intensity, and character of the pain, as well as nonverbal signs, such as grimacing; muscle tension; apparent dozing; changes in pulse or blood pressure; rapid, shallow respirations. *The client may assume that pain is to be expected or tolerated or may fear becoming addicted to analgesic medications. Careful questioning and assessment can provide accurate information about pain status, allowing better control of discomfort.*

- Ask client to rate pain using a pain scale. Document the level of pain. *Pain is a subjective experience. Clients perceive and respond to pain differently. Religion and ethnic background may affect the response to pain.*
- Assess analgesic effectiveness 30 minutes after administration. Monitor for pain relief and adverse effects. *The method of delivery, dosage, or medication itself may need to be adjusted to provide adequate pain relief.*
- Assess the incision for inflammation or swelling; assess drainage catheters and tubes for patency. *Poorly controlled pain or pain that changes may be related to organ distention from an obstructed nasogastric tube, urinary catheter, or wound drain, or may indicate an infection.*
- Assess the abdomen for distention, tenderness, and bowel sounds. *Intra-abdominal bleeding, peritonitis, or paralytic ileus can cause pain that may be confused with incisional pain.*
- Administer analgesia prior to an activity or procedure. *Adequate pain relief reduces muscle tension, allowing for more comfortable participation in activities.*
- Assist with adjunctive relief measures, such as positioning, diversional activities, management of environmental stimuli, guided imagery, and teaching relaxation techniques. *These measures enhance the effects of analgesia by reducing muscle tension.*
- Splint incision with a pillow, and teach the client how to self-splint when coughing and deep breathing, *to prevent respiratory complications related to fear of pain.*

### Imbalanced Nutrition: Less Than Body Requirements

Bowel preparation for diagnostic procedures and surgery, surgery, radiation therapy, and chemotherapy place the client with colorectal cancer at risk for nutritional deficiencies. Fluid and electrolyte replacement is provided following surgery, along with possible total parenteral nutrition (see Chapter 20). ⚭ Adequate kcal and nutrient intake is necessary for healing after surgery. Additionally, if the tumor is advanced, metabolic needs may be increased and the appetite decreased.

- Assess nutritional status, using data such as height and weight, skinfold measurements, body mass index (BMI) calculation (see Chapter 20), and laboratory data including serum albumin level. Refer to dietitian or nutritionist for dietary management. *The client who is malnourished before beginning aggressive cancer treatment requires more vigorous nutrition management to promote healing.*
- Assess readiness for resumption of oral intake after surgery or procedures using data such as statements of hunger, presence of bowel sounds, passage of flatus, and minimal abdominal distention. *Manipulation of the bowel interrupts peristalsis of the GI tract. It is important to ensure that peristalsis has resumed prior to resumption of oral intake.*
- Monitor and document food and fluid intake. *Documentation helps determine the adequacy of kilocalories and other nutrient intake.*
- Weigh daily. *Weight fluctuation may indicate adequate or inadequate dietary intake.*

- Maintain total parenteral nutrition and central intravenous lines as ordered. *Parenteral nutrition prevents tissue catabolism and promotes healing when food intake is disrupted for more than 2 to 3 days.*
- When oral intake resumes, help the client develop a meal plan that incorporates food preferences and considers the client's schedule and environment. *Consideration of likes, dislikes, and circumstances in meal planning promotes an adequate intake.*

## Anticipatory Grieving

When a bowel resection is performed for colorectal cancer, the client needs to adjust to the loss of a major body part as well as to the diagnosis of cancer. Even when the prognosis for recovery is good, many people perceive cancer as fatal. Supporting the client and family during the initial stages of grieving can improve physical recovery as well as psychologic coping and eventual adaptation.

- Work to develop a trusting relationship with the client and family. *This increases the nurse's effectiveness in helping them work through the grieving process.*
- Listen actively, encouraging the client and family to express their fears and concerns. Assist to identify strengths, past experiences, and support systems.
  a. Demonstrate respect for cultural, spiritual, and religious values and beliefs; encourage use of these resources to cope with losses.
  b. Encourage discussion of the potential impact of loss on individual family members, family structure, and family function. Assist family members to share concerns with one another.
  c. Refer to cancer support groups, social services, or counseling as appropriate.
  *These resources can be used throughout the grieving process.*

## Risk for Sexual Dysfunction

Colorectal cancer and ostomy surgery increase the risk for sexual dysfunction, defined as a change in sexual function so that it becomes unsatisfying, unrewarding, inadequate (NANDA, 2001). Physical factors that can lead to sexual dysfunction include disruption of nerves and blood vessels that supply the genitals, radiation therapy, chemotherapy, and other medications prescribed after surgery.

Psychologically, an *ostomate* (client with an ostomy), experiences an altered body image and may develop low self-esteem. The client may feel undesirable and fear rejection. He or she may be concerned about odors or pouch leakage during sexual activity. This emotional stress can also contribute to sexual dysfunction. Self-image changes following an ostomy are addressed in the Nursing Research box below.

- Provide opportunities for the client and family to express feelings about the cancer diagnosis, ostomy, and effects of other treatments. *Encouraging verbalization of feelings about the*

## Nursing Research

### Evidence-Based Practice for Ostomies

Nurses often identify Disturbed body image as a nursing diagnosis for clients who have ostomy surgery. In a prospective study, researchers studied body image changes in clients with cancer who had an ostomy created (Jenks et al., 1997).

All study participants had primary bowel or bladder cancer and required a temporary or permanent ostomy. The majority of the participants had a permanent incontinent ostomy created. In addition, most participants were treated with chemotherapy, radiation therapy, or a combination of the two. Both quantitative and qualitative measures were used to assess participants' body image preoperatively and at 1 and 6 months postoperatively.

Body image scores were lowest in the preoperative measurement, improving postoperatively and achieving the highest scores at the 6-month measurement. Qualitative data supported cancer and its associated threat of death as the predominant concern of study subjects. At 6 months, at least some participants demonstrated reintegration of body image through qualitative statements.

### IMPLICATIONS FOR NURSING

Clients undergoing ostomy surgery for cancer may be more concerned about the effect of the cancer on their lives than the effect of the ostomy. Adaptation to a life-threatening disease and survival are more critical issues for the client and deserve higher priority for nursing care focus. As the threat of the cancer diagnosis is reduced, strategies to improve and reintegrate body image will be more effective. Nurses need to acknowledge and accept the client's feelings and behavior toward the ostomy in the initial postoperative period. Progressive involvement in stoma care is important, as is preventing major leakage accidents. Education is a key strategy to promote body image; as the client acquires new skills, self-concept is enhanced.

### Critical Thinking in Client Care

1. It is important for nurses to show acceptance of the client and the ostomy in the initial postoperative period. What behaviors by the nurse will demonstrate acceptance?
2. This study suggested that the client's overriding concern with the cancer diagnosis affected body image in the preoperative period. How might this concern also affect preoperative teaching? What can the nurse do to improve learning during this stressful period?
3. How might the results of a study such as this differ if the study participants were undergoing ostomies to treat inflammatory bowel disease such as ulcerative colitis?

*Note. From "The Influence of Ostomy Surgery on Body Image in Patients with Cancer" by J. M. Jenks, K. H. Morin, & N. Tomaselli, November 1997, Applied Nursing Research, 10(4), 174–180.*

*diagnosis, ostomy, and treatments provides an opportunity to validate that feelings of anger and depression are normal responses to the diagnosis and change in body function.*

- Provide consistent colostomy care. *An accepting attitude and consistent care that provides a secure appliance and controls odor and leakage instills a sense of confidence in the client.*
- Encourage expression of sexual concerns. Provide privacy and caregivers who have established trust with the client and family and are comfortable in discussions about sexual concerns. *Sexuality is a very private concern to most people. The client and family are not likely to express their concerns openly unless trust has been established.*
- Reassure the client and significant other that the effect of physical illness and prescribed interventions on sexuality usually is temporary. *The client and partner may misinterpret an initial decrease in libido as evidence that sexual activity will not be possible or resume following recovery.*
- Refer the client and partner to social services or a family counselor for further interventions. *Clients are often discharged from acute care settings well before concerns about sexual activity surface. Ongoing counseling provides a continuing resource.*
- Arrange for a visit from a member of the United Ostomy Association. *People who are living and coping with an ostomy can provide information and support, helping the new ostomate overcome feelings of isolation and rejection.*

## Using NANDA, NIC, and NOC

Chart 24–5 shows links between NANDA nursing diagnoses, NIC, and NOC when caring for the client with colorectal cancer.

## Home Care

During the diagnostic and preoperative periods, provide instruction about the following topics.

- Tests to be performed and preparatory procedures, including dietary restrictions, laxatives, enemas, and food and fluid restrictions just prior to the procedure
- Recommended postprocedure care and potential adverse effects to report
- Preoperative care, such as intestinal preparation and food and fluid restrictions

If a colostomy is planned, refer to an enterostomal therapist for stoma placement and initial teaching.

Once treatment has been initiated, include the following topics (as appropriate) in teaching for home care.

- Pain management
- Skin care and management of potential adverse effects of radiation therapy and/or chemotherapy (Refer to Chapter 10 for further discussion of teaching needs related to these therapies.) ⃝
- Incision and ostomy care
- Recommended diet
- Follow-up appointments and care

If the tumor is inoperable or a cure is not anticipated, provide information about pain and symptom management. Discuss the hospice philosophy and available services. Provide a referral to a local hospice or home health department.

---

### CHART 24–5  NANDA, NIC, AND NOC LINKAGES

**The Client with Colorectal Cancer**

| NURSING DIAGNOSES | NURSING INTERVENTIONS | NURSING OUTCOMES |
|---|---|---|
| • Pain | • Pain Management<br>• Patient-Controlled Analgesia (PCA) Assistance | • Comfort Level<br>• Pain Control<br>• Pain: Disruptive Effects |
| • Ineffective Health Maintenance | • Ostomy Care<br>• Teaching: Procedure/Treatment | • Bowel Elimination<br>• Self-Care: Toileting |
| • Imbalanced Nutrition: Less Than Body Requirements | • Nutrition Management<br>• Total Parenteral Nutrition (TPN) Administration | • Nutritional Status<br>• Nutritional Status: Nutrient Intake |
| • Anticipatory Grieving | • Anticipatory Guidance<br>• Family Support<br>• Support System Enhancement | • Coping<br>• Grief Resolution<br>• Psychosocial Adjustment: Life Change |
| • Risk for Sexual Dysfunction | • Body Image Enhancement<br>• Sexual Counseling | • Body Image<br>• Self-Esteem |

*Note: Data from Nursing Outcomes Classification (NOC) by M. Johnson & M. Maas (Eds.), 1997, St. Louis: Mosby; Nursing Diagnoses: Definitions & Classification 2001–2002 by North American Nursing Diagnosis Association, 2001, Philadelphia: NANDA; Nursing Interventions Classification (NIC) by J.C. McCloskey & G. M. Bulechek (Eds.), 2000, St. Louis: Mosby. Reprinted by permission.*

## Nursing Care Plan
## A Client with Colorectal Cancer

William Cunningham is a 65-year-old retired railroad employee, husband, and father of three grown children. For the past 3 months, Mr. Cunningham has noticed small amounts of blood in his stools and occasional mucus. He has a sensation of pressure in the rectum, and notices that his stools are smaller in diameter, about the size of a pencil. After palpating a mass on digital examination of the rectum, the physician orders a colonoscopy. A large sessile lesion is found in the rectum and biopsied. The pathology report shows the lesion to be adenocarcinoma. Mr. Cunningham is scheduled for an abdominoperineal resection and sigmoid colostomy.

### ASSESSMENT

Madonna Hart, RN, completes the admission assessment. Mr. Cunningham states that his bowel habits have recently changed, but denies pain or other symptoms. Physical assessment findings include T 98.4 F (36.9° C), P 82, R 18, and BP 118/78. He is 70 inches (178 cm) tall and weighs 185 lb (84 kg). Laboratory findings are normal except for the previous pathology report of adenocarcinoma of rectal lesion.

Mr. Cunningham states, "I really don't want a colostomy, but if that is what it takes to get rid of this, I'm ready to get it over with."

### DIAGNOSIS

- *Pain* related to surgical intervention
- *Risk for impaired skin integrity (peristomal)* related to fecal drainage and pouch adhesive
- *Risk for constipation/diarrhea* related to effects of surgery on bowel function
- *Risk for disturbed body image* related to colostomy
- *Risk for sexual dysfunction* related to wide rectal incision, radiation therapy, and colostomy

### EXPECTED OUTCOMES

- Report pain within an acceptable range that allows ease of movement and ambulation.

- Perform colostomy care using correct technique.
- Demonstrate willingness to discuss changes in sexual function.
- Wear clothing to enhance physical and emotional self-esteem.

### PLANNING AND IMPLEMENTATION

- Provide analgesia as ordered, evaluating its effectiveness.
- Discuss foods that cause odor and gas.
- Teach colostomy care.
- Maintain consistent nursing personnel assignment to facilitate trust.
- Refer to the local United Ostomy Association.
- Provide a list of local medical supply companies for ostomy supplies.
- Provide for privacy when teaching and discussing concerns about ostomy.

### EVALUATION

On discharge, Mr. Cunningham is able to empty and rinse out his colostomy pouch. He is changing the pouch and caring for surrounding skin appropriately. Ms. Hart has given him verbal and written instructions on colostomy care. He verbalizes understanding of phantom rectal pain, and the importance of avoiding rectal temperatures and rectal suppositories. He expresses an understanding of the need to avoid heavy lifting, and the importance of follow-up care. Ms. Hart has referred Mr. Cunningham to a home health agency in his community for further questions and follow-up care.

### Critical Thinking in the Nursing Process

1. What is the cause of phantom rectal pain?
2. Why is it important to discuss dietary concerns with a client with a colostomy, especially odor- and gas-forming foods?
3. Outline a plan to teach Mr. Cunningham how to irrigate a colostomy.
4. Develop a care plan for Mr. Cunningham for the nursing diagnosis, *Disturbed body image.*

See Evaluating Your Response in Appendix C.

# STRUCTURAL AND OBSTRUCTIVE DISORDERS

Any portion of the intestines may be affected by a structural or obstructive disorder. When the structural defect is in the bowel wall, the intestine may be directly affected, as is the case with diverticula. Defects in the abdominal wall may allow intra-abdominal contents (such as loops of bowel) to protrude, indirectly affecting bowel function. Likewise, obstructions may result from disease of the bowel itself or from obstruction of the bowel lumen by an external force.

## THE CLIENT WITH A HERNIA

A **hernia** is a defect in the abdominal wall that allows abdominal contents to protrude out of the abdominal cavity. Trauma,

surgery, and increased intra-abdominal pressure caused by such conditions as pregnancy, obesity, weight lifting, or tumors are risk factors for hernia formation.

## PATHOPHYSIOLOGY AND MANIFESTATIONS

Hernias are classified by location (Figure 24–14 ■), and may be congenital or acquired. Approximately 80% of hernias occur in the groin (inguinal or femoral hernias). Inguinal hernias often are congenital, caused by improper closure of the tract that develops as the testes descend into the scrotum during fetal development. Groin hernias may be acquired, resulting from weakness of fascia in a region called Hesselbach's area or from dilation of the femoral ring (e.g., during pregnancy and childbirth). Another 10% are ventral or incisional hernias of the

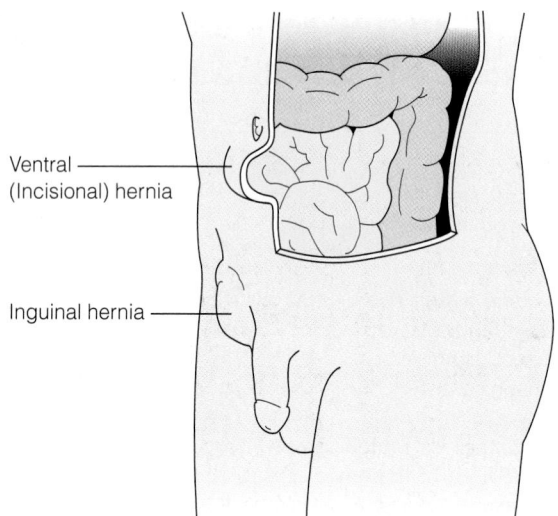

**Figure 24–14** ■ An abdominal wall (ventral or incisional) hernia and an inguinal hernia.

abdominal wall. These generally are acquired, caused by weakening of normal abdominal wall musculature. Umbilical hernias also are congenital, and usually are detected in infancy. Hiatal hernias develop in the diaphragm (see Chapter 21).

Abdominal contents (peritoneum, bowel, and other abdominal organs) can protrude through the abdominal wall to form a sac covered by skin and subcutaneous tissues. In most cases, abdominal contents move into the sac when intra-abdominal pressure increases, then return to the abdominal cavity when pressure returns to normal or when manual pressure is placed on the bulging sac. This is known as a *reducible hernia*. The risk for complications is low with a reducible hernia. If the contents of a hernia cannot be returned to the abdominal cavity, it is said to be *incarcerated*. Contents of an incarcerated hernia are trapped, usually by a narrow neck or opening to the hernia. Incarceration increases the risk of complications, including obstruction and strangulation. Obstruction occurs when the lumen of the bowel contained within the hernia becomes occluded, much like the crimping of a hose. A *strangulated hernia* develops when blood supply to bowel and other tissues in the hernia sac is compromised, leading to necrosis. The affected bowel can infarct, leading to perforation with contamination of the peritoneal cavity. Manifestations of a strangulated hernia include severe abdominal pain and distention, nausea, vomiting, tachycardia, and fever.

## Inguinal Hernias

Inguinal hernias usually affect males, and may be classified as indirect or direct inguinal hernias. *Indirect inguinal hernias* are caused by improper closure of the tract that develops as the testes descend into the scrotum before birth. A sac of abdominal contents protrudes through the internal inguinal ring into the inguinal canal. It often descends into the scrotum. Although indirect inguinal hernias are congenital defects, they often are not evident until adulthood, when increased intra-abdominal pressure and dilation of the inguinal ring allow abdominal contents to enter the channel.

*Direct inguinal hernias* are acquired defects that result from weakness of the posterior inguinal wall. Direct inguinal hernias usually affect older adults. *Femoral hernias* are also acquired defects in which a peritoneal sac protrudes through the femoral ring. These hernias usually affect obese or pregnant women.

Inguinal hernias often produce no symptoms and are discovered during routine physical examination. They may cause a lump, swelling, or bulge in the groin, particularly with lifting or straining. An inguinal hernia may cause sharp pain or a dull ache that radiates into the scrotum. A palpable mass may be present in the groin, although it may be felt only with increased intra-abdominal pressure (as occurs during coughing) and invagination of the scrotum toward the inguinal ring.

## Umbilical Hernia

Pregnancy and obesity also contribute to the development of umbilical hernias in adults. *Umbilical hernias* may be congenital and evident during infancy, or acquired as the tissue closing the umbilical ring weakens, allowing protrusion of abdominal contents. These hernias are more common in women. Other predisposing factors include multiple pregnancies with prolonged labor, ascites, and large intra-abdominal tumors.

Umbilical hernias tend to enlarge steadily and contain omentum, although they may also contain small or large bowel. The hernia may cause sharp pain on coughing or straining or a dull, aching sensation. Strangulation is a common complication of umbilical hernias.

## Incisional or Ventral Hernia

*Incisional* or *ventral hernias* occur at a previous surgical incision or following abdominal muscle tears. Inadequate healing of the incision or tear can lead to hernia development. Contributing factors include poor wound closure, postoperative infection, age or debility, obesity, inadequate nutrition, and excess incisional stress caused by vigorous coughing.

Ventral hernias are characterized by a bulge at the incisional site, often noted when the client pulls to a sitting position from a lying position. Ventral hernias often are asymptomatic, and the risk of incarceration is low because of the size of the defect.

## COLLABORATIVE CARE

The diagnosis of a hernia is made by a physical examination. The client is examined in a supine and sitting or standing position. A bulge may be seen or felt when the client coughs or bears down. No laboratory or diagnostic testing is usually required, unless bowel obstruction or strangulation is suspected.

Surgical repair, or *herniorrhaphy,* is the usual treatment of hernia. Surgery is generally well tolerated by people of all ages and carries a much lower risk than the complications of incarceration, obstruction, and strangulation. Emergency surgery is indicated for a hernia that is incarcerated, painful, or tender. In a herniorrhaphy, the abdominal wall defect is closed by suturing or with wire or mesh over the defect. If incarceration has occurred or strangulation is suspected, the abdomen is explored at the time of surgery and any infarcted bowel resected. Heavy lifting and heavy manual labor are restricted for approximately 3 weeks after surgery.

When surgery is contraindicated, the client may be taught to reduce the hernia by lying down and gently pushing against the mass. A binder or truss may be worn to prevent or control the protrusion. An incarcerated hernia should not be reduced by the client.

## NURSING CARE

### Assessment

- Health history: manifestations of hernia, such as bulging in the groin or of the abdominal wall when coughing, straining, or moving from lying to sitting; pain (abdominal, groin, or scrotal); history of hernia or abdominal surgery
- Physical examination: observe for bulging of the abdominal wall or around the umbilicus when raising head and shoulders from supine position; wearing gloves, palpate inguinal region for bulges when the client coughs or bears down (Valsalva maneuver).

### Nursing Diagnoses and Interventions

Herniorrhaphy is generally an uncomplicated procedure, usually performed as same-day surgery. Preoperative assessment and teaching and immediate postoperative care are the primary nursing care needs. Care is similar to that provided for a client with an appendectomy.

#### Risk for Ineffective Tissue Perfusion: Gastrointestinal

When providing care for a client with a known hernia, the possibility of obstruction and strangulation must be considered throughout nursing assessments. While nursing interventions may not be able to prevent these complications, rapid identification of the problem allows timely surgical treatment. Prompt treatment may prevent major complications related to infection and peritoneal contamination by bowel contents.

**PRACTICE ALERT** *Promptly report any acute increase in abdominal, groin, perineal, or scrotal pain. An abrupt increase in the intensity of pain may indicate bowel ischemia due to strangulation.* ■

- Assess bowel sounds and abdominal distention at least every 8 hours. *A change in bowel sounds—either cessation of sounds or an onset of hyperactive, high-pitched sounds—may indicate obstruction. With obstruction, abdominal girth may increase.*
- Notify primary care provider if the hernia becomes painful or tender. *Pain and tenderness may indicate incarceration and increased risk for strangulation.*
- If signs of possible obstruction or strangulation occur, notify the physician. Place client in supine position with the hips elevated and knees slightly bent. Withhold all food and fluids (NPO), and begin preparations for surgery. *This position helps relax abdominal muscles and may facilitate reduction of the hernia. Strangulation or obstruction require immediate surgical intervention.*

### Using NANDA, NIC, and NOC

Chart 24–6 shows links between NANDA nursing diagnoses, NIC and NOC for the client having a herniorrhaphy.

### Home Care

Include the following topics when teaching clients about hernias and home care.

- Rationale for examining the groin and abdomen for bulges
- The nature of hernia, risk factors, and manifestations
- Surgical intervention for hernia
- How to reduce a hernia if necessary
- The importance of seeking immediate medical intervention for signs of strangulation or obstruction
- The need to notify the physician if upper respiratory infection and cough develops preoperatively (forceful coughing is not recommended postoperatively)
- Postoperative pain management and activity restrictions

## THE CLIENT WITH INTESTINAL OBSTRUCTION

Intestinal obstruction is failure of intestinal contents to move through the bowel lumen. Intestinal obstructions may affect either the large or small bowel. The small intestine is more commonly affected; only about 15% of bowel obstructions occur in

### CHART 24–6  NANDA, NIC, AND NOC LINKAGES

#### The Client with Herniorrhaphy

| NURSING DIAGNOSES | NURSING INTERVENTIONS | NURSING OUTCOMES |
|---|---|---|
| • Pain | • Pain Management | • Pain Control |
| • Risk for Infection | • Incision Site Care | • Wound Healing: Primary Intention |
| • Urinary Retention | • Urinary Catheterization: Intermittent | • Urinary Elimination |

*Note: Data from* Nursing Outcomes Classification (NOC) *by M. Johnson & M. Maas (Eds.), 1997, St. Louis: Mosby;* Nursing Diagnoses: Definitions & Classification 2001–2002 *by North American Nursing Diagnosis Association, 2001, Philadelphia: NANDA;* Nursing Interventions Classification (NIC) *by J.C. McCloskey & G. M. Bulechek (Eds.), 2000, St. Louis: Mosby. Reprinted by permission.*

the large intestine. Obstruction is the most common reason for small bowel surgery.

## PHYSIOLOGY REVIEW

The GI tract contains layers of smooth muscle that contract in rhythmic waves. These waves of contraction, known as *peristalsis,* move along the whole length of the digestive tract to propel contents along the tract. Pacesetter cells in the smooth muscle control the rate of peristalsis.

## PATHOPHYSIOLOGY

Intestinal obstructions may be either mechanical or functional in nature. *Mechanical* obstructions may be caused by (1) problems outside the intestine, such as bands of scar tissue or hernias, (2) problems within the intestine, such as tumors or inflammatory bowel disease, or (3) obstruction of the intestinal lumen. The obstruction may be partial or complete. *Functional* obstruction occurs when peristalsis fails to propel intestinal contents although there is no mechanical obstruction. *Adynamic ileus* (also known as *paralytic ileus* or simply *ileus*) is the most common functional obstruction, and probably accounts for most intestinal obstructions altogether (Braunwald et al., 2001). Obstructions are further classified by the portion of intestine affected.

When the intestine is obstructed, gas and fluid accumulate proximal to and within the obstructed segment, distending the bowel. Swallowed air accounts for most of the gas. Ingested fluid, saliva, gastric juice, and pancreatic secretions contribute to accumulated fluid. Water and sodium are drawn into the bowel lumen, contributing to fluid accumulation, distention, and vascular fluid losses.

In some mechanical obstructions, such as a strangulated hernia, blood supply to the affected portion of bowel also is impaired, leading to necrosis and bacterial peritonitis.

Significant bowel distention, vomiting, and third spacing of fluids in the bowel and peritoneal cavity can lead to massive loss of fluids and electrolytes with resulting hypovolemia, hypokalemia, renal insufficiency, and shock.

### Small Bowel Obstruction

Adhesions, or bands of scar tissue, and hernias account for 70% to 75% of mechanical small bowel obstructions (Braunwald et al., 2001). In adults, adhesions develop following abdominal surgery or inflammatory processes. Adhesions usually produce a *simple obstruction,* or single blockage in one portion of the intestine (Figure 24-15A ■). The obstruction produced by an incarcerated hernia is a *closed-loop obstruction,* with two different portions of the bowel lumen obstructed (Figure 24-15 B).

Tumors, either intrinsic (of the bowel itself) or extrinsic (of another organ but affecting the bowel because of their size), can progressively occlude the bowel lumen and eventually obstruct it (Figure 24–15C). Other, less common causes of bowel obstruction include intussusception (rare in adults) (Figure 24–15D); volvulus, the rotation of loops of bowel about a fixed point (Figure 24–15E); foreign bodies; stricture; and inflammatory bowel disease.

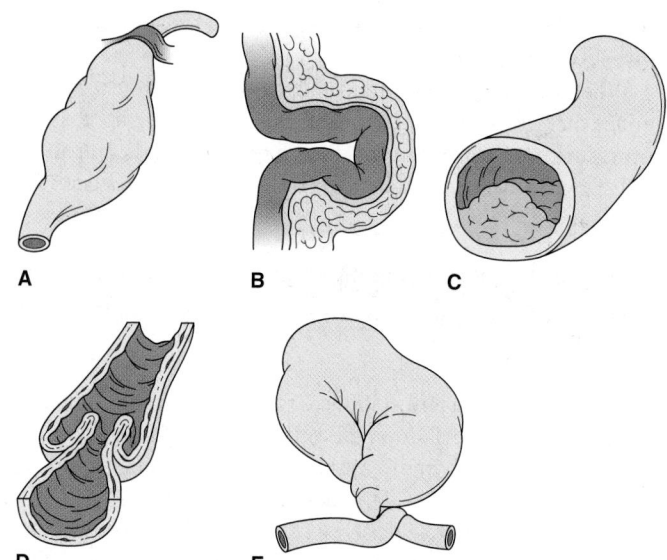

**Figure 24–15** ■ Selected causes of mechanical obstruction. *A,* Adhesions; *B,* incarcerated hernia; *C,* tumor; *D,* intussusception; *E,* volvulus.

Both volvulus and an incarcerated hernia can cause a *strangulated obstruction.* In a strangulated obstruction, not only is the lumen of the bowel obstructed, but also the blood supply to the affected portion is compromised.

In a functional obstruction or adynamic ileus, peristalsis stops due to either neurogenic or muscular impairment. The bowel lumen remains patent, but contents are not propelled forward. Temporary ileus commonly follows gastrointestinal surgery. It may also result from tissue anoxia or peritoneal irritation due to hemorrhage, peritonitis, or perforation of an organ. Other conditions that can precipitate paralytic ileus include renal colic, spinal cord injuries, uremia, and electrolyte imbalances, hypokalemia in particular. In addition, the effects of some narcotics, anticholinergic drugs, and antidiarrheal medications such as diphenoxylate can produce a functional obstruction.

### MANIFESTATIONS

The manifestations of a small bowel obstruction vary, depending on the level of obstruction and how rapidly it develops. Cramping or colicky abdominal pain that may be intermittent or increasing in intensity is common. Vomiting is common, particularly in high or proximal obstructions, because distention of the lumen stimulates the vomiting center. As bacterial fermentation occurs, vomitus becomes feculent, particularly with a low or distal obstruction. Flatus and feces already present in the lower bowel may be expelled early in the obstructive process, but this expulsion ceases as the obstruction continues.

Early in the course of a mechanical obstruction, borborygmi and high-pitched tinkling bowel sounds are present, as the intestine attempts to propel contents past the obstruction. Visible peristaltic waves may be noted in the distended loops of bowel in thin clients. In the later stages, the bowel becomes silent. With a paralytic ileus, bowel sounds are greatly diminished or absent throughout the process. Abdominal distention is minimal with proximal obstructions, but may be pronounced with distal obstruction and paralytic ileus. The abdomen may be tender to palpation as well.

In addition to abdominal and gastrointestinal manifestations, signs of fluid and electrolyte imbalance develop. Hypovolemia can develop rapidly as extracellular fluid is sequestered in the bowel and vomiting occurs. Although early vital signs may be normal, changes are noted as dehydration and hypovolemia develop. The client becomes tachycardic and tachypneic, and blood pressure falls. Temperature may be elevated. Urine output drops, and signs of hypovolemic shock may be seen.

## Complications

Hypovolemia and hypovolemic shock with multiple organ dysfunction is a significant complication of bowel obstruction and can lead to death. Renal insufficiency from hypovolemia can lead to acute renal failure. Pulmonary ventilation may be impaired as abdominal distention elevates the diaphragm and interferes with respiratory processes.

Strangulation associated with incarcerated hernia or volvulus impairs the blood supply to the bowel. Gangrene may rapidly result, causing bleeding into the bowel lumen and peritoneal cavity and eventual perforation. With perforation, bacteria and toxins from the strangulated intestine enter the peritoneum and, potentially, the circulation, resulting in peritonitis and possible septic shock.

The mortality rate in clients with obstruction of the small bowel is approximately 10%. When strangulation occurs, the mortality rate is between 20% and 75% (Braunwald et al., 2001). Delays in surgical intervention contribute to the higher mortality rate, pointing out the necessity of prompt diagnosis and intervention.

## Large Bowel Obstruction

Obstruction of the large intestine occurs much less frequently than small bowel obstruction, accounting for approximately 15% of all bowel obstructions in adults. Although any portion of the colon may be affected, obstruction usually occurs in the sigmoid segment. Cancer of the bowel is the most common cause; other causes include volvulus, diverticular disease, inflammatory disorders, and fecal impaction.

If the ileocecal valve between the small and large intestines is competent, distention proximal to the obstruction is limited to the colon itself. This is known as a *closed-loop obstruction*. It can lead to massive colon dilation as the ileum continues to empty gas and fluid into the colon. Increasing pressure within the obstructed colon impairs circulation to the bowel wall. Gangrene and perforation are potential complications. Approximately 15% of clients with large bowel obstruction have an incompetent ileocecal valve, which allows relief of colonic pressure by reflux into the ileum (Braunwald et al., 2001)

Constipation and colicky abdominal pain are usual manifestations of large bowel obstruction. The pain is often deep and cramping; severe, continuous pain may signal bowel ischemia and possible perforation. Vomiting is a late sign, if it occurs at all. The abdomen is distended, with high-pitched, tinkling bowel sounds with rushes and gurgles. On palpation, localized tenderness or a mass may be noted.

## COLLABORATIVE CARE

The management of a bowel obstruction focuses on relieving the pressure and obstruction, and providing supportive care. The intestine is decompressed, and fluid and electrolyte balance is restored. Surgery may be necessary to relieve a mechanical obstruction or if strangulation is suspected.

### Diagnostic Tests

Radiologic studies (X-rays and CT scan) are used to confirm the diagnosis of bowel obstruction. Laboratory testing is used to evaluate for the presence of infection and fluid and electrolyte imbalances.

- *WBC* often shows mild leukocytosis due to an inflammatory response to changes within the obstructed bowel lumen. With strangulation, leukocytosis is marked.
- *Serum amylase* levels may be elevated, particularly when strangulation is present.
- *Serum osmolality* and *electrolyte levels* are affected by fluid and electrolyte losses from vomiting and fluid sequestering in the bowel lumen. With hypovolemia, the serum osmolality and urine specific gravity increase. Potassium and chloride are lost through vomiting, leading to hypokalemia and hypochloremia.
- *Arterial blood gases* may reveal metabolic alkalosis (pH > 7.45, bicarbonate > 26 mEq/L, $PCO_2$ > 45 mmHg) with small bowel obstruction due to loss of hydrochloric acid from the stomach.
- *Abdominal X-ray* often shows distended loops of intestine with fluid and gas in a small bowel obstruction. Free air under the diaphragm indicates a perforation. A distended colon may be visualized with a large bowel obstruction.
- *X-ray* or *CT scan with contrast media* may be required to confirm a mechanical obstruction and assess the completeness of the obstruction. Meglumine diatrizoate (Gastrografin) is often used to provide contrast rather than barium when a bowel obstruction is suspected.

**PRACTICE ALERT**   *Unlike barium, meglumine diatrizoate contains iodine; therefore, it is vital to ask about iodine or seafood hypersensitivity prior to exam.* ■

- *Barium enema* may be used to confirm the diagnosis of large bowel obstruction and determine its location, unless perforation is suspected. See the Nursing Implications box on page 623 for nursing care related to a barium enema.
- *Sigmoidoscopy* or *colonoscopy* may be done to identify the cause when large bowel obstruction occurs. See pages 619 and 624 for nursing care related to these diagnostic studies.

### Gastrointestinal Decompression

Most partial small bowel obstructions are successfully treated with gastrointestinal decompression using a nasogastric or long intestinal tube. Functional obstructions respond to treatment with bowel rest and intestinal decompression as well. Intestinal tubes (see Figure 24–3) may be inserted through the nares or via gastrostomy. A balloon or weighted tip draws the tube from the stomach into the intestine and to the area of obstruction via peristalsis. Collected fluid and gas is removed using low suction until persitalsis resumes or the obstruction is relieved.

## Surgery

Surgical intervention is required for complete mechanical obstructions as well as for strangulated or incarcerate obstructions of the small intestine. Clients with incomplete mechanical obstruction may also require surgery if the obstruction persists.

Prior to surgery, a nasogastric tube is inserted to relieve vomiting and abdominal distention and to prevent aspiration of intestinal contents. Fluid and electrolyte balance must be restored before surgery as well. Isotonic intravenous fluids, such as normal (physiologic) saline, Ringer's solution, or other balanced electrolyte solutions, are used. Additional electrolytes may be added to the solution to correct low levels. It is particularly important to correct hypokalemia prior to surgery. Acid-base imbalances are also addressed, often using intravenous acidifiers or alkalinizing agents. If strangulation has occurred, the client may require plasma or blood replacement. Intravenous broad-spectrum antibiotics are administered prophylactically (see the section on peritonitis).

A laparotomy usually is performed to allow inspection of the small intestine and removal of infarcted or gangrenous tissue. If the obstruction was caused by adhesions, they are removed or lysed. Obstructing tumors are resected, and foreign bodies are removed. Any bowel that appears to be gangrenous is resected, usually followed by an end-to-end anastomosis of remaining intestine. If a large tumor mass or dense adhesions are found, the area of obstruction may be bypassed by anastomosis of proximal small bowel to small or large intestine distal to the obstruction. Nursing care of the client having bowel surgery is included in the box on page 671.

Obstructions of the large intestine usually necessitate surgery. The primary goal is to relieve colonic distention and prevent perforation; the secondary goal is to remove the obstructing lesion. In some cases, colonoscopy may be used to relieve the distention. If the client's condition prohibits major surgery or the obstructing tumor is advanced, laser photocoagulation may be used to enlarge the bowel lumen. Removal of the obstructing lesion is the preferred treatment. The proximal and distal bowel segments may be anastomosed, or a permanent colostomy or ileostomy may be required. (The previous section on bowel cancer discusses these surgical interventions.)

## NURSING CARE

### Health Promotion

Teach health promotion activities, such as increasing dietary fiber intake, maintaining a generous fluid intake, and exercising daily to help prevent constipation and possible large bowel obstruction, particularly in the older adult. Stress the importance of complying with dietary restrictions (such as avoiding popcorn) for clients who experience repeated small bowel obstructions.

## Assessment

Nurses may be instrumental in the early identification of intestinal obstructions in older adults, the homebound client, or the institutionalized client. Early identification and intervention significantly reduces morbidity from bowel obstruction.

- Health history: complaints of abdominal pain and bloating, constipation; previous history of bowel obstruction or risk factors such as hernia, inflammatory bowel disease, diverticulosis, or previous abdominal surgery; current medications
- Physical examination: vital signs including orthostatic blood pressure and pulse, temperature; skin color, temperature, texture, and turgor; color and moisture of mucous membranes; abdominal shape, contour, bowel sounds, presence of tenderness or masses on palpation

## Nursing Diagnoses and Interventions

In clients with a suspected or confirmed bowel obstruction, frequent assessment for complications such as fluid and electrolyte imbalance, acid-base imbalances, hypovolemic shock, perforation, and peritonitis is necessary.

### Deficient Fluid Volume

Because of the large collection of fluid in the bowel proximal to an obstruction, the accompanying vomiting, and nasogastric suction, the client with an intestinal obstruction often has a fluid volume deficit. If not corrected promptly, hypovolemic shock, acute renal failure, and multiple organ system dysfunction from poor tissue perfusion may result.

- Monitor vital signs, pulmonary artery pressures, cardiac output (CO), and central venous pressure (CVP) hourly. *A decrease in blood pressure, tachycardia, and tachypnea may indicate hypovolemia. Although invasive, hemodynamic parameters such as pulmonary artery pressures, CO, and CVP allow accurate assessment of fluid volume status.*
- Measure urinary output hourly and nasogastric drainage every 2 to 4 hours. *A urinary output of 30 mL per hour or more usually indicates an adequate glomerular filtration rate (GFR), another indicator of fluid volume. Nasogastric output provides a tool for evaluating fluid replacement needs.*

**PRACTICE ALERT** *Promptly report urine output less than 30 mL per hour. This often indicates hypovolemia and an increased risk for shock and acute renal failure.* ■

- Maintain intravenous fluids and blood volume expanders as ordered. The amount of fluid administered is calculated to meet ongoing fluid needs and replace previous and current losses. *Restoration and maintenance of blood volume is necessary to maintain cardiac output and tissue and organ perfusion.*
- Measure abdominal girth every 4 to 8 hours. Mark the level of measurement on the abdomen. *A reference mark allows consistent, accurate measurements. An increase in abdominal girth indicates increasing intestinal distention.*

- Notify the physician of changes in status. *Changes in vital signs, pain, and signs of increasing distention can indicate the need for immediate surgical intervention.*

### Ineffective Tissue Perfusion: Gastrointestinal

Perfusion of the intestinal wall and mucosa may be impaired by the obstructive process itself (e.g., strangulation or volvulus) or by significant intestinal distention. The goal is to maintain tissue perfusion and promote normal peristalsis and bowel elimination.

- Monitor vital signs hourly. Assess peripheral pulses, skin color, temperature, and capillary refill. *Cardiovascular assessment is vital to detect early signs of hypovolemic shock resulting from sequestering large volumes of fluid in the intestines. Hypovolemia and shock can convert mild bowel ischemia to infarction as the blood supply to the tissue falls.*
- Monitor urine output hourly. Report output of less than 30 mL per hour. *Urine output is a good indicator of the glomerular filtration rate (GFR) and tissue perfusion. The urine output often falls before vital sign changes are apparent in hypovolemia.*
- Monitor temperature at least every 4 hours. *An elevated temperature may be an early indication of sepsis from bowel perforation as a result of gangrene.*
- Frequently assess pain. *A change in the character of pain or a rapid increase in its intensity may signal bowel infarction or perforation.*
- Maintain NPO status until peristalsis resumes. *Enteral food or fluids may increase distention and bowel ischemia. They also are restricted until the possibility of perforation is eliminated.*

### Ineffective Breathing Pattern

Significant abdominal distention from a bowel obstruction can cause the diaphragm to flatten, impairing pulmonary ventilation. Following surgery, splinting of abdominal muscles to avoid pain can lead to shallow respirations. These factors, plus the risk of aspiration of gastrointestinal contents during vomiting, place the client at high risk for respiratory complications, particularly with a small bowel obstruction.

- Assess respiratory rate, pattern, and lung sounds at least every 2 to 4 hours. *Tachypnea, shortness of breath, or apparent dyspnea may be early signs of respiratory compromise. Diminished breath sounds, particularly in the bases of the lungs, or crackles indicate poor lung expansion and possible impaired ventilation.*
- Monitor arterial blood gas results for possible effects of altered respiratory status. *Tachypnea may lead to respiratory alkalosis as excess carbon dioxide is eliminated. Conversely, impaired chest expansion can lead to respiratory acidosis because of alveolar hypoventilation.*
- Elevate the head of the bed. *Elevating the head of the bed reduces the work of breathing and improves alveolar ventilation by reducing the pressure of abdominal distention on the diaphragm.*
- Provide a pillow or folded bath blanket to use in splinting the abdomen while coughing postoperatively. *Splinting abdominal muscles and incisions improves the ease and effectiveness of coughing postoperatively.*

- Maintain nasogastric or intestinal tube patency. *Maintaining gastrointestinal suction helps reduce abdominal distention and prevent aspiration associated with vomiting.*
- Encourage use of incentive spirometer or other assistive device hourly. *These devices encourage deep breathing, opening distal airways and preventing atelectasis.*
- Contact respiratory therapy as indicated. *The respiratory therapist may suggest or perform additional measures to maintain effective pulmonary ventilation.*
- Provide good oral care at least every 4 hours. *Dehydration and nasogastric suction dry mucous membranes of the mouth and throat, increasing the risk of bacterial growth. Many respiratory infections result from aspirated organisms.*

### Using NANDA, NIC, and NOC

Linkages between NANDA, NIC, and NOC when caring for the client with intestinal obstruction are similar to those for clients with appendicitis or peritonitis. (See Chart 24–2.)

### Home Care

Include the following topics when teaching the client with intestinal obstruction in preparation for home care.

- Wound care
- Activity level, return to work, and any other recommended restrictions
- Recommended follow-up care
- Care of temporary colostomy (if appropriate) and planned reanastamosis
- For recurrent obstructions, their cause, early identification of symptoms, and possible preventive measures

## THE CLIENT WITH DIVERTICULAR DISEASE

**Diverticula** are saclike projections of mucosa through the muscular layer of the colon (Figure 24–16 ■). Diverticula may occur anywhere in the gastrointestinal tract, excl... rectum. The vast majority, however, affect the large intestine, with 90% to 95% occurring in the sigmoid colon.

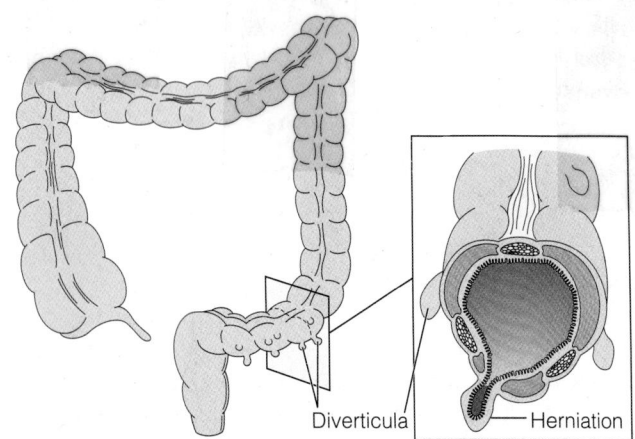

**Figure 24–16** ■ Diverticula of the colon.

People in the United States, Australia, the United Kingdom, and France have high and increasing incidence rates of diverticular disease. The disease is uncommon in Africa and Asia. Both sexes are equally affected. The incidence of diverticula increases with age: While only 5% of people under age 40 have diverticula, more than 50% of people over age 80 are affected. Millions of people have diverticular disease, but less than one-third of those affected develop symptoms (Tierney et al., 2001).

Cultural factors, diet in particular, are thought to play an important role in the development of diverticula. A diet consisting of highly refined and fiber-deficient foods is believed to be the major factor contributing to the disease. Diverticular disease was essentially unknown before grain milling (which removes two-thirds of the fiber from flour) became prevalent in the early 1900s. Decreased activity levels and postponement of defecation have been suggested as contributing factors. The increasing incidence of diverticula with aging suggests that decreased blood supply or nutrition of the bowel wall may be additional related factors (Bullock & Henze, 2000).

## PATHOPHYSIOLOGY AND MANIFESTATIONS

Diverticula form when increased pressure within the bowel lumen causes bowel mucosa to herniate through defects in the colon wall. The circular and longitudinal (teniae coli) muscles often thicken or hypertrophy in the area affected by diverticula. This narrows the bowel lumen, increasing intraluminal pressure. Deficient dietary fiber and a lack of fecal bulk contribute to muscle hypertrophy and narrowing of the bowel. Contraction of the muscles in response to normal stimuli such as meals may occlude the narrowed lumen, further increasing intraluminal pressure. The high pressure causes mucosa to herniate through the muscle wall, forming a diverticulum. Areas where nutrient blood vessels penetrate the circular muscle layer are the most common sites for diverticula formation.

### Diverticulosis

*Diverticulosis* indicates the presence of diverticula. More than two-thirds of clients with diverticulosis are asymptomatic. When manifestations such as episodic pain (usually left-sided), constipation, and diarrhea occur, they often can be attributed to irritable bowel syndrome, which commonly accompanies diverticular disease. (Irritable bowel syndrome is discussed earlier in this chapter.) As the disease progresses, abdominal cramping, narrow stools (decrease in caliber), increased constipation, occult bleeding in the stools, weakness, and fatigue may develop.

Complications of diverticulosis include hemorrhage and diverticulitis. A diverticulum may bleed, whether it is inflamed or not, possibly due to erosion of an adjacent blood vessel by a fecalith in the diverticulum.

### Diverticulitis

**Diverticulitis** is inflammation in and around the diverticular sac. It typically affects only one diverticulum, usually in the sigmoid colon. Undigested food and bacteria collect in the diverticula, forming a hard mass (*fecalith*) that impairs the mucosal blood supply, allowing bacterial invasion. Mucosal ischemia leads to perforation. With microscopic perforation, inflammation is localized. Gross perforation of a diverticulum results in more extensive bacterial contamination and can lead to abscess formation or peritonitis.

Pain is a common manifestation of diverticulitis. It is usually left-sided and may be mild to severe and either steady or cramping. The client may also experience either constipation or increased frequency of defecation. Depending on the location and severity of the inflammation, nausea, vomiting, and a low-grade fever may occur. On examination, the abdomen may be distended, with tenderness and a palpable mass in the left lower quadrant resulting from the inflammatory response.

The older adult may have less specific manifestations, complaining of vague abdominal pain. A palpable mass and signs of a large bowel obstruction may be present.

Complications associated with diverticulitis (in addition to peritonitis and abscess formation) include bowel obstruction, fistula formation, and hemorrhage. Severe or repeated episodes of diverticulitis may lead to scarring and fibrosis of the bowel wall, further narrowing the bowel lumen. This increases the risk for obstruction of the large bowel. Acutely inflamed tissue may adhere to the small bowel, increasing the potential for small bowel obstruction as well. Fistulas may form, usually between the sigmoid colon and the bladder. Urinary tract infection is the usual sign of a colovesical fistula. Fistulas may also perforate into the small intestine, ureter, vagina, perineum, or abdominal wall. Bleeding from perforation of a vessel wall can occur with diverticulitis. Although it may be significant, bleeding usually stops spontaneously.

## COLLABORATIVE CARE

Management of diverticular disease varies from no prescribed treatment to surgical resection of affected colon, depending on the severity of the disease and its complications.

### Diagnostic Tests

Diagnostic testing is used to identify diverticular disease when the disease is symptomatic or complications develop.

- *WBC count* may show leukocytosis with a left shift (an increased number of immature WBCs) due to inflammation in diverticulitis.
- *Hemoccult* or *guaiac testing* of stool may show the presence of occult blood.
- *Barium enema* may be used to confirm diverticular disease. In addition to illustrating diverticula, X-rays can reveal segmental spasm and muscular thickening with a narrowed bowel lumen. Barium enema is contraindicated in early acute diverticulitis because of the risk of barium leakage into the peritoneal cavity.
- *Abdominal X-ray* films may show free abdominal air associated with diverticulitis and perforation. When there is a risk of perforation, water-soluble contrast media may be used to illustrate an abscess, fistulas, or narrowing of the bowel lumen.

- *CT scan* may be done with or without contrast media to assess inflammation and detect an abscess or fistula.
- *Flexible sigmoidoscopy* or *colonoscopy* may be done to detect diverticulosis, assess for strictures or bleeding, and rule out tumor as the cause of the client's symptoms.

## Medications

Systemic broad-spectrum antibiotics effective against usual bowel flora are prescribed to treat acute diverticulitis. Oral antibiotics such as metronidazole (Flagyl) and ciprofloxacin (Cipro) or trimethoprim-sulfamethoxazole (Septra, Bactrim) may be prescribed if symptoms are mild. Severe, acute attacks often necessitate hospitalization and treatment with intravenous fluids and antibiotics effective against anaerobic and gram-negative bacteria. Therapy may include a second-generation cephalosporin such as cefoxitin (Mefoxin), or another antibiotic such as piperacillin-taxobactam (Zosyn) or ticarcillin-clavulanate (Timentin). Antibiotics and their nursing implications are discussed in Chapter 8.

Pentazocine (Talwin) may be prescribed for relief of pain associated with diverticulitis. This analgesic causes less increase in colonic pressure than morphine or meperidine (Demerol).

Although a stool softener such as docusate sodium (Colace) may be prescribed, it is important to note that laxatives (which can further increase intraluminal pressure in the colon) are avoided for the client with diverticular disease.

## Dietary Management

Dietary modification is central to the management of diverticular disease. It appears that dietary changes can reduce the risk of complications of diverticulosis. A high-fiber diet is recommended; it increases stool bulk, decreases intraluminal pressures, and may reduce spasm (Table 24–13). Bran is a low-cost fiber supplement that can be added to cereal, soups, salads, or other foods. Commercial bulk-forming products, such as psyllium seed (Metamucil) or methylcellulose also may be recommended. These products are discussed in the Medication Administration box on page 624. The client may be advised to avoid foods with small seeds (such as popcorn, caraway seeds, figs, or berries), which could obstruct diverticula.

| TABLE 24–13 | Foods Recommended in a High-Fiber, High-Residue Diet |
|---|---|
| **Food Group** | **Recommended Foods** |
| Cereals and grains | Wheat or oat bran; cooked cereals, such as oatmeal; dry cereals, such as bran buds or flakes, corn flakes, shredded wheat; whole-grain breads or crackers; brown rice |
| Fruits | Unpeeled raw apples, peaches, and pears; oranges |
| Vegetables | Dried beans (navy, kidney, pinto), lima beans; broccoli; peas; corn; squash; raw vegetables, such as carrots, celery, and tomatoes; potatoes (with skins) |

Bowel rest is prescribed during an acute episode of diverticulitis. The client initially may be NPO with intravenous fluids and possibly total parenteral nutrition. Feeding is resumed gradually. Initially, a clear liquid diet is prescribed with gradual advancement to a soft, low-roughage diet (i.e., a diet low in insoluble fiber) with daily added psyllium seed to soften stool and increase its bulk. Among the foods the client should avoid are wheat and corn bran, vegetable and fruit skins, nuts, and dry beans. The high-fiber diet is resumed following full recovery.

## Surgery

Clients with acute diverticulitis require surgery, usually to treat generalized peritonitis or an abscess that fails to respond to medical treatment. Hemorrhage that recurs or cannot be controlled may also necessitate surgery. Elective surgery may be performed for recurrent episodes of diverticulitis or persistent diverticulitis with continuing pain, tenderness, and a palpable mass.

The affected bowel segment is resected, and if possible an anastomosis of the proximal and distal portions is performed. When an acute infection and diverticulitis are present, a two-stage Hartmann procedure is required. A temporary colostomy is created and anastomosis delayed until the inflammation has subsided. A second surgery is performed 2 to 3 months later to reconnect the bowel and close the temporary colostomy. Refer to the boxes on pages 671 and 673 for nursing care of the client with bowel surgery and a colostomy.

## NURSING CARE

### Health Promotion

Teaching clients in many different settings about the benefits of a high-fiber diet is important primary prevention for diverticular disease. Nurses working with groups and individuals in the community should emphasize the importance of a high-fiber diet and its benefits in preventing diverticular disease and other disorders. In such facilities as residential or foster care settings, the nurse can work with dietary staff and care providers to increase the amount of fiber in residents' diets, unless this is contraindicated by a preexisting condition.

### Assessment

Because most clients with diverticular disease have few or no symptoms, nursing assessment focuses on manifestations of complications.

- Health history: abdominal pain or cramping, chronic constipation or irregular bowel habits; nausea and vomiting; history of diverticular disease or irritable bowel syndrome
- Physical examination: bowel sounds, presence of abdominal tenderness of masses and location; stool for occult blood

### Nursing Diagnoses and Interventions

Clients with acute diverticulitis are acutely ill and have multiple nursing care needs. Priority nursing diagnoses include *Impaired tissue integrity, Pain,* and *Anxiety* related to the possibility of a significant complication or possible surgery.

## Impaired Tissue Integrity: Gastrointestinal

During an acute attack of diverticulitis, inflammation and mucosal ischemia place the client at risk for perforation and peritonitis. In addition to maintaining bowel rest to reduce the risk of perforation, the nurse monitors for manifestations of perforation and possible sepsis.

- Monitor vital signs including temperature at least every 4 hours. *Tachycardia and tachypnea may be early indications of increased inflammation and resulting fluid shift. Fever greater than 101°F (38.3°C) may indicate increased or spread of inflammation. Note, however, that little temperature elevation may occur in the older client. A change in behavior or increasing lethargy may be subtle indications of infection in the older adult.*
- Assess abdomen every 4 to 8 hours or more often as indicated, including measuring abdominal girth, auscultating bowel sounds, and palpating for tenderness. Promptly report significant changes to the physician. *Increasing abdominal distention, a decrease or change in the quality of bowel sounds, and/or increasing tenderness or guarding may indicate spread of the infectious process or peritonitis.*
- Assess for evidence of lower intestinal bleeding by visual examination and guaiac testing of stools for occult blood. *Perforation of a diverticulum may produce either intestinal or intra-abdominal bleeding and require immediate treatment such as surgery.*
- Maintain intravenous fluids, total parenteral nutrition, and accurate intake and output records. *During acute diverticulitis, oral intake is usually prohibited or restricted. Intravenous fluids are given to maintain fluid and electrolyte balance; total parenteral nutrition is used to maintain nutritional status, facilitating healing and recovery.*

## Pain

Pain is a common manifestation of acute diverticulitis. It results from inflammation of the bowel and edema of affected tissues. If surgery is required, postoperative pain is managed with narcotic analgesics.

- Ask the client to rate pain using a pain scale. Document the level of pain, and note any changes in location or character of pain. *The perception and response to pain is individual and is affected by past experiences, culture, ethnic background, and many other factors. A change in the character or intensity of the pain may indicate a complication such as perforation or abscess formation.*
- Administer prescribed analgesic or maintain patient-controlled analgesia (PCA) as ordered. Assess analgesic effectiveness. Avoid administering morphine. Provide adjunctive medications as ordered, and encourage use of adjunctive techniques, such as relaxation, positioning, and distraction. Notify the physician if pain management is inadequate. *If client has not obtained adequate pain relief, further assessment and intervention are required.*
- Maintain bowel rest and total body rest (bed rest with limited activity). *Rest helps reduce inflammation and promote healing, increasing comfort.*
- Reintroduce oral foods and fluids slowly, providing a soft, low-fiber diet with bulk-forming agents. *This allows continued healing of the affected bowel while promoting soft, easily expelled stools.*

## Anxiety

The client with acute diverticulitis faces not only hospitalization, but also potential serious complications such as peritonitis and hemorrhage. Surgery and formation of a temporary colostomy may be necessary. Furthermore, episodes of acute diverticulitis are often recurrent, and the client may fear future problems.

- Assess and document level of anxiety. *Severe anxiety or panic states can interfere with the ability to respond to instructions and assist with care. Low to moderate anxiety levels enhance learning and compliance with prescribed interventions.*
- Demonstrate empathy and awareness of the perceived threat to health. *It is important to recognize and respect the client's feelings and perceptions as reality.*
- Attend to physical care needs. *This provides reassurance that these needs will be met and relieves concerns about them.*
- Spend as much time as possible with the client. *Presence of a caring nurse helps relieve fears of abandonment or that help will not be available if needed. It also enhances trust and provides opportunity for expression of fears or concerns.*
- Assess level of understanding about disease and condition. *This allows misperceptions that may contribute to anxiety to be corrected.*
- Encourage supportive family and friends to remain with the client as much as possible. *This provides a supportive environment for the client and also distracts from physical concerns.*
- Assist the client to identify and use appropriate coping mechanisms. *Coping mechanisms provide immediate relief of anxiety while the client adapts to the situation.*
- Involve the client and family (as appropriate) in care decisions. *This increases the client's sense of control over the situation.*

## Using NANDA, NIC, and NOC

Chart 24–7 shows links between NANDA nursing diagnoses, NIC and NOC when caring for the client with diverticulitis.

## Home Care

The client with diverticular disease is responsible for its day-to-day management. Discuss the following topics when preparing for home care.

- Prescribed high-fiber diet and the need to maintain the diet for life to reduce the incidence of complications, including ways to increase dietary fiber
- Complications of diverticular disease and its manifestations

Provide a referral to a dietitian for further teaching as indicated.

Prior to discharge of the client with acute diverticulitis, discuss the following:

- Food and fluid limitations, including recommendations for a low-residue diet during the initial period of healing
- Colostomy management (if a temporary colostomy has been created), including where to obtain supplies and dietary management
- Planned procedure to reanastomose the colon and revise the colostomy. Refer to community health care agencies as indicated.

CHART 24–7 NANDA, NIC, AND NOC LINKAGES

## The Client with Diverticulitis

| NURSING DIAGNOSES | NURSING INTERVENTIONS | NURSING OUTCOMES |
|---|---|---|
| • Constipation<br>• Diarrhea<br><br>• Deficient Knowledge<br>• Pain<br>• Risk for Deficient Fluid Volume | • Nutrition Management<br>• Bowel Management<br>• Diarrhea Management<br>• Teaching: Prescribed Diet<br>• Pain Management<br>• Fluid Management | • Symptom Control<br>• Bowel Elimination<br>• Symptom Severity<br>• Knowledge: Diet<br>• Comfort Level<br>• Fluid Balance |

*Note: Data from Nursing Outcomes Classification (NOC) by M. Johnson & M. Maas (Eds.), 1997, St. Louis: Mosby; Nursing Diagnoses: Definitions & Classification 2001–2002 by North American Nursing Diagnosis Association, 2001, Philadelphia: NANDA; Nursing Interventions Classification (NIC) by J.C. McCloskey & G. M. Bulechek (Eds.), 2000, St. Louis: Mosby. Reprinted by permission.*

## Nursing Care Plan
### A Client with Diverticulitis

Roseline Ukoha is a 45-year-old married school teacher who has two children. For the past 2 days, she has experienced intermittent abdominal pain and bloating. The pain increased in severity over the past 9 to 10 hours, and she developed nausea, lower back pain, and discomfort radiating into the perineal region. Mrs. Ukoha reports having had no bowel movement for the past 2 days. The emergency department nurse, Jasmine Sarino, RN, completes her admission assessment.

### ASSESSMENT

Mrs. Ukoha relates a 10-year history of chronic irritable bowel symptoms, including alternating constipation and diarrhea and intermittent abdominal cramping. She states that she thought these symptoms were due to the stress of teaching middle school, and that they never became severe enough to seek medical advice. When questioned about her diet, she calls it a typical American high-fat, fast-food diet, usually consisting of a sweet roll and coffee for breakfast, a hamburger or sandwich and soft drink for lunch, and a balanced dinner, usually including meat, a vegetable or salad, and potatoes or pasta, "except on pizza night!"

Physical assessment findings include T 101°F (38.3°C), P 92, R 24, and BP 118/70. Abdomen is slightly distended and tender to light palpation. Bowel sounds are diminished. Diagnostic tests include the following abnormal results: WBC 19,900/mm$^3$ (normal 3500 to 11,000/mm$^3$) with increased immature and mature neutrophils on differential; hemoglobin 12.8 g/dL (normal 13.3 to 17.7 g/dL); hematocrit, 37.1% (normal 40% to 52%). Abdominal X-ray films show slight to moderate distention of the large and small bowel with suggestion of possible early ileus. A small amount of free air is noted in the peritoneal cavity.

The diagnosis of probable diverticulitis with diverticular rupture is made, and Mrs. Ukoha is admitted to the medical unit for intravenous fluids, antibiotic therapy, and bowel rest.

### DIAGNOSIS

- *Pain* related to inflamed bowel and possible peritonitis
- *Risk for deficient fluid volume* related to inflammation
- *Impaired tissue integrity: Gastrointestinal* related to perforated diverticulum
- *Deficient knowledge* related to disease process and dietary management

### EXPECTED OUTCOMES

- Verbalize adequate pain relief.
- Experience no adverse effects of prescribed bed rest.
- Maintain adequate fluid balance while hospitalized, as demonstrated by balanced intake and output, stable weight, good skin turgor and mucous membrane moisture, and laboratory values within the normal range.
- Heal adequately without further evidence of peritonitis.
- Verbalize understanding of the recommended high-fiber diet and the need to increase physical activity and fluid intake to promote optimal bowel function at home.

### PLANNING AND IMPLEMENTATION

- Assess comfort status frequently, providing analgesics as needed.
- Maintain intravenous infusion as prescribed.
- Measure intake and output; weigh daily.
- Provide mouth care every 2 to 4 hours until oral intake resumes, then every 4 hours until client assumes self-care.
- Measure temperature every 4 hours.
- Advance diet from clear liquids to low-residue diet when allowed.
- Provide instruction and dietary consultation for high-fiber diet.

### EVALUATION

On discharge, Mrs. Ukoha is afebrile, and her abdomen is flat and only slightly tender to palpation. She is taking food and fluids well and has resumed a normal pattern of bowel elimination. She will continue oral antibiotic therapy for another 2 weeks at home. She verbalizes an understanding of the need to continue her low-residue diet for the next week, and maintain a high-fiber diet thereafter. She says she is glad her problem turned out to be diverticulosis instead of cancer as she had feared, and states that she can deal with this now that she knows how.

### Critical Thinking in the Nursing Process

1. Why was Mrs. Ukoha hospitalized immediately and placed on intravenous fluids and antibiotics?
2. Mrs. Ukoha reports, "I had a small bowel movement of mucus. Is this normal, or is something wrong?" What would be your response?
3. How did Mrs. Ukoha's previous diet contribute to her diverticular disease and diverticulitis? Did the symptoms of irritable bowel syndrome also contribute? How?
4. Develop a teaching plan to instruct clients with diverticular disease about dietary recommendations.

See Evaluating Your Response in Appendix C.

# ANORECTAL DISORDERS

Anorectal lesions include hemorrhoids, a normal condition common to all adults that may become enlarged and painful; anal fissure; anorectal fistulas; anorectal abscess; and pilonidal disease. Fecal incontinence also may be considered an anorectal disorder.

## THE CLIENT WITH HEMORRHOIDS

The anus and anal canal contain two superficial venous plexuses with the hemorrhoidal veins. When pressure on these veins is increased or venous return impeded, they can develop *varices,* or varicosities, thus becoming weak and distended. This condition is commonly known as **hemorrhoids,** or piles. When asymptomatic, hemorrhoids are considered to be a normal condition found in all adults.

## PATHOPHYSIOLOGY AND MANIFESTATIONS

Hemorrhoids develop when venous return from the anal canal is impaired. Straining to defecate in the sitting or squatting position increases venous pressure and is the most common cause of distended hemorrhoids. Pregnancy increases intraabdominal pressure, raising venous pressure, and is a second important cause of hemorrhoids. Other factors that may contribute to symptomatic hemorrhoids include prolonged sitting, obesity, chronic constipation, and the low-fiber diet common to Western nations.

Hemorrhoids are classed as either internal or external. *Internal* hemorrhoids affect the venous plexus above the mucocutaneous junction of the anus (Figure 24–17 ■). Internal hemorrhoids rarely cause pain, usually presenting with bleeding. Bleeding from internal hemorrhoids is bright red and unmixed with the stool. It can vary in quantity from streaks on toilet tissue to enough to color the water in the toilet. Recurrent bleeding of internal hemorrhoids may be sufficient to cause anemia. Mucus discharge and a feeling of incomplete evacuation of stool also may be manifestations of internal hemorrhoids.

*External* hemorrhoids affect the inferior hemorrhoidal plexus below the mucocutaneous junction. Bleeding is rare with external hemorrhoids. Anal irritation, a feeling of pressure, and difficulty cleaning the anal region may be manifestations of external hemorrhoids.

As they enlarge, hemorrhoids may prolapse or protrude through the anus. Initially, prolapse occurs only with defecation and the hemorrhoids spontaneously regress back into the anal canal. Eventually, the client may need to manually replace internal hemorrhoids after defecation, or they may become permanently prolapsed and replacement not possible. Symptoms of permanently prolapsed hemorrhoids include mucus discharge and clothing soilage.

"Normal" hemorrhoids are not painful. Pain is associated with ulcerated or thrombosed hemorrhoids, and it can be severe. Prolapsed hemorrhoids may become strangulated as a result of congestion and edema, leading to thrombosis. Hemorrhoidal thrombosis causes extreme pain and may lead to infarction of skin and mucosa overlying the hemorrhoid. Internal hemorrhoids associated with portal hypertension in liver disease may bleed profusely if ruptured. (See Chapter 22 ∞ for further discussion of portal hypertension.)

A *thrombosed external hemorrhoid* is a thrombosis of the subcutaneous external hemorrhoidal veins of the anal canal, rather than a true hemorrhoid. It appears as a painful bluish hematoma beneath the skin and typically occurs following a sudden increase in venous pressure, for example, heavy lifting, coughing, or straining. Pain is significant at onset but gradually subsides. Spontaneous rupture with bleeding may occur. Thrombosed external hemorrhoids resolve spontaneously without intervention.

## COLLABORATIVE CARE

Because hemorrhoids are a normal condition, management is conservative unless complications such as permanent prolapse or thrombosis occur.

Hemorrhoids are diagnosed by the client's history and by examination of the anorectal area. External hemorrhoids can be seen on visual inspection, especially if thrombosed. The client is asked to strain (Valsalva's maneuver) during the examination to detect prolapse. Internal hemorrhoids are usually not palpable or tender on digital examination of the rectum. *Anoscopic* examination is used to detect and evaluate internal hemorrhoids. For this exam, a speculum or endoscope is introduced into the anus to provide visual inspection of the tissues. Internal hemorrhoids are vascular structures that protrude into the lumen. Additional diagnostic examinations including testing of stool for occult blood and sigmoidoscopy are performed to rule

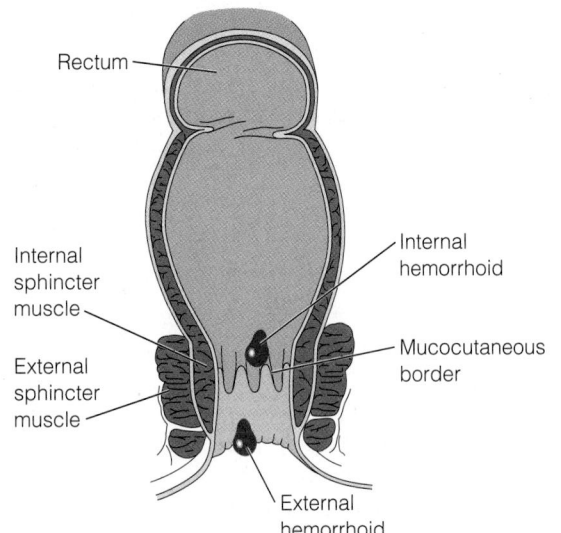

**Figure 24–17** ■ The location of internal and external hemorrhoids.

Rectum

Internal sphincter muscle

External sphincter muscle

Internal hemorrhoid

Mucocutaneous border

External hemorrhoid

out cancer of the colon or rectum, which may aggravate hemorrhoidal symptoms or produce similar manifestations. If liver disease with portal hypertension is suspected, liver function studies are ordered.

Hemorrhoids that are not permanently prolapsed or acutely thrombosed generally are treated conservatively. A high-fiber diet and increased water intake to increase stool bulk, improve its softness, and reduce straining is effective for most clients with internal or external hemorrhoids. Bulk-forming laxatives such as psyllium seed (Metamucil) or stool softeners such as docusate sodium (Colace) may be prescribed to improve constipation and reduce straining as well. Suppositories and local ointments such as Preparation H or Nupercaine have an anesthetic and astringent effect, reducing discomfort and irritation of surrounding tissues. They have little or no effect on the hemorrhoid itself. Warm sitz baths, bed rest, and local astringent compresses may be recommended to reduce the swelling of edematous prolapsed hemorrhoids after digital reduction.

Hemorrhoids that are permanently prolapsed, are thrombosed, or produce significant symptoms may be treated more aggressively. *Sclerotherapy* involves injecting a chemical irritant into tissues surrounding the hemorrhoid to induce inflammation and eventual fibrosis and scarring. It is used to treat recurrent bleeding and early prolapse of internal hemorrhoids. The treatment produces minimal pain. Enlarged or prolapsing hemorrhoids also may be treated with rubber band ligation. A rubber band is placed snugly around the hemorrhoidal plexus and surrounding mucosa, causing the tissue to necrose and slough within 7 to 10 days. Treatment is limited to one hemorrhoidal complex at a time, so repeat treatments may be necessary. Pain should be minimal if the band is placed appropriately; persistent pain following band ligation may signal an infection. Bleeding can occur as the hemorrhoid sloughs. Other procedures used to treat hemorrhoids include cryosurgery, in which hemorrhoids are necrosed by freezing with a cryoprobe, infrared photocoagulation, or electrocoagulation.

Clients with chronic symptoms, permanent prolapse, chronic bleeding and anemia, or painful thrombosed hemorrhoids may be treated surgically with a *hemorrhoidectomy*. In this procedure, hemorrhoids are surgically excised, leaving normal skin and surrounding tissues. This procedure may use conventional techniques or a laser to remove both internal and external hemorrhoids. Few complications are associated with hemorrhoidectomy.

## NURSING CARE

Primary prevention of symptomatic hemorrhoids involves education of clients of all ages. Stress the importance of maintaining an adequate intake of dietary fiber, a liberal fluid intake, and regular exercise to maintain stool bulk, softness, and regularity. Discuss the need to respond to the urge to defecate rather than postponing defecation. Teach appropriate constipation management, including the use of bulk-forming laxatives.

---

**BOX 24–4  ■ Perianal Postoperative Care**

### ASSESSMENT
- Monitor vital signs every 4 hours for 24 hours.
- Inspect rectal dressing every 2 to 3 hours for 24 hours.
- Monitor urinary output.

### PAIN CONTROL
- Assist to position of comfort, usually side-lying.
- Provide analgesics as prescribed.
- Keep fresh ice packs over the rectal dressing as ordered.
- Assist with sitz bath 3 to 4 times per day.
- Provide a flotation pad for use when sitting.

### ELIMINATION
- Give stool softeners as prescribed.
- Give an analgesic before the first postoperative bowel movement if possible.
- When tolerated, encourage fluid intake of at least 2000 mL per day.

### CLIENT AND FAMILY TEACHING
- Take sitz bath after each bowel movement for 1 to 2 weeks after surgery.
- Drink at least 2 quarts of fluid per day.
- Eat adequate dietary fiber, and exercise moderately.
- Take stool softeners as prescribed.
- Report to the physician the following symptoms: rectal bleeding, continued pain on defecation, fever greater than 101°F (38.3°C), purulent rectal drainage.

---

Most clients with hemorrhoids are treated in community settings where the primary nursing focus is educational. Discuss the appropriate use of over-the-counter preparations for the relief of minor hemorrhoidal symptoms. If necessary, teach clients how to reduce prolapsed hemorrhoids digitally.

Teach manifestations of possible hemorrhoidal complications, such as chronic bleeding, prolapse, and thrombosis. Stress the need to seek medical evaluation if symptoms persist. Discuss the link between manifestations of hemorrhoids and colorectal cancer, and urge the client to seek medical intervention for persistent, unresolved, or progressive symptoms.

When a hemorrhoidectomy is performed, the client requires more direct nursing intervention. Postoperative care of the client with perianal surgery is outlined in Box 24–4. Anal packing may be in place for the first 24 hours following the procedure. When removed, observe the client closely for bleeding. Pain is a common postoperative problem. Although the operative procedure is minor, postoperative discomfort can be significant because the anal region is richly innervated and muscle spasms may occur. In addition to systemic analgesics, sitz baths usually are ordered. These not only help promote relaxation and reduce discomfort but also clean the anal area. Use of a rubber ring or donut device minimizes pressure on the surgical site while the client sits in the bath.

The client may remain hospitalized until after the first postoperative bowel movement. Stool softeners, adequate fluids, and analgesia before defecation can reduce anxiety and discomfort. Adequate cleaning following defecation, usually with a sitz bath, is vital.

Whether caring for a client with hemorrhoids or a hemorrhoidectomy, consider the following nursing diagnoses.

- *Pain* related to inflamed anal tissues
- *Constipation* related to dietary habits and/or delay of defecation
- *Risk for infection* related to disruption of anal tissue

## THE CLIENT WITH AN ANORECTAL LESION

Unlike the rectum, which is relatively insensitive to pain, the anal canal is richly supplied with sensory nerves and highly sensitive to painful stimuli. Lesions of the anorectal area may cause significant pain, particularly with defecation. Infection is a potential complication of anorectal lesions because of contamination by fecal bacteria. The superior boundary of the anal canal (the anorectal juncture or pectinate line) contains 8 to 12 anal crypts where anorectal abscesses or fistulas can form.

### Anal Fissure

*Anal fissures* or ulcers occur when the epithelium of the anal canal over the internal sphincter becomes denuded or abraded. Irritating diarrheal stools and tightening of the anal canal with increased sphincter tension are frequent causes of anal fissures. Other factors that may contribute to their development include childbirth trauma, habitual cathartic use, laceration by a foreign body, and anal intercourse. Chronic inflammation and infection of surrounding tissues accompanies an anal fissure.

Clients with anal fissures typically have periods of exacerbation and remission. Because they occur below the mucocutaneous line, anal fissures are painful. The pain occurs with defecation and may be described as tearing, burning, or cutting. Bright red bleeding is noted with a bowel movement as well. Bleeding is typically minor and noted on toilet tissue. Because of fear of defecation, the client may develop constipation, which further disrupts normal bowel habits and aggravates symptoms.

The diagnosis of anal fissure is made on gentle digital examination of the anal canal and anoscopy using a small anoscope. Treatment is usually conservative, involving dietary changes to increase fiber intake and stool bulk, increased fluid intake and bulk-forming laxatives. A topical agent such as hydrocortisone cream may be prescribed. Surgical intervention with an internal sphincterotomy, an incision into the internal sphincter to increase its diameter, is considered when the fissure does not heal with medical intervention.

### Anorectal Abscess

Invasion of the pararectal spaces by pathogenic bacteria can lead to an *anorectal abscess*. Commonly caused by infection that extends from the anal crypt into a pararectal space, the abscess may appear small but often contains a large amount of pus. Multiple pathogens may be present, including *Escherichia coli*, *Proteus*, streptococci, and staphylococci. Other factors that may contribute to the development of an anorectal abscess include infection of a hair follicle, sebaceous gland, or sweat gland; and abrasions, fissures, or anal trauma. The incidence of anorectal abscess is higher in men.

Pain is the primary manifestation of an anorectal abscess. Sitting or walking may aggravate the pain, but it is unrelated to defecation. External swelling, redness, heat, and tenderness are apparent on examination. With a deeper abscess, swelling may not be visible, but the abscess is palpable on digital examination.

If the abscess either does not drain spontaneously or is not drained surgically, adjacent anatomic spaces will be affected. Systemic sepsis is also a potential complication.

Incision and drainage (I & D) is the treatment of choice for an anorectal abscess because it rarely resolves with antibiotic therapy alone. This treatment often leads to a persistent fistula, which is surgically closed after the infection has cleared.

### Anorectal Fistula

A fistula is a tunnel or tubelike tract with openings at each end. *Anorectal fistulas* have one opening in the anal canal with the other usually found in perianal skin. Most occur spontaneously or as a result of anorectal abscess drainage. Crohn's disease is a predisposing factor to fistula development as well.

The primary manifestation of an anorectal fistula is intermittent or constant drainage or discharge, which may be purulent. This may be accompanied by local itching, tenderness, and pain associated with defecation.

Digital and anoscopic examination with gentle probing of the fistula tract are used to establish the diagnosis. Although some fistulas may heal spontaneously, the treatment of choice is a fistulotomy. The primary opening of the fistula is removed, and the tract is opened to allow it to heal by secondary intention, from the inside outward. If the sphincter is involved, a two-stage operation may be done to preserve the muscle and prevent fecal incontinence.

### Pilonidal Disease

The client with *pilonidal disease* has an acute abscess or chronic draining sinus in the sacrococcygeal area. Underlying the abscess or sinus is a cyst with granulation tissue, fibrosis, and, often, hair tufts. This disease usually affects young hirsute (hairy) males and is probably due to hair entrapment in deep tissues of the sacrococcygeal area. Some researchers, however, believe that it is a congenital disorder.

The lesion of pilonidal disease is generally asymptomatic unless it becomes acutely infected. Manifestations of acute inflammation accompany infection, including pain, tenderness, redness, heat, and swelling of the affected area. Purulent discharge may be noted from one or more sinuses or openings in the midline.

The preferred treatment option for pilonidal disease is incision and drainage. The sinus tract and underlying cyst are excised and closed by either primary- or secondary-intention healing. The client may be instructed to remove hair from the area routinely by shaving or using a depilatory to prevent further hair entrapment and recurrence of the problem.

## NURSING CARE

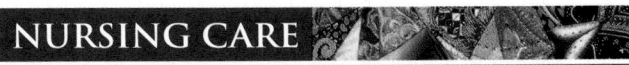

Clients with anorectal disorders are often treated in the community, and the primary nursing responsibility is education. Teach the importance of maintaining a high-fiber diet and liberal fluid intake to increase stool bulk and softness and thereby decrease discomfort with defecation. Stress the importance of responding to the urge to defecate to prevent constipation.

Following surgical treatment of any of these disorders, teach the client to keep the perianal region clean and dry. If a dressing is in place, instruct to avoid soiling it with urine or feces during elimination. Following removal of the dressing, teach to clean the area gently with soap and water following a bowel movement. Discuss the use of sitz baths for cleaning and comfort. Suggest taking an analgesic if necessary prior to defecation, but caution that some analgesics may promote constipation. Teach signs and symptoms of infection or other possible complications to report to the physician. If an antibiotic has been prescribed, provide written and verbal instructions about its use, its desired and possible adverse effects, and their management.

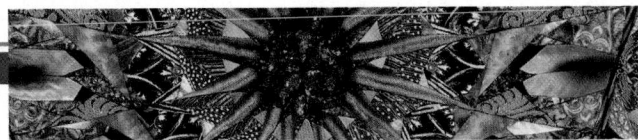

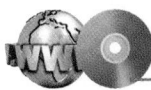

## EXPLORE MediaLink

NCLEX review questions, case studies, care plan activities, MediaLink applications, and other interactive resources for this chapter can be found on the Companion Website at www.prenhall.com/lemone.

Click on Chapter 24 to select the activities for this chapter. For animations, video clips, more NCLEX review questions, and an audio glossary, access the Student CD-ROM accompanying this textbook.

## TEST YOURSELF

1. A client presents at the urgent care clinic with complaints of diarrhea for the past week. The nurse should first:
   a. Advise the client to abstain from all food intake until the diarrhea subsides
   b. Ask the client to describe the number and character of daily stools
   c. Question the client about possible exposure to an enterotoxin or protozoal infection
   d. Recommend an over-the-counter antidiarrheal preparation such as Pepto-Bismol

2. The nurse caring for a client admitted with possible appendicitis appropriately plans which of the following?
   a. Initiate bowel preparation for a barium enema
   b. Restrict intake to clear liquids
   c. Prepare for possible immediate appendectomy
   d. Insert saline lock for intravenous antibiotic therapy

3. When teaching a client with inflammatory bowel disease about prescribed sulfasalazine, the nurse instructs the client to:
   a. Use a sunscreen while taking the drug
   b. Take the drug on an empty stomach
   c. Limit fluid intake to 1500 mL per day or less
   d. Take vitamin C while on this drug

4. A client reports frequent large, fatty, foul-smelling stools. The nurse recognizes this as:
   a. Hematochezia, a manifestation of GI bleeding
   b. Characteristic of inflammatory bowel disease
   c. A common early manifestation of colorectal cancer
   d. Steatorrhea, a manifestation of malabsorption

5. A client tells the nurse that both his father and grandfather died of colon cancer, and he is worried that he is going to die from "the same horrible disease." Which of the following does the nurse include in her recommendations?
   a. There is no genetic link seen in colon cancer, so his risk is equal to that of people with no family history of the disease
   b. He should plan for annual digital rectal exams and periodic colonoscopy (every 3 to 5 years) for early identification of possible tumors
   c. He should have annual CEA levels drawn to screen for early tumor development
   d. It is imperative that he change his diet immediately, significantly increasing his intake of dietary fiber

See Test Yourself answers in Appendix C.

# BIBLIOGRAPHY

Ackley, B.J., & Ladwig, G. B. (2002). *Nursing diagnosis handbook: A guide to planning care* (5th ed.). St. Louis: Mosby.

American Cancer Society. (2002). Cancer reference information: What are the key statistics for colon and rectum cancer? Available http://www.cancer.org

Bailey, C. (2001). Focus. Older patients' experiences of pre-treatment discussions: An analysis of qualitative data from a study of colorectal cancer. *NT Research, 6*(4), 736–746.

Baker, D. (2001). Current surgical management of colorectal cancer. *Nursing Clinics of North America, 36*(3), 579–592.

Ball, E. M. (2000). Ostomy guide, part two. A teaching guide for continent ileostomy. *RN, 63*(12), 35–36, 38, 40.

Bliss, D. Z., Jung, H., Savik, K., Lowry, A., LeMoine, M., Jensen, L., Werner, C., & Schaffer, K. (2001). Supplementation with dietary fiber improves fecal incontinence. *Nursing Research, 50*(4), 203–213.

Braunwald, E., Fauci, A. S., Kasper, D. L., Hauser, S. L., Longo, D. L., & Jameson, J. L. (2001). *Harrison's principles of internal medicine* (15th ed.). New York: McGraw-Hill.

Breeze, J. (2001). Colorectal cancer. *Nursing Times, 97*(11), 39–41.

Bullock, B. A., & Henze, R. L. (2000). *Focus on pathophysiology.* Philadelphia: Lippincott.

Burger, E. T. (2001). Preparing adult patients for international travel. *Nurse Practitioner: American Journal of Primary Health Care, 26*(5), 13–15, 19–25.

Cox, J. A., Rogers, M. A., & Cox, S. D. (2001). Treating benign colon disorders using laparoscopic colectomy. *AORN Journal, 73*(2), 375, 377–380, 382+.

Deglin, J. H., & Vallerand, A. H. (2001). *Davis's drug guide for nurses* (7th ed.). Philadelphia: F.A. Davis.

Dest, V. M. (2000). Oncology today: New horizons. Colorectal cancer. *RN, 63*(3), 53–59.

Erwin-Toth, P. (2001). Caring for a stoma is more than skin deep. *Nursing, 31*(5), 36–40.

Fontaine, K. L. (2000). *Healing practices: Alternative therapies for nursing.* Upper Saddle River, NJ: Prentice Hall Health.

Gallo, J. J., Busby-Whitehead, J., Rabins, P. V., Silliman, R. A., & Murphy, J. B. (Eds.). (1999). *Reichel's care of the elderly: Clinical aspects of aging* (5th ed.). Philadelphia: Lippincott Williams & Wilkins.

Gauf, C. L. (2000). Diagnosing appendicitis across the life span. *Journal of the American Academy of Nurse Practitioners, 12*(4), 129–133.

Heuschkel, R., Afzal, N., Wuerth, A., Zurakowski, D., Leichtner, A., Kemper, K., & Tolia, V. (2002). Complementary medicine use in children and young adults with inflammatory bowel disease. *American Journal of Gastroenterology, 97*(2), 382–388.

Jenks, J. M., Morin, K. H., & Tomaselli, N. (1997). The influence of ostomy surgery on body image in patients with cancer. *Applied Nursing Research, 10*(4), 174–180.

Joachim, G. (2000). Responses of people with inflammatory bowel disease to foods consumed. *Gastroenterology Nursing, 23*(4), 160–167.

Johnson, M., Bulechek, G., Dochterman, J. M., Maas, M., & Moorhead, S. (2001). *Nursing diagnoses, outcomes, & interventions.* St. Louis: Mosby.

Johnson, M., Maas, M., & Moorhead, S. (Eds.). (2000). *Nursing outcomes classification (NOC)* (2nd ed.). St. Louis: Mosby.

Kinney, A. Y., Choi, Y., DeVellis, B., Millikan, R., Kobetz, E., & Sandler, R. S. (2000). Attitudes toward genetic testing in patients with colorectal cancer. *Cancer Practice: A Multidisciplinary Journal of Cancer Care, 8*(4), 178–186.

Kuhn, M. A. (1999). *Complementary therapies for health care providers.* Philadelphia: Lippincott.

Langmead, L., Dawson, C., Hawkins, C., Banna, N., Loo, S., & Rampton, D. S. (2002). Antioxidant effects of herbal therapies used by patients with inflammatory bowel disease: An in vitro study. *Alimentary Pharmacologic Therapy, 16*(2), 197–205.

Lehne, R. A. (2001). *Pharmacology for nursing care* (4th ed.). Philadelphia: Saunders.

Levine, C. D. (1999). Toxic megacolon: Diagnosis and treatment challenges. *AACN Clinical Issues: Advanced Practice in Acute and Critical Care, 10*(4), 492–499.

Lord, L. M., Schaffner, R., DeCross, A. J., & Sax, H. C. (2000). Management of the patient with short bowel syndrome. *AACN Clinical Issues: Advanced Practice in Acute and Critical Care, 11*(4), 604–618.

Malarkey, L.M., & McMorrow, M.E. (2000). *Nurse's manual of laboratory tests and diagnostic procedures* (2nd ed.). Philadelphia: Saunders.

Mason, I. (2001). Inflammatory bowel disease. *Nursing Times, 97*(9), 33–35.

McCloskey, J. C., & Bulechek, G. M. (Eds.) (2000). *Nursing interventions classification (NIC)* (3rd ed.). St. Louis: Mosby.

McConnell, E. A. (2001). Appendicitis: What a pain! *Nursing, 31*(8): 32hn1–3.

_____ . (2001). What's behind intestinal obstruction? *Nursing, 31*(10), 58–63.

Meeker, M. H., & Rothrock, J. C. (1999). *Alexander's care of the patient in surgery* (11th ed.). St. Louis: Mosby.

North American Nursing Diagnosis Association. (2001). *NANDA nursing diagnoses: Definitions & classification 2001–2002.* Philadelphia: NANDA.

Olson, S. J., & Zawacki, K. (2000). Hereditary colorectal cancer. *Nursing Clinics of North America, 35*(3), 671–685.

Pontieri-Lewis, V. (2000). Colorectal cancer: Prevention and screening. *MEDSURG Nursing, 9*(1), 9–15, 20.

Porth, C. M. (2002). *Pathophysiology: Concepts of altered health states* (6th ed.). Philadelphia: Lippincott.

Rankin-Box, D. (2000). An alternative approach to bowel disorders. *Nursing Times, 96*(19), NT-plus 24, 26.

Rayhorn, N. (1999). Understanding inflammatory bowel disease. *Nursing, 29*(12), 57–61.

Sercombe, J. (2000). Inflammatory bowel disease and smoking. *Professional Nurse, 15*(7), 439–442.

_____ . (2001). Surgical therapy for inflammatory bowel disease. *Nursing Times, 97*(10), 34–36.

Shepherd, M. (2000). Treating diarrhea and constipation. *Nursing Times, 96*(6), NTplus 15–16.

Tierney, L. M., McPhee, S. J., & Papadakis, M. A. (2001). *Current medical diagnosis & treatment* (40th ed.). New York: Lange Medical Books/McGraw-Hill.

Verhoef, M. J., Rapchuk, I., Liew, T., Weir, V., & Hilsden, R. J. (2002). Complementary practitioners' views of treatment for inflammatory bowel disease. *Canadian Journal of Gastroenterology, 16*(2), 95–100.

Whitney, E. N., & Rolfes, S. R. (2002). *Understanding nutrition* (9th ed.). Belmont, CA: Wadsworth.

Wilkinson, J. M. (2000). *Nursing diagnosis handbook with NIC interventions and NOC outcomes* (7th ed.). Upper Saddle River, NJ: Prentice Hall Health.

Wood, M. C., & Ryan, C. T. (2000). Patient resources. Resources on colorectal cancer for patients. *Cancer Practice: A Multidisciplinary Journal of Cancer Care, 8*(6), 308–310.

Young, M. (2000). Caring for patients with coloanal reservoirs for rectal cancer. *MEDSURG Nursing, 9*(4), 193–197.

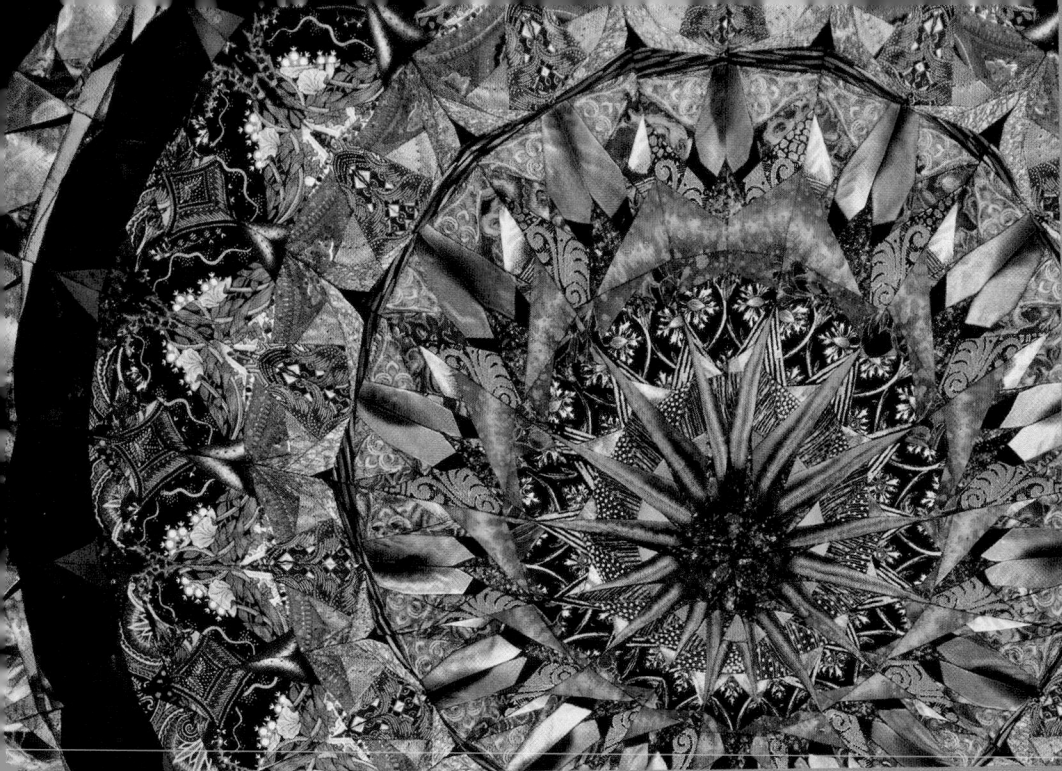

# RESPONSES TO ALTERED URINARY ELIMINATION

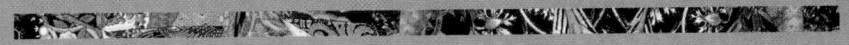

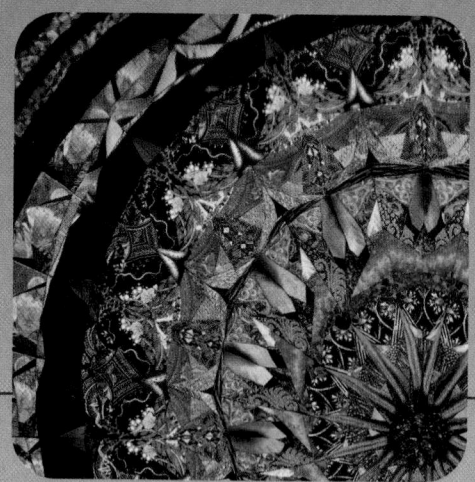

# CHAPTER 25

# Assessing Clients with Urinary System Disorders

## MediaLink

**www.prenhall.com/lemone**
Additional resources for this chapter can be found on the Student CD-ROM accompanying this textbook, and on the Companion Website at www.prenhall.com/lemone. Click on Chapter 25 to select the activities for this chapter.

**CD-ROM**
- Audio Glossary
- NCLEX Review

*Animations*
- Urinary System
- Renal Function

**Companion Website**
- More NCLEX Review
- Functional Health Pattern Assessment
- Case Study
  Renal Calculi
- MediaLink Application
  Kidney Function

## LEARNING OUTCOMES

After completing this chapter, you will be able to:

- Review the anatomy and physiology of the urinary system.

- Explain the role of the urinary system in maintaining homeostasis.

- Identify specific topics for consideration during a health history interview of the client with health problems involving the urinary system.

- Describe techniques for assessing the integrity and function of the urinary system.

- Identify abnormal findings that may indicate impairment of the urinary system.

The functions of the renal system are to regulate body fluids, to filter metabolic wastes from the bloodstream, to reabsorb needed substances and water into the bloodstream, and to eliminate metabolic wastes and water as urine. Any alteration in the structure or function of the renal system affects the whole body. In turn, healthy urinary system function depends on the health of other body systems, especially the circulatory, endocrine, and nervous systems.

## REVIEW OF ANATOMY AND PHYSIOLOGY

The organs of the urinary system are the paired kidneys, the paired ureters, the urinary bladder, and the urethra (Figure 25–1 ■). Each structure is essential to the total functioning of the urinary system.

### The Kidneys

The two kidneys are located outside the peritoneal cavity and on either side of the vertebral column at the levels of T12 through L3. These highly vascular, bean-shaped organs are approximately 4.5 inches (11.4 cm) long and 2.5 inches (6.4 cm) wide. The lateral surface of the kidney is convex; the medial surface is concave and forms a vertical cleft, the hilum. The ureter, renal artery, renal vein, lymphatic vessels, and nerves enter or exit the kidney at the level of the hilum.

The kidney is supported by three layers of connective tissue: the outer renal fascia, the middle adipose capsule, and the inner renal capsule. The renal fascia, made up of dense connective tissue, surrounds the kidney (and the adrenal gland, a discrete organ that sits on top of each kidney) and anchors it to surrounding structures. The middle adipose capsule is a fatty mass that holds the kidney in place and also cushions it against trauma. The inner renal capsule provides a barrier against infection and helps protect the kidney from trauma.

The functions of the kidney are to:

- Balance solute and water transport.
- Excrete metabolic waste products.
- Conserve nutrients.
- Regulate acid-base balance.
- Secrete hormones to help regulate blood pressure, erythrocyte production, and calcium metabolism.
- Form urine.

MediaLink | RENAL FUNCTION ANIMATION

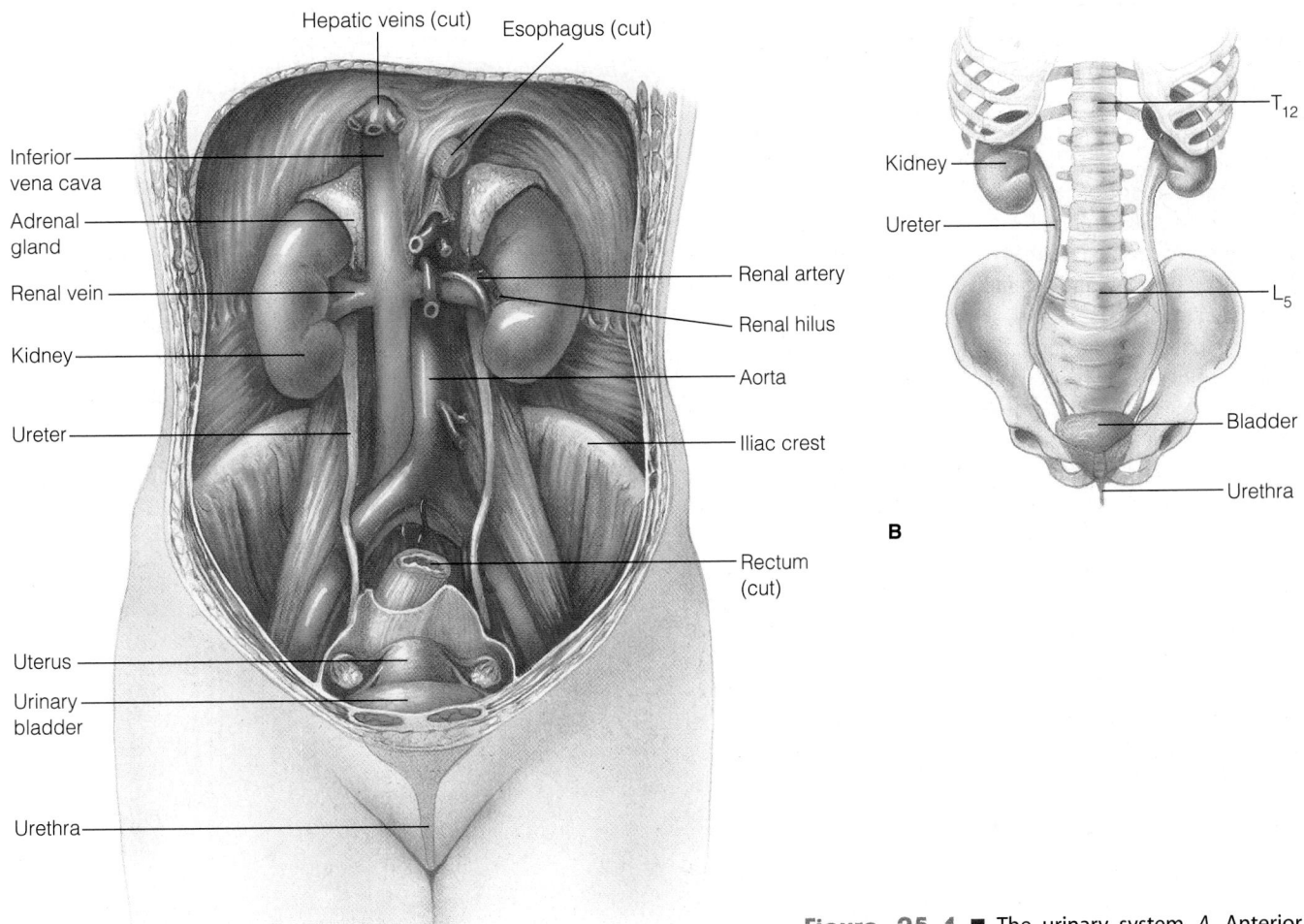

**Figure 25–1** ■ The urinary system. *A,* Anterior view of the urinary system in a female. *B,* The kidneys are shown in relation to the vertebrae and ribs.

**Figure 25–2** ■ Internal anatomy of the kidney.

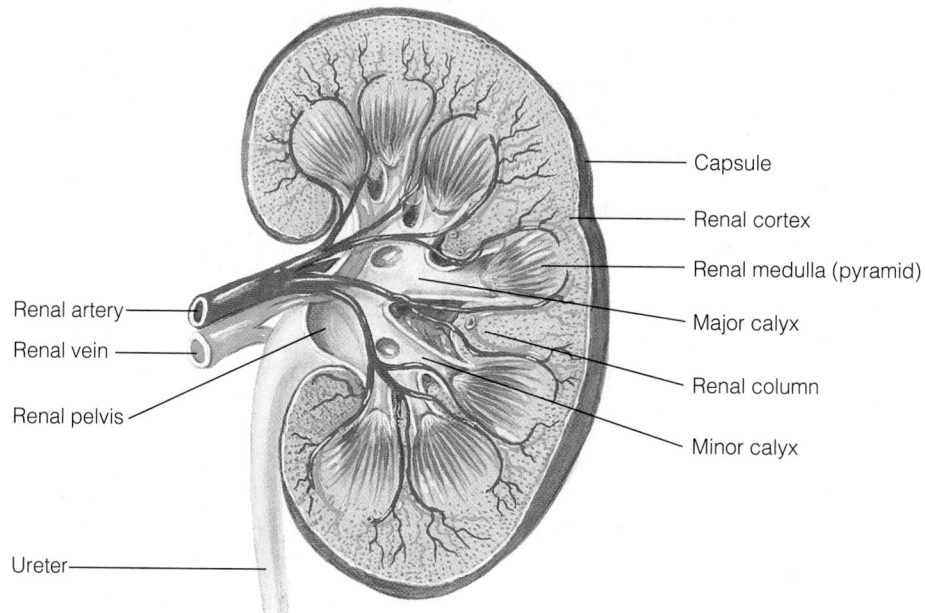

Capsule

Renal cortex

Renal medulla (pyramid)

Major calyx

Renal column

Minor calyx

Renal artery

Renal vein

Renal pelvis

Ureter

Internally, each kidney has three distinct regions: the cortex, medulla, and pelvis. The outer region, or renal cortex, is light in color and has a granular appearance (Figure 25–2 ■). This region of the kidney contains the glomeruli, small clusters of capillaries. The glomeruli bring blood to and carry waste products from the nephrons, the functional units of the kidney.

The renal medulla, just below the cortex, contains cone-shaped tissue masses called renal pyramids, formed almost entirely of bundles of collecting tubules. Areas of lighter-colored tissue called renal columns are actually extensions of the cortex and serve to separate the pyramids. The collecting tubules that make up the pyramids channel urine into the innermost region, the renal pelvis.

The renal pelvis is continuous with the ureter as it leaves the hilum. Branches of the pelvis known as the major and minor calyces extend toward the medulla and serve to collect urine and empty it into the pelvis. From the pelvis, urine is channeled through the ureter and into the bladder for storage. The walls of the calyces, the renal pelvis, and the ureter contain smooth muscle that moves urine along by peristalsis.

Each kidney contains approximately 1 million nephrons, which process the blood to make urine (Figure 25–3 ■). Each nephron contains a tuft of capillaries called the glomerulus, which is completely surrounded by the glomerular capsule (or Bowman's space). Together, the glomerulus and its surrounding capsule are called the renal corpuscle. The endothelium of the glomerulus allows capillaries to be extremely porous. Thus, large amounts of solute-rich fluid pass from the capillaries into the capsule. This fluid, called the filtrate, is the raw material of urine. Filtrate leaves the capsule and is channeled into the proximal convoluted tubule (PCT) of the nephron. Microvilli on the tubular cells increase the surface area for reabsorption of substances from the filtrate into plasma in the peritubular capillaries. Substances moved by active transport include glucose,

sodium, potassium, amino acids, proteins, and vitamins. About 70% of the water in the filtrate, as well as chloride and bicarbonate, are reabsorbed by passive transport. The filtrate then moves into the U-shaped loop of Henle and is concentrated. The descending limb of the U is relatively thin and freely per-

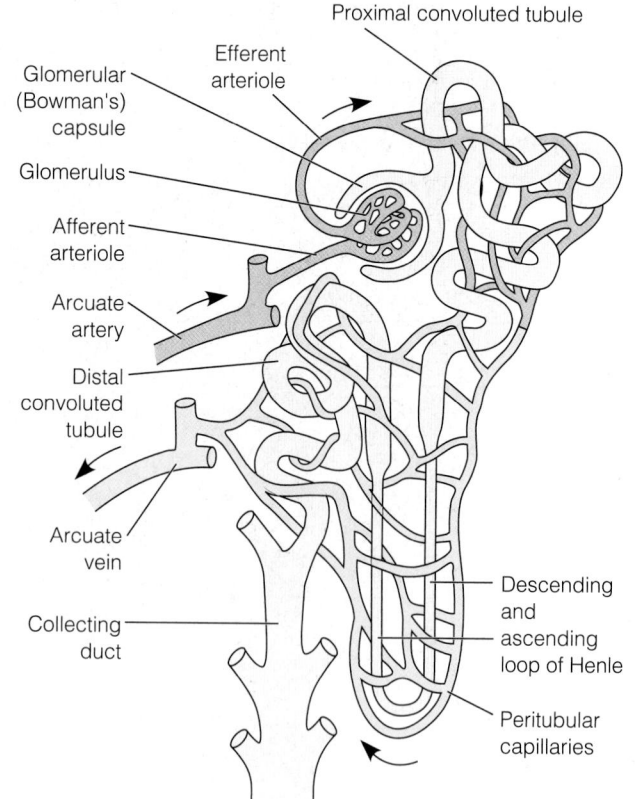

Proximal convoluted tubule

Efferent arteriole

Glomerular (Bowman's) capsule

Glomerulus

Afferent arteriole

Arcuate artery

Distal convoluted tubule

Arcuate vein

Collecting duct

Descending and ascending loop of Henle

Peritubular capillaries

**Figure 25–3** ■ The structure of a nephron, showing the glomerulus within the glomerular capsule.

meable to water, whereas the ascending segment is thick and thereby less permeable. The distal convoluted tubule (DCT) receives filtrate from the loop of Henle. Although this segment is structurally similar to the PCT, it lacks microvilli and is more involved with secreting solutes into the filtrate than in reabsorbing substances from it. The collecting duct receives the newly formed urine from many nephrons and channels urine through the minor and major calyces of the renal pelvis and into the ureter.

## The Ureters

The ureters are bilateral tubes approximately 10 to 12 inches (25 to 30 cm) long. They transport urine from the kidney to the bladder through peristaltic waves originating in the renal pelvis. The wall of the ureter has three layers: an inner epithelial mucosa, a middle layer of smooth muscle, and an outer layer of fibrous connective tissue.

## The Urinary Bladder

The urinary bladder is posterior to the symphysis pubis and serves as a storage site for urine. In males, the bladder lies immediately in front of the rectum; in females, the bladder lies next to the vagina and the uterus. Openings for the ureters and the urethra are inside the bladder: the trigone is the smooth triangular portion of the base of the bladder outlined by these three openings (Figure 25–4 ■).

The layers of the bladder wall (from internal to external) are the epithelial mucosa lining the inside, the connective tissue submucosa, the smooth muscle layer, and the fibrous outer layer. The muscle layer, called the detrusor muscle, consists of fibers arranged in inner and outer longitudinal layers and in a middle circular layer. This arrangement allows the bladder to expand or contract according to the amount of urine it holds.

The size of the bladder varies with the amount of urine it contains. In healthy adults, the bladder holds about 300 to 500 mL of urine before internal pressure rises and signals the need to empty the bladder through **micturition** (also called *urination* or voiding). However, the bladder can hold more than twice that amount if necessary. The bladder has an internal urethral sphincter that relaxes in response to a full bladder and signals the need to urinate. A second external urethral sphincter is formed by skeletal muscle and is under voluntary control.

## The Urethra

The urethra is a thin-walled muscular tube that channels urine to the outside of the body. It extends from the base of the bladder to the external urinary meatus. In females, the urethra is approximately 1.5 inches (3 to 5 cm) long, and the urinary meatus is anterior to the vaginal orifice. In males, the urethra is approximately 8 inches (20 cm) long and serves as a channel for semen as well as urine. The prostate gland encircles the urethra at the base of the bladder in males. The male urinary meatus is located at the end of the glans penis.

## FORMATION OF URINE

The complex structures of the kidneys process about 180 L (47 gal) of blood-derived fluid each day. Of this amount, only 1% is excreted as urine; the rest is returned to the circulation. (The normal characteristics of urine on laboratory analysis are listed in Table 25–1.) Urine formation is accomplished entirely by the nephron through three processes: glomerular filtration, tubular reabsorption, and tubular secretion (Figure 25–5 ■).

## Glomerular Filtration

Glomerular filtration is a passive, nonselective process in which hydrostatic pressure forces fluid and solutes through a membrane. The amount of fluid filtered from the blood into the capsule per minute is called the **glomerular filtration rate (GFR).** Three factors influence this rate: the total surface area available for filtration, the permeability of the filtration membrane, and the net filtration pressure.

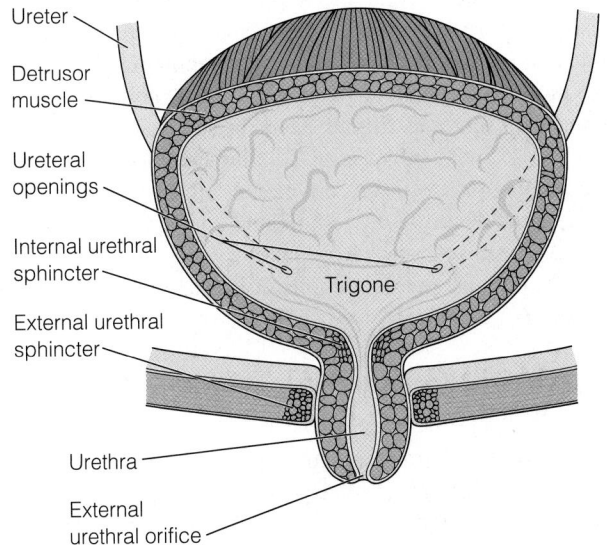

Ureter

Detrusor muscle

Ureteral openings

Internal urethral sphincter

External urethral sphincter

Trigone

Urethra

External urethral orifice

**Figure 25–4** ■ Internal view of the urinary bladder and trigone.

| TABLE 25–1 | Characteristics of Normal Urine |
|---|---|
| Color | Pale to deep yellow, clear |
| Odor | Aromatic |
| Specific gravity | 1.001–1.030 |
| pH | 4.5–8.0 |
| Protein | Negative to trace |
| Glucose | Negative |
| Ketones | Negative |
| WBCs | 0–5/high power field (hpf) |
| RBCs | 0–5/hpf |
| Casts | Negative to occasional |

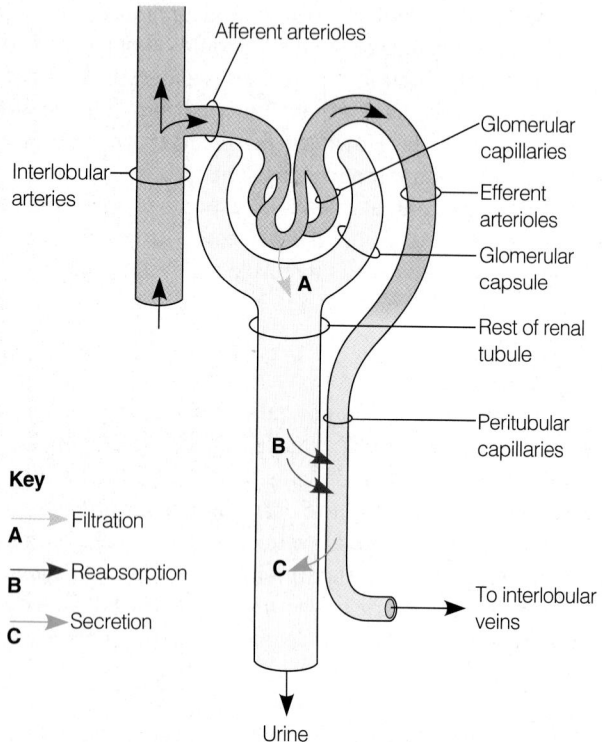

**Key**

A ——▶ Filtration

B ——▶ Reabsorption

C ——▶ Secretion

**Figure 25–5** ■ Schematic view of the three major mechanisms by which the kidneys adjust to the composition of plasma: *A*, glomerular filtration; *B*, tubular reabsorption; and *C*, tubular secretion.

The glomerulus is a far more efficient filter than most capillary beds, because the filtration membrane of the glomerulus is much more permeable to water and solutes than are other capillary membranes. In addition, the glomerular blood pressure is much higher, resulting in higher net filtration pressure.

Net filtration pressure is responsible for the formation of filtrate and is determined by two forces: hydrostatic pressure ("push") and osmotic pressure ("pull"). The glomerular hydrostatic pressure pushes water and solutes across the membrane. This pressure is opposed by the osmotic pressure in the glomerulus (primarily the colloid osmotic pressure of plasma proteins in the glomerular blood) and the capsular hydrostatic pressure exerted by fluids within the glomerular capsule. The difference between these forces determines the net filtration pressure, which is directly proportional to the GFR.

The normal GFR in both kidneys is 120 to 125 mL/min in adults. This rate is held constant under normal conditions by intrinsic controls (or renal autoregulation). The myogenic mechanism, which responds to pressure changes in the renal blood vessels, controls the diameter of the afferent arterioles, thereby achieving autoregulation. An increase in systemic blood pressure causes the renal vessels to constrict, whereas a decline in blood pressure causes the afferent arterioles to dilate. These changes adjust the glomerular hydrostatic pressure and, indirectly, maintain the glomerular filtration rate.

Another intrinsic control of the GFR is the result of the **renin-angiotensin mechanism** at work in the kidneys. Special cells known as the juxtaglomerular apparatus are located in the distal tubules and respond to slow filtrate flow by releasing chemicals that cause intense vasodilation of the afferent arterioles. Conversely, an increase in the flow of filtrate promotes vasoconstriction, decreasing the GFR. A drop in systemic blood pressure often triggers the juxtaglomerular cells to release renin. Renin acts on a plasma globulin, angiotensinogen, to release angiotensin I, which is in turn converted to angiotensin II. As a vasoconstrictor, angiotensin II activates vascular smooth muscle throughout the body, causing systemic blood pressure to rise. Thus, the renin-angiotensin mechanism is a factor in renal autoregulation, even though its main purpose is the control of systemic blood pressure.

Glomerular filtration is also under an extrinsic control mechanism through the sympathetic nervous system. During periods of extreme stress or emergency, sympathetic nervous system stimulation causes strong constriction of the afferent arterioles and inhibits filtrate formation. The sympathetic nervous system also stimulates the juxtaglomerular cells to release renin, increasing systemic blood pressure.

## Tubular Reabsorption

Tubular reabsorption is a transepithelial process that begins as the filtrate enters the proximal tubules. In healthy kidneys, virtually all organic nutrients such as glucose and amino acids are reabsorbed. However, the tubules constantly regulate and adjust the rate and degree of water and ion reabsorption in response to hormonal signals. Reabsorption may be active or passive. Substances reclaimed through active tubular reabsorption are usually moving against electrical and/or chemical gradients. These substances, including glucose, amino acids, lactate, vitamins, and most ions, require an ATP-dependent carrier to be transported into the interstitial space. In passive tubular reabsorption, which includes diffusion and osmosis, substances move along their gradient without expenditure of energy.

## Tubular Secretion

The final process in urine formation is tubular secretion, which is essentially reabsorption in reverse. Substances such as hydrogen and potassium ions, creatinine, ammonia, and organic acids move from the blood of the peritubular capillaries into the tubules themselves as filtrate. Thus, urine consists of both filtered and secreted substances. Tubular secretion is important for disposing of substances not already in the filtrate, such as medications. This process eliminates undesirable substances that have been reabsorbed by passive processes and rids the body of excessive potassium ions. It is also a vital force in the regulation of blood pH.

## MAINTAINING NORMAL COMPOSITION AND VOLUME OF URINE

Maintaining the normal composition and volume of urine involves a countercurrent exchange system. In this system, fluid flows in opposite directions through the parallel tubes of the loop of Henle and the vasa recta, tiny capillaries that run along the loop of Henle. Fluid is exchanged across these parallel membranes in response to a concentration gradient (Figure 25–6 ■). When the filtrate enters the proximal convoluted

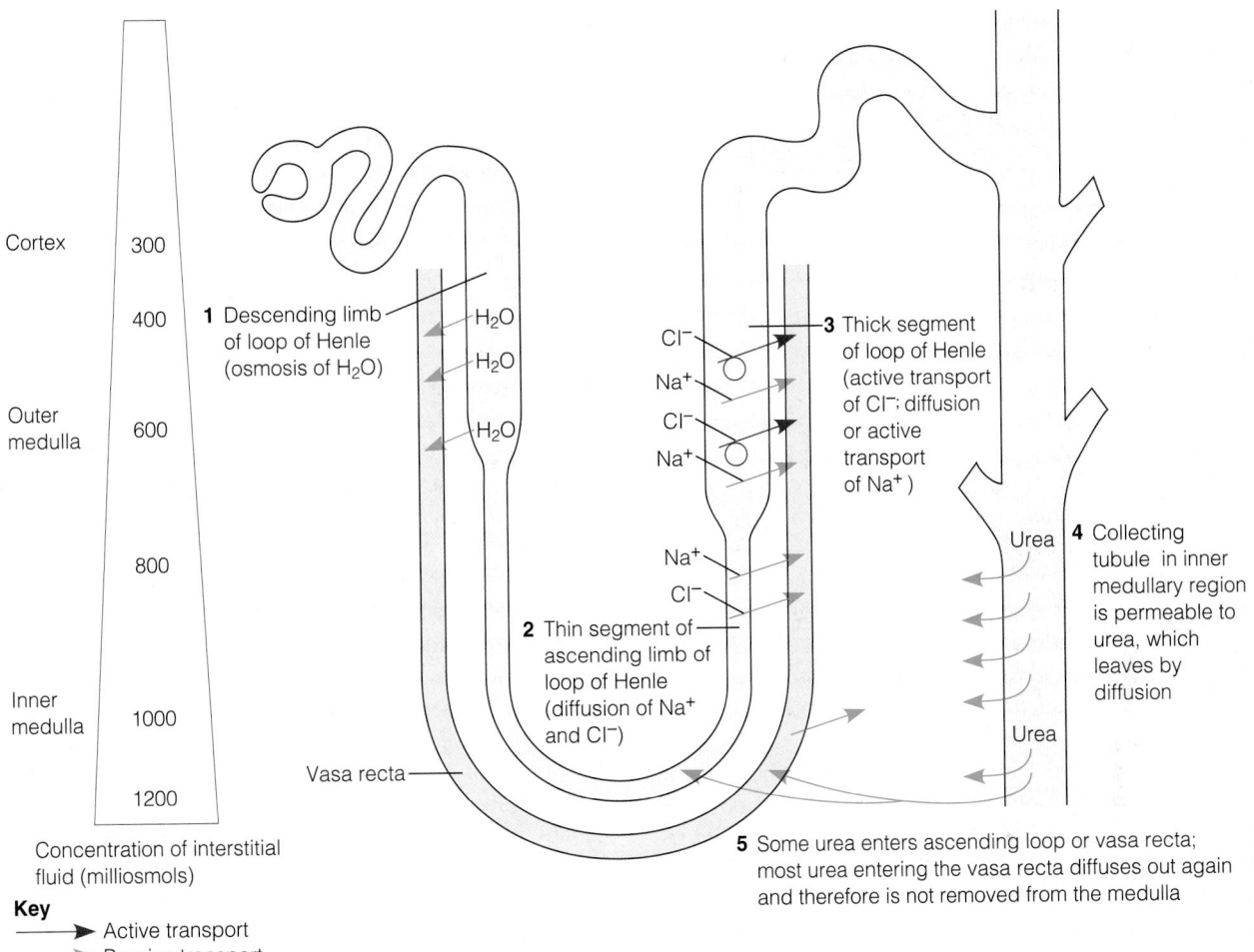

**Figure 25–6** ■ The countercurrent exchange system, responsible for establishing and maintaining an osmotic gradient necessary to the composition, volume, and pH of urine.

tubule, its osmolality (at 300 mOsm/kg) is essentially the same as that of the plasma and the interstitial fluid of the renal cortex. Note the following steps in the process.

1. The descending loop of Henle is highly permeable to water and allows chloride and sodium to enter the loop through diffusion. The hyperosmotic interstitium causes water to move out of the descending loop, so that the remaining filtrate becomes increasingly concentrated.
2. The lumen of the ascending loop of Henle is impermeable to water but allows chloride and sodium to move out into the interstitium of the medulla. As a result, the filtrate in the ascending loop becomes hypo-osmotic, and the medullary interstitium becomes hyperosmotic.
3. As the filtrate progresses through the ascending limb of the loop of Henle and enters the distal convoluted tubule, sodium and chloride are removed and water is retained. Thus, the filtrate becomes more dilute.
4. As the filtrate passes through the deep medullary regions, urea (an end product of protein metabolism and, along with water, the main constituent of urine) begins to diffuse out from the collecting tubules into the interstitial space and establishes a concentration gradient to facilitate water movement.

5. Some urea enters the ascending loop of Henle. Urea entering the vasa recta typically diffuses out again.

The dilution or concentration of urine is largely determined by the action of antidiuretic hormone (ADH), which is secreted by the posterior pituitary gland. ADH causes the pores of the collecting tubules to enlarge, so that increased amounts of water move into the interstitial space. As the end result, water is reabsorbed and urine is more highly concentrated. When ADH is not secreted, the filtrate passes through the system without further water reabsorption, so that the urine is more dilute.

Urine is composed, by volume, of about 95% water and 5% solutes. The largest component of urine by weight is urea. Other solutes normally excreted in the urine include sodium, potassium, phosphate, sulfate, creatinine, uric acid, calcium, magnesium, and bicarbonate.

## CLEARANCE OF WASTE PRODUCTS

The kidneys excrete water-soluble waste products and other chemicals or substances from the body. This process is called renal plasma clearance, which refers to the ability of the kidneys to clear (cleanse) a given amount of plasma of a particular substance in a given time (usually 1 minute). The kidneys clear 25 to 30 g of urea (a nitrogenous waste product formed in the liver from the breakdown of amino acids) each day. They also clear creatinine (an end product of creatine phosphate, found in skeletal muscle), uric acid (a metabolite of nucleic acid metabolism), and ammonia as well as bacterial toxins and water-soluble drugs. Tests of renal clearance are often used to determine the GFR and glomerular damage.

## RENAL HORMONES

Hormones either activated or synthesized by the kidneys include the active form of vitamin D, erythropoietin, and natriuretic hormone.

Vitamin D is necessary for the absorption of calcium and phosphate by the small intestine. In an inactive form, vitamin D enters the body either by dietary intake or through the action of ultraviolet rays on cholesterol in the skin. Activation occurs in two steps, the first in the liver and the second in the kidneys. The renal step is stimulated by parathyroid hormone, which in turn responds to a decreased plasma calcium level.

Erythropoietin stimulates the bone marrow to produce red blood cells in response to tissue hypoxia. The stimulus for the production of erythropoietin by the kidneys is decreased oxygen delivery to kidney cells.

The right atria of the heart releases natriuretic hormone in response to increased volume and stretch, as occurs in increased extracellular volume. This hormone inhibits ADH secretion, so that the collecting tubules are less porous and a large amount of dilute urine is produced.

## ASSESSING URINARY SYSTEM FUNCTION

The nurse conducts both a health assessment interview (to collect subjective data) and a physical assessment (to collect objective data) to assess the function of the urinary system.

## The Health Assessment Interview

This section provides guidelines for collecting subjective data through a health assessment interview specific to urinary elimination. Problems with urinary elimination may be assessed as part of the total health assessment, or may be part of a focused interview if the client has problems specific to the urinary system.

Current urinary status should include the following data.

- Color, odor, and amount of urine
- Difficulty initiating a stream of urine
- Frequency of urination
- Painful urination (**dysuria**)
- Excessive urination at night (**nocturia**)
- Blood in the urine (**hematuria**)
- Voiding scant amounts of urine (**oliguria**)
- Voiding excessive amounts of urine (**polyuria**)
- Discharge
- Flank pain

If you identify a problem with urinary elimination, analyze its onset, characteristics and course, severity, precipitating and relieving factors, and any associated symptoms, noting the timing and circumstances. For example, you may ask the following questions.

- Have you noticed any burning when you urinate?
- Do you have difficulty starting to urinate?
- When did you first notice that you were unable to control the loss of urine from your bladder?

Further explore any abnormalities in the client's current urinary status. Focus questions on changes in patterns of urination, changes in the urine, and pain.

Assess changes in patterns of urination by asking the client these questions: How many times a day do you urinate? Do you feel that you empty your bladder each time? How many times do you get up at night to urinate? Do you experience a very strong desire to urinate and feel that you just cannot wait? Have you noticed that you urinate small amounts of dark, strong-smelling urine?

Changes in the urine that should be explored include the presence of blood or a cloudy appearance of the urine. If the client has noticed blood, explore the use of medications (such as anticoagulants or dye-containing drugs) and other bleeding problems. Women may not understand that blood in the toilet after urination is normal during menstruation. Cloudy, foul-smelling urine often indicates infection (**pyuria**); ask the client about temperature elevations, chills, and general malaise. Cloudy urine in men may result from retrograde ejaculation (when semen is discharged into the bladder instead of from the penis) during intercourse.

If the client reports pain, explore its location, duration, and intensity. Kidney pain is experienced in the back and the costovertebral angle (the angle between the lower ribs and adjacent vertebrae) and may spread toward the umbilicus. Renal colic is severe, sharp, stabbing, and excruciating; often it is felt in the flank, bladder, urethra, testes, or ovaries. Bladder and urethral pain is usually dull and continuous but may be experienced as spasms. The client with a distended bladder experiences constant pain increased by any pressure over the bladder.

Information about surgeries or other treatment of previous urinary problems is essential to the health history, as is a family history of altered structure or function. A family history of renal problems may be the first clue to abnormalities in the client's urinary function. Explore information regarding family occurrence of end-stage renal disease, renal calculi, and frequent infections as well as related problems such as hypertension and diabetes mellitus.

Questions about lifestyle, diet, and work history should explore cigarette smoking, exposure to toxic chemicals, usual fluid intake, type of fluid intake, and self-care measures to replace fluids lost during work or physical activity in hot temperatures.

Interview questions and leading statements, categorized by functional health patterns, can be found on the Companion Website.

## Physical Assessment

Physical assessment of the urinary system may be performed as part of a total health assessment, as part of an abdominal assessment, or as part of the back examination (for the kidneys).

For clients with known or suspected problems of this system, assessment requires the techniques of inspection, palpation, percussion, and auscultation. Auscultate immediately after inspection because percussion or palpation may increase bowel motility and interfere with sound transmission during auscultation.

The equipment necessary to assess the urinary system is a urine specimen cup and disposable gloves. At the beginning of the assessment, the client may be sitting or lying supine. Prior to the examination, collect all necessary equipment and explain the techniques to the client to decrease anxiety.

Before beginning the assessment, ask the client to provide you with a clean-catch urine specimen and give the client a specimen cup. Assess the specimen for color, odor, and clarity before you send it to the laboratory.

Because the examination involves exposure of the genital area, give the client a gown and drape the client appropriately to minimize exposure.

Guidelines for percussion and palpation of the kidneys are outlined in the Box 25–1.

---

**BOX 25–1  ■  Guidelines for Physical Assessment of the Kidneys**

### PERCUSSION OF THE KIDNEYS
Percussion of the kidneys helps assess pain or tenderness. Assist the client to a sitting position, and stand behind the client. For indirect percussion, place the palm of your nondominant hand over the costovertebral angle (see Figure A). Strike this area with the ulnar surface of your dominant hand, curled into a fist (see Figure B). For direct percussion, also strike the area over the costovertebral angle with the ulnar surface of your dominant hand, curled into a fist. Repeat the technique for the other kidney.

You should do percussion of the kidneys with only enough force so the client feels a gentle thud. Percussion is usually done at the end of the assessment.

### PALPATION OF THE KIDNEYS
Although the technique of palpation of the kidneys is outlined here, this technique is best performed by an advanced practitioner, because it involves deep palpation. In addition, the kidneys are difficult to palpate.

Assist the client to the supine position and stand at the right side of the client. To palpate the left kidney, reach across the client and place your left hand under the client's left flank with your palm upward. Elevate the left flank with your fingers, displacing the kidney upward. Ask the client to take a deep breath and use the palmer surface of your right hand to palpate the kidney (Figure C). Repeat the technique for the right kidney.

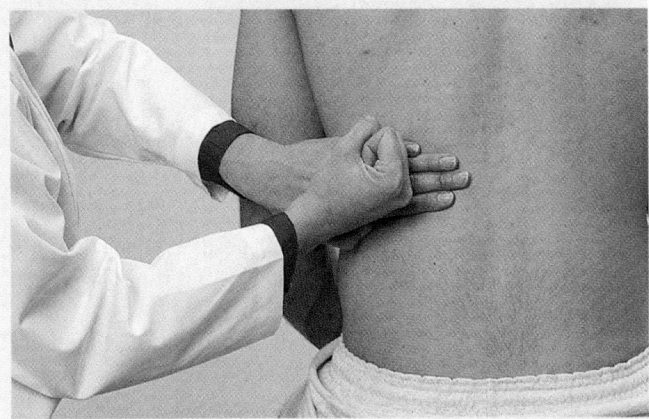

B Percussing the kidney.

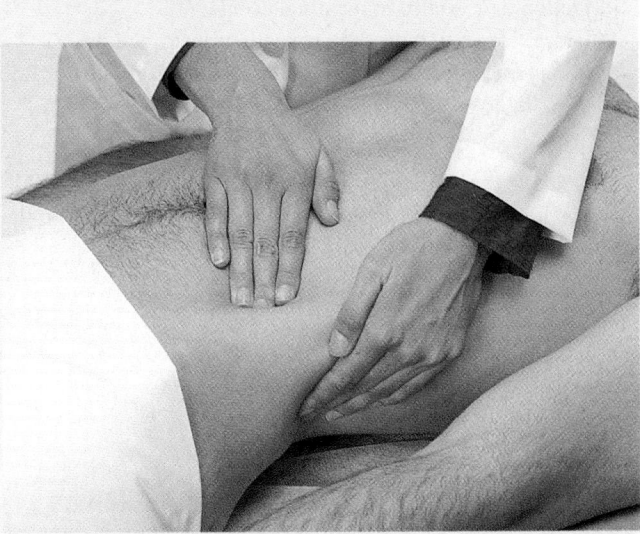

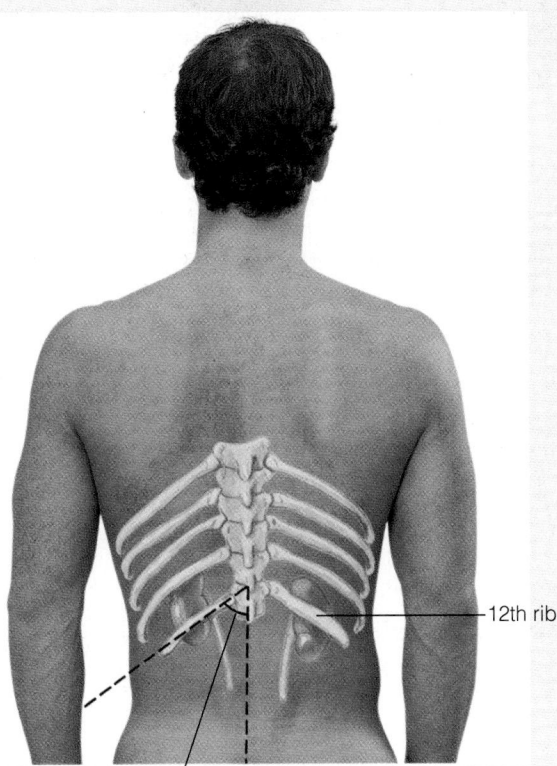

12th rib

Costovertebral angle

A Location of the kidneys and the costovertebral angle.

C Palpating the left kidney.

## Skin Assessment with Abnormal Findings (✓)

- Inspect the skin and mucous membranes, noting color, turgor, and excretions.
  - ✓ Pallor of the skin and mucous membranes may indicate kidney disease with resultant anemia.
  - ✓ Decreased turgor of the skin may indicate dehydration.
  - ✓ Edema may indicate fluid volume excess.

(Either change in turgor may indicate renal insufficiency with either excess fluid loss or retention.)

  - ✓ An accumulation of uric acid crystals, called *uremic frost*, may be seen on the skin of the client with untreated renal failure.

## Abdominal Assessment with Abnormal Findings (✓)

- Inspect the abdomen, noting size, symmetry, masses or lumps, swelling, prominent veins, distention, glistening, or skin tightness.
  - ✓ Enlargements or asymmetry may indicate a hernia or superficial mass.
  - ✓ Prominent veins may indicate renal dysfunction.
  - ✓ Distention, glistening, or skin tightness may be associated with fluid retention.
  - ✓ Ascites is an accumulation of fluid in the peritoneal cavity.

## Urinary Meatus Assessment with Abnormal Findings (✓)

(This technique is not part of a routine assessment, but it is an important component in clients with health problems of the urinary system.)

- For the male client: With the client in a sitting or standing position, compress the tip of the glans penis with your gloved hand to open the urinary meatus (Figure 25–7 ■).
- For the female client: With the client in the dorsal lithotomy position, spread the labia with your gloved hand to expose the urinary meatus.
  - ✓ Increased redness, swelling, or discharge may indicate infection or sexually transmitted disease.
  - ✓ Ulceration may indicate a sexually transmitted disease.
  - ✓ In male clients, a deviation of the meatus from the midline may suggest a congenital defect.

## Kidney Assessment with Abnormal Findings (✓)

- Auscultate the renal arteries by placing the bell of the stethoscope lightly in the areas of the renal arteries, located in the left and right upper abdominal quadrants.

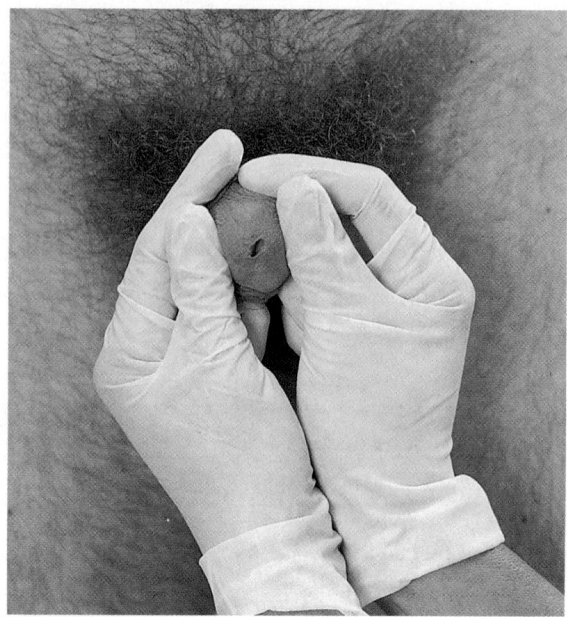

**Figure 25–7** ■ Inspecting the urinary meatus of the male.

  - ✓ Systolic bruits ("whooshing" sounds) may indicate renal artery stenosis.
- Percuss the kidneys for tenderness or pain.
  - ✓ Tenderness and pain on percussion of the costovertebral angle suggest glomerulonephritis or glomerulonephrosis.
- Palpate the kidneys.
  - ✓ A mass or lump may indicate a tumor or cyst.
  - ✓ Tenderness or pain on palpation may suggest an inflammatory process.
  - ✓ A soft kidney that feels spongy may indicate chronic renal disease.
  - ✓ Bilaterally enlarged kidneys may suggest polycystic kidney disease.
  - ✓ Unequal kidney size may indicate hydronephrosis.

## Bladder Assessment with Abnormal Findings (✓)

- Percuss the bladder for tone and position.
  - ✓ A dull percussion tone over the bladder of a client who has just urinated may indicate urinary retention.
- Palpate the bladder (over the symphysis pubis and abdomen) for distention.
  - ✓ A distended bladder may be palpated at any point from the symphysis pubis to the umbilicus and is felt as a firm, rounded organ.

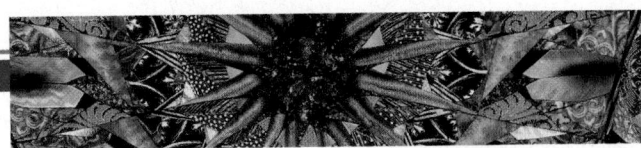

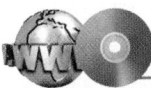 EXPLORE MediaLink

NCLEX review questions, case studies, care plan activities, MediaLink applications, and other interactive resources for this chapter can be found on the Companion Website at www.prenhall.com/lemone.

Click on Chapter 25 to select the activities for this chapter. For animations, video clips, more NCLEX review questions, and an audio glossary, access the Student CD-ROM accompanying this textbook.

## TEST YOURSELF

1. What substance primarily determines the concentration of urine?

   a. Thyroxine
   b. Renin
   c. Aldosterone
   d. ADH

2. What gland encircles the male urethra at the base of the bladder?

   a. Spleen
   b. Pancreas
   c. Prostate
   d. Adrenal

3. Your client tells you of having to get up to void several times a night. You record this finding as:

   a. Polyuria
   b. Nocturia

   c. Dysuria
   d. Hematuria

4. Before beginning the physical examination of the urinary system, you should ask the client to:

   a. Empty the bladder
   b. Take several deep breaths
   c. Collect a clean-catch urine specimen
   d. Drink several glasses of water

5. Following surgery, your client has not voided for 12 hours. What assessment should you make?

   a. Palpate for bladder distention
   b. Auscultate for bowel sounds
   c. Inspect for edema of the urethra
   d. Percuss for gastric tympany

See Test Yourself answers in Appendix C.

## BIBLIOGRAPHY

Bevan, M. (2001). Assessing renal function in older people. *Nursing Older People, 13*(2), 27–28.

Criner, J. (2001). Urinary incontinence in a vulnerable population: Older women. *Seminars in Perioperative Nursing, 10*(1), 33–37.

Edwards, S. (2000). Fluid overload and monitoring indices. *Professional Nurse, 15*(9), 568–572.

Godfrey, K. (1997). Continence: Incontinence in ethnic groups. *Community Nurse, 3*(5), 42.

Gray, M. (2000). Urinary retention. Management in the acute care setting. *American Journal of Nursing, 100*(7), 40–47.

Irwin, B. (2001). Incontinence. *Practice Nurse, 22*(4), 31–32, 43.

Johnson, S. (2000). From incontinence to confidence. *American Journal of Nursing, 100*(2), 69–76.

Kirton, C. (1997). Assessing for bladder distention. *Nursing97, 27*(4), 64.

Lyneham, J. (2001). Physical examination (abdomen, thorax, and lungs): A review. *Australian Journal of Advanced Nursing, 18*(3), 31.

Sheppard, M. (2001). Assessing fluid balance. *Nursing Times, 97* (6 Ntplus), XI–XII.

Weber, J., & Kelley, J. (2002). *Health assessment in nursing.* (2nd ed.). Philadelphia: Lippincott.

Wilson, S., & Giddens, J. (2001). *Health assessment for nursing practice.* St. Louis: Mosby.

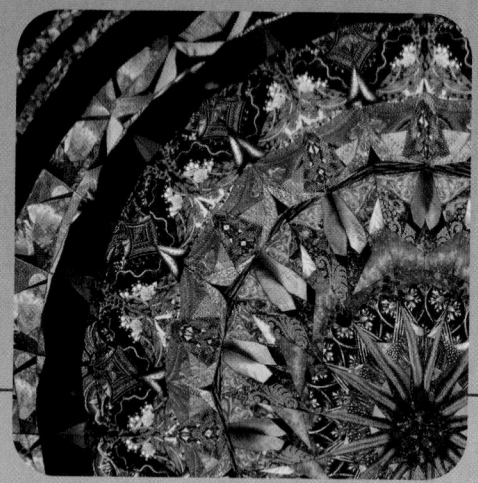

# CHAPTER 26

# Nursing Care of Clients with Urinary Tract Disorders

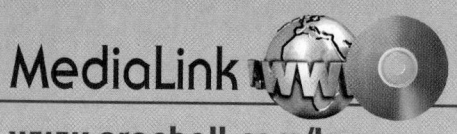

## www.prenhall.com/lemone

Additional resources for this chapter can be found on the Student CD-ROM accompanying this textbook, and on the Companion Website at www.prenhall.com/lemone. Click on Chapter 26 to select the activities for this chapter.

**CD-ROM**
- Audio Glossary
- NCLEX Review

**Companion Website**
- More NCLEX Review
- Case Study
  Urinary Tract Infection
- Care Plan Activity
  Urinary Tract Infection
- MediaLink Application
  Urinary Tract Disorders

## LEARNING OUTCOMES

After completing this chapter, you will be able to:

- Apply knowledge of the structure and function of the urinary tract to caring for clients with urinary tract disorders.

- Describe the pathophysiology of commonly occurring urinary tract disorders.

- Identify laboratory and diagnostic tests used to diagnose disorders affecting the urinary tract.

- Compare and contrast the manifestations of common urinary tract disorders.

- Discuss the nursing implications of medications prescribed for clients with urinary tract disorders.

- Provide appropriate nursing care for clients having surgery of the urinary tract.

- Use the nursing process as a framework for providing individualized care to clients with urinary tract disorders.

The urinary system includes the kidneys, ureters, urinary bladder, and urethra. This organ system can be affected by a variety of disorders, including congenital malformations, infections, obstructions, trauma, tumors, and neurologic conditions. Any portion of the system—from the kidney through the urethra—can be affected with serious or even life-threatening consequences unless the problem is appropriately diagnosed and treated. Kidney disorders can affect urine production and waste elimination directly, and are discussed in the next chapter. Disorders of the **urinary drainage system** (the kidney pelvis, ureters, bladder, and urethra) may obstruct urine flow or spread to the kidneys, affecting urine production and elimination. The anatomy and physiology and nursing assessment related to the urinary tract is presented in Chapter 25.

When caring for clients with urinary tract disorders, it is important to consider the client's modesty in voiding, possible difficulty in discussing the genitals, embarrassment about being exposed for examination and testing, and fear of changes in body image or function. These psychosocial issues may interfere with the client's willingness to seek help, discuss treatment, and learn about preventive measures.

Nursing interventions for clients with urinary tract disorders are directed toward primary prevention, early detection, and management of the disorder through health teaching and nursing care.

## THE CLIENT WITH A URINARY TRACT INFECTION

Bacterial infections of the urinary tract are a common reason for seeking health services, second only to upper respiratory infections. More than 8 million people are treated annually for urinary tract infection (UTI) (Porth, 2002). Community-acquired UTIs are common in young women, and unusual in men under the age of 50.

Most community-acquired UTIs are caused by *Escherichia coli,* a common gram-negative enteral bacteria. About 10% to 15% of symptomatic UTIs are caused by *Staphylococcus saprophyticus,* a gram-positive organism. Catheter-associated UTIs often involve other gram-negative bacteria such as *Proteus, Klebsiella, Seratia,* and *Pseudomonas.*

### PHYSIOLOGY REVIEW

The urinary tract is normally sterile above the urethra. Adequate urine volume, a free flow from the kidneys through the urinary meatus, and complete bladder emptying are the most important mechanisms maintaining sterility. Pathogens that enter and contaminate the distal urethra are washed out during voiding. Other defenses for maintaining sterile urine include its normal acidity and bacteriostatic properties of the bladder and urethral cells. The peristaltic activity of the ureters and a competent ureterovesical junction help maintain sterility of the upper urinary tract. As the ureter enters the bladder, its distal portion tunnels between the mucosa and muscle layers of the bladder wall (Figure 26–1 ■). During voiding, increased *intra-*

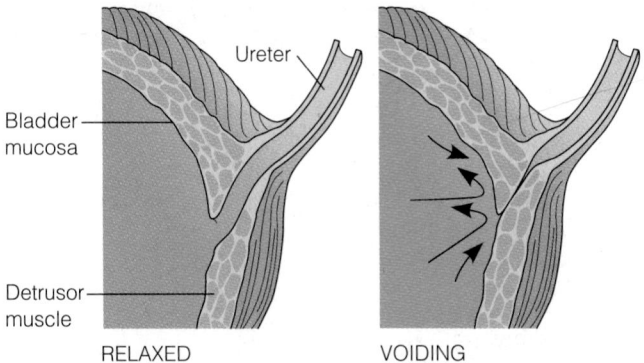

Figure 26–1  ■  A competent ureterovesical junction. Note how increased intravesicular pressure during voiding occludes the distal portion of the ureter, preventing reflux.

*vesicular* (within the bladder) pressure compresses the ureter, preventing **reflux,** or backflow of urine toward the kidneys. In males, a long urethra and the antibacterial effect of zinc in prostatic fluid also help prevent contamination of this normally sterile environment.

## PATHOPHYSIOLOGY AND MANIFESTATIONS

Pathogens usually enter the urinary tract by ascending from the mucous membranes of the perineal area into the lower urinary tract. Bacteria that have colonized the urethra, vagina, or perineal tissues are the usual source of infection (Porth, 2002). From the bladder, bacteria may continue to ascend the urinary tract, eventually infecting the *parenchyma* (functional tissue) of the kidneys (Braunwald et al., 2001). Hematogenous spread of infection to the urinary tract is rare. Infections introduced in this manner are usually associated with previous damage or scarring of the urinary tract. Bacteria introduced into the urinary tract may cause asymptomatic bacteriuria or in an inflammatory response with manifestations of UTI.

Urinary tract infections can be categorized in several ways. Anatomically, UTIs may affect the lower or the upper urinary tract. Lower urinary tract infections include *urethritis,* inflammation of the urethra; *prostatitis,* inflammation of the prostate gland (discussed in Chapter 47); and **cystitis,** inflammation of the urinary bladder. The most common upper urinary tract infection is **pyelonephritis,** inflammation of the kidney and renal pelvis. The infection may involve superficial tissues such as the bladder mucosa, or may invade other tissues such as prostate or renal tissues. Epidemiologically, UTIs are identified as community acquired or nosocomial, associated with catheterization.

Clients can be predisposed to UTI by a variety of factors (Box 26–1). Some risk factors cannot be changed (e.g., aging and the short urethra of the female). In women, sexual activity increases the risk for UTI, as bacteria are introduced into the bladder via the urethra during sexual intercourse. Use of spermicidal compounds with a diaphragm, cervical cap, or condom alters the normal bacterial flora of the vagina and perineal tissues, and further increases the risk for UTI. Some females lack a normally protective mucosal enzyme and have decreased

| BOX 26–1 ■ Risk Factors for UTI |
| --- |

**FEMALE**
- Short, straight urethra
- Proximity of urinary meatus to vagina and anus
- Sexual intercourse
- Use of diaphragm and spermicidal compounds for birth control
- Pregnancy

**MALE**
- Uncircumsized
- Prostatic hypertrophy
- Rectal intercourse

**BOTH**
- Aging
- Urinary tract obstruction
- Neurogenic bladder dysfunction
- Vesicoureteral reflux
- Genetic factors
- Catheterization

levels of cervicovaginal antibodies to enterobacteria, further increasing their risk. Prostatic hypertrophy and bacterial prostatitis are risk factors among males. Circumcision appears to have a protective effect. Anal intercourse also is a risk factor for men. Congenital or acquired factors contributing to the risk of infection include urinary tract obstruction by tumors or calculi, structural abnormalities such as strictures, impaired bladder innervation, bowel incontinence, and chronic diseases such as diabetes mellitus. Instrumentation of the urinary tract (e.g., catheterization or cystoscopy) is a major risk factor for UTI. Even when performed under strict aseptic conditions, catheterization can result in bladder infection. The placement of the catheter prevents the flushing action of voiding, and bacteria may ascend to the bladder either through the catheter lumen or via exudate between the urethral mucosa and the catheter.

Older clients have an increased incidence of UTI. The greatest degree of increase is seen in men, as the ratio of female to male UTI in older adults changes from 50:1 to less than 5:1. An increased risk of urinary stasis, chronic disease states (such as diabetes mellitus), and an impaired immune response contribute to the higher incidence of UTI in the older adult. In men, the prostate typically hypertrophies with aging, potentially resulting in urinary retention as the urethra narrows. Prostatic secretions are lessened, diminishing their protective, antibacterial effect. In older women, loss of tissue elasticity and weakening of perineal muscles often contribute to the development of a cystocele or rectocele. Resulting changes in bladder and urethral position increase the risk of incomplete bladder emptying.

## Cystitis

Cystitis, inflammation of the urinary bladder, is the most common UTI. The infection tends to remain superficial, involving the bladder mucosa. The mucosa becomes hyperemic (red) and may hemorrhage. The inflammatory response causes pus to form. This process causes the classic manifestations associated with cystitis (see the box below). Typical presenting symptoms of cystitis include **dysuria** (painful or difficult urination), urinary frequency and **urgency** (a sudden, compelling need to urinate), and **nocturia** (voiding two or more times at night). In addition, the urine may have a foul odor and appear cloudy (*pyuria*) or bloody (**hematuria**) because of mucus, excess white cells in the urine, and bleeding of the inflamed bladder wall. Suprapubic pain and tenderness also may be present.

Older clients may not experience the classic symptoms of cystitis. Instead, they often present with nonspecific manifestations such as nocturia, incontinence, confusion, behavior change, lethargy, anorexia, or "just not feeling right." Fever may be present; however, hypothermia also may develop in an older adult.

Cystitis occurs most frequently in adult females, usually because of colonization of the bladder by bacteria normally found in the lower gastrointestinal tract. These bacteria gain entry by ascending the short, straight female urethra. In addition to the risk factors listed in Box 26–1, personal hygiene practices and voluntary urinary retention can contribute to the risk for UTI in women.

Although the bacteriostatic effect of prostatic fluid and a longer urethra provide an effective barrier to bladder infection for adult males, prostatic hypertrophy commonly associated with aging increases the risk of cystitis in elderly males. An enlarged prostate can impede urine flow, leading to incomplete bladder emptying and urinary stasis. Bacteria are not completely flushed with voiding, allowing colonization of the bladder.

Cystitis is usually uncomplicated and readily responds to treatment. When left untreated, the infection can ascend to involve the kidneys. Severe or prolonged infection may lead to sloughing of bladder mucosa and ulcer formation. Chronic cystitis can lead to bladder stones (discussed later in this chapter).

## Catheter-Associated UTI

At least 10% to 15% of hospitalized clients with indwelling urinary catheters develop bacteriuria. The longer the catheter remains in place, the greater the risk for infection. Bacteria, including *E. coli, Proteus, Pseudomonas, Klebsiella,* and others, reach the bladder by either migrating through the column of urine within the catheter or by moving up the mucous sheath of the urethra outside the catheter (Braunwald et al., 2001). Bacteria enter the catheter system at the connection between the catheter and drainage system or through the emptying tube of the drainage bag. Colonization of perineal skin by bowel flora is a common source of infection in catheterized women.

Catheter-associated UTIs often are asymptomatic. Gram-negative bacteremia is the most significant complication asso-

| Manifestations of Cystitis | |
| --- | --- |
| • Dysuria | • Pyuria |
| • Frequency | • Hematuria |
| • Urgency | • Suprapubic discomfort |
| • Nocturia | |

## Nursing Research

### Evidence-Based Practice for Intermittent Catheterization

Urinary tract infection is a common complication in clients with spinal cord injury (SCI). Intermittent catheterization has significantly reduced the incidence of UTI in this client population; however, maintaining sterile technique requires using a new kit for each catheterization and may be cost prohibitive. Clean (nonsterile) intermittent catheterization is the method most frequently used to manage neurogenic bladder. The cost of nonsterile intermittent catheterization is significantly lower than that of sterile intermittent catheterization, as the catheter is cleaned and reused for up to 1 week. A study by Prieto-Fingerhut et al. (1997) found that sterile intermittent catheterization resulted in a lower rate of UTI (although the difference was not statistically significant) and reduced costs for antibiotic therapy. While the rate of infection in the nonsterile catheterization group was higher, the cost of catheterization supplies was significantly lower.

### IMPLICATIONS FOR NURSING

Several factors should be considered when choosing to use sterile versus nonsterile technique for intermittent catheterization. While the cost of sterile supplies is higher, the incidence of urinary tract infection and the need for antibiotic therapy is reduced by using sterile technique. Other factors that should be considered include the client's immune status and the potential for delaying the client's rehabilitation following SCI during UTI treatment.

### Critical Thinking in Client Care

1. Why is intermittent catheterization (using either clean or sterile technique) associated with a lower rate of UTI than that for indwelling catheters?
2. Sterile technique generally is used when catheterizing clients in acute care settings. Would clean technique be appropriate in this situation? Why or why not?

*Note. From "A Study Comparing Sterile and Nonsterile Urethral Catheterization in Patients with Spinal Cord Injury" by T. Prieto-Fingerhut, K. Banoveac, and C. M. Lynne, 1997, Rehabilitation Nursing, 22(6), 299–302.*

---

ciated with these UTIs. Most catheter-associated UTIs resolve quickly when the catheter is removed and a short course of antibiotic is administered. Intermittent catheterization carries a lower risk of infection than does an indwelling catheter, and is preferred for clients who are unable to empty their bladder by voiding (see the Nursing Research box above).

## Pyelonephritis

Pyelonephritis is inflammation of the renal pelvis and *parenchyma,* the functional kidney tissue. *Acute pyelonephritis* is a bacterial infection of the kidney; *chronic pyelonephritis* is associated with nonbacterial infections and inflammatory processes that may be metabolic, chemical, or immunologic in origin.

### Acute Pyelonephritis

Acute pyelonephritis usually results from an infection that ascends to the kidney from the lower urinary tract. Asymptomatic

## Manifestations of Acute Pyelonephritis

| URINARY | SYSTEMIC |
|---|---|
| • Urinary frequency | • Vomiting |
| • Dysuria | • Diarrhea |
| • Pyuria | • Acute fever |
| • Hematuria | • Shaking chills |
| • Flank pain | • Malaise |
| • Costovertebral tenderness | |

bacteriuria or cystitis can lead to acute pyelonephritis. Risk factors include pregnancy (because of slowed ureteral peristalsis), urinary tract obstruction, and congenital malformation. Urinary tract trauma, scarring, calculi (stones), kidney disorders such as polycystic or hypertensive kidney disease, and chronic diseases such as diabetes may also contribute to pyelonephritis. *Vesicoureteral reflux,* a condition in which urine moves from the bladder back toward the kidney, is a common risk factor in children who develop pyelonephritis and is also seen in adults when bladder outflow is obstructed.

The infection spreads from the renal pelvis to the renal cortex. The pelvis, calyces, and medulla of the kidney are primarily affected, with white blood cell infiltration and inflammation. The kidney becomes grossly edematous. Localized abscesses may develop on the cortical surface of the kidney (Bullock & Henze, 2000). As with cystitis, *E. coli* is the organism responsible for 85% of the cases of acute pyelonephritis. Other organisms commonly found include *Proteus* and *Klebsiella,* bacteria that normally inhabit the intestinal tract.

The onset of acute pyelonephritis is typically rapid, with chills and fever, malaise, vomiting, flank pain, costovertebral tenderness, urinary frequency, and dysuria (see the Manifestations box above). Symptoms of cystitis also may be present. The older adult may present with a change in behavior, acute confusion, incontinence, or a general deterioration in condition.

### Chronic Pyelonephritis

Chronic pyelonephritis involves chronic inflammation and scarring of the tubules and interstitial tissues of the kidney (Bullock & Henze, 2000). It is a common cause of chronic renal failure. It may develop as a result of UTIs or other conditions that damage the kidneys, such as hypertension or vascular conditions, severe vesicoureteral reflux, or obstruction of the urinary tract.

The client with chronic pyelonephritis may be asymptomatic or have mild manifestations such as urinary frequency, dysuria, and flank pain. Hypertension can develop as kidney tissue is destroyed.

## COLLABORATIVE CARE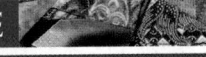

Treatment of UTI focuses on eliminating the causative organism, preventing relapse or reinfection, and identifying and correcting any contributing factors. Drug treatment with antibiotics and urinary anti-infectives is commonly used. In some cases, surgery may be indicated to correct contributing factors.

## Diagnostic Tests

Laboratory testing for UTI includes:

- *Urinalysis* to assess for pyuria, bacteria, and blood cells in the urine. A bacteria count greater than 100,000 ($10^5$) per milliliter is indicative of infection. Rapid tests for bacteria in the urine include using a *nitrite dipstick* (which turns pink in the presence of bacteria) and the *leukocyte esterase test,* an indirect method of detecting bacteria by identifying lysed or intact white blood cells (WBCs) in the urine.

  Urine should be a midstream clean-catch specimen; if necessary, straight catheterization or "mini-cath," with strict aseptic technique may be used. Catheterization is avoided if possible to reduce the risk of further infection.
- *Gram stain of the urine* may be done to identify the infecting organism by shape and characteristic (Gram positive or negative).
- *Urine culture and sensitivity* tests may be ordered to identify the infecting organism and the most effective antibiotic. Culture requires 24 to 72 hours, so treatment to eliminate the most common organisms often is initiated without culture.
- *WBC with differential* may be done to detect typical changes associated with infection, such as *leukocytosis* (elevated WBC) and increased numbers of neutrophils.

In men and in adult women with recurrent infections or persistent bacteriuria, additional diagnostic testing may be ordered to evaluate for structural abnormalities and other contributing factors.

- *Intravenous pyelography (IVP),* also known as *excretory urography,* is used to evaluate the structure and excretory function of the kidneys, ureters, and bladder. As the kidneys clear an intravenously injected contrast medium from the blood, the size and shape of the kidneys, their calices and pelvises, the ureters, and the bladder can be evaluated, and structural or functional abnormalities, such as vesicoureteral reflux, may be detected.
- *Voiding cystourethrography* involves instilling contrast medium into the bladder, then using X-rays to assess the bladder and urethra when filled and during voiding. This study can detect structural or functional abnormalities of the bladder and urethral strictures. This test has a lower risk of allergic response to the contrast dye than IVP.
- *Cystoscopy,* direct visualization of the urethra and bladder through a cystoscope, may be used to diagnose conditions such as prostatic hypertrophy, urethral strictures, bladder calculi, tumors, polyps or diverticula, and congenital abnormalities. A tissue biopsy may be obtained during the procedure, and other interventions performed (e.g., stone removal or stricture dilation).
- *Manual pelvic* or *prostate examinations* are done to assess for structural changes of the genitourinary tract, such as prostatic enlargement, cystocele, or rectocele.

Nursing implications for these diagnostic procedures are presented in the following box.

## Nursing Implications for Diagnostic Tests

### The Client with UTI

#### INTRAVENOUS PYELOGRAPHY (IVP)
**Preparation**
- Assess knowledge and understanding of procedure, clarifying information as needed.
- Schedule IVP prior to any ordered barium test or gallbladder studies using contrast material.
- Ask about allergy to seafood, iodine, or radiologic contrast dye. Notify physician or radiologist if allergies are known.
- Verify the presence of a signed consent for the procedure.
- Assess renal and fluid status, including serum osmolality, creatinine, and blood urea nitrogen (BUN) levels. Notify the physician of any abnormal values.
- Instruct the client to complete ordered pretest bowel preparation, including prescribed laxative or cathartic (see page 624) the evening before the test, and an enema or suppository the morning of the test. Withhold food for 8 hours prior to the test; clear liquids are allowed.
- Obtain baseline vital signs and record.

**After the Test**
- Monitor vital signs and urine output.
- Report manifestations of delayed reaction to the contrast media such as dyspnea, tachycardia, itching, hives, or flushing.

**Client and Family Teaching**
- X-rays and a dye that is rapidly excreted in the urine are used to show the structures of the kidney, ureters, and bladder. The test takes about 30 minutes.
- A laxative and possibly an enema or suppository are used before the test to clear the bowel of feces and gas. Do not eat after the ordered time the evening before the test; you may drink clear fluids such as water, coffee, or tea (without creamer).
- As the dye is injected, you may feel a transient flushing or burning sensation, along with possible nausea and a metallic taste.
- Notify your doctor immediately if you develop a rash, difficulty breathing, rapid heart rate, or hives during or after the test.
- Increase fluid intake after the test is completed.

#### VOIDING CYSTOURETHROGRAPHY
**Preparation**
- Assess knowledge and understanding of the procedure, clarifying information as needed.
- Verify the presence of a signed consent for the procedure.
- Ask about allergy to seafood, iodine, or radiologic contrast dye. Notify physician or radiologist if allergies are known. Because the dye is not injected, allergic reactions are rare, and allergy does not contraindicate the examination.
- Instruct to consume only clear liquids the morning of the exam, or as recommended by radiology.
- Insert indwelling catheter if ordered.

**Client and Family Teaching**
- The bladder is filled with dye solution and X-rays are taken of the filled bladder and of the bladder and urethra during urination.

## Nursing Implications for Diagnostic Tests

### The Client with UTI (continued)

- This procedure causes little or no discomfort and takes approximately 30 to 45 minutes to complete.
- After the procedure, increase your fluid intake to help eliminate the contrast dye and to reduce burning on urination.
- Report signs of infection, such as frequency, urgency, painful urination, cloudy or bloody urine, or malodorous urine.

### CYSTOSCOPY

#### Preparation

- Assess knowledge and understanding of the procedure, clarifying information as needed.
- Verify the presence of a signed consent for the procedure.
- Instruct in pretest preparation as ordered, including prescribed laxatives the evening prior to the test and any ordered food or fluid restrictions.
- Administer sedation and other medications as ordered prior to the test.

#### Client and Family Teaching

- Cystoscopy is performed in a special cystoscopy room, using local or general anesthesia. You may feel some pressure or a need to urinate as the scope is inserted through the urethra into the bladder. The procedure takes approximately 30 to 45 minutes.
- Do not attempt to stand without assistance immediately after the procedure as you may feel dizzy or faint.
- Burning on urination for a day or two after the procedure is to be expected.
- Immediately notify the physician if your urine remains bloody for more than three voidings after the procedure, or if you develop bright bleeding, low urine output, abdominal or flank pain, chills, or fever.
- Warm sitz baths, analgesic agents, and antispasmodic medications may relieve discomfort after the procedure.
- Increase fluid intake to decrease pain and difficulty voiding and reduce the risk of infection.
- Laxatives may be ordered after the procedure to prevent constipation and straining, which may cause urinary tract bleeding.

## Medications

Most uncomplicated infections of the lower urinary tract can be treated with a short course of antibiotic therapy. Upper urinary tract infections, in contrast, usually require longer treatment (2 or more weeks) to eradicate the infecting organism.

Short-course therapy (either a single antibiotic dose or a 3-day course of treatment) reduces treatment cost, increases compliance, and has a lower rate of side effects. Single dose therapy is associated with a higher rate of recurrent infection and continued vaginal colonization with *E. coli*, making a 3-day course of treatment the preferred option for uncomplicated cystitis. Oral trimethoprim-sulfamethoxazole (TMP-SMZ), TMP, or a quinolone antibiotic such as ciprofloxacin (Cipro) or enoxacin (Penetrex) may be ordered.

Men and women with pyelonephritis, urinary tract abnormalities or stones, or a history of previous infections with antibiotic-resistant infections require a 7 to 10 day course of TMP-SMZ, ciprofloxacin, ofloxacin (Floxin), or an alternate antibiotic. The client with severe illness may need hospitalization. Intravenous ciprofloxacin, gentamicin, ceftriaxone (Rocephin), or ampicillin may be prescribed for severe illness or sepsis associated with UTI. See Chapter 8 for the nursing implications for antibiotic therapy.

The outcome of treatment for UTI is determined by follow-up urinalysis and culture. *Cure*, as evidenced by no pathogens present in the urine, is the desired outcome. When therapy fails to eradicate bacteria in the urine, it is known as *unresolved bacteriuria*. *Persistent bacteriuria* or *relapse* occurs when a persistent source of infection causes repeated infection after initial cure. *Reinfection* is the development of a new infection with a different pathogen following successful UTI treatment (Tierney et al., 2001).

Clients who experience frequent symptomatic UTIs may be treated with prophylactic antibiotic therapy with a drug such as TMP-SMZ, TMP, or nitrofurantoin (Furadantin, Nitrofan). TMP and nitrofurantoin do not achieve effective plasma concentrations at recommended doses, but do reach effective concentrations in the urine. Nitrofurantoin also may be used to treat UTI in pregnant women. Nursing implications for these urinary anti-infectives and for phenazopyridine (Pyridium), a urinary analgesic, are outlined on page 710.

Antibiotics and urinary anti-infectives are not generally recommended to treat asymptomatic bacteriuria in catheterized clients. The preferred treatment for catheter-associated UTI is removal of the indwelling catheter followed by a 10 to 14 day course of antibiotic therapy to eliminate the infection.

## Surgery

Surgery may be indicated for recurrent UTI if diagnostic testing indicates calculi, structural anomalies, or strictures that contribute to the risk of infection. Table 26–1 lists major causes of urinary tract obstruction that may contribute to UTI.

**TABLE 26–1  Major Causes of Urinary Tract Obstruction by Location**

| Location | Obstructive Process |
|---|---|
| Kidney pelvis | Calculi<br>Polycystic kidney disease<br>Infection and scarring |
| Ureters | Calculi<br>Scarring and stricture<br>Congenital defects or strictures<br>External processes such as pregnancy, tumors, lymph node enlargement |
| Bladder | Neurogenic bladder<br>Tumors<br>Calculi and other foreign bodies |
| Urethra | Benign prostatic hypertrophy<br>Tumors<br>Scarring and stricture<br>Trauma |

# Medication Administration
## Urinary Anti-Infectives and Analgesics

### URINARY ANTI-INFECTIVES

Nitrofurantoin (Furadantin; Macrodantin)
Trimethoprim (Proloprim, Trimpex)

Urinary anti-infectives are usually used prophylactically to prevent recurrence of UTI in clients with frequent symptomatic infections. Nitrofurantoin also may be used to treat UTI in pregnant women.

### Nursing Responsibilities

- Ensure adequate fluid intake (1500 to 2000 mL per day) to maintain a urine output of at least 1500 mL of urine per 24 hours. Do not overhydrate.
- Administer with meals to minimize GI side effects, such as nausea, gastric upset, and abdominal cramping.
- Trimethoprim is contraindicated for use in clients with renal or hepatic impairment; nitrofurantoin is contraindicated for clients with impaired renal function. Report abnormal laboratory values such as elevated creatinine or BUN, bilirubin, alanine aminotransferase (ALT), aspartate aminotransferase (AST), and lactic dehydrogenase (LDH).
- Use with caution in older or chronically ill clients. Monitor closely for adverse effects.
- Do not administer trimethoprim to pregnant women because of possible adverse effects on the fetus.
- Monitor the client taking nitrofurantoin for an acute or chronic pulmonary reaction with manifestations of dyspnea, cough, chills, fever, and chest pain. Discontinue the drug and notify the physician.
- Nitrofurantoin may cause peripheral neuropathy, especially in older clients and adult diabetics. Notify the physician if symptoms develop.
- Nitrofurantoin oral suspension may stain the teeth; have the client rinse the mouth thoroughly after administering.
- Monitor for signs of phenytoin toxicity (sedation, ataxia, and increased blood levels) if trimethoprim is given concurrently. Phenytoin doses may need to be reduced.

### Client and Family Teaching

- These drugs are used along with hygiene practices to prevent recurrent UTI. Take as directed, even when no symptoms are present.

- Drink six to eight glasses of water or fluid per day while taking these drugs.
- Take the drug with meals or food to reduce gastric effects; however, avoid milk products because they may interfere with absorption.
- Trimethoprim should not be taken during pregnancy. Contact your physician before attempting to become pregnant.
- Contact your doctor if you develop any of the following: chest pain, difficulty breathing, cough, chills, and fever; numbness and tingling or weakness of the extremities; rash or pruritus (itching).
- If you are taking an oral suspension of nitrofurantoin, rinse your mouth thoroughly after each dose to avoid staining the teeth.
- Nitrofurantoin turns the urine brown. This is not harmful and subsides when the drug is discontinued.
- If you are taking trimethoprim along with phenytoin (Dilantin) or a related anticonvulsant, contact your doctor if you become sedated or begin to stagger.

### URINARY ANALGESIC

Phenazopyridine (Pyridium)

Phenazopyridine is a urinary tract analgesic that may be used for symptomatic relief of the pain, burning, frequency, and urgency associated with UTI during the first 24 to 48 hours of therapy. Its use is somewhat controversial, because it does not treat the infection and may delay effective treatment in the client with recurrent UTI who saves a dose or two "for the next time."

### Nursing Responsibilities

- Monitor renal function (urine output, weight, serum creatinine, and BUN) during treatment; report changes.
- Stop the drug and contact the physician if sclera or skin become yellow-tinged. This may indicate reduced excretion and toxicity.

### Client and Family Teaching

- Take with meals to minimize gastric upset.
- This drug turns urine orange or red. Protect your clothing from staining.
- Promptly contact your doctor if symptoms of UTI recur; do not take phenazopyridine before you seek medical treatment.
- If you notice a yellow tinge to your skin or eyes, stop taking the drug and notify the physician.

---

Stones, or *calculi,* in the renal pelvis or in the bladder are an irritant and provide a matrix for bacterial colonization. Treatment may include surgical removal of a large calculus from the renal pelvis or cystoscopic removal of bladder calculi. *Percutaneous ultrasonic pyelolithotomy* or *extracorporeal shock wave lithotripsy (ESWL)* (described in the next section of this chapter) may be used instead of surgery to crush and remove stones. (See page 709 for nursing care related to cystoscopy.)

**Ureteroplasty,** surgical repair of a ureter, may be indicated for structural abnormality or stricture of a ureter. This may be combined with a ureteral reimplantation if vesicoureteral reflux is present. The client returns from these surgeries with an indwelling urinary catheter (Foley or suprapubic) and a **ureteral stent** (a thin catheter inserted into the ureter to provide for urine flow and ureteral support), which remains in place for 3 to 5 days. Care of the client with a ureteral stent is outlined in the box on the next page.

## Complementary Therapies

Complementary therapies such as aromatherapy or herbal preparations may be used in conjunction with antibiotics to treat UTI. Adding bergamot, sandalwood, lavender, or juniper oil to bath water helps relieve the discomfort of UTI. Herbal supplements such as saw palmetto have a urinary antiseptic

# NURSING CARE OF THE CLIENT WITH A URETERAL STENT

Ureteral stents are used to maintain patency and promote healing of the ureters (see figure below). A stent may be temporary, used during and after a surgical procedure, or it may be used for longer periods in clients with ureteral obstruction due to tumors, strictures, or other causes.

Stents may be positioned during surgery or cystoscopy. They are made of a nontoxic material such as silicone or polyurethane,

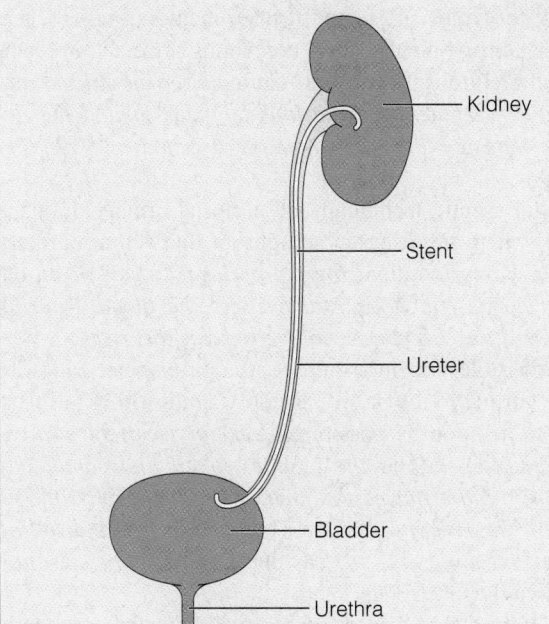

Kidney

Stent

Ureter

Bladder

Urethra

with side drainage holes placed along the length of the stent. Stents are radiopaque for easy radiographic identification. One or both ends of the stent may be pigtail or J-shaped to prevent migration.

- Label all drainage tubes including stents for easy identification. Attach each catheter and stent to a separate closed drainage system. *Careful labeling allows close monitoring of output from all sources and reservoirs. Separate drainage systems minimize the risk of infection.*
- If the stent has been brought to the surface, secure it and maintain its position. *The stent is usually placed in the renal pelvis. It is important to secure it well to prevent trauma to the kidney, inadvertent removal of the stent, and ureter obstruction.*
- Monitor urine output, including color, consistency, and odor. Monitor for signs of infection or bleeding: fever, tachycardia, pain, hematuria, and cloudy or malodorous urine. *The stent facilitates urine flow but may become obstructed because of bleeding, calculi, or sediment. Obstruction may result in hydronephrosis and kidney damage. The stent itself is a foreign body in the urinary tract and can increase the risk of UTI.*
- Maintain fluid intake, encouraging fluids that acidify urine, such as apple and cranberry juice. *The stent can precipitate calculus formation as well as UTI. Increasing fluid intake and acidifying the urine help prevent these complications.*
- For an indwelling stent, stress the need for regular follow-up to monitor for and prevent complications such as UTI and calculi. *The client with an indwelling stent may tend to forget that the stent is in place and become lax in compliance with follow-up and preventive measures.*

effect, and may be beneficial in treating or preventing UTI. Consult a qualified herbologist for recommended doses and appropriate use.

# NURSING CARE

## Health Promotion

Teach measures to prevent UTI to all clients, particularly to young, sexually active women. Encourage clients to maintain a generous fluid intake of 2.0 to 2.5 quarts per day, increasing intake during hot weather or strenuous activity. Discuss the need to avoid voluntary urinary retention, emptying the bladder every 3 to 4 hours. Instruct women to cleanse the perineal area from front to back after voiding and defecating. Teach to void before and after sexual intercourse to flush out bacteria introduced into the urethra and bladder. Teach measures to maintain the integrity of perineal tissues: Avoid bubble baths, feminine hygiene sprays, and vaginal douches; wear cotton briefs, avoid synthetic materials; if postmenopausal, use hormone replacement therapy or estrogen cream. Unless contraindicated, suggest measures to maintain acid urine: Drink two glasses of cran-

berry juice daily; take ascorbic acid (vitamin C), and avoid excess intake of milk and milk products, other fruit juices, and sodium bicarbonate (baking soda).

## Assessment

Focused assessment data for the client with a UTI includes the following:

- Health history: current symptoms, including frequency, urgency, burning on urination, voidings per night; color, clarity, and odor of urine; other manifestations such as lower abdominal, back, or flank pain, nausea or vomiting, fever; duration of symptoms and any treatment attempted; history of previous UTIs and their frequency; possibility of pregnancy and type of birth control used; chronic diseases such as diabetes; current medications and any known allergies
- Physical examination: general health; vital signs including temperature; abdominal shape, contour, tenderness to palpation (especially suprapubic); percuss for costovertebral tenderness (see Box 25–1)

See Chapter 25 ⊙ for complete nursing assessment of the urinary system.

## Nursing Diagnoses and Interventions

The client's general health, abilities for self-care, and risk factors that may contribute to UTI are considered when planning and implementing nursing care for the client with a UTI. Priority nursing diagnoses focus on comfort, urinary elimination, and teaching/learning needs.

### Pain

Pain is a common manifestation of both lower and upper UTI. Urinary tract pain is caused primarily by distention and increased pressure within the tract. The severity of the pain is related to the rate at which inflammation and distention develop, not their degree.

In cystitis, inflammation causes a sensation of fullness; dull, constant suprapubic pain; and possibly low back pain. The inflamed bladder wall and urethra cause dysuria, pain, and burning on urination. Bladder spasms may develop, causing periodic severe, stabbing discomfort. Pain associated with pyelonephritis is often steady and dull, localized to the outer abdomen or flank region. Urologic disorders rarely cause central abdominal pain.

- Assess pain: timing, quality, intensity, location, duration, and aggravating and alleviating factors. *A change in the nature, location, or intensity of the pain could indicate an extension of the infection or a related but separate problem.*

**PRACTICE ALERT** *The older adult with a UTI may not complain of dysuria with a UTI. Be alert for other manifestations of UTI such as incontinence, cloudy, or malodorous urine. Inflammatory and immune responses tend to diminish with aging, reducing the irritative symptoms of UTI.* ■

- Teach or provide comfort measures such as warm sitz baths, warm packs or heating pads, balanced rest and activity. Systemic analgesics, urinary analgesics, or antispasmodic medication may be used as ordered. *Warmth relaxes muscles, relieves spasms, and increases local blood supply. Because pain can stimulate a stress response and delay healing, it should be relieved when possible.*
- Increase fluid intake unless contraindicated. *Increased fluid dilutes urine, reducing irritation of the inflamed bladder and urethral mucosa.*

### Impaired Urinary Elimination

Inflammation of the bladder and urethral mucosa affects the normal process and patterns of voiding, causing frequency, urgency, and burning on urination, as well as nocturia. Urine may be blood-tinged, cloudy, and malodorous. The client with short- or long-term urinary retention (see the section on urinary retention later in this chapter) requires additional measures to assess for and prevent UTI.

- Monitor (or instruct the client to monitor) color, clarity, and odor of urine. *Urine should return to clear yellow*

*within 48 hours, unless drug therapy causes a change in the color of urine. If clarity does not return, further investigation may be necessary.*

**PRACTICE ALERT** *Provide for easy access to a bedpan, urinal, commode, or bathroom. Make sure that lighting is adequate and that pathways are free of obstacles. Frequency, urgency, and nocturia increase the risk of urinary incontinence and of injury due to falls, particularly in the older or debilitated client.* ■

- Instruct to avoid caffeinated drinks, including coffee, tea, and cola; citrus juices, drinks containing artificial sweeteners; and alcoholic beverages. *Caffeine, citrus juices, and artificial sweeteners irritate bladder mucosa and the detrusor muscle, and can increase urgency and bladder spasms.*
- Use strict aseptic technique and a closed urinary drainage system when inserting a straight or indwelling urinary catheter. *Bacteria colonizing the perineal tissues or on the nurse's hands can be introduced into the bladder during catheterization. Aseptic technique reduces this risk.*
- When possible, use intermittent straight catheterization to relieve urinary retention. Remove indwelling urinary catheters as soon as possible. *Using intermittent straight catheterization allows the bladder to fill and completely empty in a more normal manner, maintaining physiologic function. The risk of infection associated with an indwelling catheter is about 3% to 5% per day of catheterization* (Braunwald et al., 2001).
- Maintain the closed urinary drainage system, and use aseptic technique when emptying catheter drainage bag. Maintain gravity flow, preventing reflux of urine into the bladder from the drainage system. *Bacteria can enter the drainage system when its integrity is interrupted (e.g., disconnecting the catheter from the drainage system) or during emptying of the drainage bag. These bacteria can ascend the column of urine to the bladder, causing UTI.*
- Provide perineal care on a regular basis and following defecation. Use antiseptic preparations only as ordered. *Regular cleansing of perineal tissues reduces the risk of colonization by bowel or other bacteria. While antiseptic solutions may be ordered for catheter care, they can dry perineal tissues and reduce normal flora, increasing the risk of colonization by pathogens, and should not routinely be used.*

### Ineffective Health Maintenance

The client with a urinary tract infection is at an increased risk for future UTI and needs to understand the disease process, risk factors, measures to prevent recurrent infection, diagnostic procedures, and home care. In addition, once the manifestations of UTI are relieved, motivation to continue the treatment plan declines. Failure to complete the full course of therapy and recommended follow-up can lead to continued bacteriuria and recurrent infections.

- Teach how to obtain a midstream clean-catch urine specimen. *Cleansing of the urinary meatus and perineal area reduces contamination of the specimen by external cells and bacteria. Ninety percent of urethral bacteria are cleared in the first 10 mL of voided urine; a midstream specimen is representative of urine in the bladder.*
- Assess knowledge about the disease process, risk factors, and preventive measures. *The client may have little understanding of UTI, its causes, and contributing factors.*
- Discuss the prescribed treatment plan and the importance of taking all prescribed antibiotics.

**PRACTICE ALERT** *Symptoms are largely relieved within 24 to 48 hours of starting antibiotic therapy; however, bacteria may remain in the urinary tract. Completing the prescribed regime is important to prevent recurrent infections and resistant bacteria.* ■

- Help the client develop a plan for taking medications, such as taking them with meals (unless contraindicated) or setting out all doses for the day in the morning. *Missed doses of antibiotic can result in subtherapeutic blood levels and reduced effectiveness. Taking medication in association with a regular daily activity such as meals helps clients remember doses.*
- Instruct to keep appointments for follow-up and urine culture. *Follow-up urine culture, often scheduled 7 to 14 days after completion of antibiotic therapy, is vital to ensure complete eradication of bacteria and prevent relapse or recurrence.*
- Teach measures to prevent future UTI (see the preceding Health Promotion section). *Keeping urine dilute and acidic, and voiding regularly flush bacteria out of the bladder and urethra. The proximity of the female urethral meatus to the vagina and anus increases the risk of bacterial contamination, especially during intercourse. Bubble baths, feminine hygiene sprays, synthetic fibers, and douches may dry and irritate perineal tissues, promoting bacterial growth.*

## Using NANDA, NIC, and NOC

Chart 26–1 shows links between NANDA nursing diagnosis, NIC and NOC for the client with UTI.

## Home Care

Because both upper and lower urinary tract infections are usually managed in the community, teaching is the most important nursing intervention. Provide instruction on the following topics.

- Risk factors for UTI and how to minimize or eliminate these factors through increased fluid intake, regular elimination, and personal hygiene measures
- Early manifestations of UTI and the importance of seeking medical intervention promptly
- Maintaining optimal immune system function by attending to physical and psychosocial stressors, such as lack of adequate rest, poor nutrition, and high levels of emotional stress
- The importance of completing the prescribed treatment and keeping follow-up appointments
- Minimizing the risk of UTI when an indwelling urinary catheter is necessary:
  1. Use alternatives to an indwelling catheter when possible. For urinary incontinence, try scheduled toileting, incontinence pads or diapers, and external catheters if possible. For urinary retention, teach the client or a family member to perform straight catheterization every 3 to 4 hours using clean technique.
  2. Teach care measures such as perineal care, managing and emptying the collection chamber, maintaining a closed system, and bladder irrigation or flushing if ordered when an indwelling catheter is necessary.

## CHART 26–1  NANDA, NIC; AND NOC LINKAGES

### The Client with UTI

| NURSING DIAGNOSES | NURSING INTERVENTIONS | NURSING OUTCOMES |
| --- | --- | --- |
| • Pain | • Medication Management | • Comfort Level |
| • Impaired Urinary Elimination | • Urinary Elimination Management | • Urinary Elimination |
| • Ineffective Health Maintenance | • Health Education | • Knowledge: Health Behaviors |
| | • Teaching: Procedure/Treatment | • Knowledge: Treatment Regimen |

*Note. Data from Nursing Outcomes Classification (NOC) by M. Johnson & M. Maas (Eds.), 1997, St. Louis: Mosby; Nursing Diagnoses: Definitions & Classification 2001–2002 by North American Nursing Diagnosis Association, 2001, Philadelphia: NANDA; Nursing Interventions Classification (NIC) by J.C. McCloskey & G. M. Bulechek (Eds.), 2000, St. Louis: Mosby. Reprinted by permission.*

## Nursing Care Plan
## A Client with Cystitis

Miija Waisanen is a 25-year-old second-year nursing student. She was recently married, and she and her husband live in an apartment near the college she attends. Mrs. Waisanen has never been pregnant, and she is using a diaphragm for birth control. She presents at the local urgent care clinic complaining of low back pain, frequency, urgency, and burning on urination that began the day before.

### ASSESSMENT

Patrice Ramiros, RN, admits Mrs. Waisanen to the clinic. Mrs. Waisanen denies having had similar symptoms in the past or ever having been diagnosed with a urinary tract infection. She describes her pain as a constant, dull ache that does not change with movement. She feels the need to urinate almost constantly, but experiences difficulty in starting her stream, and burning pain and cramping when voiding. She reports getting up four times the night before to urinate. She denies painful intercourse and states that her last menstrual period began only 2 weeks ago. Physical examination reveals: BP 112/68; P 90 and regular, afebrile. Suprapubic tenderness noted but no flank or costovertebral angle tenderness. Clean-catch urine specimen shows hematuria, multiple WBCs, and a bacteria count greater than $10^5$ per milliliter.

The nurse practitioner prescribes trimethoprim-sulfamethoxazole (TMP-SMZ) 160 mg/800 mg PO bid for 3 days, and aspirin or acetaminophen gr x PO every 4 hours as needed for pain. Mrs. Waisanen is instructed to return to the clinic in 7 days for a follow-up urine culture, or sooner if her symptoms do not improve.

### DIAGNOSIS

- *Pain* related to infection and inflammatory process in the urinary tract
- *Impaired urinary elimination* related to inflammation as evidenced by frequency, urgency, nocturia, and dysuria
- *Deficient knowledge* related to lack of information about risk factors for UTI

### EXPECTED OUTCOMES

- Report relief of low back pain and burning on urination.
- Regain a normal voiding pattern without frequency, urgency, nocturia, and abnormal urine characteristics.

- Verbalize understanding of the disease process, related risk factors, follow-up instructions, and symptoms of recurrence indicating the need for medical attention.

### PLANNING AND IMPLEMENTATION

- Teach comfort measures: warm sitz baths, a heating pad on low heat applied to her lower back or abdomen, rest, increased fluid intake, avoiding caffeinated beverages, and aspirin or acetaminophen as ordered.
- Advise to refrain from sexual intercourse until infection and inflammation have cleared to avoid further irritation of inflamed tissues.
- Discuss the possible relationship between using a diaphragm for birth control and UTI in women.
- Discuss dietary and hygiene practices to prevent UTI, symptoms indicating the need for further intervention, and the risks of undertreatment.

### EVALUATION

Six months later, Mrs. Waisanen rotates through the urgent care clinic for her community-based nursing experience. Ms. Ramiros asks how she is doing. Mrs. Waisanen reports that her symptoms and urine cleared within about a day after starting the antibiotic and she has had no further problems. She has seen her women's health care nurse practitioner to change her birth control to oral contraceptives, increased her intake of fluid and vitamin C, and no longer puts off urinating until she "has time to go!"

### Critical Thinking in the Nursing Process

1. What physiologic and psychosocial factors put Mrs. Waisanen at risk for developing a UTI?
2. Compare and contrast the benefits and drawbacks to short-course therapy versus conventional therapy for UTI.
3. Why was it appropriate for the nurse practitioner to use short-course therapy with the advice to return if symptoms did not clear?
4. Develop a care plan for Mrs. Waisanen for the nursing diagnosis *Ineffective health maintenance*.

See Evaluating Your Response in Appendix C.

## THE CLIENT WITH URINARY CALCULI

**Urinary calculi,** stones in the urinary tract, are the most common cause of upper urinary tract obstruction (Porth, 2002). The term **lithiasis** means "stone formation"; when the stones form in the kidney, it is known as *nephrolithiasis;* when they form elsewhere in the urinary tract (for example, the bladder), it is called *urolithiasis.* Stones may form and obstruct the urinary tract at any point (Figure 26–2 ■). In the United States and other industrialized countries, renal or kidney stones are the most common.

Urolithiasis affects up to 720,000 people annually in the United States (Tierney et al., 2001). In the United States, the incidence varies by region, with the highest frequency in southern and midwestern states. Males are affected more often than females by a 4:1 ratio (Porth, 2002). Calculi are more common among whites than blacks. Most people affected are in young or middle adulthood.

Although the majority of stones are idiopathic (having no demonstrable cause), a number of risk factors have been identified. The greatest risk factor for stone formation is a prior personal or family history of urinary calculi. A genetic predisposi-

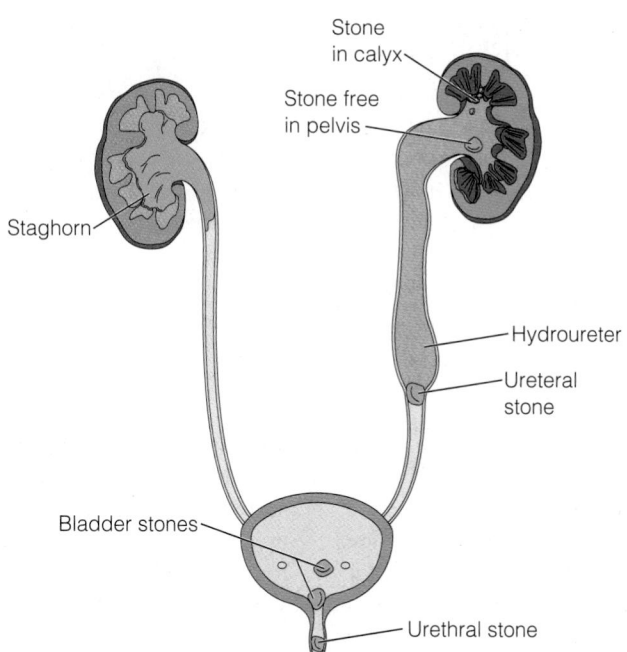

**Figure 26–2** ■ Development and location of calculi within the urinary tract.

tion toward the accumulation of certain mineral substances in the urine or a congenital lack of protective factors may explain the familial link. Other identified risk factors include dehydration with resultant increased urine concentration, immobility, and excess dietary intake of calcium, oxalate, or proteins. Gout, hyperparathyroidism, and urinary stasis or repeated infections also contribute to calculus formation.

## PHYSIOLOGY REVIEW

Normally, a balance exists in the kidneys between the need to conserve water and eliminate poorly soluble materials such as calcium salts. This balance is affected by factors such as diet, environmental temperature, and activity. Protective inorganic and organic substances in the urine, such as pyrophosphate, citrate, and glycoproteins, normally inhibit stone formation.

## PATHOPHYSIOLOGY

Three factors contribute to urolithiasis: supersaturation, nucleation, and lack of inhibitory substances in the urine.

When the concentration of an insoluble salt in the urine is very high, that is, when the urine is supersaturated, crystals may form. Usually, these crystals disperse and are eliminated because the bonds holding them together are weak. However, a nucleus of crystals may develop stable bonds to form a stone. More often, crystals form around an organic matrix or mucoprotein nucleus to become a stone. The stimulus required to initiate crystallization in supersaturated urine may be minimal. Ingesting a meal high in insoluble salt, or decreased fluid intake as occurs during sleep, allows the concentration to increase to the point where precipitation occurs and stones are formed and grow. When fluid intake is adequate, no stone growth occurs. The acidity or alkalinity of the urine and the presence or absence of calculus-inhibiting compounds also affect lithiasis.

Most (75% to 80%) kidney stones are *calcium stones,* composed of calcium oxalate and/or calcium phosphate. These stones are generally associated with high concentrations of calcium in the blood or urine. *Uric acid stones* develop when the urine concentration of uric acid is high. They are more common in men, and may be associated with gout. Genetic factors contribute to the development of uric acid stones and calcium stones. *Sturvite stones* are associated with UTI caused by urease-producing bacteria such as *Proteus.* These stones can grow to become very large, filling the renal pelvis and calyces. They often are called *staghorn stones* because of their shape. *Cystine stones* are rare, associated with a genetic defect. The types of renal calculi, contributing factors, and recommended dietary modifications are listed in Table 26–2.

| TABLE 26–2 | Risk Factors and Interventions for Renal Calculi | |
| --- | --- | --- |
| **Stone Type and Incidence** | **Risk Factors** | **Management** |
| Calcium phosphate and/or oxalate 75%–80% | Hypercalciuria and hypercalcemia: hyperparathyroidism, immobility, bone disease, vitamin D intoxication, multiple myeloma, renal tubular acidosis, prolonged steroid intake<br>Alkaline urine<br>Dehydration<br>Inflammatory bowel disease | Pharmacology: Thiazide diuretics, phosphates, calcium-binding agents<br>Dietary: Limit foods high in calcium and oxalate, increase foods that acidify urine<br>Other: Increase hydration, exercise |
| Sturvite 15%–20% | UTIs, especially *Proteus* infections | Pharmacology: Antibiotic therapy for UTI<br>Other: Surgical intervention or lithotripsy to remove stone |
| Uric acid 5%–10% | Gout, increased purine intake, acid urine | Pharmacology: Potassium citrate, allopurinol<br>Dietary: Low purine diet<br>Other: Increase hydration |
| Cystine (uncommon) | Genetic defect, acid urine | Pharmacology: Penicillamine, sodium bicarbonate<br>Dietary: Sodium restriction<br>Other: Increase hydration |

## Manifestations of Urinary Calculi

**KIDNEY STONES**
- Often asymptomatic
- Dull, aching flank pain
- Microscopic hematuria
- Manifestations of UTI

**URETERAL STONES**
- Renal colic
  - Acute, severe flank pain on affected side
  - Often radiates to suprapubic region, groin, and external genitals
- Nausea, vomiting, pallor, and cool, clammy skin

**BLADDER STONES**
- May be asymptomatic
- Dull suprapubic pain, possibly associated with exercise or voiding
- Gross or microscopic hematuria
- Manifestations of UTI

## Manifestations of Acute and Chronic Hydronephrosis

| **Acute** | **Chronic** |
|---|---|
| • Acute, colicky pain; may radiate into groin | • Dull, aching flank pain |
| • Hematuria, pyuria | • Hematuria, pyuria |
| • Fever | • Fever |
| • Nausea, vomiting, abdominal pain | • Palpable flank mass |

## MANIFESTATIONS

The symptoms caused by urinary calculi vary with their size and location (see the box above). Manifestations develop as a result of obstructed urine flow with resulting distention, and tissue trauma caused by passage of the rough-edged, crystalline stone.

Calculi affecting the kidney calices and pelvis may cause few symptoms. If the stone has gradually or partially obstructed urinary flow, dull, aching flank pain may be present, but renal calculi often are silent, without symptoms. Bladder calculi may cause few symptoms other than dull suprapubic pain with exercise or after voiding.

**Renal colic,** acute, severe flank pain on the affected side, develops when a stone obstructs the ureter, causing ureteral spasm. The pain of renal colic may radiate to the suprapubic region, groin, and external genitals (the scrotum or labia). The severity of the pain often causes a sympathetic response with associated nausea, vomiting, pallor, and cool, clammy skin.

Manifestations of UTI, including chills and fever, frequency, urgency, and dysuria, may accompany urinary calculi at any level. Trauma to the urinary tract by the calculi may cause gross or microscopic hematuria. Gross hematuria is often the only sign of bladder stones.

## Complications

### Obstruction

Stones can obstruct the urinary tract at any point from the calyces of the kidney to the distal urethra, impeding the outflow of urine. If the obstruction develops slowly, there may be few or no symptoms, whereas sudden obstruction (e.g., blockage of a ureter by a passing stone) may cause severe manifestations. Urinary tract obstruction can ultimately lead to renal failure. The degree of obstruction, its location, and the duration of impaired urine flow determine the effect on renal function.

### Hydronephrosis

The kidneys continue to produce urine, causing increased pressure and distention of the urinary tract behind the obstruction. **Hydronephrosis,** distention of the renal pelvis and calyces, and *hydroureter,* distention of the ureter, are possible results. If the pressure is unrelieved, the collecting tubules, proximal tubules, and glomeruli of the kidney are damaged, causing a gradual loss of renal function.

Acute hydronephrosis typically causes colicky pain on the affected side. The pain may radiate into the groin. Chronic hydronephrosis develops slowly, and may have few manifestations other than dull, aching back or flank pain. When hydronephrosis is significant, a palpable mass may be felt in the flank region. Hematuria and signs of UTI such as pyuria, fever, and discomfort may occur. Gastrointestinal symptoms such as nausea, vomiting, and abdominal pain may accompany hydronephrosis (see the box above).

**INFECTION.** The urinary stasis associated with partial or complete obstruction increases the risk of urinary tract infection. Either upper or lower UTI may develop.

## COLLABORATIVE CARE

Management of urinary calculi focuses on relieving acute symptoms, destroying or removing stones, and preventing further stone formation. Asymptomatic stones (those not causing pain, infection, or obstruction) are treated conservatively.

## Diagnostic Tests

Laboratory and diagnostic tests that may be ordered when urinary calculi are suspected include the following:

- *Urinalysis* to assess for hematuria and the possible presence of WBCs and crystal fragments. The urine pH is helpful in identifying the type of stone.
- *Chemical analysis* of any stones passed in the urine determines the type of stone and suggests measures to prevent further stone formation. Retrieving stones or teaching the client to do so is a nursing responsibility. All urine is strained and may be saved. Any visible stones or sediment are sent for analysis.
- *Urine calcium, uric acid,* and *oxalate* measure the amount of these substances excreted over a 24-hour period, and may be assessed to help identify possible causes of lithiasis. Elevated

## Nursing Implications for Diagnostic Tests

### 24-Hour Urine Specimen Collection

#### Preparation of the Client

- Check for ordered diet or medication regimen modifications during the collection period. Notify appropriate individuals and departments.
- Obtain a specimen container with preservative (if indicated). Label the container with identifying data, test, time started, and time of completion.
- Obtain a clean commode, bedpan, or urine-collection device for the toilet and place it in the room.
- Post notices—on the chart, in the Kardex file, on the door, over the bed, and over the toilet—alerting all personnel to save all urine.
- When collection is to begin, instruct client to completely empty the bladder and discard this urine.
- Save all urine produced during the 24-hour period in a container, refrigerating it or keeping it on ice as indicated.
- When the collection period is to end, have client empty the bladder completely and save this specimen as part of the total. Take the full specimen with requisition to the lab for analysis.
- Chart appropriately.

#### Client and Family Teaching

- This test requires you to collect all your urine over 24 hours.
- You may have to follow some dietary or medication modifications.
- Urinate (and save your urine) before you move your bowels; do not discard any toilet tissue in the urine container.

calcium levels occur in hyperparathyroidism, Cushing's syndrome, and osteoporosis, all of which may contribute to lithiasis. Uric acid levels may be elevated in clients with gout and those at risk for forming uric acid calculi. Urine oxalate excretion may help to differentiate calcium oxalate from calcium phosphate stones. See the box above for nursing responsibilities for collecting a 24-hour urine specimen.

- *Serum calcium, phosphorus,* and *uric acid* levels may be obtained to help identify factors contributing to calculus formation.
- *KUB* (kidneys, ureters, and bladder) is a flat-plate X-ray of the lower abdomen that requires no special preparation. Calculi may be identified as opacities in the kidneys, ureters, and bladder.
- *Renal ultrasonography* is a noninvasive test that uses reflected sound waves to detect stones and evaluate the kidneys for possible hydronephrosis (see the box that follows).
- *Computed tomography (CT scan)* of the kidney, with or without contrast medium, uses X-rays directed at the kidney from many angles to provide a computer-generated photograph that shows calculi, ureteral obstruction, and other renal disorders.
- *IVP* may be done to visualize the kidneys, ureters, and bladder after injection of a contrast medium. IVP may be done

## Nursing Implications for Diagnostic Tests

### Urolithiasis

#### RENAL ULTRASOUND
#### Preparation of the Client

- No special preparation is indicated; however, barium in the bowel may interfere with results. If both studies are ordered, the renal ultrasound should be scheduled first.

#### Client and Family Teaching

- This test is noninvasive and does not use radiation. You should feel no discomfort.
- Food, fluids, and ordered medications are not restricted prior to this test.
- The test takes approximately 30 to 60 minutes to complete. During this time, you need to remain relatively still.
- A conductive paste or gel (which may be cold) is applied to your back and flank to allow sound wave transmission. Then a transducer is passed over the skin, producing pictures of the reflected sound waves.

#### COMPUTED TOMOGRAPHY (CT SCAN) OF THE KIDNEY
#### Preparation of the Client

- Verify the presence of a signed informed consent.
- Check for allergies to iodine, X-ray contrast dye, and seafood. Inform the radiology department if such an allergy exists.
- Prepare the client as ordered: NPO 4 hours prior to examination; laxatives and/or enemas may be ordered to remove gas, fecal material, or retained barium from the bowel.

#### Client and Family Teaching

- The test requires 30 to 60 minutes to complete, and you must lie still during the procedure.
- Lie flat on your back during the test while a doughnut-shaped scanner revolves around your body. This can cause a sensation of claustrophobia. The machine emits loud clicking sounds as it rotates.
- The radiology technician is not in the room, but you can communicate through an intercom system at all times.
- If contrast medium is used, you may experience a flushing sensation and nausea as it is injected.

when KUB, renal ultrasonography, and CT scan fail to demonstrate clear evidence of urinary calculi.

- *Cystoscopy* is used to visualize and possibly remove calculi from the urinary bladder and distal ureters.

## Medications

An acute episode of renal colic is treated with analgesia and hydration. A narcotic analgesic such as morphine sulfate is given, often intravenously, to relieve pain and reduce ureteral spasm. Indomethacin, a nonsteroidal anti-inflammatory drug (NSAID), given as a suppository, may reduce the amount of narcotic analgesia required for acute renal colic. Oral or intravenous fluids reduce the risk of further stone formation and promote urine output.

After analysis of the calculus, various medications may be ordered to inhibit or prevent further lithiasis. A thiazide diuretic, frequently prescribed for calcium calculi, acts to reduce urinary calcium excretion and is very effective in preventing further stones. Potassium citrate alkalinizes urine (raises the pH), and is often prescribed to prevent stones that tend to form in acidic urine (uric acid, cystine, and some forms of calcium stones). See Table 26–2 for other preparations related to types of stones. Nursing responsibilities focus on teaching the client about the prescribed medication, its importance in preventing further stone formation, and potential adverse effects.

## Dietary Management

Diet modifications are often prescribed to change the character of the urine and prevent further lithiasis.

Increased fluid intake of 2.5 to 3.0 L per day is recommended, regardless of stone composition. A fluid intake to ensure the production of approximately 2.0 to 2.5 L of urine a day prevents the stone-forming salts from becoming concentrated enough to precipitate. Fluid intake should be spaced throughout the day and evening. Some authorities recommend that clients drink one to two glasses of water at night to prevent concentration of urine during sleep.

Recommended dietary changes may include reduced intake of the primary substance forming the calculi. For calcium stones, dietary calcium and vitamin D enriched foods are limited. Limiting vitamin D inhibits the absorption of calcium from the GI tract. Calcium stones may be either a calcium phosphate salt, calcium oxalate, or a combination of both; therefore, phosphorus and/or oxalate may also be limited in the diet.

The client with uric acid stones requires a diet low in purines. Organ meats, sardines, and other high-purine foods are eliminated from the diet. Foods with moderate levels of purines, such as red and white meats and some seafoods, may be limited.

In addition to limiting certain foods, the diet may be modified to maintain a urinary pH that does not promote lithiasis. Uric acid and cystine stones tend to form in acid urine. Foods which tend to alkalinize the urine may be recommended. Because alkaline urine promotes formation of calcium stones and urinary tract infections, the diet may be modified to lower the pH of the urine. Foods that affect urinary pH and foods high in various stone components are summarized in Table 26–3.

## Surgery

Treatment of existing calculi depends on the location of the stone, the extent of obstruction, renal function, the presence or absence of UTI, and the client's general state of health. In general, the stone is removed if it is causing severe obstruction, infection, unrelieved pain, or serious bleeding (Braunwald et al., 2001).

**Lithotripsy,** using sound or shock waves to crush a stone, is the preferred treatment for urinary calculi. Several techniques are available. **Extracorporeal shock wave lithotripsy (ESWL)** is a noninvasive technique for fragmenting kidney stones using shock waves generated outside the body. Acoustic shock waves are aimed under fluoroscopic guidance at the stone (Figure 26–3 ■). These shock waves travel through soft tissue without causing damage, but shatter the stone as its

| TABLE 26–3 | Examples of Food and Fluids for Teaching Clients with Urolithiasis |
| --- | --- |
| Foods high in calcium | Beans and lentils, chocolate and cocoa, dried fruits, canned or smoked fish except tuna, flour, milk and milk products |
| Foods high in oxalate | Asparagus, beer and colas, beets, cabbage, celery, chocolate and cocoa, fruits, green beans, nuts, tea, tomatoes |
| Purine-rich foods | Goose, organ meats, sardines and herring, venison; moderate in beef, chicken, crab, pork, salmon, veal |
| Acidifying foods | Cheese, cranberries, eggs, grapes, meat and poultry, plums and prunes, tomatoes, whole grains |
| Alkalinizing foods | Green vegetables, fruit (except as noted above), legumes, milk and milk products, rhubarb |

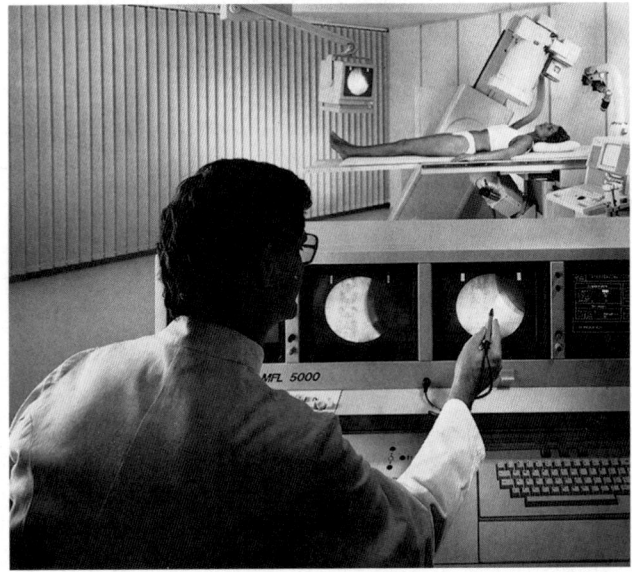

**Figure 26–3 ■** Extracorporeal shock wave lithotripsy. Acoustic shock waves generated by the shock wave generator travel through soft tissue to shatter the urinary stone into fragments, which are then eliminated in the urine.

*Courtesy of Dormier Medical Products.*

greater density stops their progress. Repeated shock waves pulverize the stone into fragments small enough to be eliminated in the urine. The procedure may require 30 minutes to 2 hours to complete. Intravenous or oral sedation or a transcutaneous electrical nerve stimulator (TENS unit) are used to maintain comfort during the procedure (Meeker & Rothrock, 1999). See the box on the next page for nursing care of the client undergoing a lithotripsy procedure.

Lithotripsy also may be performed using a percutaneous ultrasonic or laser technique. *Percutaneous ultrasonic lithotripsy* uses a nephroscope inserted into the kidney pelvis through a small flank incision (Figure 26–4 ■). The stone is fragmented using a small ultrasonic transducer, and the fragments are re-

# NURSING CARE OF THE CLIENT HAVING LITHOTRIPSY

## PREOPERATIVE CARE

- Assess knowledge and understanding of the procedure, providing information as needed. *Anxiety is reduced, and recovery is enhanced and hastened when the client is fully prepared for surgery.*
- Follow directions from the radiology department, physician, or anesthetist for withholding food and fluids and for bowel preparation prior to surgery. *Conscious sedation, general anesthesia, or spinal anesthesia may be required, depending on the procedure. Fecal material in the bowel may impede fluoroscopic visualization of the kidney and stone.*

## POSTOPERATIVE CARE

- In the initial period, monitor vital signs frequently. *The kidney is highly vascular; therefore, hemorrhage and resulting shock are potential complications of lithotripsy. Bleeding may be internal or retroperitoneal and difficult to detect.*

- Monitor amount, color, and clarity of urine output. *Urine is often bright red initially, but bleeding should diminish within 48 to 72 hours. Cloudy urine may indicate the presence of an infection.*
- Maintain placement and patency of urinary catheters. Anchor ureteral catheters or nephrostomy tubes securely. Irrigate gently if ordered. *A kinked or plugged catheter may result in hydroureter, hydronephrosis, and kidney damage. Decreased urinary output and flank pain are possible symptoms of obstructed urine flow. Excessive force in irrigation may cause trauma and bleeding.*
- Prepare for discharge by teaching care of indwelling catheter, urine-collection device, and incision site (if present). Teach signs and symptoms to report: urine leakage from incision for more than 4 days, symptoms of infection, pain, bright hematuria. *Many clients are discharged with dressings and catheters in place. The client and family need necessary information to provide self-care.*
- Teach measures to reduce the risk of further lithiasis. *Many clients have repeated episodes of lithiasis and renal colic. Prevention of stone formation is important to preserve renal function.*

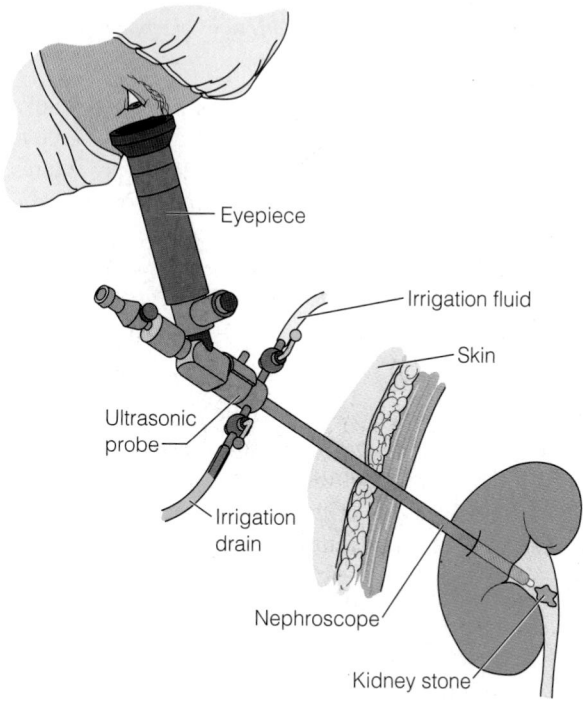

**Figure 26–4** ■ Percutaneous ultrasonic lithotripsy. A nephroscope is inserted into the renal pelvis, and ultrasonic waves are used to fragment the stone. The fragments then are removed through the nephroscope.

moved through the nephroscope. *Laser lithotripsy* is an alternative to ultrasonic lithotripsy. Laser beams are used to disintegrate the stone, without damaging soft tissue. A nephroscope or a ureteroscope (passed up the ureter from the bladder during cystoscopy) is used to guide the laser probe into direct contact with the stone (Meeker & Rothrock, 1999).

A double J stent may be inserted into the affected ureter to maintain its patency following ESWL or other lithotripsy pro-

cedures. See the box on page 711 for nursing care of the client with a ureteral stent.

On rare occasions, surgical intervention is necessary to remove a calculus in the renal pelvis or ureter. *Ureterolithotomy* is incision in the affected ureter to remove a calculus. *Pyelolithotomy* is incision into and removal of a stone from the kidney pelvis. A staghorn calculus which invades the calices and renal parenchyma, may require a *nephrolithotomy* for removal. See Chapter 7 ⊖ for care of the surgical client.

Bladder stones may be removed using an instrument passed through a cystoscope to crush the stones. The remaining stone fragments are then irrigated out of the bladder using an acid solution to counteract the alkalinity that precipitated stone formation.

# NURSING CARE

Nursing care for the client with urolithiasis is directed at providing for comfort during acute renal colic, assisting with diagnostic procedures, ensuring adequate urinary output, and teaching the client information necessary to prevent future stone formation.

## Health Promotion

Discuss the importance of maintaining an adequate fluid intake with all clients. Stress the need to increase fluid intake during warm weather and strenuous exercise or physical labor. Discuss the relationship between weight-bearing activity and retention of calcium in the bones. Encourage all clients to remain as physically active as possible to prevent bone resorption and possible hypercalciuria.

Instruct clients with known gout to maintain a generous fluid intake so as to produce at least 2 L of urine every day. Discuss the risk of lithiasis with clients who have frequent UTIs, and teach measures to reduce the incidence of UTI and the risk for lithiasis.

## Assessment

Obtain subjective and objective assessment data specific to urolithiasis.

- Health history: complaints of flank, back, or abdominal pain, radiation, characteristics and timing, aggravating or relieving factors; other symptoms such as nausea and vomiting; possible contributing factors such as dehydration; previous or family history of kidney stones; current or previous treatment measures
- Physical examination: general appearance including position, vital signs; skin color, temperature, moisture, turgor; abdominal, flank, or costovertebral tenderness; amount, color, and characteristics of urine (presence of hematuria, bacteria, pyuria, pH)

## Nursing Diagnoses and Interventions

### Acute Pain

Pain is the primary outward manifestation of urolithiasis, particularly when a stone lodges within a ureter, causing acute obstruction and distention. Invasive and noninvasive procedures to remove or crush stones also may be painful. Clients undergoing surgery also experience incisional pain.

**PRACTICE ALERT** *The intensity of renal colic pain can cause a vasovagal response with resulting hypotension and syncope. Always provide for the client's safety.* ■

- Assess pain using a standard pain scale and its characteristics. Administer analgesia as ordered and monitor its effectiveness. *The intensity, type of pain, and its responsiveness to analgesia provide valuable clues as to its cause. Regular administration of prescribed analgesics controls pain more effectively than waiting until pain becomes intolerable. Administering an ordered NSAID on a routine schedule may significantly reduce the need for narcotic analgesia in clients with renal colic.*
- Unless contraindicated, encourage fluid intake and ambulation in the client with renal colic. *Increased fluids and ambulation increase urinary output, facilitating movement of the calculus through the ureter and decreasing pain.*
- Use nonpharmacologic measures such as positioning, moist heat, relaxation techniques, guided imagery, and diversion as adjunctive therapy for pain relief. *Adjunctive pain relief measures can enhance the effectiveness of analgesics and other prescribed treatment.*
- If surgery has been performed, monitor urinary output, catheters, incision, and wound drainage. *Pain may be a symptom of proximal distention due to a blocked catheter. Infection or hematoma at the surgical site can significantly increase perceived pain.*

### Impaired Urinary Elimination

Obstruction of the urinary tract is the primary problem associated with urolithiasis. Obstruction can ultimately lead to stasis, infection, or irreversible renal damage.

- Monitor amount and character of urine output. If catheterized, measure output hourly. Document any hematuria, dysuria, frequency, urgency, and pyuria. Strain all urine for stones, saving any recovered stones for laboratory analysis. *The amount of urine output helps determine possible urinary tract obstruction and adequacy of hydration. Hematuria, gross or microscopic, is often associated with calculi and with procedures used to remove stones, such as cystoscopy or lithotripsy. A change in the amount of hematuria may indicate stone passage or a complication. Dysuria, frequency, urgency, and cloudy urine are symptoms of UTI, often associated with urolithiasis. Antibiotic therapy may be required. Analysis of stones recovered from the urine can direct measures to prevent further lithiasis.*

**PRACTICE ALERT** *A stone that completely obstructs the ureter can lead to hydronephrosis and kidney damage on the affected side. Report symptoms of hydronephrosis such as dull flank pain or aching and changes in renal function studies (BUN and serum creatinine). Because the other kidney continues to function, urine output may not fall significantly with obstruction of one ureter. A rising BUN and serum creatinine may be early signs of renal failure.* ■

- Maintain patency and integrity of all catheter systems. Secure catheters well, label as indicated, and use sterile technique for all ordered irrigations or other procedures. *A kinked or plugged catheter, particularly a ureteral catheter or nephrostomy tube, may damage the urinary system. Labeling catheters can prevent mistakes, such as inappropriate irrigation or clamping. Any catheter increases the risk of infection; aseptic technique in all procedures reduces this risk.*

### Deficient Knowledge

The client with urolithiasis has multiple learning needs. These include information about the disease and its possible consequences, any diagnostic or therapeutic procedures performed, and strategies to prevent future lithiasis.

- Assess understanding and previous learning. *Relating information to previously learned material enhances retention and understanding.*
- Present all material in a manner appropriate to knowledge base, developmental and educational level, and current needs. *Learning is an active process that requires the client's participation. Tailoring teaching to the individual increases involvement.*
- Teach about all diagnostic and treatment procedures. *Knowing what to expect reduces anxiety, enhances compliance, and hastens recovery.*
- If the client will be managed in the community, teach to:
  a. Collect and strain all urine, saving any stones.
  b. Report stone passage to the physician and bring the stone in for analysis.
  c. Report any changes in the amount or character of urine output to physician.

*When pain can be managed with oral analgesics, urinary stones are managed in the community. The client needs to know how and why to collect the calculus and indicators of complications, such as reduced urine output and cloudy or bloody urine.*

- Teach measures to prevent further urolithiasis.
  a. Increase fluid intake to 2500 to 3500 mL per day.
  b. Follow recommended dietary guidelines.
  c. Maintain activity level to prevent urinary stasis and bone resorption.
  d. Take medications as prescribed.
  *The risk of recurrent lithiasis is approximately 50%; however, this risk can be reduced by measures to prevent conditions favoring stone formation.*
- Teach about the relationship between urinary calculi and UTI, emphasizing preventive measures and the importance of prompt treatment. *Urinary tract infection promotes urolithiasis and thus requires prompt treatment to reduce this risk.*

## Using NANDA, NIC, and NOC

Chart 26–2 shows links between NANDA nursing diagnoses, NIC, and NOC for the client with urinary calculi.

## Home Care

The client with urinary calculi needs to know how to manage existing stones and what to do to reduce the risk of future stone formation. Discuss the following topics to prepare the client and family for home care.

- Importance of maintaining a fluid intake adequate to produce 2.0 to 2.5 quarts of urine per day
- Prescribed medications, their management, and potential adverse effects
- Dietary recommendations
- Prevention, recognition, and management of UTI
- Any further diagnostic or treatment measures planned

When the client is to be discharged with dressings, a nephrostomy tube, or a catheter, teach the client and family about the following:

- How to change dressings, maintaining aseptic technique
- Assessment of the wound and skin for healing and possible complications such as infection or skin breakdown
- How to manage drainage systems and maintain their patency
- Emptying drainage bags and assessing urine output
- When to contact the physician and recommendations for follow-up care

---

### CHART 26–2 NANDA, NIC, AND NOC LINKAGES

#### The Client with Urinary Calculi

| NURSING DIAGNOSES | NURSING INTERVENTIONS | NURSING OUTCOMES |
|---|---|---|
| • Acute Pain | • Pain Management<br>• Analgesic Administration | • Pain Control<br>• Pain: Disruptive Effects |
| • Impaired Urinary Elimination | • Fluid Management<br>• Specimen Management | • Urinary Elimination |
| • Deficient Knowledge | • Teaching: Disease Process<br>• Teaching: Procedure/Treatment | • Knowledge: Illness Care<br>• Knowledge: Treatment Regimen |

*Note. Data from Nursing Outcomes Classification (NOC) by M. Johnson & M. Maas (Eds.), 1997, St. Louis: Mosby; Nursing Diagnoses: Definitions & Classification 2001–2002 by North American Nursing Diagnosis Association, 2001, Philadelphia: NANDA; Nursing Interventions Classification (NIC) by J.C. McCloskey & G. M. Bulechek (Eds.), 2000, St. Louis: Mosby. Reprinted by permission.*

---

## Nursing Care Plan
## A Client with Urinary Calculi

Richard Leton, age 44, owns a small business. He is admitted to the medical unit from the emergency department after awakening at 4:00 A.M. with severe right-sided pain. His CBC is normal, and urinalysis reveals microscopic hematuria, but no protein or bacteria. A renal ultrasound shows a 4 to 5 mm stone partially obstructing the right ureter.

Stephen Phillips, Mr. Leton's admitting nurse, notes that he is pale, diaphoretic, and very anxious. He complains of nausea and asks for an emesis basin. Mr. Leton received 4 mg of intravenous morphine sulphate shortly after admission to the ED, approxi-

mately 2.5 hours ago. He denies pain at this time, but says, "I'm scared to death that it'll come back—I couldn't even move, it hurt so bad."

### ASSESSMENT

Mr. Leton's history reveals no previous episodes of renal calculi. He felt well until the pain awakened him during the night. He admits that he has been working under a deadline to complete a construction project and that he probably has not been drinking

(continued on page 722)

## Nursing Care Plan
### A Client with Urinary Calculi *(continued)*

enough fluids "considering how hot it's been." Physical assessment findings include T 100.4°F (38.0°C) PO, P 98, R 24, and BP 160/86. Color is pale to ashen, skin cool and moist. Abdomen firm with moderate tenderness in the right upper outer quadrant. The ED physician orders an IV of 5% dextrose in 1/2 normal saline at 200 mL/hr until nausea relieved, then PO fluids of at least 3000 mL/24 hr; morphine sulfate (MS) 2 to 10 mg IV prn severe pain; indomethacin (Indocin) 50 mg per rectal suppository q8h; promethazine (Phenergan) 25 mg PO or per suppository q6h prn nausea; activity to tolerance; and strain all urine, sending recovered stones for analysis.

### DIAGNOSIS

- *Anxiety* related to anticipation of recurrent severe pain
- *Risk for imbalanced nutrition: Less than body requirements,* related to nausea
- *Acute pain* related to partial obstruction of right ureter by calculus
- *Impaired urinary elimination* related to partial obstruction of ureter by calculus
- *Deficient knowledge* related to lack of information about disease process, contributing factors, and management

### EXPECTED OUTCOMES

- Demonstrate reduced anxiety by relaxed facial expression, vital signs within his normal range, and ability to rest when not disturbed.
- Consume at least 50% of diet and 100% of ordered fluids without nausea or vomiting.
- Request analgesia as needed at onset of pain; report effective pain relief.
- Maintain urine output of 2500 mL/24 hr with no signs of infection or obstruction (such as increased pain, dysuria, pyuria, or hematuria).
- Relate an understanding of the process of urolithiasis and contributing factors.
- Verbalize dietary, fluid intake, and other measures to reduce risk of future stone formation.

### PLANNING AND IMPLEMENTATION

- Reassure that measures to prevent further episodes of renal colic are being implemented, and that medication is available to relieve pain promptly.
- Assess the effectiveness of analgesia and its adverse effects, especially nausea.
- Maintain IV as ordered until oral fluid intake exceeds 200 mL of fluid per hour while awake.
- Measure and strain all urine. Assess urine for color, clarity, and odor.
- Teach about urolithiasis and its risk factors, especially as they relate to Mr. Leton.
- Teach the importance of maintaining a high fluid intake, especially when working outdoors in hot weather; recommended dietary modifications and their rationale; ordered medications and their effects; how to identify and prevent UTI; and symptoms that should be reported to the physician.

### EVALUATION

Mr. Leton passed the obstructing stone the evening after admission and is discharged the following day. On discharge, he denies pain or nausea, his urine is clear and pale yellow, and urinalysis is normal. Laboratory analysis shows that the calculus was calcium. Mr. Leton is able to state the importance of continuing a high fluid intake. He verbalizes that he will reduce his intake of calcium-rich foods, such as milk and milk products, and that he will increase his intake of foods to acidify his urine. He is able to list foods to include in his diet. He states, "You'd better believe I'll follow my diet, drink my water, and make sure I don't get an infection. I hope to never feel pain like that again!"

### Critical Thinking in the Nursing Process

1. What factors contributed to the onset and timing of Mr. Leton's ureteral colic?
2. What is the rationale for administering indomethacin, an NSAID, to a client with ureteral colic?
3. Why did Mr. Phillips include a nursing intervention to assess for a relationship between Mr. Leton's nausea, his pain, and the ordered analgesic agent?

See Evaluating Your Response in Appendix C.

## THE CLIENT WITH A URINARY TRACT TUMOR

A malignancy can develop in any part of the urinary tract; however, 90% develop in the bladder, about 8% develop in the renal pelvis, and only 2% in the ureter or urethra (Braunwald et al., 2001). When diagnosed early, the 5-year survival rate for bladder cancer is 94% (American Cancer Society [ACS], 2002).

An estimated 56,500 new cases of bladder cancer were diagnosed in the United States in 2002, and 12,600 people died as a result of the disease. The incidence of bladder cancer is about 4 times higher in men than it is in women, and about twice as high in whites as it is in blacks (ACS, 2002). Most people who develop bladder cancer are over age 60.

Two major factors are implicated in the development of bladder cancer: the presence of carcinogens in the urine and chronic inflammation or infection of bladder mucosa (See Box 26–2). Cigarette smoking is the primary risk factor for bladder cancer. The risk in smokers is twice that of nonsmokers (ACS, 2002). The chemicals and dyes used in the plastics, rubber, and cable industries; substances in the work environment of textile workers, leather finishers, spray painters, hair dressers, and petroleum workers; and the chronic use of phenacetin-containing analgesic agents also are associated with a higher risk. Additional risk factors for bladder cancer include residence in an urban area, chronic UTIs, and bladder calculi. The parasite *Schistosoma haematocium,* endemic to Egypt and the Sudan, also increases the risk for bladder cancer (Porth, 2002).

## PATHOPHYSIOLOGY

Most urinary tract malignancies arise from epithelial tissue. Transitional epithelium lines the entire tract from the renal pelvis through the urethra. Carcinogenic breakdown products of certain chemicals and from cigarette smoke are excreted in the urine and stored in the bladder, possibly causing a local influence on abnormal cell development. Squamous cell carcinoma of the urinary tract occurs less frequently than transitional epithelial cell tumors.

Urinary tract tumors begin as nonspecific cellular alterations that develop into either flat or papillary lesions. These lesions may be either superficial or invasive. About 75% of bladder tumors are papillary lesions (*papillomas*), a polyplike structure attached by a stalk to the bladder mucosa (Figure 26–5 ■). Papillomas are generally superficial, noninvasive tumors that bleed easily and frequently recur (Braunwald et al., 2001). They rarely progress to become invasive, and the prognosis for recovery is good.

Carcinoma in situ (CIS), which occurs less frequently, is a poorly differentiated flat tumor that invades directly and is associated with a poorer prognosis. Bladder tumors are rated by their cell type and grade. Grade I tumors are highly differentiated and rarely progress to become invasive, whereas grade III tumors are poorly differentiated and usually progress (Braunwald et al., 2001). The staging of bladder tumors is outlined in Table 26–4. See Chapter 10 ⊂⊃ for more information about tumor grading and staging. When metastasis oc-

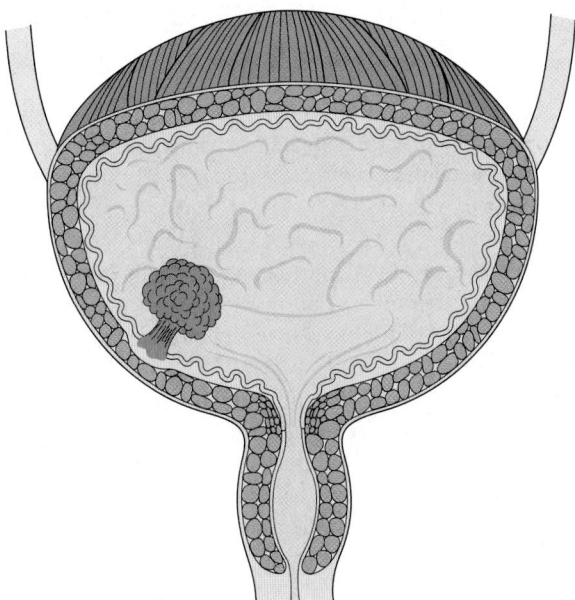

**Figure 26–5** ■ A papillary transitional cell carcinoma of the urinary bladder with minimal invasion of the bladder wall.

curs, the pelvic lymph nodes, lungs, bones, and liver are most commonly involved.

## MANIFESTATIONS

Painless hematuria is the presenting sign in 75% of urinary tract tumors. Hematuria may be gross or microscopic and is often intermittent, causing delay in seeking treatment (Porth, 2002). Inflammation surrounding the tumor occasionally causes manifestations of a urinary tract infection, including frequency, urgency, and dysuria. Ureteral tumors may cause colicky pain from obstruction. Tumors of the urinary tract typically cause few outward signs and may not be discovered until obstructed urine flow causes flank pain or renal failure.

## COLLABORATIVE CARE

Treatment of the client with a tumor of the urinary tract focuses on removal or destruction of the cancerous tissue, prevention of further invasion or metastasis, and maintenance of renal and urinary function.

## TABLE 26–4  Bladder Tumor Staging

| Depth of Involvement | TNM (Tumor, Node, Metastasis) Stage | Tumor Involvement |
|---|---|---|
| Superficial | $T_a$ | Limited to the bladder mucosa |
| | $T_1$ | Involvement of the bladder mucosa and submucosal layers |
| Invasive | $T_2$ | Invasion of superficial muscle of bladder wall |
| | $T_{3a}$ | Deep muscle invasion |
| | $T_{3b}$ | Involvement of perivesicular fat |
| | $T_{3-4}N_+$ | Regional (pelvic) lymph node involvement |
| | $T_{3-4}M_1$ | Metastasis to distant lymph nodes or organs |

## Diagnostic Tests

When a urinary tract tumor is suspected, the following diagnostic tests may be ordered.

- *Urinalysis* is done to evaluate for hematuria. Gross or microscopic hematuria is often the first indicator of a neoplasm in the urinary tract.
- *Urine cytology,* microscopic examination of cells in the urine, is performed to identify abnormal cells (tumor or pretumor cells). Periodic urine cytology is recommended for clients at high risk for bladder cancer or its recurrence due to carcinogen exposure.
- *Ultrasound of the bladder* is a noninvasive test to detect bladder tumors. No dye is required, and the client is not exposed to radiation.
- *Intravenous pyelography* is used to evaluate the structure and function of the kidneys, ureters, and bladder. IVP may reveal a rigid deformity of the bladder wall, obstruction of urine flow at the point of the tumor, or bladder filling or emptying defects.
- *Cystoscopy* and *ureteroscopy* allow direct visualization, assessment, and biopsy of lesions of the urethra, bladder, or ureters using a lighted scope inserted through the urethra. Cystoscopy or ureteroscopy with biopsy allow definitive diagnosis of urinary tract tumors.
- *Computed tomography (CT scan)* or *magnetic resonance imaging (MRI)* are primarily used to evaluate tumor invasion or metastasis.

See the box on pages 708–709 for nursing implications of these diagnostic studies.

## Medications

Immunologic or chemotherapeutic agents administered by intravesical instillation (into the bladder) may be used either as the primary treatment for bladder cancer or to prevent recurrence following endoscopic tumor removal. Bacille Calmette-Guérin (BCGLive, TheraCys) is a suspension of attenuated *Mycobacterium bovis* used to treat CIS and recurrent bladder tumors. Instillation into the bladder causes a local inflammatory reaction that eliminates or reduces superficial tumors. Systemic mycobacterial infection is a rare complication of intravesical BCG therapy that may require antituberculin treatment (Tierney et al., 2001). Other chemotherapeutic agents also may be administered intravesically, including doxorubicin and mitomycin C. Bladder irritation, frequency, dysuria, and contact dermatitis are possible adverse reactions to intravesical chemotherapy.

## Radiation Therapy

Radiation is another adjunctive therapy used in the treatment of urinary tumors. Although radiation alone is not curative, it can reduce tumor size prior to surgery and is used as palliative treatment for inoperable tumors and clients who cannot tolerate surgery. Radiation therapy also is used in combination with systemic chemotherapy to improve local and distant relapse rates (Tierney et al., 2001) (see Chapter 10). ⊖⊙

## Surgery

A number of surgical procedures, ranging from simple resection of noninvasive tumors to removal of the bladder and surrounding structures, are used to treat urinary tract tumors. Indications for each procedure and specific nursing implications are outlined in Table 26–5.

Transurethral tumor resection may be performed by excision, *fulguration* (destruction of tissue using electric sparks generated by high-frequency current) or *laser photocoagulation* (use of light energy to destroy abnormal tissue). Laser surgery carries the lowest risk of bleeding and perforation of the bladder wall. Following cystoscopic tumor resection, clients are followed at 3-month intervals for tumor recurrence. Recurrences may develop anywhere in the urinary tract, including the renal pelvis, ureter, or urethra (Braunwald et al., 2001).

**Cystectomy,** surgical removal of the bladder, is necessary to treat invasive cancers. Partial cystectomy may be done to remove a solitary lesion; however, radical cystectomy is the standard treatment for invasive tumors. The bladder and adjacent muscles and tissues are removed. In men, the prostate and seminal vessels are also removed, resulting in impotence. In women, a total hysterectomy and bilateral salpingo-

| TABLE 26–5 Surgical Procedures Used to Treat Bladder Tumors | | |
|---|---|---|
| **Procedure** | **Indications** | **Nursing Implications** |
| Transurethral resection of bladder tumor | Diagnose and treat superficial bladder tumors having low rate of recurrence; control bleeding | Maintain continuous bladder irrigation postoperatively; monitor for excessive bleeding; ensure catheter patency. Increase fluids to 2500-3000 mL per day. Give stool softeners to prevent straining. |
| Partial cystectomy | Resect solitary, isolated tumor at stage B or C not involving trigone | Maintain patency of urethral and/or suprapubic catheter to make sure suture lines are free of pressure; monitor for excess bleeding. |
| Complete or radical cystectomy | Remove large, invasive tumors; involvement of trigone | Permanent urinary diversion is required. Maintain patency and position of stents; urethral catheter may be in place to drain pelvic cavity. |

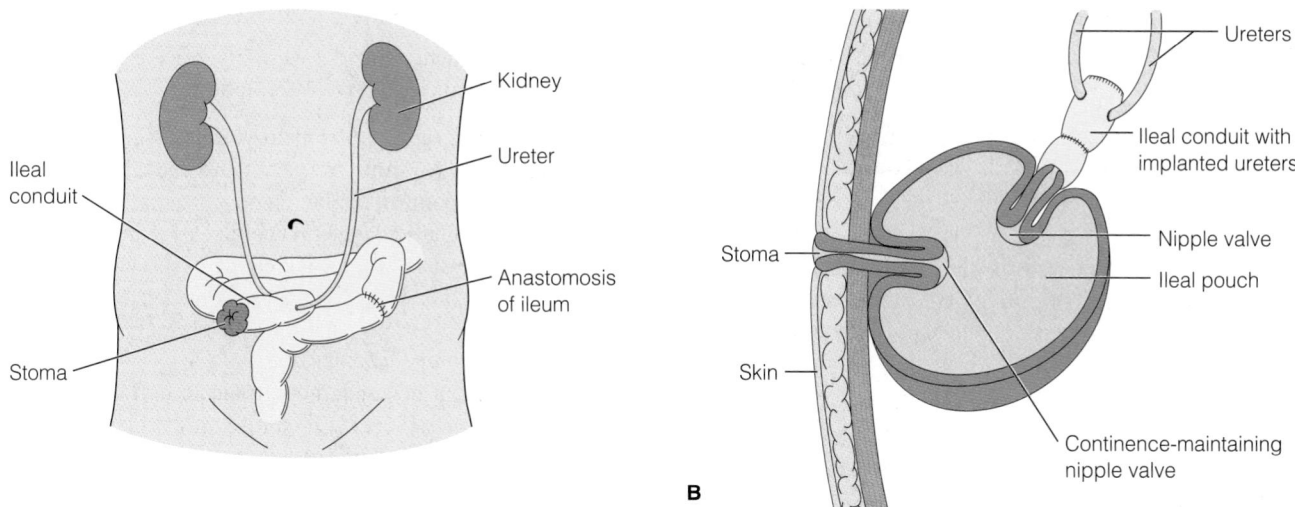

**Figure 26–6** ■ Common urinary diversion procedures. *A,* Ileal conduit. A segment of ileum is separated from the small intestine and formed into a tubular pouch with the open end brought to the skin surface to form a stoma. The ureters are connected to the pouch. *B,* A continent urinary diversion. A segment of ileum is separated from the small intestine and formed into a pouch. Nipple valves are formed at each end of the pouch by intussuscepting tissue backward into the reservoir to prevent leakage.

oophorectomy (removal of the uterus, uterine tubes, and ovaries) accompanies the procedure, causing sterility. At the time of surgery, a **urinary diversion** is created to provide for urine collection and drainage. Either an *ileal conduit* (Figure 26–6A■) or a *continent urinary diversion* (Figure 26–6B) is created to collect and drain urine. Table 26–6 describes the most frequently used urinary diversion techniques.

Surgical procedures to remove tumors involving other portions of the urinary tract vary according to the site and stage of the tumor. When the distal ureter is involved, the tumor may be resected and the ureter implanted into the opposite ureter to provide for drainage. A proximal ureteral tumor necessitates removal of the ureter and kidney on the affected side.

## TABLE 26–6   Urinary Diversion Procedures

| Procedure | Description | Nursing Considerations |
|---|---|---|
| Ileal conduit | Portion of ileum is isolated from small intestine, leaving vascular, lymphatic, and neural connections intact; ileum is formed into pouch with open end brought to surface to form a stoma; ureters are inserted into pouch. | Most common urinary diversion. Continuous urine drainage necessitates appliance. Postoperative edema may interfere with urine output. Risk of infection is less than for cutaneous ureterostomy, but potential for reflux is high. Good skin care vital because of constant contact with urine. |
| Continent internal ileal reservoir or continent ileal bladder conduit (Kock's pouch) | Pouch is created as for ileal conduit but nipple valves are formed by intussuscepting tissue backward into a reservoir to connect pouch to the skin and the ureters to the pouch; filling pressure closes valves, preventing leakage and reflux. | Drainage collection device not necessary. Client must be willing and able to perform clean intermittent self-catheterization every 2 to 4 hours. Continence valve mechanism may fail, requiring surgery for revision. |
| Indiana continent urinary reservoir | A portion of the terminal ileum, ascending colon, and cecum is isolated from the bowel with vascular and neural connections intact. Reservoir is formed from colon and cecum; portion of the ileum is brought to the surface to form nipple valve and stoma or is attached to urethral stump. | As for Kock's pouch. Client must be able and motivated to manage self-catheterization. Reservoir may absorb urea and electrolytes, resulting in imbalances. Significant portion of bowel is required to form pouch and stoma. |
| Ileocystoplasty or Camey procedure | Section of the ileum is isolated and formed into U shape. Ureters are implanted in upper portion of the U. Urethra is anastamosed to central section. | Appropriate for men only because urethra is removed with cystectomy in women. Allows client to void by relaxing pelvic muscles and using Valsalva maneuver. |

See the box below for nursing care of the client undergoing tumor resection and a urinary diversion.

# NURSING CARE

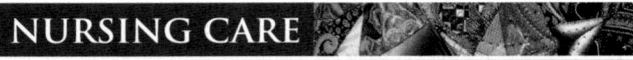

The client who undergoes treatment for a tumor of the urinary tract has many nursing care needs because of alterations in the functional health patterns of elimination, health perception/health management, cognitive/perceptual, self-perception/self-concept, role/relationship, and coping/stress tolerance.

## Health Promotion

Encourage all clients not to smoke. Provide referral to smoking cessation programs or clinics for clients who wish to quit smoking. Encourage clients at high risk for developing bladder cancer (see Box 26–2 on page 723) to have periodic examinations, including urinalysis and possible urine cytology.

## Assessment

Nursing assessment related to urinary tract cancer includes both subjective and objective information.

- Health history: risk factors; history of hematuria or manifestations of UTI (dysuria, frequency, urgency, pyuria); lower abdominal discomfort or flank pain
- Physical examination: general health; abdominal tenderness; urine for analysis.

## Nursing Diagnoses and Interventions

### Impaired Urinary Elimination

Whether the client has undergone transurethral resection of a bladder tumor or radical cystectomy with urinary diversion, urinary elimination is altered at least temporarily.

- Monitor urine output from all catheters, stents, and tubes for amount, color, and clarity hourly for the first 24 hours postoperatively, then every 4 to 8 hours. *Decreased urine output*

---

# NURSING CARE OF THE CLIENT HAVING CYSTECTOMY AND URINARY DIVERSION

## PREOPERATIVE CARE

- Provide routine preoperative care as outlined in Chapter 7. ⊂⊃
- Assess knowledge of the proposed surgery and its long-term implications, clarifying misunderstandings and discussing concerns. *Clients having surgery for cancer of the urinary tract are trying to cope with diagnosis of cancer and may not fully understand the surgery and its potential effects. Open discussion can facilitate postoperative recovery and adjustment.*
- Begin teaching about postoperative tubes and drains, self-care of stoma, and control of drainage and odor. *Postoperative physiologic and psychologic stressors may interfere with learning. A basic understanding of what to expect in the way of tubes, drains, and procedures reduces stress in the immediate postoperative period. Preoperative teaching can enhance recall and postoperative learning.*
- Assist in identifying stoma site, avoiding folds of skin, bones, scar tissue, and the waistline or belt area. Be sure to consider the client's occupation and style of clothing. The site should be visible to the client and accessible for manipulation. *Stoma placement is a vital component of adjustment and self-care. Care is taken to place the stoma away from areas of constant irritation by clothing or movement. It should be located so that the client can cover and disguise the collecting device, maintain the seal to prevent leakage, and effectively cleanse and maintain the site.*
- Perform bowel-preparation activities as ordered. *Bowel preparation is done to prevent fecal contamination of the peritoneal cavity and to decompress the bowel during surgery.*

## POSTOPERATIVE CARE

- Provide routine postoperative care (See Chapter 7).
- Monitor intake and output carefully, assessing urine output every hour for the first 24 hours, then every 4 hours or as ordered. Call the physician if urine output is less than 30 mL per hour. *Tissue edema and bleeding may interfere with urinary output from stoma, catheters, or drains. Maintenance of urine out-*

*flow is vital to prevent hydronephrosis and possible renal damage. A urine output of at least 30 mL per hour is necessary for effective renal function.*
- Assess color and consistency of urine. Expect pink or bright red urine fading to pink and then clearing by the third postoperative day. Urine may be cloudy due to mucus production by bowel mucosa. *Bright red blood in the urine from a urinary diversion may indicate hemorrhage, necessitating further surgery. Excessive cloudiness or malodorous urine may indicate infection.*
- Assess size, color, and condition of the stoma and surrounding skin every 2 hours for the first 24 hours, then every 4 hours for 48 to 72 hours. Expect the stoma to appear bright red and slightly edematous initially. Slight bleeding during cleansing is normal. *Compromised circulation causes the stoma to appear pale, gray, or cyanotic or blanch when touched. Other complications, such as infection or impaired healing may be evidenced by a change in the appearance of the stoma or incision.*
- Irrigate the ileal diversion catheter with 30 to 60 mL of normal saline every 4 hours or as ordered. *Mucus produced by the bowel wall may accumulate in the newly devised reservoir or obstruct catheters.*
- Monitor serum electrolyte values, acid-base balance, and renal function tests such as BUN and serum creatinine. *Reabsorption of electrolytes from reservoirs created by portions of bowel may result in electrolyte imbalance and metabolic acidosis. Optimal renal function is necessary to maintain a normal state of homeostasis.*
- Teach the client and family about stoma and urinary diversion care, including odor management, skin care, increased fluid intake, pouch application and leakage prevention, self-catheterization for clients with continent reservoirs, and signs of infection and other complications. *The ability to provide self-care is a significant factor in the adjustment to a changed body image. Teaching family members facilitates acceptance and adjustment. The family also needs this knowledge in case illness or disability interferes with the self-care capacity.*

*may indicate impaired catheter or drainage system patency. Prompt intervention is necessary to prevent hydronephrosis. A change in color or clarity may indicate a complication such as hemorrhage or infection.*

**PRACTICE ALERT** *Promptly report urine output of less than 30 mL per hour, which may indicate low vascular volume or renal insufficiency. Prompt intervention is vital to restore cardiac output and prevent acute renal failure.* ■

- Label all catheters, stents, and their drainage containers. Maintain separate closed gravity drainage systems for each. *Clear identification of each tube can prevent errors in irrigating and calculating outputs. Separate closed systems minimize the risk and extent of potential bacterial contamination and resultant infection.*

**PRACTICE ALERT** *Use aseptic techniques and strictly follow guidelines for irrigating catheters. Catheters placed in the kidney pelvis are irrigated using gentle pressure and small amounts of fluid (10 to 15 mL) to avoid damaging renal tissues.* ■

- Secure ureteral catheters and stents with tape; prevent kinking or occlusion; and maintain gravity flow by keeping drainage bag below level of kidneys. *Impaired urine flow can lead to urinary retention and distention of the bladder, a newly created reservoir, or the renal pelvis (hydronephrosis).*
- Encourage fluid intake of 3000 mL per day. *Increased fluid intake maintains a high urinary output, reducing the risk of infection. Dilute urine is less irritating to the skin surrounding the stoma site. Electrolyte reabsorption from reservoirs may increase risk of calculi; high fluid intake and urine output reduce this risk.*

**PRACTICE ALERT** *Monitor urine output closely for first 24 hours after stents or ureteral catheters are removed. Edema or stricture of ureters may impede output, leading to hydronephrosis and kidney damage.* ■

- Encourage activity to tolerance. *Ambulation promotes drainage of urine from reservoirs and helps prevent calcium loss from bones, which could precipitate calculus formation.*

## Risk for Impaired Skin Integrity

The skin surrounding the stoma site of an ileal conduit is at risk for irritation and breakdown. Because urine is acidic and contains high concentrations of electrolytes, it has a corrosive effect on skin. In addition, adhesives and sealants used to prevent pouch leakage may irritate the skin.

- Assess peristomal skin for redness, excoriation, or signs of breakdown. Assess for urine leakage from catheters, stents, or drains. Keep the skin clean and dry. Change wet dressings. *Intact skin is the first line of defense against infection. Impaired skin integrity may lead to local or systemic infection and impaired healing.*

---

| BOX 26–3 ■ Urinary Stoma Care |
| --- |

- Gather all supplies: a clean, disposable pouch; liquid skin barrier or barrier ring; 4-by-4 gauze squares; stoma guide; adhesive solvent; clean gloves; and a clean washcloth.
- Assess knowledge, learning needs, and ability and willingness to assist with procedure. Explain the procedure as needed.
- Use standard precautions.
- Remove old pouch, pulling gently away from skin. Warm water or adhesive solvent may be used to loosen the seal if necessary.
- Assess stoma. Normally the stoma is bright red and appears moist. Report a dark purple, black, or very pale stoma to the physician. Slight bleeding with cleansing is normal, especially in the immediate postoperative period.
- Prevent urine flow during cleaning by placing a rolled gauze square or tampon over the stoma opening.
- Cleanse skin around the stoma with soap and water, rinse, and pat or air dry.
- Use the stoma guide to determine correct size for the bag opening and/or protective ring seal. Trim the bag or seal as needed.
- Apply skin barrier; allow to dry.
- Apply the bag with an opening no more than 1 to 2 mm wider than outside of stoma. Allow no wrinkles or creases where the bag contacts the skin.
- Connect bag to the urine-collection device. Dispose of old pouch, used supplies, and gloves appropriately. Wash hands.
- Chart procedure, including stoma appearance and response of the client.

---

- Ensure gravity drainage of urine collection device or empty bag every 2 hours. *Overfilling of the collection bag may damage the seal, allowing leakage and contact of urine with skin.*
- Change urine collection appliance as needed, removing any mucus from stoma. See Box 26–3 for care of a urinary drainage stoma. *Meticulous care and protection of skin surrounding stoma can maintain integrity and prevent breakdown.*

## Disturbed Body Image

A radical cystectomy and urinary diversion affect the client's body image. In most cases, an abdominal stoma is created, requiring either a drainage appliance or regular catheterization of the stoma to drain urine. Removal of the prostate and seminal vesicles or the uterus and ovaries leaves the client sterile. If radiation or chemotherapy is planned as adjunctive therapy, the client may experience hair loss, stomatitis, nausea and vomiting, or other disturbing side effects of therapy.

- Use therapeutic communication techniques, actively listening and responding to the client's and family's concerns. *Clients must know their feelings and concerns are respected and valued. Denial, anger, guilt, bargaining, or depression are common during grieving and normal for a client undergoing a significant change in body image.*
- Recognize and accept behaviors that indicate use of coping mechanisms, encouraging adaptive mechanisms. *The client may initially use defensive coping mechanisms such as denial, minimization, and dissociation from the immediate*

*situation to reduce anxiety and maintain psychologic integrity. Adaptive mechanisms include learning as much as possible about the surgery and its effects, practicing procedures, setting realistic goals, and rehearsing various alternative outcomes.*

- Encourage looking at, touching, and caring for the stoma and appliance as soon as possible. Allow the client to proceed gradually, providing support and encouragement. *Accepting the stoma as part of the self is vital to adapting to the changed body image and is indicated by a willingness to provide self-care.*

- Discuss concerns about returning to usual activities, perceived relationship changes, and resumption of sexual relations. Provide referral to support group or provide for contact with someone who has successfully adjusted to a urinary diversion. *Clients and families may be reluctant to discuss topics of concern. An atmosphere of openness and acceptance facilitates expression of concerns and anxieties related to the changed body image.*

### Risk for Infection

Diagnostic instrumentation procedures, surgical manipulation, and disruption of normal urinary tract defense mechanisms increase the risk of ascending urinary tract infection. When an ileal conduit or artificial bladder is created using bowel tissue, the normal bacteriostatic activity of bladder mucosa is lost. In addition, the peristaltic action of the ureters may be disrupted, and the ureterovesical junction no longer prevents urine reflux. Adjunctive chemotherapy or radiation treatments may impair normal immune function and further increase the risk of infection.

- Maintain separate closed drainage systems, keeping drainage bags lower than the kidney, and prevent loops or kinks in drainage tubing, which impede urine flow. *Although urine is sterile when it leaves the kidney, bacteria grow rapidly in urine. Prevention of urine reflux is essential to preventing UTI.*

- Monitor for signs of infection: elevated temperature, cloudy or foul-smelling urine, hematuria, general malaise, back or abdominal pain, and nausea and vomiting. *Infection undermines*

**PRACTICE ALERT** *Impaired immune function (due to aging or the effects of chemotherapy) and urine cloudiness (related to the effects of urine on ileal mucosa) can mask usual signs of UTI such as fever and altered urine clarity. Be alert for more generalized manifestations such as increased fatigue and malaise.* ■

*the healing process. Early detection and treatment help prevent long-term consequences such as chronic pyelonephritis.*

- Teach signs and symptoms of infection and self-care measures to prevent UTI. *The client with a cystectomy and ileal diversion, urostomy, or continent reservoir is at risk of UTI for life because of impaired urinary defense mechanisms. Using clean or aseptic technique in providing care, increasing fluid intake, and using measures to acidify urine minimize this risk to a certain degree but do not eliminate it.*

### Using NANDA, NIC, and NOC

Chart 26–3 shows links between NANDA nursing diagnoses, NIC, and NOC for the client with a urinary tract tumor.

### Home Care

The need for individual and family teaching for the client who has had surgery to treat a urinary tract tumor is significant. For many clients, surgery means a lifelong change in urinary elimination. Even the client who has undergone transurethral excision of bladder tumors requires follow-up cystoscopy on a regular basis and needs to be alert for signs of tumor recurrence.

The client who has had a urinary diversion needs teaching about care of the stoma and surrounding skin, prevention of urine reflux and infection, signs and symptoms of UTI and renal calculi, and, in some cases, self-catheterization using clean technique.

### CHART 26–3 NANDA, NIC, AND NOC LINKAGES

#### The Client with Bladder Cancer

| NURSING DIAGNOSES | NURSING INTERVENTIONS | NURSING OUTCOMES |
|---|---|---|
| • Disturbed Body Image | • Coping Enhancement <br> • Grief Work Facilitation | • Body Image <br> • Grief Resolution |
| • Ineffective Management of Therapeutic Regimen | • Teaching: Procedure/Treatment <br> • Self-Responsibility Facilitation | • Treatment Behavior: Illness or Injury <br> • Knowledge: Treatment Regimen <br> • Participation: Health Care Decisions |
| • Risk for Impaired Skin Integrity | • Skin Surveillance <br> • Wound Care | • Tissue Integrity: Skin and Mucous Membranes <br> • Wound Healing: Primary Intention |
| • Sexual Dysfunction | • Teaching: Sexuality | • Sexual Functioning |

*Note. Data from Nursing Outcomes Classification (NOC) by M. Johnson & M. Maas (Eds.), 1997, St. Louis: Mosby; Nursing Diagnoses: Definitions & Classification 2001–2002 by North American Nursing Diagnosis Association, 2001, Philadelphia: NANDA; Nursing Interventions Classification (NIC) by J.C. McCloskey & G. M. Bulechek (Eds.), 2000, St. Louis: Mosby. Reprinted by permission.*

## Nursing Care Plan
### A Client with a Bladder Tumor

Ben Hussain is a 61-year-old automobile salesman. He is married and has five children, all of whom are grown and living away from home. One week ago, Mr. Hussain became alarmed when his urine became bright red. Even though he had no other symptoms, he called his physician. The physician ordered a urinalysis and urine cytology, revealing gross hematuria and poorly differentiated abnormal cells. Cystoscopy and tissue biopsy confirm a stage C tumor involving the bladder trigone. Mr. Hussain is admitted for a radical cystectomy and continent urinary diversion.

### ASSESSMENT

Mr. Hussain's admission history, obtained by Tara Mills, RN, his primary nurse, indicates that he has lost 10 to 15 pounds over the last few months. He smoked two to three packs of cigarettes per day for 40 years, but cut back to a pack a day about a year ago. He says he could not quit smoking entirely. He drinks five to six cups of coffee daily and consumes a moderate amount of alcohol, averaging three to four drinks a day. Mr. Hussain says that he is "a little nervous about surgery and what they're going to find." Ms. Mills notes that he fidgets and talks rapidly throughout their interview. He also expresses concern about how he will handle the pain after surgery, because he has never been hospitalized before his cystoscopy. Physical assessment findings include T 98.2°F (36.7°C) PO, P 84, R 18, and BP 154/86. Examinations of the skin, neuromuscular, and cardiac systems are within normal limits. Scattered expiratory crackles are noted on auscultation of lung fields. Bowel sounds are very active; Mr. Hussain explains that he began taking his bowel-preparation laxative the day before admission. Slight tenderness is noted in the suprapubic region. Mr. Hussain's urine is clear and bright pink. Complete blood count (CBC) and chemistry screening results are within normal limits. Surgery is planned for 9:00 A.M. the following day.

### DIAGNOSIS

- *Anxiety* related to undetermined extent of disease and fear of pain
- *Deficient knowledge* related to care and management of continent urinary diversion
- *Impaired urinary elimination* related to cystectomy and urinary diversion
- *Risk for impaired gas exchange* related to smoking history and effects of anesthesia

### EXPECTED OUTCOMES

- Verbalize decreased feelings of anxiety.
- Demonstrate appropriate postoperative pain relief through subjective reports of pain severity and objective findings.
- Be able to care for urinary diversion and surrounding skin, prior to discharge.
- Demonstrate self-catheterization of stoma using appropriate technique prior to discharge.
- Maintain normal urine output with acceptable color and clarity and no signs of infection.

- Maintain adequate gas exchange as evidenced by good skin color, $O_2$ saturation greater than 95%, and clear lung sounds upon auscultation.

### PLANNING AND IMPLEMENTATION

- Spend as much time as possible with Mr. Hussain and his family preoperatively, answering questions fully and encouraging expression of fears.
- Provide written and verbal explanations when feasible.
- Administer analgesia on a regular basis for the first 48 to 72 hours. Monitor for objective signs of unrelieved pain.
- Explain all procedures related to stoma and diversion care as they are being performed.
- Encourage Mr. Hussain to look at stoma and touch it when ready.
- Teach stoma and skin care, as well as self-catheterization, emphasizing measures to prevent skin irritation and urinary tract infection.
- Monitor urine output, color, clarity, and consistency every hour for first 24 hours, then every 4 hours for 24 hours, then every 8 hours. Report output of less than 30 mL per hour, bright bleeding, excessively cloudy or malodorous urine.
- Assist with use of incentive spirometer every hour while awake. Ambulate as soon as possible. Assess lung sounds every 4 hours, reporting increased crackles or diminished breath sounds.
- Refer Mr. and Mrs. Hussain to local stoma group on discharge.

### EVALUATION

On discharge, Mr. Hussain has performed self-catheterization and stoma and skin care several times. His wife also is able to catheterize the stoma and demonstrate skin care. His urine is pale yellow and slightly cloudy. Mr. Hussain is ambulating independently and using oxycodone (Percocet) twice a day for pain relief. His lungs are clear, and he is very proud of having "survived" 7 days without a cigarette. He says, "Now I'm going to shoot for 7 weeks, then 7 months, then 7 years without a smoke!" A home health referral is made to continue teaching Mr. Hussain to care for his diversion and appliance.

### Critical Thinking in the Nursing Process

1. How does cigarette smoking contribute to the increased risk of urinary tract tumors?
2. Suppose Mr. Hussain had become confused, disoriented, and tremorous and had begun to experience visual hallucinations 2 to 3 days postoperatively. What would you suspect the cause to be? What would be the appropriate response?
3. Develop a care plan for Mr. Hussain for the nursing diagnosis, *Risk for sexual dysfunction*.

See Evaluating Your Response in Appendix C.

## THE CLIENT WITH URINARY RETENTION

**Urinary retention,** incomplete emptying of the bladder, can lead to overdistention of the bladder, poor detrusor muscle contractility, and inability to urinate. If the problem persists, hydroureter and hydronephrosis can result.

## PHYSIOLOGY REVIEW

Normally, bladder emptying is controlled by the interaction of muscle tone and the autonomic nervous system. The sympathetic nervous system (SNS) relaxes the detrusor muscle, allowing the bladder to fill with urine. The internal sphincter, a continuation of the detrusor muscle, remains closed during filling. Pressures within the bladder remain low during filling, in contrast to high sphincter and urethral pressures. Voluntary muscles of the external sphincter and pelvic floor help maintain these high pressures. When the bladder contains 150 to 300 mL of urine, signals from stretch receptors in the bladder wall are transmitted to the spinal cord and cerebral cortex. Reflexive bladder emptying can be consciously inhibited. During *micturition* (bladder emptying), parasympathetic stimulation causes the detrusor muscle of the bladder fundus to contract, opening the internal sphincter. The external sphincter then relaxes, allowing urine to flow out.

## PATHOPHYSIOLOGY

Either mechanical obstruction of the bladder outlet or a functional problem can cause urinary retention. *Benign prostatic hypertrophy (BPH)* is a common cause; difficulty initiating and maintaining urine flow is often the presenting complaint in men with BPH. Acute inflammation associated with infection or trauma of the bladder, urethra, or vulvovaginal tissues may also interfere with micturition. Scarring due to repeated urinary tract infection can lead to urethral stricture and a mechanical obstruction. Bladder calculi may also obstruct the urethral opening from the bladder.

Surgery, particularly abdominal or pelvic surgery, may disrupt detrusor muscle function, leading to urine retention. Drugs also may interfere with its function. Anticholinergic medications such as atropine, glycopyrrolate (Robinul), propantheline bromide (Pro-Banthine), scopolamine hydrochloride (Transderm-Scop), and others can lead to acute urinary retention and bladder distention. Many other drug groups have anticholinergic side effects and may cause urinary retention. Among these are antianxiety agents such as diazepam (Valium), antidepressant and tricyclic drugs such as imipramine (Tofranil), antiparkinsonian drugs, antipsychotic agents, and some sedative/hypnotic drugs. In addition, antihistamines common in over-the-counter cough, cold, allergy, and sleep-promoting drugs have anticholinergic effects and may interfere with bladder emptying. Diphenhydramine (Benadryl) is an example of a nonprescription antihistamine.

Voluntary urinary retention (particularly common among nurses!) may lead to overfilling of the bladder and a loss of detrusor muscle tone.

The client with urinary retention is unable to empty the bladder completely. Overflow voiding or incontinence may occur, with 25 to 50 mL of urine eliminated at frequent intervals. Assessment reveals a firm, distended bladder that may be displaced to one side of midline. Percussion of the lower abdomen reveals a dull tone, reflective of fluid in the bladder.

## COLLABORATIVE CARE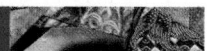

Mechanical obstructions are treated by removing or repairing the obstruction when possible. Resection of the prostate gland may be done for urinary retention related to BPH. Bladder calculi are removed, and measures to prevent their formation are instituted.

An indwelling urinary catheter or intermittent straight catheterization can prevent urinary retention and overdistention of the bladder. Cholinergic medications such as bethanechol chloride (Urecholine), which promote detrusor muscle contraction and bladder emptying, may be used. A medication with no anticholinergic side effects may be substituted when urinary retention is related to drug therapy.

## NURSING CARE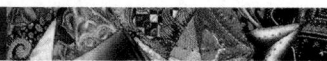

Health promotion measures to prevent urinary retention include monitoring urine output in at-risk clients and evaluating drug regimens for medications known to interfere with detrusor muscle function. Pay particular attention to elimination when these drugs are ordered (or used by) a client with BPH or other mechanical obstruction of urine flow.

### Impaired Urinary Elimination

Nursing measures to promote urination include placing the client in normal voiding position and providing for privacy. Additional measures include running water, placing the client's hands in warm water, pouring warm water over the perineum, or taking a warm sitz bath.

In acute urinary retention, catheterization may be necessary to relieve bladder distention and prevent hydronephrosis. Use a relatively small catheter (16 Fr. for a man, 14 Fr. for a woman). A coudé-tipped catheter is passed more easily in the older man with an enlarged prostate. Using 2% lidocaine gel (10 mL injected into the male urethra or lubrication of the catheter with the gel for a woman) reduces discomfort during catheterization and promotes pelvic muscle relaxation (Gray, 2000b). Carefully observe the client as the distended bladder drains.

**PRACTICE ALERT** *Some clients may experience a vasovagal response, becoming pale, sweaty, and hypotensive if the bladder is rapidly drained. Draining urine in 500 mL increments, clamping the catheter for 5 to 10 minutes between increments, may prevent this response. Hematuria also may occur with rapid bladder decompression. Promptly notify the physician if hematuria develops (Gray, 2000b).* ■

Home care for the client with urinary retention varies, depending on the cause. Some clients may be taught intermittent self-catheterization. Instruct all clients who have experienced urinary retention to avoid over-the-counter drugs that affect micturition, especially those with an anticholinergic effect (allergy and cold medications, many nonprescription sleep aids). Other home care measures include double-voiding (urinate, remain on the toilet for 2 to 5 minutes, then urinate again), scheduled voiding, or, when other measures fail, an indwelling catheter. When an indwelling catheter is necessary, teach the client and family to use clean technique when changing from overnight bag to leg bag, and to promptly report signs of UTI to the primary care provider.

## THE CLIENT WITH NEUROGENIC BLADDER

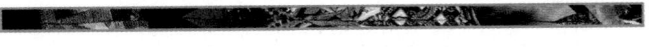

The neurologic connections influencing bladder filling, the perception of fullness and the need to void, and bladder emptying are complex. Disruption of the central or peripheral nervous systems may interfere with normal mechanisms, causing **neurogenic bladder.**

### PATHOPHYSIOLOGY

As noted in the physiology section of urinary retention, bladder filling and emptying is controlled by the central nervous system (CNS). This neurologic control can be disrupted at any level: the cerebral cortex (voluntary impulses); the micturition center of the midbrain; the spinal cord tracts; or the peripheral nerves of the bladder itself.

### Spastic Bladder Dysfunction

A simple reflex arc exists between the bladder and the spinal cord at levels S2 through S4. The stimulus of more than 400 mL of urine in the bladder causes reflex contraction of the detrusor muscle and bladder emptying unless voluntary control (cerebral input) is used to suppress it. Disruption of CNS transmission above the sacral spinal cord segment typically leads to *spastic neurogenic bladder.* Both sensory and voluntary control of urination are interrupted partially or totally, while the sacral reflex arc remains intact. The stimuli generated by bladder filling cause frequent spontaneous detrusor muscle contraction and involuntary bladder emptying. Spinal cord injury above the sacral segment is the most common cause of a spastic bladder. Other causes include stoke, multiple sclerosis, and other CNS lesions (Porth, 2002).

### Flaccid Bladder Dysfunction

Damage to the sacral spinal cord at the level of the reflex arc, the cauda equina, or the sacral nerve roots causes loss of detrusor muscle tone and a *flaccid neurogenic bladder.* The perception of bladder fullness is lost, and the bladder becomes overdistended, with weak and ineffective detrusor muscle contractions. Flaccid neurogenic bladder is seen with myelomeningocele and during the spinal shock phase of a spinal cord injury above the sacral region. During the spinal shock phase, all reflex activity below the level of spinal cord injury is suppressed.

Peripheral neuropathies may also cause bladder atony and overfilling. Either sensory or motor pathways (or both) may be disrupted, leading to incomplete bladder emptying and large residual volumes after voiding (Porth, 2002). Diabetes mellitus is the most common cause of peripheral bladder neuropathy. Other causes include multiple sclerosis, chronic alcoholism, and prolonged overdistention of the bladder.

## COLLABORATIVE CARE

Management of neurogenic bladder focuses on maintaining continence and avoiding complications associated with overfilling or incomplete emptying of the bladder. Because self-care is the goal, teaching is a primary intervention for the health care team.

### Diagnostic Tests

The following diagnostic tests may be ordered for the client with a neurogenic bladder.

- *Urine culture* to detect possible urinary tract infection related to impaired bladder function.
- *Urinalysis* and *serum BUN* and *creatinine* to evaluate renal function. Ascending infection or hydronephrosis resulting from bladder overfilling and vesicoureteral reflux can damage the kidneys. Impaired renal function may lead to blood cells or protein in the urine, and elevated BUN and creatinine levels.
- *Postvoid catheterization* to measure residual urine. After voiding, the bladder normally contains less than 50 mL of urine. Amounts greater than 50 mL may indicate ineffective detrusor muscle contractions, common in neurogenic bladder.
- *Cystometrography* to evaluate bladder filling and the detrusor muscle tone and function.

### Medications

Medications may be prescribed to increase or decrease the contractility of the detrusor muscle, increase or decrease the tone of the internal sphincter, or to relax the external urethral sphincter.

Bethanechol, a cholinergic drug, stimulates detrusor muscle contraction in flaccid neurogenic bladder. It is generally used to manage short-term urinary retention (e.g., following surgery or childbirth). It may used in combination with bladder-training techniques to promote complete emptying of a neurogenic bladder. Anticholinesterase drugs such as neostigmine (Prostigmin) and pyridostigmine (Mestinon) also may be used to increase detrusor muscle tone.

Anticholinergic drugs (parasympathetic blockers) relax the detrusor muscle and contract the internal sphincter, increasing bladder capacity in clients with spastic bladder dysfunction. Oxybutynin (Ditropan) and tolterodine (Detrol) inhibit the muscarinic effects of acetylcholine on smooth muscle, reducing detrusor muscle spasticity and promoting bladder filling. Other anticholinergic drugs also may be used, including propantheline (Pro-Banthine) or flavoxate (Urispas). Dry mouth, blurred vision, and constipation are potential adverse effects of anticholinergic medications. See the Medication Administration box on page 732 for drugs used to modify detrusor muscle activity.

## Medication Administration
### The Client with Neurogenic Bladder

**CHOLINERGIC DRUGS TO STIMULATE MICTURITION**

Bethanechol chloride (Urocholine)

Bethanechol stimulates the parasympathetic nervous system, increasing detrusor muscle tone and producing a contraction strong enough to initiate micturition. It is used primarily to treat acute postoperative and postpartum urinary retention.

**Nursing Responsibilities**
- Assess for contraindications, including hypersensitivity, hyperthyroidism, peptic ulcer disease, asthma, significant bradycardia or hypotension, coronary heart disease, epilepsy, and parkinsonism.
- Do not give to clients who have had recent gastrointestinal or bladder surgery or those with possible gastrointestinal or urinary tract obstruction.
- Give oral forms on an empty stomach to reduce the risk of nausea and vomiting.
- Administer parenteral bethanechol subcutaneously. Keep atropine, the antidote for bethanechol overdose or toxicity, available.
- Observe for desired effect within 30 to 60 minutes after oral administration, 5 to 15 minutes after injection.
- Assess for adverse effects such as malaise, headache, abdominal cramping, nausea, hypotension with reflex tachycardia, wheezing, and dyspnea.

**Client and Family Teaching**
- Take the medication 1 hour before or 2 hours after meals.
- Use caution when rising from a recumbent or sitting position; you may feel dizzy or lightheaded.

**ANTICHOLINERGIC DRUGS TO TREAT SPASTIC BLADDER**

Oxybutynin (Ditropan)
Tolterodine (Detrol)
Propantheline bromide (Pro-Banthine)
Flavoxate hydrochloride (Urispas)

Anticholinergic drugs inhibit the response to acetylcholine, relaxing the detrusor muscle and increasing internal sphincter tone. The combination of detrusor relaxation and internal sphincter contraction increases the bladder capacity of clients with spastic or hyperreflexive neurogenic bladder. Of these medications, tolterodine has the most specific effects on the detrusor muscle with fewer anticholinergic side effects.

**Nursing Responsibilities**
- Assess for contraindications, such as glaucoma, gastrointestinal or urinary tract obstruction, severe ulcerative colitis or toxic megacolon, unstable cardiovascular status, or myasthenia gravis.
- Observe for the desired effect of increased bladder capacity with decreased incontinence and spasm.
- Monitor for possible interaction with other drugs such as narcotic analgesics, antidysrhythmic medications, antihistamines, antidepressants, or psychoactive drugs.
- Monitor heart rate and blood pressure, especially when given to clients with known cardiovascular disease.
- Assess for adverse effects such as urinary hesitancy or retention, dysrhythmias, mental status changes, and gastrointestinal disturbances.

**Client and Family Teaching**
- Promptly report eye pain, rapid heart beat, difficulty breathing, rash or hives, or changes in mental function to your primary care provider.
- These drugs may cause drowsiness or blurred vision. Use caution when driving, operating machinery, or performing other tasks requiring mental acuity.
- Hard candies help relieve dry mouth associated with these drugs.
- Do not use alcohol or nonprescription antihistamines while taking these drugs.

## Treatments

### Dietary

Dietary measures to reduce the risk for UTI and urinary calculi may be suggested for the client with neurogenic bladder. A moderate to high fluid intake and a diet that acidifies the urine are helpful. Cranberry juice is recommended to maintain urine acidity. See Table 26–3 for additional foods to include or avoid in the diet to help prevent UTI and urolithiasis. The timing of fluid intake may be regulated to promote continence.

### Bladder Retraining

Clients with spastic neurogenic bladder may use measures to stimulate reflex voiding, allowing scheduled toileting. Techniques include using trigger points, for example, stroking or pinching the abdomen, inner thigh, or glans penis. Pulling pubic hairs, tapping the suprapubic region, or inserting a gloved finger into the rectum and gently stretching the anal sphincter can also stimulate urination.

The *Credé's method* (applying pressure to the suprapubic region with the fingers of one or both hands), manual pressure on the abdomen, and the Valsalva maneuver (bearing down while holding one's breath) promote bladder emptying for the client with a spastic or flaccid bladder.

**PRACTICE ALERT** *Increasing lower abdominal and bladder pressure with the Credé's method can stimulate autonomic dysreflexia in some clients with spinal cord injuries. Autonomic dysreflexia is a medical emergency in which the blood pressure rises rapidly due to SNS stimulation.* ■

See Chapter 41 for a discussion of autonomic dysreflexia. ⬭

The client with a flaccid bladder may require catheterization to completely empty the bladder. An indwelling catheter may be used initially, but intermittent catheterization is preferred. Clean intermittent self-catheterization is performed every 3 to 4 hours to prevent overdistention of the bladder (see Procedure 41–1). ∞

## Surgery

Surgery may be required when urination cannot be effectively managed using more conservative measures. *Rhizotomy,* or destruction of the nerve supply to the detrusor muscle or the external sphincter, may be used for clients with hyperreflexia or spasticity. Urinary diversion is another surgical technique used when conservative management fails. Implantation of an artificial sphincter may be useful for some clients with neurogenic bladder. See Table 26–6 for urinary diversion techniques and page 726 nursing care of the client undergoing a urinary diversion.

## NURSING CARE

Nursing care of the client with a neurogenic bladder is directed toward promoting urinary drainage and continence, preventing complications, and teaching the client and family self-care techniques.

### Assessment

Nursing assessment for neurogenic bladder includes obtaining a complete nursing history, focusing on information related to CNS or spinal cord injury or disease, as well as disorders that affect the peripheral nervous system (e.g., diabetes). Ask about measures used to stimulate or control urination. Inspect and palpate the lower abdomen and suprapubic region for tenderness or bladder distention. Percuss the suprapubic region for a dull percussion tone indicative of a full bladder. Dullness up to the level of the umbilicus indicates at least 500 mL of urine in the bladder (Gray, 2000). Assess urine for color, clarity, and odor. Collect a specimen for analysis as indicated.

### Nursing Diagnoses and Interventions

Although each client has individual nursing care needs, examples of nursing diagnoses appropriate for the client with a neurogenic bladder include the following:

- *Impaired urinary elimination* related to impaired bladder innervation
- *Self-Care deficit: Toileting* related to neurologic injury
- *Risk for impaired skin integrity* related to urinary incontinence
- *Risk for infection* related to impaired urination reflex

### Home Care

Include the following in teaching for the client with neurogenic bladder and family members.

- Measures to stimulate reflex voiding and promote bladder emptying
- Use of prescribed medications, including desired and adverse effects, and interactions with other drugs
- Manifestations of UTI or urolithiasis, and measures to reduce the risk of these complications

## THE CLIENT WITH URINARY INCONTINENCE

The most common manifestation of impaired bladder control is **urinary incontinence,** or involuntary urination. Incontinence can have significant impact, leading to physical problems such as skin breakdown, infection, and rashes. Psychosocial consequences include embarrassment, isolation and withdrawal, feelings of worthlessness and helplessness, and depression.

Approximately 13 million people in the United States have some degree of urinary incontinence. The estimated cost of managing incontinence is $10 billion yearly. Urinary incontinence is especially common among older clients (see the box below). Up to 30% of older women living in the community experience urinary incontinence. In long-term care, foster care, and homebound populations, the incidence is about 50% (Gallo et al., 1999; Tierney et al., 2001). The actual prevalence of urinary incontinence is nearly impossible to determine. Embarrassment and the availability of products to protect clothing and prevent detection contribute to clients' not seeking evaluation of and treatment for incontinence.

## Nursing Care of the Older Adult

### MINIMIZING THE RISK FOR UTI AND UI

Older adults have a higher incidence of two common urinary tract disorders: urinary tract infection (UTI) and urinary incontinence (UI).

#### URINARY TRACT INFECTION

Aging affects normal protective mechanisms to prevent UTI. The pH of urine increases with aging, allowing bacteria to grow and multiply more readily. Glucosuria, more common in older adults due to the higher incidence of diabetes, facilitates bacterial growth. Incomplete bladder emptying and urinary retention are more common due to problems such as prostatic hypertrophy in men, bladder prolapse in women, and neurogenic bladder in both sexes. Changes in vaginal pH in women and decreased prostatic secretions in men may also contribute to an increased incidence of UTI.

While many UTIs in older adults are asymptomatic and self-limited, infections can lead to bacteremia, sepsis, and shock. Manifestations of UTI in the elderly include dysuria, urgency, frequency, incontinence, occasional hematuria, and confusion. Symptoms such as fever, chills, and flank pain and tenderness may be absent. Dementia may make diagnosis more difficult.

#### URINARY INCONTINENCE

Urinary incontinence, the involuntary loss of urine, is a common problem in older adults. While incontinence should never be considered a *normal* consequence of aging, age-related changes contribute to its development. Bladder capacity tends to decline with

*(continued on page 734)*

## Nursing Care of the Older Adult

### MINIMIZING THE RISK FOR UTI AND UI (continued)

age and involuntary bladder muscle contractions are more common. In women, decreased estrogen levels and pelvic muscle relaxation decrease bladder outlet and urethral resistance pressures. Decreased estrogen also causes atrophic vaginitis and urethritis, with manifestations of dysuria and urgency. Other risk factors for UI in older adults include impaired mobility and chronic degenerative diseases, impaired cognition, medications, low fluid intake, diabetes, and stroke.

#### Assessing for Home Care

Assessment for urinary problems in the older adult focuses on risk factors, the extent and manifestations of the disorder, and contributing factors. Using clear language, ask about problems with urine loss, its frequency, and any contributing factors. Inquire about frequency, urgency, and burning on urination. Identify current medications and the time of day each is taken. Assess patterns of fluid intake and output. Assess the abdomen for evidence of bladder distention or tenderness. Perform a mental status examination if indicated.

Assess the home environment (whether in the community or a residential living facility) for possible barriers to urinary elimination:

- Inadequate lighting, particularly at night
- Narrow doorways that may interfere with access to the toilet
- Inadequate toilet facilities
- The need for mobility aids such as safety bars, a raised toilet seat, or a bedside commode

#### Teaching for Home Care

Discuss the following points to help prevent UTI and UI in the older adult.

- Maintain a generous fluid intake. Reduce or eliminate fluid intake after the evening meal to reduce nocturia.
- Wear comfortable clothing that is easy to remove for toileting.
- Maintain good hygiene, but do not bathe more often than necessary; frequent bathing and feminine hygiene sprays or douches may dry perineal tissues, increasing the risk of UTI or UI.
- Perform pelvic muscle exercises (Kegel exercises) several times a day to increase perineal muscle tone.
- Reduce consumption of caffeine-containing beverages (coffee, tea, colas), citrus juices, and artificially sweetened beverages containing Nutra-Sweet.
- Use behavioral techniques such as scheduled toileting, habit training, and bladder training to reduce the frequency of incontinence. *Scheduled toileting* is toileting at regular intervals (e.g., every 2 to 4 hours). *Habit training* is toileting the client on a schedule that corresponds with the normal pattern. *Bladder training* gradually increases the bladder capacity by increasing the intervals between voidings and resisting the urge to void.
- See your primary care provider regularly for a pelvic or prostate exam.
- For women, discuss possible benefits and risks of hormone replacement therapy, physical therapy, or surgery to treat incontinence.
- Report a change in urine color, odor, or clarity or symptoms such as burning, frequency, or urgency to your primary care provider.

#### Resources for Home Care

National Association for Continence
P.O. Box 8310
Spartanburg, SC 29305-8310
864-579-7900
Website: http://www.nafc.org

## PATHOPHYSIOLOGY

Urinary continence requires a bladder able to expand and contract and sphincters that can maintain a urethral pressure higher than that in the bladder. Incontinence results when the pressure within the urinary bladder exceeds urethral resistance, allowing urine to escape. Any condition causing higher than normal bladder pressures or reduced urethral resistance can potentially result in incontinence. Relaxation of the pelvic musculature, disruption of cerebral and nervous system control, and disturbances of the bladder and its musculature are common contributing factors.

Incontinence may be an acute, self-limited disorder, or it may be chronic. The causes may be congenital or acquired, reversible or irreversible. Congenital disorders associated with incontinence include *epispadias* (absence of the upper wall of the urethra), and *meningomyelocele* (a neural tube defect in which a portion of the spinal cord and its surrounding meninges protrude through the vertebral column). Central nervous system or spinal cord trauma, stroke, and chronic neurologic disorders such as multiple sclerosis and Parkinson's disease are examples of acquired, irreversible causes of incontinence. Reversible causes include acute con-

fusion, medications such as diuretics or sedatives, prostatic enlargement, vaginal and urethral atrophy, UTI, and fecal impaction.

Incontinence is commonly categorized as stress incontinence, urge incontinence (also known as overactive bladder), overflow incontinence, and functional incontinence. Table 26–7 summarizes each type with its physiologic cause and associated factors. *Mixed incontinence*, with elements of both stress and urge incontinence, is common. *Total incontinence* is loss of all voluntary control over urination, with urine loss occurring without stimulus and in all positions.

Incontinence is associated with an increased risk for falls, fractures, pressure ulcers, urinary tract infection, and depression. It contributes to the stress of caregivers, and may be a factor in institutionalizing the client.

## COLLABORATIVE CARE

Urinary incontinence management is directed at identifying and correcting the cause if possible. If the underlying disorder cannot be corrected, techniques to manage urine output can often be taught.

**TABLE 26-7  Types of Urinary Incontinence**

| | Description | Pathophysiology | Contributing Factors |
|---|---|---|---|
| **Stress** | Loss of urine associated with increased intra-abdominal pressure during sneezing, coughing, lifting. Quantity of urine lost is usually small. | Relaxation of pelvic musculature and weakness of urethra and surrounding muscles and tissues leads to decreased urethral resistance | • Multiple pregnancies<br>• Decreased estrogen levels<br>• Short urethra, change in angle between bladder and urethra<br>• Abdominal wall weakness<br>• Prostate surgery<br>• Increased intra-abdominal pressure due to tumor, ascites, obesity |
| **Urge** | Involuntary loss of urine associated with a strong urge to void | Hypertonic or overactive detrusor muscle leads to increased pressure within bladder and inability to inhibit voiding | • Neurologic disorders such as stroke, Parkinson's disease, multiple sclerosis; peripheral nervous system disorders<br>• Detrusor muscle overactivity associated with bladder outlet obstruction, aging, or disorders such as diabetes |
| **Overflow** | Inability to empty bladder, resulting in overdistention and frequent loss of small amounts of urine | Outlet obstruction or lack of normal detrusor activity leads to overfilling of bladder and increased pressure | • Spinal cord injuries below S2<br>• Diabetic neuropathy<br>• Prostatic hypertrophy<br>• Fecal impaction<br>• Drugs, especially those with anticholinergic effect |
| **Functional** | Incontinence resulting from physical, environmental, or psycho-social causes | Ability to respond to the need to urinate is impaired | • Confusion or dementia<br>• Physical disability or impaired mobility<br>• Diuretic therapy or sedation<br>• Depression<br>• Regression |

Evaluation for incontinence begins with a complete history, including the duration, frequency, volume, and associated circumstances of urine loss. A voiding diary (Figure 26-7 ■) is often used to collect detailed information. The history also includes information about chronic or acute illnesses, previous surgeries, and current medication use, both prescription and over the counter.

Physical assessment includes abdominal, rectal, and pelvic assessment as well as evaluation of mental and neurologic status, mobility, and dexterity. Findings often associated with incontinence in women include weak abdominal and pelvic muscle tone, cystocele or urethrocele, and atrophic vaginitis. In men, an enlarged prostate gland is the physical finding most commonly associated with incontinence.

See page 736 for a research model for diagnosing urge incontinence using specific client assessment data.

## Diagnostic Tests

• *Urinalysis* and *urine culture* using a clean-catch specimen are done to rule out infection and other acute causes of incontinence.
• *Postvoiding residual (PVR) volume* is measured to determine how completely the bladder empties with voiding. Less than 50 mL PVR is expected; when 100 mL or more is obtained, further testing is indicated.
• *Cystometrography* is used to assess neuromuscular function of the bladder by evaluating detrusor muscle function, pressure within the bladder, and the filling pattern of the bladder. The client describes sensations and any urge to void as sterile water or saline is instilled into the bladder. Normally, the urge to void is perceived at 150 to 450 mL, and the bladder feels full at 300 to 500 mL. Bladder pressure and volume are recorded on a graph. When the bladder is full, the client voids, and intravesical pressure is noted during voiding.
• *Uroflowmetry* is a noninvasive test used to evaluate voiding patterns. The uroflowmeter, contained in a funnel, measures the rate of urine flow, the continuous flow time, and the total voiding time.
• *Intravenous pyelography* may be ordered to evaluate structure and function of the upper and lower urinary tract.
• *Cystoscopy* or *ultrasonography* may be ordered to identify structural disorders contributing to incontinence, such as an enlarged prostate or a tumor.

Nursing implications for the specialized studies for urinary incontinence are outlined in the box on page 736.

## Medications

Both stress and urge incontinence may improve with drug treatment.

Drugs that contract the smooth muscles of the bladder neck may reduce episodes of mild stress incontinence. Phenylpropanolamine (Acutrim, Allerest, Contac, others), a commonly used decongestant and nonprescription diet aid, is an effective preparation. Adverse effects such as hypertension, palpitations, and nervousness may limit its use.

**Your Daily Voiding Diary**                                           Date _____

This diary will help you and your health care team identify factors causing bladder control problems. Choose a 24-hour period when you can record your fluid intake (type and amount), urine output and episodes of urine leakage, any strong urge to void just prior to leaking, and your activity when leak episodes occur. The line below illustrates how to use your diary.

| Time 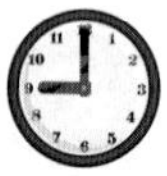 | 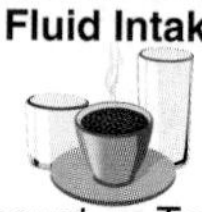 Fluid Intake | | Urine Output 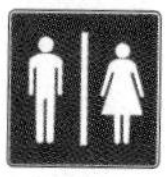 | | | Leaks 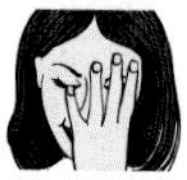 | | | Urge | Activity |
|---|---|---|---|---|---|---|---|---|---|---|
| | Amount | Type | | | | | | | Yes   No | |
| 7 am | 2 cups | coffee | sm | (med) | lg | (sm) | med | lg | Yes | walking |
| | | | sm | med | lg | sm | med | lg | | |
| | | | sm | med | lg | sm | med | lg | | |
| | | | sm | med | lg | sm | med | lg | | |
| | | | sm | med | lg | sm | med | lg | | |
| | | | sm | med | lg | sm | med | lg | | |
| | | | sm | med | lg | sm | med | lg | | |
| | | | sm | med | lg | sm | med | lg | | |
| | | | sm | med | lg | sm | med | lg | | |
| | | | sm | med | lg | sm | med | lg | | |
| | | | sm | med | lg | sm | med | lg | | |
| | | | sm | med | lg | sm | med | lg | | |
| | | | sm | med | lg | sm | med | lg | | |
| | | | sm | med | lg | sm | med | lg | | |
| | | | sm | med | lg | sm | med | lg | | |
| | | | sm | med | lg | sm | med | lg | | |
| | | | sm | med | lg | sm | med | lg | | |

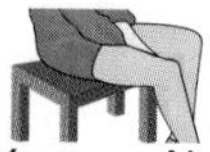

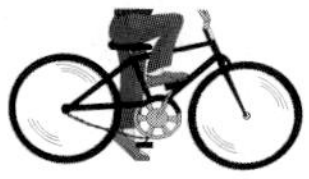

I used____ pads today.  I used ____ diapers today.

Questions to ask my health care team: _____

_____

**Figure 26–7 ■** A sample voiding diary.

*Source: Adapted: from Your Daily Bladder Diary, National Kidney and Urologic Diseases Information Center, National Institute of Diabetes and Digestive and Kidney Disease (NIDDK), National Institutes of Health.*

## Nursing Implications for Diagnostic Tests
### Urinary Incontinence

**POSTVOIDING RESIDUAL VOLUME**

**Preparation of the Client**

- Instruct the client to notify the nurse when the urge to void (urinate) is felt.
- Have client void into a collection device. Instruct to empty bladder as completely as possible. Provide for privacy to avoid "shy-bladder" syndrome.
- Immediately after voiding, catheterize using aseptic technique and a straight catheter. Drain bladder completely of residual urine.
- Record time; amount voided; amount obtained on catheterization; color, clarity, and odor of urine; and any other significant data.

**Client and Family Teaching**

- This test is used to determine how completely you empty your bladder with voiding.
- Residual urine (urine left in the bladder after urination) increases the risks of urinary infection and incontinence.

- This test poses a slight risk of infection. Report symptoms of frequency, urgency, pain on urination, nocturia, and cloudy, bloody, or malodorous urine.

**CYSTOMETROGRAM (CMG)**

**Preparation of the Client**

- Verify a signed consent for the test.
- Check for UTI as indicated by urinalysis or manifestations; infection may interfere with test results.
- No food or fluid restriction is required for this test.

**Client and Family Teaching**

- This test evaluates bladder capacity, and the motor (contraction) and sensory functions of the bladder.
- You will be given privacy during the procedure and will not be unnecessarily exposed.
- Do not strain to void during the test; straining may invalidate the results

*(continued on page 737)*

## Nursing Implications for Diagnostic Tests

### Urinary Incontinence *(continued)*

- .• You will be asked to describe sensations as the bladder is filled, including the first urge to void, the sensation of being unable to delay urination any longer, and others such as pain, sweating, or nausea.
- The test requires about 45 minutes to complete.
- Report persistent hematuria or signs of infection to the physician.
- A warm tub or sitz bath may help to relieve discomfort after testing.

### UROFLOWMETRY
#### Preparation of the Client
- Withhold medications that may interfere with test results.

#### Client and Family Teaching
- This is a rapid, simple test to measure the volume of urine voided per second.
- Privacy is provided during testing. Male clients void while standing; females, while sitting.
- You will urinate into a funnel.
- Drugs affecting bladder and sphincter tone, movement during testing, and straining during voiding may invalidate test results.
- Increase your fluid intake and do not urinate for several hours prior to the test to ensure a full bladder and a strong urge to void during testing.
- No discomfort or risk is associated with this test.

---

When incontinence is associated with postmenopausal atrophic vaginitis, estrogen therapy may be effective. Both systemic estrogens and local creams are used.

Clients with urge incontinence may be treated with preparations that increase bladder capacity. The primary drugs used to inhibit detrusor muscle contractions and increase bladder capacity include oxybutinin (Ditropan), an anticholinergic drug, and tolterodine (Detrol), a more specific antimuscarinic agent. These drugs can be taken once or twice a day, and have fewer side effects than less specific anticholinergic drugs. Drugs with anticholinergic effects are contraindicated for the client with acute glaucoma. Urinary retention is a potential side effect that must be considered when these drugs are used (see the Medication Administration box on page 732).

### Surgery

Surgery may be used to treat stress incontinence associated with cystocele or urethrocele and overflow incontinence associated with an enlarged prostate gland.

Suspension of the bladder neck, a technique that brings the angle between the bladder and urethra closer to normal, is effective in treating stress incontinence associated with urethrocele in 80% to 95% of clients. A laparoscopic, vaginal, or abdominal approach may be used to perform this surgery. Care of the client with a bladder neck suspension is outlined in the Nursing Care box on page 738.

Prostatectomy, using either the transurethral or suprapubic approach, is indicated for the client who is experiencing

## Nursing Research

### Evidence-Based Practice for Urinary Incontinence

While an accurate diagnosis of stress urinary incontinence often is made based on clinical data, motor urge incontinence has been more difficult to accurately diagnose without urodynamic testing. This presents difficulty for nurses and nurse practitioners planning care for incontinent clients when urologic testing is not feasible or readily available. A model developed by Gray, McClain, Peruggia, Patrie, and Steers (2001) may be useful to address this problem in cognitively intact adults. By comparing client data with urolodynamic testing results, this team of researchers identified factors predictive of motor urge incontinence. These factors included age, gender, and three key symptoms: diurnal frequency (urinating more often than every 2 hours while awake), nocturia (awakening with urge to urinate more than once per night if under age 65, twice per night if over age 65), and urge incontinence (urine loss associated with a strong desire to urinate). The presence of all three symptoms was more than 92% predictive of motor urge incontinence in study participants of all ages (range 18 to 89; median 61) and both genders.

#### Implications for Nursing
Asking specific questions about urinary tract symptoms can facilitate accurate identification of the nursing diagnosis, *Urge urinary*

*incontinence*. Accurate diagnosis is vital to planning and implementing appropriate care measures, and achieving the desired outcome of continence. Successful treatment promotes self-esteem and provides positive reinforcement for continuing planned strategies.

#### Critical Thinking in Client Care
1. What nursing care measures and client teaching will you provide for the client with stress incontinence that may not be appropriate or necessary for the client with urge incontinence? For the client with urge incontinence but not stress incontinence?
2. Identify circumstances in which it may not be possible or feasible to have the client undergo urodynamic testing to differentiate stress, urge, or mixed (stress and urge) incontinence.
3. The clients in this study lived independently in the community and were cognitively intact. Can the data in this study be generalized to clients residing in a long-term care facility? Can the results be applied to all types of incontinence? Why or why not?

---

*Note. From "A Model for Predicting Motor Urge Urinary Incontinence" by M. Gray et al., 2001, Nursing Research, 50(2), p. 116–122.*

## NURSING CARE OF THE CLIENT HAVING A BLADDER NECK SUSPENSION

### PREOPERATIVE CARE

- Provide routine preoperative care and teaching as outlined in Chapter 7. ⚭
- Discuss the need to avoid straining and the Valsalva maneuver postoperatively. Suggest measures such as increasing fluid and fiber intake and using a stool softener to prevent postoperative constipation. *Straining and increased abdominal pressure during the Valsalva maneuver may place excessive stress on suture lines and interfere with healing.*

### POSTOPERATIVE CARE

- Provide routine postoperative care as outlined in Chapter 7.
- Monitor urine output, including quantity, color, and clarity. Expect urine to be pink initially, gradually clearing. *Bright red urine, excessive vaginal drainage, or incisional bleeding may indi-*

*cate hemorrhage. Instrumentation of the urinary tract increases the potential for UTI; cloudy urine may be an early sign.*
- Maintain stability and patency of suprapubic and/or urethral catheters. Secure catheters in position. *Maintaining bladder decompression eliminates pressure on suture lines. Preventing movement or pulling on catheters reduces the risk for resultant pressure on surgical incisions.*
- Carefully monitor urine output after catheter removal. *Difficulty voiding is common following catheter removal. Early intervention to prevent bladder distention is important to prevent pressure on suture lines.*
- If the urethral or suprapubic catheter will remain in place on discharge, teach proper care to the client and family members as needed. *Appropriate self-care and early recognition of problems reduce the risk for significant complications.*

---

overflow incontinence as a result of an enlarged prostate gland and urethral obstruction. Care of the client with a prostatectomy is outlined in Chapter 47. ⚭

Other surgical procedures of potential benefit in the treatment of incontinence include implantation of an artificial sphincter, formation of a urethral sling to elevate and compress the urethra, and augmentation of the bladder with bowel segments to increase bladder capacity.

## Complementary Therapies

Biofeedback and relaxation techniques may help reduce episodes of urinary incontinence. Biofeedback uses electronic monitors to teach conscious control over physiologic responses of which the individual is not normally aware. Developing awareness of perceptible information allows the client to gain voluntary control over urination. Biofeedback is widely used to manage urinary incontinence.

## NURSING CARE

## Health Promotion

Although urinary incontinence rarely causes serious physical effects, it frequently has significant psychosocial effects, and can lead to lowered self-esteem, social isolation, and even institutionalization. Get the word out—inform all clients that UI is not a normal consequence of aging and that treatments are available. To reduce the incidence of UI, teach all women to perform pelvic floor exercises (Box 26–4) to improve perineal muscle tone. Advise women to seek advice from their women's health care or primary care practitioner about using topical or systemic hormone therapy during menopause to maintain perineal tissue integrity. Advise older men to have routine prostate examinations to prevent urethral obstruction and overflow incontinence.

### BOX 26–4 ■ Pelvic Floor (Kegel) Exercises

- Identify the pelvic muscles with these techniques:
  a. Stop the flow of urine during voiding and hold for a few seconds.
  b. Tighten the muscles at the vaginal entrance around a gloved finger or tampon.
  c. Tighten the muscles around the anus as though resisting defecation.
- Perform exercises by tightening pelvic muscles, holding for 10 seconds, and relaxing for 10 to 15 seconds. Continue the sequence (tighten, hold, relax) for 10 repetitions.
- Keep abdominal muscles and breathing relaxed while performing exercises.
- Initially, exercises should be performed twice per day, working up to four times a day.
- Encourage exercising at a specific time each day or in conjunction with another daily activity (such as bathing or watching the news). Establish a routine because these exercises should be continued for life.
- Assistive devices, such as vaginal cones and biofeedback, may be useful for clients who have difficulty identifying appropriate muscle groups.

## Assessment

Nursing assessment for the client with urinary incontinence includes both subjective and objective data.

- Health history: voiding diary; frequency of incontinent episodes, amount of urine loss and activities associated with incontinence; methods used to deal with incontinence; use of Kegel exercises or medications; any chronic diseases, related surgeries, etc.; effects of incontinence on usual activities, including social activities
- Physical examination: physical and mental status, including any physical limitations or impaired cognition; inspect, palpate, and percuss abdomen for bladder distention; inspect perineal tissues for redness, irritation, or tissue breakdown;

observe for bulging of bladder into vagina when bearing down; assess pelvic muscle tone as indicated

## Nursing Diagnoses and Interventions

In planning nursing care, consider the client's mental status, mobility, and motivation. Behavioral techniques can be effective, but require long-term commitment and the physical and mental capability to use them.

Nursing care and modification of routines can restore continence fully or partially even in the institutionalized client. Scheduled toileting, bladder training, and prompted voiding combined with positive reinforcement such as praise can reduce the need for diapers, incontinence pads, and indwelling catheters.

### Urinary Incontinence: Stress and/or Urge

Exercises to strengthen pelvic floor muscles, dietary modifications, and bladder training programs often are effective to restore and maintain continence.

- Instruct to keep a voiding diary, recording the time and amount of all fluid intake and urinary output, status at the time of voiding (dry or wet) and on arising from sleep, and activities. *Voiding diaries provide valuable information for identifying the type of incontinence and possible measures to reduce or eliminate incontinent episodes.*
- Teach pelvic floor muscle exercises (Box 26–4). Instruct to consciously tighten pelvic muscles when the need to void is perceived and to relax the abdomen while walking to the bathroom. *Improved pelvic muscle strength helps retain urine and prevent stress incontinence by increasing urethral pressure. Exercises also decrease abnormal detrusor muscle contractions, decreasing pressure within the bladder.*

**PRACTICE ALERT** *Do not advise clients who have difficulty emptying the bladder completely to stop urine flow while voiding to identify pelvic floor muscles. Repeated interruption of micturition can interfere with complete bladder emptying and increase the risk for UTI.* ■

- Using the client's voiding diary, suggest dietary and fluid intake modifications to reduce stress and urge incontinence. Include limiting caffeine, alcohol, citrus juice, and artificial sweetener consumption; limiting fluid intake to no less than 1.5 to 2.0 L per day; and limiting evening fluid intake. *Caffeine, alcohol, and citrus juices are bladder irritants and tend to promote detrusor instability, increasing the risk of urge incontinence. Artificial sweeteners may also irritate the bladder. Fluid intake of 1.5 to 2.0 L per day is adequate to maintain health for most clients; excess fluid may increase stress incontinence if bathroom facilities are not readily available.*

**PRACTICE ALERT** *Limiting total fluid intake to less than 1.5 to 2.0 L per day is not recommended for clients with urinary incontinence. Inadequate fluid increases urine concentration, leading to bladder wall irritation and possibly increasing problems of urge incontinence.* ■

### Self-Care Deficit: Toileting

Functional incontinence may be the predominant problem in an institutionalized older adult. Limited mobility, impaired vision, dementia, lack of access to facilities and privacy, and tight staffing patterns increase the risk for incontinence in previously continent residents. The primary problem in functional incontinence is an outside factor that interferes with the ability to respond normally to the urge to void. An immobilized client may wet the bed if a call light is not within reach; a client with Alzheimer's disease may perceive the urge to void but be unable to interpret its meaning or respond by seeking a bathroom. For these clients, self-care deficit in toileting is a primary problem.

- Assess physical and mental abilities and limitations, usual voiding pattern, and ability to assist with toileting. *A thorough assessment allows planned interventions to address specific needs and promote independence.*
- Provide assistive devices as needed to facilitate independence, such as raised toilet seats, grab bars, a bedside commode, or night lights. *Fostering independence in toileting bolsters self-concept and maintains a positive body image.*
- Plan a toileting schedule based on the client's normal elimination patterns to achieve approximately 300 mL of urine output with each voiding. *Allowing the bladder to fill to a point at which the urge to void is experienced and then emptying it completely helps maintain normal bladder capacity and bacteriostatic functions.*
- Position for ease of voiding—sitting for females, standing for males—and provide privacy. *Normal positioning, usual toileting facilities, and privacy enhance the ability to void on schedule and empty the bladder completely.*
- Adjust fluid intake so that the majority of fluids are consumed during times of day when the client is most able to remain continent. Unless fluids are restricted, maintain a fluid intake of at least 1.5 to 2.0 L per day. *An adequate fluid intake is vital to promote hydration and urinary function. Overly concentrated urine can irritate the bladder, increasing incontinence.*
- Assist with clothing that is easily removed (e.g., elastic-waisted pants or loose dresses). Velcro and zipper fasteners may be easier to use than snaps and buttons. *Clothing that is difficult to remove can increase the risk of incontinence in the client with mobility problems or impaired dexterity.*

### Social Isolation

Urinary incontinence increases the risk for social isolation due to embarrassment, fear of not having ready access to a bathroom, body odor, or other factors. Social isolation, in turn, can increase problems of incontinence, because normal cues and relationships are lost, and the need to remain dry is less strongly felt.

- Assess reasons for and extent of social isolation. Verify the degree of social isolation with the client or significant other. *Do not assume that social isolation is only related to urinary incontinence. Other problems frequently associated with aging (such as a hearing deficit) may be primary or contributing factors.*

- Refer client for urologic examination and incontinence evaluation. *Clients who assume that urinary incontinence is a normal part of the aging may not be aware of treatment options.*
- Explore alternative coping strategies with client, significant other, staff, and other health team members. *Protective pads or shields, good perineal hygiene, scheduled voiding, and clothing that does not interfere with toileting can enhance continence.*

## Using NANDA, NIC, and NOC

Chart 26–4 shows links between NANDA nursing diagnoses, NIC and NOC when caring for the client with urinary incontinence.

## Home Care

Because urinary incontinence is a contributing factor in the institutionalization of many older people, client and family teaching can have a significant impact on maintaining independence and residence in the community. Address possible causes of incontinence and appropriate treatment measures. Refer for urologic examination if not already completed. Discuss fluid intake management, perineal care, and products for clothing protection.

## CHART 26–4  NANDA, NIC, AND NOC LINKAGES

### The Client with Urinary Retention or Incontinence

| NURSING DIAGNOSES | NURSING INTERVENTIONS | NURSING OUTCOMES |
|---|---|---|
| • Urinary Retention | • Urinary Bladder Training<br>• Urinary Catheterization: Intermittent<br>• Urinary Retention Care | • Urinary Continence<br>• Urinary Elimination |
| • Functional Urinary Incontinence | • Prompted Voiding<br>• Urinary Habit Training<br>• Urinary Elimination Management | • Urinary Continence<br>• Urinary Elimination<br>• Tissue Integrity: Skin & Mucous Membranes |
| • Stress Urinary Incontinence | • Pelvic Muscle Exercise<br>• Urinary Incontinence Care<br>• Weight Management | • Urinary Continence |
| • Urge Urinary Incontinence | • Fluid Management<br>• Medication Management | • Urinary Continence |

*Note. Data from Nursing Outcomes Classification (NOC) by M. Johnson & M. Maas (Eds.), 1997, St. Louis: Mosby; Nursing Diagnoses: Definitions & Classification 2001–2002 by North American Nursing Diagnosis Association, 2001, Philadelphia: NANDA; Nursing Interventions Classification (NIC) by J.C. McCloskey & G. M. Bulechek (Eds.), 2000, St. Louis: Mosby. Reprinted by permission.*

## Nursing Care Plan
## A Client with Urinary Incontinence

Anna Giovanni, a 76-year-old retired teacher, has been widowed for 10 years and lives alone. Mrs. Giovanni's eldest daughter expresses concern that her mother seems increasingly reluctant to leave her apartment to visit friends and family. She reports a strong odor of urine throughout her mother's apartment and that her mother's bed is often wet. She expresses worry about needing to place her mother in a nursing home if she cannot continue to live independently.

### ASSESSMENT

Jane Oberle, RN, a nurse practitioner, examines Mrs. Giovanni who admits that she has problems with urine leakage when laughing and coughing, and a strong urge to void on hearing the sound of running water. At night, her urge to void is so strong that she often cannot reach the bathroom in time. Mrs. Giovanni denies a history of UTIs, neurologic disorders, or difficulty with her bowels. She had a hysterectomy at age 52 and was on hormone replacement therapy for about 10 years afterward. She is taking digoxin 0.125 mg daily, furosemide 40 mg twice daily, and potassium chloride 20 mEq 3 times daily for mild heart failure.

Physical assessment reveals a moderate cystourethrocele and atrophy of vaginal and vulvar tissues. Moderate perineal dermatitis is noted. Pelvic floor strength is weak. Urinalysis is within normal limits, and postvoiding residual urine is 5 mL.

Analysis of Mrs. Giovanni's voiding diary shows moderate consumption of tea and juices throughout the day, nine daytime voidings and four night voidings with an average volume of about 250 mL per void. She notices urine leakage most often in the late afternoon and at night. Ms. Oberle identifies a diagnoses of stress incontinence with an urgency component and decides to try a conservative approach before referring Mrs. Giovanni for further testing and possible cystourethrocele repair. She prescribes estrogen cream, tolterodine (Detrol), and a barrier cream to treat Mrs. Giovanni's vulvitis.

## Nursing Care Plan

### A Client with Urinary Incontinence *(continued)*

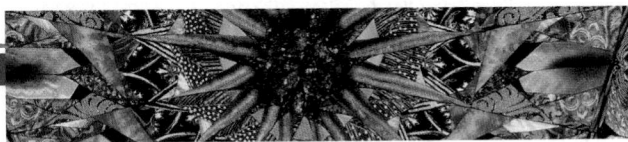

#### DIAGNOSIS

- *Stress urinary incontinence* related to weak pelvic floor musculature and tissue atrophy
- *Urge urinary incontinence* related to excess intake of caffeine and citrus juices
- *Impaired skin integrity* related to constant contact of urine with perineal tissues
- *Ineffective coping* related to inability to control urine leakage

#### EXPECTED OUTCOMES

- Remain dry between voidings and at night.
- Demonstrate improved perineal muscle strength.
- Regain and maintain perineal skin integrity.
- Return to her previous level of social activity.

#### PLANNING AND IMPLEMENTATION

- Teach how to identify pelvic floor muscles and how to perform Kegel exercises.
- Suggest drinking decaffeinated tea and noncitrus fruit juices (grape, apple, and cranberry).
- Encourage to minimize fluid intake after evening meal.
- Change afternoon dose of furosemide from 9:00 P.M. to 3:00 P.M.
- Instruct to void by the clock, gradually increasing intervals from every 45 to 60 minutes to every 2 to 2.5 hours. Advise to maintain shorter voiding intervals for 2 to 3 hours after furosemide doses.
- Teach to cleanse perineal area, wiping front to back, after each voiding or incident of urine leakage.
- Introduce commercial products available for clothing and furniture protection, encouraging experimentation to identify the most helpful product(s).

- Provide a commode for bedside at night and adequate lighting to prevent injury.
- Schedule follow-up visits and evaluations to reinforce teaching.

#### EVALUATION

Three months after her initial visit, Mrs. Giovanni states that she is doing very well, experiencing occasional leakage of small amounts of urine, primarily when sneezing, coughing, or laughing. She finds a minipad adequate for protection and is often able to remain dry all day. She has had no further problems with enuresis since changing her evening furosemide dose to late afternoon and limiting her fluids after dinner. She can make it to the bathroom and no longer needs the bedside commode. Her perineal tissue is intact, and she demonstrates improved muscle strength. Anna's daughter says her mother is beginning to resume her normal social activities, and that she is no longer worried about her mother's ability to care for herself independently.

#### Critical Thinking in the Nursing Process

1. What factors in Mrs. Giovanni's past medical history and current medication regimen contributed to her nighttime incontinence?
2. What is the rationale for including an intervention to teach Mrs. Giovanni about perineal cleansing as part of her care plan?
3. Develop a care plan for Mrs. Giovanni for the nursing diagnosis, *Situational low self-esteem* related to urinary incontinence.

See Evaluating Your Response in Appendix C.

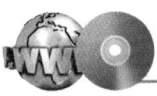

## EXPLORE MediaLink

NCLEX review questions, case studies, care plan activities, MediaLink applications, and other interactive resources for this chapter can be found on the Companion Website at www.prenhall.com/lemone.

Click on Chapter 26 to select the activities for this chapter. For animations, video clips, more NCLEX review questions, and an audio glossary, access the Student CD-ROM accompanying this textbook.

## TEST YOURSELF

1. A 23-year-old woman presents to the urgency clinic with symptoms of a urinary tract infection. The nursing history reveals that the client was treated 3 months previously for a UTI. Additional questions the nurse should ask include

   a. Did you complete your antibiotic prescription for your first UTI?

   b. What form of birth control are you using?
   c. Does your partner have similar symptoms?
   d. How much fluid do you drink each day?

2. Recognizing the risk for urolithiasis in the immobilized client, the nurse appropriately plans to:

   a. Administer a calcium supplement
   b. Regularly monitor urine pH
   c. Maintain an indwelling urinary catheter
   d. Increased fluid intake to 3,000 mL per day

3. The nurse teaching a group of community members about wellness and disease prevention includes which of the following as a measure to reduce the risk for bladder cancer?

   a. Do not start smoking; if you smoke, stop
   b. Avoid using hair dyes and pesticides in the home
   c. Limit your intake of coffee and other caffeinated beverages
   d. Empty your bladder every two hours

4. The nurse evaluates her teaching as effective when the client with a newly created continent ileal diversion is able to:

   a. Demonstrate care for the collection device
   b. State the importance of promptly reporting cloudy urine to the physician
   c. Demonstrate self catheterization of the stoma
   d. Identify factors contributing to his risk for bladder cancer

5. The nurse identifies which of the following as a high priority goal for a client with stress incontinence?

   a. Can identify products for protecting clothing and furniture
   b. States chronic and benign nature of the disorder
   c. Performs pelvic floor muscle exercises as taught at least twice a day
   d. Limits intake of beverages containing caffeine and artificial sweeteners

See Test Yourself answers in Appendix C.

# BIBLIOGRAPHY

Ackley, B. J., & Ladwig, G. B. (2002). *Nursing diagnosis handbook: A guide to planning care* (5th ed.). St. Louis: Mosby.

Ahya, S. N., Flood, K., & Paranjothi, S. (Eds.). (2001). *The Washington manual of medical therapeutics* (30th ed.). Philadelphia: Lippincott Williams & Wilkins.

American Cancer Society. (2002). *Cancer facts and figures 2002*. Atlanta: Author.

Bardsley, A. (1999). Assessment of incontinence. *Elder Care, 11*(9), 36–39.

Baxter, A. (1999). Bladder cancer: Its diagnosis and treatment. *Nursing Times, 95*(41), 42–44.

Braunwald, E., Fauci, A. S., Kasper, D. L., Hauser, S. L., Longo, D. L., & Jameson, J. L. (2001). *Harrison's principles of internal medicine* (15th ed.). New York: McGraw-Hill.

Bullock, B. A., & Henze, R. L. (2000). *Focus on pathophysiology*. Philadelphia: Lippincott.

Fontaine, K. L. (2000). *Healing practices: Alternative therapies for nursing*. Upper Saddle River, NJ: Prentice Hall Health.

Gallo, J. J., Busby-Whitehead, J., Rabins, P. V., Silliman, R. A., & Murphy, J. B. (Eds.). (1999). *Reichel's care of the elderly: Clinical aspects of aging* (5th ed.). Philadelphia: Lippincott Williams & Wilkins.

Gray, M. (2000a). Urinary retention: Management in the acute care setting. Part 1. *American Journal of Nursing, 100*(7), 40–47.

_____. (2000b). Urinary retention: Management in the acute care setting. Part 2. *American Journal of Nursing, 100*(8), 36–43.

Gray, M., McClain, R., Peruggia, M., Patrie, J., & Steers, W. D. (2001). A model for predicting motor urge urinary incontinence. *Nursing Research, 50*(2), 116–122.

Hanchett, M. (2002). Techniques for stabilizing urinary catheters. *American Journal of Nursing, 102*(3), 44–48.

Johnson, M., Bulechek, G., Dochterman, J. M., Maas, M., & Moorhead, S. (2001). *Nursing diagnoses, outcomes, & interventions*. St. Louis: Mosby.

Johnson, M., Maas, M., & Moorhead, S. (Eds.). (2000). *Nursing outcomes classification (NOC)* (2nd ed.). St. Louis: Mosby.

Johnson, S. T. (2000). From incontinence to confidence. *American Journal of Nursing, 100*(2), 69–70, 72–75.

Lekan-Rutledge, D. (2000). Diffusion of innovation. A model for implementation of prompted voiding in long-term care settings. *Journal of Gerontology Nursing, 26*(4), 25–33.

Lyons, S. S., & Specht, J. K. (2000). Prompted voiding protocol for individuals with urinary incontinence. *Journal of Gerontology Nursing, 26*(6), 5–13.

Malarkey, L.M., & McMorrow, M.E. (2000). *Nurse's manual of laboratory tests and diagnostic procedures* (2nd ed.). Philadelphia: Saunders.

Maloney, C., & Cafiero, M. R. (1999). Urinary incontinence. Noninvasive treatment options. *Advance for Nurse Practitioners, 7*(6), 36–42.

McCloskey, J. C., & Bulechek, G. M. (Eds.) (2000). *Nursing interventions classification (NIC)* (3rd ed.). St. Louis: Mosby.

McConnell, E. A. (2001). Myths & facts ... about kidney stones. *Nursing, 31*(1), 73.

Meeker, M. H., & Rothrock, J. C. (1999). *Alexander's care of the patient in surgery* (11th ed.). St. Louis: Mosby.

National Kidney and Urologic Diseases Information Clearinghouse. (1998). Urinary incontinence in women. National Institute of Diabetes and Digestive and Kidney Diseases (NIDDK), National Institutes of Health. Available www.niddk.nih.gov/health/urolog/pubs/uiwomen/uiwomen.htm

Nicolle, L. E. (2001). Urinary tract infections in long-term care facilities. *Infections Control & Hospital Epidemiology, 22*(3), 167–175.

North American Nursing Diagnosis Association. (2001). *NANDA nursing diagnoses: Definitions & classification 2001–2002*. Philadelphia: NANDA.

Porth, C. M. (2002). *Pathophysiology: Concepts of altered health states* (6th ed.). Philadelphia: Lippincott.

Prieto-Fingerhut, T., Banovac, K., & Lynne, C. M. (1997). A study comparing sterile and nonsterile urethral catheterization in patients with spinal cord injury. *Rehabilitation Nursing, 22*(6), 299–302.

Ratliff, C. R., & Donovan, A. M. (2001). Frequency of peristomal complications. *Ostomy & Wound Management, 47*(8), 26–29.

Springhouse. (1999). *Nurse's handbook of alternative & complementary therapies*. Springhouse, PA: Author.

Suchinski, G. A., Piano, M. R., Rosenberg, N., & Zerwic, J. J. (1999). Treating urinary tract infections in the elderly. *Dimensions of Critical Care Nursing, 18*(1), 21–27.

Tierney, L. M., McPhee, S. J., & Papadakis, M. A. (2001). *Current medical diagnosis & treatment* (40th ed.). New York: Lange Medical Books/McGraw-Hill.

Vinsnes, A. G., Harkless, G. E., Haltbakk, J., Bohm, J., & Hunskaar, S. (2001). Healthcare personnel's attitudes towards patients with urinary incontinence. *Journal of Clinical Nursing, 10*(4), 455–462.

Young. J. (2000). Action stat. Kidney stone. *Nursing, 30*(7), 33.

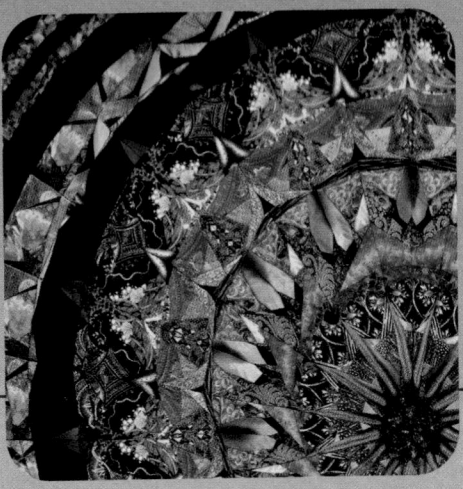

# CHAPTER 27

# Nursing Care of Clients with Kidney Disorders

MediaLink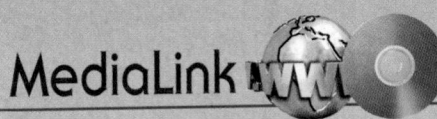

**www.prenhall.com/lemone**
Additional resources for this chapter can be found on the Student CD-ROM accompanying this textbook, and on the Companion Website at www.prenhall.com/lemone. Click on Chapter 27 to select the activities for this chapter.

**CD-ROM**
- Audio Glossary
- NCLEX Review

*Animation*
- Furosemide

**Companion Website**
- More NCLEX Review
- Case Study
    Acute Glomerulonephritis
- Care Plan Activity
    Acute Glomerulonephritis
- MediaLink Application
    Kidney Disorders

## LEARNING OUTCOMES

After completing this chapter, you will be able to:

- Relate the pathophysiology of common kidney disorders to normal renal physiology (see Chapter 25).

- Relate manifestations of kidney disease to the pathophysiology of the disorder.

- Discuss diagnostic studies used to identify disorders of the kidneys.

- Discuss the nursing implications for medications used to treat clients with kidney disorders.

- Identify specific dietary modifications ordered for clients with kidney disorders.

- Compare and contrast dialysis procedures used to manage acute and chronic renal failure.

- Discuss nursing care of the client undergoing dialysis.

- Provide appropriate nursing care for the client who has had kidney surgery or a renal transplant.

- Use the nursing process to plan and provide individualized care to clients with renal disorders.

The internal environment of the body normally remains in a relatively constant or *homeostatic* state. The kidneys help maintain homeostasis by regulating the composition and volume of extracelluar fluid. They excrete excess water and solutes and also can conserve water and solutes when deficits occur. In addition, the kidneys help regulate acid-base balance and they excrete metabolic wastes. Regulation of blood pressure is also a key function of the kidneys.

Both primary kidney disorders (such as glomerulonephritis) and systemic diseases (such as diabetes mellitus) can affect renal function. In North America, more than 20 million people are affected by kidney and urinary tract diseases. Every year, approximately 1 in every 1000 people in the United States develops end-stage renal disease (ESRD), the final phase of chronic renal failure in which little or no kidney function remains. Chronic renal disease accounts for about 80,000 deaths per year and is a major cause of lost work time and wages. Ironically, the increased prevalence of chronic renal disease in recent years is partially related to the success of dialysis and transplantation.

## AGE-RELATED CHANGES IN KIDNEY FUNCTION

Glomeruli in the renal cortex (see Chapter 25 ⬬ for a review of normal kidney structure and function) are lost with aging, reducing kidney mass. Because of the large functional reserve of the kidneys, however, renal function remains adequate unless additional stressors affect the renal system. The **glomerular filtration rate (GFR),** the amount of filtrate made by the kidneys per minute, declines due to age-related factors affecting the renovascular system (such as arteriosclerosis, decreased renal vascularity, and decreased cardiac output). By age 80, the GFR may be less than half of what it was at age 30.

Age-related changes in renal function have significant implications. The kidneys are less able to concentrate urine and compensate for increased or decreased salt intake. When combined with diminished effectiveness of antidiuretic hormone

(ADH) and a reduced thirst response, both common in aging, this decreased ability to concentrate urine increases the risk for dehydration. Potassium excretion may be decreased because of lower aldosterone levels. As a result, fluid and electrolyte imbalances are more common and potentially critical in the older client.

Decreased GFR in the older adult also reduces the clearance of drugs excreted through the kidneys. This reduced clearance prolongs the half-life of drugs and may necessitate lower drug doses and longer dosing intervals. Common medications affected by decreased GFR include:

- Cardiac drugs: digoxin, procainamide
- Antibiotics: aminoglycosides, tetracyclines, cephalosporins
- Histamine $H_2$ antagonists: cimetidine
- Antidiabetic agents: chlorpropamide

When caring for older adults, it is especially important to monitor drugs that are toxic to the renal tubules. Radiologic dyes and aminoglycoside, tetracycline, and the cephalosporin antibiotics are part of this group.

Age-related changes in renal function and related nursing implications are summarized in Table 27–1.

## THE CLIENT WITH A CONGENITAL KIDNEY MALFORMATION

Congenital kidney disorders can affect the form and/or function of the kidney. Functional congenital kidney disorders are usually identified in childhood or adolescence. If function is not affected, congenital malformations may be detected only coincidentally. Malformations include agenesis, hypoplasia, alterations in kidney position, and horseshoe kidney.

*Agenesis,* absence of the kidney, and *hypoplasia,* underdevelopment of the kidney, typically affect only one of these paired organs. Renal function remains normal unless the unaffected kidney is compromised. Abnormal kidney position af-

| TABLE 27–1 | Nursing Implications of Age-Related Changes in Kidney Function | |
| --- | --- | --- |
| **Functional Change** | **Effect** | **Implications** |
| Decreased glomerular filtration rate (GFR) | Decreased clearance of drugs excreted primarily through the kidneys increases drug half-life and blood levels, and risk of drug toxicity. | Monitor carefully for signs of toxicity, especially when administering digoxin, aminoglycoside antibiotics, tetracycline, vancomycin, chlorpropamide, procainamide, cimetidine, and cephalosporin antibiotics. |
| Decreased number of functional nephrons; lower levels of aldosterone; increased resistance to ADH | Decreased ability to conserve water and sodium; impaired potassium excretion; and decreased hydrogen ion excretion, resulting in reduced ability to compensate for acidosis. | Monitor for dehydration and hyponatremia; maintain fluid intake of 1500 to 2500 mL/day unless contraindicated; monitor for hyperkalemia, especially if taking a potassium-sparing diuretic, heparin, angiotensin-converting enzyme (ACE) inhibitor, beta-blocker, or NSAID; increased risk for acidosis. |
| Reduced numbers of functional nephrons | Decreased renal reserve with increased risk of failure. | Avoid giving nephrotoxic drugs if possible; monitor urine output and blood chemistries for early signs of renal failure. |

fects the ureters and urine flow, potentially leading to urinary stasis, increased risk of urinary tract infection (UTI), and lithiasis, or stone formation (see Chapter 26).

One in every 500 to 1000 people has *horseshoe kidney,* making it one of the most common renal malformations (Porth, 2002). Failure of the embryonic kidneys to ascend normally can result in a single, horseshoe-shaped organ. The two kidneys are fused at either the upper or lower pole (usually the lower). This malformation does not typically affect renal function; however, because the ureters cross the fused poles, there is an increased risk for *hydronephrosis,* or distention of the renal pelvis and calyces with urine (see Chapter 26). Recurrent UTI and renal calculi are also common in clients with horseshoe kidney.

Renal ultrasonography and intravenous pyelography are used to diagnose horseshoe kidney. Correction of the abnormality is rarely necessary, although surgical resection of the isthmus (connection between the kidneys) may be done to relieve ureteral obstruction or allow access to the abdominal aorta, which lies behind it.

Nursing care for clients with horseshoe kidney or other congenital malformations is primarily educational. Because abnormal kidney shape or position increases the risk of infection and stone formation, teach the client to maintain a fluid intake of at least 2500 mL per day. Emphasize the importance of avoiding dehydration by increasing fluids during hot weather and strenuous exercise. Teach hygiene practices such as perineal cleansing and voiding before and after intercourse to help prevent UTI. Teach the early manifestations of UTI and instruct to seek treatment promptly to prevent infection of the kidney. See Chapter 26.

## THE CLIENT WITH POLYCYSTIC KIDNEY DISEASE

**Polycystic kidney disease,** a hereditary disease characterized by cyst formation and massive kidney enlargement, affects both children and adults. This disease has two forms: The autosomal dominant form affects adults; the autosomal recessive form is present at birth (Bullock & Henze, 2000; Porth, 2002). Autosomal recessive polycystic kidney disease is rare. It usually is diagnosed prenatally or in infancy. Renal failure generally develops during childhood, necessitating kidney transplant or dialysis. Autosomal dominant polycystic kidney disease is relatively common, affecting 1 in every 300 to 1000 people and accounting for approximately 10% of clients with ESRD in the United States (Braunwald et al., 2001). This section focuses on autosomal dominant polycystic kidney disease, the more common, adult form of the disorder.

### PATHOPHYSIOLOGY

Renal cysts are fluid-filled sacs affecting the nephron, the functional unit of the kidneys. They develop in the tubular epithelium of the nephron, filling with straw-colored glomerular filtrate. The cysts may range in size from microscopic to several centimeters in diameter and affect the renal cortex and

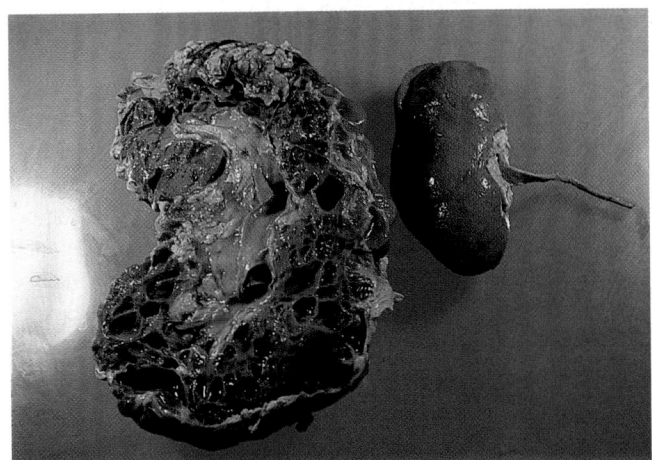

**Figure 27–1** ■ A polycystic kidney. The functional tissue of the kidneys is gradually destroyed and replaced with fluid-filled cysts.

*Source: A. Glauberman/Photo Researchers, Inc.*

medulla of both kidneys. As the cysts fill, enlarge, and multiply, the kidneys also enlarge. Renal blood vessels and nephrons are compressed and obstructed, and functional tissue destroyed (Figure 27–1 ■). The renal parenchyma atrophies and becomes fibrotic and scarred (Braunwald et al., 2001).

People affected by polycystic kidney disease often develop cysts elsewhere in the body, including the liver, spleen, pancreas, and other organs. Up to 10% of people affected experience subarachnoid hemorrhage from a type of congenital intracranial aneurysm. People with polycystic kidney disease also have an increased incidence of incompetent or "floppy" cardiac valves.

### MANIFESTATIONS

Polycystic kidney disease is slowly progressive. Symptoms usually develop by age 40 to 50. Common manifestations include flank pain, microscopic or gross **hematuria** (blood in the urine), **proteinuria** (proteins in the urine), and *polyuria* and *nocturia,* as the concentrating ability of the kidney is impaired. Urinary tract infection and renal calculi are common, as cysts interfere with normal urine drainage. Most clients develop hypertension from disruption of renal vessels. The kidneys become palpable, enlarged, and knobby. Symptoms of renal insufficiency and chronic renal failure typically develop by age 60 to 70.

### COLLABORATIVE CARE

Diagnostic tests used to determine the extent of polycystic kidney disease include the following:

• *Renal ultrasonography* is the diagnostic procedure of choice for polycystic kidney disease. Reflected sound waves are used to assess kidney size and to identify, locate, and differentiate renal masses such as cysts, tumors, and calculi. (See the box on page 717 for the nursing implications for renal ultrasound.)

• *Intravenous pyelography (IVP),* a radiologic examination, is used to evaluate the structure and excretory function of the kidneys, ureters, and bladder. An intravenously injected contrast medium illuminates kidney size and shape, the calyces and pelvis, the ureters, and the bladder as it is cleared from the blood. Cysts can be detected and sized, and the extent of kidney involvement determined. (See the Nursing Implications box on page 708 for an IVP.)

- *Computed tomography (CT scan)* of the kidney uses X-rays passed through the kidneys at many angles to create a detailed picture of renal tissue densities and composition. CT may be done with or without contrast media. Kidney CT is used to detect and differentiate renal masses such as cystic disease or tumors. (See the Nursing Implications box on page 717.)

Management of adult polycystic kidney disease is largely supportive. Care is taken to avoid further renal damage by nephrotoxic substances, UTI, obstruction, or hypertension. A fluid intake of 2000 to 2500 mL per day is encouraged to help prevent UTI and lithiasis. Hypertension associated with polycystic disease is generally controlled using angiotensin-converting enzyme (ACE) inhibitors or other antihypertensive agents (see Chapter 33). Ultimately, dialysis or renal transplantation is required. Clients with polycystic kidney disease are typically good candidates for transplantation because of the absence of associated systemic disease.

## NURSING CARE

For those with adult polycystic kidney disease, an autosomal dominant disorder, discuss genetic counseling and screening of family members for evidence of the disease. This is particularly important if renal transplantation is contemplated and family members are potential donors. Consider the following nursing diagnoses when planning care for the client with polycystic kidney disease.

- *Excess fluid volume* related to impaired renal function
- *Anticipatory grieving* related to potential loss of kidney function
- *Deficient knowledge* regarding measures to help preserve kidney function
- *Risk for ineffective coping* related to potential genetic transmission of the disorder to offspring

Teach the client with polycystic kidney disease about the disease, its genetic nature, and usual course. Discuss measures to maintain optimal renal function. Instruct to maintain a fluid intake of at least 2500 mL per day. Include additional information about preventing UTI (such as hygiene measures) and early manifestations of UTI. Stress the importance of seeking treatment to prevent further kidney damage. Advise to avoid drugs that are potentially toxic to the kidneys and to check with primary care provider before taking any new drug.

## THE CLIENT WITH A GLOMERULAR DISORDER

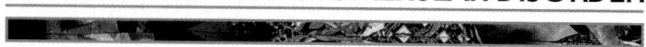

Disorders and diseases involving the glomerulus are the leading cause of chronic renal failure in the United States. They are the underlying disease process for half of those people needing dialysis and result in 12,000 deaths per year.

Glomerular disorders may be either primary, involving mainly the kidney, or secondary to a multisystem disease or hereditary condition. Primary glomerular disease is often immunologic or idiopathic in origin. Diabetes mellitus, systemic lupus erythematosus (SLE), and Goodpasture's syndrome are frequently implicated in secondary glomerular disorders.

### PHYSIOLOGY REVIEW

The glomerulus is a tuft of capillaries surrounded by a thin, double-walled capsule (Bowman's capsule). (See Figure 25–3) About 20% of the resting cardiac output flows through the glomeruli of the kidneys, forming approximately 180 L of plasma ultrafiltrate. More than 99% of this filtrate is reabsorbed in the renal tubules. The rate of glomerular filtration (GFR) is controlled by opposing forces: The pressure and amount of blood flowing through the glomeruli promote filtration, and the pressure in Bowman's capsule and colloid osmotic pressure of the blood oppose it. The total surface area of glomerular capillaries also affects the GFR. The glomerular capillary membrane has three layers: the capillary endothelial layer, the basement membrane, and the capsule epithelial layer. Water and the smallest solutes (such as electrolytes) pass freely across this membrane, while larger molecules (such as plasma proteins) are retained in the blood.

### PATHOPHYSIOLOGY

Glomerular disease affects both the structure and function of the glomerulus, disrupting glomerular filtration. The capillary membrane becomes more permeable to plasma proteins and blood cells. This increased permeability in the glomerulus causes the manifestations common to glomerular disorders: hematuria, proteinuria, and edema. The GFR falls, leading to **azotemia** (increased blood levels of nitrogenous waste products), and hypertension. Glomerular involvement may be diffuse, involving all glomeruli, or focal, involving some glomeruli while others remain essentially normal.

Both hematuria and proteinuria are caused by glomerular capillary membrane damage, which allows blood cells and proteins to escape from the blood into the glomerular filtrate. Hematuria may be either gross or microscopic. Proteinuria is considered to be the most important indicator of glomerular injury, because it increases progressively with increased glomerular damage. Loss of plasma proteins leads to *hypoalbuminemia* (low serum albumin levels), which in turn reduces the plasma oncotic pressure (osmotic pressure created by plasma proteins), leading to edema.

As plasma proteins are lost, the forces opposing filtration diminish, and the amount of filtrate increases. The increased flow of filtrate stimulates the renin-angiotensin-aldosterone mechanism (see Chapter 25), producing vasoconstriction and a fall in GFR. Increased aldosterone production causes salt and water retention which further contribute to edema. As the GFR falls, filtration and elimination of nitrogenous wastes, including urea, decreases, causing azotemia. **Oliguria,** urine output of less than 400 mL in 24 hours, may result from the decreased GFR. Hypertension results from fluid retention and disruption of the renin-angiotensin system, a key regulator of blood pressure.

The major primary glomerular disorders include acute glomerulonephritis, rapidly progressive glomerulonephritis, chronic glomerulonephritis, and nephrotic syndrome. Diabetic nephropathy and lupus nephritis are the most common secondary forms of glomerular disease.

## Acute Glomerulonephritis

**Glomerulonephritis** is inflammation of the glomerular capillary membrane. Acute glomerulonephritis can result from systemic diseases or primary glomerular diseases, but acute poststreptococcal glomerulonephritis (also known as acute proliferative glomerulonephritis) is the most common form. Infection of the pharynx or skin with group A β-hemolytic streptococcus is the usual initiating event for this disorder. Staphylococcal or viral infections, such as hepatitis B, mumps, or varicella (chickenpox), can lead to a similar postinfectious acute glomerulonephritis (Porth, 2002). This primarily childhood disease also can affect adults.

In acute glomerulonephritis, circulating antigen-antibody immune complexes formed during the primary infection become trapped in the glomerular membrane, leading to an inflammatory response. The complement system is activated, and vasoactive substances and inflammatory mediators are released. Endothelial cells proliferate, and the glomerular membrane swells and becomes permeable to plasma proteins and blood cells (Figure 27–2 ■). Renal involvement is diffuse, spread throughout the kidneys.

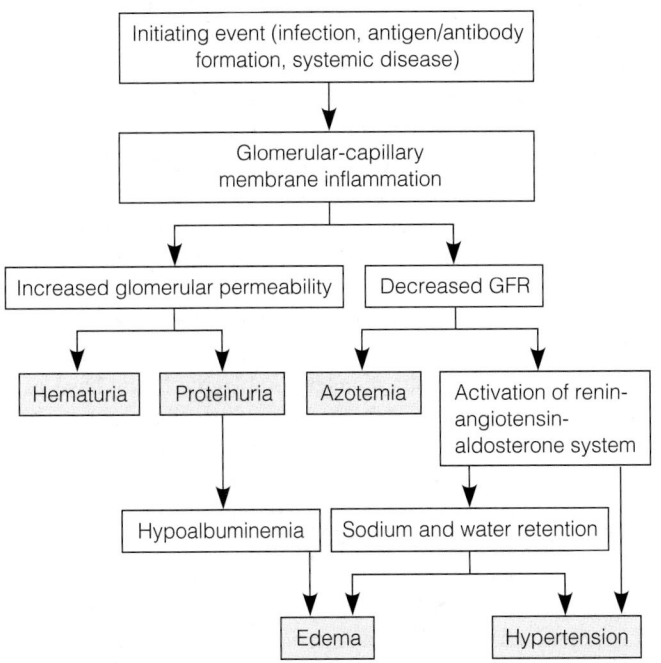

**Figure 27–2** ■ The pathogenesis of glomerulonephritis.

## MANIFESTATIONS AND COMPLICATIONS

Acute glomerulonephritis is characterized by an abrupt onset of hematuria, proteinuria, salt and water retention, and evidence of azotemia occurring 10 to 14 days after the initial infection. The urine often appears brown or cola-colored. Salt and water retention increase extracellular fluid volume, leading to hypertension and edema. The edema is primarily noted in the face, particularly around the eyes (*periorbital* edema). Dependent edema, affecting the hands and upper extremities in particular, may also be noted. Other manifestations may include fatigue, anorexia, nausea and vomiting, and headache (see the box below).

The older adult may have less apparent symptoms. Nausea, malaise, arthralgias, and proteinuria are common manifestations; hypertension and edema are seen less often. Pulmonary infiltrates may occur early in the disorder, often due to worsening of a preexisting condition such as heart failure.

The prognosis for adults with acute glomerulonephritis is less favorable than it is for children. The symptoms may resolve spontaneously within 10 to 14 days. Full recovery is usual in children, whereas 60% or more affected adults recover completely. The remainder have persistent symptoms, and some have permanent kidney damage (Porth, 2002).

## Rapidly Progressive Glomerulonephritis

*Rapidly progressive glomerulonephritis (RPGN)* is characterized by manifestations of severe glomerular injury without a specific, identifiable cause. This type of glomerulonephritis often progresses to renal failure within months. It may be idiopathic (primary), or secondary to a systemic disorder such as SLE or Goodpasture's syndrome. It affects people of all ages.

In RPGN, glomerular cells proliferate and, together with macrophages, form crescent-shaped lesions that obliterate Bowman's space (Porth, 2002). Glomerular damage is diffuse, leading to a rapid, progressive decline in renal function. Irreversible renal failure often develops over weeks to months (Braunwald et al., 2001; Bullock & Henze, 2000).

Clients with RPGN typically present with complaints of weakness, nausea, and vomiting. Some may relate a history of a flulike illness preceding the onset of the glomerulonephritis. Other symptoms include oliguria and abdominal or flank pain. Moderate hypertension may develop. On urinalysis, hematuria and massive proteinuria are noted.

### Manifestations of Acute Glomerulonephritis

- Hematuria, cola-colored urine
- Proteinuria
- Salt and water retention
- Edema, periorbital and facial, dependent
- Hypertension
- Azotemia
- Fatigue
- Anorexia, nausea, and vomiting
- Headache

MediaLink | ACUTE GLOMERULONEPHRITIS CASE STUDY

## Goodpasture's Syndrome

*Goodpasture's syndrome* is a rare autoimmune disorder of unknown etiology. It is characterized by formation of antibodies to the glomerular basement membrane. These antibodies also may bind to alveolar basement membranes, damaging alveoli and causing pulmonary hemorrhage. Goodpasture's syndrome usually affects young men between 18 and 35, although it can occur at any age and affect women as well.

Although the glomeruli may be nearly normal in appearance and function in Goodpasture's syndrome, extensive cell proliferation and crescent formation characteristic of rapidly progressive glomerulonephritis are more common. Renal manifestations include hematuria, proteinuria, and edema. Rapid progression to renal failure may occur. Alveolar membrane damage can lead to mild or life-threatening pulmonary hemorrhage. Cough, shortness of breath, and hemoptysis (bloody sputum) are early respiratory manifestations.

## Chronic Glomerulonephritis

Chronic glomerulonephritis is typically the end stage of other glomerular disorders such as RPGN, lupus nephritis, or diabetic nephropathy. In many cases, however, no previous glomerular disease has been identified.

Slow, progressive destruction of the glomeruli and a gradual decline in renal function are characteristic of chronic glomerulonephritis. The kidneys decrease in size symmetrically, and their surfaces become granular or roughened. Eventually, entire nephrons are lost.

Symptoms develop insidiously, and the disease is often not recognized until signs of renal failure develop. Chronic glomerulonephritis may also be diagnosed when hypertension and impaired renal function are found coincidentally during a routine physical examination or treatment for an unrelated disorder. Viral or bacterial infectious diseases can exacerbate the disorder, prompting its diagnosis.

The course of chronic glomerulonephritis varies, with years to decades between the diagnosis and the development of end-stage renal failure.

## Nephrotic Syndrome

**Nephrotic syndrome** is a group of clinical findings as opposed to a specific disorder. It is characterized by massive proteinuria, hypoalbuminemia, hyperlipidemia, and edema. A number of disorders can affect the glomerular capillary membrane, changing its porosity and allowing plasma proteins to escape into the urine. *Minimal change disease (MCD)* is the most common cause of nephrotic syndrome in children and accounts for 20% of adults with nephrotic syndrome (Braunwald et al., 2001). In MCD, the size and form of glomeruli appear normal by light microscopy. The prognosis for MCD is good. In adults, *membranous glomerulonephropathy* is the most common cause of idiopathic nephrotic syndrome. The glomerular basement membrane thickens, although no inflammation is present. This form of nephrotic syndrome also occurs with some systemic diseases such as SLE and hepatitis B, and with drugs such as gold or penicillamine. *Focal sclerosis,* in which scarring (sclerosis) of glomeruli occurs, and *membran-*

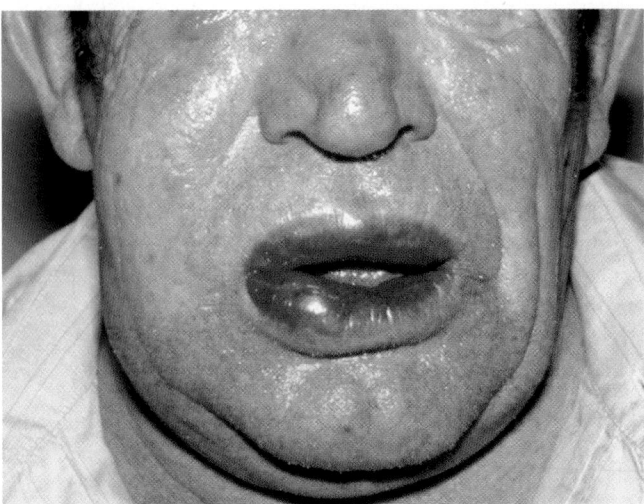

**Figure 27–3 ■** Severe edema characteristic of nephrotic syndrome.

*Source: Science Photo Library/Library Researcher, Inc.*

*oproliferative glomerulonephritis,* caused by thickening and proliferation of glomerular basement membrane cells, are additional forms of nephrotic syndrome.

With plasma protein loss in the urine and resulting hypoalbuminemia, the oncotic pressure of the plasma falls. Fluid shifts from the vascular compartment to interstitial spaces, causing the edema characteristic of nephrotic syndrome. Salt and water retention, possibly due to activation of the renin-angiotensin system, contribute to the edema. Edema may be severe, affecting the face and periorbital area as well as dependent tissues (Figure 27–3 ■).

Loss of plasma proteins stimulates the liver to increase albumin production and lipoprotein synthesis. As a result, serum triglyceride and low-density lipoprotein (LDL) levels increase, as do urine lipids (*lipiduria*). Hyperlipidemia increases the risk for atherosclerosis in clients with nephrotic syndrome.

Thromboemboli (mobilized blood clots) are a relatively common complication of nephrotic syndrome. Loss of clotting and anticlotting factors along with plasma proteins are thought to disrupt the coagulation system, increasing the risk for renal vein thrombosis, deep vein thrombosis, and pulmonary embolism. Renal vein thrombosis can cause flank or groin pain on one or both sides, gross hematuria, and a reduced GFR (Porth, 2002).

Nephrotic syndrome usually resolves without long-term effects in children. The prognosis for adults is less optimistic. Less than 50% of adults recover completely. Many have persistent proteinuria and may develop progressive renal impairment. As many as 30% of adults with nephrotic syndrome develop end-stage renal failure.

## Diabetic Nephropathy

*Diabetic nephropathy,* kidney disease common in the later stages of diabetes mellitus (DM), is the leading cause of end-stage renal disease in North America. Thirty percent of clients with type 1 DM and about 20% of type 2 diabetic clients develop nephropathy. ESRD resulting from diabetic nephropathy is seen more frequently in blacks with type 2 DM, and in whites with type 1 DM (Braunwald et al., 2001).

Initial evidence of microproteinuria indicating renal damage is typically seen within 10 to 15 years after the onset of diabetes. Overt proteinuria and nephropathy generally develop within 15 to 20 years of the initial diagnosis.

The characteristic lesion of diabetic nephropathy is glomerulosclerosis and thickening of the glomerular basement membrane. Arteriosclerosis, a common feature of long-term diabetes and hypertension, contributes to the disease, as do nephritis and tubular lesions. Pyelonephritis, inflammation of the kidney, is also implicated in the development of diabetic nephropathy. A further discussion is found in Chapter 18.

## Lupus Nephritis

Systemic lupus erythematosus (SLE) is an inflammatory autoimmune disorder affecting the connective tissue of the body. Between 40% and 85% of clients with SLE develop manifestations of nephritis (Braunwald et al., 2001). Immune complexes that form within the glomerular capillary wall are the usual trigger for glomerular injury in SLE. Manifestations of lupus nephritis range from microscopic hematuria to massive proteinuria. Its progression may be slow and chronic or *fulminant,* with a sudden onset and the rapid development of renal failure. Most clients with minimal or mild lesions survive for at least 10 years. Improved management of the underlying disease, immunotherapy, dialysis, and renal transplantation have significantly improved the prognosis in recent years.

## COLLABORATIVE CARE

Management of all types of glomerulonephritis, acute and chronic, primary and secondary, focuses on identifying the underlying disease process and preserving kidney function. In most glomerular disorders, there is no specific treatment to achieve a cure. Treatment goals are to maintain renal function, prevent complications, and support the healing process.

## Diagnostic Tests

Laboratory and diagnostic testing are valuable to identify the cause of glomerulonephritis and evaluate kidney function.

The following studies may be ordered to help identify the underlying cause or etiology.

- *Throat or skin cultures* detect infection by group A β-hemolytic streptococci. Although poststreptococcal glomerulonephritis typically follows the acute infection by 1 to 2 weeks, treatment to eradicate any remaining organisms is initiated to minimize antibody production.
- *Antistreptolysin O (ASO) titer* and other tests detect streptococcal *exoenzymes* (bacterial enzymes that stimulate the immune response in acute poststreptococcal glomerulonephritis). Other titers such as antistreptokinase (ASK) or antideoxyribonuclease B (ADNAase B) may be obtained as well.
- *Erythrocyte sedimentation rate (ESR)* is a general indicator of inflammatory response. It may be elevated in acute poststreptococcal glomerulonephritis and in lupus nephritis.

- *KUB* (kidney, ureter, bladder) *abdominal X-ray* may be done to evaluate kidney size and rule out other causes of the client's manifestations. The kidneys may be enlarged in acute glomerulonephritis, whereas bilateral small kidneys are typical of late chronic glomerulonephritis.
- *Kidney scan,* a nuclear medicine procedure, allows visualization of the kidney after intravenous administration of a radioisotope. In glomerular diseases, the uptake and excretion of the radioactive material are delayed.
- *Biopsy,* microscopic examination of kidney tissue, is the most reliable diagnostic procedure for glomerular disorders. Biopsy helps determine the type of glomerulonephritis, the prognosis, and appropriate treatment. Renal biopsy is usually done percutaneously, by inserting a biopsy needle through the skin into the kidney to obtain a tissue sample. Open biopsy, which requires surgery, may also be done.

See the box on page 750 for the nursing implications for diagnostic tests used to evaluate glomerular disorders.

The following studies are used to evaluate kidney function:

- *Blood urea nitrogen (BUN)* measures urea nitrogen, the end product of protein metabolism. It is created by the breakdown and metabolism of both dietary and body proteins. Urea is eliminated from the body by filtration in the glomerulus; minimal amounts are reabsorbed in the renal tubules. Glomerular diseases interfere with filtration and elimination of urea nitrogen, causing blood levels to rise. Increased protein catabolism (destruction), which may occur with GI bleeding or tissue breakdown, can also raise the BUN. Normal BUN values are listed in Table 27–2. Levels up to 50 mg/dL or 17.7 mmol/L indicate mild azotemia, and levels higher than 100 mg/dL or 35.7 mmol/L indicate severe renal impairment.
- *Serum creatinine* measures the amount of creatinine in the blood. Creatinine is also a metabolic by-product, produced in relatively constant amounts by skeletal muscles. It is excreted entirely by the kidneys, making the serum creatinine a good indicator of kidney function. Normal values (see Table 27–2) are lower in the older adult because of decreased muscle mass. Levels greater than 4 mg/dL indicate serious impairment of renal function.
- *Urine creatinine* also is an indicator of renal function and the GFR. Urine creatinine levels decrease when renal function is impaired as it is not effectively eliminated from the body.
- *Creatinine clearance* is a specific indicator of renal function used to evaluate the GFR. The *clearance,* or amount of blood cleared of creatinine in 1 minute, depends on the amount and pressure of blood being filtered and the filtering ability of the glomeruli. Levels normally decline with aging as the GFR decreases in the older adult. Disorders such as glomerulonephritis affect glomerular filtration, decreasing the creatinine clearance.
- *Serum electrolytes* are evaluated because impaired kidney function alters their excretion. Monitoring serum electrolytes is particularly important to prevent complications associated with imbalances.

## Nursing Implications for Diagnostic Tests
### Glomerular Disease

### CREATININE CLEARANCE
#### Preparation of the Client
- Obtain a 24-hour urine specimen container without preservative.
- Instruct to begin the specimen collection at the designated time by voiding and discarding this initial specimen. Collect all urine voided for the next 24 hours, emptying the bladder at the end of the collection time and saving the specimen. Do not discard toilet paper in the specimen container.
- Instruct to void and save the specimen prior to defecating to prevent contamination or loss of urine.
- Refrigerate or keep the urine specimen on ice during the collection period.
- Post signs in the client's room and bathroom indicating the hours of urine collection to prevent inadvertent discarding of the urine.
- Collect or have laboratory personnel collect a venous blood sample during the 24-hour urine collection period.
- Note the client's name, age, weight, and height on the laboratory requisition.

#### Client and Family Teaching
- Generally, no special diet is required during the test.
- Follow instructions for 24-hour specimen collection if the test is being done on an outpatient basis.

### KIDNEY SCAN (RENAL SCAN)
#### Preparation of the Client
- Informed consent is required. Provide teaching and answer questions as needed.
- Make sure that the client is well hydrated prior to the procedure. Provide two to three glasses of water before the procedure if indicated.
- Obtain weight (used to calculate the amount of radioisotope to be injected).
- Have void prior to the procedure.
- After the procedure, increase fluid intake to promote excretion of the radioisotope.
- No special radioactivity precautions are indicated; instruct to flush the toilet immediately after voiding and to wash hands thoroughly.
- Because of the slight potential for harm to a developing fetus, pregnant personnel should not be assigned to care for clients during the first 24 hours after this procedure.

#### Client and Family Teaching
- Increase fluid intake before and after the renal scan.
- No special diet or other preparation is required.
- The test takes 1 to 4 hours.
- No anesthesia is required, and you will experience no pain or discomfort other than that associated with remaining still for a period of time.

### RENAL BIOPSY
#### Preparation of the Client
- Informed consent is required for a kidney biopsy. Answer questions and provide additional information as needed.
- Maintain npo status from midnight before the procedure.
- Note hemoglobin and hematocrit prior to the procedure.
- If the procedure is to be performed at the bedside, obtain biopsy tray and other necessary supplies.
- Following procedure, apply a pressure dressing and position supine to help maintain pressure on the biopsy site.
- Monitor closely for bleeding during the first 24 hours after the procedure:
  a. Check vital signs frequently. Notify the physician of tachycardia, hypotension, or other signs of shock.
  b. Monitor biopsy site for bleeding.
  c. Check hemoglobin and hematocrit, comparing with preprocedure values.
  d. Observe for and report complaints of flank or back pain, shoulder pain (caused by diaphragmatic irritation if hemorrhage occurs), pallor, lightheadedness.
  e. Monitor urine output for quantity and hematuria. Initial hematuria should clear within 24 hours.
- Monitor for other potential complications such as inadvertent penetration of the liver or bowel. Report abdominal pain, guarding, and decreased bowel sounds.
- Encourage fluids during the initial postprocedure period.

#### Client and Family Teaching
- Local anesthesia is used at the injection site. The procedure may be uncomfortable but should not be painful.
- When the needle is inserted, you will be instructed not to breathe to prevent kidney motion.
- The entire procedure takes approximately 10 minutes.
- Avoid coughing during the first 24 hours after the procedure. Strenuous activity such as heavy lifting may be prohibited for approximately 2 weeks after the procedure.
- Report any signs and symptoms of complications, such as hemorrhage or urinary tract infection, to the physician.

---

- *Urinalysis* often shows red blood cells and proteins in the urine of clients with a glomerular disorder. These substances, normally too large to enter glomerular filtrate, escape due to increased porosity of glomerular capillaries in glomerular disorders. A 24-hour urine specimen is used to determine the amount of protein in the urine.

## Medications

Although no drugs are available to cure glomerular disorders, medications are used to treat underlying disorders, reduce inflammation, and manage the symptoms.

Antibiotics are prescribed for the client with poststreptococcal glomerulonephritis to eradicate any remaining bacteria,

| TABLE 27-2 | Changes in Laboratory Values Associated with Kidney Disease | |
|---|---|---|
| **Test** | **Normal Value** | **Value in Renal Disease** |
| Blood urea nitrogen (BUN) | 5–20 mg/dL Slightly higher in older adult | 20–50 mg/dL or higher |
| Creatinine, serum | Female: 0.5–1.1 mg/dL Male: 0.6–1.2 mg/dL Slightly lower in older adult | Elevated; levels >4 mg/dL indicate severe impairment of renal function |
| Creatinine clearance | Female: 88–128 mL/min Male: 97–137 mL/min Values decline in older adult | Reduced renal reserve: 32.5–90.0 mL/min Renal insufficiency: 6.5–32.5 mL/min Renal failure: <6.5 mL/min |
| Serum albumin | 3.2–5 g/dL; 3.2–4.8 g/dL in older adult | Decreased in nephrotic syndrome |
| Serum electrolytes | Potassium: 3.5–5.0 mEq/L Sodium: 136–145 mEq/L Calcium: 4.5–5.5 mEq/L or 8.2–10.5 mg/dL Phosphorus: 3.0–4.5 mg/dL | Increased in renal insufficiency Decreased in nephrotic syndrome Decreased in renal failure Increased in renal failure |
| Red blood cell count | Female: 4.0–5.5 million/mm³ Male: 4.5–6.2 million/mm³ | Decreased in chronic renal failure |
| Urine creatinine | Female: 600–1800 mg/24 hours Male: 800–2000 mg/24 hours | Decreased in disorders of impaired renal function |
| Urine protein | Resting: 50–80 mg/24 hours Ambulatory: <150–250 mg/24 hours | Increased in disorders of impaired renal function |
| Urine red blood cells | <2–3/HPF; no RBC casts | Present in glomerular disorders |

removing the stimulus for antibody production. Nephrotoxic antibiotics, such as the aminoglycoside antibiotics, streptomycin, and some cephalosporins, are avoided.

Aggressive immunosuppressive therapy is used to treat acute inflammatory processes such as rapidly progressive glomerulonephritis, Goodpasture's syndrome, and exacerbations of SLE. When begun early, immunosuppressive therapy significantly reduces the risk of end-stage renal disease and renal failure. Prednisone, a glucocorticoid, is prescribed in relatively large doses of 1 mg per kilogram of body weight per day (e.g., a 160-pound man would receive 70 to 75 mg per day). Other immunosuppressive agents such as cyclophosphamide (Cytoxan) or azathioprine (Imuran) are prescribed in conjunction with corticosteroids. Corticosteroid use in poststreptococcal glomerulonephritis may actually worsen the condition, so is avoided.

Oral glucocorticoids such as prednisone also are used in high doses to induce remission of nephrotic syndrome. When glucocorticoids alone are ineffective, other immunosuppressive agents such as cyclophosphamide or chlorambucil (Leukeran) may be used to induce or maintain remission. See Chapter 9 ⊕ for more information about corticosteroids and other immunosuppressive drugs.

ACE inhibitors may be ordered to reduce protein loss associated with nephrotic syndrome. These drugs reduce proteinuria and slow the progression of renal failure. They have a protective effect on the kidney in clients with diabetic nephropathy. Nonsteroidal anti-inflammatory drugs (NSAIDs) also reduce proteinuria in some clients, but can increase salt and water retention (Braunwald et al., 2001).

Antihypertensives may be prescribed to maintain the blood pressure within normal levels. Blood pressure management is important because systemic and renal hypertension are associated with a poorer prognosis in clients with glomerular disorders.

## Treatments

Bed rest may be ordered during the acute phase of poststreptococcal glomerulonephritis. When the edema of nephrotic syndrome is significant or the client is hypertensive, sodium intake may be restricted to 1 to 2 g per day. Dietary protein may be restricted if azotemia is present. When proteins are restricted, those included in the diet should be complete or high-value proteins. Complete proteins supply the essential amino acids required for growth and tissue maintenance. Complete and incomplete proteins are compared in Table 27–3.

Plasma exchange therapy (**plasmapheresis**), a procedure to remove damaging antibodies from the plasma, is used in

| TABLE 27-3 | Complete and Incomplete Protein Sources | |
|---|---|---|
| | **Complete Proteins** | **Incomplete Proteins** |
| **Definition** | Provide all essential amino acids needed for growth and tissue maintenance | Lack one or more essential amino acids or contain inadequate proportions |
| **Examples** | Milk, eggs, cheese, meats, poultry, fish, and soy | Vegetables, breads, cereals and grains, legumes, seeds, and nuts |

conjunction with immunosuppressive therapy to treat RPGN and Goodpasture's syndrome. Plasma and glomerular-damaging antibodies are removed using a blood cell separator. The red blood cells are then returned to the client along with albumin or human plasma to replace the plasma removed. This procedure is usually done in a series of treatments. It is not without risk, and informed consent is required. Potential complications of plasma exchange therapy include those associated with intravenous catheters, fluid volume shifts, and altered coagulation.

Renal failure resulting from a glomerular disorder may necessitate dialysis to restore fluid and electrolyte balance and remove waste products from the body. Dialysis procedures and related nursing care are explained in the acute renal failure section later in this chapter.

## NURSING CARE

### Health Promotion

Discuss the importance of effectively treating streptococcal infections in all age groups to help reduce the risk for acute glomerulonephritis. Stress the importance of completing the full course of antibiotic therapy to eradicate the infecting bacteria. Teach clients with diabetes mellitus and SLE about potential renal effects of their disease. Discuss measures to reduce the risk of associated nephritis, such as effectively managing the disease, treating hypertension, and avoiding drugs and substances that are potentially toxic to the kidneys.

### Assessment

Review Chapter 25 ⊖⊙ for complete assessment of the renal and urinary systems. Focused assessment data related to glomerular disorders includes the following:

- Health history: complaints of facial or peripheral edema or weight gain, fatigue, nausea and vomiting, headache, general malaise, abdominal or flank pain; cough or shortness of breath; changes in amount, color, or character of urine (e.g., frothy urine); history of skin or pharyngeal streptococcal infection, diabetes, SLE, or kidney disease; current medications
- Physical examination: General appearance; vital signs; weight; presence of periorbital, facial, or peripheral edema; skin for lesions, infection; inspect throat, obtain culture as indicated; urine specimen for color, character, odor

### Nursing Diagnoses and Interventions

Nursing care is supportive and educational. Monitoring renal function and fluid volume status are key components of care, as is protecting the client from infection. Both manifestations of glomerular disorders and their treatment can interfere with a client's ability to maintain usual roles and responsibilities.

### Excess Fluid Volume

Excess fluid volume and resulting edema are common manifestations of glomerular disorders. When proteins are lost in the urine, the oncotic pressure of plasma falls, and fluid shifts into the interstitial spaces. The body responds to this fluid shift by retaining sodium and water to maintain intravascular volume, leading to excess fluid volume.

- Monitor vital signs, including blood pressure, apical pulse, respirations, and breath sounds, at least every 4 hours. Report significant changes. *Excess fluid increases the cardiac workload and the blood pressure. Tachycardia may result. Associated electrolyte imbalances can cause dysrhythmias. Increased pulmonary vascular pressure can lead to pulmonary edema, tachypnea, dyspnea, and crackles (rales) in the lungs.*
- Record intake and output every 4 to 8 hours, or more frequently as indicated. *Accurate intake and output records help determine fluid volume status.*

**PRACTICE ALERT** *Weigh daily, using consistent technique (time of day, scale, and clothing). Accurate daily weights are the best indicator of approximate fluid balance (Wise et al., 2000).* ■

- Monitor serum electrolytes, hemoglobin and hematocrit, BUN, and creatinine. *Glomerular disorders affect fluid balance and may alter electrolyte balance as well, potentially leading to complications such as cardiac dysrhythmias (see Chapter 5).* ⊖⊙ *Increased intravascular volume can result in low hemoglobin and hematocrit values. BUN and creatinine provide information about renal function.*
- Maintain fluid restriction as ordered. Offer ice chips (in limited and measured amounts) and frequent mouth care to relieve thirst. With the client, develop a fluid intake schedule. *Fluids may be restricted to reduce fluid overload, edema, and hypertension. Ice chips and frequent mouth care moisten mucous membranes and help relieve thirst while maintaining oral tissue integrity. Including the client in planning fluid intake promotes a sense of control and understanding of the treatment regimen.*

**PRACTICE ALERT** *Carefully monitor and regulate intravenous infusions; include fluid used to dilute IV medications as intake. Significant "hidden" fluid intake can occur with intravenous medication administration.* ■

- Arrange dietary consultation regarding sodium or protein-restricted diets. *Including the client and dietitian in planning allows individualization of the diet to client preferences. The glomerular disorder may reduce appetite; considering food preferences can help maintain adequate nutrition.*
- Monitor for desired and adverse effects of prescribed medications. *Diuretic therapy helps reduce excess fluid volume; however, glomerular disorders can affect the client's response to treatment. In addition, diuretics can exacerbate electrolyte imbalances and muscle weakness often associated with glomerular disorders.*
- Provide frequent position changes and good skin care. *Perfusion may be altered by tissue edema, increasing the risk of breakdown.*

### Fatigue

Fatigue is a common manifestation of glomerular disorders. Anemia, loss of plasma proteins, headache, anorexia, and nausea compound this fatigue. The ability to maintain usual physical and mental activities may be impaired.

- Document energy level. *As glomerular function improves, fatigue begins to resolve, and energy increases.*
- Schedule activities and procedures to provide adequate rest and energy conservation. Prevent unnecessary fatigue. *Adequate rest and energy conservation reduce fatigue and improve the client's ability to tolerate and cope with required treatments and activities.*
- Assist with ADLs as needed. *The goal is to conserve limited energy reserves.*
- Discuss the relationship between fatigue and the disease process with client and family. *Understanding the nature of the disease and associated fatigue helps the client and family cope with reduced energy and comply with prescribed rest.*
- Reduce energy demands with frequent, small meals and short periods of activity. Limit the number of visitors and visit length. *Small, frequent meals reduce the energy needed for eating and digestion. Limiting visitors and visit length helps conserve energy. In addition, nurses can assist the fatigued client who may be reluctant to ask visitors to leave.*

## Ineffective Protection

The effects of both the glomerular disorder and treatment with anti-inflammatory and cytotoxic drugs can depress the immune system, increasing the risk for infection. The anti-inflammatory effect of corticosteroids may also mask early manifestations of infection.

**PRACTICE ALERT** *Monitor vital signs, temperature, and mental status every 4 hours. An elevated temperature may indicate infection; anti-inflammatory drugs may moderate this response, however. Tachycardia, increasing lethargy, or confusion may be the initial signs of infection.* ■

- Assess frequently for other signs of infection such as purulent wound drainage, productive cough, adventitious breath sounds, and red or inflamed lesions. Monitor for manifestations of UTI, such as dysuria, frequency and urgency, and cloudy, foul-smelling urine. *Early identification and treatment of infection is important to prevent systemic complications in the susceptible client.*
- Monitor CBC, focusing on the WBC and differential. *An elevated WBC and increased numbers of immature WBCs in the blood (left shift) may be early indicators of infection.*
- Use good handwashing technique. Protect from cross-infection by providing a private room and restricting ill visitors. *Clients with decreased resistance to infection need increased protection.*
- Avoid or minimize invasive procedures. *Maintaining the protective skin barrier is especially important for the client with altered immune status.*
- If catheterization is required, use sterile intermittent straight catheterization or maintain a closed drainage system for an indwelling catheter. Prevent urine reflux from the drainage system to the bladder or the bladder to the kidneys by ensuring a patent, gravity system. *The urinary tract is a frequent entry point for infection, particularly in the hospitalized or institutionalized client. Maintaining strict asepsis during catheterization is vital. Intermittent catheterization is associated with a lower risk of UTI than an indwelling catheter.*
- Provide a nutritionally sound diet with complete proteins. *A well-balanced, nutritionally sound diet is important to maintain nutritional status and support immune function.*
- Teach measures to prevent infection. *Care often is provided in the home, requiring the client and family to use appropriate infection control measures.*

## Ineffective Role Performance

The manifestations and treatment of glomerular disorders can affect the ability to maintain usual roles and activities. Fatigue and muscle weakness may limit physical and social activities. Bed rest or activity limitations may be ordered to minimize the degree of proteinuria. If azotemia is present, malaise, nausea, and mental status changes can interfere with role function. Facial and periorbital edema affect the client's self-esteem and may lead to isolation.

- Establish a strong therapeutic relationship. *It is important to gain the client's trust and confidence.*
- Encourage self-care and participation in decision making. *Increased autonomy helps restore self-confidence and reduce powerlessness.*
- Provide for time for verbalization of thoughts and feelings; listen actively, acknowledging and accepting fears and concerns. *Adequate time and active listening encourage expression of concerns and the affect of the disease or treatments on daily life. This helps the client deal with the illness, its treatment, and associated losses.*
- Support coping skills, helping the client identify personal strengths. *This support helps the client gain confidence.*
- When possible, enlist the support of family, other clients, and friends. *These people can provide physical, psychologic, emotional, and social support.*
- Discuss the effect of the disease and treatments on roles and relationships, helping identify potential changes in roles, relationships, and lifestyle. Help the client and family develop a plan for alternative behaviors and relationships, encouraging the client to maintain usual roles to the extent possible. *Developing a plan helps reduce the strain of role changes and maintain a sense of dignity and control.*
- Provide accurate and optimistic information about the disorder and its short- and long-term effects. *The client and family need accurate information to plan for the future.*
- Evaluate the need for additional support and social services for the client and family. Provide referrals as indicated. *Depending on client and family strengths, the severity of the disorder, and its treatment and prognosis, ongoing social support services may be necessary to facilitate coping and adaptation.*

## Using NANDA, NIC, and NOC

Chart 27–1 shows links between NANDA nursing diagnoses, NIC, and NOC when caring for the client with a glomerular disorder.

## CHART 27-1 NANDA, NIC, AND NOC LINKAGES

### The Client with a Glomerular Disorder

| NURSING DIAGNOSES | NURSING INTERVENTIONS | NURSING OUTCOMES |
|---|---|---|
| • Excess Fluid Volume | • Fluid Management<br>• Fluid Monitoring | • Fluid Balance |
| • Fatigue | • Energy Management | • Energy Conservation |
| • Imbalanced Nutrition: Less than Body Requirements | • Nutrition Management<br>• Nutrition Monitoring | • Nutritional Status: Nutrient Intake |
| • Ineffective Role Performance | • Coping Enhancement | • Coping<br>• Psychosocial Adjustment: Life Change |

Note. Data from Nursing Outcomes Classification (NOC) by M. Johnson & M. Maas (Eds.), 1997, St. Louis: Mosby; Nursing Diagnoses: Definitions & Classification 2001–2002 by North American Nursing Diagnosis Association, 2001, Philadelphia: NANDA; Nursing Interventions Classification (NIC) by J.C. McCloskey & G. M. Bulechek (Eds.), 2000, St. Louis: Mosby. Reprinted by permission.

## Home Care

Glomerular disorders may be self-limited or progressive. In either case, the course is lengthy, ranging from months to years. Self-management is essential. Provide instructions for the client and family, including the following topics.

• Information about the disease and the prognosis

• Prescribed treatment, including activity and diet restrictions; the use and potential effects, both beneficial and adverse, of all medications
• Risks, manifestations, prevention, and management of complications such as edema and infection
• Signs, symptoms, and implications of improving or declining renal function
• Measures to prevent further kidney damage, such as nephrotoxic drugs to avoid

## Nursing Care Plan

### A Client with Acute Glomerulonephritis

Jung-Lin Chang is a 23-year-old graduate student in biology. He presents at the university health center, with brown and foamy urine. The physician there admits him to the infirmary and orders a throat culture, ASO titer, CBC, BUN, serum creatinine, and urinalysis.

### ASSESSMENT

Connie King, the nurse admitting Mr. Chang, notes that his history is essentially negative for past kidney or urinary problems. He relates having had a "pretty bad" sore throat a couple of weeks before admission. However, it was during midterms, so he took a few antibiotics he had from a previous bout of strep throat, increased his fluids, and did not see a doctor. The sore throat resolved, and he felt well until noticing the change in his urine. He admits that his eyes seemed a little puffy, but he thought this was due to lack of sleep and fatigue. He has eaten little the past 2 days, but was not alarmed because his food intake is irregular most of the time.

Physical assessment findings include: T 98.8° F (37.1° C) PO, P 98, R 18, and BP 136/90. Weight 165 pounds (75 kg), up from his normal of 160 (72.5 kg). Moderate periorbital edema and edema of hands and fingers noted.

Throat culture is negative, but the ASO titer is high. CBC essentially normal. BUN 42 mg/dL, serum creatinine 2.1 mg/dL. Urinalysis reveals the presence of protein, red blood cells, and RBC casts. A subsequent 24-hour urine protein analysis shows 1025 mg of protein (normal 30 to 150 mg/24 hours).

The physician diagnoses acute poststreptococcal glomerulonephritis and places Mr. Chang on bed rest with bathroom privileges. He orders fluid restriction (1200 mL/day) and a restricted sodium and protein diet.

### DIAGNOSIS

• *Excess fluid volume* related to plasma protein deficit and sodium and water retention
• *Risk for imbalanced nutrition: Less than body requirements* related to anorexia
• *Anxiety* related to prescribed activity restriction
• *Risk for ineffective therapeutic regimen management* related to lack of information about glomerulonephritis and treatment

### EXPECTED OUTCOMES

• Maintain blood pressure within normal limits.
• Return to usual weight with no evidence of edema.
• Consume adequate calories following prescribed dietary limitations.
• Verbalize reduced anxiety regarding ability to continue studies.
• Demonstrate an understanding of acute glomerulonephritis and prescribed treatment regimen.

### PLANNING AND IMPLEMENTATION

• Vital signs every 4 hours; notify physician of significant changes.
• Weigh daily; intake and output every 8 hours.
• Schedule fluids allowing 650 mL on day shift, 450 mL on evening shift, and 100 mL on night shift.

## Nursing Care Plan
### A Client with Acute Glomerulonephritis (continued)

- Arrange dietary consultation to plan a diet that includes preferred foods as allowed.
- Provide small meals with high-carbohydrate between-meal snacks.
- Encourage Mr. Chang to talk about his condition and its potential effects.
- Assist with problem solving and exploring options for maintaining studies.
- Enlist friends and family to listen and provide support.
- Teach Mr. Chang and his family about acute glomerulonephritis and prescribed treatment.
- Instruct in appropriate antibiotic use.

### EVALUATION

Mr. Chang is released from the infirmary after 4 days. He decides to return to his parents' home for the 6 to 12 weeks of convalescence prescribed by his doctor. Mr. Chang's renal function gradually returns to normal with no further azotemia and minimal proteinuria after 4 months. He verbalizes understanding of the relationship between the strep throat, his inappropriate use of antibiotics, and the glomerulonephritis. He says, "I may not always remember to take every pill on time in the future, but I sure won't save them for the next time again!"

### Critical Thinking in the Nursing Process

1. How did Mr. Chang's use of "a few" previously prescribed antibiotics to treat his sore throat affect his risk for developing poststreptococcal glomerulonephritis?
2. What additional risk factors did Mr. Chang have for developing glomerulonephritis?
3. The initial manifestations of acute poststreptococcal glomerulonephritis and rapidly progressive glomerulonephritis are very similar. What diagnostic test would the physician use to make the differential diagnosis? Develop a plan of care for a client undergoing this examination.

See Evaluating Your Response in Appendix C.

## THE CLIENT WITH A VASCULAR KIDNEY DISORDER

Renal function is dependent on an adequate supply of blood. Blood supports renal cell metabolism and is vital to kidney function, the nephron in particular. The kidney can regulate fluid, electrolyte, and acid-base balance and serve as a major organ of excretion only when its blood supply is sufficient. Vascular disorders, therefore, can have a significant impact on renal function.

### HYPERTENSION

*Hypertension*, sustained elevation of the systemic blood pressure, can result from or cause kidney disease.

Prolonged hypertension damages the walls of arterioles and accelerates the process of atherosclerosis. This damage primarily affects the heart, brain, kidneys, eyes, and major blood vessels. In the kidney, arteriosclerotic lesions develop in the *afferent* (leading into) and *efferent* (going out of) arterioles and the glomerular capillaries. The glomerular filtration rate declines and tubular function is affected, resulting in proteinuria and microscopic hematuria. Approximately 10% of deaths attributed to hypertension result from renal failure (Braunwald et al., 2001).

*Malignant hypertension* is a rapidly progressive form of hypertension that may develop in clients with untreated primary hypertension. The diastolic pressure is in excess of 120 mmHg and may be as high as 150 to 170 mmHg. Malignant hypertension affects less than 1% of hypertensive clients; it is more common in African Americans than in people of European ancestry. Untreated, malignant hypertension causes a rapid decline in renal function due to vessel changes, renal ischemia, and infarction.

Approximately 5% to 10% of hypertensive clients have *secondary hypertension*, which is actually a manifestation of an underlying disease. Renal vascular disease and diseases of the renal parenchyma, such as diabetic nephropathy, are commonly associated with secondary hypertension.

Management of hypertension to maintain the blood pressure within normal limits is vital to prevent kidney damage. When hypertension is secondary to kidney disease, adequate blood pressure control can slow the decline in renal function. Hypertension and its management is discussed in depth in Chapter 33. ∞

### RENAL ARTERY OCCLUSION

Renal arteries can be occluded by either a primary process affecting the renal vessels or by emboli, clots, or other foreign material. Risk factors for *acute renal artery thrombosis* (formation of a blood clot in the renal artery) include severe abdominal trauma, vessel trauma from surgery or angiography, aortic or renal artery aneurysms, and severe aortic or renal artery atherosclerosis. Emboli from the left side of the heart can travel via the aorta to occlude the renal artery. Emboli may form as a result of atrial fibrillation (irregular and uncoordinated electrical activity of the atria), following myocardial infarction, as vegetative growths on heart valves associated with bacterial endocarditis, or from fatty plaque in the aorta.

Renal arterial occlusion may be asymptomatic when the occlusion develops slowly and the affected vessels are small. Acute occlusion leading to ischemia and infarction typically causes sudden, severe localized flank pain, nausea and vomiting, fever, and hypertension. Hematuria and oliguria may occur. In the older client, the new onset of hypertension or worsening of previously controlled hypertension may signal renal artery thrombosis.

Laboratory studies reveal leukocytosis (elevated WBC), and elevated renal enzyme levels, including aspartate transaminase (AST) and lactic dehydrogenase (LDH). These enzymes, normally present in renal cells, are released into the circulation when cells necrose and die. With bilateral arterial occlusion and infarction, renal function deteriorates rapidly, leading to acute renal failure (Braunwald et al., 2001).

Surgery to restore blood flow to the affected kidney may be indicated for acute occlusion. Management usually is more conservative, using anticoagulant therapy, hypertension control, and supportive treatment.

## RENAL VEIN OCCLUSION

A thrombus (clot) formed in a renal vein can occlude the vessel. The cause of the thrombus often is unclear. In adults, renal vein thrombosis usually occurs with nephrotic syndrome. Other predisposing factors include pregnancy, oral contraceptive use, and certain malignancies.

Gradual or acute deterioration of renal function may be the only manifestation of renal vein occlusion. If the thrombus breaks loose, it can become a pulmonary embolism. The definitive diagnosis is made by visualizing the thrombus through renal venography.

Thrombolytic drugs such as streptokinase or tPA may be given to dissolve or break up the thrombus. Anticoagulant therapy also is used to prevent further clotting and pulmonary emboli. Renal function often improves with treatment.

## RENAL ARTERY STENOSIS

**Renal artery stenosis** (narrowing) causes 2% to 5% of all cases of hypertension (Braunwald et al., 2001). It can affect one or both kidneys.

Atherosclerosis with gradual occlusion of the renal artery lumen by plaque is the primary cause of renal artery stenosis in men. In younger women, the most common cause is fibromuscular dysplasia, structural abnormalities involving the intimal, medial, or adventitial layers of the arterial wall.

Renal artery stenosis is suspected when hypertension develops before age 30 or after age 50 with no prior history of high blood pressure. An epigastric bruit (murmur) and other manifestations of vascular insufficiency may also be present. The affected kidney appears small and atrophied on renal ultrasound. The captopril test for renin activity and renal angiography are used to confirm the diagnosis. Clients with renovascular hypertension show higher levels of renin activity following administration of captopril, an ACE inhibitor drug (see Chapter 33) than clients with essential or primary hypertension (Braunwald et al., 2001). Renal angiography uses radiologic contrast dye injected into the renal arteries to allow visualization of renal blood vessels.

The preferred treatment for renal artery stenosis is dilation of the stenotic vessel by percutaneous transluminal angioplasty. In this procedure, a balloon-tipped catheter is inserted via the femoral artery and aorta to dilate the renal artery. It relieves symptoms immediately in 90% of clients with fibromuscular dysplasia. One year after treatment, 60% remain symptom-free. Some clients require a bypass graft of the renal artery. A section of saphenous vein or hypogastric artery is grafted from the aorta to the renal artery beyond the stenosis.

The blood pressure may not return to normal following treatment, but is more easily managed using medications.

## THE CLIENT WITH KIDNEY TRAUMA

The kidneys are relatively well protected by the rib cage and back muscles, but trauma due to blunt force or penetrating injury may inflict damage. Many renal injuries heal uneventfully, but prompt diagnosis and immediate treatment can be life-saving in the event of major damage.

## PATHOPHYSIOLOGY AND MANIFESTATIONS

Blunt force is the most common cause of kidney injury. Falls, motor vehicle accidents, and sports injuries can damage the kidney. The injury may be minor, causing a contusion or small hematoma, or more serious, resulting in laceration or other damage. The kidney may fragment or "shatter," causing significant blood loss and urine extravasation. Tearing of the renal artery or vein may cause rapid hemorrhage, with shock and possible death.

Gunshot wounds, knife wounds, impalement injuries, and fractured ribs can penetrate the kidney. Minor penetrating injuries may lacerate the capsule or renal cortex. Major injuries include laceration or destruction of renal parenchyma or the vascular supply. Renal artery, renal vein, and renal pelvis lacerations are critical injuries.

The primary manifestations of kidney trauma are hematuria (gross or microscopic), flank or abdominal pain, and oliguria or anuria. There may be localized swelling, tenderness, or ecchymoses in the flank region. Retroperitoneal bleeding from the kidney may cause Turner's sign, a bluish discoloration of the flank. Signs of shock may be present, including hypotension, tachycardia, tachypnea, cool and pale skin, and an altered level of consciousness.

## COLLABORATIVE CARE

Hemoglobin and hematocrit levels fall in significant renal injury with hemorrhage. Hematuria is typically noted on urinalysis. AST levels rise within 12 hours of significant renal trauma. Renal ultrasonography is used to diagnose bleeding and kidney damage. A CT scan and IVP to visualize renal structures may be done to establish a definitive diagnosis. Renal arteriography is used when major injury is suspected and surgery is anticipated.

Treatment of minor kidney injuries is generally conservative, including bed rest and observation. In these injuries, bleeding is typically minor and self-limiting. With major or critical trauma, immediate treatment focuses on controlling hemorrhage and treating or preventing shock. Surgery or percutaneous arterial embolization during angiography may be required to stop the bleeding. Major lacerations may require surgical repair, partial nephrectomy, or total **nephrectomy** (removal) of the affected kidney.

## NURSING CARE

Nursing care for the client who has experienced renal trauma focuses on timely and accurate assessment and appropriate intervention to preserve life and prevent complications. Obtain a urine specimen for analysis when kidney trauma is suspected. Monitor level of consciousness, vital signs, skin color and temperature, and urine output for possible signs of shock. See Chapter 6 ∞ for additional nursing care measures for the client who has had a traumatic injury or who develops shock.

## THE CLIENT WITH A RENAL TUMOR

Renal tumors may be either benign or malignant, primary or metastatic. Benign renal tumors are infrequent and are often found only on autopsy. Primary renal malignancies account for about 2% of adult cancers and approximately 12,000 deaths per year. Most primary renal tumors arise from renal cells; a primary tumor also may develop in the renal pelvis, although less frequently. Metastatic lesions to the kidney are associated with lung and breast cancer, melanoma, and malignant lymphoma.

Males are affected by renal cancer more than females by a 2:1 ratio. The highest incidence is seen in people over the age of 55 years. Smoking and obesity are risk factors; chronic irritation associated with renal calculi may also contribute. Some renal cancers are associated with genetic factors. Clients with end-stage renal disease also may develop renal cancer.

### PATHOPHYSIOLOGY AND MANIFESTATIONS

Most (85% to 95%) primary renal tumors are renal cell carcinomas (Braunwald et al., 2001; Porth, 2002). These tumors arise from tubular epithelium and can occur anywhere in the kidney. The tumor, which can range in size up to several centimeters, has clearly defined margins and contains areas of ischemia, necrosis, and hemorrhage. Renal tumors tend to invade the renal vein, and often have metastasized when first identified. Metastasis tend to occur in the lungs, bone, lymph nodes, liver, and brain (Bullock & Henze, 2000).

Renal tumors are often silent, with few manifestations. The classic triad of symptoms, gross hematuria, flank pain, and a palpable abdominal mass, is seen in only about 10% of people with renal cell carcinoma. Hematuria, often microscopic, is the most consistent symptom. Systemic manifestations include fever without infection, fatigue, and weight loss. See the box above.

The tumor may produce hormones or hormonelike substances, including parathyroid hormone, prostaglandins, prolactin, renin, gonadotropins, and glucocorticoids. These substances produce *paraneoplastic syndromes,* with additional manifestations such as hypercalcemia, hypertension, and hyperglycemia. The progression of renal cell carcinomas varies from prolonged periods of stable disease to very aggressive. Table 27–4 outlines the staging and prognosis for renal cell cancers.

## Manifestations of Renal Tumors

- Microscopic or gross hematuria
- Flank pain
- Palpable abdominal mass
- Fever
- Fatigue
- Weight loss
- Anemia or polycythemia

## COLLABORATIVE CARE

Hematuria is often the only initial manifestation of renal cancer; its presence indicates a need for further diagnostic studies, including:

- *Renal ultrasonography* to detect renal masses and differentiate cystic kidney disease from renal carcinoma.
- *CT scan* to determine tumor density, local extension of the tumor, and regional lymph node or vascular involvement.
- *IVP* and *MRI* may be done to evaluate renal structure and function.
- *Renal angiography, aortography,* and *inferior venacavography* may be used to evaluate the extent of vascular involvement prior to surgery.
- *Chest X-ray, bone scan, and liver function studies* to identify potential metastases.

*Radical nephrectomy* is the treatment of choice for kidney tumors. In a radical nephrectomy, the adrenal gland, upper ureter, fat and fascia surrounding the kidney, as well as the entire kidney,

| TABLE 27–4 | Renal Cell Cancer Staging | |
|---|---|---|
| **Stage** | **Extent of Tumor** | **Prognosis** |
| I | Confined to the kidney capsule | 66% 5-year survival |
| II | Invasion through the capsule but confined to local fascia | 64% 5-year survival |
| III | Regional lymph node, ipsilateral renal vein, or inferior vena cava involvement | 42% 5-year survival |
| IV | Locally invasive or distant metastases | 11% or less 5-year survival |

*Note. Adapted from* Harrison's Principles of Internal Medicine *(15th ed.) by E. Braunwald et al. (Eds.), 2001, New York: McGraw-Hill.*

## NURSING CARE  OF THE CLIENT HAVING A NEPHRECTOMY

### PREOPERATIVE CARE

- Provide routine preoperative care as outlined in Chapter 7.
- Report abnormal laboratory values to the surgeon. *Bacteriuria, blood coagulation abnormalities, or other significant abnormal values may affect surgery and postoperative care.*
- Discuss operative and postoperative expectations as indicated, including the location of the incision (Figure 27–4) and anticipated tubes, stents, and drains. *Preoperative teaching about postoperative expectations reduces anxiety for the client and family during the early postoperative period.*

### POSTOPERATIVE CARE

- Provide routine postoperative care as described in Chapter 7.
- Frequently assess urine color, amount, and character, noting any hematuria, pyuria, or sediment. Promptly report oliguria or anuria, as well as changes in urine color or clarity. *Preserving function of the remaining kidney is critical; frequent assessment allows early intervention for potential problems.*
- Note the placement, status, and drainage from ureteral catheters, stents, nephrostomy tubes, or drains. Label each clearly. Maintain gravity drainage; irrigate only as ordered. *Maintaining drainage tube patency is vital to prevent potential hydronephrosis. Bright bleeding or unexpected drainage may indicate a surgical complication.*
- Support the grieving process and adjustment to the loss of a kidney. *Loss of a major organ leads to a body image change and grief response. When renal cancer is the underlying diagnosis, the client may also grieve the loss of health and potential loss of life.*

- Provide the following home care instructions for the client and family.
  a. The importance of protecting the remaining kidney by preventing UTI, renal calculi, and trauma. See Chapter 26 for measures to prevent UTI and calculi. *Damage to the remaining kidney by UTI, renal calculi, or trauma can lead to renal failure.*
  b. Maintain a fluid intake of 2000 to 2500 mL per day. *This important measure helps prevent dehydration and maintain good urine flow.*
  c. Gradually increase exercise to tolerance, avoiding heavy lifting for a year after surgery. Participation in contact sports is not recommended to reduce the risk of injury to the remaining kidney. *Lifting is avoided to allow full tissue healing. Trauma to the remaining kidney could seriously jeopardize renal function.*
  d. Care of the incision and any remaining drainage tubes, catheters, or stents. *This routine postoperative instruction is vital to prepare the client for self-care and prevent complications.*
  e. Report signs and symptoms to the physician, including manifestations of UTI (dysuria, frequency, urgency, nocturia, cloudy, malodorous urine) or systemic infection (fever, general malaise, fatigue), redness, swelling, pain, or drainage from the incision or any catheter or drain tube site. *Prompt treatment of postoperative infection is vital to allow continued healing and prevent compromise of the remaining kidney.*

---

are removed. Regional lymph nodes may also be resected. Although nephrectomy can be done using a laparoscopic approach, laparotomy primarily is used for radical nephrectomy. Nursing care for the client having a nephrectomy is summarized above.

No effective treatment is available for advanced renal carcinoma with metastases. Biologic therapies such as interferon α or interleukin-2 have been used, but rarely achieve a durable effect. No chemotherapy drug consistently causes tumor regression in more than 20% of clients (Braunwald et al., 2001).

## NURSING CARE

### Nursing Diagnoses and Interventions

Nursing care for the client with renal cancer focuses on needs related to the cancer diagnosis and to the surgical intervention. Postoperative pain may be significant and the risk for respiratory complications is high. The remaining kidney must be protected from damage to preserve renal function. Psychologically, the client may grieve the loss of a major organ and the diagnosis of cancer.

### Pain

The size and location of the incision used for a radical nephrectomy (Figure 27–4 ■) make pain management a challenge. Intercostal blocks, patient-controlled analgesia (PCA), or routine analgesic administration can effectively relieve the discomfort. Nursing care focuses on assessing pain relief, providing supportive measures to enhance analgesia, and ensuring that pain or the fear of pain does not lead to respiratory complications.

- Assess frequently for adequate pain relief. Use a standard pain scale and nonverbal signs such as grimacing, tense body position, apparent dozing, elevated pulse, change of blood pressure, or rapid, shallow respirations. Notify the physician of inadequate pain relief. *The client may assume that pain is to be expected or may fear becoming addicted to analgesics. Careful questioning and assessment allow effective pain management. Responses to analgesics are individual, and the prescribed dose may need to be adjusted.*
- Assess the incision for inflammation or swelling and drainage catheters and tubes for patency. *An obstructed catheter can lead to hydronephrosis, hematoma, or abscess, increasing incisional pain.*

**PRACTICE ALERT** *Assess for adominal distention, tenderness, and bowel sounds. Intra-abdominal bleeding, peritonitis, or paralytic ileus can cause pain that may be confused with incisional pain.* ■

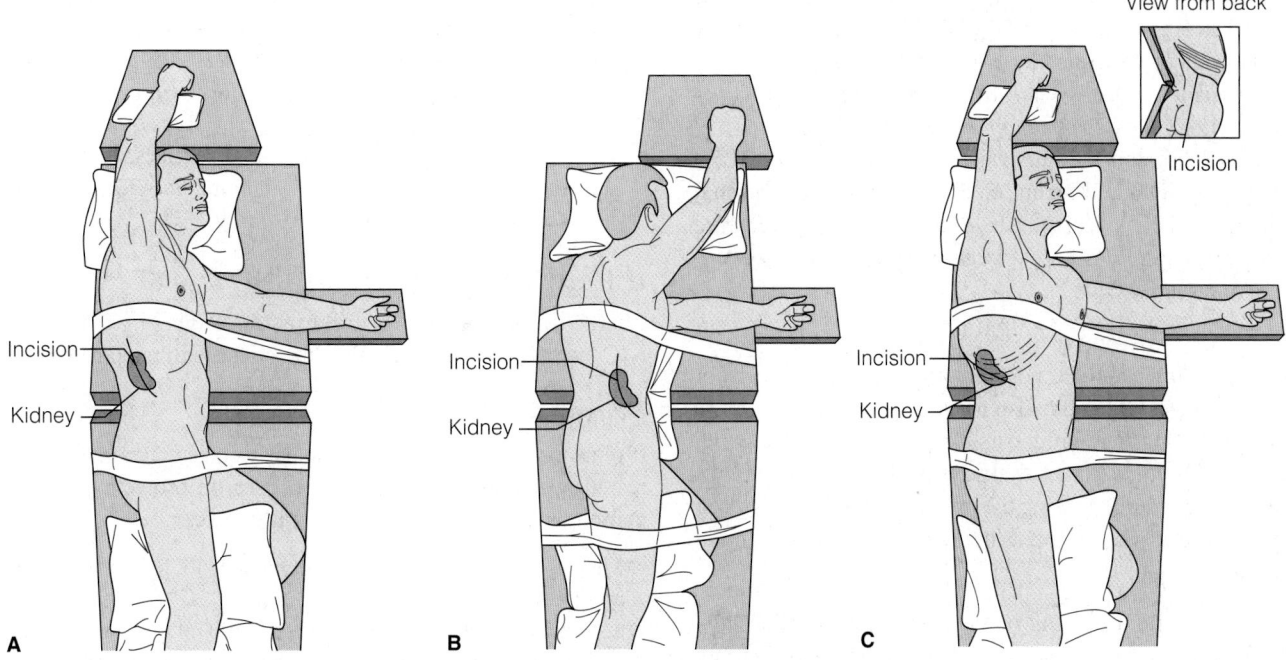

**Figure 27–4** ■ Incisions used for kidney surgery. *A,* Flank. *B,* Lumbar. *C,* Thoracoabdominal.

- Use adjunctive pain relief measures such as positioning, diversional activities, management of environmental stimuli, guided imagery, and relaxation techniques. *These can enhance the effects of analgesia.*

### Ineffective Breathing Pattern

The location of the incision combined with respiratory depressant effects of narcotic analgesics increases the risk for respiratory complications in the client who has had a nephrectomy.

- Position to promote respiratory excursion, using semi-Fowler's position and side-lying positions as allowed and tolerated. *Lung expansion is improved in semi-Fowler's and Fowler's positions.*

> **PRACTICE ALERT** *Assess respiratory status frequently, including rate and depth, cough, breath sounds, oxygen saturation, and temperature. Pneumothorax on the operative side is common. Early identification and intervention can prevent major respiratory complications.* ■

- Change position frequently, ambulate as soon as possible. *These measures promote lung expansion and the movement of mucus out of airways.*
- Encourage frequent (every 1 to 2 hours) deep breathing, spirometer use, and coughing. Assist to splint the incision. *These measures promote alveolar ventilation, gas exchange, and airway clearance.*

### Risk for Impaired Urinary Elimination

Surgery involving the urinary tract increases the risk for altered renal function and urine elimination. In addition, removal of

one kidney dictates extra caution to maintain renal circulation, a sterile urinary tract, and free urine flow.

- Monitor vital signs, CVP, and urine output every 1 to 2 hours initially, then every 4 hours. *Hypovolemia due to hemorrhage, diuresis, or fluid sequestering (third spacing) reduces blood flow to the kidney and increases the risk of renal ischemia with possible acute tubular necrosis and acute renal failure.*
- Frequently assess the amount and nature of drainage on surgical dressings and from drainage tubes, stents, and catheters. Measure and record output from each drain or catheter separately. *Frequent and accurate assessment of drainage helps to identify excess bleeding, abnormal fluid loss, infection, or other potential surgical complications.*

> **PRACTICE ALERT** *Prevent kinking, twisting, or tension on drains and tubes. Do not clamp. Irrigate carefully and only with a physician's order. Notify the physician immediately if any tube becomes dislodged. It is vital to maintain the patency of drains, particularly any affecting the remaining kidney, to prevent excess pressure of hydronephrosis.* ■

- Maintain fluid intake with intravenous fluids until oral intake is resumed. Encourage an intake of 2000 to 2500 mL per day as soon as the client tolerates oral liquids. *A liberal fluid intake prevents dehydration, helps to dilute any nephrotoxic substances, and promotes good urinary output.*
- Use strict aseptic technique in caring for all urinary catheters, tubes, stents, drains, and incisions. *Asepsis is vital to prevent infection and possible compromise of the remaining kidney.*

- Following catheter removal, assess frequently for urinary retention. Notify the physician if the client is unable to void within 4 to 6 hours or if manifestions of retention (distended bladder, discomfort, urinary dribbling) develop. *Maintenance of urine output is vital to prevent stasis and possible complications such as infection and hydronephrosis.*
- Monitor laboratory results, including urinalysis, BUN, serum creatinine, and serum electrolytes. Report abnormal findings to the physician. *Abnormal values may indicate early acute renal failure; prompt intervention is necessary to preserve renal function.*

### Anticipatory Grieving

The client having a radical nephrectomy for renal cancer not only loses a major organ but also has to adjust to the diagnosis of cancer. Although the prognosis for recovery may be good, many people perceive cancer as always fatal. Providing support for the client and family during the initial stages of grieving can improve physical recovery, psychologic coping, and eventual adaptation.

- Work to develop a trusting relationship with the client and family. *Trust increases the nurse's effectiveness in helping them work through the process of grieving.*
- Listen actively, encouraging the client and family to express fears and concerns. *As they begin to express their concerns, client and family can begin to deal more effectively with them.*
- Assist the client and family to identify strengths, past experiences, and support systems. *These resources can be employed in working through the grieving process.*
- Demonstrate respect for cultural, spiritual, and religious values and beliefs; encourage use of these resources to cope with losses. *Value and belief systems can provide a structure and form for dealing with the grieving process.*

- Encourage discussion of the potential impact of loss on the client and the family structure and function. Assist family members to share concerns with one another. *Sharing of fears and concerns among family members promotes involvement and support of the entire family unit so that the individual is not left to cope alone.*
- Refer to cancer support groups, social services, or counseling as appropriate. *Support groups and counseling services provide additional resources for coping.*

## Using NANDA, NIC, and NOC

Chart 27–2 shows links between NANDA nursing diagnoses, NIC, and NOC when caring for the client with renal cancer.

## Home Care

If renal cancer was detected at an early stage and cure is anticipated, teaching for home care focuses on protecting the remaining kidney. Include the following topics.

- Measures to prevent infection, renal calculi, hydronephrosis, and trauma
  a. Maintain a fluid intake of 2000 to 2500 mL per day, increasing the amount during hot weather or strenuous exercise.
  b. Urinate when the urge is perceived, and before and after sexual intercourse.
  c. Properly clean the perineal area.
  d. Manifestations of UTI, and the importance of early and appropriate evaluation and intervention.
  e. If the client is an older adult male, manifestations of prostatic hypertrophy, a major cause of urinary tract obstruction, and the importance of routine screening examinations.
  f. Avoid contact sports such as football or hockey; use measures to prevent motor vehicle accidents and falls, which could damage the kidney.

## CHART 27–2  NANDA, NIC, AND NOC LINKAGES

### The Client with Renal Cancer

| NURSING DIAGNOSES | NURSING INTERVENTIONS | NURSING OUTCOMES |
| --- | --- | --- |
| • Acute Pain | • Medication Management<br>• Patient-Controlled Analgesia (PCA) Assistance | • Pain: Disruptive Effects<br>• Pain Level |
| • Ineffective Breathing Pattern | • Cough Enhancement<br>• Positioning<br>• Respiratory Monitoring | • Respiratory Status: Airway Patency<br>• Respiratory Status: Ventilation |
| • Risk for Impaired Urinary Elimination | • Urinary Elimination Management | • Urinary Elimination |
| • Anticipatory Grieving | • Coping Enhancement<br>• Grief Work Facilitation | • Coping<br>• Grief Resolution |

*Note. Data from Nursing Outcomes Classification (NOC) by M. Johnson & M. Maas (Eds.), 1997, St. Louis: Mosby; Nursing Diagnoses: Definitions & Classification 2001–2002 by North American Nursing Diagnosis Association, 2001, Philadelphia: NANDA; Nursing Interventions Classification (NIC) by J.C. McCloskey & G. M. Bulechek (Eds.), 2000, St. Louis: Mosby. Reprinted by permission.*

# RENAL FAILURE

**Renal failure** is a condition in which the kidneys are unable to remove accumulated metabolites from the blood, leading to altered fluid, electrolyte, and acid-base balance. The cause may be a primary kidney disorder, or renal failure may be secondary to a systemic disease or other urologic defects. Renal failure may be either acute or chronic. **Acute renal failure** has an abrupt onset and with prompt intervention is often reversible. **Chronic renal failure** is a silent disease, developing slowly and insidiously, with few symptoms until the kidneys are severely damaged and unable to meet the excretory needs of the body. Both forms of renal failure are characterized by azotemia, increased levels of nitrogenous wastes in the blood.

Renal failure is common and costly. In 1999, approximately 89,000 new clients began receiving treatment for **end-stage renal disease (ESRD).** Annually, more than 243,000 clients with ESRD undergo dialysis, about 13,500 have kidney transplants, and another 53,000 are awaiting kidney transplants. The annual cost of ESRD treatment (in 1999 dollars) is $17.87 billion. The cost is also measured in lives and lifestyle. The 5-year survival rate for clients undergoing dialysis is 31.3 % (National Kidney and Urologic Diseases Information Clearinghouse [NKUDIC], 2001). Although many clients report satisfaction with their quality of life, often clients on dialysis are unable to work, and the family structure may disintegrate under the strain of treatment.

## THE CLIENT WITH ACUTE RENAL FAILURE

Acute renal failure (ARF) is a rapid decline in renal function with azotemia and fluid and electrolyte imbalances. Approximately 5% of all hospitalized clients develop ARF; the incidence jumps to as much as 30% in critical and special care units (Braunwald et al., 2001). The mortality rate for ARF in seriously ill clients is up to 88%. This high death rate is probably more related to the populations affected by ARF—older clients and the critically ill—than to the disorder itself (Porth, 2002).

Major trauma or surgery, infection, hemorrhage, severe heart failure, severe liver disease, and lower urinary tract obstruction are risk factors for ARF. Drugs and radiologic contrast media that are toxic to the kidney (*nephrotoxic*) also increase the risk for ARF. Older adults develop ARF more frequently due to their higher incidence of serious illness, hypotension, major surgeries, diagnostic procedures, and treatment with nephrotoxic drugs. The older adult also may have some degree of preexisting renal insufficiency associated with aging.

The most common causes of acute renal failure are ischemia and nephrotoxins. The kidney is particularly vulnerable to both because of the amount of blood that passes through it. A fall in blood pressure or volume can cause ischemia of kidney tissues. Nephrotoxins in the blood damage renal tissue directly.

## PHYSIOLOGY REVIEW

The functional unit of the kidneys, the nephron (Figure 25–3), produces urine through three processes: glomerular filtration, tubular reabsorption, and tubular secretion. In the *glomerulus,* a filtrate of water and small solutes is formed. The solute concentration of this filtrate is equal to that of plasma, with the exception of large molecules such as plasma proteins and blood cells. The glomerular filtration rate (GFR), the amount of filtrate formed per minute, is affected by blood volume and pressure, the autonomic nervous system, and other factors. From the glomerulus, the filtrate flows into the *tubules,* where its composition is changed by the processes of *tubular reabsorption* and *tubular secretion.* Most water and many filtered solutes such as electrolytes and glucose are reabsorbed. Metabolic waste products such as urea, hydrogen ion, ammonia, and some creatinine are secreted into the tubule for elimination. By the time urine exits the collecting duct into the renal pelvis, 99% of the filtrate has been reabsorbed.

## PATHOPHYSIOLOGY

The causes of acute renal failure are commonly categorized as prerenal, intrarenal, and postrenal. Prerenal causes account for 55% to 60% of ARF, intrarenal for 35% to 40%, and postrenal for less than 5%. Table 27–5 summarizes the causes of acute renal failure.

### Prerenal ARF

Prerenal causes of ARF affect renal blood flow and perfusion. Any condition that significantly decreases vascular volume, cardiac output, or systemic vascular resistance can affect renal blood flow. The kidneys normally receive 20% to 25% of the cardiac output to maintain the GFR. A drop in renal blood flow to less than 20% of normal causes ischemic changes in kidney tissue and a fall in GFR. If renal perfusion is rapidly restored, these changes are reversible. Continued ischemia can lead to tubular cell necrosis and significant nephron damage (Porth, 2002). Intrarenal ARF may result.

### Intrarenal ARF

Intrarenal failure is characterized by acute damage to the renal parenchyma and nephrons. Intrarenal causes include diseases of the kidney itself and acute tubular necrosis, the most common intrarenal cause of ARF.

In acute glomerulonephritis, glomerular inflammation can reduce renal blood flow and cause ARF. Vascular disorders affecting the kidney, such as vasculitis (inflammation of the blood vessels), malignant hypertension, and arterial or venous occlusion, can damage nephrons sufficiently to result in acute renal failure.

### Acute Tubular Necrosis

Nephrons are especially susceptible to injury from ischemia or exposure to nephrotoxins. **Acute tubular necrosis (ATN),**

## TABLE 27–5 Causes of Acute Renal Failure

| | Cause | Examples |
|---|---|---|
| **Prerenal** | Hypovolemia | Hemorrhage, dehydration, excess fluid loss from GI tract, burns, wounds |
| | Low cardiac output | Heart failure, cardiogenic shock |
| | Altered vascular resistance | Sepsis, anaphylaxis, vasoactive drugs |
| **Intrarenal** | Glomerular / microvascular injury | Glomerulonephritis, DIC, vasculitis, hypertension, toxemia of pregnancy, hemolytic uremic syndrome |
| | Acute tubular necrosis | Ischemia due to conditions associated with prerenal failure; toxins such as drugs, heavy metals; hemolysis, rhabdomyolysis (muscle cell breakdown) |
| | Interstitial nephritis | Acute pyelonephritis, toxins, metabolic imbalances, idiopathic |
| **Postrenal** | Ureteral obstruction | Calculi, cancer, external compression |
| | Urethral obstruction | Prostatic enlargement, calculi, cancer, stricture, blood clot |

destruction of tubular epithelial cells, causes an abrupt and progressive decline of renal function. Prolonged ischemia is the primary cause of ATN. When ischemia and nephrotoxin exposure occur concurrently, the risk for ATN and tubular dysfunction is especially high. See *Pathophysiology Illustrated* on the next page for the pathogenesis of acute renal failure due to ATN. Risk factors for ischemic ATN include major surgery, severe hypovolemia, sepsis, trauma, and burns. The impact of ischemia resulting from vasodilation and fluid loss in sepsis, trauma, and burns often is compounded by toxins released by bacteria or from damaged tissue.

Ischemia lasting more than 2 hours causes severe and irreversible damage to kidney tubules with patchy cellular necrosis and sloughing. The GFR is significantly reduced as a result of (1) ischemia, (2) activation of the renin-angiotensin system, and (3) tubular obstruction by cellular debris, which raises the pressure in the glomerular capsule.

Common nephrotoxins associated with ATN include the aminoglycoside antibiotics and radiologic contrast media. Many other drugs (e.g., nonsteroidal anti-inflammatory drugs and some chemotherapy drugs), heavy metals such as mercury and gold, and some common chemicals such as ethylene glycol (antifreeze) are also potentially toxic to the renal tubule. The risk for ATN is higher when nephrotoxic drugs are given to older clients or clients with preexisting renal insufficiency, and when used in combination with other nephrotoxins. Dehydration increases the risk by increasing the toxin concentration in nephrons.

Nephrotoxins destroy tubular cells by both direct and indirect effects. As tubular cells are damaged and lost through necrosis and sloughing, the tubule becomes more permeable. This increased permeability results in filtrate reabsorption, further reducing the ability of the nephron to eliminate wastes.

*Rhabdomyolysis* may cause up to 25% of all cases of ARF (Wallace, 2001). It is caused by release of excess myoglobin from injured skeletal muscles. Myoglobin is a protein that acts as the oxygen reservoir for muscle fibers, much as hemoglobin does for the blood. Muscle trauma, strenuous exercise, hyperthermia or hypothermia, drug overdose, infection, and other factors can precipitate rhabdomyolysis. The myoglobin clogs renal tubules causing ischemic injury, and contains an iron pig-

ment that directly damages the tubules. *Hemolysis*, red blood cell destruction, releases hemoglobin into the circulation, with much the same effect as rhabdomyolysis.

### Postrenal ARF

Obstructive causes of acute renal failure are classified as postrenal. Any condition that prevents urine excretion can lead to postrenal ARF. Benign prostatic hypertrophy is the most common precipitating factor. Others include renal or urinary tract calculi and tumors. See Chapter 25 for further discussion of urinary tract obstruction.

## COURSE AND MANIFESTATIONS

The course of acute renal failure typically includes three phases: initiation, maintenance, and recovery.

### Initiation Phase

The *initiation phase* may last hours to days. It begins with the initiating event (e.g., hemorrhage) and ends when tubular injury occurs. If ARF is recognized and the initiating event is effectively treated during this phase, the prognosis is good. The initiation phase of ARF has few manifestations; in fact, it is often identified only when manifestations of the maintenance phase develop.

### Maintenance Phase

The *maintenance phase* of ARF is characterized by a significant fall in GFR and tubular necrosis. Oliguria may develop, although many clients continue to produce normal or near normal amounts of urine (nonoliguric ARF). Even though urine may be produced, the kidney cannot efficiently eliminate metabolic wastes, water, electrolytes, and acids from the body during the maintenance phase of ARF. Azotemia, fluid retention, electrolyte imbalances, and metabolic acidosis develop. These abnormalities are more severe in the oliguric client than in the nonoliguric one, leading to a poorer prognosis with oliguria.

During the maintenance phase, salt and water retention cause edema, increasing the risk for heart failure and pulmonary edema. Impaired potassium excretion leads to hyperkalemia.

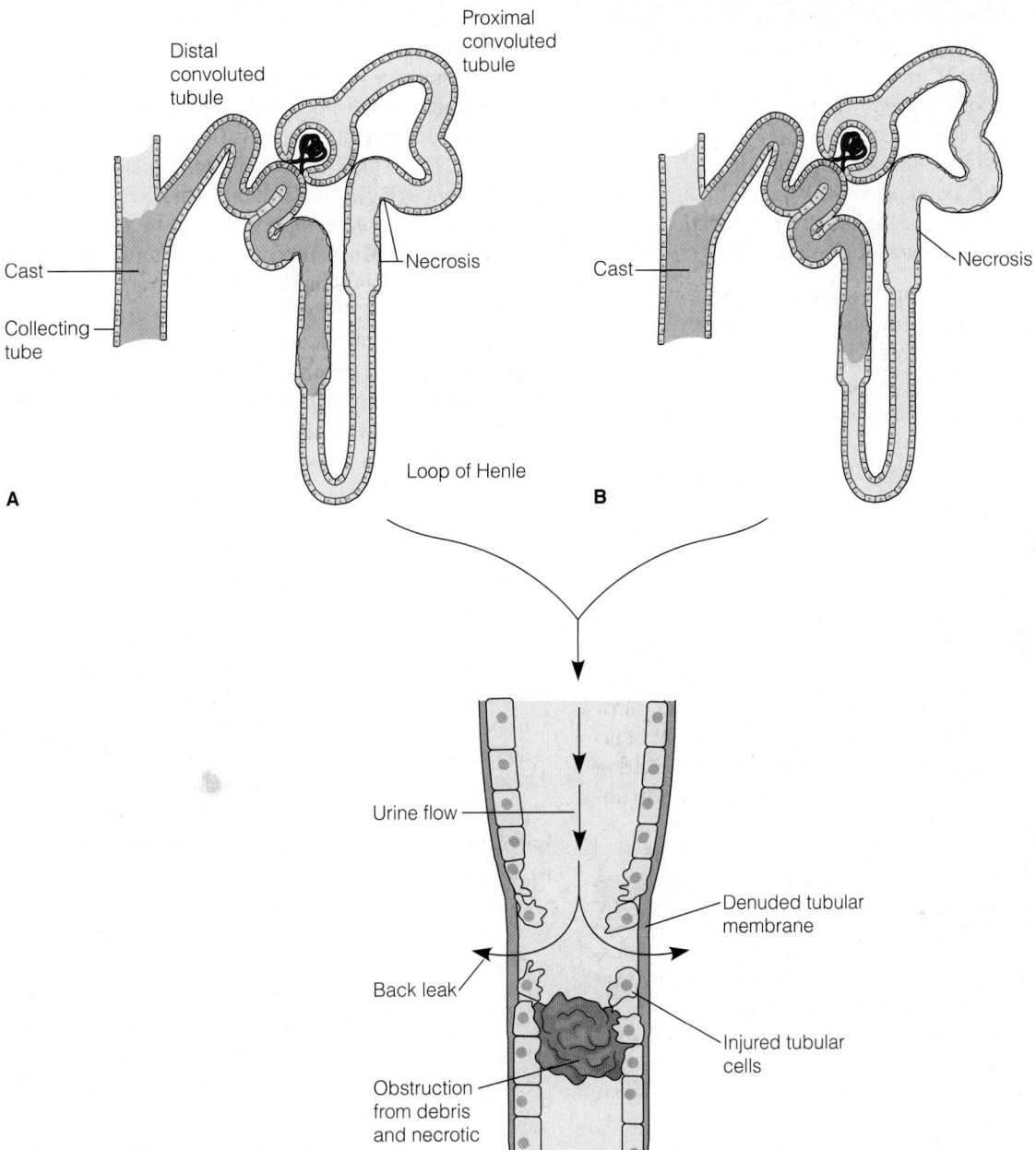

Distal convoluted tubule

Proximal convoluted tubule

Cast

Necrosis

Collecting tube

Loop of Henle

A

B

Cast

Necrosis

Urine flow

Denuded tubular membrane

Back leak

Obstruction from debris and necrotic cells

Injured tubular cells

C

Intrarenal (or intrinsic) causes of acute renal failure have the greatest effect on renal function because the functional unit of the kidney, the nephron, is damaged. The course of intrinsic renal failure often is longer, and recovery is prolonged. Acute tubular necrosis (ATN) accounts for 75% of intrinsic acute renal failure. In ATN, tubular epithelial cells are destroyed by either ischemic or toxic injury.

1. Severe hypotension, hypovolemia, and shock lead to ischemia of tubular epithelium. Renal tubular cells are very sensitive to anoxia. Cellular ATP is depleted, calcium accumulates within the cells, and free radicals damage cell membranes. Ischemia causes patchy necrosis and rupture of the basement membrane in the proximal convoluted tubule and ascending limb of the loop of Henle (Figure A).

2. Nephrotoxins include some drugs (the aminoglycoside antibiotics, in particular), radiologic dyes, pesticides, and heavy metals. Hemoglobin (e.g., released by hemolysis resulting from transfusion reaction) and myoglobin (released by muscle cells due to trauma, extreme exercise, hypo- or hyperthermia) also are nephrotoxic. Nephrotoxins damage tubular cells by their direct effects on the cell itself, or by indirect effect (e.g., vasoconstriction and ischemia). Nephrotoxic damage primarily affects the proximal tubule in a uniform pattern. It frequently is less severe than ischemic damage (Figure B).

3. Injured tubular cells release intracellular debris, which combines with proteins within the tubules to form casts. These casts, together with sloughed necrotic cells occlude the tubular lumen, increasing tubular pressure and disrupting the flow of glomerular filtrate. Glomerular filtration slows. The increased pressure pushes filtrate out of the damaged tubule into interstitial tissues (backleak). Renal blood flow and glomerular filtration may be further reduced by intrarenal angiotensin II release and vasoconstriction (Figure C).

4. Impaired tubular function affects the ability to eliminate salt, water, and metabolic waste products. As a result, oliguria, hyperkalemia, azotemia, and metabolic acidosis develop, causing the manifestations of acute renal failure.

When the serum potassium level is greater than 6.0 to 6.5 mEq/L, manifestations of its effect on neuromuscular function develop. These include muscle weakness, nausea and diarrhea, electrocardiographic changes, and possible cardiac arrest. Other electrolyte imbalances include hyperphosphatemia and hypocalcemia. Metabolic acidosis results from impaired hydrogen ion elimination by the kidneys.

Anemia develops after several days of ARF due to suppressed erythropoietin secretion by the kidneys. Immune function may be impaired, increasing the risk for infection. Other manifestations of the maintenance phase include:

- Edema and hypertension due to salt and water retention.
- Confusion, disorientation, agitation or lethargy, hyperreflexia, and possible seizures or coma due to azotemia, electrolyte and acid-base imbalances.
- Anorexia, nausea, vomiting, and decreased or absent bowel sounds.
- Uremic syndrome if ARF is prolonged (see the section on chronic renal failure that follows).

## Recovery Phase

The recovery phase of ARF is characterized by a process of tubule cell repair and regeneration and gradual return of the GFR to normal or pre-ARF levels. Diuresis may occur as the nephrons and GFR recover, and retained salt, water, and solutes are excreted. Serum creatinine, BUN, potassium, and phosphate levels remain high and may continue to rise in spite of increasing urine output. Renal function improves rapidly during the first 5 to 25 days of the recovery phase, and continues to improve for up to 1 year.

## COLLABORATIVE CARE

Preventing acute renal failure is a goal in caring for all clients, especially those in high-risk groups. Maintaining an adequate vascular volume, cardiac output, and blood pressure is vital to preserve kidney perfusion. Nephrotoxic drugs are avoided if possible. When a nephrotoxic drug or substance must be used, the risk of ARF can be reduced by using the minimum effective dose, maintaining hydration, and eliminating other known nephrotoxins from the medication regimen.

Treatment goals for acute renal failure are to (1) identify and correct the underlying cause, (2) prevent additional kidney damage, (3) restore the urine output and kidney function, and (4) compensate for renal impairment until kidney function is restored. Fluid and electrolyte balance is a key component in managing ARF.

The client's history and physical assessment can provide clues about the initiating event for ARF. Impaired perfusion for as few as 30 minutes may cause significant renal ischemia.

## Diagnostic Tests

Diagnostic tests are used to identify the cause of acute renal failure and monitor its effects on homeostasis.

- *Urinalysis* often shows the following abnormal findings in acute renal failure.

a. A fixed specific gravity of 1.010 (equal to the specific gravity of plasma) as the tubules are unable to concentrate the filtrate
b. Proteinuria if glomerular damage is the cause of ARF
c. The presence of red blood cells (due to glomerular dysfunction), white blood cells (related to inflammation), and renal tubular epithelial cells (indicating ATN)
d. Cell casts, which are protein and cellular debris molded in the shape of the tubular lumen (In ARF, RBC, WBC, and renal tubular epithelial casts may be present. Brownish pigmented casts and positive tests for occult blood indicate hemoglobinuria or myoglobinuria.)

- *Serum creatinine* and *BUN* are used to evaluate renal function. In ARF, serum creatinine levels increase rapidly, within 24 to 48 hours of the onset. Creatinine levels generally peak within 5 to 10 days. Creatinine and BUN levels tend to increase more slowly when urine output is maintained. The onset of recovery is marked by a halt in the rise of the serum creatinine and BUN.
- *Serum electrolytes* are monitored to evaluate the fluid and electrolyte status. The serum potassium rises at a moderate rate and is often used to indicate the need for dialysis. Hyponatremia is common, due to the water excess associated with ARF.
- *Arterial blood gases* often show a metabolic acidosis due to the kidneys' inability to adequately eliminate metabolic wastes and hydrogen ions (see Chapter 5).
- *Complete blood count* shows reduced RBCs, moderate anemia, and a low hematocrit. ARF affects erythropoietin secretion and RBC production. Iron and folate absorption may also be impaired, further contributing to anemia.

Laboratory findings associated with kidney disease are summarized in Table 27–2.

- *Renal ultrasonography* is used to identify obstructive causes of renal failure, and to differentiate acute renal failure from end-stage chronic renal failure. In ARF, the kidneys may be enlarged, whereas they typically appear small and shrunken in chronic renal failure. (See page 717 for nursing care of the client having a renal ultrasound or CT scan.)
- *Computed tomography (CT)* scan also may be done to evaluate kidney size and identify possible obstructions.
- *Intravenous pyelography (IVP), retrograde pyelography,* or *antegrade pyelography* may also be used to evaluate kidney structure and function. Radiologic contrast media are used with extreme caution because of their potential nephrotoxicity. Retrograde pyelography, in which contrast dye is injected into the ureters, and antegrade pyelography, in which the contrast medium is injected percutaneously into the renal pelvis, are preferred because they have fewer nephrotoxic effects than IVP. (See the Nursing Implications box on page 708.)
- *Renal biopsy* may be necessary to differentiate between acute and chronic renal failure (see the Nursing Implications box for diagnostic tests on page 750)

## Medications

The primary focus in drug management for acute renal failure is to restore and maintain renal perfusion and to eliminate drugs that are nephrotoxic from the treatment regimen.

Intravenous fluids and blood volume expanders are given as needed to restore renal perfusion. Dopamine (Intropin), administered in low doses by intravenous infusion, increases renal blood flow. Dopamine is a sympathetic neurotransmitter that improves cardiac output and dilates blood vessels of the mesentery and kidneys when given in low therapeutic doses.

If restoration of renal blood flow does not improve urinary output, a potent loop diuretic such as furosemide (Lasix) or an osmotic diuretic such as mannitol may be given with intravenous fluids. The purpose is twofold. First, if nephrotoxins are present, the combination of fluids and potent diuretics may, in effect, "wash out" the nephrons, reducing toxin concentration. Second, establishing urine output may prevent oliguria, and reduce the degree of azotemia and fluid and electrolyte imbalances. Furosemide also may be used to manage salt and water retention associated with ARF.

Aggressive hypertension management limits renal injury when ARF is associated with disorders such as toxemia and pregnancy-induced hypertension. ACE inhibitors or other antihypertensive medications are used to control arterial pressures.

All drugs that are either directly nephrotoxic or that may interfere with renal perfusion (such as potent vasoconstrictors) are discontinued. NSAIDs, nephrotoxic antibiotics, and other potentially harmful drugs are avoided throughout the course of acute renal failure.

The client in acute renal failure has an increased risk of gastrointestinal bleeding, probably related to the stress response and impaired platelet function. Regular doses of antacids, histamine $H_2$-receptor antagonists (e.g., famotidine or ranitidine), or a proton-pump inhibitor such as omeprazole (Prilosec) are often ordered to prevent GI hemorrhage.

Hyperkalemia may require active intervention as well as restricted potassium intake. Serum levels of greater than 6.5 mEq/L are treated to prevent cardiac effects of hyperkalemia. With significant hyperkalemia, calcium chloride, bicarbonate, and insulin and glucose may be given intravenously to reduce serum potassium levels by moving potassium into the cells. A potassium-binding exchange resin such as sodium polystyrene sulfonate (Kayexalate, SPS Suspension) may be given orally or by enema. This agent removes potassium from the body by exchanging sodium for potassium, primarily in the large intestine. When given orally, it is often combined with sorbitol to prevent constipation. Rectally, it is instilled as a retention enema, allowed to remain in the bowel for approximately 30 to 60 minutes, and then irrigated out using a tap-water enema.

Aluminum hydroxide (AlternaGEL, Amphojel, Nephrox), an antacid, is used to control hyperphosphatemia in renal failure. It binds with phosphates in the GI tract, which are then excreted in the feces.

Because many drugs are eliminated from the body by the kidney, drug dosages may need to be adjusted. Doses within the usual range can lead to potentially toxic blood levels, because their elimination is slowed and half-life prolonged. Nursing implications for medications commonly prescribed for the client in ARF are summarized in the box below.

---

## Medication Administration

### The Client with Acute Renal Failure

#### LOOP DIURETICS
Bumetanide (Bumex)
Ethacrynic acid (Edecrin)
Furosemide (Lasix)
Torsemide (Demadex)

The loop diuretics, named for their primary site of action in the loop of Henle, are *high-ceiling diuretics:* The response increases with increasing doses. These are highly effective diuretics used in early ARF to reestablish urine flow and convert oliguric renal failure to nonoliguric renal failure. Loop diuretics may be given with intravenous dopamine to promote renal blood flow. In ATN due to a nephrotoxin, loop diuretics are used to clear the toxin from the nephrons more rapidly. Loop diuretics cause potassium wasting, which is generally not a concern in ARF because renal failure impairs normal potassium elimination.

#### Nursing Responsibilities
- Assess weight and vital signs for baseline data.
- Monitor intake and output, daily weight (or more frequently as ordered), vital signs, skin turgor, and other indicators of fluid volume status frequently.
- Assess for orthostatic hypotension as these potent diuretics can lead to hypovolemia.
- Monitor laboratory results, especially serum electrolyte, glucose, BUN, and creatinine levels.

- Administer by mouth or, if ordered, by intravenous injection:
  a. Furosemide undiluted at a rate of no more than 20 mg per minute
  b. Ethacrynic acid 50 mg diluted with 50 mL of normal saline at a rate of no more than 10 mg per minute
  c. Bumetanide undiluted over at least 1 minute or diluted in lactated Ringer's solution, normal saline, or 5% dextrose in water for infusion
  d. Torsemide undiluted over at least 2 minutes.
- Assess response. Urine output typically increases within 10 minutes after intravenous administration.
- Monitor hearing and for complaints such as tinnitus. High doses of loop diuretics increase the risk of ototoxicity especially with ethacrynic acid. These effects may be reversible if detected early and the drug is discontinued.
- Avoid administering concurrently with other ototoxic agents, such as aminoglycoside antibiotics and cisplatin.

#### Client and Family Teaching
- Unless contraindicated, maintain a fluid intake of 2 to 3 quarts per day.
- Rise slowly from lying or sitting positions, because a fall in blood pressure may cause lightheadedness.

*(continued on page 766)*

## Medication Administration

### The Client with Acute Renal Failure (continued)

- Take in the morning and, if ordered twice a day, late afternoon to avoid sleep disturbance.
- Take with food or milk to prevent gastric distress.
- Nonsteroidal anti-inflammatory drugs (NSAIDs) interfere with the effectiveness of loop diuretics and should be avoided.

### OSMOTIC DIURETICS

Mannitol (Osmitrol, Isotol)
Urea (Ureaphil)

The osmotic diuretics act by increasing the osmotic draw in the blood and urine. In the blood, the effect is to pull extracellular water into the vascular system, increasing the GFR. These substances are then freely filtered in the glomerulus and increase the osmotic draw of the urine, inhibiting water reabsorption. The effect is to increase urine volume and flow. In addition, osmotic diuretics dilute waste products in the urine, decreasing the risk of renal damage due to excess concentrations.

#### Nursing Responsibilities

- Assess urine output. Osmotic diuretics are used in early renal failure to maintain urine output but are contraindicated in anuria. A test dose may be administered; urine output of 30 mL per hour following the test dose shows an adequate response.
- Do not give these diuretics to clients who have heart failure, or who are severely dehydrated. They increase vascular volume and may worsen heart failure. These drugs are not effective unless extracellular volume is adequate.
- Administer mannitol intravenously, diluting before use if indicated. Check solution for crystallization. Dissolve crystals by warming the solution slightly. Infuse 15% to 25% mannitol solutions through a filter over 30 to 90 minutes.
- Administer urea intravenously, diluting in 100 mL of 5% or 10% dextrose in water for every 30 g of urea. Administer no faster than 4 mL per minute through a filter.
- Monitor vital signs, breath sounds, and urinary output.
- Discontinue the drug if signs of heart failure or pulmonary edema develop or if renal function continues to decline.

#### Client and Family Teaching

- Report shortness of breath, headache, chest pain, or dizziness immediately.

### ELECTROLYTES AND ELECTROLYTE MODIFIERS

Calcium chloride
Calcium gluconate
Sodium bicarbonate
Sodium polystyrene sulfonate (Kayexalate)

Calcium chloride or gluconate and sodium bicarbonate are administered intravenously in the initial management of hyperkalemia. Calcium is also administered to correct hypocalcemia and reduce hyperphosphatemia (calcium and phosphate have a reciprocal relationship in the body; as the level of one rises, the level of the other falls). Sodium bicarbonate helps correct acidosis and move potassium back into the intracellular space. Sodium polystyrene sulfonate is not used to replace an electrolyte, but to remove excess potassium from the body by exchanging sodium for potassium in the large intestine.

#### Nursing Responsibilities

- Assess serum electrolyte levels prior to and during therapy. Report rapid shifts or adverse responses to the physician.
- Administer as appropriate:
  a. Intravenous calcium choride at less than 1 mL per minute; intravenous calcium gluconate at 0.5 mL per minute. Inject into a large vein through a small-bore needle; avoid infiltration because extravasation of intravenous solution will cause tissue necrosis.
  b. Intravenous sodium bicarbonate infusion over 4 to 8 hours; oral tablets as prescribed.
  c. Sodium polystyrene sulfonate as an oral solution mixed with sorbitol to prevent constipation, or as a retention enema mixed with warm water. Leave in the bowel for 30 to 60 minutes, irrigate using a small tap-water enema.
- Monitor for adverse reactions, such as dysrhythmias, electrolyte imbalances, and metabolic alkalosis.

#### Client and Family Teaching

- Intravenous calcium may make you lightheaded; remain in bed for at least 30 minutes after administration.
- Chew sodium bicarbonate tablets and follow with 8 ounces of water. Do not take with milk.
- Retain the sodium polystyrene sulfonate enema as long as possible.

## Fluid Management

Once vascular volume and renal perfusion are restored, fluid intake is usually restricted. The allowed daily fluid intake is calculated by allowing 500 mL for insensible losses (respiration, perspiration, bowel losses) and adding the amount excreted as urine (or lost in vomitus) during the previous 24 hours. For example, if a client with ARF excretes 325 mL of urine in 24 hours, the client is allowed a fluid intake (including oral and intravenous fluids) of 825 mL for the next 24 hours. Fluid balance is carefully monitored, using accurate weight measurements and the serum sodium as the primary indicators.

## Dietary Management

Renal insufficiency and the underlying disease process increase the rate of *catabolism* (the breakdown of body proteins) and decrease the rate of *anabolism* (body tissue repair). The client with ARF needs adequate nutrients and calories to prevent catabolism. Proteins are limited to 0.6 g per kilogram of body weight per day to minimize the degree of azotemia. Dietary proteins should be of high biologic value (rich in essential amino acids). Carbohydrates are increased to maintain adequate calorie intake and provide a protein-sparing effect.

Parenteral nutrition providing amino acids, concentrated carbohydrates, and fats may be instituted when the client cannot consume an adequate diet (e.g., due to nausea, vomiting, or underlying critical illness). The disadvantages of parenteral nutrition in the client with ARF are the high volume of fluid required and the risk for infection through the venous line.

## Dialysis

Manifestations of uremia, severe fluid overload, hyperkalemia, or metabolic acidosis in a client with renal failure indicate a need to replace renal function. **Dialysis** is the diffusion of solute molecules across a semipermeable membrane from an area of higher solute concentration to one of lower concentration. It is used to remove excess fluid and metabolic waste products in renal failure. Early use of dialysis can reduce the rate of complications. Dialysis may also be used to rapidly remove nephrotoxins in acute tubular necrosis. While dialysis compensates for lost renal elimination functions, it does not replace lost erythropoietin production. Anemia is a continuing problem for the client receiving dialysis.

In dialysis, blood is separated from a dialysis solution (**dialysate**) by a semipermeable membrane. Either **hemodialysis,** a procedure in which blood passes through a semipermeable membrane filter outside the body, or **peritoneal dialysis,** which uses the peritoneum surrounding the abdominal cavity as the dialyzing membrane, may be used for the client with ARF. **Continuous renal replacement therapy (CRRT),** in which blood is continuously circulated through a highly porous hemofilter from artery to vein or vein to vein, is a newer form of dialysis that may be used to treat ARF.

### Hemodialysis

Hemodialysis uses the principles of diffusion and ultrafiltration to remove electrolytes, waste products, and excess water from the body. Blood is taken from the client via a vascular access and pumped to the dialyzer (Figure 27–5 ■). The porous membranes of the dialyzer unit allow small molecules such as water, glucose, and electrolytes to pass through, but block larger molecules such as serum proteins and blood cells. The dialysate, a solution of approximately the same composition and temperature as normal extracellular fluid, passes along the other side of the membrane. Small solute molecules move freely across the membrane by diffusion. The direction of movement for any substance is determined by the concentrations of that substance in the blood and the dialysate. Electrolytes and waste products such as urea and creatinine diffuse from the blood into the dialysate. If it is necessary to add something to the blood, such as calcium to replace depleted stores,

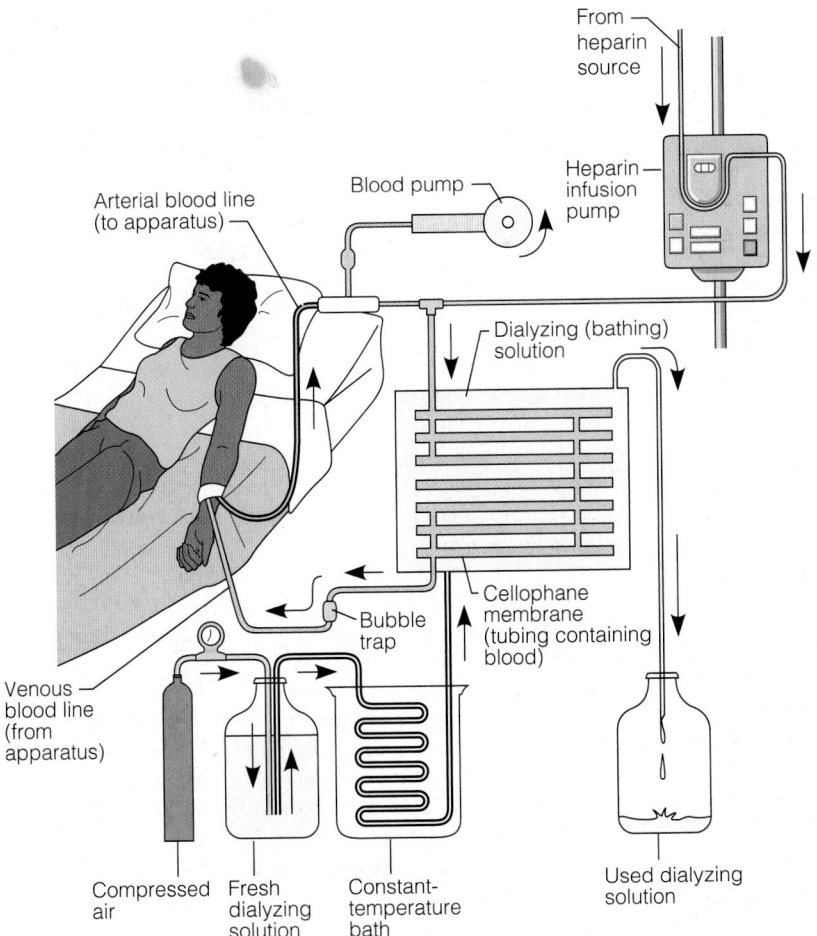

**Figure 27–5** ■ A hemodialysis system.

it can be added to the dialysate to diffuse into the blood. Excess water is removed by creating a higher hydrostatic pressure of the blood moving through the dialyzer than of the dialysate, which flows in the opposite direction. This process is known as **ultrafiltration.**

Initially, clients with ARF typically undergo daily hemodialysis, then three to four sessions per week as indicated. Hemodialysis is not used if the client is hemodynamically unstable (e.g., with hypotension or low cardiac output). Following are complications associated with hemodialysis.

- Hypotension, the most frequent complication during hemodialysis, is related to changes in serum osmolality, rapid removal of fluid from the vascular compartment, vasodilation, and other factors.
- Bleeding is related to altered platelet function associated with uremia and the use of heparin during dialysis.
- Infection (local or systemic) is related to WBC damage and immune system suppression. *Staphylococcus aureus* septicemia is commonly associated with contamination of the vascular access site. Clients on chronic hemodialysis have higher rates of hepatitis B, hepatitis C, cytomegalovirus, and HIV infection than the general population.

See the box below for nursing care for the client undergoing hemodialysis.

## Continuous Renal Replacement Therapy

Clients with acute renal failure may be unable to tolerate hemodialysis and rapid fluid removal if their cardiovascular status is unstable (e.g., due to trauma, major surgery, heart failure). Continuous renal replacement therapy (CRRT), which allows more gradual fluid and solute removal, often is used for these clients. In CRRT, blood is continuously circulated from an artery to a vein or a vein to a vein through a highly porous hemofilter for a period of 12 or more hours. Excess water and solutes such as electrolyes, urea, creatinine, uric acid, and glucose drain into a collection device. Fluid may be replaced with normal saline or a balanced electrolyte solution as needed during CRRT (Figure 27–6 ■). This

# NURSING CARE OF THE CLIENT UNDERGOING HEMODIALYSIS

## PREDIALYSIS CARE

- Assess vital signs, including orthostatic blood pressures (lying, sitting, and standing), apical pulse, respirations, and lung sounds. *These data provide baseline information to help evaluate the effects of hemodialysis. Hypertension may indicate excess fluid volume. The client who is hypotensive may not tolerate rapid fluid volume changes during dialysis. Abnormal heart sounds (e.g., a gallop or murmur) and changes in heart rate or rhythm may indicate excess fluid volume or electrolyte imbalance. Fluid overload may also cause dyspnea, tachypnea, and rales or crackles in the lungs.*
- Record weight. *Weight changes are an effective indicator of fluid volume.*
- Assess vascular access site for a palpable pulsation or vibration and an audible bruit and for inflammation. *Infection and thrombus formation are the most common problems affecting the access site in hemodialysis clients.*
- Alert all personnel to avoid using the extremity with the vascular access site (or the nondominant arm, if long-term access has not been established) for blood pressures or venipuncture. *These procedures may damage vessels and lead to failure of the AV fistula.*

## POSTDIALYSIS CARE

- Assess and document vital signs, weight, and vascular access site condition. *Rapid fluid and solute removal during dialysis may lead to orthostatic hypotension, cardiopulmonary changes, and weight loss.*
- Monitor BUN, serum creatinine, serum electrolyte, and hematocrit levels between dialysis treatments. *These values help determine the effectiveness of the treatment, the need for fluid and diet restrictions, and the timing of future dialysis sessions. The anemia associated with renal failure does not improve with*

*dialysis, and iron and folate supplements or periodic blood transfusions may be needed.*
- Assess for dialysis disequilibrium syndrome, with headache, nausea and vomiting, altered level of consciousness; and hypertension. *Rapid changes in BUN, pH, and electrolyte levels during dialysis may lead to cerebral edema and increased intracranial pressure.*
- Assess for other adverse responses to dialysis, such as dehydration, nausea and vomiting, muscle cramps, or seizure activity. Treat as ordered. *Excess fluid removal and rapid changes in electrolyte balance can cause fluid deficit, nausea, vomiting, and seizure activity.*
- Assess for bleeding at the access site or elsewhere. Use standard precautions at all times. *Renal failure and heparinization during dialysis increase the risk for bleeding. Frequent exposure to blood and blood products increase the risk for hepatitis B or C or other bloodborne diseases.*
- If a transfusion is given during dialysis, monitor for possible transfusion reaction (e.g., chills and fever; dyspnea; chest, back, or arm pain; and urticaria or itching). *Clients in renal failure may receive multiple transfusions, increasing the risk of transfusion reaction. Close monitoring during and after the transfusion is important to identify early signs of a reaction.*
- Provide psychologic support and listen actively. Address concerns and accept responses such as anger, depression, and noncompliance. Reinforce client and family strengths in coping with renal failure and hemodialysis. *Grieving is a normal response to loss of organ function. The client may feel hopeless or helpless and resent dependence on a machine. The nurse can help the client and family work through these responses and focus on positive aspects of living.*
- Refer to social services and counseling as indicated. *Clients with renal failure may need additional support services to help them adapt to and live with their disease.*

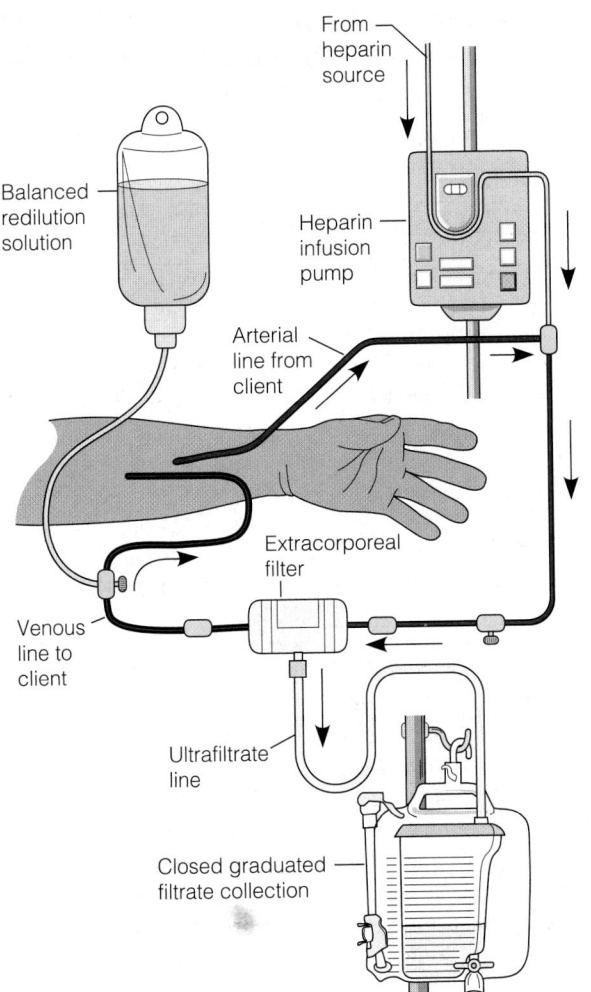

Figure 27–6 ■ Continuous arteriovenous hemofiltration (CAVH).

## Vascular Access

Acute or temporary vascular access for hemodialysis or CRRT usually is gained by inserting a double-lumen catheter into the subclavian, jugular, or femoral vein. The double-lumen catheter has a central partition separating the blood withdrawal side of the catheter from the return side. Blood is drawn into the catheter through small openings in the proximal portion of the catheter, and returned to the circulation through an opening in the distal end of the catheter to avoid withdrawing the blood that has just been dialyzed.

For longer-term vascular access, an *arteriovenous (AV) fistula* (Figure 27–7 ■) is created. In preparation for fistula formation, the nondominant arm is not used for venipuncture or blood pressure measurement during renal failure. The fistula is created by surgical anastomosis of an artery and vein, usually the radial artery and cephalic vein. It takes about a month for the fistula to mature so that it can be used for taking and replacing blood during dialysis. A functional AV fistula has a palpable pulsation and a bruit on auscultation. Venipunctures and blood pressures are avoided on the arm with the fistula.

In chronic renal failure, an *arteriovenous graft* is most often used for vascular access. The graft, a tube made of Gortex, is surgically implanted and connects the artery and the vein. Blood flows through the graft from the artery to the vein. Occasionally, an *external AV shunt* connecting a peripheral artery with a peripheral vein is used for vascular access.

slower process helps maintain hemodynamic stability and avoid complications associated with rapid changes in ECF composition. The most common CRRT techniques are outlined in Table 27–6.

CRRT is typically performed in an intensive care unit or specialized nephrology unit. Both arterial and venous lines are required for some types of CRRT; for others, a double-lumen venous catheter is used. Strict aseptic technique is vital in caring for vascular access sites to reduce the risk of infection.

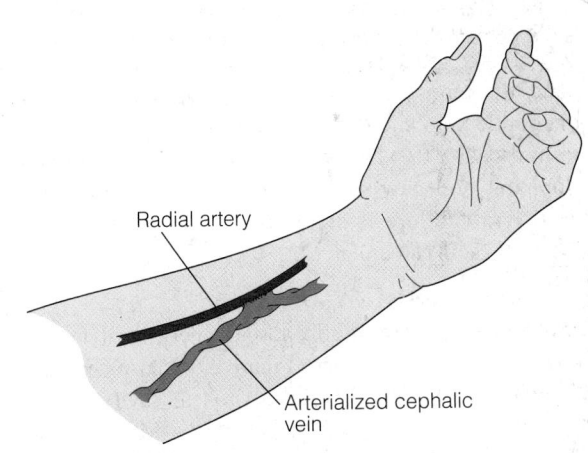

Figure 27–7 ■ An arteriovenous fistula.

| TABLE 27–6 Continuous Renal Replacement Therapies | | |
|---|---|---|
| **Type** | **Indications** | **Description** |
| Continuous arteriovenous hemofiltration (CAVH) | Remove fluid and some solutes | Arterial blood circulates through a hemofilter, then returns to client through venous line; ultrafiltrate collects in a drainage bag. |
| Continuous arteriovenous hemodialysis (CAVHD) | Remove fluid and waste products | Arterial blood circulates through a hemofilter surrounded by dialysate, then returns to client through venous line; ultrafiltrate collects in a drainage bag. |
| Continuous venovenous hemodialysis (CVVHD) | Remove fluid and waste products | Venous blood circulates through a hemofilter surrounded by dialysate, then returns to client through double-lumen venous catheter; ultrafiltrate collects in a drainage bag. |

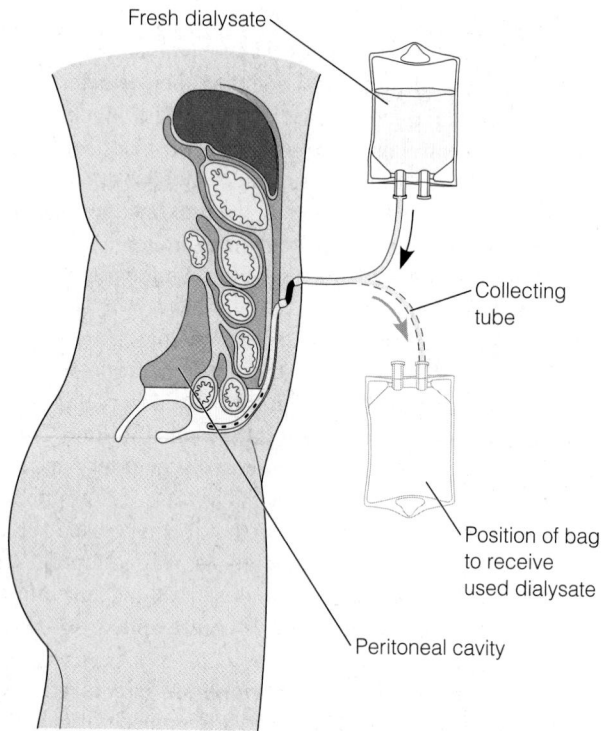

Fresh dialysate

Collecting tube

Position of bag to receive used dialysate

Peritoneal cavity

**Figure 27–8 ■** Peritoneal dialysis.

Localized AV fistula, graft, or shunt problems can occur. Infection and clotting or thrombosis are the most common shunt problems. Aneurysms may also develop. Both infection and thrombosis can lead to systemic manifestations such as septicemia and embolization. These local complications may cause the fistula or graft to fail, necessitating development of a new site. The psychologic impact of AV fistula or graft failure is significant, often causing depression and low self-esteem.

### Peritoneal Dialysis

In peritoneal dialysis, the highly vascular peritoneal membrane serves as the dialyzing surface (Figure 27–8 ■). Warmed sterile dialysate is instilled into the peritoneal cavity through a catheter inserted into the peritoneal cavity. Metabolic waste products and excess electrolytes diffuse into the dialysate while it remains in the abdomen. Water movement is controlled using dextrose as an osmotic agent to draw it into the dialysate. The fluid is then drained by gravity out of the peritoneal cavity into a sterile bag. This process of dialysate infusion, dwell time of the solution in the abdomen, and drainage is repeated at prescribed intervals.

Because excess fluid and solutes are removed more gradually in peritoneal dialysis, it poses less risk for the unstable client; however, this slower rate of metabolite removal can be a disadvantage in ARF. Peritoneal dialysis increases the risk for developing peritonitis. It is contraindicated for clients who have had recent abdominal surgery, significant lung disease, or peritonitis. See the box on the following page for nursing care for the client having peritoneal dialysis.

## NURSING CARE

### Health Promotion

Acute renal failure often can be prevented by measures that maintain fluid volume and cardiac output and reduce the risk of exposure to nephrotoxins. Carefully monitor critically ill, postoperative, and other at-risk clients for early signs of hypovolemia (low urine output, altered mental status, changes in vital signs, skin color or temperature). Promptly report a fall in urine output to less than 30 mL per hour and other evidence of decreased cardiac output. Maintain intravenous fluids as ordered. Alert the physician if the client is receiving more than one nephrotoxic drug or if a nephrotoxic drug is ordered for a dehydrated client. Closely observe clients receiving blood or blood cells for early signs of transfusion reaction and intervene appropriately.

### Assessment

Both subjective and objective data are useful when assessing the client with acute renal failure.

- Health history: complaints of anorexia, nausea, weight gain, or edema; recent exposure to a nephrotoxin such as an aminoglycoside antibiotic or radiologic procedure using an injected contrast medium; previous transfusion reaction; chronic diseases such as diabetes, heart failure, or kidney disease
- Physical examination: vital signs including temperature; urine output (amount, color, clarity, specific gravity, presence of blood cells or protein); weight; skin color, peripheral pulses; presence of edema (periorbial or dependent); lung sounds, heart sounds, and bowel tones

See page 772 for assessment of the older adult with ARF.

### Nursing Diagnoses and Interventions

The client with acute renal failure has numerous nursing care needs related not only to the renal failure but also to the underlying condition that precipitated it. Priority nursing care needs relate to fluid volume alterations, appetite and nutrition, and teaching/learning.

### Excess Fluid Volume

In acute renal failure, the kidneys often cannot excrete adequate urine to maintain a normal extracellular fluid balance. Fluid retention is greater in oliguric renal failure than in nonoliguric failure. Rapid weight gain and edema indicate fluid retention. In addition, heart failure and pulmonary edema may develop. In the older adult or severely debilitated client, fluid retention can present a significant management problem.

- Maintain hourly intake and output records. *Accurate intake and output records help guide therapy, especially fluid restrictions.*
- Weigh daily or more frequently, as ordered. Use standard technique (same scale, clothing, or coverings) to ensure accuracy. *Rapid weight changes are an accurate indicator of fluid volume status, particularly in the oliguric client.*
- Assess vital signs at least every 4 hours. *Hypertension, tachycardia, and tachypnea may indicate excess fluid volume.*

# NURSING CARE OF THE CLIENT UNDERGOING PERITONEAL DIALYSIS

## PREDIALYSIS CARE

- Document vital signs including temperature, orthostatic blood pressures (lying, sitting, and standing), apical pulse, respirations, and lung sounds. *These baseline data help assess fluid volume status and tolerance of the dialysis procedure. Hypertension, abnormal heart or lung sounds, or dyspnea may indicate excess fluid volume. Poor respiratory function may affect the ability to tolerate peritoneal dialysis. Temperature measurement is vital, because infection is the most common complication of peritoneal dialysis.*
- Weigh daily or between dialysis runs as indicated. *Weight is an accurate indicator of fluid volume status.*
- Note BUN, serum electrolyte, creatinine, pH, and hematocrit levels prior to peritoneal dialysis and periodically during the procedure. *These values are used to assess the efficacy of treatment.*
- Measure and record abdominal girth. *Increasing abdominal girth may indicate retained dialysate, excess fluid volume, or early peritonitis.*
- Maintain fluid and dietary restrictions as ordered. *Fluid and diet restrictions help reduce hypervolemia and control azotemia.*
- Have the client empty the bladder prior to catheter insertion. *Emptying the bladder reduces the risk of inadvertent puncture.*
- Warm the prescribed dialysate solution to body temperature (98.6°F or 37°C) using a warm water bath or heating pad on low setting. *Dialysate is warmed to prevent hypothermia.*
- Explain all procedures and expected sensations. *Knowledge helps reduce anxiety and elicit cooperation.*

## INTRADIALYSIS CARE

- Use strict aseptic technique during the dialysis procedure and when caring for the peritoneal catheter. *Peritonitis is a common complication of peritoneal dialysis; sterile technique reduces the risk.*
- Add prescribed medications to the dialysate; prime the tubing with solution and connect it to the peritoneal catheter, taping connections securely and avoiding kinks. *This allows dialysate to flow freely into the abdominal cavity and prevents leaking or contamination.*
- Instill dialysate into the abdominal cavity over a period of approximately 10 minutes. Clamp tubing and allow the dialysate to remain in the abdomen for the prescribed dwell time. Keep drainage tubing clamped at all times during instillation and dwell time. *Dialysate should flow freely into the abdomen if the peritoneal catheter is patent. Dialysis, the exchange of solutes and water between the blood and dialysate, occurs across the peritoneal membrane during the dwell time.*

- During instillation and dwell time, observe closely for signs of respiratory distress, such as dyspnea, tachypnea, or crackles. Place in Fowler's or semi-Fowler's position and slow the rate of instillation slightly to relieve respiratory distress if it develops. *Respiratory compromise may result from overly rapid filling or overfilling of the abdomen or from a diaphragmatic defect that allows fluid to enter the thoracic cavity.*
- After prescribed dwell time, open drainage tubing clamps and allow dialysate to drain by gravity into a sterile container. Note the clarity, color, and odor of returned dialysate. *Blood or feces in the dialysate may indicate organ or bowel perforation; cloudy or malodorous dialysate may indicate an infection.*
- Accurately record amount and type of dialysate instilled (including any added medications), dwell time, and amount and character of the drainage. *When more dialysate drains than has been instilled, excess fluid has been lost (output). If less dialysate is returned than has been instilled, a fluid gain has occurred (intake).*
- Monitor BUN, serum electrolyte, and creatinine levels. *These values are used to assess the effectiveness of dialysis.*
- Troubleshoot for possible problems during dialysis.
  a. Slow dialysate instillation. Increase the height of the container and reposition the client. Check tubing and catheter for kinks. Check abdominal dressing for wetness, indicating leakage around the catheter. *Slow dialysate flow may be related to a partially obstructed tube or catheter.*
  b. Excess dwell time. *Prolonged dwell time may lead to water depletion or hyperglycemia.*
  c. Poor dialysate drainage. Lower the drainage container, reposition, check for tubing kinks. Check abdominal dressing. *Tubing or catheter obstruction can also interfere with dialysate drainage.*

## POSTDIALYSIS CARE

- Assess vital signs, including temperature. *Comparison of pre- and postdialysis vital signs helps identify beneficial and adverse effects of the procedure.*
- Time meals to correspond with dialysis outflow. *Scheduling meals while the abdomen is empty of dialysate enhances intake and reduces nausea.*
- Teach the client and family about the procedure. *The client may elect to use peritoneal dialysis at home to manage end-stage renal disease and prevent uremia.*

---

**PRACTICE ALERT** *Frequently assess breath and heart sounds, neck veins for distention, and back and extremities for edema. Report abnormal findings. Adventitious breath sounds (crackles), abnormal heart sounds such as an S3 or S4 gallop, distended neck veins, and peripheral edema may indicate hypervolemia, heart failure, or pulmonary edema.* ■

- If not contraindicated, place in semi-Fowler's position, *to enhance cardiac and respiratory function.*
- Report abnormal serum electrolyte values and manifestations of electrolyte imbalance. The client with ARF is at particular risk for the following electrolyte imbalances:
  a. *Hyperkalemia* due to impaired potassium excretion. Manifestations include irritability, nausea, diarrhea,

## Nursing Care of the Older Adult

### RENAL FAILURE

Structural and functional changes occur in the aging kidney. Structurally, the number of nephrons decreases. The glomerular filtration rate (GFR) decreases, resulting in decreased renal clearance of drugs. Urine concentrating ability decreases, and the kidney is less able to conserve sodium. Renal compensation for acid-base imbalances takes longer. Despite these changes, the kidney retains its ability to regulate fluid and electrolyte homeostasis remarkably well unless additional stresses are added. Any additional stressors such as hypotension, exposure to nephrotoxic drugs, or an inflammatory process such as glomerulonephritis may precipitate renal failure in the older adult.

The manifestations of renal failure often are missed in aging clients (e.g., edema may be attributed to heart failure or high blood pressure to preexisting hypertension). Serum creatinine levels may rise slowly. Because older adults have less muscle mass, they produce less creatinine, a by-product of muscle cell metabolism. Likewise, the BUN may remain within normal limits.

The same measures are used to treat renal failure in older adults as in younger people. Hemodialysis, peritoneal dialysis, and renal transplantation are appropriate if necessary. Treatment options (including conservative treatment or no treatment) and their potential benefits and ramifications should be clearly explained.

### Assessing for Home Care

A number of factors should be considered in assessing the older adult's ability to manage treatment such as dialysis at home:

- Does the client have reasonable access to a dialysis center or outpatient unit? Is transportation available?
- Would home hemodialysis be appropriate? Is a caregiver available to be trained to manage dialysis? Does the client's home have appropriate electrical and plumbing fixtures?
- Would continuous ambulatory peritoneal dialysis be appropriate? Does the client have the manual dexterity, will, and cognitive ability to manage dialysis infusions? If not, would intermittent peritoneal dialysis using a dialyzing machine be more appropriate?
- Are family members or other support persons available to provide assistance to the client as needed?

### Resources for Home Care

The following resources may be useful for clients with kidney disease.

- American Association of Kidney Patients
  3505 E. Frontage Rd., Suite 315
  Tampa, FL 33607
  800-749-2257
  www.aakp.org
- American Kidney Fund
  6110 Executive Blvd., Suite 1010
  Rockville, MD 20852
  800-638-8299
  www.akfinc.org
- National Kidney Foundation
  30 E. 33rd Street, Suite 1100
  New York, NY 10016
  800-622-9010
  www.kidney.org

*MediaLink | KIDNEY DISORDERS*

---

abdominal cramping, cardiac dysrhythmias, and ECG changes.

b. *Hyponatremia* due to water retention. Manifestations include nausea, vomiting, and headache, with possible CNS manifestations of lethargy, confusion, seizures, and coma.

c. *Hyperphosphatemia* due to decreased phosphate excretion. Manifestations include hyperreflexia, paresthesias, and possible tetany.

*ARF impairs electrolyte and water excretion, causing multiple electrolyte imbalances.*

- Restrict fluids as ordered. Provide frequent mouth care and encourage using hard candies to decrease thirst. If ice chips are allowed, include the water content (approximately one-half of the total volume) as intake. *Fluids are restricted to minimize fluid retention and complications of fluid volume excess.*
- Administer medications with meals. *Giving oral medications with meals minimizes ingestion of excess fluids.*
- Turn frequently and provide good skin care. *Edema decreases tissue perfusion and increases the risk of skin breakdown, especially in the older or debilitated client.*

### Imbalanced Nutrition: Less Than Body Requirements

Anorexia and nausea associated with renal failure often interfere with food intake and nutrition. In addition, the disease process leading to ARF may contribute to increased nutritional needs for healing and decreased food intake.

- Monitor and record food intake, including the amount and type of food consumed. *A detailed intake record helps guide decisions about nutritional status and necessary supplements.*
- Weigh daily. *Weight changes over time (days to weeks) reflect nutritional status, while rapid weight changes are more reflective of fluid volume status. In ARF, weight may remain stable or increase due to fluid retention even though tissue mass is being lost.*
- Arrange for dietary consultation to plan meals within prescribed limitations that consider the client's food preferences. *Diets restricted in protein, salt, and potassium can be unpalatable; including preferred foods as allowed increases intake.*
- Engage the client in planning daily menus. *Participation in meal planning increases the client's sense of control and autonomy.*
- Allow family members to prepare meals within dietary restrictions. Encourage family members to eat with the client. *Familiar foods and social interaction encourage eating and increase enjoyment of meals.*
- Provide frequent, small meals or between-meal snacks. *These measures promote food intake in the fatigued or anorectic client.*

- Administer antiemetics as ordered and provide mouth care prior to meals. *Nausea and a metallic taste in the mouth, common manifestations of uremia, can decrease food intake.*
- Administer parenteral nutrition as ordered if the client is unable to eat or tolerate enteral nutrition. *Preventing or slowing tissue catabolism is important for the client with ARF.*

**PRACTICE ALERT** *Intravenous lines and parenteral nutrition solutions can increase the risk for infection. Monitor sites carefully for signs of infection or inflammation.* ■

### Deficient Knowledge

The client with ARF has multiple learning needs. These include information about ARF, diagnostic and laboratory studies, management strategies, and implications for the recovery period.

- Assess anxiety level and ability to comprehend instruction. Tailor information and presentation to developmental level and physical, mental, and emotional status. *The client with ARF may be critically ill or have uremic effects that hinder learning. During the initial stages of ARF it may be necessary to limit information to immediate concerns.*
- Assess knowledge and understanding. *To enhance understanding and retention, relate information presented to previous learning.*
- Teach about diagnostic tests and therapeutic procedures. *Teaching reduces anxiety and improves understanding and cooperation.*
- Discuss dietary and fluid restrictions. *These measures may be continued after discharge.*
- If the client is discharged prior to the recovery phase of ARF, teach the signs and symptoms of complications, such as fluid volume excess or deficit, heart failure, and electrolyte imbalances. *As kidney function returns, urine output increases, but the concentrating ability of the nephrons and electrolyte*

*excretion remain impaired. This impaired function increases the risk of excess fluid loss, possible dehydration, orthostatic hypotension, and electrolyte imbalance.*

- Teach how to monitor weight, blood pressure, and pulse. *These are important means of assessing fluid status.*
- Instruct to avoid nephrotoxic drugs and chemicals for up to 1 year following an episode of ARF. *During recovery, nephrons are vulnerable to damage by nephrotoxins such as NSAIDs, some antibiotics, radiologic contrast media, and heavy metals. Because alcohol can increase the nephrotoxicity of some materials, discourage alcohol ingestion.*

## Using NANDA, NIC, and NOC

Chart 27–3 shows links between NANDA nursing diagnoses, NIC, and NOC for the client with ARF.

## Home Care

Often the client is critically ill when ARF develops. Critical illness and the resulting state of client and family crisis can impair learning and retention of information. Include family members in teaching during the initial stages to promote understanding of what is happening and the reasons for specific treatment measures. Inclusion of the family reduces their anxiety, and provides a valuable resource for reinforcing client teaching about care after discharge.

Client teaching needs for home care include:

- Avoiding exposure to nephrotoxins, particularly those in over-the-counter products.
- Preventing infection and other major stressors that can slow healing.
- Monitoring weight, blood pressure, and pulse.
- Manifestations of relapse.
- Continuing dietary restrictions.
- Knowing when to contact the physician.

**CHART 27–3  NANDA, NIC, AND NOC LINKAGES**

### The Client with Acute Renal Failure

| NURSING DIAGNOSES | NURSING INTERVENTIONS | NURSING OUTCOMES |
|---|---|---|
| • Anxiety | • Active Listening<br>• Anxiety Reduction | • Anxiety Control<br>• Coping |
| • Decreased Cardiac Output | • Hemodynamic Regulation<br>• Shock Management | • Cardiac Pump Effectiveness |
| • Excess Fluid Volume | • Fluid Management<br>• Fluid / Electrolyte Management | • Electrolyte and Acid-Base Balance<br>• Fluid Balance |
| • Imbalanced Nutrition: Less than Body Requirements | • Enteral Tube Feeding<br>• Nutrition Management<br>• Nutrition Monitoring | • Nutritional Status: Food and Fluid Intake |
| • Impaired Urinary Elimination | • Urinary Elimination Management | • Urinary Elimination |

*Note. Data from Nursing Outcomes Classification (NOC) by M. Johnson & M. Maas (Eds.), 1997, St. Louis: Mosby; Nursing Diagnoses: Definitions & Classification 2001–2002 by North American Nursing Diagnosis Association, 2001, Philadelphia: NANDA; Nursing Interventions Classification (NIC) by J.C. McCloskey & G. M. Bulechek (Eds.), 2000, St. Louis: Mosby. Reprinted by permission.*

# Nursing Care Plan
## A Client with Acute Renal Failure

Judy Devak is driving home late one evening when she loses control of her car trying to avoid hitting a deer in the road. Her car strikes a tree and rolls into a deep ditch beside the road, out of sight of passing cars. The wreck is not discovered until 2 hours later. On arrival at the accident scene, the paramedics find Ms. Devak hypotensive: BP 90/60, P 120, and R 24. She is alert and in severe pain, with a fractured right femur. After immobilizing Ms. Devak's neck and back and extricating her from the car, they apply a traction splint to her leg and transport her to the local hospital.

## ASSESSMENT

Katie Leaper, RN, obtains a nursing history on Ms. Devak's admission to the intensive care unit. Ms. Devak indicates that she has been healthy, having experienced only minor illnesses and chickenpox as a child. She has never been hospitalized, and knows of no allergies to medications. Ms. Devak is not currently taking prescription or nonprescription drugs. Physical assessment findings include T 97.4° F (36.3° C) PO, P 100, R 18, and BP 124/68. Skin pale, cool, and dry, with multiple scrapes, minor abrasions, and bruises on face and extremities. A linear bruise is noted on her chest and abdomen from the seat belt. Lung sounds clear, heart tones normal, and abdomen tender but soft to palpation. Right leg alignment maintained with skeletal traction. One unit of whole blood was infused prior to ICU admission, a second unit is currently infusing. An indwelling urinary catheter and a nasogastric tube are in place.

During the first few hours after admission, Ms. Leaper notes that Ms. Devak's hourly output has dropped from 55 mL to 45 mL to 28 mL of clear yellow urine. The physician orders a 500 mL intravenous fluid challenge, STAT urinalysis, BUN, and serum creatinine. The fluid challenge elicits only a slight increase in urine output. Urinalysis results show a specific gravity of 1.010 and the presence of WBCs, red and white cell casts, and tubular epithelial cells in the sediment. Ms. Devak's BUN is 28 mg/dL; her serum creatinine, 1.5 mg/dL. The physician diagnoses probable acute renal failure and orders a nephrology consultation. In addition, the physician orders aluminum hydroxide, 10 mL every 2 hours per nasogastric tube, and ranitidine 50 mg intravenously every 8 hours.

## DIAGNOSIS

- *Acute pain* related to injuries sustained in accident
- *Anxiety* related to being in the intensive care unit
- *Risk for excess fluid volume* related to impaired renal function
- *Impaired physical mobility* related to skeletal traction
- *Ineffective protection* related to injuries and invasive procedures

## EXPECTED OUTCOMES

- Report adequate pain control.
- Verbalize reduced anxiety.
- Maintain stable weight and vital signs within normal range.

- Maintain skin integrity.
- Use the trapeze appropriately to adjust position in bed while maintaining body alignment.
- Remain free of infection, bleeding, or respiratory distress.

## PLANNING AND IMPLEMENTATION

- Maintain patient-controlled analgesia.
- Assess frequently for pain control and response to analgesia.
- Encourage expression of thoughts, feelings, and fears about condition and placement in ICU.
- Document vital signs and heart and lung sounds at least every 4 hours.
- Weigh every 12 hours.
- Document hourly intake and output.
- Restrict fluids as ordered, including diluent for all intravenous medications as intake.
- Assist with mouth care every 3 to 4 hours; allow frequent rinsing of mouth and ice chips as allowed.
- Assist with position changes at least every 2 hours; teach use of the overhead trapeze.
- Monitor frequently for signs of infection, bleeding, or respiratory distress.

## EVALUATION

After just over 3 days of oliguria, Ms. Devak's urine output increases. By the end of the fourth day she is excreting 60 to 80 mL/hour of urine. Although her BUN, serum creatinine, and potassium levels remain high, they never reach a critical point, and dialysis is not required. She is transferred from the ICU on the fifth day after admission. When Ms. Devak is able to begin eating, she is placed on a low-potassium diet, restricted to 50 g of protein. Her renal function gradually improves. By discharge, results of her renal function studies, including BUN and serum creatinine, are nearly normal. Ms. Devak verbalizes an understanding of the need to avoid nephrotoxins such as NSAIDs until allowed by her physician.

## Critical Thinking in the Nursing Process

1. What was the most likely specific precipitating factor for Ms. Devak's acute renal failure? Did anything else contribute to her risk?
2. Why did the physician prescribe aluminum hydroxide and ranitidine? Consider both the acute renal failure and Ms. Devak's placement in the intensive care unit.
3. Ms. Devak is at risk for respiratory distress related to potential fluid volume excess. How does her fractured femur further contribute to risk for respiratory distress?
4. Develop a care plan for Ms. Devak for the nursing diagnosis, *Diversional activity deficit.*

See Evaluating Your Response in Appendix C.

# THE CLIENT WITH CHRONIC RENAL FAILURE

Although the kidneys usually recover from acute injury, many chronic conditions can lead to progressive renal tissue destruction and loss of function. Nephron units are lost and renal mass decreases, with progressive deterioration of glomerular filtration, tubular secretion, and reabsorption. This process of chronic renal failure (CRF) may progress slowly for many years without being recognized. Eventually, the kidneys are unable to excrete metabolic wastes and regulate fluid and electrolyte balance adequately, a condition known as end-stage renal disease (ESRD), the final stage of CRF.

The incidence of ESRD is increasing, particularly in older adults. In 1999, more than 89,000 people started treatment for ESRD for a total of about 424,000 people undergoing ESRD treatment (NKUDIC, 2001). Native Americans have the highest incidence of ESRD, followed by African Americans, Asians and European Americans (United States Renal Data System [USRDS], 2001).

Conditions causing CRF typically involve diffuse, bilateral disease of the kidneys with progressive destruction and scarring of the entire nephron. As indicated in Figure 27–9 ■, diabetes is the leading cause of ESRD in all population groups in the United States. Hypertension closely follows diabetes as a major cause of ESRD (USRDS, 2001).

## PATHOPHYSIOLOGY AND MANIFESTATIONS

The pathophysiology of CRF involves a gradual loss of entire nephron units. In the early stages, as nephrons are destroyed, remaining functional nephrons hypertrophy. Glomerular capillary flow and pressure increase in these nephrons, and more solute particles are filtered to compensate for lost renal mass. This increased demand predisposes the remaining nephrons to glomerular sclerosis (scarring), resulting in their eventual destruction. This process of continued loss of nephron function may continue even after the initial disease process has resolved (Braunwald et al., 2001). Table 27–7 outlines common pathologic processes leading to nephron destruction and ESRD.

The course of CRF is variable, progressing over a period of months to many years. In the early stage, known as *decreased renal reserve*, unaffected nephrons compensate for the lost nephrons. The glomerular filtration rate (GFR) is about 50% of normal, and the client is asymptomatic with normal BUN and serum creatinine levels. As the disease progresses and the GFR falls to 20% to 50% of normal, azotemia and some manifestations of *renal insufficiency* may be seen. Any further insult to the kidneys at this stage (such as infection, dehydration, exposure to nephrotoxins, or urinary tract obstruction) can further reduce function and precipitate the onset of *renal failure* or overt uremia. This stage is characterized by a GFR of less than 20% of

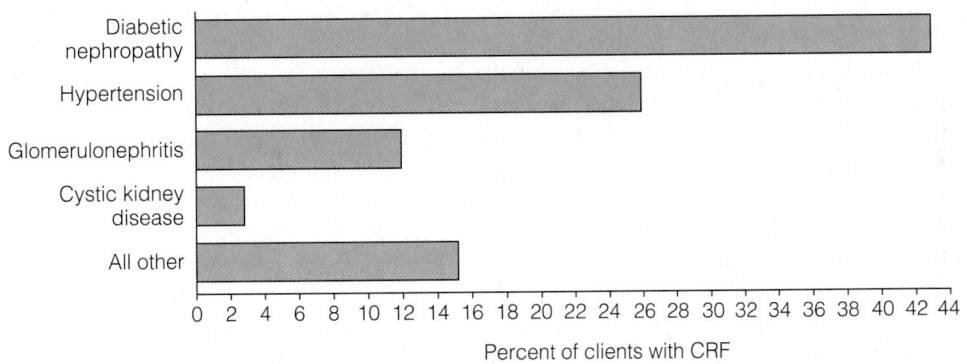

Figure 27–9 ■ The most common causes of chronic renal failure (USRDS, 2001).

TABLE 27–7  Pathophysiology of Chronic Renal Failure

| Cause | Examples |
|---|---|
| Diabetic nephropathy | Changes in the glomerular basement membrane, chronic pyelonephritis, and ischemia lead to sclerosis of the glomerulus and gradual destruction of the nephron |
| Hypertensive nephrosclerosis | Long-standing hypertension leads to renal arteriosclerosis and ischemia resulting in glomerular destruction and tubular atrophy |
| Chronic glomerulonephritis | Bilateral inflammatory process of the glomeruli leading to ischemia, nephron loss, and shrinkage of the kidney |
| Chronic pyelonephritis | Chronic infection commonly associated with an obstructive or neurologic process and vesicoureteral reflux leading to reflux nephropathy (renal scarring, atrophy, and dilated calyces) |
| Polycystic kidney disease | Multiple bilateral cysts gradually destroy normal renal tissue by compression |
| Systemic lupus erythematosus | Basement membrane damage by circulating immune complexes leading to focal, local, or diffuse glomerulonephritis |

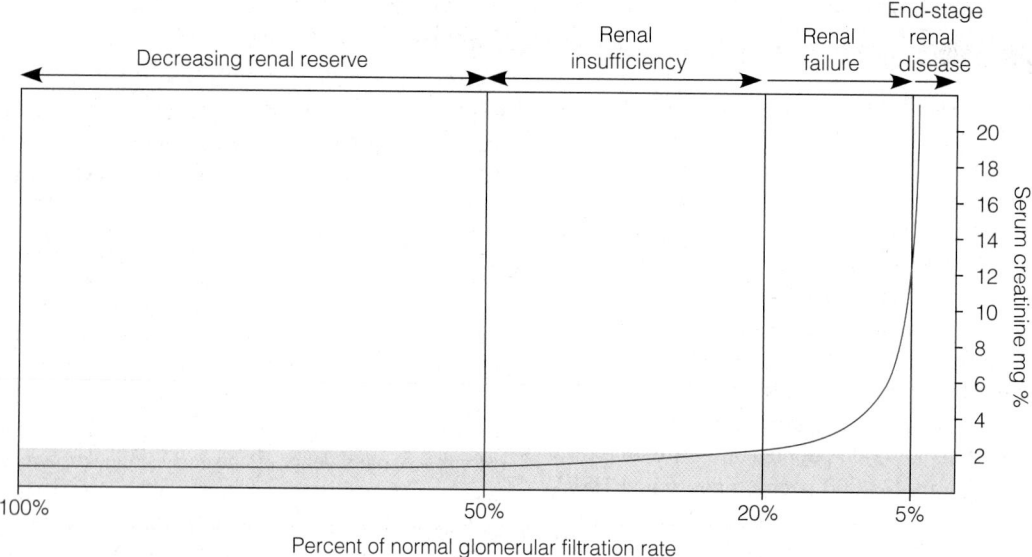

**Figure 27–10** ■ The relationship of renal function to BUN and serum creatinine values through the course of chronic renal failure.

normal. The serum creatinine and BUN levels rise sharply (Figure 27–10 ■), the client becomes oliguric, and manifestations of uremia are seen. In ESRD, the final stage of CRF, the GFR is less than 5% of normal and renal replacement therapy is necessary to sustain life (Braunwald et al., 2001; Porth, 2002). Table 27–8 summarizes the stages of chronic renal failure.

Chronic renal failure often is not identified until its final, uremic stage is reached. **Uremia,** which literally means "urine in the blood," refers to the syndrome or group of symptoms associated with ESRD. In uremia, fluid and electrolyte balance is altered, the regulatory and endocrine functions of the kidney are impaired, and accumulated metabolic waste products affect essentially every other organ system (Braunwald et al., 2001; Porth 2002).

Early manifestations of uremia include nausea, apathy, weakness, and fatigue, symptoms that are dismissed as a viral infection or influenza. As the condition progresses, frequent vomiting, increasing weakness, lethargy, and confusion develop (Porth, 2002). The *Multisystem Effects of Uremia* are illustrated on the next page.

## Fluid and Electrolyte Effects

Loss of functional kidney tissue impairs its ability to regulate fluid, electrolyte, and acid-base balance. In the early stages of CRF, impaired filtration and reabsorption lead to proteinuria, hematuria, and decreased urine concentrating ability. Salt and water are poorly conserved, and risk for dehydration increases. Polyuria, nocturia, and a fixed specific gravity of 1.008 to 1.012 are common (Porth, 2002). As the GFR decreases and renal function deteriorates further, sodium and water retention are common, necessitating salt and water restrictions.

Hyperkalemia develops as renal failure progresses. Manifestations of hyperkalemia, such as muscle weakness, paresthesias, and ECG changes, are not usually seen until the GFR is less than 5 mL/min. Phosphate excretion is also impaired, leading to hyperphosphatemia and hypocalcemia. Reduced calcium absorption due to impaired vitamin D activation also contributes to hypocalcemia. Hypermagnesemia develops with advancing renal failure; magnesium-containing antacids are avoided for this reason.

As renal failure advances, hydrogen-ion excretion and buffer production are impaired, leading to metabolic acidosis. Respiratory rate and depth increase (Kussmaul's respirations) to compensate for metabolic acidosis. Although metabolic acidosis is often asymptomatic, other possible manifestations include general malaise, weakness, headache, nausea and vomiting, and abdominal pain (see Chapter 5). ☍

## TABLE 27–8 Stages of Chronic Renal Failure

| Stage | Glomerular Filtration Rate | Manifestations |
|---|---|---|
| Decreased renal reserve | Approximately 50% of normal | None; normal BUN and creatinine |
| Renal insufficiency | 20% to 50% of normal | Polyuria with low, fixed specific gravity; azotemia; anemia; hypertension |
| Renal failure | <20% of normal | Increasing azotemia; edema, metabolic acidosis, hypercalcemia; possible uremia |
| End-stage renal disease | <5% of normal | Kidney atrophy and fibrosis; overt uremia |

# Multisystem Effects of Uremia

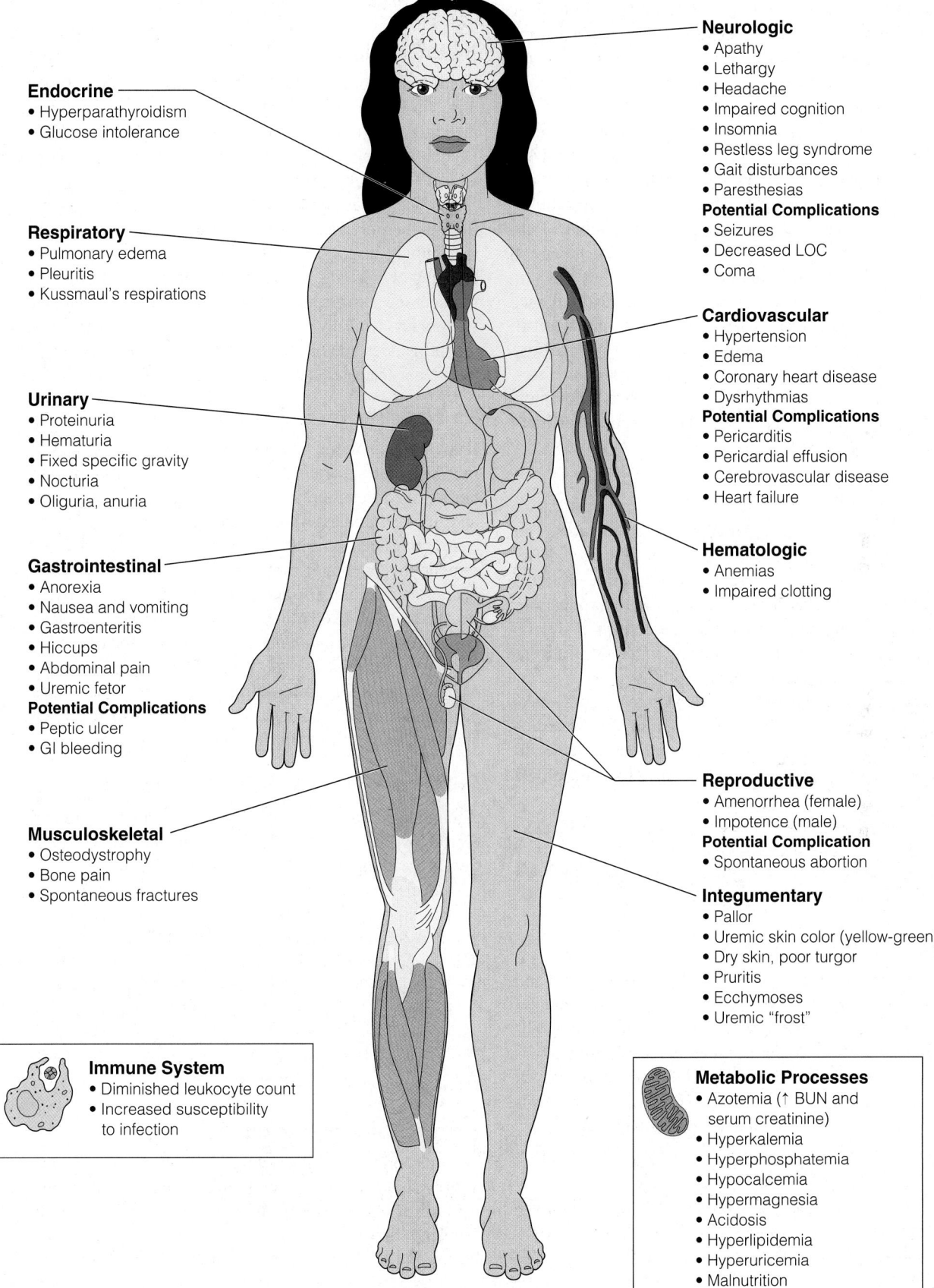

**Endocrine**
- Hyperparathyroidism
- Glucose intolerance

**Respiratory**
- Pulmonary edema
- Pleuritis
- Kussmaul's respirations

**Urinary**
- Proteinuria
- Hematuria
- Fixed specific gravity
- Nocturia
- Oliguria, anuria

**Gastrointestinal**
- Anorexia
- Nausea and vomiting
- Gastroenteritis
- Hiccups
- Abdominal pain
- Uremic fetor
**Potential Complications**
- Peptic ulcer
- GI bleeding

**Musculoskeletal**
- Osteodystrophy
- Bone pain
- Spontaneous fractures

**Immune System**
- Diminished leukocyte count
- Increased susceptibility to infection

**Neurologic**
- Apathy
- Lethargy
- Headache
- Impaired cognition
- Insomnia
- Restless leg syndrome
- Gait disturbances
- Paresthesias
**Potential Complications**
- Seizures
- Decreased LOC
- Coma

**Cardiovascular**
- Hypertension
- Edema
- Coronary heart disease
- Dysrhythmias
**Potential Complications**
- Pericarditis
- Pericardial effusion
- Cerebrovascular disease
- Heart failure

**Hematologic**
- Anemias
- Impaired clotting

**Reproductive**
- Amenorrhea (female)
- Impotence (male)
**Potential Complication**
- Spontaneous abortion

**Integumentary**
- Pallor
- Uremic skin color (yellow-green)
- Dry skin, poor turgor
- Pruritis
- Ecchymoses
- Uremic "frost"

**Metabolic Processes**
- Azotemia (↑ BUN and serum creatinine)
- Hyperkalemia
- Hyperphosphatemia
- Hypocalcemia
- Hypermagnesia
- Acidosis
- Hyperlipidemia
- Hyperuricemia
- Malnutrition

## Cardiovascular Effects

Cardiovascular disease is a common cause of death in ESRD, and results from accelerated atherosclerosis. Hypertension, hyperlipidemia, and glucose intolerance all contribute to the process. Cerebral and peripheral vascular manifestations of atherosclerosis are also seen.

Systemic hypertension is a common complication of ESRD. Hypertension results from excess fluid volume; increased rennin-angiotensin activity, increased peripheral vascular resistance, and decreased prostaglandins. Increased extracellular fluid volume also can lead to edema and heart failure. Pulmonary edema may result from heart failure and increased permeability of the alveolar capillary membrane.

Retained metabolic toxins can irritate the pericardial sac, causing an inflammatory response and signs of pericarditis. *Cardiac tamponade,* a potential complication of pericarditis, occurs when inflammatory fluid in the pericardial sac interferes with ventricular filling and cardiac output. Once a common complication of uremia, pericarditis is less common when dialysis is initiated early.

## Hematologic Effects

Anemia is common in uremia, caused by multiple factors. The kidneys produce erythropoietin, a hormone that controls RBC production. In renal failure, erythropoietin production declines. Retained metabolic toxins further suppress RBC production, and contribute to a shortened RBC life span. Nutritional deficiencies (iron and folate) and increased risk for blood loss from the GI tract also contribute to anemia.

Anemia contributes to manifestations such as fatigue, weakness, depression, and impaired cognition. It also affects cardiovascular function, and may be a major contributing factor to coronary heart disease and heart failure associated with ESRD (Porth, 2002).

Renal failure impairs platelet function, increasing the risk of bleeding disorders such as epistaxis and GI bleeding. The mechanism of impaired platelet function associated with renal failure is poorly understood.

## Immune System Effects

Uremia increases the risk for infection. High levels of urea and retained metabolic wastes impair all aspects of inflammation and immune function. The WBC declines, humoral and cell-mediated immunity are impaired, and phagocyte function is defective. Both the acute inflammatory response and delayed hypersensitivity responses are affected (Porth, 2002). Fever is suppressed, often delaying the diagnosis of infection.

## Gastrointestinal Effects

Anorexia, nausea, and vomiting are the most common early symptoms of uremia. Hiccups also are commonly experienced. Gastroenteritis is frequent. Ulcerations may affect any level of the GI tract and contribute to an increased risk of GI bleeding. Peptic ulcer disease is particularly common in uremic clients. *Uremic fetor,* a urinelike breath odor often associated with a metallic taste in the mouth, may develop. Uremic fetor can further contribute to anorexia.

## Neurologic Effects

Uremia alters both central and peripheral nervous system function. CNS manifestations occur early and include changes in mentation, difficulty concentrating, fatigue, and insomnia. Psychotic symptoms, seizures, and coma are associated with advanced uremic encephalopathy.

Peripheral neuropathy is also common in advanced uremia. Both the sensory and motor tracts are involved. The lower limbs are initially affected. "Restless leg syndrome," sensations of crawling or creeping, prickling, or itching of the lower legs with frequent leg movement, increases during rest. Paresthesias and sensory loss typically occur in a "stocking-glove" pattern. As uremia progresses, motor function is also impaired, causing muscle weakness, decreased deep tendon reflexes, and gait disturbances.

## Musculoskeletal Effects

Hyperphosphatemia and hypocalcemia associated with uremia stimulates parathyroid hormone secretion. Parathyroid hormone causes increased calcium resorption from bone. In addition, osteoblast (bone-forming) and osteoclast (bone-destructing) cell activity is affected. This bone resorption and remodeling, combined with decreased vitamin D synthesis and decreased calcium absorption from the GI tract, leads to *renal osteodystrophy,* also known as renal rickets. Osteodystrophy is characterized by *osteomalacia,* softening of the bones, and *osteoporosis,* decreased bone mass. Bone cysts may develop. Manifestations of osteodystrophy include bone tenderness, pain, and muscle weakness. The client is at increased risk for spontaneous fractures (Porth, 2002).

## Endocrine and Metabolic Effects

Accumulated waste products of protein metabolism are a primary factor involved in the effects and manifestations of uremia. Serum creatinine and BUN levels are significantly elevated. Uric acid levels are increased, contributing to an increased risk of gout.

Tissues become resistant to the effects of insulin in uremia, leading to glucose intolerance. High blood triglyceride levels and lower than normal high-density lipoprotein (HDL) levels contribute to the accelerated atherosclerotic process.

Reproductive function is affected. Pregnancies are rarely carried to term, and menstrual irregularities are common. Reduced testosterone levels, low sperm counts, and impotence affect the male client with ESRD.

## Dermatologic Effects

Anemia and retained pigmented metabolites cause pallor and a yellowish hue to the skin in uremia. Dry skin with poor turgor, a result of dehydration and sweat gland atrophy, is common. Bruising and excoriations are frequently seen. Metabolic wastes not eliminated by the kidneys may be deposited in the skin, contributing to itching or pruritus. In advanced uremia, high levels of urea in the sweat may result in *uremic frost,* crystallized deposits of urea on the skin.

## COLLABORATIVE CARE

Early management of CRF focuses on eliminating factors that may further decrease renal function and measures to slow the progression of the disease to ESRD. Additional treatment goals are to:

- Maintain nutritional status while minimizing the accumulation of toxic waste products and manifestations of uremia.
- Identify and treat complications of CRF.
- Prepare for renal replacement therapies such as dialysis or renal transplant.

### Diagnostic Tests

Diagnostic testing is used both to identify CRF and to monitor kidney function. A number of tests may be performed to determine the underlying renal disorder. Once the diagnosis is established, renal function is monitored primarily through blood levels of metabolic wastes and electrolytes.

- *Urinalysis* is done to measure urine specific gravity and detect abnormal urine components. In CRF, the specific gravity may be fixed at approximately 1.010, equivalent to that of plasma. This fixed specific gravity is due to impaired tubular secretion, reabsorption, and urine concentrating ability. Abnormal proteins, blood cells, and cellular casts may also be noted in the urine.
- *Urine culture* is ordered to identify any urinary tract infection that may hasten the progress of CRF.
- *BUN* and *serum creatinine* are obtained to evaluate kidney function in eliminating nitrogenous waste products. Levels of both are monitored to assess the progress of renal failure. A BUN of 20 to 50 mg/dL signals mild azotemia; levels greater than 100 mg/dL indicate severe renal impairment. Uremic symptoms are seen when the BUN is around 200 mg/dL or higher. Serum creatinine levels of greater than 4 mg/dL indicate serious renal impairment.
- *Creatinine clearance* evaluates the GFR and renal function. In early CRF (renal insufficiency), the GFR is more than 20% of normal and the creatinine clearance 25 mL/min or greater. As the disease progresses and the stage of renal failure is reached, the GFR is reduced to less than 20% of normal and the creatinine clearance to 10 to 30 mL/min. In ESRD, the GFR is less than 5% of normal and the creatinine clearance is 5 to 10 mL/min or less. Nursing implications for creatinine clearance are outlined in the box on page 750.
- *Serum electrolytes* are monitored throughout the course of CRF. The serum sodium may be within normal limits or low because of water retention. Potassium levels are elevated but usually remain below 6.5 mEq/L. Serum phosphate is elevated, and the calcium level is decreased. Metabolic acidosis is identified by a low pH, low $CO_2$, and low bicarbonate levels.
- *CBC* reveals moderately severe anemia with a hematocrit of 20% to 30% and a low hemoglobin. The number of red blood cells and platelets is reduced.
- *Renal ultrasonography* is done to evaluate kidney size. In CRF, kidney size decreases as nephrons are destroyed and kidney mass is reduced. Preparation of the client and nursing implications for renal ultrasonography are outlined in the box on page 717.
- *Kidney biopsy* may be done to identify the underlying disease process if this is unclear. It is also used to differentiate acute from chronic failure. Kidney biopsy may be performed in surgery or done percutaneously using needle biopsy. The box on page 750 outlines nursing care for a client having a renal biopsy.

### Medications

Chronic renal failure affects both the pharmacokinetic and pharmacodynamic effects of drug therapy. Most medications are excreted primarily by the kidney. The half-life and plasma levels of many drugs increase in chronic renal failure. Drug absorption may be decreased when phosphate-binding agents are administered concurrently. Proteinuria can significantly reduce plasma protein levels, leading to manifestations of toxicity when highly protein-bound drugs are given. In addition, any potentially nephrotoxic agent is avoided or used with extreme caution. Drugs such as meperidine, metformin (Glucophage), and other oral hypoglycemic agents eliminated by the kidney are avoided entirely (Braunwald et al., 2001).

Diuretics such as furosemide or other loop diuretics may be prescribed to reduce extracellular fluid volume and edema. Diuretic therapy also can reduce hypertension and cause potassium wasting, lowering serum potassium levels. Other antihypertensive agents are used to maintain the blood pressure within normal levels, slow the progress of renal failure, and prevent complications of coronary heart disease and cerebral vascular disease. Angiotensin-converting enzyme (ACE) inhibitors are preferred, although any class of antihypertensive agent may be prescribed (see Chapter 33).

Other drugs may be used to manage electrolyte imbalances and acidosis. Sodium bicarbonate or calcium carbonate may be used to correct mild acidosis. Oral phosphorus binding agents such as calcium carbonate or calcium acetate are given to lower serum phosphate levels and normalize serum calcium levels. Aluminum hydroxide may be used in acute treatment of hyperphosphatemia. Its use is limited to short term by complications such as encephalopathy and osteodystrophy associated with long-term administration of aluminum-containing preparations (Tierney et al., 2001). Vitamin D supplements may be given to improve calcium absorption.

If the serum potassium rises to dangerously high levels, a combination of bicarbonate, insulin, and glucose may be given intravenously to promote potassium movement into the cells. Sodium polystyrene sulfonate (Kayexalate), a potassium-ion exchange resin, can be given either orally or rectally (as an enema).

Folic acid and iron supplements are given to combat anemia associated with chronic renal failure. A multiple vitamin preparation is also often prescribed, because anorexia, nausea, and dietary restrictions may limit nutrient intake.

### Dietary and Fluid Management

As renal function declines, the elimination of water, solutes, and metabolic wastes is impaired. Accumulation of these wastes in the body leads to uremic symptoms. Instituted early in the course of CRF, dietary modifications can slow the progress of nephron destruction, reduce uremic symptoms, and help prevent complications.

Unlike carbohydrates and fats, the body is unable to store excess proteins. Unused dietary proteins are degraded into urea and other nitrogenous wastes, which are then eliminated by the kidneys. Protein-rich foods also contain inorganic ions such as hydrogen ion, phosphate, and sulfites that are eliminated by the kidneys. Research has shown that restricting dietary protein intake slows the progression of CRF and reduces uremic symptoms (Braunwald et al., 2001). A daily protein intake of 0.6 g/kg of body weight, or approximately 40 g/day for an average male client, provides the amino acids necessary for tissue repair. Proteins should be of high biologic value, rich in the essential amino acids. Carbohydrate intake is increased to maintain energy requirements and provide approximately 35 kcal/kg per day.

Water and sodium intake is regulated to maintain the extracellular fluid volume at normal levels. Water intake of 1 to 2 L per day is generally recommended to maintain water balance. Sodium is restricted to 2 g per day initially. More stringent water and sodium restrictions may be necessary as renal failure progresses. The client is instructed to monitor weight daily and report any weight gain in excess of 5 pounds over a 2-day period.

When the GFR falls to less than 10 to 20 mL/min, potassium and phosphorus intake is also restricted. Potassium intake is limited to less than 60 to 70 mEq/day (normal intake is about 100 mEq/day) (Tierney et al., 2001). The client is cautioned to avoid using salt substitutes, which typically contain high levels of potassium chloride. Foods high in phosphorus include eggs, dairy products, and meat.

## Renal Replacement Therapies

When pharmacologic and dietary management strategies are no longer effective to maintain fluid and electrolyte balance and prevent uremia, dialysis or kidney transplantation is considered.

A number of considerations affect the choice of long-term treatment. Hemodialysis and peritoneal dialysis each have advantages and disadvantages. Establishing vascular access for hemodialysis may take several months. Planning ahead to develop the access before dialysis is necessary can ease the transition to dialysis. Established access is not a consideration for peritoneal dialysis. The peritoneal catheter can be placed and treatment initiated as soon as it is indicated. When dialysis treatments will be performed at home, initiating instruction before it is required can result in more effective learning. If a family member will serve as a dialysis helper, training begins prior to the onset of uremia.

If transplantation is considered, tissue typing and identification of potential living related donors can be done prior to the onset of ESRD. To make an informed decision, both the client and the potential donor need to understand the risks, benefits, and options available. If the decision for transplant is made early, dialysis can potentially be avoided. The client's age, concurrent health problems, donor availability, and personal preference influence the choice of renal replacement therapy.

### Dialysis

Approximately 80% of all people being treated for ESRD in the United States are receiving dialysis at an average maintenance cost of about $35,000 per year (USRDS, 2001). For the client who is not a candidate for renal transplantation or who has had a transplant failure, dialysis is life sustaining.

The most common therapies for ESRD in the United States are hemodialysis performed in a dialysis center, followed by peritoneal dialysis and kidney transplant (NKUDIC, 2001). Both hemodialysis and peritoneal dialysis can be done in the home, but few clients use home hemodialysis. Of the two, peritoneal dialysis is typically the choice for at-home treatment. As the morbidity and mortality for each are comparable, factors such as the desire and ability to manage home care, employment, and availability of a dialysis center become the primary factors influencing the choice of hemodialysis or peritoneal dialysis.

Clients on long-term dialysis have a higher risk for complications and death than the general population. Many have other severe diseases along with ESRD. Infection and cardiovascular disease are common causes of illness and death. The 1-year survival rate for clients receiving dialysis is more than 78%; long-term survival, however, falls to 31% at 5 years and less than 9% at 10 years (NKUDIC, 2001).

The decision to initiate dialysis is not easy. Like insulin therapy for the diabetic, dialysis manages the symptoms of ESRD but does not cure it. Dialysis is a constant factor of life, requiring thinking and planning ahead at all times. Clients on dialysis may not be able to maintain a job. Families often fall apart with the day-to-day stress. Even with dialysis, the client may have constant flulike symptoms, never feeling truly well. Clients on hemodialysis may feel powerless because of their dependence on others for treatment. On the other hand, home peritoneal dialysis places a continuing burden on the client to maintain treatment. In the end, the client may choose to discontinue treatment, preferring death over continued dialysis.

Hemodialysis for ESRD typically is done three times a week for a total of 9 to 12 hours. The amount of dialysis needed (or *dialysis dose*) is individually determined by factors such as body size and residual renal function, dietary intake, and concurrent illness. Hypotension and muscle cramps are common complications during hemodialysis treatments. Infection and vascular access problems are common long-term complications of hemodialysis. Cardiovascular disease is the leading cause of death for clients receiving hemodialysis. The death rate from cardiovascular disease is higher in clients on hemodialysis than those on peritoneal dialysis or who have had a kidney transplant for reasons that are unclear (Braunwald et al., 2001). See the previous section on ARF and the box on page 768 for more information about hemodialysis and related nursing care.

Peritoneal dialysis is currently used by less than 10% of people who require long-term dialysis in the United States. In Canada and Europe, 35% to 45% of clients with ESRD are treated with peritoneal dialysis. In third-world countries, peritoneal dialysis is used to treat the majority of clients with ESRD.

*Continuous ambulatory peritoneal dialysis (CAPD)* is the most common form of peritoneal dialysis used. Dialysate (2 L) is instilled into the peritoneal cavity, and the catheter is sealed. The client can then continue normal daily activities, emptying the peritoneal cavity and replacing the dialysate every 4 to 6 hours. No special equipment is needed. A variation of CAPD is *continuous cyclic peritoneal dialysis (CCPD)*, which uses a delivery device during nighttime hours and a continuous dwell during the day. CAPD can be performed anywhere, and CCPD allows for home treatment at night, leaving the client free during the day.

Peritoneal dialysis has several advantages over hemodialysis. Heparinization and vascular complications associated with an AV fistula are avoided. The clearance of metabolic wastes is slower but more continuous, avoiding rapid fluctuations in extracellular fluid composition and associated symptoms. More liberal intake of fluids and nutrients is often allowed for the client on CAPD. While glucose absorbed from dialysate can increase blood glucose levels in the diabetic, regular insulin can be added to the infusion to manage hyperglycemia. The client on peritoneal dialysis is better able to self-manage the treatment regimen, reducing feelings of helplessness.

The major disadvantages of peritoneal dialysis include less effective metabolite elimination and risk of infection (peritonitis). Peritoneal dialysis may not be effective for large clients with no residual kidney function. Serum triglyceride levels increase with peritoneal dialysis. Finally, the presence of an indwelling peritoneal catheter may cause a body image disturbance. See the previous section of this chapter and the box on page 771 for more information about and nursing care for the client undergoing peritoneal dialysis.

## Kidney Transplant

Kidney transplant has become the treatment of choice for many clients with ESRD. Kidneys are the solid organ most commonly transplanted, and to date kidney transplantation is the most successful of transplantation procedures. The first kidney transplant was performed in 1954; the donor and recipient were identical twins. Kidney transplant as a treatment for ESRD is limited primarily by availability of organs. In 2001, more than 15,000 people received a kidney transplant; however, there currently are more than 52,000 awaiting a transplant (United Network of Organ Sharing [UNOS], 2002b).

Kidney transplant improves both survival and quality of life for the client with ESRD. The client on dialysis has a 62.8% probability of surviving after 2 years of dialysis; the transplant recipient has a greater than 91.5% probability of survival after 2 years. At 5 years, the difference is even greater: 31.3% for dialysis compared with 80.4% for transplant (NKUDIC, 2001). The transplant client is no longer tethered to a dialysis catheter, machine, or center. Dietary and fluid restrictions are reduced, and the body image is more "whole."

Most transplanted kidneys are obtained from cadavers; however, transplants from living donors are increasing. In 2001, of transplanted kidneys, 37.4% came from living donors, most of whom were related to the recipient (UNOS, 2002c). With both cadaver and living donor transplants, a close match between blood and tissue type is desired. Human leukocyte antigens (HLA) are compared between the donor and recipient; six antigens in common is considered to be a "perfect" match. The success of well-matched living-donor transplants is better than for cadaver organ transplants, with a 1-year graft survival of 94% compared to 89% for cadaver transplants (NKUDIC, 2001). Close tissue matching probably accounts for the better outcome with living donors. People with normal kidneys who are in good physical health may donate a kidney. Predonation counseling is vital: Nephrectomy is major surgery and involves a risk of trauma or disease damaging the remaining kidney in the future. If the transplant fails, the psychologic impact on the donor can be significant. Nursing care of the client having a nephrectomy is summarized in the box on page 758.

Cadaver kidneys are obtained from people who meet the criteria for brain death, are less than 65 years old, and are free of systemic disease, malignancy, or infection, including HIV and hepatitis B or C. Kidneys are removed after brain death has been determined, and are preserved by hypothermia or a technique called continuous hypothermic pulsatile perfusion. A kidney preserved by hypothermia is transplanted within 24 to 48 hours. Continuous pulsatile perfusion allows up to 3 days before transplantation. The system used to allocate cadaver kidneys for transplantation is outlined in Box 27–1.

---

## BOX 27–1  ■  How Cadaver Kidneys Are Allocated for Transplant

The scarcity of organs for transplant raises questions about how cadaver kidneys are allocated—who receives a kidney and who does not. Past inequities in the allocation process (e.g., more men than women, more Caucasians than people of color, more rich than poor, and more young than old) led to the development of the United Network for Organ Sharing (UNOS) in 1986. UNOS has policies for organ distribution, including kidneys, hearts, livers, and other transplanted organs.

UNOS maintains national, regional, and local lists of clients awaiting transplants. When an organ becomes available, donor information is entered into the UNOS computer. The computer then runs a match program, generating a list of clients ranked by criteria such as blood and tissue type, organ size, and medical urgency of the client. Factors such as time on the waiting list and distance between the donor and the transplant center also are considered. A candidate with a perfect match (six human leukocyte antigens in common) and compatible blood type gets priority for the kidney, regardless of region or geographic area. Otherwise, the list of clients in the local area is checked first, then the regional list of clients awaiting transplant. If no match is found in the region, the organ becomes available to clients nationwide.

The UNOS allocation system, standardized fees, and Medicare coverage for transplantation have done much to ensure equitable access to available kidneys. Still, controversy exists. Clients with resources for travel may register in several different regions for an organ. Up to 10% of clients receiving a transplant in any center may be foreign nationals competing with U.S. citizens for scarce organ resources. A transplant center can accept or reject a candidate for transplant who has lost a kidney because of noncompliance.

As long as the demand for kidneys exceeds the supply of donor organs, it is likely that controversy will exist regarding their allocation. Nurses can help by identifying potential donors and contacting the transplant coordinator. In addition, nurses can inform the public about organ donation and allocation system, and encourage donation.

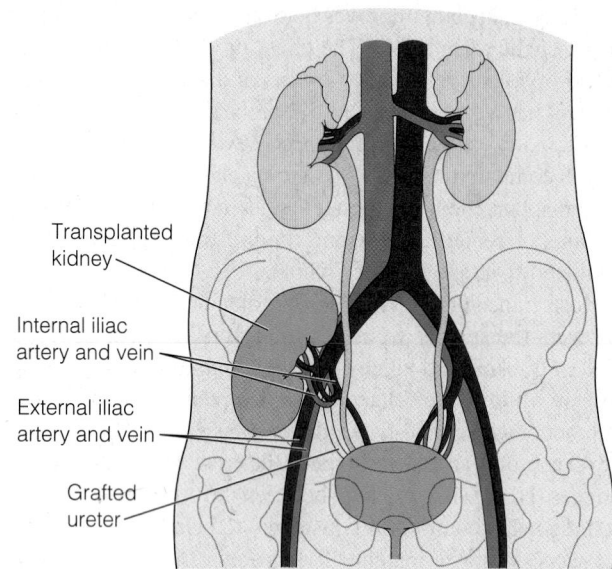

**Figure 27–11** ■ Placement of a transplanted kidney in the iliac fossa with anastomosis to the hypogastric artery, iliac vein, and bladder.

The donor kidney is placed in the lower abdominal cavity of the recipient, and the renal artery, vein, and ureter are anastomosed (Figure 27–11 ■). The renal artery of the donor kidney is connected to the hypogastric artery, and the renal vein to the iliac vein. The ureter is connected to one of the recipient's ureters or directly to the bladder, using a tunnel technique to prevent reflux. Nursing care for the client having a kidney transplant is outlined in the box on the next page.

Unless the donor and recipient are identical twins, the grafted organ stimulates an immune response to reject the transplanted organ. Immunosuppressive drugs minimize this response. Azathioprine or mycophenolate mofetil are commonly used, often in combination with prednisone, a corticosteroid. Cyclosporine, a potent immunosuppressive, also may be used. These drugs suppress a portion of the immune system and the inflammatory response, increasing the risk for infections and cancers with long-term therapy. The nursing implications of immunosuppressive therapy are outlined in Chapter 9. ○○

Glucocorticoids such as prednisone and methylprednisolone are used for both maintenance immunosuppression and to treat acute rejection episodes. Side effects of long-term corticosteroid use include impaired wound healing, emotional disturbances, osteoporosis, and cushingoid effects on glucose, protein, and fat metabolism.

Azathioprine inhibits both cellular and humoral immunity. Because this drug is rapidly metabolized by the liver, the dose may not need to be altered in the presence of renal failure. Bone marrow suppression, abnormalities of liver function, and alopecia are the primary significant adverse effects for azathioprine. The action of mycophenolate mofetil is similar to that of azathioprine. Its advantages are minimal bone marrow suppression and increased potency in preventing or reversing rejection of the transplanted organ (Braunwald et al., 2001).

Cyclosporine primarily affects cellular immunity, the helper T cells in particular. Among its many adverse effects, which include hepatotoxicity and hirsutism, nephrotoxicity is a primary concern for the kidney transplant client.

Even with immunosuppressive therapy, the transplanted kidney can be rejected at any time. Either acute or chronic rejection may develop. *Acute rejection* develops within months of the transplant. It is caused by a cellular immune response with T-lymphocyte proliferation (Porth, 2002). Few manifestations may be apparent other than a rise in serum creatinine and possible oliguria. Methylprednisolone, a glucocorticoid, and OKT3 monoclonal antibody (see Chapter 9) are used to manage acute rejection episodes. OKT3 can cause severe systemic reactions, including chills, fever, hypotension, headache, and possible pulmonary edema (Braunwald et al., 2001). *Chronic rejection,* which may develop months to years following the transplant, is a major cause of graft loss. Both humoral and cellular immune responses are involved in chronic rejection. It does not respond to increased immunosuppression. The presenting manifestations of chronic rejection—progressive azotemia, proteinuria, and hypertension—are those of progressive renal failure.

Hypertension is a possible complication of kidney transplant, resulting from graft rejection, renal artery stenosis, or renal vasoconstriction. Clients may develop glomerular lesions and manifestations of nephrosis. Hypertension and altered blood lipids (increased LDLs and decreased HDLs) increase the risk of death from myocardial infarction and stroke following transplant (Braunwald et al., 2001).

Long-term immunosuppression has adverse effects as well. Infection is a continuing threat. Bacterial and viral infections may develop, as well as fungal infections of the blood, lungs, and central nervous system. Tumors are also common, with carcinoma in situ of the cervix, lymphomas, and skin cancers most prevalent. The risk of congenital anomalies is increased in infants whose mothers have undergone immunosuppressive therapy. Corticosteroid use may lead to bone problems, gastrointestinal disorders such as peptic ulcer disease, and cataract formation.

## NURSING CARE

### Health Promotion

Measures to reduce the risk of CRF focus on preventing kidney disease and appropriately managing diabetes and hypertension. Promote early and effective treatment of all infections, particularly skin and pharyngeal infections caused by streptococcal bacteria. Discuss measures to reduce the risk for urinary tract infections, and stress the importance of prompt treatment to eradicate the infecting organism. Discuss the relationship between diabetes, hypertension, and kidney disease. Emphasize that maintaining blood glucose levels and the blood pressure within the recommended ranges reduces the risk of adverse effects on the kidneys. Ensure that all clients with less than optimal renal function are well hydrated, particularly when a nephrotoxic drug is prescribed or anticipated.

# NURSING CARE OF THE CLIENT HAVING A KIDNEY TRANSPLANT

## PREOPERATIVE CARE

- Provide routine preoperative care as outlined in Chapter 7. ⊂⊃
- Assess knowledge and feelings about the procedure, answering questions and clarifying information as needed. Listen and address concerns about surgery, the source of the donor organ, and possible complications. *Addressing concerns and reducing preoperative anxiety improve postoperative recovery.*
- Continue dialysis as ordered. *Continued renal replacement therapy is necessary to manage fluid and electrolyte balance and prevent uremia prior to surgery.*
- Administer immunosuppressive drugs as ordered before surgery. *Immunosuppression is initiated before transplantation to prevent immediate graft rejection.*

## POSTOPERATIVE CARE

- Provide routine postoperative care as outlined in Chapter 7.
- Maintain urinary catheter patency and a closed system. *Catheter patency is vital to keep the bladder decompressed and prevent pressure on suture lines. A closed drainage system minimizes the risk for urinary tract infection.*
- Measure urine output every 30 to 60 minutes initially. *Careful assessment of urine output helps determine fluid balance and transplant function. Acute tubular necrosis (ATN) is a common early complication, usually due to tissue ischemia during the period between removal of the kidney from the donor and transplantation. Oliguria is an early sign.*
- Monitor vital signs and hemodynamic pressures closely. *Diuresis may occur immediately, resulting in hypovolemia, low cardiac output, and impaired perfusion of the transplanted kidney.*
- Maintain fluid replacement, generally calculated to replace urine output over the previous 30 or 60 minutes, milliliter for milliliter. *Fluid replacement is vital to maintain vascular volume and tissue perfusion.*
- Administer diuretics as ordered. *Loop and/or osmotic diuretics such as furosemide or mannitol may be used to promote postoperative diuresis.*
- Remove the catheter within 2 to 3 days or as ordered. Encourage to void every 1 to 2 hours and assess frequently for signs of urinary retention following catheter removal. *The bladder may have atrophied prior to surgery, reducing its capacity. Urinary retention places stress on suture lines and increases the risk of infection.*
- Monitor serum electrolytes and renal function tests. *These tests are used to monitor graft function and fluid and electrolyte status. Electrolyte imbalances may develop as the transplanted kidney begins to function and diuresis occurs. Elevated serum creatinine and BUN levels may be early signs of rejection or graft failure.*

- Monitor for possible complications:
  a. *Hemorrhage* from an arterial or venous anastomosis can be either acute or insidious. Indicators include swelling at the operative site, increased abdominal girth, and signs of shock, including changes in vital signs and level of consciousness. *Hemorrhage is a surgical emergency, requiring prompt recognition and treatment to preserve the graft.*
  b. *Ureteral anastomosis failure* causes urine leakage into the peritoneal cavity. It may be marked by decreased urine output with abdominal swelling and tenderness. *Failure of the ureteral anastomosis requires surgical intervention.*
  c. *Renal artery thrombosis* is characterized by an abrupt onset of hypertension and reduced GFR. *Renal artery thrombosis can result in transplant failure.*
  d. *Infection* due to immunosuppression is an immediate and continuing risk. The inflammatory response is blunted, and infection may not significantly elevate the temperature. Monitor for signs such as change in level of consciousness, cloudy or malodorous urine, or purulent drainage from the incision. *Prevention and prompt treatment of infections is particularly important in the immunosuppressed client.*
- Include the following in predischarge teaching for the client and family:
  a. The use and effects of prescribed medications, including antihypertensive medications, immunosuppressive agents, prophylactic antibiotics, and others as ordered.
  b. Monitoring vital signs (including temperature) and weight.
  c. Manifestations of organ rejection, such as swelling and tenderness over the graft site, fever, joint aching, weight gain, and decreased urinary output. Stress the importance of promptly reporting signs and symptoms to the physician.
  d. Ordered or recommended dietary restrictions such as restricted carbohydrate and sodium intake, and increased protein intake.
  e. Measures to prevent infection, such as avoiding crowds and obviously ill individuals.
  *The client and family will manage care after discharge, and therefore need a good understanding of what to expect, how to monitor graft status, and measures to reduce the adverse effects of medications.*
- Provide psychologic support, address concerns, and provide information as needed. *The client knows that transplant success is not guaranteed. In addition, the client has often been managing a chronic disease independently and is used to having a degree of control. Providing information and allowing the client to retain control relieves anxiety and improves recovery.*

Finally, encourage the client with ESRD to investigate options for early transplantation to avoid long-term dialysis.

## Assessment

Both subjective and objective data are used to assess the client with CRF.

- Health history: complaints of anorexia, nausea, weight gain, or edema; current treatment (if any), including type and frequency of dialysis or previous kidney transplant; chronic diseases such as diabetes, heart failure, or kidney disease
- Physical examination: mental status; vital signs including temperature, heart and lung sounds, and peripheral pulses;

urine output (if any); weight; skin color, moisture, condition; presence of edema (periorbial or dependent); bowel tones; presence and location of an AV fistula, shunt, or graft, or peritoneal catheter

See the box on page 772 for assessment of the older adult with ESRD.

## Nursing Diagnoses and Interventions

Whether the client with ESRD is facing long-term dialysis or renal transplantation, a number of nursing care needs can be identified. This section focuses on nursing care related to impaired renal function, nutritional deficits due to dietary restrictions and nausea, increased risk for infection, and changes in body image.

### Impaired Tissue Perfusion: Renal

Capillaries are an integral part of the nephron. As nephrons are destroyed, kidney perfusion progressively declines. As renal perfusion and nephron function falls, the kidney is less able to maintain fluid and electrolyte balance and eliminate waste products from the body.

- Monitor intake and output, vital signs including orthostatic blood pressures, and weight. *These provide important data to identify changes in fluid volume.*

**PRACTICE ALERT** *Weight changes are a more accurate indicator of fluid volume status in the oliguric or anuric client than intake and output measurements.* ■

- Restrict fluids as ordered. *As renal function declines, the ability to eliminate excess fluid is impaired.*
- Monitor respiratory status, including lung sounds, every 4 to 8 hours. *Fluid volume overload may lead to heart failure and possible pulmonary edema.*
- Monitor BUN, serum creatinine, pH, electrolytes, and CBC. Report significant changes. *As renal function declines, progressive azotemia with increasing BUN and serum creatinine is seen. Metabolic acidosis develops as the kidney is unable to eliminate hydrogen ions and conserve bicarbonate. Hyponatremia, hyperkalemia, hyperphosphatemia, and hypocalcemia are associated with renal failure. The RBC count, hemoglobin, and hematocrit decline due to deficient erythropoietin to stimulate cell production in the bone marrow. An acute fall in hemoglobin and hematocrit may indicate GI bleeding, a risk in clients with ESRD.*
- Report manifestations of electrolyte imbalances, such as cardiac dysrhythmias and other ECG changes, muscle tremors and possible tetany, and Kussmaul's respirations. *Manifestations of electrolyte imbalance may indicate the need for intervention.*
- Administer medications to treat electrolyte imbalances as ordered. *Medications may be prescribed to help maintain electrolyte and acid-base balance and prevent adverse effects of imbalances.*

**PRACTICE ALERT** *Monitor carefully for desired and adverse effects of all medications. Impaired renal function affects drug elimination and increases the risk for toxic effects.* ■

- Administer antihypertensive medications as ordered. *Hypertension management is an important factor in slowing the progression of CRF.*
- Time activities and procedures to allow rest periods. *The anemia associated with CRF may cause significant fatigue and activity intolerance.*

### Imbalanced Nutrition: Less Than Body Requirements

Anorexia, nausea, and vomiting are common manifestations of ESRD and uremia. The client often has a metallic taste and bad breath, which also diminish appetite. A diet restricted in protein and sodium will compound these problems. Food intake may be insufficient to meet metabolic needs. Catabolism, the breakdown of body proteins to meet energy needs, exacerbates azotemia and uremia.

- Monitor food and nutrient intake as well as episodes of vomiting. *Careful monitoring helps determine the adequacy of intake.*
- Weigh daily before breakfast. *This provides the most accurate measurement. Remember that a gain of 2 pounds or more over a 24-hour period is more likely to reflect fluid retention than a gain in body mass.*
- Administer antiemetic agents 30 to 60 minutes before eating. *Antiemetics reduce nausea and the risk of vomiting with food intake.*
- Assist with mouth care prior to meals and at bedtime. *Mouth care improves taste, stimulates the appetite, and maintains the integrity of oral mucous membranes.*
- Serve small meals and provide between-meal snacks. *Small meals are less likely to prompt nausea and help improve food intake.*
- Arrange for a dietary consultation. Provide preferred foods to the extent possible, and involve the client in planning daily menus. Encourage family members to bring food as dietary restrictions allow. *Providing preferred foods within restrictions promotes intake.*
- Monitor nutritional status by tracking weight, laboratory values such as serum albumin and BUN, and anthropometric measurements (see Chapters 19 ∞ and 20). *Indicators of impaired nutrition develop gradually and may be subtle. Careful assessment is important.*
- Administer parenteral nutrition as prescribed. Routinely monitor blood glucose levels, and use strict aseptic technique when handling the solution and venous access site. *Parenteral nutrition may be necessary to prevent catabolism and increasing azotemia. Hyperglycemia and infection are risks associated with parenteral nutrition (see Chapter 20). Immune system suppression associated with renal failure further increases the risk for infection.*

### Risk for Infection

Chronic renal failure affects the immune system and leukocyte function, increasing susceptibility to infection. Invasive devices required for hemodialysis or peritoneal dialysis add to this risk. The client who has had a kidney transplant remains on immunosuppressive therapy for life, further depressing the immune system and increasing the risk for infection.

- Use standard precautions and good handwashing technique at all times. *Handwashing is a primary means of preventing the transfer of organisms. Clients who are on hemodialysis or who have had multiple blood transfusions to treat anemia have an increased risk for hepatitis B, hepatitis C, and HIV infection.*

**PRACTICE ALERT** *Use strict aseptic technique when managing ports, catheters, and incisions, to reduce the risk of introducing infectious organisms when immune responses are impaired.* ■

- Monitor temperature and vital signs at least every 4 hours. *A low-grade fever or increased pulse rate may indicate an infection in the immunosuppressed client.*
- Monitor WBC count and differential. *Increased WBCs may indicate a bacterial infection; decreased WBCs may indicate viral infection. A shift in the differential showing more immature WBCs (bands) in circulation is another indicator of infection.*
- Culture urine, peritoneal dialysis fluid, and other drainage as indicated. *Culture is done to verify the presence of pathogens.*

**PRACTICE ALERT** *Monitor clarity of dialysate return. Dialysate should return clear in the client undergoing peritoneal dialysis. Cloudy dialysate may indicate peritonitis, the most common complication of peritoneal dialysis, and should be reported and cultured.* ■

- Provide good respiratory hygiene including position changes, coughing, and deep breathing. *These measures improve clearance of respiratory secretions, reducing the risk for infection.*
- Restrict visits from obviously ill people. Teach the client and family about the risk for infection and measures to reduce the spread of infection. *The client's resistance to infection is impaired, necessitating extra caution in preventing unnecessary exposures.*

## Disturbed Body Image

Chronic disease and impaired kidney function can affect the client's body image. Hemodialysis requires an arteriovenous fistula or shunt; a permanent peritoneal catheter is required for peritoneal dialysis. While kidney transplant can restore an image of wholeness, a visible scar remains and the organ may be perceived as "foreign."

- Involve the client in care, including meal planning, dialysis, and catheter, port, or incision care to the extent possible. *Involvement improves acceptance and stimulates discussion about the effect of the disease and treatment measures on the client's life.* See the Nursing Research box below.
- Encourage expression of feelings and concerns, accepting perceptions and feelings without criticism. *Self-expression enhances the client's self-worth and acceptance.*
- Include the client in decision making and encourage self-care. *Increased autonomy enhances the client's sense of control, independence, and self-worth.*
- Support positive gains, but do not support denial. *The client may have difficulty accepting the renal failure, but adaptation to the loss is important.*
- Help the client develop and achieve realistic goals. *Realistic goals allow the client to see progress.*
- Provide positive reinforcement and feedback. *These measures support growth and adaptation.*
- Reinforce effective coping strategies. *Reinforcement helps the client develop positive versus negative strategies for coping.*
- Facilitate contact with a support group or other community members affected by renal failure. *The client benefits by*

## Nursing Research

### Evidence-Based Practice For the Client on Hemodialysis

In a study of clients undergoing hemodialysis for CRF, researchers in Sweden looked at suffering on three levels: related to sickness and treatment, related to care provided, and related to the client's unique life experience and existence (Hagren, Pettersen, Severinsson, Lutzen, & Clyne, 2001). The study included 15 clients between age 50 and 86.

The researchers identified dependence on the hemodialysis machine and dependence on caregivers as the primary sources of suffering in these clients. This dependence and the loss of freedom associated with hemodialysis affected marital and family relationships and social lives of the sufferers. Accepting dependence on the hemodialysis machine and being seen as an individual by caregivers, thus promoting autonomy, relieved clients' suffering.

### IMPLICATIONS FOR NURSING

Treating all clients with ESRD holistically, respecting their individual and unique characteristics and experience, is vital to promote acceptance and autonomy. Listen carefully, responding to each person's concerns. Discuss the effects of the disease and its treatment on the client's life, marital and family relationships, and socialization. Suggest strategies to maintain independence and provide relief for caregivers. When appropriate, discuss alternatives to hemodialysis for treating ESRD, such as kidney transplant or peritoneal dialysis. Peritoneal dialysis may be managed independently by the client, reducing dependence on others and time spent in treatment.

### Critical Thinking

1. Identify assessment tools and data you could use to evaluate degree of suffering in the client receiving long-term hemodialysis.
2. In addition to the above, what interventions can you, as the nurse, implement to promote autonomy and acceptance of hemodialysis in the client with ESRD?
3. Develop a teaching plan for families and significant others to help them promote acceptance and autonomy in the client undergoing long-term hemodialysis.

## CHART 27–4 NANDA, NIC, AND NOC LINKAGES

### The Client with End-Stage Renal Disease

| NURSING DIAGNOSES | NURSING INTERVENTIONS | NURSING OUTCOMES |
|---|---|---|
| • Chronic Sorrow | • Coping Enhancement<br>• Mood Mangement | • Acceptance: Health Status<br>• Depression Control |
| • Excess Fluid Volume | • Fluid Management<br>• Fluid / Electrolyte Management | • Electrolyte and Acid-Base Balance<br>• Fluid Balance |
| • Fatigue | • Energy Management<br>• Environmental Management | • Activity Tolerance<br>• Energy Conservation |
| • Nausea | • Nausea Management<br>• Nutritional Monitoring | • Nutritional Status: Food and Fluid Intake |
| • Risk for Infection | • Infection Protection<br>• Wound Care | • Infection Status |

*Note. Data from Nursing Outcomes Classification (NOC) by M. Johnson & M. Maas (Eds.), 1997, St. Louis: Mosby; Nursing Diagnoses: Definitions & Classification 2001–2002 by North American Nursing Diagnosis Association, 2001, Philadelphia: NANDA; Nursing Interventions Classification (NIC) by J.C. McCloskey & G. M. Bulechek (Eds.), 2000, St. Louis: Mosby. Reprinted by permission.*

*providing and receiving support in a group of people going through similar circumstances.*
- Refer for mental health counseling as indicated or desired. *Counseling can help the client develop effective coping and adaptation strategies.*

## Using NANDA, NIC, and NOC

Chart 27–4 shows links between NANDA nursing diagnoses, NIC, and NOC when caring for the client with ESRD.

## Home Care

Chronic renal failure and ESRD are long-term processes that require client management. No matter what treatment option is chosen (hemodialysis, peritoneal dialysis, or renal transplantation), day-to-day management falls to the client and family. Teaching for home care includes the following topics.

- Nature of the kidney disease and renal failure, including expected progression and effects
- Monitoring weight, vital signs, and temperature

- Prescribed dietary and fluid restrictions (Involve the client, a dietitian, and the family member usually responsible for cooking. Include strategies to manage nausea and relieve thirst within allowed fluid limits.)
- How to assess and protect a fistula or shunt for hemodialysis (or the extremity to be used if one is anticipated)
- Peritoneal catheter care and the procedure for peritoneal dialysis as indicated (Include a family member or significant other, in case the client is unable to perform the procedure independently at some time.)
- Following kidney transplant, prescribed medications, adverse effects and their management, infection prevention, graft protection, and manifestations of organ rejection

Refer to a dietitian for diet planning and counseling. If home hemodialysis is planned, refer the designated dialysis helper for formal training. Both the National Kidney Foundation and the American Association of Kidney Patients may be able to provide support and educational materials for the client with ESRD (see the box on page 772). Local and state chapters of these organizations can provide additional support.

## Nursing Care Plan

### A Client with End-Stage Renal Disease

Walter Cohen, 45 years old, is the print shop manager at a local community college. He has been a type 1 diabetic since the age of 20, and was diagnosed with diabetic nephropathy 10 years ago. Despite blood pressure control with antihypertensive medications and frequent blood glucose monitoring with insulin coverage, he developed overt proteinuria 5 years ago and has now progressed to end-stage renal disease. He enters the nephrology unit for temporary he-

modialysis to relieve uremic symptoms. While there, a CAPD catheter will be inserted. Mr. Cohen's desire to continue working is the primary factor in his choice of CAPD over hemodialysis.

### ASSESSMENT

Richard Gonzalez, Mr. Cohen's care manager, obtains a nursing assessment. Mr. Cohen states that his diabetes has always been difficult to control. He has had numerous hypoglycemic episodes and

## Nursing Care Plan

## A Client with End-Stage Renal Disease (continued)

has been hospitalized "four or five times" for ketoacidosis. Recently he has developed symptoms of peripheral neuropathy and increasing retinopathy. He attributed his lack of appetite, nausea, vomiting, and fatigue over the past month to "a touch of the flu." His weight remained stable, so he did not worry about not eating much.

Physical assessment findings include T 97.8°F (36.5°C) PO, P 96, R 20, and BP 178/100. Skin cool and dry, with minor excoriations on forearms and lower legs. Breath odor fetid. Scattered fine rales noted in bilateral lung bases. Soft $S_3$ gallop noted at cardiac apex. Bilateral pitting edema of lower extremities to just below the knees; fingers and hands also edematous. Abdominal assessment essentially normal, with hypoactive bowel sounds. Urinalysis shows a specific gravity of 1.011, gross proteinuria, and multiple cell casts. CBC results: RBC 2.9 mill/mm³; hemoglobin 9.4 g/dL; hematocrit 28%. Blood chemistry abnormalities include BUN 198 mg/dL; creatinine 18.5 mg/dL; sodium 125 mEq/L; potassium 5.7 mEq/L; calcium 7.1 mg/dL; phosphate 6.8 mg/dL. A temporary jugular venous catheter will be placed for hemodialysis the next day, followed by peritoneal catheter insertion later in the week.

### DIAGNOSIS

- *Excess fluid volume* related to failure of kidneys to eliminate excess body fluid
- *Imbalanced nutrition: Less than body requirements* related to effects of uremia
- *Impaired skin integrity of lower extremities* related to dry skin and itching
- *Risk for infection* related to invasive catheters and impaired immune function

### EXPECTED OUTCOMES

- Adhere to the prescribed fluid restriction of 750 mL per day.
- Demonstrate reduced extracellular fluid volume by weight loss, decreased peripheral edema, clear lung sounds, and normal heart sounds.
- Consume and retain 100% of prescribed diet, including snacks.
- Demonstrate healing of lower extremity skin lesions.
- Remain free of infection.
- Demonstrate appropriate peritoneal catheter care and CAPD.

### PLANNING AND IMPLEMENTATION

- Space fluids, allowing 400 mL from 0700 to 1500, 200 mL from 1500 to 2300, and 100 mL from 2300 to 0700.
- Provide mouth care at least every 4 hours and before every meal.

- Keep sugarless hard candy and ice chips at the bedside; include ice consumed as fluid intake.
- Weigh daily before breakfast; monitor vital signs, and heart and lung sounds every 4 hours.
- Document intake and output every 4 hours.
- Arrange dietary consultation for menu planning.
- Administer prescribed antiemetic 1 hour before meals.
- Monitor food intake, noting percentage and types of food consumed.
- Clean lesions on lower extremities every 8 hours and assess healing.
- Teach CAPD procedure and peritoneal catheter care.
- Assist to identify strengths and needs in health regimen management.

### EVALUATION

Mr. Cohen was hospitalized for 2 weeks, undergoing four hemodialysis sessions to reduce uremic symptoms. An arteriovenous fistula has been created in his left arm in case he should need hemodialysis in the future. He begins peritoneal dialysis the second week, and by discharge he is able to manage the catheter care and dialysis runs with the help of his wife. His heart and lung sounds are normal, and he has minimal peripheral edema on discharge. The excoriations on his legs have healed. His temperature is normal, and no evidence of infection is noted. Mr. Cohen remains anorectic and slightly nauseated, but is eating most of his prescribed diet and snacks. He has lost 10 pounds with excess fluid removal by dialysis, but his weight remains stable during the second week. Mr. Cohen and his wife have been introduced to another client who has been on CAPD for several years and promises to help them with problem solving.

### Critical Thinking in the Nursing Process

1. How does diabetes mellitus damage the kidneys and lead to ESRD? Why is this more significant for a client with type 1 diabetes than for someone with type 2 diabetes (see Chapter 18)?
2. Why do high levels of urea in the blood often cause changes in cognition and mental status? What manifestations of encephalopathy would you expect to see?
3. How might Mr. Cohen's insulin dosage and diet need to be changed with the institution of peritoneal dialysis? Why?
4. Develop a care plan for the nursing diagnosis, *Disturbed body image.*

See Evaluating Your Response in Appendix C.

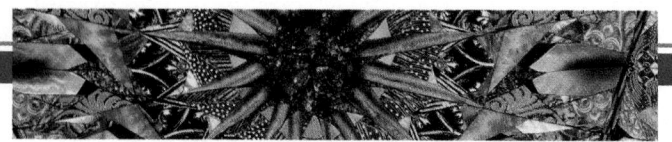

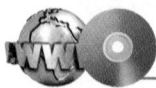 EXPLORE MediaLink

NCLEX review questions, case studies, care plan activities, MediaLink applications, and other interactive resources for this chapter can be found on the Companion Website at www.prenhall.com/lemone.

Click on Chapter 27 to select the activities for this chapter. For animations, video clips, more NCLEX review questions, and an audio glossary, access the Student CD-ROM accompanying this textbook.

## TEST YOURSELF

1. In obtaining a nursing history from a 22-year-old client admitted with a diagnosis of acute glomerulonephritis, the nurse specifically asks the client about a recent history of which of the following?

   a. Urinary tract infection
   b. Strep throat
   c. X-ray using contrast media
   d. Illicit drug use

2. Appropriate postoperative nursing interventions for the client who has had a partial or total nephrectomy include:

   a. Connecting all catheters and drains to a single collection device
   b. Routine irrigation of all catheters with sterile normal saline
   c. Administering cough suppressant medication as needed
   d. Labeling and securing all catheters, tubes, and drains

3. Important nursing interventions to prevent acute renal failure in the critically ill client include:

   a. Maintaining fluid volume and cardiac output
   b. Avoiding all potentially nephrotoxic drugs

   c. Administering antihypertensive drugs
   d. Assessing for a history of diabetes or systemic lupus erythematosus

4. The nurse evaluates her teaching as effective when the client recovering from acute renal failure states that he will:

   a. Limit his fluid intake to 1500 mL or less per day
   b. Consume only vegetable proteins
   c. Avoid taking drugs that may be nephrotoxic
   d. Self-catheterize for residual urine at least once a week

5. An appropriate goal of nursing care for a client with end-stage renal disease is the client will be able to:

   a. Identify a live-in caregiver
   b. State the advantages and disadvantages of hemodialysis, peritoneal dialysis, and kidney transplant as renal replacement therapies
   c. Demonstrate the ability to independently perform hemodialysis in the home
   d. Relate the hospice philosophy and identify indicators of the need for hospice care

See Test Yourself answers in Appendix C.

## BIBLIOGRAPHY

Ackley, B.J., & Ladwig, G. B. (2002). *Nursing diagnosis handbook: A guide to planning care* (5th ed.). St. Louis: Mosby.

American Cancer Society. (2002). *Cancer facts and figures 2002*. Atlanta: Author.

Bartucci, M. R. (1999). Kidney transplantation: State of the art. *AACN Clinical Issues: Advanced Practice in Acute and Critical Care, 10*(2), 153–163.

Braunwald, E., Fauci, A. S., Kasper, D. L., Hauser, S. L., Longo, D. L., & Jameson, J. L. (2001). *Harrison's principles of internal medicine* (15th ed.). New York: McGraw-Hill.

Bullock, B. A., & Henze, R. L. (2000). *Focus on pathophysiology*. Philadelphia: Lippincott.

Deglin, J. H., & Vallerand, A. H. (2001). *Davis's drug guide for nurses* (7th ed.). Philadelphia: F.A. Davis.

Fontaine, K. L. (2000). *Healing practices: Alternative therapies for nursing*. Upper Saddle River, NJ: Prentice Hall Health.

Fox, H. L., & Swann, D. (2001). Goodpasture syndrome: Pathophysiology, diagnosis, and management. *Nephrology Nursing Journal, 28*(3), 305–312.

Gallo, J. J., Busby-Whitehead, J., Rabins, P. V., Silliman, R. A., & Murphy, J. B. (Eds.). (1999). *Reichel's care of the elderly: Clinical aspects of aging* (5th ed.). Philadelphia: Lippincott Williams & Wilkins.

Hagren, B., Pettersen, I. M., Severinsson, E., Lutzen, K., & Clyne, N. (2001). The haemodialysis machine as a lifeline: Experiences of suffering from end-stage renal disease. *Journal of Advanced Nursing, 34*(2), 196–202.

Hayes, D. D. (2000). Caring for your patient with a permanent hemodialysis access. *Nursing, 30*(3), 41–46.

Johnson, M., Bulechek, G., Dochterman, J. M., Maas, M., & Moorhead, S. (2001). *Nursing diagnoses, outcomes, & interventions*. St. Louis: Mosby.

Johnson, M., Maas, M., & Moorhead, S. (Eds.). (2000). *Nursing outcomes classification (NOC)* (2nd ed.). St. Louis: Mosby.

King, B. (2000). Meds and the dialysis patient. *RN, 63*(7), 54–59.

Kostadaras, A. (2001). Erythropoietin for the anemia of chronic renal failure. *Home Health Care Consultant, 8*(7), 27–31.

Lang, M. M., & Towers, C. (2001). Identifying poststreptococcal glomerulonephritis. *Nurse Practitioner: American Journal of Primary Health Care, 26*(8), 34, 37–38, 40–42+.

Lehne, R. A. (2001). *Pharmacology for nursing care* (4th ed.). Philadelphia: Saunders.

Little, C. (2000). Renovascular hypertension. *American Journal of Nursing, 100*(2), 46–51.

Mackenzie, D. L. (1999). When *E. coli* turns deadly. *RN, 62*(7), 28–31.

Malarkey, L.M., & McMorrow, M.E. (2000). *Nurse's manual of laboratory tests and diagnostic procedures* (2nd ed.). Philadelphia: Saunders.

Mallick, N., & El Marasi, A. (1999). Chronic renal failure. *Care of the Critically Ill, 15*(3), 80, 82–84.

McCann, K., & Boore, J. R. (2000). Fatigue in persons with renal failure who require maintenance haemodialysis. *Journal of Advanced Nursing, 32*(5), 1132–1142.

McCloskey, J. C., & Bulechek, G. M. (Eds.) (2000). *Nursing interventions classification (NIC)* (3rd ed.). St. Louis: Mosby.

Meeker, M. H., & Rothrock, J. C. (1999). *Alexander's care of the patient in surgery* (11th ed.). St. Louis: Mosby.

Meister, J., & Reddy, K. (2002). Rhabdomyolysis: An overview. *American Journal of Nursing, 102*(2), 75, 77, 79.

Myhre, M. J. (2000). Herbal remedies, nephropathies, and renal disease. *Nephrology Nursing Journal, 27*(5), 473–480.

National Kidney and Urologic Diseases Information Clearinghouse. (2001). *Kidney and urologic disease statistics for the United States.* NIH Publication No. 02-3895. Available www.niddk.nih.gov/health/kidney/pubs/kustats

North American Nursing Diagnosis Association. (2001). *NANDA Nursing diagnoses: Definitions & classification 2001–2002.* Philadelphia: NANDA.

Porth, C. M. (2002). *Pathophysiology: Concepts of altered health states* (6th ed.). Philadelphia: Lippincott.

Ross, C. A. (2000). Emergency. Dialysis disequilibrium syndrome. *American Journal of Nursing, 100*(2), 53–54.

Schmelzer, M., & Stam, M. A. (2000). A hidden menace: Hemolytic uremic syndrome. *American Journal of Nursing, 100*(11), 26–32.

Seaton-Mills, D. (1999). Acute renal failure: Causes and considerations in the critically ill patient. *Nursing in Critical Care, 4*(6), 293–297.

Sprauve, D. (2000). Understanding chronic renal failure. *Nursing, 30*(4), Hosp Nurs 32hn12, 32hn14.

Tierney, L. M., McPhee, S. J., & Papadakis, M. A. (2001). *Current medical diagnosis & treatment* (40th ed.). New York: Lange Medical Books/McGraw-Hill.

United Network for Organ Sharing. (2002a). *All about UNOS.* Available www.unos.org/Newsroom/allabout_main.htm

———. (2002b). *Critical data. U. S. facts about transplantation.* Available www.unos.org/Newsroom/critdata_main.htm

———. (2002c). *Living donation outpaces cadaveric in 2001.* Available www.unos.org/Newsroom/archive_story_20020426_2001donornumbers.htm

Urden, L. D., Stacy, K. M., & Lough, M. E. (2002). *Thelan's critical care nursing: Diagnosis and management* (4th ed.). St. Louis: Mosby.

U. S. Renal Data System. (2001). *USRDS 2001 annual data report: Atlas of end-stage renal disease in the United States.* Bethesda, MD: National Institute of Diabetes and Digestive and Kidney Diseases (NIDDK).

Welch, J. L., & Davis, J. (2000). Self-care strategies to reduce fluid intake and control thirst in hemodialysis patients. *Nephrology Nursing Journal, 27*(4), 393–395.

Whitney, E. N., & Rolfes, S. R. (2002). *Understanding nutrition* (9th ed.). Belmont, CA: Wadsworth.

Wise, L. C., Mersch, J., Racioppi, J., Crosier, J., & Thompson, C. (2000). Evaluating the reliability and utility of cumulative intake and output. *Journal of Nursing Care Quality, 14*(3), 37–42.

Wallace, L. S. (2001). Rhabdomyolysis: A case study *Medsurg Nursing, 10*(3), 113–120.

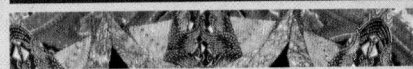

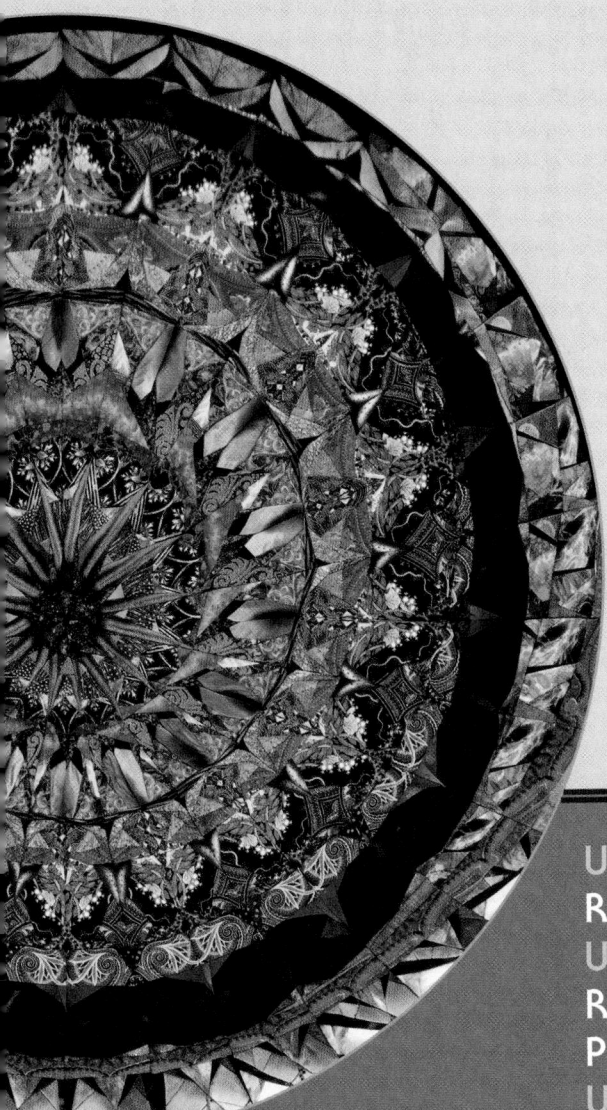

# ACTIVITY AND EXERCISE PATTERNS

# Functional Health Patterns with Related Nursing Diagnoses

## HEALTH PERCEPTION HEALTH MANAGEMENT
- Perceived health status
- Perceived health management
- Health care behaviors: health promotion and illness prevention activities, medical treatments, follow-up care

## VALUE-BELIEF
- Values, goals, or beliefs (including spirituality) that guide choices or decisions
- Perceived conflicts in values, beliefs, or expectations that are health related

## COPING-STRESS-TOLERANCE
- Capacity to resist challenges to self-integrity
- Methods of handling stress
- Support systems
- Perceived ability to control and manage situations

## NUTRITIONAL-METABOLIC
- Daily consumption of food and fluids
- Favorite foods
- Use of dietary supplements
- Skin lesions and ability to heal
- Condition of the integument
- Weight, height, temperature

## Part 4
### Activity and Exercise Patterns
### NANDA Nursing Diagnoses

- Activity Intolerance
- Risk for Activity Intolerance
- Bathing/Hygiene Self-Care Deficit
- Dressing/Grooming Self-Care Deficit
- Impaired Bed Mobility
- Risk for Disuse Syndrome
- Deficient Diversional Activity
- Fatigue
- Risk for Falls
- Impaired Home Maintenance
- Impaired Physical Mobility
- Impaired Wheelchair Mobility
- Impaired Transfer Ability
- Impaired Walking
- Delayed Surgical Recovery
- Decreased Cardiac Output
- Ineffective Breathing Pattern
- Ineffective Airway Clearance
- Impaired Gas Exchange
- Risk for Peripheral Neurovascular Dysfunction
- Impaired Tissue Perfusion
- Ineffective Tissue Perfusion
- Impaired Spontaneous Ventilation
- Dysfunctional Ventilatory Weaning Response

## SEXUALITY-REPRODUCTIVE
- Satisfaction with sexuality or sexual relationships
- Reproductive pattern
- Female menstrual and perimenopausal history

## ELIMINATION
- Patterns of bowel and urinary excretion
- Perceived regularity or irregularity of elimination
- Use of laxatives or routines
- Changes in time, modes, quality or quantity of excretions
- Use of devices for control

## ROLE-RELATIONSHIP
- Perception of major roles, relationships, and responsibilities in current life situation
- Satisfaction with or disturbances in roles and relationships

## ACTIVITY-EXERCISE
- Patterns of personally relevant exercise, activity, leisure, and recreation
- ADLs which require energy expenditure
- Factors that interfere with the desired pattern (e.g., illness or injury)

## SELF-PERCEPTION–SELF-CONCEPT
- Attitudes about self
- Perceived abilities, worth, self-image, emotions
- Body posture and movement, eye contact, voice and speech patterns

## SLEEP-REST
- Patterns of sleep and rest-/relaxation in a 24-hr period
- Perceptions of quality and quantity of sleep and rest
- Use of sleep aids and routines

## COGNITIVE-PERCEPTUAL
- Adequacy of vision, hearing, taste, touch, smell
- Pain perception and management
- Language, judgment, memory, decisions

*Reprinted from Nursing Diagnosis: Process and Application, 3rd ed., by M. Gordon, pp. 80–96, Copyright © 1994, with permission from Elsevier Science.*

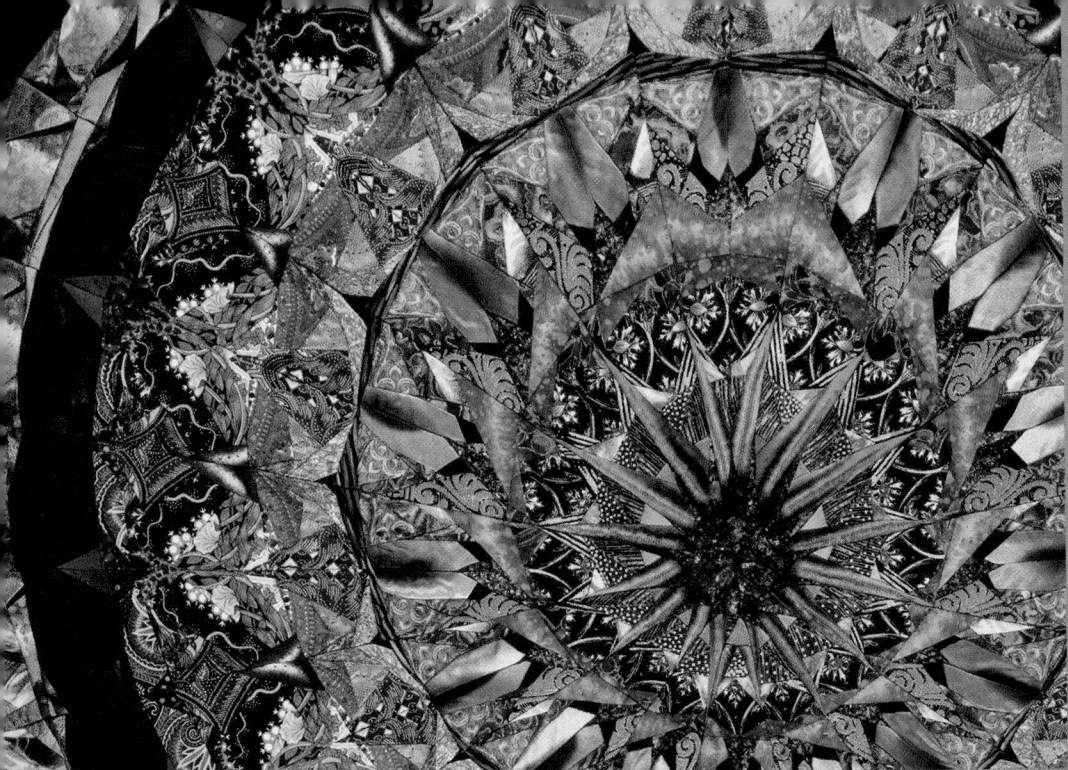

# RESPONSES TO ALTERED CARDIAC FUNCTION

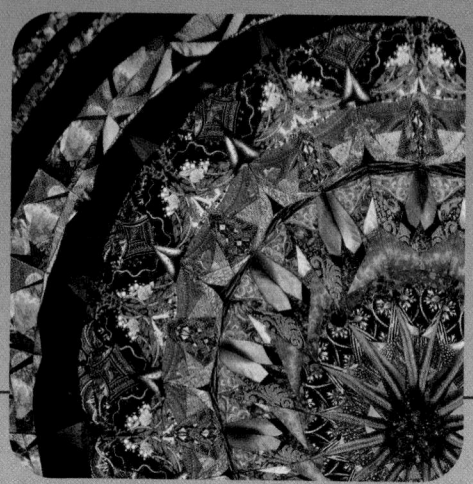

# Assessing Clients with Cardiac Disorders

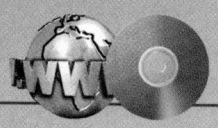

## MediaLink
### www.prenhall.com/lemone

Additional resources for this chapter can be found on the Student CD-ROM accompanying this textbook, and on the Companion Website at www.prenhall.com/lemone. Click on Chapter 28 to select the activities for this chapter.

**CD-ROM**
• Audio Glossary
• NCLEX Review

***Animations***
• Cardiac A&P
• Dysrhythmias

**Companion Website**
• More NCLEX Review
• Functional Health Pattern Assessment
• Case Study
    Chest Pain
• MediaLink Application
    Heart Sounds

## LEARNING OUTCOMES

After completing this chapter, you will be able to:

▪ Review the anatomy and physiology of the heart.

▪ Trace the circulation of blood through the heart and coronary vessels.

▪ Identify the normal heart sounds and relate them to the corresponding events in the cardiac cycle.

▪ Name and locate the elements of the heart's conduction system.

▪ Define cardiac output and explain the influence of various factors in its regulation.

▪ Identify specific topics for consideration during a health history interview of the client with health problems involving cardiac function.

▪ Describe physical assessment techniques for cardiac function.

▪ Identify abnormal findings that may indicate cardiac malfunction.

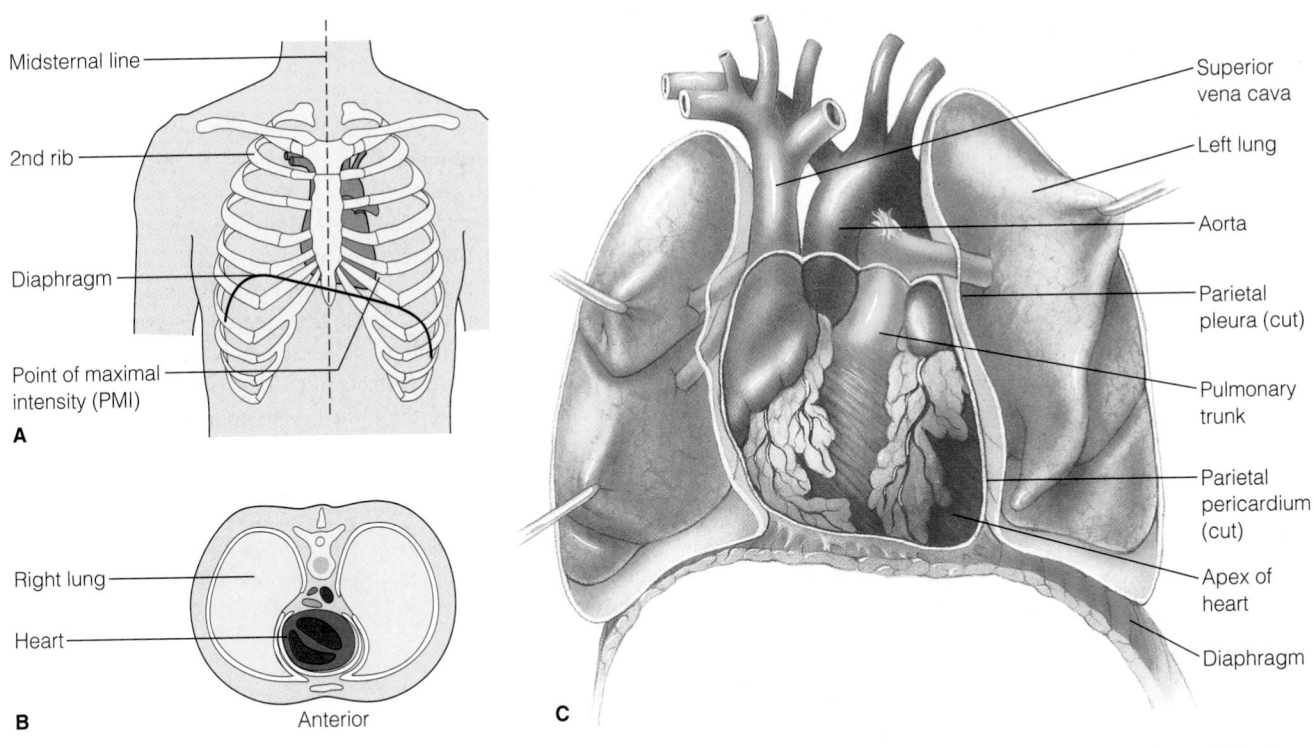

**Figure 28–1** ■ Location of the heart in the mediastinum of the thorax. *A,* Relationship of the heart to the sternum, ribs, and diaphragm. *B,* Cross-sectional view showing relative position of the heart in the thorax. *C,* Relationship of the heart and great vessels to the lungs.

The heart, a muscular pump, beats an average of 70 times per minute, or once every 0.86 seconds, every minute of a person's life. This continuous pumping moves blood through the body, nourishing tissue cells and removing wastes. Deficits in the structure or function of the heart affect all body tissues. Changes in cardiac rate, rhythm, or output may limit almost all human functions, including self-care, mobility, and the ability to maintain fluid volume status, respirations, tissue perfusion, and comfort. Cardiac changes may also affect self-concept, sexuality, and role performance.

## REVIEW OF ANATOMY AND PHYSIOLOGY

The heart is a hollow, cone-shaped organ approximately the size of an adult's fist, weighing less than 1 lb. It is located in the mediastinum of the thoracic cavity, between the vertebral column and the sternum, and is flanked laterally by the lungs. Two-thirds of the heart mass lies to the left of the sternum; the upper base lies beneath the second rib, and the pointed apex is approximate with the fifth intercostal space, midpoint to the clavicle (Figure 28–1 ■).

## The Pericardium

The heart is covered by a double layer of fibroserous membrane, the pericardium (Figure 28–2 ■). The pericardium encases the heart and anchors it to surrounding structures, forming the pericardial sac. The snug fit of the pericardium prevents the heart from overfilling with blood. The *parietal pericardium* is the outermost layer. The *visceral pericardium* (or *epicardium*)

**Figure 28–2** ■ Coverings and layers of the heart.

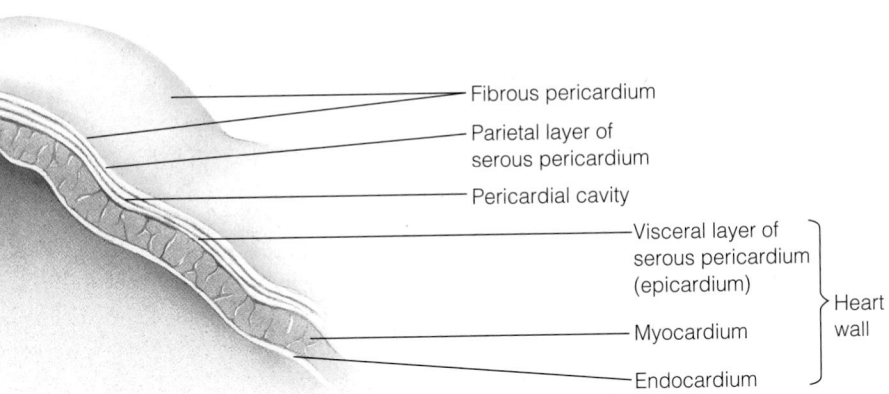

adheres to the heart surface. The small space between the visceral and parietal layers of the pericardium is called the pericardial cavity. A serous lubricating fluid produced in this space cushions the heart as it beats.

## Layers of the Heart Wall

The heart wall consists of three layers of tissue: the epicardium, the myocardium, and the endocardium (see Figure 28–2). The outermost epicardium is the same structure as the visceral pericardium. The middle layer of the heart wall, the myocardium, consists of specialized cardiac muscle cells (myofibrils) that provide the bulk of contractile heart muscle. The innermost layer, the endocardium, is a sheath of endothelium that lines the inside of the heart's chambers and great vessels.

## Chambers and Valves of the Heart

The heart has four hollow chambers, two upper atria and two lower ventricles. They are separated longitudinally by the interventricular septum (Figure 28–3 ■).

The right atrium receives deoxygenated blood from the veins of the body: The superior vena cava returns blood from the body area above the diaphragm, the inferior vena cava returns blood from the body below the diaphragm, and the coronary sinus drains blood from the heart. The left atrium receives freshly oxygenated blood from the lungs through the pulmonary veins.

The right ventricle receives deoxygenated blood from the right atrium and pumps it through the pulmonary artery to the lungs for oxygenation. The left ventricle receives the freshly oxygenated blood from the left atrium and pumps it out the aorta to the arterial circulation.

Each of the heart's chambers is separated by a valve which allows unidirectional blood flow to the next chamber or great vessel (see Figure 28–3). The atria are separated from the ventricles by the two atrioventricular (AV) valves; the tricuspid valve is on the right side, and the bicuspid (or mitral) valve is on the left. The flaps of each of these valves are anchored to the papillary muscles of the ventricles by the *chordae tendineae*. These structures control the movement of the AV valves to prevent backflow of blood.

The ventricles are connected to their great vessels by the semilunar valves. On the right, the pulmonary valve joins the right ventricle with the pulmonary artery. On the left, the aortic valve joins the left ventricle to the aorta.

Closure of the AV valves at the onset of contraction produces the first heart sound, or $S_1$ (characterized by the syllable "lub"); closure of the semilunar valves at the onset of relaxation produces the second heart sound, or $S_2$ (characterized by the syllable "dub").

## Systemic and Coronary Circulation

Because each side of the heart both receives and ejects blood, the heart is often described as a double pump. Pulmonary circulation begins with the right heart. Deoxygenated blood from the venous system enters the right atrium through two large veins, the superior and inferior venae cavae, and is transported to the lungs via the pulmonary artery and its branches

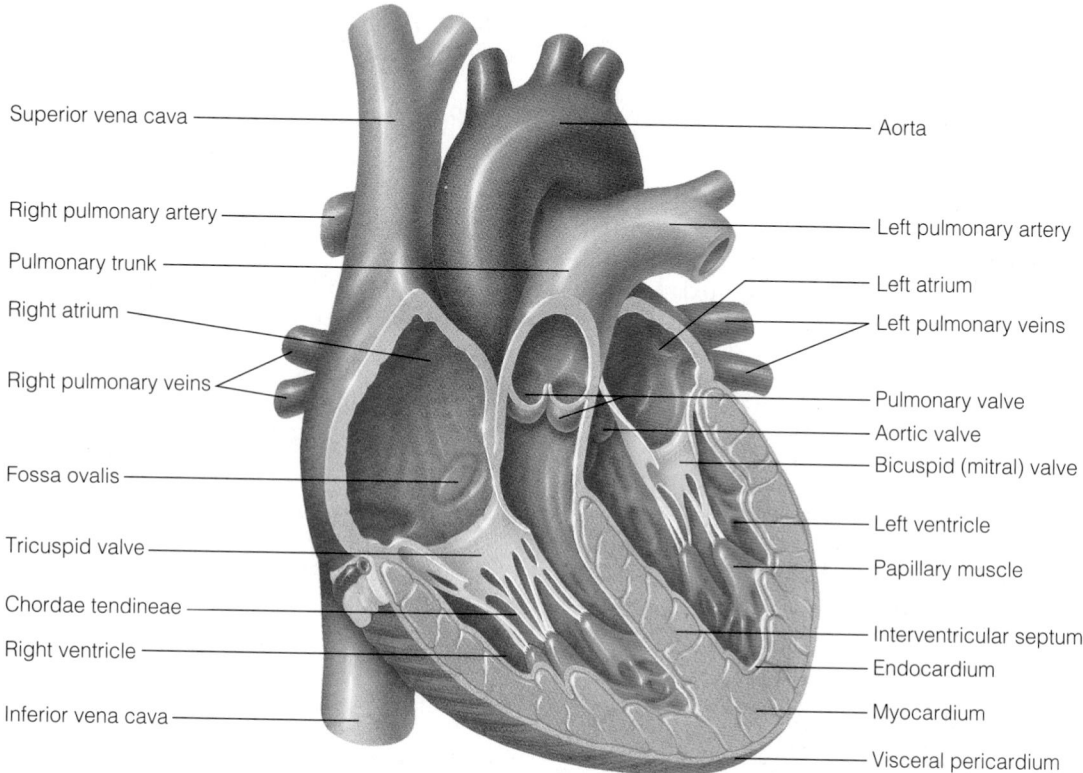

Superior vena cava

Right pulmonary artery

Pulmonary trunk

Right atrium

Right pulmonary veins

Fossa ovalis

Tricuspid valve

Chordae tendineae

Right ventricle

Inferior vena cava

Aorta

Left pulmonary artery

Left atrium

Left pulmonary veins

Pulmonary valve

Aortic valve

Bicuspid (mitral) valve

Left ventricle

Papillary muscle

Interventricular septum

Endocardium

Myocardium

Visceral pericardium

**Figure 28–3** ■ The internal anatomy of the heart, frontal section.

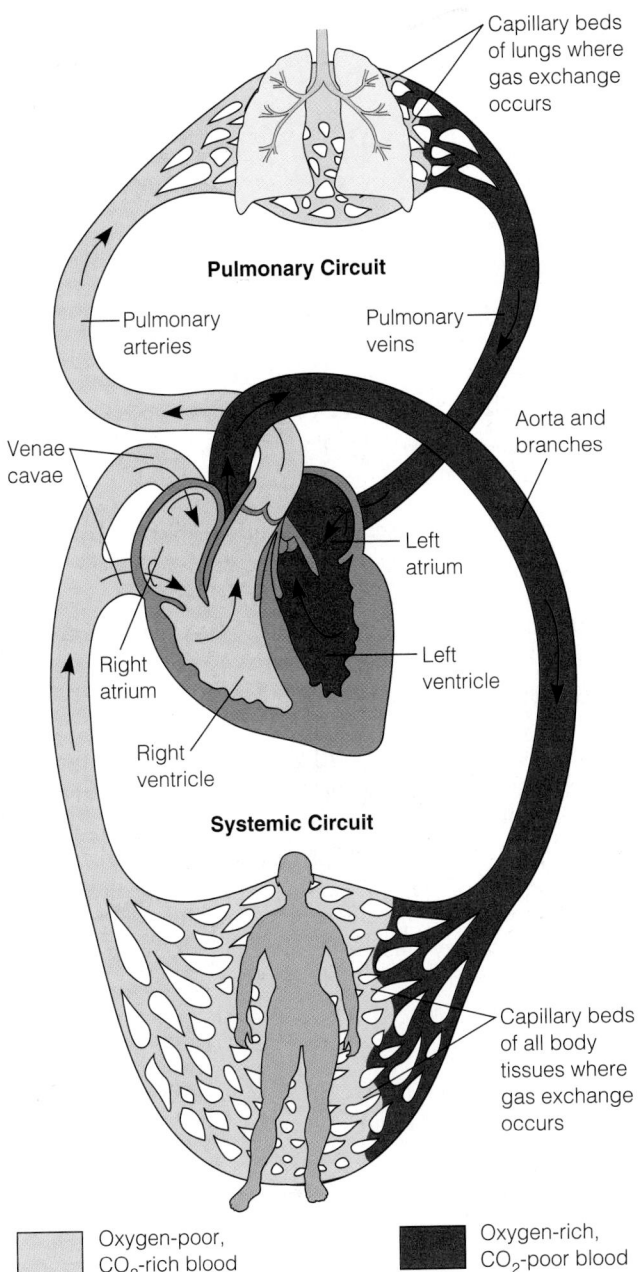

**Figure 28–4** ■ Pulmonary and systemic circulation. The left side of the heart pumps oxygenated blood into the arteries. Deoxygenated blood returns via the venous system into the right side of the heart.

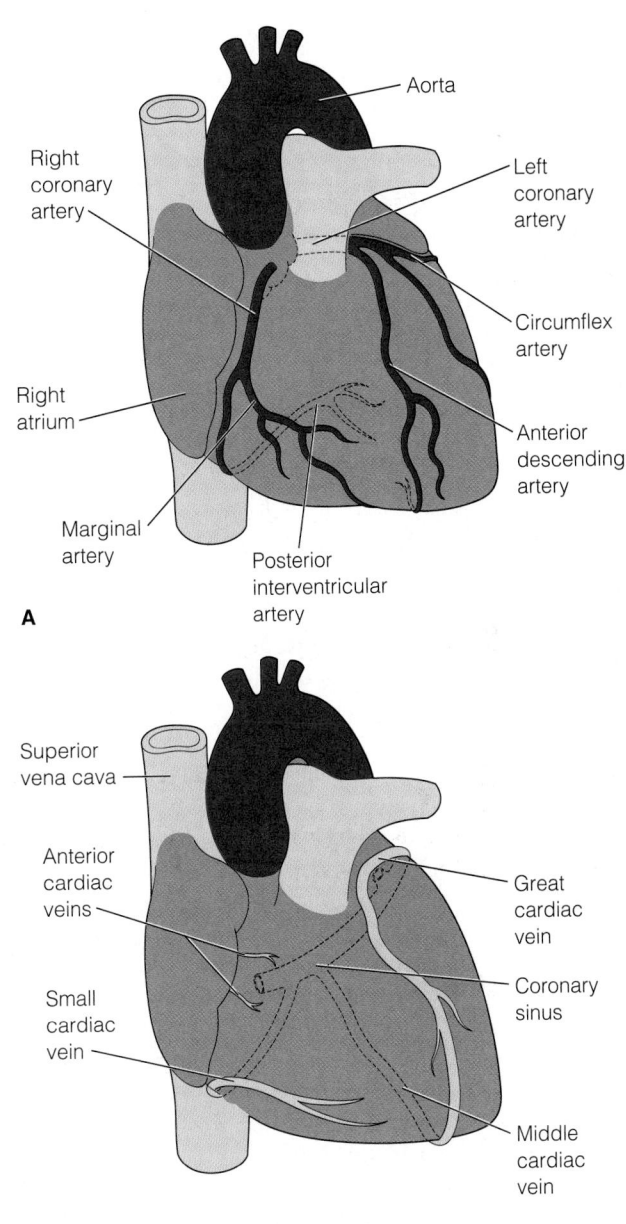

**Figure 28–5** ■ Coronary circulation. *A,* coronary arteries; *B,* coronary veins.

(Figure 28–4 ■). After oxygen and carbon dioxide are exchanged in the capillaries of the lungs, oxygen-rich blood returns to the left atrium through several pulmonary veins. Blood is then pumped out of the left ventricle through the aorta and its major branches to supply all body tissues. This second circuit of blood flow is called the systemic circulation.

While this continuous circulation of blood through the heart meets the body's oxygen needs, the heart muscle itself is supplied by its own network of vessels through the coronary circulation. The left and right coronary arteries originate at the base of the aorta and branch out to encircle the myocardium

(Figure 28–5A■). While ventricular contraction delivers blood through the pulmonary and systemic circuits as described above, it is during ventricular relaxation that the coronary arteries fill with oxygen-rich blood. Then, after the blood perfuses the heart muscle, the cardiac veins drain the blood into the coronary sinus, which empties into the right atrium of the heart (Figure 28–5B).

## The Cardiac Cycle and Cardiac Output

The contraction and relaxation of the heart constitutes one heartbeat and is called the **cardiac cycle** (Figure 28–6 ■). Ventricular filling is followed by ventricular **systole,** a phase during which the ventricles contract and eject blood into the pulmonary and systemic circuits. Systole is followed by a

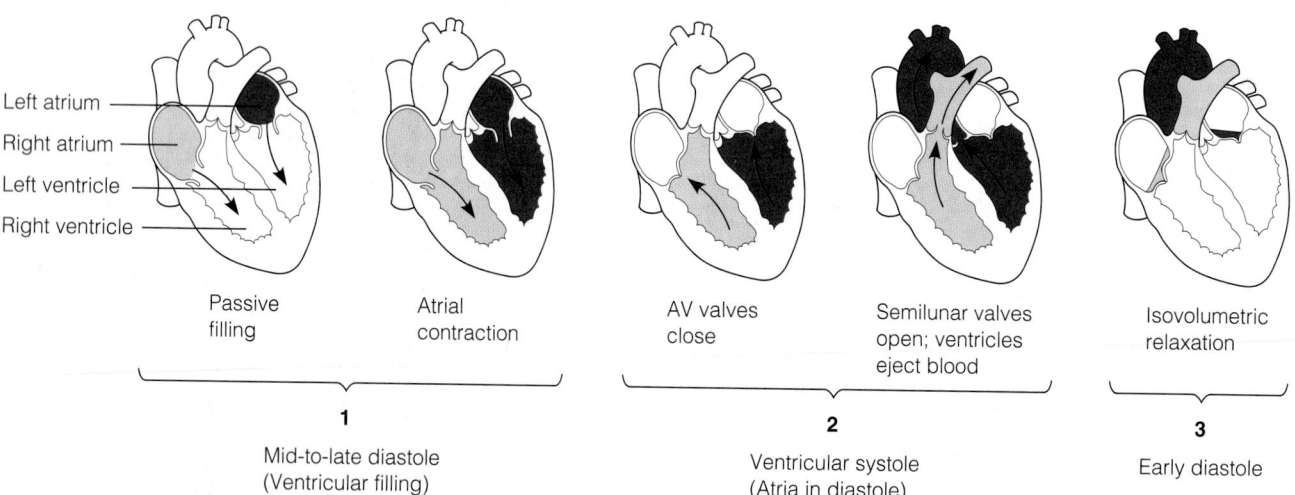

Passive filling    Atrial contraction    AV valves close    Semilunar valves open; ventricles eject blood    Isovolumetric relaxation

**1**
Mid-to-late diastole
(Ventricular filling)

**2**
Ventricular systole
(Atria in diastole)

**3**
Early diastole

**Figure 28–6** ■ The cardiac cycle has three events: (1) ventricular filling in mid-to-late diastole, (2) ventricular systole, and (3) isovolumetric relaxation in early diastole.

relaxation phase known as **diastole,** during which the ventricles refill, the atria contract, and the myocardium is perfused. Normally, the complete cardiac cycle occurs about 70 to 80 times per minute, measured as the heart rate (HR).

Each contraction ejects a certain volume of blood, called the **stroke volume (SV).** Stroke volume ranges from 60 to 100 mL/beat and averages about 70 mL/beat in an adult. The **cardiac output (CO)** is the amount of blood pumped by the ventricles into the pulmonary and systemic circulations in 1 minute. Multiplying the stroke volume by the heart rate determines the cardiac output: CO × HR = SV.

The average adult cardiac output ranges from 4 to 8 L/min. **Ejection fraction (EF)** is the percentage of total blood in the ventricle at the end of the diastole ejected from the heart with each beat. The normal ejection fraction ranges from 50% to 70%. Cardiac output is an indicator of how well the heart is functioning as a pump: If the heart cannot pump effectively, cardiac output and tissue perfusion are decreased. Body tissues that do not receive enough blood and oxygen (carried in the blood on hemoglobin) become **ischemic** (deprived of oxygen). If the tissues do not receive enough blood flow to maintain the functions of the cells, the cells die.

Activity level, metabolic rate, physiologic and psychologic stress responses, age, and body size all influence cardiac output. In addition, cardiac output is determined by the interaction of four major factors: heart rate, preload, afterload, and contractility. Changes in each of these variables influence cardiac output intrinsically, and each also can be manipulated to affect cardiac output. The heart's ability to respond to the body's changing need for cardiac output is called **cardiac reserve.**

## Heart Rate

Heart rate is affected by both direct and indirect autonomic nervous system stimulation. Direct stimulation is accomplished through the innervation of the heart muscle by sympathetic and parasympathetic nerves. The sympathetic nervous system increases the heart rate, whereas the parasympathetic vagal tone slows the heart rate. Reflex regulation of heart rate

in response to systemic blood pressure also occurs through activation of sensory receptors known as baroreceptors or pressure receptors located in the carotid sinus, aortic arch, venae cavae, and pulmonary veins.

If heart rate increases, cardiac output increases (up to a point) even if there is no change in stroke volume. However, rapid heart rates decrease the amount of time available for ventricular filling during diastole. Cardiac output then falls because decreased filling time decreases stroke volume. Coronary artery perfusion also decreases because the coronary arteries fill primarily during diastole. Cardiac output decreases during bradycardia if stroke volume stays the same, because the number of cardiac cycles is decreased.

## Preload

**Preload** is the amount of cardiac muscle fiber tension, or stretch, that exists at the end of diastole, just before contraction of the ventricles. Preload is influenced by venous return and the compliance of the ventricles. It is related to the total volume of blood in the ventricles: The greater the volume, the greater the stretch of the cardiac muscle fibers, and the greater the force with which the fibers contract to accomplish emptying. This principle is called *Starling's law of the heart.*

This mechanism has a physiologic limit. Just as continuous overstretching of a rubber band causes the band to relax and lose its ability to recoil, overstretching of the cardiac muscle fibers eventually results in ineffective contraction. Disorders such as renal disease and congestive heart failure result in sodium and water retention and increased preload. Vasoconstriction also increases venous return and preload.

Too little circulating blood volume results in a decreased venous return and therefore a decreased preload. A decreased preload reduces stroke volume and thus cardiac output. Decreased preload may result from hemorrhage or maldistribution of blood volume, as occurs in third spacing (see Chapter 5).

## Afterload

**Afterload** is the force the ventricles must overcome to eject their blood volume. It is the pressure in the arterial system ahead of the ventricles. The right ventricle must generate enough tension to open the pulmonary valve and eject its volume into the low-pressure pulmonary arteries. Right ventricle afterload is measured as pulmonary vascular resistance (PVR). The left ventricle, in contrast, ejects its load by overcoming the pressure behind the aortic valve. Afterload of the left ventricle is measured as systemic vascular resistance (SVR). Arterial pressures are much higher than pulmonary pressures; thus, the left ventricle has to work much harder than the right ventricle.

Alterations in vascular tone affect afterload and ventricular work. As the pulmonary or arterial blood pressure increases (e.g., through vasoconstriction), PVR and/or SVR increases, and the work of the ventricles increases. As workload increases, consumption of myocardial oxygen also increases. A compromised heart cannot effectively meet this increased oxygen demand, and a vicious cycle ensues. By contrast, a very low afterload decreases the forward flow of blood into the systemic circulation and the coronary arteries.

### Contractility

**Contractility** is the inherent capability of the cardiac muscle fibers to shorten. Poor contractility of the heart muscle reduces the forward flow of blood from the heart, increases the ventricular pressures from accumulation of blood volume, and reduces cardiac output. Increased contractility may overtax the heart.

## The Conduction System of the Heart

The cardiac cycle is perpetuated by a complex electrical circuit commonly known as the intrinsic conduction system of the heart. Cardiac muscle cells possess an inherent characteristic of self-excitation, which enables them to initiate and transmit impulses independent of a stimulus. However, specialized areas of myocardial cells typically exert a controlling influence in this electrical pathway.

One of these specialized areas is the sinoatrial (SA) node, located at the junction of the superior vena cava and right atrium (Figure 28–7 ■). The SA node acts as the normal "pacemaker" of the heart, usually generating an impulse 60 to 100 times per minute. This impulse travels across the atria via internodal pathways to the atrioventricular (AV) node, in the floor of the interatrial septum. The very small junctional fibers of the AV node slow the impulse, slightly delaying its transmission to the ventricles. It then passes through the bundle of His at the atrioventricular junction and continues down the interventricular septum through the right and left bundle branches and out to the Purkinje fibers in the ventricular muscle walls.

This path of electrical transmission produces a series of changes in ion concentration across the membrane of each cardiac muscle cell. The electrical stimulus increases the permeability of the cell membrane, creating an action potential (electrical potential). The result is an exchange of sodium, potassium, and calcium ions across the cell membrane, which changes the intracellular electrical charge to a positive state. This process of depolarization results in myocardial contraction. As the ion exchange reverses and the cell returns to its resting state of electronegativity, the cell is repolarized, and cardiac muscle relaxes. The cellular action potential serves as the basis for electrocardiography (ECG), the recording of the electrical impulses that immediately precede contraction of the heart muscle.

Cardiac conduction and electrocardiography are discussed in greater detail in Chapter 29. ∽

## Clinical Indicators of Cardiac Output

For many critically ill clients, invasive hemodynamic monitoring catheters are used to measure cardiac output in quantifiable numbers. However, advanced technology is not the only way to identify and assess compromised blood flow. Because cardiac output perfuses the body's tissues, clinical indicators of low

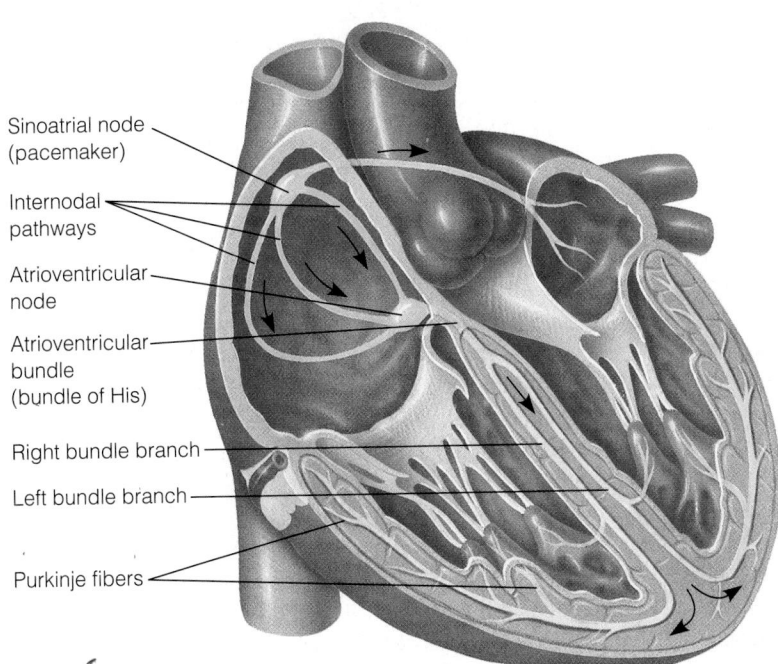

Sinoatrial node
(pacemaker)

Internodal
pathways

Atrioventricular
node

Atrioventricular
bundle
(bundle of His)

Right bundle branch

Left bundle branch

Purkinje fibers

**Figure 28–7** ■ The intrinsic conduction system of the heart.

cardiac output may be manifested by changes in organ function that result from compromised blood flow. For example, a decrease in blood flow to the brain presents as a change in level of consciousness. Other clinical manifestations of decreased cardiac output are discussed in Chapters 5 and 29. 🔗

*Cardiac index (CI)* is the cardiac output adjusted for the client's body size, also called the client's body surface area (BSA). Because it takes into account the client's BSA, the cardiac index provides more meaningful data about the heart's ability to perfuse the tissues and therefore is a more accurate indicator of the effectiveness of the circulation.

BSA is stated in square meters ($m^2$), and cardiac index is calculated as CO divided by BSA. Cardiac measurements are considered adequate when they fall within the range of 2.5 to 4.2 L/min/$m^2$. For example, two clients are determined to have a cardiac output of 4 L/min. This parameter is within normal limits. However, one client is 5 feet, 2 inches (157 cm) tall and weighs 120 lb (54.5 kg), with a BSA of 1.54 $m^2$. This client's cardiac index is 4 ÷ 1.54, or 2.6 L/min/$m^2$. The second client is 6 feet, 2 inches (188 cm) tall and weighs 280 lb (81.7 kg), with a BSA of 2.52 $m^2$. This client's cardiac index is 4 ÷ 2.52, or 1.6 L/min/$m^2$. The cardiac index results show that the same cardiac output of 4 L/min is adequate for the first client but grossly inadequate for the second client.

## ASSESSING CARDIAC FUNCTION

Conduct both a health assessment interview to collect subjective data and a physical assessment to collect objective data.

### The Health Assessment Interview

This section provides guidelines for collecting subjective data through a health assessment interview specific to cardiac function. A health assessment interview to determine problems with cardiac function may be conducted as part of a health screening or as part of a total health assessment, or it may focus on a chief complaint (such as chest pain). If the client has a problem with cardiac function, analyze its onset, characteristics, course, severity, precipitating and relieving factors, and any associated symptoms, noting the timing and circumstances. For example, ask the client:

- What is the location of the chest pain you experienced? Did it move up to your jaw or into your left arm?
- What type of activity brings on your chest pain?
- Have you noticed any changes in your energy level?
- Have you felt lightheaded during the times your heart is racing?

The interview begins by exploring the client's chief complaint (e.g., chest pain, palpitations, or shortness of breath). Describe the client's symptoms in terms of location, quality or character, timing, setting or precipitating factors, severity, aggravating and relieving factors, and associated symptoms (Table 28–1).

Explore the client's history for heart disorders such as angina, heart attack, congestive heart failure (CHF), hypertension (HTN), and valvular disease. Ask the client about previous heart surgery or illnesses, such as rheumatic fever, scarlet fever, or recurrent streptococcal throat infections. Also ask about the presence and treatment of other chronic illnesses such as dia-

| TABLE 28–1 | Assessing Chest Pain |
|---|---|
| **Characteristic** | **Examples** |
| Location | Substernal, precordial, jaw, back Localized or diffuse Radiation to neck, jaw, shoulder, arm |
| Character/quality | Pressure; tightness; crushing, burning, or aching quality; heaviness; dullness; "heartburn" or indigestion |
| Timing: onset, duration, and frequency | Onset: Sudden or gradual? Duration: How many minutes does the pain last? Frequency: Is the pain continuous or periodic? |
| Setting/precipitating factors | Awake, at rest, sleep interrupted? With activity? With eating, exertion, exercise, elimination, emotional upset? |
| Intensity/severity | Can range from 0 (no pain) to 10 (worst pain ever felt) |
| Aggravating factors Relieving factors | Activity, breathing, temperature Medication (nitroglycerine, antacid), rest; there may be no relieving factors |
| Associated symptoms | Fatigue, shortness of breath, palpitations, nausea and vomiting, sweating, anxiety, lightheadedness or dizziness |

betes mellitus, bleeding disorders, or endocrine disorders. Review the client's family history for coronary artery disease (CAD), HTN, stroke, hyperlipidemia, diabetes, congenital heart disease, or sudden death.

Ask the client about past or present occurrence of various cardiac symptoms, such as chest pain, shortness of breath, difficulty breathing, cough, palpitations, fatigue, lightheadedness or dizziness, fainting, heart murmur, blood clots, or swelling. Because cardiac function affects all other body systems, a full history may need to explore other related systems, such as respiratory function and/or peripheral vascular function.

Review the client's personal habits and nutritional history, including body weight; eating patterns; dietary intake of fats, salt, fluids; dietary restrictions; hypersensitivities or intolerances to food or medication; and the use of caffeine and alcohol. If the client uses tobacco products, ask about type (cigarettes, pipe, cigars, snuff), duration, amount, and efforts to quit. If the client uses street drugs, ask about type, method of intake (e.g., inhaled or injected), duration of use, and efforts to quit. Include questions about the client's activity level and tolerance, recreational activities, and relaxation habits. Assess the client's sleep patterns for interruptions in sleep due to dyspnea, cough, discomfort, urination, or stress. Ask how many pillows the client uses when sleeping. Also consider psychosocial factors that may affect the client's stress level: What is the client's marital status, family composition, and role within the family? Have there been any changes? What is the client's occupation, level of education, and socioeconomic level? Are resources for support available? What is the client's emotional disposition and personality type? How does the client perceive his or her state of health or illness, and how able is the client to comply with treatment?

Further interview questions and leading statements, categorized by functional health patterns, can be found on the Companion Website.

## Physical Assessment

Physical assessment of cardiac function may be performed either as part of a total assessment or alone for clients with suspected or known problems with cardiac function. Assess the heart through inspection, palpation, and auscultation over the precordium (the area of the chest wall overlying the heart).

The equipment needed for an examination of the heart includes a stethoscope with a diaphragm and a bell, a good light source, and a ruler. Before the examination, collect all the equipment, and explain the examination to the client to decrease anxiety. A quiet environment is essential to hear and assess heart sounds accurately.

The client may sit or lie in the supine position. Movements over the precordium may be more easily seen with tangential lighting (in which the light is directed at a right angle to the area being observed, producing shadows). Assess the following types of movements.

- **Apical impulse** is a normal, visible pulsation (thrust) in the area of the midclavicular line in the left fifth intercostal space. It can be seen on inspection in about half of the adult population.
- **Retraction** is a pulling in of the tissue of the precordium; a slight retraction just medial to the midclavicular line at the area of the apical impulse is normal and is more likely to be visible in thin clients.
- **Lift** is a more sustained thrust than normal.
- **Heave** is an excessive thrust.

### Apical Impulse Assessment with Abnormal Findings (✓)

- First using palmar surface and then repeating with finger pads, palpate the precordium for symmetry of movement and the apical impulse for location, size, amplitude, and duration. The sequence for palpation is shown in Figure 28–8 ■. To locate the apical impulse, ask the client to assume a left lateral recumbent position. Simultaneous palpation of the carotid pulse may also be helpful. The apical impulse is not palpable in all clients.
  - ✓ An enlarged or displaced heart is associated with an apical impulse lateral to the midclavicular line (MCL) or below the fifth left intercostal space (ICS).
  - ✓ Increased size, amplitude, and duration of the point of maximal impulse (PMI) are associated with left ventricular volume overload (increased preload) in conditions such as HTN and aortic stenosis, and in pressure overload (increased afterload) in conditions such as aortic or mitral regurgitation.
  - ✓ Increased amplitude alone may occur with hyperkinetic states, such as anxiety, hyperthyroidism, and anemia.
  - ✓ Decreased amplitude is associated with a dilated heart in cardiomyopathy.
  - ✓ Displacement alone may also occur with dextrocardia, diaphragmatic hernia, gastric distention, or chronic lung disease.
  - ✓ A **thrill** (a palpable vibration over the precordium or an artery) may accompany severe valve stenosis.
  - ✓ A marked increase in amplitude of the PMI at the right ventricular area occurs with right ventricular volume overload in atrial septal defect.
  - ✓ An increase in amplitude and duration occurs with right ventricular pressure overload in pulmonic stenosis and pulmonary hypertension. A lift or heave may also be seen in these conditions (and in chronic lung disease).
  - ✓ A palpable thrill in this area occurs with ventricular septal defect.
- Palpate the subxiphoid area with the index and middle finger.
  - ✓ Right ventricular enlargement may produce a downward pulsation against the fingertips.
  - ✓ An accentuated pulsation at the pulmonary area may be present in hyperkinetic states.
  - ✓ A prominent pulsation reflects increased flow or dilation of the pulmonary artery.
  - ✓ A thrill may be associated with aortic or pulmonary stenosis, aortic stenosis, pulmonary HTN, or atrial septal defect.
  - ✓ Increased pulsation at the aortic area may suggest aortic aneurysm.
  - ✓ A palpable second heart sound ($S_2$) may be noted with systemic HTN.

### Cardiac Rate and Rhythm Assessment with Abnormal Findings (✓)

- Auscultate heart rate.
  - ✓ A heart rate exceeding 100 beats per minute (BPM) is **tachycardia.** A heart rate less than 60 BPM is **bradycardia.**
- Simultaneously palpate the radial pulse while listening to the apical pulse.
  - ✓ If the radial pulse falls behind the apical rate, the client has a **pulse deficit,** indicating weak, ineffective contractions of the left ventricle.

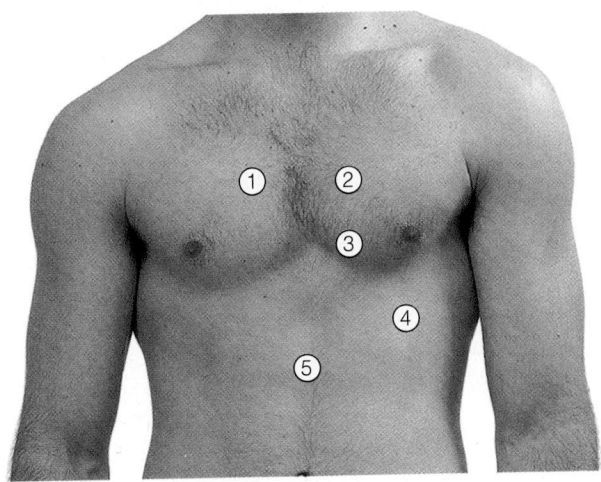

**Figure 28–8** ■ Areas for inspection and palpation of the precordium, indicating the sequence for palpation.

- Auscultate heart rhythm.
  - ✓ **Dysrhythmias** (abnormal heart rate or rhythm) may be regular or irregular in rhythm; their rates may be slow or fast. Irregular rhythms may occur in a pattern (e.g., an early beat every second beat, called *bigeminy*), sporadically, or with frequency and disorganization (e.g., atrial fibrillation). A pattern of gradual increase and decrease in heart rate that is within normal heart rate and that correlates with inspiration and expiration is called sinus arrhythmia.

### Heart Sounds Assessment with Abnormal Findings (✓)

See guidelines for cardiac auscultation in Box 28–1.

- Identify $S_1$ (first heart sound) and note its intensity. At each auscultatory area, listen for several cardiac cycles. See Figure 28–9 ■ for auscultation areas.
  - ✓ An accentuated $S_1$ occurs with tachycardia, states in which cardiac output is high (fever, anxiety, exercise, anemia, hyperthyroidism), complete heart block, and mitral stenosis.
  - ✓ A diminished $S_1$ occurs with first-degree heart block, mitral regurgitation, CHF, coronary artery disease, and pulmonary or systemic HTN. The intensity is also decreased with obesity, emphysema, and pericardial effusion. Varying intensity of $S_1$ occurs with complete heart block and grossly irregular rhythms.
- Listen for splitting of $S_1$.
  - ✓ Abnormal splitting of $S_1$ may be heard with right bundle branch block and premature ventricular contractions.
- Identify $S_2$ (second heart sound) and note its intensity.
  - ✓ An accentuated $S_2$ may be heard with HTN, exercise, excitement, and conditions of pulmonary HTN such as mitral stenosis, CHF, and cor pulmonale.

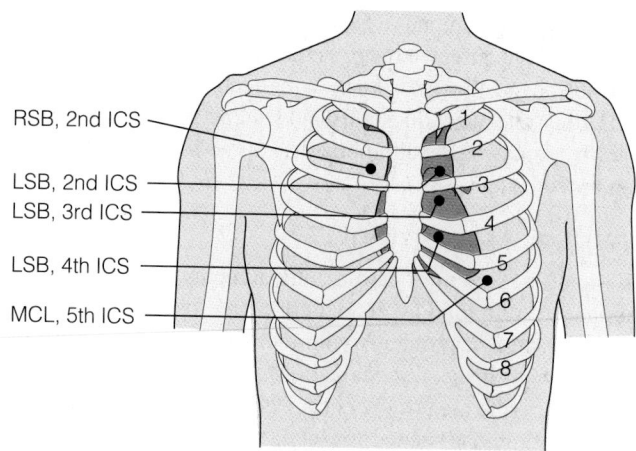

RSB, 2nd ICS
LSB, 2nd ICS
LSB, 3rd ICS
LSB, 4th ICS
MCL, 5th ICS

**Figure 28–9** ■ Areas for auscultation of the heart.

  - ✓ A diminished $S_2$ occurs with aortic stenosis, a fall in systolic blood pressure (shock), pulmonary stenosis, and increased anterioposterior chest diameter.
- Listen for splitting of $S_2$.
  - ✓ Wide splitting of $S_2$ is associated with delayed emptying of the right ventricle resulting in delayed pulmonary valve closure (e.g., mitral regurgitation, pulmonary stenosis, and right bundle branch block).
  - ✓ Fixed splitting occurs when right ventricular output is greater than left ventricular output and pulmonary valve closure is delayed (e.g., with atrial septal defect and right ventricular failure).
  - ✓ Paradoxical splitting occurs when closure of the aortic valve is delayed (e.g., left bundle branch block).
- Identify extra heart sounds in systole.
  - ✓ Ejection sounds (or clicks) result from the opening of deformed semilunar valves (e.g., aortic and pulmonary stenosis).
  - ✓ A midsystolic click is heard with mitral valve prolapse (MVP).
- Identify the presence of extra heart sounds in diastole.
  - ✓ An opening snap results from the opening sound of a stenotic mitral valve.
  - ✓ A pathologic $S_3$ (a third heart sound that immediately follows $S_2$), or *ventricular gallop*, results from myocardial failure and ventricular volume overload (e.g., CHF, mitral or tricuspid regurgitation).
  - ✓ An $S_4$ (a fourth heart sound that immediately precedes $S_1$), or *atrial gallop*, results from increased resistance to ventricular filling after atrial contraction (e.g., HTN, CAD, aortic stenosis, and cardiomyopathy).
  - ✓ A less common right-sided $S_4$ occurs with pulmonary HTN and pulmonary stenosis.
  - ✓ A combined $S_3$ and $S_4$ is called a summation gallop and occurs with severe CHF.
- Identify extra heart sounds in both systole and diastole.
  - ✓ A pericardial friction rub results from inflammation of the pericardial sac, as with pericarditis.

### Murmur Assessment with Abnormal Findings (✓)

- Identify any **murmurs.** Note location, timing, presence during systole or diastole, and intensity. Use the following scale to grade murmurs:

---

**BOX 28–1 ■ Guidelines for Cardiac Auscultation**

1. Locate the major auscultatory areas on the precordium (see Figure 28–9).
2. Choose a sequence of listening. Either begin from the apex and move upward along the sternal border to the base, or begin at the base and move downward to the apex. One suggested sequence is shown in Figure 28–9.
3. Listen first with the client in the sitting or supine position. Then ask the client to lie on the left side, and focus on the apex. Lastly, ask the client to sit up and lean forward. These position changes bring the heart closer to the chest wall and enhance auscultation. Carry out the following steps when the client assumes each of these positions:
   a. First, auscultate each area with the diaphragm of the stethoscope to listen for high-pitched sounds: $S_1$, $S_2$, murmurs, pericardial friction rubs.
   b. Next, auscultate each area with the bell of the stethoscope to listen for lower-pitched sounds: $S_3$, $S_4$, murmurs.
   c. Listen for the effect of respirations on each sound; while the client is sitting up and leaning forward, ask the client to exhale and hold the breath while you listen to heart sounds.

I = Barely heard
II = Quietly heard
III = Clearly heard
IV = Loud
V = Very loud
VI = Loudest; may be heard with stethoscope off the chest. A thrill may accompany murmurs of grade IV to grade VI.

- Note pitch (low, medium, high), and quality (harsh, blowing, or musical). Note pattern/shape, crescendo, decrescendo, and radiation/transmission (to axilla, neck).
  ✓ Midsystolic murmurs are heard with semilunar valve disease (e.g., aortic and pulmonary stenosis) and with hypertrophic cardiomyopathy.

✓ Pansystolic (holosystolic) murmurs are heard with AV valve disease (e.g., mitral and tricuspid regurgitation, ventricular septal defect).
✓ A late systolic murmur is heard with MVP.
✓ Early diastolic murmurs occur with regurgitant flow across incompetent semilunar valves (e.g., aortic regurgitation).
✓ Middiastolic and presystolic murmurs, such as with mitral stenosis, occur with turbulent flow across the AV valves.
✓ Continuous murmurs throughout systole and all or part of diastole occur with patent ductus arteriosus.

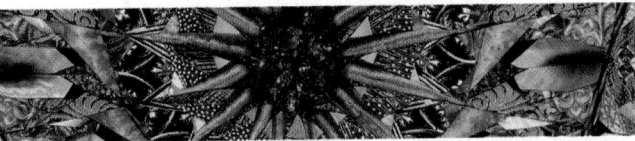

## EXPLORE MediaLink

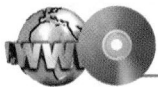

NCLEX review questions, case studies, care plan activities, MediaLink applications, and other interactive resources for this chapter can be found on the Companion Website at www.prenhall.com/lemone.

Click on Chapter 28 to select the activities for this chapter. For animations, video clips, more NCLEX review questions, and an audio glossary, access the Student CD-ROM accompanying this textbook.

## TEST YOURSELF

1. Which circulatory process supplies the heart with blood?
   a. The systemic circulation
   b. The pulmonary circulation
   c. The coronary circulation
   d. The hepatic circulation

2. The amount of blood pumped by the ventricles in 1 minute is known as:
   a. Heart rate
   b. Ventricular contraction
   c. Stroke volume
   d. Cardiac output

3. The intensity of chest pain may be assessed by asking which question?
   a. "Did the pain move into your left arm?"
   b. "Was your pain relieved by resting?"
   c. "On a scale of 0 to 10, what number was your pain?"
   d. "Was the pain a pressure, a burning, or a tightness?"

4. At what anatomic location would you assess the apical impulse?
   a. Left midclavicular, 5th intercostal space
   b. Left substernal, 6th intercostal space
   c. Right midaxillary, 2nd intercostal space
   d. Right nipple line, any intercostal space

5. Your client's pulse rate is 50. You would document this as:
   a. Tachycardia
   b. Bradycardia
   c. Hypertension
   d. Hypotension

See Test Yourself answers in Appendix C.

## BIBLIOGRAPHY

Farla, S., & Flannery, J. (1999). Assessment of the patient in heart failure. *Home Care Provider, 4*(5), 184–188.

Kirton, C. (1996). Assessing normal heart sounds. *Nursing96, 26*(2), 56–57.

———. (1997a). Assessing a heart murmur. *Nursing97, 27*(9), 51.

———. (1997b). Assessing S₃ and S₄ heart sounds. *Nursing97, 27*(7), 52–53.

Ludwig, L. (1998). Cardiovascular assessment for home healthcare nurses: Part 1. *Home Healthcare Nurse, 16*(7), 450–456.

McAvoy, J. (2000). Cardiac pain: Discover the unexpected. *Nursing, 30*(3), 34–40.

McGrath, A., & Cox, C. (1998). Cardiac and circulatory assessment in intensive care units. *Intensive & Critical Care Nursing, 14*(6), 283–287.

Norrie, P. (1999). The parameters that cardiothoracic intensive care nurses use to assess the progress or deterioration of their patients. *Nursing in Critical Care, 4*(3), 133–137.

O'Hanlon-Nichols, T. (1997). Basic assessment series: The adult cardiovascular system. *American Journal of Nursing, 97*(12), 34–40.

Scrima, D. (1997). Foundations of arrhythmia interpretation. *MEDSURG Nursing, 6*(4), 193–202.

Weber, J., & Kelley, J. (2002). *Health assessment in nursing* (2nd ed.). Philadelphia: Lippincott.

Wilson, S., & Giddens, J. (2001). *Health assessment for nursing practice*. St. Louis: Mosby.

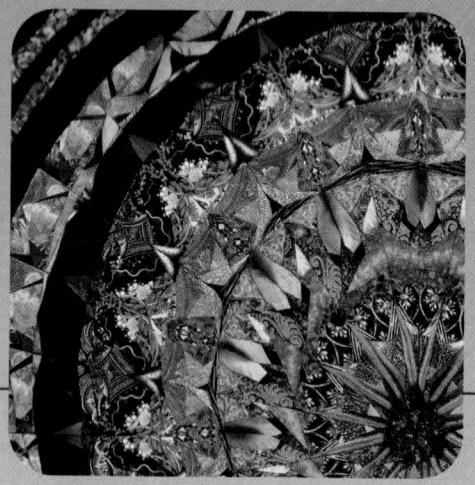

# CHAPTER 29

# Nursing Care of Clients with Coronary Heart Disease

## MediaLink

**www.prenhall.com/lemone**

Additional resources for this chapter can be found on the Student CD-ROM accompanying this textbook, and on the Companion Website at www.prenhall.com/lemone. Click on Chapter 29 to select the activities for this chapter.

### CD-ROM
- Audio Glossary
- NCLEX Review

### Animations
- Coronary Heart Disease
- Nifedipine
- Propranolol

### Companion Website
- More NCLEX Review
- Case Study
  Myocardial Infarction
- Care Plan Activity
  Perioperative Pacemaker Care
- MediaLink Application
  Women and Heart Attacks

## LEARNING OUTCOMES

After completing this chapter, you will be able to:

- Use knowledge of the normal anatomy and physiology of the heart in caring for clients with coronary heart disease.

- Discuss the coronary circulation and electrical properties of the heart.

- Compare and contrast the pathophysiology and manifestations of coronary heart disease and common cardiac dysrhythmias.

- Identify diagnostic tests and procedures used for clients with coronary heart disease and/or dysrhythmias.

- Discuss nursing implications for drugs used to prevent and treat coronary heart disease and dysrhythmias.

- Describe nursing care for the client undergoing diagnostic testing, an interventional procedure, or surgery for coronary heart disease or a dysrhythmia.

- Use the nursing process to plan and implement individualized nursing care and teaching for clients with coronary heart disease or dysrhythmias.

Changes in the conduction of electrical impulses through the heart, impaired blood flow to the myocardium, and structural changes in the heart itself affect the heart's ability to fulfill its major purpose: to pump enough blood to meet the body's demand for oxygen and nutrients. Disruptions in cardiac function affect other organ systems as well, potentially leading to organ system failure and death.

**Cardiovascular disease (CVD)** is a generic term for disorders of the heart and blood vessels. CVD is the leading cause of death and disability in the United States. Over 60 million people have some type of cardiovascular disease. The economic costs of CVD, both direct and indirect, to the nation are estimated at $329 billion annually (National Heart, Lung, and Blood Institute [NHLBI], 2002).

On an encouraging note, however, the incidence of new CVD cases per year is decreasing. Public education aimed at reducing fat intake, increasing exercise, and lowering cholesterol levels have made people more aware of risk factors associated with CVD. The mortality rate from heart disease peaked in 1963 and has shown a slow but steady decline since that time.

This chapter focuses on disorders of myocardial blood flow (coronary heart disease) and cardiac rhythm. Disorders of cardiac structure and function are discussed in Chapter 30. Review the normal anatomy and physiology and nursing assessment of the heart in Chapter 28 before proceeding with this chapter.

# DISORDERS OF MYOCARDIAL PERFUSION

## THE CLIENT WITH CORONARY HEART DISEASE

**Coronary heart disease (CHD),** or *coronary artery disease (CAD),* affects 12.6 million people in the United States and causes more than 500,000 deaths annually (NHLBI, 2002). CHD is caused by impaired blood flow to the myocardium (Porth, 2002). Accumulation of atherosclerotic plaque in the coronary arteries is the usual cause. Coronary heart disease may be asymptomatic, or may lead to angina pectoris, myocardial infarction (MI or heart attack), dysrhythmias, heart failure, and even sudden death.

Many risk factors for CHD can be controlled through lifestyle modification. In fact, with increased public awareness of risk factors related to CHD, mortality rates are declining by about 3.3% per year. Nevertheless, CHD remains a major public health problem. Heart disease is the leading cause of death for all U.S. ethnic groups except Asian females (NHBLI, 2002). Nurses are in a prime position to encourage and support positive lifestyle changes by teaching and promoting healthy living practices. Individual choices can and do affect health.

The highest incidence of CHD is in the Western world, mainly in white males age 45 and older. Both men and women are affected by coronary heart disease; in women, however, the onset is about 10 years later because of the heart-protective effects of estrogen. After menopause, women's risk is equal to that of men.

The causes of atherosclerosis are not known, but certain risk factors have been linked with the development of atherosclerotic plaques. The Framingham Heart Study provided vital research into the relationship between risk factors and the development of heart disease (Box 29–1). Research into CHD is ongoing, looking at causative factors, manifestations, and protective measures for many populations.

## RISK FACTORS

Risk factors for CHD are frequently classified as *nonmodifiable,* or factors that cannot be changed, and *modifiable,* those factors that can be changed (Table 29–1).

### Nonmodifiable

*Age* is a nonmodifiable risk factor. Over 50% of heart attack victims are 65 or older; 80% of deaths due to myocardial infarction occur in this age group. *Gender, race,* and *genetic factors* also are nonmodifiable risk factors for CHD. Men are affected by CHD at an earlier age than women. African Americans have a higher incidence of hypertension, which contributes to more rapid development of atherosclerosis.

### Modifiable

Modifiable risk factors include lifestyle factors and pathologic conditions that predispose the client to developing CHD. Pathologic conditions often can be controlled. Behavioral or lifestyle factors can be controlled or completely eliminated. Lifestyle changes require significant commitment by the client; ongoing support from the health care team is vital for success.

#### Pathologic Conditions

Disease conditions that contribute to CHD include hypertension, diabetes mellitus, and hyperlipidemia. Elevated homocystine levels and the metabolic syndrome are emerging risk factors. Although these conditions are not a matter of choice, they are modifiable risk factors that can often be controlled through medication, weight control, diet, and exercise.

*Hypertension* is consistent blood pressure readings greater than 140 mmHg systolic or 90 mmHg diastolic. Hypertension is common, affecting more than one-third of people over age 50 in the United States. Its prevalence is higher in African Americans than in Hispanics, and higher in Hispanics than in white Americans (NHLBI, 2002).

MediaLink | CORONARY HEART DISEASE ANIMATION

## BOX 29–1 ■ The Framingham Heart Study

The Framingham Heart Study (FHS) is an ongoing, significant clinical research study that has provided data about cardiovascular disease for over 50 years. The study was initiated in 1948 with an original study group of 5209 participants in the town of Framingham, Massachusetts. Every 2 years, this original group is evaluated for cardiovascular "events" via their medical history, physical findings, and diagnostic testing. Children of the original group have also been studied as part of the Framingham Offspring Study. It was in reports of the Framingham study that the term "risk factor" first appeared.

### IMPLICATIONS FOR NURSING

The data collected from both the Framingham Heart Study and the Framingham Offspring Study provide a rich database from which to develop evidence-based approaches for clients with heart disease. A major application of these research findings to practice is in primary preventive education, for example, through community cardiovascular health programs. As noted in the text, although research shows that increased public awareness of cardiovascular risk factors has lowered morbidity and mortality from heart disease, heart disease remains the number-one killer in the

United States. Education about the effects of lifestyle on the cardiovascular system must begin in the early school years and be reinforced throughout the formative years. When healthy choices become habit, cardiac disease will be reduced.

A second application of these findings is in collaborative treatment. Nurses should keep up to date on the latest strategies for medical treatment so that they can provide accurate rationales to clients and formulate effective nursing treatment plans that complement medical management strategies. The result is better communication, a sense of collegiality and teamwork, and positive client outcomes.

### Critical Thinking in Client Care

1. What kinds of strategies can be used in elementary school settings to teach cardiovascular health in a fun, informative manner?
2. Which health care providers should be included in a multidisciplinary effort to encourage clients to modify their lifestyles?
3. What changes do you need to make in your lifestyle to role model heart healthy living?

### TABLE 29–1 Risk Factors for Coronary Heart Disease

| Nonmodifiable | Modifiable | |
| --- | --- | --- |
| | Pathophysiologic | Lifestyle |
| Age<br>Gender<br>Race/ethnic background<br>Heredity | Hypertension<br>Diabetes mellitus<br>Hyperlipidemia<br>Elevated homocystine levels<br>Metabolic syndrome<br>Women only: premature menopause | Cigarette smoking<br>Obesity<br>Physical inactivity<br>Diet<br>Women only: use of oral contraceptives, hormone replacement therapy |

### TABLE 29–2 Classification of Serum Cholesterol Values*

| | Total Cholesterol (mg/dL) | LDL Cholesterol (mg/dL) |
| --- | --- | --- |
| Optimal | | Less than 100 |
| Desirable | Under 200 | 100–129 |
| Borderline High | 200 to 239 | 130 to 159 |
| High | 240 or higher | 160 or higher |
| Very High | | >190 |

*As defined by the National Blood, Lung, and Heart Institute's National Cholesterol Education Program.

*Diabetes mellitus* contributes to CHD in several ways. Diabetes is associated with higher blood lipid levels, a higher incidence of hypertension, and obesity—all risk factors in their own right. In addition, diabetes affects blood vessels, contributing to the process of atherosclerosis. Hyperglycemia, altered platelet function, and elevated fibrinogen levels also are thought to play a role.

*Hyperlipidemia* is an abnormally high level of blood lipids and lipoproteins. Lipoproteins carry cholesterol in the blood. Low-density lipoproteins (LDLs) are the primary carriers of cholesterol. High levels of LDL (Memory cue: LDLs = **l**ess **d**esirable **l**ipoproteins) promote atherosclerosis because LDL deposits cholesterol on artery walls. Table 29–2 lists desirable and high-risk levels for total and LDL cholesterol. In contrast, high-density lipoproteins (HDLs = **h**ighly **d**esirable **l**ipoproteins) help clear cholesterol from the arteries, transporting it to the liver for excretion. HDL levels above 35 mg/dL appear to reduce the

risk of CHD. Triglycerides, compounds of fatty acids bound to glycerol and used for fat storage by the body, are carried on very low-density lipoprotein (VLDL) molecules. Elevated triglycerides also contribute to the risk for CHD.

Recent research demonstrates a link between elevated serum *homocysteine levels* and CHD. Until menopause, women have lower homocysteine levels than men, which may partially explain their lower risk for CHD. Homocysteine levels are negatively correlated with serum folate and dietary folate intake; that is, increasing folate intake lowers homocysteine levels.

*Metabolic syndrome* is another emerging risk factor for CHD. Metabolic syndrome is a group of related risk factors occurring in the same individual: abdominal obesity, hyperlipidemia, hypertension, insulin resistance, and an increased tendency toward clotting and inflammation. The metabolic syndrome appears to significantly increase the risk for premature CHD.

## Nursing Research

### Evidence-Based Practice for Postmenopausal Women

The Women's Health Initiative (WHI) is studying the risks and benefits of strategies to reduce the incidence of heart disease, breast and colorectal cancer, and fractures in postmenopausal women (Writing Group, 2002). A group of 161,809 postmenopausal women between age 50 and 79 were originally enrolled in WHI trials. Of these women, a subgroup of 16,608 women with intact uteri became part of a randomized trial to assess the risks and benefits of HRT, using the most frequently prescribed combined hormone (estrogen and progestin [Prempro]) replacement in the United States.

After a mean of 5.2 years of follow-up, this study was stopped due to convincing evidence that the risk for invasive breast cancer exceeded the benefits of HRT. The study also demonstrated increased risks for coronary heart disease, stroke, deep vein thrombosis, and pulmonary embolism, although overall mortality was not affected. HRT reduced the risk for colorectal cancer and hip fracture in this study group. The risk for CHD appears to be independent of other CHD risk factors such as age, ethnicity, hypertension, diabetes, smoking, obesity, and other identified risk factors.

### IMPLICATIONS FOR NURSING

Nurses often are in position of advising women about menopause, its manifestations, and hormone replacement therapy. While HRT does reduce unpleasant menopausal effects such as night sweats and hot flashes, and it reduces the risk of osteoporosis and subsequent fractures, it carries associated risks. Advise each client about the risks and benefits of HRT, clearly presenting the evidence. Suggest alternative strategies to reduce menopausal symptoms, such as complementary medicines (see Chapter 48). ⬡ Encourage measures such as weight-bearing exercise, calcium supplements, and a diet high in fiber and antioxidants to reduce the risks for osteoporosis, fracture, and colorectal cancer. Ultimately, each client will make her own decision about postmenopausal HRT.

### Critical Thinking in Client Care

1. What factors might you suggest that a client consider when deciding whether to use HRT for menopausal manifestations and risks?
2. In this study, the increased risk for CHD was not related to the duration of time taking HRT, whereas the increased risk for stroke and invasive breast cancer emerged more than 1 year after randomization (stroke in the second through fifth year of the study, breast cancer within several years following randomization). Will this data affect your advice to menopausal women inquiring about HRT? If so, how?

---

Risk factors unique to women include *premature menopause, oral contraceptive use,* and *hormone replacement therapy (HRT).* At menopause, serum HDL levels drop and LDL levels rise, increasing the risk of CHD. Early menopause (natural or surgically induced) increases the risk of CHD and MI. Women who have bilateral oophorectomy before age 35 without hormone replacement are 8 times more likely to have an MI than women experiencing natural menopause. Estrogen replacement therapy reduces the risk of CHD and MI in these women. Oral contraceptives, by contrast, increase the risk for myocardial infarction, particularly in women who also smoke. This increased risk is due to the tendency of oral contraceptives to promote clotting, and their effects on blood pressure, serum lipids, and glucose tolerance (Woods, Froclicher, & Motzer, 2000). The Women's Health Initiative randomized trial of HRT showed an increased risk for CHD in previously healthy women taking a commonly prescribed combination of estrogen and progestin (Writing Group, 2002). This well-controlled research study (see the box above) was terminated early when it showed a small but significant increase risk for CHD, stroke, pulmonary embolism, and invasive breast cancer in women taking HRT.

### Lifestyle Factors

*Cigarette smoking* is an independent risk factor for CHD, responsible for more deaths from CHD than from lung cancer or pulmonary disease (Woods et al., 2000). The male cigarette smoker has 2 to 3 times the risk of developing heart disease than the nonsmoker; the female who smokes has up to 4 times the risk. For both men and women who stop smoking, the risk of mortality from CHD is reduced by half. Second-hand (or environmental) tobacco smoke also increases the risk of death from CHD, by as much as 30% (Woods et al., 2000). Tobacco smoke promotes CHD in several ways. Carbon monoxide damages vascular endothelium, promoting cholesterol deposition. Nicotine stimulates catecholamine release, increasing blood pressure, heart rate, and myocardial oxygen use. Nicotine also constricts arteries, limiting tissue perfusion (blood flow and oxygen delivery). Further, nicotine reduces HDL levels and increases platelet aggregation, increasing the risk of thrombus formation.

*Obesity* (body weight greater than 30% over ideal body weight), increased body mass index (BMI), and fat distribution affect the risk for CHD. Obese people have higher rates of hypertension, diabetes, and hyperlipidemia. In the Framingham study, obese men over age 50 had twice the incidence of CHD and acute MI of those who were within 10% of their ideal weight. Central obesity, or intra-abdominal fat, is associated with an increased risk for CHD. The best indicator of central obesity is the waist circumference. A waist-to-hip ratio of greater than 0.8 (women) or 0.9 (men) increases the risk for CHD.

*Physical inactivity* is associated with higher risk of CHD. Research data indicate that people who maintain a regular program of physical activity are less prone to developing CHD than sedentary people. Cardiovascular benefits of exercise include increased availability of oxygen to the heart muscle, decreased oxygen demand and cardiac workload, and increased myocardial function and electrical stability. Other positive effects of regular physical activity include decreased blood pressure, blood lipids, insulin levels, platelet aggregation, and weight.

*Diet* may be a risk factor for CHD, independent of fat and cholesterol intake. Diets high in fruits, vegetables, whole

Coronary heart disease usually is due to *athero-sclerosis*, occlusion of the coronary arteries by fibrous, fatty plaque. Coronary heart disease is manifested by *angina pectoris* and/or *myocardial infarction*. Risk factors for coronary heart disease include age (over 50 years), heredity, smoking, obesity, high serum cholesterol levels, hypertension, and diabetes mellitus. Other factors, such as diet and lack of exercise, also contribute to the risk of CHD.

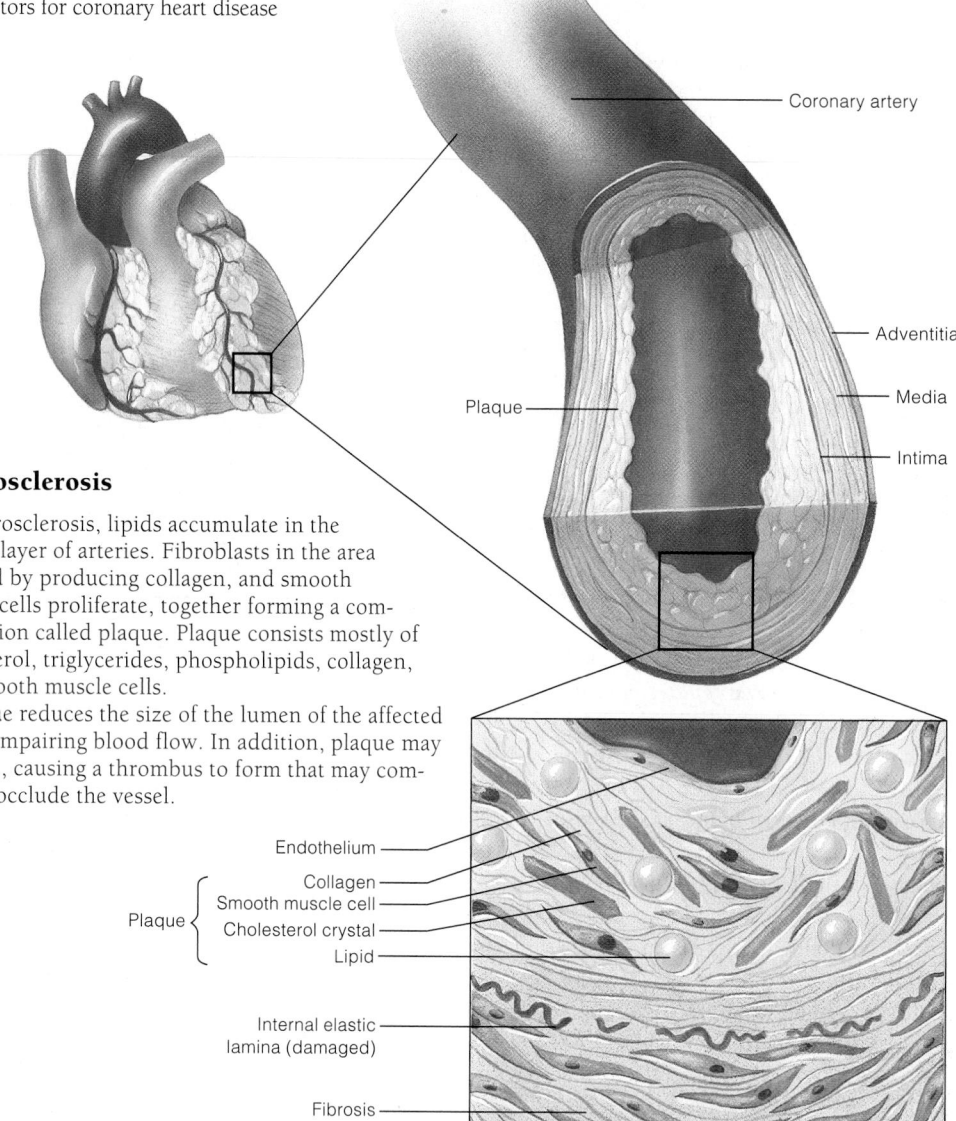

Coronary artery

Adventitia

Media

Intima

Plaque

### Atherosclerosis

In atherosclerosis, lipids accumulate in the intimal layer of arteries. Fibroblasts in the area respond by producing collagen, and smooth muscle cells proliferate, together forming a complex lesion called plaque. Plaque consists mostly of cholesterol, triglycerides, phospholipids, collagen, and smooth muscle cells.

Plaque reduces the size of the lumen of the affected artery, impairing blood flow. In addition, plaque may ulcerate, causing a thrombus to form that may completely occlude the vessel.

Endothelium

Collagen

Smooth muscle cell

Cholesterol crystal

Lipid

Plaque

Internal elastic lamina (damaged)

Fibrosis

grains, and unsaturated fatty acids appear to have a protective effect. The underlying factors are not clear, but probably relate to nutrients such as antioxidants, folic acid, other B vitamins, omega-3 fatty acids, and other unidentified micronutrients (National Cholesterol Education Program, 2001).

## PHYSIOLOGY REVIEW

The two main coronary arteries, the left and the right, supply blood, oxygen, and nutrients to the myocardium. They originate in the root of the aorta, just outside the aortic valve. The *left main coronary artery* divides to form the anterior descending and circumflex arteries. The *anterior descending* artery supplies the anterior interventricular septum and the left ventricle. The *circ-*umflex* branch supplies the left lateral wall of the left ventricle. The *right coronary artery* supplies the right ventricle and forms the posterior descending artery. The *posterior descending* artery supplies the posterior portion of the heart (see Figure 28-4).

Blood flow through the coronary arteries is regulated by several factors. Aortic pressure is the primary factor. Other factors include the heart rate (most flow occurs during diastole, when the muscle is relaxed), metabolic activity of the heart, blood vessel tone (constriction), and collateral circulation. Although there are no connections between the large coronary arteries, small arteries are joined by **collateral channels.** If large vessels are gradually occluded, these channels enlarge, providing alternative routes for blood flow (Porth, 2002).

### Angina Pectoris

Angina is characterized by episodes of chest pain, usually precipitated by exercise and relieved by rest. When myocardial oxygen needs are greater than partially occluded vessels can supply, myocardial cells become ischemic and shift to anaerobic metabolism. Anaerobic metabolism produces lactic acid that stimulates nerve endings in the muscle, causing pain. The pain subsides when the oxygen supply again meets myocardial demand.

### Myocardial Infarction

Myocardial infarction occurs when complete obstruction of a coronary artery interrupts blood supply to an area of myocardium. Affected tissue becomes ischemic and eventually dies (infarcts) if the blood supply is not restored. The necrotic area is bordered by an area of injured or damaged tissue, which is in turn surrounded by an area of ischemic tissue.

As myocardial cells die, they lyse and release various cardiac isoenzymes into the circulation. Elevated serum levels of creatinine kinase (CK) and cardiac-specific troponins are specific indicators of myocardial infarction.

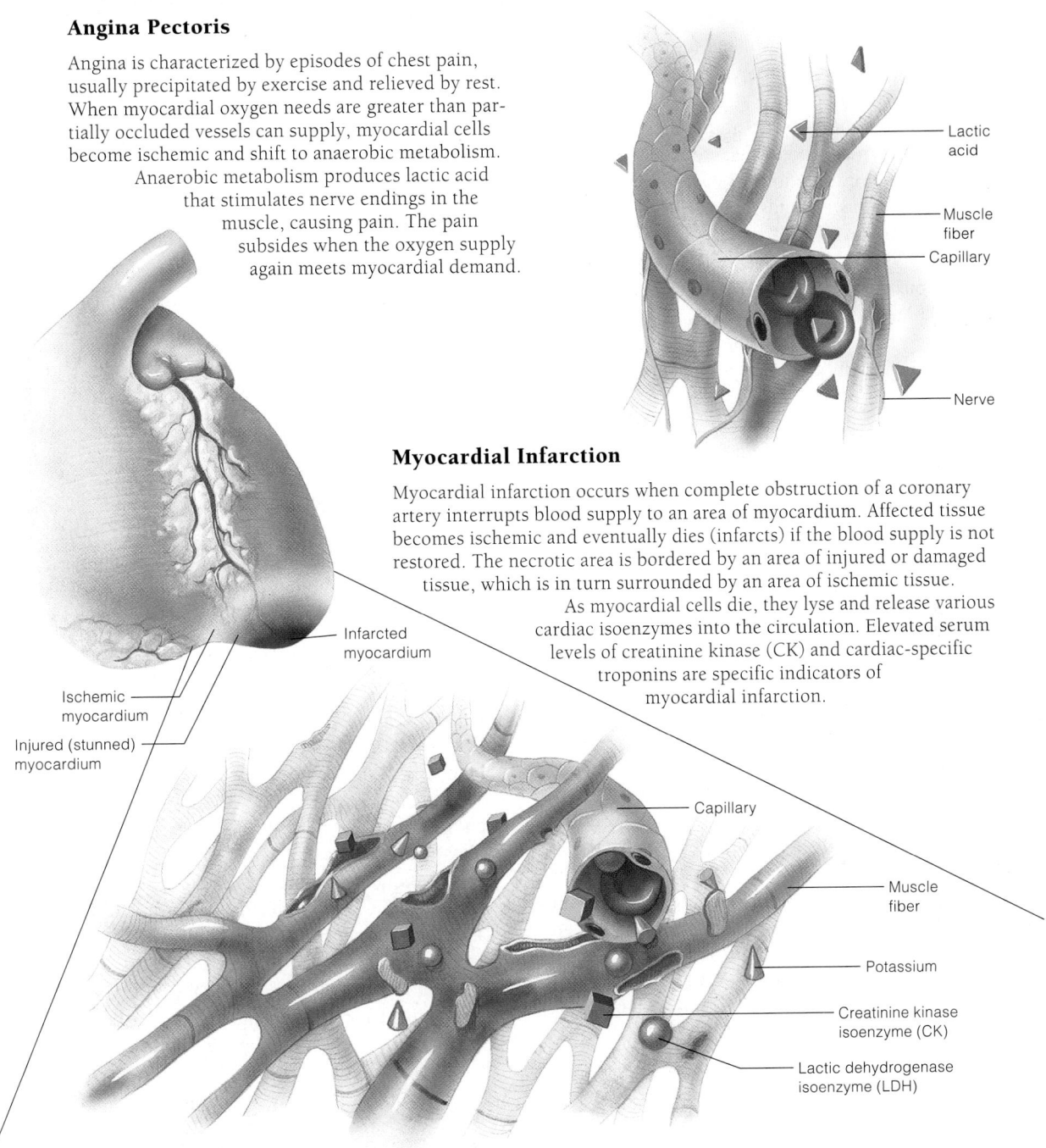

## PATHOPHYSIOLOGY

### Atherosclerosis

Coronary atherosclerosis is the most common cause of reduced coronary blood flow. **Atherosclerosis** is a progressive disease characterized by *atheroma* (plaque) formation, which affects the intimal and medial layers of large and midsize arteries. See *Pathophysiology Illustrated,* above.

Atherosclerosis is initiated by unknown precipitating factors that cause lipoproteins and fibrous tissue to accumulate in the arterial wall. Although the precise mechanisms are unknown, the most accepted theory is that atherosclerosis begins with an injury to or inflammation of endothelial cells lining the artery. Endothelial damage promotes platelet adhesion and aggregation, and attracts leukocytes to the area.

At the injury site, *atherogenic* (atherosclerosis-promoting) lipoproteins collect in the intimal lining of the artery. Macrophages migrate to the injured site as part of the inflammatory process. Contact with platelets, cholesterol, and other blood components stimulates smooth muscle cells and connective tissue within the vessel wall to proliferate abnormally. Although blood flow is not affected at this stage, this early lesion appears as a yellowish fatty streak on the inner lining of the artery. Fibrous plaque develops as smooth muscle cells enlarge, collagen fibers proliferate, and blood lipids accumulate. The lesion protrudes into the arterial lumen and is fixed to the inner wall of the intima. It may invade the muscular media layer of the vessel as well. The developing plaque not only gradually occludes the vessel lumen but also impairs the vessel's ability to dilate in response to increased oxygen demands. Fibrous plaque lesions often develop at arterial bifurcations or curves or in areas of narrowing. As the plaque expands, it can produce severe stenosis or total occlusion of the artery.

The final stage of the process is the development of *atheromas,* complex lesions consisting of lipids, fibrous tissue, collagen, calcium, cellular debris, and capillaries. These calcified lesions can ulcerate or rupture, stimulating thrombosis. The vessel lumen may be rapidly occluded by the thrombus, or it may embolize to occlude a distal vessel.

Plaque formation may be *eccentric,* located in a specific, asymmetric region of the vessel wall, or *concentric,* involving the entire vessel circumference. Manifestations of the process usually do not appear until about 75% of the arterial lumen has been occluded.

## Myocardial Ischemia

Myocardial cells become ischemic when the oxygen supply is inadequate to meet metabolic demands. The critical factors in meeting metabolic demands of cardiac cells are coronary perfusion and myocardial workload (Copstead & Banasik, 2000). The oxygen content of the blood is a contributing factor. Table 29–3 lists factors that may lead to myocardial ischemia.

Myocardial cells have limited supplies of adenosine triphosphate (ATP) for energy storage. When myocardial workload increases or the supply of blood and oxygen falls, cellular ATP stores are quickly depleted, affecting their contractility. Cellular metabolism switches from an efficient aerobic process to anaerobic metabolism. Lactic acid accumulates, and cells are damaged. If blood flow is restored within 20 minutes, aerobic metabolism and contractility are restored, and cellular repair begins (McCance & Huether, 2002). Continued ischemia results in cell necrosis and death (infarction).

Coronary heart disease is generally divided into two categories, chronic ischemic heart disease and acute coronary syndromes. *Chronic ischemic heart disease* includes stable and vasospastic angina, and silent myocardial ischemia. *Acute coronary syndromes* range from unstable angina to myocardial infarction (Porth, 2002). These disorders are discussed in the following sections of this chapter.

## COLLABORATIVE CARE

Care of clients with coronary heart disease focuses on aggressive risk factor management to slow the atherosclerotic process and maintain myocardial perfusion. Until manifestations of chronic or acute ischemia are experienced, the diagnosis often is presumptive, based on history and the presence of risk factors.

### Diagnostic Tests

Laboratory testing is used to assess for risk factors such as an abnormal blood lipid profile (elevated triglyceride and LDL levels and decreased HDL levels).

- *Total serum cholesterol* is elevated in hyperlipidemia. A *lipid profile* includes triglyceride, HDL, and LDL levels as well, and enables calculation of the ratio of HDL to total cholesterol. The ratio should be at least 1:5, with 1:3 being the ideal ratio. Elevated lipid levels are associated with an increased risk of atherosclerosis (see Table 29–2). For the most accurate results, dietary cholesterol intake should be consistent for 3 weeks prior to testing, and the client should fast for 10 to 12 hours before the sample is drawn. Alcohol intake and many medications can affect results.

Diagnostic tests to identify subclinical (asymptomatic) CHD may be indicated when multiple risk factors are present.

- *C-reactive protein* is a serum protein associated with inflammatory processes. Recent evidence suggests that elevated blood levels of this protein may be predictive of CHD.
- The *ankle-brachial blood pressure index (ABI)* is an inexpensive, noninvasive test for peripheral vascular disease that may be predictive of CHD. See Chapter 33 ⟳ for more information about this test.
- *Exercise ECG testing* may be performed. ECGs are used to assess the response to increased cardiac workload induced by exercise. The test is considered "positive" for CHD if myocardial ischemia is detected on the ECG (depression of the ST segment by greater than 3 mm; see Figure 29–1), the client develops chest pain, or the test is stopped due to excess fatigue, dysrhythmias, or other symptoms before the predicted maximal heart rate is achieved.
- *Electron beam computed tomography (EBCT)* creates a three-dimensional image of the heart and coronary arteries that can reveal plaque and other abnormalities. This noninvasive test requires no special preparation, and can identify clients at risk for developing myocardial ischemia.

| TABLE 29–3 Factors Contributing to Myocardial Ischemia | | |
|---|---|---|
| **Coronary Perfusion** | **Myocardial Workload** | **Blood Oxygen Content** |
| • Atherosclerosis<br>• Thrombosis<br>• Vasospasm<br>• Poor perfusion pressure | • Rapid heart rate<br>• Increased preload, afterload, or contractility<br>• Increased metabolic demands (e.g., hyperthyroidism) | • Reduced atmospheric oxygen pressure<br>• Impaired gas exchange<br>• Low red blood cells and hemoglobin content |

- *Myocardial perfusion imaging* (see the section on angina that follows) may be used to evaluate myocardial blood flow and perfusion, both at rest and during stress testing (exercise or mental stress). These diagnostic tests are further explained in the section on angina. Perfusion imaging studies are costly, and therefore not recommended for routine CHD risk assessment.

## Risk Factor Management

Conservative management of CHD focuses on risk factor modification, including smoking, diet, exercise, and management of contributing conditions.

### Smoking

Smoking cessation rapidly reduces the risk for CHD and improves cardiovascular status. People who quit reduce their risk by 50%, regardless of how long they smoked before quitting. For women, the risk becomes equivalent to a non-smoker within 3 to 5 years of smoking cessation (Woods et al., 2000). In addition, stopping smoking improves HDL levels, lowers LDL levels, and reduces blood viscosity. All smokers are advised to quit. Health promotion activities focus on preventing children, teenagers, and adults from starting to smoke.

### Diet

Dietary recommendations by the National Cholesterol Education Program (2001) include reduced saturated fat and cholesterol intake, and strategies to lower LDL levels (Table 29–4). Most fats are a mixture of saturated and unsaturated fatty acids. The highest proportions of saturated fat are found in whole-milk products, red meats, and coconut oil. Nonfat dairy products, fish, and poultry as primary protein sources are recommended. Solidified vegetable fats (e.g., margarine, shortening) contain *trans* fatty acids, which behave more like saturated fats. Soft margarines and vegetable oil spreads contain low levels of

trans fatty acids, and should be used instead of butter, stick margarine, and shortening. Monounsaturated fats, found in olive, canola, and peanut oils, actually lower LDL and cholesterol levels. Certain cold-water fish, such as tuna, salmon, and mackerel, contain high levels of omega-3 (or n-3) fatty acids, which help raise HDL levels, and decrease serum triglycerides, total serum cholesterol, and blood pressure.

In addition, increased intake of soluble fiber (found in oats, psyllium, pectin-rich fruit, and beans) and insoluble fiber (found in whole grains, vegetables, and fruit) is recommended. Folic acid and vitamins $B_6$ and $B_{12}$ affect homocystine metabolism, reducing serum levels. Leafy green vegetables (e.g., spinach and broccoli) and legumes (e.g., black-eyed peas, dried beans, and lentils) are rich sources of folate. Meat, fish, and poultry are rich in vitamins $B_6$ and $B_{12}$. Vitamin $B_6$ also is found in soy products; $B_{12}$ is in fortified cereals. Increased intake of antioxidant nutrients (vitamin E, in particular) and foods rich in antioxidants (fruits and vegetables) appears to increase HDL levels and have a protective effect on CHD.

In middle-aged and older adults, moderate alcohol intake may reduce the risk for CHD (National Cholesterol Education Program, 2001). Consumption of no more than two drinks per day for men or one drink per day for women is recommended. A drink is 5 ounces of wine, 12 ounces of beer, or 1 1/2 ounces of whiskey. People who do not drink alcohol, however, should not be encouraged to start consuming it as a heart-protective measure.

People who are overweight or obese are encouraged to lose weight through a combination of reduced calorie intake (maintaining a nutritionally sound diet) and increased exercise. High-protein, high-fat weight loss programs are not recommended for weight reduction.

### Exercise

Regular physical exercise reduces the risk for CHD in several ways. It lowers VLDL, LDL, and triglyceride levels, and raises HDL levels. Regular exercise reduces the blood pressure and insulin resistance. Unless contraindicated, all clients are encouraged to participate in at least 30 minutes of moderate-intensity physical activity 5 to 6 days each week.

### Hypertension

Although hypertension often cannot be prevented or cured, it can be controlled. Hypertension control (maintaining a blood pressure lower than 140/90 mmHg) is vital to reduce its atherosclerosis-promoting effects and to reduce the workload of the heart. Management strategies include reducing sodium intake, increasing calcium intake, regular exercise, stress management, and medications. Hypertension management is discussed in Chapter 33. 🔗

### Diabetes

Diabetes increases the risk of CHD by accelerating the atherosclerotic process. Weight loss (if appropriate), reduced fat intake, and exercise are particularly important for the diabetic client. Because hyperglycemia apparently also contributes to atherosclerosis, consistent blood glucose management is vital.

TABLE 29–4 Dietary Recommendations to Reduce Total Cholesterol, LDL Levels, and CHD Risk

| Nutrient | Recommendation |
| --- | --- |
| Total fat | 25%–35% of total calories |
| • Saturated fats | • <7% of total calories |
| • Polyunsaturated fat | • Up to 10% of total calories |
| • Monounsaturated fat | • Up to 20% of total calories |
| • Cholesterol | • <200 mg/day |
| Carbohydrate (primarily complex carbohydrates, such as whole grains, fruits, and vegetables) | 50%–60% of total calories |
| Dietary fiber | 20–30 g/day |
| Protein | About 15% of total calories |

*Note: Compiled from* Adult Treatment Panel III Report *by the National Cholesterol Education Program, 2001.*

## Medications

Drug therapy to lower total serum cholesterol and LDL levels and to raise HDL levels now is an integral part of CHD management. It is used in conjunction with diet and other lifestyle changes, and is based on the client's overall risk for CHD.

Drugs used to treat hyperlipidemia act specifically by lowering LDL levels. The goal of treatment is to achieve an LDL level of < 130 mg/dL. Medications to treat hyperlipidemia are not inexpensive; the cost–benefit ratio needs to be considered, as long-term treatment may be required. The four major classes of cholesterol-lowering drugs are statins, bile acid sequestrants, nicotinic acid, and fibrates. The nursing implications and client teaching for these drug classes are outlined in the Medication Administration box on the next page.

The statins, including lovastatin (Mevacor), pravastatin (Pravachol), simvastatin (Zocor), and others, are first-line drugs for treating hyperlipidemia. They effectively lower LDL levels and may also increase in HDL levels. The statins can cause myopathy; all clients are instructed to report muscle pain and weakness or brown urine. Liver function tests are monitored during therapy, as these drugs may increase liver enzyme levels.

The other cholesterol-lowering drugs, such as the bile acid sequestrants, nicotinic acid, and fibrates, are primarily used when combination therapy is required to effectively lower serum cholesterol levels. They also may be used for selected clients, such as younger adults, women who wish to become pregnant, or to specifically lower triglyceride levels.

Clients at high risk for MI are often started on prophylactic low-dose aspirin therapy. The dose ranges from 80 to 325 mg/day (Tierney et al., 2001). Aspirin is contraindicated, however, for clients who have a history of aspirin sensitivity, bleeding disorders, or active peptic ulcer disease. Angiotensin-converting enzyme (ACE) inhibitors also may be prescribed for high-risk clients, including diabetics with other CHD risk factors.

## Complementary Therapies

Diet and exercise programs that emphasize physical conditioning and a low-fat diet rich in antioxidants have been shown to be effective in managing CHD (Box 29–2). Supplements of vitamins C, E, $B_6$, and $B_{12}$, and folic acid may be beneficial. Other potentially helpful complementary therapies include herbals such as ginkgo biloba, garlic, curcumin, and green tea; and consumption of red wine, foods containing bioflavonoids, and nuts. Behavioral therapies of benefit for clients with CHD include relaxation and stress management, guided imagery, treatment of depression, anger/hostility management, and meditation, tai chi, and yoga.

## NURSING CARE

### Health Promotion

Present information about healthy lifestyle habits to community and religious groups, school children (grades K through 12), and through the print media. In promoting healthy lifestyle habits, nurses can positively affect the incidence, morbidity, and mortality from CHD.

---

**BOX 29–2 ■ Complementary Therapies: Diet for CHD**

Two diet programs have been shown to have a beneficial effect on CHD. The *Pritikin diet* is basically vegetarian, high in complex carbohydrates and fiber, low in cholesterol, and extremely low in fat (< 10% of daily calories). Egg whites and limited amounts of nonfat dairy or soy products are allowed. The Pritikin program requires 45 minutes of walking daily and recommends multivitamin supplements, including vitamins C and E and folate.

The *Ornish diet* also is vegetarian, although egg whites and a cup of nonfat milk or yogurt per day are allowed. No oil or fat is permitted, even for cooking. Two ounces of alcohol a day are permitted. The Ornish program also calls for stress reduction, emotional social support systems, daily stretching, and walking for 1 hour three times a week.

---

Strongly encourage all clients to avoid smoking in the first place, and to stop all forms of tobacco use. Discuss the adverse effects of smoking and the benefits of quitting. Provide information about dietary recommendations to maintain a healthy weight and optimal cholesterol levels. Discuss the benefits and importance of regular exercise. Finally, encourage clients with cardiovascular risk factors to undergo regular screening for hypertension, diabetes, and hyperlipidemia.

### Assessment

Nursing assessment for CHD focuses on identifying risk factors.

- Health history: current manifestations such as chest pain or heaviness, shortness of breath, weakness; current diet, exercise patterns, and medications; smoking history and pattern of alcohol intake; history of heart disease, hypertension, or diabetes; family history of CHD or other cardiac problems
- Physical examination: current weight and its appropriateness for height; body mass index; waist-to-hip ratio; blood pressure; strength and equality of peripheral pulses

### Nursing Diagnoses and Interventions
#### Imbalanced Nutrition: More than Body Requirements

This nursing diagnosis may be appropriate for clients who are obese, have a waist-to-hip ratio greater than 0.8 (female) or 0.9 (male), or whose diet history or serum cholesterol levels indicate a need to reduce fat and cholesterol intake. See Chapters 19 and 20 ⬡⬡ for more information about assessing obesity.

- Encourage assessment of food intake and eating patterns to help identify areas that can be improved. *Clients often are unaware of their fat and cholesterol intake, particularly when many meals are eaten away from home. Careful assessment increases awareness and allows the client to make conscious changes.*
- Discuss American Heart Association and therapeutic lifestyle change (TLC) dietary recommendations, emphasizing the role of diet in heart disease. Provide guidance regarding specific food choices with healthy alternatives. *Specific diet information and suggestions help the client make better food choices.*

# Medication Administration
## Cholesterol-Lowering Drugs

### STATINS

Lovastatin (Mevacor)
Pravastatin (Pravachol)
Simvastatin (Zocor)
Fluvastatin (Lescol)
Atorvastatin (Lipitor)

Statins inhibit the enzyme HMG-CoA reductase in the liver, lowering LDL synthesis and serum levels. The statins are first-line treatment for elevated LDL, used in conjunction with diet and lifestyle changes. Although their side effects are minimal, they may cause increased serum liver enzyme levels and myopathy.

### Nursing Responsibilities

- Monitor serum cholesterol and liver enzyme levels before and during therapy. Report elevated liver enzyme levels.
- Assess for muscle pain and tenderness. Monitor CPK level if present.
- If taking digoxin concurrently, monitor for and report digoxin toxicity.

### Client and Family Teaching

- Promptly report muscle pain, tenderness, or weakness; skin rash or hives, or changes in skin color; abdominal pain, nausea, or vomiting.
- Do not use these drugs if you are pregnant or plan to become pregnant.
- Inform your doctor if you are taking any other medications concurrently.

### BILE ACID SEQUESTRANTS

Cholestyramine (Questran)
Colestipol (Colestid)
Colesevelam (Welchol)

Bile acid sequestrants lower LDL levels by binding bile acids in the intestine, reducing its reabsorption and cholesterol production in the liver. They are used in combination therapy regimens and for women who are considering pregnancy. Their primary disadvantages are inconvenience of administration due to bulk and gastrointestinal side effects such as constipation.

### Nursing Responsibilities

- Mix cholestyramine and colestipol powders with 4 to 6 oz of water or juice; administer once or twice a day as ordered with meals.
- Store in a tightly closed container.

### Client and Family Teaching

- Promptly report constipation, severe gastric distress with nausea and vomiting, unexplained weight loss, black or bloody stools, or sudden back pain to your doctor.
- Drinking ample amounts of fluid while taking these drugs reduces problems of constipation and bloating.
- Do not omit doses as this may affect the absorption of other drugs you are taking.

### NICOTINIC ACID

Niacin (Nicobid, Nicolar, Niaspan, others)

Nicotinic acid in both prescription and nonprescription forms lowers total and LDL cholesterol and triglyceride levels. The crystalline form and Niaspan, a prescription extended release tablet, also raise HDL levels. Because the doses required to achieve significant cholesterol-lowering effects are associated with multiple side effects, nicotinic acid generally is used in combination therapy, particularly with the statin drugs.

### Nursing Responsibilities

- Give oral preparations with meals and accompanied by a cold beverage to minimize GI effects.
- Administer with caution to clients with active liver disease, peptic ulcer disease, gout, or type 2 diabetes.
- Monitor blood glucose, uric acid levels, and liver function tests during treatment.

### Client and Family Teaching

- Flushing of face, neck, and ears may occur within 2 hours following dose; these effects generally subside as treatment continues. Alcohol use during nicotinic acid therapy may worsen this effect.
- Report weakness or dizziness with changes in posture (lying to sitting; sitting to standing) to your doctor. Change positions slowly to reduce the risk of injury.

### FIBRIC ACID DERIVATIVES

Gemfibrozil (Lopid)
Fenofibrate (Tricor)
Clofibrate (Atromid-S)

The fibrates are used to lower serum triglyceride levels; they have only a slight to modest effect on LDL. They affect lipid regulation by blocking triglyceride synthesis. They are used to treat very high triglyceride levels, and may be used in combination with statins.

### Nursing Responsibilities

- Monitor serum LDL and VLDL levels, electrolytes, glucose, liver enzymes, renal function tests, and CBC during therapy. Report abnormal values.
- Up to 2 months of treatment may be required to achieve a therapeutic effect; rebound, with decreasing benefit, may occur in the second or third month of treatment.

### Client and Family Teaching

- Take with meals if the drug causes gastric distress.
- Promptly report flulike symptoms (fatigue, muscle aching, soreness, or weakness) to your doctor.
- Do not use this drug if you are pregnant or plan to become pregnant. Use reliable birth control measures while taking this drug.
- Contact your doctor before stopping this drug and before taking any over-the-counter preparations.

- Refer to clinical dietitian for diet planning and further teaching. Suggest cookbooks that offer low-fat recipes to encourage healthier eating, and provide American Heart Association and American Cancer Society recipe pamphlets and information on low-fat eating. *These resources provide tools for the client to use as eating patterns change.*
- Encourage gradual but progressive dietary changes. *Drastic changes in eating patterns may cause frustration and discourage the client from maintaining a healthy diet over the long term.*
- Discourage use of high-fat, low-carbohydrate, or other fad diets for weight loss. *These diets may adversely affect serum cholesterol and triglyceride levels, and often are too drastic to maintain over the long term.*
- Encourage reasonable goals for weight loss (e.g., 1.0 to 1.5 lb per week and a 10% weight loss over 6 months). Provide information about weight loss programs and support groups such as Weight Watchers and Take Off Pounds Sensibly (TOPS). *Gradual but steady weight loss is more likely to be sustained. Recognized programs that emphasize healthy eating provide support and incentive for making lifetime dietary changes.*

### Ineffective Health Maintenance

Clients with risk factors for CHD may be unable to identify or independently manage their risk factors.

- Discuss risk factors for CHD, stressing that changing or managing those factors that can be modified reduces the client's overall risk for the disease. *Clients with significant nonmodifiable risk factors may be discouraged, reducing their ability to eliminate or control modifiable risk factors.*
- Discuss the immediate benefits of smoking cessation. Provide resource materials from the American Heart Association, the American Lung Association, and the American Cancer Society. Refer to a structured smoking cessation program to increase the likelihood of success in quitting. *Long-time smokers may assume that the damage from smoking has already been done, and quitting would not be "worth the price."*
- Help the client identify specific sources of psychosocial and physical support for smoking cessation, dietary, and lifestyle changes. *Support persons, groups, and aids such as nicotine patches help the client achieve success and provide encouragement during difficult times (such as withdrawal symptoms).*
- Discuss the benefits of regular exercise for cardiovascular health and weight loss. Help identify favorite forms of exercise or physical activity. Encourage planning for 30 minutes of continuous aerobic activity (i.e., walking, running, bicycling, swimming) four to five times a week. Encourage identification of an "exercise buddy" to help maintain motivation. *Engaging in preferred activities with a partner maintains motivation and increases the likelihood of maintaining an exercise program. Encourage continuation of the plan, even when days are missed. Exercise is cumulative, so increasing the duration of exercise on subsequent days can "make up" for a lost day.*
- Provide information and teaching about prescribed medications such as cholesterol-lowering drugs. Discuss the rela-

tionship between hypertension, diabetes, and CHD. *Teaching is important to promote understanding of and compliance with the prescribed drug regimen.*

## Home Care

Encourage participation in some form of cardiac rehabilitation program. Formal programs provide comprehensive assessment of, interventions for, and teaching of clients with cardiac disease. Monitored exercise and information about risk factors help clients identify ways to lower their risk for CHD.

Because clients themselves are primarily responsible for maintaining the lifestyle changes necessary to reduce the risk of CHD, provide teaching and support as outlined in the previous section. Assist the client to make healthy choices and reinforce positive changes. Emphasize the importance of regular follow-up appointments to monitor progress.

## THE CLIENT WITH ANGINA PECTORIS

**Angina pectoris,** or *angina,* is chest pain resulting from reduced coronary blood flow, which causes a temporary imbalance between myocardial blood supply and demand. The imbalance may be due to coronary heart disease, atherosclerosis, or vessel constriction that impairs myocardial blood supply. Hypermetabolic conditions such as exercise, thyrotoxicosis, stimulant abuse (e.g., cocaine), hyperthyroidism, and emotional stress can increase myocardial oxygen demand, precipitating angina. Anemia, heart failure, or pulmonary diseases may affect blood and oxygen supplies as well, causing angina.

## PATHOPHYSIOLOGY

The imbalance between myocardial blood supply and demand causes temporary and reversible myocardial ischemia. **Ischemia,** deficient blood flow to tissue, may be caused by partial obstruction of a coronary artery, coronary artery spasm, or a thrombus. Obstruction of a coronary artery deprives cells in the region of the heart normally supplied by that vessel of oxygen and nutrients needed for metabolic processes. Cellular processes are compromised. Reduced oxygen causes cells to switch from aerobic metabolism to anaerobic metabolism. Anaerobic metabolism causes lactic acid to build up in the cells. It also affects cell membrane permeability, releasing substances such as histamine, kinins, and specific enzymes that stimulate terminal nerve fibers in the cardiac muscle and send pain impulses to the central nervous system. The pain radiates to the upper body because the heart shares the same dermatome as this region. Return of adequate circulation provides the nutrients needed by cells, and clears the waste products. More than 30 minutes of ischemia irreversibly damages myocardial cells (necrosis).

Three types of angina have been identified:

- *Stable angina* is the most common and predictable form of angina. It occurs with a predictable amount of activity or stress, and is a common manifestation of CHD. Stable angina usually occurs when the work of the heart is increased by physical exertion, exposure to cold, or by stress. Stable angina is relieved by rest and nitrates.

- *Prinzmetal's (variant) angina* is atypical angina that occurs unpredictably (unrelated to activity), and often at night. It is caused by coronary artery spasm with or without an atherosclerotic lesion. The exact mechanism of coronary artery spasm is unknown. It may result from hyperactive sympathetic nervous system responses, altered calcium flow in smooth muscle, or reduced prostaglandins to promote vasodilation.
- *Unstable angina* occurs with increasing frequency, severity, and duration. Pain is unpredictable and occurs with decreasing levels of activity or stress and may occur at rest. Clients with unstable angina are at risk for myocardial infarction.
- *Silent myocardial ischemia,* or asymptomatic ischemia, is thought to be common in people with CHD. Silent ischemia may occur with either activity or with mental stress. Mental stress increases the heart rate and blood pressure, increasing myocardial oxygen demand (McCance & Huether, 2002).

## MANIFESTATIONS

The cardinal manifestation of angina is chest pain. The pain typically is precipitated by an identifiable event, such as physical activity, strong emotion, stress, eating a heavy meal, or exposure to cold. The classic sequence of angina is activity–pain, rest–relief. The client may describe the pain as a tight, squeezing, heavy pressure, or constricting sensation. It characteristically begins beneath the sternum and may radiate to the jaw, neck, or arm. Less characteristically, the pain may be felt in the jaw, epigastric region, or back. Anginal pain usually lasts less than 15 minutes and is relieved by rest. Additional manifestations of angina include dyspnea, pallor, tachycardia, and great anxiety and fear. The manifestations of angina are summarized in the box below.

## COLLABORATIVE CARE

Acute angina care focuses on relieving pain and restoring coronary blood flow. Long-term management is directed at the causes of impaired myocardial blood supply. As for CHD, risk factor management is a vital component of care for the client with angina (see the preceding section of this chapter).

### Manifestations of Angina

- Chest pain: Substernal or precordial (across the chest wall); may radiate to neck, arms, shoulders, or jaw
- Quality: Tight, squeezing, constricting, or heavy sensation; may also be described as burning, aching, choking, dull, or constant
- Associated manifestations: Dyspnea, pallor, tachycardia, anxiety, and fear
- Precipitating factors: Exercise or activity, strong emotion, stress, cold, heavy meal
- Relieving factors: Rest, position change; nitroglycerine

## Diagnostic Tests

The diagnosis of angina is based on past medical history and family history, a comprehensive description of the chest pain, and physical assessment findings. Laboratory tests may confirm the presence of risk factors, such as an abnormal blood lipid profile and elevated blood glucose. Diagnostic tests provide information about overall cardiac function.

Common diagnostic tests to assess for coronary heart disease and angina include electrocardiography, stress testing, nuclear medicine studies, echocardiography (ultrasound), and coronary angiography.

### Electrocardiography

A resting ECG may be normal, may show nonspecific changes in the ST segment and T wave, or may show evidence of previous myocardial infarction. Characteristic ECG changes are seen during anginal episodes. During periods of ischemia, the ST segment is depressed or downsloping, and the T wave may flatten or invert (Figure 29–1 ■). These changes reverse when ischemia is relieved. For more details about the ECG, its waveforms, and its uses, see the section of this chapter about dysrhythmias.

### Stress Electrocardiography

Stress electrocardiography (exercise stress test) uses ECGs to monitor the cardiac response to an increased workload during progressive exercise. See the previous section on coronary heart disease for more information about exercise stress tests.

### Radionuclide Testing

Radionuclide testing is a safe, noninvasive technique to evaluate myocardial perfusion and left ventricular function. The

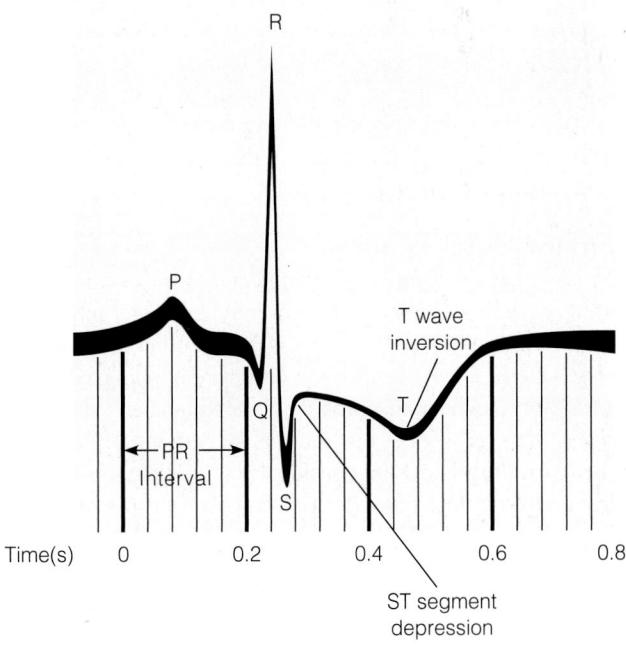

**Figure 29–1** ■ ECG changes during an episode of angina. Note characteristic T wave inversion and ST segment depression of myocardial ischemia.

amount of radioisotope injected is very small; no special radiation precautions are required during or after the scan. Thallium-201 or a technetium-based radiocompound is injected intravenously, and the heart is scanned with a radiation detector. Ischemic or infarcted cells of the myocardium do not take up the substance normally, appearing as a "cold spot" on the scan. If the ischemia is transient, these spots gradually fill in, indicating the reversibility of the process. With severe ischemia or a myocardial infarction, these areas may remain devoid of radioactivity.

Left ventricular function can also be evaluated. Whereas the ejection fraction, or portion of blood ejected from the left ventricle during systole, normally increases during exercise, it may actually decrease in coronary heart disease and stress-induced ischemia.

Radionuclide testing may be combined with pharmacologic stress testing for clients who are physically unable to exercise or to detect subclinical myocardial ischemia. A vasodilator is injected to induce the same ischemic changes that occur with exercise in the diseased heart. Coronary arteries unaffected by atherosclerosis dilate in response to the drugs, increasing blood flow to already well-perfused tissue. This reduces flow to ischemic muscle, called *myocardial steal syndrome.*

### Echocardiography

*Echocardiography* is a noninvasive test that uses ultrasound to evaluate cardiac structure and function. High-frequency sound waves emitted from a transducer are reflected off of heart structures back to the transducer as echoes. These echoes are displayed on a screen. Echocardiography is usually performed with the transducer held to the chest wall. It may be done at rest, during supine exercise, or immediately following upright exercise to evaluate movement of the myocardial wall and assess for possible ischemia or infarction.

*Transesophageal echocardiography (TEE)* uses ultrasound to identify abnormal blood flow patterns as well as cardiac structures. In TEE, the probe is on the tip of an endoscope inserted into the esophagus, positioning it close to the posterior heart (especially the left atrium and the aorta). It avoids interference by breasts, ribs, or lungs.

### Coronary Angiography

*Coronary angiography* is the gold standard for evaluating the coronary arteries. Guided by fluoroscopy, a catheter introduced into the femoral or brachial artery is threaded into the coronary artery. Dye is injected into each coronary opening, allowing visualization of the main coronary branches and any abnormalities, such as stenosis or obstruction. Narrowing of the vessel lumen by more than 50% is considered significant; most lesions that cause symptoms involve more than 70% narrowing. Vessel obstructions are noted on a coronary artery "map" that provides a guide for tracking disease progression and for elective treatment with angioplasty or cardiac surgery. During angiogram, the drug ergonovine maleate may be injected to induce coronary artery spasm and diagnose Prinzmetal's angina. Nursing care of the client undergoing a coronary angiogram is summarized in the box on the next page.

## Medications

Drugs may be used for both acute and long-term relief of angina. The goal of drug treatment is to reduce oxygen demand and increase oxygen supply to the myocardium. Three main classes of drugs are used to treat angina: nitrates, beta blockers, and calcium channel blockers.

### Nitrates

Nitrates, including nitroglycerin and longer-acting nitrate preparations, are used to treat acute anginal attacks and prevent angina.

Sublingual nitroglycerin is the drug of choice to treat acute angina. It acts within 1 to 2 minutes, decreasing myocardial work and oxygen demand through venous and arterial dilation, which in turn reduce preload and afterload. It may also improve myocardial oxygen supply by dilating collateral blood vessels and reducing stenosis. Rapid-acting nitroglycerin is also available as a buccal spray in a metered system. For some clients, this may be easier to handle than small nitroglycerin tablets.

Longer-acting nitroglycerin preparations (oral tablets, ointment, or transdermal patches) are used to prevent attacks of angina, not to treat an acute attack. The primary problem with long-term nitrate use is the development of *tolerance,* a decreasing effect from the same dose of medication. Tolerance can be limited by a dosing schedule that allows a nitrate-free period of at least 8 to 10 hours daily. This is usually scheduled at night, when angina is less likely to occur.

Headache is a common side effect of nitrates, and may limit their usefulness. Nausea, dizziness, and hypotension are also common effects of therapy.

### Beta Blockers

Beta blockers, including propranolol, metoprolol, nadolol, and atenolol, are considered first-line drugs to treat stable angina. They block the cardiac-stimulating effects of norepinephrine and epinephrine, preventing anginal attacks by reducing heart rate, myocardial contractility, and blood pressure, thus reducing myocardial oxygen demand. Beta blockers may be used alone or with other medications to prevent angina.

Beta blockers are contraindicated for clients with asthma or severe COPD (see Chapter 36 ⌾ ) because they may cause severe bronchospasm. They are not used in clients with significant bradycardia, or AV conduction blocks, and are used cautiously in heart failure, Beta blockers are not used to treat Prinzmetal's angina because they may make it worse.

### Calcium Channel Blockers

Calcium channel blockers reduce myocardial oxygen demand and increase myocardial blood and oxygen supply. These drugs, which include verapamil, diltiazem, and nifedipine, lower blood pressure, reduce myocardial contractility, and, in some cases, lower the heart rate, decreasing myocardial oxygen demand. They are also potent coronary vasodilators, effectively increasing oxygen supply. Like beta blockers, calcium channel blockers act too slowly to effectively treat an acute attack of angina; they are used for long-term prophylaxis. Because they may actually increase ischemia and mortality in clients with heart failure or left ventricular dysfunction, these drugs are not usually prescribed in

## NURSING CARE  OF THE CLIENT HAVING CORONARY ANGIOGRAPHY

### PREOPERATIVE CARE

- Assess the client's and family's knowledge and understanding of the procedure. Provide additional information as needed. Explain that the client will be awake during the procedure, which takes 1 to 2 hours to complete. A sensation of warmth (a "hot flash") and a metallic taste may occur as the dye is injected. A rapid pulse or a few "skipped beats," also are common and expected during the procedure. *A good understanding of the procedure and expected sensations reduces anxiety and improves cooperation during the procedure.*

- Provide routine preoperative care as ordered (see Chapter 7). *Although the client remains awake, sedation may be given. Signed consent is required, and preprocedure fasting may be ordered.*

- Administer ordered cardiac medications with a small sip of water unless contraindicated. *Regularly ordered medications are continued to prevent cardiac compromise or dysrhythmias during the procedure.*

- Assess for hypersensitivity to iodine, radiologic contrast media, or seafood. *An iodine-based radiologic contrast dye is typically used for an angiogram. Iodine or seafood allergy increases the risk for anaphylaxis and requires an alternative dye or special precautions.*

- Record baseline assessment data, including vital signs, height, and weight. Mark the locations of peripheral pulses; document their equality and amplitude. *The data provide a baseline for evaluating changes after the procedure.*

- Instruct to void prior to going to the cardiac catheterization laboratory, *to promote comfort.*

### POSTOPERATIVE CARE

- Assess vital signs, catheterization site for bleeding or hematoma, peripheral pulses, and neurovascular status every 15 minutes for first hour, every 30 minutes for the next hour, then hourly for 4 hours or until discharge. *The data provide vital information about the client's status and potential complications such as bleeding, hematoma, or thrombus formation.*

- Maintain bed rest as ordered, usually for 6 hours if the femoral artery is used, or 2 to 3 hours if the brachial site is used. The head of the bed may be raised to 30 degrees. *Bed rest reduces movement of and pressure in the affected artery, reducing the risk of bleeding or hematoma.*

- Keep a pressure dressing, sandbag, or ice pack in place over the arterial access site. Check frequently for bleeding (if the access site is in the groin, check for bleeding under the buttocks). *Arteries are high-pressure systems. The risk for significant bleeding after an invasive procedure is high.*

- Instruct to avoid flexing or hyperextending the affected extremity for 12 to 24 hours. *Minimizing movement of the affected joint allows the artery to effectively seal and promotes blood flow, reducing the risk of bleeding, hematoma, or thrombus formation.*

- Unless contraindicated, encourage liberal fluid intake. *An increased fluid intake promotes excretion of the contrast medium, reducing the risk of toxicity (particularly to the kidneys).*

- Promptly report diminished peripheral pulses, formation of a new hematoma or enlargement of an existing one, severe pain at the insertion site or in the affected extremity, chest pain, or dyspnea. *While the risk of complications is low, myocardial infarction or insertion site complications may occur. These necessitate prompt intervention.*

- Provide instructions about dressing changes, follow-up appointments, and potential complications prior to discharge.

---

the initial treatment of angina. They are used cautiously in clients with dysrhythmias, heart failure, or hypotension.

The nursing implications of antianginal medications are summarized in the Medication Administration box on page 818.

### Aspirin

The client with angina, particularly unstable angina, is at risk for myocardial infarction because of significant narrowing of the coronary arteries. Low-dose aspirin (80 to 325 mg/day) is often prescribed to reduce the risk of platelet aggregation and thrombus formation.

### Revascularization Procedures

Several procedures may be used to restore blood flow and oxygen to ischemic tissue. Nonsurgical techniques include transluminal coronary angioplasty, laser angioplasty, coronary atherectomy, and intracoronary stents. Coronary artery bypass grafting (CABG) is a surgical procedure that may be used.

### Percutaneous Coronary Revascularization

*Percutaneous coronary revascularization (PCR)* are procedures used to restore blood flow to the ischemic myocardium in clients with CHD. Approximately 600,000 PCR procedures are done annually in the United States. PCR is used to treat clients with:

- Moderately severe, chronic stable angina unrelieved by medical therapy.
- Mild angina but objective evidence of coronary ischemia.
- Unstable angina.
- Acute myocardial infarction (Braunwald et al., 2001).

PCR procedures are similar to the procedure used for coronary angiography. A catheter introduced into the arterial circulation is guided into the opening of the narrowed coronary artery. A flexible guidewire is inserted through the catheter lumen into the affected vessel. The guidewire is then used to thread an angioplasty balloon, arterial stent, or other therapeutic device into the narrowed segment of the artery. The procedure is performed

# Medication Administration

## Antianginal Medications

### ORGANIC NITRATES

Nitroglycerin (Nitropaste, Nitro-Dur, Nitro-Bid, Nitrol,
Transderm-Nitro, Nitrogard, Nitrodisc, Tridil)
Isosorbide dinitrate (Isordil)
Isosorbide mononitrate (ISMO)
Amyl nitrite

Nitrates dilate both arterial and venous vessels, depending on the dose. Coronary artery vasodilation increases blood flow and myocardial oxygen supply. Venous dilation allows peripheral blood pooling, reducing venous return, preload, and cardiac work. Arterial dilation reduces vascular resistance and afterload, also reducing cardiac work. Sublingual nitroglycerin (NTG) tablets are used to treat and prevent acute anginal attacks (when taken prophylactically before activity). Nitrates are administered sublingually, by buccal spray, or intravenously for immediate effect; or orally or topically for sustained effect.

### Nursing Responsibilities

- Dilute intravenous nitroglycerin before infusing; use only glass bottles for the mixture. Nitroglycerin adheres to PVC bags and tubing, affecting the amount of drug that is delivered. Use non-PVC infusion tubing.
- Wear gloves when applying nitroglycerin paste or ointment to prevent absorbing the drug through the skin. Measure dose carefully and spread evenly in a 2-by-3 inch area.
- Remove nitroglycerin patches or ointment at night to help prevent tolerance.

### Client and Family Teaching

- Use only the sublingual, buccal, and spray forms of nitrates to treat acute angina.
- If the first nitrate dose does not relieve angina within 5 minutes, take a second dose. After 5 more minutes, you may take a third dose if needed. If the pain is unrelieved or lasts for 20 minutes or longer, seek medical assistance immediately.
- Carry a supply of nitroglycerin tablets with you. Dissolve sublingual nitroglycerin tablets under the tongue or between the upper lip and gum. Do not eat, drink, or smoke until the tablet is completely dissolved.
- Keep sublingual tablets in their original amber glass bottle to protect them from heat, light, and moisture. Replace your supply every 6 months.
- You may experience a burning or tingling sensation under the tongue and develop a transient headache when you take the drug. These are expected; the headache will diminish over time.
- Use caution when standing from a sitting position; nitroglycerine may make you lightheaded.
- Rotate ointment or transdermal patch application sites. Apply to a hairless area; spread ointment evenly without rubbing or massaging. Remove the patch or residual ointment at bedtime daily. Apply a fresh dose in the morning.
- If you are using a long-acting nitrate, keep a supply of immediate-acting nitrates to treat acute angina.

### BETA BLOCKERS

Atenolol (Tenormin)
Metoprolol (Lopressor)
Propranolol (Inderal)
Nadolol (Corgard)

Beta blockers decrease cardiac workload by blocking beta receptors on the heart muscle, decreasing heart rate, contractility, myocardial oxygen consumption, and blood pressure. Beta blockers also reduce *reflex tachycardia,* which may develop with other antianginal drugs. Beta blockers are frequently prescribed as antianginal and antihypertensive agents.

### Nursing Responsibilities

- Document heart rate and blood pressure before administering the medication. Withhold drug if the heart rate is below 50 BPM or the blood pressure is below prescribed limits. Notify the physician.
- Assess for and report possible contraindications to therapy, including heart failure, bradycardia, AV block, asthma, or COPD.
- Do not abruptly discontinue these drugs after long-term therapy, as this can increase heart rate, contractility, and blood pressure, and cause fatal dysrhythmia, myocardial infarction, or stroke.

### Client and Family Teaching

- Beta blockers help prevent angina but will not relieve an acute attack. Keep a supply of fast-acting nitrates on hand for acute anginal attacks.
- Do not suddenly stop taking this medication. Discuss discontinuing this medication with your doctor.
- Take your pulse daily. Do not take the drug, and contact your doctor if your heart rate is below 50 BPM. Check your blood pressure frequently.
- Report a slow or irregular pulse, swelling or weight gain, or difficulty breathing to your doctor.

### CALCIUM CHANNEL BLOCKERS

Nifedipine (Adalat, Procardia)
Diltiazem (Cardizem)
Verapamil (Isoptin, Calan)
Bepridil (Vascor)
Felodipine (Plendil)
Isradipine (DynaCirc)
Nicardipine (Cardene)
Nimodipine (Nimotop)

Calcium channel blockers are used to control angina, hypertension, and dysrhythmias. By blocking the entry of calcium into cells, these drugs reduce contractility, slow the heart rate and conduction, and cause vasodilation. Calcium channel blockers increase myocardial oxygen supply by dilating the coronary arteries; they decrease the workload of the heart by lowering vascular resistance and oxygen demand. Calcium channel blockers are often prescribed for clients with coronary artery spasm (Prinzmetal's angina).

### Nursing Responsibilities

- Do not mix verapamil in any solution containing sodium bicarbonate. Administer IV push verapamil over 2 to 3 minutes.
- Document blood pressure and heart rate before administering the drug. Withhold the drug if the heart rate is below 50 BPM. Notify the physician.

## Medication Administration

### Antianginal Medications *(continued)*

- The nifedipine capsule may be punctured and administered by extracting the liquid with a syringe and squirting the dose under the client's tongue (discard the needle first!).
- Use caution when giving a calcium channel blocker with other cardiac depressants, such as beta blockers. Concomitant administration with nitrates may cause excessive vasodilation.
- Manifestations of toxicity include nausea, generalized weakness, signs of decreased cardiac output, hypotension, bradycardia, and AV block. Report these findings immediately. Maintain intravenous access, and slowly administer intravenous calcium chloride. Do not infuse large volumes of fluid to treat hypotension as heart failure may result.

### Client and Family Teaching

- Take your pulse before taking the drug. Do not take the drug and notify physician if your heart rate drops below 50 BPM.
- Keep a fresh supply of immediate-acting nitrate available to treat acute anginal attacks. Calcium channel blockers will not work fast enough to relieve an acute attack.

---

in the cardiac catheterization laboratory using local anesthesia. The hospital stay is short (1 to 2 days), minimizing costs.

For *balloon angioplasty* (also called percutaneous transluminal coronary angioplasty or PTCA), a balloon-tipped catheter is threaded over the guidewire, with the balloon positioned across the area of narrowing (Figure 29–2 ■). The balloon is inflated in a step-by-step fashion for about 30 seconds to 2 minutes to compress the plaque against the arterial wall, with a goal of reducing the vessel obstruction to less than 50% of the arterial lumen. When used alone, balloon angioplasty is associated with a relatively high risk of abrupt vessel closure and restenosis. Its primary current use is in combination with stent placement or atherectomy.

*Intracoronary stents* are metallic scaffolds used to maintain an open arterial lumen. Stents reduce the rate of restenosis following angioplasty by about one-third, and are now used in 70% to 80% of all PCR procedures (Braunwald et al., 2001). The stent is placed over a balloon catheter, guided into position, and expanded as the balloon is inflated (Figure 29–3 ■). It then remains in the artery as a prop after the balloon is removed. Endothelial cells will completely line the inner wall of the stent to produce a smooth inner lining. Antiplatelet medications (aspirin and ticlopidine) are given following stent insertion to reduce the risk of thrombus formation at the site.

In contrast to balloon and stent procedures which enlarge the artery by displacing plaque, *atherectomy* procedures remove plaque from the identified lesion. The directional atherectomy catheter shaves the plaque off vessel walls using a rotary cutting head, retaining the fragments in its housing and removing them from the vessel. Rotational atherectomy catheters pulverize plaque into particles small enough to pass through the coronary microcirculation. Laser atherectomy devices use laser energy to remove plaque.

Complications following PCR procedures include hematoma at the catheter insertion site, pseudoaneurysm, embolism, hypersensitivity to contrast dye, dysrhythmias, bleeding, vessel perforation, and restenosis, or reocclusion of the treated vessel.

Nursing care of the client undergoing PCR is outlined in the box on the next page.

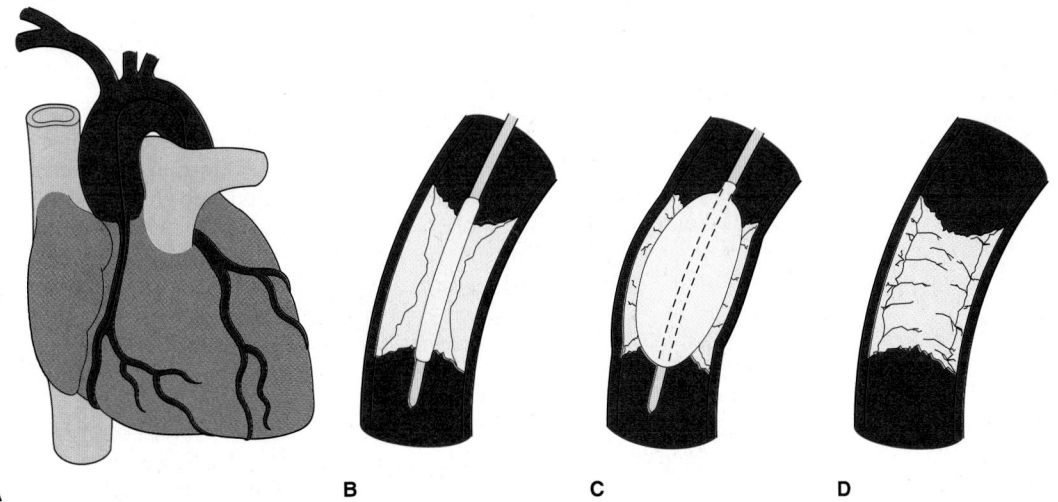

**A**    **B**    **C**    **D**

**Figure 29–2** ■ Balloon Angioplasty. *A*, The balloon catheter is threaded into the affected coronary artery. *B*, The balloon is positioned across the area of obstruction. *C*, The balloon is then inflated, flattening the plaque against the arterial wall, *D*.

**Figure 29–3** ■ Placement of the balloon expandable intracoronary stent. *A,* The stainless steel stent is fitted over a balloon-tipped catheter. *B,* The stent is positioned along the blockage and expanded. *C,* The balloon is deflated and removed, leaving the stent in place.

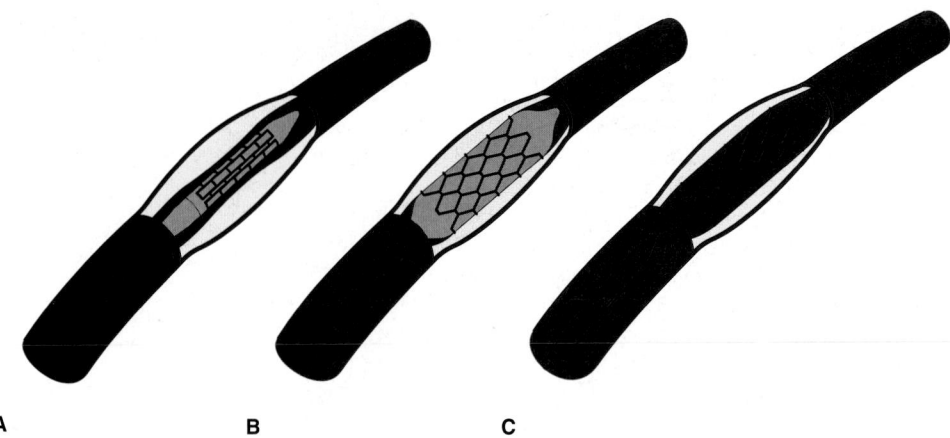

A        B        C

## Coronary Artery Bypass Grafting

Surgery for coronary heart disease involves using a section of a vein or an artery to create a connection (or bypass) between the aorta and the coronary artery beyond the obstruction (Figure 29–4 ■). This then allows blood to perfuse the ischemic portion of the heart. The internal mammary artery in the chest and the saphenous vein from the leg are the vessels most commonly used for coronary artery bypass grafting (CABG).

Bypass grafts are safe and effective. Angina is totally relieved or significantly reduced in 90% of clients who undergo

## NURSING CARE | OF THE CLIENT HAVING PCR

### BEFORE THE PROCEDURE

- Assess knowledge of the procedure and expectations of treatment. *This allows information to be tailored to the client's needs and provides an opportunity to clarify misconceptions.*
- Describe the cardiac catheterization laboratory and the planned PCR procedure, including:
  - Preoperative preparation (see Chapter 7). ☉
  - Planned anesthesia or sedation to be used.
  - Drugs that may be given during the procedure, such as anticoagulants to reduce the risk of thrombus formation, and intravenous nitroglycerine and a calcium channel blocker to dilate coronary arteries and prevent anginal pain.
- Discuss possible sensations during the procedure, including flushing or warmth and a metallic taste in the mouth as the contrast dye is injected, and a feeling of pressure or chest pain during balloon inflation. *Advanced preparation for expected sensations reduces anxiety and improves outcomes.*

### AFTER THE PROCEDURE

- Complete a head-to-toe assessment. Note any complaints of chest pain, or evidence of decreased cardiac output or myocardial infarction. *Assessment provides a baseline for subsequent assessments and allows early identification of possible complications.*
- Monitor vital signs and cardiac rhythm continuously. Treat dysrhythmias as ordered. Obtain a 12-lead ECG if signs of ischemia develop, and notify physician. *Vital signs reflect cardiac output. Dysrhythmias may develop with reperfusion of the ischemic myocardium. ECG changes may indicate infarction or restenosis of the affected vessel.*
- Maintain intravenous nitroglycerin infusion. Administer anticoagulant and antiplatelet medications, nitrates, and calcium channel blockers as ordered. *These drugs decrease oxygen de-*

*mand and increase oxygen supply by dilating the coronary arteries and systemic vasculature. They also reduce the risk of thrombus formation.*

- Monitor for and treat or report chest pain as indicated. *Chest pain may indicate ischemia and possible myocardial infarction.*
- Maintain bed rest as ordered with the head of the bed at 30 degrees or less. Prevent flexion of the leg on the affected side. Following sheath removal, follow protocol for pressure dressing or device or sandbag placement. *A large puncture wound occurs at the insertion site. Immobilization allows the wound to seal; a pressure dressing helps prevent bleeding.*
- Monitor distal pulses, color, movement, sensation, and temperature of the affected leg, and insertion site every 15 minutes for the first hour, every 30 minutes for the next hour, every hour for the next 8 hours, then every 4 hours. *A clot may form at the site, reducing perfusion of the affected leg. The site and dressing are monitored for excessive bleeding hematoma formation, or pseudoaneurysm. Pseudoaneurysm occurs as a result of inadequate hemostasis after catheter removal.*
- Monitor intake and output, serum electrolytes, blood urea nitrogen (BUN), creatinine, complete blood count (CBC), partial thromboplastin time (PTT), and cardiac enzymes. Report abnormal results to the physician. *Contrast dye causes osmotic diuresis and may cause renal damage or a hypersensitivity reaction. Electrolyte imbalances increase the risk of dysrhythmias. Cardiac enzymes are monitored for indications of possible myocardial damage during the procedure. The PTT monitors the effectiveness of heparin therapy.*
- Monitor for bradycardia, lightheadedness, hypotension, diaphoresis, and loss of consciousness during sheath removal. Keep atropine at bedside during sheath removal. *Bradycardia and signs of decreased cardiac output may occur during sheath removal because of a vasovagal reaction. Atropine decreases vagal tone and increases heart rate.*

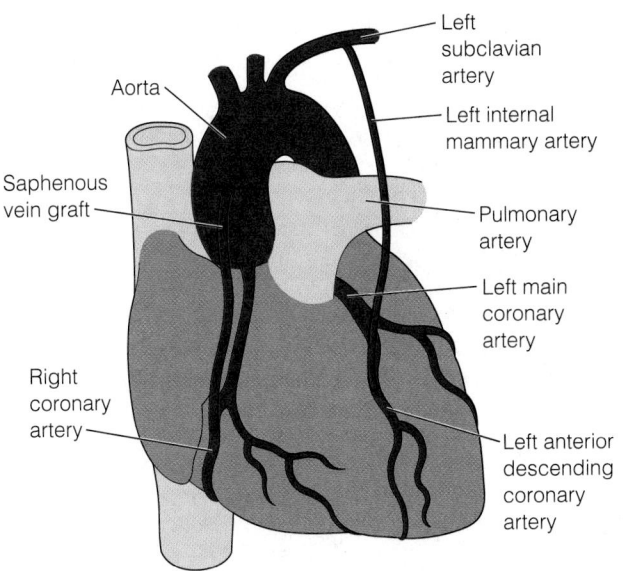

**Figure 29–4** ■ Coronary artery bypass grafting using the internal mammary artery and a saphenous vein graft.

complete revascularization. While anginal pain may recur within 3 years, it rarely is as severe as before surgery. Coronary artery bypass graft has a positive effect on mortality in many cases. It is recommended for clients who have multiple vessel disease and impaired left ventricular function or diabetes, and for clients who have significant obstruction of the left main coronary artery (Braunwald et al., 2001).

A median sternotomy is used to access the heart. The heart is usually stopped during surgery. The *cardiopulmonary bypass (CPB) pump* is used to maintain perfusion to the rest of the organs during open-heart surgery. Venous blood is removed from the body through a cannula placed in the right atrium or the superior and inferior venae cavae. Blood then circulates through the CPB pump, where it is oxygenated, its temperature regulated, and is filtered. Oxygenated blood is returned to the body through a cannula in the ascending aorta (Figure 29–5 ■). Cardiopulmonary bypass enables surgeons to operate on a quiet heart and a relatively bloodless field. Hypothermia can be maintained to reduce the metabolic rate and decrease oxygen demand during surgery.

When the saphenous vein is used, it is excised from its normal attachments in the leg, flushed with a cold heparinized saline solution, and then reversed so that its valves do not interfere with blood flow. It is *anastomosed* (grafted) to the aorta and the coronary artery, distal to the occlusion (see Figure 29–5). This provides a bridge or conduit for blood flow past the obstruction. If the internal mammary artery (IMA) is used, its distal end is excised and anatomosed to the coronary artery distal to the obstruction. The IMA often is used to revascularize the left coronary artery because of the greater oxygen demand of the left ventricle.

Once grafting is completed, cardiopulmonary bypass is discontinued and the client is rewarmed. Rewarming stimulates the heart to resume beating. Temporary pacing wires are sutured in place and passed through the chest wall in case temporary pacing is necessary. Chest tubes are placed in the pleural space

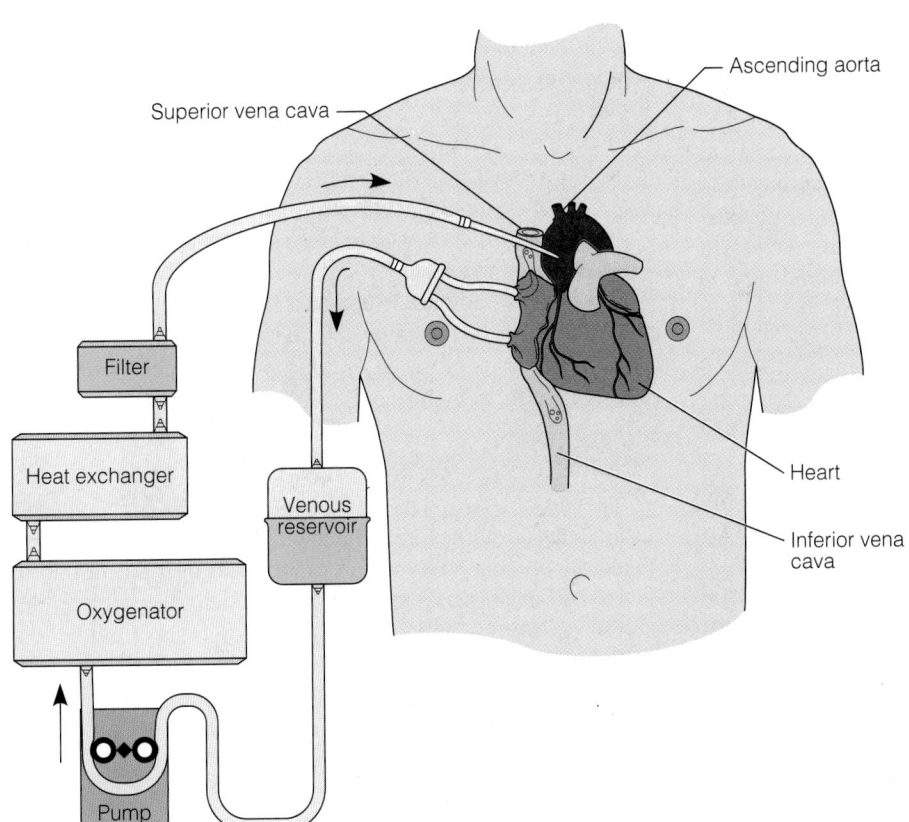

**Figure 29–5** ■ A diagrammatic representation of cardiopulmonary bypass. A cannula in the superior and inferior venae cavae removes venous blood, which is then pumped through an oxygenator and heat exchanger. After filtering, oxygenated blood is returned to the ascending aorta.

and mediastinum to drain blood and reestablish negative pressure in the thoracic cavity. The sternum is closed using heavy wires and bone wax, the skin is closed with sutures or staples, and sterile dressings are applied over sternal and leg incisions.

Pre- and postoperative nursing care and teaching for the client having a coronary artery bypass graft or other open-heart surgery are outlined on pages 823–825.

### Minimally Invasive Coronary Artery Surgery

*Minimally invasive coronary artery surgery* is a potential future alternative to CABG. Two approaches may be used: *port-access coronary artery bypass* uses several small holes, or "ports" in the chest wall to access vessels for connection to the CPB pump and the surgical site; CPB is avoided altogether using the *minimally invasive coronary artery bypass (MIDCAB)* approach. With MIDCAB, a small surgical incision and several chest wall ports are used to graft a chest wall artery to the affected coronary vessel while the heart continues to beat.

### Transmyocardial Laser Revascularization

A new development in myocardial revascularization techniques is called *transmyocardial laser revascularization (TMLR)*. In this procedure, a laser is used to drill tiny holes into the myocardial muscle itself to provide collateral blood flow to ischemic muscle. Clients whose coronary artery obstructions are too diffuse to bypass are candidates for this new surgical treatment.

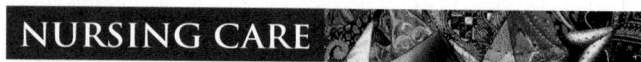

## NURSING CARE

### Health Promotion

In addition to health promotion measures identified for CHD, emphasize the importance of active CHD risk factor management to slow progression of the disease. Encourage clients to stop smoking. Discuss the use of cholesterol-lowering drug therapy with clients who have hypercholesterolemia. Encourage regular aerobic exercise and a diet based on American Heart Association or National Cholesterol Education Program guidelines.

### Assessment

Focused assessment data for the client with angina includes the following:

- Health history: chest pain, including type, intensity, duration, frequency, aggravating factors and relief measures; associated symptoms; history of other cardiovascular disorders, peripheral vascular disease, or stroke; current medications and treatment; usual diet, exercise, and alcohol intake patterns; smoking history; use of other recreational drugs
- Physical assessment: vital signs and heart sounds; strength and equality of peripheral pulses; skin color and temperature (central and peripheral); physical appearance during pain episode (e.g., shortness of breath, apparent anxiety, color, diaphoresis)

## Nursing Diagnoses and Interventions

The focus of nursing care for clients with angina is similar to the collaborative care focus: to reduce myocardial oxygen demand and improve the oxygen supply. Angina usually is treated in community settings; the primary nursing focus is education. High-priority nursing problems for clients with angina include ineffective cardiac tissue perfusion and management of the prescribed therapeutic regimen.

### Ineffective Tissue Perfusion: Cardiac

The pain of angina results from impaired blood flow and oxygen supply to the myocardium. Nursing interventions can both prevent ischemia and shorten the duration of pain.

- Keep prescribed nitroglycerin tablets at the client's side so one can be taken at the onset of pain. *Anginal pain indicates myocardial ischemia. Nitroglycerin reduces cardiac work and may improve myocardial blood flow, relieving ischemia and pain.*
- Start oxygen at 4 to 6 L/min per nasal cannula or as prescribed. *Supplemental oxygen reduces myocardial hypoxia.*
- Space activities to allow rest between them. *Activity increases cardiac work and may precipitate angina. Spacing of activities allows the heart to recover.*
- Teach about prescribed medications to maintain myocardial perfusion and reduce cardiac work. Emphasize that long-acting nitrates, beta blockers, and calcium channel blockers are used to *prevent* anginal attacks, not to *treat* an acute attack. *It is important for the client to understand the purpose and use of prescribed drugs to maintain optimal myocardial perfusion.*
- Instruct to take sublingual nitroglycerin before engaging in activities that precipitate angina (e.g., climbing stairs, sexual intercourse). *This prophylactic dose of nitroglycerin helps maintain cardiac perfusion when increased work is anticipated, preventing ischemia and chest pain.*
- Encourage to implement and maintain a progressive exercise program under the supervision of the primary care provider or a cardiac rehabilitation professional. *Exercise slows the atherosclerotic process and helps develop collateral circulation to the heart muscle.*
- Refer to a smoking cessation program as indicated. *Nicotine causes vasoconstriction and increases the heart rate, decreasing myocardial perfusion and increasing cardiac workload.*

### Risk for Ineffective Therapeutic Regimen Management

Denial may be strong in the client with angina pectoris. Because many people think of the heart as the locus of life itself, problems such as angina remind people of their mortality, an uncomfortable fact. Denial may lead to "forgetting" to take prescribed medications or to attempting activities that will precipitate angina. Some clients, by contrast, may become "cardiac cripples," afraid to engage in activities because of anticipated chest pain. Their inactivity may actually hasten the atherosclerotic process and inhibit collateral circulation development, worsening angina.

# NURSING CARE OF THE CLIENT HAVING A CORONARY ARTERY BYPASS GRAFT

## PREOPERATIVE CARE

- Provide routine preoperative care and teaching as outlined in Chapter 7. 🔗
- Verify presence of laboratory and diagnostic test results in the chart, including CBC, coagulation profile, urinalysis, chest X-ray, and coronary angiogram. *These baseline data are important for comparison of postoperative results and values.*
- Type and crossmatch four or more units of blood as ordered. *Blood is made available for use during and after surgery as needed.*
- Provide specific client and family teaching related to procedure and postoperative care. Include the following topics.
  - Cardiac recovery unit; sensory stimuli, personnel; noise and alarms; visiting policies
  - Tubes, drains, and general appearance
  - Monitoring equipment, including cardiac and hemodynamic monitoring systems
  - Respiratory support: ventilator, endotracheal tube, suctioning; communication while intubated
  - Incisions and dressings
  - Pain management
  *Preoperative teaching reduces anxiety and prepares the client and family for the postoperative environment and expected sensations.*

## POSTOPERATIVE CARE

- Provide routine postoperative care as outlined in Chapter 7. In addition to the care needs of all clients having major surgery, the cardiac surgery client has specific care needs related to open-heart and thoracic surgery. These are outlined under the nursing diagnoses identified below.

### Decreased Cardiac Output

Cardiac output may be compromised postoperatively due to bleeding and fluid loss; depression of myocardial function by drugs, hypothermia, and surgical manipulation; dysrhythmias; increased vascular resistance; and a potential complication, *cardiac tamponade,* compression of the heart due to collected blood or fluid in the pericardium

- Monitor vital signs, oxygen saturation, and hemodynamic parameters every 15 minutes. Note trends and report significant changes to the physician. *Initial hypothermia and bradycardia are expected; the heart rate should return to the normal range with rewarming. The blood pressure may fall during rewarming as vasodilation occurs. Hypotension and tachycardia, however, may indicate low cardiac output. Pulmonary artery pressure (PAP), pulmonary artery wedge pressure (PAWP), cardiac output, and oxygen saturation are monitored to evaluate fluid volume, cardiac function, and gas exchange. Hemodynamic monitoring is further discussed in Chapter 30.*
- Auscultate heart and breath sounds on admission and at least every 4 hours. *A ventricular gallop, or S₃, is an early sign of heart failure; an S₄ may indicate decreased ventricular compliance. Muffled heart sounds may be an early indication of cardiac tamponade. Adventitious breath sounds (wheezes, crackles, or rales) may be a manifestation of heart failure or respiratory compromise.*
- Assess skin color and temperature, peripheral pulses, and level of consciousness with vital signs. *Pale, mottled, or cyanotic coloring, cool and clammy skin, and diminished pulse amplitude are indicators of decreased cardiac output.*
- Continuously monitor and document cardiac rhythm. *Dysrhythmias are common, and may interfere with cardiac filling and contractility, decreasing the cardiac output.*
- Measure intake and output hourly. Report urine output less than 30 mL/h for 2 consecutive hours. *Intake and output measurements help evaluate fluid volume status. A fall in urine output may be an early indicator of decreased cardiac output.*
- Record chest tube output hourly. *Chest tube drainage greater than 70 mL/hr or that is warm, red, and free flowing indicates hemorrhage and may necessitate a return to surgery. A sudden drop in chest tube output may indicate impending cardiac tamponade.*
- Monitor hemoglobin, hematocrit, and serum electrolytes. *A drop in hemoglobin and hematocrit may indicate hemorrhage that is not otherwise obvious. Electrolyte imbalances, potassium, calcium, and magnesium in particular, affect cardiac rhythm and contractility.*
- Administer intravenous fluids, fluid boluses, and blood transfusions as ordered. *Fluid and blood replacement helps ensure adequate blood volume and oxygen-carrying capacity.*
- Administer medications as ordered. *Medications ordered in the early postoperative period to maintain the cardiac output include inotropic drugs (e.g., dopamine, dobutamine) to increase the force of myocardial contractions; vasodilators (e.g., nitroprusside or nitroglycerin) to decrease vascular resistance and afterload; and antidysrhythmics to correct dysrhythmias that affect cardiac output.*
- Keep a temporary pacemaker at the bedside; initiate pacing as indicated. *Temporary pacing may be needed to maintain the cardiac output with bradydysrhythmias, such as high-level AV blocks.*

**PRACTICE ALERT** *Assess for signs of cardiac tamponade: increased heart rate, decreased BP, decreased urine output, increased central venous pressure, a sudden decrease in chest tube output, muffled/distant heart sounds, and diminished peripheral pulses. Notify physician immediately. Cardiac tamponade is a life-threatening complication that may develop postoperatively. Cardiac tamponade interferes with ventricular filling and contraction, decreasing cardiac output. Untreated, cardiac tamponade leads to cardiogenic shock and possible cardiac arrest.* ∎

### Hypothermia

Hypothermia is maintained during cardiac surgery to reduce the metabolic rate and protect vital organs from ischemic damage. Although rewarming is instituted on completion of the surgery, the client often remains hypothermic on admission to cardiac recovery. Gradual rewarming is necessary to prevent peripheral vasodilation and hypotension.

*continued on page 824*

# NURSING CARE OF THE CLIENT HAVING A CORONARY ARTERY BYPASS GRAFT (continued)

- Monitor core body temperature (e.g., tympanic membrane, pulmonary artery, bladder) for the first 8 hours following surgery. *Oral and rectal temperature measurements are not reliable indicators of core body temperature during this period.*
- Institute rewarming measures (e.g., warmed intravenous solutions or blood transfusion, warm blankets, warm inspired gases, radiant heat lamps) as needed to maintain a temperature above 96.8 F (36° C). Administer thorazine, morphine, or diltiazem as ordered to relieve shivering. *Low body temperature may cause shivering, increasing oxygen demand and consumption. Hypothermia also increases the risk for hypoxia, metabolic acidosis, vasoconstriction and increased cardiac work, altered clotting, and dysrhythmias.*

## Acute Pain

Following a CABG, pain is experienced due to both the thoracic incision and removal of the saphenous vein from the leg. Dissection of the internal mammary artery (usually the left IMA) from the chest wall also causes chest pain on the affected side. Chest tube sites are also uncomfortable. The leg from which the saphenous vein graft was obtained may be more painful than the chest incision.

- Frequently assess for pain, including its location and character. Document its intensity using a standard pain scale. Assess for verbal and nonverbal indicators of pain. Validate pain cues with the client. *Pain is subjective, and differs among individuals. Incisional pain is expected; however, anginal pain also may develop. It is important to differentiate the type of pain.*

### PRACTICE ALERT
*Promptly report anginal or cardiac pain. Cardiac pain may indicate a perioperative or postoperative myocardial infarction.* ■

- Administer analgesics on a scheduled basis, by PCA, or by continuous infusion for the first 24 to 48 hours. *Research demonstrates that adequate pain management in the immediate postoperative period reduces complications from sympathetic stimulation and allows faster recovery. Pain causes muscle tension and vasoconstriction, impairing circulation and tissue perfusion, slowing wound healing, and increasing cardiac work.*
- Premedicate 30 minutes before activities or planned procedures. *Premedication and the subsequent reduction of pain improves client participation and cooperation with care.*

## Ineffective Airway Clearance/Impaired Gas Exchange

Atelectasis due to impaired ventilation and airway clearance is a common pulmonary complication of cardiac surgery. Gas exchange may also be affected by blood loss and decreased oxygen-carrying capacity following surgery. Phrenic nerve paralysis is a potential complication of cardiac surgery which may also contribute to impaired ventilation and gas exchange.

- Evaluate respiratory rate, depth, effort, symmetry of chest expansion, and breath sounds frequently. *Pain, anxiety, excess fluid volume, surgical injury, narcotics and anesthesia, and altered homeostasis can affect respiratory rate, depth, and effort postoperatively. Decreased chest expansion or asymmetrical movement may indicate impaired ventilation of one lung, and needs further evaluation.*
- Note endotracheal tube (ETT) placement on chest X-ray. Mark tube position and secure in place. Insert an oral airway if an oral ETT is used. *The chest X-ray documents correct ETT placement above the bifurcation to the right and left mainstem bronchus. Marking its appropriate placement allows evaluation of potential tube movement. Secure the tube firmly in place to prevent slippage or inadvertent removal. An oral airway helps prevent obstruction of an oral ETT by biting.*
- Maintain ventilator settings as ordered. Monitor arterial blood gases (ABGs) as ordered. *Mechanical ventilation promotes optimal lung expansion and oxygenation postoperatively. ABGs are used to evaluate oxygenation and acid-base balance.*
- Suction as needed. *Suctioning is performed only as indicated to clear airway secretions.*
- Prepare for ventilator weaning and extubation, as appropriate. *The client is removed from the ventilator and extubated as soon as possible to reduce complications associated with mechanical ventilation and intubation.*
- After extubation, teach use of the incentive spirometer, and encourage use every 2 hours. Encourage deep breathing; advise against vigorous coughing. Teach use of a "cough pillow" to splint chest incision and decrease pain. Frequently turn and encourage movement. Dangle on postoperative day 1. *Deep breathing, controlled coughing, and position changes improve ventilation and airway clearance and help prevent complications. Vigorous coughing may excessively increase intrathoracic pressure and cause sternal instability.*

## Risk for Infection

Following an open chest procedure, a sternal infection may develop that can progress to involve the mediastinum. Clients with IMA grafts, who are diabetic, are older, or malnourished are at high risk: Harvesting of IMA disrupts blood supply to the sternum, and these clients have impaired immune responses and healing.

- Assess sternal wound every shift. Document redness, warmth, swelling, and/or drainage from the site. Note wound approximation. *These assessments provide indicators of inflammation and healing.*
- Maintain a sterile dressing for the first 48 hours, then leave the incision open to air. Use Steri-Strips as needed to maintain approximation of the wound edges. *The sterile dressing prevents early contamination of the wound, whereas exposing the incision after 48 hours promotes healing.*
- Report signs of wound infection: a swollen, reddened area that is hot and painful to the touch; drainage from the wound; impaired healing, or healed areas that reopen. *Evidence of infection or impaired healing requires further evaluation and treatment.*
- Culture wound drainage as indicated. *Identifying the infective organism facilitates appropriate antibiotic therapy.*
- Collaborate with the dietitian to promote nutrition and fluid intake. *Good nutritional status is vital to healing and immune function.*

continued on page 825

## NURSING CARE OF THE CLIENT HAVING A CORONARY ARTERY BYPASS GRAFT *(continued)*

### Disturbed Thought Processes

Many factors affect neuropsychologic function after CABG, including the length of cardiopulmonary bypass, age, presurgery organic brain dysfunction, severity of illness, and decreased cardiac output. Sensory overload and deprivation, sleep disruption, and numerous drugs also affect thinking and mental clarity.

- Frequently reorient during initial recovery period. State that surgery is over and that the client is in the recovery area. *Frequent reorientation provides emotional support and reality checks.*
- Explain all procedures before performing them. Speak in a clear, calm voice. Encourage questions, and give honest answers. *These measures provide information, decrease anxiety, and establish trust.*
- Secure all intravenous lines and invasive catheters/tubes (e.g., ETT, Foley catheter, nasogastric tube). *Disoriented clients may tug or pull at invasive equipment, disrupting them and increasing the risk of injury.*
- Note verbal responses to questions. Correct misconceptions immediately (e.g., "Mr. Snow, look at all the special equipment in this room. Does this room look like your bedroom at home?"). *Helping the client recognize differences in the hospital environment offers a basis for continual reality checks.*
- Maintain a calendar and clock within the client's view. *This provides current information regarding day, date, and time.*
- Involve family members in providing reorientation. Place familiar objects and photographs within view. Encourage family presence. *The family provides reassurance and contact with the familiar, assisting with orientation.*
- Promote client participation in care and decision making as appropriate. *This allows the client to maintain a degree of power and control and enables the client to take an active role in recovery.*
- Report signs of hallucinations, delusions, depression, or agitation. *These may indicate progressive deterioration of mental status.*
- Administer sedatives cautiously. *Mild sedation may help prevent injury. Some sedatives may, however, have adverse effects, increasing confusion and disorientation.*
- Reevaluate neurologic status every shift. *These data allow evaluation of the effect of interventions.*

- Assess knowledge and understanding of angina. *Assessment allows tailoring of teaching and interventions to the needs of the client.*
- Teach about angina and atherosclerosis as needed, building on current knowledge base. *This can help the client understand that angina is a manageable disease and that pain can usually be controlled and the disease progress slowed.*
- Provide written and verbal instructions about prescribed medications and their use. *Written instructions reinforce teaching and are available to the client for future reference.*
- Stress the importance of taking chest pains seriously while maintaining a positive attitude. *Although it is vital to recognize the significance of chest pain and deal with it appropriately, it is also important to maintain a positive outlook.*
- Refer to a cardiac rehabilitation program or other organized activities and support groups for clients with coronary artery disease. *Programs such as these help the client develop risk factor management strategies, maintain a program of supervised activity, and gain coping skills.*

## Using NANDA, NIC, and NOC

Chart 29–1 shows links between NANDA nursing diagnoses, NIC, and NOC when caring for the client with angina.

### CHART 29–1 NANDA, NIC, AND NOC LINKAGES

#### The Client with CHD and Angina

| NURSING DIAGNOSES | NURSING INTERVENTIONS | NURSING OUTCOMES |
|---|---|---|
| • Activity Intolerance<br>• Ineffective Coping | • Cardiac Care: Rehabilitative<br>• Coping Enhancement<br>• Emotional Support | • Activity Tolerance<br>• Coping<br>• Role Performance |
| • Ineffective Health Maintenance | • Health Education<br>• Risk Identification<br>• Self-Responsibility Facilitation | • Health-Promoting Behavior<br>• Risk Detection<br>• Health-Seeking Behavior |
| • Ineffective Sexuality Patterns<br>• Ineffective Tissue Perfusion: Cardiopulmonary | • Anticipatory Guidance<br>• Cardiac Care<br>• Cardiac Precautions<br>• Medication Administration | • Role Performance<br>• Cardiac Pump Effectiveness<br>• Circulation Status<br>• Tissue Perfusion: Cardiac |

*Note. Data from Nursing Outcomes Classification (NOC) by M. Johnson & M. Maas (Eds.), 1997, St. Louis: Mosby; Nursing Diagnoses: Definitions & Classification 2001–2002 by North American Nursing Diagnosis Association, 2001, Philadelphia: NANDA; Nursing Interventions Classification (NIC) by J.C. McCloskey & G. M. Bulechek (Eds.), 2000, St. Louis: Mosby. Reprinted by permission.*

## Home Care

Many clients with stable angina manage their pain effectively, continuing to live active and productive lives. To promote effective management of this disorder, include the following topics in teaching for home care.

- Coronary heart disease and the processes that cause chest pain, including the relationship between the pain and reduced blood flow to the heart muscle
- Use and effects (desired and adverse) of prescribed medications; importance of not discontinuing medications abruptly
- Nitroglycerine use for acute angina: Always carry several tablets (not the entire supply); prophylactic use before activities that often cause chest pain; take tablet at first indication of pain rather than waiting to see if the pain develops; seek immediate medical assistance if three nitroglycerin tablets over 15 to 20 minutes do not relieve the pain
- The importance of calling 911 or going to the emergency department immediately for unrelieved chest pain
- Appropriate storage of nitroglycerin: This unstable compound needs to be stored in a cool, dry, dark place; no more than a 6-month supply should be kept on hand

For the client who has undergone cardiac surgery, also include the following:

- Respiratory care, activity, and pain management
- The importance of actively participating in rehabilitation
- Manifestations of infection or other potential complications and their management

## Nursing Care Plan
## A Client with Coronary Artery Bypass Surgery

Six weeks ago, John Clements, age 50, was discharged from the hospital after emergency triple bypass surgery. Despite having emergency surgery, his postoperative recovery was uneventful, and he was discharged 6 days after admission. He returns to the clinic for a postoperative stress test and to discuss his cardiac rehabilitation program. Anne Wagner, RN, CNS, a cardiac clinical nurse specialist and the program coordinator, meets Mr. Clements to obtain specific information regarding his medical status.

### ASSESSMENT

Mr. Clements's medical history reveals significant CHD, an anterior wall myocardial infarction that led to his emergency triple bypass, and hyperlipidemia. Current medications include Cardizem, Isordil, Ecotrin, and Transderm-Nitro 5. The ECG reveals sinus rhythm with some ST segment and T wave flattening. Resting heart rate 68, and blood pressure 136/84.

Mr. Clements has a strong family history of CHD. He does not smoke and uses alcohol occasionally in social situations. He enjoys "good Southern-style cooking" and watching television. Mr. Clements states his only regular exercise used to be an evening of dancing with his wife and friends about once a month, "But I get short of breath walking around the block now, so I guess I can't go dancing anymore!"

Mr. Clements owns his own contracting business and states that he typically works about 50 to 60 hours per week. He tells Ms. Wagner, "I don't know what this program is supposed to do for me. I have got to get back to work! You just can't sit around in my business—you have to make sure that the work is getting done on time, and you have to check on supplies and equipment and the like. But I feel like a weakling—I need to get my energy back!"

### DIAGNOSES

- Activity intolerance related to general weakness and fatigue
- Ineffective role performance related to health crisis

### EXPECTED OUTCOMES

- Verbalize an understanding of the definition and components of his structured cardiac rehabilitation program.
- Verbalize a desire to make lifestyle changes.
- Identify resources available in the community to assist with lifestyle changes.
- Participate in his activity program without suffering any complications.
- Verbalize an increase in energy after 6 weeks on the program.
- Accept the reality of the temporary change in his usual work responsibilities.

### PLANNING AND IMPLEMENTATION

- Define the purpose and components of a cardiac rehabilitation program.
- Enroll in "heart health" classes, including cardiac anatomy, physiology, and coronary heart disease; exercise and activity prescriptions; lifestyle modifications, including diet counseling and stress management; emotional reactions to CAD; sexual activity; use of cardiac medications; and self-responsibility for health.
- Plan an exercise program based on stress test results, physical examination, and interview.
- Encourage to schedule rest periods before and after activity/ exercise.
- Review signs and symptoms of overexertion.
- Provide information about community resources for emotional and educational support.
- Assist to identify strategies for dealing with concerns about his business role.

### EVALUATION

Mr. Clements decides to "give the rehab program a try." Ms. Wagner and an exercise physiologist work with him to plan an individualized exercise/activity program. A registered dietitian provides dietary counseling. Ms. Wagner emphasizes stress management strategies. Mr. Clements is able to list manifestations of overexertion and states that he realizes the need for gradual activity progression.

After 6 weeks, Mr. Clements has reported a significant increase in energy and strength. "I am feeling much stronger, and have been sleeping better. Mary and I are taking evening walks around the neighborhood. My chest soreness is also gone." He has completed the 12-week cardiac rehabilitation program, and another stress test indicates that his cardiac function is adequate. Mr.

## Nursing Care Plan

## A Client with Coronary Artery Bypass Surgery (continued)

Clements has joined the local Mended Hearts support group and states that he is now incorporating "heart-healthy" considerations into his daily routines.

### Critical Thinking in the Nursing Process

1. Develop a personalized risk factor reduction plan for Mr. Clements.
2. How might denial affect Mr. Clements's ability to (a) accept the need for cardiac rehabilitation, (b) comply with the proposed lifestyle changes, and (c) make permanent adjustments to his daily life?

3. How does spousal support influence a client's compliance with a structured cardiac rehabilitation program?
4. Mr. Clements tells you that since the surgery, his wife has been afraid that sexual activity will induce another heart attack. How would you respond to these concerns?

See Evaluating Your Response in Appendix C.

## THE CLIENT WITH ACUTE MYOCARDIAL INFARCTION

An **acute myocardial infarction (AMI),** necrosis (death) of myocardial cells, is a life-threatening event. If circulation to the affected myocardium is not promptly restored, loss of functional myocardium affects the heart's ability to maintain an effective cardiac output. This may ultimately lead to cardiogenic shock and death.

Heart disease remains the leading cause of death in the United States. Of the major heart diseases, myocardial infarction (MI) or *heart attack,* and other forms of ischemic heart disease cause the majority of deaths. Annually, approximately 650,000 people in the United States experience their first MI; another 450,000 suffer an MI subsequent to the initial one. Nearly 530,000 people died of coronary heart disease in 2000, with most of these deaths related to MI (NHLBI, 2002).

The majority of deaths from MI occur during the initial period after symptoms begin: approximately 60% within the first hour, and 40% prior to hospitalization. Heightening public awareness of the manifestations of MI, the importance of seeking immediate medical assistance, and training in cardiopulmonary resuscitation (CPR) techniques are vital to decrease deaths due to MI.

Myocardial infarction rarely occurs in clients without preexisting coronary heart disease. While no specific cause has been identified, the risk factors for MI are those for coronary heart disease: age, gender, heredity, race; smoking, obesity, hyperlipidemia, hypertension, diabetes, sedentary lifestyle, diet, and others. See the previous section of this chapter on coronary heart disease for further discussion of these risk factors.

## PATHOPHYSIOLOGY

Atherosclerotic plaque may form stable or unstable lesions. *Stable* lesions progress by gradually occluding the vessel lumen, whereas *unstable* (or *complicated*) lesions are prone to

rupture and thrombus formation. Stable lesions often cause angina (discussed in the previous section); unstable lesions often lead to **acute coronary syndromes,** or acute ischemic heart diseases. Acute coronary syndromes include unstable angina, myocardial infarction, and sudden cardiac death (McCance & Huether, 2002).

Myocardial infarction occurs when blood flow to a portion of cardiac muscle is blocked, resulting in prolonged tissue ischemia and irreversible cell damage. Coronary occlusion is usually caused by ulceration or rupture of a complicated atherosclerotic lesion. When an atherosclerotic lesion ruptures or ulcerates, substances are released that stimulate platelet aggregation, thrombin generation, and local vasomotor tone. As a result, a thrombus (clot) forms, occluding the vessel and interrupting blood flow to the myocardium distal to the obstruction.

Cellular injury occurs when the cells are denied adequate oxygen and nutrients. When ischemia is prolonged, lasting more than 20 to 45 minutes, irreversible hypoxemic damage causes cellular death and tissue necrosis. Oxygen, glycogen, and ATP stores of ischemic cells are rapidly depleted. Cellular metabolism shifts to an anaerobic process, producing hydrogen ions and lactic acid. Cellular acidosis increases cells' vulnerability to further damage. Intracellular enzymes are released through damaged cell membranes into interstitial spaces.

Cellular acidosis, electrolyte imbalances, and hormones released in response to cellular ischemia affect impulse conduction and myocardial contractility. The risk of dysrhythmias increases, and myocardial contractility decreases, reducing stroke volume, cardiac output, blood pressure, and tissue perfusion.

The subendocardium suffers the initial damage, within 20 minutes of injury, because this area is the most susceptible to changes in coronary blood flow. If blood flow is restored at this point, the infarction is limited to subendocardial tissue (a *subendocardial* or *non Q wave infarction*). The damage progresses to the epicardium within 1 to 6 hours. When all layers of the myocardium are affected, it is known as a *transmural infarction*. A significant Q wave develops with a transmural infarction, so this also may be called a *Q wave MI*. Complications

MediaLink | MYOCARDIAL INFARCTION CASE STUDY

such as heart failure are more frequently associated with Q wave MIs; however, clients with non Q wave MIs frequently experience recurrent ischemia or subsequent MI within weeks or months of the event (Woods et al., 2000).

The necrotic, infarcted tissue is surrounded by regions of injured and ischemic tissues. Tissue in this ischemic area is potentially viable; restoration of blood flow minimizes the amount of tissue lost. This surrounding tissue also undergoes metabolic changes. It may be *stunned,* its contractility impaired for hours to days following reperfusion, or *hibernating,* a process that protects myocytes until perfusion is restored. *Myocardial remodeling* also may occur, with cellular hypertrophy and loss of contractility in regions distant from the infarction. Rapid restoration of blood flow limits these changes (McCance & Huether, 2002).

When a larger artery is compromised, *collateral vessels* connecting smaller arteries in the coronary system dilate to maintain blood flow to the cardiac muscle. The degree of collateral circulation helps determine the extent of myocardial damage from ischemia. Acute occlusion of a coronary artery without any collateral flow results in massive tissue damage and possible death. Progressive narrowing of the larger coronary arteries allows collateral vessels to develop and enlarge, meeting the demand for blood flow. Good collateral circulation can limit the size of an MI.

Myocardial infarction usually affects the left ventricle because it is the major "workhorse" of the heart; its muscle mass is greater, as are its oxygen demands.

Myocardial infarctions are described by the damaged area of the heart. The coronary artery that is occluded determines the area of damage. Occlusion of the left anterior descending (LAD) artery affects blood flow to the anterior wall of the left ventricle (an *anterior MI*) and part of the interventricular septum. Occlusion of the left circumflex artery (LCA) causes a *lateral MI. Right ventricular, inferior,* and *posterior infarcts* involve occlusions of the right coronary artery (RCA) and posterior descending artery (PDA). Occlusion of the left main coronary artery is the most devastating, causing ischemia of the entire left ventricle, and a grave prognosis. Identifying the infarct site helps predict possible complications and determine appropriate therapy.

### Cocaine-Induced MI

Acute myocardial infarction may develop due to cocaine intoxication. Cocaine increases sympathetic nervous system activity by both increasing the release of catecholamines from central and peripheral stores and interfering with the reuptake of catecholamines. This increased catecholamine concentration stimulates the heart rate and increases its contractility, increases the automaticity of cardiac tissues and the risk of dysrhythmias, and causes vasoconstriction and hypertension. The client with cocaine-induced MI may present with an altered level of consciousness, confusion and restlessness, seizure activity, tachycardia, hypotension, increased respiratory rate, and respiratory crackles.

## MANIFESTATIONS

Pain is a classic manifestation of myocardial infarction. Chest pain due to MI is more severe than anginal pain. However, it is not the intensity of the chest pain that distinguishes MI from angina, but its duration and its continuous nature. The onset of pain is sudden and usually is not associated with activity. In fact, most MIs occur in the early morning. Clients with a history of angina may have more frequent anginal attacks in the days or weeks prior to an MI. Chest pain may be described as crushing and severe; as a pressure, heavy, or squeezing sensation; or as chest tightness or burning. The pain often begins in the center of the chest (*substernal*), and may radiate to the shoulders, neck, jaw, or arms. It lasts more than 15 to 20 minutes and is not relieved by rest or nitroglycerin.

Women and older adults often experience atypical chest pain, presenting with complaints of indigestion, heartburn, nausea, and vomiting (see the box below). Up to 25% of clients with acute MI deny chest discomfort (Woods et al., 2000).

Compensatory mechanisms cause many of the other symptoms of MI. Sympathetic nervous system stimulation causes anxiety, tachycardia, and vasoconstriction. This results in cool, clammy, mottled skin. Pain and blood chemistry changes stimulate the respiratory center, causing tachypnea. The client often has a sense of impending doom and death. Tissue necrosis causes an inflammatory reaction that increases the white blood cell count and elevates the temperature. Serum cardiac enzyme levels rise as enzymes are released from necrotic cardiac cells.

## Meeting Individualized Needs

### RECOGNIZING A MYOCARDIAL INFARCTION IN WOMEN AND OLDER ADULTS

Women and older adults often present with atypical manifestations of MI. However, heart disease is the number one cause of death in both groups, making early recognition and aggressive treatment vital.

Women are more likely than men to have a "silent" or unrecognized heart attack. They often experience epigastric pain and nausea, causing them to blame their discomfort on heartburn. Shortness of breath is common, as is fatigue and weakness of the shoulders and upper arms.

Older people often seek treatment for vague complaints of difficulty breathing, confusion, fainting, dizziness, abdominal pain, or cough. They often attribute their symptoms to a stroke. The prevalence of silent ischemia is greater in older adults.

Stress the importance of seeking medical help promptly for atypical manifestations of MI. Prompt diagnosis and intervention reduces the mortality and morbidity of MI in women and older adults, just as it does in men. Despite this fact, both women and older adults are more likely to delay seeking treatment and are less likely to be accurately diagnosed and aggressively treated for CHD.

## Manifestations of Acute Myocardial Infarction

- Chest pain: substernal or precordial (across the entire chest wall); may radiate to neck, jaw, shoulder(s), or left arm
- Tachycardia, tachypnea
- Dyspnea, shortness of breath
- Nausea and vomiting
- Anxiety, sense of impending doom
- Diaphoresis
- Cool, mottled skin; diminished peripheral pulses
- Hypotension or hypertension
- Palpitations, dysrhythmias
- Signs of left heart failure
- Decreased level of consciousness

Other manifestations may vary, depending on the location and amount of infarcted tissue. Hypertension, hypotension, or signs of heart failure may develop. Vagal stimulation may cause nausea and vomiting, bradycardia, and hypotension. Hiccuping may develop due to diaphagmatic irritation. If a large vessel is occluded, the first sign of MI may be sudden death. Typical manifestations of MI are listed in the box above.

The risk of complications associated with myocardial infarction is related to the size and location of the MI.

### Dysrhythmias

**Dysrhythmias,** disturbances or irregularities of heart rhythm, are the most frequent complication of MI. Dysrhythmias are discussed in detail in the next section of this chapter.

Infarcted tissue is *arrhythmogenic;* that is, it affects the generation and conduction of electrical impulses in the heart, increasing the risk of dysrhythmias. Premature ventricular contractions (PVCs) are common following an MI, developing in more than 90% of clients with an acute MI. While not dangerous in themselves, they may be predictive of more dangerous dysrhythmias such as ventricular tachycardia or ventricular fibrillation (Woods et al., 2000). The risk of ventricular fibrillation is greatest the first hour after MI; it is a frequent cause of sudden cardiac death associated with acute MI. Its incidence declines with time. If the infarct affects a conduction pathway, electrical conduction may be affected. Any degree of atrioventricular (AV) block may occur following MI, especially when the anterior wall is infarcted. First-degree and Mobitz I (Wenckebach) blocks are most common, although complete heart block may develop. Bradydysrhythmias (abnormal slow rhythms) also may develop, particularly when the inferior wall of the ventricle is affected.

### Pump Failure

Myocardial infarction reduces myocardial contractility, ventricular wall motion, and compliance. Impaired contractility and filling may produce heart failure. The risk of heart failure is greatest when large portions of the left ventricle are infarcted. Heart failure may be more severe with an anterior infarction. Loss of 20% to 30% of the left ventricular muscle mass may cause manifestations of left-sided heart failure, including dyspnea, fatigue, weakness, and respiratory crackles on auscultation. Inferior or right ventricular MI may lead to right-sided heart failure with manifestations such as neck vein distention and peripheral edema. Hemodynamic monitoring is often initiated for clients with evidence of heart failure. Heart failure and its manifestations are discussed in greater depth in Chapter 30.

*CARDIOGENIC SHOCK.* *Cardiogenic shock,* impaired tissue perfusion due to pump failure, results when functioning myocardial muscle mass decreases by more than 40%. The heart is unable to pump enough blood to meet the needs of the body and maintain organ function. Low cardiac output due to cardiogenic shock also impairs perfusion of the coronary arteries and myocardium, further increasing tissue damage. Mortality from cardiogenic shock is greater than 70%, although this can be reduced by prompt intervention with revascularization procedures. See Chapter 6 for a more extensive discussion of cardiogenic shock.

### Infarct Extension

Approximately 10% of clients experience extension or reinfarction in the area of the original infarction during the first 10 to 14 days after an MI. *Extension* of the MI is characterized by increased myocardial necrosis from continued blood flow impairment and ongoing injury. *Expansion* of the MI is described as a permanent expansion of the infarcted area from thinning and dilation of the muscle. Infarct extension and expansion may cause manifestations such as continuing chest pain, hemodynamic compromise, and worsening heart failure.

### Structural Defects

Necrotic muscle is replaced by scar tissue that is thinner than the ventricular muscle mass. This can lead to such complications as ventricular aneurysm, rupture of the interventricular septum or papillary muscle, and myocardial rupture. A *ventricular aneurysm* is an outpouching of the ventricular wall. It may develop when a large section of the ventricle is replaced by scar tissue. Because it does not contract during systole, stroke volume decreases. Blood may pool within the aneurysm, causing clots to form. Ischemia of the papillary muscle or chordae tendineae may cause structural damage leading to papillary muscle dysfunction or rupture. This affects AV valve function (usually the mitral valve), causing *regurgitation,* backflow of blood into the atria during systole. The interventricular septum may perforate or rupture due to ischemia and infarction. Myocardial rupture is a risk between days 4 and 7 after MI, when the injured tissue is soft and weak. This potential complication of MI is often fatal.

### Pericarditis

Tissue necrosis prompts an inflammatory response. *Pericarditis,* inflammation of the pericardial tissue surrounding the heart, may complicate AMI, usually within 2 to 3 days. Pericarditis causes chest pain that may be aching or sharp and stabbing, aggravated by movement or deep breathing. A *pericardial friction rub* may be heard on auscultation of heart sounds.

*Dressler's syndrome,* thought to be a hypersensitivity response to necrotic tissue or an autoimmune disorder, may develop days to weeks after AMI. It is a symptom complex characterized by fever, chest pain, and dyspnea. Dressler's syndrome may spontaneously resolve or recur over several months, causing significant discomfort and distress.

## COLLABORATIVE CARE

Immediate treatment goals for the MI client are to:

- Relieve chest pain.
- Reduce the extent of myocardial damage.
- Maintain cardiovascular stability.
- Decrease cardiac workload.
- Prevent complications.

Slowing the process of coronary heart disease and reducing the risk of future MI is a major long-term management goal for the client.

Rapid assessment and early diagnosis is important in treating AMI. "Time is muscle" is a medical truism for the client with AMI. The evolution of an AMI is dynamic: The quicker the artery is reopened (medically, surgically, or spontaneously), the more myocardium can be salvaged. Survival and long-term outcomes following AMI are improved by rapidly restoring blood flow to the "stunned" myocardium surrounding the infracted tissue, reducing myocardial oxygen demand and limiting the accumulation of toxic by-products of necrosis and reperfusion (Braunwald et al., 2001). The American Heart Association (AHA) recommends initiation of definitive treatment within 1 hour of entry into the health care system.

The major problem interfering with timely reperfusion is delay in seeking medical care following the onset of symptoms. Up to 44% of clients with symptoms of chest discomfort or pain wait more than 4 hours before seeking treatment. Many factors are cited as reasons for treatment delay, including advanced age, the perception of the seriousness of symptoms, denial, access to medical care, the availability of an emergency response system, and in-hospital delays (see the Nursing Research box below). Immediate evaluation of the client presenting with manifestations of myocardial infarction is essential to early diagnosis and treatment.

### Diagnostic Tests

Diagnostic testing is used to establish the diagnosis of AMI.

### Serum Cardiac Markers

*Serum cardiac markers* are proteins released from necrotic heart muscle. The proteins most specific for diagnosis of MI are the creatine phosphokinase (CK or CPK) and cardiac-specific troponins (see Table 29–5).

## Nursing Research

### Evidence-Based Practice for the Client Experiencing Acute Myocardial Infarction

Delay in seeking treatment significantly affects the mortality and morbidity of clients experiencing AMI. Research indicates that the sooner clients seek treatment after the onset of symptoms the greater the degree of myocardial salvage. However, many clients with AMI do not receive prompt treatment because they delay seeking medical care. In one study, researchers used the Health Belief Model as a framework for their study of variables associated with treatment delay in clients experiencing cardiac symptomatology (Dracup & Moser, 1997).

These researchers were interested in internal and/or external motivators that affected the client's decision to seek medical care. Seventy-seven subjects with a diagnosis of suspected or confirmed MI made up the sample. The study sample consisted of mainly white (82%) males (71%) with a mean age of 58.6 (+11.7) years; ages ranged from 35 to 80. Data were collected via a client questionnaire and chart review.

In this study, 60% of the sample delayed seeking treatment for longer than 3 hours. The median delay for the entire sample was 5 hours. Findings revealed that (1) clients over the age of 60 were more likely to delay treatment than younger clients, (2) the presence of family members increased the delay time, possibly because of a "shared denial" of the seriousness of the symptoms, and (3) the client's interpretation of the symptoms as not serious added to the delay.

#### IMPLICATIONS FOR NURSING

Efforts to educate the public in the seriousness of cardiac symptomatology must be continued and expanded. Programs should emphasize the warning signs of myocardial ischemia and infarction, the negative consequences of delay in seeking treatment, the benefits associated with early treatment of acute MI, and how and when to access the emergency response system.

Nurses should recognize that clients over age 60 may need extra attention and reinforcement of emergency information. Teaching individualized to the cardiac history and other existing disease processes may help the client to distinguish manifestations that require treatment from those that are associated with chronic problems. Refusal to acknowledge the warnings of cardiac disease was shown to correlate with treatment delay. Therefore, every opportunity must be taken to educate the public to make appropriate decisions during a potential cardiac event. Including the family in this teaching is encouraged. This data showed that clients who had family members present during the cardiac event delayed an average of 9 hours, compared to a 2-hour delay for clients who were alone during the experience.

#### Critical Thinking in Client Care

1. In what settings, other than the hospital, can nurses provide cardiac education classes to the public?
2. How does the concept of denial affect the client's decision to seek medical care?
3. How does the Health Belief Model offer a framework for the purposes of this study?
4. What is the extent of the emergency response system in your area, and how is it accessed?
5. What is the average length of time from activation of the system to arrival at the emergency center? How does this affect the overall onset-to-treatment goal of 60 minutes?

TABLE 29–5   Cardiac Markers

| Marker | Normal Level | Primary Tissue Location | Significance of Elevation | Changes Occuring with MI | | |
|---|---|---|---|---|---|---|
| | | | | Appears | Peaks | Duration |
| CK (CPK) | Male: 12 to 80 U/L Female: 10 to 70 U/L | Cardiac muscle, skeletal muscle, brain | Injury to muscle cells | 3 to 6 hours | 12 to 24 hours | 24 to 48 hours |
| CK-MB | 0% to 3% of total CK | Cardiac muscle | MI, cardiac ischemia, myocarditis, cardiac contusion, defibrillation | 4 to 8 hours | 18 to 24 hours | 72 hours |
| $cT_nT$ | < 0.2 mcg/L | Cardiac muscle | Acute MI, unstable angina | 2 to 4 hours | 24 to 36 hours | 10 to 14 days |
| $cT_nI$ | < 3.1 mcg/L | Cardiac muscle | Acute MI, unstable angina | 2 to 4 hours | 24 to 36 hours | 7 to 10 days |

- *Creatine phosphokinase* is an important enzyme for cellular function found principally in cardiac and skeletal muscle and the brain. CK levels rise rapidly with damage to these tissues, appearing in the serum 4 to 6 hours after AMI, peaking within 12 to 24 hours, and then declining over the next 48 to 72 hours. The CK level correlates with the size of the infarction; the greater the amount of infarcted tissue, the higher the serum CK level.
- *CK-MB* (also called MB-bands) is a subset of CK specific to cardiac muscle. This isoenzyme of CK is considered the most sensitive indicator of MI. Elevated CK alone is not specific for MI; elevated CK-MB greater than 5% is considered a positive indicator of MI. CK-MB levels do not normally rise with chest pain from angina or causes other than MI.
- Cardiac muscle troponins, *cardiac-specific troponin T ($cT_nT$)* and *cardiac-specific troponin I ($cT_nI$),* are proteins released during myocardial infarction that are sensitive indicators of myocardial damage. These proteins are part of the actin-myocin unit in cardiac muscle and normally are not detectable in the blood. With necrosis of cardiac muscle, troponins are released and blood levels rise. The specificity of $cT_nT$ and $cT_nI$ to cardiac muscle necrosis makes these markers particularly useful when skeletal muscle trauma contributes to elevated CK levels (e.g., when CPR has been performed or traumatic injury occurred at the time of the MI). They are sensitive enough to detect very small infarctions that do not cause significant CK elevation. Both $cT_nT$ and $cT_nI$ remain in the blood for 10 to 14 days after an MI, making them useful to diagnose MI when medical treatment is delayed.

Serum levels of cardiac markers are ordered on admission and for 3 succeeding days. Serial blood levels help establish the diagnosis and determine the extent of myocardial damage.

Other laboratory tests may include the following:

- *Myoglobin* is one of the first cardiac markers to be detectable in the blood after an MI. It is released within a few hours of symptom onset. Its lack of specificity to cardiac muscle and rapid excretion (blood levels return to normal within 24 hours) limit its use, however (Braunwald et al., 2001).
- *Complete blood count (CBC)* shows an elevated white blood cell (WBC) count due to inflammation of the injured myocardium. The *erythrocyte sedimentation rate (ESR)* also rises because of inflammation.
- *Arterial blood gases (ABGs)* may be ordered to assess blood oxygen levels and acid-base balance.

Electrocardiography, echocardiography, and myocardial nuclear scans are the most common diagnostic tests performed when AMI is suspected. With the exception of the ECG, the timing of these tests depends on the client's immediate condition. Hemodynamic monitoring may be initiated in the unstable client following MI.

- The *electrocardiogram* reflects changes in conduction due to myocardial ischemia and necrosis. Characteristic ECG changes seen in AMI include T wave inversion, elevation of the ST segment, and formation of a Q wave. Ischemic changes in the heart are seen as depression of the ST segment or inversion of the T wave (see Figure 29–2). With myocardial injury, elevation of the ST segment occurs (Figure 29–6A ■). Significant Q wave development (Figure 29–6B) indicates a transmural, or full-thickness infarction. Myocardial damage can be localized using the 12-lead ECG. See the next section of this chapter for more information about ECGs.
- *Echocardiography* is a noninvasive test to evaluate cardiac wall motion and left ventricular function. Images are produced as ultrasound waves strike cardiac structures and are reflected back through a transducer. Echocardiography can be done at the bedside.
- *Radionuclide imaging* may be done to evaluate myocardial perfusion. These studies cannot differentiate between an acute MI and old scar tissue, but do help identify the specific area of myocardial ischemia and damage. Several isotopes may be used. Thallium-201 collects in normally perfused myocardium; ischemic areas appear blue or as "cold" spots when the heart is scanned for radioactivity. In contrast, technetium-99m pyrophosphate, another commonly used radioisotope, accumulates in ischemic tissue and appears red, or "hot."
- *Hemodynamic monitoring* may be initiated when AMI significantly affects cardiac output and hemodynamic status. These invasive procedures are described in Chapter 30.

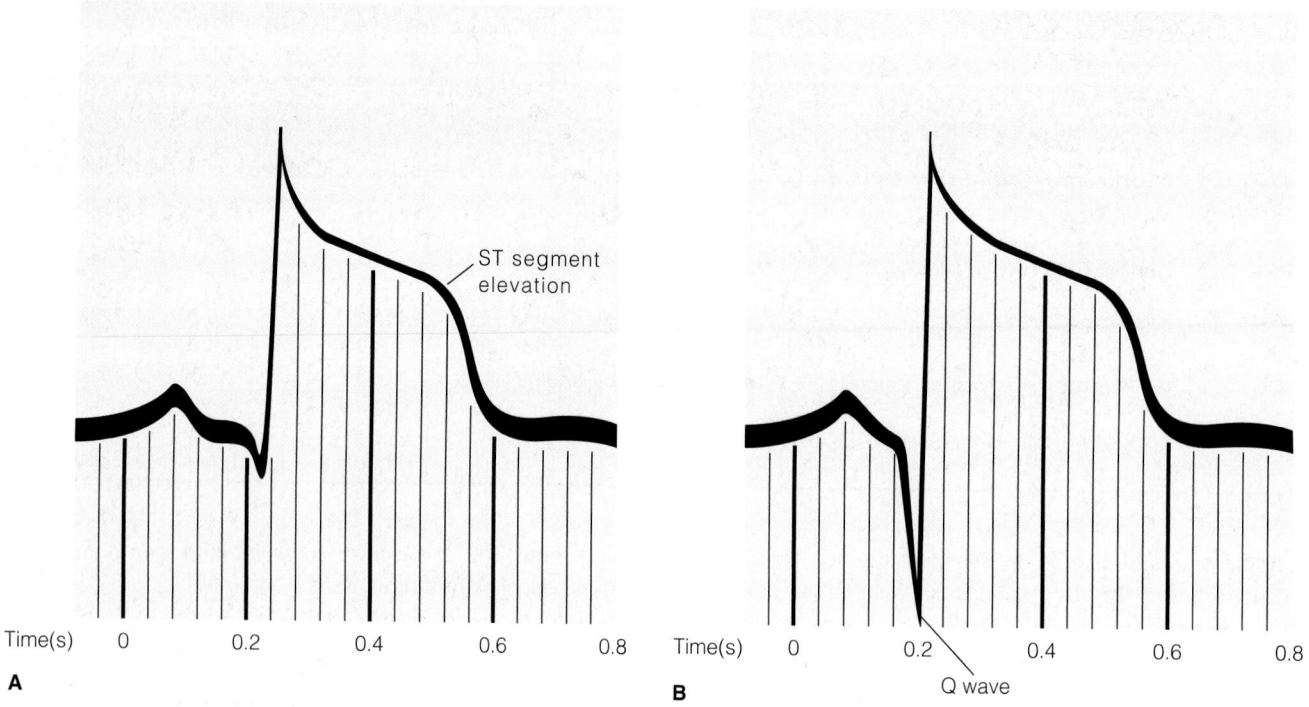

**Figure 29–6** ■ ECG changes characteristic of MI. *A*, ST segment elevation characteristic of myocardial injury. *B*, Clinically significant Q wave characteristic of a transmural infarction.

## Medications

Aspirin, a platelet inhibitor, is now considered an essential part of treating AMI. A 160 to 325 mg aspirin tablet is given by emergency personnel, with the instructions that it is to be chewed (for buccal absorption). This initial dose is followed by a daily oral dose of 160 to 325 mg of aspirin.

Other medications are used to help reduce oxygen demand and increase oxygen supply. Thrombolytic agents, analgesics, and antidysrhythmic agents are among the principal classes of drugs used.

### Thrombolytic Therapy

Thrombolytic agents, drugs that dissolve or break up blood clots, are first-line drugs used to treat acute MI. These drugs activate the fibrinolytic system to lyse or destroy the clot, restoring blood flow to the obstructed artery. Early thrombolytic administration (within the first 6 hours of MI onset) limits infarct size, reduces heart damage, and improves outcomes. Activation of the fibrinolytic system can cause multiple complications; approximately 0.5% to 5% of clients receiving thrombolytic drugs experience serious bleeding complications. Not every client is a candidate for thrombolytic therapy; for example, it is contraindicated in clients with known bleeding disorders, history of cerebrovascular disease, uncontrolled hypertension, pregnancy, or recent trauma or surgery of the head or spine (Tierney et al., 2001).

Four thrombolytic agents are commonly used today. Among the four, little difference in effectiveness has been demonstrated; there are, however, big differences in cost. Streptokinase, a biologic agent derived from group C *Streptococcus* organisms, is the least expensive of the drugs. Its primary drawback is the risk of a severe hypersensitivity reaction, in-cluding anaphylaxis. Streptokinase is administered by intravenous infusion. Anisoylated plasminogen streptokinase activator complex (APSAC) is a related drug that can be administered by bolus over 2 to 5 minutes. It has many of the same effects as streptokinase, but is considerably more expensive. Tissue plasminogen activator (t-PA) and reteplase are more effective in reestablishing myocardial perfusion, especially when the pain developed more than 3 hours previously. These drugs, however, are the most expensive. Nursing care of the client receiving a thrombolytic agent is outlined on the next page.

### Analgesia

Pain relief is vital in treating the client with AMI. Pain stimulates the sympathetic nervous system, increasing the heart rate and blood pressure and, in turn, myocardial workload. Sublingual nitroglycerin may be given (up to three 0.4-mg doses at 5-minute intervals). In addition to pain relief, nitroglycerin may decrease myocardial oxygen demand and increase the supply of oxygen to the myocardium by dilating collateral vessels. Morphine sulfate is the drug of choice for pain and sedation. Following an initial intravenous dose of 4 to 8 mg, small doses (2 to 4 mg) may be repeated intravenously every 5 minutes until pain is relieved. It is important to assess frequently for pain relief and possible adverse effects of analgesia, such as excessive sedation. See Chapter 4 ⬯ for more details about morphine administration. Antianxiety agents such as diazepam (Valium) may also be administered to promote rest.

### Antidysrhythmics

Dysrhythmias are a common complication of AMI, particularly in the first 12 to 24 hours. Antidysrhythmic medications are used as needed to treat dysrhythmias. They also may be given

# NURSING CARE OF THE CLIENT RECEIVING THROMBOLYTIC THERAPY

## PREINFUSION CARE

- Obtain nursing history, and perform a physical assessment. *Information obtained from the history and physical exam helps determine whether thrombolytic therapy is appropriate. The goal is to initiate thrombolytic therapy within 30 minutes of arrival.*
- Evaluate for contraindications to thrombolytic therapy: recent surgery or trauma (including prolonged CPR), bleeding disorders or active bleeding, cerebral vascular accident, neurosurgery within the last 2 months, gastrointestinal ulcers, diabetic hemorrhagic retinopathy, and uncontrolled hypertension. *Thrombolytic agents dissolve clots and therefore may precipitate intracranial, internal, or peripheral bleeding.*
- Inform the client of the purpose of the therapy. Discuss the risk of bleeding and the need to keep the extremity immobile during and after the infusion. *Minimal movement of the extremity is necessary to prevent bleeding from the infusion site.*

## DURING THE INFUSION

- Assess and record vital signs and the infusion site for hematoma or bleeding every 15 minutes for the first hour, every 30 minutes for the next 2 hours, and then hourly until the intravenous catheter is discontinued. Assess pulses, color, sensation, and temperature of both extremities with each vital sign check. *Vital signs and the site are frequently assessed to detect possible complications.*
- Remind the client to keep the extremity still and straight. Do not elevate head of bed above 15 degrees. *Extremity immobilization helps prevent infusion site trauma and bleeding. Hypotension may develop; keeping the bed flat helps maintain cerebral perfusion.*
- Maintain continuous cardiac monitoring during the infusion. Keep antidysrhythmic drugs and the emergency cart readily available for treatment of significant dysrhythmias. *Ventricular dysrhythmias commonly occur with reperfusion of the ischemic myocardium.*

## POSTINFUSION CARE

- Assess vital signs, distal pulses, and infusion site frequently as needed. *The client remains at high risk for bleeding following thrombolytic therapy.*
- Evaluate response to therapy: normalization of ST segment, relief of chest pain, reperfusion dysrhythmias, early peaking of the CK and CK-MB. *These are signs that the clot has been dissolved and the myocardium is being reperfused.*
- Maintain bed rest for 6 hours. Keep the head of the bed at or below 15 degrees. Reinforce the need to keep the extremity straight and immobile. Avoid any injections for 24 hours after catheter removal. *Precautions such as these are important to prevent bleeding.*
- Assess puncture sites for bleeding. On catheter removal hold direct pressure over the site for at least 30 minutes. Apply a pressure dressing to any venous or arterial sites as needed. Perform routine care in a gentle manner to avoid bruising or injury. *Thrombolytic therapy disrupts normal coagulation. Peripheral bleeding may occur at puncture sites, and there may not be sufficient fibrin to form a clot. Direct or indirect pressure may be needed to control the bleeding.*
- Assess body fluids, including urine, vomitus, and feces, for evidence of bleeding; frequently assess for changes in level of consciousness and manifestations of increased intracranial pressure, which may indicate intracranial bleeding. Assess surgical sites for bleeding. Monitor hemoglobin and hematocrit levels, prothrombin time (PT), and partial thromboplastin time (PTT). *These provide additional means of assessing for bleeding.*
- Administer platelet-modifying drugs (e.g., aspirin, dipyridamole) as ordered. *Platelet inhibitors decrease platelet aggregation and adhesion and are used to prevent reocclusion of the artery.*
- Report manifestations of reocclusion, including changes in the ST segment, chest pain, or dysrhythmias. *Early recognition of reocclusion is vital to save myocardial tissue.*

---

prophylactically to prevent dysrhythmias. Ventricular dysrhythmias are treated with a class I or class III antidysrhythmic drug (see the Medication Administration box on page 854). Symptomatic bradycardia (bradycardia with associated hypotension and other signs of low cardiac output) is treated with intravenous atropine, 0.5 to 1 mg. Intravenous verapamil or the short-acting beta blocker esmolol (Brevibloc) may be ordered to treat atrial fibrillation or other supraventricular tachydysrhythmias.

## Other Medications

Beta blockers such as propranolol (Inderal), atenolol (Tenormin), and metoprolol (Lopressor) reduce pain, limit infarct size, and decrease the incidence of serious ventricular dysrhythmias in AMI. These drugs decrease the heart rate, reducing cardiac work and myocardial oxygen demand. Initial doses are given intravenously. Oral beta blocker therapy is continued to reduce the risk of reinfarction and death related to cardiovascular causes (Braunwald et al., 2001).

Angiotensin-converting enzyme (ACE) inhibitors also reduce mortality associated with AMI. These drugs reduce ventricular remodeling following an MI, reducing the risk for subsequent heart failure. They also may reduce the risk of reinfarction (Braunwald et al., 2001).

Intravenous nitroglycerin may be administered for the first 24 to 48 hours to reduce myocardial work. Nitroglycerin is a peripheral and arterial vasodilator that reduces afterload. It dilates coronary arteries and collateral channels in the heart, increasing coronary blood flow to save myocardial tissue at risk. Nitrates may, however, cause reflex tachycardia or excessive hypotension, so close monitoring is necessary during administration. See the Medication Administration box on page 818 for the nursing implications of these drugs.

Anticoagulants and other antiplatelet medications often are prescribed to maintain coronary artery patency following thrombolysis or a revascularization procedure. Abciximab (ReoPro) suppresses platelet aggregation and reduces the risk of reocclusion following angioplasty. It also improves vessel opening with thrombolytic therapy, permitting lower doses of thrombolytic drugs (Lehne, 2001). Standard or low-molecular-weight heparin preparations often are given to clients with AMI. Heparin helps establish and maintain patency of the affected coronary artery. It also is used, along with long-term warfarin, to prevent systemic or pulmonary embolism in clients with significant left ventricular impairment or atrial fibrillation following AMI. See Chapter 33 ⊖⊃ for more information about anticoagulant therapy.

Clients with pump failure and hypotension may receive intravenous dopamine, a vasopressor. At low doses (less than 5 mg/kg/min), it improves blood flow to the kidneys, preventing renal ischemia and possible acute renal failure (see Chapter 27). With increasing doses, dopamine increases myocardial contractility and causes vasoconstriction, improving blood pressure and cardiac output.

Antilipemic agents are used for the client with hyperlipidemia. A stool softener such as docusate sodium is prescribed to maintain normal bowel function and reduce straining.

## Medical Management

The client with a suspected or confirmed MI is monitored continuously. Care is provided in the intensive coronary care unit for the first 24 to 48 hours, after which time less intensive monitoring (e.g., telemetry) may be required. An intravenous line is established to allow rapid administration of emergency medications.

Bed rest is prescribed for the first 12 hours to reduce the cardiac workload. The bedside commode generally is allowed; studies have shown this to be less stressful than using a bedpan. If the client's condition is stable, sitting in a chair at the bedside is permitted after 12 hours. Activities are gradually increased as tolerated. A quiet, calm environment with limited outside stimuli is preferred. Visitors are limited to promote rest. Oxygen is administered by nasal cannula at 2 to 5 L/min to improve oxygenation of the myocardium and other tissues.

A liquid diet is often prescribed for the first 4 to 12 hours to reduce gastric distention and myocardial work. Following that, a low-fat, low-cholesterol, reduced-sodium diet is allowed. Sodium restrictions may be lifted after 2 to 3 days if no evidence of heart failure is present. Small, frequent feedings are often recommended. Drinks containing caffeine, and very hot and cold foods may also be limited.

## Revascularization Procedures

Many clients with AMI are treated with immediate or early percutaneous coronary revascularization (PCR) such as angioplasty and stent placement. PCR may follow thrombolytic therapy or be used in place of thrombolytic therapy to restore blood flow to ischemic myocardium. When compared with thrombolytic therapy, prompt PCR reduces hospital mortality (Braunwald et al., 2001). In some cases, CABG surgery may be performed. The choice of procedure depends on the client's age and immediate condition, the time elapsed from the onset of manifestations, and the extent of myocardial disease and dam-

age. These procedures and related nursing care are covered in more depth in the preceding section on angina.

## Other Invasive Procedures

For clients with large MIs and evidence of pump failure, invasive devices may be used to temporarily take over the function of the heart, allowing the injured myocardium to heal. The intra-aortic balloon pump is widely used to augment cardiac output. Ventricular assist devices are indicated for clients requiring more or longer term artificial support than the intra-aortic balloon pump provides.

### Intra-Aortic Balloon Pump

The *intra-aortic balloon pump (IABP)*, also called intra-aortic balloon counterpulsation, is a mechanical circulatory support device that may be used after cardiac surgery or to treat cardiogenic shock following AMI. The IABP temporarily supports cardiac function, allowing the heart gradually to recover by decreasing myocardial workload and oxygen demand and increasing perfusion of the coronary arteries.

A catheter with a 30 to 40 mL balloon is introduced into the aorta, usually via the femoral artery. The balloon catheter is connected to a console that regulates the inflation and deflation of the balloon. The IABP catheter inflates during diastole, increasing perfusion of the coronary and renal arteries, and deflates during systole, decreasing afterload and cardiac workload (Figure 29–7 ■). The inflation–deflation sequence is triggered by the ECG pattern. During the most acute period, the balloon inflates and deflates with each heart beat (1:1 ratio), providing maximal assistance to the heart. As the client's condition improves, the IABP is weaned to inflate–deflate at varying intervals (e.g., 1:2, 1:4, 1:8). This provides a continually decreasing amount of support as the heart muscle recovers. When mechanical assistance is no longer required, the IABP catheter is removed.

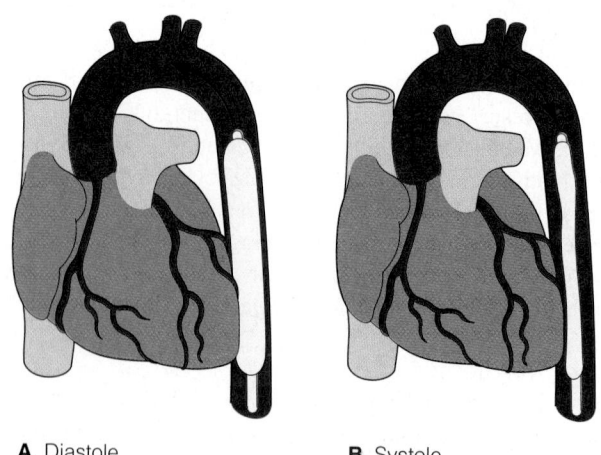

**A** Diastole  **B** Systole

**Figure 29–7** ■ The intra-aortic balloon pump. *A,* When inflated during diastole, the balloon supports cerebral, renal, and coronary artery perfusion. *B,* The balloon deflates during systole, so cardiac output is unimpeded.

## Ventricular Assist Devices

Use of *ventricular assist devices (VADs)* to aid the failing heart is becoming more common with advances in technology. Whereas the IABP can supplement cardiac output by approximately 10% to 15%, the VAD temporarily takes partial or complete control of cardiac function, depending on the type of device used. VADs may be used as temporary or complete assist in AMI and cardiogenic shock when there is a chance for recovery of normal heart function after a period of cardiac rest. The device also may be used as a bridge to heart transplant. Nursing care for the client with a VAD is supportive and includes assessing hemodynamic status and for complications associated with the device. Clients with VAD are at considerable risk for infection; strict aseptic technique is used with all invasive catheters and dressing changes. Pneumonia also is a risk due to immobility and ventilatory support. Mechanical failure of the VAD is a life-threatening event that requires immediate intervention (Urden, Stacy, & Lough 2002).

## Cardiac Rehabilitation

**Cardiac rehabilitation** is a long-term program of medical evaluation, exercise, risk factor modification, education, and counseling designed to limit the physical and psychological effects of cardiac illness and improve the client's quality of life (Woods et al., 2000). Cardiac rehabilitation begins with admission for a cardiac event such as AMI or a revascularization procedure. Phase 1 of the program is the inpatient phase. A thorough assessment of the client's history, current status, risk factors, and motivation is obtained. During this phase, activity progresses from bed rest to independent performance of activities of daily living (ADLs) and ambulation within the facility. Both subjective and objective responses to increasing activity levels are evaluated. Excess fatigue, shortness of breath, chest pain, tachypnea, tachycardia, or cool, clammy skin indicate activity intolerance. Phase 2, immediate outpatient cardiac rehabilitation, begins within 3 weeks of the cardiac event. The goals for the outpatient program are to increase activity level, participation, and capacity; improve psychosocial status and treat anxiety or depression; and provide education and support for risk factor reduction. Continuation programs, phase 3 of cardiac rehabilitation, are directed at providing a transition to independent exercise and exercise maintenance. During this final phase, the client may "check in" every 3 months to evaluate risk factors, quality of life, and exercise habits (Woods et al., 2000).

## NURSING CARE

## Health Promotion

Health promotion activities to prevent acute myocardial infarction are those outlined for coronary heart disease and angina in previous sections of this chapter. In addition, discuss risk factor management, use of prescribed medications, and cardiac rehabilitation to reduce the risk of complications or future infarctions.

## Assessment

Nursing assessment for the client with AMI must be both timely and ongoing. Assessment data related to AMI includes the following:

- Health history: complaints of chest pain, including its location, intensity, character, radiation, and timing; associated symptoms such as nausea, heartburn, shortness of breath, and anxiety; treatment measures taken since onset of pain; past medical history, especially cardiac related; chronic diseases; current medications and any known allergies to medications; smoking history and use of recreational drugs and alcohol
- Physical examination: general appearance including obvious signs of distress; vital signs; peripheral pulses; skin color, temperature, moisture; level of consciousness; heart and breath sounds; cardiac rhythm (on beside monitor); bowel sounds, abdominal tenderness

## Nursing Diagnoses and Interventions

Priorities of nursing care include relieving chest pain, reducing cardiac work, and promoting oxygenation. Psychosocial support is especially important, because an acute myocardial infarction can be devastating, bringing the client face-to-face with his or her own mortality for the first time.

### Acute Pain

Chest pain occurs when the oxygen supply to the heart muscle does not meet the demand. Myocardial ischemia and infarction cause pain, as does reperfusion of an ischemic area following thrombolytic therapy or emergent PTCA. Pain stimulates the sympathetic nervous system, increasing cardiac work. Pain relief is a priority of care for the client with AMI.

- Assess for verbal and nonverbal signs of pain. Document characteristics and the intensity of the pain, using a standard pain scale. Verify nonverbal indicators of pain with the client. *Frequent, careful pain assessment allows early intervention to reduce the risk of further damage. Pain is a subjective experience; its expression may vary with location and intensity, previous experiences, and cultural and social background. Pain scales provide an objective tool for measuring pain and a way to assess pain relief or reduction.*
- Administer oxygen at 2 to 5 L/min per nasal cannula. *Supplemental oxygen increases oxygen supply to the myocardium, decreasing ischemia and pain.*
- Promote physical and psychologic rest. Provide information and emotional support. *Rest decreases cardiac workload and sympathetic nervous system stimulation, promoting comfort. Information and emotional support help decrease anxiety and provide psychologic rest.*
- Titrate intravenous nitroglycerin as ordered to relieve chest pain, maintaining a systolic blood pressure greater than 100 mmHg. *Nitroglycerin decreases chest pain by dilating peripheral vessels, reducing cardiac work, and dilating coronary vessels, including collateral channels, improving blood flow to ischemic tissue.*

**PRACTICE ALERT** *Intravenous nitroglycerine causes peripheral vasodilation, which may lead to hypotension, reduced coronary blood flow, and tachycardia. Reduce the nitro flow rate and notify the physician if this occurs.* ∎

- Administer 2 to 4 mg morphine by intravenous push for chest pain as needed. *Morphine is an effective narcotic analgesic for chest pain. It decreases pain and anxiety, acts as a venodilator, and decreases the respiratory rate. The resulting reduction in preload and sympathetic nervous system stimulation reduces cardiac work and oxygen consumption.*

**PRACTICE ALERT** *Reassess for relief of chest pain. The goal of care is to achieve pain relief, not simply a reduction in pain to a "manageable" level.* ∎

### Ineffective Tissue Perfusion

Cardiac muscle damage affects its compliance, contractility, and the cardiac output. The extent of the effect on tissue perfusion depends on the location and amount of damage. Anterior wall infarcts have a greater effect on cardiac output than do right ventricular infarcts. Infarcted muscle also increases the risk for cardiac dysrhythmias, which can also affect the delivery of blood and oxygen to the tissues.

- Assess and document vital signs. Report increases in heart rate and changes in rhythm, blood pressure, and respiratory rate. *Decreased cardiac output activates compensatory mechanisms that may cause tachycardia and vasoconstriction, increasing cardiac work.*
- Assess for changes in level of consciousness (LOC); decreased urine output; moist, cool, pale, mottled or cyanotic skin; dusky or cyanotic mucous membranes and nail beds; diminished to absent peripheral pulses; delayed capillary refill. *These are manifestations of impaired tissue perfusion. A change in LOC is often the first manifestation of altered perfusion because brain tissue and cerebral function depends on a continuous supply of oxygen.*
- Auscultate heart and breath sounds. Note abnormal heart sounds (e.g., an $S_3$ or $S_4$ gallop or a murmur) or adventitious lung sounds. *Abnormal heart sounds or adventitious lung sounds may indicate impaired cardiac filling or output, increasing the risk for decreased tissue perfusion.*
- Monitor ECG rhythm continuously. *Dysrhythmias can further impair cardiac output and tissue perfusion.*

**PRACTICE ALERT** *Obtain a 12-lead ECG to assess complaints of chest pain. Report marked changes to the physician. Continued or unrelieved chest pain may indicate further myocardial ischemia and extension of the infarct; an ECG during episodes of chest pain provides a valuable diagnostic tool to assess myocardial perfusion.* ∎

- Monitor oxygen saturation levels. Administer oxygen as ordered. Obtain and assess ABGs as indicated. *Oxygen saturation is an indicator of gas exchange, tissue perfusion, and the*

effectiveness of oxygen administration. ABGs provide a more precise measurement of blood oxygen levels and allow assessment of acid-base balance.
- Administer antidysrhythmic medications as needed. *Dysrhythmias affect tissue perfusion by altering cardiac output.*
- Obtain serial CK, isoenzyme, and troponin levels as ordered. *Levels of cardiac markers, CK isoenzymes in particular, correlate with the extent of myocardial damage.*
- Plan for invasive hemodynamic monitoring. *Hemodynamic monitoring facilitates AMI management and treatment evaluation by providing a means of assessing pressures in the systemic and pulmonary arteries, the relationship between oxygen supply and demand, cardiac output, and cardiac index.*

**PRACTICE ALERT** *Continuously evaluate the response to interventions such as thrombolytic therapy, drugs to improve cardiac output and tissue perfusion, and drugs to reduce cardiac work. Adverse effects of therapy may reduce the effectiveness of treatment. Bleeding due to thrombolytic therapy may affect vascular volume and cardiac output; reperfusion dysrhythmias also may affect cardiac output. Drugs used to improve cardiac output may also increase cardiac work, whereas those given to reduce cardiac work may significantly affect contractility and cardiac output.* ∎

### Ineffective Coping

Coping mechanisms help a person deal with a life-threatening event or with acute changes in health. However, certain coping mechanisms may be detrimental to restoring health, particularly if the client relies on them for a prolonged period. Denial, for example, is a common coping mechanism among post–MI clients. In the initial stages, denial can reduce anxiety. Continued denial, however, can interfere with learning and compliance with treatment.

- Establish an environment of caring and trust. Encourage the client to express feelings. *Establishing a trusting nurse–client relationship provides a safe environment for the client to discuss feelings of helplessness, powerlessness, anxiety, and hopelessness. The nurse may then be able to provide additional resources to meet the client's needs.*
- Accept denial as a coping mechanism, but do not reinforce it. *Denial may initially help by diminishing the psychological threat to health, decreasing anxiety. However, its prolonged use can interfere with acceptance of reality and cooperation, possibly delaying treatment and hindering recovery.*
- Note aggressive behaviors, hostility, or anger. Document any failure to comply with treatments. *These signs can indicate anxiety and denial.*
- Help the client identify positive coping skills used in the past (e.g., problem-solving skills, verbalization of feelings, asking for help, prayer). Reinforce use of positive coping behaviors. *Coping behaviors that have been successful in the past can help the client deal with the current situation. These familiar methods can decrease feelings of powerlessness.*
- Provide opportunities for the client to make decisions about the plan of care, as possible. *This promotes self-confidence*

*and independence. Participating in care planning gives the client a sense of control and the opportunity to use positive coping skills.*

- Provide privacy for the client and significant other to share their questions and concerns. *Privacy provides an opportunity for the client and partner to share their feelings and fears, offer support and encouragement to one another, relieve anxiety, and establish effective coping methods.*

### Fear

The fear of death and disability can be a paralyzing emotion that adversely affects the client's recovery from acute myocardial infarction.

- Identify the client's level of fear, noting verbal and nonverbal signs. *This information enables the nurse to plan appropriate interventions. Clients may not voice concerns; attention to nonverbal indicators is important. Controlling fear helps decrease sympathetic nervous system responses and catecholamine release that may increase feelings of fear and anxiety.*
- Acknowledge the client's perception of the situation. Allow to verbalize concerns. *A sudden change in health status causes anxiety and fear of the unknown. Verbalizing these fears may help the client cope with change and allow the health care team to provide information and correct misconceptions.*
- Encourage questions and provide consistent, factual answers. Repeat information as needed. *Accurate and consistent information can reduce fear. Honest explanations help strengthen the client-nurse relationship and help the client develop realistic expectations. Anxiety and fear decrease the ability to concentrate and retain information; therefore, information may need to be repeated.*
- Encourage self-care. Allow the client to make decisions regarding the plan of care. *This promotes personal responsi-*

*bility for health and allows some control over the situation. Clients' confidence increases as their dependence decreases.*

- Administer antianxiety medications as ordered. *These medications promote rest and relaxation and decrease feelings of anxiety, which may act as barriers to health restoration.*
- Teach nonpharmacologic methods of stress reduction (e.g., relaxation techniques, mental imagery, music therapy, breathing exercises, meditation, massage). *Stress management techniques can help reduce tension and anxiety, provide a sense of control, and enhance coping skills.*

## Using NANDA, NIC, and NOC

Chart 29–2 shows links between NANDA nursing diagnoses, NIC, and NOC for the client with acute myocardial infarction.

## Home Care

Cardiac rehabilitation begins with admission to the health care facility and continues through the inpatient stay and after discharge into the rehabilitative period. The emphasis is on realistic application of information to maintain lifestyle changes.

Assessing readiness to learn is an important first step in preparing for home care. The client in strong denial may not identify any relevance to the information being taught. Evaluate ability to learn, assessing physiologic and psychologic health, beliefs regarding personal responsibility for health, and expectations of the health care system. Also assess developmental level, ability to perform psychomotor skills, cognitive function, learning disabilities, existing knowledge base, and the influence of previous learning experiences. Provide written material to supplement teaching and encourage questions.

Include the following topics in teaching for home care.

- The normal anatomy and physiology of the heart, and the specific area of heart damage

---

### CHART 29–2 NANDA, NIC, AND NOC LINKAGES

#### The Client with Acute Myocardial Infarction

| NURSING DIAGNOSES | NURSING INTERVENTIONS | NURSING OUTCOMES |
|---|---|---|
| • Acute Pain | • Analgesic Administration<br>• Medication Management | • Pain Control<br>• Pain: Disruptive Effects |
| • Anxiety | • Anxiety Reduction<br>• Coping Enhancement | • Anxiety Control<br>• Coping |
| • Decreased Cardiac Output | • Cardiac Care: Acute<br>• Hemodynamic Regulation<br>• Shock Management: Cardiac | • Cardiac Pump Effectiveness<br>• Circulation Status<br>• Tissue Perfusion: Peripheral<br>• Vital Signs Status |
| • Ineffective Family Coping | • Coping Enhancement<br>• Family Involvement Promotion | • Family Coping |
| • Ineffective Tissue Perfusion: Cardiopulmonary | • Bleeding Precautions<br>• Dysrhythmia Management<br>• Cardiac Care: Rehabilitative | • Cardiac Pump Effectiveness<br>• Tissue Perfusion: Cardiac |

*Note. Data from Nursing Outcomes Classification (NOC) by M. Johnson & M. Maas (Eds.), 1997, St. Louis: Mosby; Nursing Diagnoses: Definitions & Classification 2001–2002 by North American Nursing Diagnosis Association, 2001, Philadelphia: NANDA; Nursing Interventions Classification (NIC) by J.C. McCloskey & G. M. Bulechek (Eds.), 2000, St. Louis: Mosby. Reprinted by permission.*

- The process of CHD and implications of MI
- Purposes and side effects of prescribed medications
- The importance of complying with the medical regimen and cardiac rehabilitation program and of keeping follow-up appointments
- Information about community resources, such as the local chapter of the American Heart Association

After discharge, follow up by telephone within 1 week and periodically thereafter during the recovery period. Provide telephone numbers of resource personnel who are available to respond to questions and concerns after discharge. Because the client who has had an MI is at high risk for sudden cardiac death; encourage family members to learn CPR and provide information about community resources for CPR training.

## Nursing Care Plan
## A Client with Acute Myocardial Infarction

Betty Williams, a 62-year-old psychologist, is admitted to the emergency department with complaints of severe substernal chest pain. Mrs. Williams states that the pain began after lunch, about 4 hours ago. She initially attributed the pain to indigestion. She described the pain, which now radiates to her jaw and left arm, as "really severe heartburn." It is accompanied by a "choking feeling," severe shortness of breath, and diaphoresis. The pain is unrelieved by rest, antacids, or three sublingual nitroglycerin tablets (0.4 mg).

Oxygen is started per nasal cannula at 5 L/min. Central and peripheral intravenous lines are inserted. A 12-lead ECG and the following labwork are obtained: cardiac troponins, CK and CK isoenzymes, ABGs, CBC, and a chemistry panel. Morphine sulfate relieves Mrs. Williams's pain.

Mrs. Williams's medical history includes type 2 diabetes, angina, and hypertension. She has a 45-year history of cigarette smoking, averaging 1.5 to 2 packs per day. Family history reveals that Mrs. Williams's father died at age 42 of AMI, and her paternal grandfather died at age 65 of AMI. Mrs. Williams is taking the following medications: tolbutamide (Orinase), hydrochlorothiazide, and isosorbide (Isordil).

Based on ECG changes and cardiac markers, an acute anterior MI is diagnosed. Mrs. Williams has no contraindications to thrombolytic therapy and is deemed a good candidate. Intravenous alteplase (t-PA, Activase) is given by bolus followed by intravenous infusions of alteplase and heparin. She is transferred to the coronary care unit (CCU).

### ASSESSMENT

Dan Morales, RN, is Mrs. Williams's primary care nurse. Mrs. Williams is alert and oriented to person, place, and time. Vital signs are T 99.6° F (37.5° C), P 118, R 24 with adequate depth, and BP 172/92. Auscultation reveals an $S_4$ and fine crackles in the bases of both lungs. The ECG shows sinus tachycardia with occasional PVCs. Her skin is cool and slightly diaphoretic. Capillary refill is less than 3 seconds, and peripheral pulses are strong and equal. Her nail beds are pink.

A triple-lumen central line is in place. Nitroglycerin is infusing at 200 mcg/min in the distal lumen; the alteplase infusion is in the middle lumen; and a heparin infusion is in the proximal lumen. The peripheral intravenous line has a saline lock. Mrs. Williams states, "The pain is better since the nurse in the ER gave me a shot. But it has been coming and going. I would rate it a 4 right now, but it was terrible before. The doctor told me that this drug I'm getting will quickly open up the artery that is blocked. I hope it works! Do many people get this drug?"

### DIAGNOSES

- *Acute pain* related to ischemic myocardial tissue
- *Anxiety and fear* related to change in health status
- *Ineffective protection* related to the risk of bleeding secondary to thrombolytic therapy
- *Risk for decreased cardiac output* related to altered cardiac rate and rhythm

### EXPECTED OUTCOMES

- Rate chest pain as 2 or lower on a pain scale of 0 to 10.
- Verbalize reduced anxiety and fear.
- Demonstrate no signs of internal or external bleeding.
- Maintain an adequate cardiac output during and following reperfusion therapy.

### PLANNING AND IMPLEMENTATION

The following interventions are planned and implemented during the immediate phase of Mrs. Williams's hospitalization.

- Instruct to report all chest pain. Monitor and evaluate pain using a scale of 0 to 10. Titrate intravenous nitroglycerin infusion for chest pain; stop infusion if systolic BP is below 100 mmHg. Administer 2 to 4 mg morphine intravenously for chest pain unrelieved by nitroglycerin infusion.
- Encourage verbalization of fears and concerns. Respond honestly, and correct misconceptions about the disease, therapeutic interventions, or prognosis.
- Assess knowledge of CHD. Explain the purpose of thrombolytic therapy to dissolve the fresh clot and reperfuse the heart muscle, limiting heart damage.
- Explain the need for frequent monitoring of vital signs and potential bleeding.
- Assess for manifestations of internal or intracranial bleeding: complaints of back or abdominal pain, headache, decreased level of consciousness, dizziness, bloody secretions or excretions, or pallor. Test all stools, urine, and vomitus for occult blood. Notify physician immediately of any abnormal findings.
- Monitor for signs of reperfusion: decreased chest pain, return of ST segment to baseline, reperfusion dysrhythmias (e.g., PVCs, bradycardia, and heart block).
- Continuously monitor ECG for changes in cardiac rate, rhythm, and conduction. Assess vital signs.
- Treat dangerous dysrhythmias or other cardiac events per protocol. Notify the physician.
- Discuss continuing cardiac care and rehabilitation.

## Nursing Care Plan

## A Client with Acute Myocardial Infarction (continued)

### EVALUATION

The initial morphine dose reduces Mrs. Williams's chest pain from a rating of 8 to 4. The nitroglycerin infusion and thrombolytic therapy further reduce her pain to 2. The nitroglycerin infusion is gradually discontinued after 24 hours. As her pain subsides, Mrs. Williams states that she feels "much better now that the pain is gone. I was afraid it would just get worse." She verbalizes an understanding of thrombolytic therapy to limit myocardial damage. No indication of bleeding problems are noted. Reperfusion is indicated by relief of chest pain, return of the ST segment to baseline on the ECG; early peaking of CK levels; and increased frequency of PVCs but no significant dysrhythmias. Mrs. Williams remains in CCU for 36 hours and is transferred to the floor.

### Critical Thinking in the Nursing Process

1. How would the initial plan of care have changed if Mrs. Williams were not a candidate for thrombolytic therapy?
2. Two days after her initial therapy, Mrs. Williams complains of palpitations. You notice frequent PVCs on the ECG monitor. What do you do?
3. What health promotion topics would you teach Mrs. Williams before discharge?
4. Mrs. Williams states, "I've been smoking for over 45 years, and I'm not going to stop now! Besides, it calms me down when I'm anxious." How would you respond to this statement?

See Evaluating Your Response in Appendix C.

# CARDIAC RHYTHM DISORDERS

Heart muscle contracts in response to electrical stimulation. In the normal heart, electrical stimulation produces a synchronized, rhythmic heart muscle contraction that propels blood into the vascular system. Changes in cardiac rhythm affect this synchronized activity and the heart's ability to effectively pump blood to body tissues.

## THE CLIENT WITH A CARDIAC DYSRHYTHMIA

A cardiac **dysrhythmia** is a disturbance or irregularity in the electrical system of the heart. Cardiac dysrhythmias may be benign or have lethal consequences. Prompt recognition of a lethal dysrhythmia and quick action can be life saving.

Dysrhythmias develop for many reasons. Not all are pathologic; some alterations in cardiac rhythm occur in response to events such as exercise or fear. For example, a rapid heart rate due to exercise, fever, or excitement is a normal response to the body's demand for oxygen or to stimulation of the sympathetic nervous system. Slow heart rates also may be normal. *Athletic heart syndrome,* which results from long-term training on the heart muscle, allows the heart to beat more slowly and forcefully while maintaining cardiac output and tissue perfusion. Many athletes have a heart rate of less than 60 beats per minute. Aging affects cardiac rhythm as well (see the box on page 840).

Regardless of cause, a dysrhythmia can significantly affect cardiac performance, depending on heart muscle health. The client's response to the dysrhythmia is key in determining the urgency and type of treatment needed.

## PHYSIOLOGY REVIEW

Cardiac muscle is unique. Unlike skeletal muscle tissue, cardiac muscle can generate an electrical impulse and contraction independent of the nervous system.

## Conduction Pathways

Electrical activity of the heart is normally controlled by the *cardiac conduction system,* a network of specialized cells and conduction pathways that initiate and spread electrical impulses that cause the heart to beat (see Figure 28–7). *Pacemaker cells* spontaneously generate electrical impulses at a regular rate. Specialized conduction tissue rapidly transmits these impulses to myocardial cells. Myocardial muscle cells contract in response to the impulse. Electrical stimulation of heart muscle always precedes mechanical contraction.

Pacemaker cells are found throughout the heart. The *sinoatrial (SA)* or *sinus node* is the primary pacemaker of the heart. It usually fires at a regular rate of 60 to 100 BPM, initiating impulses that are conducted throughout the heart. The sinus node impulse spreads through the atria via the *interatrial pathways.* Conduction fibers narrow through the *atrioventricular (AV) node,* briefly delaying impulse conduction. This delay allows atrial muscle to contract, delivering an extra bolus of blood to the ventricles before they contract (the **atrial kick**). The AV node also controls the number of impulses that reach the ventricles, preventing extremely rapid heart rates. From the AV node, the impulse travels down the *bundle of His,* the *right and left bundle branches,* and to the *Purkinje fibers* of the ventricular conduction system. The Purkinje fibers terminate in ventricular muscle, prompting mechanical contraction, or *systole.*

If the sinus node fails, secondary pacemakers in the AV node (with an intrinsic rate of 40 to 60 BPM), and the Purkinje fibers (intrinsic rate of 15 to 40 BPM) take over as the pacemaker at a slower rate. This provides backup mechanism for electrical stimulation of the heart.

## Electrophysiologic Properties

Four unique properties of cardiac cells allow effective heart function. Three properties are electrical; the fourth is cardiac muscle's mechanical response to electrical stimulation.

## Nursing Care of the Older Adult

### CARDIAC DYSRHYTHMIAS

Aging affects the heart and the cardiac conduction system, increasing the incidence of dysrhythmias and conduction defects. Older adults may experience dysrhythmias even when no evidence of heart disease is found.

Older adults have a higher incidence of both ventricular and supraventricular dysrhythmias without detrimental effects than younger people. Ectopic beats, including short runs of ventricular tachycardia, occur more commonly during exercise in older adults. These dysrhythmias do not affect cardiac morbidity or mortality. Fibrosis of the bundle branches can lead to atrioventricular blocks; a prolonged PR interval is common in clients over the age of 65. Older adults also have a higher incidence of diseases that may affect heart rhythm. An elderly client with hyperthyroidism, for example, may present with atrial fibrillation, syncope, and confusion instead of the usual manifestations of goiter, tremor, and exophthalmos.

### ASSESSING FOR HOME CARE

Assessing older adults for problems related to cardiac dysrhythmias focuses on the effect of the dysrhythmia on functional health status.

- Ask about a history of cardiovascular disease and current medications.
- Inquire about symptoms such as episodes of dizziness, lightheadedness, fainting, palpitations, chest pain, or shortness of breath.

- Ask about relationship of symptoms such as palpitations to intake of certain foods and caffeine-containing beverages.
- Evaluate for other contributing factors such as smoking or alcohol intake.
- Inquire about a history of falls, particularly those occurring without apparent reason.

### TEACHING FOR HOME CARE

Teach measures to reduce the risk of cardiac dysrhythmias and potential adverse consequences of dysrhythmias,

- Emphasize the importance of taking medications as prescribed. Discuss possible effects of over-the-counter medications on the heart.
- Encourage reducing or eliminating caffeine intake. Caffeine increases the risk of ectopic beats and rapid heart rates.
- Encourage participation in a smoking cessation program and reduce or eliminate alcohol intake if appropriate.
- Encourage engaging in regular exercise. Discuss the beneficial effects of exercise to maintain muscle mass, including cardiac muscle, and cardiovascular health.
- Instruct to contact primary care provider for evaluation of symptoms such as dizziness, fainting, frequent palpitations, shortness of breath, unexplained falls, or chest pain.

---

- *Automaticity* is the ability of pacemaker cells to spontaneously initiate an electrical impulse. The SA node, the dominant pacemaker, normally generates impulses at the fastest rate, 60 to 100 times a minute. Myocardial muscle cells do not possess this ability.
- *Excitability* is the ability of myocardial cells to respond to stimuli generated by pacemaker cells.
- *Conductivity* is the ability to transmit an impulse from cell to cell. When one cell is stimulated, the impulse rapidly spreads throughout the heart muscle.
- *Contractility* is the ability of myocardial fibers to shorten in response to a stimulus. Heart muscle responds in an *all-or-nothing* manner: Stimulation of one muscle fiber causes the entire muscle mass to contract to its fullest extent as one unit.

## The Action Potential

Movement of ions across cell membranes causes the electrical impulse that stimulates muscle contraction. This electrical activity, called the *action potential*, produces the waveforms represented on ECG strips.

In the resting state, positive and negative ions align on either side of the cell membrane, producing a relatively negative charge within the cell and a positive extracellular charge (Figure 29–8 ■). The cell is said to be *polarized*. The negative resting membrane potential is maintained at about −90 millivolts (mV) by the sodium-potassium pump in the cell membrane.

When the resting cell is stimulated by an electrical charge from a neighboring cell or by a spontaneous event, its cell membrane permeability changes. Sodium ions enter the cell rapidly through openings called *fast sodium channels. Slow calcium-sodium channels* also open, allowing calcium into the cell. The membrane becomes less permeable to potassium ions. Addition of these positively charged ions to intracellular fluid changes the membrane potential from negative to slightly positive at +20 to +30 mV. This change in the electrical charge across the cell membrane is called **depolarization.**

As the cell becomes more positive, it reaches a point called the *threshold potential.* When the threshold potential is reached, an action potential is generated. The action potential causes a chemical reaction of calcium within the cell. This, in turn, causes actin and myosin filaments to slide together, producing cardiac muscle contraction. The action potential spreads to surrounding cells, causing a coordinated muscle contraction. As soon as the myocardium is completely depolarized, repolarization begins.

**Repolarization** returns the cell to its resting, polarized state. During *rapid repolarization,* fast sodium channels close abruptly, and the cell begins to regain its negative charge. During the *plateau phase,* muscle contraction is prolonged as slow calcium-sodium channels remain open. When these channels close, the sodium-potassium pump restores ion concentration to normal resting levels. The cell membrane is then polarized, ready for the cycle to start again. Each heartbeat represents one

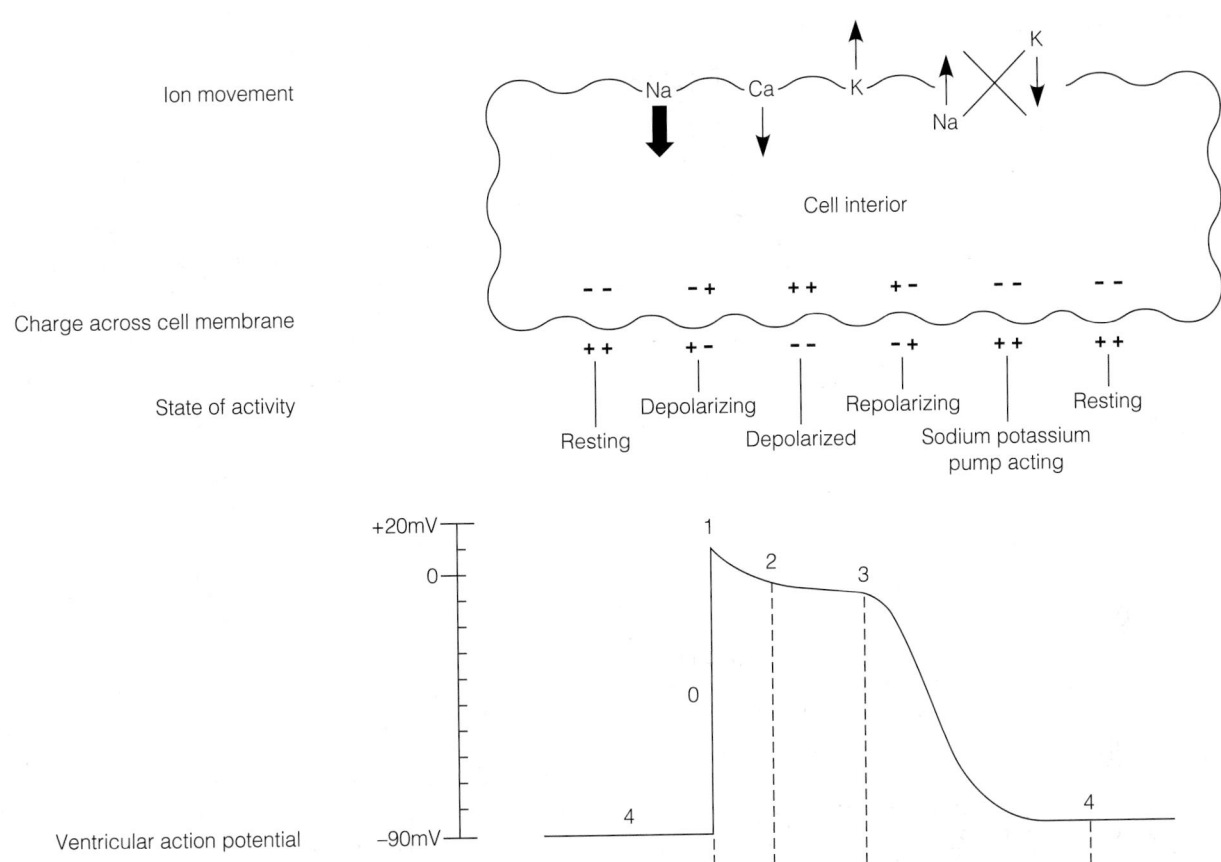

**Figure 29–8** ■ Action potential of a cardiac cell. In the resting state (phase 4), the cell membrane is polarized: the cell's interior has a negative charge compared to that of extracellular fluid. On depolarization (phase 0), sodium ions diffuse rapidly across the cell membrane into the cell, and calcium channels open. In the fully depolarized state (phase 1), the cell's interior has a net positive charge compared to its exterior. During the plateau period (phase 2), calcium moves into the cell and potassium diffusion slows, prolonging the action potential. In phase 3, calcium channels close, the sodium-potassium pump removes sodium from the cell, and the cell membrane again becomes polarized with a net negative charge.

cardiac cycle, with one depolarization and repolarization cycle and one complete cardiac muscle contraction and relaxation (systole and diastole).

Normally, only pacemaker cells demonstrate automaticity. Pacemaker cells have a resting potential that is much less negative (−70 to −50 mV) than other cardiac muscle cells. Their threshold potential also is lower than that of other myocardial cells. These differences result from constant leakage of sodium and potassium ions into the cell.

Myocardial cells have a unique protective property, the **refractory period,** during which they resist stimulation. This property protects cardiac muscle from spasm and tetany. During the *absolute refractory period,* depolarization will not occur no matter how strongly the cell is stimulated. It is followed by the *relative refractory period,* during which a greater than normal stimulus is required to generate another action potential. During the *supernormal period* that follows, a mild stimulus will cause depolarization. Many cardiac dysrhythmias are triggered during the relative refractory and supernormal periods.

## Electrocardiography

**Electrocardiography** is the graphic recording of the heart's electrical activity detected through electrodes placed on the surface of the body. Electrical activity is shown as a series of waveforms on a visual display, a strip recorder (graphic record), or both. ECG waveforms and patterns are examined to detect dysrhythmias as well as myocardial damage, the effects of drugs, and electrolyte imbalances.

The *electrocardiogram (ECG)* is a graphic record of this activity. *Electrodes* applied to the body surface are used to obtain a graphic representation of cardiac electrical activity. These electrodes detect the magnitude and direction of electrical currents produced in the heart. They attach to the electrocardiograph by an insulated wire called a *lead.* The electrocardiograph converts the electrical impulses it receives into a series of waveforms which represent cardiac depolarization and repolarization. Placement of electrodes on different parts of the body allows different views of this electrical activity, much like turning the head while holding a camera provides different views of the scenery.

Both bipolar and unipolar leads are used in recording the ECG. A *bipolar lead* uses two electrodes of opposite polarity (negative and positive). In a *unipolar* lead, one positive electrode and a negative reference point at the center of the heart are used. The electrical potential between the two monitoring points is graphically recorded as the ECG waveform.

**Figure 29–9** ■ Planes of the heart. *A,* the frontal plane. *B,* the horizontal plane.

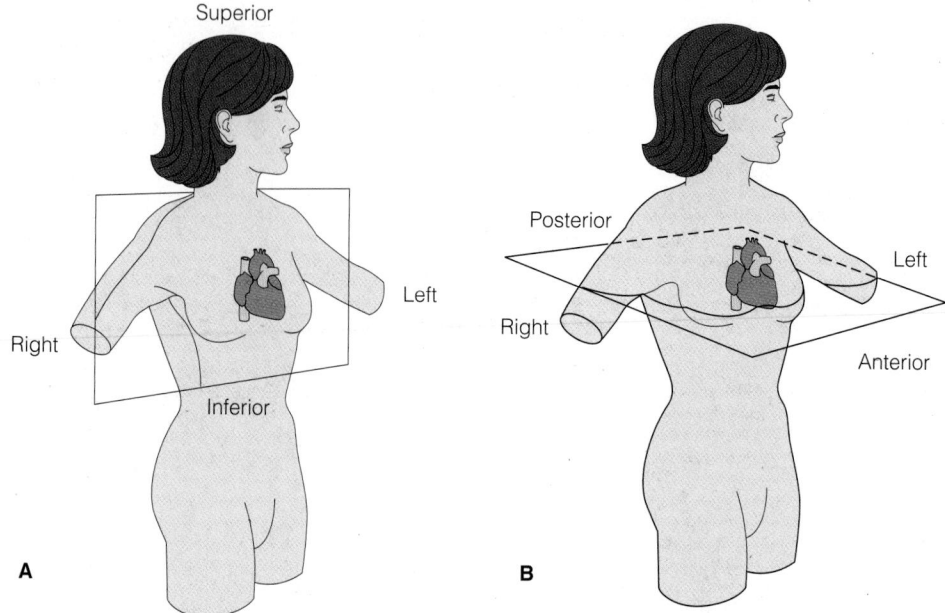

A

B

The heart can be viewed from both the *frontal plane* and the *horizontal plane* (Figure 29–9 ■). Each plane provides a unique perspective of the heart muscle. The frontal plane is an imaginary cut through the body that views the heart from top to bottom (superior–inferior) and side to side (right–left). This perspective of the heart is analogous to a paper doll cutout. It provides information about the inferior and lateral walls of the heart. The horizontal plane is a cross-sectional view of the heart from front to back (anterior–posterior) and side to side (right–left). Information regarding the anterior, septal, and lateral walls of the heart, as well as the posterior wall, are obtained from this view.

A standard 12-lead ECG provides a simultaneous recording of six limb leads and six precordial leads (Figure 29–10 ■). The *limb leads* provide information about the heart in the frontal plane and include three bipolar leads (I, II, III) and three unipolar leads (aV$_R$, aV$_L$, and aV$_F$). The bipolar limb leads measure electrical activity between a negative lead on one extremity and a positive lead on another. The unipolar limb leads (called *augmented leads*) measure the electrical activity between a single positive electrode on a limb (right arm [R], left arm [L], or left leg [F for foot]), and the center of the heart.

The *precordial leads,* also known as chest leads or V leads, view the heart in the horizontal plane. They include six unipolar leads (V$_1$, V$_2$, V$_3$, V$_4$, V$_5$, and V$_6$), which measure electrical activity between the center of the heart and a positive electrode on the chest wall.

ECG waveforms reflect the direction of electrical flow in relation to a positive electrode. Current flowing toward the positive electrode produces an upward (positive) waveform; current flowing away from the positive electrode produces a downward (negative) waveform. Current flowing perpendicular to the positive pole produces a *biphasic* (both positive and negative) waveform. Absence of electrical activity is represented by a straight line called the *isoelectric line.*

ECG waveforms are recorded by a heated stylus on heat-sensitive paper. The paper is marked at standard intervals that represent time and voltage or amplitude (Figure 29–11 ■). Each small box is 1 mm$^2$. The recording speed of the standard ECG is 25 mm/second, so each small box represents 0.04 second. Five small boxes horizontally and vertically make one large box, equivalent to 0.20 second. Five large boxes represent 1 full second. Measured vertically, each small box represents 0.1 millivolt (mV).

The cardiac cycle is depicted as a series of waveforms, the P, Q, R, S, and T waves (Figure 29–12 ■). The *P wave* represents atrial depolarization and contraction. The impulse is from the sinus node. The P wave precedes the QRS complex and is normally smooth, round, and upright. P waves may be absent when the SA node is not acting as the pacemaker. Atrial repolarization occurs during ventricular depolarization and usually is not seen on the ECG.

The *PR interval* represents the time required for the sinus impulse to travel to the AV node and into the bundle branches. This

**Figure 29–10** ■ Leads of the 12-lead ECG. *A,* Bipolar limb leads I, II, III. *B,* Unipolar limb leads aV$_R$, aV$_L$, aV$_F$. *C,* Unipolar precordial leads V$_1$ to V$_6$.

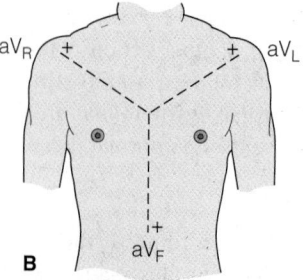

A

B

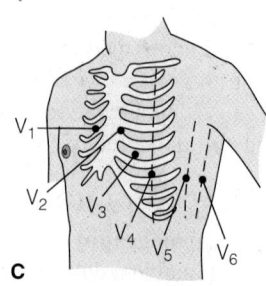

C

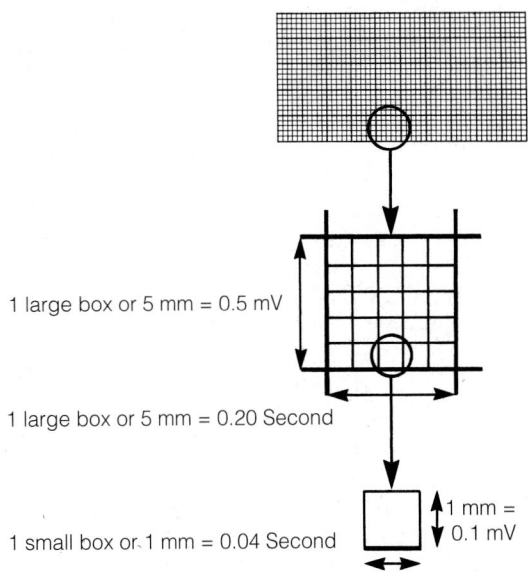

**Figure 29–11** ■ Time and voltage measurements on ECG paper at a recording speed of 25 mm/second.

interval is measured from beginning of P wave to beginning of QRS complex. If no Q wave is seen, the beginning of the R wave is used. The PR interval is normally 0.12 to 0.20 second (up to 0.24 second is considered normal in clients over age 65). PR intervals greater than 0.20 second indicate a delay in conduction from the SA node to the ventricles.

The *QRS complex* represents ventricular depolarization and contraction. The QRS complex includes three separate waves: The Q wave is the first negative deflection, the R wave is the positive or upright deflection, and the S wave is the first negative deflection after the R wave. Not all QRS complexes have all three waves; nonetheless, the complex is called a QRS complex. The normal duration of a QRS complex is from 0.06 to 0.10 second. QRS complexes greater than 0.10 second indicate delays in transmitting the impulse through the ventricular conduction system.

The *ST segment* signifies the beginning of ventricular repolarization. The ST segment, the period from the end of the QRS complex to the beginning of the T wave, should be isoelectric. An abnormal ST segment is displaced (elevated or depressed) from the isoelectric line.

The *T wave* represents ventricular repolarization. It normally has a smooth, rounded shape that is usually less than 10 mm tall. It usually points in the same direction as the QRS complex. Abnormalities of the T wave may indicate myocardial ischemia or injury, or electrolyte imbalances.

The *QT interval* is measured from the beginning of the QRS complex to the end of the T wave. It represents the total time of ventricular depolarization and repolarization. Its duration varies with gender, age, and heart rate; usually, it is 0.32 to 0.44 second long. Prolonged QT intervals indicate a prolonged relative refractory period and a greater risk of dysrhythmias. Shortened QT intervals may result from medications or electrolyte imbalances.

The *U wave* is not normally seen. It is thought to signify repolarization of the terminal Purkinje fibers. If present, the U wave follows the same direction as the T wave. It is most commonly seen in hypokalemia.

Interpreting an ECG strip to determine the cardiac rhythm is a skill that takes practice to learn and master. Many methods are used to analyze ECGs. One sequence of steps to evaluate an ECG strip is listed in Box 29–3. It is important to use a consistent method for ECG analysis. The data obtained can then be used to determine cardiac rhythm. Identifying and interpreting complex dysrhythmias requires advanced skills and knowledge obtained through further training.

## PATHOPHYSIOLOGY

Dysrhythmias arise through two major mechanisms: altered impulse formation (automaticity) and altered conductivity.

Dysrhythmias due to altered impulse formation include changes in rate and rhythm and the development of ectopic beats. This category includes *tachydysrhythmias* (rapid heart rates), *bradydysrhythmias* (slow heart rates), and ectopic rhythms. These dysrhythmias result from a change in the automaticity of cardiac cells. Impulse formation may abnormally increase or decrease. Aberrant (abnormal) impulses may originate outside normal conduction pathways, causing **ectopic beats.** Ectopic beats interrupt the normal conduction sequence; depending on the site and of abnormal impulses, they may have little effect on the client or pose a significant threat.

Conduction abnormalities result from failure or delay of impulse transmission. They cause varying degrees of **heart block,** a block in the normal conduction pathways. Myocardial injury or infarction can obstruct or delay impulse conduction. Bundle branch blocks are common in acute myocardial infarction.

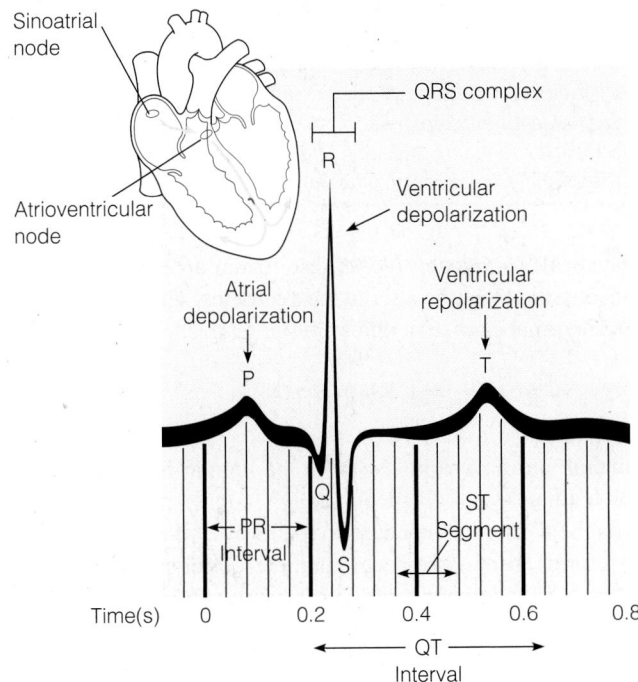

**Figure 29–12** ■ Normal ECG waveform and intervals.

## BOX 29–3  ■ ECG Rhythm Analysis

■ *Step 1: Determine rate.* Assess heart rate. Use P waves to determine the atrial rate and R waves for the ventricular rate. Several approaches can determine the heart rate.

- Count the number of complexes in a 6-second rhythm strip (the top margin of ECG paper is marked at 3-second intervals), and multiply by 10. This provides an estimate of the rate and is particularly valuable if rhythms are irregular.

- Count the number of large boxes between two consecutive complexes, and divide 300 (the number of large boxes in 1 minute) by this number. For example, there are 6 large boxes between two R waves; 300 divided by 6 equals a ventricular rate of 50 BPM. Memorize the following sequence for rapid rate determination: 300, 150, 100, 75, 60, 50, 43. One large box between complexes equals a rate of 300; two, a rate of 150; three, a rate of 100; and so on.

- Count the number of small boxes between two consecutive complexes, and divide 1500 (the number of small boxes in 1 minute) by this number. For example, there are 19 small boxes between two R waves; 1500 divided by 19 equals a ventricular rate of 79 BPM. This is the most precise measurement of heart rate.

■ *Step 2: Determine regularity.* Regularity is the consistency with which the P waves or QRS complexes occur. In a regular rhythm, all waves occur at a consistent rate. Rhythm regularity is determined by measuring the interval between consecutive waves. Place one point of an ECG caliper (a measuring device) on the peak of the P wave (for atrial rhythm) or the R wave (for ventricular rhythm). Adjust the other point to the peak of the next wave, P to P or R to R (see the figure in this box). Keeping the calipers set at this distance, evaluate intervals between consecutive waves. The rhythm is *regular* if all caliper points fall on succeeding wave peaks. Alternately, use a strip of blank paper on top of the ECG strip, marking the peaks of two or three consecutive waves. Then move the paper along the strip to consecutive waves. Wave peaks that vary by more than one to three small boxes (depending on the rate) are *irregular*. Irregular rhythms may be *irregularly irregular* (if the intervals have no pattern) or *regularly irregular* (if a consistent pattern to the irregularity can be identified).

■ *Step 3: Assess P wave.* The presence or absence of P waves helps determine origin of the rhythm. All the P waves should be alike

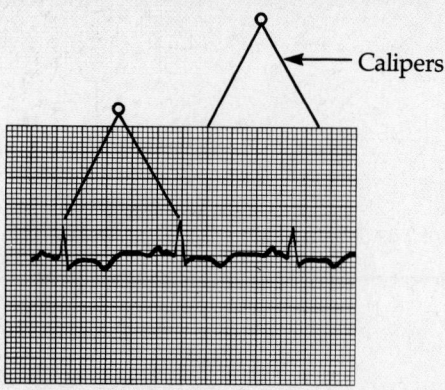

Calipers

in size and shape (*morphology*). If P waves are not seen or they differ in shape, the rhythm may not originate in the sinus node.

■ *Step 4: Assess P to QRS relationship.* Determine the relationship between P waves and QRS complexes. There should be one and only one P wave for every QRS complex, because the normal stimulus for ventricular contraction originates in the sinus node.

■ *Step 5: Determine interval durations.* To evaluate impulse transmission through the cardiac conduction system, measure the PR interval, QRS duration, and QT interval. To measure, count the number of small boxes from the beginning of the interval to the end, and multiply by 0.04 second. Then determine whether the interval duration is within its normal limits. For example, the PR interval is 3.5 small boxes wide, or 0.14 second. This is within the normal limits of 0.12 to 0.20 second. This interval should be consistent, not varying from beat to beat. A PR interval greater than 0.20 second or one that varies from beat to beat is abnormal.

The QRS complex duration is normally between 0.06 and 0.10 second. A QRS complex greater than 0.12 second indicates delayed ventricular conduction.

The QT interval is normally 0.32 to 0.44 second. It varies inversely with the heart rate: The faster the heart rate, the shorter the QT interval. As a general rule, the QT interval should be no more than half the previous R–R interval. A prolonged QT interval indicates a prolonged relative refractory period of the heart.

■ *Step 6: Identify abnormalities.* Note the presence and frequency of *ectopic* (extra) beats, deviation of the ST segment above or below the baseline, and abnormalities in waveform shape and duration.

---

The *reentry phenomenon*, a phenomenon of normal and slow conduction, is a major cause of tachydysrhythmias. A stimulus such as an ectopic beat triggers the reentry phenomenon. The impulse is delayed in one area of the heart but conducted normally through the rest. Muscle that has been depolarized by the normally conducted impulse is repolarized by the time the impulse traveling through the area of slow conduction reaches it, thus initiating another cycle of depolarization (Porth, 2002). The result is a dysrhythmia that propagates itself.

Cardiac rhythms are classified according to the site of impulse formation or the site and degree of conduction block. *Supraventricular rhythms* arise above the ventricles. These rhythms usually produce a QRS complex within the normal range. Sinus rhythms, atrial rhythms, and junctional (arising from the AV junction) rhythms are all supraventricular rhythms. *Ventricular rhythms* originate in the ventricles and may prove fatal if left untreated. *AV conduction blocks* result from a defect in impulse transmission from the atria to the ventricles. The major normal and abnormal cardiac rhythms are summarized in Table 29–6.

## Supraventricular Rhythms

### Normal Sinus Rhythm

**Normal sinus rhythm (NSR)** is the normal heart rhythm, in which impulses originate in the SA (sinus) node and travel through all normal conduction pathways without delay. All waveforms are of normal configuration, look alike, and have consistent (fixed) durations. The rate is between 60 and 100 BPM.

### Sinus Node Dysrhythmias

Sinus node dysrhythmias may occur as a normal compensatory response (e.g., to exercise) or because of altered automaticity. In these rhythms, as in NSR, the initiating impulse is from the

TABLE 29-6 Characteristics of Selected Cardiac Rhythms and Dysrhythmias

| Rhythm/ECG Appearance | ECG Characteristics | Management |
|---|---|---|
| **Supraventricular Rhythms**<br>*Normal sinus rhythm (NSR)*<br>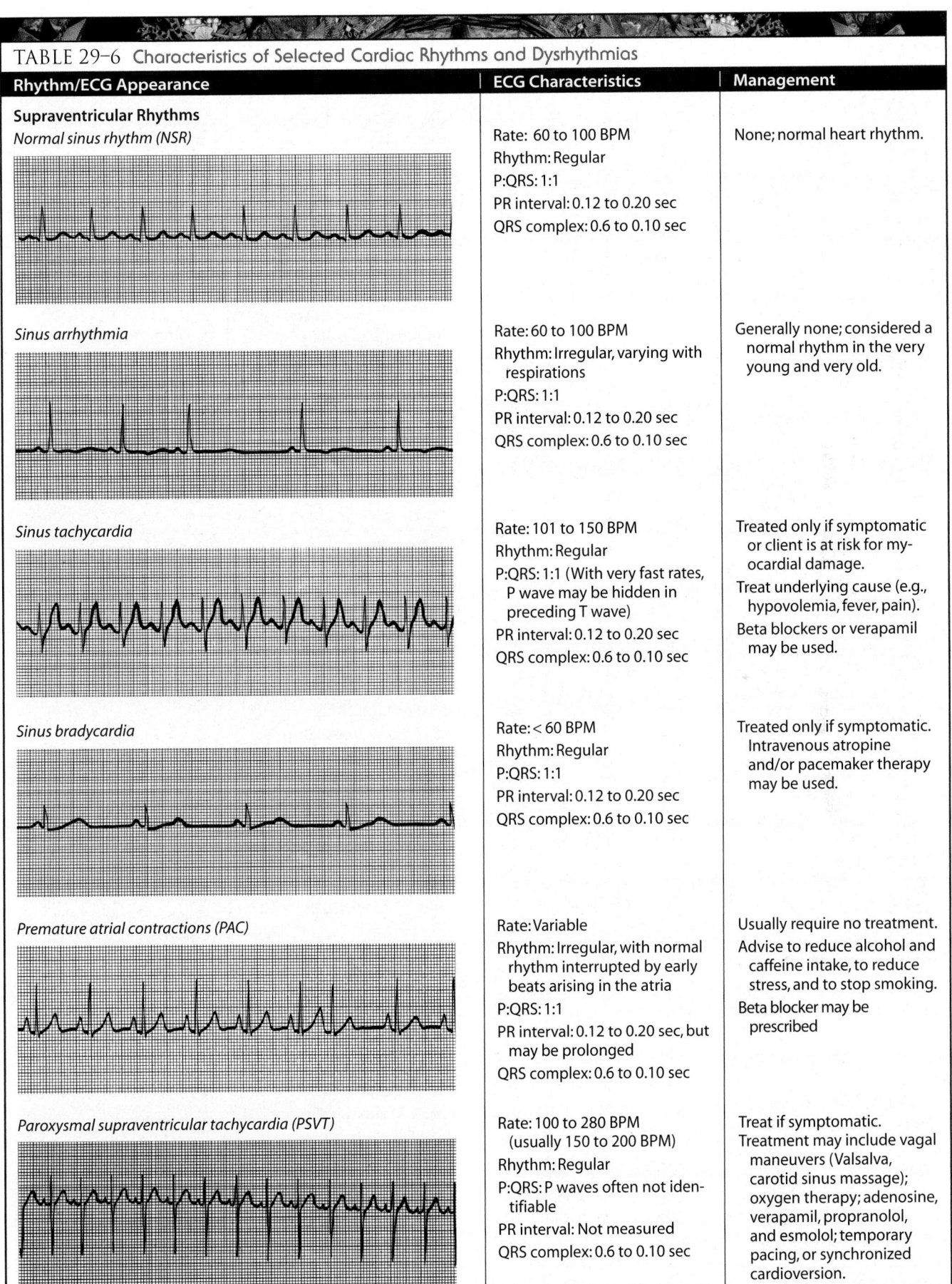 | Rate: 60 to 100 BPM<br>Rhythm: Regular<br>P:QRS: 1:1<br>PR interval: 0.12 to 0.20 sec<br>QRS complex: 0.6 to 0.10 sec | None; normal heart rhythm. |
| *Sinus arrhythmia* | Rate: 60 to 100 BPM<br>Rhythm: Irregular, varying with respirations<br>P:QRS: 1:1<br>PR interval: 0.12 to 0.20 sec<br>QRS complex: 0.6 to 0.10 sec | Generally none; considered a normal rhythm in the very young and very old. |
| *Sinus tachycardia* | Rate: 101 to 150 BPM<br>Rhythm: Regular<br>P:QRS: 1:1 (With very fast rates, P wave may be hidden in preceding T wave)<br>PR interval: 0.12 to 0.20 sec<br>QRS complex: 0.6 to 0.10 sec | Treated only if symptomatic or client is at risk for myocardial damage.<br>Treat underlying cause (e.g., hypovolemia, fever, pain).<br>Beta blockers or verapamil may be used. |
| *Sinus bradycardia* | Rate: < 60 BPM<br>Rhythm: Regular<br>P:QRS: 1:1<br>PR interval: 0.12 to 0.20 sec<br>QRS complex: 0.6 to 0.10 sec | Treated only if symptomatic. Intravenous atropine and/or pacemaker therapy may be used. |
| *Premature atrial contractions (PAC)* | Rate: Variable<br>Rhythm: Irregular, with normal rhythm interrupted by early beats arising in the atria<br>P:QRS: 1:1<br>PR interval: 0.12 to 0.20 sec, but may be prolonged<br>QRS complex: 0.6 to 0.10 sec | Usually require no treatment. Advise to reduce alcohol and caffeine intake, to reduce stress, and to stop smoking.<br>Beta blocker may be prescribed |
| *Paroxysmal supraventricular tachycardia (PSVT)* | Rate: 100 to 280 BPM (usually 150 to 200 BPM)<br>Rhythm: Regular<br>P:QRS: P waves often not identifiable<br>PR interval: Not measured<br>QRS complex: 0.6 to 0.10 sec | Treat if symptomatic. Treatment may include vagal maneuvers (Valsalva, carotid sinus massage); oxygen therapy; adenosine, verapamil, propranolol, and esmolol; temporary pacing, or synchronized cardioversion. |

*(continued on page 846)*

## TABLE 29-6   Characteristics of Selected Cardiac Rhythms and Dysrhythmias (continued)

| Rhythm/ECG Appearance | ECG Characteristics | Management |
| --- | --- | --- |
| *Atrial flutter*<br> | Rate: Atrial 240 to 360 BPM; ventricular rate depends on degree of AV block and usually is <150 BPM<br>Rhythm: Atrial regular; ventricular usually regular<br>P:QRS: 2:1, 4:1, 6:1; may vary<br>PR interval: Not measured<br>QRS complex: 0.6 to 0.10 sec. | Synchronized cardioversion; medications to slow ventricular response such as a beta blocker or calcium channel blocker (verapamil), followed by ibutilide, quinidine, procainamide, flecainide, or amiodarone. |
| *Atrial fibrillation*<br> | Rate: Atrial 300 to 600 BPM (too rapid to count); ventricular 100 to 180 BPM in untreated clients<br>Rhythm: Irregularly irregular<br>P:QRS: Variable<br>PR interval: Not measured<br>QRS complex: 0.06 to 0.10 sec | Synchronized cardioversion; medications to reduce ventricular response rate: verapamil, propranolol, or digoxin; anticoagulant therapy to reduce risk of clot formation and stroke. |
| *Junctional escape rhythm*<br> | Rate: 40 to 60 BPM; junctional tachycardia 60 to 140 BPM<br>Rhythm: Regular<br>P:QRS: P waves may be absent, inverted and immediately preceding or succeeding QRS complex, or hidden in QRS complex<br>PR interval: <0.10 sec<br>QRS complex: 0.06 to 0.10 sec | Treat cause if symptomatic. |
| **Ventricular Rhythms**<br>*Premature ventricular contractions (PVC)*<br> | Rate: Variable<br>Rhythm: Irregular, with PVC interrupting underlying rhythm and followed by a compensatory pause<br>P:QRS: No P wave noted before PVC<br>PR interval: Absent with PVC<br>QRS complex: Wide (>0.12 sec) and bizarre in appearance; differs from normal QRS complex | Treat if symptomatic or in presence of severe heart disease. Advise against stimulant use (caffeine, nicotine). Beta blockers, or class I of II antidysrhythmic agents (see the box on page 854) may be used. |
| *Ventricular tachycardia (VT or V tach)*<br> | Rate: 100 to 250 BPM<br>Rhythm: Regular<br>P:QRS: P waves usually not identifiable<br>PR interval: Not measured<br>QRS complex: 0.12 sec or greater; bizarre shape | Treat if VT is sustained, symptomatic, or associated with organic heart disease. Treatment includes intravenous procainamide or lidocaine and/or immediate cardioversion if unconscious or unstable. Surgical ablation or antitachycardia pacing with an implanted cardioverter/defibrilator (ICD) for repeated episodes. |

## TABLE 29–6 Characteristics of Selected Cardiac Rhythms and Dysrhythmias (continued)

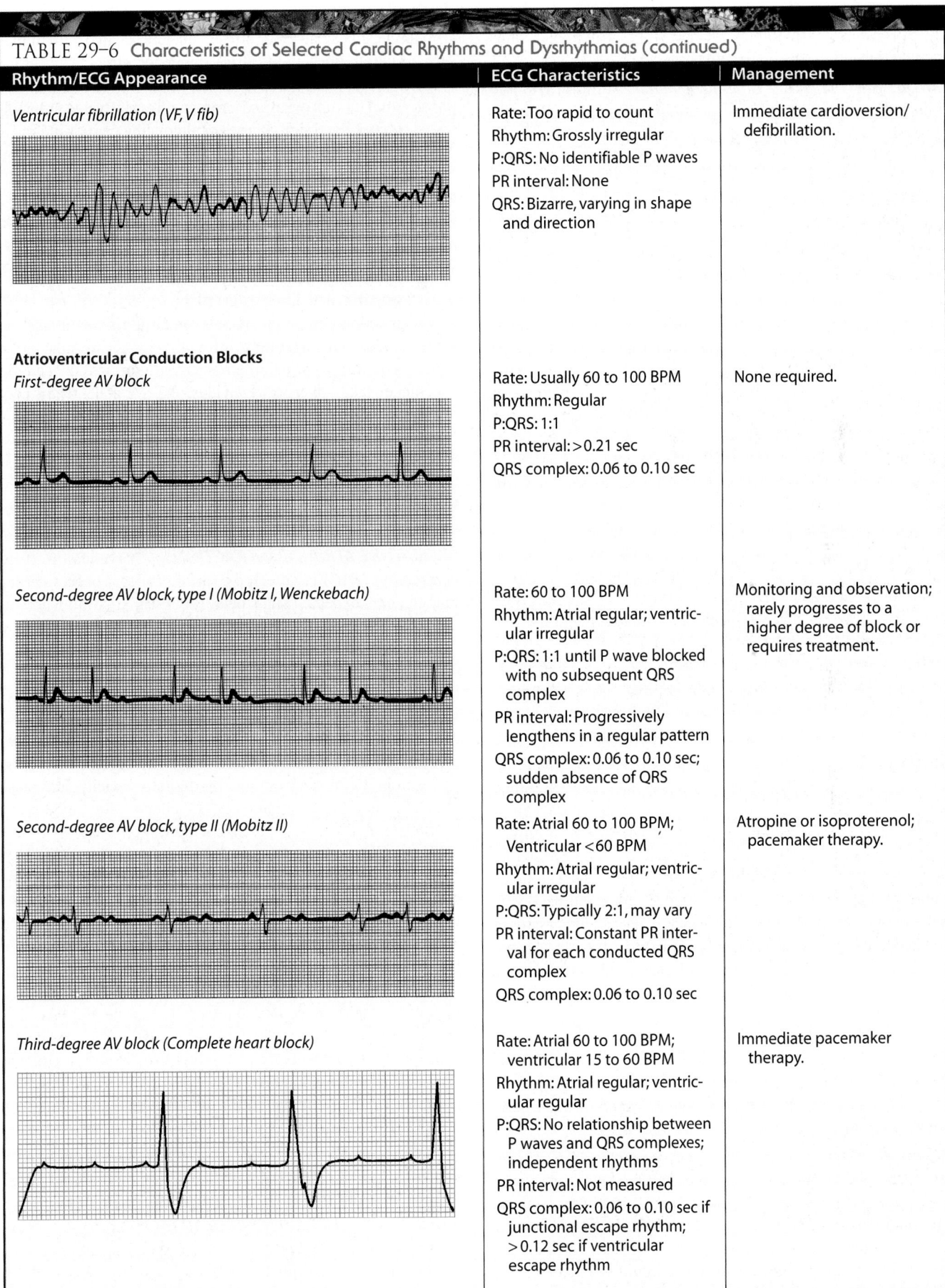

| Rhythm/ECG Appearance | ECG Characteristics | Management |
|---|---|---|
| *Ventricular fibrillation (VF, V fib)* | Rate: Too rapid to count<br>Rhythm: Grossly irregular<br>P:QRS: No identifiable P waves<br>PR interval: None<br>QRS: Bizarre, varying in shape and direction | Immediate cardioversion/ defibrillation. |
| **Atrioventricular Conduction Blocks**<br>*First-degree AV block* | Rate: Usually 60 to 100 BPM<br>Rhythm: Regular<br>P:QRS: 1:1<br>PR interval: >0.21 sec<br>QRS complex: 0.06 to 0.10 sec | None required. |
| *Second-degree AV block, type I (Mobitz I, Wenckebach)* | Rate: 60 to 100 BPM<br>Rhythm: Atrial regular; ventricular irregular<br>P:QRS: 1:1 until P wave blocked with no subsequent QRS complex<br>PR interval: Progressively lengthens in a regular pattern<br>QRS complex: 0.06 to 0.10 sec; sudden absence of QRS complex | Monitoring and observation; rarely progresses to a higher degree of block or requires treatment. |
| *Second-degree AV block, type II (Mobitz II)* | Rate: Atrial 60 to 100 BPM; Ventricular <60 BPM<br>Rhythm: Atrial regular; ventricular irregular<br>P:QRS: Typically 2:1, may vary<br>PR interval: Constant PR interval for each conducted QRS complex<br>QRS complex: 0.06 to 0.10 sec | Atropine or isoproterenol; pacemaker therapy. |
| *Third-degree AV block (Complete heart block)* | Rate: Atrial 60 to 100 BPM; ventricular 15 to 60 BPM<br>Rhythm: Atrial regular; ventricular regular<br>P:QRS: No relationship between P waves and QRS complexes; independent rhythms<br>PR interval: Not measured<br>QRS complex: 0.06 to 0.10 sec if junctional escape rhythm; >0.12 sec if ventricular escape rhythm | Immediate pacemaker therapy. |

sinus node. They differ from NSR in rate or regularity of the rhythm. Sinus dysrhythmias include sinus arrhythmia, sinus tachycardia, and sinus bradycardia.

### SINUS ARRHYTHMIA.

*Sinus arrhythmia* is a sinus rhythm in which the rate varies with respirations, causing an irregular rhythm. The rate increases during inspiration and decreases with expiration. Sinus arrhythmia is common in the very young and the very old. It can be caused by an increase in vagal tone, by digitalis toxicity, or by morphine administration.

### SINUS TACHYCARDIA.

*Sinus tachycardia* has all of the characteristics of NSR, except that the rate is greater than 100 BPM. Tachycardia arises from enhanced automaticity in response to changes in the internal environment. Sympathetic nervous system stimulation or blocked vagal (parasympathetic) activity increases the heart rate. Tachycardia is a normal response to any condition or event that increases the body's demand for oxygen and nutrients, such as exercise or hypoxia. In the client on bed rest, tachycardia is an ominous sign. Sinus tachycardia may be an early sign of cardiac dysfunction, such as heart failure. Tachycardia is detrimental in clients with cardiac disease because it increases cardiac work and oxygen use.

Common causes of sinus tachycardia include exercise, excitement, anxiety, pain, fever, hypoxia, hypovolemia, anemia, hyperthyroidism, myocardial infarction, heart failure, cardiogenic shock, pulmonary embolism, caffeine intake, and certain drugs, such as atropine, epinephrine (Adrenalin), or isoproterenol (Isuprel).

Manifestations of sinus tachycardia include a rapid pulse rate. The client may complain of feeling that the heart is "racing," shortness of breath, and dizziness. In the presence of heart disease, sinus tachycardia may precipitate chest pain.

### SINUS BRADYCARDIA.

*Sinus bradycardia* has all of the characteristics of NSR, but the rate is less than 60 BPM. Sinus bradycardia may result from increased vagal (parasympathetic) activity or from depressed automaticity due to injury or ischemia to the sinus node. Sinus bradycardia may be normal (e.g., in clients with athletic heart syndrome). The heart rate also normally slows during sleep because the parasympathetic nervous system is dominant at this time. Other causes of sinus bradycardia include pain, increased intracranial pressure, sinus node disease, acute myocardial infarction (especially with inferior wall damage), hypothermia, acidosis, and certain drugs.

Sinus bradycardia may be asymptomatic; it is important to assess the client before treating the rhythm. Manifestations of decreased cardiac output, such as decreased level of consciousness, syncope (faintness), or hypotension indicate a need for intervention.

### SICK SINUS SYNDROME.

*Sick sinus syndrome (SSS)* results from sinus node disease or dysfunction that causes problems with impulse formation, transmission, and conduction. Sick sinus syndrome is often found in older adults. It may be caused by direct injury to sinus tissue, fibrosis of conduction fibers associated with aging, and such drugs as digitalis, beta blockers, and calcium channel blockers.

ECG characteristics of SSS include sinus bradycardia, sinus arrhythmia, sinus pauses or arrest, and atrial tachydysrhythmias such as atrial fibrillation, atrial flutter, or atrial tachycardia. Bradycardia-tachycardia syndrome, characterized either by **paroxysmal** (abrupt onset and termination) atrial tachycardia followed by prolonged sinus pauses or alternating periods of bradycardia and tachycardia also may indicate sinus node dysfunction.

Manifestations of sinus node dysfunction often are intermittent, related to a drop in cardiac output caused by the irregular rhythm. Fatigue, dizziness, lightheadedness, and syncope are common. The heart rate may not increase in response to stressors such as exercise or fever.

### Supraventricular Dysrhythmias

When an action potential originates in atrial tissue outside the sinus node, the resulting rhythm is classified as a *supraventricular rhythm.* In these dysrhythmias, an ectopic pacemaker takes over, or overrides, the SA node. They may also occur when the SA node fails; an *escape rhythm* develops as a fail-safe mechanism to maintain the heart rate. The most common supraventricular dysrhythmias are premature atrial contractions, paroxysmal supraventricular tachycardia, atrial flutter, and atrial fibrillation. These rhythms may be paroxysmal, that is, occur in bursts with an abrupt beginning and end.

### PREMATURE ATRIAL CONTRACTIONS.

A *premature atrial contraction (PAC)* is an ectopic atrial beat that occurs earlier than the next expected sinus beat. PACs can arise anywhere in the atria. They are usually asymptomatic and benign, but they may initiate paroxysmal supraventricular tachycardia in susceptible individuals. PACs are common in older adults, often occurring without an obvious cause. Strong emotions, excessive alcohol intake, tobacco, and stimulants such as caffeine can precipitate PACs. They also may be associated with myocardial infarction, heart failure and other cardiac disorders, hypoxemia, pulmonary embolism, digitalis toxicity, and electrolyte or acid-base imbalances. In clients with underlying heart disease, PACs may precede a more serious dysrhythmia.

The ECG tracing shows interruption of the underlying rhythm by a premature complex that looks similar to the underlying beats. The ectopic impulse of the PAC is usually conducted normally, leading to depolarization of cardiac muscle and a normal QRS complex. Because the impulse arises above the ventricles, it follows normal conduction pathways through the ventricles. The QRS complex is narrow or matches those of the underlying rhythm. The shape of the P wave of a PAC differs from normal P waves because its impulse arises outside the sinus node. A *noncompensatory pause* usually follows, as the PAC resets the SA node rhythm. Occasionally, the ectopic impulse may not be conducted through the heart, resulting in a lone P wave without a QRS, or a nonconducted PAC.

PACs cause few manifestations. If frequent, they may cause palpitations or a fluttering sensation in the chest. Early beats may be noted on auscultating or palpating the pulse.

### PAROXYSMAL SUPRAVENTRICULAR TACHYCARDIA.

*Paroxysmal supraventricular tachycardia (PSVT)* is tachycardia of sudden onset and termination. PSVT is usually initiated by a reentry loop in or around the AV node; that is, an impulse reenters the same section of tissue over and over, causing repeated depolarizations.

PSVT occurs more frequently in women. Sympathetic nervous system stimulation and stressors such as fever, sepsis, and hyperthyroidism may precipitate PSVT. It also may be associated with heart diseases such as CHD, myocardial infarction, rheumatic heart disease, myocarditis, or acute pericarditis. Abnormal conduction pathways associated with Wolff-Parkinson-White (WPW) syndrome may account for PSVT.

PSVT affects ventricular filling and cardiac output, and decreases coronary artery perfusion. Its manifestations include complaints of palpitations and a "racing" heart, anxiety, dizziness, dyspnea, anginal pain, diaphoresis, extreme fatigue, and polyuria (urine output may reach up to 3 L in the first few hours after PSVT onset).

**ATRIAL FLUTTER.** *Atrial flutter* is a rapid and regular atrial rhythm thought to result from an intra-atrial reentry mechanism. Causes include sympathetic nervous system stimulation due to anxiety, caffeine and alcohol intake; thyrotoxicosis; coronary heart disease or myocardial infarction; pulmonary embolism; and abnormal conduction syndromes, such as WPW syndrome. Older persons with rheumatic heart disease and/or valvular disease are especially vulnerable.

Clients with atrial flutter may complain of palpitations or a fluttering sensation in the chest or throat. If the ventricular rate is rapid, manifestations of decreased cardiac output, such decreased level of consciousness, hypotension, decreased urinary output, and cool clammy skin, may be noted. The atrial kick (additional ventricular filling with atrial contraction) is lost because of inadequate atrial filling.

ECG characteristics include a "sawtooth" or "picket fence" appearance of P waves, which are labeled flutter (F) waves. The atrial rate is rapid, usually around 300 BPM. As a protective mechanism, many impulses are blocked at the AV node, and the ventricular rate is rarely greater than 150 to 170 BPM. Usually, atrial impulses are evenly conducted through the AV node, for example, two impulses to one QRS complex (2:1), four impulses to one QRS complex (4:1), or six impulses to one QRS complex (6:1). A constant conduction ratio results in a regular ventricular rhythm; the ventricular rhythm is irregular if the conduction ratio varies. The ventricular rate usually ranges from 150 to 170 BPM in 2:1 conduction and 60 to 75 BPM for lower conduction ratios. The T wave is usually hidden by overriding F waves; some F waves may be hidden in the QRS complex.

**ATRIAL FIBRILLATION.** *Atrial fibrillation* is a common dysrhythmia characterized by disorganized atrial activity without discrete atrial contractions. Extremely rapid atrial impulses bombard the AV node, resulting in an irregularly irregular ventricular response. Atrial fibrillation may occur suddenly and recur, or it may persist as a chronic dysrhythmia. Atrial fibrillation is commonly associated with heart failure, rheumatic heart disease, coronary heart disease, hypertension, and hyperthyroidism.

Manifestations of atrial fibrillation relate to the rate of the ventricular response. With rapid response rates, manifestations of decreased cardiac output such as hypotension, shortness of breath, fatigue, and angina may develop. Clients with extensive heart disease may develop syncope or heart failure. Peripheral pulses are irregular and of variable amplitude (strength).

The specific ECG characteristics of atrial fibrillation include an irregularly irregular rhythm and the absence of identifiable P waves. The atrial rate is so rapid that it is not measurable. The ventricular rate varies.

Atrial fibrillation increases the risk for formation of thromboemboli. Organ infarction may occur as a result; the incidence of stroke is high.

## Junctional Dysrhythmias

Rhythms that originate in AV nodal tissue are termed *junctional*. The AV junction includes the AV node and the bundle of His, which branches into the right and left bundle branches. An impulse arising from the AV junction may occur in response to failure of higher pacemakers, as in a *junctional escape rhythm*, or it may result from an abnormal mechanism, such as altered automaticity. An impulse arising from the AV junction may or may not be conducted back up to the atria. This conduction against the normal flow or pattern is called *retrograde conduction*. The resulting atrial wave, called a P′ wave, may be found before, during, or after the QRS complex, depending on the speed of conduction. The P′ wave is inverted in some ECG leads because the impulse moves from the AV node up to the atria instead of from the SA node down toward the AV node. In addition, the P′R interval is shorter than normal (less than 0.12 sec). The QRS complex is typically narrow.

A junctional rhythm may be due to drug toxicity (e.g., digitalis, beta blockers, or calcium channel blockers), or other causes such as hypoxemia, hyperkalemia, increased vagal tone or damage to the AV node, myocardial infarction, and heart failure. Loss of synchronized atrial contraction and the atrial kick may affect cardiac output, leading to manifestations of decreased cardiac output and impaired myocardial tissue perfusion. Heart failure may develop.

*Premature junctional contractions (PJCs)* occur before the next expected beat of the underlying rhythm. Isolated PJCs may occur in healthy people and are insignificant. *Junctional tachycardia* is a junctional rhythm with a rate greater than 60 BPM. It is caused by increased automaticity of AV nodal tissue. The ventricular rate is usually less than 140 BPM. Both rhythms are most commonly associated with digitalis toxicity, hypoxia, ischemia, or electrolyte imbalances.

## Ventricular Dysrhythmias

Ventricular dysrhythmias originate in the ventricles. Because the ventricles pump blood into the pulmonary and systemic vasculature, any disruption of their rhythm can affect cardiac output and tissue perfusion. A wide and bizarre QRS complex (greater than 0.12 sec) is a characteristic feature of ventricular dysrhythmias. This occurs because ventricular ectopic impulses begin and travel outside normal conduction pathways. Other characteristics include no relationship of the QRS complex to a P wave, increased amplitude of the QRS complex, an abnormal ST segment, and a T wave deflected in the opposite direction from the QRS complex.

## Premature Ventricular Contractions

*Premature ventricular contractions (PVCs)* are ectopic ventricular beats that occur before the next expected beat of the underlying rhythm. They usually do not reset the atrial rhythm and are followed by a full compensatory pause. PVCs often have no significance in people without heart disease. Frequent, recurrent, or multifocal PVCs may be associated with an increased risk for lethal dysrhythmias. PVCs result from either enhanced automaticity or a reentry phenomenon. They may be triggered by anxiety or stress; tobacco, alcohol, or caffeine use; hypoxia, acidosis, and electrolyte imbalances; sympathomimetic drugs; coronary heart disease; heart failure; and mechanical stimulation of the heart (e.g., the insertion of a cardiac catheter); or reperfusion after thrombolytic therapy. The incidence and significance of PVCs is greatest after myocardial infarction.

PVCs may be isolated or occur in a specific pattern. Two PVCs in a row are called a *couplet* or *paired* PVCs. Three consecutive PVCs (a *triplet* or *salvo*) is a short run of ventricular tachycardia. *Ventricular bigeminy* is characterized by a PVC following each normal beat; a PVC noted every third beat is called *ventricular trigeminy*. When the ventricular impulse arises from one ectopic site, all PVCs look the same (*monomorphic*) and are called *unifocal* PVCs. *Multifocal* PVCs arise from different ectopic sites and appear different from one another on the ECG (*polymorphic*).

The frequency and patterns of PVCs can be indicative of myocardial irritability and the risk for a lethal dysrhythmia. The following are considered warning signs in the client with acute heart disease (e.g., an acute MI).

- PVCs that develop within the first 4 hours of an MI
- Frequent PVCs (six or more per minute)
- Couplets or triplets
- Multifocal PVCs
- R-on-T phenomenon (PVCs falling on the T wave)

In people without heart disease, isolated PVCs usually are insignificant and do not require treatment. Clients may complain of feeling their hearts "skip a beat" or of palpitations. In clients with preexisting heart disease, PVCs may indicate a drug toxicity or an increased risk for lethal dysrhythmias and cardiac arrest. The risk is greatest following acute MI.

## Ventricular Tachycardia

*Ventricular tachycardia (VT; V tach)* is a rapid ventricular rhythm defined as three or more consecutive PVCs. Ventricular tachycardia may occur in short bursts, or "runs," or may persist for more than 30 seconds (sustained ventricular tachycardia). The rate is greater than 100 BPM, and the rhythm is usually regular. Reentry is the usual electrophysiologic mechanism responsible for VT. Myocardial ischemia and infarction are the most common predisposing factors for VT. It also is associated with cardiac structural disorders such as valvular disease, rheumatic heart disease, or cardiomyopathy. It may occur in the absence of heart disease, and with anorexia nervosa, metabolic disorders, and drug toxicity.

Nonsustained VT may occur paroxysmally and convert back to an effective rhythm spontaneously. The client may ex-perience a fluttering sensation in the chest or complain of palpitations and brief shortness of breath. Clients in sustained VT generally develop signs and symptoms of decreased cardiac output and hemodynamic instability, including severe hypotension, a weak or nonpalpable pulse, and loss of consciousness. Allowed to continue, VT can deteriorate into ventricular fibrillation. Sustained ventricular tachycardia is a medical emergency that requires immediate intervention, particularly in clients with cardiac disease.

## Ventricular Fibrillation

*Ventricular fibrillation (VF; V fib)* is extremely rapid, chaotic ventricular depolarization causing the ventricles to quiver and cease contracting; the heart does not pump. This is known as **cardiac arrest;** it is a medical emergency requiring immediate intervention with cardiopulmonary resuscitation (CPR). Death will follow the onset of VF within 4 minutes if the rhythm is not recognized and terminated and an effective perfusing rhythm reestablished.

Ventricular fibrillation is usually triggered by severe myocardial ischemia or infarction. It occurs without warning 50% of the time. It is the terminal event in many disease processes or traumatic conditions. Ventricular fibrillation may be precipitated by a single PVC or may follow VT. Other causes of VF include digitalis toxicity, reperfusion therapy, antidysrhythmic drugs, hypokalemia and hyperkalemia, hypothermia, metabolic acidosis, mechanical stimulation (as with the insertion of cardiac catheters or pacing wires), and electric shock.

Clinically, loss of ventricular contractions results in absence of a palpable or audible pulse. The client loses consciousness and stops breathing as perfusion ceases. The ECG shows grossly irregular, bizarre complexes with no discernable rate or rhythm.

## Atrioventricular Conduction Blocks

Conduction defects that delay or block transmission of the sinus impulse through the AV node are called *atrioventricular (AV) conduction blocks*. Impaired conduction may result from tissue injury or disease, increased vagal (parasympathetic) tone, drug effects, or a congenital defect. AV conduction blocks vary in severity from benign to severe.

### First-Degree AV Block

*First-degree AV block* is a benign conduction delay that generally poses no threat, has no symptoms, and requires no treatment. Impulse conduction through the AV node is slowed, but all atrial impulses are conducted to the ventricles. It may result from injury or infarct of the AV node, other cardiac diseases, or drug effects. The ECG shows all characteristics of NSR, except the PR interval is greater than 0.20 second.

### Second-Degree AV Block

*Second-degree AV block* is characterized by failure to conduct one or more impulses from the atria to the ventricles. Two patterns of second-degree AV block are seen, identified as type I and type II.

***SECOND-DEGREE AV BLOCK—TYPE I.*** *Type I second-degree AV block (Mobitz type I* or *Wenckebach phenomenon)* is char-acterized by a repeating pattern of increasing AV conduction delays until an impulse fails to conduct to the ventricles. On the ECG, PR intervals progressively lengthen until one QRS complex is not conducted, or dropped. The ventricular rate remains adequate to maintain cardiac output, and the client usually is asymptomatic. Mobitz type I AV block usually is transient, associated with acute MI or drug intoxication (e.g., digitalis, beta blockers, or calcium channel blockers). It rarely progresses to complete heart block.

**SECOND-DEGREE AV BLOCK—TYPE II.** *Type II second-degree AV block (Mobitz type II)* involves intermittent failure of the AV node to conduct an impulse to the ventricles without preceding delays in conduction. The PR interval remains constant, but not all P waves are followed by QRS complexes (e.g., there may be two P waves for every QRS). Conduction through the His-Purkinje system usually is delayed as well, causing a widened QRS complex (Braunwald et al., 2001). Mobitz type II block is frequently associated with acute anterior wall MI and a high rate of mortality (Porth, 2002). Manifestations of Mobitz type II block depend on the ventricular rate. Pacemaker therapy may be required to maintain the cardiac output

### Third-Degree AV Block

*Third-degree AV block (complete heart block)* occurs when atrial impulses are completely blocked at the AV node, and fail to reach the ventricles. As a result, the atria and ventricles are controlled by different and independent pacemakers, with separate rates and rhythms. The ventricular impulse arises from either junctional fibers (with a rate of 40 to 60 BPM) or a ventricular pacemaker at a rate of less than 40 BPM. The width of the QRS complex depends on the location of the escape pacemaker. The QRS is wide and the rate is slow when the rhythm arises distal to the bundle of His.

Third-degree block is frequently associated with an inferior or anteroseptal myocardial infarction. Other causes include congenital conditions, acute or degenerative cardiac disease or damage, drug effects, and electrolyte imbalances. The slow escape rhythm significantly affects cardiac output, causing manifestations such as syncope (known as a *Stokes-Adams attack*), dizziness, fatigue, exercise intolerance, and heart failure. Third-degree AV block is life threatening and requires immediate intervention to maintain adequate cardiac output.

### AV Dissociation

Complete dissociation of atrial and ventricular rhythms can occur in conditions other than third-degree AV block. The two primary factors leading to AV dissociation are severe sinus bradycardia and a lower pacemaker (junctional or ventricular) that competes with or exceeds the normal sinus rhythm (Braunwald et al., 2001). AV dissociation may result from acute myocardial ischemia or infarction, cardiac surgery, or drug effects. The ECG shows separate and competing atrial (P waves) and ventricular (QRS complexes) rhythms.

### Ventricular Conduction Blocks

Once the impulse enters the ventricles, its conduction through the right and left bundle branches may be impaired (*bundle branch block*). As a result, the impulse is conducted more slowly than normal through the ventricles. On the ECG, the QRS complex is prolonged. Its appearance varies, depending on the affected bundle (right or left). Typically, no clinical manifestations are associated with bundle branch block unless it occurs in conjunction with an AV block.

## COLLABORATIVE CARE

Cardiac dysrhythmias may be either benign or critical: Recognizing lethal dysrhythmias is a matter of life and death. Major goals of care include identifying the dysrhythmia, evaluating its effect on physical and psychosocial well-being, and treating underlying causes. This may involve correcting fluid and electrolyte or acid-base imbalances; treating hypoxia, pain, or anxiety; administering antidysrhythmic medications; or mechanical and surgical interventions.

### Diagnostic Tests

Diagnostic tests for dysrhythmias include the electrocardiogram, cardiac monitoring, and electrophysiology studies. Laboratory tests such as serum electrolytes, drug levels, and arterial blood gases may be done to help identify the cause of the dysrhythmia.

#### Electrocardiogram

The 12-lead ECG may be required to accurately diagnose a dysrhythmia. It also provides information about underlying disease processes, such as myocardial infarction or other cardiac disease. The ECG may also be used to monitor the effects of treatment.

#### Cardiac Monitoring

Cardiac monitoring allows continuous observation of the cardiac rhythm. It is used in many different circumstances (Box 29–4). Different types of ECG monitoring are employed for different situations.

---

**BOX 29–4 ■ Indications for Cardiac Monitoring**

- Perioperative monitoring of heart rate and rhythm
- Detecting and identifying dysrhythmias
- Monitoring the effects of cardiac and noncardiac diseases on the heart
- Monitoring clients with potentially life-threatening conditions:
  a. Major trauma (especially cardiac trauma)
  b. Dissecting aneurysm
  c. Acute myocardial infarction
  d. Heart failure
  e. Shock
  f. Other emergency conditions
- Evaluating responses to procedures and interventions:
  a. Drug therapies
  b. Diagnostic procedures
  c. Ablative techniques
  d. Angioplasty or cardiac catheterization
  e. Cardiac surgery
  f. Pacemaker function
  g. Automatic implantable cardioverter-defibrillator function

**CONTINUOUS CARDIAC MONITORING.**   Continuous monitoring of the cardiac rhythm is provided by bedside and central monitoring stations. Electrodes placed on the client's chest attach to cables connected to a monitor. The heart rate and rhythm is visually displayed on a bedside monitor connected to a central monitoring station. The central station allows simultaneous monitoring of multiple clients within a nursing unit. Alarms on both bedside and central monitors warn of potential problems such as very rapid or very slow heart rates. Alarm limits are preset by the nurse for the individual client. Procedure 29–1 describes how to place a client on cardiac monitoring.

*Telemetry* may be used in acute care settings when the client is ambulatory. Chest electrodes are connected to a portable transmitter worn around the neck or waist; the ECG is transmitted electronically to a central monitoring station for continuous monitoring.

**HOME MONITORING.**   Clients often complain of palpitations or other heart symptoms but are asymptomatic during evaluation in a hospital or community-based setting. Ambulatory or Holter monitoring may be used to identify intermittent dysrhythmias, to detect silent ischemia, to monitor the effects of treatment, and to assess pacemaker or automatic cardioverter-defibrillator function. Electrodes are applied and the leads attached to the portable telemetry monitor that records and stores all electrical activity. Clients are instructed to leave the electrode pads in place during monitoring, record any cardiac symptoms or events in a journal (such as chest pain, palpitations, syncope), and are told when to return to the clinic. After the prescribed period, usu-

---

## Procedure 29–1 — Initiating Cardiac Monitoring

### SUPPLIES

- Bedside monitor and cable or telemetry unit with fresh battery
- Electrodes—self-adherent, pregelled, disposable
- Lead wires
- Washcloth, soap, and towel
- Alcohol prep pads
- Dry gauze pads or ECG prep pads

### BEFORE THE PROCEDURE

Explain the reason for ECG monitoring. Reassure client that changes in heart rhythm can be noted and immediately treated if necessary. Explain that loose or disconnected lead wires, poor electrode contact, excessive movement, electrical interference, or equipment malfunction may trigger alarms and alert the staff, allowing correction of the problem. Reassure that movement allowed, within activity restrictions, while on the monitor. Explain skin preparation procedure. Provide for privacy, and drape appropriately.

### PROCEDURE

1. Follow standard precautions
2. Check equipment for damage (i.e., fraying, bent, or broken wires). Connect lead wires to cable, and secure connections.
3. Select electrode sites on the chest wall, avoiding areas of excessive movement, joints, skin creases, scar tissue, or other lesions.
4. Clean sites with soap and water, and dry thoroughly. Alcohol may be used to remove skin oils; allow the skin to dry for 60 seconds after use.
5. Gently rub the site with a dry gauze pad or ECG prep pad to remove dead skin cells, debris, and residue.
6. Open the electrode package; peel the backing from the electrode, and check to ensure that the center of the pad is moist with conductive gel.
7. Apply electrode pads, pressing firmly to ensure contact (see figure).
8. Attach leads and position cable with sufficient slack for comfort. Place the telemetry unit (if used) in gown pouch or pocket.
9. Assess ECG tracing on the monitor, adjusting settings as needed.
10. Set monitor alarm limits typically at 20 BPM higher and lower than the client's baseline rate. Turn alarms on, and leave on at all times. Assess immediately if an alarm is triggered.
11. Time and date pads with every change.

### AFTER THE PROCEDURE

Monitor periodically for comfort. Assess electrode and lead wire connections as needed. Remove and apply new pads every 24 to 48 hours or whenever the pad becomes dislodged or nonadherent. Clean gel residue from previous site, and document skin condition under the pads. Choose an alternative site if the skin appears irritated or blistered. Document ECG strips according to unit policy and/or physician's order, as well

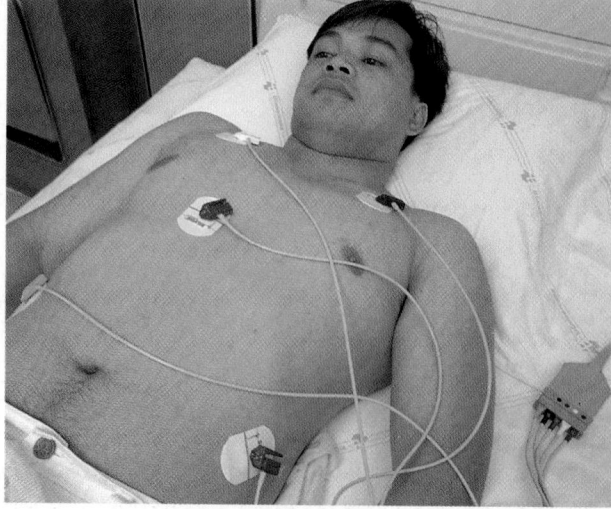

when the cardiac rhythm or the client's condition changes (especially with complaints of chest pain, decreased level of consciousness, or changes in vital signs). Note the date, time, client identification, monitor lead, duration of PR and QT intervals, and rhythm interpretation on each ECG strip.

ally 48 to 72 hours, the client returns and the monitor is removed. Diary entries are compared to the recorded heart rhythms to identify the effects of dysrhythmias.

### Electrophysiology Studies

Diagnostic cardiac *electrophysiology (EP) procedures* are used to identify dysrhythmias and their causes. EP studies are used to analyze components of the conduction system, identify sites of ectopic stimulation, and evaluate the effectiveness of treatment. EP procedures can be used for both diagnosis and as a therapeutic intervention.

In the electrophysiology laboratory, electrode catheters are guided by fluoroscopy into the heart through the femoral or brachial vein. The timing and sequence of electrical activation during normal and abnormal (aberrant) rhythms is observed and measured. Electrical stimulation may be used to induce dysrhythmias similar to the client's clinical dysrhythmia (Woods et al., 2000). Following diagnosis, an EP procedure may be used to treat the dysrhythmia, for example, by overdrive pacing (stimulating the client's heart rate to a rate faster than that of the tachydysrhythmia) to break the dysrhythmia's cycle, or to perform ablative therapy to destroy the ectopic site. See the section on ablative techniques for further information.

Nursing care for the client undergoing an EP procedure is similar to that for a coronary angiogram (see the box on page 817). The procedure and expected sensations are explained. The client remains awake during the procedure; antianxiety medications or sedatives are given to reduce apprehension. Intravenous heparin may be given during the procedure to reduce the risk of thromboembolism.

Complications of EP procedures are infrequent, but include fatal ventricular fibrillation, cardiac perforation, and major venous thrombosis (Woods et al., 2000). Careful postprocedure monitoring is vital.

### Medications

The goal of drug therapy is to suppress dysrhythmia formation. No drug has been found to be completely safe and effective. Antidysrhythmic drugs may be used for acute treatment of dysrhythmias or to manage chronic conditions. The overall goal of therapy is to maintain an effective cardiac output by stabilizing cardiac rhythm.

It is important to remember that virtually all antidysrhythmic drugs also have *prodysrhythmic* effects; that is, they can worsen existing dysrhythmias and precipitate new ones. Because of this tendency, studies that demonstrate higher mortality rates in clients receiving antidysrhythmic medications, and the increasing safety and availability of interventional techniques, the use of antidysrhythmic medications is declining.

Most antidysrhythmic drugs are classified by their effects on the cardiac action potential. Most are class I drugs, or fast sodium channel blockers. By blocking sodium channels, these drugs slow impulse conduction in the atria and ventricles. This class is further divided into subclasses A, B, and C. Class II drugs are beta blockers, which decrease SA node automaticity, AV conduction velocity, and myocardial contractility. Class III agents block potassium channels, delaying repolarization and prolong-

ing the relative refractory period. Class IV drugs are calcium channel blockers. Their effect is similar to that of beta blockers. Adenosine and digoxin do not fit within the major classes. Both drugs reduce SA node automaticity and slow AV conduction. Ibutilide and magnesium also fall outside the major classes, but are used to treat dysrhythmias. See the Medication Administration box on page 854 for identifies common antidysrhythmic drugs within each class and the nursing implications in caring for clients receiving antidysrhythmic drugs.

Drugs that affect the autonomic nervous system may also be used to treat dysrhythmias. Sympathomimetics, such as epinephrine, stimulate the heart, increasing both heart rate and contractility. Anticholinergic agents such as atropine are used to decrease vagal tone and increase the heart rate. Magnesium sulfate is an unclassified drug that has been shown to be safe and effective in treating ventricular tachycardias.

### Countershock

*Countershock* is used to interrupt cardiac rhythms that compromise cardiac output and the client's welfare. Delivery of a direct current charge depolarizes all cardiac cells at the same time. This simultaneous depolarization may stop a tachydysrhythmia and allow the sinus node to recover control of impulse formation. There are two types of countershock: synchronized cardioversion and defibrillation.

### Synchronized Cardioversion

*Synchronized cardioversion* delivers direct electrical current synchronized with the client's heart rhythm. Synchronization of the shock with the QRS complex prevents ventricular fibrillation by avoiding current delivery during the vulnerable period of repolarization. Cardioversion is usually done as an elective procedure to treat supraventricular tachycardia, atrial fibrillation, atrial flutter, or even a hemodynamically stable ventricular tachycardia.

The nurse assists with cardioversion by preparing the client before the procedure; obtaining any laboratory tests ordered; obtaining and documenting ECG strips prior to, during, and after treatment; setting up the equipment; and monitoring the client's response. Procedure 29–2 describes synchronized cardioversion.

Clients in atrial fibrillation are at high risk for thromboembolism following cardioversion. Loss of atrial contractions with atrial fibrillation leads to blood pooling in the atria, increasing the risk of clot formation. When the atria begin to contract following successful cardioversion, clots may be dislodged, embolizing to the pulmonary or systemic circulation. If possible, anticoagulants are given for several weeks before cardioversion is attempted.

### Defibrillation

Unlike carefully synchronized cardioversion, *defibrillation* is an emergency procedure that delivers direct current without regard to the cardiac cycle. Ventricular fibrillation is immediately treated as soon as the dysrhythmia is recognized. Early defibrillation has been shown to improve survival in clients experiencing VF.

Defibrillation can be delivered by external or internal paddles or pads. Conductive gel pads or paste is applied, and external paddles or pads are placed on the chest wall at the apex and

## Medication Administration
### Antidysrhythmic Drugs

### CLASS I DRUGS: SODIUM CHANNEL BLOCKERS
#### Class IA

Quinidine (Cardioquin, Quinidex, Quinaglute)
Procainamide (Pronestyl, Procan SR)
Disopyramide (Norpace, Norpace CR)

Class IA decrease the flow of sodium into the cell and prolong the action potential. This decreases automaticity, slows the rate of impulse conduction, and prolongs refractoriness. They are used to treat both supraventricular and ventricular tachycardias.

#### Class IB

Lidocaine (Xylocaine)        Tocainide (Tonocard)
Mexiletine (Mexitil)         Phenytoin (Dilantin)

Class IB, or lidocaine-like, drugs decrease the refractory period but have little effect on automaticity. Drugs in this class are used primarily to treat ventricular dysrhythmias, including PVCs and ventricular tachycardia.

#### Class IC

Flecainide (Tambocor)        Propafenone (Rythmol)

Class IC drugs slow impulse conduction velocity but have little effect on refractoriness. They are used to reduce or eliminate tachydysrhythmias associated with reentry. Their significant prodysrhythmic effects limit their usefulness, but they may be used to treat supraventricular tachycardia.

### CLASS II DRUGS: BETA-BLOCKERS

Esmolol (Brevibloc)
Propranolol (Inderal)
Acebutolol (Sectral)

Class II drugs are beta blockers that decrease automaticity and conduction through the AV node. They also reduce the heart rate and myocardial contractility. They are used to treat supraventricular tacycardia and to slow the ventricular response rate to atrial fibrillation. These drugs may cause bronchospasm and are contraindicated for clients with asthma, chronic obstructive pulmonary disease (COPD), or other restrictive or obstructive lung diseases.

### CLASS III DRUGS: POTASSIUM CHANNEL BLOCKERS

Sotalol (Betapace)           Bretylium (Bretylol)
Amiodarone (Cordarone)       Ibutilide (Corvert)

Class III drugs block potassium channels, prolonging repolarization and the refractory period. Drugs in this class are used primarily to treat ventricular tachycardia and ventricular fibrillation. Amiodarone may also be used for supraventricular tachycardias.

### CLASS IV DRUGS: CALCIUM CHANNEL BLOCKERS

Verapamil (Calan, Isoptin, Verelan)
Diltiazem (Cardizem, Dilacor XR)

Calcium channel blockers decrease automaticity and AV nodal conduction. They are used to manage supraventricular tachycardias. Like the beta blockers, calcium channel blockers reduce myocardial contractility.

### OTHER DRUGS

Adenosine (Adenocard)            Digoxin

Adenosine and digoxin decrease conduction through the AV node and are used to treat supraventricular tachycardias.

### Nursing Responsibilities
- Obtain baseline data including vital signs, cardiac rhythm (including rate, PR and QT intervals, and QRS duration), and physical assessment (especially cardiac, neurologic, and respiratory status).
- Assess medication regimen to identify drugs that may interfere with antidysrhythmic therapy.
- Monitor ECG to evaluate the effectiveness of therapy and to assess for possible dysrhythmias precipitated by treatment.
- Immediately report manifestations of drug toxicity:
  - Procainimide—signs of heart failure; conduction delays or ventricular dysrhythmias; skin rash, myalgias or arthralgias, flulike symptoms.
  - Disopyramide—urinary retention, heart failure, eye pain
  - Lidocaine—changes in neurologic status, such as agitation, confusion, dizziness, nervousness
  - Amiodarone—pulmonary fibrosis (increasing dyspnea, cough, hepatic dysfunction—changes in liver function tests, jaundice); vision changes, photosensitivity
  - Digoxin—anorexia, nausea, vomiting; blurred, or double vision; yellow green halos; new-onset dysrhythmias
- Use an infusion pump to administer intravenous infusions. Monitor the dose and assess its appropriateness (in mg/min or µg/kg/min).

### Client and Family Teaching
- Take the drug exactly as prescribed. Do not skip or double doses. Check with your physician if a dose is missed.
- Take your pulse and record the rate daily before rising. Count the pulse for 1 full minute. Bring the record with you to each office or clinic visit
- Report the following to the physician: irregular pulse rate or rhythm, dizziness, eye pain, changes in vision, skin rashes or color changes, wheezing or other respiratory problems, changes in behavior.

base of the heart (Figure 29–13 ■). Internal paddles are applied directly on the heart, and may be used in surgery, the emergency department, or critical care. Internal defibrillation is done only by a physician; external defibrillation may be performed by any health care provider who has been trained in the procedure. Automatic external defibrillators (AEDs) are available on most hospital units to allow early defibrillation for cardiac arrest. (See Procedure 29–3.)

## Pacemaker Therapy

A **pacemaker** is a pulse generator used to provide an electrical stimulus to the heart when the heart fails to generate or conduct its own at a rate that maintains the cardiac output. The pulse generator is connected to *leads* (insulated wires) passed intravenously into the heart or sutured directly to the epicardium. The leads sense intrinsic electrical activity of the heart and provide an electrical stimulus to the heart when necessary (pacing).

## Procedure 29–2 — Elective Synchronized Cardioversion

### SUPPLIES

- Cardioverter-defibrillator with ECG cable and monitor
- Conductive gel pads or paste
- Dry gauze pads
- Emergency drug kit and resuscitation equipment
- IV Supplies (catheter, solution, administration set)

### PREPROCEDURE

Explain the purpose of the procedure (to restore an effective cardiac rhythm). Describe the procedure in simple, non-threatening terms. Advise that some discomfort may be felt with each countershock, but a sedative will be given to minimize discomfort. Witness the signature on an informed consent form for this procedure. Document preprocedure rhythm on an ECG strip. Ensure a patent intravenous access site for emergency drug administration. Keep NPO as specified prior to the procedure. Assess acid-base and electrolyte levels (especially potassium, magnesium, and calcium) and drug levels if appropriate. Report abnormalities to the physician prior to the procedure. Document vital signs, level of consciousness, and peripheral pulses. Administer the prescribed sedative, and provide for safety. Remove any medication patches from the chest and all metallic objects. Place in supine position, and provide for privacy.

### PROCEDURE

1. Use standard precautions.
2. Turn on the cardioverter-defibrillator and ECG monitor.
3. Connect the client's ECG cable to the cardioverter. Select a lead with prominent R waves for monitoring.
4. Set cardioverter to "synchronize" mode. Observe the ECG waveform on the monitor for indications of synchronization, such as a flashing bold line or a blip. Many units also display the message "synchronized mode" on the monitor.
5. Place conductive pads on the chest below the right clavicle to the right of the sternum and in the midaxillary line on the left. If using conductive paste, spread it evenly on the defibrillator paddles.
6. Turn on the ECG recording strip for a continuous printout during the procedure.
7. Charge the paddles to the prescribed energy dose. The machine will beep to indicate that the selected energy level has been reached and that the paddles are ready for discharge.
8. The paddles are applied firmly to the chest over the conductive pads by the physician.
9. Turn oxygen off and remove it.
10. Ensure that no one is touching the client or the bed prior to discharge of the electrical shock. There may be a slight delay in shock delivery as the machine synchronizes with the R wave.
11. Assess client status and ECG rhythm. Assure a patent airway and the presence of a pulse.
12. The procedure may be repeated if unsuccessful. The energy level may be increased with each attempt.
13. Remove conductive pads. Using a dry gauze pad, clean paste from the chest and the paddles.

### POSTPROCEDURE

Assess client for return of consciousness from sedative or cardioversion. Evaluate neurologic, cardiovascular, and respiratory status. Assess for possible complications, including emboli (especially cerebral), respiratory depression, and dysrhythmias. Document postcardioversion rhythm strip. Assess skin for burns. Document the procedure and the client's response in the medical record.

---

Pacemakers are used to treat both acute and chronic conduction defects such as third-degree AV block. They also may be used to treat bradydysrhythmias and tachydysrhythmias.

*Temporary pacemakers* use an external pulse generator (Figure 29–14 ■) attached to a lead threaded intravenously into the right ventricle, to temporary pacing wires implanted during cardiac surgery, or to external conductive pads placed on the chest wall for emergency pacing.

*Permanent pacemakers* use an internal pulse generator placed in a subcutaneous pocket in the subclavian space or abdominal wall. The generator connects to leads sewn directly onto the heart (*epicardial*) or passed transvenously into the heart (*endocardial*). Epicardial pacemakers (Figure 29–15 ■) require surgical exposure of the heart. Leads may be placed during cardiac surgery, or using a small subxiphoid incision to expose on the heart. Transvenous pacemaker leads are positioned in the right heart via the cephalic, subclavian, or jugular vein (Figure 29–16 ■). Local anesthesia can be used for permanent pacer insertion.

Pacemakers are programmed to stimulate the atria or the ventricles (*single-chamber pacing*), or both (*dual-chamber pacing*). Table 29–7 defines terms used to describe pacemaker modes and functions. The most commonly used pacemakers either: (a) sense activity in and pace the ventricles only; or (b) sense activity in and pace both the atria and the ventricles. Dual-chamber or *atrioventricular sequential pacing* stimulates both chambers of the heart in sequence. AV pacing imitates the normal sequence of atrial contraction followed by ventricular contraction, improving cardiac output.

Pacing is detected on the ECG strip by the presence of pacing artifact (Figure 29–17 ■ on page 858). A sharp spike is noted before the P wave with atrial pacing, and before the QRS complex with ventricular pacing. Pacing spikes are seen before both the P wave and QRS complex in AV sequential pacing. Capture is noted if there is a contraction of the chamber immediately following the pacer spike. Problems in sensing, pacing, and capture are noted in Table 29–8 (on page 859).

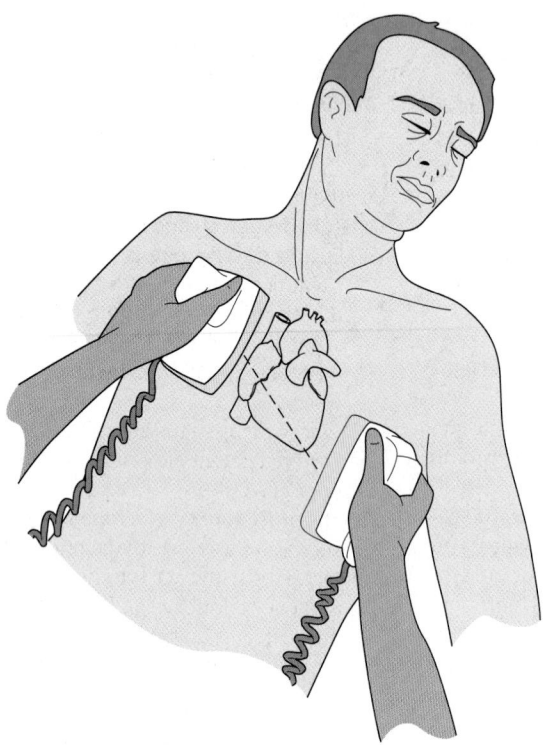

**Figure 29–13** ■ Placement of paddles for defibrillation.

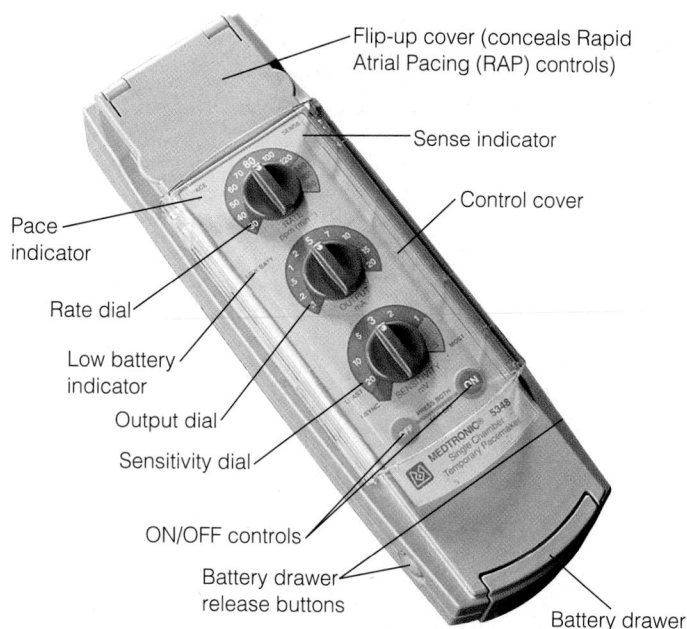

**Figure 29–14** ■ Programmable settings on a temporary pacemaker.

*Courtesy of Medtronics, Inc.*

Care of the client with a temporary or permanent pacemaker focuses on monitoring for pacemaker malfunctioning, maintaining safety (Box 29–5), and preventing infection and postoperative complications. Nursing care for the client having a pacemaker implant is outlined on page 860.

## Implantable Cardioverter-Defibrillator

Sudden cardiac death claims more than 300,000 lives per year in the United States (Woods et al., 2000). The *implantable cardioverter-defibrillator (ICD)* detects life-threatening changes in the cardiac rhythm and automatically delivers an electric shock to convert the dysrhythmia back

---

### Procedure 29–3        Emergency External Defibrillation

#### SUPPLIES

- Automatic external defibrillator or defibrillator with ECG cable and monitor
- Conductive gel pads or paste
- Dry gauze pads
- Emergency medications and cart with pacemaker, airway management equipment, and oxygen supplies.

#### PREPROCEDURE

Verify the lethal dysrhythmia, such as pulseless VT, VF, or asystole. Initiate the cardiac arrest (code) procedure, and obtain the defibrillator. If one is not immediately available, begin CPR until the emergency cart and defibrillator are brought to the bedside. Place client in supine position on a firm surface.

#### PROCEDURE

1. Turn on the defibrillator. Set it in *defibrillation* mode.
2. Turn ECG recording on for a continuous printout of events during the procedure.
3. Set the energy level and charge the paddles. Initial defibrillation is usually performed at 200 joules.
4. Place conductive pads on the chest, or spread conductive paste evenly on the paddles.
5. Position the paddles, holding them firmly on the chest wall.
6. **Ensure that no one is touching the client or the bed. State, "All clear."**
7. Depress the button on each paddle simultaneously to discharge the energy.
8. Evaluate cardiac rhythm and for a pulse after each defibrillation attempt.

9. If the first attempt is unsuccessful, repeat the procedure, increasing the energy level to 300 joules and 360 joulesfor successive attempts. Reapply conductive paste as necessary.
10. If unsuccessful after three defibrillation attempts, implement ACLS protocols.

#### POSTPROCEDURE

If the dysrhythmia is successfully converted, evaluate and support neurologic, cardiovascular, and respiratory status. Monitor and titrate any intravenous infusions as ordered. Maintain ventilatory support as needed. Evaluate skin for burns. Obtain blood for laboratory analysis as ordered. Monitor vital signs and ECG continuously. Transfer to the intensive care unit (ICU) as indicated. Provide support and information to the client and family.

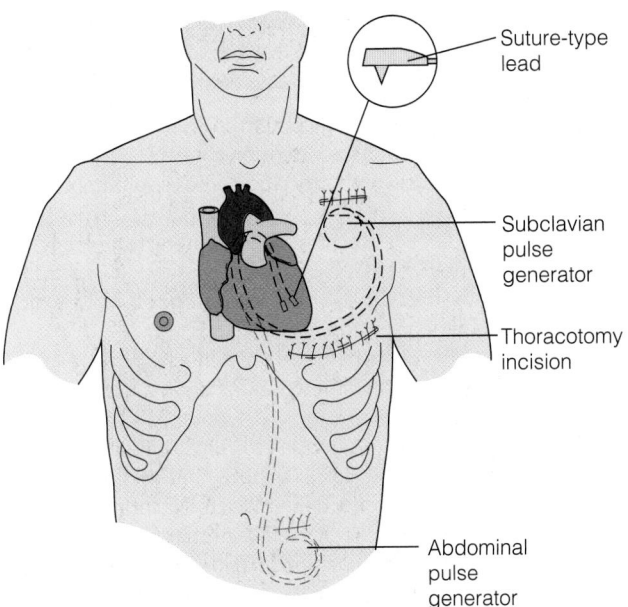

Suture-type lead

Subclavian pulse generator

Thoracotomy incision

Abdominal pulse generator

**Figure 29–15** ■ A permanent epicardial pacemaker. The pulse generator may be placed in subcutaneous pockets in the subclavian or abdominal regions.

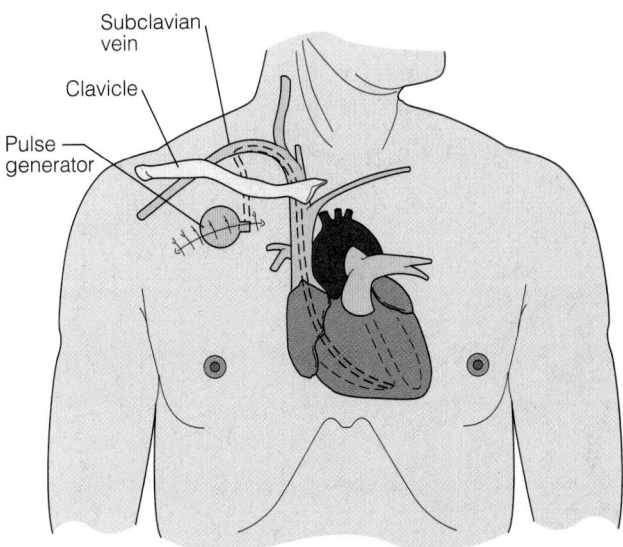

Subclavian vein

Clavicle

Pulse generator

**Figure 29–16** ■ A permanent transvenous (endocardial) pacemaker with the lead placed in the right ventricle via the subclavian vein.

into a normal rhythm. ICDs are used for sudden death survivors, clients with recurrent ventricular tachycardia, and clients with demonstrated risk factors for sudden death. ICDs can deliver a shock as needed, provide pacing on demand, and can store ECG records of tachycardic episodes (Woods et al., 2000).

A pulse generator connected to lead electrodes for rhythm detection and current delivery is implanted in the left pectoral region. The lead is threaded transvenously to the apex of the right ventricle. The ICD is programmed to sense a change in heart rate or rhythm. When it detects a potentially lethal rhythm, it shocks the heart to convert the rhythm. The device can be programmed or reprogrammed at the bedside as necessary. The ICD may be tested prior to discharge.

Local or general anesthesia is used, and the client may be discharged within 24 hours. The lithium-powered battery must be surgically replaced every 5 years. Complications and nursing care are similar to that for a client having a permanent pacemaker implant (see the Nursing Care box on page 860).

## Cardiac Mapping and Catheter Ablation

Cardiac mapping and catheter ablation are used to locate and destroy an ectopic focus. These diagnostic and therapeutic measures use electrophysiology techniques, and can be performed in the cardiac catheterization laboratory. *Cardiac mapping* is used to identify the site of earliest impulse formation in the atria or the ventricles. Intracardiac and extracardiac catheter electrodes and computer technology are used to pinpoint the ectopic site on a map of the heart. These same catheters can be used to deliver the ablative intervention.

*Ablation* destroys, removes, or isolates an ectopic focus. In most instances, radio frequency energy produced by high-frequency alternating current is used to create heat as it

### TABLE 29–7 Terms Used to Describe Pacemaker Functions

| Term | Definition |
|------|-----------|
| Asynchronous pacing | Pacemaker delivers a pacing stimulus at a set rate regardless of intrinsic cardiac activity. |
| Base rate | Rate at which the pacemaker paces when no cardiac activity is sensed. |
| Capture | The ability of the pacing stimulus to generate a cardiac depolarization. |
| Demand pacing | Pacemaker delivers a pacing stimulus only when the intrinsic rate falls below the pacemaker's base rate. |
| Dual-chamber pacing | Allows both the atria and the ventricles to be paced; most frequently used permanent pacing mode. |
| Lead | An insulated wire that senses intrinsic cardiac activity and delivers a pacing stimulus as programmed. |
| Output | The electrical stimulus delivered by the pulse generator. |
| Pacing spike | A small vertical spike noted on the ECG with every pacemaker stimulus. |
| Sensing | The pacemaker's ability to identify and respond to intrinsic cardiac activity. |
| Single-chamber pacing | Pacing of only the atria or the ventricles, not both; most common temporary pacing mode used. |

*Note. Adapted from Cardiac Nursing (4th ed.) by S. L. Woods, E. S. S. Froelicher, & S. U. Motzer, 2000, Philadelphia: Lippincott.*

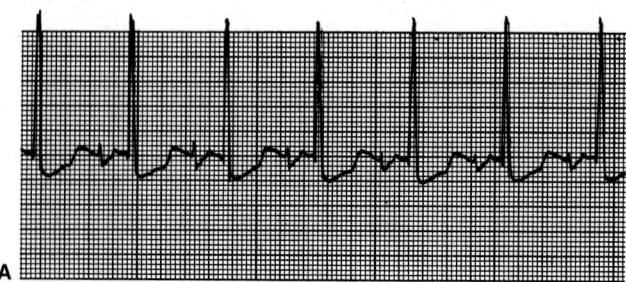

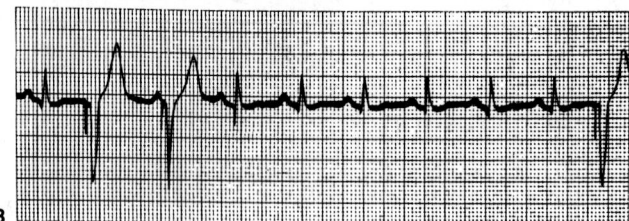

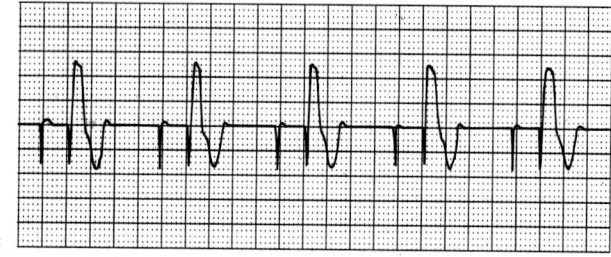

**Figure 29–17** ■ Pacing artifacts. *A,* Atrial pacing and ventricular sensing. Note the pacer spike preceding the P wave. *B,* Ventricular demand pacing. Note the absence of pacer spikes when the client's natural rhythm predominates. *C,* Atrioventricular pacing. Note the pacer spikes preceding both P waves and QRS complexes.

passes through tissue. Catheter ablation is used to treat supraventricular tachycardias, atrial fibrillation and flutter, and, in some cases, paroxysmal ventricular tachycardia (Woods et al., 2000).

Anticoagulant therapy may be started after catheter ablation to reduce the risk of clot formation at the ablation site.

## Other Therapies

In addition to medications and interventional techniques, other measures may be used to treat selected dysrhythmias. Vagal maneuvers that stimulate the parasympathetic nervous system may be used to slow the heart rate in supraventricular tachycardias. These maneuvers include *carotid sinus massage* and the *Valsalva maneuver.* Carotid sinus massage is performed only by a physician during continuous cardiac monitoring. Excessive slowing of the heart rate may result. The Valsalva maneuver, forced exhalation against a closed glottis (e.g., bearing down) increases intrathoracic pressure and vagal tone, slowing the pulse rate.

## NURSING CARE

Caring for the client with cardiac dysrhythmias requires the ability to recognize, identify, and, in some cases, promptly treat the dysrhythmia. The urgency of intervention is determined by

---

**BOX 29–5** ■ **Safety Measures for Clients with a Temporary Pacemaker**

- Ensure that all electrical equipment in use has a grounded plug; do not use adapters or extension cords.
- Encourage the use of battery-powered equipment (e.g., electric razor).
- Remove any damaged electrical equipment from the unit, including equipment that
  a. Has been abused (e.g., has been dropped or in which liquid has been spilled).
  b. From which anyone has received a shock.
  c. Has frayed, worn, or otherwise damaged electrical cords or plugs.
  d. Has other evidence of impaired function, such as a hot smell during use or control knobs that are loose or do not consistently produce the expected response.
- Wear gloves when handling pacer electrodes or wires.
- Insulate pacemaker terminals and pacing wires with nonconductive, moistureproof material (e.g., a rubber glove).
- Test the pacemaker battery prior to use.
- Keep a spare pacemaker, cable, batteries, and battery tester available at all times.
- Immediately report any apparent deviation from expected pacemaker function.

the effects of the dysrhythmia on the client. Nursing care focuses on maintaining cardiac output, monitoring the response to therapy, and teaching.

## Health Promotion

Health promotion measures to prevent coronary heart disease also reduce the risk for dysrhythmias. In most cases, dysrhythmias develop as a result of ischemic or structural changes in the heart, rather than in isolation. Advise clients who are at risk or who complain of occasional palpitations or "flutters" in their chest to reduce their intake of caffeine and other sympathetic nervous system stimulants, such as excess chocolate.

## Assessment

Assessment is vital before treating any suspected dysrhythmia. What appears to be ventricular tachycardia on the monitor may be the client scratching or brushing the teeth. Apparent asystole on the monitor may be due to a loose electrode patch. Similarly, a heart rate of 52 BPM may not affect the overall cardiac output in some clients. Review Chapter 28 for complete assessment of the client with a cardiac problem.

- Health history: complaints of palpitations (ask for further definition of palpitations), "fluttering" sensations, or a sensation of the heart racing; episodes of dizziness, lightheadedness, or syncope (fainting); timing (duration, time of day); correlation with food or beverage intake, activity; presence of chest pain, shortness of breath, or other associated symptoms; history of heart or endocrine disease (such as hyperthyroidism); current medications
- Physical examination: level of consciousness (LOC); vital signs, including apical pulse for a full minute; regularity and

## TABLE 29-8  Potential Pacemaker Problems and Corrective Strategies

| Problem | Possible Causes | Corrective Measures |
|---|---|---|
| **Undersensing**<br>Device fails to detect existing cardiac depolarizations, therefore competes with the native rhythms.<br><br>Undetected R waves<br><br><br><br>Competing pacer spikes | Lead disconnected from pacer or from viable myocardium.<br>Sensitivity set too low.<br>Lead fracture.<br>Low battery. | Check connection of lead to pacer.<br>Increase sensitivity.<br>Reposition or change lead.<br>Change battery. |
| **Oversensing**<br>Device detects noncardiac electrical events and interprets them as cardiac depolarizations, therefore is wrongly inhibited from pacing.<br><br>When artifact ceases, pacing resumes<br><br><br><br>Pacer interprets artifact as cardiac activity and fails to fire | Sensitivity set too high.<br><br>Interference from electrical sources (ungrounded equipment, short circuits) is detected and misinterpreted by the device.<br>Lead disconnected from pacer or from viable myocardium. | Decrease sensitivity (turn sensing control to a LARGER number).<br>Remove all ungrounded electrical equipment or have it evaluated by hospital engineers.<br><br>Check connection of lead to pacer. |
| **Noncapture**<br>Device emits stimuli which fail to depolarize the myocardium.<br><br><br><br>Pacer stimuli which fail to initiate myocardial depolarization | Output set too low in the noncaptured chamber.<br>Lead fracture.<br>High pacing threshold due to medication or metabolic changes.<br>Low battery. | Increase output in the noncaptured chamber.<br>Reposition or change lead.<br>Alter medication regimen, correct metabolic changes.<br>Change battery. |

Note. From "Cardiac Rhythm Control Devices" (p. 92) by C. L. Witherell, 1994, *Critical Care Nursing Clinics of North America,* 6(1).

# NURSING CARE OF THE CLIENT HAVING A PERMANENT PACEMAKER IMPLANT

## PREOPERATIVE CARE

- Provide routine preoperative care and teaching as outlined in Chapter 7. 
- Assess knowledge and understanding of the procedure, clarifying and expanding on existing knowledge as needed. *Clarifying knowledge, providing information, and conveying emotional support reduces anxiety and fear and allows the client to develop a realistic outlook regarding pacer therapy.*
- Place ECG monitor electrodes away from potential incision sites. *This helps preserve skin integrity.*
- Teach range-of-motion (ROM) exercises for the affected side. *ROM exercises of the affected arm and shoulder prevent stiffness and impaired function following pacemaker insertion.*

## POSTOPERATIVE CARE

- Provide postoperative monitoring, analgesia, and care as outlined in Chapter 7.
- Obtain a chest X-ray as ordered. *A postoperative chest X-ray is used to identify lead location and detect possible complications, such as pneumothorax or pleural effusion.*
- Position for comfort. Minimize movement of the affected arm and shoulder during the initial postoperative period. *Restricting movement minimizes discomfort on the operative side and allows the leads to become anchored, reducing the risk of dislodging.*
- Assist with gentle ROM exercises at least three times daily, beginning 24 hours after pacemaker implantation. *ROM exercises help restore normal shoulder movement and prevent contractures on the affected side.*
- Monitor pacemaker function with cardiac monitoring or intermittent ECGs. Report pacemaker problems to the physician:
  - Failure to pace. *This may indicate battery depletion, damage or dislodgement of pacer wires, or inappropriate sensing.*
  - Failure to capture (the pacemaker stimulus is not followed by ventricular depolarization). *The electrical output of the pacemaker may not be adequate, or the lead may be dislodged.*
  - Improper sensing (the pacemaker is firing or not firing, regardless of the intrinsic rate). *This increases the risk for decreased cardiac output and dysrhythmias.*
  - Runaway pacemaker (a pacemaker firing at a rapid rate). *This may by due to generator malfunction or problems with sensing.*
  - Hiccups. *A lead positioned near the diaphragm can stimulate it, causing hiccups. Hiccups may occur in extremely thin clients or may indicate a medical emergency with perforation of the right ventricle by the pacing electrode tip.*
- Assess for dysrhythmias and treat as indicated. *Until the catheter is "seated" or adheres to the myocardium, its movement*

*may cause myocardial irritability and dysrhythmias. Fibrotic tissue develops within 2 to 3 days.*
- Document the date of pacemaker insertion, the model and type, and settings. *This information is important for future reference.*
- Immediately report signs of potential complications, including myocardial perforation, cardiac tamponade, pneumothorax or hemothorax, emboli, skin breakdown, bleeding, infection, endocarditis, or poor wound healing (see Chapter 30 for more information about cardiac tamponade and endocarditis, and Chapter 36 for pneumothorax and hemothorax ). *Early identification of complications allows for aggressive intervention.*
- Provide a pacemaker identification card including the manufacturer's name, model number, mode of operation, rate parameters, and expected battery life. *This card provides a reference for the client and future health care providers.*

## HOME CARE

Provide appropriate teaching for the client and family about:

- Placement of the pacemaker generator and leads in relation to the heart.
- How the pacemaker works and the rate at which it is set.
- Battery replacement. Most pacemaker batteries last 6 to 12 years. Replacement requires a outpatient surgery to open the subcutaneous pocket and replace the battery.
- How to take and record the pulse rate. Instruct to assess pulse daily before arising and notify the physician if 5 or more BPM slower than the preset pacemaker rate.
- Incision care and signs of infection. Bruising may be present following surgery.
- Signs of pacemaker malfunction to report, including dizziness, fainting, fatigue, weakness, chest pain, or palpitations.
- Activity restrictions as ordered. This usually is limited to contact sports (which may damage the generator) and avoiding heavy lifting for 2 months after surgery.
- Resume sexual activity as recommended by the physician. Avoid positions that cause pressure on the site.
- Avoid tight-fitting clothing over the pacemaker site to reduce irritation and avoid skin breakdown.
- Carry the pacemaker identification card at all times, and wear a MedicAlert bracelet or tag.
- Notify all care providers of the pacemaker.
- Do not hold or use certain electrical devices over the pacemaker site, including household appliances or tools, garage door openers, antitheft devices, or burglar alarms. Pacemakers will set off airport security detectors; notify security officials of its presence.
- Maintain follow-up care with the physician as recommended.

amplitude of peripheral pulses; color; presence of dyspnea, adventitious lung sounds; ECG rhythm analysis; oxygen saturation levels

## Nursing Diagnoses and Interventions

The effect of the dysrhythmia on cardiac output is the priority of nursing care. Other potential nursing diagnoses related to

dysrhythmias may include *Ineffective tissue perfusion, Activity intolerance,* and *Fear* or *Anxiety.*

### Decreased Cardiac Output

Dysrhythmias can affect cardiac output. Bradycardias decrease cardiac output if the stroke volume does not increase to compensate for the slow heart rate. Tachycardia reduces diastolic filling time, affecting stroke volume and coronary artery perfusion. Loss of the atrial kick in junctional rhythms, atrial fibrillation, and AV blocks also decreases ventricular filling and cardiac output. In ventricular fibrillation, loss of ventricular contractions causes cardiac arrest and no cardiac output.

**PRACTICE ALERT** *Before treating any dysrhythmia, assess the client, not just the monitor! Loose electrode pads, disconnected leads or cables, and muscle movement can simulate critical dysrhythmias. The client's condition is the best indicator of the need for treatment.* ■

- Assess for decreased cardiac output: decreased LOC; tachycardia; tachypnea; hypotension; low oxygen saturation; diaphoresis; low urine output; cool, clammy, mottled skin; pallor or cyanosis; diminished peripheral pulses. *Initial signs of decreased cardiac output may be subtle, such as decreased LOC. Early recognition of the dysrhythmia's effect on cardiac output facilitates appropriate treatment and may prevent further adverse effects.*
- Monitor ECG; post ECG strip every shift and when rhythm changes occur. *Documenting cardiac rhythm provides a record of disease progression and treatment effectiveness.*

**PRACTICE ALERT** *Assess vital signs, ECG, and oxygen saturation every 5 to 15 minutes during acute dysrhythmic episodes and during antidysrhythmic drug infusions. These data provide a record of cardiac output during the dysrhythmia. Antidysrhythmic drugs can adversely affect heart rate, rhythm, and blood pressure, further decreasing cardiac output.* ■

- Assess for underlying causes of dysrhythmias, such as hypovolemia, hypoxia, anemia, vagal stimulation, or medications. *Sinus tachycardia often develops in response to tissue hypoxia. Vagal stimulation (such as the Valsalva maneuver) can precipitate bradycardia.*
- Assess serum electrolytes (especially potassium, calcium, and magnesium) and digitalis and antidysrhythmic drug levels as indicated. Report abnormal values. *Electrolyte imbalances affect cardiac depolarization and repolarization and may cause dysrhythmias. Toxic levels of digitalis and antidysrhythmic drugs can precipitate further dysrhythmias. Impaired renal or hepatic function increases the risk for toxicity, as does aging.*
- Be prepared to administer antidysrhythmic medications as indicated. Implement Advanced Cardiac Life Support (ACLS) protocols as needed. *Emergency drugs should be readily available, especially on units with high-risk clients. See Table 29-6 and the Medication Administration box on page 854 for drugs used to treat common dysrhythmias that may affect cardiac output.*
- If appropriate, instruct to perform the Valsalva maneuver (bear down as if straining or coughing) for supraventricular tachycardia or ventricular tachycardia without angina. *Vagal maneuvers stimulate the parasympathetic system and may terminate some dysrhythmias. The Valsalva maneuver is contraindicated if chest pain occurs with the dysrhythmia.*

- Prepare to assist with cardioversion. Prepare the client per orders or hospital protocol (see Procedure 29–2). Explain the procedure to reduce anxiety. Have emergency equipment readily available. *Elective or emergency cardioversion is a treatment of choice for certain dysrhythmias.*

**PRACTICE ALERT** *On recognizing ventricular fibrillation and cardiac arrest, begin emergency procedures. Call for help. Obtain defibrillator and immediately defibrillate. If the defibrillator will be brought by another health care provider, begin CPR. Initiate ACLS protocols and assist with resuscitation measures as directed. Cardiac output ceases with ventricular fibrillation. Immediate or early defibrillation has been shown to have the greatest impact on survival following cardiac arrest.* ■

- After cardiac arrest, transfer to critical care. Perform and document head-to-toe assessment; obtain laboratory tests, 12-lead ECG, and chest X-ray as ordered; monitor and maintain oxygenation and intravenous infusions; and monitor vital signs and cardiac rhythm. *The period following resuscitation is critical, necessitating careful monitoring. Post-arrest assessment allows comparison of the client's condition with prearrest status and may identify CPR-related injuries. Correcting electrolyte disturbances, hypoxia, and acid-base imbalances is important to prevent further dysrhythmias and potential adverse effects on cardiac output. Intravenous access is crucial to maintain drug infusions. Hemodynamic monitoring may be instituted. The 12-lead ECG documents myocardial status, and the chest X-ray provides information about pulmonary status and and possible thoracic injury due to CPR.*
- Notify the family of significant changes in the client's condition or cardiac arrest, providing up-to-date information. Prepare family members prior to visits by explaining interventions (such as invasive tubes, a ventilator, or additional equipment) implemented since the last visit. *Concern for the family and significant others is part of holistic nursing. Researchers studying the needs of families have found that one of the most important needs was information about their loved one's condition. Clients and families need and appreciate honest communication and compassionate care. Preparing the family for critical changes in the client's condition and plan of care helps them to cope with a situational crisis.*

## Using NANDA, NIC, and NOC

Chart 29–3 shows links between NANDA nursing diagnoses, NIC, and NOC when caring for the client with a dysrhythmia.

## Home Care

Dysrhythmias have a significant physical and psychologic impact on the client and all family members. Many of these clients and their families are under a great deal of stress from frequent hospitalizations, experimentation with therapies, frustration, and the fear of sudden cardiac death. A major teaching effort focuses on coping strategies and lifestyle changes, as

## CHART 29–3 NANDA, NIC, AND NOC LINKAGES

### The Client with a Dysrhythmia

| NURSING DIAGNOSIS | NURSING INTERVENTIONS | NURSING OUTCOMES |
|---|---|---|
| • Activity Intolerance | • Energy Management<br>• Self-Care Assistance | • Activity Tolerance<br>• Self-Care: ADL |
| • Anxiety | • Anxiety Reduction | • Anxiety Control |
| • Decreased Cardiac Output | • Cardiac Care: Acute<br>• Cardiac Precautions | • Cardiac Pump Effectiveness<br>• Circulation Status |
| • Deficient Knowledge | • Teaching: Disease Process<br>• Teaching: Procedure/Treatment | • Knowledge: Disease Process<br>• Knowledge: Treatment Procedure(s) |
| • Ineffective Tissue Perfusion | • Dysrhythmia Management<br>• Vital Signs Monitoring | • Cardiac Pump Effectiveness<br>• Vital Signs Status |

*Note. Data from Nursing Outcomes Classification (NOC) by M. Johnson & M. Maas (Eds.), 1997, St. Louis: Mosby; Nursing Diagnoses: Definitions & Classification 2001–2002 by North American Nursing Diagnosis Association, 2001, Philadelphia: NANDA; Nursing Interventions Classification (NIC) by J.C. McCloskey & G. M. Bulechek (Eds.), 2000, St. Louis: Mosby. Reprinted by permission.*

well as specific management of prescribed therapies. Include the following topics as appropriate when teaching the client and family for home care.

- Function, maintenance, precautions, and signs of malfunction or complications of any implanted device such as a pacemaker or ICD
- Monitoring pulse rate and rhythm
- Activity or dietary restrictions, and any potential effects of the dysrhythmia or its treatment on lifestyle
- Medication management to reduce the risk of dysrhythmias, including the desired and potential adverse effects of antidysrhythmic drugs

- Specific instructions related to planned diagnostic tests or procedures
- The importance of follow-up visits with the cardiologist
- The importance of and where to obtain CPR training for the client and family members

In addition, discuss fears related to treatment or implanted devices, such as that of shocking a significant other during close contact or sexual activity. Explain that if a shock occurs, the partner may feel a slight buzz or tingling but should not be harmed. Refer to and encourage the client and family to attend a peer support group for the specific condition.

## Nursing Care Plan

### A Client with Supraventricular Tachycardia

Elisa Vasquez, 53 years old, is admitted to the cardiac unit with complaints of palpitations, light-headedness, and shortness of breath. Her history reveals rheumatic fever at age 12 with subsequent rheumatic heart disease and mitral stenosis. An intravenous line is in place and she is receiving oxygen. Marcia Lewin, RN, is assigned to Ms. Vasquez.

#### ASSESSMENT

Ms. Lewin's assessment reveals that Ms. Vasquez is moderately anxious. Her ECG shows supraventricular tachycardia (SVT) with a rate of 154. Vital signs: T 98.8° F (37.1° C), R 26, BP 95/60. Peripheral pulses weak but equal, mucous membranes pale pink, skin cool and dry. Fine crackles noted in both lung bases. A loud $S_3$ gallop and a diastolic murmur are noted. Ms. Vasquez is still complaining of palpitations and tells Ms. Lewin, "I feel so nervous and weak and dizzy." Ms. Vasquez's cardiologist orders 2.5 mg of verapamil to be given slowly via intravenous push and tells Ms. Lewin to prepare to assist with synchronized cardioversion if drug therapy does not control the ventricular rate.

#### DIAGNOSIS

- *Decreased cardiac output* related to inadequate ventricular filling associated with rapid tachycardia
- *Ineffective tissue perfusion: cerebral/cardiopulmonary/peripheral* related to decreased cardiac output
- *Anxiety* related to unknown outcome of altered health state

#### EXPECTED OUTCOMES

- Maintain adequate cardiac output and tissue perfusion.
- Demonstrate a ventricular rate within normal limits and stable vital signs.
- Verbalize reduced anxiety.
- Verbalize an understanding of the rationale for the treatment measures to control the heart rate.

#### PLANNING AND IMPLEMENTATION

- Provide oxygen per nasal cannula at 4 L/min.
- Continuously monitor ECG for rate, rhythm, and conduction. Assess vital signs and associated symptoms with changes in ECG. Report findings to physician.

## Nursing Care Plan

### A Client with Supraventricular Tachycardia (continued)

- Explain the importance of rapidly reducing the heart rate. Explain the cardioversion procedure and encourage questions.
- Encourage verbalization of fears and concerns. Answer questions honestly, correcting misconceptions about the disease process, treatment, or prognosis.
- Administer intravenous diazepam as ordered before cardioversion.
- Document pretreatment vital signs, level of consciousness, and peripheral pulses.
- Place emergency cart with drugs and airway management supplies in client unit.
- Assist with cardioversion as indicated.
- Assess LOC, level of sedation, cardiovascular and respiratory status, and skin condition following cardioversion.
- Document procedure and postcardioversion rhythm, and response to intervention.

### EVALUATION

Intravenous verapamil lowers Ms. Vasquez's heart rate to 138 for a short time, after which it increases to 164 with BP of 82/64. Her cardiologist, Dr. Mullins, performs carotid sinus massage. The ventricular rate slows to 126 for 2 minutes, revealing atrial flutter waves, and then returns to a rate of 150. Dr. Mullins explains the treatment options, including synchronized cardioversion. Ms. Vasquez agrees to the procedure.

Ms. Vasquez is lightly sedated and synchronized cardioversion is performed. One countershock converts Ms. Vasquez to regular sinus rhythm at 96 BPM with BP 112/60.

Ms. Vasquez is sleepy from the sedation but recovers without incident. She states that she feels "much better," and her vital signs return to her normal levels. She remains in NSR with a rate of 86 to 92 for the remainder of her hospital stay. Dr. Mullins places Ms. Vasquez on furosemide to treat manifestations of mild heart failure.

### Critical Thinking in the Nursing Process

1. What is the scientific basis for using carotid massage to treat supraventricular tachycardias? Was this an appropriate maneuver in the case of Ms. Vasquez?
2. What other treatment options might the physician have used to treat Ms. Vasquez's supraventricular tachycardia if she had been asymptomatic with stable vital signs?
3. Develop a teaching plan for Ms. Vasquez related to her prescription for furosemide.

See Evaluating Your Response in Appendix C.

## THE CLIENT WITH SUDDEN CARDIAC DEATH

**Sudden cardiac death (SCD)** is defined as unexpected death occurring within 1 hour of the onset of cardiovascular symptoms. It usually is caused by ventricular fibrillation and cardiac arrest. *Cardiac arrest* is the sudden collapse, loss of consciousness, and cessation of effective circulation that precedes biologic death. Nearly half of all cardiac arrest victims die before reaching the hospital; only 25% to 30% of out-of-hospital cardiac arrest victims survive to be discharged (Woods et al., 2000).

Almost 50% of all deaths due to coronary heart disease are attributed to SCD. Coronary heart disease causes up to 80% of all sudden cardiac deaths in the United States. Other cardiac pathologies such as cardiomyopathy and valvular disorders also may lead to SCD. Noncardiac causes of sudden death include electrocution, pulmonary embolism, and rapid blood loss from a ruptured aortic aneurysm.

Ventricular fibrillation is the most common dysrhythmia associated with sudden cardiac death, accounting for 65% to 80% of cardiac arrests. Sustained severe bradydysrhythmias, *asystole* or cardiac standstill, and pulseless electrical activity (organized cardiac electrical activity without a mechanical response) are responsible for most remaining SCDs (Braunwald

et al., 2001). Selected cardiac and noncardiac causes of sudden cardiac death are listed in Box 29–6.

Risk factors for SCD are those associated with coronary heart disease (see the first section of this chapter). Advancing age and male gender are powerful risk factors. After age 65, the gap between male and female incidence of SCD narrows (Braunwald et al., 2001). Clients with dysrhythmias such as recurrent VT may have a higher risk of SCD.

### PATHOPHYSIOLOGY

Evidence of coronary heart disease with significant atherosclerosis and narrowing of two or more major coronary arteries is found in 75% of SCD victims. Although most have had prior myocardial infarction, only 20% to 30% have recent acute myocardial infarction. An acute change in cardiovascular status precedes cardiac arrest by up to 1 hour; however, often the onset is instantaneous or abrupt. Tachycardia develops, and the number of PVCs increase. This is followed by a run of ventricular tachycardia that deteriorates into ventricular fibrillation (Braunwald et al., 2001).

Abnormalities of myocardial structure or function also contribute. Structural abnormalities include infarction, hypertrophy, myopathy, and electrical anomalies. Functional deviations are caused by such factors as ischemia followed by reperfusion, altered homeostasis, autonomic nervous system

## BOX 29–6 ■ Selected Causes of Sudden Cardiac Death

### CARDIAC CAUSES

- Coronary heart disease
- Reperfusion following ischemia
- Myocardial hypertrophy
- Cardiomyopathy
- Inflammatory myocardial disorders
- Valve disorders
- Primary electrical disorders
- Dissecting or ruptured aortic or ventricular aneurysm
- Cardiac drug toxicity

### NONCARDIAC CAUSES

- Pulmonary embolism
- Cerebral hemorrhage
- Autonomic dysfunction
- Choking
- Electrical shock
- Electrolyte and acid-base imbalances

and hormone interactions, and toxic effects. The interactions of the two cause myocardial instability and may precipitate fatal dysrhythmias.

## COLLABORATIVE CARE

The goal of collaborative care is to restore cardiac output and tissue perfusion. Treatment measures are initiated as soon as clinical cardiac arrest is verified by the absence of respirations and carotid or femoral pulses. Basic and advanced cardiac life support measures must be instituted within 2 to 4 minutes of cardiac arrest to prevent permanent neurologic damage and ischemic injury to other organs.

## Basic Life Support

Basic life support (BLS) begins with identification of the cardiac arrest and initiation of an emergency response.

Providers trained in use of the *automated external debrillator (AED)* should immediately defibrillate the client in VF. Self-adhesive conductive pads attached to connecting cables are positioned on the chest (Figure 29–18 ■). The AED analyzes the rhythm, and advises the provider to charge the device if VF is detected. After warning all personnel to stand clear, the shock button is depressed to deliver a shock. Following the shock, press the analyze button to reevaluate the rhythm. Up to three shocks may be delivered before proceeding with ACLS protocol. If the AED advises against shock, CPR is initiated.

*Cardiopulmonary resuscitation (CPR)* is a mechanical attempt to maintain tissue perfusion and oxygenation using oral resuscitation and external cardiac compressions. All health care providers need to be proficient in CPR. The technique should be performed according to American Heart Association guidelines and hospital protocol. (See Box 29–7.)

CPR carries a high risk for both cardiac and noncardiac trauma. CPR-related complications include injuries to the skin, thorax, upper airway, abdomen, lungs, heart, and great vessels. These complications can be minimized by adhering to accepted CPR techniques.

## Advanced Life Support

Advanced life support (ALS), provided by specially trained health care personnel, includes endotracheal intubation to maintain the airway and oxygenation, use of intravenous drugs following specific protocols, and additional interventions such as repeated defibrillation procedures and cardiac pacing. Epinephrine, sodium bicarbonate, and antidysrhythmic drugs such as amiodarone, bretylium, lidocaine, procainamide, magnesium sulfate, and atropine are used to attempt to restore and maintain an effective cardiac rhythm.

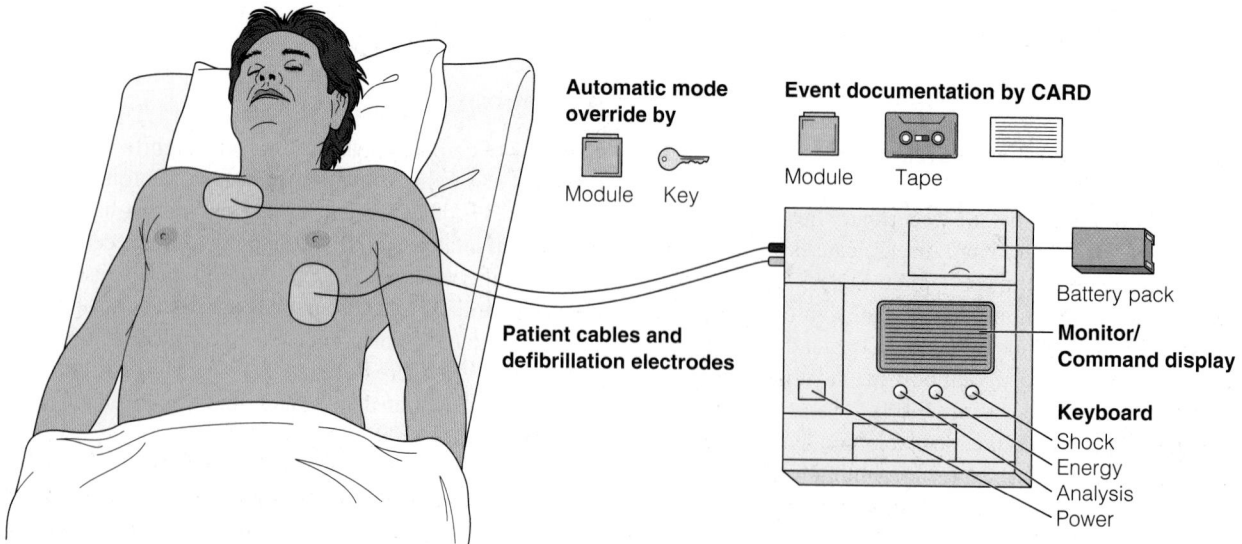

**Figure 29–18** ■ Schematic of an automated external defibrillator (AED) attached to a client.

## BOX 29–7 ■ Cardiopulmonary Resuscitation

1. Assess for responsiveness; shake the client and shout.
2. Call for help. Dial 911 (if outside the health care facility) or initiate the institutional code or cardiac arrest procedure.
3. Check for breathing; look and listen. Inspect the chest for rise and fall with respirations; listen and feel for air movement through the nose or mouth.
4. Open the airway using the-head-tilt, chin-lift maneuvers. Simultaneously press down on the forehead with one hand while lifting the chin upward with the other (part A of the accompanying figure).
5. Reassess for breathing.
6. If not breathing, begin rescue breathing using a pocket mask, mouth shield, or bag-valve mask (see part B of the figure). Administer two full breaths.
7. Check the carotid or femoral artery for a pulse.
8. If a pulse is present, continue rescue breathing until help arrives or spontaneous respirations resume Recheck the carotid pulse every 12 breaths.
9. If no pulse is present, analyze rhythm and defibrillate or initiate external cardiac compressions. Place on a firm surface. Position hands as follows:
   a. Locate the lower margin of the rib cage with the fingers of the hand closer to the legs.
   b. Move the fingers up the rib margin to locate the sternal notch.
   c. Place the heel of the hand nearer the head on the lower half of the sternum (part C of the figure), taking care to avoid positioning the hand directly over the xiphoid process.
   d. Then place the first hand in a parallel position over the second hand with the fingers either extended or interlocked.
10. Initiate cardiac compressions, pressing straight down to depress the sternum 1.5 to 2 inches, keeping the elbows locked and positioning the shoulders directly over the hands (part D of the figure). Release pressure completely between compressions but do not lift the hands from the chest.
11. Compress the chest at a rate of 80 to 100 times per minute (one-and-two-and . . . ).
    a. With one-rescuer CPR, provide 2 breaths after each 15 compressions. Assess the pulse after 4 complete cycles of 15 compressions and 2 breaths; continue CPR until help arrives.
    b. With two-rescuer CPR, provide 1 breath after every 5 compressions. Assess the pulse every minute for 5 to 10 seconds. If no pulse is present, continue CPR until help arrives.

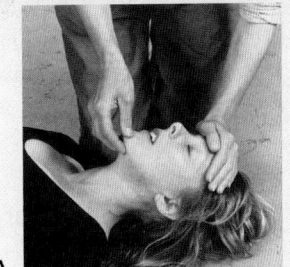

A

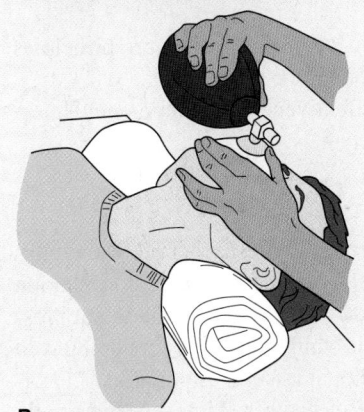

B

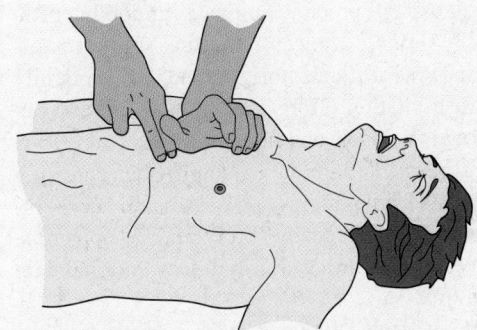

C

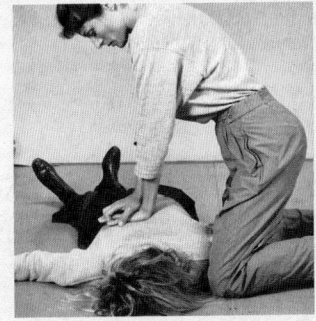

D

A, Head-tilt, chin-lift maneuver. B, Using a bag-valve mask. C, Placement of hands on lower portion of sternum above the xiphoid process. D, Arm, hand, and shoulder position for cardiac massage.

*Source: Adapted from Cardiac Nursing (4th ed.) by S. L. Woods, E.S.S. Froelicher, and S.U. Motzer, 2002, Philadelphia: Lippincott.*

## Postresuscitation Care

Clients who experience sudden cardiac death associated with ventricular fibrillation and acute MI have the best prognosis (Braunwald et al., 2001). The client is transferred to a coronary care unit and MI treatment measures are instituted. Antidysrhythmic drugs are continued for 24 to 48 hours to reduce the risk of subsequent episodes of VF.

Because the risk for recurrent SCD is significant in survivors, extensive diagnostic testing and interventions such as angioplasty or surgical revascularization of the myocardium, ablation, or an implantable cardioverter-defibrillator may be indicated.

# NURSING CARE

Nursing care of the client experiencing sudden cardiac death requires prompt recognition of the event and immediate initiation of BLS and ALS protocols. As noted before, early defibrillation of unstable VT and VF is the most important key to survival of cardiac arrest victims. Important concepts of emergency cardiac care follow.

- Treat the client, not the monitor. Recognize signs and symptoms of cardiac compromise early.
- Activate the emergency medical services system (i.e., call a code or call 911).
- Begin and continue basic cardiac life support principles throughout the resuscitation effort.
- Continually assess the effectiveness of emergency interventions.
- Defibrillate pulseless VT or VF as soon as possible.
- Initiate ALS protocols early.

The family is not forgotten during resuscitation. If the family is present, they are usually offered a private consultation room in which to await the outcome. If the family is not present, they are notified that their family member is not doing well and asked to come to the hospital as soon as possible. The situation is presented in a careful manner to prevent the family from racing to the hospital, precipitating an automobile crash. Pastoral care or the family's choice of spiritual support is offered to help during this difficult time. Attendance of family members during resuscitation efforts is controversial, and depends on institutional protocols and family desires.

After successful resuscitation, the nurse provides care specific to the client's underlying disease processes and needs. Intravenous infusions such as lidocaine, bretylium, or dopamine may be ordered to prevent further dysrhythmias and maintain hemodynamic stability.

If the client does not survive the arrest, the nurse provides postmortem care and emotional and spiritual support to the family.

Nursing diagnoses to consider for the client experiencing SCD include the following:

- *Ineffective tissue perfusion: Cerebral* related to ineffective cardiac output
- *Impaired spontaneous ventilation* related to cardiac arrest
- *Spiritual distress* related to unexplained sudden cardiac death
- *Disturbed thought processes* related to compromised cerebral circulation
- *Fear* related to risk for future episodes of sudden cardiac death

The risk for a future episode of sudden cardiac death requires careful and effective teaching for home care prior to discharge. Discuss the following topics with the client and family.

- Risk factor reduction for coronary heart disease
- Planned diagnostic studies to identify the cause of SCD, and possible interventions
- The risks and benefits of an ICD if appropriate
- The importance of carrying a card at all times listing all current medications and the health care provider
- Early manifestations or warning signs of cardiac arrest

- The importance of CPR training and maintaining proficiency in performing CPR (Provide referral to local CPR training providers or scheduled classes through the American Heart Association or American Red Cross.)

Nurses can impact death rates from cardiac arrest through community teaching as well. Survival rates from sudden cardiac death improve in communities in which a significant portion of the population is trained in CPR and early response by EMS agencies is stressed. Work with community groups and individuals can help create a population of people able to perform effective CPR.

## SPECIAL FOCUS: ADVANCE DIRECTIVES AND THE DO-NOT-RESUSCITATE ORDER

Most if not all hospitals have formal policies and procedures for resuscitation of clients who experience cardiac or respiratory arrest. *Advance directives* provide for the client's right to self-determination, that is, the client's right to make treatment decisions and to be responsible for the outcomes of those decisions. The living will and the durable power of attorney for health care are types of available advance directives. Both enable the client to state his or her wishes for medical treatments in end-of-life decisions. Nurses can assist clients to understand the purpose of advance directives.

Classification systems identifying the extent of resuscitative measures employed for clients who suffer a cardiac or respiratory arrest may include the following:

- *Full code:* Involves all resuscitative measures necessary to revive the client: defibrillation, CPR, respiratory, and pharmacologic support.
- *Partial code (varies by institution and client preference):* May involve full resuscitative measures with daily reassessment of code status, or may limit measures to be used in case of cardiac arrest.
- *No code:* The third classification may prohibit all resuscitative measures or limit measures to drug treatment without defibrillation, CPR, or intubation.
- *Comfort care:* Some institutions have a fourth class that allows discontinuation of all treatment except for pain and comfort measures.

Clients are usually considered a full code on hospital admission, unless an advance directive is in place. Without a written DNR order or advance directive, the nurse is obligated to begin resuscitation measures if indicated by the client's condition. This can create an ethical dilemma for nurses caring for critically ill or terminal clients should cardiac arrest ensue. Nurses should be aware of institutional policies and procedures regarding code status and advance directives.

DNR orders do not mean withdrawing care. Optimal nursing care is provided to these clients and their families. Health care providers collaborate to design an individualized plan of care for the client. The team approach, encouraging discussion of these issues between clients, families, and health care providers, allows information sharing and facilitates compassionate care planning. More information on DNRs, advance directives, and care of the family experiencing a loss is provided in Chapter 11. ∞

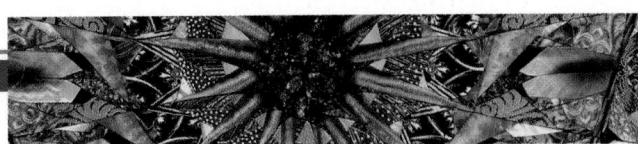

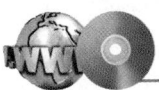 **EXPLORE MediaLink**

NCLEX review questions, case studies, care plan activities, MediaLink applications, and other interactive resources for this chapter can be found on the Companion Website at www.prenhall.com/lemone.

Click on Chapter 29 to select the activities for this chapter. For animations, video clips, more NCLEX review questions, and an audio glossary, access the Student CD-ROM accompanying this textbook.

## TEST YOURSELF

1. The nurse evaluates her teaching as effective when a client identifies which of the following modifiable risk factors for coronary heart disease (CHD) as contributing to the greatest extent?
   a. Obesity
   b. Diet
   c. Smoking
   d. Stress

2. When assessing a client with stable angina, the nurse would expect to find:
   a. Persistent ECG changes
   b. Correlation between activity level and pain
   c. Increasing nocturnal pain
   d. Evidence of impaired cardiac output such as weak peripheral pulses

3. In planning care for the client with acute myocardial infarction, (AMI) the nurse identifies the highest priority goal of care as:
   a. Stable ECG rhythm
   b. Ability to verbalize causes and effects of CHD

   c. Compliance with prescribed bed rest
   d. Relief of pain

4. Which of the following nursing diagnoses is of highest priority for the client undergoing thrombolytic therapy?
   a. *Ineffective protection*
   b. *Ineffective health maintenance*
   c. *Risk for powerlessness*
   d. *Anxiety*

5. The nurse recognizes second-degree AV block, type II (Mobitz II), and intervenes appropriately when he:
   a. Records the finding in the chart
   b. Prepares for temporary pacemaker insertion
   c. Administers a class IB antidysrhythmic drug
   d. Places the client in Fowler's position

See Test Yourself answers in Appendix C.

## BIBLIOGRAPHY

Ackley, B. J., & Ladwig, G. B. (2002). *Nursing diagnosis handbook: A guide to planning care* (5th ed.). St. Louis: Mosby.

Artinian, N. T. (2001). Perceived benefits and barriers of eating heart healthy. *MEDSURG Nursing, 10*(3), 129–138

Ayers, D. M. M. (2002). EBCT: Beaming in on coronary artery disease. *Nursing, 32*(4), 81.

Beattie, S. (2000). A portrait of postop a-fib. *RN, 63*(3), 26–29.

Braunwald, E., Fauci, A. S., Kasper, D. L., Hauser, S. L., Longo, D. L., & Jameson, J. L. (2001). *Harrison's Principles of internal medicine* (15th ed.). New York: McGraw-Hill.

Bubien, R. S. (2000). A new beat on an old rhythm. *American Journal of Nursing, 100*(1), 42–50.

Bullock, B. A., & Henze, R. L. (2000). *Focus on pathophysiology.* Philadelphia: Lippincott.

Copstead, L. C., and Banasik, J. L. (2000). *Pathophysiology: Biological and behavioral perspectives* (2nd ed.). Philadelphia: Saunders.

Cowan, M. J., Pike, K. C., & Budzynski, H. K. (2001). Psychosocial nursing therapy following sudden cardiac arrest: Impact on

two-year survival. *Nursing Research, 50*(2), 68–76.

Crumlish, C. M., Bracken, J., Hand, M. M., Keenan, K., Ruggiero, H., & Simmons, D. (2000). When time is muscle. *American Journal of Nursing, 100*(1), 26–33.

Deglin, J. H., & Vallerand, A. H. (2003). *Davis's drug guide for nurses* (8th ed.). Philadelphia: F.A. Davis.

Dracup, K., & Moser, D. K. (1997). Beyond sociodemographics: Factors influencing the decision to seek treatment for symptoms of acute myocardial infarction. *Heart & Lung, 26*(4), 253–262.

Fontaine, K. L. (2000). *Healing practices: Alternative therapies for nursing.* Upper Saddle River, NJ: Prentice Hall Health.

Gallo, J. J., Busby-Whitehead, J., Rabins, P. V., Silliman, R. A., & Murphy, J. B. (Eds.). (1999). *Reichel's care of the elderly: Clinical aspects of aging* (5th ed.). Philadelphia: Lippincott Williams & Wilkins.

Glessner, T. M., & Walker, M. K. (2001). Standardized measures: Documenting processes and

outcomes of care for patients undergoing coronary artery bypass grafting. *MEDSURG Nursing, 10*(1), 23–29.

Goodman, D. (2001). Automatic external defibrillation. *MEDSURG Nursing, 10*(5), 251–253, 276, 278.

Granger, B. B., & Miller, C. M. (2001). Acute coronary syndrome. *Nursing, 31*(11), 36–43.

Humphreys, D. R. (2001). Enhanced external counter pulsation: Beating angina. *Nursing, 31*(10), 54–55.

Incredibly easy! Understanding chest pain. (2001). *Nursing, 31*(12), 28.

Johnson, M., Bulechek, G., Dochterman, J. M., Maas, M., & Moorhead, S. (2001). *Nursing diagnoses, outcomes, & interventions.* St. Louis: Mosby.

Johnson, M., Maas, M., & Moorhead, S. (Eds.). (2000). *Nursing outcomes classification (NOC)* (2nd ed.). St. Louis: Mosby.

Kuhn, M. A. (1999). *Complementary therapies for health care providers.* Philadelphia: Lippincott.

Lehne, R. A. (2001). *Pharmacology for nursing care* (4th ed.). Philadelphia: Saunders.

Malarkey, L. M., & McMorrow, M. E. (2000). *Nurse's manual of laboratory tests and diagnostic procedures* (2nd ed.). Philadelphia: Saunders.

Mancini, M. E., & Kaye, W. (1999). AEDs: Changing the way you respond to cardiac arrest. *American Journal of Nursing, 99*(5), 26–30.

McAvoy, J. A. (2000). Cardiac pain: Discover the unexpected. *Nursing, 30*(1), 34–39.

McCance, K. L., & Huether, S. E. (2002). *Pathophysiology: The biologic basis for disease in adults and children* (4th ed.). St. Louis: Mosby.

McCloskey, J. C., & Bulechek, G. M. (Eds.) (2000). *Nursing interventions classification (NIC)* (3rd ed.). St. Louis: Mosby.

Meeker, M. H., & Rothrock, J. C. (1999). *Alexander's care of the patient in surgery* (11th ed.). St. Louis: Mosby.

National Cholesterol Education Program. (2001). *Adult treatment panel III report.* National Cholesterol Education Program Expert Panel on Detection, Evaluation, and Treatment of High Blood Cholesterol in Adults.

National Heart, Lung, and Blood Institute. National Institutes of Health. (2002). *Morbidity & mortality: 2002 chart book of cardiovascular, lung, and blood diseases.* Bethesda, MD: Author.

Navuluri, R. (2001). Antiplatelet and fibrinolytic therapy. *American Journal of Nursing, 101*(10), Hospital Extra 24A, 24D.

North American Nursing Diagnosis Association. (2001). *NANDA nursing diagnoses: Definitions & classification 2001–2002.* Philadelphia: NANDA.

Palatnik, A. M. (2001). Critical care. Acute coronary syndrome: New advances and nursing strategies. *Nursing, 31*(5), 32cc1–32cc2, 32cc4, 32cc6.

Photo guide. How to perform 3- or 5-lead monitoring. (2002). *Nursing, 32*(4), 50–52.

Porth, C. M. (2002). *Pathophysiology: Concepts of altered health states* (6th ed.). Philadelphia: Lippincott.

Robinson, A. W. (1999). Getting to the heart of denial. *American Journal of Nursing, 99*(5), 38–42.

Shaffer, R. S. (2002). ICD therapy: The patient's perspective. *American Journal of Nursing, 102*(2), 46–49.

Siomko, A. J. (2000). Demystifying cardiac markers. *American Journal of Nursing, 100*(1), 36–40.

Snowberger, P. (2001). VT or SVT? You can tell at the bedside. *RN, 64*(2), 26–31.

Steinke, E. E. (2000). Sexual counseling after myocardial infarction. *American Journal of Nursing, 100*(12), 38–43.

Sullivan, C. (2000). Critical care. Easing severe angina with laser surgery. *Nursing, 30*(4), 32cc1–32cc2, 32cc4

Tierney, L. M., McPhee, S. J., & Papadakis, M. A. (2001). *Current medical diagnosis & treatment* (40th ed.). New York: Lange Medical Books/McGraw-Hill.

Urden, L. D., Stacy, K. M., & Lough, M. E. (2002). *Thelan's critical care nursing: Diagnosis and management* (4th ed.). St. Louis: Mosby.

U. S. Preventive Services Task Force. (2002). Aspirin for the primary prevention of cardiovascular events: Recommendations and rationale. *American Journal of Nursing, 102*(3), 67, 69–70.

———. (2002). Screening for lipid disorders in adults: Recommendations and rationale. *American Journal of Nursing, 102*(6), 91, 93, 95.

Whitney, E. N., & Rolfes, S. R. (2002). *Understanding nutrition* (9th ed.). Belmont, CA: Wadsworth.

Wilkinson, J. M. (2000). *Nursing diagnosis handbook with NIC interventions and NOC outcomes* (7th ed.). Upper Saddle River, NJ: Prentice Hall Health.

Woods, S. L., Froelicher, E. S. S., & Motzer, S. U. (2000). *Cardiac nursing* (4th ed.). Philadelphia: Lippincott.

Writing Group for the Women's Health Initiative Investigators. (2002). Risks and benefits of estrogen plus progestin in healthy postmenopausal women. [On-line]. *JAMA, 288*(3). Available: http://jama.ama-assn.org/issues/v288n3/fffull/joc21036.html

# CHAPTER 30

# Nursing Care of Clients with Cardiac Disorders

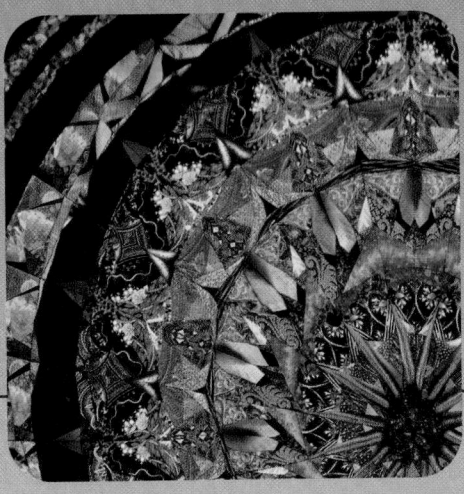

## MediaLink

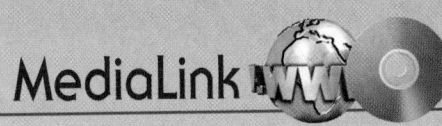

### www.prenhall.com/lemone

Additional resources for this chapter can be found on the Student CD-ROM accompanying this textbook, and on the Companion Website at www.prenhall.com/lemone. Click on Chapter 30 to select the activities for this chapter.

**CD-ROM**
- Audio Glossary
- NCLEX Review

***Animations***
- Cardiac A&P
- Digoxin
- Dopamine

**Companion Website**
- More NCLEX Review
- Case Study
    Rheumatic Fever
- Care Plan Activity
    Acute Pulmonary Edema
- MediaLink Application
    Heart Failure

## LEARNING OUTCOMES

After completing this chapter, you will be able to:

- Apply knowledge of normal cardiac anatomy and physiology and assessment techniques in caring for clients with cardiac disorders.

- Compare and contrast the pathophysiology and manifestations of common cardiac disorders, including heart failure, structural disorders, and inflammatory disorders.

- Identify common diagnostic tests used for cardiac disorders and their nursing implications.

- Discuss indications for and management of clients with hemodynamic monitoring.

- Discuss nursing implications for medications commonly prescribed for clients with cardiac disorders.

- Describe nursing care for the client undergoing cardiac surgery or cardiac transplant.

- Use the nursing process to provide individualized care for clients with cardiac disorders.

- Provide appropriate teaching and home care for clients with cardiac disorders and their families.

Cardiac disorders affect the structure and/or function of the heart. These disorders interfere with the heart's primary purpose: to pump enough blood to meet the body's demand for oxygen and nutrients. Disruptions in cardiac function affect the functioning of other organs and tissues, potentially leading to organ system failure and death.

Heart failure is the most common cardiac disorder. Other cardiac disorders discussed in this chapter include structural cardiac disorders, such as valve disorders and cardiomyopathy, and inflammatory cardiac disorders, such as endocarditis and pericarditis. Before continuing with this chapter, please review the heart's anatomy and physiology and nursing assessment in Chapter 28.

# HEART FAILURE

**Heart failure,** the inability of the heart to pump enough blood to meet the metabolic demands of the body, is the end result of many conditions. Frequently, it is a long-term effect of coronary heart disease and myocardial infarction when left ventricular damage is extensive enough to impair cardiac output (see Chapter 29). Other diseases of the heart also may cause heart failure, including structural and inflammatory disorders. In normal hearts, failure can result from excessive demands placed on the heart. Heart failure may be acute or chronic.

## THE CLIENT WITH HEART FAILURE

As mentioned, heart failure is the inability of the heart to function as a pump to meet the needs of the body. As a result, cardiac output falls, leading to decreased tissue perfusion. The body initially adjusts to reduced cardiac output by activating inherent compensatory mechanisms to restore tissue perfusion. These normal mechanisms may result in vascular congestion—and hence, the commonly used term *congestive heart failure (CHF)*. As these mechanisms are exhausted, heart failure ensues, with increased morbidity and mortality.

Heart failure is a disorder of cardiac function. It frequently is due to *impaired myocardial contraction,* which may result from coronary heart disease and myocardial ischemia or infarct or from a primary cardiac muscle disorder such as cardiomyopathy or myocarditis. Structural cardiac disorders, such as valve disorders or congenital heart defects, and hypertension also can lead to heart failure when the heart muscle is damaged by the long-standing *excessive workload* associated with these conditions. Other clients without a primary abnormality of myocardial function may present with manifestations of heart failure due to *acute excess demands* placed on the myocardium,

such as volume overload, hyperthyroidism, and massive pulmonary embolus (Table 30–1). Hypertension and coronary heart disease are the leading causes of heart failure in the United States. The high prevalence of hypertension in African Americans contributes significantly to their risk for and incidence of heart failure.

Nearly 5 million people in the United States are currently living with heart failure; approximately 550,000 new cases of heart failure are diagnosed annually (American Heart Association [AHA], 2001). Its incidence and prevalence increase with age: Less than 5% of people between ages 55 and 64 have heart failure, whereas 6% to 10% of people older than 65 are affected (see the box on the following page) (Hunt et al., 2001). The prognosis for a client with heart failure depends on its underlying cause and how effectively precipitating factors can be treated. Most clients with heart failure die within 8 years of the diagnosis. The risk for sudden cardiac death is dramatically increased, occurring at a rate 6 to 9 times that of the general population (AHA, 2001).

### PHYSIOLOGY REVIEW

The mechanical pumping action of cardiac muscle propels the blood it receives to the pulmonary and systemic vascular systems for reoxygenation and delivery to the tissues. *Cardiac output (CO)* is the amount of blood pumped from the ventricles in 1 minute. Cardiac output is used to assess cardiac performance, especially left ventricular function. Effective cardiac output depends on adequate functional muscle mass and the ability of the ventricles to work together. Cardiac output normally is regulated by the oxygen needs of the body: As oxygen use increases, cardiac output increases to maintain cellular function. *Cardiac reserve* is the ability of the heart to increase CO to meet metabolic demand. Ventricular damage reduces the cardiac reserve.

| TABLE 30–1 Selected Causes of Heart Failure | | |
|---|---|---|
| **Impaired Myocardial Function** | **Increased Cardiac Workload** | **Acute Noncardiac Conditions** |
| • Coronary heart disease | • Hypertension | • Volume overload |
| • Cardiomyopathies | • Valve disorders | • Hyperthyroidism |
| • Rheumatic fever | • Anemias | • Fever, infection |
| • Infective endocarditis | • Congenital heart defects | • Massive pulmonary embolus |

## Nursing Care of the Older Adult

### HEART FAILURE

Heart failure is common in older adults, affecting nearly 10% of people over the age of 75 years.

Aging affects cardiac function. Diastolic filling is impaired by decreased ventricular compliance. With aging, the heart is less responsive to sympathetic nervous system stimulation. As a result, maximal heart rate, cardiac reserve, and exercise tolerance are reduced. Concurrent health problems such as arthritis that affect stamina or mobility often contribute to a more sedentary lifestyle, further decreasing the heart's ability to respond to increased stress.

### Assessing for Home Care

The older adult with heart failure may not be dyspneic, instead presenting with weakness and fatigue, somnolence, confusion, disorientation, or worsening dementia. Dependent edema and respiratory crackles may or may not indicate heart failure in older adults.

Assess the diet of the older adult. Decreased taste may lead to increased use of salt to bring out food flavors. Limited mobility or visual acuity may cause the older adult to rely on prepared foods that are high in sodium such as canned soups and frozen meals. Discuss normal daily activities and assess sleep and rest patterns. It is also important to assess the environment for:

- Safe roads or neighborhoods for walking
- Access to pharmacy, medical care, and assistive services such as a cardiac rehabilitation program or structured exercise programs designed for older adults

### Client and Family Teaching

Teaching for the older adult with heart failure focuses on maintaining function and promptly identifying and treating episodes of heart failure. Teach clients how to adapt to changes in cardiovascular function associated with aging, such as:

- Allowing longer warm-up and cool-down periods during exercise
- Engaging in regular exercise such as walking 3 to 4 times a week
- Resting with feet elevated (e.g., in a recliner) when fatigued
- Maintaining adequate fluid intake
- Preventing infection through pneumococcal and influenza immunizations

---

Cardiac output is a product of heart rate and stroke volume. *Heart rate* affects cardiac output by controlling the number of ventricular contractions per minute. It is influenced by the autonomic nervous system, catecholamines, and thyroid hormones. Activation of a stress response (e.g., hypovolemia or fear) stimulates the sympathetic nervous system, increasing the heart rate and its contractility. Elevated heart rates increase cardiac output. Very rapid heart rates, however, shorten ventricular filling time (diastole), reducing stroke volume and cardiac output. On the other hand, a slow heart rate reduces cardiac output simply because of fewer cardiac cycles.

*Stroke volume* is the volume of blood ejected with each heartbeat; it is determined by preload, afterload, and myocardial contractility. *Preload* is the volume of blood in the ventricles at end-diastole (just prior to contraction). The blood in the ventricles exerts pressure on the ventricle walls, stretching muscle fibers. The greater the blood volume, the greater force with which the ventricle contracts to expel the blood. End-diastolic volume (EDV) depends on the amount of blood returning to the ventricles (*venous return*), and the distensibility or stiffness of the ventricles (*compliance*). See Box 30–1.

*Afterload* is the force needed to eject blood into the circulation. This force must be great enough to overcome arterial pressures within the pulmonary and systemic vascular systems. The right ventricle must generate enough force to open the pulmonary valve and eject its blood into the pulmonary artery. The left ventricle ejects its blood into the systemic circulation by overcoming the arterial resistance behind the aortic valve. Increased systemic vascular resistance increases afterload, impairing stroke volume and increasing myocardial work.

*Contractility* is the natural ability of cardiac muscle fibers to shorten during systole. Contractility is necessary to overcome arterial pressures and eject blood during systole. Impaired contractility affects cardiac output, by reducing stroke volume.

### BOX 30–1 ■ Explaining Physiologic Terms Using Practical Examples

The concepts of preload, the Frank-Starling mechanism, compliance, and afterload can be difficult to understand and to explain to clients. Use common analogies to make these concepts easier to understand.

- *Preload:* Think about a new rubber band. As you stretch the rubber band further, it snaps back into shape with greater force.
- *Frank-Starling mechanism:* When you repeatedly stretch that rubber band beyond a certain limit, it loses some elasticity and fails to return to its original shape and size.
- *Compliance:* Use a new rubber balloon to illustrate this concept. A new balloon is not very compliant—it takes a lot of work (force) to inflate it. As the balloon is repeatedly stretched, it becomes more compliant, expanding easily with less force.
- *Afterload:* When a hose is crimped or plugged, more force is required to eject a stream of water out its end.

The *ejection fraction (EF)* is the percentage of blood in the ventricle that is ejected during systole. A normal ejection fraction is approximately 60%.

## PATHOPHYSIOLOGY

When the heart begins to fail, mechanisms are activated to compensate for the impaired function and maintain the cardiac output. The primary compensatory mechanisms are (1) the Frank-Starling mechanism; (2) neuroendocrine responses including activation of the sympathetic nervous system and the renin-angiotensin system; and (3) myocardial hypertrophy. These mechanisms and their effects are summarized in Table 30–2.

### TABLE 30-2 Compensatory Mechanisms For Heart Failure

| Mechanism | Physiology | Effect on Body Systems | Complications |
|---|---|---|---|
| Frank-Starling mechanism | The greater the stretch of cardiac muscle fibers, the greater the force of contraction. | • Increased contractile force leading to increased CO | • Increased myocardial oxygen demand<br>• Limited by overstretching |
| Neuroendocrine response | Decreased CO stimulates the sympathetic nervous system and catecholamine release. | • Increased HR, BP, and contractility<br>• Increased vascular resistance<br>• Increased venous return | • Tachycardia with decreased filling time and decreased CO<br>• Increased vascular resistance<br>• Increased myocardial work and oxygen demand |
| | Decreased CO and decreased renal perfusion stimulate renin/angiotensin system. | • Vasoconstriction and increased BP | • Increased myocardial work<br>• Renal vasoconstriction and decreased renal perfusion |
| | Angiotensin stimulates aldosterone release from adrenal cortex. | • Salt and water retention by the kidneys<br>• Increased vascular volume | • Increased preload and afterload<br>• Pulmonary congestion |
| | ADH is released from posterior pituitary. | • Water excretion inhibited | • Fluid retention and increased preload and afterload<br>• Pulmonary congestion |
| | Atrial natriuretic factor is released. | • Increased sodium excretion<br>• Diuresis | |
| | Blood flow is redistributed to vital organs (heart and brain). | • Decreased perfusion of other organ systems<br>• Decreased perfusion of skin and muscles | • Renal failure<br>• Anaerobic metabolism and lactic acidosis |
| Ventricular hypertrophy | Increased cardiac workload causes myocardial muscle to hypertrophy and ventricles to dilate. | • Increased contractile force to maintain CO | • Increased myocardial oxygen demand<br>• Cellular enlargement |

Decreased cardiac output initially stimulates aortic baroreceptors, which in turn stimulate the sympathetic nervous system (SNS). SNS stimulation produces both cardiac and vascular responses through the release of norepinephrine. Norepinephrine increases heart rate and contractility by stimulating cardiac beta receptors. Cardiac output improves as both heart rate and stroke volume increase. Norepinephrine also causes arterial and venous vasoconstriction, increasing venous return to the heart. Increased venous return increases ventricular filling and myocardial stretch, increasing the force of contraction (the Frank-Starling mechanism). Overstretching the muscle fibers past their physiologic limit results in an ineffective contraction.

Blood flow is redistributed to the brain and the heart to maintain perfusion of these vital organs. Decreased renal perfusion causes renin to be released from the kidneys. Activation of the renin-angiotensin system produces additional vasoconstriction and stimulates the adrenal cortex to produce aldosterone and the posterior pituitary to release antidiuretic hormone (ADH). Aldosterone stimulates sodium reabsorption in renal tubules, promoting water retention. ADH acts on the distal tubule to inhibit water excretion and causes vasoconstriction. The effect of these hormones is significant vasoconstriction and salt and water retention, with a resulting increase in vascular volume. Increased ventricular filling increases the force of contraction, improving cardiac output. The increased vascular volume and venous return also increase atrial pressures, stimulating the release of an additional hormone, *atrial natriuretic factor (ANF)* or *atriopeptin*. Atrial natriuetic factor balances the effects of the other

hormones to a certain extent, promoting sodium and water excretion and inhibiting the release of norepinephrine, renin, and ADH. This hormone is thought to be a natural preventive that delays severe cardiac decompensation.

*Ventricular remodeling* occurs as the heart chambers and myocardium adapt to fluid volume and pressure increases. The chambers dilate to accommodate excess fluid resulting from increased vascular volume and incomplete emptying. Initially, this additional stretch causes more effective contractions. *Ventricular hypertrophy* occurs as existing cardiac muscle cells enlarge, increasing their contractile elements (actin and myosin) and force of contraction.

Although these responses may help in the short-term regulation of cardiac output, it is now recognized that they hasten the deterioration of cardiac function. The onset of heart failure is heralded by *decompensation,* the loss of effective compensation. Heart failure progresses due to the very mechanisms that initially maintained circulatory stability.

The rapid heart rate shortens diastolic filling time, compromises coronary artery perfusion, and increases myocardial oxygen demand. Resulting ischemia further impairs cardiac output. Beta-receptors in the heart become less sensitive to continued SNS stimulation, decreasing heart rate and contractility. As the beta-receptors become less sensitive, norepinephrine stores in the cardiac muscle become depleted. In contrast, alpha-receptors on peripheral blood vessels become increasingly sensitive to persistent stimulation, promoting vasoconstriction and increasing afterload and cardiac work.

Initially, ventricular hypertrophy and dilation increase cardiac output, but chronic distention causes the ventricular wall eventually to thin and degenerate. The purpose of hypertrophy is thus defeated. In addition, chronic overloading of the dilated ventricle eventually stretches the fibers beyond the optimal point for effective contraction. The ventricles continue to dilate to accommodate the excess fluid, but the heart loses the ability to contract forcefully. The heart muscle may eventually become so large that the coronary blood supply is inadequate, causing ischemia.

Chronic distention exhausts atrial stores of ANF. The effects of norepinephrine, renin, and ADH prevail, and the renin-angiotensin pathway is continually stimulated. This mechanism ultimately raises the hemodynamic stress on the heart by increasing both preload and afterload. As heart function deteriorates, less blood is delivered to the tissues and to the heart itself. Ischemia and necrosis of the myocardium further weaken the already failing heart, and the cycle repeats.

In normal hearts, the cardiac reserve allows the heart to adjust its output to meet metabolic needs of the body, increasing the cardiac output by up to 5 times the basal level during exercise. Clients with heart failure have minimal to no cardiac reserve. At rest, they may be unaffected; however, any stressor (e.g., exercise, illness) taxes their ability to meet the demand for oxygen and nutrients. Manifestations of activity intolerance when the person is at rest indicate a critical level of cardiac decompensation.

## Classifications

Heart failure is commonly classified in several different ways, depending on the underlying pathology. Classifications include systolic versus diastolic failure, left-sided versus right-sided failure, high-output versus low-output failure, and acute versus chronic failure.

### Systolic Versus Diastolic Failure

*Systolic failure* occurs when the ventricle fails to contract adequately to eject a sufficient blood volume into the arterial system. Systolic function is affected by loss of myocardial cells due to ischemia and infarction, cardiomyopathy, or inflammation. The manifestations of systolic failure are those of decreased cardiac output: weakness, fatigue, and decreased exercise tolerance.

*Diastolic failure* results when the heart cannot completely relax in diastole, disrupting normal filling. Passive diastolic filling decreases, increasing the importance of atrial contraction to preload. Diastolic dysfunction results from decreased ventricular compliance due to hypertrophic and cellular changes and impaired relaxation of the heart muscle. Its manifestations result from increased pressure and congestion behind the ventricle: shortness of breath, tachypnea, and respiratory crackles if the left ventricle is affected; distended neck veins, liver enlargement, anorexia, and nausea if the right ventricle is affected. Many clients have components of both systolic and diastolic failure.

### Left-Sided Versus Right-Sided Failure

Depending on the pathophysiology involved, either the left or the right ventricle may be primarily affected. In chronic heart failure, however, both ventricles typically are impaired to some degree. Coronary heart disease and hypertension are common causes of *left-sided heart failure,* whereas *right-sided heart failure* often is caused by conditions that restrict blood flow to the lungs, such as acute or chronic pulmonary disease. Left-sided heart failure also can lead to right-sided failure as pressures in the pulmonary vascular system increase with congestion behind the failing left ventricle.

As left ventricular function fails, cardiac output falls. Pressures in the left ventricle and atrium increase as the amount of blood remaining in the ventricle after systole increases. These increased pressures impair filling, causing congestion and increased pressures in the pulmonary vascular system. Increased pressures in this normally low-pressure system increase fluid movement from the blood vessels into interstitial tissues and the alveoli (Figure 30–1 ■).

The manifestations of left-sided heart failure result from pulmonary congestion and decreased cardiac output. Fatigue and activity intolerance are common early manifestations. Dizziness and syncope also may result from decreased cardiac output. Pulmonary congestion causes dyspnea, shortness of breath, and cough. The client may develop *orthopnea* (difficulty breathing while lying down), prompting use of two or

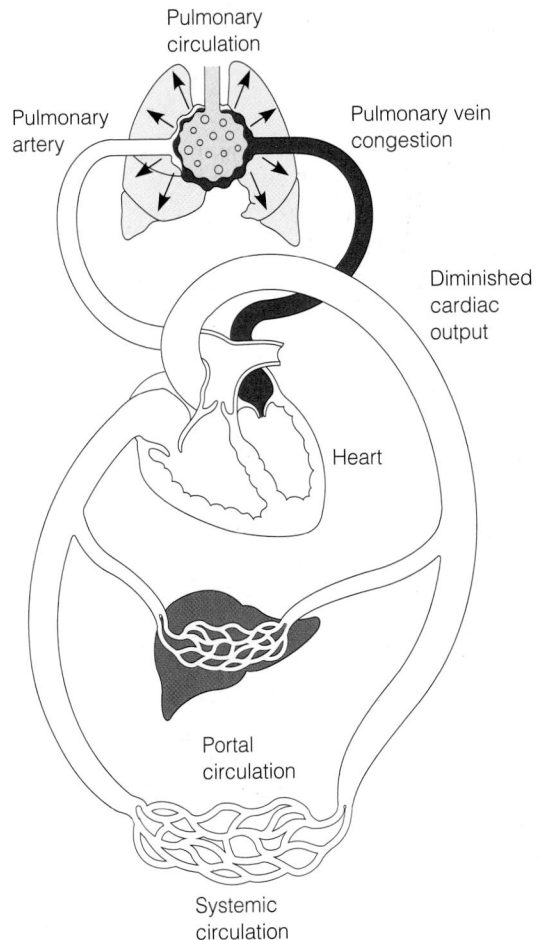

**Figure 30–1** ■ The hemodynamic effects of left-sided heart failure.

three pillows or a recliner for sleeping. Cyanosis from impaired gas exchange may be noted. On auscultation of the lungs, inspiratory crackles (rales) and wheezes may be heard in lung bases. An S₃ gallop may be present, reflecting the heart's attempts to fill an already distended ventricle.

In right-sided heart failure, increased pressures in the pulmonary vasculature or right ventricular muscle damage impair the right venticle's ability to pump blood into the pulmonary circulation. The right ventricle and atrium become distended, and blood accumulates in the systemic venous system. Increased venous pressures cause abdominal organs to become congested and peripheral tissue edema to develop (Figure 30–2 ■).

Dependent tissues tend to be affected because of the effects of gravity; edema develops in the feet and legs, or if the client is bedridden, in the sacrum. Congestion of gastrointestinal tract vessels causes anorexia and nausea. Right upper quadrant pain may result from liver engorgement. Neck veins distend and become visible even when the client is upright due to increased venous pressure.

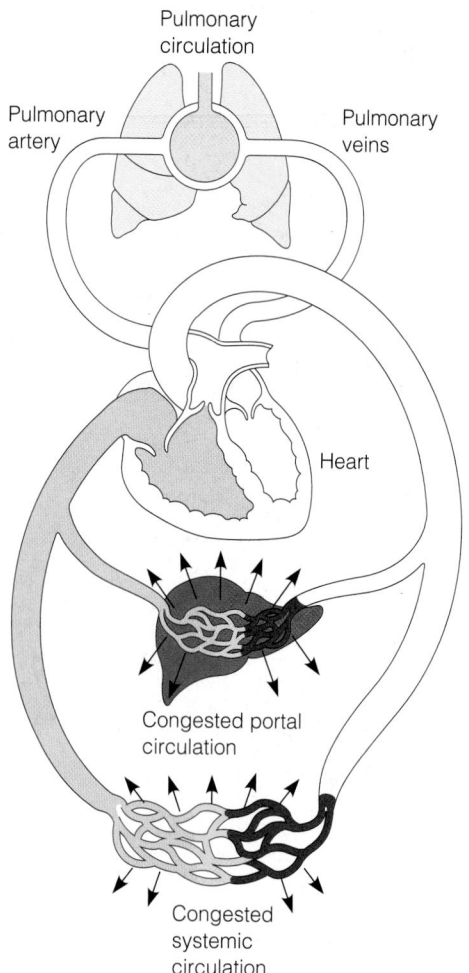

**Figure 30–2** ■ The hemodynamic effects of right-sided heart failure.

### High-Output Failure

Clients in hypermetabolic states (e.g., hyperthyroidism, infection, anemia, or pregnancy) require increased cardiac output to maintain blood flow and oxygen to the tissues. If the increased blood flow cannot meet the oxygen demands of the tissues, compensatory mechanisms are activated to further increase cardiac output, which in turn further increases oxygen demand. Thus, even though cardiac output is high, the heart is unable to meet increased oxygen demands. This condition is known as *high-output failure*.

### Acute Versus Chronic Failure

*Acute failure* is the abrupt onset of a myocardial injury (such as a massive MI) resulting in suddenly decreased cardiac function and signs of decreased cardiac output. *Chronic failure* is a progressive deterioration of the heart muscle due to cardiomyopathies, valvular disease, or CHD.

## MANIFESTATIONS AND COMPLICATIONS

In addition to the previous manifestations for the various classifications of heart failure, other signs and symptoms commonly are seen.

A fall in cardiac output activates mechanisms that cause increased salt and water retention. This causes weight gain and further increases pressures in the capillaries, resulting in edema. *Nocturia*, voiding more than one time at night, develops as edema fluid from dependent tissues is reabsorbed when the client is supine. **Paroxysmal nocturnal dyspnea (PND),** a frightening condition in which the client awakens at night acutely short of breath, also may develop. Paroxysmal nocturnal dyspnea occurs when edema fluid that has accumulated during the day is reabsorbed into the circulation at night, causing fluid overload and pulmonary congestion. Severe heart failure may cause dyspnea at rest as well as with activity, signifying little or no cardiac reserve. Both an S₃ and an S₄ gallop may be heard on auscultation.

The compensatory mechanisms initiated in heart failure can lead to complications in other body systems. Congestive hepatomegaly and splenomegaly caused by engorgement of the portal venous system results in increased abdominal pressure, ascites, and gastrointestinal problems. With prolonged right-sided heart failure, liver function may be impaired. Myocardial distention can precipitate dysrhythmias, futher impairing cardiac output. Pleural effusions and other pulmonary problems may develop. Major complications of severe heart failure are cardiogenic shock (described in Chapter 6) ⊙⊃ and acute pulmonary edema, a medical emergency described in the next section of this chapter.

See page 875 for the *Multisystem Effects of Heart Failure.*

## COLLABORATIVE CARE

The main goals for care of heart failure are to slow its progression, reduce cardiac workload, improve cardiac function, and control fluid retention. Treatment strategies are based on the evolution and progression of heart failure (Table 30–3).

# Multisystem Effects of Heart Failure

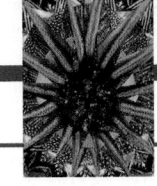

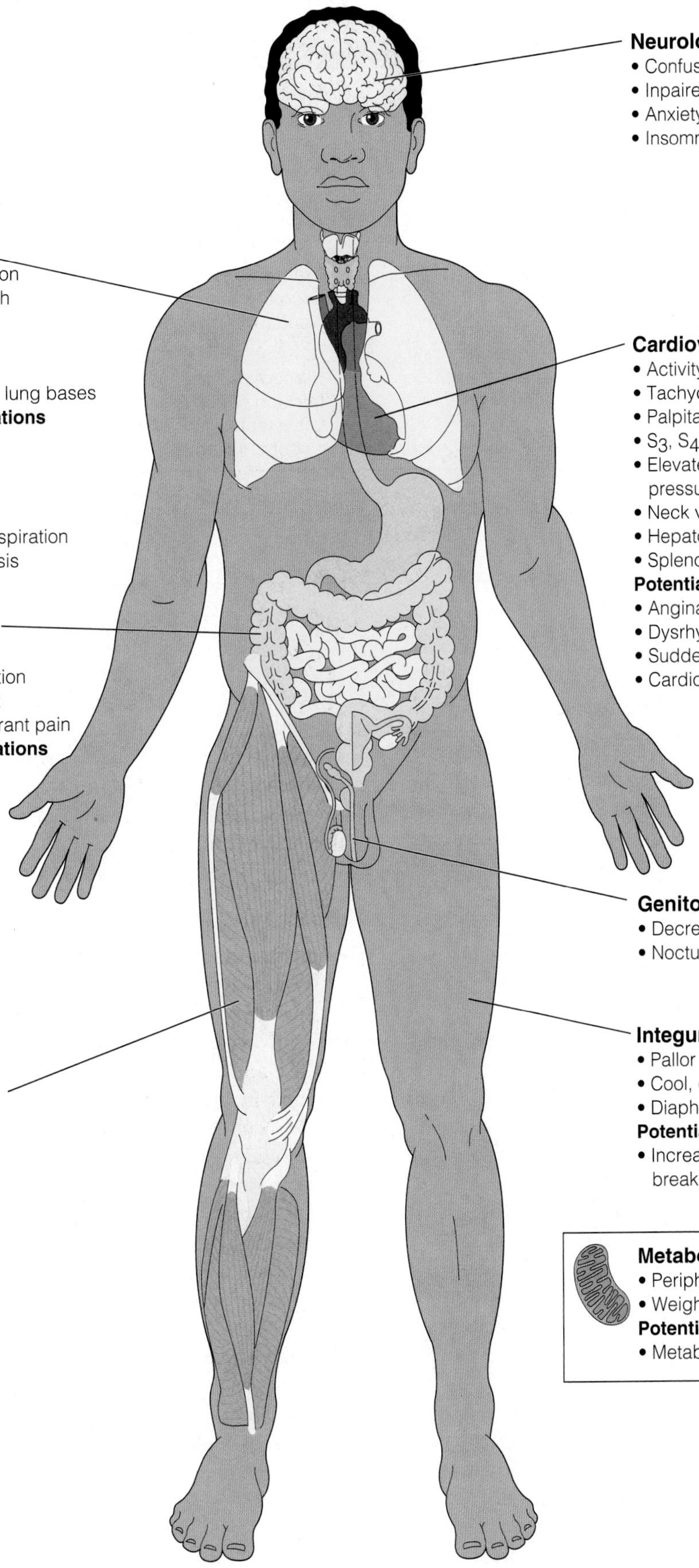
Neurologic
• Confusion
• Inpaired memory
• Anxiety, restlessness
• Insomnia
Respiratory
• Dyspnea on exertion
• Shortness of breath
• Tachypnea
• Orthopnea
• Dry cough
• Crackles (rales) in lung bases
Potential Complications
• Pulmonary edema
• Pneumonia
• Cardiac asthma
• Pleural effusion
• Cheyne-Stokes respiration
• Respiratory acidosis
Cardiovascular
• Activity intolerance
• Tachycardia
• Palpitations
• $S_3$, $S_4$ heart sounds
• Elevated central venous pressure
• Neck vein distention
• Hepatojugular reflux
• Splenomegaly
Potential Complications
• Angina
• Dysrhythmias
• Sudden cardiac death
• Cardiogenic shock
Gastrointestinal
• Anorexia, nausea
• Abdominal distention
• Liver enlargement
• Right upper quadrant pain
Potential Complications
• Malnutrition
• Ascites
• Liver dysfunction
Genitourinary
• Decreased urine output
• Nocturia
Integumentary
• Pallor or cyanosis
• Cool, clammy skin
• Diaphoresis
Potential Complications
• Increased risk for tissue breakdown
Musculoskeletal
• Fatigue
• Weakness
Metabolic Processes
• Peripheral edema
• Weight gain
Potential Complication
• Metabolic acidosis

TABLE 30–3  Stages of Heart Failure

| Stage | Description | Selected Treatment Measures |
|---|---|---|
| A | Clients at high risk for developing heart failure, but without identified structural or functional impairment | Treat underlying risk factors (e.g., hypertension, CHD) <br> ACE inhibitor therapy <br> Exercise <br> Salt restriction |
| B | Clients with structural heart disease but no manifestations of heart failure | As for stage A <br> ACE inhibitor or beta-blocker therapy <br> Valve replacement if indicated |
| C | Clients with current or prior symptoms of heart failure associated with underlying structural heart disease | As for stages A and B <br> Drug therapy with a diuretic, ACE inhibitor, beta blocker, and (usually) digitalis |
| D | Clients with advanced structural heart disease and manifestations of heart failure at rest despite aggressive treatment (end-stage heart failure) | As for stages A, B, and C as appropriate <br> Hemodynamic monitoring <br> Infusion of positive inotropic agents <br> Valve replacement, cardiac transplant, partial left ventriculectomy as indicated |

Note. Adapted from "ACC/AHA Guidelines for the Evaluation and Management of Chronic Heart Failure in the Adult: Executive Summary: A Report of the American College of Cardiology/American Heart Association Task Force on Practice Guidelines (Committee to Revise the 1995 Guidelines) for the Evaluation and Management of Heart Failure" by S. A. Hunt, D. W. Baker, M. H. Chin, M. P. Ciquegrani, A. M. Feldman, G. S. Francis, T. G. Ganiats, S. Goldstein, G. Gregoratos, M. L. Jessup, R. J. Noble, M. Packer, M. A. Silver, and L. W. Stevenson, 2001 Circulation, 104, pp. 2996–3007.

## Diagnostic Tests

Diagnosis of heart failure is based on the history, physical examination, and diagnostic findings.

- *Atrial natriuretic factor (ANF),* also called *atrial natriuretic hormone (ANH),* and *B-type natriuretic peptide (BNP)* are hormones released by the heart muscle in response to changes in blood volume. Blood levels of these hormones increase in heart failure.
- *Serum electrolytes* are measured to evaluate fluid and electrolyte status. Serum osmolarity may be low due to fluid retention. Sodium, potassium, and chloride levels provide a baseline for evaluating the effects of treatment.
- *Urinalysis, blood urea nitrogen (BUN),* and *serum creatinine* are obtained to evaluate renal function.
- *Liver function tests* including ALT, AST, LDH, serum bilirubin, and total protein and albumin levels, are obtained to evaluate possible effects of heart failure on liver function.
- In acute heart failure, *arterial blood gases (ABGs)* are drawn to evaluate gas exchange in the lungs and tissues.
- *Chest X-ray* may show pulmonary vascular congestion and cardiomegaly in heart failure.
- *Electrocardiography* is used to identify ECG changes associated with ventricular enlargement and to detect dysrhythmias, myocardial ischemia, or infarction.
- *Echocardiography with Doppler flow studies* are performed to evaluate left ventricular function. Echocardiography uses ultrasound waves reflected off cardiac structures to produce images of the heart. The transducer which generates and receives the reflected waves may be placed on the chest wall (*transthoracic echocardiography*). For more accurate evaluation of the posterior surface of the heart, the transducer may

be on the distal end of an endoscope inserted into the esophagus (*transesophageal echocardiography*). Doppler flow studies use ultrasound waves reflecting off red blood cells to measure the velocity of blood flow across valves, within cardiac chambers, and through the great vessels.
- *Radionuclide imaging* is used to evaluate ventricular function and size (see Chapter 29).

## Hemodynamic Monitoring

**Hemodynamics** is the study of forces involved in blood circulation. Hemodynamic monitoring is used to assess cardiovascular function in the critically ill or unstable client. The main goals of invasive hemodynamic monitoring are to evaluate cardiac and circulatory function and the response to interventions.

Hemodynamic parameters include heart rate, arterial blood pressure, central venous pressure, pulmonary pressures, and cardiac output. *Direct* hemodynamic parameters are obtained straight from the monitoring device (e.g., heart rate, arterial and venous pressures). *Indirect* or *derived* measurements are calculated using the direct data (e.g., the cardiac index, mean arterial blood pressure [MAP], and stroke volume). Invasive hemodynamic monitoring is routinely used in critical care units.

Hemodynamic monitoring systems measure the pressure within a vessel and convert this signal into an electrical waveform that is amplified and displayed. The electrical signal may be graphically recorded on graph paper and displayed digitally on the monitor. System components include an invasive catheter threaded into an artery or vein connected to a transducer by stiff, high-pressure tubing. The pressure transducer translates pressures into an electrical signal that is relayed to the monitor. Additional components of the system include

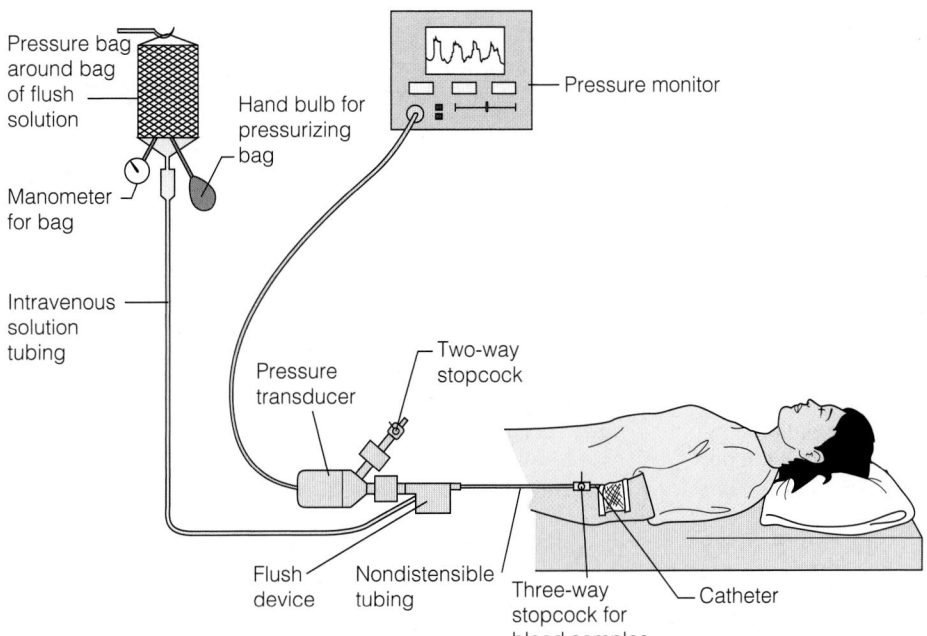

**Figure 30–3** ■ A hemodynamic monitoring setup.

Labels (clockwise from upper left): Pressure bag around bag of flush solution; Hand bulb for pressurizing bag; Pressure monitor; Manometer for bag; Intravenous solution tubing; Pressure transducer; Two-way stopcock; Flush device; Nondistensible tubing; Three-way stopcock for blood samples; Catheter.

stopcocks and a continuous flush system with normal saline or heparinized saline and an infusion pressure bag to prevent clots from forming in the catheter. Figure 30–3 ■ illustrates a pressure transducer and typical hemodynamic monitoring system.

Hemodynamic pressure monitoring may be used to measure peripheral arterial pressures, or central pressures, such as central venous pressure (CVP) and pulmonary artery pressure (PAP). Although the information obtained from invasive monitoring is valuable, the procedure is not without risk. Nursing care of the client undergoing hemodynamic monitoring is outlined on page 878. Box 30–2 lists potential complications of central pressure monitoring.

### Intra-Arterial Pressure Monitoring

Intra-arterial pressure monitoring is commonly used in intensive and coronary care units. An indwelling arterial line, commonly called an *art line* or an *A line,* allows direct and continuous monitoring of systolic, diastolic, and mean arterial blood pressure and provides easy access for arterial blood sampling. Arterial lines are used to assess blood volume, monitor the effects of vasoactive drugs, and to obtain frequent arterial blood gas determinations. Because the invasive catheter is inserted directly into the artery, it offers immediate access for blood gas measurements and blood testing.

The arterial blood pressure reflects the cardiac output and the resistance to blood flow created by the elastic arterial walls (*systemic vascular resistance, SVR*). Cardiac output is determined by the blood volume and the ability of the ventricles to fill and effectively pump that blood. Systemic vascular resistance is primarily determined by vessel diameter and distensibility (compliance). Factors such as sympathetic nervous system input, circulating hormones (e.g., epinephrine, norepinephrine, atrial natriuretic factor, and vasopressin), and the renin-angiotensin system affect SVR.

The systolic blood pressure, normally about 120 mmHg in healthy adults, reflects the pressure generated during ventricular systole. During diastole, elastic arterial walls keep a minimum pressure within the vessel (diastolic blood pressure) to maintain blood flow through the capillary beds. The average diastolic pressure in a healthy adult is 80 mmHg. The **mean arterial pressure (MAP)** is the average pressure in the arterial circulation throughout the cardiac cycle. It reflects the driving pressure, or perfusion pressure, an indicator of tissue perfusion. The formula MAP = CO × SVR often is used to show the relationships between factors determining the blood pressure. Mean arterial pressures of 70 to 90 mmHg are desirable. Perfusion to vital organs is severely jeopardized at MAPs of 50 or less; MAPs greater than 105 mmHg may indicate hypertension or vasoconstriction.

### Central Venous Pressure Monitoring

*Central venous pressure (CVP)* is a measure of blood volume and venous return. CVP also reflects right heart filling pressures. It is elevated in right-sided heart failure. CVP is primarily used to monitor fluid volume status. To measure CVP, a catheter is inserted in the internal jugular or subclavian vein. The distal tip of the catheter is positioned in the superior vena cava just above the right atrium. CVP may be measured in either centimeters of water (cm $H_2O$) or in millimeters of mercury

| BOX 30–2 ■ **Potential Complications of Central Catheters** | |
| --- | --- |
| ■ Bleeding | ■ Venospasm |
| ■ Hematoma | ■ Infection |
| ■ Pneumothorax | ■ Air embolism |
| ■ Hemothorax | ■ Thromboembolism |
| ■ Arterial puncture | ■ Brachial nerve injury |
| ■ Dysrhythmias | ■ Thoracic duct injury |

## NURSING CARE OF THE CLIENT UNDERGOING HEMODYNAMIC MONITORING

- Calibrate and level the system at least once a shift using the right atrium as a constant reference level. Relevel the transducer after a change in position. Mark the right atrial position (at the fourth intercostal space, midaxillary line) on the chest wall, and use this as a reference point for all readings. *Calibration and leveling ensure that accurate pressures are recorded. Marking the right atrial level provides a consistent reference point for all caregivers.*
- Measure all pressures between breaths. *This ensures that intrathoracic pressure does not influence pressure readings.*
- Maintain 300 mmHg of pressure on the flush solution at all times. *This ensures a continuous flow of flush solution through the pressure tubing and catheter to prevent clot formation and catheter occlusion.*
- Monitor pressure trends rather than individual readings. *Individual readings may not reflect the client's true status. Trends in pressure readings along with clinical observations provide a better overall picture of the client's status.*
- Obtain a chest X-ray before infusing intravenous fluid into any newly placed central line. *Chest X-ray verifies the location of the catheter and helps prevent pulmonary complications of incorrect catheter placement such as pneumothorax.*
- Set alarm limits for monitored hemodynamic variables. Turn alarms on. *Alarms warn of hemodynamic instability. Always investigate alarms. They may be temporarily silenced to change tubing or draw blood but should never be turned off.*
- Use aseptic technique during catheter insertion and site care. *Aseptic technique is important to prevent infection.*

- Assess and document appearance of the insertion site at least every shift; observe for signs of infiltration, infection, or phlebitis. *Frequent assessment allows early detection and prompt treatment of complications.*
- Change intravenous solutions every 24 hours, site dressing every 48 hours, and tubing to the insertion site every 72 hours. Label solution, tubing, and dressing with date and time of change. *These measures help prevent infection.*
- Thoroughly flush stopcock ports after drawing blood samples from the pressure line. *Flushing prevents colonization of bacteria and occlusion of the catheter.*
- Assess pulse and perfusion distal to the monitoring site. *Frequent assessment is vital to ensure perfusion of the distal extremity.*
- When discontinuing the pressure line, apply manual pressure to the insertion site as soon as the catheter tip is out. Hold pressure for 5 to 15 minutes or until the bleeding stops. *This is particularly important for arterial lines to prevent bleeding and hematoma formation.*
- Secure all connections and stopcocks. *This is done to prevent disconnection of the invasive line and potential hemorrhage.*
- Ensure that electrical equipment is grounded, intact, and operating as expected. *This helps prevent electrical injury.*
- Loosely restrain the affected extremity if the client pulls on the catheter or connections. *Restraints may be necessary to prevent injury from accidental or intentional disconnection or discontinuation of invasive lines (i.e., if the client has dementia or is agitated).*
- Keep tubing free of kinks and tension. *This prevents the catheter from becoming clotted or inadvertently dislodged.*

(mmHg). A water manometer is a clear tube with calibrated markings that is attached between a central catheter and the intravenous fluid bag. Pressure in the venous system causes fluid in the manometer to rise or fall. The CVP is recorded by noting the fluid level in the manometer. If the central line is connected to a pressure transducer, venous pressure is displayed digitally in millimeters of mercury.

The normal range for CVP is 2 to 8 cm $H_2O$ or 2 to 6 mmHg, but CVP varies in individual clients. Hypovolemia and shock decrease the CVP; fluid overload, vasoconstriction, and cardiac tamponade increase CVP.

### Pulmonary Artery Pressure Monitoring

The pulmonary artery (PA) catheter is a flow-directed, balloon-tipped catheter first used in the early 1970s. The PA catheter is often called a *Swan-Ganz catheter,* after the physicians who developed it. The PA catheter is used to evaluate left ventricular and overall cardiac function. The PA catheter is inserted into a central vein, usually the internal jugular or subclavian vein, and threaded into the right atrium. A small balloon at the tip of the catheter allows the catheter to be drawn into the right ventricle and from there into the pulmonary artery. The inflated balloon carries the catheter forward until the balloon wedges in a small branch of pulmonary vasculature. Once in place, the balloon is deflated, and multiple lumens of the

catheter allow measurement of pressures in the right atrium, pulmonary artery, and left ventricle. The normal PA pressure is around 25/10 mmHg; normal mean pulmonary artery pressure is about 15 mmHg. Pulmonary artery pressure is increased in left-sided heart failure.

Inflation of the balloon effectively blocks pressure from behind the balloon and allows measurement of pressures generated by the left ventricle. This is known as pulmonary artery wedge pressure (PAWP or PWP) and is used to assess left ventricular function. The normal pulmonary artery wedge pressure is 8 to 12 mmHg. PAWP is increased in left ventricular failure and pericardial tamponade, and decreased in hypovolemia.

Cardiac output also can be measured with the PA catheter using a technique called thermodilution. Cardiac output and the cardiac index are used to assess the heart's ability to meet the body's oxygen demands. Because body size affects overall cardiac output, the cardiac index is a more precise measure of heart function. The *cardiac index* is a calculation of cardiac output per square meter of body surface area. The normal cardiac index is 2.8 to 4.2 L/min/m$^2$.

### Medications

Clients with heart failure often receive multiple medications to reduce cardiac work and improve cardiac function. The main drug classes used to treat heart failure are the angiotensin-converting enzyme (ACE) inhibitors, beta blockers, diuretics, inotropic medications (including digitalis, sympathomimetic agents, and phosphodiesterase inhibitors), direct vasodilators, and antidysrhythmic drugs. Nursing implications for ACE inhibitors, diuretics, and inotropic medications are found in the Medication Administration box below.

ACE inhibitors and beta blockers interfere with the neurohormonal mechanisms of sympathetic activation and the renin-angiotensin system. ACE inhibitors interrupt the conversion of angiotensin I to angiotensin II by inhibiting the enzyme that mediates the conversion (angiotensin-converting enzyme). Angiotensin II causes intense vasoconstriction, increasing afterload and ventricular wall stress and increasing preload and ventricular dilation. It also stimulates aldosterone and ADH production, causing fluid retention. ACE inhibitors block this renin-angiotensin system activity, decreasing cardiac work and increasing cardiac output. They reduce the progression and manifestations of heart failure, thus reducing the number and frequency of hospital admissions, decreasing mortality rates, and preventing cardiac complications (Braunwald et al., 2001).

## Medication Administration

### Heart Failure

#### ANGIOTENSIN-CONVERTING ENZYME (ACE) INHIBITORS

| | |
|---|---|
| Enalapril (Vasotec) | Lisinopril (Prinivil, Zestril) |
| Captopril (Capoten) | Fosinopril (Monopril) |
| Moexipril (Univasc) | Quinapril (Accupril) |
| Ramipril (Altace) | Trandolapril (Mavik) |

ACE inhibitors prevent acute coronary events and reduce mortality in heart failure. ACE inhibitors interfere with production of angiotensin II, resulting in vasodilation, reduced blood volume, and prevention of its effects in the heart and blood vessels. In heart failure, ACE inhibitors reduce afterload and improve cardiac output and renal blood flow. They also reduce pulmonary congestion and peripheral edema. ACE inhibitors suppress myocyte growth and reduce ventricular remodeling in heart failure.

#### Nursing Responsibilities

- Do not give these drugs to women in the second and third trimesters of pregnancy.
- Carefully monitor clients who are volume depleted or who have impaired renal function.
- Use an infusion pump when administering ACE inhibitors intravenously.
- Monitor blood pressure closely for 2 hours following first dose and as indicated thereafter.
- Monitor serum potassium levels; ACE inhibitors can cause hyperkalemia.
- Monitor white blood cell (WBC) count for potential neutropenia. Report to the physician.

#### Client and Family Teaching

- Take the drug at the same time every day to ensure a stable blood level.
- Monitor your blood pressure and weight weekly. Report significant changes to your doctor.
- Avoid making sudden position changes; for example, rise from bed slowly. Lie down if you become dizzy or lightheaded, particularly after the first dose.
- Report any signs of easy bruising and bleeding, sore throat or fever, edema, or skin rash. Immediately report swelling of the face, lips, or eyelids, and itching or breathing problems.
- A persistent, dry cough may develop. Contact your doctor if this becomes a problem.
- Take captopril or moexipril 1 hour before meals.

#### DIURETICS

| | |
|---|---|
| Chlorothiazide (Diuril) | Spironolactone (Aldactone) |
| Furosemide (Lasix) | Triamterene (Dyrenium) |
| Ethacrynic acid (Edecrin) | Amiloride (Midamor) |
| Bumetanide (Bumex) | Acetazolamide (Diamox) |
| Hydrochlorothiazide (HydroDIURIL) | |

Diuretics act on different portions of the kidney tubule to inhibit the reabsorption of sodium and water and promote their excretion. With the exception of the potassium-sparing diuretics—spironolactone, triamterene, and amiloride—diuretics also promote potassium excretion, increasing the risk of hypokalemia. Spironolactone, an aldosterone receptor blocker, reduces symptoms and slows progression of heart failure. Aldosterone receptors in the heart and blood vessels promote myocardial remodeling and fibrosis, activate the sympathetic nervous system, and promote vascular fibrosis (which decreases compliance) and baroreceptor dysfunction (Lehne, 2001).

#### Nursing Responsibilities

- Obtain baseline weight and vital signs.
- Monitor blood pressure, intake and output, weight, skin turgor, and edema as indicators of fluid volume status.
- Assess for volume depletion, particularly with loop diuretics (furosemide, ethacrynic acid, and bumetanide): dizziness, orthostatic hypotension, tachycardia, muscle cramping.
- Report abnormal serum electrolyte levels to the physician. Replace electrolytes as indicated.
- Do not administer potassium replacements to clients receiving a potassium-sparing diuretic.
- Evaluate renal function by assessing urine output, BUN, and serum creatinine.
- Administer intravenous furosemide slowly, no faster than 20 mg/minute. Evaluate for signs of ototoxicity. Do not administer this drug or ethacrynic acid concurrently with aminoglycoside antibiotics (e.g., gentamycin) which are also ototoxic.

#### Client and Family Teaching

- Drink at least 6 to 8 glasses of water per day.
- Take your diuretic at times that will be the least disruptive to your lifestyle, usually in the morning and early afternoon if a second dose is ordered. Take with meals to decrease gastric upset.

(continued on page 880)

# Medication Administration

## Heart Failure (continued)

- Monitor your blood pressure, pulse, and weight weekly. Report significant weight changes to your doctor.
- Report any of the following to your doctor: severe abdominal pain, jaundice, dark urine, abnormal bleeding or bruising, flulike symptoms, signs of hypokalemia, hyponatremia, and dehydration (thirst, salt craving, dizziness, weakness, rapid pulse). See Chapter 5 ⊂⊃ for manifestations of electrolyte imbalances.
- Avoid sudden position changes. You may experience dizziness, lightheadedness, or feelings of faintness.
- Unless you are taking a potassium-sparing diuretic, integrate foods rich in potassium into your diet (see Chapter 5 ). ⊂⊃ Limit sodium use.

### POSITIVE INOTROPIC AGENTS

### Digitalis Glycosides

Digoxin (Lanoxin)

Digitalis improves myocardial contractility by interfering with ATPase in the myocardial cell membrane and increasing the amount of calcium available for contraction. The increased force of contraction causes the heart to empty more completely, increasing stroke volume and cardiac output. Improved cardiac output improves renal perfusion, decreasing renin secretion. This decreases preload and afterload, reducing cardiac work. Digitalis also has electrophysiologic effects, slowing conduction through the AV node. This decreases the heart rate and reduces oxygen consumption.

### Nursing Responsibilities

- Assess apical pulse before administering. Withhold digitalis and notify the physician if heart rate is below 60 BPM and/or manifestations of decreased cardiac output are noted. Record apical rate on medication record.
- Evaluate ECG for scooped (spoon-shaped) ST segment, AV block, bradycardia, and other dysrhythmias (especially PVCs and atrial tachycardias).
- Report manifestations of digitalis toxicity: anorexia, nausea, vomiting, abdominal pain, weakness, vision changes (diplopia, blurred vision, yellow-green or white halos seen around objects), and new-onset dysrhythmias.
- Assess potassium, magnesium, calcium, and serum digoxin levels before giving digitalis. Hypokalemia can precipitate toxicity even when the serum digitalis level is in the "normal" range.
- Monitor clients with renal insufficiency or renal failure and older adults carefully for digitalis toxicity.
- Prepare to administer digoxin immune fab (Digibind) for digoxin toxicity.

### Client and Family Teaching

- Take your pulse daily before taking your digoxin. Do not take the digoxin if your pulse is below 60 or if you are weak, fatigued, lightheadeded, dizzy, short of breath, or having chest pain. Notify your physician immediately.
- Contact your doctor if you develop manifestations of digitalis toxicity: palpitations, weakness, loss of appetite, nausea, vomiting, abdominal pain, blurred or colored vision, double vision.
- Avoid using antacids and laxatives; they decrease digoxin absorption.
- Notify your physician immediately if you develop manifestations of potassium deficiency: weakness, lethargy, thirst, depression, muscle cramps, or vomiting.
- Incorporate foods high in potassium into your diet: fresh orange or tomato juice, bananas, raisins, dates, figs, prunes, apricots, spinach, cauliflower, and potatoes.

### Sympathomimetic Agents

Dopamine (Inotropin)                     Dobutamine (Dobutrex)

Sympathomimetic agents stimulate the heart, improving the force of contraction. Dobutamine is preferred in managing heart failure because it does not increase the heart rate as much as dopamine, and it has a mild vasodilatory effect. These drugs are given by intravenous infusion and may be titrated to obtain their optimal effects.

### Phosphodiesterase Inhibitors

Amrinone (Inocor)                     Milrinone (Primacor)

Phosphodiesterase inhibitors are used in treating acute heart failure to increase myocardial contractility and cause vasodilation. The net effects are an increase in cardiac output and a decrease in afterload.

### Nursing Responsibilities

- Use an infusion pump to administer these agents. Monitor hemodynamic parameters carefully.
- Avoid discontinuing these drugs abruptly.
- Change solutions and tubing every 24 hours.
- Amrinone is given as an intravenous bolus over 2 to 3 minutes, followed by an infusion of 5 to 10 mg/kg/min.
- Amrinone may be infused full strength or diluted in normal saline or half-strength saline. Do not mix this drug with dextrose solutions. After dilution, amrinone can be piggybacked into a line containing a dextrose solution.
- Monitor liver function and platelet counts; amrinone may cause hepatotoxicity and thrombocytopenia.

### Client and Family Teaching

- Notify the nursing staff if you experience abdominal pain or notice a skin rash or bruising.

---

Beta blockers improve cardiac function in heart failure by inhibiting SNS activity. This prevents the long-term deleterious effects of sympathetic stimulation. Because beta blockers reduce the force of myocardial contraction and may actually worsen symptoms, they are used in low doses. The combination of ACE inhibitors and beta blockers improves client outcomes. Beta blockers are discussed on page 818.

Clients with symptomatic heart failure often are treated with diuretics as well. Diuretics relieve symptoms related to fluid retention. They may, however, cause significant electrolyte imbalances and rapid fluid loss. Clients with severe heart failure are often treated with a loop, or high-ceiling, diuretic such as furosemide (Lasix), bumetanide (Bumex), torsemide (Demadex), or ethacrynic acid (Edecrin). These drugs have a rapid onset of action, inhibiting chloride reabsorption in the ascending loop of Henle, prompting sodium and water excretion. Their major drawback is their efficacy in promoting diuresis; loss of vascular volume can stimulate the SNS. Thiazide diuretics may be used for clients with less severe manifestations of heart failure. These agents promote fluid excretion by blocking sodium reabsorption in the terminal loop of Henle and the distal tubule.

Vasodilators relax smooth muscle in blood vessels, causing dilation. Arterial dilation reduces peripheral vascular resistance and afterload, reducing myocardial work. Venous dilation reduces venous return and preload. Pulmonary vascular relaxation reduces pulmonary capillary pressure, allowing reabsorption of fluid from interstitial tissues and the alveoli. Vasodilators include nitrates, hydralazine, and prazosin, an alpha-adrenergic blocker. See Chapter 33 ⨀ for more information about vasodilators.

Nitrates produce both arterial and venous vasodilation. They may be given by nasal spray or the sublingual, oral, or intravenous route. Sodium nitroprusside is a potent vasodilator that may be used to treat acute heart failure. It can cause excessive hypotension, so is often given along with dopamine or dobutamine to maintain the blood pressure. Isosorbide or nitroglycerin ointment may be used in long-term management of heart failure. See page 818.

Digitalis glycosides are used judiciously in symptomatic heart failure. Digitalis has a *positive inotropic effect* on the heart, increasing the strength of myocardial contraction by increasing the intracellular calcium concentrations. Digitalis also decreases SA node automaticity and slows conduction through the AV node, increasing ventricular filling time.

Digitalis has a narrow therapeutic index; in other words, therapeutic levels are very close to toxic levels. Early manifestations of digitalis toxicity include anorexia, nausea and vomiting, headache, altered vision, and confusion. A number of cardiac dysrhythmias are also associated with digitalis toxicity, including sinus arrest, supraventricular and ventricular tachycardias, and high levels of AV block. Low serum potassium levels increase the risk of digitalis toxicity, as do low magnesium and high calcium levels. Older adults are at particular risk for digitalis toxicity.

Digitalis levels may be affected by a number of other drugs; check for potential interactions.

Dysrhythmias are common in clients with heart failure. Although PVCs are may be frequent, they are often not associated with an increased risk of ventricular tachycardia and fibrillation. Because many antidysrhythmic medications depress left ventricular function, PVCs are frequently left untreated in heart failure. Amiodarone is the drug of choice to treat nonsustained ventricular tachycardia, which is associated with a poor prognosis. See page 854.

## Diet and Activity

A sodium-restricted diet is recommended to minimize sodium and water retention. Intake is generally limited to 1.5 to 2 g of sodium per day, a moderate restriction. Box 5–4 lists high-sodium foods to avoid; Box 5–5 includes client teaching regarding sodium-restricted diet. Activity may be restricted to bed rest during acute episodes of heart failure to reduce cardiac workload and allow the heart to recompensate. Prolonged bed rest and continued activity limitations, however, are not recommended. A moderate, progressive activity program is prescribed to improve myocardial function.

## Other Treatments

In end-stage heart failure, devices to provide circulatory assistance or surgery may be required. Surgery may be used to treat the underlying cause of failure (e.g., replacement of diseased valves) or to improve quality of life. Valve replacement is discussed later in this chapter. Heart transplant is currently the only clearly effective surgical treatment for end-stage heart failure; its use is limited by the availability of donor hearts.

### Circulatory Assistance

Devices such as the intra-aortic balloon pump or a left-ventricular assist device may be used when the client is expected to recover or as a bridge to transplant. (see Chapter 29). Newer devices that will allow longer term support outside the hospital are in the developmental stages. These devices will serve either as a bridge to transplant or allow the myocardium to heal over an extended period of time.

### Cardiac Transplantation

Heart transplant is the treatment of choice for end-stage heart disease. Survival rates are good: 85% at 1 year and 70% at 5 years (Braunwald et al., 2001). The most frequently used transplant procedure leaves posterior walls of the atria, the superior and inferior vena cavae, and pulmonary veins of the recipient intact (Figure 30–4A ■). The atrial walls of the donor heart are then anatomosed to the recipient's atria (Figure 30–4B). The donor pulmonary artery and aorta are anatomosed to the recipient vessels (Figure 30–4C). Care is taken to avoid damaging the sinus node of the donor heart. Donor organs typically are obtained from young accident victims with no evidence of cardiac trauma.

Nursing care of the heart transplant client is similar to care of any cardiac surgery client (see page 823). Infection and rejection are major postoperative concerns; these are the chief causes of mortality in transplant clients. Immunosuppressive drugs are given to prevent rejection of the transplanted organ, even when the tissue match is good (see Chapter 9). ⨀ Although immunosuppressive medications help prevent organ rejection, they impair the client's defenses against infection. The donor heart is also denervated during the transplant procedure. Lack of innervation by the autonomic nervous system affects its response to position changes, stress, exercise, and certain drugs.

### Other Procedures

Other surgical procedures such as cardiomyoplasty and ventricular reduction surgery do not improve the prognosis or quality of life in clients with end-stage heart failure. *Cardiomyoplasty* involves wrapping the latissimus dorsi muscle around the heart to support the failing myocardium. The muscle is stimulated in synchrony with the heart, providing a more

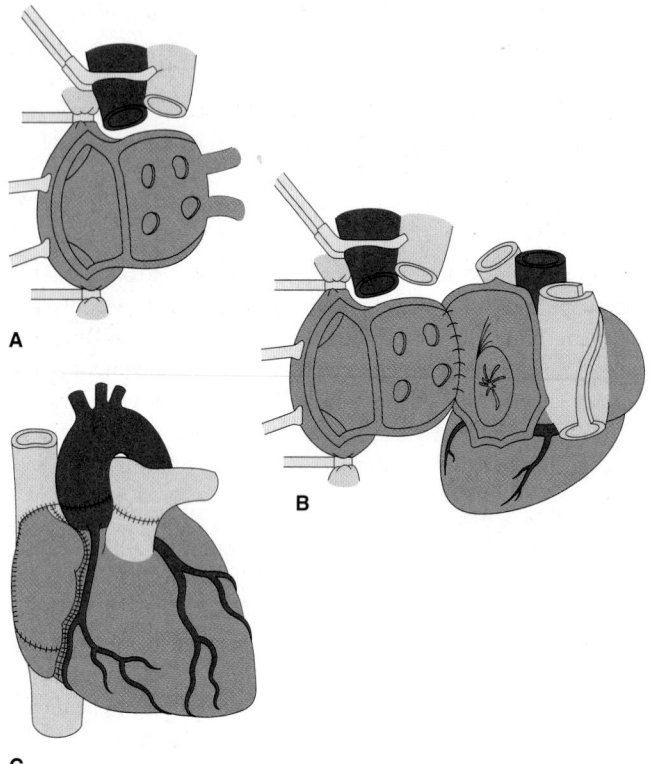

**Figure 30–4** ■ Cardiac transplantation. *A,* The heart is removed, leaving the posterior walls of the atria intact. The donor heart is anastomosed to the atria, *B,* and the great vessels, *C.*

forceful contraction and increasing cardiac output. In ventricular reduction surgery (or *partial ventriculectomy*), a portion of the anteriolateral left ventricular wall is resected to improve cardiac function (Tierney et al., 2001).

## Complementary Therapies

Strong evidence supports the use of several complementary therapies for heart failure. Hawthorn, a shrubby tree, contains natural cardiotonic ingredients in its blossoms, leaves, and fruit. It increases the force of myocardial contraction, dilates blood vessels, and has a natural ACE inhibitor. Hawthorn should never be used without consulting an experienced herb practitioner and advising the physician (Fontaine, 2000). Nutritional supplements of coenzyme Q10, magnesium, and thiamine may be used in conjunction with other treatments. Coenzyme Q10 improves mitochrondria function and energy production. Researchers in Japan linked lower levels of coenzyme Q10 with a higher mortality rate in clients with heart failure (Kuhn, 1999).

## End of Life Care

Unless a cardiac transplant is performed, chronic heart failure is ultimately a terminal disease. The client and family need honest discussions about the anticipated course of the disease and treatment options. It is important to discuss advance directives such as the living will and medical power of attorney, differentiating potential acute events from which recovery would be anticipated (e.g., reversible exacerbation of heart failure,

sudden cardiac arrest) from prolonged life support without reasonable expectation of functional recovery. Hospice services are available for clients with heart failure, and should be offered when appropriate. Severe dyspnea is common in the final stages of the disease. It may be managed with narcotic analgesics or with frequent intravenous diuretics and continuous infusion of a positive inotropic agent (Hunt et al., 2001).

## NURSING CARE

### Health Promotion

Health promotion activities to reduce the risk for and incidence of heart failure are directed at the risk factors. Teach clients about coronary heart disease, the primary underlying cause of heart failure. Discuss CHD risk factors, and ways to reduce those risk factors (see Chapter 29).

Hypertension also is a major cause of heart failure. Routinely screen clients for elevated blood pressure, and refer clients to a primary care provider as indicated. Discuss the importance of effectively managing hypertension to reduce the future risk for heart failure. Likewise, stress the relationship between effective diabetes management and reduced risk of heart failure.

### Assessment

Obtain both subjective and objective data when assessing the client with heart failure.

- Health history: complaints of increasing shortness of breath, dyspnea with exertion, decreasing activity tolerance, or paroxysmal nocturnal dyspnea; number of pillows used for sleeping; recent weight gain; presence of a cough; chest or abdominal pain; anorexia or nausea; history of cardiac disease, previous episodes of heart failure; other risk factors such as hypertension or diabetes; current medications; usual diet and activity and recent changes
- Physical examination: general appearance; ease of breathing, conversing, changing positions; apparent anxiety; vital signs including apical pulse; color of skin and mucous membranes; neck vein distension, peripheral pulses, capillary refill, presence and degree of edema; heart and breath sounds; abdominal contour, bowel sounds, tenderness; right upper abdominal tenderness, liver enlargement

### Nursing Diagnoses and Interventions

Heart failure impacts quality of life, interfering with such daily activities as self-care and role performance. Reducing the oxygen demand of the heart is a major nursing care goal for the client in acute heart failure. This includes providing rest and carrying out prescribed treatment measures to reduce cardiac work, improve contractility, and manage symptoms.

#### Decreased Cardiac Output

As the heart fails as a pump, stroke volume and tissue perfusion decrease.

- Monitor vital signs and oxygen saturation as indicated. *Decreased cardiac output stimulates the SNS to increase the heart rate in an attempt to restore CO. Tachycardia at rest is common. Diastolic blood pressure may initially be elevated because of vasoconstriction; in late stages, compensatory mechanisms fail, and BP falls. Oxygen saturation levels provide a measure of gas exchange and tissue perfusion.*

- Auscultate heart and breath sounds regularly. *$S_1$ and $S_2$ may be diminished if cardiac function is poor. A ventricular gallop ($S_3$) is an early sign of heart failure; atrial gallop ($S_4$) may also be present. Crackles are often heard in the lung bases; increasing crackles, dyspnea, and shortness of breath indicate worsening failure.*

**PRACTICE ALERT** *Report manifestations of decreased cardiac output and tissue perfusion: changes in mentation; decreased urine output; cool, clammy skin; diminished pulses; pallor or cyanosis; dysrhythmias. These are manifestations of decreased tissue perfusion to organ systems.* ■

- Administer supplemental oxygen as needed. *This improves oxygenation of the blood, decreasing the effects of hypoxia and ischemia.*
- Administer prescribed medications as ordered. *Drugs are used to decrease the cardiac workload and increase the effectiveness of contractions.*
- Encourage rest, explaining the rationale. Elevate the head of the bed to reduce the work of breathing. Provide a bedside commode, and assist with ADLs. Instruct to avoid the Valsalva maneuver. *These measures reduce cardiac workload.*

**PRACTICE ALERT** *Promote psychologic rest and decrease anxiety. Maintain a quiet environment, encourage expression of fears and feelings. Explain care measures and their purpose. Psychologic rest decreases oxygen consumption and improves cardiac function.* ■

### Excess Fluid Volume

As cardiac output falls, compensatory mechanisms cause salt and water retention, increasing blood volume. This increased fluid volume places additional stress on the already failing ventricles, making them work harder to move the fluid load.

- Assess respiratory status and auscultate lung sounds at least every 4 hours. Notify the physician of significant changes in condition. *Declining respiratory status indicates worsening left heart failure.*

**PRACTICE ALERT** *Immediately notify the physician if the client develops air hunger, an overwhelming sense of impending doom or panic, tachypnea, severe orthopnea, or a cough productive of large amounts of pink, frothy sputum. Acute pulmonary edema, a medical emergency, can develop rapidly, necessitating immediate intervention to preserve life.* ■

- Monitor intake and output. Notify the physician if urine output is less than 30 mL/h. Weigh daily. *Careful monitoring of fluid volume is important during treatment of heart failure. Diuretics may reduce circulating volume, producing hypovolemia despite persistent peripheral edema. A fall in urine output may indicate significantly reduced cardiac output and renal ischemia. Weight is an objective measure of fluid status: 1 L of fluid is equal to 2.2 lb of weight.*
- Record abdominal girth every shift. Note complaints of a loss of appetite, abdominal discomfort, or nausea. *Venous congestion can lead to ascites and may affect gastrointestinal function and nutritional status.*
- Monitor and record hemodynamic measurements. Report significant changes and negative trends. *Hemodynamic measurements provide a means of monitoring condition and response to treatment.*
- Restrict fluids as ordered. Allow choices of fluid type and timing of intake, scheduling most fluid intake during morning and afternoon hours. Offer ice chips and frequent mouth care; provide hard candies if allowed. *Providing choices increases the client's sense of control. Ice chips, hard candies, and mouth care relieve dry mouth and thirst and promote comfort.*

### Activity Intolerance

Clients with heart failure have little or no cardiac reserve to meet increased oxygen demands. As the disease progresses and cardiac function is further compromised, activity intolerance increases. The low cardiac output and inability to participate in activities may hinder self-care.

**PRACTICE ALERT** *Monitor vital signs and cardiac rhythm during and after activities. Tachycardia, dysrhythmias, increasing dyspnea, changes in blood pressure, diaphoresis, pallor, complaints of chest pain, excessive fatigue, or palpitations indicate activity intolerance. Instruct to rest if manifestations are noted. The failing heart is unable to increase cardiac output to meet increased oxygen demands associated with activity. Assessing response to activities helps evaluate cardiac function. Decreasing activity tolerance may signal deterioration of cardiac function, not overexertion.* ■

- Organize nursing care to allow rest periods. *Grouping activities together allows adequate time to "recharge."*
- Assist with ADLs as needed. Encourage independence within prescribed limits. *Assisting with ADLs helps ensure that care needs are met while reducing cardiac workload. Involving the client promotes a sense of control and reduces helplessness.*
- Plan and implement progressive activities. Use passive and active ROM exercises as appropriate. Consult with physical therapist on activity plan. *Progressive activity slowly increases exercise capacity by strengthening and improving cardiac function without strain. Activity also helps prevent skeletal muscle atrophy. ROM exercises prevent complications of immobility in severely compromised clients.*

- Provide written and verbal information about activity after discharge. *Written information provides a reference for important information. Verbal information allows clarification and validation of the material.*

### Deficient Knowledge: Low-Sodium Diet

Diet is an important part of long-term management of heart failure to manage fluid retention.

- Discuss the rationale for sodium restrictions. *Understanding fosters compliance with the prescribed diet.*
- Consult with dietitian to plan and teach a low-sodium and, if necessary for weight control, low-kcal diet. Provide a list of high-sodium, high-fat, high-cholesterol foods to avoid. Provide American Heart Association materials. *Dietary planning and teaching increases the client's sense of control and participation in disease management. Food lists are useful memory aids.*

**PRACTICE ALERT** *Teach how to read food labels for nutritional information. Many processed foods contain "hidden" sodium, which can be identified by careful label reading.* ■

- Assist the client to construct a 2-day meal plan choosing foods low in sodium. *This allows learning assessment, clarification of misunderstandings, and reinforcement of teaching.*
- Encourage small, frequent meals rather than three heavy meals per day. *Small, frequent meals provide continuing energy resources and decrease the work required to digest a large meal.*

## Using NANDA, NIC, and NOC

Chart 30–1 shows links between NANDA nursing diagnoses, NIC, and NOC for the client with heart failure.

## Home Care

Heart failure is a chronic condition requiring active participation by the client and family for effective management. In teaching for home care, include the following topics:

- The disease process and its effects on the client's life
- Warning signals of cardiac decompensation that require treatment
- Desired and adverse effects of prescribed drugs; monitoring for effects; importance of compliance with drug regimen to prevent acute and long-term complications of heart failure
- Prescribed diet and sodium restriction; practical suggestions for reducing salt intake; recommend American Heart Association materials and recipes
- Exercise recommendations to strengthen the heart muscle and improve aerobic capacity (Box 30–3)
- The importance of keeping scheduled follow-up appointments to monitor disease progression and effects of therapy.

Provide referrals for home health care and household assistance (shopping, transportation, personal needs, and housekeeping) as indicated. Referrals to community agencies, such as local cardiac rehabilitation programs, heart support groups, or the AHA, can provide with additional materials and psychosocial support.

## CHART 30–1 NANDA, NIC, AND NOC LINKAGES

### The Client with Heart Failure

| NURSING DIAGNOSES | NURSING INTERVENTIONS | NURSING OUTCOMES |
|---|---|---|
| • Activity Intolerance | • Cardiac Care: Rehabilitative<br>• Energy Management<br>• Self-Care Assistance | • Activity Tolerance<br>• Energy Conservation<br>• Self-Care: Activities of Daily Living (ADLs) |
| • Decreased Cardiac Output | • Cardiac Care: Acute<br>• Hemodynamic Regulation<br>• Vital Signs Monitoring | • Cardiac Pump Effectiveness<br>• Circulation Status<br>• Vital Signs Status |
| • Fatigue | • Activity Therapy<br>• Environmental Management<br>• Nutrition Management | • Endurance<br>• Energy Conservation<br>• Nutritional Status: Energy |
| • Excess Fluid Volume | • Fluid Management<br>• Invasive Hemodynamic Monitoring<br>• Medication Management | • Electrolyte and Acid-Base Balance<br>• Fluid Balance |
| • Ineffective Health Maintenance | • Discharge Planning<br>• Teaching: Prescribed Activity/Exercise<br>• Teaching: Prescribed Diet<br>• Decision-Making Support | • Knowledge: Health Resources<br>• Knowledge: Treatment Regimen<br>• Participation: Health Care Decisions |

*Note. Data from Nursing Outcomes Classification (NOC) by M. Johnson & M. Maas (Eds.), 1997, St. Louis: Mosby; Nursing Diagnoses: Definitions & Classifications 2001–2002 by North American Nursing Diagnosis Association, 2001, Philadelphia: NANDA; Nursing Interventions Classification (NIC) by J.C. McCloskey & G. M. Bulechek (Eds.), 2000, St. Louis: Mosby. Reprinted by permission.*

| BOX 30–3 | ■ Home Activity Guidelines for the Client with Heart Failure |
|---|---|

■ Perform as many activities as independently as you can.

■ Space your meals and activities.

   a. Eat six small meals a day.

   b. Allow time during the day for periods of rest and relaxation.

■ Perform all activities at a comfortable pace.

   a. If you get tired during any activity, stop what you are doing and rest for 15 minutes.

   b. Resume activity only if you feel up to it.

■ Stop any activity that causes chest pain, shortness of breath, dizziness, faintness, excessive weakness, or sweating. Rest. Notify your physician if your activity tolerance changes and if symptoms continue after rest.

■ Avoid straining. Do not lift heavy objects. Eat a high-fiber diet and drink plenty of water to prevent constipation. Use laxatives or stool softeners, as approved by your physician, to avoid constipation and straining during bowel movements.

■ Begin a graded exercise program. Walking is good exercise that does not require any special equipment (except a good pair of walking shoes). Plan to walk twice a day at a comfortable, slow pace for the first couple of weeks at home, and then gradually increase the distance and pace. Below is a suggested schedule—but progress at your own speed. Take your time. Aim for walking at least 3 times per week (every other day).

| | | |
|---|---|---|
| Week 1 | 200 to 400 ft (1/4 mile) | Twice a day, slow leisurely pace |
| Week 2 | 1/4 mile | 15 min, minimum of 3 times per week |
| Weeks 2 to 3 | 1/2 mile | 30 min, minimum of 3 times per week |
| Weeks 3 to 4 | 1 mile | 30 min, minimum of 3 times per week |
| Weeks 4 to 5 | 1 1/2 mile | 30 min, minimum of 3 times per week |
| Weeks 5 to 6 | 2 miles | 40 min, minimum of 3 times per week |

## Nursing Care Plan
## A Client with Heart Failure

One year ago, Arthur Jackson, 67 years old, had a large anterior wall MI and underwent subsequent coronary artery bypass surgery. On discharge, he was started on a regimen of enalapril (Vasotec), digoxin, furosemide (Lasix), coumadin, and a potassium chloride supplement. He is now in the cardiac unit complaining of severe shortness of breath, hemoptysis, and poor appetite for 1 week. He is diagnosed with acute heart failure.

### ASSESSMENT

Mr. Jackson refuses to settle in bed, preferring to sit in the bedside recliner in high Fowler's position. He states, "Lately, this is the only way I can breathe." Mr. Jackson states that he has not been able to work in his garden without getting short of breath. He complains of his shoes and belt being too tight.

When Ms. Takashi, RN, Mr. Jackson's nurse, obtains his nursing history, Mr. Jackson insists that he takes his medications regularly. He states that he normally works in his garden for light exercise. In his diet history, Mr. Jackson admits fondness for bacon and Chinese food and sheepishly admits to snacking between meals "even though I need to lose weight."

Mr. Jackson's vital signs are: BP 95/72 mmHg, HR 124 and irregular, R 28 and labored, and T 97.5°F (36.5°C). The cardiac monitor shows atrial fibrillation. An $S_3$ is noted on auscultation; the cardiac impulse is left of the midclavicular line. He has crackles and diminished breath sounds in the bases of both lungs. Significant jugular venous distention, 3+ pitting edema of feet and ankles, and abdominal distention are noted. Liver size is within normal limits by percussion. Skin cool and diaphoretic. Chest X-ray shows cardiomegaly and pulmonary infiltrates.

### DIAGNOSES

• *Excess fluid volume* related to impaired cardiac pump and salt and water retention

• *Activity intolerance* related to impaired cardiac output

• *Impaired health maintenance* related to lack of knowledge about diet restrictions

### EXPECTED OUTCOMES

• Demonstrate loss of excess fluid by weight loss and decreases in edema, jugular venous distention, and abdominal distention.

• Demonstrate improved activity tolerance.

• Verbalize understanding of diet restrictions.

### PLANNING AND IMPLEMENTATION

• Hourly vital signs and hemodynamic pressure measurements.

• Administer and monitor effects of prescribed diuretics and vasodilators.

• Weigh daily; strict intake and output.

• Enforce fluid restriction of 1500 mL/24 hours: 600 mL day shift, 600 mL evening shift, 300 mL at night.

• Auscultate heart and breath sounds every 4 hours and as indicated.

• Administer oxygen per nasal cannula at 2 L/min. Monitor oxygen satururation continuously. Notify physician if less than 94%.

• High Fowler's or position of comfort.

• Notify physician of significant changes in laboratory values.

• Teach about all medications and how to take and record pulse. Provide information about anticoagulant therapy and signs of bleeding.

• Design an activity plan with Mr. Jackson that incorporates preferred activities and scheduled rest periods.

• Instruct about sodium-restricted diet. Allow meal choices within allowed limits.

*(continued on page 886)*

## Nursing Care Plan
## A Client with Heart Failure (continued)

• Consult dietitian for planning and teaching Mr. and Mrs. Jackson about low-sodium diet.

### EVALUATION

Mr. Jackson is discharged after 3 days in the cardiac unit. He has lost 8 pounds during his stay and states it is much easier to breathe and his shoes fit better. He is able to sleep in semi-Fowler's position with only one pillow. His peripheral edema has resolved. Mr. and Mrs. Jackson met with the dietitian, who helped them develop a realistic eating plan to limit sodium, sugar, and fats. The dietitian also provided a list of high-sodium foods to avoid. Mr. Jackson is relieved to know that he can still enjoy Chinese food prepared without monosodium glutamate (MSG) or added salt. Ms. Takashi and the physical therapist designed a progressive activity plan with Mr. Jackson that he will continue at home. He remains in atrial fibrillation, a chronic condition. His knowledge of digoxin and coumadin has been assessed and reinforced. Ms. Takashi confirms that he is able to accurately check his pulse and can list signs of digoxin toxicity and excessive bleeding.

### Critical Thinking in the Nursing Process

1. Mr. Jackson's medication regimen remains the same after discharge. What specific teaching does he need related to potential interactions of these drugs?
2. Mr. Jackson tells you, "Talk to my wife about my medications—she's Tarzan and I'm Jane now." How would you respond?
3. Design an exercise plan for Mr. Jackson to prevent deconditioning and conserve energy.
4. Mr. Jackson tells you, "Sometimes I forget whether I have taken my aspirin, so I'll take another just to be sure. After all, they are only baby aspirin. One or two extra a day shouldn't hurt, right?" What is your response?
5. Mr. Jackson is admitted to the neuro unit 6 months later with a cerebral vascular accident (CVA). What is the probable cause of his stroke?

See Evaluating Your Response in Appendix C.

## THE CLIENT WITH PULMONARY EDEMA

**Pulmonary edema** is an abnormal accumulation of fluid in the interstitial tissue and alveoli of the lung. Both cardiac and noncardiac disorders can cause pulmonary edema. Cardiac causes include acute myocardial infarction, acute heart failure, and valvular disease. *Cardiogenic pulmonary edema,* the focus of this section, is a sign of severe cardiac decompensation. Noncardiac causes of pulmonary edema include primary pulmonary disorders, such as acute respiratory distress syndrome (ARDS), trauma, sepsis, drug overdose, or neurologic sequelae. Pulmonary edema due to ARDS is discussed in Chapter 36. ↩

Pulmonary edema is a medical emergency: The client is literally drowning in the fluid in the alveolar and interstitial pulmonary spaces. Its onset may be acute or gradual, progressing to severe respiratory distress. Immediate treatment is necessary.

### PATHOPHYSIOLOGY

In cardiogenic pulmonary edema, the contractility of the left ventricle is severely impaired. The ejection fraction falls as the ventricle is unable to eject the blood that enters it, causing a sharp rise in end-diastolic volume and pressure. Pulmonary hydrostatic pressures rise, ultimately exceeding the osmotic pressure of the blood. As a result, fluid leaking from the pulmonary capillaries congests interstitial tissues, decreasing lung compliance, and interfering with gas exchange. As capillary and interstitial pressures increase further, the tight junctions of the alveolar walls are disrupted, and the fluid enters the alveoli, along with large red blood cells and protein molecules. Ventilation and gas exchange are severely disrupted, and hypoxia worsens.

### MANIFESTATIONS

The client with acute pulmonary edema presents with classic manifestations (see box below). Dyspnea, shortness of breath, and labored respirations are acute and severe, accompanied by orthopnea, inability to breathe when lying down. Cyanosis is present, and the skin is cool, clammy, and diaphoretic. A productive cough with pink, frothy sputum develops due to fluid, RBCs, and plasma proteins in the alveoli and airways. Crackles are heard throughout the lung fields on auscultation. As the condition worsens, lung sounds become harsher. The client often is restless and highly anxious, although severe hypoxia may cause confusion or lethargy.

As noted earlier, pulmonary edema is a medical emergency. Without rapid and effective intervention, severe tissue hypoxia and acidosis will lead to organ system failure and death.

### Manifestations of Pulmonary Edema

**RESPIRATORY**
- Tachypnea
- Labored respirations
- Dyspnea
- Orthopnea
- Paroxysmal nocturnal dyspnea
- Cough productive of frothy, pink sputum
- Crackles, wheezes

**CARDIOVASCULAR**
- Tachycardia
- Hypotension
- Cyanosis
- Cool, clammy skin
- Hypoxemia
- Ventricular gallop

**NEUROLOGIC**
- Restlessness
- Anxiety
- Feeling of impending doom

## COLLABORATIVE CARE

Immediate treatment for acute pulmonary edema focuses on restoring effective gas exchange and reducing fluid and pressure in the pulmonary vascular system. The client is placed in an upright sitting position with the legs dangling to reduce venous return by trapping some excess fluid in the lower extremities. This position also facilitates breathing.

Diagnostic testing is limited to assessment of the acute situation. *Arterial blood gases (ABGs)* are drawn to assess gas exchange and acid-base balance. Oxygen tension ($Pao_2$) is usually low. Initially, carbon dioxide levels ($Paco_2$) may also be reduced because of rapid respirations. As the condition progresses, the $Paco_2$ rises and respiratory acidosis develops (see Chapter 5). ⊂⊃ *Oxygen saturation* levels also are continuously monitored. The *chest X-ray* shows pulmonary vascular congestion and alveolar edema. Provided the client's condition allows, *hemodynamic monitoring* is instituted. In cardiogenic pulmonary edema, the pulmonary artery wedge pressure (PAWP) is elevated, usually over 25 mmHg. Cardiac output may be decreased.

Morphine is administered intravenously to relieve anxiety and improve the efficacy of breathing. It also is a vasodilator that reduces venous return and lowers left atrial pressure. Although morphine is very effective for clients with cardiogenic pulmonary edema, naloxone, its antidote, is kept readily available in case respiratory depression occurs.

Oxygen is administered using a positive pressure system that can achieve a 100% oxygen concentration. A continuous positive airway pressure (CPAP) mask system may be used, or the client may be intubated and mechanical ventilation employed (see Chapter 36). ⊂⊃ Positive pressure increases alveolar pressures and gas exchange while decreasing fluid diffusion into the alveoli.

Potent loop diuretics such as furosemide, ethacrynic acid, or bumetanide are administered intravenously to promote rapid diuresis. Furosemide is also a venous dilator, reducing venous return to the heart. Vasodilators such as intravenous nitroprusside are given to improve cardiac output by reducing afterload. Dopamine or dobutamine and possibly digoxin are administered to improve the myocardial contractility and cardiac output. Intravenous aminophylline may be used cautiously to reduce bronchospasm and decrease wheezing.

When the client's condition has stabilized, further diagnostic tests may be done to determine the underlying cause of pulmonary edema, and specific treatment measures directed at the cause instituted.

## NURSING CARE

Nursing care of the client with acute pulmonary edema focuses on relieving the pulmonary effects of the disorder. Interventions are directed toward improving oxygenation, reducing fluid volume, and providing emotional support.

The nurse often is instrumental in recognizing early manifestations of pulmonary edema and initiating treatment. As with many critical conditions, emergent care is directed toward the ABCs: airway, breathing, and circulation.

## Nursing Diagnoses and Interventions

### Impaired Gas Exchange

Accumulated fluid in the alveoli and airways interfere with ventilation of and gas exchange within the alveoli.

- Ensure airway patency.

**PRACTICE ALERT** *Assess the effectiveness of respiratory efforts and airway clearance. Pulmonary edema increases the work of breathing. This increased effort can lead to fatigue and decreased respiratory effort.* ■

- Assess respiratory status frequently, including rate, effort, use of accessory muscles, sputum characteristics, lung sounds, and skin color. *The status of a client in acute pulmonary edema can change rapidly for the better or worse.*
- Place in high-Fowler's position with the legs dangling. *The upright position facilitates breathing and decreases venous return.*
- Administer oxygen as ordered by mask, CPAP mask, or ventilator. *Supplemental oxygen promotes gas exchange; positive pressure increases the pressure within the alveoli, airways, and thoracic cavity, decreasing venous return, pulmonary capillary pressure, and fluid leak into the alveoli.*
- Encourage to cough up secretions; provide nasotracheal suctioning if necessary. *Coughing moves secretions from smaller airways into larger airways where they can be suctioned out if necessary.*

**PRACTICE ALERT** *Have emergency equipment readily available in case of respiratory arrest. Be prepared to assist with intubation and initiation of mechanical ventilation. Fatigue, impaired gas exchange, and respiratory acidosis can lead to respiratory and cardiac arrest.* ■

### Decreased Cardiac Output

Cardiogenic pulmonary edema usually is caused by either an acute decrease in myocardial contractility or increased workload that exceeds the ability of the left ventricle.

- Monitor vital signs, hemodynamic status, and rhythm continuously. *Acute pulmonary edema is a critical condition, and cardiovascular status can change rapidly.*
- Assess heart sounds for possible $S_3$, $S_4$, or murmurs. *These abnormal heart sounds may be due to excess work or may indicate the cause of the acute pulmonary edema.*
- Initiate an intravenous line for medication administration. Administer morphine, diuretics, vasodilators, bronchodilators, and positive inotropic medications (e.g., digoxin) as ordered. *These drugs reduce cardiac work and improve contractility.*

**PRACTICE ALERT** *Insert an indwelling catheter; record output hourly. Urine output of less than 30 mL/hr indicates severely impaired cardiac output and a risk for renal failure or other complications.* ■

- Keep accurate intake and output records. Restrict fluids as ordered. *Fluids may be restricted to reduce vascular volume and cardiac work.*

## Fear

Acute pulmonary edema is a very frightening experience for everyone (including the nurse).

- Provide emotional support for the client and family members. *Fear and anxiety stimulate the sympathetic nervous system, which can lead to ineffective respiratory patterns and interfere with cooperation with care measures.*
- Explain all procedures and the reasons to the client and family members. Keep information brief and to the point. Use short sentences and a reassuring tone. *Anxiety and fear interfere with the ability to assimilate information; brief, factual information and reassurance reduce anxiety and fear.*

- Maintain close contact with the client and family, providing reassurance that recovery from acute pulmonary edema is often as dramatic as its onset.
- Answer questions, and provide accurate information in a caring manner. *Knowledge reduces anxiety and psychologic stress associated with this critical condition.*

## Home Care

During the acute period, teaching is limited to immediate care measures. Once the acute episode of pulmonary edema has resolved, teach the client and family about its underlying cause and prevention of future episodes. If pulmonary edema follows an acute MI, include information related to CHD and the AMI, as well as information related to heart failure. Review the teaching and home care for clients with these disorders for further information.

# INFLAMMATORY HEART DISORDERS

Any layer of cardiac tissue—the endocardium, myocardium, or pericardium—can become inflamed, thus damaging the heart valves, heart muscle, or pericardial lining. Manifestations of inflammatory heart disorders range from very mild to life threatening. This section discusses the causes and management of rheumatic heart disease, endocarditis, myocarditis, and pericarditis.

## THE CLIENT WITH RHEUMATIC FEVER AND RHEUMATIC HEART DISEASE

**Rheumatic fever** is a systemic inflammatory disease caused by an abnormal immune response to pharyngeal infection by group A beta-hemolytic streptococci. The peak incidence of rheumatic fever is between ages 5 and 15; although it is rare after age 40, it may affect people of any age. Rheumatic fever usually is a self-limiting disorder, although it may become recurrent or chronic. Although the heart commonly is involved in the acute inflammatory process, only about 10% of people with rheumatic fever develop rheumatic heart disease (Porth, 2002). Rheumatic heart disease frequently damages the heart valves and is a major cause of mitral and aortic valve disorders discussed in the next section of this chapter.

In the United States and other industrialized nations, rheumatic fever and its sequelae are rare. About 3% of people with untreated group A streptococcal pharyngitis develop rheumatic fever (Braunwald et al., 2001). Rheumatic fever and rheumatic heart disease remain significant public health problems in many developing countries. Highly virulent strains of group A streptococci have caused scattered outbreaks in the United States in recent years (McCance & Huether, 2002).

Risk factors for streptococcal infections of the pharynx include environmental and economic factors such as crowded living conditions, malnutrition, immunodeficiency, and poor

access to health care. Evidence also suggests an unknown genetic factor in susceptibility to rheumatic fever.

## PATHOPHYSIOLOGY

The pathophysiology of rheumatic fever is not yet totally understood. It is thought to result from an abnormal immune response to M proteins on group A β-hemolytic streptococcal bacteria. These antigens can bind to cells in the heart, muscles, and brain. They also bind with receptors in synovial joints, provoking an autoimmune response (McCance & Huether, 2002). The resulting immune response to the bacteria also leads to inflammation in tissues containing these M proteins. Inflammatory lesions develop in connective tissues on the heart, joints, and skin. The antibodies may remain in the serum for up to 6 months following the initiating event. See Chapters 8 and 9 ⬤ for more information about the immune system and inflammatory response.

*Carditis,* inflammation of the heart, develops in about 50% of people with rheumatic fever. The inflammatory process usually involves all three layers of the heart—the pericardium, myocardium, and endocardium. *Aschoff bodies,* localized areas of tissue necrosis surrounded by immune cells, develop in cardiac tissues. Pericardial and myocardial inflammation tends to be mild and self-limiting. Endocardial inflammation, however, causes swelling and erythema of valve structures and small vegetative lesions on valve leaflets. As the inflammatory process resolves, fibrous scarring occurs, causing deformity.

**Rheumatic heart disease (RHD)** is slowly progressive valvular deformity that may follow acute or repeated attacks of rheumatic fever. Valve leaflets become rigid and deformed; commissures (openings) fuse, and the chordae tendineae fibrose and shorten. This results in stenosis or regurgitation of the valve. In **stenosis,** a narrowed fused valve obstructs forward blood flow. **Regurgitation** occurs when the valve fails to close properly (an *incompetent* valve), allowing blood to flow

## Manifestations of Rheumatic Fever

### CARDIAC
- Chest pain
- Friction rub
- Heart murmur

### MUSCULOSKELETAL
- *Migratory polyarthritis:* redness, heat, swelling, pain, and tenderness of more than one joint
- Usually affects large joints of extremities

### SKIN
- *Erythema marginatum:* transitory pink, nonpruritic, macular lesions on trunk or inner aspect of upper arms or thighs
- *Subcutaneous nodules* over extensors of wrist, elbow, ankle, and knee joints

### NEUROLOGIC
- *Sydenham's chorea:* irritability, behavior changes; sudden, jerky, involuntary movements

back through it. Valves on the left side of the heart are usually affected; the mitral valve is most frequently involved.

## MANIFESTATIONS

Manifestations of rheumatic fever typically follow the initial streptococcal infection by about 2 to 3 weeks. Fever and migratory joint pain are often initial manifestations. The knees, ankles, hips, and elbows are common sites of swelling and inflammation. *Erythema marginatum* is a temporary nonpruritic skin rash characterized by red lesions with clear borders and blanched centers usually found on the trunk and proximal extremities. Neurologic symptoms of rheumatic fever, although rare in adults, may range from irritability and an inability to concentrate to clumsiness and involuntary muscle spasms.

Manifestations of carditis include chest pain, tachycardia, a pericardial friction rub, or evidence of heart failure. On auscultation, an $S_3$, $S_4$, or a heart murmur may be heard. Cardiomegaly or pericardial effusion may develop. Other manifestations of rheumatic fever are listed in the box above.

## COLLABORATIVE CARE

Management of the client with rheumatic heart disease focuses on eradicating the streptococcal infection and managing the manifestations of the disease. Carditis and resulting heart failure are treated with measures to reduce the inflammatory process and manage the heart failure. Activities are limited, but bed rest is not generally ordered.

### Diagnostic Tests

In addition to the history and physical examination, a number of laboratory and diagnostic tests may be ordered for the client with suspected rheumatic fever. Table 30–4 identifies tests and values indicative of carditis associated with rheumatic fever.

| TABLE 30–4 | Diagnostic Tests for Rheumatic Heart Disease |
|---|---|
| **Test** | **Values Characteristic of Rheumatic Heart Disease** |
| White blood cell count (WBC) | Greater than 10,000/mm³ |
| Red blood cell count (RBC) | Less than 4 million/mm³ |
| Erythrocyte sedimentation rate (ESR) | More than 20 mm/h |
| C-reactive protein | Positive |
| Antistreptolysin (ASO) titer | Above 250 IU/mL |
| Throat culture | Usually positive for group A beta-hemolytic streptococci |
| Cardiac enzymes | Elevated in severe carditis |
| ECG changes | Prolonged PR interval |
| Chest X-ray | May show cardiac enlargement |
| Echocardiogram | May show valvular damage, enlarged chambers, decreased ventricular function, or pericardial effusion |

- *Complete blood count (CBC)* and *erythrocyte sedimentation rate (ESR)* are indicators of the inflammatory process. The white blood cell count is elevated, and the number of red blood cells may be low due to the inflammatory inhibition of erythropoiesis. The ESR, a general indicator of inflammation, is elevated.
- *C-reactive protein (CRP)* is positive in an active inflammatory process.
- *Antistreptolysin (ASO) titer* is a test for streptococcal antibodies. It rises within 2 months of the onset and is positive in most clients with rheumatic fever.
- Throat culture is positive for group A β-hemolytic streptococcus in only 25% to 40% of clients with acute rheumatic fever (Braunwald et al., 2001).

## Medications

As soon as rheumatic fever is diagnosed, antibiotics are started to eliminate the streptococcal infection. Penicillin is the antibiotic of choice to treat group A streptococci. Antibiotics are prescribed for at least 10 days. Erythromycin or clindamycin is used if the client is allergic to penicillin. Prophylactic antibiotic therapy is continued for 5 to 10 years to prevent recurrences. Recurrences after 5 years or age 25 are rare (Tierney et al., 2001). Penicillin G, 1.2 million units injected intramuscularly every 3 to 4 weeks, is the prophylaxis of choice. Oral penicillin, amoxicillin, sulfadiazine, or erythromycin may also be used.

Joint pain and fever are treated with salicylates (e.g., aspirin), ibuprofen, or another nonsteroidal anti-inflammatory drug (NSAID); corticosteroids may be used for severe pain due to inflammation or carditis. See Chapter 9 ⊙ for information about the use of these anti-inflammatory medications.

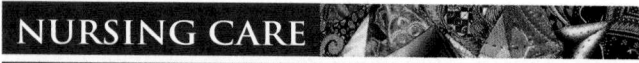

## NURSING CARE

### Health Promotion

Rheumatic fever is preventable. Prompt identification and treatment of streptococcal throat infections helps decrease spread of the pathogen and the risk for rheumatic fever. Characteristics of streptococcal sore throat include a red, fiery-looking throat, pain with swallowing, enlarged and tender cervical lymph nodes, fever range of 101° to 104°F (38.3° to 40.0°C), and headache. Emphasize the importance of finishing the complete course of medication to eradicate the pathogen.

### Assessment

Assess clients at risk for rheumatic fever (prolonged, untreated or recurrent pharyngitis) for possible manifestations.

- Health history: complaints of recent sore throat with fever, difficulty swallowing, and general malaise; treatment measures; previous history of strep throat or rheumatic fever; history of heart murmur or other cardiac problems; current medications
- Physical examination: vital signs including temperature; skin color, presence of rash on trunk or proximal extremities; mental status; evidence of inflamed joints; heart and lung sounds

### Nursing Diagnoses and Interventions

The nursing care focus for the client with RHD is on providing supportive care and preventing complications. Teaching to prevent recurrence of rheumatic fever is extremely important. *Pain* and *Activity intolerance* are priority nursing diagnoses for the client with rheumatic fever and RHD.

#### Acute Pain

Joint and chest pain due to acute inflammation is common in rheumatic fever. Pain and inflammation may interfere with rest and healing.

- Administer anti-inflammatory drugs as ordered. Promptly report manifestations of aspirin toxicity, including tinnitus, vomiting, and gastrointestinal bleeding. Give aspirin and other NSAIDs with food, milk, or antacids to minimize gastric irritation. *Joint pain and fever may be treated with anti-inflammatory agents such as aspirin and NSAIDs. When used for its anti-inflammatory effect, aspirin doses may be high, and it is given around the clock (e.g., every 4 hours). Steroids may be prescribed for severe carditis.*
- Provide warm, moist compresses for local pain relief of acutely inflamed joints. *Moist heat helps relieve pain associated with inflamed joints by reducing inflammation.*
- Auscultate heart sounds as indicated (every shift or each home visit). Notify the physician if a pericardial friction rub or a new murmur develops. *A friction rub is produced as inflamed pericardial surfaces rub against each other. This also stimulates pain receptors, and may increase discomfort.*

#### Activity Intolerance

The client with acute carditis or RHD may develop heart failure if the heart is unable to supply enough oxygen to meet the body's demand. Manifestations of fatigue, weakness, and dyspnea on exertion may result.

- Explain the importance of activity limitations and reinforce teaching as needed. *Activities are limited during the acute phase of carditis to reduce the workload of the heart. Understanding the rationale improves cooperation with the limitations.*
- Encourage social and diversional activities such as visits with friends and family, reading, playing cards or board games, watching television, and listening to music or talking books. *Diversional activities provide a focus for the client whose physical activities must be limited.*
- Encourage gradual increases in activity, monitoring for evidence of intolerance or heart failure. Consult a cardiac rehabilitation specialist to help design an activity progression schedule. *Gradual activity progression is encouraged as the client's condition improves. Activity tolerance is monitored and activities modified as needed.*

### Home Care

Most clients with rheumatic fever and carditis do not require hospitalization. Teaching for home care focuses on both acute care and preventing recurrences and further tissue damage. Include the following topics.

- The importance of completing the full course of antibiotic therapy and continuing antibiotic prophylaxis as prescribed For the client with chronic RHD, include the importance of antibiotic prophylaxis for invasive procedures (e.g., dental care, endoscopy, or surgery) to prevent bacterial endocarditis. Pamphlets on endocarditis prevention are helpful reminders, and are available from the American Heart Association.
- Preventive dental care and good oral hygiene to maintain oral health and prevent gingival infections, which can lead to recurrence of the disease
- Early recognition of streptococcal sore throat and appropriate treatment for both the client and family members
- Early manifestations of heart failure to report to the physician
- Prescribed medications, including their dosage, route, intended and potential adverse effects, and manifestations to report to the physician
- Dietary sodium restriction if ordered or recommended. A high-carbohydrate, high-protein diet may be recommended to facilitate healing and combat fatigue.

Refer for home health services or household assistance as indicated.

## THE CLIENT WITH INFECTIVE ENDOCARDITIS

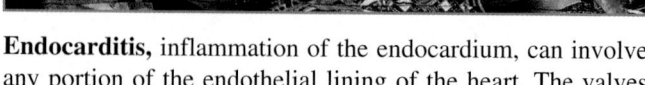

**Endocarditis,** inflammation of the endocardium, can involve any portion of the endothelial lining of the heart. The valves usually are affected. Endocarditis is usually infectious in nature, characterized by colonization or invasion of the endocardium and heart valves by a pathogen.

| TABLE 30-5 | Classifications of Infective Endocarditis | |
|---|---|---|
| | **Acute Infective Endocarditis** | **Subacute Infective Endocarditis** |
| Onset | Sudden | Gradual |
| Usual organism | *Staphylococcus aureus* | *Streptococcus viridans*, enterococci, gram-negative and gram-positive bacilli, fungi, yeasts |
| Risk factors | Usually occurs in previously normal heart; intravenous drug use, infected intravenous sites | Usually occurs in damaged or deformed hearts; dental work, invasive procedures, and infections |
| Pathologic process | Rapid valve destruction | Valve destruction leading to regurgitation; embolization of friable vegetations |
| Presentation | Abrupt onset with spiking fever and chills; manifestations of heart failure | Gradual onset of febrile illness with cough, dyspnea, arthralgias, abdominal pain |

Endocarditis is relatively uncommon, with an incidence of 1.5 to 6.2 cases per 100,000 people in developed countries (Braunwald et al., 2001). The greatest risk factor for endocarditis is previous heart damage. Lesions develop on deformed valves, on valve prostheses, or in areas of tissue damage due to congential deformities or ischemic disease. The left side of the heart, the mitral valve in particular, is usually affected. Intravenous drug use also is a significant risk factor. The right side of the heart usually is affected in these clients. Other risk factors include invasive catheters (e.g., a central venous catheter, hemodynamic monitoring, or an indwelling urinary catheter), dental procedures or poor dental health, and recent heart surgery.

Endocarditis is classified by its acuity and disease course (Table 30–5). *Acute infective endocarditis* has an abrupt onset and is a rapidly progressive, severe disease. Although almost any organism can cause infective endocarditis, virulent organisms such as *Staphylococcus aureus* cause a more abrupt onset and destructive course. *S. aureus* is commonly the infective organism in acute endocarditis. In contrast, *subacute infective endocarditis* has a more gradual onset, with predominant systemic manifestations. It is more likely to occur in clients with preexisting heart disease. *Streptococcus viridans,* enterococci, other gram-negative and gram-positive bacilli, yeasts, and fungi tend to cause the subacute forms of endocarditis (Porth, 2002).

*Prosthetic valve endocarditis (PVE)* may occur in clients with a mechanical or tissue valve replacement. This infection may develop in the early postoperative period (within 2 months after surgery) or late. Prosthetic valve endocarditis accounts for 10% to 20% of endocarditis cases. It usually affects males over the age of 60, and is more frequently associated with aortic valve prostheses than with mitral valve replacements. Early PVE is usually due to prosthetic valve contamination during surgery or perioperative bacteremia. Its course often is rapid, and mortality is high. Late-onset PVE more closely resembles subacute endocarditis.

## PATHOPHYSIOLOGY

Entry of pathogens into the bloodstream is required for infective endocarditis to develop. Bacteria may enter through oral lesions, during dental work or invasive procedures, such as intravenous catheter insertion, surgery, or urinary catheterization; during intravenous drug use; or as a result of infectious processes such as urinary tract or upper respiratory infection.

The initial lesion is a sterile platelet-fibrin vegetation formed on damaged endothelium (Figure 30–5 ■). In acute infective endocarditis, these lesions develop on healthy valve structures, although the mechanism is unknown. In subacute endocarditis, they usually develop on already damaged valves or in endocardial tissue that has been damaged by abnormal pressures or blood flow within the heart.

Organisms that have invaded the blood colonize these vegetations. The vegetation enlarges as more platelets and fibrin are attracted to the site and cover the infecting organism. This covering "protects" the bacteria from quick removal by immune defenses such as phagocytosis by neutrophils, antibodies, and complement. Vegetations may be singular or multiple. They expand while loosely attached to edges of the valve. Friable vegetations can break or shear off, embolizing and traveling through the bloodstream to other organ systems. When they lodge in small vessels, they may cause hemorrhages, infarcts, or abscesses. Ultimately, the vegetations scar and deform the valves and cause turbulence of blood flowing through the heart. Heart valve function is affected, either obstructing forward blood flow, or closing incompletely.

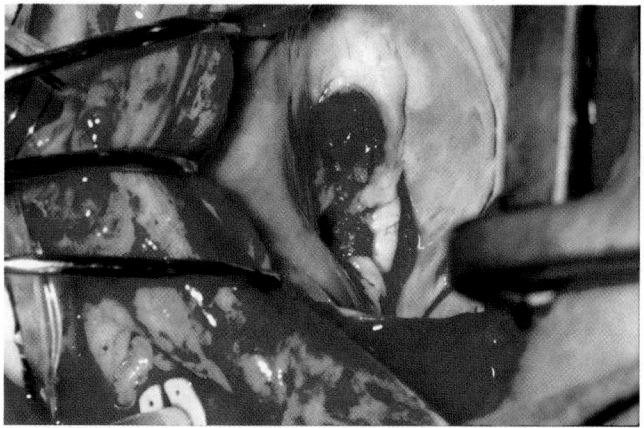

**Figure 30–5** ■ A vegetative lesion of bacterial endocarditis.

*Source: M. English/Custom Medical Stock Photo, Inc.*

## Manifestations of Infective Endocarditis

- Chills and fever
- General malaise, fatigue
- Arthralgias
- Cough, dyspnea
- Heart murmur
- Anorexia, abdominal pain
- Petechiae, splinter hemorrhages
- Splenomegaly

## MANIFESTATIONS AND COMPLICATIONS

The manifestations of infective endocarditis often are non-specific (see the box above). A temperature above 101.5°F (39.4°C) and flulike symptoms develop, accompanied by cough, shortness of breath, and joint pain. The presentation of acute staphylococcal endocarditis is more severe, with a sudden onset, chills, and a high fever. Heart murmurs are heard in 90% of persons with infective endocarditis. An existing murmur may worsen, or a new murmur may develop.

Embolic complications may affect any organ system, particularly the lungs, brain, kidneys, and the skin and mucous membranes. Splenomegaly is common in chronic disease. Peripheral manifestations of infective endocarditis result from microemboli or circulating immune complexes. These manifestations include:

- *Petechiae,* small, purplish-red hemorrhagic spots on the trunk, conjunctiva, and mucous membranes.
- *Splinter hemorrhages,* hemorrhagic streaks under the fingernails or toenails.
- *Osler's nodes,* small, reddened, painful raised growths on finger and toe pads.
- *Janeway lesions,* small, nontender, purplish-red macular lesions on the palms of the hands and soles of the feet.
- *Roth's spots,* small, whitish spots (cotton-wool spots) seen on the retina.

Infective endocarditis often causes complications such as heart failure, infarction of other organs from embolization of vegetative fragments, abscess, and aneurysms due to infiltration of the arterial wall by organisms. Without treatment, endocarditis is almost universally fatal; fortunately, antibiotic therapy is usually effective to treat this disease.

## COLLABORATIVE CARE

Eradicating the infecting organism and minimizing valve damage and other adverse consequences of infective endocarditis are the priorities of care.

### Diagnostic Tests

There are no definitive tests for infective endocarditis, but diagnostic tests help establish the diagnosis.

- *Blood cultures* usually are positive for bacteria or other pathogens. Blood cultures are considered positive when a typical infecting organism is identified from two or more separate blood cultures (drawn from different sites and/or at different times, e.g., 12-hour intervals).
- *Echocardiography* allows visualization of vegetations and evaluation of valve function. Transthoracic echocardiography (TTE) is noninvasive and can be done at the client's bedside; however, it is less sensitive than transesophageal echocardiography (TEE). The ultrasound transducer is combined with an endoscope in TEE. See page 548 for nursing care of the client undergoing an upper endoscopy. Echocardiography can be diagnostic for infective endocarditis when combined with positive blood cultures.
- *Serologic immune testing* for circulating antigens to typical infective organisms may be done.

Other diagnostic tests may include the CBC, ESR, serum creatinine, chest X-ray, and an electrocardiogram.

### Medications

Preventing endocarditis in clients at high risk is important. Antibiotics are commonly prescribed for clients with preexisting valve damage or heart disease prior to high risk procedures (Table 30–6).

### TABLE 30–6  Antibiotic Prophylaxis for Infective Endocarditis

| Indications for Prophylaxis | Selected Procedures for Which Prophylaxis Is Recommended | Suggested Antibiotics |
| --- | --- | --- |
| Prosthetic valves | Dental procedures in which bleeding is likely, including cleaning | Amoxicillin |
| Previous episode(s) of infective endocarditis | Most surgeries | Erythromycin |
| Rheumatic heart disease | Bronchoscopy | Ampicillin |
| Hypertrophic cardiomyopathy | Cystoscopy | Clindamycin |
| Mitral valve prolapse with regurgitation and murmur | Urinary catheterization when infection is present | Vancomycin |
| Sclerotic aortic valve | Incision and drainage of infected tissue | (*Note:* choice of antibiotic depends on procedure) |
| Most congenital heart malformations | Vaginal delivery if infection is present | |

Antibiotic therapy effectively treats infective endocarditis in most cases. The goal of therapy is to eradicate the infecting organism from the blood and vegetative lesions in the heart. The fibrin covering that protects colonies of organisms from immune defenses also protects them from antibiotic therapy. Therefore, an extended course of multiple intravenous antibiotics is required.

Following blood cultures, antibiotic therapy is initiated with drugs known to be effective against the most common infecting organisms: staphylococci, streptococci, and enterococci. The initial regimen may include nafcillin or oxacillin, penicillin or ampicillin, and gentamicin. Once the organism has been identified, therapy is tailored to that organism. Streptococcal and enterococcal infections are treated with a combination of penicillin and gentamicin. If the client is allergic to penicillin, ceftriaxone, cefazolin, or vancomycin may be used. Staphyloccoal infections are treated with nafcillin or oxacillin and gentamicin; cefazolin or vancomycin may be used if penicillin allergy is present. Intravenous drug therapy is continued for 2 to 8 weeks, depending on the infecting organism, the drugs used, and the results of repeat blood cultures. See Chapter 8 for the nursing implications for antibiotic therapy. 🔗

The client with prosthetic valve endocarditis requires extended treatment, usually 6 to 8 weeks. Combination therapy using vancomycin, rifampin, and gentamicin is used to treat these resistant infections.

## Surgery

Some clients with infective endocarditis require surgery to:

- Replace severely damaged valves.
- Remove large vegetations at risk for embolization
- Remove a valve that is a continuing source of infection that does not respond to antibiotic therapy.

The most common indication for surgery is valvular regurgitation that causes heart failure and does not respond to medical therapy. When the infection has not responded to antibiotic therapy within 7 to 10 days, the infected valve may be replaced to facilitate eradication of the organism. Clients with fungal endocarditis usually require surgical intervention. More information on valve replacement surgery is provided in the section on valve disorders.

## NURSING CARE

## Health Promotion

Prevention of endocarditis is vital in susceptible people. Education is a key part of prevention. Use every opportunity to educate individuals and the public about the risks of intravenous drug use, including endocarditis. Discuss preventive measures with all clients with specific risk factors, such as a heart murmur or known heart disease.

## Assessment

Assessment related to ineffective endocarditis includes identifying risk factors and manifestations of the disease.

- Health history: complaints of persistent flulike symptoms, fatigue, shortness of breath, and activity intolerance; history of recent dental work or other invasive procedures; known heart murmur, valve or other heart disorder; recent intravenous drug use
- Physical examination: Vital signs including temperature; apical pulse and heart sounds; rate and ease of respirations, lung sounds; skin color, temperature, and presence of petechiae or splinter hemorrhages

## Nursing Diagnoses and Interventions

Nursing care focuses on managing the manifestations of endocarditis, administering antibiotics, and teaching the client and family members about the disorder. In addition to the diagnoses identified below, nursing diagnoses and interventions for heart failure also may be appropriate for clients with infective endocarditis.

### Risk for Imbalanced Body Temperature

Fever is common in clients with infective endocarditis. It may be acutely elevated and accompanied by chills, particularly with acute infective endocarditis. The inflammatory process initiates a cycle of events that affects the regulation of temperature and causes discomfort.

- Record temperature every 2 to 4 hours. Report temperature above 101.5°F (39.4°C). Assess for complaints of discomfort. *Fever is usually low grade (below 101.5°F [39.4°C]) in infective endocarditis; higher temperatures may cause discomfort. The temperature usually returns to normal within 1 week after initiation of antibiotic therapy. Continued fever may indicate a need to modify the treatment regimen.*
- Obtain blood cultures as ordered, before initial antibiotic dose. *Initial blood cultures are obtained before antibiotic therapy is started to obtain adequate organisms to culture and identify. Follow-up cultures are used to assess the effectiveness of therapy.*
- Provide anti-inflammatory or antipyretic agents as prescribed. *Fever may be treated with anti-inflammatory or antipyretic agents such as aspirin, ibuprofen, or acetaminophen.*
- Administer antibiotics as ordered; obtain peak and trough drug levels as indicated. *Intravenous antibiotics are given to eradicate the pathogen. Peak and trough levels are used to evaluate the dose effectiveness in maintaining a therapeutic blood level.*

### Risk for Ineffective Tissue Perfusion

Embolization of vegetative lesions can threaten tissue and organ perfusion. Vegetations from the left heart may lodge in arterioles or capillaries of the brain, kidneys, or peripheral tissues, causing infarction or abscess. A large embolism can cause manifestations of stroke or transient ischemic attack, renal failure, or tissue ischemia. Emboli from the right side of the heart become entrapped in pulmonary vasculature, causing manifestations of pulmonary embolism.

- Assess for, document, and report manifestations of decreased organ system perfusion:
  a. Neurologic: changes in level of consciousness, numbness or tingling in extremities, hemiplegia, visual disturbances, or manifestations of stroke

b. Renal: decreased urine output, hematuria, elevated BUN or creatinine
c. Pulmonary: dyspnea, hemoptysis, shortness of breath, diminished breath sounds, restlessness, sudden chest or shoulder pain
d. Cardiovascular: chest pain radiating to jaw or arms, tachycardia, anxiety, tachypnea, hypotension

*All major organs and tissues, and the microcirculation may be affected by emboli when vegetations break off due to turbulent blood flow. Emboli may cause manifestations of organ dysfunction. The most devastating effects of emboli are in the brain and the myocardium, with resulting infarctions. Intravenous drug users have a high risk of pulmonary emboli as a result of right-sided endocardial fragments.*

- Assess and document skin color and temperature, quality of peripheral pulses, and capillary refill. *Peripheral emboli affect tissue perfusion, with a risk for tissue necrosis and possible extremity loss.*

### Ineffective Health Maintenance

The client with endocarditis often is treated in the community. Teaching about disease management and prevention of possible recurrences of endocarditis is vital.

- Demonstrate intravenous catheter site care and intermittent antibiotic administration if the client and family will manage therapy. Have the client and/or significant other redemonstrate appropriate techniques. *Intermittent antibiotic infusions may be managed by the client or family members, or the client may go to an outpatient facility to receive the infusions. Appropriate site care is necessary to reduce the risk of trauma and infection.*
- Explain the actions, doses, administration, and desired and adverse effects of prescribed drugs. Identify manifestations to be reported to the physician. Provide practical information about measures to reduce the risk of superinfection (e.g., consuming 8 oz of yogurt or buttermilk containing live bacterial cultures daily). *Careful compliance with prescribed drug therapy is vital to eradicate the infecting organism. Antibiotic therapy can, however, cause superinfections such as candidiasis due to elimination of normal body flora.*
- Teach about the function of heart valves and the effects of endocarditis on heart function. Include a simple definition of endocarditis, and explain the risk for its recurrence. *Information helps the client and family understand endocarditis, its treatment, and its effects. Understanding increases compliance.*
- Describe the manifestations of heart failure to be reported to the physician. *Evidence of heart failure may necessitate modification of the treatment regimen or replacement of infected valves.*

**PRACTICE ALERT** *Stress the importance of notifying all care providers of valve disease, heart murmur, or valve replacement before undergoing invasive procedures. Invasive procedures provide a portal of entry for bacteria. A history of valve disease increases the risk for the development or recurrence of endocarditis.* ■

- Encourage good dental hygiene and mouth care and regular dental checkups. Teach how to prevent bleeding from the gums and avoid developing mouth ulcers (e.g., gentle toothbrushing, ensuring that dentures fit properly, and avoiding toothpicks, dental floss, and high-flow water devices). *The oropharynx harbors streptococci, which are common causes of endocarditis. Bleeding gums offer an opportunity for bacteria to enter the bloodstream.*
- Encourage the client to avoid people with upper respiratory infections. *Streptococci are normal pathogens in the upper respiratory tract; exposure to people with upper respiratory infections may increase the risk of infection.*
- If anticoagulant therapy is ordered, explain its actions, administration, and major side effects. Identify manifestations of bleeding to be promptly reported to the physician. *Clients with valve disease or a prosthetic valve following infective endocarditis may require continued anticoagulant therapy to prevent thrombi and emboli. Knowledge is vital for appropriate management of anticoagulant therapy and prevention of complications.*

### Home Care

When preparing the client with infective endocarditis for home care, provide teaching as outlined for the nursing diagnosis, *Ineffective health maintenance*. In addition, discuss the following topics.

- Although serious and frightening, infective endocarditis can usually be treated effectively with intravenous antibiotics.
- The importance of promptly reporting any unusual manifestation, such as a change in vision, sudden pain, or weakness, so that interventions to control complications can be promptly implemented.
- The rationale for all treatments and procedures.
- Preventing recurrences of infective endocarditis.
- The importance of maintaining contact with the physician for follow-up care and monitoring for long-term effects such as progressive valve damage and dysfunction.
- If appropriate, explain the risks associated with intravenous drug use.

Provide educational materials on infective endocarditis from the American Heart Association. Refer as appropriate to home health or home intravenous therapy services. Refer the client and family members or significant others as appropriate to a drug or substance abuse treatment program or facility. Provide follow-up care to ensure compliance with the referral and treatment plan.

## THE CLIENT WITH MYOCARDITIS

**Myocarditis** is inflammation of the heart muscle. It usually results from an infectious process, but also may occur as an immunologic response, or due to the effects of radiation, toxins, or drugs. In the United States, myocarditis is usually viral, caused by coxsackievirus B. Approximately 10% of people with HIV disease develop myocarditis due to infiltration of the myocardium by the virus. Bacterial myocarditis, much less common, may be associated with endocarditis caused by *Staphylococcus aureus,* or with diphtheria. Parasitic infections caused by *Trypanosoma cruzi* (Chagas' disease) are common in Central and South America (Braunwald et al., 2001).

Myocarditis may occur at any age, and it is more common in men than women. Factors that alter immune response (e.g., malnutrition, alcohol use, immunosuppressive drugs, exposure to radiation, stress, and advanced age) increase the risk for myocarditis. It also is a common complication of rheumatic fever and pericarditis. Viral myocarditis usually is self-limited; it may progress, however, to become chronic, leading to dilated cardiomyopathy (see the section of this chapter that follows).

## PATHOPHYSIOLOGY AND MANIFESTATIONS

In myocarditis, myocardial cells are damaged by an inflammatory process that causes local or diffuse swelling and damage. Infectious agents infiltrate interstitial tissues, forming abscesses. Autoimmune injury may occur when the immune system destroys not only the invading pathogen but also myocardial cells. The extent of damage to cardiac muscle ultimately determines the long-term outcome of the disease.

The manifestations of myocarditis depend on the degree of myocardial damage. The client may be asymptomatic. Nonspecific manifestations of inflammation such as fever, fatigue, general malaise, dyspnea, palpitations, and arthralgias may be present. A nonspecific febrile illness or upper respiratory infection often precedes the onset of myocarditis symptoms. Abnormal heart sounds such as muffled $S_1$, an $S_3$, murmur, and pericardial friction rub may be heard. Severe myocarditis may lead to heart failure. In some cases, manifestations of myocardial infarction, including chest pain, may occur.

## COLLABORATIVE CARE

Myocarditis treatment focuses on resolving the inflammatory process to prevent further damage to the myocardium.

Diagnostic studies may be ordered to help diagnose myocarditis.

- *Electrocardiography* may show transient ST segment and T wave changes, as well as dysrhythmias and possible heart block.
- *Cardiac markers,* such as the creatinine kinase, troponin T, and troponin I, may be elevated, indicating myocardial cell damage.
- *Endomyocardial biopsy* to examine myocardial cells is necessary to establish a definitive diagnosis; patchy cell necrosis and the inflammatory process can be identified.

If appropriate, antimicrobial therapy is used to eradicate the infecting organism. Antiviral therapy with interferon-α may be instituted. Immunosuppressive therapy with corticosteroids or other immunosuppressive agents (see Chapter 9 ⊂⊃ ) may be used to minimize the inflammatory response. Heart failure is treated as needed, using ACE inhibitors and drugs. Clients with myocarditis often are particularly sensitive to the effects of dig-

italis, so it is used with caution. Other medications used in treating myocarditis include antidysrhythmic agents as to control dysrhythmias and anticoagulants to prevent emboli.

Bed rest and activity restrictions are ordered during the acute inflammatory process to reduce myocardial work and prevent myocardial damage. Activities may be limited for as long as 6 months to a year (Porth, 2002).

## NURSING CARE

Nursing care is directed at decreasing myocardial work and maintaining cardiac output. Both physical and emotional rest are indicated, because anxiety increases myocardial oxygen demand. Hemodynamic parameters and the ECG are monitored closely, especially during the acute phase of the illness. Activity tolerance, urine output, and heart and breath sounds are frequently assessed for manifestations of heart failure. Consider the following nursing diagnoses for the client with myocarditis.

- *Activity intolerance* related to impaired cardiac muscle function
- *Decreased cardiac output* related to myocardial inflammation
- *Fatigue* related to inflammation and impaired cardiac output
- *Anxiety* related to possible long-term effects of the disorder
- *Excess fluid volume* related to compensatory mechanisms for decreased cardiac output

### Home Care

Include the following topics when preparing the client with myocarditis for home care.

- Activity restrictions and other prescribed measures to reduce cardiac workload
- Early manifestations of heart failure to report to the physician
- The importance of following the prescribed treatment regimen
- Any recommended dietary modifications (such as a low-sodium diet for heart failure)
- Prescribed medications, their purpose, doses, and possible adverse effects
- The importance of adhering to the treatment plan and recommended follow-up appointments to reduce the risk of long-term consequences such as cardiomyopathy

## THE CLIENT WITH PERICARDITIS

The pericardium is the outermost layer of the heart. It is a two-layered membranous sac with a thin layer of serous fluid (normally no more than 30 to 50 mL) separating the layers. It protects and cushions the heart and the great vessels, provides a barrier to infectious processes in adjacent structures, prevents displacement of the myocardium and blood vessels, and prevents sudden distention of the heart.

**Pericarditis** is the inflammation of the pericardium. Pericarditis may be a primary disorder or develop secondarily to another cardiac or systemic disorder. Some possible causes of

| BOX 30–4 | Selected Causes of Pericarditis |
|---|---|

**INFECTIOUS**
- Viruses
- Bacteria
- Tuberculosis
- Fungi
- Syphilis
- Parasites

**NONINFECTIOUS**
- Myocardial and pericardial injury
- Uremia
- Neoplasms
- Radiation
- Trauma or surgery
- Myxedema
- Autoimmune disorders
- Rheumatic fever
- Connective tissue diseases
- Prescription and nonprescription drugs
- Postcardiac injury

pericarditis are listed in Box 30–4. Acute pericarditis is usually viral and affects men (usually under the age of 50) more frequently than women (Tierney et al., 2001). Pericarditis affects 40% to 50% of clients with end-stage renal disease and uremia. Postmyocardial infarction pericarditis and postcardiotomy (following open-heart surgery) pericarditis also are common.

## PATHOPHYSIOLOGY

Pericardial tissue damage triggers an inflammatory response. Inflammatory mediators released from the injured tissue cause vasodilation, hyperemia, and edema. Capillary permeability increases, allowing plasma proteins, including fibrinogen, to escape into the pericardial space. White blood cells amass at the site of injury to destroy the causative agent. Exudate is formed, usually fibrinous or serofibrinous (a mixture of serous fluid and fibrinous exudate). In some cases, the exudate may contain red blood cells or, if infectious, purulent material. The inflammatory process may resolve without long-term effects, or scar tissue and adhesions may form between the pericardial layers.

Fibrosis and scarring of the pericardium may restrict cardiac function. Pericardial effusions may develop as serous or purulent exudate (depending on the causative agent) collects in the pericardial sac. Pericardial effusion may be recurrent. Chronic inflammation causes the pericardium to become rigid.

## MANIFESTATIONS AND COMPLICATIONS

Classic manifestations of acute pericarditis include chest pain, a pericardial friction rub, and fever. Chest pain, the most common symptom, has an abrupt onset. It is caused by inflammation of nerve fibers in the lower parietal pericardium and pleura covering the diaphragm. The pain is usually sharp, may be steady or intermittent, and may radiate to the back or neck. The pain can mimic myocardial ischemia; careful assessment is important to rule out myocardial infarction. Pericardial pain is aggravated by respiratory movements (i.e., deep inspiration and/or coughing), changes in body position, or swallowing. Sitting upright and leaning forward reduces the discomfort by moving the heart away from the diaphragmatic side of the lung pleura.

Although not always present, a *pericardial friction rub* is the characteristic sign of pericarditis. A pericardial friction rub is a leathery, grating sound produced by the inflamed pericardial layers rubbing against the chest wall or pleura. It is heard most clearly at the left lower sternal border with the client sitting up or leaning forward. The rub is usually heard on expiration and may be constant or intermittent.

A low-grade fever (below 100°F [38.4°C]) often develops due to the inflammatory process. Dyspnea and tachycardia are common.

Pericardial effusion, cardiac tamponade, and constrictive pericarditis are possible complications of acute pericarditis.

## Pericardial Effusion

A *pericardial effusion* is an abnormal collection of fluid between the pericardial layers that threatens normal cardiac function. The fluid may consist of pus, blood, serum, lymph, or a combination. The manifestations of a pericardial effusion depend on the rate at which the fluid collects. Although the pericardium normally contains about 30 to 50 mL of fluid, the sac can stretch to accommodate a gradual accumulation of fluid. Over time, the pericardial sac can accommodate up to 2 L of fluid without immediate adverse effects. Conversely, a rapid buildup of pericardial fluid (as little as 100 mL) does not allow the sac to stretch and can compress the heart, interfering with myocardial function. This compression of the heart is known as **cardiac tamponade.** Slowly developing pericardial effusion is often painless and has few manifestations. Heart sounds may be distant or muffled. The client may have a cough or mild dyspnea.

## Cardiac Tamponade

Cardiac tamponade is a medical emergency that must be aggressively treated to preserve life. Cardiac tamponade may result from pericardial effusion, trauma, cardiac rupture, or hemorrhage. Rapid collection of fluid in the pericardial sac interferes with ventricular filling and pumping, critically reducing cardiac output.

Classic manifestations of cardiac tamponade result from rising intracardiac pressures, decreased diastolic filling, and decreased cardiac output. A hallmark of cardiac tamponade is a paradoxical pulse, or *pulsus paradoxus*. A paradoxical pulse markedly decreases in amplitude during inspiration. Intrathoracic pressure normally drops during inspiration, enhancing venous return to the right heart. This draws more blood into the right side of the heart than the left, causing the interventricular septum to bulge slightly into the left ventricle. When ventricular filling is impaired by excess fluid in the pericardial sac, this bulging of the interventricular septum decreases cardiac output during inspiration. On palpation of the carotid or femoral artery, the pulse is diminished or absent during inspiration. A drop in systolic blood pressure of more than 10 mmHg during inspiration also indicates pulsus paradoxus.

Other manifestations of cardiac tamponade include muffled heart sounds, dyspnea and tachypnea, tachycardia, a narrowed pulse pressure, and distended neck veins (see the box on the next page).

## Manifestations of Cardiac Tamponade

- Paradoxical pulse
- Narrowed pulse pressure, hypotension
- Tachycardia
- Weak peripheral pulses
- Distant, muffled heart sounds
- Jugular venous distention
- High central venous pressure
- Decreased level of consciousness
- Low urine output
- Cool, mottled skin

## Chronic Constrictive Pericarditis

Chronic pericardial inflammation can lead to scar tissue formation between the pericardial layers. This scar tissue eventually contracts, restricting diastolic filling and elevating venous pressure. Constrictive pericarditis may follow viral infection, radiation therapy, or heart surgery. Its manifestations include progressive dyspnea, fatigue, and weakness. Ascites is common; peripheral edema may develop. Neck veins are distended, and may be particularly noticeable during inspiration (*Kussmaul's sign*). This occurs because the right atrium is unable to dilate to accommodate increased venous return during inspiration.

## COLLABORATIVE CARE

Care for the client with pericarditis focuses on identifying its cause if possible, reducing inflammation, relieving symptoms, and preventing complications. The client is closely monitored for early manifestations of cardiac tamponade so that it can be treated promptly.

### Diagnostic Tests

There are no specific laboratory tests to diagnose pericarditis, but tests are often performed to differentiate pericarditis from myocardial infarction.

- *CBC* shows elevated WBCs and an ESR greater than 20 mm/h indicating acute inflammation.
- *Cardiac enzymes* may be slightly elevated because the inflammatory process extends to involve the epicardial surface of the heart. Cardiac enzymes are typically much lower in pericarditis than in myocardial infarction.
- *Electrocardiography* shows typical changes associated with pericarditis, such as diffuse ST segment elevation in all leads. This resolves more quickly than changes of acute MI and is not associated with the QRS complex and T wave changes typically seen in MI. With a large pericardial effusion, the QRS amplitude may be decreased. Atrial dysrhythmias may occur in acute pericarditis.
- *Echocardiography* is used to assess heart motion, for pericardial effusion, and the extent of restriction.
- *Hemodynamic monitoring* may be used in acute pericarditis or pericardial effusion to assess pressures and cardiac output.

Elevated pulmonary artery pressures and venous pressures occur with impaired filling due to pericardial effusion or constrictive pericarditis.

- *Chest X-ray* may show cardiac enlargement if a pericardial effusion is present.
- *Computed tomography (CT scan)* or *magnetic resonance imaging (MRI)* may be used to identify pericardial effusion or constrictive pericarditis.

### Medications

Drug treatment for pericarditis addresses its manifestations. Aspirin and acetaminophen may be used to reduce fever. Nonsteroidal anti-inflammatory drugs (NSAIDs) are used to reduce inflammation and promote comfort. In severe cases or with recurrent pericarditis, corticosteroids may be given to suppress the inflammatory response.

### Pericardiocentesis

*Pericardiocentesis* may be done to remove fluid from the pericardial sac for diagnostic or therapeutic purposes (Figure 30–6 ■). The physician inserts a large (16 to 18 gauge) needle to the left of the xiphoid process into the pericardial sac and withdraws excess fluid. The needle is attached to an ECG monitoring lead to help determine if the needle is touching the epicardial surface, which helps prevent piercing the myocardium. Pericardiocentesis may be an emergency procedure for the client with cardiac tamponade. Nursing implications for pericardiocentesis are outlined in the box on page 898.

### Surgery

For recurrent pericarditis or recurrent pericardial effusion, a rectangular piece of the pericardium, or "window," may be excised to allow collected fluid to drain into the pleural space. Constrictive pericarditis may necessitate a partial or total *pericardiectomy,* removal of part or all of the pericardium, to relieve the ventricular compression and allow adequate filling.

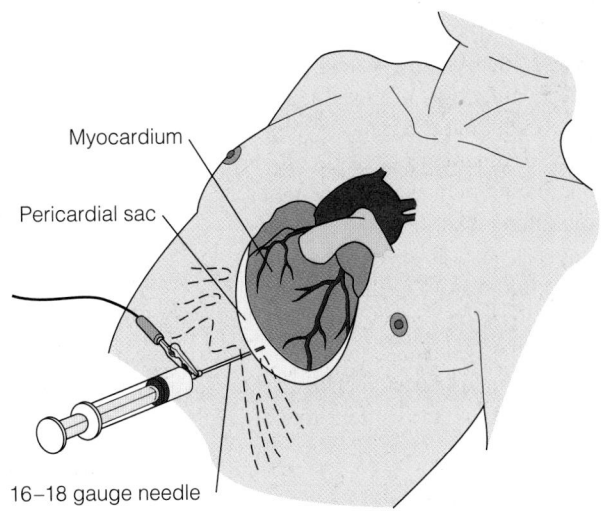

Myocardium

Pericardial sac

16–18 gauge needle

**Figure 30–6 ■** Pericardiocentesis.

## Nursing Implications for Diagnostic Tests

### Pericardiocentesis

**BEFORE THE PROCEDURE**

- Gather all supplies:
  a. Pericardiocentesis tray
  b. ECG machine and electrode patches
  c. Emergency cart with defibrillator
  d. Dressing
  e. Culture bottles (if indicated)
- Reinforce teaching and answer questions about the procedure or associated care. Provide emotional support.
- Ensure that informed consent has been obtained.
- Provide for privacy.
- Obtain and document baseline vital signs.
- Connect the client to a cardiac monitor; obtain a baseline rhythm strip for comparison during and after the procedure.
- Connect the precordial ECG lead to the hub of the aspiration needle using an alligator clamp.

**PROCEDURE**

- Follow standard precautions.
- Position seated at a 45- to 60-degree angle. Place a dry towel under the rib cage to catch blood or fluid leakage.

- Observe the ST segment for elevation and the ECG monitor for signs of myocardial irritability (PVCs) during the procedure; these indicate that the needle is touching the myocardium and should be withdrawn slightly.
- Notify the physician of changes in cardiac rhythm, blood pressure, heart rate, level of consciousness, and urine output. These may indicate cardiac complications.
- Monitor central venous pressure (CVP) and blood pressure closely. As the effusion is relieved, CVP will decrease, and BP will increase.

**AFTER THE PROCEDURE**

- Document the procedure and the client's response to and tolerance of the procedure.
- Continue to monitor vital signs and cardiac rhythm every 15 min during the first hour, every 30 min during the next hour, every hour for the next 24 hours.
- Record the amount of fluid removed as output on the intake and output record.
- If indicated, send a sample of aspirated fluid for culture and sensitivity and laboratory analysis.
- Assess heart and breath sounds.

## NURSING CARE

### Health Promotion

While it may not yet be possible to identify many clients at risk for and to prevent acute pericarditis, early identification and treatment of the disorder can reduce the risk of complications. Promptly report a pericardial friction rub or other manifestations of pericarditis in clients with recent AMI, cardiac surgery, or systemic diseases associated with a risk for pericarditis.

### Assessment

Assessment data to collect from the client with suspected pericarditis includes:

- Health history: complaints of acute substernal or precordial chest pain, effect of movement and breathing on discomfort, pain radiation, associated symptoms; recent AMI, heart surgery, or other cardiac disorder; current medications; chronic conditions such as renal failure or a connective tissue or autoimmune disorder
- Physical examination: vital signs including temperature, variation in systolic BP with respirations; strength of peripheral pulses, variations with respiratory movement; apical pulse, clarity, changes with respiratory movement, presence of a friction rub; neck vein distension; level of consciousness, skin color, and other indicators of cardiac output

### Nursing Diagnoses and Interventions

Nursing care for the client with pericarditis may occur in the acute or community setting. Closely observe for early manifestations of increasing effusion or cardiac tamponade. Priority nursing diagnoses relate to comfort, the risk for tamponade, and effects of the acute inflammatory process.

### Acute Pain

Inflamed pericardial layers rubbing against each other and the lung pleura stimulate phrenic nerve pain fibers in the lower portion of the parietal pericardium. Pain is usually acute and may be severe until inflammation resolves.

- Assess chest pain using a standard pain scale and noting the quality and radiation of the pain. Note nonverbal cues of pain (grimacing, guarding behaviors), and validate with the client. *Careful assessment helps identify the cause of pain. The pain of pericarditis may radiate to the neck or back and is aggravated by movement, coughing, or deep breathing. A pain scale allows evaluation of the effectiveness of interventions.*
- Auscultate heart sounds every 4 hours. *Presence of a pericardial friction rub often correlates with the location and severity of the pain.*
- Administer NSAIDs on a regular basis as prescribed with food. Document effectiveness. *NSAIDs reduce fever, inflammation, and pericardial pain. They are most effective when administered around the clock on a consistent basis. Administering the medications with food helps decrease gastric distress.*
- Maintain a quiet, calm environment, and position of comfort. Offer back rubs, heat/cold therapy, diversional activity, and emotional support. *Supportive interventions enhance the effects of the medication, may decrease pain perception, and convey a sense of caring.*

## Ineffective Breathing Pattern

Respiratory movement intensifies pericardial pain. In an effort to decrease pain, the client often breathes shallowly, increasing the risk for pulmonary complications.

**PRACTICE ALERT** *Document respiratory rate, effort, and breath sounds every 2 to 4 hours. Report adventitious or diminished breath sounds. Shallow, guarded respirations may lead to increased respiratory rate and effort. Poor ventilation of peripheral alveoli may lead to congestion or atelectasis.* ■

- Encourage deep breathing and use of the incentive spirometer. Provide pain medication before respiratory therapy, as needed. *Deep breathing and an incentive spirometer promote alveolar ventilation and prevent atalectasis. Analgesia prior to respiratory treatments improves their effectiveness by decreasing guarding.*
- Administer oxygen as needed. *Supplementary oxygen promotes optimal gas exchange and tissue oxygenation.*
- Place in Fowler's or high-Fowler's position. Assist to a position of comfort. *Appropriate positioning reduces the work of breathing and decreases chest pain due to pericarditis.*

## Risk for Decreased Cardiac Output

The acute inflammatory process of pericarditis can lead to significant pericardial effusion and cardiac tamponade. This potentially fatal complication can also occur with chronic pericardial effusion if the amount of fluid exceeds the ability of the pericardial sac to expand. Constrictive pericarditis increases the risk for decreased cardiac output because of restricted cardiac filling.

- Document vital signs hourly during the acute inflammatory processes. *Frequent assessment allows early recognition of manifestations of decreased cardiac output, such as tachycardia, hypotension, or changes in pulse pressure.*

**PRACTICE ALERT** *Assess heart sounds and peripheral pulses, and observe for neck vein distention and paradoxical pulse hourly. Promptly report distant, muffled heart sounds, new murmurs or extra heart sounds, decreasing quality of peripheral pulses, and distended neck veins. Acute pericardial effusion interferes with normal cardiac filling and pumping, causing venous congestion and decreased cardiac output. As the amount of fluid increases in the pericardial sac, heart sounds are obscured. A drop in systolic blood pressure of more than 10 mmHg on inspiration signifies an abnormal response to changes in intrathoracic pressure.* ■

- Report significant changes or trends in hemodynamic parameters and dysrhythmias. *Compression of the heart interferes with venous return, increasing CVP and right atrial pressures; dysrhythmias may also occur.*
- Promptly report other signs of decreased cardiac output: decreased level of consciousness; decreased urine output; cold, clammy, mottled skin; delayed capillary refill; and weak peripheral pulses. *These signs of decreased organ and tissue perfusion indicate a significant drop in cardiac output.*

- Maintain at least one patent intravenous access site. *The client in cardiac tamponade may require rapid intravenous fluid infusion to restore blood volume and administration of emergency drugs to support the circulation.*
- Prepare for emergency pericardiocentesis and/or surgery as necessary. Provide appropriate explanations and reassurance. Observe for adverse responses during pericardiocentesis. *Excess pericardial fluid must be rapidly evacuated to prevent further compromise of cardiac output and death. Emotional support and explanations reduce the client's and family's anxiety and promote a caring atmosphere.*

## Activity Intolerance

In chronic constrictive pericarditis, pericardial adhesions and scarring restrict pericardial compliance, restricting heart filling and movement. Restricted filling and ineffective cardiac contraction decrease the cardiac output. The heart cannot compensate for increased metabolic demands by increasing cardiac output, and cardiac reserve falls significantly.

- Document vital signs, cardiac rhythm, skin color, and temperature before and after activity. Note any subjective complaints of fatigue, shortness of breath, chest pain, palpitations, or other symptoms with activity. *These parameters help determine the response to increased cardiac work. Increased heart rate and respiratory rate and effort, decreased blood pressure, and dysrhythmias are indicators of activity intolerance. Pallor or cyanosis and cool, clammy, mottled skin are signs of decreased tissue perfusion. Complaints of weakness, shortness of breath, fatigue, dizziness, or palpitations are further evidence of activity intolerance.*
- Work with the client and physical therapist to develop a realistic, progressive activity plan. Monitor response. Encourage independence, but provide assistance as needed. *Client involvement in planning increases the likelihood of success, as well as the client's self-esteem and sense of control. Promoting self-care provides additional control and independence and enhances self-image. Activity that significantly increases the heart rate (more than 20 BPM over resting) should be stopped and reassessed for intensity.*
- Plan interventions and care activities to allow uninterrupted rest and sleep. *This supports healing and restoration of physical and emotional health.*

## Using NANDA, NIC, and NOC

Chart 30–2 shows links between NANDA nursing diagnoses, NIC, and NOC for the client with pericarditis.

## Home Care

Include the following topics when teaching the client and family in preparation for home care.

- The importance of continuing anti-inflammatory medications as ordered Advise to take NSAIDs with food, milk, or antacids to minimize gastric distress, and to notify the physician if unable to tolerate the drug. Instruct to avoid aspirin or preparations containing aspirin while taking NSAIDs because it may interfere with activity.

- Prescribed medications, including dose, desired and possible adverse effects, and interactions with other drugs or food
- Monitoring weight twice weekly because NSAIDs may cause fluid retention.
- Maintaining fluid intake of at least 2500 mL per day to minimize the risk of renal toxicity due to NSAID use.

- Measures to maintain activity restriction if ordered. Activity will be gradually increased once the inflammatory process has resolved.
- Manifestations of recurrent pericarditis, and the importance of reporting these manifestations promptly to the physician.

## CHART 30–2  NANDA, NIC, AND NOC LINKAGES

### The Client with Pericarditis

| NURSING DIAGNOSES | NURSING INTERVENTIONS | NURSING OUTCOMES |
|---|---|---|
| • Activity Intolerance | • Energy Management<br>• Nutrition Management<br>• Self-Care Assistance | • Endurance<br>• Energy Conservation<br>• Self-Care: Activities of Daily Living (ADLs) |
| • Acute Pain | • Medication Management<br>• Positioning | • Comfort Level<br>• Pain: Disruptive Effects |
| • Deficient Knowledge | • Teaching: Disease Process<br>• Teaching: Procedure/Treatment | • Knowledge: Disease Process<br>• Knowledge: Treatment Regimen |
| • Risk for Decreased Cardiac Output | • Cardiac Care: Acute<br>• Invasive Hemodynamic Monitoring<br>• Vital Signs Monitoring | • Cardiac Pump Effectiveness<br>• Circulation Status<br>• Vital Signs Status |

*Note. Data from Nursing Outcomes Classification (NOC) by M. Johnson & M. Maas (Eds.), 1997, St. Louis: Mosby; Nursing Diagnoses: Definitions & Classification 2001–2002 by North American Nursing Diagnosis Association, 2001, Philadelphia: NANDA; Nursing Interventions Classification (NIC) by J.C. McCloskey & G. M. Bulechek (Eds.), 2000, St. Louis: Mosby. Reprinted by permission.*

# DISORDERS OF CARDIAC STRUCTURE

## THE CLIENT WITH VALVULAR HEART DISEASE

Proper heart valve function ensures one-way blood flow through the heart and vascular system. **Valvular heart disease** interferes with blood flow to and from the heart. Acquired valvular disorders can result from acute conditions, such as infective endocarditis, or from chronic conditions, such as rheumatic heart disease. Rheumatic heart disease is the most common cause of valvular disease (McCance & Huether, 2002). Acute myocardial infarction also can damage heart valves, causing tearing, ischemia, or damage to the papillary muscles that affects valve leaflet function. Congenital heart defects may affect the heart valves, often with no manifestations until adulthood. Aging affects heart structure and function, and also increases the risk for valvular disease.

### PHYSIOLOGY REVIEW

The heart valves direct blood flow within and out of the heart. The valves are fibroelastic tissue supported by a ring of fibrous tissue (the annulus) which provides support.

The atrioventricular (AV) valves, the **mitral** (or *bicuspid*) **valve** on the left and the **tricuspid valve** on the right, separate the atria from the ventricles. These valves normally are fully open during diastole, allowing blood to flow freely from the atria into the ventricles. Rising pressure within the ventricles at the onset of systole (contraction) closes the AV valves, creating the $S_1$ heart sound ("lub"). The leaflets of the AV valves are connected to ventricular papillary muscles by fibrous *chordae tendineae*. The chordae tendineae prevent the valve leaflets from bulging back into the atria during systole.

The semilunar valves, the **aortic** and **pulmonic valves,** separate the ventricles from the great vessels. They open during systole, allowing blood to flow out of the heart with ventricular contraction. As the ventricle relaxes and intraventricular pressure falls at the beginning of diastole, the higher pressure within the great vessels (the aorta and pulmonary artery) closes these valves, creating the $S_2$ heart sound ("dup").

### PATHOPHYSIOLOGY AND MANIFESTATIONS

Valvular heart disease occurs as two major types of disorders: stenosis and regurgitation. **Stenosis** occurs when valve leaflets fuse together and cannot fully open or close. The valve open-

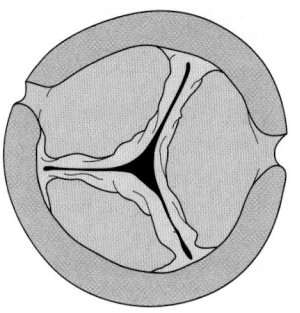 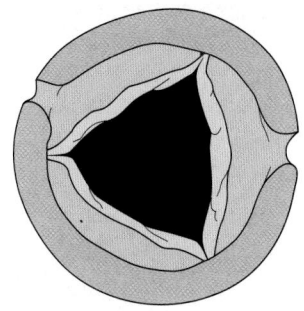

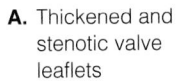

**A.** Thickened and stenotic valve leaflets

**B.** Retracted fibrosed valve openings

**Figure 30–7** ■ Valvular heart disorders. *A,* Stenosis of a heart valve. *B,* An incompetent or regurgitant heart valve.

ing narrows and becomes rigid (Figure 30–7A ■). Scarring of the valves from endocarditis or infarction, and calcium deposits can lead to stenosis. Stenotic valves impede the forward flow of blood, decreasing cardiac output because of impaired ventricular filling or ejection and stroke volume. Because stenotic valves also do not close completely, some backflow of blood occurs when the valve should be fully closed.

Regurgitant valves (also called *insufficient* or *incompetent* valves) do not close completely (Figure 30–7B). This allows **regurgitation,** or backflow of blood, through the valve into the area it just left. Regurgitation can result from deformity or erosion of valve cusps caused by the vegetative lesions of bacterial endocarditis, by scarring or tearing from myocardial infarction, or by cardiac dilation. As the heart enlarges, the valve *annulus* (supporting ring of the valve) is stretched, and the valve edges no longer meet to allow complete closure.

Valvular disease causes hemodynamic changes both in front of and behind the affected valve. Blood volume and pressures are reduced in front of the valve, because flow is obstructed through a stenotic valve and backflow occurs through a regurgitant valve. By contrast, volumes and pressures characteristically increase behind the diseased valve. These hemodynamic changes may lead to pulmonary complications or heart failure. Higher pressures and compensatory changes to maintain cardiac output lead to remodeling and hypertrophy of the heart muscle.

Stenosis increases the work of the chamber behind the affected valve as the heart attempts to move blood through the narrowed opening. Excess blood volume behind regurgitant valves causes dilation of the chamber. In mitral stenosis, for example, the left atrium hypertrophies to generate enough pressure to open and deliver its blood through the narrowed mitral valve. Not all of the blood is delivered before the valve closes, leaving blood to accumulate in the left atrium. This chamber dilates to accommodate the excess volume.

Eventually, cardiac output falls as compensatory mechanisms become less effective. The normal balance of oxygen supply and demand is upset, and the heart begins to fail. In-

creased muscle mass and size increase myocardial oxygen consumption. The size and workload of the heart exceed its blood supply, causing ischemia and chest pain. Eventually, necrosis occurs and functional muscle is lost. Contractile force, stroke volume, and cardiac output decrease. High pressures on the left side of the heart are reflected backward into the pulmonary system, causing pulmonary edema, pulmonary hypertension, and, eventually, right ventricular failure.

Valvular disorders interfere with the smooth flow of blood through the heart. The flow becomes turbulent, causing a **murmur,** a characteristic manifestation of valvular disease. Table 30–7 describes the murmurs associated with various types of valvular disorders.

Blood forced through the narrowed opening of a stenotic valve or regurgitated from a higher pressure chamber through an incompetent valve creates a jet stream effect (much like water spurting out of a partially occluded hose opening). The physical force of this jet stream damages the endocardium of the receiving chamber, increasing the risk for infective endocarditis.

The higher pressures on the left side of the heart subject its valves (the mitral and aortic valves) to more stress and damage than those on the right side of the heart (the tricuspid and pulmonic). Pulmonic valve disease is the least common of the valvular disorders.

## Mitral Stenosis

*Mitral stenosis* narrows the mitral valve, obstructing blood flow from the left atrium into the left ventricle during diastole. It is usually caused by rheumatic heart disease or bacterial endocarditis; it rarely results from congenital defects. It affects females more frequently (66%) than males (Braunwald et al., 2001). Mitral stenosis is chronic and progressive.

In mitral valve stenosis, fibrous tissue replaces normal valve tissue, causing valve leaflets to stiffen and fuse. Resulting changes in blood flow through the valve lead to calcification of the valve leaflets. As calcium is deposited in and on the valve, the leaflets become more rigid and narrow the opening further. As the valve leaflets become less mobile, the chordae tendineae fuse, thicken, and shorten. Thromboemboli may form on the calcified leaflets.

The narrowed mitral opening impairs blood flow into the left ventricle, reducing end-diastolic volume and pressure, and decreasing stroke volume. The narrowed opening also forces the left atrium to generate higher pressure to deliver blood to the left ventricle. This leads to left atrial hypertrophy. The left atrium also dilates as obstructed blood flow increases its volume. As the resistance to blood flow increases, high atrial pressures are reflected back into the pulmonary vessels, increasing pulmonary pressures (Figure 30–8 ■). Pulmonary hypertension increases the workload of the right ventricle, causing it to dilate and hypertrophy. Eventually, heart failure occurs.

Mitral stenosis may be asymptomatic or cause severe impairment. Its manifestations depend on cardiac output and

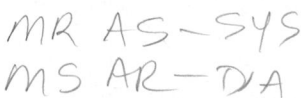

MR AS—SYS
MS AR—DIA

## TABLE 30-7  Heart Murmurs Timing and Characteristics

| Murmur | Cardiac Cycle Timing | Auscultation Site | Configuration of Sound | Continuity |
|---|---|---|---|---|
| Mitral stenosis | Diastole | Apical | $S_2$ —— $S_1$ | Rumble that increases in sound toward the end, continuous |
| Mitral regurgitation | Systole | Apex | $S_1$ —— $S_2$ | Holosystolic (occurs throughout systole), continuous |
| Aortic stenosis | Midsystolic | Right sternal border (RSB) 2nd intercostal space (ICS) | $S_1$ —— $S_2$ | Crescendo-decrescendo, continuous |
| Aortic regurgitation | Diastole (early) | 3rd ICS, LSB | $S_2$ —— $S_1$ | Decrescendo, continuous |
| Tricuspid stenosis | Diastole | Lower LSB | $S_2$ —— $S_1$ | Rumble that increases in sound toward the end, continuous |
| Tricuspid regurgitation | Systole | 4th ICS, LSB | $S_1$ —— $S_2$ | Holosystolic, continuous |

pulmonary vascular pressures. Dyspnea on exertion (DOE) is typically the earliest manifestation. Others include cough, hemoptysis, frequent pulmonary infections such as bronchitis and pneumonia, paroxysmal nocturnal dyspnea, orthopnea, weakness, fatigue, and palpitations. As the stenosis worsens, manifestations of right heart failure, including jugular venous distension, hepatomegaly, ascites, and peripheral edema develop. Crackles may be heard in the lung bases. In severe mitral stenosis, cyanosis of the face and extremities may be noted. Chest pain is rare but may occur.

On auscultation, a loud $S_1$, a split $S_2$, and a mitral opening snap may be heard. The opening snap reflects high left atrial pressure. The murmur of mitral stenosis occurs during diastole, and is typically low-pitched, rumbling, crescendo-decrescendo. It is heard best with the bell of the stethoscope in the apical region. It may be accompanied by a palpable thrill (vibration).

Atrial dysrhythmias, particularly atrial fibrillation, are common due to chronic atrial distention. Thrombi may form and subsequently embolize to the brain, coronary arteries, kidneys, spleen, and extremities—potentially devastating complications.

Women with mitral stenosis may be asymptomatic until pregnancy. As the heart tries to compensate for increased circulating volume (30% more in pregnancy) by increasing cardiac output, left atrial pressures rise, tachycardia reduces ventricular filling and stroke volume, and pulmonary pressures increase. Sudden pulmonary edema and heart failure may threaten the lives of the mother and fetus.

## Mitral Regurgitation

*Mitral regurgitation* or *insufficiency* allows blood to flow back into the left atrium during systole because the valve does not close fully. Rheumatic heart disease is a common cause of mitral regurgitation. Men develop mitral regurgitation more frequently than women. Degenerative calcification of the mitral annulus may cause mitral regurgitation in older women. Processes that dilate the mitral annulus or affect the supporting structures, papillary muscles, or the chordae tendineae may cause mitral regurgitation (e.g., left ventricular hypertrophy and MI). Congenital defects also may cause mitral regurgitation.

In mitral regurgitation, blood flows into both the systemic circulation and back into the left atrium through the deformed valve during systole. This increases left atrial volume (Figure 30–9 ■). The left atrium dilates to accommodate its extra volume, pulling the posterior valve leaflet further away from the valve opening and worsening the defect. The left ventricle dilates to accommodate its increased preload and low cardiac output, further aggravating the problem.

Mitral regurgitation may be asymptomatic or cause symptoms such as fatigue, weakness, exertional dyspnea, and orthopnea. In severe or acute regurgitation, manifestations of left-sided heart failure develop, including pulmonary congestion and edema. High pulmonary pressures may lead to manifestations of right-sided heart failure.

The murmur of mitral regurgitation is usually loud, high pitched, rumbling, and holosystolic (occurring throughout sys-

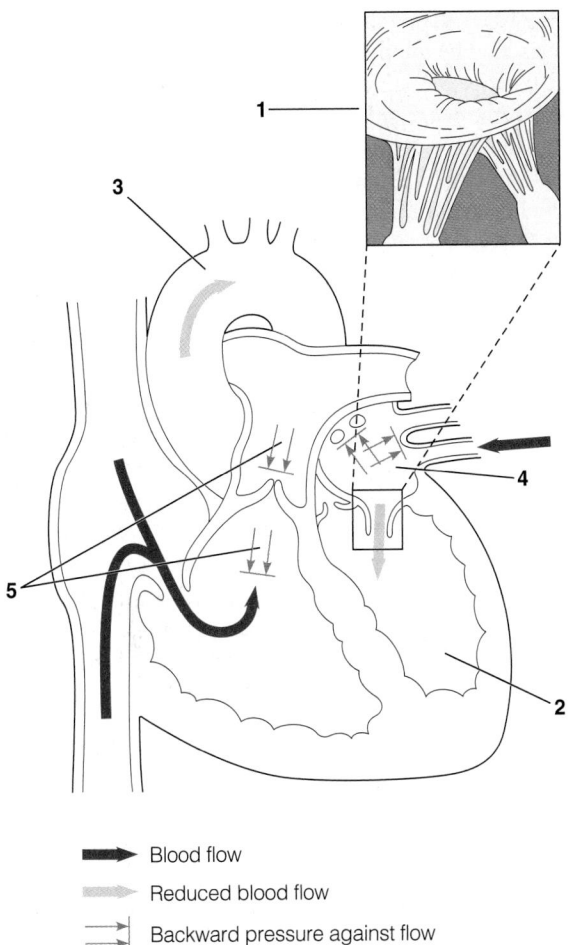

Blood flow

Reduced blood flow

Backward pressure against flow

**Figure 30-8** ■ Mitral stenosis. Narrowing of the mitral valve orifice (1), reduces blood volume to left ventricle (2), reducing cardiac output (3). Rising pressure in the left atrium (4) causes left atrial hypertrophy and pulmonary congestion. Increased pressure in pulmonary vessels (5), causes hypertrophy of the right ventricle and right atrium.

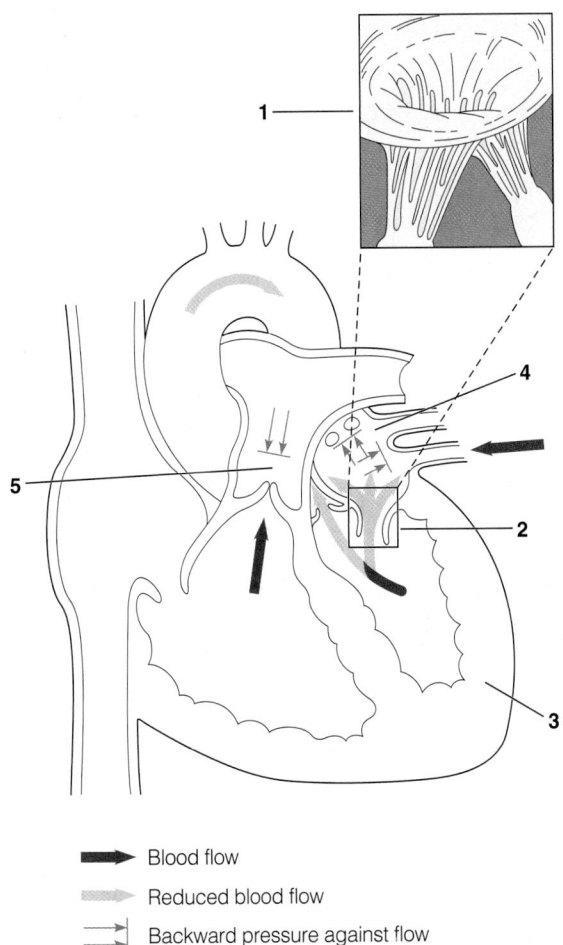

Blood flow

Reduced blood flow

Backward pressure against flow

**Figure 30-9** ■ Mitral regurgitation. The mitral valve closes incompletely (1), allowing blood to regurgitate during systole from the left ventricle to the left atrium (2). Cardiac output falls; to compensate, the left ventricle hypertrophies (3). Rising left atrial pressure (4) causes left atrial hypertrophy and pulmonary congestion. Elevated pulmonary artery pressure (5) causes slight enlargement of the right ventricle.

tole). It is often accompanied by a palpable thrill and is heard most clearly at the cardiac apex. It may be characterized as a cooing or gull-like sound or have a musical quality (Braunwald et al., 2001).

## Mitral Valve Prolapse

*Mitral valve prolapse (MVP)* is a type of mitral insufficiency that occurs when one or both mitral valve cusps billow into the atrium during ventricular systole. MVP is more common in young women between ages 14 and 30; its incidence declines with age. Its cause often is unclear. It also can result from acute or chronic rheumatic damage, ischemic heart disease, or other cardiac disorders. It commonly affects people with inherited connective tissue disorders such as Marfan syndrome (see the Meeting Individual Needs box to the right). Mitral valve prolapse usually is benign, but about 0.01% to 0.02% of people with MVP have thickened mitral leaflets and a significant risk of morbidity and sudden death.

### Meeting Individualized Needs

#### CLIENTS WITH MARFAN SYNDROME

Marfan syndrome is a genetic (autosomal dominant) connective tissue disorder that affects the skeleton, eyes, and cardiovascular system. Skeletal characteristics include a long, thin body, with long extremities and long, tapering fingers, sometimes called *arachnodactyly* (spider fingers) (Copstead & Banasik, 2000). Joints are hyperextensible, and skeletal deformities such as kyphosis, scoliosis, pigeon chest, or pectus excavatum are common. The potentially life-threatening cardiovascular effects of Marfan syndrome include mitral valve prolapse, progressive dilation of the aortic valve ring, and weakness of arterial walls. People with Marfan syndrome frequently die young, between 30 and 40 years, often due to dissection and rupture of the aorta (Porth, 2002).

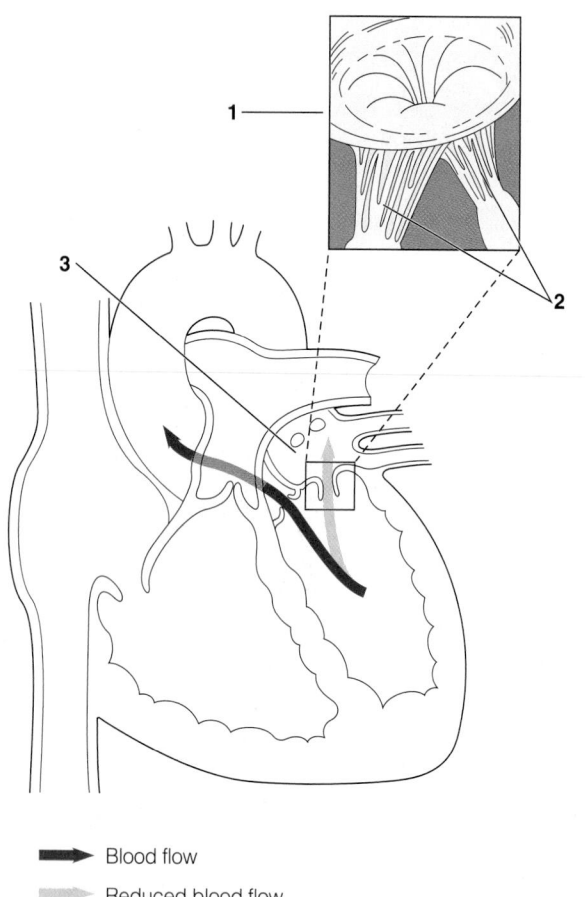

Blood flow

Reduced blood flow

**Figure 30–10 ■** Mitral valve prolapse. Excess tissue in the valve leaflets (1) and elongated cordae tendineae (2) impair mitral valve closure during systole. Some ventricular blood regurgitates into the left atrium (3).

Excess collagen tissue in the valve leaflets and elongated cordae tendineae impair closure of the mitral valve, allowing the leaflets to billow into the left atrium during systole. Some ventricular blood volume regurgitates into the left atrium (Figure 30–10 ■).

Mitral valve prolapse usually is asymptomatic. A midsystolic ejection click or murmur may be audible. A high-pitched late systolic murmur, sometimes described as a "whoop" or "honk," due to the regurgitation of blood through the valve, may develop in MVP. Atypical chest pain is the most common symptom of MVP. It may be left sided or substernal, and is frequently related to fatigue, not exertion. Tachydysrhythmias may develop with MVP, causing palpitations, lightheadedness, and syncope. Increased sympathetic nervous system tone may cause a sense of anxiety (Woods et al., 2000).

Mitral valve prolapse increases the risk for bacterial endocarditis. Progressive worsening of regurgitation can lead to heart failure. Thrombi may form on prolapsed valve leaflets; embolization may cause transient ischemic attacks (TIAs).

## Aortic Stenosis

*Aortic stenosis* obstructs blood flow from the left ventricle into the aorta during systole. Aortic stenosis is more common in

males (80%) than females (Braunwald et al., 2001). Aortic stenosis may be idiopathic, or due to a congenital defect, rheumatic damage, or degenerative changes. When rheumatic heart disease is the cause, mitral valve deformity is also often present. Rheumatic heart disease destroys aortic valve leaflets, with fibrosis and calcification causing rigidity and scarring. In the older adult, calcific aortic stenosis may result from degenerative changes associated with aging. Constant "wear and tear" on this valve can lead to fibrosis and calcification. Idiopathic calcific stenosis generally is mild and does not impair cardiac output.

As aortic stenosis progresses, the valve annulus decreases in size, increasing the work of the left ventricle to eject its volume through the narrowed opening into the aorta. To compensate, the ventricle hypertrophies to maintain an adequate stroke volume and cardiac output (Figure 30–11 ■). Left ventricular compliance also decreases. The additional workload increases myocardial oxygen consumption, which can precipitate myocardial ischemia. Coronary blood flow may also decrease in aortic stenosis. As left ventricular end-diastolic pressure increases because of reduced stroke volume, left atrial pressures increase. These pressures also affect the pulmonary vascular system; pulmonary vascular congestion and pulmonary edema may result.

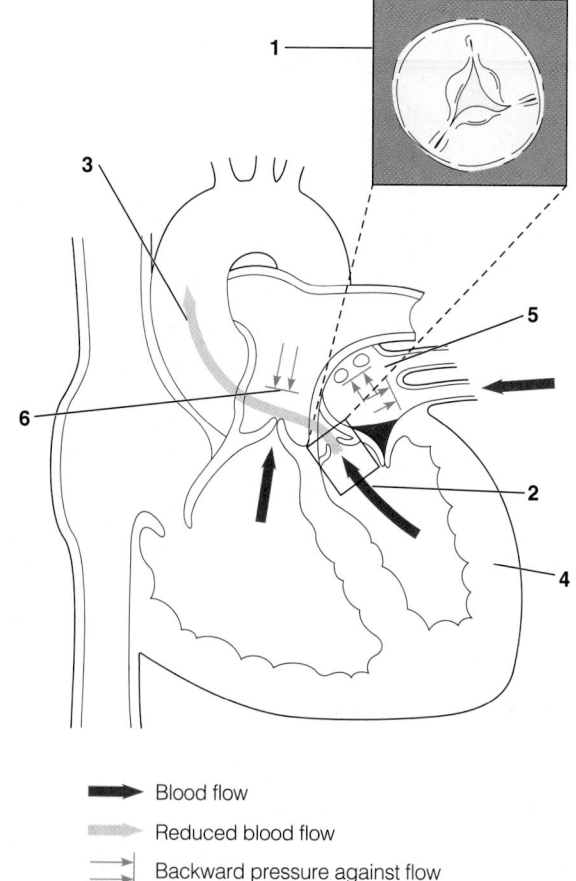

Blood flow

Reduced blood flow

Backward pressure against flow

**Figure 30–11 ■** Aortic stenosis. The narrowed aortic valve orifice (1), decreases the left ventricular ejection fraction during systole (2), and cardiac output (3). The left ventricle hypertrophies (4). Incomplete emptying of left atrium (5) causes backward pressure through pulmonary veins and pulmonary hypertension. Elevated pulmonary artery pressure (6) causes right ventricular strain.

Aortic stenosis may be asymptomatic for many years. As the disease progresses and compensation fails, usually between age 50 and 70 years, obstructed cardiac output causes manifestations of left ventricular failure. Dyspnea on exertion, angina pectoris, and exertional syncope are classic manifestations of aortic stenosis. Pulse pressure, an indicator of stroke volume, narrows to 30 mmHg or less. Hemodynamic monitors show increased left atrial pressure and pulmonary artery wedge pressure, as well as decreased stroke volume and cardiac output.

Aortic stenosis produces a harsh systolic murmur best heard in the second intercostal space to the right of the sternum. This crescendo-decrescendo murmur is produced by turbulence of blood entering the aorta through the stenotic valve. A palpable thrill is often felt. The murmur may radiate to the carotid arteries. Ventricular hypertrophy displaces the cardiac impulse to the left of the midclavicular line. As aortic stenosis progresses, $S_3$ and $S_4$ heart sounds may be heard, indicating heart failure and reduced left ventricular compliance.

As cardiac output falls, tissue perfusion decreases. Late in the disease, pulmonary hypertension and right ventricular failure develop. Untreated, symptomatic aortic stenosis has a poor prognosis; 10% to 20% of these clients experience sudden cardiac death (Braunwald et al., 2001).

## Aortic Regurgitation

*Aortic regurgitation,* also called *aortic insufficiency,* allows blood to flow back into the left ventricle from the aorta during diastole. It is more common in males (75%) in its "pure" form; in females, it is commonly associated with coexisting mitral valve disease. Most aortic regurgitation (67%) results from rheumatic heart disease (Braunwald et al., 2001). Other causes include congenital disorders, infective endocarditis, blunt chest trauma, aortic aneurysm, syphilis, Marfan syndrome, and chronic hypertension.

In aortic regurgitation, thickened and contracted valve cusps, scarring, fibrosis, and calcification impede complete valve closure. Chronic hypertension and aortic aneurysm may dilate and stretch the aortic valve opening, increasing the degree of regurgitation.

In aortic regurgitation, volume overload affects the left ventricle as blood from the aorta adds to blood received from the atrium during diastole. This increases diastolic left ventricular pressure. Increased preload causes more forceful contractions and a high stroke volume (Figure 30–12 ■). With time, muscle cells hypertrophy to compensate for increased cardiac work and afterload; eventually this hypertrophy compromises cardiac output and increases regurgitation.

High left-ventricular pressures increase left atrial workload and pressure. This pressure is transmitted to the pulmonary vessels causing pulmonary congestion. The workload of the right ventricle increases as a result, and right-sided heart failure may develop. Acute aortic regurgitation from traumatic injury or infective endocarditis causes a rapid decline in hemodynamic status from acute heart failure and pulmonary edema, because compensatory mechanisms do not have time to develop.

Aortic regurgitation may be asymptomatic for many years, even when severe. The increased stroke volume may cause

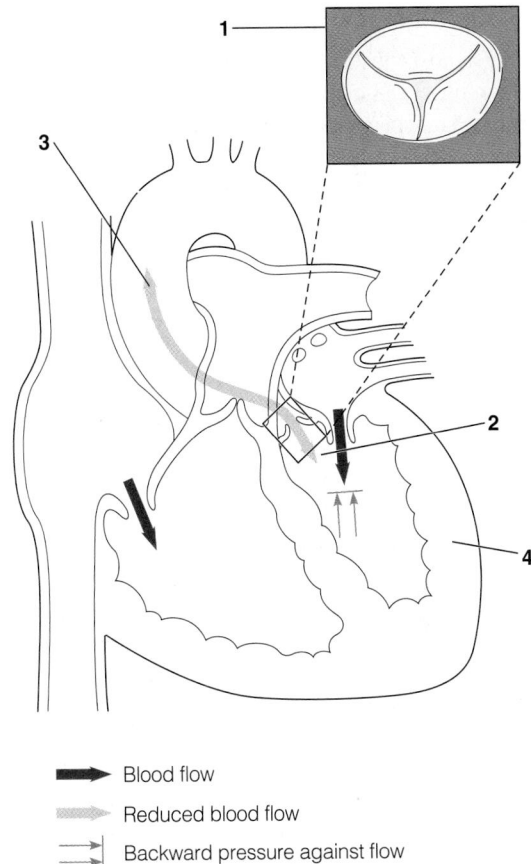

> Blood flow
> Reduced blood flow
> Backward pressure against flow

**Figure 30–12 ■** Aortic regurgitation. The cusps of the aortic valve widen and fail to close during diastole (1). Blood regurgitates from the aorta into the left ventricle (2) increasing left ventricular volume and decreasing cardiac output (3). The left ventricle dilates and hypertrophies (4) in response to the increase in blood volume and workload.

complaints of persistent palpitations, especially when recumbent. A throbbing pulse may be visible in arteries of the neck; the force of contraction may cause a characteristic head bob (Musset's sign) and shake the whole body. Other symptoms include dizziness, and exercise intolerance.

Fatigue, exertional dyspnea, orthopnea, and paroxysmal nocturnal dyspnea are common in aortic regurgitation. Anginal pain may result from excessive cardiac work and decreased coronary perfusion. Unlike CAD, angina often occurs at night and may not respond to conventional therapy.

The murmur of aortic regurgitation is heard during diastole as blood flows back into the left ventricle from the aorta. It is a "blowing," high-pitched sound heard most clearly at the third left intercostal space. A palpable thrill and ventricular heave may be noted. An $S_3$ and $S_4$ may be heard as the heart fails and ventricular compliance diminishes. The apical impulse is displaced to the left.

High systolic and low diastolic pressures cause a widened pulse pressure. The arterial pressure waveform has a rapid upstroke and quickly collapsing downstroke, known as a *water-hammer pulse.* It is caused by the force of rapid and early delivery of the stroke volume into the aorta.

## Tricuspid Valve Disorders

*Tricuspid stenosis* obstructs blood flow from the right atrium to the right ventricle. It usually results from rheumatic heart disease; mitral stenosis often occurs concurrently with tricuspid stenosis.

Fibrosed, retracted tricuspid valve cusps and fused leaflets narrow the valve orifice and prevent complete closure. Right ventricular filling is impaired during diastole, and during systole, some blood regurgitates back into the right atrium. Pressure in the right atrium increases, and it enlarges in response to the increased pressure and workload. This increased right atrial pressure is reflected backward into the systemic circulation. Right ventricular stroke volume decreases, reducing the volume delivered to the pulmonary system and left heart. Stroke volume, cardiac output, and tissue perfusion fall.

Manifestations of tricuspid stenosis relate to systemic congestion and right-sided heart failure. They include increased central venous pressure, jugular venous distention, ascites, hepatomegaly, and peripheral edema. Low cardiac output causes fatigue and weakness. The low-pitched, rumbling diastolic murmur of tricuspid stenosis is most clearly heard in the fourth intercostal space at the left sternal border or over the xiphoid process.

*Tricuspid regurgitation* usually occurs secondarily to right ventricular dilation. Stretching distorts the valve and its supporting structures, preventing complete valve closure. Left ventricular failure is the usual cause of right ventricular overload; pulmonary hypertension is another cause. The valve may also be damaged by rheumatic heart disease, infective endocarditis, inferior MI, trauma, or other conditions.

Tricuspid regurgitation allows blood to flow back into the right atrium during systole, increasing right atrial pressures. Increased right atrial pressure causes manifestations of right-sided heart failure, including systemic venous congestion and low cardiac output. Atrial fibrillation due to atrial distention is common. The retrograde flow of blood over the deformed tricuspid valve causes a high-pitched, blowing systolic murmur heard over the tricuspid or xiphoid area.

## Pulmonic Valve Disorders

*Pulmonic stenosis* obstructs blood flow from the right ventricle into the pulmonary system. It usually is a congenital disorder, although rheumatic heart disease or cancer also may cause pulmonic stenosis. The right ventricle hypertrophies to generate the pressure needed to pump blood into the pulmonary system. The right atrium also hypertrophies to overcome the high pressures generated in the right ventricle. Right-sided heart failure occurs when the ventricle can no longer generate adequate pressure to force blood past the narrowed valve opening.

Pulmonic stenosis typically is asymptomatic unless severe. Dyspnea on exertion and fatigue are early signs. As the condition progresses, right-sided heart failure develops, with peripheral edema, ascites, hepatomegaly, and increased venous pressures. Turbulent blood flow caused by the narrowed valve generates a harsh, systolic crescendo-decrescendo murmur heard in the pulmonic area, the second left intercostal space.

*Pulmonic regurgitation* is more common than pulmonary stenosis. It is a complication of pulmonary hypertension, which stretches and dilates the pulmonary orifice, causing incomplete valve closure. Infective endocarditis, pulmonary artery aneurysm, and syphilis also may cause pulmonic regurgitation.

Incomplete valve closure allows blood to flow back into the right ventricle during diastole, decreasing blood flow to the pulmonary circuit. The extra blood increases right ventricular end-diastolic volume. When the ventricle can no longer compensate for the increased volume, right-sided heart failure develops. The murmur of pulmonic regurgitation is a high-pitched, decrescendo, blowing sound heard along the left sternal border during diastole.

## COLLABORATIVE CARE

A heart murmur identified during routine physical examination often is the initial indication of valvular disease. If no symptoms are present, close observation for disease progression and prophylactic therapy to prevent infection of the diseased heart may be the only treatment.

Manifestations of heart failure are treated with diet and medications (see the preceding section on heart failure). When medical management is no longer effective, surgery is considered.

### Diagnostic Tests

The following diagnostic tests help to identify and diagnose valvular disease.

- *Echocardiography* is used routinely to diagnose valvular disease. Thickened valve leaflets, vegetations or growths on valve leaflets, myocardial function, and chamber size can be determined, and pressure gradients across valves and pulmonary artery pressures can be estimated. Either transthoracic or transesophageal echocardiography may be used.
- *Chest X-ray* can identify cardiac hypertrophy, chamber and great vessel enlargement, and dilation of the pulmonary vasculature. Calcification of the valve leaflets and annular openings may also be visible.
- *Electrocardiography* can demonstrate atrial and ventricular hypertrophy, conduction defects, and dysrhythmias associated with valvular disease.
- *Cardiac catheterization* may be used to assess contractility and to determine the pressure gradients across the heart valves, in the heart chambers, and in the pulmonary system.

### Medications

Heart failure resulting from valvular disease is treated with diuretics, ACE inhibitors, vasodilators, and possibly digitalis glycosides. Digitalis increases the force of myocardial contraction to maintain cardiac output. Diuretics, ACE inhibitors, and vasodilators reduce preload and afterload. (See the Medication Administration box on page 879).

In clients with valvular disorders, atrial distention often causes atrial fibrillation. Digitalis or small doses of beta blockers are given to slow the ventricular response (see Chapter 29 for more information about atrial fibrillation and its treatment). Anticoagulant therapy is added to prevent clot and embolus formation, a common complication of atrial fibrillation as blood pools in the noncontracting atria. Anticoagulant therapy also is required following insertion of a mechanical heart valve. See Chapter 33 ⬡⬡ for more information about anticoagulant therapy.

Valvular damage increases the risk for infective endocarditis as altered blood flow allows bacterial colonization. Antibiotics are prescribed prophylactically prior to any dental work, invasive procedures, or surgery to minimize the risk of bacteremia (bacteria in the blood) and subsequent endocarditis.

## Percutaneous Balloon Valvuloplasty

*Percutaneous balloon valvuloplasty* is an invasive procedure performed in the cardiac catheterization laboratory. A balloon catheter similar to that used in coronary angioplasty procedures is inserted into the femoral vein or artery. Guided by fluoroscopy, the catheter is advanced into the heart and positioned with the balloon straddling the stenotic valve. The balloon is then inflated for approximately 90 seconds to divide the fused leaflets and enlarge the valve orifice (Figure 30–13 ■). Balloon valvuloplasty is the treatment of choice for symptomatic mitral valve stenosis. It is used to treat children and young adults with aortic stenosis, and may be indicated for older adults who are poor surgical risks, and as a "bridge to surgery" when heart function is severely compromised (Braunwald et al., 2001). Nursing care of the client with a balloon valvuloplasty is similar to that of the client following coronary revascularization (see page 820).

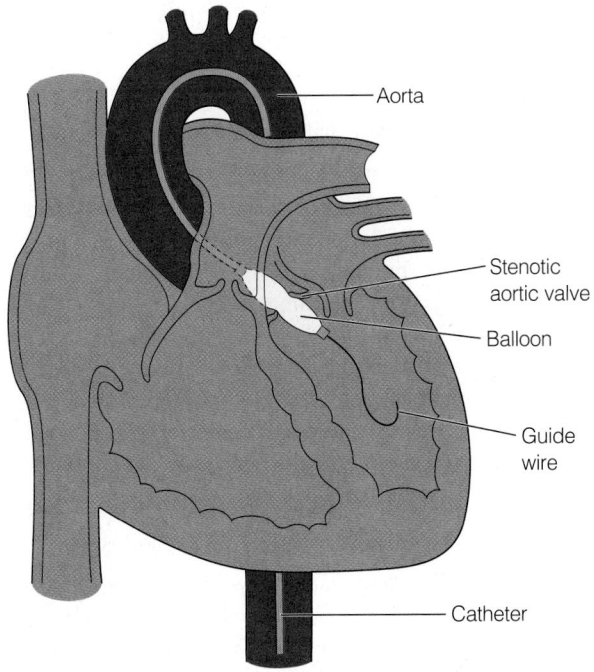

**Figure 30–13 ■** Balloon valvuloplasty. The balloon catheter is guided into position straddling the stenosed valve. The balloon is then inflated to increase the size of the valve opening.

Labels: Aorta; Stenotic aortic valve; Balloon; Guide wire; Catheter

## Surgery

Surgery to repair or replace the diseased valve may be done to restore valve function, alleviate symptoms, and prevent complications and death. Ideally, diseased valves are repaired or replaced before cardiopulmonary function is severely compromised. The diseased valve is repaired when possible, because the risk for surgical mortality and complications is lower than with valve replacement.

### Reconstructive Surgery

*Valvuloplasty* is a general term for reconstruction or repair of a heart valve. Methods include "patching" the perforated portion of the leaflet, resecting excess tissue, debriding vegetations or calcification, and other techniques. Valvuloplasty may be used for stenotic or regurgitant mitral and tricuspid valves, mitral valve prolapse, and aortic stenosis. Common valvuloplasty procedures include the following:

- *Open commissurotomy,* surgical division of fused valve leaflets, is done to open stenotic valves. Fused commissures (junctions between valve leaflets or cusps) are incised, and calcium deposits are debrided as needed.
- *Annuloplasty* repairs a narrowed or an enlarged or dilated valve annulus, the supporting ring of the valve. A prosthetic ring may be used to resize the opening, or stitches and purse-string sutures may be used to reduce and gather excess tissue. Annuloplasty may be used for either stenotic or regurgitant valves.

### Valve Replacement

Valve replacement is indicated when manifestations of valve dysfunction develop, preferably before left heart function is seriously impaired. In general, three factors determine the outcome of valve replacement surgery: (1) heart function at the time of surgery: (2) intraoperative and postoperative care, and (3) characteristics and durability of the replacement valve.

Many different prosthetic heart valves are available, including mechanical and biologic tissue valves. Selection depends on the valve hemodynamics, resistance to clot formation, ease of insertion, anatomic suitability, and client acceptance (Meeker & Rothrock, 1999). The client's age, underlying condition, and contraindications to anticoagulation (such as a desire to become pregnant) also are considered in selecting the appropriate prosthesis. Table 30–8 lists the advantages and disadvantages of biologic and mechanical valves.

Biologic tissue valves may be *heterografts,* excised from a pig (Figure 30–14A ■) or made of calf pericardium, or *homografts* from a human (obtained from a cadaver or during heart transplant). Biologic valves allow more normal blood flow and have a low risk of thrombus formation. As a result, long-term anticoagulation rarely is necessary. They are less durable, however, than mechanical valves. Up to 50% of biologic valves must be replaced by 15 years.

Mechanical prosthetic valves have the major advantage of long-term durability. These valves are frequently used when life expectancy exceeds 10 years. Their major disadvantage is the need for lifetime anticoagulation to prevent the development of clots on the valve.

### TABLE 30-8   Advantages and Disadvantages of Prosthetic Heart Valves

| Category | Types | Advantages | Disadvantages |
|---|---|---|---|
| Mechanical valves | Ball-and-cage<br>Tilting disc | Long-term durability<br>Good hemodynamics | Lifetime anticoagulation<br>Audible click<br>Risk of thromboembolism<br>Infections are harder to treat |
| Biologic tissue valves | Porcine heterograft<br>Bovine heterograft<br>Human aortic homograft | Low incidence of<br>  thromboembolism<br>No long-term anticoagulation<br>Good hemodynamics<br>Quiet<br>Infections are easier to treat | Prone to deterioration<br>Frequent replacement is<br>  required |

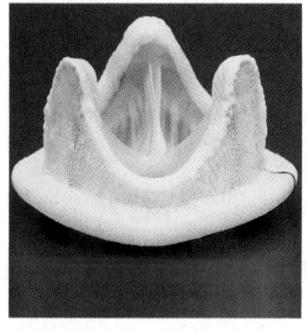 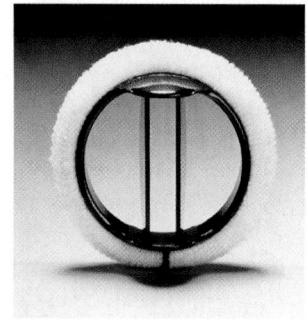 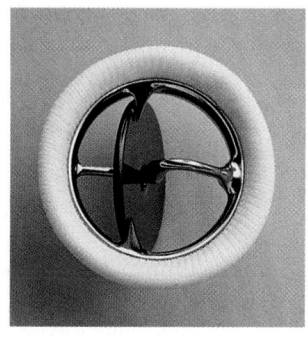 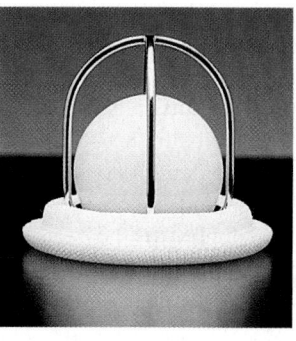

**A**          **B**          **C**          **D**

**Figure 30–14** ■ Prosthetic heart valves. *A,* Carpentier-Edwards porcine xenograft. *B,* St. Jude Medical valve. *C,* Medtronic Hall prosthetic valve. *D,* Starr-Edwards prosthetic valve.

*Courtesy of Baxter (A and D); St. Jude Medical (B); and Medtronics, Inc. (C).*

Most mechanical valves are either a tilting disk or a ball and cage design (Figures 30–14B, C, and D). The tilting-disc valve designs are frequently used because they have a lower profile than the caged-ball types, allowing blood to flow through the valve with less obstruction. The St. Jude bileaflet design has good hemodynamics and low risk for clot formation. Both biologic and mechanical valves increase the risk of endocarditis, although its incidence is fairly low.

## NURSING CARE

### Health Promotion

Preventing rheumatic heart disease is a key element in preventing heart valve disorders. Rheumatic heart disease is a consequence of rheumatic fever (see the previous section of this chapter), an immune process that may be a sequela to β-hemolytic streptococcal infection of the pharynx (strep throat). Early treatment of strep throat prevents rheumatic fever. Teach individual clients, families, and communities about the importance of timely and effective treatment of strep throat. Emphasize the importance of completing the full prescription of antibiotics to prevent development of resistant bacteria. Prophylactic antibiotic therapy before invasive procedures to prevent infectious endocarditis is an important health promotion measure for clients with preexisting heart disease.

### Assessment

Assessment data related to valvular heart disease includes the following:

- Health history: complaints of decreasing exercise tolerance, dyspnea on exertion, palpitations; history of frequent respiratory infections; previous history of rheumatic heart disease, endocarditis, or a heart murmur
- Physical examination: vital signs; skin color and temperature, evidence of clubbing or peripheral edema; neck vein distention; breath sounds; heart sounds and presence of $S_3$, $S_4$, or murmur; timing, grade, and characteristics of any murmur; palpate for cardiac heave and thrills; abdominal contour, liver and spleen size

### Nursing Diagnoses and Interventions

Nursing priorities include maintaining cardiac output, managing manifestations of the disorder, teaching about the disease process and its management, and preventing complications. Nursing care of the client undergoing valve surgery is similar to that of the client having other types of open-heart surgery (see page 823), with increased attention to anticoagulation and preventing endocarditis.

## Decreased Cardiac Output

Nearly all valve disorders affect ventricular filling and/or emptying, reducing cardiac output. Stenosis of the AV valves impairs ventricular filling and increases atrial pressures. Regurgitation of these valves reduces cardiac output as a portion of the blood in the ventricle regurgitates into the atria during systole. Stenosis of the semilunar valves obstructs ventricular outflow to the great vessels; regurgitation allows blood to flow back into the ventricles, creating higher filling pressures. When compensatory measures fail, heart failure develops.

- Monitor vital signs and hemodynamic parameters, reporting changes from the baseline. *A fall in systolic blood pressure and tachycardia may indicate decreased cardiac output. Increasing pulmonary artery and pulmonary wedge pressures may also indicate decreased cardiac output, causing increased congestion and pressure in the pulmonary vascular system.*

**PRACTICE ALERT** *Promptly report changes in level of consciousness; distended neck veins; dyspnea or respiratory crackles; urine output less than 30 mL/h; cool, clammy, or cyanotic skin; diminished peripheral pulses; or slow capillary refill. These findings indicate decreased cardiac output and impaired tissue and organ perfusion.* ∎

- Monitor intake and output; weigh daily. Report weight gain of 3 to 5 lb within 24 hours. *Fluid retention is a compensatory mechanism that occurs when cardiac output decreases; 2.2 lb (1 kg) of weight equals 1 L of fluid.*
- Restrict fluids as ordered. *Fluid intake may be restricted to reduce cardiac workload and pressures within the heart and pulmonary circuit.*
- Monitor oxygen saturation continuously and arterial blood gases as ordered. Report oxygen saturation less than 95% (or as specified) and abnormal ABG results. *Oxygen saturation levels and ABGs allow assessment of oxygenation.*
- Elevate the head of the bed. Administer supplemental oxygen as ordered. *These measures improve alveolar ventilation and oxygenation.*
- Provide for physical, emotional, and mental rest. *Physical and psychologic rest decreases the cardiac workload.*
- Administer prescribed medications as ordered to reduce cardiac workload. *Diuretics, ACE inhibitors, and direct vasodilators may be prescribed to reduce fluid volume and afterload, reducing cardiac work.*

## Activity Intolerance

Altered blood flow through the heart impairs delivery of oxygen and nutrients to the tissues. As the heart muscle fails and is unable to compensate for altered blood flow, tissue perfusion is further compromised. Dyspnea on exertion is often an early symptom of valvular disease.

- Monitor vital signs before and during activities. *A change in heart rate of more than 20 BPM, a change of 20 mmHg or more in systolic BP, and complaints of dyspnea, shortness of breath, excessive fatigue, chest pain, diaphoresis, dizziness, or syncope may indicate activity intolerance.*

- Encourage self-care and gradually increasing activities as allowed and tolerated. Provide for rest periods, uninterrupted sleep, and adequate nutritional intake. *Gradual progression of activities avoids excessive cardiac stress. Encouraging self-care increases the client's self-esteem and sense of power. Adequate rest and nutrition facilitate healing, decrease fatigue, and increase energy reserves.*
- Provide assistance as needed. Suggest use of a shower chair, sitting while brushing hair or teeth, and other energy-saving measures. *Reducing energy expenditure helps maintain a balance of oxygen supply and demand.*
- Consult with cardiac rehabilitation specialist or physical therapist for in-bed exercises and an activity plan. *In-bed exercises may help improve strength.*
- Discuss ways to conserve energy at home. *Information provides practical ways to deal with activity limitations and empowers the client to manage these limitations.*

## Risk for Infection

Damaged and deformed valve leaflets and turbulent blood flow through the heart significantly increase the risk of infective endocarditis. Invasive diagnostic and monitoring lines (e.g., cardiac catheterization, hemodynamic monitoring) and disrupted skin with surgery also increase the risk of infection.

- Use aseptic technique for all invasive procedures. *Invasive procedures breach the body's protective mechanisms, potentially allowing bacteria to enter. Aseptic technique reduces this risk.*

**PRACTICE ALERT** *Record temperature every 4 hours; notify physician if temperature exceeds 100.5°F (38.5°C). Fever may be an early indication of infection.* ∎

- Assess wounds and catheter sites for redness, swelling, warmth, pain, or evidence of drainage. *These signs of inflammation may signal infection.*
- Administer antibiotics as ordered. Ensure completion of the full course. *Antibiotics are used to prevent and treat infection. Completion of the full course of therapy prevents drug-resistant organisms from multiplying.*
- Monitor WBC and differential. Notify physician of leukocytosis or leukopenia. *A high WBC and increased percentage of immature WBCs (bands) may indicate bacterial infection; a low WBC count may indicate an impaired immune response and increased susceptibility to infection.*

## Ineffective Protection

Anticoagulant therapy commonly is prescribed for clients with chronic atrial fibrillation, a history of emboli, and following valve replacement surgery. Although chronic anticoagulant therapy decreases the risk of clots and emboli, it increases the risk for bleeding and hemorrhage.

**PRACTICE ALERT** *Monitor the International Normalized Ratio (INR) or prothrombin time (PT or protime). Report an INR > 3.5 or a PT > 2.5 times the normal to the physician. An excessively high INR or PT indicate excessive anticoagulation and an increased risk for bleeding.* ∎

- Test stools and vomitus for occult blood. *Bleeding due to excessive anticoagulation may not be apparent.*
- Instruct to avoid using aspirin or other nonsteroidal anti-inflammatory drugs (NSAIDs). Encourage reading ingredient labels on over-the-counter drugs; many contain aspirin. *Aspirin and other NSAIDs interfere with clotting and may potentiate the effects of the anticoagulant therapy.*
- Advise using a soft-bristled toothbrush, electric razor, and gentle touch when cleaning fragile skin. *These measures decrease the risk of skin or gum trauma and bleeding.*

**PRACTICE ALERT** *Monitor hemoglobin, hematocrit, and platelet count as ordered. Notify the physician of decreasing hemoglobin and hematocrit levels or if the platelet count falls below 50,000/mm³. Low hemoglobin and hematocrit indicate blood loss. Platelet counts below 50,000/mm³ significantly increase the risk of bleeding.* ∎

## Using NANDA, NIC, and NOC

Chart 30–3 shows links between NANDA nursing diagnoses, NIC, and NOC for the client with valvular heart disease.

## Home Care

For most clients, valvular disease is a chronic condition. The client has primary responsibility for managing effects of the disorder. To prepare the client and family for home care, discuss the following topics.

- Management of symptoms, including any necessary activity restrictions or lifestyle changes
- The importance of adequate rest to prevent fatigue
- Diet restrictions to reduce fluid retention and symptoms of heart failure

- Information about prescribed medications, including purpose, desired and possible adverse effects, scheduling, and possible interactions with other drugs
- The importance of keeping follow-up appointments to monitor the disease and its treatment
- Notifying all health care providers about valve disease or surgery to facilitate prescription of prophylactic antibiotics before invasive procedures or dental work
- Manifestations to immediately report to the health care provider: increasing severity of symptoms, especially of worsening heart failure or pulmonary edema; signs of transient ischemic attacks or other embolic events; evidence of bleeding, such as joint pain, easy bruising, black and tarry stools, bleeding gums, or blood in the urine or sputum

Provide referrals to community resources such as home maintenance services, home health services, and structured cardiac rehabilitation programs. Refer the client and family (especially the primary food preparer) to a dietitian or nutritionist for teaching and assistance with menu planning.

## THE CLIENT WITH CARDIOMYOPATHY

The **cardiomyopathies** are disorders that affect the heart muscle itself. They are a diverse group of disorders that affect both systolic and diastolic functions. Cardiomyopathies may be either primary or secondary in origin. Primary cardiomyopathies are idiopathic; their cause is unknown. Secondary cardiomyopathies occur as a result of other processes, such as ischemia, infectious disease, exposure to toxins, connective tissue disorders, metabolic disorders, or nutritional deficiencies. In many cases, the cause of cardiomyopathy is

| CHART 30–3 | NANDA, NIC, AND NOC LINKAGES | |
|---|---|---|
| **The Client with Valvular Heart Disease** | | |
| **NURSING DIAGNOSES** | **NURSING INTERVENTIONS** | **NURSING OUTCOMES** |
| • Activity Intolerance | • Energy Management<br>• Self-Care Assistance | • Activity Tolerance<br>• Energy Conservation |
| • Decreased Cardiac Output | • Cardiac Care: Rehabilitative<br>• Hemodynamic Regulation<br>• Fluid Management | • Cardiac Pump Effectiveness<br>• Tissue Perfusion: Peripheral |
| • Fatigue | • Teaching: Prescribed Activity / Exercise<br>• Energy Management<br>• Nutrition Management | • Endurance<br>• Energy Conservation<br>• Nutritional Status: Energy |
| • Ineffective Health Maintenance | • Teaching: Disease Process<br>• Coping Enhancement<br>• Decision-Making Support | • Treatment Behavior: Illness or Injury<br>• Participation: Health Care Decisions |

*Note. Data from Nursing Outcomes Classification (NOC) by M. Johnson & M. Maas (Eds.), 1997, St. Louis: Mosby; Nursing Diagnoses: Definitions & Classification 2001–2002 by North American Nursing Diagnosis Association, 2001, Philadelphia: NANDA; Nursing Interventions Classification (NIC) by J.C. McCloskey & G. M. Bulechek (Eds.), 2000, St. Louis: Mosby. Reprinted by permission.*

## Nursing Care Plan

## A Client with Mitral Valve Prolapse

Julie Snow, a 22-year-old college student, sees a nurse practitioner at the college health clinic for a physical examination after experiencing palpitations, fatigue, and a headache during midterm examinations. Ms. Snow tells Lakisha Johnson, FNP, "I'm scared that something is wrong with me."

Over the last few months, Ms. Snow has had occasional palpitations that she describes as "feeling like my heart is doing flip-flops." Rarely, these palpitations have been accompanied by a sharp, stabbing pain in her chest that lasts only a few seconds. She initially attributed her symptoms to stress, but she is increasingly concerned because the "attacks" are becoming more frequent. Ms. Snow states that she has "always been healthy," does not smoke, uses alcohol socially, and exercises, albeit intermittently. Ms. Snow admits that she has been drinking a lot of coffee and cola and eating a lot of "junk food" lately.

### ASSESSMENT

Ms. Johnson's assessment of Ms. Snow documents the following: height 66 in. (168 cm), weight 140 lb (63.6 kg), T 99.3, BP 118/64, P 82, and R 18. Slightly anxious but in no acute distress. Systolic click and soft crescendo murmur grade II/VI noted on auscultation. Apical impulse at fifth ICS left MCL. Lungs clear to auscultation. Review of remaining systems reveals no apparent abnormalities. An ECG shows sinus rhythm with occasional PACs. Based on the admission history, manifestations, and physical assessment, Ms. Johnson suspects mitral valve prolapse (MVP).

### DIAGNOSES

- *Anxiety* related to fear of heart disease and implications for lifestyle
- *Powerlessness* related to unpredictability of symptoms
- *Risk of infection (endocarditis)* related to altered valve function

### EXPECTED OUTCOMES

- Verbalize an understanding of MVP and its management.
- Discuss ways to decrease or relieve MVP symptoms.
- Acknowledge the risk for endocarditis and identify precautions to prevent it.

### PLANNING AND IMPLEMENTATION

- Consult with and refer to cardiologist for continued monitoring and follow-up.
- Teach about MVP, including heart valve anatomy, physiology, and function, common manifestations of MVP, and treatment rationale.
- Discuss symptoms of progressive mitral regurgitation, and the need to report these to the cardiologist.
- Discuss recommended follow-up care and its rationale.
- Allow to verbalize feelings and share concerns about MVP. Encourage to attend an MVP support group meeting.

- Discuss the prognosis for MVP, emphasizing that most clients live normal lives using diet and lifestyle management.
- Instruct to keep a weekly record of symptoms and their frequency for 1 month.
- Discuss lifestyle changes to manage symptoms: aerobic exercise with warmup and cooldown periods; maintaining adequate fluid intake, especially during hot weather or exercise; relaxation techniques (e.g., meditation, deep-breathing exercises, music therapy, yoga, guided imagery, heat therapy, or progressive muscle relaxation) to perform daily; avoiding caffeine and crash diets; forming healthy eating habits.
- Teach about infective endocarditis risk and prevention with prophylactic antibiotics. Encourage notifying dentist and other health care providers of MVP before dental or any invasive procedure.

### EVALUATION

After several educational sessions at the college health clinic, Ms. Snow verbalizes an understanding of MVP by explaining heart valve function, listing common manifestations of MVP, and describing indications of deteriorating heart function. She states she will report these manifestations to her cardiologist if they occur. She is given a booklet on MVP for additional reading. She also verbalizes understanding of the risk of endocarditis, and states that she will notify her doctors of her MVP and the need for antibiotics before invasive procedures. Ms. Snow is attending a monthly MVP support group (led by a cardiology clinical nurse specialist) on campus and states, "I am so glad to know I'm not alone! It really helps to know that others are living well with MVP." Her weekly symptom log shows her symptoms are associated with late-night studying and drinking large amounts of coffee and cola. Ms. Snow has moderated her caffeine intake and increased her fluids, relieving her symptoms. In addition, Ms. Snow is taking a relaxation music therapy class. Ms. Snow states that she realizes that she has "the ability to control my life through the choices I make."

### Critical Thinking in the Nursing Process

1. Develop an action plan for Ms. Snow that outlines specific activities she can use to manage symptoms of MVP.
2. Why are clients with symptomatic MVP encouraged to include regular exercise in their health habits?
3. How does the support of family, friends, and other people with MVP assist MVP clients in managing their condition?
4. What manifestations would indicate a progressive worsening of Ms. Snow's mitral regurgitation?

See Evaluating Your Response in Appendix C.

unknown. In 1999, more than 27,000 deaths were directly attributed to cardiomyopathy. Mortality associated with cardiomyopathy is higher in older adults, men, and African Americans (AHA, 2001).

## PATHOPHYSIOLOGY AND MANIFESTATIONS

The cardiomyopathies are categorized by their pathophysiology and presentation into three groups: dilated, hypertrophic, and restrictive. Table 30–9 compares the causes, pathophysiology, manifestations, and management of the cardiomyopathies.

## Dilated Cardiomyopathy

*Dilated cardiomyopathy* is the most common type of cardiomyopathy, accounting for 87% of cases (AHA, 2001). The cause of dilated cardiomyopathy is unknown, although alcohol and cocaine abuse, chemotherapeutic drugs, pregnancy, and

systemic hypertension may contribute to its development. Some cases of dilated cardiomyopathy are genetic; it can be transmitted in an autosomal dominant, autosomal recessive, or X-linked pattern (Porth, 2002).

In dilated cardiomyopathy, heart chambers dilate and ventricular contraction is impaired. Both end-diastolic and end-systolic volumes increase, and the left ventricular ejection fraction is substantially reduced, decreasing cardiac output. Left ventricular dilation is prominent; left ventricular hypertrophy is usually minimal. The right ventricle also may be enlarged. Extensive interstitial fibrosis (scarring) is evident; necrotic myocardial cells also may be seen (Braunwald et al., 2001).

Manifestations of dilated cardiomyopathy develop gradually. Heart failure often presents years after the onset of dilation and pump failure. Both right- and left-sided failure occur, with dyspnea on exertion, orthopnea, paroxysmal nocturnal dys-

### TABLE 30-9  Classifications of Cardiomyopathy

| | Dilated | Hypertrophic | Restrictive |
|---|---|---|---|
| | | | |
| Causes | Usually idiopathic; may be secondary to chronic alcoholism or myocarditis | Hereditary; may be secondary to chronic hypertension | Usually secondary to amyloidosis, radiation, or myocardial fibrosis |
| Pathophysiology | Scarring and atrophy of myocardial cells<br>Thickening of ventricular wall<br>Dilation of heart chambers<br>Impaired ventricular pumping<br>Increased end-diastolic and end-systolic volumes<br>Mural thrombi common | Hypertrophy of ventricular muscle mass<br>Small left ventricular volume<br>Septal hypertrophy may obstruct left ventricular outflow<br>Left atrial dilation | Excess rigidity of ventricular walls restricts filling<br>Myocardial contractility remains relatively normal |
| Manifestations | Heart failure<br>Cardiomegaly<br>Dysrhythmias<br>$S_3$ and $S_4$ gallop; murmur of mitral regurgitation | Dyspnea, anginal pain, syncope<br>Left ventricular hypertrophy<br>Dysrhythmias<br>Loud $S_4$<br>Sudden death | Dyspnea, fatigue<br>Right-sided heart failure<br>Mild to moderate cardiomegaly<br>$S_3$ and $S_4$<br>Mitral regurgitation murmur |
| Management | Management of heart failure<br>Implantable cardioverter-defibrillator (ICD) as needed<br>Cardiac transplantation | Beta-blockers<br>Calcium channel blockers<br>Antidysrhythmic agents<br>ICD, dual-chamber pacing<br>Surgical excision of part of the ventricular septum | Management of heart failure<br>Exercise restriction |

pnea, weakness, fatigue, peripheral edema, and ascites. Both $S_3$ and $S_4$ heart sounds are commonly heard, as well as an AV regurgitation murmur. Dysrhythmias are common, including supraventricular tachycardias, atrial fibrillation, and complex ventricular tachycardias. Untreated dysrhythmias can lead to sudden death (Porth, 2002). Mural thrombi (blood clots in the heart wall) may form in the left ventricular apex and embolize to other parts of the body.

The prognosis of dilated cardiomyopathy is grim; most clients get progressively worse and 50% die within 5 years after the diagnosis; 75% die within 10 years (AHA, 2001).

## Hypertrophic Cardiomyopathy

*Hypertrophic cardiomyopathy* is characterized by decreased compliance of the left ventricle and hypertrophy of the ventricular muscle mass. This impairs ventricular filling, leading to small end-diastolic volumes, and low cardiac output. About half of all clients with hypertrophic cardiomyopathy have a family history of the disease. It is genetically transmitted in an autosomal dominant pattern (Braunwald et al., 2001).

The pattern of left ventricular hypertrophy is unique in that the muscle may not hypertrophy "equally." In a majority of clients, the interventricular septal mass, especially the upper portion, increases to a greater extent than the free wall of the ventricle. The enlarged upper septum narrows the passageway of blood into the aorta, impairing ventricular outflow. For this reason, this disorder is also known as *idiopathic hypertrophic subaortic stenosis (IHSS)* or *hypertrophic obstructive cardiomyopathy (HOCM)*.

Hypertrophic cardiomyopathy may be asymptomatic for many years. Symptoms typically occur when increased oxygen demand causes increased ventricular contractility. They may develop suddenly during or after physical activity; in children and young adults, sudden cardiac death may be the first sign of the disorder. Hypertrophic cardiomyopathy is the probable or definite cause of death in 36% of young athletes who die suddenly (AHA, 2001). It is hypothesized that sudden cardiac death is due to ventricular dysrhythmias or hemodynamic factors. Predictors of sudden cardiac death in this population include age of less than 30 years, a family history of sudden death, syncopal episodes, severe ventricular hypertrophy, and ventricular tachycardia seen on ambulatory ECG monitoring (Braunwald et al., 2001). For a brief synopsis of a nursing research study regarding family presence during CPR and invasive procedures, see the box below.

The usual manifestations of hypertrophic cardiomyopathy are dyspnea, angina, and syncope. Angina may result from ischemia due to overgrowth of the ventricular muscle, coronary artery abnormalities, or decreased coronary artery perfusion. Syncope may occur when the outflow tract obstruction severely decreases cardiac output and blood flow to the brain. Ventricular dysrhythmias are common; atrial fibrillation also may develop. Other manifestations of hypertrophic cardiomyopathy include fatigue, dizziness, and palpitations. A harsh, crescendo-decrescendo systolic murmur of variable intensity heard best at the lower left sternal border and apex is characteristic in hypertrophic cardiomyopathy. An $S_4$ may also be noted on auscultation.

## Nursing Research

### Evidence-Based Practice for Sudden Cardiac Death

When cardiac arrest occurs or invasive procedures are performed, family members typically are asked to leave the client's care unit. The traditional rationale for this practice is fear of disrupted clinical interventions, trauma of the witnesses, and risk for increased hospital liability. However, in 1995, the Emergency Nurses Association (ENA) adopted a position supporting family presence during invasive procedures, including resuscitation efforts (CPR), as a means of "preserving the wholeness, dignity, and integrity of the family unit from birth to death" (Myers et al., 2000, p. 33). This study evaluated the responses of families, nurses, and physicians to family presence during invasive procedures and CPR.

Results of the study showed that families saw their presence as a positive experience and their right. They viewed themselves as active care partners, and being present met their needs for information and providing comfort and connection with the client. Nurses overwhelmingly supported family presence; attending physicians also demonstrated a positive response. Physician residents were the least supportive of family presence.

#### IMPLICATIONS FOR NURSING

Family members often are asked to leave the client's side during invasive procedures and CPR with the intention of protecting them from the trauma of witnessing painful or distressing events.

This study clearly showed being present as a positive experience, even when the ultimate outcome was the client's death.

Offering the opportunity to be present and providing information, psychologic and emotional support to an appropriate family member during invasive procedures and CPR supports the family unit and the client during times of crisis. Screening is important: People who are combative, emotionally unstable, or have altered mental status (e.g., dementia, alcohol intoxication) probably are not appropriate. It also is important to allow families to decline the invitation without guilt.

#### Critical Thinking In Client Care

1. Identify procedures and situations in which family members are often asked to leave the client's side. When would it be appropriate to allow at least one significant other to remain with the client?
2. How would you present the option and prepare a family member for being present during a traumatic event such as CPR following the sudden death of a young adult with undiagnosed hypertrophic cardiomyopathy?
3. You support family presence during traumatic events and procedures, but your charge nurse does not. What steps might you use to effect a change in policy on your unit?

## Restrictive Cardiomyopathy

The least common form of cardiomyopathy, *restrictive cardiomyopathy* is characterized by rigid ventricular walls that impair diastolic filling. Causes of restrictive cardiomyopathy include myocardial fibrosis and infiltrative processes, such as amyloidosis. Fibrosis of the myocardium and endocardium causes excessive stiffness and rigidity of the ventricles. Decreased ventricular compliance impairs filling, with decreased ventricular size, elevated end-diastolic pressures, and decreased cardiac output. Contractility is unaffected, and the ejection fraction is normal.

The manifestations of restrictive cardiomyopathy are those of heart failure and decreased tissue perfusion. Dyspnea on exertion and exercise intolerance are common. Jugular venous pressure is elevated, and $S_3$ and $S_4$ are common. The prognosis for restrictive cardiomyopathy is poor. Most clients die within 3 years, and the systemic nature of the underlying disease process precludes effective treatment.

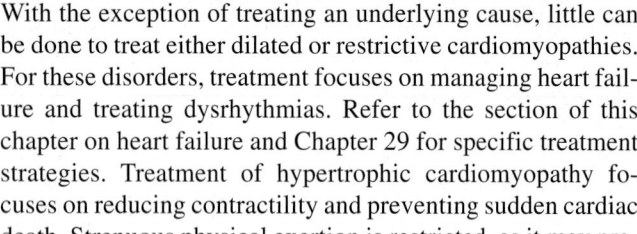

## COLLABORATIVE CARE

With the exception of treating an underlying cause, little can be done to treat either dilated or restrictive cardiomyopathies. For these disorders, treatment focuses on managing heart failure and treating dysrhythmias. Refer to the section of this chapter on heart failure and Chapter 29 for specific treatment strategies. Treatment of hypertrophic cardiomyopathy focuses on reducing contractility and preventing sudden cardiac death. Strenuous physical exertion is restricted, as it may precipitate dysrhythmias or sudden cardiac death. Dietary and sodium restrictions may help diminish the manifestations.

### Diagnostic Tests

Diagnosis begins with a history and physical assessment to rule out known causes of heart failure. Other tests may include the following:

- *Echocardiography* is done to assess chamber size and thickness, ventricular wall motion, valvular function, and systolic and diastolic function of the heart.
- *Electrocardiography* and *ambulatory ECG monitoring* demonstrate cardiac enlargement and detect dysrhythmias.
- *Chest X-ray* shows cardiomegaly, enlargement of the heart, and any pulmonary congestion or edema.
- *Hemodynamic studies* are used to assess cardiac output and pressures in the cardiac chambers and pulmonary vascular system.
- *Radionuclear scans* help identify changes in ventricular volume and mass, as well as perfusion deficits.
- *Cardiac catheterization* and *coronary angiography* may be done to evaluate coronary perfusion, the cardiac chambers, valves, and great vessels for function and structure, pressure relationships, and cardiac output.
- *Myocardial biopsy* uses the tranvenous route to obtain myocardial tissue for biopsy. The cells are examined for infiltration, fibrosis, or inflammation.

## Medications

The drug regimen used to treat heart failure also is used for dilated or restrictive cardiomyopathy. This includes ACE inhibitors, vasodilators, and digitalis (see the previous section of this chapter). Beta blockers also may be used with caution in clients with dilated cardiomyopathy. Anticoagulants are given to reduce the risk of thrombus formation and embolization. Antidysrhythmic drugs are avoided if possible due to their tendency to precipitate further dysrhythmias (Braunwald et al., 2001).

Beta blockers are the drugs of choice to reduce anginal symptoms and syncopal episodes associated with hypertrophic cardiomyopathy. The negative inotropic effects of beta blockers and calcium channel blockers decrease the myocardial contractility, decreasing obstruction of the outflow tract. Beta blockers also decrease heart rate and increase ventricular compliance, increasing diastolic filling time and cardiac output. Vasodilators, digitalis, nitrates, and diuretics are contraindicated. Amiodarone may be used to treat ventricular dysrhythmias (Braunwald et al., 2001).

## Surgery

Without definitive treatment, clients with cardiomyopathy develop end-stage heart failure. Cardiac transplant is the definitive treatment for dilated cardiomyopathy. Ventricular assist devices may be used to support cardiac output until a donor heart is available. Transplantation is not a viable option for restrictive cardiomyopathy, because transplantation does not eliminate the underlying process causing infiltration or fibrosis, and eventually the transplanted organ is affected as well. See the section on heart failure for more information about cardiac transplantation.

In severely symptomatic clients with obstructive hypertrophic cardiomyopathy, excess muscle may be surgically resected from the aortic valve outflow tract. The septum is incised, and tissue is removed. This procedure provides lasting improvement in about 75% of clients (Braunwald et al., 2001).

An implantable cardioverter-defibrillator (ICD) often is inserted to treat potentially lethal dysrhythmias, reducing the need for antidyrhythmic medications. A dual-chamber pacemaker also may be used for to treat hypertrophic cardiomyopathy.

## NURSING CARE

Nursing assessment and care for clients with dilated and restrictive cardiomyopathy is similar to that for clients with heart failure. Teaching about the disease process and its management is vital. Some degree of activity restriction often is necessary; assist to conserve energy while encouraging self-care. Support coping skills and adaptation to required lifestyle changes. Provide information and support for decision making about cardiac transplantation if that is an option. Discuss the toxic and vasodilator effects of alcohol, and encourage abstinence. See the nursing care section for heart failure for nursing diagnoses and suggested interventions.

The client with hypertrophic cardiomyopathy requires care similar to that provided for myocardial ischemia; nitrates and other vasodilators, however, are avoided. If surgery is performed, nursing care is similar to that for any client undergoing open-heart surgery or cardiac transplant. Discuss the genetic transmission of hypertrophic cardiomyopathy, and suggest screening of close relatives (parents and siblings).

Provide pre- and postoperative care and teaching as appropriate for clients undergoing invasive procedures or surgery for cardiomyopathy.

Nursing diagnoses that may be appropriate for clients with cardiomyoapathy include:

- *Decreased cardiac output* related to impaired left ventricular filling, contractility, or outflow obstruction
- *Fatigue* related to decreased cardiac output
- *Ineffective breathing pattern* related to heart failure
- *Fear* related to risk for sudden cardiac death
- *Ineffective role performance* related to decreasing cardiac function and activity restrictions
- *Anticipatory grieving* related to poor prognosis

## Home Care

Cardiomyopathies are chronic, progressive disorders generally managed in home and community care settings unless surgery or transplant are planned or end-stage heart failure develops. When teaching the client and family for home care, include the following topics.

- Activity restrictions and dietary changes to reduce manifestations and prevent complications
- Prescribed drug regimen, its rationale, intended and possible adverse effects
- The disease process, its expected ultimate outcome, and treatment options
- Cardiac transplantation, including the procedure, the need for lifetime immunosuppression to prevent transplant rejection, and the risks of postoperative infection and long-term immunosuppression
- Symptoms to report to the physician or for which immediate care is needed.
- Cardiopulmonary rescusitation procedures and available training sites

Refer the client and family for home and social services and counseling as indicated. Provide community resources such as support groups or the AHA.

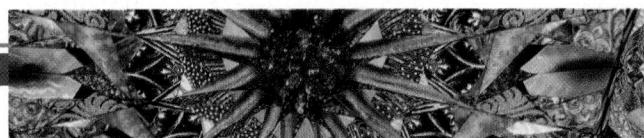

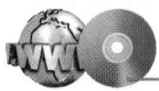

## EXPLORE MediaLink

NCLEX review questions, case studies, care plan activities, MediaLink applications, and other interactive resources for this chapter can be found on the Companion Website at www.prenhall.com/lemone.

Click on Chapter 30 to select the activities for this chapter. For animations, video clips, more NCLEX review questions, and an audio glossary, access the Student CD-ROM accompanying this textbook.

## TEST YOURSELF

1. In reviewing the physician's admitting notes for a client with heart failure, the nurse notes that the client has an ejection fraction of 25%. The nurse recognizes this as meaning:
   a. Ventricular function is severely impaired
   b. The amount of blood being ejected from the ventricles is within normal limits
   c. 25% of the blood entering the ventricle remains in the ventricle after systole
   d. Cardiac output is greater than normal, overtaxing the heart

2. In assessing a client admitted 24 hours previously with heart failure, the nurse notes that the client has lost 2.5 lb (1 kg) of weight, his heart rate is 88 (HR was 105 on admission), and he now has crackles in the bases of his lung fields only. The nurse correctly interprets this data as indicating:
   a. The client's condition is unchanged from admission
   b. A need for more aggressive treatment

   c. The treatment regimen is achieving the desired effect
   d. No further treatment is required at this time as the failure has resolved

3. Morphine 2 to 5 mg IV as needed for pain and dyspnea is ordered for a client in acute pulmonary edema. The nurse appropriately:
   a. Questions this order because no time intervals have been specified
   b. Administers the drug as ordered, monitoring respiratory status
   c. Withholds the drug until the client's respiratory status improves
   d. Administers the drug only when the client complains of chest pain

4. An appropriate goal of nursing care for the client with acute infective endocarditis would be:

a. "Will resume usual activities within 1 week of treatment."
b. "Will relate the benign and self-limiting nature of the disease."
c. "Will consider cardiac transplantation as a viable treatment option."
d. "Will state the importance of continuing intravenous antibiotic therapy as ordered."

5. An expected assessment finding in a client with mitral stenosis being admitted for a valve replacement would be:

a. Muffled heart sounds
b. $S_3$ and $S_4$ heart sounds
c. Diastolic murmur heard at the apex
d. Cardiac heave

See Test Yourself answers in Appendix C.

# BIBLIOGRAPHY

Ackley, B. J., & Ladwig, G. B. (2002). *Nursing diagnosis handbook: A guide to planning care* (5th ed.). St. Louis: Mosby.

American Heart Association. (2001). *2002 heart and stroke statistical update.* Dallas, TX: Author.

Ammon, S. (2001). Managing patients with heart failure. *American Journal of Nursing, 101*(12), 34–40.

Baptiste, M. M. (2001). Aortic valve replacement. *RN, 64*(1), 58–63.

Bither, C. J., & Apple, S. (2001). Home management of the failing heart. *American Journal of Nursing, 101*(12), 41–45.

Braunwald, E., Fauci, A. S., Kasper, D. L., Hauser, S. L., Longo, D. L., & Jameson, J. L. (2001). *Harrison's principles of internal medicine* (15th ed.). New York: McGraw-Hill.

Bullock, B. A., & Henze, R. L. (2000). *Focus on pathophysiology.* Philadelphia: Lippincott.

Capriotti, T. (2002). Current concepts and pharmacologic treatment of heart failure. *MEDSURG Nursing, 11*(2), 71–83.

Carelock, J., & Clark, A. P. (2001). Heart failure: Pathophysiologic mechanisms. *American Journal of Nursing, 101*(12), 26–33.

Copstead, L. C., and Bansik, J. L. (2000). *Pathophysiology: Biological and behavioral perspectives* (2nd ed.). Philadelphia: Saunders.

Deglin, J. H., & Vallerand, A. H. (2003). *Davis's drug guide for nurses* (8th ed.). Philadelphia: F.A. Davis.

Fontaine, K. L. (2000). *Healing practices: Alternative therapies for nursing.* Upper Saddle River, NJ: Prentice Hall Health.

Gallo, J. J., Busby-Whitehead, J., Rabins, P. V., Silliman, R. A., & Murphy, J. B. (Eds.). (1999). *Reichel's care of the elderly: Clinical aspects of aging* (5th ed.). Philadelphia: Lippincott Williams & Wilkins.

Hunt, S. A., Baker, D. W., Chin, M. H., Ciquegrani, M. P., Feldman, A. M., Francis, G. S., Ganiats, T. G., Goldstein, S., Gregoratos, G.,

Jessup, M. L., Noble, R. J., Packer, M., Silver, M. A., and Stevenson, L. W. (2001) ACC/AHA guidelines for the evaluation and management of chronic heart failure in the adult: Executive summary: A report of the American College of Cardiology / American Heart Association Task Force on Practice Guidelines (Committee to Revise the 1995 Guidelines for the Evaluation and Management of Heart Failure). *Circulation, 104,* 2996–3007.

Johnson, M., Bulechek, G., Dochterman, J. M., Maas, M., & Moorhead, S. (2001). *Nursing diagnoses, outcomes, & interventions.* St. Louis: Mosby.

Johnson, M., Maas, M., & Moorhead, S. (Eds.). (2000). *Nursing outcomes classification (NOC)* (2nd ed.). St. Louis: Mosby.

Kearney, K. (2000). Emergency. Digitalis toxicity. *American Journal of Nursing, 100*(6), 51–52.

Kuhn, M. A. (1999). *Complementary therapies for health care providers.* Philadelphia: Lippincott.

Lehne, R. A. (2001). *Pharmacology for nursing care* (4th ed.). Philadelphia: Saunders.

Malarkey, L.M., & McMorrow, M.E. (2000). *Nurse's manual of laboratory tests and diagnostic procedures* (2nd ed.). Philadelphia: Saunders.

McCance, K. L., & Huether, S. E. (2002). *Pathophysiology: The biologic basis for disease in adults and children* (4th ed.). St. Louis: Mosby.

McCloskey, J. C., & Bulechek, G. M. (Eds.) (2000). *Nursing interventions classification (NIC)* (3rd ed.). St. Louis: Mosby.

Meeker, M. H., & Rothrock, J. C. (1999). *Alexander's care of the patient in surgery* (11th ed.). St. Louis: Mosby.

Miracle, V. A. (2001). Put the brakes on pericarditis. *Nursing, 31*(4), 44–45.

Myers, T. A., Eichhorn, D. J., Guzzetta, C. E., Clark, A. P., Klein, J. D., Taliaferro, E., & Calvin, A. (2000). Family presence during invasive procedures and resuscitation: The experi-

ence of family members, nurses, and physicians. *American Journal of Nursing, 100*(2), 32–42.

National Heart, Lung, and Blood Institute. National Institutes of Health. (2002). *Morbidity & mortality: 2002 chart book of cardiovascular, lung, and blood diseases.* Bethesda, MD: Author.

North American Nursing Diagnosis Association. (2001). *NANDA nursing diagnoses: Definitions & classification 2001–2002.* Philadelphia: NANDA.

Porth, C. M. (2002). *Pathophysiology: Concepts of altered health states* (6th ed.). Philadelphia: Lippincott.

Pugh, L. C., Havens, D. S., Xie, S., Robinson, J. M., & Blaha, C. (2001). Case management for elderly persons with heart failure: The quality of life and cost outcomes. *MEDSURG Nursing, 10*(2), 71–75.

Springhouse. (1999). *Nurse's handbook of alternative & complementary therapies.* Springhouse, PA: Author.

Tierney, L. M., McPhee, S. J., & Papadakis, M. A. (2001). *Current medical diagnosis & treatment* (40th ed.). New York: Lange Medical Books/McGraw-Hill.

Urden, L. D., Stacy, K. M., & Lough, M. E. (2002). *Thelan's critical care nursing: Diagnosis and management* (4th ed.). St. Louis: Mosby

Way, L. W., & Dahoerty, G. M. (2003). *Current surgical diagnosis & treatment* (11th ed.). New York: Lange Medical/McGraw-Hill.

Wilkinson, J. M. (2000). *Nursing diagnosis handbook with NIC interventions and NOC outcomes* (7th ed.). Upper Saddle River, NJ: Prentice Hall Health.

Woods, S. L., Froelicher, E. S. S., & Motzer, S. U. (2000). *Cardiac nursing* (4th ed.). Philadelphia: Lippincott.

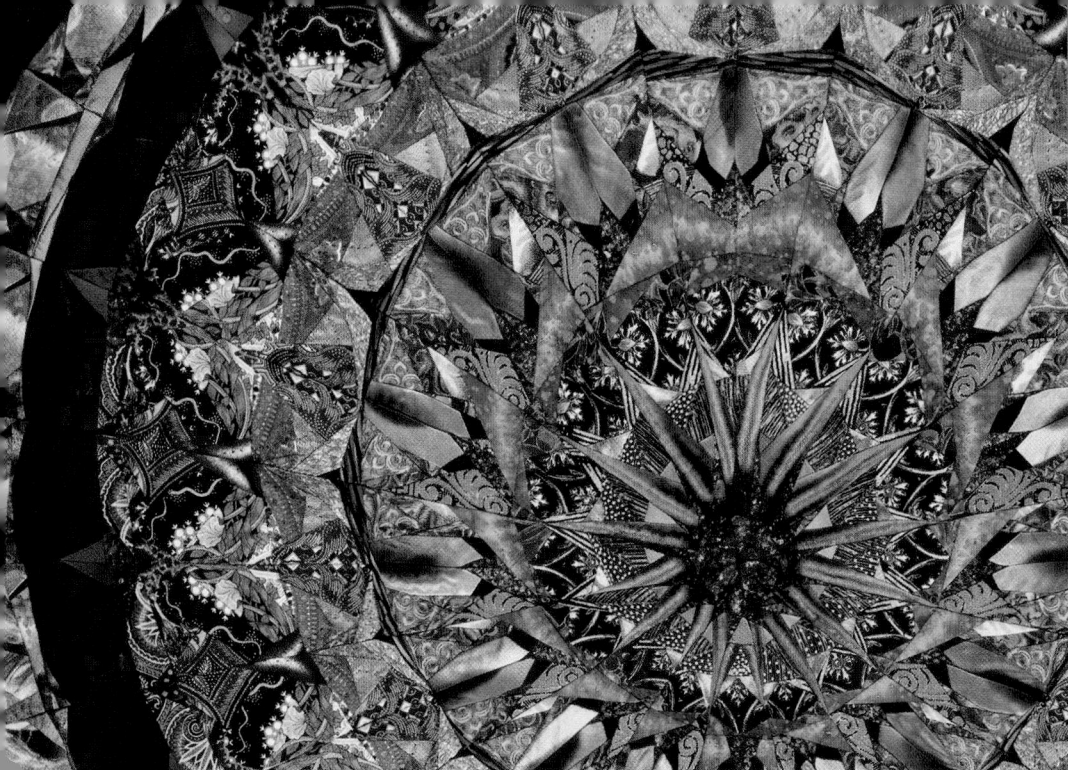

# UNIT 9

# RESPONSES TO ALTERED PERIPHERAL TISSUE PERFUSION

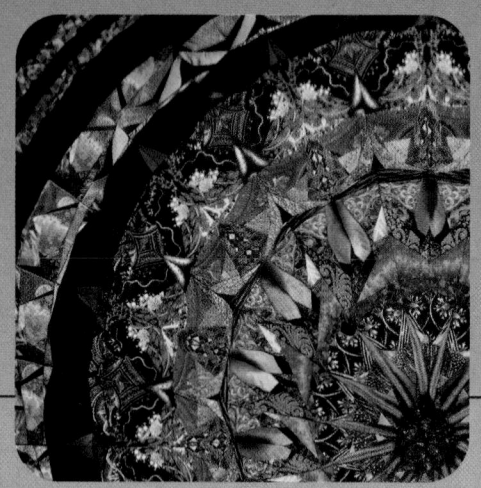

# Assessing Clients with Hematologic, Peripheral Vascular, and Lymphatic Disorders

## MediaLink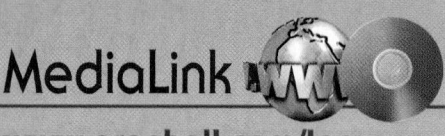

### www.prenhall.com/lemone

Additional resources for this chapter can be found on the Student CD-ROM accompanying this textbook, and on the Companion Website at www.prenhall.com/lemone. Click on Chapter 31 to select the activities for this chapter.

**CD-ROM**
- Audio Glossary
- NCLEX Review

*Animations*
- Lymphatic System
- The Immune Response

**Companion Website**
- More NCLEX Review
- Functional Health Pattern Assessment
- Case Study
  Arterial Blood Pressure

## LEARNING OUTCOMES

After completing this chapter, you will be able to:

- Review the structures and functions of the arterial and venous networks of the peripheral vascular system and the lymphatic system.

- Describe the physiologic dynamics of blood flow, peripheral resistance, and blood pressure.

- Describe the major factors influencing arterial blood pressure.

- Identify interview questions pertinent to the assessment of the peripheral vascular and lymphatic systems.

- Describe physical assessment techniques for peripheral vascular and lymphatic function.

- Identify manifestations of impairment in the function of the peripheral vascular and lymphatic systems.

As the heart ejects blood with each beat, a closed system of blood vessels transports oxygenated blood to all body organs and tissues and then returns it to the heart for reoxygenation in the lungs. This branching network of vessels is called the peripheral vascular system. Systemic circulation is made possible by the vessels of the peripheral vascular system: the arteries, veins, and capillaries. The lymphatic system is a special vascular system that helps maintain sufficient blood volume in the cardiovascular system by picking up excess tissue fluid and returning it to the bloodstream.

## REVIEW OF ANATOMY AND PHYSIOLOGY

### Arterial and Venous Networks

The two main components of the peripheral vascular system are the arterial network and the venous network. The arterial network begins with the major arteries that branch from the aorta. The major arteries of the systemic circulation are illustrated in Figure 31–1 ■. These major arteries branch into successively smaller arteries, which in turn subdivide into the smallest of the arterial vessels, called arterioles. The smallest arterioles feed into beds of hairlike capillaries in the body's organs and tissues.

In the capillary beds, oxygen and nutrients are exchanged for metabolic wastes, and deoxygenated blood begins its journey back to the heart through venules, the smallest vessels of the venous network. Venules join the smallest of veins, which in turn join larger and larger veins. The blood transported by the veins empties into the superior and inferior venae cavae entering the right side of the heart. The major veins of the systemic circulation are shown in Figure 31–2 ■.

### Structure of Blood Vessels

The structure of blood vessels reflects their different functions within the circulatory system (Figure 31–3 ■). Except for the tiniest vessels, blood vessel walls have three layers: the tunica intima, the tunica media, and the tunica adventitia. The tunica intima, the innermost layer, is made of simple squamous epithelium (the endothelium); this provides a slick surface to facilitate the flow of blood. In arteries, the middle layer, or tunica media, is made of smooth muscle and is thicker than the tunica media of veins. This makes arteries more elastic than veins and allows the arteries to alternately expand and recoil as the heart contracts and relaxes with each beat, producing a pressure wave, which can be felt as a **pulse** over an artery. The smaller arterioles are less elastic than arteries but contain more smooth muscle, which promotes their constriction (narrowing) and dilation (widening). In fact, arterioles rather than arteries exert the major control over arterial blood pressure. The tunica adventitia, or outermost layer, is made of connective tissue and serves to protect and anchor the vessel. Veins have a thicker tunica adventitia than do arteries.

Blood in the veins travels at a much lower pressure than blood in the arteries. Veins have thinner walls, a larger lumen, and greater capacity, and many are supplied with valves that help blood flow against gravity back to the heart (see Figure 31–3). The "milking" action of skeletal muscle contraction (called the *muscular pump*) also supports venous return. When skeletal muscles contract against veins, the valves proximal to the contraction open, and blood is propelled toward the heart. The abdominal and thoracic pressure changes that occur with breathing (called the *respiratory pump*) also propel blood toward the heart.

The tiny capillaries, which connect the arterioles and venules, contain only one thin layer of tunica intima that is permeable to the gases and molecules exchanged between blood and tissue cells. Capillaries typically are found in interwoven networks. They filter and shunt blood from terminal arterioles to postcapillary venules.

## Physiology of Arterial Circulation

The factors that affect arterial circulation are blood flow, peripheral vascular resistance, and blood pressure. **Blood flow** refers to the volume of blood transported in a vessel, in an organ, or throughout the entire circulation over a given period of time. It is commonly expressed as liters or milliliters per minute or cubic centimeters per second.

**Peripheral vascular resistance (PVR)** refers to the opposing forces or impedance to blood flow as the arterial channels become more and more distant from the heart. Peripheral vascular resistance is determined by three factors:

- *Blood viscosity:* The greater the viscosity, or thickness, of the blood, the greater its resistance to moving and flowing.
- *Length of the vessel:* The longer the vessel, the greater the resistance to blood flow.
- *Diameter of the vessel:* The smaller the diameter of a vessel, the greater the friction against the walls of the vessel and, thus, the greater the impedance to blood flow.

Blood pressure is the force exerted against the walls of the arteries by the blood as it is pumped from the heart. It is most accurately referred to as mean arterial pressure (MAP). The highest pressure exerted against the arterial walls at the peak of ventricular contraction (systole) is called the systolic blood pressure. The lowest pressure exerted during ventricular relaxation (diastole) is the diastolic blood pressure.

Mean arterial blood pressure is regulated mainly by cardiac output (CO) and peripheral vascular resistance (PVR), as represented in this formula: $MAP = CO \times PVR$. For clinical use, the MAP may be estimated by calculating the diastolic blood pressure plus one-third of the pulse pressure (the difference between the systolic and diastolic blood pressure).

## Factors Influencing Arterial Blood Pressure

Blood flow, peripheral vascular resistance, and blood pressure, which influence arterial circulation, are in turn influenced by various factors. The sympathetic and parasympathetic nervous systems are the primary mechanisms that regulate blood pressure. Stimulation of the sympathetic nervous system exerts a major effect on peripheral resistance by causing vasoconstriction of the arterioles, thereby increasing blood pressure. Parasympathetic stimulation causes vasodilation of the arterioles, lowering blood pressure. Baroreceptors and chemoreceptors in the aortic arch, carotid sinus, and other large vessels are sensitive to pressure and chemical changes and cause reflex

MediaLink | ARTERIAL BLOOD PRESSURE CASE STUDY

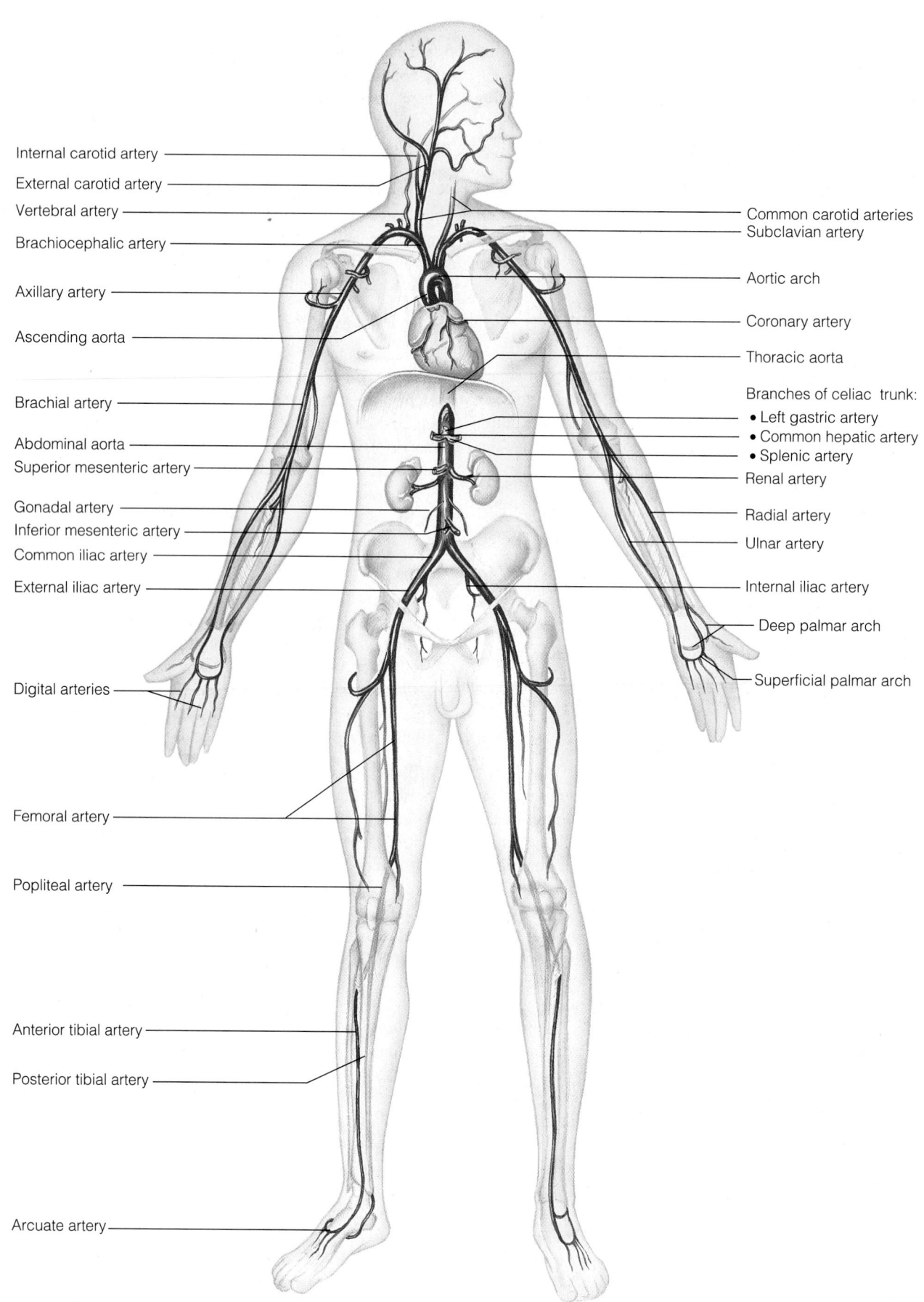

Internal carotid artery

External carotid artery

Vertebral artery

Brachiocephalic artery

Axillary artery

Ascending aorta

Brachial artery

Abdominal aorta

Superior mesenteric artery

Gonadal artery

Inferior mesenteric artery

Common iliac artery

External iliac artery

Digital arteries

Femoral artery

Popliteal artery

Anterior tibial artery

Posterior tibial artery

Arcuate artery

Common carotid arteries

Subclavian artery

Aortic arch

Coronary artery

Thoracic aorta

Branches of celiac trunk:
• Left gastric artery
• Common hepatic artery
• Splenic artery

Renal artery

Radial artery

Ulnar artery

Internal iliac artery

Deep palmar arch

Superficial palmar arch

**Figure 31–1** ■ Major arteries of the systemic circulation.

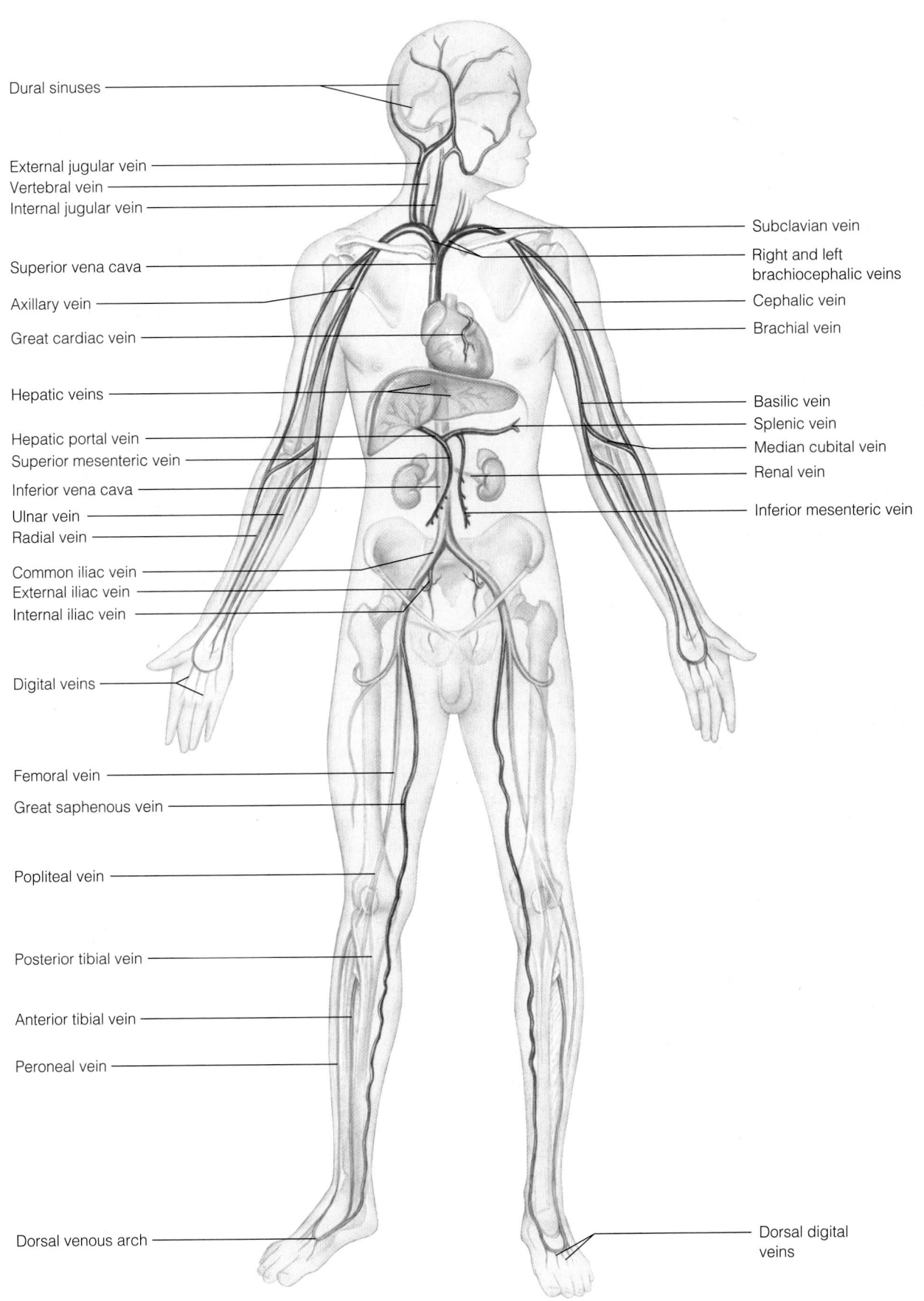

Dural sinuses

External jugular vein
Vertebral vein
Internal jugular vein

Superior vena cava

Axillary vein

Great cardiac vein

Hepatic veins

Hepatic portal vein
Superior mesenteric vein

Inferior vena cava

Ulnar vein
Radial vein

Common iliac vein
External iliac vein
Internal iliac vein

Digital veins

Femoral vein

Great saphenous vein

Popliteal vein

Posterior tibial vein

Anterior tibial vein

Peroneal vein

Dorsal venous arch

Subclavian vein

Right and left
brachiocephalic veins

Cephalic vein

Brachial vein

Basilic vein
Splenic vein

Median cubital vein

Renal vein

Inferior mesenteric vein

Dorsal digital
veins

**Figure 31–2** ■ Major veins of the systemic circulation.

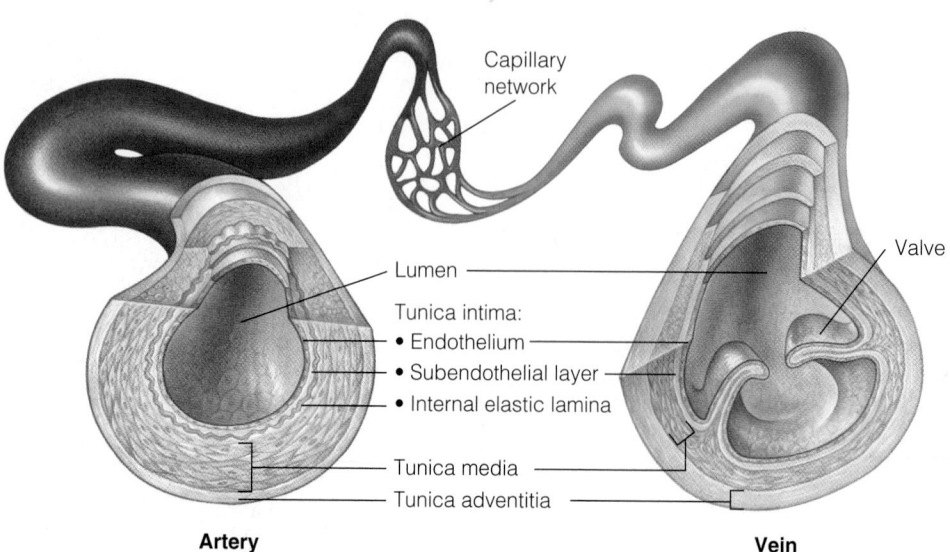

**Figure 31-3** ■ Structure of arteries, veins, and capillaries. Capillaries are composed of only a fine tunica intima. Notice that the tunica media is thicker in arteries than in veins.

sympathetic stimulation, resulting in vasoconstriction, increased heart rate, and increased blood pressure.

The kidneys help maintain blood pressure by excreting or conserving sodium and water. When blood pressure decreases, the kidneys initiate the renin-angiotensin mechanism. This stimulates vasoconstriction, resulting in the release of the hormone aldosterone from the adrenal cortex, increasing sodium ion reabsorption and water retention. In addition, pituitary release of antidiuretic hormone (ADH) promotes renal reabsorption of water. The net result is an increase in blood volume and a consequent increase in cardiac output and blood pressure.

Temperatures may also affect peripheral resistance: Cold causes vasoconstriction, whereas warmth produces vasodilation. Many chemicals, hormones, and drugs influence blood pressure by affecting cardiac output and/or peripheral vascular resistance. For example, epinephrine causes vasoconstriction and increased heart rate; prostaglandins dilate blood vessel diameter (by relaxing vascular smooth muscle); endothelin, a chemical released by the inner lining of vessels, is a potent vasoconstrictor; nicotine causes vasoconstriction; and alcohol and histamine cause vasodilation.

Dietary factors, such as intake of salt, saturated fats, and cholesterol, elevate blood pressure by affecting blood volume and vessel diameter. Race, gender, age, weight, time of day, position, exercise, and emotional state may also affect blood pressure. These factors influence the arterial pressure; systemic venous pressure, though it is much lower, is also influenced by such factors as blood volume, venous tone, and right atrial pressure.

## The Lymphatic System

The structures of the lymphatic system include the lymphatic vessels and several lymphoid organs (Figure 31-4 ■). The lymphatic vessels, or lymphatics, form a network around the arterial and venous channels and interweave at the capillary beds.

They collect and drain excess tissue fluid, called lymph, that "leaks" from the cardiovascular system and accumulates at the venous end of the capillary bed. The lymphatics return this fluid to the heart through a one-way system of lymphatic venules and veins that eventually drain into the right lymphatic duct and left thoracic duct, both of which empty into their respective subclavian veins. Lymphatics are a low-pressure system without a pump; their fluid transport depends on the rhythmic contraction of their smooth muscle and the muscular and respiratory pumps that assist venous circulation.

The organs of the lymphatic system are the lymph nodes, the spleen, the thymus, the tonsils, and the Peyer's patches of the small intestine. Lymph nodes are small aggregates of specialized cells that assist the body's immune system by removing foreign material, infectious organisms, and tumor cells from lymph. Lymph nodes are distributed along the lymphatic vessels, forming clusters in certain body regions such as the neck, axilla, and groin (see Figure 31-4). The spleen, the largest lymphoid organ, is in the upper left quadrant of the abdomen under the thorax. The main function of the spleen is to filter the blood by breaking down old red blood cells and storing or releasing to the liver their by-products (such as iron). The spleen also synthesizes lymphocytes, stores platelets for blood clotting, and serves as a reservoir of blood. The thymus gland is in the lower throat and is most active in childhood, producing hormones (such as thymosin) that facilitate the immune action of lymphocytes. The tonsils of the pharynx and Peyer's patches of the small intestine are lymphoid organs that protect the upper respiratory and digestive tracts from foreign pathogens.

## ASSESSING PERIPHERAL VASCULAR AND LYMPHATIC FUNCTION

The nurse conducts both a health assessment interview to collect subjective data and a physical assessment to collect objective data.

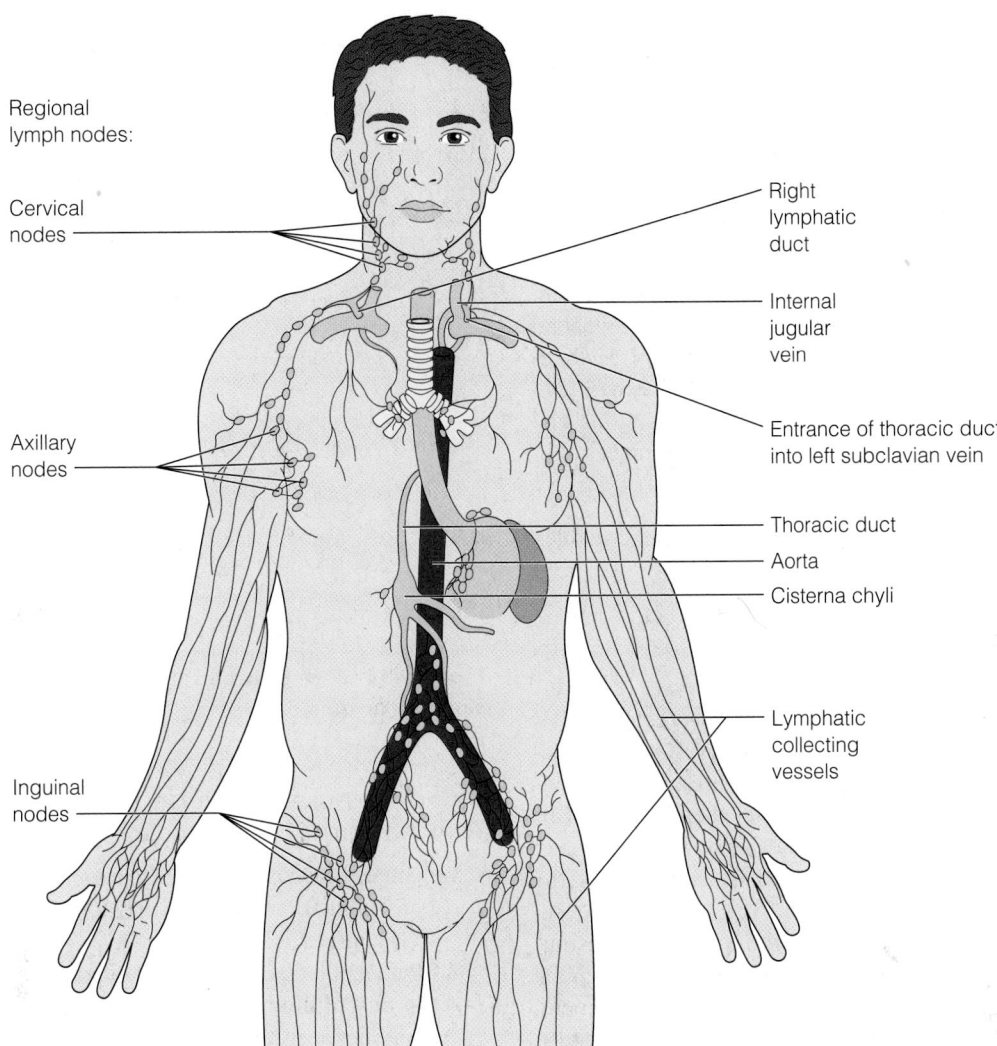

**Figure 31–4** ■ The lymphatic system.

## The Health Assessment Interview

This section provides guidelines for collecting subjective data through a health assessment interview specific to the functions of the peripheral vascular system and the lymphatic system.

### The Peripheral Vascular System

The health assessment of the peripheral vascular system may focus on the client's chief complaint (such as swelling or pain in the legs), or it may be part of a full cardiovascular assessment. If the client has a chief complaint, analyze its onset, characteristics and course, severity, precipitating and relieving factors, and any associated symptoms, noting the timing and circumstances. For example, ask the client the following:

- Does the leg pain occur only with activities such as walking, or also during rest?
- Do your ankles swell at the end of the day, after sitting for prolonged periods, or after sleeping all night?
- Does temperature or the position of your body affect the symptoms?

Next explore the client's medical and family history for any cardiovascular disorders, such as heart disease, arteriosclerosis, peripheral vascular disease (PVD), stroke, hypertension (HTN), hyperlipidemia (elevated fat in blood) and blood clots, or other chronic illnesses (e.g., diabetes). Ask about past surgery of the heart or blood vessels or tests to evaluate their function and about any medications that affect circulation or blood pressure.

Continue the assessment interview with a review of symptoms. Ask the client about past or present pain, burning, numbness, or tingling in the limbs or digits; leg fatigue or cramps; changes in skin color or temperature, texture of hair, ulcers or skin irritation, varicose veins, phlebitis (inflamed veins) or edema (swelling). Explore the client's nutritional history for intake of protein, vitamins and minerals, salt, fats, and fluid. Quantify any consumption of caffeine and alcohol and history of smoking (in pack years) or other tobacco use. Assess the client's activity level for exercise habits and tolerance.

It is important to consider socioeconomic factors that may precipitate or aggravate circulatory problems (e.g., inadequate clothing, shoes, or shelter) and occupational factors, such as prolonged standing or sitting or exposure to temperature extremes. Also assess psychosocial factors that may affect the client's stress level and emotional state.

Other questions and leading statements, categorized by functional health patterns, can be found on the Companion Website.

## The Lymphatic System

The health assessment of the lymphatic system includes a review of specific lymphatic findings, such as lymph node enlargement or swollen glands, as well as other more general complaints about infection or impaired immunity, such as fever, fatigue, or weight loss. If a health problem exists, analyze its onset, characteristics, severity, and precipitating and relieving factors, noting the timing and circumstances. For example, ask the client the following:

- Did you notice that the glands in your neck became swollen after an infection?
- Have you noticed increased fatigue or weakness?
- Have you ever been exposed to radiation?

Explore the client's history for chronic illnesses (e.g., cardiovascular disease, renal disease, cancer, tuberculosis, HIV infection), predisposing factors (e.g., surgery, trauma, infection, blood transfusions, intravenous drug use), and environmental exposure (e.g., radiation, toxic chemicals, travel-related infectious disease). Review the family history for any incidence of cancer, anemia, or blood dyscrasias. Ask the client about past or present bleeding (e.g., from the nose, gums, or mouth; from vomiting; from the rectum; bruising) and associated symptoms (e.g., pallor, dizziness, fatigue, difficulty breathing); lymph node changes (e.g., enlargement, pain or tenderness, itching, warmth); swelling of extremities; and recurrent irritations or infections. Lastly, an assessment of the client's socioeconomic status, lifestyle, intravenous drug use, and sexual practices may be significant in determining risk for diseases associated with impaired lymphatic function.

Other questions and leading statements, categorized by functional health patterns, can be found on the Companion Website.

## Physical Assessment: The Peripheral Vascular System

Physical assessment of the peripheral vascular system can be performed as part of the full cardiovascular assessment or alone for clients who have known or suspected peripheral vascular disease or who are at risk for circulatory complications (e.g., clients who have undergone surgery or are immobile). The techniques used to assess the peripheral vascular system include auscultation of blood pressure, palpation of the major pulse points of the body (Figure 31–5 ■), and inspection of the skin for such changes as edema, ulcerations, or alterations in color and temperature. Recommended equipment for this assessment includes a stethoscope, a tape measure, and a metric ruler. The client may be assessed in the supine, sitting, and standing positions. Box 31–1 reviews guidelines for blood pressure measurement.

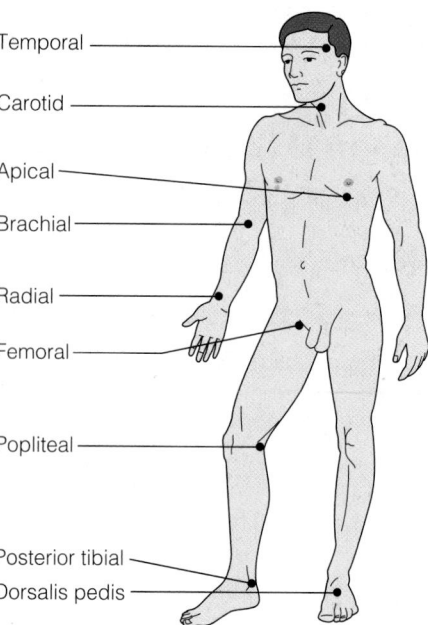

**Figure 31–5** ■ Body sites at which peripheral pulses are most easily palpated.

## Blood Pressure and Pulse Pressure Assessment with Abnormal Findings (✓)

- Auscultate blood pressure in each arm with the client seated.
  - ✓ Consistent BP readings over 140/90 in adults under age 40 is considered hypertension.
  - ✓ BP under 90/60 is considered hypotension.
  - ✓ An **auscultatory gap**—a temporary disappearance of sound between the systolic and diastolic BP—may be a normal variation, or it may be associated with systolic HTN or a drop in diastolic BP due to aortic stenosis.
  - ✓ **Korotkoff's sounds** (see Box 31–1) may be heard down to zero with cardiac valve replacements, hyperkinetic states, thyrotoxicosis, and severe anemia, as well as after vigorous exercise.
  - ✓ The sounds of aortic regurgitation may obscure the diastolic BP.
  - ✓ A difference of over 10 mmHg between arms suggests arterial compression on the side of the lower reading, aortic dissection, or coarctation of the aorta.
- Auscultate blood pressure in each arm with the client standing. If orthostatic changes occur, measure the BP with the client supine, legs dangling, and again with the client standing, 1 to 3 minutes apart.
  - ✓ A decrease in systolic BP of over 10 to 15 mmHg and a drop in diastolic BP on standing is called **orthostatic hypotension.** Causes include antihypertensive medications, volume depletion, peripheral neurovascular disease, prolonged bed rest, and aging.
- Observe the pulse pressure. The **pulse pressure** is the difference between the systolic and diastolic BP. For example, if the BP is 140/80, the pulse pressure is 60. A normal pulse pressure is one-third the systolic measurement.

## BOX 31–1  ■ Guidelines for Blood Pressure Measurement

### REVIEW OF KOROTKOFF'S SOUNDS

The first sound heard is the systolic pressure; at least two consecutive sounds should be clear. If the sound disappears and then is heard again 10 to 15 mm later, an auscultatory gap is present; this may be a normal variant, or it may be associated with hypertension. The first diastolic sound is heard as a muffling of the Korotkoff's sound and is considered the best approximation of the true diastolic pressure. The second diastolic sound is the level at which sounds are no longer heard.

The American Heart Association recommends documenting all three readings when measuring blood pressure, for example, 120/72/64. If only two readings are documented, the systolic and the second diastolic pressure are taken, for example, 120/64.

### TECHNIQUE REMINDERS

- Choose a cuff of an appropriate size: The cuff should snugly cover two-thirds of the upper arm, and the bladder should completely encircle the arm. The bladder should be centered over the brachial artery, with the lower edge 2 to 3 cm above the antecubital space.
- The client's arm should be slightly flexed and supported (on a table or by the examiner) at heart level.
- To determine how high to inflate the cuff, palpate the brachial pulse, and inflate the cuff to the point on the manometer at which the pulse is no longer felt; then, add 30 mmHg to this reading, and use the sum as the target for inflation. Wait 15 seconds before reinflating the cuff to auscultate the BP.
- To recheck a BP, wait at least 30 seconds before attempting another inflation.
- Always inflate the cuff completely, then deflate it. Once deflation begins, allow it to continue; do not try to reinflate the cuff if the first systolic sound is not heard or if the cuff inadvertently deflates.
- The bell of the stethoscope more effectively transmits the low-pitched sounds of BP.

### SOURCES OF ERROR

- Falsely high readings can occur if the cuff is too small, too loose, or if the client supports his or her own arm.
- Falsely low readings can occur if a standard cuff is used on a client with thin arms.

- Inadequate inflation may result in underestimation of the systolic pressure or overestimation of the diastolic pressure if an auscultatory gap is present.
- Rapid deflation and repeated or slow inflations (causing venous congestion) can lead to underestimation of the systolic BP and overestimation of the diastolic BP.

### FACTORS ALTERING BLOOD PRESSURE

- A change from the horizontal to upright position causes a slight decrease (5 to 10 mm) in systolic BP; the diastolic BP remains unchanged or rises slightly.
- BP taken in the arm is lower when the client is standing.
- If the BP is taken with the client in the lateral recumbent position, a lower BP reading may be obtained in both arms; this is especially apparent in the right arm with the client in the left lateral position.
- Factors that increase BP include exercise, caffeine, cold environment, eating a large meal, painful stimuli, and emotions.
- Factors that lower BP include sleep (by 20 mmHg) and very fast, slow, or irregular heart rates.
- BP tends to be higher in taller or heavier clients.

### ALTERNATIVE METHODS OF BLOOD PRESSURE MEASUREMENT

- The palpatory method may be necessary if severe hypotension is present and the BP is inaudible. Palpate the brachial pulse, and inflate the cuff 30 mm above the point where the pulse disappears; deflate the cuff, and note the point on the manometer where the pulse becomes palpable again. Record this as the palpatory systolic BP.
- Leg BP measurement may be needed when there is injury of the arms or to rule out coarctation of the aorta or aortic insufficiency when arm diastolic BP is over 90 mmHg. Place the client in the prone or supine position with the leg slightly flexed. Place a large leg cuff on the thigh with the bladder centered over the popliteal artery. Place the bell of the stethoscope over the popliteal space. Normal leg systolic BP is higher than arm BP; diastolic BP should be equal to or lower than arm BP. Abnormally low leg BP occurs with aortic insufficiency and coarctation of the aorta.

---

✓ A widened pulse pressure with an elevated systolic BP occurs with exercise, arteriosclerosis, severe anemia, thyrotoxicosis, and increased intracranial pressure.

✓ A narrowed pulse pressure with a decreased systolic BP occurs with shock, cardiac failure, and pulmonary embolus.

### Skin Assessment with Abnormal Findings (✓)

- Inspect the color of the skin.
  ✓ Pallor reflects constriction of peripheral blood flow (e.g., due to syncope or shock) or decreased circulating oxyhemoglobin (e.g., due to anemia).
  ✓ Central cyanosis of the lips, earlobes, oral mucosa, and tongue suggests chronic cardiopulmonary disease. (See Box 31–2 for abnormal findings associated with peripheral vascular and lymphatic assessment.)

### Artery and Vein Assessment with Abnormal Findings (✓)

- Palpate the temporal arteries.
  ✓ Redness, swelling, nodularity, and variations in pulse amplitude may occur with temporal arteritis.
- Inspect and palpate the carotid arteries. Note symmetry, the pulse rate, rhythm, volume, and amplitude. Note any variation with respiration. Describe all pulses as increased, normal, diminished, or absent. Scales ranging from 0 to 4+ are sometimes used as follows:

  0 = Absent
  1+ = Diminished
  2+ = Normal
  3+ = Increased
  4+ = Bounding

## BOX 31–2 ■ Abnormal Findings Associated with Peripheral Vascular and Lymphatic Assessment

■ *Pallor* is an absence of color of the skin. The degree of pallor depends on the client's normal skin color and health status. Dark skin may appear ashen or have a yellowish tinge.

■ *Cyanosis* is a bluish discoloration of the skin and mucous membranes in people with light skin. In people with dark skin, cyanosis may be difficult to observe. Inspect the nail beds and conjunctiva.

■ *Edema* is an abnormal accumulation of fluid in the interstitial spaces of body tissues. It is often most apparent in the lower extremities.

■ *Varicose veins* are tortuous and dilated veins that have incompetent valves. The saphenous veins of the legs are most commonly affected.

■ *Enlarged lymph nodes* result from infection or malignancy.

■ *Atrophic changes* are changes in size or activity of body tissues as the result of pathology or injury. Decreased blood flow and oxygenation of the lower extremities often cause atrophic changes of loss of hair, thickened toe nails, changes in pigmentation, and ulcerations.

■ *Gangrene* is the necrosis (or death) of tissue, most often the result of loss of blood supply and infection. Gangrene often begins in the most distal of the tissues of the extremities.

■ *Pressure ulcers,* also called decubitus ulcers or bed sores, are the result of ischemia and hypoxia of tissue following prolonged pressure. These ulcers often are located over bony prominences. If untreated, the tissue changes proceed from red skin to deep, craterlike ulcers.

## BOX 31–3 ■ Types of Pulse Patterns

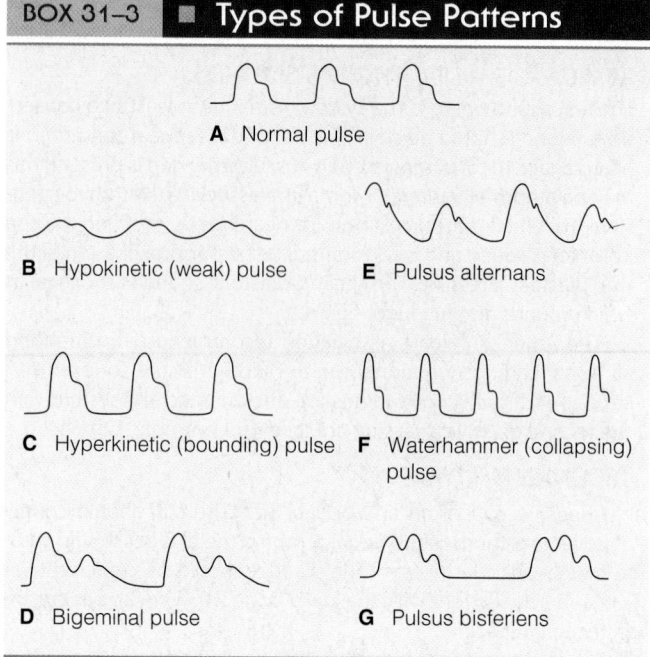

**A** Normal pulse

**B** Hypokinetic (weak) pulse

**C** Hyperkinetic (bounding) pulse

**D** Bigeminal pulse

**E** Pulsus alternans

**F** Waterhammer (collapsing) pulse

**G** Pulsus bisferiens

Pulse waveforms are shown in Box 31–3.

✓ A unilateral pulsating bulge is seen with a tortuous or kinked carotid artery.

✓ Alterations in pulse rate or rhythm are due to cardiac dysrhythmias.

✓ An absent pulse indicates arterial occlusion.

✓ A hypokinetic (weak) pulse is associated with decreased stroke volume (Box 31–3B). This may be due to congestive heart failure (CHF), aortic stenosis, or hypovolemia; to increased peripheral resistance, which may result from cold temperatures; or to arterial narrowing, commonly found with atherosclerosis.

✓ A hyperkinetic (bounding) pulse occurs with increased stroke volume and/or decreased peripheral resistance (Box 31–3C). This may result from states in which cardiac output is high or from aortic regurgitation. It also may occur with anemia, hyperthyroidism, bradycardia, or reduced compliance, as with atherosclerosis.

✓ A bigeminal pulse is marked by decreased amplitude of every second beat (Box 31–3D). This may be due to premature contractions (usually ventricular).

✓ Pulsus alternans is a regular pulse with alternating strong and weak beats (Box 31–3E). This may be due to left ventricular failure and severe HTN.

✓ The waterhammer pulse (collapsing pulse) has a greater than normal amplitude with a sharp rise and fall (Box 31–3F). It occurs with aortic insufficiency.

✓ Pulsus bisferiens has two main peaks in amplitude ("double beat") and occurs with combined aortic stenosis and regurgitation, pericardial effusion, and constructive pericarditis (Box 31–3G).

✓ Pulsus paradoxus is a pulse in which the amplitude is diminished or absent during inspiration and exaggerated during expiration. Pulsus paradoxus occurs with cardiac tamponade, constrictive pericarditis, and severe chronic lung disease.

✓ A palpable thrill over the carotid artery suggests arterial narrowing, as with atherosclerosis.

• Auscultate the carotid arteries, using the bell of the stethoscope.

✓ A murmuring or blowing sound heard over stenosed peripheral vessels is known as a bruit. A bruit heard over the middle to upper carotid artery suggests atherosclerosis.

• Inspect and palpate the internal and external jugular veins for venous pressure. See Box 31–4 for guidelines for assessing jugular venous pressure.

✓ An increase in jugular venous pressure over 3 cm and located above the sternal angle reflects increased right atrial pressure. This occurs with right ventricular failure or, less commonly, with constrictive pericarditis, tricuspid stenosis, and superior venae cavae obstruction.

• If venous pressure is elevated, assess the hepatojugular reflex. (Compress the liver in the right upper abdominal quadrant with the palm of the hand for 30 to 60 seconds while observing the jugular veins.)

✓ A decrease in venous pressure reflects reduced left ventricular output or blood volume.

## BOX 31-4 ■ Assessing Jugular Venous Pressure

When a client with normal venous pressure lies in the supine position, full neck veins are normally visible, but as the head of the bed is elevated, the pulsations disappear. In the client with greatly elevated venous pressure, visible pulsations of the jugular vein are present even in the upright position. To conduct the inspection:

1. Remove clothing from the client's neck and chest. Elevate the head of the the bed 30 to 45 degrees, and turn the client's head to the opposite side. Shine a light tangentially across the neck to increase shadows. If the external jugular veins are distended, they will be visible vertically between the mandible and outer clavicle.

2. If jugular distention is present, assess the jugular venous pressure (JVP) by measuring from the highest point of visible distention to the sternal angle (the point at which the clavicles meet) on both sides of the neck (see the accompanying figure). Bilateral measurements above 3 cm are considered elevated and indicate increased venous pressure; distention on only one side may indicate obstruction.

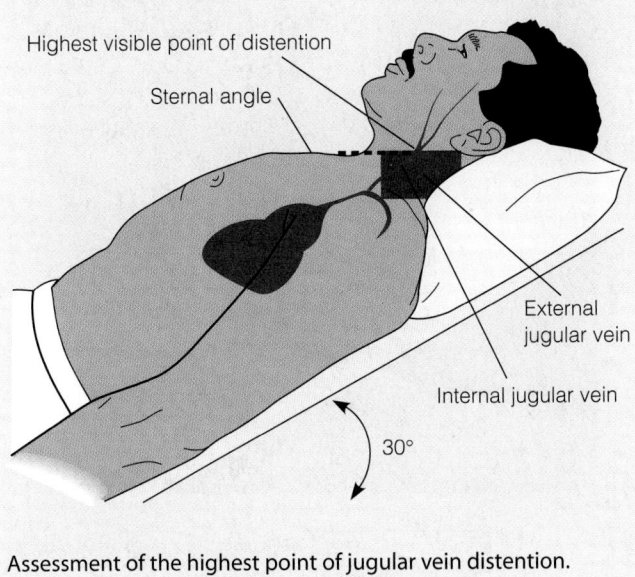

Highest visible point of distention
Sternal angle
External jugular vein
Internal jugular vein
30°

Assessment of the highest point of jugular vein distention.

✓ Unilateral neck vein distention suggests local compression or anatomic anomaly.
✓ A rise in the column of neck vein distention over 1 cm with liver compression indicates right heart failure.

## Upper Extremity Assessment with Abnormal Findings (✓)

• Inspect and palpate the arms, noting size and symmetry, skin color, and temperature.
  ✓ Unilateral swelling with venous prominence occurs with venous obstruction.
  ✓ Extreme localized pallor of the fingers is seen with Raynaud's disease.

✓ Cyanosis of the nailbeds reflects chronic cardiopulmonary disease.
✓ Cold temperature of the hands and fingers occurs with vasoconstriction.
• Palpate the nail beds for capillary refill. (Apply pressure to the client's fingertips. Watch for blanching of the nail beds. Release the pressure. Note the time it takes for capillary refill, indicated by the return of pink color on release of the pressure.)
  ✓ Capillary refill that takes more than 2 seconds reflects circulatory compromise, such as hypovolemia or anemia.
• Assess venous pattern and pressure. (Elevate one of the client's arms over the head for a few seconds. Slowly lower the arm. Observe the filling of the client's hand veins.)
  ✓ Distention of hand veins at elevations over 9 cm above heart level reflects an increase in systemic venous pressure.
• Palpate the radial and brachial pulses. Note rate, rhythm, volume amplitude, symmetry, variations with respiration.
  ✓ Alterations in pulse rate or rhythm are due to cardiac dysrhythmias (such as atrial fibrillation, atrial flutter, and premature ventricular contractions). A pulse rate over 100 beats per minute is tachycardia; a pulse rate below 60 BPM is bradycardia.
  ✓ A pulse deficit (slower radial rate than apical rate) occurs with dysrhythmias and CHF.
  ✓ Irregularities of rhythm produce early beats and pauses (skipped beats) in the pulse, which may be regular in pattern, sporadic, or grossly irregular.
  ✓ Diminished or absent radial pulses may be due to thromboangitis obliterans (Buerger's disease) or acute arterial occlusion.
  ✓ A weak and thready pulse, often with tachycardia, reflects decreased cardiac output.
  ✓ A bounding pulse occurs with hyperkinetic states and atherosclerosis.
  ✓ Unequal pulses between extremities suggest arterial narrowing or obstruction on one side.
  ✓ In sinus dysrhythmia (a normal variant, especially in young adults), the pulse rate increases with inspiration and decreases with expiration.
• If arterial insufficiency is suspected, palpate the ulnar pulse and perform the Allen test:
  • Have the client make a tight fist.
  • Compress both the radial and ulnar arteries.
  • Have the client open the hand to a slightly flexed position.
  • Observe for pallor and manifestations of pain.
  • Release the ulnar artery and observe for the return of pink color within 3 to 5 seconds.
  • Repeat the procedure on the radial artery.
  ✓ The normal ulnar artery may or may not have a palpable pulse.
  ✓ Persistent pallor with the Allen test suggests ulnar artery occlusion.
• Inspect and palpate each leg, noting size, shape, and symmetry; arterial pattern; skin color, temperature, and texture; hair

pattern; pigmentation; rashes; ulcers, sensation; and capillary refill.

✓ Chronic arterial insufficiency may be due to arteriosclerosis or autonomic dysfunction, or to acute occlusion resulting from thrombosis, embolus, or aneurysm.

✓ Signs of arterial disruption include pallor, dependent rubor (dusky redness); cool to cold temperature; and atrophic changes, such as hair loss with shiny and smooth texture, thickened nails, sensory loss, slow capillary refill, and muscle atrophy.

✓ Ulcers with symmetric margins, a deep base, black or necrotic tissue, and absence of bleeding may occur at pressure points on or between the toes, on the heel, on the lateral malleolar or tibial area, over the metatarsal heads, or along the side or sole of the foot.

✓ Gangrene due to complete arterial occlusion presents as black, dry, hard skin; pregangrenous color changes include deep cyanosis and purple-black discoloration.

## Lower Extremity Assessment with Abnormal Findings (✓)

• With the client supine, assess the venous pattern of the legs. Repeat with the client standing.

✓ Signs of venous insufficiency include swelling, thickened skin, cyanosis, stasis dermatitis (brown pigmentation, erythema, and scaling), and superficial ankle ulcers located predominantly at the medial malleolus with uneven margins, ruddy granulation tissue, and bleeding. Varicose veins appear as dilated, tortuous, and thickened veins, which are more prominent in a dependent position.

• Palpate the femoral, popliteal, posterior tibial, and dorsalis pedis pulses for volume, amplitude, and symmetry.

✓ Diminished or absent leg pulses suggest partial or complete arterial occlusion of the proximal vessel and are often due to arteriosclerosis obliterans.

✓ Increased and widened femoral and popliteal pulsations suggest aneurysm.

✓ Absence of a posterior tibial pulse with signs and symptoms of arterial insufficiency is usually due to acute occlusion by thrombosis or embolus.

✓ Diminished or absent pedal pulses are often due to popliteal occlusion associated with diabetes mellitus.

• If pulses are diminished, observe for postural color changes. Elevate both legs 60 degrees, and observe the color of the soles of the feet. Have the client sit and dangle the legs; note the return of color to the feet.

✓ Extensive pallor on elevation is suggestive of arterial insufficiency.

✓ Rubor (dusky redness) of the toes and feet along with delayed venous return (over 45 seconds) suggests arterial insufficiency.

• If arterial insufficiency is suspected, auscultate the femoral arteries.

✓ Femoral bruits suggest arterial narrowing due to arteriosclerosis.

• Inspect and gently palpate the calves.

✓ Redness, warmth, swelling, tenderness, and cords along a superficial vein suggest thrombophlebitis or deep vein thrombosis (DVT).

• Inspect and palpate for edema. Use your thumb to compress the dorsum of the client's foot, around the ankles, and along the tibia (Figure 31–6A ■). A depression in the skin that does not immediately refill is called pitting edema. Edema can be graded on a scale of from 1+ to 4+ (Figure 31–6B):

| 1+ (−2mm depression) | No visible change in the leg; slight pitting |
| 2+ (−4mm depression) | No marked change in the shape of the leg; pitting slightly deeper |
| 3+ (−6mm depression) | Leg visibly swollen; pitting deep |
| 4+ (−8mm depression) | Leg very swollen; pitting very deep |

✓ Edema may be caused by disease of the cardiovascular system such as CHF; by renal, hepatic, or lymphatic problems; or by infection.

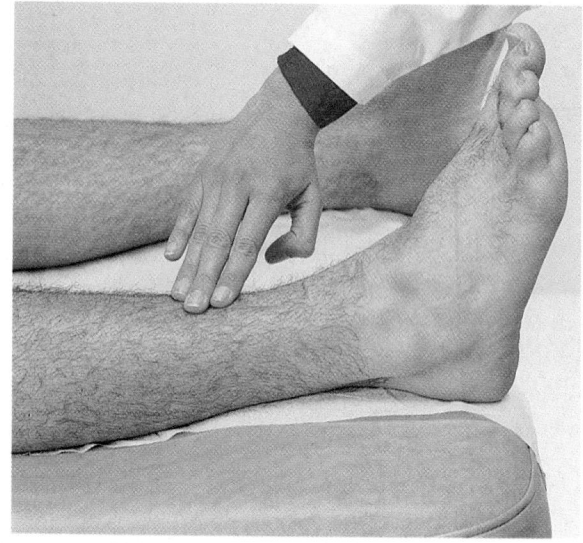

A

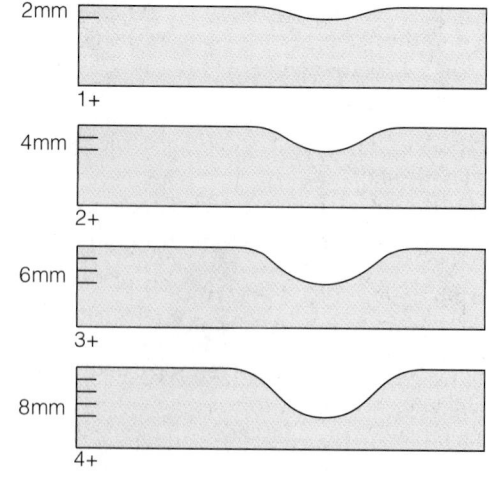

B

**Figure 31–6** ■ Evaluation of edema. *A,* Palpating for edema over the tibia. *B,* Four-point scale for grading edema.

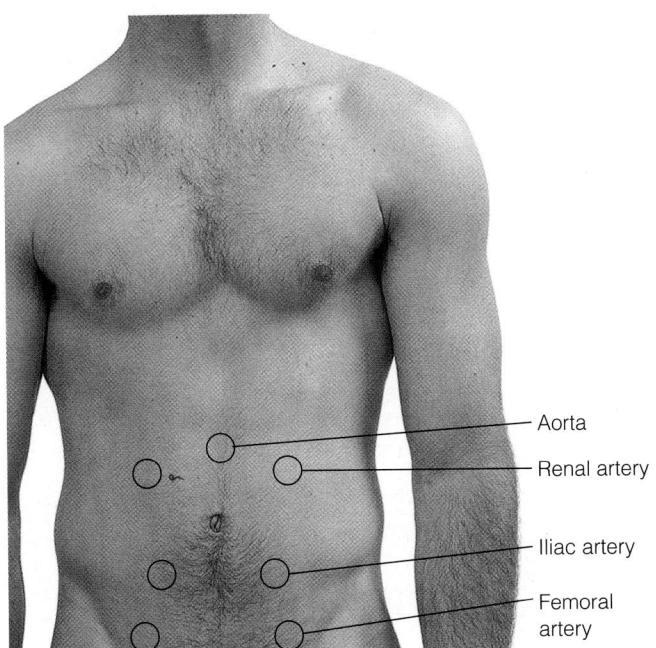

**Figure 31–7** ■ Auscultation sites of the abdominal aorta and its branches.

✓ Venous distention suggests venous insufficiency or incompetence.

## Abdominal Assessment with Abnormal Findings (✓)

- Inspect and palpate the abdominal aorta. Note size, width, and any visible pulsations or bulging.
  - ✓ A pulsating mass in the upper abdomen suggests an aortic aneurysm, particularly in the older adult.
  - ✓ An aorta greater than 2.5 to 3 cm in width reflects pathologic dilation, most likely due to arteriosclerosis.
- Auscultate the epigastrium and each abdominal quadrant, using the bell of the stethoscope (Figure 31–7 ■).
  - ✓ Abdominal bruits reflect turbulent blood flow associated with partial arterial occlusion.
  - ✓ A bruit heard over the aorta suggests an aneurysm.
  - ✓ A bruit heard over the epigastrium and radiating laterally, especially with HTN, suggests renal artery stenosis.
  - ✓ Bruits heard in the lower abdominal quadrants suggest partial occlusion of the iliac arteries.

## Physical Assessment: The Lymphatic System

Physical assessment of the lymphatic system is usually integrated into the assessment of other body systems. For example, the tonsils are observed with the pharynx during the head and neck assessment; the regional lymph nodes are evaluated with corresponding body regions (e.g., occipital, auricular, and cervical nodes are evaluated with assessment of the head and neck, axillary nodes with assessment of the breast or thorax, epitrochlear node with assessment of the peripheral vascular exam of the arms, and inguinal nodes with assessment of the

abdomen); the spleen can be palpated during the abdominal assessment. The techniques of inspection and palpation are used for the lymphatic examination; a tape measure and metric ruler may be helpful.

## Skin Assessment with Abnormal Findings (✓)

- Inspect the skin of the extremities and over the regional lymph nodes, noting any edema, erythema, red streaks, or skin lesions.
  - ✓ **Lymphangitis** (inflammation of a lymphatic vessel) may produce a red streak with induration (hardness) following the course of the lymphatic collecting duct; infected skin lesions may be present, particularly between the digits.
  - ✓ **Lymphedema** (swelling due to lymphatic obstruction) occurs with congenital lymphatic anomaly (Milroy's disease) or with trauma to the regional lymphatic ducts from surgery or metastasis (e.g., arm lymphedema after radical mastectomy with axillary node removal).
  - ✓ Edema of lymphatic origin is usually not pitting, and the skin may be thickened; one example is the taut swelling of the face and body that occurs with myxedema, associated with hypothyroidism.

## Lymph Node Assessment with Abnormal Findings (✓)

- Palpate the regional lymph nodes of the head and neck, axillae, arms, and groin.
  Use firm, circular movements of the finger pads and note size, shape, symmetry, consistency, delineation, mobility, tenderness, sensation, and condition of overlying skin.
  - ✓ **Lymphadenopathy** refers to the enlargement of lymph nodes (over 1 cm) with or without tenderness. It may be caused by inflammation, infection, or malignancy of the nodes or the regions drained by the nodes.
  - ✓ Lymph node enlargement with tenderness suggests inflammation (lymphadenitis). With bacterial infection, the nodes may be warm and matted with localized swelling.
  - ✓ Malignant or metastatic nodes may be hard, indicating lymphoma; rubbery, indicating Hodgkin's disease; or fixed to adjacent structures. Usually they are not tender.
  - ✓ Ear infections and scalp and facial lesions, such as acne, may cause enlargement of the preauricular and cervical nodes.
  - ✓ Anterior cervical nodes are enlarged and infected with streptococcal pharyngitis and mononucleosis.
  - ✓ Lymphadenitis of the cervical and submandibular nodes occurs with herpes simplex lesions.
  - ✓ Brain tumors may metastasize to the occipital nodes.
  - ✓ Enlargement of supraclavicular nodes, especially the left, is highly suggestive of metastatic disease from abdominal and thoracic cancer.
  - ✓ Axillary lymphadenopathy is associated with breast cancer.
  - ✓ Lesions of the genitals may produce enlargement of the inguinal nodes.
  - ✓ Persistent generalized lymphadenopathy is associated with acquired immune deficiency syndrome (AIDS) and AIDS-related complex (ARC).

## Spleen Assessment with Abnormal Findings (✓)

- Palpate for the spleen, in the upper left quadrant of the abdomen.
  - ✓ A palpable spleen in the left upper abdominal quadrant of an adult may indicate abnormal enlargement (splenomegaly) and may be associated with cancer, blood dyscrasias, and viral infection, such as mononucleosis.
- Percuss for splenic dullness in the lowest left intercostal space (ICS) at the anterior axillary line or in the ninth to tenth ICS at the midaxillary line (Figure 31–8 ■).
  - ✓ A dull percussion note in the lowest left ICS at the anterior axillary line or below the tenth rib at the midaxillary line suggests splenic enlargement.

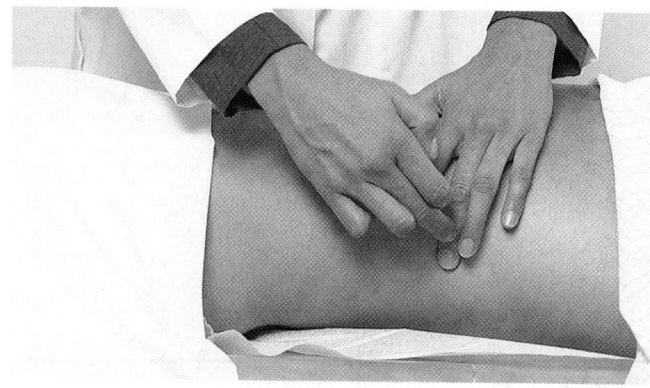

Figure 31–8 ■ Percussing the spleen.

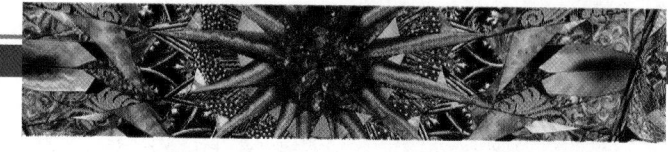

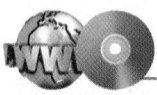 **EXPLORE MediaLink**

NCLEX review questions, case studies, care plan activities, MediaLink applications, and other interactive resources for this chapter can be found on the Companion Website at www.prenhall.com/lemone.

Click on Chapter 31 to select the activities for this chapter. For animations, video clips, more NCLEX review questions, and an audio glossary, access the Student CD-ROM accompanying this textbook.

## TEST YOURSELF

1. What part of the peripheral vascular system has the major control of blood pressure?
   a. Veins
   b. Capillaries
   c. Arteries
   d. Arterioles

2. Which of the following components of the lymphatic system is/are the largest?
   a. Spleen
   b. Tonsils
   c. Thymus
   d. Peyer's patches

3. What method would be most appropriate to assess the carotid arteries?
   a. Inspect for absence of movement
   b. Auscultate with the bell of the stethoscope

   c. Palpate with firm pressure
   d. Percuss lightly over each artery

4. When auscultating the abdominal aorta, you hear a murmuring or blowing sound. You would document this sound as a:
   a. Hypokinetic pulse
   b. Bigeminal pulse
   c. Bruit
   d. Dysrhythmia

5. Swelling of a body part as a result of lymphatic obstruction is labeled:
   a. Lymphedema
   b. Lymphadenopathy
   c. Atrophic change
   d. Central cyanosis

See Test Yourself answers in Appendix C.

## BIBLIOGRAPHY

Andresen, G. (1998). Assessing the older patient. *RN, 61*(3), 46–56.

Ayello, E. (2000). On the lookout for peripheral vascular disease. *Nursing, 30*(6 Home Health), 64hh1–2, 64hh4.

Ayello, E. (2001). Why is pressure ulcer risk assessment so important? *Nursing, 31*(11), 74–80.

Faria, S. (1999). Assessment of peripheral arterial pulses. *Home Care Provider, 4*(4), 140–141.

Hoskins, M. (1997). Using dopplers. *Community Nurse, 3*(3), 17–18.

MacLaren, J. (2001). Skin changes in lymphoedema: Pathophysiology and management options. *International Journal of Palliative Nursing, 7*(8), 381–382, 384–388.

McConnell, E. A. (1997). Performing Allen's test . . . whether ulnar and radial arteries are patent. *Nursing, 17*(11), 26.

Watson, R. (2000). Assessing cardiovascular functioning in older people. *Nursing Older People, 12*(6), 27–28.

Weber, J., & Kelley, J. (2002). *Health assessment in nursing* (2nd ed.). Philadelphia: Lippincott.

Willis, K. (2001). Gaining perspective on peripheral vascular disease. *Nursing, 31*(2 Hospital Nursing), 32hn1–4.

Wilson, S., & Giddens, J. (2001). *Health assessment for nursing practice.* St. Louis: Mosby.

Young, T. (2001). Leg ulcer assessment. *Practice Nurse, 21*(7), 50, 52.

# CHAPTER 32

# Nursing Care of Clients with Hematologic Disorders

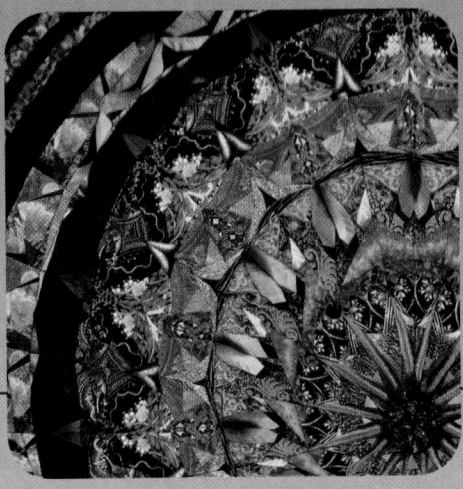

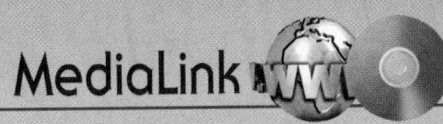

## www.prenhall.com/lemone

Additional resources for this chapter can be found on the Student CD-ROM accompanying this textbook, and on the Companion Website at www.prenhall.com/lemone. Click on Chapter 32 to select the activities for this chapter.

**CD-ROM**
- Audio Glossary
- NCLEX Review

*Animation*
- Sickle Cell Anemia

**Companion Website**
- More NCLEX Review
- Case Study
  Immune Thrombocytopenic Purpura
- Care Plan Activity
  Acute Myelocytic Leukemia
- MediaLink Applications
  Stem Cell Transplant
  Sickle Cell Anemia

## LEARNING OUTCOMES

After completing this chapter, you will be able to:

- Relate the physiology and assessment of the hematologic system and related systems (see Chapter 31) to commonly occurring hematologic disorders.

- Describe the pathophysiology of common hematologic disorders.

- Identify diagnostic tests commonly used for hematologic disorders.

- Discuss nursing implications for medications prescribed for hematologic disorders.

- Discuss nursing implications for bone marrow transplantation, chemotherapy, and radiation for hematologic disorders.

- Compare and contrast bleeding disorders.

- Describe the major types of leukemia and the most common treatment modalities and nursing interventions.

- Differentiate Hodgkin's disease from non-Hodgkin's lymphomas.

- Use the nursing process to provide individualized care to clients with hematologic disorders.

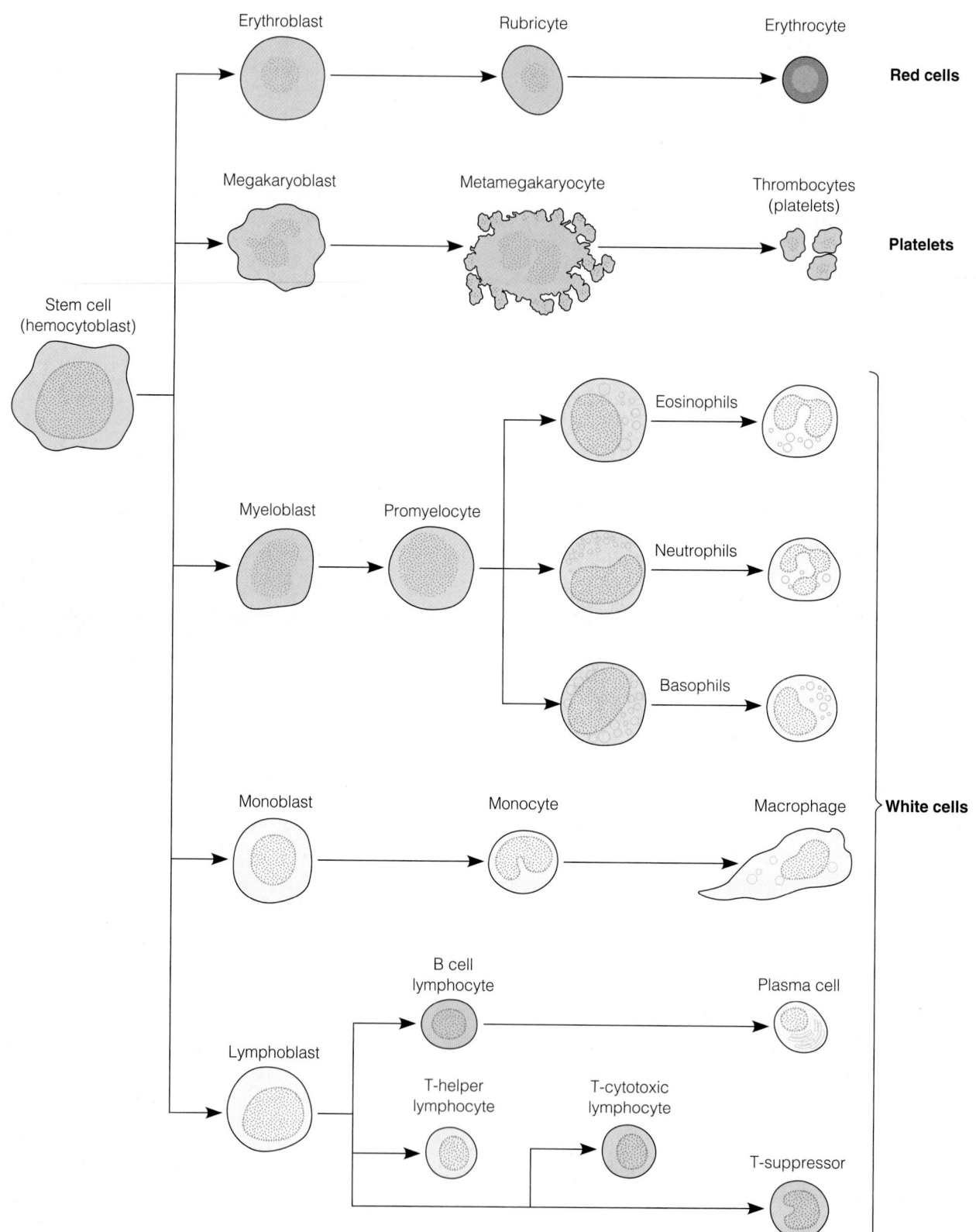

**Figure 32–1** ■ Blood cell formation from stem cells. Regulatory factors control the differentiation of stem cells into blasts. Each of the five kinds of blasts is committed to producing one type of mature blood cell. Erythroblasts, for example, can differentiate only into RBCs; megakaryoblasts can differentiate only into platelets.

Disorders affecting the blood and blood-forming organs have effects that range from minor disruptions in daily activities to major life-threatening crises. Clients with hematologic disorders need holistic nursing care, including emotional support and care for problems involving major body systems.

Blood is an exchange medium between the external environment and the body's cells. Blood consists of plasma, solutes (e.g., proteins, electrolytes, and organic constituents), red blood cells, white blood cells, and platelets, which are fragments of cells.

The *hematopoietic* (blood-forming) system includes the bone marrow (myeloid) tissues, where blood cells form, and the lymphoid tissues of the lymph nodes, where white blood cells mature and circulate. All blood cells originate from cells in the bone marrow called **stem cells,** or *hemocytoblasts*. Regulatory mechanisms cause stem cells to differentiate into families of parent cells, each of which gives rise to one of the formed elements of the blood (red blood cells, platelets, and white cells). The origin of the cellular components of blood is illustrated in Figure 32–1 ■.

This chapter focuses on health changes resulting from changes in red cells, white cells, platelets, and clotting factors. An overview of each type of blood cell is provided before the disorders are presented to facilitate understanding the effects of, responses to, and care of clients with hematologic disorders.

# RED BLOOD CELL DISORDERS

**Red blood cells (RBCs)** and the hemoglobin molecules they contain are required for oxygen transport to body tissues. Hemoglobin also binds with some carbon dioxide, carrying it to the lungs for excretion. Abnormal numbers of RBCs, changes in their size and shape, or altered hemoglobin content or structure can adversely affect health. Anemia, the most common RBC disorder, is an abnormally low RBC count or reduced hemoglobin content. Polycythemia is an abnormally high RBC count.

## PHYSIOLOGY REVIEW OF RED BLOOD CELLS

The red blood cell (**erythrocyte**) is shaped like a biconcave disk (Figure 32–2 ■). This unique shape increases the surface area of the cell and allows the cell to pass through very small capillaries without disrupting the cell membrane. RBCs are the most common type of blood cell.

Hemoglobin is the oxygen-carrying protein within RBCs. It consists of the heme molecule and globin, a protein molecule. Globin is made of four polypeptide chains—two alpha chains and two beta chains (Figure 32–3 ■). Each of the four polypeptide chains contains a heme unit containing an iron atom. The iron atom binds reversibly with oxygen, allowing it to transport oxygen as *oxyhemoglobin* to the cells. Hemoglobin is synthesized within the RBC. The rate of synthesis depends on the availability of iron (Porth, 2002).

Normal adult laboratory values for red blood cells are defined and identified in Table 32–1. The size, color, and shape of stained RBCs also may be analyzed. RBCs may be *normocytic* (normal size), smaller than normal (*microcytic*), or

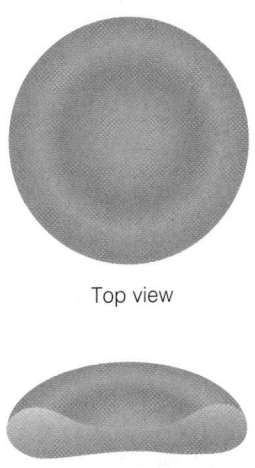

Top view

Side view

**Figure 32–2** ■ Top and side view of a red blood cell (erythrocyte). Note the distinctive concave shape.

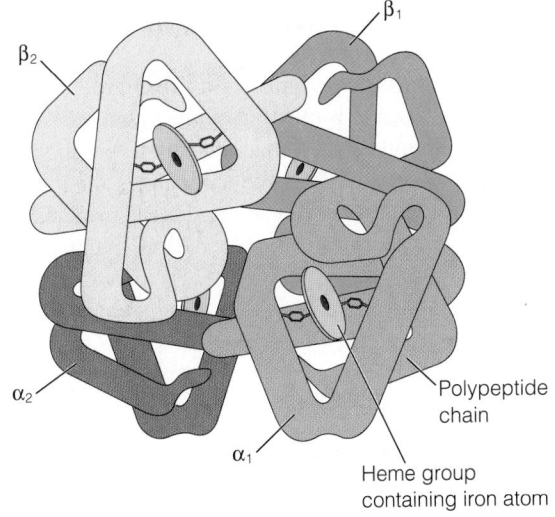

$\beta_1$

$\beta_2$

$\alpha_2$

$\alpha_1$

Polypeptide chain

Heme group containing iron atom

**Figure 32–3** ■ The hemoglobin molecule includes globin (a protein) and heme, which contains iron. Globin is made of four subunits, two alpha and two beta polypeptide chains. A heme disk containing an iron atom (red dot) nests within the folds of each protein subunit. The iron atoms combine reversibly with oxygen, transporting it to the cells.

| TABLE 32–1 | Normal Laboratory Values for Red Blood Cells | |
|---|---|---|
| **Laboratory Test** | **Normal Range** | **Definition** |
| Red blood cell (RBC) count<br>• Men<br>• Women | 4.2–5.4 million/mm³<br>3.6–5.0 million/mm³ | Number of circulating RBCs per mm³ of blood |
| Reticulocytes | 1.0%–1.5% of total RBC | Number of immature RBCs per mm³ of blood |
| Hemoglobin (Hgb)<br>• Men<br>• Women | 14–16.5 g/dL<br>12–15 g/dL | Amount of hemoglobin per dL (100 mL) of blood |
| Hematocrit (Hct)<br>• Men<br>• Women | 40%–50%<br>37%–47% | Packed volume of RBCs in 100 mL of blood expressed as a percentage |
| Mean corpuscular volume (MCV) | 85–100 fL/cell | Average volume of individual RBCs |
| Mean corpuscular hemoglobin concentration (MCHC) | 31–35 g/dL | Average concentration or percentage of hemoglobin per RBC |
| Mean corpuscular hemoglobin (MCH) | 27–34 pg/cell | Calculated average weight of hemoglobin per RBC |

larger than normal (*macrocytic*). Their color may be normal (*normochromic*) or diminished (*hypochromic*).

## Red Blood Cell Production and Regulation

In adults, RBC production (**erythropoiesis**) (Figure 32–4 ■) begins in red bone marrow of the vertebrae, sternum, ribs, and pelvis, and is completed in the blood or spleen. *Erythroblasts* begin forming hemoglobin while they are in the bone marrow, a process that continues throughout RBC lifespan. Erythroblasts differentiate into *normoblasts*. As these slightly smaller cells mature, their nucleus and most organelles are ejected, eventually causing normoblasts to collapse inward and assume the characteristic biconcave shape of RBCs. The cells enter the circulation as *reticulocytes,* which fully mature in about 48 hours. The complete sequence from stem cell to RBC takes 3 to 5 days.

Tissue hypoxia is the stimulus for RBC production. The hormone *erythropoietin* is released by the kidneys in response to hypoxia. It stimulates the bone marrow to produce RBCs. However, the process of RBC production takes about 5 days to maximize. During periods of increased RBC production, the percentage of reticulocytes in the blood exceeds that of mature cells.

## Red Blood Cell Destruction

RBCs have a life span of about 120 days. Old or damaged RBCs are *lysed* (destroyed) by phagocytes in the spleen, liver, bone marrow, and lymph nodes. The process of RBC destruction is called **hemolysis.** Phagocytes save and reuse amino acids and iron from heme units in the lysed RBCs. Most of the heme unit is converted to bilirubin, an orange-yellow pigment that is removed from the blood by the liver and excreted in the bile.

During disease processes causing increased hemolysis or impaired liver function, bilirubin accumulates in the serum, causing a yellowish appearance of the skin and sclera (*jaundice*).

## THE CLIENT WITH ANEMIA

**Anemia** is an abnormally low number of circulating RBCs, low hemoglobin concentration, or both. Decreased numbers of circulating RBCs is the usual cause of anemia. This may result from blood loss, inadequate RBC production, or increased RBC destruction. Insufficient or defective hemoglobin within RBCs contributes to anemia. Depending on its severity, anemia may affect all major organ systems.

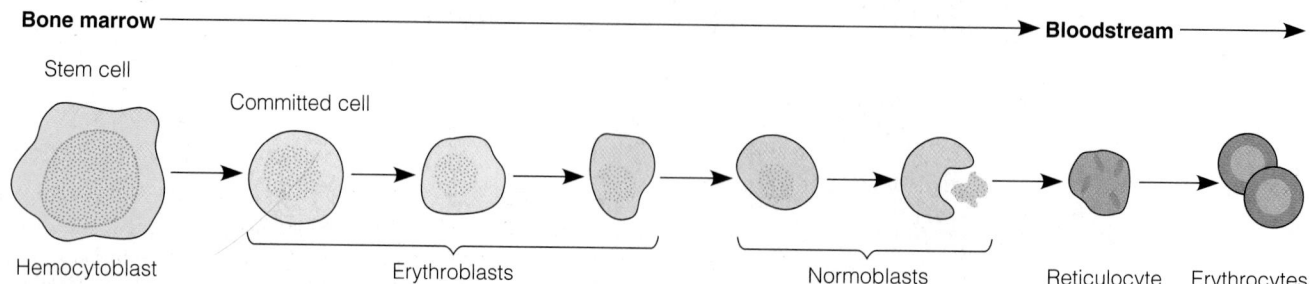

**Figure 32–4** ■ Erythropoiesis. RBCs begin as erythroblasts within the bone marrow, maturing into normoblasts, which eventually eject their nucleus and organelles to become reticulocytes. Reticulocytes mature within the blood or spleen to become erythrocytes.

## PATHOPHYSIOLOGY AND MANIFESTATIONS

A number of different pathologic mechanisms can lead to anemia (Box 32–1). Regardless of the cause, every type of anemia reduces the oxygen-carrying capacity of the blood, leading to tissue hypoxia. The resulting manifestations depend on the severity of the anemia, how quickly it develops, and other factors such as age and health status.

When anemia develops gradually and the RBC reduction is moderate, successful compensatory mechanisms may result in few symptoms except when the oxygen needs of the body increase due to exercise or infection. Symptoms develop as RBCs are further reduced. Pallor of the skin, mucous membranes, conjunctiva, and nail beds develops as a result of blood redistribution to vital organs and lack of hemoglobin. As tissue oxygenation decreases, the heart and respiratory rates rise. Tissue hypoxia may cause angina, fatigue, dyspnea on exertion, and night cramps. It also stimulates erythropoietin release; increased erythropoietin activity may cause bone pain. Cerebral hypoxia can lead to headache, dizziness, and dim vision. Heart failure may develop in severe anemia.

With rapid blood loss, blood volume is decreased as well as the oxygen-carrying capacity of the blood. Signs of circulatory shock may occur. With chronic bleeding, fluid shifts from the interstitial spaces into the vessels, maintaining blood volume. Blood viscosity is reduced, which may result in a systolic heart murmur. See page 936 for *Multisystem Effects of Anemia*.

Anemia is categorized by cause: blood loss, nutritional, hemolytic, and bone marrow suppression. The pathophysiology of these types of anemias follows.

## Blood Loss Anemia

When anemia results from acute or chronic bleeding, RBCs and other blood components are lost from the body. With acute blood loss, circulating volume decreases, increasing the risk for shock and circulatory failure (see Chapter 6).  Fluid shifts from the interstitial spaces into the vascular compartment to maintain blood volume, diluting the cellular components of the blood and reducing its viscosity. In acute blood loss, circulating RBCs are of normal size and shape, but the hemoglobin and hematocrit are reduced. If sufficient iron is available, the number of circulating RBCs returns to normal within 3 to 4 weeks after the bleeding episode. Chronic blood loss, on the other hand, depletes iron stores as RBC production attempts to maintain the RBC supply. The resulting RBCs are microcytic (small) and hypochromic (pale).

## Nutritional Anemias

Nutritional anemias result from nutrient deficits that affect RBC formation (erythropoiesis) or hemoglobin synthesis. The nutrient deficit may be caused by inadequate diet, malabsorption, or an increased need for the nutrient. The most common types of nutritional anemias are iron deficiency anemia, vitamin $B_{12}$ anemia, and folic acid deficiency anemia. Vitamin $B_{12}$ and folic acid anemias are sometimes called megaloblastic anemias, as enlarged nucleated RBCs called megaloblasts are seen in these anemias.

### Iron Deficiency Anemia

**Iron deficiency anemia** is the most common type of anemia. It develops when the supply of iron is inadequate for optimal RBC formation. The body cannot synthesize hemoglobin without iron. Iron deficiency anemia results in fewer numbers of RBCs, microcytic and hypochromic RBCs, as well as malformed RBCs (poikilocytosis).

Excessive iron loss due to chronic bleeding is the usual cause of iron deficiency anemia in adults. Menstrual blood loss is the most common cause in adult females. Iron deficiency anemia also may result from inadequate dietary iron intake (less than 1 mg/day), malabsorption, or the increased iron requirements associated with pregnancy and lactation. Box 32–2 summarizes common causes of iron deficiency anemia.

Iron deficiency anemia is particularly common in older adults. Chronic, occult (hidden) blood loss may occur from slowly bleeding ulcers, gastrointestinal inflammation, hemorrhoids, and cancer. Inadequate dietary iron intake also contributes to anemia in the older adult. Access to transportation may limit fresh food consumption, a factor contributing to poor iron intake among all adults, especially people with limited or fixed incomes.

---

### BOX 32–1 ■ Pathophysiologic Mechanisms of Anemia

#### DECREASED RBC PRODUCTION

- Altered hemoglobin synthesis
  - Iron deficiency
  - Thalassemias
  - Chronic inflammation
- Altered DNA synthesis
  - Vitamin $B_{12}$ or folic acid malabsorption or deficiency
- Bone marrow failure
  - Aplastic anemia (stem cell dysfunction)
  - Red cell aplasia
  - Myeloproliferative leukemias
  - Cancer metastasis, lymphoma
  - Chronic infection or inflammation, physical and emotional fatigue

#### INCREASED RBC LOSS OR DESTRUCTION

- Acute or chronic blood loss
  - Hemorrhage or trauma
  - Chronic gastrointesinal bleeding, menorrhagia
- Increased hemolysis
  - Hereditary cell membrane disorders
  - Defective hemoglobin—Sickle cell anemia or trait
  - Pyruvate kinase (PK) or G6PD deficiency affecting glycolysis or cell oxidation
  - Immune mechanisms and disorders (e.g., blood reaction, hypersensitivity responses, autoimmune disorders)
  - Splenomegaly and hypersplenism
  - Infection
  - Erythrocyte trauma (e.g., due to cardiopulmonary bypass, hemolytic uremic syndrome)

# Multisystem Effects of Anemia

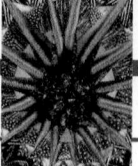

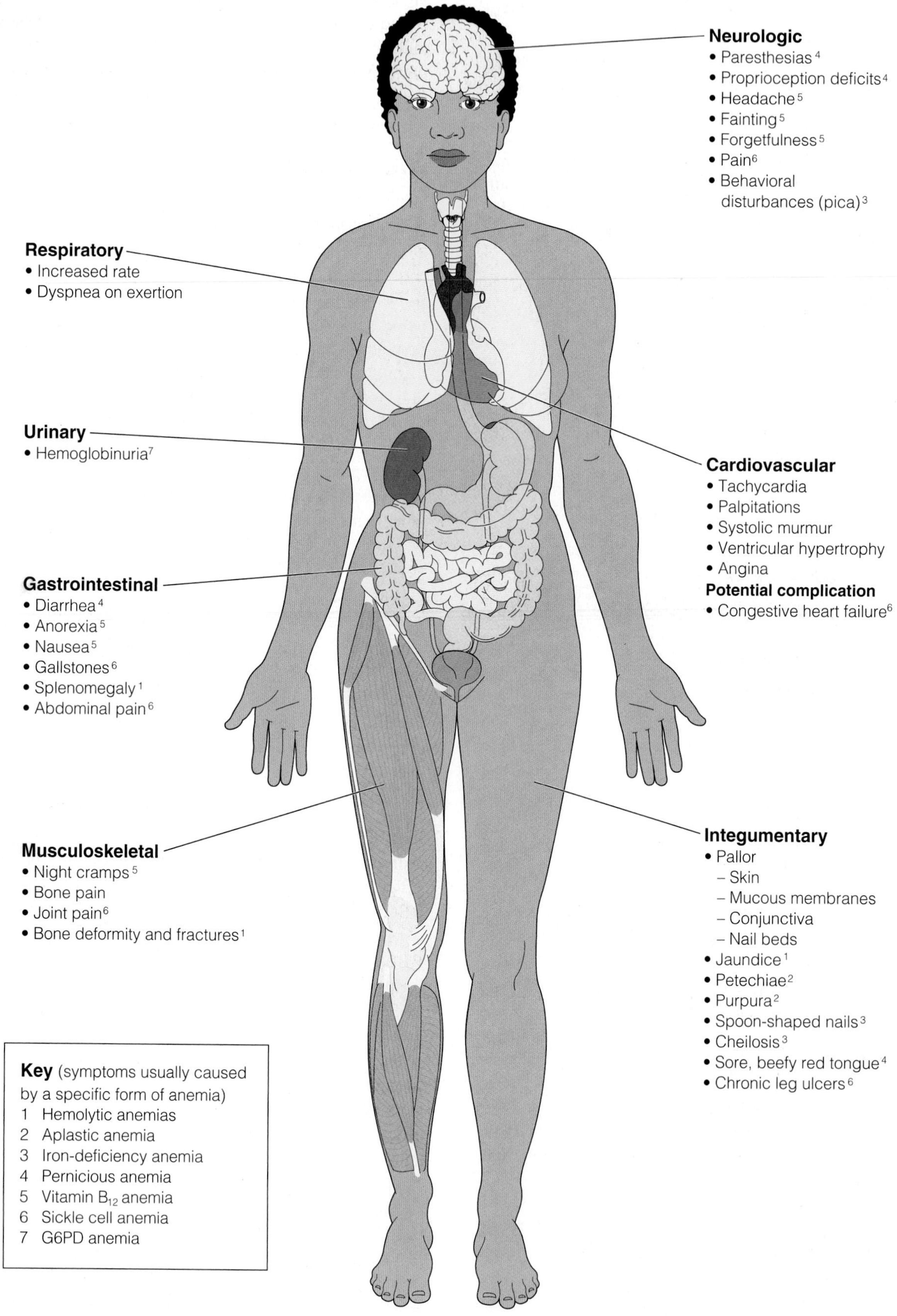
Neurologic
• Paresthesias [4]
• Proprioception deficits [4]
• Headache [5]
• Fainting [5]
• Forgetfulness [5]
• Pain [6]
• Behavioral disturbances (pica) [3]
Respiratory
• Increased rate
• Dyspnea on exertion
Urinary
• Hemoglobinuria [7]
Cardiovascular
• Tachycardia
• Palpitations
• Systolic murmur
• Ventricular hypertrophy
• Angina
Potential complication
• Congestive heart failure [6]
Gastrointestinal
• Diarrhea [4]
• Anorexia [5]
• Nausea [5]
• Gallstones [6]
• Splenomegaly [1]
• Abdominal pain [6]
Musculoskeletal
• Night cramps [5]
• Bone pain
• Joint pain [6]
• Bone deformity and fractures [1]
Integumentary
• Pallor
– Skin
– Mucous membranes
– Conjunctiva
– Nail beds
• Jaundice [1]
• Petechiae [2]
• Purpura [2]
• Spoon-shaped nails [3]
• Cheilosis [3]
• Sore, beefy red tongue [4]
• Chronic leg ulcers [6]
Key (symptoms usually caused by a specific form of anemia)
1 Hemolytic anemias
2 Aplastic anemia
3 Iron-deficiency anemia
4 Pernicious anemia
5 Vitamin $B_{12}$ anemia
6 Sickle cell anemia
7 G6PD anemia

## BOX 32-2 ■ Causes of Iron Deficiency Anemia

- Dietary deficiencies
- Decreased absorption
  a. Partial or total gastrectomy
  b. Chronic diarrhea
  c. Malabsorption syndromes
- Increased metabolic requirements
  a. Pregnancy
  b. Lactation
- Blood loss
  a. Gastrointestinal bleeding (especially due to ulcers or chronic aspirin use)
  b. Menstrual losses
- Chronic hemoglobinuria

In addition to the general manifestations of anemia described earlier, chronic iron deficiency may lead to brittle, spoon-shaped nails; cheilosis (cracks at the corners of the mouth); a smooth, sore tongue; and pica (a craving for unusual substances, such as clay or starch).

The primary treatment for iron deficiency anemia is increased dietary intake of iron-rich foods and oral or parenteral iron supplements.

### Vitamin B$_{12}$ Deficiency Anemia

Vitamin B$_{12}$ is necessary for DNA synthesis and is almost exclusively found in foods derived from animals. **Vitamin B$_{12}$ deficiency** occurs when inadequate vitamin B$_{12}$ is consumed, or, more commonly, when it is poorly absorbed from the gastrointestinal tract. Deficiency of this vitamin impairs cell division and maturation, especially in rapidly proliferating red blood cells. As a result, macrocytic, misshapen (oval rather than concave) RBCs with thin membranes are produced. Great numbers of these large, immature RBCs enter the circulation. These cells are fragile, incapable of carrying adequate amounts of oxygen, and have a shortened life span.

Failure to absorb dietary vitamin B$_{12}$ is called **pernicious anemia.** It develops due to lack of *intrinsic factor,* a substance secreted by the gastric mucosa. Intrinsic factor binds with vitamin B$_{12}$ and travels with it to the ileum, where the vitamin is absorbed. In the absence of intrinsic factor, vitamin B$_{12}$ cannot be absorbed into the body.

Vitamin B$_{12}$ deficiency may also result from other malabsorption disorders and dietary factors. Resection of the stomach or ileum, loss of pancreatic secretions, and chronic gastritis can affect vitamin B$_{12}$ absorption. Dietary deficiencies of vitamin B$_{12}$ are rare, usually occurring only among strict vegetarians.

Manifestations of vitamin B$_{12}$ deficiency anemia develop gradually as bodily stores of the vitamin are depleted. Pallor or slight jaundice and weakness develop. In pernicious anemia, a smooth, sore, beefy red tongue and diarrhea may occur. Because vitamin B$_{12}$ is important for neurologic function, *paresthesias* (altered sensations, such as numbness or tingling) in the ex-

tremities and problems with *proprioception* (the sense of one's position in space) develop. These manifestations may progress to difficulty maintaining balance due to spinal cord damage. Central nervous system manifestations of relatively short duration (6 months or less) are reversible with treatment, but may be permanent if treatment is delayed (Tierney et al, 2001).

When the anemia results from insufficient dietary intake of vitamin B$_{12}$, clients are instructed to increase their intake of foods containing the vitamin, such as meats, eggs, and dairy products. Vitamin B$_{12}$ supplements may be ordered for severe anemia or for clients who are strict vegetarians. Parenteral vitamin B$_{12}$ replacement is required when malabsorption disorders or lack of intrinsic factor is the cause. Parenteral replacement therapy must be continued for life.

### Folic Acid Deficiency Anemia

Like vitamin B$_{12}$, folic acid is required for DNA synthesis and normal maturation of red blood cells. **Folic acid deficiency anemia** is characterized by fragile, megaloblastic cells. Folic acid is found in green leafy vegetables, fruits, cereals, and meats, and is absorbed from the intestines.

Folic acid deficiency anemia due to inadequate intake is more common among people who are chronically undernourished. This includes older adults, alcoholics, and the drug addicted. Alcoholics are especially at risk because alcohol suppresses folate metabolism, which forms folic acid. Increased folic acid requirements also may lead to anemia. Pregnant women are at the greatest risk. Infants and teenagers can develop temporary folic acid deficiencies during periods of rapid growth. Impaired folic acid absorption and metabolism can cause folic acid deficiency anemia. Malabsorption disorders such as celiac sprue (a hereditary gastrointestinal disorder characterized by inability to metabolize amino acids found in gluten), and certain medications, such as methotrexate and some chemotherapeutic agents, may be implicated. Causes of folic acid deficiency anemia are summarized in Box 32–3.

## BOX 32-3 ■ Causes of Folic Acid Deficiency Anemia

- Inadequate dietary intake
  *At risk:*
  a. Older adults
  b. Alcoholics
  c. Clients receiving total parenteral nutrition
- Increased metabolic requirements
  *At risk:*
  a. Pregnant women
  b. Infants and teenagers
  c. Clients undergoing hemodialysis
  d. Clients with forms of hemolytic anemia
- Folic acid malabsorption and impaired metabolism
  a. Celiac sprue
  b. Chemotherapeutic agents, folate antagonists (methotrexate, pentamidine), or anticonvulsants
  c. Alcoholism

The manifestations develop gradually as folic acid stores are depleted. Signs and symptoms may include pallor, progressive weakness and fatigue, shortness of breath, and heart palpitations. Manifestations similar to those associated with vitamin $B_{12}$ anemia, such as glossitis, cheilosis, and diarrhea, are common. No neurologic symptoms occur with folic acid deficiency anemia, helping differentiate it from vitamin $B_{12}$ deficiency anemia. These two nutritional anemias do, however, sometimes coexist.

Among the undernourished, adding foods containing folic acid to the diet usually corrects the anemia. Other clients often require oral folic acid supplements. Depending on the cause of the deficiency, folate replacement may continue for a short or an expended period of time. Folate supplements are recommended for all women who can become pregnant and during pregnancy. Folate deficiency is strongly associated with neural tube defects such as meningomyelocele. The neural tube develops early in the process of fetal development, often before pregnancy is recognized.

## Hemolytic Anemias

**Hemolytic anemias** are characterized by premature destruction (*lysis*) of RBCs. When RBCs break down, iron and other by-products of their destruction remain in the plasma. RBC lysis may occur within the circulatory system or due to phagocytosis by cells of the reticuloendothelial system. In response to hemolysis, the hematopoietic activity of bone marrow increases, leading to increased reticulocytes in circulating blood. Most types of hemolytic anemia are characterized by normocytic and normochromic RBCs.

There are many different causes of hemolytic anemias (Box 32–4). The cause may be *intrinsic*, arising from disorders within the RBC itself, or *extrinsic*, originating outside the RBC. Intrinsic disorders include cell membrane defects, defects in hemoglobin structure and function, and inherited enzyme deficiencies. Extrinsic causes of hemolytic anemia include drugs, bacterial and other toxins, and trauma. This section discusses sickle cell anemia, thalassemia, acquired hemolytic anemia, and glucose-6-phosphate dehydrogenase anemia.

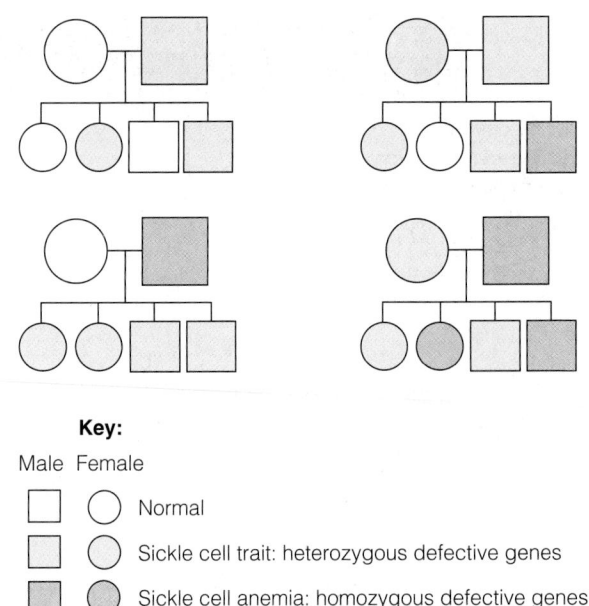

**Key:**

Male Female

- □ ○ Normal
- □ ○ Sickle cell trait: heterozygous defective genes
- □ ○ Sickle cell anemia: homozygous defective genes

**Figure 32–5** ■ Inheritance pattern for sickle cell anemia.

### Sickle Cell Anemia

**Sickle cell anemia** is a hereditary, chronic hemolytic anemia. It is characterized by episodes of *sickling,* during which RBCs become abnormally crescent shaped. The disorder is transmitted as an autosomal recessive genetic defect (Figure 32–5 ■). This defect causes synthesis of an abnormal form of hemoglobin (HbS) within red blood cells. Sickle cell anemia can significantly shorten life span, with most deaths occurring due to infection (McCance & Huether, 2002).

The disease is most common among people of African descent (see Focus on Diversity box on page 939). In the United States, 7% to 13% of blacks carry the defective gene, having inherited it from one parent (McCance & Huether, 2002). These people have *sickle cell trait.* About 40% of their hemoglobin is HbS (Porth, 2002). They are likely to remain asymptomatic unless stressed by severe hypoxia. Less than 1% of African Americans are homozygous for the disorder; that is, they have inherited a defective gene from both parents. These people have *sickle cell disease;* nearly all their hemoglobin is HbS (Porth, 2002). They are at risk for **sickle cell crisis,** severe episodes of fever and intense pain that are the hallmark of this disorder.

The HbS gene changes the structure of the beta chain of the hemoglobin molecule. When hypoxemia develops and HbS is deoxygenated, it crystallizes into rodlike structures. Clusters of these rods form long chains that deform the erythrocyte into a crescent or sickle shape. The sickled cells tend to clump together and obstruct capillary blood flow, causing ischemia and possible infarction of surrounding tissue. See *Pathophysiology Illustrated* on page 940.

When normal oxygen tension is restored, the sickled RBCs resume their normal shape; that is, they "unsickle." Repeated episodes of sickling and unsickling weaken RBC mem-

### BOX 32–4 ■ Causes of Hemolytic Anemia

#### INTRINSIC

- RBC cell-membrane defects
- Hemoglobin structure defects (e.g., sickle cell anemia, thalassemia)
- Inherited enzyme defects (e.g., G6PD deficiency)

#### EXTRINSIC

- Drugs, chemicals
- Toxins and venoms
- Bacterial and other infections
- Trauma, burns
- Mechanical damage (prosthetic heart valves)

## Focus on Diversity

### SICKLE CELL ANEMIA

Sickle cell anemia tends to affect people whose origins are in equatorial countries, particularly those in central Africa, the Near East, the Mediterranean region, and parts of India. Hispanics from the Caribbean and Central and South America also may have the HbS gene. This gene may protect against lethal forms of malaria, an endemic disease in many equatorial regions.

The gene for HbS is transmitted in an autosomal recessive pattern from parent to offspring. A parent with one HbS gene (heterozygous) has a 50% risk of transmitting the gene to each child (see Figure 32–5). If both parents carry the gene, each child has a 25% risk of inheriting the gene from both parents. A person who carries both HbS genes (homozygous) is likely to develop sickle cell disease.

Sickle cell anemia is a serious chronic and recurrent disease. The stress of the disease is compounded by the risk for its transmission to offspring. Recommend that all clients with sickle cell trait or disease obtain genetic counseling as part of their family planning process.

branes. The weakened RBCs are hemolyzed and removed. Consequently, the normal life span of RBCs is greatly reduced in sickle cell anemia, increasing the demand for RBC production. Conditions likely to trigger sickling include hypoxia, low environmental or body temperature, excessive exercise, anesthesia, dehydration, infections, or acidosis.

The acute and chronic manifestations of sickle cell anemia arise from episodes of RBC sickling. Sickling causes general manifestations of hemolytic anemia, including pallor, fatigue, jaundice, and irritability. Extensive sickling can precipitate a crisis due to occluded circulation, impaired erythropoiesis, or sequestration of large amounts of blood in the liver or spleen.

A vasoocclusive or thrombotic crisis occurs when sickling develops in the microcirculation. Obstruction of blood flow triggers vasospasm that halts all blood flow in the vessel. Lack of blood flow leads to tissue ischemia and infarction. Vasoocclusive crises are painful and last an average of 4 to 6 days. Infarction of small vessels in the extremities causes painful swelling of the hands and feet; large joints also may be affected. Priapism (persistent, painful erection of the penis) may develop. Abdominal pain may signal infarction of abdominal organs and structures. Stroke may result from cerebral vessel occlusion (McCance & Huether, 2002). Repeated infarcts associated with sickling can affect the structure and function of nearly every organ system.

Compromised erythropoiesis can lead to profound *aplastic anemia* in sickle cell disease due to the shortened RBC life span. *Sequestration crises* are marked by pooling of large amounts of blood in the liver and spleen. This sickle cell crisis only occurs in children.

There is no cure for this disease; treatment is primarily supportive. Treatment for sickle cell crisis includes rest, oxygen,

and analgesics for pain. Adequate hydration is essential to improve blood flow, reduce pain, and prevent renal damage. Precipitating factors are treated, and folic acid supplements may be given to meet the increased demands for RBC production. Blood transfusions may be necessary during surgery or pregnancy. Genetic counseling is recommended for people at risk for sickle cell anemia.

### Thalassemia

**Thalassemia** is an inherited disorder of hemoglobin synthesis in which either the alpha or beta chains of the hemoglobin molecule are missing or defective. This leads to deficient hemoglobin production and fragile hypochromic, microcytic RBCs called *target cells* because of their distinctive bull's-eye appearance.

Thalassemia usually affects certain populations. People of Mediterranean descent (southern Italy and Greece) are more likely to have beta-defect thalassemias (often called *Cooley's anemia* or Mediterranean anemia). People of Asian ancestry, especially from Thailand, the Philippines, and China, more often have alpha-defect thalassemia. Africans and African Americans may have both alpha- and beta-defect thalassemia. As with sickle cell anemia, only one defective beta chain-forming gene may be present (*beta-thalassemia minor*), causing mild symptoms or both may be defective (*beta-thalassemia major*), leading to more severe symptoms. Children with thalassemia major rarely reach adulthood, although repeated blood transfusions may extend their lifespan (McCance & Huether, 2002). Four genes are responsible for alpha chain formation; one, two, three, or all four may be defective. In the latter case (*alpha-thalassemia major*), death is inevitable and usually occurs in utero. Genetic studies and counseling are recommended for people at risk for this illness.

People with thalassemia minor often are asymptomatic. When manifestations do occur, they include mild to moderate anemia, mild splenomegaly, bronze skin coloring, and bone marrow hyperplasia. The major form of the disease causes severe anemia, heart failure, and liver and spleen enlargement from increased red cell destruction. Fractures of the long bones, ribs, and vertebrae may result from bone marrow expansion and thinning due to increased hematopoiesis. Accumulation of iron in the heart, liver, and pancreas following repeated transfusions for treatment may eventually cause failure of these organs.

### Acquired Hemolytic Anemia

*Acquired hemolytic anemia* results from hemolysis due to factors outside of the RBC. Causes of acquired hemolytic anemias include:

- Mechanical trauma to RBCs produced by prosthetic heart valves, severe burns, hemodialysis, or radiation
- Autoimmune disorders
- Bacterial or protozoal infection
- Immune-system-mediated responses, such as transfusion reactions
- Drugs, toxins, chemical agents, or venoms

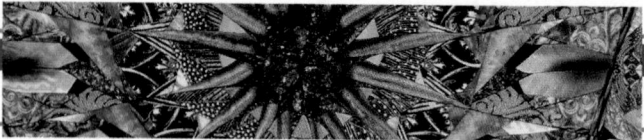

### Hemoglobin S and Red Blood Cell Sickling

Sickle cell anemia is caused by an inherited autosomal recessive defect in Hb synthesis. Sickle cell hemoglobin (HbS) differs from normal hemoglobin only in the substitution of the amino acid valine for glutamine in both beta chains of the hemoglobin molecule.

When HbS is oxygenated, it has the same globular shape as normal hemoglobin. However, when HbS off-loads oxygen, it becomes insoluble in intracellular fluid and crystallizes into rodlike structures. Clusters of rods form polymers (long chains) that bend the erythrocyte into the characteristic crescent shape of the sickle cell.

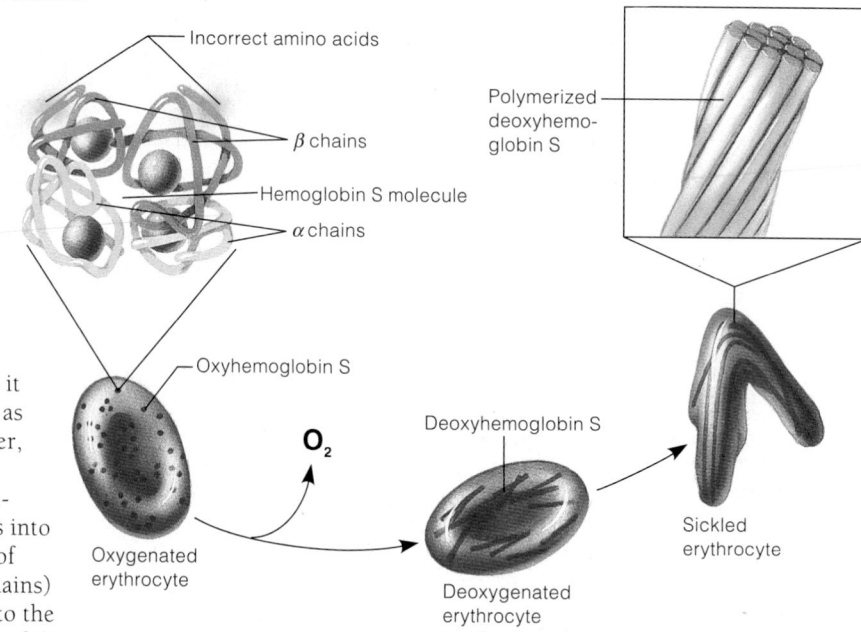

### The Sickle Cell Disease Process

Sickle cell disease is characterized by episodes of acute painful crises. Sickling crises are triggered by conditions causing high tissue oxygen demands or that affect cellular pH. As the crisis begins, sickled erythrocytes adhere to capillary walls and to each other, obstructing blood flow and causing cellular hypoxia. The crisis accelerates as tissue hypoxia and acidic metabolic waste products cause further sickling and cell damage.

Sickle cell crises cause microinfarcts in joints and organs, and repeated crises slowly destroy organs and tissues. The spleen and kidneys are especially prone to sickling damage.

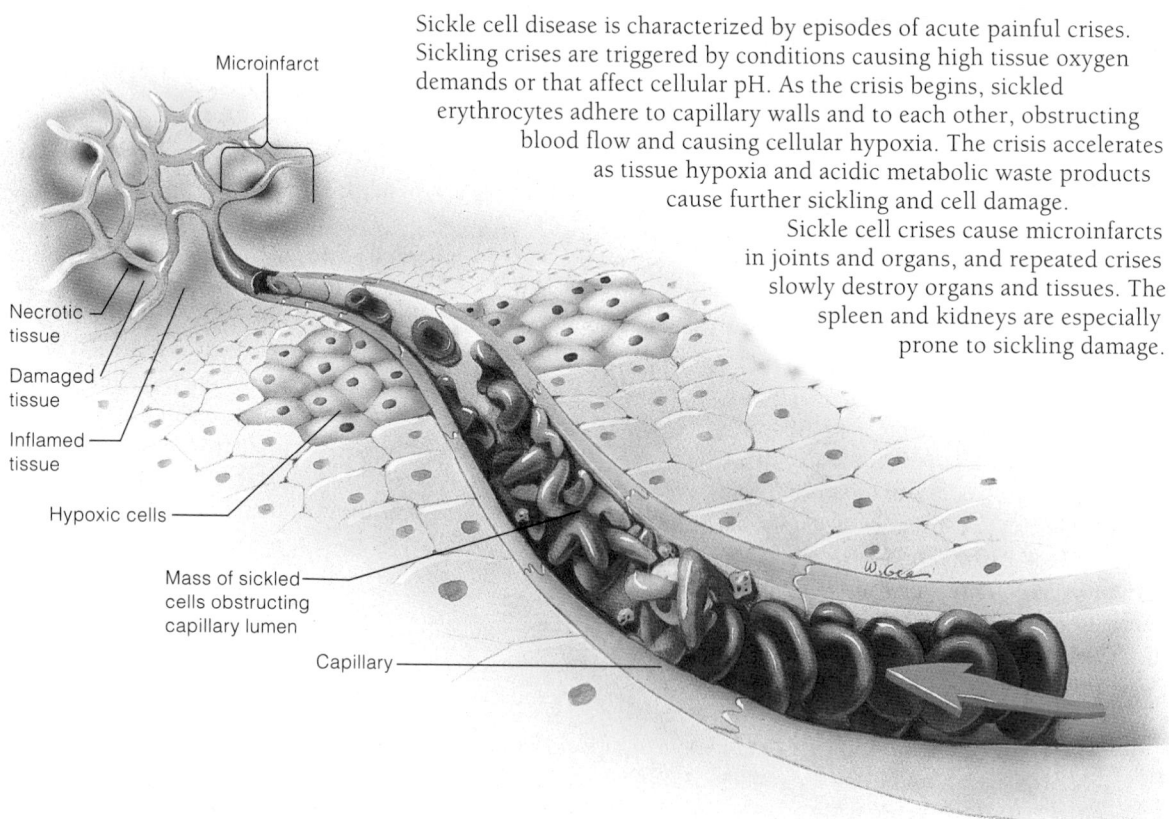

The manifestations of acquired hemolytic anemia depend on the extent of hemolysis and the body's ability to replace destroyed RBCs. The anemia itself often is mild to moderate as erythropoiesis increases to replace the destroyed RBCs. The spleen enlarges as it removes damaged or destroyed RBCs. If the breakdown of heme units exceeds the liver's ability to conjugate and excrete bilirubin, jaundice develops. When the condition is severe, bone marrow expands, and bones may be deformed or may develop pathologic fractures. The severity of generalized manifestations of anemia (tachycardia, pallor, etc.) depends on the degree of anemia and deficiency of tissue oxygenation.

### Glucose-6-Phosphate Dehydrogenase (G6PD) Anemia

*Glucose-6-phosphate dehydrogenase (G6PD) anemia* is caused by a hereditary defect in RBC metabolism. It is relatively common in people of African and Mediterranean descent. The defective gene is located on the X chromosome and therefore affects more males than females. There are many variations of this genetic defect.

G6PD is an enzyme that catalyzes glycolysis, the process in which an RBC derives cellular energy. A defect in G6PD action causes direct oxidation of hemoglobin, damaging the RBC. Hemolysis usually occurs only when the affected person is exposed to stressors (e.g., drugs such as aspirin, sulfonamides, or vitamin K derivatives) that increase the metabolic demands on RBCs. The G6PD deficiency impairs the necessary compensatory increase in glucose metabolism and causes cellular damage. Damaged RBCs are destroyed over a period of 7 to 12 days.

When exposed to a stressor triggering G6PD anemia, symptoms develop within several days. These may include pallor, jaundice, hemoglobinuria (hemoglobin in the urine), and an elevated reticulocyte count. As new RBCs develop, counts return to normal.

## Aplastic Anemia

In **aplastic anemia,** the bone marrow fails to produce all three types of blood cells, leading to *pancytopenia.* Normal bone marrow is replaced by fat. Fortunately, aplastic anemia is rare. *Fanconi anemia* is a rare aplastic anemia caused by defects of DNA repair. The underlying cause of about 50% of acquired aplastic anemia is unknown (*idiopathic aplastic anemia*). Other cases follow stem cell damage caused by exposure to radiation or certain chemical substances such as benzene, arsenic, nitrogen mustard, certain antibiotics (especially chloramphenicol), and chemotherapeutic drugs (McCance & Huether, 2002). Aplastic anemia also may occur with viral infections such as mononucleosis, hepatitis C, and HIV disease (Porth, 2002). Anemia develops as the bone marrow fails to replace RBCs that have reached the end of their life span. Remaining RBCs are normochromic and normocytic.

Manifestations of aplastic anemia vary with the severity of the pancytopenia. Its onset usually is insidious, but may be sudden. Manifestations include fatigue, pallor, progressive weakness, exertional dyspnea, headache, and ultimately tachycardia

and heart failure. Platelet deficiency leads to bleeding problems. A deficiency of white blood cells increases the risk of infection, causing manifestations such as fever.

Treatment focuses on removing the causative agent, if known, and using blood transfusions. Transfusions may be discontinued as soon as the bone marrow resumes blood cell production. Complete recovery may take months. Bone marrow transplant may be the treatment of choice in some instances.

## COLLABORATIVE CARE

Ensuring adequate tissue oxygenation is the priority of care in treating anemia. Specific therapy is determined by the underlying cause of the disorder. Usual treatments include medications, dietary modifications, blood replacement, or supportive interventions.

## Diagnostic Tests

When anemia is suspected, the following laboratory and diagnostic tests may be ordered.

- *Complete blood count (CBC)* is done to determine blood cell counts, hemoglobin, hematocrit, and red blood cell indices (see Table 32–1).
- *Iron levels* and *total iron-binding capacity* are performed to detect iron deficiency anemia. A low serum iron concentration and elevated total iron-binding capacity are indicative of iron deficiency anemia.
- *Serum ferritin* is low due to depletion of the total iron reserves available for hemoglobin synthesis. Ferritin is an iron-storage protein produced by the liver, spleen, and bone marrow. Ferritin mobilizes stored iron when metabolic needs are higher than dietary intake.
- *Sickle cell test* is a screening test to evaluate hemolytic anemia and detect HbS.
- *Hemoglobin electrophoresis* separates normal hemoglobin from abnormal forms. It is used to evaluate hemolytic anemia, diagnose thalassemia, and differentiate sickle cell trait from sickle cell disease (Malarkey & McMorrow, 2000).
- *Schilling test* measures vitamin $B_{12}$ absorption before and after intrinsic factor administration to differentiate between pernicious anemia and intestinal malabsorption of the vitamin. A 24-hour urine sample is collected following administration of radioactive vitamin $B_{12}$. Lower than normal levels of the tagged $B_{12}$ when intrinsic factor is given concurrently indicate malabsorption rather than pernicious anemia.
- *Bone marrow examination* is done to diagnose aplastic anemia. In aplastic anemia, normal marrow elements are significantly decreased as they are replaced by fat cells. Nursing implications for bone marrow collection are described on page 942.
- *Quantitative assay of G6PD* may be performed to confirm a diagnosis of glucose-6-phosphate dehydrogenase deficiency.

## Nursing Implications for Diagnostic Tests

### Bone Marrow Studies

Bone marrow specimens are obtained by either aspiration or biopsy. The preferred site for bone marrow aspiration is the posterior iliac crest; the sternum may also be used. The procedure is performed by inserting a needle into the bone and drawing out a sample of the blood in the marrow. A bone marrow biopsy is performed by making a small incision over the bone and screwing a core biopsy instrument into the bone to obtain a specimen. Bone marrow studies are used to diagnose leukemias, metastatic cancer, lymphoma, aplastic anemia, and Hodgkin's disease.

#### Preparation of the Client
- Explain the purpose and procedure of the test.
- Record vital signs. Assure presence of a signed consent for the procedure.
- Ask the client to void.
- Place in supine position if the specimen will be obtained from the sternum or anterior iliac crest; prone position if the posterior iliac crest will be used.
- Assist in remaining still during the procedure.

#### After the Procedure
- Apply pressure to the puncture site for 5 to 10 minutes.
- Assess vital signs, and compare results to preprocedure readings.
- Apply a dressing to the puncture site, and monitor for bleeding and infection for 24 hours.

#### Client and Family Teaching
- The procedure (either aspiration or biopsy) takes about 20 minutes.
- A sedative may be given prior to the procedure.
- It is important to remain very still during the procedure to prevent accidental injury.
- Although the area will be anesthetized with a local anesthetic, insertion of the needle will be painful for a short time. Taking deep breaths may make this part of the procedure less painful.
- The aspiration site may ache for 1 or 2 days.
- Report any unusual bleeding immediately.

## Medications

Medications used to treat anemia depend on its cause. Iron replacement therapy is ordered for iron deficiency anemia. Supplemental iron may be given by mouth or intramuscularly. Parenteral vitamin $B_{12}$ is given when malabsorption or lack of intrinsic factor leads to vitamin $B_{12}$ deficiency anemia. Folic acid is ordered for women of childbearing age, pregnant women, and clients with folic acid deficiency or sickle cell anemia to meet the increased demands of the bone marrow. Hydroxyurea, a drug that promotes fetal hemoglobin production, may be prescribed for clients with sickle cell disease. Resulting increased levels of fetal hemoglobin interfere with the sickling process and reduce the incidence of painful crises (Braunwald et al., 2001). Nursing implications for clients receiving iron, vitamin $B_{12}$, and folic acid are found in the Medication Administration box on page 943.

Immunosuppressive therapy with antithymocyte globulin (ATG), corticosteroids, and cyclosporine may be used to treat aplastic anemia. Androgens may stimulate blood cell production in some clients with aplastic anemia. See Chapter 9 for more information about immunosuppression.

## Dietary Therapy

Dietary modifications are recommended for nutritional deficiency anemias, such as iron deficiency anemia, vitamin $B_{12}$ deficiency anemia, or folic acid deficiency anemia. Box 32–5 identifies good sources of dietary iron, vitamin $B_{12}$, and folic acid.

## Blood Transfusion

Blood transfusions may be indicated to treat anemias resulting from major blood loss, such as from trauma or major surgery, and severe anemia regardless of cause. Blood transfusions are fully discussed in Chapter 6.

---

### BOX 32–5 ■ Dietary Sources of Iron, Folic Acid, and Vitamin $B_{12}$

#### IRON
Iron in the diet comes from two sources. *Heme iron* makes up about one-half of the iron from animal sources. *Nonheme iron* includes the remaining iron from animal sources and all the iron from plants, legumes, and nuts. Heme iron promotes absorption of nonheme iron from other foods when both forms are consumed at the same time. Absorption of nonheme iron is also enhanced by vitamin C and inhibited by tea and coffee.

#### SOURCES OF HEME IRON
- Beef
- Chicken
- Egg yolk
- Clams, oysters
- Pork loin
- Turkey
- Veal

#### SOURCES OF NONHEME IRON
- Bran flakes
- Brown rice
- Whole-grain breads
- Dried beans
- Dried fruits
- Greens
- Oatmeal

#### SOURCES OF FOLIC ACID
- Green leafy vegetables
- Broccoli
- Organ meats
- Eggs
- Wheat germ
- Asparagus
- Liver
- Milk
- Yeast
- Kidney beans

#### SOURCES OF VITAMIN $B_{12}$
- Liver
- Fresh shrimp and oysters
- Eggs
- Milk
- Kidney
- Meats (muscle)
- Cheese

# Medication Administration

## Drugs to Treat Anemia

### IRON SOURCES

> Ferrous sulfate (Feosol, Fer-in-sol)
> Ferrous gluconate (Fergon, Ferralet, Fertinic)
> Iron dextran injection (Imferon)
> Iron polysaccharide

Iron preparations are normally taken by mouth and are absorbed from the gastrointestinal tract. They are given to treat anemias resulting from iron deficiency or blood loss. When absorbed, iron combines with transferrin. This complex then is transported to the bone marrow and incorporated into hemoglobin.

### Nursing Responsibilities

- Prior to giving the drug, assess for use of drugs that might interact with iron (e.g., antacids, allopurinol, chloramphenicol, tetracyclines, vitamin E), gastrointestinal bleeding, and manifestations of anemia.
- Administer iron preparations with orange juice to enhance absorption.
- If using an elixir, give it through a straw to prevent staining the teeth.
- Monitor for manifestations of iron toxicity: nausea, diarrhea, or constipation; symptoms of anaphylactic shock (extreme cases).
- Monitor hemoglobin and reticulocyte counts.
- If the client is also taking tetracyclines, schedule the dose of iron 2 hours before tetracycline (iron reduces the absorption of tetracycline).

### Client and Family Teaching

- Gastrointestinal side effects may be reduced by taking iron with food (but not milk, which decreases absorption).
- Stools may be dark green or black; this is harmless.
- Increase fluids and fiber in diet to decrease constipation.

### VITAMIN B$_{12}$ SOURCES

> Cyanocobalamin (Kaybovite [oral], Anacobin [parenteral], Bedoz)

> Cyanocobalamin is used to treat vitamin B$_{12}$ deficiencies or malabsorption and pernicious anemia. It is rapidly absorbed when

administered orally or by injection, and it is stored in the liver. Intrinsic factor is necessary for absorption from the gastrointestinal tract.

### Nursing Responsibilities

- Do not expose crystalline injection to light.
- Assess for other drugs that might interfere with the therapeutic response: chloramphenicol, cimetidine, colchicine, and timed-release potassium decrease its effectiveness.
- Do not mix cyanocobalamin in a syringe with other medications.
- Administer parenteral doses intramuscularly or deep subcutaneously to decrease local irritation.
- Monitor hemoglobin, RBC counts, reticulocyte counts, and potassium levels.

### Client and Family Teaching

- A burning sensation with injection is temporary.
- Avoid alcohol, which interferes with absorption.
- If used to treat pernicious anemia, the medication must be taken for life.

### FOLIC ACID SOURCES

> Folic acid (Folvite, novofolacid)

Synthetic folic acid is used to treat folic acid deficiency and megaloblastic or macrocytic anemia. It is absorbed from the gastrointestinal tract and stored in the liver.

### Nursing Responsibilities

- Prior to giving the medication, assess for use of drugs that alter its effect: corticosteroids, methotrexate, oral contraceptives, phenytoin, sulfonamides.
- Do not mix folic acid with other medications in the same syringe.
- Monitor for possible hypersensitivity response of skin rash.

### Client and Family Teaching

- Large doses of folic acid may cause the urine to become darker yellow.
- Excess alcohol intake increases folic acid requirements.

## Complementary Therapies

Complementary health care practitioners may recommend specific plant enzymes to treat nutritional anemias. Plant enzymes are believed to aid digestion of proteins, fats, and carbohydrates, facilitating absorption of their nutrients. Therapy is determined by the specific type of anemia. Plant enzymes should not be used alone to treat anemia, and it is important to check for possible interactions with prescribed medications before starting therapy.

# NURSING CARE

## Health Promotion

Nursing measures to prevent anemia focus on teaching good dietary habits to all clients, regardless of age. Stress the impor-

tance of consuming adequate amounts of iron, folate, and the B vitamins. Provide a list of dietary sources of these nutrients. Discuss alternate iron sources with vegetarian clients, and teach them that foods high in vitamin C enhance the absorption of iron from grains, legumes, and other sources. Emphasize the importance of adequate iron intake in women of childbearing age and older adults. Stress the increased need for these nutrients during pregnancy, and discuss strategies to ensure an adequate intake.

## Assessment

Assessment data to collect for clients with suspected anemia includes:

- Health history: complaints of shortness of breath with activity, fatigue, weakness, dizziness or fainting, palpitations; history of previous anemia, bleeding episodes;

menstrual history (if appropriate); medications; chronic diseases; usual diet and patterns of alcohol intake or cigarette smoking
- Physical examination: general appearance, skin color; vital signs including temperature; heart and lung sounds; peripheral pulses, capillary refill; abdominal tenderness; obvious bleeding or bruising

## Nursing Diagnoses and Interventions

Anemia affects circulating oxygen levels and tissue oxygenation. Priority nursing diagnoses include activity intolerance, altered oral mucous membranes, and self-care deficits. With acute blood-loss anemia, risk for insufficient cardiac output also is a priority. Clients with sickle cell disease have specific needs related to the effects of the disease on tissue perfusion; see the section on disseminated intravascular coagulation (DIC) later in this chapter for nursing interventions appropriate to ineffective tissue perfusion, associated pain, and maintaining oxygenation.

### Activity Intolerance

Anemia causes weakness and shortness of breath on exertion. These symptoms are due to decreased circulating oxygen levels secondary to low hemoglobin levels. Weakness, fatigue, and/or vertigo may occur even during activities of daily living, including those associated with self-care, home life, job performance, and social roles.

- Help identify ways to conserve energy when performing necessary or desired activities. *Modifying the approach to a particular activity may reduce cardiorespiratory symptoms and activity-related fatigue. Alternative ways of performing tasks (e.g., sitting when performing hygiene care and kitchen tasks) may reduce oxygen demands. In some cases, assistance from others is necessary to conserve energy and reduce symptoms.*
- Help the client and family establish priorities for tasks and activities. *Because family members may need to assume responsibility for additional tasks, the plan's success depends on mutually established goals.*
- Assist to develop a schedule of alternating activity and rest periods throughout the day. *Rest periods decrease oxygen needs, reducing strain on the heart and lungs, and allowing restoration of homeostasis before further activities.*
- Encourage 8 to 10 hours of sleep at night. *Rest decreases oxygen demands and increases available energy for morning activities.*
- Monitor vital signs before and after activity. *Vital signs provide a measure of activity tolerance. Increased heart and respiratory rates or a change in blood pressure may indicate intolerance of the activity.*
- Discontinue activity if any of the following occurs.
    a. Complaints of chest pain, breathlessness, or vertigo
    b. Palpitations or tachycardia that does not return to normal within 4 minutes of resting
    c. Bradycardia
    d. Tachypnea or dyspnea
    e. Decreased systolic blood pressure

*These changes may signify cardiac decompensation due to insufficient oxygenation. The intensity, duration, or frequency of the activity needs to be reduced.*
- Instruct the client not to smoke. *Smoking causes vasoconstriction and increases carbon monoxide levels in the blood, interfering with tissue oxygenation.*

### Impaired Oral Mucous Membrane

Glossitis and cheilosis may occur with nutritional deficiencies of iron, folate, and vitamin $B_{12}$. The tongue and lips become very red, and fissures or cracks may form at the corners of the mouth.

- Monitor condition of lips and tongue daily. *Glossitis and cheilosis increase the risk for bleeding and infection and may require medical treatment. Pain and discomfort may interfere with oral intake, further worsening the nutritional deficiency.*
- Use a mouthwash of saline, saltwater, or half-strength peroxide and water to rinse the mouth every 2 to 4 hours. Avoid alcohol-based mouthwashes. *This cleanses and soothes oral mucous membranes. Alcohol-based mouthwashes further irritate and dry oral tissues.*
- Provide frequent oral hygiene (after each meal and at bedtime) with a soft bristle toothbrush or sponge. *Removing food debris from painful fissures promotes comfort. A soft toothbrush reduces irritation or bleeding of oral mucosa. Keeping the oral cavity clean also reduces the risk of infection.*
- Apply a petroleum-based lubricating jelly or ointment to the lips after oral care. *Lubricating ointment helps to retain moisture, facilitate healing, and protect the lips from other drying agents.*
- Instruct to avoid hot, spicy, or acidic foods. *Such foods may further irritate and dry mucous membranes.*
- Encourage soft, cool, bland foods. *Foods that are soothing to the mucous membranes promote comfort and help maintain adequate food and fluid intake. Minimizing oral pain may also promote compliance with oral care routines.*
- Encourage eating four to six small meals daily with high protein and vitamin content. *Small, frequent meals may be better tolerated, increasing intake. Nutrient-rich meals promote healing of the mucous membranes.*

### Risk for Decreased Cardiac Output

Cardiac output may be affected by acute bleeding and volume loss or by heart failure resulting from severe anemia. In addition, impaired tissue oxygenation leads to an increased respiratory rate and dyspnea.

- Monitor vital signs, breath sounds, and apical pulse. *Increased cardiac workload can affect the blood pressure, heart, and respiratory rates. Increased blood flow can lead to heart murmur or abnormal heart sounds such as $S_3$ or $S_4$. Tachypnea and dyspnea may affect the depth of respirations, alveolar ventilation, and blood and tissue oxygenation.*
- Assess for pallor, cyanosis, and dependent edema. *Blood is shunted to the vital organs, causing vasoconstriction of skin vessels. This, in addition to lower levels of hemoglobin, cause pallor. Cyanosis, especially of the lips and nail beds, indicates inadequate oxygenation of blood. Dependent edema occurs in response to right ventricular failure.*

**PRACTICE ALERT** *Report signs of decreased cardiac output to the physician. Severe anemia can lead to heart failure, necessitating additional treatment.* ■

### Self-Care Deficit

Energy expenditures for activities of daily living (ADLs) may cause oxygen demands to exceed supply in the client with severe anemia.

- Assist with ADLs, such as bathing, grooming, and eating, as needed. *Assistance decreases energy expenditures and tissue requirements for oxygen, reducing cardiac workload.*
- Discuss the importance of rest periods prior to such activities as dressing. *Rest reduces oxygen demand and cardiac workload. The person who is able to perform self-care in activities of daily living maintains independence, self-esteem, and morale.*

## Using NANDA, NIC, and NOC

Chart 32–1 shows links between NANDA nursing diagnoses, NIC, and NOC for the client with anemia.

## Home Care

With the exception of anemia resulting from acute hemorrhage, most clients with anemia are treated in the home and community setting. Include the following topics when preparing the client and family for home care.

- Nutritional strategies to address deficiencies
- Prescribed medications, vitamins, or mineral supplements and their appropriate use, intended effect, possible adverse effects, and interactions with food or other medications
- Energy conservation strategies
- Other recommended treatment measures and follow-up
- If the anemia is genetically transmitted, such as sickle cell anemia, include inheritance patterns of the disorder, symptoms of crisis, and manifestations to report to the physician

Provide referrals for counseling to facilitate decisions about pregnancy as indicated. Also refer for nutritional assistance and teaching, home health care, or assistance with self-care and home maintenance activities as indicated. Older adults with nutritional anemias may benefit from community services such as senior meals or Meals-on-Wheels.

---

### CHART 32–1 NANDA, NIC, AND NOC LINKAGES

#### The Client with Anemia

| NURSING DIAGNOSES | NURSING INTERVENTIONS | NURSING OUTCOMES |
|---|---|---|
| • Activity Intolerance | • Energy Management<br>• Nutrition Management | • Activity Tolerance<br>• Endurance |
| • Fatigue<br>• Ineffective Health Maintenance | • Environmental Management<br>• Health Education<br>• Self-Responsibility Facilitation<br>• Teaching: Procedure/Treatment | • Energy Conservation<br>• Health-Seeking Behavior<br>• Knowledge: Health Behaviors<br>• Knowledge: Treatment Regimen |
| • Impaired Oral Mucous Membrane | • Oral Health Restoration<br>• Oral Health Maintenance | • Oral Health<br>• Tissue Integrity: Skin and Mucous Membranes |

*Note. Data from Nursing Outcomes Classification (NOC) by M. Johnson & M. Maas (Eds.), 1997, St. Louis: Mosby; Nursing Diagnoses: Definitions & Classification 2001–2002 by North American Nursing Diagnosis Association, 2001, Philadelphia: NANDA; Nursing Interventions Classification (NIC) by J.C. McCloskey & G. M. Bulechek (Eds.), 2000, St. Louis: Mosby. Reprinted by permission.*

---

## THE CLIENT WITH POLYCYTHEMIA

**Polycythemia,** or *erythrocytosis,* is an excess of red blood cells characterized by a hematocrit higher than 55%. The two major types of polycythemia are primary and secondary. *Primary polycythemia,* also called *polycythemia vera,* is an uncommon disorder of increased RBC production. This condition more commonly affects men of European Jewish ancestry between age 40 and 70. *Secondary polycythemia* occurs in response to elevated erythropoietin levels. This commonly is a compensatory response to hypoxia, often due to living at a high altitude, smoking, or chronic lung disease. A third type of polycythemia, *relative polycythemia,* is not due to an excess of RBCs but to fluid deficit. The total red blood cell count is normal, but fluid loss increases cell concentration, thus raising the hematocrit. Relative polycythemia is corrected by rehydration.

## Nursing Care Plan
## A Client with Folic Acid Deficiency Anemia

Sheri Matthews is a 76-year-old widow who lives alone. She tells Lisa Apana, RN, the nurse in her care provider's office, that she liked to cook when her husband was alive, but preparing an entire meal just for herself seems senseless. She relates that her typical day's menu includes coffee for breakfast, a bologna sandwich and coffee for lunch, and a hot dog or two, a few cookies, and a glass of milk for dinner.

### ASSESSMENT

Mrs. Matthews's nursing history includes a 20 lb (9 kg) weight loss since her husband died 8 months ago. She states that she sometimes has heart palpitations and always feels weak. Physical assessment shows: T 98.8°F (37.1°C), P 110, R 22, BP 90/52. Skin warm, pale, and dry. Diagnostic tests indicate folic acid deficiency anemia, and Mrs. Matthews is started on an oral folic acid supplement and instructed about foods containing folic acid.

### DIAGNOSES

- *Activity intolerance* related to weakness secondary to decreased tissue oxygenation
- *Imbalanced nutrition: Less than body requirements* related to lack of motivation to cook and understanding of nutritional needs, as manifested by weight loss of 20 lb, and folic acid deficiency
- *Deficient knowledge* related to lack of information about a well-balanced diet and foods containing folic acid

### EXPECTED OUTCOMES

- Verbalize the importance of taking folic acid supplements and eating a balanced diet.
- Gain at least 1 lb (0.45 kg) per week.
- Return to previous level of physical energy.
- Consume a balanced diet, including foods containing folic acid.

### PLANNING AND IMPLEMENTATION

- Discuss foods required for a well-balanced diet, as well as dietary sources of folic acid.
- Develop a dietary plan with Mrs. Matthews which includes food preferences and foods that are easy and quick to prepare.
- Discuss the importance of taking the folic acid supplement. Advise to continue taking it even after she begins to feel better.
- Help Mrs. Matthews develop a schedule of activities that provides adequate rest and energy for cooking.

### EVALUATION

Mrs. Matthews gained 1 lb (0.45 kg) during the first week of treatment. She has met with a nutritionist and has a better understanding of nutritional needs. She states that she can prepare hot meals when she schedules a rest period before and after lunch. Ms. Apana has provided written and verbal information about the folic acid supplement and diet. Mrs. Matthews verbalizes understanding, stating, "I will continue to take the folic acid until the doctor tells me to stop. I'm beginning to enjoy cooking again, now that I have a reason to cook!" Ms. Apana contacts the local senior services representative to determine if Mrs. Matthews is able to participate in the local Meals-on-Wheels program.

### Critical Thinking in the Nursing Process

1. What is the pathophysiologic basis for Mrs. Matthews's abnormal vital signs during her initial assessment?
2. Design a week's menu that includes foods high in folic acid.
3. Why was Mrs. Matthews placed on a folic acid supplement in addition to dietary modifications?
4. Why is the older adult at increased risk for developing folic acid deficiency anemia? Consider physiologic, economic, and social factors.

See Evaluating Your Response in Appendix C.

## PATHOPHYSIOLOGY AND MANIFESTATIONS

### Primary Polycythemia

Primary polycythemia, or polycythemia vera (PV), is a neoplastic stem cell disorder characterized by overproduction of RBCs and, to a lesser extent, white blood cells and platelets. It is classified as a myeloproliferative disorder. Its cause is unknown. In PV, colonies of endogenous erythroid stem cells develop. These colonies produce RBCs in the absence of erythropoietin, leading to excess RBC production.

Initially, PV is asymptomatic, and the diagnosis may be made during routine blood tests. Its manifestations are caused by increased blood volume and viscosity. Hypertension is common, and may lead to complaints of headaches, dizziness, and vision and hearing disruptions. Venous stasis causes *plethora*, a ruddy, red color of the face, hands, feet, and mucous membranes. This often is accompanied by severe, painful itching of the fingers and toes. Retinal and cerebral vessels may be engorged. Hypermetabolism develops, causing weight loss and night sweats. Mental status may be altered, leading to drowsiness or delirium.

Thrombosis and hemorrhage are potential complications of PV. Thrombosis may cause transient ischemic attacks, angina, or manifestations of peripheral vascular disease. Gastrointestinal bleeding may occur, and portal hypertension may develop.

### Secondary Polycythemia

Secondary polycythemia, or erythrocytosis, is increased numbers of RBCs in response to excess erythropoietin secretion or prolonged hypoxia. Secondary polycythemia is the most common form of polycythemia.

## Manifestations of Polycythemia

- Hypertension
- Headache, tinnitus, blurred vision
- Plethora: dark redness of the lips, feet, ears, fingernails, and mucous membranes
- Splenomegaly (polycythemia vera)
- Severe pruritus, extremity pain
- Weight loss, night sweats
- Gastrointestinal bleeding
- Intermittent claudication
- Symptoms from thrombosis within various organs

Abnormally high erythropoietin levels can result from kidney disease or erythropoietin-secreting tumors (e.g., renal cell carcinoma). Chronic hypoxia that stimulates erythropoietin release is a more common cause of secondary polycythemia. People living at high altitudes where the atmospheric oxygen pressure is lower develop a degree of polycythemia, as do people with chronic heart or lung disease and smokers. Abnormal hemoglobin that forms tighter bonds with oxygen also may lead to secondary polycythemia.

The manifestations of secondary polycythemia are similar to those of primary polycythemia. Splenomegaly, however, does not develop. Early symptoms often are overshadowed by the manifestations of the underlying disorder. For the manifestations of polycythemia see the box above.

## COLLABORATIVE CARE

In PV, serum erythropoietin levels are low. Bone marrow studies show hyperplasia of all hematopoietic elements. With secondary polycythemia, serum erythropoietin levels usually are high, and bone marrow studies show only red stem cell hyperplasia.

For secondary polycythemia, treatment focuses on the underlying cause of the disorder. It is a physiologic response in people living at high altitudes, and unless the hematocrit is too high or oxygen saturation levels are low, no treatment is usually necessary. Smokers are urged to quit. Measures to raise oxygen saturation levels and reduce tissue hypoxia often will relieve the polycythemia. Clients with both primary and secondary polycythemia benefit from periodic phlebotomy, removing 300 to 500 mL of blood, to keep blood volume and viscosity within normal levels. For PV, chemotherapeutic agents such as hydroxyurea may be used to suppress marrow function but may increase the risk of developing leukemia (discussed later in this chapter). Pruritus may be relieved by antihistamines, or may require more aggressive treatment with interferon alpha or other treatments. One 325 mg aspirin tablet daily may be ordered to control thrombosis without increasing the risk of bleeding.

## NURSING CARE

Preventing polycythemia begins with educating children and adults about the dangers of smoking. Measures to reduce risk factors for cardiovascular disease also may be beneficial.

This chronic condition is managed in community-based settings unless a complication develops. Teach the client and family the importance of maintaining adequate hydration, increasing fluid intake during hot weather and when exercising. Discuss measures to prevent blood stasis: elevating legs and feet when sitting, using support stockings, and continuing treatment measures. Instruct to report manifestations of thrombosis (leg or calf pain, chest pain, neurologic symptoms) or bleeding (black, tarry stools, vomiting blood or coffee-ground emesis) immediately. Monitor the hematocrit and cell counts throughout treatment.

Examples of nursing diagnoses appropriate for the client with polycythemia follow:

- *Decisional conflict regarding smoking cessation* related to addictive effects
- *Pain* related to effects of altered blood flow in distal extremities
- *Risk for ineffective tissue perfusion* related to sluggish blood flow and increased risk for thrombosis

# PLATELET AND COAGULATION DISORDERS

Platelet and coagulation disorders affect **hemostasis,** control of bleeding. Hemostasis is a series of complex interactions between platelets and clotting mechanisms that maintains a relatively steady state of blood volume, blood pressure, and blood flow through injured vessels.

## PHYSIOLOGY REVIEW

### Platelets

**Platelets,** or **thrombocytes,** are cell fragments that have no nucleus and cannot replicate. They are metabolically active, however, producing ATP and releasing mediators required for clotting. Platelets are formed in the bone marrow as pinched-off portions of large megakaryocytes (see Figure 32–1). Platelet production is controlled by *thrombopoietin,* a protein produced by the liver, kidney, smooth muscle, and bone marrow. The number of circulating platelets controls thrombopoietin release. Once released from the bone marrow, platelets remain in the spleen for about 8 hours before entering the circulation. Platelets live up to 10 days in circulation. There are about 250,000 to 400,000 platelets in each milliliter of blood. An excess of platelets is *thrombocytosis.* A deficit of platelets is *thrombocytopenia.*

## Hemostasis

**Hemostasis,** or blood clotting, is a complex process that controls bleeding and clotting. The five stages to hemostasis are (1) vessel spasm, (2) formation of the platelet plug, (3) development of an insoluble fibrin clot, (4) clot retraction, and (5) clot dissolution.

### Vessel Spasm

When a blood vessel is damaged, thromboxane $A_2$ ($TXA_2$) is released from platelets and cells, causing *vessel spasm.* This spasm constricts the damaged vessel for about 1 minute.

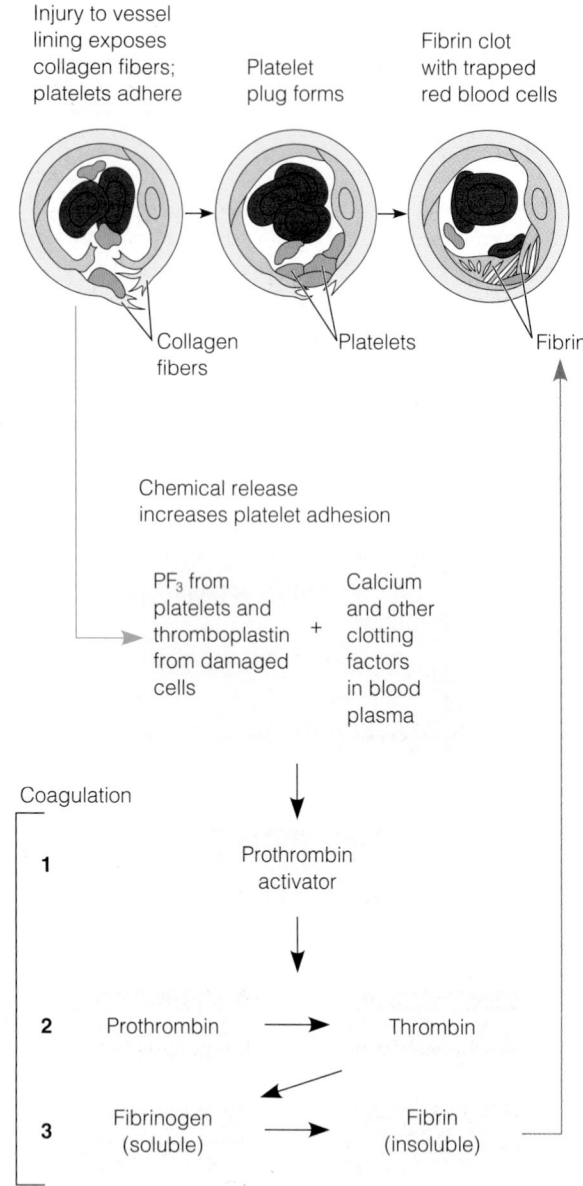

**Figure 32-6** ■ Platelet plug formation and blood clotting. The flow diagram summarizes the events leading to fibrin clot formation. $PF_3$ (blue arrow) released from damaged tissue combines with other clotting factors to release prothrombin activator, the first step of coagulation. Second, prothrombin is converted into thrombin. Finally, thrombin transforms soluble fibrinogen into insoluble fibrin (red arrow) to form a clot.

### Formation of the Platelet Plug

Platelets attracted to the damaged vessel wall change from smooth disks to spiny spheres. Receptors on the activated platelets bind with *von Willebrand's factor,* a protein molecule, and exposed collagen fibers at the site of injury to form the *platelet plug* (Figure 32–6 ■). The platelets release adenosine diphosphate (ADP) and $TXA_2$ to activate nearby platelets, adhering them to the developing plug. Activation of the clotting pathway on the platelet surface converts fibrinogen to fibrin. Fibrin, in turn, forms a meshwork that binds the platelets and other blood cells to form a stable plug (Figure 32–7 ■).

### Blood Coagulation

The process of **coagulation** creates a meshwork of fibrin strands that cements the blood components to form an insoluble clot. Coagulation requires many interactive reactions and two clotting pathways (Figure 32–8 ■). The slower intrinsic pathway is activated when blood contacts collagen in the injured vessel wall; the faster extrinsic pathway is activated when blood is exposed to tissues. The final outcome of both pathways is fibrin clot formation. Each procoagulation substance is activated in sequence; the activation of one coagulation factor activates another in turn. Table 32–2 lists known factors, their origin, and their function or pathway. A deficiency of one or more factors or inappropriate inactivation of any factor alters normal coagulation.

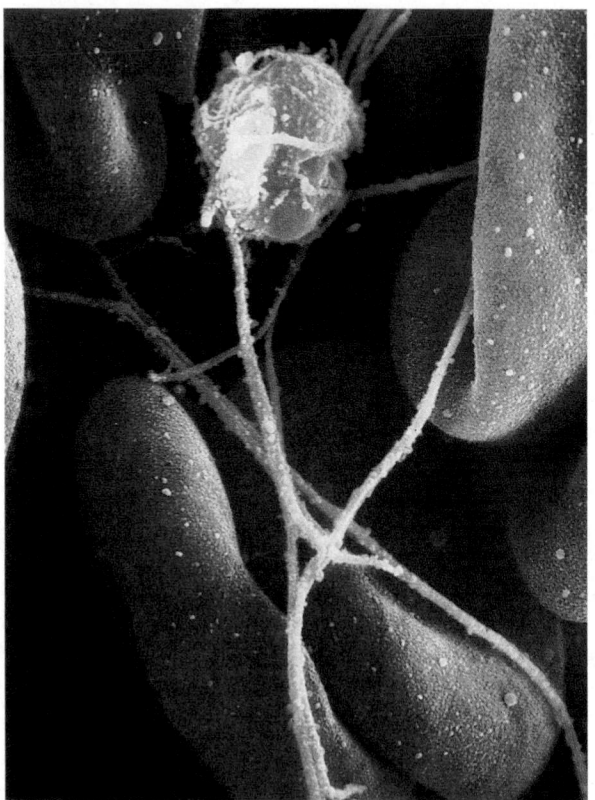

**Figure 32-7** ■ Scanning electron micrograph of a RBC trapped in a fibrin mesh. The spherical gray object at top is a platelet.

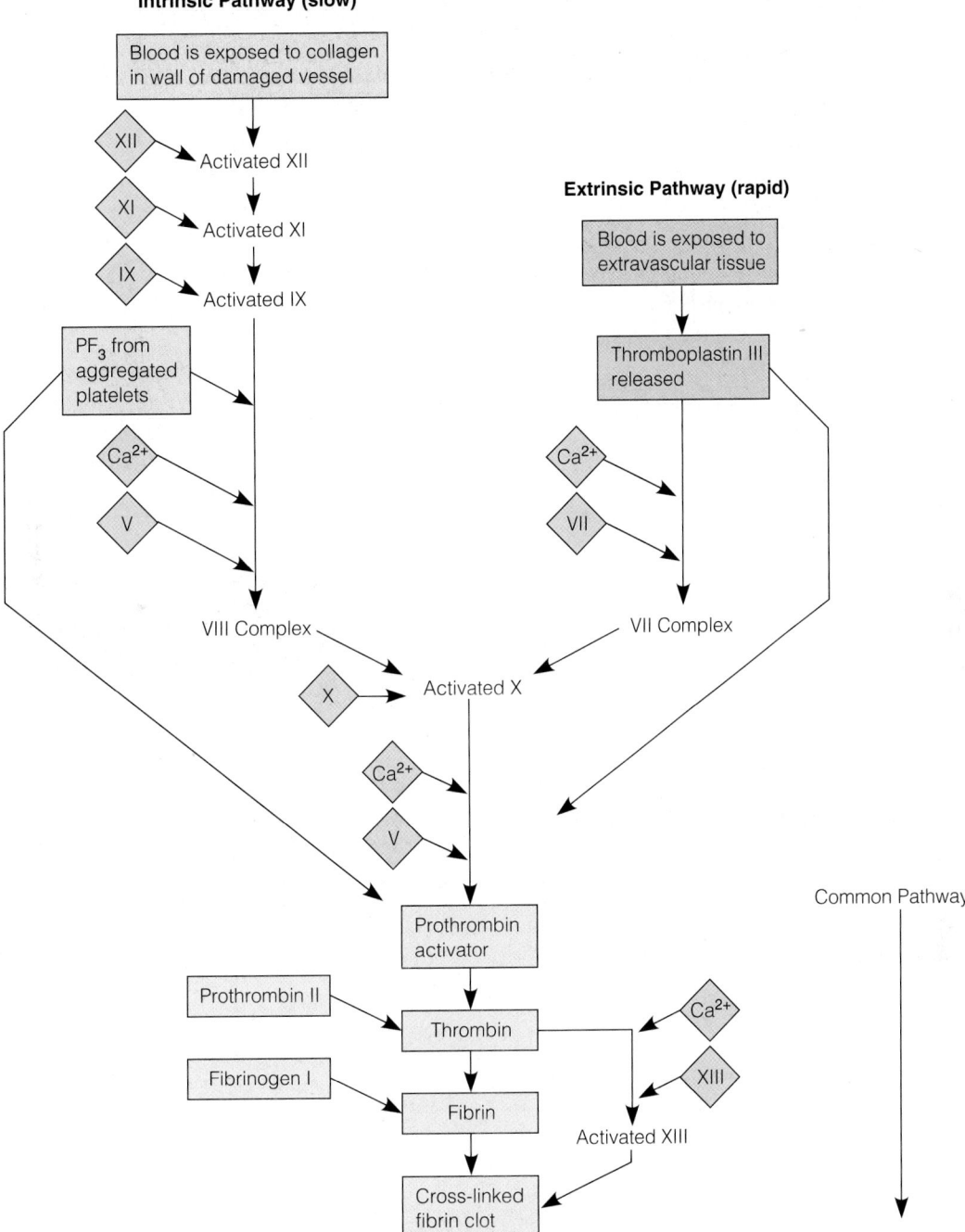

**Figure 32–8 ■** Clot formation. Both the slower intrinsic pathway and the more rapid extrinsic pathway activate factor X. Factor X then combines with other factors to form prothrombin activator. Prothrombin activator transforms prothrombin into thrombin, which then transforms fibrinogen into long fibrin strands. Thrombin also activates factor XIII, which draws the fibrin strands together into a dense meshwork. The complete process of clot formation occurs within 3 to 6 minutes after blood vessel damage.

## Clot Retraction

After the clot is stabilized (within about 30 minutes), trapped platelets contract, much like muscle cells. Platelet contraction squeezes the fibrin strands, pulling the broken portions of the ruptured blood vessel closer together. Growth factors released by the platelets stimulate cell division and tissue repair of the damaged vessel.

## Clot Dissolution

*Fibrinolysis,* the process of clot dissolution, begins shortly after the clot has formed, restoring blood flow and promoting tissue repair. Like coagulation, fibrinolysis requires a sequence of interactions between activator and inhibitor substances. Plasminogen, an enzyme that promotes fibrinolysis, is converted into plasmin, its active form, by chemical mediators released

## TABLE 32–2 Blood Coagulation Factors

| Factor | Name | Function or Pathway |
|---|---|---|
| I | Fibrinogen | Converted to fibrin strands |
| II | Prothrombin | Converted to thrombin |
| III | Thromboplastin | Catalyzes conversion of thrombin |
| IV | Calcium ions | Needed for all steps of coagulation |
| V | Proaccelerin | Extrinsic/intrinsic pathways |
| VII | Serum prothrombin conversion accelerator | Extrinsic pathway |
| VIII | Antihemophilic factor | Intrinsic pathway |
| IX | Plasma prothrombin component | Intrinsic pathway |
| X | Stuart factor | Extrinsic/intrinsic pathways |
| XI | Plasma prothrombin antecedent | Intrinsic pathway |
| XII | Hageman factor | Intrinsic pathway |
| XIII | Fibrin stabilizing factor | Cross-links fibrin strands to form insoluble clot |

from vessel walls and the liver. Plasmin dissolves the clot's fibrin strands and certain coagulation factors. Stimuli such as exercise, fever, and vasoactive drugs promote plasminogen activator release. The liver and endothelium also produce fibrinolytic inhibitors.

## THE CLIENT WITH THROMBOCYTOPENIA

**Thrombocytopenia** is a platelet count of less than 100,000 per milliliter of blood. It can lead to abnormal bleeding. A continuing decline in circulating platelets to less than 20,000/mL can lead to spontaneous bleeding and hemorrhage from minor trauma. Bleeding due to platelet deficiency usually occurs in small vessels, causing manifestations such as *petechiae* (small red or purple spots that do not blanch with pressure) and *purpura* (purple bruising). The mucous membranes of the nose, mouth, GI tract, and vagina often bleed. Serious and potentially fatal bleeding occurs when the platelet count is less than 10,000/mL.

Thrombocytopenia results from one of three mechanisms: decreased production, increased sequestration in the spleen, or accelerated destruction. Primary thrombocytopenia that leads to increased platelet destruction is discussed below. Secondary thrombocytopenia may be caused by aplastic anemia, bone marrow malignancy, infection, radiation therapy, or drug therapy (Box 32–6). Platelet sequestration usually is due to an enlarged spleen. Up to 80% of platelets may be removed from circulation with significant splenomegaly (Porth, 2002). Finally, thrombocytopenia may result from premature platelet destruction associated with disseminated intravascular coagulation (DIC).

## PATHOPHYSIOLOGY AND MANIFESTATIONS

The two types of primary thrombocytopenia are immune thrombocytopenic purpura and thrombotic thrombocytopenic purpura.

### BOX 32–6 ■ Selected Causes of Secondary Thrombocytopenia

**DISEASES**
- Vitamin-B$_{12}$ anemia
- Folic acid anemia
- Aplastic anemia
- Leukemia
- Alcoholism
- DIC
- Infectious mononucleosis
- Viral infections
- HIV disease

**DRUGS**
- Thiazide diuretics
- Aspirin
- Ibuprofen
- Indomethacin
- Naproxen
- Sulfonamides
- Quinidine
- Cimetidine
- Digitalis
- Furosemide
- Heparin
- Morphine

**TREATMENTS**
- Radiation therapy
- Chemotherapy

### Immune Thrombocytopenic Purpura

*Immune thrombocytopenic purpura (ITP),* also known as *idiopathic thrombocytopenic purpura,* is an autoimmune disorder in which platelet destruction is accelerated. In its chronic form, ITP typically affects young adults between age 20 and 40; women are affected more often than men. Acute ITP is more common in children, and often follows a viral illness. Acute ITP typically lasts only 1 to 2 months (McCance & Huether, 2002).

In ITP, proteins on the platelet cell membrane stimulate autoantibody production, usually IgG antibodies. These autoantibodies adhere to the platelet membrane. Although the platelets function normally, the spleen reacts to them as being foreign and destroys the altered platelets after only 1 to 3 days of circulation.

The manifestations of ITP are due to bleeding from small vessels and mucous membranes. Petechiae and purpura develop, often on the anterior chest, arms, neck, and oral mucous membranes. Bruising also may be apparent. As bleeding progresses, epistaxis (nosebleed), hematuria, excess menstrual bleeding, and bleeding gums occur. Spontaneous intracranial bleeding is rare but does occur. Associated symptoms include weight loss, fever, and headache.

## Thrombotic Thrombocytopenic Purpura

*Thrombotic thrombocytopenic purpura (TTP)* is a rare disorder in which thrombi occlude arterioles and capillaries of the microcirculation. Many organs are affected, including the heart, kidneys, and brain. The incidence of TTP is increasing (McCance & Huether, 2002). Its cause is unknown. Platelet aggregation is a key feature of the disorder. As RBCs circulate through partially occluded vessels, they fragment, leading to hemolytic anemia (Porth, 2002).

TTP may be acute, the more common and severe form, or chronic. Acute idiopathic TTP may be fatal within months if untreated. The manifestations of TTP include purpura and petechiae, and neurologic symptoms such as headache, seizures, and altered consciousness.

# COLLABORATIVE CARE

The diagnosis of thrombocytopenia is based on history, manifestations, and diagnostic test results. Management focuses on treating or removing any causative factors and treating the platelet deficiency.

## Diagnostic Tests

The following diagnostic tests are used to identify thrombocytopenia.

- *CBC* evaluates all cellular components of the blood, as well as the hemoglobin and hematocrit.
- *Platelet count* is decreased.
- *Antinuclear antibodies (ANA)* are measured to assess for autoantibodies.
- *Serologic studies* for hepatitis viruses, cytomegalovirus (CMV), Epstein-Barr virus, toxoplasma, and HIV may be done.
- *Bone marrow examination* evaluates for aplastic anemia and megakaryocyte production.

## Medications

Oral glucocorticoids, such as prednisone, are prescribed to suppress the autoimmune response. Many clients who respond to glucocorticoid treatment relapse when the drug is withdrawn, however. Immunosuppressive drugs such as azathioprine, cyclophosphamide, and cyclosporine may be used.

## Treatments

*Platelet transfusions* may be required to treat acute bleeding due to thrombocytopenia. Platelets are prepared from fresh whole blood; one unit contains 30 to 60 mL of platelet concentrate. The expected increase in platelets after one unit is infused is 10,000/mL. *Plasmapheresis,* or *plasma exchange therapy,* is the primary treatment for acute thrombotic thrombocytopenic purpura. The client's plasma is removed and replaced with fresh frozen plasma to remove autoantibodies, immune complexes, and toxins.

## Surgery

A *splenectomy* (surgical removal of the spleen) is the treatment of choice if the client with ITP relapses when glucocorticoids are discontinued. The spleen is the site of platelet destruction and antibody production. This surgery often cures the disorder, although relapse may occur years after splenectomy.

# NURSING CARE

## Assessment

- Health history: complaints of bruising with minor or no trauma, bleeding gums, nosebleed, heavy or prolonged menstrual periods, black, tarry, or bloody stools, hematemesis, headache, fever, or neurologic symptoms; recent weight loss; recent viral or other illness; current and recent medications; exposure to toxins
- Physical examination: skin and mucous membranes for color, temperature, petechiae, purpura, or bruises; vital signs; weight; mental status and level of consciousness; heart and breath sounds; abdominal exam; body fluids for occult blood

## Nursing Diagnoses and Interventions

Inadequate platelets impair hemostasis, placing the client at risk for bleeding. Bleeding gums, an early sign of the disorder, affects oral mucous membrane integrity as well.

### Ineffective Protection

Bleeding is a serious complication associated with thrombocytopenia. As platelet counts (measured in cubic millimeters) decrease, the risk of bleeding increases: The risk is minimal with counts greater than 50,000 mm$^3$; moderate when the count is between 20,000 and 50,000 mm$^3$; and significant when the count falls below 20,000 mm$^3$.

- Monitor vital signs, heart and breath sounds every 4 hours. Frequently assess for other manifestations of bleeding:
  a. Skin and mucous membranes for petechiae, ecchymoses, and hematoma formation
  b. Gums, nasal membranes, and conjunctiva for bleeding
  c. Overt or occult blood in emesis, urine, or stool
  d. Vaginal bleeding
  e. Prolonged bleeding from puncture sites
  f. Neurologic changes: headache, visual changes, altered mental status, decreasing level of consciousness, seizures
  g. Abdominal: epigastric pain, absence of bowel sounds, increasing abdominal girth, abdominal guarding or rigidity

*Early identification of bleeding is important to prevent serious blood loss and shock.*

**PRACTICE ALERT** *Avoid invasive procedures such as rectal temperatures, urinary catheterization, and parenteral injections to the extent possible. Diagnostic procedures such as biopsy or lumbar puncture should be avoided if the platelet count is less than 50,000 mm³. Invasive procedures can cause tissue trauma and bleeding. Procedures that use large-bore needles should be delayed until the platelet count is increased.* ■

- Apply pressure to puncture sites for 3 to 5 minutes; apply pressure to arterial blood gas sites for 15 to 20 minutes. *Pressure promotes hemostasis and clot formation.*
- Instruct to avoid forcefully blowing the nose or picking crusts from the nose, straining to have a bowel movement, and forceful coughing or sneezing. *These activities increase the risk of external and internal bleeding.*

### Impaired Oral Mucous Membranes

Thrombocytopenia frequently leads to bleeding of the gums and oral mucosa. As a result, risk for infection and impaired nutrition increases.

- Frequently assess the mouth for bleeding. Inquire about oral pain or tenderness. *Breakdown of oral mucous membranes increases the risk of infection and bleeding, and causes discomfort with eating.*
- Encourage use of a soft-bristle toothbrush or sponge to clean teeth and gums. *Hard bristles may abrade oral mucosa, causing bleeding and increasing the risk of infection.*
- Instruct to rinse the mouth with saline every 2 to 4 hours. Apply petroleum jelly to lips as needed to prevent dryness and cracking. *Saline mouth rinses and petroleum jelly help maintain oral tissue integrity and promote cleansing and healing.*
- Instruct to avoid alcohol-based mouthwashes, very hot foods, alcohol, and crusty foods. Teach to drink cool liquids at least every 2 hours. *Avoiding foods and liquids that traumatize oral mucosa increases comfort; fluid intake prevents dehydration and helps maintain mucous membrane integrity.*

### Home Care

In the adult, ITP often is a chronic disorder that the client and family must learn to manage. Secondary thrombocytopenia may be either acute or chronic. Discuss the following topics when preparing the client and family for home care.

- Nature of the disorder, its usual course, and the treatment plan
- Use, desired and potential adverse effects of prescribed medications
- Risks and benefits of surgery or treatments such as plasma replacement therapy
- The importance of follow-up tests and visits for care
- Measures to reduce the risk of bleeding: safety measures such as a soft-bristle toothbrush, electric razor, avoidance of contact sports and hazardous activities, and avoiding medications that further interfere with platelet function (Box 32–7)

Refer for home health or other community services (e.g., housekeeping, shopping) as indicated.

---

**BOX 32–7   ■ Medications That May Interfere with Platelet Function**

#### OVER-THE-COUNTER MEDICATIONS

- Aspirin and salicylates, including:
  - Alka-Seltzer
  - Bufferin
  - Doan's Pills
  - Ecotrin
  - Excedrin
  - Midol
  - Pepto-Bismol
  - Vanquish
- NSAIDS such as
  - Advil
  - Aleve
  - Nuprin
  - Pamprin IB

#### PRESCRIPTION MEDICATIONS

- Aspirin-containing analgesics
- Chemotherapy drugs
- Antibiotics such as penicillin
- Carbamazapine (Tegretol)
- Colchicine
- Dipyridamole (Persantine)
- Gold salts
- Heparin
- Quinine derivatives
- Sulfonamides
- Thiazide diuretics

---

## THE CLIENT WITH DISSEMINATED INTRAVASCULAR COAGULATION

**Disseminated intravascular coagulation (DIC)** is a disruption of hemostasis characterized by widespread intravascular clotting and bleeding. It may be acute and life threatening or relatively mild. DIC is a clinical syndrome that develops as a complication of a wide variety of other disorders (Box 32–8). Sepsis is the most common cause of DIC. Gram-negative and gram-positive bacteria as well as viruses, fungi, and protozoal infections may lead to DIC (McCance & Huether, 2002).

---

**BOX 32–8   ■ Conditions That May Precipitate Disseminated Intravascular Coagulation**

#### TISSUE DAMAGE

- Trauma: burns, gunshot wounds, frostbite, head injury
- Obstetric complications: septic abortion, abruptio placentae, amniotic fluid embolus, retained dead fetus
- Neoplasms: acute leukemia, adenocarcinomas
- Hemolysis
- Fat embolism

#### VESSEL DAMAGE

- Aortic aneurysm
- Acute glomerulonephritis
- Hemolytic uremic syndrome

#### INFECTIONS

- Bacterial infection or sepsis
- Viral or mycotic infections
- Parasitic or rickettsial infection

## PATHOPHYSIOLOGY

DIC is triggered by endothelial damage, release of tissue factors into the circulation, or inappropriate activation of the clotting cascade by an endotoxin. Both the intrinsic and the extrinsic clotting cascade may be activated, although the extrinsic cascade usually is the one activated. Extensive thrombin entering the systemic circulation overwhelms natural anticoagulants, leading to unrestricted clot formation (McCance & Huether, 2002). Clotting may be localized to an individual organ, or widespread with deposition of small thrombi and emboli throughout the microvasculature (Braunwald et al., 2001). The widespread clotting consumes clotting factors and activates fibrinolytic processes with anticoagulant production. As a result, hemorrhage occurs (Figure 32–9 ■).

The sequence of DIC follows:

1. Endothelial damage, tissue factors, or toxins stimulate the clotting cascade.
2. Excess thrombin within the circulation overwhelms naturally occurring anticoagulants.
3. Widespread clotting occurs within the microvasculature.
4. Thrombi and emboli impair tissue perfusion, leading to ischemia, infarction, and necrosis.
5. Clotting factors (including platelets) are consumed faster than they can be replaced.
6. Clotting activates fibrinolytic processes which begin to break down clots.

7. Fibrin degradation products (*FDPs,* potent anticoagulants) are released, contributing to bleeding.
8. Clotting factors are depleted, the ability to form clots is lost, and hemorrhage occurs.

## MANIFESTATIONS

The manifestations of DIC result from both clotting and bleeding, although bleeding is more obvious, especially in acute DIC. Bleeding ranges from oozing blood following an injection to frank hemorrhage from every body orifice (see box below). Chronic DIC may be asymptomatic, or may present with peripheral cyanosis, thrombosis, and pregangrenous changes in the fingers and toes, nose, and genitalia (Braunwald et al., 2001).

### Manifestations of DIC

- Frank hemorrhage from incisions
- Oozing of blood from punctures, intravenous catheter sites
- Purpura, petechiae, bruising
- Cyanosis of extremities
- Gastrointestinal bleeding or hemorrhage
- Dyspnea, tachypnea, bloody sputum
- Tachycardia, hypotension
- Hematuria, oliguria, acute renal failure
- Manifestations of increased intracranial pressure: decreased level of consciousness, papillary, motor, and sensory changes
- Mental status changes

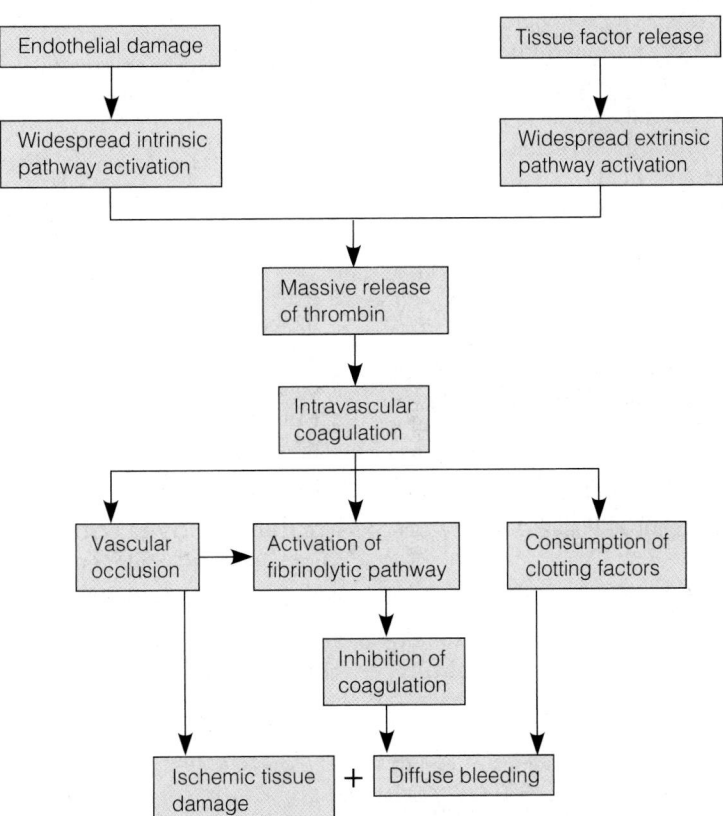

**Figure 32–9** ■ Disseminated intravascular coagulation (DIC). Endothelial cell injury or release of tissue factors activate the intrinsic or extrinsic clotting pathway (or both). As a result, numerous microthrombi form throughout the vasculature, causing ischemic tissue damage. Simultaneously, rapid consumption of clotting factors and activation of fibrinolytic mechanisms trigger widespread bleeding.

## COLLABORATIVE CARE

Treatment of DIC is directed toward treating the underlying disorder and preventing further bleeding or massive thrombosis. Treatment stabilizes the client, reduces complications, and allows recovery to occur; it does not cure DIC (Braunwald et al., 2001).

### Diagnostic Tests

Diagnostic tests are used to confirm the diagnosis of DIC and evaluate the risk for hemorrhage.

- *CBC* and *platelet count* are used to evaluate the hemoglobin, hematocrit, and number of circulating platelets. *Schistocytes*, fragmented RBCs, may be noted due to cell trapping and damage within fibrin thrombi. The platelet count is decreased.
- *Coagulation studies* show prolonged *prothrombin time (PT)*, *partial thromboplastin time (PTT)*, and *thrombin time*, and a low *fibrinogen level* due to depletion of clotting factors. The fibrinogen level helps predict bleeding in DIC: As it falls, the risk of bleeding increases (Braunwald et al., 2001).
- *Fibrin degradation products (FDPs)* or *fibrin split products (FSPs)* are increased due to the fibinolysis that occurs with DIC.

### Treatments

When bleeding is the major manifestation of DIC, fresh frozen plasma and platelet concentrates are given to restore clotting factors and platelets. Heparin, although controversial, may be administered. Heparin interferes with the clotting cascade and may prevent further clotting factor consumption due to uncontrolled thrombosis. It is used when bleeding is not controlled by plasma and platelets, as well as when the client has manifestations of thrombotic problems such as acrocyanosis and possible gangrene. Long-term heparin therapy (administered by injection or continuous infusion using a portable pump) may be necessary for clients with chronic DIC

## NURSING CARE

### Assessment

Nurses can be instrumental in identifying early manifestations of DIC, facilitating timely intervention. Focused nursing assessment for DIC includes:

- Health history: recent abortion (spontaneous or therapeutic) or current pregnancy; presence of a known malignant tumor; history of abnormal bleeding episodes or a hematologic disorder
- Physical examination: bleeding from puncture wounds (e.g., injections), IV sites, incisions; hematuria, obvious or occult blood in emesis or stool, epistaxis, other abnormal bleeding; vital signs; heart and breath sounds; abdominal assessment including girth, contour, bowel sounds, tenderness or guarding to palpation; color, temperature, skin condition of hands, feet, and digits; petechiae or purpura of skin, mucous membranes

### Nursing Diagnoses and Interventions

Clients with acute DIC often are critically ill, with multiple nursing care needs. Priority nursing diagnoses discussed in this section focus on impaired tissue perfusion and gas exchange, pain, and fear. Septic shock may precipitate DIC; hemorrhagic shock may occur as a complication of DIC. See Chapter 6 ⬡ for nursing diagnoses and interventions related to these problems.

### Ineffective Tissue Perfusion

Thrombi and emboli forming throughout the microcirculation affect the perfusion of multiple organs and tissues. Additionally, bleeding due to clotting factor consumption affects cardiac output and blood flow to these tissues.

- Assess extremity pulses, warmth, and capillary refill. Monitor level of consciousness (LOC) and mental status. *Monitoring central and peripheral tissue perfusion facilitates early treatment of impaired perfusion.*

**PRACTICE ALERT** *Promptly report complaints of chest pain, changes in mental status, LOC, tissue perfusion, respirations, gastrointestinal function, and urinary output. Chest pain or respiratory changes (tachypnea, dyspnea, orthopnea) may be due to angina, pulmonary embolism, or bleeding into lung tissue. Changes in mentation or LOC can indicate cerebral ischemia. A painful, pale, and cold extremity with no or diminished pulses indicates arterial occlusion. Prompt intervention is critical to save the extremity. Acute abdominal pain, decreased bowel sounds, and GI bleeding may indicate mesenteric occlusion, a surgical emergency. Decreased urine output may signify renal artery thrombosis; renal failure may develop.* ■

- Carefully reposition at least every 2 hours. *Position changes facilitate circulation and tissue perfusion, as well as provide an opportunity to assess for purpura, pallor, and bleeding.*
- Discourage crossing the legs, and do not elevate the knees on the bed or with a pillow. *These positions may impair arterial and venous flow to the lower legs and feet, increasing vascular stasis and the risk for thrombosis.*
- Minimize use of tape on the skin, using binders, nonadhesive dressings, and other devices as needed. *Preventing skin trauma reduces the risk for bleeding and potential infection.*

### Impaired Gas Exchange

Microclots in the pulmonary vasculature are likely to interfere with gas exchange in the client with DIC.

- Monitor oxygen saturation continuously. Administer oxygen as ordered. *Oxygen saturation levels are a noninvasive means of assessing gas exchange. Supplemental oxygen promotes gas exchange and reduces cardiac work, relieving dyspnea.*
- Place in Fowler's or high-Fowler's position as tolerated. *Elevating the head of the bed improves diaphragmatic excursion and alveolar ventilation.*
- Maintain bed rest. *Bed rest reduces oxygen demands and cardiac work.*

- Encourage deep breathing and effective coughing. *Increased respiratory depth and clearance of secretions from airways improves alveolar ventilation and oxygenation.*
- Cautious nasotracheal suctioning may be instituted if cough is ineffective or an endotracheal tube is in place. *Removal of secretions facilitates ventilation and oxygenation. However, care must be used to minimize suction-induced hypoxia and airway trauma.*

**PRACTICE ALERT** *Monitor arterial blood gas results; report abnormal results to the physician. Low $Pao_2$ and rising $Paco_2$ levels indicate impaired gas exchange and may signify the need for additional treatment.* ■

- Administer analgesics and antianxiety drugs as needed to control pain and anxiety. Provide reassurance and comfort measures. *Pain and anxiety increase the respiratory rate and decrease the depth of respirations, reducing effective ventilation and gas exchange.*

### Pain

Both the underlying cause of DIC and tissue ischemia from microvascular clots can cause pain. Identifying the etiology of pain is important to identify potential complications or harmful effects of DIC and to institute effective treatment.

- Use a standard pain scale chart to evaluate and monitor pain and analgesic effectiveness. *Monitoring pain and response to medication facilitates development of an appropriate and effective treatment plan.*

**PRACTICE ALERT** *Notify the physician promptly of new or a sudden increase in pain, especially when accompanied by changes in assessment findings. New or increased complaints of pain may signify increased circulatory impairment and ischemic changes in tissues such as the heart, bowel, or extremities. Circulation to a painful, pale or cyanotic, or cold extremity may be occluded by an arterial clot. Prompt intervention is necessary to save the extremity. Acute abdominal pain may signify mesenteric occlusion, a surgical emergency. Anginal pain may indicate occlusion of coronary arteries.* ■

- Handle extremities gently. *Gentle handling reduces the risk of further injury to and pain in ischemic tissues.*
- Apply cool compresses to painful joints. *Application of cold decreases pain through the gate-control mechanism, inhibiting the dorsal horn of the spinal cord and reducing the sensation of pain.*

**PRACTICE ALERT** *Continuously monitor effects of analgesics, mental and respiratory status. Analgesics may mask manifestations of neurologic impairment due to thromboembolism, and may depress the respiratory center, further impairing gas exchange. Judicious analgesic administration with careful monitoring is vital to safely provide effective pain relief.* ■

### Fear

The underlying serious illness and a complication such as DIC results in an uncertain prognosis, often accompanied by fear.

- Encourage the client and family to verbalize concerns. *This helps the client and family identify their concerns and frame questions.*
- Answer questions truthfully. *Providing honest answers is vital to developing a therapeutic nurse-client relationship. Accurate responses allow the client and family to set priorities as they plan for an uncertain future.*
- Help the client and family identify coping strategies to manage this significant situational stressor. *Implementing past effective coping methods may provide the skills to manage the current crisis.*
- Provide emotional support. *The presence of a caring nurse helps reduce the fear and anxiety associated with a crisis.*
- Maintain a calm environment. *A calm environment provides reassurance that the situation is in control, reduces anxiety, and promotes rest.*
- Respond promptly when the client calls for help. *Prompt responses to expressed needs helps develop a trusting relationship and a sense of security that assistance is readily available.*
- Teach relaxation techniques. *Relaxation techniques can reduce muscle tension and other signs of anxiety. Gaining control over physical responses can help the client gain a sense of control over the situation.*

### Home Care

Although the immediate crisis of acute DIC is resolved prior to discharge, the client may have some continuing effects of the disorder, such as impaired tissue integrity of distal extremities. Teach the client and family about specific care needs, such as foot care (see Box 33–4) or dressing changes. Provide instruction about any continuing medications and follow-up care. ⊙⊙

Clients with chronic DIC may require continuing heparin therapy, using either intermittent subcutaneous injections or a portable infusion pump. Teach the client and family members how to administer the injection or manage the infusion pump. Provide a referral to home health care or a home intravenous management service for assistance. Discuss the manifestations of excessive bleeding or recurrent clotting that need to be reported to the physician.

## THE CLIENT WITH HEMOPHILIA

**Hemophilia** is a group of hereditary clotting factor disorders that lead to persistent and sometimes severe bleeding. Although often considered a disease of children, hemophilia may be diagnosed in adults. Deficiencies of three clotting factors, VIII, IX, and XI, account for 90% to 95% of the bleeding disorders collectively called hemophilia (McCance & Huether, 2002).

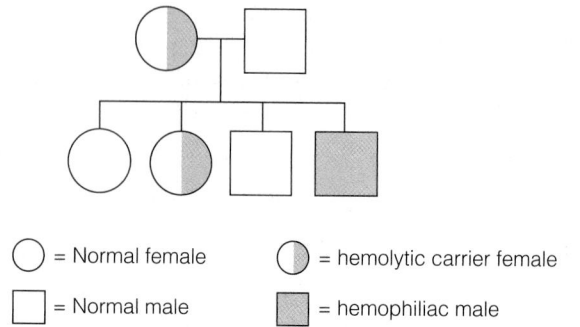

= Normal female        = hemolytic carrier female

= Normal male         = hemophiliac male

**Figure 32–10** ■ The inheritance pattern of hemophilia A and B. Both are transmitted as X-linked recessive disorders. Females may be carriers, but only males develop these disorders.

## PATHOPHYSIOLOGY

**Hemophilia A** (or *classic hemophilia*) is the most common type of hemophilia, caused by deficiency or dysfunction of clotting factor VIII. The estimated incidence of hemophilia A is 1 in 10,000 male births. It is transmitted as an X-linked recessive disorder from mothers to sons (Figure 32–10 ■). The genetic defect of hemophilia A on the X chromosome may cause deficient factor VIII production or a defective form of the protein. When the concentration of the clotting factor is 5% to 35% of normal, the disease is *mild*. Bleeding is infrequent, and usually associated with trauma. Concentrations of 1% to 5% of normal result in *moderate* disease. Again, bleeding usually occurs secondarily to trauma. *Severe* hemophilia occurs when concentrations are less than 1% of normal. Bleeding is frequent, often occurring without trauma (Braunwald et al., 2001; McCance & Huether, 2002).

**Hemophilia B** (also called *Christmas disease*), accounts for about 15% of cases, and is caused by a deficiency in factor IX. Despite the difference in clotting factor deficits, hemophilia A and B are clinically identical. Hemophilia B also is transmitted from mother to son as an X-linked recessive disorder.

**Von Willebrand's disease,** often considered as a type of hemophilia, is the most common hereditary bleeding disorder (Porth, 2002). It is caused by a deficit of or defective von Willebrand (vW) factor, a protein that mediates platelet adhesion (Tierney et al., 2001). Reduced levels of factor VIII often also are present, because vW factor carries factor VIII. This clotting disorder is transmitted in an autosomal dominant pattern, and affects men and women equally. Bleeding associated with von Willebrand's disease rarely is severe. It often is diagnosed when prolonged bleeding follows surgery or a dental extraction.

*Factor XI deficiency* (or *hemophilia C*) is inherited in an autosomal recessive pattern, and most often affects Ashkenazi Jews (Braunwald et al., 2001). It is usually a mild disorder, identified when postoperative bleeding is prolonged. A comparison of the types of hemophilia is found in Table 32–3.

People with hemophilia form a platelet plug at the site of bleeding, but the clotting factor deficit impairs formation of a stable fibrin clot. The effect of vW factor deficiency is somewhat different, in that platelet aggregation at the site of injury is impaired. In either case, prolonged or extensive bleeding may result. Often bleeding occurs in response to injury or as a result of surgery. However, a severe clotting factor deficit can lead to spontaneous bleeding into the joints (*hemarthrosis*), deep tissues, and central nervous system. Hemarthrosis often causes joint deformity and disability, usually of the elbows, hips, knees, and ankles.

## MANIFESTATIONS

The following are manifestations of hemophilia.

- Hemarthrosis
- Easy bruising and cutaneous hematoma formation with minor trauma (e.g., an injection)
- Bleeding from the gums and prolonged bleeding following minor injuries or cuts
- Gastrointestinal bleeding, with hematemesis (vomiting blood), occult blood in the stools, gastric pain, or abdominal pain
- Spontaneous hematuria or epistaxis (nosebleed)
- Pain or paralysis due to the pressure of hematomas on nerves

Intracranial hemorrhage is a potentially life-threatening manifestation of hemophilia.

| TABLE 32–3 | Types of Hemophilia | | |
|---|---|---|---|
| **Type/Name** | **Deficiency** | **Characteristics** | **Treatment** |
| Hemophilia A (Classic hemophilia) | Factor VIII | Transmitted by females; occurs primarily in males; bleeding time normal; coagulation time prolonged | Factor VIII concentrate or cryoprecipitate |
| Hemophilia B | Factor IX | Transmitted by females; occurs primarily in males; bleeding time normal; coagulation time prolonged | Factor IX (Christmas disease concentrate) |
| von Willebrand's disease | vW factor Factor VIII | Occurs in both females and males; bleeding time and coagulation time are both prolonged | Cryoprecipitate and DDAVP |
| Factor XI deficiency | Factor XI | Occurs in both males and females; the activated partial thromboplastin time is prolonged | Fresh frozen plasma |

## COLLABORATIVE CARE

Treatment of hemophilia focuses on preventing and/or treating bleeding, primarily by replacing deficient clotting factors. Specific treatment depends on the severity of the disorder and the specific factor deficiency. Care may be complicated by hepatitis or HIV disease in people with hemophilia treated with clotting factor concentrates prepared from multiple units of donated blood. Today, routine testing of all blood, improved blood donor screening, and current methods of treating hemophilia have significantly reduced the risk for these bloodborne diseases.

### Diagnostic Tests

The following laboratory tests may be ordered.

- *Serum platelet levels* are measured and are usually normal.
- *Coagulation studies* such as APTT, bleeding time, and prothrombin time are used to screen for hemophilia when abnormal bleeding occurs. APTT is increased in all types of hemophilia. Prothrombin time is unaffected in these disorders but may be measured to rule out other disorders. Bleeding time is prolonged in von Willebrand's disease but normal in hemophilia A and B.
- *Factor assays* are performed; factor VIII is decreased in hemophilia A and often in von Willebrand's disease, factor IX is decreased in hemophilia B, and factor XI in hemophilia C.
- *Amniocentesis* or *chorionic villus sampling* are used to identify the genetic defect of hemophilia when there is a known family history of the disease.

### Medications

Deficient clotting factors are replaced regularly, as a prophylactic measure before surgery and dental procedures, and to control bleeding. Clotting factors may be given as fresh-frozen plasma, cryoprecipitates, or concentrates. Factor levels are measured on a regular basis to determine whether the treatment is adequate. Clotting factors are often self-administered and may be taken either on a regular or intermittent schedule.

Fresh-frozen plasma replaces all clotting factors (including both factor VIII and factor IX) except platelets. When the cause of bleeding is not yet determined, fresh-frozen plasma may be administered intravenously until a definitive diagnosis is made.

Hemophilia A is usually treated with either heat-treated factor VIII concentrate (heat treating reduces the risk of transmitting disease) or recombinant factor VIII. Although recombinant factor VIII, produced using recombinant DNA technology, eliminates the risk of viral disease transmission, its use is limited by cost. The dose of factor VIII is determined by the severity of the deficit and the presence or prospect of active bleeding (e.g., planned surgery).

Desmopressin acetate (DDAVP, Stimate) may be given to people with mild hemophilia A or von Willebrand's disease prior to minor surgeries. This drug causes release of factor VIII and will raise blood levels by two- or threefold for several hours, reducing the risk of bleeding and the need for clotting factor concentrate (Tierney et al., 2001).

Factor IX concentrate (administered intravenously) is used to treat hemophilia B. Because factor IX concentrates also contain a number of other proteins, there is risk of thrombosis with recurrent use. They are used judiciously, only when needed. Products produced by recombinant technology or that are monoclonally purified carry a lower risk of stimulating thrombus formation (Braunwald et al., 2001). Fresh-frozen plasma replaces factor XI and is used when necessary. It may be given daily until the risk for bleeding decreases.

Factor VIII concentrates contain functional vW factor, and may be used to treat von Willebrand's disease. Aspirin is avoided in all types of hemophilia.

## NURSING CARE

### Health Promotion

Encourage clients with a family history of hemophilia or bleeding disorders to seek genetic counseling during their family planning process. Although tests are available for the hemophilia gene, the technology to correct the disorder in utero does not yet exist.

### Assessment

While severe hemophilia usually is diagnosed in childhood, milder cases may not be identified until surgery, invasive dental work, or a traumatic injury causes extensive or prolonged bleeding. Focused assessment related to hemophilia includes the following:

- Health history: previous bleeding episodes with or without trauma; history of easy bruising, hematomas, epistaxis, bleeding gums, hematuria, vomiting blood, or joint pain; aspirin use; family history of hemophilia or bleeding disorders
- Physical examination: vital signs; bruising or bleeding of skin or mucous membranes; mental status; abdominal assessment; presence of joint deformity, decreased range of motion

### Nursing Diagnoses and Interventions

Impaired blood clotting, the need for continuing care and disease management, and the risk for genetic transmission of hemophilia are priority problems for the client with hemophilia.

#### Ineffective Protection

The inability to form stable clots and stem bleeding from injured blood vessels creates a significant risk for the client with hemophilia. Nursing care measures focus on preventing injury and protecting the skin from damage.

- Monitor for signs of bleeding, including hematomas, ecchymoses, and purpura, as well as surface oozing or bleeding. Check emesis and stool for occult blood. *Bleeding may occur in cutaneous tissues as well as internal organs. Bleeding in the upper gastrointestinal tract may not be readily apparent in the stool.*
- Notify the physician of any apparent bleeding. *Prompt intervention with administration of clotting factor concentrate decreases the risk of hemorrhage and subsequent hypovolemia.*

- Avoid intramuscular injections, rectal temperatures, and enemas. *These can pose a risk of tissue and vascular trauma, which can precipitate bleeding.*
- Use safety measures in personal care. For example, use an electric razor rather than a razor blade to shave. *Use of an electric razor minimizes the opportunity to develop superficial cuts that may result in bleeding.*
- If bleeding occurs, control blood loss using gentle pressure, ice, or a topical hemostatic agent, such as absorbable gelatin sponge, microfibrillar collagen hemostat, or topical thrombin. *Direct pressure occludes bleeding vessels. Ice, a vasoconstrictor, may facilitate bleeding control, as do topical hemostatic agents.*
- Instruct to avoid activities that increase the risk of trauma, including contact sports, physical exertion associated with job performance, and to eliminate safety hazards in the home. *Depending on the severity of the clotting factor deficit, even minor trauma can lead to serious bleeding episodes. Safer activities such as noncontact sports (e.g., swimming, golf) and occupations that do not require physical labor may be substituted.*

### Risk for Ineffective Health Maintenance

Hemophilia is a chronic disorder, requiring active management to prevent and control bleeding and complications. Frequent visits to the physician or clinic may be necessary. In addition, the client may need to learn to self-administer clotting factors and measures to prevent complications. The lifelong nature of the disorder may interfere with compliance, especially during early adulthood.

- Assess knowledge of disorder and the related treatments. *Assessment allows identification of knowledge gaps and provides a basis on which to provide additional information. Impaired disease management may be due to lack of knowledge or a conscious decision not to follow the recommendations of the health care provider.*
- Provide information about the bleeding disorder and prescribed medications and treatments. *Individualized instruction is more effective than general, possibly irrelevant information.*
- Provide emotional support, expressing confidence in the client's self-care abilities. *Emotional support helps the client incorporate the care regimen into his or her lifestyle.*
- Provide supervised learning and practice opportunities for administering clotting factors and topical hemostatic agents. *Successful practice sessions instill confidence in the ability to manage care and provide an opportunity for questions and exploring alternatives.*

## Using NANDA, NIC, and NOC

Chart 32–2 shows links between NANDA nursing diagnoses, NIC, and NOC for the client with hemophilia.

## Home Care

Discuss the following topics when preparing the client with a bleeding disorder and the family for home care.

- Recognizing the manifestations of internal bleeding: pallor, weakness, restlessness, headache, disorientation, pain, swelling. These manifestations require emergency medical care and should be reported immediately.
- Applying cold packs and immobilizing the joint for 24 to 48 hours if hemarthrosis occurs
- Using analgesics for pain; avoiding prescription and over-the-counter drugs containing aspirin
- Ensuring a safe home environment (e.g., padding sharp edges of furniture, using transition lighting or a night light; avoiding scatter rugs, and wearing protective gloves when working in the house or yard)
- Using safe grooming practices such as electric razors
- Wearing a MedicAlert bracelet in case of accident
- Practicing good dental hygiene to decrease potential tooth decay and extractions. If dental procedures are necessary, discuss the need for prophylactic factor administration with the dentist and physician.

---

## CHART 32–2 NANDA, NIC, AND NOC LINKAGES

### The Client with Hemophilia

| NURSING DIAGNOSES | NURSING INTERVENTIONS | NURSING OUTCOMES |
|---|---|---|
| • Impaired Physical Mobility | • Exercise Therapy: Joint Mobility<br>• Pain Management | • Joint Movement: Active<br>• Mobility Level |
| • Ineffective Health Maintenance | • Health Education<br>• Self-Responsibility Facilitation<br>• Teaching: Procedure/Treatment | • Health-Seeking Behavior<br>• Knowledge: Health Behaviors<br>• Knowledge: Treatment Regimen |
| • Ineffective Protection | • Bleeding Precautions<br>• Blood Products Administration | • Coagulation Status |
| • Pain | • Medication Management<br>• Positioning | • Comfort Level |

*Note. Data from Nursing Outcomes Classification (NOC) by M. Johnson & M. Maas (Eds.), 1997, St. Louis: Mosby; Nursing Diagnoses: Definitions & Classification 2001–2002 by North American Nursing Diagnosis Association, 2001, Philadelphia: NANDA; Nursing Interventions Classification (NIC) by J.C. McCloskey & G. M. Bulechek (Eds.), 2000, St. Louis: Mosby. Reprinted by permission.*

- Following safer-sex practices
- Preparing and administering intravenous medications

Refer the client and family to a local hemophilia or bleeding disorders support group. Provide contact information for national organizations and information clearinghouses, such as:

National Hemophilia Foundation
112 West 32nd Street
New York, NY 10001
1-800-42-handi
www.hemophilia.org

## Nursing Care Plan
## A Client with Hemophilia

Jermiel Cruise is a 20-year-old student at the community college. He is admitted to the emergency department with a nosebleed that began when he fell during a touch football game. It has continued to bleed for over an hour.

### ASSESSMENT

Mr. Cruise states that he has hemophilia and realizes that playing contact sports "is probably a dumb thing to do." He adds that he has not had any recent bleeding episodes. An icebag and manual pressure are applied in the emergency department. The physician orders factor VIII concentrate to be administered. Physical assessment findings are: T 97.2°F (36.2°C), BP 118/64, R 18. Skin pale but warm. Laboratory tests reveal a prolonged APTT and a normal bleeding time and PT. Following treatment, Mr. Cruise's bleeding subsides.

### DIAGNOSES

- *Risk for aspiration* related to uncontrolled nosebleed
- *Noncompliance* with activity recommendations
- *Ineffective protection* related to lack of clotting factor VIII

### EXPECTED OUTCOMES

- Exhibit no further signs of bleeding.
- Maintain vital signs within his usual range.
- Maintain an open airway.
- Identify sports and recreation activities in which he can safely participate.
- Verbalize self-care measures to control bleeding.

### PLANNING AND IMPLEMENTATION

- Monitor vital signs and for further signs of bleeding.
- Assess airway and auscultate breath sounds.

- Review emergency measures to help stop bleeding.
- Reiterate the importance of seeking prompt medical attention if bleeding should occur.
- Advise regarding the importance of wearing a MedicAlert bracelet identifying him as a hemophiliac.
- Discuss alternative noncontact sports and recreational activities.

### EVALUATION

On discharge, Mr. Cruise has no further signs of bleeding, shock, or aspiration. He is able to verbalize methods to help stop local bleeding and the importance of seeking medical attention promptly when bleeding continues. Mr. Cruise agrees to stop at a local drug store on the way home to order a MedicAlert bracelet. In addition, Mr. Cruise verbalizes an understanding of the importance of avoiding contact sports and has identified swimming and golf as alternative leisure activities that he might enjoy.

### Critical Thinking in the Nursing Process

1. What is the pathophysiologic basis for the bleeding that occurs in hemophilia A and B?
2. What was Mr. Cruise's priority nursing diagnosis? Why?
3. Why is family planning a special consideration with a client who has hemophilia?
4. Outline a plan to teach the family of a client diagnosed with hemophilia how to administer an intravenous infusion.
5. Develop a care plan for Mr. Cruise for the nursing diagnosis, *Impaired social interaction*. Consider Mr. Cruise's age and developmental level in creating the plan.

See Evaluating Your Response in Appendix C.

# WHITE BLOOD CELL AND LYMPHOID TISSUE DISORDERS

Disorders of the white blood cells and lymphoid tissue include infectious mononucleosis, the leukemias, multiple myeloma, and malignant lymphomas (Hodgkin's disease and non-Hodgkin's lymphoma). A review of the physiology of white blood cells and lymphoid tissues precedes discussion of the diseases.

## PHYSIOLOGY REVIEW

### White Blood Cells

**White blood cells (WBCs),** also called leukocytes, are a part of the body's defense against microorganisms. On average, there are 5,000 to 10,000 WBCs per cubic millimeter of blood,

accounting for about 1% of total blood volume. **Leukocytosis** is a higher than normal WBC count; **leukopenia** is a WBC count that is lower than normal.

WBCs originate from hemopoietic stem cells in the bone marrow. These stem cells differentiate into the various types of white blood cells (see Figure 32–1).

The two basic types of WBCs are granular leukocytes (or *granulocytes*) and nongranular leukocytes. Granulocytes have horseshoe-shaped nuclei and contain large granules in the cytoplasm. Stimulated by granulocyte-macrophage colony-stimulating factor (GM-CSF) and granulocyte colony-stimulating factor (G-CSF), granulocytes mature fully in the bone marrow before being released into the bloodstream. Following are the three types of granulocytes.

- *Neutrophils* (also called polymorphonuclear [*PMNs*] or segmented [*segs*] leukocytes) comprise 60% to 70% of the total circulating WBCs. Their nuclei are divided into three to five lobes. Neutrophils are active phagocytes, the first cells to arrive at a site of injury. Their numbers increase during inflammation. Immature forms of neutrophils (*bands*) are released during inflammation or infections. Neutrophils have a life span of only about 10 hours and are constantly being replaced.
- *Eosinophils* comprise 1% to 3% of circulating WBCs, but are found in large numbers in the mucosa of the intestines and lungs. Their numbers increase during allergic reactions and parasitic infestations.
- *Basophils,* which comprise less than 1% of the WBC count, contain histamine, heparin, and other inflammatory mediators. Basophils increase in numbers during allergic and inflammatory reactions.

Nongranular WBCs (agranulocytes) include the monocytes and lymphocytes. They enter the bloodstream before final maturation.

- *Monocytes* are the largest of the WBCs. They comprise approximately 3% to 8% of the total WBC count. Monocytes contain powerful bactericidal substances and proteolytic enzymes. They are phagocytic cells that mature into macrophages. Macrophages dispose of foreign and waste material, especially in inflammation. They are an active part of the immune response.
- *Lymphocytes* comprise 20% to 30% of the WBC count. Lymphocytes mature in lymphoid tissue into B cells and T cells. B cells are involved in the humoral immune response and antibody formation, whereas T cells take part in the cell-mediated immunity process (see Chapter 9). ⊙⊃ Plasma cells (which arise from B cells) are lymphoid cells found in bone marrow and connective tissue; they also are involved in immune reactions.

Table 32–4 lists normal laboratory values for WBCs.

## Lymphoid Tissues and Organs

**Lymphoid tissues** are connective tissues that contain billions of lymphocytes. *Lymphoid organs* include the bone marrow, thymus, lymph nodes, associated lymphoid tissues, and the spleen. New lymphocytes are created and differentiated in the *central* or *primary* lymphoid organs, the bone marrow and thymus. Lymphocytes and other WBCs are formed in the bone marrow. While still immature, some lymphocytes migrate to the thymus. In the thymus, they further differentiate to become active immune cells (T cells or T lymphocytes).

The *peripheral* or *secondary* lymphoid organs (the lymph nodes, associated lymphoid tissues, and spleen) have an active role in immune function (see Chapter 9). ⊙⊃ The lymph circulation returns interstitial fluids to the circulatory system. Lymph nodes filter and process lymph drainage. They contain multiple lymphocytes and macrophages, so all lymph is exposed to many immunocompetent cells. Lymphoid tissue also is found in many organs, such as the gastrointestinal tract, tonsils, adenoids, and airways. This tissue, called mucosa-associated lymphoid tissue (MALT), helps prevent microorganisms from entering the body.

The spleen is the largest lymphatic organ. It stores and processes blood, removing aged RBCs and processing their hemoglobin. The spleen contains phagocytic cells that help clear bloodborne pathogens.

## THE CLIENT WITH NEUTROPENIA

*Leukopenia* is a decrease in the total circulating white blood cell count. Although any type of WBC may be affected, neutrophils, which make up the majority of WBCs, are affected most often. *Neutropenia* is a decrease in circulating neutrophils, usually less than 1500 cells/µm. Neutropenia may be either congenital or acquired, developing secondarily to prolonged infection, hematologic disorders, starvation, or autoimmune disorders (such as rheumatoid arthritis). *Agranulocytosis* is severe neutropenia, with less than 200 cells/µm. Numbers of other granulocytes also are reduced. It is usually due to impaired leukocyte formation in the bone marrow or increased cell destruction in circulating blood. Chemotherapy and other drugs can suppress the bone marrow. Agranulocytosis significantly increases the risk for infection. *Aplastic anemia* affects production of all blood cells, resulting in anemia, thrombocytopenia, and agranulocytosis.

Neutrophils are an integral component of the immune response. The manifestations of neutropenia reflect the resulting impaired immunity and inflammatory response. Opportunistic bacterial, fungal, and protozoal infections develop, commonly affecting the respiratory tract and mucosa of the mouth, GI tract, and vagina. Malaise, chills, and fever with extreme weakness and fatigue are common manifestations.

Hematopoietic growth factors such as GM-CSF are administered to stimulate granulocyte maturation and differentiation. Infections are treated with antibiotic therapy.

The primary nursing care focus is protecting the client from infection. See Risk for Infection in the leukemia section that follows for specific nursing interventions.

| TABLE 32–4 | Normal Laboratory Values for White Blood Cells |
|---|---|
| **Laboratory Test** | **Value** |
| WBC count | 5000–10,000/mm³ |
| Differential WBC count | |
|   Neutrophils | 60–70% or 3000–7000/mm³ |
|   Eosinophils | 1–3% or 50–400/mm³ |
|   Basophils | 0.3–0.5% or 25–200/mm³ |
|   Lymphocytes | 20–30% or 1000–4000/mm³ |
|   Monocytes | 3–8% or 100–600/mm³ |

## THE CLIENT WITH INFECTIOUS MONONUCLEOSIS

*Infectious mononucleosis* is characterized by invasion of B cells in the oropharyngeal lymphoid tissues by the Epstein-Barr virus (EBV). This disease is usually benign and self-limiting. It often affects young adults between the ages of 15 and 30. The virus is present in saliva, which appears to be the primary mode of transmission. As a result, infectious mononucleosis is often called the "kissing disease."

When the virus enters the body, unaffected B cells produce antibodies against the virus, and T cells directly attack the virus. Infected B cells are destroyed as the virus replicates. The proliferation of B and T cells, as well as the removal of dead and damaged leukocytes, is responsible for the swelling of lymphoid tissues.

The incubation period for infectious mononucleosis is 4 to 8 weeks. Its onset is insidious, with headache, malaise, and fatigue. Fever, sore throat, and cervical lymphadenopathy (lymph node enlargement and pain) lasting 1 to 3 weeks is common. Symptom severity varies from person to person. Lymph node involvement may be generalized; about 50% of people with infectious mononucleosis develop an enlarged spleen (splenomegaly).

Laboratory findings include increased lymphocytes and monocytes, with about 20% of the cells atypical in form. Early in the infection, the WBC count usually is normal or low, but by the second week it increases and remains elevated for 4 to 8 weeks. Platelet counts are often low during the illness.

Recovery occurs in 2 to 3 weeks; however, debility and lethargy may last for up to 3 months. The treatment includes bed rest and analgesic agents to alleviate the symptoms. Nursing care is primarily educational to prevent further spread of the disease.

## THE CLIENT WITH LEUKEMIA

**Leukemia** (literally, "white blood") is a group of chronic malignant disorders of white blood cells and white blood cell precursors. In leukemia, the usual ratio of red to white blood cells is reversed. Leukemias are characterized by replacement of bone marrow by malignant immature white blood cells, abnormal immature circulating WBCs, and infiltration of these cells into the liver, spleen, and lymph nodes throughout the body.

Although leukemia is often thought of as a childhood disease, it is diagnosed 10 times more often in adults than children. An estimated 30,800 new cases of leukemia occur yearly; approximately half are chronic leukemia and half are acute leukemia. In 2002, approximately 21,700 people died of leukemia (American Cancer Society [ACS], 2002a). The highest incidence of leukemia is found in the United States, Canada, Sweden, and New Zealand (McCance & Huether, 2002).

Although the cause of most leukemias is unknown, certain risk factors have been identified. The incidence of leukemia is higher in people with Down syndrome and certain other genetic disorders. Exposure to ionizing radiation and certain chemicals such as benzene (present in gasoline and cigarette smoke) increases the risk for leukemia, as does treatment for other cancers. Some leukemias are known to be caused by a retrovirus, human T-cell leukemia/lymphoma virus-1 (HTLV-1) (ACS, 2002).

Leukemias are classified by their acuity and by the predominant cell type involved. The *acute* leukemias are characterized by an acute onset, rapid disease progression, and immature or undifferentiated blast cells. *Chronic* leukemias, on the other hand, have a gradual onset, prolonged course, and abnormal mature-appearing cells. *Lymphocytic* (or *lymphoblastic*) leukemias involve immature lymphocytes and their precursor cells in the bone marrow. Lymphocytic leukemias infiltrate the spleen, lymph nodes, CNS, and other tissues. *Myelocytic* (or *myeloblastic*) leukemias involve myeloid stem cells in the bone marrow, interfering with the maturation of all types of blood cells, including granulocytes, RBCs, and thrombocytes (Porth, 2002). Acute lymphoblastic leukemia is the most common type of leukemia in children. In adults, acute myeloblastic leukemia and chronic lymphocytic leukemia are the most common types (McCance & Huether, 2002). In summary, the general types of leukemia are as follows:

- Acute lymphocytic (lymphoblastic) leukemia (ALL)
- Chronic lymphocytic leukemia (CLL)
- Acute myelocytic (myeloblastic) leukemia (AML)
- Chronic myelocytic (myelogenous) leukemia (CML)

This general system of classifying leukemias does not differentiate subtypes of acute leukemias. The French-American-British (FAB) system for classifying acute leukemias further differentiates acute leukemias by the predominant cell involved and the degree of cell differentiation (Table 32–5).

Without treatment, leukemia is invariably fatal, usually due to complications of leukemic cell infiltration of bone marrow or vital organs. With treatment, prognosis varies. The 5-year survival rate is 46% (ACS, 2002). The types, pathology, manifestations, and treatment for the major leukemias are outlined in Table 32–6.

### PATHOPHYSIOLOGY AND MANIFESTATIONS

Leukemia begins with malignant transformation of a single stem cell. Leukemic cells proliferate slowly, but do not differentiate normally. They have a prolonged life span and accumulate in the bone marrow. As they accumulate, they compete with the proliferation of normal cells. Leukemic cells do not function as mature WBCs, and are ineffective in the inflammatory and immune processes. Leukemic cells replace normal hematopoietic elements in the marrow. Because erythrocyte- and platelet-producing cells are crowded out, severe anemia, splenomegaly, and bleeding difficulties result.

Leukemic cells leave the bone marrow and travel through the circulatory system, infiltrating other body tissues such as the central nervous system, testes, skin, gastrointestinal tract, and the lymph nodes, liver, and spleen. Death usually is due to internal hemorrhage and infections.

TABLE 32–5   FAB Classification of Acute Leukemia

| Type | Class | Predominant Cells | Prognosis |
|------|-------|-------------------|-----------|
| Acute Lymphocytic Leukemia (ALL) | $L_1$ | Immature lymphoblasts | >90% remission rate in children |
| | $L_2$ | Mature lymphoblasts | Relapse common after 2 or more years of remission |
| Acute Myelocytic Leukemia | $M_0$ | Undifferentiated cells | Poor |
| | $M_1$ | Immature myeloblasts | Good; complete response in 65% or more |
| | $M_2$ | Mature myeloblasts | Good for 2 or more years of remission |
| | $M_3$ | Promyelocytes | Good in adults |
| | $M_4$ | Myelocytes and monocytes | Poorest in adults |
| | $M_5$ | Poorly or well-differentiated monocytes | Poor |
| | $M_6$ | Predominant eythroblasts | Variable |
| | $M_7$ | Megakaryocytes | |

The general manifestations of leukemia (regardless of type) result from anemia, infection, and bleeding. These include pallor, fatigue, tachycardia, malaise, lethargy, and dyspnea on exertion. Infection may cause fever, night sweats, oral ulcerations, and frequent or recurrent respiratory, urinary, integumentary, or other infections. Increased bleeding due to thrombocytopenia leads to bruising; petechiae; bleeding gums; and bleeding within specific organs and tissues. *Multisystem Effects of Leukemia* can be seen on page 963.

Other manifestations result from leukemic cell infiltration, increased metabolism, and increased leukocyte destruction. Infiltration of the liver, spleen, lymph nodes, and bone marrow causes pain and tissue swelling in the involved areas. Meningeal infiltration may cause manifestations of increased intracranial pressure, such as headache, altered level of consciousness, cranial nerve impairment, nausea, and vomiting. Infiltration of the kidneys may affect renal function, with decreased urine output and increased blood urea nitrogen and creatinine. Increased metabolism causes heat intolerance, weight loss, dyspnea on exertion, and tachycardia. Destruction of large numbers of WBCs releases substantial amounts of uric acid into the circulation; uric acid crystals may obstruct renal tubules, causing renal insufficiency.

## Acute Myelocytic Leukemia

**Acute myelocytic leukemia (AML)** is characterized by uncontrolled proliferation of myeloblasts (the precursors of granulocytes) and hyperplasia of the bone marrow and spleen. AML accounts for most acute leukemia in adults. Treatment induces complete remission in 70% of clients, although only about 25% achieve cure or long-term remission (Porth, 2002).

The manifestations of AML result from neutropenia and thrombocytopenia. Decreased neutrophils lead to recurrent severe infections, such as pneumonia, septicemia, abscesses, and mucous membrane ulceration. The manifestations of thrombocytopenia include petechiae, purpura, and ecchymoses (bruising), epistaxis (nosebleeds), hematomas, hematuria, and gastrointestinal bleeding. Bone infarctions or subperiosteal infiltrates of

TABLE 32–6   Major Types of Leukemia

| Classification | Characteristics | Manifestations | Treatment |
|----------------|-----------------|----------------|-----------|
| Acute lymphoblastic leukemia (ALL) | Primarily affects children and young adults; leukemic cells may infiltrate CNS | Recurrent infections; bleeding; pallor, bone pain, weight loss, sore throat, fatigue, night sweats, weakness | Chemotherapy; bone marrow transplant (BMT), or stem cell transplant (SCT) |
| Chronic lymphocytic leukemia (CLL) | Primarily affects older adults; insidious onset and slow, chronic course | Fatigue; exercise intolerance; lymphadenopathy and splenomegaly; recurrent infections, pallor, edema, thrombophlebitis | Often requires no treatment; chemotherapy; BMT |
| Acute myelocytic leukemia (AML) | Common in older adults, may affect children and young adults. Strongly associated with toxins, genetic disorders, and treatment of other cancers | Fatigue, weakness, fever; anemia; headache, bone and joint pain; abnormal bleeding and bruising; recurrent infection; lymphadenopathy, splenomegaly, and hepatomegaly | Chemotherapy; SCT |
| Chronic myelocytic leukemia (CML) | Primarily affects adults; early course slow and stable, progressing to aggressive phase in 3–4 years | Early: Weakness, fatigue, dyspnea on exertion; possible splenomegaly<br>Later: fever, weight loss, night sweats | Interferon-$\alpha$; chemotherapy, SCT |

# Multisystem Effects of Leukemia

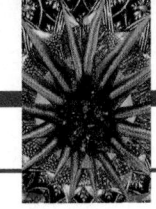

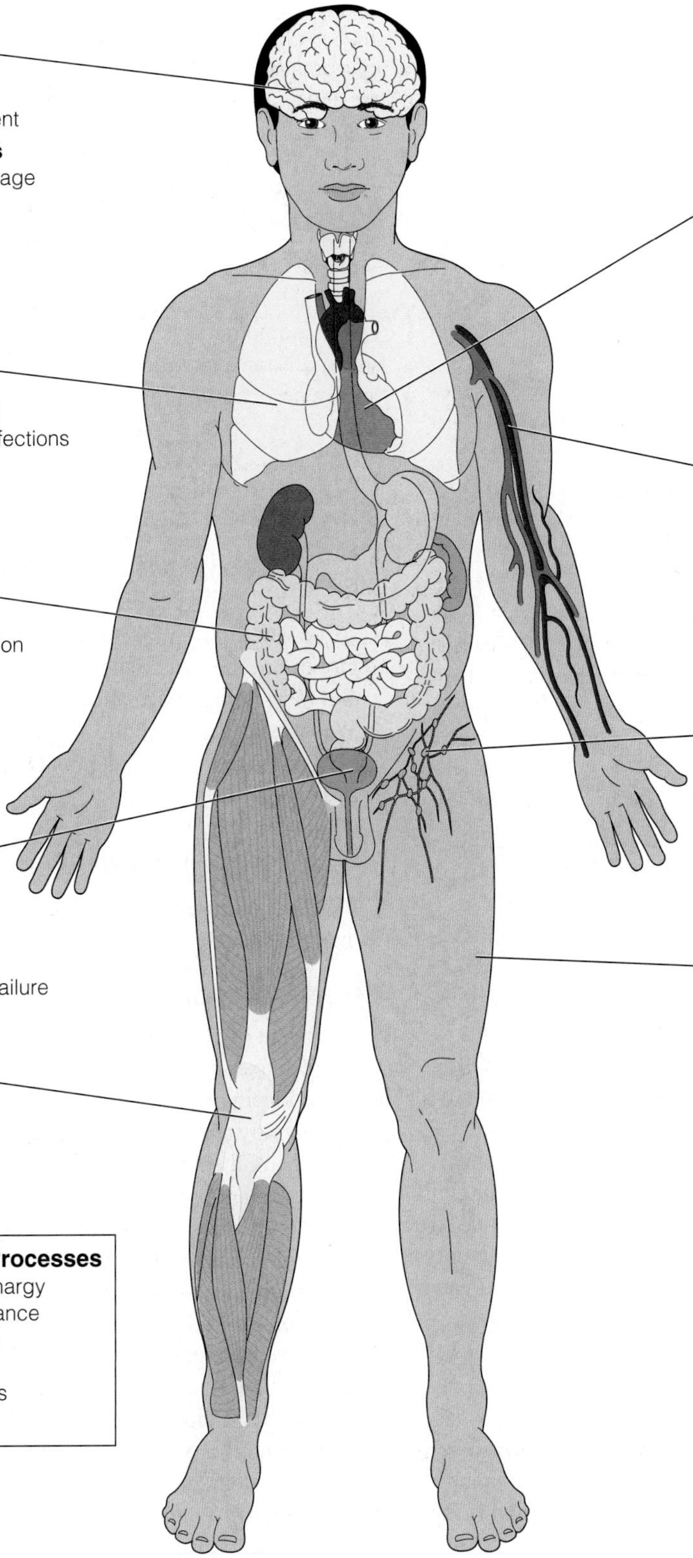

**Neurologic**
- Headache
- Altered LOC
- Cranial nerve impairment

**Potential complications**
- Subarachnoid hemorrhage
- Retinal hemorrhage
- Seizures, coma

**Respiratory**
- Dyspnea on exertion
- Pharyngitis, sore throat
- Frequent respiratory infections

**Potential complication**
- Pulmonary bleeding

**Gastrointestinal**
- Anorexia, nausea
- Oral ulcerations, infection
- Bleeding gums
- Gingival hyperplasia (gum overgrowth)
- Abdominal pain
- Hepatomegaly
- Occult GI bleeding

**Urinary**
- Urinary tract infection
- Hematuria

**Potential complication**
- Renal insufficiency or failure

**Musculoskeletal**
- Weakness
- Bone tenderness, pain
- Joint pain

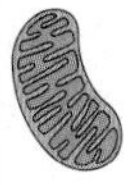

**Metabolic Processes**
- Malaise, lethargy
- Heat intolerance
- Diaphoresis
- Chills, fever
- Night sweats
- Weight loss

**Cardiovascular**
- Tachycardia, palpitations
- Orthostatic hypotension
- Heart murmurs
- Hematomas
- Edema

**Potential complications**
- Hemorrhage
- Thrombophlebitis

**Hematologic**
- Anemia
- Thrombocytopenia
- Leukopenia
- Bleeding (epistaxis)
- Splenomegaly

**Potential complication**
- DIC

**Immunologic**
- Frequent or recurrent infections
- Lymphadenopathy

**Potential complications**
- Abscesses
- Septicemia

**Integumentary**
- Skin and mucous membrane pallor
- Petechiae
- Bruising, purpura
- Ulcerations
- *Chloromas* (skin infiltrations near bony prominences)

leukemic cells may cause bone pain. Anemia is a late manifestation, causing fatigue, headaches, pallor, and dyspnea on exertion. Death usually results from infection or hemorrhage.

Bone marrow aspiration shows a proliferation of immature WBCs. The CBC shows thrombocytopenia and normocytic, normochromic anemia.

## Chronic Myelocytic Leukemia

**Chronic myelocytic leukemia (CML)** is characterized by abnormal proliferation of all bone marrow elements. CML is usually associated with a chromosome abnormality called the Philadelphia chromosome, a translocation of chromosome 22 to chromosome 9. This type of leukemia constitutes approximately 20% of adult leukemias. It usually affects clients over age 50; its incidence is higher in men than in women. Ionizing radiation and exposure to chemicals are implicated as causes of CML.

People with CML are often asymptomatic in the early stages and, in fact, are often diagnosed when a routine blood test reveals abnormal cell counts. Anemia causes weakness, fatigue, and dyspnea on exertion. The spleen often is enlarged, causing abdominal discomfort. Within 3 to 4 years, disease progresses to a more aggressive phase. Rapid cell proliferation and hypermetabolism cause fatigue, weight loss, sweating, and heat intolerance. Finally, the disease evolves to acute leukemia, with blast cell proliferation and constitutional symptoms. Survival following the onset of this final stage averages only 2 to 4 months (Porth, 2002).

## Acute Lymphocytic Leukemia

**Acute lymphocytic leukemia (ALL)** is the most common type of leukemia in children and young adults. ALL causes abnormal proliferation of lymphoblasts in the bone marrow, lymph nodes, and spleen.

The onset of ALL is usually rapid. Lymphoblasts proliferating in bone marrow and peripheral tissues crowd the growth of normal cells. Normal hematopoiesis is suppressed, leading to thrombocytopenia, leukopenia, and anemia. Manifestations of infections, bleeding, and anemia develop. Bone pain resulting from rapid generation of marrow elements, lymphadenopathy, and liver enlargement are also common. Infiltration of the central nervous system causes headaches, visual disturbances, vomiting, and seizures.

The CBC shows an elevated WBC count with increased lymphocytes on the differential. RBC and platelet counts are decreased. Bone marrow studies reveal a hypercellular marrow with growth of lymphoblasts. Combination chemotherapy produces complete remission in 80% to 90% of adults with ALL.

## Chronic Lymphocytic Leukemia

**Chronic lymphocytic leukemia (CLL)** is characterized by proliferation and accumulation of small, abnormal, mature lymphocytes in the bone marrow, peripheral blood, and body tissues. The abnormal cells are usually B-lymphocytes that are unable to produce adequate antibodies to maintain normal immune function. CLL occurs more commonly in adults, especially in older adults (median age 65). CLL is the least common type of the major leukemias.

CLL has a slow onset and is often diagnosed during a routine physical examination. If symptoms are present, they usually include vague complaints of weakness or malaise. Possible clinical findings include anemia, infection, and enlarged lymph nodes, spleen, and liver. As in other leukemias, bone marrow hyperplasia is present. Erythrocyte and platelet counts are reduced. Leukocyte counts may either be elevated or reduced, but abnormal cells are always present. In CLL, years may elapse before treatment is required. Survival of this disease averages approximately 7 years.

## COLLABORATIVE CARE

Treatment for leukemia focuses on achieving remission or cure and relieving symptoms. The methods of treatment may include chemotherapy, radiation therapy, and bone marrow or stem cell transplantation. Cure is more often achieved in children with acute leukemia than in adults, although long-term remissions (disease-free periods with no signs or symptoms) often can be achieved.

### Diagnostic Tests

The following diagnostic tests are ordered when leukemia is suspected.

- *CBC* with differential is done to evaluate cell counts, hemoglobin and hematocrit levels, and the number, distribution, and morphology (size and shape) of WBCs.
- *Platelets* are measured to identify possible thrombocytopenia secondary to the leukemia and the risk of bleeding.
- *Bone marrow examination* provides information about cells within the marrow, the type of erythropoiesis, and the maturity of erythropoietic and leukopoietic cells.

Table 32–7 outlines usual diagnostic test results in the various forms of leukemia.

### Chemotherapy

Single agent or combination chemotherapy is used to treat most types of leukemia, with the goal of eradicating leukemic cells and producing remission. Table 32–8 outlines typical chemotherapy regimens for different types of leukemia. Combination chemotherapy reduces drug resistance and toxicity, and interrupts cell growth at various stages of the cell cycle, producing complimentary effect of the drugs used. Cancer treatment with chemotherapy is discussed in detail in Chapter 10. ∞

Chemotherapy for leukemia generally is divided into the induction phase and postremission therapy. During *induction,* drug doses are high to eradicate leukemic cells from the bone marrow. These high doses often also damage stem cells and interfere with production of normal blood cells. Circulating mature blood cells are not affected because they are no longer dividing. The degree of bone marrow suppression is influenced by a number of factors, including age, nutritional status, concurrent chronic diseases such as impaired liver or renal function, the drug and drug dose, and prior treatment.

*Colony-stimulating factors (CSFs),* also called hematopoietic growth factors, often are administered to "rescue" the bone marrow following induction chemotherapy. CSFs are cytokines

**TABLE 32-7 Diagnostic Findings by Type of Leukemia**

| Test | AML | CML | ALL | CLL |
|---|---|---|---|---|
| RBC count | Low | Low | Low | Low |
| Hemoglobin | Low | Low | Low | Low |
| Hematocrit | Low | Low | Low | Low |
| Platelet count | Very low | High early, low late | Low | Low |
| WBC count | Varies | Increased | Varies | Increased |
| Myeloblasts | Present | | | |
| Neutrophils | Decreased | Increased | Decreased | Normal |
| Lymphocytes | | Normal | | Increased |
| Monocytes | | Normal/low | | |
| Blasts | Present | Present (crisis) | Present | |
| Bone marrow | Hypercellular | | Hypercellular | |
| Myeloblasts | Present | | | |
| Lymphoblasts | | | Present | |
| Lymphocytes | | | | Present |

that regulate the growth and differentiation of blood cells. Factors that support neutrophil maturation, *granulocyte-macrophage CSF (GM-CSF)* and *granulocyte CSF (G-CSF)* are commonly used. Bone pain is a common side effect of therapy with these agents. Clients also may experience fevers, chills, anorexia, muscle aches, and lethargy (Braunwald et al., 2001).

Once remission has been achieved, postremission chemotherapy is continued to eradicate any additional leukemic cells, prevent relapse, and prolong survival. A single chemotherapeutic agent, combination therapy, or bone marrow transplant may be used for postremission treatment.

**TABLE 32-8 Chemotherapeutic Regimens Used to Treat Leukemia**

| | |
|---|---|
| Acute myelocytic leukemia | • Cytarabine (Cytoxan, an alkylating agent), *with* daunorubicin (Cerubidine, an antitumor antibiotic), or idarubicin (Idamycin, an antitumor antibiotic)<br>• All-*trans* retinoic acid (ATRA) added for clients with promyelocytic leukemia |
| Chronic myelocytic leukemia | • Imatinib mesylate (STI571, Gleevec), a Bcr-Abl tyrosine kinase (enzyme) inhibitor<br>• Hydroxyurea (a DNA inhibitor) *or* homoharringtonine (HHT, a plant alkaloid) |
| Acute lymphocytic leukemia | • Daunorubicin (Cerubidine, an antitumor antibiotic) *with* vincristine (Oncovin, a plant alkaloid) *with* prednisone *with* asparaginase (Elspar) |
| Chronic lymphocytic leukemia | • Fludarabine (Fludara, an antimetabolite) *or* chlorambucil (Chloromycetin, an antitumor antibiotic)<br>• Cyclophosphamide (Cytoxan, an alkylating agent), vincristine, and prednisone<br>• Cyclophosphamide, doxorubicin (Adriamycin, an antitumor antibiotic), vincristine, and prednisone |

## Radiation Therapy

Radiation therapy damages cellular DNA. While the cell continues to function, it cannot divide and multiply. Cells that divide rapidly, such as bone marrow and cancer cells (radiosensitive cells), respond quickly to radiation therapy. Although normal cells are affected, they are better able to recover from the damage caused by the radiation than are cancer cells. The types of delivery, effects, and toxicities of radiation are discussed in greater detail in Chapter 10.

## Bone Marrow Transplant

**Bone marrow transplant (BMT)** is the treatment of choice for some types of leukemia (see Table 32–6). BMT often is used in conjunction with or following chemotherapy or radiation. There are two major categories of BMT: In allogeneic BMT, the bone marrow of a healthy donor is infused into the client with the illness; in autologous BMT, the client is infused with his or her own bone marrow.

### Allogeneic BMT

*Allogeneic BMT* uses bone marrow cells from a donor (often from a sibling with closely matched tissue antigens; closely matched unrelated donors also may be used). Prior to allogeneic BMT, high doses of chemotherapy and/or total body irradiation are used to destroy leukemic cells in the bone marrow. Then donor marrow is infused through a central venous line. Prior to BMT and reestablishment of bone marrow function, the client is critically ill and at significant risk for infection and bleeding due to depletion of WBCs and platelets.

Allogeneic BMT may precipitate *graft-versus-host disease (GVHD)*, which develops in 25% to 60% of all clients receiving an allogeneic BMT. In GVHD, immune cells of the donated bone marrow identify the recipient's body tissue as foreign. Consequently, T lymphocytes in the donated marrow attack the liver, skin, and gastrointestinal tract, causing skin rashes progressing to desquamation (loss of skin), diarrhea, gastrointestinal bleeding, and liver damage. GVHD is treated with antibiotics and steroids; immunosuppressant drugs such as thalidomide and immunotoxin (Xomazyme) may be used if necessary.

## Autologous BMT

*Autologous BMT* uses the client's own bone marrow to restore bone marrow function after chemotherapy or radiation. This procedure is often called *bone marrow rescue.* In autologous BMT, about 1 L of bone marrow is aspirated (usually from the iliac crests) during a period of disease remission. The bone marrow is then frozen and stored for use after treatment. If relapse occurs, lethal doses of chemotherapy or radiation are given to destroy the immune system and malignant cells, and to prepare space in the bone marrow for new cells. The filtered bone marrow is then thawed and infused intravenously through a central line. The infused marrow cells slowly become a part of the client's bone marrow, the neutrophil count increases, and normal hematopoiesis takes place.

As in allogeneic BMT, the client is critically ill during the period of bone marrow destruction and immunosuppression. The client is hospitalized in a private room for 6 to 8 weeks or more. Potential complications include malnutrition, infection, and bleeding.

## Stem Cell Transplant

Allogeneic **stem cell transplant (SCT)** is an alternative to bone marrow transplant. SCT results in complete and sustained replacement of the recipient's blood cell lines (WBCs, RBCs, and platelets) with cells derived from the donor stem cells.

Donors must have tissue that is closely matched with that of the recipient. Prior to harvesting, hematopoietic growth factors, including G-CSF and GM-CSF, are administered to the donor for 4 to 5 days. This increases the concentration of stem cells in peripheral blood, allowing it to be used for the transplant instead of bone marrow. Peripheral blood is removed and white cells are separated from the plasma, then administered via a large central venous catheter. Large concentrations of stem cells also are present in umbilical cord blood. This may be stored and used in some cases (Braunwald et al., 2001).

The recipient undergoes similar treatment prior to SCT as for BMT. The risks for infection and other complications, as well as GVHD, are similar.

## Biologic Therapy

Cytokines such as interferons and interleukins are biologic agents that may be used to treat some leukemias. These agents modify the body's response to cancer cells; in some cases they are cytotoxic as well. Interferons are a complex group of messenger proteins normally produced in response to antigens such as viruses (see Chapter 9). ☞ They have multiple effects, including moderating immune function and inhibiting abnormal cell proliferation and growth. Interferon-α may be used to treat some leukemias, particularly CML. Side effects commonly associated with interferon therapy include flulike symptoms, persistent fatigue and lethargy, weight loss, and muscle and joint pain.

## Complementary Therapies

Although many complementary and alternative medicine therapies have been purported to treat cancer in general, at this time none have been shown to have sustained benefit in treating leukemia.

## NURSING CARE

### Health Promotion

Health promotion activities related to leukemia include teaching about leukemia risk factors, particularly those that can be controlled. Discuss the potential dangers of exposure to ionizing radiation and certain chemicals such as benzene. Encourage all clients to avoid smoking cigarettes. Discuss genetic counseling with clients at high risk for having a child with Down syndrome (over age 35).

### Assessment

Focused assessment data related to leukemia includes:

- Health history: complaints of fatigue, weakness, dyspnea on exertion, frequent infections, sore throat, night sweats, bleeding gums, or nose bleeds; recent weight loss; exposure to ionizing radiation (multiple X-rays, residence near a site of radiation or atomic testing) or chemicals (occupational); prior treatment for cancer; history of an immune disorder
- Physical examination: skin and mucous membranes for bruising, purpura, petechiae, ulcers or lesions; pallor; vital signs including orthostatic vitals; heart and lung sounds; abdominal examination; stool for occult blood

### Nursing Diagnoses and Interventions

When caring for the client with leukemia, the nurse considers the chronic and life-threatening nature of the disease as well as the effects of treatment. See the Nursing Research box on the following page. Priority nursing problems may include *Risk for infection, Imbalanced nutrition, Impaired oral mucous membranes, Impaired protection (bleeding),* and *Grieving.*

### Risk for Infection

Changes in white blood cell function impair the immune and inflammatory responses in leukemia, increasing the risk for infection. WBCs may be immature and ineffective, or, in some cases, deficient. Chemotherapy or radiation therapy further depresses bone marrow function, and increases the risk for infection.

- Promptly report manifestations of infection: fever, chills, throat pain, cough, chest pain, burning on urination, purulent drainage, and itching and burning in vaginal or rectal areas. *Prompt reporting allows timely intervention to prevent overwhelming infection and sepsis.*
- Institute infection protection measures.
  a. Maintain protective isolation as indicated.
  b. Ensure meticulous handwashing among all people in contact with the client.
  c. Assist as needed with appropriate hygiene measures.
  d. Restrict visitors with colds, flu, or infections.
  e. Provide oral hygiene after every meal.
  f. Avoid invasive procedures when possible, including injections, intravenous catheters, catheterizations, and rectal and vaginal procedures. When necessary, use strict aseptic technique for all invasive procedures and monitor carefully for infection.

## Nursing Research

### Evidence-Based Practice for Clients with Acute Leukemia and Lymphoma

Clients with acute leukemia and malignant lymphoma experience a number of distressing manifestations of their disease, including malaise and fatigue, fever, night sweats, infections, and possible hemorrhage. Treatments such as radiation therapy and chemotherapy often have numerous adverse effects as well, including anorexia and nausea, stomatitis, lethargy, malaise, and fatigue. In this study, clients in remission from acute leukemia or malignant lymphoma were surveyed regarding physical problems, their view of help they received and who was of most help during treatment, and the impact of the disease and treatment on their current life (Persson, Hallberg, & Ohlsson, 1997).

Clients identified energy loss and nutritional problems as being most troublesome during disease treatment. In general, clients with more physical problems were less satisfied with the nursing care they received, suggesting that nurses were less effective in meeting the needs of the sickest clients. Clients continued to experience reduced psychological and sexual energy and a significant need for intimate help and counseling during remission. While family relationships improved, work and finances were negatively impacted by their disease.

### IMPLICATIONS FOR NURSING

This study points out the need for nurses to actively focus their care on the physical problems experienced during treatment, especially energy loss and nutritional problems. Overwhelming fatigue interferes with the client's ability to provide self-care, but its effects may not be readily apparent to nurses. The long-term effects of reduced psychological and sexual energy, as well as continued susceptibility to infections, indicate a need for continued follow-up care, teaching, and possibly referral to counseling services.

### Critical Thinking in Client Care

1. Explain the physiologic responses to malignancies and cancer treatments that cause fatigue, malaise, and nutritional problems.
2. Clients undergoing treatment for leukemia, malignant lymphoma, and other cancers may have few outward manifestations of their disease or responses to treatment. Discuss how this apparent well-being may affect the nurses' perception of care needs.
3. How may continued problems of fatigue and lack of psychologic and sexual energy affect family relations?
4. Develop a nursing care plan for a client with acute leukemia to address the problem: Ineffective sexuality patterns related to fatigue and lack of energy.

---

*These precautions minimize exposure to bacterial, viral, and fungal pathogens. Infection is the major cause of death in clients with leukemia. Mucous membranes are especially susceptible to breakdown and infection as a result of tissue damage from chemotherapy or radiation.*

- Monitor vital signs including temperature and oxygen saturation every 4 hours. Report temperature spikes with chilling, tachypnea, tachycardia, restlessness, change in $Pao_2$, and hypotension. *The inflammatory response may be impaired in leukemia, masking signs of infection until sepsis develops, indicated by manifestations such as those above.*

- Monitor neutrophil levels (measured in cubic millimeters) for relative risk for infection:

  2000 to 2500: no risk
  1000 to 2000: minimal risk
  500 to 1000: moderate risk
  Below 500: severe risk

  *Neutrophils are the first line of defense against infection. As levels decrease, the risk for infection increases.*

- Explain infection precautions and restrictions and their rationale; explain that these measures are usually temporary. *Client and family understanding increases compliance and lowers the risk of infection.*

### Imbalanced Nutrition:
### Less Than Body Requirements

The client with leukemia may have difficulty meeting nutritional needs due to increased metabolism, fatigue, loss of appetite from radiation, nausea and vomiting from chemotherapy, or painful oral mucous membranes that make chewing and swallowing difficult and/or painful.

- Weigh regularly and evaluate weight loss over time to determine degree of malnutrition. A weight loss of 10% to 20% may indicate malnutrition. *A minimum intake of nutrients is necessary for health and tissue repair; cancer increases metabolic needs over this basal requirement. Weight loss occurs when metabolic requirements are not met. Both the disease process and its treatment can interfere with nutrient intake.*

- Address causative or contributing factors to inadequate food and fluid intake.
  a. Provide mouth care before and after meals; use a soft toothbrush or sponges as necessary.
  b. Provide liquids with different textures and tastes.
  c. Increase liquid intake with meals.
  d. Reduce intake of milk and milk products, which makes mucus more tenacious.
  e. Assist to a sitting position for eating.
  f. Ensure that the environment is clean and odor-free.
  g. Provide medications for pain or nausea 30 minutes before meals, if prescribed.
  h. Provide rest periods before meals.
  i. Offer small, frequent meals including low-fat, high kcal foods throughout the day.
  j. Provide commercial supplements, such as Ensure.
  k. Avoid painful or unpleasant procedures immediately before or after meals.

MediaLink | ACUTE MYELOCYTIC LEUKEMIA CARE PLAN

l. Suggest measures to improve food tolerance, such as eating dry foods when arising, consuming salty foods if allowed, and avoiding very sweet, rich, or greasy foods. *Anorexia, nausea and vomiting, diarrhea, stomatitis, taste changes, and dysphagia often make eating difficult during cancer treatment when good nutrition is most important. Maintaining nutritional status decreases morbidity and mortality by preventing weight loss, improving the response to treatment, minimizing adverse effects, and improving quality of life. Small, frequent meals are often better tolerated, especially high-protein, high-kcal foods.*

## Impaired Oral Mucous Membrane

*Stomatitis,* inflammation and ulceration of the oral mucous membrane, is common in leukemia. Chemotherapy can further impair the integrity of constantly dividing oral tissues.

- Inspect the buccal region, gums, sublingual area, and the throat daily for swelling or lesions. Ask about oral pain or burning. *Breakdown of the oral mucous membrane increases the risk of infection and bleeding, causes pain and discomfort with eating and swallowing, and may cause swelling that interferes with the airway.*
- Culture any oral lesions. *Herpes simplex virus and* Candida *(yeast) are more common in clients with neutropenia. Herpes lesions are usually red, raised, fluid-filled blisters;* Candida *causes a white coating and patches of white plaque.*
- Assist with mouth care and oral rinses with saline or a solution of hydrogen peroxide and water (1:1 or 1:3 hydrogen peroxide and water) every 2 to 4 hours. Apply petroleum jelly to the lips to prevent dryness and cracking. *These measures help prevent infection and increase comfort.*
- Encourage use of soft-bristle toothbrush or sponge to clean teeth and gums. *Toothbrushes with hard bristles may abrade inflamed mucosa, causing bleeding and increasing the risk of infection.*
- Administer medications as ordered to treat infection or relieve pain. *Topical antifungal agents such as nystatin may be prescribed to treat* Candida *infections. Topical anesthetics such as lidocaine may be prescribed to relieve comfort and facilitate good oral care.*
- Instruct to avoid alcohol-based mouthwashes, citrus fruit juices, spicy foods, very hot or very cold foods, alcohol, and crusty foods. Suggest bland, cool foods and cool liquids at least every 2 hours. *Avoiding mucosa-traumatizing foods and liquids increases comfort; bland, cool foods and liquids cause the least pain. Intake of adequate fluids is necessary to prevent dehydration.*

## Ineffective Protection

Bleeding is the second most common cause of leukemia deaths. As platelet counts decrease, the risk of bleeding increases (see the preceding section on thrombocytopenia).

- Assess vital signs every 4 hours and body systems every shift for bleeding.
  a. Skin and mucous membranes for petechiae, ecchymoses, and purpura
  b. Gums, nasal membranes, and conjunctiva for bleeding

  c. Vomitus, stool, and urine for visible or occult blood
  d. Vaginal bleeding
  e. Prolonged bleeding from puncture sites
  f. Neurologic changes such as headache, visual changes, altered mentation, decreased level of consciousness, seizures
  g. Abdomen for complaints of epigastric pain, diminished bowel sounds, increasing abdominal girth, rigidity or guarding

*Early identification of bleeding helps prevent significant blood loss and potential shock. Internal hemorrhage may lead to tachycardia, hypotension, pallor, and diaphoresis. Bleeding into the lungs may cause dyspnea; bleeding into the abdomen causes increased girth, pain, and guarding. Intracranial bleeding affects mental status and level of consciousness.*

- Avoid invasive procedures such as rectal temperatures and suppositories, vaginal douches, suppositories, or tampons, urinary catheterization, and parenteral injections if possible. Diagnostic procedures such as biopsy or lumbar puncture should not be done if the platelet count is less than 50,000. *Invasive procedures can cause tissue trauma and bleeding. Procedures that use large-bore needles should be delayed until the platelet count is increased.*
- Apply pressure to injection sites for 3 to 5 minutes, and to arterial punctures for 15 to 20 minutes. *Pressure prevents prolonged bleeding by prompting hemostasis and clot formation.*
- Instruct to avoid forcefully blowing or picking the nose, forceful coughing or sneezing, and straining to have a bowel movement. *These activities can damage mucous membranes, increasing the risk for bleeding.*

## Anticipatory Grieving

The diagnosis of cancer and a potentially life-threatening illness causes actual or perceived losses, such as loss of function, independence, normal appearance, friends, self-esteem, and self. Grieving is the emotional response to those losses. The adaptive process of mourning a loss and resolving grief is called grief work; grief work cannot begin until a loss is acknowledged. See Chapter 11 ⊂⊃ for a detailed discussion of grief and loss.

- Discuss roles of the client and family and ways in which they managed stressful situations in the past. Assess coping strategies and their effectiveness. Help identify sources of strength and support. Discuss changing roles resulting from leukemia diagnosis, and its effect on spiritual, social, and economic status, and usual lifestyle. Evaluate cultural or ethnic factors that affect grief reactions. *Grieving is a normal response to a real or potential loss that begins at the time of diagnosis. The timing, duration, and intensity of grief and responses to grief may differ among family members. Share information on diagnosis, role change, and physical loss among all family members to build the foundation for mutual understanding and trust.*
- Use therapeutic communication skills to facilitate open discussion of losses and provide permission to grieve. *Encouraging discussion of the meaning of the loss helps decrease some of the anxiety associated with loss. This in turn allows*

## CHART 32–3 NANDA, NIC, AND NOC LINKAGES

### The Client with Leukemia

| NURSING DIAGNOSES | NURSING INTERVENTIONS | NURSING OUTCOMES |
|---|---|---|
| • Fatigue | • Energy Management<br>• Nutrition Management<br>• Self-Care Assistance | • Endurance<br>• Energy Conservation<br>• Nutritional Status: Energy |
| • Ineffective Protection | • Bleeding Precautions<br>• Infection Protection<br>• Neurologic Monitoring | • Coagulation Status<br>• Immune Status<br>• Neurological Status: Consciousness |
| • Imbalanced Nutrition: Less than Body Requirements | • Nutrition Management<br>• Nutrition Monitoring | • Nutritional Status<br>• Nutritional Status: Food and Fluid Intake |
| • Impaired Oral Mucous Membrane | • Oral Health Restoration<br>• Oral Health Maintenance | • Oral Health<br>• Tissue Integrity: Skin and Mucous Membranes |

*Note.* Data from Nursing Outcomes Classification (NOC) *by M. Johnson & M. Maas (Eds.), 1997, St. Louis: Mosby;* Nursing Diagnoses: Definitions & Classification 2001–2002 *by North American Nursing Diagnosis Association, 2001, Philadelphia: NANDA;* Nursing Interventions Classification (NIC) *by J.C. McCloskey & G. M. Bulechek (Eds.), 2000, St. Louis: Mosby. Reprinted by permission.*

*the client and family to examine the current situation and compare it with past situations that they have coped with successfully.*

• Provide information about agencies that may help in resolving grief, and make referrals as indicated. Consider self-help groups, cancer support groups, and bereavement groups. *Participating in support groups with others who are anticipating or experiencing a similar loss can decrease feelings of isolation.*

## Using NANDA, NIC, and NOC

Chart 32–3 shows links between NANDA nursing diagnoses, NIC, and NOC for the client with leukemia.

## Home Care

Client and family teaching for home care after treatment for leukemia focuses on encouraging self-care, providing information about the disease and the treatment, preventing infection and injury, and promoting nutrition. Teaching topics for each of these areas are as follows.

### Encouraging Self-Care

• Hygiene measures and energy conservation during self-care activities
• Oral hygiene including using a soft-bristle toothbrush several times daily; avoid flossing
• Reporting lesions, bleeding, or signs of infection promptly
• Maintaining a balance of rest and activity

### Information about Leukemia and Treatment

• Bone marrow function, the pathophysiology of leukemia, and potential complications of leukemia
• Prognosis for the specific type of leukemia
• Treatment measures such as chemotherapy, radiation, bone marrow or stem cell transplant, their purpose and effects,

where treatment is available, and potential adverse effects or risks
• Community, regional, and national resources for people with leukemia

### Preventing Infection and Injury

• Handwashing and other measures to reduce exposure to pathogens such as avoiding people who are ill and avoiding crowds
• Avoiding foodborne illnesses by washing fruits and vegetables, proper food storage
• Dental hygiene measures
• Avoiding immunizations
• Manifestations to report: fever, chills, burning on urination, foul-smelling urine, vaginal or rectal discharge, skin lesions
• Avoiding contact sports or strenuous exercise if platelet count is low
• Using an electric razor for shaving, avoiding rectal or vaginal suppositories, vaginal tampons, or enemas
• Increasing dietary fiber and using a bulk-forming laxative as needed to prevent straining
• Avoiding over-the-counter or prescription drugs that interfere with platelet function (see Box 32–6)
• The importance of reporting any bleeding (nosebleeds, rectal bleeding, vomiting blood, excessive menstrual periods, blood in the urine, bleeding gums, bruises, or collections of blood under the skin) or changes in behavior to the health care provider

### Promoting Nutrition

• Eating several small, low-fat, high-calorie meals and drinking five to eight glasses of water daily
• Reporting continued weight loss, loss of appetite, or inability to eat for 24 hours
• Discussing dietary needs with the dietitian

## Nursing Care Plan
## A Client with Acute Myelocytic Leukemia

Catherine Cole is a 37-year-old secretary who lives with her husband, Ray, and teenage daughter, Amy, in an apartment in a large metropolitan area. About 2 months ago, Mrs. Cole began to tire easily and experience night sweats several times a week. She also noted that she was pale, bruised easily, and was having heavier menstrual periods. Blood tests ordered by her primary care provider are abnormal. She is admitted for a bone marrow biopsy.

### ASSESSMENT

Mary Losapio, RN, obtains a nursing history and physical assessment for Mrs. Cole. Mrs. Cole tells her, "I'm so tired, and I have these bruises all over me. I'm so afraid of the results of the bone marrow examination. I don't know what we will do if I have cancer." Mrs. Cole clutches her husband's hand and then begins to cry. Physical assessment data include: Height 64 inches (156 cm), weight 106 lb (48.1 kg); vital signs T 100°F, P 102, R 22, BP 130/82. Numerous petechiae scattered over trunk and arms; ecchymoses noted on lower right arm and right calf. Oral mucosa is red, with several small ulcerations in buccal areas.

Blood count shows reduced RBCs, hemoglobin, and hematocrit levels. The WBC is high, with myeloblasts seen on differential. The platelet count is very low. A tentative diagnosis of acute myelogenous leukemia is made.

### DIAGNOSES

- *Risk for infection* related to altered WBC production and immune function
- *Ineffective protection* related to reduced platelet count and risk for bleeding
- *Impaired oral mucous membrane* secondary to anemia and reduced platelets
- *Fatigue* related to anemia
- *Anxiety* related to fear of leukemia diagnosis

### EXPECTED OUTCOMES

- Remain free of infection.
- Experience no significant bleeding.
- Have intact oral mucous membranes.
- Manage self-care activities despite fatigue.
- Verbalize decreased anxiety.

### PLANNING AND IMPLEMENTATION

- Place in a private room.
- Limit visitors to immediate family for the present.

- Instruct all staff, the family, and client to carefully wash hands. Post a sign over the washbasin in the room as a reminder.
- Record vital signs every 4 hours.
- Avoid invasive procedures unless absolutely necessary.
- Monitor for bleeding every 4 hours, including skin, oral mucosa, abdominal assessment, body fluids, and menstrual pad count.
- Instruct to perform oral hygiene every 2 to 4 hours, using a soft-bristle toothbrush.
- Ask the dietitian to work with Mrs. Cole to identify preferred foods. Instruct to avoid foods that may damage oral mucosa, such as very hot, very cold, or highly acidic or spicy foods.
- Provide for periods of rest alternating with activity.
- Teach about the bone marrow biopsy. Allow time for questions and to verbalize fears.
- Refer to the oncology nurse specialist for further teaching and support.

### EVALUATION

The bone marrow biopsy confirms the diagnosis of acute myelogenous leukemia. Mrs. Cole is very upset, but calms as the physician and the oncology nurse discuss treatment plans and the possibility of remission. She decides to have outpatient chemotherapy. During her hospital stay, Mrs. Cole remained free of infection or further bleeding. She tells Ms. Losapio that her mouth feels better, although it is still painful. During routine assessment, Mrs. Cole remarks, "You know, I was so scared when I came here, but I think I am a little less so now. Sometimes not knowing what is wrong is worse than knowing."

### Critical Thinking in the Nursing Process

1. Describe how alterations in WBCs can increase a person's susceptibility to infection.
2. List sources of potential infection for the hospitalized client.
3. What is the rationale for having the client do her own oral and physical hygiene?
4. Outline a teaching plan for this client and her family for home care to prevent infection.
5. Develop a care plan for Mrs. Cole for the nursing diagnosis, *Activity intolerance*.

See Evaluating Your Response in Appendix C.

---

Assistance with physical care, finances, and transportation may be required following discharge. Refer the client and family to social services, support groups, home care services as needed, and other agencies that can provide needed services (such as local chapters of the American Cancer Society, which can provide hospital beds and transportation for outpatient cancer treatment).

## THE CLIENT WITH MULTIPLE MYELOMA

**Multiple myeloma** is a malignancy in which plasma cells multiply uncontrollably and infiltrate the bone marrow, lymph nodes, spleen, and other tissues. *Plasma cells* are B-cell lymphocytes that develop to produce antibodies (immunoglobins).

The incidence of multiple myeloma is increasing, with an estimated 48,100 cases diagnosed annually. It affects blacks more than twice as often as whites, and men more frequently than women. The incidence of multiple myeloma increases with age, rarely occurring before age 40. Its cause is unknown (McCance & Huether, 2002). Possible contributing factors include genetic predisposition, oncogenic virus, inflammatory stimuli, and chronic antigenic stimulation.

## PATHOPHYSIOLOGY AND MANIFESTATIONS

Malignant plasma cells arise from one clone of B cells that produce abnormally large amounts of a particular immunoglobin called the *M protein*. This abnormal protein interferes with normal antibody production and impairs the humoral immune response. It also increases blood viscosity and may damage kidney tubules. As myeloma cells proliferate, they replace the bone marrow and infiltrate the bone itself. Cortical bone is progressively destroyed by tumor growth and enzymes produced by myeloma cells. These enzymes facilitate bone destruction, its infiltration by tumor cells, development of new blood vessels to sustain the tumor, and growth of myeloma cells (McCance & Huether, 2002). Affected bones (primarily the vertebrae, ribs, skull, pelvis, femur, clavicle, and scapula) are weakened and may break without trauma (*pathologic fracture*).

The disease develops slowly. Manifestations of multiple myeloma are due to its effects on the bone and the impaired immune response due to M protein production. Bone pain is the most common presenting symptom. With progression of the disease, the pain may increase in severity and become more localized. Rapid bone destruction releases calcium from the bone, leading to hypercalcemia and manifestations of neurologic dysfunction, such as lethargy, confusion, and weakness.

As functional antibody formation decreases and the humoral immune response is suppressed, recurrent infections develop. Cell-mediated immunity remains intact. *Bence Jones proteins* are found in the urine in multiple myeloma. These proteins are toxic to the renal tubules, and may lead to renal failure with azotemia and uremia (see Chapter 27 ⬤⬤ for more information about renal failure).

About 15% of clients with multiple myeloma die within 3 months of the diagnosis. More frequently, the disease course is chronic, progressing more rapidly with each relapse after remission. The acute terminal stage of the disease is marked by pancytopenia and widespread organ infiltration by myeloma cells (Braunwald et al., 2001).

## COLLABORATIVE CARE

Diagnostic tests for multiple myeloma include the following:

- *X-rays* and other radiologic studies of the bone may reveal multiple punched-out lesions.
- *Bone marrow examination* shows an abnormal number of immature plasma cells.
- *CBC* shows moderate to severe anemia.

- *Urinalysis* shows Bence Jones protein in the urine.
- *Biopsy* of myeloma lesions confirms the diagnosis of multiple myeloma.

There is no cure for multiple myeloma. Treatment includes systemic chemotherapy to control progression of the disease and supportive care to reduce complications of the disease and their effects.

Combination chemotherapy with an alkylating agent (melphalan [Alkeran], cyclophosphamide [Cytoxan], or chlorambucil [Chloromycetin]) and prednisone administered for 4 to 7 days every 4 to 6 weeks is commonly used. Chemotherapy typically reduces bone pain, hypercalcemia, anemia, and the number of infections (Braunwald et al., 2001). Localized radiation therapy may be used to treat painful bone lesions.

Supportive care may include treatment of hypercalcemia with hydration, possible biphosphonate therapy to reduce bone loss (see Chapter 39 ⬤⬤), and calcium, vitamin D, and fluoride supplements to support bone structure. Plasma exchange therapy (plasmapheresis) to remove circulating M proteins is used as needed to treat acute renal failure. Infections are treated promptly when they develop.

## NURSING CARE

### Assessment

Focused assessment data for the client with multiple myeloma includes the following:

- Health history: complaints of back or bone pain, onset, duration, and intensity; complaints of weakness, fatigue, anorexia; history of frequent or recurrent infections; neurologic symptoms such as numbness and tingling or clumsiness
- Physical examination: level of consciousness and mental status; mobility, gait; localized tenderness or pain, bony crepitus with movement or palpation; movement and sensation in extremities

### Nursing Diagnoses and Interventions

Nursing care of the client with multiple myeloma focuses on problems of chronic pain, impaired mobility, and the risk for injury. Risk for infection is a major nursing care focus; see the previous section on leukemia for specific interventions to reduce this risk. Other nursing care needs are similar to those of clients with other cancers and chronic pain. See Chapters 4 and 10 ⬤⬤ for additional specific nursing interventions for these problems.

### Chronic Pain

Clients with multiple myeloma typically experience chronic back pain and deep bone pain as myeloma cells saturate the bone marrow and invade the bone structure. Pathologic fractures are a common and reoccurring problem.

- Assess pain, including intensity (use a standard pain scale), onset, duration, precipitating factors, and effective relief measures. *Identifying the intensity, causes, and precipitating factors of pain helps determine and evaluate effective pain relief measures.*

- Determine position of greatest comfort, and assist as needed into this position. *The client is best able to identify positions that minimize pain, but may need assistance with repositioning.*
- Support position with pillows. *Bony prominences may be painful due to infiltrates. Pillows can help relieve pressure on these prominences, thus reducing pain.*
- Provide uninterrupted rest periods. *Adequate rest facilitates pain relief and improves pain tolerance.*
- Teach adjunctive pain relief strategies such as relaxation or guided imagery. *A combination of pharmacologic and non-pharmacologic methods provides better management of chronic pain, especially bone pain.*
- Teach effective analgesic use, including the family in instruction. *Analgesics are most effective when taken before pain becomes severe. Clients and their families may be reluctant to use prescription analgesics on a regular basis.*
- Report unrelieved pain to the physician. *A different analgesic or addition of an adjunctive medication such as a nonsteroidal anti-inflammatory drug (NSAID) may be needed to effectively control pain.*

### Impaired Physical Mobility

Painful bony infiltrates and pathologic fractures may limit mobility. A brace or splint may be used to protect extremities or support the back. In addition, persistent weakness associated with the cancer and anemia may limit the client's ability to participate in usual activities.

**PRACTICE ALERT** *Gently support extremities during repositioning. Weakened extremities due to infiltration of bone by myeloma cells and muscle atrophy from lack of use increase the risk for pathologic fractures.* ■

- Assist to change position at least every 2 hours. *Assistance with repositioning is necessary due to weakness. Frequent repositioning improves comfort and reduces the risk for impaired skin and tissue integrity.*
- Provide a trapeze to assist in repositioning. *A trapeze provides better leverage, allowing the client to assist with repositioning and providing a degree of independence. The ability to participate in self-care improves self-esteem.*

### Risk for Injury

The bone involvement of multiple myeloma places the client at high risk for pathologic and traumatic fractures. Pathologic fractures can occur with simple activities such as turning or reaching for an item. The spine usually is affected; the ribs and bones of the extremities also may be at risk for fracture.

- Place needed items close at hand. *Straining to reach objects increases the risk of falling or sustaining other injury.*
- Provide safety measures to prevent falls from bed: Place the bed in a low position, use side rails as indicated, and place the call bell within reach. *Safety measures help prevent accidental injury. A secure environment minimizes risk and helps prevent falls.*

- Provide shoes with nonskid soles, a clear pathway, adequate lighting, and a level surface free of scatter rugs or other hazards when ambulating. Provide a walker as needed for support and security. *Weightbearing exercise promotes bone repair. Safety measures, such as an unobstructed pathway and a firm walking surface, help prevent falls.*

### Home Care

When teaching clients and their families for home care, include the following topics.

- Strategies for home maintenance management
- Signs and symptoms of complications to be reported to the physician (e.g., symptoms of vertebral and extremity fractures)
- Manifestations of infection to report: fever and chills; increased malaise, fatigue, or weakness; cough with or without sputum; sore throat; dysuria, nocturia, frequency, urgency, or malodorous urine

Provide referrals for home health and home maintenance services, physical or occupational therapy, social services, and hospice care as appropriate.

## THE CLIENT WITH MALIGNANT LYMPHOMA

**Lymphomas** are malignancies of lymphoid tissue. They are characterized by the proliferation of lymphocytes, histiocytes (resident monocytes or macrophages), and their precursors or derivatives. Although there are many types of malignant lymphoid cells, at this time lymphomas commonly are identified as Hodgkin's disease or non-Hodgkin's lymphoma.

Malignant lymphomas are the sixth leading cause of cancer deaths in the United States. Approximately 60,900 new cases of lymphoma were diagnosed in 2002, and 25,800 deaths were attributed to the disease. The incidence of non-Hodgkin's lymphoma has nearly doubled since 1970, but currently has stabilized except among black females. The incidence of Hodgkin's disease has declined since the late 1980s (ACS, 2002a).

While the cause of lymphoma is unknown, some risk factors have been identified. Immunosuppression due to drug therapy following organ transplant or to HIV disease increases the risk for non-Hodgkin's lymphoma. Infectious agents such as human T-cell leukemia/lymphoma virus-1 (HTLV-1) and the Epstein-Barr virus (EBV) also have been identified as risk factors. Others may include occupational herbicide or chemical exposure (ACS, 2002a).

## PATHOPHYSIOLOGY

### Hodgkin's Disease

*Hodgkin's disease* is a lymphatic cancer, occurring most often in people between the ages of 15 and 35 or over age 50. It is somewhat more common in men than women. Approximately 7000 new cases of Hodgkin's disease were diagnosed in 2002 (ACS, 2002). The exact cause of Hodgkin's disease is unknown, but both EBV infection and genetic factors appear to play a role

**TABLE 32-9** Subtypes of Hodgkin's Disease

| Subtype | Incidence | Prognosis |
|---|---|---|
| Lymphocyte predominant | More common in adults and in males | Disease usually localized at diagnosis; excellent prognosis |
| Nodular sclerosing | Most common form; usually affects adolescents and young adults; more common in females | Good if diagnosed early |
| Mixed cellularity | Common in adults; more common in males | Poorer prognosis with 50% to 60% 5-year survival |
| Lymphocyte depleted | Least common form; usually affects older adults and people with HIV disease | Poor prognosis with 5-year survival rate of less than 50% |

in its development. Hodgkin's disease is one of the most curable cancers. As many as 60% to 90% of people with localized disease achieve cure with a normal life span (Porth, 2002).

Hodgkin's disease develops in a single lymph node or chain of nodes, spreading to adjoining nodes. Involved lymph nodes contain *Reed-Sternberg cells* (malignant cells) surrounded by host inflammatory cells. These malignant cells secrete inflammatory mediator substances, attracting inflammatory cells to the tumor site. They may invade almost any tissue in the body. The spleen often is involved; as the disease progresses, the liver, lungs, digestive tract, and CNS may be affected (Porth, 2002). Rapid proliferation of abnormal lymphocytes impairs the immune response, especially cell-mediated immune responses. Infections are common. Four subtypes of Hodgkin's disease have been identified, based on the predominant cells. Table 32–9 outlines these subtypes.

### Manifestations

The most common symptom of Hodgkin's disease is one or more painlessly enlarged lymph nodes, usually in the cervical or subclavicular region. Systemic manifestations such as persistent fever, night sweats, fatigue, and weight loss are associated with a poorer prognosis for the disease. Late symptoms such as malaise, pruritus, and anemia indicate spread of the disease (Porth, 2002). The spleen may be enlarged, and other organ systems such as the lungs and gastrointestinal tract are occasionally involved.

### Non-Hodgkin's Lymphoma

*Non-Hodgkin's lymphoma* is a diverse group of lymphoid tissue malignancies that do not contain Reed-Sternberg cells. Non-Hodgkin's lymphomas tend to arise in peripheral lymph nodes and spread early to tissues throughout the body. Non-Hodgkin's lymphoma is more common than Hodgkin's disease, affecting an estimated 53,900 people annually and causing about 24,400 deaths in 2002 (ACS, 2002). Older adults are more often affected, and it occurs more frequently in men than in women. Like Hodgkin's disease, its cause is unknown, although both genetic and environmental factors (e.g., viral infections such as EBV, HTLV-1 and HTLV-2, and HIV) are thought to play a role.

As in most malignancies, non-Hodgkin's lymphoma begins as a single transformed cell; it may arise from T cells, B cells, or tissue macrophages (histocytes). Different cell types of non-Hodgkin's lymphoma develop in different regions of the lymph node. It tends to spread early and unpredictably to other lymphoid tissues and organs. Extranodal spread may involve the nasopharynx, gastrointestinal tract, bone, CNS, thyroid, testes, and soft tissue.

The prognosis for non-Hodgkin's lymphoma ranges from excellent to poor, depending on the identified cell type and grade of differentiation. Low grade tumors (better differentiated) tend to be less aggressive and more curable. Higher grade tumors often are disseminated at the time of diagnoses, and have a poorer prognosis (Copstead & Banasik, 2000).

### Manifestations

The early manifestations of non-Hodgkin's lymphoma are similar to those for Hodgkin's disease. Painless lymphadenopathy may be localized or widespread. Systemic manifestations such as fever, night sweats, fatigue, and weight loss may be present, but are less common in non-Hodgkin's lymphoma. Organ system involvement may cause symptoms such as abdominal pain, nausea, and vomiting. Headaches, peripheral or cranial nerve symptoms, altered mental status, or seizures may signal CNS involvement.

The manifestations and clinical features of Hodgkin's disease and non-Hodgkin's lymphoma are compared in Table 32–10.

## COLLABORATIVE CARE

Chemotherapy and radiation therapy, either alone or in combination, are the primary treatments for Hodgkin's and non-Hodgkin's lymphomas. Use of monoclonal antibodies to the lymphoma cells, and bone marrow and peripheral stem cell transplants are under investigation for treating lymphomas as well. See the previous section on treatment of leukemia for more information about these transplants.

### Diagnostic Tests

The following diagnostic tests may be ordered for lymphomas.

- *CBC* often shows a mild normochromic, normocytic anemia in Hodgkin's disease; other findings in Hodgkin's disease may include leukocytosis with high neutrophil and eosinophil counts, and an elevated sed rate. In non-Hodgkin's lymphoma, the CBC typically remains normal until late in the disease, when pancytopenia may develop.

### TABLE 32–10 Features and Manifestations of Hodgkin's Disease and Non-Hodgkin's Lymphoma

| Feature or Manifestation | Hodgkin's Disease | Non-Hodgkin's Lymphoma |
|---|---|---|
| Lymphadenopathy | Localized to a single node or chain, often cervical, subclavicular, or mediastinal | Multiple peripheral nodes, nodes of the mesentery often involved |
| Spread | Orderly and continuous | Diffuse and unpredictable |
| Extranodal involvement | Rare | Early and common |
| Bone marrow involvement | Uncommon | Common |
| Fever, night sweats, weight loss | Common | Uncommon until disease is extensive |
| Other manifestations | Fatigue, pruritus, splenomegaly; anemia, neutrophilia | Abdominal pain, nausea, vomiting; dyspnea, cough; CNS symptoms; lymphocytopenia |

- *Chest X-ray* is done to identify possible enlarged mediastinal lymph nodes and pulmonary involvement.
- *Chest* or *abdominal CT scan* may be done to identify abnormal or enlarged nodes.
- *Bipedal lymphangiography* uses radiographic dye injected into the lymphatic channels of the lower legs to identify the extent of iliac, para-aortic, and abdominal lymph node involvement.
- *Biopsy* of the largest, most central enlarged lymph node is done to establish the diagnosis for both Hodgkin's disease and non-Hodgkin's lymphoma. The presence of Reed-Sternberg cells confirms the diagnosis of Hodgkin's disease.

## Staging

Staging is used to determine the extent of the disease and appropriate treatment. The Ann Arbor Staging System may be used to assess the extent and severity of lymphomas. The newer Cotswold Staging Classification System is used for Hodgkin's disease. The stages are similar in both systems:

Stage I: involvement of a single lymph node region, lymphoid structure, or extralymphatic site
Stage II: involvement of two or more lymph node regions on the same side of the diaphragm, or localized extralymphatic involvement
Stage III: involvement of lymph node regions or structures on both sides of the diaphragm; may involve the spleen or localized extranodal disease
Stage IV: diffuse or disseminated extralymphatic disease

The presence or absence of systemic symptoms is indicated by either an A (no systemic symptoms) or B (systemic symptoms of fever, night sweats, weight loss).

## Chemotherapy

Combination chemotherapy is used to treat both Hodgkin's disease and non-Hodgkin's lymphoma. In both cases, chemotherapy often is followed by radiation therapy to involved lymph node regions. The choice of drug combination depends on the stage of the disease as well as the client's age and general condition. The usual combination used in the United States is the ABVD regimen (doxorubicin, bleomycin, vinbalstine, and deacarbazine). The MOPP regimen (nitrogen mustard, vincristine, procarbazine, and prednisone) also is commonly used.

More than 75% of clients with Hodgkin's disease who do not have systemic symptoms achieve complete remission with treatment. A number of other combination regimens also are effective in treating lymphoma, some of which produce fewer adverse effects.

## Radiation Therapy

Radiation therapy is the primary treatment for early-stage Hodgkin's disease. In later stages and in non-Hodgkin's lymphoma it usually is combined with chemotherapy. Many lymphomas are highly responsive to radiation. The involved lymph node region is treated, with careful shielding to protect unaffected areas and minimize the extent of radiation burn and normal cell destruction. If the disease is advanced, total nodal irradiation may be done (Figure 32–11 ■).

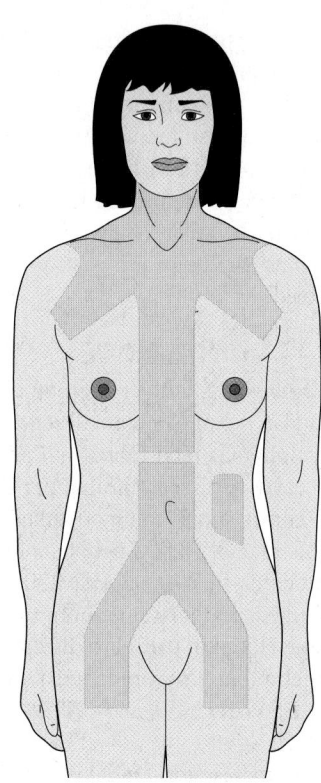

**Figure 32–11** ■ Total nodal or extended field radiation for lymphoma.

## Complications of Treatment

Both chemotherapy and radiation therapy may have long-term effects. Permanent sterility is common, especially in older adults. Bone marrow depression can lead to immunosuppression, anemia, and bleeding. Secondary cancers and cardiac injury are the most serious late adverse effects of treatment. Chemotherapy regimens using the MOPP or a related protocol carry a risk of acute leukemia. Cancers such as breast or lung cancer may develop 10 or more years after thoracic radiation. Thoracic radiation also increases the risk for coronary heart disease and hypothyroidism (Braunwald et al., 2001).

## NURSING CARE

### Assessment

Focused assessment of the client with Hodgkin's disease or non-Hodgkin's lymphoma includes:

- Nursing history: complaints of enlarged lymph node(s), fever, night sweats, weight loss, fatigue or general malaise, abdominal pain, respiratory symptoms, numbness or tingling of extremities, visual changes, or changes in mentation; history of infectious mononucleosis, HIV disease, or other immunosuppressive disorders
- Physical examination: mental status exam; inspect and palpate lymph nodes (cervical, subclavicular, axillary, and inguinal) for enlargement, tenderness; heart and lung sounds; abdominal examination for tenderness, masses, liver or spleen enlargement

### Nursing Diagnoses and Interventions

Nursing care of the client with malignant lymphoma involves both physical and emotional support during diagnosis and treatment. Common nursing care problems include impaired protection due to bone marrow suppression, fatigue, nausea, and altered body image. See the nursing care section for leukemia for specific nursing interventions for *Ineffective protection*.

### Fatigue

General malaise and fatigue may accompany malignant lymphoma and are side effects of chemotherapy. In addition, the physical and psychologic stress of dealing with a chronic, debilitating disease and its treatment may cause fatigue.

- Inquire about feelings of malaise (a vague feeling of body weakness or discomfort) and fatigue (a pervasive, drained feeling that cannot be eliminated). *Both malaise and fatigue are subjective experiences with physiologic, situational, and psychologic components.*
- Encourage verbalization of feelings about the impact of the disease and fatigue on lifestyle. *Discussion of feelings helps the client clarify values and may assist in identifying priorities.*
- Encourage enjoyable but quiet activities, such as reading, listening to music, or hobbies. *Enjoyable activities help decrease feelings of fatigue. Quiet activities conserve energy while yielding a sense of accomplishment.*

- Encourage to establish priorities and include rest periods or naps when scheduling daily activities. *This provides a sense of control over activities and helps maintain self-esteem. Scheduled rest periods help restore energy and decrease fatigue.*
- Encourage delegation of some responsibilities to family members. *Delegation helps maintain the client's involvement and role in family decisions and responsibilities, while conserving energy for those activities identified as high priority by the client.*
- Identify and encourage the client to use energy-saving equipment. *Performing tasks with less exertion and in less time helps conserve energy.*
- Encourage a diet high in carbohydrates and fluids. *A high-carbohydrate diet helps maintain muscle glycogen stores. A liberal fluid intake promotes excretion of metabolic by-products that may contribute to malaise and fatigue.*

### Nausea

The effects of malignant lymphoma and its treatment with chemotherapy and/or radiation therapy can contribute to nausea and interfere with nutritional status. Nausea, a sensation of abdominal fullness, and fear of vomiting often limit food intake. See also the nursing diagnosis, *Imbalanced nutrition,* in the section on leukemia for additional interventions.

- Assess precipitating factors for nausea and/or vomiting, the frequency of vomiting, and relief measures used by the client. *Careful assessment allows development of interventions tailored to the client's situation and needs.*

**PRACTICE ALERT** *Provide ordered antiemetics before chemotherapy is started. Administering prescribed antiemetics before chemotherapy helps prevent nausea and the psychological association of nausea with chemotherapy.* ■

- Teach measures to prevent or relieve nausea and vomiting.
  a. Eat soda crackers and suck on hard candy.
  b. Eat soft, bland foods that are cold or at room temperature.
  c. Avoid unpleasant odors, and get fresh air.
  d. Eat prior to but not immediately before chemotherapy.
  e. Use distraction or progressive muscle relaxation when nauseated.
  f. If vomiting occurs, gradually resume oral intake with frequent sips of clear liquids or ice, progressing to bland foods. *Crackers and hard candy often relieve queasiness, whereas hot, spicy, sweet, or strong smelling foods may increase nausea. Alternative nausea relief measures may be effective.*
- Provide small feedings of high-kcal, high-protein foods and fluids. *This increases nutritional intake.*
- Assist with oral care, general hygiene, and environmental control of temperature, appearance, and odors. *These measures enhance appetite.*
- Identify and provide preferred foods. *This promotes nutritional intake.*
- Assist to a sitting position during and immediately after meals. *The sitting position helps decrease early feelings of fullness.*

## Disturbed Body Image

The diagnosis of cancer is often devastating to the sense of trust in and the perception of one's body. Radiation and chemotherapy lead to changes in appearance and body function (e.g., hair loss, reduced libido, and infertility), further altering body image. Reactions to this diagnosis vary and may include refusal to look in a mirror, discuss the effects of the disease or treatment, unwillingness to participate in rehabilitation, inappropriate treatment decisions, increasing dependence on others or refusal to provide self-care, hostility, withdrawal, and signs of grieving.

- Assess perception of body image through subjective information such as:

  What the client likes most and least about his or her body.

  Pre-illness perception of sick or disabled people.

  Current understanding of health and limitations imposed by illness or treatment.

  Feelings about the illness and its effect on perception of self and others.

  *Body image is one's mental idea or picture of the body. It is based on past and present experiences and includes components of one's actual body and emotional responses to that body. Body image changes constantly. There is often a time lag between an actual body change and the changed body image; during this time, the diagnosis, teaching, and treatment may be rejected.*

- Discuss the risk for and measures to cope with alopecia. Suggest wearing wigs, scarves, hats, or caps. Teach proper scalp care using baby shampoo or mild soap, a soft brush, sunscreen, and mineral oil to reduce itching. If eyelashes and eyebrows are lost, teach eye protection, such as wearing eyeglasses and caps with wide brims. *Chemotherapeutic agents attack rapidly dividing cells such as those responsible for hair growth. Hair loss usually begins 1 to 2 weeks after initiation of chemotherapy, with maximum loss 1 to 2 months later. Alopecia may range from thinning to total hair loss.*

*Regrowth depends on the treatment schedule and doses; however, it usually begins 2 to 3 months after treatment ends. New hair may be softer, more curly, and slightly different in color. Teaching and emotional support help the client anticipate hair loss, discuss its potential effect on body image, and learn self-care techniques.*

- Discuss available resources for financial assistance with purchase of wigs, including local American Cancer Society chapters and insurance plans. *A well-matched wig (or one the color the client has always wished for!) can help maintain a positive body image.*

## Sexual Dysfunction

Sexual dysfunction may result from the malignancy and the effects of radiation and chemotherapy. Reproductive tissues are made of rapidly dividing cells, and cancer treatment may cause temporary or permanent sterility, changes in menstruation, and changes in libido.

- Encourage discussion of actual or potential sexual dysfunction or sterility with the client and significant other. *Clients may be reluctant to discuss this unintended effect of treatment unless encouraged.*
- Assess knowledge, provide information, and clarify misconceptions. Discuss realistic measures for coping (e.g., sperm banking prior to chemotherapy or radiation therapy). *Clients and their partners may be unclear about expected effects on sexuality, reproduction, and the permanency of these effects.*
- Refer for counseling as indicated. *Sexual counseling can help the client and partner develop alternative strategies for expressing their sexuality.*

## Risk for Impaired Skin Integrity

Malignant lymphomas may cause significant pruritus and drenching night sweats. As a result, skin integrity may be impaired. In addition, radiation therapy can cause superficial burns, which also may affect skin integrity.

---

### CHART 32–4  NANDA, NIC, AND NOC LINKAGES

**The Client with Malignant Lymphoma**

| NURSING DIAGNOSES | NURSING INTERVENTIONS | NURSING OUTCOMES |
|---|---|---|
| • Disturbed Body Image | • Active Listening<br>• Emotional Support<br>• Spiritual Support | • Body Image<br>• Psychosocial Adjustment: Life Change |
| • Impaired Skin Integrity | • Radiation Therapy Management<br>• Skin Surveillance | • Tissue Integrity: Skin and Mucous Membranes |
| • Nausea | • Medication Management<br>• Nausea Management | • Comfort Level<br>• Nutritional Status: Food and Fluid Intake |
| • Sexual Dysfunction | • Coping Enhancement<br>• Sexual Counseling | • Self-Esteem<br>• Sexual Functioning |

*Note. Data from Nursing Outcomes Classification (NOC) by M. Johnson & M. Maas (Eds.), 1997, St. Louis: Mosby; Nursing Diagnoses: Definitions & Classification 2001–2002 by North American Nursing Diagnosis Association, 2001, Philadelphia: NANDA; Nursing Interventions Classification (NIC) by J.C. McCloskey & G. M. Bulechek (Eds.), 2000, St. Louis: Mosby. Reprinted by permission.*

- Frequently assess skin, especially in areas undergoing radiation. *Early identification of lesions allows timely treatment and can prevent further disruption of this important line of defense against infection.*
- Provide and teach measures to promote comfort and relieve itching: Use cool water and a mild soap to bathe; blot (rather than rub) dry skin; apply plain cornstarch or non-perfumed lotion or powder to the skin unless contraindicated; use lightweight blankets and clothing; maintain adequate humidity and a cool room temperature; wash bedding and clothes in mild detergent, and put them through second rinse cycle. *Pruritus is aggravated by excessive warmth, excessive dryness, rough fabrics, fatigue, and stress. Lotions and some powders may be contraindicated during radiation therapy.*

## Using NANDA, NIC, and NOC

Chart 32–4 shows links between NANDA nursing diagnoses, NIC, and NOC for the client with malignant lymphoma.

## Home Care

When teaching the client and family for home care, include the following topics in addition to those previously identified for specific nursing diagnoses.

- Information about the illness, planned treatment, and anticipated side effects of treatment
- Skin care and measures to relieve itching and protect areas of radiation
- Symptoms to report to the physician, including those of vertebral compression (decreased sensation or strength in lower extremities)

---

## Nursing Care Plan
## A Client with Hodgkin's Disease

Albin Quito, age 28, is the nurse manager of a thoracic intensive care unit in a large teaching hospital. Lately he has been more tired than usual, often wakes up at night covered with sweat, and just does not feel well. He had thought that his symptoms were due to a viral illness and his busy work schedule. However, yesterday morning Albin noticed a large swollen area on the right side of his neck. He made an appointment with his primary health provider who found a large cervical lymph node. A biopsy of the node and a CT scan of the chest were scheduled.

### ASSESSMENT

David Herzog, the nurse in charge of the outpatient clinic, obtains a nursing history and assessment on Mr. Quito. His physical examination is essentially normal, with the exception of the enlarged node, which is not tender to palpation. When Mr. Quito is weighed, he tells Mr. Herzog that he has lost 7 lb (3.2 kg) in the past 2 months. In reviewing the results of the blood studies, Mr. Herzog notes mild anemia and an increased neutrophil count. The lymph node biopsy shows Reed-Sternberg cells. The clinic physician and Mr. Herzog tell Mr. Quito that the findings indicate stage 1-B Hodgkin's disease but that the prognosis is very good. The physician recommends a short course of combination chemotherapy followed by radiation therapy to involved sites.

### DIAGNOSES

- *Anxiety* related to the diagnosis of Hodgkin's disease and effects of treatment on job performance
- *Risk for infection* related to potential bone marrow depression due to chemotherapy
- *Fatigue* related to effects of cancer, chemotherapy, and radiation therapy

### EXPECTED OUTCOMES

- Verbalize reduced anxiety.
- Remain free of infection.
- Identify and use methods to preserve energy.

### PLANNING AND IMPLEMENTATION

- Encourage to consider a leave of absence from work during course of treatment.
- Discuss joining a support group for people with cancer.
- Provide information about the illness, combination chemotherapy, and radiation therapy.
- Reinforce knowledge of actions to decrease the risk of infection.
- Discuss ways to decrease fatigue and maintain energy:
  - Take a 1- to 2-hour nap once or twice a day.
  - Avoid overexertion during weekends and time off.
  - Maintain a well-balanced diet.

### EVALUATION

When Mr. Quito returns the following week to begin chemotherapy, he brings his friend Nancy to meet Mr. Herzog and asks him to discuss his treatment with her. Mr. Quito says, "I am still really scared, but being able to talk about this with Nancy will help a lot." Mr. Quito has made arrangements to take a 4-month leave from work, with the understanding that his job will be held for him. He states that he will have some problems with money but is working them out. He also says he feels that taking a nap is silly but that he will rest to maintain his energy level. Mr. Quito and Nancy express confidence that he will be cured and say they plan to be active members of the cancer support group—even after recovery.

### Critical Thinking in the Nursing Process

1. Discuss the rationale for treating Hodgkin's disease with chemotherapy and radiation.
2. Design a teaching plan to help Mr. Quito prevent infection while he is at home.
3. What effect does the diagnosis of cancer have on the developmental tasks of a young adult?
4. Develop a care plan for Mr. Quito for the diagnosis, *Ineffective role performance.*

See Evaluating Your Response in Appendix C.

- Use of analgesics and alternative relief strategies for abdominal pain and peripheral neuropathies
- Respiratory care if mediastinal nodes are enlarged or lungs or pleurae are involved
- Planning activities of daily living to ensure adequate rest and exercise
- Measures to relieve nausea and maintain adequate nutrition

Refer clients and family members to the local chapter of the American Cancer Society for information, assistance, and counseling. A list of state and local agencies that offer information about malignant lymphoma and financial assistance can be obtained from the Leukemia Society of America.

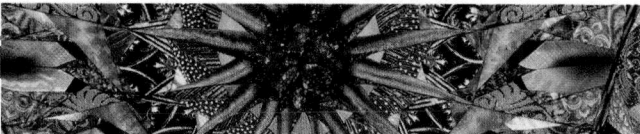

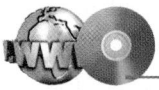 **EXPLORE MediaLink**

NCLEX review questions, case studies, care plan activities, MediaLink applications, and other interactive resources for this chapter can be found on the Companion Website at www.prenhall.com/lemone.

Click on Chapter 32 to select the activities for this chapter. For animations, video clips, more NCLEX review questions, and an audio glossary, access the Student CD-ROM accompanying this textbook.

## TEST YOURSELF

1. In assessing a female client with moderate anemia, the nurse would expect to find which of the following?

   a. Hematocrit 45%
   b. Pulse rate 140
   c. Complains of shortness of breath with exercise
   d. WBC 14,000/μL

2. The nurse administering platelets to a client with disseminated intravascular coagulation (DIC) understands that the intended effect of this treatment is to:

   a. Replace specific clotting factors
   b. Promote intravascular clotting
   c. Restore tissue oxygenation
   d. Replace depleted platelets

3. A client whose husband has hemophilia asks if her newborn baby girl could have the disease. The nurse's response is based on the knowledge that:

   a. The most common forms of hemophilia are transmitted as sex-linked recessive disorders; her daughter is at risk for carrying the defective gene
   b. Because hemophilia is a sex-linked recessive disorder carried on the Y chromosome, her daughter has no risk of having or carrying the disease
   c. Hemophilia is an autosomal dominant disorder; therefore, her daughter has a 50% chance of having the disorder

   d. Although hemophilia is genetically transmitted, its pattern of inheritance is unknown, and her daughter will need to be tested for the defective gene

4. Which of the following nursing diagnoses would be of highest priority for the client hospitalized for a bone marrow transplant to treat relapse of acute myelocytic leukemia?

   a. *Disturbed body image*
   b. *Ineffective protection*
   c. *Anxiety*
   d. *Imbalanced nutrition: Less than body requirements*

5. A client with non-Hodgkin's lymphoma tells the nurse, "I might as well give up on dating. No woman will want me now." What is the most appropriate response?

   a. "It sounds like you are concerned about the effects of this disease and the proposed treatment plan."
   b. "Don't worry. Malignant lymphomas are very treatable when caught in an early state of the disease."
   c. "Well, you may never be able to have children all right, but there are other ways to have a satisfying relationship with a woman."
   d. "Lots of women find bald men attractive; besides, your hair may grow back soft and curly."

See Test Yourself answers in Appendix C.

## BIBLIOGRAPHY

Ackley, B. J., & Ladwig, G. B. (2002). *Nursing diagnosis handbook: A guide to planning care* (5th ed.). St. Louis: Mosby.

Alcoser, P. W., & Burchett, S. (1999). Bone marrow transplantation: Immune system suppression and reconstitution. *American Journal of Nursing, 99*(6), 26–31.

American Cancer Society. (2002a). *Cancer facts and figures 2002*. Atlanta: Author.

———. (2002b). *Gleevec's new successes show growing promise of targeted therapies*. Available: www.cancer.org/eprise/main/docroot/NWS/content/NWS_1_1x_Gleevec

Braunwald, E., Fauci, A. S., Kasper, D. L., Hauser, S. L., Longo, D. L., & Jameson, J. L. (2001). *Harrison's principles of internal medicine* (15th ed.). New York: McGraw-Hill.

Bullock, B. A., & Henze, R. L. (2000). *Focus on pathophysiology*. Philadelphia: Lippincott.

Copstead, L. C., & Banasik, J. L. (2000). *Patho-physiology: Biological and behavioral perspectives* (2nd ed.). Philadephia: Saunders.

Day, S. W., & Wynn, L. W. (2000). Sickle cell pain & hydroxyurea. *American Journal of Nursing, 100*(11), 34–38.

Druker, B. J., Sawyers, C. L., Capdeville, R., Ford, J. M., Baccarani, M., & Goldman, J. M. (2001). Chronic myelogenous leukemia. *Hematology (American Society of Hematology Education Program),* 87–113. Abstract from National Cancer Institute. Available: www.nci.nih.gov/cancerinformation/doc_cit.aspx?args= 22; 11722980

Fontaine, K. L. (2000). *Healing practices: Alternative therapies for nursing.* Upper Saddle River, NJ: Prentice Hall Health.

Gorman, K. (1999). Sickle cell disease. *American Journal of Nursing, 99*(3), 38–43.

Gutaj, D. (2000). Oncology today: Lymphoma. *RN, 63*(8), 32–37.

Johnson, M., Bulechek, G., Dochterman, J. M., Maas, M., & Moorhead, S. (2001). *Nursing diagnoses, outcomes, & interventions.* St. Louis: Mosby.

Johnson, M., Maas, M., & Moorhead, S. (Eds.). (2000). *Nursing outcomes classification (NOC)* (2nd ed.). St. Louis: Mosby.

Kuhn, M. A. (1999). *Complementary therapies for health care providers.* Philadelphia: Lippincott.

Lea, D. H., & Williams, J. K. (2002). Genetic testing and screening. *American Journal of Nursing, 102*(7), 36–43.

Lehne, R. A. (2001). *Pharmacology for nursing care* (4th ed.). Philadelphia: Saunders.

Malarkey, L. M., & McMorrow, M. E. (2000). *Nurse's manual of laboratory tests and diagnostic procedures* (2nd ed.). Philadelphia: Saunders.

McCance, K. L., & Huether, S. E. (2002). Patho-physiology: *The biologic basis for disease in adults & children* (4th ed.). St. Louis: Mosby.

McCloskey, J. C., & Bulechek, G. M. (Eds.) (2000). *Nursing interventions classification (NIC)* (3rd ed.). St. Louis: Mosby.

Medoff, E. (2000). Oncology today: Leukemia. *RN, 63*(9), 42–49.

Mitchell, R. (1999). AJN Clinical Snapshot. Sickle cell anemia. *American Journal of Nursing, 99*(5), 36.

National Heart, Lung, and Blood Institute, National Institutes of Health. (2002). *Morbidity & mortality: 2002 chart book of cardiovascular, lung, and blood diseases.* Bethesda, MD: Author.

Navuluri, R. (2001). Understanding hemostasis. *American Journal of Nursing, 101*(9), Hospital extra: 24B, 24C.

North American Nursing Diagnosis Association. (2001). *NANDA nursing diagnoses: Definitions & classification 2001–2002.* Philadelphia: NANDA.

Persson, L., Hallberg, I. R., & Ohlsson, O. (1997). Survivors of acute leukemia and highly malignant lymphoma—retrospective views of daily life problems during treatment and when in remission. *Journal of Advanced Nursing, 25*(1), 68–78.

Porth, C. M. (2002). *Pathophysiology: Concepts of altered health states* (6th ed.). Philadelphia: Lippincott.

Spahis, J. (2002). Human genetics: Constructing a family pedigree. *American Journal of Nursing, 102*(7), 44–49.

Spatto, G. R., & Woods, A. L. (2003). *2003 edition PDR® nurse's drug handbook.* Clifton Park, NY: Delmar.

Springhouse. (1999). *Nurse's handbook of alternative & complementary therapies.* Springhouse, PA: Author.

Thompson, K. A. (1999). Adolescent health: Detecting Hodgkin's disease. *American Journal of Nursing, 99*(5), 61–64.

Tierney, L. M., McPhee, S. J., & Papadakis, M. A. (2001). *Current medical diagnosis & treatment* (40th ed.). New York: Lange Medical Books/McGraw-Hill.

U. S. Food and Drug Administration, Center for Drug Evaluation and Research. (2001). *Drug information. Gleevec (imatinib mesylate) questions and answers.* Available: www.fda.gov/cder/drug/infopage/gleevec/qa.htm

Wilkinson, J. M. (2000). *Nursing diagnosis handbook with NIC interventions and NOC outcomes* (7th ed.). Upper Saddle River, NJ: Prentice Hall Health.

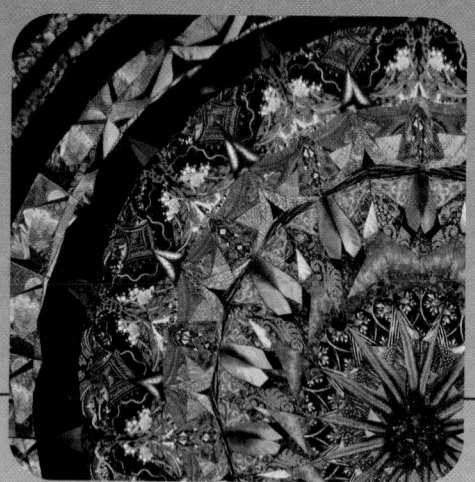

# CHAPTER 33

# Nursing Care of Clients with Peripheral Vascular and Lymphatic Disorders

## MediaLink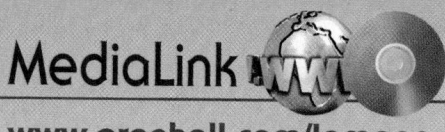

### www.prenhall.com/lemone

Additional resources for this chapter can be found on the Student CD-ROM accompanying this textbook, and on the Companion Website at www.prenhall.com/lemone. Click on Chapter 33 to select the activities for this chapter.

**CD-ROM**
- Audio Glossary
- NCLEX Review

***Animations***
- Lisinopril
- Warfarin

**Companion Website**
- More NCLEX Review
- Case Study
    Abdominal Aortic Aneurysm
- Care Plan Activity
    Lymphedema
- MediaLink Application
    Peripheral Vascular Disease

## LEARNING OUTCOMES

After completing this chapter, you will be able to:

- Relate the anatomy, physiology, and assessment of the peripheral vascular and lymphatic systems discussed in Chapter 31 to common disorders of these systems.

- Describe the pathophysiology of common peripheral vascular and lymphatic disorders.

- Identify tests used to diagnose and assess peripheral vascular and lymphatic disorders.

- Explain the nursing implications for medications used to treat clients with peripheral vascular and lymphatic disorders.

- Describe preoperative and postoperative nursing care of clients having vascular surgery.

- Provide client and family teaching to promote, maintain, and restore health in clients with common peripheral vascular and lymphatic disorders.

- Use the nursing process to plan and provide individualized care for clients with peripheral vascular and lymphatic disorders.

The major processes that interfere with peripheral blood flow and that of lymphatic fluid include constriction, obstruction, inflammation, and vasospasm. These conditions lead to disorders of blood pressure regulation, peripheral artery function, aortic structure, venous circulation, and lymphatic circulation.

A holistic approach is important when caring for clients with disorders of the peripheral vascular and lymphatic systems.

The focus of care is on teaching long-term care measures, pain relief, improving peripheral blood and lymphatic circulation, preventing tissue damage, and promoting healing. The prescribed treatment may have emotional, social, and economic effects on the client and family.

# DISORDERS OF BLOOD PRESSURE REGULATION

Blood flows through the circulatory system from areas of higher pressure to areas of lower pressure. The amount of pressure in any portion of the vascular system is affected by a number of factors, including blood volume, vascular resistance, and cardiac output. The **blood pressure** is the tension or pressure exerted by blood against arterial walls. A certain amount of pressure within the system is necessary to maintain open vessels, capillary perfusion, and oxygenation of all body tissues. Excess pressure, however, has harmful effects, increasing the workload of the heart, altering the structure of the vessels, and affecting sensitive body tissues such as the kidneys, eyes, and central nervous system.

This section focuses on **hypertension,** or excess pressure in the arterial portion of systemic circulation. Excessively low blood pressure, *hypotension,* is discussed in the shock section of Chapter 6. Altered pulmonary vascular pressures are discussed in Chapter 36.

## PHYSIOLOGY REVIEW

Blood flow through the circulatory system requires *sufficient blood volume* to fill the blood vessels and *pressure differences* within the system that allow blood to move forward. The arterial, or supply side, of the circulation has relatively high pressures created by the thick elastic walls of the arteries and arterioles. The venous, or return side of the system, on the other hand, is a low pressure system of thin-walled, distensible veins. Blood flows through the capillaries linking these two systems from the higher pressure arterial side to the lower pressure venous side.

The arterial blood pressure is created by the ejection of blood from the heart during systole (*cardiac output* or *CO*) and the tension, or resistance to blood flow, created by the elastic arterial walls (*systemic vascular resistance* or *SVR*). The blood pressure rises as the heart contracts during systole, ejecting its blood. This pressure wave, or the **systolic blood pressure,** is felt as the peripheral pulse and heard as the Korotkoff's sounds during blood pressure measurement. In healthy adults the average systolic pressure is 120 mmHg. During diastole, or cardiac relaxation and filling, elastic arterial walls maintain a minimum pressure, the **diastolic blood pressure,** to maintain blood flow through the capillary beds. The average diastolic pressure in a healthy adult is 80 mmHg. The difference between the systolic and diastolic pressure, normally about 40 mmHg, is known as the **pulse pressure.** The **mean arterial pressure**

**(MAP)** is the average pressure in the arterial circulation throughout the cardiac cycle. The formula MAP = CO × SVR often is used to show the relationships between factors determining the blood pressure.

Cardiac output is determined by the blood volume and the ability of the ventricles to fill and effectively pump that blood. A number of factors contribute to systemic vascular resistance, including vessel length, blood viscosity, and vessel diameter and distensibility (compliance). While vessel length and blood viscosity remain relatively constant, vessel diameter and compliance are subject to normal regulatory activities and disease.

The arterioles normally determine the SVR as their diameter changes in response to a variety of stimuli:

- *Sympathetic nervous system (SNS)* stimulation. Baroreceptors in the aortic arch and carotid sinus signal the SNS via the cardiovascular control center in the medulla when the MAP changes. A drop in MAP stimulates the SNS, increasing the heart rate, cardiac output, and constricting arterioles (except in skeletal muscle). As a result, BP rises. A rise in MAP has the opposite effect, decreasing the heart rate and cardiac output, and causing arteriolar vasodilation.
- *Circulating epinephrine and norepinephrine* from the adrenal cortex (e.g., the fight-or-flight response) have the same effect as SNS stimulation.
- *Renin-angiotensin-aldosterone system* responds to renal perfusion. A drop in renal perfusion stimulates renin release. Renin converts angiotensinogen to angiotensin I, which is subsequently converted to angiotensin II in the lungs by angiotensin-converting enzyme (ACE). Angiotensin II is a potent vasoconstrictor. It also promotes sodium and water retention both directly and by stimulating the adrenal medulla to release aldosterone. Both SVR and CO increase, raising BP.
- *Atrial natriuretic peptide* is released from atrial cells in response to stretching by excess blood volume. It promotes vasodilation and sodium and water excretion, lowering BP.
- *Adrenomedullin* is a peptide synthesized and released by endothelial and smooth muscle cells in blood vessels. It is a potent vasodilator.
- *Vasopressin* or *antidiuretic hormone* (from the posterior pituitary gland) promotes water retention and vasoconstriction, raising BP.
- *Local factors* such as inflammatory mediators and various metabolites can promote vasodilation, affecting BP.

**Figure 33–1** ■ Factors affecting blood pressure.

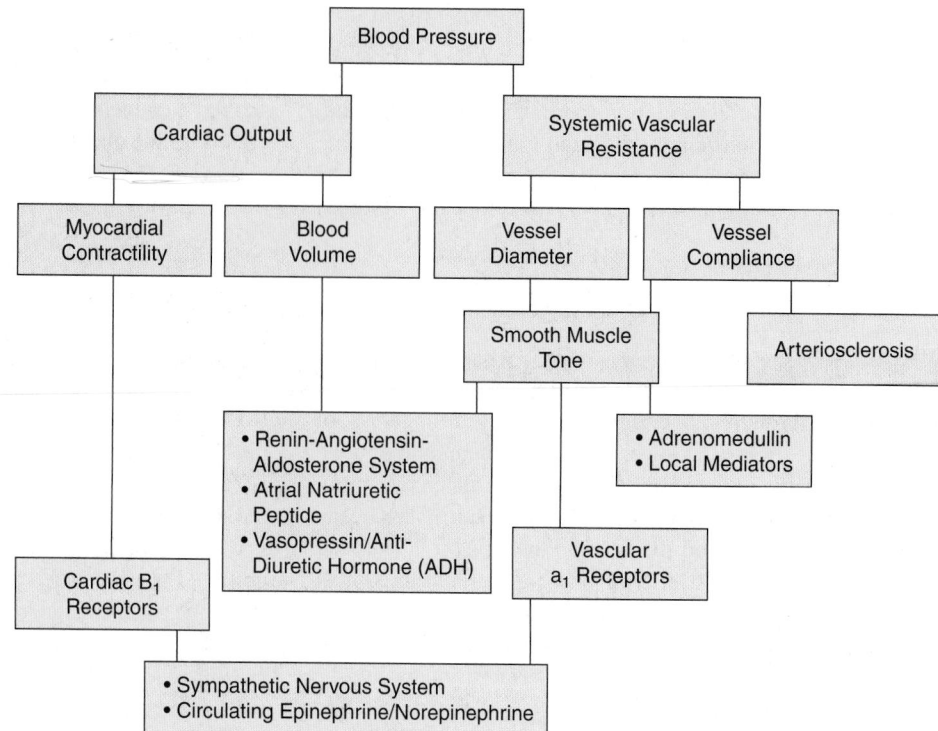

In addition to the above, the primary factor affecting vessel compliance is the extent of arteriosclerosis (hardening of the arteries) and atherosclerosis (plaque accumulation). Figure 33–1 ■ summarizes the interrelationships of major factors regulating blood pressure.

## THE CLIENT WITH PRIMARY HYPERTENSION

**Primary hypertension,** also known as *essential hypertension,* is a persistently elevated systemic blood pressure. About 50 million people in the United States have hypertension. More than 90% of these have primary hypertension, which has no identified cause.

Hypertension primarily affects middle-aged and older adults: 38% of people age 50 to 59 and 71% of people age 80 and older are hypertensive (National Heart, Lung, and Blood Institute [NHLBI], 2002). Hypertension is often called a "silent killer," because affected people often have no symptoms of the disease. Awareness and effective treatment of hypertension have significantly improved. Thirty years ago, only 51% of people with hypertension were aware of their condition and only 16% were effectively treated and controlled. In 1994, 88% of people with hypertension were aware of the disease, and 65% were effectively treated and controlled (NHLBI, 2002).

The prevalence of hypertension is significantly higher in blacks than in whites and Hispanics. More than 35% of black adults are hypertensive, whereas less than 25% of adult white and Hispanic people are affected. In whites and Hispanics, more males than females are hypertensive; in blacks the prevalence in men and women is nearly equal (NHLBI, 2002). Essential hypertension affects people of all income groups, having great financial effects because of its effects on other body systems: cerebrovascular accident (stroke), coronary artery disease, and chronic renal failure.

Hypertension is defined as systolic blood pressure of 140 mmHg or higher, or diastolic pressure of 90 mmHg or higher, based on the average of three or more readings taken on separate occasions (NHLBI, 2002). Exceptions include clients being treated for hypertension and an initial reading of a systolic pressure of 210 mmHg or higher and/or a diastolic blood pressure of 120 mmHg or higher. Table 33–1 identifies classifications of blood pressure for adults age 18 and older as defined by the Joint National Committee.

A number of risk factors have been identified for primary hypertension (Box 33–1). Genetics play a role, as do environmental factors.

- *Family history.* Studies show a genetic link in 30% to 40% of primary hypertension (Porth, 2002). Genes involved in the renin-angiotensin-aldosterone system and others that affect vascular tone, salt and water transportation in the kidney, obesity, and insulin resistance are likely involved in the development of hypertension.
- *Age.* The incidence of hypertension rises with increasing age. Aging affects baroreceptors involved in blood pressure regulation as well as arterial compliance. As the arteries become less compliant, pressure within the vessels increases. This is often most apparent as a gradual increase in the systolic pressure with aging. Systolic hypertension increases the risk for cerebrovascular accident (stroke). See the Nursing Care of the Older Adult box on page 983.
- *Race.* Essential hypertension is more common and more severe in blacks than in people of other ethnic backgrounds.

## TABLE 33–1 Classification of Blood Pressure for Adults Age 18 and Older*

| Category | Systolic (mmHg) | | Diastolic (mmHg) |
|---|---|---|---|
| Optimal | <120 | and | <80 |
| Normal | <130 | and | <85 |
| High-normal | 130–139 | or | 85–89 |
| Hypertension‡ | | | |
|    Stage 1 | 140–159 | or | 90–99 |
|    Stage 2 | 160–179 | or | 100–109 |
|    Stage 3 | ≥180 | or | ≥110 |

*When systolic and diastolic blood pressures fall into different categories, the higher category is used to classify blood pressure status.

‡Based on the average of two or more readings taken at each of two or more visits after an initial screening.

Note. Adapted from The Sixth Report of the Joint National Committee on Prevention, Detection, Education, and Treatment of High Blood Pressure, NIH Publication No. 98-4080 by NHLBI, 1997, Bethesda, MD: National Institutes of Health. Available: http://www.nhlbi.nih.gov/guidelines/hypertension

---

### BOX 33–1 ■ Factors Contributing to Hypertension

#### MODIFIABLE FACTORS

■ High sodium intake
■ Low potassium, calcium, and magnesium intake
■ Obesity
■ Excess alcohol consumption
■ Smoking
■ Glucose intolerance

#### NONMODIFIABLE FACTORS

■ Family history
■ Age
■ Race

---

This may relate to the genes controlling the renin-angiotensin-aldosterone system, although the exact mechanism for this increased risk is not yet understood.

- *Mineral intake.* High sodium intake often is associated with fluid retention. Although salt and water retention increase blood volume and cardiac output, it is not clear how salt intake contributes to the onset of hypertension or why some people are affected but others are not. Increased sodium intake does not cause hypertension, nor does the blood pressure fall with salt restriction in all hypertensive clients. Low potassium, calcium, and magnesium intakes also contribute to hypertension by unknown mechanisms. The ratio of sodium to potassium intake appears to play a role; possibly through the effects of increased potassium intake on sodium excretion. Potassium also may reduce vasoconstriction related to norepinephrine and other vasoactive substances (Porth, 2002). The link between low calcium and magnesium intakes and hypertension is unclear.

- *Obesity.* Central obesity (fat cell deposits in the abdomen), determined by an increased waist-to-hip ratio, has a stronger correlation with hypertension than body mass index or skin-fold thickness. Although a clear correlation exists between obesity and hypertension, the relationship may be one of common cause: Genetic factors appear to play a role in the common triad of obesity, hypertension, and insulin resistance.

- *Insulin resistance.* Insulin resistance, with resulting hyper-insulinemia, is linked with hypertension by an unknown mechanism. Activation of the sympathetic nervous system, vascular smooth muscle growth due to excess insulin, the effect of insulin on renal regulation of sodium and water, and changes in cell membrane transport of sodium and calcium have been proposed as mechanisms in this relationship.

- *Excess alcohol consumption.* Regular consumption of three or more drinks a day increases the risk of hypertension.

---

## Nursing Care of the Older Adult

### HYPERTENSION

Controlling high blood pressure is as important in the older adult as in younger adults. In the United States, 60% of non-Hispanic whites, 61% of Mexican Americans, and 71% of African Americans age 60 and older have high blood pressure (NHLBI, 1997). Isolated systolic hypertension is common, as is an elevated pulse pressure (systolic BP minus diastolic BP), indicating decreased compliance of large arteries.

The Framingham Heart Study shows that cardiovascular deaths are 2 to 5 times more common in older adults with isolated systolic hypertension than in people with normal blood pressures. Stroke also is more common in older adults with systolic hypertension. These findings appear to relate to changes in blood vessels associated with aging: decreased compliance and decreased baroreceptor sensitivity. Decreased compliance impairs the ability of the vessels to expand and contract with varying amounts of blood, increasing peripheral vascular resistance and decreasing renal blood flow.

To obtain accurate blood pressure readings for older clients, slightly different procedures may be required. Palpation of the artery during cuff inflation is recommended to prevent inaccurate systolic readings due to an auscultatory gap, present in many older adults. The reflexes that maintain blood pressure during position changes diminish with aging. Allow the older client to sit upright or stand for 2 to 5 minutes before evaluating the blood pressure for true orthostatic readings.

Decreasing or discontinuing alcohol consumption reduces the blood pressure, particularly systolic readings. Lifestyle factors associated with excessive alcohol intake (obesity and lack of exercise) may contribute to hypertension as well.

- *Smoking.* In recent years, a relationship between serum norepinephrine levels (elevated by smoking) and hypertension has been documented. The goal of ongoing research is to clarify the long-term effects of smoking on blood pressure.
- *Stress.* Physical and emotional stress cause transient elevations of blood pressure, but the role of stress in primary hypertension is less clear. Blood pressure normally fluctuates throughout the day, increasing with activity, discomfort, or emotional responses such as anger. Frequent or continued stress may cause vascular smooth muscle hypertrophy or affect central integrative pathways of the brain (Porth, 2002).

## PATHOPHYSIOLOGY

Primary hypertension is thought to develop from a complex interaction of factors that regulate cardiac output and systemic vascular resistance. These interactions may include:

- Sympathetic nervous system overactivity with overstimulation of α- and β-adrenergic receptors, resulting in vasoconstriction and increased cardiac output.
- Renin-angiotensin-aldosterone system overactivity affects vasomotor tone and salt and water excretion. In addition, angiotensin II mediates arteriolar remodeling which permanently increases SVR.
- Other chemical mediators of vasomotor tone and blood volume such as atrial natriuretic peptide (factor) also play a role by affecting vasomotor tone and sodium and water excretion.
- The interaction between insulin resistance and endothelial function may be a primary cause of hypertension. Insulin resistance decreases the release of nitric oxide and other endogenous vasodilators, affects renal function, and increases sympathetic nervous system activity (McCance & Huether, 2002).

The result is sustained increases in blood volume and peripheral resistance. The cardiovascular system adapts to increased blood volume by increasing cardiac output. Autoregulatory mechanisms in the systemic arteries react to the increased volume, causing vasoconstriction. The increased systemic vascular resistance causes hypertension. Sustained hypertension, in turn, affects the cardiovascular system. The rate of atherosclerosis accelerates, increasing the risk for coronary heart disease and stroke. The workload of the left ventricle increases, leading to ventricular hypertrophy, which then increases the risk for coronary heart disease, dysrhythmias, and heart failure. Hypertension also can lead to nephrosclerosis and renal insufficiency (Porth, 2002).

## MANIFESTATIONS

The early stages of primary hypertension typically are asymptomatic, marked only by elevated blood pressure. Blood pressure elevations are initially transient but eventually become permanent. When symptoms do appear, they are usually vague. Headache, usually in the back of the head and neck, may be present on awakening, subsiding during the day. Other symptoms result from target organ damage, and may include nocturia, confusion, nausea and vomiting, and visual disturbances. Examination of the retina of the eye may reveal narrowed arterioles, hemorrhages, exudates, and papilledema (swelling of the optic nerve).

## COLLABORATIVE CARE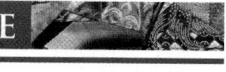

Hypertension management focuses on reducing the blood pressure to less than 140 mmHg systolic and 90 mmHg diastolic. The *Sixth Report of the Joint National Committee on Prevention, Detection, Evaluation, and Treatment of High Blood Pressure* (NHLBI, 1997) recommends a treatment plan based on cardiovascular disease risk factors, the presence or absence of target organ damage, and blood pressure levels (Table 33–2). Emphasis is placed on adherence to the treatment plan to prevent long-term consequences of hypertension (e.g., stroke, heart failure, and renal failure). Both pharmacologic and nonpharmacologic approaches are used. There is no cure for hypertension, but it can be controlled.

### TABLE 33–2  Recommended Hypertension Treatment

| Stage | Risk Group A* | Risk Group B** | Risk Group C*** |
|---|---|---|---|
| High-normal (130–139/85–89) | Lifestyle modification | Lifestyle modification | Drug therapy plus lifestyle modification |
| Stage 1 (140–159/90–99) | Lifestyle modification for up to 12 months, then drug therapy | Lifestyle modification for up to 6 months, then drug therapy | Drug therapy plus lifestyle modification |
| Stages 2 and 3 (>160/>100) | Drug therapy plus lifestyle modification | Drug therapy plus lifestyle modification | Drug therapy plus lifestyle modification |

*Risk Group A: High normal blood pressure or stage 1, 2, or 3 hypertension; no clinical cardiovascular disease, target organ damage, or other risk factors

**Risk Group B: Hypertension; no clinical cardiovascular disease or target organ damage, one or more major risk factors such as smoking, hyperlipidemia, older age (>60 years), male gender or postmenopausal female, family history of cardiovascular disease

***Risk Group C: Hypertension; clinical cardiovascular disease or target organ damage; presence of diabetes with or without other risk factors

*Note. Adapted from The Sixth Report of the Joint National Committee on Prevention, Detection, Evaluation, and Treatment of High Blood Pressure NIH Publication No. 98-4080 by the NHLBI, 1997, Bethesda, MD: National Institutes of Health. Available: http://www.nhlbi.nih.gov/guidelines/hypertension*

| BOX 33–2 ■ Lifestyle Modifications for Hypertension |
| --- |

- Lose weight if overweight.
- Dietary modifications.
  - Reduce sodium intake.
  - Maintain adequate dietary potassium intake.
  - Maintain adequate dietary calcium and magnesium intake.
  - Reduce intake of saturated fat and cholesterol.
- Limit alcohol intake to no more than 1 oz per day.
- Stop smoking.
- Engage in aerobic exercise for 30 to 45 minutes most days of the week.
- Use stress management techniques such as relaxation therapy.

| BOX 33–3 ■ DASH Diet Recommendations |
| --- |

- Grains—7 to 8 servings per day
- Vegetables—4 to 5 servings per day
- Fruits—4 to 5 servings per day
- Nonfat/lowfat milk—2 to 3 servings per day
- Lean meat (including fish and poultry)—2 or less servings per day
- Nuts, seeds, and dry beans—4 to 5 servings per week
- Calories—2000 per day

## Diagnostic Tests

There are no specific diagnostic tests for essential hypertension. Diagnostic testing focuses on identifying possible causes of secondary hypertension (discussed later in this section) and determining target organ damage and other cardiovascular risk factors. Routine laboratory tests such as urinalysis, complete blood count, and blood chemistries (including electrolytes, glucose, and cholesterol levels) are done before treatment is started.

## Lifestyle Modifications

Lifestyle modifications generally are recommended for all clients with high normal blood pressure or intermittent or sustained hypertension. These modifications include weight loss, dietary changes, restricted alcohol use and cigarette smoking, increased physical activity, and stress reduction (Box 33–2).

### Diet

Dietary approaches to managing hypertension focus on reducing sodium intake, maintaining adequate potassium and calcium intakes, and reducing total and saturated fat intake. A mild to moderate sodium restriction (no added salt) lowers blood pressure and potentiates the effect of antihypertensive drugs for most hypertensive clients. The DASH (Dietary Approaches to Stop Hypertension) diet has proven beneficial effects in lowering blood pressure. This diet (Box 33–3) focuses on whole foods rather than individual nutrients. It is rich in fruits and vegetables (up to 10 servings per day), and low in total and saturated fats.

Weight loss is recommended for clients who are obese. A balanced diet such as the DASH diet is recommended for weight loss.

### Alcohol and Cigarette Use

The recommended alcohol intake for clients with hypertension is no more than 15 mL of ethanol per day. This translates to 12 oz of beer, 5 oz of wine, or 1 oz of whiskey. Women and lighter-weight people should reduce this limit by half. Although alcohol withdrawal may increase blood pressure, this is usually temporary and diminishes as abstinence or restricted intake continues.

Although nicotine is a vasoconstrictor, substantial data linking smoking to hypertension are lacking. A definitive link exists between smoking and heart disease, however. Clients who smoke are strongly urged to quit. Smoking also reduces the effect of some antihypertensive medications such as propranolol (Inderal). Smoking cessation aids such as nicotine patches and gum contain lower amounts of nicotine and usually do not raise blood pressure.

### Physical Activity

Regular exercise (such as walking, cycling, jogging, or swimming) reduces blood pressure and contributes to weight loss, stress reduction, and feelings of overall well-being. Previously sedentary clients are encouraged to engage in aerobic exercise for 30 to 45 minutes per day most days of the week. Isometric exercise (such as weight training) may not be appropriate, as it can raise the systolic blood pressure.

### Stress Reduction

Stress stimulates the sympathetic nervous system, increasing vasoconstriction, systemic vascular resistance, cardiac output, and the blood pressure. Regular, moderate exercise is the treatment of choice for reducing stress in hypertensive clients. Relaxation techniques such as biofeedback, therapeutic touch, yoga, and meditation to relax both mind and body may also lower blood pressure, although their effect has not been proven in hypertension management.

## Medications

Current pharmacologic treatment of hypertension involves using one or more of the following drug classes: diuretics, beta-adrenergic blockers, centrally acting sympatholytics, vasodilators, angiotensin-converting enzyme (ACE) inhibitors, and calcium channel blockers. These drug classes have different sites of action (Figure 33–2 ■)

Treatment usually is initiated using a single antihypertensive drug at a low dose. The dose is slowly increased until optimal blood pressure control is achieved. If the drug does not effectively lower the blood pressure or has troubling side effects, a different drug from another class of antihypertensive medications is substituted. If, on the other hand, the drug is tolerated well but has not lowered blood pressure to the desired level, a second drug from another class may be added to the treatment regimen.

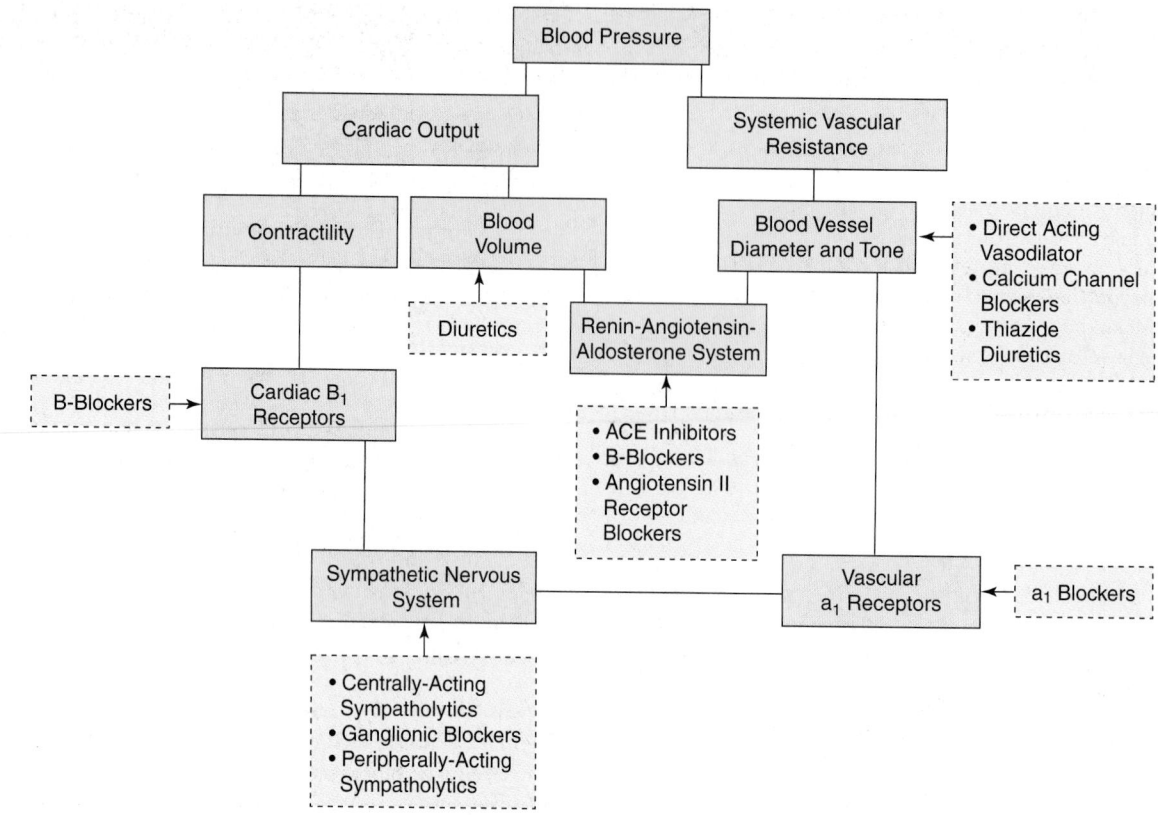

**Figure 33–2** ■ Sites of Antihypertensive Drug Action.

A diuretic or a beta blocker often is prescribed initially for uncomplicated hypertension. These drugs lower blood pressure and reduce the risk of complications such as heart failure and stroke. Diuretics are the preferred treatment for isolated systolic hypertension in older adults. ACE inhibitors also are commonly used in initial treatment of hypertension, particularly for clients who are diabetic or who have heart failure or a history of MI.

Other factors considered in selecting drugs for treating hypertension include demographic characteristics of the client, concurrent conditions, quality of life, cost, and possible interactions among prescribed drugs. In general, diuretics and calcium channel blockers are more effective for treating hypertension in blacks than beta blockers or ACE inhibitors. Beta blockers are preferred to treat hypertension with concurrent coronary heart disease and angina, but are contraindicated for clients who have asthma or depression. Beta blockers also reduce exercise tolerance and may adversely affect lifestyle for some clients. Nursing implications for administration of antihypertensive drugs (other than diuretics) are outlined on pages 987–988.

Thiazide diuretics, such as hydrochlorothiazide (Hydro-DIURIL), are widely used to control hypertension. In major clinical studies, single therapy with diuretics controlled blood pressure in about 50% of the clients and reduced hypertension-linked morbidity and mortality related to coronary heart disease. Diuretics control hypertension primarily by preventing tubular reabsorption of sodium, thus promoting sodium and water excretion and reducing blood volume. Thiazide diuretics also reduce systemic vascular resistance through an unknown mechanism. Diuretics are particularly effective in blacks and in clients who are obese, older, or who have increased plasma volume or low renin activity. The adverse effects of diuretics generally are dose related. In addition to hypokalemia, diuretics may affect serum levels of glucose, triglycerides, uric acid, low-density lipoproteins, and insulin. More information about diuretics can be found in Chapters 5 and 27. ⊶

Treatment of clients in risk group C generally is more aggressive to minimize the risk of MI, heart failure, or stroke. When the average blood pressure is greater than 200/120, immediate therapy, and possible hospitalization, is vital.

After a year of effective hypertension control, an effort may be made to reduce the dosage and number of drugs. This is known as step-down therapy. It is more successful in clients who have made lifestyle modifications. Careful blood pressure monitoring is necessary during and after step-down therapy, as the blood pressure often rises again to hypertensive levels.

## NURSING CARE

### Health Promotion

Health promotion teaching and activities focus on the modifiable risk factors for hypertension. Advise all clients (as well as children and adolescents) to stop or never start smoking. Discuss the risks of obesity, excess alcohol intake, and a sedentary

# Medication Administration

## Antihypertensive Drugs

### ALPHA-ADRENERGIC BLOCKERS

Doxazosin (Cardura)
Prazosin (Minipress)
Terazosin (Hytrin)

Alpha-adrenergic blocking agents block alpha receptors in vascular smooth muscle, decreasing vasomotor tone and vasoconstriction. They also reduce serum levels of low-density (LDL) and very low-density lipoproteins (VLDL). However, vasodilation may cause orthostatic hypotension and reflex stimulation of the heart, resulting in tachycardia and palpitations. A beta blocker may be ordered to minimize this effect.

#### Nursing Responsibilities

- Give the first dose at bedtime to minimize risk of fainting (called "first-dose syncope"). If the first dose is given in the daytime (or if the dose is increased), instruct to remain in bed for 3 to 4 hours.
- Assess blood pressure and apical pulse before each dose and as indicated thereafter.

#### Client and Family Teaching

- There is a risk of fainting after taking the first dose of this drug. Take the drug at bedtime to reduce this risk, and do not drive or engage in other hazardous activities for 12 to 24 hours after the first dose.
- This drug may cause dizziness or lightheadedness. Change positions slowly, and sit down if you become dizzy or lightheaded.
- Notify your primary care provider if you develop nasal congestion or impotence while taking this drug.
- Notify your primary care provider before discontinuing this medication.

### ANGIOTENSIN-CONVERTING ENZYME (ACE) INHIBITORS

Benazepril (Lotensin)          Moexipril (Univasc)
Captopril (Capoten)            Perindopril (Aceon)
Enalapril (Vasotec)            Quinapril (Accupril)
Fosinopril (Monopril)          Ramipril (Altace)
Lisinopril (Zestril)           Trandolapril (Mavik)

### Angiotensin II Receptor Blockers

Eprosartan (Teveten)           Losartan (Cozaar)
Irbersartan (Avapro)           Valsartan (Diovan)
Candesartan (Atacand)

The ACE inhibitors lower blood pressure by preventing conversion of angiotensin I to angiotensin II. This in turn prevents vasoconstriction and sodium and water retention. Angiotensin II receptor blockers (ARBs) have the same effect, but they act by blocking the effect of angiotensin II on receptors. Both ACE inhibitors and ARBs are less effective in black clients and are contraindicated in pregnancy (Lehne, 2001). Their primary adverse effects are persistent cough, first-dose hypotension, and hyperkalemia.

#### Nursing Responsibilities

- Assess blood pressure and WBC before giving the first dose. Monitor blood pressure for 2 hours after the first dose and regularly thereafter.
- Administer PO 1 hour before meals; tablets may be crushed.

- Report changes in WBC or differential, hyperkalemia, or changes in BUN or serum creatinine to the primary care provider.
- Do not administer to clients with renal artery stenosis or who are pregnant.
- Immediately report and treat manifestations of angioedema (giant wheals and edema of the tongue, glottis, and pharynx). Initiate resuscitation measures as needed. Discontinue drug immediately and do not use in the future.

#### Client and Family Teaching

- Report peripheral edema, signs of infection, or difficulty breathing to your primary care provider.
- Change position (lying to sitting and sitting to standing) slowly to prevent dizziness; sit down if dizziness or lightheadedness develops.
- Do not take a potassium supplement or use a potassium-based salt substitute while taking this drug unless prescribed by your physician.
- Notify your physician if you become pregnant while taking this drug. Although it is safe early in pregnancy, taking the drug during the second and third trimesters may harm the fetus.

### BETA-ADRENERGIC BLOCKING AGENTS

Acebutolol (Sectral)           Nadolol (Corgard)
Atenolol (Tenormin)            Penbutolol (Levatol)
Betaxolol (Kerlone)            Pindolol (Visken)
Bisoprolol (Zebeta)            Propranolol (Inderal)
Carteolol (Cartrol)            Timolol (Blocadren)
Metoprolol tartrate (Lopressor)

Beta-adrenergic blockers are commonly used to control hypertension. Beta blockers reduce blood pressure by preventing beta-receptor stimulation in the heart, thereby decreasing heart rate and cardiac output. Beta blockers also interfere with renin release by the kidneys, decreasing the effects of angiotensin and aldosterone. Potential adverse effects of beta blockers include bronchospasm, fatigue, sleep disturbances, nightmares, bradycardia, heart block, worsening of heart failure, gastrointestinal disturbances, impotence, and increased triglyceride levels.

#### Nursing Responsibilities

- Before giving initial dose, assess for contraindications to beta blockers such as asthma, chronic lung disease, bradycardia, or heart block.
- Assess blood pressure and apical pulse before giving; notify primary care provider if vital signs are outside established parameters.
- Report adverse effects such as bradycardia, decreased cardiac output (fatigue, dyspnea with exertion, hypotension, decreased level of consciousness), heart failure, heart block, bronchoconstriction (wheezing, dyspnea), or altered blood glucose levels (in diabetic clients).
- Carefully monitor responses of the older client.

#### Client and Family Teaching

- Monitor blood pressure and pulse daily as instructed.
- Change position (lying to sitting and sitting to standing) slowly to prevent dizziness and possible falls.
- Report effects such as fatigue, lethargy, and impotence to your primary care provider.

(continued on page 988)

MediaLink | LISINOPRIL ANIMATION

# Medication Administration

## Antihypertensive Drugs (continued)

- Notify your physician if you become short of breath or develop a cough or swelling of your extremities.
- If you have diabetes, check blood glucose levels more frequently as hypoglycemia may develop with few symptoms.
- Talk to your primary care provider before taking any over-the-counter medications.
- Carry an adequate supply of the drug when traveling. Do not stop taking this drug without notifying your primary care provider.

### CALCIUM CHANNEL BLOCKERS

Amlodipine (Norvasc)          Nifedipine (Procardia)
Diltiazem (Cardizem)          Nimodipine (Nimotop)
Felodipine (Plendil)          Nisoldipine (Sular)
Isradipine (DynaCirc)         Verapamil (Isoptin)
Nicardipine (Cardene)

Calcium channel blockers inhibit the flow of calcium ions across the cell membrane of vascular tissue and cardiac cells. In doing so, they relax arterial smooth muscle, lowering peripheral resistance through vasodilation. Calcium channel blockers can cause reflex tachycardia, and some (e.g., verapamil and diltiazem) may impair cardiac function, worsening heart failure.

### Nursing Responsibilities

- Assess blood pressure, apical pulse, and liver and renal function tests prior to giving these drugs.
- Calcium channel blockers may be given orally or intravenously.
- Do not administer verapamil or diltiazem to clients with severe hypotension, sinus, or atrioventricular blocks. Administer with caution to clients also taking digoxin or a beta blocker.
- Periodically monitor blood pressure and apical pulse during therapy. Promptly report signs of bradycardia, AV block, or heart failure to the physician.

### Client and Family Teaching

- Take blood pressure and pulse daily as taught. Notify your physician if your pulse is less than 60 BPM or your blood pressure is not within the specified range.
- This drug may cause constipation. Drink six to eight glasses of water each day, and increase fiber in diet.
- Report shortness of breath, weight gain, or swelling in feet or ankles to your primary care provider.

### CENTRALLY ACTING SYMPATHOLYTICS

Clonidine (Catapres)          Guanfacine (Tenex)
Guanabenz (Wytensin)          Methyldopa (Aldomet)

The centrally acting sympatholytics stimulate the $\alpha_2$ receptors in the CNS to suppress sympathetic outflow to the heart and blood vessels. A fall in cardiac output and vasodilation result, reducing blood pressure. Dry mouth and sedation are common adverse effects. Severe reflex hypertension may occur if abruptly discontinued. Clonidine is contraindicated during pregnancy; methyldopa is contraindicated for clients with active liver disease.

### Nursing Responsibilities

- Assess for contraindications to therapy. Obtain baseline blood pressure, CBC, Coomb's test, and liver function studies.
- Administer oral doses at bedtime to minimize effects of sedation.

- Methyldopa may be given intravenously for hypertensive emergencies.
- Apply transdermal clonidine patch to dry, hairless area of intact skin on the chest or upper arm. Assess for rash, which indicates allergy, at area of application.
- Promptly report changes in laboratory values to the physician. Discontinue methyldopa if manifestations of liver dysfunction develop.

### Client and Family Teaching

- Relieve dry mouth by sipping water or chewing sugarless gum.
- Take with meals if gastric upset or nausea develop.
- Change position (lying to sitting and sitting to standing) slowly to prevent dizziness and possible falls.
- Do not suddenly discontinue medication or skip doses; this could cause serious hypertension.
- Report mental depression or decreased mental acuity to your health care provider.
- Side effects (such as dry mouth, nausea, and dizziness) tend to diminish over time.
- Do not drive a car if the medications cause drowsiness.

### VASODILATORS

Hydralazine (Apresoline)
Minoxidil (Loniten)

Vasodilators reduce blood pressure by relaxing vascular smooth muscle (especially in the arterioles), and decreasing peripheral vascular resistance. These drugs are often prescribed in combination with a diuretic or beta blocker, because they can cause reflex tachycardia and fluid retention. Because these drugs can have significant toxic effects, they are not routinely used to manage chronic hypertension.

### Nursing Responsibilities

- Hydralazine may be given orally or intravenously; minoxidil is given orally.
- Assess blood pressure and pulse before giving the drug and monitor during therapy as indicated. Report tachycardia or hypotension to the physician.
- Report peripheral edema and manifestations of volume overload and heart failure.
- Immediately report muffled heart sounds or paradoxical pulse as pericardial effusion and possible cardiac tamponade may develop during minoxidil therapy.
- Discontinue hydralazine and report manifestations of a SLE-like syndrome: muscle or joint pain, fever, or symptoms of nephritis or pericarditis.

### Client and Family Teaching

- Change position (lying to sitting and sitting to standing) slowly to prevent dizziness and possible falls.
- Report muscle, joint aches, and fever to your health care provider.
- Headache, palpitations, and rapid pulse may develop but should abate in about 10 days.
- Do not discontinue the medication without talking to your health care provider.
- Minoxidil may cause excessive hair growth. Contact your physician if this becomes troublesome.

TABLE 33–3    Recommended Blood Pressure Follow-Up

| Category | Blood Pressure (mm Hg) | Recommended Follow-Up |
|---|---|---|
| Optimal | <120/80 | Recheck in 2 years |
| Normal | <130/85 | Recheck in 2 years |
| High-normal | 130–139/85–89 | Recheck in 1 year |
| Stage 1 hypertension | 140–159/90–99 | Confirm within 2 months |
| Stage 2 hypertension | 160–179/100–109 | Evaluate or refer to care provider within 1 month |
| Stage 3 hypertension | ≥180/≥110 | Evaluate or refer to care provider immediately or within 1 week as indicated |

*Note. Adapted from* The Sixth Report of the Joint National Committee on Prevention, Detection, Education, and Treatment of High Blood Pressure, *NIH Publication No. 98-4080, by NHLBI, 1997, Bethesda, MD: National Institutes of Health. Available: http://www.nhlbi.nih.gov/guidelines/hypertension*

lifestyle with clients. Encourage all clients to eat a diet rich in fruits and vegetables and low in total and saturated fat. Discuss the potential benefits of maintaining an adequate calcium and potassium intake and provide lists of foods containing these nutrients. Advise all clients to remain active and engage in aerobic exercise 4 or more days a week. Discuss the stress-reducing benefits of exercise.

Offer blood pressure screening, and refer clients for follow-up as indicated (Table 33–3).

## Assessment

Focused assessment of the client with hypertension includes:

- Health history: complaints of morning headache, cervical pain; cardiovascular or central nervous system manifestations; history of hypertension, renal disease, diabetes; family history of high blood pressure, heart failure, or kidney disease; current medications
- Physical examination: vital signs including blood pressure in both arms, apical and peripheral pulses; ophthalmologic exam of retinal fundus

## Nursing Diagnoses and Interventions

All clients with primary hypertension and their families need significant teaching to manage this chronic condition. Health maintenance is a high-priority problem. Depending on the stage of hypertension and concurrent illnesses, other appropriate nursing diagnoses may include imbalanced nutrition, fluid volume excess, and risk for noncompliance.

### Ineffective Health Maintenance

Unhealthy lifestyle and behaviors can lead to health problems such as hypertension. When hypertension has been identified, knowledge of the disease and its management is vital for the client. Willingness to take responsibility for hypertension management is central to effective blood pressure control. Adopting healthy lifestyle changes enhances drug therapy; in some cases, the need for medications may be eliminated or reduced. Because hypertension is often an asymptomatic disease and many antihypertensive drugs have unpleasant side effects, it is vital that the client understand the chronic progressive nature of the disease and its long-term consequences.

- Assist with identifying current behaviors that contribute to hypertension. *The client must first identify contributory behaviors before he or she can change them. Using knowledge of hypertension risk factors, the nurse can help identify behaviors and factors contributing to hypertension that can be changed. Including the family in this process is important to reduce potential sabotage of the client's efforts to adopt healthier behaviors.*
- Assist in developing a realistic health maintenance plan. *Preparing a health maintenance plan for the client does little to encourage personal responsibility for health. However, nurses can guide clients in developing realistic goals and expectations for the treatment plan and modifying risk factors such as smoking, exercise, diet, and stress.*
- Help the client and family identify strengths and weaknesses in maintaining health. *Discussing areas of the health maintenance plan that are working well and those that present difficulties can help to identify necessary changes in the plan and additional strategies for implementing it.*

### Risk for Noncompliance

Noncompliance, or failure to follow the identified treatment plan, is a continuing risk for any client with a chronic disease. Recommended lifestyle changes such as diet, exercise, restricted alcohol intake, stress reduction, and smoking cessation often are difficult to maintain on a continuing basis. In addition, prescribed medications may have undesirable effects whereas hypertension itself often has no symptoms or noticeable effects.

- Inquire about reasons for noncompliance with recommended treatment plan. Listen openly and without judging. *Nonthreatening discussion of factors contributing to noncompliance validates the client's self-esteem and partnership in the treatment plan.*

**PRACTICE ALERT** *Work with the client to develop mutual outcomes for the treatment plan. Discuss measures to improve compliance. The client has absolute control over compliance with the treatment plan. Demonstrating respect and involving the client in decision making and planning can improve compliance.* ∎

- Evaluate knowledge of hypertension, its long-term effects, and treatment. Provide additional information and reinforce teaching as needed. *Knowledge increases the sense of control, which also increases the likelihood of compliance with treatment.*

**PRACTICE ALERT** *Assess factors contributing to non-compliance, such as adverse drug effects. Suggest measures to manage adverse effects or, if indicated, contact the primary care provider about possible alternative drugs. Some adverse effects of antihypertensive drugs, such as gastric upset, lightheadedness, or nocturia may be easily managed by changing the timing of the drug dose. Others, such as fatigue, decreased exercise tolerance, or impotence may interfere with lifestyle and life roles to the extent that the client finds them intolerable.* ■

- Assist to develop realistic short-term goals for lifestyle changes. *Attempting to lose weight, exercise daily, stop smoking, and dramatically change the diet all at the same time may be overwhelming, leading to a sense of failure. Smaller, gradual changes are more easily incorporated into lifestyle and daily activities, improving compliance.*
- Help the client identify cues and develop reminders (e.g., written notes, a medication box filled weekly) to assist with maintaining a schedule for exercise and medications. *Cues and other devices provide helpful reminders of activities and schedules until they are incorporated into habits.*
- Reassure the client that relapse into old habits and behaviors is common. Encourage avoiding feelings of guilt associated with relapse, and use the circumstance to renew efforts to comply with treatment. *Guilt and feelings of failure can lead to further noncompliance unless the event is used to identify reasons for noncompliance and ways to prevent it from recurring in the future.*

## Imbalanced Nutrition:
## More Than Body Requirements

The relationship between obesity, excess alcohol intake, and hypertension is well documented. Hypertension is particularly associated with central obesity, identified by waist circumference greater than hip circumference. While weight loss is difficult and takes commitment to changing eating and exercise habits, it is possible for most clients to achieve.

- Assess usual daily food intake, and discuss possible contributing factors to excess weight, such as sedentary lifestyle, or using food as a reward or stress reliever. Inquire about diversional activities, exercise patterns, and previous weight reduction efforts (e.g., participation in weight reduction programs or using fad or crash diets). *Assessment data provides clues about contributing factors to obesity, the client's knowledge base about the relationship between eating and exercise habits and weight, and safe weight loss strategies. This provides direction for further teaching and for developing a realistic weight reduction plan.*
- Mutually determine with the client a realistic target weight (e.g., loss of 10% of current body weight over a 6-month period). Regularly monitor weight. Encourage a system of nonfood rewards for achieving small, incremental goals. *Setting weight loss goals helps formalize the process and provides motivation for continued progress. Developing realistic goals may be difficult; unrealistic goals, however, set the client up for failure. Continuous incremental weight loss provides reassurance that it can be achieved and promotes permanent weight reduction.*

- Refer to a dietitian for information about low-fat, low-calorie foods and eating plans. Focus on changing eating habits as opposed to "following a diet." *Focusing on changing eating habits promotes the sense that low-fat, low-calorie eating patterns should become a part of lifestyle rather than a short-term measure to be endured until the weight loss goal is achieved.*
- Recommend participating in an approved weight loss program such as Weight Watchers, Overeaters Anonymous, or Take off Pounds Sensibly (TOPS). *Organized weight loss programs provide structure for a balanced weight reduction program, as well as mutual support from others trying to lose weight.*

## Excess Fluid Volume

Excess fluid volume often contributes to hypertension by increasing the cardiac output. A number of factors associated with hypertension can cause excess fluid volume, including sodium retention and disruption of the renin-angiotensin-aldosterone system. In addition, some antihypertensive drugs, such as calcium channel blockers and vasodilators, can contribute to excess fluid in the interstitial spaces and peripheral edema.

**PRACTICE ALERT** *Monitor blood pressure and other vital signs as indicated: every 1 to 2 hours or more frequently during acute hypertensive states; once a week or more frequently during initial treatment in the community. Vital signs are an indicator of fluid balance and the effectiveness of treatment. An elevated blood pressure, pulse, and respiratory rate may indicate fluid retention, whereas orthostatic hypotension and tachycardia may indicate fluid volume deficit.* ■

- Monitor intake and output, and weigh daily (if in an acute or long-term care facility) or weekly (in the community). *Rapid weight changes (over days) more accurately reflect fluid balance than intake and output records. One liter of fluid weighs 1 kg (2.2 lb). Weight changes and intake and output records help monitor the effects of therapy.*
- Monitor for peripheral edema (sacral edema in the bedridden client). *Drugs such as vasodilators can cause fluid accumulation in interstitial tissues, leading to peripheral or dependent edema. Adding a diuretic to the treatment plan may be necessary.*

**PRACTICE ALERT** *Monitor laboratory values, such as blood urea nitrogen (BUN), urine specific gravity, creatinine, electrolytes, and hematocrit and hemoglobin. Hypertension can alter renal perfusion and function, leading to fluid retention and altered laboratory values. Changes in BUN and creatinine indicate impaired renal function, whereas changes in hematocrit and hemoglobin often reflect changes in fluid volume.* ■

- Refer to a dietitian for teaching about a restricted sodium diet. Discuss the relationship between sodium intake and fluid retention. Provide opportunities to choose low-sodium foods from simulated menus. Support efforts, and reassure that lifestyle changes such as consuming less sodium take time. *Knowledge provides the power to take control of sodium intake. Patience and perseverance are needed to succeed; positive reinforcement of efforts to change long-standing dietary patterns is important.*

- Discuss the importance of adhering to treatment plans such as dietary restrictions and medication schedules. *Understanding the rationale for treatment measures promotes the client's sense of control and encourages compliance with the treatment regimen.*

## Using NANDA, NIC, and NOC

Chart 33–1 shows links between NANDA nursing diagnoses, NIC, and NOC for the client with hypertension.

## Home Care

Effective control of hypertension requires the client to not only participate in the plan of care, but also to take an active role in managing the disease. Treatment is managed in community settings, with regular visits to a clinic or office to monitor blood pressure and effects of treatment measures. Include the following topics when teaching the client and family about hypertension:

- Specific lifestyle changes recommended for the client and suggestions for implementing them. For example:
  - Increase activity gradually. Develop a realistic exercise program that is enjoyable and fits into lifestyle. Identify an exercise buddy for additional motivation. Activity and exercise, through a gradual conditioning of muscles and blood vessels, lower blood pressure by reducing peripheral vascular resistance. As the heart becomes conditioned and pumps more efficiently, kidney perfusion improves and intravascular volume falls, further reducing blood pressure.

Exercise also reduces stress and contributes to weight loss and maintenance. Aerobic exercise, such as walking, jogging, swimming, and cycling are appropriate; isometric activities (such as weight lifting) should be avoided without physician approval.

- Adopt healthy eating patterns, following a low-fat, low-cholesterol, moderate sodium diet that also is rich in fruits and vegetables and includes at least two servings of low-fat milk or milk products daily. Do not give up if you slip into old eating habits on occasion; use such occasions to identify ways to avoid future lapses.

- Stop smoking. Participating in organized smoking cessation programs or using aids such as nicotine patches can help.

- Use alcohol in moderation if at all, consuming no more than 1 oz of hard liquor, 5 oz of wine, or 12 oz of beer per day.

- Use stress-reducing techniques such as meditation, relaxation, deep breathing, and exercise to manage stress. Anger and hostility intensify vasoconstriction; channeling these emotions into more positive responses such as using a change process to modify factors that provoke these emotions can reduce their harmful effects on blood pressure.

- Prescribed medications, their intended effect, dose and timing, interactions, and possible adverse effects. Discuss effects that should be reported to the physician, and those that can be managed by the client or that will diminish over time.

- The importance of monitoring blood pressure and regular visits to the primary care provider or hypertension clinic to monitor treatment. During follow-up visits, assess the blood pressure and specific laboratory work (such as serum creatinine, BUN, and/or serum electrolytes) to evaluate the disease and the effects of antihypertensive medications.

Refer the client to community blood pressure clinics, and to home health services as needed for regular follow-up and reinforcement of teaching. Refer to a dietitian or to an organized weight loss program as indicated for further teaching and weight loss support.

## CHART 33–1 NANDA, NIC, AND NOC LINKAGES

### The Client with Hypertension

| NURSING DIAGNOSES | NURSING INTERVENTIONS | NURSING OUTCOMES |
|---|---|---|
| • Decisional Conflict | • Mutual Goal Setting<br>• Decision-Making Support | • Decision Making<br>• Information Processing |
| • Imbalanced Nutrition: More than Body Requirements | • Teaching: Prescribed Diet<br>• Weight Reduction Assistance | • Nutritional Status: Nutrient Intake<br>• Weight Control |
| • Ineffective Health Maintenance | • Self-Modification Assistance<br>• Self-Responsibility Facilitation | • Health-Promoting Behavior<br>• Treatment Behavior: Illness or Injury |
| • Noncompliance | • Health Education | • Adherence Behavior |

*Note. Data from* Nursing Outcomes Classification (NOC) *by M. Johnson & M. Maas (Eds.), 1997, St. Louis: Mosby;* Nursing Diagnoses: Definitions & Classification 2001–2002 *by North American Nursing Diagnosis Association, 2001, Philadelphia: NANDA;* Nursing Interventions Classification (NIC) *by J.C. McCloskey & G. M. Bulechek (Eds.), 2000, St. Louis: Mosby. Reprinted by permission.*

## Nursing Care Plan

## A Client with Hypertension

Margaret Spezia is a married, 49-year-old Italian American with eight children whose ages range from 3 to 18 years. For the past 2 months, Mrs. Spezia has had frequent morning headaches, and occasional dizziness and blurred vision. At her annual physical examination 1 month ago, her blood pressure was 168/104 and 156/94. She was instructed to reduce her fat and cholesterol intake, to avoid using salt at the table, and to start walking for 30 to 45 minutes daily. Mrs. Spezia returns to the clinic for follow-up.

### ASSESSMENT

While escorting Mrs. Spezia to the exam room and obtaining her weight, blood pressure, and history, Lisa Christos, RN, notices that Mrs. Spezia seems restless and upset. Ms. Christos says, "You look upset about something. Is everything OK?" Mrs. Spezia responds, "Well, my head is throbbing, and I'm sort of dizzy. I think I'm just overdoing it and not getting enough rest. You know, raising eight children is a lot of work and expense. I just started working part time so we wouldn't get behind in our bills. I thought the extra money might relieve some of my stress, but I'm not so sure that's really happening. I'm not getting any better and I'm worried that I'll lose my job or become disabled and that my husband won't be able to manage the children by himself. I really need to go home, but first, I want to get rid of this awful headache. Would you please get me a couple of aspirin or something?"

Mrs. Spezia's history shows a steady weight gain over the past 18 years. She has no known family history of hypertension. Physical findings include height 63 inches (160 cm), weight 225 lb (102 kg), T 99°F (37.2°C), P 100 regular, R 16, BP 180/115 (lying), 170/110 (sitting), 165/105 (standing), average 10-point difference in readings between right and left arm (lower on left). Skin cool and dry, capillary refill 4 seconds right hand, 3 seconds left hand. Mrs. Spezia's total serum cholesterol is 245 mg/dL (normal < 200 mg/dL). All other blood and urine studies are within normal limits. Based on analysis of the data, Mrs. Spezia is started on enalapril 5 mg and hydrochlorothiazide 12.5 mg in a combination drug (Vaseretic), and placed on a low-fat low-cholesterol, no-added-salt diet.

### DIAGNOSIS

- *Fatigue* related to effects of hypertension and stresses of daily life
- *Imbalanced nutrition: More than body requirements* related to excessive food intake
- *Ineffective health maintenance* related to inability to modify lifestyle
- *Deficient knowledge* related to effects of prescribed treatment

### EXPECTED OUTCOMES

- Reduce blood pressure readings to less than 150 systolic and 90 diastolic by return visit next week.

- Incorporate low-sodium and low-fat foods from a list provided into her diet.
- Develop a plan for regular exercise.
- Verbalize understanding of the effects of prescribed drug, dietary restrictions, exercise, and follow-up visits to help control hypertension.

### PLANNING AND IMPLEMENTATION

- Teach to take own blood pressure daily and record it, bringing the record to scheduled clinic visits.
- Teach name, dose, action, and side effects of her antihypertensive medication.
- Instruct to walk for 15 minutes each day this week, and to investigate swimming classes at the local pool.
- Discuss strategies for achieving a realistic weight loss goal.
- Refer for a dietary consultation for further teaching about fat and sodium restrictions.
- Discuss stress-reducing techniques, helping identify possible choices.

### EVALUATION

Mrs. Spezia returns to the clinic 1 week later. Her average blood pressure is now 148/88 mmHg. She has lost 1.5 lb, and states that her oldest daughter has suggested that they join a weight reduction program together. Mrs. Spezia is walking for an average of 20 minutes at a local mall each day. She verbalizes an understanding of her medication, and is taking it in the morning and before dinner each day. She met with the dietitian and discussed ways to reduce the sodium and fat in her diet. The dietitian provided a list of low-fat, low-sodium foods and recommended cookbooks to help Mrs. Spezia modify her cooking. Mrs. Spezia tells Ms. Christos, "I just can't believe how much better I feel already. My headaches are gone, and I've actually lost some weight—and I feel motivated to keep going. If I had only known how much better I could feel! I don't expect I'll ever go back to my old habits again; it's just not worth it!"

### Critical Thinking in the Nursing Process

1. Identify the factors that contributed to Mrs. Spezia's hypertension. Which were modifiable and which were not?
2. What is the rationale for reducing sodium and fat in Mrs. Spezia's diet?
3. Suppose your hypertensive client is homeless and has no source of income. How could you help ensure your client would follow the treatment plan? What would you do if the client did not follow it?
4. Discuss the role of stress in hypertension. What factors in Mrs. Spezia's life contribute to her stress level?
5. Develop a plan of care for the diagnosis, *Low self-esteem* related to obesity.

See Evaluating Your Response in Appendix C.

# THE CLIENT WITH SECONDARY HYPERTENSION

**Secondary hypertension** is elevated blood pressure resulting from an identifiable underlying process. It accounts for only 5% to 10% of identified cases of hypertension. Kidney disease and coarctation of the aorta are common causes of secondary hypertension. In older adults, renovascular disease is the most common cause of sudden hypertension. The pathophysiology of selected causes of secondary hypertension are summarized below.

- *Kidney disease.* Any disease that affects renal blood flow (e.g., renal artery stenosis) or renal function (e.g., glomerulonephritis, renal failure) can lead to hypertension. Disruption of the blood supply stimulates the renin-angiotensin-aldosterone system, with resulting vasoconstriction and sodium and water retention. Altered kidney function affects the elimination of water and electrolytes, leading to hypertension.

- *Coarctation of the aorta.* Coarctation of the aorta is narrowing of the aorta, usually just distal to the subclavian arteries. Reduced renal and peripheral blood flow stimulates the renin-angiotensin-aldosterone system and local vasoconstrictive responses, raising the blood pressure. A marked difference between pressures in the upper and lower extremities is common, with weak pulses and poor capillary refill in the lower extremities.

- *Endocrine disorders.* Adrenal gland disorders such as Cushing's syndrome and primary aldosteronism can cause hypertension. A rare tumor of the adrenal medulla, *pheochromocytoma*, causes persistent or intermittent hypertension. Other endocrine disorders such as hyperthyroidism and pituitary disorders also can lead to hypertension.

- *Neurologic disorders.* Increased intracranial pressure causes an elevated blood pressure as the body attempts to maintain cerebral blood flow. Disorders that interfere with autonomic nervous system regulation (such as high spinal cord injury) may allow the sympathetic nervous system to predominate, increasing systemic vascular resistance and blood pressure.

- *Drug use.* Estrogen and oral contraceptive use may lead to hypertension, possibly by prompting sodium and water retention and affecting the renin-angiotensin-aldosterone system. Stimulant drugs, such as cocaine and methamphetamines, increase systemic vascular resistance and cardiac output, resulting in hypertension.

- *Pregnancy.* About 10% of all pregnant women are hypertensive. Hypertension may predate pregnancy or occur as a direct response to the pregnancy. The mechanism of pregnancy-induced hypertension (PIH) is unclear. It is a significant cause of maternal and fetal morbidity and mortality and requires careful perinatal management.

The pattern of secondary hypertension varies, depending on its cause. Pheochromocytoma may cause attacks of hypertension that last for minutes to hours, accompanied by anxiety, palpitations, diaphoresis, pallor, and nausea and vomiting. Primary aldosteronism may cause hypertension, weakness, paresthesias, polyuria, and nocturia (see Chapter 17). ⊂⊃ Symptoms of kidney disease accompany hypertension when a renal disorder is the cause.

The following diagnostic tests may be ordered to differentiate primary from secondary hypertension.

- *Renal function studies* and *urinalysis* to identify renal causes of hypertension. Elevated serum creatinine and BUN, reduced creatinine clearance, and hematuria, proteinuria, and casts often indicate kidney disease.
- *Serum potassium* is decreased in hyperaldosteronism.
- *Blood chemistries,* including serum electrolytes, glucose, and lipid studies are done to detect abnormalities indicative of endocrine or cardiovascular disease.
- *Intravenous pyelography (IVP), renal ultrasonography, renal arteriography,* and *CT* or *MRI* may be done when secondary hypertension is suspected.

Collaborative and nursing care for the client with secondary hypertension is the same as that for primary hypertension, discussed in the previous section. In addition, the underlying process is treated. See chapters covering specific disorders for more information about treatment measures.

# THE CLIENT WITH HYPERTENSIVE CRISIS

Some clients with hypertension may, for reasons not clearly understood, develop rapid, significant elevations in systolic and/or diastolic pressures. In a *hypertensive emergency,* the systolic pressure may be greater than 240 mmHg and the diastolic pressure higher than 130 mmHg. Immediate treatment (within 1 hour) is vital to prevent cardiac, renal, and vascular damage, and reduce morbidity and mortality. Most hypertensive emergencies occur when clients suddenly stop taking their medications or their hypertension is poorly controlled. Manifestations of hypertensive emergencies are listed in the box below.

**Malignant hypertension** is a hypertensive emergency, marked by a diastolic pressure greater than 120 mmHg. It most commonly affects younger clients (30 to 50 years old), African American men, pregnant women with toxemia, and people with collagen and/or renal disease (Porth, 2002). Malignant hypertension must be rapidly diagnosed and aggressively (yet carefully) treated to prevent encephalopathy and irreversible renal and cardiac failure (Tierney et al., 2001). Intense cerebral artery spasms help protect the brain from excess pressure; however, cerebral edema often develops. It may cause manifestations such as headache, confusion, swelling of the optic nerve

## Manifestations of Hypertensive Emergencies

- Rapid onset
- Blurred vision, papilledema
- Systolic pressure >240 mmHg
- Diastolic pressure >130 mmHg
- Headache
- Confusion
- Motor and sensory deficits

**TABLE 33-4  Intravenous Drugs Used to Treat Hypertensive Emergencies**

| Type | Name | Onset | Duration | Nursing Tips |
|------|------|-------|----------|-------------|
| Vasodilator | Nipride | seconds | 3 to 5 min | • Most effective drug<br>• Easy to titrate |
| Vasodilator | Nitroglycerin | 2 to 5 min | 3 to 5 min | • Tolerances may develop |
| Vasodilator | Diazoxide (Hyperstat) | 1 to 2 min | 4 to 24 hr | • Avoided in clients with coronary artery disease<br>• Used with beta-blockers and diuretics<br>• Painful if it enters tissues |
| Vasodilator | Fenoldopam (Corlopam) | <5 min | 30 min | • Do not use concurrently with beta blockers<br>• Monitor for heart failure, ischemic heart disease (angina, MI) |
| Vasodilator | Hydralazine (Apresoline) | 10 to 30 min | 2 to 6 hr | • Avoided in clients with coronary artery disease |
| Beta/alpha blocker | Labetalol (Trandate) | 5 to 10 min | 3 to 6 hr | • Avoided in clients with heart failure and asthma |
| Beta blocker | Esmolol (Brevibloc) | 1 to 2 min | 10 to 30 min | • Avoided in clients with heart failure and asthma |
| ACE inhibitor | Enalaprilat (Vasotec) | 15 min | 6 hr or more | • Watch for hypotension |
| Diuretic | Furosemide (Lasix) | 15 min | 4 hr | • Watch for hypotension<br>• Watch for hypokalemia |
| Calcium channel blocker | Nicardipene (Cardene) | 1 to 5 min | 3 to 6 hr | • Watch for signs of myocardial ischemia |

(papilledema), blurred vision, restlessness, and motor and sensory deficits (Porth, 2002). Prolonged malignant hypertension damages walls of the arterioles and renal blood vessels, and may lead to intravascular coagulation and acute renal failure.

The goal of care in hypertensive emergencies is to reduce the blood pressure by no more than 25% within minutes to 2 hours, then toward 160/100 within 2 to 6 hours. It is important to avoid rapid or excessive blood pressure decreases that may lead to renal, cerebral, or cardiac ischemia (NHLBI, 1997). Blood pressure is monitored frequently (every 5 to 30 minutes) during a hypertensive emergency. The BUN, serum creatinine, calcium, and total protein levels are carefully monitored to help determine the prognosis for recovery. Drug treatment for malignant hypertension includes parenteral administration of a rapidly acting antihypertensive, such as the potent vasodilator sodium nitroprusside (Nipride). Other medications that may be used are outlined in Table 33-4. Management also focuses on treating any underlying or coexisting heart, kidney, and CNS disorders.

Nursing care for the client with a hypertensive emergency focuses on continuous monitoring of the blood pressure and titrating drugs (administered by intravenous bolus or infusion) as ordered to achieve desired blood pressure. Avoiding excessive or very rapid blood pressure reductions is as important as achieving the desired blood pressure readings. Reassure the client and family of the rapid effect of prescribed drugs. Provide psychologic and emotional support as needed. Maintain an attitude of confidence that the treatment will achieve the desired effect. Following resolution of the hypertensive crisis, review causes of the crisis. Teach the client and family measures to effectively manage hypertension and prevent future hypertensive emergencies.

# DISORDERS OF THE AORTA AND ITS BRANCHES

The aorta and its branches may be affected by occlusions, aneurysms, and inflammations. These disorders may be chronic or acute and life threatening (e.g., a thoracic dissection). This section focuses on aneurysms of the aorta and its branches.

## THE CLIENT WITH AN ANEURYSM

An **aneurysm** is an abnormal dilation of a blood vessel, commonly at a site of a weakness or a tear in the vessel wall.

Aneurysms commonly affect the aorta and peripheral arteries, because of the high pressure in these vessels. An aneurysm also may develop in the ventricular wall, usually affecting the left ventricle. Most arterial aneurysms are caused by arteriosclerosis or atherosclerosis; trauma also may lead to aneurysm formation.

Arterial aneurysms are most common in men over age 50, most of whom are asymptomatic at the time of diagnosis. Hypertension is a major contributing factor in the development of some types of aortic aneurysms.

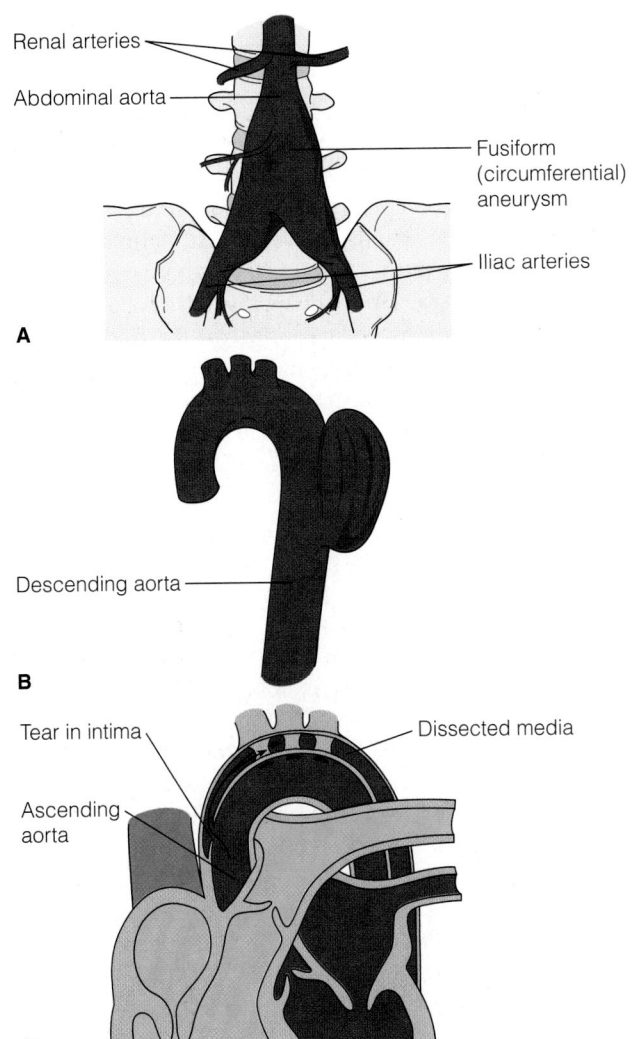

Renal arteries
Abdominal aorta
Fusiform (circumferential) aneurysm
Iliac arteries

**A**

Descending aorta

**B**

Tear in intima
Dissected media
Ascending aorta

**C**

**Figure 33–3** ■ Aortic aneurysms. *A,* Fusiform aneurysm of the abdominal aorta and iliac arteries. *B,* Saccular aneurysm of the descending thoracic aorta. *C,* Dissection of the ascending thoracic aorta.

*Source: Bullock & Henze,* Focus on Pathology *(2000). Philadelphia: Lippincott, Williams & Wilkins. Reprinted with permission.*

## PATHOPHYSIOLOGY AND MANIFESTATIONS

Aneurysms form due to weakness of the arterial wall. *True aneurysms* are caused by slow weakening of the arterial wall due to the long-term, eroding effects of atherosclerosis and hypertension. True aneurysms affect all three layers of the vessel wall, and most are fusiform and circumferential. *Fusiform aneurysms* are spindle shaped and taper at both ends (Figure 33–3A■). *Circumferential* aneurysms involve the entire diameter of the vessel. They generally grow slowly but progressively. Their length and diameter vary considerably among clients. A large fusiform aneurysm may affect most of the ascending aorta as well as a large portion of the abdominal aorta.

*False aneurysms,* also known as traumatic aneurysms, are caused by a traumatic break in the vessel wall rather than weakening of the vessel. They often are *saccular,* shaped like small outpouchings (sacs) on a portion of the vessel wall (Figure 33–3B). A *berry aneurysm* is a type of saccular aneurysm. They are often small (less than 2 cm in diameter), caused by congenital weakness in the tunica media of the artery. Berry aneurysms are commonly found in the circle of Willis.

*Dissecting aneurysms* are unique, developing when a break or tear in the tunica intima and media allows blood to invade or *dissect* the layers of the vessel wall. The blood usually is contained by the adventitia, forming a saccular or longitudinal aneurysm (Figure 33–3C).

Aneurysms affect different segments of the aorta and its branches. Their manifestations generally are due to pressure of the aneurysm on adjacent structures. Table 33–5 summarizes the manifestations and complications of various types of aortic aneurysms.

### Thoracic Aortic Aneurysms

*Thoracic aortic aneurysms* account for about 10% of aortic aneurysms. They usually result from weakening of the aortic wall by arteriosclerosis and hypertension (Tierney et al., 2001). Other causes include trauma, coarctation of the aorta, tertiary

| Type or Location | Manifestations | Complications |
|---|---|---|
| **TABLE 33–5** | Manifestations and Complications of Aortic Aneurysms | |
| Thoracic | • May be asymptomatic<br>• Back, neck, or substernal pain<br>• Dyspnea, stridor, or brassy cough if pressing on trachea<br>• Hoarseness and dysphagia if pressing on esophagus or laryngeal nerve<br>• Edema of the face and neck<br>• Distended neck veins | • Ruptured and hemorrhage |
| Abdominal | • Pulsating abdominal mass<br>• Aortic calcification noted on X-ray<br>• Mild to severe midabdominal or lumbar back pain<br>• Cool, cyanotic extremities if iliac arteries are involved<br>• Claudication (ischemic pain with exercise, relieved by rest) | • Peripheral emboli to lower extremities<br>• Rupture and hemorrage |
| Aortic dissection | • Abrupt, severe, ripping or tearing pain in area of aneurysm<br>• Mild or marked hypertension early<br>• Weak or absent pulses and blood pressure in upper extremities<br>• Syncope | • Hemorrhage<br>• Renal failure<br>• MI, heart failure, cardiac tamponade<br>• Sepsis<br>• Weakness or paralysis of lower extremities |

syphilis, fungal infections, and Marfan syndrome. The syphilis spirochete can invade and weaken aortic smooth muscle, causing an aneurysm to develop as long as 20 years after the primary infection. Marfan's syndrome fragments elastic fibers of the aortic media, weakening the vessel wall. (See the box on page 903 for more information about Marfan syndrome.)

Thoracic aneurysms frequently are asymptomatic. When present, symptoms vary by the location, size, and growth rate of the aneurysm. Substernal, neck, or back pain may occur. Pressure on the trachea, esophagus, laryngeal nerve, or superior vena cava may cause dyspnea, stridor, cough, difficult or painful swallowing, hoarseness, edema of the face and neck, and distended neck veins.

Aneurysms of the ascending aortic arch typically cause angina. Aneurysms of the aortic arch often cause dysphagia, dyspnea, hoarseness, confusion, and dizziness. Aneurysms of the thoracic aorta tend to enlarge progressively and may rupture, causing death.

## Abdominal Aortic Aneurysms

*Abdominal aortic aneurysms* are associated with arteriosclerosis and hypertension. Increasing age and smoking are believed to contribute as well. Most abdominal aortic aneurysms are found in adults over age 70. The vast majority (over 90%) develop below the renal arteries, usually where the abdominal aorta branches to form the iliac arteries.

Most abdominal aneurysms are asymptomatic, but a pulsating mass in the mid and upper abdomen and a bruit over the mass are found on exam. When pain is present, it may be constant or intermittent, usually felt in the midabdominal region or lower back. Its intensity may range from mild discomfort to severe pain. Pain intensity often correlates with the size and severity of the aneurysm. Severe pain may indicate impending rupture.

Sluggish blood flow within the aneurysm may cause thrombi (blood clots) to form. These can become emboli (circulating clots), traveling to the lower extremities and occluding peripheral arteries. The aneurysm may also rupture, with hemorrhage and hypovolemic shock. Rupture causes death before hospitalization in up to 50% of all clients; others die before surgery. Only about 10% to 20% of clients survive rupture of an abdominal aortic aneurysm.

## Popliteal and Femoral Aneurysms

Most popliteal and femoral aneurysms are due to arteriosclerosis. They are often bilateral and usually affect men.

*Popliteal aneurysms* may be asymptomatic. Manifestations, if any, are due to decreased blood flow to the lower extremity and include **intermittent claudication** (cramping or pain in the leg muscles brought on by exercise and relieved by rest), rest pain, and numbness. A pulsating mass may be palpable in the popliteal fossa (behind the knee). Thrombosis and embolism are complications; gangrene may result, often necessitating amputation.

A *femoral aneurysm* usually is detected as a pulsating mass in the femoral area. The manifestations are similar to those of popliteal aneurysms, resulting from impaired blood flow. Femoral aneurysms may rupture.

## Aortic Dissections

**Dissection** is a life-threatening emergency caused by a tear in the intima of the aorta with hemorrhage into the media. The hemorrhage dissects or splits the vessel wall, forming a blood-filled channel between its layers. Dissection can occur anywhere along the aorta. *Type A dissection* (also called *proximal dissection*) affects the ascending aorta; *type B dissection* (*distal dissection*) is limited to the descending aorta.

Hypertension is a major predisposing factor for aortic dissection. Other risk factors include male gender, advancing age, Marfan syndrome, pregnancy, congenital defects of the aortic valve, coarctation of the aorta, and inflammatory aortitis (Braunwald et al., 2001).

Dissection of the thoracic aortic walls progresses along the length of the vessel, moving both proximally and distally. As the aneurysm expands, pressure may prevent the aortic valve from closing or may occlude the branches of the aorta. Descending aortic dissection may extend into the renal, iliac, or femoral arteries.

The primary symptom of an aortic dissection is sudden, excruciating pain. The pain, often described as a ripping or tearing sensation, is usually over the area of dissection. Thoracic dissections cause chest or back pain. Other symptoms may include syncope, dyspnea, and weakness. The blood pressure may initially be increased, but rapidly falls and is often inaudible as the dissection occludes blood flow. Peripheral pulses are absent for the same reason.

Complications develop if major arteries are affected. Obstruction of the carotid artery causes neurologic symptoms such as weakness or paralysis. The myocardium, kidneys, or bowel may become ischemic or infarct. Acute aortic regurgitation may develop with dissection of the ascending aorta. With treatment, the long-term prognosis is generally good, although the in-hospital mortality rate following surgery is 15% to 20% (Braunwald et al., 2001).

## COLLABORATIVE CARE

Most aneurysms are asymptomatic, detected through a routine physical examination. Treatment depends on the size of the aneurysm. Small, asymptomatic aneurysms are often not treated; large aneurysms at risk for rupture require surgery.

## Diagnostic Tests

Diagnostic studies done to establish the diagnosis and determine the size and location of the aneurysm may include:

- *Chest X-ray* to visualize thoracic aortic aneurysms.
- *Abdominal ultrasonography* to diagnose abdominal aortic aneurysms.
- *Transesophageal echocardiography* to identify the specific location and extent of a thoracic aneurysm and to visualize a dissecting aneurysm.

- *Contrast-enhanced CT* or *MRI* allows precise measurements of aneurysm size.
- *Angiography* uses contrast solution injected into the aorta or involved vessel to visualize the precise size and location of the aneurysm.

## Medications

Thoracic aortic aneurysms are treated with long-term beta-blocker therapy and additional antihypertensive drugs as needed to control heart rate and blood pressure.

Clients with aortic dissection are initially treated with intravenous beta blockers such as propranolol (Inderal), metoprolol (Lopressor), labetalol (Normodyne), or esmolol (Brevibloc) to reduce the heart rate to about 60 BPM. Sodium nitroprusside (Nipride) infusion is started concurrently to reduce the systolic pressure to 120 mmHg or less. Calcium channel blockers also may be used. Direct vasodilators such as diazoxide (Hyperstat) and hydralazine (Apresoline) are avoided as they may actually worsen the dissection (Braunwald et al., 2001). Constant monitoring of vital signs, hemodynamic pressures (via Swan-Ganz catheter; see Chapter 30 ⊙⊙ for more information about hemodynamic hydrostatic pressure monitoring), and urine output are vital to ensure adequate perfusion of vital organs.

Following surgical correction of an aneurysm, anticoagulant therapy may be initiated. Heparin therapy is used initially, with conversion to oral anticoagulation prior to discharge. Many clients are maintained indefinitely on anticoagulant therapy; others may use lifelong, low-dose aspirin therapy to reduce the risk of clot formation.

## Surgery

Operative repair of aortic aneurysms is indicated when the aneurysm is symptomatic or expanding rapidly. Thoracic aneurysms more than 6 cm in diameter are surgically repaired; asymptomatic abdominal aneurysms greater than 5 cm in diameter may be repaired, depending on the client's operative risk factors. Type A dissections are repaired as soon as feasible; type B dissections may be surgically repaired, depending on the extent of involvement and risk for rupture (Braunwald et al., 2001).

An open surgical procedure in which the aneurysm is excised and replaced with a synthetic fabric graft is the standard treatment for expanding abdominal aortic aneurysms. Although the aneurysm walls may be excised, they usually are left intact and used to cover the graft (Figure 33–4 ■). Surgical repair of thoracic aneurysms is similar but more complex due to major vessels exiting at the aortic arch. Cardiopulmonary bypass is required if the ascending aorta is involved. The aortic valve also may be replaced during surgery. See the box on page 998 for nursing care of the client having surgery on the aorta.

Endovascular stent grafts are increasingly being used to treat abdominal aortic aneurysms. The stent, which consists of a metal sheath covered with polyester fabric, is placed percutaneously using fluoroscopy to guide its placement. Both straight and bifurcated grafts are available. This option may be pre-

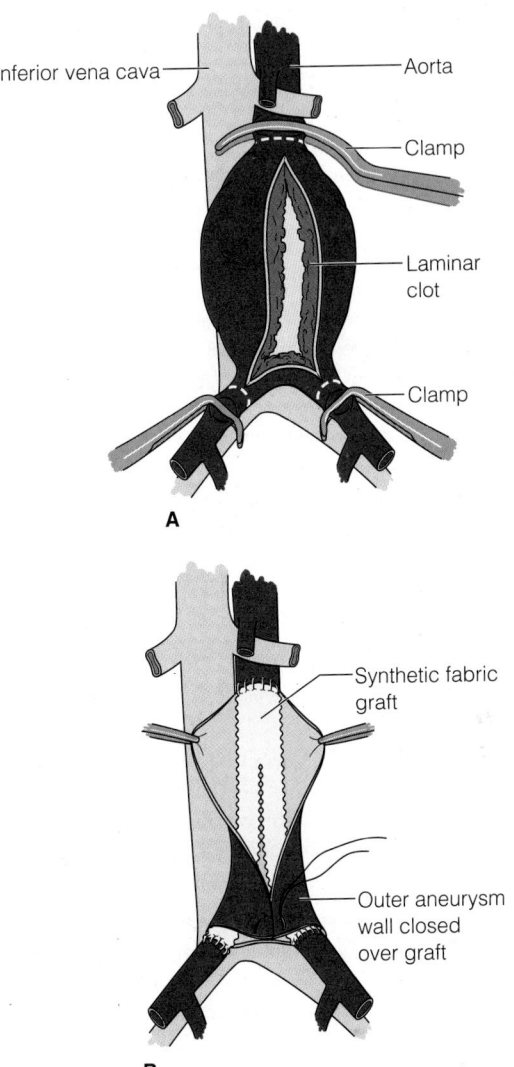

**Figure 33–4** ■ Repair of an abdominal aortic aneurysm. *A,* The aorta is exposed and clamped between the renal and iliac arteries. Atherosclerotic plaque and thrombotic material is removed. *B,* A synthetic graft is used to replace the aneurysm. The aneurysm walls are then sutured around the graft.

ferred in clients who have a high surgical risk (Meeker & Rothrock, 1999).

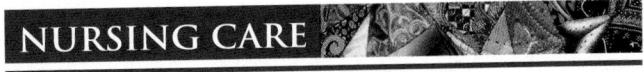

## NURSING CARE

### Assessment

Focused assessment for the client with a suspected aortic aneurysm includes:

- Health history: complaints of chest, back, or abdominal pain; extremity weakness; shortness of breath, cough, difficult or painful swallowing, hoarseness; history of hypertension, coronary heart disease, heart failure, or peripheral vascular disease

# NURSING CARE OF THE THE CLIENT HAVING SURGERY OF THE AORTA

## PREOPERATIVE CARE

- As time permits, provide routine preoperative care and teaching as outlined in Chapter 7. ⊕ *Clients having vascular surgery have similar preoperative nursing care needs to other clients having major abdominal or thoracic surgery. If emergent surgery is required, time for preoperative care and teaching may be limited.*
- Implement measures to reduce fear and anxiety:
  a. Orient to the intensive care unit, if appropriate.
  b. Describe and explain the reason for all equipment and tubes, such as cardiac monitors, ventilators, nasogastric tubes, urinary catheters, intravenous lines and fluids, and intra-arterial lines.
  c. Explain what to expect following surgery (sights, sounds, frequency of taking vital signs, dressings, pain relief measures, communication strategies).
  d. Allow time for questions and expression of fears and concerns.
  *These explanations provide a sense of control for the client and family.*

## POSTOPERATIVE CARE

- Provide routine postoperative care and specific measures as ordered by the physician. *Clients undergoing aneurysm repair require nursing care similar to that provided to all clients with major thoracic or abdominal surgery, in addition to specific measures related to vascular surgery.*

### PRACTICE ALERT

*Monitor for and report manifestations of graft leakage:*
  a. *Ecchymoses of the scrotum, perineum, or penis; a new or expanding hematoma*
  b. *Increased abdominal girth*
  c. *Weak or absent peripheral pulses; tachycardia; hypotension*

  d. *Decreased motor function or sensation in the extremities*
  e. *Fall in hemoglobin and hematocrit*
  f. *Increasing abdominal, pelvic, back, or groin pain*
  g. *Decreasing urinary output (less than 30 mL/ hour)*
  h. *Decreasing CVP, pulmonary artery pressure, or pulmonary artery wedge pressure*

*These manifestations may signal graft leakage and possible hemorrhage. Pain may be due to pressure from an expanding hematoma or bowel ischemia. Decreased renal perfusion causes the glomerular filtration rate and urine output to fall.* ■

- Maintain fluid replacement and blood or volume expanders as ordered. Promptly report changes in vital signs, level of consciousness, and urine output. *Hypovolemic shock may develop due to blood loss during surgery, third spacing, inadequate fluid replacement, and/or hemorrhage if graft separation or leakage occurs.*
- Report manifestations of lower extremity embolism: pain and numbness in lower extremities, decreasing pulses, and pale, cool, or cyanotic skin. *Pulses may be absent for 4 to 12 hours postoperatively due to vasospasm; however, absent pulses with pain, changes in sensation, and a pale, cool extremity are indicative of arterial occulsion.*
- Report manifestations of bowel ischemia or gangrene: abdominal pain and distention, occult or fresh blood in stools, and diarrhea. *Bowel ischemia may result from an embolism or occur as a complication of surgery.*
- Report manifestations of impaired renal function: urine output less than 30 mL per hour, fixed specific gravity, increasing BUN and serum creatinine levels. *Hypovolemia or clamping of the aorta during surgery may impair renal perfusion, leading to acute renal failure.*
- Report manifestations of spinal cord ischemia: lower extremity weakness or paraplegia. *Impaired spinal cord perfusion may lead to ischemia and impaired function.*

- Physical examination: vital signs including blood pressure in upper and lower extremities; peripheral pulses; skin color and temperature; neck veins; abdominal exam including gentle palpation for masses and auscultation for bruits; neurologic exam including level of consciousness, sensation, and movement of extremities

## Nursing Diagnoses and Interventions

Nursing care for clients with an aneurysm of the aorta or its branches focuses on monitoring and maintaining tissue perfusion, relieving pain, and reducing anxiety. Nursing care usually is acute, precipitated by a complication or surgical repair of the aneurysm.

## Risk for Ineffective Tissue Perfusion

Clients with aortic aneurysms are at risk for impaired tissue perfusion due to aneurysm rupture with resulting hemorrhage and lack of blood flow to tissues distal to the rupture. In addition, thrombi often form within the aneurysm and may become emboli, obstructing distal arterial blood flow.

### PRACTICE ALERT

*Immediately report manifestations of impending rupture, expansion, or dissection of the aneurysm: increased pain; discrepancy between upper and lower extremity blood pressures and peripheral pulses; increased mass size; change in LOC or motor or sensory function; laboratory results. Rapid expansion may indicate increased risk for rupture, with resulting hemorrhage, shock, and possible death. Elective or planned surgery may rapidly become emergency surgery to prevent complications.* ■

- Implement interventions to reduce the risk of aneurysm rupture:
  a. Maintain bed rest with legs flat.
  b. Maintain a calm environment, implementing measures to reduce psychologic stress.
  c. Prevent straining during defecation and instruct to avoid holding the breath while moving.
  d. Administer beta blockers and antihypertensives as prescribed.

*Activity, stress, and the Valsalva maneuver increase blood pressure, increasing the risk of rupture. Elevating or crossing the legs restricts peripheral blood flow and increases pressure in the aorta or iliac arteries. Beta blockers and antihypertensives often are ordered to reduce pressure in the dilated vessel.*

**PRACTICE ALERT** *Report manifestations of arterial thrombosis or embolism: absent peripheral pulses; a pale or cyanotic, cool extremity; severe, diffuse abdominal pain with guarding; or increased groin, lumbar, or lower extremity pain. Sluggish blood flow within the aneurysm often causes thrombi to form. These thrombi can break loose, becoming emboli that can occlude peripheral arteries or arteries to the kidneys or mesentery. Arterial occlusion may necessitate emergency surgery to restore blood flow and prevent tissue infarct or gangrene.* ■

- Continuously monitor cardiac rhythm. Report complaints of chest pain or changes in ECG tracing. Administer oxygen as indicated. *Aortic dissection and repair place the client at significant risk for myocardial infarction (MI), a major cause of postoperative mortality and morbidity (Braunwald et al., 2001). Rapid identification and treatment of this complication can reduce the risk of death or long-term adverse effects of MI.*

**PRACTICE ALERT** *Immediately report changes in mental status or symptoms of peripheral neurologic impairment (weakness, paresthesias, paralysis). The expanding aneurysm or dissection can affect carotid and cerebral blood flow or spinal cord perfusion, leading to neurologic symptoms. Immediate restoration of blood flow is vital to prevent permanent neurologic deficits.* ■

### Risk for Injury

Potent antihypertensive drugs often are given intravenously to reduce the pressure on an expanding or dissecting aneurysm. Continuous monitoring of infusions and hemodynamic parameters such as arterial pressure, pulmonary pressures, and cardiac output is vital to ensure that adequate tissue perfusion is maintained during infusions of these potent drugs.

**PRACTICE ALERT** *Use an infusion control device for all drug infusions. These devices prevent accidental or inadvertent changes in the rate of the infusion and dose of the drug.* ■

- Continuously monitor arterial pressure and hemodynamic parameters as indicated. Promptly report results outside the specified parameters to the physician. *Many of the drugs used are effective within minutes. Responses vary among individuals, particularly in the older adult, necessitating continuous monitoring.*
- Monitor urine output hourly. Report output less than 30 mL/hr. *The kidneys are very sensitive to reduced perfusion pressure; inadequate renal blood flow can lead to acute renal failure.*

### Anxiety

Clients with aortic aneurysms often are highly anxious because of the urgent nature of the disorder. The nurse must manage the anxiety levels of both the client and family members to effectively address physiologic care needs. Stress reduction also is necessary to help maintain the blood pressure within desired limits.

- Explain all procedures and treatments, using simple and understandable terms. *Simplified explanations are necessary when anxiety levels interfere with learning and understanding.*
- Respond to all questions honestly, using a calm, empathetic, but matter-of-fact manner. *Honesty with the client and family promotes trust and provides reassurance that the true nature of the situation is not being "hidden" from them.*
- Provide care in a calm, efficient manner. *Using a calm manner even during preparations for emergency surgery reassures the client and family that although the situation is critical, the staff is prepared to handle things effectively.*
- Spend as much time as possible with the client. Allow supportive family members to remain with the client when possible. *The presence of a health professional and supportive family member reassures the client that he or she is not alone in facing this crisis.*

### Home Care

Topics to discuss when preparing clients and their families for home care depend on the treatment plan. Discuss the following topics when surgical repair is not immediately planned and the aneurysm will be monitored.

- Measures to control hypertension, including lifestyle and prescribed drugs
- The benefits of smoking cessation
- Manifestations of increasing aneurysm size or complications to report to the physician

Following surgery, discuss the following topics in preparing the client and family for home care.

- Wound care and preventing infection; manifestations of impaired healing or infection to be reported
- Prescribed antihypertensive and anticoagulant medications and their expected and unintended effects
- The importance of adequate rest and nutrition for healing
- Measures to prevent constipation and straining at stool (such as increasing fluid and fiber in the diet)
- The importance of avoiding prolonged sitting, lifting heavy objects, engaging in strenuous exercise, and having sexual intercourse until approved by the physician (usually 6 to 12 weeks)
- Signs and symptoms of complications to report to the physician

Provide referrals to a home health agency or community health service as necessary. Referrals are especially important for older adults and their caregivers, who may require additional assistance with the complex care needs.

# DISORDERS OF THE PERIPHERAL ARTERIES

Disorders that impair peripheral arterial blood flow may be *acute* (e.g., arterial thrombosis) or *chronic* (e.g., peripheral arteriosclerosis). Chronic occlusive disorders may be due to structural defects of the arterial walls or spasm of affected arteries. Impaired peripheral arterial circulation limits the availability of oxygen and nutrients to the tissues, and can have significant adverse effects. This section focuses on acute and chronic disorders affecting peripheral arteries.

## PHYSIOLOGY REVIEW

Peripheral arteries are the part of the systemic circulation that delivers oxygen and nutrients to the skin and the extremities. Arterial walls have three layers: the intima, which includes the endothelium and a layer of connective tissue and the basement membrane; the media, composed of smooth muscle and elastic fibers; and the adventitia, a thin layer of connective tissue that contains elastic and collagenous fibers. The muscular peripheral arteries control blood flow as their smooth muscle contracts and relaxes. Contraction narrows the vessel lumen (**vasoconstriction**), whereas smooth muscle relaxation expands the vessel (**vasodilation**). Peripheral arteries become progressively smaller; arterioles are less than 0.5 mm in diameter and are primarily smooth muscle. The arterioles control blood flow through the capillary beds where gas, nutrient, and waste product exchange occurs. Capillary walls are very thin, consisting of a single layer of endothelial cells surrounded by a thin basement membrane.

Blood flows from an area of higher pressure to an area of lower pressure. *Resistance* opposes blood flow. Resistance is created by friction of the blood itself, although the primary determinants of vascular resistance are the diameter and length of the blood vessel. See the physiology review section under "The Client with Hypertension" for more information about factors that determine vessel resistance.

## THE CLIENT WITH ACUTE ARTERIAL OCCLUSION

A peripheral artery may be acutely occluded by development of a thrombus (blood clot) or by an embolism. Blood flow to tissues supplied by the artery is impaired, resulting in acute tissue ischemia and a risk for necrosis and gangrene.

## PATHOPHYSIOLOGY
### Arterial Thrombosis

A **thrombus** is a blood clot that adheres to the vessel wall. Thrombi tend to develop in areas where intravascular factors stimulate coagulation (e.g., where a vessel lumen is partially obstructed and its wall is damaged and roughened by atherosclerosis). Other disorders, such as infection or inflammation of the vessel wall or pooling of blood (e.g., in an aneurysm)

also can prompt coagulation and thrombus formation (Mc-Cance & Huether, 2002). A developing thrombus can occlude arterial blood flow through the vessel, leading to ischemia of tissues supplied by that artery. The extent of ischemia depends on the size of the affected artery and the degree of collateral circulation. In gradual processes of arterial occlusion such as atherosclerosis, collateral vessels often develop to compensate for impaired arterial flow. The extent of collateral circulation affects the degree of tissue ischemia distal to the thrombus.

### Arterial Embolism

An **embolism** is sudden obstruction of a blood vessel by debris. A thrombus can break loose from the arterial wall to become a **thromboembolus.** Other substances also can become emboli: atherosclerotic plaque, masses of bacteria, cancer cells, amniotic fluid, bone marrow fat, and foreign objects such as air bubbles or broken intravenous catheters. Regardless of cause, an embolus eventually lodges in a vessel that is too small to allow it to pass.

Arterial emboli often originate in the left side of the heart. They are associated with myocardial infarction, valvular heart disease, left-sided heart failure, atrial fibrillation, or infectious heart diseases. Emboli from the left heart often enter the carotid arteries and become trapped in the cerebral circulation, causing neurologic deficits (see Chapter 41). Thromboemboli that develop in the aorta or peripheral arterial circulation tend to lodge in areas where the arterial lumen is narrowed by atherosclerotic plaque and at arterial bifurcations.

### Manifestations

The manifestations of arterial thrombosis and embolism are those of tissue ischemia. Ischemic tissues are painful, pale, and cool or cold. Distal pulses are absent. Paresthesias (numbness and tingling) develop in the extremity. Cyanosis and mottling are common. Paralysis and muscle spasms may develop in the affected extremity. A line of demarcation between normal and ischemic tissue may be seen, particularly with embolism. Tissue below the line is cool or cold, and pale, cyanotic, or mottled. See the box below.

Arterial occlusion can result in permanent vessel and limb damage. Complete arterial occlusion leads to tissue necrosis and gangrene unless blood flow is promptly restored.

---

### Manifestations of Arterial Thrombosis and Embolus

- Pain
- Pallor or mottling
- Paresthesias (numbness and tingling)
- Cool or cold skin
- Pulselessness distal to the blockage
- Possible paralysis, weakness, or muscle spasms
- Possible line of demarcation; with pallor, cyanosis, and cooler skin distal to the blockage (especially with arterial embolism)

## COLLABORATIVE CARE

Acute arterial occlusions may require emergency treatment to preserve the limb if the obstructed vessel is large or collateral circulation is minimal. If the limb is not in jeopardy, more conservative management may be initiated.

### Diagnostic Tests

The diagnosis of acute arterial occlusion often is apparent by the signs and symptoms. *Arteriography* is used to confirm the diagnosis, locate the occlusion, and determine its extent.

### Medications

Anticoagulation with intravenous heparin is initiated to prevent further clot propagation and recurrent embolism. Anticoagulation is continued with oral anticoagulants after discharge. See the section on deep vein thrombosis later in this chapter for more information about anticoagulant therapy.

Arterial thrombosis may be treated with intra-arterial thrombolytic therapy using streptokinase, urokinase, or tissue plasminogen activator (t-PA) (see Chapter 29). ⊂⊃ Lysis of the thrombus or embolus is achieved in 50% to 80% of the cases (Tierney et al., 2001). Local intra-arterial injection of the thrombolytic drug allows use of lower doses and reduces the bleeding risk associated with thrombolytic drugs.

### Surgery

Immediate *embolectomy* (within 4 to 6 hours) is the treatment of choice for acute arterial occlusion by an embolus to prevent tissue necrosis and gangrene. When the involved vessel is in an extremity, local anesthesia and a special balloon-tipped catheter known as a Fogarty catheter may be used for high surgical risk clients (Tierney et al., 2001). An embolus in the mesenteric circulation necessitates emergency laparotomy. The risk of complications and limb loss increases significantly if surgery is delayed by 12 or more hours. Potential major complications include compartment syndrome (see Chapter 38), acute respiratory distress syndrome (Chapter 36), or acute renal failure (Chapter 27). ⊂⊃

Arterial thrombosis also may be treated surgically, although the required surgery may be more extensive due to the length of the vessel involved. *Thromboendarterectomy* is done to remove the thrombus and plaque in the artery. An arterial graft may be required. Nursing care for clients who have undergone embolectomy or thrombus removal is discussed in the nursing care section that follows.

## NURSING CARE

### Assessment

Nursing assessment for the client with an acute arterial occlusion is highly focused due to the emergency nature of the problem.

- Health history: complaints of pain, numbness, tingling, or weakness in the involved extremity; history of atheroscle-

rotic vessel disease, heart disease, or recent invasive procedure (e.g., angiography, percutaneous revascularization procedure)
- Physical examination: vital signs; peripheral pulses in both extremities; color, temperature, sensation, and movement of involved extremity; skin condition; presence of a line of demarcation

### Nursing Diagnoses and Interventions

Nursing care related to acute arterial occlusion focuses on protecting the affected extremity, managing anxiety, and reducing the risk of complications related to anticoagulant therapy.

#### Ineffective Tissue Perfusion: Peripheral

Protecting ischemic tissue from injury prior to surgery or medical thrombolysis is vital. Following surgery, there is a risk for thrombosis at the graft site or impaired perfusion due to edema of the surgical site.

> **PRACTICE ALERT**   *Monitor extremity perfusion, comparing affected and unaffected extremities. Assess peripheral pulses (using the Doppler stethoscope as needed), skin temperature and color, capillary refill, movement, and sensation every 1 to 4 hours. Promptly report changes or complaints of increased or unrelieved pain. Propagation of a thrombus can further obstruct arterial flow, increasing tissue ischemia. Following surgery, arterial spasms may cause a cyanotic, pulseless extremity; normal color and pulses should return within 12 hours. A thrombus may form at the surgical site or within a graft, causing tissue ischemia with pain and other manifestations of arterial occlusion. Further measures to restore circulation may be necessary.* ∎

- Maintain intravenous fluids as ordered. *Adequate circulating blood volume is necessary to maintain cardiac output and tissue perfusion.*
- Protect the extremity, keeping it horizontal or lower than the heart. Use a cradle to keep bedclothes off the extremity and sheepskin or foam pad to protect it from hard or abrasive surfaces. Do not apply heat or cold. *Keeping the extremity lower than the heart promotes collateral blood flow. Ischemic tissue is easily damaged by minimal trauma such as shearing by bed linens, or heat or cold application.*
- Following surgery, avoid raising the knee gatch, placing pillows under the knees, or sitting with 90-degree hip flexion. *These activities may impair blood flow through the affected vessel.*

#### Anxiety

Clients with an acute arterial occlusion often are very anxious. The rapid and intense nature of preoperative activities can be overwhelming, increasing anxiety about the disorder and its outcome. Manifestations of anxiety may include trembling, palpitations, restlessness, dry mouth, helplessness, inability to relax, irritability, forgetfulness, and lack of awareness of surroundings. Nursing measures focus on establishing trust and minimizing the effects of anxiety to decrease surgical risk and improve recovery.

- Spend as much time as possible with the client. Provide opportunities to verbalize anxiety; offer reassurance and support. Support adaptive coping mechanisms. *The presence of a caring nurse provides a safe environment for expressing fears and anxieties. Coping mechanisms reduce the immediate perceived threat and increase the ability to deal with the situational crisis.*

- Perform required measures in an expedient but calm manner. *Calm, confident performance of treatment measures reassures the client and family that appropriate care is being given to treat the problem at hand.*

- Assess anxiety level at least every 8 hours; more often as needed. Intervene as indicated to reduce anxiety. *Assessment helps determine the intensity of anxiety, the client's ability to control it, and directs interventions to reduce it.*

- Decrease sensory stimuli as much as possible. *Reducing environmental stimuli provides the client a degree of control over anxiety.*

- Speak slowly and clearly and avoid unnecessary interruptions when listening. Give concise directions, focusing on the present. Involve the client in simple tasks and decisions to the extent possible. *High levels of anxiety interfere with learning. Keeping interactions focused on the present situation directs the client's focus and provides reassurance that it is the most important focus of the nurse as well. Providing opportunities for self-care and decision making reinforces the client's importance and power to control the situation.*

### Altered Protection

Thombolytic and/or anticoagulant therapy used to dissolve existing clots and prevent further clot formation increase the risk for bleeding. Close monitoring of physical status and laboratory data is vital, as are measures to reduce the risk for injury and bleeding.

**PRACTICE ALERT** *Assess for and report manifestations of impaired clotting, including excessive incisional bleeding; prolonged oozing from injection sites; bleeding gums, nose bleed, or hematuria; petechiae, bruising, or purpura. Anticoagulants and thrombolytics interfere with the clotting cascade and may cause abnormal bleeding.* ■

- Monitor activated partial thromboplastin time (APTT) during heparin therapy and prothrombin time (PT) or international normalized ratio (INR) during oral anticoagulant therapy. Report values outside desired range. *The APTT, PT, and INR are prolonged by anticoagulant therapy. Values higher than the desired range may indicate an increased risk for bleeding; values below the target may indicate inadequate anticoagulation.*

- Protect from injury: Use side rails or other measures as needed to prevent falls; avoid parenteral injections and other invasive procedures as much as possible; hold firm pressure over injection and intravenous sites for 5 minutes and over arterial punctures for 20 minutes; use a soft toothbrush or sponge for oral care; use an electric razor for shaving. *Minor trauma can lead to extensive bleeding, particularly in the client who has received a thrombolytic drug.*

## Home Care

When preparing the client and family for home care related to an acute arterial occlusion, discuss the following topics as indicated.

- Care of the incision
- Manifestations of complications to be reported, including symptoms of infection or occlusion of the graft or artery
- Long-term anticoagulant therapy, including the reason, prescribed dose, follow-up laboratory testing and appointments, interactions with other drugs, and manifestations of excessive bleeding
- Any activity restrictions or dietary modifications
- Lifestyle modifications to slow atherosclerosis and control hypertension
- Measures to promote peripheral circulation and maintain tissue integrity (see the discussion of peripheral atherosclerosis that follows)

Refer for home care services (nursing care, physical therapy, housekeeping services) as indicated.

## THE CLIENT WITH PERIPHERAL ATHEROSCLEROSIS

*Arteriosclerosis* is the most common chronic arterial disorder, characterized by thickening, loss of elasticity, and calcification of arterial walls. **Atherosclerosis** is a form of arteriosclerosis in which deposits of fat and fibrin obstruct and harden the arteries. In the peripheral circulation, these pathologic changes impair the blood supply to peripheral tissues, particularly the lower extremities. This is known as **peripheral vascular disease (PVD)**.

PVD usually affects people in their 60s and 70s; men are more often affected than women. Deaths attributed to peripheral arterial disease are about the same for black and white males, but are higher among black women than white women (NHLBI, 2002).

Risk factors for PVD are similar to those for atherosclerosis and coronary heart disease (see Chapter 29). ⊖⊃ Diabetes mellitus, hypercholesterolemia, hypertension, cigarette smoking, and high homocystine levels are clear risk factors for PVD (Brauwald et al., 2001).

## PATHOPHYSIOLOGY

The pathophysiology of atherosclerosis is detailed in Chapter 29. ⊖⊃ Atherosclerotic lesions involve both the intima and the media of the involved arteries. Lesions typically develop in large and midsize arteries, particularly the abdominal aorta and iliac arteries (30% of symptomatic clients), the femoral and popliteal arteries (80% to 90% of clients), and more distal arteries (40% to 50% of clients) (Braunwald et al., 2001). Arteriosclerosis in the abdominal aorta leads to the development of aneurysms as plaque erodes the vessel wall.

Plaque tends to form at arterial bifurcations. The vessel lumen is progressively obstructed, decreasing blood flow to the

## Manifestations of Peripheral Atherosclerosis

- Intermittent claudication
- Rest pain
- Paresthesias (numbness, decreased sensation)
- Diminished or absent peripheral pulses
- Pallor with extremity elevation, dependent rubor when dependent
- Thin, shiny, hairless skin; thickened toenails
- Areas of discoloration or skin breakdown

lower extremities. Tissue hypoxia or anoxia results. With gradual obstruction of the vessel, collateral circulation often develops. However, it is usually not adequate to supply tissue needs, especially when metabolic demand increases (e.g., during exercise). Manifestations typically develop only when the vessel is occluded by 60% or more.

## MANIFESTATIONS AND COMPLICATIONS

Pain is the primary symptom of peripheral atherosclerosis. **Intermittent claudication,** a cramping or aching pain in the calves of the legs, the thighs, and the buttocks that occurs with a predictable level of activity, is characteristic of PVD. The pain is often accompanied by weakness and is relieved by rest.

*Rest pain,* in contrast, occurs during periods of inactivity. It is often described as a burning sensation in the lower legs. Rest pain increases when the legs are elevated and decreases when the legs are dependent (e.g., hanging over the side of the bed). The legs also may feel cold or numb along with the pain. Sensation is diminished and the muscles may atrophy.

Peripheral pulses may be decreased or absent. A bruit may be heard over large affected arteries, such as the femoral artery and the abdominal aorta. The legs are pale when elevated, but often are dark red (*dependent rubor*) when dependent. The skin often is thin, shiny, and hairless, with discolored areas. Toenails may be thickened. Areas of skin breakdown and ulceration may be evident. Edema may develop with severe PVD. See the box above for manifestations of peripheral atherosclerosis.

Complications of peripheral atherosclerosis include gangrene and extremity amputation, rupture of abdominal aortic aneurysms, and possible infection and sepsis.

## COLLABORATIVE CARE

Management of peripheral atherosclerosis focuses on slowing the atherosclerotic process and maintaining tissue perfusion.

### Diagnostic Tests

Although PVD often can be diagnosed by the history and physical examination, diagnostic tests may be ordered to evaluate its extent. Noninvasive studies often are sufficient.

- *Segmental pressure measurements* use sphygmomanometer cuffs and a Doppler device to compare blood pressures between the upper and lower extremities (normally similar)

and within different segments of the affected extremity. In PVD, the BP may be lower in the legs than in the arms.
- *Stress testing* using a treadmill provides functional assessment of limitations. In PVD, pressure at the ankle may decline even further with exercise, confirming the diagnosis. Evaluation for coronary heart disease may be done simultaneously during exercise testing (Braunwald et al., 2001).
- *Doppler ultrasound* uses sound waves reflected off moving red blood cells within a vessel to evaluate blood flow. The impulses may be translated into an audible signal or a graphic waveform. With significant PVD, the waveform becomes progressively flatter as the transducer is moved distally along the affected vessel. Segmental pressures may be used to locate the site of obstruction.
- *Duplex Doppler ultrasound* combines the audible or graphic Doppler ultrasound with ultrasound imaging to identify arterial or venous abnormalities. Ultrasonic imaging provides views of the affected vessel while Doppler ultrasound evaluates blood flow. *Color-flow Doppler ultrasound (CDU)* provides color images of the vessel and blood flow.
- *Transcutaneous oximetry* evaluates oxygenation of tissues.
- *Angiography* or *magnetic resonance angiography* is done before revascularization procedures to locate and evaluate the extent of arterial obstruction. For angiography, a contrast medium is injected and vessels are visualized using fluoroscopy and X-rays. Magnetic resonance angiography does not require injection of a contrast medium and may replace angiography.

### Medications

Drug treatment of peripheral atherosclerosis is less effective than with coronary heart disease. Medications to inhibit platelet aggregation, such as aspirin or clopidogrel (Plavix) are ordered to reduce the risk of arterial thrombosis. Cilostazol (Pletal), a platelet inhibitor with vasodilator properties, improves claudication. Pentoxifylliune (Trental) decreases blood viscosity and increases red blood cell flexibility, increasing blood flow to the microcirculation and tissues of the extremities. Parenteral vasodilator prostaglandins may be given on a long-term basis to decrease pain and facilitate healing in clients with severe limb ischemia (Braunwald et al., 2001).

### Treatments

Smoking cessation is vital. Nicotine not only promotes atherosclerosis, but also causes vasospasm, further reducing blood flow to the extremities.

Meticulous foot care is vital to prevent ulceration and infection (Box 33–4). Elastic support hose, which reduce circulation to the skin, are avoided. Elevating the head of the bed on blocks may help relieve rest pain. Regular, progressively strenuous exercise, such as 30 to 45 minutes of walking daily, is important. The client is taught to rest at the onset of claudication, resuming activity when the pain resolves.

Other measures to slow the process of atherosclerosis, such as controlling diabetes and hypertension, lowering cholesterol levels, and weight loss, also are recommended (see Chapter 29). See the box on page 1004 for care of the older adult.

| BOX 33–4 | ■ Foot Care for the Client with Peripheral Atherosclerosis |

1. Keep legs and feet clean, dry, and comfortable.
   - Wash legs and feet daily in warm water, using mild soap.
   - Pat dry using a soft towel; be sure to dry between the toes.
   - Apply moisturizing cream to prevent drying.
   - Use powder on the feet and between the toes.
   - Buy shoes in the afternoon (when feet are largest); never buy shoes that are uncomfortable. Be sure toes have adequate room.
   - Wear a clean pair of cotton socks each day.
2. Prevent accidents and injuries to the feet.
   - Always wear shoes or slippers when getting out of bed.
   - Walk on level ground and avoid crowds, if possible.
   - Do not go barefoot.
   - Inspect legs and feet daily; use a mirror to examine backs of legs and bottoms of feet.
   - Have a professional foot care provider trim toenails and care for corns, calluses, ingrown toenails, or athlete's foot.
   - Always check the temperature of the water before stepping into the tub.
   - Do not get the legs or tops of the feet sunburned.
   - Report leg or foot problems (increased pain, cuts, bruises, blistering, redness, or open areas) to your health care provider.
3. Improve blood supply to the legs and feet.
   - Do not cross legs.
   - Do not wear garters or knee stockings.
   - Do not swim or wade in cold water.

## Revascularization

Revascularization may be done if symptoms are progressive, severe, or disabling. Other indications for surgery include symptoms that significantly interfere with activities of daily living, rest pain, and pregangrenous or gangrenous lesions. Either nonsurgical revascularization procedures or surgery may be performed.

Nonsurgical procedures include percutaneous transluminal angioplasty (PTA), stent placement, or atherectomy. Techniques may include balloon angioplasty to dilate the narrowed lumen, mechanical atherectomy to remove plaque, or laser or thermal angioplasty to vaporize the occluding material. Iliac and femoral-popliteal PTA initially reestablish good blood flow and relieve symptoms in more than 80% of clients. While the 3-year success rate is lower, stent placement improves the duration of symptom relief (Braunwald et al., 2001). See Chapter 29 ⊚⊃ for more information about revascularization procedures.

Surgical options include endarterectomy to remove occlusive plaque from the artery and bypass grafts. Knitted Dacron bypass grafts are commonly used. Both immediate and long-term graft patency is better with bypass grafting than with nonsurgical revascularization procedures, but the risk for operative complications such as myocardial infarction, stoke, infection, and peripheral embolization is higher (Braunwald et al., 2001). Nursing care for the client having revascularization surgery is similar to that provided for clients having an aortic aneurysm repair (see the box on page 998).

## Complementary Therapies

Complementary therapies for peripheral vascular disease include interventions to improve circulation and to reduce stress. A number of complementary therapies may improve peripheral circulation, including aromatherapy with rosemary or vetiver; biofeedback; healing or therapeutic touch and massage; herbals such as ginko, garlic, cayenne, hawthorn, and bilberry; and exercise including yoga. Aromatherapy and yoga also may reduce stress, as can breathing exercises, meditation, and counseling. In addition, complementary therapies to reduce atherosclerosis and lower cholesterol levels may slow the progress of PVD. Measures such as a very low-fat or vegetarian diet, including antioxidant nutrients or using vitamin C, vitamin E, or garlic supplements, and traditional Chinese medicine may be useful.

## NURSING CARE

### Health Promotion

Discuss healthy lifestyle habits with community and religious groups, school children (grades K through 12), and through the print media to reduce the incidence and slow the progression of atherosclerosis.

Strongly encourage all clients to avoid smoking in the first place, and to stop all forms of tobacco use. Discuss the adverse effects of smoking and the benefits of quitting. Provide information about dietary recommendations to maintain a healthy

## Nursing Care of the Older Adult

### PERIPHERAL ATHEROSCLEROSIS

With aging, blood vessels thicken and become less compliant. These changes reduce oxygen delivery to the tissues and impair carbon dioxide and waste product removal from the tissues. When normal effects of aging combine with an increased risk of atherosclerosis, the risk of peripheral vascular disease is high.

The older adult with peripheral atherosclerosis requires the same care and teaching as other clients. However, visual deficits and osteoarthritis may make foot care more difficult. Long-standing smoking habits are difficult to break. Mobility may be impaired by arthritis or the effects of neurologic disorders. The client who lives alone may resist walking. Periodic visits by a community or home health nurse may be helpful, as may be encouraging the client to join a support group for stopping smoking, changing eating habits, and taking part in regular activity.

weight and optimal cholesterol levels. Discuss the benefits and importance of regular exercise. Finally, encourage clients with cardiovascular risk factors to undergo regular screening for hypertension, diabetes, and hyperlipidemia.

## Assessment

Focused assessment related to peripheral atherosclerosis includes the following:

- Health history: complaints of pain, its relationship to exercise or rest, timing, associated symptoms, and relief measures; history of coronary heart disease, peripheral vascular disease, hyperlipidemia, hypertension, or diabetes; current medications; smoking history; usual diet and activity patterns
- Physical examination: vital signs; strength and equality of peripheral pulses of all extremities; capillary refill; skin color, temperature, hair distribution, presence of any discolorations or lesions; movement and sensation of lower extremities

## Nursing Diagnoses and Interventions

Impaired tissue perfusion is an obvious problem in peripheral atherosclerosis. Acute and chronic pain may interfere with activities of daily living, and ambulation may be limited. The possibility of losing a lower extremity is frightening. For a summary of clients' concerns about peripheral atherosclerosis see the Nursing Research box below.

### Ineffective Tissue Perfusion: Peripheral

Impaired blood flow to the lower extremities affects gas, nutrient, and waste product exchange between the capillaries and cells. Oxygen and nutrient deprivation impairs cell function and tissue integrity, causing pain and impaired healing. Pain develops with exercise and when extremities are elevated.

- Assess peripheral pulses, pain, color, temperature, and capillary refill every 4 hours and as needed. Use a Doppler device if pulses are not palpable. Mark pulse locations with an indelible marker. *Assessment data provide a baseline for evaluating the effectiveness of interventions and identifies changes in arterial blood flow.*
- Position with extremities dependent. *Gravity promotes arterial flow to the dependent extremity, increasing tissue perfusion and relieving pain.*

**PRACTICE ALERT** *Instruct to avoid smoking. If necessary, obtain an order for a nicotine patch or gum from the physician. Nicotine is a potent vasoconstrictor that further impairs arterial blood flow. Smoking cessation is a vital component of care. Nicotine patches and gum contain less nicotine than cigarettes, and can help reduce the stress of smoking cessation.* ∎

- Discuss the benefits of regular exercise. *Exercise promotes development of collateral circulation to ischemic tissues and slows the process of atherosclerosis.*
- Use a foot cradle and lightweight blankets, socks, and slippers to keep extremities warm. Avoid electric heating pads or hot water bottles. *Keeping extremities warm conserves heat, prevents vasospasm, and promotes arterial flow. External heating devices are avoided to reduce the risk of burns in the client with impaired sensation. The foot cradle protects tissues from compression by linens.*
- Encourage frequent position changes. Instruct to avoid crossing legs or using a pillow under the knees. *Position changes promote blood flow and reduce damage caused by pressure. Leg crossing and excessive flexion of the hip or knee joints can compress partially obstructed arteries and impair blood flow to distal tissues.*

## Nursing Research

### Evidence-Based Practice for the Client with Peripheral Atherosclerosis

Peripheral vascular disease (PVD) affects millions of people in the United States. Peripheral atherosclerosis, a common type of PVD, develops insidiously as the arteries of the legs are gradually occluded by atherosclerotic plaque, causing symptoms such as intermittent claudication, ulceration, and gangrene. This study explored the lived experience of PVD, identifying key themes and categories through one-to-one interviews with a group of clients who had vascular bypass surgery within the past 18 months (Gibson & Kenrick, 1998). Major and minor categories and their interrelationships were identified. Powerlessness related to the direct effects of PVD and its treatment was a common theme. Clients often had unrealistic expectations of treatment measures such as surgery. Unrealistic expectations, in turn, led to the sense of powerlessness.

#### IMPLICATIONS FOR NURSING

Nurses may assume that clients with PVD understand the chronicity of their condition and the need to continue strategies to slow the process of atherosclerosis following bypass surgery. Clients, in contrast, may see surgery as curative, and the need to continue following a low-fat diet, smoking abstinence, and skin care precautions as indicative of failure. Nursing interventions to promote independence, manage pain, and reduce anxiety are vital. Teaching self-management and providing psychologic support can reduce the sense of powerlessness and improve quality of life.

#### Critical Thinking in Client Care

1. Teaching about leg and foot care is an important intervention for clients with PVD. What normal changes of aging (such as decreased visual acuity) might necessitate adaptations of a teaching plan?
2. React to the statement: Decreased mobility means decreased independence. What aspects of independent living are threatened if this statement is true?
3. You are providing immediate postoperative care to a client who has had abdominal surgery and also has peripheral arterial occlusive disease. How will the latter affect your assessments and interventions for this client?
4. While making a home visit, your client tells you he is very worried that his leg might be amputated. How would you respond?

## Pain

Impaired blood flow results in tissue ischemia. Metabolism shifts from an efficient aerobic process to an anaerobic process. Lactic acid and metabolic waste products accumulate in tissues, causing pain. Severe and cramping pain generally occurs with exercise early in the disease. Rest initially produces relief, similar to the process of angina (see Chapter 29). ⊂⊃ As the disease progresses, pain develops with less exercise and often occurs even at rest. Rest pain disrupts sleep, the sense of well-being, and has significant disruptive effects on life roles.

- Assess pain at least every 4 hours; using a standard pain scale more often as needed. *Pain is a subjective experience. Using a standard pain scale allows evaluation of treatment measures in relieving pain and restoring blood flow.*
- Keep extremities warm. *Cooling leads to vasoconstriction, increasing pain. Warming the extremities promotes vasodilation and improves arterial flow, reducing pain.*
- Teach pain relief and stress reduction techniques such as relaxation, meditation, and guided imagery. *Pain increases stress. The stress response leads to vasoconstriction, increasing pain. Stress reduction techniques, when combined with other measures to promote blood flow, can help reduce pain.*

## Impaired Skin Integrity

Clients with PVD are at risk for impaired skin integrity as a result of oxygen and nutrient deprivation. Chronic tissue ischemia leads to dry, scaly, and atrophied skin. Pruritus can lead to scratching; minor injuries may go unnoticed due to impaired sensation. Impaired tissue healing can lead to ulceration, infection, and potential gangrene.

**PRACTICE ALERT** *Assess and document skin condition at least every 8 hours a with each home visit; more frequently as indicated. Tissue ischemia increases the risk for damage, even with minor trauma such as pressure from poorly fitting shoes or bed linens. Frequent inspection and documentation of skin condition is vital to identify early indicators of impaired skin integrity and reduce the risk of complications such as infection.* ∎

- Provide meticulous daily skin care, keeping the skin clean and dry. Apply a moisturizing cream to dry or scaly areas. *Intact skin is the body's first defense against bacterial invasion. Ischemic tissues of the injured extremity provide an excellent medium for microorganism growth. Clean, dry, supple skin decreases the risk of breakdown.*
- Apply a bed cradle. *The bed cradle suspends bed linens over the legs, preventing them from placing pressure on extremities and injured tissues. Minimizing pressure on the tissues promotes capillary blood flow.*
- Provide an egg crate mattress, flotation pad, sheepskin, or heel protectors. *Ischemic tissues may be damaged by minor trauma such as that created by the shearing forces of skin against bed linens.*

## Activity Intolerance

Pain and impaired perfusion of peripheral tissues may limit the client's ability to engage in desired activities, even impairing self-care.

- Assist with care activities as needed. *Severe claudication or rest pain may limit activities. Muscle atrophy of affected extremities is common, leading to fatigue and weakness.*
- Unless contraindicated, encourage gradual increases in duration and intensity of exercise. Teach to rest with extremities dependent when claudication develops, resuming activity after pain has abated. *Gradual increases in the duration and intensity of exercise promote development of collateral circulation, improve exercise tolerance, provide a sense of well-being, and support self-esteem.*
- Provide diversional activities during periods of prescribed bed rest. Encourage relaxation techniques to reduce muscle tension. *Diversional activities help prevent boredom and stress associated with enforced rest. Relaxation techniques reduce vasoconstriction induced by stress, improving peripheral circulation.*
- Encourage frequent position changes and active range-of-motion exercises. Encourage self-care to the extent possible. *Position changes relieve pressure on tissues, improving capillary circulation and reducing tissue ischemia. Range-of-motion exercises help prevent muscle atrophy and joint contractures. Self-care supports self-esteem.*

## Using NANDA, NIC, and NOC

Chart 33-2 shows links between NANDA nursing diagnoses, NIC, and NOC for the client with peripheral atherosclerosis.

## Home Care

Discuss the following topics when preparing the client and family for home care.

- Smoking cessation strategies and ways to avoid second-hand smoke
- Prescribed medications and anticoagulants, their purpose, doses, desired and adverse effects
- Signs of excess bleeding to report to the physician
- Skin surveillance and foot care (see Box 33–4)
- Recommended diet and exercise
- Weight loss strategies if appropriate

If revascularization or surgery has been performed, include the following topics as appropriate.

- Incision care
- Manifestations of complications (e.g., infection, graft leakage, or thrombosis) to be reported to the physician
- Activity limitations

Provide referrals to home health services, physical or occupational therapy, and home maintenance assistance services as indicated. Consider resources such as Meals-on-Wheels for clients who are severely limited by their disease.

## CHART 33–2   NANDA, NIC, AND NOC LINKAGES

### The Client with Peripheral Atherosclerosis

| NURSING DIAGNOSES | NURSING INTERVENTIONS | NURSING OUTCOMES |
|---|---|---|
| • Activity Intolerance | • Exercise Promotion<br>• Self-Care Assistance<br>• Home Maintenance Assistance | • Activity Tolerance<br>• Self-Care: Instrumental Activities of Daily Living |
| • Chronic Pain | • Coping Enhancement<br>• Positioning<br>• Medication Management | • Comfort Level<br>• Pain: Disruptive Effects |
| • Ineffective Health Maintenance | • Behavior Modification<br>• Self-Responsibility Facilitation<br>• Teaching: Prescribed Activity/Exercise | • Health-Promoting Behavior<br>• Knowledge: Treatment Regimen<br>• Self-Direction of Care |
| • Ineffective Tissue Perfusion: Peripheral | • Circulatory Care: Arterial Insufficiency<br>• Positioning<br>• Neurologic Monitoring<br>• Skin Surveillance | • Tissue Integrity: Skin and Mucous Membranes<br>• Tissue Perfusion: Peripheral |

*Note. Data from* Nursing Outcomes Classification (NOC) *by M. Johnson & M. Maas (Eds.), 1997, St. Louis: Mosby;* Nursing Diagnoses: Definitions & Classification 2001–2002 *by North American Nursing Diagnosis Association, 2001, Philadelphia: NANDA;* Nursing Interventions Classification (NIC) *by J.C. McCloskey & G. M. Bulechek (Eds.), 2000, St. Louis: Mosby. Reprinted by permission.*

## Nursing Care Plan

## A Client with Peripheral Atherosclerosis

William Duffy, age 69, is retired. His wife convinces him to see his primary care provider for increasing leg pain with walking and other exercise.

### ASSESSMENT

Katie Kotson, RN, obtains Mr. Duffy's history before he sees his physician. He states that he can only walk about a block before the pain in his calves gets so bad that he has to stop and rest. As a result, he has been less and less active, spending most of his time the past few months watching sports on television. He denies rest pain. He was diagnosed with type 2 diabetes about 15 years ago, which he manages with daily glyburide (DiaBeta), an oral hypoglycemic. He also has stable angina, for which he takes atenolol (Tenormin) and an occasional nitroglycerin tablet. His alcohol intake is moderate, averaging 1 to 2 beers per day, and he smokes about a pack of cigarettes per day. He states he tried to quit smoking after developing angina, but "after nearly 50 years of smoking, I think that's impossible!"

Physical exam findings include: height 68 inches (173 cm), weight 235 lb (107 kg), BP 168/78, P 66, R 16, T 97.6°F (36.5°C); upper extremities warm and pink, normal hair distribution, pulses strong and equal; lower extremities below knees cool and ruddy when dependent, pale to pink when elevated, skin shiny, scant hair; posterior tibial pulses weak bilaterally; weak pedal pulse on R, unable to palpate on L; 1+ to 2+ edema both feet and ankles.

The physician finds that Mr. Duffy's systolic blood pressure in his legs is an average of 28 mmHg lower than in his arms. He

makes the diagnosis of peripheral atherosclerosis, and schedules Mr. Duffy for an exercise stress test with ankle pressure measurements before and after exercise and a color-flow Doppler ultrasound. Mr. Duffy is to return in 3 weeks after these studies have been completed.

### DIAGNOSIS

- *Activity intolerance* related to poor blood flow to lower extremities
- *Ineffective health maintenance* related to smoking and lack of information about disease management
- *Risk for impaired skin integrity* related to ischemic tissues of legs and feet
- *Risk for peripheral neurovascular dysfunction* related to impaired peripheral blood flow to lower extremities

### EXPECTED OUTCOMES

- Walk for at least 15 minutes three to four times per day, gradually increasing his pace and duration of exercise.
- Relate the benefits of smoking cessation.
- Identify strategies to improve chances for success in stopping smoking.
- Meet with dietitian before next visit to discuss dietary measures to promote weight loss and slow atherosclerosis.
- Verbalize an understanding of appropriate foot care measures.
- Identify measures to prevent inadvertent injury of feet and legs.

*(continued on page 1008)*

## Nursing Care Plan
### A Client with Peripheral Atherosclerosis (continued)

### PLANNING AND IMPLEMENTATION

- Teach about peripheral atherosclerosis and its relationship to Mr. Duffy's symptoms.
- With Mr. and Mrs. Duffy, plan strategies to start and maintain a program of regular exercise.
- Instruct to warm up slowly, and to stop exercise and rest for 3 minutes (or until pain is relieved) when claudication develops, then resume exercising.
- Discuss the effects of smoking on blood vessels.
- Help Mr. Duffy identify smoking cessation strategies such as support groups, clinics, and nicotine patches.
- Schedule an appointment with the dietitian to develop a low-calorie, low-fat, and low-cholesterol ADA diet that includes preferred foods and considers usual eating patterns.
- Reinforce and supplement previous foot care teaching.
- Discuss effects of impaired circulation on sensation in feet and legs and measures to prevent injury.

### EVALUATION

When Mr. Duffy returns to the office 3 weeks later, his diagnosis has been confirmed by the diagnostic studies. The physician decides to continue conservative therapy, now prescribing atorvastatin (Lipitor) to lower Mr. Duffy's serum cholesterol level, and cilostazol (Pletal) to reduce the risk of thrombosis and improve symptoms of claudication. Mr. Duffy also asks his physician for a prescription for nicotine patches, saying he is ready to quit smoking, but thinks he needs help to be successful. Mr. and Mrs. Duffy tell Miss Kotson that they are walking before every meal and really enjoying being outside more. They plan to walk in the local shopping mall when the weather gets worse. Mrs. Duffy has bought an American Heart Association cookbook, and is carefully planning their meals. Both Mr. and Mrs. Duffy have lost 5 lb since the previous visit. Mr. Duffy's skin on his legs and feet remains intact, and he identifies the measures he is using to protect his lower extremities from injury.

### Critical Thinking in the Nursing Process

1. What additional lifestyle changes related to peripheral atherosclerosis might be appropriate to suggest to Mr. Duffy at this time? Why?
2. Explain the relationship between physical exercise and pain in the client with peripheral atherosclerosis. Compare this relationship to that between exercise and angina.
3. Mr. Duffy uses a beta blocker, atenolol, to prevent angina. Why is this drug not effective in preventing claudication?
4. Develop a nursing care plan for the diagnosis, *Imbalanced nutrition: More than body requirements.*

See Evaluating Your Response in Appendix C.

## THE CLIENT WITH THROMBOANGIITIS OBLITERANS

**Thromboangiitis obliterans** (also called *Buerger's disease*) is an occlusive vascular disease in which small and midsize peripheral arteries become inflamed and spastic, causing clots to form. This disease may affect either the upper or lower extremities; it often affects a leg or foot. Its exact etiology is unknown.

Thromboangiitis obliterans primarily affects men under age 40 who smoke. Cigarette smoking is the single most significant cause of Buerger's disease. The disease is more prevalent in Asians and people of Eastern European descent. The incidence of HLA-B5 and 2A9 antigens is higher in people with Buerger's disease, suggesting a genetic link.

The course of the disease is intermittent with dramatic exacerbations and marked remissions. The disease may remain dormant for periods of weeks, months, or years. As the disease progresses, collateral vessels are more extensively involved. Consequently, subsequent episodes are more intense and prolonged. Prolonged periods of tissue hypoxia increase the risk for tissue ulceration and gangrene.

### PATHOPHYSIOLOGY AND MANIFESTATIONS

Inflammatory cells infiltrate the wall of small and midsize arteries in the feet and possibly the hands. This inflammatory process is accompanied by thrombus formation and vasospasms of arterial segments that impair blood flow. Adjacent veins and nerves also may be affected. As the disease progresses, affected vessels become scarred and fibrotic.

Pain in the affected extremities is the primary manifestation of thromboangiitis obliterans. Both claudication, cramping pain in calves and feet or the forearms and hands, and rest pain in the fingers and toes may occur. Sensation is diminished. Eventually, the skin becomes thin and shiny and the nails are thickened and malformed. On examination, the involved digits and/or extremities are pale, cyanotic, or ruddy, and cool or cold to touch. Distal pulses (e.g., the dorsalis pedis, posterior tibial, ulnar, or radial) are either difficult to locate or absent, even with a Doppler device.

Painful ulcers and gangrene may develop in the fingers and toes, as a result of severely impaired blood flow. Amputation may be necessary to remove necrotic tissue.

## COLLABORATIVE CARE

Thromboangiitis obliterans usually is diagnosed by the history and physical examination. Doppler studies may be used to locate and determine the extent of the disease. Angiography and magnetic resonance imaging may also be used to evaluate the extent of the disease, but usually are unnecessary.

The one most important component in managing this disease is smoking cessation. While stopping smoking does not cure the disease, it may slow its extension to other vessels. With continued smoking, attacks become increasingly intense and last much longer, significantly increasing the risk for ulcerations and gangrene.

Additional conservative measures are used to prevent vasoconstriction, improve peripheral blood flow, and prevent complications of chronic ischemia. These measures include keeping extremities warm, managing stress, keeping affected extremities in a dependent position, preventing injury to affected tissues, and regular exercise. Walking for 20 or more minutes several times a day is recommended.

There are no specific drugs for thromboangiitis obliterans. A calcium channel blocker such as diltiazem (Cardizem) or verapamil (Isoptin), or pentoxifylline (Trental), which decreases blood viscosity and increases red blood cell flexibility to improve peripheral blood flow, may provide some symptom relief.

Surgical approaches for thromboangiitis obliterans include sympathectomy or arterial bypass graft. Sympathectomy interrupts sympathetic nervous system input to affected vessels, reducing vasoconstriction and spasm. Arterial bypass grafts may be useful when larger vessels are affected by the disease. Amputation of an affected digit or extremity may be necessary if gangrene develops (see Chapter 38 for more information about amputation). Only portions of digits or of limbs (e.g., below the knee) may be amputated, to preserve as much healthy tissue as possible.

The prognosis for thromboangiitis obliterans depends significantly on the client's ability and willingness to stop smoking. With smoking cessation and good foot care, the prognosis for saving the extremities is good, even though no cure is available.

## NURSING CARE

Health promotion activities to prevent thromboangiitis obliterans focus on preventing smoking, especially in high-risk populations. Nursing assessment and care for clients with this disease is similar to that provided for clients with other arterial occlusive diseases. Nursing care focuses on promoting arterial circulation and preventing prolonged tissue hypoxia. Because inflammatory, spastic episodes may be unpredictable, care focuses on smoking cessation and relieving acute manifestations. In addition, postsurgical care is necessary if surgery has been performed. See the nursing care section for peripheral atherosclerosis as well as nursing care of the postsurgical client (Chapter 7) and following amputation (Chapter 38).

### Home Care

Discuss the following topics when preparing clients with thromboangiitis obliterans and their families for home care.

- Absolute necessity of smoking cessation
- Foot care
- Protecting affected extremities from injury
- Purpose, dose, desired and adverse effects, interactions, and any precautions associated with prescribed medications
- Signs and symptoms to report to the physician

## THE CLIENT WITH RAYNAUD'S DISEASE

**Raynaud's disease** and **phenomenon** are characterized by episodes of intense vasospasm in the small arteries and arterioles of the fingers and sometimes the toes (Porth, 2002). Raynaud's disease and phenomenon differ only in terms of cause. Raynaud's disease has no identifiable cause; Raynaud's phenomenon occurs secondarily to another disease (such as collagen vascular diseases like scleroderma and rheumatoid arthritis), other known causes of vasospasm, or long-term exposure to cold or machinery (McCance & Huether, 2002; Porth, 2002).

Raynaud's disease primarily affects young women between the ages of 20 and 40. Genetic predisposition may play a role in its development, although the actual cause is unknown. Table 33–6 compares thromboangiitis obliterans and Raynaud's disease.

## PATHOPHYSIOLOGY AND MANIFESTATIONS

Raynaud's disease and phenomenon are characterized by spasms of the small arteries in the digits. The arterial spasms limit arterial blood flow to the fingers and possibly the toes. Initial attacks may involve only the tips of one or two fingers; with disease progression, the entire finger and all fingers may be affected.

The manifestations of Raynaud's occur intermittently when spasms develop. Raynaud's disease has been called "the blue-white-red disease," because affected digits initially turn blue as blood flow is reduced due to vasospasm, then white as circulation is more severely limited, and finally very red as the fingers are warmed and the spasm resolves. Sensory changes may occur during attacks, including numbness, stiffness, decreased sensation, and aching pain.

The attacks tend to become more frequent and prolonged over time. With repeated attacks (and resultant decrease in oxygenation), the fingertips thicken and the nails become brittle. Ulceration and gangrene are serious complications that rarely occur.

## COLLABORATIVE CARE

Raynaud's disease and phenomenon are primarily diagnosed by the history and physical examination. There are no specific diagnostic tests for these disorders.

Vasodilators may be prescribed to provide symptomatic relief. Low doses of a sustained release calcium channel blocker such as nifedipine (Procardia) or diltiazem (Cardizem) may be prescribed. The α-adrenergic blocker prazosin (Minipress) also may reduce the frequency and severity of attacks. Transdermal nitroglycerine (or longer-acting oral nitrates) helps some clients by decreasing the amount of time necessary for the hands to return to normal following an attack (Tierney et al., 2001).

Conservative measures are a mainstay of treatment. Clients are instructed to keep their hands warm, wearing gloves when outside in cold weather and kitchen gloves when handling cold items (for instance, when preparing and serving cold foods and cleaning the refrigerator). Measures to avoid injury to the hands are taught. Sometimes attacks can be stopped by

| TABLE 33–6 Comparison of Raynaud's Disease and Thromboangiitis Obliterans | | |
|---|---|---|
| **Topic** | **Raynaud's Disease** | **Thromboangiitis Obliterans** |
| Etiology | • Unknown<br>• Possible genetic predisposition | • Cigarette smoking most probable single cause<br>• Possible autoimmune response |
| Incidence/course of the disease | • Onset commonly between 15 and 45 years of age<br>• Usually affects young women<br>• Becomes progressively worse over time | • Occurs predominantly in men under 40<br>• More common in Asians and people of European heritage<br>• Intermittent course with exacerbations and remissions<br>• Increase severity and duration of attacks over time |
| Triggering stimuli | • Emotional stress<br>• Exposure to cold | • Cigarette smoking |
| Assessment findings | • Usually affects hands, sometimes toes<br>• Pain becomes more severe and prolonged as disease progresses<br>• "Blue-white-red" changes in color of hands with accompanying changes in skin temperature | • Claudication and pain<br>• Numbness or diminished sensation<br>• Cool, pale or cyanotic skin<br>• Shiny, thin skin and white, malformed nails in affected extremities<br>• Distal pulses difficult to find or absent<br>• Trophic changes to nail beds<br>• Ulceration and gangrene in later stages<br>• Small, red, tender vascular cords in affected extremities |
| Management | • Avoid unnecessary cold exposure<br>• Emphasize smoking cessation<br>• Medications such as calcium channel or alpha adrenergic blockers as indicated<br>• Teach stress management | • Stop smoking (crucial)<br>• Regular exercise<br>• Protect extremities from cold injury<br>• Teach stress management |

swinging the arms back and forth, increasing perfusion pressure in the small arteries by centrifugal force.

Smoking cessation is important. Stress reduction measures such as exercise, relaxation techniques, massage therapy, hobbies, aroma therapy, and counseling are taught or suggested. Additional lifestyle habits that contribute to vascular health are encouraged, such as reducing dietary fat, increasing activity level, and maintaining normal body weight.

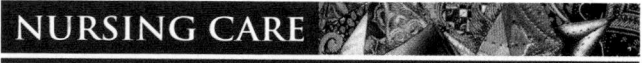

## NURSING CARE

Nursing care for the client with Raynaud's disease or phenomenon is primarily educative and supportive. Protecting the hands and feet from exposure to cold and trauma is the major

teaching topic. Nursing diagnoses and interventions previously outlined for peripheral atherosclerosis also are appropriate for clients with Raynaud's.

## Home Care

Reassure clients with Raynaud's phenomenon that most people with the disorder experience only mild, infrequent episodes. Discuss the following topics in preparing the client for managing the disorder.

• Dress warmly, keeping the trunk and hands warm.
• Avoid unnecessary exposure to cold.
• Stop smoking or do not start.
• The use, purpose, desired and potential adverse effects of prescribed medications, if any.

# DISORDERS OF VENOUS CIRCULATION

The two primary categories of venous system disorders are occlusive disorders and those related to ineffective venous blood flow. Impaired venous blood flow can lead to stasis and clotting, as well as tissue changes associated with venous congestion.

## PHYSIOLOGY REVIEW

The venous system is a low-pressure system in comparison with the arterial circulation. Veins and venules are thin-walled, distensible vessels. While they contain smooth muscle that al-

lows them to contract or expand, the media (muscle layer) of veins is significantly thinner than that of arteries. The low pressures in the venous system allow it to serve as a reservoir for blood. Stimulation by the sympathetic nervous system causes veins to contract, helping maintain vascular volume. The low pressure venous system relies on skeletal muscle contractions and pressure changes in the abdomen and thorax to facilitate blood return to the heart. Unlike arteries, veins of the extremities contain valves to prevent retrograde blood flow.

# THE CLIENT WITH VENOUS THROMBOSIS

**Venous thrombosis** (also known as *thrombophlebitis*) is a condition in which a blood clot (thrombus) forms on the wall of a vein, accompanied by inflammation of the vein wall and some degree of obstructed venous blood flow.

Venous thrombi are more common than arterial thrombi because of lower pressures and flow within the venous system (McCance & Huether, 2002). Thrombi can form in either superficial or deep veins. **Deep venous thrombosis (DVT)** is a common complication of hospitalization, surgery, and immobilization. Obstetric and orthopedic procedures carry a higher risk for venous thrombosis; it may develop in more than 50% of clients having orthopedic surgery, particularly surgeries involving hip or knee (Braunwald et al., 2001). Other significant risk factors for venous thrombosis include abdominal or thoracic surgery, certain cancers, trauma, pregnancy, and use of oral contraceptives or hormone replacement therapy. See Box 33–5.

## PATHOPHYSIOLOGY AND MANIFESTATIONS

Three pathologic factors, called *Virchow's triad,* are associated with thrombophlebitis: stasis of blood, vessel damage, and increased blood coagulability. Vessel trauma stimulates the clotting cascade. Platelets aggregate at the site, particularly when venous stasis is present. Platelets and fibrin form the initial clot. Red blood cells are trapped in the fibrin meshwork, and the thrombus propagates (grows) in the direction of blood flow. The inflammatory response is triggered, causing tenderness,

| BOX 33–5 | ■ Factors Associated with Thrombophlebitis |
|---|---|

- Immobilization: myocardial infarction, heart failure, stroke, postoperative
- Surgery: orthopedic, thoracic, abdominal, genitourinary
- Cancer: pancreatic, lung, ovary, testes, urinary tract, breast, stomach
- Trauma: fractures of the spine, pelvis, femur, tibia; spinal cord injury
- Pregnancy and delivery
- Hormone therapy: oral contraceptives, hormone replacement therapy
- Coagulation disorders

swelling, and erythema in the area of the thrombus. Initially the thrombus floats within the vein. Pieces of the thrombus may break loose and travel through the circulation as emboli. Fibroblasts eventually invade the thrombus, scarring the vein wall and destroying venous valves. Although patency of the vein may be restored, valve damage is permanent, affecting directional flow (Tierney et al., 2001).

## Deep Vein Thrombosis

The deep veins of the legs, primarily in the calf, and the pelvis provide the most hospitable environment for venous thrombosis. Approximately 80% of deep vein thromboses begin in the deep veins of the calf, often propagating into the popliteal and femoral veins (Figure 33–5 ■) (Tierney et al., 2001). DVT

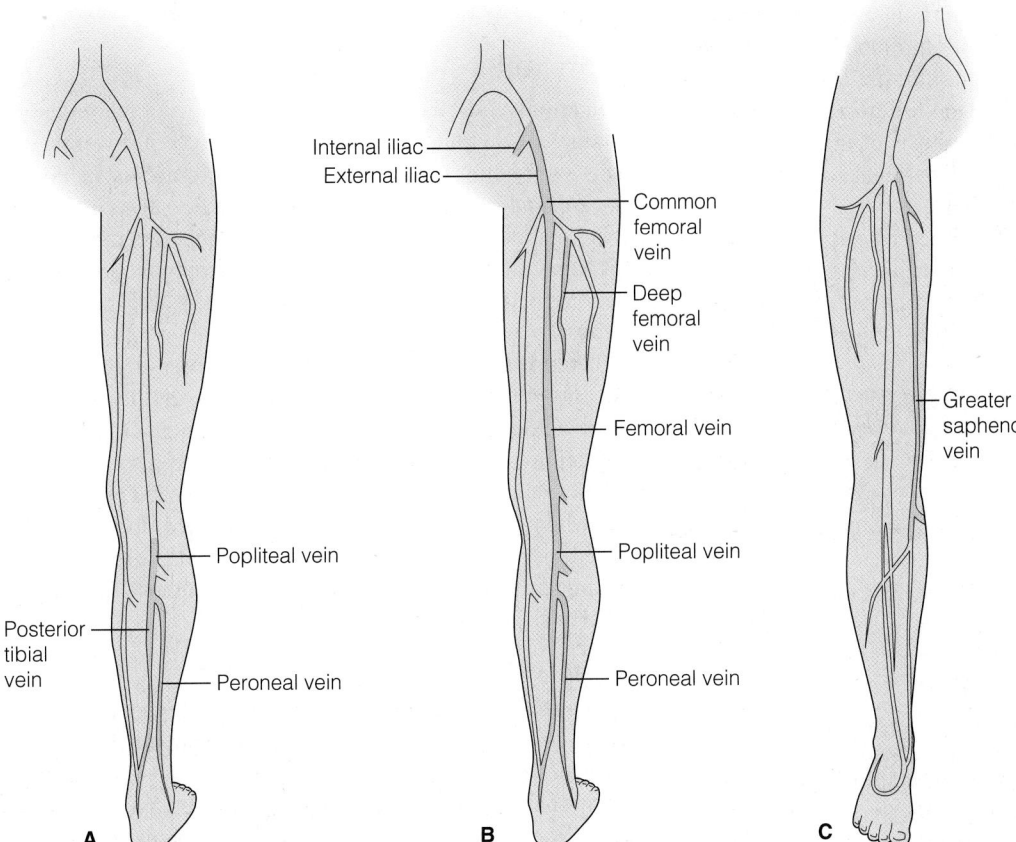

**Figure 33–5** ■ Common locations of venous thrombosis. *A,* The most common sites of deep vein thrombosis. *B,* DVT extending from the calf to the iliac veins. *C,* superficial venous thrombosis.

usually is asymptomatic; in some clients, a pulmonary embolism may be the first indication.

When present, the manifestations of DVT are primarily due to the inflammatory process accompanying the thrombus. Calf pain, which may be described as tightness or a dull, aching pain in the affected extremity, particularly upon walking, is the most common symptom. Tenderness, swelling, warmth, and erythema may be noted along the course of involved veins. The affected extremity may be cyanotic and often is edematous. Rarely, a cord may be palpated over the affected vein. A positive Homan's sign (pain in the calf when the foot is dorsiflexed) is an unreliable indicator of DVT. See the box below for a summary of the manifestations of deep and superficial venous thrombosis.

## Complications

The major complications of deep vein thrombosis are chronic venous insufficiency (see the next section of this chapter) and pulmonary embolism. Pulmonary embolism occurs when the clot fragments or breaks loose from the vein wall. As the clot travels, it moves through progressively larger veins and into the right side of the heart. From there it enters the pulmonary circulation, where it eventually occludes arterial flow to a portion of the lungs. The result is a mismatch between ventilation (air flow) and perfusion (blood flow) in a portion of the lungs. The effect on gas exchange depends on the size of the embolism and the vessel it occludes. See Chapter 36 ⊕⊘ for more information about pulmonary emboli.

## Superficial Vein Thrombosis

Venous catheters and infusions are the primary risk factors for superficial venous thrombosis. Superficial vein thrombosis also may develop in conjunction with thromboangitis obliterans, varicose veins, or deep vein thrombosis. It may develop spontaneously in pregnant women or following delivery. In some cases, superficial venous thrombosis of the long saphenous vein is the earliest sign of an abdominal cancer such as pancreatic cancer (Tierney et al., 2001).

Superficial vein thrombosis is marked by pain and tenderness at the site of the thrombus. A reddened, warm, tender cord extending along the affected vein can be palpated. The area surrounding the vein may be swollen and red (see the box below).

---

### Manifestations of Venous Thrombosis

**DEEP VEIN THROMBOSIS**
- Usually asymptomatic
- Dull, aching pain in affected extremity, especially when walking
- Possible tenderness, warmth, erythema along affected vein
- Cyanosis of affected extremity
- Edema of affected extremity

**SUPERFICIAL VEIN THROMBOSIS**
- Localized pain and tenderness over the affected vein
- Redness and warmth along the course of the vein
- Palpable cordlike structure along the affected vein
- Swelling and redness of surrounding tissue

---

## COLLABORATIVE CARE

It is important to differentiate venous thrombosis from other causes of extremity pain, such as cellulitis, muscle strain, contusion, and lymphedema. The history, physical examination, and diagnostic tests are used to establish the diagnosis. Treatment focuses on preventing further clotting or extension of the clot and addressing underlying causes.

### Diagnostic Tests

- *Duplex venous ultrasonography* is a noninvasive test used to visualize the vein and measure the velocity of blood flow in the veins. Although the clot often cannot be visualized directly, its presence can be inferred by an inability to compress the vein during the examination.
- *Plethysmography* is a noninvasive test that measures changes in blood flow through the veins. It is often used in conjunction with Doppler ultrasonography. Plethysmography is most valuable in diagnosing thromboses of larger or more superficial veins.
- *Magnetic resonance imaging (MRI)* is another noninvasive means of detecting deep vein thrombosis. It is particularly useful when thrombosis of the vena cavae or pelvic veins is suspected.
- *Ascending contrast venography* uses an injected contrast medium to assess the location and extent of venous thrombosis. Although invasive, expensive, and uncomfortable, contrast venography is the most accurate diagnostic tool for venous thrombosis. It is used when the results of less invasive tests leave the diagnosis unclear (Tierney et al., 2001).

### Prophylaxis

Medications and other measures are used to prevent venous thrombosis when the risk is high. Low-molecular-weight heparins (see below) prevent deep vein thrombosis in clients who are undergoing general or orthopedic surgery, experiencing acute medical illness, or on prolonged bed rest. Oral anticoagulation also may be used as a prophylactic measure in clients with fractures or who are undergoing orthopedic surgery.

Elevating the foot of the bed with the knees slightly flexed promotes venous return. Early mobilization and leg exercises such as ankle flexion and extension assist venous flow by muscle compression. Intermittent pneumatic compression devices applied to the legs are effective to prevent DVT. They also are used when anticoagulation is contraindicated due to the increased risk for bleeding (Braunwald et al., 2001). Elastic stockings are used to prevent venous thrombosis as well in clients at risk.

### Medications

Anticoagulants to prevent clot propagation and enable the body's own lytic system to dissolve the clot are the mainstay of treatment for venous thrombosis. Thrombolytic drugs such as streptokinase or tissue plasminogen activator (t-PA) may accelerate the process of clot lysis and prevent damage to venous valves. There is, however, no evidence that thrombolytic therapy is more effective in preventing pulmonary embolism than anticoagulants (Braunwald et al., 2001). It also significantly increases the risk for bleeding and hemorrhage.

Nonsteroidal anti-inflammatory agents such as indomethacin (Indocin) or naproxen (Naprosyn) may be ordered to reduce inflammation in the veins and provide symptomatic relief, particularly for clients with superficial vein thrombosis.

## Anticoagulants

Anticoagulants are given to prevent clot extension and reduce the risk of subsequent pulmonary embolism. Anticoagulation is initiated with unfractionated heparin or low-molecular-weight (LMW) heparin. Following an initial intravenous bolus of 7,500 to 10,000 units of unfractionated heparin, a continuous heparin infusion of 1000 to 1500 IU per hour is started. The dosage is calculated to maintain the activated partial thromboplastin time (aPTT) at approximately twice the control or normal value. An infusion pump is used to deliver the prescribed dosage. Frequent monitoring of the infusion is an important nursing responsibility. Subcutanous heparin injections may be used as an alternate to intravenous infusion in some instances.

LMW heparins are increasingly used to prevent and treat venous thrombosis. They do not require the close laboratory monitoring of unfractionated heparins. LMW heparin is administered subcutaneously in fixed doses once or twice daily, allowing the option of outpatient treatment. LMW heparins have additional advantages, in that they are more effective and carry lower risks for bleeding and thrombocytopenia than conventional, unfractionated heparins.

Oral anticoagulation with warfarin may be initiated concurrently with heparin therapy. Overlapping heparin and warfarin therapy for 4 to 5 days is important because the full anticoagulant effect of warfarin is delayed, and it may actually promote clotting during the first few days of therapy (Tierney et al., 2001). Warfarin doses are adjusted to maintain the international normalized ratio (INR) at 2.0 to 3.0 (Braunwald et al., 2001).

Once this level is achieved, the heparin is discontinued and a maintenance dose of warfarin is prescribed to prevent recurrent thrombosis. Anticoagulation generally is continued for at least 3 months. When DVT is recurrent or risk factors such as altered coagulability or cancer are present, anticoagulant therapy may be prolonged. Regular follow-up is necessary to be sure prothrombin times (INR) remain within the desirable range for anticoagulation. See the Medication Administration box below for the nursing implications for anticoagulant therapy.

# Medication Administration

## Anticoagulant Therapy

### HEPARIN

Heparin interferes with the clotting cascade by inhibiting the effects of thrombin and preventing the conversion of fibrinogen to fibrin. This prevents the formation of a stable fibrin clot. At therapeutic levels, heparin prolongs the thrombin time, clotting time, and activated partial thromboplastin time. When given intravenously, its effect is immediate. Given subcutaneously, its onset of action is within 1 hour. When heparin is discontinued, clotting times return to normal within 2 to 6 hours (Spratto & Woods, 2003).

### Nursing Responsibilities

- Assess for history of unexplained or active bleeding. Assess laboratory results for abnormal clotting profile or evidence of active bleeding.
- Give a test dose as indicated to clients with a history of multiple allergies or a history of asthma.
- Administer by deep subcutaneous injection; abdominal sites are preferred. Avoid injecting within 2 inches of the umbilicus. Rotate sites. Do not aspirate prior to injecting or massage after the injection.
- Intravenous solutions may be diluted with dextrose, normal saline, or Ringer's solution. Use an infusion pump.
- Keep protamine sulfate, a heparin antagonist, available to treat excessive bleeding.
- Monitor and report abnormal laboratory results and aPTT values outside the desired range.
- Promptly report evidence of bleeding such as hematemesis, hematuria, bleeding gums, or unexplained abdominal or back pain.

### Client and Family Teaching

- Report unusual bleeding or excessive menstrual flow.
- Use an electric razor and a soft-bristle toothbrush; prevent injury by clearing pathways, using a night light, and other measures. Do not consume alcohol.
- Avoid contact sports while on anticoagulant therapy.
- Do not consume large amounts of food rich in vitamin K (yellow and dark green vegetables).
- Do not use aspirin or NSAIDs while on heparin therapy unless advised to do so by your physician.
- Wear a MedicAlert tag and advise all health care providers (including dentists and podiatrists) of therapy.

### LOW-MOLECULAR-WEIGHT HEPARINS

| | |
|---|---|
| Ardeparin (Normiflo) | Enoxaparin (Lovenox) |
| Dalteparin (Fragmin) | Tinzaparin (Innohep) |

LMW heparins are the most bioavailable fraction of heparin. They provide a more precise and predictable anticoagulant effect than unfractionated heparins. Like unfractionated heparin, LMW heparin prevents conversion of prothrombin to thrombin, liberation of thromboplastin from platelets, and formation of a stable clot. LMW heparins cannot be used interchangeably with each other or with unfractionated heparin.

### Nursing Responsibilities

- Assess for evidence of active bleeding, a history of bleeding disorders or thrombocytopenia, or sensitivity to heparin, sulfites, or pork products.

*(continued on page 1014)*

## Medication Administration

### Anticoagulant Therapy (continued)

- Monitor for unusual or masked bleeding. PT and aPTT levels may be within normal levels even in the presence of hemorrhage.
- Administer by deep subcutaneous injection into abdominal wall, thigh, or buttocks. Rotate sites. Do not aspirate or massage.

#### Client and Family Teaching

- Subcutaneous self-administration technique, timing of doses, and site rotation. Do not rub site after administering to minimize bruising.
- Do not take aspirin, NSAIDs, or other over-the-counter drugs unless recommended by your physician.
- Promptly report excessive bruising or bleeding, chest pain, difficulty breathing, itching, rash, or swelling to your health care provider.
- Keep follow-up appointments as scheduled.

#### ORAL ANTICOAGULANT

Warfarin (Coumadin)

Warfarin interferes with synthesis of vitamin K–dependent clotting factors by the liver, leading to depletion of these factors. It has no effect on already circulating clotting factors or on existing clots. Warfarin inhibits extension of existing thrombi and the formation of new clots. Its action is cumulative and more prolonged than that of heparin.

#### Nursing Responsibilities

- Assess laboratory results and history for evidence of abnormal bleeding.
- Multiple drugs affect the metabolism and protein binding of warfarin; note all medications and assess for interactions with warfarin.

- Do not give during pregnancy as warfarin may cause congenital malformations.
- Oral tablets may be crushed and given without regard to meals.
- Dilute intravenous warfarin with supplied diluent; administer within 4 hours by direct intravenous injection at a rate of 25 mg/min.
- Keep vitamin K available to reverse effects of warfarin in the event of excessive bleeding or hemorrhage.
- Monitor PT or INR; report values outside the desired range.

#### Client and Family Teaching

- Do not take your prescribed dose and notify your physician immediately if bleeding occurs (hematemesis, bright red or black tarry feces, hematuria, bleeding gums, excessive bruising, etc.). Report rash or manifestations of hepatitis (dark urine, malaise, yellow skin or sclera).
- Take your warfarin at the same time every day; do not change brands as their effects may differ.
- Menstrual bleeding may be slightly increased; contact your health care provider if it increases significantly. Use reliable birth control to prevent pregnancy while taking warfarin. Immediately contact your health care provider if you think you may be pregnant.
- Take precautions to prevent injury and bleeding: use a soft toothbrush and electric razor, wear shoes, and use a night light. Avoid participating in contact sports.
- Do not smoke, use alcohol, or take any over-the-counter drugs unless specifically recommended by your health care provider. Notify all health care providers, including dentists and podiatrists, of therapy. Wear a MedicAlert tag.
- Obtain lab tests as scheduled and keep all scheduled follow-up appointments.

WARFARIN ANIMAITON

MediaLink

## Treatments

Treatment of venous thrombosis also includes measures to relieve symptoms and reduce inflammation. With superficial vein thrombosis, applying warm, moist compresses over the affected vein, extremity rest, and anti-inflammatory agents usually provide relief of symptoms.

Bed rest may be ordered for deep vein thrombosis. The duration of bed rest typically is determined by the extent of leg edema. The legs are elevated 15 to 20 degrees, with the knees slightly flexed, above the level of the heart to promote venous return and discourage venous pooling. Elastic antiembolism stockings (TEDS) or pneumatic compression devices are also frequently ordered to stimulate the muscle-pumping mechanism that promotes the return of blood to the heart. When permitted, walking is encouraged while avoiding prolonged standing or sitting. Crossing the legs also is avoided, as are tight-fitting garments or stockings that bind.

## Surgery

Venous thrombosis usually is effectively treated with conservative measures and anticoagulation. In some cases, however, surgery is required to remove the thrombus, prevent its extension into deep veins, or prevent the effects of embolization.

*Venous thrombectomy* is done when thrombi lodge in the femoral vein and their removal is necessary to prevent pulmonary embolism or gangrene. Successful thrombus removal rapidly improves venous circulation. The duration of this effect varies.

When venous thrombosis is recurrent and anticoagulant therapy is contraindicated, a filter may be inserted into the vena cava to capture emboli from the pelvis and lower extremities, preventing pulmonary embolism. Several different filters are available (Figure 33–6 ■). The Greenfield filter is widely used for its ability to trap emboli within its apex while maintaining patency of the vena cava. The filter can be inserted under fluoroscopy with local anesthesia. Mortality and morbidity associated with the filter are very low (Meeker & Rothrock, 1999).

Extensive thrombosis of the saphenous vein may necessitate ligation and division of the saphenous vein where it joins the femoral vein to prevent clot extension into the deep venous system. A vein affected by septic venous thrombosis is excised to control the infection. Antibiotic therapy also is initiated.

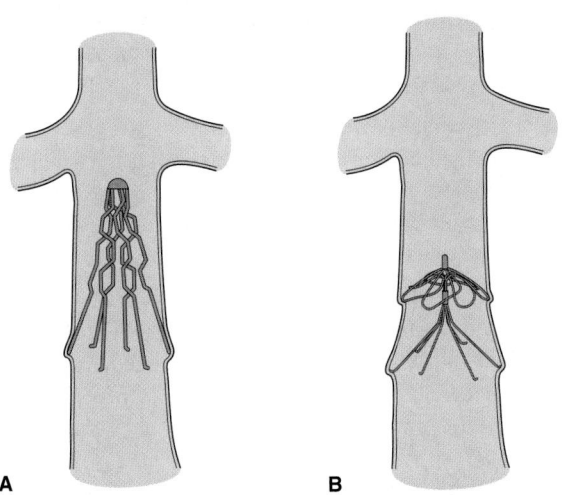

**Figure 33–6** ■ Venal caval filters. *A,* Greenfield filter. *B,* Nitinol filter.

## NURSING CARE

### Health Promotion

Prevention of venous thrombosis is an important component of nursing care for all at-risk clients. Position clients to promote venous blood flow from the lower extremities, with the feet elevated and the knees slightly bent. Avoid placing pillows under the knees and positions in which the hips and knees are sharply flexed. Use a recliner chair or foot stool when sitting. Ambulate clients as soon as possible, and maintain a regular schedule of ambulation throughout the day. Teach ankle flexion and extension exercises, and frequently remind clients to perform them. Apply elastic hose and pneumatic compression devices when appropriate. Instruct clients to avoid crossing legs when in bed or sitting. Inquire about possible prophylactic heparin or warfarin therapy for clients undergoing orthopedic surgery or other high-risk procedures. Frequently assess intravenous sites. Change the site and catheter as dictated by agency protocol and if evidence of local inflammation is noted.

### Assessment

Assess clients at risk for venous thrombosis for manifestations and risk factors.

- Health history: complaints of leg or calf pain, its duration and characteristics, and the effect of walking on the pain; history of venous thrombosis or other clotting disorders; current medications
- Physical examination: inspect affected extremity for redness, edema; palpate for tenderness, warmth, cordlike structures; body temperature

### Nursing Diagnoses and Interventions

In addition to the preventive measures identified earlier, priority nursing diagnoses for the client with venous thrombosis relate to pain, maintenance of tissue perfusion and integrity, and the potential adverse effects of prescribed treatments.

### Pain

The pain associated with venous thrombosis results from inflammation of the involved vein. It may be aggravated by use of the involved extremity. Associated edema and swelling may contribute to discomfort. Measures to reduce the inflammation often help relieve the pain.

- Regularly assess pain location, characteristics, and level using a standardized pain scale. Report increasing pain or changes in its location or characteristics. *Tissue substances released during the inflammatory process can stimulate pain receptors. In addition, localized swelling presses on pain-sensitive structures in the area of the inflammation, contributing to discomfort. As inflammation and swelling are reduced, pain should abate. Continued or increasing pain may indicate extension of the thrombosis. Sudden chest pain may indicate a pulmonary embolism, necessitating immediate intervention.*
- Measure calf and thigh diameter of the affected extremity on admission and daily thereafter. Report increases promptly. *The inflammatory process causes vasodilation and increases vessel permeability, causing edema of the affected extremity. Baseline and subsequent measurements provide a measure of treatment effectiveness.*
- Apply warm, moist heat to affected extremity at least four times daily, using warm, moist compresses or an aqua-K pad. *Moist heat penetrates tissues to a greater depth. Warmth promotes vasodilation, allowing reabsorption of excess fluid into the circulation. Vasodilation also reduces resistance within the affected vessel, reducing pain. As edema subsides, pressure on surrounding tissues is relieved, thereby reducing pain.*
- Maintain bed rest as ordered. *Using leg muscles during walking exacerbates the inflammatory process and increases edema. This, in turn, increases venous compression and pain.*

### Ineffective Tissue Perfusion: Peripheral

As thrombi develop, they occlude the lumen of the vein and obstruct blood flow. In addition, the accompanying inflammatory response may precipitate vessel spasms, further impairing arterial and venous blood flow and tissue perfusion. Impaired tissue perfusion, in turn, deprives tissues of nutrients and oxygen. As a result, distal tissues of the affected extremity are at risk for ulceration and infection.

**PRACTICE ALERT** *Assess peripheral pulses, skin integrity, capillary refill times, and color of extremities at least every 8 hours. Report changes promptly. Assessment of both extremities allows comparison of the affected and unaffected limbs. Weak or absent pulses, impaired capillary refill, or significant color changes in the affected extremity may indicate extension of the thrombus or a possible complication.* ■

- Assess skin of the affected lower leg and foot at least every 8 hours; more often as indicated. *Frequent assessment is important to rapidly detect early signs of tissue breakdown and implementation of measures to protect vulnerable tissues. Early intervention allows healing and restoration of tissue integrity; allowed to continue, the process can lead to necrosis and potential gangrene.*
- Elevate extremities at all times, keeping knees slightly flexed and legs above the level of the heart. *Elevation of the extremities promotes venous return and reduces peripheral edema. Knee flexion promotes muscle relaxation.*

**PRACTICE ALERT** *Remove antiembolic stockings or pneumatic compression device for 30 to 60 minutes during daily hygiene. Antiembolic stockings (e.g., TED hose) and pneumatic compression devices exert pressure on the extremity and promote venous return. They can, however, impair perfusion of the dermis. Removing them periodically allows assessment of the underlying tissue and restores perfusion of the dermis, reducing the risk for skin breakdown. Their use may be continued following discharge to reduce the risk of recurrent venous thrombosis.* ■

- Use mild soaps, solutions, and lotions to clean the affected leg and foot daily. Pat dry after washing, and apply a nonalcohol-based lotion or moisturizing cream. *Daily hygiene with nondrying soaps and solutions removes potential pathogens from the skin surface, and maintains skin integrity and the first line of defense against infection. Caustic or harsh soaps or solutions can dry and crack the skin. Dry, cracked skin permits bacteria and other microorganisms to enter and infect the tissue, potentially leading to ulceration and venous gangrene.*
- Use egg crate mattress or sheepskin on the bed as needed. *Egg crate mattresses and sheepskins distribute weight more evenly, preventing excess pressure on affected tissues.*
- Encourage frequent position changes, at least every 2 hours while awake. *Frequent position changes reduce pressure on bony prominences and edematous tissue, reducing the risk of tissue breakdown.*

## Ineffective Protection

Anticoagulant therapy interferes with the body's normal clotting mechanisms, increasing the risk for bleeding and hemorrhage.

**PRACTICE ALERT** *Assess for and promptly report evidence of bleeding, such as petechiae, bruising, bleeding gums, obvious or occult blood in vomitus, stool, or urine, unexplained back or abdominal pain. Anticoagulants interfere with the ability to form a stable clot and prevent excessive bleeding. Even minor trauma such as toothbrushing or bumping into furniture can result in bleeding.* ■

- Monitor laboratory results, including the INR (prothrombin time), aPTT, hemoglobin, and hematocrit as indicated. Report values outside the normal or desired range. *Coagulation studies are used to monitor the effect of anticoagulant medications. Values within the desired range prevent further clot*

*development while carrying a low risk for bleeding and hemorrhage. A fall in the hemoglobin and hematocrit may indicate undetected bleeding.*

## Impaired Physical Mobility

Although prolonged bed rest rarely is required, it is associated with many problems, including constipation, joint contractures, muscle atrophy, and boredom. Nursing care goals include maintaining joint range of motion, minimizing muscle atrophy, and reducing boredom.

- Encourage active range-of-motion exercises at least every 8 hours. Provide passive range of motion as needed. *Range-of-motion exercises maintain joint mobility and prevent contractures. Active range of motion (performed by the client) also helps prevent muscle atrophy and preserve function. While passive range-of-motion exercises do not prevent muscle atrophy, they do maintain joint mobility.*
- Encourage frequent position changes, deep breathing, and coughing. *Prolonged immobility can lead to impaired airway clearance and respiratory complications, such as atelectasis or pneumonia. Turning, coughing, and deep breathing facilitate expulsion of secretions from the respiratory tract, airway clearance, and alveolar ventilation.*
- Encourage increased fluid and dietary fiber intake. *Constipation is a frequent complication of immobility due to decreased gastrointestinal motility and loss of abdominal muscle strength. Increasing fluid and fiber intake helps maintain soft, easily expelled stools.*
- Assist with and encourage ambulation as allowed. *Ambulation promotes venous blood flow, helps maintain muscle tone and joint mobility, and increases the sense of well-being.*
- Encourage diversional activities such as reading, handiwork or other hobbies, television or video games, and socializing. *Boredom may lead to dozing and inertia, with little physical movement or mental stimulation, increasing the risk for complications of immobility.*

## Risk for Ineffective Tissue Perfusion: Cardiopulmonary

A thrombus that forms in the deep veins of the legs or pelvis may break loose or fragment, becoming an embolism. Emboli that originate in the venous system usually become trapped in the pulmonary circulation (pulmonary embolism). Gas exchange in the affected area is impaired as blood flow ceases or is reduced to an area of the lungs that is well ventilated (see Chapter 36). ⊙⊙

- Frequently assess respiratory status, including rate, depth, ease, and oxygen saturation levels. *A mismatch of ventilation and perfusion can significantly affect gas exchange, leading to rapid, shallow respirations, dyspnea and air hunger, and a fall in oxygen saturation levels.*

**PRACTICE ALERT** *Immediately report complaints of chest pain and shortness of breath, anxiety, or a sense of impending doom. The manifestations of pulmonary embolism are similar to those of myocardial infarction. Prompt intervention to restore pulmonary blood flow can reduce the risk of significant adverse effects.* ■

## CHART 33–3 NANDA, NIC, AND NOC LINKAGES

### The Client with Venous Thrombosis

| NURSING DIAGNOSES | NURSING INTERVENTIONS | NURSING OUTCOMES |
|---|---|---|
| • Impaired Physical Mobility | • Exercise Therapy: Joint Mobility<br>• Environmental Management: Safety | • Joint Movement: Active<br>• Ambulation: Walking |
| • Ineffective Health Maintenance | • Teaching: Prescribed Activity/Exercise<br>• Teaching: Prescribed Medication | • Knowledge: Health Behaviors<br>• Knowledge: Treatment Regimen |
| • Ineffective Protection<br>• Ineffective Tissue Perfusion: Peripheral | • Bleeding Precautions<br>• Circulatory Care: Venous Insufficiency<br>• Positioning | • Coagulation Status<br>• Tissue Integrity: Skin and Mucous Membranes<br>• Tissue Perfusion: Peripheral |
| • Pain | • Heat/Cold Application<br>• Coping Enhancement | • Comfort Level<br>• Pain: Disruptive Effects |

*Note. Data from Nursing Outcomes Classification (NOC) by M. Johnson & M. Maas (Eds.), 1997, St. Louis: Mosby; Nursing Diagnoses: Definitions & Classification 2001–2002 by North American Nursing Diagnosis Association, 2001, Philadelphia: NANDA; Nursing Interventions Classification (NIC) by J.C. McCloskey & G. M. Bulechek (Eds.), 2000, St. Louis: Mosby. Reprinted by permission.*

• Initiate oxygen therapy, elevate the head of the bed, and re-assure the client who is experiencing manifestations of pulmonary embolism. *Oxygen therapy and elevating the head of the bed promote ventilation and gas exchange in those alveoli that are well perfused, helping maintain tissue oxygenation. Reassurance helps reduce anxiety and slow the respiratory rate, promoting greater respiratory depth and alveolar ventilation.*

## Using NANDA, NIC, and NOC

Chart 33–3 shows links between NANDA nursing diagnoses, NIC, and NOC for the client with venous thrombosis.

## Home Care

Treatment measures for venous thrombosis may be initiated and carried out on an outpatient basis or continued for an ex-

tended period of time following hospital discharge. Include the following topics when teaching for home care.

• Explanation of the disease process
• Treatment measures, including laboratory tests and their purposes, medications and adverse effects that should be reported
• Appropriate methods of heat application
• Prescribed activity restrictions
• Measures to prevent future episodes of venous thrombosis
• The importance of follow-up visits and laboratory tests as scheduled

Refer clients for community nursing services for continued assessment and reinforcement of teaching. Provide referrals for assistance with ADLs and home maintenance services as indicated. Consider referral for physical therapy if needed.

## Nursing Care Plan
## A Client with Deep Vein Thrombosis

Mrs. Opal Hipps, age 75, lives alone with her dog, Chester, in her family home in the suburbs. She retired from her job as a postal clerk 10 years ago and now spends a lot of time reading and watching television. Over the past week she has developed a vague aching pain in her right leg. She ignored the pain until last night when it developed into a much more severe pain in her right calf. She noticed that her right lower leg seemed larger than the left, and it was very tender to the touch. After seeing her physician and undergoing Doppler ultrasound studies, Mrs. Hipps is admitted to the hospital with the diagnosis of deep vein thrombosis in the right leg. She is placed on bed rest, and intravenous heparin. Michael Cookson, RN, is assigned to admit and care for Mrs. Hipps.

### ASSESSMENT

Mr. Cookson notices that Mrs. Hipps was admitted 14 months ago for repair of a fractured femur. Mrs. Hipps says, "This business about a blood clot really has me worried." She also tells Mr. Cookson that she is worried about who will care for her dog while she is in the hospital. Physical findings include: height 62 inches (157 cm), weight 149 lb (68 kg), T 99.2 F (37.3°C); vital signs within normal limits otherwise. Her left leg is warm and pink, with strong peripheral pulses and good capillary refill. Her right calf is dark red, very warm, and dry to touch. It is tender to palpation. The right femoral and popliteal pulses are strong, but the pedal and posterior tibial pulses are difficult to locate. The right calf diameter is 0.5 inch (1.27 cm) larger than the left.

*(continued on page 1018)*

## Nursing Care Plan
## A Client with Deep Vein Thrombosis (continued)

### DIAGNOSIS

- *Pain* related to inflammatory response in affected vein
- *Anxiety* related to unexpected hospitalization and uncertainty about the seriousness of her illness
- *Ineffective tissue perfusion: Peripheral* related to decreased venous circulation in the right leg
- *Risk for impaired skin integrity* related to pooling of venous blood in the right leg

### EXPECTED OUTCOMES

- Verbalize relief of right leg pain by day of discharge.
- Verbalize reduced anxiety by the second day of her hospitalization.
- Demonstrate reduced right leg diameter by 0.25 inch (0.64 cm) by the fifth day of hospitalization.
- Maintain intact skin in the right foot throughout the hospital stay.

### PLANNING AND IMPLEMENTATION

- Elevate legs, maintaining slight knee flexion, while in bed.
- Apply warm, moist compresses to right leg using a 2-hour-on, 2-hour-off schedule around the clock.
- Administer prescribed analgesics and evaluate effectiveness.
- Spend time with Mrs. Hipps to explain venous thrombosis and its treatment.
- Arrange for a friend or neighbor to care for Mrs. Hipps's dog.
- Apply antiembolism stockings as ordered; remove for 30 minutes every 8 hours.
- Monitor laboratory values to assess effect of anticoagulant therapy; report values outside desired range.

- Assist with progressive ambulation when allowed.
- Inspect legs and feet and record findings every 8 hours.

### EVALUATION

Seven days after admission, the pain in Mrs. Hipps's right leg has subsided and the diameter of her right calf is equal to her left calf. Mrs. Hipps admits to Mr. Cookson that her fears really relate to a cousin who was hospitalized for a similar problem and had his leg amputated. After talking about her condition and the steps she can take to prevent its recurrence, she is much less anxious. Before discharge, Mr. Cookson reviews instructions for antiembolism stockings, daily walking, warfarin schedule, and scheduled follow-up appointment. Her neighbor, Kate, came to pick her up. As Mr. Cookson was helping Mrs. Hipps into the car, Kate handed her a small brown dog and said, "I took good care of Chester for you, but he's missed you." Mrs. Hipps smiled, and assured Mr. Cookson that she would call the number he provided if she had any questions.

### Critical Thinking in the Nursing Process

1. Describe the pathophysiologic reasons for the pain in Mrs. Hipps's right leg.
2. How would you respond if Mrs. Hipps tells you she does not have the money to buy the prescribed anticoagulant when she goes home?
3. How would you change your teaching and discharge planning if Mrs. Hipps had difficulty caring for herself?
4. Design a plan of care for Mrs. Hipps for the diagnosis, *Activity intolerance.*

See Evaluating Your Response in Appendix C.

---

## THE CLIENT WITH CHRONIC VENOUS INSUFFICIENCY

**Chronic venous insufficiency** is a disorder of inadequate venous return over a prolonged period. Deep vein thrombosis is the most frequent cause of chronic venous insufficiency. Other conditions, such as varicose veins or leg trauma, may contribute; in some instances, it develops without an identified precipitating cause (Braunwald et al., 2001; Tierney et al., 2001).

## PATHOPHYSIOLOGY

Following DVT, large veins may remain occluded, increasing the pressure in other veins of the extremity. This increased pressure distends the veins, separating valve leaflets and impairing their ability to close. DVT also damages valve leaflets, causing them to thicken and contract. The result is impaired unidirectional blood flow and deep vein emptying (Porth, 2002).

When venous valves are incompetent, the muscle-pumping action produced during activity cannot propel blood back to the heart. Venous blood collects and stagnates in the lower leg (*venous stasis*). Venous pressures in the calf and lower leg increase, particularly during ambulation. This increased pressure impairs arterial circulation to the lower extremities as well. The body's ability to provide sufficient oxygen and nutrients to the cells and remove metabolic waste products diminishes. Eventually, there is so little oxygen and nutrients that cells begin to die. The skin atrophies, and subcutaneous fat deposits necrose. Breakdown of red blood cells in the congested tissues causes brown skin pigmentation (Porth, 2002). Venous stasis ulcers develop. Congested tissues impair the body's ability to increase the supply of oxygen, nutrients, and metabolic energy to heal the ulcer. As a result, the condition worsens and, over time, the ulcers enlarge. The congested venous circulation also prevents the blood from mounting effective inflammatory and immune responses, significantly increasing the risk for infection in the ulcerated tissue (McCance & Huether, 2002).

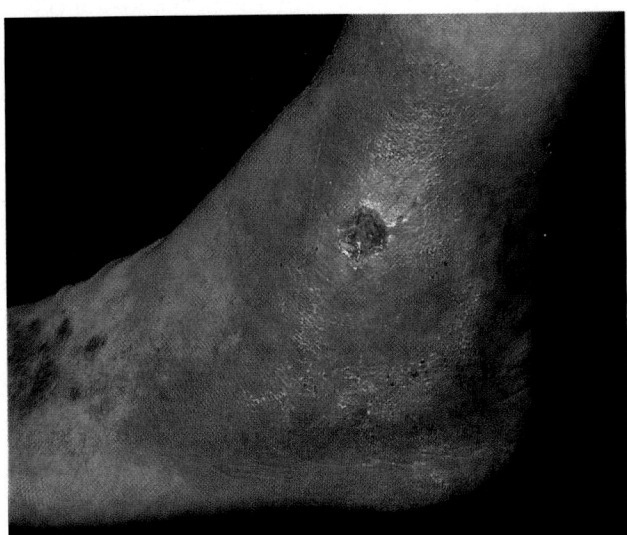

**Figure 33–7** ■ Chronic venous insufficiency. Note the discoloration of the ankle and the stasis ulcer.

*Source: Camera M. D. Studios. Carroll H. Weiss, Director. 8290 N. W. 26th Place. Sunrise, FL 33322.*

## MANIFESTATIONS

Manifestations of chronic venous insufficiency include lower leg edema, itching, and discomfort of the affected extremity that increase with prolonged standing. The extremity is cyanotic. Recurrent stasis ulcers develop (Figure 33–7 ■), usually forming just above the ankle, on the medial or anterior aspect of the leg. They heal poorly, forming scar tissue that breaks down easily. Tissue surrounding the ulcer is shiny, atrophic, and cyanotic, and there is a brownish pigmentation to the skin. Other skin changes may develop as well, such as eczema or stasis dermatitis. Necrosis and fibrosis of subcutaneous tissue causes the affected area of the leg to feel hard and somewhat leathery to the touch, but even the slightest trauma to the area can produce serious tissue breakdown. See the box on this page for the manifestations of chronic venous insufficiency. Table 33–7 compares venous and arterial ulcers.

### Manifestations of Chronic Venous Insufficiency

- Lower extremity edema that worsens with standing
- Itching, dull leg discomfort or pain that increases with standing
- Thin, shiny, atrophic skin
- Cyanosis and brown skin pigmentation of lower leg and foot
- Possible weeping dermatitis
- Thick, fibrous (hard) subcutaneous tissue
- Recurrent ulcerations of medial or anterior ankle

## COLLABORATIVE CARE

Collaborative care for the client with venous insufficiency focuses on relieving symptoms, promoting adequate circulation, and healing and preventing tissue damage.

The history and physical examination often establish the diagnosis of chronic venous insufficiency. Because a history of deep vein thrombosis is a major risk factor, careful evaluation of the past medical history and questioning of the client is important. There are no specific diagnostic tests to confirm the diagnosis of chronic venous insufficiency.

Conservative management of venous insufficiency focuses on reducing edema and treating ulcerations. Prolonged standing or sitting is discouraged. Graduated compression hosiery is ordered for daytime use, and frequent elevation of the legs and feet during the day is recommended. At night, the legs and feet should be elevated above the level of the heart by raising the foot of the mattress.

Treatment of associated stasis dermatitis varies, based on the duration of the condition. Wet compresses of boric acid, buffered aluminum actetate (Burrow's solution), or isotonic saline solution are applied to acute weeping dermatitis four times a day for 1-hour periods. Following the compress, a topical corticosteroid (such as 0.5% hydrocortisone cream) is applied. Bed rest is prescribed during the acute period. Stasis dermatitis that is subsiding or chronic may be treated with a topical

| TABLE 33-7 | Comparison of Arterial and Venous Leg Ulcers | |
| --- | --- | --- |
| **Factor** | **Arterial Ulcers** | **Venous Ulcers** |
| Location | Toes, feet, shin | Over medial or anterior ankle |
| Ulcer appearance | Deep, pale | Superficial, pink |
| Skin appearance | Normal to atrophic<br>Pallor on elevation<br>Rubor on dependency | Brown discoloration<br>Stasis dermatitis<br>Cyanosis on dependency |
| Skin temperature | Cool | Normal |
| Edema | Absent or mild | May be significant |
| Pain | Usually severe<br>Intermittent claudication<br>Rest pain | Usually mild<br>Aching pain |
| Gangrene | May occur | Does not occur |
| Pulses | Decreased or absent | Normal |

corticosteroid, zinc oxide ointment, or a topical broad-spectrum antifungal cream such as clotrimazole (Lotrimin) cream or miconazole (Monistat) cream (Tierney et al., 2001).

Isotonic saline compresses or wet-to-dry dressings are applied to stasis ulcers to promote healing. A dilute topical antibiotic solution also may be used (Braunwald et al., 2001). The ulcer may be treated by using a semirigid boot applied to the foot and lower leg. This device may be made of Unna's paste or Gauzetex bandage. Bony prominences must be well padded. The boot must be changed every 1 to 2 weeks, depending on the amount of drainage from the ulcer. This device often allows ambulatory treatment.

A very large, chronic ulcer may require surgery. In this case, the incompetent veins are ligated, the ulcer is excised, and the area is covered with a skin graft (see Chapter 14).

## NURSING CARE

Nursing care for the client with chronic venous insufficiency is primarily educative and supportive. Client teaching includes the following recommendations.

- Elevate the legs while resting and during sleep. See the box below for a nursing research study that suggests the supine position for resting.
- Walk as much as possible, but avoid sitting or standing for long periods of time.
- When sitting, do not cross your legs or allow pressure on the back of the knees (such as sitting on the side of the bed).
- Do not wear anything that pinches your legs (such as knee-high hose, garters, or girdles).

- Wear elastic hose as prescribed. The elastic hose should be tighter over the feet than at the top of the leg. Be sure the tops of the elastic hose do not cut into your legs. Put on the hose after you have had your legs elevated.
- Keep the skin on your feet and legs clean, soft, and dry.
- Follow guidelines in Box 33–4 for care of the legs and feet.

The following nursing diagnoses may apply to the client with chronic venous insufficiency.

- *Disturbed body image* related to edema and stasis ulcers on lower leg
- *Ineffective health maintenance* related to lack of knowledge about disorder and prescribed treatments
- *Risk for infection* related to ulcerations
- *Impaired physical mobility* related to pain and edema in lower legs
- *Impaired skin integrity* related to presence of stasis ulcers
- *Ineffective tissue perfusion: Peripheral* related to incompetent venous valves

See other sections of this chapter for specific nursing interventions related to many of these diagnoses. See the box on page 1021 for nursing care for the older adult with chronic venous stasis.

## THE CLIENT WITH VARICOSE VEINS

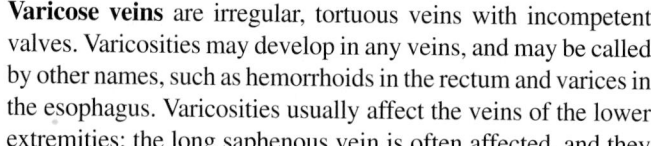

**Varicose veins** are irregular, tortuous veins with incompetent valves. Varicosities may develop in any veins, and may be called by other names, such as hemorrhoids in the rectum and varices in the esophagus. Varicosities usually affect the veins of the lower extremities; the long saphenous vein is often affected, and they also may develop in the short saphenous vein (Figure 33–8 ■).

## Nursing Research

### Evidence-Based Practice for the Client with Venous Leg Ulcers

Chronic leg ulcers due to venous insufficiency are a challenge to treat and heal. Oxygen is necessary for tissue repair and to prevent infection; however, peripheral perfusion to deliver oxygen to the tissues is impaired in clients with chronic venous insufficiency. Using measurements of transcutaneous tissue oxygen ($TcPo_2$), a group of nurse researchers evaluated the effects of four different positions and supplemental oxygen on a small group of subjects with venous ulcers (Wipke-Tevis, Stotts, Williams, Froelicher, & Hunt, 2001). Not surprisingly, these researchers found lower extremity resting $TcPo_2$ levels in clients with venous ulcers than in healthy adults. Changes in position resulted in minimal $TcPo_2$ changes in tissue surrounding the ulcer. When supplemental oxygen was given, $TcPo_2$ levels were higher in the supine position than with the legs elevated, sitting, or standing. These results suggest that control of peripheral circulation and tissue oxygenation may be impaired in clients with venous ulcers.

### IMPLICATIONS FOR NURSING
The results of this study support advising clients with chronic venous ulcers to stay off their feet and rest in bed as much as possi-

ble to promote healing of venous ulcers. Remove compression stockings and devices while the client is in bed to promote perfusion of subcutaneous tissues and of the region surrounding the ulcer itself. Discuss the effects of position on peripheral tissue perfusion with clients, and encourage frequent rest periods during the day. Consider discussing the option of supplemental oxygen therapy for a client with delayed ulcer healing with the primary care provider.

### Critical Thinking in Client Care

1. What is the usual response of blood vessels to changing positions from supine or sitting to standing? How does this compare with the results found here?
2. What is required for tissue healing? What measures can the nurse take to promote tissue healing in a client with impaired peripheral tissue perfusion?
3. How do the measures used to treat arterial and venous ulcers compare? Explain the rationale for differing treatment measures.

## Nursing Care of the Older Adult

### CHRONIC VENOUS STASIS

Disorders of venous stasis are common after the fifth decade of life. Aging affects vessels and tissues, increasing the risk for venous insufficiency and varicose veins. In addition, mobility frequently declines with aging, reducing the effect of the muscle pump in promoting venous return.

Regular exercise, walking in particular, is an important part of the treatment plan. Safety when walking is an important issue for older clients. Assess the client's mobility and stability during ambulation. If appropriate, suggest using a walker and quad-cane as needed. Assist older clients holding jobs that require prolonged standing to identify strategies to minimize standing and incorporate periods of activity into their work.

Following surgery or during treatment for stasis ulcers, older clients may need additional assistance with home care and maintenance. Initiate referral to social services as needed to arrange for home nursing care, meals, assistance with ADLs, and home maintenance services as indicated. In some instances, temporary placement in an extended care facility is necessary until the client and family can assume care.

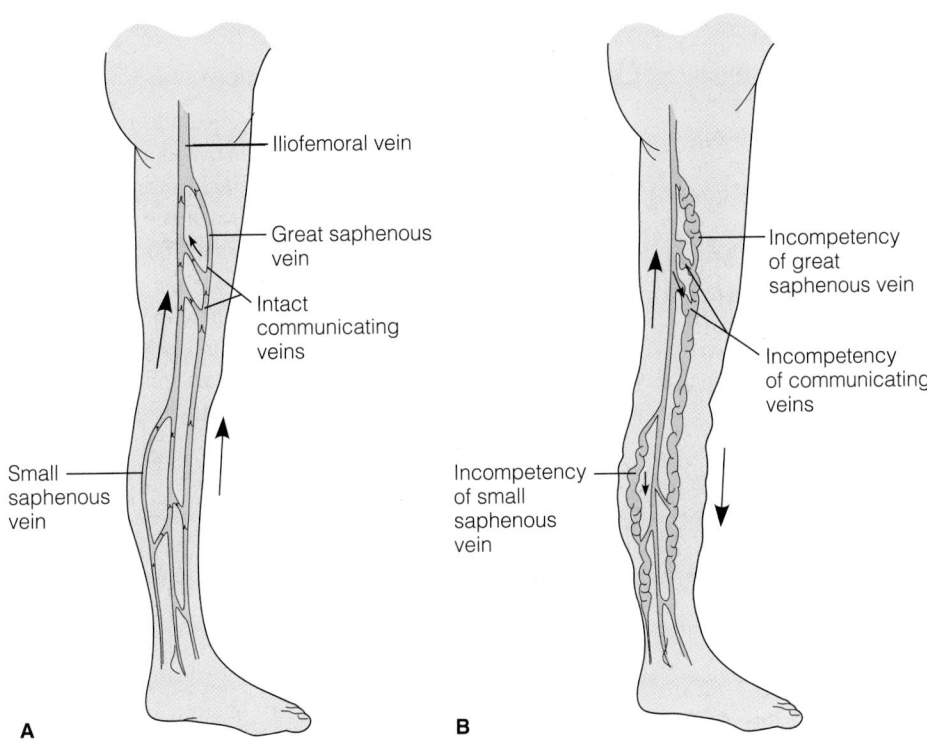

**Figure 33–8** ■ *A*, The normal venous structure of the leg. *B*, Varicose veins resulting from incompetent valves.

Varicose veins affect about 2% of people in industrialized nations. They are more common in women over age 35. Studies also suggest that the increased risk for varicose veins in women may relate to venous stasis during pregnancy. Aging is a risk factor, possibly related to decreased exercise and other factors that contribute to venous stasis. People in occupations that involve prolonged standing (such as beauticians, salespeople, and nurses) also have an increased incidence of varicose veins. Race is a risk factor: Whites are more frequently affected than blacks.

Most varicosities occur in the deep veins of the legs. Contributing causes include obesity, venous thrombosis, congenital arteriovenous malformations, or sustained pressure on abdominal veins (as in pregnancy and/or the presence of abdominal tumors). The effects of gravity, produced by long periods of standing, are a major causative factor.

## PATHOPHYSIOLOGY AND MANIFESTATIONS

Varicose veins are classified as primary (with no involvement of deep veins) or secondary (caused by the obstruction of deep veins). In both cases, long-standing increased venous pressure stretches the vessel wall. This sustained stretching impairs the ability of the venous valves to close, causing them to become incompetent.

The erect position produces a twofold negative effect on the veins. When standing, the leg veins resemble vertical columns and must withstand the full force of venous blood pressure. Prolonged standing, the force of gravity, lack of leg exercise, and incompetent venous valves all weaken the muscle-pumping mechanism, reducing venous blood return to the heart. As standing continues, the amount of blood pooled in the veins increases, further stretching the vessel wall. The venous valves become increasingly incompetent.

## Manifestations of Varicose Veins

- Severe, aching pain in the leg
- Leg fatigue, heaviness
- Itching of the affected leg (stasis dermatitis)
- Feelings of warmth in the leg
- Visibly dilated veins
- Thin, discolored skin above the ankles
- Stasis ulcers

Although varicose veins may be asymptomatic, most cause manifestations such as severe aching leg pain, leg fatigue, leg heaviness, itching, or feelings of heat in the legs. The degree of valvular incompetence does not seem to correlate well with the extent of symptoms. The menstrual cycle tends to worsen symptoms, suggesting a possible correlation with hormonal factors in women. Assessment reveals obvious dilated, tortuous veins beneath the skin of the upper and lower leg. If varicose veins are long-standing, the skin above the ankles may be thin and discolored, with a brown pigmentation. See the box above.

Complications of varicose veins include venous insufficiency and stasis ulcers. Chronic stasis dermatitis may also develop. Superficial venous thrombosis may develop in varicose veins, especially during and after pregnancy, following surgery, and in clients on estrogen therapy (oral contraceptives or hormone replacement therapy).

## COLLABORATIVE CARE

Varicose veins usually can be managed using conservative measures, although surgery may be required if symptoms are severe, when complications develop, or for cosmetic reasons.

### Diagnostic Tests

While varicose veins often are diagnosed by the history and physical examination, diagnostic tests may be ordered.

- *Doppler ultrasonography* or *duplex Doppler ultrasound* may be performed to identify specific locations of incompetent valves. This test is particularly useful before surgery to identify valves that allow reflux of blood from the femoral, popliteal, or peripheral deep veins into the superficial veins (Tierney et al., 2001).
- *Trendelenburg test* may be performed to determine the underlying cause of superficial venous insufficiency. The leg is elevated, then an elastic tourniquet is placed around the distal thigh. The varicosities then are observed as the client stands. When valves of the deep veins are incompetent, the veins remain flat on standing; they rapidly distend when the superficial venous valves are the underlying cause.

### Treatments

Although there is no real cure for varicose veins, conservative measures are the core of treatment for most clients with un-complicated varicose veins. These measures often relieve symptoms and prevent complications by improving venous circulation and relieving pressure on venous tissues. Properly fitted graduated compression stockings are commonly prescribed. They compress the veins, propelling blood back to the heart. Compression stockings augment the muscle pumping action of the legs. When worn during times of prolonged standing and in combination with frequent leg elevation, compression stockings often prevent progression of the condition and development of complications.

Regular, daily walking also is important. Prolonged sitting and standing are discouraged, although elevating the legs for specified periods during the day is beneficial. Leg elevation promotes venous return, prevents venous stasis, and decreases leg heaviness and fatigue.

### Compression Sclerotherapy

In compression sclerotherapy, a sclerosing solution is injected into the varicose vein and a compression bandage is applied for a period of time. This obliterates the vein. Venous blood is rerouted through healthy vessels whose valves are not compromised. Compression sclerotherapy may be used to treat small, symptomatic varicosities. It may be the primary treatment, or it may be used in conjunction with varicose vein surgery. While compression sclerotherapy may be done for cosmetic reasons, complications such as phlebitis, tissue necrosis, or infection may occur and need to be considered prior to the procedures.

### Surgery

Surgical treatment of varicose veins generally is reserved for clients who are very symptomatic, experience recurrent superficial venous thrombosis, and/or develop stasis ulcers. The objective of surgery is to remove the diseased veins. It may be considered for cosmetic reasons.

Surgery usually involves extensive ligation and stripping of the greater and lesser saphenous veins (Braunwald et al., 2001). The evening before surgery, the surgeon marks all incompetent superficial and perforating varicose veins with a permanent ink marker. Under either regional or general anesthesia, the greater saphenous vein is removed and the connected smaller tributaries that have not naturally clotted off are tied off. Multiple small incisions may be made over the varicosities, allowing removal of the affected segments of the vein. Incompetent tributaries that communicate with larger vessels also are ligated. For clients with less extensive disease or clients seeking cosmetic improvement, surgery may involve only the removal of the lesser saphenous vein through an incision in the popliteal fossa.

Postoperative care includes applying pressure bandages for a minimum of 6 weeks, elevating the extremities to minimize postoperative edema, and gradually increasing amounts of ambulation. Sitting and standing are prohibited during the initial recovery period, and are gradually reintroduced as deemed appropriate by the surgeon.

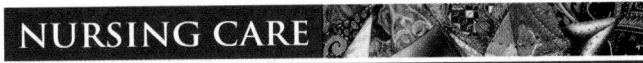

## NURSING CARE

### Health Promotion

Health promotion activities to reduce the incidence of varicose veins include teaching all clients, particularly young women, the benefits of regular exercise continued over the lifetime. Discuss the effect of prolonged sitting or standing on the legs, and encourage the client whose occupation involves these activities to periodically get up and move or to sit with the legs elevated. Encourage all clients to maintain normal weight for their height.

### Assessment

Focused assessment of the client with varicose veins includes the following:

- Health history: complaints of leg pain, aching, heaviness, or fatigue; ankle swelling; history of venous thrombosis
- Physical examination: visible, dilated, tortuous superficial veins in lower extremities

### Nursing Diagnoses and Interventions

In planning and providing nursing care for clients with varicose veins, emphasis is placed on the importance of health teaching to manage the symptoms of varicose veins, particularly because there is no cure for the disease. Nursing care for clients who have undergone surgical treatment for varicose veins focuses on assessing and promoting wound healing and preventing infection. Nursing diagnoses may include those related to pain, impaired tissue perfusion and skin integrity, and a risk for impaired neurovascular function.

### Chronic Pain

Varicose veins can lead to pooling of venous blood in the lower extremities. Venous congestion can cause a dull ache or feeling of pressure in the legs, particularly after prolonged standing. As venous pressure rises, arterial circulation and delivery of oxygen and nutrients to tissues is impaired. Tissue ischemia contributes to the pain. The pain associated with varicose veins tends to be chronic, developing and progressing gradually over a long period of time.

- Assess pain, including its intensity, duration, and aggravating and relieving factors. *Pain assessment allows collaborative planning with the client to identify appropriate interventions.*
- Inquire about current measures being used by the client to manage pain and its effects. Ask about the effectiveness of current management strategies and the desire to change. *Chronic pain management ultimately falls to the client. Strategies to address the pain must meet the client's needs.*

**PRACTICE ALERT**   *Suggest keeping a diary of pain intensity, timing, precipitating events, and effectiveness of relief measures. Systematic tracking of pain is an important measure in improving its management.* ■

- Teach and reinforce nonpharmacologic pain management strategies such as progressive relaxation, imagery, deep breathing, distraction, and meditation. *The effectiveness of such strategies is well documented. Nonpharmacologic measures provide a variety of options for controlling pain while maintaining independence. These measures also can reduce reliance on analgesics.*
- Collaborate with the client to establish a pain control plan. *Collaborative planning for pain management increases the client's sense of control and reduces powerlessness. This, in turn, enhances the ability to cope with pain and its effects.*
- Regularly evaluate the effectiveness of planned interventions and pain management strategies. *Regular evaluation allows modification of the care plan as needed, as well as providing a measure of disease progression. Increasing or poorly controlled pain may necessitate additional collaborative interventions to manage the disorder.*

### Ineffective Tissue Perfusion: Peripheral

Varicose veins and venous stasis impair delivery of nutrients and oxygen to peripheral tissues as elevated venous pressures interfere with blood flow through the capillary beds. Improving venous blood flow reduces venous pressures and promotes arterial flow to peripheral tissues.

- Assess peripheral pulses, capillary refill, skin color and temperature, and extent of edema. *Assessment of arterial flow and tissue perfusion provide baseline and continuing data for evaluating the effectiveness of interventions.*
- Teach application and use of properly fitted elastic graduated compression stockings. *Elastic compression stockings compress the veins, promoting venous return from the lower extremities. During ambulation, the stockings enhance the blood-pumping action of the muscles. Because elastic stockings inhibit blood flow through small superficial vessels, they should be removed at least once each day for at least 30 minutes.*

**PRACTICE ALERT**   *Instruct to maintain a program of regular exercise, such as walking for 20 to 30 minutes several times a day. Exercise stimulates circulation and promotes blood flow through the vascular system. When ambulation is restricted, active range-of-motion exercises help maintain muscle tone, joint mobility, and venous return.* ■

- Advise to elevate the legs for 15 to 20 minutes several times a day and to sleep with the legs elevated above the level of the heart. *Elevating the legs promotes venous return, reducing tissue congestion and improving arterial circulation. Improved venous return also increases the cardiac output and renal perfusion, promoting elimination of excess fluid and decreasing peripheral edema.*

### Risk for Impaired Skin Integrity

Ineffective venous valve function impairs venous return and increases venous pressures. These increased pressures oppose arterial blood flow and the delivery of oxygen and nutrients to the cells. As a result, tissues are vulnerable to any additional insult, and may break down.

- Assess lower extremity color, temperature, moisture, and for evidence of pressure or breakdown on admission and at each visit. *Initial and continuing assessment allows timely detection of early signs of skin and tissue breakdown. This, in turn, allows early institution of measures to prevent further tissue damage and promote healing.*
- Teach foot and skin care measures such as daily cleansing with nondrying soap, gentle drying, and lotions to prevent skin dryness and cracking. *Cleansing removes potentially harmful microorganisms and stimulates circulation. Care is taken to keep the skin moist and supple, promoting its function as the first line of defense against infection.*
- Discuss the importance of adequate nutrition and fluid intake. *Adequate nutrients are necessary to maintain tissue integrity and promote healing. A diet high in protein, carbohydrates, and vitamins and minerals promotes growth and maintenance of skin cells, provides energy, and helps prevent skin breakdown. Adequate hydration helps maintain the moisture and turgor of skin, reducing the risk of drying and breakdown.*

### Risk for Peripheral Neurovascular Dysfunction

Severe varicose veins can lead to chronic venous insufficiency, impaired arterial circulation, and ultimately, disrupted sensation in the affected extremity. Impaired neurologic function increases the client's risk for injury and infection of the extremity, as minor trauma may go unnoticed.

- Assess circulation, sensation, and movement of the lower extremities. *Disrupted circulation and venous congestion may interfere with sensory and motor function of the affected extremity. The potential for nerve and muscle involvement is especially high in clients with venous stasis ulcers.*

**PRACTICE ALERT** *Instruct to report signs of neurovascular dysfunction, such as numbness, coldness, pain, or tingling of an extremity. Early recognition of neurovascular dysfunction facilitates institution of interventions to prevent complications. Because the postoperative hospital stay following varicose vein surgery or venous stasis ulcer repair is brief, manifestations of neurovascular dysfunction may initially be detected by the client. Careful assessment and prompt reporting helps prevent potential complications such as skin breakdown, infection, and nerve damage.* ■

- Teach measures to protect the extremities from injury, such as always wearing shoes or firm slippers, cotton socks to absorb moisture, and testing the temperature of bath water with a thermometer or the upper extremities before stepping in. *Sensation in the lower extremities may be affected by poor circulation, necessitating additional measures to protect the legs and feet from injury.*

### Home Care

Most clients with varicose veins provide self-care at home. Include the following topics when preparing the client and family for home care.

- Leg elevation and exercise program
- Application and use of graduated elastic compression stockings
- Foot and leg care (see Box 33–4)
- Measures to avoid injury and skin breakdown
- Symptoms or potential complications to report to the physician

Provide information about suppliers for elastic stockings and any other required supplies. If venous stasis ulcers have developed, consider referral to home health services for regular assessment of healing and additional teaching.

## DISORDERS OF THE LYMPHATIC SYSTEM

The lymphatic system, which includes the lymphatic vessels and the lymph nodes, is a unique part of the circulatory system. The lymphatic system returns plasma and plasma proteins filtered out of the capillaries from interstitial tissues to the bloodstream. This fluid is called *lymph*. The lymphatic system consists of closed capillaries leading to larger lymphatic venules and lymphatic veins. These vessels contain smooth muscle and one-way valves that help move fluid toward the heart. Lymphatic vessels share the same sheath as arteries and veins; arterial pulsations and skeletal muscle contractions compress the lymphatic vessels to assist in maintaining lymph flow. As lymph moves through the lymphatic system, it is filtered through thousands of bean-shaped lymph nodes clustered along the vessels. Within these nodes, phagocytes remove foreign material from the lymph, preventing it from entering the bloodstream.

### THE CLIENT WITH LYMPHADENOPATHY

*Lymphadenopathy*, enlarged lymph nodes, may be localized or generalized. Localized lymphadenopathy usually results from an inflammatory process (e.g., streptococcal pharyngitis or an infected wound). The node enlarges as lymphocytes and monocytes proliferate within the node to destroy infectious material. Palpable lymph nodes often develop in response to minor trauma or a localized infection. Generalized lymphadenopathy usually is associated with malignancy or disease. Malignant cells or other abnormal cells invade the node, causing it to enlarge.

*Lymphangitis*, inflammation of the lymph vessels draining an infected area of the body, is characterized by a red streak along the inflamed vessels, pain, heat, and swelling. Fever and chills also may be present. Local lymph nodes are swollen and tender.

Treatment for lymphadenopathy and lymphangitis focuses on identifying and treating the underlying condition. Elevating the body part and applying heat to inflamed lymphatic vessels help reduce swelling and promote blood flow to the affected area.

## THE CLIENT WITH LYMPHEDEMA

**Lymphedema** may be a primary or a secondary disorder, resulting from inflammation, obstruction, or removal of lymphatic vessels. It is characterized by extremity edema due to accumulation of lymph. *Primary lymphedema* is uncommon, affecting about 1 in 10,000 people. It affects females more frequently than males, and may be associated with a genetic disorder (Braunwald et al., 2001).

*Secondary lymphedema* is an acquired condition, resulting from damage, obstruction, or removal of lymphatic vessels. The most common worldwide cause of secondary lymphedema is *filariasis,* infestation of the lymphatic vessels by filaria, a nematode worm. Other important causes of secondary lymphedema include recurrent episodes of bacterial lymphangitis, obstruction of lymph vessels by tumors, and surgical or radiation treatment for breast cancer (Braunwald et al., 2001).

## PATHOPHYSIOLOGY AND MANIFESTATIONS

Obstruction of lymph drainage prevents fluid and protein molecules from interstitial tissues from returning to the circulation. The protein molecules increase the osmotic pressure in interstitial tissues, drawing in additional fluid that causes edema in the soft tissues. One or both extremities may be affected.

The edema begins distally, progressing up the limb to involve the entire extremity (Figure 33–9 ■). Initial edema is soft and pitting; with chronic congestion, subcutaneous tissues become fibrotic, causing thick, rough skin and a woody texture of the limb (*brawny edema*). In contrast, the edema associated with venous disorders is softer, and the skin often is hyperpigmented with evidence of stasis dermatitis. Lymphedema generally is painless, although the limb may feel heavy.

## COLLABORATIVE CARE

Collaborative care for the client with lymphedema focuses on relieving edema and preventing or treating infection. The disorder may be difficult to treat effectively, and can lead to progressive disability due to the weight and awkwardness of the affected extremity.

### Diagnostic Tests

Abdominal or pelvic ultrasound and computed tomography (CT) scans are used to detect obstructing lesions. Magnetic resonance imaging (MRI) can show edema and identify lymph nodes and enlarged lymphatic vessels. More invasive procedures such as lymphangiography and radioactive isotope studies may occasionally be necessary to identify the lymphatic defect causing lymphedema.

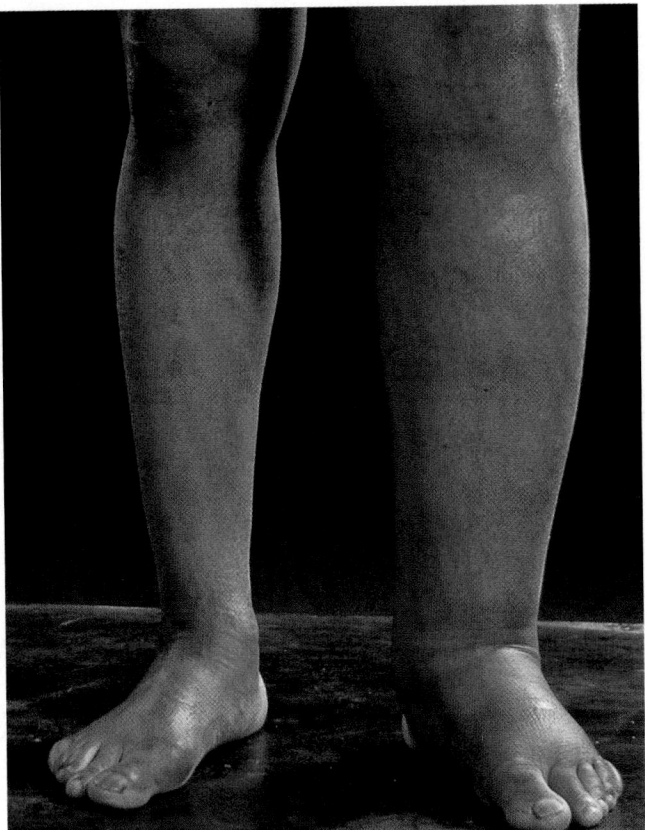

**Figure 33–9** ■ Severe lymphedema of the lower extremity.

*Source: MSNB/Custom Medical Stock Photo, Inc.*

- *Lymphangiography* uses injected contrast media to illustrate lymphatic vessels on X-rays. Organic dyes are used to identify a distal lymphatic vessel, and then a contrast medium is injected into the vessel for visualization of the lymphatic system of the limb. In primary lymphedema, lymph vessels are absent or hypoplastic (underdeveloped). In secondary lymphedema, lymph channels often are dilated; it may be possible to determine the level of obstruction (Braunwald et al., 2001).
- *Lymphoscintigraphy* involves injecting a radioactively tagged substance into distal subcutaneous tissues of the extremity, then mapping its flow through the lymphatic system. The pattern of lymph fluid distribution and transport is abnormal in clients with lymphedema.

### Treatments

Meticulous skin and foot care is vital to prevent infection in the affected extremity. Shoes should always be worn to reduce the risk of injury. Careful cleansing and use of emollient lotions are recommended to prevent drying of the skin. Exercise is encouraged, as are frequent periods of leg elevation. The foot of the bed is raised by 15 to 20 degrees at night to promote lymph flow. Elastic graduated compression stockings may be ordered for use during the day. In some cases, an intermittent pneumatic compression device to reduce edema may be prescribed for home use.

Antibiotics are given to prevent and treat infection, which can be recurrent and difficult to eradicate. Diuretic therapy may be used intermittently, particularly when primary lymphedema is exacerbated by the menstrual cycle or seasonal variability (Tierney et al., 2001).

Clients who do not respond to conservative treatment measures or who experience recurrent episodes of cellulitis and lymphangitis may require surgical treatment. Microvascular techniques may be used to create anatomoses between obstructed lymphatic vessels and adjacent veins, providing channels to redirect lymph into the venous system. Successful surgery may improve both extremity function and its cosmetic appearance (Tierney et al., 2001).

# NURSING CARE

Nursing care for clients with lymphatic disorders focuses on reducing edema, preventing tissue damage related to the edema, and promoting effective coping with the effect of the disorder on body image and function.

## Nursing Diagnoses and Interventions

Nursing diagnoses for the client with lymphedema may include *Impaired tissue integrity, Excess fluid volume,* and *Disturbed body image.*

### Impaired Tissue Integrity

Obstructed lymphatic flow leads to fluid congestion of the interstitial spaces of subcutaneous tissue. The resulting edema compresses and damages tissues of the affected extremity. Subcutaneous tissues become fibrotic, reducing their protective functions of shock absorption and insulation. In addition, obstructed lymphatic flow reduces the effectiveness of lymph nodes in filtering and removing foreign material and pathogens from the body. This increases the risk for local tissue infection such as *cellulitis,* a diffuse bacterial infection of the skin. Cellulitis increases the risk for skin and tissue breakdown and, if not effectively treated, can lead to sepsis.

**PRACTICE ALERT** *Frequently inspect the skin of the affected extremity, documenting condition with each assessment. Promptly report areas of pallor, redness, or apparent inflammation. Breaks in the skin surface allow microbial invasion, and increase the risk for infection. Prompt identification and treatment of any lesions is vital to prevent further tissue breakdown and infection.* ■

- Apply well-fitting elastic graduated compression stockings or intermittent pneumatic pressure devices as ordered. *Elastic stockings and/or pneumatic pressure devices oppose the movement of fluid out of capillaries and improve its reabsorption into vascular spaces for transportation back to the heart.*

**PRACTICE ALERT** *Remove elastic stockings and intermittent pressure devices every 8 hours or at each home visit to inspect the underlying skin for evidence of redness, irritation, dryness, or breakdown. Elastic graduated compression stockings, antiembolic stockings, and pneumatic compression devices compress small vessels nourishing the skin and subcutaneous tissue. Periodic removal not only allows inspection of the underlying skin, but also allows restoration of blood flow to these small vessels and the tissues.* ■

- Instruct to elevate the extremities while seated and during sleep. *Elevation of the extremities diminishes venous congestion, promotes venous return, facilitates arterial circulation and tissue perfusion, and helps reduce the accumulation of excess fluids in interstitial spaces of the affected extremity.*

**PRACTICE ALERT** *Use preventive skin care devices as indicated. Collected fluid in the affected extremity increases its weight and interferes with regular movement. The increased weight places greater pressure on surfaces of the limb that come in contact with furniture. Protective devices such as egg crate foam, sheepskin, pillows, or padding help prevent tissue compression, promoting circulation and reducing the risk of skin and tissue breakdown.* ■

- Keep skin clean and dry, especially in interdigital spaces. Teach skin and foot care to the client and family. *Clean, dry skin provides the first line of defense against infection. Significant limb edema can interfere with reaching the distal extremity and cleaning interdigital spaces. The dark, moist spaces between the toes are an excellent environment for bacterial growth. Teaching fosters self-care and independence, as well as preparing the client and family to manage this often chronic condition.*
- Discuss the importance of adhering to the therapeutic regimen. *Lymphedema generally is a chronic condition; effective management requires active client participation in planning and implementing care to reduce edema and maintain tissue integrity.*

### Excess Fluid Volume

In lymphedema, obstruction, destruction, or congenital malformation of lymphatic vessels interferes with the normal circulation of lymphatic fluid. As a result, lymph collects in the subcutaneous tissues of the affected extremity, causing excess fluid volume of that extremity. Some clients may benefit from intermittent diuretic therapy and dietary sodium restriction.

- Discuss the rationale for restricted sodium intake if ordered. Teach ways to maintain the recommended sodium restriction, and assist to choose foods that are low in sodium. *Sodium causes retention of extracellular water; restricting dietary sodium may help prevent additional fluid accumulation in interstitial spaces.*

**PRACTICE ALERT** *Monitor intake and output and/or weight (daily or weekly). Use consistent scales, timing, and clothing for accurate weight measurements. Intake and output records and short-term changes in weight reflect fluid balance. Measures of fluid balance permit evaluation of the effectiveness of interventions such as restricted sodium intake and diuretic therapy.* ■

- During acute periods, assess the affected extremity daily for increased edema; measure girth of the extremity using consistent technique. *The size of the affected extremity provides a measure of the effectiveness of ordered interventions and progression of the disorder.*

### Disturbed Body Image

The disproportionate size of an extremity or extremities due to lymphedema can profoundly affect body image. During early stages of the disease, conservative measures may effectively reduce the edema and size of the affected limb. However, as the disease progresses, conservative measures may become less effective, leading to more permanent disfigurement. Mobility may be impaired, and the client may develop an increasingly negative self-perception.

- Encourage discussions about usual coping patterns and perception of self. *Knowledge of existing coping patterns and behaviors helps the nurse assess the client's ability to cope with the current situation. This knowledge is then used to reinforce effective coping mechanisms and help develop more effective coping strategies. This exchange also allows the client to voice feelings related to actual or perceived changes in body image.*
- Accept the client's perception of self and of the impact of the changes in appearance. *Nonjudgmental acceptance of the client's view of self and of the effects of changes in appearance builds trust and promotes rapport. A trusting relationship promotes the client's ability to take an active role in managing the disorder, participate in health care decisions, and adhere to the plan of care. Nonjudgmental listening also promotes mutual respect and demonstrates caring and compassion.*
- Encourage active participation in self-care. Assist with identifying alternative self-care strategies when the extent of

edema interferes with performing some aspects of self-care such as trimming toenails or washing feet. *The client initially may have difficulty viewing or touching the affected body part. Gentle encouragement and support from the nurse helps the client assume self-care and accept the affected body part. Brainstorming to identify alternative care strategies promotes the client's independence even when total self-care is not feasible.*

### Home Care

When preparing the client with chronic lymphedema and family to manage the disorder, include the following teaching topics.

- Recommended program of exercise and elevation of the extremity
- Foot and skin care
- Use of elastic graduated compression stockings and/or intermittent pressure devices
- Importance of wearing elastic stockings during the majority of waking hours, removing them once during the daytime and while sleeping
- Measures to prevent infection in the affected extremity, such as wearing gloves while gardening
- Signs and symptoms to report to the health care provider (e.g., manifestations of tissue breakdown or infection, increasing edema, or evidence of compromised circulation)
- Use and precautions associated with any prescribed medications
- Sodium-restricted diet if ordered

Provide information about contacts for questions, and make referrals as needed. Evaluate the need for home health, home maintenance assistance, and other services such as physical or occupational therapy.

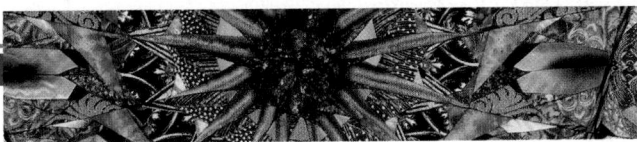

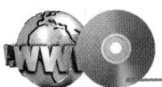 **EXPLORE MediaLink**

NCLEX review questions, case studies, care plan activities, MediaLink applications, and other interactive resources for this chapter can be found on the Companion Website at www.prenhall.com/lemone.

Click on Chapter 33 to select the activities for this chapter. For animations, video clips, more NCLEX review questions, and an audio glossary, access the Student CD-ROM accompanying this textbook.

## TEST YOURSELF

1. A potential blood donor whose blood pressure is found to average 180/106 on two different readings tells the nurse, "I don't understand how it could be so high—I feel just fine." The appropriate response by the nurse is:

   a. "This is probably just a false reading due to 'white coat syndrome.' Don't worry about it."

   b. "It is unusual that you are not having some symptoms such as severe headaches and nosebleeds."

   c. "High blood pressure often has few or no symptoms; that's why it is called the 'silent killer.'"

   d. "You probably should have your blood pressure rechecked in 3 months or so and then follow up with your primary care provider if it is still high."

2. A client is complaining of new onset calf and foot pain. The nurse notes that the leg below the knee is cool, pale, and dorsalis pedis and posterior tibial pulses are absent. The nurse should:

   a. Immediately notify the physician
   b. Elevate the leg and apply a warm blanket
   c. Provide the ordered analgesic
   d. Apply antiembolism (TED) stockings

3. An expected assessment finding in a client with peripheral atherosclerosis would be:

   a. Pallor of the legs and feet when dependent
   b. Increased hair growth on the affected extremity
   c. Higher blood pressure readings in the affected extremity
   d. Impaired sensation in the affected extremity

4. The nurse evaluates her teaching of a client admitted with deep vein thrombosis as effective when the client states:

   a. "I'll use a hard-backed, upright chair when sitting instead of my recliner."
   b. "I'll get my blood drawn as scheduled and notify the doctor if I have any unusual bleeding or bruising."
   c. "I understand why I am not allowed to exercise for the next 6 weeks and will take it easy."
   d. "I'll have my wife buy a low-cholesterol cookbook and we'll make an appointment with the dietician to learn about a low-fat, low-cholesterol diet."

5. A client with visible varicose veins tells the nurse that she wants to have surgery to remove them, because "my legs ache every evening and they are really ugly!" The most appropriate response would be:

   a. "Often measures such as elevating your legs and elastic stockings can relieve the discomfort associated with varicose veins."
   b. "Surgery will have a good cosmetic effect, but will not relieve the discomfort associated with varicose veins."
   c. "All varicose veins should be surgically removed to restore adequate blood flow to your legs and prevent gangrene."
   d. "Surgery is never indicated unless the varicose veins are interfering with circulation. Have you tried cosmetic measures to cover them up?"

See Test Yourself answers in Appendix C.

# BIBLIOGRAPHY

Ackley, B. J., & Ladwig, G. B. (2002). *Nursing diagnosis handbook: A guide to planning care* (5th ed.). St. Louis: Mosby.

Braunwald, E., Fauci, A. S., Kasper, D. L., Hauser, S. L., Longo, D. L., & Jameson, J. L. (2001). *Harrison's principles of internal medicine* (15th ed.). New York: McGraw-Hill.

Breen, P. (2000). DVT: What every nurse should know. *RN, 63*(4), 58–62.

Chase, S. L. (2000). Hypertensive crisis. *RN, 63*(6), 62–67.

Church, V. (2000). Staying on guard for DVT & PE. *Nursing, 30*(2), 34–42.

Deglin, J. H., & Vallerand, A. H. (2003). *Davis's drug guide for nurses* (8th ed.). Philadelphia: F.A. Davis.

Ferguson, M., Cook, A., Rimmasch, H., Bender, S., & Voss, A. (2000). Pressure ulcer management: The importance of nutrition. *MEDSURG Nursing, 9*(4), 163–175.

Fontaine, K. L. (2000). *Healing practices: Alternative therapies for nursing.* Upper Saddle River, NJ: Prentice Hall Health.

Gallo, J. J., Busby-Whitehead, J., Rabins, P. V., Silliman, R. A., & Murphy, J. B. (Eds.). (1999). *Reichel's care of the elderly: Clinical aspects of aging* (5th ed.). Philadelphia: Lippincott Williams & Wilkins.

Gibson, J. M., & Kenrick, M. (1998). Pain and powerlessness: The experience of living with peripheral vascular disease. *Journal of Advanced Nursing, 27*(4), 737–745.

Hess, C. T. (2001). Putting the squeeze on venous ulcers. *Nursing, 31*(9), 58–63.

Johnson, M., Bulechek, G., Dochterman, J. M., Maas, M., & Moorhead, S. (2001). *Nursing diagnoses, outcomes, & interventions.* St. Louis: Mosby.

Johnson, M., Maas, M., & Moorhead, S. (Eds.). (2000). *Nursing outcomes classification (NOC)* (2nd ed.). St. Louis: Mosby.

Kuhn, M. A. (1999). *Complementary therapies for health care providers.* Philadelphia: Lippincott.

Lehne, R. A. (2001). *Pharmacology for nursing care* (4th ed.). Philadelphia: Saunders.

Malarkey, L. M., & McMorrow, M. E. (2000). *Nurse's manual of laboratory tests and diagnostic procedures* (2nd ed.). Philadelphia: Saunders.

McCance, K. L., & Huether, S. E. (2002). *Pathophysiology: The biologic basis for disease in adults and children* (4th ed.). St. Louis: Mosby.

McCloskey, J. C., & Bulechek, G. M. (Eds.) (2000). *Nursing interventions classification (NIC)* (3rd ed.). St. Louis: Mosby.

McConnell, E. A. (2002). Clinical do's & don'ts. Applying antiembolism stockings. *Nursing, 32*(4), 17.

Meeker, M. H., & Rothrock, J. C. (1999). *Alexander's care of the patient in surgery* (11th ed.). St. Louis: Mosby.

Miracle, V. A. (2001). Act fast during a hypertensive crisis. *Nursing, 31*(9), 50–51.

National Heart, Lung, and Blood Institute: National High Blood Pressure Education Program. (1997). *The sixth report of the Joint National Committee on Prevention, Detection, Evaluation, and Treatment of High Blood Pressure.* Bethesda, MD: National Institutes of Health.

National Heart, Lung, and Blood Institute, National Institutes of Health. (2002). *Morbidity & mortality: 2002 chart book of cardiovascular, lung, and blood diseases.* Bethesda, MD: Author.

Navuluri, R. (2001a). Anticoagulant therapy. *American Journal of Nursing, 101*(11), 24A–24D.

Navuluri, R. (2001b). Nursing implications of anticoagulant therapy. *American Journal of Nursing, 101*(12), 24A–B.

North American Nursing Diagnosis Association. (2001). *NANDA nursing diagnoses: Definitions & classification 2001–2002.* Philadelphia: NANDA.

Patel, C. T. C., Kinsey, G. C., Koperski-Moen, K. J., & Bungum, L. D. (2000). Vacuum-assisted wound closure. *American Journal of Nursing, 100*(12), 45–48.

Porth, C. M. (2002). *Pathophysiology: Concepts of altered health states* (6th ed.). Philadelphia: Lippincott.

Spratto, G. R., & Woods, A. L. (2003). *2003 edition PDR® nurse's drug handbook™.* Clifton Park, NY: Delmar Learning.

Tierney, L. M., McPhee, S. J., & Papadakis, M. A. (2001). *Current medical diagnosis & treatment* (40th ed.). New York: Lange Medical Books/McGraw-Hill.

Wipke-Tevis, D. D., Stotts, N. A., Williams, D. A., Froelicher, E. S., & Hunt, T. K. (2001). Tissue oxygenation, perfusion, and position in patients with venous leg ulcers. *Nursing Research, 50*(1), 24–32.

Woods, S. L., Froelicher, E. S. S., & Motzer, S. U. (2000). *Cardiac nursing* (4th ed.). Philadelphia: Lippincott.

Woods, A. (2002). Patient education series. High blood pressure (hypertension). *Nursing, 32*(4), 54–55.

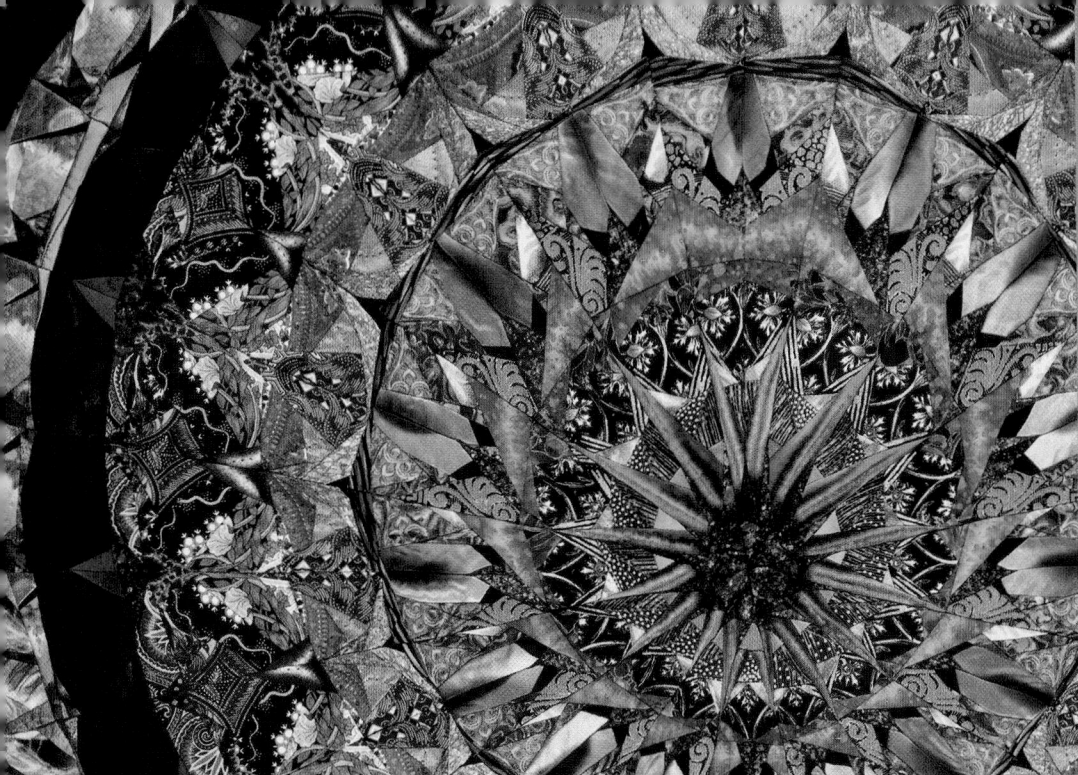

# RESPONSES TO ALTERED RESPIRATORY FUNCTION

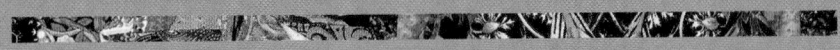

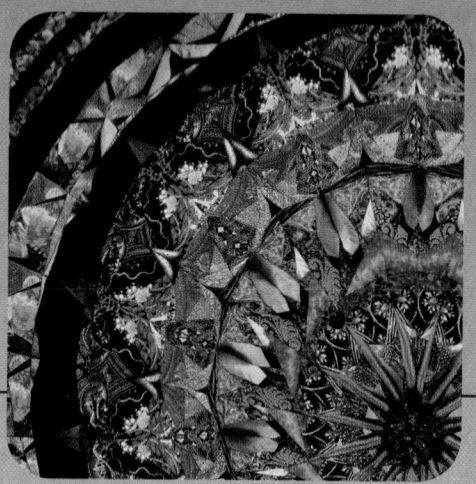

# Assessing Clients with Respiratory Disorders

## LEARNING OUTCOMES

After completing this chapter, you will be able to:

- Review the anatomy and physiology of the respiratory system.

- Explain the mechanics of ventilation.

- Describe factors affecting respiration.

- Identify specific topics for consideration during a health history interview of the client with health problems involving the respiratory system.

- Describe physical assessment techniques for respiratory function.

- Identify abnormal findings that may indicate impairment in the function of the respiratory system.

The respiratory system provides the cells of the body with oxygen and eliminates carbon dioxide, formed as a waste product of cellular metabolism. The events in this process, called respiration, are:

- *Pulmonary ventilation:* Air is moved into and out of the lungs.
- *External respiration:* Exchange of oxygen and carbon dioxide occurs between the alveoli and the blood.
- *Gas transport:* Oxygen and carbon dioxide are transported to and from the lungs and the cells of the body via the blood.
- *Internal respiration:* Exchange of oxygen and carbon dioxide is made between the blood and the cells.

## REVIEW OF ANATOMY AND PHYSIOLOGY

Although the system functions as a whole, this unit contains separate chapters dealing with the upper respiratory system (the nose, pharynx, larynx, and trachea) and the lower respiratory system (the lungs).

## The Upper Respiratory System

The upper respiratory system serves as a passageway for air moving into the lungs and carbon dioxide moving out to the external environment (Figure 34–1 ■). As air moves through these structures, it is cleaned, humidified, and warmed.

### The Nose

The nose is the external opening of the respiratory system. The external nose is given structure by the nasal, frontal, and maxillary bones as well as plates of hyaline cartilage. The nostrils (also called the external nares) are two cavities within the nose, separated by the nasal septum. These cavities open into the nasal portion of the pharynx through the internal nares. The nasal cavities just behind the nasal openings are lined with skin that contains hair follicles, sweat glands, and sebaceous glands. The nasal hairs filter the air as it enters the nares. The rest of the cavity is lined with mucous membranes that contain olfactory neurons and goblet cells that secrete thick mucus. The mucus not only traps dust and bacteria but also contains lysozyme, an enzyme that destroys bacteria as they enter the nose. As mucus and debris accumulate, mucosal ciliated cells move it toward the pharynx, where it is swallowed. The mucosa is highly vascular, warming air that moves across its surface.

Three structures project outward from the lateral wall of each nasal cavity: the superior, middle, and inferior turbinates. The turbinates cause air entering the nose to become turbulent and also increase the surface area of mucosa exposed to the air. As air moves through this area, heavier particles of debris drop out and are trapped in the mucosa of the turbinates.

### The Sinuses

The nasal cavity is surrounded by paranasal sinuses (Figure 34–2 ■). These openings are located in the frontal, sphenoid, ethmoid, and maxillary bones. Sinuses lighten the skull, assist in speech, and produce mucus that drains into the nasal cavities to help trap debris.

### The Pharynx

The pharynx, a funnel-shaped passageway about 5 inches (13 cm) long, extends from the base of the skull to the level of the C6 vertebra. The pharynx serves as a passageway for both air and food. It is divided into three regions: the nasopharynx, the oropharynx, and the laryngopharynx.

The nasopharynx serves only as a passageway for air. Located beneath the sphenoid bone and above the level of the soft palate, the nasopharynx is continuous with the nasal cavities. This segment is lined with ciliated epithelium, which continues

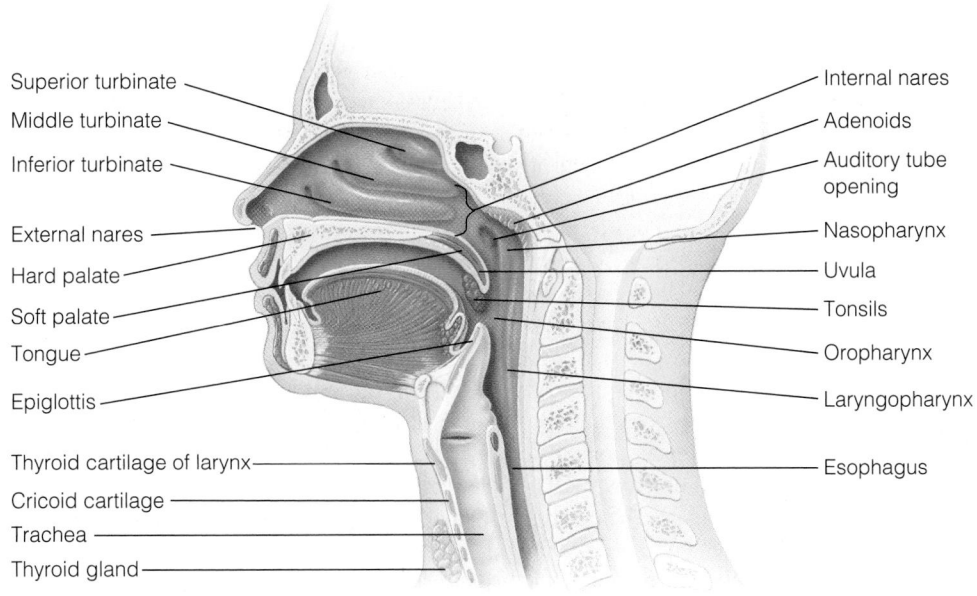

Superior turbinate
Middle turbinate
Inferior turbinate

External nares
Hard palate
Soft palate
Tongue
Epiglottis

Thyroid cartilage of larynx
Cricoid cartilage
Trachea
Thyroid gland

Internal nares
Adenoids
Auditory tube opening
Nasopharynx
Uvula
Tonsils
Oropharynx
Laryngopharynx

Esophagus

**Figure 34–1** ■ The upper respiratory system.

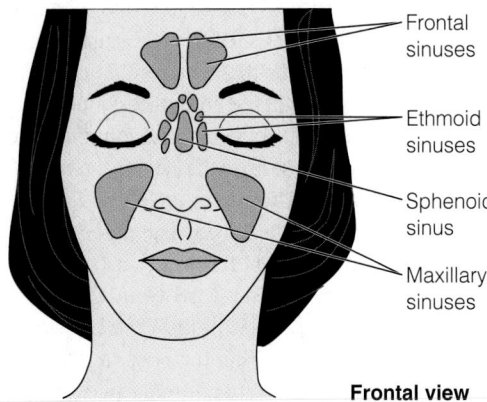
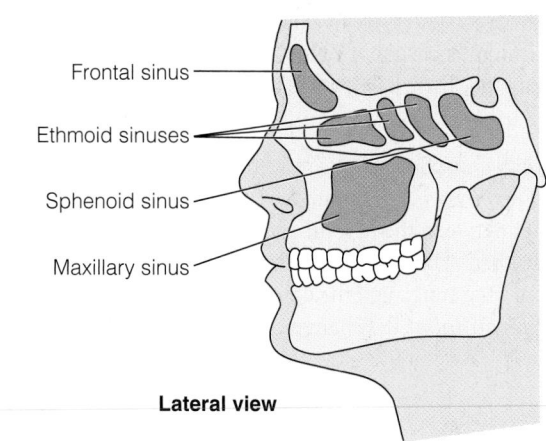

**Frontal view**

**Lateral view**

**Figure 34–2** ■ Sinuses, frontal and lateral views.

to move debris from the nasal cavities to the pharynx. Masses of lymphoid tissue (the tonsils and adenoids) are located in the mucosa high in the posterior wall; these tissues trap and destroy infectious agents entering with the air. The auditory (eustachian) tubes also open into the nasopharynx, connecting it with the middle ear.

The oropharynx lies behind the oral cavity and extends from the soft palate to the level of the hyoid bone. It serves as a passageway for both air and food. An upward rise of the soft palate prevents food from entering the nasopharynx during swallowing. The oropharynx is lined with stratified squamous epithelium that protects it from the friction of food and damage from the chemicals found in food and fluids.

The laryngopharynx extends from the hyoid bone to the larynx. It is also lined with stratified squamous epithelium, and serves as a passageway for both food and air. Air does not move into the lungs while food is being swallowed and moved into the esophagus.

### The Larynx

The larynx is about 2 inches (5 cm) long. It opens superiorly at the laryngopharynx and is continuous inferiorly with the trachea. The larynx provides an airway and routes air and food into the proper passageway. As long as air is moving through the larynx, its inlet is open; however, the inlet closes during swallowing. The larynx also contains the vocal cords, necessary for voice production.

The larynx is framed by cartilages, connected by ligaments and membranes. The thyroid cartilage is formed by the fusion of two cartilages; the fusion point is visible as the Adam's apple. The cricoid cartilage lies below the thyroid cartilage; other pairs of cartilages form the walls of the larynx. The epiglottis, also a cartilage, is covered with mucosa that contains taste buds. This structure normally projects upward to the base of the tongue; however, during swallowing, the larynx moves upward and the epiglottis tips to cover the opening to the larynx. If anything other than air enters the larynx, a cough reflex expels the foreign substance before it can enter the lungs. This protective reflex does not work if the person is unconscious.

### The Trachea

The trachea begins at the inferior larynx and descends anteriorly to the esophagus to enter the mediastinum, where it divides to become the right and left primary bronchi of the lungs. The trachea is about 4 to 5 inches (12 to 15 cm) long and 1 inch (2.5 cm) in diameter. It contains 16 to 20 C-shaped rings of cartilage joined by connective tissue. The mucosa lining the trachea consists of pseudostratified ciliated columnar epithelium containing seromucous glands that produce thick mucus. Dust and debris in the inspired air are trapped in this mucus, moved toward the throat by the cilia, and then either swallowed or coughed out through the mouth.

## The Lower Respiratory System

The lower respiratory system includes the lungs and the bronchi (Figures 34–3 ■ and 34–4 ■).

### The Lungs

The center of the thoracic cavity is filled by the *mediastinum*, which contains the heart, great blood vessels, bronchi, trachea, and esophagus. The mediastinum is flanked on either side by the lungs (see Figure 34–3). Each lung is suspended in its own pleural cavity, with the anterior, lateral, and posterior lung surfaces lying close to the ribs. The hilus, on the mediastinal surface of each lung, is where blood vessels of the pulmonary and circulatory systems enter and exit the lungs. The primary bronchus also enters in this area. The apex of each lung lies just below the clavicle, whereas the base of each lung rests on the diaphragm. The lungs are elastic connective tissue, called stroma, and are soft and spongy.

The two lungs differ in size and shape. The left lung is smaller and has two lobes, whereas the right lung has three lobes. Each of the lung lobes contains a different number of bronchopulmonary segments. These segments are separated by connective tissue. There are eight segments in the two lobes of the left lung and ten segments in the three lobes of the right lung.

The vascular system of the lungs consists of the pulmonary arteries, which deliver blood to the lungs for oxygenation, and the pulmonary veins, which deliver oxygenated blood to the heart. Within the lungs, the pulmonary arteries branch into a

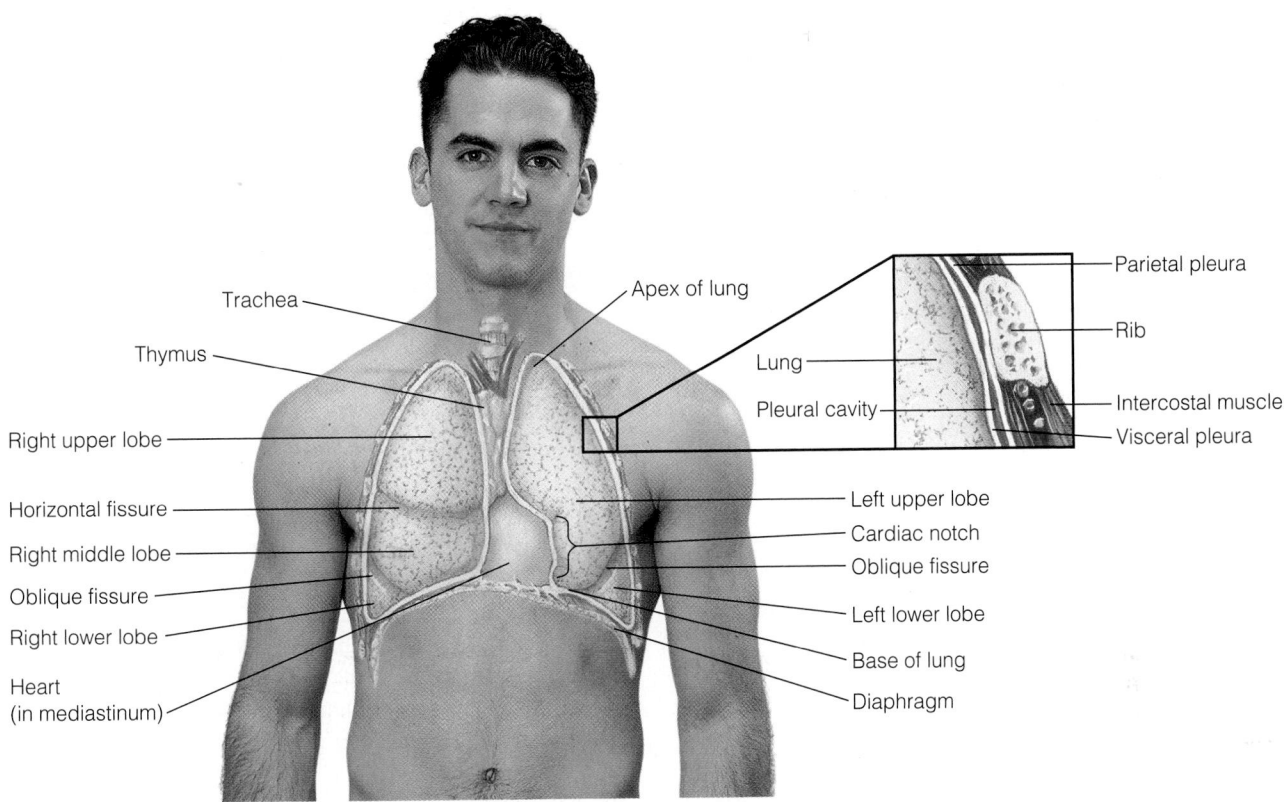

**Figure 34–3 ■** The lower respiratory system, showing the location of the lungs, the mediastinum, and layers of visceral and parietal pleura.

pulmonary capillary network that surrounds the avleoli. Lung tissue receives its blood supply from the bronchial arteries and drains by the bronchial and pulmonary veins.

## The Pleura

The pleura is a double-layered membrane that covers the lungs and the inside of the thoracic cavities (see Figure 34–3). The *parietal pleura* lines the thoracic wall and mediastinum. It is continuous with the *visceral pleura*, which covers the external lung surfaces. The pleura produces pleural fluid, a lubricating, serous fluid that allows the lungs to move easily over the thoracic wall during breathing. The pleura's two layers also cling tightly together and hold the lungs to the thoracic wall. The structure of the pleura creates a slightly negative pressure in the pleural space (which is actually a potential rather than an actual space), necessary for lung function.

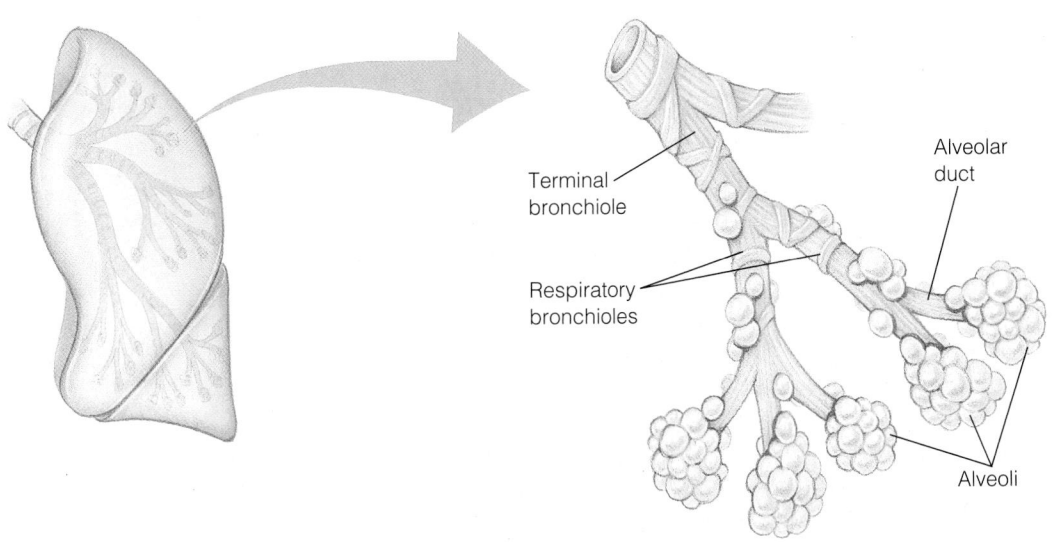

**Figure 34–4 ■** Respiratory bronchi, bronchioles, alveolar ducts, and alveoli.

## The Bronchi and Alveoli

The trachea divides into right and left primary bronchi. These main bronchi subdivide into the secondary (lobar) bronchi, then branch into the tertiary (segmental) bronchi, and then into smaller and smaller bronchioles, ending in the terminal bronchioles, which are extremely small (see Figure 34–4). These branching passageways collectively are called the bronchial or respiratory tree. From the terminal bronchioles, air moves into air sacs (called respiratory bronchioles), which further branch into alveolar ducts that lead to alveolar sacs and then to the tiny alveoli. During inspiration, air enters the lungs through the primary bronchus and then moves through the increasingly smaller passageways of the lungs to the alveoli, where oxygen and carbon dioxide exchange occurs in the process of external respiration. During expiration, the carbon dioxide is expelled.

Alveoli cluster around the alveolar sacs, which open into a common chamber called the atrium. There are millions of alveoli in each lung, providing an enormous surface for gas exchange. Alveoli have extremely thin walls of a single layer of squamous epithelial cells over a very thin basement membrane. The external surface of the alveoli are covered with pulmonary capillaries. The alveolar and capillary walls form the respiratory membrane. Gas exchange across the respiratory membrane occurs by simple diffusion. The alveolar walls also contain cells that secrete a surfactant-containing fluid, necessary for maintaining a moist surface and reducing the surface tension of the alveolar fluid to help prevent collapse of the lungs.

## The Rib Cage and Intercostal Muscles

The lungs are protected by the bones of the rib cage and the intercostal muscles. There are 12 pairs of ribs, which all articulate with the thoracic vertebrae (Figure 34–5 ■). Anteriorly, the first 7 ribs articulate with the body of the sternum. The eighth, ninth, and tenth ribs articulate with the cartilage immediately above the ribs. The eleventh and twelfth ribs are called floating ribs, because they are unattached.

The sternum has three parts: the manubrium, the body, and the xiphoid process. The junction between the manubrium and the body of the sternum is called the manubriosternal junction or the angle of Louis. The depression above the manubrium is called the suprasternal notch.

The spaces between the ribs are called the intercostal spaces. Each intercostal space is named for the rib immediately above it (e.g., the space between the third and fourth ribs is designated as the third intercostal space). The intercostal muscles between the ribs, along with the diaphragm, are called the inspiratory muscles.

## Mechanics of Ventilation

Pulmonary ventilation depends on volume changes within the thoracic cavity. A change in the volume of air in the thoracic cavity leads to a change in the air pressure within the cavity. Because gases always flow along their pressure gradients, a change in pressure results in gases flowing into or out of the lungs to equalize the pressure.

The pressures normally present in the thoracic cavity are the intrapulmonary pressure and the intrapleural pressure. The intrapulmonary pressure, within the alveoli of the lungs, rises and falls constantly as a result of the acts of ventilation (inhalation and exhalation). The intrapleural pressure, within the pleural space, also rises and falls with the acts of ventilation, but it is always less than (or negative to) the intrapulmonary pressure. Intrapulmonary and intrapleural pressures are necessary not only to expand and contract the lungs, but also to prevent their collapse.

Pulmonary ventilation has two phases: inspiration, during which air flows into the lungs; and expiration, during which gases flow out of the lungs. The two phases make up a single breath, and normally occur from 12 to 20 times each minute. A single inspiration lasts for about 1 to 1.5 seconds, whereas an expiration lasts for about 2 to 3 seconds.

During inspiration, the diaphragm contracts and flattens out to increase the vertical diameter of the thoracic cavity

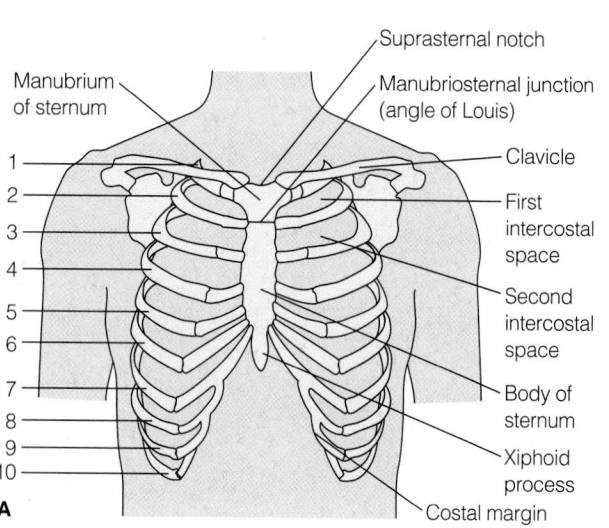
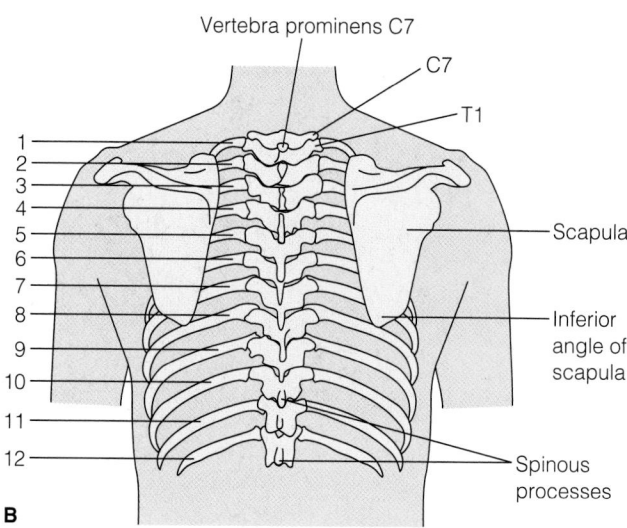

**Figure 34–5** ■ *A,* Anterior rib cage, showing intercostal spaces. *B,* Posterior rib cage.

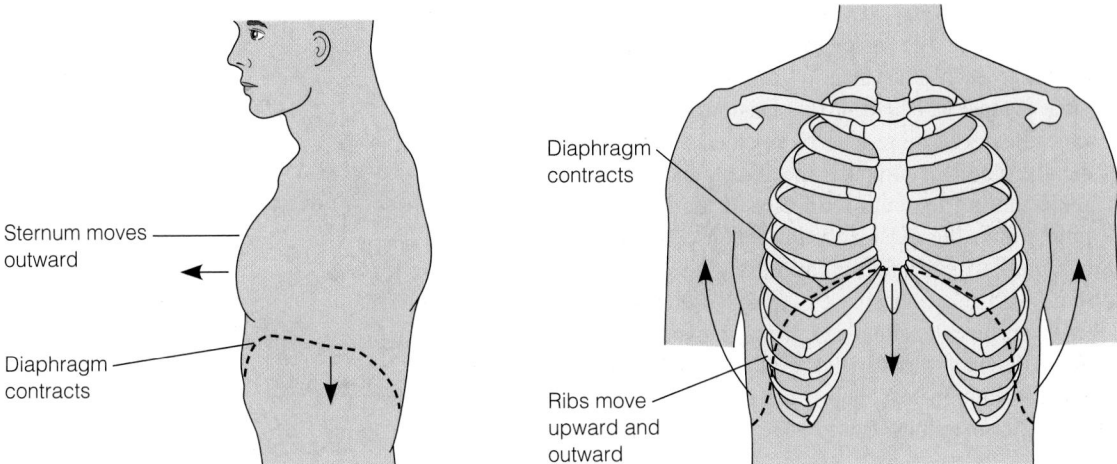

**Figure 34–6 ■** Respiratory inspiration: lateral and anterior views. Note the volume expansion of the thorax as the diaphragm flattens.

(Figure 34–6 ■). The external intercostal muscles contract, elevating the rib cage and moving the sternum forward to expand the lateral and anteroposterior diameter of the thoracic cavity, decreasing intrapleural pressure. The lungs stretch and the intrapulmonary volume increases, decreasing intrapulmonary pressure slightly below atmospheric pressure. Air rushes into the lungs as a result of this pressure gradient until the intrapulmonary and atmospheric pressures equalize.

Expiration is primarily a passive process that occurs as a result of the elasticity of the lungs (Figure 34–7 ■). The inspiratory muscles relax, the diaphragm rises, the ribs descend, and the lungs recoil. Both the thoracic and intrapulmonary pressures increase, compressing the alveoli. The intrapulmonary pressure rises to a level greater than atmospheric pressure, and gases flow out of the lungs.

## FACTORS AFFECTING RESPIRATION

The rate and depth of respirations are controlled by respiratory centers in the medulla oblongata and pons of the brain and by chemoreceptors located in the medulla and in the carotid and aortic bodies. The centers and chemoreceptors respond to changes in the concentration of oxygen, carbon dioxide, and hydrogen ions in arterial blood. For example, when carbon dioxide concentration increases or the pH decreases, the respiratory rate increases.

In addition, respiratory passageway resistance, lung compliance, lung elasticity, and alveolar surface tension forces affect respiration.

- Respiratory passageway resistance is created by the friction encountered as gases move along the respiratory passageways, by constriction of the passageways (especially the larger bronchioles), by accumulations of mucus or infectious material, and by tumors. As resistance increases, gas flow decreases.
- Lung compliance is the distensibility of the lungs. It depends on the elasticity of the lung tissue and the flexibility of the rib cage. Compliance is decreased by factors that decrease the elasticity of the lungs, block the respiratory passageways, or interfere with movement of the rib cage.
- Lung elasticity is essential for lung distention during inspiration and lung recoil during expiration. Decreased elasticity from disease such as emphysema impairs respiration.

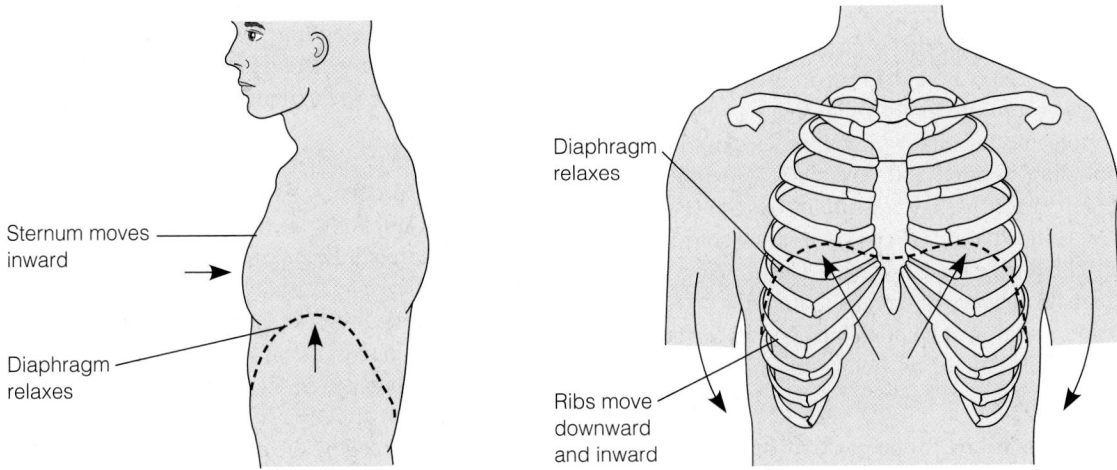

**Figure 34–7 ■** Respiratory expiration: lateral and anterior views.

- A liquid film of mostly water covers the alveolar walls. At any gas-liquid boundary, the molecules of liquid are more strongly attracted to each other than to gas molecules. This produces a state of tension, called surface tension, that draws the liquid molecules even more closely together. The water content of the alveolar film compacts the alveoli and aids in the lungs' recoil during expiration. In fact, if the alveolar film were pure water, the alveoli would collapse between breaths. Surfactant, a lipoprotein produced by the alveolar cells, interferes with this adhesiveness of the water molecules, reducing surface tension, and helping expand the lungs. With insufficient surfactant, the surface tension forces can become great enough to collapse the alveoli between breaths, requiring tremendous energy to reinflate the lungs for inspiration.

## Respiratory Volume and Capacity

Respiratory volume and capacity are affected by gender, age, weight, and health status.

- Tidal volume (TV) is the amount of air (approximately 500 mL) moved in and out of the lungs with each normal, quiet breath.
- Inspiratory reserve volume (IRV) is the amount of air (approximately 2100 to 3100 mL) that can be inhaled forcibly over the tidal volume.
- Expiratory reserve volume (ERV) is the approximately 1000 mL of air that can be forced out over the tidal volume.
- The residual volume is the volume of air (approximately 1100 mL) that remains in the lungs after a forced expiration.
- Vital capacity refers to the sum of TV + IRV + ERV and is approximately 4500 mL in the healthy client.
- About 150 mL of air never reaches the alveoli (the amount remaining in the passageways) and is called anatomical dead space volume.

## Oxygen Transport and Unloading

Oxygen is carried in the blood either bound to hemoglobin or dissolved in the plasma. Oxygen is not very soluble in water, so almost all oxygen that enters the blood from the respiratory system is carried to the cells of the body by hemoglobin. This combination of hemoglobin and oxygen is called *oxyhemoglobin.*

Each hemoglobin molecule is made of four polypeptide chains, with each chain bound to an iron-containing heme group. The iron groups are the binding sites for oxygen; each hemoglobin molecule can bind with four molecules of oxygen.

Oxygen binding is rapid and reversible. It is affected by temperature, blood pH, partial pressure of oxygen ($PO_2$), partial pressure of carbon dioxide ($PCO_2$), and serum concentration of an organic chemical called 2,3-DPG. These factors interact to ensure adequate delivery of oxygen to the cells.

The relative saturation of hemoglobin depends on the $PO_2$ of the blood, as illustrated in the oxygen-hemoglobin dissociation curve (Figure 34–8 ■).

- Under normal conditions, the hemoglobin in arterial blood is 97.4% saturated with oxygen. Hemoglobin is almost fully saturated at a $PO_2$ of 70 mmHg. As arterial blood flows

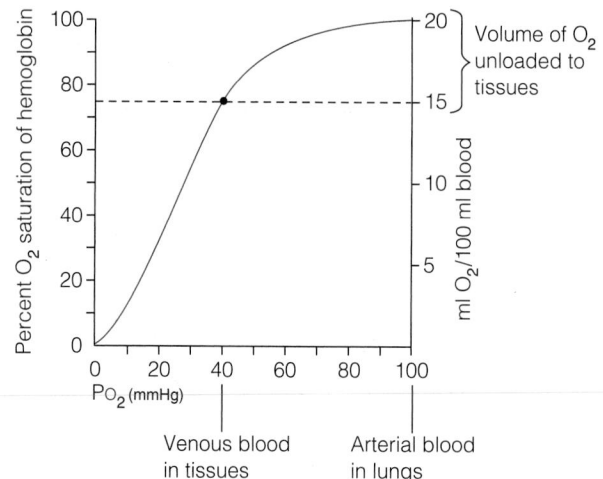

**Figure 34–8 ■** Oxygen-hemoglobin dissociation curve. The percent $O_2$ saturation of hemoglobin and total blood oxygen volume are shown for different oxygen partial pressures ($PO_2$). Arterial blood in the lungs is almost completely saturated. During one pass through the body, about 25% of hemoglobin-bound oxygen is unloaded to the tissues. Thus, venous blood is still about 75% saturated with oxygen. The steep portion of the curve shows that hemoglobin readily off-loads or on-loads oxygen at $PO_2$ levels below about 50 mmHg.

through the capillaries, oxygen is unloaded, so that the oxygen saturation of hemoglobin in venous blood is 75%.
- The affinity of oxygen and hemoglobin decreases as the temperature of body tissues increases above normal. As a result, less oxygen binds with hemoglobin, and oxygen unloading is enhanced. Conversely, as the body is chilled, oxygen unloading is inhibited.
- The oxygen-hemoglobin bond is weakened by increased hydrogen ion concentrations. As blood becomes more acidotic, oxygen unloading to the tissues is enhanced. The same process occurs when the partial pressure of carbon dioxide increases because this decreases the pH.
- The organic chemical 2,3-DPG is formed in red blood cells and enhances the release of oxygen from hemoglobin by binding to it during times of increased metabolism (as when body temperature increases). This binding alters the structure of hemoglobin to facilitate oxygen unloading.

## Carbon Dioxide Transport

Active cells produce about 200 mL of carbon dioxide each minute; this amount is exactly the same as that excreted by the lungs each minute. Excretion of carbon dioxide from the body requires transport by the blood from the cells to the lungs. Carbon dioxide is transported in three forms: dissolved in plasma, bound to hemoglobin, and as bicarbonate ions in the plasma (the largest amount is in this form).

The amount of carbon dioxide transported in the blood is strongly influenced by the oxygenation of the blood. When the $PO_2$ decreases, with a corresponding decrease in oxygen saturation, increased amounts of carbon dioxide can be carried in the blood. Carbon dioxide entering the systemic circulation from the cells causes more oxygen to dissociate from hemoglobin, in turn allowing more carbon dioxide to combine with hemoglobin and more bicarbonate ions to be generated. This situation is reversed in the pulmonary circulation, where the uptake of oxygen facilitates the release of carbon dioxide.

## ASSESSING RESPIRATORY FUNCTION

The nurse assesses the respiratory system both during a health assessment interview to collect subjective data and a physical assessment to collect objective data.

### The Health Assessment Interview

This section provides guidelines for collecting subjective data through a health assessment interview specific to the function of the respiratory system. A health assessment interview to determine problems of the respiratory system may be done as part of a health screening or as part of a total health assessment. Alternatively, the interview may focus on a chief complaint (such as difficulty breathing). If the client has a problem of any part of the respiratory system, analyze its onset, characteristics and course, severity, precipitating and relieving factors, and any associated symptoms, noting the timing and circumstances. For example, you may ask the client the following:

- What problems are you having with your breathing? Is your breathing more difficult if you lie flat? Is it painful to breathe in or out?
- When did you first notice that your cough was becoming a problem? Do you cough up mucus? What color is the mucus?
- Have you had nosebleeds in the past?

During the interview, carefully observe the client for difficulty in breathing, pausing to breathe in the middle of a sentence, hoarseness, changes in voice quality, and cough. Ask about present health status, medical history, family health history, and risk factors for illness. These areas of the client's health status include information about the nose, throat, and lungs.

To determine present health status, ask about pain in the nose, throat, or chest. Information about cough includes what type of cough, when it occurs, and how it is relieved. The client should describe any sputum associated with the cough. Is the client experiencing any dyspnea (difficult or labored breathing)? How is the dyspnea associated with activity levels and time of day? Is the client having chest pain? How is this related to activity and time of day? Note the severity, type, and location of the pain. Explore problems with swallowing, smelling, or taste. Also ask about nosebleeds and nasal or sinus stuffiness or pain, and about current medication use, aerosols or inhalants, and oxygen use.

Document past medical history by asking questions about a history of allergies, asthma, bronchitis, emphysema, pneumonia, tuberculosis, or congestive heart failure. Other questions include a history of surgery or trauma to the respiratory structures and a history of other chronic illnesses such as cancer, kidney disease, and heart disease. If the client has a health problem involving the respiratory system, ask about medications used to relieve nasal congestion, cough, dyspnea, or chest pain. Document a family history of allergies, tuberculosis, emphysema, and cancer.

The client's personal lifestyle, environment, and occupation may provide clues to risk factors for actual or potential health problems. Question the client about a history of smoking and/or exposure to environmental chemicals (including smog), dust, vapors, animals, coal dust, asbestos, fumes, or pollens. Other risk factors include a sedentary lifestyle and obesity. Also ask the client about use of alcohol and substances that are injected (such as heroin) or inhaled (such as cocaine or marijuana).

Other questions and leading statements, categorized by functional health patterns, can be found on the Companion Website.

### Physical Assessment

Physical assessment of the respiratory system may be performed as part of a total assessment, or alone for a client with known or suspected problems. Assess the respiratory system through inspection, palpation, percussion, and auscultation of the nose, throat, thorax, and lungs. In addition, note the client's level of consciousness and assess the color of the lips, nail beds, nose, ears, and tongue for signs of respiratory distress.

The equipment needed to assess the respiratory system includes a tongue blade, penlight, nasal speculum, metric ruler, marking pen, and stethoscope with diaphragm. The room should be warm and well lighted. Ask the client to remove all clothing above the waist; give female clients a gown to wear during the examination. Conduct the examination with the client in the sitting position. Prior to the examination, collect all necessary equipment and explain the techniques to the client to decrease anxiety.

The three different types of normal breath sounds are vesicular, bronchovesicular, and bronchial. Assessment of these sounds is discussed in Table 34–1.

#### Nasal Assessment with Abnormal Findings (✓)

- Inspect the nose for changes in size, shape, or color.
  - ✓ The nose may be asymmetrical as a result of previous surgery or trauma.
  - ✓ The skin around the nostrils may be red and swollen in allergies.
- Inspect the nasal cavity. Use an otoscope with a broad, short speculum. Gently insert the speculum into each of the nares and assess the condition of the mucous membranes and the turbinates.
  - ✓ The septum may be deviated.
  - ✓ Perforation of the septum may occur with chronic cocaine abuse.
  - ✓ Red mucosa indicates infection.
  - ✓ Purulent drainage indicates nasal or sinus infection.
  - ✓ Allergies may be indicated by watery nasal drainage, pale turbinates, and polyps on the turbinates.
- Assess ability to smell. Ask the client to breathe through one nostril while pressing the other one closed. Ask the client to close his or her eyes. Place a substance with an aromatic odor

| Type of Breath Sound | Characteristics |
|---|---|
| Vesicular | • Soft, low-pitched, gentle sounds<br>• Heard over all areas of the lungs except the major bronchi<br>• Have a 3:1 ratio for inspiration and expiration, with inspiration lasting longer than expiration |
| Bronchovesicular | • Medium pitch and intensity of sounds<br>• Have a 1:1 ratio, with inspiration and expiration being equal in duration<br>• Heard anteriorly over the primary bronchus on each side of the sternum, and posteriorly between the scapulae |
| Bronchial | • Loud, high-pitched sounds<br>• Gap between inspiration and expiration<br>• Have a 2:3 ratio for inspiration and expiration, with expiration longer than inspiration<br>• Heard over the manubrium |

**TABLE 34–1  Normal Breath Sounds**

under the client's nose (use ground coffee or alcohol) and ask the client to identify the odor. Test each nostril separately. This test is usually done only if the client has problems with the sense of smell.
✓ Changes in the ability to smell may be the result of damage to the olfactory nerve or to chronic inflammation of the nose.
✓ Zinc deficiency may also cause a loss of the sense of smell.

## Thoracic Assessment with Abnormal Findings (✓)

- Assess respiratory rate.
  ✓ **Tachypnea** (rapid respiratory rate) is seen in **atelectasis** (collapse of lung tissue following obstruction of the bronchus or bronchioles), pneumonia, asthma, pleural effusion, pneumothorax, and congestive heart failure.
  ✓ Damage to the brainstem from a stroke or head injury may result in either tachypnea or **bradypnea** (low respiratory rate).
  ✓ Bradypnea is seen with some circulatory disorders, lung disorders, as a side effect of some medications, and as a response to pain.
  ✓ **Apnea,** cessation of breathing lasting from a few seconds to a few minutes, may occur following a stroke or head trauma, as a side effect of some medications, or following airway obstruction.
- Inspect the anteroposterior diameter of the chest. The anteroposterior diameter of the chest should be less than the transverse diameter. Normal ratios vary from 1:2 to 5:7.
  ✓ The anteroposterior diameter is equal to the transverse diameter in barrel chest, which typically occurs with emphysema.
- Inspect for intercostal retraction.
  ✓ Retraction of intercostal spaces may be seen in asthma.
  ✓ Bulging of intercostal spaces may be seen in pneumothorax.
- Inspect and palpate for chest expansion. Place your hands with the fingers spread apart palm down on the client's posterolateral chest. Gently press the skin between your thumbs (Figure 34–9 ■). Ask the client to breathe deeply. As the client inhales, watch your hands for symmetry of movement.
  ✓ Thoracic expansion is decreased on the affected side in atelectasis, pneumonia, pneumothorax, and pleural effusion.

✓ Bilateral chest expansion is decreased in emphysema.
- Gently palpate the location and position of the trachea.
  ✓ The trachea shifts to the unaffected side in pleural effusion and pneumothorax and shifts to the affected side in atelectasis.
- Palpate for tactile fremitus. Ask the client to say "ninety-nine" as you palpate at three different levels for a vibratory sensation called tactile fremitus, which occurs as sound waves from the larynx travel through patent bronchi and lungs to the chest wall.
  ✓ Tactile fremitus is decreased in atelectasis, emphysema, asthma, pleural effusion, and pneumothorax. It is increased in pneumonia if the bronchus is patent.
- Percuss the lungs for dullness over shoulder apices and over anterior, posterior, and lateral intercostal spaces (Figure 34–10 ■).
  ✓ Dullness is heard in clients with atelectasis, lobar pneumonia, and pleural effusion.
  ✓ Hyperresonance is heard in those with chronic asthma and pneumothorax.
- Percuss the posterior chest for diaphragmatic excursion. Systematic percussion of the posterior chest from a level of lung resonance to the level of diaphragmatic dullness reveals

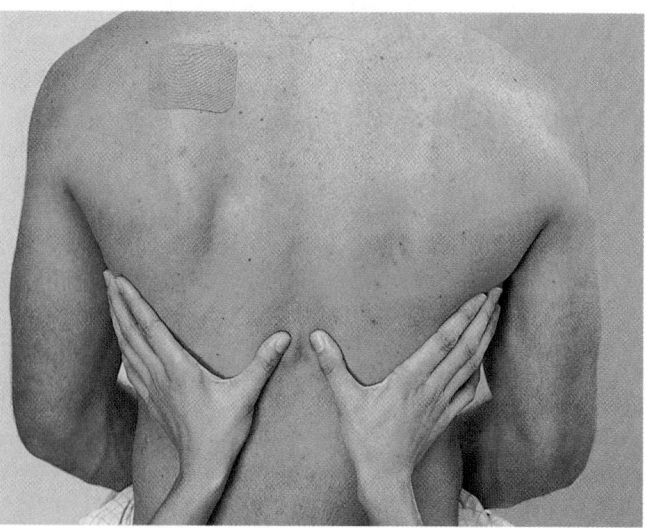

**Figure 34–9 ■** Palpating for chest expansion.

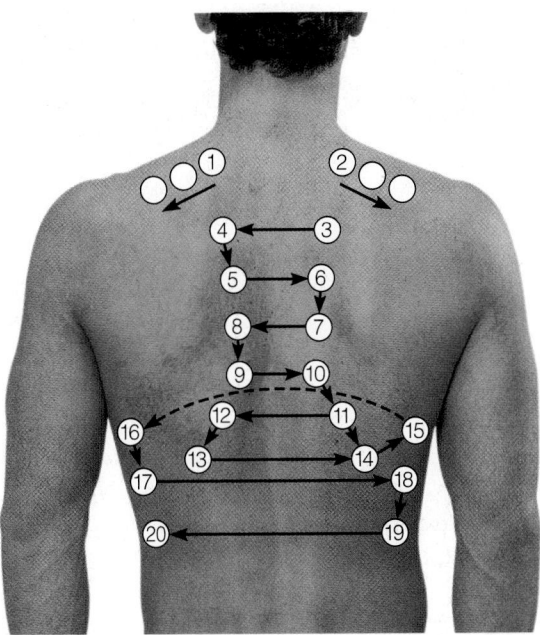

**Figure 34–10** ■ Sequence for lung percussion.

diaphragmatic excursion, a measurement of the level of the diaphragm. First percuss downward over the posterior thorax while the client exhales fully and holds the breath. Mark the spot at which the sound changes from resonant to dull. Then ask the client to inhale and hold the breath while you percuss downward again to note the descent of the diaphragm. Again mark the spot where the sound changes. Measure the difference, which normally varies from about 3 to 5 cm (Figure 34–11 ■).

✓ Diaphragmatic excursion is decreased in emphysema, on the affected side in pleural effusion, and in pneumothorax.

✓ A high level of dullness or a lack of excursion may indicate atelectasis or pleural effusion.

## Breath Sound Assessment with Abnormal Findings (✓)

- Auscultate the lungs for breath sounds with the diaphragm of the stethoscope by having the client take slow deep breaths through the mouth. Listen over anterior, posterior, and lateral intercostal spaces (Figure 34–12 ■).

  ✓ Bronchial breath sounds (expiration > inspiration) and bronchovesicular breath sounds (inspiration = expiration) are heard over lungs filled with fluid or solid tissue.

  ✓ Breath sounds are decreased over atelectasis, emphysema, asthma, pleural effusion, and pneumothorax.

  ✓ Breath sounds are increased over lobar pneumonia.

  ✓ Breath sounds are absent over collapsed lung, pleural effusion, and primary bronchus obstruction.

- Auscultate for crackles, wheezes, and friction rubs. If crackles or wheezes are heard, ask the client to cough and note if adventitious sound is cleared.

  ✓ Crackles (short, discrete, crackling or bubbling sounds) may be noted in pneumonia, bronchitis, and congestive heart failure.

  ✓ Wheezes (continuous, musical sounds) may be heard in clients with bronchitis, emphysema, and asthma.

  ✓ A friction rub is a loud, dry, creaking sound that indicates pleural inflammation.

- Auscultate voice sounds where any abnormal breath sound is noted by having client say "ninety-nine" (bronchophony); whisper "one, two, three" (whispered pectoriloquy); and say "ee" (egophony). Normally, these sounds are heard by the examiner, but are muffled.

  ✓ Voice sounds are decreased or absent over areas of atelectasis, asthma, pleural effusion, and pneumothorax.

  ✓ Voice sounds are increased and clearer over lobar pneumonia.

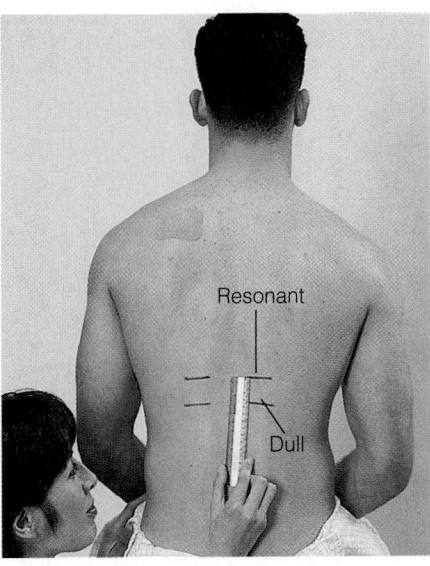

**Figure 34–11** ■ Measuring diaphragmatic excursion.

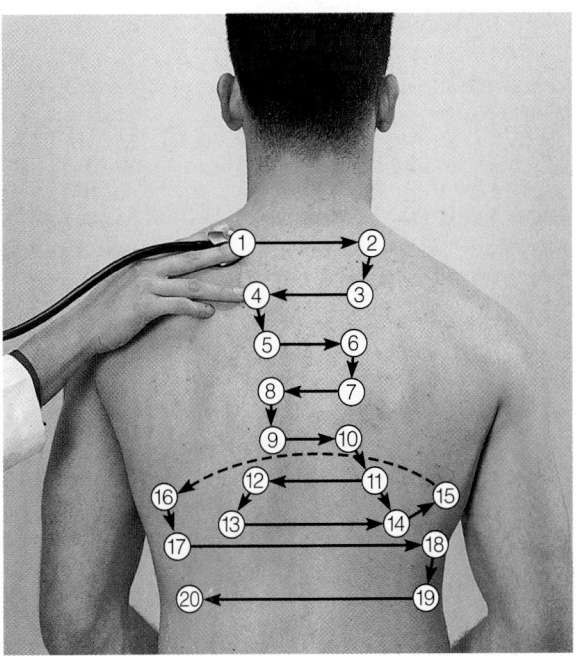

**Figure 34–12** ■ Sequence for lung auscultation.

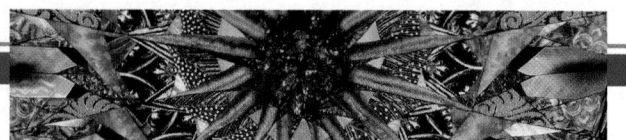

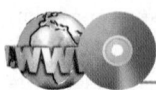

## EXPLORE MediaLink

NCLEX review questions, case studies, care plan activities, MediaLink applications, and other interactive resources for this chapter can be found on the Companion Website at www.prenhall.com/lemone.

Click on Chapter 34 to select the activities for this chapter. For animations, video clips, more NCLEX review questions, and an audio glossary, access the Student CD-ROM accompanying this textbook.

## TEST YOURSELF

1. Where is the apex of each lung located?

   a. In the mediastinum
   b. Resting on the diaphragm
   c. Within the parietal pleura
   d. Just below the clavicle

2. What physiologic process is involved in gas exchange at the respiratory membrane?

   a. Facilitates transport
   b. Active transport
   c. Simple diffusion
   d. Hydrostatic pressure

2. While auscultating your client's breath sounds, you note continuous musical sounds. You document these sounds as:

   a. Murmurs
   b. Wheezes
   c. Crackles
   d. Rales

3. Your client has had a lung removed. What type of breath sound would you expect to assess over this area?

   a. Hyperresonance
   b. Crackles
   c. Bronchovesicular
   d. Absent

4. What would you ask the client to do as you auscultate the lungs?

   a. "Hold your breath."
   b. "Repeat the numbers 99 several times."
   c. "Take slow deep breaths through your mouth."
   d. " Breathe in and out through your nose."

See Test Yourself answers in Appendix C.

## BIBLIOGRAPHY

Andresen, G. (1998). Assessing the older patient. *RN, 61*(3), 46–56.

Basfield-Holland, E. (1997). Assessing pulmonary status: It's more than listening to breath sounds. *Nursing, 27*(8), 1–2, 4–9.

Connolly, M. (2001). Chest x-rays: Completing the picture. *RN, 64*(6), 56–62, 64.

Jevon, P., & Ewens, B. (2001). Assessment of a breathless patient. *Nursing Standard, 15*(16), 48–53.

Kirton, C. (1996). Assessing breath sounds. *Nursing, 26*(6), 50–51.

Lyneham, J. (2001). Physical examination (abdomen, thorax and lungs): A review. *Australian Journal of Advanced Nursing, 18*(3), 31.

O'Hanlon-Nichols, T. (1998). Basic assessment series: The adult pulmonary system. *American Journal of Nursing, 98*(2), 39–45.

Walton, J., & Miller, J. (1998). Evaluating physical and behavioral changes in older adults. *MEDSURG Nursing, 7*(2), 85–90.

Watson, R. (2000). Assessing pulmonary function in older people. *Nursing Older People, 12*(8), 27–28.

Weber, J., & Kelley, J. (2002). *Health assessment in nursing* (2nd ed). Philadelphia: Lippincott.

Wilson, S., & Giddens, J. (2001). *Health assessment for nursing practice.* St. Louis: Mosby.

# CHAPTER 35

# Nursing Care of Clients with Upper Respiratory Disorders

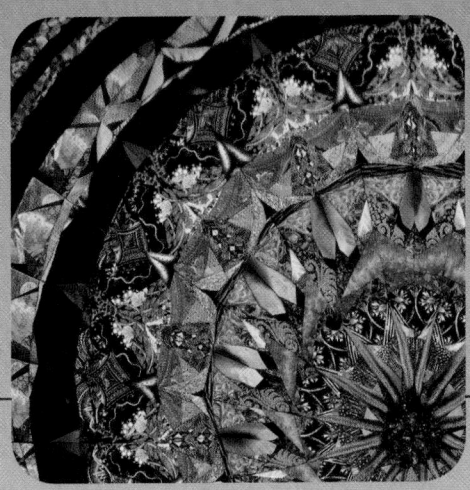

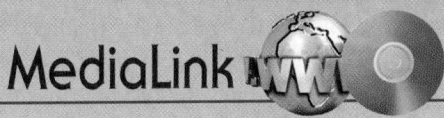

## MediaLink

**www.prenhall.com/lemone**

Additional resources for this chapter can be found on the Student CD-ROM accompanying this textbook, and on the Companion Website at www.prenhall.com/lemone. Click on Chapter 35 to select the activities for this chapter.

**CD-ROM**
- Audio Glossary
- NCLEX Review

**Companion Website**
- More NCLEX Review
- Case Study
  Sleep Apnea
- Care Plan Activity
  Epistaxis
- MediaLink Application
  Laryngectomy

## LEARNING OUTCOMES

After completing this chapter, you will be able to:

- Relate anatomy, physiology, and assessment of the upper respiratory tract to commonly occurring disorders.

- Describe the pathophysiology of common upper respiratory tract disorders, relating their manifestations to the pathophysiologic process.

- Discuss nursing implications for diagnostic tests, medications, and other collaborative care measures to treat upper respiratory disorders.

- Provide care for clients having surgery involving the upper respiratory system.

- Identify nursing care needs for the client with a tracheostomy.

- Use the nursing process to assess needs, plan and implement individualized care, and evaluate responses for clients with upper respiratory disorders.

Upper respiratory disorders may affect the nose, paranasal sinuses, tonsils, adenoids, larynx, and pharynx. See Chapter 34 to review the anatomy and physiology of these structures as well as their assessment. ᑫᑏ Upper respiratory disorders may be very minor, such as the common cold. However, a patent upper airway is necessary for effective breathing. Acute and even life-threatening problems develop when upper airway patency is affected (e.g., by laryngeal edema). Upper respiratory disorders can affect breathing, communication, and body image. When breathing is compromised because of swelling, bleeding, or accumulation of secretions, fear and anxiety develop.

Nursing care focuses on maintaining the airway, managing pain and symptoms, promoting effective communication, and providing psychologic support for the client and family.

# INFECTIOUS OR INFLAMMATORY DISORDERS

Constant exposure of the upper respiratory tract to the environment makes it vulnerable to a variety of infectious and inflammatory conditions. Although most upper respiratory infections and inflammations are minor, complications may result. In the frail older adult, the risk of serious problems following an upper respiratory infection can be significant.

**Rhinitis,** inflammation of the nasal cavities, is the most common upper respiratory disorder. Rhinitis may be either acute or chronic. *Acute viral rhinitis,* or the common cold, is discussed below. Chronic rhinitis includes allergic, vasomotor, and atrophic rhinitis. *Allergic rhinitis,* or hay fever, results from a sensitivity reaction to allergens such as plant pollens. It tends to occur seasonally. The etiology of *vasomotor rhinitis* is unknown. Although its manifestations are similar to those of allergic rhinitis, it is not linked to allergens. *Atrophic rhinitis* is characterized by changes in the mucous membrane of the nasal cavities.

## THE CLIENT WITH VIRAL UPPER RESPIRATORY INFECTION

Viral upper respiratory infections (URIs or the common cold) are the most common respiratory tract infections and are among the most common human diseases. URIs are highly contagious and are prevalent in schools and work environments. The incidence of acute URI peaks during September and late January, coinciding with the opening of schools, as well as toward the end of April. Most adults experience two to four colds each year (Porth, 2002).

## PATHOPHYSIOLOGY

More than 200 strains of virus cause URI, including rhinoviruses, adenoviruses, parainfluenza viruses, coronaviruses, and respiratory syncytial virus. Occasionally, more than one virus may be present. Viruses causing acute URI spread by aerosolized droplet nuclei during sneezing or coughing or by direct contact. The virus usually spreads when the hands and fingers pick it up from contaminated surfaces and carry it to the eyes and mucous membranes of the susceptible host. Infected clients are highly contagious, shedding virus for a few days prior to and after the appearance of symptoms. Although immunity is produced to the individual virus strain, the number of viruses causing URI ensures that most people continue to experience colds throughout their lifetime.

Viscous mucus secretions in the upper respiratory tract trap invading organisms, preventing contamination of more vulnerable areas. Cells of the upper respiratory tract are infected when the virus attaches to receptors on the cell. Local immunologic defenses, such as secretory IgA antibodies in respiratory secretions, then attempt to inactivate the antigen, producing a local inflammatory response. The mucous membranes of the nasal passages swell and become hyperemic and engorged. Mucus-secreting glands become hyperactive. These responses to the virus produce the typical manifestations of viral URI.

## MANIFESTATIONS

Acute viral upper respiratory infection often presents as the common cold. Nasal mucous membranes appear red (*erythematous*) and *boggy* (swollen). Swollen mucous membranes, local vasodilation, and secretions cause nasal congestion. Clear, watery secretions lead to **coryza** or *rhinorrhea,* profuse nasal discharge. Sneezing and coughing are common. Sore throat is common, and may be the initial symptom. Systemic manifestations of acute viral URI may include low-grade fever, headache, malaise, and muscle aches. Symptoms generally last for a few days up to 2 weeks. Although acute viral URI is typically mild and self-limited, its effects on the immune defenses of the upper respiratory tract can increase the risk for more serious bacterial infections, such as sinusitis or otitis media.

## COLLABORATIVE CARE

Because most acute viral upper respiratory infections are self-limiting, self-care is appropriate and encouraged. Medical treatment is usually required only when complications such as sinusitis or otitis media develop.

Diagnosis of acute viral URI is usually based on the history and physical examination. Diagnostic testing may be indicated if a complication such as bacterial infection is suspected. A white blood count (WBC) may be ordered to assess for leukocytosis (an elevated WBC). Cultures of purulent discharge may also be obtained.

Treatment is symptomatic. Adequate rest, maintaining fluid intake, and avoiding chilling help relieve systemic symptoms such as fever, malaise, and muscle ache. Instruct clients to cover the mouth and nose with tissue when coughing or sneezing, and to dispose of soiled tissues properly. Additionally, avoiding crowds helps prevent spread of the infection to others.

## Medications

Medications may be recommended to shorten the duration of the illness and relieve symptoms. Mild decongestants or over-the-counter antihistamines may help relieve coryza and nasal congestion. Warm saltwater gargles, throat lozenges, or mild analgesics may be used for sore throat. Although no specific antiviral therapy has been shown to be effective, experimental vaccines to prevent acute viral URI are in developmental stages. For the nursing implications of decongestants and common antihistamines see the box below.

## Complementary Therapies

Complementary therapies are appropriate for treating most acute viral URI. Herbal remedies such as Echinacea and garlic have antiviral and antibiotic effects. Taken at the first sign of infection, Echinacea may reduce the duration and symptoms. The recommended dose of Echinacea varies, depending on the part of the plant used in the preparation. It should not be used for longer than 2 weeks. It is contraindicated for use during pregnancy and lactation, and in people who have an autoimmune disease such as rheumatoid arthritis.

Aromatherapy with essential oils such as basil, cedarwood, eucalyptus, frankincense, lavender, marjoram, peppermint, or rosemary can reduce congestion, and promote comfort and recovery. Teach clients that these essential oils are to be used only for inhalation, not for internal consumption.

---

# Medication Administration
## Decongestants and Antihistamines

### DECONGESTANTS

Phenylephrine (Neo-Synephrine, others)
Phenylpropanolamine (Comtrex, Ornade, Triaminic, others)
Pseudoephedrine (Sudafed, Actifed, others)

Decongestants promote vasoconstriction, reducing the inflammation and edema of nasal mucosa and relieving nasal congestion. They are very effective when applied topically (by nasal spray) because of their rapid onset of action. However, the duration of effect is short, followed by vasodilation and rebound congestion. Because of their rapid effect and short duration, these preparations are habit-forming. Chronic use may lead to *rhinitis medicamentosa,* a rebound phenomenon of drug-induced nasal irritation and inflammation.

### Nursing Responsibilities
- Assess for contraindications, such as hypertension or chronic heart disease. These drugs stimulate the sympathetic nervous system, increasing peripheral vascular resistance, blood pressure, and heart rate.
- Evaluate medication regimen for potential interactions such as antihypertensive medications and monoamine oxidase (MAO) inhibitors.

### Client and Family Teaching
- Do not use more than the recommended dose.
- Check with the physician before taking decongestants if you are taking any prescription medications or are being treated for high blood pressure or heart disease.
- Use nasal sprays for no more than 3 to 5 days.
- Increase fluid intake to relieve mouth dryness.
- These drugs may cause nervousness, shakiness, or difficulty sleeping. Stop the drug if these effects occur.

### ANTIHISTAMINES

Brompheniramine (Dimetane, others)
Chlorpheniramine (Chlor-Trimeton, others)
Clemastine (Tavist)
Dexchlorpheniramine (Dexchlor, others)
Triprolidine (Actidil, Myidil)

### *Nonsedating*

Cetirizine (Zyrtec)
Fexofenadine (Allegra)
Loratadine (Claritin)

Antihistamines are widely available with and without a prescription. They are frequently combined with decongestants in over-the-counter cold and allergy preparations. Antihistamines relieve the systemic effects of histamine and dry respiratory secretions through an anticholinergic effect. Most antihistamines cause drowsiness; nonsedating forms are less likely to interfere with alertness.

### Nursing Responsibilities
- Before administering or recommending these drugs, assess for possible contraindications, including the following:
  - Acute asthma or lower respiratory disease that may be aggravated by drying of secretions
  - Hypersensitivity to antihistamines
  - Glaucoma (increased intraocular pressure)
  - Impaired gastrointestinal motility or obstruction
  - Prostatic hypertrophy or other urinary tract obstruction
  - Heart disease
- For clients who must remain alert while on antihistamine therapy, recommend nonsedating forms.

### Client and Family Teaching
- Do not drive or operate machinery while taking over-the-counter or prescription forms of antihistamines known to be sedating.
- Stop the drug and notify your doctor immediately if you develop confusion, excessive sedation, chest tightness, wheezing, bleeding, or easy bruising while taking antihistamines.
- Do not use alcohol or other CNS depressants while taking antihistamines.
- Hard candy, gum, ice chips, and liquids help relieve mouth dryness caused by antihistamines.

## NURSING CARE

### Health Promotion

Clients can limit their incidence of acute viral URI by frequent handwashing and avoiding exposure to crowds. Maintaining good general health and stress-reducing activities support the immune system and help prevent acute viral URI (see the box below). Teach the client that chilling or going out in the rain do not cause colds, and that URI are more likely to occur during periods of physical or psychologic stress.

### Home Care

The primary nursing role in caring for clients with acute viral URI is educational. Self-care is appropriate for most clients unless the problem is recurrent or a complication occurs. Acute viral URI may interfere with work and recreational activities. Unless limited by symptoms, normal daily activities and roles usually can be maintained. Additional rest during the acute phase of illness is recommended. Additional fluid intake and a well-balanced diet help support the immune response, hastening recovery.

## Nursing Research

### Evidence-Based Practice for the Older Adult

A volunteer population of healthy older adults participated in a 3-year study to determine the effects of moderate exercise on the incidence of respiratory tract infections. Participants walked for 30 to 35 minutes at least three times a week, with 10-minute warmup and cooldown sessions. Stress levels as perceived by the study participants were considered an additional variable, because previous studies have shown an increased incidence of upper respiratory infections in people who have high levels of stress. After just 1 year of the study, 79% of the subjects reported reduced stress and fewer symptoms of respiratory infections. Preliminary data also indicated that the majority of volunteers maintained a low incidence of upper and lower respiratory infections.

### IMPLICATIONS FOR NURSING

Nurses can play an important role in educating older adults about the beneficial effects of regular moderate exercise such as walking. The client is likely not only to reduce the incidence of respiratory infections but also to realize other benefits, such as improved cardiac and respiratory function, and improved musculoskeletal strength, endurance, and flexibility.

### Critical Thinking in Client Care Level

1. How does stress level affect susceptibility to infection of the upper respiratory tract?
2. Why is regular exercise beneficial in reducing the perceived level of stress?
3. Plan an exercise program to meet the needs of a mixed group of older adults living in a rural area of the Pacific Northwest. Consider probable access to facilities, weather (usually cool and rainy), age range, and possible gender differences.

Include the following topics in teaching for home care:

- Using disposable tissues to cover the mouth and nose while coughing or sneezing to reduce airborne spread of the virus.
- Blowing the nose with both nostrils open to prevent infected matter from being forced into the eustachian tubes.
- Washing hands frequently, especially after coughing or sneezing, to limit viral transmission.
- Using over-the-counter preparations for symptomatic relief; precautions related to the sedating effects of antihistamines.
- Limiting use of nasal decongestants to every 4 hours for only a few days at a time to prevent rebound effect.

## THE CLIENT WITH INFLUENZA

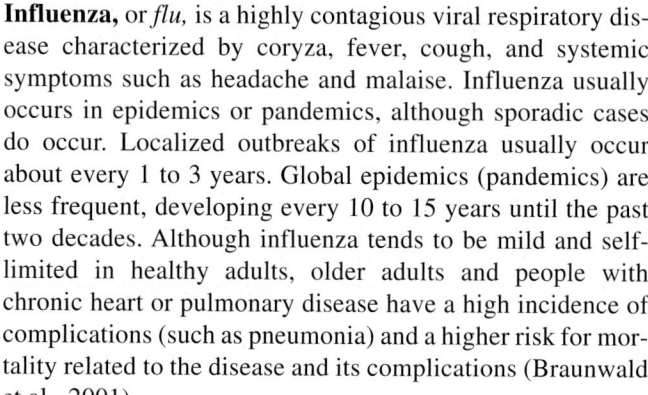

**Influenza,** or *flu,* is a highly contagious viral respiratory disease characterized by coryza, fever, cough, and systemic symptoms such as headache and malaise. Influenza usually occurs in epidemics or pandemics, although sporadic cases do occur. Localized outbreaks of influenza usually occur about every 1 to 3 years. Global epidemics (pandemics) are less frequent, developing every 10 to 15 years until the past two decades. Although influenza tends to be mild and self-limited in healthy adults, older adults and people with chronic heart or pulmonary disease have a high incidence of complications (such as pneumonia) and a higher risk for mortality related to the disease and its complications (Braunwald et al., 2001).

### PATHOPHYSIOLOGY

Influenza virus is transmitted by airborne droplet and direct contact. Three major strains of the virus have been identified as influenza A virus, influenza B virus, and influenza C virus. Influenza A is responsible for most infections and the most severe outbreaks of influenza. This is primarily due to its ability to alter its surface antigens, bypassing previously developed immune defenses to the virus. New strains of influenza virus are named according to the strain, geographic origin, and year (e.g., A/Taiwan/89). Outbreaks of influenza B virus are generally less extensive and less severe than those caused by influenza A virus. Illness associated with influenza C virus is mild and often goes unrecognized.

The incubation period for influenza is short, only 18 to 72 hours. The virus infects the respiratory epithelium. It rapidly replicates in infected cells and is released to infect neighboring cells. Inflammation leads to necrosis and shedding of serous and ciliated cells of the respiratory tract. This allows extracellular fluid to escape, producing rhinorrhea. With recovery, serous cells are replaced more rapidly than ciliated cells, leading to continued cough and coryza. Systemic manifestations of influenza likely are caused by release of inflammatory mediators such as tumor necrosis factor α and interleukin 6 (Braunwald et al., 2001).

The respiratory epithelial necrosis caused by influenza increases the risk for secondary bacterial infections. Sinusitis and otitis media are frequent complications of influenza. Tracheobronchitis, inflammation of the trachea and bronchi, may develop. While tracheobronchitis is not a serious health risk, its manifestations may persist for up to 3 weeks.

Influenza is clearly linked to an increased risk for pneumonia, particularly in older adults. Changes in respiratory function associated with aging, including decreased effectiveness of cough and increased residual lung volume, pose little risk in the healthy older adult but greatly increase the risk for pneumonia associated with influenza. Viral pneumonia is a serious complication that may be fatal. It typically develops within 48 hours of the onset of influenza, often in clients with preexisting heart valve or pulmonary disease. Influenza pneumonia progresses rapidly and can cause hypoxemia and death within a few days. Bacterial pneumonia is more likely to occur in older at-risk adults but also may affect otherwise healthy adults. It usually presents as a relapse of influenza, with a productive cough and evidence of pneumonia on the chest X-ray. See Chapter 36 for more information about pneumonia. 

*Reye's syndrome* is a rare but potentially fatal complication of influenza. Although it is more likely to affect children, it also has been identified in older adults. It is most often associated with influenza B virus. Reye's syndrome develops within 2 to 3 weeks after the onset of influenza. It has a 30% mortality rate. Hepatic failure and encephalopathy develop rapidly in clients with Reye's syndrome.

## MANIFESTATIONS

Infection with influenza virus produces one of three syndromes: uncomplicated nasopharyngeal inflammation, viral upper respiratory infection followed by bacterial infection, or viral pneumonia. The onset is rapid; profound malaise may develop in a matter of minutes.

Manifestations of influenza include abrupt onset of chills and fever, malaise, muscle aches, and headache. Respiratory manifestations include dry, nonproductive cough, sore throat, substernal burning, and coryza (see the box below). Acute symptoms subside within 2 to 3 days, although fever may last as long as a week. The cough may be severe and productive. Along with fatigue and weakness, the cough can persist for days or several weeks.

### Manifestations of Influenza

**RESPIRATORY MANIFESTATIONS**

- Coryza
- Cough, initially dry becoming productive
- Substernal burning
- Sore throat

**SYSTEMIC MANIFESTATIONS**

- Fever and chills
- Malaise
- Muscle aches
- Fatigue

## COLLABORATIVE CARE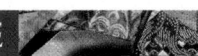

Preventing influenza by immunizing at-risk populations is an important aspect of care. Immunization with polyvalent (containing antigens of several viral strains) influenza virus vaccine is about 85% effective in preventing influenza infection for several months to a year (Tierney et al., 2001). Annual immunization is recommended for at-risk clients, including people over the age of 65, residents of nursing homes, adults and children with chronic cardiopulmonary disorders (e.g., asthma) or chronic metabolic diseases such as diabetes, and health care workers who have frequent contact with high-risk clients. Additionally, family members of at-risk clients should be vaccinated to reduce the client's risk of exposure. The vaccine is given in the fall, prior to the annual winter outbreak. (See the box below.) Medical treatment of influenza focuses on establishing the diagnosis, providing symptomatic relief, and preventing complications.

### Nursing Research
#### Evidence-Based Practice to Prevent Influenza

Older adults are disproportionately affected by influenza and related disorders: approximately 80% to 90% of all influenza-related deaths in the United States occur in people who are 65 or older (Hughes & Tartasky, 1996). Additionally, costs associated with influenza-related hospitalizations during epidemics are staggering. Previous studies have found that older adults are most likely to use strategies such as dressing warmly, ensuring adequate nutrition and taking vitamins to prevent influenza, with only 38% of participants getting influenza immunization. Few identify pneumonia as a possible consequence of influenza and upper respiratory infection. Hughes & Tartasky (1996) describe developing and implementing an immunization program for home-bound elders using the Health Belief Model as a theoretical framework.

#### IMPLICATIONS FOR NURSING
The population at highest risk for serious sequelae from colds or influenza is older adults. Nurses can have a positive influence on client outcomes by teaching appropriate prevention strategies and symptom management. It is important to include information about possible adverse consequences and indicators for medical attention when teaching self-care. Nurses in community-based settings and those providing home care should plan immunization clinics to reach older adults in accessible settings such as homes, senior centers, assisted living facilities, and grocery stores.

#### Critical Thinking in Client Care
1. Identify five common reasons given for not getting an influenza immunization.
2. For each reason given, identify at least one nursing strategy to encourage at-risk clients to seek immunization.
3. What additional measures can nurses take to reduce the risk of an influenza epidemic in their communities?

## Diagnostic Tests

The diagnosis of influenza is based on history, clinical findings, and knowledge of an influenza outbreak in the community. A chest X-ray and white blood cell (WBC) count may be done to rule out complications such as pneumonia. The WBC is commonly decreased in influenza; bacterial infections usually cause increased WBCs.

## Medications

Yearly immunization with influenza vaccine is the single most important measure to prevent or minimize symptoms of influenza. Although the vaccine is readily available and inexpensive, only about 30% of at-risk clients are vaccinated each year. Many may fear a reaction from the vaccine, although the vaccines are highly purified and reactions are rare. About 5% of people experience mild symptoms of low-grade fever, malaise, or myalgia for up to 24 hours after vaccination. Because the vaccine is produced in eggs, it should not be given to people who are allergic to egg protein. Serious adverse reactions to influenza vaccine are rare. *Guillain-Barré syndrome,* an acute neurologic disorder characterized by muscle weakness and distal sensory loss, has been associated with certain batches of vaccine.

Amantadine (Symmetrel) or rimantadine (Flumadine) may be used for prophylaxis in unvaccinated people who are exposed to the virus. If the drug is given before or within 48 hours of exposure, it inhibits viral shedding and prevents or decreases the symptoms of influenza. If possible, unvaccinated people should receive the vaccine along with the antiviral drug. The drug is continued for several weeks or for the duration of the influenza outbreak.

Amantadine, rimantadine, and the antiviral drugs zanamivir (Relenza), oseltamivir (Tamiflu), and ribavirin (Virazole) also may be used to reduce the duration and severity of flu symptoms. Both zanamivir and ribavirin are administered by inhalation; the other drugs are given orally. See Chapter 8 ⊂⊃ for nursing implications for antiviral drugs.

Over-the-counter analgesics such as aspirin, acetaminophen, or NSAIDs provide symptomatic relief of fever and muscle ache. Antitussives may decrease cough, promoting rest. Antibiotics are not indicated unless secondary bacterial infection occurs.

## NURSING CARE

### Health Promotion

Stress the importance of yearly influenza vaccination for clients in high-risk groups and their families. Teach about spread of the disease, including measures to reduce the risk of contracting influenza, such as avoiding crowds and people who are ill.

### Assessment

Unless there is a known outbreak of influenza in the community, it can be difficult to differentiate the manifestations of influenza from those of other URI.

- Health history: known exposure to virus; current symptoms, their onset and duration; presence of dyspnea, chest pain, productive cough, facial pain or pressure in sinus areas; current medications, history of influenza vaccine; chronic diseases such as heart disease, chronic obstructive pulmonary disease (COPD), or diabetes; known medication allergies.
- Physical examination: general appearance; vital signs including temperature; skin color; lung sounds; abdominal exam

## Nursing Diagnoses and Interventions

Although the symptoms of influenza are distressing, most people with the illness provide self-care and do not contact a health care provider. Recommendations to rest in bed during the acute phase of the illness and limit activities until recovery are appropriate for influenza.

Severe disease or complications of influenza may necessitate hospitalization for respiratory support and management. For these clients, nursing care focuses on maintaining airway clearance, breathing patterns, and adequate rest.

### Ineffective Breathing Pattern

Muscle aches, malaise, and elevated temperature may increase the respiratory rate and alter the depth of respirations, decreasing effective alveolar ventilation. Shallow respirations also increase the risk of *atelectasis,* lack of ventilation in an area of lung.

**PRACTICE ALERT** *Monitor respiratory rate and pattern. Tachypnea and/or rapid, shallow respirations may impair effective alveolar ventilation and gas exchange.* ■

- Pace activities to provide for periods of rest. *Tachypnea increases the work of breathing, causing fatigue; fatigue, in turn, can further impair ventilation and reduce the effectiveness of coughing.*
- Elevate the head of the bed. *The upright position improves lung excursion and reduces the work of breathing by lowering the diaphragm, moving abdominal contents downward, creating less resistance to diaphragmatic excursion, and slightly decreasing venous return.*

### Ineffective Airway Clearance

Swelling and congestion of mucous membranes, extracellular fluid exudate, and impaired ciliary action due to cell damage increase the risk of impaired airway clearance in influenza. The older adult is at particular risk because of normally reduced ciliary activity and increased lung compliance.

**PRACTICE ALERT** *Monitor the effectiveness of cough and ability to remove airway secretions. Fatigue and general malaise may impair the ability to cough effectively and mobilize secretions.* ■

## CHART 35–1 NANDA, NIC, AND NOC LINKAGES

### The Client with Influenza

| NURSING DIAGNOSES | NURSING INTERVENTIONS | NURSING OUTCOMES |
|---|---|---|
| • Ineffective Breathing Pattern | • Cough Enhancement<br>• Respiratory Monitoring | • Respiratory Status: Ventilation |
| • Deficient Fluid Volume | • Fluid Management | • Hydration |
| • Hyperthermia | • Fever Treatment | • Thermoregulation |
| • Health-Seeking Behaviors | • Health Education<br>• Immunization/Vaccination Management | • Health-Promoting Behavior<br>• Immunization Behavior |

*Note. Data from Nursing Outcomes Classification (NOC) by M. Johnson & M. Maas (Eds.), 1997, St. Louis: Mosby; Nursing Diagnoses: Definitions & Classification 2001–2002 by North American Nursing Diagnosis Association, 2001, Philadelphia: NANDA; Nursing Interventions Classification (NIC) by J.C. McCloskey & G. M. Bulechek (Eds.), 2000, St. Louis: Mosby. Reprinted by permission.*

- Maintain adequate hydration. Assess mucous membranes and skin turgor for evidence of dehydration. *Fever and decreased oral fluid intake may lead to dehydration and increased viscosity of secretions. Thick, viscous secretions are more difficult to expectorate.*
- Increase the humidity of inspired air with a bedside humidifier. *Increasing the water content of inhaled air helps loosen thick secretions and soothe mucous membranes.*
- Teach effective cough techniques. Administer analgesics as ordered. *The huff cough is effective to maintain open airways and spares energy (see Chapter 36 ⬭ for client teaching of this technique). Relieving muscle ache increases the ability to cough effectively.*

### Disturbed Sleep Pattern

Airway congestion, malaise, muscle aches, and persistent cough may interfere with the ability to rest, increasing fatigue and prolonging recovery.

- Assess sleep patterns using subjective and objective information. *The client may appear to be sleeping but not achieving normal sleep patterns because of influenza symptoms. Both subjective and objective data are important to accurately assess sleep.*
- Provide antipyretic and analgesic medications at or shortly before bedtime. *These drugs promote comfort by reducing fever and relieving muscle aches.*

**PRACTICE ALERT** *If necessary, request a cough suppressant for nighttime use. Cough suppressants are not recommended during the day because coughing promotes airway clearance. They may, however, be necessary at night to allow rest.* ■

### Using NANDA, NIC, and NOC

Chart 35–1 shows links between NANDA nursing diagnoses, NIC, and NOC for the client with influenza.

## Home Care

Encourage appropriate self-care for clients with influenza. Discuss the following topics related to home care:

- Increase rest during the acute, febrile phase of the illness.
- Maintain a liberal fluid intake even if anorexic.
- Appropriately use over-the-counter medications for symptom relief.
- Employ hygiene measures such as using disposable tissues and frequent handwashing to reduce spread of the disease.
- Know manifestations of potential complications of influenza to report to the primary care provider.

## THE CLIENT WITH SINUSITIS

**Sinusitis** is inflammation of the mucous membranes of one or more of the sinuses (see Figure 34–2). Sinusitis is a common condition that usually follows an upper respiratory infection such as acute viral upper respiratory infection or influenza. Common causative organisms include streptococci, *S. pneumoniae, Haemophilus influenzae,* and staphylococci. The risk of sinusitis is higher when the immune system is suppressed by immunosuppressive drugs or HIV infection. Sinusitis is common and difficult to treat in people who have AIDS.

### PHYSIOLOGY REVIEW

The sinuses (or *paranasal sinuses*) are air-filled cavities in the facial bones that open into the turbinates of the nasal cavity. They are lined with ciliated mucous membranes that help move fluid and microorganisms out of the sinuses into the nasal cavity. The sinuses normally are sterile. Air within the sinuses has a lower oxygen content than inspired air.

### PATHOPHYSIOLOGY

Sinusitis develops when nasal mucous membranes swell or other disorders obstruct sinus openings, impairing drainage. Mucus secretions collect in the sinus cavity, serving as a medium for bacterial growth. The nasal and sinus mucous membranes are continuous; therefore, bacteria generally spread to the sinuses via the opening into the nasal turbinates. The inflammatory response provoked by bacterial invasion draws serum and leukocytes to the area to combat the infection, increasing swelling and pressure.

Any process that impairs drainage from the sinuses may precipitate sinusitis. These include nasal polyps, deviated septum, rhinitis, tooth abscess, or swimming or diving trauma. In hospitalized clients, sinusitis may develop following prolonged nasotracheal intubation. Usually more than one sinus is infected. The frontal and maxillary sinuses are usually involved in adults.

Sinusitis may be acute or chronic. Chronic sinusitis results when acute sinusitis is untreated or inadequately treated. With continued infection, bacteria can become isolated, producing chronic inflammation. Over time, mucous membranes become thickened. Fungal infections may cause chronic infections, especially in immunosuppressed clients. Other factors that may contribute to chronic sinusitis are smoking, a history of allergy, and habitual use of nasal sprays or inhalants.

Complications develop when the infection spreads to surrounding structures (Box 35–1). These include periorbital abscess, or cellulitis, cavernous sinus thrombosis, meningitis, brain abscess, or sepsis. Eustachian tube edema may lead to hearing loss.

## MANIFESTATIONS

The client with acute sinusitis often looks sick. Manifestations of sinusitis include pain and tenderness across the infected sinuses, headache, fever, and malaise. The pain usually increases with leaning forward. When the maxillary sinuses are involved, pain and pressure are felt over the cheek. The pain may be referred to the upper teeth. Frontal sinusitis causes pain and tenderness across the lower forehead. Infection of the ethmoid sinus produces retro-orbital pain and pain over the high lateral aspect of the nose. Sphenoid sinusitis, the rarest form, may cause pain in the occiput, vertex, or middle of the head. Symptoms often worsen for 3 to 4 hours after awakening and then become less severe in the afternoon and evening as secretions drain. The intensity and location of headache pain may change as sinuses drain. In acute sinusitis, the pain is usually constant and severe. In chronic sinusitis, the pain is described as dull and may be constant or intermittent.

---

| BOX 35–1 | ■ Potential Complications of Sinusitis |
|---|---|

### LOCAL COMPLICATIONS

- Orbital cellulitis
- Subperiosteal abscess
- Orbital abscess
- Cavernous sinus thrombosis
- Mucocele
- Osteomyelitis

### INTRACRANIAL COMPLICATIONS

- Meningitis
- Epidural abscess
- Subdural abscess
- Brain abscess
- Venous sinus thrombosis

---

Other symptoms include nasal congestion, purulent nasal discharge, and bad breath. The nasal mucous membrane is red and swollen. Purulent drainage may be noted at the opening to the middle turbinate. This may be the only sign of chronic sinusitis. Swallowed secretions irritate and inflame the throat, and may cause nausea or vomiting.

## COLLABORATIVE CARE

Treatment of sinusitis focuses on restoring drainage of obstructed sinuses, controlling infection, relieving pain, and preventing complications.

### Diagnostic Tests

The diagnosis of acute sinusitis usually can be made using the history and physical exam.

- *Sinus X-rays* are evaluated. Sinuses are normally translucent because they are filled with air; affected sinuses appear cloudy or opaque. A visible air-fluid level or thickening of the sinus mucosa may be seen in infected sinuses.
- *CT scan* is a more sensitive indicator of acute and chronic sinusitis and often is performed without preceding X-rays.
- *Magnetic resonance imaging (MRI)* may be ordered if malignancy of the sinus is suspected.

### Medications

Antibiotic therapy directed at the usual organisms causing sinusitis typically is prescribed. Amoxicillin (possibly combined with clavulanate [Augmentin]), trimethoprim-sulfamethoxazole (Bactrim, Septra), cefuroxime (Ceftin), cefaclor (Ceclor), ciprofloxacin (Cipro), or clarithromycin (Biaxin) are commonly used antibiotics for sinusitis. Antibiotic therapy is continued for a full 2-week course; occasionally a longer course is prescribed to prevent relapse. If the sinusitis does not respond to treatment with oral antibiotics, hospitalization and intravenous antibiotic therapy may be required. See Chapter 8 for nursing care related to antibiotic therapy. ⊝⊙

Oral or topical (in the form of nasal sprays) decongestants such as pseudoephedrine or phenylephrine are also prescribed to reduce mucosal edema and promote sinus drainage. Antihistamines may decrease nasal congestion and facilitate sinus drainage, but they also tend to increase the viscosity of secretions and hinder drainage. For this reason, they may not be as effective as decongestants. Saline nose drops or sprays promote sinus drainage, as does inhalation of warm steam. To administer topical drugs, the client's head is tilted backward and to the side on which the drops are to be instilled. The client may need to remain in position for 5 minutes to allow the drops to reach the posterior nares. Systemic mucolytic agents such as guaifenesin may be useful to liquefy secretions, promoting sinus drainage. Aerobic exercise also promotes mucous flow and may be recommended.

### Surgery

Clients who do not respond to pharmacologic measures and who experience persistent facial pain, headache, or nasal congestion may require *endoscopic sinus surgery*. Detailed evaluation of the sinuses by CT scan is done prior to surgery. Under local or general anesthesia, a fiberoptic nasal endoscope is inserted to visualize the sinus opening. If obstruction is present, it can be removed, restoring patency and drainage. This surgery is most effective for local disease, recurrent acute sinusitis, and for removing anatomic obstructions (Way & Doherty, 2003). Clients who have endoscopic sinus surgery usually do not require nasal packing postoperatively. Instead, frequent nasal cleaning and irrigation with normal saline are performed. The client is instructed to sneeze with the mouth open and avoid blowing the nose, lifting, or straining for a week following surgery.

*Antral irrigation* can be done in the physician's office under local anesthesia. A 16-gauge needle is inserted under the inferior turbinate of the nose into the maxillary sinus on the affected side. Saline solution is instilled to irrigate the area and wash out the sinus of purulent exudate. The client is seated with the head forward and mouth open to allow drainage of the solution through the nose and mouth. A culture of the exudate may be obtained to determine appropriate antibiotic therapy.

The *Caldwell-Luc procedure* may be necessary if endoscopic sinus surgery is unsuccessful. It is performed under local or general anesthesia. An incision is made under the upper lip into the maxillary sinus, and diseased mucous membrane and periosteum are removed. An opening between the maxillary sinus and lateral nasal wall, a "nasal antral window," is created to increase aeration of the sinus and promote drainage into the nasal cavity. The area is packed with gauze for 24 to 48 hours postoperatively. The gauze packing obstructs nasal breathing while it is in place. As the maxillary sinus heals, exposed bone is covered by mucosa. The upper lip and teeth may be numb for several months after the procedure because of nerve trauma. Chewing may be impaired on the affected side. Only liquids are given for the first 24 hours, followed by a soft diet. The client is instructed to avoid wearing dentures and the Valsalva maneuver (no blowing the nose, coughing, or straining at stool) for about 2 weeks after the packing has been removed to prevent bleeding.

In *external sphenoethmoidectomy,* an incision along the side of the nose from the middle of the eyebrow is used to open and remove diseased tissue from the sphenoid or ethmoid sinuses (Figure 35–1 ■). Nasal polyps may also be removed using this approach. Nasal packing is inserted, and an eye pressure patch is applied to decrease periorbital edema. Care is similar to that following the Caldwell-Luc procedure.

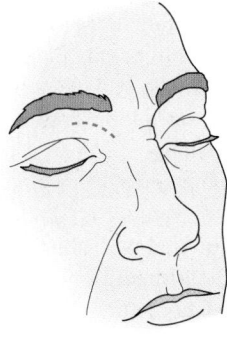

**Figure 35–1 ■** Incision to access ethmoid and frontal sinuses. Resulting scar is nearly invisible in folds of the eye.

## NURSING CARE

### Assessment

Focused assessment of the client with suspected sinusitis includes the following:

- Health history: complaints of frontal or periorbital headache, cheek, teeth, or ear pain; timing of pain and changes in intensity over course of the day; nasal discharge or postnasal drip; other symptoms; previous sinus problems; current medications, known medication allergies
- Physical examination: general appearance, vital signs including temperature; inspect nasal and pharyngeal mucous membranes; percuss sinuses for tenderness

### Nursing Diagnoses and Interventions

The client with sinusitis is often acutely uncomfortable. Obstructed and congested sinuses cause pain and pressure that increase with position changes and leaning forward. Treatment usually is community based, making education the key nursing role. When the client is hospitalized for intravenous antibiotic therapy or sinus surgery, *Pain* and *Imbalanced nutrition* are priority nursing diagnoses.

### Pain

Although sinus surgery is relatively minor, both the incision and postoperative swelling can cause discomfort. Nasal packing, if used, contributes to the discomfort.

- Assess pain using a standardized pain scale. Administer analgesics as ordered. *Relief of pain promotes a feeling of well-being and enhances recovery.*
- Apply ice packs to the nose. *Cold compresses reduce swelling, control bleeding, and provide local analgesia.*
- Elevate the head of the bed to Fowler's or high-Fowler's position for 24 to 48 hours after surgery. *Elevating the operative site minimizes tissue swelling and promotes comfort.*

### Imbalanced Nutrition: Less Than Body Requirements

Postoperatively, the sense of smell, an appetite stimulus, is diminished by nasal packing. Mouth discomfort from the incision and numbness of the upper teeth also may impact appetite and eating.

- Provide clear liquid diet progressing to soft foods as tolerated. High-calorie dietary supplements may be used. *A progressive diet is used to assess the ability to swallow without choking and allay fears. Foods high in calories and nutritional value provide for metabolic and healing requirements.*
- Monitor intake, output, and weight. *This information allows assessment of overall fluid balance and the adequacy of dietary intake.*
- Elevate the head of the bed during meals. *The upright position facilitates swallowing and minimizes risk of aspiration.*

## Home Care

Teaching for clients with sinusitis and their families focuses on following through with appropriate treatment and promoting comfort. Discuss the following topics when preparing for home care:

- The importance of completing the entire course of prescribed antibiotics to achieve cure and prevent the development of antibiotic-resistant bacteria. Assist in developing a schedule that helps ensure all doses are taken.
- Measures to prevent superinfections (such as vaginitis or oral thrush) during the prolonged course of treatment (e.g., consume 8 oz of yogurt containing live bacterial cultures daily while on antibiotics).
- Use systemic or topical decongestants to promote sinus drainage.
- Maintain a liberal fluid intake to reduce the viscosity of mucous drainage.
- Use a humidifier or steam inhalation to promote sinus drainage.
- Sleep with the head of the bed elevated to a 45-degree angle and on the unaffected side to promote drainage of affected sinuses.
- Application of a warm, moist pack to the area of pain and tenderness to promote comfort.
- Notify the physician if symptoms do not improve with treatment or if signs of a complication develop, such as increased pain, and redness and swelling on the side of the nose or around the eyes.
- Postoperative instructions to prevent bleeding, such as avoiding blowing the nose for 7 to 10 days and avoiding strenuous activity such as heavy lifting for about 2 weeks.
- Use saline nasal sprays postoperatively to keep the nasal mucosa moist.

## THE CLIENT WITH PHARYNGITIS OR TONSILLITIS

**Pharyngitis,** acute inflammation of the pharynx, is one of the most commonly identified clinical problems. Although it is usually viral in origin, pharyngitis may also be caused by bacterial infection. *Group A beta-hemolytic streptococcus* (strep throat) is the most common cause of bacterial pharyngitis. Other bacteria that may cause pharyngitis include *Neisseria gonorrheae,* a gram-negative diplococcus that is sexually transmitted, *Mycoplasma,* and *Chlamydia trachomatis.*

**Tonsillitis** is acute inflammation of the palatine tonsils. Although it is sometimes viral in origin, tonsillitis is usually due to streptococcal infection. The incidence of streptococcal infections is greatest between late fall and spring, especially in cold climates. Viral tonsillitis may occur in epidemics in people living in crowded conditions, such as military recruits.

## PATHOPHYSIOLOGY AND MANIFESTATIONS

Pharyngitis and tonsillitis are contagious and spread by droplet nuclei. Incubation varies from a few hours to several days, depending on the organism. Viral infections are communicable for 2 to 3 days. Symptoms usually resolve within 3 to 10 days after onset.

Viral pharyngitis may be attributed to the same viruses causing the common cold, rhinovirus, coronavirus, or parainfluenza virus. Pharyngitis caused by adenovirus, influenza virus, or Epstein-Barr virus (associated with infectious mononucleosis) may be particularly severe.

Although bacterial pharyngitis may be mild and indistinguishable from viral pharyngitis by its signs and symptoms, it can lead to significant complications such as abscess, scarlet fever, toxic shock syndrome, rheumatic fever, or acute post-streptococcal glomerulonephritis.

Acute pharyngitis causes pain and fever. The pain may vary from a scratchy sore throat to one so painful that swallowing is difficult. Streptococcal pharyngitis is usually marked by an abrupt onset, with fever of 101° F (38.3° C) or higher, severe sore throat with dysphagia, malaise, and often arthralgias and myalgias. Anterior lymph nodes are often enlarged and tender. Exudate (pus) may be seen on the pharynx and tonsils. In contrast, the onset of viral pharyngitis is often gradual, with manifestations of low-grade fever, sore throat, mild hoarseness, headache, and rhinorrhea. The pharyngeal membranes appear mildly red with vascular congestion. Infectious mononucleosis, caused by the Epstein-Barr virus, often presents as acute pharyngitis, with visible patches of exudate on the pharynx or tonsils (Braunwald et al., 2001). The cervical lymph nodes are enlarged and tender as well.

In tonsillitis, the tonsils appear bright red and edematous. White exudate is present on the tonsils; pressing on a tonsil may produce purulent drainage. The uvula may also be reddened and swollen. Cervical lymph nodes are usually tender and enlarged.

The client with tonsillitis complains of a sore throat, difficulty swallowing, general malaise, fever, and otalgia (pain referred to the ear). Manifestations are often more severe in adolescents and adults than in children. Infection may extend via the eustachian tubes to cause acute otitis media. This may lead to further damage such as spontaneous rupture of the eardrums and mastoiditis. See Chapter 45 ⬀ for more information about otitis media.

*Peritonsillar abscess,* or *quinsy,* is a potential complication of tonsillitis. It usually results from group A beta-hemolytic streptococcus infection extending from the tonsils to the surrounding tissue. The abscess causes pus formation behind the tonsil with marked swelling and asymmetric deviation of the uvula. The degree of swelling may make it difficult to swallow anything other than liquids. The client may exhibit thickening of the voice, drooling, and a tonic contraction of the muscles of mastication, called trismus.

Rare (1% to 3%) but serious complications of streptococcal pharyngitis and tonsillitis include acute glomerulonephritis and rheumatic fever, abnormal immune responses to the infection. Acute glomerulonephritis generally presents with sudden onset of hematuria, proteinuria, and less commonly, hypertension and edema within 7 to 10 days after the acute infection. Rheumatic fever typically presents 3 to 5 weeks after acute infection with fever, painful or swollen joints, rash, and heart murmur. Other complications of bacterial infection include sinusitis, otitis media, mastoiditis, and cervical adenitis.

## COLLABORATIVE CARE

Both viral and bacterial pharyngitis are usually self-limited diseases. However, because of the risk for serious complications associated with streptococcal sore throat, an effort is usually made to establish an accurate diagnosis and treat bacterial pharyngitis.

- *Throat swab* is obtained and examined for streptococcus antigen using the latex agglutination (LA) antigen test or enzyme immunoassay (ELISA) testing. These tests allow rapid identification of the antigen (in as little as 10 minutes for the LA test) but are not highly sensitive. When the test is positive, treatment for strep throat is initiated. If the test is negative, the swab is cultured to ensure that streptococcus organisms are not present. Even throat cultures are not always accurate, with approximately 10% false negative and 20% false positive results.
- *Complete blood count (CBC)* may be done on severely ill clients or to rule out other causes of pharyngitis. The WBC count is usually normal or low in viral infections and elevated in bacterial infections.

Antipyretics and mild analgesics such as aspirin or acetaminophen provide symptomatic relief for throat pain and associated myalgias. Penicillin is the drug of choice for group A streptococci. Erythromycin, amoxicillin, or cefuroxime (Ceftin, Kefurox) may be used if the client is allergic to penicillin. Antibiotic therapy is continued for at least 10 days. The client is no longer contagious after 24 hours of antibiotic therapy.

A peritonsillar abscess is drained by needle aspiration or by incision and drainage. The area is first sprayed with a topical anesthetic such as cetacaine and then injected with a local anesthetic. The sitting position is preferred for the procedure, because it enables expectoration of blood and pus. Tonsillectomy is done either immediately or 6 weeks after incision and drainage of peritonsillar abscess.

*Tonsillectomy* (surgical removal of the tonsils) is indicated for recurrent or chronic infections that have not responded to antibiotic therapy, hypertrophy of the tonsils with risk of airway obstruction, peritonsillar abscess, repeated attacks of purulent otitis media, and tonsil malignancy. Adenoid tissue usually is removed at the same time. Bleeding is the most significant postoperative complication of tonsillectomy.

## NURSING CARE

Because of the risk of significant complications associated with streptococcal pharyngitis, encourage all clients with symptoms that persist for several days or that include fever, lymphadenopathy, and myalgias to seek evaluation and treatment.

Home care is appropriate for acute uncomplicated pharyngitis. Treatment focuses on adequate rest and relief of symptoms. A liquid or soft diet is useful when swallowing is difficult. Increased fluid intake is encouraged, especially when febrile. Warm saline gargles, moist inhalations, and application of an ice collar are soothing to the sore throat.

Following tonsillectomy, ensure a patent airway by placing the client in semi-Fowler's position with the head turned to the side to allow secretions to drain from the mouth and pharynx. Keep the airway in place until the gag and swallowing reflexes have returned. Apply an ice collar to reduce swelling and pain. Notify the surgeon immediately if excessive bleeding or hemorrhage occurs. If there is no bleeding, allow water and cracked ice as desired. Warm saline mouthwashes are helpful in managing thick oral secretions following tonsillectomy. A liquid or semiliquid diet is recommended for several days.

### Home Care

Discuss the following topics when preparing the client for home care.

- The importance of completing the full 10 days of antibiotic therapy if prescribed
- Using warm saline gargles or throat lozenges for symptomatic relief
- Signs and symptoms of possible complications of streptococcal infection such as glomerulonephritis or rheumatic fever
- Monitoring temperature in the morning and evening until well to ensure that the infection has not spread to deeper tissues
- Proper use and disposal of tissues and frequent handwashing to prevent spreading the infection to others

For the client who has had a peritonsillar abscess drainage or tonsillectomy, provide the following instructions.

- Postoperative mouth and throat care
- Avoiding use of aspirin for 2 weeks to reduce the risk of postoperative bleeding
- Manifestations of bleeding to report to the physician (delayed hemorrhage may occur for up to 1 week post surgery)

## THE CLIENT WITH A LARYNGEAL INFECTION

The larynx, located between the upper airways and the lungs, protects the lower respiratory tract from inhaled substances other than air, and allows speech. The larynx includes the epiglottis, which covers the larynx during swallowing, and the glottis, or vocal cords. Either portion of the larynx may become inflamed.

### EPIGLOTTITIS

*Epiglottitis,* inflammation of the epiglottis, is an uncommon disorder that presents as a medical emergency. *H. influenzae* infection is the most common cause of epiglottitis. Epiglottitis is

## Nursing Care Plan
## A Client with Peritonsillar Abscess

Monica Wunderman, age 27, was recently treated for tonsillitis caused by infection by group A streptococcus. She presents to the emergency department 10 days later appearing acutely ill. She states that her throat is so sore that she has difficulty swallowing even liquids. Barbara Ironhorse, the ED nurse, completes an assessment of Ms. Wunderman.

### ASSESSMENT

Findings include T 102°F (38.8°C). An acutely swollen and reddened area of the soft palate is noted in her mouth, half occluding the orifice from the mouth into the pharynx. Yellow exudate is present. CBC reveals an elevated WBC of 16,000/mm³. A diagnosis of peritonsillar abscess is made. Needle aspiration of the abscess is performed.

### DIAGNOSIS

- *Acute pain* related to swelling
- *Risk for ineffective airway clearance* related to pain and swelling
- *Deficient fluid volume* related to fever and difficulty in swallowing fluids

### EXPECTED OUTCOMES

- Have minimal or no pain.
- Maintain a patent airway as demonstrated by normal respiratory rate and rhythm.
- Maintain optimal fluid intake as evidenced by consumption of fluids and semiliquid foods, moist mucous membranes, normal skin turgor, and normal temperature.

### PLANNING AND IMPLEMENTATION

- Teach that ice-cold fluids may be easier to swallow than hot or room-temperature beverages and may provide a local analgesic effect.
- Advise to avoid citrus juices, hot or spicy foods, and rough-textured foods for 1 week.
- Teach pain management strategies such as applying an ice collar as desired and gargling with warm saline or mouthwash solution every 1 to 2 hours for the first 24 to 48 hours after aspiration of the abscess.
- Instruct to take medications as prescribed.

### EVALUATION

When Ms. Ironhorse contacts Ms. Wunderman by telephone 2 days after her visit to the emergency department, she reports complete relief of symptoms. She is afebrile, taking fluids without difficulty, and has had no difficulty breathing. She has not experienced any pain.

### Critical Thinking in the Nursing Process

1. Describe common symptoms of infectious or inflammatory diseases of the upper airway and discuss methods of symptom relief.
2. Describe common pharmacologic interventions for these disorders.
3. What themes of nursing diagnoses emerge for these clients?

See Evaluating Your Response in Appendix C.

---

a rapidly progressive cellulitis that begins between the base of the tongue and the epiglottis. The epiglottis itself becomes swollen and inflamed; swelling of adjacent tissues pushes the epiglottis posteriorly. This swelling and edema threatens the airway. Adults usually present with a 1 to 2 day history of sore throat, *odynophagia* (painful swallowing), dyspnea, and possibly drooling and stridor.

Using a tongue blade to view the oropharynx is avoided; this may precipitate laryngospasm and airway obstruction. The epiglottis is visualized using a flexible fiberoptic laryngoscope to establish the diagnosis. The epiglottis appears red, swollen, and edematous. Nasotracheal intubation may be required to ensure airway patency. The client is admitted to a critical care unit and intravenous antibiotic therapy is initiated. Ceftriaxone (Rocephin), cefuroxime (Ceftin), or ampicillin/sulbactam (Unasyn) may be prescribed. If allergic to penicillin, a combination of clindamycin (Cleocin) and either trimethoprim-sulfamthoxazole (TMP-SMZ) or ciprofloxacin (Cipro) may be used. Dexamethasone, a systemic corticosteroid, is also given to suppress the inflammatory response and rapidly reduce swelling of the epiglottis.

Nursing care for the client with acute epiglottitis focuses on monitoring and maintaining airway patency. Monitor oxygen saturation continuously. Observe closely for signs of airway obstruction, including nasal flaring, restlessness, stridor, use of accessory muscles, and decreased oxygen saturation measurements. If the client is not intubated, supplies for emergency intubation should be kept in the unit. Epiglottitis is frightening for both the client and the nurse. Maintaining a calm, reassuring manner is an essential nursing role.

### LARYNGITIS

**Laryngitis,** inflammation of the larynx, is a common disorder that may occur alone or in conjunction with other upper respiratory infections. It is commonly associated with viral URI such as influenza. It may also occur with bronchitis, pneumonia, or other respiratory infections. Excessive use of the voice, sudden changes in temperature or exposure to dust, irritating fumes, smoke, or other pollutants can also cause acute or chronic laryngitis. It is more common in the winter and in colder climates.

In laryngitis, the mucous membrane lining the larynx becomes inflamed; the vocal cords also may become edematous.

The primary symptom of laryngitis is a change in the voice. Hoarseness or *aphonia,* complete loss of the voice, may occur. The throat is often sore and scratchy, and a dry, harsh cough may be present.

There is no specific treatment for viral laryngitis. Any identified precipitating factors such as overuse of the voice and exposure to irritants should be eliminated. Voice rest is advised, as is abstinence from tobacco and alcohol, which are chemical irritants. Treatment may also include inhaling steam or spraying the throat with antiseptic solutions. Identifying and eliminating irritants is helpful to prevent future attacks.

Impaired verbal communication is the priority nursing problem for clients with laryngitis. The meaning of messages is conveyed not only by the words used, but also by the tone and loudness of voice. Instruct to rest the voice as much as possible. Encourage speaking in short sentences or using alternate methods of communication, such as writing. Resting the voice hastens recovery and decreases throat discomfort. Advise to use soothing throat lozenges, sprays, or other comfort measures such as gargling with a warm antiseptic solution. Help identify potential irritants, such as fumes, chemicals, or cold temperature, to prevent future bouts of laryngitis.

## THE CLIENT WITH DIPHTHERIA

*Diphtheria* is an acute, contagious disease caused by *Corynebacterium diphtheriae,* a small aerobic pathogen. This disease, which primarily affects adults, is uncommon in the United States. Waning immunity due to lack of periodic booster immunizations is the primary risk factor for diphtheria in the United States.

The disease is spread through droplet nuclei and by contamination of articles such as eating utensils. Asymptomatic carriers can be a factor in spreading this infection. People who have recovered from diphtheria can harbor bacteria in their throats for up to 4 weeks. Diphtheria is easily spread in areas where sanitation is poor, living conditions are crowded, and access to health care is limited. Immunization is readily available, and infants and children are usually immunized against diphtheria, pertussis, and tetanus concurrently.

## PATHOPHYSIOLOGY AND MANIFESTATIONS

*C. diphtheriae* infects the mucous membranes of the respiratory tract and can invade skin lesions. The tonsils and pharynx are common sites of infection. Toxins released by the organism inflame mucosal surfaces of the pharynx. Exudate from inflamed tissues forms a thick, grayish, rubbery pseudomembrane over the posterior pharynx and sometimes into the trachea. This pseudomembrane adheres to inflamed, eroded surfaces and interferes with eating, drinking, and breathing. The airway may be obstructed, necessitating tracheostomy to maintain respirations. The toxins damage the heart and central nervous system and may cause myocarditis and paralysis of cranial or peripheral nerves.

Clients with diphtheria develop fever, malaise, sore throat, and malodorous breath. In severe cases, the neck may be warm and swollen because of lymphadenopathy. Isolated patches of gray or white exudate grow and extend to form a gray membrane that becomes progressively thicker. Dislodging the membrane often causes bleeding. Symptoms of airway obstruction, such as stridor and cyanosis, can develop quickly.

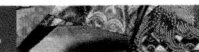
## COLLABORATIVE CARE

Collaborative care goals for diphtheria are to prevent its transmission, treat the infection, neutralize toxins, and provide respiratory support. The diagnosis is confirmed by a throat culture. Gram-stain or immunofluorescent antibody stains may also be used.

Strict isolation procedures are instituted, and all contacts are screened and immunized. Booster shots are given to people who were immunized 5 or more years previously. Unimmunized contacts are treated with immunization and antibiotics.

Diphtheria antitoxin is given to neutralize free toxin and prevent further toxin production. Diphtheria antitoxin is produced in horses; a skin test for sensitivity to horse serum should precede immunization. Anaphylaxis is a risk during antitoxin therapy; epinephrine must be readily available. Antibiotics such as penicillin or erythromycin are administered to eliminate the organism.

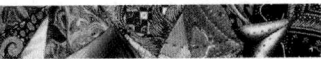
## NURSING CARE

Clients with diphtheria require intensive nursing care. The client is placed on bed rest and monitored closely for airway obstruction, cardiac manifestations, and CNS complications. Nutrition and fluid balance may be affected by difficulty swallowing. Upright positioning can promote fluid intake during the acute phase of the disease. Equipment for suction, emergency intubation, and tracheostomy are kept at the bedside.

**PRACTICE ALERT**    *Diphtheria is a reportable disease. Immediately contact the local health department and the Centers for Disease Control and Prevention of all suspected and confirmed cases.* ■

Preventing further cases of diphtheria is a nursing responsibility. Symptomatic clients are isolated and treated until two negative throat cultures are obtained. Nasopharyngeal and throat cultures are also obtained from all close contacts. Asymptomatic disease carriers are confined to home until at least 3 days of antibiotic therapy have been completed. All contacts, including hospital personnel, receive tetanus and diphtheria toxoids (Td).

## THE CLIENT WITH PERTUSSIS

**Pertussis,** or *whooping cough,* is a highly contagious acute upper respiratory infection caused by the bacterium *Bordetella pertussis*. Although it is thought to be a childhood disease that has been virtually eliminated by aggressive immunization of infants, pertussis still occurs in North America. Up to 45% of people affected by pertussis are adolescents and adults. Adults are thought to be an important reservoir for this disease (Braunwald et al., 2001).

### PATHOPHYSIOLOGY

*B. pertussis* is a gram-negative rod that is spread by respiratory droplets. The bacteria attach to ciliated epithelial cells of the nasopharynx, multiplying and invading respiratory tissues. The damage and effects of pertussis are not due to the infection itself, but to toxins produced by the bacteria. These toxins damage the mucosa and paralyze the cilia. As a result, clearance of respiratory secretions is impaired, increasing the risk for pneumonia. The toxins also prompt an inflammatory response and inhibit immune defenses.

Although immunization does not appear to confer lifetime immunity, the disease tends to be milder in adolescents, adults, and people who have been immunized. These infected individuals can, however, transmit the disease to other susceptible people, including unimmunized or underimmunized infants (Atkinson, Wolfe, Humiston, & Nelson, 2000).

Young infants have the highest risk for complications of the disease, such as pneumonia and neurologic complications. Neurologic complications are thought to result from hypoxia due to prolonged paroxysms of coughing. Complications in adolescents and adults may occur as a result of increased intrathoracic pressure during prolonged coughing spells. These may include pneumothorax, weight loss, inguinal hernia, rib fracture, and *cough syncope* (fainting due to hypoxia) (Braunwald et al., 2001).

### MANIFESTATIONS

Classic pertussis follows a predictable pattern, with typical upper respiratory infection symptoms (coryza, sneezing, low-grade fever, and mild cough) beginning 7 to 10 days after exposure. After 1 to 2 weeks, the cough becomes more frequent, occurring in paroxysms or bursts of rapid coughs, often ending with an audible whoop caused by rapid inspiration. This whoop is less common in adolescents and adults, often delaying diagnosis. Vomiting commonly follows an episode of coughing. Coughing paroxysms vary in frequency from several per hour to 5 to 10 per day, interfering with eating and sleep. This stage of the disease, called the *paroxysmal stage,* usually lasts no more than 6 weeks, after which coughing becomes less severe and gradually resolves over a period of up to 3 months.

In adolescents and adults, pertussis is suspected when an upper respiratory infection produces a cough that persists longer than 7 days, is accompanied by vomiting, and is worse at night. See the box in next column.

### Manifestations of Pertussis

**CLASSIC**
- Catarrhal phase: coryza, malaise, low-grade fever, sneezing, cough
- Paroxysmal phase: frequent spasms of sometimes violent coughing, worse at night; characteristic whoop on inspiration following cough paroxysm; vomiting, fatigue, weight loss resulting from severe cough
- Convalescent phase: gradually decreasing frequency and severity of coughing episodes

**ATYPICAL (often seen in adolescents and adults)**
- Severe, prolonged cough that may not be paroxysmal; whoop uncommon
- Vomiting with cough
- Cough at night

## COLLABORATIVE CARE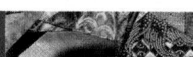

Active immunization with pertussis vaccine is the primary preventive strategy for pertussis. Acellular pertussis vaccines that are effective but produce fewer adverse reactions than traditional whole-cell vaccines are available and preferred for immunization.

The diagnosis of pertussis is established by culture of nasopharyngeal secretions. However, nasopharyngeal secretions may remain positive for the organism for only about 3 weeks after the onset of symptoms, so blood tests for antibodies to the organism may be necessary to confirm the diagnosis. Lymphocytosis (elevated lymphocyte count) may be present.

Erythromycin is the antibiotic of choice to eradicate *B. pertussis* infection. Trimethoprim-sulfamethoxazole (TMP-SMZ) may be used as an alternate to erythromycin. Hospitalization rarely is required for adults, although children and infants with severe disease often are hospitalized to prevent complications such as neurologic effects of hypoxia and malnutrition. Respiratory isolation is instituted for 5 days after antibiotic therapy is started. Prophylactic erythromycin or TMP-SMZ is prescribed for all household and close contacts of the infected client.

## NURSING CARE

Nurses are instrumental in promoting effective immunization of all infants and young children against pertussis. Education is a key nursing role related to immunization, as significant controversy currently exists about potential long-term adverse consequences of the vaccine. Recommend that all parents request acellular vaccine due to its lower risk of adverse effects.

Recommend nasopharyngeal culture for clients complaining of persistent cough, especially when the cough is accompanied by vomiting or significantly worse at night, or if other members of the household or close contacts have a similar illness.

Education is a primary nursing role related to pertussis. Adult clients usually remain in the community for treatment. Teach respiratory isolation measures to be used until the disease is no longer communicable to others. Discuss ways to control respiratory secretions, and the importance of disposing of tissues and secretions personally to prevent exposure of others. Stress the importance of prophylactic treatment for all household and close contacts. Discuss measures to maintain fluid and nutrient intake, and use of a cough suppressant at night to promote rest. Encourage increased fluid intake to promote expectoration of respiratory secretions. Teach about the prescribed antibiotic, including its potential adverse effects and measures to reduce them, such as taking erythromycin with meals to prevent gastric upset. Contact the local county health department for follow-up of contacts and compliance with prescribed treatment.

# UPPER RESPIRATORY TRAUMA OR OBSTRUCTION

## THE CLIENT WITH EPISTAXIS

The nose has a rich blood supply, receiving major arterial vessels from both the internal and external carotid artery systems. **Epistaxis,** or nosebleed, may be precipitated by a number of factors. Trauma (picking the nose or blunt trauma) can cause epistaxis, as can drying of nasal mucous membranes, infection, substance abuse (e.g., cocaine), arteriosclerosis, or hypertension. Epistaxis may also indicate a bleeding disorder related to acute leukemia, thrombocytopenia, aplastic anemia, or severe liver disease. Additionally, treatment with an anticoagulant or antiplatelet drug may cause nosebleed. In adults, men more frequently have nosebleeds than women.

### PATHOPHYSIOLOGY

Ninety percent of all nosebleeds arise in the anterior nasal septum from Kiesselbach's area, a rich vascular plexus. Because of their location, these vessels are susceptible to trauma from nose picking, drying, and infection. Posterior epistaxis more often develops secondarily to systemic disorders such as blood dyscrasias, hypertension, or diabetes. In posterior epistaxis, bleeding is from the terminal branches of the sphenopalatine and internal maxillary arteries. Posterior epistaxis tends to be more severe and occurs more frequently in the older adult.

## COLLABORATIVE CARE

The goal of treatment for epistaxis is to identify and control the source of bleeding.

Anterior bleeding can usually be managed by simple first-aid measures, such as applying pressure (pinching the nose toward the septum) for 5 to 10 minutes and applying ice packs to the nose and forehead to cause vasoconstriction. The client is placed in a sitting position to decrease blood flow to the head and reduce venous pressure. Leaning forward reduces drainage of blood backward into the nasopharynx and decreases swallowing of blood. The client is instructed to spit out the blood to help estimate the amount of bleeding and to prevent nausea and vomiting as a result of swallowed blood.

If applying pressure does not control the bleeding, medications, nasal packing, or surgery may be necessary.

### Medications

Topical vasoconstrictors such as cocaine (0.5%), phenylephrine (Neo-Synephrine) (1:1000), or adrenaline (1:1000) may be used to control anterior bleeding. These medications may be applied by nasal spray or on a cotton swab held against the bleeding site. Chemical cauterization of the bleeding vessel may be done using agents such as silver nitrate or Gelfoam. A topical anesthetic such as tetracaine, lidocaine, or cocaine may be used prior to nasal packing. If posterior nasal packing is required, prophylactic antibiotic therapy is initiated to prevent sinusitis or possible toxic shock syndrome.

### Nasal Packing

If bleeding cannot be controlled with pressure and local medications, the nasal cavity may be packed with 0.25-inch petroleum gauze. For an anterior pack, several feet of packing are placed carefully and systematically along the floor of the nasal cavity and then into the vault of the nose. Anterior nasal packs are usually left in place for 24 to 72 hours. If epistaxis is caused by a bleeding disorder, the packing may be left in place for 4 to 5 days while the disorder is treated.

Posterior nosebleeds are more difficult to control, requiring both anterior and posterior packing (Figure 35–2 ■). Posterior packs are usually left in place for 2 to 5 days. A loose anterior nasal pack may also be inserted. Posterior nasal packing is very uncomfortable, and can cause respiratory and cardiovascular complications. Hypoxemia is common; supplementary oxygen is administered. Narcotic analgesics are prescribed to manage the discomfort. Hypertension, dysrhythmias, and even acute myocardial infarction may occur in clients with severe cardiovascular disease. Toxic shock syndrome is another potential complication of posterior nasal packing. The pack may occlude

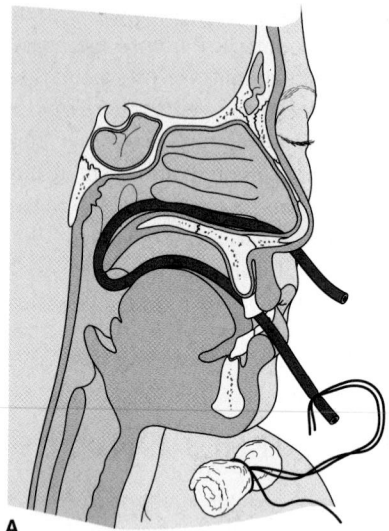

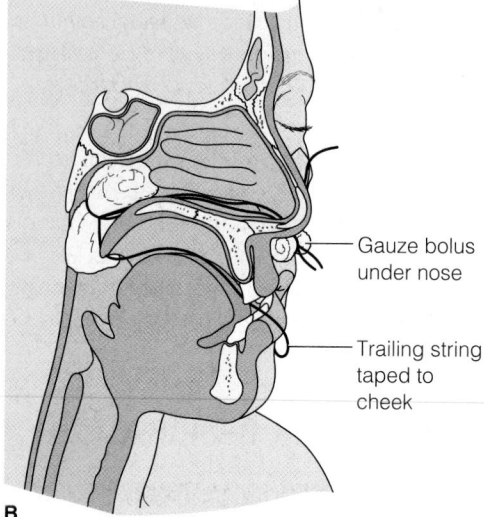

Gauze bolus under nose

Trailing string taped to cheek

**Figure 35–2** ■ Posterior nasal packing. *A,* A rubber catheter is inserted through the nose and out the mouth and attached to the packing. *B,* The catheter is withdrawn through the nose to position the packing in the posterior nasopharynx. Ties exiting through the nose and mouth are used to stabilize the packing in position and remove it when it is no longer needed.

the eustachian tube and sinus openings, resulting in ear discomfort, possible otitis media, or sinusitis. Oral and nasal dryness can be minimized by use of a high-humidity face tent. Nursing care of the client with nasal packing is outlined in the box below.

A Foley catheter or inflatable nasal balloons may be used as an alternative to posterior nasal packing for effective tamponade. The catheter or nasal balloon is inserted through the nose into the nasopharynx, inflated, and left in place for 2 to 3 days.

## Surgery

Chemical or surgical cautery procedures may be used to sclerose involved vessels in the anterior aspect of the nose. The resulting scab must be left undisturbed until the mucosa has healed, or further bleeding may occur.

Surgical procedures to control bleeding are often preferred to posterior nasal packing for posterior bleeding. The bleeding vessel may be cauterized using an endoscopic approach. In some cases, surgery is required to occlude the internal maxil-

# NURSING CARE OF THE CLIENT WITH NASAL PACKING

- Continuously monitor oxygen saturation. Administer supplementary oxygen as ordered. *Posterior nasal packing causes hypoxemia. Supplemental oxygen is given to maintain tissue oxygenation.*
- Frequently monitor vital signs and respiratory rate or pattern. *Posterior nasal packing increases the risk for respiratory and cardiovascular complications. Tachycardia and tachypnea may be early signs of cardiac or respiratory compromise.*
- Inspect the mouth and oropharynx. Notify the physician if the packing is seen in the oropharynx. *Misplacement of nasal packing can obstruct the upper airway.*
- Elevate the head of the bed. *Elevating the head of the bed facilitates ventilation.*
- Encourage deep, slow breathing through the mouth. Provide psychologic support, reassurance, and teaching. *Inability to breathe through the nose causes anxiety and fear.*

- Check for blood at the back of the throat and frequent swallowing. *Visible blood or frequent swallowing could indicate posterior bleeding.*
- Report hematemesis. *Bleeding from the posterior portion of the nose often drains down the nasopharynx and is swallowed. Hematemesis may indicate continued bleeding.*
- Apply cold compresses to nose. *An ice or cold compress decreases pain and promotes vasoconstriction, decreasing bleeding and swelling.*
- Provide for rest. *Rest reduces the metabolic demands and oxygen consumption.*
- Ensure adequate oral fluid intake. *Fluid intake helps maintain fluid balance and decreases dryness of oral mucous membranes because of mouth breathing.*
- Provide frequent oral hygiene. Use a bedside humidifier. *These measures reduce drying of oral mucous membranes and promote comfort.*

lary artery by ligation (tying off) or embolization. These procedures may be done under either conscious sedation and local anesthesia or general anesthesia. Facial paralysis, paresthesias, facial pain, and dental injury are potential complications (Way & Doherty, 2003).

## NURSING CARE

### Assessment

Nursing assessment of the client with a nosebleed focuses on the immediate problem and possible underlying conditions.

- Health history: duration of current bleed; any identified precipitating factors such as trauma; history of prior nosebleeds; current medications; chronic conditions such as hypertension, bleeding disorders, etc.
- Physical examination: estimated amount of bleeding; presence of blood in oropharynx; vital signs; evidence of facial or nasal trauma

### Nursing Diagnoses and Interventions

Nosebleeds can be frightening, particularly when they occur without preceding trauma. Nurses provide care for clients with epistaxis in outpatient and emergency settings, and may care for hospitalized clients with nasal packing. Support, reassurance, and education are important nursing roles related to epistaxis. Priority nursing diagnoses include *Anxiety* and *Risk for aspiration.*

#### Anxiety

The amount of blood lost in a nosebleed can be frightening. The sensation of blood draining down the throat and inability to breathe through the nose contribute to anxiety. Spontaneous epistaxis may lead to fear of a major health problem such as high blood pressure.

> **PRACTICE ALERT** *Maintain an attitude of calm reassurance. By remaining calm and confident, the nurse reassures the client that the nosebleed is not a life-threatening event.* ■

- Instruct the client to pinch the nares together at the bridge of the nose. *Most nosebleeds are anterior in origin; direct pressure usually stops the bleeding. Having the client place pressure on the nose provides a focus and helps restore a sense of control, reducing anxiety.*
- Encourage slow, deep breathing through the mouth. *Controlled mouth breathing maintains lung ventilation and reduces anxiety.*
- Provide a basin and tissues; encourage the client to expectorate blood, not swallow it. *These measures give the client greater control and reduce the fear of choking on blood.*

> **PRACTICE ALERT** *Assess the client with nasal packing frequently for adequate oxygenation. Maintain supplemental oxygen as ordered. Cerebral hypoxia produces a sense of apprehension and fear.* ■

#### Risk for Aspiration

Anxiety and blood draining into the nasopharynx increase the risk for aspiration of blood into the trachea. When nasal packing is in place, the client is unable to breathe through the nose, increasing the risk of aspiration when food or fluids are consumed.

> **PRACTICE ALERT** *Position upright with the head forward. Provide a basin for expectorating blood. These measures minimize the amount of blood draining down the nasopharynx and swallowed, reducing the risk of aspiration and minimizing nausea from swallowed blood. Vomiting of swallowed blood increases the risk of aspiration.* ■

- Apply ice or a cold compress to the nose. *Cold causes vasoconstriction, reducing bleeding.*

> **PRACTICE ALERT** *Position the client with nasal packing with the head elevated and on the side when asleep. This position reduces the risk of aspiration of oral secretions.* ■

### Home Care

Following an episode of epistaxis, teaching for home care focuses on measures to prevent further bleeding. Include the following teaching topics.

- Avoid strenuous exercise for several days or weeks, depending on the severity of the nosebleed and its treatment.
- Do not blow the nose or engage in activities such as heavy lifting or bending that could increase pressure and dislodge the crust; sneeze with the mouth open to avoid increasing pressure in nasal vessels.
- For an anterior nose bleed, use petroleum jelly, a water-soluble lubricant, or bacitracin ointment to lubricate nasal mucosa and reduce the risk of spontaneous bleeding.
- Use a humidifier or vaporizer to minimize dryness of the mucous membranes.
- Do not forcefully blow the nose or pick the nose.
- For spontaneous nose bleed, seek medical evaluation for any possible underlying problem, such as hypertension or a bleeding disorder.

## THE CLIENT WITH NASAL TRAUMA OR SURGERY

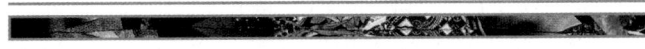

The nose is the most commonly broken bone of the face. A nasal fracture (broken nose) usually is caused by a sports injury or trauma related to violence or motor vehicle crashes. The nasal septum normally divides the nose into two equal parts. Deviation of the septum can result from nasal trauma. Soft tissue trauma commonly accompanies nasal fracture.

MediaLink | EPISTAXIS CARE PLAN

## Manifestations of Nasal Fracture

- Epistaxis
- Deformity or displacement to one side
- Crepitus
- Periorbital edema and ecchymosis
- Nasal bridge instability

## PATHOPHYSIOLOGY AND MANIFESTATIONS

One or both sides of the nose may be broken. A *unilateral fracture* involves only one side of the nose. It causes little displacement or cosmetic deformity. It is usually not serious, but septal deviation and swelling can obstruct the airway. *Bilateral fractures* are more common, with depression or displacement of both nasal bones to one side. The nose appears flattened or deviated with an S or C configuration. *Complex fractures* may also involve the septum, ascending processes of the maxilla, and frontal bones of the face.

Soft-tissue trauma commonly accompanies nasal fracture. Mucous membrane tears cause epistaxis. Soft-tissue hematomas (black eye) are also frequent. Swelling develops rapidly following the injury and may obscure the fracture. Boney crepitus may be felt on gentle palpation. Septal hematoma may develop, increasing the risk for infection. The manifestations of nasal fracture are listed in the box above.

Potential complications of nasal fracture include septal hematoma and abscess formation, septal perforation or deviation, and cerebrospinal fluid (CSF) leakage. Septal hematoma can lead to complete and bilateral nasal obstruction. If undrained, hematoma increases the risk of staphylococcal abscess, which can lead to necrosis of septal cartilage and *saddle nose deformity.*

Septal deviation causes varying degrees of nasal obstruction. The septal cartilage bulges or deviates to one side, partially or totally obstructing the nares. Mild deviation is generally asymptomatic. Partial obstruction of air flow through one side may cause noisy breathing while awake and snoring during sleep. Major deviations can cause pain because of sinus obstruction or infection. They may also cause nosebleeds due to dryness of the nasal mucosa. Occasionally, the defect is severe enough to cause cosmetic deformity. Perforations are usually not serious and do not usually require repair unless obstruction or external deformity occur.

Fractures of other facial bones may accompany a broken nose, particularly when facial trauma is severe. Fractures in the nasoethmoidal or frontal region can disrupt the dura, causing CSF leakage or rhinorrhea. CSF rhinorrhea is suspected by watery nasal drainage tests positive for glucose.

## COLLABORATIVE CARE

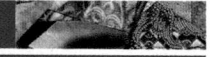

The major treatment goals for nasal fractures are to maintain a patent airway and prevent deformity. Respirations are closely monitored.

## Diagnostic Tests

Head and facial X-rays are done to identify the fracture and assess for other facial fractures. The intranasal cavity is examined using a nasal speculum to rule out septal hematoma. If a CSF leak is suspected, a CT scan is done. A radiopaque substance or fluorescein dye may be instilled into the intrathecal or lumbar subarachnoid space to identify the site of leakage.

## Treatments

Ideally, the fracture is reduced early, before significant edema develops. Nasal fractures heal rapidly. Simple reduction may be done in the emergency department with local anesthesia. An external splint may be applied for 7 to 10 days to maintain proper alignment until healing occurs. The splint is padded to prevent skin breakdown. Ice may be gently applied to the face and nose to control edema and bleeding. Nasal packing may be used to control epistaxis.

## Surgery

Complex nasal fractures, nasal septal deviation, or persistent CSF leakage may require surgical repair or realignment of nasal bones. Rhinoplasty with concurrent septoplasty is the most common procedure used to repair nasal fracture or a deviated nasal septum.

**Rhinoplasty** is surgical reconstruction of the nose. It is done to relieve airway obstruction and repair visible deformity of the nose following fracture. If edema is excessive after nasal fracture, surgery is delayed for 7 to 10 days to allow swelling to subside. Using an intranasal incision, the nasal skin is lifted and the framework of the nose reshaped by removing, rearranging, or augmenting bone or cartilage. The skin is then repositioned over the reconstructed frame. Prosthetic implants may help reshape the nose. Either local or general anesthesia may be used; hospitalization is often unnecessary. Following surgery, nasal packing is left in place for up to 72 hours to minimize bleeding and provide tissue support. A temporary plastic splint molded to the shape of the nose is removed in 3 to 5 days. The splint protects the reshaped nose and helps to control swelling. Most swelling and bruising subside within 10 to 14 days; normal sensation returns within several months following surgery. Rhinoplasty generally has few complications.

Either a septoplasty or a submucous resection (SMR) may be done under local anesthesia to correct a deviated septum. *Septoplasty* involves incising one side of the septum, elevating the mucous membrane, and removing or straightening the deviated portion of septal cartilage. In a *submucous resection,* bone and cartilage are removed. In both procedures, packing is applied to both sides of the nose to prevent bleeding and to keep the septal mucosa in midline position.

Small defects in the cribriform plate, fovea ethmoidalis, or sphenoid sinus associated with persistent CSF leakage may require endoscopic repair. Either a tissue graft or fibrin glue may be used to repair the defect. The graft or glue is held in place with an absorbable packing. Large defects may require craniotomy for repair (Way & Doherty, 2003).

## NURSING CARE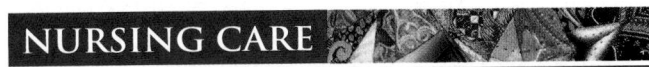

### Health Promotion

Teach all people, children and adolescents in particular, about the importance of wearing helmets and facial protectors when participating in high-risk sports such as football, hockey, and baseball catching. Promote the use of seatbelts with shoulder harness and airbags in vehicles to reduce the risk of facial injury in motor vehicle crashes.

### Assessment

Focused nursing assessment for the client with a suspected nasal fracture includes:

- Health history: nature and circumstances of the injury; pain; ability to breathe through the nose
- Physical examination: evident trauma, swelling, ecchymosis, or deformity of the nose; vital signs, respiratory rate and ease; gently palpate nose and facial bones for crepitus; inspect oropharynx for drainage; test nasal discharge for glucose

### Nursing Diagnoses and Interventions

Nursing care for clients with nasal fracture focuses on controlling pain, bleeding, and swelling. Airway management is a priority. Most nasal fractures are managed on an outpatient basis, and education is a vital nursing function.

#### Ineffective Airway Clearance

Immediately following nasal trauma and fracture, the airway is at risk for obstruction by bleeding and edema. Deformity resulting from inappropriate fracture position during healing also can impair nasal airway clearance. This is a consideration when inserting nasogastric tubes or suctioning clients with septal deviation.

**PRACTICE ALERT**  *Monitor airway patency. Edema and bleeding may obstruct the airway, causing signs of respiratory distress such as tachypnea, dyspnea, shortness of breath, tachycardia, and use of accessory muscles.* ■

- Monitor cough effectiveness and ability to clear airway secretions. *Pain, edema, and nasal bleeding may impair the ability to cough effectively.*

**PRACTICE ALERT**  *Have suction equipment available. Airway patency is a priority; oropharyngeal suctioning may be necessary to remove secretions and maintain a clear airway. Suctioning of the nasopharynx is avoided to prevent additional tissue trauma.* ■

- Maintain adequate hydration. Assess mucous membranes and skin turgor for evidence of dehydration. *Decreased oral fluid intake may lead to dehydration and thick, viscous secretions that are more difficult to expectorate.*

- Assess patency of both nares before inserting a nasogastric tube or feeding tube. If airflow is obstructed through one side, insert the tube through the unobstructed nare. Carefully monitor respiratory status following tube insertion. *The nasogastric tube is inserted through the unobstructed nare to avoid mucosal trauma; however, a large gastric tube may interfere with nasal breathing, necessitating close monitoring.*

#### Risk for Infection

The client with a nasal fracture is at increased risk for infection. The nasal mucosa is a natural barrier to infection, and trauma increases the risk for invasion by pathogens. Septal hematoma can lead to abscess formation and staphylococcal infection. A CSF leak indicates disruption of the dura, increasing the risk of ascending infection and meningitis.

**PRACTICE ALERT**  *Test watery, clear fluid dripping from the ear or nose for glucose. CSF will test positive for glucose on a Dextrostrip.* ■

- Avoid suctioning if possible. *Suctioning catheters could introduce microorganisms and cause additional trauma to tissues.*
- Monitor vital signs every 4 hours. *A rise in temperature may indicate infection.*
- Administer antibiotics as ordered. *Antibiotics may be prescribed to prevent abscess formation, and, if CSF leakage is present, to prevent meningitis.*

### Home Care

Provide the following teaching when preparing the client with a nasal fracture for home care.

- Elevate the head of the bed with blocks and apply ice or cold packs to the nose for 20 minutes four times a day to reduce swelling.
- Swelling usually subsides in several days; bruising may persist for several weeks.
- It is difficult to determine the final cosmetic outcome until swelling has subsided.
- If indicated by delayed fracture reduction or malformation, discuss rhinoplasty and its potential benefits.

  If CSF leakage is present, also include the following instructions.

- Rest in bed with the head of the bed elevated to 30 to 45 degrees.
- Restrict fluid intake as ordered and take the prescribed diuretic to reduce intracranial pressure and CSF leakage.
- Distribute allowed fluids throughout the day.
- List name, purpose, effects, and precautions for any prescribed medication.
- Avoid straining, blowing the nose, sneezing, or vigorous coughing until allowed by the physician.
- Immediately report manifestations of infection, including stiff neck, headache, and fever to the physician.

Following rhinoplasty or septoplasty, provide the following instructions.

- Apply ice packs to the nose to relieve discomfort and reduce swelling.
- Elevate the head of the bed on blocks to decrease local edema.

- Do not blow the nose for 48 hours after the packing is removed to prevent bleeding.
- Vigorous coughing or straining at stool may cause bleeding and should be avoided.
- Clean teeth and mouth frequently and increase fluid intake to decrease oral dryness due to mouth breathing.
- Bruising around the eyes and nose will last for several days.

---

## Nursing Care Plan
### A Client with Nasal Trauma

Clifton Kavanaugh is a 36-year-old mailman who broke his nose when he was hit in the face by a baseball. He is admitted to the emergency department accompanied by a friend.

#### ASSESSMENT

Mr. Kavanaugh presents with obvious deformity of the nose. It is swollen, bloody, and deviated to one side. The nose is bleeding slightly. Mr. Kavanaugh rates the pain as a 6 on a scale of 1 to 10. Vital signs are BP 132/70, P 120 and regular, R 22, T 98.6°F (37°C) axillary.

Mr. Kavanaugh is breathing through his mouth and holding an ice compress to his nose. Boney crepitus and edema are felt on palpation. There is no evidence of CSF leak from either nose or ears. X-ray confirms a nasal fracture.

#### DIAGNOSES

- *Acute pain* related to nasal fracture
- *Ineffective breathing pattern* related to nasal swelling and bleeding
- *Anxiety* related to pain and need for emergency care
- *Disturbed body image* related to nasal deformity

#### EXPECTED OUTCOMES

- Verbalize relief of pain.
- Maintain a patent airway and normalize his breathing pattern.
- Demonstrate reduced anxiety.
- Express concerns about potential body image change.

#### PLANNING AND IMPLEMENTATION

- Administer analgesics as ordered.
- Apply ice compress to nose.
- Inspect oropharynx for evidence of bleeding.
- Encourage deep, slow breathing through the mouth.
- Provide oral hygiene.
- Discuss concerns regarding injury.
- Assist with nasal splint application.

#### EVALUATION

Following treatment, Mr. Kavanaugh reports his pain has decreased to a level of 2 on a scale of 1 to 10. He appears more relaxed, no longer grimacing and with a relaxed posture. His respirations are easy at 18. The nasal splint is intact. Mr. Kavanaugh is able to look in a mirror and state with a laugh, "I look like a raccoon." He is admitted to the hospital for rhinoplasty.

#### Critical Thinking in the Nursing Process

1. A client in the emergency department with nasal trauma becomes extremely panicky because of blood draining down his throat. How would you intervene to reduce this client's anxiety without using nasal suction? Why is it important to avoid suctioning the nasopharynx in the client with nasal trauma?
2. Develop a plan of care for the client with a leak of CSF from a nasal fracture.
3. Compare immediate versus delayed rhinoplasty for the client with nasal fracture.

See Evaluating Your Response in Appendix C.

---

## THE CLIENT WITH LARYNGEAL OBSTRUCTION OR TRAUMA

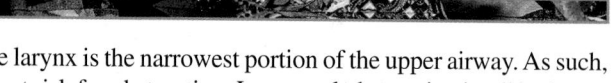

The larynx is the narrowest portion of the upper airway. As such, it is at risk for obstruction. Laryngeal obstruction is a life-threatening emergency. Blows to the neck or other traumatic injuries may damage the larynx, interfering with its patency and function.

## PATHOPHYSIOLOGY AND MANIFESTATIONS
### Laryngeal Obstruction

The larynx may be partially or fully obstructed by aspirated food or foreign objects, or by laryngospasm or edema due to inflammation, injury, or anaphylaxis. Anything that occludes the larynx can obstruct the airway. The most common cause of obstruction in adults is ingested meat that lodges in the airway (the so-called *café coronary*). Risk factors for food aspiration include ingesting large boluses of food and chewing them insufficiently, consuming excess alcohol, and wearing dentures. A foreign body in the larynx causes pain, laryngospasm, dyspnea, and inspiratory stridor. Aspirated foreign bodies may pass through the larynx into the trachea and lungs, causing pneumonitis.

Laryngospasm occurs due to repeated or traumatic intubation attempts, chemical irritation, or hypocalcemia. An acute type I hypersensitivity response may cause anaphylaxis with release of inflammatory mediators leading to angioedema of upper airways and severe laryngeal edema.

The most common manifestations of laryngeal obstruction are coughing, choking, gagging, obvious difficulty breathing with use of accessory muscles, and inspiratory stridor. As the airway is obstructed, signs of asphyxia become apparent. Respirations are labored and noisy with wheezing and stridor. Cyanosis may develop. Respiratory arrest and death may result without prompt treatment.

## Laryngeal Trauma

Trauma to the larynx can occur in motor vehicle crashes or assaults (e.g., blows to the neck or attempted strangulation). The larynx also may be traumatized during endotracheal intubation or tracheotomy. Trauma may fracture thyroid and/or cricoid cartilage, resulting in loss of airway patency. Soft-tissue injuries can cause swelling that further impairs the airway. Manifestations of laryngeal trauma may include subcutaneous emphysema or crepitus, voice change, dysphagia and pain with swallowing, inspiratory stridor, hemoptysis, and cough.

## COLLABORATIVE CARE

The treatment goal is to maintain an open airway. If airway obstruction is partial and the client is able to cough and move air in and out of the lungs, radiologic and laryngoscopic examination may be done to locate the foreign body. An endotracheal tube may be inserted to maintain airflow through the larynx in spasm or an edematous larynx. For anaphylaxis, epinephrine may be administered to reduce laryngeal edema and relieve obstruction.

When airway obstruction is complete, the Heimlich maneuver is performed immediately to clear the obstruction. For the conscious person, the rescuer wraps his or her arms around the victim from behind, places one fist between the umbilicus and xiphoid process, covers the fist with the other hand and forcefully thrusts the hands upward (Figure 35–3A■). For the unconscious victim, the rescuer straddles the victim's thighs and delivers thrusts upward and inward on the upper abdomen

(Figure 35–3B). These moves are continued until the obstruction is relieved or more definitive care can be given. Endotracheal intubation may be attempted. If intubation is unsuccessful, an immediate cricothyrotomy or tracheotomy must be performed to open the airway.

CT scan is used to identify laryngeal fractures; however, emergency treatment may be required prior to diagnosis to ensure airway patency and preserve life. Soft-tissue injuries may be managed conservatively with bedside humidifier, intravenous fluids, antibiotics, and corticosteroids to reduce edema. More severe injuries require endotracheal intubation or immediate tracheostomy.

## NURSING CARE

**PRACTICE ALERT**   *The priority of nursing care in laryngeal obstruction or trauma is restoring a patent airway to prevent cerebral anoxia and death. Laryngeal obstruction and trauma are medical emergencies requiring immediate intervention.* ■

Closely monitor clients at risk for laryngeal obstruction (e.g., following neck trauma, newly extubated clients, and people receiving medications with a high risk of anaphylaxis, such as intravenous antibiotics or radiologic dyes) for manifestations of obstruction, including dyspnea, nasal flaring, tachypnea, anxiety, wheezing, and stridor. Suction the airway as needed; small aspirated foreign bodies might possibly be removed by suctioning. If obstruction is complete, initiate a cardiopulmonary arrest procedure and perform the Heimlich maneuver until the obstruction is relieved or the emergency response team arrives. Prepare to assist with emergency intubation or tracheotomy as needed. Provide emotional support, reassurance, and teaching for the client and family to reduce anxiety.

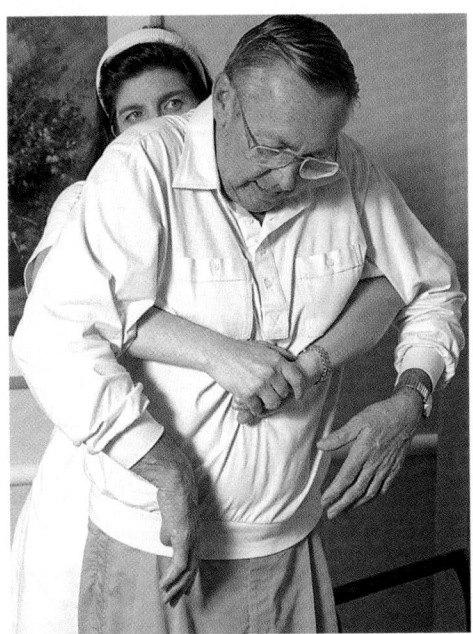
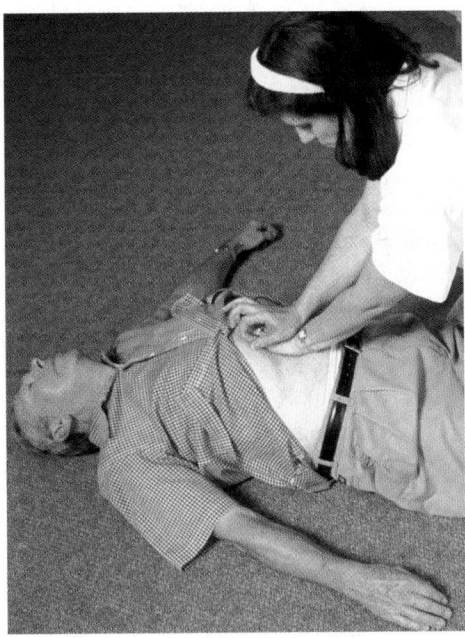

**Figure 35–3** ■ Administering abdominal thrusts (the Heimlich maneuver) to *A*, a conscious victim, and *B*, an unconscious victim.

**A**          **B**

Health promotion and teaching for home care focus on preventing laryngeal obstruction and early intervention techniques. Everyone should be aware of the risk factors for adult aspiration. Caution clients who wear dentures to take small bites, chewing each bite carefully before swallowing. Discuss the relationship between excess alcohol intake and food aspiration. Participate in promoting training of the general public in CPR and the Heimlich maneuver. The more people who are adequately trained in emergency procedures, the more likely it is that emergency procedures will be initiated in a timely manner. Clients with a known risk for anaphylaxis, such as people with a previous anaphylactic response and those allergic to bee venom, should wear a MedicAlert tag and carry a bee-sting kit to allow early intervention to prevent severe laryngeal edema and spasm.

# THE CLIENT WITH OBSTRUCTIVE SLEEP APNEA

**Sleep apnea,** intermittent absence of airflow through the mouth and nose during sleep, is a serious and potentially life-threatening disorder. It affects at least 2% of middle-aged women and 4% of middle-aged men. Sleep apnea is a leading cause of excessive daytime sleepiness, and may contribute to other problems such as poor work performance and motor vehicle crashes (Braunwald et al., 2001; McCance & Huether, 2002).

Types of sleep apnea include obstructive and central. In *obstructive sleep apnea,* the more common type, the respiratory drive remains intact, but airflow ceases due to occlusion of the oropharyngeal airway. *Central sleep apnea* is a neurologic disorder that involves transient impairment of the neurologic drive to respiratory muscles.

In addition to male gender, risk factors for obstructive sleep apnea include increasing age and obesity. Large neck circumference (>17 inches in men and >16 inches in women) also is a known risk factor for obstructive sleep apnea (Porth, 2002). Use of alcohol and other central nervous system depressants may contribute to sleep apnea.

## PATHOPHYSIOLOGY

During sleep, skeletal muscle tone decreases (except the diaphragm). The most significant decrease occurs during rapid eye movement (REM) sleep (Porth, 2002). Loss of normal pharyngeal muscle tone permits the pharynx to collapse during inspiration as pressure within the airways becomes negative in relation to atmospheric pressure. The tongue is also pulled against the posterior pharyngeal wall by gravity during sleep, causing further obstruction. Obesity or skeletal or soft-tissue changes that decrease inspiratory tone, such as a relatively large tongue in a relatively small oropharynx, contribute to the problem. Airflow obstruction causes the oxygen saturation, $Po_2$, and pH to fall, and the $Pco_2$ to rise. This progressive asphyxia causes brief arousal from sleep, which restores airway patency and airflow. Sleep can be severely fragmented as these episodes may occur hundreds of times each night.

> ## Manifestations of Obstructive Sleep Apnea
>
> - Loud, cyclic snoring
> - Periods of apnea lasting 15 to 120 seconds during sleep
> - Gasping or choking during sleep
> - Restlessness, thrashing during sleep
> - Daytime fatigue and sleepiness
> - Morning headache
> - Personality changes, depression
> - Intellectual impairment
> - Impotence
> - Hypertension

Recurrent episodes of apnea and arousal during sleep have secondary physiologic effects. Sleep fragmentation and loss of slow-wave sleep are thought to contribute to neurologic and behavior problems such as excessive daytime sleepiness, impaired intellect, memory loss, and personality changes. Recurrent nocturnal asphyxia and negative intrathoracic pressure due to airway obstruction increase the workload of the heart. People with coronary heart disease may develop myocardial ischemia and angina. Dysrhythmias such as significant bradycardia and dangerous tachydysrhythmias may develop. Left ventricular function may be impaired and heart failure may occur. Systemic blood pressure remains high during sleep and may contribute to systemic hypertension that affects more than 50% of people with obstructive sleep apnea (Braunwald et al., 2001). Pulmonary hypertension also may develop. Sudden cardiac death is believed to be a potential fatal complication of obstructive sleep apnea.

## MANIFESTATIONS

Narrowed upper airways produce loud snoring during sleep, often years before obstructive sleep apnea occurs. Excessive daytime sleepiness, headache, irritability, and restless sleep also are common manifestations. See the box above.

## COLLABORATIVE CARE

The goal of care for obstructive sleep apnea is to restore airflow and prevent the adverse effects of the disorder. Sustained weight loss may cure obstructive sleep apnea.

### Diagnostic Tests

The diagnosis of obstructive sleep apnea is based on *polysomnography,* an overnight sleep study. Several variables are recorded during the study, including:

- Electroencephalogram and measurements of ocular activity and muscle tone
- Recordings of ventilatory activity and airflow
- Continuous arterial oxygen saturation readings
- Heart rate

Transcutaneous arterial $Pco_2$ readings also may be monitored during the study. Because sleep studies are time consuming and expensive, overnight monitoring of oxygen saturation by pulse

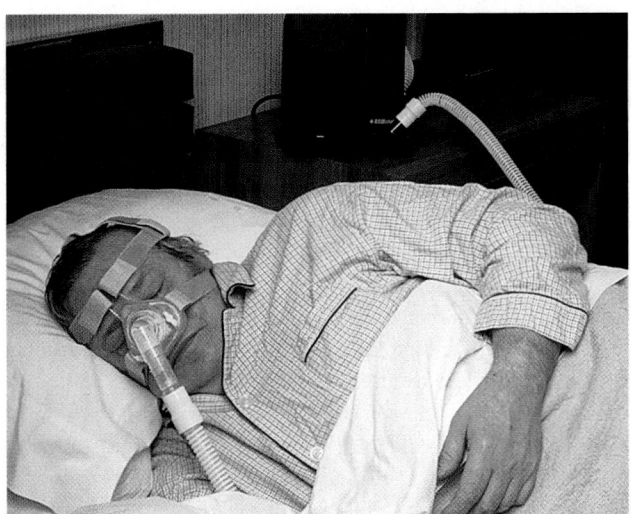

**Figure 35–4** ■ A client using a nasal mask and CPAP to treat sleep apnea.

*Courtesy of Respironics, Inc.*

oximetry may be used to confirm the diagnosis of sleep apnea when symptoms indicate a high probability of the disorder (Braunwald et al., 2001).

## Treatments

Mild to moderate obstructive sleep apnea may be treated by weight reduction, alcohol abstinence, improving nasal patency, and avoiding the supine position for sleep. Although weight reduction often cures the disorder, maintaining optimal weight is difficult. Oral appliances designed to keep the mandible and tongue forward also may be prescribed.

Nasal continuous positive airway pressure (CPAP) is the treatment of choice for obstructive sleep apnea. Positive pressure generated by an air compressor and administered through a tight-fitting nasal mask (Figure 35–4 ■) splints the pharyngeal airway, preventing collapse and obstruction. With proper training, this device is well tolerated by the client. Nasal airways can become dry and irritated with CPAP, so in-line humidifier or a room humidifier is recommended. A newer device, the BiPaP ventilator, delivers higher pressures during inhalation and lower pressures during expiration, providing less resistance to exhaling.

## Surgery

Tonsillectomy and adenoidectomy may relieve upper airway obstruction in some clients. Excision of obstructive tissue from the soft palate, uvula, and posterior lateral pharyngeal wall may be accomplished by *uvulopalatopharyngoplasty* (*UPPP*). Although only about 50% of these surgeries are successful in treating sleep apnea, UPPP is useful in selected cases. In severe cases, tracheostomy may also be performed to bypass the area of obstruction.

## NURSING CARE

Obstructive sleep apnea usually is treated in the home. Nursing care focuses on teaching the client and family about equipment use and strategies to decrease contributing factors such as obesity and alcohol intake. The following nursing diagnoses are appropriate for clients with sleep apnea.

- *Disturbed sleep pattern* related to repeated apneic episodes
- *Fatigue* related to interrupted sleep patterns
- *Ineffective breathing pattern* related to obstruction of upper airway during sleep
- *Impaired gas exchange* related to altered lung ventilation during obstructive episodes
- *Risk for injury* related to daytime somnolence and altered judgment
- *Risk for sexual dysfunction* related to impotence resulting from sleep apnea

## Home Care

Effective sleep apnea management depends on the client's willingness to participate in care. Provide teaching about the following topics.

- Relationship between obesity and sleep apnea
- Plans, resources, and referrals as needed for weight loss (e.g., programs such as Weight Watchers to provide additional support)
- Relationship of alcohol and sedatives to sleep apnea; referral to an alcohol treatment program or Alcoholics Anonymous as indicated
- How to use CPAP if ordered
- The importance of using CPAP continuously at night
- Measures to reduce airway dryness, including supplemental humidity and an adequate fluid intake to maintain moist mucous membranes

If a support group for people with sleep apnea syndrome is available in the local area, refer the client and family to the group.

# UPPER RESPIRATORY TUMORS

Although tumors of the upper respiratory tract are relatively uncommon, they have the potential to impair the upper airways and interfere with breathing and ventilation of the lungs. Of the upper respiratory tract structures, the larynx is affected by abnormal growths most often.

## THE CLIENT WITH NASAL POLYPS

*Nasal polyps* are benign grapelike growths of the mucous membrane lining the nose. These benign tumors can interfere with air movement through nasal passages or obstruct sinus openings, leading to sinusitis. They usually affect people who have chronic allergic rhinitis or asthma.

## PATHOPHYSIOLOGY AND MANIFESTATIONS

Chronic irritation and swelling of the mucous membranes from allergic rhinitis may cause slow polyp formation. Polyps form in areas of dependent mucous membrane, presenting as pale, edematous masses covered with mucous membrane. They are usually bilateral and have a stemlike base, making them fairly moveable. Polyps can continue to enlarge, eventually becoming larger than a grape. Polyps may be asymptomatic, although large polyps may cause nasal obstruction, rhinorrhea, and loss of sense of smell. Manifestations of sinusitis may develop. The voice may have a nasal tone. Asthmatics who have nasal polyps may have an associated aspirin allergy of which they are not aware.

## COLLABORATIVE CARE

When polyps occur in conjunction with an acute upper respiratory infection, they may regress spontaneously with resolution of the infection. When symptomatic, polyps may be managed with topical corticosteroid nasal sprays or low-dose oral corticosteroids to shrink the edematous polyps and manage allergic symptoms. However, polyps continue to enlarge when corticosteroid therapy is discontinued.

Surgery may be required to restore normal breathing. Surgical removal of polyps (*polypectomy*) often is done in the physician's office under local anesthesia. A wire snare is used to clip the polyps from their stemlike base. Nasal packing is inserted to control bleeding after removal. Alternatively, laser surgery may be used to remove polyps. Healing is more rapid following laser intervention, and the risk of bleeding is reduced. Because polyps tend to recur, repeated surgeries may be necessary.

## NURSING CARE

Teaching about home care following polypectomy is the primary nursing responsibility for the client with nasal polyps. Provide postoperative care instructions, and discuss measures to reduce the risk of bleeding.

a. Apply ice or cold compresses to the nose to decrease swelling, promote comfort, and prevent bleeding.
b. Avoid blowing the nose for 24 to 48 hours after nasal packing is removed.
c. Avoid straining at stool, vigorous coughing, and strenuous exercise.

Discuss manifestations of possible bleeding, such as frequent swallowing or visible blood at the back of the throat. Swallowed blood may cause nausea and vomiting. Encourage the client to rest for 2 to 3 days after surgery to reduce the risk of bleeding. Instruct to increase fluid intake and clean mouth frequently to reduce oral dryness associated with mouth breathing while nasal packing is in place.

## THE CLIENT WITH A LARYNGEAL TUMOR

Laryngeal tumors may be either benign or malignant. Benign tumors of the larynx include papillomas, nodules, and polyps. People who chronically shout, project, or vocalize in an abnormally high or low tone, abusing the voice, are at risk for developing benign laryngeal tumors. In adults, vocal cord nodules are often referred to as "singer's nodules"; cheerleaders and public speakers may also develop them. Voice abuse also contributes to the development of vocal cord polyps, as does cigarette smoking and chronic irritation from industrial pollutants.

Malignancy, or cancer of the larynx is uncommon and is often curable if detected early. However, an estimated 3700 people died from laryngeal cancer in 2002; and 8900 new cases were diagnosed (ACS, 2002a). Men are affected more than 3 times as often as women. Cancer of the larynx usually develops between age 50 and 70. Cigarette smoking is the major risk factor for laryngeal cancer: The risk of developing laryngeal cancer is 5 to 35 times greater in smokers than in nonsmokers. Alcohol consumption is a significant cofactor in increasing the risk. When combined with smoking, the risk increases significantly, perhaps as much as 100 times (ACS, 2002b). Other risk factors include poor nutrition, human papillomavirus infection, exposure to asbestos and other occupational pollutants, and race (laryngeal cancer is more common in African Americans than among whites).

## PATHOPHYSIOLOGY AND MANIFESTATIONS
### Benign Tumors

Papillomas are small, wartlike growths believed to be viral in origin. Polyps and nodules may develop on the vocal cords of the larynx as a result of voice abuse. Nodules occur as paired lesions on the free edges of the vocal cords. Hoarseness and a breathy voice quality are manifestations of benign vocal cord tumors.

### Laryngeal Cancer

Squamous cell carcinoma is the most common malignancy of the larynx. Changes in the laryngeal mucosa occur over time as it is subjected to noxious irritants such as cigarette smoke. White, patchy, precancerous lesions known as *leukoplakia* appear. Red, velvety patches, called *erythroplakia,* are thought to represent a later stage of carcinoma development. The initial cancerous lesion, carcinoma in situ (CIS), is superficial. Malignant cells replace the lining layer, but do not invade into deeper tissues. Untreated, about 30% of CIS lesions develop into squamous cell cancer (ACS, 2002b). Laryngeal cancer spreads by both direct invasion of surrounding tissues and metastasis. It may metastasize to the lungs; however, metastases of other cancers to the larynx are rare.

Laryngeal cancer may develop in any of the three areas of the larynx—the glottis, the supraglottis, and the subglottis. Manifestations vary according to site of the lesion.

Lesions of the true vocal cords or glottis account for nearly 65% of all laryngeal cancers (Figure 35–5 ■). Fortunately, these cancers tend to be well differentiated and slow growing. Metastasis occurs late in the course of the disease because of a

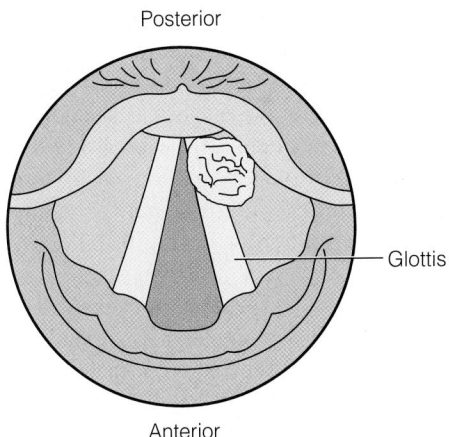

**Figure 35–5** ■ Cancer of the larynx. Most lesions form along the edges of the glottis.

limited lymphatic supply. The usual symptom of glottic cancer is hoarseness, or a change in the voice because the tumor prevents complete closure of the vocal cords during speech.

Approximately 35% of laryngeal cancers develop in the supraglottic area, which includes the epiglottis, aryepiglottic folds, arytenoid muscles and cartilage, and false vocal cords. Lymphatic supply to this region of the larynx is rich; tumors often invade locally and metastasize early. Symptoms often do not develop until the tumor is relatively large, delaying diagnosis. Manifestations of supraglottic cancer include painful swallowing, sore throat, or a feeling of a lump in the throat. Later manifestations include dyspnea, foul breath, and pain that radiates to the ear.

Subglottic tumors (below the vocal cords) are the least common. They often are asymptomatic until the enlarging tumor obstructs the airway.

Common manifestations of laryngeal cancer are listed in the box on this page.

## COLLABORATIVE CARE

Benign laryngeal tumors may resolve with correction of the underlying problem, such as voice training with a speech thera-

---

### Manifestations of Laryngeal Cancer

- Hoarseness
- Change in the voice
- Painful swallowing
- Dyspnea
- Foul breath
- Palpable lump in neck
- Earache

---

pist or smoking cessation. Treatment of laryngeal malignancy varies with the extent of the cancer. Early diagnosis and treatment are important: 80% to 95% of early stage tumors can be cured, whereas 50% to 80% of people with advanced laryngeal cancer die of the disease.

### Diagnostic Tests

- *Direct* or *indirect laryngoscopy* is used for initial evaluation when laryngeal cancer is suspected. A fiberoptic laryngoscope is used for direct laryngoscopy; mirrors are used to visualize the larynx in indirect laryngoscopy.
- *Biopsy* is obtained from suspicious lesions to examine the cells. Biopsy is usually obtained under general anesthesia. Tissue may be obtained via endoscopy or by fine needle aspiration of the mass.
- *Imaging studies* such as CT scan, MRI, and chest X-ray are obtained to evaluate the size of the mass, possible extension into deeper tissues, involvement of lymph nodes, and possible metastasis to the lungs. A barium swallow may be done to evaluate the effects of the tumor on swallowing.

### Treatments

An inhaled steroid spray may be used for vocal cord polyps. In some cases, surgical excision of benign nodules or polyps is required. This usually is performed via laryngoscopy, using microforceps or a laser. A biopsy of the tumor is done to rule out malignancy.

Laryngeal cancer treatment is determined by *staging* the cancer. Information such as tumor size and location (T), number of involved lymph nodes (N), and presence or absence of metastases (M) is combined to assign a stage, designated by Roman numerals I to IV. Table 35–1 outlines laryngeal cancer stages.

---

| TABLE 35–1 | Staging of Laryngeal Tumors |
|---|---|
| Stage 0 | • Carcinoma in situ<br>• No lymph node involvement or metastasis |
| Stage I | • Tumor confined to site of origin with normal vocal cord mobility<br>• No lymph node involvement or metastasis |
| Stage II | • Tumor involves adjacent tissues<br>• No lymph node involvement or metastasis |
| Stage III | • Tumor confined to larynx with fixation of vocal cords; immediately surrounding supraglottic tissues may be involved<br>• No lymph node involvement or a single positive node on the side of the tumor<br>• No metastasis |
| Stage IV | • Massive tumor that extends beyond boundaries of larynx to involve surrounding tissues<br>• Single or multiple lymph nodes may be involved<br>• Distant metastasis may be present |

## Radiation Therapy

Radiation therapy is often the treatment of choice for early laryngeal cancer. Radiation disrupts the DNA of the cell, causing it to die. External radiation may be used, or implants of iridium seeds can be placed into hollow plastic needles that are inserted directly into or near the tumor site during surgery to deliver radiation. Radiation therapy is extremely effective for treating glottic cancer, with cure rates equal to those achieved by surgery. Radiation therapy preserves the voice, although the tone or timber of the voice may be affected.

Radiation therapy may be used in combination with chemotherapy to treat more advanced laryngeal cancers. Nearly two-thirds of clients with locally invasive cancers can avoid total laryngectomy when treated with combination radiation and chemotherapy. Survival rates are equal to those achieved with total laryngectomy (Way & Doherty, 2003).

Radiation therapy also may be used in conjunction with surgery to destroy any remaining cancerous cells, or as a palliative treatment for advanced tumors. See Chapter 10 for more information about radiation therapy and its nursing implications.

## Chemotherapy

Chemotherapy is used in combination with radiation therapy as the primary treatment for some laryngeal cancers. It also is used to treat distant metastasis and for palliation when the tumor is unresectable. The most commonly used chemotherapy drugs to treat laryngeal cancer are cisplatin (Platinol) and 5-fluorouracil (5-FU). Other drugs that may be used include methotrexate (Mexate), bleomycin sulfate (Blenoxane), and carboplatin (Paraplatin). A multiple-drug treatment regimen may be employed to maximize therapeutic effects. See Chapter 10 for the nursing implications for chemotherapy.

## Surgery

The type of surgery used to treat laryngeal cancer is based on site, size, and invasiveness of the tumor into the larynx. The goals of surgery are to remove the malignancy, maintain airway patency, and achieve optimal cosmetic appearance.

Carcinoma in situ, vocal cord polyps, and early vocal cord cancers may be removed by laser during a laryngoscopy procedure. The cure rate for early tumors using this method is excellent. This surgery may be performed on an outpatient basis. The degree of trauma to the vocal cords varies, depending on the size of the lesion. The voice is preserved, but total voice rest with whispering only may be ordered for a week or more following surgery. In some cases, a temporary tracheostomy may be done at the time of surgery to ensure that swelling does not interfere with airway patency. Once the tracheostomy tube is removed and the opening is closed, the client can eat, speak, and breathe normally.

**Laryngectomy,** removal of the larynx, may be necessary. A *partial laryngectomy* (hemilaryngectomy, vertical partial laryngectomy) may be used for tumors localized to a portion of the larynx with limited extension beyond the larynx. In a partial laryngectomy, 50% or more of the larynx is removed. The voice generally is well preserved, although it may be

changed by the surgery. A tracheostomy tube may be inserted for early postoperative airway management. It is usually removed in 5 to 7 days as postoperative swelling subsides, and the stoma is allowed to close. Normal speaking, breathing, and swallowing are restored. If the epiglottis has been removed, careful monitoring for aspiration is necessary. Enteral tube feedings or parenteral nutrition may be required for several weeks after surgery. Swallowing techniques to prevent aspiration are taught.

A *total laryngectomy* is required for cancers that extend beyond the vocal cords. The entire larynx is removed, along with the epiglottis, thyroid cartilage, several tracheal rings, and the hyoid bone. Because the trachea and the esophagus are permanently separated by this surgery (Figure 35–6 ■), there is no risk of aspiration during swallowing. Normal speech is lost, and a permanent tracheostomy is created in a total laryngectomy. The tracheostomy tube inserted during surgery may be left in place for several weeks and then removed, leaving a natural stoma, or it may be left in place permanently. See page 1067 for nursing care of the client undergoing a total laryngectomy. Procedure 35–1 on page 1068 outlines tracheostomy care.

If cervical lymph nodes are involved but there is no evidence of distal metastasis, *radical* or *modified neck dissection* may be performed along with total laryngectomy. In a radical neck dissection, all soft tissue from the lower edge of the mandible down

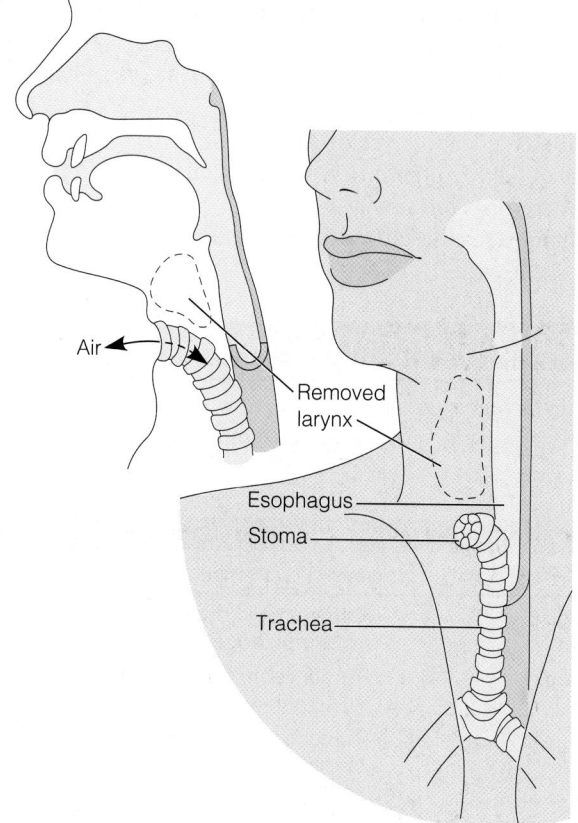

**Figure 35–6 ■** Following a total laryngectomy, the client has a permanent tracheostomy. No connection between the trachea and esophagus remains.

---

# NURSING CARE OF THE CLIENT HAVING A TOTAL LARYNGECTOMY

## PREOPERATIVE CARE

- Assess knowledge and understanding of the diagnosis and proposed surgery. Clarify information and reinforce previous teaching as needed. *A clear understanding by the client and family of the purpose, anticipated benefits, and consequences of total laryngectomy prior to surgery is vital to promote postoperative recovery.*
- Provide routine preoperative care and teaching as explained in Chapter 7. 🔗
- Assess anxiety levels of the client and family related to the diagnosis and proposed surgery. *High levels of anxiety interfere with learning and the ability to cooperate in care. Interventions to reduce anxiety may be required prior to teaching and providing preoperative instructions.*
- Without increasing fear, emphasize that total laryngectomy results in a loss of speech and that the client will breathe through a permanent stoma in the neck. *Although clients and family members may verbalize an understanding of the loss of speech following surgery, they may believe that verbal communication will still be possible through the stoma.*
- Establish a means of communicating postoperatively, using a magic slate, alphabet board, eye or hand signals, or other strategies. *Learning techniques for communicating preoperatively decreases the client's and family's postoperative anxiety. Long-term speech rehabilitation measures, such as the tracheoesophageal puncture are not appropriate for use in the immediate postoperative period.*
- Point out that surgery will affect the sense of taste and smell, and eating in the initial postoperative period. Reassure that nutritional and fluid needs will be met with intravenous or enteral feedings until eating can be resumed. *The client may not be prepared for the effect of surgery on taste and smell, and therefore the enjoyment of food.*
- If possible and desired by the client and family, arrange a visit by a postlaryngectomy client who effectively uses an alternate form of verbal communication. *The client and family may feel more comfortable expressing their fears and asking questions of someone who has gone through the same experience they are facing.*

## POSTOPERATIVE CARE

- Provide routine postoperative nursing care and monitoring as explained in Chapter 7.

- Frequently monitor airway patency and respiratory status, including respiratory rate and pattern; lung sounds; oxygen saturation. *Excessive or retained respiratory secretions can impair gas exchange, increase the work of breathing, and lead to complications such as pneumonia.*
- Encourage deep breathing and coughing. *Deep breathing helps ensure adequate ventilation of lower airways; coughing helps to move secretions out of airways.*
- Elevate the head of the bed. *The upright position promotes effective ventilation of the lungs, and reduces edema and swelling of the neck.*
- Maintain humidification of inspired gases. *With a tracheostomy, humidification of inspired air in the upper airways is lost. Humidified air helps maintain moist mucous membranes and secretions, promoting secretion removal by coughing or suctioning.*
- Maintain an adequate fluid intake (intravenously, enteral, and oral when allowed). *Adequate hydration keeps secretions liquid and mucous membranes moist.*
- Suction via tracheostomy using sterile technique as needed. *Surgery, impaired nutrition, and the effects of radiation therapy may cause fatigue and a weak cough effort. Suctioning may be necessary to clear secretions and maintain airway patency.*
- Provide tracheostomy care as needed. See Procedure 35–1. *Periodic cleaning of the tracheostomy tube is necessary to remove accumulated secretions and maintain airway patency.*
- Teach to protect the stoma from particulate matter in the air with a gauze square or other stoma protector. *Permanent tracheostomy results in loss of the protective mechanisms of the upper airway that prevent foreign material from entering the lungs.*
- Instruct to support the head when moving in bed. *Additional head support reduces the strain on tissues in the operative area.*
- Place the call light within easy reach at all times; answer the call light promptly. *The client who is unable to speak needs reassurance that help is within reach at all times.*
- Encourage family members to remain present when possible. *Supportive family presence helps reassure the client that he or she will not be left alone or helpless.*
- Spend as much time as possible with the client. When leaving the room, specify the time when you will return. *These measures help establish trust and relieve anxiety.*

---

to the clavicle is removed, including cervical lymph nodes, the sternocleidomastoid muscle, internal jugular vein, cranial nerve XI (spinal accessory), and submaxillary salivary gland. Extensive tissue dissection can result in significant deformity. Skin grafts or flaps may be used to close the wound. Hemovac drains are placed in the wound to prevent hematoma and extensive edema formation. After surgery, the client may have difficulty lifting and turning the head because of muscle loss. Resection of the spinal accessory nerve causes shoulder drop on the affected side. In a modified neck dissection, neck contents are removed, with the exception of the sternocleidomastoid muscle, internal jugular vein, and spinal accessory nerve.

## Speech Rehabilitation

Various techniques may be used to restore speech after total laryngectomy. *Tracheoesophageal puncture (TEP)* is the usual method used to restore speech. A small fistula is created between the posterior tracheal wall and the anterior esophagus. A small, one-way shunt valve is fitted into the fistula (Figure 35–7 ■). Occluding the tracheostomy stoma with a finger forces exhaled air through the valve into the esophagus and hypopharynx, creating vibration and sound. The muscles of speech are used to form words. The one-way valve prevents aspiration from the esophagus into the trachea. An external tracheostoma valve may be used to avoid using the hand to

## Procedure 35-1

## Providing Tracheostomy Care

### GATHER ALL SUPPLIES

- Tracheostomy cleaning kit
- Sterile suction catheter and glove kit
- Cleaning solutions, e.g., hydrogen peroxide and sterile normal saline
- Sterile 4×4 gauze dressings (not cotton-filled) or precut dressing
- Sterile cotton-tipped applicators
- Cotton twill ties
- Scissors
- Clean exam gloves

### BEFORE THE PROCEDURE

Provide for privacy. Explain the procedure. Provide for a means of communication (e.g., eye blinking or raising a finger to indicate distress). If condition permits, provide a pencil and paper or magic slate for questions. Place in semi-Fowler's or Fowler's position to facilitate lung ventilation. Assess lung sounds; suction the tracheostomy using sterile technique as needed.

### PROCEDURE

- Use standard precautions.
- Wearing a clean disposable glove, remove the tracheostomy dressing. Dispose of the glove and dressing.
- Open sterile supplies, pouring hydrogen peroxide and normal saline into separate containers. Don sterile gloves.
- Using sterile applicators or gauze dressings moistened with normal saline, clean around the incision, using each applicator or gauze dressing only once. Hydrogen peroxide may be used to remove crusted secretions; thoroughly rinse the area with gauze moistened with normal saline afterward to prevent skin irritation from hydrogen peroxide.
- If the tracheostomy tube has an inner cannula that can be removed for cleaning, remove the tube and place it in the hydrogen peroxide. Cleanse the flange of the outer cannula in the same manner as the incision.
- Clean the inner cannula using a small brush, pipe cleaners (provided in the tracheostomy care kit), or cotton-tipped applicators.

- Rinse the inner cannula thoroughly in normal saline. Tap it gently against the inner aspect of the sterile bowl to remove excess liquid.
- Suction the outer cannula using sterile technique.
- Replace the inner cannula into the tracheostomy tube.
- Replace the dressing, using either a commercially prepared tracheostomy dressing or an opened gauze 4×4 refolded into a V shape (see the accompanying figure). Do not cut the dressing or use a cotton-filled dressing to prevent aspiration of foreign material into the respiratory tract.
- Apply clean tracheostomy ties using either the one- or two-strip method.

*One-Strip Method*

a. Cut a length of twill tape 2.5 times the length needed to go around the client's neck from one tube flange to the other.
b. Thread one end of the tape through one flange of the tracheostomy tube. Bring the other end around the back of the client's neck, then thread it through the other flange and back around the back of the neck to meet the first end. Tie the loose ends securely using a square knot and allowing one or two fingers' breadth of slack between the tie and the client's neck.

*Two-Strip Method*

a. Cut a length of twill tape about 1.5 times the distance from flange to flange under the client's neck. Divide this into two unequal pieces (approximately 1/3, 2/3).
b. Make a small slit approximately 2 to 3 cm from one end of each piece. Thread the end of the tape with the slit through the flange, then thread the other end of the tape through the slit to secure it. Repeat with the other portion of tape.
c. Position the longer tape behind the client's neck and tie the free ends of tape securely, using a square knot and allowing a small amount of slack as before.

- Once the clean ties are secured, remove the old ties.
- Pad the knot to reduce skin irritation.

### AFTER THE PROCEDURE

Assess breathing and tolerance of the procedure. Dispose of supplies and used solutions. Wash hands. Chart the procedure and any observations made during the procedure such as amount, color, and consistency of sputum and appearance of the incision.

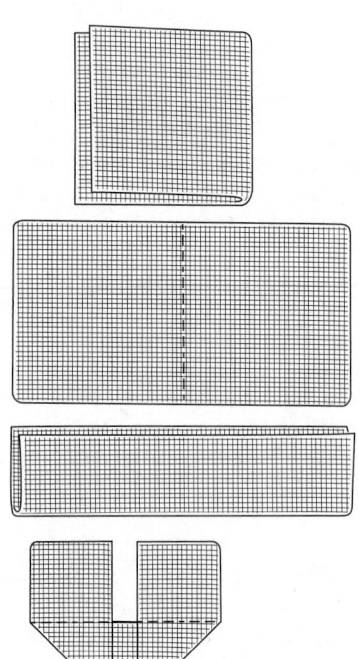

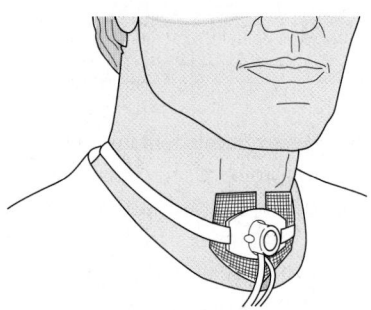

Steps of folding a gauze 4×4 into a tracheostomy dressing

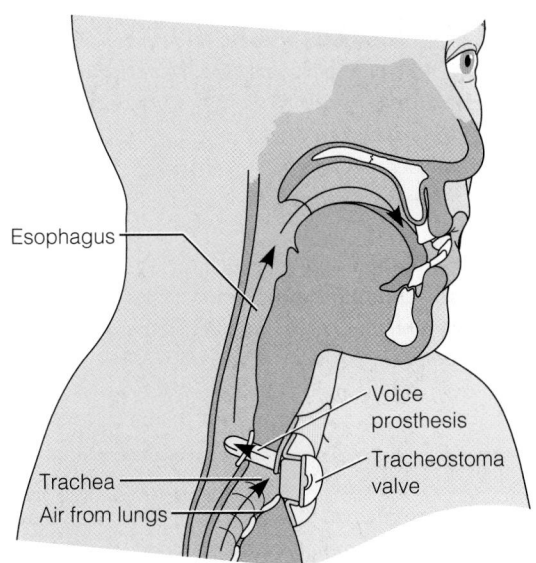

**Figure 35–7** ■ The tracheoesophageal prosthesis (TEP) allows diversion of air from the trachea through a one-way valve into the esophagus and oropharynx, producing speech when the tracheostomy stoma is occluded. The one-way valve prevents food from entering the trachea.

occlude the stoma. This device covers the entire tracheal stoma and closes during exhalation, forcing air directly into the voice prosthesis. Not all postlaryngectomy clients are candidates for this device, because its use requires motivation and manual dexterity.

*Esophageal speech* uses swallowed air to create sound and form words as it is expelled in a controlled belch. The pharyngoesophageal segment vibrates with the belch, creating sound. Muscles of the mouth and tongue are used to control the sound and form words. This form of speech takes practice, and fluent speech may not be restored.

Several speech generators (electrolarynx) are available. One type is held to the neck and creates vibrations that are transmitted to the neck and into the mouth (Figure 35–8A■). The transmitted vibrations are formed into words using the normal muscles of speech. Another device delivers a tone into the mouth via a plastic tube inserted into the corner of the mouth (Figure 35–8B). The lips, tongue, and mouth muscles are used to form the sound into words.

## NURSING CARE

Nurses can be instrumental in early identification and treatment of laryngeal disorders by emphasizing the need for clients with new chronic hoarseness to seek treatment.

## Health Promotion

Health promotion activities to prevent laryngeal cancer focus on preventing smoking among children, adolescents, and young adults, and promoting smoking cessation in people who do smoke. Activities to promote abstinence or moderate alcohol use also are beneficial in reducing a significant risk factor for laryngeal cancer.

## Assessment

Nurses can be instrumental in identifying early signs of laryngeal cancer, facilitating early diagnosis and treatment.

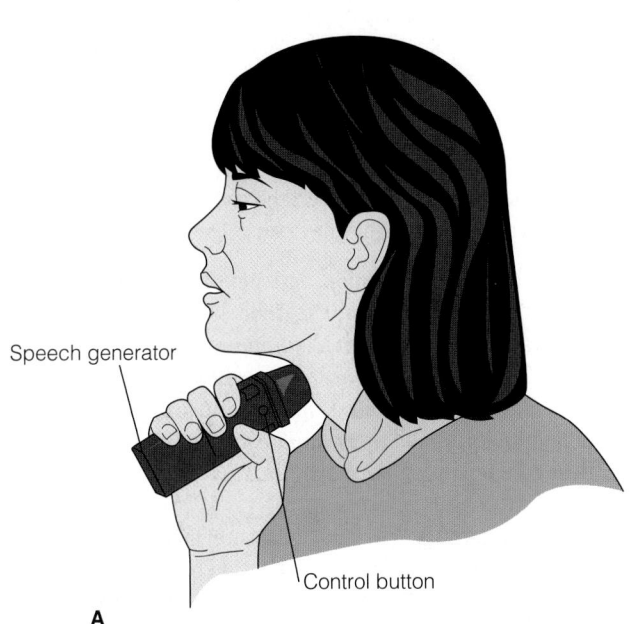

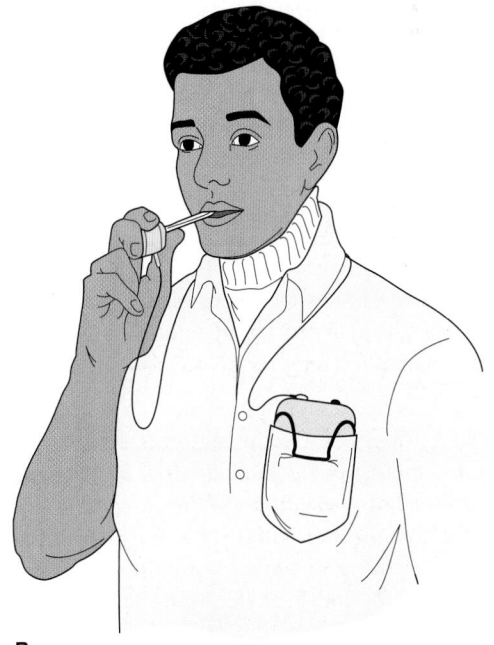

A                                                    B

**Figure 35–8** ■ Speech generators. *A,* The client holds the vibrating tip of the speech generator against the throat, using the mouth to form words. *B,* A plastic handpiece of the generator is held in the corner of the mouth. The audible tone produced by the generator is formed into words.

- Health history: current symptoms, including voice change, difficulty swallowing, throat pain; risk factors such as voice abuse, family history of cancer, occupational exposures; smoking history, use of alcohol and amount.
- Physical examination: voice character; general appearance and apparent state of health; swallowing ability; visible or palpable mass in neck.

## Nursing Diagnoses and Interventions

Nursing care for the client with a benign tumor of the larynx focuses on maintaining a patent airway and teaching about the disorder and strategies to prevent its recurrence. The client with laryngeal cancer has multiple nursing care needs. The risk for impaired verbal communication is significant. Dysphagia may interfere with swallowing and nutrition. Nutrition also may be impaired by radiation, chemotherapy, and surgery. The diagnosis of cancer is frightening for most clients, no matter what the potential for cure is with treatment.

### Risk for Impaired Airway Clearance

Following resection of a benign or malignant vocal cord nodule, local tissue edema may interfere with airway patency.

**PRACTICE ALERT** *During the immediate postoperative period, closely monitor for signs of airway obstruction, such as labored breathing or inspiratory stridor. The larynx is the narrowest portion of the upper airways. Tissue edema following surgery can further restrict the airway, interfering with lung ventilation and gas exchange.* ■

- Apply cold packs to the neck as ordered or indicated. *Cold application constricts local blood vessels and reduces edema development.*
- Withhold food and fluids until the cough and gag reflexes have returned. *Local anesthesia used during removal of benign tumors and nodules impairs the cough and gag reflexes, increasing the risk for aspiration.*

### Impaired Verbal Communication

Treatment of laryngeal cancer often alters the quality of the voice, results in short-term restriction on speaking, or, in the case of total laryngectomy, causes loss of the voice. The client ultimately determines treatment choices for laryngeal cancer; some choose to forgo laryngectomy to avoid voice loss when the chance for long-term success and cancer cure is minimal.

- Prior to surgery, assess for additional obstacles to communication. *Communication may be impaired by hearing loss, illiteracy, or weakness associated with the disease process, altering the ability to use alternative communication strategies.*
- Assess the importance of verbal communication to self-concept, occupation, and lifestyle. *Many factors influence adaptation to the loss of normal verbal communication. If the ability to speak is central to an occupation (e.g., elementary school teacher, singer) or self-concept (e.g., a politician or attorney), adapting to a total laryngectomy may be difficult. For these clients, laryngectomy may mean a loss of employment or career.*

**PRACTICE ALERT** *Prior to surgery, introduce nonverbal communication strategies such as pencil and paper, magic slate, or an alphabet board. Encourage the client to practice using each method and to choose the most acceptable one. Having the client determine a means of communication prior to surgery helps to alleviate anxiety and increases the sense of control.* ■

- Arrange consultation with a speech therapist about alternate forms of oral communication prior to surgery if possible. *Determining a means of communicating on a continuing basis prior to surgery helps to relieve fear of inability to communicate and may guide the choice of a surgical procedure.*

**PRACTICE ALERT** *After surgery, assess frequently. Place the call bell at hand. The presence of a caring nurse helps to decrease anxiety and promotes communication. Knowing that help is readily available enhances feelings of security and decreases anxiety.* ■

- Reinforce teaching about alternative communication strategies. *Anxiety or information overload may impair the ability to retain information; reinforcement facilitates learning.*
- Maintain a positive attitude about postoperative communication, but do not promote unrealistic expectations. *Not all clients are able to use all alternative methods of verbal communication after the laryngectomy. Some clients remain nonverbal.*
- If desired, arrange a visit by a rehabilitated laryngectomy client who has mastered an alternative form of verbal communication and has a positive attitude about rehabilitation. *Many clients and their families find that they are better able to communicate their fears with someone who has gone through the same experience they are facing.*

### Impaired Swallowing

Disruption of laryngeal structures by the tumor itself or due to radiation or surgery can impair the swallowing mechanism. Additionally, even when a total laryngectomy has been performed and a connection between the oropharynx and trachea no longer exists, swallowing may cause fear of choking.

- Maintain intravenous fluids and enteral feedings or parenteral nutrition until adequate food and fluids can be ingested orally. *It is important to maintain nutritional and fluid balance until normal eating can be resumed.*
- Postoperatively, initiate oral intake with soft foods, not liquids. *Soft foods are easier to handle and swallow initially. As recovery progresses, thickened liquids can be swallowed and, eventually, a normal diet.*
- Following total laryngectomy, reassure that choking is not possible, because there is no connection between the esophagus and trachea. *Clients often fear that swallowing will result in choking and they will be unable to cough effectively.*
- Instruct to initiate a swallow by placing a small amount of food on the back of the tongue, flex the head forward, and then think "swallow." *Swallowing is no longer an automatic function and needs to be relearned.*

*Provide for privacy during initial attempts at eating. Eating in the presence of others may cause embarrassment until confidence in eating is regained. Privacy also reduces distractions, allowing concentration on swallowing.* ■

## Imbalanced Nutrition: Less Than Body Requirements

Large laryngeal tumors often place pressure on the esophagus and may cause dysphagia (difficulty swallowing) or odynophagia (painful swallowing). In either case, difficulty eating may ultimately impair nutrition. Additionally, cancer often produces a hypermetabolic state, increasing calorie requirements. If surgery is performed, difficulty swallowing and a fear of aspiration in the early postoperative period also interfere with eating. Enteral or parenteral feedings are usually needed initially to meet nutritional status. After a total laryngectomy, the senses of taste and smell are disrupted. Although the sense of taste may be partially recovered, clients may complain that eating no longer is pleasurable.

- Assess nutritional status using height and weight charts, reported weight loss, and anthropometric measurements such as skinfolds. *Thorough assessment of nutritional status is important in planning to meet current and anticipated calorie needs.*

*Monitor food and fluid intake and urinary output. Pain or fatigue, rather than a sensation of fullness, may prompt the decision to stop eating, resulting in inadequate intake.* ■

- Evaluate current and preferred eating habits and foods, as well as understanding of nutrition. *This evaluation provides additional information about nutrition as well as a basis for future planning.*

*Weigh daily. Daily weight is an accurate measure of both fluid balance and nutritional status.* ■

- Refer to a dietitian for further evaluation, planning, and education. *A professional can identify nutritional needs and help plan a diet that will meet them.*
- Encourage experimentation with foods of different textures and temperatures. *Very cold foods or foods of a soft texture may be easier to swallow.*
- Encourage frequent, small meals rather than three large meals per day. *Frequent, small quantities of food improve overall intake when dysphagia, odynophagia, or fatigue interfere with nutrition.*
- Recommend liquid supplements such as Ensure when calorie needs are not being met. Provide information about where to obtain nutritional supplements. *Liquid dietary supplements provide balanced nutrition as well as additional calories and are an effective way of increasing intake. They are available without prescription in major supermarkets.*

- Provide mouth care before meals and supplemental feedings. Provide a topical anesthetic such as viscous lidocaine before eating for stomatitis or esophagitis related to radiation or chemotherapy. *The tumor or its treatment may cause bad breath or a foul taste in the mouth, which suppresses appetite. Inflamed mucosa may make eating uncomfortable. A topical anesthetic may relieve this discomfort and thus promote food intake.*
- Provide an antiemetic 30 minutes before eating as needed to relieve nausea. *Nausea interferes with food intake. An antiemetic can relieve nausea and make eating possible.*
- Suggest enteral (tube) feedings via nasogastric or gastrostomy tube if the client is unable to consume enough food to maintain weight and nutritional status. *Both cancer and surgery increase calorie needs. Supplemental enteral feedings may be necessary to prevent catabolism and to promote healing and recovery.*

*Following laryngectomy, place in semi-Fowler's or Fowler's position. Elevating the head of the bed facilitates swallowing of oral secretions and helps prevent regurgitation of tube feedings.* ■

- Instruct to perform mouth rinses before initiating feeding postoperatively. *Rinsing helps clean the mouth and also provides practice in using tongue and cheek muscles to control fluid in the mouth.*
- Refer to a physical or speech therapist for swallowing rehabilitation following laryngectomy. *Because surgery changes the relationship of the trachea, esophagus, and oropharynx, swallowing needs to be relearned before eating.*
- Reinforce swallowing instructions. *Reinforcement promotes learning.*

## Anticipatory Grieving

The client with laryngeal cancer faces not only the diagnosis of cancer, which is often perceived as a death sentence, but also the prospect of mutilating surgery. If laryngectomy is necessary, the client grieves the loss of both a body part and an important function, speech, a vital aspect of social interaction and often necessary for one's career. It also enables people to express their needs when they cannot meet them alone. The loss of speech, therefore, is a major loss. In addition, the tracheal stoma changes the manner in which the client breathes. If radical neck dissection is required, loss of neck musculature and function also alters body image and self-concept.

- Provide opportunities for expressing feelings of grief, anger, or fear about the diagnosis of cancer, the impending surgery, and the anticipated loss of speech. *The client with laryngeal cancer needs the opportunity (and may need permission) to grieve anticipated losses. A cancer diagnosis may precipitate grieving for unfulfilled plans and expectations, even though a cure may be anticipated. Laryngectomy causes a major change in body image, with loss of a vital body part and creation of a stoma. The client also grieves the loss of speech. This loss can have a significant impact on occupation and social interaction.*

**PRACTICE ALERT** *Provide a calm, supportive environment with adequate privacy and emotional support for the client and family members as they work through the grieving process. It is important for the client and family to know that their feelings of loss are real and accepted by caregivers.* ■

- Help the client and family discuss the potential impact of the loss on family structure and function. *Discussion helps family members understand each other's feelings and support one another.*
- Refer for psychologic or spiritual counseling as appropriate. *Counseling and spiritual guidance can help the client and family deal with the diagnosis and proposed treatment, and help prevent a sense of defeat and hopelessness.*
- Help identify additional resources, such as coping strategies that have been successfully used in the past to deal with crises. *This exercise helps the client and family identify strengths they can use to deal with the present situation.*

## Using NANDA, NIC, and NOC

Chart 35–2 shows links between NANDA nursing diagnoses, NIC, and NOC for the client with laryngeal cancer.

## Home Care

Teaching for the client with a benign laryngeal tumor emphasizes management of contributing factors. Stress the importance of not yelling or screaming. Refer clients, particularly singers, to a speech therapist for voice training. Emphasize the need to keep the voice within its normal range to reduce vocal cord stress. Encourage smoking cessation, particularly if the client is also a singer. Discuss the relationship of industrial pollutants to laryngeal tumors and help explore ways of reducing pollutant exposure.

Teaching the client and family about laryngeal cancer, treatment options, and home care related to those treatments is an important nursing responsibility. Include the following topics when teaching.

- Clarification of treatment options, including risks and benefits
- Importance of early intervention to reduce the risk of local spread and metastasis
- If a total laryngectomy is proposed, options for communication after surgery, including the pros and cons of each:
  a. The tracheoesophageal puncture device requires some manual dexterity to manipulate.
  b. Only about 30% of clients are able to master esophageal speech.
  c. A trial of the speech generator prior to surgery may reduce frustration in learning to use it postoperatively.
- Care related to radiation therapy, including skin and mouth care, management of secretions (see Chapter 10 ⊂⊃ for more information about radiation therapy and its effects)
- Strategies and resources for smoking cessation and alcohol abstinence
- Ways to achieve and maintain optimal nutrition.
- Tracheostomy stoma care and preventing respiratory infection. Provide opportunities to practice and redemonstrate techniques. Clean technique (rather than sterile) is used; the tracheostomy tube may not be needed once the stoma is fully healed. Discuss these additional measures.
  a. Using a humidifier or vaporizer to add humidity to inspired air.

## CHART 35–2 NANDA, NIC, AND NOC LINKAGES

### The Client with Laryngeal Cancer

| NURSING DIAGNOSES | NURSING INTERVENTIONS | NURSING OUTCOMES |
|---|---|---|
| • Impaired Verbal Communication | • Communication Enhancement: Speech Deficit<br>• Anxiety Reduction<br>• Support System Enhancement | • Communication Ability<br>• Communication: Expressive Ability<br>• Coping |
| • Ineffective Airway Clearance | • Airway Management<br>• Airway Suctioning<br>• Artificial Airway Management | • Respiratory Status: Ventilation<br>• Knowledge: Treatment Regimen |
| • Impaired Swallowing | • Aspiration Precautions<br>• Swallowing Therapy<br>• Enteral Tube Feeding<br>• Positioning | • Aspiration Control<br>• Swallowing Status<br>• Nutritional Status: Food and Fluid Intake |

*Note. Data from* Nursing Outcomes Classification (NOC) *by M. Johnson & M. Maas (Eds.), 1997, St. Louis: Mosby;* Nursing Diagnoses: Definitions & Classification 2001–2002 *by North American Nursing Diagnosis Association, 2001, Philadelphia: NANDA;* Nursing Interventions Classification (NIC) *by J.C. McCloskey & G. M. Bulechek (Eds.), 2000, St. Louis: Mosby. Reprinted by permission.*

b. Increasing fluid intake to maintain mucosal moisture and loosen secretions.

c. Shielding the stoma with a stoma guard, such as a gauze square on a tie around the neck, to prevent particulate matter from entering the lower respiratory tract.

d. Promptly removing secretions from skin surrounding the stoma to prevent irritation and skin breakdown.

e. Water sports are contraindicated with a permanent tracheostomy; there is no restriction on other activities although lifting may be more difficult because of inability to hold the breath (the Valsalva maneuver).

f. Showering and bathing (without submerging the neck or head) are allowed; protect the stoma with a cupped hand or washcloth.

• Manifestations of potential complications of laryngectomy to be reported to the physician, including loss of hearing or facial expression due to auditory or facial nerve injury, or shoulder drop due to damage to the spinal accessory nerve.

The client and family need emotional and motivational support through this trying time. Refer to local support groups such as a laryngectomy club or lost cord club. If the client and family are having difficulty adjusting to the diagnosis of cancer and the effects of treatment, provide referral to counseling.

## Nursing Care Plan
## A Client with Total Laryngectomy

David Tom is a 61-year-old accountant who is divorced and has two adult children. He has smoked two packs of cigarettes daily since high school, and usually has three or four cocktails each evening. After several months of persistent sore throat and hoarseness, Mr. Tom was diagnosed with cancer of the larynx. He has been admitted to the surgical care unit from the ICU 2 days post total laryngectomy.

### ASSESSMENT

Mr. Tom's vital signs are stable: BP 146/84, P 92 and regular, R 18, T 98°F (36.7°C) axillary. A tracheostomy tube is sutured in place, and he is receiving humidified oxygen at 28% per tracheostomy collar. Pulse oximetry is 94%. He is receiving continuous tube feeding per nasogastric feeding tube. Two Hemovac wound drains are present in the right neck area. A moderate amount of edema is noted in the right facial and submandibular area. Mr. Tom is ambulatory within the room.

### DIAGNOSIS

• *Risk for ineffective airway clearance* related to postoperative edema
• *Risk for ineffective breathing pattern* related to pain and anxiety
• *Disturbed body image* related to total laryngectomy and presence of tracheostomy stoma
• *Impaired verbal communication* related to total laryngectomy
• *Pain* related to surgical procedure
• *Risk for imbalanced nutrition: Less than body requirements* related to difficulty eating after surgery

### EXPECTED OUTCOMES

• Maintain clear airways and lung sounds.
• Maintain oxygen saturation level greater than 92%.
• Demonstrate interest in providing incision and stoma care.
• Accept information about potential communication strategies.
• Communicate effective pain management.
• Maintain appropriate body weight, intake, and output.

### PLANNING AND IMPLEMENTATION

• Assess respiratory status including rate, pattern, lung sounds, and cough effectiveness at least every 4 hours.
• Monitor quantity, color, and odor of secretions.
• Assess vital signs and pain at least every 4 hours. Administer analgesics as ordered.
• Schedule time to sit with Mr. Tom and discuss his concerns and feelings at least three times per day.
• Provide written information as requested.
• Monitor intake, output, and daily weight.
• Arrange dietary consultation to determine caloric requirements.

### EVALUATION

Mr. Tom reports in writing that his pain is adequately controlled. His respiratory status is stable with clear breath sounds throughout and an oxygen saturation of 94%. He is afebrile. Mr. Tom is tolerating tube feedings well and expresses a desire to begin eating. The dietitian has visited and assisted in planning to begin oral feedings. Intake and output are stable, as is his weight. Mr. Tom has been receptive to receiving information about follow-up care and exploration of various modalities of speech.

### Critical Thinking in the Nursing Process

1. Compare and contrast advantages and disadvantages of various methods to allow speech following total laryngectomy.
2. Develop a plan of care for Mr. Tom for the nursing diagnosis, *Disturbed body image.*
3. Discuss nursing interventions to provide wound care for the client with laryngectomy and radical neck dissection.
4. List strategies to optimize ventilation.

See Evaluating Your Response in Appendix C.

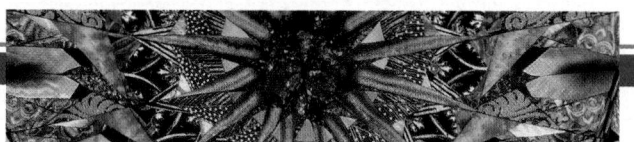

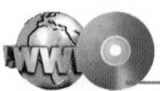 EXPLORE MediaLink

NCLEX review questions, case studies, care plan activities, MediaLink applications, and other interactive resources for this chapter can be found on the Companion Website at www.prenhall.com/lemone.

Click on Chapter 35 to select the activities for this chapter. For animations, video clips, more NCLEX review questions, and an audio glossary, access the Student CD-ROM accompanying this textbook.

## TEST YOURSELF

1. Which of the following health promotion activities planned by a nurse working with a group of community-dwelling senior citizens would be most likely to prevent influenza and pneumonia?

   a. Indoor exercise programs during winter months
   b. Influenza vaccine clinics at the senior center
   c. Teaching effective handwashing
   d. Advising seniors to avoid crowds

2. A client in the emergency department following facial trauma complains that his nose "just keeps dripping." The drainage appears like watery blood. The most appropriate nursing action would be to:

   a. Provide a box of tissues
   b. Reassure the client that this is expected with a nasal fracture
   c. Suction the nasopharynx
   d. Obtain a specimen for glucose testing

3. An expected finding in a client with obstructive sleep apnea would be:

   a. Confusion and signs of dementia
   b. Enlarged tongue
   c. Complaints of daytime sleepiness
   d. Decreased oxygen saturation levels while awake

4. The nurse in a physician's office notes that a regular client's voice is hoarse, a change from previous visits. The most appropriate question to ask the client would be:

   a. "How long has your voice been hoarse?"
   b. "Do you smoke?"
   c. "Do you have a sore throat?"
   d. "Would you like a prescription for throat lozenges?"

5. The nurse evaluates his teaching as effective when a client with stage 1 laryngeal cancer states:

   a. "I'm glad I don't have to worry about treating this cancer now because it is so early."
   b. "I hate to think about eventually losing the ability to speak, but I'd rather treat it aggressively than lose my life to cancer."
   c. "I'm glad this was diagnosed early, when it can be treated with radiation so I won't lose my voice."
   d. "Thank goodness this type of cancer usually doesn't spread anywhere else."

See Test Yourself answers in Appendix C.

## BIBLIOGRAPHY

Ackley, B. J., & Ladwig, G. B. (2002). *Nursing diagnosis handbook: A guide to planning care* (5th ed.). St. Louis: Mosby.

American Cancer Society. (2002a). *Cancer facts and figures 2002*. Atlanta: Author.

———.(2002b). *Laryngeal and hypopharyngeal cancer*. Available: www.cancer.org

Atkinson, W., Wolfe, C., Humiston, S., & Nelson, R. (Eds.). (2000). *Epidemiology and prevention of vaccine-preventable diseases* (6th ed.) Atlanta: Centers for Disease Control and Prevention.

Braunwald, E., Fauci, A. S., Kasper, D. L., Hauser, S. L., Longo, D. L., & Jameson, J. L. (2001). *Harrison's principles of internal medicine* (15th ed.). New York: McGraw-Hill.

Bullock, B. A., & Henze, R. L. (2000). *Focus on pathophysiology*. Philadelphia: Lippincott.

Conn, V. (1991). Self-care actions taken by older adults for influenza and colds. *Nursing Research, 40*(3), 176–181.

Deglin, J. H., & Vallerand, A. H. (2001). *Davis's drug guide for nurses* (7th ed.). Philadelphia: F.A. Davis.

Fontaine, K. L. (2000). *Healing practices: Alternative therapies for nursing*. Upper Saddle River, NJ: Prentice Hall Health.

Hakemi, A. (2001). Diagnosing and managing rhinosinusitis. *Physician Assistant, 25*(11), 16–25.

Hughes, D. L., & Tartasky, D. (1996). Implementation of a flu immunization program for homebound elders: A graduate student practicum. *Geriatric Nursing, 17*(5), 217–221.

Johnson, M., Bulechek, G., Dochterman, J. M., Maas, M., & Moorhead, S. (2001). *Nursing diagnoses, outcomes, & interventions*. St. Louis: Mosby.

Johnson, M., Maas, M., & Moorhead, S. (Eds.). (2000). *Nursing outcomes classification (NOC)* (2nd ed.). St. Louis: Mosby.

Kearney, K. (2001). Emergency. Epiglottitis. *American Journal of Nursing, 101*(8), 37–38.

Kirchner, J. T. (1999). Manifestations of pertussis in immunized children and adults. *American Family Physician, 60*(7), 2148–2149.

Klein, L. (2001). Sinusitis: When to treat and how. *RN, 64*(1), 42–44, 46, 48.

Kuhn, M. A. (1999). *Complementary therapies for health care providers*. Philadelphia: Lippincott.

Lehne, R. A. (2001). *Pharmacology for nursing care* (4th ed.). Philadelphia: Saunders.

Loud, B. (2001). A water pick to clear sinuses? *RN, 64*(1), 48–49.

Malarkey, L. M., & McMorrow, M. E. (2000). *Nurse's manual of laboratory tests and diagnostic procedures* (2nd ed.). Philadelphia: Saunders.

Marchiondo, K. (2000). Pickwickian syndrome: The challenge of severe sleep apnea. *MEDSURG Nursing, 9*(4), 183–188.

McCloskey, J. C., & Bulechek, G. M. (Eds.). (2000). *Nursing interventions classification (NIC)* (3rd ed.). St. Louis: Mosby.

Meeker, M. H., & Rothrock, J. C. (1999). *Alexander's care of the patient in surgery* (11th ed.). St. Louis: Mosby.

Merritt, S. L. (2000). Putting sleep disorders to rest. *RN, 63*(7), 26–30.

North American Nursing Diagnosis Association. (2001). *NANDA nursing diagnoses: Definitions & classification 2001–2002.* Philadelphia: NANDA.

Porth, C. M. (2002). *Pathophysiology: Concepts of altered health states* (6th ed.). Philadelphia: Lippincott.

Seay, S. J., Gay, S. L., & Strauss, M. (2002). Emergency. Tracheostomy emergencies. *American Journal of Nursing, 102*(3), 59, 61, 63.

Shellenbarger, T., & Wolfe, S. (2000). Nosebleeds: Not just kids' stuff. *RN, 63*(2), 50–55.

Springhouse. (1999). *Nurse's handbook of alternative & complementary therapies.* Springhouse, PA: Author.

Tierney, L. M., McPhee, S. J., & Papadakis, M. A. (2001). *Current medical diagnosis & treatment* (40th ed.). New York: Lange Medical Books/McGraw-Hill.

Urden, L. D., Stacy, K. M., & Lough, M. E. (2002). *Thelan's critical care nursing: Diagnosis and management* (4th ed.). St. Louis: Mosby.

The Voice Center. (2002). Speech after a total laryngectomy. Available: www.voice-center.com/alaryngeal_speech.htm

Way, L. W., & Doherty, G. M. (2003). *Current surgical diagnosis and treatment* (11th ed.). New York: McGraw-Hill.

Whitney, E. N., & Rolfes, S. R. (2002). *Understanding nutrition* (9th ed.). Belmont, CA: Wadsworth.

Wilkinson, J. M. (2000). *Nursing diagnosis handbook with NIC interventions and NOC outcomes* (7th ed.). Upper Saddle River, NJ: Prentice Hall Health.

Yantis, M. A. (2002). Pain control. Obstructive sleep apnea syndrome. *American Journal of Nursing, 102*(6), 83, 85.

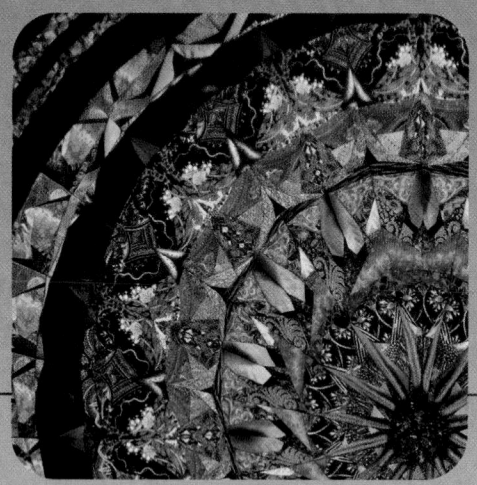

# CHAPTER 36

# Nursing Care of Clients with Lower Respiratory Disorders

## MediaLink

**www.prenhall.com/lemone**

Additional resources for this chapter can be found on the Student CD-ROM accompanying this textbook, and on the Companion Website at www.prenhall.com/lemone. Click on Chapter 36 to select the activities for this chapter.

**CD-ROM**
- Audio Glossary
- NCLEX Review

*Animation*
- ARDS
- Asthma
- Salmeterol

**Companion Website**
- More NCLEX Review
- Case Study
  Acute Asthma Attack
- Care Plan Activity
  Pneumonia
- MediaLink Application
  Respiratory Disorders

## LEARNING OUTCOMES

After completing this chapter, you will be able to:

- Relate anatomy, physiology, and assessment of the lower respiratory tract and its function to common disorders affecting the lower respiratory system.

- Describe the pathophysiology and manifestations of common lower respiratory disorders.

- Identify tests used to diagnose disorders of the lower respiratory system.

- Discuss nursing implications for medications and treatments prescribed for lower respiratory disorders.

- Provide appropriate care for the client having thoracic surgery.

- Effectively teach clients with lower respiratory disorders and their families.

- Use the nursing process to assess, plan and implement individualized care, and evaluate responses for a client with a lower respiratory disorder.

Many clients in acute care, long-term care, and the community experience acute or chronic disorders affecting the lower respiratory system. These disorders often lead to lost work time and account for a significant portion of health care costs.

Normal function of the lower respiratory system depends on several organ systems: the central nervous system, which stimulates and controls breathing; chemoreceptors in the brain, aortic arch, and carotid bodies, which monitor the pH and oxygen content of blood; the heart and circulatory system, which provide for blood supply and gas exchange; the musculoskeletal system, which provides an intact thoracic cavity capable of expanding and contracting; and the lungs and bronchial tree, which allow air movement and gas exchange. Impaired function of any of these systems affects ventilation and respiration. As a result, tissues may become *hypoxic,* with inadequate oxygen to support metabolic activity.

Disorders of the lower respiratory tract have both local and systemic effects. Local effects include cough, excess mucus production, shortness of breath or **dyspnea** (difficult or labored breathing), **hemoptysis** (bloody sputum), and chest pain. Systemic effects may include fever, anorexia and malaise, **cyanosis** (gray to blue or purple skin color caused by deoxygenated hemoglobin), **clubbing** of fingers and toes (enlargement and blunting of terminal digits), and other manifestations of impaired gas exchange.

Disorders of the lower respiratory system discussed in this chapter include infectious or inflammatory conditions, obstructive and restrictive lung diseases, pulmonary vascular disorders, lung cancer, chest and respiratory trauma, and respiratory failure. Before continuing, review the anatomy, physiology, and assessment of the lower respiratory system in Chapter 34.

## INFECTIONS AND INFLAMMATORY DISORDERS

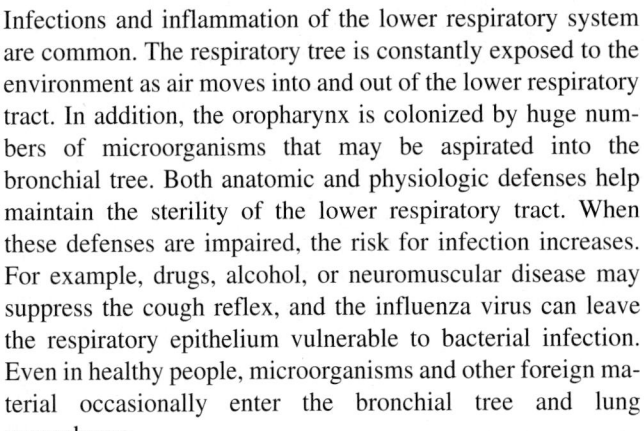

Infections and inflammation of the lower respiratory system are common. The respiratory tree is constantly exposed to the environment as air moves into and out of the lower respiratory tract. In addition, the oropharynx is colonized by huge numbers of microorganisms that may be aspirated into the bronchial tree. Both anatomic and physiologic defenses help maintain the sterility of the lower respiratory tract. When these defenses are impaired, the risk for infection increases. For example, drugs, alcohol, or neuromuscular disease may suppress the cough reflex, and the influenza virus can leave the respiratory epithelium vulnerable to bacterial infection. Even in healthy people, microorganisms and other foreign material occasionally enter the bronchial tree and lung parenchyma.

### THE CLIENT WITH ACUTE BRONCHITIS

**Bronchitis,** inflammation of the bronchi, may be either an acute or a chronic condition. Acute bronchitis is relatively common in adults. Impaired immune defenses and cigarette smoking increase the risk for acute bronchitis. In otherwise healthy adults, it typically follows a viral upper respiratory infection. Chronic bronchitis is a component of chronic obstructive pulmonary disease (COPD) and is discussed later in this chapter.

### PATHOPHYSIOLOGY AND MANIFESTATIONS

Infectious bronchitis can be caused by either viruses or bacteria that damage the respiratory mucosa. Inhalation of toxic gases or chemicals can lead to inflammatory bronchitis. In either case, the inflammatory response causes vasodilation and edema of the mucosal lining of the bronchi. Mucosal irritation increases mucus production and initiates the cough reflex.

Acute bronchitis is typically heralded by a nonproductive cough that later becomes productive. The cough often occurs in paroxysms, and may be aggravated by cold, dry, or dusty air. Chest pain, often substernal, is common. Other manifestations include moderate fever and general malaise.

### COLLABORATIVE CARE

The diagnosis of acute bronchitis typically is based on the history and clinical presentation. A chest X-ray may be ordered to rule out pneumonia, because the presenting manifestations can be similar. Other diagnostic testing is rarely indicated. Treatment is symptomatic and includes rest, increased fluid intake, and the use of aspirin or acetaminophen to relieve fever and malaise. Many physicians prescribe a broad-spectrum antibiotic such as erythromycin or penicillin, because approximately 50% of acute bronchitis is bacterial in origin. An expectorant cough medication is recommended for use during the day and a cough suppressant for night to facilitate rest.

### NURSING CARE

Nursing interventions for clients with acute bronchitis are primarily educational. Include the following teaching topics.

- Increase fluid intake to keep mucus thin and meet increased needs related to fever.
- Use over-the-counter analgesics and cough preparations containing dextromethorphan for symptom relief.
- Use and effects of any prescribed medications.
- The importance of smoking cessation (as appropriate).

## THE CLIENT WITH PNEUMONIA

Inflammation of the lung parenchyma (the respiratory bronchioles and alveoli) is known as **pneumonia.** Despite significant advances in antibiotic therapy, pneumonia remains the sixth leading cause of death in the United States, and the leading cause of death from infectious disease (Porth, 2002). In 1999, nearly 64,000 deaths in the United States were attributed to pneumonia (NHLBI, 2002). Its incidence and mortality are highest in older adults and people with debilitating diseases. Pneumonia currently accounts for about 10% of adult hospital admissions in the United States.

Pneumonia may be either infectious or noninfectious. Bacteria, viruses, fungi, protozoa, and other microbes can lead to infectious pneumonia. Noninfectious causes include aspiration of gastric contents and inhalation of toxic or irritating gases. Pneumonias often are classified as community acquired, nosocomial (hospital acquired), or opportunistic. Different organisms are implicated in each of these classifications (Table 36–1). The most common causative organism for community-acquired pneumonia is *Streptococcus pneumoniae* (also called pneumococcus), a gram-positive bacterium. This organism causes 70% to 75% of all diagnosed cases of pneumonia. *Mycoplasma pneumoniae, Haemophilus influenzae,* and the influenza virus are also leading causes of community-acquired pneumonia. *Staphylococcus aureus* and gram-negative bacteria such as *Klebsiella pneumoniae, Pseudomonas aeruginosa,* and enteric bacilli, including *Escherichia coli,* are often implicated as nosocomial causes of pneumonia. Organisms such as *Pneumonocystis carinii* generally cause infections only in immunocompromised people (opportunistic infections).

## PHYSIOLOGY REVIEW

The lower respiratory tract normally is sterile. A number of defense mechanisms help maintain this sterile environment. Infectious particles trapped by the mucous membranes of the nose are removed by sneezing, while those deposited in the nasopharynx usually are swallowed or expectorated. Reflex closure of the epiglottis and the branching bronchial tree present anatomic barriers to entry of microorganisms and other possible contaminants. The cilia and mucus that line the respiratory tract, and the cough reflex, serve to trap and eliminate foreign matter that enters the lower respiratory tract. Organisms that make it past these barriers usually are rapidly phagocytized in the alveolus by resident macrophages, then attacked by the in-

### Nursing Care of the Older Adult

#### PNEUMONIA

Several changes associated with aging and disease affect respiratory function and airway clearance. The number of cilia decreases, and the cough weakens. Gag and cough reflexes diminish. The older adult is at greater risk for dehydration, leading to thick, viscous mucus that is difficult to expectorate. Immune function declines with aging. These factors increase the risk of pulmonary infection and reduce the older adult's ability to respond effectively to infectious processes.

Other factors also may increase the risk for and severity of lower respiratory infections in the older adult: immobility, smoking history, surgical procedures, use of multiple medications, malnutrition, and such diseases as chronic obstructive pulmonary disease (COPD) and heart disease.

flammatory and immune defenses of the body. Aging impairs these immune responses, increasing the risk for pneumonia (see the box above).

## PATHOPHYSIOLOGY

The most common means of entry of pathogens into the lung is aspiration of oropharyngeal secretions containing microbes. Microorganisms also may be inhaled after having been released when an infected person coughs, sneezes, or talks. Contaminated aerosolized water also may be inhaled, an important means of spread for viral and some other types of pneumonia. Finally, bacteria may spread to the lungs through the bloodstream from infection elsewhere in the body.

When the invading microorganisms colonize the alveoli, an inflammatory and immune response is initiated. The antigen-antibody response and endotoxins released by some organisms damage bronchial and alveolar mucous membranes, causing inflammation and edema. Infectious debris and exudate can fill alveoli, interfering with ventilation and gas exchange.

The pathologic process, anatomic location, and manifestations of pneumonias vary according to the infective organism.

### Acute Bacterial Pneumonia

Of the bacterial pneumonias, the pathogenesis of pneumococcal (*Streptococcus pneumoniae*) pneumonia is best understood (Figure 36–1 ■). These bacteria reside in the upper respiratory tract of up to 70% of adults. They may be spread by direct person-to-person contact via droplets. In many cases, infection results from aspiration of resident bacteria. In the lower respi-

| TABLE 36–1 | Common Organisms Causing Pneumonia in Adults | |
| --- | --- | --- |
| **Community Acquired** | **Hospital Acquired** | **Opportunistic** |
| • *Streptococcus pneumoniae* <br> • *Mycoplasma pneumoniae* <br> • *Haemophilus influenzae* <br> • Influenza virus <br> • *Chlamydia pneumoniae* <br> • *Legionella pneumophila* | • *Staphylococcus aureus* <br> • *Pseudomonas aeruginosa* <br> • *Klebsiella pneumoniae* <br> • *Escherichia coli* | • *Pneumocystis carinii* <br> • *Mycobacterium tuberculosis* <br> • Cytomegalovirus (CMV) <br> • Atypical mycobacteria <br> • Fungi |

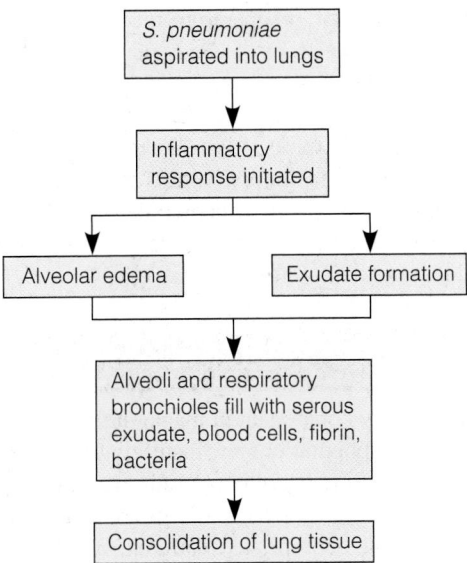

**Figure 36–1** ■ The pathogenesis of pneumococcal pneumonia.

ratory tract, the inflammatory response initiated by these organisms causes alveolar edema and the formation of exudate. As alveoli and respiratory bronchioles fill with serous exudate, blood cells, fibrin, and bacteria, *consolidation* (solidification) of lung tissue occurs. The lower lobes of the lungs are usually affected because of gravity. Consolidation of a large portion of an entire lung lobe is known as *lobar pneumonia*. This is the typical pattern for pneumococcal pneumonia. *Bronchopneumonia* is patchy consolidation involving several lobules. Other bacterial pneumonias often present with the patchy involvement of bronchopneumonia; pneumococcal pneumonia may also follow this pattern. The process resolves when macrophages predominate, digesting and removing inflammatory exudate from the infected lung.

## MANIFESTATIONS AND COMPLICATIONS

The presentation of bacterial pneumonia is usually acute, with rapid onset of shaking chills, fever, and cough productive of rust-colored or purulent sputum. Chest aching or *pleuritic pain* (sharp localized chest pain that increases with breathing and coughing) is common. Limited breath sounds and fine crackles or rales are heard over the affected area of lung. A pleural friction rub may be audible. If the involved area is large and gas exchange is impaired, dyspnea and cyanosis may be noted.

A more insidious onset with low-grade fever, cough, and scattered crackles is more typical of bronchopneumonia. Dyspnea is less commonly seen. The older adult or debilitated client may have atypical manifestations of pneumonia, with little cough, scant sputum, and minimal evidence of respiratory distress. Fever, tachypnea, and altered mentation or agitation may be the primary presenting symptoms.

Pneumococcal pneumonia typically resolves uneventfully; normal lung structure is restored on completion of the process. Local extension of the infection to involve the pleura (*pleuritis*) is the most common complication. Bacteremia can spread the

infection to other tissues, leading to meningitis, endocarditis, or peritonitis, and increasing the risk of mortality.

Pneumonias caused by *Staphylococcus aureus* and gram-negative bacteria often cause extensive parenchymal damage with necrosis, lung abscess, and empyema. **Empyema** is accumulation of purulent exudate in the pleural cavity. Progressive destruction of lung tissue and functional impairment is a possible consequence of *Klebsiella* pneumonia.

### Legionnaires' Disease

Legionnaires' disease is a form of bronchopneumonia caused by *Legionella pneumophila*, a gram-negative bacterium widely found in water, particularly warm standing water. Legionnaires' disease occurs sporadically and in outbreaks, such as that which occurred at an American Legion convention in 1976, when the disease was first recognized. Contaminated water-cooled air-conditioning systems and other water sources have been implicated in its spread.

Smokers, older adults, and people with chronic diseases or impaired immune defenses are most susceptible to Legionnaires' disease. Symptoms develop gradually, beginning 2 to 10 days after exposure. Dry cough, dyspnea, general malaise, chills and fever, headache, confusion, anorexia and diarrhea, myalgias and arthralgias are common manifestations. Consolidation of lung tissue is patchy or lobar. The mortality rate in Legionnaires' disease is up to 31% without treatment in otherwise healthy people and up to 80% in people who are immunocompromised (Braunwald et al., 2001).

### Primary Atypical Pneumonia

Pneumonia caused by *Mycoplasma pneumoniae* is generally classified as *primary atypical pneumonia,* because its presentation and course significantly differ from other bacterial pneumonias. Mycoplasma infection often causes pharyngitis or bronchitis. When pneumonia develops, patchy inflammatory changes in the alveolar septum and interstitial tissue of the lung occur. Alveolar exudate and consolidation of lung tissue are not features of atypical pneumonia.

Young adults—college students and military recruits in particular—are the primary affected population. Primary atypical pneumonia is highly contagious. Its manifestations resemble those of viral pneumonia; systemic manifestations of fever, headache, myalgias, and arthralgias often predominate. The cough associated with atypical pneumonia is dry, hacking, and nonproductive. Because of the typically mild nature and predominant systemic manifestations, mycoplasmal and viral pneumonia are often referred to as "walking pneumonias."

### Viral Pneumonia

Approximately 10% of pneumonias in adults are viral. Influenza and adenovirus are the most common organisms; however, the incidence of cytomegalovirus (CMV) pneumonia is increasing in immunocompromised people. Other viruses such as herpesviruses and measles virus also may cause viral pneumonia. As in primary atypical pneumonia, lung involvement in viral pneumonia is limited to the alveolar septum and interstitial spaces.

Viral pneumonia is typically a mild disease that often affects older adults and people with chronic conditions. It usually occurs in community epidemics. Flulike symptoms of headache, fever, fatigue, malaise, and muscle aching are common, along with a dry cough.

## Pneumocystis carinii Pneumonia

As many as 75% to 80% of people with acquired immune deficiency syndrome (AIDS) develop an opportunistic pneumonia caused by *Pneumocystis carinii,* a common parasite found worldwide. Immunity to *P. carinii* is nearly universal, except in immunocompromised people. Opportunistic infection may develop in people treated with immunosuppressive or cytotoxic drugs for cancer or organ transplant and in people with genetic or acquired immunodeficiency.

Infection with *P. carinii* produces patchy involvement throughout the lungs, causing affected alveoli to thicken, become edematous, and fill with foamy, protein-rich fluid. Gas exchange is severely impaired as the disease progresses.

*P. carinii* pneumonia (PCP) has an abrupt onset with fever, tachypnea and shortness of breath, and a dry, nonproductive cough. Respiratory distress can be significant, with intercostal retractions and cyanosis.

Table 36–2 compares the manifestations of infectious pneumonias.

## Aspiration Pneumonia

Aspiration of gastric contents into the lungs results in a chemical and bacterial pneumonia known as *aspiration pneumonia.* Major risk factors for aspiration pneumonia include emergency surgery or obstetric procedures, depressed cough and gag reflexes, and impaired swallowing. Older surgical clients are at significant risk. Enteral nutrition by either nasogastric or gastric tube also increases the risk for aspiration pneumonia. Vomiting is not always apparent; silent regurgitation of gastric contents may occur when the level of consciousness is decreased. Measures to reduce the risk for aspiration pneumonia include

minimizing the use of preoperative medications, promoting anesthetic elimination from the body, and preventing nausea and gastric distention.

The low pH of gastric contents causes a severe inflammatory response when aspirated into the respiratory tract. Pulmonary edema and respiratory failure may result. Common complications of aspiration pneumonia include abscesses, bronchiectasis (chronic dilation of the bronchi and bronchioles), and gangrene of pulmonary tissue.

## COLLABORATIVE CARE

Prevention is a key component in managing pneumonia. Identifying vulnerable populations and instituting preventive strategies are measures to reduce the mortality and morbidity associated with pneumonia. With early identification of the infecting organism, appropriate treatment, and support of respiratory function, most clients recover uneventfully. However, pneumonia remains a serious disease with significant mortality, especially in aged and debilitated populations.

### Diagnostic Tests

Diagnostic testing for pneumonia focuses on establishing a diagnosis, determining the extent of lung involvement, and identifying the causative organism.

- *Sputum gram stain* rapidly identifies the infecting organisms as gram-positive or gram-negative bacteria. Antibiotic therapy can then be directed at the predominant type of organism until culture and sensitivity results are obtained.
- *Sputum culture and sensitivity* is ordered to identify the infecting organism and determine the most effective antibiotic therapy. When obtaining sputum for culture, it is important to obtain secretions from the lower respiratory tract, not the mouth and nasal passages. See Procedure 36–1.
- *Complete blood count (CBC) with white blood cell (WBC) differential* shows an elevated WBC (11,000/mm³ or higher)

## TABLE 36-2  Manifestations of Infectious Pneumonias

| Type | Onset | Respiratory Manifestations | Systemic Manifestations |
|------|-------|----------------------------|-------------------------|
| Pneumococcal or lobar pneumonia | Abrupt | Cough productive of purulent or rust-colored sputum; pleuritic or aching chest pain; decreased breath sounds and crackles over affected area; possible dyspnea and cyanosis | Chills and fever |
| Bronchopneumonia | Gradual | Cough, scattered crackles; minimal dyspnea and respiratory distress | Low-grade fever |
| Legionnaires' disease | Gradual | Dry cough; dyspnea | Chills and fever; general malaise; headache; confusion; anorexia and diarrhea; myalgias and arthralgias |
| Primary atypical pneumonia | Gradual | Dry, hacking, nonproductive cough | Fever, headache, myalgias, and arthralgias predominate |
| Viral pneumonia | Sudden or gradual | Dry cough | Flulike symptoms |
| *Pneumocystis carinii* pneumonia | Abrupt | Dry cough; tachypnea and shortness of breath; significant respiratory distress | Fever |

## Procedure 36–1 — Obtaining a Sputum Specimen

### SUPPLIES

- Sterile sputum container, specimen cup, or mucus trap
- Mouth care supplies
- Sterile suction kit, if necessary
- Gloves

### BEFORE THE PROCEDURE

If the sputum specimen is to establish the initial diagnosis, obtain the specimen before starting oxygen and/or antibiotic therapy. Antibiotics reduce the bacterial count, making it difficult to identify the infecting organism. Oxygen therapy dries mucous membranes, making it more difficult to obtain a specimen. Unless otherwise instructed, obtain the specimen early in the morning, just after awakening. Respiratory secretions tend to pool during sleep; it is easier to obtain a specimen before normal coughing and daily activity has cleared them.

Provide for privacy, and explain the procedure. Emphasize the importance of coughing deeply to obtain sputum from the lower respiratory tract, avoiding expectoration of saliva. Increasing fluid intake prior to obtaining the specimen can help liquefy secretions, making them easier to expectorate.

### DURING THE PROCEDURE

1. Use standard precautions.
2. Provide for mouth care prior to obtaining the specimen to reduce contamination by oral flora.
3. Instruct to cough deeply several times, expectorating mucus into the container.
4. Close the container securely using aseptic technique.
5. Label the container with name and other identifying data, time and date, and any special conditions, such as antibiotic or oxygen therapy. Enclose specimen container in a clean plastic bag, and take to the laboratory or refrigerate as ordered to preserve the specimen.
6. To obtain a specimen by suctioning:
   - Provide mouth care as indicated above.
   - Obtain a sterile mucus trap. Using aseptic technique, attach the trap to the suction apparatus between the suction catheter and tubing.
   - Preoxygenate for suctioning as needed.
   - Perform tracheal suctioning using aseptic technique via either the nasotracheal route, endotracheal tube, or tracheostomy. Lubricate the catheter with sterile normal saline. Apply no suction as the catheter is being inserted into the trachea; apply suction for no longer than 10 seconds while withdrawing the catheter.
   - Detach the mucus trap; close and label. Clear the suction catheter and tubing with normal saline after removing the mucus trap. Dispose of equipment appropriately.
7. A sputum specimen also may be obtained during bronchoscopy procedure.

### AFTER THE PROCEDURE

Provide mouth care as needed. Teach the importance of completing all ordered antibiotic prescriptions to ensure complete eradication of microorganisms. Document the time and date that the specimen was obtained; and note color, consistency, and odor of sputum.

---

with increased circulating immature leukocytes (a left shift) in response to the infectious process. White blood cell changes are minimal in viral and other pneumonias.

- *Arterial blood gases (ABGs)* may be ordered to evaluate gas exchange. Alveolar inflammation can interfere with gas exchange across the alveolar-capillary membrane, especially if exudate or consolidation is present. Respiratory secretions or pleuritic pain also can interfere with alveolar ventilation. An arterial oxygen tension ($Po_2$) of less than 75 to 80 mmHg indicates impaired gas exchange or alveolar ventilation.
- *Pulse oximetry,* a noninvasive method of measuring arterial oxygen saturation, is ordered to continuously monitor gas exchange. The $Sao_2$ is the percentage of arterial hemoglobin that is saturated or combined with oxygen; it normally is 95% or higher. An $Sao_2$ of less than 95% may indicate impaired alveolar gas exchange.
- *Chest X-ray* is obtained to determine the extent and pattern of lung involvement. Fluid, infiltrates, consolidated lung tissue, and atelectasis (areas of alveolar collapse) appear as densities on the film.
- *Fiberoptic bronchoscopy* may be done to obtain a sputum specimen or remove secretions from the bronchial tree (Figure 36–2 ■). In this procedure, a flexible bronchoscope

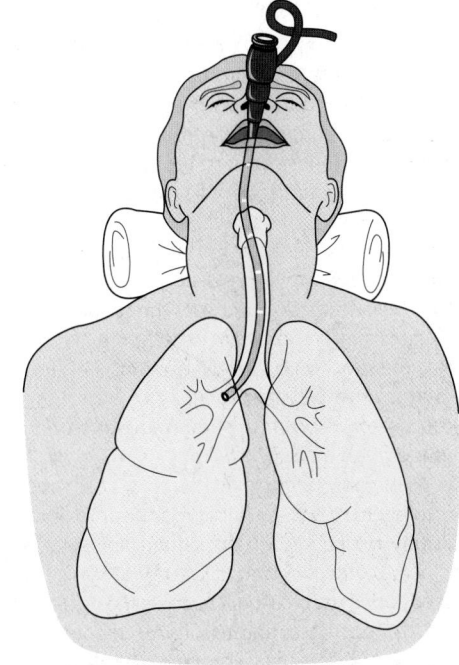

**Figure 36–2 ■** Fiberoptic bronchoscopy.

is inserted through the mouth and larynx into the tracheo-bronchial tree, allowing direct visualization of tissues and collection of specimens for analysis. Nursing responsibilities related to bronchoscopy are summarized in the box below.

## Immunization

Vaccines offer some degree of protection against the most common bacterial and viral pneumonias.

Pneumococcal vaccine, made of antigens from 23 types of pneumococcus, usually imparts lifetime immunity with a single dose. The vaccine is recommended for people who have a high risk of adverse outcome from bacterial pneumonias: people over age 65; those with chronic cardiac or respiratory conditions, diabetes mellitus, alcoholism, or other chronic diseases; and immunocompromised people.

Influenza vaccine is also recommended for high-risk populations. The predominant strain of influenza virus varies from year to year. A new vaccine formulation is prepared yearly, incorporating antigens of the influenza strains predicted to be the most prevalent for the upcoming flu season (typically the winter months). Vulnerable populations for whom yearly vaccine is recommended include those listed above as well as health care workers and residents of long-term care facilities. The vaccine contains egg protein, and is not recommended for people who have a severe allergy to eggs or who have previously experienced a severe hypersensitivity response to the vaccine.

## Medications

Medications used to treat pneumonia may include antibiotics to eradicate the infection and bronchodilators to reduce bronchospasm and improve ventilation.

Initial antibiotic therapy is based on the results of sputum Gram stain and the pattern of lung involvement shown on the chest X-ray. Typically, a broad-spectrum antibiotic such as a penicillin, cephalosporin, erythromycin, or aminoglycoside is ordered until the results of sputum culture and sensitivity tests are available. Table 36–3 lists commonly prescribed antibiotics for selected pneumonias; nursing implications for selected antibiotics are summarized on pages 224–226.

When an inflammatory response to the infection causes bronchospasm and constriction, bronchodilators may be ordered to improve ventilation and reduce hypoxia. Bronchodilators generally belong to one of two major groups: the sympathomimetic drugs, such as albuterol sulfate (Proventil) and metaproterenol (Alupent); or the methylxanthines, such as theophylline and aminophylline. Use of these drugs and related nursing implications are discussed in detail in the section on asthma.

An agent to "break up" mucus or reduce its viscosity may be prescribed. Acetylcysteine (Mucomyst), potassium iodide, and guaifenesin (a common ingredient in expectorant cough syrups), help to liquefy mucus, making it easier to expectorate. For many clients, however, increasing fluid intake is an effective means of liquefying mucus.

---

# Nursing Implications for Diagnostic Tests

## Bronchoscopy

### Nursing Responsibilities

- Provide routine preoperative care as ordered. *Bronchoscopy is an invasive procedure requiring conscious sedation or anesthesia. Care provided prior to the procedure is similar to that provided before many minor surgical procedures.*
- Provide mouth care just prior to bronchoscopy. *Mouth care reduces oral microorganisms and the risk of introducing them into the lungs.*
- Bring resuscitation and suction equipment to the bedside. *Laryngospasm and respiratory distress may occur following the procedure. The anesthetic suppresses the cough and gag reflexes, and secretions may be difficult to expectorate.*
- Following the procedure, closely monitor vital signs and respiratory status. *Possible complications of bronchoscopy include laryngospasm, bronchospasm, bronchial perforation with possible pneumothorax or subcutaneous emphysema, hemorrhage, hypoxia, pneumonia or bacteremia, and cardiac stress.*
- Instruct to avoid eating or drinking for approximately 2 hours or until fully awake with intact cough and gag reflexes. *Suppression of the cough and gag reflexes by systemic and local anesthesia used during the procedure increase the risk for aspiration.*
- Provide an emesis basin and tissues for expectorating sputum and saliva. *Until reflexes have returned, the client may be unable to swallow sputum and saliva safely.*

- Monitor color and character of respiratory secretions. *Secretions normally are blood tinged for several hours following bronchoscopy, especially if biopsy has been obtained.* Notify the physician if sputum is grossly bloody. *Grossly bloody sputum may indicate a complication such as perforation.*
- Collect postbronchoscopy sputum specimens for cytologic examination as ordered. *Cells in the sputum may be examined if a tumor is suspected.*

### Client and Family Teaching

- Fiberoptic bronchoscopy requires 30 to 45 minutes to complete. It may be done at the bedside, in a special procedure room, or in the surgical suite.
- The procedure usually causes little pain or discomfort, because an anesthetic is given. You will be able to breathe during the bronchoscopy.
- Some voice hoarseness and a sore throat are common following the procedure. Throat lozenges or warm saline gargles may help relieve discomfort.
- You may develop a mild fever within the first 24 hours following the procedure. This is a normal response.
- Persistent cough, bloody or purulent sputum, wheezing, shortness of breath, difficulty breathing, or chest pain may indicate a complication. Notify your physician if they develop.

TABLE 36-3 Antibiotic Therapy for Selected Pneumonias

| Causative Organism | Antibiotic of Choice | Alternative Antibiotics |
|---|---|---|
| *Streptococcus pneumoniae* | Penicillin G or V; doxycycline; amoxicillin | Erythromycin, cephalosporins, fluoroquinolone, vancomycin |
| *Staphylococcus aureus* | Penicillinase-resistant penicillin (e.g., nafcillin); vancomycin for methicillin-resistant organisms | Cephalosporins, vancomycin, clindamycin; ciprofloxacin, fluoroquinlones, TMP-SMZ* |
| *Mycoplasma pneumoniae* | Erythromycin | Doxycycline, clarithromycin, azithromycin, fluoroquinolone |
| *Klebsiella pneumoniae* | Third-generation cephalosporin (with aminoglycoside if severe); methronidazole | Aztreonam, imipenem-cilastatin, fluoroquinolone |
| *Legionella pneumophila* | Erythromycin + rifampin; fluoroquinolone | TMP-SMZ*, azithromycin, clarithromycin, ciprofloxacin |
| *Pneumocystis carinii* | TMP-SMZ*, pentamidine | Dapsone + trimethoprim, clindamycin + primaquine, trimetrexate + folinic acid |

* Trimethoprim-sulfamethoxazole

## Treatments

When mucous secretions are thick and viscous, increasing fluid intake to 2500 to 3000 mL per day helps liquefy secretions, making them easier to cough up and expectorate. If the client is unable to maintain an adequate oral intake, intravenous fluids and nutrition may be required.

Incentive spirometry may be used to promote deep breathing, coughing, and clearance of respiratory secretions. Endotracheal suctioning may be required if the cough is ineffective. This invasive technique is discussed in the section describing nursing care for the client with acute respiratory failure. On occasion, bronchoscopy is used to perform pulmonary toilet and remove secretions.

### Oxygen Therapy

Oxygen therapy may be indicated for the client who is tachypneic or hypoxemic.

Inflammation of the alveolar-capillary membrane interferes with diffusion of gases across the membrane. Diffusion is affected by several other factors, including the partial pressure of gases on each side of the membrane. Increasing the percentage of inspired oxygen above that of room air (21%) increases the partial pressure of oxygen in the alveoli and enhances its diffusion into the capillaries. Supplemental oxygen therefore improves oxygenation of the blood and tissues in clients with pneumonia.

Depending on the degree of hypoxia, oxygen may be administered by either a low-flow or high-flow system. Low-flow systems include the nasal cannula, simple face mask, partial rebreathing mask, and nonrebreathing mask (Figure 36–3 ■). A nasal cannula can deliver 24% to 45% oxygen concentrations with flow rates of 2 to 6 L/min. The nasal cannula is comfortable and does not interfere with eating or talking. A simple face mask delivers 40% to 60% oxygen concentrations with flow rates of 5 to 8 L/min. Up to 100% oxygen can be delivered by the nonrebreather mask, the highest concentration possible without mechanical ventilation. When the amount of oxygen delivered must be precisely regulated, a high-flow

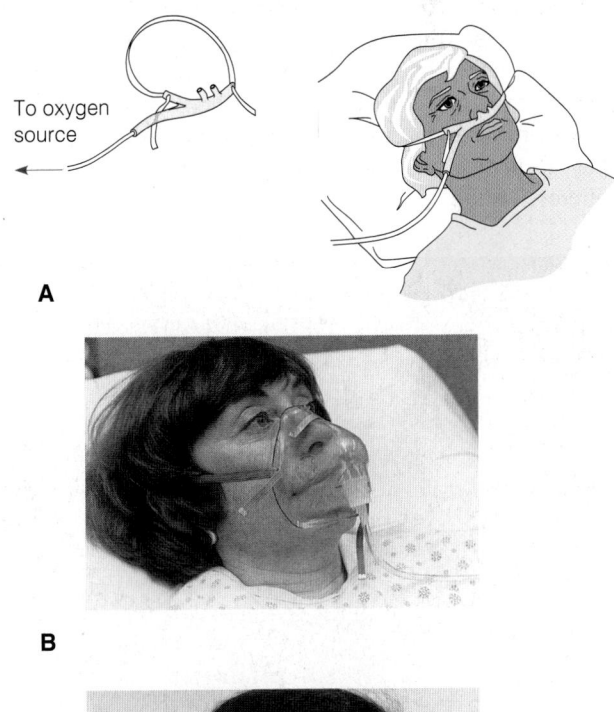

To oxygen source

**A**

**B**

**C**

Figure 36–3 ■ Low-flow oxygen delivery devices: *A,* nasal cannula; *B,* simple face mask; *C,* nonrebreather mask.

*Source: NMSB, Custom Medical Stock Photos, Inc.*

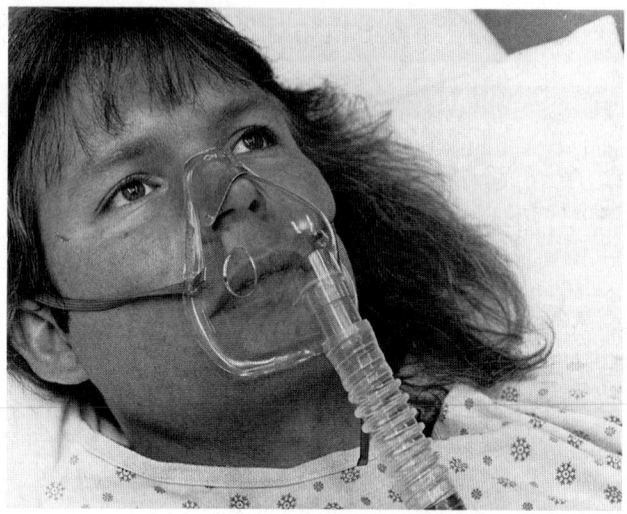

**Figure 36–4** ■ Venturi mask, a high-flow oxygen delivery system.

system such as a Venturi mask is used (Figure 36–4 ■). The Venturi mask regulates the ratio of oxygen to room air, allowing precise regulation of the oxygen percentage delivered, from 24% to 50%. Severe hypoxia may necessitate intubation and mechanical ventilation. Endotracheal intubation and methods of mechanical ventilation are discussed in the section on respiratory failure.

## Chest Physiotherapy

Chest physiotherapy, including percussion, vibration, and postural drainage, may be prescribed to reduce lung consolidation and prevent atelectasis. *Percussion* is performed by rhythmically striking or clapping the chest wall with cupped hands (Figure 36–5A ■), using rapid wrist flexion and extension. Cupping traps air between the palm and the client's skin, setting up vibrations through the chest wall that loosen respiratory secretions. The trapped air also provides a cushion, preventing injury. When performed correctly, percussion produces a hollow, popping sound. Percussion may also be done using a mechanical percussion cup. The breasts, sternum, spinal column, and kidney regions are avoided during percussion.

*Vibration* facilitates secretion movement into larger airways. It usually is combined with percussion, although it may be used when percussion is contraindicated or poorly tolerated. Vibration is performed by repeatedly tensing the arm and hand muscles while maintaining firm but gentle pressure over the affected area with the flat of the hand (Figure 36–5B).

Percussion and vibration are done in conjunction with *postural drainage,* which uses gravity to facilitate removal of secretions from a particular lung segment. The client is positioned with the segment to be drained superior to or above the trachea or mainstem bronchus. Drainage of all lung segments requires a variety of positions (Figure 36–6 ■); rarely do all segments require drainage. Bronchodilators or nebulizer treat-

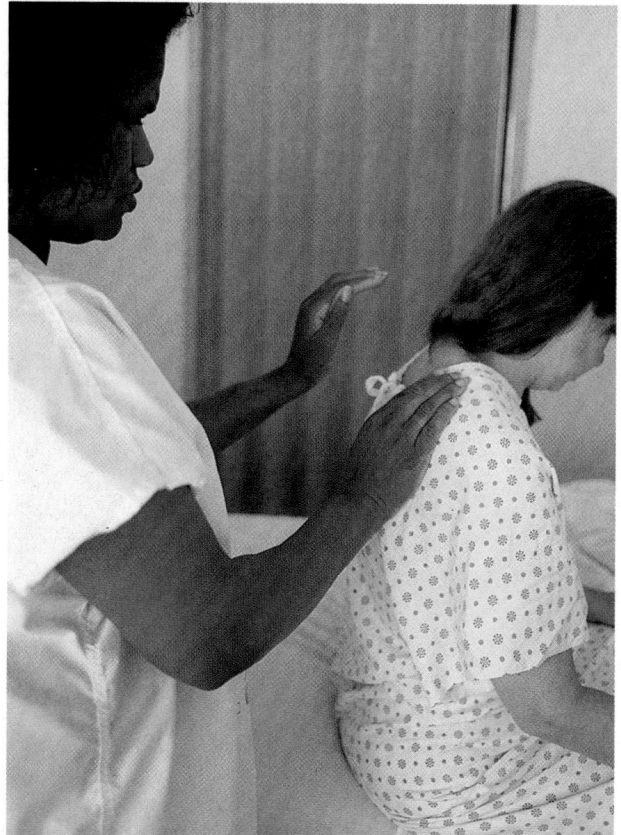

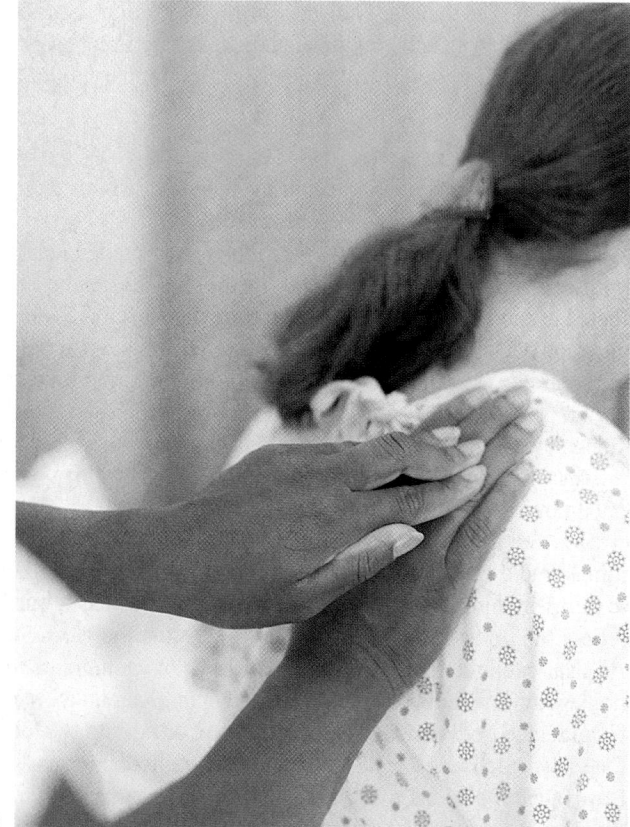

**A**

**B**

**Figure 36–5** ■ *A,* Percussing (clapping) the upper posterior chest. Notice the cupped position of the nurse's hands. *B,* Vibrating the upper posterior chest.

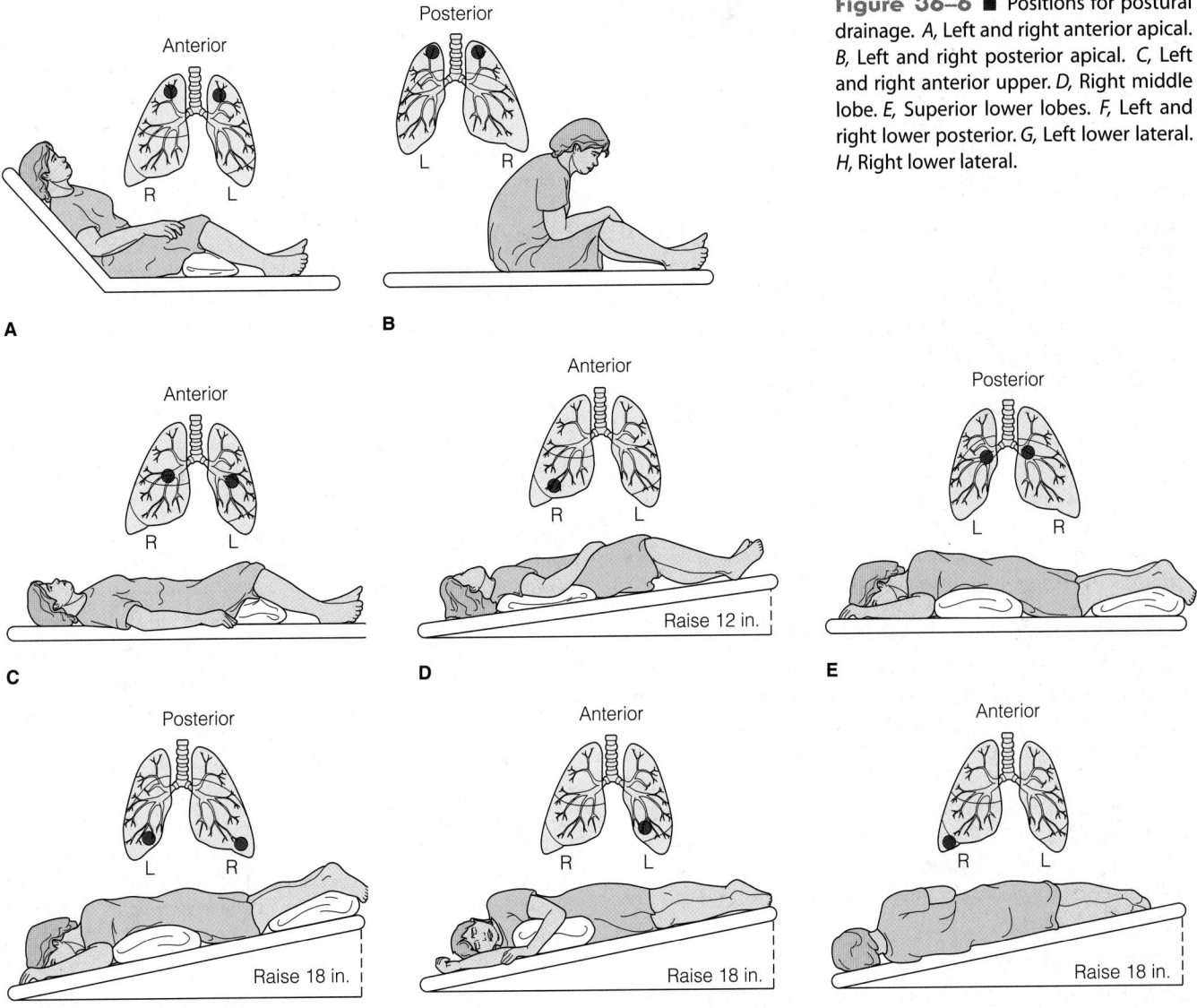

**Figure 36–6** ■ Positions for postural drainage. *A,* Left and right anterior apical. *B,* Left and right posterior apical. *C,* Left and right anterior upper. *D,* Right middle lobe. *E,* Superior lower lobes. *F,* Left and right lower posterior. *G,* Left lower lateral. *H,* Right lower lateral.

ments are administered as ordered prior to postural drainage. It is best to perform postural drainage before meals to avoid nausea and vomiting.

## Complementary Therapies

Although complementary therapies do not replace conventional treatment for pneumonia, they often promote comfort and speed recovery. The herb Echinacea is widely used to stimulate immune function and treat upper respiratory infections (URIs). Because viral URIs often precede pneumonia, it may be helpful in preventing pneumonia. Goldenseal, which often is sold in combination with Echinaciea, is used to treat bacterial, fungal, and protozoal infections of the mucous membranes of the respiratory tract (Lehne, 2001). Ma huang contains the active ingredient ephedra, which may help relieve bronchospasm and ease breathing. Because the pharmacology of ephedra is identical to ephedrine, this herb should not be used by clients with heart disease, hypertension, diabetes, or prostatic hypertrophy (Lehne, 2001).

## NURSING CARE

### Health Promotion

Health promotion activities focus on pneumonia prevention. Make clients in high-risk groups aware of the benefits of immunizations against influenza and pneumococcal pneumonia. A single dose of pneumococcus vaccine usually produces immunity to most strains of pneumococcal pneumonia, although repeat doses may be needed for older adults and people who are immunosuppressed. (Pneumococcus vaccine is contraindicated for people receiving immunosuppressive therapy.) Annual influenza vaccine helps prevent pneumonia, because pneumonia often occurs as a sequella to influenza.

**PRACTICE ALERT** *Inquire about allergic responses to eggs or previous influenza vaccinations prior to administering influenza vaccine. A significant hypersensitivity response may occur in clients who are allergic to egg protein.* ■

Additional measures to screen for and detect pneumonia in older adults are appropriate. Frequent pulmonary assessment and aggressive interventions help prevent problems. Restoring and maintaining mobility improves ventilation and helps mobilize secretions. Promoting adequate fluid intake liquefies secretions, making them easier to expectorate.

## Assessment

Focused assessment of the client with pneumonia includes the following:

- Health history: current symptoms and their duration; presence of shortness of breath or difficulty breathing, chest pain and its relationship to breathing; cough, productive or nonproductive, color, consistency of sputum; other symptoms; recent upper respiratory or other acute illness; chronic diseases such as diabetes, chronic lung disease, or heart disease; current medications; medication allergies
- Physical examination: presentation, apparent distress, level of consciousness; vital signs including temperature; skin color, temperature; respiratory excursion, use of accessory muscles of respiration; lung sounds

## Nursing Diagnoses and Interventions

Clients with lower respiratory disorders such as pneumonia may have multiple nursing care needs, depending on the severity of the illness. Alveolar ventilation and the process of alveolar respiration can be affected by inflammation and secretions. **Hypoxemia,** low levels of oxygen in the blood, and tissue hypoxia may result. Nursing care focuses on supporting optimal respiratory function and promoting rest to reduce metabolic and oxygen needs. Priority nursing diagnoses include *Ineffective airway clearance, Ineffective breathing pattern,* and *Activity intolerance.*

### Ineffective Airway Clearance

The inflammatory response to infection causes tissue edema and exudate formation. In the lungs, the inflammatory response can narrow and potentially obstruct bronchial passages and alveoli. Assessment findings supporting this nursing diagnosis include adventitious breath sounds such as crackles (rales), rhonchi, and wheezes; dyspnea and tachypnea; coughing; and indicators of hypoxia such as cyanosis, reduced $SaO_2$ levels, anxiety, and apprehension.

- Assess respiratory status, including vital signs, breath sounds, $SaO_2$, and skin color at least every 4 hours. *Early identification of respiratory compromise allows intervention before tissue hypoxia is significant.*
- Assess cough and sputum (amount, color, consistency, and possible odor). *Assessment of the cough and nature of sputum produced allow evaluation of the effectiveness of respiratory clearance and the response to therapy.*
- Monitor arterial blood gas results; report increasing hypoxemia and other abnormal results to the physician. *Blood gas changes may be an early indicator of impaired gas exchange due to airway narrowing or obstruction.*
- Place in Fowler's or high-Fowler's position. Encourage frequent position changes and ambulation as allowed. *The up-*

*right position promotes lung expansion; position changes and ambulation facilitate the movement of secretions.*
- Assist to cough, deep breathe, and use assistive devices. Provide endotracheal suctioning using aseptic technique as ordered. *Coughing, deep breathing, and suctioning help clear airways.*
- Provide a fluid intake of at least 2500 to 3000 mL per day. *A liberal fluid intake helps liquefy secretions, facilitating their clearance.*
- Work with the physician and respiratory therapist to provide pulmonary hygiene measures, such as postural drainage, percussion, and vibration. *These techniques help mobilize and clear secretions.*
- Administer prescribed medications as ordered, and monitor their effects. *If the infecting organism is resistant to the prescribed antibiotic, little improvement may be seen with treatment. Bronchodilators help maintain open airways but may have adverse effects such as anxiety and restlessness.*

### Ineffective Breathing Pattern

Pleural inflammation often accompanies pneumonia, causing sharp localized pain that increases with deep breathing, coughing, and movement, which can lead to rapid and shallow breathing. Distal airways and alveoli may not expand optimally with each breath, increasing the risk for atelectasis and decreasing gas exchange. Fatigue from the increased work of breathing is an additional problem in pneumonia. This, too, can lead to decreased lung inflation and an ineffective breathing pattern.

**PRACTICE ALERT** *Assess respiratory rate, depth, and lung sounds at least every 4 hours. Tachypnea and diminished or adventitious breath sounds may be early indicators of respiratory compromise.* ■

- Provide for rest periods. *Rest reduces metabolic demands, fatigue, and the work of breathing, promoting a more effective breathing pattern.*
- Assess for pleuritic discomfort. Provide analgesics as ordered. *Adequate pain relief minimizes splinting and promotes adequate ventilation.*
- Provide reassurance during periods of respiratory distress. *Hypoxia and respiratory distress produce high levels of anxiety, which tends to further increase tachypnea and fatigue and decrease ventilation.*
- Administer oxygen as ordered. *Oxygen therapy increases the alveolar oxygen concentration and facilitates its diffusion across the alveolar-capillary membrane, reducing hypoxia and anxiety.*
- Teach slow abdominal breathing. *This breathing pattern promotes lung expansion.*
- Teach use of relaxation techniques, such as visualization and meditation. *These techniques help reduce anxiety and slow the breathing pattern.*

### Activity Intolerance

Impaired airway clearance and gas exchange interfere with oxygen delivery to body cells and tissues. At the same time,

MediaLink | PNEUMONIA CARE PLAN

the infectious process and the body's response to it increase metabolic demands on the cells. The net result of this imbalance between oxygen delivery and oxygen demand is a lack of physiologic energy to maintain normal daily activities.

- Assess activity tolerance, noting any increase in pulse, respirations, dyspnea, diaphoresis, or cyanosis. *These assessment findings may indicate limited or impaired activity tolerance.*
- Assist with self-care activities, such as bathing. *Assistance with ADLs reduces energy demands.*
- Schedule activities, planning for rest periods. *Rest periods minimize fatigue and improve activity tolerance.*
- Provide assistive devices, such as an overhead trapeze. *These assistive devices facilitate movement and reduce energy demands.*
- Enlist the family's help to minimize stress and anxiety levels. *Stress and anxiety increase metabolic demands and can decrease activity tolerance.*
- Perform active or passive ROM exercises. *Exercises help maintain muscle tone and joint mobility, and prevent contractures if bed rest is prolonged.*
- Provide emotional support and reassurance that strength and energy will return to normal when the infectious process has resolved and the balance of oxygen supply and demand is restored. *The client may be concerned that activity intolerance will continue to be a problem after the acute infection is resolved.*

## Using NANDA, NIC, and NOC

Chart 36–1 shows links between NANDA nursing diagnoses, NIC, and NOC for the client with pneumonia.

## Home Care

Clients with pneumonia usually are treated in the community, unless their respiratory status is significantly compromised. Discuss the following topics when preparing the client and family for home care.

- The importance of completing the prescribed medication regimen as ordered; potential drug side effects and their management, including manifestations that necessitate stopping the drug and notifying the physician
- Recommendations for limiting activities and increasing rest
- Maintaining adequate fluid intake to keep mucus thin for easier expectoration
- Ways to maintain adequate nutritional intake, such as small, frequent, well-balanced meals
- The importance of avoiding smoking or exposure to second-hand smoke to prevent further irritation of the lungs
- Manifestations to report to the physician, such as increasing shortness of breath, difficulty breathing, increased fever, fatigue, headache, sleepiness, or confusion
- The importance of keeping all follow-up appointments to ensure disease cure

Clients with severe respiratory compromise or who are elderly or debilitated may require home care assistance to remain at home. Provide referrals to home intravenous services, home health nursing services, and home maintenance services as indicated. Community services such as Meals-on-Wheels can provide support to reduce the energy demands of meal preparation.

## CHART 36–1   NANDA, NIC, AND NOC LINKAGES

### The Client with Pneumonia

| NURSING DIAGNOSES | NURSING INTERVENTIONS | NURSING OUTCOMES |
|---|---|---|
| • Activity Intolerance | • Energy Management<br>• Environmental Management<br>• Self-Care Assistance | • Activity Tolerance<br>• Energy Conservation<br>• Self-Care: Activities of Daily Living (ADLs) |
| • Deficient Knowledge | • Infection Protection<br>• Teaching: Disease Process<br>• Teaching: Prescribed Medication | • Knowledge: Health Behaviors<br>• Knowledge: Energy Conservation<br>• Knowledge: Illness Care |
| • Impaired Gas Exchange | • Anxiety Reduction<br>• Oxygen Therapy<br>• Respiratory Monitoring | • Respiratory Status: Gas Exchange |
| • Ineffective Airway Clearance | • Cough Enhancement<br>• Chest Physiotherapy<br>• Positioning | • Respiratory Status: Airway Patency<br>• Respiratory Status: Ventilation |

*Note. Data from* Nursing Outcomes Classification (NOC) *by M. Johnson & M. Maas (Eds.), 1997, St. Louis: Mosby;* Nursing Diagnoses: Definitions & Classification 2001–2002 *by North American Nursing Diagnosis Association, 2001, Philadelphia: NANDA;* Nursing Interventions Classification (NIC) *by J.C. McCloskey & G. M. Bulechek (Eds.), 2000, St. Louis: Mosby. Reprinted by permission.*

## Nursing Care Plan
## A Client with Pneumonia

Mary O'Neal is a 35-year-old executive assistant and a part-time college student. On returning home from class one evening, she begins to chill. She alternates between chills and sweats all night. Staying home from work, she remains in bed most of the next day. Her fever continues, and she develops a cough and dull aching chest pain. When the cough becomes productive of rust-colored sputum the following day, she seeks medical treatment from her family doctor.

### ASSESSMENT

Debby Kowalski, RN, the family practice clinic nurse, admits Mrs. O'Neal to the clinic and obtains the nursing assessment. Mrs. O'Neal denies any previous history of respiratory diseases "other than the usual colds, flu, and such." She also denies any history of smoking or medication allergies. She says her symptoms began abruptly with the onset of the chills. She describes her chest pain as a dull ache that was initially substernal but now is localized in her lower lateral right chest. The pain increases with deep breathing, coughing, and moving. Her cough is increasing in frequency and severity, and her sputum appears rusty brown. Her vital signs are BP 116/74, P 104 and regular, R 26, T 101.8°F (38.7°C). Skin warm and flushed, with no evidence of cyanosis. Respirations shallow, unlabored; respiratory excursion equal. Diminished breath sounds in bases bilaterally, crackles noted in right posterior and lateral base. Faint pleural rub heard at right midaxillary line.

A STAT CBC shows a WBC of 18,900/mm³; differential shows increased numbers of neutrophils and immature WBCs (bands). Ms. Kowalski has Mrs. O'Neal rinse with an antiseptic mouthwash and collect a sputum specimen for culture and Gram stain prior to seeing the physician.

The physician orders a chest X-ray after examining Mrs. O'Neal. Based on her history, examination, and the chest X-ray, he makes the diagnosis of acute bacterial pneumonia, probably pneumococcal. He prescribes oral penicillin V, 500 mg every 6 hours for 10 days. He asks Mrs. O'Neal to return for a follow-up appointment in 10 days and refers her back to Ms. Kowalski for appropriate teaching.

### DIAGNOSIS

- *Ineffective breathing pattern* related to pleuritic chest pain
- *Hyperthermia* related to inflammatory process
- *Deficient knowledge* about pneumonia and its treatment

### EXPECTED OUTCOMES

- Maintain normal pulmonary function.
- Describe measures to minimize elevations in body temperature.
- Identify a schedule for taking her medication that will facilitate compliance with the regimen.

- Describe manifestations that should be reported to the physician.

### PLANNING AND IMPLEMENTATION

- Assess knowledge and understanding of pneumonia and its effects.
- Assist to develop a medication schedule that coordinates with normal daily routine.
- Teach about the following:
  a. Importance of avoiding use of a cough suppressant except at night to facilitate rest
  b. Ways to increase fluid intake to reduce fever and maintain thin mucus for easy expectoration
  c. Beneficial effects of rest, especially during the acute phase of her illness
  d. Safe use of aspirin and acetaminophen to reduce fever
  e. Importance of taking all prescribed medication doses as scheduled
  f. Common side effects of penicillin V and their management
  g. Early manifestations of penicillin allergy that necessitate stopping the medication and notifying the physician
  h. Signs of complications of pneumonia or worsening pneumonia to report

### EVALUATION

The sputum culture confirms *S. pneumoniae* as the cause of Mrs. O'Neal's pneumonia. When she returns for her follow-up appointment, she reports that she began to feel better after 2 days on the penicillin and returned to work the following Monday. Her examination reveals good breath sounds throughout with no adventitious sounds. The follow-up sputum culture is free of pathogens.

### Critical Thinking in the Nursing Process

1. Do any of the factors identified in the case study increase Mrs. O'Neal's risk for acute bacterial pneumonia?
2. Mrs. O'Neal's WBC differential showed increased neutrophil and band counts. Describe the reason for and effect of this change.
3. Even though Mrs. O'Neal has no history of medication allergies, anaphylactic shock remains a potential risk. Describe the sequence of events leading to anaphylactic shock, its initial symptoms, and immediate nursing interventions.
4. Had Mrs. O'Neal required hospitalization to treat her acute pneumonia, interruption of her usual activities and responsibilities could lead to anxiety. Develop a care plan for this situation, using the nursing diagnosis, *Altered role performance* related to hospitalization.

See Evaluating Your Response in Appendix C.

## THE CLIENT WITH SEVERE ACUTE RESPIRATORY SYNDROME

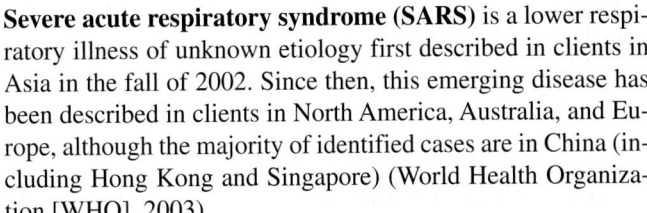

**Severe acute respiratory syndrome (SARS)** is a lower respiratory illness of unknown etiology first described in clients in Asia in the fall of 2002. Since then, this emerging disease has been described in clients in North America, Australia, and Europe, although the majority of identified cases are in China (including Hong Kong and Singapore) (World Health Organization [WHO], 2003).

The primary population affected by SARS is previously healthy adults age 25 to 70 years. Recent travel (within 10 days of the onset of symptoms) to an area with documented or suspected community transmission of SARS or close contact with a person known or suspected to have SARS are the primary risk factors for this disease.

## PATHOPHYSIOLOGY AND MANIFESTATIONS

Although not yet proven, the infective agent responsible for SARS is thought to be a newly identified coronavirus. This virus appears to spread by close person-to-person contact. Other potential sources of the infection are through direct contact with an infected person or contaminated object, and exposure of the eyes or mucous membranes to respiratory secretions (Centers for Disease Control and Prevention [CDC], 2003c).

The incubation period for SARS is generally 2 to 7 days, although it may be as long as 10 days in some people. Fever higher than 100.4°F (38°C) is typically the initial manifestation of the disease. The high fever may be accompanied by chills, headache, malaise, and muscle aches. After 3 to 7 days, respiratory manifestations of SARS develop, including nonproductive cough, shortness of breath, dyspnea, and possible hypoxemia.

While the majority of people with SARS recover, up to 20% of affected clients require intubation and mechanical ventilation (see the section on respiratory failure). About 3 in 100 clients with SARS die.

## COLLABORATIVE CARE

Prompt identification of SARS, infection control measures, and reporting of the disease are vital to control this potentially deadly disease. Health care providers and public health personnel should report cases of SARS to state and local health departments.

### Diagnostic Tests

At this time, no laboratory test is available to diagnose SARS. Initial diagnostic testing for a client with suspected SARS may include the following:

- *Serology tests* for antibodies to the new coronavirus may be available in some research centers.
- *Chest X-ray* may be normal or show interstitial infiltrates in a focal or generalized patchy pattern. In late stages of SARS, consolidation may be evident.

- *Pulse oximetry (oxygen saturation)* often shows hypoxemia in the respiratory phase of the illness.
- *Complete blood count (CBC)* often demonstrates a low lymphocyte count early in the disease. Leukopenia and thrombocytopenia may develop at the peak of the respiratory illness.
- *Creatinine phosphokinase (CPK or CK), ALT,* and *AST* levels may be markedly increased in SARS.
- *Sputum specimen* is obtained. Gram stain and culture are performed on the specimen to rule out other causes of pneumonia.
- *Blood culture* may be done to identify possible bacteremia.

### Medications

At this time, no medications have been shown to be consistently effective in treating SARS. Antibiotic and/or antiviral therapy targeted at community-acquired forms of pneumonia may be administered.

### Infection Control

Because health care workers are at risk for developing SARS after caring for infected clients, infection control precautions should be immediately instituted when SARS is suspected. Standard precautions (see Appendix A 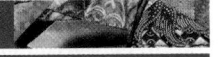 ) are implemented along with contact and airborne precautions. The Centers for Disease Control and Prevention (2003b) recommends hand hygiene, gown, gloves, eye protection, and an N95 respirator to prevent transmission of SARS in healthcare settings.

When clients with SARS are managed in the community, they are advised to remain home for 10 days after the fever has resolved and until respiratory symptoms are absent or minimal. Members of the household are advised to wash hands frequently or use alcohol-based hand rubs. The client is advised to cover the mouth and nose with tissue when coughing or sneezing and to wear a surgical mask during close contact with uninfected people. Sharing of utensils, towels, and bedding should be avoided. Routine cleaning (e.g., washing with soap and hot water) is adequate to disinfect objects and no special precautions are necessary for disposing of waste.

### Treatments

Care of the client with SARS is supportive. Oxygen may be administered to treat hypoxemia. Intubation and mechanical ventilation may be required if respiratory failure or acute respiratory distress syndrome (ARDS) develops.

## NURSING CARE

Nursing care of the client with SARS focuses on preventing spread of the disease to others and providing respiratory support.

### Health Promotion

Advise clients planning elective or nonessential travel to mainland China and Hong Kong, Singapore, and Hanoi, Vietnam, that they may wish to postpone their trips. Use respiratory and contact infection control precautions in addition to standard precautions when caring for all clients with suspected SARS to prevent spread of the disease to health care workers or other clients.

## Assessment

Focused assessment data for the client with suspected SARS include the following. For more complete respiratory assessment, see Chapter 34.

- Health history: current symptoms, including fever, malaise, shortness of breath, and cough; onset of symptoms; recent international travel or exposure to a person known to have SARS
- Physical assessment: vital signs including temperature; respiratory status, including respiratory rate, depth, and effort; presence of cough; adventitious lung sounds

## Nursing Diagnoses and Interventions

The client with SARS poses a risk for spread of the infection to health care workers and others. In addition, while many people with this disease experience only mild symptoms and recover fully and uneventfully, others develop severe respiratory distress and may require significant respiratory support. Gas exchange may be impaired, leading to significant hypoxemia. In addition to the nursing diagnoses discussed in the previous section on pneumonia, *Impaired gas exchange* and *Risk for infection* are priority nursing diagnoses.

### Impaired Gas Exchange

Although the pathophysiology of SARS is not fully understood, this disorder is known to cause hypoxemia of varying degrees in some clients. Significant hypoxemia may necessitate intubation and mechanical ventilation to support cellular function until recovery occurs.

- Monitor vital signs, color, oxygen saturation, and arterial blood gases. Assess for manifestations such as anxiety or apprehension, restlessness, confusion or lethargy, or complaints of headache. *These assessment data alert the nurse and care providers to potential hypoxemia or hypercapnia due to impaired gas exchange.*

**PRACTICE ALERT** *Promptly report signs of respiratory distress, including tachypnea, tachycardia, nasal flaring, use of accessory muscles, intercostal retractions, cyanosis, increasing restlessness, anxiety, or decreased level of consciousness. These may be early manifestations of respiratory failure and inability to maintain ventilatory effort.* ■

- Promptly report worsening arterial blood gases and oxygen saturation levels. *Close assessment of these values allows timely intervention as needed.*
- Maintain oxygen therapy and mechanical ventilation as ordered. Hyperoxygenate prior to suctioning. *Oxygen and mechanical ventilation support alveolar gas exchange. Hyperoxygenation prior to suctioning reduces the degree of hypoxemia that occurs during suctioning.*

- Place in Fowler's or high Fowler's position. *Sitting positions decrease pressure on the diaphragm and chest, improving lung ventilation and decreasing the work of breathing.*
- Minimize activities and energy expenditures by assisting with ADLs, spacing procedures and activities, and allowing uninterrupted rest periods. *Rest is vital to reduce oxygen and energy demands.*

**PRACTICE ALERT** *Avoid sedatives and respiratory depressant drugs unless mechanically ventilated. These medications can further depress the respiratory drive, worsening respiratory failure.* ■

- If intubation and mechanical ventilation is necessary, explain the procedure and its purpose to the client and family, providing reassurance that this *temporary* measure improves oxygenation and reduces the work of breathing. Alert that talking is not possible while the endotracheal tube is in place, and establish a means of communication. *Thorough explanation is important to relieve anxiety.*

See the section on respiratory failure later in this chapter for more information about caring for a client who is intubated and mechanically ventilated.

### Risk for Infection

The spread of SARS is a risk both in the health care facility and the community in which the client resides. Respiratory and contract precautions are recommended to prevent the spread of SARS via respiratory secretions or contact with the virus.

- Place the client in a private room with airflow control that prevents air within the room from circulating into the hallway or other rooms. A negative flow room in which air is diluted by at least six fresh-air exchanges per hour is recommended. *A negative flow room and multiple fresh-air exchanges dilute the concentration of virus within the room and prevent its spread to adjacent areas.*
- Use standard precautions and respiratory and contact isolation techniques as recommended by the CDC, including wearing respirators, gowns, and eye protection when caring for clients with SARS. *These measures are important to prevent the spread of SARS to others.*
- Discuss the reasons for and importance of respiratory and contact isolation procedures during treatment. *Maintenance of infection control precautions during and immediately following the febrile and respiratory phases of SARS is vital to prevent its spread to health care workers and the community.*
- Place a mask on the client when transporting to other parts of the facility for diagnostic or treatment procedures. *Covering the client's nose and mouth during transport minimizes air contamination and the risk to visitors and personnel.*
- Inform all personnel having contact with the client of the diagnosis. *This allows personnel to take appropriate precautions.*
- Assist visitors to mask prior to entering the room. *Providing visitors with appropriate masks or respirators reduces their risk of infection.*

- Teach the client how to limit transmitting the disease to others:
  a. Always cough and expectorate into tissues.
  b. Dispose of tissues properly, placing them in a closed bag.
  c. Wear a mask if sneezing or unable to control respiratory secretions.
  d. Do not share eating utensils, towels, bedding, or other objects with others, as this disease may also be spread by contact with contaminated objects.

*Teaching appropriate precautions helps prevent the spread of SARS to others while allowing as much freedom from restraints as possible.*

## Home Care

Many clients with SARS experience only mild symptoms and are appropriately cared for in the community. Teaching about home care and infection control precautions is vital to prevent spread of this disease to the community. Include the following topics when teaching for home care.

- The disease, its origin, and how it is spread
- Manifestations of impaired respiratory status to report to the physician
- Preventing spread of the disease to others:
  1. Cover the mouth and nose with tissues when coughing or sneezing. Personally dispose of tissues in a paper bag or the garbage. Wear a surgical mask during close contact with other members of the household.
  2. Limit interactions outside the home; do not go to work, school, or other public areas until you have been free of fever for 10 days and your respiratory symptoms are resolving.
  3. Remind all members of the household to wash hands (or use an alcohol-based hand sanitizer) frequently, particularly after direct contact with body fluids.
  4. Do not share eating utensils, towels, or bedding with others. These items can be cleaned with soap and hot water between uses. Clean contaminated surfaces with a household disinfectant.
- Monitoring uninfected members of the household for signs of the illness (Instruct to report fever or respiratory symptoms to the physician.)

## THE CLIENT WITH LUNG ABSCESS

A **lung abscess** is a localized area of lung destruction or necrosis and pus formation. The most common cause of lung abscess is aspiration and resulting pneumonia. Risk factors, therefore, are those for aspiration: decreased level of consciousness due to anesthesia, injury or disease of the central nervous system, seizure, excessive sedation, or alcohol abuse; swallowing disorders; dental caries; and debilitation secondary to cancer or chronic disease. Lung abscess also may occur as a complication of some types of pneumonia, including those due to *Staphylococcus aureus*, *Klebsiella*, and *Legionella*.

## PATHOPHYSIOLOGY AND MANIFESTATIONS

A lung abscess forms after lung tissue becomes consolidated (i.e., after alveoli become filled with fluid, pus, and microorganisms). Consolidated tissue becomes necrotic. This necrotic process can spread to involve the entire bronchopulmonary segment and progress proximally until it ruptures into a bronchus. With rupture, the contents of the abscess empty into the bronchus, leaving a cavity filled with air and fluid, a process known as *cavitation*. If purulent material from the abscess is not expectorated, the infection may spread, leading to diffuse pneumonia or a syndrome similar to acute respiratory distress syndrome (ARDS, discussed later in this chapter).

Manifestations of lung abscess typically develop about 2 weeks after the precipitating event (aspiration, pneumonia, and so on). Their onset may be either acute or insidious. Early symptoms are those of pneumonia: productive cough, chills and fever, pleuritic chest pain, malaise, and anorexia. The temperature may be significantly elevated, 103°F (39.4°C) or higher. When the abscess ruptures, the client may expectorate large amounts of foul-smelling, purulent, and possibly blood-streaked sputum. Breath sounds are diminished, and crackles may be noted in the region of the abscess. A dull percussion tone is also present.

## COLLABORATIVE CARE

The diagnosis of lung abscess usually is based on the history and presentation. The CBC may indicate leukocytosis. Sputum culture may not show the organism involved unless rupture occurs. Chest X-ray shows a thick-walled, solitary cavity with surrounding consolidation, although differentiating lung abscess from consolidation can be difficult until cavitation occurs.

Lung abscess is treated with antibiotic therapy, usually intravenous clindamycin (Cleocin), amoxicillin-clavulanate (Augmentin), or penicillin (Tierney et al., 2001). Postural drainage may be ordered to relieve obstruction and promote drainage. In some cases, bronchoscopy is used to drain the abscess. If the pleural space becomes involved, a chest tube (tube thoracostomy) may be used to drain the abscess. See the section on pneumothorax for further discussion of chest tubes.

## NURSING CARE

Although most clients with lung abscess recover fully with appropriate antibiotic treatment, rupture and drainage of the abscess into a bronchus is a frightening experience. Nursing care needs of the client relate primarily to maintaining a patent airway and adequate gas exchange. The following nursing diagnoses may be appropriate for the client with lung abscess.

- *Risk for ineffective airway clearance* related to large amounts of purulent drainage in bronchi
- *Impaired gas exchange* related to necrotic and consolidated lung tissue

- *Hyperthermia* related to infectious process
- *Anxiety,* related to copious amounts of purulent sputum

Client and family teaching focuses on the importance of completing the prescribed antibiotic therapy. Most lung abscesses are successfully treated with antibiotics; however, treatment may last up to 1 month or more. Emphasize the importance of completing the entire course of therapy to eliminate the infecting organisms. Teach about the medication, including its name, dose, desired and adverse effects. Stress the need to contact the physician if symptoms do not improve or if they become worse. Infection from lung abscess can spread not only to lung and pleural tissue but systemically, causing sepsis. If postural drainage is ordered, teach the client and family how to perform this procedure. When procedures such as bronchoscopy or thoracostomy are performed to drain the abscess, provide preoperative teaching and instruction on postoperative care.

## THE CLIENT WITH TUBERCULOSIS

**Tuberculosis (TB)** is a chronic, recurrent infectious disease that usually affects the lungs, although any organ can be affected. This disease, caused by *Mycobacterium tuberculosis,* is uncommon in the United States, especially among young adults of European descent. Its incidence fell steadily until the mid-1980s, thanks to improved sanitation, surveillance, and treatment of people with active disease. The late 1980s and early 1990s saw a resurgence of the disease, attributed primarily to the HIV/AIDS epidemic, the emergence of multiple-drug-resistant (MDR) strains of TB, and social factors such as immigration, poverty, homelessness, and drug abuse. Today, the number of people affected by TB in the United States continues to decline, with a total of 15,989 cases reported in 2001 (National Center for HIV, STD, and TB Prevention, 2002). This decline can be attributed to TB-control programs that emphasize promptly identifying new cases and initiating and completing appropriate therapy.

Worldwide, TB continues to be an important health problem. An estimated 8 million cases of TB develop annually, with the vast majority (90%) occurring in developing countries of Asia, Africa, the Middle East, and Latin America. TB accounts for an estimated 2 million deaths each year (Braunwald et al., 2001).

Today, TB in the United States is a disease primarily affecting immigrants, those infected with HIV, and disadvantaged populations. The TB case rate for foreign-born U.S. residents is more than 8 times higher than that for people born in the United States (NCHSTP 2002). Minority populations are affected to a greater extent than whites—the case rates for blacks, Hispanics, and Native Americans are 7 to 8 times that for whites; for Asians and Pacific Islanders living in the United States, it is more than 20 times higher. Poor urban areas are hit the hardest—areas that are also affected by the epidemics of injection drug use, homelessness, malnutrition, and poor living conditions. Overcrowded institutions also contribute to the spread of TB; transmission in hospitals, homeless shelters,

drug treatment centers, prisons, and residential facilities has been documented. People with altered immune function, including older adults (see the box on page 1093) and people with AIDS are at particular risk for tuberculosis. Some strains of *M. tb* have become resistant to drugs used to treat the disease.

*M. tuberculosis* is a relatively slow-growing, slender, rod-shaped, acid-fast organism with a waxy outer capsule, which increases its resistance to destruction. Although the lungs are usually infected, tuberculosis can involve other organs as well. It is transmitted by *droplet nuclei,* airborne droplets produced when an infected person coughs, sneezes, speaks, or sings. The tiny droplets can remain suspended in air for several hours. Infection may develop when a susceptible host breathes in air containing droplet nuclei and the contaminated particle eludes the normal defenses of the upper respiratory tract to reach the alveoli.

The risk for infection is affected by characteristics of the infectious person, the extent of air contamination, duration of exposure, and susceptibility of the host. The number of microbes in the sputum, frequency and force of coughing, and behaviors such as covering the mouth when coughing affect the production of droplet nuclei. In a small, closed, or poorly ventilated space, droplet nuclei become more concentrated, increasing the risk of exposure. Prolonged contact, such as living in the same household, increases the risk. Less-than-optimal immune function, a problem for people in lower socioeconomic groups, injection drug users, the homeless, alcoholics, and people with HIV infection, increases the susceptibility of the host.

## PATHOPHYSIOLOGY
### Pulmonary Tuberculosis

Minute droplet nuclei containing one to three bacilli that elude upper airway defense systems to enter the lungs implant in an alveolus or respiratory bronchiole, usually in an upper lobe. As the bacteria multiply, they cause a local inflammatory response. The inflammatory response brings neutrophils and macrophages to the site. These phagocytic cells surround and engulf the bacilli, isolating them and preventing their spread. *M. tb* continues to slowly multiply; some enter the lymphatic system to stimulate a cellular-mediated immune response (see Chapter 9 ⊂⊃ to review immune responses). Neutrophils and macrophages isolate the bacteria but cannot destroy them. A granulomatous lesion called a *tubercle,* a sealed-off colony of bacilli, is formed. Within the tubercle, infected tissue dies, forming a cheeselike center, a process called *caseation necrosis.*

If the immune response is adequate, scar tissue develops around the tubercle, and the bacilli remain encapsulated. These lesions eventually calcify and are visible on X-ray. The client, while infected by *M. tb,* does not develop tuberculosis disease. If the immune response is inadequate to contain the bacilli, the disease of tuberculosis can develop. Occasionally, the infection can progress, leading to extensive destruction of lung tissue. In *primary tuberculosis,* granulomatous tissue may erode into a bronchus or into a blood vessel, allowing the disease to spread

## Nursing Care of The Older Adult

# TUBERCULOSIS

Up to 30% of all newly diagnosed tuberculosis cases occur among people over 65 years of age. Of these cases, approximately 90% occur due to reactivation the dormant bacterium. Older adults are at increased risk for reactivation tuberculosis due to age-related decreases in cell-mediated immunity. Chronic illnesses, poor nutrition, gastrectomy, alcoholism, or the long-term use of steroids and immunosuppressive agents may also reactivate dormant TB lesions.

Presenting symptoms of tuberculosis in the older adult are often vague, including coughing, weight loss, anorexia, or periodic fevers. These signs and symptoms should not be dismissed as a normal part of aging.

Residents of nursing homes are at increased risk for acquiring tuberculosis because of group living. Yearly tuberculin skin testing with purified protein derivative (PPD) is often required by state health departments. If the initial test is negative, a repeat PPD in 1 to 2 weeks is recommended. This improves sensitivity to the test so that silent cases of tuberculosis are not missed. A chest X-ray and sputum culture for acid-fast bacilli are obtained if the PPD is positive.

Successful treatment for tuberculosis includes taking at least two drugs for at least 6 to 9 months to totally eradicate the organism. Older adults usually do not develop drug-resistant forms of tuberculosis, because they acquired the disease prior to emergence of drug-resistant strains.

## Assessing for Home Care

Community-dwelling older adults are susceptible to tuberculosis as well as those in care facilities. The older adult with respiratory symptoms often is treated presumptively for pneumonia, without a sputum smear and Gram stain. Older adults living in the community may not have had a tuberculin test or chest X-ray for many years.

Assess risk factors for tuberculosis:

- General health and nutritional status, including intake of specific nutrients such as vitamin D (lack of vitamin D is associated with a higher risk of developing active tuberculosis)
- Presence of a chronic disease such as silicosis, diabetes, alcoholism, or HIV infection; past history of a gastrectomy
- Past history of a positive tuberculin test that now has converted to negative
- Medications such as corticosteroids or other immunosuppressive drugs

Assess living and social situation:

- Natural light and ventilation in the home
- Access to clean water, cooking facilities, grocery stores, and other services
- Possible exposure to infected people, e.g., sharing a household with someone with active TB, crowded living facilities, homelessness, frequent participation in senior activities, volunteer work in residential care facilities or other institutional settings
- Access to health care

Tuberculosis is typically treated in the community; hospitalization or institutionalization rarely is necessary or desirable. For the older adult being treated for active TB in the community, assess:

- Knowledge and understanding of the disease and the prescribed treatment regimen
- Mental status and ability to follow prescribed regimen and precautions to avoid exposing others to the disease
- Transportation and ability to access health care services on a regular basis
- Financial resources to complete treatment and follow-up care
- Need for home health or social services to ensure adequate treatment

## Teaching for Home Care

Teaching focuses on improving the older adult's ability to self-manage the disease and treatment. Teach about tuberculosis and how it is spread. Emphasize the importance of taking all medications as prescribed and complying with follow-up appointments and testing. Discuss the importance of:

- Using disposable tissues to contain respiratory secretions, especially during the first 2 weeks of treatment when the disease may be transmitted to others
- Avoiding exposure to crowds or people with infectious diseases
- Eating a well-balanced diet with adequate nutrients
- Getting adequate rest, sleep, and exercise to maintain good general health
- Ensuring that housemates or others having frequent contact with the client are tested and receive prophylactic treatment if indicated

Teach about possible side effects of the prescribed medications and the importance of reporting these to health care providers:

- Peripheral neuropathy (numbness, tingling, or a burning sensation of the extremities) may occur with isoniazid (INH). Pyridoxine (vitamin $B_6$) often is prescribed to prevent this adverse effect.
- Both INH and rifampin may cause hepatitis. Avoid alcohol while taking these drugs, and report any manifestations such as nausea and anorexia, jaundice, a change in urine or stool color, or pain in the upper right quadrant.
- Rifampin may cause an orange-red coloration of saliva and urine.
- Streptomycin can affect hearing and balance; promptly report any changes, as they may be irreversible.
- Ethambutol may affect red-green color discrimination and visual acuity. Use caution when driving or walking in unfamiliar areas and promptly report any vision changes.

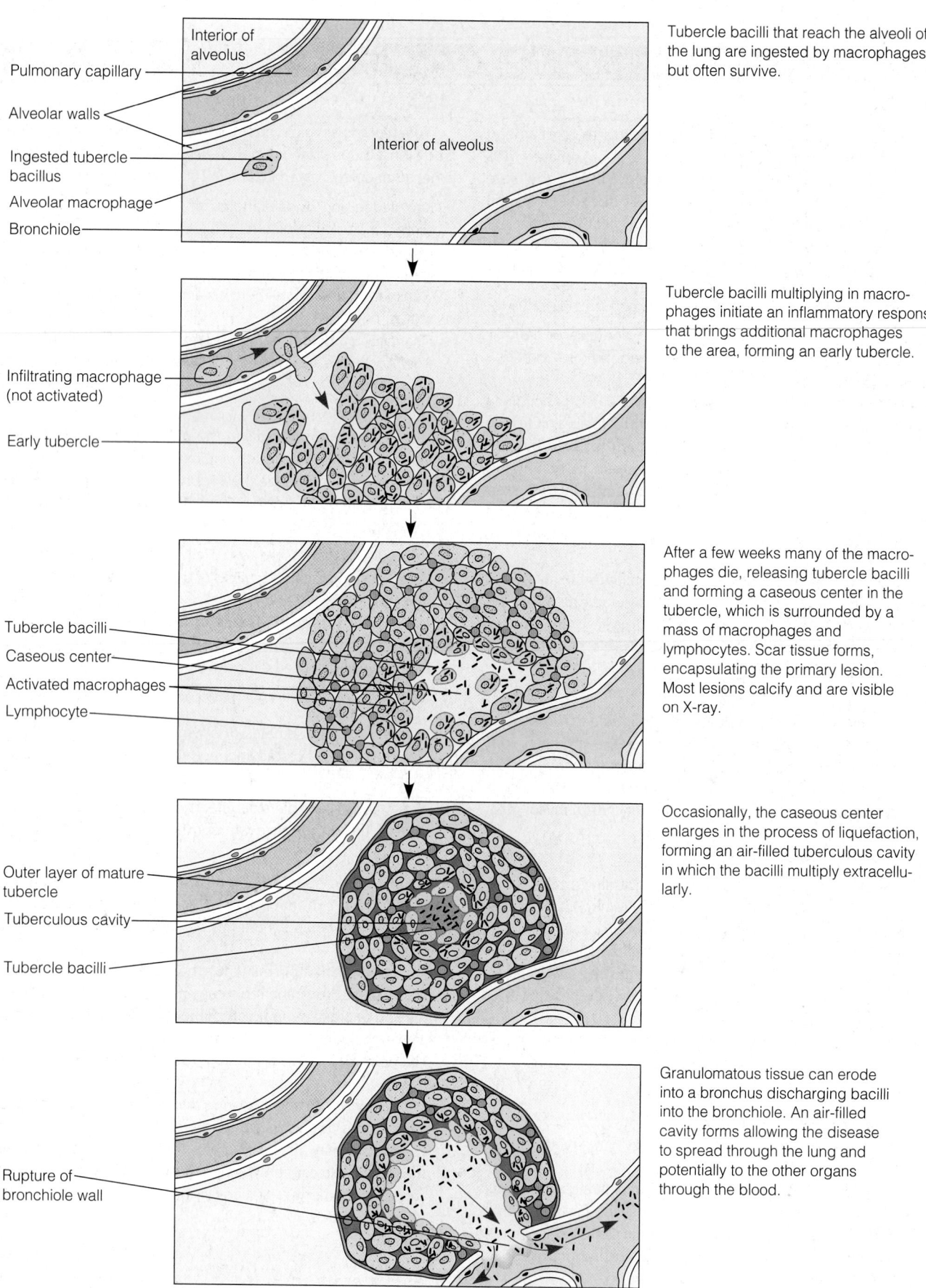

Interior of alveolus

Pulmonary capillary

Alveolar walls

Ingested tubercle bacillus

Alveolar macrophage

Bronchiole

Interior of alveolus

Tubercle bacilli that reach the alveoli of the lung are ingested by macrophages but often survive.

Infiltrating macrophage (not activated)

Early tubercle

Tubercle bacilli multiplying in macrophages initiate an inflammatory response that brings additional macrophages to the area, forming an early tubercle.

Tubercle bacilli

Caseous center

Activated macrophages

Lymphocyte

After a few weeks many of the macrophages die, releasing tubercle bacilli and forming a caseous center in the tubercle, which is surrounded by a mass of macrophages and lymphocytes. Scar tissue forms, encapsulating the primary lesion. Most lesions calcify and are visible on X-ray.

Outer layer of mature tubercle

Tuberculous cavity

Tubercle bacilli

Occasionally, the caseous center enlarges in the process of liquefaction, forming an air-filled tuberculous cavity in which the bacilli multiply extracellularly.

Rupture of bronchiole wall

Granulomatous tissue can erode into a bronchus discharging bacilli into the bronchiole. An air-filled cavity forms allowing the disease to spread through the lung and potentially to the other organs through the blood.

**Figure 36–7** ■ The pathogenesis of tuberculosis.

throughout the lung or other organs. This severe form of tuberculosis is uncommon in adults (Braunwald et al., 2001).

A previously healed tuberculosis lesion may be reactivated. *Reactivation tuberculosis* occurs when the immune system is suppressed due to age, disease, or use of immunosuppressive drugs. The extent of lung disease can vary from small lesions to extensive cavitation of lung tissue. Tubercles rupture, spreading bacilli into the airways to form satellite lesions and produce tuberculosis pneumonia. Without treatment, massive lung involvement can lead to death, or a more chronic process of tubercle formation and cavitation may result. People with chronic disease continue to spread *M. tb* into the environment, potentially infecting others. Figure 36–7 ■ illustrates the pathogenesis of tuberculosis.

Clients with HIV disease are at high risk for developing active tuberculosis, due to primary infection or reactivation. HIV infection suppresses cellular immunity, which is vital to limiting the replication and spread of *M. tb*.

## MANIFESTATIONS AND COMPLICATIONS

The initial infection causes few symptoms and typically goes unnoticed until the tuberculin test becomes positive or calcified lesions are seen on chest X-ray. Manifestations of primary progressive or reactivation tuberculosis often develop insidiously and are initially nonspecific (see the box below). Fatigue, weight loss, anorexia, low-grade afternoon fever, and night sweats are common. A dry cough develops, which later becomes productive of purulent and/or blood-tinged sputum. It is often at this stage that the client seeks medical attention.

Tuberculosis empyema and bronchopleural fistula are the most serious complications of pulmonary tuberculosis. When a tuberculosis lesion ruptures, bacilli may contaminate the pleural space. Rupture also may allow air to enter the pleural space from the lung, causing pneumothorax.

### Extrapulmonary Tuberculosis

When primary disease or reactivation allows live bacilli to enter the bronchi, the disease may spread through the blood and lymph system to other organs. These distant disease metastases may produce an active lesion, or they may become dormant and reactivate at a later time. Extrapulmonary tuberculosis is especially prevalent in people with HIV disease.

### Miliary Tuberculosis

*Miliary tuberculosis* results from hematogenous spread (through the blood) of the bacilli throughout the body. Miliary tuberculosis causes chills and fever, weakness, malaise, and progressive dyspnea. Multiple lesions evenly distributed throughout the lungs are noted on X-ray. The sputum rarely contains organisms. The bone marrow is usually involved, causing anemia, thrombocytopenia, and leukocytosis. Without appropriate treatment, the prognosis is poor.

### Genitourinary Tuberculosis

The kidney and genitourinary tract are common extrapulmonary sites for tuberculosis. The organism spreads to the kidney through the blood, initiating an inflammatory process similar to that which occurs in the lungs. Reactivation can occur years after the original infection. As the lesion then enlarges and caseates, a large portion of the renal parenchyma is destroyed. The infection then can spread to rest of the urinary tract, including the ureters and bladder. Scarring and strictures commonly result. In men, the prostate, seminal vesicles, and epididymis may be involved. In women, tuberculosis may affect the fallopian tubes and ovaries.

Manifestations of genitourinary tuberculosis develop insidiously. Symptoms of a urinary tract infection, including malaise, dysuria, hematuria, and pyuria, develop. Flank pain may be present. Men may develop manifestations of epididymitis or prostatitis: perineal, sacral, or scrotal pain and tenderness; difficulty voiding; and fever. Women may have manifestations of pelvic inflammatory disease, impaired fertility, or ectopic pregnancy.

### Tuberculosis Meningitis

Tuberculosis meningitis results when tuberculosis spreads to the subarachnoid space. In the United States, this complication most often affects older adults, usually from reactivation of latent disease. Manifestations develop gradually, with listlessness, irritability, anorexia, and fever. Headache and behavior changes are common early symptoms in the older adult. As the disease progresses, the headache increases in intensity, vomiting develops, and the level of consciousness decreases. Convulsions and coma may follow. Without appropriate treatment, neurologic effects may become permanent.

### Skeletal Tuberculosis

Tuberculosis of the bones and joints is most likely to occur during childhood, when bone epiphyses are open and their blood supply is rich. The organisms spread via the blood to vertebrae, the ends of long bones, and joints. Immune and inflammatory processes isolate the bacilli, and the disease often becomes evident years or decades later.

Tuberculous spondylitis usually involves the thoracic vertebrae, eroding vertebral bodies and causing them to collapse. Significant kyphosis develops, and the spinal cord may be compressed. The large, weight-bearing joints (hips and knees) are most often affected by tuberculous arthritis, although other joints may be affected, particularly if they have been previously damaged. The involved joint is painful, warm, and tender.

## COLLABORATIVE CARE

Tuberculosis was a major public health concern earlier in this century, before the development of effective sanitation measures and drug treatment. Developing drug-resistant strains,

---

### Manifestations of Pulmonary Tuberculosis

- Fatigue
- Weight loss
- Anorexia
- Low-grade afternoon fever and night sweats
- Cough: initially dry, later productive of purulent and/or blood-tinged sputum

susceptibility of people with HIV disease, and inadequate access to health care for high-risk populations contribute to the continuing significance of tuberculosis as a significant public health threat. Collaborative care, therefore, focuses on the following:

- Early detection
- Accurate diagnosis
- Effective disease treatment
- Preventing tuberculosis spread to others

Hospitalization is rarely required to treat tuberculosis. With appropriate treatment, clients become noninfective to others fairly rapidly. However, a client with active tuberculosis may be admitted for a concurrent problem or a complication of the disease. Nurses and other health care workers are at risk for exposure if the disease has not yet been diagnosed. When a client with tuberculosis is institutionalized, maintain respiratory isolation to minimize the risk of infection to other clients and to the health care workers.

Noncompliance with prescribed treatment is a major problem in treating active tuberculosis: The client can continue transmitting the disease to others, and drug-resistant strains of bacteria can develop when treatment is incomplete. Tuberculosis must be reported to local and state public health departments; contacts are identified and examined. People who share living or work environments with the client are tested and receive prophylactic treatment. Continuing contact with clients who have active TB is vital to ensure effective cure.

## Screening

The tuberculin test is used to screen for tuberculosis infection. A cellular, or delayed hypersensitivity, response to *M. tuberculosis* develops within 3 to 10 weeks after the infection. Injecting a small amount of *purified protein derivative (PPD)* of tuberculin any time thereafter activates this response, attracting macrophages to the area and causing a pronounced local inflammatory response. The amount of induration surrounding the injection site is used to determine infection (see Table 36–4 and Figure 36–8 ■). It is important to remember that a positive response indicates that infection and a cellular (T-cell) response have developed; however, it does not mean that active disease is present or that the client is infectious to others.

Several methods are currently available for tuberculin testing:

- *Intradermal PPD (Mantoux) test:* 0.1 mL of PPD (5 tuberculin units, or TU) is injected intradermally into the dorsal aspect of the forearm. This test is read within 48 to 72 hours, the peak reaction period, and recorded as the diameter of induration (raised area, not erythema) in millimeters.
- *Multiple-puncture (tine) test:* A multiple-puncture device is used to introduce tuberculin into the skin. This test is less accurate than other testing methods. A vesicular reaction is considered positive; any other reaction must be confirmed using a Mantoux test.

Although it is impractical and unnecessary to screen the entire population, the Centers for Disease Control and Preven-

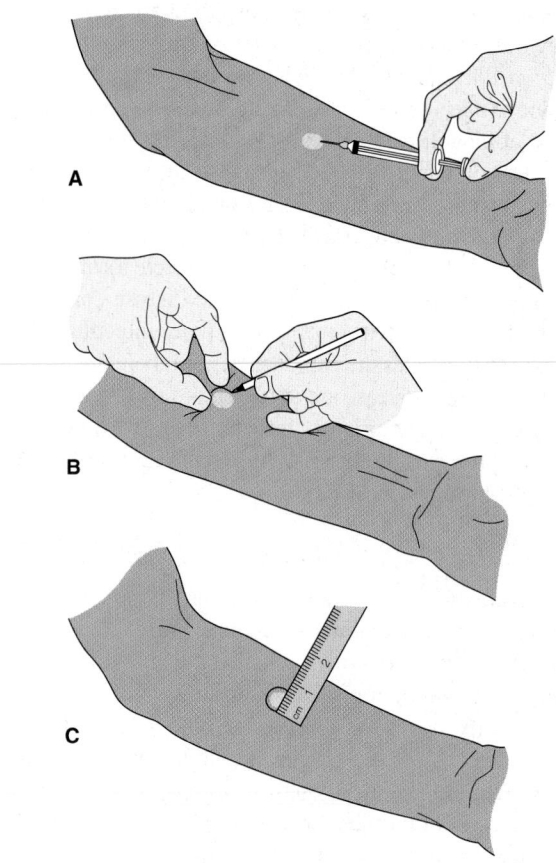

**Figure 36–8** ■ *A,* Intradermal injection for tuberculin testing. *B,* The injection causes a local inflammatory response (wheal). *C,* Measurement of induration following tuberculin testing.

| TABLE 36–4 | Interpreting Tuberculin Test Results |
|---|---|
| **Area of Induration** | **Significance** |
| Less than 5 mm | Negative response; does not rule out infection. |
| 5 to 9 mm | Positive for people who:<br>• Are in close contact with a client with infective TB.<br>• Have an abnormal chest X-ray.<br>• Have HIV infection.<br>Negative for all others. |
| 10 to 15 mm | Positive for people who have other risk factors:<br>• Birth in a high-incidence country<br>• Low socioeconomic status<br>• African American, Hispanic, Asian American in poverty areas<br>• Injection drug use<br>• Residence in a long-term care facility<br>• Identified local risk factors |
| Greater than 15 mm | Positive for all people |

tion (CDC) recommends screening people in the following risk groups.

- People with or at high risk for HIV infection
- Close contacts of people who have or are suspected of having infectious TB
- People with medical risk factors, such as silicosis, chronic malabsorption, end-stage renal failure, diabetes mellitus, immunosuppression, and hematologic and other malignancies
- People born in countries with a high prevalence of TB
- Medically underserved low-income populations, including racial and ethnic minorities
- Alcoholics and injection drug users
- Residents and staff of long-term residential facilities, such as long-term care facilities, correctional institutions, and mental health facilities

False-negative responses are common in people who are immunosuppressed. A two-step procedure may be necessary to elicit a positive response. If the first test elicits a negative response, a second PPD test is given 1 week later. If the second test also is negative, the client either is free of infection or is *anergic* (unable to react to common antigens). This two-step procedure is recommended for long-term care residents and workers.

## Diagnostic Tests

A positive tuberculin test alone does not indicate active disease. Sputum tests for the bacillus and chest X-rays are routinely used to diagnose and evaluate active disease. A series of three consecutive early-morning sputum specimens is typically examined for bacilli (see Procedure 36–1). Use special procedures or personal protective devices when obtaining sputum specimens. If possible, collect specimens in a room equipped with airflow control devices, ultraviolet light, or both. Alternatively, have the client step outside to collect the specimen. Wear a mask capable of filtering droplet nuclei when collecting sputum specimens. Aerosol therapy, percussion, and postural drainage may help the client produce sputum. Occasionally, endotracheal suctioning, bronchoscopy, or gastric lavage may be necessary to obtain a specimen. See the box on page 1082 for nursing care related to bronchoscopy.

- *Sputum smear* is microscopically examined for *acid-fast bacilli. M. tuberculosis* resists decolorizing chemicals after staining. This property is called "acid-fast." The acid-fast smear provides a rapid indicator of the tubercle bacillus.
- *Sputum culture* positive for *M. tuberculosis* provides the definitive diagnosis. However, *M. tuberculosis* is slow growing, requiring 4 to 8 weeks before it can be detected using traditional culture techniques. Automated radiometric culture systems (such as Bactec) allow detection of *M. tuberculosis* in several days.
- Once the organism is detected, *sensitivity testing* is performed to identify appropriate drug therapy.
- *Polymerase chain reaction (PCR)* permits rapid detection of DNA from *M. tuberculosis.*

- *Chest X-ray* is ordered to diagnose and evaluate TB. Typical findings in pulmonary TB include dense lesions in the apical and posterior segments of the upper lobe and possible cavity formation.

Prior to initiating antituberculosis drug therapy, several additional diagnostic tests may be done to establish baseline data for monitoring potential adverse effects of the drugs.

- *Liver function tests* are obtained prior to treatment with isoniazid (INH) as this drug is hepatotoxic.
- A thorough *vision examination* is done prior to treatment with ethambutol, a commonly used antituberculosis medication. Optic neuritis is a potential adverse effect of this drug. Periodic eye examinations are scheduled during the course of therapy.
- *Audiometric testing* is performed before streptomycin therapy is initiated. Ototoxicity is a significant adverse effect of streptomycin and other aminoglycoside antibiotics. Hearing also is evaluated periodically during the course of therapy to detect any hearing loss.

## Medications

Chemotherapeutic medications are used both to prevent and treat tuberculosis infection. Goals of the pharmacologic treatment of TB are to:

- Make the disease noncommunicable to others.
- Reduce symptoms of the disease.
- Effect a cure in the shortest possible time.

Prophylactic treatment is used to prevent active tuberculosis. Clients with a recent skin test conversion from negative to positive are often started on prophylactic therapy, especially when other risk factors are present. Prophylactic therapy also is used for people in close household contact with a person whose sputum is positive for bacilli. Single-drug therapy is effective for prophylactic treatment, whereas treatment of active disease always involves two or more chemotherapeutic medications. For adults, isoniazid (INH), 300 mg per day for a period of 6 to 12 months, is commonly used to prevent active TB.

When isoniazid prophylaxis is contraindicted, bacilli Calmette-Guérin (BCG) vaccine may be prescribed. This vaccine is widely used in developing countries. BCG is made from an attenuated strain of *M. bovis,* a closely related bacillus that causes tuberculosis in cattle. In the United States, BCG vaccine is recommended only for infants, children, and health care workers with a negative tuberculin test who are repeatedly exposed to untreated or ineffectively treated people with active disease. After vaccination with BCG, a positive reaction to tuberculin testing is common. Periodic chest X-rays may be required for screening purposes.

The tuberculosis bacillus mutates readily to drug-resistant forms when only one anti-infective agent is used. Active disease is always treated with concurrent use of at least two antibacterial medications to which the organism is sensitive. The primary antituberculosis drugs can prevent development of resistance because all act by different mechanisms. However, the

### TABLE 36–5  Antituberculosis Medications

| Drug and Dosage | Adverse Effects | Nursing Implications |
|---|---|---|
| Isoniazid (INH), oral:<br>  300 mg daily or<br>  900 mg twice weekly | Peripheral neuropathy<br>Hepatitis | Administer pyridoxine (vitamin B$_6$) concurrently.<br>Monitor liver function studies (AST and ALT); avoid other hepatotoxins. |
| Rifampin (RMP), oral:<br>  600 mg daily or<br>  twice weekly | Hepatitis<br>Flulike syndrome; fever<br><br>Colors body fluids—including sweat, urine, saliva, tears, and cerebrospinal fluid (CSF)—orange-red | As for INH.<br>Do not miss or skip doses; flulike syndrome and fever occur when drug is resumed.<br>Contact lenses may become discolored and should not be worn. |
| Pyrazinamide (PZA), oral:<br>  15 to 30 mg/kg, up to 2 g daily;<br>  or 30 to 70 mg/kg twice weekly | Hyperuricemia<br>Hepatotoxicity | Monitor uric acid levels.<br>Monitor AST and ALT; avoid other hepatotoxins. |
| Ethambutol (EMB), oral:<br>  15 to 25 mg/kg, up to 2.5 g daily;<br>  or 50 mg/kg twice weekly | Optic neuritis | Monitor red-green color discrimination and visual acuity. |
| Streptomycin (SM), intramuscular:<br>  15 mg/kg, up to 1 g daily;<br>  or 25 to 30 mg/kg twice weekly | Ototoxicity, vertigo<br>Nephrotoxicity | Have periodic audiometric examinations conducted.<br>Monitor renal function studies, including BUN and serum creatinine. |

organism is protected within the tubercule, and 6 or more months of treatment is necessary to eradicate it.

Newly diagnosed tuberculosis is typically treated with an initial regimen of three oral antitubercular drugs, isoniazid (INH), rifampin, and pyrazinamide, daily for the first 2 months of treatment. This initial regimen is followed by at least 4 additional months of therapy with isoniazid and rifampin, given daily or two or three times weekly. In the presence of HIV infection, treatment is continued for at least 9 months. The most common antituberculosis drugs are outlined in Table 36–5; their nursing implications are outlined in the box below.

If a drug-resistant strain is suspected, therapy is tailored to the resistance. In some cases, four or more anti-infective drugs may be used.

Antitubercular medications have many adverse and toxic effects. Close monitoring during therapy is necessary. Most have some degree of, or risk for, hepatotoxicity. For this reason, clients should avoid using alcohol and other drugs (such as acetaminophen) or chemicals that can damage the liver. Baseline liver and renal function studies are done prior to initiating therapy. Audiometric testing also may be done before treatment is started, because several commonly used medications can affect hearing. Regular visits to a health care provider are necessary to evaluate regularly for adverse effects. Although none of these drugs have been proved to be teratogenic, potential adverse effects on the fetus are weighed against the benefit to the mother before they are prescribed during pregnancy.

Compliance with the prescribed regimen also is evaluated during follow-up visits. The urine can be examined for color changes characteristic of rifampin and tested for metabolites of INH. When compliance is a problem, medications are administered under direct supervision. Twice-weekly therapy is more cost-effective in this instance, with a public health nurse watching the client take and swallow the prescribed medication.

Repeat sputum specimens and chest X-rays are used to evaluate the effectiveness of therapy. In most cases, sputum cultures for *M. tuberculosis* are negative within 2 months of therapy; virtually all clients have negative sputum cultures within 3 months. If cultures remain positive at 3 months and beyond, treatment failure and drug resistance are suspected. In this case, cultures of the organism are tested for susceptibility to antitubercular agents, and two or three previously unused drugs are added to the treatment regimen (Braunwald et al., 2001).

## Medication Administration

### Antituberculosis Drugs

#### ISONIAZID (INH, LANIAZID, NYDRAZID)

Isoniazid is the drug of choice for tuberculosis prophylaxis and a first-line drug for treating active disease. It is effective against both intracellular and extracellular organisms. Isoniazid is used alone as a prophylactic medication and in combination with rifampin, ethambutol, or both. A fixed-dose combination form with 150 mg of INH and 300 mg of rifampin (Rifamate) is available as well.

#### Nursing Responsibilities

- Administer on an empty stomach 1 hour before or 2 hours after meals for maximal effect if tolerated; May be given with meals to reduce gastrointestinal effects.
- Monitor for adverse effects.
  a. Numbness and tingling of the extremities (most likely to occur in malnourished, alcoholic, or diabetic clients)

# Medication Administration

## Antituberculosis Drugs (continued)

b. Hepatotoxicity, as evidenced by abnormal liver function studies and scleral jaundice

c. Hypersensitivity reactions, such as rash, drug fever, or evidence of anemia, bruising, bleeding, or infection related to agranulocytosis

- Isoniazid interferes with the metabolism of diazepam (Valium), phenytoin (Dilantin), and carbamazepine. Doses of these drugs may need to be reduced to prevent toxicity.

### Client and Family Teaching

- Take the medication as prescribed for the entire treatment period to prevent incomplete eradication of the bacteria and development of resistant strains.
- Take the medication on an empty stomach. If nausea and vomiting occur, take with meals.
- If anorexia, nausea, vomiting, and jaundice (yellowing of the skin and the whites of the eyes) develop, notify your doctor immediately.
- Take pyridoxine as prescribed to prevent peripheral neuropathy.
- Avoid alcohol and other agents that may be harmful to the liver.
- Notify your doctor if you develop signs of an allergic reaction, such as rash, fever, easy bruising, bleeding gums, or fatigue.
- Use measures to prevent pregnancy while taking INH; this drug may be harmful to the developing fetus.

### RIFAMPIN (RIFADIN, RIMACTANE)

Rifampin is commonly used in combination with INH and other antitubercular drugs. It is relatively low in toxicity, although it can cause hepatitis, a flulike immune response, and, rarely, renal failure. Rifampin stimulates the microsomal enzymes of the liver, increasing the rate of metabolism of many drugs and decreasing their effectiveness.

### Nursing Responsibilities

- Administer on an empty stomach.
- Monitor CBC, liver function studies, and renal function studies for evidence of toxicity.
- Rifampin reduces the effect of oral contraceptives, quinidine, corticosteroids, warfarin, methadone, digoxin, and hypoglycemics. Monitor for the effectiveness of these drugs.

### Client and Family Teaching

- Rifampin causes body fluids, including sweat, urine, saliva, and tears, to turn red-orange. This is not harmful. Avoid wearing soft contact lenses because they may be permanently stained.
- Aspirin may interfere with rifampin absorption and should not be taken concurrently.
- Fever, flulike symptoms, excessive fatigue, sore throat, or unusual bleeding may indicate an adverse reaction to the drug and should be reported to your doctor.

### PYRAZINAMIDE (TEBRAZID)

Pyrazinamide typically is given with INH and rifampin for the first 2 months of tuberculosis treatment. Concurrent use of pyrazinamide allows a shorter course of therapy. As with many of the antitubercular agents, pyrazinamide is toxic to the liver. Its other principal adverse effect is hyperuricemia. Gout, however, rarely develops.

### Nursing Responsibilities

- Administer with meals to reduce gastrointestinal side effects.
- Monitor liver function studies and serum uric acid levels. Notify the physician if changes are noted.

### Client and Family Teaching

- Notify your doctor if you develop loss of appetite, nausea, vomiting, jaundice, or symptoms of gout (a painful, red, hot, swollen joint, often the great toe or elbow).
- While taking this drug, avoid using alcohol or other substances that may be harmful to the liver.

### ETHAMBUTOL (MYAMBUTOL)

Ethambutol is added to the initial treatment regimen or substituted for INH when an INH-resistant strain of TB is suspected. Ethambutol is a bacteriostatic drug that reduces the development of resistance to the bactericidal first-line agents. Its principal toxic effect is optic neuritis; fortunately, this is reversible. Early signs of optic neuritis include decreased visual acuity and loss of red-green discrimination. This drug may be safe for use in pregnancy.

### Nursing Responsibilities

- Record a baseline visual examination prior to therapy. Schedule periodic eye exams during the course of treatment.
- Administer with meals to reduce gastrointestinal side effects.
- Monitor liver and renal function studies and neurologic status while taking this drug. Notify the physician of abnormal findings or significant changes.

### Client and Family Teaching

- Monitor vision daily by reading newspapers and looking at the same blue object (using usual corrective lenses, if appropriate). Notify your doctor if changes in vision or color perception occur.

### STREPTOMYCIN

An aminoglycoside antibiotic, streptomycin is highly effective in treating most mycobacterial infection. Resistance may develop if it is used alone. There are two primary drawbacks to streptomycin: (1) It must be administered parenterally because it is not absorbed in the gastrointestinal tract, and (2) it has toxic effects on the kidneys and ears.

### Nursing Responsibilities

- Administer by deep intramuscular injection into a large muscle mass, rotating sites to minimize tissue trauma.
- Monitor urine output, weight, and renal function studies (including BUN and serum creatinine) to detect early signs of nephrotoxicity. Report significant changes to the physician.
- Maintain fluid intake at 2000 to 3000 mL per day to minimize the concentration of drug in the kidney tubules.
- Assess hearing and balance frequently. Have audiometric testing performed as indicated.

### Client and Family Teaching

- Maintain a daily fluid intake of at least 2½ to 3 quarts.
- Weigh yourself on the same scale at least twice a week; report any significant weight gain to your doctor.
- Notify your doctor if hearing acuity decreases, ringing or buzzing sensations in the ear develop, or dizziness occurs.

With adherence to prescribed treatment, virtually all clients should have negative sputum cultures for *M. tuberculosis* within 3 months. The relapse rate for current treatment regimens is less than 5%. The principal cause of treatment failure is noncompliance (Tierney et al., 2001).

## NURSING CARE

### Health Promotion

Tuberculosis today presents a greater threat to public health than it does to individuals. Nurses play a key role in maintaining public health. Education and tuberculosis screening are major nursing strategies to prevent TB. Public health teaching includes increasing awareness of tuberculosis as a reemerging threat. Teach clients in all settings how to reduce the spread of TB by covering their mouths when coughing or sneezing and disposing of sputum appropriately. The benefit of screening programs to identify infected (though not necessarily infective) people also needs to be included in public health education.

The best tuberculosis prevention is early diagnosis of infections and appropriate treatment to achieve cure. BCG vaccine is recommended for infants born in countries where tuberculosis is prevalent, but is not widely used in the United States. It may be administered to health care workers in settings where the risk of infection with MDR strains of *M. tb* is high despite rigorous infection control measures (Braunwald et al., 2001).

The primary preventive strategy used in the United States is treating people with latent tuberculosis infection demonstrated by a positive tuberculin test. A 9- to 10-month course of treatment with isoniazid reduces the risk of active TB by 90% or more (Braunwald et al., 2001). Isoniazid also is prescribed prophylactically for people with HIV infection who have been exposed to TB.

### Assessment

Focused assessment for the client with suspected TB includes the following:

- Health history: complaints of fatigue, weight loss, night sweats, difficulty breathing, cough (productive or nonproductive), bloody sputum, or chest pain; known exposure to TB; most recent tuberculin test and results; living circumstances; alcohol and other recreational drug use
- Physical examination: vital signs including temperature; general appearance; respiratory rate and lung sounds

### Nursing Diagnoses and Interventions

Nursing care related to tuberculosis focuses primarily on infection control and compliance with prescribed treatment.

#### Deficient Knowledge

Adequate knowledge and information are necessary to manage the disease and prevent its transmission to others. The client needs to understand reasons for prolonged drug therapy and the importance of complying with treatment and follow-up. Anti-

tuberculosis drugs are relatively toxic. The client needs to know how to minimize toxicity.

- Assess knowledge about the disease process; identify misperceptions and emotional reactions. *Teaching based on previous learning enhances understanding and retention of information.*
- Assess ability and interest in learning, developmental level, and obstacles to learning. *Assessment allows presentation of information in a manner tailored to the learning needs and style of the client, promoting learning.*
- Identify support systems, and include significant others in teaching. *A knowledgeable significant other provides reinforcement of learning, confirmation of understanding, and encouragement for the client. Including significant others also reduces the risk of inadvertent sabotage of the treatment plan.*
- Establish a relationship of mutual trust with the client and significant others. *An atmosphere of trust increases receptiveness to teaching and learning.*
- Develop mutually acceptable learning goals with the client and significant other. *Working together to identify learning needs and establish goals increases the client's "ownership" and interest in the process.*
- Select appropriate teaching strategies, using learning aids such as literature and visual materials that are appropriate for age, level of education, and intellect. *Teaching tailored to the client is more effective and results in better learning.*
- Teach about tuberculosis and the prescribed treatment, including:
  a. Nature of the disease and its spread.
  b. Purpose of treatment and follow-up procedures.
  c. Measures to prevent spreading the disease to others.
  d. Importance of maintaining good general health by eating a well-balanced, high-protein, high-carbohydrate diet; balancing exercise with rest; and avoiding crowds and people with upper respiratory infections.
  e. Names, doses, purposes, and adverse effects of prescribed medications.
  f. Importance of avoiding alcohol and other substances that may damage the liver while taking chemotherapeutic drugs.
  g. Fluid intake needs of 2.5 to 3.0 quarts of fluid per day.
  h. Manifestations to report to the physician: chest pain, hemoptysis, difficulty breathing; anorexia, nausea, or vomiting; yellow tint to skin or sclera; sudden weight gain, swollen feet, ankles, legs, or hands; hearing loss, tinnitus, or vertigo; change in vision or difficulty discriminating colors.
  *Tuberculosis is a chronic disease requiring lengthy treatment with antitubercular medications. A good understanding of the disease, its treatment, and potential adverse effects of therapy prepares the client to manage care.*
- Document teaching and level of understanding. Reinforce teaching and learning as needed. *Teaching is not complete until the client can demonstrate learning of the information.*

#### Ineffective Therapeutic Regimen Management

The populations at highest risk for developing active tuberculosis—the homeless and members of lower socioeconomic groups—are also at high risk for being unable to manage its complex treatment regimen. Three or more costly medications that may have unpleasant or even dangerous side effects are prescribed. Frequent medical follow-up is required. Infectious diseases such as TB carry a stigma that may lead to denial of the disease or its seriousness. Alcoholics and IV drug users need to withdraw from their addiction to be successful in treating the disease. The client with HIV infection faces a potentially fatal disease and costly treatment that may well override concerns about tuberculosis management.

- Assess self-care abilities and support systems. *Assessment is used to help determine the client's ability to follow the prescribed regimen.*
- Assess knowledge and understanding of the disease, its complications, treatment, and risks to others. Provide additional teaching and reinforcement as indicated. *Lack of understanding is a barrier to compliance with and management of the treatment regimen.*
- Work collaboratively to identify barriers or obstacles to managing the prescribed treatment. *Working collaboratively with the client and other members of the health care team provides insight for overcoming identified barriers to effective treatment.*
- Assist the client, significant others (if available), and health care team members to develop a plan for managing the prescribed regimen. *Including the client in developing a plan to manage care increases the sense of control and ownership and helps ensure that personal, cultural, and lifestyle factors are considered. This increases the likelihood of compliance.*
- Provide verbal and written instructions that are clear and appropriate for level of literacy, knowledge, and understanding. *Clearly written directions provide support and reinforcement for the client.*
- Provide active intervention for homeless people, including shelter placement or other housing and ongoing follow-up by easily accessed health care providers (clinics and public health workers in the neighborhood that do not present transportation or access problems, either real or perceived). *Simple referral will not ensure compliance, especially among disenfranchised populations. Active intervention is needed to help ensure treatment compliance.*
- Refer clients who are unlikely to comply with the treatment regimen to the public health department for management and follow-up. *Because tuberculosis presents a significant public health risk, public health follow-up is essential. In some cases, it is necessary for nurses to administer medications, observing the client swallow all pills.*

### Risk for Infection

The spread of tuberculosis is a risk in any facility housing many people. It is especially high in residential care facilities for older clients and for people with AIDS. The increasing incidence of TB among homeless people and members of lower socioeconomic groups increases the risk in hospitals, emergency departments, and public and urgent care clinics. Respiratory precautions are necessary to prevent the spread of TB

via microscopic airborne droplets to other clients and to health care workers.

- Place the client in a private room with airflow control that prevents air within the room from circulating into the hallway or other rooms. A negative flow room in which air is diluted by at least six fresh-air exchanges per hour is recommended. *A negative flow room and multiple fresh-air exchanges dilute the concentration of droplet nuclei within the room and prevent their spread to adjacent areas.*
- Use standard precautions and tuberculosis isolation techniques as recommended by the CDC, including wearing masks and gowns when caring for clients who do not reliably cover the mouth when coughing. *These measures are important to prevent the spread of tuberculosis to others.*

**PRACTICE ALERT** *Use personal protective devices to reduce the risk of transmission during client care. The Occupational Safety and Health Administration (OSHA) requires use of a HEPA-filtered respirator for protection against occupational exposure to tuberculosis. Surgical masks are ineffective to filter droplet nuclei, necessitating the use of protective devices capable of filtering bacteria and particles smaller than 1 micron.* ■

- Discuss the reasons for and importance of respiratory isolation procedures during initial hospitalization. When treatment is provided as an outpatient, instruct to avoid crowds and close physical contact and maintain ventilation in living facilities, particularly during the first 3 weeks of treatment. *These measures help protect others during initial treatment, when sputum is still likely to contain significant numbers of bacilli.*
- Place a mask on the client when transporting to other parts of the facility for diagnostic or treatment procedures. *Covering the client's nose and mouth during transport minimizes air contamination and the risk to visitors and personnel.*
- Inform all personnel having contact with the client of the diagnosis. *This allows personnel to take appropriate precautions.*
- Assist visitors to mask prior to entering the room. *Providing visitors with appropriate masks or respirators reduces their risk of infection.*
- Teach the client how to limit transmitting the disease to others:
  a. Always cough and expectorate into tissues.
  b. Dispose of tissues properly, placing them in a closed bag.
  c. Wear a mask if you are sneezing or unable to control respiratory secretions.
  d. The disease is not spread by touching inanimate objects, so no special precautions are required for eating utensils, clothing, books, or other objects used.

  *Teaching appropriate precautions helps prevent the spread of tuberculosis to others while allowing as much freedom from restraints as possible.*
- Teach how to collect sputum specimens. If necessary, have the client step outside to collect a sputum specimen. *This minimizes the risk of exposure to health care personnel and provides for rapid dilution of any droplet nuclei produced and their exposure to ultraviolet light (which kills the bacteria).*

## CHART 36–2 NANDA, NIC, AND NOC LINKAGES

### The Client with Tuberculosis

| NURSING DIAGNOSES | NURSING INTERVENTIONS | NURSING OUTCOMES |
| --- | --- | --- |
| • Fatigue | • Energy Management<br>• Nutrition Management | • Activity Tolerance<br>• Endurance |
| • Deficient Knowledge | • Health System Guidance<br>• Teaching: Disease Process<br>• Teaching: Prescribed Medication | • Knowledge: Health Resources<br>• Knowledge: Infection Control<br>• Knowledge: Medication |
| • Ineffective Therapeutic Regimen Management | • Learning Facilitation<br>• Patient Contracting<br>• Self-Responsibility Facilitation | • Compliance Behavior<br>• Treatment Behavior: Illness or Injury |
| • Risk for Infection | • Health Screening<br>• Infection Control | • Immune Status<br>• Infection Status |

*Note. Data from Nursing Outcomes Classification (NOC) by M. Johnson & M. Maas (Eds.), 1997, St. Louis: Mosby; Nursing Diagnoses: Definitions & Classification 2001–2002 by North American Nursing Diagnosis Association, 2001, Philadelphia: NANDA; Nursing Interventions Classification (NIC) by J.C. McCloskey & G. M. Bulechek (Eds.), 2000, St. Louis: Mosby. Reprinted by permission.*

• Teach the importance of complying with prescribed treatment for the entire course of therapy. *Completion of the entire treatment regimen is important to reduce the risk of relapse and creation of drug-resistant organisms.*

## Using NANDA, NIC, and NOC

Chart 36–2 shows links between NANDA nursing diagnoses, NIC, and NOC for the client with tuberculosis.

## Home Care

Most clients with TB are managed in community settings; few require institutionalization. In addition to the teaching topics and strategies identified above, discuss the following topics when preparing the client and significant others for home care.

• Importance of screening close contacts for infection and possibly prophylactic treatment

• Effect, dose, and timing for all medications, and potential side effects and their management
• Importance of long-term therapy in eradicating the disease
• Principles of good nutrition, dietary guidelines for a client with TB, and other measures to help maintain good health, such as balancing rest with exercise
• Signs and symptoms of complications to report to the physician or health care provider.

Provide referrals as appropriate:

• Smoking cessation clinics or support groups
• Alcohol treatment facilities, Alcoholics Anonymous, other treatment programs or support groups
• Drug treatment facilities, Narcotics Anonymous, other outpatient or inpatient treatment programs or support groups
• Low-cost community clinics and incentive programs for people with TB
• Counseling, support groups, and other community resources that provide additional assistance and support

## Nursing Care Plan
### A Client with Tuberculosis

Harry Facée, age 53, arrives at a metropolitan public health clinic complaining of aching chest pain that has lasted for the past few days. He says that his sputum also is bloody. He is afraid he might have lung cancer, so he came in to see a doctor.

### ASSESSMENT

Raj Kamil, RN, the public health nurse at the clinic, obtains an admission history and physical examination of Mr. Facée. Mr. Kamil notes that Mr. Facée is a homeless person who has lived on the streets and in various shelters for the past "10 years or so." He usually prefers to sleep outdoors, taking refuge in shelters only during very cold or very wet weather. He has a small disability income, but usually scrounges for food or eats with other homeless people at soup kitchens. Mr. Facée states that he has had a cough for a long time, which has become worse recently. It is now productive, especially in the mornings. He also admits that he has recently been waking up drenched with sweat in the middle of the night and is more tired than usual.

Although Mr. Facée's clothes are tattered, he is fairly clean. He answers questions appropriately and intelligently. Mr. Kamil does not detect any odor of alcohol on his breath. He is very thin, almost

## Nursing Care Plan
### A Client with Tuberculosis (continued)

emaciated. Mr. Facée's vital signs are BP 152/86, P 92, R 20, and T 100.2°F (37.8°C).

Suspecting tuberculosis, Mr. Kamil obtains a sputum specimen for Gram stain and culture, administers a tuberculin test, and sends Mr. Facée for a chest X-ray before he sees the clinic physician. Although the chest X-ray is inconclusive, the Gram stain is positive for acid-fast bacilli. The diagnosis of probable active pulmonary tuberculosis is made. The physician prescribes isoniazid, 300 mg orally; rifampin, 600 mg orally; and pyrazinamide, 1500 mg orally daily for 2 months, to be followed by twice weekly isoniazid 900 mg orally and rifampin 600 mg orally. The physician also orders weekly sputum cultures for the first month.

### DIAGNOSES
- *Ineffective health maintenance* related to homelessness
- *Risk for noncompliance with prescribed treatment* related to lack of understanding and resources
- *Imbalanced nutrition: Less than body requirements* related to increased metabolic needs associated with infection
- *Risk for disturbed sensory perception: Kinesthetic* related to effects of isoniazid therapy

### EXPECTED OUTCOMES
- Keep all follow-up appointments as scheduled.
- Verbalize an understanding of his disease and its treatment.
- Follow the prescribed plan of care.
- Demonstrate measures to prevent spread of the organism to others.
- Gain 1 to 2 lb of weight per week.
- Promptly report symptoms of peripheral neuropathy, including numbness, tingling, or burning sensations.

### PLANNING AND IMPLEMENTATION
- Teach about tuberculosis, and provide a client education pamphlet about the disease.
- Instruct about the prescribed medications, potential adverse effects, and the importance of completing the entire prescribed regimen.
- Emphasize the importance of continued follow-up.
- Teach and demonstrate sputum and droplet control measures.
- Escort to the local incentive shelter program for directly observed medical therapy and meals.
- Identify verbally and in writing manifestations to report to the physician.

### EVALUATION
Mr. Kamil successfully enrolls Mr. Facée in the local incentive shelter program. In this program, a health care worker administers Mr. Facée's medications daily, watching him swallow them. He is assigned a small individual room and can eat three daily meals at the shelter. He still prefers to sleep outside when the weather permits, but he complies with the requirement for supervised medication administration because he "likes the food there." Always a clean person, Mr. Facée is able to demonstrate appropriate sputum control measures and practices them faithfully. The sputum culture done after 2 months of treatment is negative for tubercle bacilli, and his chest X-ray indicates no disease progression.

### Critical Thinking in the Nursing Process
1. Many homeless people have schizophrenia or other mental diseases. How would you adapt the care plan for a homeless schizophrenic client with active tuberculosis?
2. Mr. Kamil was fortunate in having access to an incentive shelter with health care workers to supervise medication compliance. Identify available resources in your area for homeless clients infected with tuberculosis.
3. Develop a care plan for the nursing diagnosis, *Ineffective airway clearance* related to mucopurulent sputum and weak cough.

See Evaluating Your Response in Appendix C.

## THE CLIENT WITH INHALATION ANTHRAX

*Inhalation anthrax* is a relatively new potential threat in the United States. This disease rarely affects humans in nature, even though both wild and domestic animals can be infected. However, *Bacillus anthracis,* the spore-forming rod responsible for causing anthrax, has been identified as an agent likely to be used as a biologic weapon. Anthrax spores can be aerosolized so they remain suspended in the air, allowing them to be inhaled into the lungs. Person-to-person transmission does not occur.

Inhalation anthrax causes initial flulike symptoms, including malaise, dry cough, and fever. This is followed by an abrupt onset of severe dyspnea, stridor, and cyanosis. Lymph nodes in the mediastinum and thorax become inflamed and enlarged. Septic shock and/or meningitis may develop. Untreated, death results from hemorrhagic thoracic lymphadenitis and hemorrhagic mediastinitis (Persell et al., 2002).

Blood cultures and chest X-ray are used to diagnose inhalation anthrax. However, because death can quickly result from the disease, people who are known or suspected to have been exposed to anthrax spores often are treated prophylactically. Ciprofloxacin (Cipro) is used to both prevent and treat inhalation anthrax. Doxycycline (Vibramycin) is an alternative to ciprofloxacin. Although an anthrax vaccine exists, its use at this time is considered experiemental (Persell et al., 2002). See the section on bioterrorism in Chapter 8 ⚮ for more information about anthrax and the section of this chapter on respiratory failure for nursing care measures for the client with inhalation anthrax.

# THE CLIENT WITH A FUNGAL INFECTION

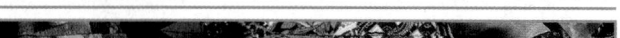

Fungal spores are endemic, present in the air everyone breathes. Normal respiratory defense mechanisms allow few of these spores to reach the lungs. If they reach the lungs, pulmonary macrophages and neutrophils efficiently remove them in most people. When they do cause infection, it is typically mild and self-limiting. Most fungi are opportunistic, able to cause infection only in people who are immunocompromised. For this reason, clients with AIDS, renal failure, leukemia, burns, or chronic diseases, as well as people receiving corticosteroids or immunosuppressants, are particularly susceptible to fungal diseases.

Many fungal lung diseases have a geographic distribution pattern. Histoplasmosis and blastomycosis are more common in the southeastern, mid-Atlantic, and central states. California, Arizona, and western Texas are the primary sites for coccidioidomycosis, also known as San Joaquin valley fever (Braunwald et al., 2001).

The course and manifestations of fungal lung diseases resemble those of tuberculosis. Lung lesions are slow to develop, and symptoms are mild. The fungus can disseminate from the lung to other organs.

## PATHOPHYSIOLOGY

### Histoplasmosis

Histoplasmosis, an infectious disease caused by *Histoplasma capsulatum,* is the most common fungal lung infection in the United States. The organism is found in the soil and is linked to exposure to bird droppings and bats. Infection occurs when the spores are inhaled and reach the alveoli. Most infections develop into *latent asymptomatic disease,* much like tuberculosis, or *primary acute histoplasmosis,* a mild, self-limiting influenzalike illness. Initial chest X-rays are nonspecific; later ones show areas of calcification. *Chronic progressive disease,* usually seen in older adults, typically is limited to the lung but may involve any organ. Progressive lung changes and cavitation occur, with increasing dyspnea and eventual disabling pulmonary disease.

Regional lymph vessels spread the organism from the lungs to other parts of the body, much like the process that occurs in tuberculosis. In the healthy host, normal immune responses inactivate and remove the organism. In the immunocompromised host, however, macrophages remove the fungi but are unable to destroy them, resulting in *disseminated histoplasmosis.* This type of histoplasmosis is often fatal. Manifestations of fever, dyspnea, cough, weight loss, and muscle wasting are usual. Ulcerations of the mouth and oropharynx may be present, and the liver and spleen are enlarged.

## Coccidioidomycosis

Coccidioidomycosis is an infectious disease caused by the fungus *Coccidioides immitis.* This mold grows in the soil of the arid Southwest, Mexico, and Central and South America. When inhaled, the fungus typically causes an acute, self-limiting pulmonary infection that often is asymptomatic and goes unrecognized. If manifestations do occur, they resemble those of influenza, with malaise, fever, body aches, and cough. Pleuritic pain, skin rash, and arthritis of the knees and ankles also may develop. Disseminated disease, which may affect the lymph nodes, meninges, spleen, liver, kidney, skin, and adrenal glands, is rare in immunocompetent people. When it does occur, the mortality rate is high. Meningitis is the usual cause of death.

## Blastomycosis

The fungus *Blastomyces dermatitidis* causes the infectious disease blastomycosis. It occurs primarily in the south central and midwestern regions of the United States and in Canada. Men are affected more frequently than women. The lungs are the primary site for the disease, although it may spread to involve the skin, bones, genitourinary system, and, rarely, the central nervous system. Pulmonary symptoms include fever, dyspnea, pleuritic chest pain, and cough, which may become productive of bloody or purulent sputum. If untreated, the disseminated disease is slowly progressive and ultimately fatal.

## Aspergillosis

*Aspergillus* spores are common in the environment, but rarely cause disease except in the immunocompromised. When they do cause infection, *Aspergillus* species invade blood vessels and produce hyphae that branch at acute angles, frequently causing venous or arterial thrombosis. In the lungs, aspergillosis can cause an acute, diffuse, self-limited pneumonitis. The manifestations of pulmonary aspergillosis include dyspnea, nonproductive cough, pleuritic chest pain, chills, and fever. If the organism invades a pulmonary blood vessel, hemoptysis or massive pulmonary hemorrhage can occur. In clients with underlying lung disease, balls of *Aspergillus* hyphae may form within cysts or cavities, usually in the upper lobes of the lung. Symptoms often are milder and more insidious in onset, with fever, weight loss, night sweats, and cough (Braunwald et al., 2001; Morrison & Lew, 2001).

## COLLABORATIVE CARE

Most fungal lung infections can be diagnosed by microscopic examination of a sputum specimen for the fungus. Blood cultures also may be done, as well as cultures of cerebrospinal fluid if indicated. Chest X-ray may show typical changes in lung tissue or widening of the mediastinum, depending on the infecting organism.

Acute pulmonary histoplasmosis and acute pulmonary coccidioidomycosis usually resolve without treatment, although antifungal drugs may be given to shorten the disease course. Oral itraconazole (Sporanox), a broad-spectrum antifungal agent, is commonly prescribed to treat histoplasmosis. Other fungal lung diseases and clients who are immunocompromised are often treated with intravenous amphotericin B. Surgery (lobectomy) may be indicated for clients with severe hemoptysis associated with aspergillosis.

## NURSING CARE

Clients with fungal lung infections have different nursing care needs, depending on the disease and their immune status. For most clients, nursing care focuses on education. People living in high-prevalence areas or who have specific risk factors such as exposure to bird droppings (for example, by cleaning chicken coops, pigeon lofts, or barns where birds roost), decomposed vegetation, rotting wood, or stored grain need to be aware of the risk, common symptoms, and measures to reduce the risk. Clients with latent histoplasmosis may need education to maintain good general health to prevent reactivation. Teach clients receiving antifungal drugs about the specific drug, its intended and adverse effects, the duration of therapy, and symptoms to report to the physician. Include teaching about any specific precautions such as drug or food interactions. Itraconazole interacts with many medications; verify the safety of concurrent usage with all other prescribed drugs. Its use is contraindicated during pregnancy and lactation; emphasize the importance of effective birth control and of notifying the physician immediately if pregnancy occurs. Amphotericin B is a toxic drug. Administer the intial intravenous dose slowly after premedicating with an antihistamine and antiemetic as ordered to manage its adverse effects. Monitor carefully during infusion and therapy for changes in vital signs, hydration, nutrition, weight, or urine output.

# OBSTRUCTIVE DISORDERS OF THE AIRWAYS

Many pulmonary disorders and diseases can affect the airways. Although their pathophysiology differs, these diseases are characterized by limited airflow. Airflow is limited when:

- Elastic recoil of the lungs is reduced, decreasing the force to push air out.
- Airway lumen are obstructed by secretions, increasing resistance.
- Airway walls are thickened.
- Smooth muscle of the airways is activated, causing bronchoconstriction.
- Interstitial support necessary to maintain airway distention and patency is lost.

Aging contributes to airflow limitation. The number of alveoli decrease, and emphysematous changes (senile emphysema) reduce the surface area for gas exchange. Alveoli become less elastic, causing increased air trapping and dead space.

Limited airflow increases the work of breathing and the residual volume of the lungs as air is trapped behind narrowed or collapsed airways. Inspired air mixes with an abnormally large volume of residual air, effectively reducing the amount of oxygen available in the alveoli. Decreased alveolar ventilation further reduces oxygen available for exchange.

## THE CLIENT WITH ASTHMA

**Asthma** is a chronic inflammatory disorder of the airways characterized by recurrent episodes of wheezing, breathlessness, chest tightness, and coughing. Inflammation causes increased responsiveness of the airways to multiple stimuli. The widespread airflow obstruction that occurs during acute episodes usually reverses either spontaneously or with treatment.

In the United States, approximately 11 million people experienced at least one asthma attack in the year 2000. Although it is more common in children than adults, about 4% of the adult population is affected. After several years of increase, the prevalence of asthma currently is relatively stable. Asthma is a serious disease, causing more than 4000 deaths in the United States in 1999. Mortality due to asthma is higher in blacks than in whites and higher in females than in males (NHLBI, 2002).

A number of risk factors can be identified for asthma, although many clients develop the disease in the absence of known risk factors. Allergies play a strong role in childhood asthma, although less so in adults. There is a strong genetic component to the disease, although a specific pattern of inheritance has not been identified. Environmental factors, including air pollution and occupational exposure to industrial compounds, may contribute. Respiratory viruses such as rhinovirus and influenza can precipitate asthma attacks. Other contributory factors include exercise (particularly in cold air) and emotional stress.

### PHYSIOLOGY REVIEW

Airways within the lungs contain crisscrossing strips of smooth muscle that control their diameter. This muscle is innervated by the autonomic nervous system. Parasympathetic (cholinergic) stimulation leads to bronchoconstriction, or narrowing of the airways. Sympathetic stimulation through $\beta_2$-adrenergic receptors causes bronchodilation, or expansion of the airways. Slight bronchoconstriction normally predominates. However, when increased airflow is necessary (e.g., during exercise), the parasympathetic system is inhibited, and stimulation of the sympathetic system causes bronchodilation. Inflammatory mediators (such as histamine) released during an antigen-antibody response act directly on bronchial smooth muscle to produce bronchoconstriction.

## PATHOPHYSIOLOGY

During symptom-free periods, airway inflammation in asthma is subacute or quiet. An acute inflammatory response may be triggered by a variety of factors. Common triggers for an acute asthma attack include exposure to allergens, respiratory tract infection, exercise, inhaled irritants, and emotional upsets.

Childhood asthma (which may continue into adulthood) is most often linked to inhalation of allergens such as pollen, animal dander, or household dust. Clients with allergic asthma often have a history of other allergies. Environmental pollutants, such as tobacco smoke and irritant gases (e.g., sulfur dioxide, nitrogen dioxide, and ozone) can provoke asthma. Exposure to secondhand smoke as a child is associated with a higher risk for and increased severity of asthma. Agents found in the workplace, such as noxious fumes and gases, chemicals, and dusts, may cause occupational asthma.

Respiratory infections, viral in particular, are a common internal stimulus for an asthmatic attack. Exercise-induced asthma attacks also are common, affecting 40% to 90% of people with bronchial asthma (Porth, 2002). Loss of heat or water from the bronchial surface may contribute to exercise-induced asthma. Exercising in cold, dry air increases the risk of an asthma attack in susceptible people.

Emotional stress is a significant etiologic factor for attacks in as many as half of clients with asthma. Common pharmacologic triggers include aspirin and other NSAIDs, sulfites (which are used as preservatives in wine, beer, fresh fruits, and salad), and beta blockers.

When a trigger such as inhalation of an allergen or irritant occurs, an *acute* or *early response* develops in the hyperreactive airways predisposed to bronchospasm. Sensitized mast cells in the bronchial mucosa release inflammatory mediators such as histamine, prostaglandins, and leukotrienes. These mediators stimulate parasympathetic receptors and bronchial smooth muscle to produce bronchoconstriction. They also increase capillary permeability, leading to mucosal edema, and stimulate mucus production.

The attack is prolonged by the *late phase response,* which develops 4 to 12 hours after exposure to the trigger. Inflammatory cells such as basophils and eosinophils are activated, which damage airway epithelium, produce mucosal edema, impair mucociliary clearance, and produce or prolong bronchoconstriction. The degree of hyperreactivity depends on the extent of inflammation. Together, bronchoconstriction, edema and inflammation, and mucous secretion narrow the airway. Airway resistance increases, limiting airflow, and increasing the work of breathing (Figure 36–9 ■).

Limited expiratory airflow traps air distal to the spastic airways. Trapped air mixes with inspired air in the alveoli, reducing its oxygen tension and gas exchange across the alveolar-capillary membrane. Blood flow is reduced to distended alveoli, further affecting gas exchange. As a result, hypoxemia develops. Hypoxemia and increased lung volume due to trapping stimulate the respiratory rate. As a result, the $PaCO_2$ falls, leading to respiratory alkalosis. (See Chapter 5 ⊂⊃ for more information about acid-base imbalances.)

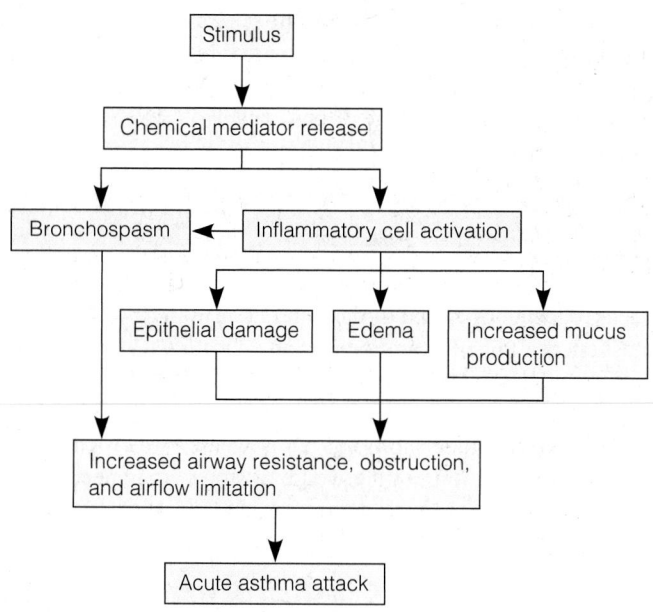

**Figure 36–9 ■** The pathogenesis of an acute episode of asthma.

### Manifestations of Acute Asthma

- Chest tightness
- Dyspnea
- Wheezing
- Cough
- Tachypnea and tachycardia
- Anxiety and apprehension

## MANIFESTATIONS AND COMPLICATIONS

An asthma attack is characterized by a subjective sensation of chest tightness, dyspnea, wheezing, and cough (see the box above). The onset of symptoms may be either abrupt or insidious, and an attack may subside rapidly or persist for hours or days. During an attack, tachycardia, tachypnea, and prolonged expiration are common. Diffuse wheezing is heard on auscultation. With more severe attacks, use of accessory muscles of respiration, intercostal retractions, loud wheezing, and distant breath sounds may be noted. Fatigue, anxiety, apprehension, and severe dyspnea that allows speaking only one or two words between breaths, may occur with persistent severe episodes. The onset of respiratory failure is marked by inaudible breath sounds with reduced wheezing and an ineffective cough. Without careful assessment, this apparent relief of symptoms can be misinterpreted as an improvement.

The frequency of attacks and severity of symptoms vary greatly from person to person. Although some people have infrequent, mild episodes, others have nearly continuous manifestations of cough and wheezing with periodic severe exacerbations (Table 36–6).

**Status asthmaticus** is severe, prolonged asthma that does not respond to routine treatment. Without aggressive therapy, status asthmaticus can lead to respiratory failure with hypox-

| TABLE 36-6 | Classification of Asthma Severity | |
|---|---|---|
| **Classification** | **Symptom Frequency** | **Nighttime Symptoms** |
| Mild intermittent | • No more than twice a week<br>• Brief attacks (hours to days) of varied intensity<br>• Asymptomatic and normal peak expiratory flow (PEF) rate between attacks | No more than twice a month |
| Mild persistent | • More than twice a week but less than once a day<br>• Exacerbations may affect activity | More than twice a month |
| Moderate persistent | • Daily symptoms<br>• Daily short-acting bronchodilator use<br>• Exacerbations affect activity<br>• Exacerbations more than twice a week, may last for days | More than once a week |
| Severe persistent | • Continual symptoms<br>• Limited physical activity<br>• Frequent exacerbations | Frequent |

*Note. Adapted from* Expert Panel Report 2: Guidelines for the Diagnosis and Management of Asthma, *Publication No. 97-4051 by National Education and Prevention Program, 1997, Bethesda, MD: National Institutes of Health.*

emia, hypercapnia, and acidosis. Endotracheal intubation, mechanical ventilation, and aggressive drug treatment may be necessary to sustain life.

In addition to acute respiratory failure, other complications associated with acute asthma include dehydration, respiratory infection, atelectasis, pneumothorax, and cor pulmonale.

## COLLABORATIVE CARE

The diagnosis of asthma is based primarily on the history and manifestations. Treatment goals are twofold. Daily management focuses on controlling symptoms and preventing acute attacks. During an acute attack, therapy is directed toward restoring airway patency and alveolar ventilation.

### Diagnostic Tests

Diagnostic tests are used to determine the degree of airway involvement during and between acute episodes and identify causative factors such as allergens.

- *Pulmonary function tests (PFTs)* are used to evaluate the degree of airway obstruction. Pulmonary function testing done before and after use of an aerosolized bronchodilator helps determine the reversibility of airway obstruction. The residual volume (RV) of the lungs may be increased and vital capacity decreased or normal even during periods of remission. The forced expiratory volume ($FEV_1$) and peak expiratory flow rate (PEFR) are the most valuable pulmonary function studies to evaluate the severity of an asthma attack and the effectiveness of treatment measures. See Box 36–1.
- *Challenge or bronchial provocation testing* uses an inhaled substance such as methacholine or histamine with PFTs to confirm the diagnosis of asthma by detecting airway hyperresponsiveness.

- *ABGs* are drawn during an acute attack to evaluate oxygenation, carbon dioxide elimination, and acid-base status. ABGs initially show hypoxemia with a low $PO_2$, and mild respiratory alkalosis with an elevated pH and low $PCO_2$ due to tachypnea. Severe airflow obstruction causes significant hypoxemia and respiratory acidosis (pH less than 7.35 and $PCO_2$ greater than 42 mmHg), indicative of respiratory failure and the need for mechanical ventilation.
- *Skin testing* may be done to identify specific allergens if an allergic trigger is suspected for asthma attacks.

### Disease Monitoring

*Peak expiratory flow rate (PEFR)* is used on a day-to-day basis to evaluate the severity of bronchial hyperresponsiveness. Small, inexpensive meters to measure PEFR are available. Readings taken at varying times of day over several weeks are used to establish the client's personal best or normal PEFR. This value is then used to evaluate the severity of airway obstruction. Traffic signal colors are used for simplicity: *green* (80% to 100% of personal best) indicates asthma that is under control; *yellow* (50% to 80%) is caution, indicating a need for further medication or treatment; and *red* (50% or less) signals an immediate need for a bronchodilator and medical treatment if the level does not immediately return to the yellow range (Porth, 2002).

### Preventive Measures

Asthma attacks often can be prevented by avoiding allergens and environmental triggers. Modifying the home environment by controlling dust, removing carpets, covering mattresses and pillows to reduce dust mite populations, and installing air filtering systems may be useful. Pets may need to be removed from the household. Eliminating all tobacco smoke in the home is vital. Wearing a mask that retains humidity and warm air while exercising in cold weather may help prevent attacks of exercise-induced asthma. Early treatment of respiratory infections is vital to prevent asthma exacerbations.

## BOX 36–1 ■ Pulmonary Function Tests

Pulmonary function tests (PFTs) are performed in a pulmonary function laboratory. After preparing the client, a nose clip is applied and the unsedated client breathes into a spirometer or body plethysmograph, a device for measuring and recording lung volume in liters versus time in seconds. The client is instruced how to breathe for specific tests: for example, to inhale as deeply as possible and then exhale to the maximal extent possible. Using measured lung volumes, respiratory capacities are calculated to assess pulmonary status. The specific values determined by PFT and illustrated in the figure include the following:

■ *Total lung capacity (TLC)* is the total volume of the lungs at their maximum inflation. Four values are used to calculate TLC:
   a. *Tidal volume ($V_T$)*, the volume inhaled and exhaled with normal quiet breathing.
   b. *Inspiratory reserve volume (IRV)*, the maximum amount that can be inhaled over and above a normal inspiration.
   c. *Expiratory reserve volume (ERV)*, the maximum amount that can be exhaled following a normal exhalation.
   d. *Residual volume (RV)*, the amount of air remaining in the lungs after maximal exhalation.
■ *Vital capacity (VC)* is the total amount of air that can be exhaled after a maximal inspiration. It is calculated by adding together the IRV, $V_T$, and the ERV.

■ *Inspiratory capacity* is the total amount of air that can be inhaled following a normal quiet exhalation. It is calculated by adding the $V_T$ and IRV.
■ *Functional residual capacity (FRC)* is the volume of air left in the lungs after a normal exhalation. The ERV and RV are added to determine the FRC.
■ *Forced expiratory volume ($FEV_1$)* is the amount of air that can be exhaled in 1 second.
■ *Forced vital capacity (FVC)* is the amount of air that can be exhaled forcefully and rapidly after maximum air intake.
■ *Minute volume (MV)* is the total amount or volume of air breathed in 1 minute.

In older clients, residual capacity is increased, and vital capacity is decreased. These age-related changes result from the following:

■ Calcification of the costal cartilage and weakening of the intercostal muscles, which reduce movement of the chest wall.
■ Vertebral osteoporosis, which decreases spinal flexibility and increases the degree of kyphosis, further increasing the anterior-posterior diameter of the chest.
■ Diaphragmatic flattening and loss of elasticity.

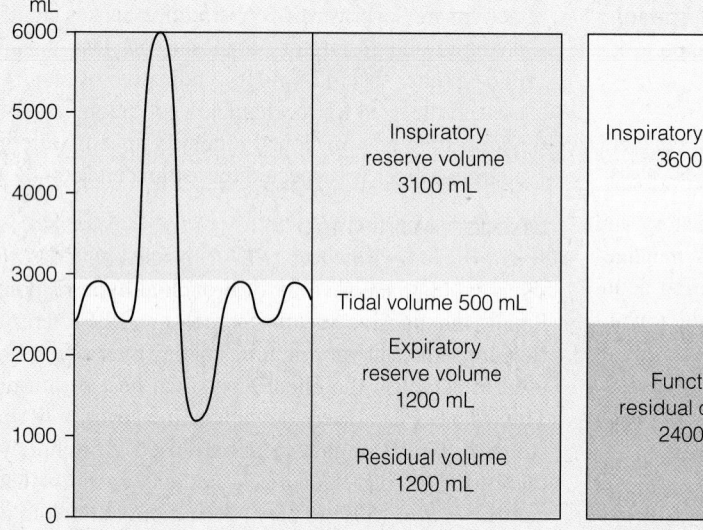
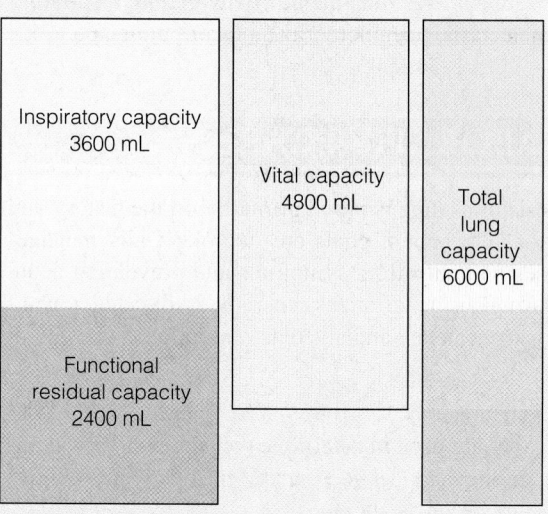

The relationship of lung volumes and capacities. Volumes (mL) shown are for an average adult male.

## Medications

Medications are used to prevent and control asthma symptoms, reduce the frequency and severity of exacerbations, and reverse airway obstruction. Drugs used for long-term control of asthma are taken daily to maintain control of the disease. The primary drugs in this group are anti-inflammatory agents, long-acting bronchodilators, and leukotriene modifiers. Quick-relief medications provide prompt relief of bronchoconstriction and airflow obstruction with associated wheezing, cough, and chest tightness. Short-acting adrenergic stimulants (rapid-acting bronchodilators), anticholinergic drugs, and methylxanthines fall into this category.

## Bronchodilators

Most asthmatics need bronchodilator therapy to control their symptoms. Inhalation of nebulized medication is the preferred means of administration. The primary bronchodilators used include adrenergic stimulants, methylxanthines, and anticholinergic agents.

Adrenergic stimulants affect receptors on smooth muscle cells of the respiratory tract, causing smooth muscle relaxation and bronchodilation. Long-acting adrenergic stimulants such as inhaled salmeterol and oral sustained-release albuterol are used in conjunction with anti-inflammatory drugs to control symptoms, but are not appropriate to treat an acute episode of

## BOX 36-2  ■  Client Teaching: Using a Metered-Dose Inhaler

- Firmly insert a charged metered-dose inhaler (MDI) canister into the mouthpiece unit.
- Remove mouthpiece cap. Shake canister vigorously for 3 to 5 seconds.
- Exhale slowly and completely.
- Holding the canister upside down, place the mouthpiece in the mouth, closing lips around it, or directly in front of the mouth.
- Press and hold the canister down while inhaling deeply and slowly for 3 to 5 seconds (see figure).
- Hold breath for 10 seconds, release pressure on the container, remove from mouth, and exhale. Wait 20 to 30 seconds before repeating the procedure for a second puff.
- Rinse the mouth after using the inhaler to minimize systemic absorption and drying the mucous membranes.
- Rinse the inhaler mouthpiece at least once a day.

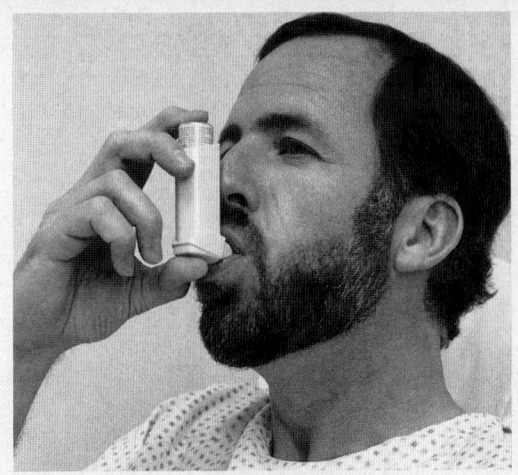

Use of a metered-dose inhaler.

asthma. Inhaled short-acting beta-adrenergic agonists such as albuterol, bitolterol, pirbuterol, and terbutaline, administered by metered-dose inhalers (MDIs), are the treatment of choice for quick relief (Box 36–2). They act within minutes, but their duration generally is short, lasting only 4 to 6 hours. Tachycardia and muscle tremors, common side effects of adrenergic agonists, are minimal with inhalation therapy.

Anticholinergic medications prevent bronchoconstriction by blocking parasympathetic input to bronchial smooth muscle. Ipratropium bromide, an anticholinergic drug administered by metered-dose inhaler, is useful when asthma symptoms are poorly controlled by adrenergic stimulants alone. Anticholinergic drugs act more slowly than adrenergic stimulants, requiring up to 60 to 90 minutes to achieve maximal effect.

Theophylline is a methylxanthine used as adjunctive treatment for asthma. It relaxes bronchial smooth muscle and may also inhibit the release of chemical mediators of the inflammatory response. Monitoring of serum theophylline levels is necessary because of wide individual variations in metabolism and elimination of the drug and its toxic effects. Serum levels of 10 to 20 µg/mL or lower are recommended. Theophylline may be used as a long-term bronchodilator, given once or twice daily. A related drug, aminophylline, may be administered intravenously to treat an acute, severe exacerbation of the disease.

### Anti-Inflammatory Agents

Corticosteroids and two nonsteroidal anti-inflammatory agents, cromolyn sodium and nedocromil, are used to suppress airway inflammation and reduce asthma symptoms.

Corticosteroids block the late response to inhaled allergens and reduce bronchial hyperresponsiveness. The preferred route of administration is by metered-dose inhaler to minimize systemic absorption and reduce the adverse effects of prolonged steroid use (cushingoid effects). For a severe acute attack, corticosteroids may be given systemically to alleviate symptoms and induce remission.

Cromolyn sodium and nedocromil are used to prevent acute episodes of asthma. They reduce airway hyperreactivity and inhibit the release of mediator substances. These drugs are used for long-term control of asthma, not quick relief. They have a wide margin of safety and few side effects.

### Leukotriene Modifiers

Leukotriene modifiers, zafirlukast (Accolate) and zileuton (Zyflo Filmtab), are new oral medications that reduce the inflammatory response in asthma. They appear to improve lung function, diminish symptoms, and reduce the need for short-acting bronchodilators. These drugs affect the metabolism and excretion of other medications such as warfarin and theophylline and may cause liver toxicity.

Nursing implications for medications used to treat asthma are outlined on pages 1110–1111.

### Complementary Therapies

A number of herbal preparations and other complementary therapies have been shown to be helpful in treating asthma. Herbal preparations may include atopa belladonna (the natural form of atropine) or ephedra (also called ma huang), an herb that contains ephedrine. These herbals have effects similar to those of drugs used to treat asthma, and should not be used in combination with sympathetic stimulants or anticholinergic preparations. The safety of ephedra is currently in question; advise clients to always check with a physician before using preparations containing ephedra. Capsaicin also may relieve acute asthma symptoms. Other herbal preparations include quercetin and grape seed extract. Refer clients interested in using natural preparations to a qualified herbalist, and emphasize the importance of talking to the physician before using these preparations along with conventional treatment.

In addition to herbals, other complementary therapies such as biofeedback, yoga, breathing techniques, acupuncture, homeopathy, and massage have been found to alleviate or help control asthma symptoms.

# Medication Administration

## Asthma

### ADRENERGIC STIMULANTS

> Epinephrine
> Isoproterenol (Isuprel)
> Metaproterenol (Alupent, Metaprel)
> Terbutaline (Brethaire, Brethine)
> Isoetharine (Bronkosol, Bronkometer)
> Albuterol (Proventil, Ventolin)
> Bitolterol (Tornalate)
> Pirbuterol (Maxair)
> Salmeterol (Serevent)

Adrenergic stimulants affect sympathetic receptors in the respiratory tract, resulting in smooth muscle relaxation and bronchodilation. Administered by metered-dose inhalers, these drugs are the treatment of choice for acute bronchial asthma. Oral forms may be used for prophylaxis but are not effective in treating an acute attack because of their slow onset. When administered orally or parenterally, their effect on the sympathetic nervous system can produce undesirable side effects such as nervousness, irritability, tachycardia, and cardiac dysrhythmias.

### Nursing Responsibilities

- Use with caution in clients with hypertension, cardiovascular disease or dysrhythmias, hyperthyroidism, or diabetes.
- When given to a client who is hypoxemic and acidotic, these drugs may cause potentially dangerous cardiac stimulation.
- When given by MDI wait 1 to 2 minutes between puffs to allow airways to dilate, permitting the second dose to reach distal airways.
- Observe for desired effect of reduced dyspnea and wheezing. Central nervous system stimulation (anxiety, irritability, and insomnia) and tremor are common side effects.

### Client and Family Teaching

- Use the prescribed inhaler or nebulizer as directed.
- If you are taking a bronchodilator along with another medication by inhalation, use the bronchodilator first to open airways and enhance the effectiveness of the second medication.
- Rinse the mouth after using inhalers to reduce systemic absorption of the medication.
- Keep a log to track your bronchodilator use. If the drug becomes less effective, or if you need a higher dosage or more frequent doses than prescribed, contact your physician.
- Report palpitations, irregular pulse, and other side effects to the physician.

### METHYLXANTHINES

> Theophylline (Bronkotabs, Quibron, Slo-Phyllin Theolair, Theo-Dur, others)
> Aminophylline (Somophyllin)

The methylxanthines are chemically related to caffeine. Once the drugs of choice for preventing and treating asthma attacks, they are now are used primarily to prevent nocturnal asthma in affected adult clients. Theophylline has a narrow margin of safety and high potential for toxicity. Because the metabolism and excretion of theophylline vary significantly from person to person—affected by such factors as age, smoking, genetic factors, alcoholism, and other chronic diseases—monitoring of serum levels is vital.

### Nursing Responsibilities

- The therapeutic blood level for theophylline is 10 to 20 µg/mL.
- Monitor for manifestations of toxicity. Anorexia, nausea, vomiting, restlessness, insomnia, cardiac dysrhythmias, and seizures are early manifestations. Other manifestations include epigastric pain, hematemesis, diarrhea, headache, irritability, muscle twitching, palpitations, tachycardia, flushing, and circulatory failure.
- Administer with meals or a full glass of water or milk to minimize gastric irritation.
- Monitor effect closely when administering concurrently with other medications such as barbiturates, anticonvulsants, thyroid hormone, beta blockers, bronchodilators, and others.
- Aminophylline is incompatible with many other intravenous drugs. Use a separate line or flush the line with normal saline before and after administering any other preparation.

### Client and Family Teaching

- Oral methylxanthines are ineffective to treat an acute asthma attack; do not delay other treatment by using these drugs.
- Check with the physician before taking any over-the-counter medications or other prescription drugs while on theophylline.
- Do not smoke while using this drug.
- Report adverse effects to the physician.

### ANTICHOLINERGICS

> Atropine
> Ipratropium bromide (Atrovent)

Anticholinergics are potent bronchodilators, blocking input from the parasympathetic nervous system. Atropine is used infrequently because of its tendency to dry secretions of the mucous membranes and other side effects. Ipratropium bromide is available as an inhaler and has fewer side effects than atropine.

### Nursing Responsibilities

- Assess for possible contraindications to the drug, including hypersensitivity, glaucoma, prostatic hypertrophy, or bladder-neck obstruction.
- Assess for desired and/or adverse effects: improving or worsening symptoms; nausea, vomiting, abdominal cramping, anxiety, dizziness; headache.
- Provide ice chips, fluids, or hard candy to relieve dry mouth.

### Client and Family Teaching

- To prevent overdose, take no more than the prescribed number of doses per day.
- If the drug becomes less effective over time, notify the physician; an adjustment in dosage may be needed.

### CORTICOSTEROIDS

> Beclomethasone dipropionate (Vanceril, Beclovent)
> Triamcinalone acetonide (Azmacort)
> Flunisolide (AeroBid)
> Dexamethasone sodium phosphate (Decadron Phosphate Respihaler)

The anti-inflammatory effect of corticosteroids helps both prevent and treat acute episodes. Corticosteroids are used to reduce

# Medication Administration

## Asthma (continued)

the frequency and severity of asthma attacks and allow reduced dosages of other drugs. The cushingoid side effects of corticosteroids, always a major concern with their use, are minimized when they are inhaled.

### Nursing Responsibilities
- Administer inhaler doses after bronchodilators to facilitate transit of the medication to distal airways.
- Assess for common side effects: sore throat; hoarseness; and oropharyngeal or laryngeal *Candida albicans* infection.
- Administer antifungal medications or gargles as ordered.

### Client and Family Teaching
- Rinse the mouth after using the inhaler and maintain good oral hygiene to reduce the risk of fungal infections.
- These medications should not be used to alleviate the symptoms of an acute attack.
- Several weeks of continued therapy may be required before a beneficial effect is noticed.
- Notify the physician if you develop weight gain, fluid retention, muscle weakness, redistribution of fat, or mood changes.

## MAST CELL STABILIZERS

Cromolyn sodium (Intal, Nasalcrom)
Nedocromil (Tilade)

Cromolyn sodium and nedocromil inhibit inflammatory cells in the airway, blocking early and late responses to inhaled antigens. Both also prevent bronchoconstriction in response to inhaling cold air. They are administered by metered-dose inhaler, and have a wide margin of safety. Clients using nedocromil may complain of an unpleasant taste.

### Nursing Responsibilities
- Evaluate for potential adverse effects of wheezing and bronchoconstriction.

### Client and Family Teaching
- Gargling or sipping water can decrease the throat irritation associated with nebulizer treatment.
- Use appropriate technique. Inhale deeply with head tipped back to open airways, hold breath, and then exhale. Repeat until all of the drug has been inhaled.
- These drugs are used only to prevent asthma attacks; they are not effective in treating an acute attack.
- Several weeks may be required before a beneficial effect is noted.

## LEUKOTRIENE MODIFIERS

Zafirlukast (Accolate)
Zileuton (Zyflo)

Leukotriene modifiers interfere with the inflammatory process in the airways, improving airflow, decreasing symptoms, and reducing the need for short-acting bronchodilators. They are used for maintenance therapy in adults and children over the age of 12 as an alternative to inhaled corticosteroid therapy. They are not used to treat an acute attack.

### Nursing Responsibilities
- Administer at least 1 hour before or 2 hours after meals.
- These drugs inhibit some liver enzymes, affecting the metabolism of warfarin and possibly terfenadine and theophylline. Monitor prothrombin times and theophylline blood levels.
- Monitor liver enzymes, as these drugs may be toxic to the liver.

### Client and Family Teaching
- Take the drugs as prescribed on an empty stomach.
- Notify the physician if a change in color of stools or urine is noted or if jaundice develops.

---

# NURSING CARE

Nurses encounter clients with asthma both in the acute care setting during an acute exacerbation and as outpatients or in homes. The priority nursing care needs differ with each setting.

## Health Promotion

Although specific measures to prevent asthma have not yet been identified, the link between parental smoking and childhood asthma is strong. Discuss this link with young people and families with children. Encourage all clients to not start smoking, and if they do smoke, to quit. Provide referrals to smoking cessation clinics, help groups, or a care provider for nicotine patches as needed to facilitate quitting.

## Assessment

Assessment of the client experiencing an acute asthma attack must be very focused and timely.

- Health history: current symptoms, including chest tightness, shortness of breath, dyspnea; duration of current attack; measures used to relieve symptoms and their effect; identified precipitating factors for the attack; frequency of attacks; current medications; known allergies
- Physical examination: apparent level of distress; color; vital signs; respiratory rate and excursion, breath sounds throughout lung fields; apical pulse

## Nursing Diagnoses and Interventions

An acute asthma attack causes fear as breathing becomes increasingly difficult and hypoxemia develops. Anxiety in turn tends to increase the severity and manifestations of the attack. Priority nursing care needs during an acute attack focus on improving airway clearance and reducing fear and anxiety. Teaching about prevention of future attacks and home management must be postponed until adequate ventilation is restored.

### Ineffective Airway Clearance

Bronchospasm and bronchoconstriction, increased mucus secretion, and airway edema narrow the airways and impair airflow during an acute attack of asthma. Both inspiratory and expiratory volume are affected, decreasing the oxygen available at the alveolus for the process of respiration. Narrowed air passages increase the work of breathing, increasing the metabolic rate and tissue demand for oxygen.

**PRACTICE ALERT** *Frequently assess respiratory status (at least every 1 to 2 hours): respiratory rate and depth, chest movement or excursion, breath sounds, and peak expiratory flow rate. Respiratory status can change rapidly during an acute asthma attack and its treatment. Decreasing PEFRs indicate worsening airflow restriction. Slowed, shallow respirations with significantly diminished breath sounds and decreased wheezing may indicate exhaustion and impending respiratory failure. Immediate intervention is necessary.* ∎

- Monitor skin color and temperature and level of consciousness. *Cyanosis, cool clammy skin, and changes in level of consciousness (agitation, lethargy, or confusion) indicate worsening hypoxia.*
- Assess arterial blood gas results and pulse oximetry readings; notify the physician of abnormal values or changes in status. *These values provide information about gas exchange and the adequacy of alveolar ventilation. A fall in oxygen saturation levels is an early indicator of impaired gas exchange.*

**PRACTICE ALERT** *Assess cough effort and sputum for color, consistency, and amount. Ineffective cough may also signal impending respiratory failure.* ∎

- Place in Fowler's, high-Fowler's, or orthopneic (with head and arms supported on the overbed table) position to facilitate breathing and lung expansion. *These positions reduce the work of breathing and increase lung expansion, especially of basilar areas.*
- Administer oxygen as ordered. If a mask is used, monitor closely for feelings of claustrophobia or suffocation. *Supplemental oxygen reduces hypoxemia. Although the mask is a very effective oxygen delivery system, it may increase anxiety.*
- Administer nebulizer treatments and provide humidification as ordered. *Nebulizer treatments are used to administer bronchodilators and other medications; humidity helps loosen secretions.*
- Initiate or assist with chest physiotherapy, including percussion and postural drainage. *Percussion and postural drainage facilitate the movement of secretions and airway clearance.*
- Increase fluid intake. *Increasing fluids helps keep secretions thin.*
- Provide endotracheal suctioning as needed. *Endotracheal suctioning may be necessary to remove secretions and improve ventilation if the client is unable to clear secretions by coughing.*

## Ineffective Breathing Pattern

The physiologic changes in lung ventilation that occur during an acute asthma attack impair both lung expansion and emptying. Anxiety caused by hypoxia and dyspnea compounds the problem by increasing the respiratory rate. Collaborative and nursing interventions can help restore a more normal breathing pattern and adequate lung ventilation.

**PRACTICE ALERT** *Frequently assess respiratory rate, pattern, and breath sounds. Note manifestations of ineffective breathing, including rapid rate, shallow respirations, nasal flaring, use of accessory muscles, intercostal retractions, and diminished or absent breath sounds. Early identification of ineffective respirations allows timely initiation of interventions.* ∎

- Monitor vital signs and laboratory results. *Tachypnea, tachycardia, an elevated blood pressure, and increasing hypoxemia and hypercapnia are signs of compromised respiratory status.*
- Assist with ADLs as needed. *This conserves energy and reduces fatigue.*
- Provide rest periods between scheduled activities and treatments. *Scheduled rest is important to prevent fatigue and reduce oxygen demands.*
- Teach and assist to use techniques to control breathing pattern:
  a. Pursed-lip breathing
  b. Abdominal breathing
  c. Relaxation techniques including visualization, meditation, and others
  *Pursed-lip breathing helps keep airways open by maintaining positive pressure, and abdominal breathing improves lung expansion. Relaxation techniques reduce anxiety and its effect on the respiratory rate.*
- Administer medications, including bronchodilators and antiinflammatory drugs, as ordered. Monitor for desired and possible adverse effects. *Medications are used to improve airway status and facilitate breathing.*

## Anxiety

Acute exacerbations of asthma can produce significant anxiety. Fear of being unable to breathe and feelings of suffocation associated with acute asthma are significant. Financial or other concerns may cause the client to want to avoid hospitalization. Increasingly frequent and severe episodes may cause fear for the future. Hypoxia contributes to anxiety as well, stimulating the sympathetic nervous system and the fight-or-flight response.

- Assess level of anxiety. *Interventions for severe anxiety or panic differ from those for mild or moderate anxiety.*
- Assist to identify coping skills that have been successful in the past. *Successful coping helps the client regain control of the situation, reducing anxiety.*

**PRACTICE ALERT** *Provide physical and emotional support. Remain with the client during episodes of severe anxiety; schedule time every 1 to 2 hours to be with the mildly or moderately anxious client. Answer call lights promptly. The severely anxious client may fear being alone or believe that he or she will die if someone is not on hand. Knowing that the nurse is readily available and will return regardless if help is needed reduces anxiety.* ∎

- Listen actively to concerns; do not deny or negate the fear of dying or of being unable to breathe. *Active listening promotes trust and helps the client express concerns.*

> **PRACTICE ALERT** *Provide clear, concise directions and explanations about procedures. Avoid presenting more information than the client is able to assimilate. Anxiety interferes with the ability to learn. Explanations may need to be repeated frequently.* ■

- Include the client in care planning and decisions as appropriate, without making excessive demands. *Participating in decision making increases the client's sense of control. Because high levels of anxiety interfere with the ability to make decisions, it is important to avoid placing demands on the client that may further increase the level of anxiety.*
- Reduce excessive environmental stimuli, and maintain a calm demeanor. *This promotes rest.*
- Allow supportive family members to remain with the client. *Significant others provide additional support and can help reduce anxiety.*
- Assist to use relaxation techniques, such as guided imagery, muscle relaxation, and meditation. *These techniques help restore psychologic balance and reduce sympathetic stimulation and responses.*

### Ineffective Therapeutic Regimen Management

Once acute asthma is under control and effective respirations have been reestablished, it is important to help the client identify contributing factors to the attack. This helps the client prevent future episodes.

- Assess level of understanding about asthma and the prescribed treatment regimen. Provide additional information and teaching as indicated. *Assessment helps to identify and clarify misperceptions and difficulties with disease management.*
- Discuss the client's perception of the illness and its effect on his or her lifestyle. *Open discussion can help identify conflicts between lifestyle and the treatment regimen.*

> **PRACTICE ALERT** *Assist to identify factors that contributed to the acute episode. Identifying contributing factors increases the client's awareness of the disease and strategies to prevent future exacerbations.* ■

- Assist the client and significant others to identify problems or difficulties integrating the treatment regimen into their lifestyle. *Asthma and its management may necessitate lifestyle modifications to prevent acute exacerbations. This can significantly impact family members, for example, eliminating cigarette smoking or pets from the household, removing carpets, or daily damp-dusting to remove dust mites.*
- Assess knowledge and understanding of prescribed medications and use of over-the-counter preparations. *This is important to determine misperceptions or possible misuse of medications.*

- Provide verbal and written instructions. *Written instructions reinforce teaching and allow future reference.*
- Refer to counseling, support groups, or self-help organizations. *Counseling, support groups, and self-help organizations can help the client and family adapt to living with asthma and the treatment regimen.*

## Home Care

Asthma is a chronic disease that is best managed by the client with assistance from medical personnel. Teaching for home care focuses on promoting the highest level of wellness and preventing and managing acute episodes and exacerbations of the disease. Topics to include in teaching are as follows:

- Suggestions for lifestyle changes to avoid specific triggers for asthma attacks, for example:
  - Warm up slowly before exercising in cold weather; wear a special mask or scarf to retain air warmth and humidity while exercising.
  - Substitute indoor exercises during cold, dry weather.
  - Reduce the risk for respiratory infections (e.g., adequate rest, good nutrition, and stress management to maintain immune function, yearly influenza vaccines and immunization against pneumococcal pneumonia).
  - Use techniques to reduce or manage physical and psychologic stress.
- Using PEFR meter to monitor airway status; how to manage the disease based on results
- Using prescribed medications, including:
  - Name, frequency, dose, and desired effect.
  - Potential adverse effects and their management, including effects to report to the physician.
  - Potential interactions with other drugs (including over-the-counter herbal preparations) or foods.
  - If tolerance is a potential risk, how to identify it and steps to take.

Provide referrals to local or regional resources for further teaching and support as needed. Consider the need for home health services, home respiratory care services, and others as needed. See Box 36–3 for selected national resource agencies.

---

**BOX 36–3** ■ **Home Care Resources for Clients with Asthma**

American Lung Association
800-LUNG-USA (800-586-4872)
www.lungusa.org

Asthma and Allergy Foundation of America
800-7-ASTHMA (800-727-8462)

Asthma Information Center
www.mdnet.de/asthma

National Asthma Education and Prevention Program
National Heart, Lung, and Blood Institute Information Center
301-251-1222
www.nhlbi.nih.gov

# THE CLIENT WITH CHRONIC OBSTRUCTIVE PULMONARY DISEASE

Clients with chronic airflow obstruction due to chronic bronchitis and/or emphysema are said to have **chronic obstructive pulmonary disease (COPD).**

In 2000, approximately 11.4 million Americans were affected by COPD. It is more common in whites than in blacks and affects men more frequently than women. It is the fourth leading cause of death in the United States. The death rate from COPD continues to rise, particularly among black males and females of all ethnic groups. In the year 2000, COPD and other chronic obstructive lung diseases accounted for over 123,500 deaths (NHLBI, 2002). In addition, COPD morbidity is significant. In people under age 65, COPD is second only to heart disease as a cause of disability, resulting in an estimated 250 million lost work hours yearly.

Obstructive lung disease typically affects middle-aged and older adults. Cigarette smoking is clearly implicated as the primary cause of COPD, even though it develops in only 10% to 15% of smokers. Cigarette smoke and the irritants it contains impair ciliary movement, inhibit the function of alveolar macrophages, and cause mucus-secreting glands to hypertrophy. It also produces emphysema or airway destruction and constricts smooth muscle, increasing airway resistance. Other contributing factors include air pollution, occupational exposure to noxious dusts and gases, airway infection, and familial and genetic factors.

## PATHOPHYSIOLOGY AND MANIFESTATIONS

COPD is characterized by slowly progressive obstruction of the airways. The disease is one of periodic exacerbations, often related to respiratory infection, with increased symptoms of dyspnea and sputum production. Unlike acute processes in which lung tissues recover, airways and lung parenchyma do not return to normal following an exacerbation; instead, they demonstrate progressive destructive changes.

Although one or the other may predominate, COPD typically includes components of both chronic bronchitis and emphysema, two distinctly different processes. Chronic asthma is also often present. Through different mechanisms, these processes cause airways to narrow, resistance to airflow to increase, and expiration to become slow or difficult (Figure 36–10 ■). The result is a mismatch between alveolar ventilation and blood flow or perfusion, leading to impaired gas exchange.

The clinical presentation of COPD varies from simple chronic bronchitis without disability to chronic respiratory failure and severe disability. Manifestations are typically absent or minor early in the disease. When the client finally seeks care, productive cough, dyspnea, and exercise intolerance often have been present for as long as 10 years. The cough typically occurs in the mornings and often is attributed to "smoker's cough." Initially, dyspnea occurs only on extreme exertion; as the disease progresses, dyspnea becomes more severe and accompanies mild activity. Manifestations characteristic of chronic bronchi-

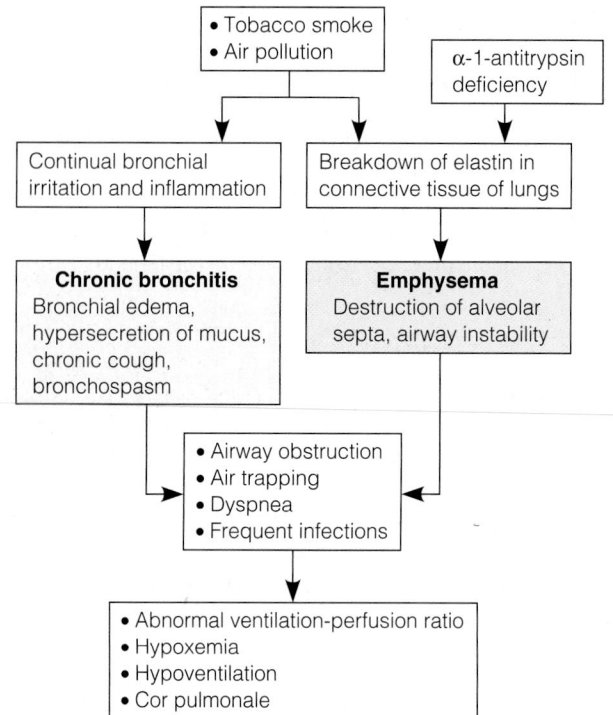

**Figure  36–10** ■ The pathogenesis of chronic obstructive pulmonary disease.

tis and emphysema develop. The clinical features and manifestations of COPD are summarized in Table 36–7.

## Chronic Bronchitis

**Chronic bronchitis** is a disorder of excessive bronchial mucus secretion. It is characterized by a productive cough lasting 3 or more months in 2 consecutive years (Porth, 2002). Cigarette smoke is the major factor implicated in the development of chronic bronchitis.

Inhaled irritants lead to a chronic inflammatory process with vasodilation, congestion, and edema of the bronchial mucosa. Thick, tenacious mucus is produced in increased amounts. Narrowed airways and excess secretions obstruct airflow; expiration is affected first, then inspiration. Because ciliary function is impaired, normal defense mechanisms are unable to clear the mucus and any inhaled pathogens. Recurrent infection is common in chronic bronchitis. An imbalance between ventilation and perfusion leads to hypoxemia, hypercapnia, and pulmonary hypertension. Pulmonary hypertension often leads to right-sided heart failure.

Manifestations of chronic bronchitis are a cough productive of copious amounts of thick, tenacious sputum, cyanosis, and evidence of right-sided heart failure, including distended neck veins, edema, liver engorgement, and an enlarged heart. Adventitious sounds, including loud rhonchi and possible wheezes, are prominent on auscultation.

## Emphysema

**Emphysema** is characterized by destruction of the walls of the alveoli, with resulting enlargement of abnormal air spaces. As

| TABLE 36–7 | Clinical Features and Manifestations of COPD | | |
|---|---|---|---|
| | **Feature** | **Chronic Bronchitis** | **Emphysema** |
| **History** | Onset | After age 35; recurrent respiratory infections | After age 50; insidious progressive dyspnea |
| | Smoking | Usual | Usual |
| | Cough | Persistent, productive of copious mucopurulent sputum | Absent or mild with scant clear sputum, if any |
| **Physical Examination** | Appearance | Often obese; edematous and cyanotic; distended neck veins and other symptoms of right-sided heart failure | Usually thin and cachectic; barrel chest; prominent accessory muscles of respiration |
| | Chest | Adventitious sounds with wheezing and rhonchi; normal percussion note | Distant or diminished breath sounds; hyperresonant percussion note |
| **Other Features** | Blood gases | Hypercapnia and hypoxemia; respiratory acidosis | Normal or mild hypoxemia; normal pH |
| | Pulmonary function studies | Normal or decreased total lung capacity; moderately increased residual volume | Increased total lung capacity; markedly increased residual volume |
| | Pulmonary hypertension | May be severe | Only when advanced |

in chronic bronchitis, cigarette smoking is strongly implicated as a causative factor in most cases of emphysema. Deficiency of alpha$_1$-antitrypsin, an enzyme that normally inhibits the activity of proteolytic enzymes and tissue destruction in the lungs, leads to an early onset of emphysema, often before age 40 (Braunwald et al., 2001).

Alveolar wall destruction causes alveoli and air spaces to enlarge with loss of corresponding portions of the pulmonary capillary bed. As a result, the surface area for alveolar-capillary diffusion is reduced, affecting gas exchange. Elastic recoil is lost, reducing the volume of air that is passively expired. The loss of support tissue also affects airways, increasing the risk of expiratory collapse and further air trapping. Anatomically, either respiratory bronchioles or alveoli may be the primary tissue involved.

Emphysema is insidious in onset. Dyspnea is the initial symptom. Initially occurring only with exertion, dyspnea may progress to become severe even at rest. Cough is minimal or absent. Air trapping and hyperinflation increase the anterior-posterior chest diameter, causing *barrel chest*. The client often is thin, tachypneic, uses accessory muscles of respiration and often assumes a position of sitting and leaning forward (Figure 36–11 ■). The expiratory phase of the respiratory cycle is prolonged. On auscultation, breath sounds are diminished, and the percussion tone is hyperresonant.

## COLLABORATIVE CARE

Although COPD can be prevented in most people, it cannot be cured. Smoking abstinence is the only certain way to prevent COPD and to slow its progression. To a certain extent, airway obstruction can be reversed and disability minimized early in the disease. Treatment generally focuses on relieving symptoms, minimizing obstruction, and slowing disability.

## Diagnostic Tests

Diagnostic tests are used to help establish the diagnosis of chronic obstructive pulmonary disease and identify the predominant component, emphysema or chronic bronchitis. These procedures also are used to assess respiratory status and monitor treatment effectiveness.

• *Pulmonary function testing* is performed to establish the diagnosis and evaluate the extent and progress of COPD (see Box 36–1). Fasting is not required for this noninvasive test; however, tobacco products, bronchodilators, and eating a heavy meal should be avoided for 4 to 6 hours prior to testing. Results are based on calculated norms for each person

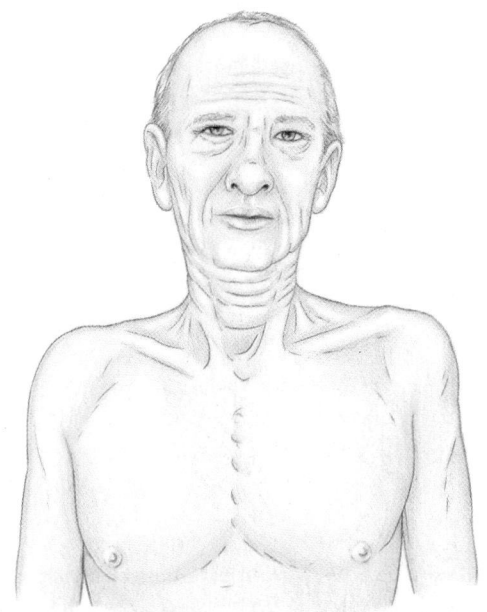

**Figure 36–11** ■ Typical appearance of a client with emphysema.

by age, height, sex, and weight; note these as well as all current medications on the requisition. In COPD, the total lung capacity and residual volume typically are increased. The forced expiratory volume ($FEV_1$) and forced vital capacity (FVC) are decreased due to narrowed airways and resistance to airflow.

- *Ventilation-perfusion scanning* may be performed to determine the extent of ventilation/perfusion mismatch—that is, the extent to which lung tissue is ventilated but not perfused (dead space), or perfused but inadequately ventilated (physiologic shunting). A radioisotope is injected or inhaled to illustrate areas of shunting and absent capillaries (Figure 36–12 ■).
- *Serum alpha$_1$-antitrypsin levels* may be drawn to screen for deficiency, particularly in clients with a family history of obstructive airway disease, those with an early onset, women, and nonsmokers. Normal adult serum alpha$_1$-antitrypsin levels range from 80 to 260 mg/dL. Fasting is not required prior to this test.
- *Arterial blood gases (ABGs)* are drawn to evaluate gas exchange, particularly during acute exacerbations of COPD. Clients with predominant emphysema often have mild hypoxemia and normal or low carbon dioxide tension. Respiratory alkalosis may be present due to an increased respiratory rate. Predominant chronic bronchitis and airway obstruction may cause marked hypoxemia and hypercapnia with respiratory acidosis. Oxygen saturation levels are low due to marked hypoxemia. See page 122 for steps to interpret ABGs.

**PRACTICE ALERT** *Hypercapnia (elevated $Paco_2$ levels) often is chronic in clients with COPD. This reduces the stimulatory effect of the $Paco_2$ and pH on the respiratory center; instead, breathing is driven by a fall in arterial oxygen levels. Administering oxygen can lead to respiratory arrest because the drive to breathe is suppressed.* ■

- *Pulse oximetry* is used to monitor oxygen saturation of the blood. Marked airway obstruction and hypoxemia often causes oxygen saturation levels less than 95%. Pulse oximetry may be continuously monitored to assess the need for supplemental oxygen.
- *Exhaled carbon dioxide (capnogram* or *$ETco_2$)* may be measured to evaluate alveolar ventilation. The normal $ETco_2$ reading is 35 to 45 mmHg; it is elevated when ventilation is inadequate, and decreased when pulmonary perfusion is impaired. $ETco_2$ monitoring can reduce the frequency of ABG determinations.
- *CBC with WBC differential* often shows increased RBCs and hematocrit (erythrocytosis) as chronic hypoxia stimulates increased erythropoiesis to increase the oxygen-carrying capacity of the blood. *Polycythemia*, increased numbers of all blood cells, may be evident. Increased WBC count and a higher percentage of immature WBCs (bands) are often indicative of bacterial infection.
- *Chest X-ray* may show flattening of the diaphragm due to hyperinflation and evidence of pulmonary infection if present.

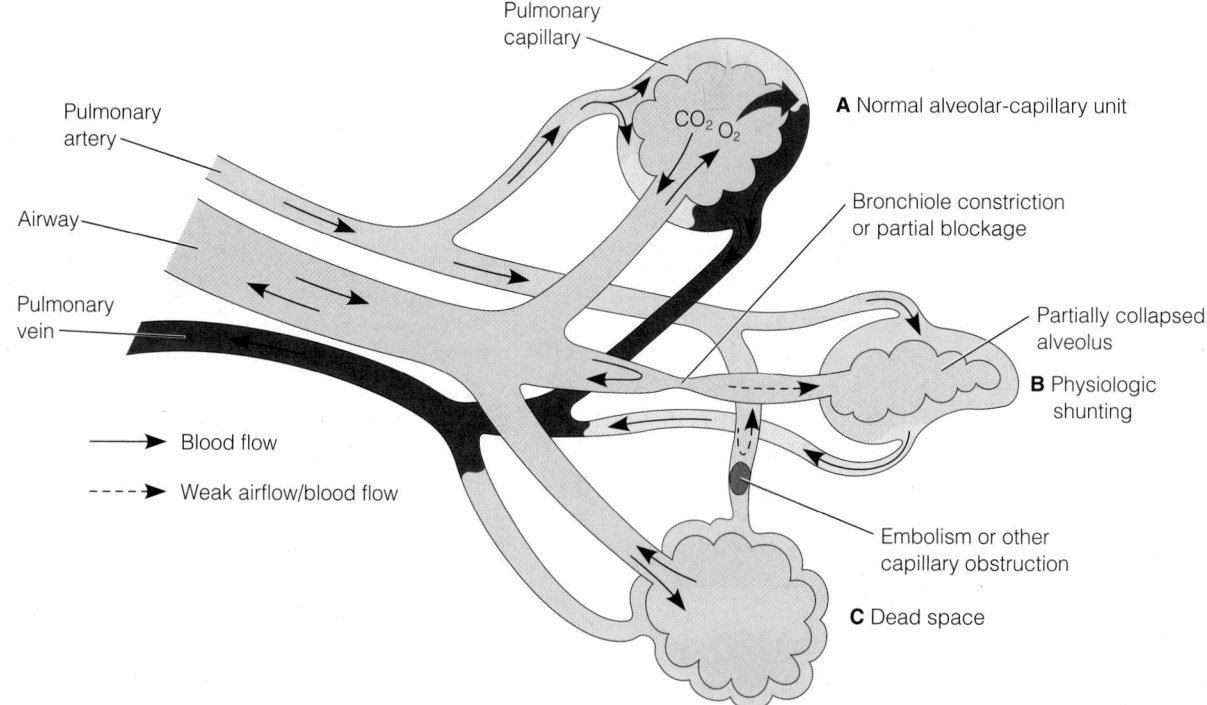

**Figure 36–12** ■ Ventilation-perfusion relationships. *A,* Normal alveolar-capillary unit with an ideal match of ventilation and blood flow. Maximum gas exchange occurs between alveolus and blood. *B,* Physiologic shunting: A unit with adequate perfusion but inadequate ventilation. *C,* Dead space: A unit with adequate ventilation but inadequate perfusion. In the latter two cases, gas exchange is impaired.

## Smoking Cessation

Smoking cessation can not only prevent COPD from developing, but also can improve lung function once the disease has been diagnosed. Forced expiratory volume ($FEV_1$) improves, and survival is prolonged, largely due to lower rates of lung cancer and heart disease. Sustained quitting is difficult; only 6% of smokers succeed in long-term abstinence from smoking (Braunwald et al., 2001). Use of nicotine patches or gum and an antidepressant such as bupropion (Wellbutrin, Zyban) improve the chances of success.

## Medications

Immunization against pneumococcal pneumonia and yearly influenza vaccine are recommended to reduce the risk of respiratory infections. A broad-spectrum antibiotic is prescribed if infection is suspected. Recent studies indicate that clients with purulent sputum and increased dyspnea will likely benefit from antibiotic therapy, even if no other signs of infection are present. Prophylactic antibiotics may be ordered for clients who experience four or more disease exacerbations per year (Braunwald et al., 2001).

Bronchodilators improve airflow and reduce air trapping in COPD, resulting in improved dyspnea and exercise tolerance. Bronchodilators may be given by metered-dose inhaler (MDI), by nebulizer, or orally. Oral administration may promote adherence, but is associated with much higher rates of adverse effects. A spacer or holding chamber may facilitate effective use of an MDI. Ipratropium bromide, an anticholinergic agent administered by MDI, is frequently prescribed. It has a longer duration of action than the short-acting $\beta_2$-adrenergic stimulant bronchodilators and few side effects. Salmeterol, a longer-acting $\beta_2$ agonist, may be used in combination therapy. Oral theophylline, a methylxanthine, is a weak bronchodilator and has a narrow therapeutic range, but often is prescribed for its other effects. Theophylline stimulates the respiratory drive, strengthens diaphragmatic contractions, and improves cardiac output. As a result, dyspnea, exercise tolerance, and quality of life improve for the client with COPD. Bronchodilators are discussed in further detail in the section on asthma, and their nursing implications are outlined in the box on page 1110.

Corticosteroid therapy may be used when asthma is a major component of COPD. It also improves symptoms and exercise tolerance, and may reduce the severity of exacerbations and the need for hospitalization. Oral corticosteroids, such as prednisone, are used initially. If a beneficial response occurs, the amount is reduced to the lowest effective dose. Every-other-day dosing or administration by inhaler is preferred to minimize steroid side effects, such as cushingoid effects and an increased risk for osteoporosis and vertebral fractures.

Alpha$_1$-antitrypsin ($\alpha_1$AT) replacement therapy is available for clients with emphysema due to a genetic deficiency of the enzyme. Although expensive and inconvenient ($\alpha_1$AT is administered weekly by intravenous infusion), it has been shown to reduce the rate of airflow decline and mortality.

## Treatments

In addition to refraining from smoking, exposure to other airway irritants and allergens should be avoided. The client should remain indoors during periods of significant air pollution to prevent exacerbations of the disease. Air filtering systems or air conditioning may be useful.

Pulmonary hygiene measures, including hydration, effective cough, percussion, and postural drainage, are used to improve clearance of airway secretions. Maintaining adequate systemic hydration is essential to keep secretions thin. Forceful coughing is often less effective than leaning forward and repeatedly "huffing," with relaxed breathing between huffs. Percussion and postural drainage may be necessary if the client is unable to clear secretions by usual means. Cough suppressants and sedatives generally are avoided as they may cause retention of secretions.

Unless disabling cardiac disease is present, a regular exercise program is beneficial in:

- Improving exercise tolerance.
- Enhancing ability to perform activities of daily living.
- Preventing deterioration of physical condition.

A program of regular aerobic exercise (e.g., walking for 20 minutes at least three times weekly) designed to gradually increase exercise tolerance is recommended. Activities that strengthen the muscles used for breathing and ADLs, such as swimming and golf, also are beneficial. See the Nursing Research box on page 1118.

Breathing exercises are used to slow the respiratory rate and relieve accessory muscle fatigue. Pursed-lip breathing slows the respiratory rate and helps maintain open airways during exhalation by keeping positive pressure in the airways. Abdominal breathing relieves the work of accessory muscles of respiration.

### Oxygen

Long-term oxygen therapy is used for severe and progressive hypoxemia. Oxygen therapy improves exercise tolerance, mental functioning, and quality of life in advanced COPD. It also reduces the rate of hospitalization and increases length of survival. Oxygen may be used intermittently, at night, or continuously. For severely hypoxemic clients, the greatest benefit is seen with continuous oxygen. Home oxygen may be supplied as liquid oxygen, compressed gas cylinders, or oxygen concentrators.

An acute exacerbation of COPD may necessitate oxygenation and inspiratory positive-pressure assistance with a face mask or intubation and mechanical ventilation. Oxygen administered without intubation and mechanical ventilation requires caution: Chronic elevated carbon dioxide levels in the blood inhibit this normal stimulus to breathe, leaving only the stimulus of low blood oxygen tension. Oxygen administered at high flow rates or a high percentage can reduce this stimulus, leading to respiratory insufficiency or arrest.

### Surgery

When medical therapy is no longer effective, lung transplantation may be an option. Both single and bilateral transplants

## Nursing Research

### Evidence-Based Practice for the Client with COPD

The correlation between physical activity and performance of essential activities of daily living, quality of life, and higher level functioning is well established. This is particularly true for the elderly and people with disease-related impairment in physical abilities. Physical inactivity is both a cause and an effect of declining physical function in the elderly. A study by Belza, Steele, Hunziker, Lakshminaryan, Holt, and Buchner (2001) sought to describe the relationships between functional performance measured as physical activity, functional capacity, symptoms, and health-related quality of life in a group of clients with chronic obstructive pulmonary disease.

A number of variables were used to evaluate physical activity and functional capacity (degree of airways obstruction, exercise capacity, and self-sufficiency in walking). Physical activity was not found to correlate well with self-reported functional status. A 6-minute walk test was, however, identified as a good predictor of physical activity and symptom severity.

### IMPLICATIONS FOR NURSING

Although this study is preliminary and replication of the results is necessary to generalize its findings, it supports a program of regular physical activity as a measure to maintain functional status and reduce symptom progression. Encourage COPD clients to enroll in a pulmonary rehabilitation program if one is available. If there is no organized program in the area, work with a pulmonologist, respiratory therapist, and physical therapist to develop an exercise program for clients with COPD.

### Critical Thinking in Nursing

1. Why do you think the 6-minute walk test was found to be a better measure of physical activity than the clients' self-reports?
2. Use the physiologic and psychologic effects of regular exercise to explain the correlation between the 6-minute walk test and improved symptoms in the client with COPD.
3. Consider the age of most clients with COPD. What other physical or psychosocial factors commonly limit physical activity in this population? How can you use this information in designing an appropriate exercise program?

have been performed successfully, with a 2-year survival rate of 75%. Lung reduction surgery is an experimental surgical intervention for advanced diffuse emphysema and lung hyperinflation. The procedure reduces the overall volume of the lung, reshapes it, and improves elastic recoil. As a result, pulmonary function and exercise tolerance improve and dyspnea is reduced. See the box on page 1140 for nursing care of the client undergoing lung surgery.

## Complementary Therapies

Complementary therapies may be useful to help manage symptoms of COPD. Dietary measures such as minimizing intake of dairy products and salt may help reduce mucous production and to keep mucus more liquefied. Be sure to recommend measures to replace the protein and calcium in dairy products to help maintain nutritional balance.

Herbal teas made with peppermint and yarrow, coltsfoot, or comfrey may act as expectorants to help relieve chest congestion. Licorice root, which may be taken in several forms, also has expectorant and anti-inflammatory effects that may be beneficial. Licorice root can, however, cause toxicity when used for extended periods of time. Refer clients to a qualified herbalist for treatment.

Acupuncture may help the client with smoking cessation, and also has been used to treat asthma and other respiratory conditions. Hypnotherapy and guided imagery are used to assist with smoking cessation. These techniques also can help the client control anxiety and breathing patterns. Refer clients to a trained professional. Nurses, physicians, psychologists, counselors, social workers and others can take professional training in hypnotherapy and guided imagery (Fontaine, 2000).

## NURSING CARE

### Health Promotion

Not smoking—never start, or quit—is the best preventive measure for chronic obstructive pulmonary disease. Even in clients with COPD, smoking cessation improves lung function and increases survival. Educate all clients, including preschool and school-age children, about the risks of smoking. See Box 36–4.

### Assessment

Focused assessment for the client with chronic obstructive pulmonary disease includes:

- Health history: current symptoms, including cough, sputum production, shortness of breath or dyspnea, activity tolerance; frequency of respiratory infections and most recent episode; previous diagnosis of emphysema, chronic bronchitis, or asthma; current medications; smoking history (in pack years—packs per day times number of years smoked), history of exposure to secondhand smoke, occupational or other pollutants
- Physical examination: general appearance, weight for height, mental status; vital signs including temperature; skin color and temperature; anterior-posterior:lateral chest diameter, use of accessory muscles, nasal flaring or pursed-lip breathing; respiratory excursion and diaphragmatic excursion; percussion tone; breath sounds throughout; neck veins, apical pulse and heart sounds, peripheral pulses, edema

## BOX 36–4 ■ Cigarette Smoking and Tobacco Use

The use of tobacco reaches back to early civilizations, when it was used in religious ceremonies and as an offering of friendship. At one time, tobacco was thought to have medicinal qualities effective against all common diseases. Widespread use of tobacco among the male population of the industrialized world began during World War I.

Tobacco is now recognized as the leading cause of preventable illness in the world. In spite of this knowledge, aggressive marketing of the product continues, and its worldwide use is increasing, especially in underdeveloped countries.

The link between tobacco use and lung cancer was reported as early as 1912. In 1987, lung cancer became the leading cause of cancer-related death in the United States among both men and women.

Cigarette smoke contains approximately 4000 chemicals, including nicotine. Nicotine is a highly addictive psychoactive substance that is relatively cheap and readily available. It produces euphoria, which acts as a positive reinforcer for continued use. In North American society, tobacco is more acceptable than many other dependency-producing drugs.

Tar is the particulate matter in cigarette smoke that is responsible for most of its carcinogenic and pathologic effects on the lungs. Smoke also paralyzes the cilia, reducing their ability to remove tars from contact with the respiratory epithelium. The risk for cancer and other lung diseases is dose related, affected by the age at which smoking began, the number of cigarettes smoked per day, and the number of years smoked. Smoking cessation reduces the risks associated with tobacco use. For some, such as the risk of coronary heart disease, quitting smoking yields rapid benefits. For others, the degree of risk reduction is less immediate, but still significant.

Nurses need to do more than simply advise clients to quit smoking and talk about the risks of smoking. Nurses can take an active role in smoking cessation. Identify smoking habits, smoking-related illnesses, and previous efforts to quit. Work with the client to identify barriers and obstacles to quitting. Educate about the addictive nature of nicotine, and explain the manifestations of nicotine withdrawal (anxiety, irritability, headache, and disturbed sleep). Develop a plan with the client that specifies a target date to quit and includes ways to deal with obstacles to quitting, withdrawal symptoms, and the temptation to resume smoking. Offer self-help material at an appropriate reading level. Refer to a counselor, physician, self-help group, or smoking cessation clinic. If a relapse occurs, accept it as a normal part of rehabilitation from any addictive substance. Continue to provide support and encouragement, helping the client avoid further relapses.

Nurses can be especially effective in primary prevention of cigarette smoking and the diseases associated with it. Just as tobacco companies direct advertising at women and teens, nurses can target these populations and younger children for programs to prevent smoking. In addition, nurses need to become active in reducing minors' access to tobacco products, especially cigarettes and chewing tobacco (often the first product used by teens).

Nursing diagnoses that may be appropriate related to smoking include the following:

- *Ineffective health maintenance* related to tobacco use
- *Decisional conflict* related to tobacco use
- *Ineffective denial* related to acknowledgment of substance abuse and dependence

## Nursing Diagnoses and Interventions

Clients with chronic obstructive pulmonary disease, whether hospitalized or in the community, have multiple nursing care needs. Because of the obstructive nature of the disease, airway clearance is a high priority. Nutritional deficit is common, particularly when emphysema is predominant. Because this chronic disease affects all functional health patterns, psychosocial issues are also of concern in planning nursing care.

### Ineffective Airway Clearance

Both chronic bronchitis and emphysema affect the ability to maintain open airways. In chronic bronchitis, copious amounts of thick, tenacious mucus are produced. Ciliary action is impaired, making it difficult to clear mucus from the airways. The loss of supporting tissue caused by emphysema increases the the risk for airway collapse. In both cases, air is trapped distally, and less oxygen is available to the alveoli for diffusion. Normal respiratory defense mechanisms are impaired, and mucus-plugged airways provide an ideal environment for bacterial growth. Respiratory infection further impairs airway clearance and is often the cause of an acute exacerbation.

- Assess respiratory status every 1 to 2 hours or as indicated. Assess rate and pattern; cough and secretions (color, amount, consistency, and odor); and breath sounds, both normal and adventitious. *Frequent assessment is vital to monitor current status and response to treatment. Adventitious sounds should decrease with effective intervention. Diminished or absent breath sounds may indicate increasing airway obstruction and possible atelectasis.*

**PRACTICE ALERT** *Promptly report changes in oxygen saturation, skin color, or mental status. A drop in oxygen saturation levels, increasing cyanosis, or altered level of consciousness indicate hypoxemia, possibly related to airway obstruction.* ■

- Monitor arterial blood gas results. *Increasing hypoxemia, hypercapnia, and respiratory acidosis may indicate increasing airway obstruction.*
- Weigh daily, monitor intake and output, and assess mucous membranes and skin turgor. *Dehydration causes respiratory secretions to become thicker, more tenacious, and difficult to expectorate; fluid overload can further compromise respiratory status.*
- Encourage a fluid intake of at least 2000 to 2500 mL per day unless contraindicated. *Adequate fluid intake helps keep mucous secretions thin.*

- Place in Fowler's, high-Fowler's, or orthopneic position; encourage movement and activity to tolerance. *Upright positions improve ventilation and reduce the work of breathing. Activity helps mobilize secretions and prevent them from pooling.*
- Assist with coughing and deep breathing at least every 2 hours while awake. Position seated upright, leaning forward during coughing. *The upright position promotes chest expansion, increasing the effectiveness of coughing and reducing the work involved.*
- Provide tissues and a paper bag to dispose of expectorated sputum. *This important infection control measure reduces the spread of respiratory organisms to other people.*
- Refer to a respiratory therapist, and assist with or perform percussion and postural drainage as needed. *Percussion helps loosen secretions in airways; postural drainage facilitates movement of these secretions out of the respiratory tract.*

**PRACTICE ALERT** *Provide endotracheal, oral, or nasopharyngeal suctioning as necessary. Suctioning may be necessary to stimulate cough and help clear secretions.* ■

- Provide rest periods between treatments and procedures. *The client with COPD fatigues easily; adequate rest is important to conserve energy and reduce fatigue.*
- Administer expectorant and bronchodilator medications as ordered. Correlate timing with respiratory treatments. *Using expectorants and bronchodilators prior to coughing, percussion, and postural drainage increases their effectiveness in clearing airways.*
- Provide supplemental oxygen as ordered. *Supplemental oxygen helps maintain adequate blood and tissue oxygenation.*

**PRACTICE ALERT** *Prepare for intubation and mechanical ventilation if respiratory status deteriorates (increasing hypoxemia and hypercapnia, decreased level of consciousness, cyanosis, or worsening airway obstruction). Respiratory failure is a possible complication of an acute exacerbation of COPD and requires immediate intervention to preserve life.* ■

## Imbalanced Nutrition:
## Less Than Body Requirements

With advanced COPD, minimal activity, including eating, can cause fatigue and dyspnea. The client may be unable to consume a full meal without resting. At the same time, the increased work of breathing increases metabolic demands, and more calories are required. The client may appear cachectic (thin and wasted). Poor nutritional status further impairs immune function and increases the risk of a complicating infection.

- Assess nutritional status, including diet history, weight for height (use reference tables of desired weights), and anthropometric (skinfold) measurements. *It is important to differentiate nutritional status from body type rather than assume a nutritional impairment.*
- Observe and document food intake, including types, amounts, and caloric intake. *This information can provide direction for supplementation, if needed.*

- Monitor laboratory values, including serum albumin and electrolyte levels. *These values provide information about the adequacy of nutritional intake, including protein.*
- Consult with a dietitian to plan meals and nutritional supplements that meet caloric needs. *More concentrated sources of high-energy foods may be required to maintain caloric intake without excess fatigue. A diet high in proteins and fats without excess carbohydrates is recommended to minimize carbon dioxide production during metabolism (carbohydrates are metabolized to form $CO_2$ and water).*
- Provide frequent, small feedings with between-meal supplements. *Frequent, small meals help maintain intake and reduce fatigue associated with eating.*
- Place seated or in high-Fowler's position for meals. *An upright position promotes lung expansion and reduces dyspnea.*
- Assist to choose preferred foods from the menu; encourage family members to bring food from home if allowed. *Providing preferred foods encourages eating.*
- Keep snacks at the bedside. *Snacks provide additional caloric intake.*
- Provide mouth care prior to meals. *This helps enhance the appetite.*
- If unable to maintain oral intake, consult with the physician about enteral or parenteral feedings. *Maintenance of caloric and nutrient intake is vital to prevent catabolism.*

## Compromised Family Coping

Chronic illness affects the entire family structure. Roles and relationships change; additional demands are placed on the family. Family members may blame the client for causing the illness or have distorted perceptions about it, even denying its existence. They may refuse to assist or participate in care. The client may develop an attitude of helplessness or dependence or may demonstrate anger, hostility, or aggression.

- Assess interactions between client and family. *Assessment helps identify desired and potential destructive behaviors.*
- Assess the effect of the illness on the family. *Assessment of family interactions, roles, and relationships assists in planning appropriate interventions.*
- Help the client and family identify strengths for coping with the situation. *Identifying personal and family strengths helps the family regain a sense of control.*
- Provide information and teaching about COPD. *Education helps the family gain an understanding of the client's condition and needs.*
- Encourage expression of feelings. Avoid judging feelings expressed or family members as "good" or "bad," "right" or "wrong." *It is important that the nurse remain objective to maintain the therapeutic relationship.*
- Help family members recognize behaviors and attitudes that may hinder effective treatment, such as continuing to smoke in the house. *Family members may be unaware of the effect of their behavior on the client's ability to change habits and cope with a disabling disease.*
- Encourage family members to participate in care. *This helps develop skills for use at home.*

- Initiate a care conference involving the client, family, and health care team members from a variety of disciplines. *A wide range of perspectives and areas of expertise aids in problem solving and facilitates communication.*
- If dysfunctional family relationships interfere with measures to enhance coping, advocate for the client, reaffirming his or her right to make decisions. *Dysfunctional family relationships are not likely to change simply because of illness. The nurse can better meet the client's needs by accepting his or her limitations in dealing with family members.*
- Refer the client and family to support groups and pulmonary rehabilitation programs, as available. *Support groups and structured rehabilitation programs enhance coping abilities.*
- Arrange a social services consultation. *This can help the client and family identify care and support service needs.*
- Refer community agencies or services such as home health, homemaker services, or Meals-on-Wheels as appropriate. *Agencies or community services can provide additional support beyond the family's means or capability.*

### Decisional Conflict: Smoking

Smoking is more than a habit; it is an addiction. The client who must quit is facing a significant loss, not only of nicotine but also of a lifestyle. Although the client may fully comprehend the consequences of continuing to smoke, the decision to give up a part of his or her life is not easy. This fear may be expressed in such concerns as "I'll gain weight," or "What will I do with my hands?" In addition to providing practical information, a plan, and assistance with nicotine withdrawal, the nurse must support the client's decision-making process to comply with an order to stop smoking.

- Assess knowledge and understanding of the choices involved and possible consequences of each. *The decision to quit smoking ultimately belongs to the client. He or she needs a full understanding of the consequences of quitting or continuing to smoke.*
- Acknowledge concerns, values, and beliefs; listen nonjudgmentally. *The nurse needs to avoid imposing his or her values and beliefs about smoking on the client.*
- Spend time with the client, encouraging expression of feelings. *This demonstrates acceptance of the client and his or her right to make the decision.*
- Help plan a course of action for quitting smoking and adapt it as necessary. *When the client develops the plan, he or she has more ownership in it and interest in making it work.*
- Demonstrate respect for decisions and the right to choose. *Respect supports self-esteem and the ability to cope.*
- Provide referral to a counselor or other professional as needed. *Counselors or other people trained to assist with smoking cessation can help with decision making.*

### Using NANDA, NIC, and NOC

Chart 36–3 shows links between NANDA nursing diagnoses, NIC, and NOC for the client with COPD.

### Home Care

As with any chronic disease, the client and family will have primary responsibility for disease management. Teaching is vital to promote optimal health and slow disease progression. Teaching for home care focuses on effective coughing and breathing techniques, preventing exacerbations, and managing prescribed therapies.

---

### CHART 36–3   NANDA, NIC, AND NOC LINKAGES

#### The Client with COPD

| NURSING DIAGNOSES | NURSING INTERVENTIONS | NURSING OUTCOMES |
|---|---|---|
| • Anxiety | • Anxiety Reduction<br>• Coping Enhancement | • Anxiety Control<br>• Coping |
| • Decisional Conflict | • Decision-Making Support<br>• Health System Guidance | • Decision Making<br>• Participation: Health Care Decisions |
| • Imbalanced Nutrition: Less than Body Requirements | • Nutrition Management<br>• Weight Gain Assistance | • Nutritional Status: Food and Fluid Intake |
| • Ineffective Airway Clearance | • Airway Management<br>• Cough Enhancement<br>• Oxygen Therapy<br>• Respiratory Monitoring | • Respiratory Status: Airway Patency<br>• Respiratory Status: Gas Exchange |
| • Ineffective Breathing Pattern | • Energy Management<br>• Positioning | • Respiratory Status: Ventilation<br>• Vital Signs Status |
| • Ineffective Health Maintenance | • Self-Responsibility Facilitation<br>• Teaching: Disease Process | • Self-Direction of Care<br>• Treatment Behavior: Illness or Injury |

*Note. Data from Nursing Outcomes Classification (NOC) by M. Johnson & M. Maas (Eds.), 1997, St. Louis: Mosby; Nursing Diagnoses: Definitions & Classification 2001–2002 by North American Nursing Diagnosis Association, 2001, Philadelphia: NANDA; Nursing Interventions Classification (NIC) by J.C. McCloskey & G. M. Bulechek (Eds.), 2000, St. Louis: Mosby. Reprinted by permission.*

Pursed-lip and diaphragmatic breathing techniques help minimize air trapping and fatigue. Pursed-lip breathing helps maintain open airways by maintaining positive pressures longer during exhalation. Teach the client to:

1. Inhale through the nose with the mouth closed.
2. Exhale slowly through pursed lips, as though whistling or blowing out a candle, making exhalation twice as long as inhalation.

Diaphragmatic or abdominal breathing helps conserve energy by using the larger and more efficient muscles of respiration. Teach the client to:

1. Place one hand on the abdomen, the other on the chest.
2. Inhale, concentrating on pushing the abdominal hand outward while the chest hand remains still.
3. Exhale slowly, while the abdominal hand moves inward and the chest hand remains still.

Repeat these exercises as often as necessary until the techniques become incorporated into normal breathing.

Several different coughing techniques may be useful. For controlled cough technique, teach the client to:

1. Following prescribed bronchodilator treatment, inhale deeply, and hold breath briefly.
2. Cough twice, the first time to loosen mucus, the second to expel secretions.
3. Inhale by sniffing to prevent mucus from moving back into deep airways.
4. Rest. Avoid prolonged coughing to prevent fatigue and hypoxemia.

For huff coughing, teach the client to:

1. Inhale deeply while leaning forward.
2. Exhale sharply with a "huff" sound, to help keep airways open while mobilizing secretions.

In addition, include the following topics when teaching for home care.

- Maintaining adequate fluid intake, at least 2.0 to 2.5 quarts of fluid daily
- Avoiding respiratory irritants, including cigarette smoke, both primary and secondary, other smoke sources, dust, aerosol sprays, air pollution, and very cold dry air
- Preventing exposure to infection, especially upper respiratory infections
- Importance of pneumococcal vaccine and annual influenza immunization
- Prescribed exercise program, maintaining ADLs, and balancing rest and exercise
- Maintaining nutrient intake (e.g., eating small frequent meals and using nutritional supplements to provide adequate calories)
- Ways of reducing sodium intake if prescribed
- Identifying early signs of an infection or exacerbation and the importance of seeking medical attention for the following: fever, increased sputum production, purulent (green or yellow) sputum, upper respiratory infection, increased shortness of breath or difficulty breathing, decreased activity tolerance or appetite, increased need for oxygen
- Prescribed medications, including purpose, proper use, and expected effects
- Avoiding use of over-the-counter medications unless approved by the physician.
- Other prescribed therapies, such as use of home oxygen, percussion, postural drainage, and nebulizer treatments
- Use, cleaning, and maintenance of any required special equipment
- Importance of wearing an identification band and carrying a list of medications at all times in case of an emergency.

Provide referrals to home care services such as home health, assistance with ADLs as needed, home maintenance services, respiratory therapy and home oxygen services, and other agencies such as Meals-on-Wheels and senior services as indicated.

## Nursing Care Plan
## A Client with COPD

Anna Mercurio, known as "Happy" by all her friends, is an 83-year-old widow who lives with her two adult sons. Over the past 15 years, Mrs. Mercurio has become increasingly short of breath while gardening and walking, two favorite activities. She also has developed a chronic cough that is particularly bad in the mornings. Ten years ago, her family physician told her that she had emphysema. She is admitted to the hospital with possible pneumonia and acute exacerbation of COPD.

### ASSESSMENT
Jeff Harris, RN, admits Mrs. Mercurio to the medical unit. In the nursing history, Mr. Harris notes that she denies ever smoking, but says that her husband and two sons have been smokers "for practically their whole lives." She says she lived an active life before developing lung disease, but now her breathing and cough have progressed so that she now must rest after just a few minutes of housework or other activity. Her cough is productive of moderate to large amounts of sputum, particularly in the mornings. She

## Nursing Care Plan

### A Client with COPD *(continued)*

developed increasing shortness of breath and sputum 2 days ago; this morning, she could not complete her morning activities without resting, so she contacted her doctor.

On physical examination, Mr. Harris notes the following: skin very warm and dry, color dusky. Pauses frequently while speaking to breathe. Respiratory rate 36, fairly shallow; coughs frequently, producing large amounts of thick, tenacious green sputum. Other vital signs: P 115 and irregular, BP 186/60, T 102.4°F (39°C). Appears very thin; weight 96 lb (43.6 kg), height 63 inches (160 cm). Anteroposterior:lateral chest diameter approximately 1:1; moderate kyphosis noted. Chest hyperresonant to percussion. Auscultation reveals distant breath sounds with scattered wheezes and rhonchi throughout lung fields. Chest X-ray shows flattening of diaphragm, slight cardiac enlargement, prominent vascular and bronchial markings, and patchy infiltrates. Initial laboratory work reveals moderate erythrocytosis, leukocytosis, and low serum albumin. Arterial blood gas results: pH 7.19; $Po_2$ 54 mmHg; $Pco_2$ 59 mmHg; $Hco_3^-$ 30 mg/dL, and $O_2$ saturation 88%. Admitting orders include sputum specimen for culture; intravenous penicillin G, 2 million units every 4 hours; ipratropium bromide (Atrovent) inhaler, two puffs every 6 hours; beclomethasone diproprionate (Vanceril) inhaler, two puffs every 6 hours; bed rest with bathroom privileges; oxygen per nasal cannula at 2 L continuously; and regular diet.

### DIAGNOSES

- *Ineffective airway clearance* related to pneumonia and COPD
- *Impaired gas exchange* related to acute and chronic lung disease
- *Risk for impaired spontaneous ventilation* related to loss of hypoxemic respiratory drive and respiratory muscle fatigue
- *Impaired home maintenance* related to activity intolerance

### EXPECTED OUTCOMES

- Expectorate secretions effectively.
- Return to level of pulmonary function prior to acute exacerbation.
- Demonstrate improved arterial blood gas and oxygen saturation values.
- Maintain spontaneous respirations without excess fatigue.
- Verbalize willingness to allow sons or a housekeeper to assist with daily household tasks.

### PLANNING AND IMPLEMENTATION

- Assess respiratory status and level of consciousness every 1 to 2 hours until stable, then at least every 4 hours.
- Closely monitor response to oxygen therapy, including skin color, oxygen saturation, sputum consistency, and respiratory drive.
- Increase fluid intake to at least 2500 mL per day and provide bedside humidifier.
- Elevate head of bed to at least 30 degrees at all times.

- Teach "huff" coughing technique.
- Administer medications as ordered; providing ipratropium inhaler before beclomethasone inhaler. Provide mouth care after inhalers.
- Contact respiratory therapy for percussion and postural drainage following inhaler treatments.
- Provide for uninterrupted rest periods following treatments and procedures.
- Meet with Mrs. Mercurio and her sons to develop a postdischarge care plan.
- Refer to home health department for nursing follow-up.
- Refer to social services for possible assistance with home maintenance.

### EVALUATION

After the first day in the hospital, Mrs. Mercurio's condition begins to improve slowly. On discharge 6 days later, she is able to provide self-care with less fatigue and dyspnea. She is using oxygen at night only, admitting that it is just for security. Although a few scattered wheezes and rhonchi are still present in her lungs, Mrs. Mercurio's sputum is thinner, white, and easily expectorated. She will continue taking oral penicillin V for an additional 10 days at home. She will also continue using the Atrovent and Vanceril inhalers as prescribed at home. Although Mrs. Mercurio's sons admit they will probably never be able to quit smoking, they have agreed to smoke only in the garage or outside. A home health nurse will initially evaluate Mrs. Mercurio's progress three times weekly. Arrangements have been made for a housekeeper to come twice a week for cleaning and laundry. Mrs. Mercurio is glad to be returning home and grateful for the arrangements that have been made.

### Critical Thinking in the Nursing Process

1. Mrs. Mercurio has never been a smoker but had long-term exposure to secondhand smoke. How does secondhand smoke contribute to lung diseases in adults and children?
2. Mr. Harris's nursing care plan included the nursing diagnosis, *Risk for impaired spontaneous ventilation* related to loss of hypoxemic respiratory drive and respiratory muscle fatigue. Identify the normal physiologic events that stimulate breathing, and describe how these differ for the client with chronic hypoxemia and hypercapnia.
3. The client with an acute exacerbation of COPD is at risk for respiratory failure. What changes in Mrs. Mercurio's assessment findings could indicate this complication?
4. Develop a nursing care plan for Mrs. Mercurio for the nursing diagnosis, *Deficient diversional activities* related to inability to continue preferred activities.

See Evaluating Your Response in Appendix C.

## THE CLIENT WITH CYSTIC FIBROSIS

**Cystic fibrosis (CF)** is an autosomal recessive disorder that affects epithelial cells of the respiratory, gastrointestinal, and reproductive tracts and leads to abnormal exocrine gland secretions. Although it can affect many organ systems, CF is particularly damaging to the lungs, leading to COPD in childhood and early adulthood. Respiratory manifestations of CF are the usual cause of morbidity and death from this disease. The gastrointestinal tract also is affected significantly; exocrine pancreatic insufficiency is characteristic of CF. Abnormally high sweat electrolytes also occur in CF.

CF is the most common lethal genetic disease in Caucasian Americans, affecting about 1 in 2500 live births. It is less common in African Americans and rare in Asians. About 5% of Caucasians in the United States carry the CF trait. Although the manifestations of CF develop in childhood, improved disease management has prolonged the life span for people with CF. Adults now make up about one-third of the CF population in the United States, with many clients surviving into their 30s (Braunwald et al., 2001).

## PATHOPHYSIOLOGY

An abnormal gene on the long arm of chromosome 7 causes a lack or abnormality of a protein involved in transporting chloride across the surfaces of epithelial cells. Defective chloride transport causes more water and sodium reabsorption than normal. Secretions in affected organs become thick and viscous, obstructing glands and ducts. This obstruction causes dilation of secretory glands and damage to exocrine tissue. The hallmark pathophysiologic effects of CF include:

- Excess mucus production in the respiratory tract with impaired ability to clear secretions and progressive COPD.
- Pancreatic enzyme deficiency and impaired digestion.
- Abnormal elevation of sodium and chloride concentrations in sweat.

In the lungs, viscous mucus plugs small airways and impairs mucociliary clearance, leading to atelectasis, infection, bronchiectasis, and dilation of distal airways. Lower respiratory infections with *Staphyococcus aureus* and *Pseudomonas* are common (Porth, 2002). Acute and chronic damage to lung parenchyma causes tissue loss and extensive scarring and fibrosis. The upper lobes are involved to a greater extent than the lower lobes. Severe airway obstruction and chronic hypoxemia lead to pulmonary hypertension, right ventricular hypertrophy, and eventual cor pulmonale. Death usually results from a combination of cardiovascular changes and respiratory failure.

Pancreatic insufficiency is a frequent component of CF. It can range from slight pancreatic dysfunction to complete absence of function due to obstruction of pancreatic ducts with thick mucus and degenerative and fibrotic changes. Pancreatic insufficiency and impaired enzyme secretion leads to impaired digestion and absorption of proteins, carbohydrates, and fats.

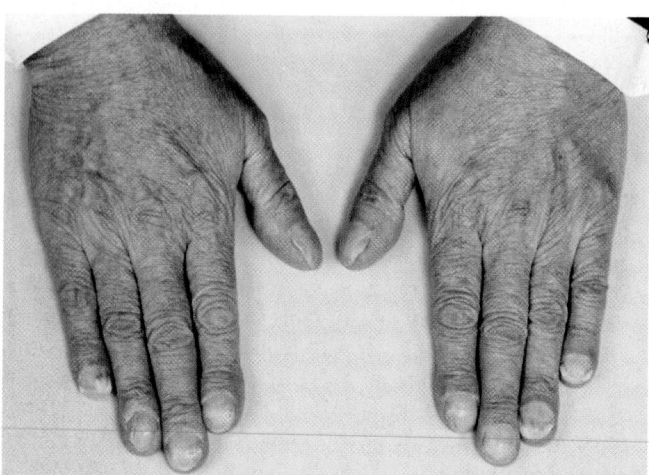

**Figure 36–13** ■ Clubbing of fingers caused by chronic hypoxemia.

*Source: John Radcliffe Hospital/Science Photo Library/Photo Researchers, Inc.*

About 8% of clients with CF develop diabetes mellitus (Porth, 2002). Liver failure is another potential complication of the disease (McCance & Huether, 2002). Because the genetic defect also affects cells of the reproductive tract, males with CF usually are sterile. While females may have difficulty conceiving, pregnancies usually are carried to term (Braunwald et al., 2001).

## MANIFESTATIONS

Manifestations of CF in a young adult include a history of chronic lung disease. Recurrent pneumonia, exercise intolerance, and chronic cough are typical. Other pulmonary manifestations include *clubbing* of the fingers and toes (Figure 36–13 ■), increased anteroposterior chest diameter (barrel chest), hyperresonant percussion tone, and basilar crackles on auscultation. Distended neck veins, ascites, and peripheral edema accompany right-sided heart failure. Abdominal pain and *steatorrhea* (excess fat in the stools, causing frequent, bulky, foul-smelling stool) commonly result from associated pancreatic insufficiency. Growth and development are often retarded, resulting in small stature.

## COLLABORATIVE CARE

Cystic fibrosis typically is diagnosed in infancy, but in some cases may not be diagnosed until adolescence or early adulthood. The treatment plan is multidisciplinary, with the goals of preventing or treating respiratory complications and maintaining adequate nutrition. Psychosocial care is vital, as is genetic and occupational counseling.

### Diagnostic Tests

Although evidence of lung disease and pancreatic insufficiency suggest CF, the pilocarpine iontophoresis sweat chloride test is used to establish the diagnosis. Pilocarpine (a parasympathomimetic agent) and a small electric current are used to increase sweat production on the forearm. Absorbent paper or gauze is used to collect the sweat for analysis. In CF, sodium and chloride levels in sweat are significantly elevated.

ABGs and oxygen saturation levels show hypoxemia. Pulmonary function studies reveal reduced air flow, reduced forced vital capacity (see Box 36–1), and reduced total lung capacity. Alveolar-capillary diffusion also is typically reduced.

## Medications

Immunization against respiratory infections is vital to promote optimal health. Yearly influenza vaccine is recommended, along with measles and pertussis boosters as needed.

Bronchodilator inhalers may be used to control airways constriction. Acute pulmonary infections are treated with appropriate antibiotic therapy as determined by sputum culture and sensitivity tests. A prolonged treatment course or multiple antibiotics may be required to eradicate pulmonary infections. Dornase alfa, recombinant human DNAse, breaks down the excess DNA in the sputum of clients with CF, decreasing its viscosity and making it easier to clear. Dornase alfa, administered by aerosol, reduces the frequency of hospitalizations and the need for antibiotics for some clients.

## Treatments

Chest physiotherapy with percussion and postural drainage is used to promote airway clearance. Newer airway clearance techniques include the use of the "huff" cough technique with specified breathing cycles or patterns. In one technique, a valved mask or mouthpiece is used to maintain positive expiratory pressure (PEP) for approximately 20 breaths, followed by 3 to 5 "huff" coughs. This cycle is repeated for a total of 20 minutes. The autogenic drainage technique, a form of biofeedback, involves controlled breathing at specific lung volumes and patterns to facilitate the movement of mucus into larger airways, where it can be cleared with the "huff" cough. A flutter valve device, which looks like a fat pipe, contains a steel ball within an inner cone. The weight of the ball provides intermittent PEP, which vibrates airway walls to loosen secretions (Goodfellow & Jones, 2002).

Oxygen therapy may be required for hypoxemia. A liberal fluid intake helps reduce the viscosity of mucus secretions. A diet high in protein, fat, and calories may be necessary to maintain weight. Vitamins and minerals are supplemented to counteract excess losses in the sweat and stools. Enteral or parenteral nutrition may be required during acute exacerbations of the disease.

Genetic screening of family members of a CF client can detect 70% to 75% of carriers of the CF gene. Screening for the CF gene is not recommended for the general population. Gene therapy is being explored as a treatment for CF.

Lung transplantation currently offers the only definitive treatment for CF. Lung transplantation lengthens life span and improves quality of life. Single-lung, double-lung, and heart-lung transplants have been successfully completed. Because the donor lungs do not have the CF gene, they do not develop the pathophysiologic changes of CF. Although the other defects characteristic of CF remain, these can be managed with pharmacologic therapy.

## NURSING CARE

Nursing care for the client with cystic fibrosis is much the same as that for any chronic obstructive lung disease. The genetic component of the disease and the client's age are important considerations. Adults with CF are just entering their productive years and face a life span that is likely to be shortened significantly. Females who do conceive face the prospect of transmitting the defective gene to their offspring.

The following nursing diagnoses are all appropriate for the client with CF:

- *Ineffective Airway Clearance*
- *Ineffective Breathing Pattern*
- *Anxiety*
- *Ineffective Therapeutic Regimen Management*
- *Imbalanced Nutrition: Less Than Body Requirements*
- *Compromised Family Coping*

Suggested interventions for these diagnoses are included in the nursing care sections for asthma and COPD.

Other diagnoses that should be considered for the client with CF follow:

- *Interrupted Family Processes* related to chronic genetic disease
- *Hopelessness* related to limited career options and opportunities
- *Delayed Growth and Development* related to gastrointestinal and respiratory effects of CF
- *Anticipatory Grieving* related to probable shortened lifespan

### Home Care

Education of the client and family affected by cystic fibrosis is essential to maintaining optimal health. The adult whose disease was diagnosed in infancy or childhood has grown up with the disease and often has a much greater knowledge level than many caregivers. However, when the initial diagnosis is made as an adolescent or young adult, teaching needs are significant. Include the following topics when teaching for home care:

- Respiratory care techniques, including percussion, postural drainage, and controlled cough techniques.
- Specific breathing and coughing exercises and procedures.
- The importance of avoiding respiratory irritants, such as cigarette smoke, air pollution, and occupational dusts and gases.
- Measures to prevent respiratory infection, such as maintaining immunizations and optimal general health, and avoiding exposure to large crowds and infected people.

Refer to a dietitian for planning and teaching to maintain adequate nutrition and minimize gastrointestinal symptoms. Referral to community agencies and support groups is also helpful.

Discuss the genetic transmission of cystic fibrosis and refer for counseling and possible genetic testing. Help the client and family sort through the impact of the disease on future pregnancies and generations. Remember that the possibility of CF may present an ethical dilemma regarding future pregnancies. Provide support as needed.

## THE CLIENT WITH ATELECTASIS

**Atelectasis** is not a disease but a condition associated with many respiratory disorders. It is a state of partial or total lung collapse and airlessness. It may be acute or chronic. The most common cause of atelectasis is obstruction of the bronchus ventilating a segment of lung tissue. The affected segment may be small or an entire lobe. Other causes include compression of the lung by pneumothorax, pleural effusion, or tumor; or loss of pulmonary surfactant and inability to maintain open alveoli.

The manifestations of atelectasis depend on its size. Diminished breath sounds over the affected area may be the only sign of a small atelectasis. If a large lung segment is affected, manifestations may include tachycardia, tachypnea, dyspnea, cyanosis, and other signs of hypoxemia. Chest expansion may be reduced and breath sounds absent on the affected side. Fever and other manifestations of infection may be present.

Chest X-ray shows an area of airless lung. CT scan may help determine the cause of atelectasis.

The primary therapy for atelectasis is prevention. High risk clients, such as those with COPD, smokers undergoing surgery, and people on prolonged bed rest or mechanical ventilation, should have vigorous chest physiotherapy to maintain open airways. Frequently assess respiratory status, including rate, breath sounds, and spirometry readings for early detection and treatment.

When atelectasis develops, treatment focuses on the underlying cause. Vigorous coughing and chest therapy may relieve obstruction by a mucus plug. Bronchoscopy may be necessary to remove the obstruction. Antibiotic therapy is ordered to treat infectious causes.

Nursing care to prevent and treat atelectasis is directed toward airway clearance. Position the client with atelectasis on the unaffected side to promote gravity drainage of affected segment. Encourage frequent position changes, ambulation, coughing, and deep breathing. Unless contraindicated, encourage fluids to help liquefy secretions. Teach the client at high risk for developing atelectasis about pulmonary care measures, fluid intake, and preventing pulmonary infections.

## THE CLIENT WITH BRONCHIECTASIS

**Bronchiectasis** is characterized by permanent abnormal dilation of one or more large bronchi and destruction of bronchial walls. Infection often is present. The destructive process of bronchiectasis is initiated by inflammation, usually due to recurrent airways infection. About half of all cases of bronchiectasis are related to cystic fibrosis. Other causes include infections, such as severe pneumonia, tuberculosis, or fungal infections; lung abscess; exposure to toxic gases; abnormal lung or immunologic defenses; and localized airway obstruction due to a foreign body or tumor. Inflammation and airway obstruction are common to all these processes. Bronchial walls become weakened and dilated as a result, leading to pooling of secretions and further infection and inflammation.

A chronic cough productive of large amounts of mucopurulent sputum is characteristic. Other manifestations of bronchiectasis include hemoptysis, recurrent pneumonia, wheezing and shortness of breath, malnutrition, right-sided heart failure, and cor pulmonale.

Collaborative care for bronchiectasis focuses on maintaining optimal pulmonary function and preventing progression of the disorder. The diagnosis is typically based on the history and physical examination. Chest X-ray and CT scan may be ordered to help confirm the diagnosis and determine the extent of lung damage.

Antibiotics are prescribed at the first indication of infection and may also be used prophylactically. Inhaled bronchodilators may be ordered. Chest physiotherapy is a vital component of continuing care for bronchiectasis. Percussion and postural drainage help mobilize secretions. Oxygen may be prescribed. Bronchoscopy may be used to clear retained secretions or obstruction or to evaluate hemoptysis. If lung destruction is localized and unresponsive to conservative management, surgical lung resection may be necessary.

Nursing care of the client with bronchiectasis is similar to that for clients with other obstructive lung diseases. Airway clearance is a primary problem, as is ineffective breathing pattern. Other applicable nursing diagnoses may include Impaired Gas Exchange, Imbalanced Nutrition: Less Than Body Requirements and Self-Care Deficit.

# INTERSTITIAL PULMONARY DISORDERS

Many lung diseases damage the interstitial or connective tissue of the lung. Occupational lung diseases and sarcoidosis are interstitial lung diseases. Toxic drugs and radiation also cause interstitial damage. Table 36–8 identifies common causes of interstitial lung disorders.

These disorders may be acute or insidious. Their rate of progression varies from person to person, as does the degree of disability they produce.

## THE CLIENT WITH AN OCCUPATIONAL LUNG DISEASE

Occupational lung diseases are a diverse group of disorders directly related to inhalation of noxious substances in the work environment. There are two major classifications of occupational lung diseases:

| TABLE 36-8 | Selected Causes of Interstitial Lung Disorders |
|---|---|
| **Cause** | **Examples** |
| Inorganic dusts | Silica (silicosis), asbestos (asbestosis), coal (coal workers' pneumoconioses), talc (talcosis) |
| Organic dusts | Cotton (byssinosis), sugar cane (bagassosis), moldy hay (farmer's lung) |
| Drugs | Antineoplastic agents, antibiotics, gold salts, phenytoin |
| Radiation | External radiation or inhaled radioactive materials |
| Infections | Widespread TB or fungal infections, viral or *Pneumocystis carinii* pneumonia |
| Poisons and noxious gases | Paraquat, nitrogen dioxide, chlorine, ammonia, sulfur dioxide |
| Systemic diseases | Uremia, pulmonary edema |
| Unknown causes | Sarcoidosis, idiopathic pulmonary fibrosis, connective tissue disorders |

- *Pneumoconioses*, chronic fibrotic lung diseases caused by inhalation of inorganic dusts and particulate matter
- *Hypersensitivity pneumonitis*, allergic pulmonary diseases caused by exposure to inhaled organic dusts

## PHYSIOLOGY REVIEW

Lung tissue contains elastin and collagen fibers. Elastin fibers are easily stretched, facilitating lung expansion. Collagen fibers, in contrast, resist stretching. This increases the work of breathing. Both elastin and collagen affect lung compliance, or the ease with which the lungs are inflated. Other factors affecting compliance include the water content of lung tissue and surface tension (Porth, 2002).

## PATHOPHYSIOLOGY

When a noxious substance is inhaled, the response to that substance depends on:

- The size of particulates;
- Its nature (organic or inorganic);
- Where it deposits in the respiratory tract; and
- The susceptibility of the individual.

Relatively large particles, larger than 6 microns, are too big to reach lower airways and often are deposited in the nose. Smaller particles can be carried with inspired air into the alveoli. Normal lung defenses, including alveolar macrophages, lymph channels, and the mucociliary escalator, attempt to remove particulate matter from the alveoli. Cigarette smoking, alcohol ingestion, or hypersensitivity reactions can impair these defenses.

The inhaled substance damages alveolar epithelium, leading to an inflammatory process of the alveoli and interstitial tissue of the lung. The inflammatory response produces further damage, and abnormal fibrotic (scar) tissue replaces the elastin fibers of normal lung tissue. As a result, the lungs become stiff and noncompliant. Lung volumes decrease, the work of breathing increases, and alveolar-capillary diffusion is impaired, leading to hypoxemia.

## Asbestosis

Inhalation of asbestos fibers is a common cause of occupational lung disease. *Asbestosis* is a diffuse interstitial fibrotic disease involving the terminal airways, alveoli, and pleurae. Exposure to asbestos fibers occurs during mining, milling, manufacturing, and application of asbestos products. Although symptoms may not become apparent until 20 years after exposure, they tend to progress, even when further exposure has been halted. Asbestosis is also associated with an increased risk of bronchogenic carcinoma, especially in cigarette smokers, malignant mesothelioma (an uncommon tumor of membranes such as the pleura and peritoneum), and pleural plaques (Tierney et al., 2001).

The manifestations of asbestosis include exertional dyspnea, exercise intolerance, and inspiratory crackles. Diffuse, small, irregular or linear opacities appear on chest X-ray, primarily in the lower lobes. As the disease progresses, respiratory failure and marked hypoxemia may develop.

## Silicosis

Inhalation of silica dust by hard-rock miners, foundry workers, sandblasters, pottery makers, and granite cutters can lead to *silicosis*, a nodular pulmonary fibrosis. Silicosis affects 1.2 to 3 million workers in the United States. Although generally associated with long-term exposure to silica, it can develop in as little as 10 months of intense exposure (Braunwald et al., 2001). In silicosis, macrophages are destroyed as they engulf silica particles, releasing substances that damage lung tissue and lead to fibrosis and scarring.

Simple silicosis is asymptomatic with no demonstrable respiratory impairment. Complicated silicosis, in contrast, is characterized by large conglomerate densities in the upper lungs. These clients may be severely dyspneic and have a productive cough. Pulmonary function testing shows both restrictive and obstructive changes. Increasing size of conglomerate masses can lead to severe disability, cor pulmonale, and death.

## Coal Worker's Pneumoconiosis

Ingestion of coal dust by alveolar macrophages causes "coal macules" to form, leading to *coal worker's pneumoconiosis*, or *"black lung disease."* This occupational lung disease affects 12% of all miners, with a higher incidence in the eastern United States than in the West (Braunwald et al., 2001). Coal macules appear on chest X-ray as diffuse, small opacities primarily affecting the upper lungs.

Simple coal worker's pneumoconiosis (CWP) generally is asymptomatic. A small percentage of clients (1% to 2%) develop progressive massive fibrosis which destroys the pulmonary vascular bed and airways of the upper lungs. This progressive form of the disease causes symptoms similar to those of complicated silicosis.

## Hypersensitivity Pneumonitis

Workers exposed to organic dusts and gases may develop *hypersensitivity pneumonitis,* an allergic pulmonary disease affecting the airways and alveoli. Byssinosis, resulting from cotton dust exposure, bagassosis, due to exposure to moldy sugar cane fiber, farmer's lung, and bird-fancier's lung are examples of hypersensitivity pneumonitis.

Either acute or subacute illness can occur. Acute illness occurs 4 to 8 hours after exposure and is heralded by sudden onset of malaise, chills and fever, dyspnea, cough, and nausea. The subacute syndrome is characterized by an insidious onset of chronic cough, progressive dyspnea, anorexia, and weight loss. Diffuse fibrosis occurs after repeated exposure to the organic material, leading to respiratory insufficiency.

## COLLABORATIVE CARE

Prevention is a key strategy for all occupational lung diseases. Containing dust and wearing personal protective devices that limit the amount of inhaled particles are essential for people who work in industries with known risks.

Chest X-ray, pulmonary function studies, bronchoscopy, and possibly lung biopsy are used to establish the diagnosis of pneumoconioses. Characteristic patterns are seen for each disorder on X-ray. Pulmonary function testing shows restrictive impairment of lung ventilation, with reduced vital capacity and reduced total lung capacity. The diffusing capacity of the lungs is also decreased. Blood gas analysis reveals hypoxemia, especially with exercise. Bronchoscopy may be performed to obtain tissue for biopsy. Specialized lung scans may be used to determine the extent of fibrosis.

Eliminating further exposure to the offending agent is an important part of disease management. There is no specific therapy. Anti-inflammatory drugs, such as corticosteroids, may reduce the inflammatory response and slow the progression of the disease. Preventing exposure to other damaging substances such as cigarette smoke and pollution is vital. Pneumococcal vaccine and annual influenza immunizations are recommended to reduce the risk of lower respiratory infections. Other care is supportive, similar to that for COPD.

## NURSING CARE

### Health Promotion

Teaching about the dangers of occupational lung diseases and ways to reduce their risk needs to begin early, before the disease develops. Nurses in industrial and public health settings can begin by recognizing potential dangers and teaching workers about measures to reduce dust in their work area and the use of personal protective devices such as masks. Nurses working with affected families have an excellent opportunity to begin educating children about the risks associated with the occupation.

### Nursing Diagnoses and Interventions

Nursing care for clients with occupational lung diseases is similar to that for clients with COPD. Activity intolerance is a high-priority problem for many clients. Severe dyspnea can significantly interfere with ADLs. Nursing measures to reduce energy expenditures and provide for rest are essential. Caregiver role strain, either actual or potential, must be considered when the client with severe disability is being cared for at home.

Both client and family coping may be compromised. Many of these diseases develop after 20 to 30 years of exposure to the hazardous material. Clients who entered the industry following high school may develop evidence of disease in their 40s and face the possibility of changing their occupation or developing significant disability. The resulting role strain affects all members of the family.

Other nursing diagnoses to consider for the client with an occupational lung disease follow:

- *Ineffective Breathing Pattern* related to restrictive lung disease
- *Anticipatory Grieving* related to potential loss of employment and income
- *Low Self-Esteem: Situational* related to change of occupation

### Home Care

The affected client and family need teaching in preparation for home care, including:

- Prevention of further lung damage, e.g., avoiding cigarette smoke and heavy air pollution.
- Recommendations for pneumococcal and annual influenza immunizations; yearly tuberculin testing for clients with silicosis.
- Pulmonary hygiene measures, such as liberal fluid intake, coughing, and deep-breathing exercises.
- Use and care of oxygen therapy equipment if required
- Use and effects of any prescribed or recommended over-the-counter medications.

## THE CLIENT WITH SARCOIDOSIS

**Sarcoidosis** is a chronic, multisystem disease characterized by an exaggerated cellular immune response in involved tissues. This abnormal immune response leads to granuloma formation in the lungs, lymph nodes, liver, eyes, skin, and other organs. Its cause is unknown. Sarcoidosis primarily affects young adults between the ages of 20 and 40. In the United States, the incidence is highest in African Americans. Women are affected at a slightly higher rate than men (Braunwald et al., 2001).

In sarcoidosis, multiple granulomas form; these lesions may resolve spontaneously or proceed to fibrosis. The lungs are affected in about 90% of clients with sarcoidosis. Sarcoidosis has a low mortality rate—less than 3%—but a relatively high rate (approximately 10%) of serious disability from ocular, respiratory, or other organ damage. Pulmonary hemorrhage and cardiac and respiratory failure from pulmonary fibrosis are the leading causes of death from sarcoidosis.

The manifestations of sarcoidosis vary, depending on the organ system affected. It may be asymptomatic, diagnosed by characteristic findings on routine chest X-ray. Symptoms may be insidious, with anorexia, fatigue, weight loss, fever, dyspnea, arthralgias, and myalgias. Skin lesions, uveitis, lymphadenopathy, hepatomegaly, or other manifestations may also develop.

Leukopenia, eosinophilia, and an elevated erythrocyte sedimentation rate (ESR) typically are noted in sarcoidosis. The chest X-ray helps to determine the extent of pulmonary involvement. Biopsy of a granulomatous lesion may be required to confirm the diagnosis. Pulmonary function tests reveal decreased compliance and impaired diffusing capacity.

Sarcoidosis often resolves spontaneously, therefore treatment is indicated only when symptoms are severe or disabling. Corticosteroid therapy is prescribed to suppress the inflammatory process when indicated. Relapse frequently occurs when corticosteroids are discontinued. Other anti-inflammatory or immune-modifier medications may also be used, including chloroquine, indomethacin, azathioprine, and methotrexate.

Nursing care for clients with sarcoidosis is directed by involved organ systems and related manifestations. Respiratory care is supportive and includes avoiding respiratory irritants and maintaining adequate ventilation. Refer for smoking cessation assistance as needed.

Teach clients with limited symptoms about the disease and symptoms to report to a health care provider, including shortness of breath, tearing and eye inflammation, chest pain or irregular pulse, skin lesions, and swollen and painful joints. If corticosteroid therapy is prescribed, teach the importance of taking the drug as prescribed and not stopping it abruptly. Include information about managing the side effects of corticosteroids by limiting sodium and increasing potassium in the diet, taking the medication with food or milk to minimize gastric irritation, and identifying early signs of infection.

# PULMONARY VASCULAR DISORDERS

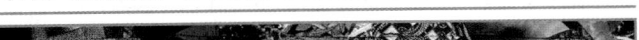

The cardiovascular and respiratory systems are closely interrelated. As blood flows through the capillary network of the pulmonary vascular system, oxygen diffuses into it, and carbon dioxide diffuses out. An effective match of alveolar ventilation and capillary perfusion is essential to maintain this process and, ultimately, tissue oxygenation and function of all organ systems. Both vascular and alveolar changes can alter gas exchange. Arteriosclerotic changes in pulmonary vasculature reduce blood flow to the alveolus. Nearly all lower respiratory system disorders potentially can affect ventilation. Many also have a secondary effect on lung perfusion, because breakdown or fibrosis of alveolar walls destroys the capillary network as well. This section focuses on primary disorders of the pulmonary vascular system.

## THE CLIENT WITH PULMONARY EMBOLISM

A **pulmonary embolism** is obstruction of blood flow in part of the pulmonary vascular system by an embolus. *Thromboemboli,* or blood clots, that develop in the venous system or right side of the heart are the most frequent cause of pulmonary embolism. Other sources of emboli include tumors that have invaded venous circulation, fat or bone marrow entering the circulation due to fracture or other trauma, amniotic fluid released into the circulation during childbirth, and intravenous injection of air or other foreign substances.

Pulmonary embolism causes an estimated 50,000 deaths annually, making it the third leading cause of death in hospitalized clients (Tierney et al., 2001). Although many substances can become emboli, thrombus arising from the deep veins of the legs is the leading cause of pulmonary embolism. *Deep venous thrombosis (DVT)* develops in approximately 5 million people per year in the United States. The risk factors for pulmonary embolus are those for DVT: stasis of venous blood flow, vessel wall damage, and altered blood coagulation.

Prolonged immobility; trauma, including hip and femur fractures; surgery (orthopedic, pelvic, and gynecologic surgery in particular); myocardial infarction and heart failure; obesity; and advanced age are risk factors for DVT. Women who use oral contraceptives or estrogen therapy are at risk, as are women during pregnancy and childbirth. See Chapter 33 for more information about DVT.

Pulmonary embolism is a medical emergency. Fifty percent of deaths from pulmonary embolism occur within the first two hours following embolization. In many cases, DVT has not been recognized or treated; often embolization also goes undetected. Prevention is the most effective treatment strategy for pulmonary embolism.

## PHYSIOLOGY REVIEW

The right heart receives deoxygenated blood from the systemic venous circulation. The entire output of the right ventricle enters the pulmonary circulation via the pulmonary artery. This artery branches into successively smaller arteries, arterioles, and capillaries of the pulmonary vascular system. Each alveolus of the lungs is surrounded by a meshwork of capillaries; capillaries within the septa between alveoli are exposed to the gases in alveoli on both sides of the septum. The respiratory membrane, where gas exchange occurs, consists of the squamous cell lining of the alveolus, the epithelial cell lining of the capillary, and a thin basement membrane between the alveolar and capillary cells. Oxygen and carbon dioxide readily diffuse across this very thin membrane. Diffusion is driven by a concentration gradient: The partial pressure of oxygen in the alveolus is greater than that in the capillary, therefore it diffuses into the blood. Carbon dioxide, in contrast, diffuses from the capillaries into the alveoli, driven by the higher pressure of dissolved carbon dioxide in venous blood.

A match between blood flow through the pulmonary vascular system (perfusion) and lung ventilation is necessary for effective *respiration* (the exchange of gases between the organism and the environment). Local factors regulate ventilation and perfusion to maintain this match. A low alveolar $Po_2$ causes alveolar capillary constriction, directing blood flow to areas of the lung where the alveolar $Po_2$ is higher. Likewise, high alveolar $Pco_2$ levels cause local bronchodilation, increasing airflow and eliminating excess carbon dioxide.

## PATHOPHYSIOLOGY

Thrombi affecting only the deep veins of the calf rarely embolize to the pulmonary circulation. However, thrombi often propogate proximally to the popliteal and ileofemoral veins. From there, they may break loose to become an embolus. As vessels of the venous system become progressively larger, the embolus rarely is trapped until it enters the pulmonary arterial system with its progressively smaller vessels leading to the pulmonary capillary beds.

The impact of a pulmonary embolus depends on the extent to which pulmonary blood flow is obstructed, the size of the embolus, its nature, and secondary effects of the obstruction. The effects can range widely:

- Occlusion of a large pulmonary artery with sudden death. Gas exchange is significantly reduced or prevented, and cardiac output falls dramatically as blood fails to move through the pulmonary vascular system and return to the left heart.
- Lung tissue infarction due to occlusion of a significant portion of pulmonary blood flow. Fewer than 10% of pulmonary emboli result in pulmonary infarction.
- Obstruction of a small segment of the pulmonary circulation with no permanent lung injury.
- Chronic or recurrent small emboli which may be multiple.

Obstruction of pulmonary blood flow by an embolus affects both perfusion and ventilation. Neurohumoral reflexes triggered by obstruction cause vasoconstriction, increasing pulmonary vascular resistance. In severe cases, this can lead to pulmonary hypertension and right ventricular heart failure. Systemically, hypotension and a drop in cardiac output may develop. Bronchoconstriction occurs in the affected area of lung. Dead space (areas of the lung that are ventilated but not perfused) increases. Alveolar surfactant decreases, increasing the risk for atelectasis.

If infarction does not occur, the fibrinolytic system (see Chapter 32) ultimately dissolves the clot, and pulmonary function returns to normal. Infarcted tissue becomes scarred and fibrotic.

Fat emboli are the most common nonthrombotic pulmonary emboli. A fat embolism usually occurs after fracture of long bone (typically the femur) releases bone marrow fat into the circulation. Adipose tissue or liver trauma may also lead to fat emboli.

## MANIFESTATIONS

The manifestations of pulmonary embolism depend on its size and location. Small emboli may be asymptomatic. Manifestations usually develop abruptly, over a period of minutes. The most common symptoms are dyspnea and pleuritic chest pain. Anxiety, a sense of impending doom, and cough are also common. See the box below. Diaphoresis and hemoptysis may develop. Massive pulmonary embolus can cause syncope and cyanosis. On examination, tachycardia and tachypnea are noted. Crackles may be heard on auscultation of the chest, and a cardiac gallop ($S_3$ and possibly $S_4$) may be noted. A low-grade fever may develop. It is difficult to differentiate pulmonary embolism from myocardial infarction or pneumonia by manifestations.

Characteristic manifestations of fat emboli include sudden onset of cardiopulmonary and neurologic symptoms: dyspnea, tachypnea, tachycardia, confusion, delirium, and decreased level of consciousness. Petechiae often develop on the chest and arms.

## COLLABORATIVE CARE

Because deep venous thrombosis may not be identified until pulmonary embolism occurs, prevention is the primary goal in treating pulmonary embolism.

Early ambulation of medical and surgical clients is an effective means of preventing venous stasis and reducing the incidence of pulmonary embolism. External pneumatic compression of the legs is also effective for clients undergoing neurosurgery, urologic surgery, or major surgery of the hip or knee, or when anticoagulant therapy is contraindicated. Other preventive measures include elevating the legs and active and passive leg exercises.

When pulmonary embolism occurs, treatment is supportive. Oxygen therapy is initiated, and analgesics may be ordered to relieve severe pleuritic pain and anxiety. Pulmonary artery and wedge pressures are monitored with a balloon (Swan-Ganz) catheter. Cardiac outputs also may be assessed. Cardiac rhythm is monitored to detect dysrhythmias.

### Manifestations of Pulmonary Embolism

**COMMON**

- Dyspnea and shortness of breath
- Chest pain
- Anxiety and apprehension
- Cough
- Tachycardia and tachypnea
- Crackles (rales)
- Low-grade fever

**LESS COMMON**

- Diaphoresis
- Hemoptysis
- Syncope
- Cyanosis
- $S_3$ and/or $S_4$ gallop

## Diagnostic Tests

The studies performed to identify DVT differ from those used to diagnose a pulmonary embolism. See Chapter 33 for diagnostic studies for venous thrombosis.

- *Plasma D-dimer levels* are highly specific to the presence of a thrombus. D-dimer is a fragment of fibrin formed during lysis of a blood clot; elevated blood levels indicate thrombus formation and lysis (e.g., DVT and pulmonary embolism).
- *Lung scans,* including perfusion and ventilation scans are performed, alone or in combination, to diagnose pulmonary embolism. In a perfusion lung scan, radiotagged albumin is injected intravenously and distributed in the lungs by the pulmonary blood flow. The lungs are then scanned for distribution of the isotope. An area of lung in which the isotope is undetectable is suggestive of occluded blood flow and pulmonary embolism (Figure 36–14 ■). For a ventilation scan, a radiotagged gas such as krypton or xenon-133 is inhaled. The lungs are scanned for gas distribution. Combined perfusion and ventilation scans allow identification of areas of the lungs that are ventilated but not perfused, a characteristic of pulmonary embolism.
- *Pulmonary angiography* is the definitive test for pulmonary embolism when other, less invasive tests are inconclusive. It is possible to detect very small emboli with angiography. A contrast medium injected into the pulmonary arteries illustrates the pulmonary vascular system on X-ray.
- *Chest X-ray* often shows pulmonary infiltration and occasionally pleural effusion.
- *Electrocardiogram (ECG)* is ordered to rule out acute myocardial infarction as the cause of symptoms. ECG findings commonly associated with pulmonary embolism include tachycardia and nonspecific T wave changes.
- *ABGs* usually show hypoxemia ($PO_2$ less than 80 mmHg), and often respiratory alkalosis (pH >7.45, $PCO_2$ <38 mmHg) due to tachypnea and hyperventilation.
- *Exhaled carbon dioxide ($ETCO_2$)* may be measured to evaluate alveolar perfusion. The normal $ETCO_2$ reading is 35 to 45 mmHg; it is decreased when pulmonary perfusion is impaired.
- *Coagulation studies* are ordered to monitor the response to therapy. The *activated partial thromboplastin time (aPTT or PTT)* is used to assess the intrinsic clotting pathway and the response to heparin therapy. Desired levels with anticoagulant therapy are 1.5 to 2 times the control value. The risk of recurrent thromboembolism is high at levels less than 1.5 times the control; the risk of bleeding increases at levels greater than 2 times the control. The *prothrombin time (PT or Pro-time)* or *International Normalized Ratio (INR)* is used to assess the extrinsic clotting system and oral anticoagulation with warfarin (Coumadin). The goal of anticoagulant therapy is to achieve a prothrombin time 1.25 to 1.5 times the control time. The therapeutic range for the INR is 2.0 to 3.0.

## Medications

Anticoagulant therapy is the standard treatment to prevent pulmonary emboli. It is often instituted in high-risk clients who have no evidence of pulmonary embolism, to prevent possible devastating effects. In the client with DVT or a pulmonary embolus, anticoagulants are administered to prevent further clotting and embolization. See Chapter 33 for more information about anticoagulant therapy to prevent and treat DVT. See the Medication Administration box on pages 1013 and 1014 for the nursing implications for anticoagulant therapy.

For pulmonary embolus, heparin therapy is initiated with an intravenous bolus of 5,000 to 10,000 units of heparin, followed by continuous infusion at the rate of 1000 to 1500 units per hour. The aPTT or PTT is monitored frequently until stabilized. Heparin therapy is typically continued for about 5 days or until oral anticoagulant therapy has become fully effective.

Oral anticoagulant therapy with warfarin sodium (Coumadin) is initiated at the same time as heparin. Warfarin alters the synthesis of vitamin K–dependent clotting factors and requires 5 to 7 days to be fully effective. Anticoagulant therapy is continued for 2 to 3 months when few risk factors for thromboemboli exist; long-term therapy is used when chronic disorders that increase the risk of thromboemboli are present.

Bleeding is a risk associated with anticoagulant therapy. Although major hemorrhage is uncommon, it occurs in approximately 5% of clients receiving intravenous heparin. Cardiac, hepatic, and renal disease increase the risk of significant bleeding, as does age over 60 years. Protamine, a protein that combines with heparin to inactivate it, is used to stop its anticoagulant effect if major bleeding occurs. Vitamin K is given to treat bleeding associated with Coumadin therapy.

Thrombolytic therapy may be used to treat massive pulmonary embolus and hypotension. Streptokinase, urokinase, or tissue plasminogen activator (t-PA) are used to *lyse* (disintegrate) the embolus, restore pulmonary blood flow, and reduce pulmonary artery and right heart pressures. Although thrombolytic therapy may not reduce mortality associated with pulmonary embolus, it may reduce the incidence of pulmonary hypertension, which develops 3 to 5 years after an embolism. Thrombolysis significantly increases the risk of bleeding, particularly cerebral bleeding. Contraindications to thrombolysis include intracranial disease, recent stroke, active bleeding or a bleeding disorder, pregnancy, severe hypertension, and recent

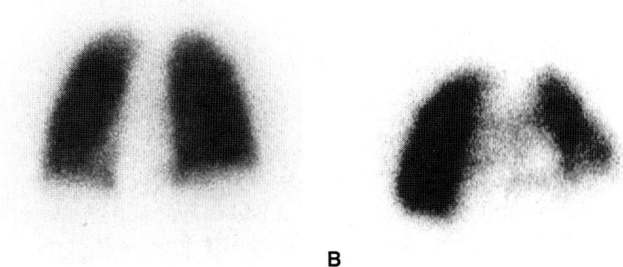

**Figure 36–14 ■** *A,* Normal perfusion lung scan showing smooth outlines and complete lung fields. *B,* Perfusion lung scan of a client with pulmonary embolus showing uneven densities in right lung, indicating impaired blood flow.

*Courtesy of University of California, Davis Medical Center.*

surgery or trauma. Because of the increased risk of hemorrhage, invasive procedures are avoided after thrombolysis. See Chapter 29 ⊝⊃ for further discussion of thrombolytic therapy and its nursing implications.

## Surgery

When anticoagulant therapy fails to prevent recurrent emboli or is contraindicated, an umbrellalike filter may be inserted into the inferior vena cava to trap large emboli while allowing continued blood flow (see Figure 33-6). The filter usually is inserted percutaneously, via either the femoral or jugular vein.

## NURSING CARE

### Health Promotion

Nurses are key in preventing pulmonary embolism. Encouraging clients to ambulate after surgery or illness, applying compression stockings or pneumatic compression devices, teaching and encouraging leg exercises, discouraging the use of pillows under the knees—all these measures help prevent DVT and subsequent pulmonary emboli.

Teach clients to reduce the risks associated with long periods of immobility, stopping every 1 to 2 hours during long automobile trips for a brief stretch and walk, getting up every hour or so and doing leg exercises while seated during long flights, and avoiding crossing the legs to prevent venous stasis and pooling. Regular exercise such as walking also reduces the risk of DVT. Instruct clients who stand for long periods to use well-fitted elastic stockings, being careful to avoid hose that bind around the knee or thigh.

### Assessment

Because pulmonary embolus can be a medical emergency, assessment may be very focused. In other instances, when emboli are small and not life threatening, a more extensive nursing assessment may be done.

- Health history: chest pain, shortness of breath, other symptoms, including onset, severity, precipitating factors; history of recent surgery, venous thrombosis, or other risk factor such as childbirth or malignancy; current medications
- Physical examination: level of consciousness, presence of respirations and pulse; color, skin temperature and moisture; vital signs including apical pulse and temperature; breath sounds and heart sounds; oxygen saturation level; neck vein distention, peripheral edema

### Nursing Diagnoses and Interventions

A large pulmonary embolus can cause a significant mismatch between pulmonary ventilation and circulation. Impaired gas exchange is a priority problem and focus for interventions. Cardiac output may be significantly affected by obstructed pulmonary blood flow. Thrombolytic and anticoagulant therapy affect the clotting process, increasing the risk for bleeding. Anxiety accompanies pulmonary embolism almost universally.

### Impaired Gas Exchange

Pulmonary embolism results in areas of the lung that are ventilated but not perfused; they receive no capillary blood flow. If the embolus is large and a major segment of the lung is unperfused, gas exchange is significantly affected. Nursing interventions are directed toward compensating for impaired gas exchange.

- Frequently assess respiratory status, including rate, depth, effort, lung sounds, and oxygen saturation. *Impaired ventilation will further compromise gas exchange and worsen hypoxemia. Oxygen saturation can be monitored continuously and noninvasively to evaluate gas exchange.*

**PRACTICE ALERT** *Monitor and record level of consciousness, mental status, and skin color. Hypoxemia often causes confusion and agitation; hypercapnia may reduce level of consciousness. Cyanosis indicates significant hypoxemia.* ■

- Place in Fowler's or high-Fowler's position, with the lower extremities dependent. *This position facilitates maximal lung expansion and reduces venous return to the right side of the heart, lowering pressures in the pulmonary vascular system.*

**PRACTICE ALERT** *Start oxygen per nasal cannula or mask. Obtain a physician's order if one has not been written. Supplemental oxygen increases alveolar and arterial oxygenation. Oxygen is a drug and must be prescribed by the physician. It may, however, be initiated by the nurse in an emergency to prevent tissue hypoxia.* ■

- Monitor arterial blood gas results, reporting abnormal findings as indicated. *ABGs are used to assess gas exchange and tissue oxygenation. An arterial line may be inserted for monitoring arterial pressure and arterial blood sampling.*
- Maintain bed rest. *Bed rest reduces metabolic demands and tissue needs for oxygen.*

### Decreased Cardiac Output

The impact of a large pulmonary embolus on hemodynamic status can be significant. Pressures in the pulmonary vascular system and right heart increase; blood return to the left heart and cardiac output may significantly decrease. Nursing interventions focus on preserving an adequate blood pressure and organ function until cardiopulmonary status stabilizes.

**PRACTICE ALERT** *Assess and record vital signs and cardiopulmonary status every 15 to 30 minutes initially, then every 2 to 4 hours as condition stabilizes. Frequent assessment facilitates timely interventions to maintain cardiovascular status and preserve organ function.* ■

- Auscultate heart sounds every 2 to 4 hours, reporting any abnormalities. *Sounds such as an $S_3$ or $S_4$ gallop may indicate cardiac compromise.*

**PRACTICE ALERT** *Record intake and output hourly. Decreased urinary output often is an early indicator of decreased cardiac output. Maintaining renal perfusion is vital to preserve renal function and prevent acute renal failure.* ■

- Assess skin color and temperature. *These assessments monitor tissue perfusion.*
- Monitor cardiac rhythm. *A drop in cardiac output and other hemodynamic alterations resulting from pulmonary embolism can precipitate dysrhythmias. Dysrhythmias, in turn, can further impair cardiac output.*
- Administer vasopressors and other medications as ordered. Carefully monitor the response to prescribed medications. *Drugs may be prescribed to maintain adequate arterial pressure and tissue perfusion. Potent drugs such as vasopressors require careful monitoring for desired and adverse effects.*
- Monitor pulmonary artery pressures, neck vein distension, and peripheral edema. Report findings as indicated. *Right-sided heart failure is a potential complication of pulmonary embolism because of increased pulmonary artery pressures.*
- Maintain intravenous and arterial access sites as well as central lines. *The client may be in unstable and critical condition, potentially needing immediate interventions to maintain life.*

**PRACTICE ALERT** *Provide frequent skin care. Impaired tissue perfusion and oxygenation increase the risk of skin and tissue breakdown.* ■

- Instruct to report chest pain or other symptoms. *Decreased cardiac output and an increased workload due to pulmonary hypertension may cause anginal pain.*

### Ineffective Protection

Thrombolytics and anticoagulant therapy impair normal clotting mechanisms, increasing the risk for bleeding and hemorrhage. This risk is particularly acute during the first 24 to 48 hours following thrombolytic drug administration.

- Assess frequently for overt and covert signs of bleeding: bleeding gums; hematuria; obvious or occult blood in stool or vomitus; incisional bleeding, bleeding or bruising of injection sites or with minor trauma; joint pain or immobility; abdominal or flank pain. *Careful monitoring is necessary to identify early signs of abnormal bleeding and prevent potential hemorrhage.*

**PRACTICE ALERT** *Promptly report changes in neurologic status. Although cerebral bleeding is not evident externally, changes in level of consciousness and other neurologic signs suggest it and should be reported immediately.* ■

- Report coagulation study results outside the desired range for anticoagulant therapy. *Levels less than the target range may indicate an increased risk for further clot development and pulmonary emboli; levels above the target range indicate an increased risk for bleeding.*

- Keep protamine sulfate available for heparin therapy and vitamin K available for warfarin (Coumadin) therapy. *Bleeding or hemorrhage due to excess anticoagulant may require antidote administration to rapidly reverse anticoagulant effects.*
- Assess medication regimen for possible drug interactions that could potentiate or inhibit anticoagulant effects. *Drug interactions can increase the risk for hemorrhage or further embolus formation.*
- Avoid invasive procedures, injections, and venous punctures when possible, particularly during and following thrombolytic therapy. *Invasive procedures increase the risk of tissue trauma and bleeding.*
- Maintain firm pressure on injection and venipuncture sites. Maintain pressure for 30 minutes following arterial puncture. *Firm pressure reduces the risk for bleeding into the tissues.*

**PRACTICE ALERT** *Use an infusion device to administer heparin infusion. Using an infusion pump or device helps prevent administration of excess medication.* ■

- Maintain adequate fluid intake. Administer stool softeners as ordered. *These measures help prevent constipation and straining, which may precipitate bleeding of hemorrhoids.*

### Anxiety

Pulmonary embolism is a physiologic and psychologic threat to safety and integrity. It is a major physiologic stressor, eliciting a strong neuroendocrine stress response. The feeling of suffocation and inability to catch one's breath that accompanies a pulmonary embolus is also a strong psychologic stressor. Fear, anxiety, and apprehension are common responses.

- Assess anxiety level. *Appropriate interventions are determined by the level of anxiety.*

**PRACTICE ALERT** *Provide reassurance and emotional support, listening to fears. Do not negate the fear of dying, but reassure that treatment usually restores effective respiratory function. The fear of death is very real and must not be discounted; however, it is important to provide reassurance to alleviate excess anxiety.* ■

- Remain with the client as much as possible. *The presence of a caring nurse helps reduce fear.*
- Explain procedures and treatments, using short, simple sentences. *Providing clearly understood, simple instructions reduces fear of the unknown.*
- Reduce environmental stimuli, and use a calm, reassuring manner. *These measures help reduce anxiety (for both the nurse and the client).*
- Allow supportive family members to remain with the client as much as possible. *Calm, supportive family members provide further reassurance.*
- Administer morphine sulfate as ordered. *Morphine is given to reduce pain and anxiety.*

## Home Care

Discuss the following topics when preparing the client with pulmonary embolism and family members for home care.

- Use of prescribed anticoagulant, including drug interactions, scheduled laboratory testing, and manifestations of bleeding to report to the primary care provider
- Using a soft toothbrush and electric razor to reduce the risk of bleeding
- Avoiding aspirin (unless prescribed) and other over-the-counter medications without approval by the physician
- Importance of wearing a MedicAlert tag for anticoagulant use
- Health promotion measures to reduce the risk of recurrent pulmonary embolism
- Symptoms of recurrent pulmonary embolism, such as sudden chest pain, shortness of breath, and possibly bloody sputum

# THE CLIENT WITH PULMONARY HYPERTENSION

The pulmonary vascular system is normally a high-flow, low-pressure, low-resistance system that can accommodate large increases in blood flow when necessary (e.g., during exercise). The normal mean arterial pressure in the pulmonary system is 12 to 15 mmHg (25 to 28 systolic/8 diastolic). **Pulmonary hypertension** is abnormal elevation of the pulmonary arterial pressure.

## PATHOPHYSIOLOGY AND MANIFESTATIONS

Pulmonary hypertension can develop as a primary disorder, but usually occurs secondarily to another condition.

### Primary Pulmonary Hypertension

*Primary pulmonary hypertension* is an uncommon disorder characterized by increased pulmonary vascular pressure and resistance with no apparent cause. Its etiology is unknown. It affects primarily women in their 30s or 40s. The manifestations of primary pulmonary hypertension are progressive dyspnea, fatigue, angina, and syncope with exertion. This progressive disorder generally causes a steady decline to death within 3 to 4 years.

### Secondary Pulmonary Hypertension

*Secondary pulmonary hypertension* is more common than primary. Its usual cause is reduced size of the pulmonary vascular bed, which may be due to vasoconstriction or widespread vessel destruction or obstruction. Hypoxemia is a potent pulmonary vasoconstrictor and a common initiating factor in pulmonary hypertension. Chronic lung diseases, sleep apnea, and hypoventilation due to obesity or neuromuscular disease can lead to hypoxemia. Alveolar wall destruction associated with emphysema leads to loss of pulmonary capillaries. Large or multiple pulmonary emboli may cause significant vessel obstruction. Other factors such as left ventricular failure or mitral stenosis also can lead to elevated pulmonary pressures. Once initiated, pulmonary hypertension becomes self-sustaining, because pulmonary vessels undergo changes that further narrow the pulmonary bed.

Manifestations of secondary pulmonary hypertension often are masked by those of the underlying disease. Dyspnea and dull, retrosternal chest pain are typical, as well as fatigue and syncope on exertion.

### Cor Pulmonale

**Cor pulmonale** is a condition of right ventricular hypertrophy and failure resulting from long-standing pulmonary hypertension. Chronic obstructive pulmonary disease is the most common cause of cor pulmonale.

The manifestations of cor pulmonale are those of the underlying pulmonary disorder and right-sided heart failure. Chronic productive cough, progressive dyspnea, and wheezing are common. With right-sided heart failure, peripheral edema and distended neck veins are seen. Skin is warm, moist, and both ruddy and cyanotic because of increased numbers of RBCs and hypoxemia.

# COLLABORATIVE CARE

The CBC commonly shows *polycythemia,* increased numbers of red blood cells. ABGs and oxygen saturation measurements reveal hypoxemia. The chest X-ray shows right heart enlargement and dilation of central pulmonary arteries. Typical ECG changes are those of right ventricular hypertrophy. An echocardiogram may be done to identify cardiac changes occurring either as a cause or result of pulmonary hypertension. Doppler ultrasonography is a noninvasive means of estimating pulmonary artery pressure, but cardiac catheterization may be required for definitive diagnosis. See page 817 for nursing care of the client undergoing cardiac catheterization.

Treatment for primary pulmonary hypertension is not particularly effective to reverse or slow the course of the disease. The calcium channel blockers nifedipine (Procardia) or diltiazem (Cardizem) may be given to reduce pulmonary vascular resistance and improve cardiac output. Short-acting direct vasodilators such as intravenous adenosine, inhaled nitric oxide, or intravenous prostacyclin may be used for severe disability. Bilateral lung or heart-lung transplant is the most effective long-term treatment for primary pulmonary hypertension.

Treatment of secondary pulmonary hypertension is directed toward the underlying disease process. Pulmonary hypertension often is advanced at the time of diagnosis and resistant to treatment. Supplemental oxygen may be ordered to reduce hypoxemia. Long-term anticoagulation or calcium channel blockers may be prescribed. If polycythemia is present, phlebotomy is performed to reduce the viscosity of the blood.

When cor pulmonale is present, salt and water restrictions as well as diuretic therapy are added to the above regimen to manage the right-sided heart failure.

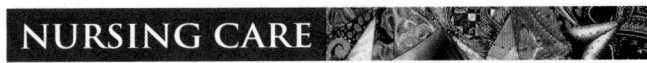

## NURSING CARE

Nursing care for the client with pulmonary hypertension or cor pulmonale is largely supportive. The focus is toward the underlying lung disease. Impaired gas exchange due to contraction of the pulmonary vascular system is a significant problem that causes many secondary problems, such as activity intolerance, anxiety, fatigue, and others. Nursing interventions for impaired gas exchange are directed toward maintaining adequate alveolar ventilation, oxygenation, and perfusion. The following measures may be included.

- Monitoring breath sounds, respiratory rate, skin color, and use of accessory muscles
- Positioning for optimal lung expansion
- Coughing, deep breathing, and chest physiotherapy
- Administering prescribed vasodilators

It is important to assess fatigue and dyspnea with activities and to plan frequent rest periods. Assist with self-care as needed to conserve energy.

With primary pulmonary hypertension, *Anticipatory grieving* and *Hopelessness* are additional potential nursing diag-

noses. When cor pulmonale is present, *Decreased cardiac output, Excess fluid volume,* and *Ineffective individual coping* must be considered.

### Home Care

Most care for these chronic conditions is provided in the home and community settings. Teaching is directed both at the underlying lung disease, if present, and the resulting hypertensive process. Refer to the section on COPD for teaching related to this disease, the most frequent underlying cause of cor pulmonale.

In addition, provide teaching about the following topics for the client and family.

- Disease process, its management, and the prognosis
- Manifestations or changes in condition to report to the physician, such as a change in activity tolerance, increased edema, and signs of respiratory infection or exacerbation
- Importance of planned rest periods between activities and measures to conserve energy, such as using a shower chair
- Importance of not smoking due to its irritant and vasoconstrictive effects
- Prescribed medications, including their use and effects

# LUNG CANCER

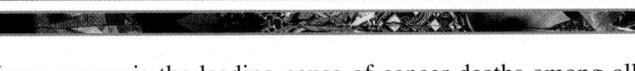

## THE CLIENT WITH LUNG CANCER

Lung cancer is the leading cause of cancer deaths among all racial groups in the United States, accounting for 31% of all cancer deaths in men and 25% of all cancer deaths in women. In 2002, nearly 155,000 people died from lung cancer in the United States; an estimated 169,400 new cases were diagnosed in that same year (ACS, 2002). It is a major health problem with a grim prognosis: Most people with lung cancer die within 1 year of the initial diagnosis.

The incidence of lung cancer varies from state to state and among nations. It increases with age, occurring most commonly in clients over age 50. Cigarette smoke, which contains 43 known chemical carcinogens and cancer promoters, is clearly the most significant cause of lung cancer. More than 80% of lung cancer cases are related to smoking, and the disease is 10 times more common in smokers than nonsmokers. There is a dose-response relationship between smoking and lung cancer; the more the person smokes and the longer the person smokes, the greater the risk. Exposure to ionizing radiation and inhaled irritants, asbestos in particular, is also recognized as a risk factor for lung cancer (Porth, 2002).

At the time of diagnosis, cancer of the lung typically is well advanced, with distant metastasis present in 55% of clients and regional lymph node involvement in another 25%. The prognosis is generally poor: The overall 5-year survival rate is only 15% (ACS, 2002).

## PATHOPHYSIOLOGY

The vast majority of primary lung lesions are *bronchogenic carcinoma,* tumors of the airway epithelium. These tumors are further differentiated by cell type: small-cell carcinoma, adenocarcinoma, squamous cell carcinoma, and large-cell carcinoma. For clinical purposes, the latter three cell types frequently are classified together as non-small-cell carcinomas. *Small-cell carcinomas,* which account for approximately 25% of lung cancers, grow rapidly and spread early. These tumors have paraneoplastic properties; that is, they produce manifestations at sites that are not directly affected by the tumor. Small-cell lung carcinomas can synthesize bioactive products and hormones such as adrenocorticotropic hormones (ACTH), antidiuretic hormone (ADH), a parathormone-like hormone, and gastrin-releasing peptide. *Non-small-cell carcinoma* accounts for about 75% of lung cancers. Each cell type differs in its incidence, presentation, and manner of spread. Table 36–9 outlines the incidence and unique characteristics of each cell type.

Bronchogenic cancer, regardless of cell type, tends to be aggressive, locally invasive, and have widespread metastatic lesions. Tumors begin as mucosal lesions that grow to form masses which obstruct the bronchi or invade adjacent lung tissue. All types frequently spread via the lymph system to nodes and other organs such as the brain, bones, and liver. *Superior vena cava syndrome,* partial or complete obstruction of the superior vena cava, is a potential complication of lung cancer, particularly when the tumor involves the superior mediastinum or the mediastinal lymph nodes.

TABLE 36-9  Comparison of Lung Cancer Cell Types

| | Cell Type and Prevalence | Presentation and Associated Manifestations | Spread |
|---|---|---|---|
| | Small-cell (oat cell) carcinoma 20% to 25% of all lung cancers | Central lesion with hilar mass common, early mediastinal involvement, no cavitation; SIADH, Cushing's syndrome, thrombophlebitis | Aggressive tumor; more than 40% of clients have distant metastasis at time of presentation |
| | Adenocarcinoma 20% to 40% of all lung cancers | Peripheral mass involving bronchi; few local symptoms; hypertrophic pulmonary osteoarthropathy | Early metastasis to central nervous system, skeleton, and adrenal glands |
| | Squamous cell carcinoma 30% to 32% of all lung cancers | Central lesion located in large bronchi; client presents with cough, dyspnea, atelectasis, and wheezing; hypercalcemia common | Spreads by local invasion |
| | Large-cell carcinoma 10% to 15% of all lung cancers | Usually, peripheral lesion that is larger than that associated with adenocarcinoma and tends to cavitate; gynecomastia, thrombophlebitis | Early metastasis |

## MANIFESTATIONS

The manifestations of lung cancer are related to the location and spread of the tumor. Clients may present with symptoms related to the primary tumor, manifestations of metastatic disease, or with systemic symptoms. Initial symptoms often are attributed to smoking or chronic bronchitis. Chronic cough is common, as is hemoptysis. Wheezing and shortness of breath occur as a result of airway obstruction. Dull, aching chest pain occurs as the tumor spreads to the mediastinum; pleuritic pain occurs when the pleura is invaded. Hoarseness and/or dysphagia indicates pressure of the tumor on the trachea or esophagus.

Systemic and paraneoplastic manifestations of lung cancer include weight loss, anorexia, fatigue, and weakness; bone pain, tenderness, and swelling; clubbing of the fingers and toes; and various endocrine, neuromuscular, cardiovascular, and

hematologic symptoms. The *Multisystem Effects of Lung Cancer* are illustrated on the next page.

Confusion, impaired gait and balance, headache, and personality changes may indicate brain metastasis. Bone metastases cause bone pain, pathologic fractures, and possible spinal cord compression, as well as thrombocytopenia and anemia if bone marrow is invaded. When the liver is affected, symptoms of liver dysfunction and biliary obstruction—including jaundice, anorexia, and upper right quadrant pain—are evident.

Symptoms of superior vena cava syndrome (edema of the neck and face, headache, dizziness, vision disturbances, and syncope) may develop acutely or more gradually. Veins of the upper chest and neck are dilated; flushing occurs, followed by cyanosis. Cerebral edema may affect the level of consciousness; laryngeal edema may impair respirations.

# Multisystem Effects of Lung Cancer

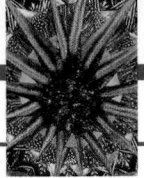

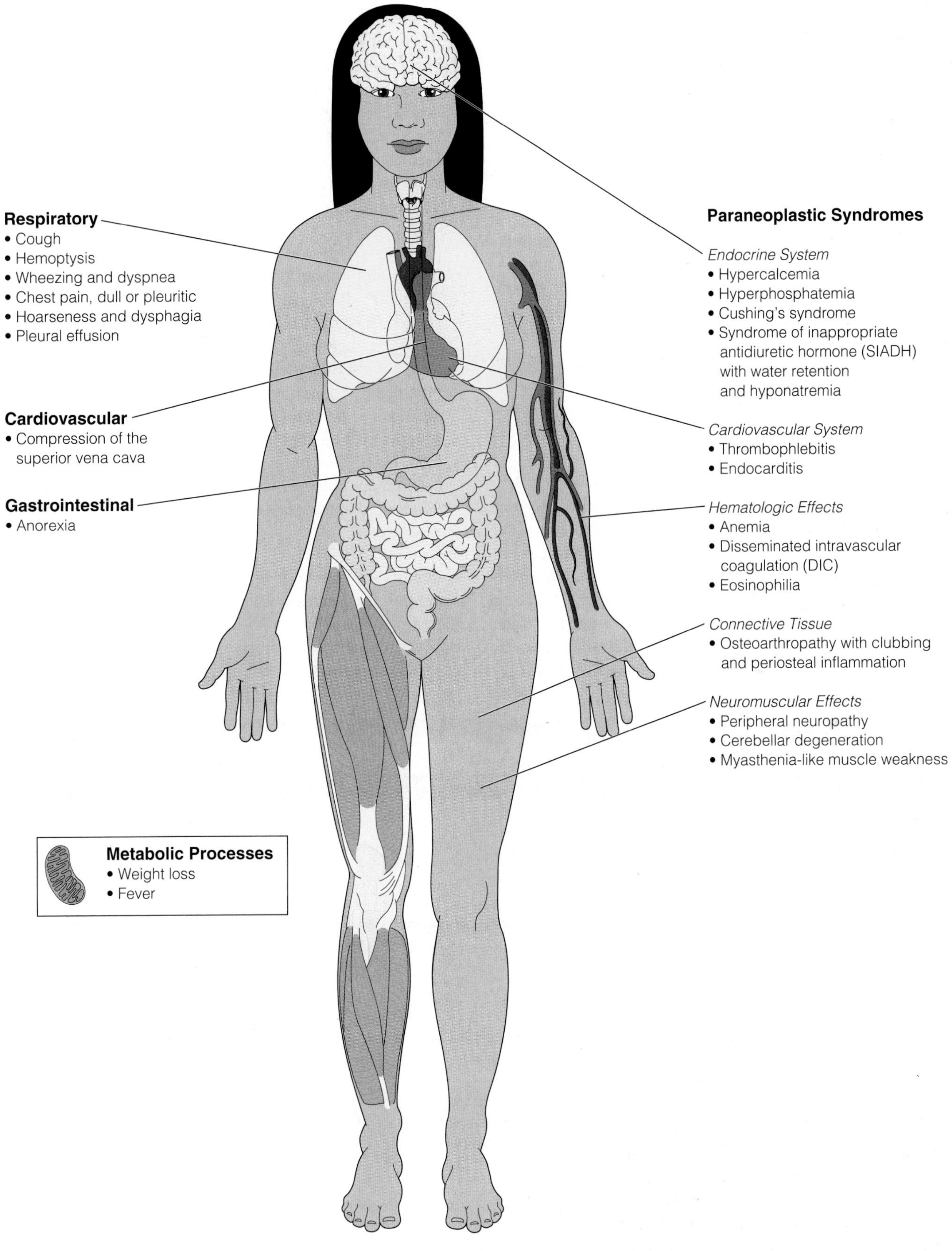

Respiratory
• Cough
• Hemoptysis
• Wheezing and dyspnea
• Chest pain, dull or pleuritic
• Hoarseness and dysphagia
• Pleural effusion
Cardiovascular
• Compression of the superior vena cava
Gastrointestinal
• Anorexia
Metabolic Processes
• Weight loss
• Fever
Paraneoplastic Syndromes
Endocrine System
• Hypercalcemia
• Hyperphosphatemia
• Cushing's syndrome
• Syndrome of inappropriate antidiuretic hormone (SIADH) with water retention and hyponatremia
Cardiovascular System
• Thrombophlebitis
• Endocarditis
Hematologic Effects
• Anemia
• Disseminated intravascular coagulation (DIC)
• Eosinophilia
Connective Tissue
• Osteoarthropathy with clubbing and periosteal inflammation
Neuromuscular Effects
• Peripheral neuropathy
• Cerebellar degeneration
• Myasthenia-like muscle weakness

## COLLABORATIVE CARE

Because lung cancer typically is advanced when diagnosed and the prognosis generally is poor, prevention of the disease must be a primary goal for all health care providers. With 80% of lung cancer related to cigarette smoking, reducing tobacco use can have a significant impact on the death rate from lung cancer—a far greater impact than advances in treatment. Unfortunately, declines in adult tobacco use have slowed in recent years and its use among teenagers increased significantly during the 1990s (ACS, 2002).

Establishing an accurate diagnosis is the first step in treating lung cancer. Treatment decisions are based on the tumor location, type of cancer cell, staging of the tumor, and the client's ability to tolerate treatment. Lung cancer is staged by the tumor size, location, degree of invasion of the primary tumor, and the presence of metastatic disease. Lung cancer staging is summarized in Table 36–10. Surgery is the treatment of choice for most forms of lung cancer.

### Diagnostic Tests

- *Chest X-ray* usually provides the first evidence of lung cancer. It is particularly reliable as a diagnostic tool when compared with previous chest X-ray. In high-risk populations, the chest X-ray may be used as a screening tool for lung cancer.
- *Sputum specimen* is sent for *cytologic examination* to establish the diagnosis of lung cancer. The sputum sample is collected on arising in the morning. If malignant cells are found in the sputum, more expensive and invasive examinations may be unnecessary. However, a sputum sample negative for malig-

nant cells does not rule out lung cancer; it may simply indicate that the tumor is not shedding cells into mucous secretions.
- *Bronchoscopy* is frequently done to visualize and obtain tissue for biopsy from the tumor. A flexible fiberoptic bronchoscope is inserted through the mouth into the bronchus. When a tumor mass or suspicious tissue is identified visually, a cable-activated instrument is used to obtain a biopsy specimen. If the tumor cannot be seen, the airways may be flushed with a saline solution (bronchial washing) to obtain cells for cytologic examination. Nursing care of the client undergoing a bronchoscopy is included in the box on page 1080.
- *CT scan* is used to evaluate and localize tumors, particularly tumors in the lung parenchyma and pleura. It also is done prior to needle biopsy to localize the tumor. CT scanning can also detect distant tumor metastasis and evaluate tumor response to treatment.
- Cells or tissue for *cytologic examination and biopsy* may be obtained by aspirating fluid from a pleural effusion, percutaneous needle biopsy, and lymph node biopsy. These procedures may be done in an outpatient or a surgical setting.
- *CBC, liver function studies,* and *serum electrolytes* including calcium are obtained to evaluate for evidence of metastatic disease or paraneoplastic syndromes.

### Medications

Combination chemotherapy is the treatment of choice for small-cell lung cancer because of its rapid growth, dissemination, and sensitivity to cytotoxic drugs. Used in combination, chemotherapeutic drugs allow tumor cells to be attacked at different parts of the cell cycle and in different ways, in-

| TABLE 36–10 | Lung Cancer Staging | | |
|---|---|---|---|
| | **Primary Tumor (T-Stage)** | **Regional Lymph Nodes (N)** | **Distant Metastasis (M)** |
| **Stage 0** | $T_0$–No evidence of primary tumor<br><br>$T_X$–Malignant cells in bronchopulmonary secretions, but no tumor visualized | | $M_X$–Presence of distant metastasis cannot be assessed |
| **Stage I** | $T_1S$–Carcinoma in situ<br><br>$T_1$–Tumor that is 3 cm diameter or less, with no evidence of invasion | $N_0$–No regional lymph node metastasis | $M_0$–No distant metastasis |
| **Stage II** | $T_2$–Tumor that is greater than 3 cm diameter, or invades visceral pleura, or has associated atelectasis or pneumonitis | $N_1$–Metastasis or direct extension to peribronchial or ipsilateral hilar nodes | |
| **Stage III** | $T_3$–Tumor with direct extension into an adjacent structure, or any tumor with associated pleural effusion or atelectasis or pneumonitis of entire lung | $N_2$–Metastasis to ipsilateral mediastinal or subcarinal nodes | |
| **Stage IV** | $T_4$–Tumor that invades mediastinum or involves the heart, great vessels, trachea, esophagus, vertebral body, or carina; presence of malignant pleural effusion | $N_3$–Metastasis to contralateral mediastinal, scalene, or supraclavicular nodes | $M_1$–Distant metastasis present |

creasing the effectiveness of therapy. Fifty percent of clients with tumors at early stages achieve complete tumor remission with combination chemotherapy. When a complete tumor response is achieved in the first few cycles of chemotherapy, the chances for long-term survival are much greater.

Combination chemotherapy is used also as an adjunct to surgery or radiation therapy for lung cancer. It may be used to reduce the size of advanced local tumors prior to surgery, and to lengthen survival when distant metastases are present. See Chapter 10 ⊖ for further discussion of chemotherapy.

Bronchodilators may be prescribed to reduce airway obstruction. Analgesics and pain management strategies are vital when the cancer is advanced. See Chapter 4 ⊖ for more information about postoperative and cancer pain management.

## Surgery

Surgery offers the only real chance for a cure in non-small-cell lung cancer. Unfortunately, most tumors are inoperable or only partially resectable at the time of diagnosis. The 5-year survival rate for clients with resectable tumors is between 20% and 50%, depending on the size of the tumor and the extent of lymph node involvement (Braunwald et al., 2001). The type of surgery performed depends on the location and size of the tumor, as well as the client's pulmonary and general health. The goal of surgery is to remove all involved tissue while preserving as much functional lung as possible. Table 36–11 outlines various surgical procedures used to treat lung cancer. Nursing care for the client having lung surgery is outlined in the box on page 1140.

## Radiation Therapy

Radiation therapy is used alone or in combination with surgery or chemotherapy for lung cancer. The treatment goal may be either cure or symptom relief (palliative). Prior to surgery, radiation therapy is used to "debulk" tumors. When cancer has spread by direct extension to other thoracic structures and surgery is not feasible, radiation therapy may be the treatment of choice. It also may be used to relieve manifestations such as cough, hemoptysis, pain due to bone metastasis, and dyspnea from bronchial obstruction. Complications of lung cancer, such as superior vena cava syndrome, may be treated with radiation.

Radiation therapy may be delivered by external beam to the primary tumor site or by intraluminal radiation, or brachytherapy. Radiation therapy and related nursing care is discussed further in Chapter 10. Specific nursing measures for the client undergoing radiation therapy for lung cancer are outlined in the Nursing Care box on page 1141.

## NURSING CARE

### Health Promotion

The incidence of lung cancer is decreasing as the use of tobacco products declines. Teach people of all ages, particularly children and teenagers, about the link between cigarette smoking and lung cancer. Not smoking and avoiding exposure to secondhand smoke is the primary preventive measure for lung cancer. In addition, explain the risk of lung cancer to clients with occupational risk factors, exposure to asbestos products in particular.

### Assessment

Nursing assessment related to lung cancer focuses on identifying risk factors for the disease, early manifestations of lung cancer, and respiratory function in the client undergoing treatment.

- Health history: current symptoms, including chronic cough, shortness of breath, blood-tinged sputum; systemic manifestations such as recent weight loss, fatigue, anorexia, bone pain; smoking history; occupational exposure to carcinogens; chronic diseases such as COPD
- Physical examination: general appearance; skin color, evidence of clubbing; weight and height; vital signs; respiratory rate, depth, excursion; lung sounds to percussion and auscultation

| TABLE 36–11 | Types of Lung Surgery for Lung Cancer | |
|---|---|---|
| **Procedure** | **Description** | **Used for** |
| Laser bronchoscopy | Bronchoscopy-guided laser used to resect tumor | Tumors localized in a main bronchus |
| Mediastinoscopy | Visualization of the mediastinum using an endoscope passed through a suprasternal incision | Evaluation and biopsy of a mediastinal tumor and lymph nodes |
| Thoracotomy | Incision into the chest wall | Access the lung and thoracic cavity for surgery |
| Wedge resection | Removal of a small section (wedge) of peripheral lung tissue | Small, peripheral lung tumors |
| Segmental resection | Removal of an individual bronchovascular segment of a lobe | Peripheral lung tumor with no evidence of extension to the chest wall or metastasis |
| Sleeve resection (bronchoplastic reconstruction) | Resection of a section of a major bronchus with reconstruction of remaining normal bronchus | Small lesion of a major bronchus |
| Lobectomy | Removal of a single lung lobe | Tumors confined to a single lobe |
| Pneumonectomy | Removal of an entire lung | Tumor widespread throughout the lung, involving the main bronchus, or fixed to the hilum |

## NURSING CARE OF THE CLIENT HAVING LUNG SURGERY

### PREOPERATIVE CARE

- Provide routine preoperative nursing care as outlined in Chapter 7. 🔗
- Note any history of smoking, respiratory and cardiac diseases, and other chronic conditions in the nursing history. *These factors may affect the response to surgery and the risk for postoperative complications.*
- Provide emotional and psychologic support for the client and family. *In addition to facing surgery, the client may be adjusting to a new diagnosis of cancer and the possibility that surgical intervention will be only partially successful.*
- Instruct about postoperative procedures, including respiratory therapy, breathing exercises, and coughing techniques. Allow practice time. *Learning will be easier in the preoperative period, when pain and analgesia are not affecting mental function.*
- If the client will return from surgery with an endotracheal tube and mechanical ventilation, establish a means of communication using hand or eye signals or a magic slate. *Establishing a means of communication prior to surgery reduces postoperative anxiety at being unable to speak.*
- If the client will return to ICU, introduce the client and family to the unit and any machines, such as ventilators and monitors, that will be used. *The knowledge that this is an expected part of surgical recovery reduces the client's and family's postoperative anxiety.*

### POSTOPERATIVE CARE

- Assess and provide routine postoperative care as outlined in Chapter 7.
- Assess for adequate pain control, and provide analgesics as needed. *Incisional pain commonly causes altered breathing patterns in the client who has undergone lung surgery.*
- Frequently assess respiratory status, including color, oxygen saturation, respiratory rate and depth, chest expansion, lung sounds, percussion tone, and arterial blood gases. *Maintaining adequate ventilation and gas exchange postoperatively is vital to reduce mortality and morbity. Gas exchange may be impaired by complications of lung surgery, including pneumothorax, atelectasis, bronchospasm, pulmonary embolus, bronchopleural fistula, and acute respiratory distress syndrome (ARDS).*
- Assist with effective coughing techniques, postural drainage, and incentive spirometry. Perform endotracheal suctioning as needed while intubated. *Surgical manipulation and anesthesia can increase the mucous production, leading to airway obstruction. Aggressive pulmonary hygiene is important to prevent this complication.*
- Monitor and maintain effective mechanical ventilation. *This is vital to ensure adequate ventilation and gas exchange in the early postoperative period.*
- Maintain patent chest tubes and a closed drainage system. Monitor chest tube output every hour initially, then every 2 to 4 or 8 hours as indicated. Notify the physician if chest tube output exceeds 70 mL per hour and/or is bright red, warm, and free flowing. *Maintaining a patent, intact chest drainage system is vital to reestablish negative pressure within the chest cavity and reexpansion of the lungs. Increased amounts of warm, free-flowing blood indicate intrathoracic hemorrhage that may necessitate surgical intervention.*
- Assess for signs of infection involving the incision or chest tube site(s). Use strict aseptic technique in caring for incisions and invasive monitoring devices. *The postoperative client is at risk for incisional infections, empyema in the chest cavity, and pneumonia.*
- Assist with turning and to ambulate as soon as possible. *Early mobility is important to prevent possible complications, such as pneumonia or pulmonary embolus.*
- Assess and maintain nutritional status. Initiate enteral or parenteral nutrition early if intubation and mechanical ventilation will be required for an extended period. Provide frequent small feedings once extubated. *Maintaining nutritional status promotes wound healing and prevents negative nitrogen balance. Frequent small feedings reduce the fatigue associated with eating.*

## Nursing Diagnoses and Interventions

The client with lung cancer is facing invasive treatments with undesirable side effects, possibly surgery, and typically a poor prognosis for long-term survival. Nursing care needs are diverse, related to respiratory status, the cancer itself and possible metastases, and the treatment plan. Priority nursing diagnoses related to respiratory function include ineffective breathing pattern and activity intolerance. Pain and anticipatory grieving also are likely to be high-priority problems.

### Ineffective Breathing Pattern

Breathing pattern and ventilation may be affected by the tumor itself or by treatment of the tumor. Thoracic surgery increases the risk due to the incision and disruption of the muscles of respiration. Maintaining effective lung ventilation is particularly important postoperatively to reexpand remaining lung tissue and prevent surgical complications.

- Assess and document respiratory rate, depth, and lung sounds at least every 4 hours; evaluate more frequently in the immediate postoperative period or as indicated by condition. *Early detection of signs of respiratory compromise or adventitious lung sounds is vital for effective intervention.*

**PRACTICE ALERT** *Monitor oxygen saturation, exhaled carbon dioxide, and/or blood gas results, reporting changes from normal. Changes in levels of blood oxygen or exhaled $CO_2$ may be early indications of respiratory compromise.* ■

- Frequently assess and document pain level (using a standard pain scale); provide analgesics as needed. *Pain and attempting to avoid chest movement to prevent additional pain can lead to rapid, shallow respirations and ineffective ventilation.*

## NURSING CARE OF THE CLIENT RECEIVING RADIATION THERAPY

Although radiation therapy is well controlled and specifically directed toward the tumor cells, some normal cells are also damaged in the process of treatment. Nursing care and client teaching help the client cope with uncomfortable side effects associated with radiation therapy.

### Nursing Responsibilities

- Monitor for potential complications:
  a. Radiation pneumonitis—dyspnea on exertion, dry cough, fever
  b. Pericarditis—chest pain, pericardial friction rub; muffled heart sounds, paradoxical pulse, ECG abnormalities (Notify the physician if symptoms develop.)
  c. Esophagitis—pain, sore throat, difficulty swallowing
- Encourage adequate fluid intake to liquefy respiratory secretions.
- Provide local analgesics and local anesthetics such as viscous lidocaine as ordered to relieve dysphagia and sore throat.
- Offer small frequent meals of soft, cool foods and liquids to maintain nutritional status.

### Client and Family Teaching

- If dyspnea or pneumonitis develop, teach positioning, pursed-lip techniques, and relaxation exercises to facilitate breathing.
- Reassure that pneumonitis is generally a self-limiting process and should resolve when the course of radiotherapy is completed.
- Teach the manifestations of pericarditis, which may develop during treatment or up to 1 year after its completion. Chest pain or pressure, rapid heartbeat, and fever may signal pericarditis; increasing fatigue, dyspnea, and lightheadedness can indicate a chronic process with pericardial effusion and possible cardiac tamponade.
- Instruct to eliminate hot, spicy, or acidic foods from the diet if esophagitis is a problem. Alcohol and tobacco should also be avoided.
- Adequate rest and nutrition are important to alleviate the symptoms of radiation fatigue, which is common in clients receiving radiation therapy for lung cancer. The fatigue is generally temporary.

---

- Elevate the head of the bed to 60 degrees. *Elevating the head of the bed reduces pressure on the diaphragm and permits optimal lung expansion.*
- Assist to turn, cough, and deep breathe and use incentive spirometry. Help splint the chest with a pillow or blanket when coughing. *These measures promote airway clearance.*
- Suction airway as needed. *Suctioning may be required to remove secretions that the client is unable to cough up and expectorate.*

**PRACTICE ALERT** *Maintain chest tube integrity and patency by ensuring uninterrupted gravity flow. Chest tubes help reestablish negative pressure in the thoracic cavity, allowing the lung to fully reexpand.* ■

- Provide chest physiotherapy with percussion and postural drainage as needed or ordered. *Percussion and postural drainage help maintain airway patency and effective respirations.*
- If mechanical ventilation is instituted, work with respiratory therapy and use analgesia or sedation as needed to synchronize respirations with the ventilator. *Coordination of the client's respiratory effort with ventilator-delivered breaths is important for fully effective mechanical ventilation.*
- Provide reassurance and emotional support. *These measures help relieve anxiety and promote an effective breathing pattern.*

### Activity Intolerance

Both resectional lung surgery and inoperable lung cancer reduce the amount of functional lung tissue and surface area for gas diffusion. This can lead to activity intolerance if the oxygen supply is insufficient to meet the body's oxygen demand.

**PRACTICE ALERT** *Assess and document physiologic responses to activity, including pulse, respiratory rate, dyspnea, and fatigue. These assessments are good indicators of activity tolerance.* ■

- Plan rest periods between activities and procedures. *Rest periods reduce oxygen demands and fatigue.*
- Assist the postoperative client to increase activities gradually. *Increasing activity levels gradually improves exercise tolerance.*
- Teach measures to conserve energy while performing ADLs, such as sitting while showering and dressing and wearing slip-on shoes. *These energy-conserving measures reduce oxygen demand and allow the client to remain independent as long as possible.*
- Keep frequently used objects within easy reach. *This helps conserve energy.*
- Administer oxygen as prescribed. Teach the client and family about home oxygen use if appropriate. *Supplemental oxygen can help improve activity and exercise tolerance.*
- Encourage maintenance of physical activity to tolerance. *Maintaining activity levels to the degree possible improves physical and emotional well-being.*
- Allow family members to provide assistance as needed. *This helps the client conserve energy and allows the family to retain a sense of usefulness.*

### Pain

Pain is a priority problem in both the postoperative period as well as in the terminal stages of cancer. Poorly managed pain prolongs recovery from surgery. In the terminal cancer client, chronic and acute pain must be managed effectively to allow a peaceful death.

- Assess and document pain using a standardized pain scale and objective data. *Pain is a subjective experience, best evaluated by the client. Changes in vital signs, guarded movement, or unwillingness to move may indicate unreported pain.*

- Provide analgesics as needed to maintain comfort. *Postoperative recovery and restoration of function is facilitated by adequate pain management.*
- For cancer pain, maintain an around-the-clock medication schedule using narcotic, nonsteroidal anti-inflammatory drugs, and other medications as ordered. *Addiction is not a concern in terminal cancer; providing adequate pain relief that does not allow "breakthrough" pain is important.*
- Provide or assist with comfort measures, such as massage, positioning, distraction, and relaxation techniques. *These techniques promote relaxation and enhance pain relief.*
- Assist the client and family to plan and engage in activities that distract from pain such as reading, watching television, and engaging in social interactions. *Distraction helps the client focus away from the pain.*
- Spend as much time with the client as possible; allow family members to remain with the client. *Physical presence of the nurse and family provides emotional support for the client.*

## Anticipatory Grieving

Because lung cancer often is advanced when diagnosed, the client faces the very real prospect of dying from the disease. Grieving for the anticipated loss of life is a normal response as the client and family begin to adapt to the diagnosis. Nursing care goals are to promote expression of feelings and thoughts about the loss, and to help the client and family initiate grief work, make decisions, and use appropriate resources and coping mechanisms to deal with the loss.

- Spend time with the client and family. *Time is necessary to develop a trusting, therapeutic relationship.*

- Answer questions honestly; do not deny the probable outcome of the disease. *Honesty reinforces reality and provides a sense of control over decisions to be made.*
- Encourage the client and family to express their feelings, fears, and concerns. *Open expression of feelings helps to promote understanding and acceptance.*
- Assist with understanding the grieving process and acceptance of feelings as normal. *Feelings of guilt, anger, or depression may cause the client to withdraw from others. Explanation of the grieving process enhances understanding and ability to cope.*
- Help identify strengths and coping measures that have been used effectively in the past. Provide positive reinforcement for effective coping behavior. *Past effective coping measures can help the client and family deal with the present situation and regain a sense of control.*
- Help the client and family make decisions regarding treatment and care. *This also is important to give them a sense of control.*
- Encourage use of other support systems, such as spiritual and social groups. Refer the client and family to support groups, social support services, and hospice care as indicated. Provide American Cancer Society literature and information as appropriate. *These support systems provide emotional support and help the client and family cope with the diagnosis.*
- Discuss advance directives (the living will) and power of attorney for health care with the client and family. *These documents give the client and family a sense of control over medical care provided if the client is no longer able to express his or her own wishes.*

## Using NANDA, NIC, and NOC

Chart 36–4 shows links between NANDA nursing diagnoses, NIC, and NOC for the client with lung cancer.

## CHART 36–4 NANDA, NIC, AND NOC LINKAGES

### The Client with Lung Cancer

| NURSING DIAGNOSES | NURSING INTERVENTIONS | NURSING OUTCOMES |
|---|---|---|
| • Activity Intolerance | • Energy Management<br>• Self-Care Assistance | • Activity Tolerance<br>• Energy Conservation |
| • Acute and/or Chronic Pain | • Pain Management<br>• Patient-Controlled Analgesia (PCA) Assistance | • Comfort Level<br>• Pain Control<br>• Pain: Disruptive Effects |
| • Anticipatory Grieving | • Grief Work Facilitation<br>• Family Support | • Coping<br>• Family Coping |
| • Ineffective Breathing Pattern | • Airway Management<br>• Respiratory Monitoring | • Respiratory Status: Ventilation |
| • Ineffective Coping | • Coping Enhancement<br>• Decision-Making Support<br>• Support System Enhancement | • Coping<br>• Decision Making<br>• Social Support |

*Note. Data from Nursing Outcomes Classification (NOC) by M. Johnson & M. Maas (Eds.), 1997, St. Louis: Mosby; Nursing Diagnoses: Definitions & Classification 2001–2002 by North American Nursing Diagnosis Association, 2001, Philadelphia: NANDA; Nursing Interventions Classification (NIC) by J.C. McCloskey & G. M. Bulechek (Eds.), 2000, St. Louis: Mosby. Reprinted by permission.*

## Home Care

A primary teaching need to prepare the client and family affected by lung cancer for home care is information about the disease itself, expected prognosis, and planned treatment strategies. Provide honest information; do not promote false hope. Include the following additional topics in teaching for home care.

- Importance of quitting smoking, especially if surgery has been performed (The client with lung cancer may have difficulty recognizing the need to stop smoking. Include information about the effects of nicotine and the tars in cigarette smoke on healing and already compromised lung tissue.)
- Planned treatments such as chemotherapy or radiation therapy, including expected effects and usual side effects of each
- Strategies to cope with noxious effects of radiation or chemotherapy

- Activities and exercises to improve strength and regain function for the postoperative client
- The need to continue coughing and deep-breathing exercises at home
- Symptoms to report to the physician: fever, increasing or continued shortness of breath, cough, increased or purulent sputum, redness, pain, swelling, or incisional drainage
- Use of prescribed medications, including desired and potential side effects and interactions with other drugs or foods
- Use of analgesics and other pain relief measures for postoperative or cancer pain
- Information about hospice services, home health, local cancer support groups for clients and caregivers, and American Cancer Society services

Refer the client and family for home health services including nursing care, assistance with ADLs, respiratory care, and respite care as needed.

## Nursing Care Plan
## A Client with Lung Cancer

After coughing up bloody sputum one morning, James Mueller, a 68-year-old retired millworker, sees his physician. A chest X-ray shows a suspicious density in the central portion of his right lung. Mr. Mueller is admitted to the hospital the following Monday for diagnostic tests.

### ASSESSMENT

Anita Sarros, RN, admits Mr. Mueller to the oncology unit and obtains a nursing history. Mr. Mueller is married and has three grown children. He worked in a local paper mill for 35 years before retiring at age 62. He describes himself as "pretty healthy," except for a chronic smoker's cough. He started smoking as a young man in the army. He has a 50 pack-year smoking history, having smoked a pack a day for 50 years, since age 18. Mr. Mueller says he briefly quit smoking following a small heart attack 3 years ago, but started again after 4 months. On further questioning, Mr. Mueller says his cough has been productive for the past few months, especially in the morning, and that he is shorter of breath than usual with activity.

Mr. Mueller's examination data includes BP 162/86, P 78 and regular, R 20, and T 98.4°F (36.9 C). Color good, skin warm and dry. Inspiratory and expiratory wheezes noted in right chest but good breath sounds throughout. No other abnormal findings are noted on examination. The physician orders early-morning sputum specimens times 3 days for cytologic examination and schedules a CT scan of the chest the morning after admission.

Mr. Mueller's CBC shows mild anemia, but remaining routine laboratory tests are essentially normal. Sputum cytology is positive for small-cell bronchogenic cancer. The CT scan shows a central mass approximately 4 cm in diameter with involved mediastinal and subclavicular lymph nodes. A small mass is also noted on the lumbar spine. After conferring with his physician and an oncologist, Mr. Mueller decides to undergo a trial course of chemotherapy.

### DIAGNOSIS

- *Ineffective airway clearance* related to tumor mass
- *Risk for imbalanced nutrition: Less than body requirements* related to effects of chemotherapy
- *Risk for compromised family coping* related to new diagnosis of lung cancer
- *Deficient knowledge* about lung cancer and aids to smoking cessation

### EXPECTED OUTCOMES

- Maintain a patent airway.
- Maintain current weight.
- Express feelings and concerns about the effect of cancer on the family unit.
- Participate in care.
- Contact appropriate support groups.
- Verbalize an understanding of the disease, its treatment, and prognosis.
- Develop a plan to stop smoking.

### PLANNING AND IMPLEMENTATION

- Teach coughing, deep breathing, and hydration measures to facilitate airway clearance.
- Discuss symptoms to report to the physician: increased dyspnea or hemoptysis, severe stridor or wheezing, chest pain.
- Discuss measures to relieve nausea associated with chemotherapy, including premedication with a prescribed antiemetic.
- Have dietitian consult with Mr. and Mrs. Mueller to develop a diet plan for maintaining ideal weight.
- Discuss possible effects of lung cancer with Mr. and Mrs. Mueller.
- Encourage Mr. and Mrs. Mueller to call a family conference to discuss the disease with their children and grandchildren.

(continued on page 1144)

## Nursing Care Plan
### A Client with Lung Cancer (continued)

- Evaluate family members' knowledge and understanding of lung cancer, correcting misinformation and teaching as needed.
- Have an American Cancer Society volunteer contact the family.
- Refer to local cancer support group.
- Refer to home health department for follow-up and further teaching.
- Work with Mr. Mueller to develop a plan to stop smoking.
- Ask the physician for a prescription for nicotine patches or gum for Mr. Mueller.

### EVALUATION

Mr. Mueller had his first chemotherapy treatment in the hospital and was discharged 4 days after admission. After 3 months of chemotherapy, his tumor shows little regression, and a liver scan reveals further metastasis. He and his wife decide to stop chemotherapy, a decision with which the children reluctantly agree. Mr. and Mrs. Mueller are referred to hospice services. With

the help of hospice nurses and volunteers, Mr. Mueller is able to remain at home. His pain is managed initially with oral MS Contin, a sustained-release form of morphine sulfate, and later with an intravenous morphine infusion. Mr. Mueller dies at home with his family at his side 9 months after his diagnosis of lung cancer.

### Critical Thinking in the Nursing Process

1. The oncologist prescribed a chemotherapy regimen of cyclophosphamide, doxorubicin, and vincristine. Describe how each of these drugs works against cancer cells, and discuss the rationale for using this combination.
2. Develop a care plan to deal with the specific side effects for the above treatment regimen.
3. Mr. Mueller had small-cell (oat cell) cancer. How would his presentation and treatment differ if the diagnosis had been non-small-cell adenocarcinoma, stage $T_2N_2M_0$?

See Evaluating Your Response in Appendix C.

# DISORDERS OF THE PLEURA

The *pleura* is a thin membrane with two layers: the visceral pleura, which overlies the lung surface, and the parietal pleura, which lines the inner chest wall. Between the layers of pleura is a potential space, the *pleural cavity,* which contains a thin layer of serous fluid. As the thoracic cavity expands during inspiration, the pressure in this space becomes negative in relation to atmospheric and alveolar pressure. The expansible lung is drawn out, and air rushes into the alveoli. When the pleura is inflamed or affected by disease or injury, air or fluid can collect in the pleural cavity, restricting lung expansion and air movement.

## Pleuritis

**Pleuritis,** or inflammation of the pleura, irritates sensory fibers of the parietal pleura, causing characteristic pain. Pleural inflammation usually occurs secondarily to another process, such as a viral respiratory illness, pneumonia, or rib injury.

The onset of pleuritis is typically abrupt. The pain is unilateral and well localized; it is usually sharp or stabbing in nature. Pain may be referred to the neck or the shoulder. Deep breathing, coughing, and movement aggravate the pain. Respirations are rapid and shallow, and chest wall movement is limited on the affected side. Breath sounds are diminished, and a pleural friction rub may be heard over the site.

The diagnosis of pleuritis is based on its manifestations. Chest X-ray and ECG may be ordered to rule out other causes of chest pain. Treatment for pleuritis is symptomatic. Analgesics and NSAIDs, indomethacin (Indocin) in particular, help relieve the pain. Codeine may be ordered, both to relieve pain and to suppress the cough.

Nursing care for the client with pleuritis is directed toward promoting comfort, including administration of NSAIDs and analgesics. Positioning and splinting the chest while coughing

also are helpful. Although wrapping the chest with 6-inch-wide elastic bandages may help relieve pain, this may excessively restrict chest motion, increasing the risk of impaired airway clearance.

Teach the client and family that pleuritis is generally self-limited and of short duration. Discuss symptoms to report to the physician: increased fever, productive cough, difficulty breathing, or shortness of breath. Provide information about prescription and nonprescription NSAIDs and analgesics, including the drug ordered, how to use it, and its desired and possible adverse effects.

## THE CLIENT WITH A PLEURAL EFFUSION

The pleural space normally contains only about 10 to 20 mL of serous fluid. **Pleural effusion** is collection of excess fluid in the pleural space. Pleural effusions result from either systemic or local disease. Systemic disorders that may lead to pleural effusion include heart failure, liver or renal disease, and connective tissue disorders, such as rheumatoid arthritis and systemic lupus erythematosus. Pneumonia, atelectasis, tuberculosis, lung cancer, and trauma are local conditions that may cause pleural effusion.

## PATHOPHYSIOLOGY AND MANIFESTATIONS

Excess pleural fluid may be either *transudate,* formed when capillary pressure is high or plasma proteins are low, or *exudate,* the result of increased capillary permeability. Other pleural fluid collections include *empyema,* pus in the pleural cavity; *hemothorax,* the presence of blood in the cavity; and *hemorrhagic pleural effusion,* a mixture of blood and pleural fluid.

A large pleural effusion compresses adjacent lung tissue. This causes the characteristic manifestation of dyspnea. Pain may develop, although with inflammatory processes pleuritic pain often is relieved by formation of an effusion. Breath sounds are diminished or absent, and a dull percussion tone is heard over the affected area. Chest wall movement may be limited.

## COLLABORATIVE CARE

Chest X-ray often provides the first evidence of a pleural effusion. Because fluid typically collects in dependent regions, it is seen at the base of the affected lung on an upright chest X-ray, and along the lateral wall when the client is positioned on the affected side. CT scans and ultrasonography also are used to localize and differentiate pleural effusions.

If the cause of pleural effusion is not apparent, a thoracentesis is done. **Thoracentesis** is an invasive procedure in which fluid (or occasionally air) is removed from the pleural space with a needle. Aspirated fluid is analyzed for appearance, cell counts, protein and glucose content, the presence of enzymes such as LDH and amylase, abnormal cells, and culture.

When pleural effusion is significant and interferes with respirations, thoracentesis is the treatment of choice to remove the fluid (Figure 36–15 ■). Thoracentesis may be performed at the bedside, in a procedure room, or in an outpatient setting. Local anesthesia is used, and the procedure requires less than 30 minutes to complete. Percussion, auscultation, radiography, or ultrasonography are used to locate the effusion and needle in-

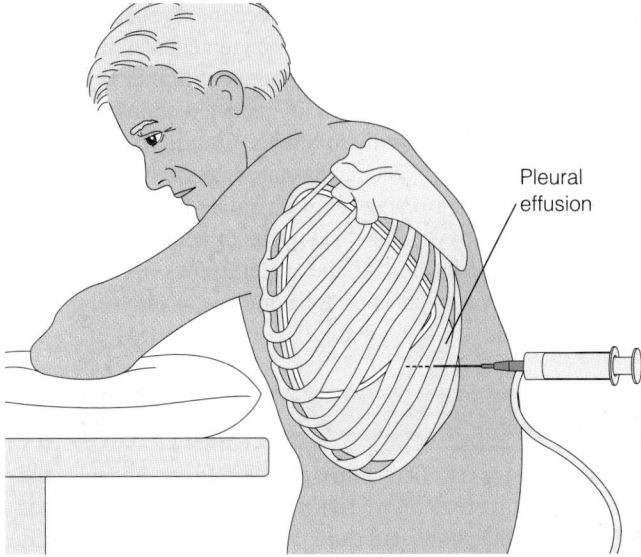

Pleural effusion

**Figure 36–15 ■** Thoracentesis. With the client seated, a needle is inserted between the ribs into the pleural space to withdraw accumulated fluid.

sertion site. The amount of fluid removed is limited to 1200 to 1500 mL at one time to reduce the risk of cardiovascular collapse from rapid removal of too much fluid. Pneumothorax is a possible complication of thoracentesis if the visceral pleura is punctured or a closed drainage system not maintained during the procedure. Nursing care for the client undergoing a thoracentesis is outlined in the box below.

## NURSING CARE OF THE CLIENT HAVING A THORACENTESIS

### PREPROCEDURE CARE

- Verify a signed informed consent for the procedure. *This invasive procedure requires informed consent.*
- Assess knowledge and understanding of the procedure and its purpose; provide additional information as needed. *An informed client will be less apprehensive and more able to cooperate during the thoracentesis.*
- Preprocedure fasting or sedation is not required. *Only local anesthesia is used in this procedure, and the gag and cough reflexes remain intact.*
- Administer a cough suppressant if indicated. *Movement and coughing during the procedure may cause inadvertent damage to the lung or pleura.*
- Obtain a thoracentesis tray, sterile gloves, injectable lidocaine, povidone-iodine, dressing supplies, and an extra overbed table or mayo stand. *These supplies are used by the physician performing the procedure.*
- Position the client upright, leaning forward with arms and head supported on an anchored overbed table. *This position spreads the ribs, enlarging the intercostal space for needle insertion.*
- Inform the client that although local anesthesia prevents pain as the needle is inserted, a sensation of pressure may be felt. *A pressure sensation occurs as the needle punctures the parietal pleura to enter the pleural space.*

### POSTPROCEDURE CARE

- Monitor pulse, color, oxygen saturation, and other signs during thoracentesis. *These are indicators of physiologic tolerance of the procedure.*
- Apply a dressing over the puncture site, and position on the unaffected side for 1 hour. *This allows the pleural puncture to heal.*
- Label obtained specimen with name, date, source, and diagnosis; send specimen to the laboratory for analysis. *Fluid obtained during thoracentesis may be examined for abnormal cells, bacteria, and other substances to determine the cause of the pleural effusion.*
- During the first several hours after thoracentesis, frequently assess and document vital signs; oxygen saturation; respiratory status, including, respiratory excursion, lung sounds, cough, or hemoptysis; and puncture site for bleeding or crepitus. *Frequent assessment is important to detect possible complications of thoracentesis, such as pneumothorax.*
- Obtain a chest X-ray. *Chest X-ray is ordered to detect possible pneumothorax.*
- Normal activities generally can be resumed after 1 hour if no evidence of pneumothorax or other complication is present. *The puncture wound of thoracentesis heals rapidly.*

Because pleural effusion usually occurs secondarily to another disease or disorder, medical management also focuses on treating the underlying condition to prevent further fluid accumulation. An empyema may require repeated drainage, as well as high doses of parenteral antibiotics. Occasionally, thoracotomy and surgical excision may be necessary. Recurrent pleural effusions, often due to cancer, may be prevented by instilling an irritant, such as doxycycline bleomycin, or talc, into the pleural space to cause adhesion of the parietal and visceral pleura (*pleurodesis*). Water-seal chest tube drainage is often employed for hemothorax.

## NURSING CARE

Nursing care for the client with a pleural effusion is directed toward supporting respiratory function and assisting with procedures to evacuate collected fluid. With a large pleural effusion and partial lung collapse, impaired gas exchange and activity intolerance are high-priority nursing problems. Risk for impaired gas exchange is also a priority problem during the initial period following thoracentesis.

Teaching for home care focuses on symptoms of recurrent effusion or complications following a thoracentesis to report to the physician: Increasing dyspnea or shortness of breath, cough, and hemoptysis. Pleuritic pain may be an early sign of effusion and also should be reported. Further teaching about an underlying condition also may be necessary; for example, the client with heart failure may need teaching about a salt-restricted diet.

## THE CLIENT WITH PNEUMOTHORAX

Accumulation of air in the pleural space is called **pneumothorax.** Pneumothorax can occur spontaneously, without apparent cause, as a complication of preexisting lung disease, as a result of blunt or penetrating trauma to the chest, or from an iatrogenic cause (e.g., following thoracentesis).

## PATHOPHYSIOLOGY AND MANIFESTATIONS

Pressure in the pleural space is normally negative in relation to atmospheric pressure. This negative pressure is vital to the process of breathing. Contraction of the diaphragm and the intercostal muscles enlarges the thoracic space. Negative intrapleural pressure draws the lung outward, increasing its volume so air rushes in to fill the expanded lung space.

When either the visceral or parietal pleura is breached, air enters the pleural space, equalizing this pressure. Lung expansion is impaired, and the natural recoil tendency of the lung causes it to collapse to a greater or lesser extent, depending on the size and rapidity of air accumulation. Table 36–12 illustrates the classifications of pneumothorax.

### Spontaneous Pneumothorax

*Spontaneous pneumothorax* develops when an air-filled bleb, or blister, on the lung surface ruptures. Rupture allows air from the airways to enter the pleural space. Air accumulates until pressures are equalized or until collapse of the involved lung section seals the leak. Spontaneous pneumothorax may be either *primary* (*simple*) or *secondary* (*complicated*).

Primary pneumothorax affects previously healthy people, usually tall, slender men between ages 16 and 24 (Way & Doherty, 2003). The cause of primary pneumothorax is unknown. Risk factors include smoking and familial factors. Air-filled blebs tend to form in the apices of the lungs. This is considered to be a benign condition, although recurrences are common. Certain activities also increase the risk of spontaneous pneumothorax, such as high altitude flying and rapid decompression during scuba diving.

Secondary pneumothorax, generally caused by overdistention and rupture of an alveolus, is more serious and potentially life threatening. It develops in clients with underlying lung disease, usually COPD. Middle-age and older adults are primarily affected. Secondary pneumothorax also may be associated with asthma, cystic fibrosis, pulmonary fibrosis, tuberculosis, acute respiratory distress syndrome (ARDS), and other lung diseases. Rarely, a form of secondary pneumothorax called *catamenial pneumothorax* can develop in affected women within 24 to 48 hours of the onset of menstrual flow.

The manifestations of spontaneous pneumothorax depend on the size of pneumothorax, extent of lung collapse, and any underlying lung disease. Typically, pleuritic chest pain and shortness of breath begin abruptly, often while at rest. The respiratory and heart rates increase as gas exchange is affected. Chest wall movement may be asymmetrical, with less movement on the affected side than the unaffected side. The affected side is hyperresonant to percussion, and breath sounds may be diminished or absent. Hypoxemia may develop, although normal mechanisms that shunt blood flow to the unaffected lung often maintain normal oxygen saturation levels. Hypoxemia is more pronounced in secondary pneumothorax.

### Traumatic Pneumothorax

Blunt or penetrating trauma of the chest wall and pleura can cause pneumothorax. Blunt trauma, for example, due to a motor vehicle crash, fall, or during cardiopulmonary resuscitation (CPR), can lead to a *closed pneumothorax*. Fractured ribs penetrating the pleura are the leading cause of pneumothorax due to blunt trauma. Fracture of the trachea and a ruptured bronchus or esophagus also may result from blunt trauma, leading to closed pneumothorax.

*Open pneumothorax* (*sucking chest wound*) results from penetrating chest trauma such as a stab wound, gunshot wound, or impalement injury. With open pneumothorax, air moves freely between the pleural space and the atmosphere through the wound. Pressure on the affected side equalizes with the atmosphere, and the lung collapses rapidly. The result is significant hypoventilation.

*Iatrogenic pneumothorax* may result from puncture or laceration of the visceral pleura during central-line placement, thoracentesis, or lung biopsy. During bronchoscopy, bronchi or lung tissue can be disrupted. Alveoli can become overdistended and rupture during anesthesia, resuscitation procedures, or mechanical ventilation.

## TABLE 36-12  Types of Pneumothorax

| Type | Pathophysiology | Manifestations |
|---|---|---|
| **Spontaneous** Normal lung — Pleural space | Rupture of a bleb on the lung surface allows air to enter pleural space from airways. • *Primary pneumothorax* affects previously healthy people. • *Secondary pneumothorax* affects people with preexisting lung disease (e.g., COPD). | • Abrupt onset • Pleuritic chest pain • Dyspnea, shortness of breath • Tachypnea, tachycardia • Unequal lung excursion • Decreased breath sounds and hyperresonant percussion tone on affected side |
| **Traumatic** Puncture wound through chest wall | Trauma to the chest wall or pleura disrupts the pleural membrane. • *Open* occurs with penetrating chest trauma that allows air from the environment to enter the pleural space. • *Closed* occurs with blunt trauma that allows air from the lung to enter the pleural space. • *Iatrogenic* involves laceration of visceral pleura during a procedure such as thoracentesis or central-line insertion. | • Pain • Dyspnea • Tachypnea, tachycardia • Decreased respiratory excursion • Absent breath sounds in affected area • Air movement through an open wound |
| **Tension** Mediastinal shift to unaffected side — Chest wound allows air to enter pleural space but prevents escape. | Air enters pleural space through chest wall or from airways but is unable to escape, resulting in rapid accumulation. Lung on affected side collapses. As intrapleural pressure increases, heart, great vessels, trachea, and esophagus shift toward the unaffected side. | • Hypotension, shock • Distended neck veins • Severe dyspnea • Tachypnea, tachycardia • Decreased respiratory excursion • Absent breath sounds on affected side • Tracheal deviation toward unaffected side |

With traumatic pneumothorax, manifestations of pain and dyspnea may be masked or missed due to other injuries. Tachypnea and tachycardia may be attributed to the primary injury. Focused assessment for evidence of pneumothorax is vital. Chest wall movement on the affected side is diminished, and breath sounds are absent. If a penetrating wound is present, air may be heard and felt moving through it with respiratory efforts. Hemothorax frequently accompanies traumatic pneumothorax. The manifestations of iatrogenic pneumothorax are similar to those of spontaneous pneumothorax.

## Tension Pneumothorax

*Tension pneumothorax* develops when injury to the chest wall or lungs allows air to enter the pleural space but prevents it from escaping. Pressure within the pleural space becomes positive in relation to atmospheric pressure as air rapidly accumulates with each breath. The lung on the affected side collapses, and pressure on the mediastinum shifts thoracic organs to the unaffected side of the chest, placing pressure on the opposite lung as well. Ventilation is severely compromised, and venous return to the heart is impaired. Tension pneumothorax is a medical emergency requiring immediate intervention to preserve respiration and cardiac output.

In addition to manifestations of pneumothorax, hypotension and distended neck veins are evident as venous return and cardiac output are affected. The trachea is displaced toward the unaffected side as a result of the mediastinal shift. Signs of shock may be present. See Chapter 6 ⬤⬤ for the manifestations and treatment of shock.

## COLLABORATIVE CARE

Treatment for pneumothorax depends on the severity of the problem. A small simple pneumothorax may require no treatment other than monitoring with serial X-rays. Air is absorbed from the pleural space, allowing most small pneumothoraces to resolve spontaneously. A large pneumothorax or significant symptoms usually requires treatment with *thoracostomy,* or the placement of chest tubes. Surgical intervention may be necessary to prevent recurrent spontaneous pneumothorax.

### Diagnostic Tests

Oxygen saturation measurements are obtained to evaluate the effect of pneumothorax on gas exchange. ABGs may be obtained to further assess gas exchange.

The chest X-ray is an effective diagnostic tool for pneumothorax. In tension pneumothorax, air is evident on the affected side, and mediastinal structures are shifted toward the opposite or unaffected side.

### Treatments

#### Chest Tubes

The treatment of choice for significant pneumothorax is placement of a closed-chest catheter to allow the lung to reexpand. When a tube is placed in the pleural cavity to remove air or fluid, it must be sealed to prevent air from also entering the

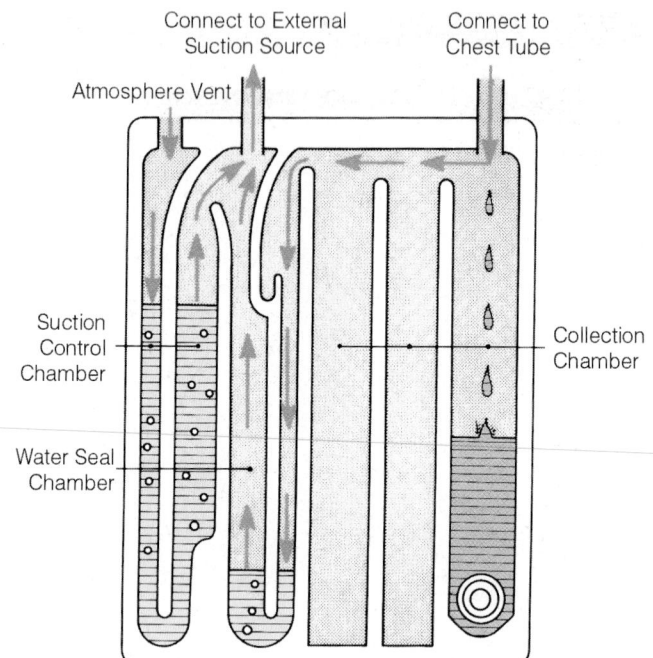

**Figure 36–16** ■ A closed-chest drainage system.

tube and, in essence, creating an open pneumothorax. Chest tubes are sealed with a Heimlich (one-way) valve or connected to a closed drainage system with a "water seal." The valve or water seal prevent air from entering the chest cavity during inspiration and allow air to escape during expiration. Applying a low level of suction to the system helps to reestablish negative pressure in the pleural space, allowing the lung to reexpand.

A number of closed-drainage chest tube systems are available. Most are self-contained disposable systems (Figure 36–16 ■). Drainage from the chest tube is collected in the first collection chamber. This sealed chamber is connected to a water-seal chamber, which is in turn connected to the suction-control chamber. Nursing care of the client with chest tubes is discussed in the box on page 1149.

A large-bore needle or plastic intravenous catheter may be inserted through the chest wall as emergency treatment of a tension pneumothorax. This allows air to escape from the affected side, relieving pressure on mediastinal structures and the opposite lung.

### Pleurodesis

Although controversial, *pleurodesis,* or creation of adhesions between the parietal and visceral pleura, may be used to prevent recurrent pneumothorax. This procedure involves instilling a chemical agent such as doxycycline into the pleural space. The subsequent inflammatory response creates scar tissue and adhesions between the pleural layers. This procedure reduces the recurrence rate to as low as 2% but can make subsequent surgery more difficult (Way & Doherty, 2003).

### Surgery

The risk for recurrence of spontaneous pneumothorax increases with each attack. Clients at high risk for recurrent pneumothorax may have surgery to reduce the risk of future

## NURSING CARE OF THE CLIENT WITH CHEST TUBES

### PREPROCEDURE CARE

- Ensure a signed informed consent for chest tube insertion. *This invasive procedure requires informed consent.*
- Provide additional information as indicated. Explain that local anesthesia will be used but that pressure may be felt as the trochar is inserted. Reassure that breathing will be easier once the chest tube is in place and the lung reexpands. *The client may be extremely dyspneic and anxious and may need reassurance that this invasive procedure will provide relief.*
- Gather all needed supplies, including thoracostomy tray, injectable lidocaine, sterile gloves, chest tube drainage system, sterile water, and a large sterile catheter-tipped syringe to use as a funnel for filling water-seal and suction chambers. *These supplies are used during the insertion procedure to establish a water-seal drainage system.*
- Position as indicated for the procedure. *Either an upright position (as for thoracentesis) or side-lying position may be used, depending on the site of the pneumothorax.*
- Assist with chest tube insertion as needed. The procedure may be performed in a procedure room, in the surgical suite, or at the bedside. *Although chest tube insertion is a relatively simple procedure, nursing assistance is necessary to support the client and rapidly establish a closed drainage system.*

### POSTPROCEDURE CARE

- Assess respiratory status at least every 4 hours. *Frequent assessment is necessary to monitor respiratory status and the effect of chest tube.*
- Maintain a closed system. Tape all connections, and secure the chest tube to the chest wall. *These measures are important to prevent inadvertent tube removal or disruption of the system integrity.*
- Keep the collection apparatus below the level of the chest. *Pleural fluid drains into the collection apparatus by gravity flow.*
- Check tubes frequently for kinks or loops. *These could interfere with drainage.*
- Check the water seal frequently. The water level should fluctuate with respiratory effort. If it does not, the system may not be patent or intact. Periodic air bubbles in the water-seal chamber are normal and indicate that trapped air is being removed from the chest. *Frequent assessment of the system is important to ensure appropriate functioning.*
- Measure drainage every 8 hours, marking the level on the drainage chamber. Report drainage that is cloudy, in excess of 70 mL per hour, or red, warm, and free flowing. *Red, free-flowing drainage indicates hemorrhage; cloudiness may indicate an infection. Emptying the drainage would disrupt integrity of the closed system.*
- Periodically assess water level in the suction control chamber, adding water as necessary. *Adequate water in the suction control chamber prevents excess suction from being placed on delicate pleural tissue.*
- Assist with frequent position changes and sitting and ambulation as allowed. *Chest tubes should not prevent performance of allowed activities. Care is needed to prevent inadvertent disconnection or removal of the tubes.*
- When the chest tube is removed, immediately apply a sterile occlusive petroleum jelly dressing. *An occlusive dressing prevents air from reentering the pleural space through the chest wound.*

---

ruptures. A thoracotomy is done to excise or oversew blebs (usually at the apices of the lungs). The overlying pleura is then roughened or irritated to induce scarring and adhesion to the surface of the lung. In some cases, the parietal pleura may be partially excised. These procedures can be done using video-assisted thoracoscopic surgery (VATS), a minimally invasive surgical technique (Way & Doherty, 2003).

## NURSING CARE

### Health Promotion

Health promotion activities to prevent spontaneous and traumatic pneumothorax primarily involve health teaching. Initiate and participate in programs to prevent smoking among children and teenagers. Teach safe behaviors such as always wearing a seat beat in an automobile, driving safely, and using precautions to prevent falls when working or recreating in high places.

### Assessment

The client with pneumothorax may be in acute respiratory distress, necessitating rapid and focused assessment.

- Health history: current symptoms and their duration; precipitating factors or activities if known; previous episodes of pneumothorax; smoking history; chronic pulmonary diseases such as COPD
- Physical assessment: general appearance and degree of apparent respiratory distress; evidence of chest trauma; vital signs, oxygen saturation, skin color, level of consciousness; respiratory excursion, percussion tone, and breath sounds anterior and posterior chest; neck vein inspection, position of trachea; peripheral pulses

### Nursing Diagnoses and Interventions

Maintaining or restoring adequate alveolar ventilation and gas exchange is of highest priority for the client with a pneumothorax. Chest tubes may interfere with physical mobility, contributing to a high risk for injury.

#### Impaired Gas Exchange

Loss of negative pressure in the pleural cavity and the resulting collapse of lung tissue can cause poor chest expansion and loss of alveolar ventilation. As the pneumothorax is removed or reabsorbed, ventilation and gas exchange improve.

- Assess and document vital signs and respiratory status, including rate, depth, lung sounds, and oxygen saturation at least every 4 hours. *Frequent assessment is important to monitor the adequacy of respirations and lung expansion.*

**PRACTICE ALERT** *Evaluate chest wall movement, position of the trachea, and neck veins frequently. Early identification of tension pneumothorax and appropriate interventions are vital to preserve cardiorespiratory function.* ■

- Place in Fowler's or high-Fowler's position. *This position facilitates lung expansion.*
- Administer oxygen as ordered. *Supplemental oxygen is given to improve oxygenation of the blood and tissues.*

**PRACTICE ALERT** *Provide emotional support, particularly in early stages and during chest tube insertion. Dyspnea and hypoxemia can cause extreme anxiety and apprehension, impairing the ability to cooperate with procedures.* ■

- Assess chest tube, system function, and drainage at least every 2 hours. *The system must remain patent and intact to function effectively.*
- Provide for rest. *Adequate rest is important to conserve energy and reduce oxygen demand.*

### Risk for Injury

Pain and the presence of chest tubes can reduce the perceived ability to ambulate and provide self-care. Moderate activity is encouraged unless respiratory function is significantly impaired. Caution is taken to maintain integrity of the chest tube system. If the tube is inadvertently pulled out or system integrity is disrupted, the pneumothorax may increase or infection may develop.

**PRACTICE ALERT** *Avoid placing tension on chest tubes during positioning, ambulation, and care activities. The chest tubes are minimally secured to the chest wall and can be dislodged if tension is placed on them.* ■

- Secure a loop of drainage tubing to the sheet or gown. *Looping the drainage tubing prevents direct pressure on the chest tube itself.*
- When turning to the affected side, ensure that neither the chest tube nor drainage tubing is kinked or occluded under the client. *This maintains patency of the system.*
- Teach the client how to ambulate with the drainage system, keeping the system lower than the chest. In most cases, suction can be discontinued during ambulation. *Ambulation facilitates lung ventilation and expansion. Drainage systems are portable to allow ambulation while chest tubes are in place. Keeping the drainage system lower than the chest promotes drainage and prevents reflux.*
- Observe insertion site for redness, swelling, pain, or drainage. Report any signs of infection, including fever, to the physician. *Interruption of skin integrity by chest tube insertion increases the risk for infection.*

- If a connection comes loose, reconnect it as soon as possible. *A closed, sealed system is vital to prevent air from entering the pleural space and an open pneumothorax.*

**PRACTICE ALERT** *Seal the wound of an open pneumothorax or from inadvertent tube removal as soon as possible with a sterile occlusive dressing, such as gauze impregnated with petroleum jelly. If a sterile dressing is not available, other occlusive material such as foil or plastic wrap can be used. Tape the dressing on three sides only. An occlusive dressing taped on three sides prevents the development of a tension pneumothorax by inhibiting air from entering the wound during inhalation but allowing it to escape during exhalation.* ■

## Home Care

Clients who have experienced spontaneous pneumothorax need education about their future risk. After a single episode of spontaneous pneumothorax, the risk of recurrence is 40% to 50%. This risk increases with subsequent episodes (Way & Doherty, 2003). Stress the importance of quitting smoking to reduce the risk. Other activities that can precipitate recurrent episodes include mountain climbing or those involving exposure to high altitudes, flying in unpressurized aircraft, and scuba diving (Tierney et al., 2001). The client may be advised to avoid contact sports.

Following a pneumothorax, instruct the client to gradually increase exercise and activity to previous levels. Stress the importance of follow-up care and monitoring. Discuss manifestations to report to the physician: upper respiratory infections; fever, cough, or difficulty breathing; sudden, sharp chest pain; or redness, pain, swelling, tenderness, or drainage from the chest tube puncture wound.

## THE CLIENT WITH HEMOTHORAX

**Hemothorax,** or blood in the pleural space, usually occurs as a result of chest trauma, surgery, or diagnostic procedures. Tumors, pulmonary infarction, and infections such as tuberculosis also can cause hemothorax. When blood collects in the pleural space, pressure on the affected lung impairs ventilation and gas exchange. With significant hemorrhage, a risk of shock exists.

Hemothorax causes symptoms similar to those of pneumothorax. Lung sounds are diminished, and a dull percussion tone is noted over the collected blood, typically at the base of the lung. Chest X-ray is used to confirm the diagnosis of hemothorax.

Thoracentesis or thoracostomy with chest tube drainage is used to remove blood from the pleural space. With significant hemorrhage (e.g., due to trauma or surgery), the blood may be collected for subsequent autotransfusion. Blood for autotransfusion should be collected and reinfused within 4 hours. Strict aseptic technique is used in collecting the blood. It is collected through a gross particulate filter into a container primed with anticoagulant and reinfused when the container is full or when transfusion is necessary. Air is removed from the blood container prior to reinfusion and a filter used to eliminate debris, such as degenerating blood cells, fat particles, and fibrin.

Priority nursing care for the client with hemothorax focuses on assessing and maintaining adequate respiratory function and cardiac output. The priority of care depends on the rate and extent of hemothorax. In a large, slow-developing hemothorax, ventilatory status may be affected significantly. In this instance, impaired gas exchange and ineffective breathing pattern are priority nursing diagnoses. When hemothorax develops rapidly and hemorrhage is significant, additional priority nursing diagnoses include *Decreased cardiac output* and *Risk for deficient fluid volume.*

When preparing the client for home care following a hemothorax, discuss the importance of avoiding smoking and preventing respiratory infection. Include symptoms to report to the physician. If trauma or infection caused the hemothorax, discuss measures to prevent future trauma and continuing treatment for the infection as indicated.

# TRAUMA OF THE CHEST OR LUNG

Chest injury is a leading cause of death from trauma. It is commonly associated with motor vehicle crashes, violent crime, and falls. Chest injuries can range from mild, such as a simple rib fracture, to severe and fatal. Traumatic injury to the chest may involve both the chest wall and underlying thoracic structures, including the lungs, heart, great vessels, and esophagus. Chest and lung injury can result from several different mechanisms: penetrating trauma, such as a stab or gunshot wound; blunt trauma, such as a fall, motor vehicle crash, vehicle-pedestrian impact, or crush injury; or inhalation injury, such as smoke inhalation or near drowning.

Rapid and continuing assessment of the airway, breathing, and circulation (ABCs) is vital in chest or lung injuries. Chest trauma can disrupt any or all of these functions. Chest injuries that may be life threatening include airway obstruction, tension pneumothorax, open pneumothorax, massive hemothorax, and flail chest with pulmonary contusion.

## THE CLIENT WITH A THORACIC INJURY

Thoracic injuries may be minor and have little effect on respiratory status, for example, simple rib fracture in a previously healthy client. When pain or chest wall instability impair breathing or the underlying lung tissue is damaged, the risk is more significant. Thoracic trauma usually is caused by motor vehicle crashes or falls.

## PATHOPHYSIOLOGY AND MANIFESTATIONS

Acceleration-deceleration injury and direct mechanisms of injury (e.g., crush injuries) are the most common mechanisms of thoracic injuries. Acceleration-deceleration injuries are caused by a rapid change in velocity as occurs in a motor vehicle crash or fall. The body stops suddenly, but the tissues and organs within the chest cavity continue to move forward until they impact with the chest wall. Injuries sustained can be significant, depending on the velocity (speed) of the vehicle or body at the point of impact, the surface with which the body impacts, and individual characteristics (e.g., size and bone structure).

## Rib Fracture

Simple rib fracture, usually involving a single rib, is the most common chest wall injury. Rib fracture generally is tolerated well and heals rapidly in a young, previously healthy person. In an older adult or person with preexisting lung disease, however, a fractured rib may lead to significant complications, such as pneumonia, atelectasis, and, potentially, respiratory failure. Displaced fractured ribs can penetrate the pleura, leading to pneumothorax and possible hemothorax. Fractures of certain ribs are more frequently associated with underlying tissue damage. Intrathoracic vessels may be damaged or torn with fractures of the first and second ribs. Fractures of the seventh through tenth ribs may cause liver or spleen injuries (Urden, Stacy, & Lough, 2002).

Rib fracture causes pain on inspiration and coughing. This leads to voluntary splinting, with rapid, shallow respirations and inhibited cough. Bruising may be seen over the fracture, and crepitus may be palpated with respiratory movement. Breath sounds are diminished, especially in the bases, due to splinting. If pneumothorax develops, chest wall movement on the affected side may be reduced, and breath sounds absent or significantly diminished. A hyperresonant percussion tone usually is noted. Hemothorax also causes diminished or absent breath sounds on the affected side, with a dull percussion note.

## Flail Chest

Multiple rib fractures may impair chest wall stability and normal chest wall function. When two or more consecutive ribs are fractured in multiple places, a free-floating segment of the chest wall, or **flail chest,** results. Physiologic function of the chest wall is impaired as the flail segment is sucked inward during inhalation and moves outward with exhalation. This is known as *paradoxic movement* (Figure 36–17 ■). Lung expansion is impaired and the work of breathing increases. Flail chest is frequently associated with underlying pulmonary contusion, which may lead to respiratory failure.

Flail chest causes dyspnea and pain, especially on inspiration. Paradoxic chest movement is evident with inspection. Chest expansion is unequal, and palpable crepitus is present. Breath sounds are diminished, and crackles may be heard on auscultation.

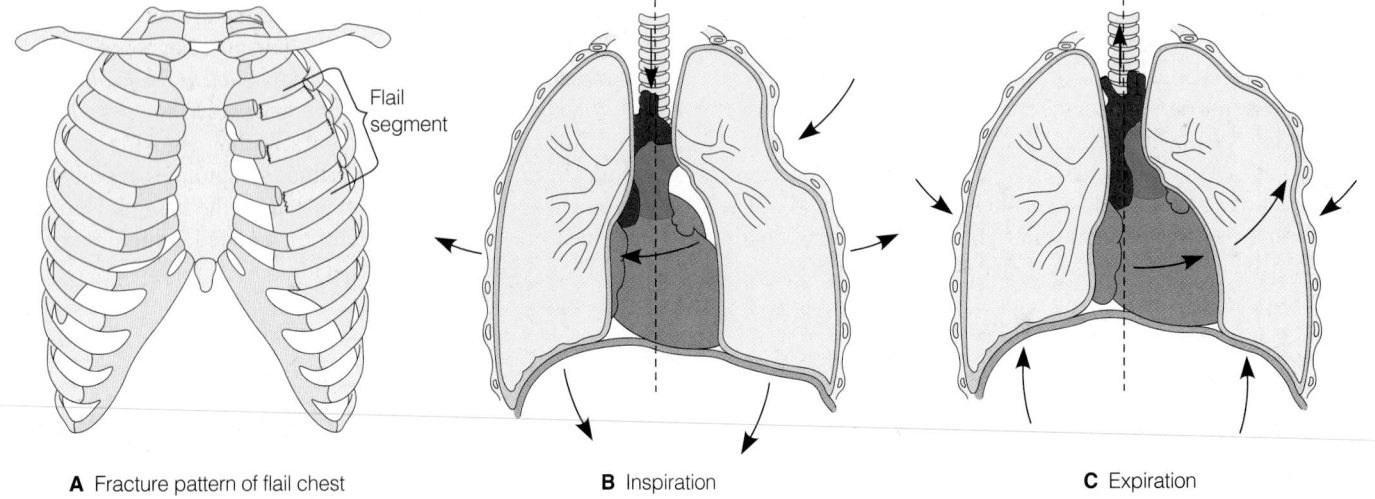

**A** Fracture pattern of flail chest      **B** Inspiration      **C** Expiration

**Figure 36-17** ■ Flail chest with paradoxic movement.

## Pulmonary Contusion

Pulmonary contusion, or lung tissue injury, is frequently associated with flail chest and other blunt chest trauma. It may occur unilaterally or bilaterally. Pulmonary contusion often results from abrupt chest compression followed by sudden decompression, as can occur with an MVC, significant fall, or crush injury. Alveoli and pulmonary arterioles rupture, causing intra-alveolar hemorrhage and interstitial and bronchial edema. The resulting inflammatory response increases capillary permeability, leading to edema which may be localized to the damaged lung tissue or more generalized. Inflammation and edema impair the production of surfactant within the alveoli, decreasing compliance. Pulmonary vascular resistance increases and blood flow decreases. Airway obstruction, atelectasis, and impaired gas diffusion result. Associated chest wall injury impairs the ability to clear secretions effectively, and the work of breathing is significantly increased.

Manifestations of pulmonary contusion may not be apparent until 12 to 24 hours after the injury. Increasing shortness of breath, restlessness, apprehension, and chest pain are early signs. Copious sputum, which may be blood tinged, is present. Later manifestations include tachycardia, tachypnea, dyspnea, and cyanosis. Even with appropriate treatment, pulmonary contusion can lead to acute respiratory distress and potential death.

## COLLABORATIVE CARE

Chest X-ray is used to identify most chest wall injuries. Rib fractures are evident on X-ray. Pulmonary contusion may show as initial patchy opacifications progressing to diffuse opacification, or "white-out." Changes in oxygen saturation and arterial blood gases depend on the degree to which ventilation and gas exchange are affected by the injury.

Simple rib fractures typically heal uneventfully. Providing adequate analgesia to promote breathing, coughing, and movement is the primary intervention. With multiple rib fractures, an intercostal nerve block may be used to ensure adequate ventilation. Rib belts, binders, and taping to stabilize the rib cage are not recommended, because they may interfere with ventilation and lead to atelectasis. Even with simple rib fracture, older clients and clients with preexisting lung disease require close monitoring to prevent and detect atelectasis, pneumonia, and other complications.

Intercostal nerve blocks or continuous epidural analgesia may be employed to manage the pain associated with flail chest. For a small flail chest, analgesia combined with supplemental oxygen therapy may be adequate. In some cases, internal or external fixation of the flail segment may be done.

The preferred treatment for flail chest is intubation and mechanical ventilation. Positive-pressure ventilation provides support and stabilization of the flail segment and improves ventilation and gas exchange. The work of breathing is decreased and healing improved.

Clients with pulmonary contusion often are critically ill, requiring intensive care management. Treatment is supportive, directed at maintaining adequate ventilation and alveolar gas exchange. Endotracheal intubation and mechanical ventilation are necessary in most cases. Repeated bronchoscopy may be done to remove secretions and cellular debris, preventing atelectasis. Although adequate hydration is necessary to prevent shock, overhydration can increase pulmonary edema. Pulmonary arterial pressure monitoring with a Swan-Ganz catheter and frequent arterial blood gas measurement is required for optimal fluid replacement and management of ventilatory support. See Chapter 30 ⊕ for more information about pulmonary artery pressure monitoring.

Unilateral pulmonary contusion may present a unique management problem. Mechanical ventilation with positive end-expiratory pressure (PEEP) to maintain open alveoli and adequate gas exchange can damage the unaffected lung. Intubation with a double-lumen endotracheal tube which permits independent ventilation of each lung may be used.

## NURSING CARE

Chest wall trauma can interfere with adequate chest expansion and alveolar ventilation. When a pulmonary contusion is also present, gas exchange is affected as well. Priorities for nursing management include controlling pain, ensuring adequate ventilation, and promoting gas exchange.

### Acute Pain

With many thoracic injuries, pain interferes with lung expansion and coughing, leading to such complications as pneumonia and atelectasis. Adequate pain management is a key component of medical and nursing management for these clients.

- Frequently assess pain, using a standard pain scale and objective data. *Increased respiratory rate, shallow respirations, diminished breath sounds, and reluctance to move and cough may indicate inadequate pain control in a thoracic injury.*
- Administer analgesics by patient-controlled analgesia or on a schedule to maintain pain control. *Analgesics are more effective when pain is not allowed to become intense.*

**PRACTICE ALERT** *Assess for possible respiratory depression due to narcotic analgesia. Respiratory depression can further compromise ventilation in the client with thoracic injury.* ■

- Notify the physician if pain relief is inadequate or excess sedation and respiratory depression occur. *An intercostal nerve block may be done to reduce the need for narcotic analgesia. Assess for bleeding and adequate ventilation following a nerve block.*

### Ineffective Airway Clearance

Aggressive respiratory hygiene may be necessary to maintain open airways and adequate ventilation.

- Assess lung sounds and respiratory rate, depth, and effort frequently. Encourage to cough, deep breathe, and change position every 1 to 2 hours, and use the incentive spirometer. *Frequent assessment and measures to maintain airway patency are vital to prevent complications in the client with thoracic injury.*
- Teach how to splint the affected area with a blanket or pillow when coughing. *Splinting reduces movement and discomfort of the affected area.*
- Suction airway as indicated. Work with respiratory therapy to maintain optimal mechanical ventilation. Secure the endotracheal tube to maintain appropriate position and lung ventilation. *Endotracheal tube security is particularly important when a double-lumen endotracheal tube is in place, because malposition can occlude one main bronchus and prevent ventilation of the affected lung.*

- Elevate the head of the bed. *Elevating the head of the bed facilitates lung expansion and reduces the work of breathing.*

**PRACTICE ALERT** *Promptly report to the physician signs of complications, such as diminished breath sounds, increasing crackles (rales) or rhonchi, dull or hyperresonant percussion tones, unequal chest movement, hemoptysis, chills or fever, or changes in vital signs. Prompt intervention for complications is vital to promote healing and recovery.* ■

### Impaired Gas Exchange

Impaired gas exchange is of particular concern in pulmonary contusion. Alveolar damage and pulmonary edema can significantly impair oxygenation of the blood and removal of carbon dioxide.

- Monitor vital signs, color, oxygen saturation, and arterial blood gases. Assess for manifestations such as anxiety or apprehension, restlessness, confusion or lethargy, or complaints of headache. *These assessment data alert the nurse and care providers to potential hypoxemia or hypercapnia due to impaired gas exchange.*
- Maintain oxygen therapy and mechanical ventilation as ordered. Hyperoxygenate prior to suctioning. *Oxygen and mechanical ventilation support alveolar gas exchange. Hyperoxygenation prior to suctioning reduces the degree of hypoxemia that occurs during suctioning.*
- Monitor intake and output, weigh daily, and monitor central venous pressure and pulmonary artery pressure as ordered. Maintain any ordered fluid restriction. *Fluid volume status is monitored to reduce the effects of pulmonary edema on lung tissues.*
- Maintain bed rest or activity restriction as ordered. Space activities to allow periods of uninterrupted rest. *Rest reduces the metabolic rate and oxygen consumption.*

### Home Care

Simple rib fracture and minor chest wall injuries often are managed on an outpatient basis. Include the following topics when teaching for home care.

- Pain management and its importance in preventing respiratory complications
- Importance of coughing and deep breathing; how to splint the rib cage during coughing
- Reasons for not taping or wrapping the chest continuously
- Symptoms to report to the physician: chills and fever, productive cough, purulent or bloody sputum, shortness of breath or difficulty breathing, and increasing chest pain
- Importance of avoiding respiratory irritants, such as cigarette smoke and occupational or environmental pollutants

Significant pulmonary contusion can result in long-term respiratory insufficiency. Discuss activity modifications and occupational changes with the client and family as indicated. Refer to home care services such as respiratory therapy and home health if needed.

## THE CLIENT WITH INHALATION INJURY

The internal environment of the lungs normally is protected from noxious substances by respiratory defense mechanisms. If these defenses are breached, inhaled agents, such as gases, fumes, toxins, and water, can cause internal trauma to the lungs.

## PATHOPHYSIOLOGY AND MANIFESTATIONS

### Smoke Inhalation

Pulmonary injury due to inhalation of hot air, toxic gases, or particulate matter is the leading cause of death in burn injury (Braunwald et al., 2001). Smoke inhalation affects up to one-third of clients admitted to burn units. Smoke inhalation can significantly affect normal respiratory function through three different mechanisms:

- Thermal damage to the airways, leading to impaired ventilation
- Carbon monoxide or cyanide poisoning, resulting in tissue hypoxia
- Chemical damage to the lung from noxious gases, which can impair gas exchange

Smoke inhalation is suspected whenever a burn occurs in a closed space; if there are burns to the face or upper torso or singed nasal hairs; if sputum contains ashlike material; and when manifestations such as dyspnea, wheezing, rales, or rhonchi develop.

The lower airways of the lungs typically are protected from thermal damage by cooling of the inhaled gases in the upper airway and laryngeal spasm. Upper airway obstruction due to tissue edema and laryngeal spasm can occur quickly, however, resulting in **asphyxiation,** or oxygen deprivation, without lung damage. Steam inhalation can cause thermal damage to tissues of the lower respiratory tract.

Inhalation of carbon monoxide or cyanide gas poses an immediate threat to life. Carbon monoxide is a colorless, odorless gas produced in a fire. It binds readily with hemoglobin. The affinity of carbon monoxide for hemoglobin is 200 to 250 times stronger than that of oxygen. Hemoglobin bound to carbon monoxide reduces the oxygen-carrying capacity of blood and oxygen delivery to cells of the body. Carbon monoxide poisoning is suspected if the burn occurred in a closed space, if there is evidence of inhalation injury, or if dyspnea develops.

The manifestations of carbon monoxide poisoning depend on the level of carboxyhemoglobin saturation. When hemoglobin is 10% to 20% saturated with carbon monoxide, symptoms include headache, dizziness, dyspnea, and nausea. A characteristic "cherry-red" color of the skin and mucous membranes may be seen. With increasing levels, confusion, visual disturbances, irritability, hallucinations, hypotension, seizures, and coma develop. Permanent neurologic deficit can occur in survivors of severe acute carbon monoxide poisoning.

Many other toxic chemicals may be present in smoke, especially in a house fire or industrial plant fire. Hydrogen cyanide can be lethal when inhaled. Inhalation of toxic chemicals causes bronchospasm and edema of the airways and alveoli. Acute respiratory distress syndrome may develop within 1 to 2 days. Sloughing of damaged mucosa leads to airway obstruction and atelectasis. Pneumonia is common following smoke inhalation.

### Near-Drowning

Drowning is a leading preventable cause of accidental death in the United States. Approximately 5500 people die of drowning every year in the United States. Alcohol ingestion is a factor in 25% to 33% of adult drowning deaths (Tierney et al., 2001). Asphyxiation and aspiration are the primary problems associated with drowning and near-drowning. About 10% of victims do not aspirate water; instead, laryngeal spasm causes asphyxia. This is known as "dry drowning." In most cases, however, asphyxia and hypoxemia are the result of fluid aspiration. The effects of hypoxemia occur rapidly; loss of consciousness can occur within 3 to 5 minutes after total immersion. Circulatory impairment, brain injury, and brain death can occur within 5 to 10 minutes. Immersion in very cold water and the *dive reflex,* a protective mechanism that slows the heartbeat, constricts peripheral vessels, and shunts blood to the brain and heart, may prolong survival.

Water aspiration can cause delayed death from near-drowning. Respiratory and systemic effects differ, depending on whether freshwater or saltwater has been aspirated. Freshwater is hypotonic; when aspirated, it is rapidly absorbed from the alveoli, leading to hypervolemia and hemodilution. Hemolysis occurs as blood cells are subjected to a hypotonic environment, and serum electrolytes are diluted. Electrolyte imbalances can cause cardiac dysrhythmias and death. Hemolysis can lead to acute tubular necrosis and acute renal failure. Aspiration of freshwater impairs pulmonary surfactant and damages the alveolar-capillary membrane. Respiratory failure can result.

Nearly the opposite effects occur with saltwater aspiration. As a hypertonic fluid, saltwater draws fluid into the alveoli, resulting in hypovolemia and hemoconcentration. Hemolysis is insignificant, and small elevations in serum sodium and chloride levels rarely cause life-threatening effects. With either type of near-drowning episode, inhaled microorganisms and debris can lead to pneumonia. The pathophysiologic changes associated with freshwater and saltwater near-drowning are illustrated in Figure 36–18 ■.

Manifestations of near-drowning may include altered level of consciousness, restlessness, and apprehension. The client may complain of headache or chest pain. Other signs include vomiting, possible cyanosis, apnea, tachypnea, and wheezing. If pulmonary edema is present, pink froth may be visible in the mouth and nose. Other manifestations include tachycardia, dysrhythmias, hypotension, shock, and cardiac arrest. Hypothermia may be present.

The near-drowning victim who never loses consciousness or is conscious on admission to the emergency department has a good prognosis for recovery. The prognosis is less optimistic when neurologic damage has occurred.

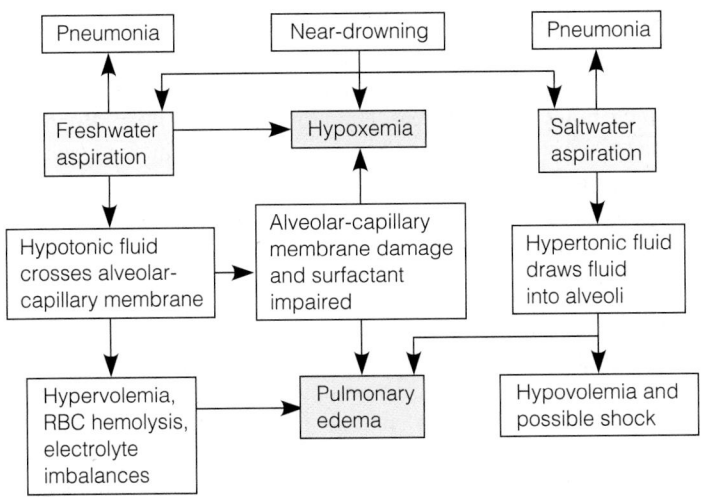

**Figure 36–18** ■ The pathogenesis of near-drowning, freshwater and saltwater.

## COLLABORATIVE CARE

With inhalation injuries, the most effective treatment is prevention. A working smoke detector (with functioning batteries) could prevent the majority of deaths from smoke inhalation occurring in the home. The line, "A smoke detector was found, but the batteries had been removed," is all too familiar in news reports of fire-related deaths.

To prevent drowning, life preservers and flotation vests or jackets should be worn on the body, not stored in the hold of the boat. These devices are designed to keep the head above water. Even accomplished swimmers should never enter the water alone in unguarded areas. Just as alcohol and driving do not mix, neither do alcohol and boating or other water sports.

The second most important line of defense against death or permanent injury from inhalation injuries is removing the victim from the area of the fire or water and administering effective cardiopulmonary resuscitation. In many cases, immediate restoration of effective breathing and circulation is key to preserving life. Hypoxemia progresses rapidly until breathing is restored; reversal of tissue hypoxia depends on adequate circulation. In both smoke inhalation and near drowning, intubation may be necessary to establish an airway. Oxygen is administered as soon as possible. Attempts to drain water from the lungs of the near-drowning victim waste time and are generally ineffective in restoring alveolar ventilation. External cardiac defibrillation may be necessary to reestablish an effective cardiac rhythm and circulation. When the victim is hypothermic, resuscitation measures are continued until the core body temperature reaches approximately 90°F (32°C). The basic rule in hypothermia is that the client is not declared dead until the body has been rewarmed and life signs remain absent.

### Diagnostic Tests

When inhalation injury is known or suspected, the following diagnostic tests may be done.

- *ABGs* are drawn to evaluate gas exchange and the degree of hypoxemia. Combined respiratory and metabolic acidosis may be apparent. With effective ventilation and supplemental oxygen, acidosis may reverse quickly. With carbon monoxide poisoning, arterial $PO_2$ may be normal, but oxyhemoglobin saturation is less than normal.
- *Carboxyhemoglobin levels* are drawn in suspected carbon monoxide poisoning. Normal levels are less than 5% in nonsmokers and less than 10% in smokers. Higher levels indicate carbon monoxide poisoning. Levels less than 20% are considered mild poisoning; between 20% and 40% is moderate poisoning; and 40% to 60% is severe poisoning. Levels higher than 60% are generally fatal.
- *Serum electrolytes* and *osmolality levels* vary in near-drowning, depending on the type of water aspirated. In freshwater drowning, serum electrolyte levels and osmolality may be significantly reduced. With saltwater drowning, serum sodium and chloride may be somewhat high, and osmolality is increased because of hypovolemia.
- *Chest X-ray* is done, but may not show changes until 12 or more hours after the insult. Evidence of acute respiratory distress syndrome may be seen 24 to 48 hours after inhalation injury.
- *Bronchoscopy* may be ordered to inspect damaged lung tissue, particularly with smoke inhalation and possible thermal injury.

### Treatments

Treatment of inhalation injury is generally supportive. Endotracheal intubation and mechanical ventilation often are required to maintain the airway and provide adequate alveolar ventilation and oxygenation. All clients with inhalation injury require supplemental oxygen, even when intubation and ventilation are not required. *Hyperbaric oxygen therapy,* the delivery of 100% oxygen at increased atmospheric pressure, may be used to treat carbon monoxide poisoning. This treatment carries some risks, such as oxygen toxicity and potential trauma to lung tissues, sinuses, and ears due to the increased pressures (Leifer, 2001).

Other treatment measures may include bronchodilator therapy to manage bronchospasm. Bronchodilators can be administered by aerosol inhalation or intravenous infusion. Coughing and suctioning is important to remove secretions and debris. Chest physiotherapy with percussion and postural drainage may be performed.

Intravenous fluids may be ordered; if significant hemolysis has occurred, packed red blood cells may be given to improve the oxygen-carrying capacity of the blood. Fluid therapy is monitored carefully, using pulmonary artery or central venous pressures to reduce the risk of pulmonary edema.

With near-drowning victims, measures such as inducing hypothermia or barbiturate-induced coma and administering corticosteroids and osmotic diuretics may be employed to help prevent neurologic damage.

Careful monitoring for complications such as pneumonia and acute respiratory distress syndrome is vital throughout the course of treatment. Respiratory status, vital signs, and other data are frequently assessed to identify complications and allow early intervention.

# NURSING CARE

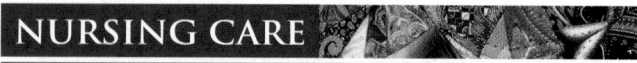

## Health Promotion

Prevention of inhalation injuries is an important nursing responsibility. Teach everyone the value of a working smoke detector, especially in the sleeping areas of the house. Encourage families to develop an escape plan in case of fire and to use fire drills to rehearse getting out of the house. Smoldering cigarettes are a leading cause of house fires; help clients develop a plan to stop smoking. Teach people to drop and roll should clothing catch fire. (Flames rise, increasing the risk of respiratory injury when upright.)

Learning to swim safely is important to prevent drowning. Teach clients never to swim alone, when fatigued, or immediately following a meal. Remind clients that knowing how to swim will not prevent drowning in very cold water or in large bodies of water, such as lakes, rivers, or the ocean. Instruct to always wear flotation devices while boating, water-skiing, surfing, or wind-surfing. Wet suits help prevent hypothermia during activities in very cold water. Advise covering or fencing swimming pools, hot tubs, and ponds to prevent inadvertent entry and drowning.

A population well trained in effective, safe cardiopulmonary resuscitation (CPR) provides the best second line of defense against inhalation injury. Rapid restoration of breathing is essential to prevent hypoxia and brain damage. Encourage all people to be trained and regularly update CPR skills. Work with communities to increase the number of trained people. Refer clients to local chapters of the American Red Cross or American Heart Association for classes.

## Assessment

Inhalation injuries may be a medical emergency, necessitating focused and timely nursing assessment.

- Health history: circumstances of the injury, including duration of exposure to smoke or time under water, explosion or fire in a closed area, type and temperature of water immersed in; resuscitation measures used; allergies, and current medical problems
- Physical examination: airway, breathing, circulation; level of consciousness; color; vital signs; heart and lung sounds; urine output; evidence of burns or soot around nares or mouth

## Nursing Diagnoses and Interventions

Nursing care priorities for the client with an inhalation injury are determined by the type of injury or tissue damage. Airway clearance is a major concern in all inhalation injuries, as is impaired gas exchange. Tissue hypoxia also can be a significant problem.

### Ineffective Airway Clearance

Nursing measures to maintain an adequate airway begin with careful and frequent assessment of respiratory status, including rate, depth, and effort as well as breath sounds. Note amount, color, and consistency of sputum. Assist to cough frequently; suction the intubated client as needed to remove secretions. El-evate the head of the bed to facilitate alveolar ventilation unless otherwise ordered. Stabilize endotracheal tube with tape and ties to prevent displacement into a mainstem bronchus, which could lead to ventilation of only one lung. Report changes in the character of secretions that may indicate complications: pink, frothy sputum suggesting pulmonary edema, or purulent sputum suggestive of pneumonia. Administer bronchodilators as ordered. Perform percussion and postural drainage as ordered.

### Impaired Gas Exchange

Support gas exchange by administering supplemental oxygen, with or without mechanical ventilation. Frequently assess oxygen saturation, skin color, and mental status. Decreasing level of consciousness may be an early sign of hypoxemia. Monitor exhaled carbon dioxide, arterial blood gases, and pulmonary artery pressures as ordered and indicated. Report changes to the physician. Maintain oxygen flow rates as ordered. Provide frequent mouth care to reduce the discomfort of dry mucous membranes and prevent tissue breakdown. Work with respiratory therapy to maintain effective oxygen delivery with mechanical ventilation. Administer sedation as required. Maintain fluid restriction if ordered.

### Ineffective Tissue Perfusion: Cerebral

Impaired cerebral tissue perfusion is a priority problem, especially with near-drowning. Hypoxia and possible hypervolemia can lead to cerebral edema and increased intracranial pressure (IICP), further impairing blood flow. Monitor vital signs and neurologic status frequently. A change in level of consciousness or behavior is typically the earliest sign of IICP. Changes noted on an intracranial pressure monitor also provide early evidence of IICP. Increasing systolic blood pressure and pulse pressure and slowed heart rate are late signs. Other manifestations may include pupillary changes and decreasing muscle strength. Report changes promptly to the physician. Elevate the head of the bed and keep the head in neutral position to promote drainage from the cranial vault. Maintain effective ventilation and oxygenation; hypercapnia and hypoxemia increase cerebral edema. Administer sedation, osmotic diuretics, or corticosteroids as ordered to reduce cerebral edema. Maintain fluid restriction. Space activities and promote rest to reduce metabolic demands.

## Home Care

Teach clients who do not require hospitalization for inhalation injury about symptoms that may indicate a complication and should be reported to the physician: increasing dyspnea, cough productive of purulent or pink frothy mucus, confusion, or other changes. Manifestations of respiratory damage may not be apparent for 24 to 48 hours following the injury.

Significant hypoxia due to near-drowning or carbon monoxide poisoning may cause permanent neurologic effects. Work with the family to develop communication techniques and identify remaining strengths. Help the family identify future care needs and means for meeting them, such as home health, personal care aides, or long-term care facilities. Provide social services and support group referrals.

# RESPIRATORY FAILURE

Many of the conditions discussed in this chapter, from pneumonia to acute respiratory distress syndrome (ARDS), can lead to respiratory failure. In **respiratory failure,** the lungs are unable to oxygenate the blood and remove carbon dioxide adequately to meet the body's needs, even at rest.

## THE CLIENT WITH ACUTE RESPIRATORY FAILURE

Respiratory failure is not a disease but a consequence of severe respiratory dysfunction. It is often defined by arterial blood gas values. An arterial oxygen level ($PO_2$) of less than 50 to 60 mmHg and an arterial carbon dioxide level ($PCO_2$) of greater than 50 mmHg are generally accepted as indicators of respiratory failure. However, clients with advanced COPD may be alert and functional with blood gas values that would indicate respiratory failure in someone whose respiratory function was previously normal. In clients with COPD, respiratory failure is indicated by an acute drop in blood oxygen levels along with increased carbon dioxide levels.

Respiratory failure can result from inadequate alveolar ventilation (hypoventilation), impaired gas exchange, or a significant ventilation-perfusion mismatch. COPD is the most common cause of respiratory failure. Other lung diseases, chest injury, inhalation trauma, neuromuscular disorders, and cardiac conditions can also lead to respiratory failure. Selected causes of acute respiratory failure are identified in Table 36–13.

### PATHOPHYSIOLOGY

Respiratory failure may be characterized by primary hypoxemia or a combination of hypoxemia and hypercapnia (Figure 36–19 ■). In hypoxemic respiratory failure, $PO_2$ is significantly

| TABLE 36–13 | Selected Causes of Respiratory Failure |
|---|---|
| **Type of Dysfunction** | **Examples** |
| **Impaired ventilation:** | |
| • Airway obstruction | Laryngospasm, foreign body aspiration, airway edema |
| • Respiratory disease | Asthma, COPD |
| • Neurologic causes | Spinal cord injury, poliomyelitis, Guillain-Barré syndrome, drug overdose, stroke |
| • Chest wall injury | Flail chest, pneumothorax |
| **Impaired diffusion:** | |
| • Alveolar disorders | Pneumonia, pneumonitis, COPD |
| • Pulmonary edema | Heart failure, acute respiratory distress syndrome (ARDS), near-drowning |
| **Ventilation-perfusion mismatch** | Pulmonary embolism |

reduced, whereas $PCO_2$ remains normal or is low due to stimulation of the respiratory center and tachypnea. Impaired diffusion across the alveolar-capillary membrane, and a ventilation-perfusion mismatch can cause a drop in arterial oxygen levels that is more rapid than the rise in carbon dioxide. Metabolic acidosis results from tissue hypoxia. The increased work of breathing can eventually lead to respiratory muscle fatigue and hypoventilation.

Hypoventilation, or reduced movement of air into and out of the lung, causes carbon dioxide retention. With significant hypoventilation, the carbon dioxide level in the blood rises rapidly, leading to respiratory acidosis. Hypoxemia develops more slowly, and responds readily to administration of oxygen unless gas exchange also is impaired.

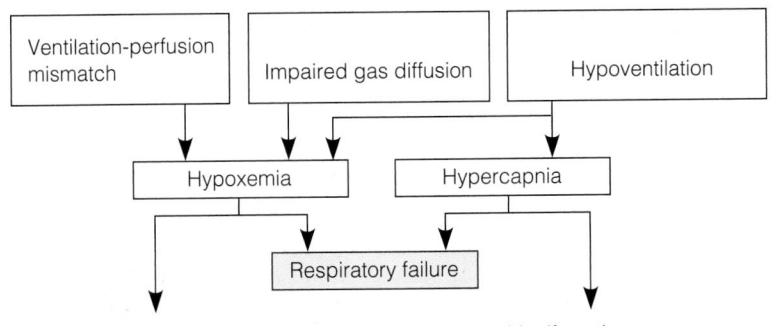

**Figure 36–19 ■** Respiratory failure, its causes and manifestations.

In summary, hypoxemia without a corresponding rise in carbon dioxide levels indicates a failure of oxygenation; hypoxemia with hypercapnia is the result of lung hypoventilation.

The prognosis for acute respiratory failure varies, depending on the underlying disease process. Respiratory failure resulting from uncomplicated drug overdose generally resolves quickly without long-term effects. When respiratory failure results from underlying lung disease, the course may be prolonged and the outcome less favorable. Among adults requiring mechanical ventilation for acute respiratory failure, it is estimated that 62% survive to be weaned from the ventilator, but only 43% survive to be discharged from the hospital, and 30% remain alive at 1 year after discharge (Tierney et al., 2001).

## MANIFESTATIONS

The manifestations of respiratory failure are caused by hypoxemia and hypercapnia, as well as the underlying disease process. Hypoxemia causes dyspnea and neurologic symptoms such as restlessness, apprehension, impaired judgment, and motor impairment. Tachycardia and hypertension develop as the cardiac output increases in an effort to bring more oxygen to the tissues. Cyanosis is present. As hypoxemia progresses, dysrhythmias, hypotension, and decreased cardiac output may develop.

Increased carbon dioxide levels depress CNS function and cause vasodilation. Dyspnea and headache are early signs. Other manifestations include peripheral and conjunctival vasodilation, papilledema, neuromuscular irritability, and decreased level of consciousness. As hypercapnia worsens, the respiratory center may be depressed, reducing dyspnea and slowing respirations. Increased carbon dioxide and hydrogen ion concentrations not longer stimulate the respiratory center; hypoxemia provides the only active breathing stimulus. Administering oxygen without ventilatory support may eliminate any drive to breathe, leading to respiratory arrest.

## COLLABORATIVE CARE

Treatment of respiratory failure focuses on correcting the underlying cause or disease, supporting ventilation, and correcting hypoxemia and hypercapnia. Care related to disorders that can precipitate respiratory failure is discussed in the sections specific to each disorder.

## Diagnostic Tests

Exhaled carbon dioxide and arterial blood gases are used to diagnose and monitor treatment of respiratory failure.

- *Exhaled carbon dioxide (ETCO$_2$)* is used to evaluate alveolar ventilation. The normal ETCO$_2$ is 35 to 45 mmHg; it is elevated when ventilation is inadequate, and decreased when pulmonary perfusion is impaired.
- *Arterial blood gases* also are used to evaluate alveolar ventilation and gas exchange. With hypoxemic respiratory failure, the PCO$_2$ may be normal, 38 to 42 mmHg, or even low due to tachypnea. A pH of less than 7.35 and low bicarbonate levels indicate metabolic acidosis, typical of hypoxemic respiratory failure.

In respiratory failure due to hypoventilation, the PCO$_2$ is elevated, usually greater than 50 mmHg. The pH is low due to respiratory acidosis. Acidosis develops rapidly in hypoxemia and hypercapnia because of increased acid production (metabolic) and decreased acid elimination (respiratory).

## Medications

Drugs used in treating respiratory failure depend on the underlying cause of the failure and the need for intubation and mechanical ventilation.

Beta-adrenergic (sympathomimetic) or anticholinergic medications may be administered by inhalation to promote bronchodilation. If mechanical ventilation is required, the drugs may be given by nebulizer attached to the ventilator. Methyxanthine bronchodilators (theophylline derivatives) may be given intravenously. See the box on page 1110 and the asthma section of this chapter for more information about bronchodilators and their nursing implications. Corticosteroids, administered by inhalation or intravenously, may be ordered to reduce airway edema. Antibiotics are given to treat any underlying infection.

Sedation and analgesia often are required during mechanical ventilation to decrease pain and anxiety. Benzodiazepines such as diazepam (Valium), lorazepam (Ativan), or midazolam (Versed) may be used for sedation and to inhibit the respiratory drive. Intravenous morphine or fentanyl provide analgesia and also inhibit the respiratory drive, allowing more effective mechanical ventilation. Occasionally, the client's respiratory drive competes with the ventilator despite sedation, decreasing its effectiveness and increasing the work of breathing. A neuromuscular blocking agent may be necessary to induce paralysis and suppress the ability to breathe. Nursing implications of neuromuscular blockers are described in the Medication Administration box on page 1159.

## Oxygen Therapy

Oxygen is administered to reverse hypoxemia in acute respiratory failure. In general, the goal is to achieve an oxygen saturation of 90% or greater without oxygen toxicity. A PO$_2$ of about 60 mmHg usually is adequate to meet the oxygen needs of body tissues. Higher levels do not significantly increase oxygen saturation and may lead to hypoventilation in clients with chronic hypercapnia. As little as 1 to 3 L of oxygen per nasal cannula or 28% oxygen per Venturi mask may correct hypoxemia in advanced COPD. Oxygen concentrations of 40% to 60% may be required when diffusion is impaired (e.g., in pneumonia or acute respiratory distress syndrome). High concentrations are used only for short periods to avoid oxygen toxicity. Both the oxygen concentration and duration of therapy contribute to oxygen toxicity. Continued high oxygen concentrations impair the synthesis of surfactant, reducing lung compliance (ease of inflation). Acute respiratory distress syndrome or absorption atelectasis may develop.

When respiratory failure is caused by hypoventilation or usual oxygen delivery systems do not correct hypoxemia, a tight-fitting mask to maintain *continuous positive airway pressure (CPAP)* may be used. CPAP increases lung volume,

## Medication Administration

### Neuromuscular Blockers

#### NONDEPOLARIZING NEUROMUSCULAR BLOCKERS

Rocuronium (Zemuron)
Pancuronium bromide (Pavulon)
Atracurium besylate (Tracrium)
Cisatracurium (Nimbex)

Nondepolarizing neuromuscular blockers competitively block the action of acetylcholine (ACh) at skeletal muscle receptors, preventing muscle depolarization and contraction. Complete muscle paralysis is achieved within minutes. Facial muscles are affected first, followed by muscles of the limbs, neck, and trunk. The muscles of respiration (the diaphragm and intercostal muscles) are least sensitive to the effects of neuromuscular blockers and are paralyzed last. When the drug is discontinued or an antagonist is given, muscles recover in reverse order, respiratory function is recovered first.

#### Nursing Responsibilities

- Prior to administering, assess endotracheal tube placement and ensure effective mechanical ventilator function. The risk of hypoxemia and organ damage is significant if respiratory muscles are paralyzed without adequate ventilatory support in place.
- Administer the drug by slow intravenous injection and/or intravenous infusion as prescribed.

- Keep an acetylcholinesterase (AChE) inhibitor such as neostigmine (Prostigmin) available at the bedside to rapidly reverse neuromuscular effects if needed.
- Administer morphine sulfate, diazepam (Valium), or other antianxiety agent or sedative as ordered. Neuromuscular blockers provide no sedation or pain relief; muscle paralysis produces extreme anxiety.
- Instill artificial tears every 2 to 4 hours.
- Suction oral cavity as needed to remove saliva.
- *Never* turn off ventilator alarms when administering neuromuscular blockers. Should the tubing become disconnected or plugged, the client is unable to breathe independently or call for help.
- Treat the client as though awake and alert. Although unable to respond, mental function is unaffected.

#### Client and Family Teaching

- Reassure that the ability to move and communicate will return when the drug is discontinued.
- Teach the family about the effects of the drug and the reason for its use. Explain that the client can hear and understand what is going on.

---

opening previously closed alveoli, improving ventilation of underventilated alveoli, and improving ventilation-perfusion relationships.

### Airway Management

If the upper airway is obstructed or positive pressure mechanical ventilation is necessary to correct hypoxemia and hypercapnia, an endotracheal tube that extends from the mouth or nose into the trachea is inserted (Figure 36–20 ■). To maintain positive pressure ventilation, the tube is cuffed with an air-filled or foam sac just above the end of the tube. When the cuff is inflated, it obstructs the upper airway, preventing air from escaping back into the nose or mouth. Excess pressure of the cuff can cause tissue ischemia and necrosis of the trachea. To minimize this risk, high-volume, low-pressure ("floppy") cuffs are used. Tubes with low-pressure cuffs may be left in place for 3 to 4 weeks.

A tracheostomy may be performed if long-term ventilatory support is required. Although a tracheostomy is more comfortable and easier to secure in place, complications such as cuff necrosis and increased risk of infection are associated with tracheostomy as well as endotracheal intubation. Table 36–14 compares the advantages, disadvantages, and possible complications of endotracheal tubes and tracheostomy.

When the client is able to maintain effective respirations and ventilatory support is no longer required, the endotracheal tube is removed (*extubation*). Gag, cough, and swallow reflexes must be intact to prevent aspiration. After oxygenation and suctioning, the cuff is deflated and the tube removed. Humidified oxygen is provided immediately following removal. Close observation for respiratory distress is vital following extubation. Inspiratory stridor within the first 24 hours indicates laryngeal edema, which may necessitate reintubation. Sore throat and a hoarse voice are common after extubation. Oral intake is reinitiated slowly, with careful assessment of swallowing.

### Mechanical Ventilation

Mechanical ventilation is indicated when alveolar ventilation is inadequate to maintain blood oxygen and carbon dioxide levels. Specific indications for mechanical ventilation include:

- Apnea or acute ventilatory failure.
- Hypoxemia unresponsive to oxygen therapy alone.
- Increased work of breathing with progressive client fatigue.

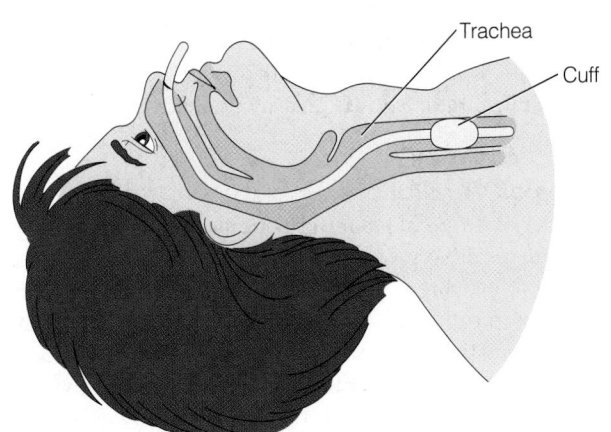

**Figure 36–20** ■ Nasal endotracheal (nasotracheal) intubation.

**TABLE 36-14    A Comparison of Endotracheal Tubes and Tracheostomy**

| | Advantages | Disadvantages | Potential Complications |
|---|---|---|---|
| Oral endotracheal tube | • More easily inserted<br>• Larger tube can be used, facilitating work of breathing, suctioning | • More difficult to secure<br>• Can be obstructed by biting<br>• Communication and mouth care more difficult<br>• Increased risk of lower respiratory infection | • Obstruction or displacement<br>• Pressure necrosis of lip<br>• Tracheoesophageal fistula |
| Nasal endotracheal tube | • More easily secured and stabilized<br>• Well tolerated by client<br>• Facilitate communication and oral hygiene | • Necessitate smaller tube which may impede removal of secretions<br>• Increased risk of lower respiratory infection | • Obstruction or displacement<br>• Pressure necrosis of nares<br>• Obstruction of sinus drainage, possible sinusitis<br>• Tracheoesphageal fistula |
| Tracheostomy | • Easily secured and stabilized<br>• Enable swallowing, speech, and oral hygiene<br>• Avoid upper airway complications | • Require surgical incision<br>• Increased risk of lower respiratory infection | • Hemorrhage due to incision or vessel erosion by tube<br>• Wound infection<br>• Subcutaneous emphysema |

Drug overdose, neural disorders, chest wall injury, and airway problems such as severe asthma or COPD can lead to acute ventilatory failure. Disorders that affect alveolar-capillary diffusion, such as pulmonary contusion, pneumonia, and ARDS, may necessitate mechanical ventilation to attain adequate oxygenation. Positive pressure ventilation increases lung volume, helps redistribute fluid from the alveolar to the interstitial space, and helps reduce the oxygen demand caused by increased work of breathing in many conditions leading to respiratory failure.

## Types of Ventilators

Two broad general classifications of mechanical ventilators are available. Negative-pressure ventilators create subatmospheric pressure externally to draw the chest outward and air into the lungs, mimicking spontaneous breathing. The iron lung, Curiass ventilator, and PulmoWrap are examples of negative-pressure ventilators (Figure 36–21 ■).

Positive-pressure ventilators are more commonly used, especially in treating acute respiratory failure (Figure 36–22 ■). These ventilators push air into the lungs, rather than drawing it in like negative-pressure ventilators. An endotracheal tube or tracheostomy is necessary for positive-pressure ventilation.

Several variables are used to trigger, cycle, and limit airflow with positive-pressure ventilators. The *trigger* prompts the ventilator to deliver a breath. The client's inspiratory effort triggers *ventilator-assisted breaths*. *Ventilator-controlled breaths* usually are triggered by a preset time interval (e.g., a breath is delivered every 5 seconds for a rate of 12 breaths per minute). The ventilator *cycle,* or duration of inspiration, can be limited by volume, pressure, flow, or time. *Volume-cycled ventilators* deliver air until a preset volume is delivered. *Pressure-cycled ventilators* cycle off when a preset pressure is achieved within the airways. *Flow-cycled ventilators* are cycled by a preset inspiratory flow rate, and *time-cycled ventila-*

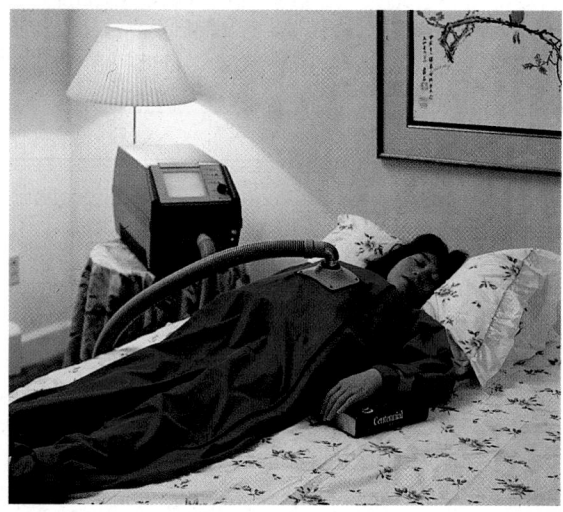

**Figure 36–21 ■** A negative-pressure ventilator.

*Courtesy of Life Care Corporation.*

*tors* deliver air for a set time interval. Airflow delivered by the ventilator also can be limited by factors such as airway pressure (e.g., a volume-cycled ventilator can be set to immediately stop inspiratory flow if airway pressure exceeds a preset value).

## Modes of Ventilation

A number of different *modes* or patterns of ventilation may be used with positive-pressure ventilators. Assist-control mode ventilation, synchronized intermittent mandatory ventilation, continuous positive airway pressure, positive end-expiratory pressure, pressure support ventilation, and pressure-control ventilation are common modes of ventilation in use today (Table 36–15).

*Assist-control mode ventilation (ACMV)* is frequently used to initiate mechanical ventilation and when the client is at risk

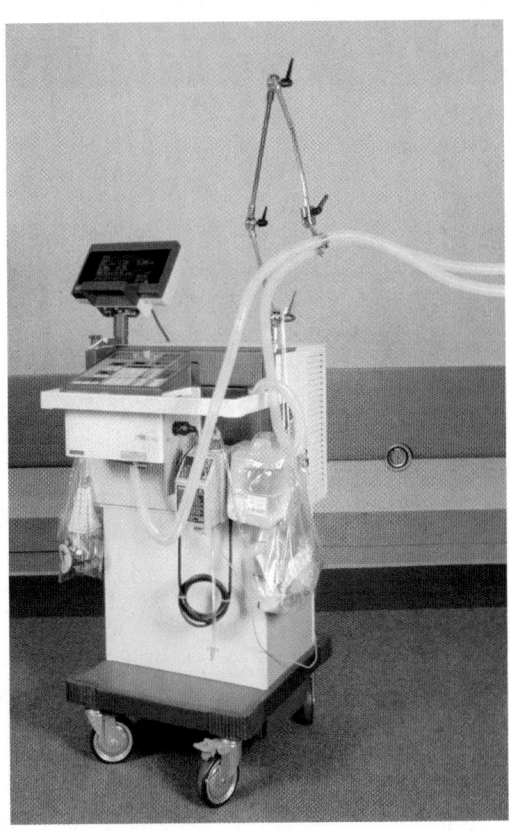
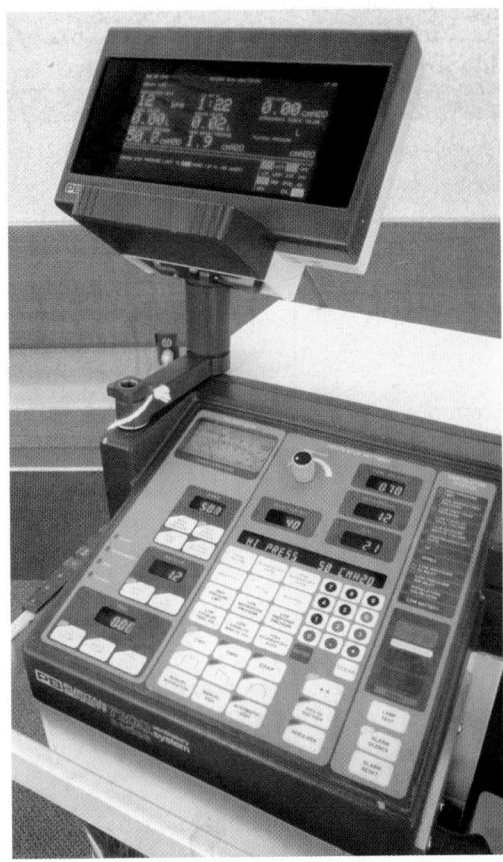

**Figure 36–22** ■ A positive-pressure ventilator and the control panel used to set the mode, rate, limits, and percentage of oxygen delivered.

for respiratory arrest (e.g., overdose or head injury). Assisted breaths are triggered by inspiratory effort; however, if the respiratory rate falls below a preset number (e.g., 14 per minute), ventilator-controlled breaths are delivered. All breaths, assisted and controlled, are delivered at a specific tidal volume or pressure and inspiratory flow rate.

*Synchronized intermittent mandatory ventilation (SIMV)* allows the client to breathe spontaneously, without ventilator assistance, between delivered ventilator breaths. Mandatory or ventilator-controlled breaths are delivered at a preset rate, volume, and/or pressure, coordinated with the client's inspiratory efforts. This mode of ventilation is used to support ventilation, to exercise respiratory muscles between ventilator-assisted breaths and during the weaning process (Braunwald et al., 2001).

*Continuous positive airway pressure (CPAP)* applies positive pressure to the airways of a spontaneously breathing client. CPAP may be used with either endotracheal intubation or a tight-fitting face mask. All breathing is spontaneous (client triggered) and pressure controlled. CPAP is used to help maintain open airways and alveoli, decreasing the work of breathing.

*Positive end-expiratory pressure (PEEP)* requires intubation and can be applied to any of the previously described ventilator modes. With PEEP, a positive pressure is maintained in the airways during exhalation and between breaths. Keeping alveoli open between breaths improves ventilation-perfusion relationships and diffusion across the alveolar-capillary membrane. This reduces hypoxemia and allows use of lower percentages of inspired oxygen. PEEP is particularly useful for treating ARDS.

In *pressure support ventilation (PSV)*, ventilator-assisted breaths are delivered when the client initiates an inspiratory effort. The cycle is flow limited; inspiration is terminated when inspiratory airflow falls below a preset rate. This mode decreases the work of breathing. It can be used in combination with SIMV when the respiratory drive is depressed. Ventilatory support can be gradually withdrawn during weaning.

*Pressure-control ventilation (PCV)*, in contrast, controls pressure within the airways to reduce the risk of airway trauma (e.g., following thoracic surgery). Ventilation is time triggered and time cycled, but pressure is limited. The ventilator maintains a preset airway pressure throughout inspiration. Because all breaths are controlled by the ventilator, heavy sedation may be required to prevent competition between inspiratory effort and ventilator control.

*Noninvasive ventilation (NIV)* provides ventilator support using a tight-fitting facemask, thus avoiding intubation. Its primary use is to support clients with impending respiratory failure (e.g., advanced COPD). The degree of success varies, primarily limited to client intolerance due to the physical and psychologic discomfort of wearing a mask when dyspneic (Braunwald et al., 2001).

## TABLE 36–15   Modes of Positive-Pressure Ventilator Operation

| Mode | Description | Pattern |
|------|-------------|---------|
| Spontaneous breathing | Client has full control of rate, tidal volume, pressures. | |
| Assist-control mode ventilation (ACMV) | Client can trigger ventilator to deliver breaths at preset volume or pressure and inspiratory flow rate; breaths will be delivered at preset rate if client does not initiate. | |
| Synchronized intermittent mandatory ventilation (SIMV) | Mandatory breaths delivered by ventilator are synchronized with client's inspiratory effort. | |
| Continuous positive airway pressure (CPAP) | Positive pressure is maintained in airways; all breaths are spontaneous. | |
| Positive end-expiratory pressure (PEEP) | Used in conjunction with other ventilator modes; positive airway pressure is maintained throughout respiratory cycle. | |
| Pressure support ventilation (PSV) | Pressurized inspiratory flow supports the client's inspiratory effort, decreasing the work of breathing. | |

## TABLE 36-16  Ventilator Settings

| Parameter | Description |
|---|---|
| Rate (f) | Number of ventilator-delivered breaths per minute: usually 12 to 15 in adults using ACMV, may be lower in SIMV |
| Tidal volume ($V_t$) | Amount of gas delivered with each ventilator breath: usually 8 to 10 mL/kg of body weight |
| Oxygen concentration ($FIO_2$) | Percentage of oxygen delivered with ventilator breaths: can be set between 21% (room air) and 100% |
| I:E ratio | Duration of inspiration to expiration: usually 1:2 to 1:1.5 |
| Flow rate | Speed at which air is delivered |
| Sensitivity | Effort required by client to initiate a ventilator-assisted breath |
| Pressure limit | Maximal pressure within airways that will terminate a ventilator breath |

## Ventilator Settings

In addition to choosing the mode of ventilation, other parameters are set to meet individual client needs when positive-pressure ventilation is used (Table 36–16).

For most adult clients, the rate is initially set between 12 and 15 breaths per minute. With ACMV or SIMV, the client's respiratory rate often is higher than the ventilator setting due to spontaneous breathing. Exhaled carbon dioxide ($ETCO_2$) or the $PCO_2$ may be used to determine the rate. A $PCO_2$ less than 38 mmHg indicates hyperventilation and respiratory alkalosis; the set rate is reduced. A $PCO_2$ above 42 mmHg or an $ETCO_2$ greater than 45 mmHg indicates hypoventilation and a need to increase the rate.

The tidal volume setting controls the amount of gas delivered with each ventilator breath. The normal adult tidal volume at rest is about 7 mL/kg of body weight, or 400 to 550 mL. The tidal volume delivered by mechanical ventilation is slightly higher (500 to 750 mL) to compensate for tubing dead space. Higher tidal volumes can cause lung tissue trauma.

The percentage of oxygen delivered with ventilator breaths is adjusted to maintain the oxygen saturation and $PO_2$ within acceptable ranges. Because prolonged delivery of high oxygen concentrations increases the risk of oxygen toxicity and pulmonary fibrosis, the $FIO_2$ is set at the lowest possible level for adequate tissue oxygenation. For most clients, the goal is to maintain an oxygen saturation greater than 90%. Lower levels may be appropriate for clients with long-standing COPD.

## Complications

Although endotracheal intubation and mechanical ventilation can be life-saving in respiratory failure, they are not without risk. Improper endotracheal tube placement or advancement of the tube into a mainstem bronchus can result in ventilation of one lung only. The inflated lung becomes overdistended and traumatized, and the uninflated lung develops atalectasis.

**NOSOCOMIAL PNEUMONIA.**  Infection is a significant risk associated with intubation and mechanical ventilation. Normal upper respiratory tract defense mechanisms are bypassed, with loss of air humidification and trapping of pathogens. Oral secretions and gastric contents can enter the respiratory tree through the open epiglottis. Often the cough reflex is inhibited or impaired by the underlying disease process and the continued presence of the endotracheal tube. Even when strict asepsis is used for suctioning and other respiratory procedures, the lower airways are contaminated within 24 hours of intubation (Urden et al., 2002). Secretions often become thick and tenacious, increasing the risk of atelectasis.

**BAROTRAUMA.**  *Barotrauma* (also called *volutrauma*) is lung injury due to alveolar overdistention. Both the volume of delivered gas and the pressures under which it is delivered can contribute to barotraumas. As a result, overdistended alveoli rupture, allowing air to escape into the pulmonary interstitial spaces and the mediastinum, pleural space, and other tissues. Subcutaneous emphysema, pneumothorax, and pneumomediastinum are possible results of barotrauma. *Subcutaneous emphysema,* or air in the subcutaneous tissue, causes tissue swelling of the chest, neck, and face. A "crackling" or air-bubble-popping sensation is felt on palpation of subcutaneous emphysema. Swelling may be massive. Once the cause is corrected, the air is gradually reabsorbed.

*Pneumothorax* is identified by signs of unequal chest expansion, a sudden loss or significant decrease in breath sounds on the affected side, and a hyperresonant percussion tone. Rapid chest tube insertion is necessary to prevent tension pneumothorax and cardiovascular compromise. *Pneumomediastinum* is the presence of air in the mediastinum, the space between the lungs that contains the heart, great vessels, trachea, and esophagus. Air in the mediastinal space can interfere with the function of all these organs and lead to such complications as pneumopericardium (air in the pericardial sac). Pneumomediastinum may have few manifestations, but the chest X-ray shows widening of the mediastinal space.

**CARDIOVASCULAR EFFECTS.**  Positive-pressure ventilation increases intrathoracic pressure, which can interfere with venous return to the heart and ventricular filling. As a result, cardiac output falls. Use of PEEP increases the effects of mechanical ventilation on cardiac output. The decreased cardiac output can affect liver and kidney function secondarily.

**GASTROINTESTINAL EFFECTS.**  Gastrointestinal complications are commonly associated with prolonged mechanical ventilation. Stress ulcers (erosive gastritis) may develop, leading to painless gastrointestinal hemorrhage. Histamine $H_2$-receptor blockers or sucralfate are often used to prevent stress ulcers. Air leaks around the endotracheal tube can cause gastric distention; a nasogastric tube often is inserted to prevent vomiting. Sedation and other medications used during mechanical ventilation can slow intestinal motility, leading to constipation.

### Weaning

The process of removing ventilator support and reestablishing spontaneous, independent respirations is called **weaning.** Weaning begins only after the underlying process causing respiratory failure has been corrected or stabilized. The process and time required for weaning depend on factors such as pre-existing lung condition, duration of mechanical ventilation, and the client's general condition, both physical and psychologic. In all cases, the vital signs, respiratory rate, extent of dyspnea, blood gases, and clinical status are used to evaluate weaning and its progress.

Following a brief period of mechanical ventilation, T-piece or CPAP may be used for weaning. In T-piece weaning, the ventilator is removed for brief periods during which oxygen is delivered using a T-piece (Figure 36–23 ■). The duration of periods off the ventilator is gradually increased until the client can maintain adequate independent respirations for several hours. Vital signs, oxygen saturation, $ETCO_2$, and $PO_2$ are carefully monitored during the process. When mechanical ventilation is no longer needed, the endotracheal tube is removed. CPAP weaning follows a similar process, with trials of spontaneous breathing supported by the ventilator in CPAP mode.

SIMV and PSV are used for weaning when the duration of mechanical ventilation has been longer and reconditioning of respiratory muscles is needed. When SIMV is used, the number of mandatory ventilator-assisted breaths is gradually decreased as ABGs, $ETCO_2$, and the respiratory rate are monitored. When the client is able to tolerate SIMV at 4 breaths per minute without rest periods of greater ventilatory support, CPAP or T-piece weaning is attempted prior to extubation (Braunwald et al., 2001).

Weaning is the primary use for pressure-support ventilation (PSV). Initially, PSV is set slightly below peak inspiratory pressures required during volume-cycled ventilation. Pressure support levels are gradually decreased, often in a cyclic pattern of periods of minimal support alternating with higher support to recondition respiratory muscles. When the PSV level is just enough to overcome endotracheal tube resistance, support is discontinued and the client is extubated (Braunwald et al., 2001).

***TERMINAL WEANING.*** When an illness is terminal or irreversible with a poor prognosis, terminal weaning may be requested by the client or family. *Terminal weaning* is the gradual withdrawal of mechanical ventilation when survival without assisted ventilation is not expected. Unlike weaning when recovery is expected which usually occurs in an intensive care unit (ICU), the client is moved to a quiet medical-surgical or hospice room or even home prior to initiating terminal weaning. Family members are encouraged to remain with the client throughout the process. If possible, decisions about sedation and analgesia prior to and during weaning are made with the client, as are decisions about hydration and nutritional support following weaning. Ventilator support is gradually withdrawn using the same modes described earlier (SIMV, PSV). Analgesia and sedation are given to promote comfort during weaning.

### Other Treatments

Attention also must be paid to fluid and electrolyte status and adequate nutrition. Mechanical ventilation promotes sodium and water retention due to its effects on cardiac output. Renal perfusion is decreased, stimulating the renin-angiotensin-aldosterone system to retain sodium and water. A Swan-Ganz catheter is often inserted to monitor pulmonary artery pressures and cardiac output. An arterial line allows repeated blood gas analysis and continuous arterial pressure monitoring. Serum electrolytes are drawn frequently, and intake, output, and daily weight are carefully monitored.

Enteral or pareteral nutrition are provided during mechanical ventilation, because the endotracheal tube prohibits eating. A nasogastric, gastrostomy, or jejunostomy feeding tube is placed for enteral nutrition. A jejunostomy tube may be used to reduce the risk of regurgitation and aspiration.

## NURSING CARE

### Health Promotion

Education is a primary strategy to prevent respiratory failure. Teach all clients and the public about the risks of smoking, water safety, the value of a working smoke detector, and measures to prevent smoke inhalation in a fire. Discuss the importance of pneumococcal vaccine and annual influenza immunizations for people who are at high risk, including those over age 65 and people with chronic diseases. Teach clients with COPD about measures to reduce their risk of respiratory infection and symptoms to report to the physician.

### Assessment

Focused assessment data related to respiratory failure includes the following:

- Health history: current manifestations, their duration, and identified precipitating factors (may need to be obtained from family members if mental status is affected); history of

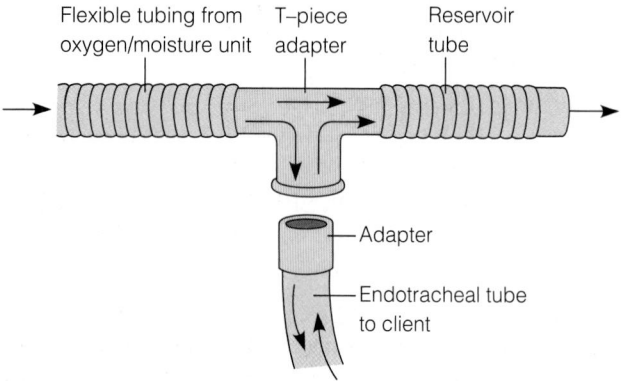

**Figure 36–23** ■ A T-piece, or "blow-by" unit, for weaning from mechanical ventilation.

previous episodes; chronic diseases such as COPD, occupational lung disease; current medications
- Physical examination: level of consciousness, mental status; vital signs; color and oxygen saturation; respiratory assessment including rate and depth, use of accessory muscles, respiratory excursion, auscultation; cardiovascular assessment including heart rate and sounds, neck vein distention, peripheral pulses, evidence of clubbing

## Nursing Diagnoses and Interventions

Clients in respiratory failure are often unstable and critically ill. They require both intensive medical care and intensive nursing care. Priority nursing needs relate to maintaining ventilation and a patent airway. Perhaps less obvious, but no less critical, nursing care needs relate to preventing injury and managing anxiety.

### Impaired Spontaneous Ventilation

In acute respiratory failure, fatigue from the work of breathing may impair the ability to maintain adequate ventilation. This is a concern both prior to initiation of mechanical ventilation and during the weaning process. See the box below.

- Assess and document respiratory rate, vital signs, and oxygen saturation every 15 to 30 minutes. *Close monitoring is vital to detect early signs of increasing respiratory distress and inability to sustain adequate breathing.*

**PRACTICE ALERT** *Promptly report signs of respiratory distress, including tachypnea, tachycardia, nasal flaring, use of accessory muscles, intercostal retractions, cyanosis, increasing restlessness, anxiety, or decreased level of consciousness. These may be early manifestations of respiratory failure and inability to maintain ventilatory effort.* ∎

- Promptly report worsening arterial blood gases and oxygen saturation levels. *Close assessment of these values allows timely intervention as needed.*
- Administer oxygen as ordered, monitoring response. Observe closely for respiratory depression, especially in the client with COPD. *Oxygen administration reduces the hypoxemic respiratory drive. Chronically high $PCO_2$ levels depress the respiratory center; hypoxemia may provide the only respiratory drive.*
- Place in Fowler's or high-Fowler's position. *Sitting positions decrease pressure on the diaphragm and chest, improving lung ventilation and decreasing the work of breathing.*
- Minimize activities and energy expenditures by assisting with ADLs, spacing procedures and activities, and allowing uninterrupted rest periods. *Rest is vital to reduce oxygen and energy demands.*

**PRACTICE ALERT** *Avoid sedatives and respiratory depressant drugs unless mechanically ventilated. These medications can further depress the respiratory drive, worsening respiratory failure.* ∎

## Nursing Research

### Evidence-Based Practice for the Client on Long-Term Mechanical Ventilation

Problems associated with long-term mechanical ventilation can further impair the client's ability to be weaned from ventilator support. These problems include symptom control, nutrition, psychologic and emotional problems, and sleep-rest deprivation. Fatigue, a psychologic and physiologic response to physical, situational, and psychologic stress, often is overlooked as a factor during weaning procedures. The client has had to relinquish control of his or her body and environment. Exposure to environmental, drug-related, mental, and emotional stressors is constant, and nutritional, sleep-rest, and activity patterns are altered for days or weeks. Technology impairs human interactions and increases vulnerability to energy depletion.

Higgins (1998) studied fatigue, nutrition, depression, and sleep-rest in a group of clients who were mechanically ventilated for at least 7 days. None of the clients had been ventilator dependent before hospital admission. They ranged in age from 24 to 79 years; 65% of the subjects had a primary diagnosis of acute respiratory failure on admission to critical care. Interestingly, five subjects declined to participate in the study because of fatigue. Descriptive and laboratory data obtained from the medical record and a questionnaire were used to measure the perception of fatigue, depression, and sleep-rest. All study participants perceived themselves as fatigued, with 45% reporting severe fatigue. Although all subjects were followed by a dietitian and received enteral nutrition, serum albumin levels fell during hospitalization. Moderate depression was noted on a standardized depression tool.

#### IMPLICATIONS FOR NURSING

The data obtained in this study suggest that clients on long-term ventilator support are malnourished, and experience fatigue, depression, and disturbed sleep-rest. Nurses need to monitor nutritional status, and actively collaborate with the physician and dietitian to maintain adequate nutrition. Fatigue and related manifestations indicate a need for energy-conserving nursing interventions. Sleep is fragmented. Consideration should be given to moving clients on long-term ventilation to an intermediate care or step-down unit as soon as possible to provide for privacy and social interaction with family and to reduce noxious environmental stimuli.

#### Critical Thinking in Client Care

1. Serum albumin and hemoglobin levels were used to evaluate the subjects' nutritional status. What other measures could be used to assess client nutrition?
2. Identify possible behavioral indicators of depression in the client who is intubated and on mechanical ventilation. What nursing measures would be appropriate related to depression in the critically ill client?
3. Develop a nursing care plan to improve the quality and duration of sleep for a client who is intubated and on mechanical ventilation.

- Prepare for endotracheal intubation and mechanical ventilation:
  a. Obtain an intubation tray with a selection of sterile endotracheal tubes and laryngoscope with a variety of adult blades.
  b. Check laryngoscope lamp; replace battery pack or bulb as needed.
  c. Set up for endotracheal suction, bringing continuous suction head, container, tubing, sterile catheter and glove kits, and sterile normal saline to the bedside.
  d. Notify respiratory therapy to set up the ventilator.
  e. Notify radiology that a portable chest X-ray will be needed on completion of intubation to verify correct placement of the endotracheal tube.

  *Intubation and mechanical ventilation may be required to maintain ventilation and gas exchange.*

- Explain the procedure and its purpose to the client and family, providing reassurance that this is a temporary measure to reduce the work of breathing and allow rest. Alert that talking is not possible while the endotracheal tube is in place, and establish a means of communication. *Thorough explanation is important to relieve anxiety.*

## Ineffective Airway Clearance

Ineffective airway clearance may either cause respiratory failure or occur as a result of interventions. Impaired ventilation frequently leads to acute respiratory failure, particularly in clients with COPD or asthma. Chest trauma also can impair airway patency as a result of pulmonary contusion and ineffective cough. Although intubation and mechanical ventilation can be life-saving measures, they also increase the risk of respiratory infection and ineffective secretion management.

**PRACTICE ALERT** *Frequently assess respiratory rate, chest movement, lung sounds, oxygen saturation, $ETco_2$, and ABGs. Intubation and mechanical ventilation do not ensure adequate oxygenation and ventilation. Displacement of the endotracheal tube or obstruction by respiratory secretions impair ventilation.* ■

- Suction as needed to maintain a patent airway. Indicators for suctioning include crackles and rhonchi on auscultation, frequent coughing or setting off the high-pressure alarm, and increasing restlessness or anxiety. Procedure 36–2 outlines endotracheal suctioning. *Although clients with a tracheostomy can usually cough up secretions, the length and diameter of endotracheal tubes makes this extremely difficult. Even with humidification, secretions often become thick and tenacious, further inhibiting their removal.*
- Obtain sputum for culture if it appears purulent or is odorous. *Culture is necessary to identify pathogens and guide antibiotic therapy.*
- Perform percussion, vibration, and postural drainage as ordered. *These techniques help loosen secretions and move them into larger airways for removal by coughing or suctioning.*

**PRACTICE ALERT** *Evaluate endotracheal tube cuff pressure by measurement (should have no more than 20 to 25 mmHg of pressure) or by auscultating the suprasternal notch for a hissing sound at the end of inspiration. The minimum effective cuff pressure to maintain alveolar ventilation is used to reduce the risk of tracheal ischemia and necrosis.* ■

- Firmly secure endotracheal or tracheostomy tube. Provide adequate slack on ventilator tubing to prevent tension on the tube when turning, positioning, or transferring to chair or stretcher. If necessary, loosely restrain hands. *These measures are important to ensure proper airway placement and prevent its inadvertent removal.*
- Assess fluid balance and maintain adequate hydration. *Adequate hydration helps liquefy secretions.*

## Risk for Injury

Many factors increase the risk for injury in acute respiratory failure. Hypoxemia and hypercapnia affect the level of consciousness and may impair mental status. Endotracheal intubation and mechanical ventilation carry risks of tracheal damage and trauma to the lungs. Neuromuscular blockade, if used, presents a significant risk for injury as the client is unable to breathe spontaneously, communicate, and move.

- Assess frequently, noting the following:
  a. Level of consciousness, orientation, and awareness
  b. Condition of mucosa of mouth and nose
  c. Respiratory: lung sounds, chest excursion, and ventilator pressures
  d. Cardiovascular: vital signs, skin color, capillary refill, and peripheral pulses
  e. Gastrointestinal: bowel sounds; test gastric secretions and feces for occult blood
  f. Genitourinary: urine output, daily weight
  g. Skin and extremities

  *Complications associated with respiratory failure and mechanical ventilation can affect many body systems. Frequent assessment allows early detection and intervention.*

**PRACTICE ALERT** *Do not bypass or turn off any ventilator alarms. The intubated client is unable to communicate verbally and cannot call for help. If neuromuscular blockers are used, the client is also unable to breathe without ventilator support.* ■

- Report condition changes such as increasing air leak around the cuff and decreased breath sounds or chest movement. *These may be manifestations of a complication of intubation and ventilation, such as tracheal necrosis, displacement of the endotracheal tube into the right mainstem bronchus, pneumothorax, or atelectasis.*
- Turn and reposition frequently, taking care to stabilize endotracheal tube during movement. *Repositioning helps maintain tissue perfusion and prevent skin and tissue breakdown.*
- Keep skin and linens clean, dry, and wrinkle-free. Protect pressure areas with padding, eggcrate, or heal and elbow protectors. *The client may not be able to perceive and report*

## Procedure 36–2  Endotracheal Suctioning

### SUPPLIES

- Suction unit with connecting tubing and connector at the bedside
- If an in-line suction catheter is not present
  a. Sterile suction catheter (size 12 to 16 Fr) and glove-kit or suction catheter and sleeve
  b. Sterile normal saline
- Personal protective devices as indicated: goggles, mask, gown

### PREPROCEDURE

Explain the procedure and why it is being done. Tell the client that although suctioning is not painful, it is uncomfortable. While suction is being applied, breathing is difficult but these periods last only 10 seconds. Stress that suctioning allows removal of secretions and stimulates coughing, which helps clear secretions from smaller airways. Establish a means of communicating; for example, tell the client to raise a finger or rapidly blink if unable to tolerate suctioning.

### PROCEDURE

1. Use standard precautions.
2. Prepare the suction unit by turning it on and regulating it to no more than −80 to −120 mmHg.
3. Open sterile saline bottle, leaving the cap loosely in place.

#### WITH AN IN-LINE CATHETER

- Wearing exam gloves, attach the catheter to suction tubing.
- Adjust the oxygen (FiO$_2$) to 100%; allow three breaths.

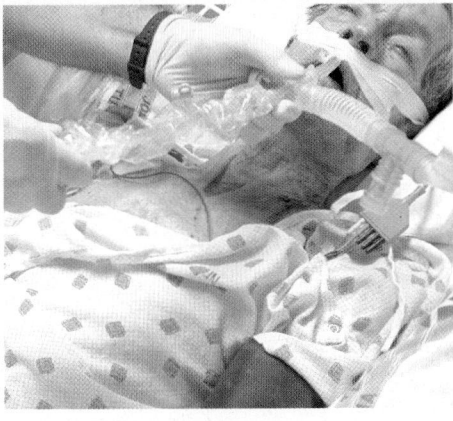

- Manipulating the catheter through the plastic shield (to maintain its sterility), insert the catheter without applying suction until resistance is met; apply suction while slowly withdrawing the catheter with a twirling motion (see figure)
- Suction for no longer than 10 seconds (count the seconds or watch the clock—the time passes more quickly than you think), then allow to rest for three to five breaths. Repeat the procedure as needed for a total of no more than three times.
- Remove suction tubing from the catheter, clear the tubing, turn off suction, and remove and discard gloves.

#### WITH A SEPARATE CATHETER-AND-GLOVE KIT

- Open suction catheter/glove kit. Remove saline cup, and fill with sterile normal saline.
- Put on sterile gloves, and attach catheter to suction tubing, keeping dominant hand sterile; lubricate catheter tip with sterile saline.

- Use the nondominant hand to adjust oxygen (FiO$_2$) to 100%; allow three breaths.
- Using the nondominant hand, disconnect ventilator tubing from the endotracheal tube. Manipulating the suction catheter with the dominant (sterile) hand and the suction control valve with the non-dominant (nonsterile) hand, insert the catheter, without applying suction until resistance is met. Then, apply suction while slowly withdrawing the catheter, using a twirling motion.
- Suction for no longer than 10 seconds. Reconnect the ventilator, and allow to rest for three to five breaths; clear suction tubing with sterile saline.
- Repeat the above two steps as needed for a total of three times.
- Reconnect ventilator tubing to the endotracheal tube.
- Clear suction tubing, turn off suction, and remove the catheter, discarding it with the gloves.
4. Provide three additional breaths at 100% oxygen, then readjust to the previous ordered level.
5. Note color, quantity, consistency, and odor of sputum.
6. Assess lung sounds and tolerance of the procedure.
7. Wash hands.

### POSTPROCEDURE

Document assessment before and after suctioning, along with the character of the sputum and the client's tolerance of the procedure. Report changes in sputum character, such as purulence or an odor that may indicate infection.

---

*pain, and move voluntarily to reduce pressure, necessitating excellent skin care.*
- Perform passive ROM exercises every 4 to 8 hours. *These exercises maintain joint flexibility and help prevent contractures associated with long-term immobility.*
- Keep side rails up and use soft restraints as needed. *These safety measures are important to prevent falls, inadvertent disconnection of the ventilator, or dislodging of the endotracheal tube.*
- Administer histamine H$_2$-blockers and sucralfate as ordered. *Stress gastritis and possible gastrointestinal hemorrhage are common, preventable complications of mechanical ventilation.*

### Anxiety

Critical illness creates anxiety for any client. In acute respiratory failure, this anxiety is compounded by the presence of an endotracheal tube or tracheostomy, mechanical ventilator, numerous monitors and equipment, and, potentially, neuromuscular blockade and paralysis of voluntary muscles. Fear of continued dependence on the mechanical ventilator and inability to return to a normal life may compound this anxiety.

**PRACTICE ALERT** *Frequently monitor anxiety level. High levels of anxiety increase oxygen use and often interfere with the ability to work with the respirator. This can increase hypoxemia and further increase anxiety; intervention is necessary to break this cycle.* ∎

- Remain with the client as much as possible. *The frequent and continuing presence of a caregiver provides reassurance that help is readily available.*
- Explain all monitors, procedures, unusual sounds, and machinery. *Understanding of the environment and various sounds and alarms reduces anxiety.*
- Provide a simple means of communication, such as a slate, picture board, or alphabet board. If neuromuscular blockade is used, use methods such as looking to the right for "yes" and left for "no." Reassure that endotracheal tube removal restores the ability to speak. *The inability to speak and call out for help is frightening for the client. Providing an alternate means of communication helps reduce anxiety.*
- Encourage frequent family visits, especially if the time of visitations is being limited. Encourage family participation in care. *Family visits help reduce anxiety and feelings of abandonment. Allowing family members to participate in care helps reduce their anxiety as well.*
- Explain to the family that the client can hear and understand. Emphasize the importance of talking to the client, not over or about the client. *The family may not understand that the client may be mentally alert although unable to respond. Talking to the client about everyday things reduces the client's sense of isolation and fear.*
- Provide distraction with radio or television if allowed. *Distraction helps reduce the focus on machines and unusual sounds of monitors and alarms.*
- Attend to physical needs promptly and completely. *This provides reassurance that needs will be met even though the client is unable to ask for assistance.*
- Reassure that intubation and mechanical ventilation is a temporary measure to allow the lungs to rest and heal. Reinforce that the client will be able to breathe independently again. *The client may fear continued dependence on mechanical ventilation.*

**PRACTICE ALERT** *Provide sedation and antianxiety medications as needed, especially when neuromuscular blockade is used. Although neuromuscular blockade paralyzes voluntary muscles, the level of consciousness is unimpaired.* ■

## Using NANDA, NIC, and NOC

Chart 36–5 shows links between NANDA nursing diagnoses, NIC, and NOC for the client with respiratory failure.

## Home Care

Prior to hospital discharge, teach the client and family about the following topics.

- Factors that precipitated respiratory failure and measures to prevent it in the future (e.g., the impact of respiratory irritants on compromised lungs)
- Measures to prevent future episodes such as remaining indoors with an air filter or air conditioning when pollution levels are high, obtaining influenza and pneumonia immunizations, and avoiding exposure to cigarette smoke
- Effective coughing and pulmonary hygiene measures such as percussion, vibration, and postural drainage

Acute respiratory failure resulting from an acute insult such as pneumonia or near-drowning often resolves with few long-term sequelae. When respiratory failure results from an underlying disease such as COPD, the prognosis is less optimistic. Clients with end-stage COPD may have repeated episodes of respiratory failure, with a gradual loss of respiratory function and reserve. These clients may choose terminal weaning rather than a future of increasing disability. Discuss what to expect during the terminal weaning process with the client and family. Discuss use of sedation prior to and during the weaning process. Explain that medications are used to reduce respiratory distress and dyspnea during weaning. Assure

## CHART 36–5 NANDA, NIC, AND NOC LINKAGES

### The Client with Respiratory Failure

| NURSING DIAGNOSES | NURSING INTERVENTIONS | NURSING OUTCOMES |
|---|---|---|
| • Impaired Spontaneous Ventilation | • Respiratory Monitoring<br>• Artificial Airway Management<br>• Mechanical Ventilation | • Respiratory Status: Gas Exchange<br>• Respiratory Status: Ventilation |
| • Dysfunctional Ventilatory Weaning Response | • Anxiety Reduction<br>• Mechanical Ventilatory Weaning<br>• Energy Management | • Anxiety Control<br>• Respiratory Status: Ventilation<br>• Energy Conservation |
| • Ineffective Airway Clearance | • Airway Suctioning<br>• Airway Insertion and Stabilization | • Respiratory Status: Airway Patency |
| • Impaired Gas Exchange | • Oxygen Therapy | • Respiratory Status: Gas Exchange |

*Note. Data from Nursing Outcomes Classification (NOC) by M. Johnson & M. Maas (Eds.), 1997, St. Louis: Mosby; Nursing Diagnoses: Definitions & Classification 2001–2002 by North American Nursing Diagnosis Association, 2001, Philadelphia: NANDA; Nursing Interventions Classification (NIC) by J.C. McCloskey & G. M. Bulechek (Eds.), 2000, St. Louis: Mosby. Reprinted by permission.*

the client and family that nursing support is continuously available during the weaning process and that family and other supporters such as clergy are allowed to remain with the client.

## THE CLIENT WITH ACUTE RESPIRATORY DISTRESS SYNDROME

**Acute respiratory distress syndrome (ARDS)** is characterized by noncardiac pulmonary edema and progressive refractory hypoxemia. First identified in 1967, ARDS has been known by various names, such as shock lung, wet lung, Vietnam lung, and adult hyaline membrane disease. It is widely recognized as a severe form of acute respiratory failure. The mortality rate associated with acute respiratory distress syndrome, while declining, remains around 50%.

Although the exact cause of ARDS is unclear, it is known that ARDS does not occur as a primary process but may follow a number of diverse conditions producing direct or indirect lung injury (see Table 36–17).

## PATHOPHYSIOLOGY

The underlying pathology in ARDS is acute lung injury resulting from an unregulated systemic inflammatory response to acute injury or inflammation. Inflammatory cellular responses and biochemical mediators damage the alveolar-capillary membrane. This damage develops rapidly, often within 90 minutes of the systemic inflammatory response and within 24 hours of the initial insult (Figure 36–24 ■). Damaged capillary membranes allow plasma and blood cells to escape into the interstitial space. Increased interstitial pressure and damage to the alveolar membrane allow fluid to enter the alveoli. Within the alveolus, the fluid dilutes and inactivates

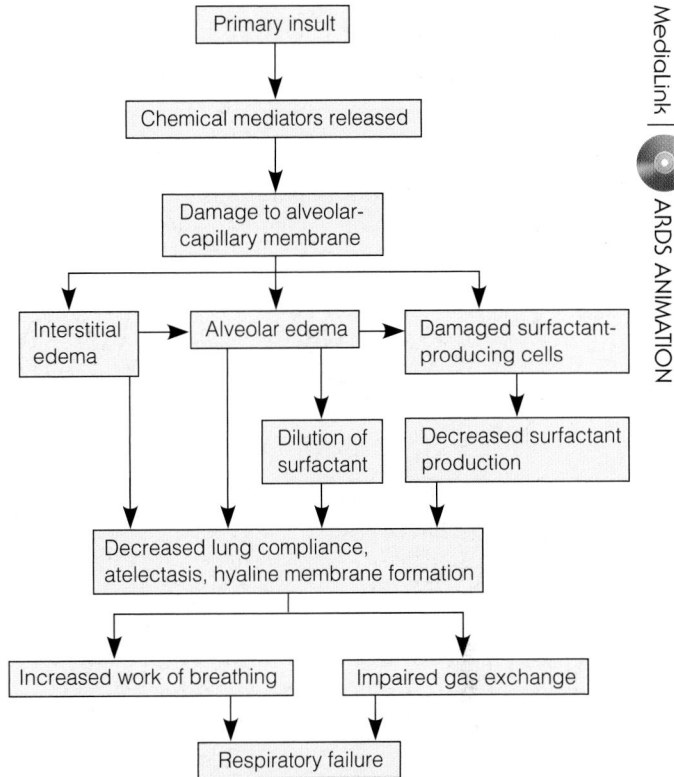

**Figure 36–24** ■ The pathogenesis of ARDS.

surfactant. Surfactant-producing cells are damaged by the inflammatory process, leading to a deficit of surfactant, increased alveolar surface tension, and alveolar collapse with atelectasis. The lungs become less compliant, and gas exchange is impaired. As the syndrome progresses, hyaline membranes form, further reducing gas exchange and compliance. Finally, fibrotic changes occur in the lungs. Intra-alveolar septa thicken, and alveolar surface area for gas exchange is reduced. Hypoxemia becomes refractory or resistant to improvement with supplemental oxygen, and the $PCO_2$ rises as diffusion is further impaired. Figure 36–24 and the *Pathophysiology Illustrated* figure on pages 1170 and 1171 illustrate the pathophysiology of ARDS.

As ARDS progresses, tissue hypoxia becomes significant, and metabolic acidosis develops. Carbon dioxide exchange is impaired as well as oxygen exchange, leading to combined respiratory and metabolic acidosis. Sepsis and multiple organ system dysfunction of the kidneys, liver, gastrointestinal tract, central nervous system, and cardiovascular system are the leading causes of death in ARDS. If the process is halted before this occurs, the long-term prognosis for recovery is good.

## MANIFESTATIONS

Initial manifestations of ARDS typically develop 24 to 48 hours after the initial insult. Dyspnea, tachypnea, and anxiety are early manifestations. Progressive respiratory distress develops, with increasing respiratory rate, intercostal retractions, and use of accessory muscles of respiration. Cyanosis develops that may not improve with oxygen administration.

| TABLE 36–17 | Conditions Associated with the Development of ARDS |
|---|---|
| **Conditions** | **Examples** |
| Shock | Hemorrhagic shock, septic shock |
| Inhalation injuries | Aspiration of gastric contents, smoke and toxic gases, near-drowning, oxygen toxicity |
| Infections | Gram-negative sepsis, viral pneumonias, *Pneumocystis cariniii* pneumonia, miliary tuberculosis |
| Drug overdose | Heroin, methadone, propoxyphene, aspirin |
| Trauma | Burns, head injury, lung contusion, fat emboli |
| Other | Disseminated intravascular coagulation (DIC), pancreatitis, uremia, amniotic fluid and air emboli, multiple transfusions, open heart surgery with cardiopulmonary bypass |

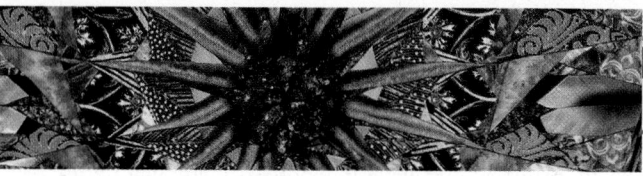

Acute respiratory distress syndrome (ARDS) is a severe form of acute respiratory failure that occurs in response to pulmonary or systemic insults. ARDS is characterized by noncardiogenic pulmonary edema caused by inflammatory damage to alveolar and capillary walls. Many disorders may precipitate ARDS, although sepsis is the most common.

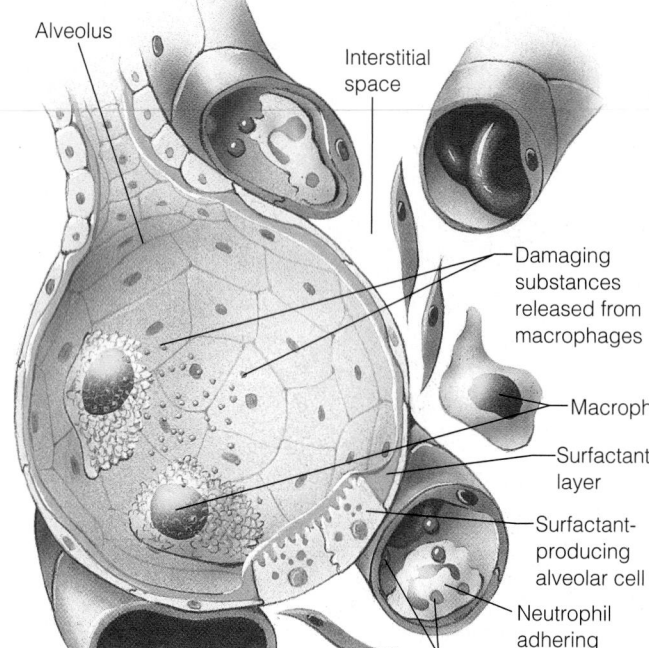

Alveolus
Interstitial space
Damaging substances released from macrophages
Macrophages
Surfactant layer
Surfactant-producing alveolar cell
Neutrophil adhering to capillary wall
Capillary
Lysosomal enzymes

### 1. Initiation of ARDS

In sepsis-induced ARDS, bacterial toxins cause macrophages and neutrophils to adhere to endothelial surfaces of the alveoli and capillaries. The macrophages release oxidants, inflammatory mediators, enzymes, and peptides that damage the capillary and alveolar walls. In response, neutrophils release lysosomal enzymes causing further damage.

### 2. Onset of Pulmonary Edema

The damaged capillary and alveolar walls become more permeable, allowing plasma, proteins, and erythrocytes to enter the interstitial space. As interstitial edema increases, pressure in the interstitial space rises and fluid leaks into alveoli. Plasma proteins accumulating in the interstitial space lower the osmotic gradient between the capillary and interstitial compartment. As a result, the balance is disrupted between the osmotic force that pulls fluid from the interstitial space into the capillaries and the normal hydrostatic pressure that pushes fluid out of the capillaries. This imbalance causes even more fluid to enter alveoli.

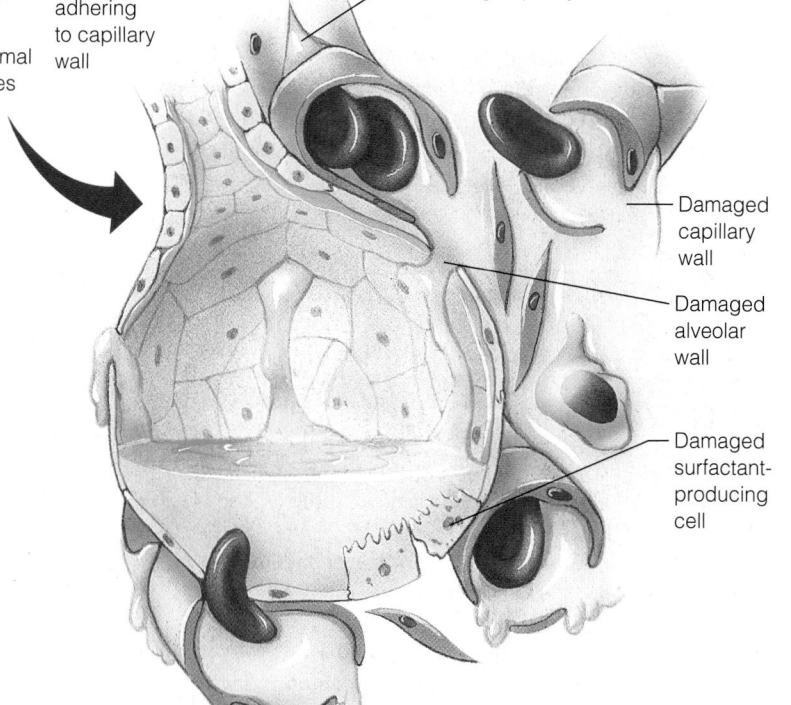

Leaking capillary wall
Damaged capillary wall
Damaged alveolar wall
Damaged surfactant-producing cell

### 4. End-Stage ARDS

Fibrin and cell debris from necrotic cells combine to form hyaline membranes, which line the interior of the alveoli and further reduce alveolar compliance and gas exchange. Because $CO_2$ cannot diffuse across hyaline membranes, $PCO_2$ levels now begin to rise while $PO_2$ levels continue to fall. Rising $PCO_2$ levels can lead to respiratory acidosis. Without respiratory support, respiratory failure will develop. Even with aggressive treatment, almost 50% of clients with ARDS die.

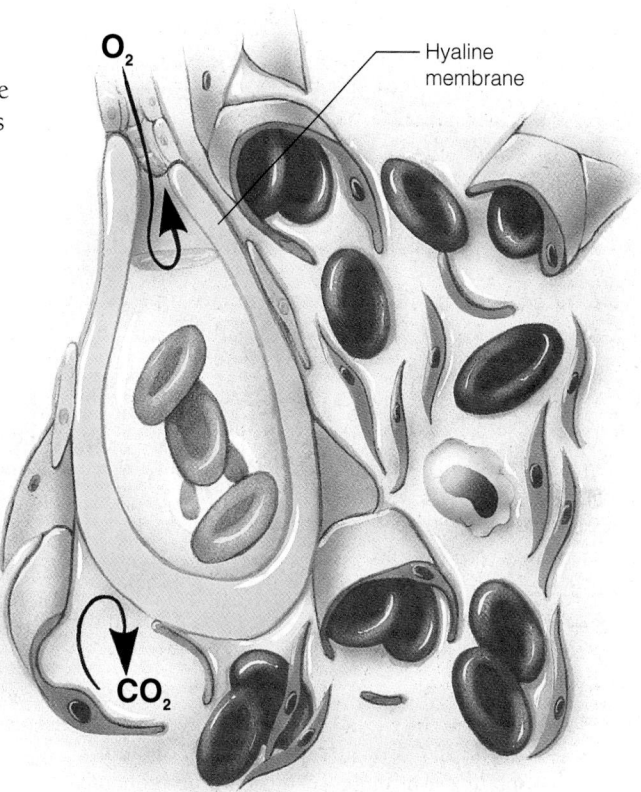

### 3. Alveolar Collapse

Protein-rich fluid accumulates in the alveoli, inactivating surfactant and damaging type II alveolar cells that produce surfactant. (Surfactant is important in maintaining alveolar compliance—the ability of tissue to stretch or distend.) As active surfactant is lost, the alveoli stiffen and collapse, leading to atelectasis, which increases breathing effort.

Decreased alveolar compliance, atelectasis, and fluid-filled alveoli interfere with gas exchange across the alveolar-capillary membrane. Blood oxygen ($PO_2$) levels fall. Because carbon dioxide diffuses more readily than oxygen, however, blood carbon dioxide ($PCO_2$) levels also fall initially as tachypnea causes more $CO_2$ to be expired.

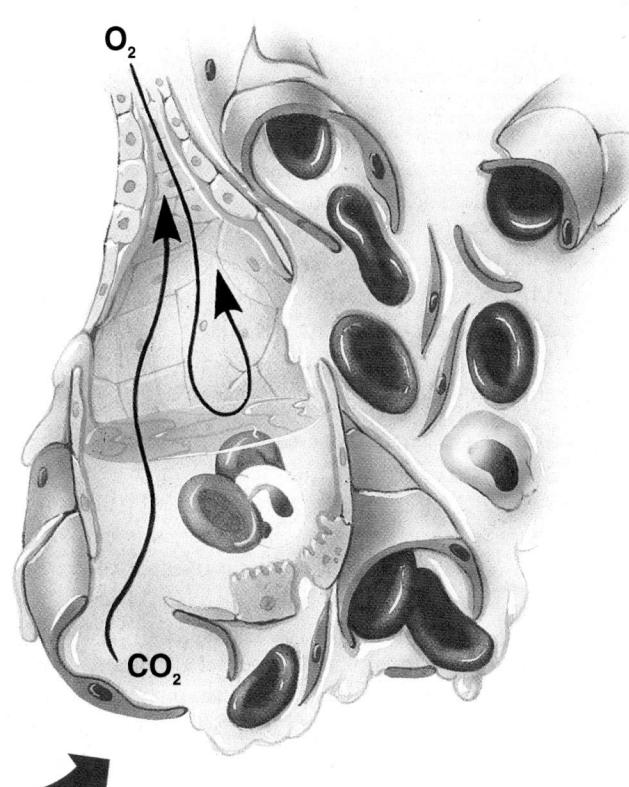

Breath sounds are initially clear, but crackles (rales) and rhonchi develop later. As respiratory failure progresses, mental status changes such as agitation, confusion, and lethargy occur.

## COLLABORATIVE CARE

ARDS management is directed toward identifying and treating its underlying cause and providing aggressive respiratory support.

### Diagnostic Tests

*Refractory hypoxemia* (hypoxemia that does not improve with oxygen administration) is the hallmark of ARDS.

- *Arterial blood gases* initially show hypoxemia with a $PO_2$ of less than 60 mmHg and respiratory alkalosis due to tachypnea.
- *Chest X-ray* changes may not be evident for as long as 24 hours after the onset of ARDS. Diffuse infiltrates are seen initially, progressing to a "white out" pattern.
- *Pulmonary function testing* shows decreased lung compliance with reduced vital capacity, minute volume, and functional vital capacity (see Box 36–1).
- *Pulmonary artery pressure monitoring* shows normal pressures in ARDS, helping distinguish ARDS from cardiogenic pulmonary edema.

### Medications

Although there is no definitive drug therapy for ARDS, a number of medications may be used. Inhaled nitric oxide reduces intrapulmonary shunting and improves oxygenation by dilating blood vessels in better-ventilated areas of the lungs. Surfactant therapy may be prescribed. Surfactant is a complex mixture of phospholipids, neutral lipids, and proteins that forms a thin layer atop a thin layer of water on the inner surface of the alveolus, reducing the surface tension within the alveoli. Surface tension tends to pull the walls of the alveoli together, increasing the likelihood of collapse during exhalation. Surfactant, by reducing surface tension, helps maintain open alveoli, decreasing the work of breathing, improving compliance and gas exchange, and preventing atelectasis.

Interventions to block the inflammatory response are under investigation, such as using nonsteroidal anti-inflammatory agents and corticosteroids. Corticosteroids may be used late in the course of ARDS to improve oxygenation and lung mechanics when fibrotic changes occur.

### Mechanical Ventilation

The mainstay of ARDS management is endotracheal intubation and mechanical ventilation. With ARDS, it is rarely possible to maintain adequate tissue oxygenation with oxygen therapy alone.

With mechanical ventilation, the $FIO_2$ is set at the lowest possible level to maintain a $PO_2$ higher than 60 mmHg and oxygen saturation of approximately 90%. When the $PO_2$ cannot be maintained with less than 50% inspired oxygen, there is a risk that oxygen toxicity will accentuate ARDS. Often it is necessary to add continuous positive airway pressure (CPAP) or positive end-expiratory pressure (PEEP) to mechanical ventilation settings to maintain blood and tissue oxygenation. Maintaining open airways and alveoli enhances gas diffusion and reduces ventilation-perfusion mismatch. PEEP decreases cardiac output and increases the risk of barotrauma, necessitating close monitoring. Either assist-control or SIMV may be used along with PEEP or CPAP in treating ARDS.

It is important to remember that mechanical ventilation does not cure ARDS; it simply supports respiratory function while the underlying problem is being identified and treated.

### Treatments

Atelectasis frequently occurs in dependent lung regions in ARDS. Prone positioning in conjunction with mechanical ventilation reduces the pressure of surrounding tissue on dependent regions and improves oxygenation.

Other management strategies include careful fluid replacement, attention to nutrition, treatment of any infection, and correction of the underlying condition. A Swan-Ganz line is placed to monitor pulmonary artery pressures and cardiac output. Fluid replacement is carefully tailored to these measurements to avoid fluid imbalances, which may worsen hypoxia and ARDS. Enteral or parenteral feeding is necessary to maintain nutritional status and prevent tissue catabolism. Infections are treated with intravenous antibiotic therapy tailored to the causative organism. Low-molecular-weight heparin may be ordered to prevent thrombophlebitis and possible pulmonary embolus or disseminated intravascular coagulation (DIC), a possible complication of ARDS.

## NURSING CARE

The nursing care needs of the client with ARDS are very similar to those of any client with acute respiratory failure. Maintaining adequate ventilation and respirations are of highest priority, along with preventing injury and managing anxiety. See the section on acute respiratory failure for nursing care related to these diagnoses. Additional high-priority nursing care concerns for the client with ARDS are related to the effects of PEEP on cardiac output and potential problems of weaning ventilatory support.

### Decreased Cardiac Output

With positive pressure ventilation, increased intrathoracic pressure decreases cardiac output. When PEEP is applied, intrathoracic pressure increases further; this can significantly decrease venous return, ventricular filling, stroke volume, and cardiac output. Manifestations of decreased cardiac output include hypotension and compensatory tachycardia as the heart attempts to maintain cardiac output despite decreased stoke volume. In the client who is already hypoxic because of ARDS, this drop in cardiac output can increase tissue damage. Urine output falls, and dysrhythmias may develop.

- Monitor and record vital signs, including apical pulse, at least every 2 hours; more frequently immediately following initiation of mechanical ventilation or addition of PEEP. *Frequent assessment is vital to detect early signs of decreased cardiac output.*

> **PRACTICE ALERT** *Record urine output hourly. Because a significant portion of the cardiac output goes directly to the kidneys, a fall in urine output to less than 30 mL per hour is often the first sign of decreased cardiac output.* ■

- Assess level of consciousness at least every 4 hours. *Altered level of consciousness, confusion, and restlessness are early signs of cerebral hypoxia due to decreased cardiac output.*
- Monitor pulmonary artery pressures, central venous pressure, and cardiac output readings every 1 to 4 hours. *Changes in these measurements may indicate worsening cardiac status.*
- Assess heart and lung sounds frequently. *Increasing crackles or abnormal heart sounds may indicate heart failure.*
- Weigh daily at the same time. *Accurate daily weights are the best indicator of fluid volume status.*
- Frequently provide good skin care, keeping skin clean and dry and protecting pressure points. *Tissue hypoxia increases the risk of skin breakdown, which in turn increases the risk of infection and sepsis.*
- Maintain intravenous fluids as ordered. *Intravenous fluids are given to maintain vascular volume and prevent dehydration.*
- Administer analgesics, sedatives, and neuromuscular blockers as needed. *These medications may be prescribed to decrease cardiac workload.*

### Dysfunctional Ventilatory Weaning Response

The client with dysfunctional ventilatory weaning response has difficulty adjusting to reduced mechanical ventilator support, prolonging the weaning process. Airway congestion, inadequate rest or nutrition, pain, anxiety, and a nonsupportive environment are factors that can contribute to difficulty weaning. With ARDS, the pathologic processes of the disease and its effects on gas exchange may be responsible for a prolonged or ineffective weaning process.

Assessment findings indicative of dysfunctional weaning include:

- Dyspnea, apprehension, or agitation.
- Decreasing oxygen saturation level.
- Cyanosis or pallor, diaphoresis.
- Increased blood pressure, pulse, and respiratory rate.
- Diminished or adventitious breath sounds, use of accessory muscles.
- Decreased level of consciousness.
- Deteriorating arterial blood gas values.
- Shallow, gasping breaths or paradoxic abdominal breathing.

Nursing interventions for dysfunctional weaning include the following:

- Assess vital signs every 15 to 30 minutes following changes in ventilator settings and during T-piece trials. *Vital signs, heart and respiratory rates in particular, can provide early signs of hypoxemia and poor tolerance of the weaning process.*

> **PRACTICE ALERT** *Frequently monitor oxygen saturation, $ET_{CO_2}$, and arterial blood gases following changes in ventilator settings. These values are used to assess the adequacy of ventilation and gas exchange during the weaning process.* ■

- Place in Fowler's or high-Fowler's position. *Fowler's position facilitates lung expansion and reduces the work of breathing.*
- Fully explain all weaning procedures, along with expected changes in breathing. *Adequate explanations help reduce anxiety and improve the ability to cooperate.*
- Remain with the client during initial periods following changes of ventilator settings or T-piece trials. *This provides reassurance and allows close monitoring of the response.*
- Limit procedures and activities during weaning periods. *Reducing energy expenditures and cardiac work facilitates the weaning process.*
- Provide diversion, such as television or radio. *Diversion helps distract the focus from breathing.*
- Begin weaning procedures in the morning, when the client is well rested and alert; weaning may be discontinued overnight to provide rest. *The work of breathing increases during the weaning process; adequate rest is important.*
- When SIMV is used for weaning, decrease the SIMV rate by increments of two breaths per minute. *Slow reduction of ventilator support allows respiratory muscle reconditioning and gradual resumption of the work of breathing.*
- Avoid administering drugs that may depress respirations during the weaning process (except as ordered at night to facilitate rest when ventilator support is provided). *Sedatives or analgesics that depress respirations can impair the weaning process.*

> **PRACTICE ALERT** *Frequently assess respiratory status following weaning and extubation. Keep an intubation kit readily available following extubation; be prepared for emergency reintubation. Laryngeal spasm or laryngeal edema may develop following extubation, necessitating reintubation to maintain respirations.* ■

- Keep oxygen at the bedside following weaning and extubation. *Supplemental oxygen may be necessary to maintain adequate blood and tissue oxygenation.*
- Provide pulmonary hygiene with percussion and postural drainage. *Maintaining patent airways and adequate alveolar ventilation is vital during the weaning process.*

### Home Care

When preparing the client who has recovered from ARDS and the family for home care, discuss the following topics.

- ARDS did not result from something they did or did not do, but developed as a consequence of serious illness. Provide factual information about ARDS.
- Maximal respiratory function following ARDS is usually achieved within 6 months; respiratory function may remain significantly impaired. This may necessitate changes in occupation, lifestyle, and family roles.

- Avoiding smoking and exposure to secondhand smoke and environmental pollutants is vital to prevent further lung damage.
- Obtain immunization for pneumococcal pneumonia and annual influenza immunizations to prevent further episodes of serious respiratory disease.

Provide referrals to home health and respiratory care services as indicated, as well as for occupational therapy and counseling as needed.

## Nursing Care Plan
## A Client with ARDS

Peggy Adamson is a 36-year-old single woman admitted to the hospital following a near-drowning in a local lake. On admission to the emergency department, Ms. Adamson is alert and oriented, having been rescued and resuscitated within 2 minutes of the accident. Rescuers report that she seemed to have aspirated "a lot" of water as she was water-skiing when the accident occurred. She is admitted to the intensive care unit for observation. Oxygen is started per nasal cannula at 6 L/min, intravenous fluids are administered to correct electrolyte imbalances, and 40 mg of furosemide (Lasix) is given intravenously for hypervolemia.

### ASSESSMENT

Nadia Mucha cares for Ms. Adamson the evening of the day after her admission. Throughout her stay, Ms. Adamson has remained alert and oriented with stable vital signs. Her respiratory rate has been 20 to 24 per minute, with scattered crackles, oxygen saturations of around 94%, and a $Po_2$ of 75 to 80 mmHg on 6 L/min of oxygen. Her pulse has been 96 to 100 and regular. On her initial assessment, Ms. Mucha notes that Ms. Adamson seems apprehensive and anxious. Although her blood pressure is 116/74, unchanged from previous levels, her heart rate is up to 106 and respiratory rate is 28 per minute. Her lungs have scattered crackles but good breath sounds throughout, unchanged from previous assessments. Ms. Adamson's oxygen saturation has dropped to 84%, so Ms. Mucha orders ABGs and increases the oxygen to 8 L/min. ABG results show $Po_2$ 65 mmHg and respiratory alkalosis pH 7.48, and $Pco_2$ 32 mmHg.

Ms. Mucha orders a portable chest X-ray and notifies the physician of the arterial blood gas results and the change in Ms. Adamson's status. The physician orders a nonrebreather mask at 8 L/min and repeat ABGs in 1 hour. The chest X-ray reveals scattered infiltrates and a normal heart size.

Ms. Adamson's oxygen saturation continues to fall, and subsequent blood gases show a $Po_2$ of 55 mmHg. The attending physician diagnoses probable ARDS and orders nasotracheal intubation and mechanical ventilation.

### DIAGNOSES

- *Ineffective breathing pattern* related to anxiety
- *Impaired gas exchange* related to effects of near-drowning
- *Anxiety* related to hypoxemia
- *Risk for decreased cardiac output* related to mechanical ventilation
- *Risk for injury* related to endotracheal intubation

### EXPECTED OUTCOMES

- Breathe effectively with the mechanical ventilator.

- Demonstrate improved oxygen saturation, $ETco_2$, and ABG values.
- Express fears related to intubation and mechanical ventilation.
- Demonstrate reduced anxiety levels (relaxed facial expression, ability to rest).
- Maintain adequate cardiac output and tissue perfusion.
- Tolerate endotracheal intubation and mechanical ventilation without evidence of infection or barotrauma.

### PLANNING AND IMPLEMENTATION

- Obtain all necessary supplies and notify respiratory therapy and radiology in preparation for intubation and mechanical ventilation.
- Explain the purpose and procedure of intubation.
- Provide an opportunity to express fears related to intubation and mechanical ventilation; answer questions and provide reassurance.
- Discuss communication strategies while intubated; obtain a magic slate.
- Administer analgesics and/or sedatives as ordered.
- Monitor oxygen saturation and $ETco_2$ levels every 30 to 60 minutes initially after instituting mechanical ventilation; report changes to the physician.
- Obtain ABGs as ordered or indicated; monitor and report results.
- Suction via endotracheal tube as needed to maintain clear airways.
- Allow periods of uninterrupted rest.
- Monitor vital signs every 1 to 2 hours.
- Assess skin color, capillary refill, and the presence of edema every 4 hours.
- Monitor urine output hourly; report output of less than 30 mL per hour.
- Assess lung sounds and chest excursion every 1 to 2 hours.

### EVALUATION

Ms. Adamson is intubated and placed on a volume-cycled ventilator at 50% $FIo_2$ and a tidal volume of 700 mL in the assist-control mode at 16 breaths per minute. She has difficulty working with the ventilator initially, so a fentanyl drip is ordered to reduce her anxiety. Ms. Adamson's oxygen saturation, $ETco_2$, and ABG results do not begin to improve until 5 mmHg of PEEP is added to ventilator settings. After 3 days of mechanical ventilation with PEEP and aggressive fluid and diuretic therapy, Ms. Adamson begins to improve. She is placed on SIMV, and over the course of another 3 days she is gradually weaned off the ventilator to a face mask with CPAP. She eventually recovers fully, with minimal apparent long-term effects.

## Nursing Care Plan

### A Client with ARDS *(continued)*

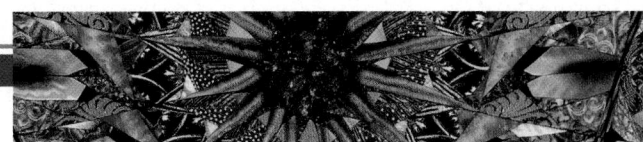

### Critical Thinking in the Nursing Process

1. Endotracheal intubation and mechanical ventilation were effective in supporting Ms. Adamson's respiratory status as she recovered from ARDS. Discuss a possible sequence of events had it not been possible to wean her from the ventilator.
2. How might the presentation and management of an acute episode of respiratory failure due to ARDS differ from respiratory failure related to COPD?
3. What measures can nurses take to prevent the development of ARDS?
4. Develop a nursing care plan for Ms. Adamson for the nursing diagnosis, *Powerlessness* related to endotracheal intubation and mechanical ventilation.

See Evaluating Your Response in Appendix C.

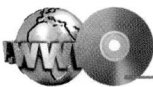

## EXPLORE MediaLink

NCLEX review questions, case studies, care plan activities, MediaLink applications, and other interactive resources for this chapter can be found on the Companion Website at www.prenhall.com/lemone.

Click on Chapter 36 to select the activities for this chapter. For animations, video clips, more NCLEX review questions, and an audio glossary, access the Student CD-ROM accompanying this textbook.

## TEST YOURSELF

1. Admitting orders for a client with acute bacterial pneumonia include an intravenous antibiotic every 8 hours, oxygen per nasal cannula at 5 L/min, continuous pulse oximetry monitoring, bedrest with bathroom privileges and chair at bedside as desired, diet as tolerated, sputum specimen for C&S, CBC, urinalysis, and chemisty panel. Which order should the nurse carry out first?

   a. Start the oxygen per nasal cannula
   b. Insert an intravenous catheter and start the prescribed antibiotic
   c. Provide a dinner tray to the client
   d. Obtain the sputum specimen

2. All of the following nursing diagnoses are appropriate for a client with an acute asthma attack. Which is of highest priority?

   a. *Anxiety* related to difficulty breathing
   b. *Ineffective airway clearance* related to bronchoconstriction and increased mucous production
   c. *Ineffective breathing pattern* related to anxiety
   d. *Ineffective health maintenance* related of lack of knowledge about attack triggers and appropriate use of medications

3. Which of the following would be an expected assessment finding in a client admitted with chronic obstructive airway disease?

   a. AP chest diameter equal to or greater than lateral chest diameter
   b. Mental confusion and lethargy
   c. Three+ pitting edema of ankles and lower legs
   d. Oxygen saturation readings of 85% or less

4. Which of the following statements made by a client with a new diagnosis of lung cancer would indicate that the nurse's teaching has been effective?

   a. "Well, since I'm going to die anyway, I may as well go home, put my affairs in order, and spend the rest of my time in the easy chair."
   b. "I understand that because the cancer has already spread, I will be undergoing aggressive cancer treatment for the next several years to beat this thing."
   c. "Even though I can't undo the damage caused by cigarette smoking, I will try to quit to prevent further damage to my lungs."
   d. "Having the 'big C' is very scary; I'm just glad it is one of the more curable forms of cancer."

5. The nurse caring for a client undergoing mechanical ventilation for acute respiratory failure plans and implements which of the following measures to help maintain effective alveolar ventilation?

   a. Keeps the client in supine position
   b. Increases the tidal volume on the ventilator
   c. Maintains ordered oxygen concentration
   d. Performs endotracheal suctioning as indicated

See Test Yourself answers in Appendix C.

# BIBLIOGRAPHY

Ackley, B. J., & Ladwig, G. B. (2002). *Nursing diagnosis handbook: A guide to planning care* (5th ed.). St. Louis: Mosby.

Adatsi, G. (1999). Health going up in smoke: How can you prevent it? *American Journal of Nursing, 99*(3), 63–64, 66, 67–68.

Adiutori, D. M. (2000). Primary pulmonary hypertension: A review for advanced practice nurses. *MEDSURG Nursing, 9*(5), 255–264.

American Cancer Society. (2002). *Cancer facts and figures 2002.* Atlanta: Author.

Belza, B., Steele, B. G., Hunziker, J., Lakshminaryan, S., Holt, L., & Buchner, D. M. (2001). Correlates of physical activity in chronic obstructive pulmonary disease. *Nursing Research, 50*(4), 195–202.

Braunwald, E., Fauci, A. S., Kasper, D. L., Hauser, S. L., Longo, D. L., & Jameson, J. L. (2001). *Harrison's principles of internal medicine* (15th ed.). New York: McGraw-Hill.

Carroll, P. (2000). Exploring chest drain options. *RN, 63*(10), 50–54.

Centers for Disease Control and Prevention. (2003a). *Guidelines and recommendations. Interim domestic guidance for management of exposures to severe acute respiratory syndrome (SARS) for healthcare and other institutional settings.* Author: Department of Health and Human Services.

_____. (2003b). *Guidelines and recommendations. Interim guidance on infection control precautions for patients with suspected severe acute respiratory syndrome (SARS) and close contacts in households.* Author: Department of Health and Human Services.

_____. (2003c). *Fact sheet. Basic information about SARS.* Author: Department of Health and Human Services.

Chernecky, C. (2001). Pulmonary complications in patients with cancer. *American Journal of Nursing, 101*(5), 24A, 24E, 24G–24H.

Deglin, J. H., & Vallerand, A. H. (2003). *Davis's drug guide for nurses* (8th ed.). Philadelphia: F. A. Davis.

Dest, V. (2000). Ocology today: Lung cancer. *RN, 63*(5), 32–34, 36, 38.

Dunn, N. A. (2001). Keeping COPD patients out of the ED. *RN, 64*(2), 33–37.

Evans, T. (2000). Neuromuscular blockade: When and how. *RN, 63*(5), 56–60.

Fontaine, K. L. (2000). *Healing practices: Alternative therapies for nursing.* Upper Saddle River, NJ: Prentice Hall Health.

Goldsmith, C., & Haban, M. (2002). Lung cancer: A preventable tragedy. *NurseWeek, 3*(2), 17–18.

Goodfellow, L. T., & Jones, M. (2002). Bronchial hygiene therapy. *American Journal of Nursing, 102*(1), 37–43.

Hayes, D. D. (2001). Stemming the tide of pleural effusions. *Nursing2001, 31*(5), 49–52.

Higgins, P. A. (1998). Patient perception of fatigue while undergoing long-term mechanical ventilation: Incidence and associated factors. *Heart & Lung, 27*(3), 177–183.

Johnson, M., Bulechek, G., Dochterman, J. M., Maas, M., & Moorhead, S. (2001). *Nursing diagnoses, outcomes, & interventions.* St. Louis: Mosby.

Johnson, M., Maas, M., & Moorhead, S. (Eds.). (2000). *Nursing outcomes classification (NOC)* (2nd ed.). St. Louis: Mosby.

Kuhn, M. A. (1999). *Complementary therapies for health care providers.* Philadelphia: Lippincott.

LaDuke, S. (2001). Terminal dyspnea & palliative care. *American Journal of Nursing, 101*(11), 26–31.

Lehne, R. A. (2001). *Pharmacology for nursing care* (4th ed.). Philadelphia: Saunders.

Leifer, G. (2001). Hyperbaric oxygen therapy. *American Journal of Nursing, 101*(8), 26–34.

Lenaghan, N. A. (2000). The nurse's role in smoking cessation. *MEDSURG Nursing, 9*(6), 298–302.

Little, C. (2001). What you need to know about chronic bronchitis. *Nursing2001, 31*(9), 52–55.

Malarkey, L. M., & McMorrow, M. E. (2000). *Nurse's manual of laboratory tests and diagnostic procedures* (2nd ed.). Philadelphia: Saunders.

Marion, B. S. (2001). A turn for the better: 'Prone positioning' of patients with ARDS. *American Journal of Nursing, 101*(5), 26–34.

Martin, B., Llewellyn, J., Faut-Callahan, M., & Meyer, P. (2000). The use of telemetric oximetry in the clinical setting. *MEDSURG Nursing, 9*(2), 71–76.

McCance, K. L., & Huether, S. E. (2002). *Pathophysiology: The biologic basis for disease in adults and children* (4th ed.). St. Louis: Mosby.

McCloskey, J. C., & Bulechek, G. M. (Eds.) (2000). *Nursing interventions classification (NIC)* (3rd ed.). St. Louis: Mosby.

Miracle, V., & Winston, M. (2000). Take the wind out of asthma. *Nursing2000, 30*(8), 34–41.

Morrison, C., & Lew, E. (2001). Aspergillosis. *American Journal of Nursing, 101*(8), 40–48.

National Center for HIV, STD, and TB Prevention, Division of Tuberculosis Elimination. (2002). *Surveillance reports. Reported tuberculosis in the United States 2001.* Atlanta, GA: Centers for Disease Control and Prevention.

National Heart, Lung, and Blood Institute, National Institutes of Health. (2002). *Morbidity & mortality: 2002 chart book of cardiovascular, lung, and blood diseases.* Bethesda, MD: Author.

North American Nursing Diagnosis Association. (2001). *NANDA nursing diagnoses: Definitions & classification 2001–2002.* Philadelphia: NANDA.

Owen, C. L. (1999). New directions in asthma management. *American Journal of Nursing, 99*(3), 26–33.

Persell, D. J., Arangie, P., Young, C., Stokes, E. N., Payne, W. C., Skorga, P., & Gilbert-Palmer, D. (2002). Preparing for bioterrorism. *Nursing, 32*(2), 37–43.

Pope, B. B. (2002). Patient education series. Asthma. *Nursing2002, 32*(5), 44–45.

Porth, C. M. (2002). *Pathophysiology: Concepts of altered health states* (6th ed.). Philadelphia: Lippincott.

Ruppert, R. A. (1999). The last smoke. *American Journal of Nursing, 99*(11), 26–32.

Schultz, T. R. (2002). Straight talk about community-acquired pneumonia. *Nursing2002, 32*(1), 46–49.

Sellers, K. F., Hargrove, B., & Jenkins, P. (2000). Asthma disease management programs improve clinical and economic outcomes. *MEDSURG Nursing, 9*(4), 201–203, 207.

Tierney, L. M., McPhee, S. J., & Papadakis, M. A. (2001). *Current medical diagnosis & treatment* (40th ed.). New York: Lange Medical Books/McGraw-Hill.

Trogger, D. A., & Brenner, P. S. (2001). Metered dose inhalers. *American Journal of Nursing, 101*(10), 26–32.

Trudeau, M. E., & Solano-McGuire, S. M. (1999). Evaluating the quality of COPD care. *American Journal of Nursing, 99*(3), 47–50.

Truesdell, S. (2000). Helping patients with COPD manage episodes of acute shortness of breath. *MEDSURG Nursing, 9*(4), 178–182.

Urden, L. D., Stacy, K. M., & Lough, M. E. (2002). *Thelan's critical care nursing: Diagnosis and management* (4th ed.). St. Louis: Mosby.

Way, L. W., & Doherty, G. M. (2003). *Current surgical diagnosis & treatment* (11th ed.). New York: Lange Medical Books/McGraw-Hill.

Whitney, E. N., & Rolfes, S. R. (2002). *Understanding nutrition* (9th ed. ). Belmont, CA: Wadsworth.

Wilkinson, J. M. (2000). *Nursing diagnosis handbook with NIC interventions and NOC outcomes* (7th ed.). Upper Saddle River, NJ: Prentice Hall Health.

Woods, S. L., Froelicher, E. S. S., & Motzer, S. U. (2000). *Cardiac nursing* (4th ed.). Philadelphia: Lippincott.

World Health Organization. (2003). Cumulative number of reported probable cases of severe acute respiratory syndrome (SARS). *Communicable disease surveillance & response (CSR).* Author.

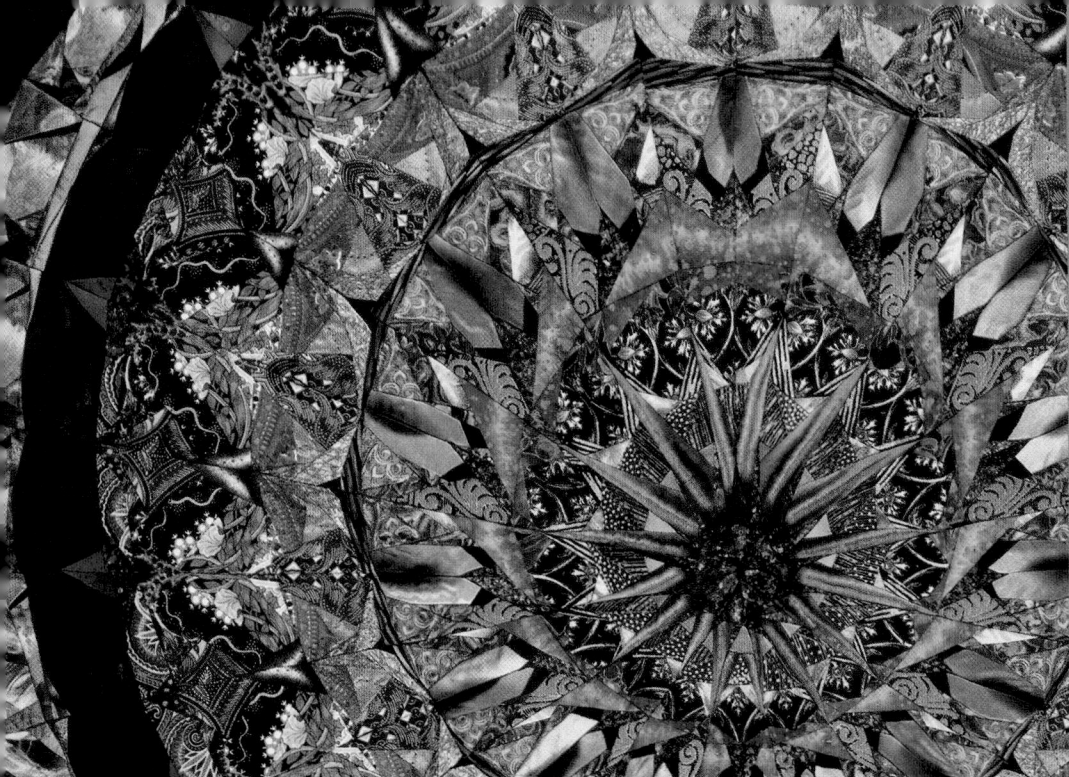

UNIT 11

# RESPONSES TO ALTERED MUSCULOSKELETAL FUNCTION

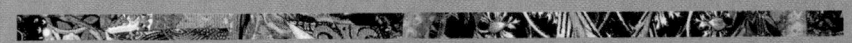

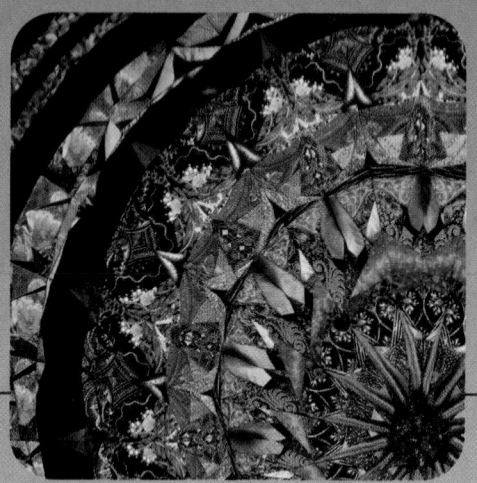

# Assessing Clients with Musculoskeletal Disorders

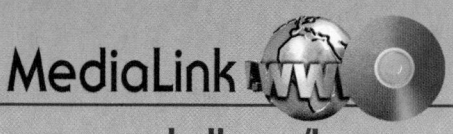

## MediaLink

**www.prenhall.com/lemone**

Additional resources for this chapter can be found on the Student CD-ROM accompanying this textbook, and on the Companion Website at www.prenhall.com/lemone. Click on Chapter 37 to select the activities for this chapter.

**CD-ROM**
- Audio Glossary
- NCLEX Review

*Animation*
- Musculoskeletal A&P

**Companion Website**
- More NCLEX Review
- Functional Health Pattern Assessment
- Case Study
  Knee Pain

## LEARNING OUTCOMES

After completing this chapter, you will be able to:

- Review the anatomy and physiology of the musculoskeletal system.

- Describe the normal movements allowed by synovial joints.

- Identify specific topics for consideration during a health history interview of the client with health problems involving the musculoskeletal system.

- Describe physical assessment techniques for musculoskeletal function.

- Identify abnormal findings that may indicate impairment of the musculoskeletal system.

The tissues and structures of the musculoskeletal system perform many functions, including support, protection, and movement. The musculoskeletal system has two subsystems: the bones and joints of the skeleton, and the skeletal muscles. These subsystems work together to allow the body to perform both gross, simple movements such as closing a door, and fine, complex movements such as repairing a watch.

## REVIEW OF ANATOMY AND PHYSIOLOGY

### The Skeleton

The human skeleton is made up of 206 bones (Figure 37–1 ■). The axial skeleton includes the bones of the skull, the ribs and sternum, and the vertebral column. The appendicular skeleton consists of all the bones of the limbs, the shoulder girdles, and the pelvic girdle.

Bones form the body's structure and provide support for soft tissues. They also protect vital organs from injury and serve to move body parts by providing points of attachment for muscles. Bones also store minerals and serve as a site for *hematopoiesis* (blood cell formation).

Bone cells include osteoblasts (cells that form bone), osteocytes (cells that maintain bone matrix), and osteoclasts (cells that resorb bone). Bone matrix is the extracellular element of bone tissue; it consists of collagen fibers, minerals (primarily calcium and phosphate), proteins, carbohydrates, and ground substance. Ground substance is a gelatinous material that facilitates diffusion of nutrients, wastes, and gases between the blood vessels and bone tissue. Bones are covered with **periosteum,** a double-layered connective tissue. The outer layer of the periosteum contains blood vessels and nerves; the inner layer is anchored to the bone.

Bones consist of a rigid connective tissue called osseous tissue, of which there are two types: Compact bone is smooth and dense; spongy bone contains spaces between meshworks of bone. Both types contain the same elements and are found in almost all bones of the body.

The basic structural unit of compact bone is the Haversian system (also called an osteon). The Haversian system consists of a central canal, called the Haversian canal; concentric layers of bone matrix, called lamellae; spaces between the lamellae, called lacunae; osteocytes within the lacunae; and small channels, called canaliculi (Figure 37–2 ■).

Spongy bone has no Haversian systems. Instead, the lamellae are arranged in concentric layers called trabeculae which branch and join to form meshworks. The spongy sections of long bones and flat bones contain tissue for hematopoiesis. In the adult, these sections, called red marrow cavities, are present in the spongy center of flat bones (especially the sternum) and in only two long bones: the humerus and the head of the femur. This red marrow is active in hematopoiesis in adults.

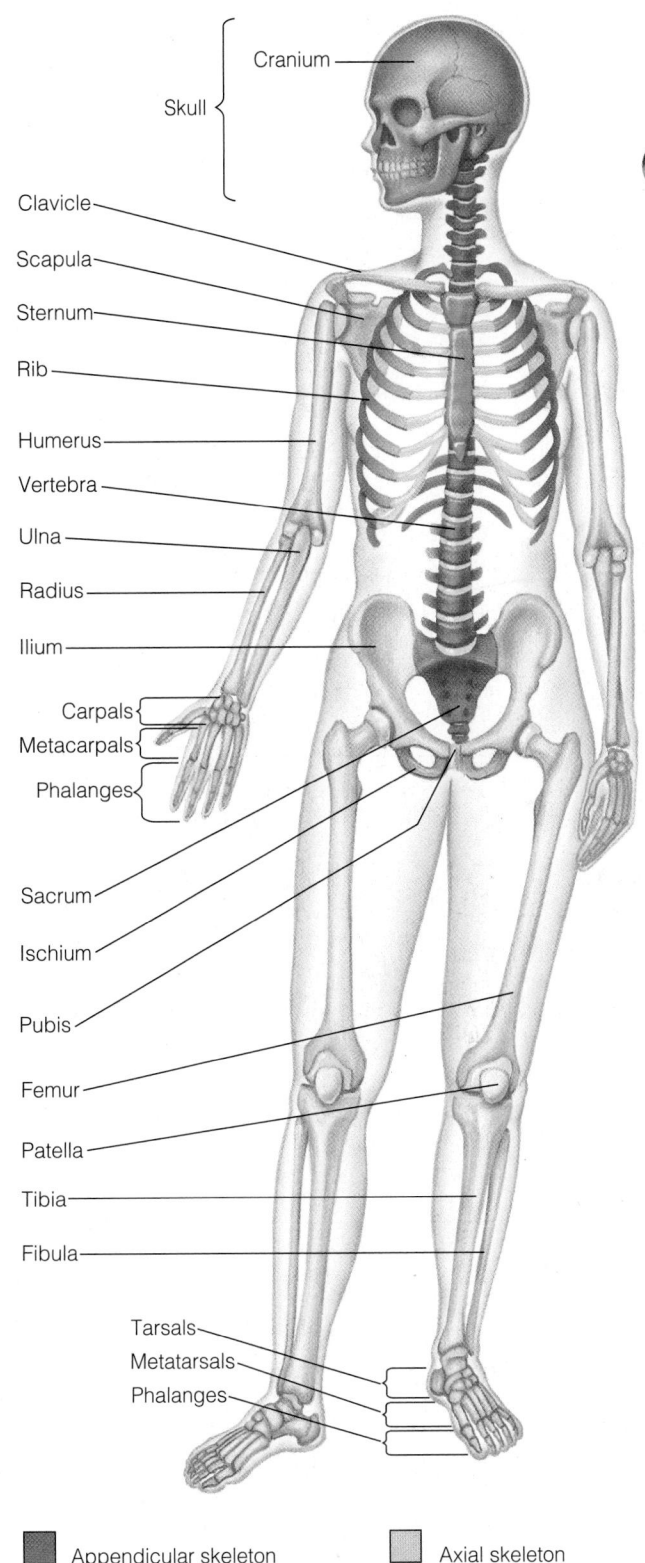

Appendicular skeleton     Axial skeleton

**Figure 37–1** ■ Bones of the human skeleton.

MediaLink | MUSCULOSKELETAL A&P ANIMATIONS

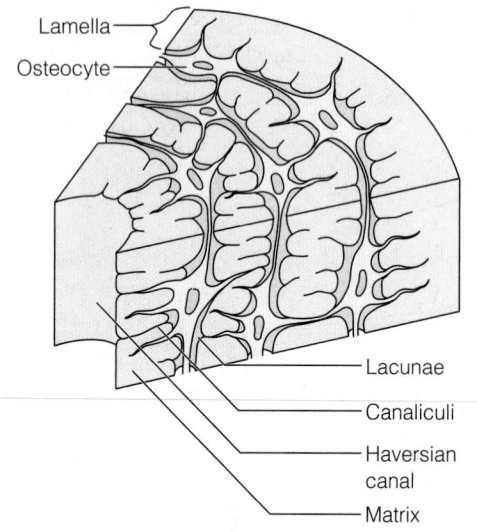

Lamella
Osteocyte
Lacunae
Canaliculi
Haversian canal
Matrix

**Figure 37-2** ■ The microscopic structure of compact bone.

Bones are classified by shape (Figure 37–3 ■):

- Long bones are longer than they are wide. They have a midportion, or shaft, called a **diaphysis** and two broad ends, called **epiphyses.** The diaphysis is compact bone and contains the marrow cavity, which is lined with endosteum. Each epiphysis is spongy bone covered by a thin layer of compact bone. Long bones include the bones of the arms and legs, fingers, and toes.
- Short bones, also called cuboid bones, are spongy bone covered by compact bone. They include the bones of the wrist and ankle.
- Flat bones are thin and flat, and most are curved. Their disclike structure consists of a layer of spongy bone between two thin layers of compact bone. Flat bones include most bones of the skull, the sternum, and the ribs.
- Irregular bones are of various shapes and sizes and, like flat bones, are plates of compact bone with spongy bone between. Irregular bones include the vertebrae, the scapulae, and the bones of the pelvic girdle.

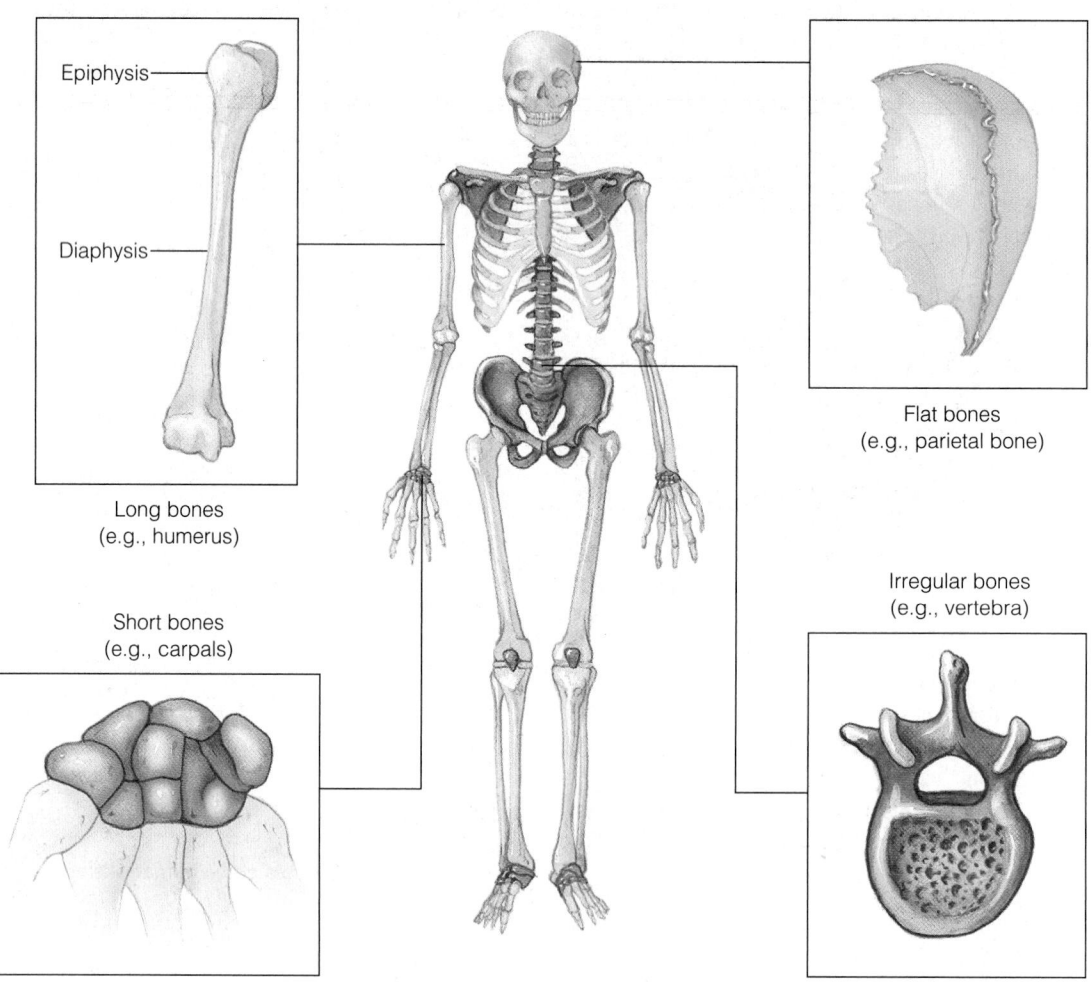

Epiphysis

Diaphysis

Long bones
(e.g., humerus)

Short bones
(e.g., carpals)

Flat bones
(e.g., parietal bone)

Irregular bones
(e.g., vertebra)

**Figure 37-3** ■ Classification of bones according to shape.

## Bone Remodeling in Adults

Although the bones of adults do not normally increase in length and size, constant remodeling of bones, as well as repair of damaged bone tissue, occurs throughout life. In the bone remodeling process, bone resorption and bone deposit occur at all periosteal and endosteal surfaces. Hormones and forces that put stress on the bones regulate this process, which involves a combined action of the osteocytes, osteoclasts, and osteoblasts. Bones that are in use, and are therefore subjected to stress, increase their osteoblastic activity to increase ossification (the development of bone). Bones that are inactive undergo increased osteoclast activity and bone resorption.

The hormonal stimulus for bone remodeling is controlled by a negative feedback mechanism that regulates blood calcium levels. This stimulus involves the interaction of parathyroid hormone (PTH) from the parathyroid glands and calcitonin from the thyroid gland. When blood levels of calcium decrease, PTH is released; PTH then stimulates osteoclast activity and bone resorption so that calcium is released from the bone matrix. As a result, blood levels of calcium rise, and the stimulus for PTH release ends. Rising blood calcium levels stimulate the secretion of calcitonin, inhibit bone resorption, and cause the deposit of calcium salts in the bone matrix. Thus, bones regulate blood calcium levels. Calcium ions are necessary for the transmission of nerve impulses, the release of neurotransmitters, muscle contraction, blood clotting, glandular secretion, and cell division. Of the body's 1200 to 1400 g of calcium, over 99% is present as bone minerals.

Bone remodeling is also regulated by the response of bones to gravitational pull and to mechanical stress from the pull of muscles. Although the exact mechanism is not fully understood, it is known that bones that undergo increased stress are heavier and larger. This finding supports Wolff's law, which states that bone develops and remodels itself to resist the stresses placed on it.

The process of bone repair following a fracture is discussed in Chapter 38.

## Joints, Ligaments, and Tendons

**Joints,** or **articulations,** are regions where two or more bones meet. Joints hold the bones of the skeleton together while allowing the body to move. Joints may be classified by function as synarthroses, amphiarthroses, or diarthroses. Table 37–1 describes each of these types.

Joints are also classified by structure as fibrous, cartilaginous, or synovial. Fibrous joints permit little or no movement, because the articulating bones are joined either by short connective tissue fibers that bind the bones together, as with the sutures of the skull, or by short cords of fibrous tissue called ligaments (discussed on the next page), which permit slight give but no true movement.

Some cartilaginous joints, such as the sternocostal joints of the rib cage, are composed of hyaline cartilage growths that fuse together the articulating bone ends. These joints are immobile. In other cartilaginous joints, such as the intervertebral discs, the hyaline cartilage fuses to an intervening plate of flex-

ible fibrocartilage. This structural feature accounts for the flexibility of the vertebral column.

Bones in synovial joints are enclosed by a cavity that is filled with synovial fluid, a filtrate of blood plasma. These joints are freely movable. Synovial joints are found at all articulations of the limbs. They have several characteristics:

- The articular surfaces are covered with articular cartilage.
- The joint cavity is enclosed by a tough, fibrous, double-layered articular capsule; internally, the cavity is lined with a synovial membrane that covers all surfaces not covered by the articular cartilage.
- Synovial fluid fills the free spaces of the joint capsule, enhancing the smooth movement of the articulating bones.

Synovial joints allow many kinds of movements, listed and described in Table 37–2.

### TABLE 37–1  Functional Classification of Joints

| Type | Description | Examples |
|------|-------------|----------|
| Synarthrosis | Immovable joint | Skull sutures<br>Epiphyseal plates<br>Joint between first rib and manubrium of sternum |
| Amphiarthrosis | Slightly movable joint | Vertebral joints<br>Joint of the pubic symphysis |
| Diarthrosis | Freely movable joint | Joints of the limbs<br>Shoulder joints<br>Hip joints |

### TABLE 37–2  Movements Allowed by Synovial Joints

| Movement | Description |
|----------|-------------|
| Abduction | Move limb away from body midline |
| Adduction | Move limb toward body midline |
| Extension | Straighten limbs at joint |
| Flexion | Bend limbs at joint |
| Dorsiflexion | Bend ankle to bring top of foot toward shin |
| Plantar flexion | Straighten ankle to point toes down |
| Pronation | Turn forearm to place palm down |
| Supination | Turn forearm to place palm up |
| Eversion | Turn out |
| Inversion | Turn in |
| Circumduction | Move in circle |
| Internal rotation | Move inward on a central axis |
| External rotation | Move outward on a central axis |
| Protraction | Move forward and parallel to ground |
| Retraction | Move backward and parallel to ground |

The fibrous capsules that surround synovial joints are supported by ligaments, dense bands of connective tissue that connect bones to bones. Ligaments limit or enhance movement, provide joint stability, and enhance joint strength. Tendons are fibrous connective tissue bands that connect muscles to the periosteum of bones and enable the bones to move when skeletal muscles contract. When muscles contract, increased pressure causes the tendon to pull, push, or rotate the bone to which it is connected.

**Bursae** are small sacs of synovial fluid that cushion and protect bony areas that are at high risk for friction, such as the knee and the shoulder. Tendon sheaths are a form of bursae, but they are wrapped around tendons in high-friction areas.

## Muscles

The three types of muscle tissue in the body are skeletal muscle, smooth muscle, and cardiac muscle (Table 37–3). This discussion focuses on skeletal muscle, the only muscle that allows musculoskeletal function.

Skeletal muscle cells have typical functional properties:

- *Excitability:* the ability to receive and respond to a stimulus. The stimulus is usually a neurotransmitter released by a neuron, and the response is the generation and transmission of an action potential along the plasma membrane of the muscle cell. (Chapter 40 discusses action potentials.)
- *Contractibility:* the ability to respond to a stimulus by forcibly shortening.
- *Extensibility:* the ability to respond to a stimulus by extending and relaxing; muscle fibers shorten when they contract and extend when they relax.
- *Elasticity:* the ability to resume its resting length after it has shortened or lengthened.

Skeletal muscles are thick bundles of parallel multinucleated contractile cells called fibers. Each single muscle fiber is itself a bundle of smaller structures called myofibrils. The myofibrils have alternating light and dark bands that give skeletal muscle its striated (striped) appearance under an electron microscope. Myofibrils are strands of smaller repeating units called sarcomeres, which consist of thick filaments of myosin and thin filaments of actin, proteins that contribute to muscle contraction.

Skeletal muscle movement is triggered when motor neurons release acetylcholine, a neurotransmitter that alters the perme-

ability of the muscle fiber. Sodium ions enter the fiber, producing an action potential that causes muscle contraction. The more fibers that contract, the stronger the contraction of the entire muscle.

Prolonged strenuous activity causes continuous nerve impulses and eventually results in a buildup of lactic acid and reduced energy in the muscle, or muscle fatigue. However, continuous nerve impulses are also responsible for maintaining muscle tone. Lack of use results in muscle atrophy, whereas regular exercise increases the size and strength of muscles.

Skeletal muscles attach to and cover the bones of the skeleton. Skeletal muscles promote body movement, help maintain posture, and produce body heat. They may be moved by conscious, voluntary control or by reflex activity. The body has approximately 600 skeletal muscles (Figure 37–4 ■).

## ASSESSING MUSCULOSKELETAL FUNCTION

The function of the musculoskeletal system is assessed by both a health assessment interview to collect subjective data and a physical assessment to collect objective data.

## Health Assessment Interview

This section provides guidelines for collecting subjective data through a health assessment interview specific to musculoskeletal function. An assessment interview to determine problems with musculoskeletal function may be conducted as part of a health screening or as part of a total health assessment, or it may focus on a chief complaint (such as pain, swelling, or limited mobility). Health problems affecting the neurologic system may manifest as musculoskeletal function problems; an assessment of both systems may be necessary. (See Chapter 40 for assessment of the neurologic system.) If the client has a health problem involving the bones or muscles, analyze its onset, characteristics and course, severity, precipitating and relieving factors, and any associated manifestations, noting the timing and circumstances. For example, ask the client:

- Describe the pain you have had in your elbow. Does the pain increase with movement? Have you noticed any redness or swelling?
- Did you injure your ankle before you began to experience difficulty walking?
- Is your pain worse in the morning, or does it get worse through the day?

The primary manifestations of altered function of the musculoskeletal system are pain and limited mobility. Specific descriptors of the pain, its location, and its nature are important. Other significant information includes associated manifestations, such as fever, fatigue, changes in weight, rash, and/or swelling. Also collect information about the client's lifestyle: type of employment, ability to carry out activities of daily living (ADLs) and provide self-care, exercise or participation in sports, use of alcohol or drugs, and nutrition. Explore past injuries and measures to self-treat pain (such as over-the-counter medications, prescribed medications, application of heat or cold, splinting, wrapping, or rest).

| TABLE 37–3 | Types of Body Muscle | |
|---|---|---|
| **Type** | **Description** | **Examples** |
| Skeletal | Striated, voluntary muscle (can consciously move) | Biceps, triceps, deltoid, gluteus maximus |
| Smooth | Nonstriated, involuntary muscle (cannot consciously move) | Muscles in the walls of the bladder, stomach, and bronchi |
| Cardiac | Striated, involuntary muscle | Heart muscle |

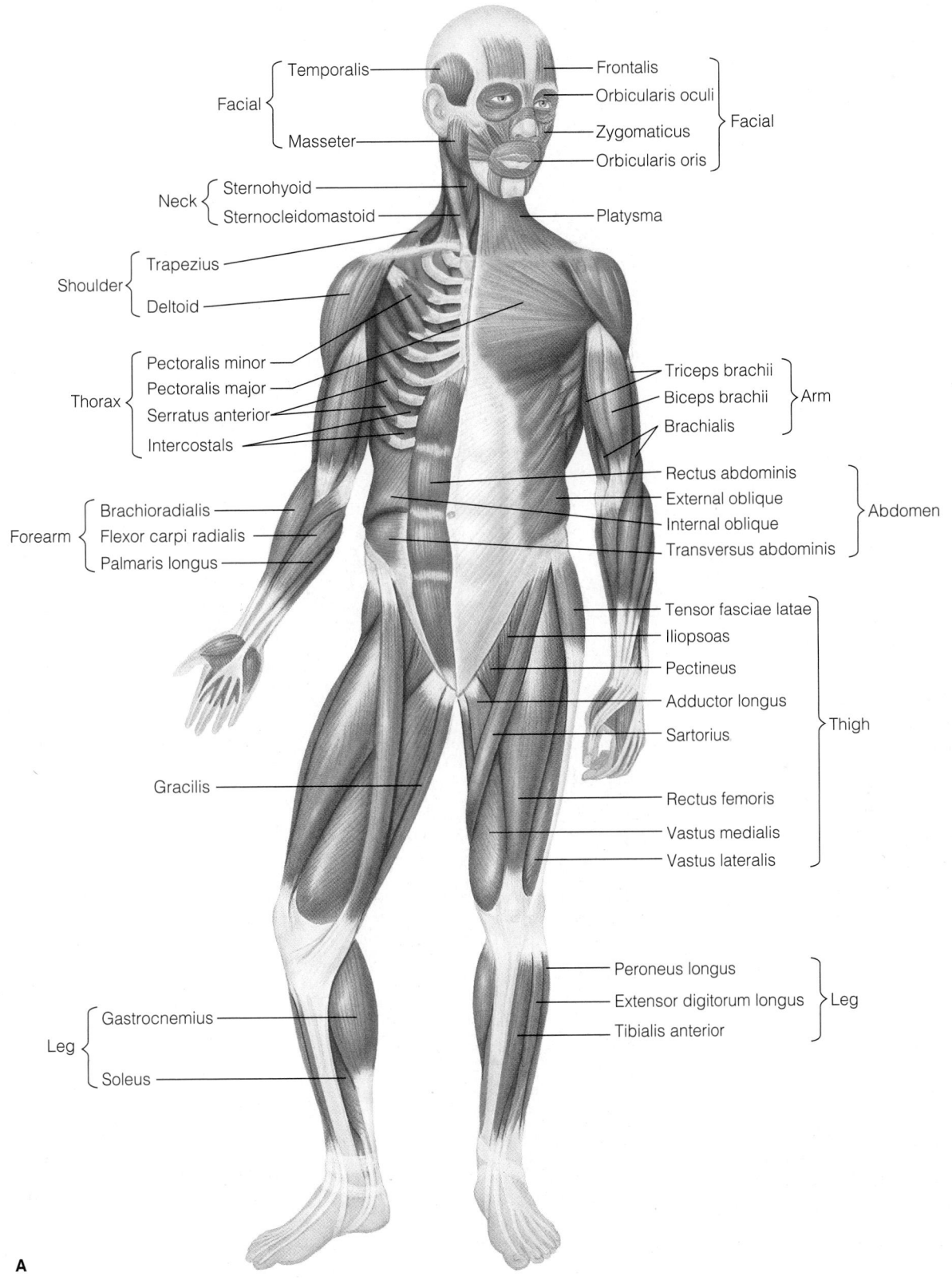

**Facial**
- Temporalis
- Masseter

**Facial**
- Frontalis
- Orbicularis oculi
- Zygomaticus
- Orbicularis oris

**Neck**
- Sternohyoid
- Sternocleidomastoid

- Platysma

**Shoulder**
- Trapezius
- Deltoid

**Thorax**
- Pectoralis minor
- Pectoralis major
- Serratus anterior
- Intercostals

**Arm**
- Triceps brachii
- Biceps brachii
- Brachialis

**Abdomen**
- Rectus abdominis
- External oblique
- Internal oblique
- Transversus abdominis

**Forearm**
- Brachioradialis
- Flexor carpi radialis
- Palmaris longus

**Thigh**
- Tensor fasciae latae
- Iliopsoas
- Pectineus
- Adductor longus
- Sartorius
- Rectus femoris
- Vastus medialis
- Vastus lateralis

- Gracilis

**Leg**
- Peroneus longus
- Extensor digitorum longus
- Tibialis anterior

**Leg**
- Gastrocnemius
- Soleus

A

**Figure 37–4** ■ *A,* Muscles of the anterior body.

*(Figure continues on page 1184)*

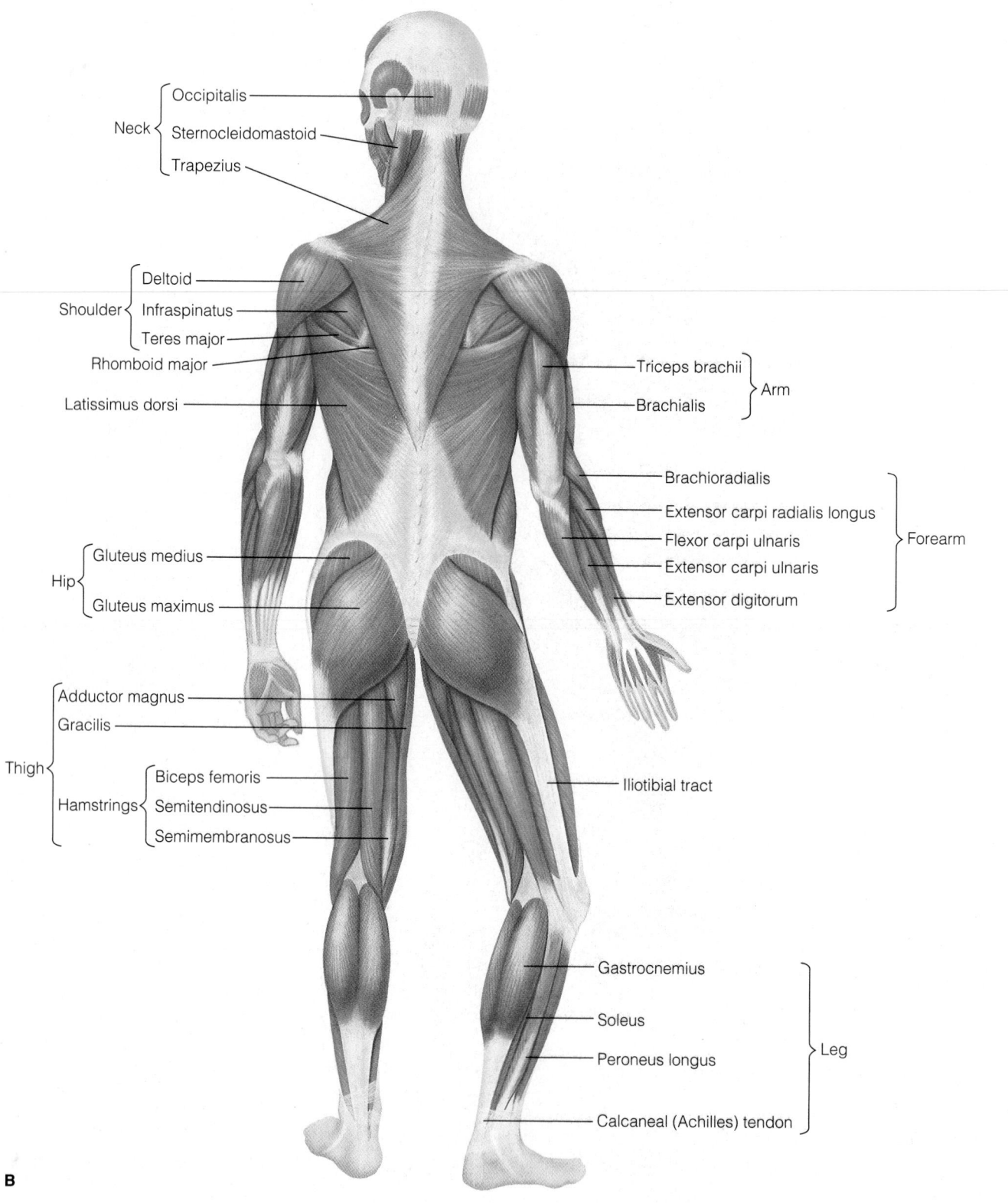

**Neck**
- Occipitalis
- Sternocleidomastoid
- Trapezius

**Shoulder**
- Deltoid
- Infraspinatus
- Teres major

Rhomboid major

Latissimus dorsi

Triceps brachii
Brachialis
**Arm**

Brachioradialis
Extensor carpi radialis longus
Flexor carpi ulnaris
Extensor carpi ulnaris
Extensor digitorum
**Forearm**

**Hip**
- Gluteus medius
- Gluteus maximus

**Thigh**

Adductor magnus

Gracilis

**Hamstrings**
- Biceps femoris
- Semitendinosus
- Semimembranosus

Iliotibial tract

Gastrocnemius
Soleus
Peroneus longus
Calcaneal (Achilles) tendon
**Leg**

**B**

**Figure 37–4** ■ (Continued)  B, Muscles of the posterior body.

Other questions and leading statements, categorized by functional health patterns, can be found on the Companion Website.

## Physical Assessment

Physical assessment of the musculoskeletal system is conducted through inspection, palpation, and measurement of muscle mass and range of motion. The client should be comfortably dressed in clothing that lets you see the movement of all joints clearly. The client may be standing, sitting, or lying down; the sequence of the examination should be such that the client does not have frequent position changes. An assessment of the older adult, the client in pain, or the client who is weak may take extra time.

The equipment necessary for assessing the musculoskeletal system is a tape measure to determine muscle size and a goniometer to measure joint range of motion (ROM). Prior to the examination, collect all equipment and explain the techniques to decrease the client's anxiety.

The general sequence for a musculoskeletal examination follows:

1. Begin the examination with an assessment of the client's gait and posture. Observe how the client walks, sits, and/or moves about in bed.
2. Inspect and palpate the client's bones for any obvious deformity or changes in size or shape. Palpation also will elicit tenderness or pain.
3. Measure the extremities for length and circumference. Before taking measurements, make sure the client is lying in a comfortable position. Remember to compare limbs bilaterally.
4. Assess muscle mass by first inspecting for obvious increase or decrease in size. Assess and document muscle strength on a scale of 0 to 5 (Table 37–4). Box 37–1 provides client instructions for testing the strength of various muscles.
5. Assess joints for swelling, pain, redness, warmth, crepitus, and ROM. Only assess the ROM of every joint if the client has a specific musculoskeletal problem; however, assessing one or more joints is a common part of nursing care. Use a goniometer for precise measurements of joint ROM (Figure 37–5 ■). This device has a pointer joined to a protractor at 0 degrees. These two arms are placed along articulating bones, and the angle of joint movement is recorded in degrees.

### TABLE 37–4 Muscle Grading Scale

| Grading Scale | Assessment Description |
|---|---|
| 0 | (No visible) contraction; paralysis |
| 1 | Can feel contraction of muscle but there is no movement of limb |
| 2 | Passive ROM |
| 3 | Full ROM against gravity |
| 4 | Full ROM against some resistance |
| 5 | Full ROM against full resistance |

### BOX 37–1 ■ Guidelines for Determining Muscle Strength

In adults, muscles are usually strong and equally strong bilaterally. However, neuromuscular diseases, disuse, metabolic disorders, or infections can cause muscle weakness. Muscle strength is expected to be greater in the dominant arm and leg. In most instances (and especially when moving digits and extremities), the nurse provides resistance by pushing in the opposite direction.

The muscles listed below are routinely tested. Instructions for clients are also provided:

| Muscle | Client Instructions |
|---|---|
| Ocular muscles and lids | Close eyes tightly. |
| Finger muscles | Shake hands. |
| | Make a fist. |
| | Spread fingers. |
| Facial muscles | Blow out cheeks. |
| | Stick out tongue. |
| Hip muscles | Raise straight leg while supine. |
| Neck muscles | Bend head forward and backward. |
| Gluteal and leg muscles | Alternately cross legs while sitting. |
| Deltoid muscles | Hold arms up. |
| Biceps muscle | Bend the arm. |
| Quadriceps muscle | Straighten leg. |
| Triceps muscle | Straighten the arm. |
| Wrist muscles | Bend hand forward and backward. |
| Ankle and foot muscles | Bend foot up and down. |

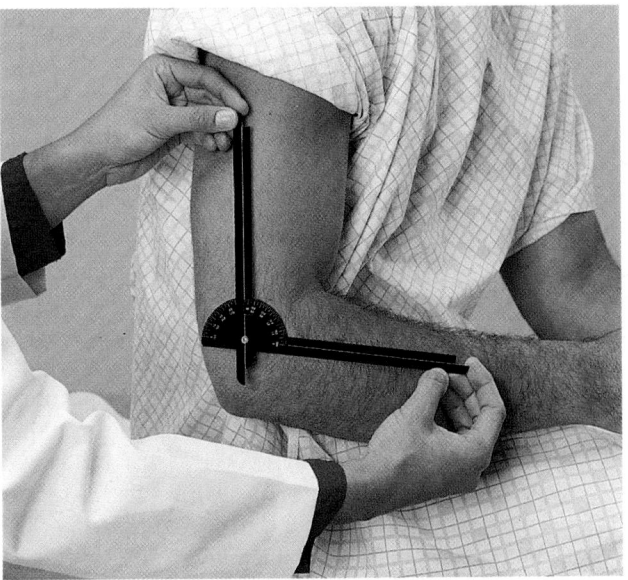

**Figure 37–5** ■ Using a goniometer to measure joint ROM.

## Gait and Body Posture Assessment with Abnormal Findings (✓)

- Inspect gait and body posture.
  - ✓ Joint stiffness, pain, deformities, and muscle weakness can cause changes in gait and posture.
- Inspect the spine for curvature. Ask the client to stand and bend back slowly as far as possible, bend slowly to the right and then to the left as far as possible, turn slowly to the right and left in a circular motion, and bend forward slowly and try to touch fingers to toes.
  - ✓ With herniated lumbar discs, the lumbar curve flattens and spinal mobility is decreased.
  - ✓ An increased lumbar curve, called **lordosis,** may be seen in obesity or pregnancy.
  - ✓ A lateral, S-shaped curvature of the spine is called **scoliosis.** Functional scoliosis usually is a compensatory response to painful paravertebral muscles, herniated discs, or discrepancy in leg length. It disappears with forward flexion. Structural scoliosis is often congenital and tends to appear during adolescence. It is accentuated with forward bending.
  - ✓ **Kyphosis** is an exaggerated thoracic curvature of the spine common in older adults.

## Joint Assessment with Abnormal Findings (✓)

- Inspect the joints for deformity, swelling, and redness.
  - ✓ Diseases of the joints may be manifested by such deformities as tissue loss, tissue overgrowth, or contractures, irreversible shortenings of muscles and tendons.
  - ✓ Edema in a joint may cause obvious bulging.
  - ✓ Redness, swelling, and pain are evidence of an inflammation or infection in the joint.
- Palpate the joints for tenderness, warmth, crepitation, consistency, and muscle mass.
  - ✓ Inflammation and injury cause joint pain.
  - ✓ Arthritis, bursitis, tendonitis, and osteomyelitis (infection of a bone) result in painful, hot joints.
  - ✓ **Crepitation** (a grating sound) is present in a joint when the articulating surfaces have lost their cartilage, such as in arthritis.

## Range-of-Motion Assessment with Abnormal Findings (✓)

Assess joint ROM by asking the client to perform activities specific to:

- *Temporomandibular joint:* "Open your mouth wide, and then close your mouth." (As the client opens and closes the mouth, palpate the temporomandibular joints with your index and middle fingers, as shown in Figure 37–6 ■.)
  - ✓ Clicking or popping noises, decreased ROM, pain, and swelling may indicate temporomandibular joint syndrome or, in rare cases, osteoarthritis.
- *Cervical spine:*
  45-degree flexion: "Touch your chin to your chest."
  55-degree extension: "Look at the ceiling."
  40-degree lateral bending: "Try to touch your right ear to your right shoulder." Repeat with the left side
  70-degree rotation: "Try to touch your chin to each shoulder."

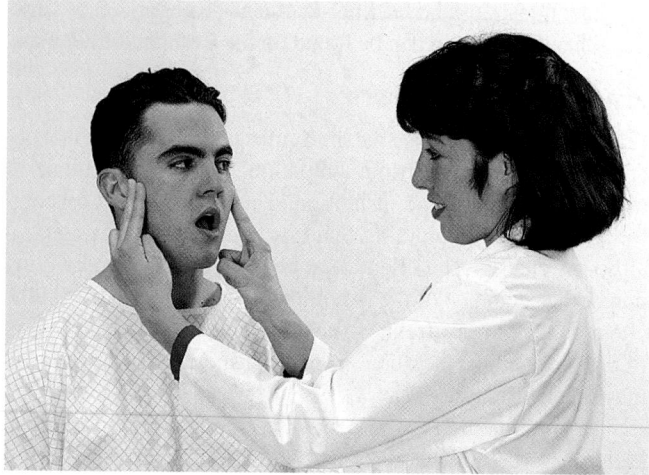

**Figure 37–6** ■ Palpating the temporomandibular joints.

  - ✓ Neck pain and limited extension with lateral bending are seen with herniated cervical discs and in cervical spondylosis.
  - ✓ An immobile neck with head and neck thrust forward is seen with ankylosing spondylitis.
- *Lumbar spine:*
  75- to 90-degree flexion: "Touch your toes with your fingers" (Figure 37–7A ■).
  30-degree extension: "Bend backward slowly."
  35-degree lateral bending: "Bend right and left" (Figure 37–7B).
  30-degree rotation: "Twist your shoulders right and left" (Figure 37–7C).
  - ✓ Decreased movement or pain with movement may indicate an abnormal spinal curvature, arthritis, herniated disc, or spasm of paravertebral muscles.
- *Fingers:*
  Flexion: "Make a fist."
  Extension: "Open your hand."
  Abduction: "Spread your fingers."
  Adduction: "Close your fingers."
  - ✓ Flexion and extension of fingers is decreased in arthritis.
  - ✓ Heberden's nodes and Bouchard's nodes are hard, nontender nodules on the dorsolateral parts of the distal and proximal interphalangeal joints, respectively. They are common in osteoarthritis.
  - ✓ Stiff, painful, swollen finger joints are seen in acute rheumatoid arthritis.
  - ✓ Boutonnière and swan-neck deformities are seen in chronic rheumatoid arthritis.
  - ✓ Swollen finger joints with a white chalky discharge may be seen in chronic gout.
- *Wrists:*
  90-degree flexion: "Bend wrist down."
  70-degree extension: "Bend wrist up."
  55-degree ulnar deviation: "Bend wrist toward little finger."
  20-degree radial deviation: "Bend wrist toward thumb."
  - ✓ Bilateral chronic swelling in the wrist is seen in arthritis.

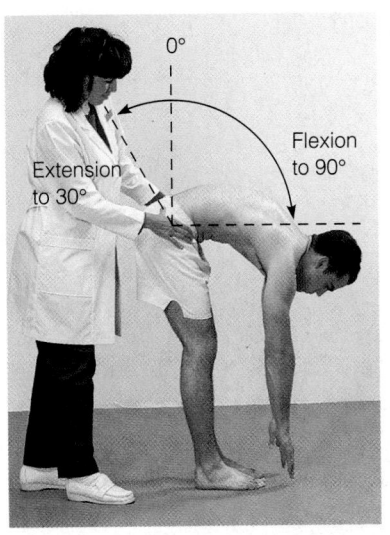
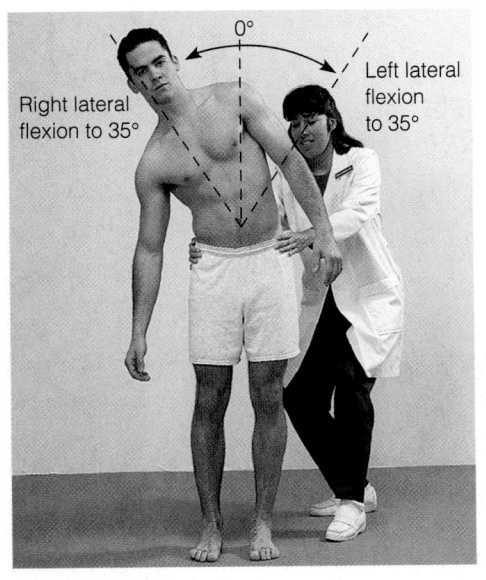
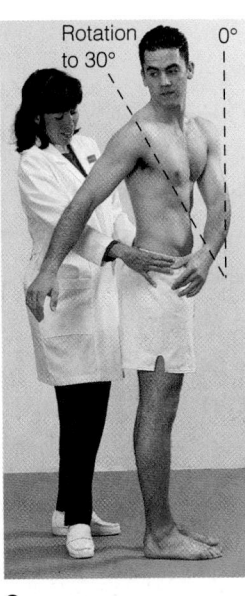

**Figure 37–7** ■ *A,* Forward flexion of spine. *B,* Lateral flexion of spine. *C,* Rotation of spine.

- *Elbows:*
  160-degree flexion: "Touch your hands to your shoulders."
  180-degree extension: "Straighten your elbows."
  90-degree supination: "Bend your elbows 90 degrees, and turn hands palm up."
  90-degree pronation: "Bend your elbows 90 degrees, and turn fists down."
  ✓ Swollen, tender, inflamed elbows are apparent in gouty arthritis and rheumatoid arthritis.
  ✓ Pain and tenderness at the lateral epicondyle occurs in tennis elbow.
- *Shoulders:*
  180-degree flexion: "Hold your arms straight up and out."
  50-degree hyperextension: "Put your straight arm behind your back."
  90-degree internal rotation: "Put your forearm behind your lower back."
  180-degree abduction: "Raise your straight arm up and out to your side."
  50-degree adduction: "Put your straight arm across your chest."
  ✓ Pain and tenderness over the biceps tendon occurs with tendinitis (inflammation of a tendon).
  ✓ The arm cannot be abducted fully when the supraspinatus tendon of the shoulder is ruptured.
  ✓ Pain and limited abduction is also seen with bursitis (inflammation of a bursa) and calcium deposits in this area.
- *Toes:*
  90-degree flexion: "Walk on your toes."
  ✓ The great toe is excessively abducted in hallux valgus.
  ✓ The joint above the great toe is swollen, inflamed, and painful in gouty arthritis.

✓ There is hyperextension of the metatarsophalangeal joint and flexion of the proximal interphalangeal joint with hammer toes.
- *Ankles:*
  20-degree dorsiflexion: "Point your foot to the ceiling."
  45-degree plantar flexion: "Point your foot to the floor."
  30-degree inversion: "Walk on the outside of your feet."
  20-degree eversion: "Walk on the inside of your feet."
  ✓ Contractures of the Achilles tendon may occur in clients with rheumatoid arthritis following prolonged bed rest.
- *Knees:*
  130-degree flexion: "Do a deep knee bend."
  180-degree extension: "Sit down and hold your legs straight out in front of you."
  ✓ Swelling over the suprapatellar pouch is seen with inflammation and fluid in the articular capsule of the knee. Synovitis is inflammation of the synovial membrane lining the articular capsule of a joint. It is common with knee trauma.
  ✓ Swelling over the patella is seen in bursitis.
- *Hips:* (The client is lying down.)
  120-degree flexion: "Bring bent knee up to your chest."
  30-degree hyperextension: "Lie on the abdomen, and lift up one leg at a time."
  45-degree abduction: "Hold your leg straight, and move it out to the side."
  40-degree internal rotation: "Bend your knee, and swing it toward your other leg."
  45-degree external rotation: "Bend your knee, and swing it out to the side."
  ✓ Movement of the hip is limited and/or painful in arthritis.

## Special Assessments with Abnormal Findings (✓)

- Perform *Phalen's test.* Ask the client to hold the wrist in acute flexion for 60 seconds (Figure 37–8 ■).

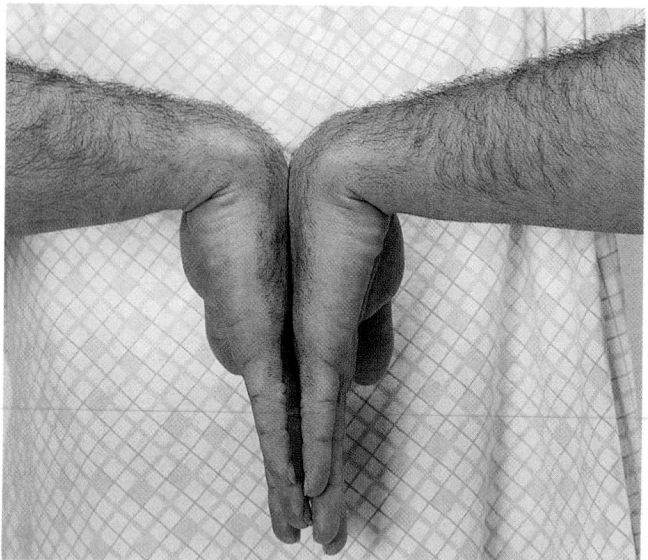

**Figure 37–8** ■ Phalen's test.

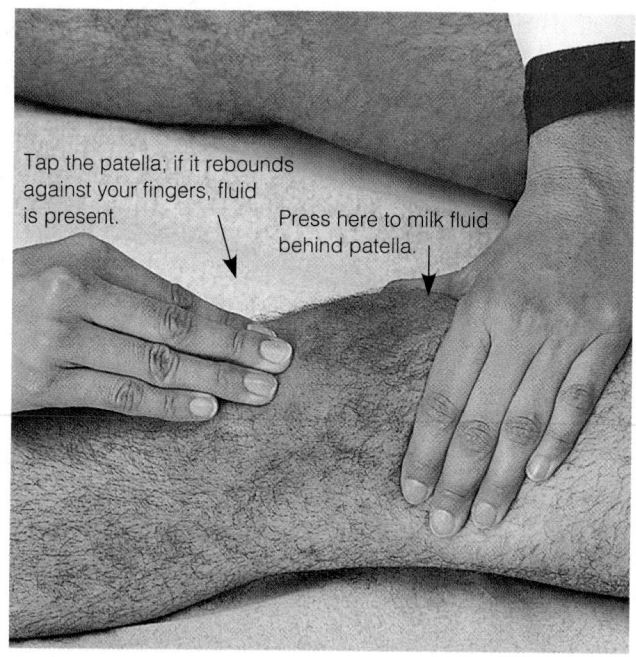

Tap the patella; if it rebounds against your fingers, fluid is present.

Press here to milk fluid behind patella.

**Figure 37–10** ■ Checking for ballottement.

✓ Numbness and burning in the fingers during Phalen's test may indicate carpal tunnel syndrome.

• Check for small amounts of fluid on the knee by assessing for a "bulge sign." Milk upward on the medial side of the knee, and then tap the lateral side of the patella (Figure 37–9 ■).

✓ A fluid bulge indicates increased fluid in the knee joint rather than soft tissue swelling.

• Check for larger amounts of fluid by assessing ballottement. Apply downward pressure on the knee with one hand while pushing the patella backward against the femur with the other hand (Figure 37–10 ■).

✓ Increased fluid will cause a tapping sound as the patella displaces the fluid and hits the femur.

• Perform *McMurray's test.* While reclining, ask the client to turn the flexed knee toward the center of the body. Stabilize the knee with one hand, and apply pressure on the lower leg with the other hand (Figure 37–11 ■).

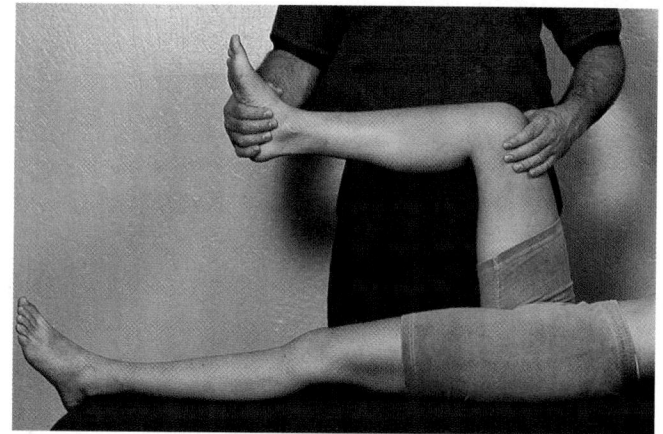

**Figure 37–11** ■ McMurray's test.

**Figure 37–9** ■ Checking for the bulge sign.

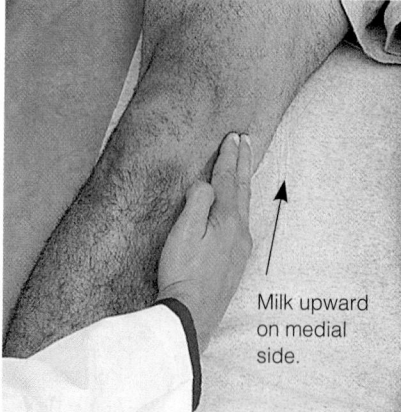

Milk upward on medial side.

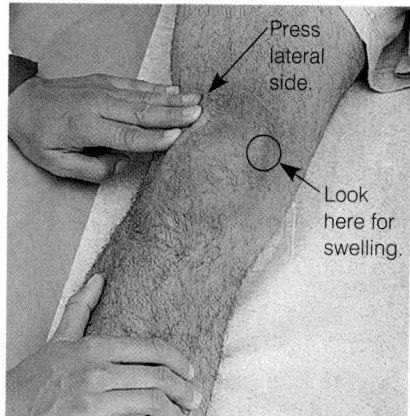

Press lateral side.

Look here for swelling.

✓ Pain, locking (inability to fully extend the knee), or a popping sound may indicate an injury to a meniscus, a disc of cartilaginous tissue in the knee.

• Perform the *Thomas test.* Ask the client to lie down and extend one leg while bringing the knee of the opposite leg to the chest (Figure 37–12 ■).

✓ A hip flexion contracture will cause the extended leg to rise off the table.

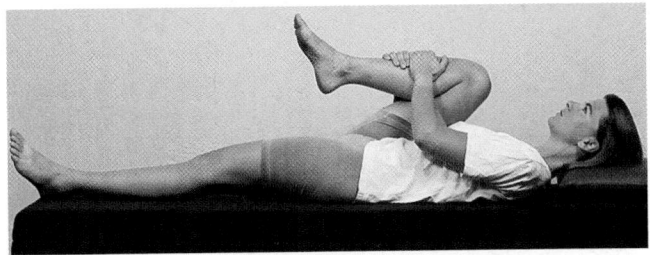

**Figure 37–12** ■ Thomas test for hip contracture.

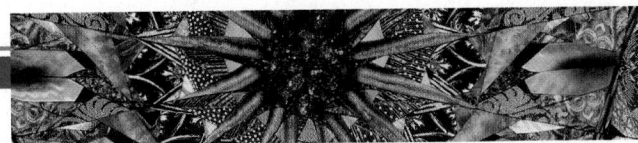

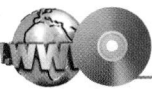

## EXPLORE MediaLink

NCLEX review questions, case studies, care plan activities, MediaLink applications, and other interactive resources for this chapter can be found on the Companion Website at www.prenhall.com/lemone.

Click on Chapter 37 to select the activities for this chapter. For animations, video clips, more NCLEX review questions, and an audio glossary, access the Student CD-ROM accompanying this textbook.

## TEST YOURSELF

1. What classification of bones has a diaphysis and epiphyses?
   a. Irregular bones
   b. Flat bones
   c. Long bones
   d. Short bones

2. The movement of a limb away from the body midline is:
   a. Abduction
   b. Adduction
   c. Extension
   d. Flexion

3. What would you ask the client to do in order to assess facial muscle strength?
   a. "Close your eyes tightly."
   b. "Stick out your tongue."
   c. "Bend your head forward."
   d. "Open your eyes widely."

4. What term is used to describe a grating sound when a joint is moved?
   a. Crackles
   b. Arthritis
   c. Synovitis
   d. Crepitation

5. What are the most common manifestations of musculoskeletal disorders?
   a. Pain and limited mobility
   b. Swelling and redness
   c. Cyanosis and decreased pulses
   d. Pallor and decreased ROM

See Test Yourself answers in Appendix C.

## BIBLIOGRAPHY

Andresen, G. (1998). Assessing the older patient. *RN, 61*(3), 46–56.

Bynum, D. (1997). Clinical snapshot: Gout. *American Journal of Nursing, 97*(7), 36–37.

Campbell-Giovaniello, K. (1997). Clinical snapshot: Plantar fasciitis. *American Journal of Nursing, 97*(9), 38–39.

Krug, B. (1997). Rheumatoid arthritis and osteoarthritis: A basic comparison. *Orthopedic Nursing, 16*(5), 73–75.

Ludwidk, R., Dieckman, B., & Snelson, C. (1999). Assessment of the geriatric orthopaedic trauma patient. *Orthopaedic Nursing, 18*(6), 11–20.

Mangini, M. (1998). Physical assessment of the musculoskeletal system. *Nursing Clinics of North America, 33*(4), 643–652.

McDougall, T. (1999). Orthopedic update: Assessment of limb injury. *Australian Emergency Nursing Journal, 2*(1), 26–28.

Neal, L. (1997). Basic musculoskeletal assessment: Tips for the home health nurse. *Home Healthcare Nurse, 15*(4), 227–235.

O'Hanlon-Nichols, T. (1998). A review of the adult musculoskeletal system: A guide to a key aspect of patient care. *American Journal of Nursing, 98*(6), 48–52.

Watson, R. (2001). Assessing the musculoskeletal system in older people. *Nursing Older People, 13*(5), 29–30.

Weber, J., & Kelley, J. (2002). *Health assessment in nursing* (2nd ed.) Philadelphia: Lippincott.

Wilson, S., & Giddens, J. (2001). *Health assessment for nursing practice.* St. Louis: Mosby.

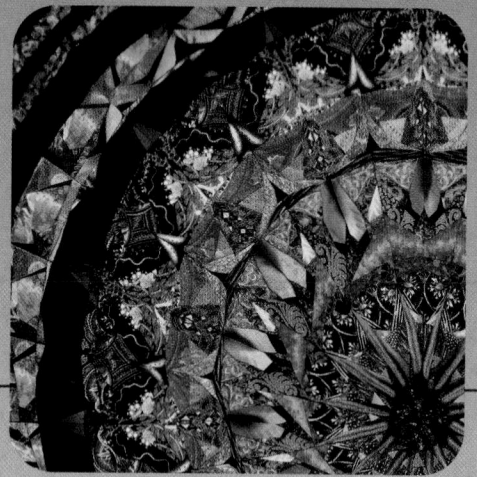

# CHAPTER 38

# Nursing Care of Clients with Musculoskeletal Trauma

## MediaLink

### www.prenhall.com/lemone

Additional resources for this chapter can be found on the Student CD-ROM accompanying this textbook, and on the Companion Website at www. prenhall.com/lemone. Click on Chapter 38 to select the activities for this chapter.

**CD-ROM**
- Audio Glossary
- NCLEX Review

*Animations*
- Bone Healing
- Fracture Repair

**Companion Website**
- More NCLEX Review
- Case Study
  A Client with Fractures
- Care Plan Activity
  Below-the-Knee Amputation
- MediaLink Application
  Preventing Musculoskeletal Injuries

## LEARNING OUTCOMES

After completing this chapter, you will be able to:

- Apply knowledge of normal anatomy, physiology, and assessments when providing care for clients with musculoskeletal trauma (see Chapter 37).

- Explain the factors that lead to musculoskeletal trauma and amputations.

- Describe the pathophysiology, manifestations, complications, and collaborative care for clients with contusions, strains, sprains, fractures, amputations, and repetitive use injury.

- Describe the stages of bone healing.

- Explain the purposes and related nursing interventions for casts, traction, and stump care.

- Use the nursing process as a framework for providing individualized care for clients who have experienced musculoskeletal trauma.

Musculoskeletal trauma is an injury to muscle, bone, or soft tissue that results from excessive external force. The external source transmits more kinetic energy than the tissue can absorb, and injury results. The severity of the trauma depends not only on the amount of force but also on the location of the impact, because different parts of the body can withstand different amounts of force. A wide variety of external sources can cause trauma, and the force involved can vary in severity (e.g., a step off the curb, a fall, being tackled in a football game, and a motor vehicle crash). See Chapter 6 ⊘⊘ for a detailed discussion of the results of different forces and types of injury from trauma.

Musculoskeletal injuries resulting from trauma include blunt tissue trauma, alterations in tendons and ligaments, and fractures of bones. Various forces that cause musculoskeletal trauma are typical for a specific environment, activity, or age group. For example, motorcycle crashes resulting in fractures of the distal tibia, midshaft femur, and radius are common in young men. Sports injuries, resulting from either overuse or acute trauma, are seen more often in adolescents and young adults. Falls are the most common cause of injury in people age 65 or older, with fractures of the vertebrae, proximal humerus, and hip seen most often (Porth, 2002).

Musculoskeletal trauma can result in mild or severe injuries. A client may experience a soft-tissue injury, a fracture, and/or a complete amputation. In addition, trauma to one part of the musculoskeletal system often produces dysfunction in adjacent structures. For example, a fracture of the femur prevents the adjacent muscles from abducting and adducting. Nursing care helps minimize the effects of trauma, prevents complications, and hastens restoration of function. The injury may require rehabilitation and temporary or permanent changes in lifestyle. This chapter discusses fractures, amputations, soft-tissue injuries, dislocations, and repetitive use injuries.

# TRAUMATIC INJURIES OF THE MUSCLES, LIGAMENTS, AND JOINTS

## THE CLIENT WITH A CONTUSION, STRAIN, OR SPRAIN

Contusion, strains, and sprains are among the most commonly reported injuries. They account for about 50% of work-related injuries, with lower back injuries the most commonly reported occupational injury. However, many sprains and strains are not work related, and often are not reported. The lower back and cervical region of the spine are the most common sites for muscle strains; the ankle is the most commonly sprained joint, usually caused by forced inversion of the foot.

## PATHOPHYSIOLOGY AND MANIFESTATIONS

A **contusion,** the least serious form of musculoskeletal injury, is bleeding into soft tissue that results from a blunt force, such as a kick or striking a body part against a hard object. The skin remains intact, but small blood vessels rupture and bleed into soft tissues. A contusion with a large amount of bleeding is referred to as a **hematoma.** The manifestations of a contusion include swelling and discoloration of the skin. The blood in the soft tissue initially results in a purple and blue color commonly referred to as a mark or bruise. As the blood begins to reabsorb, the mark becomes brown and then yellow, until it disappears.

A **strain** is a stretching injury to a muscle or a muscle-tendon unit caused by mechanical overloading. A muscle that is forced to extend past its elasticity will become strained. Lifting heavy objects without bending the knees, or a sudden acceleration-deceleration, as in a motor vehicle crash, can cause strains. The most common sites for a muscle strain are the lower back and cervical regions of the spine. The manifesta-

| BOX 38–1 | ■ Comparison of Sprains and Strains |

**Sprain**
- Defined as an injury to a ligament that results from a twisting motion.
- Can cause joint instability.
- Pain, edema, and swelling are present.
- Motion increases the joint pain.

**Strain**
- Defined as a microscopic tear in the muscle.
- Sharp or dull pain is present.
- Pain increases with isometric contraction of the muscle.
- Swelling and local tenderness are present.

tions of a strain include a sharp or dull pain that increases with isometric contraction of the muscle, swelling, and stiffness.

A **sprain** is an injury to a ligament surrounding a joint. Forces going in opposite directions cause the ligament to overstretch and/or tear. The ligaments may be incompletely or completely torn. Although any joint may be involved, sprains of the ankle and knee are most common. Manifestations include joint instability, discoloration, heat, pain, edema, and rapid swelling. Motion increases the joint pain. A comparison of sprains and strains is presented in Box 38–1.

## COLLABORATIVE CARE

Soft-tissue trauma is treated with measures that decrease swelling and alleviate pain. Severe sprains may require surgical repair. A splint may be applied to rest the injured area. Ice is applied for the first 24 to 48 hours, after which heat can be applied. A compression dressing, such as an Ace bandage, may be applied. The injured extremity should be elevated to or above the level of the heart to increase venous return and decrease swelling. Ankle sprains may be immobilized with an air cast, with no limitations on weight bearing. A knee injury also requires a knee immobilizer. If the upper extremity is injured, a sling is provided. Physical therapy may be recommended during rehabilitation.

## Diagnostic Tests

The following diagnostic tests may be ordered when soft-tissue trauma is suspected:

- *X-rays* rule out a fracture before making a diagnosis of soft-tissue injury.
- *Magnetic resonance imaging (MRI)* is used if further assessment is necessary.

## Medications

Medications used to treat soft-tissue trauma include NSAIDs and analgesics.

## NURSING CARE

The nursing care of each client is individualized. A strain or sprain may not be as devastating to an attorney as it is to a professional athlete; therefore, the nurse should determine what the injury means to the particular client.

## Nursing Diagnoses and Interventions

Nursing diagnoses focus on providing information about self-care to decrease pain and return physical mobility to preinjury levels.

### Acute Pain

The pain that results from soft-tissue trauma is due primarily to the injury to the muscle or ligament and secondarily to bleeding and edema at the injury site.

- Teach the client the acronym RICE (rest, ice, compression, elevation) to care for the injury:
  - Rest the injured extremity. *Rest allows the injured muscle or ligament to heal.*
  - Apply ice to the injured area. *Cold causes vasoconstriction and decreases the pooling of blood in the injured area. Ice may also numb the tender area.*
  - Apply a compression dressing, such as an Ace bandage. *A compression dressing can decrease the formation of edema and thereby decrease pain.*
  - Elevate the extremity above the heart. *Elevating the extremity promotes venous return and decreases edema, which will decrease pain.*
- If pain is still present after 24 to 48 hours of applying ice, instruct the client to apply heat. *Heat increases blood flow and venous return and thereby decreases edema and pain.*

### Impaired Physical Mobility

Pain causes the client to avoid using or bearing weight with the injured extremity. Always observe the client's use of assistive devices; if the device is inappropriate, the client can face a greater risk of falling. The device may be appropriate, but the client may not be using it correctly or safely. As a person ages, muscle mass in the upper extremities declines. As a result, the older client with a sprained ankle may not be able to use crutches, because crutches require that the person distribute body weight along the upper extremities. Older clients may therefore find a walker more useful.

- Teach the correct use of crutches, walkers, canes, or slings if prescribed. *The correct technique increases safety and encourages use of these devices.*
- Encourage follow-up care. *Severe sprains may require further testing to determine if surgical intervention is indicated.*

## THE CLIENT WITH A JOINT DISLOCATION

A **dislocation** of a joint is the loss of articulation of the bone ends in the joint capsule. Dislocations usually follow severe trauma, with the bone ends displaced or separated from their normal position in the joint capsule. They occur most frequently in the shoulder and acromioclavicular joints. A **subluxation** is a partial dislocation in which the bone ends are still partially in contact with each other.

## PATHOPHYSIOLOGY AND MANIFESTATIONS

Dislocations may be congenital, traumatic, or pathologic. Congenital dislocations are present at birth and are seen in the hip and knee. Traumatic dislocations result from falls, blows, or rotational injuries. Pathologic dislocations result from disease of the joint, including infection, rheumatoid arthritis, paralysis, and neuromuscular diseases. The manifestations of a dislocation include pain, deformity, and limited motion.

## COLLABORATIVE CARE

Care of the client with a dislocation focuses on relieving pain, correcting the dislocation, and preventing complications. The dislocation is diagnosed by physical examination and X-rays. The joint is reduced by means of manual traction.

Shoulder joint dislocations are reduced and immobilized in a sling for 3 weeks, after which time rehabilitation can begin. A dislocated hip requires immediate reduction in the emergency room to prevent necrosis of the femoral head and injury to the sciatic and femoral nerves. After reduction, the client is placed on bed rest. In some cases, traction is needed for several weeks. If a hip dislocation is accompanied by a fracture, the client will undergo surgery to increase mobility, decrease complications, and rapidly stabilize the joint.

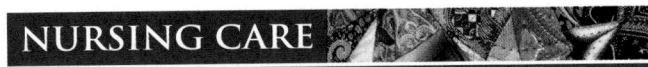

## NURSING CARE

Nursing care of the client with a dislocation or subluxation is individualized to the cause of injury, the type of dislocation, and the age of the client.

### Nursing Diagnoses and Interventions

Nursing diagnoses focus on relieving pain (see previous section) and preventing complications.

#### Risk for Injury

The client with a dislocation requires frequent assessments to ensure that neurovascular compromise does not develop.

- Monitor neurovascular status by assessing pain, pulses, pallor, paralysis, and paresthesia. *Neurovascular compromise is indicated by increased pain, decreased or absent pulses, pale skin, inability to move a body part or extremity, and changes in sensation (such as "pins and needles" sensations, or loss of sense of sharp/dull touch).*
- Maintain immobilization after reduction. *Immobilization prevents the joint from dislocating again.*

### Home Care

Joint dislocations often tend to be recurring injuries for clients actively participating in contact sports and other vigorous physical activities. Younger adults have a 60% to 80% recurrence rate for anterior shoulder dislocations. Prolonged immobilization (for several weeks after the injury) and aggressive rehabilitation following the initial dislocation can reduce the risk of recurrent dislocation. The following topics should be addressed in preparing the client for home care.

- Importance of complying with the prescribed length of immobilization
- Skin care and ways to prevent skin-to-skin contact, particularly in the axillary area
- Prescribed rehabilitation exercises that will strengthen muscles and other supportive structures in the shoulder, decreasing the risk of future dislocations
- Alternatives to activities that precipitate recurrent dislocations
- Instructions or referrals to physical therapy if needed for further teaching about using assistive devices
- Referrals to physical and occupational therapy and home health services as needed

## TRAUMATIC INJURIES OF BONES

### THE CLIENT WITH A FRACTURE

A **fracture** is any break in the continuity of a bone. Fractures vary in severity according to the location and the type of fracture. Although fractures occur in all age groups, they are more common in people who have sustained trauma and in older clients.

#### PATHOPHYSIOLOGY

Any of the 206 bones in the body can sustain a fracture. A fracture occurs when the bone is subjected to more kinetic energy than it can absorb. Fractures may result from a direct blow, a crushing force (compression), a sudden twisting motion (torsion), a severe muscle contraction, or disease that has weakened the bone (called a **pathologic fracture**). Two basic mechanisms produce fractures: direct force and indirect force. With direct force, the kinetic energy is applied at or near the site of the fracture. The bone cannot withstand the force. With indirect force, the kinetic energy is transmitted from the point of impact to a site where the bone is weaker. The fracture occurs at the weaker point.

Fractures are classified in the following ways:

- If the skin is intact, the fracture is considered a **closed** (or **simple**) **fracture.** If the skin integrity is interrupted, the fracture is considered an **open** (or **compound**) **fracture** (Figure 38–1 ■). An open fracture allows bacteria to enter the injured area and increases the risk of complications.

- The fracture line may be **oblique** (at a 45-degree angle to the bone) or **spiral** (curves around the bone). An **avulsed** fracture occurs when the fracture pulls bone and other tissues away from the point of attachment. It may also be described as **comminuted** (the bone breaks in many pieces), **compressed** (the bone is crushed), **impacted** (the broken bone

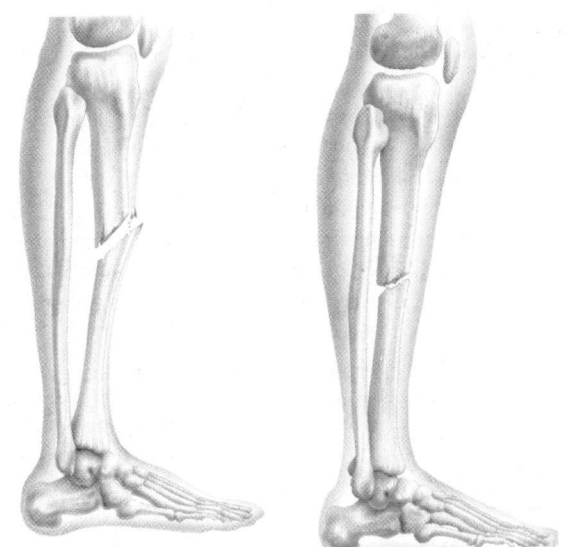

**Figure 38–1** ■ *A,* An open fracture. *B,* A closed fracture.

ends are forced into each other), or **depressed** (the broken bone is forced inward).

- **Complete fractures** involve the entire width of the bone, whereas **incomplete fractures** do not involve the entire width of the bone.
- A **stable (nondisplaced) fracture** is one in which the bones maintain their anatomic alignment. An **unstable (displaced) fracture** occurs when the bones move out of correct anatomic alignment. If a fracture is displaced, immediate interventions are required to prevent further damage to soft tissue, muscle, and bone.
- Fractures may also be classified by point of reference on the bone, such as midshaft, middle third, and distal third. The point of reference may also be specific, such as intrarticular or diaphyseal.

## MANIFESTATIONS AND COMPLICATIONS

Fractures are often accompanied by soft tissue injuries that involve muscles, arteries, veins, nerves, or skin. The degree of soft-tissue involvement depends on the amount of energy or force transmitted to the area. Fracture manifestations and their causes are outlined in Table 38–1. The section following fracture healing describes manifestations and complications, with related collaborative and nursing care, for fractures of specific bones.

### Fracture Healing

Regardless of classification or type, fracture healing progresses over three phases: the inflammatory phase, the reparative phase, and the remodeling phase. See *Pathophysiology Illustrated* on the next page. The bleeding and inflammation that develop at the site of the fracture initiate the inflammatory phase. A hematoma forms between the fractured bone ends and around the bone surfaces. The osteocytes at the bone ends die as the hematoma clots, obstructing blood flow and depriving them of oxygen and nutrients. Necrosis of the cells heightens the inflammatory response, which in turn leads to vasodilation and edema. In addition, fibroblasts, lymphocytes, macrophages, and even osteoblasts from the bone migrate to the fracture site. Fibroblasts form a fibrin meshwork and promote the growth of granulation tissue and capillary buds. The lymphocytes and macrophages wall off the area, localizing and containing the inflammation. The capillary buds invade the fracture site and supply a source of nutrients to promote the formation of collagen. The collagen allows calcium to be deposited.

Once calcium is deposited, a callus begins to form. In this reparative phase, osteoblasts promote the formation of new bone, and osteoclasts destroy dead bone and assist in the synthesis of new bone. Collagen formation and calcium deposition continues. During the remodeling phase, excess callus is removed and new bone is laid down along the fracture line. Eventually, the fracture site is calcified, and the bone is reunited.

The age, physical condition of the client, and the type of fracture sustained influence the healing of fractures. Other factors influence bone healing either positively or negatively and may be grouped according to their local or systemic influence (Box 38–2). Healing time varies with the individual. An uncomplicated fracture of the arm or foot can heal in 6 to 8 weeks. A fractured vertebra will take at least 12 weeks to heal. A fractured hip may take from 12 to 16 weeks.

| TABLE 38–1 | Manifestations of Fracture |
|---|---|
| **Manifestation** | **Cause** |
| Deformity | Abnormal position of bones secondary to fracture and muscles pulling on fractured bone |
| Swelling | Edema from localization of serous fluid and bleeding |
| Pain/tenderness | Muscle spasm, direct tissue trauma, nerve pressure, movement of fractured bone |
| Numbness | Nerve damage or nerve entrapment |
| Guarding | Pain |
| Crepitus | Grating of bones or entrance of air in an open fracture. *Note:* Do not manipulate the extremity to elicit crepitus; doing so may cause additional damage. |
| Hypovolemic shock | Blood loss or associated injuries |
| Muscle spasms | Muscle contraction near the fracture |
| Ecchymosis | Extravasation of blood into the subcutaneous tissue |

---

**BOX 38–2 ■ Factors Influencing Bone Healing**

**POSITIVE FACTORS**

**Local**
- Immobilization
- Timely correction of displacement
- Application of ice
- Electrical stimulation

**Systemic**
- Adequate amounts of growth hormone, vitamin D, and calcium
- Adequate blood supply
- Absence of infection or diseases
- Younger age
- Moderate activity level prior to injury

**NEGATIVE FACTORS**

**Local**
- Delay in correction of displacement
- Open fracture (increases risk of infection)
- Presence of foreign body at fracture site

**Systemic**
- Immunocompromised status
- Decreased circulation (as in diabetes or peripheral vascular disease)
- Malnutrition
- Osteoporosis
- Advanced age

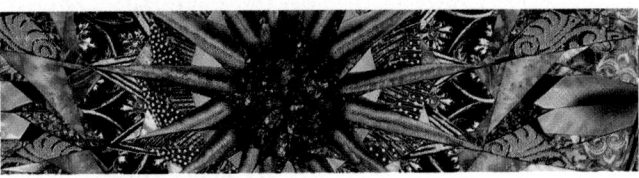

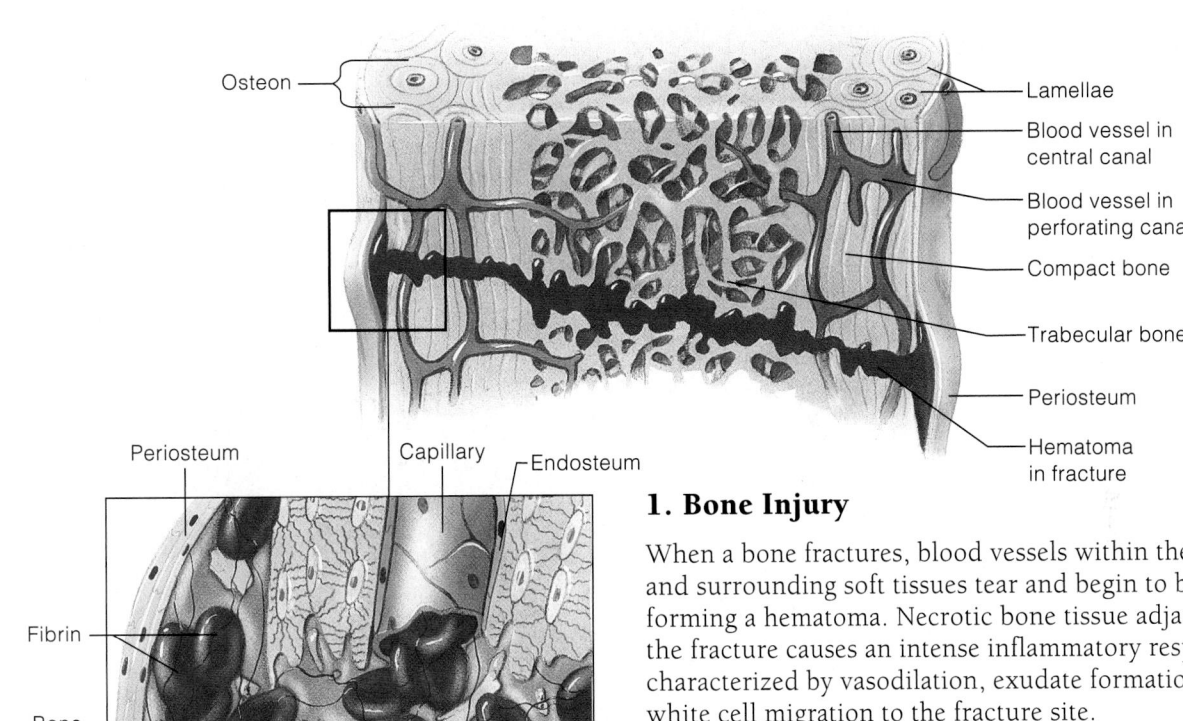

## 1. Bone Injury

When a bone fractures, blood vessels within the bone and surrounding soft tissues tear and begin to bleed, forming a hematoma. Necrotic bone tissue adjacent to the fracture causes an intense inflammatory response characterized by vasodilation, exudate formation, and white cell migration to the fracture site.

## 2. Fibrocartilaginous Callus Formation

Clotting factors within the hematoma form a fibrin meshwork. Within 48 hours, fibroblasts and new capillaries growing into the fracture form granulation tissue that gradually replaces the hematoma. Phagocytes begin to remove cell debris.

Osteoblasts, bone-forming cells, proliferate and migrate into the fracture site, forming a fibrocartilaginous callus. The osteoblasts build a web of collagen fibers from both sides of the fracture site that eventually unites to connect bone fragments, thus splinting the bone. Chondroblasts lay down patches of cartilage that provide a base for bone growth.

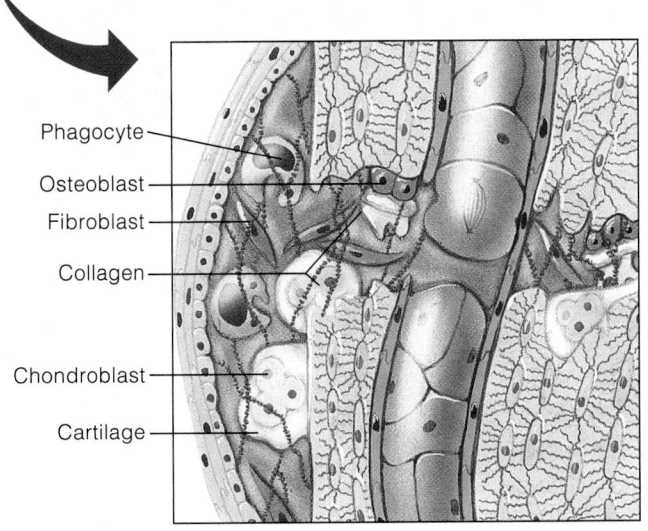

*(continued on page 1196)*

1195

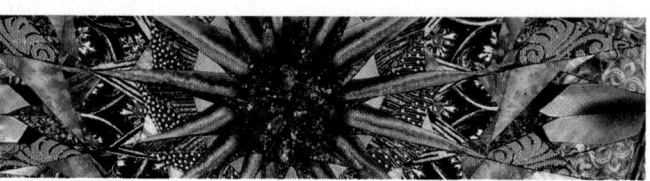

## 4. Bone Remodeling

Osteoblasts continue to form new woven bone, which is in turn organized into the lamellar structures of compact bone. Osteoclasts resorb excess callus as it is replaced by mature bone.

As the bone heals and is subjected to the mechanical stress of everyday use, osteoblasts and osteoclasts respond by remodeling the repair site along the lines of force. This ensures that the repaired section of bone eventually resembles the structure of the uninjured part.

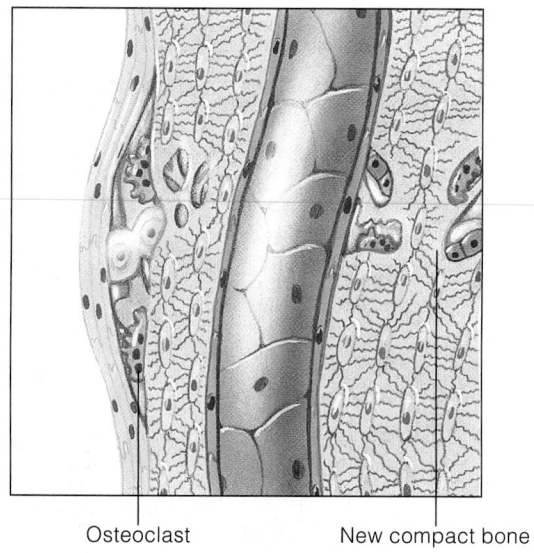

Osteoclast          New compact bone

## 3. Bony Callus Formation

Osteoblasts continue to proliferate and synthesize collagen fibers and bone matrix, which are gradually mineralized with calcium and mineral salts to form a spongey mass of woven bone. The trabeculae of woven bone bridge the fracture. Osteoclasts migrate to the repair site and begin removing excess bone in the callus. Bony callus formation usually continues for 2 to 3 months.

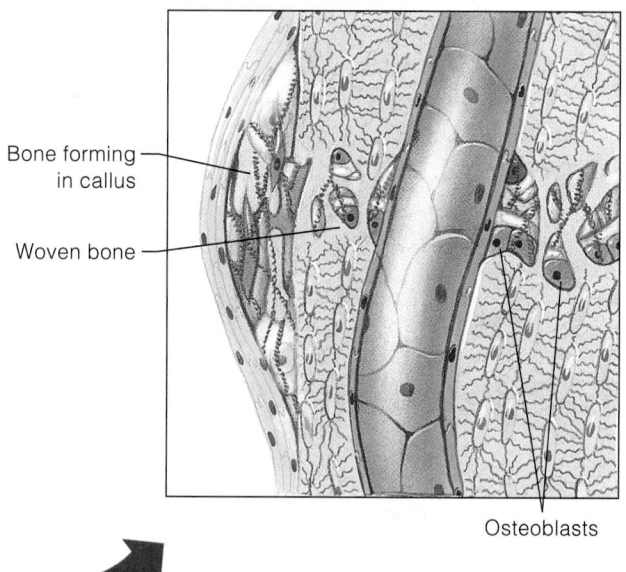

Bone forming in callus

Woven bone

Osteoblasts

## COLLABORATIVE CARE

A fracture requires treatment involving stabilizing the fractured bone(s), maintaining bone immobilization, preventing complications, and restoring function. The diagnosis of a fracture is primarily based on physical assessments and X-rays.

### Emergency Care

Emergency care of the client with a fracture includes immobilizing the fracture, maintaining tissue perfusion, and preventing infection. In the case of serious trauma, normal body alignment must be maintained and may involve cervical immobilization. Once the client is in a secure location, he or she is assessed for instability or deformity of the bone. If any deformity or instability is detected, the extremity is rapidly immobilized. Open wounds are covered with sterile dressings, and bleeding may be controlled with a pressure dressing. The extremities are assessed for the presence of pulses, movement, and sensation. The joint above and below the deformity is immobilized. Pulses, movement, and sensation are reevaluated after splinting.

The fracture is splinted to maintain normal anatomical alignment and prevent the fracture from dislocating. Splinting relieves pain and prevents further damage to the arteries, nerves, and bones. Splinting can be accomplished with air splints. If equipment is not available, the limb may be secured to the body. For example, an arm may be secured with a sling, or one leg may be strapped to the other leg.

### Diagnostic Tests

Diagnosis of a fracture begins with the history and initial assessment and usually is confirmed by radiographic tests. The following tests may be ordered:

- *X-rays* are commonly used to assess bones for fractures (Figure 38–2 ■).
- *Bone scan* may be necessary to determine if a fracture is present, indicated by an increased uptake, or a "hot spot."

- *Blood chemistry studies, complete blood count (CBC),* and *coagulation studies* may be used to assess blood loss, renal function, muscle breakdown, and the risk of excessive bleeding or clotting.

### Medications

Most clients with a fracture require pharmacologic interventions. The first and foremost intervention focuses on relieving pain. In the case of multiple fractures or fractures of large bones, narcotics are administered initially. As healing progresses, the client begins to take oral medication for pain. Pain management for the client with a fracture is described in Box 38–3.

Stool softeners may be administered to decrease the risk of constipation secondary to narcotics and immobility. Clients who have sustained trauma are often placed on antiulcer medications or antacids. NSAIDs may continue to be prescribed to decrease inflammation. Antibiotics may be administered prophylactically, particularly to clients with open or complex fractures. Anticoagulants may be prescribed to prevent deep vein thrombosis.

### Treatments

#### Surgery

Surgery is indicated in the client who has a fracture that requires direct visualization and repair, a fracture with common long-term complications, or a fracture that is severely comminuted and threatens vascular supply.

The simplest form of surgery is done by external fixation with an external fixator device. An external fixator consists of a frame connected to pins that are inserted perpendicular to the long axis of the bone (Figure 38–3 ■). The number of pins inserted varies with the type and site of the fracture, but in all cases the same number of pins is inserted above and below the fracture line. The pins require care similar to that of skeletal traction pins. The client is monitored for infection, and frequent neurovascular assessment is performed. The fixator increases independence while maintaining immobilization.

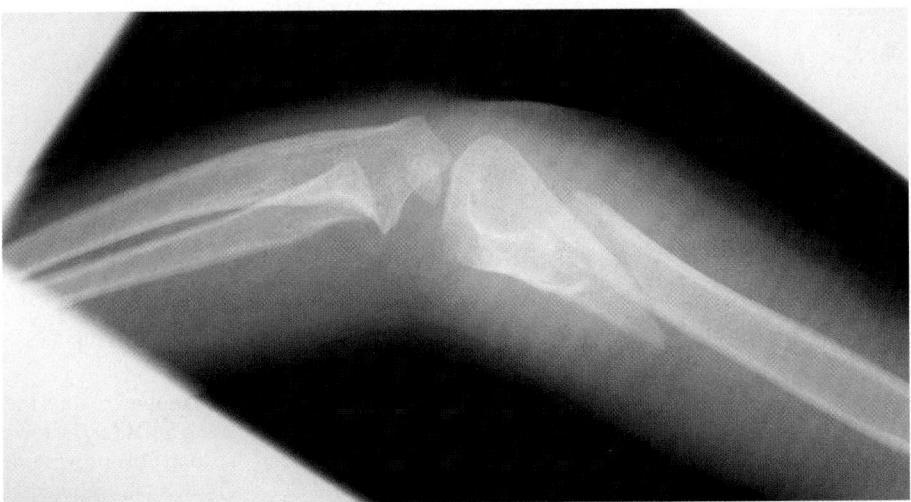

**Figure 38–2 ■** X-ray of an oblique fracture of the femur.

*Source: Charles Stewart and Associates.*

## BOX 38-3 ■ Pain Management in the Client with a Fracture

The client who has had musculoskeletal trauma from an accident or surgery experiences pain from many different causes:

- The interruption in the continuity of the bone itself
- Damage to ligaments and tendons
- Swelling of tissues around the trauma site
- Muscle spasms
- Tissue anoxia from swelling inside a cast, splint, or the muscle fascia sheath
- Hematoma formation
- Pressure over bony prominences from casts or splints

The pain is often severe and may be described as sharp, aching, or burning. Carefully assess any complaint of pain; pain may be an indication of a serious complication, such as compartment syndrome, decreased tissue perfusion and neurovascular impairment, or pressure ulcers. Do not administer analgesics until the location, character, and duration of pain has been carefully assessed. After the cause of the pain has been identified, the following nursing interventions may be implemented.

1. Administer prescribed analgesics, which may include NSAIDs and narcotic analgesics. For serious fractures or following orthopedic surgery, PCA or epidural methods of providing pain relief may be used. If medications are used on an as-needed

basis, tell the client to request the medication before the pain is severe; alternatively, offer the medications at regular intervals for the first 24 to 48 hours. Reassure the client that addiction does not result from taking medications to relieve fracture or surgical pain. Most clients require only oral analgesics by the third or fourth day after orthopedic surgery. Refer to Chapter 4 ⊂⊃ for information about narcotic and nonnarcotic pain medications.

2. Elevate the involved extremity, and apply cold (if prescribed) to help decrease swelling.
3. Monitor and drain the accumulated fluids in any drainage devices to ensure patency and to decrease the possibility of hematoma formation.
4. Encourage the client to wiggle fingers and toes on an extremity in a cast or traction to improve venous return and decrease edema.
5. Assist the client to change positions to relieve pressure and use pillows to provide support.
6. Teach the client alternative methods of pain management, such as relaxation and guided imagery.
7. Notify the physician of unrelieved pain, which may indicate a serious complication such as compartment syndrome or neurovascular impairment.

---

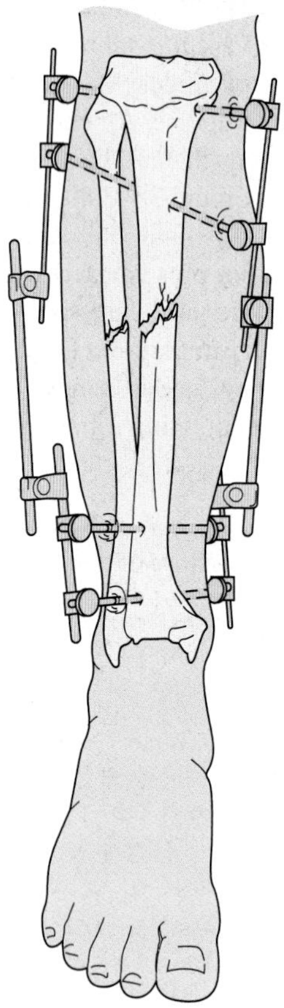

**Figure 38-3** ■ In external fixation, pins are placed through the bone above and below the fracture site to immobilize the bone. External fixation rods hold the pins in place.

Internal fixation can be accomplished through a surgical procedure called an *open reduction and internal fixation (ORIF)*. In this procedure, the fracture is reduced (placed in correct anatomic alignment) and nails, screws, plates, or pins are inserted to hold the bones in place (Figure 38-4 ■). Open fractures of the arms and legs are most commonly repaired in this way. Hip fractures in older clients are almost always repaired with ORIF to prevent complications and to allow early rehabilitation. Implications for postoperative nursing care are presented in Box 38-4.

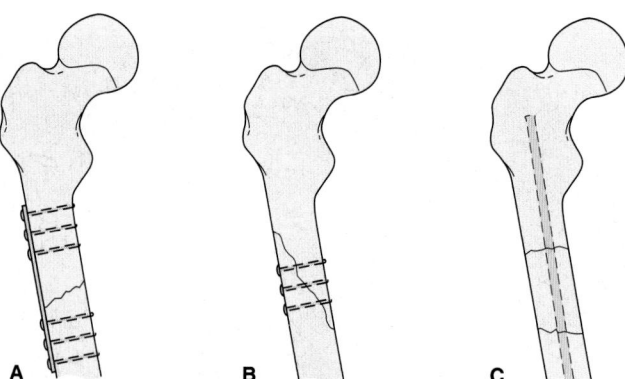

**Figure 38-4** ■ Internal fixation hardware is entirely within the body. *A,* Fixation of a short oblique fracture using a plate and screws above and below the fracture. *B,* Fixation of a long oblique fracture using screws through the fracture site. *C,* Fixation of a segmental fracture using a medullary nail.

| BOX 38–4 ■ Nursing Implications for Clients with Internal Fixation |
|---|

- Expect the client to have sutures and at least one Hemovac drain.
- Perform neurovascular assessments frequently.
- Also assess the following:
  a. Wounds for drainage
  b. Hemovac for drainage of serosanguineous fluid
  c. Bowel sounds
  d. Lung sounds

- Administer medications, such as analgesics and antibiotics, per physician's orders.
- In hip fractures, place an abductor pillow between client's legs to prevent dislocation of the hip joint.
- Arrange for physical and occupational therapy, as ordered.
- Assist with weight-bearing program, if ordered.
- Encourage early mobilization, coughing, and deep breathing, as appropriate, to help prevent complications.

## Traction

Muscle spasms usually accompany fractures and may pull bones out of alignment. **Traction** is the application of a straightening or pulling force to return or maintain the fractured bones in normal anatomic position. Weights are applied to maintain the necessary force. Types of traction are as follows:

- In **manual traction,** the hand directly applies the pulling force. Other common types of traction include straight traction, balanced suspension traction, skin traction, and skeletal traction (Figure 38–5 ■).
- **Straight traction** is a pulling force applied in a straight line to the injured body part resting on the bed. The most com-

mon type of straight traction is Buck's traction, in which the lower portion of the injured extremity is placed in a cradle-like sleeve. This sleeve is harnessed to itself, and a weight is hung from the bottom of a traction frame. The result is a force that pulls straight away from the body. This traction exerts its grabbing and pulling force through the client's skin. Therefore, this traction may be considered straight skin traction. The advantage of skin traction is the relative ease of use and ability to maintain comfort. The disadvantage is that the weight required to maintain normal body alignment or fracture alignment cannot exceed the tolerance of the skin, about 6 lb per extremity.

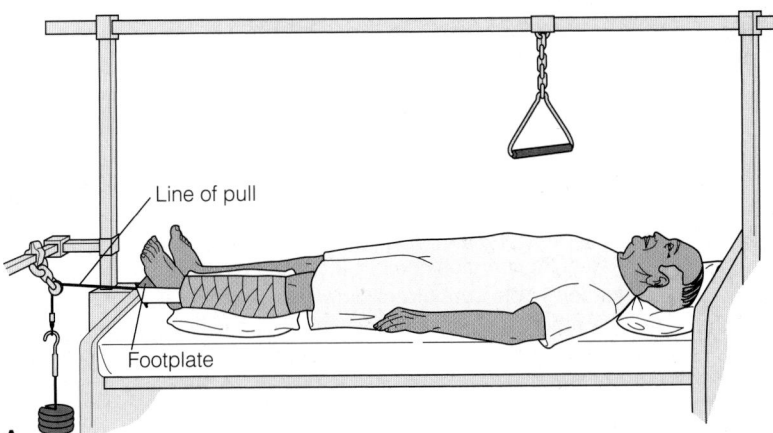

**Figure 38–5** ■ Traction is the application of a pulling force to maintain bone alignment during fracture healing. Different fractures require different types of traction. *A,* Skin traction (also called straight traction) such as Buck's traction shown here, is often used for hip fractures. *B,* Balanced suspension traction is commonly used for fractures of the femur. *C,* Skeletal traction, in which the pulling force is applied directly to the bone, may be used to treat fractures of the humerus.

Line of pull

Footplate

**A**

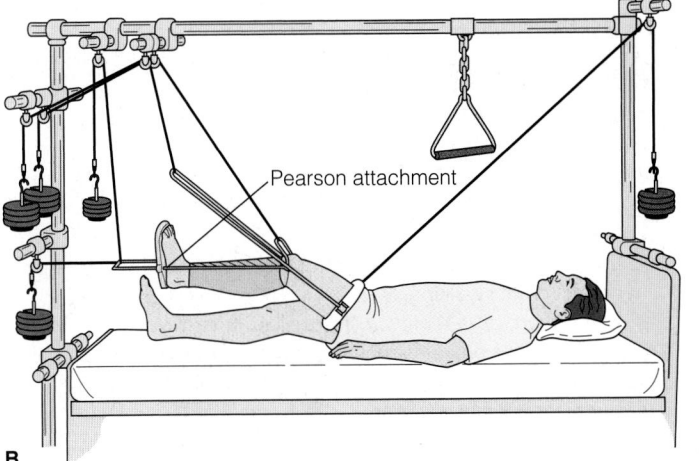

Pearson attachment

**B**

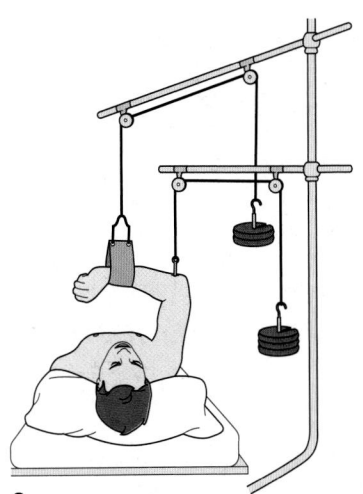

**C**

- **Balanced suspension traction** involves more than one force of pull. Several forces work in unison to raise and support the client's injured extremity off the bed and pull it in a straight fashion away from the body. The advantage of this type of traction is that it increases mobility without threatening joint continuity. The disadvantage is that the increased use of multiple weights makes the client more likely to slide in the bed.
- **Skeletal traction** is the application of a pulling force through placement of pins into the bone. The client receives local anesthetic, and the pin is inserted in a twisting motion into the bone. This type of traction must be applied under sterile conditions because of the increased risk of infection. One or more pulling forces may be applied with skeletal traction. The advantage of this type of traction is that more weight can be used to maintain the proper anatomic alignment if necessary. The disadvantages include increased anxiety, increased risk of infection, and increased discomfort. Nursing implications for clients receiving traction are presented in Box 38–5.

## Casts

A **cast** is a rigid device applied to immobilize the injured bones and promote healing. The cast is applied to immobilize the joint above and the joint below the fractured bone so that the bone will not move during healing. A fracture is first reduced manually and a cast is then applied. Casts are applied on clients who have relatively stable fractures

The cast, which may be composed of plaster or fiberglass, is applied over a thin cushion of padding and molded to the normal contour of the body. The cast must be allowed to dry before any pressure is applied to it; simply palpating a wet cast with the fingertips will leave dents that may cause pressure sores. A plaster cast may require up to 48 hours to dry, whereas a fiberglass cast dries in less than 1 hour. The type of cast applied is determined by the location of the fracture (Figure 38–6 ■). Nursing implications for clients with casts are discussed in the box below. During follow-up appointments, the physician may X-ray the bone to assess alignment and healing, and possibly remove the cast for skin assessment.

---

**BOX 38–5 ■ Nursing Implications for Clients Receiving Traction**

- In skeletal traction, never remove the weights.
- In skin traction, remove weights only when intermittent skin traction has been ordered to alleviate muscle spasm.
- For traction to be successful, a countertraction is necessary. In most instances, the countertraction is the client's weight. Therefore, do not wedge the client's foot or place it flush with the foot-board of the bed.
- Maintain the line of pull:
  a. Center the client on the bed.
  b. Ensure that weights hang freely and do not touch the floor.
- Ensure that nothing is lying on or obstructing the ropes. Do not allow the knots at the end of the rope to come into contact with the pulley.
- If a problem is detected, assist in repositioning. The area of the fracture must be stabilized when the client is repositioned.

- In skin traction:
  a. Frequently assess skin for evidence of pressure, shearing, or pending breakdown.
  b. Protect pressure sites with padding and protective dressings as indicated.
- In skeletal traction:
  a. Frequent skin assessments should include pin care per policy.
  b. Report signs of infection at the pin sites, such as redness, drainage, and increased tenderness.
  c. The client may require more frequent analgesic administration.
- Perform neurovascular assessments frequently.
- Assess for common complications of immobility, including formation of pressure ulcers, formation of renal calculi, deep vein thrombosis, pneumonia, paralytic ileus, and loss of appetite.
- Teach the client and family about the type and purpose of the traction.

---

# NURSING CARE OF THE CLIENT WITH A CAST

## NURSING RESPONSIBILITIES
- Perform frequent neurovascular assessments.
- Palpate the cast for "hot spots" that may indicate the presence of underlying infection.
- Report any drainage promptly.

## CLIENT AND FAMILY TEACHING
- Do not place any objects in the cast.
- If the cast is made of plaster, keep it dry.
- If the cast is made of fiberglass, dry it with a blow dryer on the cool setting if it becomes wet.
- Assess the injured extremity for coolness, changes in color, increased pain, increased swelling, and/or loss of sensation.

- Use a blow dryer on the cool setting to relieve itching by blowing cool air into the cast.
- If a sling is used, it should distribute the weight of the cast evenly around the neck. Do not roll the sling; this can impair circulation to the neck.
- If crutches are used, arrange for physical therapist to teach correct crutch walking.
- When the cast is removed, an oscillating cast remover will be used. A guard prevents the cast remover from penetrating past the depth of the cast, so it will not cut the client. It is noisy, and the client will feel vibration.

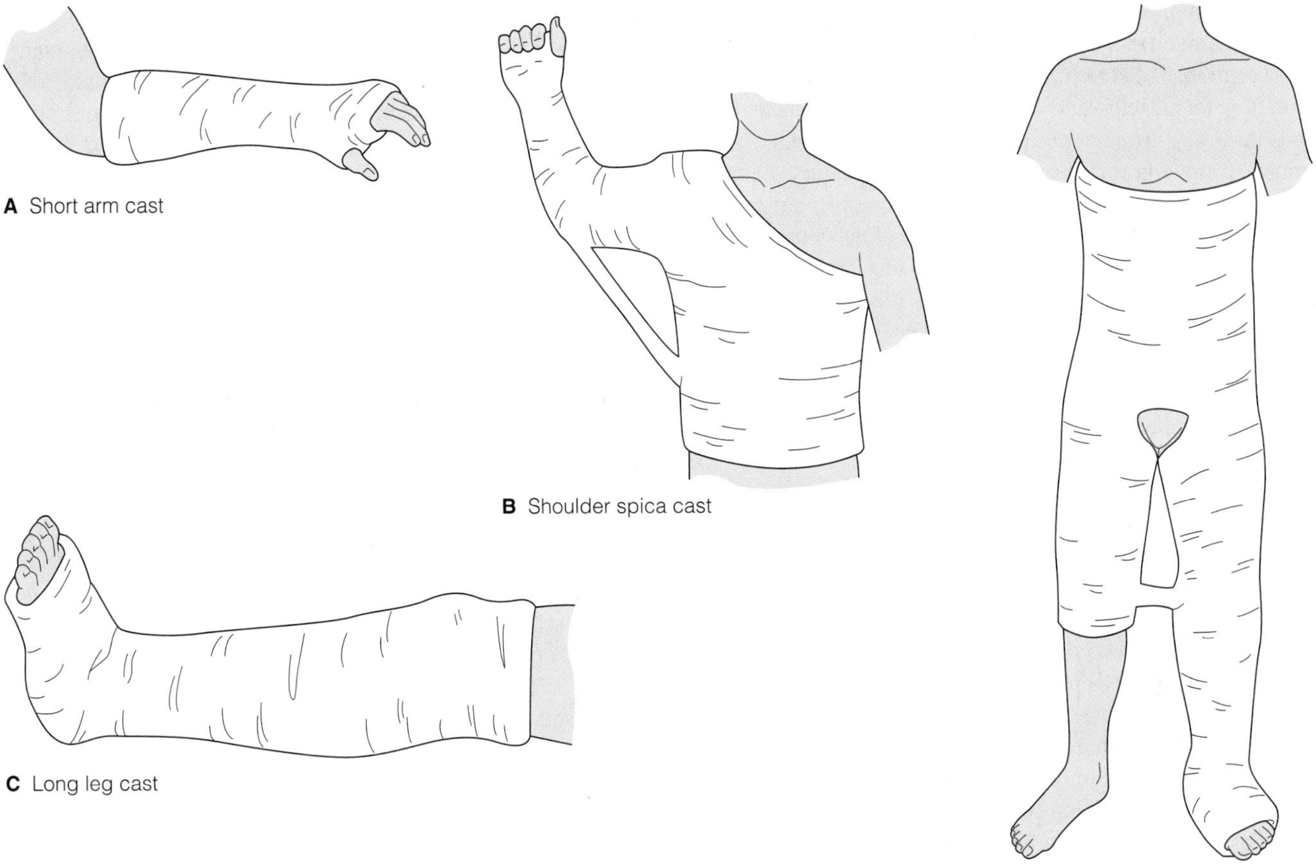

**A** Short arm cast

**B** Shoulder spica cast

**C** Long leg cast

**D** One-and-one half hip spica cast

**Figure 38–6** ■ Common types of casts used to immobilize fractures.

## Electrical Bone Stimulation

**Electrical bone stimulation** is the application of an electrical current at the fracture site. It is used to treat fractures that are not healing appropriately. The electrical stress increases the migration of osteoblasts and osteoclasts to the fracture site. Mineral deposition increases, promoting bone healing. Electrical bone stimulation can be accomplished invasively or noninvasively (Figure 38–7 ■). In invasive stimulation, the surgeon inserts a cathode and a lead wire at the fracture site. The lead wire is attached to an internal or external generator, which delivers electricity through the lead wire to the cathode 24 hours a day. In noninvasive inductive stimulation, a treatment coil encircles the cast or skin directly over the fracture site. The coil is attached to an external generator that runs on batteries. The electricity goes through the skin to the fracture site. The time period for external stimulation can vary from 3 to 10 hours per day. The client may be taught to self-administer the noninvasive electrical stimulation. Electrical bone stimulation is contraindicated in the presence of infection.

## Fracture Complications with Related Collaborative Care

Complications of musculoskeletal trauma are associated with pressure from edema and hemorrhage, development of fat emboli, deep vein thrombosis, infection, loss of skeletal integrity, or involvement of nerve fibers. Bone fragments may also result in further injury or complications.

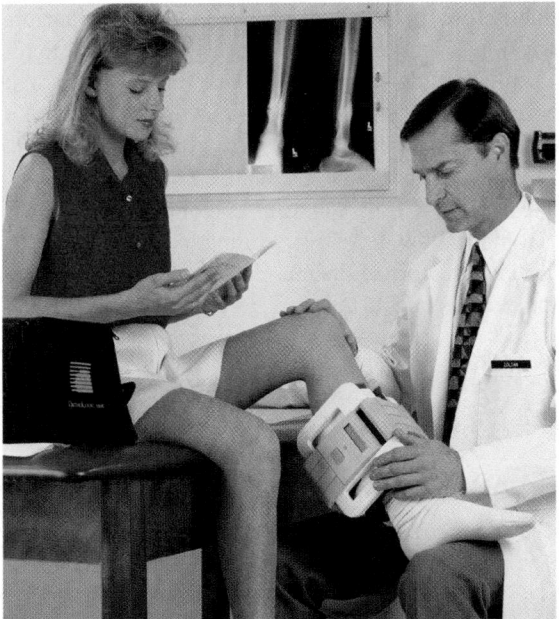

**Figure 38–7** ■ External electrical bone growth stimulator.

*Courtesy of Orthologic, Inc.*

## Compartment Syndrome

A compartment is a space enclosed by a fibrous membrane or fascia. The fascia lines the compartment within the limbs and is nonexpandable. Compartments within the limbs may enclose and support bones, nerves, and blood vessels. **Compartment syndrome** occurs when excess pressure in a limited space constricts the structures within a compartment, reducing circulation to muscles and nerves. Acute compartment syndrome may result from hemorrhage and edema within the compartment following a fracture or from a crush injury, or from external compression of the limb by a cast that is too tight. Increased pressure within the confined space of the compartment results in entrapment of nerves, blood vessels, and muscles.

Entrapment of the blood vessels limits tissue perfusion, beginning a cycle of events that may result in the loss of the limb. Inadequate oxygen supply causes cellular acidosis, which intensifies as cellular energy requirements are met through anaerobic metabolism. The capillaries inside the compartment dilate in an attempt to increase the supply of blood and oxygen. Additional blood and oxygen are not available, and plasma proteins leak out into the interstitial tissues. The interstitial tissue then pulls fluid in to balance the protein load. As a result, edema within the compartment increases. The edema causes further compression of the vascular network, and the cycle continues. Uninterrupted, this cycle threatens the client's limb and increases the risk of sepsis. Compartment syndrome usually develops within the first 48 hours of injury, when edema is at its peak. Manifestations of compartment syndrome are listed in the box below. It is important to note that arterial pulses may remain normal, even when pressure within the compartment is high enough to significantly impair tissue perfusion.

If compartment syndrome develops, interventions to alleviate pressure will be implemented; these may include removal of a tightly fitting cast. If the pressure is internal, a **fasciotomy,** a surgical intervention in which muscle fascia is cut to relieve pressure within the compartment, may be necessary. After a fasciotomy, the incision is left open, and passive ROM exercises are performed on the extremity.

Volkmann's contracture, a common complication of elbow fractures, can result from unresolved compartment syndrome. Arterial blood flow decreases, leading to ischemia, degeneration, and contracture of the muscle. Arm mobility is impaired, and the client is unable to completely extend the arm.

## Manifestations of Compartment Syndrome

### EARLY MANIFESTATIONS

- Pain
- Normal or decreased peripheral pulse

### LATER MANIFESTATIONS

- Cyanosis
- Tingling, loss of sensation (paresthesias)
- Weakness (paresis)
- Severe pain, especially when the extremity is passively flexed
- Eventual renal failure (due to release of myoglobin into the bloodstream; myoglobin molecule is too large for effective filtration and excretion by kidney and renal failure results)

## Fat Embolism Syndrome

Fat emboli occur when fat globules lodge in the pulmonary vascular bed or peripheral circulation. **Fat embolism syndrome (FES)** is characterized by neurologic dysfunction, pulmonary insufficiency, and a petechial rash on the chest, axilla, and upper arms. Long bone fractures and other major trauma are the principle risk factors for fat emboli; hip replacement surgery also poses a risk for FES.

When a bone is fractured, pressure within the bone marrow rises and exceeds capillary pressure; as a result, fat globules leave the bone marrow and enter the bloodstream. Another contributing factor may be the stress-induced release of catecholamine, which causes the rapid mobilization of fatty acids. Once the fat globules are released, they combine with platelets and travel to the brain, lungs, kidneys, and other organs, occluding small blood vessels and causing tissue ischemia.

Manifestations usually develop within a few hours to a week after injury. The manifestations result from the occlusion of the blood supply and the presence of fatty acids. Altered cerebral blood flow causes confusion and changes in level of consciousness. Pulmonary circulation may be disrupted, and free fatty acids damage the alveolar-capillary membrane. Pulmonary edema, impaired surfactant production, and atelectasis can result in significant respiratory insufficiency and manifestations of acute respiratory distress syndrome (ARDS) (see Chapter 36). Fat droplets activate the clotting cascade, causing thrombocytopenia. Petechiae (pin-sized purplish areas from bleeding under the skin) appearing on the skin, buccal membranes, and conjunctival sacs are thought to result from either microvascular clotting or the accompanying thrombocytopenia.

Early stabilization of long bone fractures is preventive for FES. Prompt identification and treatment of the syndrome are necessary to maintain adequate pulmonary function. In severe cases, the client may require intubation and mechanical ventilation to prevent hypoxia. Fluid balance is closely monitored. Corticosteroids may be administered to decrease the inflammatory response of lung tissues, stabilize lipid membranes, and reduce bronchospasm (Porth, 2002).

## Deep Vein Thrombosis

A **deep vein thrombosis (DVT)** is a blood clot that forms along the intimal lining of a large vein. Three precursors linked to DVT formation are (1) venous stasis, or decreased blood flow, (2) injury to blood vessel walls, and (3) altered blood coagulation (Table 38–2). Any or all of these precursors can cause a DVT to form. Damage to the lining of the vein causes the platelets to aggregate or clump together, forming the thrombus. Fibrin, WBCs, and RBCs begin to cling to the thrombus, and a tail forms. This tail or the entire thrombus may dislodge and move to the brain, lungs, or heart. Five percent of DVTs dislodge and enter the pulmonary circulation to form a pulmonary embolus. If the thrombus remains in the vein, venous insufficiency may result from scarring and valve damage.

The best treatment for DVT is prevention. Early immobilization of the fracture and early ambulation of the client are imperative. The extremity should be elevated above the level of

| TABLE 38–2 | Precursors of Deep Vein Thrombosis |
|---|---|
| **Precursor** | **Implications for Fractures** |
| Decreased blood flow | Common in fracture clients, who are immobilized and less active. Bed rest alone can decrease venous flow by 50%. |
| Injury to blood vessel wall | May occur as a direct result of the force that caused the fracture or from surgical manipulation. |
| Altered blood coagulation | May result from active blood loss. The body's attempt to maintain homeostasis leads to increased production of platelets and clotting factor. |

the heart. Frequent assessments of the injured extremity may lead to early recognition of DVT and prevent the formation of pulmonary embolus. Prophylactic anticoagulant administration is also beneficial. Antiembolism stockings and compression boots also increase venous return and prevent stasis of blood. Constrictive clothing should be avoided.

If a DVT is present, there may be swelling, leg pain, tenderness, or cramping. Not all clients experience manifestations, however. For this reason, diagnostic tests, such as a venogram or Doppler ultrasound of lower extremities, may be required. A venogram requires intravenous administration of dye in the radiology department, whereas a Doppler ultrasound study is noninvasive and can be performed at the client's bedside. Doppler ultrasonography uses sound waves to form an image on a computer screen.

The diagnosis of DVT requires rapid intervention. The client is placed on bed rest for 5 to 7 days to prevent dislodgment of the clot. Thrombolytic agents, which dissolve the clot, may be administered. Heparin may be administered intravenously to prevent more clots from forming. A vena cava filter may be placed to prevent the existing clot from entering the pulmonary circulation and forming a pulmonary embolus. In extreme cases in which anticoagulation therapy is contraindicated, a thrombectomy (surgical removal of the clot) may be necessary. See Chapter 33 ⟲ for further discussion of DVT.

### Infection

Infection is more likely to occur in an open fracture than a closed fracture, but any complication that decreases blood supply increases the risk of infection. Infection may result from contamination at the time of injury or during surgery. *Pseudomonas, Staphylococcus,* or *Clostridium* organisms may invade the wound or bone. *Clostridium* infection is particularly serious because it may lead to severe gas gangrene and cellulitis, but any infection may delay healing and result in **osteomyelitis,** infection within the bone that can lead to tissue death and necrosis. (See Chapter 39 for a discussion of osteomyelitis.)

### Delayed Union and Nonunion

**Delayed union** is the prolonged healing of bones beyond the usual time period. Many factors may inhibit bone healing, including poor nutrition, inadequate immobilization, prolonged reduction time, infection, necrosis, age, immunosuppression,

and severe bone trauma resulting in multiple fragments. Delayed union is diagnosed by means of serial X-ray studies. It is important to note that X-ray findings may lag 1 to 2 weeks behind the healing process; for example, a client may be completely healed by week 13, but this fact may not be apparent on the X-ray until week 14.

Delayed union may lead to **nonunion,** which can cause persistent pain and movement at the fracture site. Nonunion may require surgical interventions, such as internal fixation and bone grafting. If infection is present, the bones are surgically debrided. Electrical stimulation of the fracture site may be as effective as bone grafting.

### Reflex Sympathetic Dystrophy

**Reflex sympathetic dystrophy** may occur after musculoskeletal or nerve trauma. This term refers to a group of poorly understood posttraumatic conditions involving persistent pain, hyperesthesias, swelling, changes in skin color and texture, changes in temperature, and decreased motion. Diagnosis is made by the client's history and physical examination. X-rays may demonstrate spotty osteoporosis, and bone scans may reveal increased uptake of radionucleide. Treatment with a sympathetic nervous system blocking agent often alleviates the symptoms.

## Fractures of Specific Bones or Bony Areas

### Fracture of the Skull

The skull may be fractured as a result of either a fall or a direct blow. The client must be assessed for neurologic damage and any loss of consciousness must be documented. A complete neurologic assessment is conducted: Pupillary reaction to light, movement and strength of all extremities, complaints of nausea and vomiting, level of consciousness and orientation to person, place, and time are noted. A displaced skull fracture, which is referred to as depressed, may press on the brain and cause neurologic damage. Brain injuries related to skull fractures are discussed in Chapter 42. ⟲

### Fracture of the Face

Fracture of the facial bones may result from a direct blow. The client presents with hematomas, pain, edema, and bony deformity. Nondisplaced fractures are monitored to ensure the airway is not compromised. The client is observed for any neurologic deficits. Severely displaced or multiple facial fractures are treated with open reduction and internal fixation with wires or plates.

Nursing care focuses on maintaining the airway by helping the client clear secretions from the oropharynx. The nurse monitors the client's breathing for increased effort or tachypnea and notifies the physician immediately if these findings are noted. Pain is treated with analgesics, and body image disturbances are addressed. If the client asks to see his or her face, the nurse should plan to stay with the client and answer questions while the client looks in a mirror.

### Fracture of the Spine

The spine can be injured in many ways, including sports injuries, falls, and motor vehicle crashes. The spine can be fractured in the cervical, thoracic, lumbar, or sacral area. The most severe complication of spine fracture is injury to the spinal cord. A fracture to the vertebrae may cause the bones to become displaced and apply pressure on the spinal cord. This pressure on the spinal cord may result in permanent paralysis.

A nondisplaced cervical spinal fracture may be treated with a cervical collar or a halo immobilizing brace. The displaced cervical fracture is reduced by manual or skeletal traction and, eventually, application of a brace and/or surgical stabilization of the bones with plates and screws. Immobilization after a spinal fracture may last as long as 6 months. Chapter 41 ⊝ discusses spinal fractures and spinal cord injury.

## Fracture of the Clavicle

A fracture of the clavicle commonly results from a direct blow or a fall. The most common location is midclavicular. A person with a midclavicular fracture typically assumes a protective slumping position to immobilize the arm and prevent shoulder movement. A less common fracture occurs along the distal third of the clavicle. This type of fracture may be associated with ligament damage. Injuries to the clavicle may be associated with skull or cervical fractures. The fractured bone, if displaced, may lacerate the subclavian vessels and result in hemorrhage. The fractured bone may also puncture the lung, resulting in a pneumothorax. Malunion may occur at the fracture site and result in asymmetry of the clavicles. Injury to the brachial plexus may result in numbness and decreased movement of the arm on the affected side.

A deformity may be observed or palpated along the clavicle. Treatment focuses on immobilizing the fractured bone in normal anatomic position by applying a clavicular strap (Figure 38–8 ■), or a surgical repair may be necessary.

## Fracture of the Humerus

The exact location of the fracture, the presence of displacement, and the results of the neurovascular examination determine the severity of a fracture of the humerus and the appropriate interventions. Treatment focuses on immobilizing the fractured bone in normal anatomic position. Common complications of humeral fracture include nerve and ligament damage, frozen or stiff joints, and malunion. Early interventions and follow-up may prevent permanent damage.

Fractures of the proximal humerus are common in older adults. A simple nondisplaced fracture of the proximal humerus (near the humeral head) with a normal neurovascular assessment can be safely treated with immobilization. A more com-

plicated displaced fracture of the proximal humerus with bone fragmentation requires surgical intervention. The more severe the fracture and damage to soft tissue, the more likely the range of motion of the shoulder will be impaired. Rehabilitative measures focus on increasing ROM.

The humerus may also fracture along the shaft, usually as a direct result of trauma. If the humeral shaft fracture is simple and nondisplaced, a hanging arm cast is applied. This cast maintains alignment of the fracture by using the pulling force of gravity; therefore, the client must be instructed not to rest the cast on anything to alleviate the weight. If the client is on bed rest, a hanging arm cast is not applied, because the arm would not be able to hang freely. Instead, the fracture is immobilized with external skeletal traction. This traction places the injured arm in an upright position over the face, and weights are hung off the distal portion of the humerus (see Figure 38–6C). Nursing implications for clients with fractures of the humerus are presented in Box 38–6.

## Fracture of the Elbow

The most common location of an elbow fracture is the distal humerus. Elbow fractures usually result from a fall or direct blow to the elbow. The client guards the injured extremity, holding the arm rigidly in a flexed position or an extended position. Because the radius, ulna, or humerus may be involved in the elbow fracture, all three bones must be visualized by X-ray.

Complications of an elbow fracture include nerve or artery damage and **hemarthrosis,** a collection of blood in the elbow joint. The most serious complication of an elbow fracture is **Volkmann's contracture,** which results from arterial occlusion and muscle ischemia. The client complains of forearm pain, impaired sensation, and loss of motor function. Rapid interventions are aimed at relieving pressure on the brachial artery and nerve and preventing muscle atrophy.

Nondisplaced elbow fractures are treated by immobilizing the fracture with a posterior splint or cast. The displaced fracture is first reduced and then immobilized. Nursing interventions focus on alleviating pain, maintaining immobilization, and educating clients in neurovascular assessments.

| BOX 38–6 | ■ Nursing Implications for Clients with Fractures of the Humerus |
| --- | --- |

- Perform neurovascular assessments frequently.
- Administer prescribed medications to alleviate pain.
- Encourage exercises for clients with a hanging cast.
  a. Finger exercises: Move each finger of the affected arm through complete range of motion.
  b. Pendulum shoulder exercises: Dangle the affected arm at the side, and move it forward and backward about 30 degrees in each direction.
- If client is discharged, instruct the client and family in cast care and sling application, neurovascular assessments, exercises, prescribed pain medications, and manifestations of complications.
- If client is admitted to the hospital, provide pre-operative teaching.

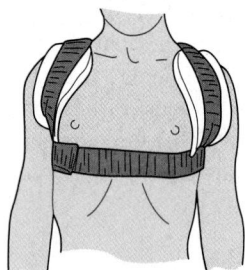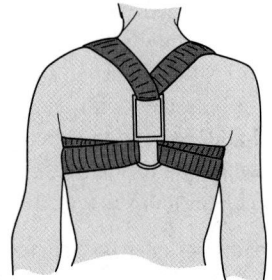

**Figure 38–8** ■ A clavicular strap is used to immobilize a clavicular fracture.

## Fracture of the Radius and/or Ulna

Fractures of the radius and ulna may occur as a result of either indirect injury, such as twisting or pulling on the arm, or direct injury, such as that resulting from a fall. The usual treatment of radius fractures depends on the location. The proximal radial head may be fractured from a fall on an outstretched hand. Blood commonly collects in the elbow joint and must be aspirated. If the fracture is nondisplaced, a sling is applied. If the fracture is displaced, surgical intervention is required. After surgical repair of a displaced fracture, the arm is splinted with a posterior plaster splint. The client avoids movement for the first week and then initiates movement gradually.

When both bones are broken, the fracture is usually displaced. The client complains of pain and inability to turn the palm of the hand up. A nondisplaced fracture is casted for about 6 weeks, and either a shorter cast or a brace is then applied for 6 more weeks. If the fracture is displaced, surgical intervention is performed. The physician reduces the fracture and may insert pins or screws to keep the bones in alignment. After the surgery, a cast is applied, and the client is encouraged to exercise the fingers.

Complications after a radius and/or ulnar fracture include compartment syndrome, delayed healing, and decreased wrist and finger movement. After surgery, the client also has an increased risk of infection. Nursing interventions focus on alleviating pain, maintaining immobilization, and educating clients in neurovascular assessments, the importance of elevation, and the need to inform the physician of changes in sensation or an increase in pain.

## Fractures in the Wrist and Hand

Wrist fractures often result from a fall onto an outstretched hand or onto the back of the hand. A common type of wrist fracture is **Colles's fracture,** in which the distal radius fractures after a fall onto an outstretched hand. The client with a wrist fracture presents with a bony deformity, pain, numbness, weakness, and decreased ROM of the fingers. The capillary refill and sensation of the hand must be assessed.

The hand is composed of many bones. Most commonly, the metacarpals and phalanges are involved in a hand fracture. The injuring mechanism in a hand fracture varies greatly from striking an object with a closed fist to closing a hand in a door. The client presents with complaints of pain, edema, and decreased ROM. The cause of the injury usually focuses the assessment on circulation, sensation, and ROM.

Comparative X-rays may be obtained to compare left and right wrists and hands. Complications of wrist and hand fractures are compartment syndrome, nerve damage, ligament damage, and delayed union. A wrist fracture is commonly treated with closed reduction, cast application, and elevation of the injured extremity. A hand fracture is splinted and elevated.

Nursing interventions focus on alleviating pain and educating the client in neurovascular assessments, the importance of elevation, and how to exercise the fingers to prevent stiffness. If the dominant hand is injured, the client will require assistance in performing ADLs.

## Fracture of the Ribs

Rib fractures commonly result from blunt chest trauma. The location of the fracture and involvement of underlying organs determine the severity of the injury. Fractures of the first through third ribs may result in injury to the subclavian artery or vein. Fractures of the lower ribs may result in spleen and liver injuries.

The client presents with a history of recent chest trauma. Typically, the client complains of pain along the lateral portion of the rib. Palpation of the rib reveals a bony deformity and increases pain. Deep inspiration also increases pain. The skin over the fracture site may be ecchymotic (bruised).

A complication of rib fractures is a **flail chest,** which results from the fracture of two or more adjacent ribs in two or more places and the formation of a free-floating segment that moves in the opposite direction of the rib cage. The bony instability impairs respirations (see Chapter 36). Treatment is aimed at stabilizing the flail segment and supporting respirations. Other complications of rib fractures include pneumothorax and/or hemothorax. The fractured rib may pierce the lung and injure it. The lower ribs may pierce the liver or spleen, resulting in intra-abdominal bleeding. Pneumonia may also develop from ineffective clearing of respiratory secretions.

A simple rib fracture is treated with pain medication and instructions for coughing, deep breathing, and splinting. The client is also instructed to return to the emergency room if shortness of breath develops. Nursing interventions focus on alleviating pain and teaching the client about splinting. Because deep inspiration increases pain, clients frequently avoid it. The client may be instructed to splint the injured rib with the hand or a pillow and take deep breaths and cough to decrease the chance of developing atelectasis. Incentive spirometry is encouraged.

## Fracture of the Pelvis

The client with a pelvic fracture presents with pain in the back or hip area. A single fracture in the pelvis is treated conservatively with bed rest on a firm mattress. Log rolling increases client comfort. A pelvic fracture with two fracture sites is considered unstable and treated with surgery. An external fixator may be applied to stabilize the pelvis. In the client who is not stable for surgery, a pelvic sling may be used. The pelvic sling stabilizes the pelvis and allows the client to move in bed with less pain. Common complications include hypovolemia, spinal injury, bladder injury, urethral injury, kidney damage, and gastrointestinal trauma.

Nursing care focuses on alleviating discomfort, maintaining immobilization, and preparing the client for surgery if necessary. The nurse monitors the client for increased heart rate, decreased blood pressure, and decreasing hemoglobin levels. These findings may indicate impending hypovolemia due to bleeding into the pelvis. Any blood in the urine should be reported to the physician; this may indicate kidney, bladder, or urethral damage.

## Fracture of the Shaft of the Femur

A large amount of force, such as from motor vehicle crashes, falls, or acts of violence, is required to fracture the shaft of the femur. Clients with femoral shaft fractures often have associated multiple trauma. A fracture of the femoral shaft is manifested by an edematous, deformed, painful thigh. The client is unable to move the hip or knee. Initial assessment focuses on the circulation and sensation present in the affected extremity. Pedal pulses and capillary refill in the affected extremity are compared to the unaffected extremity. Complications of a femoral shaft fracture include hypovolemia due to blood loss (which may be as great as 1.0 to 1.5 L), fat embolism, dislocation of the hip or knee, muscle atrophy, and ligament damage.

Treatment of fractures of the shaft of the femur initially includes skeletal traction to separate the bony fragments and reduce and immobilize the fracture. Depending on the location and severity of the fracture, traction may be followed by either external or internal fixation. Strength in the affected extremity is maintained through gluteal and quadricep exercises. ROM exercises for unaffected extremities are critical in preparation for ambulation. Although full weight bearing is usually restricted until X-rays demonstrate bone union, the client may be allowed to carry out non-weight-bearing activities with an assistive device.

The nurse assesses pulses in the extremity and compares them bilaterally. Sensation is evaluated by asking whether the client can feel touch and discriminate sharp from dull objects. Nursing interventions include providing pain medication, providing reassurance and decreasing anxiety, and assisting with exercises of the lower legs, feet, and toes.

### Fracture of the Hip

A hip fracture refers to a fracture of the femur at the head, neck, or trochanteric regions (Figure 38–9 ■). Hip fractures are classified as intracapsular or extracapsular. **Intracapsular fractures** involve the head or neck of the femur; **extracapsular fractures** involve the trochanteric region. The majority of hip fractures involve the neck or trochanteric regions. The femoral head and neck lie within the joint capsule and are not covered

in periosteum; thus, they do not have a large blood supply. Fractures here usually fragment and may further decrease blood supply, increasing the risk of nonunion and avascular necrosis. The trochanteric region is covered in periosteum and therefore has more blood supply than the head or neck.

Hip fractures are a significant problem, causing the greatest number of deaths and most serious health problems of all fractures. Most are the result of falls, which account for 87% of all fractures for people 65 years or older (CDC, 2000). Statistics for hip fractures include the following:

- Approximately 75% to 80% of hip fractures are sustained by postmenopausal women, who have the highest incidence of osteoporosis.
- Most people with hip fractures are hospitalized for 2 weeks.
- Half of all older adults hospitalized for a hip fracture cannot return home or live independently after the fracture.
- By the year 2040, the number of hip fractures is expected to exceed 500,000, which reflects society's increasing older population. Factors contributing to falls include problems with gait and balance, neurological and musculoskeletal impairments, dementia, psychoactive medications, and visual impairments.

Hip fractures are common in older adults as a result of decreases in bone mass and the increased tendency to fall. Whether the femur breaks spontaneously and causes the fall or whether the fall causes the fracture is not always clear; regardless of the cause of the fracture, however, rapid interventions are required to prevent bone necrosis. Assessment findings commonly associated with a hip fracture are pain, shortening of the affected lower extremity, and external rotation. Rarely, the fracture dislocates posteriorly; if that occurs, the extremity may internally rotate.

A hip fracture may be treated with traction to decrease muscle spasms, followed by surgery; or surgery may be performed

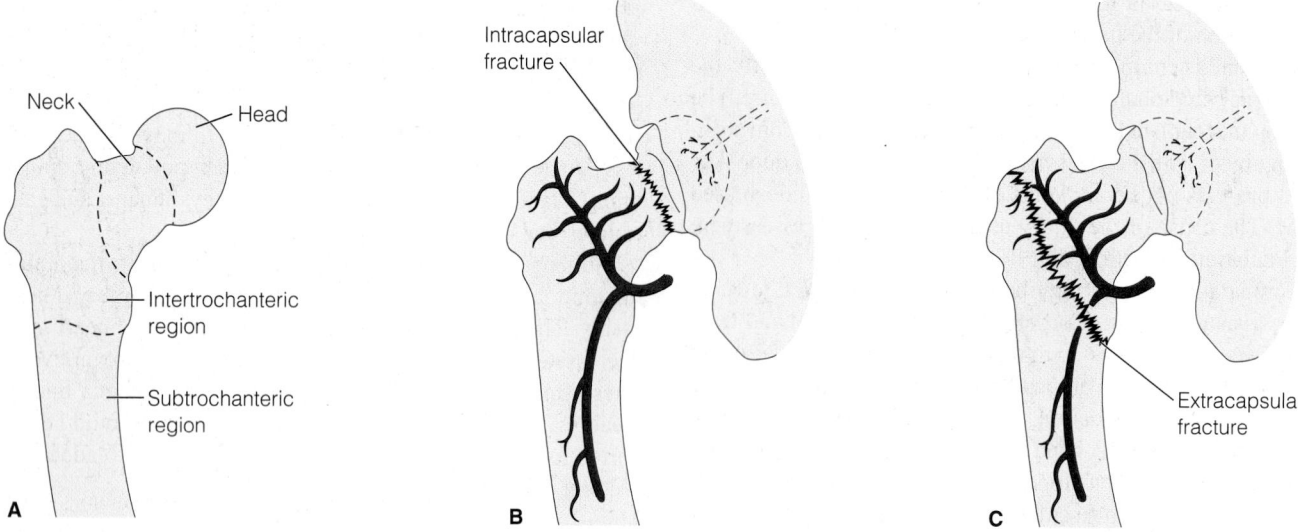

**Figure 38–9** ■ *A,* Regions where hip fractures may occur: the head of the femur, the neck of the femur, and the trochanteric regions of the femur. *B,* Intracapsular fractures occur across the head or neck of the femur. *C,* Extracapsular fractures occur across the trochanteric regions. Note how both intracapsular and extracapsular fractures disrupt the blood supply to the bone.

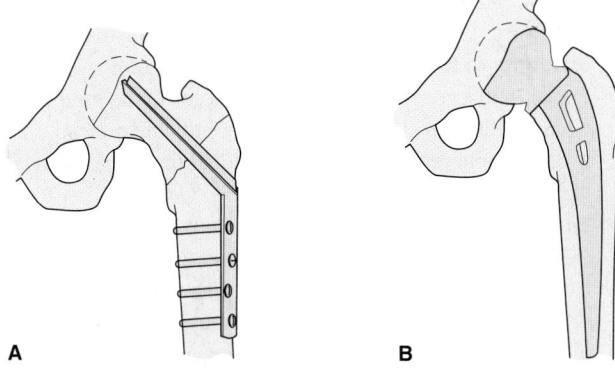

**Figure 38–10** ■ Surgical fixation of hip fractures. *A*, A surgical nail or screw used to stabilize an intertrochanteric fracture. *B*, Use of a hip prosthesis (artificial hip) to replace a damaged femoral head.

immediately or within the first 24 hours. The goal of surgery is to reduce and stabilize the fracture, thereby increasing mobility, decreasing pain, and preventing complications. Surgery usually consists of open reduction and internal fixation of the fracture. Fixation is accomplished by securing the femur in place with pins, screws, nails, or plates (Figure 38–10A ■). An open reduction and internal fixation works well for fractures in the trochanteric area. Fractures of the femoral neck frequently disrupt blood supply to the femoral head. If blood supply is disrupted, the surgeon will replace the femoral head with a prosthesis (Figure 38–10B). If the acetabulum has been damaged, the surgeon may insert a metal cup. Replacement of either the femoral head or the acetabulum with a prosthesis is called a hemiarthroplasty. Replacement of both the femoral head and the acetabulum is a total hip arthroplasty (THA), discussed in Chapter 39. Nursing care focuses on alleviating pain, maintaining circulation to the injured extremity, and increasing mobility.

### Fracture of the Tibia and/or Fibula

Fractures of the lower extremities often result from a fall on a flexed foot, a direct blow, or a twisting motion. The client presents with edema, pain, bony deformity, and a hematoma at the level of injury.

Circulation and sensation are assessed to rule out common complications of the fracture, including damage to the peroneal nerve or tibial artery, compartment syndrome, hemarthroses, and ligament damage. Peroneal nerve damage may be indicated by the client's inability to point the toe on the affected side upward. Tibial artery damage may be the cause of an absent dorsalis pedis pulse on the affected side. Compartment syndrome may be present if the client develops pain on passive movement and paresthesias. An edematous knee may indicate a collection of blood in the knee joint. Ligament damage may be present if the client cannot move the knee and/or ankle.

If the fracture is closed, a closed reduction and casting are frequently performed. A long leg cast that allows for partial weight bearing is used. Partial weight bearing usually is prescribed by the physician within 10 days of the fracture. A short leg cast will be applied in 3 to 4 weeks. If the fracture is open, either external fixation or open reduction and internal fixation

will be performed. After surgery, a cast may be applied, and weight bearing begins according to the physician's orders, usually in about 6 weeks.

Nursing care is designed to increase comfort, monitor neurovascular status, and prevent complications. The nurse instructs the client in cast care, the use of assistive devices, how to perform neurovascular assessment, and when to follow up with the physician.

### Fracture in the Ankle and Foot

The client with an ankle fracture presents with pain, limited ROM, hematoma, edema, and difficulty ambulating. Most ankle fractures are treated by closed reduction and casting. Open fractures are treated by surgical intervention and splinting.

The client with a foot fracture presents with similar symptoms; however, range of motion of the ankle is not usually affected. Most foot fractures are nondisplaced and treated with closed reduction and casting. More severe displaced foot fractures may require surgery and the placement of wires to maintain reduction of the fracture.

Nursing care focuses on increasing comfort, increasing mobility, and educating the client. Analgesia is given for pain. The extremity should be elevated, and ice can be applied. The client is taught cast care, neurovascular assessment, and crutch walking.

## NURSING CARE

In planning and implementing nursing care for the client with fractures, the nurse should consider the client's response to the traumatic experience. Although each client has individual needs, nursing care commonly focuses on client problems with pain, impaired physical mobility, impaired tissue perfusion, and neurovascular compromise.

### Health Promotion

Trauma prevention can save lives. Many communities are educating people of all ages, from grade-schoolers to older adults, in trauma prevention. Young adults face a high risk of sustaining trauma. They need to be taught the importance of safety equipment—such as automobile seat belts, bicycle helmets, football pads, proper footwear, protective eyewear, and hard hats—in preventing or decreasing the severity of injury from trauma. Older adults should have regular screenings for osteoporosis, activity levels, cognitive and affective disorders, sensory impairments, and risk for falls. Educational programs about workplace and farm safety, including information about ergonomic principles, can also help prevent musculoskeletal injuries.

Having a regular exercise program and avoiding obesity are important factors in maintaining good bone health in all adults. An adequate intake of calcium is essential to ensure proper growth, development, and maintenance of strong bones throughout life. It is important that women ensure good bone health prior to menopause, as the loss of estrogen during and after menopause decreases calcium use. Strong bones are formed by calcium intake and weight-bearing exercise, both of which are equally important in the postmenopausal woman.

## Meeting Individualized Needs

### TEACHING OLDER ADULTS TO PREVENT FALLS

- Begin a regular exercise program; lack of exercise leads to weakness and an increased chance of falling. Exercises that improve balance and coordination (such as tai chi) are the most helpful.
- Make your home safer:
  - Remove any items in your pathway, including from stairs, to avoid tripping.
  - Remove small throw rugs or use double-sided tape to keep rugs from slipping.
  - Place frequently used items within easy reach to avoid use of a step stool.
  - Install grab bars next to your toilet and in the tub or shower.
  - Use nonslip mats in the bathtub and on shower floors.
  - Improve lighting, using lamp shades or frosted bulbs to reduce glare.
  - Install handrails and lights in all staircases.
  - Wear shoes that give good support and have thin, nonslip soles. Avoid wearing slippers and athletic shoes with deep treads.
- Ask your health care provider to review your medications, including prescriptions and over-the-counter medications. Some medications or a combination of medications may cause dizziness or drowsiness, leading to falls.
- Have your vision checked by an eye doctor. Your glasses may no longer have the correct prescription, or you may have developed an eye condition such as cataracts or glaucoma that limits your vision.

Note. Adapted from *Preventing Falls Among Seniors* by Centers for Disease Control & Prevention, National Center for Injury Prevention & Control, 2002. Available www.cdc.gov/ncipc/duip/spotlite/falltips.htm

Older clients are at higher risk for musculoskeletal trauma due to falls. For these clients, home assessments must be performed and potential hazards removed. Specific teaching topics for preventing falls in older adults are outlined in the box above.

## Assessment

Collect the following data through the health history and physical examination (see Chapter 37).

- Health history: age, history of traumatic event, history of chronic illnesses, history of prior musculoskeletal injuries, medications (ask the older adult specifically about anticoagulants)
- Physical assessment: pain with movement, pulses, edema, skin color and temperature, deformity, range of motion, touch (These assessments include the five Ps of neurovascular assessment, as follows, included in both the initial assessment and ongoing focused assessments.)
  - *Pain.* Assess pain in the injured extremity by asking the client to grade it on a scale of 0 to 10, with 10 as the most severe pain.

- *Pulses.* Assess distal pulses beginning with the unaffected extremity. Compare the quality of pulses in the affected extremity to those of the unaffected extremity.
- *Pallor.* Observe for pallor and skin color in the injured extremity. Paleness and coolness may indicate arterial compromise, whereas warmth and a bluish tinge may indicate venous blood pooling.
- *Paralysis/Paresis.* Assess ability to move body parts distal to the fracture site. Inability to move indicates paralysis. Loss of muscle strength (weakness) when moving is paresis. A finding of limited range of motion may lead to early recognition of problems such as nerve damage and paralysis.
- *Paresthesia.* Ask the client if any change in sensation (paresthesia) has occurred.

## Nursing Diagnoses and Interventions

Nursing care for clients with fractures ranges from teaching for home care treatments provided in the emergency or urgent care department (such as manual reduction and cast application) to providing interventions to maintain health and decrease the risk of complications in clients with complex or multiple fractures. Teaching is also necessary for caregivers of the older adult who is discharged home or to a long-term care or rehabilitation facility following a fractured hip.

### Acute Pain

Pain is caused by soft tissue damage and is compounded by muscle spasms and swelling.

- Monitor vital signs. *Some analgesics decrease respiratory effort and blood pressure.*
- Ask the client to rate the pain on a scale of 0 to 10 (with 10 as the most severe pain) before and after any intervention. *This facilitates objective assessment of the effectiveness of the chosen pain relief strategy. Pain that increases in intensity or remains unrelieved with analgesics can indicate compartment syndrome.*
- For the client with a hip fracture, apply Buck's traction per physician's orders. *Buck's traction immobilizes the fracture and decreases pain and additional trauma.*
- Move the client gently and slowly. *Gentle moving helps to prevent the development of severe muscle spasms.*

**PRACTICE ALERT**  *Supporting the extremity above and below the fracture (in the case of fracture in an extremity) can also decrease pain and muscle spasms.* ■

- Elevate the injured extremity above the level of the heart. *Elevating the extremity promotes venous return and decreases edema, which decreases pain.*
- Encourage distraction or other noninvasive methods of pain relief, such as deep breathing and relaxation. *Distraction, deep breathing, and relaxation help decrease the focus on the pain and may lessen the intensity of pain.*
- Administer pain medications as prescribed. For home care, explain the importance of taking pain medications before the pain is severe. *Analgesics alleviate pain by stimulating opiate receptor sites.*

## Risk for Peripheral Neurovascular Dysfunction

In the client with a fracture, compartment syndrome or deep vein thrombosis can impair circulation and, in turn, tissue perfusion.

- Assess the five Ps every 1 to 2 hours. Report abnormal findings immediately. *Unrelenting pain, pallor, diminished distal pulses, paresthesias, and paresis are strong indicators of compartment syndrome.*

**PRACTICE ALERT** *Pulses may remain strong, even in the presence of compartment syndrome.* ■

- Assess nailbeds for capillary refill. *Delayed capillary refill may indicate decreased tissue perfusion.*

**PRACTICE ALERT** *It may not be possible to accurately assess capillary refill in older adults who often have thickened, discolored nails. If so, test nearby skin.* ■

- Monitor the extremity for edema and swelling. *Excessive swelling and hematoma formation can compromise circulation.*
- Assess for deep, throbbing, unrelenting pain. *Pain that is not relieved by analgesics may indicate neurovascular compromise.*
- Assess the tightness of the cast. *Edema can cause the cast to become tight; a tight-fitting cast may lead to compartment syndrome or paralysis.*
- If cast is tight, be prepared to assist the physician with **bivalving** (Figure 38–11 ■). *Bivalving, the process of splitting the cast down both sides, alleviates pressure on the injured extremity.*

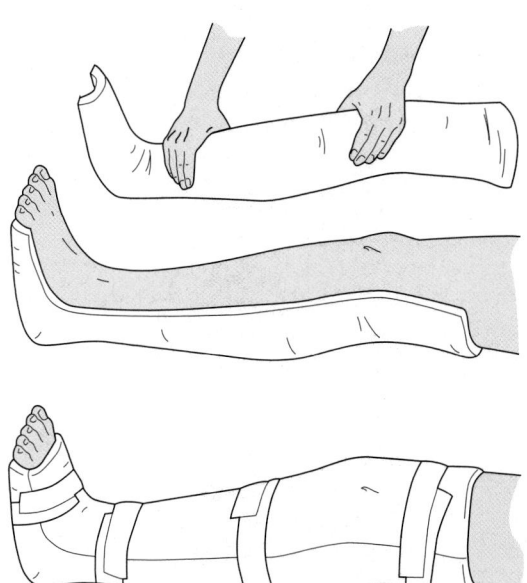

**Figure 38–11** ■ Bivalving is the process of splitting the cast down both sides to alleviate pressure on or allow visualization of the extremity.

- If compartment syndrome is suspected, assist the physician in measuring compartment pressure. Normal compartment pressure is 10 to 20 mmHg. *Compartment pressure greater than 30 mmHg indicates compartment syndrome.*
- Elevate the injured extremity above level of the heart. *Elevating the extremity increases venous return and decreases edema.*
- Administer anticoagulant per physician's order. *Prophylactic anticoagulation decreases the risk of clot formation.*

## Risk for Infection

The client who undergoes surgical repair will have a postoperative wound. Any break in skin integrity must be monitored for infection.

- Monitor vital signs and lab reports of WBCs. *Increases in pulse rate, respiratory rate, temperature, and WBCs may indicate infection.*
- Use sterile technique for dressing changes. *The initial postoperative dressing will be changed by the surgeon. The nurse must change all subsequent dressings without introducing organisms into the operative site.*
- Assess the wound for size, color, and the presence of any drainage. *Redness, swelling, and purulent drainage indicate infection.*
- Administer antibiotics per physician's orders. *Short-term prophylactic antibiotic administration inhibits bacterial reproduction and thereby helps prevent skin flora from entering the wound. Antibiotics are usually only administered for 24 hours.*

## Impaired Physical Mobility

The client who has experienced a fracture requires immobilization of the fractured bone(s). Immobilization alters normal gait and mobility. The client will need to use assistive devices such as crutches, canes, slings, or walkers.

- Teach or assist client with ROM exercises of the unaffected limbs. *ROM exercises help prevent muscle atrophy and maintain strength and joint function. Flexion and extension exercises prevent the development of foot drop, wrist drop, or frozen joints.*
- Teach isometric exercises, and encourage the client to perform them every 4 hours. *Isometric exercises help prevent muscle atrophy and force synovial fluid and nutrients into the cartilage.*
- Encourage ambulation when able; provide assistance as necessary. *Ambulation maintains and improves circulation, helps prevent muscle atrophy, and helps maintain bowel function*
- Teach and observe the client's use of assistive devices (such as canes, crutches, walkers, slings) in conjunction with the physical therapist. *Proper use of devices is necessary for safe ambulation and helps prevent the loss of joint function secondary to complications and falls.*
- Turn the client on bed rest every 2 hours. If the client is in traction, teach the client to shift his or her weight every hour. *Turning and shifting weight increase circulation and help prevent skin breakdown.*

## Risk for Disturbed Sensory Perception: Tactile

The client who has sustained a fracture is at risk for nerve injury from the initial trauma, as well as from complications such as compartment syndrome.

- Assess the ability to differentiate between sharp and dull touch and the presence of paresthesias and paralysis every 1 to 2 hours. *Paresthesias develop as a result of pressure on nerves and may indicate compartment syndrome.*

**PRACTICE ALERT** *Paralysis is a late sign of nerve entrapment and requires that the physician be notified immediately.* ■

- Elevate the injured extremity above the level of the heart. *Elevating the extremity decreases swelling and the risk of compartment syndrome and nerve entrapment.* Check the cast for fit. *A tightly fitting cast can decrease blood flow to distal tissues, compress nerves, and cause compartment syndrome.*
- Support the injured extremity above and below the fracture site when moving the client. *Supporting the injured extremity above and below the fracture site helps prevent displacement of bony fragments and decreases the risk of further nerve damage.*

## Using NANDA, NIC and NOC

Chart 38–1 shows links between NANDA nursing diagnosis, NIC, and NOC when caring for the client with a compound fracture.

## Home Care

Client and family teaching focuses on individualized needs. The type of fracture and its location determine how much teaching the client and family will require. For example, a client who has a simple nondisplaced tibial fracture may need to be taught only cast care and crutch walking. An older client who has sustained a hip fracture and requires surgical intervention, by contrast, has a wider array of teaching needs, including the use of an abduction pillow, proper bending, and proper sitting. Address the following topics for home care of the client who has fractured a hip.

- Encourage independence in ADLs (see the Nursing Research box on page 1211 for research in this area).
- Explain that the client should sit only on high chairs to prevent excess flexion of the hip; a high toilet seat can be added to a regular toilet seat.
- Encourage the client and family to equip the shower with a rail to aid stability and prevent falls.
- If a walker is needed, teach the client its proper use: Do not carry the walker, but lift it, advance it, and then take two steps, or use a rolling walker.
- If a cane is needed, instruct the client to use it on the affected side.
- Stress the importance of well-balanced meals, and explain all prescribed medications.

Clients who have experienced a fracture or who have had orthopedic surgery often require an extended period of immobilization or limited activities. Address the following topics for home care.

## CHART 38–1 NANDA, NIC, AND NOC LINKAGES

### The Client with a Compound Fracture

| NURSING DIAGNOSES | NURSING INTERVENTIONS | NURSING OUTCOMES |
|---|---|---|
| • Risk for Infection | • Infection Protection<br>• Wound Care | • Infection Status |
| • Acute Pain | • Analgesic Administration<br>• Heat/Cold Application<br>• Pain Management<br>• Simple Relaxation Therapy | • Comfort Level<br>• Symptom Severity |
| • Impaired Physical Mobility | • Exercise Promotion<br>• Self-Care Assistance<br>• Teaching: Prescribed Activity/Exercise<br>• Traction/Immobilization Care<br>• Cast Care: Wet<br>• Cast Care: Maintenance | • Mobility Level<br>• Self-Care: ADLs |
| • Risk for Peripheral Neurovascular Dysfunction | • Peripheral Sensation Management<br>• Circulatory Precautions<br>• Cast Care<br>• Embolus Precautions | • Circulation Status<br>• Neurologic Status<br>• Tissue Perfusion: Peripheral |

*Note. Data from Nursing Outcomes Classification (NOC) by M. Johnson & M. Maas (Eds.), 1997, St. Louis: Mosby; Nursing Diagnoses: Definitions & Classification 2001–2002 by North American Nursing Diagnosis Association, 2001, Philadelphia: NANDA; Nursing Interventions Classification (NIC) by J.C. McCloskey & G. M. Bulechek (Eds.), 2000, St. Louis: Mosby. Reprinted by permission.*

## Nursing Research

### Evidence-Based Practice for Care of the Older Adult with a Hip Fracture

Fracture of the hip often results in loss of independence and long-term disability. Postoperatively, helping the client regain independence in performing activities of daily living (ADLs) is a nursing care priority that often is inhibited by diminished cognitive status of the client. This study (Milisen, Abraham, & Broos, 1998) looked at the incidence of impaired cognition, its evolution, and its effects on functional status in 26 elderly clients with hip fracture. Nineteen of the 26 clients demonstrated some degree of cognitive impairment before and/or after surgery. The highest incidence of impaired cognition was seen during the postoperative period, with memory and psychomotor skills affected to the greatest degree. Additionally, clients with decreased cognition postoperatively remained more ADL-dependent than nonimpaired clients.

#### IMPLICATIONS FOR NURSING

Teaching and promoting independence in ADLs are important nursing care priorities for the client who experiences a fractured hip. However, the client who is cognitively impaired does not learn as effectively and is less able to regain the ability to independently perform ADLs following hip fracture. This study points out the importance of assessing the cognitive status of clients before and after surgery and using this information in planning nursing care activities. Nurses and other health care providers need to promote recovery in long-term care facilities as well as

more effectively meet clients' needs in the home and community. In all settings, nurses must collaborate with other nurses and with other members of the health care team to facilitate continuity of care, teaching, and rehabilitation. Teaching for clients with memory impairment needs to be very focused, presented in brief sessions, and repeatedly reinforced. Despite all best efforts, it may be unrealistic to expect some clients to resume independent function in performing ADLs, at least during the initial postoperative period.

#### Critical Thinking in Client Care

1. Many people believe that a broken hip signals the onset of an older adult's decline until death. How can nurses change this perception?
2. If your client is an older adult who lives alone and has no available caregivers, what community resources can you recommend to provide care until independence is regained?
3. What factors do you think contribute to impaired cognition in the older adult who experiences a hip fracture and surgical stabilization or replacement?
4. You are caring for an 84-year-old woman with a fractured hip who is being discharged to a long-term care facility. She begins to cry and says, "I know I will die there; please don't let them send me there." What would you say to her?

---

- Do not try to scratch under a cast with a sharp object.
- Do not get a plaster cast wet.
- Follow the physician's order for weight bearing.
- Physical therapy departments or offices often can evaluate the home environment for safety and suggest modifications as needed. Physical therapists also teach crutch walking, limited weight bearing, transferring, and other activities.
- Home care agencies can teach wound care and provide ongoing monitoring of wound healing.
- Local medical equipment and supply sources rent or sell durable equipment such as crutches, walkers, wheelchairs, overhead trapeze units, shower chairs, elevated toilet seats, grab bars, and bedside commodes. Slings or braces may be purchased through medical equipment dealers.
- Local pharmacies are good resources for dressing supplies such as antiseptic solutions or ointments, dressings, and tape.
- Fitness equipment suppliers may be useful for rehabilitation needs such as hand or ankle weights for strengthening exercises.

## THE CLIENT WITH AN AMPUTATION

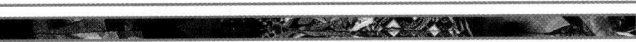

An **amputation** is the partial or total removal of a body part. Amputation may be the result of an acute process, such as a traumatic event, or a chronic condition, such as peripheral vas-

cular disease or diabetes mellitus. Regardless of the cause, an amputation is devastating to the client. It is estimated that 350,000 people with amputations live in the United States, and that 135, 000 new amputations occur each year. In the United States, the most common causes of lower extremity amputations are disease (70%), trauma (22%), congenital or birth defects (4%), and tumors (4%). Upper extremity amputation is usually due to trauma or birth defect (Moss Rehab Resource Net, 2002).

The loss of all or part of an extremity has a significant physical and psychosocial effect on the client and family. Adaptation may take a long time and require much effort. A multidisciplinary health care team is necessary to meet the client's physical, spiritual, cultural, and emotional needs.

### CAUSES OF AMPUTATION

Peripheral vascular disease (PVD) is the major cause of amputation of the lower extremities (see Chapter 33). Common risk factors for the development of PVD include hypertension, diabetes, smoking, and hyperlipidemia. Peripheral neuropathy also places the person with diabetes at risk for amputation. In peripheral neuropathy, loss of sensation frequently leads to unrecognized injury and infection. Untreated infection may lead to gangrene and the need for amputation. These risks are fully discussed in Chapter 18.

Trauma is the major cause of amputation of the upper extremities. Upper extremity amputations represent a more

## Nursing Care Plan
## A Client with a Hip Fracture

Stella Carbolito is a 74-year-old Italian American with a history of osteoporosis. She is a widow and lives alone in a two-story row home. Mrs. Carbolito is retired and depends on a pension check and social security for her income. She takes pride in making all her own food from scratch.

While walking to the market one day, Mrs. Carbolito falls and fractures her left hip. She is transported by ambulance to the nearest hospital emergency department.

### ASSESSMENT

During the initial assessment at the ED, abnormal findings are that Mrs. Carbolito's left leg is shorter than her right leg and is externally rotated. Distal pulses are present and bilaterally strong; both legs are warm. Mrs. Carbolito complains of severe pain but states that no numbness or burning is present. She is able to wiggle the toes on her left leg and has full movement of her right leg. Initial vital signs are as follows: T 98.0°F (36.6°C), P 100, R 18, BP 120/58. Diagnostic tests include CBC, blood chemistry, and X-ray studies of the left hip and pelvis. The CBC reveals a hemoglobin of 11.0 g/dL and a normal WBC count. Blood chemistry findings are within normal limits. The X-ray reveals a fracture of the left femoral neck. Mrs. Carbolito is admitted to the hospital with an order for 10 lb of straight leg traction. An open reduction and internal fixation (ORIF) is planned for the following day.

### DIAGNOSIS

- *Acute pain* related to fractured left femoral neck and muscle spasms
- *Impaired physical mobility* related to bed rest and fractured left femoral neck
- *Risk for ineffective tissue perfusion* related to unstable bones and swelling
- *Risk for disturbed sensory perception: Tactile* related to the risk of nerve impairment

### EXPECTED OUTCOMES

- Verbalize a decrease in pain.
- Verbalize the purpose of traction and surgery
- Maintain normal neurovascular assessments.
- Demonstrate postoperative exercises.

### PLANNING AND IMPLEMENTATION

- Assess pain on a scale of 0 to 10 before and after implementing measures to reduce pain.
- Administer narcotics per the physician's order.
- Perform neurovascular assessment every 2 to 4 hours, and document findings.
- Apply straight leg traction per physician's order.
- Encourage deep breathing and relaxation techniques.
- Teach the purpose of traction and surgery.
- Teach the purpose of and the procedure for performing isometric and flexion/extension exercises.

### EVALUATION

Three days after surgery, Mrs. Carbolito is out of bed and in a chair. She verbalizes a decrease in pain. There have been no abnormal neurovascular assessments. She is able to independently perform isometric and flexion/extension exercises in both lower extremities. Discharge planning included referrals for home care. A home health nurse will visit, and the social worker at the hospital has ordered a trapeze for her bed, an elevated toilet seat, an elevated cushion for her chair, and a walker.

### Critical Thinking in the Nursing Process

1. What factors placed Mrs. Carbolito at risk for a hip fracture?
2. Mrs. Carbolito says, "I don't understand why they had to put that heavy thing on my leg before I went to surgery to get my hip fixed." What would you tell her? What preoperative factors might have decreased teaching effectiveness?
3. Describe how each of the following, if manifested by Mrs. Carbolito, would increase her risk for postoperative complications: urinary incontinence, weight more than 20% under normal for her height, chronic constipation. What nursing diagnoses and interventions would you include in her plan of care to decrease the risk?

See Evaluating Your Response in Appendix C.

---

serious threat to independence, because these limbs perform more specialized functions. The incidence of traumatic amputations is highest among young men. Most amputations in this group result from motor vehicle crashes or accidents involving machinery at work. The client may present to the trauma center with an injury that may be life threatening; significant loss of blood and tissue may have already occurred, and shock may develop. (See Chapter 6 for a discussion of shock and trauma.) Other traumatic events that may necessitate an amputation are frostbite, burns, or electrocution.

Amputations result from or are necessitated by interruption in blood flow, either acute or chronic. In acute trauma situations, the limb is partially or completely severed, and tissue death ensues. Replantation of fingers, small body parts, and entire limbs has been successful.

In the chronic disease processes, circulation is impaired, venous pooling begins, proteins leak into the interstitium, and edema develops. Edema increases the risk of injury and further decreases circulation. Stasis ulcers develop and readily become infected because impaired healing and altered immune processes allow bacteria to proliferate. The presence of progressive infection further compromises circulation and ultimately leads to gangrene (tissue death), which requires amputation.

## LEVELS OF AMPUTATION

The level of amputation is determined by local and systemic factors. Local factors include ischemia and gangrene; system factors include cardiovascular status, renal function, and sever-

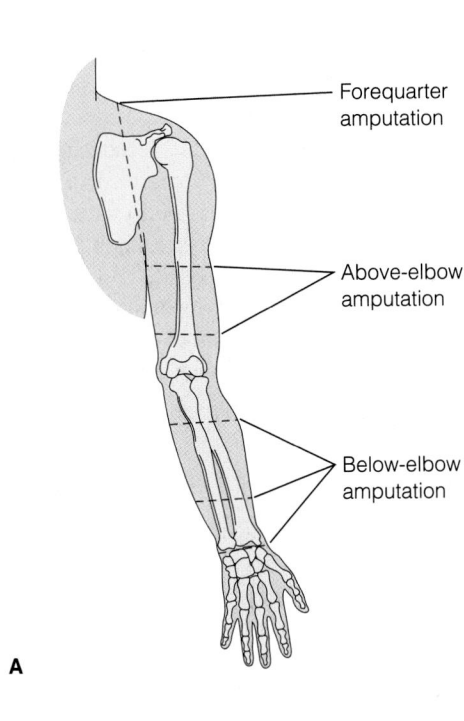

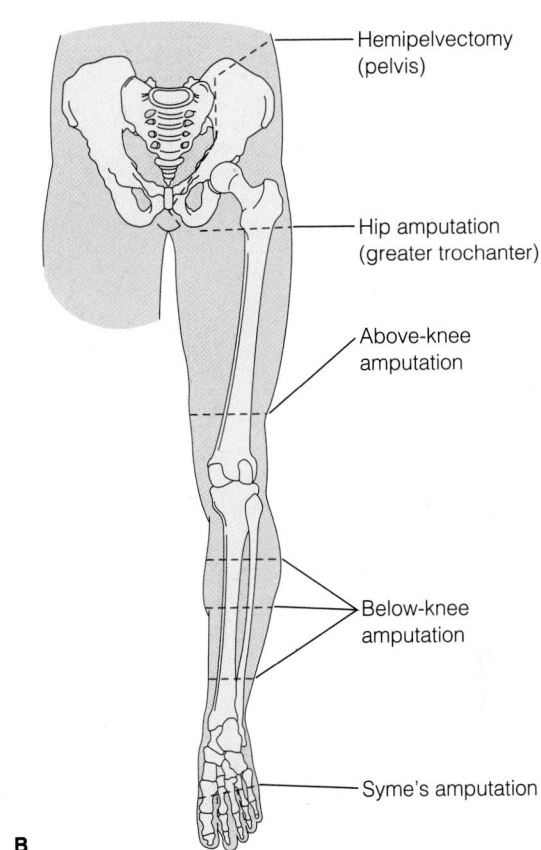

**Figure 38–12** ■ Common sites of amputation. *A,* The upper extremities. *B,* The lower extremities. The surgeon determines the level of amputation based on blood supply and tissue condition.

ity of diabetes mellitus. The goals are to alleviate symptoms, to maintain healthy tissue, and to increase functional outcome. When possible, the joints are preserved because they allow greater function of the extremity. Figure 38–12 ■ illustrates common sites of amputation.

## TYPES OF AMPUTATION

Amputations may be open (*guillotine*) or closed (*flap*). Open amputations are performed when infection is present. The wound is not closed but remains open to drain. When infection is no longer present, surgery is performed to close the wound. In closed amputations, the wound is closed with a flap of skin that is sutured in place over the stump. Terms used to refer to amputations are presented in Table 38–3.

## AMPUTATION SITE HEALING

For the prosthesis to fit well, the amputation site must heal properly. To promote healing, a rigid or compression dressing is applied to prevent infection and minimize edema. A rigid dressing is made by placing a cast on the stump and molding the stump to fit a prosthesis. A soft compression dressing is applied when frequent wound checks are necessary. When this type of dressing is used, a splint is sometimes applied to help mold the extremity to fit the prosthesis. After the wound is dressed, the client is encouraged to toughen the stump skin by

| TABLE 38–3 | Amputation Terms |
| --- | --- |
| **Term** | **Meaning** |
| Arm | Amputation of a portion of the arm, either above or below the elbow |
| Disarticulation | Amputation through a joint |
| Forequarter | Removal of the entire arm and disarticulation of the shoulder |
| Closed (flap) | Amputation in which a flap of skin is formed to cover the end of the wound |
| Open (guillotine) | Perpendicular cutting of the extremity in which the wound is left open; used when infection is present |
| Leg | Amputation below the knee (BK) |
| Thigh | Amputation above the knee (AK) |
| Finger or Toe | Amputation of one or all of the fingers or toes |
| Syme | Modified disarticulation of the ankle |
| Foot | Amputation of part of the foot and toes |

pushing it into first soft and then harder surfaces. The stump is wrapped in an Ace bandage to allow a conical shape to form and prevent edema. The bandage is applied from the distal to the proximal extremity (Figure 38–13 ■).

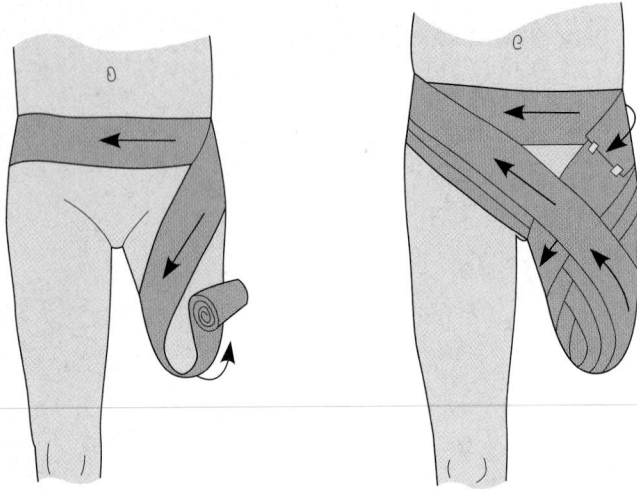

**Figure 38–13** ■ Stump dressings increase venous return, decrease edema, and help shape the stump for a prosthesis. With an above-knee amputation, a figure-eight bandage is started by bringing the bandage down over the stump and back up around the hips.

## COMPLICATIONS

Complications that may occur after an amputation include infection, delayed healing, chronic stump pain and phantom pain, and contracture.

### Infection

Generally, the client who suffers a traumatic amputation has a greater risk of infection than the person who has a planned amputation. However, even planned amputations carry a risk of infection. The client who is older, has diabetes mellitus, or suffers peripheral neurovascular compromise is at a particularly high risk for infection. Infection may present itself locally or systemically. Local manifestations of infection include drainage, odor, redness, positive wound cultures, and increased discomfort at the suture line. Systemic manifestations include fever, an increased heart rate, a decrease in blood pressure, chills, and positive wound or blood cultures.

### Delayed Healing

If infection is present or if the circulation remains compromised, delayed healing will result. Delayed healing occurs at a slower rate than expected. In older clients, other preexisting conditions can increase the risk of delayed healing. In clients of any age, electrolyte imbalances can contribute to delayed healing, as can a diet that lacks the proper nutrients to meet the body's increased metabolic demands. Smoking also compromises healing by causing vasoconstriction and decreasing blood flow to the stump. Deep vein thrombosis and compromised venous return, which may result from prolonged immobilization, are other potential factors. Decreased cardiac output decreases blood flow and thus also delays healing.

### Chronic Stump Pain and Phantom Pain

**Chronic stump pain** is the result of neuroma formation, causing severe burning pain. Interventions to relieve this pain include medications, nerve blocks, transcutaneous electrical nerve stimulation (TENS), and surgical stump reconstruction. **Phantom limb pain** is not the same as phantom limb sensation. A majority of amputees experience phantom limb sensation (sensations such as tingling, numbness, cramping or itching in the phantom foot or hand) early in the postoperative period. It is often self-limited, but may last for decades in some clients. When phantom limb sensation is painful, it is referred to as phantom limb pain. Although various theories have been proposed, the exact cause of this experience is unknown. Treatments include pain management, TENS, and a variety of surgical procedures. The management of phantom limb pain is often difficult for both clients and health care professionals. Clients with phantom limb pain often benefit from referral to a pain clinic for a comprehensive pain management program (Maher, Salmond, & Pellino, 2002).

### Contractures

A **contracture** is an abnormal flexion and fixation of a joint caused by muscle atrophy and shortening. Contracture of the joint above the amputation is a common complication. The client needs to be taught to extend the joint. The client with an above-the-knee amputation should lie prone for periods throughout the day. The client with a below-the-knee amputation should elevate the stump, keeping the knee extended. The same principles apply to the upper extremity. All joints should receive either active or passive ROM exercises every 2 to 4 hours. A trapeze frame should be added to the bed to encourage the client to change position every 2 hours. The client who has an upper extremity amputation should exercise both shoulders. Postural exercises can help prevent the client from hunching over secondary to the loss of weight on the affected side. The client with an above-the-knee amputation should not sit for prolonged periods of time; prolonged sitting can lead to hip contracture.

## COLLABORATIVE CARE

Multidisciplinary care is necessary for the client who has sustained an amputation. Physical therapy and occupational retraining are necessary, and the client may also benefit from the presence of clergy. The entire health care team must view both the positive and the negative effects of amputation; that is, they must see amputation as a means to increase the client's independence and to relieve symptoms. The client should be able to become familiar with the members of the health care team and their roles; this allows the client greater control over his or her care and rehabilitation and promotes independence.

### Diagnostic Tests

Preoperatively, the client has routine laboratory and diagnostic tests (see Chapter 7). Preoperative tests are performed to assess the circulation present in the limb at different levels and determine the level of viable tissue. Preoperative tests include:

- *Doppler flowmetry* to evaluate blood flow in the extremity.
- *Segmental blood pressure determinations* to evaluate the blood flow and vessel pressures in the extremity.

- *Transcutaneous partial pressure oxygen readings* to measure the oxygen delivery by blood vessels in the affected extremity.
- If revascularization with a bypass is planned in conjunction with the amputation, *angiography* is also performed.

Postoperative diagnostic tests include the following:

- *CBC* to determine hemoglobin and hematocrit levels. A sudden drop in these values may indicate hemorrhage. The WBC count is also monitored with a CBC; a sudden increase in the WBC may indicate the presence of infection.
- *Blood chemistries* measure electrolytes and reflect fluid balance.
- *Vascular Doppler ultrasonography* may be performed if a client is suspected of having a DVT.

## Medications

The client receives medications preoperatively, intraoperatively, and postoperatively. Preoperatively, the physician may prescribe intravenous antibiotics. Intraoperatively, anesthetic agents are administered. It also may be necessary to administer agents to control blood pressure during the surgery. Postoperatively, the client resumes any routinely prescribed medications and in addition may receive antibiotics and analgesics. Steroids may be administered to decrease swelling. A histamine $H_2$ antagonist may also be ordered to decrease the risk of peptic ulcer formation. Stool softeners may be administered to prevent constipation.

## Prosthesis

The type of prosthesis selected for the client with an amputation depends on the level of the amputation as well as the client's occupation and lifestyle. Each prosthesis is based on a detailed prosthetic prescription and is custom made for the client based on the specific characteristics of the stump. Most are made of plastic and foam materials. Many factors influence the client's use of the prosthesis, including the status of the remaining limb, cognitive status, cardiovascular status, preoperative activity level, and motivation to use the prosthesis (Maher, Salmond, & Pellino, 2002).

Clients with a lower extremity amputation are often fitted with early walking aids. These are pneumatic devices that fit over the stump and are used in the immediate postoperative period to allow early ambulation, decreased postoperative swelling, and improved morale. Clients may begin weight bearing as soon as 2 weeks after surgery. Clients with upper extremity amputations may be fitted for a prosthesis immediately after surgery. Rehabilitation of the client with an amputation is a team effort, involving the client, nurse, physician, physical therapist, occupational therapist, social worker, prosthetist, and vocational counselor.

## NURSING CARE

## Health Promotion

The goals of health promotion activities focus on preventing the progression of chronic diseases such as peripheral vascular disease and diabetes mellitus, and on safety. Clients with peripheral vascular disease from any cause need education about foot care and early recognition of decreased circulation. Education within both urban and rural populations should provide knowledge about working safely with farm and occupational machinery.

In addition, it is important that the public know what to do if a traumatic amputation occurs in the home, community, or workplace. The following guidelines may help preserve the amputated part until it can be surgically reattached:

- Keep the person in a prone position with the legs elevated.
- Apply firm pressure to the bleeding area, using a towel or article of clothing.
- Wrap the amputated part in a clean cloth. If possible, soak the cloth in saline (such as contact lens solution).
- Put the amputated part in a plastic bag and put the bag on ice. Do not let the amputated part come into direct contact with the ice or water.
- Send the amputated part to the emergency department with the injured person, and be sure the emergency personnel know what it is.

## Assessment

Collect the following data through the health history and physical examination. Further focused assessments are described in the nursing interventions below.

- Health history: mechanism of injury, current and past health problems, pain, occupation, activities of daily living, changes in sensation in the feet, cultural and/or religious guidelines for handling the amputated part
- Physical examination: bilateral neurovascular status of the extremities, bilateral capillary refill time, skin over the lower extremities (discoloration, edema, ulcerations, hair, gangrene)

## Nursing Diagnoses and Interventions

The goals of nursing care for a person with an amputation are to relieve pain, promote healing, prevent complications, support the client and family during the process of grieving and adaptation to alterations in body image, and restore mobility. Care is individualized, and the circumstances that led to the amputation (e.g., traumatic injury or disease) also must be addressed. Applying rehabilitation principles to nursing care is also important.

### Acute Pain

Pain from the surgical procedure can be compounded by muscle spasms, swelling, and phantom limb pain.

- Ask the client to rate the pain on a scale of 0 to 10 before and after any intervention. *This facilitates objective assessment of the effectiveness of the chosen pain relief strategy. Pain that increases in intensity or remains unrelieved with analgesics can indicate compartment syndrome.*
- Splint and support the injured area. *Splinting prevents additional injury by immobilizing the stump and decreasing edema while molding the stump for a good prosthetic fit.*
- Unless contraindicated, elevate the stump on a pillow for the first 24 hours after surgery. *Elevating the stump promotes venous return and decreases edema, which will decrease pain.*

*Elevating the stump for long periods after the immediate postoperative period increases the risk for hip contractures.* ■

- Move and turn the client gently and slowly. *Gentle moving and turning prevents the development of severe muscle spasms.*
- Administer pain medications as prescribed. A PCA pump may be ordered by the physician. *Analgesics alleviate pain by stimulating opiate receptor sites. PCA pumps increase client control over and allow early relief of pain before it intensifies.*
- Encourage deep breathing and relaxation exercises. *These techniques increase the effectiveness of analgesics and modify the pain experience.*
- Reposition client every 2 hours; turning from side to side and onto abdomen. *Repositioning alleviates pressure from one area and distributes it throughout the body and helps prevent cramping of muscles.*

*Lying prone prevents hip contracture.* ■

## Risk for Infection

The client who has an amputation is at risk for wound infection. Early recognition of infection can lead to early treatment and prevent wound dehiscence.

- Assess the wound for redness, drainage, temperature, edema, and suture line approximation. *Redness is normal in the immediate postoperative period; if it persists, however, it can indicate infection. A hot area over the incision or increased drainage may also indicate infection.*
- Take the client's temperature at least once every 4 hours. *Increased body temperature may indicate infection.*
- Monitor white blood cell count. *The white blood cell count rises in the presence of infection.*
- Use aseptic technique to change the wound dressing. *Aseptic technique prevents the contamination of the wound with bacteria.*
- Administer antibiotics as ordered. *Antibiotics inhibit bacterial cell replication and help prevent or eradicate infection.*
- Teach the client stump-wrapping techniques. *Correctly wrapping the stump from the distal to proximal extremity increases venous return and prevents pooling of fluid, thereby reducing the chance of infection.*

## Risk for Impaired Skin Integrity

Stump care is essential, not only in the postoperative healing period, but also throughout life with a prosthesis. A variety of skin problems may be caused by a prosthesis, including epidermoid cysts, abrasions, blisters, and hair follicle infections. The client must be taught stump care prior to discharge.

- Each day, preferably at night, wash the stump with soap and warm water and dry thoroughly. Inspect the stump for redness, irritation, or abrasions. *It is essential to maintain intact skin to ensure successful use of the prosthesis.*

- Massage the end of the stump, beginning 3 weeks after surgery. *Massage helps desensitize the remaining part of the limb and prevents scar tissue formation. If the skin adheres to the underlying tissue, it will tear when stressed by wearing a prosthesis.*
- Expose any open areas of skin on the remaining part of the limb for 1 hour four times a day. *Air exposure promotes healing.*
- Change stump socks and elastic wraps each day. Wash these in mild soap and water, and allow to completely dry before using again. *Stump socks and elastic wraps must be kept clean and dry to prevent skin breakdown.*

## Risk for Dysfunctional Grieving

The client who has lost an extremity is at risk for dysfunctional grieving. Denial of the need for surgery and the inability to discuss feelings compound this risk.

- Encourage verbalization of feelings, using open-ended questions. *Asking open-ended questions allows the client to discuss feelings and communicates the listener's willingness to listen.*
- Actively listen and maintain eye contact. *Active listening and eye contact communicate respect for what the client is expressing.*
- Reflect on the client's feelings. *Reflection statements such as, "You seem angry," allow the client to recognize feelings and perhaps develop a plan for resolution.*
- Allow the client to have unlimited visiting hours, if possible. *Unlimited visiting hours allows increased social support.*
- If desired by the client, provide spiritual support by activities such as visits from a spiritual leader, prayer, and meditation. *These activities often provide support during the grieving process.*

## Disturbed Body Image

Although amputation is a reconstructive surgery, the client's body image will be disturbed. Risk for body image disturbance is higher in young trauma clients, in whom body image is a particularly important component of self-image.

- Encourage verbalization of feelings. *This allows the client to communicate concerns and fears and lets the client know the nurse is willing to listen.*
- Allow the client to wear clothing from home. *Familiar clothing provides emotional comfort and helps the client retain a sense of his or her own identity.*
- Encourage the client to look at the stump. *Looking at and touching the stump helps the client face his or her fear of the unknown and move from denial to acceptance.*
- Encourage the client to care for the stump. *Active participation in care increases self-esteem and independence.*
- Offer to have a fellow amputee visit the client. *A support person who has experienced the same change gives the client the hope that he or she can regain independence.*
- Encourage active participation in rehabilitation. *Active participation in rehabilitation increases independence and mobility.*

## Impaired Physical Mobility

If time allows, the client should begin strengthening muscles preoperatively. If the amputation is the result of an emergency, exercises begin within 24 to 48 hours of surgery. The return of independent mobility boosts self-esteem and promotes adaptation to amputation.

- Perform ROM exercises on all joints. *ROM exercises help prevent the development of joint contractures that limit mobility.*
- Maintain postoperative stump shrinkage devices. These may be elastic bandages, shrinker socks, elastic stockinette, or a rigid plaster cast. *Postoperative dressings decrease edema and shape the stump for prosthetic wear.*
- Turn and reposition the client every 2 hours. *The client with a lower extremity amputation should lie prone every 4 hours. Repositioning increases blood flow to muscles, forces synovial fluid into joints, and helps prevent contractures.*
- Reinforce teaching by the physical therapist in crutch walking or the use of assistive devices. *These devices increase mobility by balancing the client and facilitating ambulation.*
- Encourage active participation in physical therapy. *Physical therapy will fatigue the client in the early stage of healing. Encouragement may increase the client's participation in the physical therapy regimen and thereby increase activity tolerance.*

## Using NANDA, NIC and NOC

Chart 38–2 shows links between NANDA nursing diagnoses, NIC, and NOC when caring for the client with an amputation.

## Home Care

Client and family teaching focuses on stump care, prosthesis fitting and care, medications, assistive devices, exercises, rehabilitation, counseling, support services, and follow-up appointments. The depth of teaching depends on the cause and site of the amputation and the needs of the client. See the Meeting Individualized Needs box on page 1218.

Holistic nursing care is especially important for the older client with an amputation. The normal aging process decreases renal and liver function; hence, medications have longer half-lives. Altered circulation prolongs wound healing, and slowing of reflexes and alterations in gait may disrupt balance. A walker may be more appropriate than crutches, because older clients have less strength in the upper extremities. Safety issues, such as decreasing the risk for recurrent falls, must be addressed. The nurse should also assess the client's need for in-home assistance and make appropriate referrals to visiting nurses and home health aides.

In addition, suggest the following resources:

- The Amputee Coalition of America
- Amputee Resource Foundation of America

---

## CHART 38–2 NANDA, NIC, AND NOC LINKAGES

### The Client with an Amputation

| NURSING DIAGNOSES | NURSING INTERVENTIONS | NURSING OUTCOMES |
|---|---|---|
| • Risk for Infection | • Infection Protection<br>• Wound Care<br>• Vital Signs Monitoring | • Infection Status |
| • Impaired Skin Integrity | • Incision Site Care<br>• Amputation Care<br>• Exercise Promotion<br>• Prosthesis Care<br>• Skin Surveillance<br>• Wound Care | • Wound Healing: Primary Intention<br>• Wound Healing: Secondary Intention<br>• Tissue Integrity: Skin<br>• Immobility Consequences: Physiological |
| • Chronic Pain | • Pain Management<br>• Medication Management<br>• Progressive Muscle Relaxation<br>• Simple Relaxation Therapy | • Comfort Level<br>• Pain Control Behavior<br>• Symptom Severity<br>• Well-Being |
| • Disturbed Body Image | • Body Image Enhancement<br>• Amputation Care<br>• Wound Care<br>• Coping Enhancement<br>• Grief Work Facilitation | • Body Image<br>• Grief Resolution |

*Note. Data from* Nursing Outcomes Classification (NOC) *by M. Johnson & M. Maas (Eds.), 1997, St. Louis: Mosby;* Nursing Diagnoses: Definitions & Classification 2001–2002 *by North American Nursing Diagnosis Association, 2001, Philadelphia: NANDA;* Nursing Interventions Classification (NIC) *by J.C. McCloskey & G. M. Bulechek (Eds.), 2000, St. Louis: Mosby. Reprinted by permission.*

## Meeting Individualized Needs

### THE CLIENT WITH AN AMPUTATION

Amputation of a limb has significant long-term consequences for the client. The client will grieve the loss of a body part and must adjust to a new self-image. The client's ability to perform normal activities of daily living (ADLs) and to maintain his or her usual family and social roles may be significantly affected, at least initially. Depending on the client's occupation, job performance may be affected, necessitating a change of career.

The nurse may be responsible for involving multiple members of the health care team in the client's care and rehabilitation and coordinating their activities. Following an amputation, the client may need the services of any or all of the following:

- Social services to help with rehabilitative and financial arrangements
- Physical therapists to teach ambulation techniques, and to provide deep heat or massage
- Occupational therapists to assist the client in developing adaptive techniques to deal with the loss of a limb
- Prosthetists to develop a prosthesis for the missing limb that will meet the client's needs for ADLs and other activities
- Home health services for nursing care such as assessments and wound care
- Support group services to assist in adapting to the body image change and effects of amputation on ADLs

### Assessing for Home Care

Preparing the amputee for home care includes a careful assessment of the client, family and support services, and the home for possible barriers to the client's safety and independence.

Assess the client's acceptance of the amputation and knowledge base about care needs, any activity restrictions or special needs, and resources for home care. Discuss home management—who is responsible for household activities such as cleaning and cooking. Inquire about arrangements that have been made for home care activities and ADLs. Evaluate the client's use of prescription and nonprescription medications, paying particular attention to possible interactions and drugs that may affect the client's balance, mental alertness, or appetite. Ask about social habits, such as cigarette smoking, alcohol use, or other drug use, that may affect healing or the client's ability to provide self-care.

Assess the client's home environment for possible safety hazards or barriers to ambulation, such as:

- Scatter rugs
- Stairs between living areas of the house
- Presence of grab bars to facilitate toileting and bathing
- Access to clean water and other needs for wound care

### Teaching for Home Care

The new amputee needs a great deal of teaching to learn to adapt to loss of a limb, whether it is an upper or lower extremity that has been lost. Because the client must be ready to learn before teaching can be effective, use therapeutic communication techniques to encourage the client to verbalize feelings about the amputation and its effects. Use active listening and teach the client ways to reduce anxiety and deal with feelings of helplessness and loss. Encourage the client to participate in care of the stump to build self-esteem and reinforce teaching. Include the following in teaching for home care:

- Teach the client to wrap the stump appropriately in preparation for fitting the prosthesis.
- Discuss positioning of the stump. Contractures are a particular problem for clients with an above-knee amputation, and can interfere with ability to effectively use a prosthesis.
- Teach the client how to perform stump exercises to maintain joint mobility and muscle tone of the affected limb.
- Encourage the client to resume physical activities as soon as possible. This improves the client's health and well-being, as well as the client's self-esteem.
- Discuss household modifications to promote independence, such as grab bars in the bathroom, faucets with single-handle controls for water flow and temperature, and handheld shower heads and shower chairs for bathing.

## THE CLIENT WITH A REPETITIVE USE INJURY

Repeatedly twisting and turning the wrist, pronating and supinating the forearm, kneeling, or raising arms over the head can result in repetitive use injuries. Common repetitive use injuries include carpal tunnel syndrome, bursitis, and epicondylitis. Clients with repetitive use injuries pose a challenge to the health care team. Often these clients appear puzzled as they relate a history of manifestations that have worsened over time. They deny abrupt trauma and often worry about the ability to return to work. Repetitive use injuries are common. The number of worker's compensation claims for repetitive use injuries is steadily growing. The increase is believed to be a result of technology advances in the workplace.

## PATHOPHYSIOLOGY

### Carpal Tunnel Syndrome

The carpal tunnel is a canal through which flexor tendons and the median nerve pass from the wrist to the hand. The syndrome develops from narrowing of the tunnel and irritation of the median nerve. **Carpal tunnel syndrome** involves compression of the median nerve as a result of inflammation and swelling of the synovial lining of the tendon sheaths. The client complains of numbness and tingling of the thumb, index finger, and lateral ventral surface of the middle finger. The client may also complain of pain in this area that interferes with sleep and is alleviated by shaking or massaging the hand and fingers. The affected hand may become weak and the client may be unable to hold utensils or perform activities that require precision.

## Nursing Care Plan

## A Client with a Below-the-Knee Amputation

John Rocke is a 45-year-old divorcee with no children. He has a history of type one diabetes mellitus and poor control of blood glucose levels. Mr. Rocke is unemployed and currently receives unemployment compensation. He lives alone in a second-floor apartment. Mr. Rocke had developed gangrene in the toe and failed to seek prompt medical attention; as a result, a left below-the-knee amputation was necessary.

Mr. Rocke is in his second postoperative day and his vital signs are stable. The stump is splinted and has a soft dressing. The wound is approximating well without signs of infection. He has not performed ROM exercises or turning since his surgery, complaining of severe pain. When the nurse goes into the room, he yells, "Get out! I don't want anyone to see me like this." No one has visited him since his hospitalization. He is tolerating an 1800-kcal American Diabetes Association diet and is using a urinal independently. He has an order for meperidine (Demerol), 100 mg IM every 4 hours prn for pain, and cefazolin (Ancef), 1 g IV every 8 hours. He is on blood glucose coverage with regular insulin subcutaneously.

### ASSESSMENT

Jane Simmons, RN, has just come on duty. She notes that the client is upset and angry. Mr. Rocke will not let anyone enter the room to give him medication or assess his vital signs.

### DIAGNOSIS

- *Disturbed body image* related to amputation of a left lower leg
- *Dysfunctional grieving* related to anger and loss of left lower leg
- *Situational low self-esteem* related to appearance
- *Risk for injury from infection and contractures* related to refusal of care
- *Pain* related to surgery

### EXPECTED OUTCOMES

- Verbalize his feelings about the amputation.
- Allow the staff to monitor his vital signs and administer medications.

- Be allowed to control his pain with a PCA pump.
- Verbalize a decrease in pain.
- Verbalize the importance of turning.
- Turn every 2 hours.

### PLANNING AND IMPLEMENTATION

- Encourage verbalization of feelings.
- Actively listen to the client.
- Offer to arrange a visit with a fellow amputee.
- Ask the physician if the client can be placed on a PCA pump.
- Teach the client the importance of turning every 2 hours to prevent contractures.
- Encourage turning and lying prone.
- Teach the importance of antibiotics in preventing and treating infection.

### EVALUATION

One week after his surgery, Mr. Rocke is actively participating in his care. He has apologized for his behavior and has explained to Ms. Simmons that he was angry about the loss of his leg. He states, "I thought I knew what to expect, but I didn't."

### Critical Thinking in the Nursing Process

1. Once Mr. Rocke is ready to assist with his stump care, how would you proceed? Would you give him full responsibility for care and dressings, or would you gradually increase his participation? Why?
2. What factors in Mr. Rocke's home environment and medical history may make self-care more difficult? Do you expect Mr. Rocke to follow up on care after his discharge? Why or why not?
3. Mr. Rocke states, "Why should I exercise this leg—it was already cut off!" How would you respond? What is the purpose of exercising the stump?

See Evaluating Your Response in Appendix C.

---

Carpal tunnel syndrome is one of the three most common work-related injuries. The incidence is believed to be related directly to the number of people using computers. The incidence of carpal tunnel syndrome is higher in women, especially postmenopausal women.

## Bursitis

**Bursitis** is an inflammation of a bursa. A bursa is an enclosed sac found between muscles, tendons, and bony prominences. The bursae that commonly become inflamed are in the shoulder, hip, leg, and elbow. Constant friction between the bursa and the musculoskeletal tissue around it causes irritation, edema, and inflammation. Manifestations develop as the sac becomes engorged. The area around the sac is tender, and extension and flexion of the joint near the bursa produce pain. The inflamed bursa is hot, red, and edematous. The client guards the joint to decrease pain and may point to the area of the bursa when identifying joint tenderness.

## Epicondylitis

**Epicondylitis** is the inflammation of the tendon at its point of origin into the bone. Epicondylitis is also referred to as *tennis elbow* or *golfer's elbow*. The exact pathophysiology of epicondylitis is unknown. Current theories attribute inflammation of the tendon to microvascular trauma. Tears, bleeding, and edema are thought to cause avascularization and calcification of the tendon. Manifestations of epicondylitis include point tenderness, pain radiating down the dorsal surface of the forearm, and a history of repetitive use.

## COLLABORATIVE CARE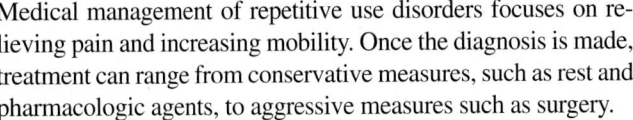

Medical management of repetitive use disorders focuses on relieving pain and increasing mobility. Once the diagnosis is made, treatment can range from conservative measures, such as rest and pharmacologic agents, to aggressive measures such as surgery.

## Diagnostic Tests

Carpal tunnel syndrome is diagnosed by the client's history and physical examination. History may reveal an occupation that involves areas such as computer work, jackhammer operation, mechanical work, or gymnastics. History of a radial bone fracture or rheumatoid arthritis also increases the risk of carpal tunnel syndrome. Tests specific for carpal tunnel include the Phalen test (see Chapter 37). Bursitis and epicondylitis are diagnosed by history and physical examination.

## Medications

The client with a repetitive use injury usually receives NSAIDs. Narcotics also may be administered for acute flare-ups and severe pain. For the client who has epicondylitis or carpal tunnel syndrome, corticosteroids may be injected into the joint.

## Treatments

### Conservative Management

The first steps in the care of all repetitive use injuries are to immobilize and rest the involved joint. The joint may be splinted, and ice may be applied in the first 24 to 48 hours to decrease pain and inflammation. Ice application may be followed by heat application every 4 hours.

### Surgery

Surgery is usually reserved for the client who does not obtain relief with conservative treatment. Surgery for carpal tunnel syndrome includes resection of the carpal ligament to enlarge the tunnel. In epicondylitis and bursitis, calcified deposits may be removed from the area surrounding the tendon or bursa.

## NURSING CARE

The nursing care of a client with a repetitive use injury focuses on relieving pain, teaching about the disease process and treatment, and improving physical mobility.

## Nursing Diagnoses and Interventions

### Acute Pain

Swelling and nerve inflammation lead to pain in the client with a repetitive use injury.

- Ask the client to rate the pain on a scale of 0 to 10 (with 10 being the most severe pain) before and after any intervention.

*This facilitates objective assessment of the effectiveness of the chosen pain relief strategy.*
- Encourage the use of immobilizers. *Splinting maintains joint alignment and prevents pain due to movement of inflamed tissues.*
- Teach the client to apply ice and/or heat as prescribed. *Ice causes vasoconstriction and decreases the pooling of blood in the inflamed area. Ice may also numb the tender area. Heat decreases swelling by increasing venous return.*
- Encourage use of NSAIDs as prescribed. *NSAIDs decrease swelling by inhibiting prostaglandins.*
- Explain why treatment should not be abruptly discontinued. *Abrupt discontinuation of treatment may cause reinflammation of the injured area.*

### Impaired Physical Mobility

Joint pain and swelling can impair mobility.

- Suggest interventions to alleviate pain (such as using immobilizer and taking pain medications). *If the joint is pain free, the client will be more likely to take an active role in therapy.*
- Refer to a physical therapist for exercises. *The physical therapist can assist the client with exercise to prevent joint stiffness.*
- Suggest consultation with an occupational therapist. *Occupational therapy can help the client learn new ways to perform tasks to prevent recurring symptoms.*

## Home Care

Address the following topics for home care.

- Causes and treatments for repetitive use injury
- Rehabilitation to allow the client to return to a state of independence
- Ways to avoid unnecessary exposure to the activities that increase risk of redeveloping the injury. Suggest evaluation of the client's work environment by an environmental risk manager who can prescribe measures to reduce the risk of repetitive use injuries. Wrist supports or an ergonomic keyboard may be useful for the client who uses a computer extensively. Appropriate desk and chair height also are important in maintaining correct anatomical position while working.
- Information about sources for braces or other assistive devices.

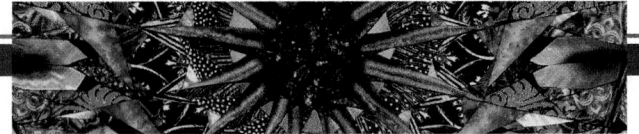

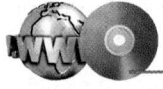 EXPLORE MediaLink

# TEST YOURSELF

1. You are teaching a young adult how to provide self-care for a sprained ankle. You explain the reason for applying ice immediately after the injury is based on the principle that ice:

   a. Increases the diameter of blood vessels
   b. Decreases the diameter of blood vessels
   c. Is helpful in increasing white blood cells
   d. Lowers the blood pressure and pulse

2. A client with a compound, open fracture has been admitted to the emergency department and is scheduled for immediate surgery. Which of the following nursing diagnoses would be most appropriate in the immediate postoperative period?

   a. *Risk for posttrauma syndrome*
   b. *Impaired transfer ability*
   c. *Risk for infection*
   d. *Risk for falls*

3. While providing care to an older woman with a cast on her left lower arm (from below the elbow to above the fingers), you perform a neurovascular assessment. Which of the following assessments indicate a possible complication?

   a. Slightly edematous fingers
   b. Warm, pink skin above the cast
   c. Pale, cold fingers
   d. Pain rating of 2 on a 1 to 10 scale

4. At what position would you place the remaining extremity following a below-the-knee amputation during the first 24 hours after surgery?

   a. Elevated above the level of the heart
   b. Lower than the rest of the body
   c. Crossed over the intact extremity
   d. Level with the rest of the body

5. Your husband is cutting wood with a circular saw. He suddenly screams that he has cut off his finger. What would you do with the amputated finger?

   a. Don't worry about it; the important thing is to get him to the hospital
   b. Put it in a storage bag filled with warm water
   c. Tape it to his hand so the emergency personnel will know where it is
   d. Wrap it in a towel, put it in a plastic bag, and lay it on ice

See Test Yourself answers in Appendix C.

# BIBLIOGRAPHY

*Amputation.* (2001). Available www.hendrickhealth.org/healthy/0037150.html

*A parents guide to first aid. Amputation.* (2002). Available www.choa.org/first_aid/amputation.shtml.

Black, C. (1997). Wound management in patients with traumatic injuries. *Journal of Wound Care, 6*(5), 209–211.

Davis, P., & Barr, L. (1999). Principles of traction. *Journal of Orthopaedic Nursing, 3*(4), 222–227.

Electrical stimulation and bone healing. (2001). *Foot & Ankle Quarterly—The Seminar Journal, 14*(1), 1–37.

*Falls and hip fractures among older adults.* (2000). National Center for Injury Prevention & Control, CDC. Available www.cdc.gov/ncipc/factsheets/falls.htm

Hager, C. A., & Brncick, N. (1998). Fat embolism syndrome: A complication of orthopaedic trauma. *Orthopaedic Nursing, 17*(2), 41–43, 46, 58.

Hess, D. (1997). Employee perceived stress. Relationship to the development of repetitive strain injury symptoms. *AAOHN Journal, 45*(3), 115–123.

Johnson, M., & Maas, M. (Eds.). (1997). *Nursing outcomes classification (NOC).* St. Louis: Mosby.

Junge, T. (2000). Fat embolism: A complication of long bone fracture. *Surgical Technologist, 32*(11), 34–41.

Love, C. (2001). Using assisted walking devices. *Journal of Orthopaedic Nursing, 5*(1), 45–53.

Maher, A., Salmond, S., & Pellino, T. (2002). *Orthopedic nursing* (3rd ed.). Philadelphia: Saunders.

McCloskey, J. C., & Bulechek, G. M. (Eds.). (2000). *Nursing interventions classification (NIC)* (3rd ed.). St. Louis: Mosby.

Milisen, K., Abraham, I. L., & Broos, P. L. (1998). Postoperative variation in neurocognitive and functional status in elderly hip fracture patients. *Journal of Advanced Nursing, 27*(1), 59–67.

Mooney, N. (2001). Pain management in the orthopaedic patient. *Pain Management Nursing, 2*(1), 4–5.

Moss Rehab Resource Net. (2002). *Amputation fact sheet.* Available www.mossresourcenet.org/amputa.htm

North American Nursing Diagnosis Association. (2001). *NANDA nursing diagnoses: Definitions and classification, 2001–2002.* Philadelphia: Author.

National Center for Injury Prevention and Control. (2000). *Preventing falls among seniors.* Atlanta: Author.

O'Neill, M. (2001). Developing a clinically effective DVT prophylaxis protocol. *Journal of Orthopaedic Nursing, 5*(4), 186–191.

Pachucki-Hyde, L. (2001). Assessment of risk factors for osteoporosis and fracture. *Nursing Clinics of North America, 36*(3), 401–408.

Parsons, L., Krau, S., & Ward, K. (2001). Orthopedic trauma: Managing secondary medical problems. *Nursing Clinics of North America, 13*(3), 433–442.

Porth, C. M. (2002). *Pathophysiology: Concepts of altered health states* (6th ed.). Philadelphia: Lippincott.

Santy, J., & Mackintosh, C. (2001). A phenomenological study of pain following fractured shaft of femur. *Journal of Clinical Nursing, 10*(4), 521–527.

Scott, J. (1998). Mending broken bones. *Nursing Times, 94*(12), 28–30.

Shannon, M., Wilson, B., & Stang, C. (2002). *Health professionals drug guide 2002.* Upper Saddle River, NJ: Prentice Hall.

Sydell, W. (1999). Care of patients in casts. *Nursing Standard, 14*(8), 55.

Thompson, J., McFarland, G., Hirsch, J., & Tucker, S. (2002). *Mosby's clinical nursing* (5th ed.). St. Louis: Mosby.

Walls, M. (2002). Orthopedic trauma. *RN, 65*(7), 53–56.

Walsh, C. R., & McBryde, A. M., Jr. (1997). A joint protocol for home skeletal traction. *Orthopaedic Nursing, 16*(3), 28–33.

Weiss, S. A., & Lindell, B. (1996). Phantom limb pain and etiology of amputation in unilateral lower extremity amputees. *Journal of Pain and Symptom Management, 11*(1), 3–17.

Williams, M. A., Hughes, S. H., Bjorklund, B. C., & Oberst, M. T. (1996). Family caregiving in cases of hip fracture. *Rehabilitation Nursing, 21*(3), 124–131, 138.

Yarnold, B. (1999). Hip fracture: Caring for a fragile population. *American Journal of Nursing, 99*(2), 36–41.

Yetzer, E. A. (1996). Helping the patient through the experience of an amputation. *Orthopaedic Nursing, 15*(6), 45–49.

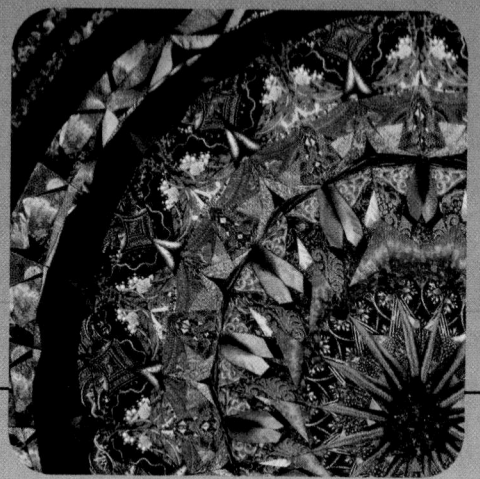

# CHAPTER 39

# Nursing Care of Clients with Musculoskeletal Disorders

## MediaLink

**www.prenhall.com/lemone**

Additional resources for this chapter can be found on the Student CD-ROM accompanying this textbook, and on the Companion Website at www.prenhall.com/lemone. Click on Chapter 39 to select the activities for this chapter.

**CD-ROM**
- Audio Glossary
- NCLEX Review

**Companion Website**
- More NCLEX Review
- Case Study
  Rheumatoid Arthritis
- Care Plan Activity
  Lower Back Pain
- MediaLink Application
  Osteoporosis Prevention

## LEARNING OUTCOMES

After completing this chapter, you will be able to:

- Apply knowledge of normal anatomy, physiology, and assessments when providing care for clients with musculoskeletal disorders (see Chapter 37).

- Explain the pathophysiology, manifestations, and complications of metabolic, degenerative, autoimmune, inflammatory, infectious, neoplastic, connective tissue, and structural musculoskeletal disorders.

- Describe the collaborative care, with related nursing care, of clients with musculoskeletal disorders.

- Provide appropriate nursing care for the client having musculoskeletal surgery.

- Use the nursing process as a framework for providing individualized care to clients with musculoskeletal disorders.

Various metabolic, autoimmune, inflammatory, degenerative, neoplastic, infectious, and structural disorders may affect the musculoskeletal system. Many of these diseases have significant physical, psychosocial, and financial consequences. When these problems occur, clients experience many different individualized responses to their altered health status. Nursing care is directed toward meeting physiologic needs, providing education, and ensuring psychologic support for the client and family.

**Arthritis,** meaning joint inflammation, and **arthralgia,** meaning joint pain, are terms used to describe many disease processes and manifestations involving the musculoskeletal system. These diseases affect not only the joints but also the connective tissues of the body. The various types of arthritis are discussed in this chapter in different sections, depending on the primary etiology of the disorder. Arthritis and other rheumatic disorders (various conditions that affect the musculoskeletal system) are widespread, affecting more than 33 million people in the United States. Arthritic disorders are a leading cause of disability; however, their very prevalence may lead the public and health care professionals to treat them as normal aging processes or discount the validity of the pain and disability experienced by the person with arthritis.

The etiology of most rheumatic disorders is not clear; in many cases, the pathophysiologic processes involved are often complex and poorly understood. Many are primary disorders; others occur as secondary processes associated with another disease. The wear and tear of aging, autoimmune processes, metabolic disorders, genetic factors, and infection are implicated as causative factors in some forms of rheumatic disease.

# METABOLIC DISORDERS

Metabolic bone disorders originate in the bone remodeling process, which normally involves a sequence of events of bone reabsorption and formation. In the adult, this process is primarily internal remodeling through replacement of trabecular bone. Adults replace about 25% of trabecular bone every 4 months through reabsorption of old bone by osteoclasts and formation of new bone by osetoblasts (Porth, 2002). Metabolic bone disorders may result from a variety of factors, including aging, calcium and phosphate imbalances, genetics, and changes in levels of hormones.

## THE CLIENT WITH OSTEOPOROSIS

**Osteoporosis,** literally defined as "porous bones," is a metabolic bone disorder characterized by loss of bone mass, increased bone fragility, and an increased risk of fractures. The reduced bone mass is caused by an imbalance of the processes that influence bone growth and maintenance. Although osteoporosis may result from an endocrine disorder or malignancy, it is most often associated with aging.

Osteoporosis is a health threat for an estimated 28 million Americans; 10 million people have osteoporosis and 18 million have low bone mass, increasing their risk for the disease (National Institute of Health [NIH], 2002). Although osteoporosis can occur at any age and in both men and women, it is most common in aging women. Approximately 50% of all women and 13% of men over the age of 50 will experience an osteoporosis-related fracture in their lifetime, most frequently in the hip, wrist, and vertebrae.

### RISK FACTORS

The risk of developing osteoporosis depends on how much bone mass is achieved between ages 25 and 35, and how much is lost later. Certain diseases, lifestyle habits, and ethnic backgrounds increase the risk of developing osteoporosis (see the Focus on Diversity box above). Many different variables affect one's risk of osteoporosis—some can be modified and others cannot. The risk factors are summarized in Box 39–1.

### Unmodifiable Risk Factors

Both men and women are susceptible to osteoporosis as they age, because the osteoblasts and osteoclasts undergo alterations

---

**Focus on Diversity**

**RISK AND INCIDENCE OF OSTEOPOROSIS IN PEOPLE AGE 50 OR OLDER**

- 20% of non-Hispanic white and Asian women are estimated to have osteoporosis; 52% have a low bone mass. In men, 7% have osteoporosis and 35% have low bone mass.
- 10% of Hispanic women are estimated to have osteoporosis, with another 49% having a low bone mass. In men, 3% have osteoporosis and 23% have low bone mass.
- 5% of African American women are estimated to have osteoporosis with an additional 35% having a lower bone mass. In men, 4% have osteoporosis; 19% have low bone mass.

---

**BOX 39–1   ■   Risk Factors for Osteoporosis**

***Unmodifiable Risk Factors***

- Age
- Female gender
- Race
- Genetic factors
- Endocrine disorders

***Modifiable Risk Factors***

- Calcium deficiency
- Estrogen deficiency
- Smoking
- High alcohol intake
- Sedentary lifestyle
- Medications

that diminish their activity. Women have a significantly higher risk for manifestations and complications of osteoporosis because their peak bone mass is 10% to 15% less than that of men. In addition, age-related bone loss begins earlier and proceeds more rapidly in women, beginning in the 30s and accelerating before menopause. Estrogen in women and testosterone in men appear to help prevent bone loss; decreasing levels of these hormones associated with aging contribute to bone loss. Age-related bone loss in men occurs 15 to 20 years later than in women and at a slower rate.

European Americans and Asians are at a higher risk for osteoporosis than African Americans, who have greater bone density (bone mass positively correlates with the amount of skin pigmentation). Premature osteoporosis is increasing in female athletes, who have a greater incidence of eating disorders and amenorrhea. Poor nutrition and intense physical training can result in a deficient production of estrogen. Decreased estrogen, combined with a lack of calcium and vitamin D, results in a loss of bone density (Porth, 2002).

Clients who have an endocrine disorder such as hyperthyroidism, hyperparathyroidism, Cushing's syndrome, or diabetes mellitus are at high risk for osteoporosis. These disorders affect the metabolism, in turn affecting nutritional status and bone mineralization.

## Modifiable Risk Factors

Modifiable risk factors include behaviors that place a person at risk for developing osteoporosis, as well as physical changes such as menopause whose contribution to osteoporosis can be modified by preventive strategies. Calcium deficiency is an important modifiable risk factor contributing to osteoporosis. Calcium is an essential mineral in the process of bone formation and other significant body functions. When there is an insufficient intake of calcium in the diet, the body compensates by removing calcium from the skeleton, weakening bone tissue. Acidosis, which may result from a high-protein diet, contributes to osteoporosis in two ways. Calcium is withdrawn from the bone as the kidneys attempt to buffer the excess acid. Acidosis also may directly stimulate osteoclast function. A high intake of diet soda with a high phosphate content also can deplete calcium stores (McCance & Huether, 2002).

With menopause and decreasing estrogen levels, bone loss accelerates in women. Estrogen promotes the activity of osteoblasts, increasing new bone formation. In addition, estrogen enhances calcium absorption and stimulates the thyroid gland to secrete calcitonin, a hormone that suppresses osteoclast activity and increases osteoblast activity. Estrogen replacement therapy (ERT) in postmenopausal women can reverse the bone changes that occur as estrogen levels decline in early menopause.

Cigarette smoking has long been identified as a risk factor for osteoporosis. Smoking decreases the blood supply to bones. Nicotine slows the production of osteoblasts and impairs the absorption of calcium, contributing to decreased bone density.

Excess alcohol intake is another risk factor for osteoporosis. Alcohol has a direct toxic effect on osteoblast activity, suppressing bone formation during periods of alcohol intoxication. In addition, heavy alcohol use may be associated with nutritional deficiencies that contribute to osteoporosis. Interestingly, moderate alcohol consumption in postmenopausal women actually may increase bone mineral content, possibly by increasing levels of estrogen and calcitonin.

Sedentary lifestyle is another modifiable risk factor that can cause osteoporosis. Weight-bearing exercise, such as walking, influences bone metabolism in several ways. The stress of this type of exercise causes an increase in blood flow to bones, which brings growth-producing nutrients to the cells. Walking causes an increase in osteoblast growth and activity.

Prolonged use of medications that increase calcium excretion, such as aluminum-containing antacids, corticosteroids, and anticonvulsants, increase the risk of developing osteoporosis. Heparin therapy increases bone resorption, and its prolonged use is associated with osteoporosis. Antiretroviral therapy for people with AIDS or HIV infection may cause decreased bone density and osteoporosis (Porth, 2002).

## PATHOPHYSIOLOGY

While the exact pathophysiology of osteoporosis is unclear, it is known to involve an imbalance of the activity of osteoblasts that form new bone and osteoclasts that resorb bone. Until age 35, when peak bone mass occurs, formation occurs more rapidly than does reabsorption. After peak bone mass is achieved, slightly more is lost than is gained (about 0.3% to 0.5% per year); this loss is accelerated if the diet is deficient in vitamin D and calcium. In women, bone loss increases after menopause (with loss of estrogen), then slows but does not stop at about age 60. Older women may have lost between 35% and 50% of their bone mass, older men may have lost between 20% and 35% (Mayo Clinic, 2002).

Osteoporosis affects the diaphysis (shaft of the bone) and the metaphysis (portion of the bone between the diaphysis and the epiphysis). The diameter of the bone increases, thinning the outer supporting cortex. As osteoporosis progresses, trabeculae are lost from cancellous bone (the spongy tissue of bone) and the outer cortex thins to the point that even minimal stress will fracture the bone (Porth, 2002).

## MANIFESTATIONS AND COMPLICATIONS

The most common manifestations of osteoporosis are loss of height, progressive curvature of the spine, low back pain, and fractures of the forearm, spine, or hip. Osteoporosis is often called the "silent disease," as bone loss occurs without symptoms.

The loss of height occurs as vertebral bodies collapse. Acute episodes generally are painful, with radiation of the pain around the flank into the abdomen. Vertebral collapse can occur with little or no stress; minimal movements such as bending, lifting, or jumping may precipitate the pain. In some clients, vertebral collapse may occur slowly, accompanied by little discomfort. Along with loss of height, characteristic dorsal kyphosis and cervical lordosis develop, accounting for the "dowager's hump" often associated with aging. The abdomen tends to protrude and knees and hips flex as the body attempts to maintain its center of gravity (Figure 39–1 ■).

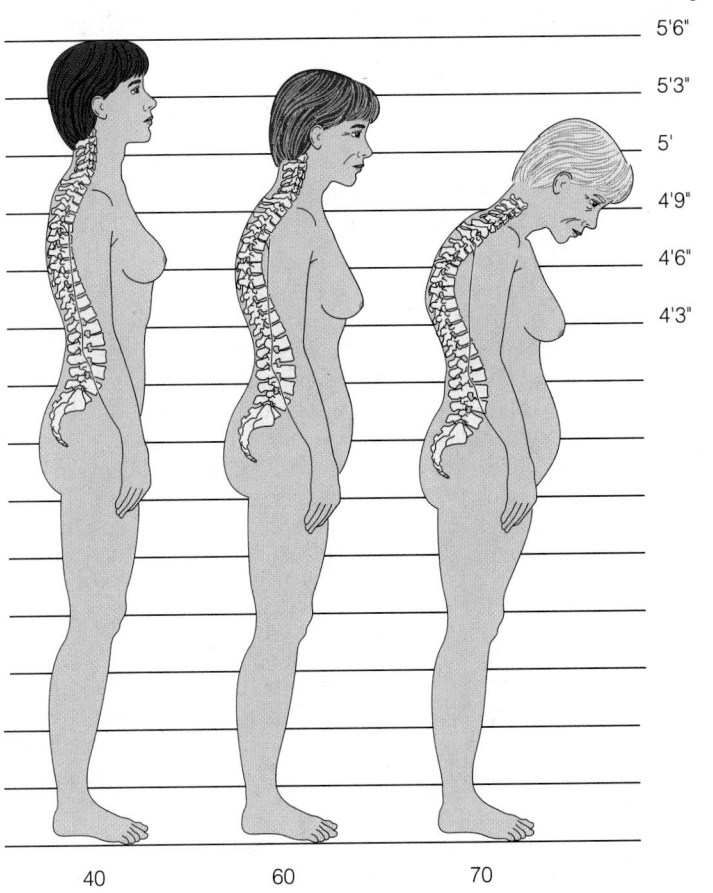

Height
5'6"
5'3"
5'
4'9"
4'6"
4'3"

Age        40          60          70

**Figure 39–1** ■ Spinal changes caused by osteoporosis. As the condition progresses, height can be reduced by as much as 7 inches.

Fractures are the most common complication of osteoporosis, with the disease being responsible for more than 1.5 million fractures each year. These include 700,000 vertebral compression fractures, 300,000 hip fractures, 250,000 wrist fractures, and 300,000 fractures at other sites (NIH, 2002). There may be no obvious manifestations of osteoporosis until fractures occur. Some fractures are spontaneous; others may result from everyday activities. While wrist and vertebral fractures have not been shown to increase disability or mortality, persistent pain and associated posture changes may restrict the client's activities or interfere with ADLs.

## COLLABORATIVE CARE

Care of the client with osteoporosis focuses on stopping or slowing the process, alleviating the symptoms, and preventing complications. Proper nutrition and exercise are important components of the treatment program.

### Diagnostic Tests

The manifestations of osteoporosis can mimic those of other bone disorders, so diagnostic tests are needed to differentiate osteoporosis from other problems

- *X-rays* provide a picture of skeletal structures; however, osteoporotic changes may not be seen until over 30% of the bone mass has been lost.

- *Quantitative computed tomography (QCT)* of the spine measures trabecular bone within vertebral bodies.
- *Dual-energy X-ray absorptiometry (DEXA)* measures bone density in the lumbar spine or hip and is considered to be highly accurate.
- *Ultrasound* transmits painless sound waves through the heel of the foot to measure bone density. This 1-minute test is not as sensitive as DEXA, but is accurate enough for screening purposes.
- *Alkaline phosphatase (AST)* may be elevated following a fracture.
- *Serum bone Gla-protein,* also called *osteocalcin,* can be used as a marker of osteoclastic activity and therefore is an indicator of the rate of bone turnover. This test is most useful to evaluate the effects of treatment, rather than as an indicator of the severity of the disease.

### Medications

Estrogen replacement therapy reduces bone loss, increases bone density in the spine and hip, and reduces the risk of fractures in postmenopausal women. It is particularly recommended for women who have undergone surgical menopause before age 50, and often is prescribed for women with other osteoporosis risk factors. Estrogen therapy alone is associated with an increased risk of endometrial cancer, so it usually is prescribed in combination with progestin (hormone replacement therapy or HRT). As discussed in Chapter 48, ⬡⬡ the

# Medication Administration
## The Client with Osteoporosis

### CALCIUM

Postmenopausal women, regardless if they take replacement estrogens, are encouraged to take calcium to prevent osteoporosis.

#### Nursing Responsibilities

- Help clients maintain an adequate dietary intake of calcium. The best dietary source is milk and other dairy products, including yogurt.
- Postmenopausal women who take estrogens need 1000 mg of calcium daily. Those who do not take estrogens need about 1500 mg daily to minimize osteoporosis.
- Identify alternate sources, such as skim milk and low-fat yogurt, oysters, canned sardines or salmon, beans, cauliflower, and dark-green leafy vegetables.

#### Client and Family Teaching

- Take calcium carbonate in divided doses 30 to 60 minutes before meals to allow for absorption.
- Take calcium citrate with meals to minimize gastrointestinal distress.

### CALCITONIN

Calcitonin-salmon injection, synthetic
Calcimar
Miacalin (injection or nasal spray)

In postmenopausal osteoporosis, calcitonin prevents further bone loss and increases bone mass if the client consumes adequate amounts of calcium and vitamin D. Calcitonin may be used in postmenopausal women who cannot or will not take estrogen.

#### Nursing Responsibilities

- Calcitonin is protein in nature; both the parenteral and nasal spray forms may cause an anaphylactic-type allergic response. Observe the client for 20 minutes after administration; have appropriate emergency equipment and drugs available to treat anaphylaxis.
- Alternate nostrils daily when administering calcitonin nasal spray.
- Review medical history for conditions that contraindicate use of calcitonin products: hypersensitivity to salmon calcitonin and lactation (calcitonin is secreted in breast milk and may inhibit lactation).

- Observe for side effects: nausea and vomiting, anorexia, mild transient flushing of the palms of the hands and the soles of the feet, and urinary frequency.
- Teach the client the proper technique for handling and injecting the drug at home.

#### Client and Family Teaching

- Take the medication in the evening to minimize side effects.
- Warm nasal spray to room temperature before using.
- Rhinitis (runny nose) is the most common side effect with calcitonin nasal spray. Other possible side effects include sores, itching, or other nasal symptoms. Report nosebleeds to your primary care provider.
- Nausea and vomiting may occur during initial stages of therapy; they disappear as treatment continues.
- While taking the medication, be sure to consume adequate amounts of calcium and vitamin D.

### FLUORIDE

Fluoride is a mineral long recognized as essential for the normal formation of dentin and tooth enamel. Fluoride appears to decrease the solubility of bone mineral and therefore the rate of bone reabsorption. Its use in preventing and treating osteoporosis is relatively new but promising.

#### Nursing Responsibilities

- Monitor serum fluoride levels every 3 months.
- Have bone mineral density studies conducted at 6-month intervals to document progress of bone growth.

#### Client and Family Teaching

- Take sodium fluoride tablets after meals, and avoid milk or dairy products; these reduce gastrointestinal absorption of the medication.
- While taking fluoride, be sure to maintain an adequate calcium intake.
- Use fluoride mouth rinse immediately after brushing teeth and just before retiring at night. Do not swallow the rinse, and avoid eating or drinking for at least 30 minutes after use.
- Notify the physician if teeth become stained or mottled after repeated use of fluoride mouth rinse.

---

risks of HRT are believed to be too high for long-term therapy. The choice of using HRT to prevent osteoporosis is one that must be made between the woman and her health care provider.

Raloxifene (Evista) is a selective estrogen receptor modulator (SERM) that appears to prevent bone loss by mimicking estrogen's beneficial effects on bone density in postmenopausal women. It does not have the risks of estrogen. Hot flashes are a common side effect, and this drug should not be taken by a woman with a history of blood clots.

Alendronate (Fosamax), risedronate (Actonel), and etidronate (Didronel) are from the class of drugs known as biphosphonates. Biphosphonates are potent inhibitors of bone resorption that may be used to prevent and treat osteoporosis. They inhibit bone breakdown, preserve bone mass, and increase bone density in the

hip and vertebrae. These are especially useful for men, young adults, and to prevent or treat steroid-induced osteoporosis. The nursing implications of biphosphonates are found in the Medication Administration box on page 1232.

Calcitonin (Miacalcin) is a hormone that increases bone formation and decreases bone resorption. Calcitonin increases spinal bone density and reduces the risk of compression fractures; it may reduce the risk of hip fracture as well. Calcitonin usually is prescribed as a nasal spray, although it also is available in parenteral form. Because calcitonin is a protein, it can precipitate anaphylactic-type allergic responses. See the box above.

Sodium fluoride stimulates osteoblast activity, increasing bone formation. When used to treat osteoporosis, bone mass of the spine increases and the risk of spinal fractures may be reduced. Fluoride therapy may, however, be associated with an increased risk of hip and other nonvertebral fractures. See the Medication Administration box on page 1226.

## NURSING CARE

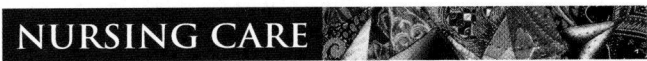

Osteoporosis is both preventable and treatable; therefore, nursing care focuses primarily on planning and implementing interventions to prevent the disease, its manifestations, and the resulting injuries. An important aspect of preventing osteoporosis is educating clients under age 35.

## Health Promotion

Health promotion activities to prevent or slow osteoporosis focus on calcium intake, exercise, and health-related behaviors.

### Diet

For clients of all ages, stress the importance of maintaining a daily calcium intake that meets NIH recommendations (see Chapter 5). ⊖⊘ This is particularly important for adolescent girls and young adult women who may avoid eating many high-calcium foods such as dairy products because of concerns about weight. Optimal calcium intake before age 30 to 35 probably increases peak bone mass. Emphasize that lowfat (or nonfat) dairy products also contain calcium, although some fat in the product may enhance calcium absorption.

Milk and milk products are the best sources of calcium. The lactose in milk facilitates calcium absorption as well. Other food sources of calcium include sardines, clams, oysters, and salmon, as well as dark green, leafy vegetables such as broccoli, collard greens, bok choy, and spinach. For clients who avoid dairy products because of lactose intolerance or a vegetarian diet, suggest alternate sources.

Calcium supplements are available in many forms. Most supplements (including Tums) provide calcium carbonate in the range of 200 to 600 mg per tablet. Other forms of calcium, including citrate, gluconate, and lactate, generally provide a lower amount of elemental calcium per tablet. A combination of calcium with vitamin D is recommended, particularly for older adults who may have a vitamin D deficiency that impairs their ability to absorb and use calcium. (Calcium supplements are discussed in Chapter 5.) ⊖⊘

### Exercise

Teach clients the importance of physical activity and weight-bearing exercises in preventing and slowing bone loss. Suggest that clients participate in regular exercise such as walking for at least 20 minutes four or more times a week. Inform clients that swimming and pool aerobic exercises are not as beneficial in maintaining bone density because of the lack of weight-bearing activity.

### Healthy Behaviors

Behaviors that help prevent osteoporosis include not smoking, avoiding excessive alcohol intake, and limiting caffeine intake to two or three cups of coffee each day.

## Assessment

Collect the following data through the health history and physical examination (see Chapter 37).

- Health history: age, risk factors, history of fractures, smoking history, alcohol intake, medications, usual diet, menstrual history including menopause, usual exercise/activity level
- Physical examination: height, spinal curves, low back pain

## Nursing Diagnoses and Interventions

Nursing care of clients who have osteoporosis focuses on teaching about the disease process, helping maintain physical mobility and nutrition, and solving problems associated with pain and injury.

### Health-Seeking Behaviors

At multiple points in the client's lifetime, nurses can provide vital information that will help clients use self-care strategies to reduce their risk of developing osteoporosis.

- Assess the client's health habits, including diet, exercise, smoking, and alcohol use. *The risk of developing osteoporosis in later life is affected by such things as diet, regular participation in weight-bearing exercise, and personal habits such as smoking and alcohol consumption.*
- Teach women and men of all ages about the importance of maintaining an adequate calcium intake. Provide a list of calcium-rich foods, and discuss the use of calcium supplements with clients who do not consume adequate dietary calcium. *Calcium needs vary during the course of a lifetime; however, many clients never consume adequate amounts of calcium. This affects their peak bone mass and the rate of bone loss with aging. Calcium in foods is more completely absorbed than that supplied by calcium supplements.*

**PRACTICE ALERT** *Recommended calcium intake increases through the adult years as follows: age 19 to 50 = 1000 mg/day; age 51 to 64 = 12000 mg/day; age 65 and older = 1500 mg/day.* ■

- Discuss the importance of maintaining a regular schedule of weight-bearing exercise, either through an exercise program or regular physical activity. *Weight-bearing exercise promotes osteoblast activity, helping maintain bone strength and integrity.*
- Refer clients to smoking-cessation programs and alcohol treatment programs as appropriate. *Smoking interferes with estrogen's protective effects on bones, promoting bone loss. Excess alcohol intake affects the nutritional status of the client, increasing the risk of calcium and vitamin D deficiency.*
- Refer clients with significant risk factors for osteoporosis to primary care providers or clinics for bone-density evaluation as indicated. *Early identification and treatment of osteoporotic changes in bones can reduce the risk and possible long-term consequences of falls and fractures.*

### Risk for Injury

Falls that would result in little or no injury in the healthy adult may cause fractures in the client with osteoporosis. Even normal movements such as twisting, bending, lifting, or rising from bed can precipitate a vertebral fracture.

- Implement safety precautions as necessary for the client who is hospitalized or in a long-term care facility. Maintain the client's bed in low position; use side rails if indicated to prevent the client from getting up alone; provide nighttime lighting to toilet facilities. *Most falls are preventable, particularly in hospitals and long-term care facilities.*
- Avoid using restraints (if hospitalized or a resident in a long-term care facility) if at all possible. *Restraints may actually increase the client's risk of falling and increase the risk of injury associated with a fall.*

**PRACTICE ALERT** *Clients may fracture osteoporotic bones when pulling against restraints.* ■

- Teach clients who are able to participate in weight-bearing exercises to perform exercises at least three times a week for a sustained period of 30 to 40 minutes. The mechanical force of weight-bearing exercises promotes bone growth. *Bones weaken and demineralize without exercise. Walking is an easy, low-impact form of exercise. Swimming (including walking on the bottom of the pool) does not provide the needed weight-bearing activity.*
- Encourage older adults to use assistive devices to maintain independence in ADLs. *Walking sticks, canes, and other assistive devices encourage client independence and support activities that promote bone growth.*
- Teach older clients about safety and fall precautions. *A simple assessment of the client's home for safety and fall risks may reduce the risk of fractures and, in turn, the cost of hospitalization and potential disability and/or death.*
- Evaluate and closely monitor the client's medications. The reasons for, types of, and dosage of the client's medications should be evaluated, especially if the person has been falling frequently or has a change in mental status. *Falls may be related to the number of both prescribed and over-the-counter medications the client is taking.*

### Imbalanced Nutrition: Less Than Body Requirements

Most Americans do not maintain their recommended daily intake of calcium. Clients must therefore be made aware of the relationship between an adequate calcium intake and maintaining strong bones.

- Teach adolescents, pregnant or lactating women, and adults through age 35 to eat foods high in calcium and to maintain a daily calcium intake of 1200 to 1500 mg. *The National Institutes of Health recommend a daily calcium intake of 1200 to 1500 mg per day for adolescents and young adults, as well as for pregnant and lactating women.*
- Encourage postmenopausal women to maintain a calcium intake of 1000 to 1500 mg daily, either through diet or a calcium supplement. *Calcium needs for postmenopausal women vary, depending on age and estrogen therapy.*
- Teach clients taking calcium supplements the importance of taking the medication at the proper time and the side effects

that may occur. *Free hydrochloric acid is needed for calcium absorption. Calcium carbonate supplement (e.g., Tums) should be taken 30 to 60 minutes before meals to allow adequate absorption. Calcium citrate supplements should be taken with meals to prevent gastrointestinal distress.*

**PRACTICE ALERT** *Calcium supplements should be taken in divided doses (two to three times daily) for improved distribution.* ■

### Acute Pain

Advanced stages of osteoporosis can result in pain and immobilization. Acute pain usually results from a complicating fracture, especially a compression fracture of the vertebrae.

- Review activity tolerance and suggest modifications in exercise schedules as indicated. *Clients with osteoporosis should remain active and participate in weight-bearing exercises; however, the client's abilities and severity of the disease may warrant a modification in the exercise regimen.*
- Suggest anti-inflammatory pain medications for treatment of both acute and chronic phases of pain. Clients should be instructed in the amount and frequency as noted on the manufacturer's labels. *Continuous administration of ibuprofen or other NSAIDs can be useful to provide relief from pain.*

**PRACTICE ALERT** *Teach clients on long-term anti-inflammatory medications to watch for bright red bleeding from the stomach or dark black bowel movements.* ■

- Suggest the application of heat to relieve pain. *A heating pad may offer temporary pain relief. To avoid the "rebound effect," the heat should be removed every 20 to 30 minutes.*

### Using NANDA, NIC, and NOC

Chart 39–1 shows links between NANDA nursing diagnoses, NIC, and NOC when caring for the client with osteoporosis.

### Home Care

The client who has osteoporosis needs education on safety and preventing falls (see Chapter 38). In addition to home safety, outdoor safety is important too. Clients should be taught to use assistive devices for added stability, to wear rubber-soled shoes for traction, to walk on the grass when sidewalks are slippery, and to sprinkle salt or kitty litter on icy sidewalks in the winter.

Address the following topics when discussing home care.

- Resources for medical supplies and assistive devices
- Diet, exercise, and medications
- Pain management
- Maintaining good posture to help prevent stress on the spine
- Helpful resources:
  - National Osteoporosis Foundation
  - Osteoporosis and Related Bone Diseases National Resource Center (National Institutes of Health)
  - National Women's Health Resource Center
  - Older Women's League

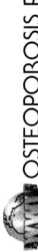

MediaLink | OSTEOPOROSIS PREVENTION APPLICATION

## CHART 39–1  NANDA, NIC, AND NOC LINKAGES

### The Client with Osteoporosis

| NURSING DIAGNOSES | NURSING INTERVENTIONS | NURSING OUTCOMES |
|---|---|---|
| • Chronic Pain | • Medication Administration<br>• Pain Management | • Comfort Level<br>• Pain: Disruptive Effects |
| • Risk for Trauma | • Environmental Management: Safety<br>• Fall Prevention<br>• Health Education<br>• Teaching: Disease Process | • Risk Control<br>• Safety Behavior: Fall Prevention<br>• Self-Care: Activities of Daily Living |
| • Knowledge Deficit: Calcium Intake | • Teaching: Disease Process<br>• Teaching: Prescribed Diet<br>• Teaching: Prescribed Medications | • Knowledge: Disease Process<br>• Knowledge: Diet<br>• Knowledge: Prescribed Medications |

*Note: Data from* Nursing Outcomes Classification (NOC) *by M. Johnson & M. Maas (Eds.), 1997, St. Louis: Mosby;* Nursing Diagnoses: Definitions & Classification 2001–2002 *by North American Nursing Diagnosis Association, 2001, Philadelphia: NANDA;* Nursing Interventions Classification (NIC) *by J.C. McCloskey & G. M. Bulechek (Eds.), 2000, St. Louis: Mosby. Reprinted by permission.*

## Nursing Care Plan
## A Client with Osteoporosis

Nancy Bauer is a 53-year-old schoolteacher. She has been married for 36 years and has two children. Mrs. Bauer says she is 65 inches tall. She has smoked one pack of cigarettes a day for 30 years and drinks one to two glasses of wine with dinner each evening. She does not routinely exercise. Mrs. Bauer has had symptoms of menopause for 8 years, including hot flashes in the early years and mood swings of late. She has never been on hormone replacement therapy.

Mrs. Bauer is currently seeking medical advice for continuous low back pain. The pain is not relieved with an over-the-counter analgesic, and she frequently wakes up during the night because of the pain.

### ASSESSMENT

The nurse practitioner notes that Mrs. Bauer's vital signs are all within normal limits. She has full range of motion of all extremities and is able to stand and bend over, but she reports discomfort when returning to the upright position. Mrs. Bauer has a slightly pronounced "hump" on her upper back and is 1 inch shorter than her stated height on admission. Her muscle strength is symmetric and strong.

### DIAGNOSIS

• *Acute pain* of the lower spine related to vertebral compression
• *Deficient knowledge* related to osteoporosis and treatment to prevent further damage
• *Imbalanced nutrition: Less than body requirements* related to inadequate intake of calcium
• *Risk for injury* related to effects of change in bone structure secondary to osteoporosis

### EXPECTED OUTCOMES

• Verbalize a decrease in back pain.
• Be able to describe ways to treat her osteoporosis and prevent further complications.
• Verbalize an understanding of the current research and treatment regarding osteoporosis.

• Verbalize how stopping smoking can help prevent further progression of osteoporosis.
• Seek consultation for supplements and medications to prevent further bone loss.
• Design a program of physical activity to prevent complications of osteoporosis.
• Verbalize safety precautions to prevent fractures due to falls.

### PLANNING AND IMPLEMENTATION

• Teach back strengthening exercises.
• Refer to an osteoporosis support group, if available.
• Provide realistic, yet optimistic, feedback about loss of height and bone integrity and the potential outcomes of treatment.
• Assess current knowledge base, and correct misconceptions regarding treatment of osteoporosis.
• Provide current educational literature regarding treatment of osteoporosis.
• Instruct in dietary and calcium supplements that help prevent effects of osteoporosis.
• Discuss physical exercises that help prevent complications due to osteoporosis.
• Review safety and fall precautions, and provide literature regarding how to create a safe home environment.

### EVALUATION

On her return visit 6 months later, Mrs. Bauer reports that she feels much better. She is no longer irritable and does not experience mood swings, because she has been taking her prescribed hormone replacements for 6 months. She is eating products rich in calcium and taking a daily supplement of calcium with vitamin D. Mrs. Bauer has reduced her wine intake to one glass in the evening and now drinks decaffeinated coffee and tea. She also states that since she stopped smoking, she has been walking 30 to 45 minutes every day.

(continued on page 1230)

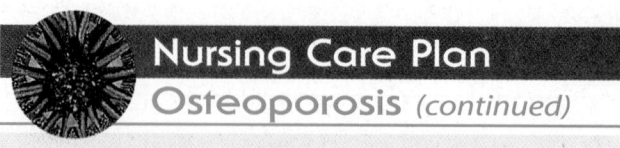

## Nursing Care Plan
### Osteoporosis *(continued)*

### Critical Thinking in the Nursing Process

1. What is the rationale for stopping smoking and limiting caffeine and alcohol intake in the treatment of osteoporosis?
2. What foods would you encourage for clients at high risk for osteoporosis whose serum cholesterol and LDL/HDL ratios indicate a high risk for cardiovascular disease?
3. What physical activities would you consider beneficial in helping to prevent the effects of osteoporosis in the female client who is wheelchair bound or has limited mobility?
4. Develop a care plan for Mrs. Bauer for the nursing diagnosis, *Risk for trauma.*

See Evaluating Your Response in Appendix C.

## THE CLIENT WITH PAGET'S DISEASE

**Paget's disease,** also called **osteitis deformans,** is a progressive skeletal disorder that results from excessive metabolic activity in bone, with abnormal bone resorption and formation. This chronic remodeling results in the affected bones being larger and softer (McCance & Huether, 2002). This disorder affects the axial skeleton, especially the femur, pelvis, vertebrae, sacrum, sternum, and skull.

Paget's disease affects about 3% of the population over age 40, and the incidence doubles each 10 years after age 50. Paget's disease occurs more frequently in whites in continental Europe, England, Australia, New Zealand, and North America. It has a familial tendency and is slightly more common in men than in women (Porth, 2002).

### PATHOPHYSIOLOGY

The cause of Paget's disease is unknown; however, several theories have been proposed, including hormonal imbalance, vascular disorder, neoplasm, autoimmune disorder, and inborn error of connective tissue. Of people affected by Paget's disease, 20% to 30% have a family history of the disorder, suggesting a genetic linkage. A slow-activating viral infection also has been theorized as a cause of Paget's disease.

Paget's disease progresses slowly. It usually follows a two-stage process: an excessive amount of osteoclastic bone resorption, followed by excessive osteoblastic bone formation. The initial phase presents with an abnormal increase in osteoclasts. The bones increase in size and thickness because of the acceleration in bone resorption and regeneration, resulting in a thick layer of coarse bone with a rough and pitted outer surface (Porth, 2002). Resorption of cancellous bone occurs rapidly. As new bone tissue tries to replace the loss, fibrous tissue forms in the bone marrow. The bone is at first hyperemic and soft, and bowing occurs. When this excessive bone cell activity decreases, the result is a gain in bone mass, but the newly formed bone becomes hard and

brittle. This brittleness may lead to fractures. Paget's disease varies in severity, and may involve one or many bones.

## MANIFESTATIONS AND COMPLICATIONS

Most clients with Paget's disease are asymptomatic, and the disease often is discovered when typical changes are seen on an incidental X-ray. Manifestations are often vague and depend on the specific area involved (see the box below). The most common complaint is localized pain of the long bones, spine, pelvis, and cranium. The pain is described as a mild to moderate deep ache that is aggravated by pressure and weight bearing. It is more noticeable at night or when the client is resting. The pain usually is due to metabolic bone activity, secondary degenerative osteoarthritis, fractures, or nerve impingement. Because of the increase in blood flow to pagetic bone, flushing and warmth of the overlying skin may be apparent.

Other complications of Paget's disease are as follows:

- Nerve palsy syndromes from involvement of the upper extremities
- Pathologic fractures from loss of bone structure
- Mental deterioration from compression of the brain when the skull is involved
- Compression of the spinal cord from affected cervical vertebra causing tetraplegia
- Cardiovascular disease, resulting from vasodilation of the vessels in the skin and subcutaneous tissues overlying the affected bones
- Osteogenic sarcoma (in about 1% of cases)

## Manifestations of Paget's Disease

### MUSCULOSKELETAL EFFECTS
- Pain (in the long bones of lower extremities or joints)
- Deformity (enlargement of skull, bowing of lower extremities, and deformity of elbows and knees)
- Chalkstick-type fractures of lower extremities
- Pathologic fractures (especially of the tibia)
- Compression fractures
- Collapse of the vertebrae, resulting in kyphosis and loss of height
- Muscle weakness

### NEUROLOGIC EFFECTS
- Hearing loss
- Spinal cord injuries
- Dementia
- Pain from spinal stenosis
- Bladder and/or bowel dysfunction

### CARDIOVASCULAR EFFECTS
- High cardiac output
- Congestive heart failure
- Increased skin temperature over affected extremities

### METABOLIC EFFECTS
- Symptoms of hypercalcemia in immobilized clients
- Hypercalciuria and renal calculi

TABLE 39–1  Differential Features of Osteoporosis, Osteomalacia, and Paget's Disease

| Differentiating Features | Osteoporosis | Osteomalacia | Paget's Disease |
|---|---|---|---|
| Pathophysiology | Resorption greater than bone formation | Inadequate mineralization of bone matrix | Excessive osteoclastic activity and formation of poor-quality bone |
| Calcium level (serum) | Normal | Low or normal | Normal or elevated (especially in immobilized clients) |
| Phosphate level (serum) | Normal | Low or normal | Normal |
| Parathyroid hormone level (serum) | Normal | High or normal | Normal |
| Alkaline phosphatase level (serum) | Normal | Elevated | Increased; not a reliable test for clients who have liver disease or are pregnant |
| Hydroxyproline (urine) | Not applicable | Not applicable | Increased |
| Radiographic findings | Osteopenia, fractures | Decreased bone density, radiolucent bands known as Looser's zones, or pseudofractures | "Punched-out" appearance of bone, increase in bone thickness, linear fractures, mosaic pattern of bone matrix |

## COLLABORATIVE CARE

Care of the client with Paget's disease focuses on relieving pain, suppressing bone cell activity if necessary, and preventing or minimizing the effects of complications. Many clients with Paget's disease are asymptomatic and do not require treatment. For more severely affected clients, pharmacologic agents are usually effective. Occasionally, surgery may be required.

### Diagnostic Tests

Many of the diagnostic tests that are useful for the diagnosis of osteoporosis are equally useful for clients with Paget's disease (Table 39–1). These include the following:

- *X-rays* illustrate localized areas of demineralization in the early stages, seen as "punched out" areas that lend a coarse, irregular appearance to the bone. In the later phase, X-rays show enlargement of the bones, tiny cracks in the long bones, and/or bowing of the weight-bearing bones.
- *Bone scan* will show areas of active Paget's disease.
- *CT scans* and *MRI* help identify possible causes of pain, including degenerative problems, spinal stenosis, or nerve root impingement.
- *Serum alkaline phosphatase* will show a steady rise as the disease progresses; the normal level (30 to 115 IU/L) may be elevated from high normal to over 3000 IU/L.
- *Urinary collagen pyridinoline testing* is a sensitive indicator of the rate of bone resorption.

### Medications

Clients who have mild symptoms often find relief using aspirin or NSAIDs, such as ibuprofen (Motrin) and indomethacin (Indocin). Clients who are experiencing manifestations and whose diagnostic test results are elevated are usually treated with an agent that retards bone resorption, such as calcitonin or a bisphosphonate.

Bisphosphonates such as alendronate (Fosamax), pamidronate (Aredia), and tiludronate (Skelid) are the primary treatments used for severe Paget's disease. These drugs inhibit bone resorption, possibly by attaching to the surface of the calcium/phosphate phase of bone and inhibiting osteoclast activity. They are safe, and usually are well tolerated by the client. In the United States, alendronate is available as an oral preparation, and pamidronate is available for intravenous administration. Oral preparations are poorly absorbed from the GI tract, and may cause gastric or esophageal irritation. Alendronate should be given with a full glass of water on an empty stomach, at least 30 minutes before other medications or food. Pamidronate is given as an intravenous infusion in D5W or normal saline. It is given for 3 successive days, generally promoting a rapid response with reduced urinary excretion of hydroxyproline and pyridinium and a fall in alkaline phosphatate. Intravenous pamidronate may cause flulike symptoms, but these generally are short-lived. Calcium supplements also are prescribed for clients receiving bisphosphonates. After bisphosphonate treatment, clients often experience remission of symptoms for a year or more. See the Medication Adminstration box on page 1232 for nursing implications.

Calcitonin inhibits osteoclastic resorption of bone. It also works as an analgesic for bone pain. The two derivatives of this medication are salmon (fish) and human. Salmon calcitonin (Calcimar) is generally preferred because it is inexpensive and widely available. Human calcitonin (Cibacalcin) is derived from human thyroid glands, which makes it more expensive and difficult to obtain. Both parenteral and nasal spray formulations of calcitonin are available (refer to the Medication Administration box on page 1226 for nursing implications).

### Surgery

Total hip or knee replacement is usually required when the client with Paget's disease develops degenerative arthritis of the hip or knee. These surgical procedures are usually performed

## Medication Administration
### The Client with Paget's Disease

**BISPHOSPHONATES**

Alendronate (Fosamax)
Pamidronate (Aredia)
Tiludronate (Skelid)

The bisphosphonates inhibit bone resorption, increasing the mineral density of bones and reducing the incidence of fractures. They are also used both in the prevention and treatment of osteoporosis. When used for Paget's disease, bisphosphonates slow the accelerated bone turnover associated with this disease. Bone pain is relieved, and the incidence of pathologic fractures is reduced. Cardiac and vascular manifestations of the disease also improve.

**Nursing Responsibilities**
- Administer alendronate with water when the client arises 30 minutes before food or other medications.
- Do not give foods high in calcium, vitamins with mineral supplements, or antacids within 2 hours of administering alendronate.
- Instruct the client to avoid lying down for 30 minutes after taking the drug.
- Assess renal function studies before initiating therapy; alendronate is not recommended for use in clients with renal insufficiency.
- Dilute the prescribed dose of pamidronate in 1000 mL of D5W or normal saline; infuse over at least 4 hours. Do not add to calcium-containing solutions such as Ringer's or lactated Ringer's solutions.
- Monitor the IV site for signs of thrombophlebitis.
- Assess the client for signs of electrolyte imbalance or other adverse responses such as a drug fever.

**Client and Family Teaching**
- Take the medication as directed with clear water only. Consuming other beverages or food within 30 minutes of taking alendronate may interfere with its absorption and effectiveness.
- Do not lie down until after you have eaten breakfast. Alendronate can irritate the esophagus.
- Report symptoms such as new or worsening heart-burn, difficulty swallowing, or painful swallowing.
- Fever with or without chills may occur while receiving intravenous pamidronate; this will subside without treatment. Flu-like symptoms also may occur; these will subside within a week or so.
- Report any abnormal symptoms such as tingling around the mouth or numbness and tingling of the fingers or toes, which may indicate an imbalance of electrolytes in the blood.
- Take calcium and vitamin D supplements as instructed by your primary care provider.
- Response to these medications is gradual, and continues for months after the drug is stopped.

---

to address severe pain during weight bearing and impaired mobility. Neurologic manifestations related to spinal stenosis or nerve root compression may also require surgery.

## NURSING CARE

### Nursing Diagnoses and Interventions

The nursing interventions for the client with symptomatic Paget's disease focus on pain control, prevention of injury or fractures, and education regarding the disease process and prescribed therapies.

### Chronic Pain

The most common manifestation of Paget's disease is bone pain. This usually is the manifestation that prompts the client to seek health care.

- Assess the location and extent of the pain to determine the bone areas involved. *Bone pain in Paget's disease is poorly localized and is frequently described as "aching and deep."*
- Teach the client to take NSAIDs or aspirin on a regular basis as prescribed. *Pain is most noticeable at night or when the client is resting. The pain can become evident when it is aggravated by pressure and weight bearing.*
- Ensure correct placement of prescribed brace or corset. The client may be required to wear a light brace or corset to relieve back pain and provide support when assuming an upright position. *The client may need instruction in the correct application of the device and in the evaluation of pressure areas that may result from wearing the device.*
- Suggest referral for heat therapy and massage. *Heat therapy and massage can alleviate mild discomfort. Care should be taken when applying massage over areas prone to pathologic fractures.*

### Impaired Physical Mobility

Clients with Paget's disease need to maintain or improve mobility so that they can perform necessary self-care activities and prevent complications of immobility.

- Provide an assistive device for use when ambulating. *During the active phase of Paget's disease, the client is prone to fractures. Bone deformities, activity intolerance, fear of falling, and pain are all factors that may make the client more prone to falls. An assistive device can provide both physical and psychologic support during ambulation, permit the client to ambulate further, and provide a device for resting during the ambulation session.*
- Teach good body mechanics. *The client with bone deformities should avoid activities that require lifting and twisting.*

**PRACTICE ALERT** *Activities as seemingly simple as lifting a heavy box may result in a fracture in the client with Paget's disease.* ■

- Reinforce information about exercise protocols and activity regimens. *Exercise and activity protocols should be planned carefully to prevent injury and to minimize fatigue.*

## Home Care

Paget's disease, once diagnosed, can be frightening for the client and family. It is important that they understand that this is a treatable disease, and that many manifestations of the disease will be relieved with treatment. Inform the client that remissions of the disease often last for a year or more after effective treatment. The Paget Foundation should be suggested as a resource. Discuss the following topics.

- The importance of following the prescribed treatment regimen and keeping scheduled follow-up appointments
- Because it may take several weeks to notice a response to treatment, the importance of continuing therapy during this time and after a response is obtained
- If bisphosphonates such as alendronate or pamidronate are ordered, the importance of taking supplemental calcium to prevent low blood calcium levels
- The importance of remaining active
- Safety in the home and outdoor environment to prevent falls
- The need to report to the primary care provider any sudden pain or disability, even if no trauma has occurred, as pathologic fractures are possible

# THE CLIENT WITH GOUT

**Gout** is a syndrome that occurs from an inflammatory response to the production or excretion of uric acid resulting in high levels of uric acid in the blood (*hyperuricemia)* and in other body fluids, including synovial fluid (McCance & Huether, 2002). This metabolic disorder is characterized by deposits of urates (insoluble precipitates) in the connective tissues of the body. Gout has an acute onset, usually at night, and often involves the first metatarsophalangeal joint (great toe). The initial acute attack is usually followed by a period of months or years without manifestations. As the disease progresses, urates are deposited in various other connective tissues. Deposits in the synovial fluids cause acute inflammation of the joint (**gouty arthritis**). Over time, urate deposits in subcutaneous tissues cause the formation of small white nodules (called **tophi**). Deposits of crystals in the kidneys can form urate kidney stones and result in kidney failure.

Gout may occur as either a primary or secondary disorder. Primary gout is characterized by elevated serum uric acid levels resulting from either an inborn error of purine metabolism or a decrease in renal uric acid excretion due to an unknown cause. Purines are part of the structure of the nuclear compounds DNA and RNA; they also may be synthesized by the body. Impaired uric acid excretion leads to hyperuricemia in the majority of people with primary gout. In secondary gout, hyperuricemia occurs as a result of another disorder or treatment with certain medications. Disorders associated with rapid cell turnover, such as some malignancies (leukemia in particular), hemolytic anemia, and polycythemia, can increase purine metabolism. Chronic renal disease, hypertension, starvation, and diabetic ketoacidosis can interfere with

uric acid excretion, as can certain drugs, including some diuretics (such as furosemide, ethacrynic acid, and chlorothiazide), pyrazinamide, cyclosporin, ethambutol, and low-dose salicylates. Ethanol ingestion appears to interfere with uric acid excretion and to accelerate its synthesis. In addition, hospitalized clients with gout are at risk for an acute attack from changes in their diet, abdominal surgery, or medications (Tierney et al., 2001).

The peak age of onset of gout in men is between 40 and 50 years. It is rare in women before menopause. The disease is more common in Pacific Islanders.

## PATHOPHYSIOLOGY

Uric acid is the breakdown product of purine metabolism. Normally, a balance exists between its production and excretion, with approximately two-thirds of the amount produced each day excreted by the kidneys and the rest in the feces. The serum uric acid level is normally maintained between 3.4 and 7.0 mg/dL in men and 2.4 and 6.0 mg/dL in women. At levels greater than 7.0 mg/dL, the serum is saturated, and monosodium urate crystals may form. It is not known exactly how crystals of monosodium urate crystals are deposited in joints. Several mechanisms may be involved:

- Crystals tend to form in peripheral tissues of the body, where lower temperatures reduce the solubility of the uric acid.
- A decrease in extracellular fluid pH and reduced plasma protein binding of urate crystals are evident.
- Tissue trauma and a rapid change in uric acid levels may also lead to crystal deposition. A rapid increase in uric acid may occur with tissue trauma and release of cellular components.

The monosodium urate crystals may form in the synovial fluid or in the synovial membrane, cartilage, or other joint connective tissues. They may also form in the heart, earlobes, and kidneys. These crystals stimulate and continue the inflammatory process, during which neutrophils respond by ingesting the crystals. The neutrophils release their phagolysosomes, causing tissue damage, which perpetuates the inflammation.

## MANIFESTATIONS AND COMPLICATIONS

The manifestations of gout are hyperuricemia, recurrent attacks of inflammation of a single joint, tophi in and around the joint, renal disease, and renal stones. Unless treated, the manifestations of gout appear in three stages: asymptomatic hyperuricemia, acute gouty arthritis, and tophaceous gout.

### Asymptomatic Hyperuricemia

The first stage is asymptomatic hyperuricemia, with serum levels averaging 9 to 10 mg/dL. Most people with hyperuricemia do not progress to further stages of the disease.

### Acute Gouty Arthritis

The second state is acute gouty arthritis. The acute attack, usually affecting a single joint, occurs unexpectedly, often beginning at night. It may be triggered by trauma, alcohol ingestion, dietary excess, or a stressor such as surgery. It is often precipitated by an abrupt or sustained increase in uric acid levels. The

## Manifestations of Gout

### ACUTE GOUTY ARTHRITIS

- Usually monoarticular, affecting metatarsophalangeal joint of great toe, instep, ankle, knee, wrist, or elbow
- Acute pain
- Red, hot, swollen, and tender joint
- Fever, chills, malaise
- Elevated WBC and sedimentation rate

### CHRONIC TOPHACEOUS GOUT

- Tophi evident on joints, bursae, tendon sheaths, pressure points, helix of ear
- Joint stiffness, limited ROM, and deformity
- Ulceration of tophi with chalky discharge

affected joint becomes red, hot, swollen, and exquisitely painful and tender.

Approximately 50% of initial attacks of acute gouty arthritis occur in the metatarsophalangeal joint of the great toe. Other sites for acute attacks include the instep of the foot, ankles, heels, knees, wrists, fingers, and elbows. The pain, often intense, peaks within several hours and may be accompanied by fever and an elevated WBC and sedimentation rate. (See the box above.) The affected joints are swollen, the skin over the joint is warm and dusky red.

Acute attacks of gouty arthritis last from several hours up to several weeks and typically subside spontaneously. There are no long-lasting sequelae, and the client enters an asymptomatic period called the intercritical period. The intercritical period may last up to 10 years; however, approximately 60% of people experience a recurrent attack within 1 year. Successive attacks tend to last longer, occur with increasing frequency, and resolve less completely than the initial attack.

## Tophaceous (Chronic) Gout

Tophaceous or chronic gout occurs when hyperuricemia is not treated. The urate pool expands, and monosodium urate crystal deposits (tophi) develop in cartilage, synovial membranes, tendons, and soft tissues. They are seen most often in the helix of the ear; in tissues surrounding joints and bursae (especially around the elbows and knees); along tendons of the finger, toes, ankles, and wrists; on ulnar surfaces of the forearms; along the shins of the legs; and on other pressure points. The skin over tophi may ulcerate, exuding chalky material containing inflammatory cells and urate crystals. Tophi can also develop in the tissues of the heart and spinal epidura. Although tophi themselves are not painful, they may restrict joint movement and cause pain and deformities of the affected joints. Tophi may also compress nerves and erode and drain through the skin.

Kidney disease may occur in clients with untreated gout, particularly when hypertension is also present. Urate crystals are deposited in renal interstitial tissue. Uric acid crystals also form in the collecting tubules, renal pelvis, and ureter, forming stones. Renal stones are 1000 times more prevalent in people with primary gout (McCance & Huether, 2002).

The stones can range in size from a grain of sand to a massive structure filling the spaces of the kidney. Uric acid stones can potentially obstruct urine flow and lead to acute renal failure.

## COLLABORATIVE CARE

The classic presentation of acute gouty arthritis is so distinctive that the diagnosis can often be based on the client's history and physical examination. Treatment is directed toward terminating an acute attack, preventing recurrent attacks, and reversing or preventing complications resulting from crystal deposition in tissues and formation of uric acid kidney stones.

### Diagnostic Tests

Diagnostic testing is performed to establish an accurate diagnosis and direct long-term therapy.

- *Serum uric acid* is nearly always elevated (usually above 7.5 mg/dL) and is indicative of hyperuricemia.
- *WBC count* shows significant elevation, reaching levels as high as 20,000/mm³ during an acute attack.
- *Eosinophil sedimentation rate (ESR or sed rate)* is elevated during an acute attack from the acute inflammatory process that accompanies deposits of urate crystals in a joint.
- A *24-hour urine specimen* is analyzed to determine uric acid production and excretion.
- *Analysis of fluid* aspirated from the acutely inflamed joint or material aspirated from a tophus shows typical needle-shaped urate crystals, providing the definitive diagnosis of gout.

### Medications

Medications are used to terminate an acute attack, prevent further attacks, and reduce serum uric acid levels to prevent long-term sequelae of the disease. It is important to treat the acute attack of gouty arthritis before initiating treatment to reduce serum uric acid levels, because an abrupt decrease in serum uric acid may lead to further acute manifestations. Pharmacologic therapy is a mainstay of treatment in achieving these goals.

#### Acute Attack

NSAIDs are the treatment of choice for an acute attack of gout. Indomethacin (Indocin) is the most frequently used NSAID for gout, although others are equally effective. During an acute attack, indomethacin is usually prescribed at 50 mg every 8 hours until the client's manifestations have resolved. Other NSAIDs which may be prescribed include ibuprofen (Motrin), naproxen (Naprosyn, Anaprox), tolmetin sodium (Tolectin), piroxicam (Feldene), and sulindac (Clinoril). While extremely effective, NSAIDs are contraindicated for clients with active peptic ulcer disease, impaired renal function, or a history of hypersensitivity reactions to the drugs. (NSAIDS are fully described in Chapter 8.) 

Colchicine can dramatically affect the course of an acute attack. Joint pain begins to diminish within 12 hours of the initiation of treatment and disappears within 2 days. Colchicine apparently acts by interrupting the cycle of urate crystal deposition and inflammation in an acute attack of gout. It has no anti-inflammatory effect in other forms of arthritis, and its use is limited to gout. The use of colchicine is limited by significant side effects. When administered orally, the majority of clients develop significant abdominal cramping, diarrhea, nausea, or vomiting. Intravenous administration is limited by potential toxic effects including local pain, tissue damage if extravasation occurs during injection, bone marrow suppression, and disseminated intravascular coagulation (DIC). It is contraindicated for clients who have significant gastrointestinal, renal, hepatic, or cardiac disease.

Corticosteroids may also be prescribed for the client with acute gouty arthritis. If possible, the intra-articular route is preferred for monoarticular arthritis to avoid the multiple systemic effects of steroid therapy. When gout is polyarticular, corticosteroids may be administered either orally or intravenously.

Analgesics may also be prescribed during an acute episode of gouty arthritis. Either codeine or meperidine (Demerol) may be administered orally every 4 hours to manage the client's pain. Aspirin is avoided because it may interfere with uric acid excretion.

### Prophylactic Therapy

In clients at high risk for future attacks of acute gout, prophylactic therapy with daily colchicine may be initiated. Prophylaxis is particularly useful during the first 1 to 2 years of treatment with antihyperuricemic agents. Although colchicine does not affect the serum uric acid directly, it reduces the frequency of attacks by preventing crystal deposition within the joint. The doses required to achieve this effect are small, and few side effects are associated with therapy.

Treatment to reduce serum uric acid levels is typically initiated for clients with recurring gout, tophi, or renal damage. Asymptomatic hyperuricemic clients require no treatment. Uricosuric agents are used for clients who do not eliminate uric acid adequately; allopurinol is prescribed for clients who produce excessive amounts of uric acid. Uricosuric drugs block the tubular reabsorption of uric acid, promoting its excretion and reducing serum levels. These drugs reduce the frequency of acute attacks, particularly when administered with colchicine. Probenecid (Benemid) and sulfinpyrazone (Aprazone, Anturane, Zynol) are the primary uricosuric drugs employed.

Allopurinol (Zyloprim) is a xanthine oxidase inhibitor that lowers plasma uric acid levels and facilitates the mobilization of tophi. Because of its effectiveness in lowering serum uric acid levels, it may trigger an attack of acute gout. The nursing implications for medications used to treat gout are included on page 1236 in the Medication Administration box.

### Dietary Management

Dietary purines contribute only slightly to uric acid levels in the body, and no specific diet may be recommended. If a low-purine diet is recommended, the client should be taught that high purine foods include all meats and seafood, yeast, beans, peas, lentils, oatmeal, spinach, asparagus, cauliflower, and mushrooms. The obese client is advised to lose weight, but fasting is contraindicated for clients with gout. Alcohol intake and specific foods that tend to precipitate attacks are avoided.

### Other Treatments

During an acute attack of gouty arthritis, bed rest is prescribed. It is continued for approximately 24 hours after the attack has subsided, because early ambulation may bring about recurrence of acute manifestations (Tierney et al., 2001). The affected joint may be elevated, and hot or cold compresses may be applied for comfort.

A liberal fluid intake to maintain a daily urinary output of 2000 mL or more is recommended to increase urate excretion and reduce the risk of urinary stone formation. Urinary alkalinizing agents, such as sodium bicarbonate or potassium citrate, may be prescribed as well to minimize the risk of uric acid stones. It is important to monitor clients receiving these preparations carefully for signs of fluid and electrolyte or acid-base imbalances.

## NURSING CARE

Clients with gout provide self-care at home. Teaching focuses on self-management of pain and altered mobility.

### Nursing Diagnoses and Interventions

Pain is a primary focus for nursing interventions in the client experiencing an acute attack of gout. The client's mobility is also impaired during an acute attack, both because of discomfort and prescribed activity limitations.

#### Acute Pain

The pain associated with an attack of acute gouty arthritis is intense and accompanied by exquisite tenderness of the affected joint. Measures to alleviate the pain are vital in the initial period until anti-inflammatory medications become effective and the acute inflammatory response is relieved. The following are important in teaching about pain relief.

- Position the affected joint for comfort. Elevate the joint or extremity (usually the foot) on a pillow, maintaining alignment. *Elevation and normal body alignment facilitate blood return from the affected joint, alleviating some of the edema.*
- Protect the affected joint from pressure, placing a foot cradle on the bed to keep bed covers off the foot. *A foot cradle keeps bed linens from applying pressure on the affected joint.*

**PRACTICE ALERT** *The affected joints are so painful that even the weight of a sheet can be unbearable.* ■

- Take anti-inflammatory and antigout medications as prescribed. In the initial period, colchicine may be given hourly. *These medications reduce the acute inflammatory response, gradually relieving discomfort.*

# Medication Administration
## The Client with Gout

### COLCHICINE

Colchicine is used to terminate an acute attack of gouty arthritis and to prevent recurrent episodes of the disease. Colchicine does not alter serum uric acid levels, but appears to interrupt the cycle of urate crystal deposition and inflammatory response. It may be administered either by mouth or intravenously. Colchicine is also available as a fixed-dose combination with a uricosuric agent, probenecid (Benemid). Only plain colchicine is used to treat an acute attack of gout; combination therapy is employed to prevent further attacks.

### Nursing Responsibilities

- Assess for possible contraindications to colchicine therapy, including serious gastrointestinal, renal, hepatic, or cardiac disease.
- Administer the following as ordered:
  - *Intravenous doses:* Give undiluted or diluted in up to 20 mL sterile normal saline for injection. Administer over a period of 2 to 5 minutes.
  - *Oral doses:* Give on an empty stomach to facilitate absorption.
- Evaluate for adverse effects, including abdominal cramping, nausea, vomiting, and diarrhea, and report promptly, because these side effects may necessitate discontinuation of the drug.

### Client and Family Teaching

- Drink 3 to 4 quarts of liquid per day.
- Report adverse responses, including gastrointestinal problems, fatigue, bleeding, easy bruising, or recurrent infections, to the physician.
- Do not drink alcohol.

### URICOSURIC DRUGS

> Probenecid (Benemid)
> Sulfinpyrazone (Anturane)

Probenecid is a uricosuric drug that inhibits the tubular reabsorption of urate, promoting the excretion of uric acid and decreasing serum uric acid levels. Sulfinpyrazone is a uricosuric drug that potentiates the renal excretion of uric acid, reducing serum uric acid levels. It is used to prevent recurrent attacks of acute gouty arthritis and treat chronic gout.

### Nursing Responsibilities

- Assess for prior hypersensitivity responses to this drug.
- Administer after meals or with milk to minimize gastric distress.
- Increase fluid intake to at least 3 L/day to prevent the formation of uric acid kidney calculi.
- Administer sodium bicarbonate or potassium citrate as ordered to maintain an alkaline urine.
- Do not administer aspirin to clients receiving probenecid because salicylates interfere with the action of the drug.
- Monitor clients receiving the following drugs concurrently with probenecid for increased or toxic effects: penicillin and related antibiotics, indomethacin, acetaminophen, naproxen, ketoprofen, meclofenamate, lorazepam, and rifampin.
- Monitor for possible adverse effects of probenecid, including headache, dizziness, hepatic necrosis, nausea and vomiting, renal colic, bone marrow depression, anaphylaxis, fever, hives, and pruritus.
- Administer sulfinpyrazone with meals or antacid to minimize gastric distress.

- Monitor clients taking sulfinpyrazone with other sulfa drugs for increased or toxic effects; monitor for hypoglycemia in clients receiving insulin or oral hypoglycemics concurrently, and monitor for bleeding or increased anticoagulant effect in clients receiving warfarin concurrently.
- Assess for contraindications to therapy with sulfinpyrazone, including active peptic ulcer disease, a history of hypersensitivity to phenylbutazone or other pyrazoles, or blood dyscrasias.

### Client and Family Teaching

- Do not take aspirin or products containing aspirin while taking probenecid. Use acetaminophen for relief of mild pain.
- Drink at least 3 quarts of fluids per day to minimize the risk of kidney stone formation.
- Take sulfinpyrazone with meals to minimize gastric distress, and report epigastric pain, nausea, or black stools to the physician promptly

### ALLOPURINOL (ZYLOPRIM)

Allopurinol acts on purine metabolism, reducing the production of uric acid and decreasing serum and urinary concentrations of uric acid. It is used for clients with manifestations of primary or secondary gout, including acute attacks, tophi, joint destruction, urinary stones, and nephropathy. It is not indicated for use in the treatment of asymptomatic hyperuricemia.

### Nursing Responsibilities

- Monitor intake and output and increase fluid intake to approximately 3 L/day.
- Monitor for desired effect of decreased serum uric acid levels, and for adverse effects such as nausea, diarrhea, and rash.
- Assess BUN and creatinine levels prior to the initiation of and during treatment with allopurinol. Report signs of impaired renal function such as an elevated BUN and creatinine, decreased urine output, and dilute or frothy urine to the physician.
- Administer with meals to minimize gastric distress.
- Monitor CBC periodically because allopurinol therapy may cause bone marrow depression.
- In clients receiving warfarin concurrently, monitor prothrombin times and be alert to evidence of bleeding, because allopurinol prolongs the half-life of warfarin.
- Monitor clients receiving chlorpropamide, cyclophosphamide, hydantoin, theophylline, vidarabine, or ACE inhibitors concurrently for increased drug effects.
- Discontinue the drug and notify the physician immediately if the client develops a rash. Rash and hypersensitivity responses occur more frequently in clients receiving ampicillin, amoxicillin, or thiazide diuretics.

### Client and Family Teaching

- Stop taking the drug and report any skin rash, painful urination, blood in the urine, eye irritation, or swelling of the lips or mouth to the physician immediately.
- Take the medication after meals to minimize gastric distress.
- Drink 3 to 4 quarts of fluid daily to maintain a urinary output greater than 2 L/day.
- Acute gouty attacks may occur during the initial stages of allopurinol therapy; continue therapy prescribed for attacks (such as colchicine) to minimize acute episodes.
- Do not take a double dose of medication if you miss a dose.

- Take analgesics as prescribed. *Supplemental analgesia may be necessary in the acute period until the inflammatory response is mediated.*
- Maintain bed rest. *It is important to immobilize the affected joint and promote rest to prevent exacerbation of joint inflammation.*

### Impaired Physical Mobility

Bed rest is prescribed to prevent further urate mobilization and joint inflammation as well as to protect the affected joint.

- Encourage active and passive ROM exercises of joints and muscle-tensing exercises on unaffected limbs. *These exercises help maintain joint mobility, muscle tone, and the client's sense of well-being.*
- When ambulation is allowed, suggest using a walker or cane as needed. *Weight bearing on the affected limb may be restricted until the inflammation is totally relieved.*
- Resume normal activities as allowed by the physician. *Initial acute attacks of gouty arthritis do not cause permanent damage to the affected joint, and the client can resume usual activities once the attack has subsided.*

## Home Care

Discuss the following topics with the client.

- *The disease and its manifestations.* Tell the client that initial attacks cause no permanent damage but that recurrent attacks can lead to permanent damage and joint destruction. Discuss other potential effects of continued hyperuricemia, including tophaceous deposits in subcutaneous and other connective tissues. Discuss the potential for kidney damage and kidney stones.
- *The rationale for and use of prescribed medication.* Stress the need to continue the medication until the physician discontinues it, even though the client is free of manifestations of gout.
- *The importance of a high intake of fluids each day and avoiding the use of alcohol.*

## THE CLIENT WITH OSTEOMALACIA

**Osteomalacia,** often referred to as *adult rickets,* is a metabolic bone disorder characterized by inadequate or delayed mineralization of bone matrix in mature compact and spongy bone. Bone mineralization requires adequate calcium and phosphate ions in extracellular fluid. When either of these ions is insufficient due to (1) inadequate calcium intake or decreased calcium absorption from the intestines because of insufficient vitamin D, and (2) increased renal losses or decreased intestinal absorption of phosphate, the bone matrix is not mineralized and cannot sustain weight bearing. Marked deformities of weight-bearing bone and pathologic fractures occur. The primary causes of osteomalacia are vitamin D deficiency and hypophosphatemia. Osteomalacia can be corrected with treatment.

Osteomalacia has been almost nonexistent in the United States because many foods are fortified with vitamin D, but its incidence is increasing among older adults, very-low-birth-weight infants, and people who adhere to strict vegetarian diets. It is a significant health problem in cultures whose diets tend to be deficient in calcium and vitamin D. Women in northern China, Japan, and northern India have a higher incidence of the disorder than men because of the combined effects of pregnancy, lactation, and more indoor confinement (Porth, 2002).

The major risk factors for vitamin D deficiency are a diet low in vitamin D, decreased endogenous production of vitamin D because of inadequate sun exposure, impaired intestinal absorption of fats (vitamin D is a fat-soluble vitamin), and disorders that interfere with the metabolism of vitamin D to its active forms. Gastrectomy and small bowel disorders may reduce the absorptive surface of the bowel to the extent that nutrients are not completely or adequately absorbed. Both vitamin D and calcium absorption may be affected. Hepatobiliary disorders that interfere with bile production and release, and chronic pancreatic insufficiency with inadequate pancreatic enzyme production, also can affect the absorption of fats and vitamin D from the bowel. Once absorbed, vitamin D is metabolized in the liver and the kidney to its active form; therefore, liver disorders such as cirrhosis and renal disorders can affect this activation. Certain drugs, such as isoniazid, rifampin, and anticonvulsants, accelerate vitamin D metabolism, resulting in less availability to the tissues. Renal excretion of vitamin D is increased in some kidney disorders such as nephrotic syndrome (Box 39–2).

---

### BOX 39–2 ■ Causes of Osteomalacia

**VITAMIN D DEFICIENCY**
- Inadequate dietary intake
- Lack of sun exposure
- Malabsorption from intestines: gastrectomy, small bowel disorders, gall bladder disease, chronic pancreatic insufficiency
- Renal or liver disorders
- Drug effects: isoniazid, rifampin, anticonvulsants

**PHOSPHATE DEPLETION**
- Inadequate intake
- Impaired absorption due to chronic antacid use
- Impaired renal tubular reabsorption due to either acquired or genetic disorders

**SYSTEMIC ACIDOSIS**
- Renal tubular acidosis
- Ureterosigmoidostomy
- Fanconi's syndrome

**BONE MINERALIZATION INHIBITORS**
- Hypophosphatasia
- Sodium fluoride or disodium etidronate (Didronel)
- Aluminum intoxication

**CHRONIC RENAL FAILURE**

**CALCIUM MALABSORPTION**

Hypophosphatemia can be the result of insufficient dietary intake, excessive losses through the urine or stool, or a shift into the cells. Alcohol abuse is the most common cause of hypophosphatemia, because of related dietary deficiencies, vomiting, antacid use, and increased renal excretion of phosphate. Ingesting large amounts of nonabsorbable antacids causes increased phosphate losses in the stool. Several acquired and genetic disorders cause increased losses of phosphate in the urine.

## PATHOPHYSIOLOGY AND MANIFESTATIONS

The two main causes of osteomalacia are (1) insufficient calcium absorption in the intestine due to a lack of calcium or resistance to the action of vitamin D and (2) increased losses of phosphorus through the urine (Porth, 2002). In its natural form, vitamin D is obtained from certain foods and ultraviolet radiation of the sun. Vitamin D maintains adequate serum levels of calcium and phosphate for normal mineralization of the bone. Vitamin D deficiency or resistance to its action disrupts the normal mineralization of the bone, causing softening of the bone.

Vitamin D is inactive when it is absorbed from the intestine or synthesized from exposure to ultraviolet light. For vitamin D to become active, a two-step process must occur. Vitamin D (and its metabolites) is transported in the blood to the liver, where it is converted to calcidiol. Calcidiol is then transported to the kidney and transformed to an active form, calcitriol.

The active form of vitamin D is needed for optimal absorption of calcium and phosphorus from the intestine. Calcium and phosphorus are transported in the blood to the bones for normal mineralization. If there is a lack of vitamin D, calcium and phosphorus are not absorbed from the intestine, and serum calcium and phosphorus levels therefore fall. A deficiency in these minerals in turn activates the parathyroid glands, with loss of calcium and phosphorus from bone. The continued loss of calcium and phosphate in the bone disrupts bone mineralization.

Impaired bone mineralization causes abnormalities in both spongy and compact bone. The osteoid (the soft, noncalcified part of the matrix) continues to be produced but is not mineralized. This abnormal buildup of demineralized bone leads to gross deformities of the long bones, spine, pelvis, and skull, because the bone is soft and unable to bear the weight and stress of body movement.

The manifestations of osteomalacia include bone pain and tenderness (see box in next column). As the disease progresses, fractures occur (Porth, 2002). In contrast to osteoporosis, osteomalacia is not associated with a significant occurrence of hip fractures. Instead, pathologic fractures occur in the commonly weakened areas (e.g., distal radius and proximal femur).

## COLLABORATIVE CARE

Once the specific cause is determined, appropriate therapy will correct the disorder. Osteomalacia may be difficult to differentiate from osteoporosis because the manifestations are very similar; however, certain diagnostic tests can help pinpoint its diagnosis.

### Manifestations of Osteomalacia

- Bone pain: May be vague and generalized at first, becoming more intense with activity as the disease progresses; occurs most frequently in the pelvis, long bones of the extremities, spine, and ribs.
- Difficulty changing from lying to sitting position, sitting to standing position, and so on.
- Muscle weakness: Frequently an early sign in severe cases.
- Waddling gait: May be due to pain and muscle weakness.
- Dorsal kyphosis: May occur in severe cases.
- Pathologic fractures

## Diagnostic Tests

A history of inadequate dietary intake, renal failure, or some malabsorption states may suggest osteomalacia. Table 39–1 compares the diagnostic findings of osteomalacia with those of osteoporosis and Paget's disease.

- *X-rays* demonstrate the effects of generalized bone demineralization: trabecular bone loss, cyst formation, compression fractures, bowing and bending deformities of the long bones, and osteoid deposits, particularly in the vertebral bodies and pelvis.
- *Serum calcium* level may be normal or low, depending on the cause of the disease. Calcium levels may be reduced when calcium absorption is impaired or in severe vitamin D deficiency. Secondary hypoparathyroidism may shift calcium from the bone into extracellular fluid, maintaining a normal serum calcium level.
- *Serum parathyroid hormone* is frequently elevated as a compensatory response to hypocalcemia in renal failure or vitamin D deficiency.
- *Serum alkaline phosphatase* level usually is elevated.

## Medications

Therapeutic management of osteomalacia depends on the cause of the disease. Because the causes are so diverse, it is difficult to generalize treatment. Most clients are placed on vitamin D therapy. Calcium and phosphate supplements also may be indicated. Radiologic evidence of healing often is apparent within weeks of initiating therapy.

## NURSING CARE

Managing the client with osteomalacia includes assessing the client's current dietary intake of vitamin D, calcium, and phosphorus and exposure to ultraviolet light. It also includes managing client responses to bone pain and tenderness, fractures, and muscle weakness.

Teaching is important not only for the client with osteomalacia, but also for people at risk for developing the disease. When milk and other dairy products began to be fortified with vitamin D, the incidence of childhood rickets decreased dramatically. Now many clients are unaware of the importance of vitamin D, calcium, and phosphorus to bone health.

Older adults as a group are at high risk for osteomalacia because of dietary deficiencies and possible physical mobility limitations that restrict their exposure to sunlight. Teach older adults about the importance of maintaining an adequate intake of milk and other dairy products that are not only rich in calcium and phosphorus, but also are fortified with vitamin D. Few other food sources provide enough vitamin D to meet recommended levels. Cod liver oil may be used as a supplement, as it contains significant amounts of vitamin D. Supplements are not recommended, however, for clients who get adequate vitamin D through dietary sources and sun exposure, because this fat-soluble vitamin may become toxic at high levels. Instruct clients who are taking supplements to report to their primary care provider symptoms such as anorexia, nausea and vomiting, frequent urination, muscle weakness, and constipation that may be indicative of hypervitaminosis D.

Instruct the client with osteomalacia about safety measures to prevent falls. Discuss the importance of eliminating scatter rugs and clutter from living areas to prevent tripping. Teach the client to place a night light in hallways and the bathroom to prevent falls associated with nighttime toileting. Suggest installing grab bars in the shower and tub and next to the toilet for safety.

Teach clients with bone pain and muscle weakness to use assistive devices such as walkers, canes, or crutches when ambulating. Provide referrals to physical therapy for teaching clients how to safely use these devices. Encourage clients to participate in a supervised exercise program such as water aerobics or tai chi to improve muscle strength and balance.

# DEGENERATIVE DISORDERS

Degenerative disorders, especially degenerative joint disease, are the most common form of arthritis in the older adult. Both primary and secondary forms are seen in adults of all ages. Primary or idiopathic osteoarthritis, the most common type, occurs without a clear precipitating factor. Secondary osteoarthritis is associated with an identifiable cause. For instance, it may be related to trauma to a joint, inflammation, skeletal disorders such as congenital hip dysplasia, or metabolic disorders. Regardless of cause, degenerative disorders of the joints and muscles can lead to impaired mobility and chronic pain. These problems may in turn cause disability, especially in the performance of ADLs by older adults.

## THE CLIENT WITH OSTEOARTHRITIS

**Osteoarthritis (OA)** (also labeled *degenerative joint disease*) is the most commonly occurring of all forms of arthritis. This disease is characterized by loss of articular cartilage in articulating joints and hypertrophy of the bones at the articular margins. OA may be idiopathic (without known cause) or secondary (associated with known risk factors). Idiopathic OA affects more than 60 million people in the United States, affecting adult men more than women until after age 55, when the incidence becomes twice as high in women (McCance & Huether, 2002) The joints most affected are in the hand, wrist, neck, lower back, hip, knee, ankles, and feet. Men are more likely than women to have hip OA, while postmenopausal women more often have hand OA.

Localized OA affects only one or two joints. Generalized OA affects three or more joints. Generalized OA may also be classified as nodal (involving the hand) or nonnodal (no hand involvement). Nodal OA may also affect the knees, hips, cer-

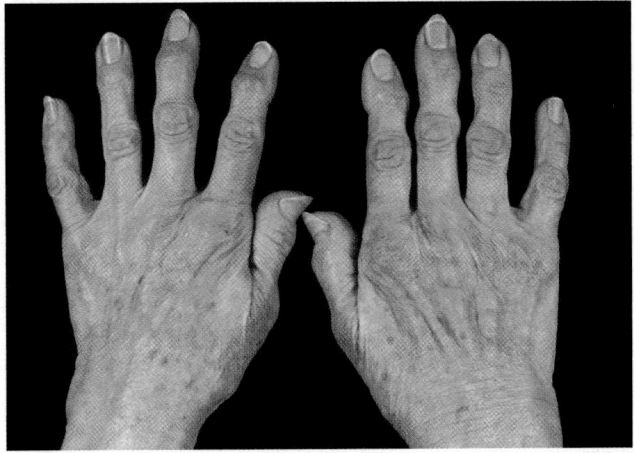

**Figure 39–2** ■ Typical interphalangeal joint changes associated with osteoarthritis.

*Source: L. Samsuri/Custom Medical Stock Photo.*

vical spine, and lumbar spine. Idiopathic OA most commonly affects the terminal interphalangeal joints (*Heberden's nodes*), and less often the proximal interphalangeal joints (*Bouchard's nodes*) (Figure 39–2 ■), the joints of the thumb, the hip, the knee, the metatarsophalangeal joint of the big toe, and the cervical and lumbar spine. Secondary OA may occur in any joint from an articular injury.

## RISK FACTORS

Idiopathic OA is associated with increasing age, with more than 90% of individuals affected by age 40 but few experiencing manifestations until after 50 or 60 (Maher, Salmond, & Pellino, 2002). It has been suggested that OA may be inherited as an autosomal recessive trait, with genetic defects that cause premature destruction of the joint cartilage. The causes of secondary OA include trauma, mechanical stress, inflammation of joint structures, joint instability, neurologic disorders, endocrine disorders, and selected medications.

Excessive weight contributes to the development of OA, especially in the hip and knee. Inactivity is another risk factor. Moderate recreational exercise has been shown to both decrease the chance of developing OA and the progression of manifestations when OA is present. People involved in strenuous, repetitive exercise (such as participating in sports) have an increased risk of developing secondary OA.

Other risk factors that are linked to OA are hormonal factors such as decreased estrogen in menopausal women, excessive growth hormone, and increased parathyroid hormone.

## PATHOPHYSIOLOGY

The cartilage that lines joints provides a smooth surface, so that the bones of the joint glide over one another without friction, and it distributes the load from one bone to the next, dissipating the mechanical stress that occurs with joint loading. This cartilage normally contains more than 70% water. More than 90% of its dry weight is collagen, which provides strength, and proteoglycans, which provide elasticity and stiffness to compression. Cartilage cells, the chondrocytes, nest in this meshwork of collagen and proteoglycans. Normal articular cartilage exudes some of its water with compression, providing lubrication for joint surfaces. This water is reabsorbed during relaxation of the joint.

In OA, proteoglycans and collagen are lost from the cartilage as a result of enzymatic degradation. The water content of the cartilage increases as the collagen matrix is destroyed. With the loss of proteoglycans and collagen fibers, the cartilage becomes yellow or brownish gray and loses its tensile strength. Surface ulcerations occur, and fissures develop in deeper layers of the cartilage. Eventually, large areas of articular cartilage are lost, and underlying bone is exposed. The bone thickens in exposed areas, reducing its ability to absorb energy in joint loading. Cysts can also develop in the bone. Cartilage-coated **osteophytes** (bony outgrowths often called "joint mice") change the anatomy of the joint. As these spurs or projections enlarge, small pieces may break off, leading to mild synovitis (inflammation of the synovial membrane).

## MANIFESTATIONS AND COMPLICATIONS

The onset of OA is usually gradual and insidious, and the course slowly progressive. Pain and stiffness in one or more joints (usually weight bearing) are the first manifestations of OA. The pain is localized to the affected joints and may be described as a deep ache. It typically is aggravated by use or motion of the joint and relieved by rest, although it may become persistent as the disease progresses. Pain at night may be accompanied by paresthesias (numbness, tingling). Pain may also be referred to other parts of the body; for example, OA of the lumbosacral spine may cause severe pain along the path of the sciatic nerve. Following periods of immobility, such as sleeping all night or after a long automobile ride, involved joints may stiffen. Usually only a few minutes of activity are neces-

| TABLE 39–2 | Manifestations of Osteoarthritis |
|---|---|
| **Affected Site** | **Manifestations** |
| Interphalangeal joints | • *Heberden's nodes*—bony enlargements of distal joints; may cause pain, redness, swelling<br>• *Bouchard's nodes*—bony enlargement of proximal joints |
| First carpometacarpal | • Swelling, tenderness at base of thumb<br>• Crepitus with movement<br>• "Squared" appearance of joint |
| Spine | • Localized pain and stiffness<br>• Muscle spasm<br>• Limited range of motion<br>• Nerve root compression with radicular pain and motor weakness |
| Hips | • Pain referred to inguinal area, buttock, thigh, or knee<br>• Loss of internal rotation<br>• Limited extension, adduction, and flexion |
| Knees | • Pain and bony enlargement<br>• Effusions<br>• Crepitus<br>• Instability and deformity with advanced disease |

sary to relieve the stiffness. Range of motion of the joint decreases as the disease progresses, and grating or crepitus may be noted during movement. Bony overgrowth may cause joint enlargement, and flexion contractures may occur because of joint instability. In OA, enlarged joints are characteristically bony-hard and cool on palpation. Manifestations specific to affected joints are outlined in Table 39–2.

OA of the spine may involve the vertebral bodies and intervertebral disks, the diarthrodial joints, or both. Spondylosis is degenerative disk disease. As the intervertebral disks degenerate, disk space between the vertebrae is lost. Degenerative disk disease may be complicated by herniated disk, the protrusion of the nucleus pulposus of the disk. Herniation usually occurs in a lateral direction, potentially compressing nerve roots and causing radicular (distributed along the nerve) pain and muscle weakness. See Chapter 41 for further discussion of disk disorders.

Disk degeneration and joint space narrowing alter the mechanics of the spinal column, promoting osteoarthritic changes in the articular processes (the facet joints) of the vertebrae. The cartilage covering the inferior and superior articular processes degenerates, causing localized pain, stiffness, muscle spasm, and limited range of motion. Osteophytes may form on articular processes, further contributing to pain and muscle spasm.

The presentation of OA in older clients is similar to that in younger adults. However, in this population, the risk of debilitation because of OA is greater, and the disease may progress faster. In addition, pain, stiffness, and limited range of motion increase the risk of falls and fractures in the older adult.

# COLLABORATIVE CARE

At this time, no treatment is available to arrest the process of joint degeneration. Appropriate management, however, is important to relieve pain and maintain the client's function and mobility.

## Diagnostic Tests

The diagnosis of OA is generally based on the client's history and physical examination and X-rays of affected joints. Characteristic changes of OA are visible in X-ray studies of affected joints. Initially, irregular joint space narrowing is seen. Progressive changes include increased density of subchondral (under cartilage) bone, osteophyte formation at the joint periphery, and the formation of cysts in the bone.

## Medications

The pain of OA often can be managed through the use of analgesics such as aspirin or acetaminophen. Acetaminophen is generally preferred for use in older clients because it has fewer toxic side effects. NSAIDs may also be prescribed. These medications are discussed in more detail in Chapter 8. ⚭ Capsaicin cream can reduce joint pain and tenderness when applied topically to affected joints.

Medications that have proven effective in decreasing the pain and stiffness of OA are the NSAID COX-2 inhibitors meloxicam (Mobic), celecoxib (Celebrex), and rofecoxib (Vioxx). These medications provide analgesic/anti-inflammatory effects comparable to conventional NSAIDS, but have fewer adverse effects on the gastrointestinal and renal systems. Clients should be taught to report any signs of gastrointestinal bleeding to their health care providers. If meloxicam is prescribed, teach the client that it may decrease the effectiveness of ACE inhibitors and diuretics, may increase lithium levels and toxicity, and there is a risk of increased bleeding if taken at the same time as aspirin, warfarin, and the herbs feverfew, garlic, ginger, and ginko.

Potent anti-inflammatory medications, such as systemic corticosteroids, are seldom prescribed for clients with OA, although intra-articular corticosteroid injections may be used. With intra-articular injections, a long-acting corticosteroid medication, often mixed with a local anesthetic such as lidocaine, is injected directly into the joint space of the affected joints. Although this procedure may provide marked pain relief, it can hasten the rate of cartilage breakdown if performed more frequently than every 4 to 6 months.

## Conservative Treatment

Conservative treatment may include any or all of the following:

- Physical therapy for ROM exercises
- Resting the involved joint
- Using a cane, crutches, or a walker
- Weight loss, if indicated
- Analgesic and anti-inflammatory medications

## Surgery

Surgical procedures can provide dramatic results for clients with significant chronic pain and loss of joint function. Although elective surgical procedures are frequently avoided in the older adult, even aged clients can benefit significantly if they do not have a chronic medical condition that contraindicates surgery.

### Arthroscopy

Although arthroscopic debridement and lavage of involved joints has been used, certain questions exist about its effectiveness and thus research is ongoing (Reuters Health, 2002).

### Osteotomy

An **osteotomy,** an incision into or transection of the bone, may be performed to realign an affected joint, particularly when significant bony overgrowth or osteophyte formation has occurred. This procedure may also be used to shift the joint load toward areas of less severely damaged cartilage. Although osteotomy does not halt the process of OA, it may have a beneficial effect on joint function and pain, delaying the need for a joint replacement by several years.

### Joint Arthroplasty

A **joint arthroplasty** is the reconstruction or replacement of a joint. Arthroplasty is usually indicated when the client has severely restricted joint mobility and pain at rest. Pain is virtually eliminated, and the function of the joint is generally improved. Arthroplasty may involve partial joint replacement or reshaping of the bones of a joint. For most clients with OA, both surfaces of the affected joint are replaced with prosthetic parts in a procedure known as a **total joint replacement.** Joints that may be replaced include the hip, knee, shoulder, elbow, ankle, wrist, and joints of the fingers and toes.

In a total joint replacement, some or all of the synovium, cartilage, and bone on both sides of the joint are removed. A metallic prosthesis is inserted to replace one joint surface (generally the load-end or distal portion of a weight-bearing joint). The other joint surface is replaced by a silicone-lined ceramic or plastic prosthesis.

Most prosthetic joints are uncemented, that is, made of porous ceramic and metal components inserted so that they fit tightly into existing bone. The implant is secured by new bone growth into the prosthesis, a process that requires approximately 6 weeks. Although a longer non-weight-bearing period is necessary initially until the prosthesis is fixed in place by the bony growth, the implant appears to have a longer useful life span than cemented prostheses. In a cemented joint replacement, methyl methacrylate (a pliable polymer that hardens to hold the prosthesis in place) is used to secure the prosthesis to existing bone. Although the client is able to resume normal activities more rapidly following a cemented joint replacement, methyl methacrylate initiates an inflammatory response, and the joint eventually loosens.

- In a *total hip replacement,* the articular surfaces of the acetabulum and femoral head are replaced. The entire head of the femur and part of the femoral neck are removed and replaced with a prosthesis (Figure 39–3 ■). The acetabulum is remodeled, and a prosthesis of high-molecular-weight polyethylene is inserted. The success rate for total hip replacement is reported to be greater than 90%. Approximately 250,000 total hip replacements are done each year in the United States; most are for treatment of OA (McCance & Huether, 2002). Potential problems associated with a total hip replacement include dislocation within the prosthesis, loosening of joint components from surrounding bone, and infection. If recurrent or ineffectively treated, these complications may necessitate removal of the prosthesis, resulting in severe shortening of the extremity and an unstable hip joint.

• *Total knee replacement* is performed if the client has intractable pain and X-ray films show evidence of arthritis of the knee. Several prosthetic devices involving removal of varying amounts of bone are available for knee joint replacement (Figure 39–4 ■). The femoral side of the joint is replaced with a metallic surface, and the tibial side with polyethylene. More than 80% of clients obtain significant or total relief of pain with a total knee replacement. They must, however, engage in a vigorous program of rehabilitation to achieve the best results. Joint failure is more common with knee replacement than with a total hip replacement. Loosened joint components, often on the tibial side, are the most common cause of failure.

• *Total shoulder replacement* is indicated for unremitting pain and marked limitation of range of motion because of arthritic involvement of both the humeral and glenoid joint surfaces of the shoulder. The joint is immobilized in a sling or abduction splint for 2 to 3 weeks following arthroplasty. Dislocation, loosening of the prosthesis, and infection are potential problems associated with total shoulder replacement.

• *Total elbow replacement* involves replacement of the humeral and ulnar surfaces of the elbow joint with a metal and polyethylene prosthesis. Pain and disabling stiffness of the joint are indications for an elbow arthroplasty. Complications, including dislocation, fracture, tricep weakness, loosening, and infection, occur frequently.

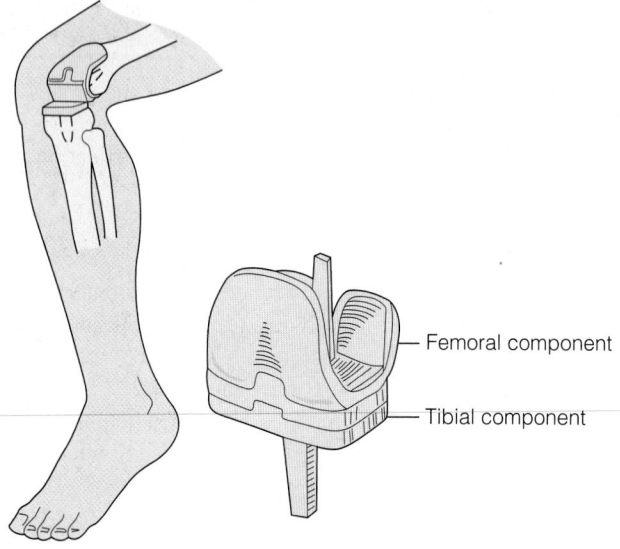

**Figure 39–4** ■ Total knee replacement.

Infection is the major complication associated with total joint replacement. Not only does infection interfere with healing and prolong recovery, but also it may necessitate removal of the prosthesis and may lead to loss of joint function. Other potential complications include circulatory impairment to the affected limb, thromboembolism, nerve damage, and dislocation of the joint.

Nursing care for the client undergoing total joint replacement is outlined on pages 1243–1244. Refer to Chapter 7 ⮾ for further discussion of care for the client undergoing surgery.

## Complementary Therapies

The following complementary therapies are examples of those that may be used by people with OA to relieve pain and stiffness (Springhouse, 1998).

• Bioelectromagnetic therapy
• Eliminating nightshade foods such as potatoes, tomatoes, peppers, eggplant, tobacco
• Taking nutritional supplements, such as boron, zinc, copper, selenium, manganese, flavonoids, evening primrose oil
• Herbal therapy
• Osteopathic manipulation
• Vitamin therapy
• Yoga

## NURSING CARE

OA is a chronic process for which there is no cure. The focus of nursing care for the client with OA is providing comfort, helping maintain mobility and ADLs, and assisting with adaptations to maintain life roles.

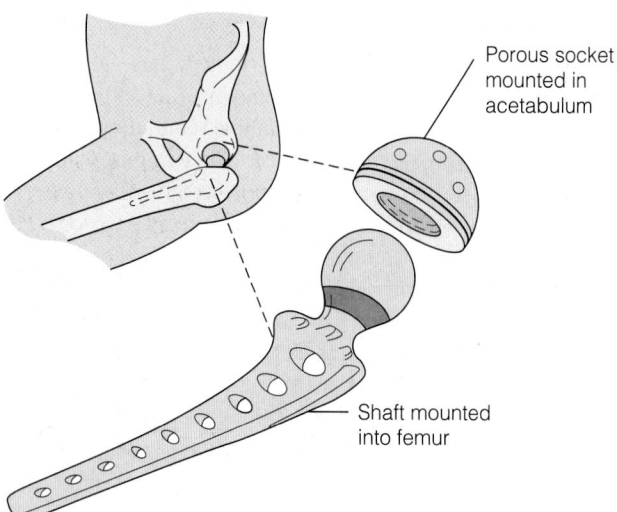

**Figure 39–3** ■ Total hip prosthesis.

# NURSING CARE OF THE CLIENT HAVING TOTAL JOINT REPLACEMENT

## PREOPERATIVE CARE

- Assess the client's knowledge and understanding of the planned operative procedure. Provide further explanations and clarification as needed. *It is important that the client have a clear and realistic understanding of the surgical procedure and expected results. Knowledge decreases anxiety and increases the client's ability to assist with postoperative care procedures.*
- Obtain a nursing history and physical assessment, including range of motion of the affected joints. *This information not only allows nurses to tailor care to the needs of the individual but also serves as a baseline for comparison of postoperative assessment data.*
- Explain necessary postoperative activity restrictions. Teach how to use the overhead trapeze for changing positions. *The client who learns and practices moving techniques before surgery can use them more effectively in the postoperative period.*
- Provide or reinforce teaching of postoperative exercises specific to the joint on which surgery is to be performed. *Exercises are prescribed postoperatively to (a) strengthen muscles providing joint stability and support, (b) prevent muscle atrophy and joint contractures; and (c) prevent venous stasis and possible thromboembolism.*
- Teach respiratory hygiene procedures such as the use of incentive spirometry, coughing, and deep breathing. *Adequate respiratory hygiene is imperative for all clients undergoing joint replacement to prevent respiratory complications associated with immobility and the effects of anesthesia. In addition, many clients undergoing total joint replacement are elderly and may have reduced mucociliary clearance.*
- Discuss postoperative pain control measures, including use of patient-controlled analgesia (PCA) or epidural infusion as appropriate. *It is important for the client to understand the purpose and use of postoperative pain control measures to allow early mobility and reduce complications associated with immobility.*
- Teach or provide prescribed preoperative skin preparation such as shower, shampoo, and skin scrub with antibacterial solution. *These measures help reduce transient bacteria that may be introduced into the surgical site.*
- Administer intravenous antibiotic as ordered. *Antibiotic therapy is initiated before or during surgery and continued postoperatively to further reduce the risk of infection.*

## POSTOPERATIVE CARE

- Check vital signs, including temperature and level of consciousness, every 4 hours or more frequently as indicated. Report significant changes to the physician. *These routine assessments provide information about the client's cardiovascular status and can give early indications of complications such as excessive bleeding, fluid volume deficit, and infection.*
- Perform neurovascular checks (color, temperature, pulses and capillary refill, movement, and sensation) on the affected limb hourly for the first 12 to 24 hours, then every 2 to 4 hours. Report abnormal findings to the physician immediately. *Surgery can disrupt the blood supply to or innervation of the af-*

fected extremity. If so, rapid intervention is important to preserve the function of the extremity.
- Monitor incisional bleeding by emptying and recording suction drainage every 4 hours and assessing the dressing frequently. *Significant blood loss can occur with a total joint replacement, particularly a total hip replacement.*
- Reinforce the dressing as needed. *The dressing is usually changed 24 to 48 hours after surgery but may need reinforcement if excess bleeding occurs.*
- Maintain intravenous infusion and accurate intake and output records during the initial postoperative period. *The client is at risk for fluid volume deficit in the initial postoperative period because of blood and fluid loss during surgery, as well as the effects of the anesthetic.*
- Maintain bed rest and prescribed position of the affected extremity using a sling, abduction splint, brace, immobilizer, or other prescribed device. *Proper positioning of the affected extremity is vital in the initial postoperative period so that the joint prosthesis does not become dislocated or displaced.*
- Help the client shift position at least every 2 hours while on bed rest. *Shifting of position helps prevent pressure sores and other complications of immobility.*
- Remind the client to use the incentive spirometer, to cough, and to breathe deeply at least every 2 hours. *These measures are important to prevent respiratory complications such as pneumonia.*
- Assess the client's level of comfort frequently. Maintain PCA, epidural infusion, or other prescribed analgesia to promote comfort. *Adequate pain management promotes healing and mobility.*
- Help the client get out of bed as soon as allowed. Teach and reinforce the use of techniques to prevent weight bearing on the affected extremity, such as the over-head trapeze, pivot turning, and toe-touch. *Early mobility prevents complications such as pneumonia and thromboembolism, but appropriate techniques must be used to prevent injury to the operative site.*
- Initiate physical therapy and exercises as prescribed for the specific joint replaced, such as quadriceps setting, leg raising, and passive and active range-of-motion exercises. *These exercises help prevent muscle atrophy and thromboembolism and strengthen the muscles of the affected extremity so that it can support the prosthetic joint.*
- Use sequential compression devices or antiembolism stockings as prescribed. *These help prevent thromboembolism and pulmonary embolus for the client who must remain immobile following surgery.*
- For the client with a total hip replacement, prevent hip flexion of greater than 90 degrees or adduction of the affected leg. Provide a seat riser for the toilet or commode. *These measures prevent dislocation of the joint.*
- Assess the client with a total hip replacement for signs of prosthesis dislocation, including pain in the affected hip or shortening and internal rotation of the affected leg.

*(continued on page 1244)*

## NURSING CARE OF THE CLIENT HAVING TOTAL JOINT REPLACEMENT (continued)

- For the client with a total knee replacement, use a continuous passive range-of-motion (CPM) device or range-of-motion exercises as prescribed. *Dislocation is not a problem with a knee replacement, and more emphasis is placed on range-of-motion exercises in the early postoperative period.*
- Maintain fluid intake and encourage a high-fiber diet. Administer stool softeners or rectal suppositories as needed. *Immobility contributes to the potential problem of constipation; these measures help maintain regular fecal elimination.*
- Encourage consumption of a well-balanced diet with adequate protein. *Adequate nutrition promotes tissue healing.*
- Teach or reinforce postdischarge exercises and activity restrictions. Emphasize the importance of scheduled follow-up physi-

cian visits. *Clients are discharged from the acute care facility before healing is complete. Exercises are prescribed and activities are resumed gradually to protect the integrity of the joint replacement and prevent contractures.*
- For those clients needing additional direct care after discharge, arrange placement in a long-term care or rehabilitation facility. *Activity restrictions may preclude discharge to home for some clients.*
- Make referrals as needed to home health agencies and physical therapy. *Clients often require home health care for both nursing care needs and continued physical therapy following discharge from acute or long-term care.*

## Health Promotion

Although OA cannot be prevented, maintaining a normal weight and having a program of regular, moderate exercise will reduce risk factors. Glucosamine and chrondroitin are popular nutritional supplements for OA that are increasingly popular and have been found to be of benefit in reducing manifestations. Clients should discuss these supplements with their health care provider before using them.

## Assessment

Collect the following data through the health history and physical examination (see Chapter 37).

- Health history: family history of OA, occupation, recreational activities, joint pain and stiffness, ability to carry out ADLs and self-care activities
- Physical assessment: height/weight; gait, joints: symmetry, size, shape, color, appearance, temperature, pain, crepitus, range of motion, Heberden's nodes, Bouchard's nodes

## Nursing Diagnoses and Interventions

### Chronic Pain

Pain is a primary manifestation of OA. As joint tissues degenerate and changes in joint structure occur, the amount of discomfort generally increases. The pain associated with OA increases with activity and tends to be relieved with rest. Nonpharmacologic comfort measures are appropriate, with mild analgesics used to supplement these as needed.

- Monitor the client's level of pain, including intensity, location, quality, and aggravating and relieving factors. *Accurate assessment of pain provides a basis for evaluation of the effect of interventions.*
- Teach clients to take prescribed analgesic or anti-inflammatory medication as needed. *Analgesics reduce the perception of pain and may decrease muscle spasm as well. Anti-inflammatory medication may be ordered to decrease local inflammatory response in affected joints.*
- Encourage rest of painful joints. *The pain of OA is often relieved by joint rest.*

- Suggest applying heat to painful joints using the shower, a tub or sitz bath, warm packs, hot wax baths, heated gloves, or diathermy, which uses high-frequency electrical currents to generate heat. *Heat application reduces accompanying muscle spasm, relieving pain. Moist heat penetrates deeper than dry heat; diathermy delivers heat directly to lesions in deeper body tissues.*
- Emphasize the importance of proper posture and good body mechanics for walking, sitting, lifting, and moving. *Good body mechanics and posture reduce stress on affected joints.*
- Encourage the overweight client to reduce. *Excess weight places abnormal stress on joints, particularly the knees.*
- Teach the client to use splints or other devices on affected joints as needed. *These assistive devices help maintain the correct anatomic position of the joint and relieve stress.*
- Encourage the client to use nonpharmacologic pain relief measures such as progressive relaxation, meditation, visualization, and distraction. *These adjunctive pain relief measures can reduce the client's reliance on analgesics and increase comfort.*

## Impaired Physical Mobility

As intra-articular cartilage degenerates and joint structures are altered, the client with OA experiences pain, stiffness, and decreased range of motion in affected joints. When the spine, large weight-bearing joints of the hips and knees, or the ankles and feet are affected, physical mobility can be significantly reduced.

- Assess the range of motion of affected joints. *Assessing joint mobility is important as a basis for planning appropriate interventions.*
- Perform a functional mobility assessment, evaluating the client's gait, ability to sit and rise from sitting, ability to step into and out of the tub or shower, and negotiation of stairs. *The functional assessment provides vital data about the client's ability to maintain ADLs.*
- Teach the client active and passive ROM exercises as well as isometric, progressive resistance, and low-impact aerobic exercises. *Active ROM exercises help maintain muscle tone and mobility of affected joints and prevent contractures.*

*Isometric and progressive resistance exercises improve muscle tone and strength; aerobic exercise improves endurance and cardiovascular fitness.*

**PRACTICE ALERT**  *The older woman with OA may be more willing to take part in weight-bearing exercises if she does so as part of a group or organized activity.* ∎

- Suggest the client take analgesics or other pain relief measures prior to exercise or ambulation. *With decreased pain, the client is able to perform exercises better and ambulate greater distances.*
- Encourage the client to plan periods of rest during the day. *Rest helps reduce fatigue, pain, and joint stress.*
- Teach the client how to use ambulatory aids such as a cane or walker as prescribed. *These devices help relieve some weight bearing and stress on affected joints.*

### Self-Care Deficit

Just as OA of the lower extremities can reduce the client's mobility, OA of the upper extremities (the wrist, hand, and finger joints in particular) can significantly interfere with performance of ADLs such as cooking and brushing the hair. When the lower extremities are affected, bathing and toileting can be difficult.

- Perform a functional assessment of the upper and lower extremities. For upper extremities, assess the ability to touch the back of the head, and to hold and use small items such as eating utensils. *The functional assessment provides important data about the client's ability to provide self-care.*
- Assess the client's home setting to determine the need for assistive devices such as handrails, grab bars, walk-in shower stall, or shower chair and handheld showerhead. *Many assistive devices are relatively easy and inexpensive to obtain and can significantly improve the client's independence in performing ADLs.*

- Assist the client in obtaining other assistive devices such as long-handled shoehorns, zipper grabbers, long-handled tongs or grippers for retrieving items from the floor, jar openers, and special eating utensils. *These devices can prolong independence in performing ADLs.*

## Using NANDA, NIC, and NOC

Chart 39–2 shows links between NANDA nursing diagnoses, NIC, and NOC when caring for the client with OA.

## Home Care

Because of the chronicity of OA, clients and their families need appropriate teaching to manage the disease and its consequences effectively. Much of the teaching focus is on preservation of joint function and mobility. Discuss the following topics.

- Safeguard against hazards to safe mobility, such as scatter rugs. Encourage installation of safety devices such as hand rails and grab bars.
- Understand the disease process and its chronic degenerative nature.
- Learn exercise techniques, including range of motion, isometric, postural, stretching, and strengthening, to maintain healthy cartilage, preserve range of motion, and develop supportive muscles and tendons. A walking program is beneficial for clients with OA of the knee.
- Do not overuse or stress affected joints with heavy lifting, excessive stair climbing or bending, or other repetitive actions.
- Balance exercise with rest of affected joints through the use of whole body rest, splints, or assistive devices. In addition, sit in a straight chair without slumping; avoid soft chairs or recliners and sleep on a firm mattress or use a bed board.
- Use pain relief measures including prescribed or over-the-counter analgesic medications, and nonpharmacologic pain relief measures such as heat, rest, massage, relaxation, and meditation.

---

### CHART 39–2  NANDA, NIC, AND NOC LINKAGES

#### The Client with Osteoarthritis

| NURSING DIAGNOSES | NURSING INTERVENTIONS | NURSING OUTCOMES |
|---|---|---|
| • Chronic Pain | • Medication Administration<br>• Pain Management<br>• Heat/Cold Application | • Comfort Level<br>• Pain: Disruptive Effects |
| • Impaired Physical Mobility | • Mobility Level<br>• Exercise Therapy: Joint Mobility<br>• Exercise Therapy: Ambulation | • Ambulation: Walking<br>• Joint Movement: Active |
| • Knowledge Deficit: Weight Loss | • Teaching: Prescribed Diet<br>• Nutrition Management<br>• Weight Management | • Knowledge: Diet |

*Note: Data from* Nursing Outcomes Classification (NOC) *by M. Johnson & M. Maas (Eds.), 1997, St. Louis: Mosby;* Nursing Diagnoses: Definitions & Classification 2001–2002 *by North American Nursing Diagnosis Association, 2001, Philadelphia: NANDA;* Nursing Interventions Classification (NIC) *by J.C. McCloskey & G. M. Bulechek (Eds.), 2000, St. Louis: Mosby. Reprinted by permission.*

## Nursing Care Plan
## A Client with Osteoarthritis

Robert Cerulli is a 72-year-old retired commercial fisherman who has experienced arthritic pain in his hips for the past 10 to 15 years. Over the past year, the pain in his right hip has become severe, prompting him to seek medical attention. Significant degenerative changes in both hip joints are noted on X-ray films. The physician recommends a total replacement of the right hip, and total replacement of the left hip to follow in 6 to 12 months. Mr. Cerulli has preoperative teaching and tests the afternoon prior to his surgery, scheduled for 0800 the following morning.

### ASSESSMENT

Christie Phlaugh, RN, completes a nursing history and examination of Mr. Cerulli on admission. Reviewing his medical record, she notes that Mr. Cerulli has mild Parkinson's disease and is taking carbidopa/levodopa (Sinemet 25-100) four times a day to control his symptoms. No other chronic medical conditions have been reported. Mr. Cerulli says he has been essentially healthy his entire life. He has no known allergies to medications, has never smoked, and consumes only small amounts of alcohol.

On examination of Mr. Cerulli, Ms. Phlaugh notes that he is alert and oriented. His vital signs are BP 116/64, P 68 regular, R 18, T 97.4°F (36.3°C) PO. Peripheral pulses are strong and equal in the upper extremities, and slightly weaker but equal in the lower extremities. His feet are cool to touch but have immediate capillary refill. He has full ROM of his shoulders, elbows, and wrists. The ROM of both hips is significantly restricted. Hip flexion beyond 90 degrees prompts pain on both sides. Both flexion and extension of the knees are limited slightly. Mr. Cerulli walks with a limp, favoring his right hip, and has a shuffling gait.

Preoperative laboratory studies including CBC, coagulation studies, chemistry panel, and urinalysis show a serum creatinine of 1.7 mg/dL and BUN of 30 mg/dL, with no other abnormal values noted. His ECG and chest X-ray show no apparent pathologies. Cefazolin (Ancef) 500 mg is to be administered intravenously at 0600 prior to surgery, and Mr. Cerulli is to shower and shampoo with antibacterial soap at bedtime. The physical therapist meets with Mr. Cerulli to evaluate his mobility and begin teaching him about postoperative weight-bearing restrictions.

### DIAGNOSIS (Postoperative)

- *Acute pain* related to surgical incision
- *Impaired physical mobility* related to activity and weight-bearing restrictions
- *Risk for infection* related to disruption in skin integrity
- *Risk for ineffective tissue perfusion, right leg* related to vascular disruption and edema

### EXPECTED OUTCOMES

- Maintain an adequate level of comfort postoperatively as demonstrated by:
  - The ability to move easily within restrictions.
  - Compliance with instructions to cough and breathe deeply.
  - Verbal expressions of comfort.
- Remain free of adverse consequences of immobility such as pneumonia, pressure areas, thromboembolism, or contracture.
- Remain free of infection.

- Maintain adequate perfusion of affected leg.
- Remain free of injury postoperatively.

### PLANNING AND IMPLEMENTATION

- Assess pain at least hourly during first 24 to 48 hours postoperatively, and as needed thereafter.
- Instruct in the use of patient-controlled analgesia (PCA) and monitor its effectiveness.
- Help change position at least every 2 hours; encourage the use of the overhead trapeze to shift positions frequently.
- Maintain sequential compression device and antiembolic stocking as ordered; remove for 1 hour daily.
- Encourage the use of the incentive spirometer hourly for first 24 hours, then at least every 2 hours while awake.
- Assist out of bed three times a day after the first 24 hours.
- Maintain abduction of the right hip with pillows.
- Perform passive ROM exercises of unaffected extremities every shift.
- Encourage frequent quadriceps-setting exercises and plantar and dorsiflexion of feet.
- Assess the surgical site frequently; report signs of excess bleeding or inflammation.
- Monitor temperature every 4 hours.
- Assess pulses, color, movement, and sensation of right foot hourly for the first 24 hours, then every 2 hours for 24 hours, then every 4 hours.

### EVALUATION

Mr. Cerulli returns to the orthopedic unit from the postanesthesia care unit. He becomes confused and disoriented during the first 36 hours after surgery, but his orientation and thought processes gradually clear. His family has stayed with him, and he has not experienced injury or other adverse consequences from his confusion. Otherwise, Mr. Cerulli has had an uneventful postoperative recovery. Six days after surgery, he is transferred to an extended care rehabilitation facility for further therapy until he is able to ambulate with partial weight bearing on his affected leg. He returns home 5 weeks after surgery, able to use a walker for ambulation. Arrangements are made for an overbed trapeze, elevated toilet seat, and shower chair in his home. A home health nurse and physical therapist visit Mr. and Mrs. Cerulli weekly for a month following his discharge. During this time he gradually resumes full weight bearing. Mr. Cerulli expresses pleasure with the relief of his hip pain and says he has no fear of having his left hip replaced in the future.

### Critical Thinking in the Nursing Process

1. Mr. Cerulli's preoperative laboratory work showed a modest elevation in his serum creatinine and BUN. What do these studies indicate? How might these changes affect nursing responsibilities related to medication administration for Mr. Cerulli?
2. Mr. Cerulli became confused postoperatively. What factors in his history might have alerted the nurses to this possibility? How might anesthesia and postoperative analgesics have contributed to his confusion?
3. Develop a care plan for Mr. Cerulli using the nursing diagnosis, *Acute confusion.*

See Evaluating Your Response in Appendix C.

- For the client who has had a total joint replacement, discuss the following:
  - Use and weight bearing of the affected limb
  - Proper use of splints, braces, slings, or other devices to maintain the desired limb position during healing
  - Appropriate environmental modifications, such as an overhead trapeze for getting out of bed, elevated toilet seats, and types of chairs to use and avoid when sitting
  - Prescribed exercises
  - Use of assistive devices for ambulation, such as crutches or a walker
  - Possible complications, including signs of infection or dislocation, and the need to notify the physician promptly if these occur.
- Make referrals to home care, physical or occupational therapy, or other community agencies as indicated.

## THE CLIENT WITH MUSCULAR DYSTROPHY

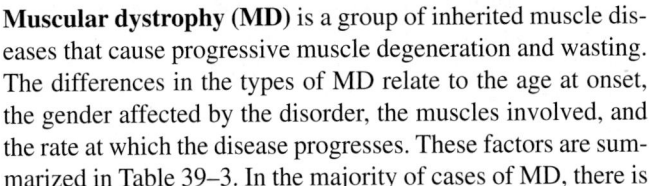

**Muscular dystrophy (MD)** is a group of inherited muscle diseases that cause progressive muscle degeneration and wasting. The differences in the types of MD relate to the age at onset, the gender affected by the disorder, the muscles involved, and the rate at which the disease progresses. These factors are summarized in Table 39–3. In the majority of cases of MD, there is a positive family history.

The most common form of MD, Duchenne's muscular dystrophy, is inherited as a recessive single gene defect on the X chromosome (a sex-linked recessive disorder), and is transmitted from the mother to male children (Porth, 2002). This disorder affects males exclusively and occurs in 1 of 3500 live male births. It can be recognized early in pregnancy in about 95% of cases by genetic studies; or in late pregnancy through amniocentesis. Genetic counseling cannot be reliably used to prevent this disease because there is no way to determine if the woman carries the defective gene. The manifestations appear in early childhood, with the average lifespan being about 15 years after onset.

Other types of MD have an onset at any age, and a slow progression with a normal lifespan.

### PATHOPHYSIOLOGY AND MANIFESTATIONS

The basic defect in MD is unknown; however, three theories have been proposed. The *vascular* and *neurogenic theories* suggest that the cause is a lack of blood supply to the muscle or a disturbance in the interaction between the nerve and muscle. The *membrane theory* suggests that an alteration in the cell membranes of the muscle causes them to degenerate. Recent genetic studies have shown a deficiency in the amount of dystrophin, a muscle membrane protein, in clients with Duchenne's MD. Dystrophin plays an important role in protecting the muscle against mechanical stresses.

All forms of MD exhibit manifestations of muscle weakness. The specific muscles involved depend on the type of MD. As the disease progresses, the person develops difficulty with ambulation and eventually becomes wheelchair-bound and finally bed-bound. Cardiac abnormalities, endocrine abnormalities, and mental retardation may also be involved.

## COLLABORATIVE CARE

Because there is no cure or specific treatment for MD, care focuses on preserving and promoting mobility. A multidisciplinary approach, involving many members of the health care team, is necessary to meet the physical and psychologic needs of these clients and their families.

TABLE 39–3　Types of Muscular Dystrophy

| Type | Sex and Age at Onset | Clinical Manifestations | Progression |
|------|----------------------|-------------------------|-------------|
| Duchenne | Males<br>Age 3 to 5 | Weakness of pelvic and shoulder girdles<br>Waddling gait<br>Toe walking<br>Lordosis<br>Cardiac abnormalities<br>Low IQ in 50% of cases | Rapid; client usually confined to wheelchair by age 15; death occurs by age 20 |
| Myotonic | Males and females<br>Any age | Myotonia of hand muscles<br>Muscular weakness of arms and legs<br>Cardiac abnormalities<br>Endocrine abnormalities<br>Mental retardation (common) | Slow; death usually occurs in early 50s |
| Becker's | Males<br>Age 5 to 20 | Weakness of pelvic and shoulder girdles | Slow; client usually confined to wheelchair at 25 years after onset; normal life span |
| Facioscapulohumeral | Males and females<br>Age 10 to 20 | Weakness of face and shoulder girdles | Slow; normal life span |
| Limb-girdle | Males and females<br>Age 20 to 40 | Weakness of shoulder and pelvic girdles | Extremely variable; usually slow |

Diagnosis and classification of the muscular dystrophies are most often based on the manifestations and the pattern of muscle involvement. Biochemical examination, muscle biopsy, and electromyography confirm the diagnosis. Tests include the following:

- *Creatine kinase* (CK-MM, the isoenzyme found in skeletal muscle) is elevated in the client with suspected MD.
- *Muscle biopsy* will show fibrous connective tissue and fatty deposits that displace functional muscle fibers.
- *Electromyogram* (EMG) readings show a decrease in amplitude.

## NURSING CARE

Nursing care for a client with MD focuses on promoting independence and mobility and providing psychologic support for both the client and family. A holistic approach is essential in planning and implementing care.

### Nursing Diagnoses and Interventions
#### Self-Care Deficit
The progressive muscle weakness that is associated with MD impairs the client's ability to perform self-care. Nursing interventions with rationales follow:

- Provide clients and family with supportive care during the progress of the disease. *The goal of treatment is to prolong each functional stage and delay or prevent deformity. When transition from ambulation to a wheelchair occurs, depression and grief may occur.*
- Promote independence. Encourage tasks the client can accomplish rather than letting the client struggle with tasks that may prove frustrating. *All forms of MD result in progressive muscle weakness. Management of the disease is directed toward keeping the client as functional as possible while preventing any deformities.*

### Home Care
Teaching of the client with MD focuses on maintaining function and independence and preventing deformities. Teach prescribed exercises such as stretching and counterposturing exercises. For the client with braces, discuss skin care and ways to prevent irritation under the brace. Because the client may have weakness involving muscles of respiration, instruct the client on ways to prevent respiratory infections, such as avoiding crowds during flu season and being immunized against pneumococcal pneumonia and influenza. Provide information about support services and organizations such as the Muscular Dystrophy Association.

# AUTOIMMUNE AND INFLAMMATORY DISORDERS

Autoimmune and inflammatory disorders of the musculoskeletal system are chronic systemic rheumatic disorders, characterized by diffuse inflammatory lesions and degenerative changes in connective tissues. The disorders have similar clinical features and may affect many of the same structures and organs.

## THE CLIENT WITH RHEUMATOID ARTHRITIS

**Rheumatoid arthritis (RA)** is a chronic systemic autoimmune disease that causes inflammation of connective tissue, primarily in the joints. It is found worldwide, affecting 1% to 2% of the total population and all races. It affects 3 times as many women as men. The onset of RA occurs most frequently between the ages of 20 and 40 years. Its course and severity are variable, and the range of manifestations is broad. Manifestations of RA may be minimal, with mild inflammation of only a few joints and little structural damage, or relentlessly progressive, with multiple inflamed joints and marked deformity. Most clients exhibit a pattern of symmetric involvement of multiple peripheral joints and periods of remission and exacerbation.

The cause of RA is unknown. A combination of genetic, environmental, hormonal, and reproductive factors are thought to play a role in its development. It is speculated that infectious agents, such as bacteria, mycoplasmas, and viruses (especially Epstein-Barr virus) may play a role in initiating the autoimmune processes present in RA.

The course of RA is variable and fluctuating. Remissions are most likely to occur in the first year of the disease. The rate at which joint deformities develop is not constant. Disease progression is fastest during the first 6 years, slowing thereafter. RA contributes to disability and a tendency to shorten life expectancy.

The incidence of RA increases with age up to about 70 years. Although the onset and manifestations of RA are much the same in older and younger clients, differentiating between RA and OA in the older adult may be difficult at times. It is important to establish an accurate diagnosis, however, because the management of these disorders differs significantly. Clinical features distinguishing RA from OA are listed in Table 39–4.

For older clients, RA is managed much as it is for younger people. However, prolonged bed rest or inactivity is not prescribed for acute episodes, because it may result in irreversible immobility in the older adult. Also, pharmacologic therapy is used with greater caution because of the increased risk of toxicity. In many cases, less emphasis is placed on preventing joint deformity and more emphasis on maintaining function for the older client with RA.

TABLE 39–4    A Comparison of the Manifestations of Rheumatoid Arthritis and Osteoarthritis

| Feature | Rheumatoid Arthritis | Osteoarthritis |
|---|---|---|
| Onset | Usually insidious, may be abrupt | Insidious |
| Course | Generally progressive, characterized by remissions and exacerbations | Slowly progressive |
| Pain and stiffness | Predominant on arising, lasting >1 hour; also occurs after prolonged inactivity | Pain with activity; stiffness following periods of immobility generally relieved within minutes |
| Affected joints | • Appear red, hot, swollen; "boggy" and tender to palpation; decreased ROM, weakness<br>• Multiple joints affected in symmetric pattern; PIP, MCP, wrists, knees, ankles, and toes often involved | • Affected joints may appear swollen; cool and bony hard on palpation; decreased ROM<br>• One or several joints affected including hips, knees, lumbar and cervical spine, PIP and DIP, wrist, and 1st MTP joint |
| Systemic manifestations | Fatigue, weakness, anorexia, weight loss, fever; rheumatoid nodules; anemia | Fatigue |

## PATHOPHYSIOLOGY

It is believed that long-term exposure to an unidentified antigen causes an aberrant immune response in a genetically susceptible host. As a result, normal antibodies (immunoglobulins) become autoantibodies and attack host tissues. These transformed antibodies, usually present in people with RA, are called **rheumatoid factors (RFs).** The self-produced antibodies bind with their target antigens in blood and synovial membranes, forming immune complexes (see Chapter 9 ⊙ for further information about autoimmune processes).

The damage to cartilage that occurs in RA is the result of at least three processes (McCance & Huether, 2002):

- Neutrophils, T cells, and other synovial fluid cells are activated and degrade the surface layer of the articular cartilage.
- Cytokines (especially interleukin-1 and tumor necrosis factor alpha) cause the chondrocytes to attack the cartilage.
- The synovium digests nearby cartilage, releasing inflammatory molecules containing interleukin-1 and tumor necrosis factor alpha.

Leukocytes are attracted to the synovial membrane from the circulation, where neutrophils and macrophages ingest the immune complexes and release enzymes that degrade synovial tissue and articular cartilage. Activation of B and T lymphocytes results in increased production of rheumatoid factors and enzymes that increase and continue the inflammatory process.

The synovial membrane is damaged by the inflammatory and immune processes. It swells from infiltration of the leukocytes and thickens as cells proliferate and abnormally enlarge. The inflammation spreads and involves synovial blood vessels. Small venules are occluded and vascular flow to the synovial tissue decreases. As blood flow decreases and metabolic needs increase (from the increased number and size of cells), hypoxia and metabolic acidosis occur. Acidosis stimulates synovial cells to release hydrolytic enzymes into surrounding tissues, starting erosion of the articular cartilage and inflammation of the supporting ligaments and tendons.

The inflammation also causes hemorrhage, coagulation, and deposits of fibrin on the synovial membrane, in the intracellu-

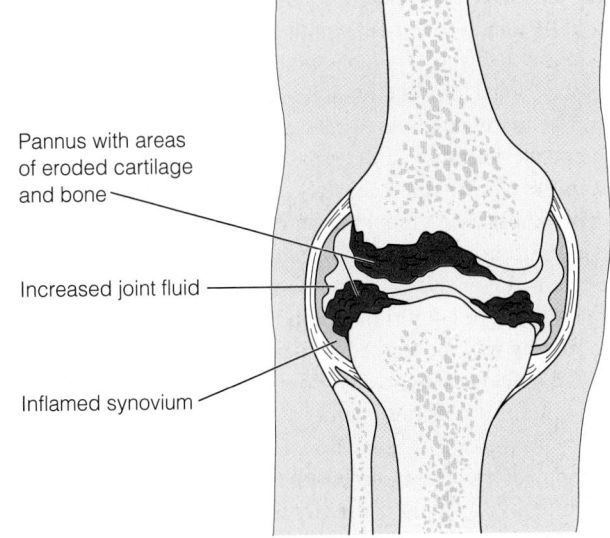

Pannus with areas of eroded cartilage and bone

Increased joint fluid

Inflamed synovium

**Figure 39–5** ■ Joint inflammation and destruction in rheumatoid arthritis. Note synovial inflammation with pannus formation and the erosion of cartilage and underlying bone.

lar matrix, and in the synovial fluid. Fibrin develops into granulation tissue (**pannus**) over denuded areas of the synovial membrane. The formation of pannus leads to scar tissue formation that immobilizes the joint (Figure 39–5 ■).

## Joint Manifestations

The onset of RA is typically insidious, although it may be acute (precipitated by a stressor such as infection, surgery, or trauma). Joint manifestations are often preceded by systemic manifestations of inflammation, including fatigue, anorexia, weight loss, and nonspecific aching and stiffness. Clients report joint swelling with associated stiffness, warmth, tenderness, and pain. The pattern of joint involvement is typically polyarticular (involving multiple joints) and symmetric. The proximal interphalangeal (PIP) and metacarpophalangeal (MCP) joints of the fingers, the wrists, the knees, the ankles, and the toes are most frequently involved, although RA can

 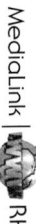

affect any joint. Stiffness is most pronounced in the morning, lasting more than 1 hour. It may also occur with prolonged rest during the day and may be more severe following strenuous activity. Swollen, inflamed joints feel "boggy" or spongelike on palpation because of synovial edema. Range of motion is limited in affected joints, and weakness may be evident.

The persistent inflammation of RA causes deformities of the joint itself and supporting structures such as ligaments, tendons, and muscles. As the joint is destroyed, ligaments, tendons, and the joint capsule are weakened or destroyed. Joint cartilage and bone are also destroyed. Weakening or destruction of these supporting structures results in lack of opposition to muscle pull, causing deformity.

Characteristic changes in the hands and fingers include ulnar deviation of the fingers and subluxation at the MCP joints. Swan-neck deformity is characterized by hyperextension of the PIP joint with compensatory flexion of the distal interphalangeal (DIP) joints. A flexion deformity of the PIP joints with extension of the DIP joint is called a boutonnière deformity (Figure 39–6 ■). The ability to effect a pinch is limited by hyperextension of the interphalangeal joint and flexion of the MCP joint of the thumb.

Wrist involvement is nearly universal, leading to limited movement, deformity, and carpal tunnel syndrome. Inflammation of the elbows often causes flexion contracture.

The knees are frequently affected in RA, with visible swelling often obliterating normal contours. Instability of the knee joint along with quadriceps atrophy, contractures, and valgus (knock-knee) deformities can lead to significant disability. Ambulation may be limited by pain and deformities when the ankles and feet are involved. Typical deformities of the feet and toes include subluxation, hallux valgus (deviation of the great toe toward the other digits of the foot), lateral deviation of the toes, and cock-up toes (turned-up toes).

Spinal involvement is usually limited to the cervical vertebrae. Neck pain is common, and neurologic complications can occur.

## Extra-Articular Manifestations

RA is a systemic disease with a variety of extra-articular manifestations. These are seen particularly in clients with high levels of circulating rheumatoid factor. Fatigue, weakness, anorexia, weight loss, and low-grade fever are common when the disease is active. Anemia resistant to iron therapy frequently affects clients with RA. Skeletal muscle atrophy is common, usually most apparent in the musculature around affected joints.

Rheumatoid nodules may develop, usually in subcutaneous tissue in areas subject to pressure: on the forearm, olecranon bursa, over the MCP joints, and on the toes. Rheumatoid nodules are granulomatous lesions that are firm and either movable or fixed. They may also be found in viscera, including the heart, lungs, intestinal tract, and dura.

Other possible extra-articular manifestations of RA include subcutaneous nodules, pleural effusion, vasculitis, pericarditis, and splenomegly (enlargement of the spleen). The *Multisystem Effects of RA* are illustrated on page 1251.

## COLLABORATIVE CARE

The diagnosis of RA is based on the client's history, physical assessment, and diagnostic tests. Diagnostic criteria developed by the American Rheumatism Association are used as well (Box 39–3). At least four of seven criteria must be present to establish the diagnosis.

Once the diagnosis of RA has been established, the goals of therapy are to:

- Relieve pain.
- Reduce inflammation.
- Slow or stop joint damage.
- Improve well-being and ability to function.

No cure currently exists for RA; the goal of treatment is to relieve its manifestations. A multidisciplinary approach is used, with a balance of rest, exercise, physical therapy, and suppression of the inflammatory processes.

Because a cure is not available and traditional therapies are not always fully effective, the client with RA is vulnerable to quackery. Many nontraditional treatments, including diets, topical preparations, vaccines, hormones, plant extracts, and copper bracelets, have been put forth. These treatments are often costly, and none has been shown to be effective.

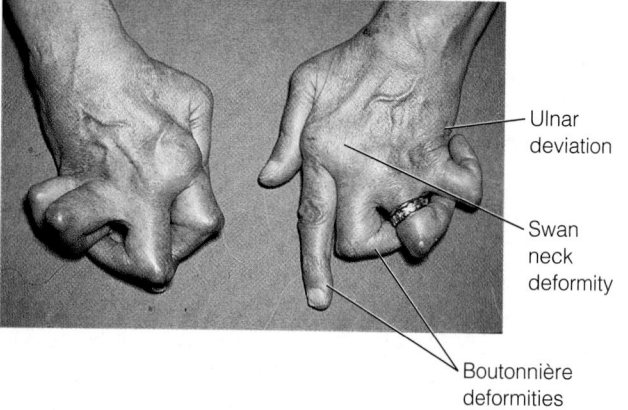

**Figure  39–6 ■** Typical hand deformities associated with rheumatoid arthritis.

Ulnar deviation

Swan neck deformity

Boutonnière deformities

*Source: Biophoto Associates/Photo Researchers, Inc.*

| BOX 39–3 | ■ Diagnostic Criteria for Rheumatoid Arthritis |
|---|---|

- Morning stiffness lasting for at least 1 hour and persisting over at least 6 weeks
- Arthritis with swelling or effusion of three or more joints persisting for at least 6 weeks
- Arthritis of wrist, MCP, or PIP joints persisting for at least 6 weeks
- Symmetric arthritis with simultaneous involvement of corresponding joints on both sides of the body
- Rheumatoid nodules
- Positive serum rheumatoid factor
- Characteristic radiologic changes of rheumatoid arthritis noted in hands and wrists

# Multisystem Effects of Rheumatoid Arthritis

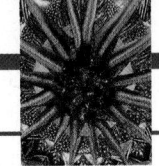

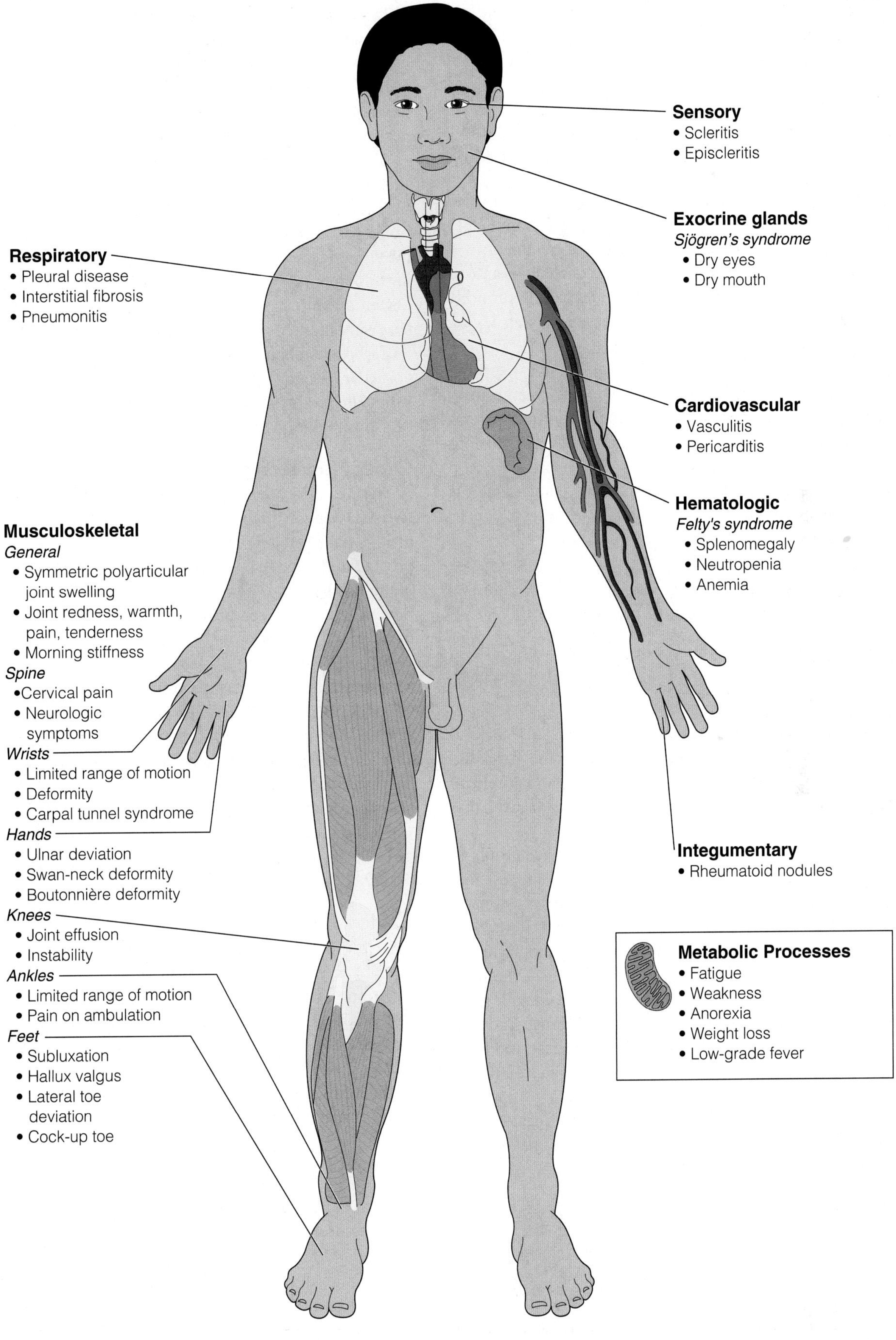
Sensory
• Scleritis
• Episcleritis
Exocrine glands
Sjögren's syndrome
• Dry eyes
• Dry mouth
Respiratory
• Pleural disease
• Interstitial fibrosis
• Pneumonitis
Cardiovascular
• Vasculitis
• Pericarditis
Hematologic
Felty's syndrome
• Splenomegaly
• Neutropenia
• Anemia
Musculoskeletal
General
• Symmetric polyarticular joint swelling
• Joint redness, warmth, pain, tenderness
• Morning stiffness
Spine
•Cervical pain
• Neurologic symptoms
Wrists
• Limited range of motion
• Deformity
• Carpal tunnel syndrome
Hands
• Ulnar deviation
• Swan-neck deformity
• Boutonnière deformity
Knees
• Joint effusion
• Instability
Ankles
• Limited range of motion
• Pain on ambulation
Feet
• Subluxation
• Hallux valgus
• Lateral toe deviation
• Cock-up toe
Integumentary
• Rheumatoid nodules
Metabolic Processes
• Fatigue
• Weakness
• Anorexia
• Weight loss
• Low-grade fever

## Diagnostic Tests

Diagnostic tests are used to help establish the diagnosis of RA, although no test specific to the disease is available. Testing is also used to rule out other forms of arthritis and connective tissue disorders.

- *Rheumatoid factors* (RFs), autoantibodies to IgG, are present in approximately 75% of people with RA. High levels of RF are often associated with severe RA.
- *Erythrocyte sedimentation rate (ESR)* is typically elevated and is often used as an indicator of disease and inflammatory activity when evaluating the effectiveness of treatment.
- *Synovial fluid examination* will demonstrate changes associated with inflammation, including increased turbidity (cloudiness), decreased viscosity, increased protein levels, and 3000 to 50,000 WBCs.
- *X-rays* of affected joints are taken, and are the most specific for diagnosis of RA. Early in the disease, few changes may be evident other than soft-tissue swelling and joint effusions. As the disease progresses, joint space narrowing and erosions are seen.
- *CBC* usually shows moderate anemia. The platelet count is often elevated.

## Treatments

The primary objectives in treating RA are to reduce pain and inflammation, preserve function, and prevent deformity.

### Medications

Four general approaches are used in the pharmacologic management of clients with RA.

- Aspirin and other NSAIDs and mild analgesics are used to reduce the inflammatory process and manage the signs and symptoms of the disease. Although these drugs may relieve manifestations of RA, they appear to have little effect on disease progression.
- The second approach uses low-dose oral corticosteroids to reduce pain and inflammation. Recent studies suggest that low-dose oral corticosteroids also may slow the development and progression of bone erosions associated with RA.
- A diverse group of drugs classified as disease-modifying or slow-acting antirheumatic drugs are employed in the third approach to treating RA. These drugs, which include gold compounds, D-penicillamine, antimalarial agents, and sulfasalazine, appear to alter the course of the disease, reducing its destruction of joints. Immunosuppressive and cytotoxic drugs are included in this category as well.
- Intra-articular corticosteroids may be used to provide temporary relief in clients for whom other therapies have failed to control inflammation.

### Aspirin

Aspirin is often the first drug prescribed in the treatment of RA unless its use is contraindicated for the client. Aspirin is an inexpensive and effective anti-inflammatory and analgesic agent. The dose of aspirin required to achieve a therapeutic blood level of 15 to 30 mg/dL and its full anti-inflammatory effect is approximately 4 g per day in divided doses (three or four 5 g [325 mg] tablets qid). This effective dose is just under the toxic dose, which produces tinnitus and hearing loss. The client may be instructed to increase the dose of aspirin gradually until either maximal improvement or toxicity occurs. If tinnitus develops, the client reduces the dose by two to three tablets per day until the tinnitus stops.

Gastrointestinal side effects and interference with platelet function are the greatest hazards of aspirin therapy. Clients are instructed to take aspirin with meals, milk, or antacids to minimize gastrointestinal distress and reduce the risk of GI bleeding. Enteric-coated forms of aspirin and nonacetylated salicylate compounds produce less gastric distress than plain or buffered aspirin and reduce the risk of gastric ulceration, but they are more expensive. Salsalate (Disalcid, Mono-Gesic, Salflex) and choline magnesium trisalicylate (Trilisate, Tricosal) are examples of nonacetylated salicylate products. All salicylate products are contraindicated for clients with a history of aspirin allergy.

### Other Nonsteroidal Anti-Inflammatory Drugs

A number of other nonsteroidal anti-inflammatory drugs (NSAIDs) are available for use in the management of RA if aspirin is not tolerated or effective. All NSAIDs act by inhibiting prostaglandin synthesis. Although the efficacy of all NSAIDs, including aspirin, is equivalent, client responses are individual. Several trials of different NSAIDs may be necessary to find the most effective drug.

Some NSAIDs are considerably more expensive than aspirin but may cause less gastrointestinal distress and require fewer doses per day. Gastric irritation, ulceration, and bleeding remain the most common toxic effects of NSAIDs. They can also affect the lower intestinal tract, leading to perforation or aggravation of inflammatory bowel disorders. All NSAIDs can also be toxic to the kidneys.

NSAIDs commonly prescribed for clients with RA are listed in Table 39–5. Nursing implications of their administration are described in Chapter 8. ᐲᐧ

### Corticosteroids

Systemic corticosteroids can dramatically relieve the symptoms of RA and appear to slow the progression of joint destruction. The long-term use of corticosteroids is associated with multiple side effects, such as poor wound healing, increased risk of infection, osteoporosis, and gastrointestinal bleeding. Severe rebound manifestations can occur when these medications are discontinued. For these reasons, the use of systemic corticosteroids is limited to low dosages daily. The nursing implications for corticosteroid therapy are discussed in Chapter 9. ᐲᐧ

### Disease-Modifying Drugs

Disease-modifying drugs are a diverse group of medications including drugs that modify immune and inflammatory responses, gold salts, antimalarial agents, sulfasalazine, and D-penicillamine (Table 39–6). They share characteristics that make them useful in the treatment of RA. Although beneficial

| Drug | Average Dose | Comments and Precautions |
|---|---|---|
| Aspirin | 600–900 mg 4 to 6 times daily | Least expensive NSAID; associated with risk of GI ulceration, bleeding, and possible hemorrhage; may cause hepatotoxicity |
| Diclofenac (Voltaren) | 50 mg tid or qid; or 75 mg bid | Expensive; risk of hepatotoxicity |
| Etodolac (Lodine) | 200–400 mg q6h | Expensive; may have less gastrointestinal toxicity |
| Fenoprofen (Nalfon) | 300–600 mg tid or qid | Should not be administered to clients with impaired renal function; risk of GU effects such as dysuria, cystitis, hematuria, acute interstitial nephritis, and nephrotic syndrome |
| Flurbiprofen (Ansaid) | 50–100 mg tid or qid, not to exceed 300 mg/day | Expensive |
| Ibuprofen (Motrin, Advil, others) | 300 mg qid; 400–800 mg tid or qid | Available in prescription and over-the-counter forms; less gastric distress reported than with aspirin or indomethacin; discontinue if visual disturbances develop |
| Indomethacin (Indocin) | 25–50 mg bid or tid | A potent NSAID used for moderate to severe RA and acute episodes of chronic disease; higher incidence of adverse GI effects and CNS effects such as headache, dizziness, and depression |
| Ketoprofen (Orudis) | 50–75 mg tid or qid | Expensive; older adults and clients with renal insufficiency require lower doses |
| Meclofenamate sodium (Meclomen) | 100 mg bid to qid | Increased risk of adverse effects in older adults; GI effects include diarrhea and abdominal pain; anemia may develop during therapy |
| Nabumetone (Relafen) | 1000–2000 mg per day | Most common adverse effects include diarrhea, dyspepsia, and abdominal pain |
| Naproxen (Aleve, Anaprox, Naprosyn) | 250–500 mg bid | Available in prescription and over-the-counter preparations |
| Oxaprozin (Daypro) | 1200 mg daily | Expensive; risk of severe hepatotoxicity; rash may occur |
| Piroxicam (Feldene) | 20 mg daily in a single or divided dose | Expensive; GI side effects including stomatitis, anorexia, and gastric distress may occur more frequently than with other NSAIDs |
| Sulindac (Clinoril) | 150–200 mg bid | May be safer for use than other NSAIDs in clients with chronic renal disease; rare fatal hypersensitivity reaction with fever, liver function abnormalities, and severe skin reaction |
| Tolmetin (Tolectin) | 200–600 mg tid | Expensive; may have higher rate of side effects including GI distress, headache, dizziness, elevated blood pressure, edema, and weight gain |

**TABLE 39–5   Examples of Nonsteroidal Anti-Inflammatory Drugs Used to Treat Rheumatoid Arthritis**

effects are not apparent for several weeks or months following the initiation of therapy, they can produce not only clinical improvement but also evidence of decreased disease activity. Because their anti-inflammatory effect is minimal, NSAIDs are continued during therapy. As many as two-thirds of clients taking disease-modifying drugs show improvement, although these drugs have not been shown to slow bone erosion or facilitate healing. All of these drugs are fairly toxic, and close monitoring is necessary during the course of therapy.

Drugs that modify the autoimmune and inflammatory responses in clients with RA include leflunomide (Arava) and etanercept (Enbrel). Leflunomide reversibly inhibits an enzyme involved in the autoimmune process and etanercept inhibits the binding of tumor necrosis factor to receptor sites.

Gold salts may be administered by mouth, but the intramuscular route is preferred because it is more effective. The mode of action of gold is unknown, but it may produce clinical remission in some clients and decrease new bony erosions. Weekly therapy is continued until significant improvement is noted unless toxic reactions occur. Clients experiencing benefit from gold therapy may be continued on monthly injections

for several years. About 30% of clients on gold therapy experience toxic reactions, including dermatitis, stomatitis, bone marrow depression, and proteinuria. Mild skin reactions do not always necessitate discontinuation of therapy. CBC and urinalysis are monitored throughout treatment with gold to assess for more severe toxic responses.

Hydroxychloroquine (Plaquenil) is an antimalarial agent sometimes employed in the treatment of RA. Three to 6 months of therapy is required to achieve the desired response, and many clients do not experience significant benefit. Although hydroxychloroquine has a relatively low toxicity, it can cause pigmentary retinitis and vision loss. Clients receiving this drug require a thorough vision examination every 6 months.

Sulfasalazine, a drug regularly prescribed for chronic inflammatory bowel disease, may also be prescribed for RA. See Chapter 23 ⊂⊃ for further discussion of this drug and its nursing implications. For clients not responding to the above preparations, penicillamine may be prescribed. Although this agent may be effective in the management of RA, toxic reactions are common and can be severe, including bone marrow suppression, proteinuria, and nephrosis.

| TABLE 39-6 | Disease-Modifying Drugs Used to Treat Rheumatoid Arthritis | | |
|---|---|---|---|
| **Class/Medications** | **Usual Dose** | **Adverse Effects** | **Comments/Nursing Responsibilities** |
| Gold salts:<br>Gold sodium thiomalate (Myochrysine)<br>Aurothioglucose (Solganal)<br>Auranofin (Ridaura Capsules) | Parenteral: 1st dose 10 mg; 2nd dose 25 mg, then 50 mg weekly IM<br>Oral: 6 mg daily | • Pruritus, dermatitis<br>• Stomatitis, metallic taste<br>• Renal toxicity<br>• Blood dyscrasias<br>• Gastrointestinal distress | • Frequent UA and CBC<br>• Monitor client after injection for flushing, fainting, dizziness, sweating, possible anaphylactic reaction |
| Antimalarial:<br>Hydroxychloroquine (Plaquenil) | 200–600 mg daily with meals | • CNS reactions including irritability, nightmares, psychoses<br>• Retinopathy<br>• Alopecia, pruritus<br>• Blood dyscrasias<br>• GI disturbances | • Should not be used during pregnancy<br>• Regular ophthalmologic examination required |
| Sulfasalazine (Azulfidine) | 2 g/day in divided doses with meals | • Anorexia, nausea, vomiting, gastric distress<br>• Decreased sperm count<br>• Headache<br>• Rash<br>• Blood dyscrasias<br>• Hypersensitivity responses including Stevens-Johnson syndrome<br>• CNS, liver, and renal toxicity | • Administer in evenly divided doses<br>• Maintain high fluid intake<br>• May cause yellow-orange skin or urine discoloration<br>• Regular CBCs necessary |
| Penicillamine (Cuprimine, Depen Titratable) | 125–250 mg/day initially, slowly increased to a total of 1000–1500 mg/day | • Skin rashes<br>• Fever<br>• Gastrointestinal distress<br>• Oral ulcers, loss of taste<br>• Fever<br>• Bone marrow depression with thrombocytopenia, leukopenia, anemia<br>• Renal toxicity<br>• May induce immune complex disorders such as Goodpasture's syndrome and myasthenia gravis | • Regular CBC and UA necessary<br>• Administer on an empty stomach<br>• Discontinue during pregnancy<br>• May require 2 to 3 months of therapy before benefit is seen |

## Immunosuppressive Therapy

Immunosuppressive or cytotoxic drugs are increasingly employed in the management of RA. Indeed, many now consider methotrexate the treatment of choice for clients with aggressive RA. Methotrexate may be used along with NSAIDs in the initial treatment plan. A weekly dose can produce a beneficial effect in as few as 2 to 4 weeks. Gastric irritation and stomatitis are the most frequent side effects associated with methotrexate. Alcoholism, diabetes, obesity, advanced age, and renal disease increase the risk of toxic effects (hepatotoxicity, bone marrow suppression, interstitial pneumonitis).

Other immunosuppressive agents such as cyclosporine, azathioprine, and monoclonal antibodies have also been employed in the treatment of clients with severe, progressive, crippling disease who have failed to respond to other measures.

## Rest and Exercise

A balanced program of rest and exercise is an important component in the management of clients with RA. During an acute exacerbation of the disease, the client may be hospitalized, or a short period of complete bed rest may be prescribed. For most clients, regular rest periods during the day are beneficial to reduce manifestations of the disease. Additionally, splinting of inflamed joints reduces unwanted motion and provides local joint rest. A variety of orthotic devices are available to reduce joint strain and help maintain function.

Rest must be balanced with a program of physical therapy and exercise to maintain muscle strength and joint mobility. Range-of-motion exercises are prescribed to maintain joint function and prevent contractures. Isometric exercises are used to improve muscle strength without increasing joint stress. Isotonic exercises also help improve muscle strength and preserve function. Low-impact aerobic exercises, such as swimming and walking, have been shown to benefit clients with RA without adversely affecting joint inflammation or prompting acute episodes.

## Physical and Occupational Therapy

Physical and occupational therapists can design and monitor individualized activity and rest programs.

## Heat and Cold

Heat and cold are used for their analgesic and muscle-relaxing effects. Moist heat is generally the most effective, and can be provided by a tub bath. Joint pain is relieved in some clients through the application of cold.

## Assistive Devices and Splints

Assistive devices, such as a cane, walker, or raised toilet seat, are most useful for clients with significant hip or knee arthritis. Splints provide joint rest and prevent contractures. Night splints for the hands and/or wrists should maintain the extremity in a position of maximum function. The best "splint" for the hip is lying prone for several hours a day on a firm bed. In general, splints should be applied for the shortest period needed, should be made of lightweight materials, and should be easily removed to perform ROM exercises once or twice a day.

## Diet

For most clients with RA, an ordinary, well-balanced diet is recommended. Some clients may benefit from substitution of usual dietary fat with omega-3 fatty acids found in certain fish oils.

## Surgery

Surgical intervention may be employed for the client with RA at a variety of disease stages. Early in the course of the disease, synovectomy, excision of synovial membrane, can provide temporary relief of inflammation, relieve pain, and slow the destructive process, helping to preserve joint function. Arthrodesis, joint fusion, may be used to stabilize joints such as cervical vertebrae, wrists, and ankles. Arthroplasty, or total joint replacement, may be necessary in cases of gross deformity and joint destruction. Total joint replacement and nursing care needs of clients undergoing this surgery are discussed in the preceding section on OA.

## Other Therapies

Several newer treatments that are not yet in widespread use may be employed in clients with progressive RA. These experimental therapies are directed toward ameliorating the underlying immunologic process. Plasmapheresis has been used to remove circulating antibodies, moderating the autoimmune response. Total lymphoid irradiation decreases total lymphocyte levels, although serious adverse effects are associated with this treatment, and its continued efficacy has not been established.

## NURSING CARE

Clients with chronic, progressive, systemic disorders such as RA have multiple nursing care needs involving all functional health patterns. Physical manifestations of the disease often result in acute and chronic pain, fatigue, impaired mobility, and difficulty performing routine tasks. The disease also has many psychosocial effects. The client has an incurable chronic disease that may lead to severe crippling. Pain and fatigue can interfere with the client's ability to perform expected roles, such as home maintenance or job responsibilities. Even though the client's hands may appear swollen, other people may not understand the systemic nature of the disease or realize the difference between RA and OA.

## Health Promotion

People with RA have control of their lives by becoming arthritis self-managers. They can help prevent deformities and the effects of arthritis by following prescriptions for exercise, rest, weight management, posture, and positioning. The following suggestions are outlined by the Moss Rehab Resource Net (2002).

- Never attempt an activity that cannot be stopped immediately if it proves to be beyond your power to complete it.
- Respect pain as a warning signal. When you experience pain, change your method of doing things, use equipment or tools if necessary, and take intermittent rest periods.
- Use the strongest joints available for an activity. For example, use the palm of your hand or the crook of your elbow instead of fingers for grasping while carrying.
- Avoid stress toward a position of deformity, such as when the fingers drift toward the little finger. For example, open a jar with your right hand and close a jar with your left hand.
- Avoid activities that need a tight grip, such as writing, wringing, and unscrewing.

## Assessment

Collect the following data through the health history and physical examination (see Chapter 37).

- Health history: pain, stiffness, fatigue, joint problems: location, duration, onset, effect on function, fever, sleep patterns, past illnesses or surgery, ability to carry out ADLs and self-care activities
- Physical assessment: height/weight; gait, joints: symmetry, size, shape, color, appearance, temperature, range of motion, pain; skin: nodules, purpura; respiratory: cough, crackles; cardiovascular: pericardial friction rub, apical bradycardia, $S_3$.

## Nursing Diagnoses and Interventions

Many nursing diagnoses may be appropriate for the client with RA. This section focuses on those related to its predominant manifestations and their effect on the client's life.

### Chronic Pain

Pain is a constant feature of RA when the disease is active. Pain accompanies both acute inflammation and lower levels of chronic inflammation. Some clients say the pain in joints and surrounding tissue is like a deep, constant toothache. Pain can significantly affect the client's ability to provide self-care and maintain daily activities. It also contributes to the client's fatigue.

- Monitor the level of pain and duration of morning stiffness. *Pain and morning stiffness are indicators of disease activity. Increased pain may necessitate changes in the therapeutic treatment plan.*
- Encourage the client to relate pain to activity level and adjust activities accordingly. Teach the importance of joint and whole-body rest in relieving pain. *Pain is an indicator of*

*excess stress on inflamed joints. Increasing pain indicates a need to decrease activity levels.*

- Teach the use of heat and cold applications to provide pain relief. The client may apply heat by showering or taking tub baths, or using warm compresses or other local applications such as paraffin dips. For clients who find that heat increases pain and swelling during periods of acute inflammation, cold packs may be more effective. *Both heat and cold have analgesic effects and can help relieve associated muscle spasms.*
- Teach about the use of prescribed anti-inflammatory medications and the relationship of pain and inflammation. *Anti-inflammatory agents reduce chemical mediators of inflammation and swelling, relieving pain.*
- Encourage using other nonpharmacologic pain relief measures such as visualization, distraction, meditation, and progressive relaxation techniques. *These techniques can reduce muscle tension and help the client focus away from the pain, decreasing the intensity of the pain experience.*

## Fatigue

The pain and chronic inflammatory processes associated with RA lead to fatigue. Other factors contribute as well. Discomfort often disrupts the client's sleep patterns. Anemia, muscle atrophy, and poor nutrition also play a role in the development of fatigue. The client with RA may experience depression or hopelessness, with associated manifestations of fatigue. (See the box in next column for related nursing research).

- Encourage a balance of periods of activity with periods of rest. *Both joint and whole-body rest are important to reduce the inflammatory response.*
- Stress the importance of planned rest periods during the day. *Rest is vital during acute exacerbations of the disease but also important to maintain the client in remission.*
- Help in prioritizing activities, performing the most important ones early in the day. *Assigning priorities helps the client avoid performing relatively unimportant activities at the expense of more meaningful and important ones.*
- Encourage regular physical activity in addition to prescribed ROM exercises. *Aerobic exercise promotes a sense of well-being and restful sleep patterns.*
- Refer to counseling or support groups. *Counseling and support groups can help the client develop effective coping strategies and deal with depression and hopelessness.*

## Ineffective Role Performance

Fatigue, pain, and the crippling effects of RA can interfere with the client's ability to pursue a career and fill other life roles, such as parent, spouse, or homemaker. As the client's role changes, so must the roles of other family members. This can contribute to changes in family processes, increased stress in the family, and further difficulty coping with the effects of the disease.

- Discuss the effects of the disease on the client's career and other life roles. Encourage the client to identify changes brought on by the disease. *Discussion helps the client to accept the changes and begin to identify strategies for coping with them.*
- Encourage the client and family to discuss their feelings about role changes and grieve lost roles or abilities. *Verbal-*

## Nursing Research

### Evidence-Based Practice for Fatigue in Clients with Rheumatoid Arthritis

Fatigue is a common systemic manifestation of rheumatoid arthritis (RA) that can interfere with clients' ability to maintain independence, their family roles, sense of well-being, and self esteem. In this study, researchers evaluated the effects of 12 weeks of low-impact aerobic exercise on fatigue, aerobic fitness, and disease activity in a group of 25 adults with rheumatoid arthritis (Neuberger et al., 1997). Study results showed that subjects who participated in aerobic exercise more frequently reported decreased fatigue, while those who participated less frequently reported increased fatigue. All subjects benefited from increased aerobic fitness, increased grip strength and decreased pain. Interestingly, measures of increased disease activity, including number of involved joints and sedimentation rate (erythrocyte sedimentation rate or ESR), remained stable or improved during the course of the study.

### IMPLICATIONS FOR NURSING

Nurses and other health care providers should encourage clients with rheumatoid arthritis to maintain a regular schedule of activities such as walking, swimming, and other activities that place relatively little stress on joints. Regular activity improves the client's overall health and general fitness. It may help reduce disease activity, and promotes comfort and restful sleep. These can reduce fatigue and improve the client's functional capacity.

### Critical Thinking in Client Care

1. How do you think regular low-impact aerobic exercise works to reduce disease activity in the client with rheumatoid arthritis?
2. Develop an exercise/activity plan for a client with RA that takes the disease manifestations into consideration and minimizes stress on affected joints.
3. What measures can the nurse recommend to promote comfort and uninterrupted, restful sleep for the client with RA?

*ization allows family members to validate and accept feelings about losses and changes, thus helping them to move into new roles.*

- Listen actively to concerns expressed by the client and family members; acknowledge the validity of concerns about the disease, prescribed treatment, and the prognosis. *Demonstrating acceptance of these feelings and concerns promotes trust and validates their reality.*

**PRACTICE ALERT** *Remember that grief resolution takes time and that clients may respond to loss with anger.* ■

- Help the client and family identify strengths they can use to cope with role changes. *Identifying strengths helps the client and family to consider role changes that maintain self-esteem and dignity.*
- Encourage the client to make decisions and assume personal responsibility for disease management. *Clients who assume*

*a personal and active role in managing their disease maintain a greater sense of self-control and self-esteem.*

- Encourage the client to maintain life roles as far as the disease allows. *Maintaining roles helps the client continue to feel useful and stay in contact with other people.*

### Disturbed Body Image

The acute and long-term effects of RA can affect the client's body image, leading to feelings of hopelessness and powerlessness, social withdrawal, and difficulty adapting to changes. When inflammation and joint deformity occur despite compliance, the client may have difficulty accepting the need to continue therapeutic measures, particularly those that have side effects or are costly or time consuming. In addition, unproven alternative treatment strategies and quackery may become increasingly attractive to the client.

- Demonstrate a caring, accepting attitude toward the client. *This attitude helps the client accept the physical changes brought on by the disease.*
- Encourage the client to talk about the effects of the disease, both physical effects and effects on life roles. *Verbalization helps the client identify feelings and gives the nurse opportunity to validate these feelings.*
- Encourage the client to maintain self-care and usual roles to the extent possible. Discuss the use of clothing and adaptive devices that promote independence. *Independence enhances the client's self-esteem.*
- Provide positive feedback for self-care activities and adaptive strategies. *Positive reinforcement encourages the client to continue adaptive measures and maintain independence.*

- Refer to self-help groups, support groups, and other agencies that provide assistive devices and literature. *These groups and agencies can help the client develop adaptive strategies to cope with the effects of RA, enhancing the client's self-concept, body image, and independence.*

## Using NANDA, NIC, and NOC

Chart 39–3 shows links between NANDA nursing diagnoses, NIC, and NOC when caring for the client with RA.

## Home Care

RA is typically a chronic, progressive disease. As with most diseases of this nature, involvement of the client and family in its management is vital. Education is an important nursing role in caring for clients with RA and their families. Address the following topics for home care of the client and for family members.

- Disease process and treatments, including rest and exercise
- Medications
- Management of stiffness and pain
- Energy conservation
- Use of assistive devices to maintain independence, including self-care aids such as handheld showers, long-handled brushes and shoe horns, and eating utensils with oversized or special handles
- Clothing options such as elastic waist pants without zippers, Velcro closures, zippers with large pull-tabs, and slip-on shoes
- How to apply splints and take care of skin
- Home and equipment modifications, such as a raised toilet seat, grab bars in the bathroom, a bath chair, or adapted counter heights for clients in a wheelchair

## CHART 39–3 NANDA, NIC, AND NOC LINKAGES

### The Client with Rheumatoid Arthritis

| NURSING DIAGNOSES | NURSING INTERVENTIONS | NURSING OUTCOMES |
|---|---|---|
| • Chronic Pain | • Medication Administration<br>• Pain Management<br>• Heat/Cold Application | • Comfort Level<br>• Pain: Disruptive Effects |
| • Fatigue | • Energy Management<br>• Sleep Enhancement | • Energy Conservation<br>• Rest |
| • Self-Care Deficit: Bathing/Hygiene; Dressing/Grooming; Feeding; Toileting | • Self-Care Assistance<br>• Teaching: Individual | • Self-Care: Activities of Daily Living<br>• Self-Care: Bathing/Hygiene; Dressing; Grooming; Eating; Toileting |
| • Powerlessness | • Emotional Support<br>• Self-Esteem Enhancement<br>• Environmental Management<br>• Self-Care Assistance<br>• Support Group | • Health Beliefs: Perceived Control<br>• Health Beliefs: Perceived Resources<br>• Social Support |
| • Ineffective Sexuality Patterns | • Teaching: Sexuality<br>• Sexual Counseling | • Body Image<br>• Self-Esteem |

*Note. Data from* Nursing Outcomes Classification (NOC) *by M. Johnson & M. Maas (Eds.), 1997, St. Louis: Mosby;* Nursing Diagnoses: Definitions & Classification 2001–2002 *by North American Nursing Diagnosis Association, 2001, Philadelphia: NANDA;* Nursing Interventions Classification (NIC) *by J.C. McCloskey & G. M. Bulechek (Eds.), 2000, St. Louis: Mosby. Reprinted by permission.*

- Physical therapy, occupational therapy, home health and homemaker services
- Helpful resources:
  - National Institute of Arthritis and Musculoskeletal and Skin Diseases

- American College of Rheumatology
- Arthritis Foundation
- American Physical Therapy Foundation
- American Chronic Pain Association

## Nursing Care Plan
## A Client with Rheumatoid Arthritis

Janice James is a 42-year-old high school science teacher who began noticing vague joint pain, fatigue, poor appetite, and general malaise, which she initially attributed to a case of the flu. However, her symptoms continued, and she reports feeling very stiff in the mornings, often taking until 10:00 or 11:00 A.M. to begin to feel "normal." She has begun to call this her "morning sickness." She then began to notice aching in her hands and wrists, which she attributed to the quilting she loves to do in the evenings. She made an appointment with her family physician when she noticed that her knuckles and finger joints are not just achy but also swollen and hot. Noting that Mrs. James has lost 10 lb since her last visit and has mild anemia and a significantly elevated sedimentation rate (ESR), the physician refers her to the rheumatology clinic for further evaluation. Following examination, laboratory, and radiologic testing, the rheumatologist establishes a diagnosis of rheumatoid arthritis and initiates a multidisciplinary team conference to plan the management of Mrs. James's rheumatoid arthritis.

### ASSESSMENT

Cathy Greenstein, RN, completes a nursing assessment of Mrs. James. She notes that Mrs. James is well groomed and answers questions readily but appears fatigued and ill. Mrs. James relates that her job has been extremely stressful because teacher layoffs have resulted in larger class sizes and fewer teaching assistants. Despite symptoms, she continues to teach full time, but says she feels unable to keep up with all her responsibilities due to her fatigue.

Mrs. James states that she is allergic to penicillin. Her past medical history reveals only the usual childhood diseases and three uncomplicated pregnancies, resulting in the births of her children, ages 14, 11, and 9. Physical assessment findings include. BP 124/78, P 82 regular, R 18, T 100.2°F (37.8°C) PO. Hands: swelling of the proximal interphalangeal (PIP) and metacarpophalangeal (MCP) joints of both hands; second and third PIP and second MCP joints on right hand are red, shiny, hot, spongy, and tender to palpation; able to extend fingers to 180 degrees but cannot make a complete fist with either hand, with flexion limited to less than 90 degrees; grip strength is weak bilaterally; wrist ROM is limited in all directions. Knees are swollen, and flexion is slightly limited; positive bulge sign in the right knee. Diagnostic findings are an ESR of 52 mm/hr, a hematocrit of 30%, and positive for rheumatoid factor. Few changes other than soft-tissue swelling are evident on hand and wrist X-rays.

### DIAGNOSIS

- *Chronic pain* related to joint inflammation
- *Impaired home maintenance* related to fatigue
- *Activity intolerance* related to the effects of inflammation
- *Deficient knowledge: Therapeutic regimen*

### EXPECTED OUTCOMES

- Verbalize effective pain management strategies.

- Use assistive devices to minimize joint stress with ADLs.
- Verbalize a plan to reduce responsibilities for home maintenance.
- Express a willingness to plan rest breaks during the day.
- Demonstrate understanding of the prescribed therapeutic regimen and its importance for both short- and long-term benefit.

### PLANNING AND IMPLEMENTATION

- Teach techniques for relieving pain and morning stiffness, including:
  - Scheduling NSAIDs at equal intervals throughout the day
  - Taking morning NSAID dose with milk and crackers approximately 30 minutes before rising
  - Performing ROM exercises in shower or bathtub
  - Applying local heat with paraffin dip or compress; using cold packs as needed
- Teach techniques to minimize joint stress while performing ADLs.
- Provide Arthritis Foundation literature and information.
- Discuss ways to delegate household tasks to other family members.
- Explore ways to incorporate 30-minute rest breaks into Mrs. James's work schedule.
- Provide information about the disease process and its manifestations, prescribed medications with desired and adverse effects, and the importance of balancing rest and activity.

### EVALUATION

The initial treatment regimen of aspirin, rest, exercise, and physical therapy succeeded in partially relieving the acute manifestations of rheumatoid arthritis in Mrs. James. Her "morning sickness" now lasts only about 45 minutes. However, complete remission has not been achieved. She has had difficulty scheduling rest periods at work and has had to struggle to delegate household tasks. "I don't look sick to the kids, and they seem to think housecleaning is a terrible imposition on their time. It's often easier to just do it myself than to fight about it. Besides, that way it gets done right." Mrs. James has faithfully followed the prescribed medication regimen and exercise routines, and she has kept her scheduled appointments and maintained contact with the treatment team.

### Critical Thinking in the Nursing Process

1. Mrs. James is 42 years old. Would your nursing interventions differ if she were 72 years old? If so, how.
2. Rheumatoid arthritis is a chronic illness. What are the physical, emotional, and economic implications of a chronic illness that results in chronic pain and deformity?
3. Develop a nursing care plan for Mrs. James using the nursing diagnosis, *Ineffective role performance*.

See Evaluating Your Response in Appendix C.

# THE CLIENT WITH ANKYLOSING SPONDYLITIS

**Ankylosing spondylitis** is a chronic inflammatory arthritis that primarily affects the axial skeleton, leading to pain and progressive stiffening and fusion of the spine. The incidence is greater in men than women and men have more severe disease. It is common in people of European ancestry and certain Native American tribes; it is rare in African Americans and people of Japanese descent. The onset of the disease is usually in the late teens and early 20s.

The cause of ankylosing spondylitis is unknown. As with the other spondylarthropathies, there is a strong genetic component. Approximately 90% of people with ankylosing spondylitis have the HLA-B27 antigen; about 8% of the general population have this antigen (Porth, 2002).

## PATHOPHYSIOLOGY AND MANIFESTATIONS

Early inflammatory changes often are first noted in the sacroiliac joints. As the cartilage erodes, joint margins ossify and are replaced by scar tissue. The joints of the spine are also affected, with inflammation of the cartilaginous joints, and gradual calcification and ossification that leads to ankylosis, or joint consolidation and immobility. Other organ systems may be affected as well, including the eyes, lungs, heart, and kidneys.

The onset of ankylosing spondylitis is usually gradual and insidious. Clients may have persistent or intermittent bouts of low back pain. The pain is worse at night, followed by morning stiffness that is relieved by activity. Pain may radiate to the buttocks, hips, or down the legs. As the disease progresses, back motion becomes limited, the lumbar curve is lost, and the thoracic curvature is accentuated (Figure 39–7 ■). In severe cases, the entire spine becomes fused, preventing any motion. Clients with ankylosing spondylitis may also experience some peripheral arthritis, primarily affecting the hip, shoulders, and knee joints. Systemic manifestations include anorexia, weight loss, fever, and fatigue. Many clients develop uveitis, inflammation of the iris and the middle, vascular layer of the eye.

For most clients with ankylosing spondylitis, the disease is intermittent with mild to moderate acute episodes. These clients have a good prognosis with little risk of severe disability.

## COLLABORATIVE CARE

Diagnostic testing shows an elevated ESR during periods of active disease and typically a positive HLA-B27 antigen. The diagnosis of ankylosing spondylitis is usually confirmed with X-ray examination of the sacroiliac joints and spine. The sacroiliac joint becomes blurred and gradually obliterated. As the disease progresses, vertebrae become squared, and disc spaces narrow.

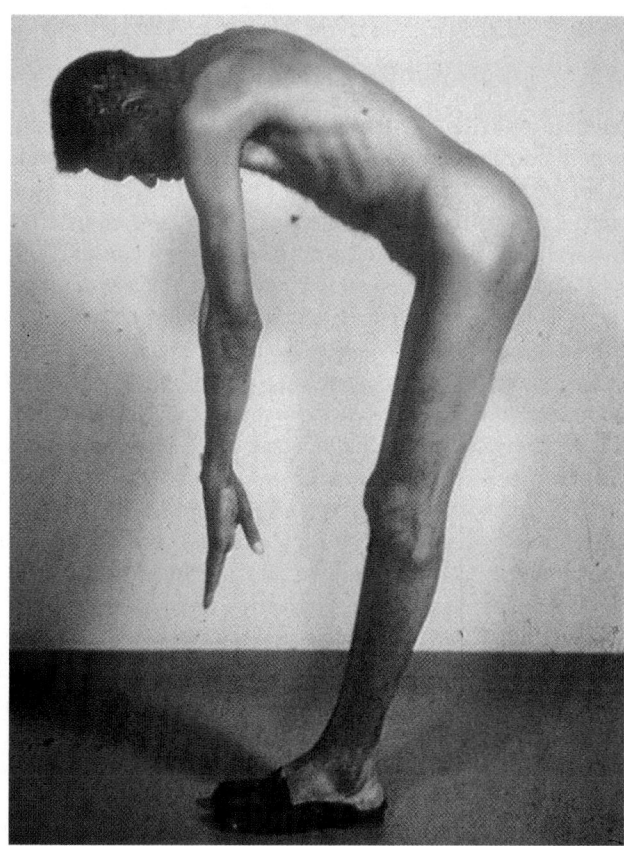

**Figure 39–7** ■ A client with ankylosing spondylitis. Note the flattened lumbar curve, exaggerated thoracic curvature, and flexion deformity of the neck.

*Source: American College of Rheumatology.*

As with other forms of arthritis, the management of ankylosing spondylitis is multidimensional. Physical therapy and daily exercises are important to maintain posture and joint range of motion. NSAIDs relieve pain and stiffness and allow the client to perform necessary exercises. Indomethacin (Indocin) is the NSAID most commonly used to treat ankylosing spondylitis. It may, however, have many adverse effects, including headache, nausea and vomiting, depression, and psychosis. Other drugs that may be prescribed include sulfasalazine (Azulfidine) and topical or intra-articular corticosteroids. Severe hip joint arthritis may necessitate total hip arthroplasty.

## NURSING CARE

The primary nursing role in ankylosing spondylitis is one of providing supportive care and education. To promote mobility, teach the client to take NSAIDs at regular intervals throughout the day with food, milk, or antacid. Encourage the client to maintain a fluid intake of 2500 mL or more per day. Suggest that the client perform exercises in the shower because warm, moist heat prompts mobility. Stress the importance of following the prescribed physical therapy and exercise program to maintain mobility.

## THE CLIENT WITH REACTIVE ARTHRITIS

**Reactive arthritis (Reiter's syndrome)** is an acute, nonpurulent inflammatory arthritis that complicates a bacterial infection of the genitourinary or gastrointestinal tracts. This type of arthritis most often affects young men who have an inherited HLA-B27 antigen. Reactive arthritis is often found in clients with HIV infection, although the reason for the association is not clear. The defining characteristics are arthropathy (usually of the lower extremity) and one of more of urethritis/cervicitis, dysentery, inflammatory eye disease, and disorders of the skin and mucous membranes (Maher, et al., 2002). Reactive arthritis is typically self-limited, although it can be recurrent or progressive.

Nonbacterial urethritis is often the initial manifestation of Reiter's syndrome. In women, urethritis and cervicitis may be asymptomatic. Conjunctivitis and inflammatory arthritis follow. The arthritis is usually asymmetric, affecting large weight-bearing joints such as the knees and ankles, the sacroiliac joints, or the spine. Mouth ulcers, inflammation of the glans penis, and skin lesions may occur. The heart and aorta may also be affected.

The diagnosis of reactive arthritis is generally based on the client's history and presenting symptoms. No test is specific for the disorder. Urethral or cervical cultures are obtained to rule out gonococcal infection. When Chlamydia is suspected, the client and sexual partner are treated with tetracycline or erythromycin. Reactive arthritis is treated symptomatically, usually with NSAIDs.

## NURSING CARE

Clients with reactive arthritis usually are seen in primary care settings such as a clinic or physician's office, making the nursing role primarily one of education. Teach the client about the association of the arthritis with the precipitating infection (if identified). Stress the importance of treating the infection effectively if it is still present. Use this opportunity to provide information about sexually transmitted diseases and protective measures to prevent their transmission. Discuss the usual self-limited nature of reactive arthritis, the appropriate use of prescribed NSAID preparations, and symptomatic relief measures such as application of heat and rest.

## THE CLIENT WITH SYSTEMIC LUPUS ERYTHEMATOSUS

**Systemic lupus erythematosus (SLE)** is a chronic inflammatory immune complex connective-tissue disease. It affects almost all body systems, including the musculoskeletal system. The manifestations of SLE are widely variable, thought to result from cell and tissue damage caused by deposition of antigen-antibody complexes in connective tissues. SLE affects multiple body systems, and it can range from a mild, episodic disorder to a rapidly fatal disease process.

Approximately 1 person in 2000 is affected by SLE, with women predominating by a ratio of 9:1 over men. The disease usually affects women of childbearing age (when the incidence is 30 times greater than in men) but it can occur at any age. It is more common in African Americans, Hispanics, and Asians than it is in Caucasians (Porth, 2002). The incidence is higher in some families.

Although the exact etiology of SLE is unknown, genetic, environmental, and hormonal factors play a role in its development. Twin studies and a familial pattern of the disease point to a genetic component, as does an increased incidence of other connective-tissue diseases in relatives of people with SLE. Certain human leukocyte antigen (HLA) genes are seen more frequently in people with SLE. Environmental factors such as viruses, bacterial antigens, chemicals, drugs, or ultraviolet light may play a role in activation of the pathologic mechanisms of the disease. In addition, it is felt that sex hormones may influence the development of SLE. Women with SLE have reduced levels of several active androgens that are known to inhibit antibody responses. Estrogens have been shown to enhance antibody responses and have an adverse effect in clients with SLE.

The course of SLE is mild and chronic in most clients, with periods of remission and exacerbation. The number and severity of exacerbations tend to decrease with time. In some clients, however, SLE is a virulent disease with significant organ system involvement.

Clients with active disease have an increased risk for infections, which are often opportunistic and severe. Infections such as pneumonia and septicemia are the leading cause of death in clients with SLE, followed by the effects of renal or central nervous system involvement.

### PATHOPHYSIOLOGY

The pathophysiology of SLE involves the production of a large variety of autoantibodies against normal body components such as nucleic acids, erythrocytes, coagulation proteins, lymphocytes, and platelets. Autoantibody production results from hyperreactivity of B cells (humoral response) because of disordered T-cell function (cellular immune response). The most characteristic autoantibodies in SLE are produced in response to nucleic acids, including DNA, histones, ribonucleoproteins, and other components of the cell nucleus.

SLE autoantibodies react with their corresponding antigen to form immune complexes, which are then deposited in the connective tissue of blood vessels, lymphatic vessels, and other tissues. The deposits trigger an inflammatory response leading to local tissue damage. The kidneys are a frequent site of complex deposition and damage; other tissues affected include the musculoskeletal system, brain, heart, spleen, lung, GI tract, skin, and peritoneum. The autoantibodies produced and their target tissue determine the manifestations of SLE.

A number of drugs can cause a syndrome that mimics lupus in clients with no other risk factors for the disease. Procainamide (Procan-SR, Pronestyl, others) and hydralazine (Apresoline, Hydralyn) are the most common drugs implicated, along with isoniazid (INH).

Renal and CNS manifestations of SLE rarely occur with drug-induced lupus, but arthritic and other systemic symptoms are common. Manifestations of drug-induced lupus usually resolve when the medication is discontinued.

## MANIFESTATIONS AND COMPLICATIONS

Typical early manifestations of SLE mimic those of rheumatoid arthritis, including systemic manifestations of fever, anorexia, malaise, and weight loss, and musculoskeletal manifestations of multiple arthralgias and symmetric polyarthritis. Joint symptoms affect more than 90% of clients with SLE. Although synovitis may be present, the arthritis associated with SLE is rarely deforming.

Most people affected by SLE have skin manifestations at some point during their disease. In fact, SLE was originally described as a skin disorder and named for the characteristic red butterfly rash across the cheeks and bridge of the nose (Figure 39–8 ■). Many clients with SLE are photosensitive; a diffuse maculopapular rash on skin exposed to the sun is also common. Other cutaneous manifestations include discoid lesions (raised, scaly, circular lesions with an erythematous rim), hives, erythematous fingertip lesions, and splinter hemorrhages. Alopecia is common in clients with SLE, although the hair usually grows back. Painless mucous membrane ulcerations may occur on the lips or in the mouth or nose.

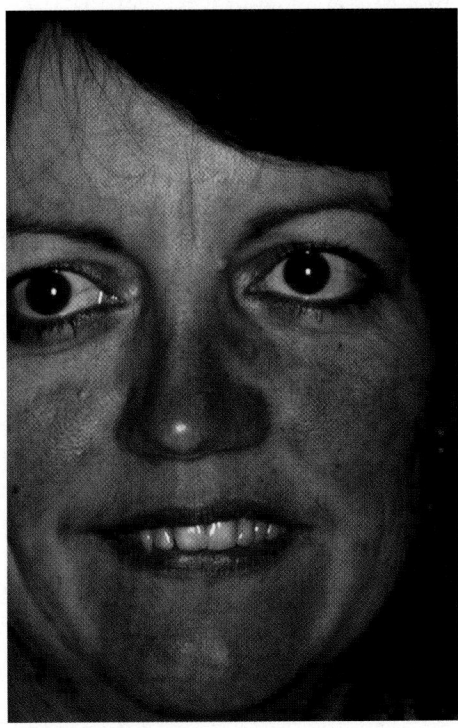

**Figure 39–8 ■** The butterfly rash of systemic lupus erythematosus.

*Source: Wellcome Trust/Custom Medical Stock Photo.*

Approximately 50% of people with SLE experience renal manifestations of the disease, including proteinuria, cellular casts, and nephrotic syndrome. Up to 10% develop renal failure as a result of the disease.

Hematologic abnormalities such as anemia, leukopenia, and thrombocytopenia are common with SLE. Cardiovascular disorders such as pericarditis, vasculitis, and Raynaud's phenomenon often occur. Less frequently, myocarditis, endocarditis, and venous or arterial thrombosis may develop. Pleurisy, pleural effusions, and lupus pneumonitis are common pulmonary manifestations of SLE.

Many clients with SLE develop transient nervous system involvement, often within the first year of the disease. Organic brain syndrome manifestations include decline in intellect, memory loss, and disorientation. Other possible neurologic manifestations include psychosis, seizures, depression, and stroke. Ocular manifestations of SLE include conjunctivitis, photophobia, and transient blindness due to retinal vasculitis.

Gastrointestinal symptoms of SLE, such as anorexia, nausea, abdominal pain, and diarrhea, may affect up to 45% of clients with the disease. The liver may be enlarged, and liver function tests may yield abnormal results.

Clients with SLE who become pregnant may experience abrupt onset of hypertension, edema, and proteinuria (a syndrome similar to pregnancy-induced hypertension). Midtrimester fetal death may result.

The *Multisystem Effects of SLE* are illustrated on page 1262.

## COLLABORATIVE CARE

Because of the diversity of organ system involvement and manifestations of SLE, diagnosis can be difficult. No one specific test is available to confirm the presence of this disease in all people suspected of having it. Instead, the diagnosis is based on the client's history and physical assessment, as well as laboratory studies.

As with rheumatoid arthritis, effective management of SLE requires teamwork, with active participation by both the client and the physician. Communication, trust, and emotional support are especially important. Although there is no cure for SLE, the 10-year survival rate is greater than 70% among clients with this disease, which was once considered fatal in most cases.

### Diagnostic Tests

The multiple autoantibodies produced in SLE cause a number of abnormalities in laboratory studies.

- *Anti-DNA antibody testing* is a more specific indicator of SLE, because these antibodies are rarely found in any other disorder.
- *Eosinophil sedimentation rate (ESR)* is typically elevated, occasionally to >100 mm/hr.
- *Serum complement levels* are usually decreased as complement is consumed or "used up" by the development of antigen-antibody complexes.

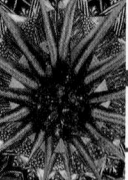

# Multisystem Effects of Systemic Lupus Erythematosus

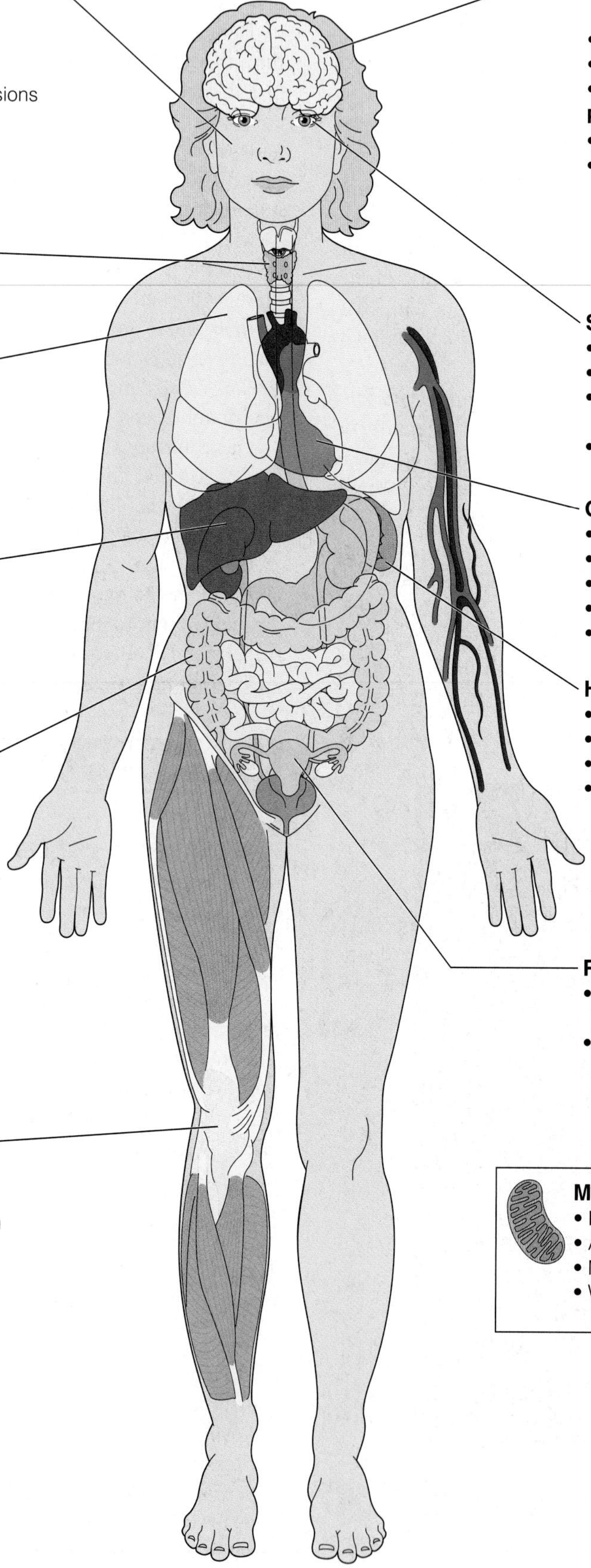

**Integumentary**
- Butterfly rash on face
- Photosensitivity
- Maculopapular rash on exposed body surfaces
- Discoid lesions
- Erythematous fingertip lesions
- Splinter hemorrhages
- Alopecia
- Ulcers (lip, mouth, nose)

**Endocrine**
- Thyroid abnormalities
- Hyperparathyroidism
- Glucose intolerance

**Respiratory**
- Pleurisy
- Pleural effusion
- Pneumonitis
- Interstitial fibrosis

**Urinary**
- Proteinuria
- Cellular casts

**Potential Complications**
- Nephrotic syndrome
- Renal failure

**Gastrointestinal**
- Anorexia
- Nausea
- Abdominal pain
- Diarrhea
- Hepatomegaly

**Musculoskeletal**
- Arthralgias
- Symmetric polyarthritis
- Joint swelling and effusion
- Morning stiffness

**Neurologic**
- Neuropathies (peripheral and central)
- Seizures
- Depression
- Psychosis

**Potential Complications**
- CVA
- Organic brain syndrome
  - Intellectual impairment
  - Memory loss
  - Personality changes
  - Disorientation

**Sensory**
- Conjunctivitis
- Photophobia
- Retinal vasculitis with transient blindness
- Cotton-wool spots on retina

**Cardiovascular**
- Pericarditis
- Myocarditis
- Endocarditis
- Vasculitis
- Venous or arterial thrombosis

**Hematologic**
- Anemia
- Leukopenia
- Thrombocytopenia
- Splenomegaly

**Reproductive**
- Pregnancy-induced hypertension, edema, and proteinuria
- Fetal loss

**Metabolic Processes**
- Low-grade fever
- Anorexia
- Malaise
- Weight loss

- *CBC abnormalities* include moderate to severe anemia, leukopenia and lymphocytopenia, and possible thrombocytopenia.
- *Urinalysis* shows mild proteinuria, hematuria, and blood cell casts during exacerbations of the disease when the kidneys are involved. *Renal function tests* including a serum creatinine and blood urea nitrogen (BUN) may also be ordered to evaluate the extent of renal disease.
- *Kidney biopsy* may be performed to assess the severity of renal lesions and guide therapy.

## Medications

The client with mild or remittent lupus erythematosus may need little or no therapy other than supportive care. Arthralgias, arthritis, fever, and fatigue can often be managed with aspirin or other NSAIDs. Aspirin is particularly beneficial for clients with SLE because its antiplatelet effects help prevent thrombosis. It may, however, cause liver toxicity and hepatitis.

Skin and arthritic manifestations of SLE may be treated with antimalarial drugs such as hydroxychloroquine (Plaquenil). Hydroxychloroquine has also been shown to be effective in reducing the frequency of acute episodes of SLE in people with mild or inactive disease. Retinal toxicity and possibly irreversible blindness are the primary concerns with this drug. For this reason, the client taking hydroxychloroquine undergoes ophthalmologic exam every 6 months.

Clients with severe and life-threatening manifestations of SLE (such as nephritis, hemolytic anemia, myocarditis, pericarditis, or CNS lupus) require corticosteroid therapy in high doses. Such clients may require 40 to 60 mg of prednisone per day initially. The dosage is tapered as rapidly as the client's disease allows, although lowering the dosage may precipitate an acute episode. Some clients with SLE require long-term corticosteroid therapy to manage symptoms and prevent major organ damage. These clients are at increased risk for corticosteroid side effects, such as cushingoid effects, weight gain, hypertension, infection, accelerated osteoporosis, and hypokalemia.

Immunosuppressive agents such as cyclophosphamide or azathioprine may be used, alone or in combination with corticosteroids, to treat clients with active SLE or lupus nephritis (see the Medication Administration box below). When these agents are used in combination, lower, less toxic doses of each drug can be used. The client receiving immunosuppressive agents is at increased risk for infection, malignancy, bone marrow depression, and toxic effects specific to the drug prescribed.

## Other Treatments

Because of the photosensitivity associated with SLE, the client should be cautioned to avoid sun exposure. Clients should use sunscreens with a sun protection factor (SPF) rating of 15 or higher when out of doors. Topical corticosteroids may be used to treat skin lesions. Some physicians recommend avoiding the use of oral contraceptives, because estrogen can trigger an acute episode.

Clients with lupus nephritis who progress to develop end-stage renal disease are treated with dialysis (hemodialysis or peritoneal dialysis) and kidney transplantation. These treatment strategies are discussed in Chapter 27. ∞

---

# Medication Administration

## Immunosuppressive Agents

### CYTOTOXIC AGENTS

Azathioprine (Imuran)
Cyclophosphamide (Cytoxan)
Cyclosporine (Sandimmune)

Certain cytotoxic or antineoplastic drugs are effective as immunosuppressive agents. They act by decreasing the proliferation of cells within the immune system and are widely used to prevent rejection following a tissue or organ transplant. They are usually administered concurrently with corticosteroid therapy, allowing lower doses of both preparations, and resulting in fewer side effects.

### Nursing Responsibilities

- Monitor blood count, with particular attention to the white blood cell (WBC) and platelet counts. Notify the physician if WBCs fall below 4000 or platelets below 75,000.
- Monitor renal and liver function studies including creatinine, BUN, creatinine clearance, and liver enzyme levels. Report any abnormal levels to the physician.
- Oral preparations should be administered with food to minimize gastrointestinal effects. Antacids may be ordered.
- Increase fluids to maintain good hydration and urinary output.
- Monitor intake and output.

- Monitor for signs of abnormal bleeding: bleeding gums, bruising, petechiae, joint pain, hematuria, and black or tarry stools.
- Use meticulous handwashing and other appropriate measures to protect the client from infection. Assess for signs of infection.
- Pulmonary fibrosis is a potential adverse effect of cyclophosphamide. Therefore, monitor the results of pulmonary function studies and be alert to clinical signs of dyspnea or cough.

### Client and Family Teaching

- Avoid large crowds and situations where you might be exposed to infections.
- Report signs of infection such as chills, fever, sore throat, fatigue, or malaise to the physician.
- Use contraceptive measures to prevent pregnancy while you are taking these drugs because they cause birth defects.
- Avoid the use of aspirin or ibuprofen while taking these drugs. Report any signs of bleeding to the physician.
- You may stop menstruating while you are taking cyclophosphamide. The menses will resume after the drug is discontinued.
- If you are taking cyclophosphamide, be sure to report difficulty breathing or cough to the physician.

# NURSING CARE

Nursing care for the client with mild SLE may be limited to teaching. The client with severe disease, however, has many diverse nursing needs, which vary according to the organ systems involved. Because of the close link between rheumatoid arthritis and SLE, many of the nursing diagnoses and interventions identified for the client with arthritis may be appropriate for the client with lupus. The client with lupus nephritis or end-stage renal disease has the nursing care needs outlined in the sections of Chapter 27 ⊂⊃ related to glomerulonephritis and chronic renal failure. This section focuses on the unique needs of the client related to the dermatologic manifestations of lupus, an increased risk for infection, and health maintenance problems.

## Nursing Diagnoses and Interventions

### Impaired Skin Integrity

Skin lesions are a common manifestation of SLE. A rash or discoid lesion interrupts the integrity of the skin and the first line of protection against infection, increasing the client's already high risk of infection. These lesions, which usually appear on exposed parts of the skin, can also be disfiguring and cause the client emotional distress.

- Assess knowledge of SLE and its possible effects on the skin. *Assessment allows the nurse to base teaching and information on the client's existing knowledge, improving learning and retention.*
- Discuss the relationship between sun exposure and disease activity, both dermatologic and systemic. *It is important for the client to understand that sun exposure may not only cause dermatologic manifestations but also trigger an acute episode.*
- Help the client identify strategies to limit sun exposure:
  - Avoid being out of doors during hours of greatest sun intensity (10:00 A.M. to 3:00 P.M.).
  - Use sunscreen with an SPF of 15 or higher when sun exposure cannot be avoided.
  - Reapply sunscreen after swimming, exercising, or bathing.
  - Wear loose clothing with long sleeves and wide-brimmed hats when out of doors.

  *These strategies can help the client maintain a normal lifestyle while helping to prevent acute episodes.*
- Keep skin clean and dry; apply therapeutic creams or ointments to lesions as prescribed. *These measures promote healing and reduce the risk of infection.*

### Ineffective Protection

Ineffective protection can be a problem for the client with SLE, who is at increased risk for infection and multiple organ system problems because of the disease. In addition, treatment with corticosteroids or immunosuppressive agents further impairs immune responses and the ability to fight infection. The following interventions are for the client who is hospitalized.

- Wash hands before and after providing direct care. *Handwashing removes transient organisms from the skin, reducing the risk of transmission to the client.*

**PRACTICE ALERT** *Hands must be washed before and after providing direct care, even if gloves are worn. A decrease in this type of medical asepsis is contributing to the increasing number of hospital-acquired infections that are resistant to antibiotics.* ■

- Use strict aseptic technique in caring for intravenous lines and indwelling urinary catheters or performing any wound care. *Aseptic technique offers protection against external and resident host microorganisms.*
- Assess frequently for signs and symptoms of infection. Monitor temperature and vital signs every 4 hours. Assess for signs of cellulitis, including tenderness, redness, swelling, and warmth. Report signs of infection to the physician promptly. *Therapy can suppress usual responses, such as elevated temperature and inflammation. The fever of infection may be mistaken for the fever commonly associated with lupus. The client receiving immunosuppressive therapy for the disease has an even higher risk for infection.*

**PRACTICE ALERT** *The client with lupus is susceptible to infection, and the usual signs and symptoms may not be evident.* ■

- Monitor laboratory values, including CBC and tests of organ function; report changes to the physician. *An elevation in the WBC count with a shift to the left (increased numbers of immature leukocytes in the blood) may be an early indication of infection. Changes in liver function studies, renal function studies, myocardial enzymes, or other laboratory values may indicate organ system involvement.*
- Initiate reverse or protective isolation procedures as indicated by the client's immune status. *These procedures provide further protection from infection for the severely immunocompromised client.*
- Instruct family members and visitors to avoid contact with the client when they are ill. *A "minor" upper respiratory infection can be a significant illness for the client with SLE.*
- Help ensure an adequate nutrient intake, offering supplementary feedings as indicated or maintaining parenteral nutrition if necessary. *Adequate nutrition is important for healing and immune system function.*
- Teach the client the importance of good handwashing after using the bathroom and before eating. *Handwashing reduces the risk of infection with endogenous organisms.*
- Provide good mouth care. *Good oral hygiene reduces the population of microorganisms in the mouth and helps to keep oral mucous membranes intact.*
- Monitor for potential adverse effects of medications including thrombocytopenia and possible bleeding, fluid retention with edema and possible hypertension, loss of bone density, osteoporosis, and possible pathologic fractures, renal or hepatic toxicity, and cardiac effects, particularly in the client with fluid retention and hypervolemia. *Medications used to treat SLE have many potential adverse effects that can impair normal protective and homeostatic mechanisms.*

## Impaired Health Maintenance

As with other chronic diseases, much of the responsibility for maintaining optimal health rests with the client. Disease manifestations such as fatigue, arthralgias, arthritis, and increased risk for infection can interfere with the client's ability to maintain health. Psychosocial issues can also be a significant factor in health maintenance for the client with lupus. These issues may include denial of the significance of the disease, poor coping, lack of financial and other resources, and an inadequate support system.

- Assess the client's ability to maintain optimal health, identifying physical and psychosocial factors that may affect health maintenance. *Before intervening to improve the client's health maintenance, the nurse must identify and understand factors affecting it.*
- Provide care and teaching in a nonjudgmental manner. *To intervene effectively, the nurse must accept the client and family as they are.*
- Encourage the client and family members to discuss the effect of the disease on their lives. *Open discussion helps the client and the nurse identify barriers to health maintenance and begin exploring alternative strategies.*
- Initiate a multidisciplinary care conference with the client and family. *In this care conference, a number of perspectives can be expressed, improving the planning of strategies for health maintenance activities.*
- Refer the client and family to counseling as needed. *Counseling may help the client and family develop the necessary coping skills to accept and deal with the disease.*
- Refer the client and family to community and social service agencies, and local support groups. *These groups and agencies are valuable resources for the client and family.*

## Home Care

Teaching is a critical factor in preparing clients with SLE to care for themselves at home. Address the following topics.

- The disease and its potential effects. Promote an optimistic outlook, stressing that the majority of clients do not require long-term corticosteroid therapy and that the disease may improve over time.
- The importance of skin care. Teach the client to avoid irritating soaps, shampoos, or chemicals (e.g., hair dyes and permanent wave solution) to prevent excessive drying of the skin. Encourage the client to use hypoallergenic products. Discuss the need to limit sun exposure, particularly between 10:00 A.M. and 3:00 P.M. Encourage the client to use sunscreen with an SPF of at least 15 and to wear long sleeves and wide-brimmed hats. For clients with hair loss, discuss the use of wigs, turbans, or other head coverings. Provide encouragement by reminding the client that the hair will grow back during periods of remission.
- The importance of avoiding exposure to infection. Encourage the client to avoid crowds and infectious individuals. Teach the client that getting adequate rest and nutrition and avoiding stress will increase resistance to infection.

- The need to follow the prescribed treatment plan, including rest and exercise, medications, and follow-up appointments. Discuss manifestations of an acute episode, including fever, chills, rash, increased fatigue and malaise, arthralgias, arthritis, urinary manifestations such as oliguria or dysuria, chest pain, cough, or neurologic symptoms. Stress the importance of contacting the physician promptly if any of these symptoms occur.
- The significance of wearing a MedicAlert tag identifying their condition and therapy such as corticosteroids or immunosuppressives.
- Family planning with the client and spouse. The use of oral contraceptives may be contraindicated for the client; if appropriate, provide information about alternative means of birth control. Pregnancy is not contraindicated for most women with lupus. However, the pregnant client requires close monitoring because acute episodes sometimes accompany pregnancy.
- Helpful resources:
  - National Institute of Arthritis and Musculoskeletal and Skin Diseases
  - Lupus Foundation of America

## THE CLIENT WITH POLYMYOSITIS

**Polymyositis** is a systemic connective-tissue disorder characterized by inflammation of connective tissue and muscle fibers leading to muscle weakness and atrophy. When muscle fiber inflammation is accompanied by skin lesions, the disease is known as dermatomyositis. Polymyositis is an autoimmune disorder of unknown cause that affects more women than men by a ratio of 2:1. The onset of the disease typically occurs between the ages of 40 and 60 years, although a childhood-onset form is also seen.

The immune mechanism causing the inflammatory response in polymyositis is not clear, but autoantibodies can be identified in the majority of people with the disease. The activation of complement is thought to contribute to the inflammatory process. Inflammation leads to muscle fiber necrosis and degeneration.

Initial manifestations of polymyositis include muscle pain, tenderness, and weakness; rash; arthralgias; fatigue; fever; and weight loss. Skeletal muscle weakness is the predominant manifestation. Its onset may be either insidious or abrupt. Muscle weakness tends to progress over weeks to months. Muscles of the shoulder and pelvic girdles are particularly affected, making it difficult for the client to get out of chairs, climb stairs, and reach overhead. Weakness of neck flexor muscles may make it difficult to raise the head from a pillow. Affected muscles may also be tender and painful. A characteristic dusky red rash may be present on the face and upper trunk. Other manifestations include Raynaud's phenomenon, dysphagia, dyspnea, and cough (due to interstitial pneumonitis). The risk of malignancy is increased, particularly in clients with dermatomyositis.

## COLLABORATIVE CARE

There is no specific test to diagnose polymyositis. Autoantibodies may be identified in blood serum. Serum levels of muscle enzymes are elevated, particularly creatine kinase (CK) and aldolase levels. Biopsy of involved muscle shows patchy muscle fiber necrosis and the presence of inflammatory cells.

A combination of rest and corticosteroid therapy is prescribed for the client with polymyositis. Long-term corticosteroid therapy may be necessary to manage the disease. Immunosuppressive agents such as methotrexate, cyclophosphamide, and azathioprine may be used for clients who do not respond well to treatment with corticosteroids.

## NURSING CARE

The nursing role in caring for the client with polymyositis is supportive. Measures to promote comfort are important. Muscle weakness may interfere with the client's ability to provide self-care and manage health and home. The client may have difficulty with speech because of pharyngeal muscle weakness. Provide alternate means of communication as needed, and use patience in listening. Observe closely while the client eats, because aspiration is a potential problem. Modify the client's diet as needed to maintain nutrition and safety.

Education of the client and family is an important component of care. Emphasize the need to balance periods of rest and activity. Discuss skin care to prevent dryness and infection. Teach the client about prescribed medications and their short- and long-term side effects. Provide information about safety measures while eating. Encourage family members to become trained in performance of the Heimlich maneuver and CPR. Discuss signs of respiratory infection and other possible complications of polymyositis, including renal failure and malignancy.

## THE CLIENT WITH LYME DISEASE

**Lyme disease** is an inflammatory disorder caused by the spirochete *Borrelia burgdorferi,* which is transmitted primarily by ticks. It is the most commonly reported tick-borne illness in the United States. Geographically, Lyme disease is more prevalent in the mid-Atlantic, northeastern, and North Central regions of the United States (Tierney et al., 2001). It has also been reported throughout Europe, Asia, and Australia. Ticks that act as vectors for Lyme disease, primarily *Ixodes dammini, Ixodes pacificus,* and *Ixodes scapularis* in the United States, are usually carried by mice or deer, although other animals may be infected. The most frequent time of onset is the summer months.

## PATHOPHYSIOLOGY AND MANIFESTATIONS

Manifestations often are seen in the skin, musculoskeletal system, and central nervous system. The typical progression of Lyme disease is initially flulike manifestations and a skin rash; followed weeks or months later by Bell's palsy or meningitis, and months to years later, arthritis. This progression is highly individualized.

*Borrelia burgdorferi* enters the skin at the site of the tick bite. After an incubation period of up to 30 days, it migrates outward in the skin, forming a characteristic lesion called erythema migrans. It may also spread via lymph or blood to other skin sites, nodes, or organs. The inflammatory joint changes associated with Lyme disease closely resemble those of rheumatoid arthritis (vascular congestion, tissue infiltration by inflammatory cells, possible pannus formation, and erosion of cartilage and bone).

Erythema migrans is the initial manifestation of Lyme disease. This flat or slightly raised red lesion at the site of the tick bite expands over several days (up to a diameter of 50 cm), with the central area clearing as it expands. Systemic symptoms such as fatigue, malaise, fever, chills, and myalgias often accompany the initial lesion. As the disease spreads, secondary skin lesions develop, as do migratory musculoskeletal symptoms, including arthralgias, myalgias, and tendinitis. Persistent fatigue is common during this stage of the disease. Headache and stiff neck are characteristic neurologic manifestations.

With untreated infection, late manifestations can develop months to years after the initial infection. Chronic recurrent arthritis, primarily affecting large joints (especially the knee), is common. Permanent disability may result. Other effects that may be seen weeks to months after the initial infection include meningitis, encephalitis, and neuropathies, as well as cardiac manifestations including myocarditis and heart block.

## COLLABORATIVE CARE

Both manifestations and laboratory studies are used to establish the diagnosis of Lyme disease. Culture of the organism from tissues and body fluids is difficult and slow. Antibodies to *B. burgdorferi* can be detected by either ELISA (enzyme-linked immunosorbent assay) or Western blot methods within 2 to 4 weeks of the initial skin lesion.

The early diagnosis and proper antibiotic treatment of Lyme disease are important to preventing the complications of infection. A number of antibiotics may be used to treat Lyme disease, including doxycycline (Doxy-Caps, Vibramycin), tetracycline, amoxicillin (Amoxil), cefuroxime axetil (Ceftin), or erythromycin. Therapy may be continued for up to 1 month to ensure eradication of the organism from affected tissues. The nursing implications for various classes of antibiotics are summarized in Chapter 8. ∞

In addition to antibiotic treatment, aspirin or another NSAID may be prescribed for relief of arthritic symptoms. The affected joint may be splinted to rest the joint. When the knee is involved, weight bearing may be restricted and the use of crutches indicated.

## NURSING CARE

Nursing care focuses on prevention of the disease. Many people do not protect themselves from tick bites. This protection is becoming increasingly important with a higher incidence of Lyme disease, due in part to an overpopulation of deer and the encroachment of the suburbs on once rural areas. Simple measures that can help prevent tick bites are as follows:

- Avoid tick-infested areas, especially in spring and summer, such as woods and rural areas with brush and tall weeds.

- Cover exposed skin with long-sleeved shirts and tuck pants into socks. Wearing high rubber boots may provide additional protection.
- Use insect repellents that contain DEET on clothing and exposed skin and apply permethrin to clothing prior to exposure.
- Inspect skin, especially in areas of tight-fitting clothing, after exposure. Transmission of the bacteria from the tick is unlikely to occur until 36 hours of tick attachment.
- Remove attached ticks with fine-tipped tweezers. Grasp the tick firmly as close to the skin as possible and pull the tick's body away from the skin. If the tick's head remains in the skin, it will not cause Lyme disease (the bacteria are in the tick's midgut). Clean the area with an antiseptic.

# INFECTIOUS DISORDERS

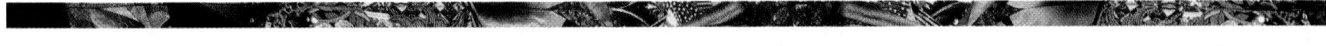

Infectious disorders are caused by a pathogen. These infections of bone and joints are often difficult to treat. Chronic infections may result in pain, deformity, and disability.

## THE CLIENT WITH OSTEOMYELITIS

**Osteomyelitis** is an infection of the bone. Osteomyelitis may occur as an acute, subacute, or chronic process. It occurs as a consequence of bacteremia (hematogenous osteomyelitis), invasion from a contiguous focus of infection, or skin breakdown in the presence of vascular insufficiency (Tierney et al., 2001).

Osteomyelitis can occur at any age, but adults over age 50 are more commonly affected. The older adult is at risk for osteomyelitis for several reasons. Immune function tends to decline with aging; the older adult also is more likely to have a chronic disease process that affects immune function. Circulatory status in the elderly often is compromised by atherosclerotic processes, impairing blood flow to the bone. Older adults have a higher risk of pressure ulcers because of circulatory, skin, sensation, and mobility changes associated with aging. Pressure ulcers that cannot be staged and treated because of eschar formation pose a particular risk. In addition, the older adult may not demonstrate typical signs of infection and inflammation, thus allowing an infectious process to become well established before it is detected.

### PATHOPHYSIOLOGY AND MANIFESTATIONS

The cause of osteomyelitis is usually bacterial; however, fungi, parasites, and viruses can also cause bone infection. *Staphylococcus aureus* is the most common infecting organism. Other organisms include *Escherichia coli, Pseudomonas, Klebsiella, Salmonella,* and *Proteus.*

Direct contamination of bone from an open wound, such as an open fracture or a gunshot or puncture wound, is the most common cause of osteomyelitis; osteomyelitis also may occur

as a complication of surgery. The third mode of entry for microorganisms that invade bone tissue is the extension from adjacent soft-tissue infection. Clients with venous stasis or arterial ulcers of the lower extremities or long-term complications of diabetes mellitus are good candidates for this type of bacterial invasion.

After entry, bacteria lodge and multiply in the bone, resulting in the inflammatory and immune system response. Phagocytes attempt to contain the infection, releasing enzymes in the process that destroy bone tissue. Pus forms, followed by edema and vascular congestion. The Haversian canals in the medullary (marrow) cavity of the bone allow the infection to travel to other segments of the bone. If the infection reaches the outer margin of the bone (Figure 39–9 ■), it raises the periosteum of the bone, spreading along the surface. Lifting of the periosteum from the cortex disrupts the blood vessels that enter the bone. Pressure increases, further compromising the vascular supply and leading to ischemia and eventual necrosis of the bone. Blood and antibiotics cannot reach the bone tissue once the pressure compromises the vascular and arteriolar systems. In addition, bacteria adhere to damaged bone, coating the underlying bone with a protective film that further impedes host defenses.

### Hematogenous Osteomyelitis

Hematogenous infections are caused by pathogens that are carried in the blood from sites of infection elsewhere in the body. Hematogenous osteomyelitis primarily affects older adults, people with sickle cell anemia, and intravenous drug users. The spine is the usual site of infection in adults. Pathogens enter the well-perfused vertebral bodies of adults via the spinal arteries. From there, the infection spreads into the disk space. The lumbar spine is involved more frequently than the thoracic or cervical spine. Urinary tract infections, soft-tissue infection, endocarditis, and infected intravenous sites are sources of pathogens.

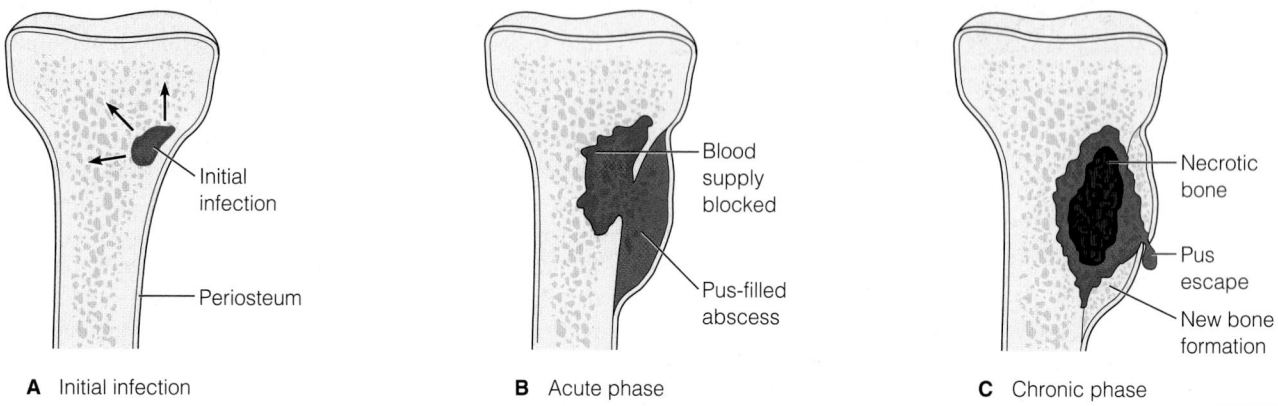

**Figure 39–9** ■ Osteomyelitis. *A*, Site of initial infection. Bacteria enter and multiply in the bone, and the inflammatory response is initiated. *B*, Acute phase, in which infection spreads to other parts of the bone. Pus forms, edema occurs, and the vascular supply is compromised. If the infection reaches the outer margin of the bone, the periosteum is lifted, and ischemia and necrosis eventually occur. *C*, Chronic phase. Necrotic bone separates, a new layer of bone forms around the necrotic bone, and a sinus develops to allow the wound to drain.

Clients with acute hematogenous osteomyelitis experience an acute onset of pain, tenderness, and fever. Soft-tissue swelling over the affected bone may be noted. The course of vertebral osteomyelitis in intravenous drug users often is subacute, with vague, dull pain in the affected region and a normal or low-grade fever. The pain intensifies over 2 to 3 months, and is accompanied by tenderness, muscle spasm, and limited range of motion.

## Osteomyelitis from a Contiguous Infection

Infections caused by an extension of infection from adjacent soft tissues fall into this category of osteomyelitis. The infection is a result of or complication of direct penetrating wounds, joint replacements, decubitus ulcers, and neurosurgery. This is the most common cause of osteomyelitis in adults.

## Manifestations of Osteomyelitis

**CARDIOVASCULAR EFFECTS**
- Tachycardia

**GASTROINTESTINAL EFFECTS**
- Nausea and vomiting
- Anorexia

**MUSCULOSKELETAL EFFECTS**
- Limp in involved extremity
- Localized tenderness, especially in epiphyseal area

**INTEGUMENTARY EFFECTS**
- Drainage and ulceration at involved site
- Swelling, erythema, and warmth at involved site
- Lymph node involvement, especially in the involved extremity

**OTHER EFFECTS**
- High temperature with chills
- Abrupt onset of pain
- Malaise

The diagnosis of osteomyelitis often is not made until the infection has become chronic because the signs of acute infection may be masked by local tissue inflammation. Failure to heal a surgical wound or fracture or a developing sinus tract may be initial indicators of infection.

## Osteomyelitis Associated with Vascular Insufficiency

People with diabetes and peripheral vascular disease are at risk for developing osteomyelitis involving the feet. Diabetic neuropathy exposes the foot to trauma and pressure sores; the client may be unaware of the infection as it spreads into the bone. When tissue perfusion is poor, normal inflammatory responses and wound healing are impaired. The infection often is diagnosed when the client seeks treatment for a nonhealing sore, swollen toe, or acute cellulitis.

Manifestations of osteomyelitis vary according to the age of the client, the cause and site of involvement, and whether the infection is acute, subacute, or chronic (see box in left column).

## COLLABORATIVE CARE

The care of the client with osteomyelitis focuses on relieving pain, eliminating the infection, and preventing or minimizing complications. Early diagnosis is important to prevent bone necrosis by early antibiotic therapy. Most clients require both debridement of bone and a long period of antibiotic administration.

### Diagnostic Tests

The diagnosis of osteomyelitis is based on bone scans, magnetic resonance imaging, blood tests, and biopsy.

- *Magnetic resonance imaging (MRI)* can show epidural abscesses and other soft-tissue processes accompanying osteomyelitis.
- *Computed tomography (CT) scan* is used to detect sequestra, sinus tracts, and soft-tissue abscesses.

## Nursing Implications for Diagnostic Tests

### Bone Scan and Gallium Scan

#### BONE SCAN

##### Client Preparation

- Assess the client's understanding of the procedure, providing explanation, clarification, and emotional support as needed.
- Radioactive material (technetium-99m phosphate) is injected intravenously for 2 to 3 hours so that it concentrates in the bone.
- Observe the injection site for redness or swelling. If a hematoma forms, apply warm soaks to the area.
- Have the client drink four to six glasses of water in the 2- to 3-hour waiting period before the procedure to facilitate renal clearance of any circulating radioactive material.
- The client is not restricted to foods or fluids prior to the exam.
- Have the client empty the bladder prior to testing; a full bladder will mask the pelvic bones and make the client uncomfortable.
- The scan takes about 30 to 60 minutes to complete. The client must remain still during the scanning.
- The client may be active during the waiting period.
- A sedative should be ordered and administered to any client who may have difficulty lying quietly.

##### Postprocedure Care

- No specific care is needed after the procedure.

##### Client and Family Teaching

- Remove jewelry or any metal objects that may hide X-ray visualization of the bones.

- The scanner machine moves over the body and detects radiation emitted by the skeleton. X-ray films are prepared, showing a two-dimensional view of the skeleton. You may have to be repositioned several times.
- The scanning machine makes a clicking sound.
- Drinking liquids and frequent activity in the first 6 hours after the procedure help reduce excess radiation to the bladder and gonads.
- Family members will not be affected by the radionuclide, nor will urine or feces need special handling before, during, or after the procedure.

#### GALLIUM SCAN

##### Client Preparation

- Prepare as for a bone scan.
- Radioactive material, gallium-67, is injected intravenously 24 to 72 hours prior to the examination.
- Gallium is used because of its high affinity for soft-tissue abscesses.

##### Postprocedure Care

- Additional imaging may be performed at 24-hour intervals to differentiate normal activity from pathologic concentrations.
- No specific care is needed after the procedure.

##### Client and Family Teaching

- Refer to bone scan discussion.
- After a gallium scan, X-ray films may be obtained in 24-hour intervals for comparative results.

---

- *Radionucleotide bone scans* help determine if infection is active and differentiate between infectious and noninflammatory bone changes. Nursing care for clients having these procedures is described in the box above.
- *Ultrasound* can detect subperiosteal fluid collections, abscesses, and periosteal thickening and elevation associated with osteomyelitis.
- *Erythrocyte sedimentation rate (ESR)* and *WBC* are elevated in an acute infection.
- *Blood and tissue cultures* (from affected bone or soft tissue) are obtained to identify the infecting organism and direct antibiotic therapy.

## Medications

Antibiotic therapy is mandatory to prevent acute osteomyelitis from progressing to the chronic phase. Parenteral antibiotic therapy begins as soon as cultures (blood and/or wound) are obtained. A penicillinase-resistant semisynthetic penicillin (e.g, methacillin, oxacillin) may be given until the culture and sensitivity results are known. These antibiotics are used initially because many cases of osteomyelitis are caused by *Staphylococcus aureus.* When the detailed sensitivity report is obtained from the cultures, more definitive antibiotics are prescribed.

For the client with acute or chronic osteomyelitis, antibiotics are continued for 4 to 6 weeks. Intravenous antibiotic adminis-

tration or oral therapy is common. Oral therapy with twice-daily ciprofloxacin has been shown to be as effective as parenteral therapy for treating adult clients with chronic osteomyelitis caused by susceptible organisms (Tierney et al., 2001).

## Surgery

Needle aspiration or percutaneous needle biopsy may be performed to obtain a specimen in acute osteomyelitis. Surgery may be performed to obtain a specimen of the infectious agent, to debride the area, or both.

Surgical debridement is the primary treatment for the client with chronic osteomyelitis. The periosteum is excised and the cortex is drilled to release the pressure from accumulated pus. During this procedure, cultures may be obtained and sent to the laboratory for analysis. The wound holes are irrigated, and the wound is then closed. The cavity may be kept clean by inserting drainage tubes that are connected to an irrigation and suction system.

Postoperatively, the nurse is responsible for instilling and removing dilute antibiotic solutions through the drainage tubes. See the Nursing Care box on page 1270 for related nursing care.

A musculocutaneous (myocutaneous) flap is another approach used for the treatment of the dead space caused by extensive debridement of the infected site. The procedure involves moving or rotating a muscle and the section of skin fed

## NURSING CARE OF THE CLIENT UNDERGOING SURGICAL DEBRIDEMENT FOR OSTEOMYELITIS

### PREOPERATIVE CARE

- Discuss the impending surgery, the client's concerns regarding surgery and its risks, and what steps will be taken if surgery is ineffective. *Open discussion and active listening are important means of gaining the client's trust and encouraging the client to express concerns about the outcome of the surgery. Surgery is frequently performed when 36 to 48 hours of antimicrobial therapy yields no improvement and when prolonged bacteremia and evidence of an abscess formation are present. The periosteum is excised, allowing access to the purulent material in the infected area. If pus is not apparent, several holes may be drilled into the bone. In some cases, irrigation tubes are inserted and connected to an elaborate system for postoperative antimicrobial therapy.*
- Clients may need extensive antimicrobial treatment postoperatively if an irrigation system is surgically implanted. Before the procedure, explain to the client that bed rest and an extended period of treatment in the hospital are imperative. *Clients who understand the events that may occur postoperatively may be more accepting of the required restrictions.*

### POSTOPERATIVE CARE

- Provide meticulous care of the dressing and/or irrigation setup. *Frequently, the irrigation tubes are connected to a 3-way stopcock, which allows irrigation and drainage of the debrided area without separating the tube from the collection device. Nurses need to be extremely cautious and adhere to strict sterile technique.*
- Assess the client for manifestations of further infection. *Although the client will receive antimicrobial agents, it is important to assess the client continually for sudden spikes in temperature, pain at the involved site, and other indications of superinfection.*

### CLIENT AND FAMILY TEACHING

- While receiving antimicrobial agents, be sure to drink adequate amounts of fluid and eat a high-calorie diet to minimize the risks for damage to the kidneys, yeast infection, and adverse gastrointestinal effects.

---

by the arteries from that muscle into the cavity created by the surgery. A skin graft is performed later.

## NURSING CARE

The client with chronic osteomyelitis faces frequent and lengthy hospitalizations and/or treatment modalities. The prognosis is uncertain, and functional deficits and amputation are a constant concern. The ongoing expenses, loss of financial support, and role changes within the family are also nursing concerns.

### Nursing Diagnoses and Interventions

Nursing diagnoses associated with acute osteomyelitis focus on preventing the transmission of infection and problems due to immobility. Providing comfort and client teaching are also very important.

### Risk for Infection

Compromised immune status places the client with osteomyelitis at risk for superinfection. An inadequate kcal intake is an additional factor that contributes to the risk.

- Maintain strict handwashing practices. *Meticulous handwashing helps prevent the spread of infection by minimizing the entry of organisms into susceptible clients.*

> **PRACTICE ALERT** *Careful handwashing before and after direct care is essential even if gloves are worn.* ■

- Administer antimicrobial therapy at specified time intervals. *Optimal blood levels of antibiotic therapy are mandatory in clients with infectious processes.*

- Maintain the client's optimal dietary kcal and protein intake. *High kcal and protein intake provide the client with sufficient nutritional support for the body's needs during the stressful event of the inflammatory process.*

### Hyperthermia

The infection and associated inflammatory process can cause fever in the client with osteomyelitis.

- Monitor temperature every 4 hours and when client reports chills and/or fever. Blood cultures are frequently ordered when an acute elevation of temperature occurs. *A sudden rise in temperature in clients with either acute or chronic osteomyelitis may indicate inadequate antimicrobial management.*
- Maintain a cool environment and provide light clothing and bedding during temperature elevation. *Proper environmental conditions and clothing enhance the evaporative process during acute temperature elevation and promote comfort.*
- Ensure a daily fluid intake of 2000 to 3000 mL. Dehydration may result from evaporative fluid losses during acute temperature elevations. Furthermore, clients taking large doses of antibiotic therapy may experience fluid loss through excessive diarrhea, as a side effect of the therapy. *Fluid replacement is necessary during this time to prevent further dehydration.*

### Impaired Physical Mobility

Pain, infection, inflammation, and the use of immobilizers can all impair the mobility of the client with osteomyelitis.

- Maintain the affected limb in functional position when immobilized. *The client may hesitate to move the involved extremity because of continuous pain; therefore, the extremity must be maintained in functional position to avoid flexion contracture.*

- Maintain rest, and avoid subjecting the affected extremity to weight-bearing activities. *The involved extremity must be immobilized to avoid pathologic fractures caused by stress on the weakened bone.*
- Ensure active or passive ROM exercises every 4 hours. *Flexion contracture occurs when the client remains immobile or when there is only minimal joint movement. Consult a physical therapist for plan of exercises to avoid contracture.*

### Acute Pain

The client with osteomyelitis experience pain due to swelling.

- Use a splint or immobilizer when the client experiences acute pain from swelling. *Splinting or immobilizing the involved extremity provides support and reduces pain caused by movement.*
- Ask the physician to order scheduled administration of narcotic and nonnarcotic analgesics on a 24-hour basis rather than as needed. *The use of 24-hour administration allows blood levels of pain-relieving medications to remain constant.*

**PRACTICE ALERT** *Clients are often reluctant to ask for a prn pain medication, allowing the pain to reach a level that is difficult to manage.* ■

- Use nonpharmacologic strategies (e.g., distraction, relaxation techniques) for pain management. *Pain of the muscles and joints may be controlled through nonpharmacologic interventions. Warm moist packs, warm baths, or heating pads to the involved extremity provide comfort due to vasodilation.*
- Avoid excessive manipulation of the involved area; handle the area gently. Carefully assess the client for guarding, limping, or unwillingness to move the affected part. Communicate to other health care professionals the client's preferences for assistive devices and means of manipulating the involved area. *Gentle handling and minimal manipulation help reduce pain.*

### Anxiety

The long-term nature of the disease can cause feelings of anxiety in the client with osteomyelitis.

- While the client is in the hospital, provide information regarding the disease process and diagnostic tests. *An understanding of the disease process and the diagnostic and treatment modalities minimizes anxiety.*
- Inform the client about ways to maximize the treatment phases for the disease process. *The nurse should enable the client to participate fully in the treatment plan so that maximum results can be obtained. Clients need to understand that their adherence to the prescribed antibiotic therapy is essential.*

### Home Care

Although clients may be hospitalized for acute treatment and surgery, most care is provided at home. Home health services can provide intravenous medications, if prescribed. Discuss the following topics for home care.

- The importance of careful handwashing, especially after toileting and dressing changes
- The importance of taking all antibiotics as prescribed. Include information about helping prevent the yeast infections (of the mouth or vagina) often associated with prolonged antibiotic therapy by eating 8 oz of live-culture yogurt each day.
- The need to take pain medications on a regular basis to prevent pain from becoming severe. Provide information about how to deal with side effects, such as constipation, by increasing fluid and fiber intake.
- How to perform wound care and sources for needed equipment and supplies
- Rest or limited weight bearing for the affected extremity or body part. Teach how to avoid complications associated with prolonged immobilization, such as frequently shifting position, keeping skin and linens clean and dry, and doing active ROM exercises for unaffected joints.
- The importance of maintaining good nutrition. An adequate supply of kilocalories, protein, and other nutrients is necessary for immune function and healing. Suggest frequent small meals and using nutritional supplements such as Ensure to help maintain nutritional intake.

## THE CLIENT WITH SEPTIC ARTHRITIS

**Septic arthritis** can develop if a joint space is invaded by a pathogen. The primary risk factors for septic arthritis are persistent bacteremia (bacteria in the blood) (e.g., due to use of injectable drugs, endocarditis) and previous joint damage (e.g., due to trauma or rheumatoid arthritis). Arthroscopic surgery and total joint replacements which allow potential direct contamination of the joint are additional risk factors (Tierney et al., 2001).

### PATHOPHYSIOLOGY AND MANIFESTATIONS

The most common bacteria implicated in septic arthritis include *gonococci, Staphylococcus aureus,* and *streptococci.* Infections by gram-negative bacteria such as *E. coli* and *Pseudomonas* are seen with increasing frequency, particularly in people who inject recreational drugs or are immunocompromised (Tierney et al., 2001).

Infection of the joint leads to inflammation with resulting synovitis and joint effusion. Abscesses may form in synovial tissues or bone underlying joint cartilage. If not treated promptly and effectively, septic arthritis can lead to destruction of the affected joint. A single joint, often the knee, is usually affected. Septic arthritis may also affect other joints such as the shoulder, wrist, hip, fingers, or elbow.

The onset of septic arthritis is typically abrupt, marked by pain and stiffness of the infected joint. The joint appears red and swollen, and is hot and tender to the touch. Effusion (increased fluid within the joint space) is usually present. Systemic manifestations of infection, such as chills and fever, often accompany local manifestations, although these may be muted if the client is taking anti-inflammatory medications.

## COLLABORATIVE CARE

Septic arthritis is a medical emergency requiring prompt treatment to preserve joint function. When it is suspected, the affected joint is aspirated and fluid sent for Gram stain and culture. Cultures also are obtained from all likely sources of the infection, including blood, sputum, or wounds. The synovial fluid culture is always positive in nongonococcal septic arthritis but often is negative for bacteria in early gonococcal arthritis. Infected synovial fluid usually is cloudy, with a high WBC count and a low glucose level. Joint X-ray films are often normal in the initial stages, but soon show demineralization, bony erosions, and joint space narrowing.

The infected joint is treated with rest, immobilization, and elevation along with systemic antibiotic therapy. Therapy with a broad-spectrum parenteral antibiotic is initiated before the results of culture are obtained. The medication may be changed or adjusted once the organism has been identified. Antibiotic therapy is continued for at least 2 weeks after inflammatory signs and symptoms have abated. Frequent joint aspirations may be performed to remove excess fluid and pus, and to evaluate for the continued presence of bacteria. Surgical drainage may be performed if the hip joint is involved (because of the difficulty of aspirating this joint) or when medical therapy does not rapidly eliminate bacteria from the synovial fluid. Physical therapy is implemented during the recovery period to ensure maintenance of optimal joint function.

## NURSING CARE

Septic arthritis can be frightening to the client who experiences a sudden onset of joint pain and swelling and is faced with the possibility of rapid functional loss of movement. Nursing care is both supportive and educative. Clients may be hospitalized for initial treatment with intravenous antibiotics. It is important to monitor the client's response to therapy, including systemic manifestations such as fever. Position the affected joint appropriately, using pillows to elevate it as needed. Splints or traction may be used to immobilize the joint. Warm compresses may be ordered for comfort. Active ROM exercises preserve joint mobility and should be initiated as soon as the physician allows.

The client with septic arthritis needs information about the disorder, its etiology, and its treatment. Teach the client how organisms may gain entry into the joint space. Discuss the role that the use of injected drugs and sexually transmitted diseases play in septic arthritis, and means to prevent infection as appropriate (e.g., using clean "works," practicing safer sex). Refer the client to a drug treatment program if necessary. Emphasize the importance of complying with all aspects of the treatment plan to prevent joint destruction and disability.

# NEOPLASTIC DISORDERS

Bone tumors, or neoplasms of skeletal tissue, may be either primary (arising in the bone itself) or metastatic (seeded from a tumor elsewhere in the body). Like other tumors, bone tumors can be either benign or malignant.

## THE CLIENT WITH BONE TUMORS

Benign bone tumors tend to grow slowly and do not often destroy surrounding tissues. Malignant tumors grow rapidly and metastasize. Primary malignant tumors of the bone are rare, accounting for only about 1% of all adult cancers (Porth, 2002). Virtually every malignant tumor can metastasize to bone. However, the most common metastatic bone tumors originate from primary tumors of the prostate, breast, kidney, thyroid, and lung.

Primary bone tumors arise from bone tissue itself, that is, cartilage (chondogenic), bone (osteogenic), collagen (collagenic), and bone marrow cells (myelogenic). The tissue type, neoplasm classification, sites, and incidence of the most common primary bone tumors are summarized in Table 39–7. The focus for discussion in this section is care of the client with a primary bone tumor.

## PATHOPHYSIOLOGY AND MANIFESTATIONS

The etiology of bone tumors is unknown, but there is a connection between increased bone activity and the development of primary bone tumors. Bone tumors frequently occur when primary bone growth is at its peak in adolescence or is overstimulated during disease, such as Paget's disease.

Primary tumors cause bone breakdown, called *osteolysis,* which weakens the bone, resulting in bone fractures. Normal bone adjacent to the tumor responds to tumor pressure by altering its normal pattern of remodeling. The bone's surface becomes altered, and the contours enlarge in the area of the tumor growth.

Malignant bone tumors invade and destroy adjacent bone tissue by producing substances that promote bone resorption or by interfering with a bone's blood supply. Benign bone tumors, unlike malignant ones, have a symmetric, controlled growth pattern. As they grow, they push against neighboring bone tissue. This weakens the bone's structure until it becomes unable to withstand the stress of ordinary use and frequently causes pathologic fracture.

The three main manifestations of bone tumors are pain, a mass, and impaired function. The manifestations of bone tu-

TABLE 39–7  Description of Common Primary Bone Tumors

| Tissue Type | Benign | Malignant | Site | Incidence |
|---|---|---|---|---|
| Chondrogenic (cartilage-forming tumors) | Osteochondroma—most common benign tumor | | Pelvis, scapula, ribs | Higher in males |
| | Chondroma | | Hands, feet, ribs, spine, sternum, or long bones | Age 30 to 50 Higher in males |
| | | Chondrosarcoma | Femur, pelvis, ribs, head (epiphysis) of long bones | 13% of malignant bone tumors Middle age and older Higher in males |
| Osteogenic (bone-forming tumors) | Osteoid Osteoma | | Shaft (diaphysis) of long bones, i.e., femur, tibia | Age 20 to 30 Higher in males |
| | | Osteosarcoma—most common malignant tumor | Long bones, knee | 38% of malignant bone tumors Predominant in adolescents and people 50 to 60 |
| Collagenic (collagen-forming tumors) | | Fibrosarcoma | Femur, tibia | 4% of malignant bone tumors Wide age distribution, but usually occurs in people 40 to 50 Higher in females |
| Myelogenic (tumors of bone marrow cells) | Giant cell tumor | | Shaft (diaphysis) of long bones, i.e., femur, tibia, radius, humerus | 4% to 5% of bone tumors Wide age distribution Higher in females |

mors are usually associated with a history of a fall or blow to the extremity that brings the mass to the client's attention. The injury, rather than the growth itself, usually causes the client to seek medical attention. Manifestations of bone tumors are listed in the box below.

## COLLABORATIVE CARE
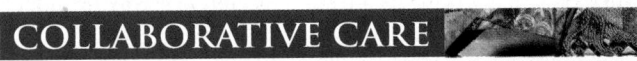

Care of the client with bone tumors focuses on prompt diagnosis, removal of the tumor, prevention of complications, and client education.

## Manifestations of Neoplasms of the Musculoskeletal System

### BONY SARCOMAS

**Site**
Upper or lower extremity or pelvis

**Manifestations**
- Worsening deep bony pain due to inflammation or weakness of bone
- Pain at night or during rest that may radiate and become severe
- Muscular weakness or atrophy due to pain

Metaphysis of distal femur, proximal tibia, proximal humerus, and pelvis
- Soft-tissue mass extending from bone with erythematous or warm skin over tissue mass
- Alternation in ability to perform activities of daily living
- Fever

### SOFT TISSUE SARCOMAS

**Site**
Upper or lower extremity and pelvis

**Manifestations**
- Enlarging firm mass with irregular borders, which causes pain in surrounding soft-tissue structures

Thigh, shoulder, and pelvis
- Erythema or warmth and venous dilation over skin
- Muscular weakness and atrophy with limited range of motion, alteration in ability to perform activities of daily living, and alteration in gait
- Paresthesia with neurologic involvement and distal swelling
- Palpable local lymph nodes resulting from inflammation of tumor

Pelvis
- Above manifestations, plus altered bowel and bladder habits or pain with intercourse
- Weakening of muscles due to lumbosacral nerve involvement

## Diagnostic Tests

The diagnosis of bone tumors is critical to the survival of the client and possible preservation of the affected limb. The following tests may be performed.

- *X-rays* show the location of the tumors and the extent of bone involvement. Benign tumors are characterized by sharp margins that are clearly separate from the surrounding normal bone. Metastatic bone destruction has a characteristic "moth-eaten" pattern in which the growth has a less-defined margin that cannot be separated from the normal bone.
- *CT scan* is useful in evaluating the extent of tumor invasion into bone, soft tissues, and neurovascular structures.
- *MRI* is used to determine the extent of tumor invasion of surrounding tissue, to determine the response of bone tumors to radiation or chemotherapy, and to detect recurrent disease.
- *Percutaneous needle biopsy* or *needle biopsy* at the time of surgery is used to determine the exact type of bone tumor.
- *Serum alkaline phosphatase* is elevated in the client with a malignant bone tumor.
- *RBC count* is elevated.
- *Serum calcium* is elevated when there is massive bone destruction.

## Chemotherapy

Chemotherapeutic agents are administered to shrink the tumor before surgery, to control recurrence of tumor growth after surgery, or to treat metastasis of the tumor. Chemotherapeutic agents used to treat bone tumors are listed in Box 39–4. See Chapter 10 ⟳ for further discussion of chemotherapy and its nursing implications.

## Radiation Therapy

Radiation therapy may be used in combination with chemotherapy. Radiation therapy is frequently applied to metastatic bone carcinomas as a method of pain control. It is also used to eliminate bony tumors or to eliminate any remaining tumor after a surgical procedure. Radiation therapy is discussed in Chapter 10.

## Surgery

The goal of surgery for the treatment of primary bone tumors is to eliminate the tumor completely. Tumors are removed either by excising the tumor itself or by amputating the affected limb. The type of procedure varies from removing the tumor only, to removing the tumor along with a small margin of normal tissue surrounding the tumor, to removing the tumor and a wide zone of normal tissue, to removing the tumor and part or all of the bone in which it lies. Cadaver allografts or metal prostheses often are used to replace missing bone, avoiding amputation. Care of the client undergoing amputation is discussed in Chapter 38.

## NURSING CARE

Nursing care for the client with bone tumors requires innovative actions from the time of diagnosis through the rehabilitation phase. In the acute phase, problems associated with pain, lack of knowledge, immobility, coping, and anxiety are foremost. If the client develops complications from treatment or if a malignancy metastasizes, problems related to home health maintenance management, self-concept, and prevention of further complications become more prominent.

## Nursing Diagnoses and Interventions

### Risk for Injury

In the client with a bone tumor, changes in bone tissue can cause pathologic fractures.

- Instruct clients in ways to avoid falls or injury to the tumor site. *Pathologic fractures may occur at the tumor site because bone destruction can weaken the area.*
- Provide referral to physical or occupational therapy for fitting of and teaching about assistive devices for ambulating, such as a cane, crutches, or a walker. *Assistive devices can reduce the risk of falling when the client has significant weakness of an extremity or when balance has been affected by treatment of the disease.*

### Acute and Chronic Pain

In the client with a bone tumor, pain may be related to direct invasion of the tumor or to pathologic fractures.

- Develop strategies for controlling both acute pain (from surgery, fracture, or inflammation) and chronic pain (from progression of the disease). *Analgesics combined with nonpharmacologic methods of pain control provide optimum relief of pain. Chronic pain, when mild in nature, is best managed with NSAIDs or aspirin. Moderate pain is best managed with a combination of codeine and NSAIDs. Severe pain is best relieved with long-acting or sustained relief narcotic analgesics.*
- Provide assistive devices (e.g., canes, walkers, crutches) when the client ambulates. *Assistive devices lessen the pain by supporting weight bearing during ambulation.*
- Provide regular rest periods between therapeutic activities. *Therapy should be performed at a time of maximum comfort for the client to increase mobility.*

### Impaired Physical Mobility

Pain, muscle wasting, or surgical procedures can impair the physical mobility of the client with a bone tumor.

- Begin muscle strengthening and active and passive ROM exercises immediately after surgery. A continuous passive motion (CPM) machine may be used after surgical proce-

---

| BOX 39–4 | ■ Chemotherapeutic Agents Used for Musculoskeletal Neoplasms |
|---|---|

**Alkylating Agents**
Ifosfamide
Cyclophosphamide

**Antibiotics**
Doxorubicin
Bleomycin

**Antimetabolites**
Methotrexate

**Plant Alkaloids**
Vincristine

**Synthetic Agents**
Cisplatin

dures to either upper or lower extremities. *Muscle strengthening exercises must be encouraged as soon as possible to prevent muscle wasting and shorten the rehabilitation period.*

- Encourage exercises that help strengthen the triceps muscles. *The triceps are the major muscles in the arms and must be strengthened to assist in use of crutches or other assistive devices.*
- For the client who has undergone an amputation of a lower extremity, encourage quadriceps and gluteal setting exercises and leg raises. *These exercises will benefit the client when the rehabilitation period begins.*
- Teach clients how to use the trapeze correctly. Clients can use the trapeze to reposition themselves while supine, get out of bed, and assist the nurse's efforts to reposition them in bed and perform other activities. *Use of the trapeze helps strengthen the biceps of the arm.*

### Decisional Conflict

Knowledge deficit about diagnosis and treatment regimen can impair the client's ability to make informed decisions about the treatment plan.

- Explain issues related to diagnosis, radiologic evaluation, biopsy, surgery, chemotherapy, radiation therapy, potential complications, alternative therapies, risks, benefits, nursing management, discharge plans, home care, and long-term treatment and follow-up. *The client requires this information in order to make informed decisions about treatment.*

### Home Care

The client with a primary bone tumor needs information about the disease, its potential consequences, and treatment options. Present information in a matter-of-fact manner, taking time to listen to and address the client's and family's concerns. Discuss expected effects and potential side effects of surgery, chemotherapy, and radiation therapy. Provide information about how to minimize side effects. Teach the postsurgical client about wound care, demonstrating dressing changes and stump care (if amputation has occurred). Provide the client with a list of local resources for obtaining supplies. Discuss activity and weight-bearing restrictions. Refer the client to physical therapy for teaching about ambulation and appropriate muscle-group strengthening exercises. Ensure that the client who has experienced an amputation is working with or has a referral to a prosthetic specialist. For the client with metastatic disease, discuss hospice services and support groups for clients with cancer.

## CONNECTIVE TISSUE DISORDERS

Connective tissue is the most abundant and widely distributed body tissue. It not only connects body parts but also provides support; forms bones, cartilage, and the walls of blood vessels; and attaches muscles to bones. Connective tissue consists of three elements: (1) long fibers embedded in a (2) noncellular ground substance, and (3) cells specific to the class of connective tissue. Fibers made up primarily of collagen, a protein, are the most abundant in connective tissue.

Connective-tissue disorders, also known as collagen diseases, are a group of immune-mediated disorders. Although they appear to have a genetic component, their cause is unknown. Because connective tissue and collagen are widely distributed in many varied tissues, these are systemic diseases with diverse manifestations.

## THE CLIENT WITH SYSTEMIC SCLEROSIS (SCLERODERMA)

**Systemic sclerosis**, also known as **scleroderma** ("hardening of the skin"), is a chronic disease characterized by the formation of excess fibrous connective tissue and diffuse fibrosis of the skin and internal organs. The cause of scleroderma is unknown, although genetic, immune, and environmental factors are thought to play a role. Although this uncommon disease is distributed worldwide, a higher incidence is noted in coal and gold miners and in people exposed to certain chemicals such as polyvinyl chloride, epoxy resins, and aromatic hydrocarbons. It affects women more often than men by a ratio of approximately 3:1. The onset of scleroderma typically occurs between the ages of 30 and 50 years (Tierney et al., 2001).

### PATHOPHYSIOLOGY

Abnormalities in cellular immune function are believed to contribute to the development of scleroderma. Abnormal proliferation of fibrous connective tissue occurs in affected tissues, including the skin, blood vessels, lungs, kidneys, and other organs.

Scleroderma may be either localized, affecting the skin only, or generalized (systemic sclerosis), with both skin and visceral organ involvement. Eighty percent of people with generalized disease have limited involvement, frequently manifested by CREST syndrome, a combination of calcinosis (abnormal calcium salt deposition in the tissues), Raynaud's phenomenon, esophageal dysfunction, sclerodactyly (localized scleroderma of the fingers), and telangiectasia (dilated, superficial blood vessels). The remainder of clients with generalized systemic sclerosis have a diffuse form of the disease and a higher risk of visceral organ involvement.

### MANIFESTATIONS AND COMPLICATIONS

The initial manifestations of systemic sclerosis are usually noted in the skin, which thickens markedly. Diffuse, nonpitting swelling also is noted. As the disease progresses, the skin begins to atrophy, becoming taut, shiny, and hyperpigmented

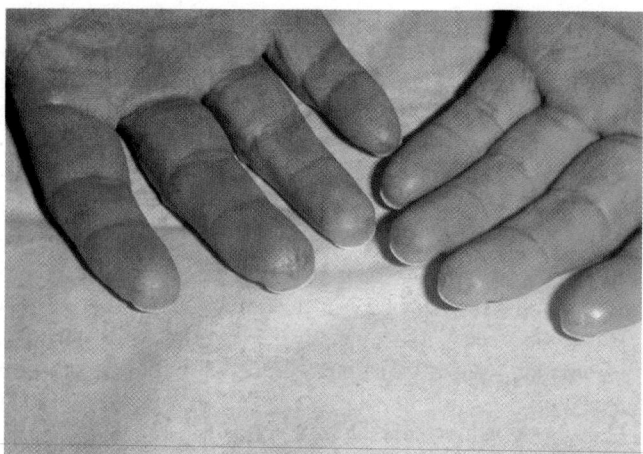

**Figure 39–10** ■ Characteristic skin changes of scleroderma.

*Source: Logical Images/Custom Medical Stock Photo.*

(Figure 39–10 ■). Facial skin tightening leads to loss of skin lines and a pursed-lip appearance. Skin tightness may limit mobility, particularly of the face and hands. Other skin manifestations include telangiectasias (flat, red areas caused by dilation of small blood vessels, usually noted on the face, hands, and in the mouth) and calcium deposits, usually noted around joints.

Arthralgias and Raynaud's phenomenon also are common early manifestations of systemic sclerosis. Raynaud's phenomenon (intermittent attacks of small artery vasospasm) is characterized by pallor of the fingers followed by cyanosis, and then reactive hyperemia with redness. Attacks are usually triggered by cold temperatures.

The client with visceral organ involvement may have varied symptoms. Dysphagia is common, because the motility of the esophagus is affected. Pulmonary involvement can lead to exertional dyspnea due to impaired gas exchange and right-sided heart failure due to pulmonary hypertension. Involvement of the heart may cause manifestations of pericarditis and dysrhythmias. Diarrhea or constipation, abdominal cramping, and malabsorption can occur when the GI tract is affected. Renal effects can lead to proteinuria, hematuria, hypertension, and renal failure.

The prognosis for localized and limited scleroderma is good; many clients have a normal life span. The course of diffuse systemic sclerosis is highly variable. This disease is usually progressive; complete remission is rare.

## COLLABORATIVE CARE

The manifestations of systemic sclerosis often allow diagnosis with little or no testing. No cure is currently available; treatment is symptomatic and supportive.

### Diagnostic Tests

No single test is specific for systemic sclerosis. The following tests may be ordered.

- *ESR* is typically elevated because of the chronic inflammatory process.

- *CBC* will typically find anemia because of the chronic disease process and its effects on various organs.
- *Gammaglobulin levels* are often high, and *antinuclear antibodies* and *rheumatoid factor* may be present in low levels.
- *Skin biopsy* may be performed to confirm the diagnosis.

### Medications

Medications to treat systemic sclerosis are chosen based on the client's symptoms. Immunosuppressive agents and corticosteroids are of limited benefit, but may be used to slow or prevent pulmonary fibrosis and in life-threatening disease. Penicillamine may be used to treat scleroderma and pulmonary fibrosis. Calcium channel blockers such as nifedipine (Procardia) or alpha-adrenergic blockers such as prazosin (Minipress) may be prescribed for clients with Raynaud's phenomenon. When manifestations of esophagitis accompany systemic sclerosis, $H_2$-receptor blockers such as cimetidine (Tagamet) or ranitidine (Zantac), antacids, or omeprazole (Prilosec), which blocks all gastric secretion, may be ordered. Tetracycline or another broad-spectrum antibiotic may be prescribed to suppress intestinal flora and relieve symptoms of malabsorption. Clients with kidney disease are usually treated with angiotensin-converting enzyme (ACE) inhibitors such as captopril (Capoten) to control hypertension and preserve renal function. End-stage kidney disease is managed with dialysis and transplantation.

### Physical Therapy

Physical therapy is an important part of the management of systemic sclerosis to maintain mobility of affected tissues, the hands and face in particular. Because the mouth opening becomes increasingly smaller as the disease progresses, stretching and strengthening of facial muscles can be vital to maintaining oral food intake.

## NURSING CARE

Nursing care needs of clients with systemic sclerosis are individualized to the effects and manifestations of the disease, with interventions summarized in the following discussion.

### Nursing Interventions

Skin manifestations are present to some degree in nearly all clients with scleroderma. Nursing care related to the skin focuses on maintaining skin integrity and flexibility. Measures to maintain supple skin are important, because elasticity cannot be regained once it is lost. Apply moisturizers to prevent dryness and cracking. Protect the skin where it is stretched taut over joints or bony prominences. Perform ROM exercises to help prevent joint contractures due to increasingly tight skin.

Difficulty swallowing and recurrent esophagitis may interfere with the client's nutritional status. Provide small, frequent meals. Consult with the dietitian and the client to determine which foods are easy to swallow. Keep the client in a sitting or Fowler's position after meals to minimize esophageal reflux. Elevate the head of the bed at night as well.

The dermatologic and systemic effects of the disease may have significant psychologic effects on the client, leading to feelings of helplessness and hopelessness, and self-esteem disturbance. Establish an atmosphere of trust with the client. Listen actively and acknowledge concerns about the disease and its effects on the client's life and appearance. Encourage the client to share these concerns with family members and significant others. Provide referral to social services or counseling as appropriate.

The client with predominant pulmonary disease has nursing care needs similar to those of other clients with restrictive respiratory disorders (see Chapter 36). If the client with systemic sclerosis has impaired renal function, nursing care is similar to that for clients with chronic renal failure (see Chapter 27).

## Home Care

Teach the client with systemic sclerosis about the disease and introduce measures to help manage its effects. Stress the importance of good skin care and physical therapy exercises to maintain mobility, particularly of the hands and face. Discuss the need to avoid chilling (local and whole body) to prevent episodes of Raynaud's phenomenon. Teach the role of proper dress: loose, warm clothing, gloves, and warm stockings in the winter. Stress the need to stop smoking because of the vasoconstrictive effect of nicotine and the respiratory effects of the disease. Provide the client with information about manifestations of disease progression and organ involvement. Teach the client to report new or worsening symptoms to the physician. In addition, suggest the following resources.

- National Arthritis and Musculoskeletal and Skin Diseases, National Institutes of Health
- Scleroderma Foundation, Inc.
- Scleroderma Research Foundation

## THE CLIENT WITH SJÖGREN'S SYNDROME

**Sjögren's syndrome** is an autoimmune disorder that causes inflammation and dysfunction of exocrine glands throughout the body. Sjögren's syndrome primarily affects women, with a ratio of women to men at 9:1 The highest incidence is between the ages of 40 and 60 years. Although it can occur as a primary disorder, Sjogren's syndrome is often associated with other rheumatic disease, including rheumatoid arthritis, systemic lupus erythematosus, primary biliary cirrhosis, scleroderma, Hashimoto's thyroiditis, and interstitial pulmonary fibrosis (Tierney et al., 2001).

## PATHOPHYSIOLOGY

In this disease, exocrine glands in many areas of the body are destroyed by the infiltration of lymphocytes and deposition of immune complexes. The salivary and lacrimal glands are particularly affected, leading to the characteristic manifestations of *xerophthalmia* (dry eyes) and *xerostomia* (dry mouth). Clients often experience dry, gritty-feeling eyes and may de-

velop corneal ulcerations. Mucosal dryness affects taste, smell, chewing, and swallowing and leads to increased dental caries. Parotid gland enlargement is common. Excess dryness can also affect the nose, throat, larynx, bronchi, vagina, and skin. Systemic effects of Sjögren's syndrome include arthritis, dysphagia, pancreatitis, pleuritis, neurologic manifestations including migraine, and vasculitis. Nephritis may occur, but renal failure rarely results. Clients with Sjögren's syndrome have a greatly increased risk of developing malignant lymphoma.

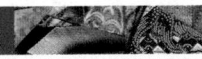
## COLLABORATIVE CARE

The diagnosis of Sjögren's syndrome is often based on the client's history and clinical presentation. Schirmer's test, which measures the quantity of tears secreted in a 5-minute period in response to irritation, ocular staining, and slit-lamp examination of the eye, may be performed. A definitive diagnosis can be made by biopsy of either the lacrimal or salivary gland.

Treatment is supportive. Artificial tears are used to decrease eye irritation and dryness. The client can keep the mouth moist by drinking fluids, using a saliva substitute, and chewing sugarless gum. Medications that increase mouth dryness, such as atropine and decongestants, should be avoided.

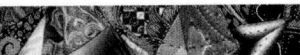
## NURSING CARE

Nurses caring for clients with Sjögren's syndrome need to promote and teach measures to protect the client's eyes and oral mucosa. Instill artificial tears as needed. Encourage the client to sip fluids throughout the day. Provide frequent oral hygiene, particularly before and after meals. Ensure that the client has sufficient fluids to drink during meals, because fluids help with chewing and swallowing.

## THE CLIENT WITH FIBROMYALGIA

**Fibromyalgia** is a common rheumatic syndrome characterized by musculoskeletal pain, stiffness, and tenderness. Fibromyalgia affects from 3% to 10% of the general population, and is found most commonly in women between 20 years and 50 years (Tierney et al., 2002). The cause is unknown, but possible etiologies include sleep disorders, depression, infections, and an altered perception of normal stimuli. Fibromyalgia can be a complication of hypothyroidism, rheumatoid arthritis, or (in men) sleep apnea. It closely resembles chronic fatigue syndrome, except that musculoskeletal pain is predominant in fibromyalgia, whereas fatigue is a more significant feature of chronic fatigue syndrome.

## PATHOPHYSIOLOGY AND MANIFESTATIONS

No inflammatory, structural, or physiologic muscle changes have been demonstrated in fibromyalgia. A gradual onset of chronic, achy muscle pain is typical, although the onset may be sudden, occasionally following a viral illness. The pain may be localized or involve the entire body. The neck, spine, shoulders, and hips are often affected. Pain is produced by palpating localized "tender points" (for example, on the trapezius, medial fat pad of the knee, and the lateral epicondyle of the elbow). Local tightness or muscle spasm may also occur. Systemic manifestations of fibromyalgia include fatigue, sleep disruptions, headaches, and an irritable bowel. Pain and fatigue are aggravated by exertion.

## COLLABORATIVE CARE

The diagnosis of fibromyalgia is based on the history and physical assessment. There are no laboratory or diagnostic tests for the disorder, although tests may be performed to rule out other rheumatic disorders, such as rheumatoid arthritis or systemic lupus erythematosus. Fibromyalgia also may occur as a complication of hypothyroidism, so thyroid function studies are performed. Criteria for diagnosis of fibromyalgia, developed by The American College of Rheumatology, are that the person must have widespread pain in combination with tenderness in at least 11 of the 18 specific tender point sites.

This disorder may resolve spontaneously or become chronic and recurrent. The client with fibromyalgia needs re-assurance of the benign nature of the disorder along with validation of its reality. Other therapeutic measures include local heat applications, massage, stretching exercises, and sleep improvement. Amitriptyline, a tricyclic antidepressant, has been shown to promote better sleep and relieve manifestations of fibromyalgia. NSAIDs have not been effective in its treatment.

## NURSING CARE

Nursing care for clients with fibromyalgia is supportive and educational, provided in community settings such as clinics and other primary care settings. It is important to validate clients' concerns and reassure them that their symptoms are not "all in the head." This syndrome is recognizable and manageable; its course is not progressive. Teach clients about the disorder, and reassure them that it resolves uneventfully in most instances. Provide verbal and written instructions about the use of heat, exercise, stress-reduction techniques, and prescribed medications to relieve its manifestations. In addition, suggest the following resources:

- Fibromyalgia Network
- National Fibromyalgia Awareness Campaign

# STRUCTURAL DISORDERS

Structural disorders of the musculoskeletal system most commonly affect the spine. The disorders discussed in this section are spinal deformities and low back pain.

## THE CLIENT WITH SPINAL DEFORMITIES

Scoliosis and kyphosis are the two most common deformities of the spinal column. **Scoliosis** is a lateral curvature of the spine. **Kyphosis** is excessive angulation of the normal posterior curve of the thoracic spine (Figure 39–11 ■).

An estimated 500,000 adults in the United States are affected by scoliosis. It usually is diagnosed in adolescence, with girls affected more than boys by an 8:1 margin. Idiopathic scoliosis is the most common form of the disorder, accounting for approximately 75% of cases. Congenital and neuromuscular disorders such as cerebral palsy, poliomyelitis, and MD account for the rest (Porth, 2002).

Kyphosis can be caused by a variety of congenital conditions or childhood disorders. Detailed discussions of the causes and treatment of scoliosis and kyphosis in younger clients can be found in pediatric nursing textbooks. This discussion focuses on the nursing care of adults with these disorders.

The manifestations of scoliosis and kyphosis are listed in the box on page 1279.

## PATHOPHYSIOLOGY AND MANIFESTATIONS
### Scoliosis

Scoliosis is classified as *postural* when the small curve corrects with bending, and *structural* when the curve does not correct with bending (Porth, 2002). Most clients requiring treatment have structural scoliosis, a curve caused by a fixed deformity.

The lateral curve that occurs in scoliosis is usually evident in the thoracic, lumbar, or thoracolumbar regions of the spine. The vertebral bodies in these spinal regions can be rotated as well as curved to one side or the other.

As scoliosis emerges, the soft tissues (muscles and ligaments) shorten on the concave side of the curvature. Over time, progressive deformities of the vertebral column and ribs develop, causing one-sided compression of the vertebral bodies. The degree of compression and twisting varies according to the location of each vertebra within the curved portion of the spine.

If the lateral curvature is less than 40 degrees when the client's spine reaches maturity, the risk of further progression during adult life is small. However, the spine becomes unstable if the lateral curvature is greater than 50 degrees, and curvature likely will worsen throughout the client's lifetime.

Scoliosis is usually first noted by the deformity it causes, such as one shoulder that is higher than the other, a prominent hip, or a projecting scapula. Pain is present in severe cases, usually in the lumbar region. Pain also may be caused by pressure on the ribs or the crest of the ilium. Shortness of breath may re-

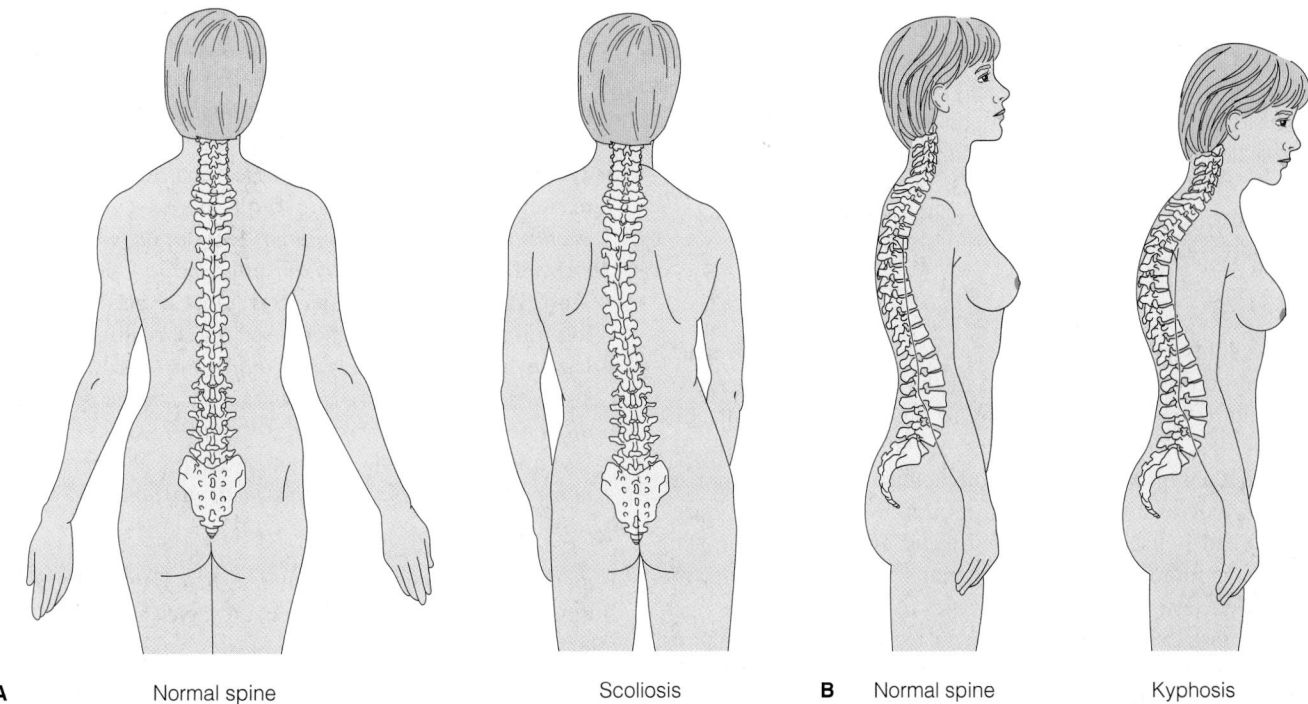

**A** Normal spine     Scoliosis     **B** Normal spine     Kyphosis

**Figure 39–11** ■ Common deformities of the spinal column: *A*, Scoliosis is a lateral curvature of the spine. *B*, Kyphosis is an exaggerated posterior curvature of the thoracic spine.

## Manifestations of Scoliosis and Kyphosis

### SCOLIOSIS

- Asymmetry of shoulders, scapulae, waist creases
- Prominence of the thoracic ribs or paravertebral muscles on forward bend
- Lateral curvature and vertebral rotation on posteroanterior X-ray film

### SEVERE SCOLIOSIS

- Back pain
- Shortness of breath
- Anorexia, nausea

### KYPHOSIS

- Posterior rounding at the thoracic level
- Kyphotic curve of over 45 degrees on X-ray film

sult from diminished chest expansion, and gastrointestinal disturbances because of crowding of the abdominal organs.

### Kyphosis

Like scoliosis, kyphosis is classified as postural or structural. Postural kyphosis is caused by a slumping posture. Structural kyphosis may result from congenital malformations or pediatric disorders such as rickets or poliomyelitis. However, kyphosis also may occur during adulthood from vertebral tuberculosis and Paget's disease or from metabolic disorders such as osteoporosis and osteomalacia. The condition can also

result from the surgical removal or radiation of intervertebral discs for the treatment of spinal cord tumors or cysts.

The manifestations of kyphosis include moderate back pain and increased curvature of the thoracic spine as viewed from the side ("hunchback"). Impaired mobility and respiratory problems may occur in cases of severe curvature.

## COLLABORATIVE CARE

Diagnosis of scoliosis and kyphosis is important to prevent severe spinal deformity in the adult. The client stands with the arms relaxed and hanging freely at the sides while the examiner evaluates the client from both the back and the front for symmetry of the shoulders, scapulae, waist creases, and the length of the arms. The client then bends forward, and the examiner observes for prominence of the thoracic ribs or vertebral muscles. The client is then viewed from the side while the screener looks for increased thoracic rounding or lumbar swayback.

A scoliometer is used to quantify the prominence of any curvatures noted during the examination. The scoliometer is placed at the apex of the curvature. A reading of greater than 10 degrees requires referral to a physician (Porth, 2002).

### Diagnostic Tests

Upright posteroanterior and lateral radiographs are used to confirm the diagnosis of curvature of the spine. For the client with scoliosis, the degree of curve is measured by determining the amount of lateral deviation to the left or right. For the client with kyphosis, anteroposterior and lateral views typically reveal wedging of the vertebrae.

## Conservative Treatment

Braces, electrical stimulation, and traction may be used to prevent progression of scoliosis and kyphosis in younger clients whose skeletons have not yet matured. Unfortunately, these approaches are ineffective in the adult client. Conservative treatment for adults with scoliosis and kyphosis may include weight reduction, active and passive exercises, and the use of braces for support.

## Surgery

For adolescents and adults, the use of surgery to correct spinal deformities depends on factors such as the degree of curvature and the client's overall physical, emotional, and neurologic status. Even with surgery, it is not possible to correct the abnormal curvature completely. The surgical procedure involves attaching metal reinforcing rods to the vertebrae, and is usually performed using an anterior approach, although more severe curvature may require both an anterior and a posterior approach. The types of straightening devices used most frequently use bilateral rods with wire hooks or screws that stabilize the spine and correct the deformity.

## NURSING CARE

Nursing interventions focus on minimizing the risk for injury and neurologic impairment.

## Nursing Diagnoses and Interventions

### Risk for Injury

Clients with spinal deformities are at risk for injury from several sources, including structural aspects of bracing both prior to and after surgical intervention, dislocation of hooks and rods resulting from improper alignment or movement of the back, and changes in body position after prolonged immobilization.

- Assess the environment for safety hazards. *The client needs to learn to use the handrail on stairways and take precautions when walking on slippery surfaces or areas with throw rugs.*

**PRACTICE ALERT** *Some braces do not allow the client to flex or hyperextend the spinal column.* ■

- Teach the clients ways to reduce irritation of skin surfaces beneath the brace: wearing a smooth cotton T-shirt or cotton tube under the brace at all times, changing undergarments at least once daily, and washing them with a mild soap. Undergarments should be changed more frequently in warmer weather. *The client wearing a brace is especially prone to skin breakdown and must take precautions to prevent it.*

**PRACTICE ALERT** *Teach the client to avoid lotion and body powders; they may irritate the skin.* ■

- Teach the client to loosen the brace during meals and for the first 30 minutes after each meal. *Clients have difficulty eating if the brace is tight. Loosening the brace after each meal will allow adequate nutritional intake and promote comfort.*
- Teach clients how to apply the brace, and explain ambulatory restrictions. *Clients requiring a brace need to learn how to apply the brace prior to ambulating. Ambulation is frequently restricted to walking rather than sitting for long periods.*
- Turn clients who have undergone spinal surgery by using the log-rolling technique. Clients require a position change at least every 2 hours. *The use of a turnsheet and sufficient assistance allow the nurse to maintain the client's proper body alignment during the turning procedure.*
- Use a fracture bedpan following surgery. *The fracture bedpan provides minimal misalignment of spine and thus ensures comfort.*

### Risk for Peripheral Neurovascular Dysfunction

Surgical procedures can lead to neurologic impairment in the client with a spinal deformity.

- Assess the movement and sensation of lower extremities every 2 hours for the first 8 hours then every shift and as needed. *Neurologic assessment related to sensation and movement of the lower extremities is necessary because the surgical procedure is in close proximity to spinal nerves. Swelling of the surgical site can impinge on the spinal nerves and cause a loss of sensation.*

## Home Care

Clients with structural scoliosis or kyphosis need reassurance that the condition was not caused by poor posture. If a brace is prescribed to relieve pain and other symptoms associated with the disorder, provide verbal and written instructions for wearing the brace, such as the number of hours per day it is to be worn and activity restrictions to follow when wearing or not wearing the brace. Teach the client how to protect and care for skin under the brace.

Surgical clients need postoperative teaching regarding site care and activities. Clients who have spinal surgery often are allowed to ambulate fairly rapidly after surgery, but sitting may be restricted because of the stresses it places on the spine. Instruct the client to notify the physician if numbness, tingling, pain, or weakness of an extremity develop after surgery.

Discuss the importance of not smoking and of avoiding respiratory infections for clients with scoliosis or kyphosis that restrict respiratory excursion. Encourage these clients to obtain pneumococcal pneumonia and influenza immunizations.

## THE CLIENT WITH LOW BACK PAIN

Acute or chronic low back pain involves the lumbar, lumbosacral, or sacroiliac areas of the back. In most cases, low back pain is due to strains in the muscles and tendons of the back caused by abnormal stress or overuse. Low back pain

## BOX 39–5 ■ Factors Associated with Back Pain

### MECHANICAL INJURY OR TRAUMA
- Muscle strain or spasm
- Compression fracture
- Lumbar disc disease

### DEGENERATIVE DISORDERS
- Spondylosis
- Spinal stenosis
- Osteoarthritis

### SYSTEMIC DISORDERS
- Osteomyelitis
- Osteoporosis or osteomalacia
- Neoplasms, primary or metastatic

### REFERRED PAIN
- Gastrointestinal disorders
- Genitourinary disorders
- Gynecologic disorders
- Abdominal aortic aneurysm
- Hip pathology

### OTHER
- Fibromyalgia
- Psychiatric syndromes
- Chronic anxiety
- Depression

## Manifestations of Low Back Pain

### ALTERATIONS IN GAIT AND FLEXION
- Walking in a stiff, flexed state
- Inability to bend at waist
- Limp, which may indicate impairment of the sciatic nerve

### NEUROLOGIC INVOLVEMENT
- When tested for light and deep touch with a pin and cotton ball, may feel sensations in both limbs but experience a stronger sensation in the unaffected side
- Loss of both bowel and bladder control due to involvement of the sacral nerve

### PAIN
- Pain in the affected leg when walking on heel or toes
- Continuous, knifelike localized pain in muscles close to the affected disk
- Pain that radiates down posterior of leg
- Sharp, burning pain in the posterior thigh or calf
- Pain in middle of buttock
- Tenderness when muscle close to the affected disc is palpated
- Severe pain with straight leg-raising maneuver

## COLLABORATIVE CARE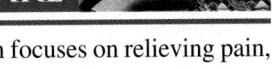

Care of the client with low back pain focuses on relieving pain, correcting the condition if possible, preventing complications, and educating the client.

### Diagnostic Tests

The choice of diagnostic tests for the client with low back pain depends on the suspected diagnoses, clinical findings, and history. Current guidelines for care recommend that radiography, CT scans, and MRI be used only with clinical signs of a potentially serious underlying condition. They also state that diagnostic testing may be considered if pain and other manifestations continue to limit the client after 4 weeks of conservative treatment.

### Medications

The medications of choice for low back pain include NSAIDs and analgesics. NSAIDs block prostaglandin production and reduce inflammation, thus relieving the pain. Muscle relaxants, such as cyclobenzaprine (Flexeril), methocarbamol (Robaxin), or carisoprodol (Soma) may be used, but little evidence supports their efficacy.

Epidural steroid injections may be used to help reduce intense, intractable pain. A steroid solution is injected into the epidural space, which helps decrease the swelling and inflammation of the spinal nerves.

### Conservative Treatment

The majority of clients with acute low back pain need only a short-term treatment regimen. Limited rest, combined with appropriate exercise and education, is often the primary method of treatment. There is no evidence that activity is harmful or aggravating to the source of pain. In fact, increased activity

---

caused by degenerative disc disease and herniated vertebral discs is covered in Chapter 41. 🔗

## PATHOPHYSIOLOGY AND MANIFESTATIONS

The pathophysiology of back pain varies with its many causes (Box 39–5). In general, the five types of back pain are as follows:

- Local pain is caused by compression or irritation of sensory nerves. Fractures, strains, and sprains are common causes of local pain; tumors also may press on pain-sensitive structures.
- Referred pain may originate from abdominal or pelvic viscera.
- Pain of spinal origin, that is, pain associated with pathology of the spine such as disk disease or arthritis, may be referred to other structures such as the buttocks, groin, or legs.
- Radicular back pain is sharp, radiating from the back to the leg along a nerve root. This pain may be aggravated by movements such as coughing, sneezing, or sitting.
- Muscle spasm pain is associated with many spine disorders, although its origin may be unclear. This type of back pain is dull and may be accompanied by abnormal posture and taut spinal muscles.

Clients with low back pain report pain ranging from mild discomfort lasting a few hours to chronic debilitating pain. Acute pain is usually caused when the client participates in an activity that is not usually pursued, such as unusual lifting or bending, playing an active sport, or shoveling snow. Manifestations are presented in the box in the next column.

promotes bone and muscle strength and may increase endorphin levels. Therefore, active rehabilitation helps to restore function and reduce pain.

Pain may be relieved by an ice bag or hot water bottle (or heating pad) applied to the back. Exercise programs are helpful provided that the client begins gradually and increases activity gradually as the recovery process continues. Physical therapy procedures include diathermy (deep heat therapy), ultrasonography, hydrotherapy, and transcutaneous electrical nerve stimluation (TENS) units. These therapies reduce the muscle spasms and pain temporarily. They are frequently used in combination with exercise to provide early mobilization for the client.

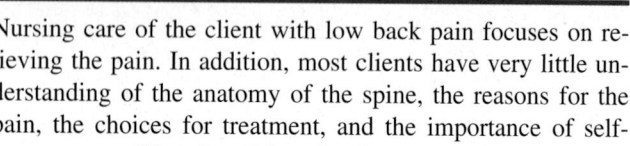

# NURSING CARE

Nursing care of the client with low back pain focuses on relieving the pain. In addition, most clients have very little understanding of the anatomy of the spine, the reasons for the pain, the choices for treatment, and the importance of self-management. Therefore, education is another essential aspect of treating low back pain.

## Health Promotion

Recommendations for preventing back pain from the National Institute of Neurological Disorders and Stroke (2001) include:

- Have a regular exercise program.
- Stretch before working in the yard, jogging, and playing sport.
- Quit smoking.
- Lose weight.
- Maintain a correct posture.
- Use supportive seats when driving.
- Lift by bending at the knees rather than at the waist.
- Reduce emotional stress that causes muscle tension.

In industrial and work settings, nurses should be alert for situations that increase the risk of back pain and injury. Office workers should have chairs with appropriate seat height and length and back support. Modifications of work space or machinery may be necessary for industrial workers to avoid excess stresses on back muscles. Finally, it is important to remember that back pain is a leading cause of lost work time for nurses themselves. Remind coworkers to use good body mechanics and to seek help when lifting or moving clients.

## Nursing Diagnoses and Interventions

### Acute Pain

Muscle spasms and inflammation are among the contributing factors of low back pain.

- Teach the client appropriate comfort measures. *Every client with low back pain has discomfort due to muscle spasms and/or inflammation due to nerve compression, surgery, or irritation from a brace.*
- Instruct the client to take NSAIDs or analgesics on a routine schedule rather than as needed. *Maintaining a constant blood level of the NSAIDs or analgesics reduces inflammation and provides continuous pain relief.*

### Deficient Knowledge

The client with low back pain requires information regarding treatment modalities.

- Encourage clients to remain on bed rest for a limited period. *There is little scientific evidence to show that bed rest is beneficial, but there is ample evidence about the adverse effects of bed rest. Prolonged rest can lead to depression, loss of work, and difficulty in initiating rehabilitation.*
- Teach the client about the "rebound phenomenon" of prolonged heat or ice therapy. *Ice remaining on the skin longer than 15 minutes or heat longer than 30 minutes causes a reverse effect known as the rebound phenomenon. For example, heat produces maximum vasodilation in 20 to 30 minutes. Continuation of the application beyond 30 to 45 minutes causes tissue congestion, and the blood vessels constrict. Likewise, with cold application, maximum vasoconstriction occurs when the skin reaches a temperature of 60°F (15°C). Prolonged cold can create a drop in temperature, at which time vasodilation occurs.*
- Provide instructions about appropriate back exercises such as partial sit-ups with the knees bent and knee-chest exercises to stretch hamstrings and spinal muscles. Each exercise should be done 5 times and gradually increased to 10 times. Advise the client to discontinue any exercise that is painful and to seek professional advice before continuing the exercise. *Repetition of prescribed back exercises, such as the pelvic tilt, partial sit-ups, and back rolls, will strengthen the muscles that protect the spine and thus prevent back strain.*

### Risk for Impaired Adjustment

In the client with low back pain, the need for lifestyle changes may lead to impaired adjustment.

- Teach the client to use appropriate body mechanics in lifting and reaching. The client should be instructed to plan the lift, keep the object being lifted close to the body, and avoid twisting when lifting. Encourage the client to obtain help when lifting. *An item is considered excessively heavy if it equals 35% of the lifter's body weight.*
- Instruct the client to modify the workplace or environment to minimize stress to the lower back. *Lumbar supports in chairs, adjustment of chair or table height, and rubber floor mats help prevent back strain or injury.*
- Encourage obese clients to lose weight. *The trunk of the body must carry excess weight when the client is obese. Obese people are farther away from the objects they lift because of their greater abdominal girth. They may also have more difficulty squatting to lift. The greater the distance between an object and the client's center of gravity, the higher the risk for straining the lower back.*
- Encourage the client to stop smoking. *Research indicates that smoking decreases blood oxygenation to the disc and thereby interferes with repair of the disc and causes premature aging and degeneration. Smokers also cough frequently,*

*which increases the number of pounds of pressure on the disc, increasing disc stress.*

- Instruct client to refrain from prolonged standing or sitting, lying prone, and wearing high heels. *These activities exacerbate back pain.*

## Home Care

Back pain is a common problem in the United States and other industrialized countries. Nurses can have an effect on this significant problem by teaching health practices to prevent back injury to clients of all ages. Teach clients how to safely lift, bend, and turn when engaging in physical activity. Stress the importance of using large muscle groups of the legs to lift rather than bending and lifting with the smaller muscles of the back. Teach other aspects of good body mechanics, including posture, sleeping on a firm mattress, and sitting in chairs that provide good support. Discuss the positive effect of maintaining optimal body weight and good physical fitness.

## THE CLIENT WITH COMMON FOOT DISORDERS

Hallux valgus, hammertoe, and Morton's neuroma are common foot disorders that cause pain or difficulty in walking. All three disorders may be caused by wearing poorly fitting or confining shoes. For this reason, these disorders are more prevalent among women.

## PATHOPHYSIOLOGY

### Hallux Valgus

**Hallux valgus,** commonly called a **bunion,** is the enlargement and lateral displacement of the first metatarsal (the great toe) (Figure 39–12 ■). Hallux valgus develops when chronic pressure against the great toe causes the connective tissue in the sole of the foot to lengthen so that the stabilizing action of the great toe is gradually lost. The toe bends laterally away from the midline of the body, and the metatarsophalangeal joint (MTP) is exposed to friction during walking and becomes en-

larged. As the deformity progresses, calluses form over the metatarsal head, and bursitis develops in the MTP. In severe cases, the lateral displacement of the great toe may approach 70 to 90 degrees, and the second toe may be forced upward, causing hammertoe. Although bunions may be a congenital disorder, most are caused by wearing pointed, narrow-toed shoes or high heels.

Hallux valgus is obvious on physical examination of the foot. The client may report an inability to fit into shoes. Often, the client may report joint pain or pain around calluses. In advanced or severe cases, the first metatarsal joint may have limited range of motion, particularly in dorsiflexion, and crepitus (crackling or popping) may occur during joint movement.

### Hammertoe

**Hammertoe** (claw toe) is the dorsiflexion of the first phalanx with accompanying plantar flexion of the second and third phalanges (Figure 39–13 ■). The condition may affect any toe, but the second toe is most commonly affected. As the deformity begins, clients experience mild inflammation of the synovial membranes of the involved joints. As the deformity progresses, the dorsiflexed joint rubs against the overlying shoe, causing painful corns to develop.

### Morton's Neuroma

**Morton's neuroma** is a tumorlike mass formed within the neurovascular bundle of the intermetatarsal spaces (Figure 39–14 ■). The neuromas usually occur in only one foot, most frequently in the third web space. Like other common foot disorders, Morton's neuroma usually is caused by wearing tight, confining shoes. The condition develops when repeated compression of the toes causes irritation and scarring of tissues surrounding the plantar digital nerve. The affected nerve becomes inflamed and swells. After repeated episodes of inflammation, the nerve fibers become fibrotic, and a neuroma forms.

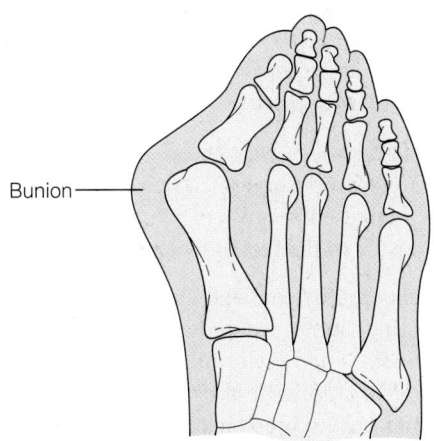

**Figure 39–12** ■ Hallux valgus (bunion).

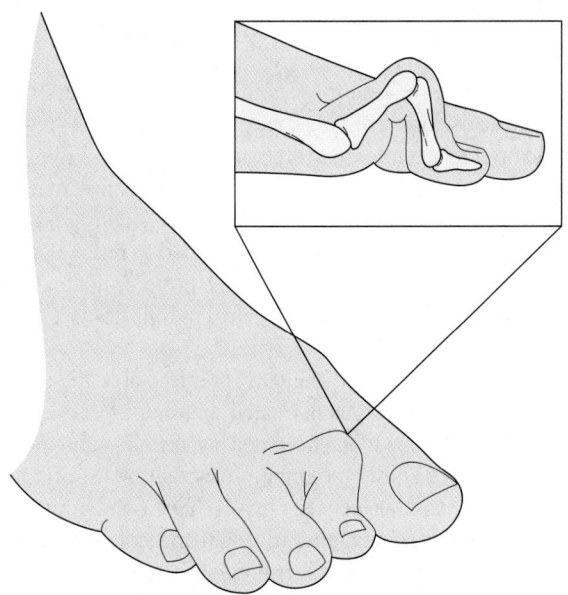

**Figure 39–13** ■ Hammertoe.

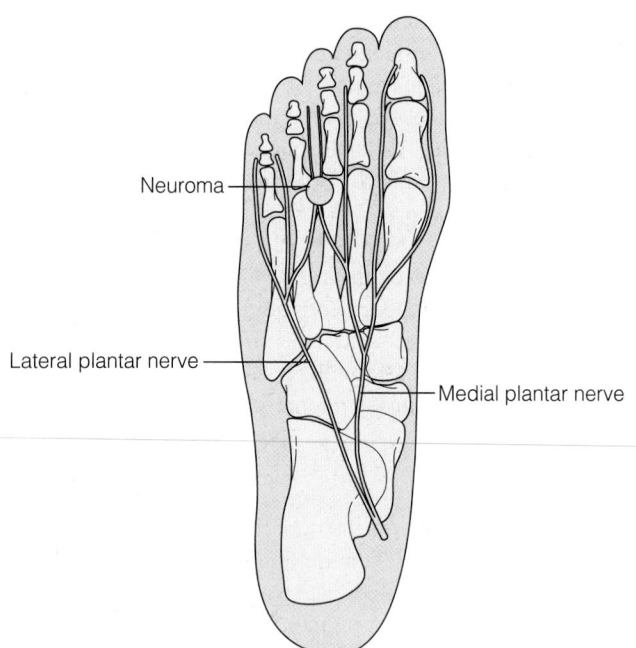

**Neuroma**

**Lateral plantar nerve**

**Medial plantar nerve**

**Figure 39–14 ■** Morton's neuroma.

Manifestations include a burning pain at the web space of the affected foot that radiates into the tips of the involved toes. Weight bearing usually worsens any symptoms; removing the shoe and massaging the foot often relieves the pain. The neuroma may present as a palpable mass between the affected toes. The area over the neuroma usually is tender.

## COLLABORATIVE CARE

Care of the client with common foot disorders such as hallux valgus, hammertoe, and Morton's neuroma focuses on relieving pain, correcting the structural deformity, and preventing reoccurrence. In most cases, all three conditions are diagnosed by inspection; X-ray films of the affected foot are taken if the need for surgery arises.

Conservative treatment for common foot disorders usually involves the use of corrective shoes. Orthotic devices that cushion and stretch the affected joints may be placed within shoes or between the client's toes. For Morton's neuroma, metatarsal pads are used to spread the client's toes and decompress the affected nerve. Analgesics may be prescribed to relieve pain and inflammation. In severe cases, corticosteroid drugs may be injected into the affected joints or surrounding tissue to relieve acute inflammation.

Surgery is reserved for clients with intractable toe deformities or pain. Hallux valgus is treated with bunionectomy; ligaments are lengthened or shortened as needed, and pins are drilled into place so the toe remains in position. Similarly, the correction of hammertoe also involves straightening the affected toe and inserting pins to retain the correction. A cast may be applied over the foot following surgery to correct toe deformities. Surgery for Morton's neuroma causes loss of sen-

sation to a portion of the foot because removing the neuroma involves cutting out a portion of the plantar nerve.

## NURSING CARE

Nursing care for clients with these foot deformities focuses on the same areas because the conservative treatment and preoperative and postoperative interventions are similar.

### Nursing Diagnoses and Interventions

Pain relief, prevention of infection, and client education are important components of the nursing care of these clients.

#### Chronic Pain

In the client with a foot deformity, constant pressure of footwear over the involved joint can cause pain.

- Instruct clients to wear corrective footwear to assist in the conservative treatment of foot problems. *Pain related to foot problems can result from improper footwear that does not provide proper toe room; in addition, heels higher than 1 inch can cause constant flexion and hyperextension problems. In some instances, the client must purchase special shoes or orthotics to ensure correct fit and relief of symptoms. Shoes that fit well and provide enough foot space laterally and dorsally, such as running shoes, are recommended.*
- Provide clients with information about available resources that can help them obtain a proper shoe fit. *Shoe stores have devices for stretching the shoe at the pressure area, but the customer must purchase the shoe before the stretching is done. Shoe repair shops charge a reasonable fee for stretching a shoe. Fabric shoes are the most comfortable shoes for the aged client with bunions because fabric stretches more readily than leather or other synthetic materials.*
- Suggest purchasing appropriate pads to wear over painful bunions, calluses/corns, and the ball of the foot. *Protective pads are manufactured for specific foot problems; these include bunion pads, corn pads, and metatarsal pads.*
- Instruct clients to remove pads and inspect the skin every other day. Clients who have difficulty reaching or observing the involved foot should ask another person to do the inspection for them. *It is very important to emphasize the need for inspection to clients who have experienced loss of sensation of the feet due to such disorders as diabetes and chronic peripheral vascular disease.*

#### Risk for Infection

Like all surgeries, foot surgery carries a risk of infection. This risk may be increased because of impaired peripheral circulation and exposure of the feet to the environment.

- Teach clients proper care and cleaning of exposed pins implanted during the surgical procedure. *Pins inserted into soft tissue of the toes and bones are prone to becoming infected and can potentially result in osteomyelitis.*
- Teach clients how to keep pins and casts dry while bathing or ambulating in inclement weather. Clients must wear a plas-

tic bag over the cast or pins when bathing or walking in rain or snow. *When casts or pins are exposed in water, infection may result.*

## Home Care

For clients in all age groups, teach the importance of well-fitting footwear. Discuss the long-term effects of wearing high-heeled shoes with constricting toes with women in particular. Suggest alternatives for stylish footwear, and encourage clients to wear supportive and nonrestrictive footwear at all times. Discuss the possible effects of bunions on balance, and talk about safety measures to prevent falls and injury. Teach clients techniques to relieve pressure on affected joints.

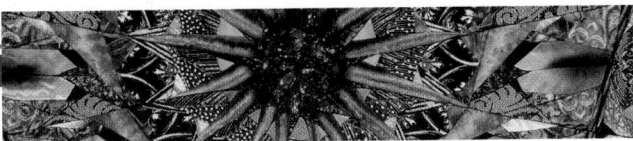

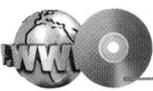

## EXPLORE MediaLink

NCLEX review questions, case studies, care plan activities, MediaLink applications, and other interactive resources for this chapter can be found on the Companion Website at www.prenhall.com/lemone.

Click on Chapter 39 to select the activities for this chapter. For animations, video clips, more NCLEX review questions, and an audio glossary, access the Student CD-ROM accompanying this textbook.

## TEST YOURSELF

1. Although all of the following nursing diagnoses are important when planning care for the client with osteoporosis, which is most significant in terms of long-term disability?

   a. *Chronic pain*
   b. *Risk for falls*
   c. *Activity intolerance*
   d. *Acute pain*

2. You are preparing a teaching plan for a woman with osteoarthritis. Which group of medications should you be prepared to discuss?

   a. Opioids
   b. Antibiotics
   c. Hormones
   d. NSAIDs

3. A postoperative nursing care plan for a client who has had a total knee replacement includes monitoring vital signs and laboratory results. The rationale for these interventions is to:

   a. Reassure the client that blood pressure and pulse are fine
   b. Promote rapport between the client and the health care providers

   c. Ensure adequate circulation to the involved extremity
   d. Prevent the progression of infection (the most common complication)

4. When comparing osteoarthritis and rheumatoid arthritis, what assessment finding would be different in the client with rheumatoid arthritis?

   a. Health history includes general feeling of sickness
   b. Abnormal joint findings are limited to the hands
   c. Stiffness is relieved by activity
   d. Herberden nodes are located on the finger joints

5. *Ineffective protection* is an appropriate nursing diagnosis for the client with SLE. What would be your most important intervention for the hospitalized client?

   a. Monitor laboratory findings
   b. Provide appropriate skin care
   c. Practice careful handwashing
   d. Administer prescribed medications

See Test Yourself answers in Appendix C.

## BIBLIOGRAPHY

Adler, P., Good, M., Roberts, B., & Snyder, S. (2000). Abstract: The effects of Tai Chi on older adults with chronic arthritis pain. *Journal of Nursing Scholarship, 32*(4), 377.

American Cancer Society. (2001). *What is bone cancer?* Available www.cancer.org

Barbieri, R. L. (1998). A step-by-step approach to osteoporosis treatment. *Patient Care, 32*(8), 138–147.

Curry, L., & Hogstel, M. (2002). Osteoporosis. *American Journal of Nursing, 102*(1), 26–33.

Delmas, P. D., & Meunier, P. J. (1997). The management of Paget's disease of bone. *The New England Journal of Medicine, 336*(8), 558–567.

Drugay, M. (1997). Breaking the silence: A health promotion approach to osteoporosis. *Journal of Gerontological Nursing, 23*(6), 36–43.

Garfin, J., & Garfin, S. (2002). Low back pain: Exercises to prevent recurrence. *Consultant, 42*(3), 357–358.

Hill, N., & Davis, P. (2000). Nursing care of total joint replacement. *Journal of Orthopaedic Nursing, 4*(1), 41–45.

Holmes, S. (1998). Osteoporosis: The hidden illness. *Nursing Times, 94*(1), 20–23.

Johnson, M., & Maas, M. (Eds.). (1997). *Nursing outcomes classification (NOC)*. St. Louis: Mosby.

Katz, W. A., & Sherman, C. (1998). Osteoporosis: The role of exercise in optimal management. *The Physician and Sportsmedicine, 26*(2), 33–41.

Kee, C. C., McCoy, S., Rouser, G., Booth, L. A., & Harris, S. (1998). Perspectives on the nursing management of osteoarthritis. *Geriatric Nursing, 19*(1), 19–26.

Kee, J. (2001). *Handbook of laboratory and diagnostic tests with nursing implications* (4th ed.). Upper Saddle River, NJ: Prentice Hall.

Krug, B. (1997). Rheumatoid arthritis and osteoarthritis: A basic comparison. *Orthopaedic Nursing, 16*(5), 73–75.

Mahat, G. (1997). Perceived stressors and coping strategies among individuals with rheumatoid arthritis. *Journal of Advanced Nursing, 25*(6), 1144–1150.

Maher, A., Salmond, S., & Pellino, T. (2002). *Orthopaedic nursing* (3rd ed.). Philadelphia: Saunders.

Mayo Clinic. (2002). *Osteoporosis.* Available www.mayoclinic.com/invoke.cfm?id=DS00128

Matula, P., & Shollenberger, D. (1999). Total joint project: Acute care to home care. *MEDSURG Nursing, 8*(2), 92–98.

McCance, K., & Huether, S. (2002). *Pathophysiology: The biologic basis for disease in adults & children* (4th ed.). St. Louis: Mosby.

McCloskey, J., & Bulechek, G. (Eds.). (2000). *Nursing interventions classification (NIC)* (3rd ed.). St. Louis: Mosby.

Mooney, N. (2001). Pain management in the orthopaedic patient. *Pain Management Nursing, 2*(1), 4–5.

Moss Rehab Resource Net. (2002). *Arthritis fact sheet.* Available www.mossresourcenet.org/arthritis.htm

National Center for Chronic Disease Prevention and Health Promotion. (2002). *Arthritis.* Available www.cdc.gov/ncedphp/arthritis/index.htm

National Center for Chronic Disease Prevention and Health Promotion. (2002). *Chronic diseases and conditions: Arthritis.* Available www.cdc.gov/needphp/major.htm

National Center for Chronic Disease Prevention and Health Promotion. (2002). *Healthy aging: Preventing disease and improving quality of life among older Americans.* Available www.cdc.gov/nccdphp/aag-aging.htm

National Institute of Arthritis and Musculoskeletal and Skin Diseases. (2002). *Questions and answers about fibromyalgia.* Available www.niams.nih.gov/i/topics/fibromyalgia/fibrofs.htm

National Institute of Neurological Disorders and Stroke. (2001). *NINDS back pain information page.* Available www.ninds.nih.gov/health_and_medical disorders/back pain_doc.htm

National Institutes of Health. (2002). *Osteoporosis overview.* Available www.osteo.org/osteo.html

Neuberger, G. B., Press, A. N., Lindsley, H. B., Hinton, R., Cagle, P. E., Carlson, K., Scott, S., Dahl, J., & Kramer, B. (1997). Effects of exercise on fatigue, aerobic fitness, and disease activity measures in persons with rheumatoid arthritis. *Research in Nursing and Health, 20*(3), 195–204.

North American Nursing Diagnosis Association. (2001). *Nursing diagnoses: Definitions and classification, 2001–2002.* Philadelphia: Author.

Overdorf, J., Pachuki-Hyde, L., Kressenich, C., McClung, B., & Lucasey, C. (2001). Osteoporosis: There's so much we can do. *RN, 64*(12), 30–35.

Pachucki-Hyde, L. (2001). Assessment of risk factors for osteoporosis and fracture. *Nursing Clinics of North America, 36*(3), 401–408.

Porth, C. M. (2002). *Pathophysiology: Concepts of altered health states* (6th ed.). Philadelphia: Lippincott.

Raak, R., & Wahren L. (2002). Background pain in fribromyalgia patients affecting clinical examination of the skin. *Journal of Clinical Nursing, 11*(1), 58–64.

Ramsburg, K. (2000). Rheumatoid arthritis. *American Journal of Nursing, 100*(11), 40–43.

Reuters Health. (2002). *Arthroscopic surgery for knee arthritis doubted.* Available www.reutershealth.com

Rizzoli, R., Schaad, M., & Uebelhart, B. (2001). Osteoporosis in men. *Nursing Clinics of North America, 36*(3), 467–479.

Rossiter, R. (2000). Understanding the special needs of the patient with scleroderma. *Australian Nursing Journal, 8*(3), Insert 1–4 (27–30).

Ryan, S. (1996). The role of the nurse in the management of scleroderma. *Nursing Standard, 10*(48), 39–42.

Sedlak, C., & Dohehy, M. (2000). Fashion tips for women with osteoporosis. *Orthopedic Nursing, 19*(5), 31–35.

Shannon, M., Wilson, B., & Stang, C. (2002). *Health professional's drug guide 2002.* Upper Saddle River, NJ: Prentice Hall.

Solomon, J. (1998). Osteoporosis. When supports weaken. *RN, 61*(5), 37–40.

Springhouse. (1998). *Nurse's handbook of alternative & complementary therapies.* Springhouse, PA: Springhouse Corp.

Tierney, L. M., McPhee, S. J., & Papadakis, M. A. (Eds.). (2001). *Current medical diagnosis & treatment (40th ed.).* Stamford, CT: Appleton & Lange.

Weinstein, R. S. (1997). Advances in the treatment of Paget's bone disease. *Hospital Practice, 32*(3), 63–76.

Wright, A. (1998). Nursing interventions with advanced osteoporosis. *Home Healthcare Nurse, 16*(3), 144–151.

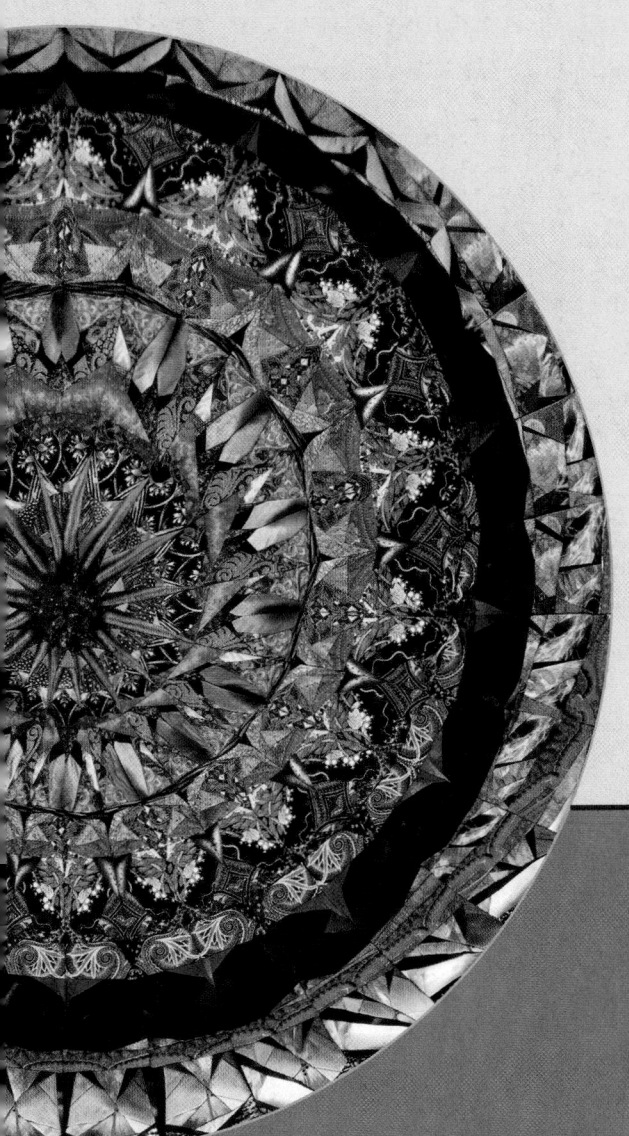

# COGNITIVE AND PERCEPTUAL PATTERNS

# Functional Health Patterns with Related Nursing Diagnoses

### HEALTH PERCEPTION HEALTH MANAGEMENT
- Perceived health status
- Perceived health management
- Health care behaviors: health promotion and illness prevention activities, medical treatments, follow-up care

### VALUE-BELIEF
- Values, goals, or beliefs (including spirituality) that guide choices or decisions
- Perceived conflicts in values, beliefs, or expectations that are health related

### COPING-STRESS-TOLERANCE
- Capacity to resist challenges to self-integrity
- Methods of handling stress
- Support systems
- Perceived ability to control and manage situations

### NUTRITIONAL-METABOLIC
- Daily consumption of food and fluids
- Favorite foods
- Use of dietary supplements
- Skin lesions and ability to heal
- Condition of the integument
- Weight, height, temperature

### Part 5
### Cognitive-Perceptual Patterns
### NANDA Nursing Diagnoses

- Acute Confusion
- Decreased Intracranial Adaptive Capacity
- Autonomic Dysreflexia
- Risk for Autonomic Dysreflexia
- Chronic Confusion
- Impaired Verbal Communication
- Acute Pain
- Chronic Pain
- Impaired Memory
- Unilateral Neglect
- Risk for Peripheral Neurovascular Dysfunction
- Risk for Post-Trauma Syndrome
- Ineffective Protection
- Disturbed Sensory Perception
- Disturbed Thought Processes
- Decisional Conflict
- Risk for Trauma
- Wandering
- Unilateral Neglect
- Impaired Environmental Interpretation Syndrome

### SEXUALITY-REPRODUCTIVE
- Satisfaction with sexuality or sexual relationships
- Reproductive pattern
- Female menstrual and perimeno-pausal history

### ELIMINATION
- Patterns of bowel and urinary excretion
- Perceived regularity or irregularity of elimination
- Use of laxatives or routines
- Changes in time, modes, quality or quantity of excretions
- Use of devices for control

### ROLE-RELATIONSHIP
- Perception of major roles, relationships, and responsibilities in current life situation
- Satisfaction with or disturbances in roles and relationships

### ACTIVITY-EXERCISE
- Patterns of personally relevant exercise, activity, leisure, and recreation
- ADLs which require energy expenditure
- Factors that interfere with the desired pattern (e.g., illness or injury)

### SELF-PERCEPTION–SELF-CONCEPT
- Attitudes about self
- Perceived abilities, worth, self-image, emotions
- Body posture and movement, eye contact, voice and speech patterns

### SLEEP-REST
- Patterns of sleep and rest-/relaxation in a 24-hr period
- Perceptions of quality and quantity of sleep and rest
- Use of sleep aids and routines

### COGNITIVE-PERCEPTUAL
- Adequacy of vision, hearing, taste, touch, smell
- Pain perception and management
- Language, judgment, memory, decisions

*Reprinted from Nursing Diagnosis: Process and Application, 3rd ed., by M. Gordon, pp. 80–96, Copyright © 1994, with permission from Elsevier Science.*

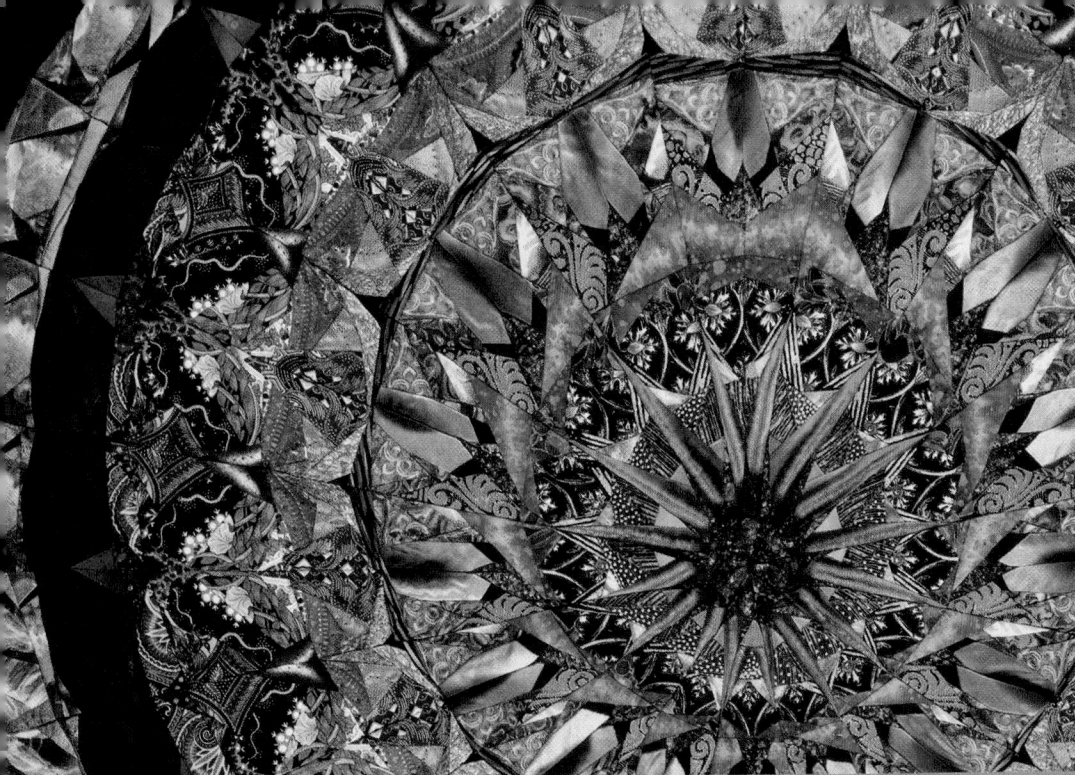

# RESPONSES TO ALTERED NEUROLOGIC FUNCTION

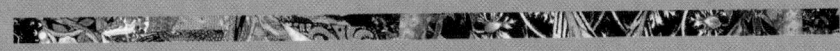

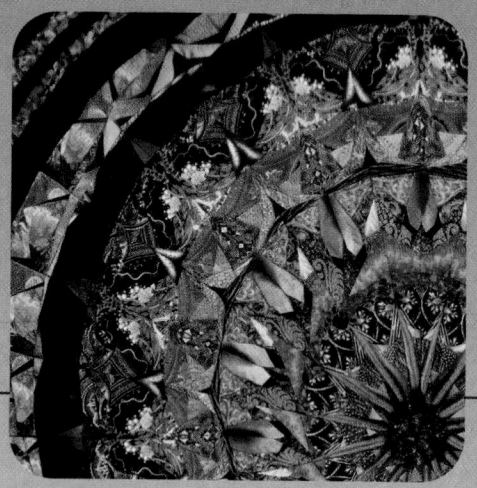

# Assessing Clients with Neurologic Disorders

## MediaLink

**www.prenhall.com/lemone**

Additional resources for this chapter can be found on the Student CD-ROM accompanying this textbook, and on the Companion Website at www. prenhall.com/lemone. Click on Chapter 40 to select the activities for this chapter.

**CD-ROM**
- Audio Glossary
- NCLEX Review

*Animation*
- Nervous System A&P

*Video*
- Extrapyramidal Signs

**Companion Website**
- More NCLEX Review
- Functional Health Pattern Assessment
- Case Study
  Assessing an Unconscious Client

## LEARNING OUTCOMES

After completing this chapter, you will be able to:

- Review the anatomy and physiology of the nervous system.

- Identify specific topics for consideration during a health history assessment interview of the client with neurologic disorders.

- Describe assessment of neurologic function, including examinations of mental status, cranial nerves, sensory nerves, motor nerves, cerebellar function, and reflexes.

- Describe special neurologic examinations for clients with suspected meningeal irritation and for comatose clients.

- Identify abnormal findings that may indicate impairment of neurologic function.

The nervous system regulates and integrates all body functions, mental abilities, and emotions. It collects information from the internal and external environments as sensory input, processes and interprets the input, and causes responses that are manifested as motor or sensory output.

## REVIEW OF ANATOMY AND PHYSIOLOGY

The nervous system is divided into two regions: the central nervous system (CNS), which consists of the brain and spinal cord, and the peripheral nervous system (PNS), which consists of the cranial nerves, the spinal nerves, and the autonomic nervous system. These two highly integrated regions consist of just two types of cells: neurons, which receive impulses and send them on to other cells, and neuroglia, which protect and nourish the neurons.

### Neurons

Each neuron consists of a dendrite, a cell body, and an axon. The dendrite is a short process (projection) from the cell body that conducts impulses toward (afferent) the cell body. Cell bodies, most of which are located within the CNS, are clustered in ganglia or nuclei. The cell bodies and dendrites comprise what is often called the gray matter of the CNS. The axon, a long process, conducts impulses away (efferent) from the cell body. Many axons are covered with a myelin sheath, a white lipid substance. It is interrupted at intervals in unmyelinated areas called nodes of Ranvier, which allow movement of ions between the axon and the extracellular fluid. The myelin sheath serves to increase the speed of nerve impulse conduction in axons and is essential for the survival of larger nerve processes. Myelinated nerve fibers comprise the white matter of the brain and spinal cord.

### Action Potentials

Action potentials are impulses (movements of electrical charge along an axon membrane) that allow neurons to communicate with other neurons and body cells. They are initiated by stimuli and propagated by the rapid movement of charged ions through the cell membrane. When a neuron reaches a certain level of stimulation, an electrical impulse is generated and conducted along the length of its axon. The movement of impulses to and from the CNS is made possible by afferent and efferent neurons. Afferent, or sensory, neurons have receptors in skin, muscles, and other organs and relay impulses to the CNS. Efferent, or motor, neurons transmit impulses from the CNS to cause some type of action.

Nerve impulses occur when a stimulus reaches a point great enough to generate a change in electrical charge across the cell membrane of a neuron. A neuron that is not involved in impulse conduction is in a resting, or polarized, state, in which the number of positive ions in the fluid outside of the cell membrane is greater than in the fluid within the cell. The chief regulators of membrane potential are sodium and potassium: Sodium is the major positive ion in the extracellular fluid, and potassium is the major positive ion in the intracellular fluid. In response to an electrical stimulus, the cell membrane becomes permeable to sodium, which moves into the cell. This changes the polar-

ity of the cell membrane, and the neuron is said to depolarize. This event stimulates an action potential, or a nerve impulse, to travel down the axon. When the charges and ions return to their original resting state, the neuron is repolarized. The events in an action potential are as follows:

- Initially, sodium permeability increases. As the membrane is depolarized, sodium channels open and sodium rushes into the cell to a point of depolarization (the inside of the cell becomes less negative in comparison to the outside of the cell).
- This is followed by a decrease in sodium permeability, lasting only about 1 millisecond. The sodium gates close and the sodium influx stops.
- The final event is an increase in potassium permeability. The potassium gates open, potassium rushes out of the cell, and the cell interior becomes progressively less positive. The membrane potential moves back to its resting state and is repolarized.

The action potential is generated only at the point of the stimulus; but once generated, it is propagated along the entire length of the axon regardless if the stimulus continues. Conduction of the impulse is rapid in myelinated fibers, with the action potential "jumping" from one node of Ranvier to the next. The conduction of the impulse is slower in unmyelinated fibers.

### Neurotransmitters

Neurotransmitters are the chemical messengers of the nervous system. When the action potential reaches the end of the axon at the presynaptic terminal, a neurotransmitter is released and travels across the synaptic cleft to bind with receptors in the postsynaptic neuron dendrite or cell body. The neurotransmitter may either be inhibitory or excitatory. The excitatory neurotransmitter is almost always acetylcholine (ACh), which is rapidly degraded by the enzyme acetylcholinesterase. Norepinephrine (NE) is another major neurotransmitter. It may be either excitatory or inhibitory.

Nerves that transmit impulses through the release of ACh are called cholinergic. Receptors that bind ACh are found in the viscera, skeletal muscle cells, and the adrenal medulla (where they stimulate the release of epinephrine). The effect of ACh binding may be either to stimulate or to inhibit a response.

Nerves that transmit impulses through the release of NE are called adrenergic. Receptors that bind NE are found in the heart, lungs, kidneys, blood vessels, and all target organs stimulated by the sympathetic division except the heart. Adrenergic receptors are further divided into alpha and beta types. Alpha-adrenergic receptors help control such varied functions as arterial vasoconstriction and pupil dilation. Beta-adrenergic fibers may be either beta$_1$ or beta$_2$ receptors. Beta$_1$ receptors are found in the heart, where they regulate the rate and force of contraction. Beta$_2$ receptors are found in receptor cells of the lungs, arteries, liver, and uterus; they help regulate bronchial diameter, arterial diameter, and glycogenesis. Generally, binding of NE to alpha receptors stimulates a response, whereas binding to beta receptors inhibits a response.

Other neurotransmitters include gamma aminobutyric acid (GABA), which inhibits CNS function; dopamine, which may be inhibitory or excitatory and helps control fine movement and emotions; and serotonin, which is usually inhibitory and controls sleep, hunger, and behavior and also affects consciousness.

## The Central Nervous System

The central nervous system (CNS) consists of the brain and spinal cord, highly evolved clusters of neurons which act to accept, interconnect, interpret, and generate a response to nerve impulses originating throughout the body.

### The Brain

The brain is the control center of the nervous system and also generates thoughts, emotions, and speech. Averaging 3 to 4 lb in weight, the brain is surrounded by the skull, a bony structure that provides support and protection. The brain has four major regions: the cerebrum, the diencephalon, the brainstem, and the cerebellum (Figure 40–1 ■). The general functions of these regions are summarized in Table 40–1.

The two hemispheres of the cerebrum account for almost 60% of brain weight. The surface of the cerebrum is folded into elevated ridges of tissue called gyri, which are separated by shallow grooves called sulci. Deep grooves called fissures further divide the surface of the cerebrum. The longitudinal fissure separates the hemispheres, and the transverse fissure separates the cerebrum from the cerebellum. In addition, each cerebral hemisphere is divided into frontal, parietal, temporal, and occipital lobes (Figure 40–2 ■).

The cerebral hemispheres are connected by a thick band of nerve fibers called the corpus callosum, which allows communication between the two hemispheres. Each hemisphere receives sensory and motor impulses from the opposite side of the body. One of the cerebral hemispheres tends to develop

| TABLE 40–1 | General Functions of the Four Regions of the Brain |
|---|---|
| **Region** | **Functions** |
| Cerebrum | Interprets sensory input. Controls skeletal muscle activity. Processes intellect and emotions. Contains skills memory. |
| Diencephalon | Conducts sensory and motor impulses. Regulates autonomic nervous system. Regulates and produces hormones. Mediates emotional responses. |
| Brainstem | Serves as conduction pathway. Serves as site of decussation of tracts. Contains respiratory nuclei. Helps regulate skeletal muscles. |
| Cerebellum | Processes information. Provides information necessary for balance, posture, and coordinated muscle movement. |

more than the other. Most people have a more highly developed left hemisphere, which is responsible for the control of language. The right hemisphere has greater control over nonverbal perceptual functions.

The cerebral cortex is the outer surface of the cerebrum. It consists of neuron cell bodies, unmyelinated fibers, neuroglia, and blood vessels. The functions of the different lobes of the cerebrum and the specific areas of the cerebral cortex are shown in Figure 40–2 and listed in Table 40–2.

The diencephalon is embedded in the cerebrum superior to the brainstem. It consists of the thalamus, hypothalamus, and epithalamus (see Figure 40–1). The thalamus begins to process sensory impulses before they ascend to the cerebral cortex. It

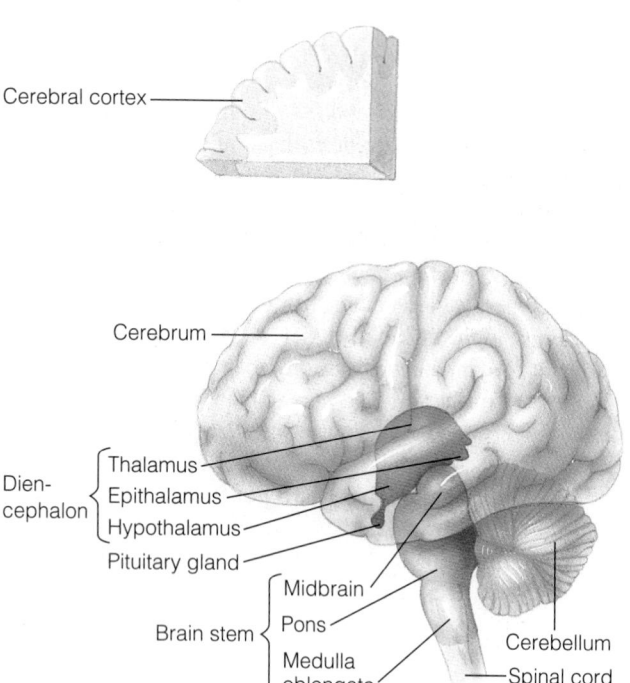

**Figure 40–1** ■ The four major regions of the brain.

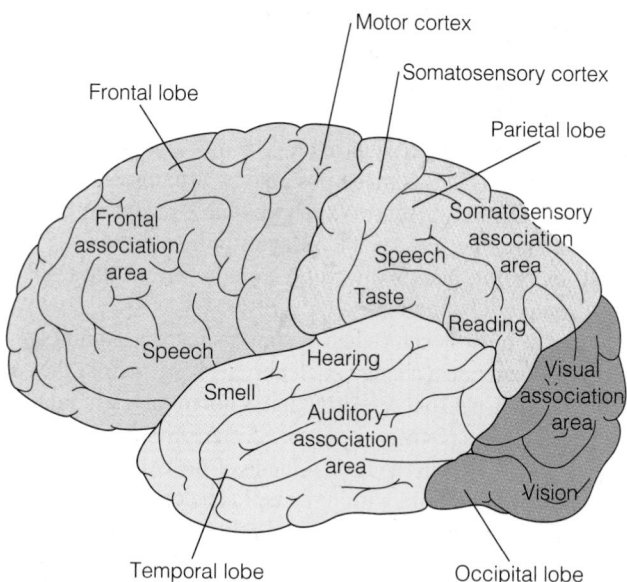

**Figure 40–2** ■ Lobes of the cerebrum and functional areas of the cerebral cortex.

TABLE 40-2 Functions of Lobes of the Cerebrum and Areas of the Cerebral Cortex

| Area | Functions |
|---|---|
| Parietal lobe (somatic sensory area of cerebral cortex) | Promotes recognition of pain, coldness, and light touch. The left side receives input from the right side of the body, and vice versa. |
| Occipital lobe | Receives and interprets visual stimuli. |
| Temporal lobe | Receives and interprets olfactory and auditory stimuli. |
| Frontal lobe | Controls movements of voluntary muscles. |
| Primary motor area | Facilitates voluntary movement of skeletal muscles. |
| Speech area | Promotes understanding of spoken and written words. |
| Motor speech area (Broca's area) | Promotes vocalization of words. |

serves as a sorting, processing, and relay station for input into the cortical region. The hypothalamus, located inferior to the thalamus, regulates temperature, water metabolism, appetite, emotional expressions, part of the sleep-wake cycle, and thirst. The epithalamus forms the dorsal part of the diencephalon and includes the pineal body, which is part of the endocrine system that affects growth and development.

***BRAINSTEM.*** The brainstem consists of the midbrain, pons, and medulla oblongata (see Figure 40–1). The midbrain is a center for auditory and visual reflexes. In addition, it functions as a nerve pathway between the cerebral hemispheres and lower brain. The pons is located just below the midbrain. It consists mostly of fiber tracts, but it also contains nuclei that control respiration. The medulla oblongata, located at the base of the brainstem, is continuous with the superior portion of the spinal cord. Nuclei of the medulla oblongata play an important role in controlling cardiac rate, blood pressure, respiration, and swallowing.

The cerebellum is connected to the midbrain, pons, and medulla. Its functions include coordination of skeletal muscle activity, maintenance of balance, and control of fine movements.

***VENTRICLES.*** The brain contains four ventricles, which are chambers filled with cerebrospinal fluid (CSF). They are linked by ducts that allow the CSF to circulate. One lateral ventricle is located within each hemisphere. These communicate with the third ventricle through the foramen of Monro. The third ventricle communicates with the fourth ventricle through the cerebral aqueduct that runs through the midbrain. The cerebral aqueduct is continuous with the central canal of the spinal cord.

***CEREBROSPINAL FLUID.*** A clear and colorless liquid, cerebrospinal fluid (CSF) is formed by the choroid plexus, which are groups of capillaries located in the brain ventricles. It consists of 99% water and contains protein, sodium, chloride, potassium, bicarbonate, and glucose. The usual amount of CSF

ranges from 80 to 200 mL, averaging about 150 mL, and is replaced several times each day. It is absorbed by arachnoid villi. CSF is normally produced and absorbed in equal amounts. CSF circulates from the lateral ventricles of the cerebral hemispheres into the third ventricle, through the midbrain, and into the fourth ventricle. Some CSF flows down the center of the spinal cord as the rest of it circulates into the subarachnoid space and returns to the blood through the arachnoid villi. CSF forms a cushion for the brain tissue, protects the brain and spinal cord from trauma, helps provide nourishment for the brain, and removes waste products of cerebrospinal cellular metabolism.

***MENINGES.*** The CNS is covered and protected by three connective tissue membranes called meninges. The meninges form divisions within the skull, enclose venous sinuses, and contain CSF. The meninges have three layers (Figure 40–3 ■). The outermost layer is attached to the inner surface of the skull, and the innermost layer is the most external brain covering. The outermost, double layer is the dura mater. The middle layer is the arachnoid mater. It forms a space that contains CSF and is the site of all major cerebral blood vessels. The innermost layer, the pia mater, clings to the brain itself and is filled with small blood vessels.

## Cerebral Circulation and the Blood-Brain Barrier

The cerebral hemispheres receive their blood supply from the anterior and middle internal cerebral arteries. These two arteries are branches of the common carotid arteries. The brainstem and cerebellum receive their blood supply from the basilar

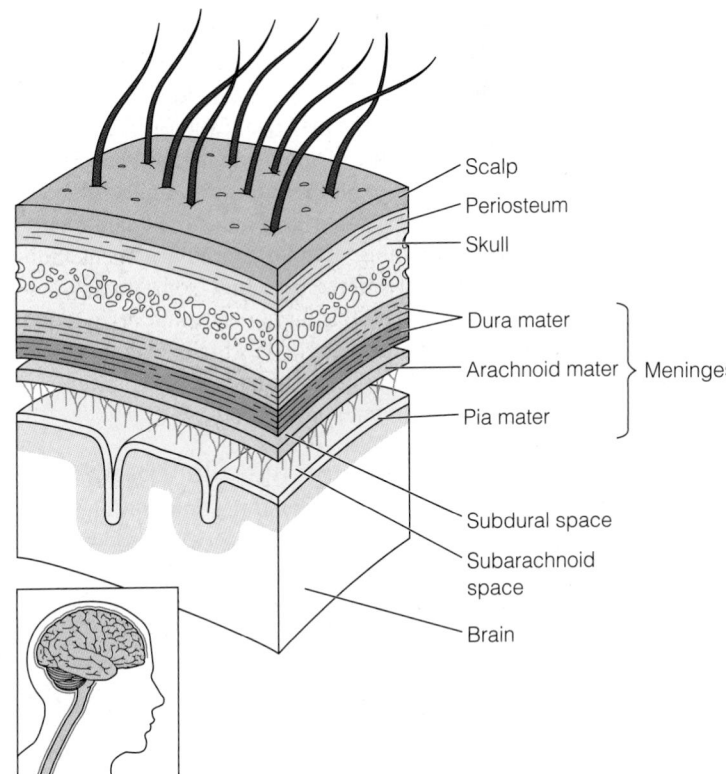

Figure 40-3 ■ Anatomy of the meninges.

**Figure 40–4 ■** Major arteries serving the brain and the circle of Willis.

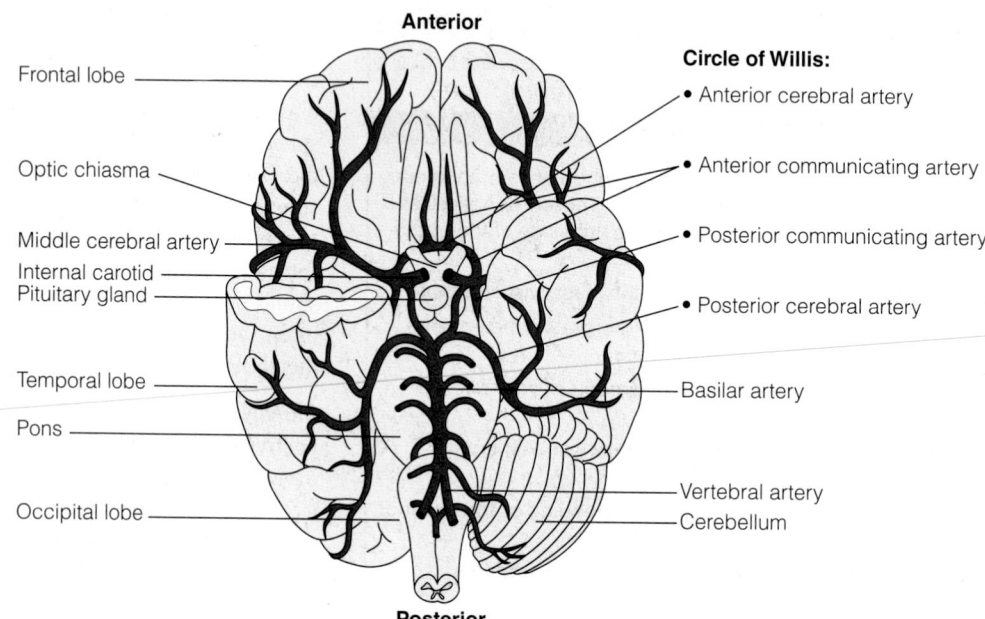

artery. The posterior cerebrum receives blood from the posterior cerebral arteries. These major arteries are connected by small anterior and posterior communicating arteries, which form a circle of connected blood vessels called the circle of Willis (Figure 40–4 ■). This circle serves as a protective device, providing alternative routes for brain tissues to receive their blood supply. The brain receives about 750 mL of blood each minute and uses 20% of the body's total oxygen uptake. The large amount of oxygen is necessary for metabolism of glucose, which is the brain's sole source of energy.

The capillaries in the brain have low permeability because the cells that compose their walls join at very tight junctions and are surrounded by a basement membrane and by the processes of supporting cells in the brain (called astrocytes). As a result, the brain is protected from many harmful substances in the blood. This blood-brain barrier allows lipids, glucose, some amino acids, water, carbon dioxide, and oxygen to pass through it, thus maintaining a controlled environment. Substances such as urea, creatinine, proteins, some toxins, and most antibiotics cannot pass this barrier and enter brain tissue. However, injury to or infection of the brain may cause increased permeability of the blood-brain barrier, altering concentrations of proteins, water, and electrolytes.

### The Limbic System and the Reticular Formation

The limbic system and the reticular formation are functional brain systems. These systems, made of networks of neurons, communicate across areas of the brain.

The limbic system consists of structures that form a ring of tissue in the medial side of each hemisphere, surrounding the upper portion of the brainstem and corpus callosum. The limbic system integrates and modulates input to make up the affective part of the brain, providing emotional and behavioral responses to environmental stimuli.

The reticular formation is located through the central core of the medulla oblongata, pons, and midbrain. This system has widespread connections throughout the brain and relays sensory input from all body systems to all levels of the brain. The reticular formation includes the reticular activating system (RAS). The RAS is a stimulating system for the cerebral cortex, keeping it alert and responsive to incoming sensory stimuli while filtering out repetitive or unwanted stimuli. The sleep center inhibits activity of the RAS and drugs and alcohol may depress it. Other parts of the reticular formation include motor nuclei that help maintain muscle tone and coordinated movements through interconnections with spinal nerves, and the vasomotor and cardiovascular regulatory centers, which are part of autonomic regulation of the cardiovascular system.

### The Spinal Cord

The spinal cord is surrounded and protected by 33 vertebrae, including 7 cervical, 12 thoracic, 5 lumbar, 5 sacral, and 4 fused vertebrae, which form the coccyx. Each vertebra consists of a body and a vertebral arch formed by projections from the body. This arch encloses a space called the vertebral foramen. The vertebral foramina of all the vertebrae form the vertebral canal through which the spinal cord passes. Intervertebral foramina are spaces between the vertebrae through which spinal nerve roots pass as they exit the vertebral column.

Intervertebral discs are located between each of the movable vertebrae. Each disc is made of a thick capsule surrounding a gelatinous core called the nucleus pulposus. Ligaments that provide mobility and protection surround the vertebral column, which is discussed in greater detail in Chapter 42. ⬤

The spinal cord extends from the medulla to the level of the first lumbar vertebra (Figure 40–5 ■). It serves as a center for conducting messages to and from the brain and as a reflex center. The spinal cord is about 17 inches (42 cm) long and 0.75 inch (1.8 cm) thick. The cord is protected by the vertebrae, the meninges, and cerebrospinal fluid. The gray matter of the cord is on the inside, and the white matter is on the outside (the reverse of the arrangement in the brain).

The roots of 31 pairs of spinal nerves, divided into the cervical, thoracic, and lumbar nerves, arise from the cord (see Figure 40–5). Each separates into posterior (sensory) and anterior (motor) roots. Damage to the posterior roots results in loss of sensation, whereas damage to the anterior root results in flaccid paralysis.

## Functions of the Spinal Cord and Spinal Roots

Messages to and from the brain are conducted via ascending (sensory) pathways and descending (motor) pathways (Figure 40–6 ■). The major ascending tracts are the lateral and anterior spinothalamic tracts, which carry sensations for pain, temperature, and crude touch; and the posterior tracts, called the fasciculus gracilis and fasciculus cuneatus, which carry sensations for fine touch, position, and vibration. The lateral and anterior corticospinal (pyramidal) tracts are descending tracts consisting of fibers that originate in the motor cortex of the brain and travel to the brainstem and then down the spinal cord. They mediate voluntary purposeful movements and stimulate certain muscular actions while inhibiting others. They also carry fibers that inhibit muscle tone. The rubrospinal, anterior and lateral reticulospinal, and tectospinal (extrapyramidal) tracts include the pathways between the cerebral cortex, basal ganglia, brainstem, and spinal cord outside the pyramidal tract. They maintain muscle tone and gross body movements.

## Upper and Lower Motor Neurons

Upper motor neurons, such as those of the corticospinal and extrapyramidal tract, carry impulses from the cerebral cortex to the anterior gray column of the spinal cord. Damage to upper motor neurons results in increased muscle tone, decreased muscle strength, decreased coordination, and hyperactive reflexes. Lower motor neurons, such as the peripheral and cranial nerves, begin in the anterior gray column of the spinal cord and end in the muscle. These are the "final common pathways." Damage to lower motor neurons results in decreased muscle tone and loss of reflexes.

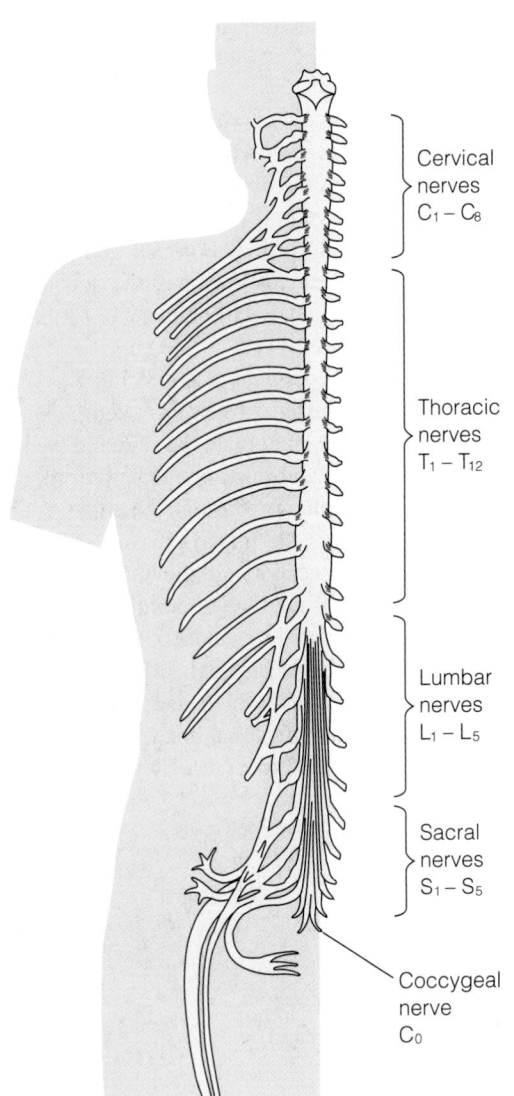

**Figure 40–5** ■ Distribution of spinal nerves.

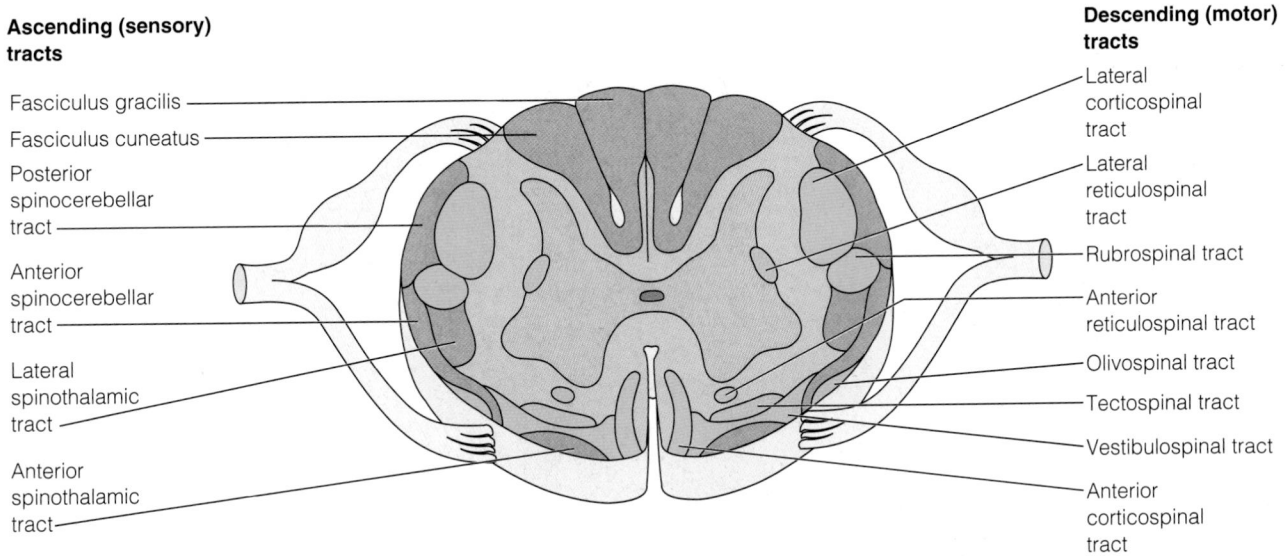

**Figure 40–6** ■ Ascending and descending tracts of the spinal cord.

## The Peripheral Nervous System

The peripheral nervous system (PNS) links the CNS with the rest of the body. It is responsible for receiving and transmitting information from and about the external environment. The PNS consists of nerves, ganglia (groups of nerve cells), and sensory receptors located outside—or peripheral to—the brain and spinal cord. The PNS is divided into a sensory (afferent) division and a motor (efferent) division. Most nerves of the PNS contain fibers for both divisions and all are classified regionally as either spinal nerves or cranial nerves.

### Spinal Nerves

The 31 pairs of spinal nerves (see Figure 40–5) are named by their location:

- Cervical nerves: 8 pairs
- Thoracic nerves: 12 pairs
- Lumbar nerves: 5 pairs
- Sacral nerves: 5 pairs
- Coccygeal nerves: 1 pair

Spinal nerves exit the vertebral column through intervertebral foramina to travel to the body regions they serve. The spinal cord does not reach the end of the vertebral column; as a result, the lumbar and sacral nerve roots travel inferiorly through the vertebral canal for some distance before exiting the vertebral column through their associated intervertebral foramina. This collection of descending nerve roots is called the cauda equina.

Each spinal nerve contains both sensory and motor fibers. The sensory fibers are located in the dorsal root, and their cell bodies are located within the dorsal root ganglion. The motor fibers are located in the ventral root, and their cell bodies are located within the spinal cord. The dorsal and ventral roots merge outside the vertebral canal just past the dorsal root ganglion, forming a spinal nerve. Each spinal nerve further divides into branches called rami.

The ventral rami of the cervical, brachial, lumbar, and sacral regions form complex clusters of nerves called plexuses. The main spinal nerve plexuses innervate the skin and the underlying muscles of the arms and legs. For example, the cervical plexus innervates the diaphragm through the phrenic nerve; the brachial plexus innervates the upper extremities through the median, ulnar, and radial nerves; and the lumbar plexus innervates the anterior thigh through the femoral nerve.

An area of skin innervated by cutaneous branches of a single spinal nerve is called a dermatome. The dorsal roots of the spinal nerves carry sensations from these specific dermatomes. Dermatomes provide anatomical landmarks that are useful for locating neurologic lesions (Figure 40–7 ■).

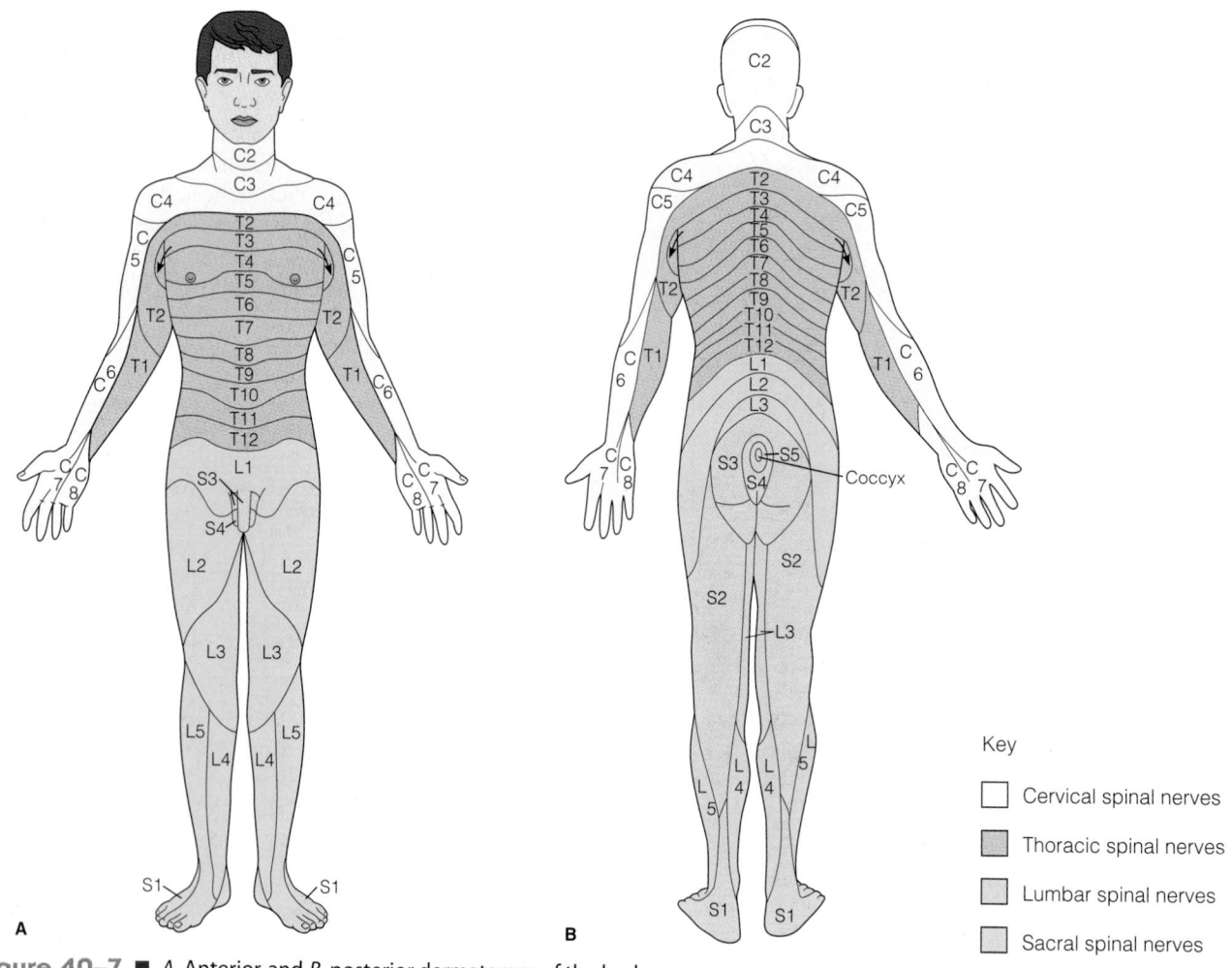

**Figure 40–7** ■ *A*, Anterior, and *B*, posterior dermatomes of the body.

**Figure 40–8** ■ Cranial nerves.

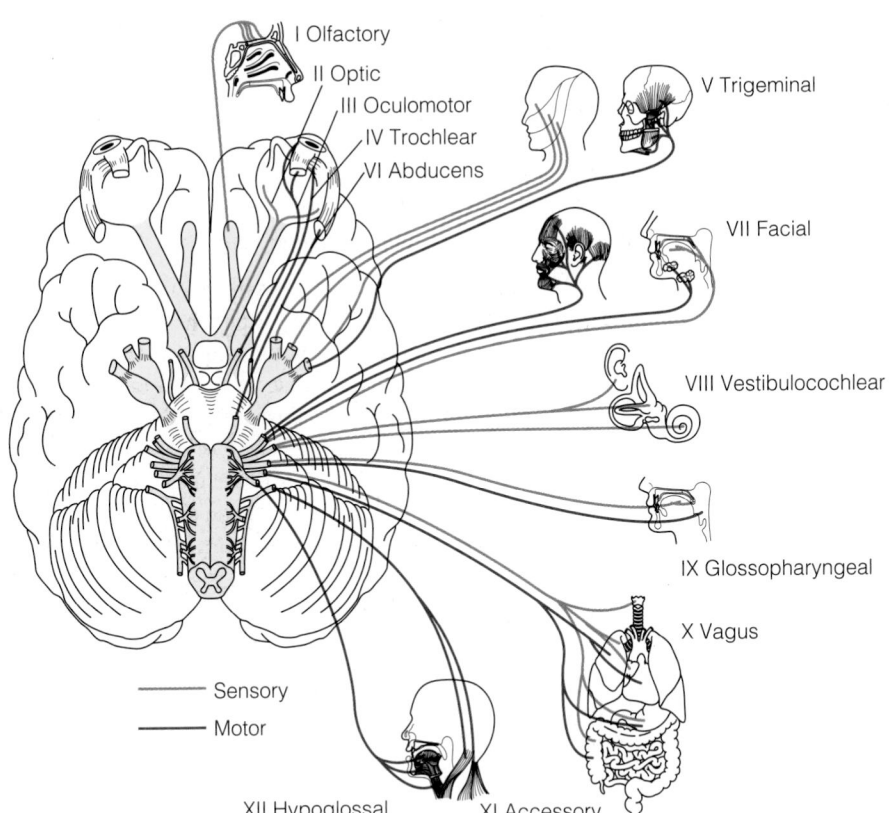

Sensory
Motor

I Olfactory
II Optic
III Oculomotor
IV Trochlear
VI Abducens
V Trigeminal
VII Facial
VIII Vestibulocochlear
IX Glossopharyngeal
X Vagus
XII Hypoglossal
XI Accessory

## Cranial Nerves

Twelve pairs of cranial nerves originate in the forebrain and brainstem (Figure 40–8 ■). The vagus nerve extends into the ventral body cavity, but the 11 other pairs innervate only head and neck regions. Although most are mixed nerves, three pairs (olfactory, optic, and vestibulocochlear) are solely sensory. The cranial nerves and their related functions are listed in Table 40–3.

## Reflexes

A reflex is a rapid, involuntary, predictable motor response to a stimulus. Reflexes are categorized as either somatic or autonomic. *Somatic reflexes* result in skeletal muscle contraction. *Autonomic reflexes* activate cardiac muscle, smooth muscle, and glands. A reflex occurs over a pathway called a reflex arc.

The essential components of a *reflex arc* are a receptor, a sensory neuron to carry afferent impulses to the CNS, an integration center in the spinal cord or brain, a motor neuron to carry efferent impulses, and an effector (the tissue that responds by contracting or secreting) (Figure 40–9 ■).

Somatic reflexes mediated by the spinal cord are called *spinal reflexes.* Many spinal reflexes occur without impulses traveling to and from the brain, with the cord serving as the integration center, while others require brain activity and modulation. *Deep-tendon reflexes (DTRs)* occur in response to muscle contraction and cause muscle relaxation and lengthening. DTRs depend on intact sensory and motor nerve roots, functional synapses in the spinal cord, a functional neuromuscular

junction, and a competent muscle. Thus, an abnormal deep-tendon reflex could indicate a variety of health problems, including a lesion of a spinal nerve. Flexor, or withdrawal, reflexes are caused by actual or perceived painful stimuli and result in withdrawal of the part of the body that is threatened. Superficial responses result from gentle cutaneous stimulation. These responses depend on functional upper motor pathways and on an intact reflex arc.

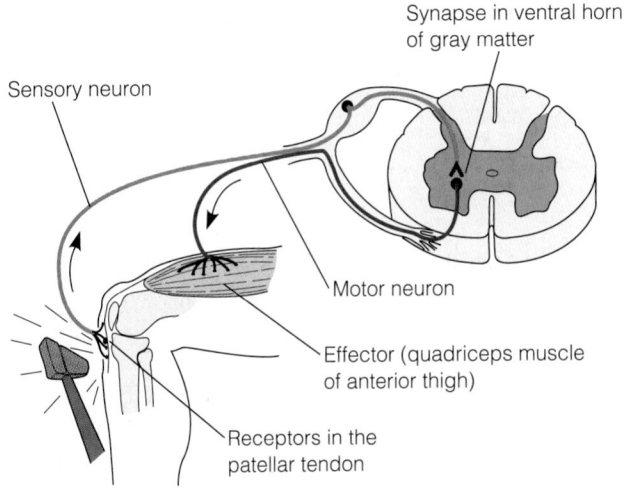

Synapse in ventral horn of gray matter
Sensory neuron
Motor neuron
Effector (quadriceps muscle of anterior thigh)
Receptors in the patellar tendon

**Figure 40–9** ■ A typical reflex arc of a spinal nerve. In the two-neuron reflex arc, the stimulus is transferred from the sensory neuron directly to the motor neuron at the point of synapse in the spinal cord.

| TABLE 40-3 Cranial Nerves | |
|---|---|
| **Name** | **Function** |
| I Olfactory | Sense of smell |
| II Optic | Vision |
| III Oculomotor | Eyeball movement<br>Raising of upper eyelid<br>Constriction of pupil<br>Proprioception |
| IV Trochlear | Eyeball movement |
| V Trigeminal | Sensation of the upper scalp, upper eyelid, nose, nasal cavity, cornea, and lacrimal gland<br>Sensation of the palate, upper teeth, cheek, top lip, lower eyelid, and scalp<br>Sensation of the tongue, lower teeth, chin, and temporal scalp<br>Chewing |
| VI Abducens | Lateral movement of the eyeball |
| VII Facial | Movement of facial muscles<br>Secretions of lacrimal, nasal, submandibular, and sublingual glands<br>Sensation of taste |
| VIII Vestibulocochlear | Sense of equilibrium<br>Sense of hearing |
| IX Glossopharyngeal | Swallowing<br>Gag reflex<br>Secretions of parotid salivary gland<br>Sense of taste<br>Touch, pressure, and pain from pharynx and posterior tongue<br>Pressure from carotid arteries<br>Receptors to regulate blood pressure |
| X Vagus | Swallowing<br>Regulation of cardiac rate<br>Regulation of respirations<br>Digestion<br>Sensation from thoracic and abdominal organs<br>Proprioception<br>Sense of taste |
| XI Accessory | Movement of head and neck<br>Proprioception |
| XII Hypoglossal | Movement of tongue for speech and swallowing |

## The Autonomic Nervous System

The autonomic nervous system (ANS) is a division of the PNS that regulates the internal environment of the body. It is also called the general visceral motor system, because it consists of motor neurons that innervate the body's viscera. Whereas skeletal muscle activity is regulated by a division of the PNS called the somatic nervous system, the ANS regulates the activity of cardiac muscle, smooth muscle, and glands.

The reticular formation in the brainstem is the primary controller of the ANS. Stimulation of centers in the medulla initiates reflexes that regulate cardiac rate, blood vessel diameter, and gastrointestinal function.

The ANS has sympathetic and parasympathetic divisions. Although fibers from both divisions affect the same structures, the actions of the two divisions are opposite in effect, and they serve to counterbalance each other. The major neurotransmitters for impulse transmission in the ANS are acetylcholine and norepinephrine. Acetylcholine is the primary neurotransmitter of the parasympathetic division. Norepinephrine is the primary neurotransmitter of the sympathetic division.

**SYMPATHETIC DIVISION.** The sympathetic division of the ANS prepares the body to handle situations that are perceived as harmful or stressful and to participate in strenuous activity. Cell bodies for this division arise in the lateral horns of the spinal cord in the area from $T_1$ through $L_2$. The fibers separate after leaving the cord, and form a chain of ganglia that extends from the neck to the pelvis. Long fibers then extend to the organs that are supplied by the sympathetic division. Stimulation of the sympathetic division can exert the following effects on target organs or tissues.

- Dilated pupils
- Inhibited secretions
- Copious production of sweat (**diaphoresis**)
- Increased rate and force of heartbeat
- Vasodilation of the coronary arteries
- Dilation of the bronchioles
- Decreased digestion
- Increased release of glucose by the liver
- Decreased urine output
- Vasoconstriction of arteries
- Vasoconstriction of abdominal and skin blood vessels
- Increased blood clotting
- Increased metabolic rate
- Increased mental alertness

**PARASYMPATHETIC DIVISION.** The parasympathetic division of the ANS operates during nonstressful situations. Cell bodies for this division are located in the brainstem (for the cranial nerves) and in the lateral gray matter of $S_2$ through $S_4$. Other than the fibers supplying the cranial nerves III, VII, IX, and X, the fibers are carried by the vagus nerve to body tissues, thoracic organs, and visceral organs. Stimulation of the parasympathetic division of the ANS produces the following effects.

- Constriction of pupils
- Stimulation of glandular secretions
- Decreased heart rate
- Vasoconstriction of coronary arteries
- Constriction of the bronchioles
- Increased peristalsis and secretion of gastrointestinal fluid

## ASSESSING NEUROLOGIC FUNCTION

The client's neurologic system is assessed by both a health assessment interview to collect subjective data and a physical assessment to collect objective data.

### Health Assessment Interview

This section provides guidelines for collecting subjective data through a health assessment interview specific to the functions

| TABLE 40-4 | Glasgow Coma Scale | |
|---|---|---|
| **Assessment** | **Response** | **Score*** |
| **Eyes open** (Record C if eyes are closed by swelling.) | Spontaneously | 4 |
| | To speech | 3 |
| | To pain | 2 |
| | No response | 1 |
| **Best motor response** (Record best upper arm response.) | Obeys commands | 6 |
| | Localizes pain | 5 |
| | Flexion-withdrawal | 4 |
| | Abnormal flexion | 3 |
| | Abnormal extension | 2 |
| | No response | 1 |
| **Best verbal response** (Record T if an endotracheal or tracheostomy tube is in place.) | Oriented | 5 |
| | Confused | 4 |
| | Inappropriate words | 3 |
| | Incomprehensible sounds | 2 |
| | No response | 1 |
| **Total Score:** | | —— |

*A higher score indicates a higher level of functioning.

of the neurologic system. If the client's level of consciousness is altered, the nurse may need to rely on family members for information. The client's level of consciousness may be assessed by using the Glasgow Coma Scale, found in Table 40–4.

An interview to assess neurologic function may focus on a chief complaint or may be done as part of a total health assessment. If the client has a health problem involving any component of neurologic function, analyze its onset, characteristics and course, severity, precipitating and relieving factors, and any associated symptoms, noting the timing and circumstances. For example, ask the client the following:

- Describe the location and intensity of the pain you have experienced in your left leg. Is it made worse by coughing, sneezing, or walking?
- When did you first notice that you were having numbness in your fingers?
- Describe the difficulty you have when you try to walk.

Questions about present health status include information about numbness, tingling sensations, tremors, problems with coordination or balance, or loss of movement in any part of the body. Ask the client about difficulty with speaking, seeing, hearing, tasting, or detecting odors. In addition, elicit information about memory, feeling state (such as anxiety or depression), recent changes in sleep patterns, ability to perform self-care and activities of daily living, sexual activity, and weight. If the client is taking prescribed or over-the-counter medications, ask about the type and purpose, as well as the frequency and duration of use.

Ask about any past history of seizures, fainting, dizziness, headaches, and any trauma, tumors, or surgery of the brain, spinal cord, or nerves. Discuss illnesses that may cause neurologic manifestations, including cardiac disease, strokes, pernicious anemia, sinus infections, liver disease, and/or renal failure. Also ask the client about family history of neurologic health

problems, diabetes mellitus, hypertension, seizures, or mental health problems.

Question the client about occupational hazards, such as exposure to toxic chemicals or materials, use of protective headgear, and the amount of time spent performing repetitive motions (e.g., data entry and assembly). Ask questions about self-care to assess the client's diet and use of tobacco, drugs, or alcohol, and ask whether the client wears a helmet when riding a bike or motorcycle or participating in contact sports.

Interview questions categorized by functional health patterns can be found on the Companion Website.

## Physical Assessment

Physical assessment of the client begins when the nurse first meets the client and makes an overall evaluation of the client's mental and physical status. The mental status examination is conducted with both the nurse and the client seated. The rest of the neurologic examination may be performed with the client either sitting or standing.

The neurologic system is assessed through inspection, palpation, and percussion (with a reflex hammer). When conducting the mental status and cognitive portions of the examination, be aware that fatigue or illness may alter findings. Provide rest periods for the client as needed. When interpreting findings, consider the client's age, educational background, and cultural orientation.

Collect the equipment necessary for this assessment: a cotton ball and safety pin, tongue blade, tuning fork, ophthalmoscope, reflex hammer, pencil and paper, printed materials, and substances to test the senses of smell and taste. The assessment should take place in a private, comfortable setting. Ask the client to remove outer clothing, shoes, and stockings. Provide a gown for the client to wear. It is important to explain to the client that the neurologic examination is lengthy and may consist of questions and requests that seem strange to the client. Explain the rationale for each part of the examination.

A brief version of this physical assessment, often referred to as a *neuro check,* may be performed in a shorter time period when a client requires frequent ongoing assessments of neurologic status (Box 40–1).

### Mental Status Assessment with Abnormal Findings (✓)

- Assess appearance.
- Observe dress, hygiene, and grooming.

| BOX 40–1 | ■ Abbreviated Neurologic Assessment (Neuro Check) |
|---|---|

1. Assess level of consciousness (response to auditory and/or tactile stimulus).
2. Obtain vital signs (BP, P, R).
3. Check pupillary response to light.
4. Assess strength of hand grip and movement of extremities bilaterally.
5. Determine ability to sense touch/pain in extremities.

Medialink | FUNCTIONAL HEALTH PATTERN ASSESSMENT

- Observe gait and posture.
  - ✓ Unilateral neglect (inattention to one side of body) may occur with some strokes of the middle cerebral artery. Poor hygiene and grooming may be seen in clients with dementing disorders.
  - ✓ Abnormal gait and posture may be seen in transient ischemic attacks (TIAs), strokes, and Parkinson's disease.
- Assess behavior.
  - Observe client's actions and affect.
  - Note the content and quality of speech.
  - Note level of consciousness. Use the Glasgow Coma Scale (see Table 40–4) to document findings. Scores may range from 3 (deeply comatose) to 15 (alert and oriented).
  - ✓ Emotional swings or changes in personality may be observed with strokes of the anterior cerebral artery.
  - ✓ The face appears masklike (very little expressive movement of facial muscles) in clients with Parkinson's disease.
  - ✓ Apathy is seen in dementing disorders.
  - ✓ Aphasia (defective or absent language function) may occur in TIAs. Receptive aphasia (inability to understand verbal or written language) is often noted in strokes of the posterior or anterior cerebral artery. Aphasias are seen with damage to the left cerebral cortex. Aphasias are more often seen with strokes of the right hemisphere than the left hemisphere.
  - ✓ Dysphonia (change in the tone of the voice) is common in strokes of the posterior inferior cerebral artery. Dysphonia is seen with paralysis of the vocal cords (cranial nerve X).
  - ✓ Dysarthria (difficulty speaking) is seen with lesions of upper and lower motor neurons, the cerebellum, and the extrapyramidal tract. It is also seen in strokes of the anterior inferior and superior cerebral arteries.
  - ✓ Damage to the brainstem and/or cerebral cortex may alter level of consciousness.
  - ✓ Drowsiness and decreased level of consciousness may be associated with brain trauma, infections, TIAs, stroke, and brain tumors.
  - ✓ Level of consciousness is usually altered and may progress to coma with stroke of the middle cerebral artery.
  - ✓ Confusion and coma may be seen in clients with strokes affecting the vertebralbasilar arteries.
- Assess cognitive function.
  - Note orientation to time, place, and person.
  - Note attention span and recent and remote memory. Ask the client to:
    1. Repeat five to seven numbers.
    2. Recall three items after 5 minutes.
    3. Recall his or her address, breakfast, or birthday.
  - Assess thought processes (both content and perceptions) by noting responses to questions.
  - Note ability to understand what is said and to express thoughts.
  - Note ability to make logical and safe judgments.
  - ✓ Disorientation to time and place may occur in clients with stroke of the right cerebral hemisphere.
  - ✓ Memory deficits are often seen with strokes of the anterior cerebral artery and vertebralbasilar artery.

- ✓ Perceptual deficits may be seen in strokes of the middle cerebral artery. These same deficits may occur following brain trauma and in dementing disorders.
- ✓ Impaired cognition is often noted with strokes of the middle cerebral artery, cerebral trauma, and brain tumors.

## Cranial Nerve Assessments with Possible Abnormal Findings (✓)

- Test CN I (olfactory).
- Note client's ability to smell scents (e.g., soap, coffee) with each nostril. This test is usually done only if a problem with the ability to smell is reported.
  - ✓ Anosmia (an inability to smell) may be seen with lesions of the frontal lobe and may also occur with impaired blood flow to the middle cerebral artery.
- Test CN II (optic).
  - Assess vision with Snellen chart (see Chapter 44 ⌘ for guidelines).
  - ✓ Blindness in one eye may be seen with strokes of the internal carotid artery or with TIAs. Impaired vision or blindness in one side of both eyes (homonymous hemianopia) is associated with blockage of the posterior cerebral artery.
  - ✓ Impaired vision may also be seen with strokes of the anterior cerebral artery and brain tumors.
  - ✓ Blindness or double vision may be noted with involvement of the vertebralbasilar arteries. Double or blurred vision may also occur with TIAs.
  - ✓ Papilledema (swelling of the optic nerve) occurs with increased intracranial pressure.
- Test CN III, IV, and VI (oculomotor, trochlear, and abducens).
  - Assess extraocular movements by asking the client to follow your finger as you write an *H* in the air (see Chapter 44).
  - Assess PERRL ("pupils equally round and reactive to light") by covering one eye at a time and shining a bright light directly into the uncovered eye (use a penlight or the ophthalmoscope). See Chapter 44 for more detailed assessment guidelines.
  - Assess for ptosis (drooping eyelids).
  - ✓ Nystagmus (involuntary eye movement) may be seen with strokes of the anterior, inferior, and superior cerebellar arteries. Constricted pupils are associated with impaired blood flow to the vertebralbasilar arteries. Ptosis (also called Horner's syndrome) occurs with strokes of the posterior inferior cerebellar artery, myasthenia gravis, and palsy of CN III.
- Test CN V (trigeminal).
  - Assess ability to feel light, dull, and sharp sensations on the face. With the client's eyes closed, check whether sensation is the same on both sides of the face. Stroke the cheek with a wisp of cotton for light touch, with a closed safety pin for dull touch, and with a tongue blade for sharp touch. If the sharp point of a safety pin is used to assess sharp touch, be sure to avoid scratching the surface of the skin, and discard the pin after it is used.
  - Assess the corneal reflex by touching the corneal surface with a wisp of cotton. This reflex is tested on unconscious clients. Normally the client blinks.

✓ Changes in facial sensations are noted with impaired blood flow to the carotid artery.

✓ Decreased sensations to the face and cornea on the same side of the body occur with strokes of the posterior inferior cerebral artery.

✓ Lip and mouth numbness occur with strokes of the vertebralbasilar artery.

✓ Loss of facial sensation or contraction of the masseter and temporal muscles is seen with lesions of CN V.

✓ Severe facial pain is seen with trigeminal neuralgia (tic douloureux).

✓ The corneal reflex may be impaired with lesions of CN V or VII.

• Test CN VII (facial).
  • Assess ability to taste sweet, sour, and salt on the anterior two-thirds of the tongue by asking the client to stick out the tongue and applying a salty, sweet, or sour substance.
  • Assess ability to frown, show teeth, blow out cheeks, raise eyebrows, smile, and close eyes tightly.
  ✓ Loss of ability to taste may occur with brain tumors or with nerve impairment.
  ✓ Asymmetry or decreased movement of facial muscles is noted with lesions of the upper and lower motor neurons.
  ✓ Paralysis of the lower motor neurons results in the inability to close eyes, a flat nasolabial fold, paralysis of lower face, and inability to wrinkle forehead.
  ✓ Paralysis of the upper motor neurons results in weakness of eyelids and paralysis of lower face.
  ✓ Pain, paralysis, and sagging of facial muscles is seen on the affected side in Bell's palsy.

• Test CN VIII (acoustic).
  • Assess ability to hear the ticking of a watch and whispered and spoken words (see Chapter 44).
  ✓ Decreased hearing or deafness may occur with strokes of the vertebralbasilar arteries and/or tumors of CN VIII.

• Test CN IX and X (glossopharyngeal and vagus).
  • Observe client swallowing a small drink of water.
  • Observe for a symmetrical rise of the soft palate and uvula as the client says "ah."
  • Assess gag reflex by touching back of client's throat with tongue blade.
  • Assess ability to taste salty, sweet, and sour substances on the posterior third of the tongue (see previous description).
  ✓ **Dysphagia** (difficulty swallowing) is common with impaired blood flow to the vertebralbasilar arteries and to the posterior inferior, anterior inferior, or superior cerebellar arteries.
  ✓ Unilateral loss of the gag reflex occurs with lesions of CN IX and X.

• Test CN XI (spinal accessory).
  • Assess the client's ability to shrug the shoulders and turn head against resistance: Ask the client to turn the head to one side against the resistance of your hand; ask the client to shrug the shoulders while you exert downward pressure. Observe symmetry, strength, and size of muscles.
  ✓ Muscle weakness is noted with lower motor neuron disease. Contralateral hemiparesis is seen with strokes affecting the middle or internal carotid artery.

• Test CN XII (hypoglossal).
  • Assess the client's ability to stick out the tongue and move the tongue from side to side against resistance of a tongue blade.
  ✓ Atrophy and **fasciculations** (twitches) of the tongue are seen in lower motor neuron disease. The tongue may deviate toward involved side of the body.

### Sensory Function Assessments with Abnormal Findings (✓)

• Assess ability to perceive various sensations.
  • Touch both sides of various parts of the body (the chest, abdomen, arms, and legs) with one or more of the following:
    1. Cotton wisp
    2. Sharp object
    3. Dull object
    4. Vibrating tuning fork placed on bony prominences
  ✓ Decreased sensation of pain occurs with injury to the spinothalamic tract.
  ✓ Decreased vibratory sensations are seen with injuries to the posterior column tract.
  ✓ Transient numbness of face, arm, or hand is seen with TIAs.
  ✓ Sensory loss on one side of the body is seen with lesions of higher pathways to the spinal cord.
  ✓ Bilateral sensory loss is seen in polyneuropathy. Sensations are impaired with strokes, brain tumors, and spinal cord trauma or compression.

• Assess sense of position (**kinesthesia**).
  • Move the client's finger or big toe up or down. Ask the client to describe the movement.
  ✓ Lesions of the posterior column of the spinal cord may affect sense of position.

• Assess ability to discriminate fine touch.
  • Ask the client to identify:
    1. Object in hand, such as a coin or key (tests stereognosis).
    2. Number written on hand (tests graphesthesia) (Figure 40–10 ■).

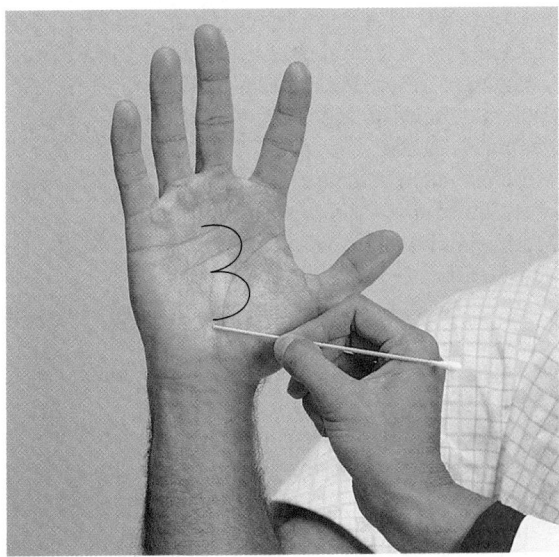

**Figure 40–10** ■ Testing graphesthesia.

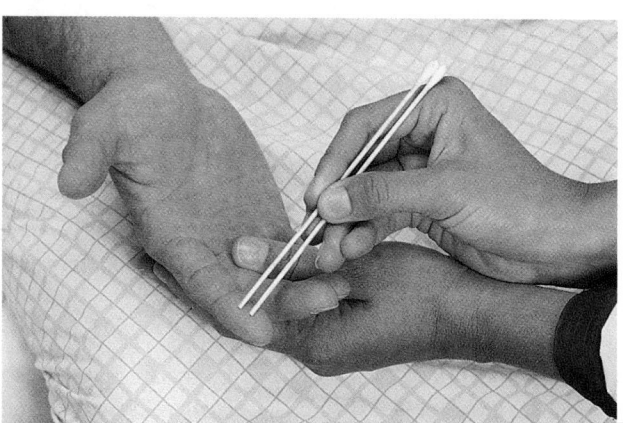

**Figure 40–11** ■ Testing two-point discrimination.

3. Two points of simultaneous pinpricks on the hand (tests two-point discrimination) (Figure 40–11 ■).
4. Where he/she is being touched (tests localization).
5. How many sensations are felt when touched simultaneously on both sides of the body (tests extinction).
✓ Inability to discriminate fine touch (stereognosis, graphesthesia, two points, point localization and extinction) may occur with injury to the posterior columns or sensory cortex.

## Motor Function Assessments with Abnormal Findings (✓)

• Assess bilateral symmetry and size of muscles.
   ✓ Atrophy of muscles is seen with disease of the lower motor neurons.
• Assess for **tremors** (rhythmic movements) and fasciculations. Observe movements as client is at rest (not making a purposeful movement) and with activity (making a purposeful movement, such as reaching for a glass of water).
   ✓ Tremors that occur with activity are seen in multiple sclerosis and disease of the cerebellar system.
   ✓ Tremors that occur at rest and disappear with movement are common in Parkinson's disease.
   ✓ Fasciculations occur in disease or trauma to the lower motor neurons, as a side effect of medications, in fever, in sodium deficiency, and in uremia.
• Assess muscle tone.
   ✓ Muscle tone is decreased (**flaccidity**) in disease or trauma of the lower motor neurons and early stroke.
   ✓ Muscle tone is increased (**spasticity**) in disease of the corticospinal motor tract.
   ✓ Muscles are rigid in disease of the extrapyramidal motor tract.
   ✓ Muscles move in small, regular jerky movements (cogwheel rigidity) in Parkinson's disease.
• Assess bilateral muscle strength and movement. The following criteria for recording the grading of muscle strength are often used.
   0 = no contraction
   1 = trace of contraction
   2 = active movement with gravity

3 = active movement against gravity
4 = active movement against gravity and resistance
5 = normal power

Ask the client to:

1. Squeeze your hands.
2. Push feet against the resistance of your hands.
3. Raise both legs off the bed.
✓ Weakness of the arms, legs, or hands is often seen with TIAs. **Hemiplegia** (paralysis of one-half of the body vertically) is noted with strokes of the internal carotid artery and posterior cerebral artery.
✓ Weakness of extremities is often noted with strokes of the vertebralbasilar arteries.
✓ Flaccid paralysis is noted with strokes of the anterior spinal artery.
✓ Paralysis or decreased movement is seen in multiple sclerosis and myasthenia gravis.
✓ There is total loss of motor function below the level of injury in complete spinal cord transection and in injuries to the anterior portion of the spinal cord.
✓ Spasticity of muscles may occur as a result of incomplete spinal cord injuries.

## Cerebellar Function Assessments with Abnormal Findings (✓)

• Assess the gait. Ask the client to walk normally, then in a heel-to-toe fashion, then on toes, and finally on heels.
• Perform Romberg's test: Ask the client to stand with the feet together and eyes closed. (Stand close to client to prevent falling). There should be minimal swaying for up to 20 seconds.
   ✓ **Ataxia** is a lack of coordination and a clumsiness of movements, with staggering, wide-based, and unbalanced gait. Ataxia is often seen with anterior strokes and cerebellar tumors. Swaying and falling is seen in cerebellar ataxia. Inability to walk on toes, then heels may indicate disease of the upper motor neurons.
   ✓ Spastic hemiparesis is often associated with strokes or upper motor neuron disease. The client walks with one leg stiffly dragging while the other leg circles out and forward. One arm is held flexed and close to the side.
   ✓ Steppage gait is noted with disease of the lower motor neurons. The client drags or lifts the foot high, then slaps the foot onto the floor. The client cannot walk on the heels.
   ✓ Sensory ataxia may be associated with polyneuropathy or damage to the posterior columns. The client walks on the heels before bringing down the toes and the feet are held wide apart. Gait worsens with the eyes closed.
   ✓ Parkinsonian gait is often seen in Parkinson's disease. The client stoops over while walking and shuffles the feet. The arms are held close to the side.
   ✓ A positive Romberg's test may be seen in cerebellar ataxia.
• Assess coordination.
   • Observe ability to pat knees, alternating front and back of hands and increasing speed.
   • Observe ability to touch each finger of one hand to the thumb.

 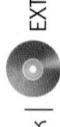

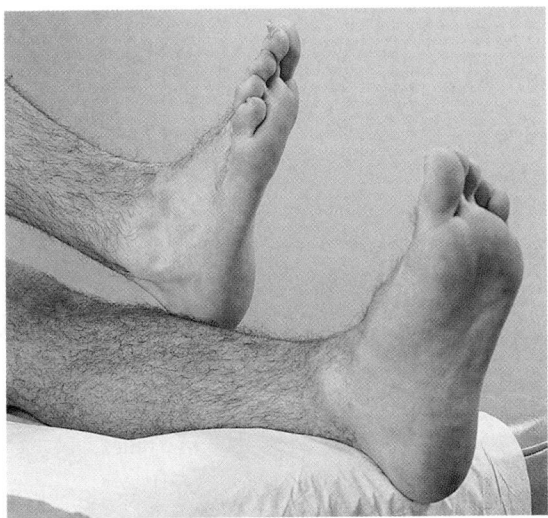

**Figure 40–12** ■ Heel-to-shin test.

- Observe ability to touch the nose, then one of your fingers, then the nose again.
- Observe ability to run each heel down each shin, while in a supine position (Figure 40–12 ■).
  ✓ Ataxic movements are apparent in cerebellar disease.

## Reflex Assessments with Abnormal Findings (✓)

A reflex hammer is used to strike the tendon of various reflex sites. To test deep-tendon reflexes, ask the client to lock the fingers of both hands together and then pull; this encourages relaxation and promotes reflexes of lower extremities. Superficial reflexes are assessed by lightly stroking the area with the end of a tongue blade. The following criteria for recording reflexes are often used. A score of 2 is considered normal.

0 = absent or no response
1 = hypoactive; weaker than normal (+)
2 = normal (++)
3 = stronger than normal (+++)
4 = hyperactive (++++)

- Assess the patellar, biceps, brachioradialis, triceps, and achilles deep-tendon reflexes (Figure 40–13 ■).
  ✓ Hyperactive reflexes are present with lesions of upper motor neurons.
  ✓ Decreased reflexes are present with lower motor neuron involvement.
- Assess for clonus by dorsiflexing the client's foot.
  ✓ **Clonus,** a hyperactive, rhythmic dorsiflexion and plantar flexion of the foot, is noted with upper motor neuron disease.

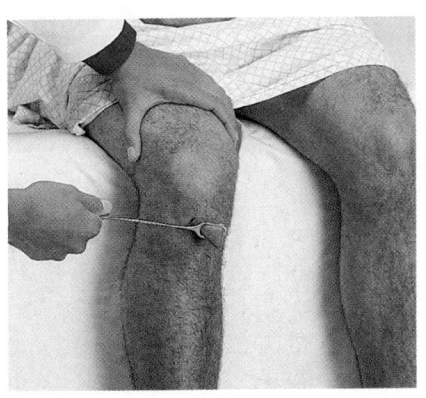

**A**

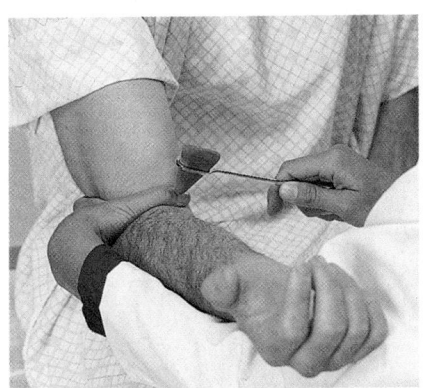

**B**

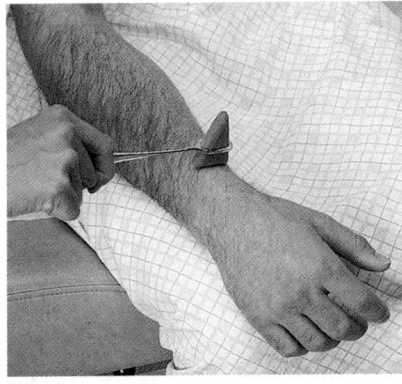

**C**

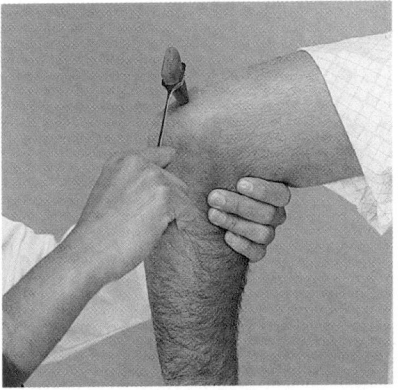

**D**

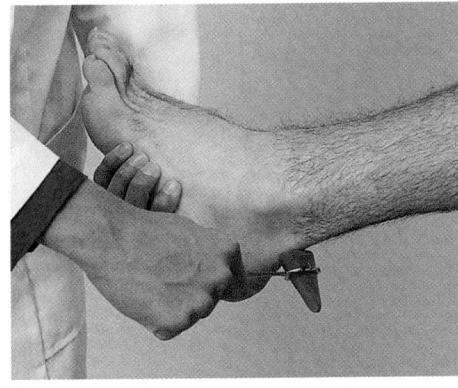

**E**

**Figure 40–13** ■ Deep-tendon reflexes. *A,* Using reinforcement technique to test the patellar reflex. *B,* Biceps reflex. *C,* Brachioradialis reflex. *D,* Triceps reflex. *E,* Achilles reflex.

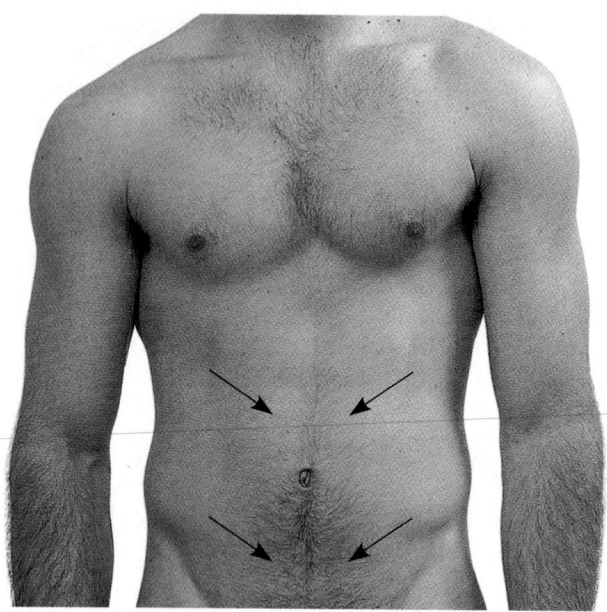

**Figure 40–14** ■ Location of superficial abdominal reflexes.

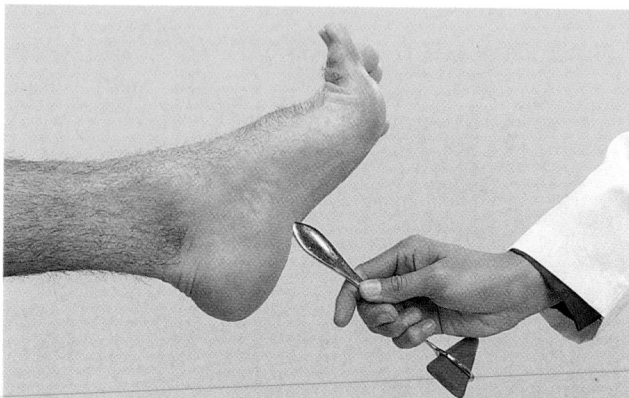

**Figure 40–15** ■ Testing for the Babinski reflex.

- Assess the superficial abdominal and cremasteric reflexes.
  - Abdominal reflex: Lightly stroke the abdomen with a tongue blade from the side to the midline. Normally the side of the abdomen being stroked will contract (Figure 40–14 ■).
  - Cremasteric reflex: Lightly stroke the inner thigh of the male client with a tongue blade. Normally, the testicle on the side being stroked will rise.
  - ✓ Superficial reflexes may be absent with disease of the lower and upper motor neurons.
- Assess the Babinski reflex (Figure 40–15 ■).
  - ✓ Dorsiflexion of the big toe and fanning of the other toes is seen with upper motor neuron disease of the pyramidal tract.

## Special Neurologic Assessments with Abnormal Findings (✓)

- Assess for Brudzinski's sign. With the client supine, flex the head to the chest (Figure 40–16 ■).
  - ✓ Pain, resistance, and flexion of hips and knees occur with meningeal irritation.
- Assess for Kernig's sign. With the client supine, flex the knees and hips, then straighten the knee (Figure 40–17 ■).
  - ✓ Excessive pain and/or resistance occurs with meningeal irritation.
- Assess for abnormal postures.
  - Observe for **decorticate posturing,** in which the upper arms are close to the sides; the elbows, wrists, and fingers are flexed; the legs are extended with internal rotation; and the feet are plantar flexed (Figure 40–18 ■).
  - Observe for **decerebrate posturing,** in which the neck is extended, with the jaw clenched; the arms are pronated, extended, and close to the sides; the legs are extended straight out; and the feet are plantar flexed (Figure 40–19 ■).
  - ✓ Decorticate posturing occurs with lesions of the corticospinal tracts.
  - ✓ Decerebrate posturing occurs with lesions of the midbrain, pons, or diencephalon.

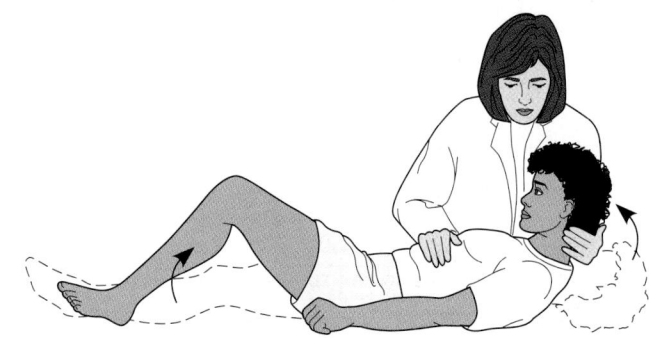

**Figure 40–16** ■ Testing for Brudzinski's sign.

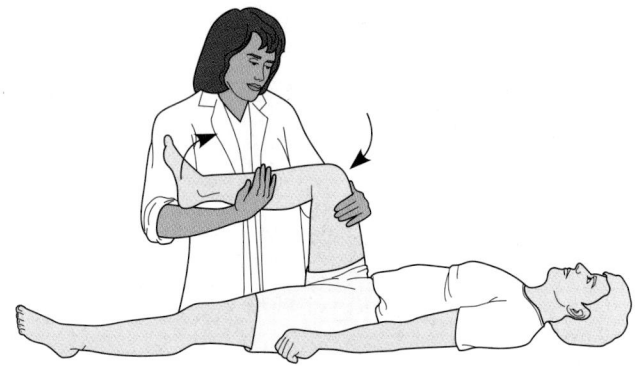

**Figure 40–17** ■ Testing for Kernig's sign.

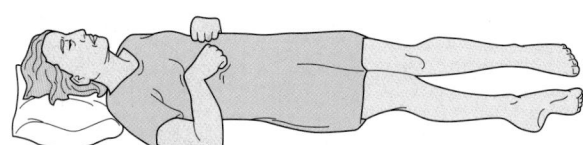

**Figure 40–18** ■ Decorticate posturing.

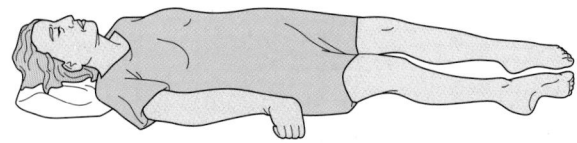

**Figure 40–19** ■ Decerebrate posturing.

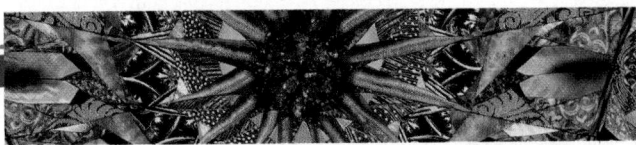

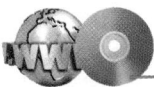 EXPLORE MediaLink

NCLEX review questions, case studies, care plan activities, MediaLink applications, and other interactive resources for this chapter can be found on the Companion Website at www.prenhall.com/lemone.

Click on Chapter 40 to select the activities for this chapter. For animations, video clips, more NCLEX review questions, and an audio glossary, access the Student CD-ROM accompanying this textbook.

## TEST YOURSELF

1. What component of the brain protects it from harmful substances?

   a. The circulation of cerebrospinal fluid
   b. The large oxygen demand
   c. The structure of neurons
   d. The blood-brain barrier

2. What pathophysiology results from damage to the lower motor neurons?

   a. Loss of cognitive ability
   b. Inability to communicate verbally
   c. Loss of reflexes
   d. Decreasing levels of consciousness

3. Which of the physical assessment techniques is **not** used in the neurologic examination?

   a. Inspection
   b. Auscultation
   c. Percussion
   d. Palpation

4. What would you need to assess function of cranial nerve V (trigeminal)?

   a. Cotton ball and safety pin
   b. Stethoscope with bell and diaphragm
   c. Measuring tape and pencil
   d. Various scents, such as coffee and vanilla

5. Which position best describes decorticate posturing?

   a. Neck extended, arms extended and pronated, feet plantar flexed
   b. Arms close to sides, elbows and wrists flexed, legs extended
   c. In prone position with arms and knees sharply flexed
   d. In supine position, spine extended, legs extended

See Test Yourself answers in Appendix C.

## BIBLIOGRAPHY

Jagoda, A., & Riggio, S. (1999). The rapid neurologic examination, part 1. History, mental status, cranial nerves. An orderly search identifies problems requiring immediate care. *Journal of Critical Illness, 14*(6), 325–331.

Maher, L. (2000). A quick neurologic examination. *Patient Care, 34*(3), 161–162, 165–168, 171–172.
O'Hanlon-Nichols, T. (1999). Neurologic assessment. *American Journal of Nursing, 99*(6), 44–50.
Riggio, S., & Jagoda A. (1999). The rapid neurologic examination, part 2: Movement, reflexes,

sensation, balance. Know the signs that lead to the site of the pathologic process. *Journal of Critical Illness, 14*(7), 368–372.
Weber, J., & Kelley, J. (2002). *Health assessment in nursing* (2nd ed.). Philadelphia: Lippincott.

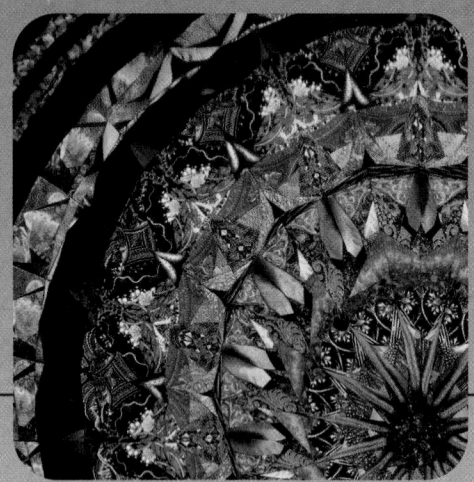

# CHAPTER 41

# Nursing Care of Clients with Cerebrovascular and Spinal Cord Disorders

 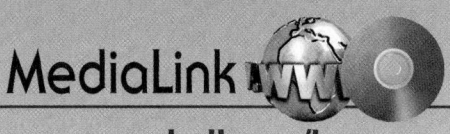
## LEARNING OUTCOMES

After completing this chapter, you will be able to:

- Apply knowledge of normal neurologic anatomy and physiology and assessments when providing nursing care for clients with cerebrovascular and spinal cord disorders (see Chapter 40).

- Identify factors responsible for disorders in cerebral blood flow.

- Explain the pathophysiologic effects, manifestations, and complications of alterations in cerebral blood flow due to thrombi, emboli, hemorrhage, aneurysm, and arteriovenous malformation.

- Identify factors responsible for spinal cord injuries.

- Discuss the pathophysiologic effects of injuries of the spinal cord by level of injury.

- Describe the causes and manifestations of cervical and lumbar herniated intervertebral disks.

- Discuss the types and manifestations of spinal cord tumors.

- Explain the collaborative care of clients with cerebrovascular and spinal cord disorders.

- Use the nursing process as a framework for providing individualized care to clients with cerebrovascular and spinal cord disorders.

The health problems discussed in this chapter result from alterations in cerebral blood flow and from disorders of the spinal cord. Disorders of the spinal cord and brain affect an estimated 50 million Americans, costing the American public more than $400 billion a year in direct health care costs and indirect lifetime costs. Clients with disorders of cerebral blood flow and the spinal cord experience a wide variety of neurologic deficits that affect cognitive and perceptual health patterns.

Nursing care for clients with these disorders is tailored to meet the needs of the client and is individualized according to the client's responses to alterations in intracranial and spinal cord structure and function. This chapter's discussion of nursing care includes consideration of acute and long-term health care needs.

# CEREBROVASCULAR DISORDERS

## THE CLIENT WITH A STROKE

A **stroke (cerebral vascular accident, CVA),** also referred to as a *brain attack,* is a condition in which neurologic deficits result from decreased blood flow to a localized area of the brain. Strokes may be *ischemic* (when blood supply to a part of the brain is suddenly interrupted by a thrombus or embolus) or *hemorrhagic* (when a blood vessel breaks open, spilling blood into spaces surrounding neurons). The neurologic deficits caused by ischemia and the resultant necrosis of cells in the brain vary according to the area of the brain involved, the size of the affected area, and the length of time blood flow is decreased or stopped. A major loss of blood supply to the brain can cause severe disability or death. When the duration of decreased blood flow is short and the anatomical area involved is small, the person may not be aware that damage has been done.

### INCIDENCE AND PREVALENCE

Strokes are the third leading cause of death in North America, where approximately 600,000 people suffer a stroke each year. Of those, 160,000 die, and many clients who survive are left with some type of functional impairment (Porth, 2002). The highest incidence occurs in people over 65 years of age. However, 28% of cerebral vascular accidents occur in people under the age of 65, and strokes occur in every age group. They occur more frequently in men than women.

### Risk Factors

Certain diseases, lifestyle habits, and ethnic backgrounds increase the risk of a stroke (see the box below), including:

## Focus on Diversity

### RISK AND INCIDENCE OF CVA

- CVAs are more common in the African American population, probably because of an increased incidence of hypertension in individuals of African descent. An additional factor is sickle cell anemia, specific to this race.
- The incidence of hemorrhagic CVAs is highest in Asians (especially the Japanese).

- *Hypertension.* Increased systolic and diastolic blood pressure is associated with damage to all blood vessels, including the cerebral vessels.
- *Diabetes mellitus.* Diabetes leads to vascular changes in both the systemic and cerebral circulation and increases the risk of hypertension.
- *Sickle cell disease.* Changes in the shape of the red blood cells increase blood viscosity and produce erythrocyte clumps that may occlude small cerebral vessels.
- *Substance abuse.* The injection of unpurified substances increases the risk for a stroke, and abuse of certain drugs can decrease cerebral blood flow and increase the risk for intracranial hemorrhage. Substances associated with strokes include alcohol, nicotine, heroin, amphetamines, and cocaine.
- *Atherosclerosis.* Occlusion of cerebral vessels by atherosclerotic plaque impairs or obstructs blood flow to specific areas of the brain.

Other risk factors include a family history of obesity, a sedentary lifestyle, hyperlipidemia, atrial fibrillation, cardiac disease, cigarette smoking, and previous transient ischemic attacks. Risk factors specific to women are oral contraceptive use, pregnancy, and menopause.

### Overview of Normal Cerebral Blood Flow

The brain, which makes up only 2% of total body weight, receives approximately 20% of the cardiac output each minute (about 750 mL) and accounts for 20% of the body's oxygen consumption. Brain function depends on a consistent blood and oxygen supply. When cerebral blood flow is decreased or interrupted, the resulting ischemia may lead to death of brain cells and pathophysiologic alterations (Porth, 2002).

The brain is supplied with blood from the internal carotid arteries (anteriorly) and the vertebral arteries (posteriorly) (see Figure 40–4 on page 1294). Two sets of veins drain cerebral blood into venous plexuses and dural sinuses and then into the internal jugular veins at the base of the skull. The veins in the cerebral system do not have valves; therefore, the direction of flow depends on gravity or pressure differences between the venous sinuses and the extracranial veins.

Activities that increase intrathoracic pressure (such as sneezing, coughing, straining to have a bowel movement, or vomiting) also briefly increase intracranial pressure. This increased intracranial pressure occurs because the increased intrathoracic pressure is transmitted through the internal jugular veins and the dural sinuses.

Cerebral blood flow, especially in the deep cerebral vessels, is largely self-regulated by the brain to meet metabolic needs. This self-regulation (also called *autoregulation*) allows the brain to maintain a constant blood flow despite changes in systemic blood pressure. However, autoregulation is not effective when systemic blood pressure falls below 50 mmHg or rises above 160 mmHg. In the latter case, the increased systemic pressure (as in hypertension) causes an increase in cerebral blood flow with resultant overdistention of cerebral vessels. Cerebral blood flow is affected by concentrations of carbon dioxide, oxygen, and hydrogen ions. Cerebral blood flow increases in response to increased carbon dioxide concentrations, increased hydrogen ion concentrations, and decreased oxygen concentrations.

## PATHOPHYSIOLOGY

A stroke is characterized by a gradual or rapid onset of neurologic deficits due to compromised cerebral blood flow. Strokes may result from a variety of problems, including transient ischemic attack (TIA), cerebral thrombosis, cerebral embolism, and cerebral hemorrhage.

When blood flow to and oxygenation of cerebral neurons are decreased or interrupted, pathophysiologic changes at the cellular level take place in 4 to 5 minutes. Cellular metabolism ceases as glucose, glycogen, and adenosine triphosphate (ATP) are depleted and the sodium-potassium pump fails. Cells swell as sodium draws water into the cell. Cerebral blood vessel walls also swell, further decreasing blood flow. Even if circulation is restored, vasospasm and increased blood viscosity can continue to impede blood flow. Severe or prolonged ischemia leads to cellular death. A central core of dead or dying cells is surrounded by a band of minimally perfused cells, called the *penumbra.* Although cells in the penumbra have impaired metabolic activities, their structural integrity is maintained. The survival of these cells depends on a timely return of adequate circulation, the volume of toxic products released by adjacent dying cells, the degree of cerebral edema, and alterations in local blood flow. The potential survival of cells in the penumbra has led to the use of thrombolytic agents in the early treatment of ischemic stroke (Porth, 2002).

The neurologic deficits that occur as a result of a stroke can often be used to identify its location. Because the sensory-motor pathways cross at the junction of the medulla and spinal cord (decussation), strokes lead to loss or impairment of sensory-motor functions on the side of the body opposite the side of the brain that is damaged. This effect, known as a **contralateral deficit,** causes a stroke in the right hemisphere of the brain to be manifested by deficits in the left side of the body (and vice versa).

### Ischemic Stroke

Ischemic strokes result from cerebrovascular obstruction by thrombosis or emboli. They include TIAs, thrombotic stroke, and embolic stroke.

### Transient Ischemic Attack

A **transient ischemic attack (TIA)** is a brief period of localized cerebral ischemia that causes neurologic deficits lasting for less than 24 hours (usually less than 1 to 2 hours) (Porth, 2002). The deficits may be present for only minutes or may last for hours. TIAs are often warning signals of an ischemic thrombotic stroke. One or many TIAs may precede a stroke, with the time between the TIA and a stroke ranging from hours to months.

The etiology of TIA includes inflammatory artery disorders, sickle cell anemia, atherosclerotic changes in cerebral vessels, thrombosis, and emboli. Transient cerebral ischemia may also occur as a result of subclavian steal syndrome, a relatively rare pathophysiologic process in which blood that normally flows from the vertebral arteries into the circulation of the brain changes direction and flows from the vertebral arteries into the arteries of the arm. This reverse flow occurs when the arm is exercised and the subclavian artery is occluded.

Neurologic manifestations of a TIA vary according to the location and size of the cerebral vessel involved. Manifestations have a sudden onset and often disappear within minutes or hours. Commonly occurring deficits include contralateral numbness or weakness of the hand, forearm, and corner of the mouth (due to middle cerebral artery involvement); aphasia (due to ischemia of the left hemisphere); and visual disturbances such as blurring (due to involvement of the posterior cerebral artery) (Porth, 2002).

### Thrombotic Stroke

A **thrombotic stroke** is caused by occlusion of a large cerebral vessel by a thrombus (a blood clot). Thrombotic CVAs most often occur in older people who are resting or sleeping. The blood pressure is lower during sleep, so there is less pressure to push the blood through an already narrowed arterial lumen, and ischemia may result.

Thrombi tend to form in large arteries that bifurcate and have narrowed lumens as a result of deposits of atherosclerotic plaque. The plaque involves the intima of the arteries, causing the internal elastic lamina to become thin and frayed with exposure of underlying connective tissue. This structural change causes platelets to adhere to the rough surface and release the enzyme adenosine diphosphate. This enzyme initiates the clotting sequence, and the thrombus forms. A thrombus may remain in place and continue to enlarge, completely occluding the lumen of the vessel, or a part of it may break off and become an embolus.

The most common locations of thrombi are the internal carotid artery, the vertebral arteries, and the junction of the vertebral and basilar arteries. Thrombotic strokes affecting the smaller cerebral vessels are called **lacunar strokes,** because the infarcted areas slough off, leaving a small cavity or "lake" in the brain tissue. A thrombotic stroke usually affects only one region of the brain that is supplied by a single cerebral artery.

A thrombotic stroke occurs rapidly but progresses slowly. It often begins with a TIA, and continues to worsen over 1 to 2 days; the condition is called a stroke-in-evolution. When maximum neurologic deficit has been reached, usually in 3 days, the condition is called a completed stroke. At that time, the damaged area is edematous and necrotic.

## Embolic Stroke

An **embolic stroke** occurs when a blood clot or clump of matter traveling through the cerebral blood vessels becomes lodged in a vessel too narrow to permit further movement. The area of the brain supplied by the blocked vessel becomes ischemic. The most frequent sites of cerebral emboli are at bifurcations of vessels, particularly those of the carotid and middle cerebral arteries. This type of stroke is typically seen in clients who are younger than those experiencing thrombotic strokes and occurs when the client is awake and active.

Many embolic strokes originate from a thrombus in the left chambers of the heart, formed during atrial fibrillation. These are referred to as *cardiogenic embolic strokes*. Emboli result when parts of the thrombus break off and are carried through the arterial system to the brain. Cerebral emboli may also be due to carotid artery atherosclerotic plaque, bacterial endocarditis, recent myocardial infarction, rheumatic heart disease, and ventricular aneurysm.

An embolic stroke has a sudden onset and causes immediate deficits. If the embolus breaks up into smaller fragments and is absorbed by the body, symptoms will disappear in a few hours to a few days. If the embolus is not absorbed, symptoms will persist. Even if the embolus is absorbed, the vessel wall where the embolus lodges may be weakened, increasing the potential for cerebral hemorrhage.

## Hemorrhagic Stroke

A **hemorrhagic stroke,** or **intracranial hemorrhage,** occurs when a cerebral blood vessel ruptures. It occurs most often in people with sustained increase in systolic-diastolic pressure. Intracranial hemorrhage usually occurs suddenly, often when the affected person is engaged in some activity. Although hypertension is the most common cause, a variety of factors may contribute to a hemorrhagic stroke, including ruptured intracranial aneurysms, trauma, erosion of blood vessels by tumors, arteriovenous malformations, anticoagulant therapy, and blood disorders. Of all forms of stroke, this form is most often fatal.

As a result of the blood vessel rupture, blood enters the brain tissue, the cerebral ventricles, or the subarachnoid space, compressing adjacent tissues and causing blood vessel spasm and cerebral edema. Blood in the ventricles or subarachnoid space irritates the meninges and brain tissue, causing an inflammatory reaction and impairing absorption and circulation of cerebral spinal fluid.

The onset of manifestations from a hemorrhagic stroke is rapid. Manifestations depend on the location of the hemorrhage, but may include vomiting, headache, seizures, hemiplegia, and loss of consciousness. Pressure on the brain tissue from increased intracranial pressure (discussed in Chapter 42) may cause coma and death.

## MANIFESTATIONS AND COMPLICATIONS

Manifestations and complications of a stroke vary according to the cerebral artery involved and the area of the brain affected.

### Manifestations of a Stroke by Involved Cerebral Vessel

**INTERNAL CAROTID ARTERY**
- Contralateral paralysis of the arm, leg, and face
- Contralateral sensory deficits of the arm, leg, and face
- If the dominant hemisphere is involved: aphasia
- If the nondominant hemisphere is involved: apraxia, agnosia, unilateral neglect
- Homonymous hemianopia

**MIDDLE CEREBRAL ARTERY**
- Drowsiness, stupor, coma
- Contralateral hemiplegia of the arm and face
- Contralateral sensory deficits of the arm and face
- Global aphasia (if dominant hemisphere involved)
- Homonymous hemianopia

**ANTERIOR CEREBRAL ARTERY**
- Contralateral weakness or paralysis of the foot and leg
- Contralateral sensory loss of the toes, foot, and leg
- Loss of ability to make decisions or act voluntarily
- Urinary incontinence

**VERTEBRAL ARTERY**
- Pain in face, nose, or eye
- Numbness and weakness of the face on involved side
- Problems with gait
- Dysphagia
- Dysarthria

Manifestations are always sudden in onset, focal, and usually one sided. The most common manifestation is weakness involving the face and arm, and sometimes the leg. Other common manifestations are numbness on one side, loss of vision in one eye or to the side, speech difficulties, and difficulties with balance. The various deficits associated with involvement of a specific cerebral artery are collectively referred to as stroke syndromes, although the deficits often overlap, as shown in the box above.

Typical manifestations and complications include motor deficits, elimination disorders, sensory-perceptual deficits, language disorders, and behavioral changes. These may be transient or permanent, depending on the degree of ischemia and necrosis as well as time of treatment. As a result of the neurologic deficits, the client with a stroke has manifestations that involve many different body systems (see the box on page 1310).

## Motor Deficits

Body movement results from a complex interaction between the brain, spinal cord, and peripheral nerves. The motor areas of the cerebral cortex, the basal ganglia, and the cerebellum initiate voluntary movement by sending messages to the spinal cord, which then transmits the messages to the peripheral nerves. A stroke may interrupt the central nervous system component of this relay system and produce effects in the contralateral side ranging from mild weakness to severe limitation of any kind of movement.

## Manifestations and Complications of Stroke by Body System

### INTEGUMENT

- Decubitus (pressure) ulcers

### NEUROLOGIC

- Hyperthermia
- Neglect syndrome
- Seizures
- Agnosias
- Communication deficits
  a. Expressive aphasia
  b. Receptive aphasia
  c. Global aphasia
  d. Agraphia
- Visual deficits
  a. Homonymous hemianopia
  b. Diplopia
  c. Decreased acuity
- Cognitive changes
  a. Memory loss
  b. Short attention span
  c. Distractibility
  d. Poor judgment
  e. Poor problem-solving ability
  f. Disorientation
- Behavioral changes
  a. Emotional lability
  b. Loss of social inhibitions
  c. Fear
  d. Hostility
  e. Anger
  f. Depression
- Increased intracranial pressure
- Alterations in consciousness
- Sensory loss (touch, pain, heat, cold, pressure)

### RESPIRATORY

- Respiratory center damage
- Airway obstruction
- Decreased ability to cough

### GASTROINTESTINAL

- Dysphagia
- Constipation
- Stool impaction

### GENITOURINARY

- Incontinence
- Frequency
- Urgency
- Urinary retention
- Renal calculi

### MUSCULOSKELETAL

- Hemiplegia
- Contractures
- Bony ankylosis
- Disuse atrophy
- Dysarthria

---

Depending on the area of the brain involved, strokes may cause weakness, paralysis, and/or spasticity. The deficits include:

- **Hemiplegia:** paralysis of the left or right half of the body (see Figure 41–1 ■).

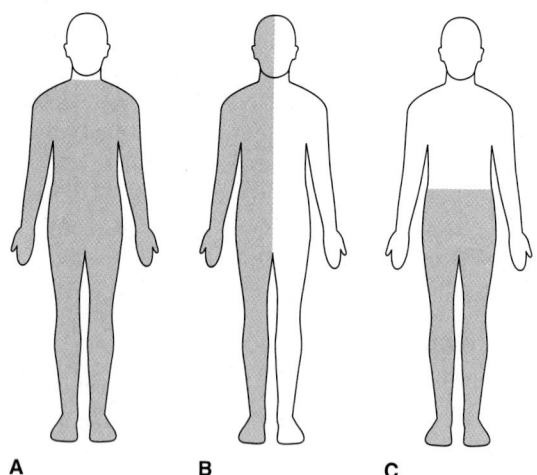

**A**      **B**      **C**

**Figure 41–1** ■ Types of paralysis. *A,* Tetraplegia is complete or partial paralysis of the upper extremities and complete paralysis of the lower part of the body. *B,* Hemiplegia is paralysis of one-half of the body when it is divided along the median sagittal plane. *C,* Paraplegia is paralysis of the lower part of the body.

- **Hemiparesis:** weakness of the left or right half of the body.
- **Flaccidity:** absence of muscle tone (hypotonia).
- **Spasticity:** increased muscle tone (hypertonia), usually with some degree of weakness. The flexor muscles are usually more strongly affected in the upper extremities and the extensor muscles are more strongly affected in the lower extremities.

When the corticospinal tract is involved, the affected arm and leg almost always are initially flaccid and then become spastic within 6 to 8 weeks. Spasticity often causes characteristic body positioning: adduction of the shoulder, pronation of the forearm, flexion of the fingers, and extension of the hip and knee. There is often foot drop, outward rotation of the leg, and dependent edema in the involved extremities.

The motor deficits may result in altered mobility, further impairing body function. The complications of immobility involve multiple body systems and include orthostatic hypotension, increased thrombus formation, decreased cardiac output, impaired respiratory function, osteoporosis, formation of renal calculi, contractures, and decubitus ulcer formation.

### Elimination Disorders

Disorders of bladder and bowel elimination are common. A stroke may cause partial loss of the sensations that trigger bladder elimination, resulting in urinary frequency, urgency, or incontinence. Control of urination may be altered as a result of cognitive deficits. Changes in bowel elimination are common; they result from changes in level of consciousness, immobility, and dehydration (Hickey, 2003).

## Sensory-Perceptual Deficits

A stroke may involve pathologic changes in neurologic pathways that alter the ability to integrate, interpret, and attend to sensory data. The client may experience deficits in vision, hearing, equilibrium, taste, and sense of smell. The ability to perceive vibration, pain, warmth, cold, and pressure may be impaired, as may proprioception (the body's sense of its position). The loss of these sensory abilities increases the risk for injury. Deficits may include:

- **Hemianopia:** the loss of half of the visual field of one or both eyes; when the same half is missing in each eye, the condition is called *homonymous hemianopia* (Figure 41–2 ■).
- **Agnosia:** the inability to recognize one or more subjects that were previously familiar; agnosia may be visual, tactile, or auditory.
- **Apraxia:** the inability to carry out some motor pattern (e.g., drawing a figure, getting dressed) even when strength and coordination are adequate.

Another form of sensory-perceptual deficit is the **neglect syndrome** (or unilateral neglect), in which the client has a disorder of attention. In this syndrome, the person cannot integrate and use perceptions from the affected side of the body or from the environment on the affected side, and ignores that part. In severe cases, the client may even deny the paralysis. This deficit is more common following a stroke of the right hemisphere where damage to the parietal lobe (a center for mediation of directed attention) results in perceptual deficits.

## Communication Disorders

Communication is a complex process, involving motor functions, speech, language, memory, reasoning, and emotions.

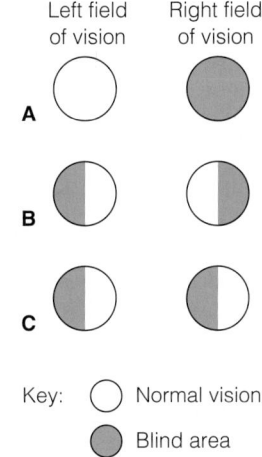

Left field of vision    Right field of vision

A

B

C

Key:   ○ Normal vision
       ● Blind area

**Figure 41–2 ■** Abnormal visual fields. *A,* Normal left field of vision with loss of vision in right field. *B,* Loss of vision in temporal half of both fields (bitemporal hemianopia). *C,* Loss of vision in nasal field of right eye and temporal field of left eye (homonymous hemianopia).

Communication problems are usually the result of a stroke affecting the dominant hemisphere. The left hemisphere is dominant in about 95% of right-handed people and 70% of left-handed people (Porth, 2002).

Many different impairments may occur, and most are partial. Disorders of communication affect both speech (the mechanical act of articulating language through the spoken word) and language (the vocal or written formulation of ideas to communicate thoughts and feelings). Language involves oral and written expression and auditory and reading comprehension. Among these disorders are:

- **Aphasia:** the inability to use or understand language; aphasia may be expressive, receptive, or mixed (global).
- Expressive aphasia: a motor speech problem in which one can understand what is being said but can respond verbally only in short phrases; also called *Broca's aphasia.*
- Receptive aphasia: a sensory speech problem in which one cannot understand the spoken (and often written) word. Speech may be fluent but with inappropriate content; also called *Wernicke's aphasia.*
- Mixed or global aphasia: language dysfunction in both understanding and expression.
- Dysarthria: any disturbance in muscular control of speech.

## Cognitive and Behavioral Changes

A change in consciousness, ranging from mild confusion to coma, is a common manifestation of a stroke. It may result from tissue damage following ischemia or hemorrhage involving either the carotid or vertebral arteries. Altered consciousness may also be the result of cerebral edema or increased intracranial pressure.

Behavioral changes include emotional lability (in which the client may laugh or cry inappropriately), loss of self-control (manifested by behavior such as swearing or refusing to wear clothing), and decreased tolerance for stress (resulting in anger or depression). Intellectual changes may include memory loss, decreased attention span, poor judgment, and an inability to think abstractly.

## COLLABORATIVE CARE

The client with a stroke may receive medical and/or surgical treatment. The focus in the acute care phase is on diagnosing the type and cause of the stroke, supporting cerebral circulation, and controlling or preventing further deficits.

### Diagnostic Tests

Diagnostic tests may be ordered to detect increased risk for a stroke or to identify pathophysiologic changes after a stroke has occurred.

- *Computed tomography (CT)* without contrast is the first imaging technique used to demonstrate the presence of hemorrhage, tumors, aneurysm, ischemia, edema, and tissue necrosis. A CT scan can also demonstrate a shift in intracranial contents and is useful in distinguishing the type of stroke (e.g., a hemorrhagic stroke results in an increase in density).

Nursing interventions for the client having a CT scan of the head are described in the box below.

- *Arteriography* of cerebral vessels is performed to demonstrate abnormal vessel structures, vasospasm, loss of vessel wall integrity, and stenosis of the carotid arteries.
- *Transcranial ultrasound Doppler (TCD)* studies are used to evaluate the velocity of the blood flow through the intracranial arteries and provide information about partial or complete occlusion.
- *Magnetic resonance imaging (MRI) test* may be conducted to detect shifting of brain tissues as a result of hemorrhage or edema. A *magnetic resonance angiography (MRA)* may be performed to detect occlusive disease of the large cerebral vessels.
- *Positron emission tomography (PET)* and *single-photon emission computed tomography (SPECT)* are used to examine cerebral blood flow distribution and metabolic activity of the brain. Both tests use very short-lived radionuclides that emit radioactive energy as they move through the circulation. PET allows the identification of the location and size of the stroke; SPECT provides information about the metabolism of and blood flow through the brain tissue affected by the stroke.

## Nursing Implications for Diagnostic Tests

### Computed Tomography (CT) of the Head

#### Preparation of Client
- Ensure a signed consent form.
- Check hospital policy on withholding food and fluids. Clients are usually on NPO status (except for the medications ordered as part of the test) for 8 hours before the test if it is done in the morning. If the test is done in the afternoon, the client may have a liquid breakfast.
- Give medications up to 2 hours before test.
- Assess for possible reaction to iodine dye (by asking about allergy to seafood). Document any allergy and inform the physician and radiology department.
- Remove metal hairpins, clips, and earrings.

#### Client and Family Teaching
- (*If applicable*) Do not drink or eat anything before the test except for the ordered medications.
- You may be given an intravenous infusion. When the contrast dye is injected, you may feel warm and have a metallic taste in the mouth.
- The exam lasts from 30 to 90 minutes.
- Your head will be positioned in a cradle, and a wide rubber strap will be applied snugly across the forehead during the test (to keep your head immobilized).
- The CT scanner is circular with a round opening. You are strapped to a special table, and the scanner revolves around the body part to be examined. The scanner makes a clicking noise.
- The test is painless.
- Someone is always immediately available during the test.

- *Lumbar puncture* may be performed to obtain cerebrospinal fluid for examination if there is no danger of increased intracranial pressure. (Removal of cerebrospinal fluid when intracranial pressure is increased can result in herniation of the brainstem.) A thrombotic stroke may elevate cerebrospinal fluid pressure; after a hemorrhagic stroke frank blood may be seen in the cerebrospinal fluid. Nursing interventions for the client having a lumbar puncture are described in the Nursing Implications box on the next page.

## Medications

Medications are administered to prevent a stroke in clients with TIAs or a previous stroke, and to treat the client during the acute phase of a stroke.

### Prevention

Antiplatelet agents are often used to treat clients with TIAs or who have had a previous stroke. Platelets are concentrated in high blood flow arteries, they adhere to endothelial tissue damaged by atherosclerosis and occlude the vessel. The drugs used to prevent clot formation and blood vessel occlusion include aspirin, clopidogrel (Plavix), dipyridamole (Persantine), pentoxifylline (Trental), and ticlopidine (Ticlid).

Daily low-dose aspirin reduces TIA occurrence and stroke risk by interfering with platelet aggregation. Ticlopidine (Ticlid) is a platelet-aggregation inhibitor that has shown reduction in thrombotic stroke risk.

### Acute Stroke

Pharmacologic agents are used to treat the client during the acute phase of an ischemic stroke to prevent further thrombosis formation, increase cerebral blood flow, and protect cerebral neurons. The type of medication used varies according to the type of stroke.

Anticoagulant drug therapy (discussed in Chapter 33) is often ordered for thrombotic stroke during the stroke-in-evolution phase but is contraindicated in completed stroke because it may increase the risk of cerebral hemorrhage. Anticoagulants are never administered to a client with a hemorrhagic stroke. Anticoagulants do not dissolve an existing clot but prevent further extension of the clot and formation of new clots. Sodium heparin may be given subcutaneously or by continuous IV drip, or warfarin sodium (Coumadin) may be given orally.

Thrombolytic therapy, using a tissue plasminogen activator such as recombinant altephase (Activase rt-pa), sometimes given concurrently with an anticoagulant, is used to treat thrombotic stroke. The drug converts plasminogen to plasmin, resulting in fibrinolysis of the clot. To be effective, it must be given within 3 hours of the onset of manifestations (Tierney et al., 2001).

Antithrombotic drugs, which inhibit the platelet phase of clot formation, have been used as a preventive measure for clients at risk for embolic and thrombotic CVA. Both aspirin and dipyridamole have been used for this purpose. These drugs are sometimes also used in combination with other drugs during acute treatment. Antiplatelet agents are contraindicated in clients with a hemorrhagic stroke.

## Nursing Implications for Diagnostic Tests

### Lumbar Puncture

#### Preparation of the Client
- Ensure a signed consent form (this consent may be obtained as part of the general consent given on admission to the hospital or agency).
- Ask the client to empty the bladder before the procedure begins.
- Help the client to assume a lateral recumbent position near the side of the bed. The client should assume the fetal position (knees flexed toward the head, head bent toward the chest), with the hands clasped around the knees.

#### Client and Family Teaching
- A local anesthetic is injected into the skin over the area of the needle insertion. This medication may cause a burning sensation.
- A long, thin needle is inserted into the lower back below the level of the spinal cord. Cerebrospinal fluid is withdrawn.
- The cerebrospinal fluid pressure is measured with a calibrated tube called a manometer.
- There may be slight pain down one leg during the procedure.
- It is important to remain still during the procedure.
- A small dressing is used to cover the place where the needle was inserted.

- After the procedure, remain flat in bed for the number of hours prescribed by the physician (this ranges from 4 to 24 hours). The nurses will take your vital signs and look under the small dressing at regular intervals.
- Drink fluids so that your body can replace the fluid that was withdrawn.
- If you have a headache or backache, ask for medications for pain.
- Notify your health care provider if you notice increased pain or drainage from the area where the procedure was done.

#### Postprocedure Nursing Care
- Take and record vital signs as indicated by agency standards.
- Monitor neurologic status at least every 4 hours for 24 hours following the procedure.
- Monitor the puncture site for leakage of cerebrospinal fluid or hematoma formation.
- Ensure that the client voids within 8 hours of the procedure.
- Encourage increased intake of fluids (up to 3000 mL in 24 hours).
- Administer analgesics as prescribed for pain.

---

Calcium channel blockers, such as nimodipine (Nimotop), are under investigation and have been used in clinical trials to reduce ischemic deficits and death from stroke. They block glutamate, an excitatory neurotransmitter, to reduce the sensitivity of neurons to ischemia.

Corticosteriods, such as prednisone or dexamethasone have been used to treat cerebral edema, but the results are not always positive. If the client has increased intracranial pressure, hyperosmolar solutions (such as mannitol) or diuretics (such as furosemide) may be administered. Anticonvulsants, such as phenytoin (Dilantin), and barbiturates may be prescribed if increased intracranial pressure causes seizures.

## Treatments

The treatments used in the medical management of a stroke include surgery, physical therapy, occupational therapy, and speech therapy.

### Surgery

Surgery may be performed to prevent the occurrence of a stroke or to restore blood flow when a stroke has already occurred. In people who have had TIAs or are in danger of having another stroke, a carotid endarterectomy at the carotid artery bifurcation may be performed to remove atherosclerotic plaque (Figure 41–3 ■). Nursing care for the client in the initial postoperative period following a carotid endarterectomy is described in the box on page 1314.

When an occluded or stenotic vessel is not directly accessible, an extracranial-intracranial bypass may be performed. Bypass of the internal carotid, middle cerebral, or vertebral arter-

ies may be required. The indications for the bypass are symptoms of ischemia caused by TIAs or a mild completed stroke. The procedure reestablishes blood flow to the affected area of the brain.

### Physical/Occupational/Speech Therapy

Physical therapy may help prevent contractures and improve muscle strength and coordination. Occupational therapy provides assistive devices and a plan for regaining lost motor skills that greatly improve quality of life after a stroke. In addition, the client with a communication disorder requires speech therapy.

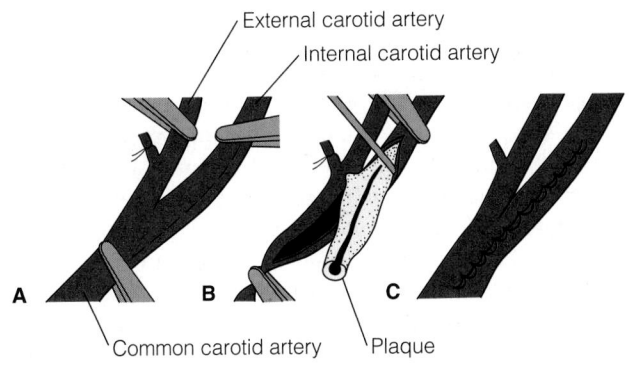

**Figure 41–3** ■ Carotid endarterectomy. *A,* The occluded area is clamped off and an incision is made in the artery. *B,* Plaque is removed from the inner layer of the artery. *C,* To restore blood flow through the artery, the artery is sutured, or a graft is completed.

## NURSING CARE OF THE CLIENT HAVING A CAROTID ENDARTERECTOMY

### POSTOPERATIVE CARE

- Position on the unoperated side and either maintain a flat position or elevate the head of the bed 30 degrees as prescribed. Maintain head and neck alignment and avoid rotating, flexing, or hyperextending head. *Pressure on the wound is undesirable. Elevating the head decreases edema in the operative site. Maintaining head and neck alignment prevents additional tension or pressure on the operative side.*
- Support the head when changing position. Teach to support the head with the hands when able to move about. *Supporting the head helps prevent stress on the operative site (which may cause bleeding and hematoma formation); it also helps reduce stress on the suture line.*
- Perform focused assessments to monitor for complications:
  a. *Hemorrhage.* Assess the dressing and the area under the neck and shoulders for drainage. Assess for increased pulse and decreased blood pressure. *The most common cause of respiratory problems is pressure on the trachea from a hematoma formation.*
  b. *Respiratory distress.* Assess respiratory rate, rhythm, depth, and effort. Observe for restlessness. Keep a tracheostomy tray at the bedside. *Respiratory distress may result from edema and hematoma formation, which may compress the trachea.*
  c. *Cranial nerve impairment.* Observe and record any facial drooping, tongue deviation, hoarseness, dysphagia, or loss of facial sensation. *Cranial nerves may be stretched during surgery, leading to temporary deficits in cranial nerve function.*
  d. *Hypertension* or *hypotension.* Take and record blood pressure at least hourly. Report any changes immediately and implement orders for medications to treat hypertension or hypotension. *About one-half of all clients having a carotid endarterectomy develop unstable blood pressure related to surgical denervation of the carotid sinus. Uncontrolled hypertension may precipitate a CVA. The most common problem is hypotension, possibly related to stimulation of the carotid body baroreceptors, which are exposed during surgery. Hypotension may result in myocardial ischemia.*

## NURSING CARE

*MediaLink | HEMORRHAGIC STROKE CARE PLAN*

Even though many people who have a stroke have full recovery, a substantial number are left with disabilities that affect their physical, emotional, interpersonal, and family status. The required nursing care is often complex and multidimensional, requiring consideration of continuity of care for clients in acute care settings, long-term care settings, rehabilitation centers, and the home.

Nurses caring for clients who have had a stroke require knowledge and skill to meet client needs during both the acute and the rehabilitative phases of care. The client often has multiple losses: loss of mobility, ability to provide self-care, communications, concept of self, and interpersonal or intimate relationships with others. Holistic, individualized nursing care is essential in all settings and focuses on promoting the achievement of maximum potential and quality of life.

The client's family is often faced with many changes. The young to middle-aged adult with a family member who has had a stroke may be faced with economic difficulties and social isolation. The middle-aged adult family member may become the caretaker for an older parent, in essence switching roles with the parent. An older adult may not be able to care for a spouse and may have to accept nursing home placement. In addition, the older adult who has no family may have to struggle alone to regain the ability to function independently. Although not all of these problems are amenable to nursing solutions, the nurse is most often the health care provider who assesses and identifies the needs of each individual and provides information and referrals to clients and families to help meet those needs.

Because a stroke has the potential to cause many different health problems, a wide variety of nursing diagnoses may be appropriate. It is important to remember that each person will be affected differently, depending on the degree of ischemia and the area of the brain involved. Nursing diagnoses discussed in this section focus on problems with cerebral tissue perfusion (specific to nursing care during the acute phase), physical mobility, self-care, communication, sensory-perceptual deficits, bowel and urine elimination, and swallowing (specific to prevention of complications and rehabilitation). See the Manifestations box on page 1310 for more information.

### Health Promotion

Health promotion activities focus on stroke prevention, especially for those people with known risk factors. It is important to discuss the importance of stopping smoking and drug use with clients of all ages. Maintaining a normal weight through diet and exercise can help reduce obesity, which increases the risk of hypertension and Type 2 diabetes mellitus (both in turn increase the risk of a stroke). Cholesterol levels should be screened regularly to monitor for hyperlipidemia. Regular health care to monitor for and treat cardiovascular disorders and to detect and treat infections such as infective endocarditis are important. It is also important to increase public awareness of the signs of a TIA or stroke and of the need to call 911 or to seek care immediately if the following warning signs or symptoms occur.

- Sudden weakness or numbness of the face, arm, or leg, especially on one side of the body
- Sudden confusion, difficulty speaking, or difficulty understanding speech
- Sudden trouble walking, dizziness, loss of coordination
- Sudden difficulty with vision in one or both eyes
- Sudden severe headache without a cause

## Nursing Care of the Older Adult

### VARIATIONS IN ASSESSMENT FINDINGS—CVA

- Response to questions is often slower.
- Sensations, reflexes, and motor coordination are decreased.
- Alternating movements may be difficult.
- Gait may be slower and more deliberate.
- Motor strength is often decreased.
- Vision, taste, and sense of smell are often decreased.

## Assessment

The following data are collected through the health history and physical examination (see Chapter 40). Further focused assessments are described with the following nursing interventions. When assessing the older client, be aware of normal changes with aging, outlined in the box above.

- Health history: risk factors, drug use (medications and illegal), smoking history, when symptoms began, severity of symptoms, presence of incontinence, level of consciousness, family support system
- Physical assessment: motor strength, coordination, communication, cranial nerves

## Nursing Diagnoses and Interventions

The acute phase of a stroke is most often the time from admission to the hospital until the client is stabilized: usually 24 to 72 hours after admission (Hickey, 2003). Depending on the severity of the stroke, the client may be admitted to the intensive care unit. Regardless of the hospital setting, the nurse provides interventions to maintain body functions and prevent complications.

### Ineffective Tissue Perfusion (Cerebral)

The initial assessment and care of the client admitted for intensive care focuses on identifying changes that may indicate altered cerebral perfusion. The client's airway, breathing, circulation, and neurologic status are monitored and interventions are provided to maintain cerebral perfusion.

- Monitor respiratory status and airway patency. Auscultate pulmonary sounds and monitor respiratory rate and results of studies of arterial blood gases.
- Suction as necessary, using care to suction no longer than 10 to 15 seconds at any one time, and using sterile technique.
- Place in a side-lying position.
- Administer oxygen as prescribed.

*The client is often unconscious and breathing may be impaired. Suctioning removes secretions that not only obstruct airflow but also pose the risk for aspiration and pneumonia. Suctioning for longer than 15 seconds at a time may increase intracranial pressure (Hickey, 2003). Respiratory complications develop rapidly, as manifested by crackles and wheezes, rapid respirations, and respiratory acidosis. The administration of oxygen decreases the risk for hypoxia and hypercapnia, which can increase cerebral ischemia and intracranial pressure.*

**PRACTICE ALERT** *Positioning the client on the side allows secretions to drain out of the mouth, helping to prevent aspiration.* ■

- Monitor neurologic status.
- Assess mental status and level of consciousness: restlessness, drowsiness, lethargy, inability to follow commands, unresponsiveness.
- Monitor strength and reflexes, and assess for pain, headache, decreased muscle strength, sluggish pupillary reflexes, absent gag or swallowing reflexes, hemiplegia, Babinski's sign, and decerebrate or decorticate posturing. *Frequent monitoring of neurologic status is necessary to detect changes. Alterations in mental status, level of consciousness, movement, strength, and reflexes indicate increased intracranial pressure, the major cause of death in the acute phase of a stroke.*
- Continuously monitor cardiac status, observing for dysrhythmias. *A stroke may cause cardiac dysrhythmias, including bradycardia, PVCs, tachycardia, and AV block. Characteristic ECG changes include a shortened PR interval, peaked T waves, and a depressed ST segment.*
- Monitor body temperature. *Hyperthermia may develop if the hypothalamus is affected.*
- Maintain accurate intake and output records; measure urinary output via a Foley catheter. *A stroke may damage the pituitary gland, resulting in diabetes insipidus and the possibility of dehydration from greatly increased urinary output.*

**PRACTICE ALERT** *Diabetes insipidus is indicated by a large output of dilute urine; dehydration is indicated by scanty amounts of dark, concentrated urine.* ■

- Monitor seizures. Pad the side rails, and administer prescribed anticonvulsants. *Seizures may be the result of cerebral tissue damage or increased intracranial pressure. Padded side rails prevent injury if a seizure occurs. Anticonvulsants prevent or treat seizures.*

### Impaired Physical Mobility

The broad goals of care for clients with impaired mobility are to maintain and improve functional abilities (by maintaining normal function and alignment, preventing edema of extremities, and reducing spasticity) and to prevent complications.

- Encourage active ROM exercises for unaffected extremities and perform passive ROM exercises for affected extremities every 4 hours during day and evening shifts and once during the night shift. Support the joint during passive ROM exercises. *Active ROM exercises maintain or improve muscle strength and endurance, and help to maintain cardiopulmonary function. Passive ROM exercises do not strengthen muscles but do help maintain joint flexibility.*

**PRACTICE ALERT** *Both active and passive exercises increase venous return, decreasing the risk of thrombophlebitis.* ■

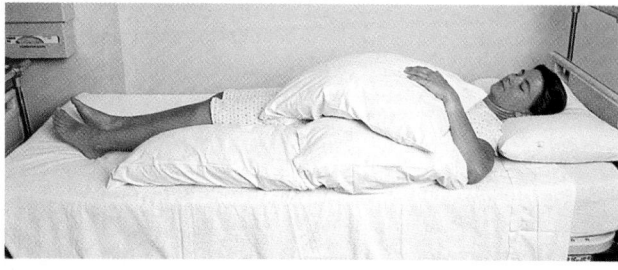

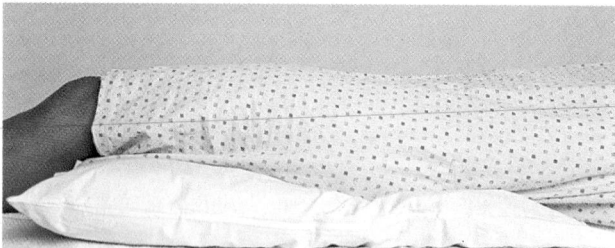

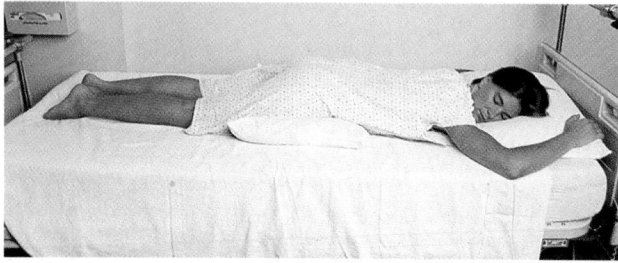

**Figure 41–4** ■ Positioning the client with hemiplegia is important in preventing deformity of the affected extremities. *A*, With the client in a supine position, place a pillow in the axilla (to prevent adduction) and under the hand and arm, with the hand higher than the elbow (to prevent flexion and edema). *B*, When the client is lying supine, use a pillow from the iliac crest to the middle of the thigh to prevent external rotation of the hip. *C*, When the client is in the prone position, place a pillow under the pelvis to promote hip hyperextension.

- Turn every 2 hours around the clock, following a posted schedule for side-to-side and supine-to-prone position changes (verify prone positioning with the physician). Maintain body alignment and support extremities in proper position with pillows. *Turning on a regular basis, accompanied by proper positioning, maintains joint function, alleviates pressure on bony prominences that can lead to skin breakdown, decreases dependent edema in hands and feet, and lessens the risk of complications resulting from immobility (Figure 41–4 ■).*

**PRACTICE ALERT** *When lying on the affected side, clients may be restless as they do not have normal sensation and feel as they may fall.* ■

- Monitor the lower extremities each shift for symptoms of thrombophlebitis. Assess for increased warmth and redness in calves; measure the circumference of the calves and thighs. *Clients on bed rest (especially those with loss of muscle strength and tone) are particularly prone to the development of deep vein thrombosis. Promptly report symptoms of thrombophlebitis.*
- Collaborate with the physical therapist as the client gains mobility, using consistent techniques to move the client from the bed to the wheelchair and to help the client ambulate. *The use of consistent techniques facilitates rehabilitation.*

### Self-Care Deficit

The client who has had a stroke may have a self-care deficit as a result of impaired mobility or mental confusion. It is important for clients to perform as much of their own physical care and grooming as possible to promote functional ability, increase independence, decrease feelings of powerlessness, and improve self-esteem.

Before establishing a plan to increase self-care, determine which hand was dominant before the stroke. If the client's dominant side is affected, self-care will be more difficult.

- Encourage use of the unaffected arm to bathe, brush teeth, comb hair, dress, and eat. *Use of the unaffected arm promotes functional ability and independence.*
- Teach the client to put on clothing by first dressing the affected extremities and then dressing the unaffected extremities. *This technique facilitates self-dressing with minimal assistance.*
- Collaborate with the occupational therapist in scheduling times for training for upper extremity functioning necessary for activities of daily living. Encourage the use of assistive devices (if required) for eating, physical hygiene, and dressing. *Following a regular schedule in daily routines promotes learning. The use of assistive devices promotes independence and decreases feelings of powerlessness. Optimal grooming facilitates positive self-concept.*

### Impaired Verbal Communication

The client who loses communication abilities requires intensive speech therapy and emotional support. It is important to determine the specific nature of the impairment when planning interventions and helping family members understand specific problem. Although the speech therapist is usually most involved with speech rehabilitation, nurses must plan interventions to meet communication needs during all phases of care.

Use the following guidelines:

- Approach and treat the client as an adult.
- Do not assume that the client who does not respond verbally cannot hear. Do not use a raised voice when addressing the client.
- Allow adequate time for the client to respond.
- Face the client and speak slowly.
- When you do not understand the client's speech, be honest and say so.
- Use short, simple statements and questions. *Accepting the client and providing dignity and respect enhances the nurse-client relationship. Allowing adequate response time and using short verbal statements or questions*

*while facing the client motivates the client to communicate and decreases frustration.*

- Accept frustration and anger as a normal reaction to the loss of function. *Anger represents the client's frustration at the inability to control the loss of function.*
- Try alternate methods of communication, including writing tablets, flash cards, and computerized talking boards. *Clients unable to communicate verbally may use other methods effectively.*

### Impaired Urinary Elimination and Risk for Constipation

Both urinary and bowel elimination may be altered because of neurologic deficits, impaired mobility, cognitive impairment, communication deficits, or preexisting problems (especially if the client is an older adult, as is usual). Other causes include changes in food and fluid intake and side effects of medications. Urinary incontinence or retention and constipation and fecal impaction are the usual manifestations.

- Assess for urinary frequency, urgency, incontinence, nocturia, and voiding in small amounts. In addition, assess the client's ability to respond to the need to void, the ability to use the call light, and the ability to use toileting equipment.

**PRACTICE ALERT**  *Voiding small amounts of urine frequently may be a manifestation of a bladder dysfunction. Assess for a distended bladder.* ■

- Encourage bladder training by having client void on schedule, such as every 2 hours, rather than in response to the urge to void.
- Teach Kegel exercises. To perform Kegel exercises, the client contracts the perineal muscles as though stopping urination, holds the contraction for 5 seconds, and then releases.
- Use positive reinforcement (verbal praise) for successful management of urinary elimination. *Voiding every 2 hours or on schedule promotes bladder tone and urine storage. Kegel exercises increase pubococcygeal muscle tone and bladder control, decreasing incontinence. Positive reinforcement can be a useful part of the teaching program.*
- Discuss prestroke bowel habits, as well as the pattern of bowel elimination since the stroke.
- If the client is able to swallow without difficulty, encourage fluids (up to 2000 mL per day) and a high-fiber diet.
- Increase physical activity as tolerated.
- Assist in using the toilet facilities at the same time each day (based on usual patterns of bowel elimination), ensuring privacy and having client sit in upright position if at all possible.
- Administer prescribed stool softeners if the client is following a bowel elimination routine or is not drinking sufficient fluids. *Increased fluids, fiber, and activity stimulate intestinal motility. Establishing a regular daily time for bowel movements in the upright position and in privacy promotes normal bowel elimination. Stool softeners help prevent the formation of hard stool that is more difficult to expel.*

### Impaired Swallowing

A stroke may impair the ability to swallow. Weakness or lack of coordination of the tongue, attention deficits, and deficits involving the swallowing reflex all play a role. Dysphagia (difficulty swallowing) may result in choking, drooling, aspiration, or regurgitation. Nursing care focuses on maintaining safety by preventing aspiration and on ensuring adequate nutrition. See the box below.

## Nursing Research

### Evidence-Based Practice for Caring for the Client at Risk for Impaired Swallowing

It is the nurse's responsibility to assess a client's swallowing, to initiate feeding, and to teach family caregivers to safely feed clients at home when impaired swallowing is a problem. However, little nursing research has been conducted on how to assess swallowing and eating before feeding. McHale et al. (1998) investigated the practical knowledge of expert nurses when they assess and feed clients who have difficulty swallowing.

The researchers found that nurses do not often use a formal method of assessment, but rather depend on obvious manifestations and practical experience. Cues used in assessment included level of consciousness, coughing, and choking. When feeding clients with impaired swallowing, the nurses were most concerned about providing nutrition to promote healing and health, and preventing aspiration. Knowing the client was identified as a critical factor in safe feeding.

### IMPLICATIONS FOR NURSING

Impaired swallowing is a response to neurologic, musculoskeletal, and aging disorders. However, in today's health care arena, feeding clients is often delegated to nonprofessionals in the acute care setting or taught to caregivers in the home setting. Clear guidelines for assessment parameters and protection from aspiration are needed to promote clients' ability to recover from illness or injury, and to prevent morbidity and mortality from aspiration complications.

### Critical Thinking in Client Care

1. Your client with a left-brain stroke has the following symptoms: drooping left cheek, loss of gag reflex on the left, aphasia, and a weak cough. Describe any further assessments you would make before initiating feeding.
2. What is the physiologic rationale for having the client with impaired swallowing in an upright position during and after feeding?
3. Describe the consistency of foods most easily swallowed.
4. The wife of your home-care client tells you that her husband drools and food falls out of his mouth when she tries to feed him. What could you suggest that might make feeding less difficult for both the client and his wife?

- Ensure safety when eating.
  - Position in upright sitting position with neck slightly flexed.
  - Order puréed or soft food.
  - Feed or teach client to eat by putting food behind the front teeth on the unaffected side of mouth and tilting the head slightly backward. Teach to swallow one bite at a time.

**PRACTICE ALERT** *After eating, check the mouth for "pocketing" of food, especially in the affected cheek.* ∎

- Have suction equipment available at the bedside in case of choking or aspiration. *Sitting upright with the head and neck first slightly flexed and then tilted back helps the client swallow. The client can usually swallow puréed or soft foods more easily than liquid or solid foods. Using the unaffected side of the mouth helps prevent food from collecting in the mouth and makes swallowing safer; in addition, food is less likely to fall out of the mouth.*
- Minimize distractions and, if necessary, give step-by-step instructions for eating. *Distractions increase the risk of aspiration. Complex activities are easier to perform when broken down into small steps.*

## Using NANDA, NIC, AND NOC

Chart 41–1 shows links between NANDA nursing diagnoses, NIC, and NOC when caring for the client with a stroke.

## Home Care

Throughout the rehabilitation process, it is important to encourage self-care as much as possible but also to involve family members in the plan of care. Stress that ADLs may take twice as long as they did before the stroke. Emphasize that physical function may continue to improve for up to 3 months, and speech may continue to improve for even longer. Address the following topics in preparing the client and family for home care.

- Physical care, medications, physical therapy
- Realistic expectations
- Time off for the caregiver, respite care services
- Distributors for equipment and supplies
- Home environment conducive to using equipment (e.g., a wheel chair or walker)
- Home and equipment modifications (e.g., a raised toilet seat, grab bars in the bathroom, a bath chair, a vise lid opener, a long-handled shoehorn)
- Home health services
- Community resources, such as Meals-on-Wheels, senior centers, eldercare, large-print telephone dials, stroke clubs, Life-line (emergency alerting systems through a local hospital or agency).
- Helpful organizational resources:
  - American Heart Association
  - National Stroke Association
  - Stroke Clubs International
  - The National Institute of Neurological Disorders and Stroke

*(Margin, vertical text: MediaLink | STROKE RESOURCES)*

---

**CHART 41–1 NANDA, NIC, AND NOC LINKAGES**

### The Client with a CVA

| NURSING DIAGNOSES | NURSING INTERVENTIONS | NURSING OUTCOMES |
|---|---|---|
| • Altered Cerebral Tissue Perfusion | • Acid-Base Management<br>• Cerebral Perfusion | • Electrolyte and Acid-Base Balance<br>• Circulation Status<br>• Cognitive Ability<br>• Neurologic Status |
| • Unilateral Neglect Management | • Unilateral Neglect<br>• Body Positioning: Self-Initiated | • Body Image |
| • Dressing/Grooming Self-Care Deficit | • Dressing<br>• Hair Care | • Self-Care: Dressing<br>• Self-Care: Grooming |
| • Powerlessness | • Self-Esteem Enhancement<br>• Self-Responsibility Enhancement | • Health Beliefs: Perceived Control<br>• Participation: Health Care Decisions |

*Note. Data from Nursing Outcomes Classification (NOC) by M. Johnson & M. Maas (Eds.), 1997, St. Louis: Mosby; Nursing Diagnoses: Definitions & Classification 2001–2002 by North American Nursing Diagnosis Association, 2001, Philadelphia: NANDA; Nursing Interventions Classification (NIC) by J.C. McCloskey & G. M. Bulechek (Eds.), 2000, St. Louis: Mosby. Reprinted by permission.*

## Nursing Care Plan
## A Client with a Stroke

Orville Boren is a 68-year-old African American who had a stroke due to right cerebral thrombosis 1 week ago. He is a history instructor at the local community college. His hobbies are wood carving and gardening. Mr. Boren is also an active member of his church. For the past 2 years, Mr. Boren has been taking medication for hypertension, but his wife Emily reports that he often forgets to take it and that his blood pressure was high at his last physical examination. Mrs. Boren tells the staff that she has never had to worry about her husband's health before and that she wants to learn everything she can to care for him at home. However, she says that her husband was always the one to make the decisions and pay the bills. Mrs. Boren adds that all the children, grandchildren, neighbors, and family pastor want to see Mr. Boren back at home as soon as possible.

### ASSESSMENT

Carol Merck, RN, the nurse assigned to Mr. Boren, completes a health history and physical assessment, with Mrs. Boren providing information for the history. Mrs. Boren reports that her husband did have several spells of dizziness and blurred vision the week before his stroke, but they lasted only a few minutes and he believed them to be due to "old age and working out in the sun." On the morning of admission, Mr. Boren woke up and could not move his left arm or leg; he also could not speak sensibly. Mrs. Boren called 911, and an ambulance took her husband to the hospital.

Physical assessment findings include the following: Mr. Boren is drowsy but responds to verbal stimuli. Although he does not respond verbally, he can nod his head to indicate "yes" when asked questions. Flaccid paralysis is present in his left arm and left leg, with no response noted to touch in those extremities (he is left-handed). Visual fields are decreased in a pattern consistent with homonymous hemianopia. A CT scan, negative on admission, is repeated on the third day after admission and confirms the medical diagnosis of a right-brain stroke due to a thrombus of the middle cerebral artery.

Mr. Boren's medical treatment includes heparin sodium administered by continuous intravenous drip, with clotting studies to be performed every 4 hours and the dose adjusted accordingly.

### DIAGNOSES

- *Feeding self-care deficit* related to loss of the ability to use the left hand and arm
- *Impaired physical mobility* related to neurologic deficits causing left hemiplegia
- *Risk for impaired skin integrity* related to inability to change position
- *Sensory/perceptual alterations: visual* related to changes in visual fields
- *Impaired verbal communication* related to cerebral injury

### EXPECTED OUTCOMES

- Learn to use his right hand to feed himself.
- Participate in exercises necessary to maintain muscle strength and tone.
- Maintain skin integrity.
- Indicate understanding that visual fields may improve in a few weeks.
- Practice and implement speech therapy activities while at the same time using alternative methods of communication.

### PLANNING AND IMPLEMENTATION

- Arrange mealtimes so that he is sitting up by the window in a clean and private environment.
- Provide adaptive devices (silverware with thick handles and nonslip plates).
- Encourage Mrs. Boren to visit at mealtimes, to assist with meals, and periodically to bring a favorite food from home.
- Provide passive ROM exercises for his left arm and leg; schedule active ROM exercises for his right extremities as well as quadriceps and gluteal sets every 4 hours during waking hours.
- Keep his skin clean and dry at all times.
- Establish and maintain a regular schedule for turning when he is in bed.
- Place objects (e.g., call bell, tissues) on unaffected side and approach him from that side.
- Support attempts to communicate verbally; when he is not understood, he prefers to use a large marker and tablet.

### EVALUATION

Mr. Boren is discharged to his home after being in the hospital for 10 days. During the first 2 months after discharge, Martha Grimes, RN, the home health nurse, visits Mr. and Mrs. Boren at home. At the end of 2 months, Mr. Boren is using his right hand to feed himself. He has regained partial use of his left arm and leg and is using a walker to move around the house and yard; he is even able to work in his flower garden. His skin has remained intact, and his vision is back to normal. He is slowly relearning speech; this has been the most difficult change for him to accept. Once he writes on his tablet, "I think God has forgotten me."

### Critical Thinking in the Nursing Process

1. Hypertension is sometimes referred to as "the silent killer." Provide justifications for this statement.
2. The functional changes Mr. Boren has experienced may make a return to teaching difficult. What other uses of his knowledge and abilities might you suggest?
3. What would be your reply if, after you had completed passive ROM on Mr. Boren's left arm, he wrote: "I just ignore that part of my body—it doesn't work anyway"?

See Evaluating your Response in Appendix C.

# THE CLIENT WITH AN INTRACRANIAL ANEURYSM

An **intracranial aneurysm** is a saccular outpouching of a cerebral artery that occurs at the site of a weakness in the vessel wall. The weakness may be the result of atherosclerosis, a congenital defect, trauma to the head, aging, or hypertension. A ruptured cerebral aneurysm is the most common cause of a hemorrhagic stroke.

## INCIDENCE AND PREVALENCE

Approximately 5 million North Americans have intracranial aneurysms; most go through life without any manifestations of bleeding. However, it is estimated that 30,000 people will have a rupture of an intracranial aneurysm each year, and two-thirds of the survivors will have serious disabilities. Intracranial aneurysms are most common in adults age 30 to 60 (Hickey, 2003; Porth, 2002).

The exact etiology is unknown, but theories of cause include (1) a developmental defect in the vessel wall and (2) degeneration or fragility of the vessel wall due to conditions such as hypertension, atherosclerosis, connective tissue disease, or abnormal blood flow. Hypertension and cigarette smoking may be predisposing factors.

## PATHOPHYSIOLOGY

Intracranial aneurysms tend to occur at the bifurcations and branches of the carotid arteries and the vertebrobasilar arteries at the circle of Willis, with most aneurysms (85%) located anteriorly. They range in size from smaller than 15 mm to larger than 50 mm. Intracranial aneurysms tend to enlarge with time, making the vessel wall thin and increasing the probability of rupture.

There are several different types of intracranial aneurysms: A *berry aneurysm* is probably the result of a congenital abnormality of the tunica media of the artery. The aneurysm usually ruptures without warning. A *saccular aneurysm* is any aneurysm with a saccular outpouching, which distends only a small portion of the vessel wall. This type of aneurysm is often caused by trauma. In a *fusiform aneurysm,* the entire circumference of a blood vessel swells to form an elongated tube. Most aneurysms of this type occur as a result of the changes of arteriosclerosis. Fusiform aneurysms act as space-occupying lesions. In a *dissecting aneurysm,* the tunica intima pulls away from the tunica media of the artery, and blood is forced between the two layers. It may result from atherosclerosis, inflammation, or trauma.

Intracranial aneurysms typically rupture from the dome rather than the base, forcing blood into the subarachnoid space at the base of the brain. The aneurysm may also rupture and force blood into brain tissue, the ventricles, or the subdural space. This discussion focuses on intracranial hemorrhages due to rupture of a cerebral aneurysm. See Chapter 42 for further discussion of types of intracranial hemorrhage.

## MANIFESTATIONS AND COMPLICATIONS

An intracranial aneurysm is usually asymptomatic until it ruptures, although very large aneurysms may cause headache and/or neurologic deficits due to pressure on adjacent intracranial structures. Small leakages of blood may occur periodically, causing headache, nausea, vomiting, and pain in the neck and back. The client may also have prodromal manifestations before the rupture occurs, such as headache, eye pain, visual deficits, and a dilated pupil.

The manifestations of a ruptured intracranial aneurysm (and subsequent subarachnoid hemorrhage) include a sudden, explosive headache; loss of consciousness; nausea and vomiting; a stiff neck and photophobia (due to meningeal irritation); cranial nerve deficits; stroke syndrome manifestations; and pituitary malfunctions (that result primarily from changes in ADH secretion).

The severity of the rupture is often inferred from the manifestations of the subarachnoid hemorrhage. In one system, severity ranges from grade I, in which the client has no symptoms or a slight headache with some stiffness of the neck, to grade V, in which the client is in a deep coma with decerebrate posturing.

Fibrin and platelets seal off the bleeding point, but the escaped blood forms a clot that irritates the brain tissue. The resulting inflammatory response causes cerebral edema, and both the edema and the hemorrhage increase intracranial pressure (Hickey, 2003). Bleeding into the subarachnoid space causes meningeal irritation. Hypothalamic dysfunction and seizures are also potential complications. The major complications of a ruptured intracranial aneurysm are rebleeding, vasospasm, and hydrocephalus.

### Rebleeding

The greatest risk for rebleeding is within the first day after the initial rupture, and again in 7 to 10 days (when the initial clot breaks down). Rebleeding is manifested by a sudden severe headache, nausea and vomiting, decreasing levels of consciousness, and new neurologic deficits (Hickey, 2003). The mortality from rebleeding is as high as from the initial rupture.

### Vasospasm

Cerebral vasospasm is a common but dangerous complication that occurs between 3 and 10 days after a subarachnoid hemorrhage. It is associated with a large number of deaths and disability. A cerebral vasospasm narrows the lumen of one or more cerebral vessels, causing ischemia and infarction of tissue supplied by the affected vessels. The actual cause is unknown, but it occurs in blood vessels surrounded by thick blood clots, suggesting that some substance in the clot initiates the spasm. The manifestations vary according to the degree of spasm and the area of brain affected. Regional alterations may cause focal deficits (such as hemiplegia), whereas global alterations cause loss of consciousness.

### Hydrocephalus

**Hydrocephalus,** an abnormal accumulation of cerebrospinal fluid (CSF) within the cranial vault and dilation of the ventricles, is a potential complication of a ruptured intracranial aneurysm. Hydrocephalus is thought to be the result of obstruction of reabsorption of CSF through the arachnoid villi. The obstruction is caused by an increased protein content of the CSF because of lysis of blood in the subarachnoid space (Porth, 2002). The accumulation of cerebrospinal fluid increases intracranial pressure. Initial manifestations of hydrocephalus are typically nonspecific but commonly include decreasing levels of consciousness.

## COLLABORATIVE CARE

The care of the client with a ruptured intracranial aneurysm includes determining the location of the aneurysm, treating the manifestations of the hemorrhage, and preventing rebleeding and vasospasm. Surgery is the treatment of choice to repair the bleeding artery.

### Diagnostic Tests

The following diagnostic tests may be conducted to identify the site and extent of a ruptured intracranial aneurysm, as well as rebleeding.

- *CT scan* of the brain demonstrates blood in the subarachnoid space in most clients within the first 24 to 48 hours after rupture.
- *Lumbar puncture* may be performed to withdraw cerebrospinal fluid for analysis. The presence of blood in the cerebrospinal fluid confirms a subarachnoid hemorrhage. However, this procedure poses a risk of rebleeding and brain herniation (Porth, 2002).
- *Bilateral carotid* and *vertebral cerebral angiography* may be conducted to determine the site and size of an aneurysm. A contrast medium (if used) is injected into an artery, and X-ray films are taken to visualize the cerebral vessels. This diagnostic test is not conducted unless the client's condition is stable enough for surgery.

### Medications

If surgery is not possible because of the client's condition, medications may be used to reduce the risk of rebleeding and vasospasm until surgery is feasible.

Aminocaproic acid (Amicar, Epsikapron) is a fibrinolysis inhibitor used to treat excessive bleeding in acute, lifethreatening situations. It prevents the lysis of any blood clot that has formed near the site of a rupture. This drug is used in the first 2 weeks after aneurysm rupture (or until the client has surgery) to reduce the risk of rebleeding. The drug is administered intravenously the first week and orally thereafter. Potential complications include pulmonary embolism, venous thrombosis, and focal ischemic neurologic deficits.

Calcium channel blockers, such as nimodipine (Nimotop), are used to improve neurologic deficits due to vasospasm following subarachnoid hemorrhage from ruptured intracranial aneurysms. The drug is administered orally for 3 weeks after the hemorrhage. It has been found to reduce the incidence of ischemic deficits from arterial spasm without side effects (Tierney et al., 2001).

Other medications that may be prescribed include:

- Anticonvulsants, such as phenytoin (Dilantin), to prevent seizures if the client has increased intracranial pressure.
- Stool softeners, such as docusate, to prevent constipation and straining with a bowel movement (which increases intracranial pressure and blood pressure). These, in turn, may cause rebleeding.
- Analgesics (e.g., acetaminophen or codeine) for headache.

### Surgery

Surgery for the treatment of intracranial aneurysm is done either to prevent rupture or to isolate the vessel to prevent further bleeding. Clients with good neurologic status may have surgery soon after the rupture. In clients with significant neurologic deficits, surgery may be delayed until they are more stable and less at risk for vasospasm.

There are several different types of surgery to repair a ruptured intracranial aneurysm or to prevent the rupture of an existing large aneurysm. The skull is opened (craniotomy), and the aneurysm is located. The neck of the aneurysm may be clipped with a metal clip (preventing the entry of blood into the aneurysm), or the involved artery may be clipped both proximally and distally to the aneurysm to isolate the affected area. Endovascular Gudlielmi detachable coils (GDCs) are used to treat aneurysms with narrow necks. The coil is inserted into the dome of the aneurysm and an electric current is passed through the coil to cause coagulation. The procedure, performed by a neuroradiologist, may be conducted either under general or local anesthesia (Bucher & Melander, 1999).

## NURSING CARE

### Nursing Diagnoses and Interventions

Nursing care is planned and implemented for the client with a ruptured intracranial aneurysm to prevent rebleeding as well as to meet needs resulting from neurologic deficits. Other appropriate nursing diagnoses and interventions are described earlier in the chapter in the discussion of nursing care for the client with a stroke.

### Ineffective Tissue Perfusion (Cerebral)

This discussion focuses on the care of the client immediately after the intracranial aneurysm ruptures. The expected outcome of care is preventing rebleeding and improving cerebral tissue perfusion.

- Institute aneurysm precautions to prevent rebleeding, as follows:
  - Keep the client in a private, quiet, darkened room. Disconnect or remove the telephone. Avoid using bright overhead lights. *A quiet environment helps prevent an increase in blood pressure, which could precipitate rebleeding. The client may experience photophobia (abnormal sensitivity to light) if hemorrhage has damaged the oculomotor nerve.*

- Elevate the head of the bed 30 to 45 degrees; follow prescribed activity orders (usually complete bed rest, but in some cases bathroom privileges may be approved). *Elevating the head of the bed promotes venous return from the brain and thus decreases intracranial pressure. Decreasing activity reduces the likelihood of increases in blood pressure.*
- Limit visitors to two family members at any one time, and limit the duration of visits. Monitor client response to visitors and decrease interactions if the client becomes agitated or upset. *Psychologic stress may increase blood pressure and the risk of rebleeding; however, social isolation may increase anxiety and stress. Each client (and family) must be individually evaluated.*
- Allow reading, watching television (if available), or listening to the radio (if available) to promote relaxation. *Although these passive activities were previously contraindicated for the client on aneurysm precautions, current therapy is based on the belief that these activities promote relaxation and help control blood pressure.*
- Prevent constipation and straining to have a bowel movement. Administer stool softeners as prescribed. Collaborate with the client and physician about use of a bedside commode or the bathroom. Do not administer enemas. *The client is at risk for constipation as a result of decreased mobility and the administration of narcotics (such as codeine) for headache. When straining to have a bowel movement, the client uses the Valsalva maneuver, which increases intracranial pressure and may precipitate rebleeding.*

**PRACTICE ALERT** *Maintaining a daily stool chart is an important assessment in preventing constipation.* ■

- If the client is alert, and depending on physician preferences, allow to feed self and provide own personal care. *In many instances, self-care causes less anxiety and stress than care provided by the nurse. The extent of care provided varies according to client condition and physician preferences.*
- Monitor vital signs and neurologic status as indicated by client condition (frequency of assessments may range from every 15 minutes to every 4 hours). *Vital signs and neurologic assessments provide ongoing data for evaluation of changes indicative of increasing intracranial pressure and decreasing neurologic function. Report any change immediately to the physician.*

**PRACTICE ALERT** *A rising blood pressure and falling pulse rate are manifestations of increased intracranial pressure.* ■

- Maintain seizure precautions: Have suction equipment and an oropharyngeal tube at the bedside, maintain the bed in the low position, and keep the side rails padded and raised. *Applying suction and inserting an oropharyngeal airway may be necessary to maintain an open airway in case of seizure. A lowered bed and padded, raised side rails prevent injury if a seizure occurs.*
- Avoid positioning and activities that increase intracranial pressure such as coughing, sneezing, vomiting, sharply flexing the neck, blowing the nose, enemas, moving self up in bed, or cigarette smoking. *These measures help to prevent increasing intracranial pressure and rebleeding.*

## THE CLIENT WITH AN ARTERIOVENOUS MALFORMATION

An **arteriovenous (AV) malformation** is a congenital intracranial lesion, formed by a tangled collection of dilated arteries and veins, that allows blood to flow directly from the arterial into the venous system, bypassing the normal capillary network. Most AV malformations (90%) are located in the cerebral hemispheres; the remainder are found in the cerebellum and brainstem.

Rupture of vessels in the malformations account for 2% of all strokes. Clients with this condition develop manifestations before 40 years of age; it affects men and women equally (Porth, 2002). The manifestations are the result of spontaneous bleeding from the lesion into the subarachnoid space or brain tissue.

## PATHOPHYSIOLOGY

AV malformations displace rather than encompass normal brain tissue (Hickey, 2003). The pathophysiologic effects of an AV malformation are the result of the shunting of blood from the arterial to the venous system and of altered perfusion of cerebral tissue near the malformation. The shunting of arterial blood directly into the venous system within the malformation transfers the higher arterial pressure directly into the lower-pressure venous system. This increased pressure is likely to cause spontaneous bleeding or progressive expansion and rupture of a blood vessel.

Altered cerebral perfusion results when blood flow through a large, high-flow malformation is diverted from the normal cerebral circulation, causing tissue ischemia of the area surrounding the malformation. This is sometimes called a vascular "steal" phenomenon.

AV malformations range in size from very small to very large. Large malformations are usually initially manifested by seizure activity. In contrast, the manifestations of a small malformation are more often due to a hemorrhage that causes neurologic deficits. In both instances, the client may have recurrent headaches that do not respond to treatment.

## COLLABORATIVE CARE

AV malformations are diagnosed with the same diagnostic tests (CT scan, MRI, angiography) used to diagnose an intracranial aneurysm.

If the malformation is accessible, the ideal treatment is excision of the malformation and removal of any hematoma.

Large malformations may be treated by embolization. In this procedure, substances such as Gelfoam or metallic pellets are introduced into the involved area of the cerebral circulation, where they form emboli and gradually obstruct blood flow in the malformation. Inaccessible malformations are also treated with radiation therapy or laser therapy, to coagulate blood in the malformation and thicken its vascular elements, eventually obstructing it. When the malformation is excised or obstructed, blood flow is no longer shunted, and cerebral perfusion improves.

## NURSING CARE

Nursing care depends on the condition of the malformation. If hemorrhage has not occurred, teach the client to avoid activities that raise blood pressure or could cause injury. The client is usually given medications to control blood pressure and prevent seizures.

If the malformation ruptures and causes an intracranial hemorrhage, nursing care is the same as for any client who has had a hemorrhagic stroke (discussed earlier in this chapter).

# SPINAL CORD DISORDERS

## THE CLIENT WITH A SPINAL CORD INJURY

Nursing care of clients with disorders of the spinal cord takes place from the acute management phase through ongoing rehabilitation in a variety of settings. Although priorities of care may change depending on the client and setting, care focuses on maximizing function to preserve quality of life. The nurse provides independent care and also collaborates with other health care professionals to meet this goal.

### INCIDENCE AND PREVALENCE

A **spinal cord injury (SCI)** is usually due to trauma. There are an estimated 250,000 to 400,000 people with SCIs living in the United States. Although SCIs occur in people of all ages, they are most often seen in young adults age 16 to 30. The majority of the injuries are due to motor vehicle accidents; other causes include falls, violence, and sports injuries (with the majority from diving). Approximately 8000 people have a SCI each year, with the greatest risk for injury being in the summer (National Spinal Cord Injury Association, 1998; Porth, 2002).

The major causes of SCI are concussion, contusion, laceration, transection, hemorrhage, and damage to blood vessels that supply the spinal cord. If vertebrae are fractured and ligaments are torn, bony fragments can damage the cord and make the spinal column unstable. Injury to blood vessels supplying the cord can cause permanent damage. The injury is identified by vertebral level. For example, a C6 spinal cord injury is at the sixth cervical vertebra.

### Risk Factors

The three major risk factors for SCIs are age, gender, and alcohol or drug abuse. Young men are more prone to take risks than women. Older adults are more likely to have a cord injury from even minor trauma as a result of age-related vertebral degeneration. Motor vehicle crashes while under the influence of alcohol or drugs are a major source of trauma to people of all ages.

## OVERVIEW OF THE NORMAL SPINAL CORD

The spinal cord runs through the vertebral canal of the vertebral column from the foramen magnum to the L1 or L2 level. The cord provides a two-way pathway for the conduction of impulses and information to and from the brain and the body, serves as a major reflex center, and (through its attached spinal nerves) is involved in the sensory and motor innervation of the entire body below the head.

The cord consists of an outer region of white matter and an inner region of gray matter. The gray matter comprises the central canal of the cord, the posterior horns, the anterior horns, and the lateral horns. It is divided into a sensory half (dorsally) and a motor half (ventrally) and innervates somatic and visceral regions of the body. The white matter consists of tracts or pathways that convey information. The ascending (sensory) pathways carry information about proprioception, fine touch, discrimination, pain, temperature, deep pressure, and touch. The descending (motor) pathways carry information about movement. The pyramidal tracts control skilled voluntary movements (such as writing). The extrapyramidal tracts (all tracts other than the pyramidal tracts) bring about all other body movements. See Chapter 40 for further information.

### PATHOPHYSIOLOGY

The primary injury causes microscopic hemorrhages in the gray matter of the cord and edema of the white matter of the cord. These initial pathologic changes are followed by the secondary injury, with mechanisms that increase the area of injury. The hemorrhages extend, eventually involving the entire gray matter. Microcirculation to the cord is impaired by edema and hemorrhage. The injured tissue releases norepinephrine, serotonin, dopamine, and histamine; these vasoactive substances cause vasospasm and further decrease microcirculation. As a result, vascular perfusion and oxygen tension of the affected area is decreased, which leads to ischemia.

When ischemia is prolonged, necrosis of both gray and white matter begins within a few hours, and within 24 hours the function of nerves passing through the injured area is lost. Although circulation returns to the white matter of the cord in about 24 hours, decreased circulation in the gray matter continues. Because edema extends the level of injury for two cord segments above and below the affected level, the extent of injury cannot be determined for up to 1 week.

Tissue repair occurs over a period of 3 to 4 weeks. Phagocytes enter the area in 36 to 48 hours after the initial injury. Neurons degenerate and are removed by microphages in the first 10 days after the injury. Red blood cells disintegrate, and the hemorrhages are reabsorbed. Eventually the area of injury is replaced by acellular collagenous tissue, and the meninges thicken.

## Forces Resulting in SCI

SCIs are the result of the application of excessive force to the spinal column. The most common cause of abnormal spinal column movements are acceleration and deceleration (forces that are applied to the body, for example, in automobile crashes and falls). *Acceleration* occurs when external force is applied in a rear-end collision; the upper torso and head are forced backward and then forward. *Deceleration* occurs in a head-on collision; the external force is applied from the front. The head and body move forward until they meet a stationary object and then are forced backward. The following forces and movements (Figure 41–5 ■) may cause a variety of spinal cord injuries, with the extent of injury depending on the amount and direction of motion, and the rate of application of force.

- *Hyperflexion,* or forcible forward bending, may compress vertebral bodies and disrupt ligaments and intervertebral disks.
- *Hyperextension,* or forcible backward bending, often disrupts ligaments and causes vertebral fractures. A whiplash injury is a less severe form of hyperextension, with injury to soft tissues but no vertebral or spinal cord damage.
- *Axial loading,* a form of compression, is the application of vertical force to the spinal column (for instance, by falling and landing on the feet or buttocks or by diving into shallow water).
- *Excessive rotation,* in which the head is excessively turned, may tear ligaments, fracture articular surfaces, and cause compression fractures.

The alteration of the spinal cord and soft tissues caused by these abnormal movements is called **deformation.** In addition, the spinal cord may be penetrated by bullets and other foreign objects (e.g., sharp objects used as weapons, shrapnel from explosions). Penetrating injuries may cause vertebral fractures, tear ligaments and muscles, or cut through a part or all of the spinal cord. Complete severing of the cord is rare.

## Sites of Pathology

Injuries occur most often in the lumbar and cervical regions. The most frequent sites of injury of the cord are at the first, second, and fourth to sixth cervical vertebrae (C1, C2, C4 to C6);

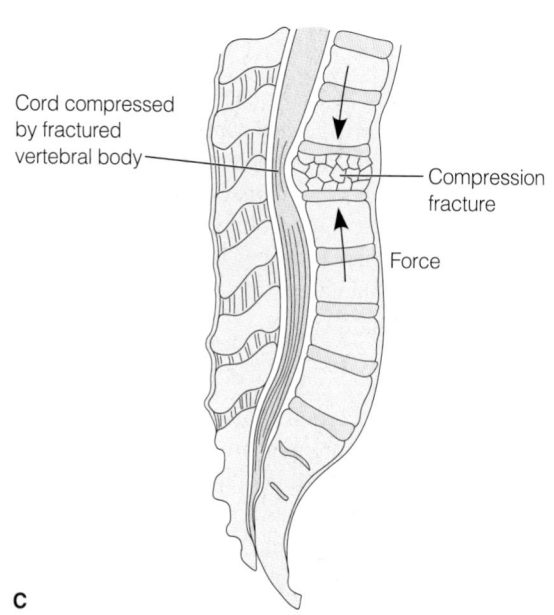

**Figure 41–5** ■ Spinal cord injury mechanisms. *A,* Hyperflexion. *B,* Hyperextension. *C,* Axial loading, a form of compression.

Torn posterior longitudinal ligaments

Cord compressed by disc and dislocated vertebra

Force

C5

Disk

Anterior dislocation of vertebra

**A**

Force

Torn anterior longitudinal ligament

Cord stretched

**B**

Cord compressed by fractured vertebral body

Compression fracture

Force

**C**

and the eleventh thoracic to second lumbar vertebrae (T11 to L2). Because the cervical spine has a wider range of movement than the rest of the spine, the cervical portion is more likely to be affected by externally applied forces. In addition, the cord fills most of the vertebral canal in the cervical and lumbar regions and thus is more easily injured. Damage to the vertebrae and ligaments causes the spinal column to become unstable, increasing the possibility of compression or stretching of the spinal cord with any further movement.

## Classification of SCI

SCIs are classified according to systems, for instance (1) as complete or incomplete cord injury, (2) by cause of injury, and (3) by level of injury. In clinical practice, these classifications often overlap. In a *complete SCI,* the motor and sensory neural pathways are completely interrupted (transected), resulting in total loss of motor and sensory function below the level of the injury. In an *incomplete SCI,* the motor and sensory pathways are only partially interrupted, with variable loss of function below the level of injury. Incomplete spinal cord injuries are further classified into syndromes as outlined in Table 41–1. The alterations in function that occur as the result of a spinal cord injury vary greatly depending on the amount of tissue damage and the level of injury.

## MANIFESTATIONS AND COMPLICATIONS

The spinal cord, the vertebrae, the intervertebral disks, the spinal nerves, the ligaments, and the surrounding soft-tissue structures are in such close anatomic proximity that any condition or injury affecting one structure may well affect any one or all of the other structures. The conditions with the most critical

effects are disorders affecting the spinal cord. Disorders and injuries of the spinal cord have the potential to affect movement, perception, sensation, sexual function, and elimination. Manifestations and complications of SCI by body system are listed in the box below.

### Manifestations and Complications of Spinal Cord Injury by Body System

**Integument**
- Decubitus (pressure) ulcers

**Neurologic**
- Pain
- Areflexia
- Hypotonia
- Autonomic dysreflexia

**Cardiovascular**
- Spinal shock
- Paroxysmal hypertension
- Orthostatic hypotension
- Cardiac dysrhythmias
- Decreased venous return
- Hypercalcemia

**Respiratory**
- Limited chest expansion
- Decreased cough reflex
- Decreased vital capacity

**Gastrointestinal**
- Stress ulcers
- Paralytic ileus
- Stool impaction
- Stool incontinence

**Genitourinary**
- Urinary retention
- Urinary incontinence
- Neurogenic bladder
- Impotence
- Testicular atrophy
- Inability to ejaculate
- Decreased vaginal lubrication

**Musculoskeletal**
- Joint contractures
- Bone demineralization
- Osteoporosis
- Muscle spasms
- Muscle atrophy
- Pathologic fractures
- Paraplegia
- Tetraplegia

### TABLE 41–1  Incomplete Spinal Cord Injury Syndromes

| Type | Cause | Location | Deficits |
|---|---|---|---|
| Central syndrome | Cord transection Hyperextension | Cervical | Spastic paralysis of the upper extremities Variable paralysis of the lower extremities Variable effects on the bowel, the bladder, and sexual function |
| Anterior syndrome | Damage to the anterior spinal artery Infarction of the anterior spinal artery Hyperflexion | Anterior two-thirds of the cord | Paralysis below the level of injury Loss of temperature and pain sensation below the level of injury |
| Posterior syndrome | Vertebral dislocation Herniated disk Compression | Nerve roots | Weakness in isolated muscle groups Tingling, pain Decreased or absent reflexes in the involved area Bowel or bladder dysfunction |
| Brown-Séquard syndrome | Penetrating trauma | Hemisection of the anterior and posterior cord | Paralysis below the level of injury on the ipsilateral (same) side of the body Contralateral loss of temperature and pain sensation below the level of injury Ipsilateral loss of proprioception below the level of injury |
| Horner's syndrome | Incomplete cord transection | Cervical sympathetic nerves | Ipsilateral ptosis of the eyelid, constricted pupil, and facial anhidrosis (inability to perspire) |

## Spinal Shock

**Spinal shock** is the temporary loss of reflex function (called **areflexia**) below the level of injury. This response begins immediately after complete transection of the spinal cord, when connections between the brain and the spinal cord are interrupted and the cord does not function at all. The response also occurs (although in varying degrees) after partial transection as well as after spinal cord contusions, compression, and ischemia.

Normal activity of the spinal cord is dependent on constant impulses from the higher centers of the brain. When damage from an injury stops these impulses, spinal shock follows. There is loss of motor function, tendon reflexes, and autonomic function. Of particular concern is the effect on pulse and blood pressure; the parasympathetic system dominates in spinal shock, causing bradycardia and hypotension.

Spinal shock may begin within 1 hour of the injury. The condition may last from a few minutes to several months (although it usually lasts from 1 to 6 weeks), and then reflex activity returns. Spinal shock ends slowly, with the gradual reappearance of reflexes, hyperreflexia (increased reflex responses), muscle spasticity, and reflex bladder emptying.

The manifestations of acute spinal shock (which vary in degree) include the following:

- Bradycardia
- Hypotension
- Flaccid paralysis of skeletal muscles
- Loss of sensations of pain, touch, temperature, and pressure
- Absence of visceral and somatic sensations
- Bowel and bladder dysfunction
- Loss of the ability to perspire

A person with a cervical cord injury may also have neurogenic shock, resulting in cardiovascular changes. These changes are due to the inability of higher centers in the brainstem to modulate reflexes. As a result, vascular beds dilate, and the cardiac accelerator reflex is suppressed. The client experiences orthostatic hypotension and bradycardia. Other symptoms may include respiratory insufficiency due to loss of innervation of the diaphragm in C1 to C4 injuries, hypothermia, paralytic ileus, urinary retention, and oliguria.

Both bradycardia and hypotension may persist even after the spinal shock resolves. In addition to losing sympathetic control of the heart rate, the client with a high-level SCI experiences decreased peripheral resistance and loss of muscle activity. These changes result in sluggish blood flow and decreased venous return, increasing the risk for thrombophlebitis.

## Upper and Lower Motor Neuron Deficits

Injuries to the spinal cord are often classified as either *upper motor neuron lesions* or *lower motor neuron lesions*. Motor neurons are functional units that carry motor impulses. The upper motor neurons (located in the cerebral cortex, thalamus, brainstem, and corticospinal and corticobulbar tracts) are responsible for voluntary movement. When these motor pathways are interrupted, the client experiences spastic paralysis and hyperreflexia and may be unable to carry out skilled movement.

Lower motor neurons (located in the anterior horn of the spinal cord, the motor nuclei of the brainstem, and the axons that reach the motor end plate of skeletal muscles) are responsible for innervation and contraction of skeletal muscles. Interruption of lower motor neurons results in muscle flaccidity and extensive muscle atrophy, with loss of both voluntary and involuntary movement. If only some of the motor neurons supplying a muscle are affected, the client experiences partial paralysis (paresis); if all motor neurons to a muscle are affected, the client experiences complete paralysis. Hyporeflexia is also present.

## Paraplegia and Tetraplegia

Two common neurologic deficits resulting from an SCI are paraplegia and tetraplegia (see Figure 41–1). **Paraplegia** is paralysis of the lower portion of the body, sometimes involving the lower trunk. Paraplegia occurs when the thoracic, lumbar, and sacral portions of the spinal cord are injured, causing loss or impairment of sensory and/or motor function. **Tetraplegia,** formerly called quadriplegia, occurs when cervical segments of the cord are injured, impairing function of the arms, trunk, legs, and pelvic organs.

## Autonomic Dysreflexia

**Autonomic dysreflexia** (also called *autonomic hyperreflexia*) is an exaggerated sympathetic response that occurs in clients with SCIs at or above the T6 level. This response, which is seen only after recovery from spinal shock, occurs as a result of a lack of control of the autonomic nervous system by higher centers. When stimuli (such as a full bladder) are unable to ascend the cord, mass reflex stimulation of the sympathetic nerves below the level of the injured cord area occurs, triggering massive vasoconstriction. In response, the vagus nerve causes bradycardia and vasodilation above the level of injury. If untreated, autonomic dysreflexia can cause seizures, a stroke, or a myocardial infarction (Hickey, 2003). The complications of untreated dysreflexia are potentially fatal.

Autonomic dysreflexia is triggered by stimuli that would normally cause abdominal discomfort (a full bladder is the most common cause), by stimulation of pain receptors, and by visceral contractions (Porth, 2002). Causes include fecal impaction, bladder infections or stones, acute abdominal disorders, intrauterine contractions, ejaculation, and stimulation from pressure ulcers or ingrown toenails.

The manifestations of this condition include pounding headache; bradycardia; hypertension (with readings as high as 300/160); flushed, warm skin with profuse sweating above the lesion and pale, cold, and dry skin below it; and anxiety (Porth, 2002). Dysreflexia is a neurologic emergency and requires immediate treatment.

# COLLABORATIVE CARE

The client with an acute SCI requires emergency assessment and care and medications; sometimes the client also requires immobilization and surgery. The client is first assessed and stabilized at the scene of the accident, initially treated in the emergency room, and then admitted to the hospital intensive care unit.

## Emergency Care at the Scene

The danger of death from SCI is greatest when there is damage to or transection of the upper cervical region. When the injury is at the C1 to C4 level, respiratory paralysis is common, and the client who survives requires ventilator assistance to breathe. Injuries below C4 may increase the risk of respiratory failure if edema ascends the cord. It is of critical importance not to complicate the initial injury by allowing the fractured vertebrae to damage the cord further during transport to the hospital. Although at one time injuries to the high cervical cord were almost always fatal, advances in trauma care have greatly improved the survival rate.

All people who have sustained trauma to the head or spine, or who are unconscious, should be treated as though they have a spinal cord injury. Prehospital management includes rapid assessment of the ABCs (airway, breathing, circulation), immobilizing and stabilizing the head and neck, removing the person from the site of injury, stabilizing other life-threatening injuries, and rapidly transporting the person to the appropriate facility. Guidelines for emergency care are as follows:

- Avoid flexing, extending, or rotating the neck.
- Immobilize the neck, using rolled towels or blankets, or apply a cervical collar before moving the client onto a backboard.
- Secure the head by placing a belt or tape across the forehead and securing it to the stretcher.
- Maintain the client in the supine position.
- Transfer directly from the stretcher with backboard still in place to the type of bed that will be used in the hospital.

## Emergency Department Management

Assessment findings at the scene of the accident or in the emergency room vary according to the level of injury. The following findings indicate cervical injury.

- Paralysis or weakness of extremities
- Respiratory distress manifested by changes in arterial blood gas studies, cyanosis, flaring of the nostrils, use of accessory muscles of respiration, and restlessness
- Pulse rate below 60 and systolic BP below 80
- Decreased peristalsis

This finding indicates thoracic and lumbar injury:

- Paralysis or weakness of extremities

These findings indicate acute spinal shock:

- Loss of skin sensation
- Flaccid paralysis, areflexia
- Absent bowel sounds
- Bladder distention
- Decreasing blood pressure
- Absence of the cremasteric reflex in males (retraction of the left or right testicle in response to stimulation of the skin of, respectively, the inner left or right thigh)

The client in the emergency department with a suspected or identified SCI is also treated for respiratory problems, par-alytic ileus, atonic bladder, and cardiovascular alterations. Respiratory distress in the client with a cervical-level injury is treated by placing the client on a ventilator. Oxygen is administered to the client with a thoracic-level injury. Paralytic ileus (obstruction of the intestines due to lack of peristalsis) is common in clients with a spinal cord injury and is treated by the insertion of a nasogastric tube with connection to suction. To prevent overdistention of an atonic bladder, an indwelling catheter is inserted and connected to dependent drainage. Cardiovascular status is assessed on a continuous basis by inserting invasive monitoring devices, such as a Swan-Ganz catheter, and attaching the client to a cardiac monitor.

High-dose steroid protocol using methylprednisolone (Medrol) must be immediately implemented on admission to the emergency room. Clinical research indicates that the use of this adrenocorticosteroid is effective in preventing secondary spinal cord damage from edema and ischemia. The medication must be administered intravenously within 8 hours of the injury to be effective in preventing secondary damage. A loading dose is administered initially and a maintenance dose is continued for 23 hours.

## Diagnostic Tests

Diagnostic tests are ordered to identify the level and extent of injury, and to detect any complications.

- *X-ray films* of the cervical spine are taken immediately after admission to establish the level of injury and extent of vertebral injury. Thoracic and lumbar spine X-rays are taken at the same time if possible.
- *CT scan* or *MRI* illustrates changes in the vertebrae, spinal cord, and tissues around the cord.
- *Arterial blood gases* are measured to establish a baseline or to identify problems due to respiratory insufficiency.
- *Somatosensory evoked potential (SEP) studies* may be done to locate the level of spinal cord injury. In these tests, peripheral nerves are stimulated and response times measured.

## Medications

The pharmacologic treatment of the client with SCI is symptomatic. It is directed primarily toward decreasing edema from the injury, treating hypotension and bradycardia, and treating spasticity.

- Corticosteroids, discussed earlier in this section, may be used to decrease or control edema of the cord.
- Vasopressors are used in the immediate critical care phase to treat bradycardia or hypotension due to spinal and neurogenic shock. Examples of drugs are dopamine (Intropin) to treat hypotension in neurogenic shock and dobutamine (Dobutrex) to support cardiac function. Atropine should be available at the bedside to treat bradycardia.
- Antispasmodics are used to treat spasticity in clients with spinal cord injury. Both baclofen (Lioresal) and diazepam (Valium) may be used. A discussion of nursing implications of treatment with antispasmodics is found in the Medication Administration box on page 1328.

## Medication Administration

### Antispasmodics in Spinal Cord Injury

Baclofen (Lioresal)
Chlorzoxazone (Paraflex)
Cyclobenzaprine hydrochloride (Flexeril)
Diazepam (Valium)
Orphenadrine citrate (Norflex)

These drugs depress the central nervous system and inhibit the transmission of impulses from the spinal cord to skeletal muscle. They are used to control muscle spasm and pain associated with acute or chronic musculoskeletal conditions. They are not always effective in controlling spasticity resulting from cerebral or spinal cord conditions.

#### Nursing Responsibilities
- Assess the client's spasticity and involuntary movements to obtain baseline data for comparison of results of therapy.

- Do not expect therapy to have effects for 1 week.
- Administer oral medications with food to decrease gastrointestinal symptoms.

#### Client and Family Teaching
- These drugs may cause drowsiness, diplopia, and impotence.
- Take your medications with meals to decrease gastric irritation.
- Physical improvement may take several weeks.
- Report slurred speech, drooling, or inability to carry out normal functions to the physician.
- Do not stop taking the medication without consulting your health care provider.

---

- Analgesics such as nonsteroidal anti-inflammatory agents and tricylic antidepressants such as amitriptyline (Elavil) and imipramine (Tofranil) are administered to reduce pain.
- Histamine $H_2$ antagonists (e.g., ranitidine [Zantac]) are often administered to prevent stress-related gastric ulcers, a common complication in SCI.
- Anticoagulants (heparin or warfarin) may be given to prevent thrombophlebitis.
- Stool softeners may be administered as part of a bowel training program.

## Treatments

The treatments used in the management of an SCI include surgery, stabilization, and immobilization.

### Surgery

Early surgical treatment may be necessary if there is evidence of compression of the spinal cord by bone fragments or a hematoma. Surgery may also be done to stabilize and support the spine. However, many clients are treated with stabilization devices and do not require surgery. Surgeries that may be performed include a decompression laminectomy, a spinal fusion, and insertion of metal rods. Surgeries of the spine are discussed later in the chapter.

### Stabilization and Immobilization

The client with an SCI as a result of one or more dislocations or fractures of the cervical vertebrae may be immobilized by being placed in some type of traction or external fixation device to stabilize the vertebral column and prevent any further damage. Traction may also be used to stabilize the spinal column for clients who are not yet in a condition to have surgery or who have severe bleeding and edema of the injured cord. The physician applies the traction or fixation device; the nurse is responsible for assessments and interventions following the application.

Although used less frequently today, various devices provide cervical traction. Gardner-Wells tongs may be used (Figure 41–6 ■). In this type of traction, the physician applies

pins to the skull, approximately 1 cm above each ear, and weights are attached to the device.

The halo external fixation device is often used to provide stabilization if there is no significant involvement of the ligaments (Figure 41–7 ■). It is most often used to provide stability for fractures of the cervical and high thoracic vertebrae without cord damage. This device allows greater mobility, self-care, and participation in rehabilitation programs. The device is secured with four pins inserted into the skull, two in the frontal bone and two in the occipital bone. The halo ring is then attached to a rigid plastic vest lined with sheepskin. Nursing interventions for the client using a halo fixation device are described in the Nursing Care box on page 1329.

## NURSING CARE

Both during the acute phase and the rehabilitative phase, the client with a SCI has complex needs that involve all members of the health care team. Because these injuries are more common in younger clients, consideration of life-long effects on both the client and the family is essential. The nurse coordi-

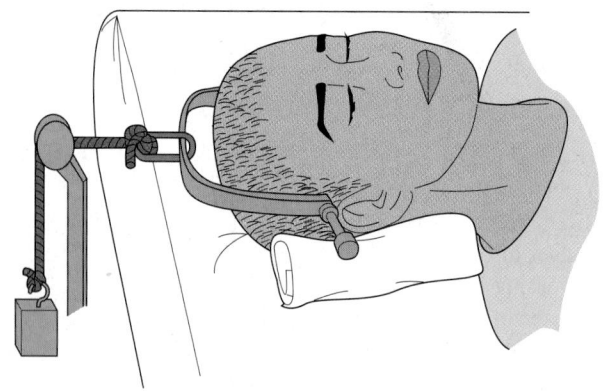

**Figure 41–6 ■** Cervical traction may be applied by several methods, including Gardner-Wells tongs.

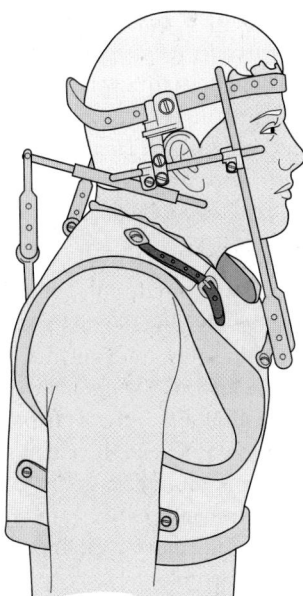

**Figure 41–7** ■ The halo external fixation device.

nates client care and develops and implements a care plan that is individualized to each client and family. The focus of the plan is to prevent the secondary complications of immobility and altered body functions, to promote self-care, and to educate the client and family.

## Health Promotion

Health promotion for SCI primarily involves preventing injuries. Nurses can provide valuable information in the community and in the workplace to prevent SCI. Programs that focus on wearing seat belts and using approved infant seats and child booster chairs in automobiles can do much to help decrease the number of SCIs each year. Educational programs that promote workplace safety and farm safety should include information to prevent falls and how to use heavy equipment safely.

## Assessment

The following data are collected through the health history and physical examination (see Chapter 40). Further focused assessments are described with nursing interventions in the next section.

- Health history: time, location, and type of accident; location, duration, quality, and intensity of pain; dyspnea; sensation; paresthesia
- Physical examination: vital signs, motor strength, movement, spinal reflexes, bowel sounds, bladder distention

## Nursing Diagnoses and Interventions

Because an SCI has many possible effects, many nursing diagnoses may be appropriate. Nursing diagnoses discussed in this section focus on problems with physical mobility, gas exchange, dysreflexia, bowel and bladder elimination, sexual dysfunction, and self-esteem.

## Impaired Physical Mobility

After the initial period of spinal shock and areflexia, the client regains spinal reflex activity and muscle tone that is not under the control of higher centers. Clients with injuries above the level of T12 experience involuntary spastic movements of skeletal muscles. These movements reach a peak about 2 years after the injury and then gradually subside (Porth, 2002). Spasms impair the ability to carry out the activities of daily life and work. In addition, the paraplegia or tetraplegia increases the potential for impaired skin integrity, thrombophlebitis, and contractures.

The goals of care for clients with impaired mobility due to a spinal cord injury are to reduce the effects of spasticity and to

## NURSING CARE OF THE CLIENT IN HALO FIXATION

### NURSING RESPONSIBILITIES

- Maintain integrity of the halo external fixation device.
  a. Inspect pins and traction bars for tightness; report loosened pins to physician.
  b. Tape the appropriate wrench to the head of the bed for emergency intervention.
  c. Never use the halo ring to lift or reposition the client.
  *Loosening of the apparatus poses the risk of further damage to the cord. It is the responsibility of the nurse to maintain the integrity of the apparatus and the safety of the client.*
- Assess muscle function and skin sensation every 2 hours in the acute phase and every 4 hours thereafter.
  a. Assess motor function on a scale of 0 to 5, with 0 being no evidence of muscle contraction and 5 being normal muscle strength with full range of motion.
  b. Assess sensation by comparing touch and pain, moving from impaired to normal areas, and testing both the right and left sides of the body.

*Monitoring muscle function and skin sensation allows early identification of potential neurologic deficits.*
- Monitor pin sites each shift and follow hospital policy for pin care. Here are some general guidelines.
  a. Assess pin sites for redness, edema, and drainage.
  b. Depending on policy, clean each pin site with a sterile applicator dipped in hydrogen peroxide, apply a topical antibiotic, and cover with sterile 2-inch split gauze squares.
  *Organisms can enter the body through the pin-insertion site; assessments and care are provided to detect signs of and prevent infection.*
- Maintain skin integrity.
  a. Turn the immobile client every 2 hours.
  b. Inspect the skin around edges of the vest every 4 hours.
  c. Change the sheepskin liner when it is soiled and at least once each week.

*These interventions prevent skin injury and irritation.*

prevent complications involving the skin, the cardiovascular system, and joint function.

- Perform passive ROM exercises for all extremities at least twice a day. Identify stimuli that cause spastic movements and either avoid the stimuli (such as certain exercises) or teach the client to expect the movements. *ROM exercises help prevent contractures and stretch spastic muscles, promoting rehabilitation.*
- Maintain skin integrity by turning every 2 hours, assessing pressure points at least once each shift, and using a special bed if necessary. The client may be placed on a regular or special bed, such as a kinetic bed. *Immobility compresses soft tissues and promotes the development of decubitus ulcers. The lack of sensory warning mechanisms and of voluntary motor control of skin dermatomes further increases the risk for altered skin integrity. Special beds allow movement or turning while keeping the spinal column in alignment.*
- Assess the lower extremities each shift for symptoms of thrombophlebitis. Observe for redness and for increased heat every shift; measure thigh and calf circumference daily. If antiembolic stockings (TEDs) are ordered, remove for 30 to 60 minutes each shift. Assess for skin impairment and provide skin care while TEDs are removed. *Clients with neurologic deficits are at high risk for deep vein thrombosis as a result of immobility, vasomotor dysfunction, and decreased venous return with venous stasis. Antiembolic stockings help to prevent the pooling of blood in the lower extremities and increase venous return, lessening the risk for venous stasis and thrombus formation.*

**PRACTICE ALERT** *Removing TED stockings each shift not only promotes healthy skin but also lets the nurse assess skin integrity.* ■

## Impaired Gas Exchange

Injuries at the level of T1 to T7 leave the phrenic nerve intact, but the innervation of intercostal muscles is affected, compromising respiratory function. In addition, because the abdominal muscles are paralyzed, the client cannot expel secretions by coughing. (Clients with cord injuries at C3 or above have paralysis of the respiratory muscles and cannot breathe without a ventilator.)

- Monitor vital capacity and respiratory effectiveness, assessing for tachycardia, restlessness, $PaO_2$ less than 60 mmHg, $PaCO_2$ greater than 50 mmHg, and vital capacity less than 1L. *Clients with cervical cord injuries frequently require ventilatory support because of reduced vital capacity and inability to expel secretions by coughing.*

**PRACTICE ALERT** *Changes in arterial blood gases and vital capacity signal respiratory insufficiency.* ■

- Monitor for signs of ascending edema of the spinal cord, including difficulty in swallowing or coughing, respiratory stridor, use of accessory muscles of respiration, bradycardia, and increased motor and sensory loss. *Hemorrhage and edema can further impair respiratory function.*
- Help the client to cough, as follows: Place the hand between the umbilicus and xiphoid process and push in and up as the client exhales and coughs. *The client who is unable to cough effectively and has decreased ventilatory capacity may develop atelectasis, pneumonia, and respiratory failure.*

## Ineffective Breathing Patterns

Respiratory function is impaired in the client with SCI in the cervical and thoracic levels if the diaphragm (innervated at C3 to C5), the intercostal muscles (innervated at T1 to T7), and the abdominal muscles are affected. In clients with injury at higher levels, assisted ventilation and a tracheostomy are necessary; when the injury is at lower levels, the client's ability to take a deep breath and cough is diminished. The goal of nursing interventions is to maintain normal respiratory rate (12 to 20 breaths per minute) and to prevent pulmonary complications such as atelectasis and pneumonia.

- Assess respiratory rate, rhythm, and depth every 4 hours (or more frequently if needed). Auscultate breath sounds as a part of respiratory assessment. *Injury to the cord in the cervical or thoracic regions can decrease respiratory function and increase the risk for respiratory problems.*

**PRACTICE ALERT** *Auscultate the lungs for crackles and wheezes.* ■

- Monitor results of oxygen saturation and arterial blood gas studies. *ABG studies provide information about gas exchange; decreasing Ph, oxygen, and oxygen saturation levels, and increasing carbon dioxide levels signal respiratory acidosis.*
- Help the client turn, cough, and deep breathe at least every 2 hours. Use assisted coughing as necessary. *Paralysis of intercostal or abdominal muscles decreases the ability to expel secretions by coughing; retained secretions increase the risk for pneumonia. The inability to breathe deeply may result in atelectasis.*
- Increase fluids given by mouth to 3000 mL per day (if oral intake is approved), according to client preference for type of liquids and predicated on the client's ability to swallow. *Increased fluid intake thins secretions, which can more easily be expelled and expectorated.*

## Dysreflexia

Autonomic dysreflexia is an emergency that requires immediate assessment and intervention to prevent complications of extremely high blood pressure (loss of consciousness, convulsions, and even death).

- Elevate the head of the client's bed and remove TEDs. *These measures increase pooling of blood in the lower extremities and decrease venous return, thus decreasing blood pressure.*
- Assess blood pressure every 2 to 3 minutes while at the same time assessing for stimuli that initiated the response (such as a full bladder, impacted stool, or skin pressure). *The most serious danger in dysreflexia is elevated blood pressure, which could precipitate a CVA, myocardial in-*

*farction, dysrhythmias, or seizures. If the client has a Foley catheter, ensure that there are no kinks in the tubing. If the client does not have a Foley catheter, drain the bladder with a straight catheter. If symptoms persist, assess for a fecal impaction. If an impaction is present, insert Nupercaine cream into the anus, wait 10 minutes, and manually remove the impaction.*

**PRACTICE ALERT** *Blood pressure readings may be as high as 300/160.* ■

- If blood pressure remains dangerously elevated, the physician may prescribe intravenous administration of diazoxide (Hyperstat). Other medications that may be used include nifedipine (Procardia) and hydralazine (Apresoline). *Diazoxide is an antihypertensive drug used in emergency situations to lower blood pressure in adults with dangerously high readings. Nifedipine and hydralazine are peripheral vasodilators that are administered to decrease the elevated blood pressure.*

## Altered Urinary Elimination and Constipation

Depending on the level of the injury, the client with a SCI may have alterations in bowel and bladder function. Clients with injuries to the cord at or above the S2 to S4 levels will have a neurogenic bladder, with deficits in control of micturition. Voluntary and involuntary bowel control is affected in the

client with a lower motor neuron injury. Both bowel and bladder retraining are possible; if not, some form of assisted elimination is necessary. Although an indwelling catheter may be used in the acute phase of care, the goal is to reestablish a catheter-free state.

- Monitor for manifestations of a full bladder. *Overdistention stretches the bladder and can lead to backflow of urine into the ureters and kidney; stasis of urine in an incompletely emptied bladder increases the risk for infection.*

**PRACTICE ALERT** *A distended bladder can be palpated over the lower abdomen above the symphysis pubis.* ■

- Teach client to use trigger voiding techniques prior to straight catheterization. These techniques include stroking the inner thigh, pulling the pubic hair, tapping on the abdomen over the bladder, and (in females) pouring warm water over the vulva. *These trigger voiding techniques stimulate parasympathetic nerve fibers to cause reflex activity and may facilitate voiding.*
- Teach self-catheterization to clients who will be able to carry out the procedure alone or with minimal assistance (Procedure 41–1). *Straight catheterization at regular intervals is part of bladder training because periodic distention and relaxation of the muscles of the bladder promote reflex bladder activity. In addition, self-care fosters independence.*

---

**Procedure 41–1** | **Client Self-Catheterization**

Self-catheterization on an intermittent basis (usually a part of self-care at home) is a clean rather than a sterile procedure. The hands should be washed before and after the procedure, and the urinary meatus should be cleaned by washing with soap and water.

### FEMALE SELF-CATHETERIZATION

- Attempt to void. If urine is not of sufficient quantity (at least 100 mL) or if you cannot void at all, do self-catheterization. *A large amount of residual urine means that more frequent catheterizations (every 4 to 6 hours) are necessary.*
- While sitting on the wheelchair or the commode, locate the urethra. Visualize the urethra by looking in a mirror, or palpate the urethra with a fingertip. *Visualization or palpation of the meatus is necessary for proper catheter insertion.*
- Lubricate the meatus with a water-soluble lubricant. *Lubrication facilitates the insertion of the catheter and reduces trauma to tissues.*

- Take a deep breath and insert the catheter tip 2 to 3 inches or until urine flows. *The catheter enters the bladder more easily when the sphincter is relaxed. The deep breath relaxes the sphincter. The female urethra is 1½ to 2½ inches long.*
- Hold the catheter securely and allow urine to drain until the flow stops. *Withdrawing and reinserting the catheter increase the risk of infection.*
- Withdraw the catheter and wash it with soap and water. Store the catheter in a clean container. *The catheter can be reused until it is too soft or too hard to be directed into and through the urinary meatus. Clean rather than sterile technique is usually used for self-catheterization at home.*

### MALE SELF-CATHETERIZATION

- Attempt to void. If urine is not of sufficient quantity (e.g., less than 100 mL) or if you cannot void at all, do self-catheterization. *A large amount of residual urine means that more frequent catheterizations (every 4 to 6 hours) are necessary.*

- Sit either on the commode or in the wheelchair. Hold the penis with slight upward tension and extend it to its full length. *Extending the penis straightens the urethra.*
- Lubricate the catheter from the tip to about 6 inches downward. *Lubrication is especially important for male catheterization because of the length of the urethra.*
- Take a deep breath and insert the catheter 6 to 7 inches or until urine flows. *The catheter enters the bladder more easily when the sphincter is relaxed. The deep breath relaxes the sphincter. The male urethra is about 6 inches long.*
- Hold the catheter securely and allow urine to drain until flow has stopped. *Withdrawing and reinserting the catheter increase the risk of infection.*
- Withdraw the catheter and wash it with soap and water. Store the catheter in a clean container. *The catheter can be reused until it is too soft or too hard to be directed into and through the urethra. Clean rather than sterile technique is usually used for self-catheterization at home.*

- Monitor residual urine throughout the bladder retraining program. *A residual urine amount of less than 80 mL after a triggered voiding is considered satisfactory.*
- Institute a bowel retraining program as follows:
  - Assess usual patterns of bowel elimination to establish best times for individualized program.
  - Maintain a high-fluid, high-fiber diet.
  - Use stool softeners as prescribed; rectal suppositories and enemas may be used 30 minutes after meals to stimulate stronger peristalsis and facilitate evacuation.
  - Maintain upright position if at all possible and ensure privacy.
  - If client is unable to evacuate, digital stimulation or manual removal on a regular basis may be the most effective long-term management.

  *A bowel retraining program to regulate the bowel through reflex activity may be instituted in clients with upper motor neuron injuries. The client with a lower motor neuron injury loses the defecation reflex, and bowel retraining is more difficult (if not impossible).*

### Sexual Dysfunction

Sexual intercourse is often still possible for the client with an SCI. In men, the general rule is that the higher the level of injury the greater the potential to have reflexogenic erections, although ejaculation or orgasm may not occur, and fertility is usually lower. However, ejaculation may be stimulated and the sperm used to inseminate the client's partner, so that fatherhood is a possibility. Men who have sacral-level injuries do not have reflexogenic erections but may have psychogenic erections. They are also more likely to remain fertile.

Women with SCI generally do not have sensation during sexual intercourse, but pregnancy is possible. However, pregnant women with an SCI are at increased risk for autonomic dysreflexia during labor and delivery. Birth control options should be discussed prior to discharge from the acute care setting.

A client with an SCI may be deeply concerned about alterations in sexual function. These concerns may lead to lowered self-esteem, altered self-image, or changes in feelings about being an attractive and desirable person. Assess concerns and provide a climate that is receptive to discussion about sexuality. Examples of objectives for sexual counseling for the client with an SCI are that the client will understand how the injury has altered sexual functioning, be aware of alternative ways of achieving sexual pleasure, and have a positive self-concept and body image.

- Include data about sexuality when obtaining the nursing history and database. *Sexuality is a private matter for most people, and the client may not discuss it unless the nurse introduces the topic.*
- Provide accurate information about the effect of the SCI on sexual function. *Accurate information gives the client a realistic picture of how the injury will affect sexuality.*
- Initiate a discussion with the client and partner of alternative means of gaining sexual satisfaction; these include the use of vibrators, and oral-genital and manual stimulation. *Alternatives to intercourse can meet sexual needs and help maintain the relationship with a significant other.*
- Refer for sexual counseling, if appropriate, or to local support groups where questions can be answered by others with similar concerns. *Knowing that others have had similar experiences can decrease social isolation and provide a means of learning alternative methods of sexual functioning.*

### Low Self-Esteem

An SCI is often the result of sudden trauma. Within moments, a formerly independent, fully functioning individual is suddenly unable to move and faces enormous adjustments in social, economic, and personal roles and relationships. Body image, self-esteem, and role performance are all affected by the damage. As a result, the client often demonstrates behaviors that may be difficult for the nurse to handle: depression, denial, and anger are often seen in the period immediately after the injury. In addition to these responses, the young adult client may act out by making sexually overt statements.

- Encourage talking about all aspects of physical function and care. *Talking provides a safe outlet for fears and frustrations and also increases self-awareness. Acceptance of self facilitates rehabilitation.*
- Encourage self-care and independent decision making. *Participating in self-care can promote positive coping; making decisions decreases feelings of powerlessness.*
- Help identify strategies to increase independence in desired roles; include both short- and long-term goals. Discuss assistive devices (such as hand-operated automobiles). *Identifying strategies to increase independence in the future fosters a positive self-concept and motivates the client to achieve rehabilitation goals.*
- Include family members and important others in discussions. *The realization that others do care and will continue to provide support is important in fostering positive self-regard.*
- Refer the client and family to support groups or for psychologic counseling. *Adjustment to change is more likely when the client and family seek peer and professional assistance.*

## Using NANDA, NIC, and NOC

Chart 41–2 shows links between NANDA nursing diagnoses, NIC, and NOC when caring for the client with an SCI.

## Home Care

Rehabilitation of the client with an SCI is an ongoing process that moves from intensive care through intermediate care to rehabilitation and then home care. Nursing interventions are necessary at all points in the process to prevent the complications of altered physical mobility and body functions, and to teach the client and family measures that promote independence in self-care.

Discharge planning should be addressed even in the initial plan of care while the client is in the critical care setting. Advance planning ensures continuity of care when the client leaves the hospital setting.

## CHART 41–2 NANDA, NIC, AND NOC LINKAGES

### The Client with a SCI

| NURSING DIAGNOSES | NURSING INTERVENTIONS | NURSING OUTCOMES |
|---|---|---|
| • Risk for Impaired Skin Integrity | • Pressure Management<br>• Pressure Ulcer Prevention | • Risk Control<br>• Tissue Perfusion: Peripheral<br>• Immobility Consequences: Physiological |
| • Risk for Injury | • Malignant Hyperthermia<br>• Surveillance: Safety<br>• Neurologic Monitoring | • Symptom Control Behavior |
| • Self-Care Deficit | • Bathing<br>• Dressing<br>• Feeding<br>• Bowel Management | • Self-Care: Bathing<br>• Self-Care: Dressing<br>• Self-Care: Eating<br>• Self-Care: Toileting |
| • Self-Esteem Disturbance<br>• Impaired Home Maintenance | • Self-Esteem Enhancement<br>• Home Maintenance Assistance<br>• Environmental Management | • Self-Esteem<br>• Mobility Level<br>• Self-Care: Instrumental Activities of Daily Living |

*Note. Data from Nursing Outcomes Classification (NOC) by M. Johnson & M. Maas (Eds.), 1997, St. Louis: Mosby; Nursing Diagnoses: Definitions & Classification 2001–2002 by North American Nursing Diagnosis Association, 2001, Philadelphia: NANDA; Nursing Interventions Classification (NIC) by J.C. McCloskey & G. M. Bulechek (Eds.), 2000, St. Louis: Mosby. Reprinted by permission.*

The following should be included in teaching the client and family about care at home.

• Self-care activities (ADLs, exercises, bowel and bladder programs, skin care)
• Mobility (use of assistive devices: wheelchair, crutches, special automobiles)
• Preparation of the home environment
  • If the client is in a wheelchair, will steps, stairs, doors, or carpeted floors present physical barriers?
  • If a special bed is necessary, have arrangements been made, and is it in the home?
• Psychologic support
• Independent activities

• Community resources, such as Life-line (emergency alerting systems through a local hospital or agency), support groups, career centers for job retraining, counseling
• Coping skills for client and caregiver
• Referral to a home health agency and physical therapist for the client who is returning home
• Helpful resources:
  • The National Spinal Cord Injury Association
  • American Paralysis Association
  • Christopher Reeve Paralysis Foundation
  • Paralyzed Veterans of America
  • Canadian Paraplegic Association
  • Australian Quadriplegic Association

## THE CLIENT WITH A HERNIATED INTERVERTEBRAL DISK

A **herniated intervertebral disk,** also called a **ruptured disk,** herniated nucleus pulposus, or a slipped disk, is a rupture of the cartilage surrounding the intervertebral disk with protrusion of the nucleus pulposus (Figure 41–8 ■). Perhaps few neuro-orthopedic disorders are as challenging as those involving the intervertebral disks. Clients with herniation (rupture) of a disk have not only excruciating pain but also limited mobility. These problems may in turn cause alterations in role function, coping, and the ability to perform activities of daily living.

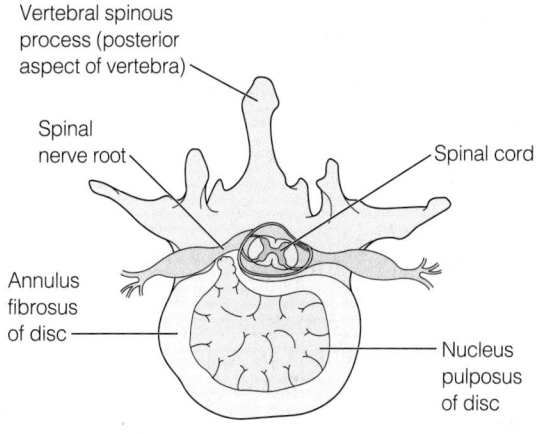

**Figure 41–8** ■ A herniated intervertebral disk. The herniated nucleus pulposus is applying pressure against the nerve root.

MediaLink | SPINAL CORD INJURY RESOURCES

## Nursing Care Plan
## A Client with a SCI

Jim Valdez, a 19-year-old college sophomore, is admitted to the hospital by ambulance following an automobile accident. His family (father, mother, and sister) live 100 miles away and cannot visit often, although they are very concerned. On admission to the hospital, a CT scan of the spine shows a fracture and partial laceration of the cord at the C7 level. Mr. Valdez is in halo traction. One night, he tells the nurse, "I wish I had just died when I got hurt. I don't think I can stand to live like this."

### ASSESSMENT

When Mr. Valdez is admitted to the intensive care unit, he has flaccid paralysis involving all extremities. He has no sensation below the clavicle or in portions of his arms and legs. His bladder is distended and bowel sounds are absent. Other assessment findings include BP 90/56, P 50, T 97°F (36.1°C), arterial blood gases Ph 7.4, Pao₂ 96, Paco₂ 37, Sao₂ 96%. Oxygen per nasal cannula is given at 2 L/min, and halo traction is applied. A Foley catheter is inserted into his bladder, and a nasogastric tube is inserted into his stomach and attached to low-pressure continuous suction.

After 7 days, Mr. Valdez is moved from the intensive care unit to the neurosurgical unit for continuing care and planning for transfer to a rehabilitation hospital in his home town. His vital signs have stabilized and are normal for his age; respirations and oxygenation are normal. Other neurologic assessments remain the same.

### DIAGNOSES

- *Impaired physical mobility* related to paralysis of lower and upper extremities secondary to C7 injury
- *Bowel incontinence* related to lack of voluntary sphincter control secondary to C7 injury
- *Grieving* related to loss of the use of his arms and legs and the effect of that loss on finishing school and getting a job

### EXPECTED OUTCOMES

- Be actively involved in exercise programs.
- Have a soft, formed stool every second or third day.
- Verbally express his grief to parents and staff.

### PLANNING AND IMPLEMENTATION

- Conduct passive exercises on all extremities four times a day.
- Provide progressive mobilization by initially raising the head of the bed 90 degrees (repeat two to three times during the first

day of movement); if blood pressure remains normal, dangle for 5 minutes before transferring him to a chair.
- His usual time for a bowel movement is after breakfast; schedule retraining program for that time.
- Encourage a diet high in fiber and fluids. Likes whole-wheat bread, orange juice, and cola; does not like water.
- Promote grief work by providing time to express feelings. Explain to the family that his denial and anger are part of the grieving process.
- Determine food likes and dislikes and order preferred foods from the menu. Encourage his friends to bring in his favorite foods periodically.
- Take and record weight every third day, using the bed scales.

### EVALUATION

By the time Mr. Valdez is transferred to the rehabilitation hospital he is looking forward to learning how to use special equipment and getting his own motorized wheelchair. He is able to sit up in a chair without dizziness or hypotension. The use of ordered stool softeners combined with a high-fiber diet and fluid intake of 2000 to 3000 mL per day has maintained bowel elimination. Mr. Valdez and his parents have spent 3 hours talking about their feelings related to the accident and the future. Although the discussion is emotionally difficult, all three say they now feel much better. Mr. Valdez still has episodes of angry outbursts and tears, but he is more optimistic about what can be done and believes he can finish college. He selects foods from the menu each day and eats most of his meals, but he especially enjoys the times his friends bring in pizza or hamburgers.

### Critical Thinking in the Nursing Process

1. Considering Mr. Valdez's age and developmental level, do you think his emotional responses to his injury were appropriate?
2. Issues of sexuality are obviously important for the client with a spinal cord injury. How would you approach Mr. Valdez about this topic?
3. What would be your response as a male or female nurse if Mr. Valdez would allow only male nurses to provide care?
4. Outline a teaching program to help Mr. Valdez meet long-term urinary elimination needs.

See Evaluating your Response in Appendix C.

## INCIDENCE AND PREVALENCE

A herniated intervertebral disk may occur at any adult age. However, it is more common as people enter middle age and age-related changes occur. The nucleus pulposus loses fluid content, and the disks are less able to absorb shocks. The disks become smaller and slip out of place more easily. Aging causes degeneration in the annulus fibrosus and the posterior longitu-

dinal ligaments, and the vertebrae and disks are less able to respond to movement and are more easily injured.

Herniated intervertebral disks are more common in men than women. Most clients are between the ages of 30 and 50. The majority of herniated disks occur in the lumbar region (L4 or L5 to S1); when disks herniate in the cervical region, they most commonly do so at C6 to C7. Multiple herniations are not common, occurring in only about 10% of all clients (Hickey, 2003).

## PATHOPHYSIOLOGY

The intervertebral disks, located between the vertebral bodies, are made of an inner nucleus pulposus and an outer collar (the annulus fibrosus). The disks allow the spine to absorb compression by acting as shock absorbers. A herniated intervertebral disk occurs when the nucleus pulposus protrudes through a weakened or torn annulus fibrosus of an intervertebral disk. This protrusion may occur anywhere along the vertebral column, but herniation of thoracic disks is uncommon. The protrusion may occur spontaneously or as a result of trauma, with trauma (such as lifting heavy objects or falling) causing about half of all cases. Rupture of the disk allows herniation of the nucleus pulposus in a posterolateral direction, with compression of the associated nerve root. The resulting pressure on adjacent spinal nerves causes characteristic manifestations, which vary with the location and the amount of protruding disk material (see the box on this page). Occasionally the herniation is central rather than posterolateral, with pressure on the spinal cord.

The herniation may be abrupt or gradual. Lifting incorrectly or suddenly twisting the spine can cause rupture with immediate intense pain and muscle spasms. Gradual herniation is the result of degenerative changes, osteoarthritis, or ankylosis spondylitis. Clients with a gradual herniation have a slow onset of pain and neurologic deficits.

### Lumbar Disk Manifestations

The classic manifestation of a ruptured lumbar disk is recurrent episodes of pain in the lower back. The pain typically radiates across the buttock and down the posterior leg, although it may be experienced only in the leg. **Sciatica** is a term used to describe lumbar back pain that radiates down the posterior leg to the ankle and is increased by sneezing or coughing (the result of pressure on nerve roots L4, L5, S1, S2, or S3, which give rise to the sciatic nerve). Sciatica may be elicited by straight-leg raising: The client feels pain when lifting one leg while dorsiflexing the foot of that leg. Sciatica pain varies in intensity, ranging from mildly uncomfortable to excruciating. It is aggravated by a variety of positions and activities, including sitting, straining, coughing, sneezing, climbing stairs, walking, and riding in a car.

Other manifestations include postural deformity, motor deficits, sensory deficits, and changes in reflexes. In about 60% of clients with ruptured lumbar disks, the normal lumbar lordosis is absent. When standing, the client typically has a slight forward tilt to the trunk, scoliosis of the lumbar spine, slight flexion of the hip and knee on the affected side, and paravertebral muscle spasms (Hickey, 2003). Motor deficits include weakness and in some clients problems with sexual function and urinary elimination. Sensory deficits include paresthesias and numbness. Knee and ankle reflexes are decreased or absent.

### Cervical Disk Manifestations

Cervical disks that herniate laterally cause pain in the shoulder, neck, and arm. Other manifestations of lateral cervical hernia-

---

## Manifestations of a Ruptured Intervertebral Disk

### L4 TO L5 LEVEL (AFFECTS FIFTH LUMBAR NERVE ROOT)

- Pain in hip, lower back, posterolateral thigh, anterior leg, dorsal surface of foot, great toe
- Muscle spasms
- Paresthesia over lateral leg and web of great toe
- Footdrop (rare)
- Decreased or absent ankle reflex
- Cauda equina syndrome (with complete nerve root compression): bowel and bladder incontinence, paralysis of lower extremities

### L5 TO S1 LEVEL (AFFECTS FIRST SACRAL NERVE ROOT)

- Pain in midgluteal region, posterior thigh, calf to heel, plantar surface of the foot to the fourth and fifth toes
- Paresthesias in posterior calf and lateral heel, foot, and toes
- Difficulty walking on toes

### C5 TO C6 LEVEL (AFFECTS SIXTH CERVICAL NERVE ROOT)

- Pain in neck, shoulder, anterior upper arm, radial area of forearm, thumb
- Paresthesia of forearm, thumb, forefinger and lateral arm
- Decreased biceps and supinator reflex
- Triceps reflex normal to hyperactive

---

tion include paresthesias, muscle spasms and stiff neck, and decreased or absent arm reflexes. Central cervical herniations result in mild, intermittent pain; however, the client may also experience lower extremity weakness, unsteady gait, muscle spasms, urinary elimination problems, altered sexual function, and hyperactive lower extremity reflexes.

## COLLABORATIVE CARE

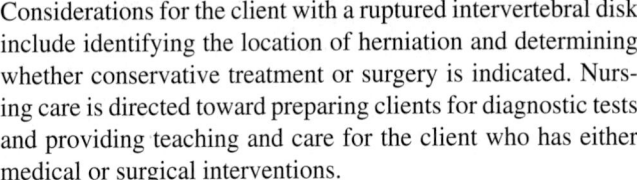

Considerations for the client with a ruptured intervertebral disk include identifying the location of herniation and determining whether conservative treatment or surgery is indicated. Nursing care is directed toward preparing clients for diagnostic tests and providing teaching and care for the client who has either medical or surgical interventions.

### Diagnostic Tests

Diagnostic tests are ordered to differentiate the cause of back pain; for example, back and leg pain is also caused by spinal tumors, degenerative processes, or abdominal disease. Assessing pain is an important part of diagnosis.

- *Flat-plate X-ray films* may be taken of the lumbosacral or cervical area to identify skeletal deformities and narrowing of the disk spaces.
- *CT scans* are used to identify disk rupture or protrusion and may provide definitive diagnosis. However, if the client has

had previous back surgery or if more than one disk is involved, a CT scan may not clearly identify the ruptured disk.

- *MRI* is used to image the vertebral elements, thecal sac, disks, cerebrospinal fluid, nerve roots, and spinal cord. This noninvasive examination is increasingly being used to provide initial diagnosis.
- *Myelography* with contrast medium illustrates areas of herniation but does not provide the detail found with CT or MRI. However, myelography is diagnostic in 80% to 90% of all cases and is used both to rule out tumors and locate the herniation.

A myelogram is a radiologic examination of the subarachnoid space of the spinal canal, using a contrast agent. A myelogram is performed to visualize the lumbar, thoracic, or cervical area, or the whole spinal axis. It is used in the diagnosis of a spinal cord tumor, a herniated intervertebral disk, or a ruptured disk. Any obstruction of the flow of the contrast medium can be seen on X-ray film.

To perform a myelogram, a lumbar puncture is performed and about 10 mL of cerebrospinal fluid (CSF) is removed. A water-based contrast medium such as iopamidol (Isovue) is injected into the subarachnoid space. When the medium is injected, it diffuses up through the CSF and penetrates the nerve root sleeves, nerve rootlets, and narrow areas of the subarachnoid space. The head of the X-ray table is kept ele-

vated at 30 degrees and the client is kept quiet to prevent rapid upward dispersion. If the contrast medium entered the cranial vault, it could cause seizures. The contrast medium is absorbed through the bloodstream and eliminated by the kidneys. Nursing implications for the care of a client having a myelogram are outlined in the box below.

- *Electromyography (EMG),* which measures electrical activity of skeletal muscles at rest and during voluntary contraction, may be conducted to identify specific muscles affected by the pressure of the herniation on the nerve roots.

## Medications

The client with a ruptured intervertebral disk is treated with medications to relieve pain and reduce swelling and muscle spasms. Pain is usually managed with nonsteroidal anti-inflammatory drugs (see Chapter 4). Muscle spasms are treated with muscle relaxants.

## Treatment

A ruptured intervertebral disk may be treated conservatively or with surgery.

### Conservative Treatment

A ruptured intervertebral disk is usually managed conservatively with bed rest and medication unless the client is experiencing severe neurologic deficits. The goals of treatment are

## Nursing Implications for Diagnostic Tests

### Myelography

#### Preparation of the Client

Ensure a signed informed consent.
- The meal prior to the procedure is usually omitted.
- The client should be well hydrated.
- Administer enemas or laxatives as ordered to ensure visualization of lumbar spine.
- Administer prescribed pretest medications, such as a sedative or diazepam (Valium).

#### Client and Family Teaching

- Remain NPO several hours before the test.
- The examination lasts about 1 hour.
- The position used to perform the examination will depend on the physician. You may have to lie on your stomach, sit and lean forward, or sit with the knees to the chest.
- A strap may be used to prevent falls, and the table will be tilted during the examination.
- A lumbar puncture ("spinal tap") is performed to inject the dye. A local anesthetic is used where the needle will be inserted. There may be a feeling of pressure during needle insertion. The needle is inserted below the level of the spinal cord.
- Tell the physician if you experience pain.
- It is important to stay in bed with the head of the bed elevated for at least 6 to 12 hours (the length of time will depend on physician preference and hospital policy).
- The nurse will check your blood pressure, pulse, and respirations. The nurse will also check your ability to feel and move at least every 4 hours (or more often) after the examination.

#### Postexamination Nursing Care

- Take and record vital signs and assess neurologic status as prescribed (and at least every 4 hours) for 24 hours postexamination. Record and report any changes.
- Assess the site of the lumbar puncture for leakage of cerebrospinal fluid or bleeding every 4 hours. Notify the physician of leakage or bleeding.
- Encourage increased intake of oral fluids to replace that withdrawn during the examination. (This may also help decrease a postmyelogram headache).
- Make sure that the client voids within 8 hours after the examination. If policy permits, allow male clients to stand at the bedside, or clients of either gender to use the bathroom. Notify the physician if the client has not voided within 8 hours.
- Administer analgesics as prescribed for postexamination pain, headache, or muscle spasms.
- Keep the client's head elevated at least 30 degrees (in bed or in a chair) for 12 hours, or as ordered.
- Resume diet if there is no nausea or vomiting.
- Force oral fluids to 2400 to 3000 mL in 24 hours, beginning immediately after the procedure.
- Administer prescribed medications for nausea.
- Do not give any phenothiazine derivatives for 48 hours (to reduce the possibility of seizures).

pain relief and healing of the involved disk by fibrosis. Conservative treatment is usually prescribed for 2 to 6 weeks. After that time, surgery may be considered. The treatment regimen depends on the severity of the manifestations but usually includes one or more of the following (Hickey, 2003):

- Decreasing activity level
- Avoiding flexion of the spine (e.g., do not lift, bend, or twist)
- Wearing a support garment, such as a corset or cervical collar
- Following a prescribed exercise program
- Using a firm mattress
- Taking prescribed medications for pain, inflammation, and muscle spasms

Some clients achieve pain relief with transcutaneous electrical stimulation (TENS) or transcutaneous neural stimulation (TNS). Another pain relief intervention is bed rest. It is important that the client use a firm mattress. The client should lie so that the pull on the affected nerve is reduced. Clients with lumbar involvement should usually flex the knees and elevate the head of the bed to about 30 degrees. After 4 days or less of bed rest, the client may begin walking and an exercise program designed by the physical therapist. This program includes teaching proper body mechanics and positioning, exercises to strengthen the back and decrease muscle spasms, massage, and the application of heat. Most clients report a good recovery after conservative management.

Medications used to treat back pain include nonnarcotic analgesics, anti-inflammatory drugs such as the nonsteroidal agents (NSAIDs), muscle relaxants, and sedative-tranquilizers.

## Surgery

Surgery is indicated for clients who do not respond to conservative management or have serious neurologic deficits. Several surgical interventions are used to treat a ruptured intervertebral disk. The type of surgery chosen depends on the location of the disk and the stability of the spinal column.

- A **laminectomy,** the type of surgery most often performed, is the removal of a part of the vertebral lamina. The surgery is done to relieve pressure on the nerves. It is often combined with removal of the protruding nucleus pulposus (*nuclectomy*). Nursing care for the client having a laminectomy is discussed in the box below. A *diskectomy* is the removal of the nucleus pulposus of an intervertebral disk. Diskectomy may be performed alone or along with a laminectomy.
- **Spinal fusion** is the insertion of a wedge-shaped piece of bone or bone chips between the vertebrae to stabilize them. The bone is usually taken from a client donor site, such as the iliac crest. A spinal fusion may also be performed through a spinal implant with a device called a BAK (a hollow titanium cylinder with holes) which is packed with grafted bone from a donor site and placed in the space where a disk is removed. Although not appropriate for all clients requiring a spinal fusion, this does require a short hospital stay and convalescence.
- *Foraminotomy* is an enlargement of the opening between the disk and the facet joint to remove bony overgrowth compressing the nerve. The location and size of the incision vary according to the surgeon's preference and the location and

---

## NURSING CARE OF THE CLIENT HAVING A POSTERIOR LAMINECTOMY

### PREOPERATIVE TEACHING

- Demonstrate and ask the client to practice logrolling; explain that it will be done by the nurses for the first day or two, and then the client can do it alone. *To ensure healing, the spinal column must remain in alignment when turning and moving.*
- Explain the importance of taking pain medications regularly and of asking for them before the pain is severe. Include information about the possibility of the pain being much the same after surgery. *Pain is easier to control if medications are taken before the pain is severe. Pain may be the same following surgery for a herniated intervertebral disk because edema due to surgery irritates and compresses the nerve roots.*
- Demonstrate the use of a fracture bedpan and ask the client to practice its use. *The client usually must remain flat in bed for a period of time following surgery. A fracture bedpan is more comfortable for clients who must lie flat.*
- Explain that the client may need to eat while lying flat. *This position prevents flexion of the spine.*
- Demonstrate and ask the client to practice deep breathing, the use of the incentive spirometer, and leg exercises. Ask the client to demonstrate these skills. *These measures prevent respiratory and circulatory complications.*

### POSTOPERATIVE CARE

- Maintain the client in a position that minimizes stress on the surgical wound. For clients with cervical laminectomy:
  a. Elevate the head of the bed slightly.
  b. Position a small pillow under the neck.
  c. Maintain the position of the cervical collar.

  For clients with lumbar laminectomy:
  a. Keep the bed flat or elevate the head of the bed slightly.
  b. Place a small pillow under the head.
  c. Place a small pillow under the knees, or use a pillow to support the upper leg when the client lies on one side.

  *These positions minimize stress on the surgical wound and suture line. A cervical collar provides stability and prevents flexing or twisting the neck.*
- Turn the client every 2 hours, using the logrolling technique. Teach the client not to use the side rails to change position. Maintain proper body alignment in all positions. *The client's body is turned as a single unit (usually with a turning sheet) to avoid movement of the operative area. Pulling on the side rails puts stress on the operative area and may also cause misalignment of the vertebral column.*

(continued on page 1338)

## NURSING CARE OF THE CLIENT HAVING A POSTERIOR LAMINECTOMY (continued)

### POSTOPERATIVE CARE (continued)

- Monitor the client for signs of nerve root compression.
  a. Cervical laminectomy: Assess hand grips and arm strength, ability to move the fingers, and ability to detect touch.
  b. Lumbar laminectomy: Assess leg strength, ability to wiggle the toes, and ability to detect touch.
  Compare bilateral findings. Report muscle weakness or sensory impairment to the physician immediately. *Loss of motor and sensory function may indicate nerve root compression.*
- Assess for hematoma formation as manifested by severe incisional pain that is not relieved by analgesics and decreased motor function. Report these findings to the surgeon immediately. *A hematoma may form at the surgical site. If untreated, it may cause irreversible neurologic deficits, including paraplegia and bowel/bladder dysfunctions (Hickey, 2003).*
- Assess for leakage of cerebrospinal fluid. Assess the dressing for increased moisture. Check the sheets for wetness when the client is lying supine; check for clear liquid running down the back when the client is sitting or standing. Gently palpate the sides of the wound to detect a bulge. Use a Dextrostrix strip to assess any leakage for the presence of glucose, a positive indicator of cerebrospinal fluid. *Although uncommon, leakage of cerebrospinal fluid greatly increases the risk for infection of the wound and of the meninges.*
- Assess for nerve root injury. Assess the client's ability to dorsiflex the foot (lumbar laminectomy) and the client's grip strength (cervical laminectomy). Assess the client who has had a cervical laminectomy for hoarseness. Report hoarseness to the physician and further assess the client's ability to swallow. *Nerve root compression may cause permanent damage, resulting in footdrop (in lumbar laminectomy clients) and hand weakness (in cervical laminectomy clients). Damage to the laryngeal nerve may cause permanent hoarseness. Impaired ability to swallow puts the client at risk for aspiration.*
- Assess for urinary retention. The client should void within 8 hours after surgery. If the physician allows, let males stand to void. Compare intake and output for each 8-hour period. *All clients who have received a general anesthetic are at risk for urinary retention. The client who has had a lumbar laminectomy*

*may have even more difficulty voiding as a result of stimulation of sympathetic nerves during surgery.*
- Assess for pain using a scale from 0 (no pain) to 10 (severe pain). Administer prescribed analgesics on a regular basis, or teach client to use PCA analgesia, if prescribed. Discuss client concerns about pain that is unrelieved by surgery. *Compression of the nerve root over time results in edema and inflammation. Because of surgery-induced edema, the client is likely to experience either the same pain or perhaps more severe pain in the period immediately after surgery. This pain usually persists for several weeks after surgery. In addition, many clients who have had a lumbar laminectomy have muscle spasms in the lower back, abdomen, and thighs for the first few days after surgery.*
- Assess for infection by taking and recording vital signs at least every 4 hours; report increased body temperature. Assess the wound and dressing for signs of infection: increased redness, drainage, pain, and pus. Use sterile technique to change dressings. *The surgical client is always at risk for infection; the client with a laminectomy is also at risk for arachnoiditis. This inflammation of the arachnoid layer of the spinal meninges results from wound infection or contamination during surgery and may cause the formation of painful adhesions.*
- Encourage deep breathing and the use of the incentive spirometer every 2 hours; coughing may be discouraged. *Anesthesia and immobility depress respiratory function. Coughing may be discouraged because it can disrupt healing tissues, especially in clients having a cervical laminectomy.*
- Increase mobility as prescribed. (The time frame for ambulation is prescribed by the physician; the routine here is representative.) Clients often sit on the side of the bed and dangle their legs the evening after surgery or the first day thereafter. Many clients ambulate the first or second postoperative day. To help the client out of bed, first elevate the head of the bed. Then bring the client's legs over the side of the bed at the same time that the upper body moves into the upright position. Clients should not ambulate without assistance until they are no longer dizzy or weak. *Early ambulation increases respiratory and circulatory function and decreases the risk of thrombophlebitis of the lower extremities. The vertebral column should remain in alignment while the client sits and stands. Safety must be considered throughout care.*

size of the ruptured disk. The posterior approach is taken for lumbar surgery. Either the posterior or the anterior approach may be taken for cervical disks.

- A *microdiskectomy,* in which microsurgical techniques are used, is performed through a very small incision. This type of surgery decreases the possibility of trauma to surrounding structures during surgery and allows early postoperative mobility and a short hospital stay.

## NURSING CARE

Nursing care for the client with a ruptured intervertebral disk may be provided through information in community and work settings, during conservative treatment, and during pre- and

postoperative treatment. The pain of the ruptured disk is often discouraging and debilitating, and may well affect the client's ability to work.

### Prevention

Proper body mechanics may help prevent the occurrence of a ruptured intervertebral disk. Teaching the proper method of lifting and moving heavy objects should begin when children enter school. This information should also be given to all workers who have lifting as part of their responsibilities; including nurses. The guidelines for proper body mechanics are as follows:

- Begin activities by spreading the feet apart to broaden the base of support.

- Use large muscles of the arms to lift and the legs to push when lifting.
- Work as closely as possible to the object that is to be lifted or moved.
- Slide, roll, push, or pull an object rather than lift it.
- When lifting, bend the knees and lift up over your center of gravity.

## Assessment

The following data are collected through the heath history and physical examination (see Chapter 40).

- Health history: type of employment, risk factors, pain (location, duration, intensity)
- Physical examination: muscle strength and coordination, sensation, reflexes

## Nursing Diagnosis and Interventions

Nursing care for clients with a herniated intervertebral disk focuses largely on pain management, both during conservative management and after surgery.

### Acute Pain

Clients with a ruptured intervertebral disk experience acute back and leg pain. Acute pain may be related to preoperative muscle spasms or nerve root compression. After surgery, the client may have pain at the site of the incision and in the surgical area.

- Encourage discussion of pain. Assess the degree of pain and identify contributing and relieving factors. *Pain is a subjective experience. The nurse needs to assess it thoroughly before initiating interventions.*
- Maintain bed rest as prescribed. Teach the client how to logroll (to turn the body without bending the spine) when changing positions. *Restricting activity and proper positioning may prevent muscle spasms.*
- Use a firm mattress or place a board under the mattress. *A firm bed supports the spinal column and muscles.*
- Teach the client to avoid turning or twisting the spinal column and to assume positions that decrease stress on the vertebral column (e.g., when in the supine position, flex the hips slightly). A small pillow may be placed under the knees (for clients with a herniated lumbar disk) or under the neck (for clients with a herniated cervical disk). *Correct body positions can decrease intradisk pressure.*
- Provide analgesic medications around the clock. *Intense pain can increase muscle spasms; maintaining serum levels of analgesics often prevents severe pain.*

**PRACTICE ALERT** *It is important to maintain a constant level of pain relief. Health care providers have the responsibility of relieving pain with adequate medications.* ■

### Chronic Pain

The client with a ruptured intervertebral disk often has pain for an extended period of time. Despite conservative treatment or previous surgery, pain may be ongoing or intermittent. If previous surgery has not relieved the pain, the client may be depressed or angry. Caring for a client with chronic pain is frustrating, and the client is often regarded as difficult.

- Treat the client's reports of pain with respect. *The client is the person experiencing the pain and is thus the expert about it.*
- Do not refer to the client as being addicted to pain medication. *All types of pain medications may be used legitimately to manage pain.*

**PRACTICE ALERT** *Although the client may develop tolerance to a narcotic analgesic, tolerance does not imply addiction.* ■

- Monitor the client carefully for any changes in condition. *Significant changes in the client's condition may go unrecognized when pain is present for a prolonged period of time.*
- Maintain written plans of care for pain management that are individualized and ensure continuity of care. *When the client makes several visits (for instance, to an emergency department or a pain clinic), written records help caregivers determine what is effective in managing pain and what is not.*
- Teach the client alternative methods of pain management. *Consider the client's coping style when recommending methods. Clients who have a passive coping style are often better able to manage pain by depending on others, taking medications, and resting. Clients with an active coping style are probably better able to manage pain by learning self-management methods, taking part in activities, and staying busy.*
- Develop effective methods of improving rest and sleep. Problems with rest and sleep make pain management more difficult. *Sleeping poorly at night contributes to decreased motivation, confused thinking, depression, and muscle aches.*
- Refer the client to a physical therapist for an exercise program, if appropriate. *The client needs to know exactly what exercises to do, how many repetitions are recommended, for how long, and how often. The client should not exercise to the point of causing increased pain.*
- Assess the need for referrals (and make them if necessary) for the client who is depressed or anxious. *Anxiety and depression often are a part of long-term chronic pain, making pain management more difficult. Suggest that referrals for help with the frustration (rather than "depression") may make a significant difference in the client's ability to manage pain.*

### Constipation

The client with a ruptured intervertebral disk often has problems with constipation because of reduced mobility and bed rest. Nursing interventions to alleviate and prevent constipation are important because straining to have a bowel movement can increase intradisk pressure, thus increasing pain.

- Assess the client's usual bowel routine, including diet, fluid intake, and the use of laxatives or enemas. *Effective interventions are based on individualized needs.*

**PRACTICE ALERT** *People who have used laxatives or enemas for long periods of time may be dependent on those methods of having a bowel movement.* ■

- Encourage a fluid intake of 2500 to 3000 mL per day unless contraindicated by the presence of renal or cardiac disease. *Adequate fluid intake facilitates the passage of feces.*
- Increase fiber and bulk in the diet. If the client is unable to tolerate increased fiber, consult with the physician about the use of stool softeners or bulk-forming agents. *Bulk and fiber promote regularity by retaining water in the large intestine.*

## Home Care

It is the nurse's responsibility to teach the client and family about chronic pain control, including specific interventions to alleviate pain. The nurse's role may be that of advocate and creative problem solver (see the Meeting Individualized Needs box on page 1341 for specific teaching topics). The following topics should be addressed:

- Often the goal is to control pain so that the client can perform normal activities of daily living, rather than to reach a pain-free state.
- Nonpharmacologic methods of pain management include relaxation techniques, guided imagery, distraction, hypnosis, and music. Joining a support group may be an effective intervention in coping with and managing pain.
- Clients may be referred to a physical therapist for education about body mechanics and back-strengthening exercises. Nurses should have the client demonstrate the exercises as a way of reinforcing teaching.

## Nursing Care Plan
## A Client with a Ruptured Intervertebral Disk

Maree Ivans is a 50-year-old lawyer who lives in Montana. She sustains ruptured intervertebral disks at C5 and C6 when she is thrown over the handlebars of her bicycle while mountain biking. Mrs. Ivans is the mother of two young adults; her husband operates a small business.

### ASSESSMENT
Immediately after the accident, Mrs. Ivans is taken to the nearest hospital by ambulance and evaluated by a neurosurgeon. Diagnostic tests include a CT scan, an MRI study, and X-ray films of the cervical vertebrae. The results demonstrate damaged ligaments and herniation of the C7 disk. Mrs. Ivans is sent home wearing a cervical collar to stabilize the area and is instructed to limit activity. Twisting or turning the neck is prohibited. After 2 weeks at home, Mrs. Ivans complains of having no appetite, being unable to sleep at night, and having acute pain in the neck and shoulders. She also has numbness and tingling in several fingers of her left (dominant) hand. A major concern is whether she will be able to return to work and resume her usual activities. A cervical laminectomy with spinal fusion is being discussed.

### DIAGNOSES
- *Acute pain* related to edema and muscle spasms
- *Impaired mobility* related to altered comfort
- *Disturbed sleep pattern* related to pain with movement
- *Risk for compromised family coping* related to altered lifestyle and lack of knowledge about the injury

### EXPECTED OUTCOMES
- State that her pain is decreased to the point of tolerance.
- Experience restful sleep as evidenced by statements of increased energy.
- Collaborate with her husband in discussing the injury and planning how best to meet household needs.

### PLANNING AND IMPLEMENTATION
- Take prescribed analgesics around the clock (when awake) to manage pain. Take prescribed muscle relaxants to control muscle spasms.
- Keep the cervical collar on at all times. Do not lift objects or bend or twist the neck.
- Follow a regular bedtime routine, sleeping on a firm mattress with a small pillow under the neck if desired.
- Drink six to eight full glasses of water each day.
- Increase fiber and bulk in the diet.

### EVALUATION
Following the acute care period, Mrs. Ivans's physical symptoms have decreased. She is able to manage her pain with oral analgesics and is sleeping better at night. She has begun a program of physical therapy and has continued to wear the cervical collar. After 2 months, Mrs. Ivans is so much improved that she begins to work half days. Her family has taken over cooking and cleaning responsibilities, and they remain supportive and understanding.

### Critical Thinking in the Nursing Process
1. Discuss the rationale for taking Mrs. Ivans to the hospital by ambulance after the bicycle accident.
2. Mrs. Ivans has grown children and a husband who provided help and support. How might the teaching you provide differ if the client who sustained this injury were a young single mother of two small children?
3. Design a teaching plan for Mrs. Ivans for the diagnosis, *Dressing/grooming self-care deficit.*

See Evaluating your Response in Appendix C.

Radiation of the spinal cord may cause the development of radiation-induced myelopathy. This complication of radiation exposure occurs over time, with manifestations of a *Brown-Séquard syndrome* developing 12 to 15 months after therapy. The manifestations may progress to paraplegia, sensory loss, and loss of bowel and bladder control (Hickey, 2003).

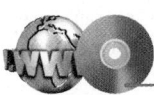

## NURSING CARE

Nursing care for the client with a spinal cord tumor is individualized in accordance with the type of tumor and the type of treatment. The client with a benign tumor that is removed by surgery has different health care needs than the client with a metastatic tumor, even though they may have similar neurologic deficits. The client with a spinal cord tumor (regardless of type) requires nursing care to monitor for neurologic changes, to provide pain management, and to manage motor and sensory deficits in order to preserve quality of life.

The assessments and nursing interventions for the client with a spinal cord tumor are similar to those described for the client with SCI or who is undergoing surgery for a ruptured intervertebral disk. The following nursing diagnoses m propriate for the client with a spinal cord tumor.

- *Anxiety* related to a diagnosis of malignant spinal cord tumor
- *Risk for constipation* related to the effects of spinal cord compression
- *Impaired physical mobility* related to weakness of lower extremities
- *Acute pain* related to compression of spinal nerve roots
- *Sexual dysfunction* related to effects of spinal cord compression
- *Urinary retention* related to the effects of spinal cord compression

Following surgical treatment, the client may be transferred to a rehabilitation center or may go home for the recovery period. Referrals for home care, occupational therapy, and physical therapy often help the client regain functional abilities. Teach family members how to move the client in the bed and from the bed to a chair. Also teach them how to provide physical care, care for any appliances (such as an indwelling catheter), and prevent or treat constipation.

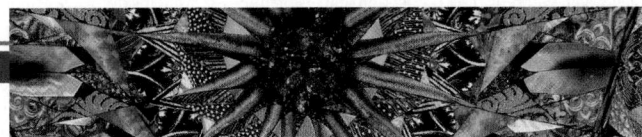

## EXPLORE MediaLink

NCLEX review questions, case studies, care plan activities, MediaLink applications, and other interactive resources for this chapter can be found on the Companion Website at www.prenhall.com/lemone.

Click on Chapter 41 to select the activities for this chapter. For animations, video clips, more NCLEX review questions, and an audio glossary, access the Student CD-ROM accompanying this textbook.

## TEST YOURSELF

1. Which of the following manifestations would alert you to the possibility that your client has had a TIA?

   a. Sudden severe pain over the left eye
   b. Numbness and tingling in the corner of the mouth
   c. Complete paralysis of the right arm and leg
   d. Loss of sensation and reflexes in both legs

2. What is the rationale for administration of a tissue plasminogen activator within the first 3 hours of a thrombotic stroke?

   a. To reduce the risk of vasospasm
   b. To decrease the risk of infection
   c. To increase platelet aggregation
   d. To cause fibrinolysis of the clot

3. Oxygen is often administered to the client who has had a stroke. Preventing hypoxia and hypercapnia through this treatment will lessen the risk of which complication?

   a. Fluid accumulation in the lungs

   b. Pulmonary emboli
   c. Increased intracranial pressure
   d. Rebleeding

4. What is the primary pathophysiologic process of spinal shock?

   a. Temporary loss of reflex function below the level of injury
   b. Loss of control of cardiovascular mechanisms
   c. Exaggerated sympathetic response
   d. Damage to the lower motor neurons

5. Your client has manifestations of autonomic dysreflexia. Which of these assessments would indicate a possible cause for this condition?

   a. Extreme hypertension
   b. Kinked catheter tubing
   c. Respiratory wheezes and stridor
   d. Skin breakdown over the coccyx

See Test Yourself answers in Appendix C.

# BIBLIOGRAPHY

Breteton, L., & Nolan, M. (2000). "You do know he's had a stroke, don't you?" Preparation for family care-giving: The neglected dimension. *Journal of Clinical Nursing, 9*(4), 498–506.

Bucher, L. & Melander, S. (1999). *Critical Care Nursing.* Philadelphia Saunders.

Buckley, D., & Guanci, M. (1999). Spinal cord trauma. *Nursing Clinics of North America, 34*(3), 661–687.

Chotikul, L. (2000). Spinal implants. *RN, 63*(5), 28–31.

Christensen, J., Cook, E., & Martin, B. (1997). Identifying denial in stroke patients. *Clinical Nursing Research, 6*(1), 105–118.

Davies, S. (1999). Dysphagia in acute strokes. *Nursing Standard, 13*(30), 49–55.

DeLisa, J., & Kirshblum, S. (1997). A review: Frustrations and needs in clinical care of spinal cord injury patients. *Journal of Spinal Cord Medicine, 20*(4), 384–390.

Duncan, P., & Lai, S. (1997). Stroke recovery. *Topics in Stroke Rehabilitation, 4*(3), 51–58.

Garner, C. (1999). Cancer-related spinal cord compression. *American Journal of Nursing, 99*(7), 34–35.

Gendreau-Webb, R. (2001). Action stat: Ischemic stroke. *Nursing, 31*(11), 120.

Gerhart, K., Charlifue, S., Weitzenkamp, D., Menter, R., & Whiteneck, G. (1997). Aging with spinal cord injury. *American Rehabilitation, 23*(1), 19–25.

Harding-Okimoto, M. (1997). Pressure ulcers, self-concept and body image in spinal cord injury patients. *SCI Nursing, 14*(4), 111–117.

Hayn, M., & Fisher, T. (1997). Stroke rehabilitation: Salvaging ability after the storm. *Nursing97, 27*(3), 40–46, 48.

Hickey, J. (2003). *The clinical practice of neurological and neurosurgical nursing* (4th ed.). Philadelphia: Lippincott.

Hock, N. (1999). Brain attack: The stroke continuum. *Nursing Clinics of North America, 34*(3), 689–723.

Huston, C. (1998). Cervical spine injury. *American Journal of Nursing, 98*(6), 33.

Identification and nursing management of dysphagia in adults with neurological impairment. *Best Practice, 4*(2), 1–6.

John, C. (1997). Time is of the essence. . . "Brain attack: Treating acute ischemic CVA." *Nursing97, 27*(6), 9–10.

Johnson, M., & Maas, M. (Eds.). (1997). *Iowa outcome project: Nursing outcomes classification (NOC).* St. Louis: Mosby.

Krause, J. (1998). Skin sores after spinal cord injury: Relationship to life adjustment. *Spinal Cord, 36*(1), 51–56.

LaFavor, K., & Ang, R. (1997). Managing autonomic dysreflexia through the use of clinical practice guidelines. *SCI Nursing, 14*(3), 83–86.

McAweeney, M., Tate, D., & McAweeney, W. (1997). Psychosocial interventions in the rehabilitation of people with spinal cord injury: A comprehensive methodologic inquiry. *SCI Psychosocial Process, 10*(2), 58–66.

McCloskey, J., & Bulechek, G. (Eds.). (2000). *Iowa intervention project: Nursing interventions classification (NIC)* (3rd ed.). St. Louis: Mosby.

McColl, M., Walker, J., Stirling, P., Wilkins, R., & Corey, P. (1997). Expectations of life and health among spinal cord injured adults. *Spinal Cord, 35*(12), 818–828.

McHale, J., Phipps, M., Horvath, K., & Schmelz, J. (1998). Expert nursing knowledge in the care of patients at risk of impaired swallowing. *Image: Journal of Nursing Scholarship, 30*(2), 137–141.

Mower, D. (1997). Brain attack: Treating acute ischemic CVA. *Nursing97, 27*(3), 34–39, 47–48.

National Spinal Cord Injury Association (1998). *Spinal cord injury statistics.* Available www.eskimo.com/~jlubin/disabled/nscia/fact02.html

Perry, L. (2001). Screening swallowing function of patients with acute stroke. Part 2. Detailed evaluation of the tool used by nurses. *Journal of Clinical Nursing, 10*(4), 474–481.

Petterson, M. (1997). Thrombolytic therapy in stroke management. *Critical Care Nurse, 17*(5), 88–93.

Porth, C. ( 2002). *Pathophysiology: Concepts of altered health states* (6th ed.). Philadelphia: Lippincott.

Routh, J. (1997). Consumer's perspective: Dressing and undressing following a stroke. *Topics in Stroke Rehabilitation, 4*(2), 94–98.

Sander, R. (1998). Stroke: The hidden problems. *Elderly Care, 10*(1), 27–32.

Shannon, M., Wilson, B., & Stang, C. (2002). *Health professionals drug guide 2002.* Upper Saddle River, NJ: Prentice Hall

Sipski, M. (1997). Sexuality and spinal cord injury: Where we are and where we are going. *American Rehabilitation, 23*(1), 26–28.

Thompson, J., McFarland, G., Hirsch, J., & Tucker, S. (2002). *Mosby's clinical nursing* (5th ed.). St. Louis: Mosby.

Tierney, L., McPhee, S., & Papadakis, M. (Eds.). (2001). *Current medical diagnosis & treatment.* Stamford, CT: Appleton & Lange.

Westergren, A., Ohlsson, O., & Halberg, I. (2001). Eating difficulties, complications, and nursing interventions during a period of three months after a stroke. *Journal of Advanced Nursing, 35*(3), 416–426.

Whipple, B., & Komisarck, B. (1997). Sexuality and women with complete spinal cord injury. *Spinal Cord, 35*(3), 136–138.

# CHAPTER 42

# Nursing Care of Clients with Intracranial Disorders

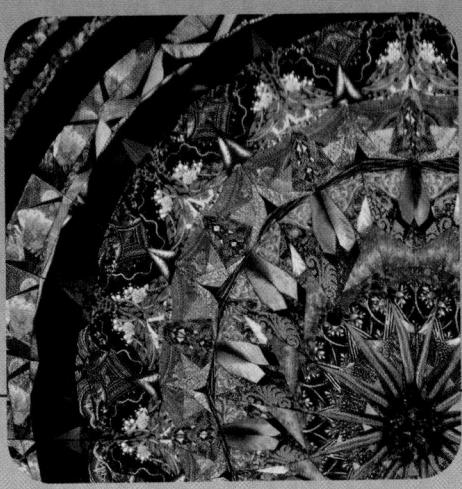

**www.prenhall.com/lemone**

Additional resources for this chapter can be found on the Student CD-ROM accompanying this textbook, and on the Companion Website at www. prenhall.com/lemone. Click on Chapter 42 to select the activities for this chapter.

**CD-ROM**
• Audio Glossary
• NCLEX Review

*Animation*
• Coup-Contrecoup Injury

**Companion Website**
• More NCLEX Review
• Care Plan Activity
  Subdural Hematoma
• MediaLink Application
  Meningitis Prevention

## LEARNING OUTCOMES

After completing this chapter, you will be able to:

▪ Apply knowledge of normal anatomy, physiology, and assessments when providing nursing care for clients with intracranial disorders (see Chapter 40).

▪ Explain the pathophysiology, manifestations, collaborative care, and nursing care of altered level of consciousness and increased intracranial pressure.

▪ Describe the pathophysiology and manifestations of seizures, headaches, traumatic brain injury, intracranial infections, and brain tumors.

▪ Identify diagnostic tests used to identify and manage intracranial disorders.

▪ Discuss nursing implications for medications used to treat intracranial disorders.

▪ Explain collaborative care for clients with intracranial disorders.

▪ Describe nursing interventions in the preoperative and postoperative care of the client having intracranial surgery.

▪ Use the nursing process as a framework for providing individualized care to clients with intracranial disorders.

The client with an intracranial disorder presents a unique challenge to the nurse. Problems the client experiences in the acute stage of the disorder are often a prelude to long-term problems requiring ongoing management. These long-term problems range from alterations in the body's basic functioning to dysfunctions in the complex processes of the human mind. Systemic problems may accompany or develop secondary to an intracranial disorder. Intracranial disorders may affect the client's quality of life and that of the client's family. This chapter first discusses altered level of consciousness and increased intracranial pressure, followed by intracranial disorders that may manifest these and other health problems. Information specific to the client with a stroke is in Chapter 41.

# ALTERED CEREBRAL FUNCTION

The manifestations of altered cerebral function occur as a result of illness or injury. Assessment of the patterns of those manifestations helps determine the extent of the cerebral dysfunction and improvement or deterioration of cerebral function. Except in the case of direct damage to the brainstem and **reticular activating system (RAS),** brain function deterioration usually follows a predictable rostral to caudal progression, that is, a pattern in which higher levels of function are impaired initially, progressing to impairment of more primitive functions. Altered level of consciousness and behavior changes are early manifestations of the deterioration of the function of the cerebral hemispheres. Structures in the midbrain and brainstem are affected sequentially, with characteristic changes in level of consciousness; patterns of respiration, pupillary and oculomotor responses; and motor function (Porth, 2002). Manifestations of progressive deterioration of cerebral function are outlined in Table 42–1.

## TABLE 42–1  Progression of Deteriorating Brain Function

| Level of Consciousness | Pupillary Response | Oculomotor Responses | Motor Responses | Breathing |
|---|---|---|---|---|
| Alert; oriented to time, place, and person | Brisk and equal; pupils regular | Eyes move as head turns Caloric testing (ear irrigation) produces nystagmus | Purposeful movement; responds to commands | Regular pattern with normal rate and depth |
| Responds to verbal stimuli; decreased concentration; agitation, confusion, lethargy; disoriented | Small and reactive | Roving eye movements; doll's eyes positive, with gaze fixed straight ahead; eye deviation away from cold caloric stimulus and toward warm stimulus | Purposeful movement in response to pain stimulus | Yawning, sighing respirations |
| Requires continuous stimulation to rouse | | | Decorticate posturing with upper extremity flexion | Cheyne-Stokes respirations with crescendo-decrescendo pattern in rate and depth followed by period of apnea |
| Reflexive positioning to pain stimulus | Pupils fixed (nonreactive) in midposition | Caloric testing produces nystagmus | Decerebrate posturing with adduction and rigid extension of upper and lower extremities | Central neurogenic hyperventilation with rapid, regular, and deep respirations; apneustic breathing with prolonged inspiration and pauses at full inspiration and following expiration |
| No response to stimuli | Pupils fixed in midposition | No spontaneous eye movement or nystagmus | Extension of upper extremities with flexion of lower extremities; flaccidity | Cluster or ataxic breathing with irregular pattern and depth of respirations; gasping respirations or apnea |

# THE CLIENT WITH ALTERED LEVEL OF CONSCIOUSNESS

**Consciousness** is a condition in which the person is aware of self and environment and is able to respond appropriately to stimuli. Full consciousness requires both normal arousal and full cognition.

- *Arousal*, or alertness, depends on the RAS, a diffuse system of neurons in the thalamus and upper brainstem.
- *Cognition* is a complex process involving all mental activities controlled by the cerebral hemispheres, including thought processes, memory, perception, problem solving, and emotion.

These two components of consciousness depend on the normal physiologic function of and connection between the arousal mechanisms of the reticular formation and the cognitive functions of the cerebral hemispheres. Because arousal and cognition are independent components of consciousness, each can act separately on stimuli. For example, the RAS reacts to the discomfort caused by a full bladder by waking the person in the middle of the night. Once awake, however, the frontal cortex alerts the person that the bladder is full and prompts the person to go to the bathroom and empty it.

The physiologic seat of consciousness, the reticular formation, is a mass of nerve cells and fibers that make up the core of the brainstem, extending from the medulla to the midbrain. The axons of reticular neurons are exceptionally long and branch outward to cells in the hypothalamus, thalamus, cerebellum, and spinal cord. A system of reticular neurons within the RAS passes steady streams of impulses through thalamic relays in order to stimulate the cerebral cortex into wakefulness. The body's sensory tracts interact with RAS neurons; this interrelationship helps control the strength of the RAS's rousing effect on the cerebrum.

Conditions that affect either the RAS or the function of the cerebral hemispheres can interfere with the normal level of consciousness. Terms describing altered level of consciousness (LOC) are listed and defined in Table 42–2. Nurses should remember that consciousness is a dynamic state: A client may pass from full consciousness to coma within hours or experience a slow diminishment of consciousness that does not become evident for weeks or months. The nurse can help provide effective care for a client with an altered level of consciousness by looking beyond the diagnostic labels of consciousness and accurately assessing the client's behavior and response to stimuli.

## PATHOPHYSIOLOGY

Level of consciousness may be altered by processes that affect the arousal functions of the brainstem, the cognitive functions of the cerebral hemispheres, or both. The major causes are (1) lesions or injuries that affect the cerebral hemispheres directly and widely or that compress or destroy the neurons of the RAS and (2) metabolic disorders.

**TABLE 42–2  Terms Used to Describe Level of Consciousness**

| Term | Characteristics of Client |
|---|---|
| Full consciousness | Alert; oriented to time, place, and person; comprehends spoken and written words |
| Confusion | Unable to think rapidly and clearly; easily bewildered, with poor memory and short attention span; misinterprets stimuli; judgment is impaired |
| Disorientation | Not aware of or not oriented to time, place, or person |
| Obtundation | Lethargic, somnolent; responsive to verbal or tactile stimuli but quickly drifts back to sleep |
| Stupor | Generally unresponsive; may be briefly aroused by vigorous, repeated, or painful stimuli; may shrink away from or grab at the source of stimuli |
| Semicomatose | Does not move spontaneously; unresponsive to stimuli, although vigorous or painful stimuli may result in stirring, moaning, or withdrawal from the stimuli, without actual arousal |
| Coma | Unarousable; will not stir or moan in response to any stimulus; may exhibit nonpurposeful response (slight movement) of area stimulated but makes no attempt to withdraw |
| Deep coma | Completely unarousable and unresponsive to any kind of stimulus, including pain; absence of brainstem reflexes, corneal, pupillary, and pharyngeal reflexes and tendon and plantar reflexes |

## Arousal

Damage to the RAS impairs the person's ability to maintain wakefulness and arousal. Stroke is the most common cause of RAS destruction. Other causes include demyelinating diseases such as multiple sclerosis, tumors, abscesses, and head injury. Function of the RAS may be suppressed by compression of the brainstem, which produces edema and ischemia. Pressure and compression of the brainstem may be due to tumors, increased intracranial pressure, hematomas or hemorrhage, or aneurysm (McCance & Huether, 2002). Although it is possible to assess level of consciousness or arousal in the client with RAS damage, the impairment in arousal may make it impossible to assess cognitive function.

The function of the brain, especially the cerebral hemispheres, depends on continuous blood flow with unimpeded supplies of oxygen and glucose. Processes that disrupt this flow of blood and nutrients may cause widespread damage to the cerebral hemispheres, impairing arousal and cognition. Bilateral hemispheric lesions, such as global ischemia, or metabolic disorders, such as hypoglycemia, are the most common causes of altered LOC related to cerebral dysfunction of the hemispheres. Localized masses, such as a hematoma or cerebral edema that displace normal structures and cause direct or indirect pressure on the opposite hemisphere or brainstem can also affect LOC. The client who has widespread damage to the cerebral hemispheres but an intact RAS has sleep-wake cycles and may rouse in response to stimuli; the client cannot be said to be alert, however, because cognition is impaired.

Both localized neurologic processes and systemic disorders can alter LOC. Processes occurring within the brain, which may directly destroy or compress neurologic structures, include the following:

- Increased intracranial pressure
- Stroke
- Hematoma
- Intracranial hemorrhage
- Tumors
- Infections
- Demyelinating disorders

Any systemic condition that affects the delivery of blood, oxygen, and glucose to the brain or alters cell membranes may also alter LOC. If cerebral blood flow is impaired or the client becomes hypoxic or hypoglycemic, cerebral metabolism is impaired and level of consciousness declines rapidly. Clients at particular risk include those with poorly controlled diabetes and those with cardiac or respiratory failure.

Other metabolic alterations that can affect LOC include fluid and electrolyte imbalances, such as hyponatremia or hyperosmolality, and acid-base alterations, such as hypercapnia (an elevated arterial carbon dioxide level). Accumulated waste products and toxins from liver or renal failure can affect neuronal and neurotransmitter function, altering LOC. Drugs that depress the central nervous system (e.g., alcohol, analgesics, anesthetics) suppress metabolic and membrane activities in the RAS and cerebral hemispheres, thereby affecting LOC.

Seizure activity, abnormal electrical discharges from a local area of the brain or from the entire brain, commonly affects LOC. It appears that the spontaneous, disordered discharge of activity that occurs during a seizure exhausts energy metabolites or produces locally toxic molecules, altering LOC for a time after the seizure. Consciousness returns when the metabolic balance of the neurons is restored.

As the impairment of brain function progresses, more stimuli are required to elicit a response from the client. Initially, the client may rouse to verbal stimuli and respond appropriately to questions, remaining oriented to time, place, and person. With deterioration of neurologic function, the client becomes more difficult to rouse and may become agitated and confused when awakened. Orientation to time is lost initially, followed by orientation to place and then to person. Continuous stimulation or vigorous shaking is required to maintain wakefulness as LOC decreases. Eventually, the client does not respond, even with deep painful stimuli.

## Patterns of Breathing

Progressive impairment of neural function also causes predictable changes in breathing patterns as respiratory centers are affected. In normal respirations, a rhythmic pattern is maintained by neural centers in the pons and medulla that respond to changes in arterial levels of oxygen ($PaO_2$) and carbon dioxide ($PaCO_2$). When there is damage to the RAS or cerebral hemispheres, neural control of these centers is lost, and lower brainstem centers regulate breathing patterns by responding only to changes in $PaCO_2$, resulting in irregular respiratory patterns. As outlined in Table 42–1 and illustrated in Table 42–3, progressive deterioration in brain function is accompanied by decreasing LOC and changes in breathing patterns. The type of respirations, by area of cerebral damage, are as follows (Porth, 2002):

- *Diencephalon:* Cheyne-Stokes respirations
- *Midbrain:* neurogenic hyperventilation (may exceed 40 per minute), the result of uninhibited stimulation of the respiratory centers
- *Pons:* apneustic respirations, characterized by sighing on midinspiration or prolonged inhalation and exhalation; results from excessive stimulation of the respiratory centers
- *Medulla:* ataxic/apneic respirations (totally uncoordinated and irregular), probably as a result of the loss of responsiveness to $CO_2$

## Pupillary and Oculomotor Responses

The brainstem areas that control arousal are adjacent to areas that control the pupils. A predictable progression of pupillary

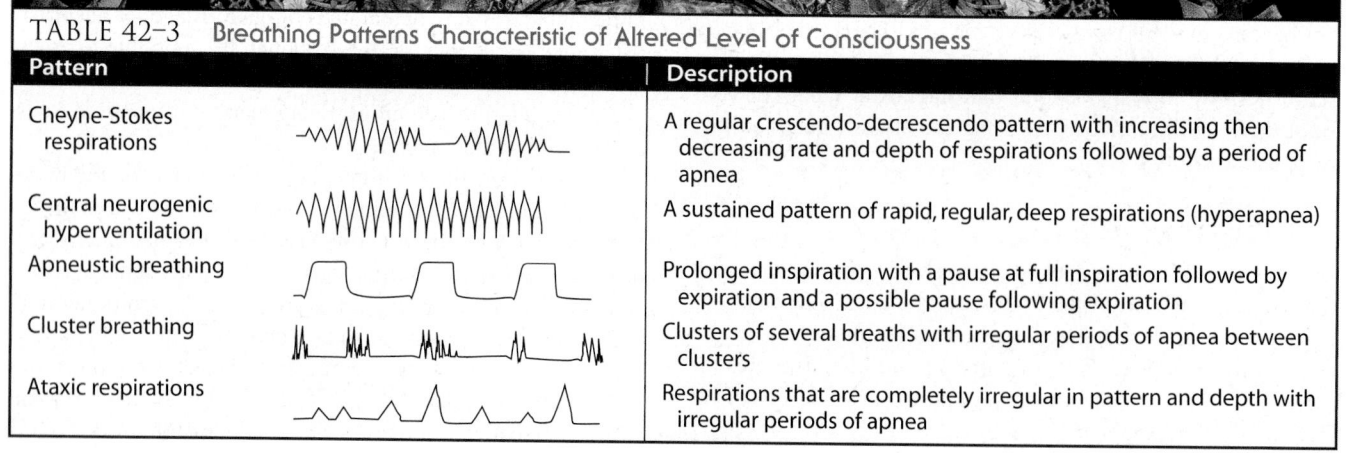

| TABLE 42–3 | Breathing Patterns Characteristic of Altered Level of Consciousness | |
|---|---|---|
| **Pattern** | | **Description** |
| Cheyne-Stokes respirations | | A regular crescendo-decrescendo pattern with increasing then decreasing rate and depth of respirations followed by a period of apnea |
| Central neurogenic hyperventilation | | A sustained pattern of rapid, regular, deep respirations (hyperapnea) |
| Apneustic breathing | | Prolonged inspiration with a pause at full inspiration followed by expiration and a possible pause following expiration |
| Cluster breathing | | Clusters of several breaths with irregular periods of apnea between clusters |
| Ataxic respirations | | Respirations that are completely irregular in pattern and depth with irregular periods of apnea |

and oculomotor responses occurs as level of consciousness deteriorates toward coma (see Table 42–1). If the lesion or process affecting neurologic function is localized, effects may initially be seen in the *ipsilateral pupil* (the pupil on the same side as the lesion). With generalized or systemic processes, pupils are affected equally. If the pupils are small and equally reactive, metabolic processes affecting LOC may be present. With compression of cranial nerve III at the midbrain, the pupils may become oval or eccentric (off center). As the level of functional impairment progresses, the pupils become fixed (unresponsive to light) and, eventually, dilated.

In deteriorating LOC and coma, spontaneous eye movement is lost and reflexive ocular movements are altered. Normally, both eyes move simultaneously in the same direction; injury to the cranial nerve nuclei in the midbrain and pons can impair normal movement. **Doll's eye movements** are reflexive movements of the eyes in the opposite direction of head rotation; they are an indicator of brainstem function (Figure 42–1 ■). As a result of the oculocephalic reflex, the eyes move upward with passive flexion of the neck and downward with passive neck extension. As brainstem function deteriorates, this reflex is lost. The eyes fail to turn together and, eventually, remain fixed in the midposition as the head is turned.

Instilling cold water into the ear canal (cold caloric testing) tests the oculovestibular response. Normally, this stimulus causes **nystagmus** (lateral tonic deviation of the eyes) toward the stimulus. This reflex is also lost as brain function deteriorates.

## Motor Responses

The level of brain dysfunction and the side of the brain affected may be assessed by motor responses. These responses are the most accurate identifier of changes in mental status. In altered LOC, motor responses to stimuli range from an appropriate response to a command (e.g., "squeeze my hand" or "push my hands away with your feet") to flaccidity (see Table 42–1). Initially, the client may be able to move purposefully away from a noxious stimulus, for example, to brush the examiner's hand away from the face. As function declines, movements become more generalized (withdrawal, grimacing) and less purposeful.

Reflexive motor responses may occur, including *decorticate* posturing with flexion of the upper extremities accompanied by extension of the lower extremities. With further decline, *decerebrate* posturing is seen, with adduction and rigid extension of the upper and lower extremities. Without intervention, the client eventually becomes flaccid, with little or no motor response to stimuli.

## COMA STATES AND BRAIN DEATH

Possible outcomes of altered LOC and coma include full recovery with no long-term residual effects, recovery with residual damage (such as learning deficits, emotional difficulties, or impaired judgment), or more severe consequences such as persistent vegetative state (cerebral death) or brain death.

### Irreversible Coma

**Irreversible coma (persistent vegetative state)** is a permanent condition of complete unawareness of self and the environment, resulting from death of the cerebral hemispheres with continued function of the brainstem and cerebellum. While the homeostatic regulatory functions of the brain continue, the ability to respond meaningfully to the environment is lost.

The client in vegetative state has sleep-wake cycles and retains the ability to chew, swallow, and cough but cannot interact with the environment. When awake, the client's eyes may wander back and forth across the room, but they cannot track an object or person. In a **minimally conscious state,** the client is aware of the environment and can follow simple commands, manipulate objects, gesture or verbalize to indicate "yes/no" responses, and make meaningful movements (such as blinking or smiling) in response to a stimulus (McCance & Huether, 2002). Vegetative state is usually the result of severe head injury or global anoxia. With appropriate supportive care, the client may remain in this state for 2 to 5 years.

### Locked-In Syndrome

**Locked-in syndrome** is distinctly different from vegetative state, in that the client is alert and fully aware of the environment and has intact cognitive abilities, but is unable to

**Head in neutral position**

**Head rotated to client's left**

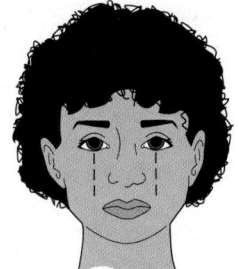

Eyes midline

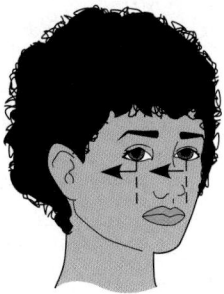

Doll's eyes present:
Eyes move right in
relation to head.

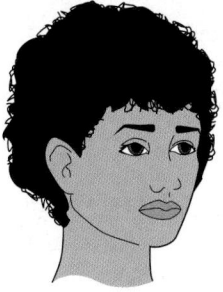

Doll's eyes absent:
Eyes do not move
in relation to head.
Direction of vision follows
head to left.

**Figure 42–1** ■ Doll's eye movements characteristic of altered level of consciousness.

communicate through speech or movement because of blocked efferent pathways from the brain. Motor paralysis affects all voluntary muscles, although the upper cranial nerves (I through IV) may remain intact, allowing the client to communicate through eye movements and blinking. In essence, the client is "locked" inside a paralyzed body in which he or she remains fully conscious of self and environment. Infarction or hemorrhage of the pons that disrupts outgoing nerve tracts but spares the RAS is the usual cause of locked-in syndrome. This condition may also result when the corticospinal tracts between the midbrain and pons are interrupted. Disorders of the lower motor neurons or muscles, such as acute polyneuritis, myasthenia gravis, or amyotrophic lateral sclerosis (ALS), may also paralyze motor responses, leading to locked-in syndrome.

## Brain Death

**Brain death** is the cessation and irreversibility of all brain functions, including the brainstem. Although the exact criteria for establishing brain death may vary somewhat from state to state, it is generally agreed that brain death has occurred when there is no evidence of cerebral or brainstem function for an extended period (usually 6 to 24 hours) in a client who has a normal body temperature and is not affected by a depressant drug or alcohol poisoning. Generally recognized criteria are:

- Unresponsive coma with absent motor and reflex movements.
- No spontaneous respiration (apnea).
- Pupils fixed (unresponsive to light) and dilated.
- Absent ocular responses to head turning and caloric stimulation.
- Flat EEG and no cerebral blood circulation present on angiography (if performed).
- Persistence of these manifestations for 30 minutes to 1 hour and for 6 hours after onset of coma and apnea.

Apnea in the comatose client is determined by the apnea test. The ventilator is removed while maintaining oxygenation by tracheal cannula and allowing the $P_{CO_2}$ to increase to 60 mmHg or higher. This level of carbon dioxide is high enough to stimulate respiration if the brainstem is functional. The electroencephalogram (EEG) may be used to establish the absence of brain activity when brain death is suspected. A flat (isoelectric) EEG over a period of 6 to 12 hours in a client who is not hypothermic or under the influence of drugs that depress the central nervous system is generally accepted as an indicator of brain death (McCance & Huether, 2002).

## PROGNOSIS

The prognosis for clients with altered levels of consciousness and coma varies according to the underlying cause and pathologic process. Age and general medical condition also play a role in determining outcome. Young adults may fully recover following deep coma from head injury, drug overdose, or other cause. Recovery of consciousness within 2 weeks is associated with a favorable outcome. In general, the prognosis is poor for clients who lack pupillary reaction or reflex eye movements 6 hours after the onset of coma.

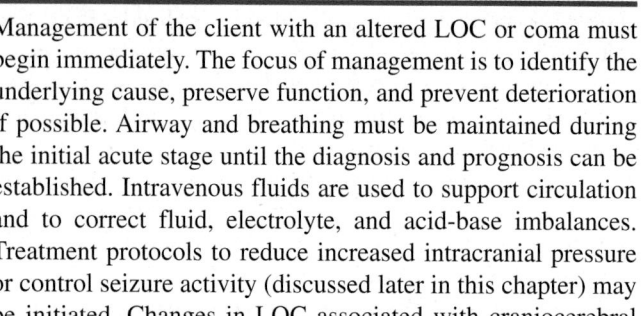

## COLLABORATIVE CARE

Management of the client with an altered LOC or coma must begin immediately. The focus of management is to identify the underlying cause, preserve function, and prevent deterioration if possible. Airway and breathing must be maintained during the initial acute stage until the diagnosis and prognosis can be established. Intravenous fluids are used to support circulation and to correct fluid, electrolyte, and acid-base imbalances. Treatment protocols to reduce increased intracranial pressure or control seizure activity (discussed later in this chapter) may be initiated. Changes in LOC associated with craniocerebral trauma, such as hematomas, often require immediate surgical intervention.

## Diagnostic Tests

Although the client's history and physical examination findings often indicate the cause of alterations in LOC, several diagnostic tests may be useful in establishing the diagnosis. The following tests may be ordered to evaluate for possible metabolic, toxic, or drug-induced disorders.

- *Blood glucose* is measured immediately when coma is of unknown origin and hypoglycemia is suspected or possible. The brain contains minimal stores of glucose and is dependent on a continuous supply for metabolism. When the blood glucose falls to less than 40 to 50 mg/dL, cerebral function declines rapidly. The client with type 1 diabetes is at particular risk for hypoglycemia-induced coma.
- *Serum electrolytes*—sodium, potassium, bicarbonate, chloride, and calcium in particular—are measured to assess for metabolic disturbances and guide intravenous therapy. Hyponatremia, in which serum sodium levels are below 115 mEq/L (normal level: 135 to 145 mEq/L), is associated with coma and convulsions, especially if it develops rapidly.
- *Serum osmolality* is evaluated. Both hyperosmolar and hypoosmolar states may be associated with coma. Hyperosmolality (above 320 mOsm/kg $H_2O$) causes cellular dehydration of brain tissue as fluid is drawn into the vascular system by osmosis. Hypo-osmolality (less than 250 mOsm/kg $H_2O$), by contrast, leads to cerebral edema and swelling, impairing consciousness.
- *ABGs* are drawn to evaluate arterial oxygen and carbon dioxide levels as well as acid-base balance. Hypoxemia is a frequent cause of altered LOC; increased levels of carbon dioxide are also toxic to the brain and can induce coma, particularly when the onset of hypercapnia is acute.
- *Serum creatinine* and *BUN* are measured to evaluate renal function.
- *Liver function tests,* including bilirubin, AST, ALT, LDH, serum albumin, and serum ammonia levels, are determined to evaluate hepatic function. High ammonia levels seen in hepatic failure interfere with cerebral metabolism and neurotransmitters, affecting level of consciousness.
- *Toxicology screening* of blood and urine is done to determine if altered LOC is the result of acute drug or alcohol toxicity. Serum alcohol levels are measured and the blood is assessed

for the presence of substances such as barbiturates, carbon monoxide, or lead.

- *CBC with differential* is done to assess for possible anemia or infectious causes of coma.
- *CT* and *MRI scanning* are done to detect neurologic damage due to hemorrhage, tumor, cyst, edema, myocardial infarction, or brain atrophy. These tests may also identify displacement of brain structures by large or expanding lesions. It is important to remember, however, that not all lesions or causes of altered LOC can be determined by CT scan or MRI.
- *EEG* is used to evaluate the electrical activity of the brain. The EEG is particularly valuable in identifying unrecognized seizure activity as a cause of altered LOC and is also useful in identifying certain infectious and metabolic causes of altered LOC. A normal EEG in an unresponsive client may identify locked-in syndrome. In addition to the baseline EEG, evoked responses may also be determined. The EEG is monitored as an auditory tone or other sensory stimulus is provided to assess the brain's responsiveness.
- *Radioisotope brain scan* is performed to identify abnormal lesions in the brain and evaluate cerebral blood flow.
- *Cerebral angiography* allows radiographic visualization of the cerebral vascular system. A radiopaque dye is injected into the carotid or vertebral arteries, followed by fluoroscopic and serial X-ray evaluation of the cerebral circulation. This exam can identify lesions such as aneurysms, occluded vessels, or tumors, and may also be used to determine cessation of cerebral blood flow and brain death.
- *Transcranial Doppler studies* use an ultrasound velocity detector that records sound waves reflected from RBCs in blood vessels to assess cerebral blood flow.
- *Lumbar puncture with CSF analysis* is performed when infection and possible meningitis are suspected as a cause of altered LOC.

## Medications

Medications are used to support homeostasis and normal function for the client with altered LOC, as well as to treat specific underlying disorders. An intravenous catheter is inserted, and fluid balance is maintained using isotonic or slightly hypertonic solutions, such as normal saline or lactated Ringer's solution. The client's response to fluid administration is monitored carefully for evidence of increased cerebral edema.

If hypoglycemia is present, 50% glucose is administered intravenously to restore cerebral metabolism rapidly. Conversely, insulin is administered to the client with hyperglycemia to reduce the blood glucose level and thus the serum osmolality. With narcotic overdose, naloxone is administered. Naloxone is a narcotic antagonist that competes for narcotic receptor sites, effectively blocking the depressant effect of the narcotic. Thiamine may be administered with glucose, particularly if the client is malnourished or known to abuse alcohol, to prevent exacerbation of Wernicke's encephalopathy, a hemorrhagic encephalopathy due to thiamine deficiency and associated with chronic alcoholism (Tierney et al., 2001).

Any underlying fluid and electrolyte imbalance is corrected by administering medications or appropriate electrolytes. For the client who is hyponatremic and has a low serum osmolality, furosemide (Lasix) or an osmotic diuretic such as mannitol may be administered to promote water excretion. Appropriate antibiotics are administered intravenously to the client with suspected or confirmed meningitis.

## Surgery

Although surgery is not indicated for most clients with altered LOC, it may be necessary if the cause of coma is a tumor, hemorrhage, or hematoma. Surgical intervention is discussed later in this chapter, in the section on brain tumors. When there is a risk of increased intracranial pressure, the client is monitored continuously. These measures are discussed in the section on increased intracranial pressure.

## Other Therapeutic Measures

Support of the airway and respirations is vital in the client with an altered LOC. The client who is drowsy but rousable may need little more than an oral pharyngeal airway. With more severe alterations in consciousness, the client may need endotracheal intubation to maintain airway patency, particularly if the cough and gag reflexes are absent. Mechanical ventilation is indicated when hypoventilation or apnea is present. Unless a do-not-resuscitate (DNR) order is in effect, mechanical ventilation should be initiated even if it has not been established that the disorder is reversible; without ventilatory support, cerebral anoxia develops rapidly, and brain death may ensue. ABGs are monitored frequently to determine the adequacy of ventilation. Hyperventilation may be used to reduce $PCO_2$ and promote cerebral vasoconstriction to reduce cerebral edema.

In clients with long-term alterations in consciousness, such as vegetative state or locked-in syndrome, measures to maintain nutritional status are initiated. Enteral feedings with a gastrostomy tube are preferred if the client is unable to take enough food by mouth without aspirating. In some cases, parenteral nutrition may be used.

### NURSING CARE

## Nursing Diagnoses and Interventions

Nursing care of the client with an altered LOC is planned and implemented for a variety of responses. Nursing diagnoses and interventions discussed in this section are directed toward the unconscious client and focus on problems with airway maintenance, skin integrity, contractures, and nutrition.

### Ineffective Airway Clearance

Ineffective airway clearance related to loss of the cough reflex and the inability to expectorate is a major problem for the unconscious client. The cough reflex may be absent or impaired when conditions that produce coma depress the function of the medullary centers.

- Assess ability to clear secretions. Monitor breath sounds, rate and depth of respirations, dyspnea, pulse oximeter, and the presence of cyanosis. *The client's ability to clear secretions serves as the initial assessment base for developing further interventions.*

- In unconscious clients or those without an intact cough reflex, maintain an open airway by periodic suctioning, limiting the time of suctioning to 10 to 15 seconds or less. *Periodic suctioning may be necessary to clear the airway of mucus, blood, or other drainage. Suctioning for more than 15 seconds in the client with increased intracranial pressure may cause hypercapnia, which in turn vasodilates cerebral vessels, increases cerebral blood volume, and increases intracranial pressure.*

**PRACTICE ALERT** *If the client has a basilar skull fracture or cerebral spinal fluid draining from the ears or nose, never suction nasally.* ■

- Turn from side to side every 2 hours, and maintain a side-lying position with the head of the bed elevated approximately 30 degrees. Do not position the unconscious client on the back. *Turning the client from side to side facilitates respirations, prevents the tongue from obstructing the airway, and helps prevent pooling of secretions in one area of the lungs (thus decreasing the risk of pneumonia).*
- If the client has a tracheostomy, provide tracheostomy care every 4 hours and suction when secretions are present (see Chapter 35 ⬜ ), *to maintain an open airway.*

### Risk for Aspiration

The unconscious client with a depressed or absent gag and swallowing reflex is at high risk for aspiration. Drainage, mucus, or blood may obstruct the airway and interfere with oxygenation. Pooling of aspiration secretions in the lungs also increases the risk of pneumonia.

- Assess swallowing and gag reflexes every shift as appropriate to the client's level of consciousness. *Deepening levels of unconsciousness may cause a loss in swallow and gag reflexes.*
- Monitor for and report manifestations of aspiration: crackles and wheezes, dullness to percussion over an area of the lungs, dyspnea, tachypnea, cyanosis. *Early recognition facilitates prompt intervention.*
- Provide interventions to prevent aspiration:
  - Maintain NPO status.
  - Place in the side-lying position.
  - Provide oral hygiene and suctioning as needed.
  *The side-lying position allows secretions to drain from the mouth rather than into the pharynx. Oral hygiene and suctioning remove secretions that might otherwise be aspirated.*

**PRACTICE ALERT** *Never give unconscious clients oral food and fluids because of the risk of aspiration.* ■

- Monitor the results of arterial blood gas analysis and pulse oximetry. Maintain records of trends. *Arterial blood gases and pulse oximetry directly measure the oxygen content of blood and are good indicators of the lungs' ability to oxygenate the blood.*

### Risk for Impaired Skin Integrity

The unconscious client is at risk for impaired skin integrity as a result of immobility and the inability to provide self-care. On average, healthy people change positions during sleep every 11 minutes; the unconscious client often cannot maintain the movement needed to prevent pressure on the skin, especially over bony prominences. As a result, the skin and subcutaneous tissues may become ischemic and prone to develop pressure ulcers. Perspiration and incontinence of urine and stool may exacerbate the problem. Nursing interventions are directed to maintaining the integrity not only of the skin, but also of the lips and mucous membranes.

- Assess skin every shift, especially over bony prominences and around genitals and buttocks. The large surface area of the skin bears weight and is in constant contact with the surface of the bed. *The skin, subcutaneous tissue, and muscles, especially those tissues over bony prominences, undergo constant pressure. This impairs normal capillary blood flow, which interferes with the exchange of nutrients and waste products. Tissue ischemia and necrosis may result and lead to the development of pressure ulcers.*
- Provide proper positioning. Reposition bed-ridden clients at least every 2 hours if this is consistent with the overall treatment goals. Keep the head of the bed elevated no higher than 30 degrees. Provide special pads and mattresses that distribute weight more evenly (e.g., silicone-filled pads, egg-crate cushions, turning frames, flotation pads). Lift the client instead of dragging the client across the sheet. *When the head of the bed is elevated above 30 degrees, the client's torso tends to slide down toward the foot of the bed. Friction and perspiration cause the skin and superficial fascia to remain fixed against the bed linens while the deep fascia and skeleton slide downward. When a person is pulled rather than lifted, the skin remains fixed to the sheet while the fascia and muscles are pulled upward. These sheering forces promote tissue breakdown.*
- Provide interventions to prevent breakdown of the skin and mucous membranes:
  - Keep bed linens clean, dry, and wrinkle free.
  - Provide daily bath with mild soap.
  - Cleanse the skin after urine and fecal soiling with a mild cleansing agent.
  - Provide oral care and lubricate the lips every 2 to 4 hours.
  - Maintain accurate intake and output records.
  - Keep the cornea moist by instilling methyl cellulose solution (0.5% to 1%) and apply protective eye shields or close the eyelids with adhesive strips if the corneal reflex is absent.
  *Keeping linens clean, dry, and wrinkle free decreases the risk of injury from the shearing force of bed rest and protects against environmental factors that cause drying. Adequate hydration of the stratum corneum appears to protect the skin against mechanical insult. Preventing dehydration maintains circulation and decreases the concentration of urine, thereby minimizing skin irritation in people who are incontinent. Proper eye care prevents corneal abrasion and irritation.*

## Impaired Physical Mobility

Clients who are unconscious are unable to maintain normal musculoskeletal movement and are at high risk for contractures related to decreased movement. Because the flexor and adductor muscles are stronger than the extensors and abductors, flexor and adductor contractures develop quickly without preventive measures. Passive ROM exercises must be performed routinely to maintain muscle tone and function, to prevent additional disability, and to help restore impaired motor function.

- Maintain extremities in functional positions by providing proper support devices. Remove support devices every 4 hours for skin care and passive ROM exercises. Provide pillows for the axillary region; rolled washcloths may be placed in elevated hands; use splints to prevent plantar flexion (footdrop). *Pillows in the axillary region help prevent adduction of the shoulder. Rolled washcloths help decrease edema and flexion contracture of the fingers. Splints are useful in preventing plantar flexion. Remove these support devices every 4 hours to increase circulation to the area.*
- Perform passive ROM exercises (unless contraindicated, as for the client with increased intracranial pressure) at least four times a day, keeping the following principles in mind:
  - Place one hand above the joint being exercised. The other hand gently moves the joint through its normal range of motion.
  - Move the body part to the point of resistance, and stop. *Placing one hand above the joint provides support against gravity and prevents unwanted movement. ROM exercises help prevent contractures by stretching muscles and tendons and maintaining joint mobility.*

## Risk for Imbalanced Nutrition: Less Than Body Requirements

The unconscious client is at risk for an alteration in nutrition related to a reduced or complete inability to eat. This is especially true for the client who is unconscious as the result of an infection or trauma, both of which increase metabolic requirements.

- Monitor nutritional status through daily weights (on bed scales) and laboratory data. *For accuracy, weigh the client at the same time each day, using the same scales. Ensure that the client wears the same clothing. Changes in laboratory data with decreased nutrition include a decrease in the levels of serum albumin and serum transferrin.*
- Assess the need for alternative methods of nutritional support (tube feeding or total parenteral nutrition) through collaboration with dietitian. *Clients unable to take oral food require parenteral nutrition or liquid feedings through a nasogastric, gastrostomy, or jejunostomy tube. Needs for protein, calories, zinc, and vitamin C increase during wound healing.*

## Support of the Family

Family members of a client with an altered level of consciousness are often very anxious. It is difficult for the family to deal with the client's uncertain prognosis. They may experience various conflicting emotions, such as guilt and anger. Reinforce information provided by the physician, and encourage the family to talk to the client as though he or she were able to understand. Explain that this communication may initially seem awkward, but in time it will feel appropriate. Evaluate the family's readiness to receive explanations regarding the client's treatment and care. The presence of many tubes (e.g., intravenous line, catheter, ventilator) may be overwhelming to the family. They may misperceive the seriousness of the situation if a thorough explanation is not given. Include the family in the client's care as much as they wish to be involved.

Allow significant others to stay with the client when possible. Reinforce the need for family members to care for themselves by encouraging adequate meals and rest. Offer to contact support services, such as friends, neighbors, and social services that the hospital may provide. Ask family members to leave a telephone number where they can be reached, and assure them that they will be called if any significant changes occur. Encourage family members to call if they have questions or concerns.

# THE CLIENT WITH INCREASED INTRACRANIAL PRESSURE

**Intracranial pressure (ICP)** is the pressure within the cranial cavity, usually measured as the pressure within the lateral ventricles (Porth, 2002). Transient increases in ICP occur with normal activities such as coughing, sneezing, straining, or bending forward. These transient increases are not harmful; however, sustained increases in intracranial pressure can result in significant tissue ischemia and damage to delicate neural tissue. Cerebral edema is the most frequent cause of sustained increases in ICP. Other causes include head trauma, tumors, abscesses, stroke, inflammation, and hemorrhage.

## OVERVIEW OF NORMAL INTRACEREBRAL BLOOD FLOW AND PERFUSION

In the adult, the rigid cranial cavity created by the skull is normally filled to capacity with three essentially noncompressible elements: the brain (80%), cerebrospinal fluid (10%), and blood (10%). A state of dynamic equilibrium exists; if the volume of any of the three components increases, the volume of the others must decrease to maintain normal pressures within the cranial cavity. This is known as the *Monro-Kellie hypothesis.* The normal intracranial pressure is 5 to 15 mmHg (measured intracranially with a pressure transducer while the client is lying with the head elevated 30 degrees) or 60 to 180 cm $H_2O$ (measured with a water manometer while the client is lying in a lateral recumbent position) (McCance & Huether, 2002).

Cerebral blood flow and perfusion are important concepts for understanding the development and effects of increased intracranial pressure. Whereas blood and CSF contribute an equal percentage to normal intracranial volume, vascular factors account for twice the amount of increase in ICP that CSF does. The brain requires a constant supply of oxygen and glucose to meet its metabolic demands; 15% to 20% of the resting cardiac output goes to the brain to meet its metabolic needs. Interruption of the cerebral blood flow leads to ischemia and disruption of the cerebral metabolism. Cerebral hemodynamics include the following:

- Cerebral blood volume is the amount of blood in the intracranial vault at any one time. Normally about 10%, most is in the venous system, and is determined by autoregulatory mechanism.
- Cerebral blood flow is normally maintained at about 750 mL/min, a rate that matches or exceeds local metabolic needs of the brain. Cerebral blood flow is regulated through vasoconstriction or vasodilation of the cerebral vessels in response to changes in arterial oxygen and carbon dioxide concentrations.
- Cerebral perfusion pressure (CPP) is the pressure required to perfuse brain cells. It is the difference between the mean arterial pressure (MAP) and the ICP. Normal cerebral perfusion pressure is 80 to 100 mmHg. CPP must be at least 50 mmHg to provide minimal blood flow to the brain.

*Autoregulation* is a compensatory mechanism in which cerebral arterioles change diameter to maintain cerebral blood flow when ICP increases. The two forms of autoregulation are pressure autoregulation and chemical or metabolic autoregulation.

In pressure autoregulation, stretch receptors within small blood vessels of the brain cause smooth muscle of the arterioles to contract. Increased arterial pressure stimulates these receptors, leading to vasoconstriction; when arterial pressure is low, stimulation of these receptors decreases, causing relaxation and vasodilation.

Chemical, or metabolic, autoregulation works in much the same way as pressure autoregulation. In this case, the stimulus is a buildup of metabolic by-products of cell metabolism, including lactic acid, pyruvic acid, carbonic acid, and carbon dioxide. Carbon dioxide and increased hydrogen ion concentration are potent cerebral vasodilators that may act locally or systemically to increase cerebral blood flow. Conversely, a fall in $PaCO_2$ causes cerebral vasoconstriction. Arterial oxygen tension ($PaO_2$) also affects cerebral blood flow, although it is a less powerful mechanism than that exerted by carbon dioxide and hydrogen ions.

## PATHOPHYSIOLOGY AND MANIFESTATIONS OF INCREASED ICP

Increased ICP (also labeled **intracranial hypertension**) may result from an increase in intracranial contents from a space-occupying lesion, cerebral edema (swelling), excess cerebrospinal fluid, or intracranial hemorrhage. Displacement of some CSF to the spinal subarachnoid space and increased CSF absorption are early compensatory mechanisms. The low-pressure venous system is also compressed, and cerebral arteries constrict to reduce blood flow. Brain tissue's ability to accommodate change is relatively restricted (Porth, 2002). The relationship between the volume of the intracranial components and intracranial pressure is known as *compliance*. When the capacity to compensate for increased intracranial pressure

is exceeded, *increased intracranial pressure (hypertension)* develops. Intracranial hypertension is a sustained state of increased ICP and is potentially life-threatening.

Autoregulatory mechanisms have a limited ability to maintain cerebral blood flow. When autoregulation fails, cerebrovascular tone is reduced and cerebral blood flow becomes dependent on changes in blood pressure. Autoregulation may be lost either locally or globally because of several factors, including increasing intracranial pressure, local or diffuse cerebral tissue ischemia or inflammation, prolonged hypotension, and hypercapnia or hypoxia.

With loss of autoregulation, intracranial pressure continues to rise and cerebral perfusion falls. Cerebral tissue becomes ischemic, and manifestations of cellular hypoxia appear. Because the neurons of the cerebral cortex are most sensitive to oxygen deficit, changes in cortical function are the earliest manifestations of increasing ICP (Porth, 2002). Behavior and personality changes occur; the client may become irritable and agitated. Memory and judgment are impaired, and speech pattern changes may be noted. The client's LOC decreases. As cerebral hypertension and hypoxia progress, the LOC continues to decrease in a predictable pattern to coma and unresponsiveness.

Pressure on the pyramidal tract often causes weakness (hemiparesis) on the contralateral side early in increased ICP. As ICP continues to increase, hemiplegia and abnormal motor responses, such as decorticate or decerebrate posturing (see Chapter 40), develop.

Altered vision is an early manifestation of increased ICP; it is caused by pressure on the visual pathways and cranial nerves. Blurred vision, decreased visual acuity, and diplopia are common. Pupillary and oculomotor responses are affected as well. Because the cause of increased ICP is often localized at first, pupillary changes, including gradual dilation and sluggish response to light, may initially be limited to the ipsilateral side.

Additional manifestations of increased ICP include headache, particularly on rising, that worsens with position changes. Headache is more common with slowly developing increased ICP and occurs because of pressure on pain-sensitive structures, such as the middle meningeal arteries, the venous sinuses, and the dura at the base of the skull. Papilledema (edema and swelling of the optic disk) may be noted on fundoscopic examination. Vomiting, often projectile and occurring without warning, may develop.

Ischemia of the vasomotor center in the brainstem triggers the CNS ischemic response, a late sign of increased ICP. Neuronal ischemia in the vasomotor center causes a marked increase in the mean arterial pressure (MAP), with a significant increase in systolic blood pressure and increased pulse pressure. The increased MAP causes reflexive slowing of the cardiac rate. This trio of manifestations (increased MAP, increased pulse pressure, and bradycardia) is known as *Cushing's response (or triad)*, and represents the brainstem's final effort to maintain cerebral perfusion (Porth, 2002). The respiratory pattern also changes, often in the predictable progression outlined in Table 42–1. Although the temperature is usually normal in early stages, as ICP continues to increase, hypothalamic function is impaired and the temperature may rise dramatically.

## Manifestations of Increased Intracranial Pressure

- Decreased level of consciousness. *Early:* Confusion, restlessness, lethargy; disorientation, first to time, then to place and person. *Late:* Comatose with no response to painful stimuli.
- Pupillary dysfunction. Sluggish response to light progressing to fixed pupils; with a localized process, pupillary dysfunction is first noted on the ipsilateral side.
- Oculomotor dysfunction. Inability to move eye(s) upward; ptosis (drooping) of the eyelid.
- Visual abnormalities. Decreased visual acuity, blurred vision, diplopia.
- Papilledema. May be late sign.
- Motor impairment. *Early:* Hemiparesis or hemiplegia of the contralateral side. *Late:* Abnormal responses such as decorticate or decerebrate positioning; flaccidity.
- Headache. Uncommon but may occur with processes that slowly increase ICP; worse on rising in the morning and with position changes.
- Projectile vomiting without nausea.
- Cushing's response. Increased systolic blood pressure, widening pulse pressure, bradycardia.
- Respirations. Altered respiratory pattern related to level of brain dysfunction.
- Temperature. May be significantly elevated as compensatory mechanisms fail.

The manifestations of increased ICP are listed in the box above.

## Cerebral Edema

**Cerebral edema** is an increase in the volume of brain tissue due to abnormal accumulation of fluid. Cerebral edema is often associated with increased intracranial pressure; it may occur as a local process in the area of a tumor or injury, or it may affect the entire brain. Three types of cerebral edema have been identified and are described as follows (Porth, 2002). The client with intracranial hypertension may have more than one type.

- *Vasogenic edema,* an increase in the capillary permeability of cerebral vessels, occurs with impairment of the blood-brain barrier, allowing diffusion of water and protein into the interstitial spaces of the brain's white matter. A variety of pathologies, such as ischemia, hemorrhage, brain tumors and injuries, and infections (such as meningitis), may cause the increase in capillary permeability. The site of the brain injury, the level of increase in capillary permeability, and the client's systemic blood pressure influence the rate and extent of the edema's spread. Vasogenic edema is manifested by focal neurologic deficits, altered levels of consciousness, and severe intracranial hypertension.
- *Cytotoxic edema,* an increase of fluid in the intracellular space (primarily in the gray matter), involves changes in the functional or structural integrity of cell membranes due to pathologies such as water intoxication or severe ischemia, intracranial hypoxia, acidosis, and brain trauma. With abnormally low cerebral perfusion, oxygen and nutrients are depleted, intracranial cells switch to anaerobic metabolism, and

the sodium-potassium pump in the cell walls is impaired. Sodium diffuses into the cells, pulling fluid after it. The cells swell, and intracranial pressure rises. Accumulated metabolic waste products, such as lactic acid, contribute to a rapid deterioration of cell function. Cytotoxic edema is a slowly progressive process that results in altered consciousness. The edema may be so severe that it causes cerebral infarction with brain tissue necrosis.

- *Interstitial cerebral edema* involves movement of CSF across the ventricular wall, resulting in water and sodium in the periventricular white space. This type is seen more often in pathologies that obstruct CSF flow through the ventricles, such as hydrocephalus or purulent meningitis.

Cerebral edema tends to be proportional to the extent of the pathology precipitating it. Brain function is not disrupted by cerebral edema unless the edema causes an increase in ICP. When it does, a vicious cycle can ensue: Cerebral edema increases ICP, which in turn decreases cerebral blood flow. Brain tissue becomes hypoxic and ischemic, increasing toxic metabolic by-products, hydrogen ion concentration, and carbon dioxide levels in the tissue. Autoregulatory mechanisms cause vasodilation and increase cerebral blood flow, further increasing cerebral edema and intracranial pressure. Without effective intervention, the client's condition can deteriorate rapidly; intracranial pressure increases to the point where brain structures herniate.

## Hydrocephalus

**Hydrocephalus** is an increase in volume of CSF within the ventricular system, which becomes dilated. Hydrocephalus may increase ICP when it develops acutely. Hydrocephalus occurs when the production of CSF exceeds its absorption. It is generally classified as either noncommunicating or communicating hydrocephalus. *Noncommunicating hydrocephalus* occurs when CSF drainage from the ventricular system is obstructed. It may develop when a mass or tumor, inflammation or hemorrhage, or congenital malformation obstructs the ventricular system. *Communicating hydrocephalus* is a condition in which CSF is not effectively reabsorbed through the arachnoid villi. It may occur secondarily to subarachnoid hemorrhage or scarring from infection. In *normal pressure hydrocephalus,* seen most often in adults age 60 or older, ventricular enlargement causes cerebral tissue compression but the CSF pressure on lumbar puncture is normal. This condition may follow cerebral trauma or surgery, or the cause may not be known. Manifestations of hydrocephalus depend on the rate of its development. They may be mild and insidious in onset, presenting as progressive cognitive dysfunctions, gait disruptions, and urinary incontinence. If the process causing hydrocephalus is an acute one, the manifestations are those of increased ICP.

## Brain Herniation

If increased ICP is not treated, cerebral tissue is displaced toward a more compliant area. This can result in **brain herniation,** the displacement of brain tissue from its normal compartment under dural folds of the falx cerebri or through the tentorial notch or incisura of the tentorium cerebelli (Porth,

2002). Herniation of the cerebellum through the tentorium exerts pressure on the brainstem, with subsequent herniation through the foramen magnum. This is a lethal complication of increased ICP because it puts pressure on the vital centers of the medulla.

Brain herniation syndromes are generally categorized as supratentorial or infratentorial, depending on their location above or below the tentorium cerebelli (Figure 42–2 ■). Supratentorial herniation syndromes include cingulate herniation, central or transtentorial herniation, and uncal or lateral transtentorial herniation.

- *Cingulate herniation* (Figure 42–2A) occurs when the cingulate gyrus is displaced under the falx cerebri. Local blood supply and cerebral tissue are compressed, resulting in ischemia and further increases in intracranial pressure.
- *Central or transtentorial* herniation is the downward displacement of brain structures, including the cerebral hemispheres, basal ganglia, diencephalon, and midbrain through the tentorial incisura (Figure 42–2B). The client's neurologic signs may deteriorate rapidly, with decreased LOC progressing to coma, Cheyne-Stokes respirations progressing to central neurogenic hyperventilation, and pupils progressing from small and reactive to midsize and fixed. The client may demonstrate abnormal motor responses with unilateral decorticate posturing.
- *Uncal or lateral transtentorial* herniation occurs when a lateral mass displaces cerebral tissue centrally, forcing the medial aspect of the temporal lobe under the edge of the tentorial incisura (Figure 42–2C). The oculomotor nerve (cranial nerve III) often becomes trapped between the uncus and the tentorium, causing ipsilateral pupillary dilation. Other manifestations include alterations in LOC, motor deficits (which

may occur on the same side as the herniation because of compression of the cerebral peduncle on the opposite side), decreased sensation, respiratory changes, abnormal positioning, and eventual respiratory arrest.

- *Infratentorial herniation* results from increased pressure within the infratentorial compartment. Herniation may occur either upward, with structures displaced through the tentorial incisura, or downward, with displacement through the foramen magnum (Figure 42–2D). Downward displacement compresses the medulla, including its centers for controlling vital functions. Manifestations associated with medullary compression include coma, altered respiratory patterns, fixed pupils, and decorticate or decerebrate posturing. Respiratory or cardiac arrest may occur.

## COLLABORATIVE CARE

Care of the client with increased ICP is directed toward identifying and treating the underlying cause of the disorder, and controlling ICP to prevent herniation syndrome. Increased ICP is a medical emergency, and there is little time to complete lengthy diagnostic tests. The diagnosis must be made on the basis of observation and neurologic assessment; even subtle changes may be clinically significant.

### Diagnostic Tests

Diagnostic tests focus on identifying the presence of increased ICP and its underlying cause. A CT scan or MRI is generally the initial test. These tests are used to identify the possible causes of increased ICP (such as space-occupying lesions or hydrocephalus) and to evaluate therapeutic options. In general, a lumbar puncture is not performed when increased ICP is suspected because the sudden release of the pressure in the skull may cause cerebral herniation.

In addition to the diagnostic tests listed in the previous section for altered LOC, the following specific tests are ordered and their results closely monitored.

- *Serum osmolality* is an indicator of hydration status in the client with increased ICP. The test measures the number of dissolved particles (electrolytes, urea, glucose) in the serum. The normal range for the adult is 280 to 300 mOsm/kg $H_2O$. In addition to the restriction of fluids in the client with increased ICP, serum osmolality is maintained at a slightly elevated level (325 mOsm/kg $H_2O$) to draw excess intracellular fluid into the vascular system.
- *ABGs* are monitored frequently to assess pH and levels of oxygen and carbon dioxide. Hydrogen ions and carbon dioxide are both potent vasodilators; hypoxemia also causes vasodilation, although to a lesser degree.

### Medications

Medications play an important role in the management of increased ICP. Diuretics, particularly osmotic diuretics, are commonly used to reduce ICP and are the mainstays of pharmacologic treatment.

Osmotic diuretics work by increasing the osmolarity of the blood, thereby drawing water out of edematous brain tissue and

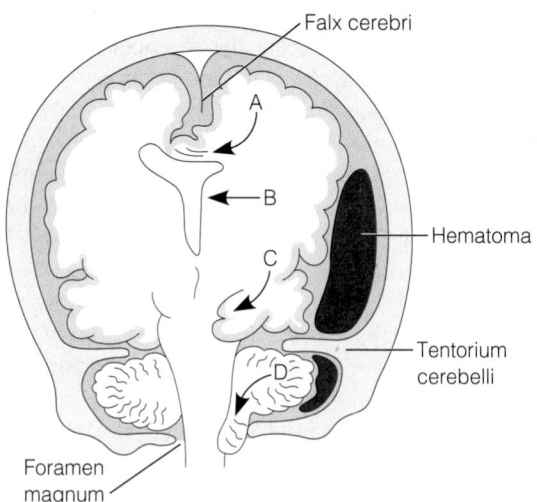

**Figure 42–2** ■ Forms of brain herniation due to intracranial hypertension. *A,* Cingulate herniation occurs when the cingulate gyrus is compressed under the falx cerebri. *B,* Central herniation occurs when a centrally located lesion compresses central and midbrain structures. *C,* Lateral herniation occurs when a lesion at the side of the brain compresses the uncus or hippocampal gyrus. *D,* Infratentorial herniation occurs when the cerebellar tonsils are forced downward, compressing the medulla and top of the spinal cord.

into the vascular system for elimination via the kidneys. The effects of these drugs vary with the type of injury. Regardless of the agent used, the optimal dose is the lowest that reduces ICP. Mannitol is the most commonly employed osmotic diuretic. Glucose, urea, and glycerol are other osmotic diuretics that may be used. Urine output by Foley catheter is monitored. Electrolyte levels are carefully assessed and potassium is replaced as indicated.

Loop diuretics, such as furosemide (Lasix) (the drug of choice) and ethacrynic acid (Edecrin), may be prescribed for some clients with increased ICP. These diuretics act on the renal tubule and are extremely effective in promoting diuresis. Additionally, loop diuretics may be used to manage the rebound effect that may occur with mannitol administration.

Antipyretics, such as acetaminophen, are used alone or in combination with a hypothermia blanket to treat hyperthermia.

Hyperthermia increases the cerebral metabolic rate and exacerbates an existing increase in ICP. Anticonvulsants are often required to manage seizure activity associated with brain injury and increased ICP. Gastrointestinal prophylaxis with histamine H$_2$ antagonists or sucralfate (Carafate) is often used, as clients with ICP are at increased risk for the development of stress ulcers.

To treat clients with severe, persistent intracranial hypertension that does not respond to other therapy, barbiturates may be used to induce coma. The mechanism of action of this controversial therapy is unclear, but it is thought to reduce metabolic demands in the injured brain. Because neurologic signs are masked, close monitoring of the client in induced coma is vital.

Nursing implications for these medications are described in the box below.

# Medication Administration

## Increased Intracranial Pressure

### OSMOTIC DIURETICS

Mannitol (Osmitrol)
Urea
Glucose

Osmotic diuretics (hyperosmotic agents) draw fluid out of brain cells by increasing the osmolality of the blood. The effects of these drugs vary with the type of injury. Mannitol therapy is often initiated if the client's ICP has exceeded 15 to 20 mmHg for at least 10 minutes. Both intravenous bolus and continuous infusion techniques are used. Repeated use of mannitol can lead to continual elevations in serum osmolality, with attendant risk of seizures and serious fluid and electrolyte imbalance. Urea is seldom administered intravenously because a severe local reaction may result if leakage occurs at the injection site. Mannitol and urea are used cautiously if renal disease is present.

**Note:** Because the client with increased intracranial pressure often has an altered level of consciousness, client and family teaching is not discussed in this box.

#### Nursing Responsibilities

- Monitor vital signs, urinary output, central venous pressure (CVP), and pulmonary artery pressures (PAP) before and every hour throughout administration.
- Assess client for manifestations of dehydration.
- Assess client for muscle weakness, numbness, tingling, paresthesia, confusion, and excessive thirst.
- Assess client for pulmonary edema while administering the medication.
- Monitor neurologic status and intracranial pressure readings.
- Monitor renal function and serum electrolytes throughout therapy.
- Do not administer the medication if crystals are present in solution. Administer with an in-line filter. Observe infusion site frequently for infiltration.
- Do not administer mannitol solution with blood.
- Do not discontinue medication abruptly. Rebound migraine headaches may occur.

### LOOP DIURETICS

Furosemide (Lasix)
Ethacrynic acid (Edecrin)

Loop diuretics such as furosemide and ethacrynic acid inhibit sodium and chloride reabsorption at the ascending loop of Henle. They cause a reduction in the rate of CSF production, thus reducing the ICP.

#### Nursing Responsibilities

- Monitor vital signs and electrolyte values closely.
- Assess fluid status throughout therapy.
- Monitor blood pressure and pulse before and during administration.
- Monitor renal laboratory studies closely.
- Use infusion pump to ensure accurate dosage.

### INTRAVENOUS FLUIDS

Keeping the client moderately dehydrated to maintain serum osmolality can be effective in reducing cerebral edema. When giving intravenous fluids, closely monitor the osmolality of the solutions; if clients with increased ICP are given hypo-osmolar solutions, increased cerebral edema can occur. Preferred solutions include 0.45% to 0.9% sodium chloride solutions.

#### Nursing Responsibilities

- Monitor fluid status closely.
- Monitor neurologic status closely.
- Avoid administering hypo-osmolar solutions, such as 5% dextrose in water.
- Half-strength normal saline (0.45% sodium chloride) is considered a suitable fluid for a client who has increased intracranial pressure.
- Take care not to restrict fluids excessively in clients receiving dehydrating agents (such as osmotic or loop diuretics).

### OTHER PHARMACOLOGIC INTERVENTIONS FOR ICP

- Antipyretics, such as acetaminophen, are used to reduce hyperthermia, thereby decreasing the high cerebral metabolism that contributes to ICP.
- Antiulcer drugs, such as histamine H$_2$ antagonists (for example, ranitidine [Zantac]) or sucralfate (Carafate), are used in clients with ICP to decrease the development of stress ulcers.
- Antihypertensive agents, such as beta-adrenergic blocking agents, may be used if the mean arterial pressure is high.
- Vasopressors may be used if the mean arterial pressure is low.
- Anticonvulsants may be given to prevent or treat seizures.

Intravenous fluids are usually necessary to maintain the client's fluid and electrolyte balance as well as vascular volume. If the client's blood pressure is unstable, vasoactive medications may be administered to maintain the MAP in a range that supports cerebral perfusion while minimizing increases in ICP. When enteral feeding is not possible, total parenteral nutrition may be administered.

## Treatments

### Surgery

Clients with increased ICP may undergo various intracranial surgical techniques to treat the underlying cause (see the discussion in the later section on brain tumors). In addition, infarcted or necrotic tissue may be resected to reduce brain mass. A drainage catheter or shunt may be inserted laterally via a burr hole into a ventricle to drain excess cerebrospinal fluid and reduce hydrocephalus. The removal of even a small amount of CSF may dramatically reduce ICP and restore cerebral perfusion pressure.

### ICP Monitoring

Intracranial pressure monitors facilitate continual assessment of ICP and are more precise than often vague clinical manifestations. With these devices, the effects of medical therapy and nursing interventions on ICP can also be monitored. In addition, cerebral perfusion pressure (the difference between MAP and ICP) can be readily calculated, allowing more precise manipulation of therapeutic measures to maintain cerebral perfusion and thereby prevent ischemia. The criteria for ICP monitoring depends on the client, but in general, clients who are comatose and have a Glasgow Coma Score of 8 or less should be monitored.

Basic monitoring systems include an intraventricular catheter, subarachnoid bolt or screw, and epidural probe (Figure 42–3 ■). Intraventricular fluid-filled catheters are placed in the anterior horn of the lateral ventricle (most often in the right side). They can both drain CSF and measure ICP. The ICP value is measured deep in the brain and is considered the most reflective of the whole brain pressure. Subarachnoid devices are placed in the subarachnoid space. Epidural catheters are usually fiberoptic pressure transducers; they do not penetrate the dura and are considered relatively noninvasive. A fiberoptic transducer-tipped catheter can be placed in the epidural, subdural, or l parenchymal space, with ICP values considered very accurate. Subarachnoid, epidural, or fiberoptic monitoring devices can drain CSF. The choice of monitor depends on both the suspected disorder and the physician's preference. Once the intracranial sensor is implanted, it is con-

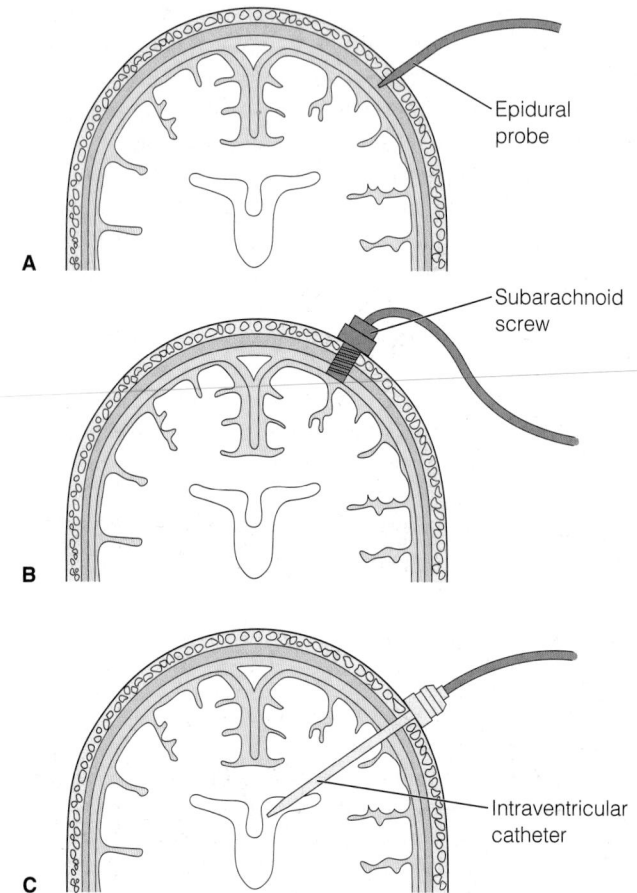

**Figure 42–3 ■** Types of intracranial pressure monitoring. *A*, Epidural probe. *B*, Subarachnoid screw. *C*, Intraventricular catheter.

nected to a transducer that converts the impulses to a signal that the recording device can translate into an oscilloscope tracing, digital value, or graphic recording. Factors that increase the risk for infection during ICP monitoring are listed in Box 42–1.

### Mechanical Ventilation

Clients who require intubation for airway management are placed on a ventilator. Mechanical ventilation may be used to maintain partial pressure of oxygen and carbon dioxide, thus preventing hypoxemia and hypercapnia, both of which can increase intracranial pressure (Hilton, 2001). It is important to maintain adequate oxygenation with a partial pressure of arterial oxygen at about 100 mmHg and a partial pressure of arterial

| BOX 42–1 ■ Risk Factors for Infection with Intracranial Pressure Monitoring | |
|---|---|
| *Factor* | *Rationale* |
| Intraventricular catheter | Is more invasive than other monitoring devices |
| Open head trauma or neurosurgery | Disrupts protective skin and skeletal barriers |
| Intracranial hemorrhage | Necessitates frequent flushing of catheter to maintain patency |
| Older adult | Tends to have impaired immune defenses |
| Monitoring for more than 3 to 5 days; or open system or frequent irrigation | Offers increased opportunity for pathogens to enter and grow |

carbon dioxide of about 35 mmHg (Bucher & Melander, 1999). The client with increased ICP and signs of impending herniation may be judiciously hyperventilated to cause cerebral vasoconstriction; however, this also increases cerebral ischemia.

## NURSING CARE

The nursing care of clients with increased ICP involves identifying those at risk and managing factors known to increase intracranial pressure. A major focus is protecting the client from sudden increases in ICP or a decrease in cerebral blood flow.

## Nursing Diagnoses and Interventions

Nursing interventions include performing neurologic assessments, maintaining the patency of the airway, ensuring adequate ventilation, positioning and moving, instituting seizure precautions, and monitoring fluids and electrolytes. Additionally, both client and family need emotional support during this period. The client with increased ICP has varied responses to actual or potential changes in physiologic processes (see the box below).

## Ineffective Tissue Perfusion: Cerebral

A number of disorders may lead to increased ICP, including cerebral edema, hydrocephalus, space-occupying lesions and hemorrhage, herniation syndromes, and changes in carbon dioxide concentrations. Increasing intracranial pressure alters cerebral perfusion and oxygenation of brain cells. The client with increased ICP requires intensive care, and often needs ventilator assistance.

- Assess for and report any of the manifestations of increasing ICP every 1 to 2 hours and as necessary. Assessment areas include level of consciousness, behavior, motor/sensory functions, pupillary size and reaction to light, and vital signs, including temperature. Look for trends, because vital signs alone do not correlate well with early deterioration. *Assessment of neurologic status establishes the client's clinical condition and provides a baseline to measure changes. Sudden changes in neurologic signs often indicate deterioration. An elevated temperature with increased oxygen consumption further increases intracranial pressure. Pupillary responses mirror the status of the midbrain and pons. Pressure on the brainstem may compromise the function of cranial nerves IX and X and protective mechanisms, such as the gag and cough reflexes.*

**PRACTICE ALERT** *Often, the earliest manifestations of a change in intracranial pressure are alterations in the level of consciousness and breathing patterns.* ■

- For the client on a ventilator: Maintain patency of the airway; preoxygenate with 100% oxygen before suctioning; limit suctioning to 10 seconds; suction gently. *Preoxygenation helps maintain oxygen levels during suctioning. Suctioning stimulates the cough reflex and Valsalva maneuver. Correct suctioning minimizes the risk of hypoxemia.*
- Monitor arterial blood gases (ABGs). *ABGs provide a reliable indicator of oxygen and carbon dioxide levels. If oxygen concentration is low, oxygen may be given or increased.*

## Nursing Research

### Evidence-Based Practice for Clients with Increased Intracranial Pressure

Nursing diagnoses are made based on the presence of defining characteristics. This study (Wall et al., 1995) was conducted to identify defining characteristics and risk factors for the nursing diagnoses of *Increased intracranial pressure* and *High risk for increased intracranial pressure*. Although this diagnosis is not listed in the NANDA taxonomy, the authors believe it should be. A national sample of nurses who care for clients with neurologic impairments were surveyed, and a number of defining characteristics were validated. The researchers concluded that the defining characteristics and risk factors identified in the literature represent these diagnoses well, although additional characteristics may be present in the clinical setting. Further clinical studies are recommended, with differentiation of characteristics specific to various settings and specialty areas.

The authors of this study believe that findings can assist nurses to identify relevant defining characteristics and risk factors, make a diagnosis, and implement appropriate interventions. Findings can also be helpful to students in learning critical thinking and diagnostic reasoning skills.

### IMPLICATIONS FOR NURSING

It is very important that nursing interventions be knowledge based. Studies such as this are important in defining the language of nursing and in facilitating the classification of nursing language. To provide safe and knowledgeable care, nurses must make accurate assessments, recognize and differentiate characteristics that support specific diagnoses, provide interventions, and evaluate outcomes of care.

### Critical Thinking in Client Care

1. Do you believe that increased intracranial pressure is a human response to an actual or a potential health problem? Can nurses select the interventions to treat this problem? Why or why not?
2. Provide a rationale for nursing assessment and monitoring of each of the following manifestations (defining characteristics) of increased intracranial pressure:
   a. Eye opening, motor and verbal responses
   b. Vital signs
   c. Pupillary responses
   d. Vomiting
   e. Headache
   f. Level of consciousness
3. Describe the rationale for administering intravenous fluids by an infusion pump to the client with a severe head injury.

- Elevate head of the bed to 30 degrees or keep flat, as prescribed; maintain the alignment of the head and neck to avoid hyperextension or exaggerated neck flexion; avoid prone position. *Keeping the head of the bed elevated facilitates venous drainage from the cerebrum. Obstruction of jugular veins can impede venous drainage from the brain (Sullivan, 2000).*
- Assess for bladder distention and bowel constipation. Administer stool softeners and use the Credé technique to empty the bladder. If the Credé technique is not effective, evaluate the pros and cons of urinary catheterization if the bladder remains distended. *Constipation and bladder distention increase intrathoracic or intra-abdominal pressure and place the client at risk for impaired venous drainage from the brain.*
- Assist in moving up in bed. Do not ask to push with heels or arms or push against a footboard. Avoid a footboard and restraints. *Moving up in bed requires pushing. Helping the client move prevents initiation of the Valsalva maneuver, which increases intracranial pressure.*
- Plan nursing care so that activities are not clustered together; avoid turning the client, getting the client on the bedpan, or suctioning within the same time period. Schedule nursing care to provide rest periods between procedures. *Multiple procedures, including certain nursing care activities, can increase ICP. Constant stimulation tends to increase ICP. Individualized nursing care ensures optimal spacing of activities and rest.*
- Provide a quiet environment, limiting noxious stimuli. Avoid jarring the bed. Try to limit situations that cause emotional upset; maintain a calm, reassuring manner; caution family members to refrain from unpleasant conversations or that may be emotionally stimulating to the client. *Noxious stimuli and emotional upsets cause an elevation in ICP.*
- Maintain fluid limitations, if prescribed. *Restricting fluids helps decrease cerebral edema by reducing total body water.*

### Risk for Infection

Although any client with an open head wound is at risk for infection, the interventions discussed here are for the client with an intracranial monitoring device. Most clinical units have written protocols for managing these systems. The following nursing actions serve only as a general guide.

- Keep dressings over the catheter dry, and change dressings on a prescribed basis (usually every 24 to 48 hours). *Wet dressings are conducive to bacterial growth.*
- Monitor the insertion site for leaking CSF, drainage, or infection. Monitor for manifestations of infection, including changes in vital signs, chills, increased WBC counts, and positive cultures of drainage. *Close monitoring helps detect the earliest signs of infection and helps prevent major complications. Fever is usually considered the key assessment. However, fever in a client with a neurologic disorder may be due to damage to the hypothalamus. Headache, generalized muscle aches, shivering, and chills may also be seen in the client with infection.*
- Use strict aseptic technique when in contact with the device. Check drainage system for loose connections. *The use of aseptic technique and monitoring drainage systems for loose connections helps prevent nosocomial infections. Most nosocomial infections are transmitted by health care workers who fail to wash their hands properly, to change gloves between clients, or to follow aseptic technique protocols. Invasive procedures provide an excellent opportunity for microbes to enter the body.*

## Client and Family Teaching

Teach the client at risk for increased ICP (and able to follow instructions) to avoid coughing, blowing the nose, straining to have a bowel movement, pushing against the bed rails, or performing isometric (muscle contracting) exercises. Advise the client to maintain head and neck alignment when turning in bed and to take rest periods.

Encourage the family to talk to the client, but maintain a quiet environment with a minimum of stimuli. Inform family members that upsetting the client may increase intracranial pressure and that they should avoid discussions that may distress the client. For clients unable to make decisions about treatment and to sign informed consent, the family must carry out these functions.

## THE CLIENT WITH A HEADACHE

**Headache** is pain within the cranial vault. Headache is one of the most common symptoms people experience, although its cause is frequently unknown. Headaches may occur as a result of benign or pathologic conditions, intracranial or extracranial conditions, diseases of other body systems, stress, musculoskeletal tension, or a combination of these factors.

Most headaches are mild, transient, and relieved by a mild analgesic. However, some headaches are chronic, intense, and recurrent. Manifestations of headache vary according to the cause, type, and precipitating symptoms.

## PATHOPHYSIOLOGY AND MANIFESTATIONS

Selected structures within the cranial vault are sensitive to pain. Pain-sensitive structures include supporting structures, such as the skin, muscles, and periosteum; the nasal cavities and sinuses; portions of the meninges, cranial nerves II, III, IV, V, VI, IX, and X; and cerebral vessels, including extracranial arteries and the venous sinuses. Most facial and scalp structures are sensitive to pain. Stretching (traction), inflammation, pressure compression, and dilation of the pain-sensitive structures of the cranial vault, scalp, and face can produce a headache. The most common types of headaches are tension, migraine, and cluster headaches (Table 42–4).

### Tension Headache

**Tension headache,** the most common type of headache, is characterized by bilateral pain, with a sensation of a band of tightness or pressure around the head. Sharply localized painful

TABLE 42–4  Comparison of Migraine, Cluster, and Tension Headaches

| Type | Risk Factors | Frequency and Duration | Description | Prodromal and Associated Manifestations |
|------|-------------|------------------------|-------------|------------------------------------------|
| Migraine | Female<br>Family history of migraine headache.<br>Age not a risk factor. | Episodic:<br>• Tends to occur with stress and crisis.<br>• Often correlates with menstrual cycle.<br>• Can last hours to days. | Slow onset; pain becomes more severe, involving one side of head more than other. | Prodromal manifestations: visual defects, confusion, paresthesias.<br>Associated manifestations: nausea, vomiting, chills, fatigue, irritability, sweating. |
| Cluster | Male<br>Use of alcohol or nitrates.<br>May begin in early childhood. | Episodes are clustered together in rapid succession for a few days or weeks with remissions that last for months.<br>Can last a few minutes to a few hours. | May begin in infraorbital region and spread to head and neck; throbbing, deep pain, often unilateral. | Prodromal manifestations: uncommon.<br>Associated manifestations: flushing, tearing of eyes, nasal congestion, sweating and swelling of temporal vessels. |
| Tension | Related to tension and anxiety.<br>No family history.<br>Often begins in adolescence. | Episodic:<br>• Varies with amount of stress.<br>• Duration also varies; can be constant. | Tight, pressing, viselike; may involve neck and shoulders. | Prodromal manifestations: uncommon.<br>Associated manifestations: sustained contraction of neck muscles. |

spots (trigger points) may be present. The onset is gradual, and the intensity, frequency, and duration of the attack vary greatly. This type of headache is caused by sustained contraction of the muscles of the head and neck. It is often precipitated by stressful situations and anxiety. Secondary causes include disorders of the eyes, ears, sinuses, or cervical vertebrae. Abnormal posture associated with occupations that require bending over a desk (e.g., office workers, students) often precipitates tension-type headache. Additionally, slouching while reading or watching television can lead to muscle contraction. Most headaches are tension-type headaches.

## Migraine Headache

**Migraine headache** is a recurring vascular headache often initiated by a triggering event and usually accompanied by a neurologic dysfunction. It affects as many as 23 million people in the United States (5 million men and 18 million women) (Lin, 2001). It is more common between the ages of 25 to 55 years. There is often a positive family history. Headaches classified as migraines may differ in intensity, duration, and frequency. The exact causes of migraine are not fully understood, but they are believed to be the result of abnormalities in cerebrovascular blood flow, a reduction in brain and electrical activity, or increased release of sensory substances such as serotonin, norepinephrine, substance P, nitric oxide, and glutamate (McCance & Huether, 2002).

The classic migraine headache has several stages, including the aura stage, the headache stage (or period of throbbing), and the postheadache stage.

• The **aura** stage is characterized by sensory manifestations, usually visual disturbances such as bright spots or flashing lights zig-zagging across the visual fields. This stage lasts from 5 to 60 minutes. Less common sensory symptoms include numbness or tingling of the face or hand, paresis of an arm or leg, mild aphasia, confusion, drowsiness, and lack of coordination. Additionally, some clients experience a premonition the day prior to an attack. They may feel nervous or have other mood changes. The aura period corresponds with the initial physiologic change of vasoconstriction.

• The headache stage is characterized by vasodilation, a decline in serotonin levels, and the onset of throbbing headache. It appears that the pain is related to increased vessel permeability and polypeptide exudation by perivascular nerve endings rather than the vasodilation itself. Cerebral arteries are dilated and distended, with walls that are edematous and rigid. Beginning unilaterally, the headache eventually may involve both sides as it increases in intensity during the next several hours. Nausea and vomiting often occur. The client may be acutely ill and is often extremely irritable. The sensory organs often become hypersensitive, and the client withdraws from sound and light. The scalp is tender. The headache may last from several hours to a day or two.

• During the postheadache phase, the headache area is sensitive to touch, and a deep aching is present. The client is exhausted. Vessel size and serotonin levels return to normal.

A variety of factors are believed to trigger the onset of a migraine headache. Rapid changes in blood glucose levels, stress, emotional excitement, fatigue, hormonal changes due to menstruation, stimuli such as bright lights, and food high in tyramine or other vasoactive substances (e.g., aged cheese, nuts, chocolate, and alcoholic beverages) have been associated with migraine attacks. Hypertension and febrile states may make the disorder worse.

Another type of migraine headache is called a *migraine without aura.* This type is the most common and is associated with hereditary factors. The aura stage is absent; clients are aware only that a headache is eminent. The headache develops gradually, lasting hours to days, and may occur during periods of premenstrual tension and fluid retention. Chills, nausea and vomiting, fatigue, and nasal congestion are often present.

## Cluster Headache

The **cluster headache** is predominantly experienced by middle-aged men. The physiologic mechanism underlying cluster headaches is not well understood, but involves a vascular disorder, a disturbance of serotonergic mechanisms, a sympathetic defect, or dysregulation of the hypothalamus.

Although the headache may occur at any time, it typically begins 2 to 3 hours after falling asleep, awakens the person, and then lasts for less than 2 hours. Prodromal signs are absent. Intense unilateral pain around or behind one eye wakes the client. The pain is accompanied by rhinorrhea, lacrimation, flushing, sweating, facial edema, and possible miosis or ptosis on the affected side. Headaches last 30 minutes to a few hours and abate abruptly.

The attacks tend to occur frequently, in clusters of 1 to 8 daily, for weeks or a few months. The headaches often occur in the spring and fall and then disappear for an extended period. The same side of the head is involved in each cluster of attacks. Attacks may be triggered by drinking alcohol or eating specific foods, or there may be no known precipitating event.

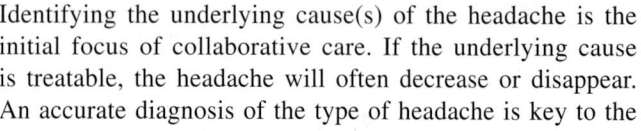

## COLLABORATIVE CARE

Identifying the underlying cause(s) of the headache is the initial focus of collaborative care. If the underlying cause is treatable, the headache will often decrease or disappear. An accurate diagnosis of the type of headache is key to the treatment.

Therapeutic management for migraine headache includes a combination of client teaching, medications, and measures to control contributing factors. Dietary changes such as eliminating caffeine, cured meats, monosodium glutamate (MSG), and foods containing tyramine (red wine, aged cheese, and others) may be necessary. Stress management or biofeedback are also part of the overall strategy. Treatment protocols for cluster headache include eliminating aggravating factors (e.g., consumption of alcohol) and using medications and oxygen inhalation. The management of tension headaches is directed toward reducing the client's level of stress and relieving pain with ice and aspirin or NSAIDs.

## Diagnostic Tests

Diagnosis and treatment are based on history, the identification of triggering or precipitating events, and the type of headache. A thorough history and physical examination are integral parts of the assessment. Neurodiagnostic testing may be done to rule out a structural disease process. Testing may

include a brain scan, MRI, X-ray studies of the skull and cervical spine, EEG, or lumbar puncture for CSF if inflammation is suspected. Serum metabolic screens and hypersensitivity testing also may be performed if systemic problems are suspected.

## Medications

Pharmacologic management depends on the type of headache. The goals of treatment are to reduce the frequency and severity of headaches and to limit or relieve a headache that is beginning or in progress.

The management of migraine headache includes administering medications to prevent pain (prophylactic therapy) as well as drugs to stop (or abort) a headache in progress. The client with frequent migraine headaches is a candidate for prophylactic therapy. Drugs used to reduce the frequency and severity of migraine follow:

- Methysergide maleate (Sansert) is a serotonin antagonist that competitively blocks serotonin receptors in the CNS and is also a potent vasoconstrictor.
- Propranolol hydrochloride (Inderal) is a beta blocker that prevents dilation of vessels in the pia mater and inhibits serotonin uptake.
- Verapamil (Isoptin) is a calcium channel blocker that is thought to prevent migraine by controlling cerebral vasospasms.

When the manifestations of migraine are recognized early, several medications may be used to abort or limit the severity and duration of the headache. Ergotamine tartrate (Cafergot) is a complex drug that reduces extracranial blood flow, decreases the amplitude of cranial artery pulsation, and decreases basilar artery hyperperfusion. Administered at the onset of an attack, ergotamine controls up to 70% of acute attacks. Sumatriptan (Imitrex) is available in oral, nasal spray, or subcutaneous injection forms. It binds with serotonin$_1$ receptors and is rapidly effective. Zolmitriptan (Zomig), a selective serotonin$_1$ receptor agonist, is administered orally and is effective in the treatment of acute headache. Once a migraine is in progress, a narcotic analgesic such as codeine or meperidine (Demerol) may be required. Antiemetics may be prescribed to control nausea and vomiting.

Many of the same medications used for migraine also prevent or treat cluster headache. Because the onset of cluster headaches is abrupt, abortive therapy is not possible. Medications such as ergotamine tartrate may be given in suppository form at bedtime to prevent headache during the episodic attacks. Clients may find that inhaling 100% oxygen at 7 L/min for 15 minutes at the onset of an attack relieves their headache (Tierney et al., 2001).

Nonnarcotic analgesics such as aspirin or acetaminophen may relieve tension headaches. Additionally, tranquilizers such as diazepam may reduce muscle tension.

Nursing implications for drugs commonly prescribed for headaches are described in the Medication Administration box on pages 1363–1364.

# Medication Administration

## Headaches

### BETA BLOCKERS

Propanolol hydrochloride (Inderal)
Nadolol (Corgard)
Atenolol (Tenormin)
Timolol maleate (Blocadren)

Beta blockers are effective in the prophylactic treatment of headache. They act by combining with beta-adrenergic receptors to block the response to sympathetic nerve impulses, circulating catecholamines, or adrenergic drugs.

### Nursing Responsibilities

- Before beginning therapy, determine pulse and blood pressure in both arms with client lying, sitting, and standing.
- Assess baseline and monitor serum glucose level, CBC, electrolytes, and liver and renal function studies.
- Note any history of diabetes or impaired renal function.
- Note the rate and quality of respirations; drugs in this category may cause dyspnea and bronchospasm.
- Administer the drug with meals to prevent gastrointestinal disturbances.
- Be alert that beta blockers cause bradycardia and the heart rate may not rise in response to stress, such as exercise or fever. Notify the primary health care provider if pulse falls below 50 or if blood pressure changes significantly.
- Teach the client or family member how to take a pulse and blood pressure reading.

### Client and Family Teaching

- Take the medication with meals to provide a coating for the gastrointestinal tract and prevent gastrointestinal disturbances.
- Return for blood work as prescribed.
- Take the last dose of the day at bedtime.
- Rise from a sitting or lying position to a standing position slowly to avoid dizziness and falls.
- Take pulse and blood pressure each day and maintain a record of readings.
- Avoid excessive intake of alcohol, coffee, tea, or cola. Consult with the health care provider before taking any over-the-counter medications.
- Report any cough, nasal stuffiness, or feelings of depression to the health care provider.

### TRICYCLIC ANTIDEPRESSANTS

Imipramine hydrochloride (Tofranil)
Amitriptyline hydrochloride (Elavil)

The tricyclic antidepressants have been successful in the prophylaxis of cluster and migraine headaches. Although the exact mechanism is not known, they do prevent the reuptake of norepinephrine or serotonin, or both. They are chemically related to the phenothiazines, and as such they exhibit many of the same pharmacologic effects (e.g., anticholinergic, antiserotonin, sedative, antihistaminic, and hypotensive effects).

### Nursing Responsibilities

- Assess baseline CBC and liver function studies, heart sounds, and neurologic status before initiating prescribed therapy.

### Client and Family Teaching

- Make position changes slowly.
- Chew sugarless gum to relieve dry mouth.
- Do not abruptly quit taking the medication.

### ERGOT ALKALOID DERIVATIVES

Methysergide maleate (Sansert)

Methysergide is an ergot alkaloid derivative structurally related to LSD. It acts by stimulating smooth muscle, leading to vasoconstriction. It is thought that methysergide prevents headaches by blocking the effects of serotonin, a powerful vasodilator believed to play a role in vascular headaches. It also inhibits the release of histamine from mast cells and prevents the release of serotonin from platelets.

### Nursing Responsibilities

- Note any history of renal or hepatic disease.
- Assess baseline eosinophil and neutrophil counts before beginning therapy.
- Administer the drug with meals or milk to minimize gastrointestinal irritation due to increased hydrochloric acid production.
- Assess for renal, central nervous system, and cardiovascular complications.
- Drug dosage should be gradually reduced over 2 to 3 weeks to prevent rebound headaches. A drug-free interval of 3 to 4 weeks is required with each 6-month course of therapy to prevent complications.
- Monitor for signs of ergotism, such as coldness or numbness of the fingers and toes, nausea, vomiting, headache, muscle pain, and weakness. Vasoconstriction may further impair peripheral circulation and increase blood pressure.

### Client and Family Teaching

- Take the medication with meals or milk to minimize gastrointestinal upset.
- Report to the primary care provider nervousness, weakness, rashes, hair loss, or swelling of the extremities.
- Weigh daily and report any unusual weight gain to the primary care provider.
- Return to the primary care provider for a checkup at least every 6 months or as instructed. Do not take the drug on a regular basis for longer than 6 months, but do not abruptly stop taking it.
- Return for follow-up blood work as ordered.

### SEROTONIN SELECTIVE AGONIST

Sumatriptan succinate injection (Imitrex)
Zolmitriptan (Zomig)
Rizatriptan Benzoate (Maxalt)

Binds to vascular receptors to vasoconstrict cranial blood vessels and relieve migraine headache.

### Nursing Responsibilities

- Assess for history of peripheral vascular disease, renal or hepatic problems, and pregnancy.
- Evaluate relief of migraine headache, and assess for side effects of photophobia, sound sensitivity, and nausea and vomiting.

*(continued on page 1364)*

## Medication Administration

### Headaches (continued)

#### Client and Family Teaching

- Do not use more than two injections in a 24-hour period, and allow at least 1 hour between injections.
- Use the autoinjector to administer the medication, and follow instructions for proper method of giving the injection and disposing of the syringe.
- Report wheezing, heart palpitations, skin rash, swelling of the eyelids or face, or chest pain to the health care provider immediately.

#### CALCIUM CHANNEL BLOCKERS

Verapamil (Isoptin)
Nifedipine (Procardia)

The calcium channel blockers may have value in controlling cerebral vasospasms by two mechanisms: inhibiting the influx of calcium into the cerebral artery and interfering with the destruction of erythrocytes and aggregation of platelets.

#### Nursing Responsibilities

- These drugs cause peripheral vasodilation. Therefore, monitor blood pressure and pulse during the initial administration of the drug. Any excessive hypotensive response and tachycardia may precipitate angina. Request written parameters for safe drug administration.
- Monitor intake and output and daily weights. Assess for manifestations of congestive heart failure: weight gain, peripheral edema, dyspnea, rales, and jugular vein distention.
- Teach client and family members how to take pulse and blood pressure readings.

#### Client and Family Teaching

- Take the medication with meals to reduce gastrointestinal irritation.
- Take pulse and blood pressure before taking medications each day at the same time, and follow instructions regarding when to withhold medication and when to contact the provider. Keep a record of pulse and blood pressure readings.
- Report any side effects, such as dizziness, vertigo, unusual flushing, facial, warmth, or headaches, to the primary care provider.
- Report immediately any swelling of the hands or feet, pronounced dizziness, or chest pain accompanied by sweating, shortness of breath, or severe headaches.

#### NONSTEROIDAL ANTI-INFLAMMATORY DRUG (NSAID): SALICYLATE

Acetylsalicylic acid (Ecotrin, Bufferin)

Acetylsalicylic acid, or aspirin, is a nonnarcotic analgesic, antipyretic, anti-inflammatory agent used to relieve headache pain.

#### Nursing Responsibilities

- Determine the type and pattern of pain. If aspirin was used in the past for pain control, note its effectiveness.
- Note any history of peptic ulcers or other conditions that may suggest potential problems with the use of salicylates.
- Assess clients receiving anticoagulant therapy for bruises, bleeding of the mucous membranes, or blood in the urine or stool.

#### Client and Family Teaching

- Take aspirin after meals or before meals with an antacid and a full glass of water to minimize gastric irritation.
- Report ringing in the ears, unusual bleeding of gums, bruising, or black tarry stools to the primary health care provider.
- Monitor blood glucose levels carefully (if you have diabetes), and report hypoglycemia if it occurs.

#### ERGOTAMINE

Caffeine-ergotamine tartrate combination (Cafergot)
Ergotamine tartrate (Gynergen)

Ergot alkaloids vasoconstrict the cerebral blood vessels, decreasing the amplitude of the pulsations of the cranial arteries. The major use of ergot alkaloids is the treatment of migraine headaches. Cafergot has the same actions as Gynergen, in addition, the caffeine it contains provides a vasoconstrictive action, enhancing the effects of ergotamine.

#### Nursing Responsibilities

- Because the drug accumulates in the body and is eliminated slowly, ergotamine poisoning may occur. Sepsis, renal and vascular disease, heavy smoking, malnutrition, pregnancy, contraceptive hormones, and fever can increase the risk of ergotamine poisoning.
- These drugs are contraindicated in clients with diabetes mellitus, sepsis, hepatic or renal disease, peripheral and coronary artery disease, hypertension, and pregnancy.

#### Client and Family Teaching

- Take the drug immediately at onset of headache.
- Report the following to your health care provider: pain in the leg muscles, weakness, and coldness or numbness of fingers or toes.
- A dose of Cafergot taken late in the day may prevent sleep because of the effects of caffeine.

## Complementary Therapies

The following complementary therapies are used to relieve the pain of headaches.

- Intake of vitamin D, elemental calcium, riboflavin (vitamin B), and magnesium
- Acupuncture
- Relaxation, guided imagery, massage
- Regular exercise
- Magnetic field therapy
- Herbal therapy
- Osteopathic manipulation

### NURSING CARE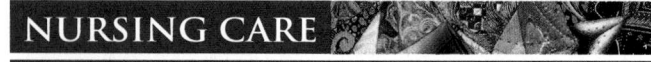

#### Health Promotion

Teach clients with tension headaches relaxation techniques, such as massage and biofeedback. Counseling for chronic anxiety may also be helpful. Triggers for migraine or cluster headache should be identified and, if possible, eliminated. For example, avoiding physical and emotional stress, having regular and consistent sleep patterns, eating meals regularly, and avoiding specific foods or alcohol can be incorporated into daily life and are helpful.

## Assessment

Collect the following data through the health history and physical examination.

- Health history: history of intracerebral trauma, tumor, or infection; detailed history and description of headache characteristics; family history; triggering factors; effects of recurring headaches on lifestyle, ADLs, and role performance
- Physical assessment: skin (diaphoresis, pallor, flushing), eyes (sensitivity to light, tearing), muscle strength and movement

## Nursing Diagnoses and Interventions

The primary response of the client requiring nursing interventions is acute pain. Develop nursing interventions to help the client identify strategies for controlling the pain and discomfort of the headache.

### Acute Pain

Headaches originate from both intracranial and extracranial sources and range in severity from benign, transient discomfort to severe, incapacitating pain. Interventions focus on teaching the client self-care measures to control or relieve the pain, and reducing any associated problems, such as nausea and vomiting or anxiety.

- Teach to maintain a diary of headaches, including duration, onset, location, relation to menstruation or food intake, and related manifestations such as factors that relieve or intensify the pain. *A thorough assessment of the headache is essential for both the client and the health care provider to identify the circumstances and patterns of headache occurrence.*
- Ask the client to rate the pain or discomfort on a scale of 0 to 10 (with 10 being the worst pain). *Using a scale to rate the pain provides an objective measure of the client's subjective experience of the pain or discomfort. The scale can also be used to evaluate the effectiveness of pain relief measures.*
- Teach to minimize light, noise, and activity and rest in a quiet, nonstimulating environment when experiencing a headache. *Manipulating the environment helps reduce noxious stimuli that may increase pain.*
- Teach to use noninvasive and nonpharmacologic pain relief measures such as deep breathing or relaxation to facilitate self-management of pain (see Chapter 4). ⊙ *Alternative strategies to control pain can help reduce tension and may help to increase the client's sense of control over the pain.*
- If appropriate, teach to apply cold compresses or dry heat to the head and neck. *The application of cold can cause vasoconstriction, which helps reduce pain in vascular headaches. Application of heat can reduce muscle tension and improve circulation.*

- Teach to follow good nutrition guidelines, get regular exercise and sleep, and minimize stress. *Headaches are more likely to occur when ill, tired, or under stress.*

## Home Care

In addition to implementing comfort measures, client education has a high priority. Develop a teaching plan to help the client learn how to limit attacks (e.g., by avoiding precipitating factors) and reduce the effects of the headache. Provide specific information about prescribed medications. Referrals for methods of stress reduction may be necessary for clients with long-term or migraine headaches.

## THE CLIENT WITH A SEIZURE DISORDER

**Seizures** are "paroxysmal motor, sensory, or cognitive manifestations of spontaneous, abnormally synchronous discharges of collections of neurons in the cerebral cortex" (Porth, 2002, p. 1189). This abnormal neuronal activity, which may involve all or part of the brain, disturbs skeletal motor function, sensation, autonomic function of the viscera, behavior, or consciousness. The term **epilepsy** is used to denote any disorder characterized by recurrent seizures. Epilepsy is categorized as a paroxysmal disorder because its manifestations are discontinuous; that is, minutes, days, weeks, or even years may elapse between seizures.

## INCIDENCE AND PREVALENCE

Epilepsy and seizures affect approximately 2.3 million Americans, costing an estimated $12.5 billion in medical expenses and lost or reduced earnings. About 10% of Americans will experience a seizure. People of all ages are affected, but particularly children and the elderly. The incidence of epilepsy is increasing. Researchers have suggested that the increase may be due to technologic advances in obstetric and pediatric care that allow extremely high-risk neonates to survive and to other technologic advances that have improved survival rates after craniocerebral trauma.

Isolated seizure episodes may occur in otherwise healthy people for a variety of reasons, including an acute febrile state, infection, metabolic or endocrine disorder (such as hypoglycemia), or exposure to toxins. Epilepsy may be idiopathic (that is, it may have no identifiable cause), or it may be secondary to birth injury, infection, vascular abnormalities, trauma, or tumors. Older adults may experience seizures as a result of vascular diseases (the most common cause in adults over 60) and degenerative disorders such as Alzheimer's disease.

## PATHOPHYSIOLOGY AND MANIFESTATIONS

Normally, when the mind is actively working, electrical activity in the brain is unsynchronized; when the mind is at rest, electrical activity is mildly synchronized. It is believed that most seizures arise from a few unstable, hypersensitive, and hyperreactive neurons in the brain. During a seizure, these neurons produce a rhythmic and repetitive hypersynchronous

# Nursing Care Plan
## A Client with a Migraine Headache

Betty Friedman is a 25-year-old grade-school teacher. Her friends and the other teachers regard Ms. Friedman as an enthusiastic person who sets high standards for herself and strives for perfection. During the spring semester, Ms. Friedman begins to miss work and sometimes appears very nervous. One day, another teacher notices Ms. Friedman running down the hall and into the restroom; the teacher finds Ms. Friedman vomiting. As she washes up, Ms. Friedman tells the other teacher that she has been having headaches since she began menstruating, but that they have never been as intense and frequent as during this past year. They even wake her from her sleep. Ms. Friedman agrees to see the nurse practitioner, Jane Schickadanz, at the school clinic for evaluation.

### ASSESSMENT
During her health history, Ms. Friedman relates that each month before her menstrual cycle she becomes nervous and sees flashing lights. She also has difficulty expressing herself and thinking clearly. The next day she develops a "sick headache." She states that the headache can last 1 to 2 days and that afterwards she cannot brush her hair because her scalp hurts. Ms. Friedman attributes these symptoms to PMS and adds that she thinks she is allergic to cheese and nuts because she gets very sick after eating them. After assessment, and in consultation with the physician, Ms. Schickadanz diagnoses Ms. Friedman's problem as a migraine with aura headache. Sumatriptan succinate (Imitrex) injections are prescribed.

### DIAGNOSES
- *Acute pain* related to vasodilation of cerebral vessels and a decreased serotonin level
- *Deficient knowledge* pain management
- *Altered role performance* related to pain

### EXPECTED OUTCOMES
- Experience reduced frequency and duration of pain.
- Identify the available resources for helping with self-management of pain.

### PLANNING AND IMPLEMENTATION
- Ask to keep a diary of her headaches for the next month, noting times of their occurrence, location and duration of pain, and factors that trigger the onset, such as her menstrual period or certain foods.
- Teach techniques for administering the subcutaneous injection and for disposing of the syringe and guidelines for administration. Teach to take the medication at the first awareness of an impending attack.
- Suggest an appointment with a counselor to learn methods of relaxation and stress relief.
- Request dietary referral for elimination of foods that might precipitate headaches.

### EVALUATION
Four weeks after beginning medication therapy with Imitrex and relaxation techniques, Ms. Friedman has noted a decrease in the intensity of the headaches. She reports that the medication has stopped the headaches, which, she has noted, tend to occur more frequently immediately before her menstrual period. She is walking for 30 minutes each day and has made changes in her usual diet. Ms. Friedman states, "I feel good about going to work with my kids at school and knowing I can control my pain."

### Critical Thinking in the Nursing Process
1. List the questions you would include in a health history that would identify stressors consistent with migraine headaches.
2. Develop a teaching plan for Ms. Friedman that includes methods of reducing fluid retention before her menstrual period, as well as a suggested diet based on the food guide pyramid.
3. Design a plan of care for Ms. Friedman for the nursing diagnosis, *Disturbed sleep pattern.*

See Evaluating Your Response in Appendix C.

---

discharge. Although the exact initiating factor for seizure activity has not been identified, several theories have been proposed (Porth, 2002):

- Alterations in the permeability of, or ion distribution across, cell membranes
- Alterations in the excitability of neurons resulting from glial scarring or decreased inhibition of activity in the cerebral cortex or thalamic region
- Imbalances of excitatory and inhibitory neurotransmitters such as acetylcholine (ACh) or gamma aminobutyric acid (GABA)

All people have a seizure threshold; when this threshold is exceeded, a seizure may result. In some people, the seizure threshold may be abnormally low, increasing their risk for seizure activity; in other people pathologic processes may alter the seizure threshold (Porth, 2002). The neurons that initiate seizure activity are called the *epileptogenic focus*. Abnormal neuronal activity may remain localized, causing a partial or focal seizure, or it may spread to involve the entire brain, causing generalized seizure activity. Seizures may also be provoked or unprovoked. *Unprovoked (primary or idiopathic) seizures* have no identifiable cause, with multiple episodes diagnosed as a seizure disorder or epilepsy. *Provoked (secondary) seizure* etiologies include febrile seizures in children, toxemia of pregnancy, rapid withdrawal from alcohol or barbiturates, systemic metabolic conditions (such as hypoglycemia, hypoxia, uremia, and electrolyte imbalances), and pathologies of the brain (such as meningitis, cerebral bleeding, or cerebral edema).

Metabolic needs of the brain increase dramatically during seizure activity. The demand for adenosine triphosphate (ATP), the energy source of the brain, increases by approximately 250%. Consequently, the demand for glucose and oxygen (which are needed to produce ATP) increases, and oxygen consumption increases by about 60%. To supply this increased oxygen need and remove carbon dioxide and other metabolic by-products, cerebral blood flow increases to about 2.5 times that of the normal rate. As long as oxygenation, blood glucose levels, and cardiac function remain normal, cerebral blood flow can respond to this increased metabolic demand of the brain. If cerebral blood flow cannot meet these needs, however, cellular exhaustion and cellular destruction may result.

Although seizures may be categorized in several different ways, the classification developed by the International League Against Epilepsy is the most useful clinically (Tierney et al., 2001). Seizures are divided into those that affect only part of the brain (partial seizures) and those that are generalized.

## Partial Seizures

**Partial seizures** involve the activation of only a restricted part of one cerebral hemisphere. A partial seizure accompanied by no alteration in consciousness is called a *simple partial seizure;* one in which consciousness is impaired is called a *complex partial seizure.*

The manifestations of simple partial seizures depend on the involved area of the brain. Manifestations may include alterations in motor function, sensory signs, or autonomic or psychic symptoms. Typically, the motor portion of the cortex is affected, causing recurrent muscle contractions of a contralateral part of the body, such as a finger or hand, or the face. This motor activity may stay confined to one area or spread sequentially to adjacent parts, a phenomenon known as a *Jacksonian march* or *Jacksonian seizure.* Manifestations of a simple partial seizure involving the sensory portion of the brain may include abnormal sensations or hallucinations. Disruptions in the function of the autonomic nervous system, with resulting tachycardia, flushing, hypotension, and hypertension, or psychic manifestations, such as a sense of déjà vu or inappropriate fear or anger, may also be experienced during a simple partial seizure.

During a complex partial seizure, consciousness is impaired and the client may engage in repetitive, nonpurposeful activity, such as lip smacking, aimless walking, or picking at clothing. These behaviors are known as *automatisms.* During the seizure, the client loses conscious contact with the environment; amnesia is common after the seizure, and several hours may elapse before the client regains full consciousness. Complex partial seizures usually originate in the temporal lobe and may be preceded by an aura, such as an unusual smell, a sense of déjà vu, or a sudden intense emotion.

## Generalized Seizures

**Generalized seizures** involve both hemispheres of the brain as well as deeper brain structures, such as the thalamus, basal ganglia, and upper brainstem. Consciousness is always impaired with generalized seizures. Absence and tonic-clonic seizures are the common forms of generalized seizure activity; they occur more frequently (especially in children) than partial seizures.

### Absence Seizures

**Absence (petit mal) seizures** are characterized by a sudden brief cessation of all motor activity accompanied by a blank stare and unresponsiveness. Absence seizures are more common in children than in adults. The seizure typically lasts only 5 to 10 seconds, although some may last for 30 seconds or more. Movements such as eyelid fluttering or automatisms such as lip smacking may occur during an absence seizure. Seizure activity may vary from occasional episodes to several hundred per day.

### Tonic-Clonic Seizures

**Tonic-clonic seizures** are the most common type of seizure activity in adults. This type of seizure activity follows a typical pattern. An aura may precede generalized seizure activity. The aura may be a vague sense of uneasiness or an abnormal sensation (such as a smell of burning rubber or seeing bright light). Often, however, the seizure occurs without warning.

The seizure begins with a sudden loss of consciousness and sharp tonic muscle contractions (the *tonic phase* of the seizure). With the muscle contraction, air is forced out of the lungs, and the client may cry out. Postural control is lost, and the client falls to the floor in the opisthotonic posture (Figure 42–4A■). Muscles are rigid, with the arms and legs extended and the jaw clenched. Urinary incontinence is common; bowel incontinence may also occur. Breathing ceases and cyanosis develops during the tonic phase of a seizure. The pupils are fixed and dilated. The tonic phase lasts an average of 15 seconds, although it may persist for up to a minute.

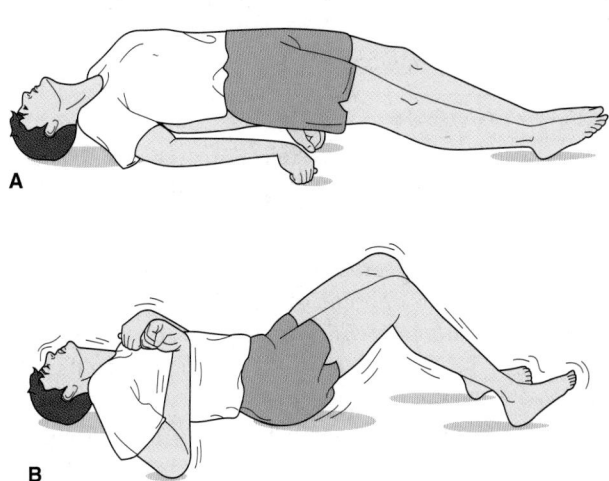

**Figure 42–4** ■ Tonic-clonic seizures in grand mal seizures. *A,* Tonic phase. *B,* Clonic phase.

The *clonic phase,* which follows the tonic phase, is characterized by alternating contraction and relaxation of the muscles in all the extremities along with hyperventilation (Figure 42–4B). The eyes roll back, and the client froths at the mouth. The clonic phase varies in duration and subsides gradually. The entire tonic-clonic portion of the seizure generally lasts no more than 60 to 90 seconds.

Following the clonic phase of seizure activity, the client remains unconscious and unresponsive to stimuli. This period is known as the *postictal period* or *phase.* The client is relaxed and breathes quietly. The client regains consciousness gradually and may be confused and disoriented on waking. Headache, muscle aches, and fatigue often follow the seizure, and the client many sleep for several hours. Amnesia of the seizure is usual; the client also may not recall events just prior to the seizure activity.

Because of the lack of warning with tonic-clonic seizures, the client may experience injury. Head injury, fractures, burns, or motor vehicle crashes may occur secondarily to seizure activity.

## Status Epilepticus

**Status epilepticus** can develop during seizure activity. In this case, the seizure activity becomes continuous, with only very short periods of calm between intense and persistent seizures. The repetitive seizures may be of any type, although they are usually generalized tonic-clonic (Porth, 2002). Repeated seizures have a cumulative effect, producing muscular contractions that can interfere with respirations. The client is in great danger of developing hypoxia, acidosis, hypoglycemia, hyperthermia, and exhaustion if the convulsive activity is not halted. Status epilepticus is considered a life-threatening medical emergency that requires immediate treatment

## COLLABORATIVE CARE

Initial treatment focuses on controlling the seizure; the long-term goal is to determine the cause and prevent future seizures. Collaborative care includes diagnostic testing, medications, and, in some cases, surgery.

## Diagnostic Tests

Diagnostic testing is performed to confirm the seizure diagnosis and to determine any treatable causes and precipitating factors. The tests include:

- *Complete neurologic exam* to determine the focal neurologic deficit or the focus or origin of seizure activity.
- *Electroencephalogram (EEG)* to help confirm the seizure diagnosis and localize any lesion(s). See the box on this page for the nursing implications of EEG.
- *Skull X-rays* to identify possible fractures, deformities in bony structures, or calcification.
- *MRI* or *CT scan* to determine the presence of a tumor, congenital lesions, edema, infarct, hemorrhage, arteriovenous malformation, or a structural deviation, such as ventricular enlargement.

### Nursing Implications for Diagnostic Tests

#### Electroencephalogram (EEG)

An EEG is used to detect abnormal brain function. It provides a graphic record of the brain's electrical activity (brain waves) and is useful in evaluating seizure activity.

##### Client Preparation

- Explain the procedure, emphasizing the importance of cooperation.
- Withhold fluids, foods, and medications (as prescribed) that may stimulate or depress brain waves. These include anticonvulsants, tranquilizers, depressants, and caffeine-containing foods (e.g., coffee, tea, colas, and chocolate). Medications are usually withheld for 24 to 48 hours before the test.
- Help the client wash the hair before the test.

##### Client and Family Teaching

- The test takes about 1 hour.
- The test is painless and will be performed while sitting in a comfortable chair or lying on a stretcher.
- The electrodes are applied to the scalp with a thick paste.
- During the test, you will first be asked to breathe in and out deeply for a few minutes. Then, you will close your eyes while a light is flashed on them and, finally, you will lie quietly with your eyes closed.
- After the test, the nurse will help you wash the paste out of your hair.

- *Lumbar puncture* to determine the presence of infection (meningitis) or elevated protein levels in the CSF.
- *Blood studies* to assess blood count, electrolytes, blood urea, and blood glucose.
- *Electrocardiogram (ECG)* to rule out underlying cardiac dysrhythmias.

## Medications

Anticonvulsant medications can reduce or control most seizure activity. These medications do not cure the disorder; they only manage its manifestations. Anticonvulsant medications generally act in one of two ways: by raising the seizure threshold or by limiting the spread of abnormal activity within the brain.

The goals of medications for epilepsy are to protect the client from harm and to reduce or prevent seizure activity without impairing cognitive function or producing undesirable side effects. Ideally, the lowest possible dose of a single medication that will control the client's seizures is prescribed; often, however, several medications must be tried before the most effective is identified, and a combination of drugs may be needed to manage the client's seizures. Therapy is individualized, based on the type of seizure activity and the client's response to the medication. Nursing implications for these drugs are described in the Medication Administration box on the page 1369; drug interactions are listed in Box 42–2. The success rate is higher in clients with partial and secondary tonic-clonic seizures when carbamazepine (Tegretol), phenytoin (Dilantin), or valproic acid (Depakote) is used. Another

# Medication Administration

## Seizures

### ANTICONVULSANTS

Examples of anticonvulsants are:

| | |
|---|---|
| Phenytoin (Dilantin) | Ethosuximide (Zarontin) |
| Phenobarbital | Clonazepam (Klonopin) |
| Primidone (Mysoline) | Gabapentin (Neurontin) |
| Carbamazepine (Tegretol) | Lamotrigine (Lamictal) |
| Valproic acid (Depakene) | Tiagabine HCL (Gabitril) |

Anticonvulsant agents are used to control chronic seizures and involuntary muscle spasms or movements characteristic of certain neurologic diseases. These drugs act in the motor cortex of the brain to reduce the spread of electrical discharges from the rapidly firing epileptic foci in this area. These agents control seizures without impairing the normal functions of the CNS. Drugs effective against one type of seizure may not be effective against another; anticonvulsant therapy must be individualized.

### Nursing Responsibilities

- Monitor blood pressure, pulse, and respirations.
- Note evidence of CNS side effects, such as blurred vision, dimmed vision, slurred speech, nystagmus, or confusion. Gingival hyperplasia may be noted in clients taking phenytoin.
- Recognize that if clients are to be on prolonged therapy, they may need a diet rich in vitamin D.
- Monitor the serum calcium level as ordered; phenytoin can contribute to demineralization of bone.
- When administering anticonvulsants intravenously, monitor closely for respiratory depression and cardiovascular collapse.

- Administer gabapentin 2 hours after antacids.
- Administer tiagabine HCL with food.

### Client and Family Teaching

- Take the exact dosage prescribed. Do not increase, decrease, or discontinue the dosage without obtaining the primary care provider's approval; doing so may lead to convulsions.
- Avoid hazardous tasks until the drug has been regulated. Anticonvulsant drugs may at first decrease mental alertness and cause drowsiness, headache, dizziness, and incoordination of muscles. These effects are usually dose related and may disappear with a change of dosage or continued therapy.
- If you are taking phenytoin (Dilantin), maintain good oral hygiene: Use a soft toothbrush, massage the gums, and floss daily.
- It is very important to obtain liver function studies regularly as ordered by the primary care provider. This will help detect early signs of hepatitis and other liver problems. Report for all scheduled laboratory studies, including complete blood count, kidney and liver function studies, and drug levels.
- Carry identification indicating the type of seizures for which you are being treated.
- Do not take gabapentin 1 hour before or less than 2 hours after an antacid.
- If you are taking lamotrigine and develop a rash, tell your health care provider.
- Take Tiagabine HCL (Gabitril) with food.

---

medication approved for partial seizures is tiagabine (Gabitril), a GABA inhibitor. If the client has been seizure free for at least 3 years, withdrawal of medications may be considered, with the dose of one drug at a time reduced over weeks or months. There is no way of predicting which clients can remain seizure free without medication, but if seizures reoccur, the same medications usually provide good control.

Status epilepticus requires immediate intervention to preserve life. Establishing and maintaining the airway is a priority. A solution of 50% dextrose is administered intravenously to prevent hypoglycemia. Diazepam (Valium) or lorazepam (Ativan) is given intravenously, and the dose repeated in 10 minutes if necessary to stop seizure activity. Phenytoin (Dilantin) is also administered intravenously for longer-term control of seizures. Phenobarbital may also be administered to clients in status epilepticus.

## Treatments

### Surgery

When all attempts to control the client's seizures fail, excision of the tissue involved in the seizure activity may be an effective and safe treatment alternative. An estimated 5% of clients with epilepsy may be candidates for surgery. The goal of surgery is to reduce the client's uncontrollable seizures.

To be selected as a candidate for surgery, the client must be highly motivated and psychologically prepared. A psychologic screening is required because the preoperative

### BOX 42–2 ■ Drug Interactions with Anticonvulsants

- *Valproic acid (Depakene) and phenobarbital.* Blood levels of phenobarbital may rise significantly when valproic acid is added to the client's medication regimen.
- *Phenobarbital and digoxin.* This combination may increase the metabolism of digoxin, resulting in decreased digoxin levels.
- *Phenobarbital and sodium warfarin (Coumadin).* Phenobarbital may decrease the absorption of sodium warfarin from the gastrointestinal tract and decrease the drug's anticoagulant response.
- *Disulfiram (Antabuse) and phenobarbital.* This combination may inhibit the metabolism of the anticonvulsant drug and increase the incidence of side effects associated with the anticonvulsant drug.
- *Carbamazepine and oral contraceptives.* Carbamazepine decreases the effectiveness of oral contraceptives.
- *Other drugs.* Other drugs reported to interact with anticonvulsant drugs include aspirin, certain antibiotics, isoniazid, acetazolamide (Diamox), antacids, folic acid, and narcotics.

preparation is extensive and time-consuming and because the surgery is long and requires that the client remain awake during surgery so that he or she can cooperate and respond to commands. The EEG is monitored during surgery to identify the epileptogenic focus and evaluate the effect of surgical intervention.

# NURSING CARE OF THE CLIENT WITH SEIZURES WHO IS HAVING SURGERY

## PREOPERATIVE CARE

- For most clients, anticonvulsant medications are withheld the morning or evening of the day before surgery. *Anticonvulsant medications may interfere with intraoperative EEG monitoring.*
- For clients with frequent and/or severe seizures, however, a partial dose of medication may be administered. *This prevents seizures or status epilepticus during surgery.*
- A low dose of analgesics is administered before surgery. *The client must remain awake throughout the lengthy procedure to respond to commands during EEG recording.*

## POSTOPERATIVE CARE

- Anticonvulsant medications are administered parenterally until the client can tolerate oral fluids; medications are then continued orally. *It is common for the client to have seizures in the early postoperative period.*
- Steroids are administered for the first 3 days after surgery and are tapered and then discontinued during the following week. *Steroids are given to decrease cerebral edema.*

General postoperative care for the client with intracranial surgery follows the nursing management guidelines outlined later in the chapter. Specific preoperative and postoperative care for a client with a seizure disorder is described in the box above.

Resective surgery, with removal of the epileptogenic focus, is an option that is still in its early stages. Candidates for this type of surgery include those who are unresponsive to medical management, who have a unilateral focus, and who have impaired quality of life from seizures. Resections of the temporal lobe are most commonly performed and are most effective for partial complex seizures.

## Vagal Nerve Stimulation

Vagal nerve stimulation is approved as a treatment for clients with partial-onset seizures who do not respond to drugs and are not candidates for surgery. The mechanism of action is unknown.

# NURSING CARE

## Health Promotion

Health promotion activities for the client with seizures focus on teaching to reduce the incidence of seizure activity and to promote safety. Stress the following:

- Know the importance of follow-up care, of keeping medical appointments, and of continuing to take anticonvulsant medications as prescribed even when no seizures are experienced.
- Review any state and local laws that apply to people with seizure disorders. Driving a motor vehicle is usually prohibited for 6 months to 2 years after a seizure episode. Usually, a driver's license can be reinstated or obtained after a seizure-free period and a letter from the nurse practitioner or physician.
- Teach client and family members measures to prevent injury at home:
  - Avoid smoking when alone or in bed.
  - Avoid alcohol.
  - Avoid becoming excessively tired.
  - Install grab bars in the shower and tub area.
  - Do not lock doors of the bedroom or bathroom.
  - Avoid an excessive intake of caffeine.

## Assessment

Collect the following data through the health history and physical examination.

- Health history: past seizures: age when the client's first seizure occurred, most recent seizure, factors precipitating a seizure, any warning signs (aura), prophylactic anticonvulsant therapy, and specific concerns the client may have about the seizures
- Physical assessment: important data used in determining an accurate diagnosis that describe manifestations obtained from nursing assessments before, during, and after a seizure (Table 42–5 lists nursing assessments with rationale.)

## Nursing Diagnoses and Interventions

Nursing care of clients with a seizure disorder focuses on providing care during and immediately after the seizure and on client teaching. The client with seizures has a wide variety of responses to actual or potential changes in health status; interventions discussed in this section focus on facilitating physical and psychologic comfort and safety.

### Risk for Ineffective Airway Clearance

During a seizure, the tongue may fall back and obstruct the airway, the gag reflex may be depressed, and secretions may pool at the back of the throat. These may put the client at risk for an obstructed airway. Most seizures occur in the home or community; also teach these interventions to the client's family.

- Provide interventions to maintain a patent airway:
  - Loosen clothing around the neck.
  - Turn on the side.
  - Do not force anything into the mouth.
  - If prescribed and available, administer oxygen by mask.
  *Although it was at one time believed that it was necessary to place a padded tongue blade in the client's mouth during a seizure, this is no longer recommended; an improperly placed tongue blade can obstruct the airway. Turning the client on the side allows secretions to drain from the mouth.*

| TABLE 42–5 | Nursing Assessments Before, During, and After a Seizure |
|---|---|
| **Assessment** | **Rationale** |
| What was the client's level of consciousness? If consciousness was lost, at what point? | Indicates area of brain involved and type of seizure. |
| What was the client doing just before the attack? | May suggest precipitating factors. |
| In what part of the body did the seizure start? | May indicate the site of seizure activity in the brain tissue; for example, if jerking movements were first observed in right hand, the seizure focus may be in left motor cortex in the area of the hand. |
| Was there an epileptic cry? | Usually indicates the tonic stage of a generalized tonic-clonic seizure. |
| Were any automatisms such as eyelid fluttering, chewing, lip smacking, or swallowing observed? | Often seen in complex, partial, and absence seizures. |
| How long did movements last? Did the location or character change (tonic to clonic)? Did movements involve both sides of the body or just one? | Indicates areas in which focal activity originated. |
| Did the head and/or eyes turn to one side and, if so, which side? | Helps localize the focus of the seizure. During the seizure, the head and eyes typically will turn away from the side of the epileptogenic focus. |
| Were there changes in pupillary reactions? | Indicates involvement of the autonomic nervous system. |
| If the client fell, was the head hit? | Skull X-ray studies may be needed to rule out subdural hematoma or fracture. |
| Was there foaming or frothing from the mouth? | Usually indicates a tonic-clonic seizure. |

- Teach family members or significant others how to care for the client during a seizure to prevent airway obstruction. *Family members are often the only people present to provide this emergency intervention.*

## Anxiety

The client with a seizure disorder is understandably anxious about the future, with questions about ability to go to school, work, have a family, and drive a car. Feelings of embarrassment about having a seizure in public and rejection by others are common and also increase the client's anxiety.

- Provide support by explaining that concerns are normal. *It is important to be sensitive to the effect of seizures on the client's self-concept and body image; alterations in these areas not only increase anxiety but also cause withdrawal from socialization with others. Demonstrating acceptance of the client's concerns allows further discussion.*
- Help identify safe leisure activities. *Worrying about being hurt if a seizure occurs may cause withdrawal from social activities that are pleasurable.*
- Provide information about sources and support groups. *Sharing information with other people with similar health problems allows for a more realistic viewpoint; accurate information can clear up misconceptions that cause anxiety.*
- Provide accurate information about hiring practices and legal limitations on driving or operating heavy or dangerous machinery. *Accurate information decreases anxiety about the unknown. The American Disabilities Act prohibits discrimination; however, there are legal limitations on driving until the person is proved free of seizures.*

## Using NANDA, NIC, and NOC

Chart 42–1 shows links between NANDA nursing diagnosis, NIC, and NOC when caring for the client with a seizure disorder.

## Home Care

Teaching follows a systematic assessment of the needs of both the client and family. Include family members so that they can learn seizure management, including the care and observations

---

## CHART 42–1  NANDA, NIC, AND NOC LINKAGES

### The Client with a Seizure Disorder

| NURSING DIAGNOSES | NURSING INTERVENTIONS | NURSING OUTCOMES |
|---|---|---|
| • Risk for Aspiration<br>• Risk for Falls<br>• Anxiety | • Aspiration Precautions<br>• Fall Prevention<br>• Anxiety Reduction | • Neurological Status<br>• Safety Behavior: Fall Prevention<br>• Anxiety Control<br>• Acceptance: Health Status |

*Note. Data from Nursing Outcomes Classification (NOC) by M. Johnson & M. Maas (Eds.), 1997, St. Louis: Mosby; Nursing Diagnoses: Definitions & Classification 2001–2002 by North American Nursing Diagnosis Association, 2001, Philadelphia: NANDA; Nursing Interventions Classification (NIC) by J.C. McCloskey & G. M. Bulechek (Eds.), 2000, St. Louis: Mosby. Reprinted by permission.*

necessary before and during a seizure. Stress the importance of safety and keeping the airway patent.

Help both the client and family adjust to a diagnosis of epilepsy. Address the following topics.

- Misconceptions, common fears, and myths about epilepsy
- The importance of wearing a MedicAlert band or carrying a medical alert card at all times
- Avoiding alcoholic beverages and limiting coffee intake

- Taking showers versus tub baths, because of safety issues during a generalized seizure
- Factors that may trigger a seizure, such as abrupt withdrawal from medication, constipation, fatigue, excessive stress, fever, menstruation, sights and sounds such as television, flashing video, and computer screens
- Helpful resources:
  - American Epilepsy Society
  - Epilepsy Foundation

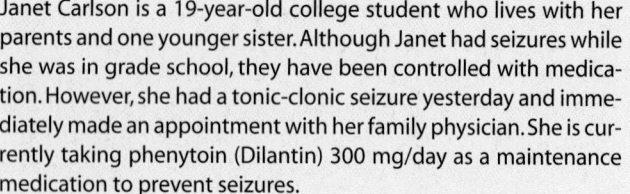

## Nursing Care Plan
## A Client with a Seizure Disorder

Janet Carlson is a 19-year-old college student who lives with her parents and one younger sister. Although Janet had seizures while she was in grade school, they have been controlled with medication. However, she had a tonic-clonic seizure yesterday and immediately made an appointment with her family physician. She is currently taking phenytoin (Dilantin) 300 mg/day as a maintenance medication to prevent seizures.

### ASSESSMENT

Evita Farias, RN, completes a health history for Ms. Carlson. During the history, she tells Ms. Farias that she has been under stress because of difficulties in completing her course requirements this semester. She has not been sleeping as many hours per night, and sometimes she forgets to take her medication. Janet's serum phenytoin level is 8 mg/mL. Therapeutic level is 10 to 20 mg/ml.

### DIAGNOSES

- *Risk for injury* related to recurrence of generalized tonic-clonic seizure activity and low serum phenytoin levels
- *Deficient knowledge* related to activities that may trigger seizure occurrence, the effect of stress on seizures, and medication information

### EXPECTED OUTCOMES

- Will verbalize precipitating and triggering factors related to the onset of seizures.
- Will verbalize the relationship between emotional and physical stress and seizures.
- Will verbalize the importance of taking anticonvulsant medications.

### PLANNING AND IMPLEMENTATION

- Teach client and her family the following:

- Current information about seizures
- Care during and after a seizure
- Medication protocols
- Factors and activities that can trigger seizures
- The importance of follow-up care
- Refer client and her family to a local epilepsy support group.
- Recommend that she purchase and wear a MedicAlert bracelet.

### EVALUATION

Ms. Carlson is instructed to continue taking Dilantin 300 mg/day. She states the importance of nutrition, rest, and measures to reduce stress. She also discusses the importance of maintaining the proper blood levels of her medication, stating that too little or too much of the medication could cause problems. Ms. Carlson recognizes that the seizure problems had recurred during a busy time in school during which she had forgotten to take her medication. She is now wearing a MedicAlert bracelet. Ms. Farias provides the Carlsons with the telephone number of the Epilepsy Foundation of America.

### Critical Thinking in the Nursing Process

1. If you were Ms. Carlson's nurse, would your teaching differ if she were living alone? If so, how?
2. Ms. Carlson tells you that although she knows she should not drive a car, she often drives her friend to work. How would you approach this problem?
3. Ms. Carlson states that "it's embarrassing to wear a MedicAlert bracelet." How would you respond, and what recommendation(s) would you make?

See Evaluating Your Response in Appendix C.

# TRAUMATIC BRAIN INJURY

**Traumatic brain injury (TBI)** is a leading cause of death and disability in the United States. The National Head Injury Foundation defines TBI as a traumatic insult to the brain capable of causing physical, intellectual, emotional, social, and vocational changes. A TBI may be classified as a *penetrating (open) head injury* (e.g., resulting from a knife, bullet, or baseball bat) or a *closed head injury* (a blunt injury to the brain that does not result in an open skull fracture).

## INCIDENCE AND PREVALENCE

The CDC estimates that each year 1 million people in the United States are treated and released from hospital emergency departments as a result of TBI: 230,000 people are hospitalized and survive: and 50,000 people die. Additionally, more than 80,000 are discharged with TBI-related injuries, and 5.3 million Americans are living today with a TBI-related disability.

## Risk Factors

Motor vehicle accidents (MVAs) are a major cause of TBI; elevated blood alcohol levels contribute significantly to the risk of MVA and subsequent injury. Other causes of head injury include falls, sports injuries, occupational injuries, assaults, and gunshot wounds. Adults age 15 to 30 are at the greatest risk, with the male to female ratio of 3:1 (McCance & Huether, 2002). Other risk factors include being over the age of 75 and living in a high-crime area.

## MECHANISMS OF CRANIOCEREBRAL TRAUMA

Specific damage following craniocerebral injuries is related to the mechanism of the injury (how it occurs), the nature of the injury (type), and the location of the injury (where it occurs).

Injuries to the head can occur through several mechanisms:

- *Acceleration injury* is sustained when the head is struck by a moving object, such as a swinging bat.
- *Deceleration injury* occurs when the head hits a stationary object, such as a concrete wall.
- *Acceleration-deceleration injury* (also called a *coup-contrecoup phenomenon*) occurs when the head hits an object and the brain "rebounds" within the skull (Figure 42–5 ■). The brain is injured at the point of impact (the coup) and on the opposite side of the impact (the countercoup). Two or more areas of the brain can be injured as a result of this phenomenon.
- *Deformation injuries* are those in which the force deforms and disrupts the integrity of the impacted body part (e.g., skull fracture).
- Head injuries can also be classified as *blunt* or *penetrating*.

Types of craniocerebral trauma include injuries to the skull (including fractures), injuries to the brain (including concussion and contusion), and intracranial hemorrhage (including hematomas). Brain injury can result either from the direct effects of the trauma on brain tissue or from secondary responses to trauma, such as cerebral edema, hematoma, swelling, or increased intracranial pressure.

## THE CLIENT WITH A SKULL FRACTURE

A **skull fracture** is a break in the continuity of the skull. It may occur with or without damage to the brain; however, intracranial trauma often results from skull fractures. The considerable force of impact significantly increases the risk of underlying hematoma formation. Disruption of the skull can also cause cranial nerve injury, allow bacteria to enter the cranial vault, or allow CSF to leak out.

## PATHOPHYSIOLOGY AND MANIFESTATIONS

Skull fractures are classified as open or closed. In an open fracture, the dura is torn, and in a closed fracture, the dura is not torn. Skull fractures are further classified into one of four categories: linear, comminuted, depressed, or basilar (Table 42–6).

*Linear fractures* are the most common, accounting for 80% of all skull fractures. They typically extend from the point of impact toward the base of the skull. Although the risk of infection or CSF leakage is minimal with this type of fracture because the dura usually remains intact, subdural or epidural hematomas (a collection of blood) frequently underlie the fracture. A hematoma (discussed later in this chapter) places pressure on underlying brain tissue, increasing both intracranial pressure and the risk of brain damage.

*Comminuted* and *depressed skull fractures* increase the risk of direct damage to brain tissue from bruising (*contusion*) and bone fragments. However, the risk of secondary brain injury may be reduced in these fractures, because in breaking the bone, the traumatic impact energy is distributed and dissipated. If the skin overlying the fracture is lacerated or the dura is torn, the risk of infection is greater.

*Basilar skull fractures* involve the base of the skull and usually are extensions of adjacent fractures, although they may occur independently. Although most basilar skull fractures are uncomplicated, they may involve the sinuses of the frontal bone or the petrous portion of the temporal bone (middle ear).

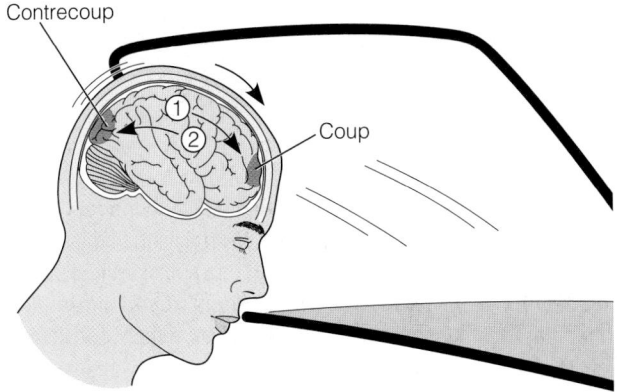

**Figure 42–5** ■ Coup-contrecoup head injury. Following the initial injury (coup), the brain rebounds within the skull and sustains additional injury (contrecoup) in the opposite part of the brain.

| TABLE 42–6 | Types of Skull Fractures |
|---|---|
| **Type** | **Description** |
| Linear (simple) | Simple, clean break in skull. Occurs with low-velocity injuries. |
| Comminuted | Bone is crushed into small, fragmented pieces. Usually seen with high-impact injuries. |
| Depressed | Inward depression of bone fragments. Usually due to a powerful blow to the skull. The dura may or may not be intact. Bone fragments may penetrate into the brain tissue. |
| Basilar | Occurs at the base of the skull. May be linear, comminuted, or depressed. |

If the dura is disrupted, CSF may leak through the tear. Manifestations of CSF leakage may include **rhinorrhea** (CSF leakage through the nose) or **otorrhea** (CSF leakage from the ear). Basilar skull fractures can be difficult to identify on X-ray film, but they have certain common manifestations. For example, blood may be visible behind the tympanic membrane (*hemotympanum*), or ecchymosis may be noted over the mastoid process (known as *Battle's sign*). Bilateral periorbital ecchymosis ("raccoon eyes") is another possible manifestation. If CSF leakage is present, the risk of infection is high. Other complications of basilar skull fractures include injury to the internal carotid artery and compression of cranial nerve II, VI, or VII.

## COLLABORATIVE CARE
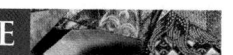

Treatment of a client with a skull fracture depends on the type and location of the fracture. Skull fracture may be only one of several head injuries.

A simple linear fracture generally requires bed rest and observation for underlying injury to brain tissue or hematoma formation. No specific treatment is required. Depressed skull fractures require surgical intervention, usually within 24 hours of the injury, to debride the wound completely and remove bone fragments, which may become embedded in brain tissue or cerebral blood vessels. If depressed deeply, the bone may be elevated. If cerebral edema is not present, a cranioplasty with insertion of acrylic bone may be performed. Basilar skull fractures do not require surgery unless CSF leakage persists. Regular neurologic assessments and observation for manifestations of meningitis are required for the hospitalized client. Antibiotics may be administered prophylactically.

## NURSING CARE

The client with a craniocerebral trauma may have a variety of responses and health care needs, depending on the location and extent of the trauma. Many of those problems with related nursing interventions are discussed in other sections of this chapter, including seizures, increased intracranial pressure, and bleeding within the brain.

## Nursing Diagnoses and Interventions

This section discusses the risk for infection, a problem common in the client with an open head wound from a skull fracture.

### Risk for Infection
The client with a skull fracture is at high risk for infection related to possible access to the cranial contents through a tear in the dura. In an open, depressed fracture, the wound may be contaminated by dirt, hair, or other debris.

- Monitor for otorrhea or rhinorrhea. *Open fractures of the skull increase the possibility of leakage of CSF from the ears or nose.*
- Test drainage of clear fluid from ear and nose for glucose by using a glucose reagent strip, such as Dextrostix. *Clear*

drainage that tests positive for glucose indicates leakage of CSF.
- Observe blood-tinged fluid for "halo" sign. *CSF dries in concentric rings on gauze or tissues.*
- Keep the nasopharynx and the external ear clean. Place a piece of sterile cotton in the ear, or tape a sterile cotton pad loosely under the nose; change dressings when they become wet. *Wet dressings facilitate movement of organisms.*
- Instruct client not to blow nose, cough, or inhibit sneeze; sneeze through open mouth. *Blowing the nose and coughing increase ICP. Withholding a sneeze forces bacteria backward.*
- Use aseptic technique at all times when changing head dressings or ICP monitor dressings and insertion sites. *Using aseptic technique reduces the possibility of introducing infection.*

## Home Care

The client and family need to be informed about the degree of injury that has occurred with the skull fracture. The client with a linear fracture, who may not be hospitalized, will need teaching that focuses on the need to monitor progress closely. To prevent complications, advise the client and family to go to the emergency room if the client experiences any of the following:

- Growing drowsiness or confusion
- Difficulty waking (instruct a family member to wake the client every 2 hours during the first night home)
- Vomiting
- Blurred vision
- Slurred speech
- Prolonged headache
- Blood or clear fluid leaking from the ears or nose
- Weakness in an arm or leg
- Stiff neck
- Seizure

## THE CLIENT WITH A FOCAL OR DIFFUSE BRAIN INJURY

Even when the skull and other structures overlying the brain remain intact, a blow to the head can cause significant brain injury. Closed head injuries may result in either diffuse or focal damage to the brain. They range in severity from mild to severe.

### PATHOPHYSIOLOGY
Brain injury results from both primary and secondary mechanisms. Primary injury results from the impact. A blow to the head, even with no break in the skull, can cause serious and diffuse brain injury. Injury to axons disrupts oligodendroglia and direct mechanical disruption is caused by debris and leakage. The immediate vascular response to the injury results in increased capillary permeability to solutes.

Secondary injury is the progression of the initial injury resulting from events that affect perfusion and oxygenation of brain cells. These events include intracranial edema, hematoma, infection, hypoxia, or ischemia. Cerebral ischemia is the most common cause of secondary brain injury (Porth, 2002). Ischemia leads to cerebral hypoxia, with consequences of increased glial permeability to sodium (cyctotoxic edema), an influx of calcium with changes in electrophysiology and release of free fatty acids and lactic acidosis.

Acute brain injury affects all body systems as well as the central nervous system. Systemic effects of acute brain injury are listed in Box 42–3.

## Focal Brain Injuries

**Focal brain injuries** are specific, grossly observable brain lesions confined to one area of the brain. The force of the impact produces contusions from direct contact with the inside of the skull that in turn may cause epidural hemorrhage and subdural and intracerebral hematomas. The mechanisms of injury are coup and/or contrecoup damage of the brain at the point of the impact and the rebound effect. The damaged brain area is surrounded by edema, contributing to increased ICP. Infarction and necrosis, multiple hemorrhages, and edema are found within the contused areas. The maximum effects of the injury peak in 18 to 36 hours (McCance & Huether, 2002).

Intracranial hemorrhage can result directly from the trauma (e.g., beneath a fracture) or from shearing forces on cerebral arteries and veins that occur with acceleration-deceleration. Depending on the site and rate of bleeding, manifestations may appear immediately or may not become evident for hours or even weeks. Intracranial hemorrhages and the hematomas they cause place pressure on surrounding structures, causing manifestations of an expanding focal lesion. They also cause increased ICP, leading to altered levels of consciousness and potential herniation syndromes. Intracranial hematomas are classified by their location as

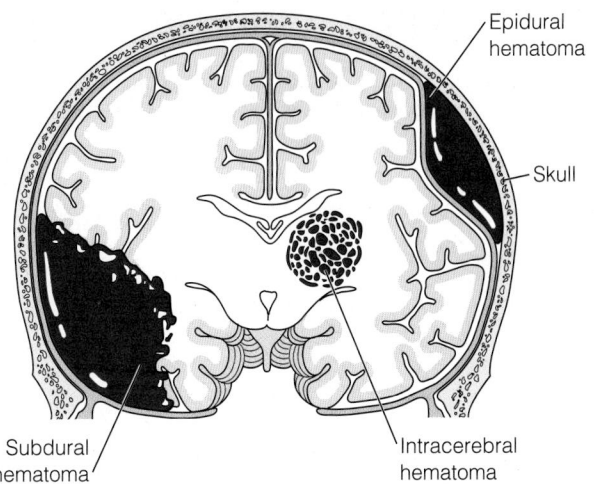

**Figure 42–6** ■ Three types of hematomas: epidural hematoma, subdural hematoma, and intracerebral hematoma.

epidural, subdural, or intracerebral. Table 42–7 compares the frequency, locations, common sites, precipitating factors, and clinical manifestations of intracranial hematomas; Figure 42–6 ■ illustrates their locations.

### Contusion

A **contusion** is a bruise of the surface of the brain, typically accompanied by small, diffuse venous hemorrhages. Both white and gray matter may have a bruised, discolored appearance. A decrease in pH, with accumulation of lactic acid and decreased oxygen consumption, may hinder cell function. Contusions (and other focal brain injuries) occur when the brain strikes the inner skull, often with a *coup* (point of impact) lesion and a *contrecoup* lesion on the opposite side of the brain. Contusions

---

| BOX 42–3 ■ Systemic Effects of Acute Brain Injury | |
|---|---|
| ***Cause*** | ***Effect*** |
| ■ Stimulation of the sympathetic nervous system, which stimulates the adrenal cortex and medulla to increase glucocorticoid and mineralocorticoid levels | ■ Increased metabolism of carbohydrates, fats, and proteins<br>■ Retention of sodium and water |
| ■ Stimulation of the sympathetic nervous system, increasing the serum catecholamine levels | ■ Hypertension<br>■ EEG changes<br>■ Dysrrhymias (bradycardia, sinus tachycardia) |
| ■ Altered release of ADH from the posterior pituitary | ■ Retention of water or diuresis and diabetes insipidus |
| ■ Neurogenic pulmonary dysfunction | ■ Abnormal respiratory patterns<br>■ Reduced residual capacity with retention of $CO_2$, vasodilation, and increased ICP<br>■ Pulmonary edema |
| ■ Stress response to trauma | ■ Hyperglycemia |
| ■ Increased platelet, plasma fibrinogen, and thromboplastin levels | ■ Decreased clotting and prothrombin times<br>■ Vascular occlusion<br>■ Disseminated intravascular coagulation<br>■ Anemia |
| ■ Immunosuppression | ■ Infection |
| ■ Decreased gastric motility and increased gastric acidity | ■ Gastritis<br>■ Gastric ulcers |

| TABLE 42–7 | Comparison of Intracranial Hematomas | | |
|---|---|---|---|
| | Location/Common Site | Precipitating Factors | Manifestations |
| **Epidural Hematoma** 2% to 6% of all types of head injuries | Located in the space between the skull and the dura mater Common site: the temporal bone (over the middle meningeal artery) | Skull fractures Contusion | Momentary loss of consciousness followed by a lucid period lasting from a few hours to 1 to 2 days Rapid deterioration in level of consciousness (drowsiness to confusion to coma) Seizures Headache Hemiparesis (may be ipsilateral or contralateral) Fixed dilated ipsilateral pupil Rise in blood pressure with decreases in pulse and respirations indicates a rapidly increasing hematoma |
| **Subdural Hematoma** Approximately 29% of all types of head injuries | Located in the space below the dural surface (between the dura and arachnoid and pia mater layers of meninges) Common site: may occur any place in cranium | Closed head injury Acceleration-deceleration injury Cerebral atrophy (seen in older adults) Chronic alcoholism Use of anticoagulants Contusion | Acute: • Headache • Drowsiness • Agitation • Slowed thinking • Confusion Subacute: • Same as those of acute subdural hematoma but develop more slowly Chronic: • Manifestations may not appear until weeks to months after injury • Confusion, slowed thinking, drowsiness |
| **Intracerebral Hematoma** 14% to 15% of all types of head injuries | Located directly in the brain tissue Common sites: frontal or temporal region | Gunshot wounds Depressed bone fractures Stab injury Long history of systemic hypertension Contusions | Headache Deteriorating consciousness to deep coma Hemiplegia on contralateral side Dilated pupil on the side of the clot |

occur most frequently near bony prominences of the skull. Cerebral edema can follow contusion, resulting in increased ICP. Contusions; small, diffuse venous hemorrhages; and brain swelling are at their peak 12 to 24 hours after injury.

Manifestations of contusion depend on the size and location of the brain injury. An initial loss of consciousness occurs; level of consciousness may remain altered, and behavior changes such as combativeness may persist for an extended period. Full consciousness may be regained extremely slowly, and residual deficits may persist; in some clients, full level of consciousness never really returns. Focal effects of the contusion may cause loss of reflexes, hemiparesis (muscular weakness of one-half of the body), or abnormal posturing. Manifestations of increased ICP may occur if cerebral edema develops. Regaining full LOC may take an extended period of time and residual deficits may persist.

### Epidural Hematoma

An **epidural hematoma** (also called an extradural hematoma) develops in the potential space between the dura and the skull, which normally adhere to one another. As the blood collects, the expanding hematoma strips the dura away from the skull. Epidural hematomas affect young to middle-aged adults more frequently than older adults, because the dura becomes more tightly attached to the skull with aging.

Epidural hematomas usually result from a skull fracture, resulting in a torn artery, often the middle meningeal artery. Because epidural hematomas are arterial in origin, they tend to develop rapidly. The client may lose consciousness with the initial injury, and then have a brief lucid period before the level of consciousness rapidly declines from drowsiness to coma as the hematoma expands, stripping the dura away from the skull and placing pressure on brain tissue. Other manifestations include headache; vomiting; a fixed, dilated pupil on the same side (ipsilateral) as the hematoma; contralateral (opposite side) hemiparesis or hemiplegia; and possible seizures. Because epidural hematomas usually develop rapidly, timely intervention is vital to prevent significant increases in ICP and herniation.

### Subdural Hematoma

**Subdural hematomas,** in which a localized mass of blood collects between the dura mater and the arachnoid mater, are more common than epidural hematomas. Acute subdural hematomas are unusually located at the top of the head, and develop within 48 hours of the initial head injury. Chronic subdural hematomas develop over weeks or months. The chronic type is seen most often in the older adult and people who have some brain atrophy with subsequent enlarged epidural space. These hematomas are often venous in origin, although they may involve bleeding from small arteries as well. Subdural hematomas may form without direct trauma or contusion; acceleration-deceleration forces may tear the bridging veins that connect veins on the surface of the cerebral cortex to the dural sinuses. As blood collects, it places direct pressure on underlying brain tissue.

Acute subdural hematomas develop rapidly following head injury. Although a lucid period may occur, the client commonly develops drowsiness, confusion, and enlargement of the ipsilateral pupil within minutes or hours of the injury. If responsive, the client may complain of a unilateral headache. Hemiparesis and respiratory pattern changes may occur.

Chronic subdural hematomas are often associated with relatively minor trauma such as a fall. Weeks to months may elapse before manifestations of the hematoma occur; the initial trauma may have been forgotten. Chronic subdural hematomas may also occur spontaneously in the older adult or in clients with bleeding disorders. Manifestations of the hematoma develop slowly and may be mistaken for the onset of dementia in the older adult. Slowed thinking, confusion, drowsiness, or lethargy are common early manifestations. Other manifestations include headache, dilation and sluggishness of the ipsilateral pupil, and possible seizures.

### Intracerebral Hematoma

**Intracerebral hematomas** may be single or multiple, and are associated with contusions. They may occur in any location but usually are found in the frontal or temporal lobes. They may result from closed head trauma, particularly contusion or shearing of small blood vessels deep within the hemispheres. Intracerebral hematomas can also accompany other types of head trauma such as lacerations. Older adults are particularly vulnerable to intracerebral hemorrhage because cerebral blood vessels are more fragile and easily torn.

The manifestations of intracerebral hematoma vary according to the location of the hematoma. Headache may develop, along with decreasing level of consciousness, hemiplegia, and dilation of the ipsilateral pupil. The expanding clot increases intracranial pressure, and herniation may occur.

## Diffuse Brain Injury (DBI)

A **diffuse brain injury (DBI)** affects the entire brain and is caused by a shaking motion, with twisting movement (rotational acceleration) the primary mechanism of injury. Shearing stresses on brain tissue cause axonal damage from shearing, tearing, or stretching of nerve fibers. The most serious axonal injuries are located farthest from the brainstem, with the frontal and temporal axonal tracts being most vulnerable to injury. Physical deficits resulting from diffuse brain injuries include spastic paralysis, peripheral nerve injury, swallowing disorders, visual and hearing impairments, and taste and smell disorders. Damage decreases the speed of information processing and responding and disrupts attention, resulting in serious cognitive and affective impairments. Cognitive deficits that may result include disorientation and confusion, short attention span, problems with memory and learning, perceptual problems, and poor judgment. Possible behavioral deficits include agitation, impulsivity, depression, and social withdrawal.

Initially, the damage involves tearing of axons, blood vessels, and brain tissue (visible only by electron microscope). The number of damaged axons progressively increases, with pathology involving the nucleii and axons. The damaged axons, which resemble sausage links, regress into round balls called *retraction balls* (visible with light microscopy). After several weeks, the retraction balls are replaced by clusters of microglia. In the final phase, astrocytosis (equivalent to scarring) occurs at the site of axonal damage, accompanied by demyelination of long axon tracts.

The categories of DBI (McCance & Huether, 2002) include mild concussion, classic cerebral concussion, and diffuse axonal injury.

### Mild Concussion

**Mild concussion** involves temporary axonal disturbances. It is defined as a momentary interruption of brain function with or without loss of consciousness (Porth, 2002). A concussion may be associated with an immediate, brief loss of consciousness on impact. Altered consciousness may last only seconds or persist for several hours. Amnesia for events immediately preceding and following the injury (*retrograde and antegrade amnesia*) is common. Other manifestations of concussion include headache, drowsiness, confusion, dizziness, and visual disturbances such as diplopia or blurred vision (see the box below).

The grades of mild concussion, with manifestations, are as follows:

- Grade I: Momentary amnesia, confusion, and disorientation
- Grade II: Momentary confusion and retrograde amnesia that develops after 5 to 10 minutes
- Grade III: Confusion and retrograde amnesia that are present from impact

### Classic Cerebral Concussion (Grade IV)

A **classic cerebral concussion** involves diffuse cerebral disconnection from the brainstem RAS. An immediate loss of consciousness occurs, lasting less than 6 hours. Both retrograde and anterograde amnesia occur. Cerebral contusions may be present. In a severe concussion, a brief seizure and respiratory

---

### Manifestations of Concussion

- Immediate loss of consciousness (lasting usually no longer than 5 minutes)
- Amnesia for events surrounding injury
- Headache
- Drowsiness, confusion, dizziness
- Visual disturbances
- Possible brief seizure activity with transient apnea, bradycardia, pallor, and hypotension

#### Postconcussion Syndrome

- Persistent headache
- Dizziness
- Irritability and insomnia
- Impaired memory and concentration, learning problems

arrest may occur; transient pallor, bradycardia, and hypotension may accompany loss of consciousness.

Following concussion, clients may develop **postconcussion syndrome** with persistent headache, dizziness, irritability, insomnia, impaired memory and concentration, and learning problems. Postconcussion syndrome may last for several weeks or, rarely, up to a year.

### Diffuse Axonal Injury

**Diffuse axonal injury (DAI)** is a brain injury in which a high-speed acceleration-deceleration injury, typically associated with motor vehicle crashes, causes widespread disruption of axons in the white matter. Focal lesions may be found in the corpus callosum, midbrain, and brainstem. An immediate loss of consciousness occurs. The prognosis is poor; most clients with severe DAI either die or remain in persistent vegetative state.

DAI may range from mild to severe. In mild DAI, coma lasts 6 to 24 hours, and cognitive, psychologic, and sensorimotor deficits may persist. In moderate DAI, injury and impairment is spread throughout the cererbral cortex and diencephalon. There is axonal tearing, coma lasting more than 24 hours, and often incomplete recovery. In severe DAI, axonal injury occurs in both cerebral hemispheres, the diencephalon, and the brainstem. Immediate autonomic dysfunction occurs, and increased ICP is manifested in 4 to 6 days. Profound cognitive and sensorimotor deficits occur, involving movement, verbal and written communication, ability to learn and reason, and ability to modulate behavior.

## COLLABORATIVE CARE

The client with a brain injury may receive medical and/or surgical treatment. Specific guidelines for the medical management of severe head injury have been developed by the Brain Trauma Foundation (1995).

## Concussion

Following a concussion, the client may be observed for 1 to 2 hours in the emergency department, and then discharged home with instructions for further observation to detect manifestations of secondary injury. If the loss of consciousness extended more than 2 minutes, the client may be admitted to the hospital for observation.

## Acute TBI

Recognition and management of acute TBI with transport to an ED is essential to client outcomes. Morbidity and mortality increase with hypotension (systolic pressure less than 90 mmHg) and hypoxia ($Pao_2$ less than 60 mmHg) (Bucher & Melander, 1999). Assessment of the client's airway, breathing, and circulation (ABCs), with management of dysfunction, is necessary to decrease the secondary effects of the brain injury. An intracranial pressure monitor probe may be inserted to assess ICP and monitor therapy to reduce cerebral edema and maintain cerebral perfusion. Osmotic diuretics such as mannitol also may be administered to reduce cerebral edema.

## Diagnostic Tests

Diagnostic testing may be done to monitor hemodynamic status and detect conditions that may contribute to cerebral edema.

- *Skull X-rays* detect skull fractures and assess penetrating objects.
- *ABGs* are analyzed, with particular attention to oxygen and carbon dioxide levels. Adequate oxygenation is vital to maintain cerebral metabolism; carbon dioxide is a potent vasodilator, and increased levels may contribute to cerebral edema and increased ICP.
- *Blood count, serum glucose and electrolyte levels,* and *serum osmolarity* are assessed to monitor for infection or conditions that can affect cerebral blood flow or metabolism.
- *CT scan* or *MRI* is ordered to detect contusions and lesions associated with diffuse axonal injury. CT scan shows normal findings in concussion but characteristic lesions with contusion and DAI.
- Other diagnostic tests may include an *EEG* and possibly a *lumbar puncture* to assess for bleeding.

## Treatments

### Management of Increased ICP

Increased ICP is managed (as described in a previous section) to reestablish equilibrium of the intracranial contents and prevent secondary brain damage. Treatments include airway management, hyperventilation (used if signs of herniation appear), fluid resuscitation, positioning, temperature regulation, and medications. Medications other than those previously discussed include a category of drugs called neuroprotectants. These drugs are used to treat or alter some of the pathologic pathways that occur in ischemia, and must be administered within a short time of the injury to be effective. Classifications of the drugs include lipid peroxidase inhibitors, free radical scavengers, receptor antagonists, calcium channel blockers, and gangliosides (Bucher & Melander, 1999).

### Surgery

Small subdural hematomas can frequently be reabsorbed and may be treated conservatively, with close observation and supportive care. However, the treatment of choice for epidural hematomas and large acute subdural hematomas is surgical evacuation of the clot. This can often be performed through *burr holes* made into the skull (Figure 42–7 ■). In an epidural hematoma, the bleeding vessel can also be ligated during this procedure, preventing further bleeding. Rebleeding may occur following evacuation of an acute subdural hematoma in older adults and clients with chronic alcoholism. A craniotomy is necessary to evacuate chronic subdural hematomas because the hematoma tends to solidify, making it difficult or impossible to remove through burr holes. Surgery is less successful in treating intracerebral hematomas because of widespread tissue damage. Supportive care to manage intracranial pressure and prevent complications is provided.

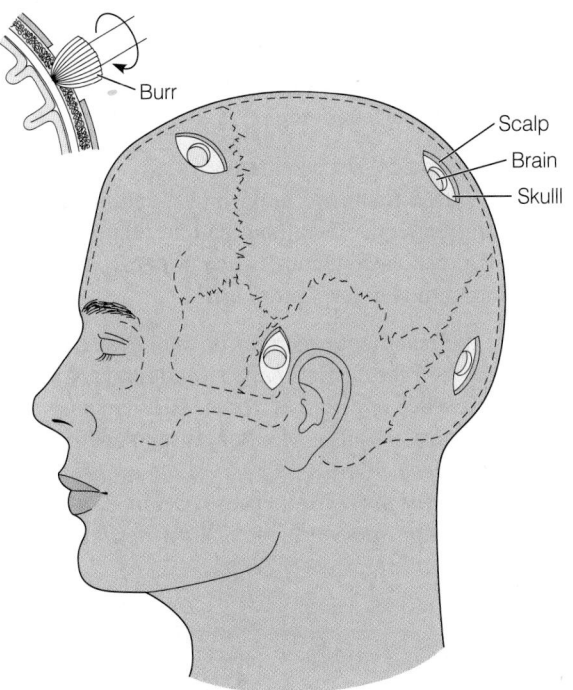

**Figure 42–7** ■ Possible locations of burr holes.

# NURSING CARE

## Health Promotion

The best way to treat any injury is to prevent it from happening. Public education must continue to stress the importance of safe driving, the dangers of driving under the influence of alcohol or drugs, and the necessity of wearing seat belts. Legislation has mandated such motor vehicle changes as seat belts, child safety seats, and airbags. Other behaviors that can reduce the morbidity and mortality associated with TBI are wearing bicycle and motorcycle helmets, learning and following gun safety rules, promoting farm safety, and teaching older adults about safety (such as preventing falls) in the home.

## Assessment

Collect the following data through the health history and physical examination (see Chapter 40). When assessing the older adult, be aware of normal changes with aging, described in Box 42–4.

- Health history: A history of the injury is helpful in understanding the nature of the craniocerebral trauma; knowledge about loss of consciousness assists the nurse in planning care
- Physical examination: neurologic assessment, including pupils, LOC, Glasgow Coma Scale, brainstem reflexes (cornea, cough, gag, extraocular movements), vital signs; skull and face (deformity, lacerations, bruising, bleeding); movement of extremities

## BOX 42–4 ■ Assessment Findings in the Older Adult

As one ages, neurons continue to die without being replaced, and the weight and mass of the brain decline. However, intellectual function continues at a nearly optimal level, unless disease impairs the function of the brain; for example, arteriosclerosis and hypertension may lead to a CVA that causes brain damage. Older people respond to questions more slowly, and sensations, reflexes, and motor coordination decline. Thus, when interviewing the older client, it is important to ask questions slowly and clearly and to allow adequate time for the client to respond. When testing the client's ability to perceive various tactile stimuli, be prepared to use more pressure before the client perceives the sensation. Although sensation may be decreased, it should be symmetrical. Other age-related changes include the following:

- All reflexes may be decreased, and the abdominal and plantar reflexes may be absent. Often, the ankle reflex is the first tendon reflex lost with aging.
- It may be difficult for the older client to perform alternating movements.
- Senile tremors at rest may be observed in the hands; the head may nod, and the tongue may protrude. However, this type of senile tremor is benign and has no associated rigidity, as occurs in Parkinson's disease.
- The older client usually walks with a gait that is slower and more deliberate than that of the younger client, and the posture may be stooped.
- Motor strength may decrease slightly.
- Vibratory sensation, especially in the feet and ankles, decreases.
- There is a progressive decrease in the ability to taste and smell.
- The pupil may respond more slowly to light.

## Nursing Diagnoses and Interventions

Nursing care of the client in the acute care phase initially focuses on maintaining an effective airway and breathing pattern. Nursing care is also directed toward continuous assessment and monitoring of neurologic function as well as other body systems. This close monitoring provides early recognition and treatment of problems and complications, and initiation of aggressive forms of therapy that may be needed.

Many nursing diagnoses associated with traumatic brain injury correspond with those outlined previously in the sections on the client with altered level of consciousness and increased intracranial pressure. Specific nursing diagnoses discussed in this section focus on problems with decreased intracranial adaptive capacity, airway clearance, and breathing patterns.

### Decreased Intracranial Adaptive Capacity

The client with a traumatic brain injury has or is at high risk for increased ICP. As the mechanisms that normally compensate for changes in intracranial pressure are compromised, intracranial pressure increases in disproportional response to a variety

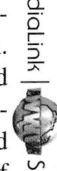

MediaLink | SUBDURAL HEMATOMA CARE PLAN

of stimuli. (See the discussion earlier in the chapter for other nursing diagnoses and interventions for the client with increased ICP).

- Monitor for manifestations of increased ICP, including eye opening response, motor response, and verbal response. *These responses evaluate the ability to integrate commands with conscious and involuntary movement.*
- Monitor for changes in vital signs: bradycardia or tachycardia, varying breathing patterns, hypertension, and/or widening pulse pressure. *Vital signs vary depending on the site of impairment. Cushing's triad (bradycardia, increased systolic blood pressure, and increased pulse pressure) indicates brainstem ischemia leading to cerebral herniation.*
- Assess for vomiting, headache, lethargy, restlessness, purposeless movements, and changes in mentation. *These manifestations may be early indicators of intracranial pressure changes.*
- Monitor temperature and initiate hypothermia treatment as prescribed. *Impaired hypothalmic function can interfere with temperature regulation. Hyperthermia may increase ICP.*
- Monitor fluid status: Regularly compare intake and output, review serum osmolality, and use infusion pump to administer IV fluids (if prescribed). *Osmotic diuretics, if used to treat cerebral edema, may cause hypotension and decreased cardiac output.*

**PRACTICE ALERT**  *Overhydration from rapid infusion of IV fluids may cause or further increase increased ICP.* ■

### Ineffective Airway Clearance

The primary objective in the care of any trauma client is maintaining a patent airway to prevent hypoxia. However, in the initial acute care phase, the risk of cervical vertebral fractures and spinal cord injury may complicate the process of establishing a patent airway. In addition, other multisystem injuries may complicate the interpretation of vital signs. In general, all unconscious people with a head injury should be intubated with an endotracheal tube to prevent aspiration. Clients with head trauma may also require a tracheostomy to provide an airway and be placed on a ventilator.

- Assess neurologic manifestations on a regular schedule. *Changes in neurologic manifestations may indicate increased ICP, with the risk of further depression of the respiratory system and respiratory arrest.*
- Maintain head and neck in neutral alignment, immobilized until injury is determined. *Head rotation and neck flexion are associated with increased ICP, decreased jugular venous outflow, and localized changes in cerebral blood flow (Sullivan, 2000). Immobilization prevents spinal cord injury in suspected or actual fractures of the cervical spine; spinal cord injury at this level would further impair respiratory function.*
- Clear the nose and mouth of mucus and blood. *This ensures patency of the upper airway.*

- Suction the airway as needed, limiting suctioning time to no more than 10 seconds at one time. Do not suction the nasal passages until a dural tear has been ruled out. *Suctioning is usually necessary to maintain a patent airway.*

### Ineffective Breathing Pattern

The client with a traumatic brain injury and hematoma is at high risk for ineffective breathing pattern related to increased ICP. If ICP increases dramatically, tentorial herniation may occur, leading to sudden respiratory arrest.

- Monitor the respiratory pattern for rate, depth, and rhythm every 2 hours if the client is not on a ventilator. Assess breath sounds, presence of cyanosis, restlessness, and use of accessory respiratory muscles. Monitor pulse oximetry and blood gas levels. *Head injuries may cause alterations in respirations. An increased respiratory rate may indicate hypoxia. A decrease in respiratory rate may be the result of depression of the medullary respiratory center.*

**PRACTICE ALERT**  *In general, an initial increase in intracranial pressure causes respirations to slow; as the pressure continues to increase, respirations become rapid.* ■

- Monitor ICP readings. *Continuous measurement of ICP is used to diagnose and monitor increased intracranial pressure. As ICP increases, herniation may occur, leading to respiratory arrest and death.*
- If the client is not intubated, prepare for oxygen administration and/or tracheal intubation if respiratory distress occurs. *Supplying oxygen prevents hypoxia until a hematoma can be evacuated, relieving pressure on the respiratory center.*
- Prepare for cranial surgery if deteriorating respiratory pattern and neurologic changes are noted. *Surgical intervention usually consists of placing several burr holes in the skull or performing a craniotomy to remove the hematoma. (Intracranial surgery is discussed later in the chapter.) However, the cerebral edema and increased intracranial pressure may cause death even if surgery is performed.*

## Using NANDA, NIC, and NOC

Chart 42–2 shows links between NANDA nursing diagnoses, NIC, and NOC when caring for the client with an acute brain injury.

## Home Care

### Concussion

Inform the client and family that a postconcussion syndrome sometimes occurs. If the client experiences persistent headaches and dizziness, is uncharacteristically emotional, seems overly tired, or has difficulty paying attention or remembering, the health care provider should be notified. Explain that these manifestations may persist for some time. Rehabilitation may help the client compensate for memory impairment and attention deficits.

## CHART 42-2   NANDA, NIC, AND NOC LINKAGES

### The Client with an Acute Brain Injury

| NURSING DIAGNOSES | NURSING INTERVENTIONS | NURSING OUTCOMES |
|---|---|---|
| • Acute Confusion | • Delirium Management<br>• Surveillance: Safety | • Cognitive Ability<br>• Neurological Status: Consciousness<br>• Memory |
| • Risk for Aspiration | • Aspiration Precautions<br>• Vomiting Management | • Neurological Status |
| • Hyperthermia | • Temperature Regulation | • Thermoregulation |
| • Impaired Memory | • Memory Training | • Memory |
| • Disturbed Sensory Perception | • Cerebral Perfusion Promotion<br>• Environmental Management<br>• Cerebral Edema Management<br>• ICP Monitoring | • Cognitive Ability<br>• Neurological Status |

*Note. Data from Nursing Outcomes Classification (NOC) by M. Johnson & M. Maas (Eds.), 1997, St. Louis: Mosby; Nursing Diagnoses: Definitions & Classification 2001–2002 by North American Nursing Diagnosis Association, 2001, Philadelphia: NANDA; Nursing Interventions Classification (NIC) by J.C. McCloskey & G. M. Bulechek (Eds.), 2000, St. Louis: Mosby. Reprinted by permission.*

### Acute Brain Injury

Clients who survive an acute brain injury will require long-term physical care and rehabilitation. Although recovery is highly individualized, many clients who regain consciousness require life-long care; others remain in a coma or vegetative state. The family often expects the client to recover fully after the coma subsides, and they need information about the real possibility of residual deficits in self-care, emotional responses, cognition, communication, and movement. Topics that should be addressed for home care include:

• The need to encourage self-care and independence as much as possible.

• Positioning, movement, and skin care to prevent contractures and pressure ulcers.
• Safety issues.
• Equipment needs, such as a wheelchair and hospital bed.
• Vocational counseling and services.
• Referral to community resources and support groups.
• Helpful resources:
  • National Head Injury Foundation
  • Brain Trauma Foundation
  • International Center for Individuals with Disabilities

## Nursing Care Plan

## A Client with a Subdural Hematoma

Wong Lee is a 50-year-old tug boat mechanic who is married and has three sons. Although Mr. Lee has been through rehabilitation twice for alcoholism, he has not been able to quit drinking. His physician has explained the physical consequences and the possible interaction between alcohol and the anticoagulant Mr. Lee is taking for chronic atrial fibrillation. While attending a family reunion, during which he eats a large meal and drinks several beers, Mr. Lee joins a game of softball. Mrs. Lee is concerned that Mr. Lee has consumed too much alcohol to play ball in the heat, but Mr. Lee is adamant and states that he wants to pitch. During the end of the second inning, the batter hits a ball that strikes Mr. Lee in the head. Mr. Lee stumbles and drops to the ground, holding his head. He does not lose consciousness and gets up on his own. His sons and wife try to persuade him to go to the hospital, but Mr. Lee insists he feels fine.

Two weeks later, after an evening of consuming several mixed drinks, Mr. Lee develops a headache. He attributes the headache

to a hangover, but instead of improving the next day, the headache becomes steadily worse. He becomes confused and disoriented. His wife, concerned that his drinking is increasing again, calls the physician, who admits Mr. Lee to the detoxification center at the local hospital. A CT scan is performed. The diagnosis of a subdural hematoma is made, and Mr. Lee is transferred to the neurosurgical unit.

### ASSESSMENT

When Saundra Knight, the nurse on the neurosurgical unit, enters the room, she notices that Mr. Lee is sitting in bed, laughing and giddy. As she begins to talk to Mr. Lee, he states, "Don't ask me anything—I can't think. My headache is getting worse." Over the next few hours, the giddiness subsides, and Mr. Lee becomes drowsy. Ms. Knight reports a Glasgow Coma Scale score of 11. An

(continued on page 1382)

## Nursing Care Plan
### A Client with a Subdural Hematoma *(continued)*

ICP monitor is inserted and reveals increased intracranial pressure. Mr. Lee is scheduled to have burr holes and hematoma evacuation that afternoon.

### DIAGNOSES
- *Risk for ineffective breathing pattern* related to pressure on respiratory center by intracranial hematoma
- *Ineffective cerebral tissue perfusion* related to increased intracranial pressure secondary to cerebral edema

### EXPECTED OUTCOMES
- Maintain a respiratory rate and rhythm within normal limits.
- Maintain adequate cerebral perfusion, as evidenced by stable vital signs, stable neurologic status, and no decrease in level of consciousness.

### PLANNING AND IMPLEMENTATION
- Perform neurologic assessment every 2 hours or as needed.
- Monitor vital signs every 2 hours or as needed.
- Explain to the family the procedure for intracranial surgery.

### EVALUATION
The first day postoperatively, Mr. Lee begins breathing on his own without ventilatory support. His respiratory rate and rhythm are within normal limits, with no signs of abnormal breath sounds. The ICP monitor readings are appropriate, and Mr. Lee shows significant improvement in level of consciousness, with a Glasgow Coma Scale score of 15. Mr. Lee continues to improve and is discharged to home 5 days after surgery.

### Critical Thinking in the Nursing Process
1. Describe the similarities and differences between Mr. Lee's disorder and the manifestations of other types of intracranial hematomas.
2. Mr. Lee kept trying to pull out his ICP line. You know he should not be restrained, because pulling against restraints increases restlessness and increases intracranial pressure. What would you do?
3. Write a care plan for Mr. Lee for the nursing diagnosis, *Acute confusion.*

See Evaluating Your Response in Appendix C.

---

# THE CLIENT WITH A CENTRAL NERVOUS SYSTEM INFECTION

The central nervous system (CNS), including the meninges, neural tissues, and blood vessels, may be directly affected by bacteria, viruses, fungi, protozoans, and rickettsiae. The CNS may also be affected by toxins from bacterial infections. The major CNS infections include meningitis, encephalitis, and brain abscesses.

## INCIDENCE AND PREVALENCE

The most common infection of the meninges is bacterial meningitis. The mortality rate is 25% in adults. Brain abscess occur 2 times more often in men than in women, with the median age for abscess formation 30 to 40 years (McCance & Huether, 2002). Meningococcal meningitis may occur in epidemics among people who are in close contact with one another, such as military recruits and students living in dormitories. Pneumococcal meningitis, in contrast, primarily affects the very young and very old.

The incidence of pathogenic infections of the CNS increases with the onset of AIDS. Clients who are HIV positive may have CNS infections caused by toxoplasmosis, cryptococcus, tuberculosis, herpes simplex, cytomegalovirus, or a polyoma virus (resulting in progressive multifocal leukoencephalopathy).

## Risk Factors

Those at highest risk are the young, frail older adults, those with debilitating diseases, and the immunosuppressed (such as clients having radiation therapy or chemotherapy treatments).

Other risk factors are having AIDS, having an infection elsewhere in the body, and having a skull fracture or invasive neurosurgery (King, 1999).

## PATHOPHYSIOLOGY AND MANIFESTATIONS

When pathogens enter the CNS and the meninges, an inflammatory process results. The pathology of CNS infections includes the invading pathogens, the subsequent inflammation, and the increase in intracranial pressure that may result from the inflammatory processes. Both the pathogenic damage and the increased ICP may result in brain damage and life-threatening complications.

### Meningitis

**Meningitis** is an inflammation of the pia mater, the arachnoid, and the subarachnoid space. Inflammation spreads rapidly throughout the CNS because of the circulation of CSF around the brain and spinal cord. Infection is the usual cause of meningitis, although chemical meningitis may also occur (Porth, 2002). Meningitis may be acute or chronic, and it may be bacterial, viral, fungal, or parasitic in origin.

In meningitis, the infecting organisms usually reach the CNS in one of two ways: by direct extension, such as can occur after cranial trauma or invasive procedures (e.g., ICP monitoring devices or neurosurgery); or through the bloodstream secondary to another infection in the body.

The organism responsible for meningitis must overcome nonspecific and specific host defense mechanisms to invade and replicate in the CSF. These defenses include the skin barrier, the blood-brain barrier, the nonspecific inflammatory response, and the immune response. Host response to the particular pathogen is responsible for the manifestations of clinical meningitis. The organisms that initiate the host response in meningitis demonstrate an affinity for the nervous system. They colonize and invade the nasopharyngeal mucosa, survive intravascularly, and penetrate the CNS if the blood-brain barrier is damaged, as can happen during surgery, the inflammatory response, or cerebral edema.

Infection of the CSF and meninges causes an inflammatory response in the pia, arachnoid, and CSF. Because the meninges and subarachnoid space are continuous around the brain, spinal cord, and optic nerves, the infection and inflammatory response is always cerebrospinal, involving both the brain and the spinal cord. Inflamed blood vessels in the area leak fluids as cell permeability increases. Purulent exudate infiltrates cranial nerve sheaths and blocks the chorioid plexus and subarachnoid villi. Increased ICP occurs as brain tissue responds to the pathogen. With an increase in ICP, cerebral perfusion decreases and cerebral autoregulation is lost.

## Bacterial Meningitis

The causative organisms of bacterial meningitis include *Neisseria meningitis,* meningococcus, *Streptococcus pneumoniae, Haemophilus influenzae,* and *E. coli.* Risk factors include head trauma with a basilar skull fracture, otitis media, sinusitis, neurosurgery, systemic sepsis, or immunocompromise (Porth, 2002).

Once the pathogen enters the central nervous system, it or its toxic products (free radicals) initiate an inflammatory response in the meninges, CSF, and ventricles. Meningeal vessels become engorged, and their permeability increases. Phagocytic white blood cells migrate into the subarachnoid space, forming a purulent exudate that thickens and clouds the CSF and interferes with its flow. Rapid exudate formation causes further inflammation and edema of meningeal cells. Blood vessel engorgement, exudate formation, impaired CSF flow, and cellular edema cause the intracranial pressure to increase.

The client with bacterial meningitis typically presents with fever and chills, headache, back and abdominal pain, and nausea and vomiting. (The older adult may not have a high fever, but may rather exhibit confusion). Meningeal irritation causes *nuchal rigidity,* with a very stiff neck and positive Brudzinski's sign (flexion of the neck that causes the hip and knee to flex) and positive Kernig's sign (inability to extend the knee while the hip is flexed at a 90-degree angle). Photophobia is present; the client may also experience diplopia. With meningococcal meningitis, a rapidly spreading petechial rash involving the skin and mucous membranes may be noted. The client may also have increased ICP, manifested by decreased LOC, seizures, changes in vital signs and respiratory pattern, and papilledema. The manifestations of bacterial meningitis are listed in the box in the following column.

Complications of bacterial meningitis include arthritis, cranial nerve damage, and hydrocephalus. Cranial nerve VIII, the auditory nerve, is frequently affected, with resulting nerve deafness. Thrombophlebitis may develop in cerebral vessels, with infarction of surrounding tissues (Porth, 2002).

## Manifestations of Bacterial Meningitis

- Restlessness, agitation, and irritability
- Severe headache
- Signs of meningeal irritation:
  a. Nuchal rigidity (stiff neck)
  b. Positive Brudzinski's sign
  c. Positive Kernig's sign
- Chills and high fever
- Confusion, altered LOC
- Photophobia (aversion to light), diplopia
- Seizures
- Signs of increased ICP (widened pulse pressure and bradycardia, respiratory irregularity, decreased LOC, headache, and vomiting)
- Petechial rash (in meningococcal meningitis)

### Viral Meningitis

Acute viral meningitis, also called aseptic meningitis, is a less severe disease than bacterial meningitis. It can be caused by numerous viruses, such as herpes simplex, herpes zoster, Epstein-Barr virus, or cytomegalovirus (CMV). Viral meningitis most often appears after a case of mumps. Although viral infection also triggers the inflammatory response, the course of the disease is benign and of short duration. Recovery is uneventful.

The manifestations of viral meningitis are similar to those of bacterial meningitis, although usually milder. The client may have a mild flulike illness prior to the onset of meningitis. Headache is intense and is accompanied by malaise, nausea, vomiting, and lethargy. Photophobia may be present. The client generally remains oriented, although possibly drowsy. Temperature is mildly elevated. Neck stiffness, positive Brudzinski's sign, and positive Kernig's sign are usually present.

## Encephalitis

**Encephalitis** is an acute inflammation of the parenchyma of the brain or spinal cord. It is almost always caused by a virus, but it may also be caused by bacteria, fungi, and other organisms. Other less common causes include ingested lead; postvaccination encephalitis (from vaccines for measles, mumps, and rabies), and HIV (Porth, 2002). See Table 42–8 for a list of the most common causes of encephalitis.

### Viral Encephalitis

Viruses depend on living tissue for reproduction and become highly destructive when they invade brain tissue. The inflammatory response extends over the cerebral cortex, the white matter, and the meninges, with degeneration of the neurons. The pathology of encephalitis includes local necrotizing hemorrhage, which ultimately becomes generalized, with prominent edema. There is progressive degeneration of nerve cell bodies. The inflammatory response in encephalitis does not cause exudate formation as it does in meningitis. Certain viruses show a propensity for specific areas of the brain (e.g., herpes simplex virus involves frontal and temporal lobes). The

### TABLE 42-8  Causes of Encephalitis

| Cause | Comments |
|---|---|
| Arboviruses | Transmitted by bites from ticks and mosquitoes.<br>Bites from ticks occur more frequently in spring.<br>Bites from mosquitoes occur in middle to late summer.<br>Most common types are St. Louis and eastern and western equine encephalitis.<br>May destroy major parts of the lobe or hemisphere.<br>Two-thirds of clients who develop eastern equine encephalitis either die or develop severe residual disabilities (e.g., seizures, blindness, deafness, speech disorders, or mental retardation).<br>The incubation is 5 to 15 days.<br>Mortality rates associated with arboviruses are higher than those associated with enteroviruses. |
| Enteroviruses, such as echovirus, coxsackievirus, poliovirus, paramyxovirus (the virus that causes mumps), and varicella-zoster (the virus that causes chickenpox) | Infection occurs more frequently in summer (except infection by the mumps virus, which occurs more frequently in early winter).<br>Some degree of protection can be afforded by immunization against measles, mumps, and poliomyelitis.<br>Mortality rates are lower than those associated with herpes simplex type 1 virus. |
| Herpes simplex type 1 virus | Most common nonepidemic encephalitis in North America.<br>Can occur any time of year and throughout the world.<br>Has an affinity for the inferomedial portions of the frontal and temporal lobes.<br>Prognosis is grave but not hopeless: Mortality rate can be as high as 40%, and client may die within 2 weeks. |
| Amebic meningoencephalitis due to infection by *Naegleria* and *Acanthamoeba* protozoa | Both protozoa are found in warm fresh water.<br>Enter the nasal mucosa of people swimming in ponds or lakes.<br>May also be found in soil and decaying vegetation.<br>Incidence of infection is increasing in North America. |
| Exogenous poisoning | May occur after ingestion of lead or arsenic or inhalation of carbon monoxide. |

virus gains access to the CNS via the bloodstream or along peripheral or cranial nerves, or it may already be present in the meninges in the client with meningitis.

The manifestations of viral encephalitis vary, depending on the organism and area of the brain affected. Usual manifestations are similar to those of meningitis, including fever, headache, seizures, stiff neck, and altered LOC. The client may be disoriented, agitated and restless, or lethargic and drowsy. As the disease progresses, the LOC deteriorates, and the client may become comatose.

### Arbovirus Encephalitis

The arboviruses are arthropod (mosquito or tick) borne agents that infect humans. They include many different types, including Western equine encephalitis, St. Louis encephalitis, and Rift Valley fever. Adults are most often infected with St. Louis encephalitis, with older adults affected more often. The arthropods may live in small mammals and birds, or may be carried by horses and deer. The newest arboviral encephalitis in the United States is West Nile encephalitis, first identified in 1999. Bird infections began in New York and are spreading across the continent.

The arthropod-borne agents cause widespread degeneration of nerve cells, and edema and necrosis with or without hemorrhage occur. Increased ICP may develop. Manifestations include fever, malaise, sore throat, nausea and vomiting, stiff neck, tremors, paralysis of extremities, exaggerated deep tendon reflexes, seizures, and altered level of consciousness.

## Brain Abscess

A **brain abscess** is an infection with a collection of purulent material within the brain tissue. Approximately 80% are found in the cerebrum and 20% are cerebellar.

The causes of a brain abscess include open trauma and neurosurgery; infections of the mastoid, middle ear, nasal cavity, or nasal sinuses; metastatic spread from distant foci (such as heart, lungs, skin, abscessed teeth, and dirty needles); and arising from other associated areas of infection. The immunocompromised are at increased risk for abscesses. The most common pathogens causing the abscess are streptococci, staphylococci, and bacteroids. Yeast and fungi may also cause brain abscess.

A brain abscess results from the presence of microorganisms in the brain tissue. If the abscess is encapsulated, it has the ability to enlarge and, therefore, behave as a space-occupying lesion within the cranium. This predisposes the client not only to the systemic effects of the inflammatory process but also to the serious consequences of increased intracranial pressure. Occasionally, the abscess does not become encapsulated; instead, it spreads through the brain tissue to the subarachnoid space and ventricular system.

Initially, the client exhibits the general symptoms associated with an acute infectious process, such as chills, fever, malaise, and anorexia. Because brain abscess generally forms after infection, the client may consider these signs to be an exacerbation of that illness. The client may experience seizures, altered level of consciousness, and manifestations of increased ICP. As the abscess enlarges, specific symptoms are related to location; for example the client with a frontal lobe abscess may have contralateral hemiparesis, expressive aphasia, focal seizures, and frontal headache.

## COLLABORATIVE CARE

Bacterial meningitis is a medical emergency that, if not treated immediately, can be fatal within days. Successful management depends on rapid diagnosis and aggressive treatment to eradicate the infecting organism and support vital functions. The client may be placed in strict or respiratory isolation until the organism has been identified, depending on hospital policy. Universal precautions apply to CSF as well as blood.

Treatment for viral meningitis focuses on managing client symptoms and is supportive. Antipyretics and analgesics may provide relief. Antibiotic therapy is not indicated, and isolation precautions are not required.

Treatment of the client with a brain abscess focuses on prompt initiation of antibiotic therapy. Other manifestations are treated symptomatically, as with the client diagnosed with meningitis or encephalitis. If pharmacologic management is not effective, the abscess may be drained or, if it is encapsulated, removed.

### Diagnostic Tests

The diagnosis of meningitis is based on manifestations and diagnostic tests results. The following diagnostic tests may be ordered.

- *Lumbar puncture* with examination of the CSF is the definitive diagnostic measure for bacterial meningitis. Data that indicate bacterial meningitis include turbid, cloudy fluid; a markedly increased white blood cell count and protein content; and a decreased glucose content. The opening pressure on the lumbar puncture is elevated. In contrast, CSF analysis in the client with encephalitis may have a normal CSF analysis and pressure or may have some lymphocytes. The client with a brain abscess will have a markedly elevated pressure with elevated protein content and elevated WBC count. Glucose content is normal. (As a lumbar puncture in the presence of a space-occupying lesion can result in brain herniation and death, a CT scan is performed first if neurologic findings support such a lesion.)
- *Gram stain* and *culture of the CSF* are performed. Gram stain is used to determine if a bacterial infection is present. Cultures are used to determine the specific agent; no bacteria are cultured from the CSF in viral meningitis. Culture results take several days.
- *Counterimmunoelectrophoresis (CIE)* is a laboratory test that may be ordered to determine the presence of viruses or protozoa.
- *Polymerase chain reaction techniques* may be used to detect viral DNA or RNA in spinal fluid. This test is especially sensitive to herpes simplex.
- *MRI* can detect focal edema and hemorrhage in encephalitis.
- *CT scan* will show an area of increased contrast surrounding a low-density core with brain abscess.

## Medications

### Meningitis

Immediate intravenous administration of a broad-spectrum antibiotic that crosses the blood-brain barrier into the subarachnoid space is instituted in cases of bacterial meningitis. Once culture reports identify the causative organism, drug therapy is continued from 7 to 21 days, using the most effective drug or drugs specific to that bacterium. The cephalosporin antibiotics are preferred. A major concern in the treatment of CNS infections is penicillin-resistant streptococci. Recommendations for treatment are for a broad-spectrum cephalosporin, such as rifampin (Rifadin), cefotaxime (Claforam), or vancomycin (Vancocin). However, as the bacteria are killed, the toxins they release increase production of inflammatory cytokines, which are potentially lethal. Steroids such as dexamethasone (Decadron) are often give with the antibiotics to suppress inflammation. The CDC recommends that the client remain on isolation for 24 hours after the start of antibiotic therapy.

### Encephalitis

Treatment for encephalitis consists of administering specific medications and preventing complications. Fungal meningitis is treated with antifungal agents, such as amphotericin-B (Amphotec), flucytosine (Ancobon), and fluconazole (Diflucan). Viral encephalitis is treated with intravenous acyclovir (Zoviran) or vidarabine (Vira-A).

### Brain Abscess

Antibiotic therapy is the primary treatment for brain abscess. A combination of broad-spectrum antibiotics is used if the infecting organism is unknown.

An intraventricular method of medication administration uses an Ommaya reservoir that has been surgically implanted into a lateral ventricle of the brain (Figure 42–8 ■). This device

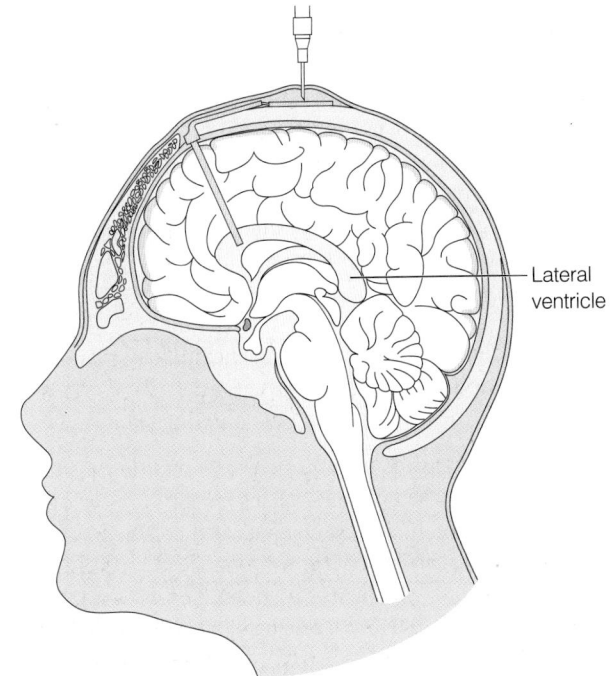

Lateral ventricle

**Figure 42–8** ■ Ommaya reservoir for medication administration.

is used to enhance CSF absorption of antibiotics and to maintain treatment over an extended period of time.

Anticonvulsant medications such as phenytoin (Dilantin) are often prescribed to prevent or control seizure activity. Antipyretic and analgesic medications may provide symptomatic relief; however, analgesics that have a depressant effect on the CNS (such as opiates) are avoided to prevent masking of early manifestations of deteriorating LOC. The client initially may require antiemetics to control nausea and vomiting. Fluid and electrolyte status is maintained through intravenous fluid replacement until the client is able to resume oral intake.

## Surgery

Surgical drainage of an encapsulated abscess may be necessary. The decision to perform surgery is based on the client's general condition, the stage of abscess development, and the site of the abscess.

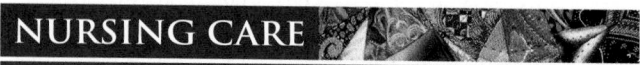

# NURSING CARE

Central nervous system infections are serious illnesses, with potentially life-threatening effects and complications. Nursing assessments and interventions are critical in identifying changes in the client's neurologic status and preventing complications from increased ICP.

## Health Promotion

The following help to prevent central nervous system infections.

- Vaccinations for meningococcal, pneumococcal, and hemophilic meningitis
- Administration of prophylactic rifampin (Rifadin) for people exposed to meningococcal meningitis
- Mosquito control with repellants, insecticides, and protective clothing
- Destruction of the insect larvae and elimination of breeding places, such as pools of stagnant water
- Vaccination against Japanese B encephalitis (recommended for summer travelers to rural East Asia)
- Prompt diagnosis and treatment of infections of the head, neck, and respiratory system
- Careful asepsis for care of any client with an open head injury or postoperative neurosurgery

## Assessment

Collect the following data through the health history and physical examination (see Chapter 40). Further focused assessments are described with nursing interventions below.

- Health history: risk factors (concurrent infections, other illnesses, travel), when manifestations began, severity of manifestations, current nausea and headache, seizures
- Physical examination: Glasgow Coma Scale, level of consciousness, vital signs, motor function, pupillary check, cranial nerves, neck ROM, Brudzinski's sign, Kernig's sign, skin (rash, petechiae, purpura), muscle movement and strength, speech

## Nursing Diagnoses and Interventions

In planning and implementing nursing care for the client with a CNS infection, the prognosis may depend on the supportive care given. The client is often very ill, and the combination of fever, dehydration, and cerebral edema may predispose the client to seizures. Airway obstruction, respiratory arrest, or cardiac dysrhythmias may occur. Nursing diagnoses and interventions previously discussed for the client with an altered LOC, increased ICP, and seizures are also appropriate for the client with a CNS infection. Nursing interventions in this section focus on altered protection and risk for fluid volume deficit.

## Ineffective Protection

Clients with CNS infections are less able to protect themselves against insults from both internal and external sources. The effects of the inflammation and resulting pathophysiologic processes may include pain, fever, altered LOC, seizures, increased ICP, and cranial nerve dysfunction. In addition, pathophysiologic effects on the brain from toxins or thrombosis of a cerebral vessel may lead to permanent neurologic deficits, such as loss of motor function or dementia.

- Assess neurologic status on a regular basis. *Many complications are evidenced by changes in neurologic manifestations.*
- Assess vital signs, including temperature, on a regular basis. *The client often has a high temperature throughout the illness, ranging from 101°F (38°C) to 105°F (40.5°C).*

**PRACTICE ALERT** *Hyperthermia may result from increased intracranial pressure, while an increased temperature can also increase ICP.* ∎

- Monitor levels of consciousness. Assess levels of orientation, memory, attention span, and response to stimuli. *Early in the infection, the client often has problems with memory and orientation. There may be problems with following commands, restlessness, irritability, and combativeness. As the illness progresses, the level of consciousness decreases to lethargy and finally into deep coma.*
- Assess for manifestations of seizure activity, and institute seizure precautions:
  - Monitor twitching of hands or face and tonic-clonic movements.
  - Have an oral airway and suction equipment readily available.
  - Pad side rails, maintain bed in low position, and keep side rails up.
  *Irritation of the cerebral cortex secondary to meningeal inflammation may cause seizures. Careful monitoring and seizure precautions are necessary to prevent injury.*
- Assess for manifestations of cranial nerve damage; monitor extraocular movements, facial movement, dizziness, ability to hear, double vision, drooping upper eyelids (*ptosis*), and pupillary changes. *Cranial nerve dysfunction may result from inflammation or vascular changes in the brain.*

- Assess for manifestations of increased intracranial pressure: decreased pulse, increased blood pressure, widening pulse pressure, respiratory changes, and vomiting. *Increased intracranial pressure results from infectious or inflammatory exudate, cerebral edema, and hydrocephalus.*
- Administer prescribed medications and maintain prescribed fluid restrictions. *Diuretics are often prescribed to prevent increases in ICP, anticonvulsants are prescribed to prevent or control seizures, and antibiotics are prescribed to eradicate the bacteria. Fluids may be restricted to help prevent increased ICP.*

### Risk for Deficient Fluid Volume

The client is at risk for fluid volume deficit related to increased metabolic rate, diaphoresis, and fluid restrictions.

- Assess for presence, or worsening, of fluid volume deficit.
  - Measure and compare intake and output every 2 to 4 hours.
  - Monitor daily body weights.
  - Monitor skin turgor.
  - Monitor condition of mucous membranes.
  - Monitor urine amount, color, and odor.
  - Monitor BUN:creatinine ratio.

*The elastic property of the skin depends partially on interstitial fluid volume. If there is a fluid volume deficit, skin flattens more slowly after a pinch is released. Mucous membranes are dry. In fluid volume deficit, urine output is decreased, urine is dark in color and concentrated with a strong odor, and urine specific gravity is greater than 1.020, and BUN will rise out of proportion to serum creatinine.*

**PRACTICE ALERT** *An acute weight loss of 1 lb represents a fluid loss of approximately 500 mL.* ■

- When administering fluids, either orally or parenterally, consider concurrent illnesses. For example, clients with increased intracranial pressure or renal failure require complex management. See Chapter 5 ⧉ for a further discussion of fluid volume deficit.

## Using NANDA, NIC and NOC

Chart 42–3 shows links between NANDA nursing diagnoses, NIC, and NOC when caring for the client with a CNS infection.

## Home Care

The importance of preventive measures, such as recognizing predisposing conditions, is a major focus for client education. People who have had close contact with the client with meningitis should be assessed for fever, headache, or neck stiffness. Some physicians believe that those closest to the client are candidates for antimicrobial prophylaxis. Also address the following topics.

- The need to report any signs or symptoms of ear infection, sore throat, or upper respiratory infection
- The names and purposes of all medications that may be prescribed
- The importance of taking all medication until completely gone, because some clients may think it is acceptable to stop the medication as soon as they feel better

---

### CHART 42–3 NANDA, NIC, AND NOC LINKAGES

#### The Client with a CNS Infection

| NURSING DIAGNOSES | NURSING INTERVENTIONS | NURSING OUTCOMES |
|---|---|---|
| • Risk for Imbalanced Body Temperature | • Temperature Regulation<br>• Vital Signs Monitoring<br>• Cerebral Edema Management | • Infection Status |
| • Acute Confusion | • Delirium Management<br>• Surveillance: Safety | • Cognitive Ability<br>• Neurological Status: Consciousness<br>• Memory |
| • Self-Care Deficit | • Self-Care Assistance | • Self-Care: ADLs<br>• Self-Care: Bathing<br>• Self-Care: Hygiene<br>• Self-Care: Eating<br>• Self-Care: Toileting |

*Note. Data from Nursing Outcomes Classification (NOC) by M. Johnson & M. Maas (Eds.), 1997, St. Louis: Mosby; Nursing Diagnoses: Definitions & Classification 2001–2002 by North American Nursing Diagnosis Association, 2001, Philadelphia: NANDA; Nursing Interventions Classification (NIC) by J.C. McCloskey & G. M. Bulechek (Eds.), 2000, St. Louis: Mosby. Reprinted by permission.*

## Nursing Care Plan
## A Client with Bacterial Meningitis

Monty Cook is a 22-year-old musician who plays in a local rock band. He is unmarried and lives with his parents. He is known by everyone in the community as a quiet, low-key, easygoing person and an excellent guitar player. During a performance 2 days ago, he had difficulty playing his guitar, complaining of bright stage lights blazing in his eyes. When he tried to keep his head down to prevent the lights from hurting his eyes, he noticed his neck was very stiff. After the performance, one of the newest members of the band remarked that it certainly was not their best performance. Monty responded angrily that maybe the new members of the group needed more practice. Then he stomped out and went home to bed.

He wakes at 4:00 A.M. with a severe headache, sweating, and chills; his temperature is 102°F, and he cannot bend his neck without severe pain. His mother recognizes that he is agitated and irritable, which is uncharacteristic. Frightened, she rushes him to the hospital emergency room. A lumbar puncture performed in the emergency room reveals turbid, cloudy fluid, a markedly increased white blood cell count, and protein with a decreased glucose content. Bacterial meningitis is the medical diagnosis. Mr. Cook is admitted to the hospital for treatment and care.

### ASSESSMENT

When the nurse, Aisha Aldi, enters Mr. Cook's isolation room, she sees him thrashing about in the bed, talking incoherently, and becoming more agitated. On assessment, Ms. Aldi notes dry mucous membranes, cracked lips, and small petechiae over the upper torso and abdomen. Mr. Cook's temperature is 104°F. Kernig's sign is positive. Intravenous broad-spectrum antibiotics are prescribed and initiated. After the first 2 hours on duty, Ms. Aldi notes a decrease in Mr. Cook's level of consciousness.

### DIAGNOSES

- *Hyperthermia* related to infection and abnormal temperature regulation by hypothalamus
- *Disturbed thought processes* related to intracranial infection
- *Ineffective protection* related to progression of illness

### EXPECTED OUTCOMES

- Have a decrease in body temperature.

- Become less restless and agitated.
- Remain free of injury.

### PLANNING AND IMPLEMENTATION

- Monitor vital signs every 2 hours.
- Provide sponge baths if temperature continues to rise.
- Provide a quiet, nonstimulating environment with the shades drawn.
- Provide oral care every 4 hours.
- Measure and compare intake and output every 2 hours.
- Perform neurologic assessments every 2 to 4 hours.
- Monitor for and report seizure activity and decreasing level of consciousness.
- Keep bed in low position with side rails elevated.
- Administer prescribed intravenous antibiotics.

### EVALUATION

After 4 days of antibiotic therapy, Mr. Cook's temperature has returned to near normal. Ms. Aldi notes that he has begun opening his eyes and visually tracking her as she moves about the room. Mr. Cook responds to a request to squeeze Ms. Aldi's fingers and after several hours asks her what had happened. On day 5, Mr. Cook states that he feels better and his headache is gone. He asks for sips of juice and begins urinating regularly. Seven days after admission, Mr. Cook is discharged and is able to go home with his mother. He has some weakness in his legs, but otherwise has no evidence of neurologic deficits.

### Critical Thinking in the Nursing Process

1. What strategies should the nurse use to decrease the environmental stimuli for Mr. Cook, and what is the rationale for doing these?
2. If you were caring for Mr. Cook in the initial phase of the illness and he became combative, what would you do?
3. Develop a plan of care for Mr. Cook for the nursing diagnosis, *Acute pain.* Consider the effect of narcotics on respiratory function in designing the plan.

See Evaluating Your Response in Appendix C.

## THE CLIENT WITH A BRAIN TUMOR

**Brain tumors** are growths within the cranium, including tumors in brain tissue, meninges, pituitary gland, or blood vessels. Brain tumors may be benign or malignant, primary or metastatic, and intracerebral or extracerebral. Regardless of type or location, brain tumors are potentially lethal as they grow within a closed cranial vault and displace or impinge on CNS structures.

### INCIDENCE AND PREVALENCE

An estimated 17,000 new cases of malignant brain tumors are diagnosed in the United States each year (American Cancer Society, 2001). In addition, more than 100,000 people die each year from metastatic brain tumors (Porth, 2002). Although brain tumors can occur in any age group, the highest incidence is among young children and among adults ages 50 to 70. In the adult population, the most common tumor is glioblastoma multiforme, followed by meningioma and cytoma. Glioblastomas represent more than 50% of all primary intracranial lesions.

The cause of many brain tumors is unknown. Although a number of chemical and viral agents can cause brain tumors in laboratory animals, there is no evidence that these agents cause tumors in humans. Other factors associated with brain tumors include heredity, cranial irradiation, and exposure to some chemicals (Porth, 2002).

## TABLE 42-9  Classification of Brain Tumors

| Tumor Type | Tumor | Characteristics |
|---|---|---|
| **Primary Tumors**<br>Intracerebral tumors<br>Account for 40% to 50% of all brain tumors<br>Originates from neuroglia and invades brain tissue<br>Most common type of brain tumor | *Glioma*<br>• Astrocytoma<br><br>• Glioblastoma multiforme<br>• Ependymoma<br><br><br>• Oligodendroglioma<br><br>• Astroblastoma | Most common glioma<br>Graded I to IV according to degree of cell differentiation<br>Most malignant form<br>Fast growing<br>Tumor that develops from lining of ventricles<br>Graded I to IV according to degree of cell differentiation<br>Slow growing<br>Rare, slow growing<br>May be encapsulated<br>Benign |
| Extracerebral tumors<br><br>Tumors arising from the supporting structures of the nervous system<br>Account for 10% to 15% of all brain tumors | Medulloblastoma<br><br><br>Meningioma<br><br><br>Acoustic neuroma | Fast growing and malignant<br>Occurs primarily in children; can occur in adults<br>Found in cerebellum<br>Slow growing<br>Develops in meninges (especially dura)<br>Firm and encapsulated<br>Slow growing<br>Benign<br>Originates from Schwann cells of the cranial nerve XIII<br>May also affect cranial nerves V, VII, IX, and X<br>Also called neurofibromatosis<br>Genetic origin due to autosomal dominant mendelian trait<br>Firm, encapsulated lesions attached to nerve |
| Congenital (developmental) tumors<br>Account for 4% to 8% of all brain tumors | Hemangioblastoma<br><br>Craniopharyngioma | Vascular tumor<br>Slow growing<br>Originates from Rathke's pouch<br>Solid or cystic tumor<br>Compresses pituitary gland<br>Presses on the third ventricle and may cause blockage of cerebrospinal fluid (CSF) |
| Pituitary adenomas<br>Slow growing<br>Account for 8% to 12% of all brain tumors | Chromophobic<br><br>Eosinophilic<br>Basophilic | Account for 90% of pituitary tumors<br>Nonsecreting tumor<br>Secreting tumors that produce growth hormone<br>Secreting tumors that produce adrenocorticotropic hormone<br>Fast growing |
| **Secondary Tumors**<br>Metastatic brain tumors<br>  Slow-growing tumors that arise from other parts of the body<br>Account for 10% of all brain tumors<br>Tumors of the lung, breast, lower gastrointestinal tract, pancreas, kidney, skin | | Usually well differentiated from the brain |

## PATHOPHYSIOLOGY AND MANIFESTATIONS

Brain tumors may be classified as benign or malignant, based on the tissue type and characteristics of the cells. The use of the term *benign* may be misleading. A tumor that is benign by histologic examination but is surgically inaccessible may continue to expand, increasing intracranial pressure and causing neurologic deficits, herniation, and finally death. In discussions of brain tumors, the term *malignant* is used to describe the lack of cell differentiation, the invasive nature of the tumor, and its ability to metastasize.

Brain tumors also may be classified as primary or metastatic, depending on their origin (Table 42–9). Primary tumors of CNS tissue arise from the cells and structures that are found within the brain, for example, neurons and neuroglia. The primary intracranial tumors that originate in the skull cavity but not from brain tissue itself arise from the supporting structures; including the meninges, pituitary gland, and pineal gland. Primary brain tumors rarely metastasize outside the central nervous system. Metastatic brain tumors originate from structures outside the brain, such as the breasts, lungs, and prostate gland.

Focal disturbances take place when there is compression of brain tissue and infiltration or direct invasion of brain parenchyma with destruction of neural tissue. As the tumor grows, edema develops in adjacent tissues. The mechanism is not completely understood, but it is thought that an osmotic gradient causes the tumor to absorb fluid. Some tumors may cause hemorrhage. Venous obstruction and edema due to breakdown of the blood-brain barrier increase intracranial volume and intracranial pressure. Obstruction of the circulation of CSF from the lateral ventricles to the subarachnoid space causes hydrocephalus.

An estimated 25% of people with cancer develop brain metastasis. Metastatic brain tumors present in the same way as primary brain tumors, with increased ICP, and focal and/or diffuse cerebral dysfunction. The most common source of intracranial metastasis is cancer of the lung. Other common primary sites are the breast, kidney, and gastrointestinal tract. The metastasis reaches the brain through the circulation. In more than 75% of cases, the tumors are multiple and are scattered through the cerebellum and cerebrum (McCance & Huether, 2002).

Multiple manifestations can develop as a result of the growth of the tumor, while others are related to the location of the lesion (see the box below). Some of the more common manifestations include changes in cognition or consciousness, headache that is usually worse in the morning, seizures, and vomiting. Compression of brain tissue and the invasion of the brain tumor into the cerebral tissue may lead to changes typi-cally seen with cerebral edema and increased ICP. Cerebral blood supply may diminish as the tumor compresses blood vessels. Shifts in brain tissue can occur, leading to brain herniation syndromes and, if untreated, death.

## COLLABORATIVE CARE

Treatment for a brain tumor may involve chemotherapy, radiation therapy, surgery, or any combination of these. Several variables are considered when selecting the appropriate treatment modality: the size and location of the tumor, the type of tumor, related symptoms (such as neurologic deficits), and the client's overall condition.

### Diagnostic Tests

The following diagnostic tests may be ordered.

- *CT scan* or *MRI* with gadolinium enhancement can locate the tumor and define its size, shape, extent to which normal anatomy is distorted, and the degree of any associated cerebral edema.
- *Arteriography* may show stretching or displacement of cerebral vessels by the tumor, as well as the presence of tumor vascularity.
- *EEG* provides information about cerebral function, may demonstrate focal or diffuse changes, and is useful if seizures are present.
- *Endocrine studies* are conducted if a pituitary tumor is suspected.

### Medications

The choice of drug for treatment is based on the type of tumor, its location, and the client's response to therapy. The use of chemotherapy to treat brain tumors is still emerging. An intraventricular method of medication administration uses an Ommaya reservoir that has been surgically implanted into a lateral ventricle of the brain (see Figure 42–8). Other medications that may be prescribed include corticosteroids and anticonvulsants.

### Treatments

#### Surgery

Surgery is used to remove tumors, to reduce the size of the tumor, or for symptom relief (*palliation*). The type of procedure, the surgical approach, and the timing of surgery (emergency versus planned procedure) influence the overall nursing management of the client having intracranial surgery.

Some of the more common intracranial neurosurgical procedures follow:

- **Burr hole.** A hole made in the skull with a special drill. The hole may facilitate the evacuation of an extracerebral clot, or a series of holes may be made in preparation of craniotomy (see Figure 42–7).
- **Craniotomy.** A surgical opening into the cranial cavity (Figure 42–9 ■). For a craniotomy, a series of burr holes are made. The bone between the holes is then cut with a special

## Manifestations of Brain Tumors

### FRONTAL LOBE TUMORS
- Inappropriate behavior
- Personality changes
- Inability to concentrate
- Impaired judgment
- Recent memory loss
- Headache
- Expressive aphasia
- Motor dysfunctions

### PARIETAL LOBE TUMORS
- Sensory deficits: paresthesia, loss of two-point discrimination, visual field deficits

### TEMPORAL LOBE TUMORS
- Psychomotor seizures

### OCCIPITAL LOBE TUMORS
- Visual disturbances

### CEREBELLUM TUMORS
- Disturbances in coordination and equilibrium

### PITUITARY TUMORS
- Endocrine dysfunction
- Visual deficits
- Headache

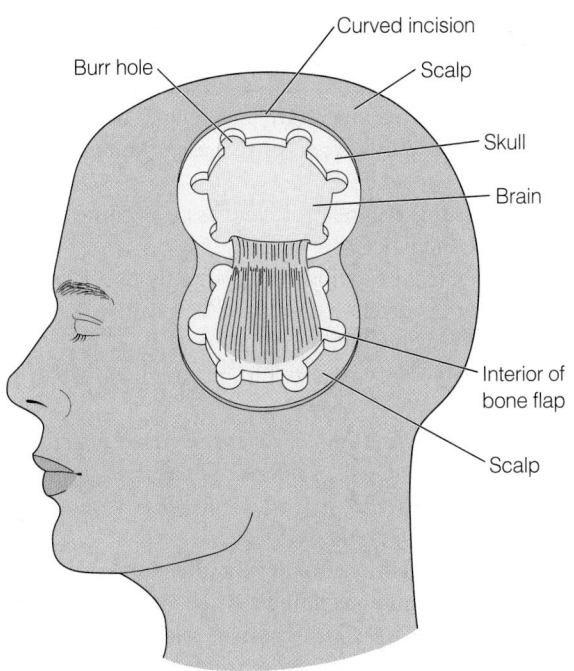

**Figure 42–9** ■ In a craniotomy, a portion of the skull and overlying scalp is removed to allow access to the brain.

saw called a craniotome. The tumor is excised, and the bone flap is turned down. A craniotomy may also be performed to repair defects associated with traumatic head injuries or to repair a cerebral aneurysm.

A *supratentorial craniotomy* refers to surgery above the tentorium. It provides access to the frontal, temporal, parietal, and occipital lobes. The incision for this procedure is usually within the hairline over the area involved.

An *infratentorial craniotomy* refers to surgery below the tentorium. Access is provided to lesions in the cerebellum and the brainstem. The incision is made at the nape of the neck, around the occipital lobe.

- **Craniectomy.** An excision of a portion of the skull and complete removal of the bone flap. This procedure may be done to provide decompression after cerebral edema. Pressure on the brain structures is lessened by providing space for expansion.
- **Cranioplasty.** Plastic repair to the skull in which synthetic material is inserted to replace the cranial bone that was removed. This procedure may be performed after a large craniectomy. The plastic repair restores the contour and integrity of the cranium.

### Radiation Therapy

Radiation therapy may be administered alone or as adjunctive therapy with surgery. Radiation is often the treatment of choice for surgically inaccessible tumors; it may also be used to decrease the size of a tumor prior to surgery. Tumors that were not completely excised by surgery may also be treated with radiation.

### Specialty Procedures

Technologic advances—including the development of special instruments, the use of stereotaxic techniques for localizing a specific target, and the use of the laser beam—have greatly advanced neurosurgical practice. Microsurgery involves an operating microscope with microinstruments and supportive illumination equipment. With stereotaxic techniques, the client is positioned to allow location of discrete areas of the brain that control specific functions and exact locations of deep brain lesions. The use of a laser beam for excision of a tumor results in less damage to surrounding tissue and less postoperative swelling. The gamma knife, which is not actually a knife but a gamma unit, consists of a heavily shielded helmet containing 201 sources of cobalt-60, which is capable of destroying deep and otherwise inaccessible lesions in a single treatment session.

## NURSING CARE

The nursing care of the client with a brain tumor includes support during the diagnostic period and specific management as directed by the selected treatment. The foundation for care is data from the health history and physical assessment, which includes identifying neurologic deficits. This information directs planning and implementing care. Many of the alterations in health commonly experienced by the client with a brain tumor have been discussed throughout this chapter, including altered level of consciousness, increased intracranial pressure, and seizures. The client will require intensive care in the immediate postoperative period.

## Nursing Diagnoses and Interventions

This section of the chapter focuses on nursing interventions for the client who has intracranial surgery. The nursing diagnoses discussed are anxiety, risk for infection, ineffective protection, acute pain, and disturbed self-esteem.

### Anxiety

The diagnosis of a brain tumor brings anxiety and feelings of uncertainty about the future. Both the client and family members are likely to be apprehensive and require education and emotional support.

- Assist through routine medical procedures, including blood work and radiologic studies. *Baseline laboratory and radiologic studies are needed to ensure that the client has no other preexisting medical condition. Explaining the procedures and assisting the client through this process helps decrease anxiety.*
- Reinforce, clarify, and repeat information. *Both client and family may have limited understanding of the scheduled diagnostic tests, procedures, and treatment modalities. The client may be confused or have altered thought processes as a result of the tumor. Information may need to be repeated or reexplained.*

- Encourage client and family to verbalize feelings, questions, and fears; provide realistic information appropriate to their level of understanding. *Verbalization helps reduce anxiety and fear.*
- Review client and family strengths and effective coping skills. *Personal strengths, support systems, and coping skills can aid in the development of appropriate strategies to reduce anxiety.*
- Arrange for a member of the clergy to visit if desired. *Faith in a higher being is often a strong source of strength and support.*
- Provide preoperative teaching, including the following information.
  - Type of anesthesia and surgery
  - Time surgery will begin and expected length of procedure and recovery room stay
  - Where the client will be taken after surgery (CCU, ICU) (If possible, show the client and family the CCU or ICU and introduce them to the nurse who will be in charge of care after the surgery.)
  - Where family can wait during and following surgery
  - Appearance of the client after surgery, which may include swollen, bruised eyelids and other facial features; a large dressing covering the head; and a tracheostomy or endotracheal tube
  - Behavior of the client after surgery, which will differ depending on the site of surgery, although cognitive and behavioral changes are common
  *Information about what to expect reduces anxiety.*
- Allow time for client and family to be together. *Clients and families need quiet time together to support each other and prepare emotionally for surgery.*

### Risk for Infection

The client who has had intracranial surgery is at risk for infection from multiple invasive lines, the scalp wound, and the risk of introduction of bacteria into the operative area. The nurse provides interventions to monitor for and prevent infection.

- Assess for leakage of CSF:
  - Presence of glucose in clear drainage from ears, nose, or wound
  - Complaints of "something dripping down the back of the throat"
  - Constant swallowing
  *These manifestations indicate an opening in the dura, which provides an avenue for an ascending infection.*
- Provide interventions to prevent contamination of area leaking CSF:
  - If leaking from the nose: Keep head of bed elevated 20 degrees unless contraindicated; do not suction nasally; do not clean nose; tell client not to put finger in nose; do not insert packing.
  - If leaking from the ear: Position client on side of leakage unless contraindicated; do not clean ear; tell client not to put finger in ear; do not insert packing.
  - Place a sterile dressing over the area of drainage and change as soon as it becomes damp.
  *Leakage of CSF indicates a break in the dura and increases the risk of an ascending infection. Surgery may be necessary*

*to repair the break; however, the leak usually heals spontaneously in about 1 week.*
- Monitor and report manifestations of infection:
  - Take and record temperature on a regular basis.
  - Assess IV insertion sites for redness, swelling, drainage, and pain.
  - Assess scalp wound for redness, swelling, bulging, drainage, and pain.
  - Assess for manifestations of meningitis: fever and chills, increasing headache, neck stiffness, positive Kernig's or Brudzinski's sign, photophobia.
  - Monitor laboratory reports for increased white blood cell count.
  *Intact skin is the first line of defense against infection. Any break in the skin increases the risk of infection. Intracranial surgery increases the risk of meningitis, with infectious agents ascending into the brain.*
- Implement interventions to prevent infection:
  - Use strict aseptic technique when changing dressings and when caring for wound drains and ICP monitor lines.
  - Keep the client's hands away from drains and dressings; use mitten restraints if necessary.
  - Administer prescribed antibiotics.
  *Sterile technique decreases the risk of introducing infection into a wound. Antibiotics are usually prescribed prophylactically to prevent infection.*

### Ineffective Protection

The client who has intracranial surgery does not have normal human defenses against changes in intracranial pressure and is also at risk from cerebral edema and a shift of intracerebral contents. In addition, the surgery may cause cerebral bleeding or hematoma formation.

- Monitor for manifestations of increased intracranial pressure:
  - Restlessness, agitation, and decreasing level of consciousness
  - Headache
  - Vomiting
  - Seizures
  - Decreasing sensory and motor function
  - Changes in pupil size and reaction
  - Changes in vital signs: altered respiratory rate or depth, increasing pulse pressure, decreasing pulse rate, increasing blood pressure
  - Abnormal posturing
  *Increasing intracranial pressure is manifested by alterations in the functions and centers controlled by the brain.*
- Implement interventions to decrease the risk of increased intracranial pressure:
  - Elevate the head of the bed 15 to 30 degrees as prescribed (unless contraindicated).
  - Avoid neck flexion or rotation; keep head in midline position unless a large bone flap or mass was removed; then position the client on unoperated side to decrease venous congestion in the operative area.
  - Do not take rectal temperatures.

- Avoid clustering activities that increase intracranial pressure: suctioning, turning, bathing.
- Administer medications to prevent vomiting.
- Do not suction for more than 10 seconds at one time.
- Teach the client (if possible) to avoid coughing, sneezing, and straining to have a bowel movement.
- Maintain fluid restrictions as prescribed.
- For internal shunts: Avoid pressure on the shunt, reservoir, or tubing. Pump the shunt as prescribed.
- For external shunts: Avoid kinks in tubing, and maintain the drainage collecting device and client's head at the prescribed levels.

*Keeping the head of the bed slightly elevated facilitates venous drainage from the brain. Neck flexion or rotation disrupts circulation to and from the brain. Rectal stimulation, suctioning, turning, bathing, coughing, sneezing, and straining to have a bowel movement all initiate Valsalva's maneuver, which constricts the jugular veins and impairs venous return from the brain. Fluid restriction may be prescribed to dehydrate the client slightly and lessen ICP.*

- Maintain (as much as possible) a quiet, calm, softly lighted environment. Avoid excessive sensory stimulation. *These interventions promote rest and decrease stimulation, thereby reducing ICP.*
- Implement interventions to prevent seizures or, if they occur, to prevent injury to the client:
  - Pad side rails of the bed.
  - Place bed in lowest position, and keep side rails up.
  - Carry out interventions to prevent and treat increased intracranial pressure.
  - Have an oral airway and suction equipment immediately available.
  - Administer prescribed anticonvulsants.
  - If a seizure occurs: Maintain a patent airway; do not restrain client; do not force anything into the client's mouth; provide physical and emotional support.

*These interventions promote safety and help prevent injury. Anticonvulsants are often prescribed prophylactically to prevent seizures after intracranial surgery.*

- Carefully monitor hydration status. Compare trends in intake and output, laboratory results of serum osmolality, and urine specific gravity and osmolality. *Changes in fluid balance and osmolality may result from excess intravenous fluids, osmotic diuretics, surgically induced diabetes insipidus or syndrome of inappropriate antidiuretic hormone secretion, fever, diarrhea, tube feedings, or hyperglycemia.*

## Acute Pain

The client who has intracranial surgery has pain, manifested as a headache, as a result of either compression or displacement of brain tissue or from increased intracranial pressure. A headache may also be a manifestation of meningitis.

- Assess the location, duration, and intensity of the pain, using a scale from 0 (no pain) to 10 (worst pain) in the client who can verbally communicate. *The client is the best source of information about pain.*

- Implement interventions to reduce the pain:
  - Raise the head of the bed slightly.
  - Reduce noise and bright lights in the room.
  - If allowed, loosen head dressing.
  - Administer narcotic analgesics with caution.

*Nonpharmacologic measures may be used to reduce increased intracranial pressure and headache.*

**PRACTICE ALERT** *Narcotic analgesics mask changes in eye signs and depress respirations.* ■

### Disturbed Self-Esteem

The client who has intracranial surgery has many alterations that affect self-esteem and body image. Physical changes include a loss of hair on the scalp, swelling and bruising in the eyelids and face, and perhaps an indentation in the skull. The client is no longer independent in self-care, but must depend on others to meet basic needs. There are often long-term neurologic deficits, affecting areas such as speech, vision, and motor abilities, which require changes in roles and relationships.

- Assess for verbal and nonverbal manifestations of negative self-esteem:
  - Denial of changes
  - Preoccupation with changes
  - Refusal to look in the mirror
  - Withdrawal from family and friends
  - Expressions of grief and loss (see Chapter 11) ⊘⊃

*Low self-esteem can be initiated by stressful situations and changes in body image.*

- Provide interventions to improve self-concept:
  - Limit negative self-assessment.
  - Help focus on positive areas of life.
  - Help identify sources of support and strength.
  - Help identify and use helpful coping methods.
  - Encourage significant others to visit.
  - Encourage independence in self-care.

*Self-esteem is derived from one's own perceptions of competence and from the responses of others. When one's self-concept and self-ideal are congruent, self-esteem is enhanced.*

### Home Care

The effect of the possible outcomes following the surgery produces fear in both client and family, interfering with their ability to retain information. Also, the client may have cognitive or neurologic deficits that interfere with learning. Family members also must be assessed for their ability to cope with the stress of the surgery. Information may have to be repeated several times.

Clients and their families who have experienced intracranial surgery require emotional support. The process of recovery is often extended and may involve adaptation to change in body image and management of any motor or sensory deficits. The family should be involved in the care of the client. If family members are willing, they may begin to assist with ADLs while the client is in the hospital, such as assisting with personal hygiene and meals. Clients should also be encouraged to

## Nursing Care Plan
### A Client with a Brain Tumor

Claire Lange is a 44-year-old television announcer. During one night's broadcast, she confuses several major news items so badly that her co-anchor tries to correct her. Ms. Lange responds angrily that she does not need any help and then rises and storms off the set. As she leaves the camera area, she limps noticeably and appears to drag her left leg. The show's producer asks her what is wrong; she screams that nothing is wrong—she simply has another headache. He follows her to her dressing room and inquires about her headaches. She tells him that they come and go but have been getting worse lately. He then asks her if she has injured her left leg; she responds that the leg was weak because she was tired. As the producer leaves the dressing room, Ms. Lange begins to shake and collapses on the floor. The producer recognizes that she is having a seizure and calls for an ambulance.

Ms. Lange is admitted to the neurology floor of the local hospital for evaluation. A CT scan, MRI study, and EEG are completed and identify an intracranial mass. A biopsy of the mass is positive for malignant cells. A glioma in the frontal lobe is identified, and surgery is scheduled for that week.

### ASSESSMENT

When Clara Rosetti, RN, enters Ms. Lange's room, she sees Ms. Lange looking at her shoulder-length hair in the mirror. Ms. Lange tells Ms. Rosetti that she has never in her life worn her hair any shorter, and "Now you're going to cut it all off!" She paces the room and makes the statement, "I guess the hair isn't really important if I survive this situation." She also says that she has a headache.

### DIAGNOSES

- *Acute pain* (headache) related to tumor and increase in intracranial pressure
- *Disturbed body image* related to upcoming hair loss and cranial incision
- *Anxiety* related to unknown future following surgery

### EXPECTED OUTCOMES

- Verbalize the causes of pain.
- Verbalize an understanding of the changes in body appearance that are associated with the scheduled intracranial surgery (e.g., shaving of the head prior to surgery, cranial incision, facial swelling postoperatively).
- Identify measures that will help minimize the effect of the hair loss.
- Verbalize a reduction in anxiety.

### PLANNING AND IMPLEMENTATION

- Assess level of discomfort using a rating scale of 0 to 10.
- Provide a quiet, nonstimulating environment.
- Position the client for comfort, keeping the head of the bed elevated to promote venous drainage.
- Assess level of consciousness for potential increases in ICP.
- Encourage to verbalize feelings about the surgery.
- Suggest measures that may help minimize the hair loss, such as the use of turbans, scarves, hats, and wigs.
- Suggest relaxation techniques to decrease anxiety.

### EVALUATION

By the time of surgery, Ms. Lange has recognized the relationship between the brain tumor and the headache. She states that lying in a flat position and coughing increase the headache. The head of the bed is kept at a 30- to 45-degree angle. Daily activities are spaced to provide periods of rest. Ms. Lange demonstrates no significant changes in level of consciousness. She has talked about the effect of the hair loss and her television responsibilities. Ms. Lange has learned that the hair preparation would be done in surgery and that the hair would be saved for her. She states she has already consulted her hair stylist and that "scarves and turbans are on the way."

### Critical Thinking in the Nursing Process

1. Outline interventions to decrease intracranial pressure both before and after surgery.
2. When making your initial assessments on the morning of surgery, you find that Ms. Lange has a decreased pulse and increased blood pressure. She tells you her headache is worse and suddenly vomits. What do you do now?
3. Ms. Lange asks you to be sure that she has absolutely no visitors after surgery, because she knows how ugly she will look. How would you respond?
4. Design a plan of care for Ms. Lange for the nursing diagnosis, *Powerlessness*.

See Evaluating Your Response in Appendix C.

---

take an active role in their own care. Discharge planning includes a discussion of the following topics: medication information; wound care; the use of wigs, turbans, hats, or colorful scarves; and the importance of follow-up visits. In addition, emphasize the importance of reporting manifestations such as stiff neck, increasing headache, elevated temperature, new motor or sensory deficits, vision changes, or seizures.

Provide information about the overall treatment plan, management of deficits and/or disabilities, and future needs. Specific teaching topics are as follows:

- Safety measures for motor deficits, sensory deficits, lack of coordination, seizures, and cognitive deficits
- Comfort measures for nausea, vomiting, and pain
- Measures for communication if aphasia is present
- Measures to improve vision if visual deficits are present
- How to buy wigs and hairpieces
- Referrals to support groups and community resources
- Helpful resources:
  - American Cancer Society
  - American Brain Tumor Association
  - National Brain Tumor Foundation

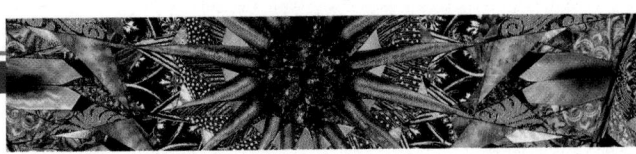

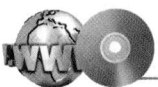 EXPLORE MediaLink

NCLEX review questions, case studies, care plan activities, MediaLink applications, and other interactive resources for this chapter can be found on the Companion Website at www.prenhall.com/lemone.

Click on Chapter 42 to select the activities for this chapter. For animations, video clips, more NCLEX review questions, and an audio glossary, access the Student CD-ROM accompanying this textbook.

## TEST YOURSELF

1. Which of the following pathophysiologic events results in irregular respiratory patterns as LOC decreases?

   a. Pressure on the meninges
   b. Reflexive motor responses
   c. Loss of the oculocephalic reflex
   d. Brainstem responds only to changes in $Paco_2$

2. The unconscious client has depressed or absent gag and swallowing reflexes. Which nursing diagnosis would be appropriate?

   a. *Decreased intracranial adaptive capacity*
   b. *Risk for aspiration*
   c. *Imbalanced nutrition: Less than body requirements*
   d. *Ineffective breathing pattern*

3. What is the rationale for the use of osmotic diuretics to treat increased ICP?

   a. Hyperthermia increases the cerebral metabolic rate and exacerbates increased ICP
   b. Increased blood osmolality draws edematous fluid into the vascular system

   c. Clients with ICP are at increased risk for gastrointestinal hemorrhage
   d. Brain injury and increased ICP often cause seizures

4. What manifestation is consistently assessed in clients with generalized seizures?

   a. Loss of consciousness
   b. Repetitive nonpurposeful activity
   c. Tonic movements
   d. Clonic movements

5. When assessing a client with a head injury, you test fluid dripping from one ear for glucose. What are you assessing for?

   a. Infection
   b. Blood
   c. CSF
   d. Serum

See Test Yourself answers in Appendix C.

## BIBLIOGRAPHY

American Cancer Society. (2001). *Cancer facts and figures–2001*. Atlanta: ACS.

Barker, E. (1998). The xenon CT: A new neuro tool. *RN, 61*(2), 22–25.

Brain Trauma Foundation and the Joint Section on Neurotrauma and Critical Care of the American Association of Neurological Surgeons and the Congress of Neurological Surgeons. (1995). *Guidelines for the management of severe head injury*. Park Ridge, IL: The Brain Trauma Foundation.

Bucher, L., & Melander, S. (1999). *Critical Care Nursing*. Philadelphia: Saunders

Chiocca, E. (1997). Action stat! Bacterial meningitis. *Nursing, 27*(9), 33.

Dodick, D. (1997). Headache as a symptom of ominous disease... what are the warning signals? *Postgraduate Medicine, 101*(5), 46–50, 55–56, 62.

Duff, D., & Wells, D. (1997). Postcomatose unawareness/vegetative state following severe brain injury: A content methodology. *Journal of Neuroscience Nursing, 29*(5), 305–307, 312–317.

Edmeads, J. (1997). Headaches in older people: How are they different in this age group? *Postgraduate Medicine, 101*(5), 91–94, 98, 100.

Fettes, I. (1997). Menstrual migraine: Methods of prevention and control. *Postgraduate Medicine, 101*(5), 67–70, 73–75, 77.

Hickey, J. (2003). *The clinical practice of neurological and neurosurgical nursing* ( 5th ed.). Philadelphia: Lippincott.

Hilton, G. (2001). Emergency: Acute head injury. *American Journal of Nursing, 101*(9), 51–52.

———.(1997). Seizure disorder in adults: Evaluation and management of new onset seizures. *Nurse Practitioner: American Journal of Primary Health Care, 22*(9), 42, 54, 49–50.

Horowitz, S., Passik, S., & Malkin, M. (1996). "In sickness and in health": A group intervention for spouses caring for patients with brain tumors. *Journal of Psychosocial Oncology, 14*(2), 43–56.

Johnson, M., & Maas, M. (Eds.). (1997). *Nursing outcomes classification (NOC)*. St. Louis: Mosby.

Kee, J. (2001). *Handbook of laboratory and diagnostic tests* (4th ed.). Upper Saddle River, NJ: Prentice Hall.

Kidd, P., & Wagner, K. (2001). *High-acuity nursing* (3rd ed.). Upper Saddle River, NJ: Prentice Hall.

King, D. (1999). Central nervous system infections. Basic concepts. *Nursing Clinics of North America, 34*(3), 761–771.

Levitt, M., Lamb, S., & Voss, B. (1996). Brain tumor support group: Content themes and mechanisms of support. *Oncology Nursing Forum, 23*(8), 1247–1356.

Lin, Jong-mi. (2001). Overview of migraine. *Journal of Neuroscience Nursing, 33*(1), 6–13.

Liporace, J. (1997). Women's issues in epilepsy: Menses, childbearing and more... *Postgraduate Medicine, 102*(1), 123–124, 127–129, 133–135.

Long, L., & McAuley, J. (1996). Epilepsy: A review of seizure types, etiologies, diagnosis, treatment, and nursing implications. *Critical Care Nurse, 16*(4), 83–92.

Long, L., & Reeves, A. (1997). The practical aspects of epilepsy: Critical components of comprehensive patient care. *Journal of Neuroscience Nursing, 29*(4), 249–254.

McCance, K., & Huether, S. (2002). *Pathophysiology: The biologic basis for disease in adults and children* (4th ed.). St. Louis: Mosby.

McCloskey, J., & Bulechek, G. (Eds.). (2000). *Nursing interventions classification (NIC)* (3rd ed.). St. Louis: Mosby.

McKenry, L., & Salerno, E. (1998). *Pharmacology in nursing* (20th ed.). St. Louis: Mosby.

McNair, N. (1999). Traumatic brain injury. *Nursing Clinics of North America, 34*(3), 637–659.

McNew, C., Hunt, S., & Warner, L. (1997). How to help your patient with epilepsy. *Nursing, 27*(9), 56–63.

Miller, L., & Chol, C. (1997). Meningitis in older patients: How to diagnose and treat a deadly infection. *Geriatrics, 52*(8), 43–44, 47–50, 55.

Myers, F. (2000). Meningitis: The fears, the facts. *RN, 63*(11), 53–57.

North American Nursing Diagnosis Association. (2001). *Nursing diagnoses: Definitions & classification 2001–2002.* Philadelphia: NANDA.

Porth, C. (2002). *Pathophysiology: Concepts of altered health states* (6th ed.). Philadelphia: Lippincott.

Schultz, R. (1997). Eggs and brains. . . the basics of head trauma. *Emergency Medical Services, 26*(4), 29–34, 75.

Shafer, P. (1999). Epilepsy and seizures. *Nursing Clinics of North America, 34*(3), 743–759.

Shannon, M., Wilson, B., & Stang, C. (2002). *Drug guide 2002.* Upper Saddle River, NJ: Prentice Hall.

Sullivan, J. (2000). Positioning of patients with severe traumatic brain injury: Research-based practice. *Journal of Neuroscience Nursing, 32*(4), 204–209.

Tierney, L., McPhee, S., & Papadakis, M. (Eds.). (2001). *Current medical diagnosis & treatment* (40th ed). New York: McGraw-Hill.

Wall, B., Howard, J., & Perry-Phillips, J. (1995). Validation of two nursing diagnoses: Increased intracranial pressure and high risk for increased intracranial pressure. In M. Rantz & P. LeMone (Eds). *Classification of nursing diagnoses: Proceedings of the 11th conference* (pp. 166–170). Glendate, CA: CINAHL.

Wright, M. (1999). Resuscitation of the multi-trauma patient with head injury. *AACN Clinical Issues, 10*(1), 32–45.

Yarbo, C., Frogge, M., Goodman, M., & Groenwald, S. (Eds.). (2001). *Cancer nursing: Principles and practice* (5th ed.). Sudbury, MA: Jones & Bartlett.

# CHAPTER 43

# Nursing Care of Clients with Neurologic Disorders

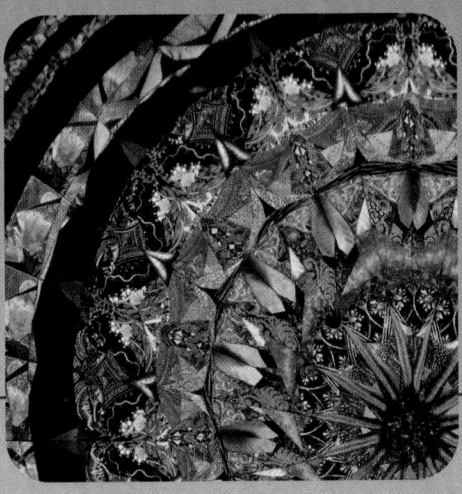

**MediaLink**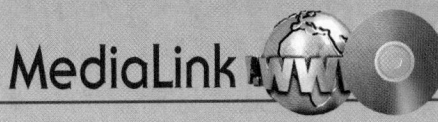

## www.prenhall.com/lemone

Additional resources for this chapter can be found on the Student CD-ROM accompanying this textbook, and on the Companion Website at www. prenhall.com/lemone. Click on Chapter 43 to select the activities for this chapter.

**CD-ROM**
- Audio Glossary
- NCLEX Review

***Animations***
- Multiple Sclerosis
- Dopamine
- Levodopa

***Videos***
- Akinesia
- Bradykinesia

**Companion Website**
- More NCLEX Review
- Case Study
    Parkinson's Disease
- Care Plan Activity
    Guillain-Barré Syndrome
- MediaLink Application
    Alzheimer's Disease

## LEARNING OUTCOMES

After completing this chapter, you will be able to:

- Apply knowledge of normal anatomy, physiology, and assessments when providing nursing care for clients with neurologic disorders (see Chapter 40).

- Explain the pathophysiology of neurologic disorders.

- Identify diagnostic tests used to diagnose selected neurologic disorders.

- Discuss the nursing implications of medications used to treat clients experiencing neurologic disorders.

- Discuss collaborative care for clients with neurologic disorders.

- Provide appropriate nursing care to clients undergoing neurologic surgery.

- Use the nursing process as a framework for providing individualized care to clients with neurologic disorders.

This chapter discusses a variety of neurologic disorders. Included are degenerative disorders, peripheral nervous system disorders, and disorders caused by neurotoxins and viruses. For many of the disorders, nursing care is based on similar nursing diagnoses. To avoid repeating those diagnoses and interventions for each disorder, they have been divided among the nursing care discussions as appropriate.

# DEGENERATIVE NEUROLOGIC DISORDERS

Degenerative neurologic disorders can affect the central nervous system and the peripheral nerves. By progressively disrupting cognitive processes or motor functions, disorders such as multiple sclerosis, Alzheimer's disease, and Parkinson's disease strike at the core of an individual's sense of personal autonomy and well-being and can be psychologically and emotionally devastating to family members and caregivers.

Ongoing medical research into degenerative neurologic disorders offers an increasing measure of hope to clients and their families. The discovery of genetic or biochemical markers associated with some of these disorders is leading to the development of effective screening and diagnostic methods. In addition, new drugs may make it possible to halt the progression of the disorders in some clients, transforming the disorders into manageable conditions.

## THE CLIENT WITH ALZHEIMER'S DISEASE

**Alzheimer's disease (AD)** (also called *dementia of Alzheimer type [DAT]* or *senile disease complex*) is a form of dementia characterized by progressive, irreversible deterioration of general intellectual functioning. **Dementia** is defined by the World Health Organization as a chronic or progressive disease of the brain in which multiple cortical functions, calculation, learning capacity, language, and judgment are disturbed. Impairments of cognitive function are usually accompanied by deterioration in emotional control, social behavior, and motivation.

Memory loss is usually the first sign of Alzheimer's disease. Memory deficits are initially subtle and family members and friends may not suspect a problem until the disease progresses and symptoms become more noticeable. Family members may also deny the symptoms and hide deficits until the person exhibits unsafe or extremely unusual behavior. Progression of the disease varies, but the course is one of deteriorating cognition and judgment with eventual physical decline and total inability to perform ADLs. With the loss of the ability to perform even the most basic ADLs, the burden of meeting the client's needs shifts to the caregiver.

## INCIDENCE AND PREVALENCE

Alzheimer's disease is the most common degenerative neurologic illness and the most common cause of cognitive impairment (Porth, 2002). It accounts for about two-thirds of cases of dementia in America, affecting adults in middle to late life.

Scientists estimate that more than 4 million people have AD, and the number of people with AD doubles every 5 years beyond age 65.

## Risk Factors and Warning Signs

As one ages, the risk of developing AD increases. With numbers of older people increasing, this type of dementia is predicted to also increase. The risk factors for AD are older age, family history, and female gender. Warning signs are:

- Memory loss that affects job skills
- Difficulty performing familiar tasks
- Problems with language
- Disorientation to time and place
- Poor or decreased judgment
- Problems with abstract thinking
- Misplacing things
- Changes in mood or behavior
- Changes in personality
- Loss of initiative

Recognizing early symptoms is important, because the cause of dementia (such as from depression or hypothyroidism) may be reversible. Dementia from AD is not reversible. Treatment, however, can maximize quality of life and allow the affected person to plan for the future.

## PATHOPHYSIOLOGY

The exact cause of AD is unknown. Theories include loss of neurotransmitter stimulation by choline acetyltransferase, mutation for encoding amyloid precursor protein, and alteration in apolipoprotein E. Other possible causes are gene defects on chromosomes 14, 19, or 21, which may lead to clumping and precipitation of insoluble amyloid as plaques. The role of protein kinase C, the link between AD and aluminum, a viral cause, an autoimmune cause, and mitochondrial defects that alter cell metabolism and protein processing are being studied (McCance & Huether, 2002).

Two types of AD exist: *Familial AD* follows an inheritance pattern and *sporadic AD* has no obvious inheritance pattern. AD is further described as early onset (occurring in people younger than 65) and late onset (occurring in people age 65 and older). Early-onset AD usually affects people ages 30 to 60, is relatively rare, and often progresses more rapidly than late-onset AD.

Several structural and chemical changes in the brain occur with AD, especially in the hippocampus and the frontal and temporal lobes of the cerebral cortex. As AD destroys neurons in the hippocampus and related structures, short-term memory fails and the ability to perform easy and familiar tasks declines. The effect of AD on neurons in the cerebral cortex is loss of language skills and judgment. Emotional outbursts and behavior changes (such as wandering and agitation) begin to occur and become more frequent as the disease progresses. Eventually, other areas of the brain are affected; all affected areas begin to atrophy, and the person becomes totally helpless and unresponsive.

Characteristic findings in the brains of AD clients are loss of nerve cells and the presence of *neurofibrillary tangles* and *amyloid plaques* (Figure 43–1 ■). Neurofibrillary tangles result when a tau, a kind of protein in the neurons, becomes distorted and twisted. Tau normally holds together the microtubles, which guide nutrients and molecules to the end of the axon. In AD, tau changes and twists into pairs of filaments, which then join to form tangles. As tau no longer maintains the transport system, communication is lost between neurons. Death of neurons may follow, contributing to the development of dementia.

Groups of nerve cells (and especially the terminal axons) degenerate and clump around an amyloid core as plaque. They are found in the spaces between the neurons of the brain. These plaques, which develop first in areas used for memory and cognition, disrupt transmission of nerve impulses. The plaques

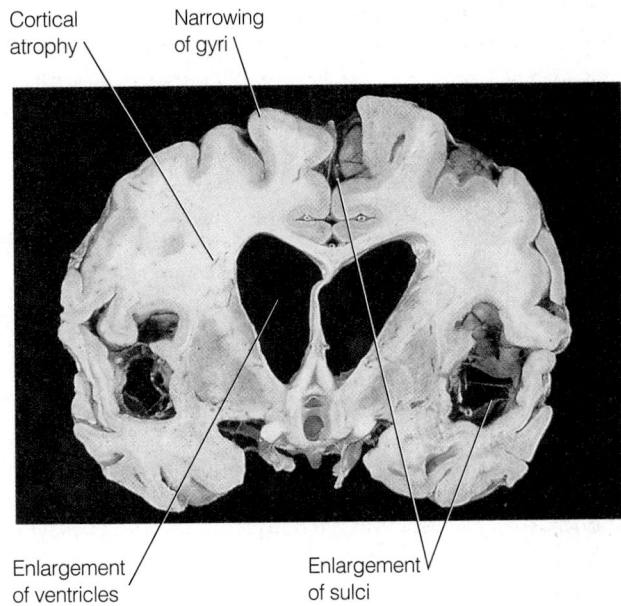

Figure 43–2 ■ Changes in neuroanatomy associated with Alzheimer's disease. Note areas of cortical atrophy, narrowing of the gyri, enlargement of sulci, and ventricular dilation.

consist primarily of insoluble deposits of beta-amyloid, a protein fragment from a larger protein called amyloid precursor protein (APP), mixed with other neurons and nonnerve cells. It is not yet known if plaque formation causes AD or if plaques are a by-product of the AD process.

Blood flow to the affected areas of the brain is decreased. The brain atrophies, and corresponding enlargement of ventricles and sulci is evident (Figure 43–2 ■). As AD progresses, more areas of the brain are affected, with symptoms correlating to those affected areas of the brain. For example, neuronal and neurotransmitter losses in the parietal lobe result in problems with perception and interpretation of environmental stimuli; deficits in the frontal lobe cause changes in personality and emotional lability.

## MANIFESTATIONS

Alzheimer's disease is classified into three stages based on the client's manifestations and abilities, as outlined in the Manifestations box on page 1400. It is important to note that the progression of AD varies for each individual and may not precisely follow the model.

### Stage I AD

In stage I, a client typically appears physically healthy and alert, and cognitive deficits can go undetected unless thorough and periodic evaluations are performed. Usually, family members are the first to notice lapses in memory, subtle changes in personality, or problems in doing simple calculations. AD clients and families may consciously or unconsciously compensate for cognitive deficits by adjusting schedules and routines. Clients may seem restless, forgetful, or uncoordinated.

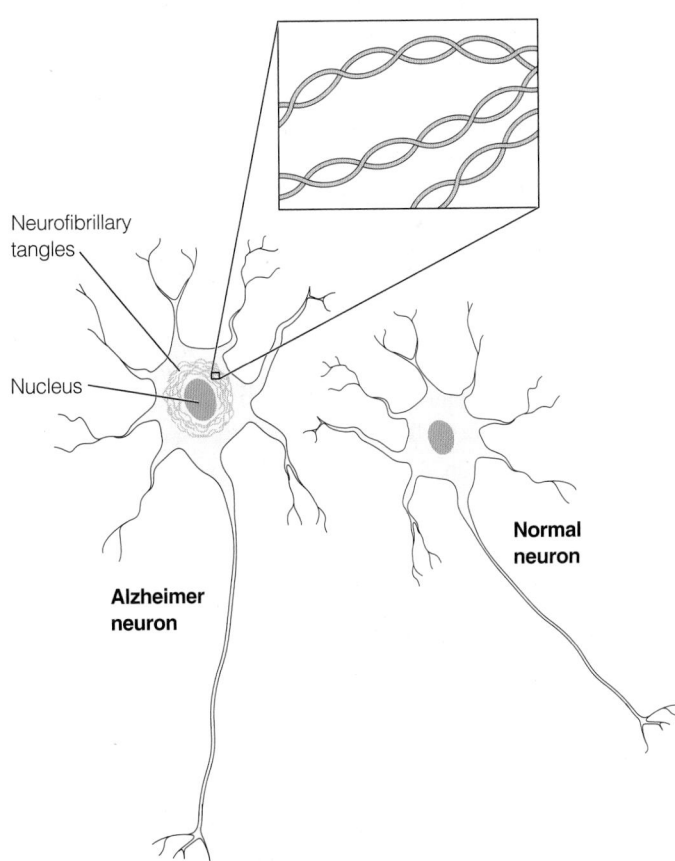

Figure 43–1 ■ Neuron with neurofibrillary tangles seen in Alzheimer's disease.

## Manifestations of Alzheimer's Disease

### STAGE I: APPROXIMATELY 2 TO 4 YEARS

- Short-term memory loss: Forgets location and names of objects and has difficulty learning new information; long-term memory is unaffected.
- Decreased attention span.
- Subtle personality changes: Lacks spontaneity; denial, irritability, and depression are possible.
- Mild cognitive deficits: Attempts to adjust to and cover up memory loss.
- Visuospatial deficits: Some problems with depth perception.

### STAGE II: APPROXIMATELY 2 TO 12 YEARS

- Impaired cognition: Obvious memory deficits and confusion; loss of abstract thinking; astereognosis and agraphia; inability to do math calculations; loss of ability to tell time and time disorientation, manifested as "sundowning"; wandering behavior.

- Personality changes: Becomes easily agitated and irritable; may have delusions or hallucinations.
- Visuospatial deficits: Is unable to dress self; has poor spatial orientation.
- Impaired motor skills: Paces and is restless at times; motor apraxia is evident when using familiar objects.
- Impaired judgment: Diminished social skills; inability to drive a car; inability to make decisions (e.g., choose clothing).

### STAGE III: APPROXIMATELY 2 TO 4 YEARS OR LONGER

- Cognitive abilities grossly decreased or absent: Is usually disoriented to time, place, and person.
- Communication skills usually absent: Is frequently mute.
- Motor skills grossly impaired or absent: Limb rigidity and posture flexion; bowel and bladder incontinence.

## Stage II AD

In stage II, memory deficits are more apparent, and the client is less able to behave spontaneously. Clients may wander and get lost, even in their own homes. Although progression of manifestations continues and orientation to place and time deteriorates, AD clients may still have periods of mental lucidity and engage in time-oriented conversations. Generally, however, clients become more confused and lose their sense of time, leading to changes in sleeping patterns, agitation, and stress. AD clients are less able to make even simple decisions and to adapt to environmental changes. Some AD clients develop severe attacks related to seemingly minor events; this reaction may result from a progressively lowered stress threshold. **Sundowning** is another behavioral change, characterized by increased agitation, time disorientation, and wandering behaviors during afternoon and evening hours; it is accelerated on overcast days.

Language deficits are common in stage II. They include *paraphasia* (using the wrong word), *echolalia* (repetition of words or phrases), and *scanning speech,* in which the client appears to search for words. Eventually, total *aphasia* (absence of speech) may occur. Frustration and depression are common among AD clients as the full extent and implications of the deficits become obvious.

The AD client slowly loses the ability to perform simple tasks required for hygiene or eating because sequencing of tasks is lost. For example, the client may open a can of soup but not remember to pour it into a pan to heat it. Instead, the client might place the can directly on the burner and leave the heat on high even after a smoke alarm sounds. The AD client may falsely interpret the smoke alarm as a telephone ringing, a tornado warning siren, or an ambulance siren. Thus, safety is a high priority for the client in stage II.

Sensorimotor deficits in stage II include *apraxia,* the inability to perform purposeful movements and use objects correctly; *astereognosis,* the inability to identify objects by touch; and *agraphia,* the inability to write. Problems related to malnutri-

tion and decreased fluid intake, such as anemia and constipation, may be evident. Sleep pattern disturbances are also common and are related to the loss of time orientation, sundowning phenomenon, and depression.

## Stage III AD

Stage III brings increasing dependence, with inability to communicate, loss of continence, and progressive loss of cognitive abilities. Common complications include pneumonia, dehydration, malnutrition, falls, depression, delusions, and paranoid reactions. The prognosis of a client with AD is poor, with an average life expectancy of 7 years from time of diagnosis. Death frequently occurs from pneumonia secondary to aspiration.

## COLLABORATIVE CARE

There is no cure for AD, and the main objective of care is to provide an environment that matches the client's functional abilities. Nurses, physicians, physical therapists, and social workers collaborate with the client's family to provide the least restrictive environment in which the client can safely function.

### Diagnostic Tests

Alzheimer's disease is diagnosed by ruling out causes for the client's manifestations. The only definitive method of diagnosis is postmortem examination of brain tissue. An extensive workup is especially important, because the dementia may be due to a reversible or treatable condition. For example, an older client's misuse of medications can lead to overdosing and resulting confusion. Other categories of conditions that may be considered and ruled out include depression, infection, hypothyroidism, dehydration, heart disease, stroke, and chronic obstructive respiratory disease.

The following diagnostic tests may be done.

- *EEG* may reveal a slowed pattern in the later stages of the disorder.

**Orientation to Time**
"What is the date?"

**Registration**
"Listen carefully. I am going to say three words. You say them back after I stop. Ready? Here they are …
HOUSE (pause), CAR (pause), LAKE (pause). Now repeat those words back to me."
[Repeat up to 5 times, but score only the first trial.]

**Naming**
"What is this?" [Point to a pencil or pen.]

**Reading**
"Please read this and do what it says." [Show examinee the words on the stimulus form.]
CLOSE YOUR EYES.

**Figure 43–3** ■ Mini Mental Status Examination Examples.

*Reproduced by special permission of the Publisher, Psychological Assessment Resources, Inc., 16204 North Florida Avenue, Lutz, Florida 33549, from the Mini Mental State Examination, by Marshal Folstein and Susan Folstein, Copyright 1975, 1998, 2001 by Mini Mental LLC, Inc. Further reproduction is prohibited without permission of PAR, Inc. The MMSE can be purchased form PAR, Inc. by calling (800) 331-8378 or (813) 968-3303.*

- *MRI* and *CT scan of the brain* demonstrates shrinkage of the hippocampus as well as changes in other parts of the brain.
- *Positron emission tomography (PET) scan* allows visualizing the activity and interactions of various parts of the brain as they are used during cognitive operations involving information processing.
- *Psychometric evaluation* using the Folstein Mini Mental Status Examination form (Figure 43–3 ■) or a similar instrument reflects the loss of memory and other cognitive skills over time.

Other tests may be performed, depending on the client's manifestations. For example, if the client has hypertension and memory changes, cerebral vascular studies are indicated to exclude multi-infarct dementia or other problems. Ruling out reversible dementia disorders requires evaluation of specific laboratory studies, such as thyroid function studies and measurement of electrolyte and vitamin levels.

Guidelines for the early recognition and assessment of AD have been established by the Agency for Healthcare Research and Quality. A diagnosis of Alzheimer's disease requires the presence of dementia, onset between age 40 and 90 years (most often after age 65), and absence of systemic or brain disorders that could cause mental changes.

## Medications

Cholinesterase inhibitors are used to treat mild to moderate dementia in AD. Tacrine hydrochloride (Cognex) was the first medication specifically approved for the treatment of AD. Donepezil hydrochloride (Aricept) is used to treat mild to moderate AD dementia with some success. Rivastigmine tartrate (Exelon) is also used to treat mild to moderate AD symptoms. It improves the ability to carry out ADLs, decreases agitation and delusions, and improves cognitive function. See the box below for information about medications used to treat AD.

## Medication Administration

### The Client with Alzheimer's Disease (AD)

#### CHOLINERGIC (PARASYMPATHOMIMETICS); CHOLINESTERASE INHIBITORS

Tacrine hydrochloride (Cognex)
Donepezil hydrochloride (Aricept)
Rivastigmine tartrate (Exelon)

In the early stages of AD, the pathologic changes in neurons result in a deficiency of acetylcholine (a key neurotransmitter involved in cognitive functioning). Cholinesterase inhibitors slow the breakdown of acetylcholine release by the remaining intact neurons. In addition, rivastigmine tartrate inhibits the $G_1$ form of acetylcholinesterase (found in higher levels in the brain of clients with AD), so less acetylcholine is degraded. The drugs are used to improve memory in mild to moderate AD dementia.

#### Nursing Responsibilities
- Administer tacrine hydrochloride 1 hour before meals, if possible.
- Administer donepezil hydrochloride at bedtime.
- Administer rivastigmine tartrate (both capsules and liquid) with food. Liquid form may be administered undiluted or mixed with water, juice, or soda. Stir to completely dissolve.

- Monitor for jaundice, increased bilirubin levels, and other signs of liver involvement, such as rising serum aminotransferase (AST, ALT) levels. Therapy is usually decreased when the enzyme level exceeds 4 times normal limits and discontinued when the level reaches 5 times normal.
- Observe for gastrointestinal bleeding and gastric ulcer pain.
- Monitor for cholinergic-related problems: bladder outlet obstruction, seizures, and slowed cardiac rate.
- Assist with ambulation as dizziness is a common side effect.
- Monitor glycemic control in clients with diabetes.
- Assess for improvement in AD symptoms, especially in reasoning, memory, and ADLs.

#### Client and Family Teaching
- Notify the physician promptly if jaundice, seizures, slowed heart rate, GI bleeding, or difficulty urinating occurs.
- Follow directions for times and instructions about administration of specific medication.
- Follow your health care provider's recommendation for periodic EEG, blood tests, and urine tests.
- These medications do not cure AD, and will at some point become ineffective as the disease progresses.

Depression often accompanies AD and is treated with the appropriate medication. Antihistamines and tricyclic antidepressants that have high anticholinergic activity are usually avoided because they can increase AD symptoms. Occasionally clients with AD require tranquilizers such as thioridazine (Mellaril) or haloperidol (Haldol) to manage severe agitation. Other therapies under study to prevent or delay the onset of AD include antioxidants such as vitamin E, anti-inflammatory agents, and estrogen replacement therapy in women.

## Complementary Therapy

The following types of complementary therapy may be used in treating the manifestations of AD.

- Massage, which decreases agitation
- Herbs
  - Ginko biloba, which is thought (among other actions) to improve cognition
  - Huperzine A, a traditional Chinese medicine, which acts as an acetylcholinesterase inhibitor
- Coenzyme Q10, an antioxidant that naturally occurs in the body
- Supplements, such as zinc, selenium, and evening primrose oil
- Therapies involving art, music, sound, and dance

## NURSING CARE

Clients with AD often require intensive, supportive nursing interventions directed at the physical and psychosocial responses to illness. Equally important, the nurse can facilitate the long-term support of these clients by providing teaching and referrals to follow-up care in the community.

## Health Promotion

Health promotion for the client with AD focuses on maintaining functional abilities and safety. If the client will be cared for at home, address safety considerations (see the box below)

as well as the caregivers' abilities to meet the client's basic needs, such as maintaining hygiene and other ADLs. Adapt nursing interventions and teaching to the client's stage of Alzheimer's disease.

## Assessment

Collect the following data through the health history and physical examination (see Chapter 40). Further focused assessments are described with nursing interventions below.

- Health history: family member/caregiver support, living arrangements, ability to carry out ADLs, drug use, work history (e.g., exposure to metals), previous history of multiple strokes, brain injury or brain infection, family history of dementia, sleep pattern, changes in cognition and memory, ability to communicate, changes in behavior
- Physical assessment: height/weight, orientation, abstract reasoning, mental status

## Nursing Diagnoses and Interventions

During the early stage of AD, nursing care focuses on helping the client make minor adaptations to his or her environment. As the client becomes progressively unable to manage self-care tasks, more adaptations are required. Equally important, the caregiver needs much support—both physical and psychosocial—as the client becomes increasingly dependent.

### Impaired Memory

Impaired memory is an appropriate nursing diagnosis in stage I AD. At this stage, techniques to help with the memory loss should be included in teaching for both the client and the caregiver.

- Suggest complementary therapies, such as meditation, massage, or exercise. *These activities can help reduce stress, which can aggravate memory loss.*
- Suggest using a calendar, keeping lists of reminders, or asking someone else to remind of appointments and events. *Written or verbal reminders are helpful if memory is impaired.*

## Meeting Individualized Needs: Safety Interventions for the Client with AD

### DECREASING THE RISK OF FALLS
- Assess usual environment for hazards, such as throw rugs, electrical cords, and slick floors.
- Observe areas of special concern, such as the bathroom, kitchen, and stairs, and modify as needed; for example, provide skidproof surfaces, and mark stairs to show depth.
- Evaluate muscle strength and gait; consult a physical therapist to plan exercises to increase strength and balance.
- Check shoes for fit and support.
- Inquire about alcohol use and medications that affect balance or cause mobility problems; for example, antihypertensive agents can cause dizziness with position changes.
- Use night-lights and increase daytime lighting in dark areas, such as hallways.
- Keep traffic areas free from clutter.

### DECREASING THE INJURIES RELATED TO COGNITIVE IMPAIRMENTS
- Secure items that may be mistakenly ingested, such as cleaning preparations and house plants.
- Modify potentially unsafe areas, such as unenclosed porches.
- Provide double lock systems to outside doors and doors to rooms that are off-limits.
- Protect from fire hazards; for example, make matches and cigarettes inaccessible.
- Fence the yard with a locked gate to prevent wandering.
- Modify the controls on the oven and stove.
- Adjust the water heater to a safe temperature.

### GENERAL SAFETY CONSIDERATIONS
- Plan a calling system for emergencies; have children call at about the same time every day as a check.
- Ensure that the cognitively impaired family member has no access to objects in the home such as knives and guns.

- Recommend using a medication box labeled with days and times. *A medication box is a good way to remember to take medications.*

**PRACTICE ALERT** *It may be necessary to teach the caregiver how to refill the medication box, or to stress the importance of spot-checking if the client fills it.* ■

- If safety is a concern (such as turning on the stove and forgetting it), suggest using alternatives such as a microwave. Program emergency numbers into the telephone. Ask client to consider a Life-line telephone program. *These measures can increase safety.*
- Suggest using cues, such as an alarm on a watch or a pocket computer, to trigger actions at designated times. *Cues are often helpful when memory loss is a problem.*

## Chronic Confusion

Clients with AD often have memory deficits that make functioning in a nonstructured environment difficult. Many of the nursing interventions for this diagnosis need to be modified over time as the client continues to lose cognitive function.

- Label rooms, drawers, and other items as needed. *Visual cues promote the highest possible degree of independence for the client.*
- Remove potential hazards (such as sharp knives or potentially harmful liquids or chemicals) from the environment. *Ensuring safety is a critical factor in providing care.*
- Keep environmental stimuli to a minimum: Decrease noise levels; speak in a calm, low voice; and take an unhurried approach. *Minimizing sensory input and maintaining a calm manner may decrease anxiety.*
- Begin each interaction by identifying self and calling client by name. See Box 43–1 for other communication techniques. *These techniques provide information for the client with memory loss.*
- Limit questions to those that require a simple yes or no response. *Questions need to be appropriate to the client's ability as decision making and verbal skills decline.*
- Orient to the environment, person, and time as able; place large, easy-to-read calendars and clocks in the client's line of vision. Make references to the season or day of the week when conversing with the client. *Orient the client according to his or her level of ability; orienting to precise time may not be possible in the later stages of AD.*
- Provide boundaries by placing red or yellow tape on the floor. *Boundaries help the client stay within safe areas.*

**PRACTICE ALERT** *Red and yellow are more easily seen by older adults.* ■

- Provide continuity in nursing staff. *This not only promotes consistency of care for the client but also allows the nurse to determine more accurately changes in the client's condition.*

---

**BOX 43–1** ■ **Communication Techniques for the Client with AD**

- Face the client and talk directly to him or her; call the client by name.
- When first approaching the client, identify yourself.
- Use simple sentences and words with few syllables.
- Speak in a calm, low voice.
- Ask one question at a time. Use questions that require only a yes or no response.
- Keep nonverbal communication relaxed and parallel to the verbal communication.
- Avoid giving the impression of being in a hurry; try to have a relaxed approach.
- Observe for anxiety—wringing hands, pacing, darting eye movements—and alter your approach to decrease anxiety.
- Avoid arguing with clients; do not insist on orienting client to reality; the client's point of reference may not be based in reality.
- Give plenty of time for the client with AD to process what you are trying to say; do not expect clients to perform skills beyond their abilities.
- Repeat explanations in simple terms.

---

- Repeat explanations simply and as needed to decrease anxiety. *Loss of short-term memory leads to loss of a point of reference; eventually, AD clients think they are experiencing everything for the first time.*

## Anxiety

Managing the AD client's behaviors associated with anxiety, restlessness, and confusion is a major challenge confronting nurses and caregivers. Frequently, clients are relatively calm in the morning hours, only to experience increasing periods of agitation in the afternoon and evening hours. The AD client may even waken from the night's sleep with confusion, fearfulness, or panic attacks.

- Monitor for early behaviors of fatigue and agitation. *Early assessment of problems results in prompt intervention to promote rest or to remove the client from the situation causing anxiety.*
- Remove from situations that are causing increased anxiety, such as noisy activities involving large groups. *High-stimulus situations may increase anxious feelings and agitation.*
- Keep daily routine as consistent as possible. *Providing a structured day enhances feelings of familiarity and decreases stress.*
- Schedule rest periods or quiet times throughout the day. *Fatigue contributes to anxiety and lowers the stress threshold.*
- Provide quiet activities, such as listening to favorite music, in the afternoon or early evening. *Quiet activities may help decrease sundowning.*
- If confusion and agitation persist or escalate, assess for physical causes such as decreased oxygenation, infections, fatigue, constipation, and electrolyte imbalance. *Physical factors can increase agitation in clients with AD.*
- Use therapeutic touch or gentle hand massage. *These activities induce relaxation and have a calming effect.*

## Hopelessness

As the client and family recognize the impact of AD on their lives, they may feel a sense of hopelessness and powerlessness. They may not have the coping skills to deal effectively with the diagnosis and anticipated problems. The increasingly degenerative, irreversible nature of the disorder tends to diminish hope; only the ability to adapt to the many problems can restore it.

- Assess the client's and family's response to the diagnosis and understanding of AD; encourage expression of feelings. *Understanding the client/family's perspective enables the nurse to dispel myths about AD.*
- Provide realistic information about the disorder; provide information at the client/family's level of understanding. *Client and family may need to have separate sessions. Factual information provides a foundation for decision making.*
- Avoid criticizing or judging expressed feelings. *An environment accepting of the expression of real feelings promotes both further expression of feelings and willingness to discuss other issues.*
- Support positive family bonds and enhance communication among family members; promote mutual positive regard. *Strong family relationships can provide direction for living and convey a willingness to share the burden.*
- Encourage the client to make as many decisions as possible. *Self-determination enhances a feeling of control over a situation and may give a sense of hope.*
- Encourage the client and family to seek spiritual guidance that previously inspired hope. *The client's church is a legitimate support system. Belief in God can inspire hope beyond present circumstances.*

## Caregiver Role Strain

Most caregivers of clients with AD are spouses or other family members. Because AD is a chronic and eventually debilitating disorder, caregivers may feel overwhelmed by their responsibilities. The caregiving spouse faces not only the responsibility for the client's multiple physical demands but also economic and psychosocial stressors. An area that must be discussed is the ability and safety of the client in driving an automobile. Although is may be necessary, the loss of independence represented by the loss of the ability to drive may further trigger anxiety and anger. Fear of the future, loss of income, loss of companionship and a mate—combined with fatigue—make the caregiver vulnerable. Caregivers may become physically and mentally exhausted and socially isolated because of the overwhelming responsibilities of providing total care to the incapacitated family member.

- Teach the caregivers self-care techniques, such as taking rest periods and avoiding fatigue. *Fatigue adds to stress and potentially leads to poor decision making.*
- Have the caregivers list and regularly take part in physical activities they enjoy, such as walking or swimming. *Regular physical exercise decreases stress.*
- Refer the caregivers to local AD support groups. Suggest books pertinent to the subject. *Explicit suggestions in locating support systems and providing specific information promotes coping.*
- Refer the caregivers to Meals-on-Wheels, home health, respite care, and other community services. *Community agencies can relieve some of the daily care burdens, thus providing time for other activities. Programs that support caregivers have been shown to delay nursing home placement.*
- Ensure the family knows that hospice care is available during the end stages of AD. *Hospice services can support the family during this difficult time.*

## Using NANDA, NIC, and NOC

Chart 43–1 shows links between NANDA nursing diagnoses, NIC, and NOC when caring for the client with AD.

## Home Care

Teaching for clients and families centers initially on explaining the disorder and exploring available support systems. Anticipate the need to reexplain the disorder and its consequences, as clients and families may be in shock or denial during the initial period of the disease.

---

### CHART 43–1 NANDA, NIC, AND NOC LINKAGES

**The Client with AD**

| NURSING DIAGNOSES | NURSING INTERVENTIONS | NURSING OUTCOMES |
|---|---|---|
| • Chronic Confusion | • Dementia Management<br>• Anxiety Reduction<br>• Family Support<br>• Environmental Management: Safety | • Cognitive Orientation<br>• Distorted Thought Control<br>• Identity<br>• Safety Behavior |
| • Disturbed Sleep Pattern | • Sleep Enhancement<br>• Security Enhancement | • Sleep<br>• Anxiety Control<br>• Comfort Level |
| • Self-Care Deficit | • Self-Care Assistance | • Cognitive Ability<br>• Anxiety Control |

*Note. Data from Nursing Outcomes Classification (NOC) by M. Johnson & M. Maas (Eds.), 1997, St. Louis: Mosby; Nursing Diagnoses: Definitions & Classification 2001–2002 by North American Nursing Diagnosis Association, 2001, Philadelphia: NANDA; Nursing Interventions Classification (NIC) by J.C. McCloskey & G. M. Bulechek (Eds.), 2000, St. Louis: Mosby. Reprinted by permission.*

In addition to explaining the anticipated changes with AD, suggest practical solutions to identified problems. It is important to evaluate both the client and caregivers; interventions must be appropriate for the family's situation and resources. Maintaining the least restrictive environment that promotes safety for the client is a major goal of teaching. Using memory cues, such as labeling drawers to indicate the specific types of clothing and labeling rooms, can help orient the client and foster independence. Consistency in the environment and daily routine is an essential part of care. Emphasizing realistic expectations means adjusting care and communication techniques to the client's level of ability.

Address the following topics for home care of the client and for the caregiver.

- Support groups and peer counseling are helpful in handling caregiver stress.
- A person with AD who is confused or agitated is not comfortable and is usually frightened.

- Plan care that matches the person's level of coping, using a consistent routine.
- Provide regular rest periods to decrease the client's stress and fatigue (these do not increase nighttime wandering).
- Plan care for the caregiver. Periodic respite care during the initial stages, with plans for increasing assistance to meet the client's daily needs as the disease progresses, may be sufficient. Referrals to the appropriate agency for long-term care, including skilled nursing facilities, may be indicated. Family members may need help adjusting to the idea of extended care but may be relieved to relinquish the physical care needs.
- Suggest the following resources:
  - Alzheimer's Association
  - Alzheimer's Disease and Related Disorders Association
  - Alzheimer's Disease Education and Referral Center
  - National Institute of Neurological and Communicative Disorders and Stroke

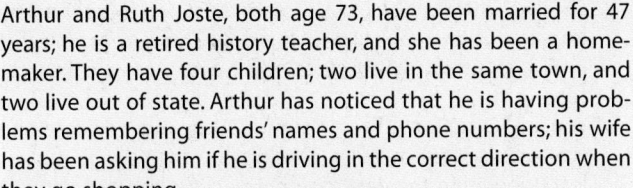

## Nursing Care Plan
## A Client with AD

Arthur and Ruth Joste, both age 73, have been married for 47 years; he is a retired history teacher, and she has been a homemaker. They have four children; two live in the same town, and two live out of state. Arthur has noticed that he is having problems remembering friends' names and phone numbers; his wife has been asking him if he is driving in the correct direction when they go shopping.

Mrs. Joste has severe osteoarthritis and is unable to lift heavy objects or perform all but light housekeeping tasks. For about 18 months, Mrs. Joste has been aware of her husband's progressive cognitive decline, including forgetting current news from last night's newspaper; miscalculating checkbook balances; neglecting his hygiene needs; and confusing their children's and grandchildren's names. The Jostes are referred to a neurologist for evaluation.

### ASSESSMENT
Martha Spital, RN, assesses Mr. Joste at the neurologist's office. She notes that he is unable to recall his home address without prompting, to name the correct date (although he does know the day of the week), to subtract serial 7s more than twice, and to recall two of three objects. He is alert to his surroundings. Mr. Joste scores 21 of a possible 30 points on the Mini Mental Status Exam. Mrs. Joste states that the problems seem to be getting worse with time and that she has had to "cover up" mistakes for her husband. Mr. Joste seems easily agitated, and his wife reports that his sleep habits are "jumbled"; he has long periods of wakefulness in the nighttime hours.

Following a thorough evaluation and diagnostic testing to rule out other possible disorders, the neurologist tells the couple that Mr. Joste has probable dementia of the Alzheimer's type. Both have feared this diagnosis; they want to know how they can be sure that Mr. Joste has this disease and what they can do to prevent further decline. Both are obviously much saddened, and they verbalize their feelings of being overwhelmed. The Jostes intend to remain in their home "for as long as we can."

### DIAGNOSES
- *Chronic confusion* related to deterioration of brain function and dementia
- *Self-care deficits* related to forgetfulness and declining physical abilities
- *Risk for injury* related to decreased orientation
- *Disturbed sleep pattern* related to time disorientation
- *Caregiver role strain* (wife) related to need to care for self and husband

### EXPECTED OUTCOMES
- Remain free of injury.
- Navigate home environment with modifications as needed.
- Participate in grooming and hygiene activities with prompting and supervision.
- Obtain a minimum of 7 uninterrupted hours of sleep a night.
- Mrs. Joste will participate in a minimum of two out-of-home activities a week.

### PLANNING AND IMPLEMENTATION
The home health nurse, Erick Montane, RN, makes a home visit to evaluate the environment, assess available support, and determine needs. He meets two of the Jostes' children, Dawn and Jay, who live in the same community and are willing to participate as much as possible in providing care and modifying the home.

Mr. Montane discusses the importance of establishing and maintaining a consistent daily routine. He emphasizes the importance of matching activities to Mr. Joste's mental abilities to avoid frustration and increased agitation. Mr. Montane recommends labeling drawers with their contents, such as Mr. Joste's sock drawer. Labeling rooms may eventually be necessary.

Because his inability to comprehend and process information distresses and agitates Mr. Joste, Mr. Montane teaches the family to modify their communications to fit Mr. Joste's cognitive ability, such as using simple, direct statements and directions.

(continued on page 1406)

## Nursing Care Plan
### A Client with AD *(continued)*

Mr. Montane recommends that family members keep background noise to a minimum because this may be a source of confusion.

After touring the home, Mr. Montane makes the following recommendations about safety:

- Remove throw rugs from hallways, and tack down any remaining carpets.
- Secure the kitchen, bathroom, and workshop cabinets as well as the controls on the oven and stove.
- Modify the doors so that negotiating locks requires a two-step system of unlocking, such as with a deadbolt and a key.
- Provide extra lighting in dark areas, especially a night-light in the bathroom.

Mr. Montane explains that Mrs. Joste will need assistance with housekeeping as Mr. Joste continues to decline. Mr. Montane provides referrals to community services, including Meals-on-Wheels, which can supply a daily meal. He also suggests that the Jostes obtain the services of a home health aide to provide daily hygiene care. Most of the remaining home maintenance needs can be met with the children's help.

Mr. and Mrs. Joste and the two children attend the weekly local support group meetings for Alzheimer's disease and related disorders for approximately 3 months; thereafter, Mrs. Joste attends with her daughter.

### EVALUATION

Six months after the initial home visit and family planning session, Mr. Joste:

- Has not had a fall, burn, or other injury.
- Has periods of confusion when outside his home, but 90% of the time is oriented to place when at home.
- Has attended several support group meetings until 3 months ago. Currently, his wife attends weekly, and a daughter occa-

sionally accompanies her. She has continued to participate in their church and maintains contact with a few friends. She is finding it harder to leave her husband unattended for even a few minutes.

- Is able to clean and dress himself with prompting; he is not able to choose his own clothing. If hygiene articles are "set up" (e.g., if the toothpaste is placed on the toothbrush), he remembers to perform the hygiene activity. The children have been replacing buttons and zippers with Velcro closures on his clothing.
- Sleeps an average of 6 hours a night with a 30-minute nap in the afternoon; this pattern is consistent with his previous sleep pattern.
- Has seemed to be more easily agitated for the past month. He wanders from room to room, apparently looking for something. These behaviors are worse in the evening and on cloudy days. Mrs. Joste acknowledges her progressive inability to care for her husband.

### Critical Thinking in the Nursing Process

1. Develop a tool to teach safety needs for the client and family with Alzheimer's disease.
2. List five interventions to decrease agitation in cognitively impaired older adults; give three additional examples of activities suited to an older adult with AD who has osteoarthritis.
3. You are caring for a client in Stage 2 Alzheimer's disease. She is 65 inches (165 cm) tall and weighs 132 lb (59.9 kg); she has lost 3 lb within the past month. The client has difficulty focusing on eating and is easily agitated. Describe your plan for ensuring that she takes in enough nutrition to meet her needs.

See Evaluating Your Response in Appendix C.

## THE CLIENT WITH MULTIPLE SCLEROSIS

**Multiple sclerosis (MS)** is a chronic demyelinating disease of the central nervous system, associated with an abnormal immune response to an environmental factor. The symptoms of MS vary according to the area of the nervous system affected. The initial onset may be followed by a total remission, making diagnosis difficult. In about 60% of clients, MS is characterized by periods of exacerbation, when symptoms are highly pronounced, followed by periods of remission. The end result, however, is progression of the disease with increasing loss of function.

### INCIDENCE AND PREVALENCE

Approximately 500,000 people in the United States have MS. Females are affected 2 times more often than males, and the incidence is highest in young adults (age 20 to 40). The disease occurs more commonly in temperate climates, including the

northern United States. This association is established by approximately age 15, and moving to or from a temperate climate after that age does not change it.

The onset of MS is usually between 20 and 50 years of age, with a peak at age 30. MS is the most prevalent CNS demyelinating disorder, and is a leading cause of neurologic disability in young adults. Although all races are affected, MS is primarily a disease of Caucasians. Although a definite genetic factor has not been established, 15% of those with MS have a relative with the disease (McCance & Huether, 2002).

### PATHOPHYSIOLOGY

MS is believed to occur as a result of an autoimmune response to a prior viral infection in a genetically susceptible person. The infection, which is thought to occur early in life, activates T cells. T cells usually move in and out of the CNS across the blood-brain barrier, but for an unknown reason, they remain in the CNS in people with MS. The T cells facilitate infiltration by other leukocytes, and an inflammatory

| BOX 43–2 | ■ Classifications of Multiple Sclerosis |
| --- | --- |

**Relapsing-remitting:** The most common clinical course of MS, characterized by exacerbations (acute attacks) with either full recovery or partial recovery with disability.

**Primary progressive:** Steady worsening of disease from the onset with occasional minor recovery.

**Secondary progressive:** Begins as with relapsing-remitting, but the disease steadily becomes worse between exacerbations.

**Progressive-relapsing:** This rare form continues to progress from the onset but also has exacerbations.

process follows. Inflammation destroys myelin and oligodendrocytes (myelin-producing cells), leading to axon dysfunction. The myelin sheaths are fatty, segmented wrappings that normally protect and insulate nerve fibers and increase the speed of transmission of nerve impulses. In multiple sclerosis, these myelin sheaths of the white matter of the spinal cord, brain, and optic nerve are destroyed in patches, called plaques, along the axon (see *Pathophysiology Illustrated* on pages 1408–1409). The **demyelination** of nerve fibers slows and distorts the conduction of nerve impulses and sometimes results in the total absence of impulse transmission. The neurons usually affected by MS are located in the spinal cord, brainstem, cerebral and cerebellar areas, and the optic nerve.

Both plaques and diffuse lesions form as demyelinating lesions. Plaques typically are scattered through the white matter of the CNS, although they may extend into adjacent gray matter. Early manifestations are the result of inflammatory edema in and around the plaque and partial demyelination. These manifestations typically disappear within weeks after the initial episode. With progression of the disease, the demyelination and plaque formation result in scarring of glia (*gliosis*) and degeneration of axons. Continued loss of function leads to permanent disability, usually over about 20 years.

There are four classifications of MS: relapsing-remitting, primary progressive, secondary progressive, and progressive-relapsing (Box 43–2). Most individuals with MS present with the relapsing-remitting type.

Various stressors have been suggested as triggers for MS. These stressors include febrile states, pregnancy, extreme physical exertion, and fatigue. These precipitating factors can also cause a relapse of the manifestations during the course of the disease.

## MANIFESTATIONS

The manifestations of MS vary according to the areas destroyed by demyelination and the affected body system (see *Multisystems Effects of MS* on page 1410). Fatigue is one of the most disabling manifestations, and affects almost all clients with MS. The manifestations, categorized by the established syndromes of MS, include:

*Mixed or Generalized Type (50% of cases)*

- Manifestations include optic nerve involvement, with visual blurring, fogginess, or haziness; and impaired color perception. There is also decreased central visual acuity, area of diminished vision in the visual fields, acquired color vision deficit (especially to red and green), and an altered pupillary reaction to light.
- Brainstem lesions (cranial nerves III to XII) are noted, with nystagmus, dysarthria, deafness, vertigo, vomiting, tinnitus, facial weakness, and decreased sensation. Other manifestations include diplopia and eye pain, and cognitive dysfunctions involving concentration, short-term memory, word finding, and planning.
- Mood alterations are manifested as depression more often than euphoria.

*Spinal Type (25% of cases)*

- Weakness and/or numbness is noted in one or both extremities (most often the legs).
- Upper motor neuron involvement is manifested by stiffness, slowness, weakness (spastic paresis).
- Bladder dyfunctions include urgency, hesitancy, and incontinence.
- Bowel dysfunction is most often seen as constipation.
- Neurogenic impotence is noted.

*Cerebellar Type (5% of cases)*

- Client shows manifestations of nystagmus, ataxia, and hyptonia.

*Amaurotic Form (5% of cases)*

- Client develops blindness.

Short-lived attacks of neurologic deficits indicate the temporary appearance or worsening of manifestations. Conditions that cause short-lived attacks include (1) minor increases in body temperature or serum calcium concentrations (both increase the leakage of current through demyelinated neurons) and (2) functional demands that exceed conduction capacity. Paroxysmal attacks are sensory or motor manifestations that occur abruptly and last for only seconds or minutes; the manifestations are paresthesias, dysarthria and ataxia, and tonic head turning. Paroxysmal attacks, which may occur many times a day, result from the direct transmission of nerve impulses between adjacent demyelinated axons (McCance & Huether, 2002).

## COLLABORATIVE CARE

Management of the client with MS varies according to the severity of the manifestations. The focus is on retaining the optimal level of functioning possible, given the degree of disability. Rehabilitation—physical, occupational/vocational, and psychosocial—is a cornerstone of a team approach to treatment. During exacerbations, the focus of interventions shifts to controlling manifestations and quickly returning to remission.

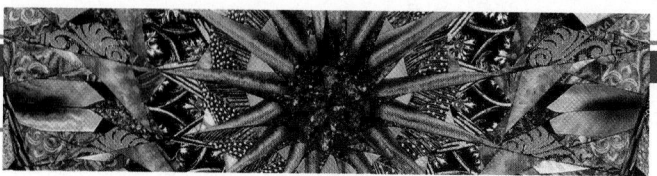

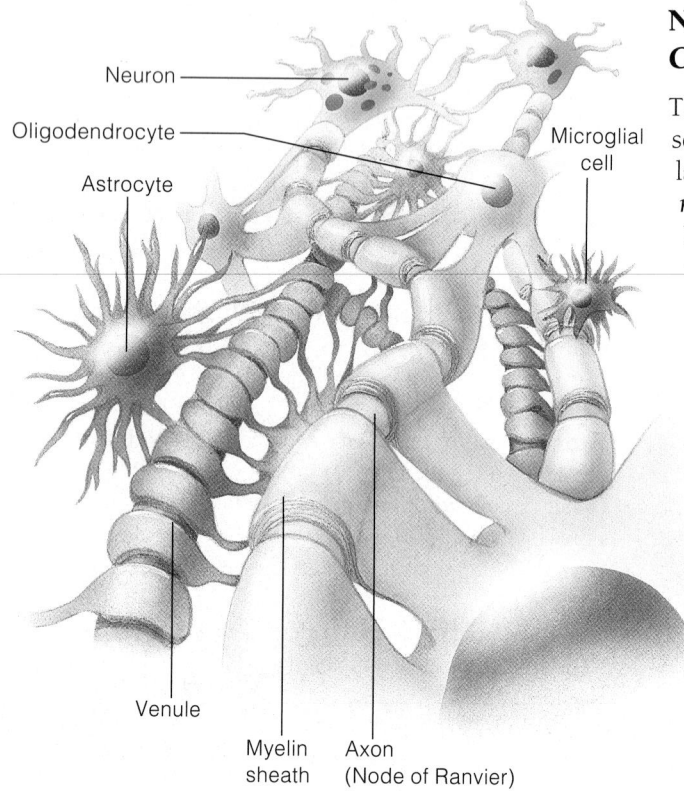

Neuron

Oligodendrocyte

Astrocyte

Microglial cell

Venule

Myelin sheath

Axon (Node of Ranvier)

## Normal Anatomy of the Central Nervous System

The central nervous system (CNS) is composed of several cell types arranged in a dense, interconnected lattice. The basic functional cell of the CNS is the *neuron*, which transmits electrochemical impulses. Dendrites, thin projections extending from the neuron body, receive impulses that are passed down the neuronal axon for transmission to other cells. Myelin, a lipid-protein substance, surrounds the axons, insulating them and speeding nerve impulse transmission.

Neurons are surrounded by a network of neuroglial cells:

- *Astrocytes* support neurons and connnect them to surrounding capillaries and venules.
- *Microglia* are motile phagocytic cells.
- *Oligodendrocytes* wrap concentric layers of myelin around nearby axons.

## Acute Attack

Multiple sclerosis (MS) is a demyelinating disease in which axonal myelin in the central nervous system is eroded, destroyed, and replaced by scar tissue.

An autoimmune process apparently triggered by genetic and environmental factors is believed to cause inflammation of venules in the CNS. This disrupts the blood–brain barrier, allowing lymphocytes to enter CNS tissue. These lymphocytes proliferate and produce IgG, an antibody that attacks and damages myelin and causes the release of inflammatory chemicals and edema. As the inflammation subsides, the myelin regenerates and manifestations of the disease subside.

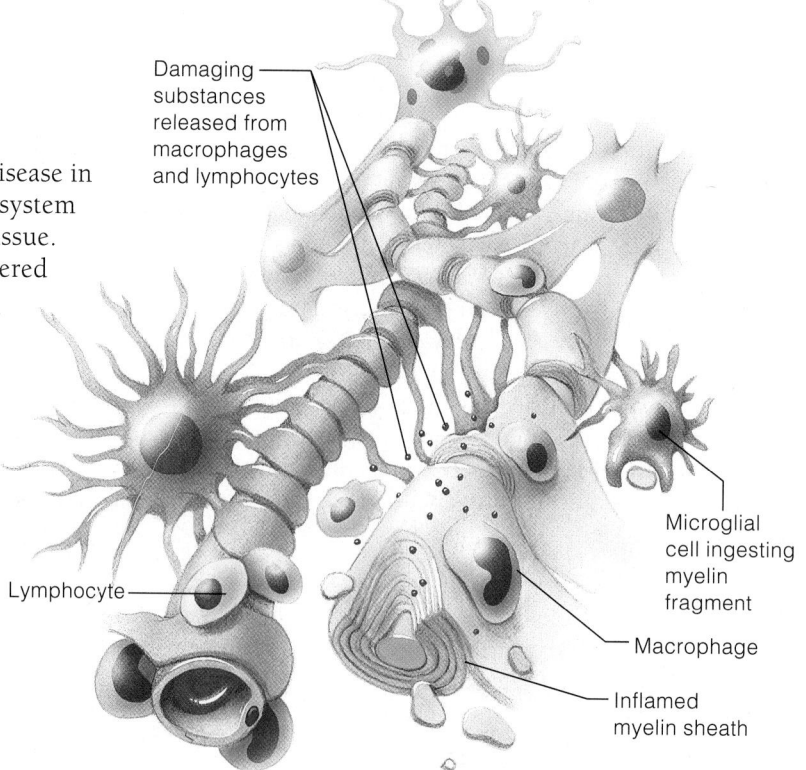

Damaging substances released from macrophages and lymphocytes

Microglial cell ingesting myelin fragment

Macrophage

Inflamed myelin sheath

Lymphocyte

## Chronic Lesion

After repeated inflammatory attacks, myelin is irreparably damaged. Segments of axons become totally demyelinated and may degenerate. Astrocytes proliferate in damaged regions of the CNS (a process call *gliosis*), forming plaques. The plaques are scattered throughout the CNS, appearing as gray or pinkish lesions. The relapsing-remitting character of MS and the scattered areas of damage within the CNS account for the variable nature of MS manifestations.

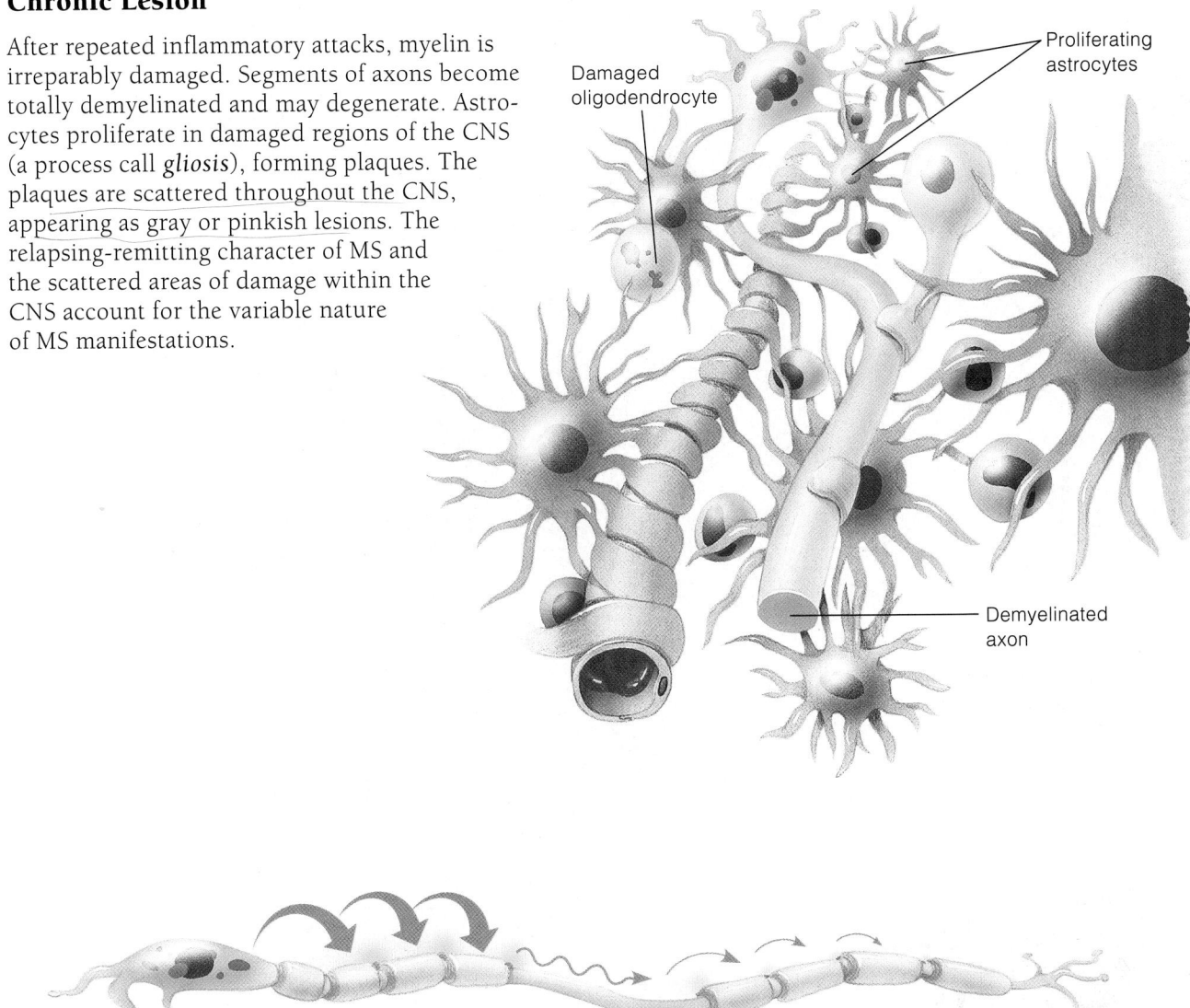

Damaged oligodendrocyte

Proliferating astrocytes

Demyelinated axon

## Abnormal Nerve Impulse Transmission

In an undamaged neuron, nerve impulses travel down the axon by "leaping" from one node of Ranvier to the next, thus greatly increasing the speed of impulse transmission. When nerve impulses travel down an axon damaged by MS, they are significantly slowed and weakened as they pass across the surface of demyelin-ated areas. Impulses may be blocked entirely when axons degenerate. The weakening or interruption of the transmission of nerve impulses and plaque formation within the CNS cause the manifestations of MS, including extremity weakness, paresthesias, visual disturbances, bladder dysfunction, and vertigo.

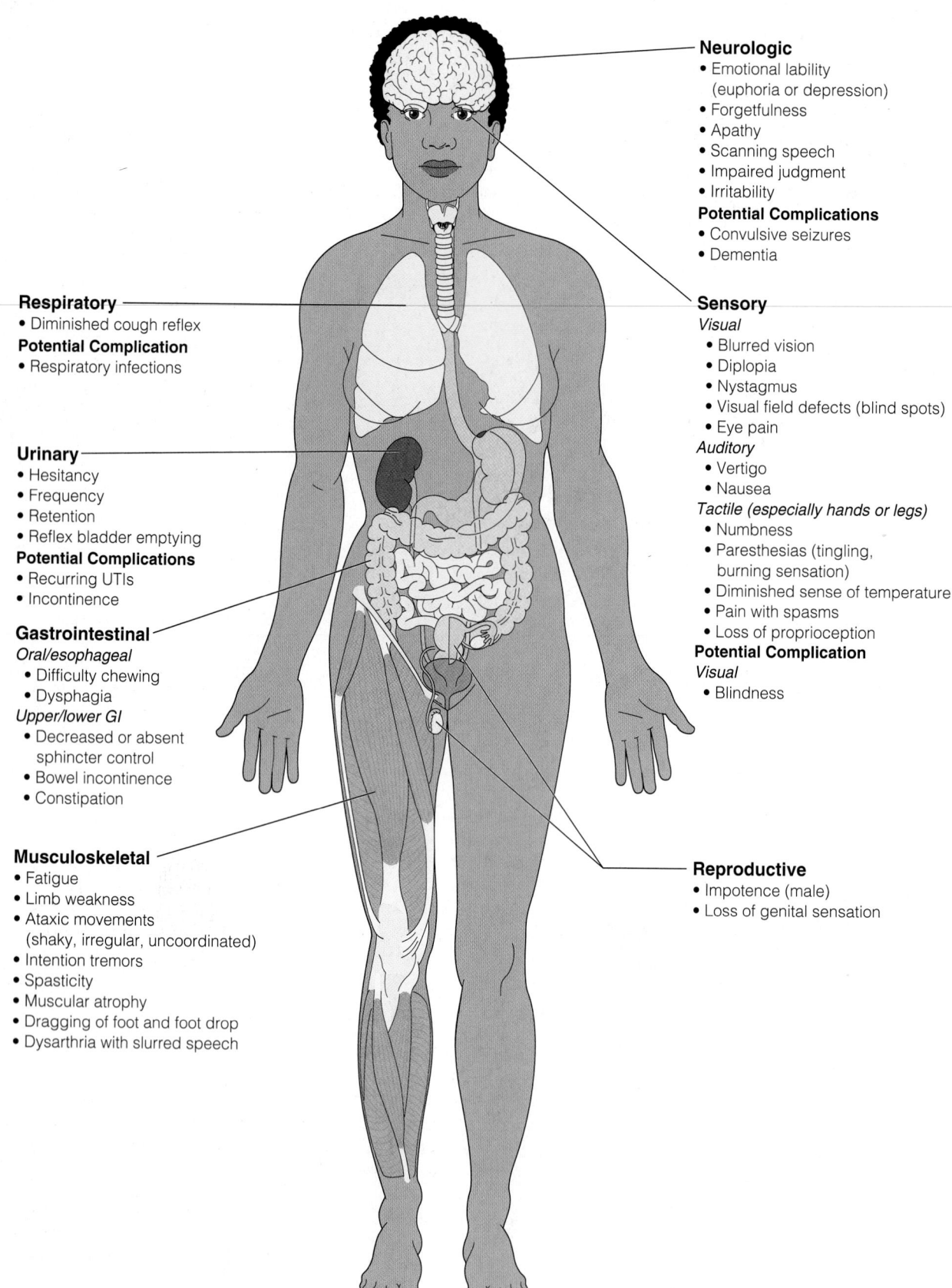

**Neurologic**
- Emotional lability (euphoria or depression)
- Forgetfulness
- Apathy
- Scanning speech
- Impaired judgment
- Irritability

**Potential Complications**
- Convulsive seizures
- Dementia

**Sensory**

*Visual*
- Blurred vision
- Diplopia
- Nystagmus
- Visual field defects (blind spots)
- Eye pain

*Auditory*
- Vertigo
- Nausea

*Tactile (especially hands or legs)*
- Numbness
- Paresthesias (tingling, burning sensation)
- Diminished sense of temperature
- Pain with spasms
- Loss of proprioception

**Potential Complication**
*Visual*
- Blindness

**Respiratory**
- Diminished cough reflex

**Potential Complication**
- Respiratory infections

**Urinary**
- Hesitancy
- Frequency
- Retention
- Reflex bladder emptying

**Potential Complications**
- Recurring UTIs
- Incontinence

**Gastrointestinal**

*Oral/esophageal*
- Difficulty chewing
- Dysphagia

*Upper/lower GI*
- Decreased or absent sphincter control
- Bowel incontinence
- Constipation

**Musculoskeletal**
- Fatigue
- Limb weakness
- Ataxic movements (shaky, irregular, uncoordinated)
- Intention tremors
- Spasticity
- Muscular atrophy
- Dragging of foot and foot drop
- Dysarthria with slurred speech

**Reproductive**
- Impotence (male)
- Loss of genital sensation

## Diagnostic Tests

Diagnosis of MS is challenging because the disease does not present uniformly. Initially, a thorough history and physical examination are completed, and their importance in establishing a diagnosis cannot be overemphasized. Diagnostic tests vary with the presenting complaints. MRI is the most definitive test available; however, it is one of several laboratory and diagnostic tests that may be performed when establishing the diagnosis.

- *Cerebral spinal fluid (CSF) analysis* reveals an increased number of T lymphocytes that are reactive with antigens, indicating the presence of an immune response in the client. Of MS patients, 80% have elevated levels of immunoglobulin G (IgG) in the CSF. IgG may not be increased during the initial period of the disease.
- *MRI studies* are performed. Cerebral MRI detects multifocal lesions in the white matter. Serial MRIs may be performed to chart the course of the disease. MRI of the spinal cord or optic nerves can detect lesions in these areas.
- *CT scan* of the brain shows atrophy and white matter lesions. In about 25% of clients with MS, enlarged ventricles are visible on CT.
- *Positron emission tomography (PET) scan* measures brain activity. In MS clients, the scan reveals areas with changes in glucose metabolism.

- *Evoked response testing* of visual, auditory, or somatosensory impulses may show delayed conduction.

## Medications

Medications slow the progression of MS and decrease the number of attacks. See the Medication Administration box on pages 1411–1412 for information about these medications.

The medications used during an exacerbation are aimed at decreasing inflammation to inhibit manifestations and induce remission. Frequently, a combination of adrenocorticotrophic hormone (ACTH) and glucocorticoids is used to decrease inflammation and suppress the immune system. Immunosuppressive agents, including azathioprine (Imuran) and cyclophosphamide (Cytoxan), are also used. Some centers administer cyclophosphamide monthly to prevent exacerbations.

Other medications treat the manifestations of MS, such as muscle spasms. Anticholinergics are sometimes administered for bladder spasticity; cholinergics are given if the client has a problem with urinary retention related to flaccid bladder.

## Treatments

Although medications are the primary method of controlling manifestations, other treatments include surgery, dietary management, and rehabilitative therapies.

---

# Medication Administration

## The Client with Multiple Sclerosis

### IMMUNOMODULATORS

Interferon beta-1a (Avonex)
Interferon beta-1b (Betaseron)
Glatiramer acetate (Copaxone, Copolymer-1)

Interferon beta-1a, interferon beta-1b, and glatiramer acetate are administered to clients with relapsing-remitting MS to prolong the time of onset to disability. Their use is based on the assumption that MS is an immunologically mediated disease. Interferon beta-1b produces a decrease in the MS lesions in some clients. Some clients, however, develop a decrease in the absolute neutrophil count and increases in the levels of liver enzymes. Anxiety, confusion, and depression with suicidal tendencies also have been reported. Other adverse reactions include pain, inflammation, hypersensitivity at the injection site, and generalized flulike manifestations. Some women experience menstrual disorders. Pregnant women should not take these medications.

### Nursing Responsibilities

- Assess baseline parameters to evaluate drug side effects: psychologic profile, liver function tests, and CBC with differential. Monitor CBC and liver function tests every 3 months or as prescribed.
- Assess injection site and report ulceration promptly (pain and redness are common reactions).
- Evaluate client's baseline neurologic, sensory, and motor function. Monitor changes in condition and function.
- Report if client is pregnant or breast-feeding.

### Client and Family Teaching

- This drug may cause depression and thoughts of suicide; report these feelings immediately to the physician.
- The medication is reconstituted and should be discarded if it becomes discolored or precipitates out. Administer the medication within 3 hours of reconstitution. Rotate injection sites, and avoid any areas that are red or show other skin reactions.
- Seek follow-up care to monitor neurologic changes, CBC, and liver function.
- Avoid prolonged exposure to sunlight.

### ADRENOCORTICOSTEROID THERAPY

Adrenocorticotropic hormone (ACTH) (Acthar)
Prednisone (Deltasone, Meticorten, Orasone)
Methylprednisolone (Medrol, Solu-Medrol)

Adrenocorticosteroids are used both to sustain a remission and to treat exacerbations of MS. ACTH is usually given to induce a remission; it is administered intravenously for 1 week and may be followed by oral prednisone therapy. Another protocol involves administering ACTH intravenously for 3 days followed by intramuscular injections every 12 hours for 1 week (Hickey, 2002). The drugs are given to suppress the immune system, implicated in the etiology of MS. If the drug is used long term, the usual steroid precautions are indicated, such as monitoring for

*(continued on page 1412)*

# Medication Administration

## The Client with Multiple Sclerosis (continued)

glucose intolerance, osteoporosis, and cataract formation. The drugs are used with caution in pregnant and lactating women.

### MUSCLE RELAXANTS

Baclofen (Lioresal)
Dantrolene (Dantrium)
Diazepam (Valium)

Muscle relaxants are given to clients with MS to relieve muscle spasms. Baclofen and diazepam act by suppressing CNS reflexes that regulate muscle activity; neither drug affects muscle strength. Baclofen therapy should be discontinued over 1 to 2 weeks; sudden withdrawal may cause seizures and paranoid ideation. In contrast to diazepam and baclofen, dantrolene acts directly on skeletal muscles, and it may affect muscle strength. Dantrolene may cause hepatotoxicity and should not be administered when hepatitis or cirrhosis is present.

### Nursing Responsibilities

- Evaluate baseline muscle strength and spasticity, ROM, and dexterity.
- Maintain safety or fall precautions; dizziness and drowsiness are common side effects.
- For the client taking dantrolene, monitor liver function tests (enzymes and bilirubin) for signs of hepatotoxicity.

### Client and Family Teaching

- These drugs may cause sedative effects. Take appropriate safety measures (e.g., avoid driving).
- Avoid CNS depressants (antihistamines, alcohol); they can increase the sedative effects of the medication.
- Continue follow-up care; if you are taking dantrolene, for example, liver function will need to be monitored.

- If you are taking baclofen, do not suddenly stop the medication.
- Increase fiber and fluids in the diet to prevent constipation.
- Change positions slowly to minimize dizziness and other effects of orthostatic hypotension.

### IMMUNOSUPPRESSANTS

Azathioprine (Imuran)
Cyclophosphamide (Cytoxan)

Immunosuppressants are given to clients with MS because of the autoimmune component of the disease. Both medications can cause bone marrow suppression and increase the risk of cancer. Azathioprine may produce hepatitis. Toxic effects of cyclophosphamide include hemorrhagic cystitis, sterility, and stomatitis.

### Nursing Responsibilities

- Monitor baseline parameters: CBC with platelet count and differential, urinalysis, liver function tests, hepatitis profile.
- Assess for anemia: fatigue, lethargy, pallor.
- Watch for signs of bleeding.
- Protect against and observe for subtle signs of infection.

### Client and Family Teaching

- Report signs of infection, bleeding, and anemia immediately.
- Drink at least 2 L (2 quarts) of fluid a day, and observe urine for blood.
- Report jaundice immediately.
- Check oral cavity daily for changes or ulcers.
- Avoid becoming pregnant while taking these drugs.
- Obtain follow-up care, including frequent blood tests.

## Surgery

Surgery may be indicated for clients who experience severe spasticity and deformity. However, physical therapy can prevent most severe problems. Foot drop from severe plantar flexion can be relieved with an Achilles tenotomy, a surgical procedure in which the Achilles tendon is transected.

## Dietary Management

Several diets involving manipulation of fats are currently under investigation. Clients with MS may be overweight because of their inability to ambulate; depression may contribute to the problem because people who are depressed tend to eat more and burn fewer calories. Ideally, the client should maintain a weight as close as possible to that recommended for the client's height and body type.

As MS progresses, the client's ability to prepare food and eat is compromised. Changes in muscle tone, tremor, weakness, and ataxia all contribute to nutritional problems. Dysphagia also is a common problem. The diet must be adapted to accommodate changes in the client's ability to chew and swallow.

## Rehabilitation

Physical and rehabilitative therapies are tailored to the client's level of functioning. The long-term goal is to enable the client to retain as much independence as possible. One major intervention is to maintain and increase existing muscle strength.

Spasticity is managed with stretching exercises, gait training, and braces, splints, or other assistive devices. To maintain balance, the client is encouraged to widen the base of support by standing with the feet slightly further apart. Walkers and canes may be weighted to provide support and balance for the ataxic client.

A team approach to rehabilitation will provide supportive services: speech therapy for problems with phonation, occupational therapy to maintain strength in the upper extremities and carry out ADLs, and occupational counseling. Consultations with a urologist are indicated for problems with urinary incontinence, urinary tract infections, retention, and impotence. Consultation with a respiratory therapist may be needed if the client develops chronic respiratory infections from inability to cough, move secretions, or breathe deeply, especially with increased debilitation.

## NURSING CARE

Because the disease most often affects young adults in the prime of life, the psychosocial and economic impact can be devastating. People with MS have to make adjustments to the body image changes while simultaneously adapting to the altered relationships and decreased earnings usually encountered with the disease. A once-healthy spouse becomes wheelchair-bound; a person once independent may eventually become dependent for even the most basic ADLs. The unpredictable course of MS is a challenge for long-term planning.

### Health Promotion

Following an overview of the disorder, the client needs to understand how to prevent fatigue and exacerbations. Teach the client to avoid stress, extremes of cold and heat, high humidity, physical overexertion, and infections. Because pregnancy can exacerbate symptoms, counseling about this risk is indicated. Also, address preventive measures to avoid risk of respiratory and urinary tract infections.

### Assessment

Collect the following data through the health history and physical examination (see Chapter 40).

- Health history: history of childhood viral illnesses, geographical residence when a child, exposure to physical or emotional stressors (pregnancy/delivery, extremes of heat), medications, symptom onset, severity of symptoms
- Physical assessment: affect, mood, speech, eye movements, gait, tremors, vision and hearing, reflexes, muscle strength and movement, sensation

### Nursing Diagnoses and Interventions

Interventions for the client with MS vary with the acuity of exacerbations and the presenting problems. Many nursing diagnoses relate to the inability to perform ADLs, for example, *Self-care deficit, Impaired home maintenance management,* and *Powerlessness.* Others reflect problems with musculoskeletal changes or altered nerve conduction, for example, *Impaired physical mobility, Ineffective breathing pattern, Social isolation, constipation,* and *Urinary incontinence.* The nursing diagnoses discussed in this section are *Fatigue* and *Self-care deficit.*

### Fatigue

Fatigue is defined by NANDA (2001) as an overwhelming sustained sense of exhaustion and decreased capacity for physical and mental work at the usual level. Fatigue affects every aspect of the MS client's life—the ability to remain independent and perform self-care, sexual function, mobility, airway clearance, and ultimately self-concept and coping. A great deal of teaching is needed to help the client and family understand fatigue and how to adapt. Clients and families need assistance managing fatigue in a society in which energy is highly valued.

- Assess degree of fatigue and identify contributing factors. *Fatigue is a subjective experience that needs to be evaluated thoroughly before planning can begin.*
- Arrange daily activities to include rest periods. *Rest is essential to manage feelings of fatigue; periods of relaxation may help replenish energy reserves.*

**PRACTICE ALERT** *It is important to remember that the fatigue from chronic illnesses such as MS is very different from being "tired," and that rest and sleep may not result in improvement.* ∎

- Ask the client to consider which activities are really necessary and to set priorities. *Prioritizing activities promotes independence and self-control.*
- Suggest performing tasks in the morning hours. *Biorhythm studies indicate that people usually have greater energy reserves in the morning hours and diminished reserves in the afternoon.*
- Advise to avoid temperature extremes, such as hot showers or exposure to cold. *Maintaining a relatively constant body temperature may avoid exacerbation of the disorder. Heat can delay impulse transmission across demyelinated nerves, which contributes to fatigue.*
- Refer to the appropriate professionals to manage fatigue: stress management groups, support groups, occupational or physical therapist, as indicated. *Support groups and therapy can facilitate self-management and improving coping.*

### Self-Care Deficits

Clients with MS may need assistance with bathing, toileting, dressing, grooming, and feeding. The help needed can range from minimal guidance to total dependence. The client's ability to perform self-care activities is the gauge by which family members and caregivers need to adjust assistance. Self-care encompasses both the decisions about care and the provision of care; most clients are capable of making decisions even after physical limitations prevent physical self-care. The need to maintain self-determination cannot be overemphasized and must be incorporated into each intervention. See the Nursing Research box on page 1414 for research findings supporting the importance of maintaining a client's quality of life.

- Assess the extent of the client's self-care deficit; refer to other health team members for assessment as appropriate. For example, refer to a speech pathologist to assess swallowing and gag reflex, if indicated. *An accurate assessment is crucial to individualizing interventions.*
- Suggest adaptive devices, such as arm or wrist braces, as needed. *Meeting hygiene needs and feeding self are essential for positive self-concept, self-esteem, and socialization.*
- Teach to use assistive devices, such as plate guards; to modify consistency of foods; and to eat when energy level is better. If unable to buy and prepare meals, provide referral to Meals-on-Wheels. *Proper nutrition is basic to health;*

## Nursing Research

### Evidence-Based Practice to Improve Quality of Life in Clients with Multiple Sclerosis

Quality of life is a critical factor in living with chronic illnesses like multiple sclerosis. Regardless of health status or functional disabilities, quality of life is made up of the same factors and relationships important to healthy people. It is experienced when basic needs are met and opportunities are available to pursue and achieve life goals. Gulick (1997) conducted a study to investigate the extent to which demographic and self-reported health and role predicted quality of life in 153 people with multiple sclerosis.

Analysis of data resulted in the following findings specific to people with MS:

- Marriage, work, and health are major contributors to a positive outlook on life.
- Living with a spouse, followed by employment, were the most important demographic variables related to quality of life.
- Depression may result from anxieties about the loss of body function; loss of normal pleasures; and loss of social, business, and personal factors of life.
- Recreation and socialization are important correlates of quality of life.

### IMPLICATIONS FOR NURSING

Nurses can help clients with MS identify aspects of their health and roles/relationships that adversely and positively affect quality of life. By identifying strengths and weaknesses, nurses can provide interventions to enhance the client's quality of life. Those interventions would include sexuality counseling, provision of assistive devices to enable greater mobility, and referral to support groups.

### Critical Thinking in Client Care

1. In reflecting on the manifestations of multiple sclerosis, what factors can you identify as potential strengths and weaknesses for a client?
2. As a person with MS ages, disabilities often become more severe. How would you adapt teaching plans for home care for the following people?
   - A 29-year-old mother of two toddlers, diagnosed 1 year ago
   - A 45-year-old man who has worked in construction all his life
   - A 60-year-old woman who is a college professor

*adapting utensils and foods can ensure that nutritional needs are met.*
- Teach interventions related to altered bowel and bladder function: fluid intake of at least 2000 mL daily, bowel routine as indicated to prevent constipation, self-catheterization skills as necessary. *Maintaining optimal bowel and bladder function decreases the risk of urinary tract infection and bowel impaction.*

### Using NANDA, NIC, and NOC

Chart 43–2 Shows links between NANDA nursing diagnoses, NIC, and NOC when caring for the client with MS.

### Home Care

The nurse adapts teaching approaches based on the MS client's needs. The inconsistent and erratic nature of the disease can make teaching difficult. Initial teaching focuses on a

### CHART 43–2  NANDA, NIC, AND NOC LINKAGESS

#### The Client with MS

| NURSING DIAGNOSES | NURSING INTERVENTIONS | NURSING OUTCOMES |
|---|---|---|
| • Impaired Physical Mobility | • Energy Management<br>• Exercise Therapy: Ambulation<br>• Exercise Therapy: Joint Mobility | • Mobility Level<br>• Ambulation: Walking<br>• Joint Movement: Active |
| • Disturbed Sensory Perception: Visual | • Communication Enhancement<br>• Environment Management<br>• Eye Care | • Neurological Status |
| • Urinary Retention | • Urinary Catheterization<br>• Urinary Retention Care | • Urinary Elimination |
| • Sexual Dysfunction | • Sexual Counseling | • Self-Esteem |
| • Interrupted Family Processes | • Family Process Promotion<br>• Emotional Support<br>• Support System Enhancement | • Role Performance |

*Note. Data from Nursing Outcomes Classification (NOC) by M. Johnson & M. Maas (Eds.), 1997, St. Louis: Mosby; Nursing Diagnoses: Definitions & Classification 2001–2002 by North American Nursing Diagnosis Association, 2001, Philadelphia: NANDA; Nursing Interventions Classification (NIC) by J.C. McCloskey & G. M. Bulechek (Eds.), 2000, St. Louis: Mosby. Reprinted by permission.*

realistic explanation of MS. Referral to a support group early in the course of the disease also is indicated. Social support can make a positive difference in a client's ability to cope with MS. Address the following topics in preparing the client for home care.

- Various treatment options and their side effects
- Information about medications, particularly steroid use, and about possible interactions with prescription or over-the-counter medications

- Ongoing care from nurses, counselors, and physical, occupational, and speech therapists, as well as the physician and community health nurse.
- Helpful resources:
  - National Multiple Sclerosis Society
  - National Institute of Neurological and Communicative Disorders and Stroke

## Nursing Care Plan
### A Client with MS

George McMurphy, a 45-year-old from northern Minnesota, was diagnosed with MS approximately 5 years ago. He states that he probably had mild symptoms as long ago as 10 years. He works as a manager for a large grocery store chain near his home. He lives at home with his wife and two children, ages 12 and 15. Recently, Mr. McMurphy has had increasing problems with urinary incontinence, lack of energy, weakness, extreme fatigue, and altered mobility from spasticity in his leg muscles. He also has a fever, chest congestion, and a cough productive of green sputum. He is admitted to the hospital for evaluation and treatment of pneumonia and exacerbation of his MS.

### ASSESSMENT

Denise Miller, RN, primary care nurse, is assigned to care for Mr. McMurphy. His major complaint is the inability to "bring up all this sputum; I feel rotten from being so congested. I hate not being able to get to work and for my wife having to tend to my personal needs." Vital signs are as follows: BP 134/84, P 94, R 30, T 102°F (38.8°C). Mr. McMurphy is admitted for an acute exacerbation of the disorder, probably triggered by pneumonia. He will be treated with ACTH and intravenous antibiotics during this admission.

### DIAGNOSES

- *Ineffective airway clearance* related to lung infection and thick mucus
- *Activity intolerance* related to fatigue and spasticity
- *Self-care deficit: Toileting, feeding, and grooming* related to muscle weakness

### EXPECTED OUTCOMES

- Be able to clear airway.
- Have breath sounds clear to auscultation and pulse oximetry readings above 95%.
- Be able to ambulate using assistive devices, if needed.
- Perform self-care activities without becoming overly fatigued and tired.
- Verbalize methods to adapt daily routine to his level of tolerance.

### PLANNING AND IMPLEMENTATION

- Initiate pulmonary hygiene measures (e.g., incentive spirometry, turning, deep breathing and coughing, breathing exercises, and postural drainage) at least every 2 hours. Assess lung sounds, oxygen saturation, and ability to clear airway.

- Teach the importance of maintaining an oral fluid intake of at least 2000 mL per day to prevent tenacious sputum and to prevent urinary tract infections. Teach signs and symptoms of urinary and respiratory infections.
- Encourage participation in decision making about care.
- Assist with ADLs only as needed, based on level of fatigue and muscle weakness.
- Plan self-care activities so that they are performed during periods of peak level of energy; intersperse rest periods throughout the day.
- Refer to an MS support group.
- Refer to physical and occupational therapists for counseling regarding control of spasticity and possible splinting of spastic muscles.
- Consult a urologist for assessment of bladder incontinence; teach intermittent catheterization. Alternatively, the use of an external condom catheter may be indicated.

### EVALUATION

Mr. McMurphy is discharged 3 days following admission. He states that he feels stronger; on discharge, he has no problem clearing his airway. Although he continues to pace his activities to avoid fatigue, his muscle strength and "tiredness" have improved. He is able to complete ADLs unassisted.

Pulmonary function has returned to normal, prehospitalization levels: ABGs and pulse oximetry are within normal limits. Both Mr. McMurphy and his wife have listed several ways to modify their daily routine to allow more rest and decreased stress. Follow-up visits to his primary care physician have been arranged, and they have been provided with information about the local MS support group.

### Critical Thinking in the Nursing Process

1. Describe approaches the nurse could take to ensure that Mr. McMurphy does not exceed his activity tolerance.
2. Develop a teaching plan for Mr. McMurphy to help prevent future respiratory infections.
3. Develop a care plan for Mr. McMurphy for the nursing diagnosis, *Risk for injury* related to fatigue, muscle weakness, and spasticity.

See Evaluating Your Response in Appendix C.

# THE CLIENT WITH PARKINSON'S DISEASE

**Parkinson's disease (PD)** is a progressive, degenerative neurologic disease characterized by *tremor at rest* (resting or **nonintention tremor**), muscle rigidity, and *akinesia* (poverty of movement). People with PD are faced with multiple problems involving independence in ADLs, emotional well-being, financial security, and relationships with caregivers.

## INCIDENCE AND PREVALENCE

Parkinson's disease is one of the most common neurologic disorders affecting older adults, affecting up to 1 million people in the United States. Although it may occur in younger people, the onset of PD is most often after age 40, with the mean age being 60. Men are affected more than women.

Parkinson's-like manifestations, called *secondary parkinsonism,* may result from other disorders such as trauma, encephalitis, tumors, toxins, and drugs. Drug-induced parkinsonism, which is usually reversible, may occur in people taking neuroleptics, antiemetics, antihypertensives, and illegal designer drugs containing the chemical MPTP (McCance & Huether, 2002). Carbon monoxide or cyanide poisoning can also cause secondary parkinsonism. This discussion focuses on primary Parkinson's disease, the cause of which is unknown.

## PATHOPHYSIOLOGY

Coordinated, voluntary body movement is achieved through the actions of neurotransmitters in the basal ganglia of the brain. Some neurotransmitters facilitate the transmission of excitatory nerve impulses, while other neurotransmitters inhibit their transmission. Together, this system allows control of movement. A disturbed balance between excitatory and inhibitory neurotransmitters causes disorders of voluntary motor function.

In PD, neurons in the cerebral cortex atrophy and are lost, and the dopaminergic nigrostriatal (pigmented) pathway degenerates. Also, the number of specific dopamine receptors in the basal ganglia decreases. These pathologic processes cause a decrease in dopamine (a neurotransmitter that helps regulate nerve impulses involved in motor function). The usual balance of dopamine (an inhibitory neurotransmitter) and acetylcholine (an excitatory neurotransmitter) in the brain is disrupted, and dopamine no longer inhibits acetylcholine. The failure to inhibit acetylcholine is the underlying basis for the manifestations of the disorder. Parkinson's disease has five stages, outlined in Box 43–3.

## MANIFESTATIONS

Parkinson's disease begins with subtle symptoms. Clients complain of feeling tired and seem to move more slowly; a slight tremor may accompany the fatigue. In a small percentage of clients, dementia is the initial presenting symptom. The manifestations of PD are presented in the box on page 1417.

---

| BOX 43–3 | ■ Stages of Parkinson's Disease |
|---|---|

I   Unilateral involvement only, usually with minimal or no functional impairment.

II  Bilateral or midline involvement, without impairment of balance.

III First sign of impaired righting reflexes, evidenced as unsteadiness as the client turns or demonstrated when the client is pushed from standing equilibrium with the feet together and eyes closed. Functionally, the client is somewhat restricted in activities but may have some employment potential, depending on the type of employment. Clients are physically capable of leading independent lives, and their disability is mild to moderate.

IV  Fully developed, severely disabling disease; the client is still able to walk and stand unassisted but is markedly incapacitated.

V   Client is confined to bed or wheelchair unless aided.

## Tremor at Rest

Tremor at rest is usually the first manifestation experienced, with upper extremities more often affected. Resting tremors of the hand show a "pill rolling" motion of the thumb and fingers (given this name as this is the way in which medicinal pills were formed in the early days of medicine). The tremor may be controlled with purposeful, voluntary movement, and is worsened by stress and anxiety. Clients have progressive impairment in performing skills that require dexterity and fine muscle control, such as writing and eating.

## Rigidity and Akinesia

Manifestations related to motor and postural effects include rigidity, akinesia, and uncoordinated movements. *Rigidity* (resulting from involuntary contraction of all skeletal muscles) makes both active and passive movement difficult. It is manifested as increased resistance to passive range of motions. Although the extremity moves, it does so in a jerky motion, called *cogwheel rigidity*. The first manifestation of rigidity may be muscle cramps in the toes or hands, but most often the client describes stiffness, heaviness, or aching in muscles.

*Akinesia* is the most common and crippling manifestation. All striated muscles are affected, including those that involve chewing, swallowing, and speaking. Slowed or delayed movements affect the eyes, mouth, and voice, causing a masklike face and softened or muffled voice. Disorders of swallowing result in problems with eating and with drooling. Clients have a staring gaze with minimal change in expression (Figure 43–4 ■). Akinetic movements include both hypokinesia and bradykinesia. *Hypokinesia* (decreased frequency or absence of associated movements) is one of the earliest manifestations. Clients describe being "frozen" in place as voluntary movement is lost, and they sit or lie in one position without movement for long periods of time. **Bradykinesia** (slow movement) is experienced as difficulty in starting, continuing, or coordinating movements. Both of these disorders

## Manifestations of Parkinson's Disease

### MANIFESTATIONS RELATED TO MOTOR DYSFUNCTION

- Nonintention tremor
- Bradykinesia or akinesia
  a. Slowed movements; inability to initiate voluntary movements
  b. Slowed speech, low amplitude
  c. Poor articulation
  d. Decreased eye movements (i.e., blinking)
  e. Masklike, expressionless face
- Rigidity
- Posture and gait disturbances
  a. Trunk tilted forward
  b. Shuffling gait, propulsive at times
  c. Retropulsion
- Complications: falls, fractures, impaired communication, social isolation

### MANIFESTATIONS RELATED TO AUTONOMIC SYSTEM DYSFUNCTION

- Skin problems
  a. Seborrhea
  b. Excess sweating on face and neck, absence of sweating of trunk and extremities
  c. Mottled skin
- Heat intolerance
- Postural hypotension
- Constipation
- Complications: skin breakdown, dizziness, falls, constipation

### MANIFESTATIONS RELATED TO COGNITIVE AND PSYCHOLOGIC DYSFUNCTION

- Dementia
  a. Memory loss
  b. Lack of insight and problem-solving ability
  c. Declining intellectual abilities
- Anxiety
- Depression
- Complications: loss of ability to function, social isolation

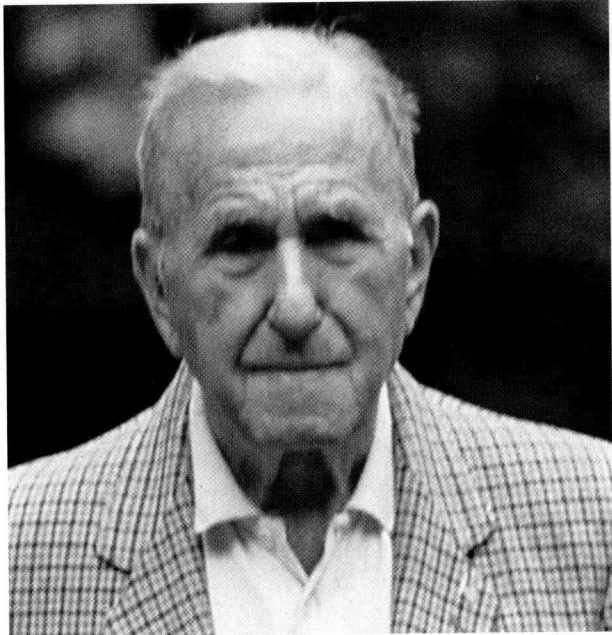

**Figure 43–4** ■ In Parkinson's disease, the client's face lacks expression or animation.

*Source: Yoav Levy/Phototake NYC.*

of movement are interspersed with freezing, which is brought about by turning, increasing the effort to move, or making visual or touch contacts.

## Abnormal Posture

The loss of normal postural reflexes results in postural abnormalities, including disorders of postural fixation, equilibrium, and righting. Involuntary flexion of the head and shoulders means the person with PD cannot maintain an upright position of the trunk when sitting or standing. This problem of postural fixation results in the characteristic stooped, leaning forward position. Disorders of equilibrium follow loss of postural fixation with an inability to make adjustments when leaning or falling. The client takes short, accelerated steps, also characteristic of PD, to try to maintain an upright position when walking.

## Autonomic and Neuroendocrine Effects

Many manifestations result from the loss of functions controlled by the autonomic nervous system. Elimination problems include constipation and urinary hesitation or frequency. Clients may experience problems related to orthostatic hypotension, including dizziness with position change. Eczematous skin changes and seborrhea are related to the increase in sweat gland activity secondary to increased sebotropic hormone production.

## Mood and Cognition

Both depression and dementia are pathologies associated with PD. Depression occurs in half of all clients and a third have dementia. Dementia, resulting from loss of cholinergic cells, loss of neurons, senile plaques, neurofibrillary tangles, and amyloid changes in small blood vessels, is seen more often in clients over the age of 70. The client manifests confusion, disorientation, memory loss, distractibility, and changes in abstraction and judgment. *Bradyphrenia* may also occur, resulting in slow thinking and a decreased ability to form thoughts, plan, and decide.

## Sleep Disturbances

Clients with PD also have sleep disturbances, although they may experience decreased manifestations during sleep in the early stages. The ability to fall and stay sleep is affected by acetylcholine. Muscle rigidity may compromise sleep because of the inability to change position. This lack of muscle movement causes the client to awaken and consciously shift position.

MediaLink | AKINESIA/BRADYKINESIA VIDEOS

## Interrelated Effects

Some of the manifestations that clients with PD experience have multiple contributing factors. For example, constipation is common because of decreased peristalsis. However, decreased peristalsis is not the only cause: Immobility, tremors (resulting in being unable to drink from a glass easily), and dietary changes from dysphagia all contribute to the problem of constipation.

The following complications are associated with Parkinson's disease.

- Oculogyric crisis, in which the eyes become fixed with a lateral and upward gaze
- Paranoia and hallucinations, which may accompany dementia
- Impaired communication due to changes in speech, handwriting, and expressiveness
- Falls from balance, posture, and motor changes
- Infections, such as pneumonia, related to immobility
- Malnutrition related to dysphagia and inability to prepare meals
- Altered sleep patterns due to loss of dopamine, l-dopa side effects (nightmares, dreams), or side effects of anticholinergics (hyperreflexia, muscle twitching), and depression
- Skin breakdown and pressure ulcers associated with urinary incontinence, malnutrition, and sweat reflex changes
- Depression and social isolation

## PROGNOSIS

Prognosis is poor, owing to the progressive degeneration that ultimately affects multiple physiologic systems and their function. Psychosocial effects are equally devastating, and the family needs more support as the client's debilitation increases. Total disability is usually seen 10 to 20 years after diagnosis. The leading cause of death is pneumonia.

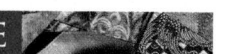

# COLLABORATIVE CARE

Diagnosis is based primarily on a thorough history and physical examination, and is made based on two of the following manifestations: tremor at rest, bradykinesia, rigidity, and postural instability. Interventions vary with the clinical stage of the disorder and include medication, surgery, and rehabilitation to retain the optimal level of functioning possible. A team approach is essential for these clients.

## Diagnostic Tests

Diagnostic studies may support a potential diagnosis of Parkinson's disease; however, no test clearly differentiates Parkinson's disease from other neurologic disorders. However, PET scan will show decreased uptake of 6-[18F]-fluorodopa. Tests are usually performed to rule out disorders that produce secondary parkinsonism. The following tests may be ordered.

- *Drug screens* determine the presence of medications or toxins that cause secondary parkinsonism, such as methyldopa, reserpine, or carbon monoxide.

- *EEG* may indicate slowed pattern and disorganization.
- *Upper GI X-ray series* with small bowel follow-through shows delayed emptying, distention, and possibly mega-colon with severe constipation.
- *CBC* may show low hemoglobin and hematocrit levels due to anemia.
- *Chemistry profile* may reflect low protein and albumin levels related to the client's inability to buy and prepare meals.

## Medications

The goal of drug therapy is to control symptoms to the extent possible. Generally, medications vary with the stage of the disease; however, response is individualized and guides the selection of medications. Types of drugs used include monoamine oxidase (MAO) inhibitors, dopaminergics, dopamine agonists, and anticholinergics. Information about these drugs is presented in the Medication Administration box on page 1419.

Initially clients are treated with selegiline (Carbex, Eldepryl), amantadine (Symmetrel), or anticholinergics. As the disease progresses, levodopa (Dopar, Larodopa) in combination with carbidopa (Lodosyn) is used in a medication named carbidopa-levodopa (Sinemet). Because levodopa eventually loses its effectiveness, dopamine agonists are added to increase the effectiveness of levodopa. Eventually, pharmacotherapeutic agents lose their efficacy, and the disease continues to progress despite treatment. Response to the drugs fluctuate; this phenomenon is called the "on-off" response.

Bromocriptine (Parlodel) and pergolide (Permax), agents that inhibit the breakdown of dopamine, are used to delay progression of the disease. COMT inhibitors (tolcapone [Tasmar] and entacapone [Comtan]) are used in conjunction with carbidopa-levodopa therapy to reduce the metabolism of levodopa, leading to more sustained dopaminergic stimulation of the brain.

Other medications may be used to treat problems related to Parkinson's disease. Antidepressants may be prescribed. Propranolol (Inderal) may be used to treat tremors; it should be used cautiously when clients have orthostatic hypotension.

## Treatments

Treatments to control manifestations and to improve function include electrical stimulation, surgery, and physical therapy, occupational therapy, and speech therapy.

### Electrical Stimulation

Activa TM tremor control therapy uses an implanted pacemaker-like device to deliver mild electrical stimulation to block the brain impulses that cause tremor. In this procedure, an insulated wire is surgically placed in the thalamus and connected to an implanted pulse generator (similar to an advanced cardiac pacemaker) near the clavicle. Clients can increase or decrease the stimulation depending on their tremor suppression needs (National Parkinson Foundation, 2001).

### Surgery

*Pallidotomy* is a surgical technique for Parkinson's disease, and its results have been helpful for many clients. In this procedure,

# Medication Administration

## The Client with Parkinson's Disease

### DOPAMINERGICS

Levodopa (Larodopa, Dopar)
Carbidopa-levodopa (Sinemet)
Amantadine (Symmetrel)

These drugs have their major effect on the akinesia of Parkinson's disease, improving mobility while decreasing muscle rigidity and tremor. Levodopa is a metabolic precursor of dopamine, but unlike dopamine, it can cross the blood–brain barrier. Levodopa is converted to dopamine in the brain by decarboxylase, a catalytic enzyme, and stimulates dopamine receptors to balance the dopamine/acetylcholine concentrations. Carbidopa prevents decarboxylase from converting levodopa to dopamine in the peripheral tissues; therefore, carbidopa is frequently given in combination with levodopa. Amantadine is used to treat dyskinesia and also elevates mood.

Levodopa is avoided in clients with narrow-angle glaucoma, severe angina pectoris, transient ischemic attacks, or melanoma. The "on-off" phenomenon occurs after the client takes levodopa for several years; this phenomenon is characterized by unexpected dyskinesias and lack of symptom control.

Common side effects are nausea and vomiting; darkening of urine and sweat; dyskinesias, especially in the first few months of therapy; dysrhythmias; orthostatic hypotension; and psychologic reactions, such as hallucinations and vivid dreams. Older adults are particularly susceptible to psychologic disturbances.

### Nursing Responsibilities

- Establish the client's baseline functional abilities in performing ADLs and administering the medication; assess motor control and coordination.
- To avoid adverse reactions, assess the client's overall health status before initiating therapy.
- Monitor medications known to cause adverse drug interactions: anticholinergics, pyridoxine, and antipsychotic agents alter the effectiveness of levodopa; MAO-B inhibitors can cause severe hypertension because of their vasoconstrictive effects.
- Withhold levodopa for 8 hours prior to administering Sinemet to avoid potentiating the effects of the circulating levodopa.

### Client and Family Teaching

- Levodopa may not take effect for several weeks to months.
- Do not alter dosages of medications; taking more of a medication may not result in better symptom control and can cause severe side effects.
- Your protein intake should be divided into equal amounts for the day's meals. Avoid foods high in pyridoxine, such as pork, beef, ham, avocado, beans, and oatmeal.
- Levodopa may cause a change in color of urine; this is harmless, however.
- To prevent side effects:
  - Prevent nausea by taking medication with food.
  - Change position slowly to avoid a drop in blood pressure and risk of falling.
  - Prevent constipation by increasing fluid intake and exercising regularly.
- Notify practitioner if you begin to have difficulty making voluntary movements or cardiac or psychologic symptoms develop.

- Watch for the "on-off" phenomenon, in which periods of symptom control alternate with periods when the drug fails to control symptoms.

### MONOAMINE OXIDASE (MAO) INHIBITORS

Selegiline (Eldepryl, Deprenyl)

Selegiline works by selectively inhibiting the enzyme that inactivates dopamine in the brain. It may be administered alone or as an adjunct therapy with levodopa: Selegiline inhibits the enzyme system that would otherwise break down and destroy dopamine. This synergistic effect lasts approximately 1 to 2 years. The combination of selegiline and levodopa increases the adverse reactions of dopamine; nurses must be alert for orthostatic hypotension, changes in movement, hallucinations, and confusion. These responses can be modified by lowering the dose of levodopa. Because it is highly selective for the MAO-A enzyme, selegiline does not have antidepressant effects like the MAO-B inhibitors. The risk of severe hypertension is low.

### Nursing Responsibilities

- Establish baseline functional abilities: motor control and movements, position changes, mental status.
- Monitor problems with insomnia.
- Assess for orthostatic hypotension; look for unsteadiness with position change and complaints of dizziness.
- Assess for hypertension, which can occur with higher than usual doses.

### Client and Family Teaching

- It is very important to take the medication as directed, especially dose and time of administration.
- Notify the practitioner if insomnia occurs.
- Report signs of dizziness when changing positions or standing, changes in ability to move, or psychologic changes.
- Change positions slowly, especially when moving from a sitting to standing position.
- Keep follow-up appointments for evaluation of the medication's effectiveness.

### DOPAMINE AGONISTS

Bromocriptine (Parlodel)          Pramipexole (Mirapex)
Pergolide (Permax)                Ropinirole (Requip)

Dopamine agonists act by directly activating dopamine receptors in the brain. They are frequently used in combination with levodopa therapy: When dopamine agonists are given with levodopa, they increase the therapeutic effects of levodopa and reduce fluctuations in motor symptoms. Adverse reactions are similar to those of levodopa: nausea, orthostatic hypotension, and psychologic disturbances are common. Nursing responsibilities and client and family teaching information are similar to those that apply to the dopaminergics.

### COMT INHIBITORS

Tolcapone (Tasmar)
Entacapone (Comtess)

COMT inhibitors inhibit catechol-O-methyltransferase (COMT), which is responsible for metabolizing dopamine. The concurrent

(continued on page 1420)

## Medication Administration

### The Client with Parkinson's Disease (continued)

administration of a COMT inhibitor with levodopa increases the amount of levodopa available to the brain to control Parkinson's disease.

#### Nursing Responsibilities

- Monitor liver function test results and manifestations of liver impairment (dark urine, jaundice).
- Administer with food.
- If given concurrently with warfarin, monitor PT and INR.

#### Client and Family Teaching

- Avoid using alcohol and sedatives.
- Rise slowly from a sitting or lying position to avoid falling.
- Nausea is common at the beginning of therapy.
- Do not abruptly stop taking the medication.
- Report increased loss of muscle control, yellow skin or eyes, dark urine, hallucinations, severe diarrhea.

#### ANTICHOLINERGICS

Trihexyphenidyl (Artane)
Benztropine (Cogentin)
Biperiden (Akineton)
Cycrimine (Pagitane)

Procyclidine (Kemadrin)
Chlorphenoxamine
   (Phenoxene)

Anticholinergics are effective in Parkinson's disease because they block the excitatory action of the neurotransmitter acetylcholine. They are frequently used during the early stages of the disease or when the client can no longer take levodopa. They may be given in combination with carbidopa-levodopa therapy. These medications ease drooling, tremors, and rigidity; however, side effects are common and may include blurred vision, dry mouth, constipa-tion, delayed gastric emptying, urinary retention, photophobia, and tachycardia. Older adults are especially susceptible to heat stroke and psychologic side effects, including confusion, depression, delusions, and hallucinations. Anticholinergics should be ta-pered slowly when discontinued to avoid enhancing parkinson-ian symptoms.

#### Nursing Responsibilities

- Perform baseline assessment for presence of glaucoma, car-diac dysfunction, and prostatic hypertrophy.
- Note other medications, including over-the-counter medica-tions that have anticholinergic effects, such as antihistamines and tricyclic antidepressants.
- Monitor for side effects, especially changes in vision, elimina-tion, gastric emptying, and mentation.

#### Client and Family Teaching

- Inform your practitioner if you begin taking any new medica-tions or notice any new symptoms.
- Avoid overexposure to heat, and take precautions to avoid heat stroke: Drink fluids, keep cool, and avoid strenuous activ-ity on hot days.
- Drink adequate amounts of fluid to minimize constipation.
- Practice home safety to prevent falls associated with blurred vision.
- Avoid taking over-the-counter antihistamines or sleeping aids; these have anticholinergic activity.
- Have the eyes examined annually to check for glaucoma; wear dark glasses if photophobia develops.
- Do not suddenly stop taking anticholinergics.

---

the neurosurgeon locates the affected areas of the globus pallidus and destroys the involved tissue. As a result, clients who could not previously ambulate are able to walk, and tremors cease. The long-term effects are still being evaluated.

*Stereotaxic thalamotomy* (an X-ray is taken during neuro-surgery to guide the insertion of a needle into a specific area of the brain) has been used only for clients who do not respond to medications—generally, younger people with extreme unilat-eral tremor. The surgeon destroys a small amount of tissue by creating a lesion in the ventrolateral nucleus of the thalamus. This surgery decreases tremors and rigidity in the contralateral extremity.

Autologous adrenal medullary transplant is another proce-dure that has been used when medications do not adequately control a client's symptoms. The client must be a good surgi-cal risk and free of dementia and end-stage cardiac, pul-monary, or renal disease. First an adrenalectomy and then a craniotomy are performed. Care of the client undergoing cran-iotomy was discussed in Chapter 42. Use of this procedure re-mains controversial.

Fetal tissue transplantation is another controversial surgical procedure limited to select medical centers. In this procedure, tissue of the substantia nigra is transplanted into the client's caudate nucleus.

### Rehabilitation

Depending on their individual needs, clients frequently benefit from rehabilitation therapy with a physical therapist, social worker, psychologist, and/or speech therapist.

Physical therapists (PT) can implement an individual exer-cise program to improve coordination, balance, gait, and transfers. Preventing contractures is an important goal of ex-ercise therapy. It is crucial that family and health care per-sonnel permit the client adequate time to perform not only exercise regimens but also ADLs. Activities should not be rushed.

An occupational therapist (OT) helps the client adapt to changing abilities pertinent to work, self-care, and recre-ational activities. Some rehabilitation centers assign OT per-sonnel the responsibility of addressing the client's upper ex-tremity functions while assigning PT personnel to manage lower extremity problems. For example, skills related to cook-ing and grooming would be supervised by the OT, whereas mobility and posture skills would be supervised by the PT.

Speech therapists frequently address not only the client's speech but also chewing and swallowing. These therapists eval-uate clients and plan treatment regimens. The challenge with clients who have PD is that they not only have vocalization problems, but also dexterity deficits; speech therapists therefore must evaluate the potential benefits of assistive devices, such as a magic slate, voice synthesizer, or computer, for each client.

## NURSING CARE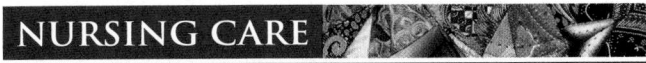

The chronic and eventually debilitating nature of PD poses many challenges to clients, families, and health care professionals. Dependence due to declining physical and mental abilities is of major concern. In the early stages, most clients are able to remain at home, with the family assisting with or providing many of the client's ADL needs. As the disease progresses and the burden of care increases, the client and family may prefer placement in a long-term care facility.

### Health Promotion

Teaching preventive measures is extremely important when caring for clients who have Parkinson's disease. Preventing malnutrition, falls and other environmental accidents, constipation, skin breakdown from incontinence or immobility, and joint contracture requires teaching and reinforcement.

In addition to incorporating information about safety needs, teach ways to prevent orthostatic hypotension when the client changes positions; some clients may also benefit from wearing elastic hose. In addition, address safety considerations about proper administration of medications.

### Assessment

Collect the following data through the health history and physical examination (see Chapter 40). Further focused assessments are described with nursing interventions below. When assessing the older client, be aware of normal changes with aging, outlined in Box 42–4 on page 1379.

- Health history: brain trauma, stroke, infection, exposure to heavy metals or carbon monoxide, medication and drug use, incontinence, constipation, weight loss, sweating, sleep problems, muscle pain, mood
- Physical assessment: affect; appearance; speech, scalp, eyelashes, and skin; drooling; tremor; coordination; posture; gait; muscle rigidity; mental status

### Nursing Diagnoses and Interventions

Clients with PD have complex and, ultimately, multisystem needs. Deficits in mobility and self-care are common. Psychosocial needs may include problems related to ineffective coping, powerlessness, and disturbed body image. Refer to the nursing care sections throughout this chapter for discussions of fatigue, self-care deficit, ineffective airway clearance, and other pertinent diagnoses. This section focuses on the nursing diagnoses related to impaired physical mobility, impaired verbal communication, imbalanced nutrition: less than body requirements, and disturbed sleep pattern.

#### Impaired Physical Mobility

Clients with PD have impaired mobility for several reasons, including tremors, gait pattern disturbances, and alterations in body positioning, such as forward bending of the trunk. Poor self-esteem may contribute to the client's lack of motivation and willingness to be mobile.

- Request the physical therapist teach caregivers how to do ROM exercises at least twice a day, emphasizing the trunk, neck, arms, hips, and legs. *Maintaining joint mobility promotes better function and strength, improving gait pattern. Consistent ROM exercises can prevent contractures.*
- Consult with a physical therapist to develop an individualized exercise program. *A program specific to the client supplies motivation as well as helping the client maintain muscle tone, flexibility, and mobility.*
- Ask caregivers to ambulate the client at least four times a day if possible. *Exercise fosters independence and self-esteem.*
- Recommend assistive devices, such as canes, splints, or braces, as indicated. *Adaptive equipment improves balance, protects joints, and promotes proper anatomic positioning.*
- To promote mobility and safety (see the Nursing Research box on page 1422):
  - Slightly elevate the back legs of chairs and raise the toilet seat to help rise from a sitting position to a standing position.
  - Wear shoes with Velcro closures.
  - Remove potential hazards, such as unanchored throw rugs.
  - Install hand rails and nonskid surfaces in bath tubs and showers.
  - Ensure adequate lighting throughout the home and in outside areas, especially in areas where transfers are common.
  *Safety measures prevent potential complications that may result from falls or other accidents and promote self-esteem through self-care.*

### PRACTICE ALERT
*Parkinson's disease is a disorder common in older adults, who are at greater risk for falls resulting from orthostatic hypotension, osteoporosis, poor vision, and other problems causing disorientation and confusion, such as Alzheimer's disease.* ■

#### Impaired Verbal Communication

Diminished vocal amplitude and loss of muscular control can impair the client's ability to speak. Both caregivers and family members must remember to give clients enough time for self-expression; an unhurried approach is recommended. Seek input from family members when determining alternative methods of communicating with the client.

- Assess current communication abilities in speech, hearing, and writing. *Communication involves both sending and receiving messages.*
- Develop methods of communication appropriate to coordination abilities, such as a magic slate; flash cards with common phrases; pointing to objects. *Individualizing a method of communication decreases anxiety and isolation.*
- Consult with a speech pathologist to develop oral exercises and interventions that will facilitate speaking. *The muscles of speech and swallowing are affected by the Parkinson's disease process.*
- Remind to speak more loudly, if possible. *A low, monotonous voice is characteristic of the client with Parkinson's disease.*

## Nursing Research

### Evidence-Based Practice for Preventing Falls in Clients with PD

Although clients with PD are at risk for and experience frequent falls, not much research has been done to identify the risk factors involved with this population. Gray and Hildebrand (2000) conducted this study to collect demographic, environmental, and medical history data. They also asked subjects to maintain a fall diary for a 3-month period. Of the 118 participants, 59% reported one or more falls (a total of 237 falls).

Analysis of data resulted in the following factors involved in an increased risk for falls in people with PD:

• Duration and severity of manifestations of PD, especially freezing, involuntary movements, and postural disorders that affected gait while walking (Clients with PD for more than 15 years were 5 times more likely to fall than those with PD for 5 years or less. Of subjects who reported episodes of freezing, 80% had falls.)
• Postural hypotension
• Using an aid to walk, such as a cane or walker
• Requiring help with ADLs
• Giving up usual activities
• Daily alcohol intake

#### IMPLICATIONS FOR NURSING

Nurses play an important role in identifying clients with PD who are at risk for falls, and in teaching clients and caregivers how to prevent them. A fall risk assessment should be an integral part of the nursing assessment. Clients and caregivers can be alerted to factors that increase the risk, and take preventive measures to reduce injuries. For example, being aware of the fall risk with turning, standing, walking, and freezing can increase attention to safety measures. In addition, stress the risk of alcohol intake, as well as intake and timing of medications and avoiding changes in the client's environment.

#### Critical Thinking in Client Care

1. How would interventions for the nursing diagnosis, *Risk for falls*, differ in a 60-year-old man who lives alone and an 88-year-old woman who is a resident in a nursing home?
2. Postural hypotension and lightheadedness may be side effects of medications for PD. Outline a teaching plan to decrease the risk for falls from these manifestations.
3. What factors would you include in a home assessment that would increase the client's risk for falls?

## Imbalanced Nutrition: Less Than Body Requirements

Tremors, altered gait, and impaired chewing and swallowing can cause nutritional problems in the client with PD. As the disorder progresses, interventions for ensuring optimal nutrition need to be adapted to the client's functional abilities. Assess the client's swallow reflex before starting any feeding program. During the initial stages of the disorder, some clients may have the nursing diagnosis, *Imbalanced nutrition: More than body requirements*, if kcal intake exceeds energy expenditure.

• Assess nutritional status and self-feeding abilities; consult with occupational or speech therapist, if needed. *An initial assessment of abilities ensures that interventions are personalized to the client's current functional abilities.*
• Teach caregivers how to prepare foods of proper consistency as determined by swallowing function. *The client may aspirate food that is too liquid.*
• Weigh weekly. *Early recognition of weight loss allows for intervention.*
• Teach eating methods to decrease tremors, such as holding a piece of bread in the hand that is not holding an eating utensil. *Nonintention tremor may be reduced through purposeful activity.*
• Encourage diet that is high in bulk and fluids. *Several anti-Parkinson's medications can cause constipation.*

## Disturbed Sleep Pattern

Rigidity and weakness can cause clients with Parkinson's disease to lose the ability to move and change positions during sleep. The resulting discomfort causes periods of wakefulness. Medications to treat Parkinson's disease contribute to sleep pattern disturbance; for example, levodopa can cause vivid dreams. Nurses can help accurately assess the sleep pattern disturbance and in planning interventions to improve or increase sleep time.

• Assess sleep pattern and existing conditions that may affect sleep, such as depression or pain. *Clients experiencing anxiety, depression, and dementia have a difficult time falling asleep and may wake up more at night.*

**PRACTICE ALERT** *Remember to assess pain status; lack of adequate pain control may interfere with sleep.* ∎

• Explain the disease process and the effects of decreased dopamine on the sleep-wake cycle. *Depending on the dosage, levodopa causes less REM sleep and deep sleep.*
• Review the client's medication. *Bromocriptine and levodopa, especially if used with an anticholinergic, can cause vivid dreams. Other medications (diuretics, theophylline, hypnotics) also may interfere with sleep.*
• Teach how to modify lifestyle activities that affect sleep:
  • Institute a routine of activities with limited rest periods during the day; avoid napping close to bedtime. Avoid strenuous exercise in the evening. *Daytime sleeping may contribute to decreased nighttime sleeping. Vigorous exercise just before bedtime may act as a stimulant.*
  • Incorporate diet modifications, such as limiting caffeine and alcohol intake. *Caffeine is a stimulant, and alcohol may cause early-morning awakenings, increased daytime sleepiness, and nightmares.*
  • Drink a glass of milk before bedtime. *Milk contains L-tryptophan, which produces sedative effects by shortening the time taken to fall asleep (sleep latency).*

## CHART 43-3 NANDA, NIC, AND NOC LINKAGES

### The Client with PD

| NURSING DIAGNOSES | NURSING INTERVENTIONS | NURSING OUTCOMES |
|---|---|---|
| • Impaired Physical Mobility | • Energy Management<br>• Exercise Therapy: Ambulation | • Mobility Level<br>• Ambulation: Walking |
| • Self-Care Deficits | • Bathing/Hygiene<br>• Dressing/Hair Care<br>• Feeding<br>• Toileting | • Self-Care: ADLs<br>• Self-Care: Bathing<br>• Self-Care: Dressing<br>• Self-Care: Feeding<br>• Self-Care: Toileting |
| • Constipation<br>• Imbalanced Nutrition: Risk for Less than Body Requirements | • Bowel Management<br>• Nutrition Management<br>• Swallowing Therapy<br>• Self-Care Assistance: Feeding | • Bowel Elimination<br>• Nutritional Status |

*Note. Data from Nursing Outcomes Classification (NOC) by M. Johnson & M. Maas (Eds.), 1997, St. Louis: Mosby; Nursing Diagnoses: Definitions & Classification 2001–2002 by North American Nursing Diagnosis Association, 2001, Philadelphia: NANDA; Nursing Interventions Classification (NIC) by J.C. McCloskey & G. M. Bulechek (Eds.), 2000, St. Louis: Mosby. Reprinted by permission.*

• Adapt the environment to aid in sleep (e.g., darken the room and decrease noises). *Reducing environmental stimuli decreases external sleep disturbances.*

## Using NANDA, NIC, and NOC

Chart 43–3 shows links between NANDA nursing diagnoses, NIC, and NOC when caring for the client with PD.

## Home Care

It is important for both the client and the family to maintain independence and self care as long as possible. To maintain function and quality of life, the following topics should be addressed.

• Realistic expectations
• Equipment suppliers
• Home environment conducive to using equipment
• Referrals to speech therapist, occupational therapist, physical therapist, dietitian

• Gait training and exercises for improving ambulation, speech, swallowing, and self-care
• Increased fluid intake of 3000 mL/day and increased fiber in every meal
• Stool softeners or laxatives as needed for bowel elimination
• Swallowing during eating and taking medications (Have suction equipment available and know the Heimlich maneuver if choking occurs.)
• Foods that can be easily swallowed (such as pureed or soft) and feed six small meals a day if possible
• Helpful resources:
  • American Parkinson's Disease Association
  • National Parkinson Foundation, Inc.
  • Parkinson's Disease Foundation
  • The National Institute of Neurological Disorders and Stroke

MediaLink | PARKINSON'S DISEASE RESOURCES

## Nursing Care Plan
### A Client with PD

Walter Avneil, age 78, was diagnosed with PD at age 64. His wife died 5 years ago and he has no other family living. Mr. Avneil worked for more than 40 years as a mechanic in a large factory. He is a resident of a long-term care facility. During his last clinic visit for a review of his medications, the following assessment was made.

#### ASSESSMENT

Elderly white male with history of PD for the past 14 years. Skin oily and damp. Tremors in both hands and the lips. Gait is slow and shuffling, with a forward leaning posture. Speech slow and slurred. Face expressionless. Has lost 10 lb since last visit 3 months ago. Has been on levodopa with carbidopa since diagnosis. States major problems are "eating problems, bowel problems, walking problems."

#### DIAGNOSIS

• *Constipation* related to lack of exercise, decreased food intake, and effects of medications
• *Impaired verbal communication* related to lip tremors, slow/slurred speech, and facial muscle involvement of PD
• *Imbalanced nutrition: Less than body requirements* related to difficulty swallowing and chewing
• *Impaired physical mobility* related to rigidity and bradykinesia

#### EXPECTED OUTCOMES

• Have a soft stool at least every other day.
• Practice exercises provided by speech therapist twice a day.

*(continued on page 1424)*

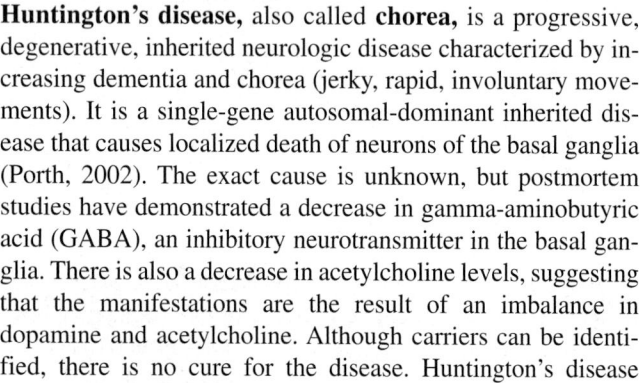

## Nursing Care Plan
## A Client with PD (continued)

- Increase number of calories, fluids, and fiber in diet provided at long-term facility.
- Improve joint mobility and ability to ambulate.

### PLANNING AND IMPLEMENTATION

- Discuss problems with bowel elimination with staff at long-term facility; suggest increasing fluids to 3000 mL per day and also increasing fiber in the diet with oatmeal for breakfast, and more fruits and vegetables at meals.
- Encourage exercises provided by speech therapist to improve speech and swallowing. If these are not effective, make a referral for another evaluation.
- Discuss diet plan with dietitian at the long-term care facility, including consistency of foods and number of calories. Suggest dietitian be a part of swallowing evaluation by the speech therapist.
- Refer for physical therapy and occupational therapy for a program to improve gait and joint mobility, and to decrease risk of falling.

### EVALUATION

In a return visit 3 months later, Mr. Avneil reports that "my bowels are working better." He has gained 7 lb, and the staff report that this is related to multiple factors, including practicing his swallow-

ing exercises, getting more exercise that stimulated his appetite, and changing his diet to six small meals a day of soft or pureed foods. The staff is offering him liquids at meals and snack times, and he usually drinks all they give him. His speech is not much improved. He posture and gait are somewhat better, and he is doing the exercises provided by the physical therapist and occupational therapist. Mr. Avneil's functional abilities have improved so much that the staff is considering training sessions specific to care of residents with PD.

### Critical Thinking in the Nursing Process

1. Although Mr. Avneil did not mention it, the staff reports that he is frustrated by not being able to dress himself. What suggestions could you make to facilitate his independence?
2. Mr. Avneil spends most of his time alone, although he enjoys the company of the other residents. List assessments and interventions you might provide to increase his diversional activity.
3. The loss of his wife and the debilitating effects of his disease increase Mr. Avneil's risk for chronic sorrow. What might you suggest the long-term staff do to reduce this risk?

See Evaluating Your Response in Appendix C.

## THE CLIENT WITH HUNTINGTON'S DISEASE

**Huntington's disease,** also called **chorea,** is a progressive, degenerative, inherited neurologic disease characterized by increasing dementia and chorea (jerky, rapid, involuntary movements). It is a single-gene autosomal-dominant inherited disease that causes localized death of neurons of the basal ganglia (Porth, 2002). The exact cause is unknown, but postmortem studies have demonstrated a decrease in gamma-aminobutyric acid (GABA), an inhibitory neurotransmitter in the basal ganglia. There is also a decrease in acetylcholine levels, suggesting that the manifestations are the result of an imbalance in dopamine and acetylcholine. Although carriers can be identified, there is no cure for the disease. Huntington's disease causes progressive chorea, speech problems, and dementia.

Because the client is usually asymptomatic until age 30 to 40, he or she may already have passed the gene to the next generation. The psychologic impact is devastating to clients and their families. The family not only experiences guilt from passing the disease from one generation to the next, but also is faced with the overwhelming long-term care needs of those affected. It is common for several family members to be afflicted with the disease.

### PATHOPHYSIOLOGY

Huntington's disease causes destruction of cells in the caudate nucleus and putamen areas of the basal ganglia. Other areas of

the brain, such as the frontal lobes, may selectively atrophy. Several neurotransmitters and their receptors are decreased, including GABA and acetylcholine. The neurotransmitter dopamine is not affected in Huntington's disease, but the decrease in acetylcholine results in a relative excess of dopamine in the basal ganglia. Whereas in Parkinson's disease a deficit of dopamine causes slow movement or lack of movement, in Huntington's disease the opposite occurs: There is a relative excess of dopamine, causing excessive, uncontrolled movement.

### MANIFESTATIONS

Manifestations primarily involve abnormal movement and progressive dementia (see the box on page 1425). The progression and sequence of manifestations varies somewhat; however, initially the psychologic manifestations are more debilitating than the choreiform movements.

Early signs of personality change include severe depression, memory loss with decreased ability to concentrate, emotional lability, and impulsiveness. The client experiences frequent mood swings ranging from uncontrollable periods of anger to apathy. Eventually, signs of dementia, including disorientation, confusion, and lack of sense of time, become evident and interfere with self-care.

Motor symptoms usually parallel personality and mood changes. The motor symptoms worsen with environmental stimuli and emotional stress but are absent when the client is sleeping. Initially, movement problems are described as "fidgeting" or restlessness, followed by progressive worsening of

## Manifestations of Huntington's Disease

### MOTOR EFFECTS

**Early**

- Restlessness
- "Fidgety" feeling
- Minor gait changes—unsteady on feet
- Posture and positioning disturbances, frequent falls
- Inability to keep the tongue from protruding
- Slurred speech with poor articulation
- Complications: increasing problem with self-care activities, such as bathing, grooming, eating

**Late**

- Chorea—severely altered gait with irregular, uncontrollable movement; the distal extremity is most affected; shoulders shrug arrhythmically
- Facial grimacing—raising of eyebrows, uncontrollable protrusion of the tongue
- Dysphagia
- Unintelligible speech
- Impaired diaphragmatic movement
- Complications: immobility, aspiration, choking, and, eventually, total dependence, poor oxygenation, emaciation, and cachexia

### PSYCHOSOCIAL EFFECTS

**Early**

- Irritability
- Outbursts of rage alternating with euphoria
- Depression
- Complication: suicide

**Late**

- Decreasing memory
- Loss of cognitive skills
- Eventual dementia
- Complication: total dependence

abnormal movements. The choreiform movements, which begin in the face and arms and then involve the entire body, are manifested by facial grimaces, tongue protrusion, jerky movement of the distal arms or legs, and a rhythmic, lurching gait that almost resembles a dance. (The term *chorea* comes from *choreia,* the Greek word meaning "dance.") Gait changes cause uncoordinated movements and contribute to frequent falls.

The muscles of swallowing, chewing, and speaking are affected, leading to dysphagia and dysarthria and associated problems with communication and nutrition. The client's constant movement and difficulty in swallowing contribute to weight loss and eventual cachexia. Breathing is impaired because the diaphragm is unable to move effectively.

The manifestations slowly progress over approximately 15 to 20 years after initial symptoms appear. Prognosis is poor, with inevitable debilitation and total dependence. Death usually results from aspiration pneumonia or another infectious process.

## COLLABORATIVE CARE

There is no cure for Huntington's disease, and treatment addresses the disease's manifestations. Nurses provide care to clients with Huntington's disease in a variety of community settings. Initially, clients and families can manage care needs at home, but as the disease progresses, the client requires constant supervision, such as that provided in day care facilities. Eventually, skilled long-term care is needed. Clients who develop acute problems may be hospitalized until the crisis is managed. Because of the inevitable total multisystem debilitation of clients with Huntington's disease, nurses and other caregivers face many challenges.

### Diagnostic Tests

Genetic testing is the only test available to diagnose clients suspected of having Huntington's disease. Both blood and amniotic fluid may be tested for the presence of chromosome 4 using DNA analysis. The test can predict with 95% accuracy which offspring have the disease.

### Medications

The following medications are given for palliation of the symptoms of Huntington's disease.

- Antipsychotics, specifically phenothiazines and butyrophenones, are effective in Huntington's disease because they block dopamine receptors in the brain. The therapeutic goal is to restore the balance among the neurotransmitters.
- Antidepressants are prescribed in the early stage of the disease; however, medications are no substitute for intense follow-up counseling for clients and families.

## NURSING CARE

Nurses are faced with a multitude of challenges when caring for families who have Huntington's disease, including physiologic, psychosocial, and ethical problems. Physiologic problems are related to the progressive and eventually debilitating nature of the disease. Psychosocial concerns occur as a result of the client's personality and mental changes, the family's responsibility for providing care, and the guilt implicit in a genetically transmitted disease. Ethical difficulties relate to the genetic nature of the disease: DNA testing for the marker on chromosome 4 can determine whether the person is a carrier of the disease before he or she begins to exhibit manifestations. Children of people with Huntington's disease are thus faced with the choice of finding out whether they will eventually be affected. If they choose not to be tested, they may pass the disease on to yet another generation; and if a fetus is affected, they may face the decision of whether to undergo an abortion.

### Nursing Diagnoses and Interventions

Initially, much of the nursing care focuses on teaching about the disease, psychologic support, and genetic counseling. As manifestations become more severe, nursing considerations center on problems related not only to immobility and altered nutrition, but also to the increasing self-care deficits. Families and clients experiencing Huntington's disease face many psychosocial issues. Nurses must be prepared to listen actively as well as to provide comfort and encouragement throughout the lengthy illness. There are many possible nursing diagnoses for the client with Huntington's disease; this section focuses on nursing diagnoses related to aspiration, nutrition, skin integrity, and communication.

### Risk for Aspiration

Uncoordinated movements and swallowing and chewing problems put the client at high risk for aspiration.

- Maintain in an upright position while the client eats; support the head. *Proper positioning may prevent aspiration during mealtime.*
- Teach the Heimlich maneuver to caregivers and family members. *Aspiration is a real possibility; caregivers must be prepared to reestablish the client's airway.*
- Provide food that is thick enough to manage, such as thick soups, mashed potatoes, stews, or casseroles. *These foods are more readily tolerated and manipulated by the tongue than liquids.*
- Make sure food is swallowed before giving another spoonful of food. *The automatic phase of swallowing may be disrupted in the client with Huntington's disease; providing adequate time and smaller bites may improve the ability to manipulate foods.*
- Provide a calm, relaxing eating environment. *Stress worsens choreiform movements and inappropriate behaviors.*

### Imbalanced Nutrition: Less Than Body Requirements

Clients with Huntington's disease have unpredictable choreiform movements of the extremities and decreased ability to control muscles involved with chewing and swallowing. Families and caregivers are challenged to provide sufficient calories to maintain the client in positive nitrogen balance.

- Evaluate current weight and nutritional status, including serum albumin and transferrin levels. *Establishing a baseline is crucial for meeting individual caloric, protein, vitamin, and mineral needs.*
- Assess ability to swallow and manipulate eating utensils. *Aspiration is an ever-present danger that must be avoided; utensils may need to be adapted to client's abilities, if client is able to assist at all.*
- Continue feeding even if the client physically turns away from the meal. *Involuntary choreiform movements should not be interpreted as a refusal to eat.*
- Provide high-kcal, nutritious foods and sufficient snacks; request input from a dietitian. *The constant movement of Huntington's disease increases caloric requirements.*
- Avoid milk; provide frequent oral hygiene. *Milk tends to thicken secretions. Decreasing thick secretions may improve ability to swallow and enable the client to ingest more calories.*

### Impaired Skin Integrity

Skin integrity is only one component of the client's general need for protection and avoidance of injury. Several factors increase the risk for impaired skin integrity, including poor nutritional status, eventual total immobility, and incontinence.

- Evaluate the skin for actual and potential areas of breakdown. *Establishing a baseline is necessary to modify care and provide prophylactic protection of high-risk pressure areas.*
- Determine nutritional status, especially serum albumin level and vitamin, mineral, and kcal intake. *Optimal nutritional status and positive nitrogen balance help prevent skin breakdown and formation of pressure ulcers.*
- Turn and inspect the skin at least every 2 hours, giving special consideration to areas that are most prone to breakdown, such as heels and coccyx. *Pressure points are particularly susceptible to skin breakdown.*
- Provide ROM exercises on a regular schedule in the daytime. *Movement stimulates circulation, which provides oxygenation and allows nutrients to reach muscles and skin.*
- Keep the skin clean and dry; pay particular attention to the perineal area if incontinent. *Skin in close proximity to perineal area, such as the sacral area, is highly susceptible to breakdown due to exposure to wet, acidic urine and fecal material.*
- Place on an alternating-pressure mattress with foot board. *Decreasing pressure on bony prominences and preventing shearing forces serve to prevent skin breakdown.*
- Pad side rails and headrests of special chairs; have the client wear a football-type helmet. *The client's violent movements can cause trauma to the head and extremities.*

### Impaired Verbal Communication

The inability to control muscles related to speech, swallowing, and facial movement contributes to problems of verbal communication. Because Huntington's disease affects fine motor movement, especially the distal portion of the extremities, the hands are not effective in communication. As the disease progresses, mental abilities are also compromised, making both receptive and expressive communication impossible.

- Choose alternative methods of communication while the client is able to participate. *Anticipatory planning may facilitate communication and decrease anxiety.*
- Continue to incorporate therapeutic communication techniques, even though client is not responsive: maintain eye contact, use touch, and talk directly to the client rather than to others in the room. *These techniques enhance the individual's dignity and worth.*
- Seek input from family about client's usual preferences and how they are communicated; be alert for subtle cues. *Nonverbal communication techniques may be individualized and more readily recognized by the family member or caregiver that usually provides care.*
- Continue talking to the client, even though there is no apparent response. *Hearing may not be impaired, even though the client cannot speak.*

## BOX 43–4 ■ Inheritance of an Autosomal Dominant Trait

■ The abnormal trait is dominant over the normal characteristics—in the case of Huntington's disease, neurologic functioning.

■ People affected usually have at least one parent who also is affected.

■ Each offspring has a 50% risk of being affected. In other words, transmission of the dominant trait is independent of number of children who may or may not already have the disease.

■ Both sexes are equally affected because the inheritance is autosomal dominant, not X-linked.

■ Children who are not affected will not genetically transmit the disease to their children.

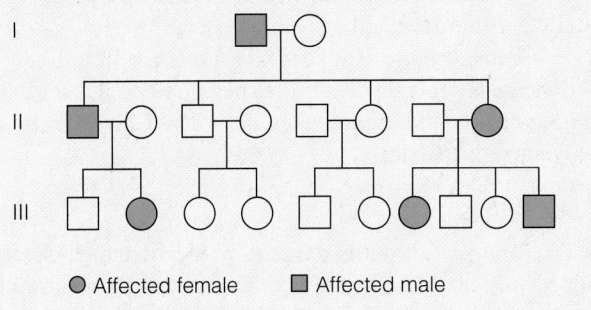

● Affected female   ■ Affected male

## Home Care

Clients with Huntington's disease and their families know how devastating the illness is as they may have cared for a parent or other close family member who has suffered through the illness. Many families are overwhelmed with just the thought of the physical and psychosocial debilitation that the disease brings. Fear, anxiety, and hopelessness leading to depression are common reactions. Teaching ways to cope effectively with the psychosocial and physical changes is an integral part of the nurse's responsibilities. Referrals to appropriate agencies, such as the Huntington's Disease Foundation and local support groups or a psychologist, should be part of the nursing plan.

Another aspect of client teaching concerns the genetic transmission of Huntington's disease; refer clients and family members to a geneticist. Nurses are frequently involved with clarifying information, especially concerning the transmission, course of illness, and prognosis. A caring, sensitive approach is crucial. Information about transmission of an autosomal-dominant trait is presented in Box 43–4.

Nurses in the community are often the professionals with whom families have the most contact. Teaching family members ways to prevent injury from falls and methods to avoid malnutrition are part of holistic care. Measures to assist with incontinence are instituted when indicated.

## THE CLIENT WITH AMYOTROPHIC LATERAL SCLEROSIS

**Amyotrophic lateral sclerosis (ALS),** or **Lou Gehrig's disease,** is a progressive, degenerative neurologic disease characterized by weakness and wasting of the involved muscles, without any accompanying sensory or cognitive changes. The name is derived from the pathophysiologic processes of muscle atrophy (*amyotrophy*) resulting from lower motor neuron involvement and lateral sclerosis of the corticospinal tract in the lateral column of the spinal cord resulting from upper motor neuron involvement. Death results in 2 to 5 years after onset of the symptoms, usually due to respiratory failure.

ALS is the most common motor neuron disease in the United States, with approximately 5000 new cases diagnosed each year (McCance & Huether, 2002). There are several types, categorized as sporadic ALS (no family history of ALS) and familial ALS (a family history of ALS). Most people are between 40 and 60 years of age at diagnosis; the incidence is higher in men in the earlier ages but becomes equal with women after menopause. Classic ALS (Lou Gehrig's disease) occurs most often in the early 50s. There is a genetic factor involved, with familial ALS linked to chromosome 21 defects. Most of the physiologic problems a client with ALS encounters are related to swallowing and managing secretions, communication, and dysfunction of the muscles used in respiration.

## PATHOPHYSIOLOGY AND MANIFESTATIONS

ALS results from the degeneration and demyelination of motor neurons in the anterior horn of the spinal cord, brainstem, and cerebral cortex. ALS involves both upper and lower motor neurons. Death of the motor neurons results in axonal degeneration, demyelination, glial proliferation, and scarring along the corticospinal tract. In the early stages of the disease, surviving motor neurons sprout new branches to reinnervate affected muscle fibers, preserving muscle strength. However, when more than half of the lower motor neurons are affected, reinnervation fails and weakness is evidenced (Ross, 1999).

Although the pathogenesis of ALS is not clear, abnormal glutamate metabolism and hydrogen peroxide production are being studied. Echovirus RNA have also been isolated in spinal cord tissue in some clients with nonfamilial ALS (McCance & Huether, 2002). Environmental factors, excess intracellular calcium, and antibodies to calcium channels are also being researched.

The initial manifestations may relate to dysfunction of upper motor neurons, lower motor neurons, or both. Dysfunction of upper motor neurons (located in the cerebral cortex and conduct impulses within the central nervous system) results in spastic, weak muscles with increased deep-tendon reflexes. Dysfunction of lower motor neurons (which originate in the gray matter of the spinal cord or the brainstem cranial nerves and innervate skeletal muscles) results in muscle flaccidity, paresis (weakness), paralysis, and atrophy.

Weakness and paresis are common early complaints. The weakness may initially affect only one muscle group. Manifestations vary according to the particular muscle group involved; **fasciculations,** or focal twitching, of involved muscles are common in the early stage of the disorder. With the loss of muscle innervation, the muscles atrophy, and paralysis results. Clinically, the muscle mass decreases, and clients complain of progressive fatigue. Typically, the disease first affects the hands, then the shoulders, upper arms, and finally the legs.

Increasing brainstem involvement causes progressive atrophy of the tongue and facial muscles with eventual dysphagia and dysarthria. Emotional lability and loss of control occur, but dementia is not part of the pathologic progression of ALS. Vision, hearing, sensation, and cognitive ability usually remain intact. A summary of manifestations is presented in the box below.

About 50% of clients die within 2 to 5 years of diagnosis, but the course of the disease varies. Eventually, the client faces total debilitation and dependence. Death frequently results from aspiration pneumonia, another infectious process, or respiratory failure.

## COLLABORATIVE CARE

Because many treatable disorders may cause manifestations similar to those that appear in the initial stage of ALS, a thorough evaluation is required. Once ALS is diagnosed, the primary goal is to support the client and family in meeting physical and psychosocial needs, particularly as the disease progresses.

Medical and nursing care for clients with ALS is primarily supportive. Referral to community health nurses for home health management is indicated. Occupational, physical, speech, and respiratory therapy are major supportive and rehabilita-

tive treatments. As the disorder progresses and swallowing becomes ineffective, a gastrostomy tube may be indicated to provide adequate nutritional intake. Ventilatory assistance should be discussed with clients before the need occurs.

### Diagnostic Tests

A number of disorders may mimic early ALS, including hyperthyroidism, hypoglycemia, compression of the spinal cord, toxic agents, infections, and neoplasms. In addition to diagnostic studies performed to rule out other suspected conditions, the following tests may be ordered.

- *EMG* is done to differentiate a neuropathy from a myopathy. Fibrillations of the muscle at rest supports the diagnosis of ALS.
- *Muscle biopsy* reflects tissue changes consistent with atrophy and loss of muscle fiber.
- *Serum creatine kinase (CK) enzyme levels* are usually elevated; however, this finding is not specific to ALS.
- *Pulmonary function studies* may be ordered if respiratory involvement is a factor.

### Medications

Riluzole (Rilutek), an antiglutamate, is the first medication developed to treat ALS. It inhibits the presynaptic release of glutamic acid in the CNS and protects neurons against the excitotoxicity of glutamic acid. This oral medication is administered without food at the same time each day. Clients are regularly monitored for liver function, blood count, blood chemistries, and alkaline phosphatase. They should be warned to report any febrile illness to their health care provider and to avoid alcohol.

## NURSING CARE

Nursing care focuses on current health problems and on anticipating future difficulties. As with other disorders causing incapacitation and dependence, individualized nursing goals and interventions relate to decreasing complications, especially those associated with loss of muscular function and immobility; promoting independence to the extent possible; initiating referrals, particularly to a support group for both client and family; and providing physical and psychosocial support as indicated.

Of special consideration is planning for the client's eventual inability to communicate. Because the client's eye muscles and movements remain intact, signals can be prearranged before the loss of speech.

### Nursing Diagnoses and Interventions

Two nursing diagnoses that frequently apply to clients with ALS are Risk for disuse syndrome and Ineffective breathing pattern.

#### Risk for Disuse Syndrome

Clients with ALS are at risk for developing problems associated with bed rest not only because they cannot move and reposition themselves but also because they frequently have altered nutritional and hydration status. Nursing interventions focus on

## Manifestations of ALS

### MUSCULOSKELETAL SYSTEM

- Weakness and fatigue
- "Heaviness" of legs
- Fasciculations
- Uncoordinated movements, loss of fine motor control in hands
- Spasticity
- Paresis
- Hyperreflexia
- Atrophy
- Problems with articulation
- Complications: paralysis, loss of ability to perform ADLs, total immobility, aspiration, loss of verbal communication

### RESPIRATORY SYSTEM

- Dyspnea
- Difficulty clearing airway
- Complications: pneumonia, eventual respiratory failure

### NUTRITIONAL EFFECTS

- Difficulty chewing
- Dysphagia
- Complication: malnutrition

### EMOTIONAL EFFECTS

- Loss of control, lability
- Complication: depression

preventing skin breakdown and infections, such as urinary tract infections.

- Assess current condition for baseline parameters, particularly skin over bony prominences, lung sounds, and vital signs. *Understanding client's current condition allows accurate future assessment and realistic planning.*
- Assess skin; provide skin care, and obtain an alternating-pressure mattress. *Pressure points are at risk for breakdown; early detection is crucial to instituting appropriate care.*
- Institute active ROM exercises, as the client is able. Perform passive ROM exercises every 2 hours, when the client is turned. *Contractures can develop within a week because extensor muscles are weaker than flexor muscles.*
- Maintain positive nitrogen balance and hydration status: Monitor albumin levels, hemoglobin and hematocrit levels, and urine specific gravity. *Adequate protein is required to maintain osmotic pressure and prevent edema; positive nitrogen balance promotes optimal body functioning.*
- Monitor for manifestations of infection; for example, assess urine, especially if a urinary catheter is present. *Urinary catheters place clients at high risk for sepsis; bed rest places the client at greater risk for urinary stasis.*

**PRACTICE ALERT** *Urinary tract infection is indicated by cloudy, foul-smelling urine, pain on urination, fever, and general malaise.* ■

### Ineffective Breathing Pattern

As the muscle weakness of ALS continues, clients become less able to breathe. The respiratory muscles are affected, and clients eventually may require ventilatory assistance. The nurse must initiate measures to support the existing respiratory effort.

- Obtain a baseline assessment of breathing pattern, air movement, and oxygen saturation. *Assessments indicating the client's current condition provide data to plan individualized interventions.*
- Turn at least every 2 hours. *Movement enhances the ability to move pulmonary secretions and prevents stasis.*
- Elevate the head of the bed at least 30 degrees, suction as indicated, and provide oxygen. *This supports ventilation and enhances lung expansion as the client's condition changes.*
- Assess temperature and lung sounds routinely; obtain sputum culture as indicated. *Early detection of a possible infectious process leads to prompt treatment.*

**PRACTICE ALERT** *A pulmonary infection is indicated by respiratory difficulty, crackles and/or wheezes, cough productive of yellow or green sputum, fever, and malaise.* ■

### Home Care

Initial teaching centers on explaining the disease process, expected course, and prognosis. Referral to a social worker to determine home care needs and financial assistance is helpful.

Counseling and referrals to a community health nurse, dietitian, and physical, speech, and occupational therapists can help the family meet the client's changing needs and abilities. The need for realistic anticipation of needs cannot be overemphasized.

As the client becomes more debilitated, family members or other care providers focus on preventing complications. For example, family members need to know how to suction the client and perform the Heimlich maneuver to prevent aspiration. Teaching the family how to prevent problems related to immobility is a primary consideration for the nurse.

Another focus of teaching is basic care needs, such as care required to meet elimination needs. Teach families methods to establish a bowel routine, considerations related to a urinary catheter, and the need to promptly report manifestations of an infection.

Throughout the early stage and continued care of the client and family with ALS, much consideration is given to psychosocial concerns. Depression, anger, and denial may be initial reactions; refer the client and family to an ALS support group, social worker, psychologist, or psychiatrist as indicated.

## THE CLIENT WITH CREUTZFELDT-JAKOB DISEASE

**Creutzfeldt-Jakob disease (CJD, spongiform encephalopathy)** is a rapidly progressive, degenerative, neurologic disease that causes brain degeneration without inflammation. The disease is transmissible and progressively fatal. The causative agent is believed to be an abnormal form of a cellular glycoprotein known as the prion protein. Transmission of the agent is by direct contamination with infected neural tissue, such as during eye and brain surgery. The injection of contaminated human growth hormone from cadaveric pituitaries has also been implicated.

A new disease, called **new variant CJD (vCJD)** is also a rare, degenerative, fatal brain disorder, but is not the same as the classic form of CJD. New variant CJD, referred to as "mad-cow disease" is believed due to consumption of cattle products contaminated with bovine spongiform encephalopathy (BSE). This form primarily affects younger people. As the illness is fatal and is associated with infected cattle, severe restrictions have been placed on the importation of cattle, sheep, and goats; and on products from these animals from countries in which BSE is known to exist. To date, no case of this cattle disease has been detected in the United States, but it has been identified in England, France, Ireland, Italy, and Canada.

In the United States, the annual incidence of the classic form of CJD is estimated to be between 0.9 and 31.3 cases per million people. It primarily affects adults over the age of 50; men and women are affected equally. The peak age for onset is between the ages of 55 and 74. The disease occurs worldwide, but clusters occur in several areas, more often in England, Chile, and Italy.

## PATHOPHYSIOLOGY AND MANIFESTATIONS

Creutzfeldt-Jakob disease is characterized by degeneration of the gray matter of the brain. The spongiform degeneration (involving the formation of tiny holes and resembling a sponge) produces severe dementia, myoclonus (muscle contractions), and characteristic changes in brain waves. On autopsy or biopsy of brain tissue, the brain shows loss of neurons and a proliferation of astrocytes (indicating destruction of nearby neurons).

The disease, which is often fatal within 3 to 12 months of diagnosis, has characteristic stages and manifestations. The onset is characterized by memory changes, an exaggerated startle reflex, sleep disturbances, and nervousness. The person then experiences rapid deterioration in motor, sensory, and language function. Tremors, hyperreflexia, rigidity, and a positive Babinski reflex are often present, and confusion progresses to dementia in almost all cases. Clients in the terminal state are comatose and exhibit decorticate and decerebrate posturing.

## COLLABORATIVE CARE

The disease is diagnosed by a thorough neurologic examination, specific EEG changes, and a CT scan. However, the final diagnosis of CJD can be made only by postmortem examination. It is often difficult to differentiate this disease from Alzheimer's disease, especially in the early stages.

There is no specific treatment available to stop or slow the progression of CJD. Collaborative interventions focus on the disease's manifestations.

## NURSING CARE

The nurse may identify the manifestations of Creutzfeldt-Jakob disease when conducting a health history and total physical assessment. Include questions about familial history, cultural and geographic risk, and high-risk occupations or procedures in the history. Assessment of mental function, reflexes, and cranial nerve function may provide information to assist in diagnosis.

Nursing care focuses on maximizing comfort, preventing injury, preventing transmission, and providing support. The following guidelines are useful in designing the plan of care.

- Although comfort is difficult to assess in clients with impaired cognitive function, interventions that provide a quiet environment and analgesia are important.
- Communication is essential, even if the client is unable to respond.
- Institute seizure precautions, and pad side rails.
- Provide skin care, changes in position, and pressure-relief mattresses to decrease the risk of pressure ulcers, venous stasis, and pneumonia.
- Use standard precautions for blood and body fluids when providing care. Disinfect surfaces with a solution of 5% bleach. Sterilize contaminated equipment by autoclave, or soak in 5% bleach solution for 1 hour. Label all specimens as biohazardous. Label lines as biohazardous. Teach staff members and family members guidelines for care, including careful handwashing. It is not necessary to place the client in isolation, however.
- Provide time for family members to verbalize grief and loss, which may be manifested as anger and frustration with the health care system.
- Provide information to family members about all procedures and the plan of care.
- Refer family members to sources of support, such as social services and the appropriate clergy.

# PERIPHERAL NERVOUS SYSTEM DISORDERS

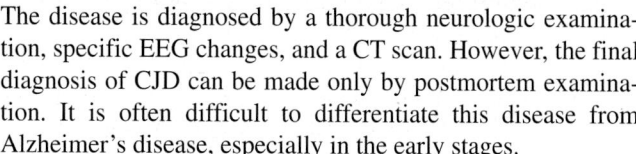

Many etiologic agents are responsible for peripheral nervous system disorders. Autoimmune disorders, viruses, environmental toxins such as heavy metals, and nutritional deficiencies can affect the peripheral nervous system.

## THE CLIENT WITH MYASTHENIA GRAVIS

**Myasthenia gravis** is a chronic neuromuscular disorder characterized by fatigue and severe weakness of skeletal muscles. Clients experience periods of remission and exacerbation, and mild forms of the disorder exist. Weakness may remain limited to a few muscle groups, especially the ocular muscles, or may become generalized with all muscles eventually becoming weakened.

Myasthenia gravis is believed to be an autoimmune disease. Women are 3 times more frequently affected than men. The age of onset for most clients is between ages 20 and 30. Treatment with anticholinesterase medications has greatly improved the prognosis and symptom management.

## PATHOPHYSIOLOGY

The axons of motor neurons divide as they enter skeletal muscles, and each axonal ending forms a neuromuscular junction. Although the axonal ending and the muscle fiber are extremely close, they are separated by the synaptic cleft. The transmission of nerve impulses from the nerve to the muscles occurs at the neuromuscular junctions. The neurotransmitter acetylcholine is released from the axonal ending, crosses the synaptic cleft, attaches to acetylcholine receptors on the muscle fiber, and stimulates the muscle.

In myasthenia gravis, antibodies destroy or block neuromuscular junction receptor sites, resulting in a decreased number of acetylcholine receptors. Structural changes also result in diminished acetylcholine uptake. The net result is a decrease in the muscle's ability to contract despite a sufficient amount of acetylcholine. A comparison of a normal neuromuscular junction and one affected by myasthenia gravis is shown in Figure 43–5 ■.

In about 75% of clients with myasthenia gravis, the thymus gland, which is usually inactive after puberty, continues to produce antibodies because of hyperplasia of the gland or because of tumors. It is believed that the thymus is a source of autoantigen that triggers an autoimmune response in myasthenia gravis. The exact mechanism and reason for the thymus gland's antibody production is unknown.

Myasthenia gravis is sometimes associated with a tumor of the thymus, thyrotoxicosis (hyperthyroidism), rheumatoid arthritis, and lupus erythematosus. The disorder is often diagnosed when a client seeks treatment for a coincidental infec-

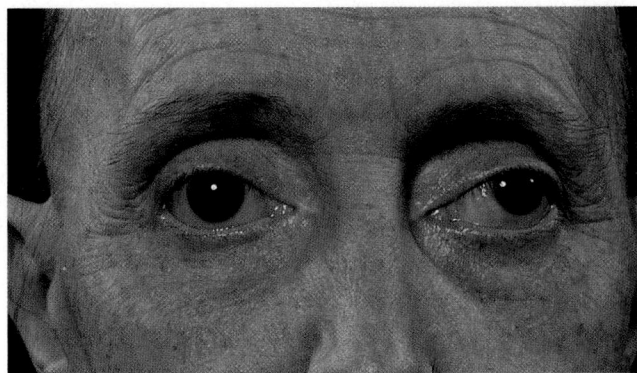

**Figure 43–6** ■ In myasthenia gravis, the client experiences unilateral weakness of the facial muscles. Note the drooping of one eyelid.

Source: Custom Medical Stock Photo, Inc.

tion that exacerbates manifestations. Exacerbations may also occur before the menstrual period and during or soon after pregnancy.

## MANIFESTATIONS AND COMPLICATIONS

The manifestations of myasthenia gravis correspond to the muscles involved. Initially, the eye muscles are affected and the client experiences either **diplopia** (unilateral or bilateral double vision) or **ptosis** (drooping of the eyelid) (Figure 43–6 ■). Next, the facial, speech, and mastication muscles become weak, and clients may have periods of dysarthria and dysphagia. Fatigue is evident even when the client tries to eat a meal; the muscles of chewing tire, and the client is forced to stop eating momentarily. A smile becomes a snarl or grimace, and the voice is weak with a muffled nasal quality. Problems performing fine motor movements of the hands, such as writing, appear early in the disease.

As the disease progresses, the muscles of the neck and extremities become affected. As the muscles of the neck become affected, the head juts forward. Deep-tendon reflexes are usually normal, however, even in weak muscles. Fatigue and weakness are exacerbated with stress, fever, overexertion, and exposure to heat and are relieved by rest. Symptoms vary on a daily basis, and the disease is characterized by remissions and exacerbations. Manifestations of myasthenia gravis are listed in the box on page 1432.

Complications are directly related to the degree of muscle weakness and the specific muscles involved. For example, when the pharyngeal and palatal muscles are affected, the client cannot manage swallowing and may aspirate food or fluids. The client is at increased risk for pneumonia because weakness of the diaphragm and muscles of respiration compromises gas exchange.

Clients with myasthenia gravis can develop life-threatening emergencies. A **myasthenic crisis** is a sudden exacerbation of motor weakness putting the client at risk of respiratory failure and aspiration. Myasthenic crisis most often is due to undermedication, missed doses of medication, or a developing infection. Manifestations of myasthenic crisis include tachycardia, tachypnea, severe respiratory distress, dysphagia, restlessness,

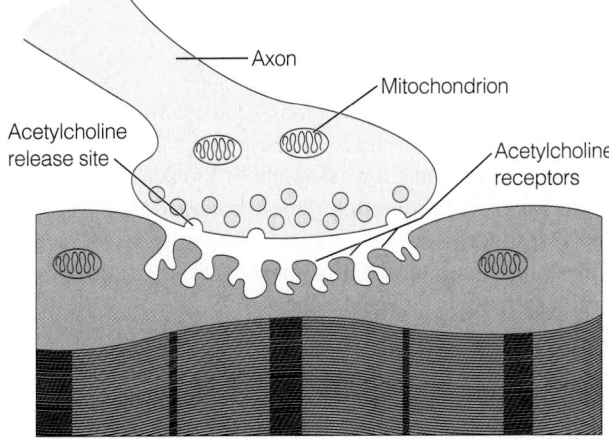

**A** Normal neuromuscular junction

Axon
Mitochondrion
Acetylcholine release site
Acetylcholine receptors

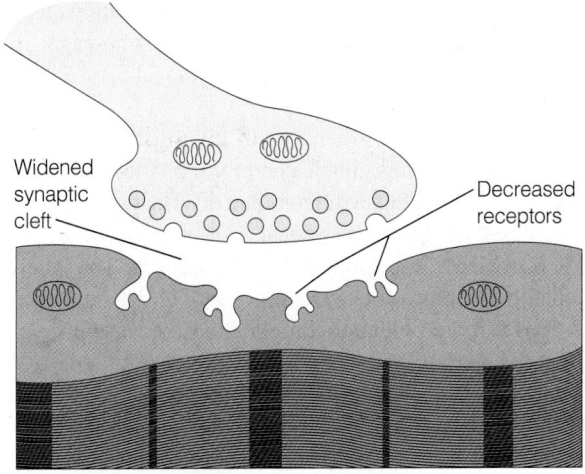

**B** Myasthenia gravis

Widened synaptic cleft
Decreased receptors

**Figure 43–5** ■ *A,* A normal neuromuscular junction and *B,* one showing the changes seen in myasthenia gravis. These changes interfere with the transmission of nerve impulses to the muscle.

## Manifestations of Myasthenia Gravis

### OCULAR AND FACIAL

- Ptosis
- Diplopia
- Facial weakness
- Dysphagia
- Dysarthria
- Complications: difficulty closing eyes, aspiration, impaired communication and nutrition

### MUSCULOSKELETAL

- Weakness and fatigue
- Decreased function of hands, arms, legs, and neck muscles
- Complications: inability to perform ADLs and self-care activities, complications related to immobility, myasthenic and cholinergic crises

### RESPIRATORY

- Weakening of intercostal muscles
- Decrease in diaphragm movement
- Breathlessness and dyspnea
- Poor gas exchange
- Complications: decreasing ability to walk, eat, and perform other ADLs, pneumonia

### NUTRITIONAL

- Inability to chew and swallow
- Decreasing ability to move tongue
- Impairment of fine motor movements: inability to feed self
- Complications: weight loss, dehydration, malnutrition, aspiration

impaired speech, and anxiety. **Cholinergic crisis** is the result of overdosage with anticholinesterase (cholinergic) medications used to treat myasthenia gravis. Gastrointestinal symptoms, severe muscle weakness, vertigo, and respiratory distress are signs of cholinergic crisis. Both types of crises are emergency, life-threatening situations; clients frequently require ventilatory assistance. Differentiation is based on the client's response to edrophonium chloride (Tensilon). In myasthenic crisis the test is positive, and in cholinergic crisis the test is negative (see the discussions following).

## COLLABORATIVE CARE

Care of the client with myasthenia gravis focuses on providing appropriate treatment, preventing complications, and supporting the client and family in meeting physical and psychosocial needs, especially as the disease progresses.

### Diagnostic Tests

Diagnostic tests are conducted following a thorough history and physical examination, with special attention to the facial, oculomotor, laryngeal, and respiratory muscles. Diagnostic tests include the following:

- *Tensilon test:* The client is injected with edrophonium chloride (Tensilon), a short-acting anticholinesterase. Clients with myasthenia gravis show a significant improvement in muscle strength that lasts approximately 5 minutes. This test is also used to differentiate myasthenic crisis (caused by insufficient medication, so the client shows improvement with the drug) from cholinergic crisis (caused by overmedication, so the client does not show improvement).
- *EMG studies* demonstrate a reduced amplitude of the action potential in response to electrical stimulation when myasthenia gravis is present.
- *Antiacetylcholine receptor antibody serum levels* are increased in about 80% of clients with myasthenia gravis; this test is also useful in follow-up of effectiveness of therapy.
- *CT scan* of the chest may demonstrate abnormalities in the thymus.
- *Single-fiber electromyography* detects delayed or failed neuromuscular transmission in muscle fibers supplied by a single nerve fiber.
- *Repetitive 2- or 3-Hz stimulation* of motor nerves helps indicate a disturbance of neuromuscular transmission.
- *Serum assay* of circulating acetylcholine receptor antibodies, if increased, is diagnostic of myasthenia gravis with a sensitivity of 80% to 90% (Tierney et al., 2001).

### Medications

The primary group of medications used to treat myasthenia gravis is the anticholinesterases. These drugs act at the neuromuscular junction and allow acetylcholine to concentrate at the receptor sites, thus promoting muscle contraction. Pyridostigmine (Mestinon) is the most commonly used acetylcholinesterase inhibitor for myasthenia gravis. The client's decrease in symptoms guides dosage.

Immunosuppression with glucocorticoids, typically prednisone, is another pharmacologic therapy aimed at improving muscle strength. Clients must be aware of the need to stay on the drug at the prescribed dose to determine the least amount required for efficacy. If clients do not respond to prednisone alone, it may be combined with other immunosuppressive agents, such as cyclosporine or azathioprine (Imuran). Medications used to treat myasthenia gravis are discussed in the box on page 1433.

### Surgery

Approximately 75% of clients with myasthenia gravis have dysplasia of the thymus gland. Therefore, thymectomy is often recommended for clients younger than 60. The two surgical approaches used are the transcervical approach, which is considered less invasive, and the transternal approach. The latter approach allows a more extensive removal of the gland; however, it also poses more potential complications because it involves splitting the sternum.

Preoperatively, clients may be tapered from steroid therapy. Usually, pyridostigmine is administered to prevent muscular manifestations during the perioperative period. Postoperative nursing care focuses on preventing complications and controlling pain. Nursing implications for the client undergoing thymectomy are presented on page 1433. Remission is obtained in about 40% of clients but may take several years to achieve. Refer to Chapter 36 for care of the client having

# Medication Administration

## The Client with Myasthenia Gravis

### ANTICHOLINESTERASES/CHOLINESTERASE INHIBITORS

Neostigmine (Prostigmin)
Ambenonium (Mytelase Caplets)
Pyridostigmine (Mestinon, Regonol)
For diagnosis: edrophonium chloride (Tensilon)

Cholinesterase inhibitors are used in myasthenia gravis to enhance the effects of acetylcholine at the remaining skeletal muscle receptors. Cholinesterase inhibitors do not cure or change the underlying pathophysiologic processes, but they can provide effective, lifelong improvement of symptoms. Because the cholinesterase inhibitors are nonselective, the neuromuscular, muscarinic, and ganglionic junctions are each affected.

Adjusting the dose to obtain maximum benefit with minimal side effects is a major consideration when administering cholinesterase inhibitors. Initially, small doses are given followed by incremental increases until optimal muscle strength is obtained. The dose may need to be adjusted when activities result in symptoms of undermedication, such as increased ptosis. Severe undermedication results in myasthenic crisis. Although a sustained release form of pyridostigmine is available for bedtime use, it should not be used during the day because of its inconsistent absorption.

When the client takes an overdose of anticholinesterase inhibitors, a cholinergic crisis occurs. Clients and family members must be taught the symptoms and actions to take in each crisis. The oral dose of neostigmine is approximately 30 times greater than parenteral doses.

Cholinesterase inhibitors should not be administered to clients experiencing obstruction of the intestinal or urinary tract. Caution is advised when administering these drugs to clients with asthma, hyperthyroidism, bradycardia, or peptic ulcer disease. Cholinesterase inhibitors can cross the placenta; reproductive counseling is indicated.

### Nursing Responsibilities
- Obtain a baseline assessment of muscle strength and abilities, concentrating on swallowing and ptosis.
- Administer the medication parenterally if the client has dysphagia.
- Check the dose of the medication carefully when changing from oral to parenteral routes.
- Evaluate the effectiveness of the medication and document the response, for example, time when fatigue occurs in relation to activities.
- Promptly recognize and respond to manifestations of excessive stimulation of muscarinic receptors: excess salivation, urinary urgency, bradycardia, gastrointestinal hypermotility, diaphoresis. Atropine can be administered to combat these manifestations. Respiratory depression and failure can occur and require mechanical ventilation.
- Have a muscarinic antagonist (e.g., physostigmine) readily available to treat poisoning.

### Client and Family Teaching
- Balancing symptom control with dosage is crucial; record time of dose and response in a journal. Note the time of day when fatigued and any adverse effects, such as excess salivation, sweating, slow heartbeat, and diarrhea.
- Take the medication about 30 minutes prior to meals to enhance swallowing and chewing.
- Report manifestations of myasthenic crisis immediately: severe muscle weakness, fast heartbeat, restlessness, difficulty breathing, increasing difficulty swallowing or speaking.
- Report slow heartbeat, increased salivation or sweating, and/or decreased blood pressure immediately:
- Review possible causes of myasthenic crisis: physical or emotional stress, infection, or reduction in the medication dosage.
- Wear or carry MedicAlert identification.

# NURSING CARE OF THE CLIENT HAVING A THYMECTOMY

## PREOPERATIVE CARE
- Reinforce the physician's explanation of the procedure, and prepare the client for chest tubes and tracheostomy. *Realistic preparation of what to expect postoperatively encourages compliance and allays anxiety.*
- Anticipate the need for alternative communication. *The client may have a tracheostomy; preoperative planning facilitates communication after surgery.*
- Allow sufficient time for questions. *Thymectomy is a major surgery requiring either a thoracotomy and sternal split or transcervical approach. The client is usually anxious, and adequate time must be allocated to preoperative instruction.*

## POSTOPERATIVE CARE
- Provide meticulous pulmonary hygiene: turning, deep breathing, and coughing at least every 2 hours; use an incentive spirometer. *Regardless of surgical approach, measures are aimed at preventing pulmonary complications of atelectasis and pneumonia.*
- Clients with a thoracotomy and sternal split procedure will require care of the anterior chest tube. Observe for complications; such as pneumothorax. *Air may enter the thoracic cavity—be alert for sudden chest pain and dyspnea, decreased breath sounds, and early signs of shock, such as restlessness.*
- Manage pain with scheduled analgesic therapy. *Maintaining a therapeutic blood level of analgesic provides better pain control than waiting until the client requests medication, as on a prn basis.*

a thoracotomy and chest tubes. A tracheostomy may be required when the diaphragm or intercostal muscles are involved.

## Plasmapheresis

Plasma exchange in myasthenia gravis may be used in conjunction with other therapies; for example, it may be performed prior to surgical intervention. The goal of therapy is to remove the antiacetylcholine receptor antibodies, thus improving severe muscle weakness, fatigue, and other symptoms. The procedure is frequently performed when respiratory muscle involvement is evident. See Figure 43–7 ■ and the box below for nursing care.

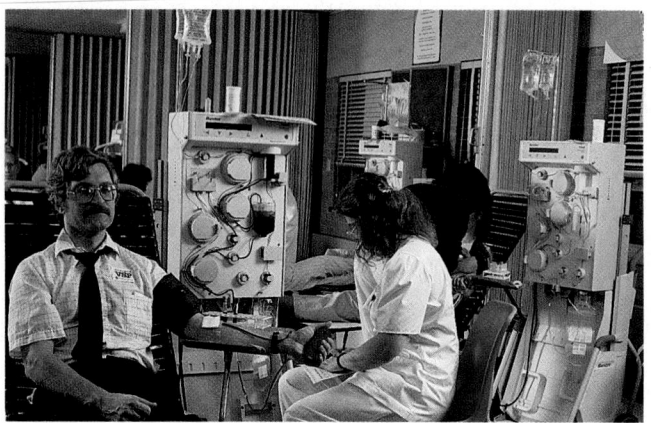

**Figure 43–7** ■ Plasmapheresis is a procedure used to separate the blood's cellular components from plasma. About 50 mL per minute is withdrawn to the centrifuge in the plasmapheresis machine. The plasma is replaced with donor plasma or colloids and returned to the client.

*Courtesy of Baxter Healthcare Corporation.*

## NURSING CARE

Because avoiding fatigue is a major part of teaching, it is important to incorporate interventions to enhance rest and conserve energy (see Box 43–5). Suggest sitting while preparing meals and while performing hygiene and grooming, for example. Anticipating problems, such as impaired communication, and developing alternative solutions can be helpful in promoting independence.

### Nursing Diagnoses and Interventions

Nursing care of clients with myasthenia gravis focuses not only on present problems but also on anticipated needs. Preventing myasthenic and cholinergic crises and providing psychologic support to clients and families are two important aspects of care. Individualized care depends on the specific therapy insti-

## NURSING CARE OF THE CLIENT TREATED WITH PLASMAPHERESIS

### PREPROCEDURE CARE

- Teach about the procedure and what to expect, including what the machine looks like, the need for arterial and venous insertion sites, and the length of time of the procedure (2 to 5 hours). *Giving information, answering questions, and addressing concerns decreases anxiety.*
- Check with physician about holding medications until after the procedure. *Medications may be removed from the body as an incidental part of the plasmapheresis process.*
- Assess vital signs and weight. *Baseline parameters are necessary to evaluate for fluid imbalances and response to therapy.*
- Assess CBC, platelet count, and clotting studies. *Clients undergoing plasmapheresis are at high risk for anemia and coagulation problems secondary to hemolysis of cells.*
- Check blood type and crossmatch for replacement blood products. *Hypersensitivity reactions can occur, and close monitoring is important.*

### CARE DURING THE PROCEDURE AND POSTPROCEDURE

- Observe for dizziness or hypotension. *Hypovolemia is a complication of plasma exchange, especially during the procedure when up to 15% of the client's blood volume is in the cell separator.*
- Apply pressure dressing to access site(s). *Direct pressure helps decrease or prevent bleeding.*
- Monitor for infection and bruises at the intravenous port site. *The site of vascular access is at risk for complications and must be routinely and carefully assessed for signs of infection and for bleeding or hematoma formation.*
- Monitor electrolytes and signs of electrolyte loss. Report imbalances, and replace electrolytes as ordered. Observe for circumoral tingling, Chvostek's and Trousseau's signs if calcium levels are low, and cardiac dysrhythmias and leg cramps if potassium levels are low. *Hypocalcemia and hypokalemia may occur. Hypocalcemia occurs because the anticoagulant citrate dextrose binds with calcium.*
- Reevaluate preprocedure laboratory data, especially CBC, platelet count, and clotting times. *The cell-separating process can damage cells; anticoagulation is part of the procedure.*

tuted. This section discusses the nursing diagnoses related to ineffective airway clearance and impaired swallowing; other nursing diagnoses that commonly apply, such as that related to fatigue, are addressed in other sections of this chapter.

### Ineffective Airway Clearance

The underlying causes for ineffective airway clearance for the person with myasthenia gravis include poor cough mechanism, decreased rib cage expansion, diminished diaphragm movement, and decreased expiratory effort. The following interventions require particular attention if the client undergoes a thymectomy.

- Assist with turning, deep breathing, and coughing at least every 2 hours. Teach proper coughing techniques; use an incentive spirometer every 2 hours while the client is awake. *Position changes promote lung expansion; coughing helps clear secretions from the tracheobronchial tree.*
- Place in a semi-Fowler's position. *This position expands the lungs and alleviates pressure from the diaphragm, especially important considerations if the client is obese.*
- Maintain hydration status and monitor for dehydration; use a humidifier as needed. If needed, teach family how to perform percussion, postural drainage, and suction. *Interventions to liquefy secretions, such as ensuring a daily fluid intake of up to 2500 mL (perhaps via feeding tube or parenteral route), help the client mobilize and expectorate sputum.*
- Assess lung sounds, the rate and character of respirations, and pulse oximetry readings at least every 4 hours or as indicated by client's condition. *Monitoring for hypoxia and worsening of client's ability to move air alerts the nurse to early signs of arteriovenous shunting.*

### Impaired Swallowing

Clients with myasthenia gravis have weakness of the laryngeal and pharyngeal muscles involved with swallowing. Alterations in swallowing place the client at risk for poor nutrition as well as for possible aspiration. Family members need to be included in teaching, particularly the person who prepares and assists with meals.

- Assess the ability to safely manage various consistencies of foods; consult with a speech pathologist for evaluation. *Dysphagic clients are at risk for aspiration; matching food consistency to the client's ability to swallow enhances safety.*
- Plan meals to promote medication effectiveness. *Pyridostigmine should be given 30 minutes before the meal to provide optimal muscle strength for swallowing and chewing.*
- Have the client eat slowly, using small bites of food. Schedule meals during periods when the client is adequately rested; develop a daily schedule incorporating rest periods. *Fatigue may add to dysphagia, putting the client at greater risk for aspiration.*
- If necessary, give cues while eating, such as: "Chew your food thoroughly; swallow." *Keeping client focused may enhance swallowing.*

- Teach caregivers the Heimlich maneuver and how to suction. *Knowing specific measures to take in case of aspiration decreases both the client's and family's anxiety and promotes confidence in managing potential problems.*

### Home Care

Teaching for the client and family with myasthenia gravis focuses on prevention and recognition of crisis situations, understanding the disorder, and methods for coping with both physical and psychosocial problems. Setting realistic goals with the client and family provides opportunities for self-assessment and promotes active participation in rehabilitation.

Address the following topics.

- The importance of maintaining consistency in medication dosage and management
- Realistic expectations
- Methods to avoid fatigue and undue stress; specific measures for avoiding upper respiratory infections and exposure to extreme heat or cold
- Birth control measures or referral for counseling (Pregnancy can exacerbate symptoms; also, medications used to control myasthenia gravis, such as neostigmine bromide (Prostigmin), cross the placenta.)
- Referral to support groups
- Helpful resources such as the Myasthenia Foundation

## THE CLIENT WITH GUILLAIN-BARRÉ SYNDROME

**Guillain-Barré syndrome (GBS)** is an acute inflammatory demyelinating disorder of the peripheral nervous system characterized by an acute onset of motor paralysis (usually ascending). The classification of Guillain-Barré subtypes includes acute inflammatory demyelinating polyradiculoneuropathy, acute axonal motor neuropathy, acute motor and sensory axonal neuropathy, and Miller-Fisher syndrome.

Guillain-Barré syndrome is one of the most common peripheral nervous system disorders. The cause is unknown, but precipitating events include a respiratory or gastrointestinal viral or bacterial infection 1 to 3 weeks prior to the onset of manifestations, surgery, viral immunizations, and other viral illnesses. In 60% of cases, *Campylobacter jejuni* is identified as the cause of the preceding infection. Approximately 80% to 90% of clients with GBS have a spontaneous recovery with little or no residual disabilities. However, the disease has a 4% to 6% mortality rate, and up to 10% of cases have permanent disabling weakness, imbalance, and sensory loss (McCance & Huether, 2002).

The disease is characterized by progressive ascending flaccid paralysis of the extremities, accompanied by paresthesias and numbness. About 20% of clients have respiratory involvement to the point that ventilatory assistance is required. GBS is often a medical emergency.

## Nursing Care Plan
## A Client with Myasthenia Gravis

Kirsten Avis, a 44-year-old homemaker and mother of two teenage sons, was diagnosed with myasthenia gravis 2 years ago. She takes an anticholinesterase medication, pyridostigmine (Mestinon), four times a day. Over the past month she has been experimenting with decreasing the dose of her pyridostigmine because she has "felt so good." She was prescribed 60 mg of pyridostigmine three times a day before meals and one-half of a long-acting 180 mg pyridostigmine tablet at night.

Three days ago, she began having chills and fever and her myasthenic symptoms became markedly worse. Mrs. Avis is easily fatigued and has been experiencing increasing weakness, bilateral ptosis, and mild dysphagia in the late afternoon and evenings.

### ASSESSMENT

Lela Silva, RN, is caring for Mrs. Avis. Physical examination of Mrs. Avis reveals severe muscle weakness bilaterally in her hands, arms, and thorax. Her voice is nasal, and she speaks slowly; the longer she speaks, the more difficult it becomes to understand her. She is anxious and dyspneic. Her complaints of weakness, dysphagia, dysarthria, problems with mobility, and ptosis are more pronounced later in the day. Vital signs are as follows: BP 138/88, P 88, R 28, T 102.4°F (39°C).

Some improvement in muscle weakness is noted following a restful night's sleep; however, the respiratory distress is more evident, and Mrs. Avis is increasingly restless. She is moved to the intensive care unit for advanced monitoring and possible ventilatory assistance. The medical diagnosis is myasthenic crisis secondary to pulmonary infection.

### DIAGNOSES

- *Impaired gas exchange* related to ineffective breathing pattern and muscle weakness
- *Risk for aspiration* related to difficulty swallowing
- *Fatigue* related to increased energy needs from muscular involvement

### EXPECTED OUTCOMES

- Pulse oximetry readings will be maintained at 92% or above.
- No aspiration will occur.
- Will verbalize decreasing fatigue when performing ADLs.
- Will state the correct method of medication dosing and demonstrate how she will maintain schedule.

### PLANNING AND IMPLEMENTATION

Mrs. Avis's manifestations improve following administration of edrophonium chloride (Tensilon) to verify myasthenic crisis. She is placed on oxygen by mask and suctioned as needed; equipment for possible intubation and ventilation is made readily available. She is placed in a semi-Fowler's position, and vital signs are assessed every 5 minutes during the acute exacerbation. The nurses in the intensive care unit remain in constant attendance throughout the crisis period and provide explanations to Mrs. Avis in an effort to decrease her stress and to avoid further severity of manifestations.

Three days after the crisis period, Mrs. Avis is moved to a progressive nursing care unit. Nurses follow up on teaching her the manifestations of both myasthenic and cholinergic crises. They discuss the need to wear MedicAlert identification and review medication administration techniques with Mrs. Avis. The nurses emphasize in particular that Mrs. Avis must not split time-released medications.

Within 5 days, Mrs. Avis's condition stabilizes, and her weakness decreases sufficiently to allow discharge home. Although her temperature has returned to normal and her respiratory status has improved, she still has a productive cough. Oral antibiotics are prescribed for 2 weeks, after which she will have a follow-up visit with her primary care provider. She is instructed to seek treatment promptly if respiratory symptoms or temperature indicate recurrence of infection.

### EVALUATION

Mrs. Avis is discharged without developing aspiration pneumonia or any symptoms of aspiration. Her airway was maintained throughout the myasthenic crisis, and her pulse oximetry readings remained above 92% once oxygen therapy was initiated. On discharge, pulse oximetry is above 95% without oxygen therapy. Mrs. Avis states that her fatigue and weakness have significantly improved.

Both Mrs. Avis and her husband are able to explain the difference between myasthenic and cholinergic crises and to identify methods to avoid both problems. Mrs. Avis correctly relates her proper medication regimen and makes an appointment for a follow-up visit with her physician.

### Critical Thinking in the Nursing Process

1. What is the rationale for administering Tensilon to evaluate a myasthenic crisis?
2. Develop a plan to teach Mrs. Avis how to avoid fatigue when preparing and eating meals.
3. Develop a nursing care plan for Mrs. Avis for the nursing diagnosis, *Ineffective role performance*.

See Evaluating Your Response in Appendix C.

## BOX 43–6 ■ Stages of Guillain-Barré Syndrome

### I. ACUTE STAGE

■ Characterized by severe and rapid weakness, especially, in the lower extremities; loss of muscle strength progressing to quadriplegia and respiratory failure; decreasing deep-tendon reflexes; decreasing vital capacity; paresthesias, numbness; pain, especially nocturnal; facial muscle involvement (inability to wrinkle forehead or change expressions).

■ Involvement of the autonomic nervous system manifested by bradycardia, sweating, fluctuating blood pressure, notably hypotension, which may last for 2 weeks.

### II. STABILIZING/PLATEAU STAGE

■ Occurs 2 to 3 weeks after initial onset.

■ Marks the end of changes in condition; characterized by a "leveling off" of symptoms.

■ Generally, the labile autonomic functions stabilize.

### III. RECOVERY STAGE

■ May take from several months to 2 years.

■ Marked by improvement in symptoms.

■ Generally, muscle strength and function return in descending order.

## PATHOPHYSIOLOGY AND MANIFESTATIONS

The primary pathophysiologic process in Guillain-Barré syndrome is the destruction of myelin sheaths covering the axons of peripheral nerves. The demyelination is thought to be the result of both a humoral- and cell-mediated immunologic response. The loss of myelin results in poor conduction of nerve impulses, causing sudden muscle weakness and loss of reflex response. Other manifestations occur when nerve conduction to various muscles is interrupted. The stages of Guillain-Barré syndrome and their usual manifestations are presented in Box 43–6.

Muscles, sensory nerves, and cranial nerves are commonly affected in clients with GBS. Most people experience symmetric muscle weakness, initially in the lower extremities. The weakness and sensory loss then ascends to the upper extremities, torso, and cranial nerves. Sensory involvement includes severe pain, paresthesia, and numbness. Cognition and level of consciousness are not affected. Facial nerve involvement results in the inability to change facial expressions and close the eyes. Muscles involved with chewing, swallowing, and speaking may be affected.

Paralysis of intercostal and diaphragmatic muscles may alter respiratory function. These clients require ventilatory assistance and supportive care. Involvement of the autonomic nervous system is characterized by fluctuating blood pressure, cardiac dysrhythmias and tachycardia, paralytic ileus, syndrome of inappropriate antidiuretic hormone (SIADH) secretion and urinary retention.

The weakness usually plateaus or improves by the fourth week. Strength then improves slowly over days or months.

Most affected individuals have full recovery. Women who have had Guillain-Barré syndrome are at increased risk for relapse in the first trimester of pregnancy.

## COLLABORATIVE CARE

Interventions during the acute phase (1 to 3 weeks) focus primarily on ensuring oxygenation via ventilatory assistance and preventing complications from immobility. Rehabilitation time to regain muscle strength and function varies; most people return to full presyndrome muscle function within 6 months to 2 years.

Care of the client with Guillain-Barré syndrome requires a team approach. From the initial acute phase through rehabilitation, many members of the health care team are involved. An accurate and rapid diagnosis is needed to ensure prompt supportive treatment, particularly if there is respiratory involvement combined with widespread paralysis.

### Diagnostic Tests

Diagnosis of Guillain-Barré syndrome is made after a thorough history and clinical examination. It must be differentiated from several disorders, among them influenza, heavy metal poisoning, Lyme disease, and cranial hemorrhage. Diagnosis is made based on manifestations, history of a recent viral infection, elevated CSF protein levels, and EMG studies. Although there is no specific test to diagnose this syndrome, several findings support and confirm the diagnosis.

* *CSF analysis* shows increased protein levels with a normal cell count. This elevation is caused by active demyelination.
* *EMG studies* reflect decreased nerve conduction with fibrillations during the severe stage of the syndrome.
* *Pulmonary function tests* and *ABGs* are performed when respiratory function is compromised. Abnormal results reflect the decreased ventilatory function.

### Medications

There are no medications available for the specific treatment of Guillain-Barré syndrome. Other medications may be prescribed to provide support or prophylaxis, or to combat concurrent problems; for example, antibiotics may be prescribed for urinary tract or respiratory infections. Morphine is commonly administered to control muscle pain. Anticoagulation therapy is usually instituted to prevent thromboembolic complications, such as deep-vein thrombosis and pulmonary embolism, which are associated with prolonged bed rest. If hypotension is a problem, vasopressors are prescribed.

### Treatments

#### Surgery

Tracheostomy is performed if respiratory failure occurs. Clients who need ventilatory support are usually able to be weaned after 2 to 3 weeks, but the time frame varies greatly. When the client's vital capacity reaches 8 to 10 mL/kg, he or she may be weaned from the ventilator (Hickey, 2002). Insertion of a temporary pacemaker may be indicated for bradycardia.

## Plasmapheresis

Plasma exchange has been beneficial, particularly when performed within the first 2 weeks of the syndrome's development. Antibodies are removed, and immunosuppressive agents are administered concurrently. Clients typically have five exchanges during an 8- to 10-day period (see the Nursing Care box on page 1434).

## Dietary Management

Nutritional support for the client who is immobilized for prolonged periods of time is crucial. Maintaining positive nitrogen balance, ensuring sufficient fluid intake and electrolyte balance, and ensuring recommended caloric intake are goals of therapy. When swallowing problems occur, total parenteral nutrition may be indicated if feeding via a nasogastric or gastrostomy tube is ineffective.

## Physical and Occupational Therapy

Long-term physical and occupational therapy is crucial to recovery. Clients with Guillain-Barré syndrome usually require prolonged rehabilitation care, which begins during the acute phase and focuses on preventing complications and limiting the effects of immobility. The severe muscle atrophy and loss of muscle tone require that clients relearn many functions and skills, such as walking. Compromise in respiratory function may delay physical rehabilitation; clients need positive reinforcement when they make even small gains in their progress. Continued attention to pain control is essential because paresthesia and pain can interfere with physical therapy.

# NURSING CARE

Many of the nursing interventions for clients with this syndrome involve assessing neurologic function, preventing problems of immobility, ensuring adequate hydration and nutrition, and promoting respiratory function. Anticipating needs of both the client and family is an important aspect of care. For example, developing an alternative method of communication before it is necessary may decrease anxiety. It is very important that nursing care focus on preventing complications that may be fatal by following a rigorous predetermined schedule for turning and pulmonary toilet, using strict aseptic technique, and providing continuous psychosocial support.

## Nursing Diagnoses and Interventions

Anxiety and powerlessness are major nursing considerations. The client is almost always admitted to the ICU for care, and is mentally alert but suddenly mute, ventilator dependent, and immobile. Refer to previous nursing care sections in this chapter for interventions related to anxiety, imbalanced nutrition, impaired swallowing, impaired verbal communication, and ineffective airway clearance. This section focuses on managing the nursing diagnoses related to pain and risk for impaired skin integrity.

## Acute Pain

Pain experienced with Guillain-Barré syndrome varies. Frequently, there is a "stocking-glove" pattern, with pain in the hands, feet, and legs. Pain and tenderness in muscles can be severe; interventions must be individualized to client needs. The intense pain combined with altered sensations leads to anxiety; nursing interventions can make a difference in breaking the cycle of increasing pain that leads to increased anxiety and in turn causes more pain.

- Listen to the description of pain; determine presence of triggers or a pattern. *Acknowledging the client's perception of pain is a basis for treatment; listening establishes trust.*
- Use a pain scale for determining extent of pain. *Consistent measurement is essential to evaluate degree of pain and effectiveness of intervention.*
- Use complementary therapies to help manage pain:
  - Application of heat/cold
  - Guided imagery
  - Relaxation techniques
  - Massage

  *Presenting options for managing pain gives the client control over the situation and helps reduce anxiety. Noninvasive interventions may augment the therapeutic benefit of medications.*
- Provide analgesics as indicated; administer on a regular schedule rather than waiting until pain becomes severe. *Anticipating and managing pain before it becomes severe decreases anxiety and averts the cycle of increased anxiety leading to increased pain.*
- Monitor for side effects of analgesics, particularly respiratory depression; assess respirations and lung sounds. Perform routine pulmonary hygiene measures and monitor for aspiration. *Clients with Guillain-Barré syndrome have a weakened thoracic musculature; frequent respiratory monitoring is indicated.*

## Risk for Impaired Skin Integrity

During the acute and plateau stages of Guillain-Barré syndrome, clients are at risk for problems related to immobility and malnutrition. Impaired skin integrity is one such problem. Preventing areas of skin breakdown is important. Prophylactic interventions will help ensure that ingested protein and calories are used to maintain ideal body weight and other body functions rather than to heal an avoidable problem. Implicit in the following interventions is maintenance of adequate nutrition.

- Inspect bony prominences and provide skin care at least every 2 hours. Reposition the client and clean, dry, and lubricate the skin as needed. *These activities stimulate circulation and ensure even distribution of body weight; baseline observations allow discovery of early signs of altered integrity.*
- Pad bony prominences, such as sacral area, heels, and elbows. *This decreases shearing tears on these pressure points.*
- Use an alternating-pressure mattress or water bed. *Relieving pressure stimulates circulation and promotes oxygenation of tissues.*
- Monitor for incontinence and provide thorough skin care following each episode of incontinence. *Urine is caustic to the skin, and the moisture promotes skin breakdown.*

## Home Care

Clients and family members are frequently stunned by the rapid deterioration of function and fear that the paralysis will be permanent. Regularly reinforce teaching because the client's high anxiety level may interfere with listening and understanding. When possible, include the client and family in decision making; for example, seek their input when planning a daily schedule of care that incorporates various therapies.

Referrals to appropriate therapists are a component of anticipating needs; speech, nutritional, occupational, and physical therapists are an integral part of rehabilitation. Another focus of care is teaching both the client and family; incorporate explanations for interventions aimed at promoting self-care. For further information, refer the client and family to the Guillain-Barré Syndrome Foundation, International.

Teaching the rationales for preventive measures reinforces the client's and family's understanding and may promote compliance during the lengthy rehabilitation. For example, because of autonomic nerve involvement, clients need to be monitored for cardiac dysrhythmias and taught to avoid changing position suddenly to prevent orthostatic hypotension.

# CRANIAL NERVE DISORDERS

Disorders of the cranial nerves may be caused by intracranial trauma or by pathologic processes. The pairs of cranial nerves, described in Chapter 40, are numbered in the order in which they arise in the brain and are named according to their anatomic characteristic or primary function. The most common cranial nerve disorders are those affecting the trigeminal (cranial nerve V) and the facial (cranial nerve VII) nerves. These disorders, discussed in the following sections, result primarily in pain or loss of sensory or motor function.

## THE CLIENT WITH TRIGEMINAL NEURALGIA

**Trigeminal neuralgia,** also called **tic douloureux,** is a chronic disease of the trigeminal cranial nerve (V) that causes severe facial pain. The trigeminal nerve has three divisions: the ophthalmic, the maxillary, and mandibular (Figure 43–8 ■). The ophthalmic division supplies the forehead, eyes, nose, temples, meninges, paranasal sinus, and part of the nasal mucosa. The maxillary division supplies the upper jaw, teeth, lip, cheeks, hard palate, maxillary sinus, and part of the nasal mucosa. The mandibular division supplies the lower jaw, teeth, lip, buccal mucosa, tongue, part of the external ear, and the meninges. Sensory fibers of the nerve conduct impulses for touch, pain, and temperature; motor fibers innervate the temporal and masseter muscles used for chewing and lateral movement of the jaw. The maxillary and mandibular divisions are the divisions of the trigeminal nerve affected in almost all cases of this disorder.

Trigeminal neuralgia occurs more commonly in middle and older adults and affects women more often than men. The actual cause is unknown; however, contributing factors include irritation from flulike illnesses, trauma or infection of the teeth or jaw, and pressure on the nerve by an aneurysm, a tumor, or arteriosclerotic changes of an artery close to the nerve (Hickey, 2002).

## PATHOPHYSIOLOGY AND MANIFESTATIONS

Trigeminal neuralgia is characterized by brief (lasting a few seconds to a few minutes), repetitive episodes of sudden severe facial pain. The pain may occur as often as hundreds of times a day to as infrequently as a few times a year. The unilateral pain is experienced over the surface of the skin. It most often begins near one side of the mouth and rises toward the ear, eye, or nostril on the same side of the face. Clients describe the pain as stabbing or lightning-like and often respond to the pain by wincing or grimacing.

Stimulating specific areas of the face, called *trigger zones,* may initiate the onset of pain. These trigger zones usually parallel the distribution of the nerve and typically follow a track leading from just over the eyebrow to the ridge of the cheekbone, along the nasolabial fold, around the corner of the mouth, and down the side of the chin. The episodes of pain are initiated by many factors, including light touch, eating, swallowing, talking, sneezing, shaving, chewing gum, brushing the teeth, or washing the face. Other factors that may trigger a pain episode include changes in temperature and exposure to wind. In an attempt to control the pain, clients may refuse to wash, shave, eat, or talk.

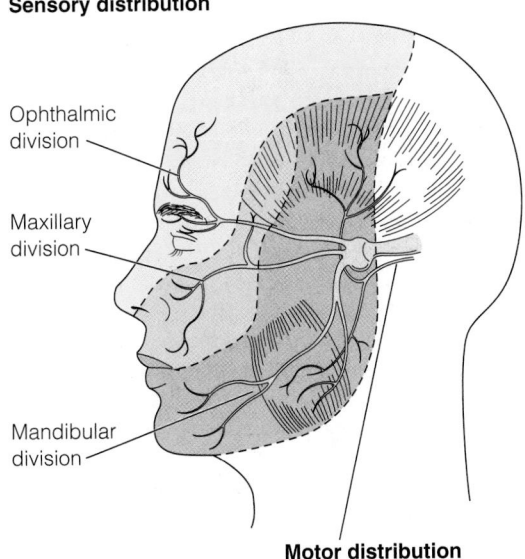

**Sensory distribution**

Ophthalmic division

Maxillary division

Mandibular division

**Motor distribution**

**Figure 43–8** ■ Sensory and motor distribution of the trigeminal nerve. The three sensory divisions are ophthalmic, maxillary, and mandibular.

The episodes of pain may recur for several weeks or months. The disease then spontaneously goes into remission, and the client is free of pain for periods lasting from days to years. As the client grows older, the remissions tend to become shorter, and a dull ache may be present between episodes of acute pain.

## COLLABORATIVE CARE

There are no specific diagnostic tests for trigeminal neuralgia. The disorder is diagnosed by the characteristic location and type of pain. The disorder is treated by pharmacologic or surgical interventions.

## Medications

The drug most useful in controlling the pain is the tricyclic anticonvulsant carbamazepine (Tegretol). If carbamazepine is ineffective, other medications such as the anticonvulsants phenytoin (Dilantin) or gabapentin (Neurontin), or the skeletal muscle relaxant baclofen (Lioresal) may be used. These drugs are administered to decrease paroxysmal afferent impulses and stop the pain. Drugs in this category may cause side effects of dizziness, nausea, and drowsiness. In addition, liver function, bone marrow function, and blood levels of the medications should be monitored on a regular basis.

## Surgery

If medications do not control the pain, surgical procedures may be performed, including various types of **rhizotomy,** the surgical severing of a nerve root. Closed surgical interventions by percutaneous rhizotomy involve inserting a needle through the cheek into the foramen ovale at the base of the brain and partially destroying the trigeminal nerve with glycerol (an alcohol), by radiofrequency-induced heat, or by balloon compression of the trigeminal ganglion. These procedures carry less risk and result in shorter hospital stays than do open procedures, but there is a possibility of recurrence of pain. Following surgery, the client may have some facial numbness, but there usually is no residual paralysis. The involved side of the face is insensitive to pain. The client will have some loss of facial sensation (e.g., to temperature and/or touch) and is at risk for loss of the corneal reflex. Closed procedures provide long-term pain relief and are well tolerated by the older adult. Nursing care of the client undergoing a percutaneous rhizotomy is presented in the box below.

It has been found that some structural abnormalities (such as an artery or vein compressing the nerve) may cause the neuralgia, and if so, decompression and separation of the blood vessel from the nerve root produces lasting relief of the pain (Tierney et al., 2001). The Jannetta procedure involves locating and lifting the involved vessel and placing a small piece of silicone sponge between the vessel and the nerve. Possible complications of the procedure include headache and facial pain.

## NURSING CARE

Nursing care for the client with trigeminal neuralgia involves teaching self-management at home after medical or surgical intervention. Primary client concerns are managing pain, maintaining nutrition, and preventing injury.

## Nursing Diagnoses and Interventions

Interventions for managing pain and improving nutritional intake are addressed here; teaching to prevent injury following surgery is discussed under client and family teaching.

### Acute Pain

The client with trigeminal neuralgia has excruciating pain and often avoids ADLs and socializing with others in an attempt to prevent the onset of pain. Pain management is fully discussed in Chapter 4. Nursing interventions for pain in clients with this disorder focus on strategies for self-management.

---

## NURSING CARE OF THE CLIENT HAVING PERCUTANEOUS RHIZOTOMY

### POSTOPERATIVE CARE

- Follow routine postoperative interventions for clients having surgery (see Chapter 7).
- Monitor cranial nerve function every 2 to 4 hours:
  a. Assess the corneal reflex by lightly touching the cornea with a wisp of cotton. If the reflex is intact, the client will blink. *Severing the ophthalmic division of the trigeminal nerve destroys the corneal reflex and leaves the cornea at risk for dryness and injury.*
  b. Assess the facial nerve by asking the client to blow out the cheeks, wrinkle the forehead, frown, wink, and close both eyes tightly. Test taste by placing bitter, salty, and sweet substances on the anterior portion of the tongue. *Facial weakness is evidenced by changes in movement in the involved side of the face. The facial nerve also innervates the anterior two-thirds of the tongue.*
  c. Assess the function of the oculomotor muscles by asking the client to follow your finger through the cardinal positions of vision (see Chapter 40). *The eyes should move together; alterations in movement indicate an abnormal response.*
  d. Assess the motor portion of the trigeminal nerve by asking the client to clench the teeth while you palpate the tightness of the contracted masseter and temporal muscles: *Loss of motor function is indicated by loss of bulk and tightness of these muscles.*
  e. Apply, as prescribed; an ice pack to the jaw on the operative site. *Cold decreases bleeding and swelling.*
  f. Teach the client to avoid rubbing the eye on the involved side. *Loss of the corneal reflex removes protection because the client no longer has the sensation of pain in the involved eye. Rubbing the eye could cause corneal abrasions.*

- Identify factors that trigger an attack, and discuss strategies to avoid these precipitating factors. *Most clients can clearly identify trigger zones and triggering factors. Identification is the first step in pain control.*
- Determine usual response to pain. *Sensitivity and reaction to pain are influenced by previous experiences with pain, age, gender, emotional factors, and cultural background.*
- Assess factors that affect the ability to influence pain tolerance, including the knowledge and cause of the pain, the meaning of the pain, the ability to control the pain, cultural background, and support systems. *Pain tolerance, which is the duration and intensity of pain a person is willing to endure, differs greatly among individuals and may also vary within particular clients in different situations.*
- Monitor the effects of the medication prescribed for the neuralgia. *If the prescribed medication does not provide relief, other medications or methods of treatment may be used to control the pain.*

### Risk for Altered Nutrition: Less Than Body Requirements

Clients often refuse to eat during periods of pain attacks, fearing that the movements of chewing may precipitate the pain. In addition, the chronic nature of the illness often causes depression, which may depress the appetite.

- Monitor dietary intake and weight at each visit, and ask the client to keep a weekly weight record. *Ongoing assessments are necessary for early detection of nutritional deficiencies.*
- Discuss the temperature and consistency of foods eaten, and suggest referral to a dietitian if necessary. *Hot or cold foods may trigger an attack; soft, warm, or cool foods are less likely to act as triggers.*
- Suggest chewing on the unaffected side of the mouth. *Chewing on the unaffected side is less likely to trigger an attack of pain and so facilitate food intake.*
- If unable to tolerate oral food, tube feedings may be necessary. *Adequate kcal and nutrients for metabolic processes are essential.*

## Home Care

The client with trigeminal neuralgia who is receiving medical treatment and providing self-care at home requires teaching about the disease process, the medication(s) being taken, and ways to reduce the incidence of attacks or pain. Diet teaching and assistance with self-management of pain are also important. For example, if the home setting is drafty and attacks of pain are triggered by wind blowing across the face, it may be necessary to encourage the client to put weather stripping around windows and doors. Family members are also included in teaching. To prevent injury to affected areas, the following topics should be addressed.

### Eye Care

- Do not rub the eyes; use artificial tears four times a day if the eyes are dry or irritated.
- Wear an eyepatch at night.

- Wear protective sunglasses or goggles when outside, when working in dusty areas, when mowing the lawn, and when using any type of spray material (e.g., hair spray, cleaning materials, paint, insecticides).
- Remember to blink frequently.
- Check your eyes for redness or swelling each day.
- Schedule regular eye examinations.

### Face and Mouth Care

- Chew on the unaffected side of the mouth.
- Avoid eating hot foods or drinking hot liquids.
- After every meal, brush your teeth and inspect the inside of your mouth for food that may collect between the gums and cheek.
- Have regular dental examinations; you will not be able to feel pain associated with gum infection or tooth decay.
- Use an electric razor to shave the face.
- Protect your face from very cold or windy conditions.

## THE CLIENT WITH BELL'S PALSY

**Bell's palsy,** also called *facial paralysis,* is a disorder of the seventh cranial (facial) nerve, characterized by unilateral paralysis of the facial muscles. The facial nerve is primarily a motor nerve that supplies all the muscles associated with expression on one side of the face. The sensory component innervates the anterior two-thirds of one side of the tongue.

This disorder can occur at any age but is seen most often in adults between 20 and 60. The incidence is equal in men and women. The exact cause of the disorder is unknown, although inflammation of the nerve and a relationship to the herpes simplex virus have been suggested (Tierney et al., 2001).

## PATHOPHYSIOLOGY AND MANIFESTATIONS

The onset of Bell's palsy is usually sudden and almost always involves one side of the face. Pain behind the ear or along the jaw may precede the paralysis. Manifestations of Bell's palsy are listed in the box below.

The client initially notices numbness or stiffness of one side of the face that distorts the appearance. As the disease progresses, the distortion becomes more obvious, and the face appears asymmetric. The facial paralysis causes the entire side of the face to droop, and the client cannot wrinkle the forehead, close the eye, or pucker the lips on the affected side. When the client attempts to smile, the lower facial muscles

### Manifestations of Bell's Palsy

- Paralysis of the facial muscles on one side of the face
- Paralysis of the upper eyelid with loss of the corneal reflex on the affected side
- Loss or impairment of taste over the anterior portion of the tongue on the affected side
- Increased tearing from the lacrimal gland on the affected side

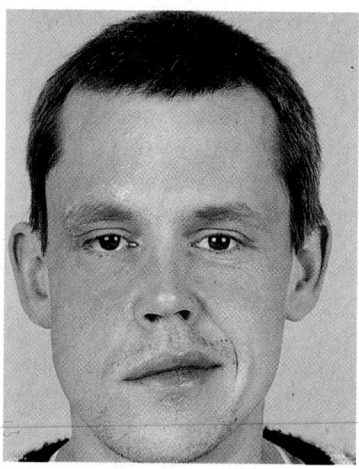

**Figure 43–9 ■** The client with Bell's palsy shows the typical drooping of one side of the face.

*Source: NIH/Phototake NYC.*

are pulled to the opposite side of the face. Some clients have only mild manifestations, whereas others have complete facial paralysis (Figure 43–9 ■). Clients often believe they have had a stroke.

Eighty percent of clients recover completely within a few weeks to a few months (and three-fourths recover without any treatment). Of those remaining, 15% recover some function but have some permanent facial paralysis; these clients are usually older, have diabetes mellitus, or have more severe manifestations, such as vertigo, a sensitivity to noise, and deep head pain.

## COLLABORATIVE CARE

There are no definitive laboratory or diagnostic tests for Bell's palsy, nor are there any specific treatments. The only medical treatment that influences outcome is the use of corticosteroids, but their use has also been questioned (Tierney et al., 2001). Care of the client with Bell's palsy is supportive, as described below.

## NURSING CARE

Although clients provide self-care at home, the nurse plays a key role in teaching the client and family about the disease and how to prevent injury and maintain nutrition. The client is often anxious about his or her appearance and may require counseling if any deficits in facial expression become permanent. The following topics should be addressed.

- Use artificial tears four times a day to lubricate the eye; wear an eye patch or tape the eye shut at night. Wear sunglasses or goggles when outside, when working in dusty conditions, and when using any type of spray.
- Massage combined with warm, moist heat often is effective in relieving the pain.
- A soft diet that does not require chewing and six small meals a day are helpful. Chew slowly on the unaffected side and avoid hot foods. Clean the mouth and carefully inspect the area between the gums and cheek for food after each meal.
- As function returns, practice wrinkling the forehead, closing the eyes, blowing air out of the puckered mouth, and whistling for 5 minutes three or four times a day.

# NEUROLOGIC DISORDERS RESULTING FROM VIRAL INFECTIONS AND NEUROTOXINS

A variety of disorders of the nervous system may have toxic or infectious causes. Although these disorders are not common, those included here require significant nursing care when they do occur.

## THE CLIENT WITH POSTPOLIOMYELITIS SYNDROME

**Postpoliomyelitis syndrome** is a complication of a previous infection by the poliomyelitis virus. This disease was epidemic in the 1940s and 1950s, but has largely been eradicated through immunization with oral live trivalent virus vaccine. However, it is thought that nearly 50% of the estimated 1.63 million people in the United States who had the disease are reexperiencing manifestations of the acute illness. These people have struggled for years to rehabilitate themselves and lead productive lives. Now, as they reach retirement age, they again experience symptoms which may be physically and psychologically incapacitating.

The poliomyelitis virus destroys some of the motor cells of the anterior horn cells of the spinal cord, causing neuromuscu-

lar effects that range from mild to severe flaccid paralysis and atrophy. The primary cause of death is respiratory arrest (Tierney et al., 2001).

Manifestations of motor neuron degeneration and weakness may emerge years after the initial infection. Most clients with postpoliomyelitis syndrome initially had a more severe case of polio and required hospitalization, contracted the disease after the age of 10, required ventilator assistance for respiration, and had paralysis in all four extremities. The incidence is slightly higher in women. As the population ages, it is projected that the number of older adults with postpoliomyelitis syndrome will increase.

## PATHOPHYSIOLOGY AND MANIFESTATIONS

The pathophysiologic process in postpoliomyelitis syndrome is not known. The manifestations include fatigue, muscle and joint weakness, loss of muscle mass, respiratory difficulties, and pain. These manifestations typically begin 25 to 35 years after the initial illness. The manifestations are most often seen in muscles affected by the initial infection, but new muscle groups may also be affected. In addition to neuromuscular manifestations, the client may experience cold intolerance, dizziness, headaches, urinary incontinence, and sleep disorders.

## COLLABORATIVE CARE

Postpoliomyelitis syndrome is diagnosed by a previous history of polio and the current manifestations. Diagnostic studies of nerve conduction, muscle strength, and pulmonary function determine current physical status. Treatment addresses the manifestations, and often involves physical therapy and pulmonary rehabilitation programs.

## NURSING CARE

The client with postpoliomyelitis syndrome faces the challenge of unexpected physical changes. Clients are often anxious about how others will react or what the future holds. Respiratory dysfunction may result in the need for oxygen. Muscular weakness and decreased pulmonary function may make walking difficult, if not impossible. Activities of daily living, independent self-care, and careers are threatened.

Many clients have not fully recovered psychologically from having polio and may respond to a recurrence of symptoms with denial and disbelief. Older clients may not know they had polio as children. Nurses are responsible for assessing and identifying the manifestations of postpoliomyelitis syndrome. It is essential to question middle to older adults about a past history of polio when conducting the health history and to ask specific questions about manifestations that the client may be experiencing.

### Home Care

The nurse individualizes teaching to meet the physical and psychosocial needs of the client and family. Provide candid explanations, and teach the client how to prevent fatigue, promote optimal respiratory function, meet self-care needs, modify ADLs, and maintain safety. Follow-up care with nurses, physicians, physical therapists, respiratory therapists, and counselors is indicated. Referral to a support group can make a positive difference in the client's and family's ability to cope with the disorder.

## THE CLIENT WITH RABIES

**Rabies** is a rhabdovirus infection of the central nervous system transmitted by infected saliva that enters the human body through a bite or an open wound. This is a critical illness that almost always causes death if untreated. The rabies virus is carried by both wild and domestic animals, including bats, skunks, foxes, raccoons, cats, and dogs. After an incubation period that may last from 10 days to many years (norm is 3 to 7 weeks), the virus travels to the brain of the infected animal via the nerves. It multiplies and migrates to the salivary glands.

## PATHOPHYSIOLOGY

The client with rabies usually has a history of an animal bite but may also become infected through an abrasion or open wound that is exposed to the infected saliva. The virus spreads from the wound to local muscle cells and then invades the peripheral nerves. It eventually travels to the central nervous system. The incubation period in humans varies according to the severity and location of the bite. For example, bites on the face may result in manifestations in 10 days to a few weeks, whereas bites on the lower extremities may incubate for as long as 1 year.

## MANIFESTATIONS

The manifestations occur in stages. During the initial, or prodromal, stage, the site of the wound is painful and then exhibits various paresthesias. The infected person is anxious, irritable, and depressed. General manifestations of infection (such as headache, loss of appetite, and sore throat) may appear. The person may also have increased sensitivity to light and sounds, and the skin is especially sensitive to changes in temperature.

The prodromal stage is followed by an excitement stage. The infected person has periods of excitement that alternate with periods of quiet. Attempts to drink cause such painful larynogospasms that the person refuses to drink (a phenomenon called hydrophobia). Large amounts of thick, tenacious mucus are present. The client experiences convulsions, muscle spasms, and periods of apnea. Death occurs approximately 7 days from the onset of manifestations and is usually due to respiratory failure.

## COLLABORATIVE CARE

Animals that bite are kept under observation, if possible, for 7 to 10 days to detect rabies manifestations. Sick animals should be euthanized and their brains examined for presence of the rabies virus, which is detected by fluorescent antibody testing. The blood of an infected person can also be tested with the same diagnostic study to demonstrate the presence of rabies antibodies.

## NURSING CARE

Nursing care for clients with rabies is provided in an intensive care unit, with the client in a quiet, darkened room to decrease stimulation as much as possible. The client requires interventions to maintain the airway, maintain oxygenation, and control seizures. Standard precautions are essential, because the rabies virus is present in the saliva of the client. If an open wound of a health care provider is contaminated with infected saliva, the provider must receive postexposure immunizations.

### Health Promotion

Client and family teaching focuses on the importance of immunizing pets, providing proper care of wounds, seeking immediate medical attention for animal bites, and obtaining treatment after any suspicious bite.

Because the untreated disease is almost always fatal, the best intervention is prevention. Preventive activities follow:

- Immunize household dogs and cats; immunize people who are exposed to animals.
- Local treatment of animal bites and scratches:
  - Carefully and thoroughly clean and flush wounds with soap and water to remove the saliva and dilute the viral exposure.
  - Immediately take the person with the bite for emergency treatment.
- Postexposure care:
  - Rabies immune globulin (RIG) is administered for passive immunization. Up to 50% of the globulin is infiltrated around the wound, and the rest is administered intramuscularly. At the same time, an inactivated human diploid cell vaccine (HDCV) is administered intramuscularly, with 1 mL given on the day of exposure and on days 3, 7, 14, and 28 after exposure (Tierney et al., 2001). Rabies immune globulin and rabies vaccine (HDCV) should never be given in the same syringe or at the same site. Local and mild systemic reactions include itching, tenderness, headaches, muscle aches, and nausea.
  - If RIG is not available, equine rabies antiserum may be administered after testing the client for horse serum sensitivity.

## THE CLIENT WITH TETANUS

**Tetanus,** more commonly called **lockjaw,** is a disorder of the nervous system caused by a neurotoxin elaborated by *Clostridium tetani.* This anaerobic bacillus lives in the soil. Spores of the bacillus enter the body through open wounds contaminated with dirt, street dust, or feces (animal or human). The wounds may result from scratches or abrasions, bee stings, abortions, surgery, trauma, burns, or intravenous drug use. Incidence is highest among people who have never been immunized, older adults whose immunity has been lost, and women. The majority of cases occur in people over age 50. Tetanus has a high mortality rate, with death occurring in over 40% of all cases. Contaminated lesions of the head and face are more dangerous than those in other parts of the body.

## PATHOPHYSIOLOGY

When the spores of *Clostridium tetani* enter the open wound, they germinate and produce a toxin called tetanospasmin. The incubation period averages 8 to 12 days but can range from 5 days to 15 weeks (Tierney et al., 2001). The toxins are absorbed by the peripheral nerves and carried to the spinal cord, where they block the action of inhibitory enzymes at spinal synapses and interfere with transmission of neuromuscular impulses. As a result, even minor stimuli cause uncontrolled muscle spasms.

## MANIFESTATIONS

The manifestations often begin with pain at the site of the infection. The infected person has stiffness of the jaw and neck and dysphagia. There is often profuse perspiration and drooling from increased salivation. As the infection progresses, the person experiences hyperreflexia, spasms of the jaw muscles (*trismus*) or facial muscles, and rigidity and spasms of the abdominal, neck, and back muscles. Generalized tonic seizures are caused by even minor stimuli, and the person assumes a typical opisthotonic position during the seizures: The head is retracted, the back is arched, and the feet are extended. The muscle spasms are painful. The person may be unable to breathe from spasms of the glottis and respiratory muscles. Despite these physical effects, the client has no change in mental status.

The complications of tetanus include urinary retention and airway obstruction from the spasms. Cardiac and respiratory failure are late, life-threatening complications.

## COLLABORATIVE CARE

There are no specific diagnostic tests for tetanus; diagnosis is based on manifestations. Tetanus is completely preventable by active immunization. Immunization for children includes tetanus toxoid, administered as part of the diphtheria-pertussis-tetanus (DPT) immunization series. In adults, immunization is obtained by administering tetanus toxoid as two doses 4 to 6 weeks apart, with a third dose in 6 to 12 months. All individuals should have a booster dose every 10 years throughout life or at the time of a major injury if the last booster dose was given more than 5 years prior to the injury.

If a wound is contaminated or if the person's immunization status is uncertain, passive immunization with tetanus immune globulin is administered. Active immunization with tetanus toxoid is begun at the same time. The wound is carefully and thoroughly debrided and antibiotics administered.

The client with tetanus requires intensive care in an area of minimal stimulation. Penicillin is administered to help destroy the toxin-producing organism. Muscle spasms and seizures are controlled by chlorpromazine (Thorazine) or diazepam (Valium), often combined with a sedative. Anticoagulants may be prescribed to prevent venous thrombosis. In severe cases, seizures and spasms are controlled with paralysis by a curare-like medication, and airway obstruction is managed by mechanical ventilation.

## NURSING CARE

Nursing care for the client with tetanus is intensive and focuses on assessments and interventions to promote safety, prevent injury, maintain nutrition, and maintain pulmonary and cardiovascular function. The client usually requires in-hospital care for 2 to 5 weeks. The nursing care plan commonly includes the following:

- Place in a quiet, darkened room to decrease stimuli that cause muscle spasms and seizures.

- Provide only necessary physical care, and do so during periods of maximal sedation to decrease tactile stimulation that causes muscle spasms.
- Maintain oxygenation through mechanical ventilator and frequent suctioning of secretions.
- Maintain intravenous access for the administration of fluids and medications.
- Administer prescribed antibiotics, anticonvulsants, and sedatives. In the case of cardiovascular complications, administer prescribed beta-adrenergic blocking agents such as propranolol (Inderal).
- Provide adequate nutrition through prescribed nutritional support, such as total parenteral nutrition.
- Monitor respiratory and cardiovascular status and provide immediate interventions for respiratory or cardiovascular failure.
- Monitor fluid and electrolyte status. Ensure adequate fluid intake to maintain hydration and urinary output.
- Monitor urinary output, which should be maintained at 1.5 to 2 L per day.
- Monitor for the hazards of immobility, including constipation, pneumonia, deep vein thrombosis, and pressure ulcers.

## Health Promotion

Tetanus is a preventable disorder, and nurses have a major role in promoting immunizations for all children and for educating adults about the need for booster doses. The older population is especially at risk for never having been immunized or for letting immunizations lapse. Information for this age group can be provided through activities such as community health fairs and programs at senior citizen groups.

It is also necessary to teach the proper care of wounds. All wounds, no matter how small, should be thoroughly washed with soap and water. All foreign material should be carefully flushed out or removed from a wound, and medical care should be sought for wounds that are more extensive or contaminated.

## THE CLIENT WITH BOTULISM

**Botulism** is food poisoning caused by ingestion of food contaminated with a toxin produced by the bacillus *Clostridium botulinum*. This anaerobic spore-forming bacillus is found in the soil. Most cases of botulism occur from eating improperly canned or cooked foods, especially home-canned vegetables and fruits, smoked meats, and vacuum-packed fish. The mortality rate is high if the disease is untreated.

## PATHOPHYSIOLOGY AND MANIFESTATIONS

The toxins liberated by *Clostridium botulinum* are absorbed by the gastrointestinal tract and bound to nerve tissues. They block the release of acetylcholine from nerve endings and thus cause respiratory paralysis due to paralysis of skeletal muscles. Manifestations usually appear 12 to 36 hours after ingestion of the contaminated food.

The manifestations of botulism usually begin with visual disturbances such as diplopia, loss of accommodation, and fixed, dilated pupils. Ptosis is often present. Gastrointestinal manifestations include nausea and vomiting, diarrhea, dysphagia, and dry mouth. Involvement of the larynx is manifested by dystonia (impaired muscle tone). Paralysis of all muscle groups progresses throughout the body, with respiratory paralysis causing death if the client is not placed on a mechanical ventilator. There is no effect on mental status.

## COLLABORATIVE CARE

Infection with the Clostridium toxin is verified by laboratory analysis of the serum and stool and of suspected food, if possible. If botulism is suspected, the state health department and the Centers for Disease Control and Prevention should be notified for assistance with laboratory assays and procuring botulism antitoxin. All people who may have eaten the contaminated food must be located and observed.

Any toxins in the gastrointestinal system are removed by cathartics, enemas, and gastric lavage. The client with respiratory paralysis is placed on a mechanical ventilator and may require a tracheostomy. Botulism antitoxin is administered to eradicate toxins in the circulation. Nutritional support is often provided with total parenteral nutrition. Intravenous fluids are administered to prevent dehydration and renal failure. If ventilation can be maintained, the client often recovers without further neurologic deficits.

## NURSING CARE

The client with botulism is hospitalized, and interventions focus on monitoring for respiratory failure and providing ventilatory assistance if necessary. Ongoing assessments are also made for manifestations of paralytic ileus and urinary retention. The client will be NPO until able to swallow and breathe; therefore, hydration and nutritional status are monitored. Teach the client and family that fatigue and weakness may persist for up to a year. During this time, the client may need to modify ADLs and take rest periods throughout the day.

## Health Promotion

Education of the public to prevent botulism is important. Address the following topics at health fairs and community programs and explain them to rural residents who do home canning.

- Home-canned foods must be processed in a pressure cooker rather than in boiling water because the organism is difficult to kill.
- Do not eat home-processed foods that have a change in color, are soft, contain gas bubbles, or have a bad odor.
- Always heat both home-processed and commercial foods at temperatures over 248° F (120 C) or boil for 10 minutes before tasting or eating them.
- Discard home-processed or commercially canned or bottled foods with defective seals.
- Discard commercially prepared canned foods that are damaged or have bulging sides or leaking contents.

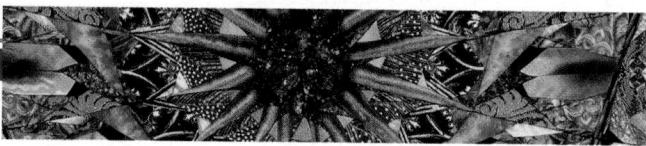

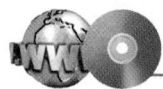 EXPLORE MediaLink

NCLEX review questions, case studies, care plan activities, MediaLink applications, and other interactive resources for this chapter can be found on the Companion Website at www.prenhall.com/lemone.

Click on Chapter 43 to select the activities for this chapter. For animations, video clips, more NCLEX review questions, and an audio glossary, access the Student CD-ROM accompanying this textbook.

## TEST YOURSELF

1. What manifestation is usually the first indication of the onset of AD?

   a. Total inability to perform ADLs
   b. Sundowning
   c. Subtle memory deficits
   d. Inability to communicate

2. Which of the following nursing diagnoses is appropriate for clients with MS, regardless of type or severity?

   a. *Fatigue*
   b. *Risk for aspiration*
   c. *Acute pain*
   d. *Impaired gas exchange*

3. The manifestations of Parkinson's disease are the result of:

   a. Autoimmune responses to a viral infection
   b. The failure of dopamine to inhibit acetylcholine

   c. Effects of a neurotoxin
   d. A genetic defect

4. What drug classification is the medication used to treat ALS?

   a. Dopamine agonist
   b. Anticholinergic
   c. Antiinflammatory
   d. Antiglutamate

5. How can the nurse prevent tetanus?

   a. Teach safe food preparation techniques
   b. Promote immunizations for all children
   c. Demonstrate proper disposal of soiled dressings
   d. Promote immunization of household pets

See Test Yourself answers in Appendix C.

## BIBLIOGRAPHY

Alzheimer's Disease and Related Disorders Association, Inc. (2000). Available www.Alzheimers.org

Andresen, G. (1998). Dx dementia. But what kind? *RN, 61*(6), 26–29.

Baker, L. (1998). Sense making in multiple sclerosis: The information needs of people during an acute exacerbation. *Qualitative Health Research, 8*(1), 106–120.

Bell, V., & Troxel, D. (2001). Spirituality and the person with dementia–A view from the field. *Alzheimer's Care Quarterly, 2*(2), 31–45.

Boyden, K. (2000). The pathophysiology of demyelination and the ionic basis of nerve conduction in multiple sclerosis: An overview. *Journal of Neuroscience Nursing, 32*(1), 49–53, 60.

Center for Disease Control. (2001). *Bovine spongiform encephalopathy and Creutzfeldt-Jakob disease.* Available www.cdc.gov/ncidod/diseases

Charles, T., & Swash, M. (2001). Amyotrophic lateral sclerosis: Current understanding. *Journal of Neuroscience Nursing, 33*(5), 245–253.

Costa, M. (1998). Trigeminal neuralgia. *American Journal of Nursing, 98*(6), 42–43.

Dewing, J. (2001). Care for older people with a dementia in acute hospital settings. *Nursing Older People, 13*(3), 18–20.

Epps, C. (2001). Recognizing pain in the institutionalized elder with dementia. *Geriatric Nursing, 22*(2), 71–79.

Fontaine, K. (2000). *Healing practices: Alternative therapies for nursing.* Upper Saddle River, NJ: Prentice Hall.

Fowler, S. (1997). Hope and a health-promoting lifestyle in persons with Parkinson's disease. *Journal of Neuroscience Nursing, 29*(2), 111–116.

Gerdner, L., & Hall. G. (2001). Chronic confusion. In M. Maas, K. Buckwalter, M. Hardy, T. Tripp-Reimer, M. Titler, & J. Specht (Eds.), *Nursing care of older adults: Diagnoses, outcomes, & interventions* (pp. 421–441). St. Louis: Mosby.

Gray, P., & Hildebrand, K. (2000). Fall risk factors in Parkinson's disease. *Journal of Neuroscience Nursing, 32*(4), 222–228.

Greenway, M., & Walker, A. (1998). Home health: Helping caregivers cope with Alzheimer's disease. *Nursing98, 28*(2), 32hh 1–2, 4–6.

Gulick, E. (1997). Correlates of quality of life among persons with multiple sclerosis. *Nursing Research, 46*(6), 305–311.

Herndon, C., Young, K., Herndon, A., & Dole, E. (2000). Parkinson's disease revisited. *Journal of Neuroscience Nursing, 32*(4), 216–221.

Hickey, J. (2002). *The clinical practice of neurological and neurosurgical nursing* (5th ed.). Philadelphia: Lippincott.

Johnson, M., & Maas, M. (Eds.). (1997). *Nursing outcomes classification (NOC).* St. Louis: Mosby.

Kee, J. (1998). *Handbook of laboratory and diagnostic tests with nursing implications* (4th ed.). Upper Saddle River, NJ: Prentice Hall.

Lisak, D. (2001). Overview of symptomatic management of multiple sclerosis. *Journal of Neuroscience Nursing, 33*(5), 224–230.

McCance, K., & Huether, S. (2002). *Pathophysiology: The biologic basis for disease in adults and children.* St. Louis: Mosby.

McCloskey, J., & Bulechek, G. (Eds.). (2000). *Nursing interventions classification (NIC)* (3rd ed.). St. Louis: Mosby.

McKenry, L., & Salerno, E. (1998). *Pharmacology in nursing* (20th ed.). St. Louis: Mosby.

McMahon-Parkes, K., & Cornock, M. (1997). Guillain-Barré syndrome: Biological basis, treatment and care. *Intensive & Critical Care Nursing, 13*(1), 42–48.

Mini-mental state exam. (1975). *J Psychiatric Research, 12,* 189–198. Oxford: Elsevier Science.

National Parkinson Foundation, Inc. (2001). New approaches for treating tremor. Available www.Parkinson.org/treatment.htm

North American Nursing Diagnosis Association. (2001). *Nursing diagnoses: Definitions & classification 2001–2002*. Philadelphia: NANDA.

O'Donnell, L. (1997). Immune-mediated neurological diseases. Management of myasthenia gravis—An overview. *Journal of Care Management, 3*(6 Disease Management Digest), 4–5, 17–18.

Porth, C. (2002). *Pathophysiology: Concepts of altered health states* (6th ed.). Philadelphia: Lippincott.

Ross, A. (1999). Neurologic degenerative disorders. *Nursing Clinics of North America, 34*(3), 725–742.

Schutte, D., Williams, J., Schutte, B., & Maas, M. (1998). Alzheimer's disease genetics: Practice and education implications for special care unit nurses. *Journal of Gerontological Nursing, 24*(1), 40–48, 58–64.

Segatore, M. (1998). Managing the surgical orthopaedic patient with Parkinson's disease. *Orthopaedic Nursing, 17*(1), 13–22.

Shannon, M., Wilson, B., & Stang, C. (2002). *Health professional's drug guide 2002*. Upper Saddle River, NJ: Prentice Hall.

Spratto, G., & Woods, A. (1998). *Delmar's therapeutic class drug guide for nurses 1998*. Albany, NY: Delmar.

Tierney, L., McPhee, S., & Papadakis, M. (Eds.). (2001). *Current medical diagnosis & treatment* (40th ed.). Stamford, CT: Appleton & Lange.

Worsham, T. (2000). Easing the course of Guilllain-Barre syndrome. *RN, 63*(3), 46–50.

Zaveruha, A., Bishop, D., St. Clair, A., & Moreau, K. (1997). Rabies update for nurse practitioners. *Clinical Excellence for Nurse Practitioners, 1*(6), 367–375.

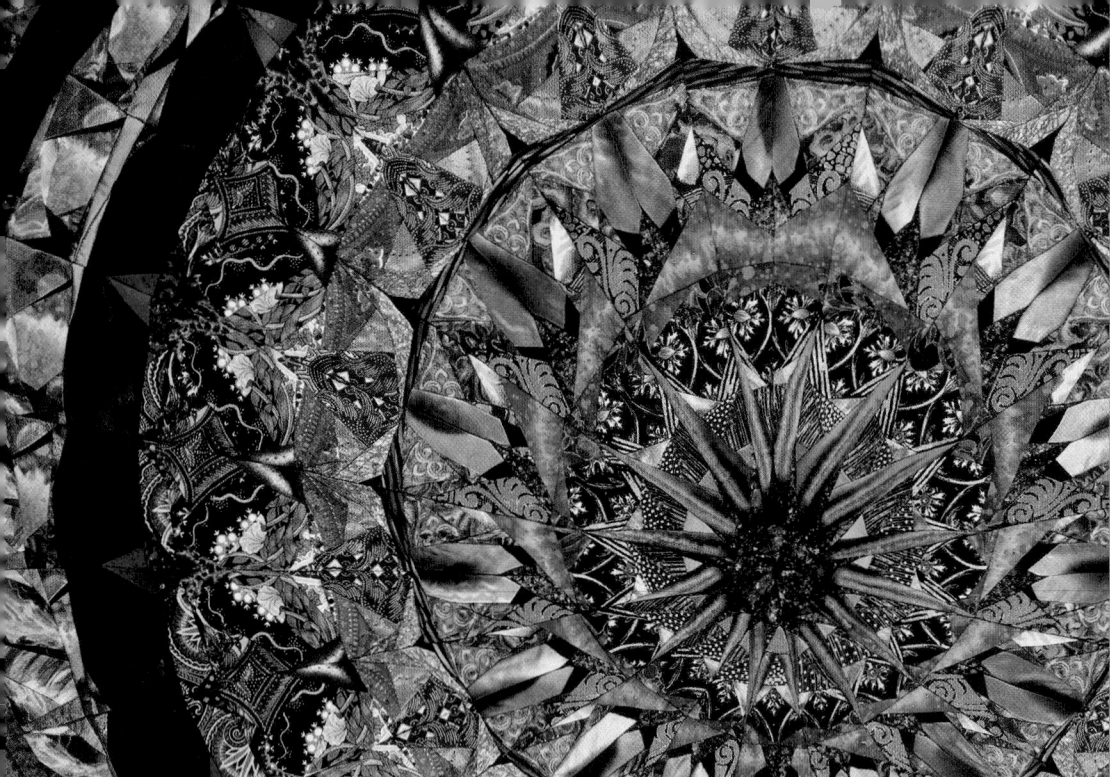

# RESPONSES TO ALTERED VISUAL AND AUDITORY FUNCTION

# CHAPTER 44

# Assessing Clients with Eye and Ear Disorders

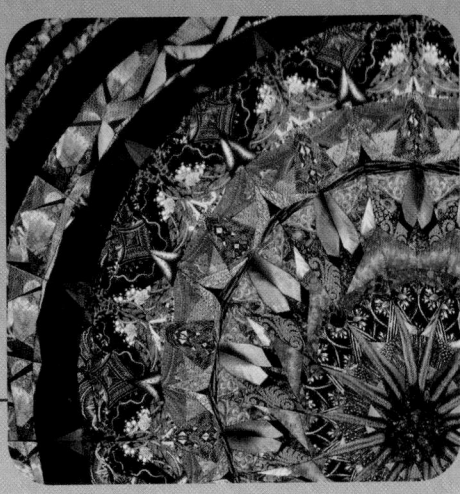

## LEARNING OUTCOMES

After completing this chapter, you will be able to:

- Review the anatomy and physiology of the eye and the ear.
- Explain the physiologic processes involved in vision, hearing, and equilibrium.
- Identify specific topics for consideration during a health history interview of the client with health problems of the eye or ear.
- Describe techniques for assessing the structure and function of the eye and ear.
- Identify abnormal findings that may indicate impairment in the function of the eye and the ear.

## MediaLink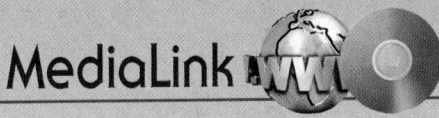

### www.prenhall.com/lemone

Additional resources for this chapter can be found on the Student CD-ROM accompanying this textbook, and on the Companion Website at www.prenhall.com/lemone. Click on Chapter 44 to select the activities for this chapter.

**CD-ROM**
- Audio Glossary
- NCLEX Review

*Animations*
- Ear Anatomy
- Eye Anatomy

**Companion Website**
- More NCLEX Review
- Functional Health Pattern Assessment
- Case Study
    Otitis Media

Vision and hearing allow us to experience the world in which we live. The eyes and ears provide pathways for visual and auditory stimuli to reach the brain. In addition, specialized structures within the ear help maintain position sense and equilibrium. Deficits in vision and hearing may limit self-care, mobility, independence, communication, and relationships with others

## REVIEW OF ANATOMY AND PHYSIOLOGY

### The Eye and Vision

The eyes are complex structures, containing 70% of the sensory receptors of the body. Each eye is a sphere measuring about 1 inch (2.5 cm) in diameter, surrounded and protected by a bony orbit and cushions of fat. The primary functions of the eye are to encode the patterns of light from the environment through photoreceptors and to carry the coded information from the eyes to the brain. The brain gives meaning to the coded information, allowing us to make sense of what we see. Both extraocular and intraocular structures are considered parts of the eye.

### Extraocular Structures

Although the extraocular structures of the eye are outside the eyeball, they are vital to its protection. These structures are the eyebrows, eyelids, eyelashes, conjunctiva, lacrimal apparatus, and extrinsic eye muscles (Figure 44–1 ■).

The eyebrows shade the eyes and keep perspiration away from them. The eyelids are thin, loose folds of skin covering the anterior eye. They protect the eye from foreign bodies, regulate the entry of light into the eye, and distribute tears by blinking. The eyelashes are short hairs that project from the top and bottom borders of the eyelids. An unexpected touch to the eyelashes initiates the blinking reflex to protect the eyes from foreign objects.

The conjunctiva is a thin, transparent membrane that lines the inner surfaces of the eyelids and also folds over the anterior surface of the eyeball. The palpebral conjunctiva lines the upper and lower eyelids, whereas the bulbar conjunctiva loosely covers the anterior sclera (the white part of the eye). The conjunctiva is a mucous membrane that lubricates the eyes. The lacrimal apparatus is composed of the lacrimal gland, the puncta, the lacrimal sac, and the nasolacrimal duct. Together, these structures secrete, distribute, and drain tears to cleanse and moisten the eye's surface.

The six extrinsic eye muscles control movement of the eye, allowing it to follow a moving object and move precisely. The muscles also help maintain the shape of the eyeball. The cranial nerves control the extrinsic muscles (Figure 44–2 ■).

### Intraocular Structures

The intraocular structures transmit visual images and maintain homeostasis of the inner eye. Those in the anterior portion of each eyeball are the sclera and the cornea (forming the outermost coat of the eye, called the fibrous tunic), the iris, the pupil, and the anterior cavity (Figure 44–3 ■).

The white sclera lines the outside of the eyeball, and protects and gives shape to the eyeball. The sclera gives way to the cornea over the iris and pupil. The cornea is transparent, avascular, and sensitive to touch. The cornea forms a window that allows light to enter the eye and is a part of its light-bending apparatus. When the cornea is touched, the eyelids blink (the *corneal reflex*) and tears are secreted.

The iris is a disc of muscle tissue surrounding the pupil and lying between the cornea and the lens. The iris gives the eye its color and regulates light entry by controlling the size of the pupil. The pupil is the dark center of the eye through which light enters. The pupil constricts when bright light enters the eye and when it is used for near vision; it dilates when light conditions are dim and when the eye is used for far vision. In response to intense light, the pupil constricts rapidly in the pupillary light reflex.

The anterior cavity is made of the anterior chamber (the space between the cornea and the iris) and the posterior chamber (the space between the iris and the lens). The anterior cavity is filled with a clear fluid, the aqueous humor. Aqueous humor is con-

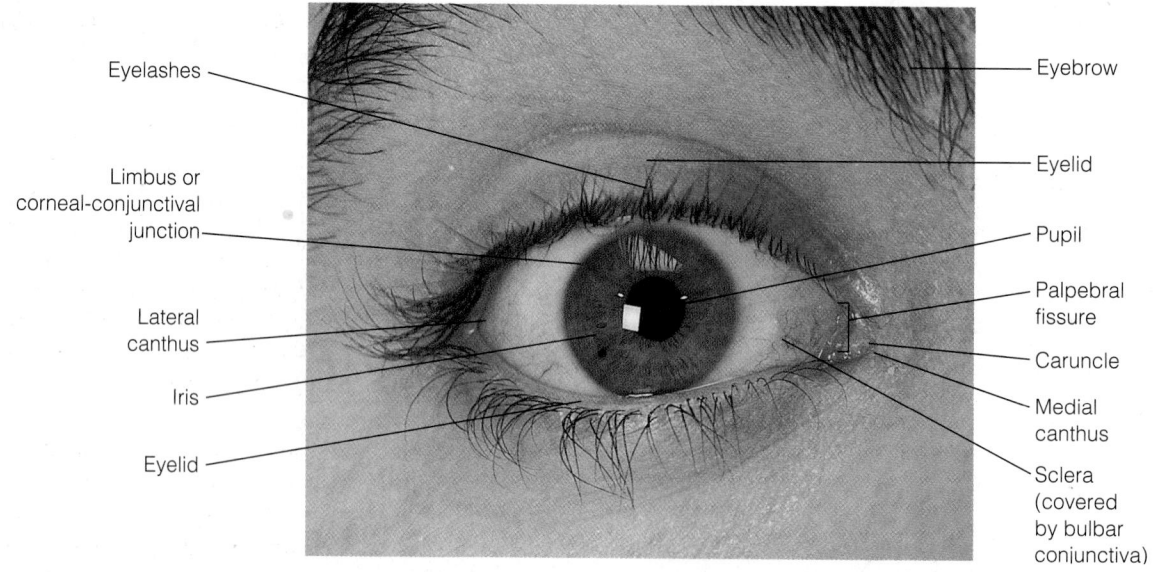

**Figure 44–1** ■ Accessory and external structures of the eye.

*Source: Todd Buck*

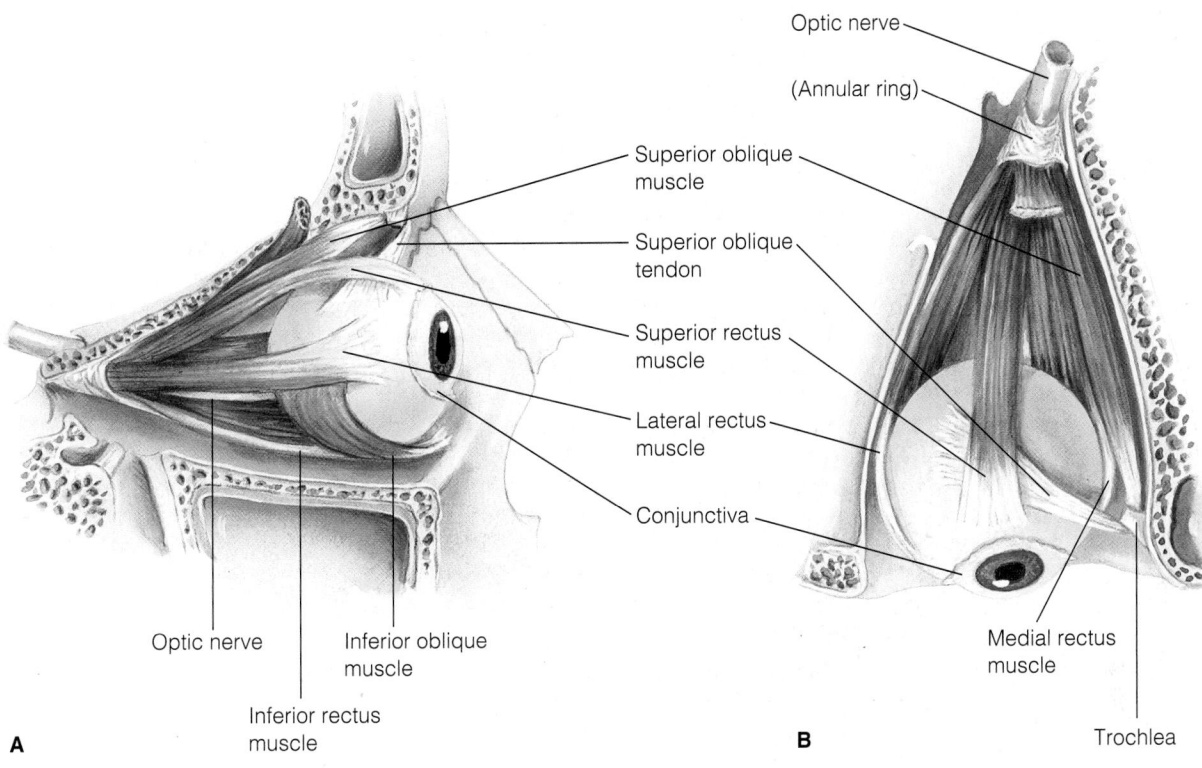

| Name | Controlling cranial nerve | Action |
|------|--------------------------|--------|
| Lateral rectus | VI (abducens) | Moves eye laterally |
| Medial rectus | III (oculomotor) | Moves eye medially |
| Superior rectus | III (oculomotor) | Elevates eye or rolls it superiorly |
| Inferior rectus | III (oculomotor) | Depresses eye or rolls it inferiorly |
| Inferior oblique | III (oculomotor) | Elevates eye and turns it laterally |
| Superior oblique | IV (trochlear) | Depresses eye and turns it laterally |

**Figure 44–2** ■ Extraocular muscles. *A*, Lateral view of the right eye. *B*, Superior view of the right eye. *C*, Innervation of the extraocular muscles by the cranial nerves.

stantly formed and drained to maintain a relatively constant pressure of from 15 to 20 mmHg in the eye. The canal of Schlemm, a network of channels that circles the eye in the angle at the junction of the sclera and the cornea, is the drainage system for fluid moving between the anterior and posterior chambers. Aqueous humor provides nutrients and oxygen to the cornea and the lens.

The intraocular structures that lie in the internal chamber of the eye are the posterior cavity and vitreous humor, the lens, the ciliary body, the uvea, and the retina.

The posterior cavity lies behind the lens. It is filled with a clear gelatinous substance, the vitreous humor, which supports the posterior surface of the lens, maintains the position of the retina, and transmits light. The lens is a biconvex, avascular, transparent structure located directly behind the pupil. It can change shape to focus and refract light onto the retina.

The uvea, also called the vascular tunic, is the middle layer of the eyeball. This pigmented layer has three components: the iris, ciliary body, and choroid. The ciliary body encircles the lens, and along with the iris, regulates the amount of light reaching the retina by controlling the shape of the lens. Most of the uvea is made up of the choroid, which is pigmented and vascular. Blood vessels of the choroid nourish the layers of the eyeball. Its pigmented areas absorb light, preventing it from scattering within the eyeball.

The retina is the innermost lining of the eyeball. It has an outer pigmented layer and an inner neural layer. The outer layer, next to the choroid, serves as the link between visual stimuli and the brain. The transparent inner layer is made up of millions of light receptors in structures called rods and cones. Rods enable vision in dim light as well as peripheral

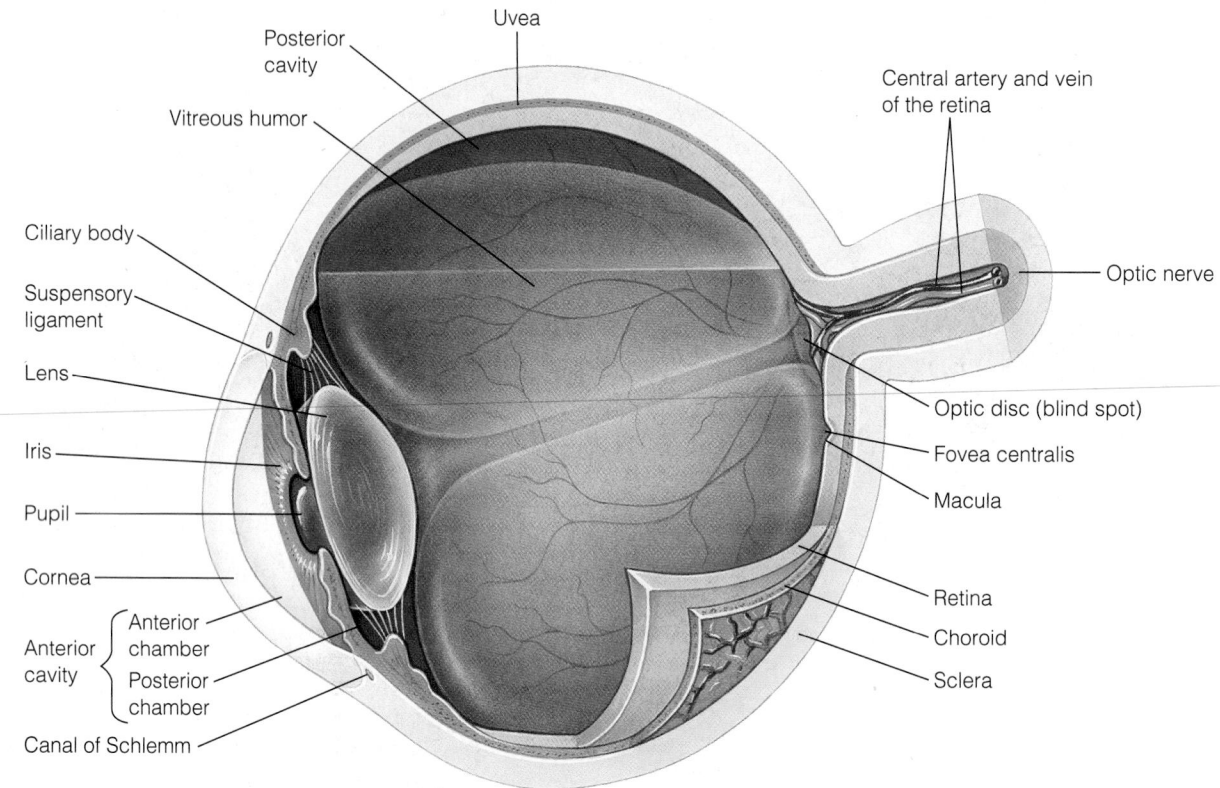

**Figure 44–3** ■ Internal structures of the eye.

vision. Cones enable vision in bright light and the perception of color. The optic disc, a cream-colored round or oval area within the retina, is the point at which the optic nerve enters the eye. The slight depression in the center of the optic disc is often called the physiologic cup. Located laterally to the optic disc is the macula, a darker area with no visible blood vessels. The macula contains primarily cones. The fovea centralis is a slight depression in the center of the macula that contains only cones and is a main receptor of detailed color vision.

## The Visual Pathway

The optic nerves are cranial nerves formed of the axons of ganglion cells. The two optic nerves meet at the optic chiasma, just anterior to the pituitary gland in the brain. At the optic chiasma, axons from the medial half of each retina cross to the opposite side to form pairs of axons from each eye. These pairs continue as the left and right optic tracts (Figure 44–4 ■). The crossing of the axons results in each optic tract carrying information from both eyes. The left optic tract carries visual information from the lateral half of the retina of the left eye and the medial

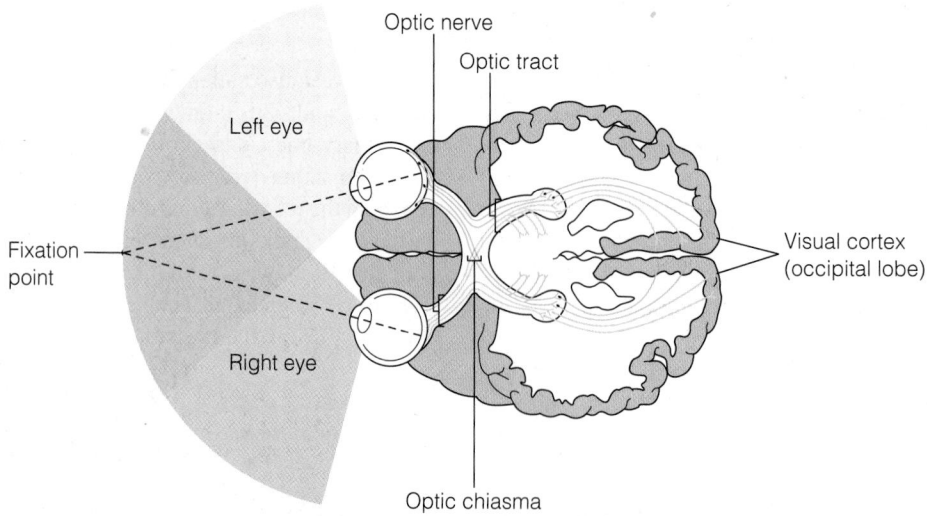

**Figure 44–4** ■ The visual fields of the eye, and the visual pathways to the brain.

half of the retina of the right eye, whereas the right optic tract carries visual information from the lateral half of the retina of the right eye and the medial half of the retina of the left eye.

The ganglion cell axons in the optic tracts travel to the thalamus and create synapses with neurons, forming pathways called optic radiations. The optic radiations terminate in the visual cortex of the occipital lobe. Here the nerve impulses that originated in the retina are interpreted.

The visual fields of each eye overlap considerably, and each eye sees a slightly different view. Because of this overlap and the crossing of the axons, information from both eyes reaches each side of the visual cortex, which then fuses the information into one image. This fusion of images accounts for the ability to perceive depth; however, depth perception depends on visual input from two eyes that both focus well.

## Refraction

Refraction is the bending of light rays as they pass from one medium to another medium of different optical density. As light rays pass through the eye, they are refracted at several points: as they enter the cornea, as they leave the cornea and enter the aqueous humor, as they enter the lens, and as they leave the lens and enter the vitreous humor. At the lens, the light is bent so that it converges at a single point on the retina. This focusing of the image is called accommodation. Because the lens is convex, the image projected onto the retina (the real image) is upside down and reversed from left to right. This real image is coded as electric signals that are sent to the brain. The brain decodes the image so that the person perceives it as it occurs in space.

The eyes are best adapted to see distant objects. Both eyes fix on the same distant image and do not require any change in accommodation. For people with *emmetropic* (normal) vision, the distance from the viewed object at which the eyes require no accommodation is 20 ft (6 m). This point is called the far point of vision. To focus for near vision, the eyes must instantly accommodate the lens, constrict the pupils, and converge the eyeballs. Accommodation is accomplished by contraction of the ciliary muscles. This contraction reduces the tension on the lens capsule so that it bulges outward to increase the curvature. This change in shape also achieves a shorter focal length, another requirement for focusing close images on the retina. The closest point on which a person can focus is called the near point of vision; in young adults with normal vision this is usually 8 to 10 inches (20 to 25 cm). Pupillary constriction helps eliminate most of the divergent light rays and sharpens focus. Convergence (the medial rotation of the eyeballs so that each is directed toward the viewed object) allows the focusing of the image on the retinal fovea of each eye.

## ASSESSING THE EYE

Data about the function of the eyes and vision are gathered both during the health assessment interview to collect subjective data and the physical assessment to collect objective data.

## Health Assessment Interview

This section provides guidelines for collecting subjective data about the functions of the eye and ear through a health assessment interview.

A health assessment interview to determine problems with the eyes and vision may be part of a health screening, may focus on a chief complaint (such as blurred vision or an eye infection), or may be part of a total health assessment. If the client has a health problem involving one or both eyes, analyze its onset, characteristics and course, severity, precipitating and relieving factors, and any associated symptoms, noting the timing and circumstances. For example, you may ask the client:

- Describe the type of pain you experience in your eyes. When did it begin? How long does it last?
- Have you noticed rings of color around streetlights at night?
- When did you first notice having difficulty reading the paper?

Throughout the interview, be alert to nonverbal behaviors (such as squinting or abnormal eye movements) that suggest problems with eye function. Explore problems such as watery, irritated eyes or changes in vision. Assess the client's use of corrective eyewear and care of eyeglasses or contact lenses. If the client uses eye medications, ask about the type and purpose as well as the frequency and duration of use. When taking the history, find out about eye trauma, surgery, or infections, as well as the date and results of the last eye examination. In addition, ask the client about a medical history of diabetes, hypertension, thyroid disorders, glaucoma, cataracts, and eye infections. Include questions about a family history of nearsightedness or farsightedness, cancer of the retina, color blindness, and any other eye or vision disorders.

Collect information about environmental or work exposure to irritating chemicals, participation in sports or hobbies that pose the risk of eye injury, and the use of protective eyewear during dangerous activities.

Further interview questions and leading statements, categorized by functional health patterns, can be found on the Companion Website.

## Physical Assessment of the Eye and Vision

Physical assessment of the eyes and of visual acuity may be performed as part of a total assessment or separately for clients with known or suspected problems of the eyes. The eyes and vision are primarily assessed through inspection of external structures and assessment of visual fields and visual acuity, extraocular muscle function, and internal structures. Palpation (e.g., of a blocked lacrimal duct) may be used if a problem is identified. Prior to the examination, collect all necessary equipment—visual acuity charts, an opaque eye cover, a pen, a penlight, a cotton-tipped applicator, and an ophthalmoscope—and explain the techniques to the client to decrease anxiety. The client may sit or stand during the assessment.

## Assessing Visual Fields

Visual fields are tested to assess the functioning of the macula and peripheral vision. The visual fields of the examiner (which must be normal to perform this assessment) are used as the standard. To measure visual fields, sit directly opposite the client at a distance of 18 to 24 inches. Ask the client to cover one eye with the opaque cover while you cover your own eye opposite to the client (for example, if the client covers the right eye, you cover your left eye). Ask the client to look directly at you. Move the penlight from the periphery toward the center from right to left, above and below, and from the middle of each of these directions. Both you and the client should see the penlight enter the field of vision at the same time.

## Vision Assessment with Abnormal Findings (✓)

Visual acuity is assessed with the Snellen chart or the E chart for testing distance vision and the Rosenbaum chart for testing near vision. The Snellen chart contains rows of letters in various sizes, with standardized numbers at the end of each row. The number at the end of the row indicates the visual acuity of a client who can read the row at a distance of 20 feet. (If the client is unable to read or does not read English, you can use the E chart to test visual acuity.) The top number at the end of the row is always 20, representing the distance between the client and the chart. The bottom number is the distance (in feet) at which a person with normal vision can read the line. A person with normal vision can read the row marked 20/20. To conduct the assessment, ask the person to stand 20 feet from the chart in a well-lit area. Ask the client to cover one eye with an opaque cover (Figure 44–5 ■). Then ask the client to read each row of letters, moving from largest letters to the smallest ones that the client can see. Measure visual acuity in the other eye in the same way, and then assess visual acuity while the client has both eyes uncovered. You may test the client who wears corrective lenses with and without the lenses.

The Rosenbaum chart is held at a distance of from 12 to 14 inches from the eyes, with visual acuity measured in the same manner as with the Snellen chart (Figure 44–6 ■). A gross estimate of near vision may also be assessed by asking the person to read from a magazine or newspaper.

- Assess distant vision, using the Snellen or E chart.
  ✓ Changes in distant vision are most commonly the result of **myopia** (nearsightedness). For example, a reading of 20/100 indicates impaired distance vision. A person has to stand 20 feet from the chart to read a line that a person with normal vision could read 100 feet from the chart.

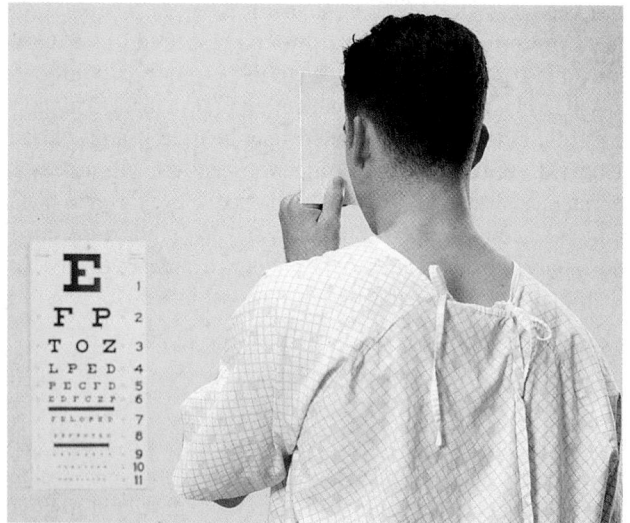

**Figure 44–5** ■ Testing distant vision using the Snellen eye chart.

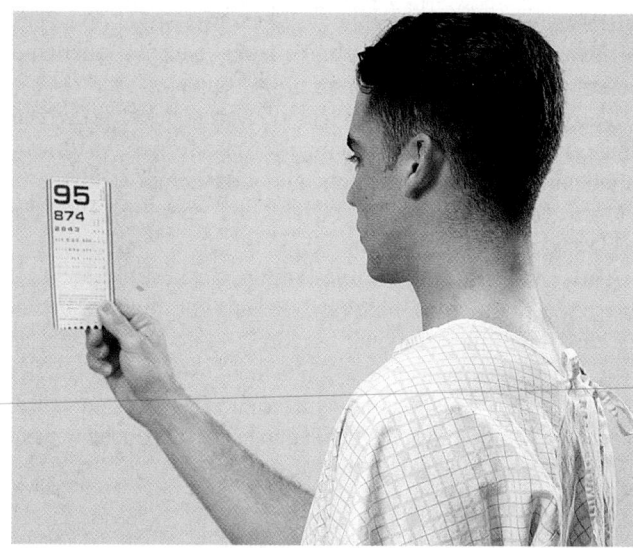

**Figure 44–6** ■ Testing near vision using Rosenbaum eye chart.

- Assess near vision, using a Rosenbaum chart or a card with newsprint held 12 to 14 inches from the client's eyes.
  ✓ Changes in near vision, especially in clients over 45, can indicate **presbyopia,** impaired near vision resulting from a loss of elasticity of the lens related to aging. In younger clients, this condition is referred to as **hyperopia** (far-sightedness).

## Eye Movement and Alignment Assessment with Abnormal Findings (✓)

- Assess the cardinal fields of vision to gain information about extraocular eye movements. Ask the client to follow a pen or your finger while keeping the head stationary. Move the pen or your finger through the six fields one at a time, returning to the central starting point before proceeding to the next field (Figure 44–7 ■). The eyes should move through each field without involuntary movements.
- The cover-uncover test is a test for strabismus, a weakening of a muscle that causes one eye to deviate from the other when the person is focusing on an object. To conduct the test, hold a pen or your finger about 1 foot from the eyes and ask the person to focus on that object. Cover one of the client's eyes and note any movement in the uncovered eye; as you remove the cover, assess for movement in the eye that was just uncovered. Repeat the procedure with the other eye.
- Assess convergence. Ask the client to follow an object as you move it toward the client's eyes; normally both eyes converge toward the center.
  ✓ Failure of the eyes to converge equally on an approaching object may indicate a neuromuscular disorder or improper eye alignment.
- Assess extraocular movements.
  ✓ Failure of one or both eyes to follow the object in any given direction may indicate extraocular muscle weakness or cranial nerve dysfunction.
  ✓ An involuntary rhythmic movement of the eyes, nystagmus, is associated with neurologic disorders and the use of some medications.

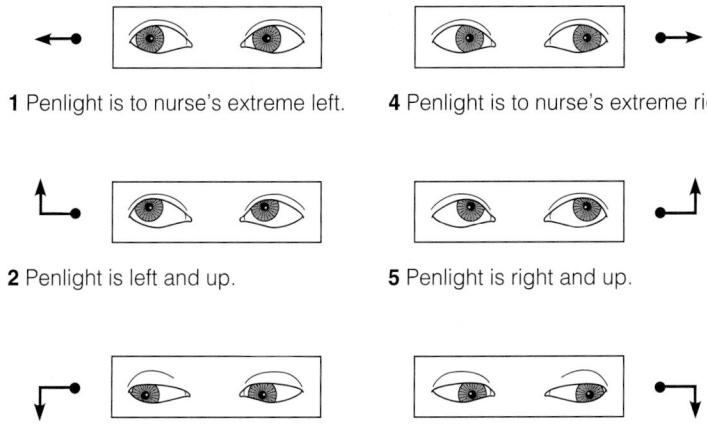

**1** Penlight is to nurse's extreme left.

**4** Penlight is to nurse's extreme right.

**2** Penlight is left and up.

**5** Penlight is right and up.

**3** Penlight is left and down.

**6** Penlight is right and down.

**Figure 44–7** ■ The six cardinal fields of vision.

- Assess the corneal light reflex. Direct a light source onto the bridge of the nose from 12 to 15 inches. Observe for equal reflection of the light from each eye.
  - ✓ Reflections of the light from different sites on the eyes reveal improper alignment.

## Pupillary Assessment with Abnormal Findings (✓)

- Observe pupil size and equality.
  - ✓ Pupils that are unequal in size may indicate a severe neurologic problem, such as increased intracranial pressure.
- Assess direct and consensual pupil response. Ask the client to look straight ahead. Shine a light obliquely into one eye at a time. Observe for constriction of the pupil in the illuminated eye. Test both eyes. To test consensual pupil response, again shine a light obliquely into one eye at a time as the client looks straight ahead. Observe constriction of the pupil in the opposite eye.
  - ✓ Failure of the pupils to respond to light may indicate degeneration of the retina or destruction of the optic nerve.
  - ✓ A client who has one dilated and unresponsive pupil may have paralysis of the oculomotor nerve.
  - ✓ Some eye medications may cause unequal dilation, constriction, or inequality of pupil size. Morphine and similar drugs may cause small, unresponsive pupils, and anticholinergic drugs such as atropine may cause dilated, unresponsive pupils.
- Test for accommodation. Hold an object at a distance of a few feet from the client. The pupils should dilate. Ask the client to follow the object as you bring it to within a few inches of the client's nose. The pupils should constrict and converge as they change focus to follow the object.
  - ✓ Failure of accommodation along with lack of pupil response to light may signal a neurologic problem.
  - ✓ Lack of response to light with appropriate response to accommodation is often seen in clients with diabetes.

## External Eye Assessment with Abnormal Findings (✓)

- Inspect the eyelids.
  - ✓ Unusual redness or discharge may indicate an inflammatory state due to trauma, allergies, or infection.

- ✓ Drooping of one eyelid, called **ptosis,** may be the result of a stroke, indicate a neuromuscular disorder, or be congenital (Figure 44–8 ■).
- ✓ Unusual widening of the lids may be due to **exophthalmos,** protrusion of the eyeball due to an increase in intraocular volume. Exophthalmos is often associated with hyperthyroid conditions (see Chapter 17).
- ✓ Yellow plaques noted most often on the lid margins are referred to as *xanthelasma* and may indicate high lipid levels.
- ✓ An acute localized inflammation of a hair follicle is known as a hordeolum (sty) and is generally caused by staphylococcal organisms (Figure 44–9 ■).

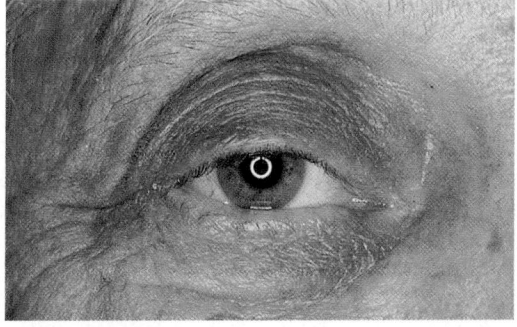

**Figure 44–8** ■ Ptosis.

*Source: Leonard Lessen/Peter Arnold, Inc.*

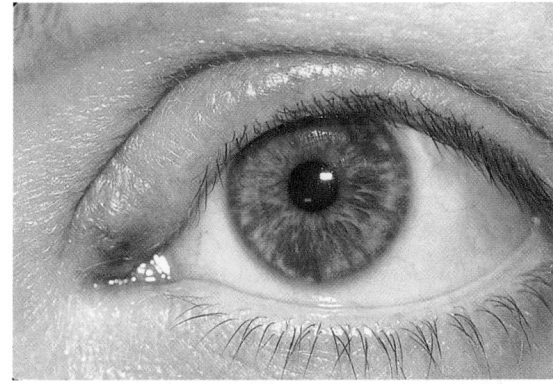

**Figure 44–9** ■ Hordeolum.

*Source: Science Photo Library/Photo Researchers, Inc.*

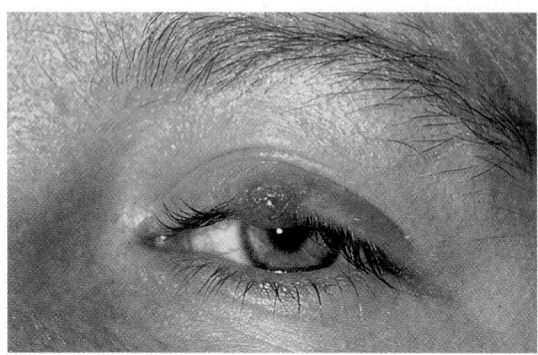

**Figure 44–10** ■ Chalazion.

Source: Custom Medical Stock Photo, Inc.

✓ A chalazion is an infection or retention cyst of the meibomian glands (Figure 44–10 ■). The swelling is firm and not painful.
- Inspect the puncta.
  ✓ Unusual redness or discharge from the puncta may indicate an inflammation due to trauma, infection, or allergies.
- Inspect the bulbar and palpebral conjunctiva.
  ✓ Increased erythema or the presence of exudate may indicate acute conjunctivitis.
  ✓ A cobblestone appearance is often associated with allergies.
  ✓ A fold in the conjunctiva, called a *pterygium,* may be seen as a clouded area that extends over the cornea. This is an abnormal growth of the bulbar conjunctiva, usually seen on the nasal side of the cornea. It may interfere with vision if it covers the pupil.
- Inspect the sclera.
  ✓ Unusual redness may indicate an inflammatory state as a result of trauma, allergies, or infection.
  ✓ Yellow discoloration of the sclera may be seen in conditions involving the liver, such as hepatitis.
  ✓ Bright red areas in the sclera are often subconjunctival hemorrhages and may indicate trauma or bleeding disorders. They may also occur spontaneously.
- Inspect the cornea.
  ✓ Dullness, opacities, or irregularities of the cornea may be abnormal.
  ✓ *Corneal arcus* is a thin, grayish white arc seen toward the edge of the cornea. It is normal in older clients.
- Assess corneal sensitivity. Lightly touch a wisp of cotton to the client's cornea. This action should cause a blink reflex.
  ✓ Failure of the blink reflex may indicate a neurologic disorder.
- Inspect the iris.
  ✓ Lack of clarity of the iris may indicate a cloudiness of the cornea.
  ✓ Constriction of the pupil accompanied by pain and circumcorneal redness indicates acute iritis.

### Internal Eye Assessment with Abnormal Findings (✓)

Assess internal structures of the eye by using the ophthalmoscope, an instrument that allows visualization of the lens, the vitreous humor, and the retina. Box 44–1 provides guidelines for using the ophthalmoscope.

- Inspect for the red reflex.
  ✓ Absence of a red reflex often indicates improper position of the ophthalmoscope, but also may indicate total opacity of the pupil by a cataract or a hemorrhage into the vitreous humor.
- Inspect the lens and vitreous body.
  ✓ A *cataract* is an opacity of the lens, often seen as a dark shadow on ophthalmoscopic examination. It may be due to aging, trauma, diabetes, or a congenital defect.
- Inspect the retina.
  ✓ Areas of hemorrhage, exudate, and white patches may be a result of diabetes or long-standing hypertension.
- Inspect the optic disc.
  ✓ Loss of definition of the optic disc, as well as an increase in the size of the physiologic cup, results from papilledema from increased intracranial pressure.
- Inspect the blood vessels of the retina.
  ✓ Glaucoma often results in displacement of blood vessels from the center of the optic disc due to increased intraocular pressure.
  ✓ Hypertension may cause an apparent narrowing of the vein where an arteriole crosses over.
  ✓ Engorged veins may occur with diabetes, atherosclerosis, and blood disorders.
- Inspect the retinal background.
  ✓ Variations in color or a pale color overall may indicate disease.
- Inspect the macula.
  ✓ Absence of the fovea centralis is common in older clients. It may indicate macular degeneration, a common cause of loss of central vision.
- Palpate over the lacrimal glands, puncta, and nasolacrimal duct.
  ✓ Tenderness over any of these areas or drainage from the puncta may indicate an infectious process. (Wear gloves if you see any drainage.)
  ✓ Excessive tearing may indicate a blockage of the nasolacrimal duct.

## REVIEW OF ANATOMY AND PHYSIOLOGY
## The Ear and Hearing

As a sensory organ, the ear has two primary functions, hearing and maintaining equilibrium. Anatomically, the ear is divided into three areas: the external ear, the middle ear, and the inner ear (Figure 44–11 ■). Each area has a unique function. All three are involved in hearing, but only the inner ear is involved in equilibrium.

### The External Ear
The external ear consists of the auricle (or pinna), the external auditory canal, and the tympanic membrane.

The auricles are elastic cartilage covered with thin skin. They contain sebaceous and sweat glands and sometimes hair.

## BOX 44–1 ■ Guidelines for Using the Ophthalmoscope

The ophthalmoscope has a head and a handle. (See the figure below.) The head contains a focus wheel (also called a lens selector dial) located on the side, lenses of varying magnification, and an opening through which the eye structures are visualized. The focus wheel adjusts the lens refraction, which is measured in diopters. The diopter measurements range from 0 to +40 when the lens is rotated clockwise, and from 0 to −25 when the lens is rotated counterclockwise. By moving the focus wheel, the examiner can converge or diverge light rays to visualize the retina.

The handle usually contains batteries that can be plugged into a wall socket for recharging.

Before the examination, explain the procedure to the client. Assemble the ophthalmoscope. Wash your hands and wear disposable gloves if the client has any drainage from the eyes. Darken the room (to allow the pupils of the client to dilate), and ask the client to look straight ahead, focusing on a fixed point such as an object on the wall. Hold the ophthalmoscope in one hand, resting the index finger on the focus wheel (see the figure at right).

1. Turn on the ophthalmoscope light, and set focus wheel to 0 diopters. Hold the ophthalmoscope in your right hand with your index finger on the focus wheel. Standing in front of the client, position yourself at a 15-degree angle to the client's line of vision.

2. Hold the opening of the ophthalmoscope up to your right eye and direct the light toward the client's right eye from a distance of about 12 inches.

3. As the beam of light falls on the client's pupil, observe for the red reflex, which appears as a sharply outlined orange glow from within the pupil. This glow is the reflection of the light from the retina.

4. Move closer to the client, turning the focus wheel clockwise toward the positive numbers as needed to maintain clear focus.

5. Examine the lens and the vitreous body, both of which should be clear.

6. Gradually rotate the focus wheel counterclockwise toward the negative numbers as needed, focusing on a structure of the retina (such as the disc or a blood vessel). Turn the focus wheel until the image is clear. Examine the structures of the retina as follows:

   a. The optic disc (see the accompanying figure). Assess for size, shape, color, distinct margins, and the physiologic cup. The disc is round to slightly oval and about 1.5 mm in diameter. It has a yellow to pink color that is lighter than the retina itself. The margins should be sharp and clear. The physiologic cup is a small depression that occupies about one-third of the optic disc, lying temporal to the center of the disc.

   b. The vessels of the retina. Assess for color, arteriolar light reflex, ratio of arterioles to veins, and arteriovenous crossings. The arterioles are red, brighter than the veins, and about one-fourth smaller. The arterioles normally have a

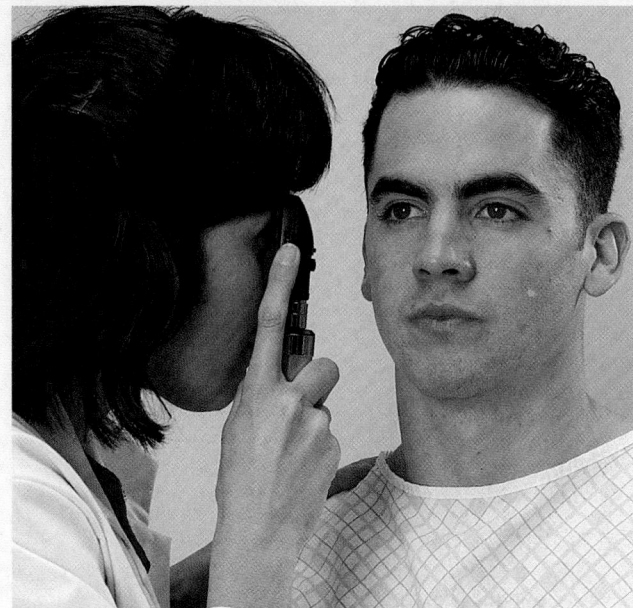

Technique for holding an ophthalmoscope.

narrow light reflex from the center of each vessel; veins do not have this light reflex. The ratio of arterioles to veins is usually 2:3 or 4:5. The vessels normally cross and become smaller toward the periphery.

   c. The retinal background. Assess color and changes in color. The retina is normally reddish orange and regular in color.

   d. The macula. Assess size and color. To assess the macula, ask the client to look directly into the ophthalmoscope light. The macula is temporal to the optic disc, appears slightly darker than the retina, and has no visible vessels. The fovea centralis may be seen as a bright spot of light. Because looking directly into the light causes some discomfort, conduct this portion of the examination last. The macula is often difficult to visualize.

7. Using the same technique, examine the left eye.

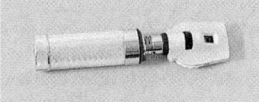

An ophthalmoscope.

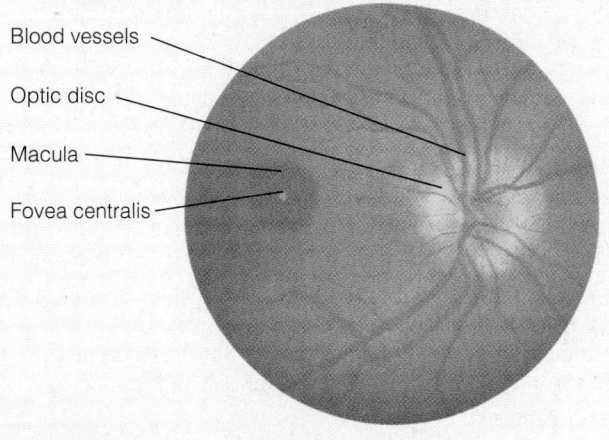

Blood vessels

Optic disc

Macula

Fovea centralis

The optic disc.

*Source: Don Wong/Science Source/Photo Researchers, Inc.*

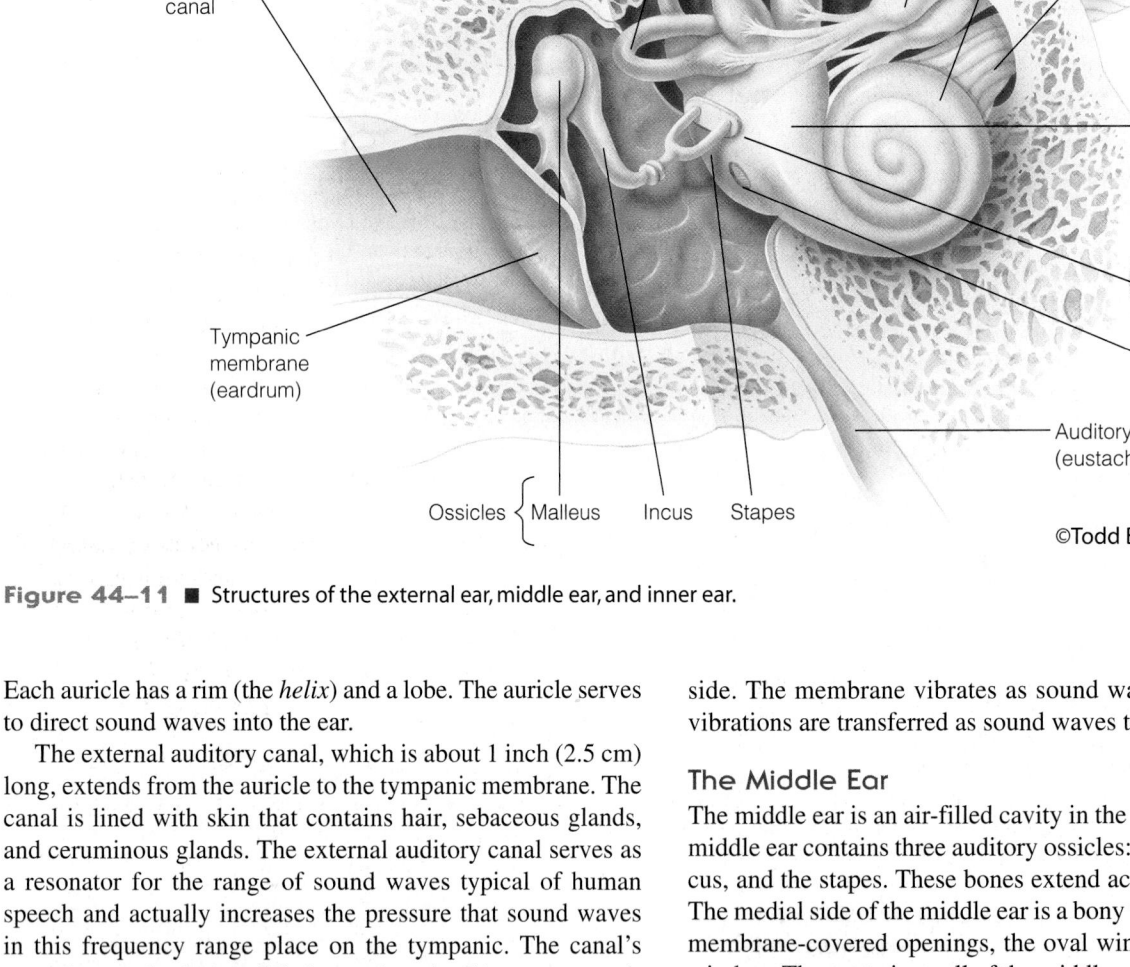

**Figure 44–11** ■ Structures of the external ear, middle ear, and inner ear.

©Todd Buck

Each auricle has a rim (the *helix*) and a lobe. The auricle serves to direct sound waves into the ear.

The external auditory canal, which is about 1 inch (2.5 cm) long, extends from the auricle to the tympanic membrane. The canal is lined with skin that contains hair, sebaceous glands, and ceruminous glands. The external auditory canal serves as a resonator for the range of sound waves typical of human speech and actually increases the pressure that sound waves in this frequency range place on the tympanic. The canal's ceruminous glands (modified apocrine glands) secrete a yellow to brown waxy substance called **cerumen** (earwax). Cerumen traps foreign bodies; it also has bacteriostatic properties, protecting the tympanic membrane and the middle ear from infections.

The tympanic membrane lies between the external ear and the middle ear. It is a thin, semitransparent, fibrous structure covered with skin on the external side and mucosa on the inner side. The membrane vibrates as sound waves strike it; these vibrations are transferred as sound waves to the middle ear.

## The Middle Ear

The middle ear is an air-filled cavity in the temporal bone. The middle ear contains three auditory ossicles: the malleus, the incus, and the stapes. These bones extend across the middle ear. The medial side of the middle ear is a bony wall containing two membrane-covered openings, the oval window and the round window. The posterior wall of the middle ear contains the mastoid antrum. This cavity communicates with the mastoid sinuses, which help the middle ear adjust to changes in pressure. It also opens into the eustachian tube, which connects with the nasopharynx. The eustachian tube helps to equalize the air pressure in the middle ear by opening briefly in response to differences between middle ear pressure and atmospheric pressure. This action also ensures that vibrations of the tympanic membrane remain adequate. The mucous membrane lining the middle ear is continuous with the mucous membranes lining the throat.

The malleus attaches to the tympanic membrane and articulates with the incus, which in turn articulates with the stapes. The stapes fits into the oval window. When the tympanic membrane vibrates, the vibrations are conducted across the middle ear to the oval window by the ossicles. The vibrations then set in motion the fluids of the inner ear, which in turn stimulate the hearing receptors. Two small muscles attached to the ossicles contract reflexively in response to sudden loud noises, thus decreasing the vibrations and protecting the inner ear.

### The Inner Ear

The inner ear, also called the labyrinth, is a maze of bony chambers located deep within the temporal bone, just behind the eye socket. The labyrinth is further divided into two parts: the bony labyrinth, a system of open channels that houses the second part, the membranous labyrinth. The bony labyrinth is filled with a fluid similar to cerebrospinal fluid called perilymph, which bathes the membranous labyrinth. Within the chambers of the membranous labyrinth is a fluid called endolymph.

The bony labyrinth has three regions: the vestibule, the semicircular canals, and the cochlea. The vestibule is the central portion of the inner ear, one side of which is a bony wall containing the oval window. Two sacs within the vestibule (the saccule and the utricle) join the vestibule with the cochlea and the semicircular canals. The saccule and the utricle contain receptors for equilibrium that respond to changes in gravity and changes in position of the head. The three semicircular canals each project into a different plane (anterior, posterior, and lateral). Each canal contains a semicircular duct that communicates with the utricle of the vestibule. Each duct has an enlarged area at one end containing an equilibrium receptor that responds to angular movements of the head.

The cochlea is a tiny bony chamber that houses the organ of Corti, the receptor organ for hearing. The organ of Corti is a series of sensory hair cells, arranged in a single row of inner hair cells and three rows of outer hair cells. The hair cells are innervated by sensory fibers from cranial nerve VIII. The organ of Corti is supported in the cochlea by the flexible basilar membrane, which has fibers of varying lengths that respond to different sound wave frequencies.

### Sound Conduction

Hearing is the perception and interpretation of sound. Sound is produced when the molecules of a medium are compressed, resulting in a pressure disturbance evidenced as a sound wave. The intensity or loudness of sound is determined by the amplitude (height) of the sound wave, with greater amplitudes causing louder sounds. The frequency of the sound wave in vibrations per second determines the pitch or tone of the sound, with higher frequencies resulting in higher sounds. The human ear is most sensitive to sound waves with frequencies between 1000 and 4000 cycles per second, but can detect sound waves with frequencies between 20 and 20,000 cycles per second.

Sound waves enter the external auditory canal and cause the tympanic membrane to vibrate at the same frequency. The os-

sicles not only transmit the motion of the tympanic membrane to the oval window but also amplify the energy of the sound wave. As the stapes moves against the oval window, the perilymph in the vestibule is set in motion. The increased pressure of the perilymph is transmitted to fibers of the basilar membrane and then to the organ of Corti (directly above the basilar membrane). The up-and-down movements of the fibers of the basilar membrane pull the hair cells in the organ of Corti, which in turn generates action potentials that are transmitted to cranial nerve VIII and then to the brain for interpretation.

Several brainstem auditory nuclei transmit impulses to the cerebral cortex. Fibers from each ear cross, with each auditory cortex receiving impulses from both ears. Auditory processing is so finely tuned that a wide variety of sounds of different pitch and loudness can be heard at any one time. In addition, the source of the sound can be localized.

### Maintenance of Equilibrium

The inner ear also provides information about the position of the head. This information is used to coordinate body movements so that equilibrium and balance are maintained. The types of equilibrium are static balance (affected by changes in the position of the head) and dynamic balance (affected by the movement of the head).

Receptors called maculae in the utricle and the saccule of the vestibule detect changes in the position of the head. Maculae are groups of hair cells; these cells have protrusions covered with a gelatinous substance. Embedded in this gelatinous substance are tiny particles of calcium carbonate called otoliths (ear stones), which make the gelatin heavier than the endolymph that fills the membranous labyrinth. As a result, when the head is in the upright position, gravity causes the gelatinous substance to bear down on the hair cells. When the position of the head changes, the force on the hair cells also changes, bending them and altering the pattern of stimulation of the neurons. Thus, a different pattern of nerve impulses is transmitted to the brain, where stimulation of the motor centers initiates actions that coordinate various body movements according to the position of the head.

The receptor for dynamic equilibrium is in the crista, a crest in the membrane lining the ampulla of each semicircular canal. The cristae are stimulated by rotatory head movement (acceleration and deceleration) as a result of changes in the flow of endolymph and of movement of hair cells in the maculae. The direction of endolymph and hair cell movement is always opposite to the motion of the body.

## ASSESSING THE EAR

Data about the function of the ears and hearing are gathered both during the health assessment interview to collect subjective data and the physical assessment to collect objective data.

### Health Assessment Interview

The health history assessment to collect subjective data about the ears and hearing may be part of a health screening, may focus on a chief complaint (such as hearing problems or pain in the ear), or may be part of a total health assessment. If the

## BOX 44–2 ■ Guidelines for Using the Otoscope

The otoscope has a handle that contains batteries for the light and various specula that fit onto the handle. (See the accompanying figure.) This instrument is used to inspect the auditory canal and the tympanic membrane. A pneumatic otoscope is used to determine the mobility of the tympanic membrane. A pneumatic otoscope has an attached rubber bulb that can be squeezed to inject air into the auditory canal, causing a normal tympanic membrane to move in and out.

Before the examination, explain the procedure to the client. Assemble the otoscope, using the largest speculum that will fit into the client's auditory canal without discomfort. Wash your hands; wear disposable gloves if the client has any drainage from the ears. Turn on the otoscope light. Ask the client to tip the head slightly toward the shoulder opposite the ear being examined. When the client is in this position, the auditory canal is aligned with the speculum.

1. Hold the handle of the otoscope in your dominant hand. If the client is restless, hold the otoscope handle upward, resting the hand against the client's head. If the client is cooperative, hold the handle downward.
2. For adult clients, grasp the superior portion of the auricle and pull up, out, and back to straighten the auditory canal. (See the accompanying figure.)
3. Insert the speculum into the ear and advance it gently. Assess the walls of the auditory canal while advancing the speculum, inspecting for color, obstructions, hair growth, and cerumen. Old cerumen is very dark and may obstruct visualization of part or all of the tympanic membrane.
4. Move the otoscope so that you can see the tympanic membrane. You may need to realign the auditory canal by gently continuing to pull up and back on the auricle. A normal membrane is semitransparent, allowing visualization of a portion of the auditory ossicles. The concave nature of the tympanic membrane and its oblique position in the auditory canal account for the triangular light reflex (cone of light) seen on otoscopic examination.
5. Note the color and surface of the membrane. The normal tympanic membrane is pearly gray, shiny, and semitransparent. The surface should be continuous, intact, and either flat or concave.
6. Identify the landmarks of the tympanic membrane (see the accompanying figure):
   a. The cone of light, located over the anteroinferior quadrant.
   b. The malleus, pars tensa, annulus, pars flaccida, and malleolar folds.
7. Assess movement of the tympanic membrane. If the auditory tube is patent, the membrane moves in and out when air is injected (or when the client performs the Valsalva maneuver).
8. Gently withdraw the speculum. If the speculum is soiled with drainage or cerumen, use a clean speculum for the other ear.
9. Using the same technique, examine the other ear.

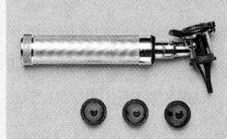

An otoscope.

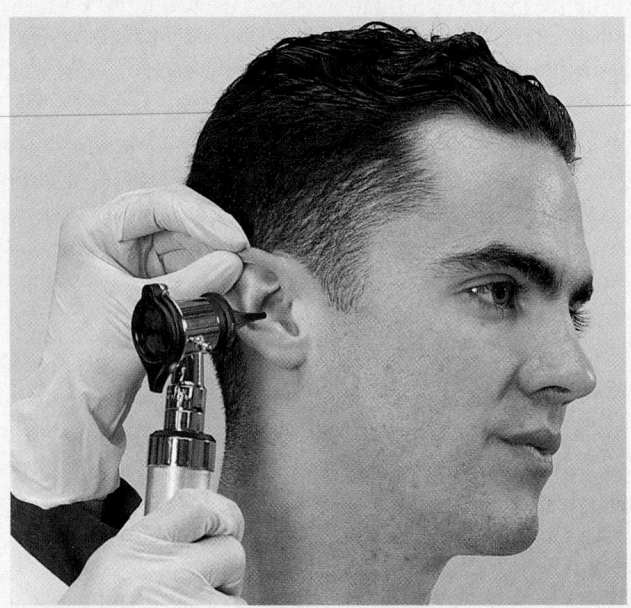

Technique for using an otoscope.

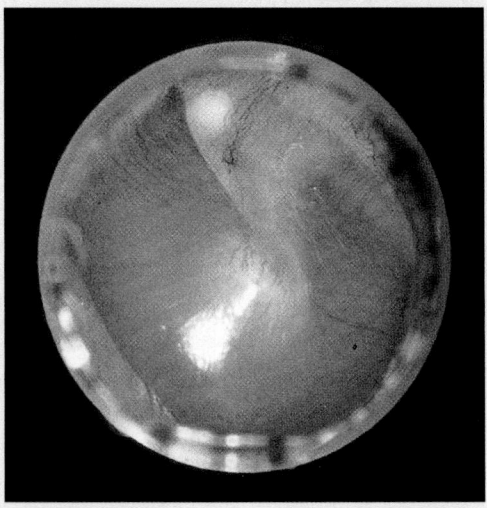

Structures of the tympanic membrane visible through the otoscope.

client has a problem involving one or both ears, analyze its onset, characteristics and course, severity, precipitating and relieving factors, and any associated symptoms, noting the timing and circumstances. For example, you may ask the following questions.

- Have you noticed any difficulty hearing high-pitched sounds, low-pitched sounds, or both?
- When did you first notice the ringing in your ears?
- Is your workplace very noisy? If so, do you wear protective ear equipment at work?

Throughout the examination, be alert to nonverbal behaviors (such as inappropriate answers or requests to repeat statements) that suggest problems with ear function. Explore changes in hearing, ringing in the ears (*tinnitus*), ear pain, drainage from the ears, or the use of hearing aids. When taking the history, ask about trauma, surgery, or infections of the ear as well as the date of the last ear examination. In addition, ask the client about a medical history of infectious diseases, such as meningitis or mumps, as well as the use of medications that may affect hearing. Because ear problems tend to run in families, ask about a family history of hearing loss, ear problems, or diseases that could result in such problems. If the client has a hearing aid, ascertain the type and assess measures for its care.

Specific questions and leading statements, categorized by functional health patterns, can be found on the Companion Website.

## Physical Assessment of the Ear and Hearing

Physical assessment of the ear and hearing may be performed as part of a total health assessment or separately for clients with known or suspected problems with the ears. The ears and hearing are assessed primarily through inspection of external structures, the external auditory canal, and the tympanic membrane. Hearing acuity is assessed by voice tests and tuning fork tests. The external structures may be palpated.

Equipment includes an otoscope and a tuning fork. The client should be sitting, and the examiner's head should be level with the head of the client. Prior to the assessment, collect all necessary equipment and explain the techniques to the client to decrease anxiety.

The auditory canal and tympanic membrane are inspected with the otoscope. Guidelines for use of the otoscope are listed on the previous page in Box 44–2.

### Hearing Assessment with Abnormal Findings (✓)
Tuning forks are used to determine whether a hearing loss is conductive or perceptive (sensorineural) (Figure 44–12 ■).

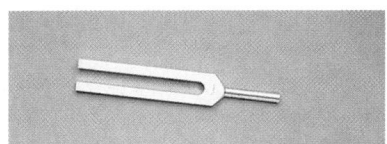

**Figure 44–12** ■ A tuning fork.

Hold the tuning fork at the base and make it ring softly by stroking the prongs or by lightly tapping them on the heel of the opposite hand. The vibrating tuning fork emits sound waves of a particular frequency, measured in Hertz (Hz). Tuning forks with a frequency of 512 to 1024 Hz are preferred for auditory evaluation, because that range corresponds to the range of normal speech.

- Perform the **Weber test.** Place the base of a vibrating tuning fork on the midline vertex of the client's head (Figure 44–13 ■). Ask whether the client hears the sound equally in both ears or better in one than the other. Sound is normally heard equally in both ears.
  - ✓ Sound heard in, or lateralized to, one ear indicates either a conductive loss in that ear or a sensorineural loss in the other ear. Conductive losses may be due to a buildup of cerumen, an infection such as otitis media, or perforation of the eardrum.
- Perform the **Rinne test.** Place the base of a vibrating tuning fork on the client's mastoid bone. Ask the client to indicate when the sound is no longer heard. When the client does so, quickly reposition the tuning fork in front of the client's ear close to the ear canal. Ask whether the client can hear the sound. If the client says yes, ask the client to indicate when the sound is no longer heard. The client with no conductive hearing loss will hear the sound twice as long by air conduction as by bone conduction (Figure 44–14 ■).
  - ✓ Bone conduction is greater than air conduction in the ear with a conductive loss. The normal pattern is AC>BC (air conduction greater than bone conduction).
- Perform the **whisper test.** Ask the client to occlude one ear with a finger. Stand 1 to 2 feet away from the client, on the

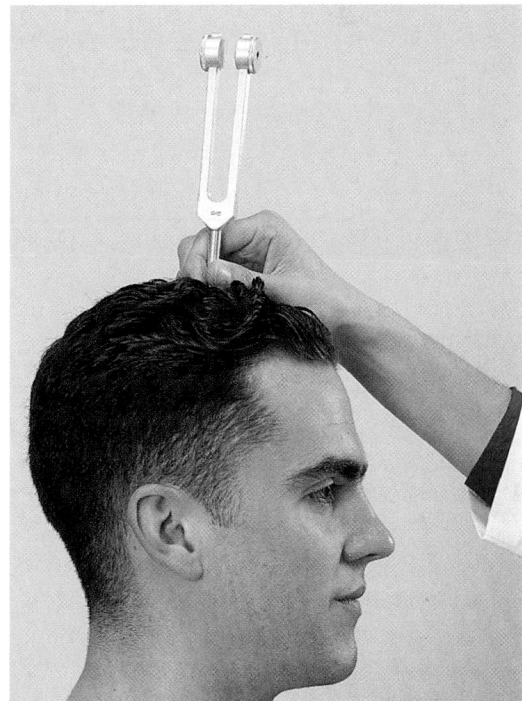

**Figure 44–13** ■ Performing the Weber test.

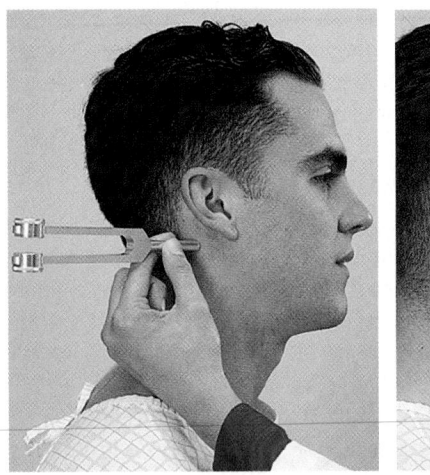
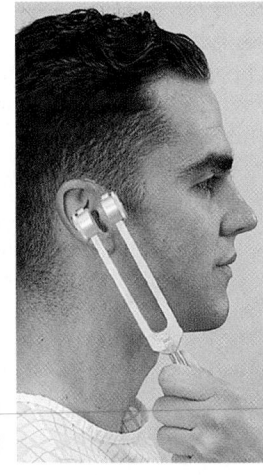

**Figure 44–14 ■** Performing the Rinne test.

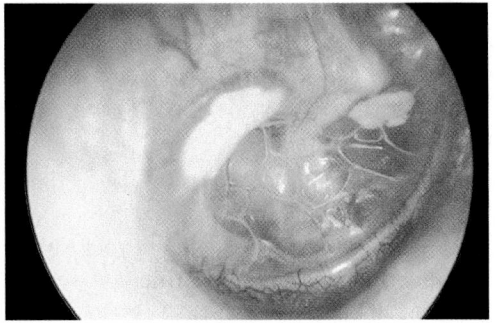

**Figure 44–15 ■** Scarring of the tympanic membrane.

*Source: Professor Tony Wright, Institute of Laryncology and Otology/SPL/Photo Researchers, Inc.*

side of the unoccluded ear. Softly whisper numbers and ask the client to repeat them. Repeat the procedure, having the client occlude the other ear. Note whether you need to raise your voice or to stand closer to make the client hear you.
✓ This is a rough estimate of hearing loss.

## External Ear Assessment with Abnormal Findings (✓)

- Inspect the auricle.
  ✓ Unusual redness or drainage may indicate an inflammatory response to infection or trauma.
  ✓ Scales or skin lesions around the rim of the auricle may indicate skin cancer.
  ✓ Small, raised lesions on the rim of the ear are known as *tophi* and indicate gout.
- Inspect the external auditory canal with the otoscope.
  ✓ Unusual redness, lesions, or purulent drainage may indicate an infection.

✓ Cerumen varies in color and texture, but hardened, dry, or foul-smelling cerumen may indicate an infection or an impaction of cerumen that requires removal. People with darker skin tend to have darker cerumen.
- Inspect the tympanic membrane.
  ✓ White, opaque areas on the tympanic membrane are often scars from previous perforations (Figure 44–15 ■).
  ✓ Inconsistent texture and color may be due to scarring from previous perforation caused by infection, allergies, or trauma.
  ✓ Bulging membranes are indicated by a loss of bony landmarks and a distorted light reflex. Such bulges may be the result of otitis media or malfunctioning auditory tubes.
  ✓ Retracted tympanic membranes are indicated by accentuated bony landmarks and a distorted light reflex. Such retraction is often due to an obstructed auditory tube.
- Palpate the auricles and over the mastoid process.
  ✓ Tenderness, swelling, or nodules may indicate inflammation of the external auditory canal or mastoiditis.

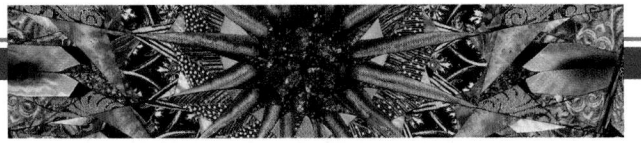

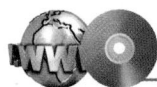 EXPLORE MediaLink

# TEST YOURSELF

1. What part of the eye covers the iris and pupil?
   a. Lens
   b. Cornea
   c. Sclera
   d. Puncta

2. What function, in addition to hearing, is provided by the inner ear?
   a. Coordinates visual pathways
   b. Integrates efferent neuron messages
   c. Provides information about head position
   d. Maintains middle ear structure and function

3. Why is the Snellen eye chart used during vision assessment?
   a. To test distant vision
   b. To test near vision
   c. To determine visual fields
   d. To examine convergence

4. Impaired near vision, especially in clients over 45, often indicates:
   a. Strabismus
   b. Nystagmus
   c. Myopia
   d. Presbyopia

5. What equipment is necessary to conduct the Weber and Rinne tests for hearing?
   a. Pen light
   b. Otoscope
   c. Tuning fork
   d. Stethoscope

See Test Yourself answers in Appendix C.

# BIBLIOGRAPHY

Andresen, G. (1998). Assessing the older patient. *RN, 61*(3), 46–56.

Darovic, G. (1997). Assessing pupillary responses. *Nursing, 27*(2), 49.

Russell, J. (1995). Ear screening. *Community Nurse, 1*(4), 14–16.

Unresponsive patient: A deaf ear? (1997). *Nursing, 27*(8), 68.

Use of eardrops. (1997). *Community Nurse, 3*(7), 29.

Waitzman, A., & Hawke, M. (1996). Otoscopic examination: What to look for in the middle ear. *Consultant, 36*(6), 1299–1303.

Weber, J., & Kelley, J. (2002). *Health assessment in nursing* (2nd ed.). Philadelphia: Lippincott.

West, G. (1997). Care of the older person: Detecting and treating eye problems in later life. *Community Nurse, 3*(5), 24, 27.

Wilson, S., & Giddens, J. (2001). *Health assessment for nursing practice.* St. Louis: Mosby.

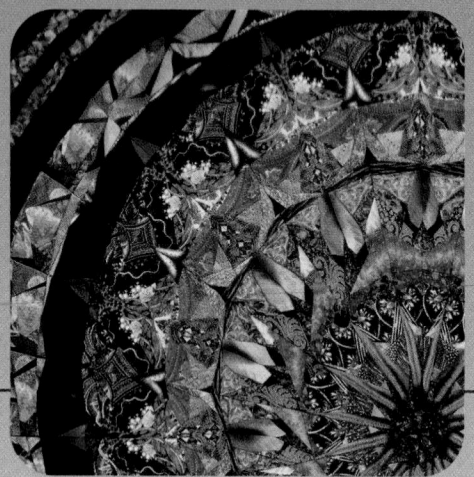

# CHAPTER 45

# Nursing Care of Clients with Eye and Ear Disorders

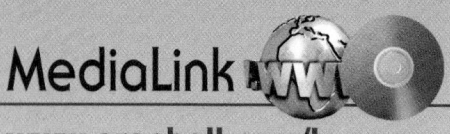

## MediaLink

**www.prenhall.com/lemone**

Additional resources for this chapter can be found on the Student CD-ROM accompanying this textbook, and on the Companion Website at www. prenhall.com/lemone. Click on Chapter 45 to select the activities for this chapter.

**CD-ROM**
• Audio Glossary
• NCLEX Review

**Animations**
• Ear Abnormalities
• Middle Ear Dynamics
• Pilocarpine

**Companion Website**
• More NCLEX Review
• Case Study
  Retinal Detachment
• Care Plan Activity
  Hearing Aid

## LEARNING OUTCOMES

After completing this chapter, you will be able to:

▪ Use knowledge of normal anatomy and physiology of the eye and ear and assessments to provide care for clients with disorders of the eyes and ears (see Chapter 44).

▪ Describe the pathophysiology of commonly occurring disorders of the eyes and ears, relating their manifestations to the pathophysiologic process.

▪ Identify diagnostic tests used to diagnose eye and ear disorders.

▪ Discuss the nursing implications for medications prescribed for clients with eye and ear disorders.

▪ Provide appropriate care for the client having eye or ear surgery.

▪ Use the nursing process as a framework for providing care to clients with impaired vision or hearing.

Vision and hearing provide the primary means of input for much of what we know about the world. The ability to receive and organize information orients us to our surroundings. These senses allow us to communicate easily, gain access to information, and derive pleasure from the sights and sounds of the world around us.

This chapter discusses conditions affecting vision and hearing as the result of eye and ear disorders. Nursing care focuses on clients with vision and hearing deficits that can result from the disorders presented.

## EYE DISORDERS

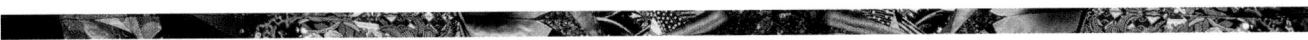

Any portion of the eye and its protective structures may be affected by an acute or chronic condition. Disorders and diseases of the outer, visible portion of the eye often cause discomfort and may have cosmetic effects. The effect on vision can often be prevented or reversed with proper treatment of the disorder. The client who has had eye surgery or minor trauma may have either temporary or permanent visual impairment. Disorders affecting the internal structures or the function of the eye are more likely to have adverse effects on vision. Although these disorders often cannot be prevented or cured, some can be controlled and vision corrected to normal or near normal. Although many eye disorders do not pose a threat to vision, the client may perceive a threat and therefore feel anxiety.

### THE CLIENT WITH AGE-RELATED CHANGES IN VISION

Not all conditions affecting the eye are pathologic; some are associated with normal aging (See Figures 45–1 ■ and 45–2 ■). The pupil decreases in size and does not dilate readily, reducing the amount of light that reaches the retina. Night vision is affected, and increased light intensity is necessary for reading and handwork. The lens becomes less elastic, making it increasingly difficult to focus for near vision. Clients notice that "their arms have become too short" to read the newspaper comfortably. With aging, the lens discolors and opacifies, causing it to absorb more of the short wavelengths of light, resulting in a decrease in color perception. This change affects the green, blue, and violet hues in particular. Clients may tend to choose brighter colors of clothing and decor as color perception changes.

Other effects of aging on the eye include changes in the vitreous humor, atrophy of the choroid, thinning of the retina, and degenerative changes in the optic nerve (Hazzard et al., 1998). Depth perception and the ability to see lines of demarcation (e.g., the edges of steps or a change in direction of walls) diminish with age.

As the aging client loses subcutaneous tissue, the eyes may recess into the eye sockets, creating tissue folds on the upper lids. These structural changes, along with a decrease in eye mobility, can limit the older adult's vision upward and to the sides. Nurses can help the client by placing signs at eye level, not above. Checking for low-hanging objects that the client may not see can prevent head injuries.

Changes of the eye and vision commonly associated with the aging process are summarized in Table 45–1.

### THE CLIENT WITH AN INFECTIOUS OR INFLAMMATORY EYE DISORDER

The extraocular structures—the eyelids, eyelashes, and conjunctiva in particular—are vulnerable to inflammation and infection because of their constant exposure to the environment. When inflamed, these normally protective structures may perform their functions less effectively and may cause discomfort and changes in the client's appearance. The corneal reflex and tears (which contain antibodies and lysozyme, an antibacterial enzyme) protect the eye against most hazards. As tear production decreases with aging, the risk of infection increases.

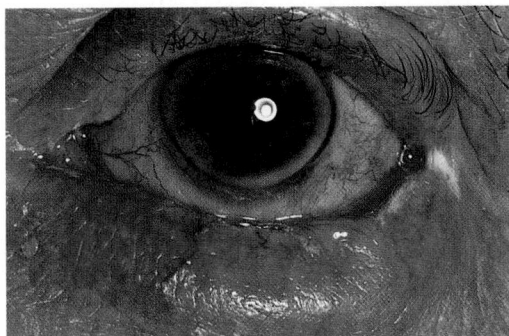

**Figure 45–1** ■ Entropion.

*Source: Science Photo Library/Photo Researchers, Inc.*

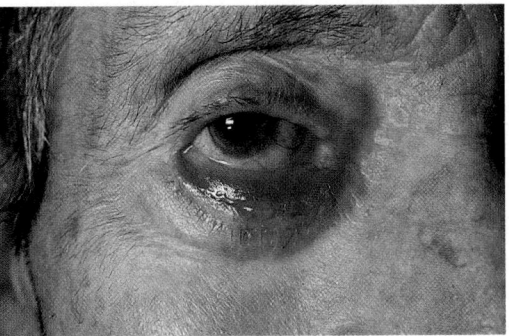

**Figure 45–2** ■ Ectropion.

*Source: Science Photo Library/Photo Researchers, Inc.*

| TABLE 45-1 Age-Related Changes in the Eye and Vision | | |
|---|---|---|
| **Physiologic Change** | **Conditions** | **Effect on Vision** |
| Changes that lead to altered protection of the eye | • Senile entropion: Inversion of the lid margins<br>• Senile ectropion: Eversion of the eyelid margin<br>• Decreased corneal sensitivity<br><br>• Decreased tear secretion | • Lashes may cause corneal irritation and damage<br>• Conjunctival exposure and possible inflammation<br>• Increased potential for damage due to foreign body or trauma<br>• Increased potential for infection or damage due to environmental pollution |
| Changes that affect vision | • Flattening of the cornea<br><br>• Pupillary constriction | • Reduced refractory power and decreased visual acuity<br>• Reduction in the amount of light reaching the retina to approximately one-third of previous amount (in younger years) |
| | • Decreased lens elasticity and increased lens density<br><br><br><br><br><br>• Loss of sensory cells at the periphery of the retina | • Decreased visual acuity, affecting close vision especially<br>• Increased problems with glare (scattering of light rays)<br>• Decreased color perception, especially in blue, green, and violet spectra<br>• Decreased visual fields (peripheral vision) |
| Mechanical changes that may affect vision | • Senile enophthalmos: Sinking in of the eyes giving a "hollow-eyed" appearance<br>• Decreased eye motility | • May limit peripheral vision in all directions: to the sides, upward, and downward<br>• Increased difficulty with looking upward and convergence |
| Cosmetic changes | • Yellowing of the sclera due to fatty deposits<br>• Arcus senilis: Formation of a grayish yellow ring at the corneal margin | • None<br>• None |

## PATHOPHYSIOLOGY AND MANIFESTATIONS
### Eyelid Infections and Inflammations

The most common disorder affecting the eyelids is **marginal blepharitis,** an inflammation of the glands and lash follicles on the margins of the eyelids. This inflammatory disorder can be caused by a staphylococcal infection or it may be seborrheic in origin; commonly, both types are present. Seborrheic blepharitis is usually associated with seborrhea (dandruff) of the scalp or eyebrows. Irritation, burning, and itching of eyelid margins are common manifestations of blepharitis. The eye appears red-rimmed with mucous discharge, and there is crusting or scaling of lid margins. Lid margins may ulcerate, resulting in a loss of eyelashes.

Infection of one or more of the sebaceous glands of the eyelid may cause a **hordeolum (sty).** Hordeolum is a staphylococcal abscess that may occur on either the external or internal margin of the lid (see Figure 44–9). An external hordeolum is characterized initially by acute pain at the lid margin and redness. A small tender raised area is visible. The client may also experience photophobia, tearing, and the sensation of a foreign body in the affected eye. Internal hordeola are seen on the conjunctival side of the lid and may have more severe manifestations.

Chronic inflammation of a meibomian gland may lead to formation of a **chalazion,** a granulomatous cyst or nodule of the lid (see Figure 44–10). It presents as a hard swelling on the lid, and surrounding conjunctival tissue is reddened. Chalazion may also follow a hordeolum that was inadequately treated. Unlike a hordeolum, a chalazion is painless. It may slowly in-

crease in size and eventually require removal, but most resolve within several months.

### Conjunctivitis

The conjunctiva lines the inner lid and covers the outer portion of the eye to the margin of the cornea. **Conjunctivitis,** inflammation of the conjunctiva, is the most common eye disease and most often results from bacterial or viral infections. These infections are usually transmitted to the eye by direct contact (e.g., hands, tissues, towels). Allergens, chemical irritants, and exposure to radiant energy such as ultraviolet light from the sun or tanning devices can also lead to this common condition. Its severity can range from mild irritation with redness and tearing to conjunctival edema, hemorrhage, or a severe necrotizing process with tissue destruction.

### Acute Conjunctivitis

Infectious conjunctivitis may be bacterial, viral, or fungal in origin. Bacterial conjunctivitis, also known as "pink eye," is highly contagious, and often is caused by *Staphylococcus* and *Haemophilus.* Adenovirus infection is the leading cause of conjunctivitis in adults. Systemic infections that may affect the eyes include herpes simplex and other viral infections. Contact with genital secretions infected with Gonococcus can cause gonococcal conjunctivitis, a medical emergency that can lead to corneal perforation.

Redness and itching of the affected eye are common manifestations of acute conjunctivitis (Figure 45–3 ■). The client may also complain of a scratchy, burning, or gritty sensation. Pain is not common; however, photophobia may occur. Tearing

The entire lens and its surrounding capsule may be removed in a procedure called intracapsular extraction (Figure 45–5A ■). Extracapsular extraction is the most common procedure presently used to treat cataracts. It involves removal of the nucleus and cortex of the lens, leaving the posterior capsule intact (Figure 45–5B). The remaining capsule supports the lens implant and protects the retina. An additional advantage to extracapsular lens removal is the smaller incision required.

After removal of the lens, the eye can no longer focus light on the retina, and vision is seriously affected. Usually a polymethylmethacrylate (PMMA or Plexiglas) intraocular lens is implanted at the time of surgery to provide for light refraction and restore visual acuity. This implant rapidly restores binocular vision and depth perception. An anterior chamber lens implant is used following intracapsular lens removal. In an anterior chamber implant, the lens is lodged in the anterior chamber of the eye, resting over the pupil. In a posterior implant, the lens is positioned in the posterior capsule to restore vision following an extracapsular lens extraction. The posterior chamber lens is positioned behind the iris and stabilized by the remaining posterior capsule.

For some clients, convex corrective glasses or contact lenses may be used instead of intraocular lens implants to correct vision after cataract removal. Although contact lenses can provide excellent vision correction following cataract surgery, they may be difficult for some clients to adapt to or manipulate. The client with a preexisting refractive error may continue to require corrective lenses and often needs a prescriptive change after surgery.

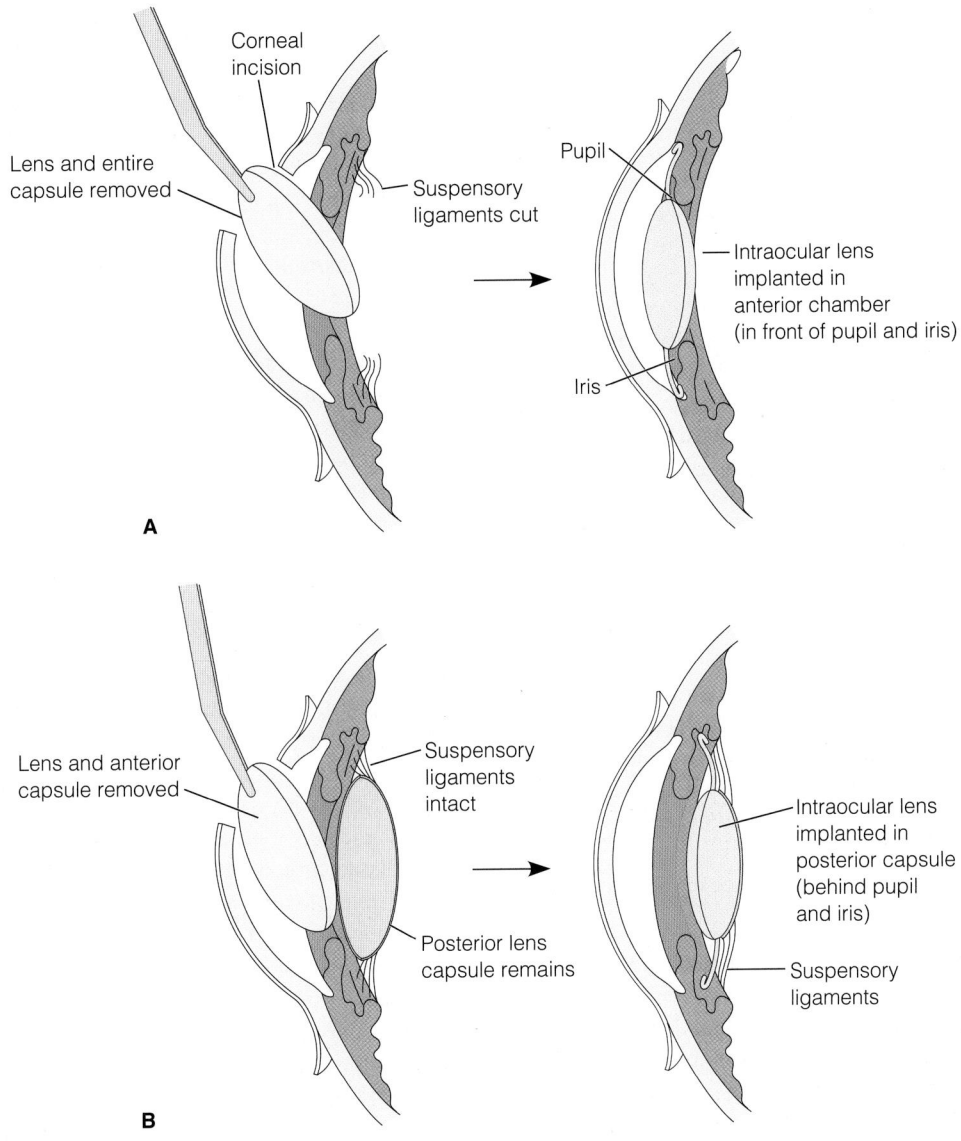

**Figure 45–5** ■ Cataract removal with intraocular lens implant. *A*, Intracapsular cataract extraction with removal of the entire lens and capsule. The intraocular lens is implanted in the eye's anterior chamber. *B*, Extracapsular cataract extraction with removal of the lens and anterior capsule, leaving the posterior capsule intact. The intraocular lens is implanted within posterior capsule.

Complications of cataract surgery are unusual and occur in less than 1% of the surgeries. Loss of vitreous humor, corneal edema, increased intraocular pressure, hemorrhage, inflammation or infection, retinal detachment, and displacement of the implanted lens are potential complications. Up to 35% of clients who undergo extracapsular extraction may develop opacification of the remaining posterior capsule. Vision can be restored using laser capsulotomy (creating an opening for light to pass through the opacified capsule) or surgical incision into the posterior capsule to allow light to reach the retina (Braunwald et al., 2001; Quillen, 1999).

## NURSING CARE

The client with cataracts has few physical care nursing needs. Patient advocacy, psychologic and emotional support, and teaching/learning needs are typically of higher priority for these clients.

With the initial diagnosis of a cataract, the nurse often becomes an important resource for the client. The nurse can explain the nonemergent nature of the condition and help the client determine the extent to which the cataract is affecting daily life. In so doing, the nurse helps the client decide when to proceed with surgery. The nurse can also provide information about cataracts and their surgical removal to assist the client with decision making. A preoperative nursing evaluation of the client's ability to perform necessary postoperative care is helpful. If the client has a chronic condition, such as arthritis, that may make administration of eye drops difficult, a family member may need teaching to perform this intervention. If visual limitations in the initial postoperative period are likely to interfere with the client's other care needs, such as insulin injections, arrangements may need to be made for home health coverage or other assistance.

Fear of blindness is second only to fear of cancer for many clients. Careful listening, teaching, and a caring, understanding attitude by the nurse can help the client deal with this fear prior to surgery.

As cataract surgery is often performed on an outpatient or same-day basis, postoperative nursing care focuses on maintaining client safety and patient teaching. If local anesthesia was used, the client is often discharged within 1 hour after surgery. Nursing care of the client having eye surgery is outlined in the box on page 1469.

The following nursing diagnoses may be appropriate for the client with cataracts.

- *Disturbed sensory perception: Visual* related to effect of lens opacification
- *Risk for injury* related to altered vision and depth perception
- *Deficient knowledge* related to lack of information about cataracts, treatment options, and postoperative care
- *Risk for ineffective therapeutic regimen management* related to difficulty in administering eye medications or inserting contact lenses

## Home Care

With the initial diagnosis of cataract, teaching focuses on the nature of the condition, indications for intervention, and options for replacement lenses following cataract removal. Teaching adaptive strategies to deal with the alteration in vision and depth perception are also useful. Clients requiring the use of the thick corrective glasses are cautioned that objects appear closer, necessitating adjustments in their living arrangements.

When the client decides to proceed with cataract surgery, the nurse teaches about surgery and postoperative care. The client and, if possible, a family member or friend are taught how to instill eye drops. The time of surgery, instructions for fasting, and other preoperative care are included in teaching.

Discuss postoperative care and include a significant other in the teaching. Reinforce the following information with written instructions:

- Limitations such as avoiding reading, lifting, strenuous activity, and sleeping on operative side
- Importance of not disturbing the eye dressing
- Prescribed medications and side effects
- Importance of follow-up appointments
- Signs and symptoms of postoperative complications such as eye pain, decreased visual acuity or other change in vision, headache, nausea, or itching and redness of the affected eye
- Instillation of eye drops, and application of eye patch or shield
- Care, insertion, and removal of contact lenses as appropriate
- Instruction in the visual changes associated with thick-lensed eyeglasses as appropriate
- Helpful resources, such as the American Society of Cataract & Refractive Surgery

## THE CLIENT WITH GLAUCOMA

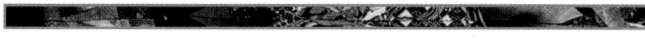

**Glaucoma** is a condition characterized by increased intraocular pressure of the eye and a gradual loss of vision. Glaucoma is a silent thief of vision. The client typically experiences no manifestations other than narrowing of the visual field, which occurs so gradually that it often goes unnoticed until late in the disease process.

Glaucoma affects about 3 million people over the age of 40 in the United States; it remains undetected in approximately 25% of these cases. Glaucoma is a leading cause of blindness worldwide and the leading cause of blindness among African Americans (Turkoski, 2000).

Glaucoma usually exists as a primary condition without identified precipitating cause. Primary glaucoma is most common in adults over the age of 60, but may be a congenital condition in infants and children. Secondary glaucoma can develop as a result of infection or inflammation of the eye, cataract, tumor, hemorrhage, or eye trauma.

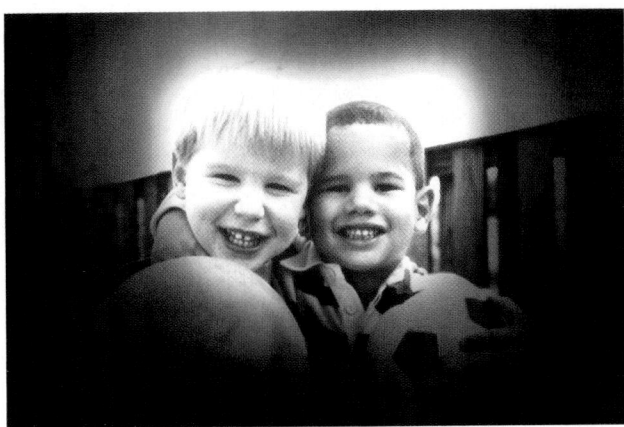

**Figure 45–6** ■ Narrowing of visual fields typical of untreated glaucoma.

*Courtesy of The National Eye Institute, National Institutes of Health.*

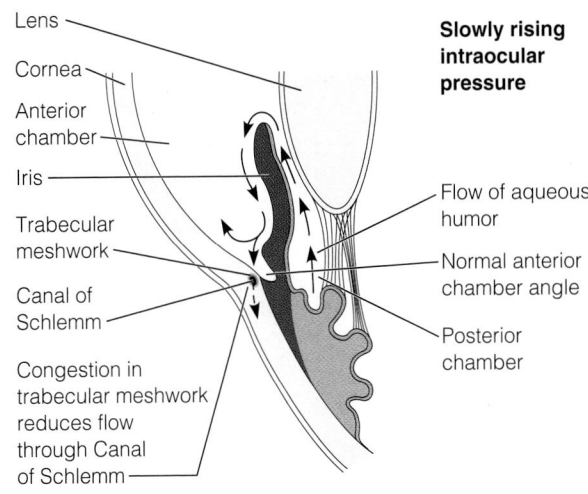

A

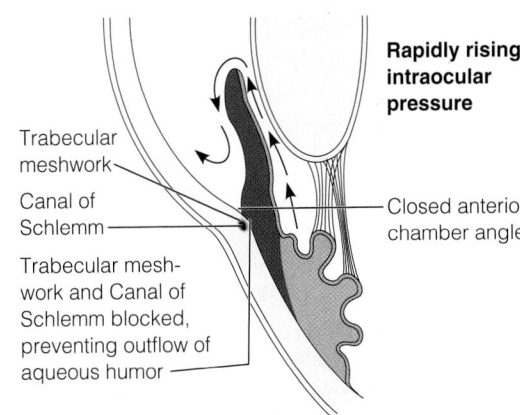

B

**Figure 45–7** ■ Forms of primary adult glaucoma. *A,* In chronic open-angle glaucoma, the anterior chamber angle remains open, but drainage of aqueous humor through the canal of Schlemm is impaired. *B,* In acute angle-closure glaucoma, the angle of the iris and anterior chamber narrows, obstructing the outflow of aqueous humor.

## PATHOPHYSIOLOGY

Aqueous humor, a thick fluid, occupies both the anterior and posterior chambers of the eye. The normal intraocular pressure of 15 to 20 mmHg is maintained by a balance between the production of aqueous humor in the ciliary body, its flow through the pupil from the posterior to the anterior chamber of the eye, and its outflow or absorption through the trabecular meshwork and canal of Schlemm (see Figure 44–3). When this balance is disrupted, usually because of a decrease in the outflow or absorption of aqueous humor, the intraocular pressure increases, causing ischemia of the neurons of the eye and degeneration of the optic nerve. The ischemic neurons die beginning at the periphery of the retina, causing a painless, progressive narrowing of the visual field (Figure 45–6 ■) and eventual blindness. Vision loss is often significant before the client seeks treatment and glaucoma is diagnosed.

Primary glaucoma in adults has two major forms: open-angle glaucoma and angle-closure glaucoma. Both terms refer to the angle formed at the point where the iris meets the cornea in the eye's anterior chamber (Figure 45–7 ■). Forms of primary glaucoma are compared in Table 45–2.

### Open-Angle Glaucoma

Open-angle glaucoma, often called chronic simple glaucoma, is the most common form in adults, accounting for approximately 90% of all glaucoma. Its cause is unknown; it is thought to have a hereditary component, but no clear inheritance pattern can be identified. Open-angle glaucoma occurs more frequently and at an earlier age in African Americans (Tierney et al., 2001).

In open-angle glaucoma, the anterior chamber angle between the iris and cornea is normal (Figure 45–7A), hence the term *open angle*. However, the flow of aqueous humor through the trabecular meshwork and into the canal of Schlemm is relatively obstructed; the cause of this obstruction is unknown. Restricted outflow leads to an increased amount of fluid in the eye and increased intraocular pressure. Open-angle glaucoma tends to be a chronic, gradually progressive disease. The trabecular meshwork increasingly inhibits the outflow of aqueous humor, and the intraocular pressure gradually increases. The result is neuronal ischemia and optic nerve degeneration, leading to gradual loss of vision.

Open-angle glaucoma typically affects both eyes, although the pressures and progression may not be symmetric.

### Manifestations

The manifestations of open-angle glaucoma are vague, and often the client is unaware of them. Along with loss of peripheral vision, the client may complain of mild headaches, have difficulty adapting to the dark, see halos around lights, and have some difficulty focusing on near objects. As intraocular pressure continues to increase, visual acuity is reduced.

TABLE 45–2  A Comparison of Open-Angle and Angle-Closure Glaucoma

|  | Open-Angle Glaucoma | Angle-Closure Glaucoma |
|---|---|---|
| Incidence | • Common<br>• Accounts for 90% of all cases of glaucoma | • Uncommon |
| Risk Factors | • Over age 35<br>• Genetic link<br>• African American ancestry | • Narrow anterior chamber angle<br>• Aging<br>• Asian ancestry |
| Pathophysiology | • Impaired aqueous outflow through the canal of Schlemm<br>• Cause unknown<br>• Gradual, consistent increase in intraocular pressure<br>• Usually bilateral | • Pupil dilation or lens accommodation causes already narrowed angle to close, blocking aqueous outflow<br>• Rapid rise in intraocular pressure<br>• Usually unilateral |
| Manifestations | • No initial manifestations<br>• Frequent lens changes in glasses<br>• Impaired dark adaptation<br>• Halos around lights<br>• Gradual reduction of visual fields with preservation of central vision until late in the disease<br>• Mild to severe increased intraocular pressure | • Abrupt onset of eye pain, headache<br>• Decreased visual acuity<br>• Nausea and vomiting<br>• Reddened conjunctiva<br>• Cloudy cornea<br>• Fixed pupil<br>• Rapid, significant increase in intraocular pressure |
| Management | • Topical medications such as miotics, betablockers, prostaglandin analogues<br>• Carbonic anhydrase inhibitors<br>• Laser trabeculoplasty, trabeculectomy | • Topical miotics or betablockers<br>• Systemic osmotic agents, carbonic anhydrase inhibitors<br>• Laser iridotomy or peripheral iridectomy |

## Angle-Closure Glaucoma

Acute angle-closure (also called narrow-angle or closed-angle) glaucoma is the other, less common form of primary glaucoma in adults. It accounts for approximately 5% to 10% of all cases of glaucoma (Porth, 2002).

Approximately 1% of people over the age of 35 have narrowed anterior chamber angles; the incidence is higher in older adults and in people of Asian ancestry. Narrowing of the anterior chamber angle occurs because of corneal flattening or bulging of the iris into the anterior chamber. When the lens thickens during accommodation or the iris thickens during pupil dilation, this angle can close completely. Closure of the angle blocks the outflow of aqueous humor through the trabecular meshwork and canal of Schlemm, and the intraocular pressure rises abruptly (Figure 45–7B). This abrupt increase in intraocular pressure damages the neurons of the retina and the optic nerve, leading to a rapid and permanent loss of vision if not treated promptly.

Episodes of angle-closure glaucoma are typically unilateral. However, in clients who have had angle-closure glaucoma of one eye, the other eye is at increased risk in the future.

Because of the effect of pupil dilation on aqueous outflow in angle-closure glaucoma, episodes often occur in association with darkness, emotional upset, or other factors that cause the pupil to dilate. Clients may have intermittent episodes lasting several hours before having a more typical prolonged attack of angle-closure glaucoma. For clients with a history of the condition, it is vital to avoid medications such as atropine and other anticholinergics, which have a mydriatic or pupil-dilating effect.

### Manifestations

Symptoms such as severe eye and face pain, general malaise, nausea and vomiting, seeing colored halos around lights, and an abrupt decrease in visual acuity are associated with acute episodes of angle-closure glaucoma. The conjunctiva of the affected eye may be reddened and the cornea clouded with corneal edema. The pupil may be fixed (nonreactive to light) at midpoint.

## COLLABORATIVE CARE

Although glaucoma cannot be predicted, prevented, or cured, in most cases it can be controlled and vision preserved if diagnosed early. Because the most prevalent type of glaucoma, open-angle, has few symptoms, routine eye examinations are recommended for early detection. Measurement of intraocular pressure, fundoscopy to assess the optic disk, and visual field testing are used for diagnosis and monitoring of treatment effectiveness.

### Diagnostic Tests

The following diagnostic studies are used to detect and evaluate for the presence, severity, type, and effects of glaucoma.

• *Tonometry* indirectly measures intraocular pressure. Either contact or noncontact tonometry may be used. In contact tonometry, the eye is anesthetized, and the force needed to produce an indentation in the cornea is measured using a Schiötz tonometer (Figure 45–8 ■) or a Goldmann applanation tonometer. Noncontact tonometry measures the time required to flatten the cornea with a puff of air to determine the

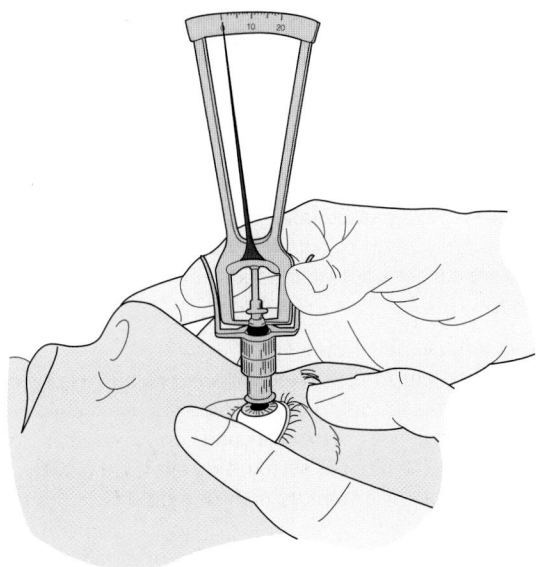

**Figure 45–8** ■ The Schiötz tonometer for measuring intraocular pressure.

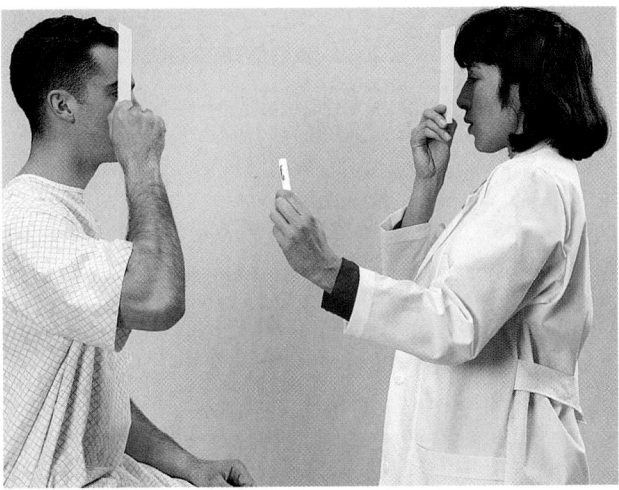

**Figure 45–9** ■ Visual field testing. Peripheral vision or visual fields are assessed by testing the client's ability to detect an object brought into the line of vision from the periphery. The client's peripheral vision is compared to the nurse examiner's. Each eye is tested separately.

intraocular pressure. No anesthesia is needed. Routine tonometry screening is recommended for all people over the age of 60. A single elevated pressure reading does not warrant a diagnosis of glaucoma; variations in intraocular pressure occur throughout the day.

- *Fundoscopy* identifies pallor and an increase in the size and depth of the optic cup on the optic disk. These changes are significant for diagnosing glaucoma.
- *Gonioscopy* uses a gonioscope to measure the depth of the anterior chamber. This test differentiates open-angle from angle-closure glaucoma.
- *Visual field testing* (Figure 45–9 ■) identifies the degree of central visual field narrowing and peripheral vision loss. The client with glaucoma may retain 20/20 central vision even though there is severe peripheral vision loss.

## Medications

Although medications cannot cure glaucoma, many clients with open-angle glaucoma can control intraocular pressure and preserve vision indefinitely with medications. Medications are used alone or in combination with the timing and dosage individually determined by pressure measurements. The primary pharmacologic agents used to treat glaucoma are the cholinergics (miotics), adrenergics (mydriatics), beta-adrenergic blocking agents, carbonic anhydrase inhibitors, and prostaglandin analogs.

Cholinergics or miotics (pilocarpine, carbachol) cause contraction of the sphincter of the iris, constricting the pupil, and contraction of the ciliary muscle that promotes accommodation for near vision. The net effect is to facilitate aqueous humor outflow by increasing drainage through the trabecular meshwork in open-angle glaucoma. In angle-closure glaucoma, pupillary constriction flattens the iris, opening the angle and the canal of Schlemm. Miotics are administered topically as

drops, with the dose and frequency dependent on the preparation prescribed and the client response.

The adrenergic agonists epinephrine and dipivefrin may be prescribed along with miotics to counteract the effect of the miotic on accommodation. Epinephrine decreases the production of aqueous humor by the ciliary body, further reducing the intraocular pressure.

Timolol (Timoptic) is a beta-adrenergic blocking agent that also acts to decrease the production of aqueous humor in the ciliary body. Beta-adrenergic blockers have a longer duration of activity than the miotics, allowing fewer doses per day. When administering beta blockers or teaching a client about their use, it is important to remember that ophthalmic preparations can produce the systemic effects of other beta blockers, including bronchospasm, bradycardia, and heart failure.

Dorzolamide (Trusopt), a carbonic anhydrase inhibitor, decreases the production of aqueous humor and reduces intraocular pressure. It is used with other drugs to control pressures and in clients for whom beta blockers are contraindicated because of heart failure or reactive airway disease. Acetazolamide (Diamox), a systemic carbonic anhydrase inhibitor, also may be used for some clients.

Prostaglandin analogs such as latanoprost (Xalatan) are a newer class of ophthalmics prescribed to increase aqueous outflow. They are similar to beta blockers in their longer duration of action, thus requiring only a daily dose.

Nursing implications for the medications used to control chronic glaucoma are outlined in the Medication Administration box on pages 1480–1481.

In acute angle-closure glaucoma, diuretics may be administered intravenously to achieve a rapid decrease in intraocular pressure prior to surgical intervention. Both the carbonic anhydrase inhibitor acetazolamide and osmotic diuretics, such

# Medication Administration

## The Client with Glaucoma

### CHOLINERGICS (MIOTICS)

Acetylcholine (Miochol)
Carbachol (Isopto Carbachol)
Pilocarpine (Isopto Carpine, Ocusert-Pilo)

Miotics constrict the pupil and block the sympathetic nervous system input, which causes the pupil to dilate in low light. They also contract the ciliary muscle; both effects reduce intraocular pressure. Pilocarpine is the most widely used of these drugs.

#### Nursing Responsibilities

- Assess the client for contraindications to therapy with miotic or parasympathomimetic agents, including bronchial asthma, intestinal obstruction, urinary retention, bradycardia, or acute iritis.
- Do not administer with anticholinergic drugs such as atropine and or drugs with anticholinergic side effects because they can block the desired effect.
- After administering drops, have the client gently squeeze the lacrimal sac for 1 to 2 minutes to increase the local effect and decrease systemic absorption.
- Follow this procedure for administering pilocarpine with the Ocusert system.
  a. Because pilocarpine may blur vision, apply at bedtime.
  b. Place Ocusert-Pilo in the conjunctival sac, preferably under the upper lid.
  c. Notify the physician if the client develops signs of conjunctival irritation, redness and increased mucous secretion that do not clear within several days of the initial use of Ocusert.
  d. Remove and replace the system weekly or if the client develops signs of an unexpected increase in drug action.
- Assess for possible side effects including increased lacrimation, brow pain, and headache.

#### Client and Family Teaching

- Follow these steps when administering eye drops:
  a. Wash your hands prior to administration.
  b. Do not touch the dropper to the eye or lid, or with the hands.
  c. Squeeze the bridge of the nose gently after administration to prevent systemic absorption.
  d. Keep the eye closed for 1 to 2 minutes after administration to enhance the effect of the medication.
- If you are using the Ocusert system, follow a special procedure. (See the procedure in the preceding section, "Nursing Responsibilities.")
- Avoid medications that may block the effect of the miotics, including many over-the-counter cold and sleep preparations.
- Visual acuity may be decreased during the initiation of therapy. Avoid tasks requiring sharp vision.
- Vision is reduced in dim light; provide night lights in halls and baths, and avoid night driving.
- Report adverse effects such as abdominal pain, wheezing, difficulty breathing, sweating, or flushing to the physician.

### ADRENERGIC AGONISTS (MYDRIATICS)

Epinephrine (Epitrate, Mytrate/Epifrin)

Epinephrine is a sympathomimetic drug acting to dilate the pupil, reduce the production of aqueous humor, and increase its absorption, effectively reducing intraocular pressure in open-angle glaucoma.

#### Nursing Responsibilities

- Assess the client for contraindications and adverse reactions to epinephrine, including acute angle-closure glaucoma, hypertension, cardiac dysrhythmias, and coronary heart disease.
- Assess for central nervous system side effects of anxiety, nervousness, and muscle tremors. If these side effects are severe, notify the physician.
- Assess for a hypersensitivity reaction, including itching, lid edema, and discharge from the eyes. Notify the physician if you notice these signs.

#### Client and Family Teaching

- Report any change in visual acuity or eye pain. (Eye pain may indicate an attack of angle-closure glaucoma and must be reported to the physician immediately.)
- Avoid over-the-counter sinus and cold medications containing pseudoephedrine and phenylephrine. They may accentuate the side effects of epinephrine.

### BETA-ADRENERGIC BLOCKERS

Betaxolol (Betoptic)
Levobunolol (Betagan)

Selected beta-adrenergic blockers reduce intraocular pressure by decreasing the production of aqueous humor. Because beta blockers do not affect pupil size and lens accommodation, they do not have the adverse effects on visual acuity that miotics and adrenergic agonists do.

#### Nursing Responsibilities

- Assess the client for allergies or contraindications to beta-blocker therapy, including asthma, chronic obstructive pulmonary disease (COPD), heart block, and heart failure.
- Maintain pressure over the lacrimal sac after administration to prevent systemic absorption.
- Assess for side effects such as bradycardia, hypotension, and depression.
- Teach about the drug, its dose, administration, and desired and side effects.

#### Client and Family Teaching

- Put pressure on the lacrimal sac, at the corner of the eye near the bridge of the nose, to keep the drug from entering your system.
- Your vision may be blurred during the initial period of therapy, but it will improve as you continue to use the drug.
- Report adverse effects, including worsening vision, difficulty breathing, reduced exercise tolerance, and sweating or flushing, to the physician.

## Medication Administration

### The Client with Glaucoma (continued)

**CARBONIC ANHYDRASE INHIBITORS**

Dorzolamide (Trusopt)
Brinzolamide (Azopt)
Acetazolamide (Diamox)

The carbonic anhydrate inhibitors lower intraocular pressure and are used primarily as adjunctive therapy. Dorzolamide and brinzolamide are administered as eye drops whereas acetazolamide may given PO, IM, or IV.

#### Nursing Responsibilities

- Assess for allergies or other contraindications to the use of carbonic anhydrase inhibitors, including known allergy to sulfa, or severe renal or hepatic disease.
- Monitor for increased drug interactions of amphetamines, procainamide, quinidine, tricyclic antidepressants, and ephedrine and pseudoephedrine.

- Assess daily weight, intake and output, serum electrolytes, and vital signs in clients taking oral or parenteral carbonic anhydrase inhibitors.
- Administer PO in the morning to prevent sleep disruption because of the diuretic effect.
- If used with another topical ophthalmic, administer 10 minutes apart.
- Teach the client about the drug, its dose, administration, and desired and side effects.

#### Client and Family Teaching

- For oral medications, maintain a fluid intake of 2 to 3 L per day and rise slowly from lying or sitting positions because you may feel dizzy when you first stand (orthostatic hypotension).
- For topical medications, notify the physician if you have prolonged eye irritation.

---

as mannitol, are used. Fast-acting miotic drops, such as acetylcholine, are also administered to constrict the pupil and draw the iris away from the angle and from the canal of Schlemm.

## Surgery

Surgical intervention is indicated for clients with acute angleclosure glaucoma and for clients with chronic open-angle glaucoma that is not effectively controlled by medication.

Surgical management of chronic open-angle glaucoma involves improving the drainage of aqueous humor from the anterior chamber of the eye. Trabeculoplasty and trabeculectomy filtration surgery are the most commonly used procedures.

In a *laser trabeculoplasty,* an argon laser is aimed through a gonioscope to create multiple laser burns spaced evenly around the trabecular meshwork. As the burns heal, the scars they create cause tension, stretching and opening the meshwork. This noninvasive technique is the treatment of choice because it requires no incision and can be performed as an outpatient procedure.

*Trabeculectomy* is a type of filtration surgery in which a permanent fistula is created to drain aqueous humor from the anterior chamber of the eye. A portion of trabecular meshwork is removed, and a flap of sclera is left unsutured to create a channel or fistula between the anterior chamber and the subconjunctival space. Aqueous humor is able to drain into the space under the conjunctiva, where it can be absorbed into the systemic circulation. A trabeculectomy is usually performed under general anesthesia and requires hospitalization.

If these procedures are not fully effective, either photocoagulation using an argon laser (heat) or cyclocryotherapy using a probe to freeze tissue may be employed to destroy portions of the ciliary body. This tissue destruction reduces the production of aqueous humor, subsequently reducing intraocular pressure. Another surgical procedure involves insertion of a glaucoma drainage device which regulates the outflow of aqueous humor.

Surgical procedures used in the treatment of acute angleclosure glaucoma include gonioplasty, laser iridotomy, and peripheral iridectomy. Because of the high risk for a future attack of angle-closure glaucoma in the unaffected eye, these procedures are often performed prophylactically.

In *gonioplasty,* the healing and scarring of microscopic lesions created at the periphery of the iris draws the iris away from the cornea, widening the anterior chamber. This widening of the chamber increases the angle and opens drainage channels for aqueous humor.

*Laser iridotomy* is a noninvasive procedure using a laser to create multiple small perforations in the iris of the eye. These perforations allow aqueous humor to drain from the posterior chamber to the anterior chamber and out through the trabecular meshwork and the canal of Schlemm. During an *iridectomy,* a small segment of the iris is removed to facilitate the flow of aqueous humor between the posterior and anterior chambers and to open the anterior chamber angle.

## NURSING CARE

When planning and implementing nursing care for the client with glaucoma, the nurse needs to consider both the specific pathophysiology and related needs affecting the client, and the actual or potential effects on the client's vision, lifestyle, safety, and psychosocial well-being. In the hospitalized client, glaucoma is typically a complicating factor rather than the primary reason for seeking care, unless the diagnosis is acute angleclosure glaucoma.

### Health Promotion

Although glaucoma cannot be prevented, its severity and potentially deleterious permanent effects can be limited with early visual screening. The nurse assumes an important role in educating the public about the risk factors for glaucoma such as increased age, and the higher incidence in African

Americans and Asians. All people over the age of 40 are encouraged to receive an eye examination every 2 to 4 years, including tonometry screening. Those with a predominant family history should be evaluated more frequently, every 1 to 2 years. After the age of 65, yearly ophthalmologic examinations are recommended.

## Assessment

Collect the following data through a health history and physical examination (see Chapter 44).

- Health history: family history; presence of altered vision, halos, and excessive tearing; sudden, severe eye pain; use of corrective lenses
- Physical examination: distant and near vision, peripheral fields, retina for optic nerve cupping

## Nursing Diagnoses and Interventions

Nursing care planning focuses on problems associated with the temporary or permanent visual impairment, the resultant increased risk for injury, and the psychosocial problems of anxiety and coping.

### Risk for Disturbed Sensory Perception: Visual

Whether glaucoma and resulting impaired vision is the client's primary problem or a preexisting condition in a client with another disorder, it must be a primary consideration in nursing care planning.

- Address by name and identify yourself with each interaction. Orient to time, place, person, and situation as indicated. State the purpose of your visit. *The client with impaired vision must rely on input from the other senses. A lack of visual cues increases the importance of verbal ones. For example, the visually impaired client cannot see the nurse checking an intravenous infusion and needs a verbal explanation of who is in the room and why. When the client's normal daily routine is disrupted by illness or hospitalization, additional sensory input such as a radio, television, and explanations of the routine and activities are useful to maintain the client's orientation.*
- Provide any visual aids that are routinely used. Keep them close, making sure that the client knows where they are and can reach them easily. *Easy access encourages the client to use these items and enhances the ability to provide self-care.*
- Orient to the environment. Explain the location of the call bell, personal items, and the furniture in the room. If able, tour client's room, including the bathroom and sink. *Visually impaired clients are usually very capable of providing self-care in a known environment.*
- Provide other tools or items that can help compensate for diminished vision:
  a. Bright, nonglare lighting
  b. Books, magazines, and instructions in large print
  c. Books on tape
  d. Telephones with oversize pushbuttons
  e. A clock with numbers and hands that can be felt

- Assist with meals by:
  a. Reading menu selections and marking choices.
  b. Describing the position of foods on a meal tray according to the clock system, for example, "On the plate, the peas are at 9 o'clock, the mashed potatoes at 1 o'clock, and the chicken breast at 6 o'clock. The milk glass is at 2 o'clock on the tray above the plate, and coffee is at 11 o'clock."
  c. Placing the utensils in a readily accessible position.
  d. Removing lids from containers, buttering the bread, and cutting meat, as needed.
  e. If the visual impairment is new or temporary, the client may need feeding or continued assistance during the meal.

*Providing assistance during eating is important to maintain the client's nutritional status. The client may be ashamed of needing help or embarrassed to request it and may respond by not eating or by claiming not to be hungry.*

- Assist with mobility and ambulation as needed:
  a. Have the client hold your arm or elbow, and walk slightly ahead as a guide. Do not hold the client's arm or elbow.
  b. Describe the surroundings and progress as you proceed. Warn in advance of potential hazards, turns, and steps.
  c. Teach to feel the chair, bed, or commode with the hands and the back of the legs before sitting.

*These measures help ensure the client's safety while providing for mobility and helping prevent complications associated with immobility.*

- If the vision loss is unilateral and recent, provide instructions related to unilateral vision loss and change in depth perception:
  a. Caution about the loss of depth perception and teach safety precautions, such as reaching slowly for objects and using visual cues as to distance, especially when driving.
  b. Teach to scan, turning the head fully toward the affected side to identify potential hazards and looking up and down to compensate for the loss of depth perception.

*The client with a unilateral vision loss is often unaware of its effect on peripheral vision and depth perception.*

### Risk for Injury

Whether the client is experiencing a sudden loss of vision due to acute angle-closure glaucoma or significant visual impairment due to inadequately managed chronic glaucoma, both are at an increased risk for injury. Clients who have had surgical interventions for glaucoma are at even greater risk.

- Assess ability to perform activities of daily living. *Clients may be reluctant to request assistance, believing that they should be able to perform these familiar tasks. Careful assessment and provision of needed assistance help prevent injury and maintain the client's self-esteem.*

**PRACTICE ALERT** *Keep traffic area free of clutter to reduce the risk for injury in visually impaired clients.* ∎

- Notify housekeeping and place a sign on the client's door to alert all personnel not to change the arrangement of the client's room. *The visually impaired client is at high risk for falling when in an unfamiliar environment. It is important to maintain a safe, familiar room when the client is hospitalized.*
- Raise two or three side rails on the client's bed. *Raised rails remind clients to ask for assistance before ambulating in an unfamiliar environment.*
- Discuss possible adaptations in the home to help the client remain as independent as possible and prevent falls or other injuries. *Often minor changes in the home environment, such as removing scatter rugs and small items of furniture, allow the client to navigate safely in this already familiar environment.*

### Anxiety

The actual or potential loss of sight threatens the client's self-concept, role functioning, patterns of interaction, and, potentially, environment. The visually impaired client who functions well in a familiar environment will feel anxious in the unfamiliar setting of a hospital or care facility.

- Assess for verbal and nonverbal indications of level of anxiety and for normal coping mechanisms. Repeated expressions of concern or denial that the vision change will affect the client's life indicate anxiety. Nonverbal indicators include tension, difficulty concentrating or thinking, restlessness, poor eye contact, and changes in vocalization (rapid speech, voice quivering). Physical indicators include tachycardia, dilated pupils, cool and clammy skin, and tremors. *The client may not recognize this feeling as anxiety. Identifying and acknowledging the anxiety state can help the client recognize and deal with it.*
- Encourage to verbalize fears, anger, and feelings of anxiety. *Verbalizing helps externalize the anxiety and allows fears to be addressed.*
- Discuss perception of the eye condition and its effects on lifestyle and roles. *Discussion provides an opportunity to correct misperceptions and introduce alternative activities and assistive devices for the visually impaired.*
- Introduce yourself when entering the room, explain all procedures fully before and as they are being performed, and use touch to convey proximity and caring. *The visually impaired client must rely on the other senses to make up for the loss of sight. Because the client cannot see what you are doing, complete explanations of even simple tasks such as refilling a water glass help to relieve anxiety.*
- Identify coping strategies that have been useful in the past and to adapt these strategies to the present situation. *Previously successful coping strategies may be employed to increase the client's sense of control.*

## Using NANDA, NIC and NOC Linkages

Chart 45–2 shows links between NANDA nursing diagnoses, NIC, and NOC when caring for the client with glaucoma.

## Home Care

Clients with glaucoma require teaching about lifetime strategies for managing their chronic disorder at home. They need to understand the importance of lifetime therapy to control the disease and prevent blindness. If a permanent visual impairment has resulted, the client needs information on achieving the maximum possible independence while maintaining safety. The following topics should be discussed with the client and family:

- Prescribed medications including proper way to instill drops
- Importance of not taking certain prescription and over-the-counter medications without consulting a physician
- Periodic eye examinations with intraocular pressure measurement
- Risks, warning signs, and management of acute angle-closure glaucoma
- Possible surgical options
- Community resources, such as Visually Impaired Society, local library, and transportation services
- Helpful resources:
  - National Glaucoma Foundation
  - Young and Under Pressure Glaucoma Foundation
  - Glaucoma Research Foundation
  - Prevention of Blindness Society

MediaLink | GLAUCOMA RESOURCES

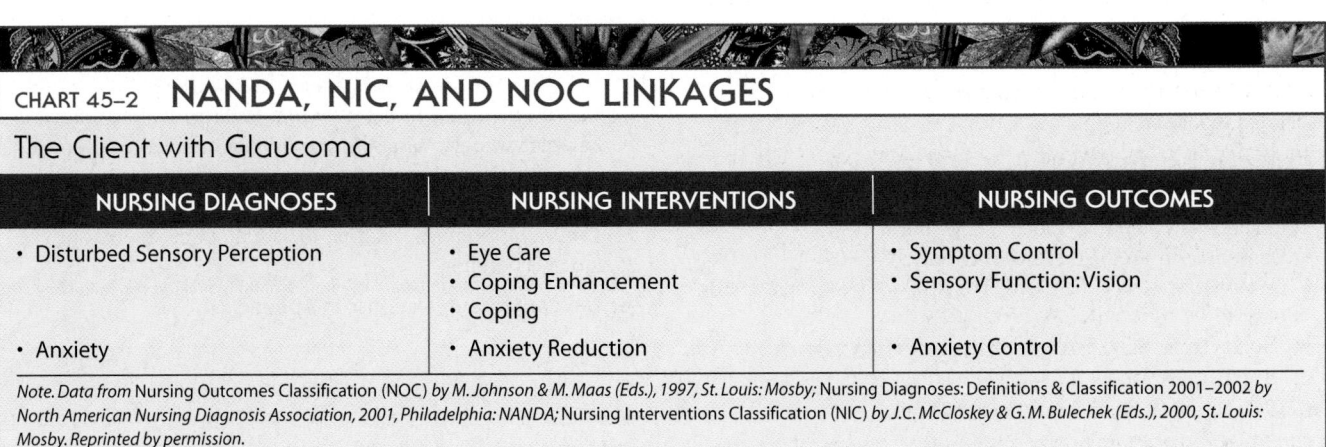

### CHART 45–2  NANDA, NIC, AND NOC LINKAGES

#### The Client with Glaucoma

| NURSING DIAGNOSES | NURSING INTERVENTIONS | NURSING OUTCOMES |
|---|---|---|
| • Disturbed Sensory Perception | • Eye Care<br>• Coping Enhancement<br>• Coping | • Symptom Control<br>• Sensory Function: Vision |
| • Anxiety | • Anxiety Reduction | • Anxiety Control |

*Note. Data from Nursing Outcomes Classification (NOC) by M. Johnson & M. Maas (Eds.), 1997, St. Louis: Mosby; Nursing Diagnoses: Definitions & Classification 2001–2002 by North American Nursing Diagnosis Association, 2001, Philadelphia: NANDA; Nursing Interventions Classification (NIC) by J.C. McCloskey & G. M. Bulechek (Eds.), 2000, St. Louis: Mosby. Reprinted by permission.*

## Nursing Care Plan
## A Client with Glaucoma and Cataracts

Lila Rainey is an 80-year-old widow who lives alone in the house she and her late husband built 50 years ago. She has worn glasses for nearsightedness since she was a young girl. She was diagnosed 4 years ago with chronic open-angle glaucoma, for which she takes timolol maleate (Timoptic) 0.5%. Recently she has noticed difficulty reading and watching television despite a new lens prescription. She has stopped driving at night because the glare of oncoming headlights makes it difficult for her to see. Mrs. Rainey's ophthalmologist has told her that she has cataracts but that they do not need to come out until they bother her. Although her glaucoma is still controlled with timolol maleate 0.5%, one drop in each eye twice a day, her intraocular pressure measurements have been gradually increasing. Mrs. Rainey has taken 325 mg of aspirin daily since a TIA 8 years ago. She is being admitted to the outpatient surgery unit for a cataract removal and intraocular lens implant in her right eye.

### ASSESSMENT

Mrs. Rainey is admitted to the eye surgery unit by Susan Schafer, RN. In her assessment, Ms. Schafer finds Mrs. Rainey to be alert and oriented, though apprehensive about her upcoming surgery. Assessment findings include BP 134/72, P 86, R 18. Mrs. Rainey's neurologic, respiratory, cardiovascular, and abdominal assessments are essentially normal. Her pupils are round and equal, and react briskly to light and accommodation. Her conjunctivae are pink; sclera and corneas, clear. Using the ophthalmoscope, Ms. Schafer notes that the red reflex in Mrs. Rainey's right eye is diminished. Ophthalmic examination shows visual acuity of 20/150 OD (right eye) and 20/50 OS (left eye) with corrective lenses. Her intraocular pressures are 21 mmHg OD and 17 mmHg OS. On fundoscopic exam, no disease of the blood vessels, retina, macula, or disc is found. Ms. Schafer reviews the operative procedure with Mrs. Rainey, answering her questions and telling her what to expect after surgery. Following preoperative protocols, Mrs. Rainey is prepared and transported to surgery.

### DIAGNOSIS

- *Disturbed sensory perception: Visual* related to myopia and lens extraction
- *Anxiety* related to anticipated surgery
- *Deficient knowledge:* lack of information regarding postoperative care
- *Impaired home maintenance* related to activity restrictions and impaired vision

### EXPECTED OUTCOMES

- Regain sufficient visual acuity to maintain ADLs, including reading and watching television for enjoyment.
- Demonstrate a reduced level of anxiety.
- Demonstrate the procedure for instilling eye drops postoperatively.

- Demonstrate knowledge of the home care she will require after surgery, signs of complications, and actions to take if complications occur.
- Use appropriate resources to assist with home maintenance until vision stabilizes and activity restrictions are lifted.

### PLANNING AND IMPLEMENTATION

- Provide a safe environment, placing the call light and personal care items within easy reach.
- Encourage Mrs. Rainey to express her fears about surgery and its potential effect on vision.
- Explain all procedures related to surgery and recovery.
- Instruct her to avoid shutting the eyelids tightly, sneezing, coughing, laughing, bending over, lifting, or straining to have a bowel movement. Teach her to wear glasses during the day and an eye shield at night to prevent injury to the surgical site.
- Explain and demonstrate the procedure for administering eye drops.
- Provide verbal and written instructions about postoperative care, including a schedule of follow-up examinations, potential complications, and actions to take in response.
- Refer Mrs. Rainey to a discharge planner or social worker to help establish a plan for home maintenance.

### EVALUATION

Mrs. Rainey is discharged the morning after her surgery. She is visibly relieved when the eye patch is removed because her vision in the operated eye is better than before surgery, even without her glasses. She is able to relate the recommended activity restrictions. Mrs. Rainey administers her own eye drops before discharge and relates an understanding of the prescribed postoperative care and safety precautions. Mrs. Rainey's daughter plans to visit her mother two to three times a week to help with laundry and vacuuming until Mrs. Rainey is able to resume all her household activities. Mrs. Rainey says that she won't "be so scared when I need my other eye done." She understands the chronic nature of her glaucoma and says that her vision is too important for her to neglect her timolol drops and routine eye exams.

### Critical Thinking in the Nursing Process

1. Why did it become more difficult to control Mrs. Rainey's intraocular pressure as her cataract matured?
2. Identify medications that are commonly prescribed following cataract surgery. What are the risks of interactions between these medications and Mrs. Rainey's timolol drops?
3. Develop a care plan for the nursing diagnosis, *Self-care deficit: Dressing/grooming,* related to visual impairment and restricted bending.

See Evaluating Your Response in Appendix C.

## THE CLIENT WITH A RETINAL DETACHMENT

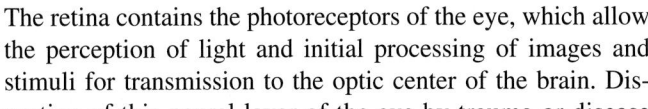

The retina contains the photoreceptors of the eye, which allow the perception of light and initial processing of images and stimuli for transmission to the optic center of the brain. Disruption of this neural layer of the eye by trauma or disease interferes with light perception and image transmission, potentially resulting in blindness.

Both primary eye conditions and systemic diseases can affect the retina and interfere with vision. Retinal tears or detachments can occur either spontaneously or as a result of trauma.

### PATHOPHYSIOLOGY AND MANIFESTATIONS

Separation of the retina or sensory portion of the eye from the choroid, the pigmented vascular layer, is known as a **retinal detachment.** Although retinal detachment may be precipitated by trauma, it usually occurs spontaneously. The vitreous humor normally adheres to the retina at the optic disk, the macula, and the periphery of the eye. With aging, the vitreous humor shrinks and may pull the retina away from the choroid. Aging therefore is a common risk factor, as are myopia and aphakia, absence of the lens (e.g., following lens removal for cataracts) (Porth, 2002; Tierney et al., 2001).

The retina may actually tear and fold back on itself, or the retina may remain intact but no longer adhere to the choroid (Figure 45–10 ■). A break or tear in the retina allows fluid from the vitreous cavity to enter the defect. This, along with fluid that escapes from choroid vessels, the pull of gravity, and traction exerted by the vitreous humor, separates the retina from the choroid. The detached area may rapidly increase in size, increasing loss of vision. Unless contact between the retina and choroid is reestablished, the neurons of the retina become ishemic and die, causing permanent vision loss. For this reason, retinal detachment is a true medical emergency, requiring prompt ophthalmologic referral and treatment.

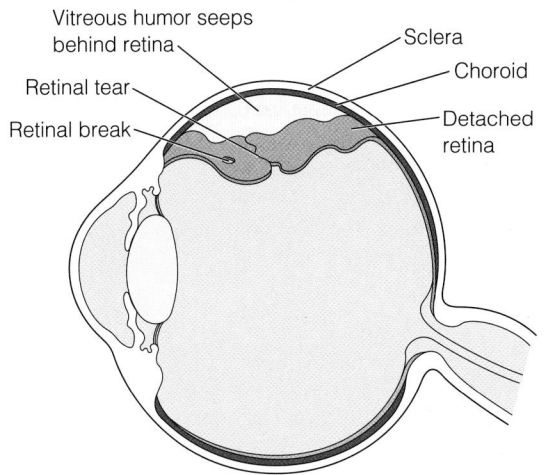

**Figure 45–10** ■ Retinal detachment.

### Manifestations of Retinal Detachment

- Floaters: irregular, dark lines or spots in the field of vision
- Flashes of light
- Blurred vision
- Progressive deterioration of vision
- Sensation of a curtain or veil being drawn across the field of vision
- If the macula is involved, loss of central vision

When the retina detaches, the client experiences floaters, or "spots," and lines or flashes of light in the visual field. Often the client describes the sensation of having a curtain drawn across the vision, much like a curtain being drawn over a window. The area of the visual field affected is directly related to the area of detachment. For example, because light rays cross as they pass through the lens, a retinal tear in the superior portion of the eye results in a deficit in the lower part of the visual field. The client feels no pain, and the eye appears normal to visual inspection. Common manifestations of retinal detachment are listed in the box above.

### COLLABORATIVE CARE

The manifestations and examination of the ocular fundus by ophthalmoscopy establish the diagnosis of retinal detachment. Early diagnosis and intervention are vital. If the condition is left untreated, the detached portion will become necrotic because of separation from the vascular supply of the choroid. The result is permanent blindness in that portion of the eye. If an ophthalmologist is not readily available, the client's head is positioned so that gravity pulls the detached portion of the retina into closer contact with the choroid.

Interventions are directed toward bringing the retina and choroid back into contact and reestablishing the blood and nutrient supply to the retina. Either cryotherapy, using a supercooled probe, or laser photocoagulation may be used to create an area of inflammation and adhesion to "weld" the layers together.

A surgical procedure called *scleral buckling* also may be used. In this procedure, an indentation or fold is created in the sclera, bringing the choroid into contact with the retina. Contact is maintained with a local implant on the sclera or an encircling strap or "buckle." Air may also be injected into the vitreous cavity, a procedure called pneumatic retinopexy. The client is positioned so that the air bubble pushes the detached portion of the retina into contact with the choroid.

With a retinal tear, it may be necessary to use surgical instruments to manipulate the detached section of retina into place. Air or a liquid is then injected into the vitreous to maintain retinal contact with the choroid, or laser therapy used to create a bond.

Medialink | RETINAL DETACHMENT CASE STUDY

# NURSING CARE

The nursing focus for the client with a detached retina is on early identification and treatment. Because early intervention is vital to preserve the client's sight, nurses must recognize early manifestations of retinal detachment and intervene appropriately to obtain definitive treatment for the client. Retinal detachment can be successfully treated on an outpatient basis, often in an ophthalmologist's office. For these clients, the nursing focus is on education.

## Ineffective Tissue Perfusion: Retinal

Restoring contact between the retina and choroid is a priority of nursing and medical care for the client with retinal detachment. Vitreous humor may leak through a retinal tear, and fluid exudate may collect behind the tear, causing further retinal detachment. If the macula is detached, central vision is lost, and the client's prognosis for full vision restoration is poorer.

### PRACTICE ALERT
*Carefully assess anyone who complains of a sudden rapid loss of vision because these are often medical emergencies.* ■

- Assess for other manifestations of eye disease. *Retinal detachment is painless and has no outward manifestations. The client with a red eye or cloudy cornea may be experiencing acute angle-closure glaucoma rather than retinal detachment.*
- Notify physician and the ophthalmologist immediately. *Immediate medical intervention is required in clients with retinal detachment to preserve vision.*
- Position so the area of detachment is inferior. For instance, for a superior temporal retinal detachment of the right eye (with corresponding vision loss in the inferior medial visual field of that eye), place supine with the head turned to the right. *Correct positioning allows the contents of the posterior portion of the eye to place pressure on the detached area, bringing the retina in closer contact with the choroid.*

## Anxiety

The client with retinal detachment has a rapid decline in vision in the affected eye, often occurring spontaneously and without pain. Unless the client has had previous episodes, he or she usually does not know what is causing the problem. Anxiety and fear of complete vision loss are common, expected reactions.

- Maintain a calm, confident attitude while carrying out priority interventions. *Administering care in a calm although urgent manner helps reassure the client that the problem is treatable and that appropriate measures are being taken.*
- Reassure that most retinal detachments are successfully treated, usually on an outpatient basis. *Reassurance can help allay the client's fear of permanent vision loss.*
- For spontaneous detachments, assure that he or she did not cause the detachment to occur. *The client may believe that the detachment is related to a specific activity and feel guilty for "causing" this loss of vision.*

- Explain all procedures fully, including the reason for positioning. *Explanations facilitate the client's understanding and help relieve anxiety in unfamiliar settings.*
- Allow supportive family members or friends to remain with the client as much as possible. *Additional support helps lower the client's anxiety level.*

## Home Care

Teaching the client undergoing surgical repair of retinal detachment is similar to that for clients experiencing other types of eye surgery (see page 1469). If the retina remains detached, the client needs instructions about the change in peripheral vision or other visual fields and changes in depth perception.

Discuss the following topics with the client and family to prepare for home care:

- Limitations on positioning the head following pneumatic retinopexy
- Activity restrictions such as no bending or straining at stool
- Use of eye shield
- Early manifestations and the importance of seeking immediate treatment
- Follow-up treatment with the ophthalmologist

# THE CLIENT WITH MACULAR DEGENERATION

The leading cause of blindness in people over the age of 65 is **macular degeneration** (Quillen, 1999). The macula is the area of the retina that receives light from the center of the visual field and that has the greatest visual acuity. Factors associated with macular degeneration include aging, smoking, hypertension, and hypercholesterolemia. The destructive changes in the macula occur most often as a response to the aging process. It affects males and females equally and is seen more frequently in people of European ancestry.

Age-related macular degeneration is thought to result from gradual failure of the outer pigmented layer of the retina (the retinal layer adjacent to the choroid), which removes cellular waste products and keeps the retina attached to the choroid. This failure causes photoreceptor (sensory) cells to be lost at an increasing rate. In addition, waste and toxins from cell breakdown further damage the cells of the outer pigmented retinal layer. Serous fluid may enter the subretinal space, leading to retinal detachments and depriving sensory cells of oxygen and nutrients, increasing cell death. The process is typically bilateral and slowly progressive.

Two forms of macular degeneration exist. *Atrophic degeneration* (dry) causes gradual and progressive vision loss because of atrophy and degeneration of the outer pigmented retinal layer. Vision loss is more rapid and severe in *exudative degeneration;* this form accounts for 90% of people who are legally blind because of macular degeneration. In exudative degeneration (wet), a proliferation of new blood vessels (neovascularization) form in the subretinal space. These vessels leak serous fluid or blood into the retina, separating the pigmented retina from the choroid or separating the neurosensory retina (innermost layer) from the pigmented retina (Tierney et al., 2001).

When the macula is damaged, central vision becomes blurred and distorted, but peripheral vision remains intact. Distortion of vision in one eye is a common initial manifestation; straight lines appear wavy or distorted (Figure 45–11A ■). With the loss of central vision, activities that require close central vision, such as reading and sewing, are particularly affected (Figure 45–11B).

There is currently no effective treatment for atrophic macular degeneration. Laser photocoagulation may slow the exudative form if performed early in the course of the disease to seal leaking capillaries and stop exudation. Large-print books and magazines, the use of a magnifying glass, and high-intensity lighting can help the client to cope with the reduced vision of macular degeneration.

Nurses should be alert for clients demonstrating new and rapid onset manifestations of macular degeneration and promptly refer these clients for ophthalmologic evaluation. Early intervention may preserve a greater degree of vision and slow the progress of the disease. For clients with slowly progressive manifestations, the nursing focus is on helping the client and family members adapt to the gradual decline in vision by recommending visual aids and other coping strategies. Client education materials should be in a large-print format.

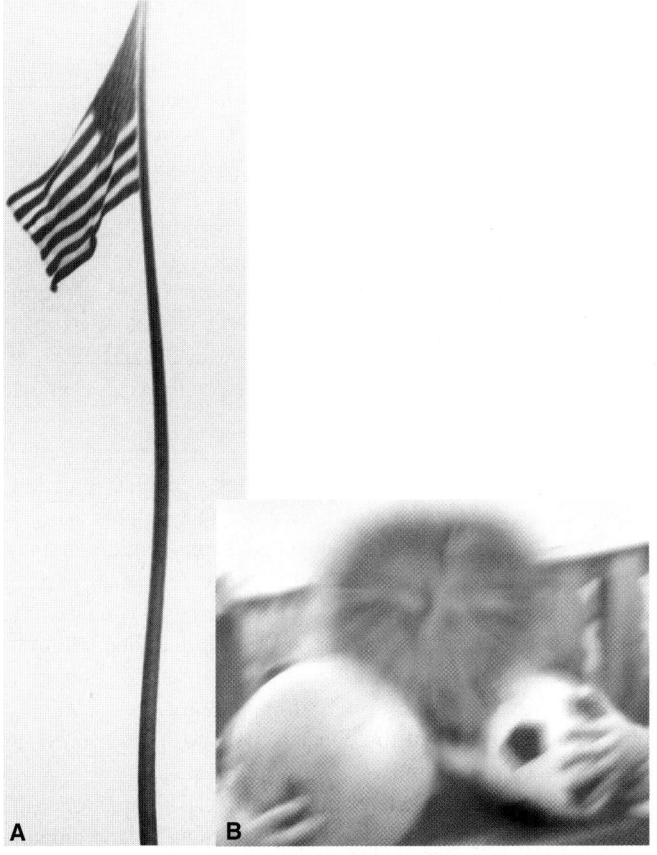

**Figure 45–11** ■ *A,* The visual distortion of straight lines typical of early macular degeneration. *B,* Loss of central vision with advanced macular degeneration.

*Courtesy of Prevent Blindness America (A); the National Eye Institute, National Institutes of Health (B).*

## THE CLIENT WITH RETINITIS PIGMENTOSA

**Retinitis pigmentosa** is a hereditary degenerative disease characterized by retinal atrophy and loss of retinal function progressing from the periphery to the central region of the retina. It is inherited as an autosomal dominant, autosomal recessive, or X-linked trait and may be associated with other genetic defects (Braunwald et al, 2001; Porth, 2002).

In retinitis pigmentosa, the genetic defect appears to cause production of an unstable form of rhodopsin, the receptor protein of rod cells in the retina. Rod cells degenerate, initially at the periphery of the retina. The areas of degeneration and cell death slowly expand, causing vision to narrow. Central vision is finally lost as well.

The initial manifestation of retinitis pigmentosa, difficulty with night vision, is often noted during childhood. As the disease progresses, there is slow loss of visual fields, photophobia, and disrupted color vision. The progression to tunnel vision and blindness is gradual; the client may be totally blind by age 40.

Currently, there is no effective treatment for retinitis pigmentosa. Research into the role that defective rhodopsin plays in the disease holds future promise for the development of therapy that may at least slow its progress.

Clients with retinitis pigmentosa may benefit from low-vision aids, much like those for the client with macular degeneration. Additionally, information about the disease and its progress is vital so the client can plan for the eventual total loss of sight. Clients with retinitis pigmentosa should be referred for genetic counseling prior to starting a family to determine the risk of transmitting the disease to their children.

## THE CLIENT WITH DIABETIC RETINOPATHY

In the United States, **diabetic retinopathy** is the leading cause of new blindness in people age 20 to 74. While approximately 85% of diabetics will develop retinopathy, the majority will not become blind (Braunwald et al, 2001). Diabetic retinopathy is a vascular disorder affecting the capillaries of the retina. The capillaries become sclerotic and lose their ability to transport sufficient oxygen and nutrients to the retina. Retinopathy is seen in both type 1 and type 2 diabetes. In the diabetic, the extent of retinopathy is reflective of the length of time the client has had the disease and the degree of control that has been maintained. Nursing care of the client with diabetes is discussed in Chapter 18. ⊝⊃

Diabetic retinopathy has two major forms: *nonproliferative* or background retinopathy and *proliferative* retinopathy. Nonproliferative retinopathy is typically the initial form seen. The venous capillaries of the eye dilate and develop microaneurysms that may then leak, causing retinal edema, or they may rupture, causing small hemorrhages into the retina. On ophthalmoscopic examination, yellow exudates, cotton-wool patches indicative of retinal ischemia, and red-dot hemorrhages

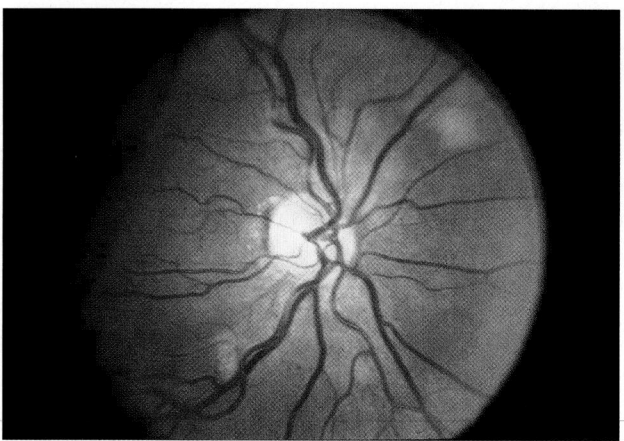

**Figure 45–12** ■ Appearance of the ocular fundus in diabetic retinopathy.

*Courtesy of the National Eye Institute, National Institutes of Health.*

are observed (Figure 45–12 ■). When the peripheral retina is involved, the client may experience few symptoms other than light glare. Edema of the macula or a large hemorrhage may cause vision loss.

Diabetic retinopathy may progress to the proliferative form. This disease is marked by large areas of retinal ischemia and the formation of new blood vessels (neovascularization) spreading over the inner surface of the retina and into the vitreous body. These vessels are fine and fragile, making them permeable and easily ruptured. Blood and blood protein leakage contribute to retinal edema, and hemorrhage into the vitreous body may occur. The vessels gradually become fibrous and firmly attached to the vitreous body, increasing the risk of retinal detachment.

Clients with diabetes should be examined yearly by an ophthalmologist. The development of any new visual manifestations is an additional indication for prompt ophthalmologic examination and possibly retinal angiography.

Laser photocoagulation is used to treat both the nonproliferative and proliferative forms of diabetic retinopathy. Leaking microaneurysms are sealed and proliferating vessels destroyed, reducing the risk of hemorrhage, retinal edema, and retinal detachment. This treatment also slows the progress of aneurysms and new vessel formation; however, it does not cure the disorder. Clients with severe proliferative retinopathy may undergo vitrectomy to remove vitreous hemorrhage or treat associated retinal detachments (Tierney et al., 2001).

As with many other eye disorders, the nursing care focus for diabetic retinopathy is primarily educational. The newly diagnosed diabetic client needs to understand the importance of regular eye examinations beginning approximately 5 years after the onset of type 1 diabetes and at the time of onset of type 2 diabetes. Changes of diabetic retinopathy may already be present when type 2 is diagnosed.

Teach the client to report promptly any new visual manifestation, including blurred vision; black spots (floaters), cobwebs, or flashing lights in the visual field; or a sudden loss of vision in one or both eyes. Emphasize to the client that careful blood glucose control may help prevent diabetic retinopathy

from developing; it may also slow its progress. The client's blood pressure should also be maintained within normal limits to prevent further damage to retinal vessels. Although diabetic retinopathy cannot be halted or cured, its progress can be slowed with aggressive management. Much of the burden for this management falls on the client, increasing the importance of good teaching.

## THE CLIENT WITH HIV INFECTION

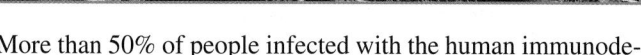

More than 50% of people infected with the human immunodeficiency virus (HIV) develop an infectious or noninfectious ocular condition, generally as a late manifestation of the disease (Braunwald et al., 2001).

HIV retinopathy, manifested as cotton-wool spots around the optic nerve, is the most common noninfectious ophthalmic lesion in AIDS. Cotton-wool spots indicate areas of retinal ischemia. Microaneurysms and dot-, blot-, or flame-shaped hemorrhages may also be seen in HIV retinopathy.

Neoplasms common in the client with AIDS can also affect the eye. Kaposi's sarcoma may affect the external surface or anterior segment of the eye or the eyelids. Kaposi's lesions vary in color (red, brown, or purple) and in size, shape, and location. Conjunctival lesions resemble a benign subconjunctival hemorrhage. Kaposi's lesions of the lid may cause **ptosis** (drooping of the lid) and abnormal lid function. Vision or eye position and movement may be affected by the tumor or by the effect of increased intracranial pressure on the cranial nerves.

The most serious and frequent opportunistic eye infection associated with HIV infection is cytomegalovirus (CMV) retinitis. CMV retinitis develops in 10% to 15% of people with AIDS, generally when CD4 cell counts drop below 50 mL. Initially unilateral, CMV retinitis commonly progresses to become bilateral because of the systemic nature of the infection. CMV invades the retina of the eye directly, producing exudate and cotton-wool spots, hemorrhage, cell death, and necrosis. Visual field deficits develop and can progress to eventual blindness.

Corneal ulcers from opportunistic bacterial, fungal, protozoal, or viral infections are also associated with HIV infection. Toxoplasmic and fungal retinal infections may occur.

The client with an HIV-associated ocular condition may complain of a change in visual acuity, blurring, floaters, or gaps in the field of vision. Extensive retinal damage may cause retinal detachment and symptoms of flashing lights, multiple floaters, and a loss of vision. Because the observed changes in the retina are nonspecific, it is important for the examining physician to know that the client is HIV positive in order to make an accurate diagnosis.

In addition to the general treatment of HIV infection with retroviral medications such as zidovudine (AZT) and didanosine (ddI), specific therapies may be directed toward the ocular manifestations of the disease. CMV retinitis is commonly treated with the antivirals ganciclovir (Cytovene) and foscarnet sodium (Foscavir).

## Procedure 45-1 — Removing and Reinserting a Prosthetic Eye

### SUPPLIES

- Gloves
- Clean basin or plastic denture cup
- Sterile normal saline or soap and water for cleaning the prosthesis
- Gauze squares or cotton cloth for cleaning the socket
- A bulb syringe for irrigation if necessary

### BEFORE THE PROCEDURE

Most clients who have an artificial eye provide self-care and require little assistance. However, it may be necessary for the nurse to remove an eye prosthesis from the unconscious or debilitated client. Explain the procedure to the client and provide for privacy.

### PROCEDURE

- Follow standard precautions.
- Wash the hands and put on clean exam gloves.
- To remove the prosthesis, either

- Pull down the lower lid and gently exert outward and upward pressure on the lower edge of the prosthesis. This pressure usually causes the prosthesis to slip out.
- Pull down the lower lid and apply a moistened suction cup to the prosthesis by squeezing the device. Twist gently to remove the prosthesis from the socket.
- Wash the prosthesis using mild soap and water or normal saline. Rinse thoroughly. Do not use abrasives or chemicals for cleaning.
- If the prosthesis is not immediately replaced in the eye socket, store it in a clearly labeled plastic container lined with a soft cloth or gauze squares. Avoid scratching or damaging the prosthesis. Store it in a safe place to prevent loss.
- If irrigation of the eye socket is ordered, have the client lean over a sink or basin if possible, or position on the affected side with a clean emesis basin to hold the irrigant as it flows out of the socket.

Gently hold the lids open and irrigate the socket using a bulb syringe and clean warm water.
- Reinsert the prosthesis.
  a. Moisten the prosthesis with warm normal saline or water.
  b. Gently hold the lids open, inserting the upper edge of the prosthesis under the upper lid first, then the lower edge under the lower lid using slight pressure.
  c. If a suction device is used, attach it to the cleaned prosthesis over the pupil. Holding the lids open, insert the prosthesis using the above procedure, then remove the suction cup by squeezing it gently and exerting slight pressure on the edge of the cup with the lower lid.

### AFTER THE PROCEDURE

Ensure that the client is comfortable. Chart the procedure and any abnormal findings, such as drainage or inflammation.

---

Although treatment of ocular Kaposi's sarcoma is usually not indicated, conjunctival lesions may be excised for comfort or cosmetic reasons. Lid lesions may be treated with radiation or intralesional chemotherapy.

## THE CLIENT WITH AN ENUCLEATION

Occasionally surgical removal of an eye is necessary because of trauma, infection, glaucoma, intractable pain, or malignancy. This procedure is known as **enucleation.**

Enucleation is performed under local or general anesthesia. After the globe is removed, the conjunctiva and eye muscles are sutured to a round implant inserted into the orbit to maintain its shape. A pressure dressing is left in place for 24 to 48 hours. The client is permitted out of bed on the day of surgery. Hemorrhage and infection are the most commonly seen complications.

Postoperative nursing care includes teaching, psychologic support, and observation for potential complications. The client may be instructed to apply warm compresses and instill antibiotic ointment or drops postoperatively.

Within 1 week, a temporary prosthesis called a conformer is fitted into the empty socket. The permanent prosthesis is individually designed to closely resemble the client's other eye. The prosthesis can be fitted 1 to 2 months after surgery. Often it is difficult to discern which eye is functional and which is

the prosthesis. Procedure 45–1 outlines the proper way to remove and reinsert an eye prosthesis when the client is unable to do so.

## THE CLIENT WHO IS BLIND

Visual impairment exists on a continuum from blindness to decreased visual acuity that can be corrected with refractive lenses to normal or near normal. The legal definition of blindness is visual acuity no better than 20/200 in the better eye with optimal correction, or a visual field of less than 20 degrees (compared to the normal of 180 degrees). Total blindness usually indicates that the client has no light perception at all. In practical terms, a person with a visual deficit sufficient to need assistive devices or aid from other people for normal activities of daily living is considered blind.

Ten to 12 million people in the United States have a visual impairment that cannot be corrected. More than 500,000 Americans are legally blind. Worldwide, between 40 and 50 million people have visual impairment significant enough to be considered blind.

The major worldwide causes of blindness are as follows:

1. Cataracts
2. Trachoma
3. Glaucoma

4. Onchocerciasis (river blindness), a parasitic infection transmitted by flies that causes opacification of the cornea, inflammation of the iris and choroid (uveitis), and eventual destruction of vision
5. Nutritional deficiencies including xerophthalmia and keratomalacia due to vitamin A deficiency
6. Trauma

## PATHOPHYSIOLOGY

Although approximately two-thirds of all cases of blindness worldwide are either preventable or curable, it continues to be prevalent because of lack of access to care, fear of surgery or other treatment, poor sanitation and nutrition, and ignorance of need. In the United States, sanitation measures, better access to health care, and a higher level of nutrition have reduced the threat of infectious disorders to vision. However, glaucoma and cataracts remain significant causes of blindness. Other major causes of blindness in the United States include retinal diseases such as diabetic retinopathy, macular degeneration, and congenital disorders.

## NURSING CARE

Blind people need to cope not only with the loss of a significant sense but often also with societal attitudes that make them feel inferior, helpless, and inadequate. The idea of losing the sense of vision is uniformly feared, leaving sighted people unable to understand the magnitude and impact of the loss in those who have experienced it. Because of this fear and confusion, sighted people are unsure of what the blind expect from them.

The adjustment of the person who is born blind and raised to become an independent member of society differs from that of the person who has been sighted and becomes blind. The person who has been blind from birth has developed numerous adaptive strategies that the newly blind person has yet to learn.

Although adaptation may be easier for the client who has experienced a gradual loss of vision than for someone with an abrupt loss, both must grieve the lost sense. The blind client needs to grieve the lost body part as well as the loss of mobility, self-sufficiency, perhaps economic security, and, to a certain extent, contact with reality as it has been perceived. The client's self-concept and self-esteem are threatened. Anger, denial, remorse, and self-pity are not uncommon in the initial period following loss of sight. Interpersonal relationships and roles are affected. Communication patterns change with the loss of the ability to perceive many nonverbal cues. Expressions of sexuality may be impaired.

Acceptance of the change from sighted to blind is characterized by releasing the hope that vision will be regained. Self-esteem increases as the client attempts and masters activities of self-sufficiency such as completing ADLs, cooking, and becoming mobile outside the known home environment.

Health professionals often confuse the role of the blind person with the role of the client, seeing the person as helpless, dependent, and lacking in personal identity and control. Although nurses need to take blindness into account in planning care and maintaining client safety, it is vital to give the blind client the same respect and decision-making power that all clients deserve. Nurses who have dealt with their own emotions and responses to vision loss are better prepared to help the client adapt.

Nurses can foster independence in the hospitalized client with a significant vision deficit by doing the following:

- Orient to the environment verbally and physically. Describe the client's room using a central point such as the bed. Lead the client around the room, identifying chairs, sink, bathroom, and other landmarks. Be sure that only the client moves objects such as chairs, personal items, and clothing. Leave doors either fully open or closed as the client wishes, but, to preserve the client's safety, do not leave doors partially open. Keep the room and hallways where the client will be ambulating free of clutter.
- Use verbal communication freely. Describe activities going on around the client. Introduce yourself as you enter the room and let the client know when you are leaving.
- Provide other sensory stimuli such as radio and television as desired by the client.
- Orient to food trays by using the face of a clock to describe the position of food items on the plate and tray (unless the client has always been blind and cannot visualize a clock face).
- When assisting with ambulation, allow to hold your arm as you walk slightly ahead. Do not hold the client's arm. Verbally describe the environment, such as, "There will be two steps up 5 feet ahead."
- Do not hesitate to ask what assistance the client desires.

For the client with a new loss of sight, refer to available services. Counseling can help the client cope with and eventually adapt to the loss of sight. People who are blind are eligible for mobility training, assistance with relearning self-care activities, education in the use of braille to communicate, and vocational and other forms of rehabilitation. Local, state, and national agencies such as the American Foundation for the Blind, National Braille Association, and National Federation for the Blind coordinate services for the blind. Many assistive devices are available, including guide or pilot dogs, computer services, talking books and tape players, and low-vision aids.

Although each client with a significant vision deficit has individualized needs, the following nursing diagnoses may be appropriate for the blind client.

- *Disturbed sensory perception: Visual* related to trauma or disease process
- *Bathing/hygiene, dressing/grooming, feeding self-care deficit* related to impaired vision
- *Deficient knowledge* related to lack of information about available resources
- *Hopelessness* related to loss of vision
- *Grieving* related to loss of a body part
- *Risk for situational low self-esteem* related to significant change in body image

# EAR DISORDERS

For a person to hear, sound waves must enter the external auditory meatus and travel through the ear canal to vibrate the tympanic membrane and bony structures of the middle ear, which in turn activate the receptors of the cochlea. Trauma or disease involving any portion of this pathway can affect hearing. **Tinnitus,** the perception of sound such as ringing, buzzing, or roaring in the ears, is another potential result of problems affecting the auditory system.

Disorders of the external ear, including the auricle, auditory meatus, and ear canal, can affect the conduction of sound waves and hearing. Obstruction of the external auditory canal or damage to the tympanic membrane, which separates the outer from the middle ear, may lead to conductive hearing loss. Infection or inflammation, trauma, and obstruction of the ear canal with cerumen (wax) or a foreign body are the most common conditions affecting the external ear.

Disorders of the middle ear may be either acute or chronic. Unless these disorders are treated promptly and effectively, damage and scarring of middle ear structures can result in a permanent conductive hearing loss. Infectious or inflammatory disorders such as otitis media and mastoiditis are the most common conditions affecting the middle ear. Otosclerosis, a genetic condition, may also affect the structures of the middle ear.

## THE CLIENT WITH EXTERNAL OTITIS

**External otitis** is inflammation of the ear canal. Commonly known as *swimmer's ear,* it is most prevalent in people who spend significant time in the water. Competitive athletes, including swimmers, divers, and surfers, are particularly prone to external otitis. Wearing a hearing aid or ear plugs, which hold moisture in the ear canal, is an additional risk factor. Although *Pseudomonas aeruginosa* or other bacterial infection is the most common cause, external otitis may also be due to fungal infection, mechanical trauma (such as cleaning the ear with hair pins), or a local hypersensitivity reaction.

## PATHOPHYSIOLOGY AND MANIFESTATIONS

Disruption of the normal environment within the external auditory canal typically precedes the inflammatory process. Retained moisture, cleaning, or drying of the ear canal remove the protective layer of cerumen, an acidic, water-repellent substance with antimicrobial properties. Its removal leaves the skin of the ear canal vulnerable to invasion and infection. For surfers, the presence of *exostoses,* bony growths in the ear canals resulting from prolonged exposure to cold, predisposes to impaction and retained moisture within the canal.

The client with external otitis often complains of a feeling of fullness in the ear. Ear pain typically is present and may be severe. The pain of otitis externa can be differentiated from that associated with otitis media by manipulation of the auricle. In external otitis, this maneuver increases the pain, whereas the client with otitis media experiences no change in pain perception. Odorless watery or purulent drainage may be present. The ear canal appears inflamed and edematous on examination.

## COLLABORATIVE CARE

Management of the client with an external ear disorder focuses on restoring the normal balance of the external ear and canal and teaching the client how to prevent future problems.

For otitis externa, the following steps are recommended in treatment.

- Thorough cleansing of the ear canal, particularly if drainage or debris is present
- Treatment of the infection with local antibiotics; if cellulitis is present, systemic antibiotics may be necessary
- Medication to relieve the pain and itching
- Teaching on the prevention of future episodes of swimmer's ear

A topical antibiotic is often prescribed for the treatment of otitis externa. A topical corticosteroid may be ordered in combination with the antibiotic to provide immediate relief of the pain, swelling, and itching. Polymyxin B-neomycin-hydrocortisone (Cortisporin Otic) is a typical combination preparation used to treat external otitis; these antibiotics are effective against *Pseudomonas.* It is important to identify known sensitivity to any of the drugs in this preparation prior to initiating therapy. Clients who are sensitive to neomycin may develop dermatitis, in which case the drug must be stopped. Other preparations such as 1% tolnaftate solution (Tinactin) may be prescribed for a fungal infection of the ear canal.

## NURSING CARE

External otitis can cause severe pain and discomfort. Although the disorder is rarely serious enough to require hospitalization, the nurse teaches the client about the disorder, comfort measures, and prevention of future episodes.

### Impaired Tissue Integrity

External otitis may result from attempts to clean the ear canal with a toothpick, cotton-tipped applicator, or other implement that damages the skin, allowing an infectious organism to invade the tissue. Even if the canal is not damaged by attempts to clean it, the cleaning process often interrupts normal mechanisms, causing cerumen and debris to collect in the canal. This collected debris, in turn, tends to trap water within the canal, causing maceration of the skin.

- Inform that ear canals rarely need cleansing beyond washing of the external meatus with soap and water. Teach clients of all ages not to clean ear canals with any implement. *"Cleaning" increases the risk of tissue damage and impairs the normal mechanism that clears the canal of accumulated cerumen and debris.*

- Teach client (and, if necessary, a family member) how to instill prescribed ear drops:
  a. Wash the hands.
  b. Warm the medication briefly by holding the container in the hand or placing it in a pocket for approximately 5 minutes before instilling the drops. *Warming the medication promotes comfort.*
  c. Lie on the unaffected side; if sitting, tilt the head toward the unaffected side. *This position allows gravity to assist in moving the medication to the inner portion of the ear canal.*
  d. Partially fill the ear dropper with medication.
  e. Using the nondominant hand, straighten the ear canal by pulling the pinna of the ear up and back. *Straightening helps the medication travel along the length of the canal.*
  f. Administer the prescribed number of drops into the ear canal. *It is important that the full amount of prescribed medication be administered to penetrate the length of the canal and achieve full effectiveness.*
  g. Remain in the side-lying position for approximately 5 minutes after the instillation of drops. *This position allows the medication to penetrate into deeper portions of the canal and prevents it from running out when the head is moved upright.*
  h. Loosely place a small piece of cotton in the auditory meatus for 15 to 20 minutes. *The cotton helps keep the medication in the canal.*
- Teach to avoid getting water in the affected ear until it is fully healed. Cotton balls may be used while showering to prevent water from entering the ear canal. The client should refrain from water sports and activities until approved by the primary care provider. *Retained moisture in the ear canal can further impair skin integrity, increasing inflammation.*

## Home Care

The client is ultimately responsible for carrying out the prescribed treatment regimen in external otitis and for implementing measures to prevent future episodes. Teaching is vital. Provide verbal and written instructions on use of the prescribed medications. Teach the client care measures to prevent recurrent episodes especially important in swimmers, divers, and surfers (Box 45–1).

Cellulitis of the surrounding tissue is a possible complication of external otitis. Instruct the client to report to the primary care provider any increase in pain, swelling, or redness of surrounding tissues; fever; or other manifestations of infection such as malaise or increased fatigue.

## THE CLIENT WITH IMPACTED CERUMEN AND FOREIGN BODIES

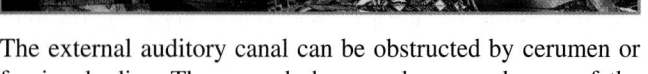

The external auditory canal can be obstructed by cerumen or foreign bodies. The curved shape and narrow lumen of the canal make it particularly vulnerable to obstruction.

---

### BOX 45–1 ■ Teaching to Prevent External Otitis

- Stay out of the water until the acute inflammatory process is completely resolved. Ideally, allow 7 to 10 days before resuming water activities.
- Take precautions to keep the ear canal dry while in the water.
  a. Use silicone earplugs, which can keep water out of the ear without reducing hearing significantly.
  b. Wear a tight-fitting swim cap or wet suit hood, especially in cold ocean water. Although these do not prevent water from entering the ear, they protect the ear from the cold and possibly slow the formation of bony growths in the ears. They also protect the ear from sand and other water debris.
- Immediately after swimming, dry the ear canal. Allow water to drain by tilting the head and jumping to shake water out of the ear. Dry the outer ear with a towel, then use a hair dryer on the lowest setting several inches from the ear to dry the canal.
- Do not insert cotton swabs or other objects into the ear canal to dry it. This removes the protective layer of cerumen and may damage the skin of the canal, increasing the risk of bacterial infection. In addition, if debris such as sand is present, the swab may actually push debris further into the canal, forming an impacted mass.
- Use a drying agent in the ear canal after swimming. A 2% acetic acid solution or 2% boric acid in ethyl alcohol is effective in drying the canal and restoring its normal acidic environment.
- If it is necessary to remove impacted debris from the ear canal, irrigate the ear with warm tap water. A bulb syringe available over the counter or a 20 mL syringe attached to a short Teflon intravenous catheter (with the needle removed) is effective. With the head tilted toward the affected side, direct a stream of warm water toward the upper wall of the ear canal, allowing the water to run out into a bowl or sink. Repeated instillations may be necessary to break up and flush out impacted wax and debris.

---

As cerumen dries, it moves down and out of the ear canal. In some individuals it tends to accumulate, narrowing the canal. Aging is a risk factor for cerumen impaction, because less is produced and it is harder and drier. The accumulation of cerumen is often aggravated by attempting to remove it using cotton-tipped swabs or hairpins, which pack it more deeply into the ear canal. A study of cerumen impaction, common ear-cleaning practices, and hearing acuity in older adults is summarized in the Nursing Research box on page 1493.

A variety of objects become foreign bodies in the ear canal. In adults, implements used to clean the ear canal may break and become lodged. Insects also may enter the ear canal and be unable to exit.

When the ear canal becomes occluded with either cerumen or a foreign body, the client experiences a conductive hearing loss in the affected ear. Manifestations include a sensation of fullness, along with tinnitus and coughing due to stimulation of the vagal nerve. The foreign body or impacted cerumen may be

## Nursing Research

### Evidence-Based Practice for Ear-Cleaning and Hearing Loss

A descriptive study of the incidence of cerumen impaction, ear-cleaning practices, and hearing loss in three groups of adults over the age of 60 included people living independently and participating in senior citizen center activities, and clients in personal care homes and nursing homes (Ney, 1993). The researchers found that individuals living independently had significantly fewer cerumen impactions than those in the other groups. This finding may reflect the higher level of activity of the independent adults, facilitating the natural drainage of cerumen from the ear canal, or better hygiene practices of that group. Approximately one-third of the subjects inserted an object (usually a cotton-tipped applicator) into the ear canal for the purpose of cleaning on a regular or periodic basis.

Some degree of hearing deficit was demonstrated in two-thirds of the subjects, with 18% of the population unable to hear any tone presented. Loss at the highest frequency was the most common deficit noted.

### IMPLICATIONS FOR NURSING

This study demonstrates the potential role nurses can play in identifying hearing deficits, preventing further conductive deficit from impacted cerumen, and teaching clients about appropriate ear-hygiene measures.

The higher incidence of impacted cerumen in residents of personal care homes and nursing homes demonstrates the need for routine assessment of the ear canal and cleaning as necessary. Clients who routinely clean the ear canals using an object such as a cotton-tipped swab, hairpin, paper clip, or nail need to be taught alternative methods. Several subjects in this study used alcohol or hydrogen peroxide to soften cerumen; only one used a commercial product specifically for that purpose. Nurses can have a positive impact by increasing awareness of acceptable alternatives.

### Critical Thinking in Client Care

1. Why is the resident of a personal care home or nursing home at higher risk for developing a cerumen impaction?
2. How can nurses in these settings prevent cerumen from accumulating to this degree?
3. How can the nurse in a long-term care setting screen the hearing of the residents to identify possible deficits?

---

visualized on otoscopy. Impacted cerumen appears as a yellow, brown, or black mass in the canal.

Treatment focuses on clearing the canal. If there is no evidence of tympanic membrane perforation, irrigation of the canal is often the initial therapy.

Impacted wax, objects, or insects may require physical removal using an ear curet, forceps, or right-angle hook inserted via an otoscope and ear speculum. Mineral oil or topical lidocaine drops are used to immobilize or kill insects prior to their removal from the ear. When an organic foreign body such as a bean or an insect is suspected, water should not be instilled into the ear canal, because it may cause the object to swell, making its removal more difficult. Smooth, round objects present the biggest challenge to remove from the ear canal. Suction applied using a piece of soft intravenous tubing may be effective.

Nurses are often involved in identifying and relieving obstructions of the ear canal, especially in outpatient and community settings. Any client with evidence of a new conductive hearing loss or complaints of discomfort and fullness in one ear should be evaluated for possible obstruction. Inability to visualize the tympanic membrane or observation of a dark, shiny mass obstructing the canal may indicate a need for an irrigation or other procedure to clear the canal. It is important to determine that the tympanic membrane is intact before irrigating; assessment by a physician or advanced practitioner may be necessary if a ruptured membrane is suspected.

Because obstruction of the ear canal with cerumen or a foreign body is generally preventable, teaching is a key component of nursing care. Clients need to know appropriate care measures for the external ear. Although the ear canal rarely needs cleaning, the client prone to cerumen impaction needs teaching about the use of mineral oil or commercial products to soften wax and of irrigation to remove it. All clients should un-

derstand the importance of not inserting anything smaller than a finger wrapped with a washcloth into the ear canal to avoid trauma to the canal or eardrum. Stress the risk of impacting cerumen against the tympanic membrane when using cotton-tipped swabs to clean the ear canal. Additionally, the swab may break and lodge in the canal. If ear drops have been prescribed, teach the client and a family member how to instill them.

## THE CLIENT WITH OTITIS MEDIA

**Otitis media,** inflammation or infection of the middle ear, primarily affects infants and young children but may also occur in adults. The tympanic membrane, which separates the middle ear from the external auditory canal, protects the middle ear from the external environment. The auditory (eustachian) tube connects the middle ear with the nasopharynx to help equalize the pressure in the middle ear with the atmospheric pressure. Unfortunately, this connecting tube also provides a route by which infectious organisms enter the middle ear from the nose and throat, causing otitis media, the most common disease of the middle ear.

## PATHOPHYSIOLOGY AND MANIFESTATIONS

There are two primary forms of otitis media: (1) serous and (2) acute or suppurative. Both forms are associated with upper respiratory infection and auditory tube dysfunction. The auditory tube is narrow and flat, normally opening only during yawning and swallowing. Allergies or upper respiratory tract infections can cause edema of the tube lining, impairing its function. Air within the middle ear is trapped and gradually absorbed, creating negative pressure in this space.

## Serous Otitis Media

Serous otitis media occurs when the auditory tube is obstructed for a prolonged time, impairing equalization of air pressure in the middle ear. Air within the middle ear space is gradually absorbed; the tube obstruction prevents more air from entering the middle ear. The resulting negative pressure in the middle ear causes sterile serous fluid to move from the capillaries into the space, forming a sterile effusion of the middle ear.

Upper respiratory infection or allergies such as hay fever predispose the client to serous otitis media. Clients with narrowed or edematous auditory tubes may also be subject to barotrauma or barotitis media. In these clients, the middle ear cannot adapt to rapid changes in barometric pressure as occur during air travel or underwater diving. Barotrauma tends to occur during descent in an airplane, because negative pressure within the middle ear causes the auditory tube to collapse and lock. However, underwater diving places even greater stress on the auditory tube and middle ear (Tierney et al., 2001).

Typical manifestations of serous otitis media include decreased hearing in the affected ear and complaints of "snapping" or "popping" in the ear. On examination, the tympanic membrane demonstrates decreased mobility and may appear retracted or bulging. Fluid or air bubbles are often visible behind the drum. Severe pressure differences as occur with barotrauma may cause acute pain, hemorrhage into the middle ear, rupture of the tympanic membrane, or even rupture of the round window with sensory hearing loss and severe **vertigo** (a sensation of whirling or rotation). *Hemotympanum*, bleeding into or behind the tympanic membrane, may be observed on otoscopic examination.

## Acute Otitis Media

The auditory tube also provides a route for the entry of pathogens into the normally sterile middle ear, resulting in acute or suppurative otitis media. Acute otitis media typically follows an upper respiratory infection. Edema of the auditory tube impairs drainage of the middle ear, causing mucus and serous fluid to accumulate. This fluid is an excellent environment for the growth of bacteria, which may enter from the oronasopharynx via the auditory tube. Although a viral upper respiratory infection may predispose the client to a middle ear infection, the bacteria *Streptococcus pneumoniae, Haemophilus influenzae,* and *Streptococcus pyogenes* account for most cases of otitis media in adults. Invasion and colonization of the middle ear by bacteria and the resultant migration of white blood cells cause pus formation. Accumulated pus can increase middle ear pressure sufficiently to rupture the tympanic membrane. The bacterial infection may also migrate internally, causing mastoiditis, brain abscess, or bacterial meningitis. A more common complication of otitis media is a persistent conductive hearing loss, which typically resolves when the middle ear effusion clears.

The client with acute otitis media experiences mild to severe pain in the affected ear. The client's temperature is often elevated. Diminished hearing, dizziness, vertigo, and tinnitus are

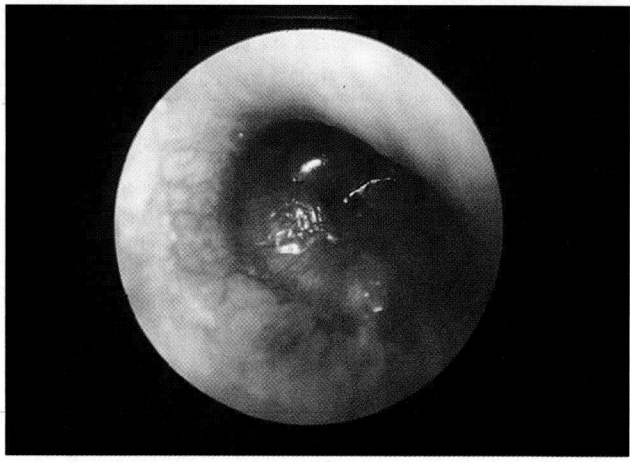

**Figure 45–13** ■ A red, bulging tympanic membrane of otitis media.

*Source: Janet Hayes/Medical Images, Inc.*

common associated complaints. Pus within the mastoid air cells often causes mastoid tenderness in acute otitis media. On otoscopic examination, the tympanic membrane appears red and inflamed or dull and bulging (Figure 45–13 ■). Decreased movement of the membrane is demonstrated by tympanometry or air insufflation. Spontaneous rupture of the tympanic membrane releases a purulent discharge. **Myringotomy** (an incision of the tympanic membrane) may be performed to relieve the pressure.

## COLLABORATIVE CARE

The diagnosis of otitis media is usually based on the history and the physical examination. The tympanic membrane may be visualized with a pneumatic otoscope that allows a puff of air to be instilled into the ear canal so that the examiner can evaluate the mobility of the tympanic membrane. Generally, the tympanic membrane moves slightly when air is instilled or the client performs the Valsalva maneuver. Less movement is seen in clients with auditory tube dysfunction and acute otitis media with effusion.

### Diagnostic Tests

- *Impedance audiometry,* also known as tympanometry, is an accurate diagnostic test for otitis media with effusion. In this test, an audiometer with a sealed probe tip is used to deliver a continuous tone to the tympanic membrane. The instrument also records the energy reflected from the surface of the tympanic membrane, allowing measurement of the compliance of the tympanic membrane and middle ear system. With middle ear effusion, compliance is reduced.
- A *CBC* may be performed to assess for an elevated WBC indicative of acute bacterial infection. If the tympanic membrane has ruptured or a tympanocentesis or myringotomy is performed, drainage is cultured to determine the infecting organism.

## Medications

Auditory tube dysfunction and serous otitis media are treated with decongestants and autoinflation of the middle ear. Decongestants are used to reduce the mucosal edema of the auditory tube and improve its patency. They may be administered either systemically or by intranasal spray. Although controversial, a short course of oral corticosteroids may be prescribed for clients with serous otitis media. (Refer to Chapter 17 ⊙⊙ for further discussion of these medications.)

The client with auditory tube dysfunction may be taught to autoinflate the middle ear by performing the Valsalva maneuver or by forcefully exhaling against closed nostrils. Additionally, the client is advised to avoid air travel and underwater diving.

Acute otitis media is treated with antibiotic therapy, especially amoxicillin, trimethoprim-sulfamethoxazole, cefaclor, or azithromycin for 5 to 10 days. This course of treatment is long enough to ensure eradication of the infective organism; yet, short enough to reduce the incidence of bacterial resistance. (See Chapter 8 ⊙⊙ for further discussion of antibiotics). Symptomatic relief may be provided by analgesics, antipyretics, antihistamines, and local application of heat.

## Surgery

A myringotomy or tympanocentesis may be performed to relieve excess pressure in the middle ear and prevent spontaneous rupture of the eardrum. To perform a tympanocentesis, the physician inserts a 20-gauge spinal needle through the inferior portion of the tympanic membrane, allowing aspiration of fluid and pus from the middle ear to relieve pressure and, if necessary, obtain a specimen for culture. *Myringotomy,* or surgical drainage of the middle ear, may be performed to relieve severe pain or when complications of acute otitis media, such as mastoiditis, are present. As soon as the pressure is released, pain subsides and hearing improves.

Clients who do not respond to antibiotic therapy may require myringotomy with insertion of ventilation (tympanostomy) tubes. Small tubes are inserted into the inferior portion of the tympanic membrane, providing for ventilation and drainage of the middle ear during healing. The tube is eventually extruded from the ear, and the tympanic membrane heals. While the tube is in place, it is important to avoid getting any water in the ear canal because it may then enter the middle ear space.

## NURSING CARE

Clients with otitis media are commonly treated in outpatient and community settings. The nursing role is primarily one of support and education.

## Health Promotion

Health promotion for otitis media focuses on educating clients about the importance of seeking medical care for prolonged, severe ear pain with or without drainage combined with an upper respiratory tract infection. Untreated or repeated attacks of otitis media can progress to a chronic form of otitis media, acute mastoiditis, or eardrum perforation.

## Assessment

Collect assessment data through a health history and physical examination (see Chapter 44).

- Health history: recent upper respiratory infection, presence of pain in affected ear, sense of fullness or pressure in the ear, change in hearing
- Physical examination: hearing test, inspect tympanic membrane

## Nursing Diagnosis and Interventions

Pain can be a significant problem for clients with otitis media, as can the risk of damage to delicate tissues of the middle ear by the infectious and inflammatory processes.

### Pain

Tissue edema, effusion of the middle ear, and the inflammatory response can affect the pain-sensitive tissues of the middle ear in otitis media, causing acute discomfort. This discomfort is increased by pressure changes, such as those that occur during air travel or underwater diving.

- Assess pain for severity, quality, and location. *A thorough assessment is important to determine the source of the pain. The pain of otitis media, unlike that of external otitis, is not aggravated by movement of the external ear.*
- Encourage the use of mild analgesics such as aspirin or acetaminophen every 4 hours as needed to relieve pain and fever. *These nonprescription medications are effective in reducing the perception of pain. Aspirin also has anti-inflammatory properties that may help relieve the inflammation of the ear.*
- Advise to apply heat to the affected side unless contraindicated. *Heat dilates blood vessels, promoting the reabsorption of fluid and reducing swelling.*
- Instruct to avoid air travel, rapid changes in elevation, or diving. *A rapid change in barometric pressure can increase the client's pain significantly.*
- Instruct to report promptly an abrupt relief of pain to the primary care provider. *Pain that subsides abruptly may indicate spontaneous perforation of the tympanic membrane with relief of pressure within the middle ear.*

## Home Care

The client who has otitis media needs teaching about the disorder, its causes and prevention, and any specific treatment recommended or prescribed. Discuss the following topics with the client and family.

- Antibiotic therapy and potential side effects
- Importance of completing all ordered doses
- Follow-up examinations in 2 to 4 weeks
- Avoid swimming, diving, or submerging the head while bathing if ventilation tubes are in place

If surgical intervention is necessary, teach the client and family members about the surgery and postoperative care. Provide instruction about any special postoperative precautions, such as avoiding water in the ear canals or avoiding sudden changes in air pressure.

## THE CLIENT WITH ACUTE MASTOIDITIS

The mastoid process is a portion of the temporal bone of the skull lying adjacent to the middle ear. It is full of air cavities called mastoid air cells or mastoid sinuses. The infection of acute otitis media always extends into the mastoid air cells; effective treatment of acute otitis media eliminates the infection from the mastoid cells as well. When treatment is ineffective, pus remains in the mastoid air cells, and acute **mastoiditis,** bacterial infection of the mastoid process, may develop.

## PATHOPHYSIOLOGY AND MANIFESTATIONS

In acute mastoiditis, the bony septa between mastoid air cells are destroyed and cells coalesce to form large spaces. Portions of the mastoid process are eroded. With chronic infection, an abscess may form, or bony sclerosis of the mastoid may result. Acute mastoiditis increases the risk of meningitis because only a very thin bony plate separates mastoid air cells from the brain. Fortunately, this complication is rare since the advent of effective antibiotic therapy for treating otitis media.

Manifestations of acute mastoiditis usually develop approximately 2 to 3 weeks after an episode of acute otitis media and include recurrent earache and hearing loss on the affected side. The pain is persistent and throbbing; tenderness is present over the mastoid process (behind the ear). It may also be red and inflamed. Swelling of the process can cause the auricle of the ear to protrude more than normal. Fever may be accompanied by tinnitus and headache. Profuse drainage from the affected ear may be noted.

## COLLABORATIVE CARE

In addition to the manifestations of acute mastoiditis, loss of septa between mastoid air cells may be noted on radiologic examination. Acute mastoiditis is treated aggressively with antibiotic therapy. Intravenous ticarcillin-clavulanate (Timentin) and gentamicin may be used initially, with therapy tailored to the specific organism once culture results are obtained. Antibiotics are continued for at least 14 days. Infections that do not respond to medical therapy or that pose a high risk of spreading to the brain may necessitate **mastoidectomy,** surgical removal of the infected mastoid air cells, bone, and pus, and inspection of the underlying dura for possible abscess. The extent of tissue destruction determines the extent of surgery required. In a modified mastoidectomy, as much tissue is preserved as possible to avoid disruption of hearing. A radical mastoidectomy involves removal of middle ear structures including the incus and malleus as well as the diseased portions of the mastoid process. Unless reconstruction is performed at the time of

surgery, this surgery results in conductive hearing loss. **Tympanoplasty,** surgical reconstruction of the middle ear, can restore or preserve hearing.

## NURSING CARE

Prevention is the primary focus of collaborative and nursing care related to mastoiditis. Adequate, effective antibiotic treatment of acute otitis media prevents mastoiditis in nearly all instances.

Following surgical intervention, carefully assess the wound and drainage for evidence of infection or other complications. The client's hearing may be temporarily or permanently affected, depending on the extent of the surgery. If the client has impaired hearing in the unaffected ear as well, develop a means of communication with the client prior to surgery. If the hearing is preserved in the unaffected ear, position the client with that ear toward the door. Speak slowly and clearly; do not shout or speak unusually loudly. Be sure that family and staff know about the client's hearing loss and use appropriate communication techniques. Assist the client with ambulation initially, because dizziness and vertigo are not unusual following surgery. Nursing care of the client having ear surgery is discussed in the box on page 1497.

### Home Care

When teaching about acute mastoiditis, stress the importance of complying with the prescribed antibiotic therapy and recommendations for follow-up. Instruct the client and family to report any adverse reactions to the primary care provider so that therapy can be adjusted. Teach the client and family how to change the surgical dressing using aseptic technique. Provide referrals to appropriate community agencies for the client with a new hearing loss resulting from mastoiditis or its treatment.

## THE CLIENT WITH CHRONIC OTITIS MEDIA

**Chronic otitis media** involves permanent perforation of the tympanic membrane, with or without recurrent pus formation and often accompanied by changes in the mucosa and bony structures (ossicles) of the middle ear. Chronic otitis media is usually a consequence of recurrent acute otitis media and auditory tube dysfunction, but may also result from trauma or other diseases.

Marginal perforations, which usually occur in the posterior-superior portion of the tympanic membrane, are associated with more complications than central perforations. With marginal perforations, squamous epithelium may migrate from the ear canal into the middle ear, where it begins to desquamate and accumulate, forming a *cholesteatoma* (a cyst or mass filled with epithelial cell debris). Its incidence is highest in young adults. The desquamating epithelium continues to accumulate and remains infected, producing collagenases (enzymes) that destroy adjacent bone. The inflammatory process compromises

# NURSING CARE OF THE CLIENT HAVING EAR SURGERY

## PREOPERATIVE CARE

- Review Chapter 7 ⊕ for routine preoperative care.
- Assess the client's hearing or verify documentation of preoperative hearing assessment. *These data are important in evaluating the results of the surgical procedure.*
- Agree on a means of communication to be used after surgery. *Hearing may be impaired after surgery.*
- Explain that blowing of the nose, coughing, and sneezing are restricted to prevent pressure changes in the middle ear and potential disruption of the surgical site. If the client needs to cough or sneeze, leaving the mouth open minimizes pressure changes in the middle ear. *Providing teaching and the opportunity to practice before surgery promotes the client's cooperation in the postoperative period.*

## POSTOPERATIVE CARE

- Review Chapter 7 for routine postoperative care.
- Assess the client for bleeding or drainage from the affected ear. *Infection and hemorrhage are possible complications.*
- Administer antiemetics as ordered to prevent vomiting. *Vomiting may increase the pressure in the middle ear, disrupting the surgical site.*
- Elevate the head of bed and have the client lie on the unaffected side. *This position minimizes the pressure in the middle ear.*
- Assess for vertigo or dizziness, especially with ambulation or movement in bed. Avoid unnecessary movements such as turning. Take measures to ensure safety when the client gets up and ambulates. *Surgery on the ear may disrupt the client's equilibrium, increasing the risk of falling.*
- Assess the client's hearing postoperatively. Stand on the client's unaffected side to communicate and use other meas-

ures such as written messages as needed for effective communication with the hearing-impaired client. Reassure the client that decreased hearing acuity immediately after surgery is expected. *Hearing improvement, if an expected result of the ear surgery, typically does not occur until ear plugs are removed, and edema and drainage at the operative site have resolved. If no reconstruction of the middle ear is done or the cochlea is involved, permanent hearing loss in the affected ear may be an expected result.*
- Remind client to avoid coughing, sneezing, or blowing the nose. *These increase pressure in the middle ear.*

## Client and Family Teaching

- Provide instructions for home care.
  a. To prevent contamination of the ear canal, avoid showers, shampooing, and immersing the head until the physician says you can do so.
  b. Keep the outer ear plug clean and dry, changing it as needed. Do not remove inner ear dressing until the physician so orders.
  c. Avoid blowing the nose; if you need to cough or sneeze, keep the mouth open.
  d. Do not swim or dive without physician approval. Check with the physician regarding air travel.
  e. Meclizine hydrochloride (Antivert) or other antiemetic/antihistamine medication may be necessary for up to 1 month following surgery.
  f. Fever, bleeding, increased drainage, increased dizziness, or decreased hearing after discharge may indicate a complication. Notify the physician if any of these occur.

---

blood supply to the stapes, causing its destruction and conductive hearing loss. Cholesteatomas are benign and slow-growing tumors, which can enlarge to fill the entire middle ear. Untreated, the cholesteatoma can progressively destroy the ossicles and erode into the inner ear, causing profound hearing loss.

Systemic antibiotics are prescribed for exacerbations of purulent otitis media. Tympanic membrane perforation is repaired with a tympanoplasty to restore sound conduction and the integrity of the middle ear. A cholesteatoma may require radical mastoidectomy to remove the tympanic membrane, ossicles, and tumor. The mastoid air cells and middle ear are converted into an open cavity, which can be inspected and cleaned as necessary.

As with other complications of acute otitis media, a priority of nursing care is prevention of chronic otitis media and cholesteatoma. Clients with chronic otitis media need to understand various treatment options and their risks and benefits, as well as the long-term risk of not treating a perforated tympanic membrane. They are also taught how to instill ear drops, to clean the external auditory meatus, and to not irrigate the ear when the tympanic membrane is perforated or if they think it might be.

If surgical treatment of chronic otitis media will affect the client's hearing, include this information in preoperative teaching. Teach the client and family how to use alternative means of communication if this will be necessary postoperatively. When an assistive device is ordered, teach the client and a family member about its use.

## THE CLIENT WITH OTOSCLEROSIS

**Otosclerosis** is a common cause of conductive hearing loss. Abnormal bone formation in the osseous labyrinth of the temporal bone causes the footplate of the stapes to become fixed or immobile in the oval window. The result is a conductive hearing loss.

Otosclerosis is a hereditary disorder with an autosomal dominant pattern of inheritance. It occurs most commonly in Caucasians and in females. The progressive hearing loss typically begins in adolescence or early adulthood and seems to be accelerated by pregnancy. Although both ears are affected, the rate of hearing loss is asymmetric. Because bone conduction of sound is retained, the client may be able to use the telephone but have difficulty conversing in person. Tinnitus may also be associated with otosclerosis.

On examination, a reddish or pinkish-orange tympanic membrane may be noted because of increased vascularity of the middle ear. The Rinne test (see Chapter 44) shows bone sound conduction to be equal to or greater than air conduction, an abnormal finding.

Clients with otosclerosis may choose conservative treatment, relying on a hearing aid to improve their ability to hear and interact with others. Sodium fluoride may be prescribed to slow bone resorption and overgrowth. Surgical treatment involves a stapedectomy and middle ear reconstruction or a stapedotomy. A *stapedectomy* is a microsurgical technique for removing the diseased stapes. A metallic prosthesis is then inserted, with one end connected to the incus and the other inserted into the oval window. *Stapedotomy* involves creation of a small hole in the footplate of the stapes and insertion of a wire or platinum ribbon prosthesis. An argon, KTP, or $CO_2$ laser may be used for surgery. Surgery usually restores hearing for the client with otosclerosis.

Education and referral of the client to appropriate community agencies are important nursing care priorities for the client with otosclerosis. For the client who chooses surgical treatment, nursing care is similar to that for other clients undergoing ear surgery. The following nursing diagnoses may be appropriate:

- *Risk for injury* related to hearing loss or postoperative vertigo
- *Disturbed sensory perception: Auditory* related to bony sclerosis of the stapes
- *Impaired verbal communication* related to hearing loss
- *Anxiety* related to concern about transmission of genetic disorder to children

## THE CLIENT WITH AN INNER EAR DISORDER

Disorders affecting the inner ear are much less common than disorders of the outer or middle ear. Inner ear disorders affect equilibrium and may also affect sensorineural hearing, the perception of sound. Labyrinthitis and Meniere's disease are the most common diseases of the inner ear. Vertigo may be a disorder of the inner ear itself or a manifestation of other disorders.

## PATHOPHYSIOLOGY AND MANIFESTATIONS

The inner ear (also called the labyrinth) contains the cochlea and the semicircular canals. The hair cells and neurons that allow sound perception and transmission to the auditory center of the brain are in the cochlea. The semicircular canals filled with endolymph are the primary organs involved in maintaining equilibrium. Disruption of this portion of the ear by an inflammatory process or excess endolymph not only affects balance but may also result in permanent hearing loss.

## Labyrinthitis

**Labyrinthitis,** also called otitis interna, is an inflammation of the inner ear. It is an uncommon disorder, because the bony protection of the membranous labyrinth makes it difficult for organisms to enter the inner ear. However, bacteria, viruses, and other organisms may enter and infect the inner ear through the oval window during acute otitis media, through the cochlear aqueduct during meningitis, or through the blood. Viral labyrinthitis is suspected when the client has a sudden onset of symptoms after an upper respiratory infection or when there is no evidence of concurrent otitis media.

Inflammation of the labyrinth typically causes vertigo, sensorineural hearing deficit, and **nystagmus** (rapid involuntary eye movements).

Vertigo, a sensation of motion when there is none, or an exaggerated sense of motion in response to movement, is the hallmark manifestation of inner ear disorders. The vertigo of labyrinthitis is severe and often accompanied by nausea and vomiting. Any movement can aggravate the vertigo, and falling is a significant risk if the client attempts to stand. Vertigo lasts days to weeks in labyrinthitis, making client education a vital component of care.

Hearing loss in the ear affected by labyrinthitis may be temporary or permanent. If inflammation destroys tissue of the membranous labyrinth, the hearing loss may be complete and permanent.

The involuntary rhythmic eye movements of nystagmus may not be present in all clients with labyrinthitis. When present, the eye movement is typically horizontal. Applying positive or negative pressure to the tympanic membrane of the affected ear may stimulate nystagmus, as will caloric testing (irrigating the ear canal with warm or cool water). Although nystagmus may also be a symptom of brainstem or cerebellar dysfunction, vertigo and hearing loss are not typically associated with those disorders.

## Meniere's Disease

**Meniere's disease,** also known as endolymphatic hydrops, is a chronic disorder of unknown cause characterized by recurrent attacks of vertigo with tinnitus and a progressive unilateral hearing loss. This disorder affects men and women equally, with adults between the ages of 35 and 60 at highest risk.

The cause of Meniere's disease is unclear. It is brought about by an overaccumulation of endolymph, the fluid in the membranous labyrinth of the inner ear. The excess fluid is thought to be caused by impaired reabsorption of endolymph in the endolymph duct or sac (Porth, 2002). The lymphatic channels dilate in response, resulting in labyrinthine dysfunction. Autonomic nervous system control of labyrinthine circulation may be impaired, or damage to the inner ear from severe otitis media or a head injury can precipitate Meniere's disease. A family history of the disease increases risk, suggesting a possible genetic link in some clients. In many clients, however, it is idiopathic, thought to be precipitated by a viral injury to the fluid transport system of the inner ear. Immune dysfunction also may contribute.

The onset of Meniere's disease may be gradual or sudden. It is characterized by recurrent attacks of vertigo, gradual loss of hearing, and tinnitus. Attacks may be preceded by a feeling of fullness in the ears, and a roaring or ringing sensation. The sensorineural hearing loss and tinnitus are usually unilateral but can become bilateral. Attacks of severe rotary vertigo occur abruptly and often unpredictably, lasting from minutes to hours. An attack may be linked to increased sodium intake, stress, allergies, vasoconstriction, or premenstrual fluid retention. As the disease continues, hearing loss progresses and the vertigo can be severe enough to cause immobility, nausea, and vomiting. Attacks are often accompanied by hypotension, sweating, and nystagmus.

## Vertigo

Normally, the integration of input from the labyrinths, eyes, muscles, joints, and neural centers maintains balance and posture. This input and integration can be affected by disorders of the labyrinth, vestibular nerve or nuclei, eyes, cerebellum, brainstem, or cerebral cortex, causing vertigo. Vertigo is a disorder of equilibrium. The sensation of whirling, rotation, or movement is described as either subjective or objective.

Clients with subjective vertigo report the sensation of being in motion in a stable environment. This is not always a sense of spinning; the client may have a sense of tumbling or falling forward or backward. The sensation is reversed in objective vertigo; clients report a sensation of stability in a moving environment. This motion may be perceived as the room spinning around the client or the ground rocking beneath the client's feet. Dizziness, which may be mistaken for vertigo, is a sensation of unsteadiness, lack of balance, lightheadedness, or movement within the head. The person who is dizzy does not have the rotational sensation felt with vertigo.

Vertigo may be disabling, resulting in falls, injury, and difficulty walking. Attacks of vertigo are often accompanied by nausea and vomiting, nystagmus, and autonomic symptoms such as pallor, sweating, hypotension, and salivation.

## COLLABORATIVE CARE

The manifestations associated with inner ear disorders are similar, making testing necessary to establish a diagnosis. Once the diagnosis is determined, collaborative care is directed toward managing symptoms and preventing permanent hearing loss.

The following diagnostic studies may be ordered.

- *Electronystagmography* evaluates the vestibulo-ocular reflex by identifying eye movements (nystagmus) in response to caloric testing. Water is instilled directly into the ear canal so that it contacts the tympanic membrane while eye motion is recorded. In clients with impaired vestibular function, the normal nystagmus response is blunted or absent. This portion of the test is contraindicated in clients who have a perforated tympanic membrane.
- *Rinne* and *Weber tests* of hearing (see Chapter 44) show decreased air and bone conduction on the affected side if a sensorineural hearing loss is present. In Meniere's disease,

audiology shows sensorineural hearing loss involving the low tones.

- *X-rays* and *CT scans* of the petrous bones are used to evaluate the internal auditory canal. In clients with Meniere's disease, the vestibular aqueducts may be shorter and straighter than normal.
- *Glycerol test* is conducted by giving the client oral glycerol to decrease fluid pressure in the inner ear. An acute temporary hearing improvement is considered diagnostic for Meniere's disease.

Once the diagnosis is established, specific treatments can be ordered. Clients with labyrinthitis or an acute attack of Meniere's disease may require hospitalization to manage the vertigo and its effects. Atropine is used to decrease the parasympathetic nervous system response. A central nervous system depressant such as diazepam (Valium) or lorazepam (Ativan) may be an alternative to atropine. Parenteral droperidol (Inapsine) provides both a sedative and antiemetic effect, making it a useful drug for acute attacks. Antivertigo/antiemetic medications such as meclizine (Antivert), prochlorperazine (Compazine), or hydroxyzine hydrochloride (Vistaril) are prescribed to reduce the whirling sensation and nausea. If the nausea and vomiting are severe, intravenous fluids may be necessary to maintain fluid and electrolyte balance. Bed rest in a quiet, darkened room with minimal sensory stimuli and minimal movement provides the most comfort for the client.

Large doses of antibiotics, often administered intravenously, are prescribed for labyrinthitis when the cause is thought to be bacterial. No specific therapy is indicated for viral labyrinthitis.

Management of the client between acute attacks of Meniere's disease is directed at preventing future attacks and preserving hearing. A low-sodium diet and an oral diuretic such as furosemide (Lasix) or hydrochlorothiazide/triamterene (Dyazide) help maintain a lower labyrinthine pressure. The Furstenberg diet, a salt-free neutral ash diet, may be prescribed if moderate sodium restriction is ineffective in controlling attacks. Clients should avoid tobacco, which causes vasoconstriction and can precipitate an attack, along with alcohol and caffeine.

When medical interventions are ineffective in controlling episodes of vertigo in Meniere's disease, surgical intervention may be necessary. Surgical *endolymphatic decompression* relieves the excess pressure in the labyrinth; a shunt is then inserted between the membranous labyrinth and the subarachnoid space to drain excess fluid away from the labyrinths and maintain lower pressure. This procedure preserves hearing for the majority of the clients. Vertigo is relieved in approximately 70% of clients, but the sensations of fullness and tinnitus remain for about 50% of people after the surgery.

Destruction of a portion of the acoustic nerve is an alternative to shunting procedures. In a *vestibular neurectomy,* the portion of the cranial nerve VIII controlling balance and sensations of vertigo is severed. This procedure relieves vertigo for up to 90% of clients. Although there is a risk of damage to the cochlear portion of the nerve and resultant hearing loss, for most clients hearing loss stabilizes after neurectomy, even improving for some.

The surgery of last resort for Meniere's disease is a **labyrinthectomy.** The labyrinth is completely removed, destroying cochlear function. This procedure is used only when hearing loss is nearly complete and vertigo is persistent. Although labyrinthectomy relieves vertigo in nearly all cases, the client may remain unsteady and have continued problems with balance.

After surgery on the inner ear, the client is positioned to minimize ear pressure and vertigo. The client's movement is restricted, and assistance is provided when the client gets up. Antiemetics and antivertigo medications are used to manage the symptoms resulting from disruption of the inner ear. Complications include infection and leakage of cerebral spinal fluid.

## NURSING CARE

The client with an inner ear disorder has multiple nursing care needs related to the manifestations of the disorder.

### Health Promotion

Health promotion focuses on identifying clients with potential inner ear disorders. Persistent episodes of dizziness, ringing in the ears, balance problems, or loss of hearing should be reported to a health care provider. Clients diagnosed early may have a lower risk for injury and can be taught strategies for maintaining as near normal as possible their work and social life.

### Assessment

Collect the following data for the client with potential inner ear disorders through a health history and physical examination. Assess the older client further for other medical causes of imbalance and dizziness. Neurologic dysfunction, musculoskeletal and cardiovascular disorders, and endocrine problems often contribute to the older client's unsteadiness.

- Health history: medication use; presence of vertigo, nystagmus, nausea and vomiting, and hearing loss; balance problems; frequency and duration of symptoms
- Physical examination: hearing, tinnitus, balance

### Nursing Diagnoses and Interventions

The risk for trauma in clients with inner ear disorders is great. Attacks of vertigo may occur without warning and can be so severe that the client is unable to remain upright. If frequent attacks are accompanied by vertigo, the client's nutrition may be compromised. Constant or intermittent tinnitus can interfere with sleep and rest. Finally, because nearly all inner ear disorders are associated with some degree of hearing loss, which may be progressive, the client has significant psychosocial needs.

### Risk for Trauma

Because of the unpredictable nature of attacks, the client with vertigo due to an inner ear disorder needs to learn strategies for dealing with an acute episode. Because vertigo tends to be chronic except in acute viral labyrinthitis, the emphasis is on

helping the client develop strategies to reduce the frequency of attacks and the risk of injury.

- Monitor for vertigo, nystagmus, nausea, vomiting, and hearing loss. *Monitoring is important to determine the severity of impairment, the duration of attacks, and the client's ability to predict an impending attack.*

**PRACTICE ALERT** *During an acute attack of vertigo, keep on bed rest with the side rails raised and the call light readily accessible.* ■

- Instruct to not get up without assistance during episodes of vertigo. *During attacks of vertigo, assistance reduces the risk of falling.*
- Teach to avoid sudden head movements or position changes. *Sudden movement may precipitate an attack of vertigo.*
- Administer prescribed medications as ordered, including antiemetics, diuretics, and sedatives. *These medications may reduce the frequency, severity, and duration of vertigo attacks.*
- Instruct that when sensing an impending attack it is best to respond by taking the prescribed medication and lying down in a quiet, darkened room. *These measures help protect the client from injury and may shorten the duration and reduce the severity of the attack.*
- Advise to pull to the side of the road and wait for the symptoms to subside if an attack occurs while the client is driving. *Perception and judgment necessary for safe driving may be impaired during an acute attack; pulling off the road is vital to protect the safety of the client and others.*
- Discuss the effect of unilateral hearing loss on the ability to identify the direction from which sounds come. To ensure safety, encourage the client to use other senses (e.g., when crossing the street). *Just as depth perception changes when vision is lost in one eye, sound perception and differentiation of direction change when hearing is lost unilaterally.*

### Sleep Pattern Disturbance

The tinnitus often associated with inner ear disorders may be loud and continuous, interfering with the client's ability to concentrate, relax, and sleep. It may be perceived as a continuous high-pitched whine, buzzing, ringing, or humming sound. In some clients, it may have a pulsatile quality.

- Refer for a complete hearing and ear examination if one has not been done. *Although most tinnitus is associated with hearing loss, often due to noise exposure, it may also be associated with treatable conditions such as impacted cerumen, hypertension, cerebrovascular disorders, and other conditions.*
- Discuss options for masking tinnitus to promote concentration and sleep.
  a. Ambient noise from a radio or sound system
  b. Masking device or white-noise machine
  c. Hearing aid that produces a tone to mask the tinnitus
  d. Hearing aid that amplifies ambient sound

## CHART 45–3  NANDA, NIC, AND NOC LINKAGES

### The Client with Inner Ear Disorders

| NURSING DIAGNOSES | NURSING INTERVENTIONS | NURSING OUTCOMES |
|---|---|---|
| • Disturbed Sensory Perception: Auditory | • Communication Enhancement: Hearing Deficit | • Hearing Compensation Behavior |
|  |  | • Risk Control: Hearing Impairment |
| • Risk for Trauma | • Environmental Management: Safety | • Safety Behavior: Fall Prevention |
| • Disturbed Sleep Pattern | • Sleep Enhancement | • Sleep |

*Note. Data from Nursing Outcomes Classification (NOC) by M. Johnson & M. Maas (Eds.), 1997, St. Louis: Mosby; Nursing Diagnoses: Definitions & Classification 2001–2002 by North American Nursing Diagnosis Association, 2001, Philadelphia: NANDA; Nursing Interventions Classification (NIC) by J.C. McCloskey & G. M. Bulechek (Eds.), 2000, St. Louis: Mosby. Reprinted by permission.*

*These techniques or devices help mask the subjective perception of tinnitus, allowing the client to focus on something other than the sound.*

- Discuss the possible risks and benefits of medications to treat tinnitus. *Many medications have been used to treat tinnitus; oral antidepressants such as nortriptyline (Aventyl, Pamelor) taken at bedtime have been shown to be most effective.*

## Using NANDA, NIC, and NOC

Chart 45–3 shows links between NANDA nursing diagnoses, NIC, and NOC when caring for the client with an inner ear disorder.

## Home Care

Because disorders of the inner ear disrupt balance, safety is a primary focus of teaching. The nurse assists the client to identify possible hazards in the home environment. Discuss the following points during the teaching session.

- Change positions slowly, especially when ambulating.
- Turn the whole body rather than just the head.
- Sit down immediately with the onset of vertigo and lie down if possible.
- Take prescribed antiemetic and antivertigo medications.
- Wear MedicAlert identification.
- If appropriate, discuss the surgical procedure, the immediate postoperative period, and the long-term effects of the surgery.
- Discuss alternative communication techniques as needed.
- Suggest the following resources.
  - Better Hearing Institute
  - Self-Help for Hard of Hearing People

## THE CLIENT WITH AN ACOUSTIC NEUROMA

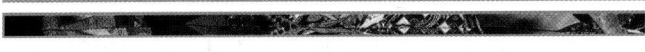

An **acoustic neuroma** or **schwannoma** is a benign tumor of cranial nerve VIII. It typically occurs in adults between the ages of 40 and 50. Acoustic neuromas are common and account for 7% to 8% of intracranial tumors (Way & Doherty, 2003).

These tumors usually occur in the internal auditory meatus, compressing the auditory nerve where it exits the skull to the inner ear. Both the vestibular and cochlear branches are af-

fected; however, the tumor arises from the vestibular division of the auditory nerve twice as often. If allowed to grow, the tumor eventually destroys the labyrinth, including the cochlea and vestibular apparatus. As the tumor expands, it erodes the wall of the internal auditory meatus. The tumor may eventually impinge on the inferior cerebellar artery, which provides blood to the lateral pons and medulla, the brainstem, and the cerebellum. An obstructive hydrocephalus can also occur. Cranial nerves VII (facial) and V (trigeminal) are often affected by the expanding tumor; the tumor frequently wraps around the facial nerve.

Early manifestations of an acoustic neuroma are those associated with disorders of the inner ear: tinnitus, unilateral hearing loss, and nystagmus. Dizziness or vertigo may occur. As the tumor expands and occupies increasing amounts of space in the closed cranium, the client experiences neurologic signs related to the area of the brain affected.

The presence of the tumor can generally be identified on CT or MRI scans. X-ray films of the petrous pyramid of the temporal bone may show erosion caused by the tumor.

The treatment of choice for an acoustic neuroma is surgical excision. In surgery, every effort is made to preserve this nerve and its function as well as other cranial nerves that may be affected. Small tumors of the vestibular division of the acoustic nerve may be excised using microsurgical techniques; hearing can often be preserved. A translabyrinthine approach provides good access to the tumor and allows the facial nerve to be preserved. However, this approach destroys hearing in the affected ear, and it is usually used only when the tumor is large or little effective hearing remains in the affected ear. Larger tumors require craniotomy for removal; facial nerve paralysis is a common result of surgery.

Postoperative nursing care focuses on preserving cerebral function. Position the client to minimize cerebral edema and monitor frequently for signs of increased intracranial pressure. Because the gag reflex may be affected, assess the client carefully before food and fluids are allowed by mouth. Speech therapy is often prescribed for the client after surgery. Because deficits may not resolve for a long time after surgery, education and support are vital components of nursing care for the client. (See Chapter 40 for care of the client undergoing craniotomy).

# THE CLIENT WITH A HEARING LOSS

Approximately 10 million adults in the United States are hearing impaired. The problem of hearing loss is particularly significant in older adults, affecting an estimated 24% of people between the ages of 65 and 74, and up to 39% of those over age 75. As many as 70% of nursing home residents have impaired hearing. Hearing loss is more prevalent in lower socioeconomic groups of older adults (Hazzard et al., 1998).

Lesions in the outer ear, middle ear, inner ear, or central auditory pathways can result in hearing loss. The process of aging also can affect the structures of the ear and hearing. Hearing loss is classified as conductive, sensorineural, or mixed, depending on what portion of the auditory system is affected. Profound deafness is often a congenital condition.

Clients with a hearing loss, whether conductive or sensorineural, may display signs that caregivers can recognize. The voice volume of the hearing-impaired client frequently increases, and the client positions the head with the better ear toward the speaker. The client frequently may ask people to repeat what they have said or respond inappropriately to questions or statements. A question may elicit a blank look if the client has not heard or understood its content.

## PATHOPHYSIOLOGY AND MANIFESTATIONS

Hearing loss impairs the ability to communicate in a world filled with sound and hearing individuals. A hearing deficit can be partial or total, congenital or acquired. It may affect one or both ears. In some types of hearing loss, the ability to perceive sound at specific frequencies is lost. In others, hearing is diminished across all frequencies.

### Conductive Hearing Loss

Anything that disrupts the transmission of sound from the external auditory meatus to the inner ear results in a conductive hearing loss. The most common cause of conductive hearing loss is obstruction of the external ear canal. Impacted cerumen, edema of the canal lining, stenosis, and neoplasms all may lead to canal obstruction. Other etiologic factors for conductive loss include a perforated tympanic membrane, disruption or fixation of the ossicles of the middle ear, fluid, scarring, or tumors of the middle ear.

With conductive hearing loss, there is an equal loss of hearing at all sound frequencies. If the level of sound is greater than the threshold for hearing, speech discrimination is good. Because of this, the client with a conductive hearing loss benefits from amplification by a hearing aid.

### Sensorineural Hearing Loss

Disorders that affect the inner ear, the auditory nerve, or the auditory pathways of the brain may lead to a sensorineural hearing loss. In this type of hearing loss, sound waves are effectively transmitted to the inner ear. In the inner ear, however, lost or damaged receptor cells, changes in the cochlear apparatus, or auditory nerve abnormalities decrease or distort the ability to receive and interpret stimuli.

A significant cause of sensorineural hearing deficit is damage to the hair cells of the organ of Corti. In the United States, noise exposure is the major cause. Exposure to a high level of noise (e.g., standing close to the stage or speakers at a rock concert) on an intermittent or continuing basis damages the hair and supporting cells of the organ of Corti. Ototoxic drugs also damage the hair cells; when combined with high noise levels, the damage is greater and resultant hearing loss more profound. Ototoxic drugs include aspirin, furosemide (Lasix), aminoglycosides, vancomycin (Vancocin), antimalarial drugs, and chemotherapy such as cisplatin (Platinol). Other potential causes of sensory hearing loss include prenatal exposure to rubella, viral infections, meningitis, trauma, Meniere's disease, and aging.

Tumors such as acoustic neuromas, vascular disorders, demyelinating or degenerative diseases, infections (bacterial meningitis in particular), or trauma may affect the central auditory pathways and produce a neural hearing loss.

Sensorineural hearing losses typically affect the perception of high-frequency tones more than of low-frequency tones. This loss makes speech discrimination difficult, especially in a noisy environment. Hearing aids are often not useful, because they amplify both speech and background noise. The increased sound intensity may actually cause discomfort for the client.

### Presbycusis

With aging, the hair cells of the cochlea degenerate, producing a progressive sensorineural hearing loss. In presbycusis, hearing acuity begins to decrease in early adulthood and progresses as long as the individual lives. Higher pitched tones and conversational speech are lost initially. Hearing aids and other amplification devices are useful for most clients with presbycusis.

Because the hearing loss of presbycusis is gradual, the client and family may not realize the extent of the deficit. The hearing-impaired individual may be described as unsociable or paranoid. The family may worry that the person is becoming increasingly forgetful, absent minded, or perhaps "senile." Depression, confusion, inattentiveness, tension, and negativism have been noted in hearing-impaired older adults. Functional problems such as poor general health, reduced mobility, and impaired interpersonal communication are also associated with hearing loss. Caregivers need to be alert for signs of impaired hearing such as cupping an ear, difficulty understanding verbal communication when the person cannot see the speaker's face, difficulty following conversation in a large group, and withdrawal from social activities.

### Tinnitus

Tinnitus is the perception of sound or noise in the ears without stimulus from the environment. The sound may be steady, intermittent, or pulsatile and is often described as a buzzing, roaring, or ringing.

Tinnitus is usually associated with hearing loss (conductive or sensorineural); however, the mechanism producing the sound is poorly understood. It is often an early symptom of noise-induced hearing damage and drug-related ototoxicity. Tinnitus is especially associated with salicylate, quinine, or quinidine toxicity. Other etiologic conditions include obstruction of the auditory meatus, presbycusis, inflammations and infections of the middle or inner ear, otosclerosis, and Meniere's disease. Most tinnitus, however, is chronic and has no pathologic importance.

Tinnitus that is intermittent or slight enough to be masked by environmental sounds is often well tolerated. When it is loud, continuous, and not responsive to treatment, tinnitus can be a significant stressor. It can interfere with activities of daily living, sleep, and rest.

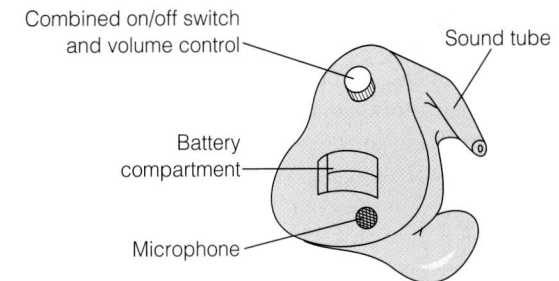

**Figure 45–14** ■ An in-ear hearing aid.

## COLLABORATIVE CARE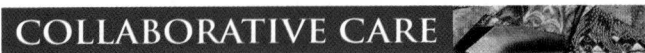

The best treatment for hearing loss is prevention. Clients need to know the potential for hearing damage and how to prevent it. Awareness of the effects of noise exposure, especially when combined with the ototoxic effects of aspirin or other drugs, is important to prevent sensorineural hearing loss.

### Diagnostic Tests

Hearing evaluation includes gross tests of hearing (such as the whisper test), the Rinne and Weber tests, and audiometry.

*   *Rinne and Weber tests* compare air and bone sound conduction. When bone conduction of sound is better than air conduction, the hearing deficit is a conductive loss. The Rinne test can identify even mild conductive hearing losses. If both air and bone conduction are impaired, a sensorineural loss is indicated. (See Chapter 44.)
*   *Audiometry* identifies the type and pattern of hearing loss. Specific sound frequencies are presented to each ear by either air or bone conduction.
*   *Speech audiometry* identifies the intensity at which speech can be recognized and interpreted.
*   *Tympanometry* is an indirect measurement of the compliance and impedance of the middle ear to sound transmission. The external auditory meatus is subjected to neutral, positive, and negative air pressure while the resultant sound energy flow is monitored.

### Amplification

A hearing aid or other amplification device can help many clients with hearing deficits. These assistive devices do nothing to prevent, minimize, or treat the hearing loss itself, but they amplify the sound presented to the hearing apparatus of the ear. Amplification may bring the level of sound above the hearing threshold for the client, allowing more accurate perception and interpretation of its meaning. For the client with distorted sound perception, the hearing aid may be less helpful, because it simply amplifies the distorted sound.

Unfortunately, less than one-fifth of older clients with a hearing deficit have a hearing aid. Denial of the deficit, other health problems, poor visual acuity, decreased manual dexterity, and cost all contribute to this low usage. Hearing aids must

be individually prescribed by an audiologist. Proper design, proper fit, and regular maintenance are necessary for their effectiveness.

Hearing aids are available in a variety of styles, each with advantages and disadvantages. The newest and least noticeable style fits entirely in the ear canal. This small and unobtrusive device allows use of the telephone and can be worn during exercise. Because of its small size, the client must have good manual dexterity to insert it, clean it, and change the batteries. For this reason, older clients or clients with impaired dexterity may be unable to use it.

The in-ear style of aid fits into the external ear and is more visible than the in-canal aid (Figure 45–14 ■). Its larger size makes manipulation somewhat easier, although it still may be difficult for less dextrous individuals. A greater degree of amplification is possible with the in-ear aid. Many have a toggle switch for telephone usage. With both the in-canal and in-ear style, cleaning is important. Small portals may become plugged with cerumen, interfering with sound transmission.

The behind-ear hearing aid allows finer adjustment of the level of amplification and is easier for the client to manipulate (Figure 45–15 ■). For the client who wears glasses, this style can be modified, with all components fitting into the temple of the eyeglasses.

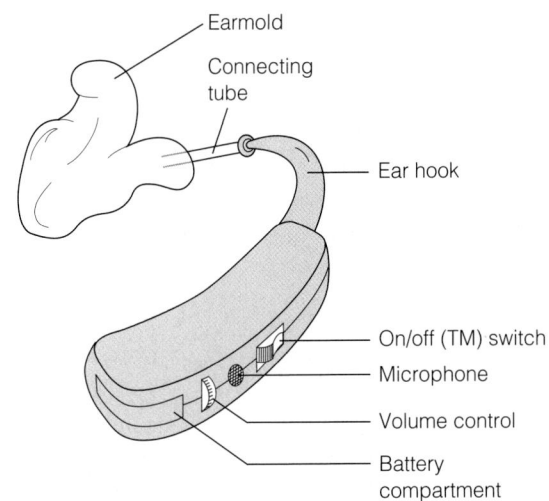

**Figure 45–15** ■ A behind-ear hearing aid.

Clients with profound hearing loss may require a body hearing aid. The microphone and amplifier of this aid are contained in a pocket-sized case that the client clips on to clothing, slips into a pocket, or carries in a harness. The receiver is attached by a cord to the case and clips onto the ear mold, which delivers the sound to the ear canal.

For the client who does not have a hearing aid, an *assistive listening device,* or "pocket talker," with a microphone and "Walkman" type earpieces, is useful. Pocket talkers are available over the counter or through an audiologist and are relatively inexpensive. The earpiece requires no special fitting, and the external microphone allows the client to focus on the desired sound rather than simply amplifying all sounds. Assistive listening devices may also be used in conjunction with a hearing aid.

Clients with tinnitus may find a white-noise masking device helpful to promote concentration and rest. These devices conduct a pleasant sound to the affected ear, allowing the client to block out the abnormal sound.

## Surgery

Reconstructive surgeries of the middle ear, such as a stapedectomy or tympanoplasty, may be useful for the client with a conductive hearing loss. Stapedectomy is the removal and replacement of the stapes. This procedure is used for clients with a conductive hearing loss related to otosclerosis.

In a tympanoplasty, the structures of the middle ear are reconstructed to improve conductive hearing deficits. Chronic otitis media with necrosis and scarring of the middle ear is a common indication for this type of surgery.

For the client with a sensorineural hearing loss, a cochlear implant may be the only hope for restoring sound perception. Two types of cochlear implant are available. The first uses an electrode implanted in the cochlea to stimulate remaining, intact, excitable auditory neurons (Figure 45–16 ■). A small

processor carried outside the body receives sound through a microphone and sends a signal to a transmitter mounted behind the ear. The transmitter then sends the signal to a receiver implanted under the skin, which in turn transmits it to the electrode implanted in the cochlea.

The second type of cochlear implant is used when no excitable auditory nerve fibers are available. The external microphone-transmitter sends the signal to an implanted receiver, which transmits the stimulus via an electrode implanted in the brainstem over the cochlear nucleus.

Cochlear prostheses provide the client with the perception of sound but not normal hearing. The client is able to recognize warning sounds such as automobiles, sirens, telephones, and doors opening or closing. They also receive stimuli to alert them to incoming communication so they can focus on the person speaking. Many clients can learn to interpret the perceived sounds as words, especially with newer implant devices.

## NURSING CARE

In planning and implementing nursing care for the client with a hearing deficit, the nurse needs to consider the type and extent of hearing loss, the client's adaptation to the loss, and the availability of assistive hearing devices and the client's ability and willingness to use them.

### Health Promotion

Health care personnel can be instrumental in preventing hearing loss through education. It is important to promote environmental noise control and the use of ear protection. The Occupational Safety and Health Administration (OSHA) requires ear protection for work environments that consistently exceed 85 decibels. Teaching for primary prevention focuses on the following:

- Care of the ears and ear canals, including cleaning and treatment of infection
- No placing of any hard objects into the ear canal
- Use of plugs to protect the ears during swimming or diving
- Protecting the hearing by avoiding intermittent or frequent exposure to loud noise
- Monitoring for side effects with ototoxic medications
- Hearing evaluation when hearing difficulty is present

### Assessment

Collect the following data through a health history and physical examination (see Chapter 44).

- Health history: ototoxic medication use; presence of upper respiratory tract infection, previous bacterial or viral infections; high noise level exposure; presence of vertigo, tinnitus, unsteadiness, or imbalance
- Physical examination: external ear, tympanic membrane; hearing, cranial nerve

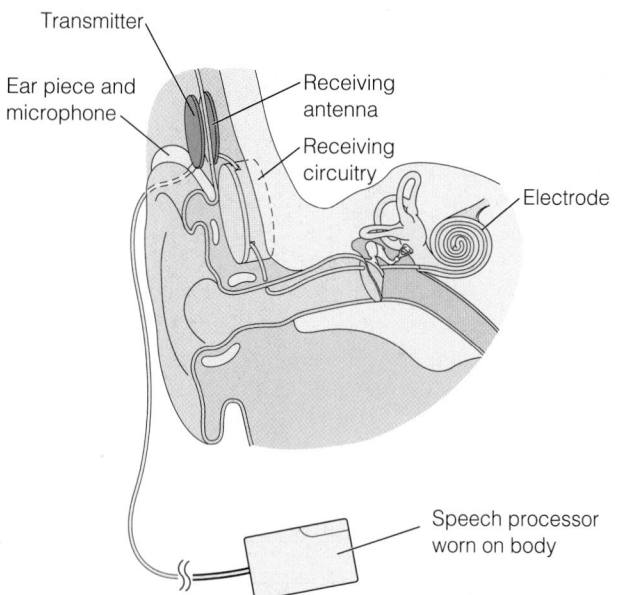

Transmitter

Ear piece and microphone

Receiving antenna

Receiving circuitry

Electrode

Speech processor worn on body

**Figure 45–16** ■ A cochlear implant for sensorineural hearing loss.

## Nursing Diagnoses and Interventions

This section focuses on the problems of having a hearing deficit, impaired communication, and social isolation for the client who is hearing impaired.

### Disturbed Sensory Perception: Auditory

Whether the client's hearing deficit is partial or total, impaired sound perception is the primary problem. The client needs to understand what causes the deficit and what to expect for the future. Nursing interventions focus on maximizing available hearing and preventing further deterioration to the extent possible.

- Encourage to talk about the loss of hearing and its effect on activities of daily living. *Hearing loss affects each individual in a different way. The client may be denying the extent of the deficit or grieving the loss. Listening to the client and providing support encourage the client to develop coping strategies.*
- Provide information about the type of hearing loss. Refer to an audiologist for evaluation of the hearing loss and possible exploration of amplification devices. *With improved understanding of the deficit, the client can plan ways to compensate.*
- Replace batteries in hearing aids regularly and as needed. *Hearing aid batteries last approximately 1 week. If a battery is old or has been improperly stored, the life may be reduced further.*
- If the hearing aid has a toggle switch for microphone/telephone, be sure it is in the appropriate position. *This ensures proper amplification with the hearing aid.*

**PRACTICE ALERT** *Check hearing aids for patency, cleaning out cerumen as necessary.* ■

### Impaired Verbal Communication

A hearing deficit impairs the client's ability to receive and interpret verbal communication. A hearing loss affects the client's ability to follow conversations, use the telephone, and enjoy television or other forms of entertainment.

- Wave the hand or tap the shoulder before beginning to speak.
- When speaking, face the client and keep the hands away from the face.
- Keep your face in full light.
- Reduce the noise in the environment before speaking.
- Use a low voice pitch with normal loudness.
- Use short sentences and pause at the end of each sentence.
- Speak at a normal rate, and do not overarticulate.
- Use facial expressions or gestures.
- Provide a magic slate for written communication.

This prepares the client to receive incoming communication. Hearing-impaired individuals often lip-read, making good visibility of the speaker's face necessary. Excessive environmental noise interferes with the ability to perceive the message. Higher tones are typically lost with presbycusis and other types of hearing loss. Using short sentences and pausing give the client time to interpret the message. Overarticulating

makes it more difficult to follow the flow and to lip-read. Nonverbal cues and written messages enhance the client's understanding.

- Be sure hearing aid is properly placed, is turned on, and has fresh batteries. *The client may not be aware that the hearing aid is not functioning well.*
- Do not place intravenous catheters in the dominant hand. *The client may need to use that hand to write.*
- Rephrase sentences when there is difficulty understanding. *Hearing losses may affect different sound tones, making some words more difficult to comprehend. Using alternative words and phrases may increase the client's ability to perceive the message.*
- Repeat important information. *The nurse makes sure that the client understands the information.*
- Inform other staff about the client's hearing deficit and effective strategies for communication. *Consistent use of effective strategies for communication decreases the client's frustration.*

### Social Isolation

The client with impaired hearing often becomes socially isolated. This isolation may be self-imposed because of the client's difficulty in communicating, especially in a group. Often, however, the isolation comes about gradually and without intention. The client finds social settings such as family dinners or community gatherings increasingly difficult. Friends and family become frustrated trying to communicate with the hearing-impaired person, and invitations to participate in social activities dwindle.

- Identify the extent and cause of the social isolation. Help to differentiate the reality of the isolation and its cause from the client's perception of isolation. *Hearing-impaired clients may be unaware that they are isolated. Identifying factors that contribute to the isolation may provide the impetus the client needs to remedy the hearing loss. Clients may also experience paranoid thinking as a result of the impaired communication and believe that friends and family have purposely begun to avoid interactions.*
- Encourage to interact with friends and family on a one-to-one basis in quiet settings. *Clients with impaired hearing are more successful in understanding conversations that take place in small groups and quiet settings.*
- Treat with dignity and remind friends and family that a hearing deficit does not mean loss of mental faculties. *Inappropriate responses due to a hearing deficit can cause others to perceive the client as "stupid" or demented.*
- Involve in activities that do not require acute hearing, such as checkers and chess. *The client has an opportunity to interact socially without the stress of straining to hear.*
- Obtain a pocket talker or encourage the client and family to do so.
- Refer the client to an audiologist for evaluation and possible hearing-aid fitting.
- Refer to resources such as support groups and senior citizen centers. *These groups provide new social outlets.*

## CHART 45–4   NANDA, NIC, AND NOC LINKAGES

### The Client with a Hearing Loss

| NURSING DIAGNOSES | NURSING INTERVENTIONS | NURSING OUTCOMES |
|---|---|---|
| • Impaired Verbal Communication<br><br>• Social Isolation | • Communication Enhancement: Hearing Deficit<br>• Social Enhancement | • Communication: Receptive Ability<br><br>• Loneliness<br>• Social Involvement<br>• Well-Being |

*Note. Data from* Nursing Outcomes Classification (NOC) *by M. Johnson & M. Maas (Eds.), 1997, St. Louis: Mosby;* Nursing Diagnoses: Definitions & Classification 2001–2002 *by North American Nursing Diagnosis Association, 2001, Philadelphia: NANDA;* Nursing Interventions Classification (NIC) *by J.C. McCloskey & G. M. Bulechek (Eds.), 2000, St. Louis: Mosby. Reprinted by permission.*

## Using NANDA, NIC, and NOC

Chart 45–4 shows links between NANDA nursing diagnoses, NIC, and NOC when caring for the client with a hearing loss.

## Home Care

For the client with a permanent hearing loss, teaching relates to managing the deficit and developing coping strategies. The nurse can refer the client to an audiologist to evaluate the usefulness of a hearing aid. In addition, discuss the following topics as appropriate for each client.

• Use, care, and maintenance of a hearing aid

• Strategies for coping with the hearing deficit
• Voicing a preference for individual visits and small group interactions rather than large social functions
• Helpful resources include the following:
  • American Deafness and Rehabilitation Association
  • International Hearing Dog, Inc.
  • National Association for the Deaf
  • National Institute on Deafness and Other Communication Disorders
  • Self-Help for Hard of Hearing People

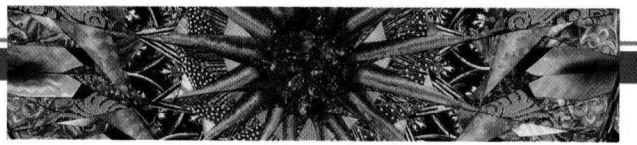

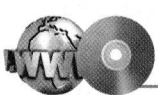 EXPLORE MediaLink

NCLEX review questions, case studies, care plan activities, MediaLink applications, and other interactive resources for this chapter can be found on the Companion Website at www.prenhall.com/lemone.

Click on Chapter 45 to select the activities for this chapter. For animations, video clips, more NCLEX review questions, and an audio glossary, access the Student CD-ROM accompanying this textbook.

## TEST YOURSELF

1. A client complains of decreasing peripheral vision and halos around lights. These manifestations are characteristic of:

   a. Retinal detachment
   b. Open-angle glaucoma
   c. Cataract
   d. Macular degeneration

2. A client with Meniere's disease experiences frequent attacks of vertigo and tinnitus. Of the following teaching points, which one has the highest priority for this client?

   a. Provide instruction about a low-sodium diet
   b. Encourage the client to stop smoking

   c. Instruct the client about antiemetic medications
   d. Teach the client to sit down immediately during an attack

3. A patient with glaucoma also has a history of bradycardia. Which medication should the nurse discuss with the physician before administering it?

   a. Pilocarpine (Isopto Carpine)
   b. Acetazolamide (Diamox)
   c. Timolol (Timoptic)
   d. Epinephrine (Epitrate)

4. During the first 24 hours after eye surgery, what is the rationale for placing the client in a semi-Fowler's position on the unaffected side?

   a. To reduce intraocular pressure in the affected eye
   b. To prevent hemorrhage in the affected eye
   c. To prevent accidental scratching of the cornea
   d. To increase retinal contact with the choroid

5. The nurse should suspect a potential hearing impairment when a client demonstrates which one of the following manifestations:

   a. Speaks in soft tones
   b. Complains of persistent ear ringing
   c. Asks for questions to be repeated
   d. Socially withdraws from group interactions

See Test Yourself answers in Appendix C.

# BIBLIOGRAPHY

Ackley, B. J., & Ladwig, G. B. (2002). *Nursing diagnosis handbook: A guide to planning care* (5th ed.). St. Louis: Mosby.

Andreoli, T. E., Bennett, J. C., Carpenter, C. C. J., & Plum, F. (1997). *Cecil essentials of medicine* (4th ed.). Philadelphia: W. B. Saunders Company.

Barnes, G. (1997). The suitability of cataract patients for day surgery. *Professional Nurse, 12*(4), 264–268.

Braunwald, E., Fauci, A. S., Kasper, D. L., Hauser, S. L., Longo, D. L, & Jameson, J. L. (2001). *Harrison's principles of internal medicine* (15th ed.). New York: McGraw-Hill.

Bullock, B. A. & Henze, R. L. (2000). *Focus on pathophysiology.* Philadelphia: Lippincott.

Coleman, A. L. (1999, November, 20). Glaucoma. *The Lancet, 354,* 1803–1810.

Copstead, L. E. & Banasik, J. L. (2000). *Pathophysiology biological and behavioral perspectives* (2nd ed.). Philadelphia: W. B. Saunders.

Demers, K. (2001). Hearing screening. *Journal of Gerontological Nursing, 27*(11), 8–9.

Duffield, P. (1997). Primary care diagnosis of acute closed-angle glaucoma. A case report. *Advance for Nurse Practitioners, 5*(11), 67.

Elfervig, L. S. (1998). Age-related macular degeneration. *Nurse Practitioner Forum, 9*(1), 4–6.

Eliopoulos, C. (2001). *Gerontological nursing* (5th ed.). Philadelphia: Lippincott.

Galant, J. J. (1997). Differential diagnosis of decreased vision: A case study. *Journal of the American Academy of Nurse Practitioners, 9*(9), 421–425.

Hazzard, W. R., Blass, J. P., Ettinger, W. H., Jr., Halter, J. B., Ouslader, J. G. (Eds.). (1998).

*Principles of geriatric medicine and gerontology* (4th ed.). New York: McGraw-Hill.

Ho-Shing, D. (2000). Treating glaucoma with drainage and pericardial grafts. *AORN, 71*(6), 1237–1251.

Johnson, M., & Maas, M. (Eds.). (2000). *Nursing outcomes classification (NOC).* St. Louis: Mosby.

Jupiter, T., & Spivey, V. (1997). Perception of hearing loss and hearing handicap on hearing aid use by nursing home residents. *Geriatric Nursing, 18*(5), 201–207.

Kupecz, D. (2001). Keeping up with recent ophthalmic drug approvals. *The Nurse Practitioner, 26*(4), 61–62, 64, 67.

McCloskey, J. C., & Bulechek, G. M. (Eds.). (2000). *Nursing interventions classification (NIC)* (3rd ed.). St. Louis: Mosby.

National Institutes of Health, National Eye Institute. (2001). National Eye Institute low vision resource list. Available www.nei.nih.gov/health/lowvision/resources.htm

_____ . (2001). National Eye Institute statement on detection of glaucoma. Available www.nei.nih.gov/nehep/statements.htm

_____ . (2001). National Eye Institute statement on vision screening in adults. Available www. nei.nih.gov/news/statements/visions_task.htm

Ney, D. F. (1993, March/April). Cerumen impaction, ear hygiene practices, and hearing acuity. *Geriatric Nursing, 14,* 70–73.

Norwood-Chapman, L., & Burchfield, S. B. (1999). Nursing home personnel knowledge and attitudes about hearing loss and hearing aids. *Gerontology and Geriatrics Education, 20*(2), 37–47.

Porth, C. M. (2002). Pathophysiology: *Concepts of altered health states* (6th ed.). Philadelphia: Lippincott.

Quillen, D. A. (1999). Common causes of vision loss in elderly patients. *American Family Physician, 60*(1), 99–107.

Ramponi, D. (2000). Go with the flow during an eye emergency. *Nursing 2000, 30*(8), 54–56.

Smith, S. C. (1998). Diabetic retinopathy. *Nurse Practitioner Forum, 9*(1), 13–18.

_____ . (1998). Aging, physiology, and vision. *Nurse Practitioner Forum, 9*(1), 19–22.

Stegbauer, C. C. (2000). Hallucinations in the vision-impaired elderly: The Charles Bonnet syndrome. *The Nurse Practitioner, 25*(8), 74–76.

Stone, C. M. (1999). Preventing cerumen impaction in nursing home residents. *Journal of Gerontological Nursing, 25*(5), 43–45.

Tierney, L. M., McPhee, S. J., & Papadakis, M. A. (Eds.). (2001). *Current medical diagnosis & treatment* (40th ed.). Stamford, CT: Appleton & Lange.

Tigges, B. B. (2000). Acute otitis media and pneumococcal resistance: Making judicious management decisions. *The Nurse Practitioner, 25*(1), 69–79.

Tolson, D., & McIntosh, J. (1997). Listening in the care environment—chaos or clarity for the hearing-impaired elderly person. *International Journal of Nursing Studies, 34*(3), 173–182.

Turkoski, B. B. (2000). Glaucoma and glaucoma medications. *Orthopaedic Nursing, 19*(5), 71–76.

Way, L. W., & Doherty, G. M. (2003). *Current surgical diagnosis & treatment* (11 th ed.) New York. McGraw-Hill.

Wingate, S. (1999). Treating corneal abrasions. *The Nurse Practitioner, 24*(6), 53–54, 57, 60, 65–66, 68.

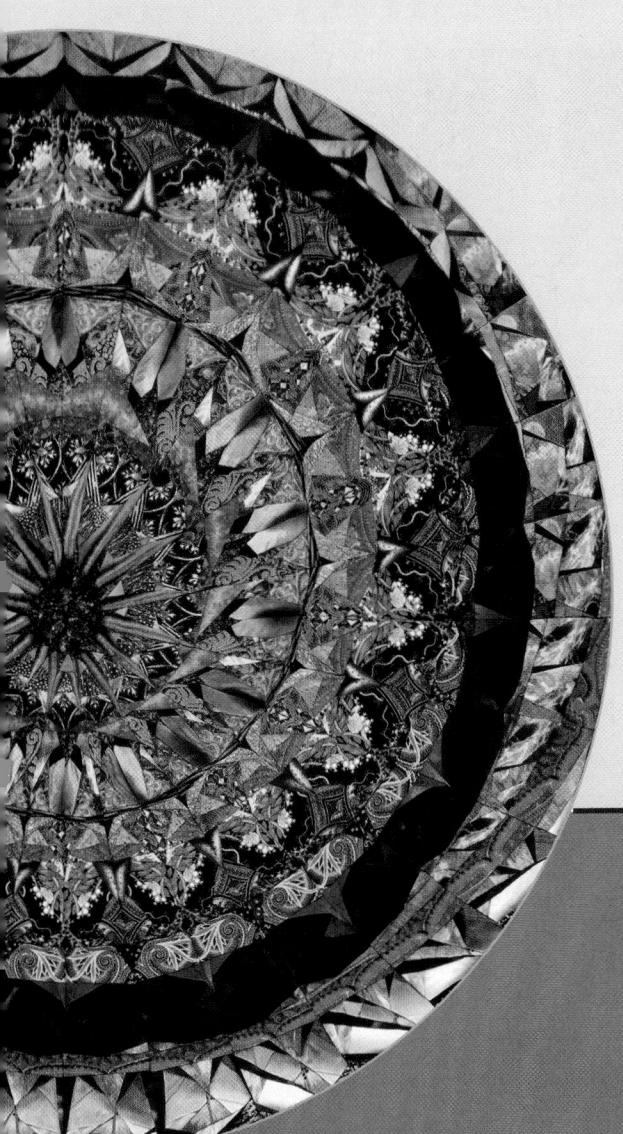

# SEXUALITY AND REPRODUCTIVE PATTERNS

**Unit 14**
**Responses to Altered Sexual and Reproductive Function**

# Functional Health Patterns with Related Nursing Diagnosis

### HEALTH PERCEPTION – HEALTH MANAGEMENT
- Perceived health status
- Perceived health management
- Health care behaviors: health promotion and illness prevention activities, medical treatments, follow-up care

### VALUE-BELIEF
- Values, goals, or beliefs (including spirituality) that guide choices or decisions
- Perceived conflicts in values, beliefs, or expectations that are health related

### COPING-STRESS-TOLERANCE
- Capacity to resist challenges to self-integrity
- Methods of handling stress
- Support systems
- Perceived ability to control and manage situations

### NUTRITIONAL-METABOLIC
- Daily consumption of food and fluids
- Favorite foods
- Use of dietary supplements
- Skin lesions and ability to heal
- Condition of the integument
- Weight, height, temperature

### Part 6
Sexuality-Reproductive Patterns
NANDA Nursing Diagnoses

- Rape-Trauma Syndrome
- Sexual Dysfunction
- Ineffective Sexuality Patterns

### SEXUALITY-REPRODUCTIVE
- Satisfaction with sexuality or sexual relationships
- Reproductive pattern
- Female menstrual and perimeno-pausal history

### ELIMINATION
- Patterns of bowel and urinary excretion
- Perceived regularity or irregularity of elimination
- Use of laxatives or routines
- Changes in time, modes, quality or quantity of excretions
- Use of devices for control

### ROLE-RELATIONSHIP
- Perception of major roles, relationships, and responsibilities in current life situation
- Satisfaction with or disturbances in roles and relationships

### ACTIVITY-EXERCISE
- Patterns of personally relevant exercise, activity, leisure, and recreation
- ADLs which require energy expenditure
- Factors that interfere with the desired pattern (e.g., illness or injury)

### SELF-PERCEPTION–SELF-CONCEPT
- Attitudes about self
- Perceived abilities, worth, self-image, emotions
- Body posture and movement, eye contact, voice and speech patterns

### SLEEP-REST
- Patterns of sleep and rest-/relaxation in a 24-hr period
- Perceptions of quality and quantity of sleep and rest
- Use of sleep aids and routines

### COGNITIVE-PERCEPTUAL
- Adequacy of vision, hearing, taste, touch, smell
- Pain perception and management
- Language, judgment, memory, decisions

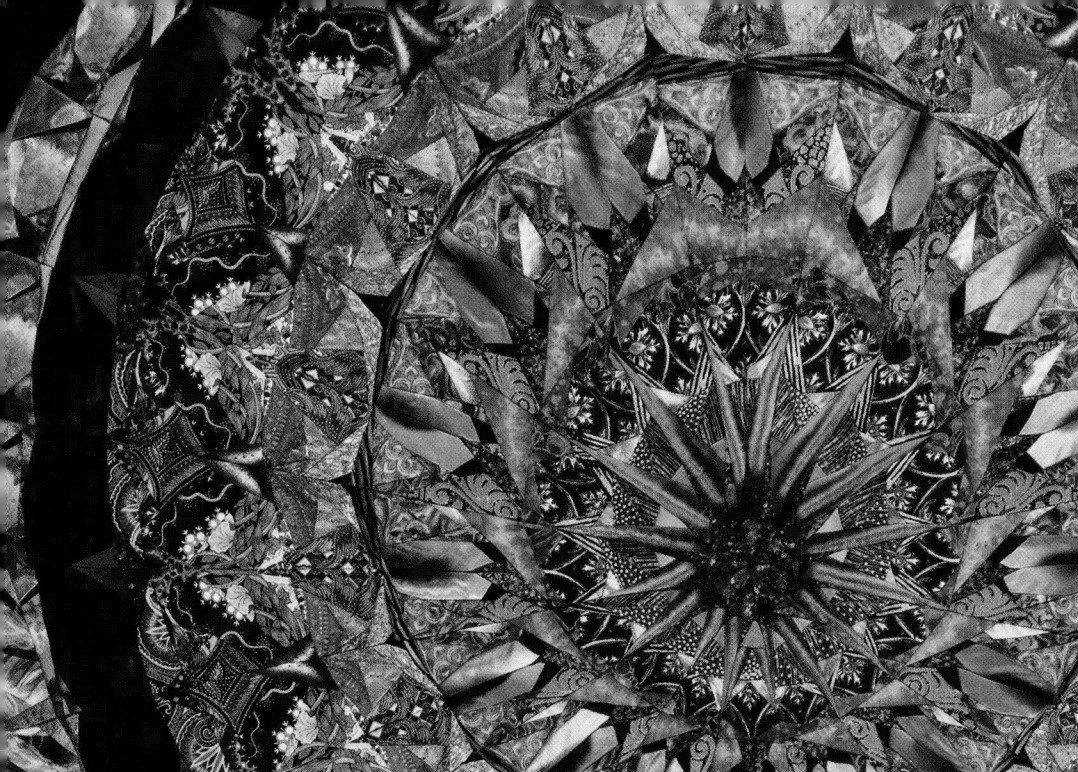

# RESPONSES TO ALTERED SEXUAL AND REPRODUCTIVE FUNCTION

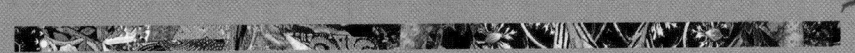

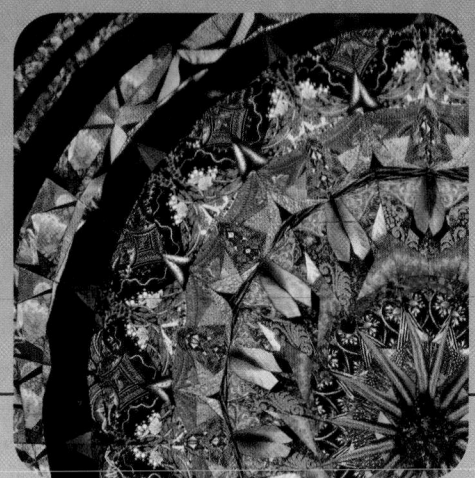

# Assessing Clients with Reproductive System Disorders

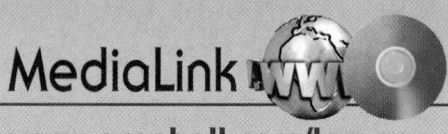

## MediaLink

**www.prenhall.com/lemone**

Additional resources for this chapter can be found on the Student CD-ROM accompanying this textbook, and on the Companion Website at www. prenhall.com/lemone. Click on Chapter 46 to select the activities for this chapter.

**CD-ROM**
- Audio Glossary
- NCLEX Review

*Animations*
- Female Reproductive System
- Male Reproductive System

**Companion Website**
- More NCLEX Review
- Functional Health Pattern Assessment
- Case Study
  Irregular Menstrual Cycle

## LEARNING OUTCOMES

After completing this chapter, you will be able to:

- Review the anatomy and physiology of the male and female reproductive systems.

- Explain the functions of the male and female sex hormones.

- Identify specific topics for consideration during a health history interview of the client with health problems involving reproductive function.

- Describe techniques for physical assessment of male and female reproductive function.

- Identify abnormal findings that may indicate impairment in reproductive function in men and women.

Although the reproductive organs in men and women are very different, they do share common functions: enabling sexual pleasure and reproduction. The reproductive organs, in conjunction with the neuroendocrine system, produce hormones important in biologic development and sexual behavior. Parts of the reproductive organs also enclose and are integral to the function of the urinary system. The assessment of the reproductive and urinary systems is often difficult for both the beginning nurse and the client and requires skill on the part of the nurse when asking questions about sensitive topics that the client may be hesitant to talk about. Skill in conducting physical examinations of an area of the body usually considered private is also required. This chapter discusses the assessment of the reproductive system for both men and women.

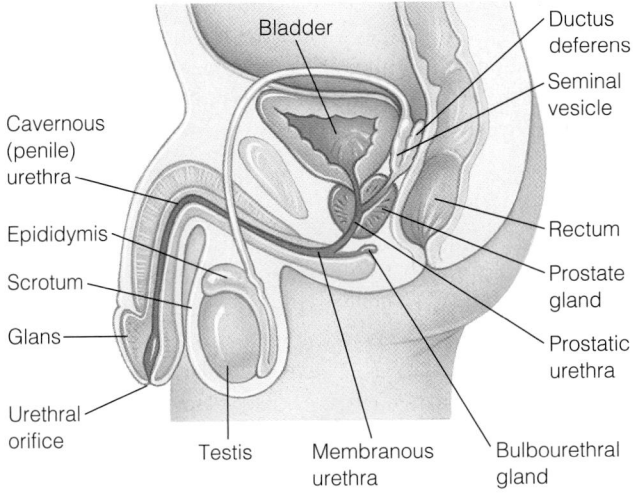

**Figure 46–1** ■ The male reproductive system.

# REVIEW OF ANATOMY AND PHYSIOLOGY

## The Male Reproductive System

The male reproductive system consists of the paired testes, the scrotum, ducts, glands, and penis (Figure 46–1 ■). The location and function of the male reproductive organs are summarized in Table 46–1.

### The Testes

The testes develop in the abdominal cavity of the fetus and then descend through the inguinal canal into the scrotum. They are homologous to the female's ovaries. These paired organs are each about 1.5 inches (4 cm) long and 1 inch (2.5 cm) in diameter. They are suspended in the scrotum by the spermatic cord. Each is surrounded by two coverings: an outer tunica vaginalis and an inner tunica albuginea. Each testis is divided into 250 to 300 lobules, with each lobule containing one to four seminiferous tubules. The testes produce sperm and testosterone.

The seminiferous tubules are responsible for sperm production. Leydig's cells (or interstitial cells) lie in the connective tissue surrounding the seminiferous tubules. They produce testosterone.

### The Ducts and Semen

The seminiferous tubules lead into the efferent ducts and become the rete testis. From the rete testis, 10,000 to 20,000 efferent ducts join the epididymis, a long coiled tube that lies over the outer surface of each testis. The epididymis is the final area for the storage and maturation of sperm. When a man is sexually excited, the epididymis contracts to propel the sperm through the vas deferens to the ampulla, where they are stored until ejaculation.

MediaLink | MALE REPRODUCTIVE SYSTEM ANIMATION

## TABLE 46–1   Location and Function of the Male Reproductive Organs

| Male Reproductive Organ | Location | Function |
|---|---|---|
| Scrotum | Hangs from body at root of penis. | Contains testes, epididymis, and portions of the vas (ductus) deferens. |
| Testes | In the scrotal sac. | Produce sperm and testosterone. |
| Epididymis | Posterolateral to upper aspect of each testis. | Stores sperm. Promotes sperm maturation. Transports sperm to vas deferens. |
| Vas deferens (ductus deferens) | Between the epididymis and the seminal vesicle forming the ejaculatory duct. | Stores sperm. Transports sperm. |
| Penis | Attached to front and sides of the pubic arch. Proximal, ventral surface is directly continuous with the scrotum. | Excretes semen and urine. Deposits sperm in female reproductive tract. |
| Urethra | Begins at bladder and passes through prostate and penis. | Serves as passageway for urine or semen. |
| Prostate gland | Encircles the urethra at the neck of the bladder. | Contributes to ejaculatory volume. Enhances sperm motility and fertility. |
| Seminal vesicles | Lie on posterior bladder wall. | Contribute to ejaculatory volume. Contain nutrients to sustain sperm and prostaglandins to facilitate sperm motility. |
| Bulbourethral (Cowper's) glands | Inferior to the prostate. | Secrete mucus into urethra. Neutralize traces of acidic urine in the urethra. |

The seminal vesicles at the base of the bladder produce about 60% of the volume of seminal fluid. Seminal fluid is also made of secretions from the accessory sex organs, the epididymis, the prostate gland, and Cowper's glands. Seminal fluid nourishes the sperm, provides bulk, and increases its alkalinity. (An alkaline pH is essential to mobilize the sperm and ensure fertilization of the ova.) Sperm mixed with this fluid is called semen. Each seminal vesicle joins its corresponding vas deferens to form an ejaculatory duct, which enters the prostatic urethra. During ejaculation, seminal fluid mixes with sperm at the ejaculatory duct and enters the urethra for expulsion.

The total amount of semen ejaculated is 2 to 4 mL, although the amount varies. The sperm count of the total ejaculate of a healthy male is from 100 to 400 million.

## The Scrotum

The scrotum is a sac or pouch made of two layers. The outer layer is continuous with the skin of the perineum and thighs. The inner layer is made of muscle and fascia. The scrotum hangs at the base of the penis, anterior to the anus, and regulates the temperature of the testes. The optimum temperature for sperm production is about 2 to 3 degrees below body temperature. When the testicular temperature is too low, the scrotum contracts to bring the testes up against the body. When the testicular temperature is too high, the scrotum relaxes to allow the testes to lie further away from the body.

## The Prostate Gland

The prostate gland is about the size of a walnut. It encircles the urethra just below the urinary bladder (see Figure 46–1). It is made of 20 to 30 tuboloalveolar glands surrounded by smooth muscle. Secretions of the prostate gland make up about one-third of the volume of the semen. These secretions enter the urethra through several ducts during ejaculation.

## The Penis

The penis is the genital organ that encloses the urethra (see Figure 46–1). It is homologous to the clitoris of the female. The penis is composed of a shaft and a tip called the glans, which is covered in the uncircumcised man by the foreskin (or prepuce). The shaft contains three columns of erectile tissue: The two lateral columns are called the corpora cavernosa, and the central mass is called the corpus spongiosum.

Erection occurs when the penile masses become filled with blood in response to a reflex that triggers the parasympathetic nervous system to stimulate arteriolar vasodilation. The erection reflex may be initiated by touch, pressure, sights, sounds, smells, or thoughts of a sexual encounter. After ejaculation, the arterioles vasoconstrict, and the penis becomes flaccid.

## Spermatogenesis

Spermatogenesis is the series of physiologic events that generate sperm in the seminiferous tubules. This process begins with puberty and continues throughout a man's life, with several hundred million sperm produced each day.

The inner layer of the seminiferous tubules consists of sustentacular cells (or Sertoli's cells), which contain the spermatocytes and sperm in different stages of development. Sertoli's cells secrete a nourishing fluid for the developing sperm, as well as enzymes that help convert spermatocytes to sperm. The events in spermatogenesis, which takes 64 to 72 days, are as follows:

1. The spermatogonia (sperm stem cells) undergo rapid mitotic division. As these cells multiply, the more mature spermatogonia divide into two daughter cells. These daughter cells grow and become the primary spermatocytes (and eventually become sperm).
2. Primary spermatocytes divide by meiosis to form two smaller secondary spermatocytes, which in turn divide to form two spermatids. This process occurs over several weeks.
3. The spermatids elongate into a mature sperm cell with a head and a tail. The head contains enzymes essential to the penetration and fertilization of the ova. The flagellar motion of the tail allows the sperm to move. The sperm cells then move to the epididymis to mature further and develop motility.

## Male Sex Hormones

The male sex hormones are called androgens. Most androgens are produced in the testes, although the adrenal cortex also produces a small amount. Testosterone, the primary androgen produced by the testes, is essential for the development and maintenance of sexual organs and secondary sex characteristics, and for spermatogenesis. It also promotes metabolism, growth of muscles and bone, and libido (sexual desire).

# The Female Reproductive System

The female reproductive system consists of the paired ovaries and fallopian tubes, uterus, vagina, mons pubis, labia majora, labia minora, and clitoris. The breasts are also a part of women's reproductive organs. In women, the urethra and urinary meatus are separated from the reproductive organs; however, they are in such close proximity that a health problem with one often affects the other. The location and function of the female reproductive organs are summarized in Table 46–2.

## The Internal Structures

The ovaries, fallopian tubes, uterus, and vagina make up the internal organs of the female reproductive system (Figure 46–2 ■). The ovaries are the primary reproductive organs in women and also produce female sex hormones. The fallopian tubes, uterus, and vagina serve as accessory ducts for the ovaries and a developing fetus.

***THE VAGINA.*** The vagina is a fibromuscular tube about 3 to 4 inches (8 to 10 cm) in length located posterior to the bladder and urethra and anterior to the rectum. The upper end contains the uterine cervix in an area called the fornix. The walls of the vagina are membranes that form folds, called rugae. These membranes are composed of mucus-secreting stratified squamous epithelial cells. The vagina serves as a route for the excretion of secretions, including menstrual fluid, and also is an organ of sexual response.

## TABLE 46–2  Location and Function of the Female Reproductive Organs

| Female Reproductive Organ | Location | Function |
|---|---|---|
| Mons pubis (mons veneris) | Anterior and superior to the pubis. | Enhances sexual sensations.<br>Protects and cushions pubic symphysis during intercourse. |
| Labia majora | Extend from mons pubis to perineum. | Protect labia minora, urethral and vaginal openings.<br>Enhance sexual arousal. |
| Labia minora | Enclosed by the labia majora. | Protect clitoris.<br>Inferiorly, merge to form posterior ring of vaginal introitus (fourchette).<br>Lubricate vulva.<br>Enhance sexual arousal. |
| Vestibule | Area enclosed by labia minora. | Contains openings for urethra, vagina, Bartholin's glands, and Skene's glands. |
| Bartholin's (greater vestibular) glands | Posterior on each side of the vaginal orifice. Open onto the sides of the vestibule in the groove between the labia minora and hymen. | Secrete clear, viscid mucus during intercourse. |
| Skene's (lesser vestibular, paraurethral) glands | Open onto the vestibule on each side of the urethra. | Drain urethral glands.<br>Produce lubricating mucus. |
| Clitoris | Small bud of erectile tissue just below the superior joining of the labia minora. | Stimulates and elevates levels of sexual arousal. |
| Perineum | Skin-covered muscular area between vaginal opening and anus. | Provides support for pelvic organs. |
| Mammary glands | Contained within breasts. Anterior to pectoral muscles of thorax. | Produce human milk.<br>Play a role in sexual arousal. |
| Ovaries | Lie on each side of the uterus below and behind the uterine tubes. | Produce and secrete ova.<br>Produce the hormones estrogen and progesterone. |
| Fallopian tubes (uterine tubes, oviducts) | One tube extends medially from the area of each ovary and empties into the upper portion (fundus) of the uterus. | Transport ova. |
| Uterus (adnexa of the uterus are composed of the uterine tubes and ovaries) | Anterior to the rectum and posterior/superior to the bladder. | Receives, retains, and nourishes the fertilized ovum.<br>Contracts rhythmically to expel infant. Cyclically sheds lining when ovum is not fertilized. |
| Cervix | Lower portion of uterus extending into the vagina. | Connects uterine cavity with vagina.<br>Opens to allow passage of menstrual flow and infant. |
| Vagina | Extends from the external orifice in the vestibule to the cervix. | Receives penis and semen during intercourse.<br>Passageway for menstrual flow and expulsion of infant at birth. |

The walls of the vagina are usually moist and maintain a pH ranging from 3.8 to 4.2. This pH is bacteriostatic and is maintained by the action of estrogen and normal vaginal flora. Estrogen stimulates the growth of vaginal mucosal cells so that they thicken and have increased glycogen content. The glycogen is fermented to lactic acid by Döderlein's bacilli (lactobacilli that normally inhabit the vagina), slightly acidifying the vaginal fluid.

**THE UTERUS.**  The uterus is a hollow pear-shaped muscular organ with thick walls located between the bladder and the rectum. It has three parts: the fundus, the body, and the cervix. It is supported in the abdominal cavity by the broad ligaments, the round ligaments, the uterosacral ligaments, and the transverse cervical ligaments. The uterus receives the fertilized ovum and provides a site for growth and development of the fetus.

The uterine wall has three layers. The *perimetrium* is the outer serous layer that merges with the peritoneum. The *myometrium* is the middle layer and makes up most of the uterine wall. This layer has muscle fibers that run in various directions, allowing contractions during **menstruation** (the periodic shedding of the uterine lining in a woman of childbearing age who is not pregnant) or childbirth and expansion as the fetus grows. The *endometrium* lines the uterus. Its outermost layer is shed during menstruation.

The cervix projects into the vagina and forms a pathway between the uterus and the vagina. The uterine opening of the cervix is called the internal os; the vaginal opening is called the

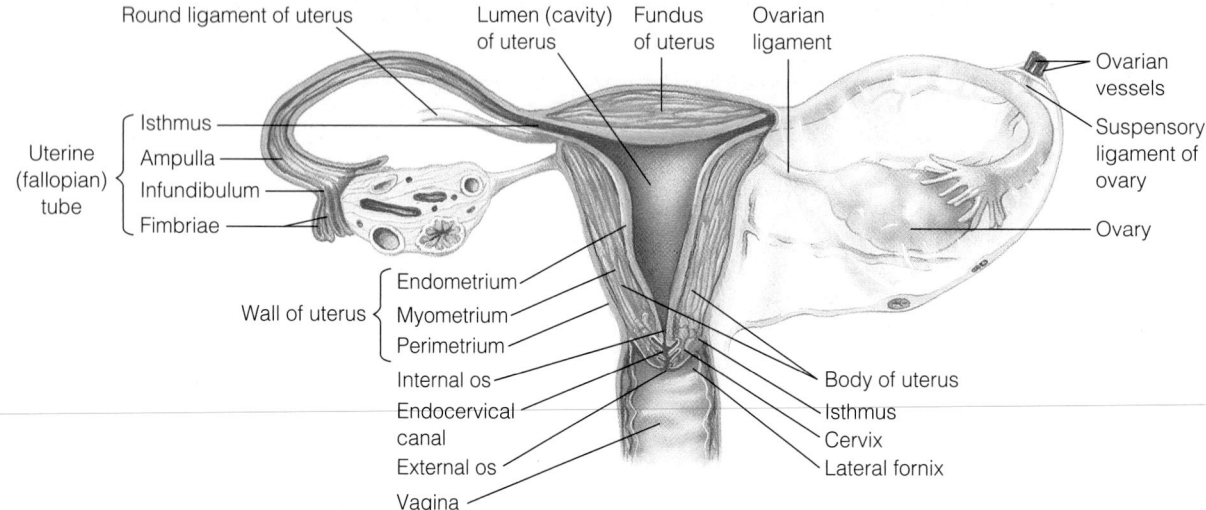

**Figure 46–2** ■ The internal organs of the female reproductive system.

external os. The space between these openings, the endocervical canal, serves as a route for the discharge of menstrual fluid and the entrance for sperm. The cervix is a firm structure that softens in response to hormones during pregnancy. It is protected by mucus that changes consistency and quantity during the menstrual cycle and during pregnancy.

**THE FALLOPIAN TUBES.**   The fallopian tubes are thin cylindrical structures about 4 inches (10 cm) long and 2.5 inches (1 cm) in diameter. They are attached to the uterus on one end and are supported by the broad ligaments. The lateral ends of the uterine tubes are open and made of projections called *fimbriae* that drape over the ovary. The fimbriae pick up the ovum after it is discharged from the ovary.

The fallopian tubes, made of smooth muscle, are lined with ciliated, mucus-producing epithelial cells. The movement of the cilia and contractions of the smooth muscle move the ovum through the tubes toward the uterus. Fertilization of the ovum by the sperm usually occurs in the outer portion of a fallopian tube.

**THE OVARIES.**   The ovaries in the adult woman are flat, almond-shaped structures located on either side of the uterus below the ends of the fallopian tubes. They are homologous to the male's testes. They are attached to the uterus by a ligament and are also attached to the broad ligament. The ovaries store the female germ cells and produce the female hormones *estrogen* and *progesterone*. A woman's total number of ova is present at birth.

Each ovary is divided into a medulla and a cortex. It contains many small structures called ovarian follicles. Each follicle contains an immature ovum, called an oocyte. Each month, several follicles are stimulated by follicle-stimulating hormone (FSH) and luteinizing hormone (LH) to mature. The developing follicles are surrounded by layers of follicle cells, with the mature follicles called graafian follicles. The graafian follicles produce estrogen, which stimulates the development of endometrium. Each month in the menstruating

woman, one or two of the mature follicles ejects an oocyte in a process called ovulation. The ruptured follicle then becomes a structure called the corpus luteum. The corpus luteum produces both estrogen and progesterone to support the endometrium until conception occurs or the cycle begins again. The corpus luteum slowly degenerates, leaving a scar on the surface of the ovary.

## The External Structures

The external genitalia collectively are called the vulva. They include the mons pubis, the labia, the clitoris, the vaginal and urethral openings, and glands (Figure 46–3 ■).

The mons pubis is a pad of adipose (fat) tissue covered with skin. It lies anterior to the symphysis pubis. After puberty, the mons is covered with hair with a diamond-shaped distribution.

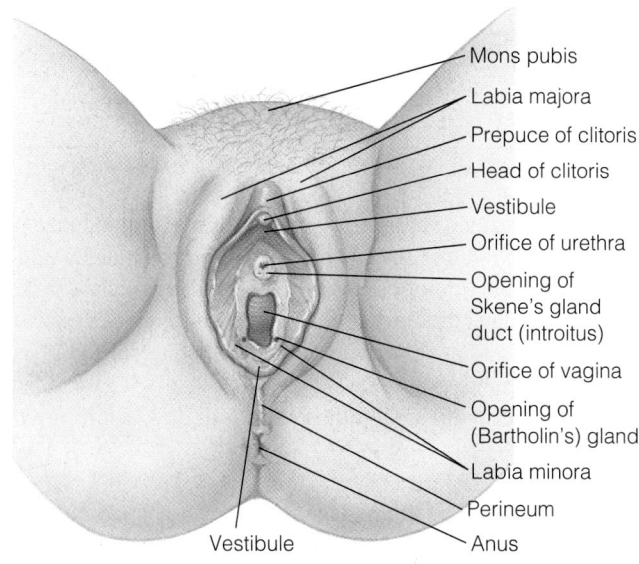

**Figure 46–3** ■ The external organs of the female reproductive system.

The labia are divided into two structures. The *labia majora,* folds of skin and adipose tissue covered with hair, are outermost; they begin at the base of the mons pubis and end at the anus. The *labia minora,* located between the clitoris and the base of the vagina, are enclosed by the labia majora. They are made of skin, adipose tissue, and some erectile tissues. They are usually light pink and hairless.

The area between the labia is called the vestibule, and contains the openings for the vagina and the urethra as well as the Bartholin's glands. Skene's glands open onto the vestibule on each side of the urethra. Bartholin's and Skene's glands secrete lubricating fluid during the sexual response cycle.

The clitoris is an erectile organ analogous to the penis in the male. It is formed by the joining of the labia minora. Like the penis, it is highly sensitive and distends during sexual arousal.

The vaginal opening, called the introitus, is the opening between the internal and the external genitals. The introitus is surrounded by a connective tissue membrane called the hymen, which determines the size and shape of the opening.

### The Breasts

The breasts (or mammary glands) are located between the third and seventh ribs on the anterior chest wall. They are supported by the pectoral muscles and are richly supplied with nerves, blood, and lymph (Figure 46–4 ■). A pigmented area called the areola is located slightly below the center of each breast and contains sebaceous glands and a nipple. The nipple is usually protrusive and becomes erect in response to cold and stimulation. The primary purpose of the breasts is to supply nourishment for the infant.

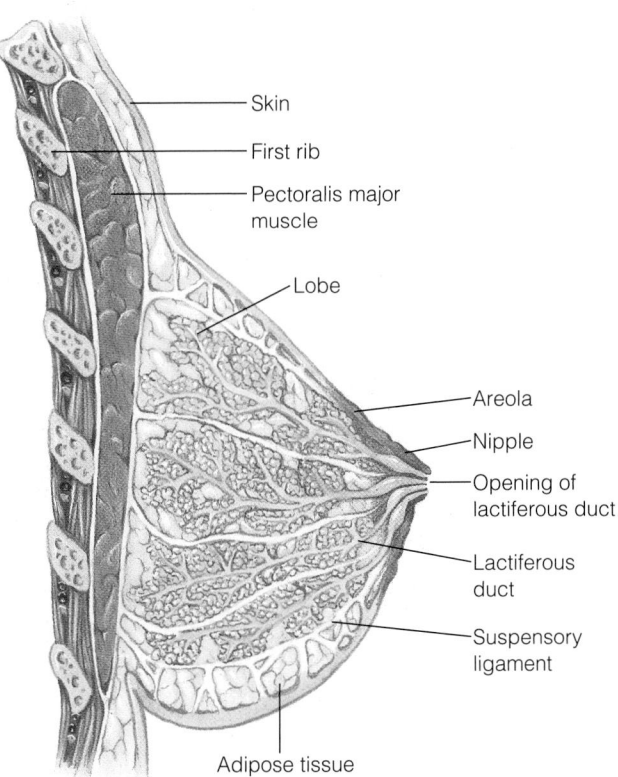

Labels: Skin; First rib; Pectoralis major muscle; Lobe; Areola; Nipple; Opening of lactiferous duct; Lactiferous duct; Suspensory ligament; Adipose tissue

**Figure 46–4 ■** Structure of the female breast.

The breasts are made of adipose tissue, fibrous connective tissue, and glandular tissue. Cooper's ligaments support the breast and extend from the outer breast tissue to the nipple, dividing the breast into 15 to 25 lobes. Each lobe is made of alveolar glands connected by ducts which open to the nipple.

### Female Sex Hormones

The ovaries produce estrogens, progesterone, and androgens in a cyclic pattern. Estrogens are steroid hormones that occur naturally in three forms: estrone ($E_1$), estradiol ($E_2$), and estriol ($E_3$). Estradiol is the most potent and is the form secreted in greatest amount by the ovaries. Although estrogens are secreted throughout the menstrual cycle, they are at a higher level during certain phases of the cycle, discussed shortly.

Estrogens are essential for the development and maintenance of secondary sex characteristics; and in conjunction with other hormones, they stimulate the female reproductive organs to prepare for growth of a fetus. Estrogens are responsible for the normal structure of skin and blood vessels. They also decrease the rate of bone resorption, promote increased high-density lipoproteins, reduce cholesterol levels, and enhance the clotting of blood. Estrogens also promote the retention of sodium and water.

Progesterone primarily affects the development of breast glandular tissue and the endometrium. During pregnancy, progesterone relaxes smooth muscle to decrease uterine contractions. It also increases body temperature. Androgens are responsible for normal hair growth patterns at puberty and may also have metabolic effects.

### Oogenesis and the Ovarian Cycle

All of a woman's ova are present as primary oocytes in primordial ovarian follicles at her birth. Each month from puberty until menopause, the remaining events of oogenesis, the production of ova, occur. Collectively, these events are known as the ovarian cycle.

The ovarian cycle has three consecutive phases that occur cyclically each 28 days (although the cycle normally may be longer or shorter). The *follicular phase* lasts from the 1st to the 10th day of the cycle; the *ovulatory phase* lasts from the 11th to the 14th day of the cycle and ends with ovulation; and the *luteal phase* lasts from the 14th to the 28th days.

During the follicular phase, the follicle develops and the oocyte matures. These processes are controlled by the interaction of FSH and LH. On day 1 of the cycle, gonadotropin-releasing hormone (GnRH) from the hypothalamus increases and stimulates increased production of FSH and LH by the anterior pituitary. FSH and LH stimulate follicular growth, and the oocyte increases in size. The structure, now called the primary follicle, becomes a multicellular mass surrounded by a fibrous capsule, the theca folliculi. As the follicle continues to increase in size, estrogen is produced and a fluid-filled space (the antrum) forms within the follicle. The oocyte is enclosed by a membrane, the zona pellucida. By about day 10, the follicle is a mature graafian follicle and bulges out from the surface of the ovary. There are always follicles at different stages of development in each ovary, but usually only one follicle becomes dominant and matures to ovulation, while the others degenerate.

The ovulatory phase begins when estrogen levels reach a level high enough to stimulate the anterior pituitary, and a surge of LH is produced. The LH stimulates meiosis in the developing oocyte, and its first meiotic division occurs. The LH also stimulates enzymes that act on the bulging ovarian wall, causing it to rupture and discharge the antrum fluid and the oocyte. The oocyte is expelled from the mature ovarian follicle in the process called ovulation.

During the luteal phase, the surge in LH also stimulates the ruptured follicle to change into a corpus luteum and then stimulates the corpus luteum to begin immediately to produce progesterone and estrogen. The increase of progesterone and estrogen in the blood has a negative feedback effect on the production of LH, inhibiting the further growth and development of other follicles.

If pregnancy does not occur, the corpus luteum begins to degenerate, and its hormone production ceases. The declining production of progesterone and estrogen at the end of the cycle allows the secretion of LH and FSH to increase, and a new cycle begins. The ovarian cycle is compared to the menstrual cycle in Figure 46–5 ■.

## The Menstrual Cycle

The endometrium of the uterus responds to changes in estrogen and progesterone during the ovarian cycle to prepare for implantation of the fertilized embryo. The endometrium is receptive to implantation of the embryo for only a brief period each month, coinciding with the time when the embryo would normally reach the uterus from the uterine tube (usually 7 days).

The cycle begins with the *menstrual phase,* lasting from days 1 to 5. The inner endometrial (functionalis) layer detaches and is expelled as menstrual fluid (fluid and blood) for 3 to 5 days. As the maturing follicle begins to produce estrogen (days 6 to 14), the proliferative phase begins. In response, the functionalis layer is repaired and thickens, while spiral arteries increase in number and tubular glands form. Cervical mucus changes to a thin, crystalline substance, forming channels to help the sperm move up into the uterus.

The final phase, lasting from days 14 to 28, is the secretory phase. As the corpus luteum produces progesterone, the rising levels act on the endometrium, causing increased vascularity, changing the inner layer to secretory mucosa, stimulating the secretion of glycogen into the uterine cavity, and causing the cervical mucus again to become thick and block the internal os. If fertilization does not occur, hormone levels fall. Spasm of the spiral arteries causes hypoxia of the endometrial cells, which begin to degenerate and slough off. As with the ovarian cycle, the process begins again with the sloughing of the functionalis layer.

## ASSESSING REPRODUCTIVE FUNCTION

The function of the reproductive systems in men and women is assessed both by a health assessment interview to collect subjective data and a physical assessment to collect objective data. When assessing the male or female reproductive systems, consider the psychologic, social, and cultural factors that affect

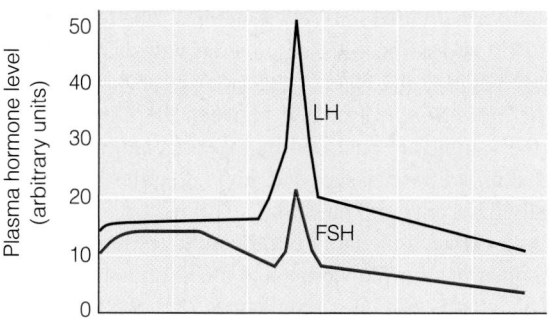

A Fluctuation of gonadotropin levels

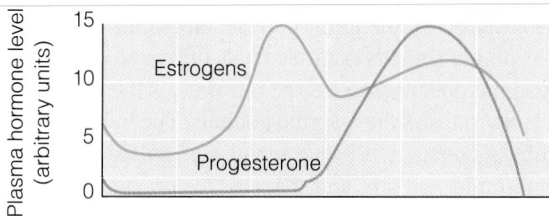

B Fluctuation of ovarian hormone levels

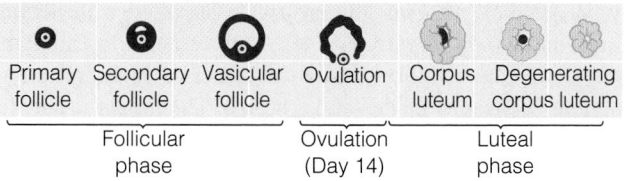

C Ovarian cycle

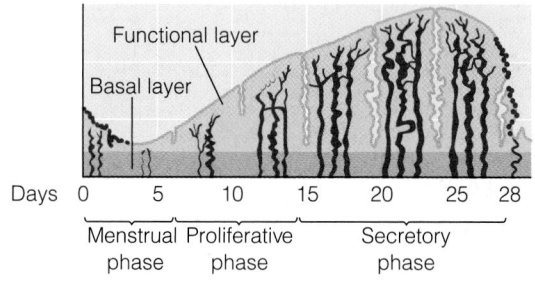

D Uterine cycle

**Figure 46–5 ■** Comparison of the ovarian and uterine cycles. *A,* Fluctuating levels of follicle-stimulating hormone (FSH) and luteinizing hormone (LH), the pituitary gonadotropins regulating the ovarian cycle. *B,* Fluctuating levels of ovarian hormones that cause endometrial changes during the uterine cycle. *C,* Changes in the ovarian follicles during the 28-day ovarian cycle. *D,* Corresponding changes in the endometrium during the uterine cycle.

sexual activity and sexuality. Use words that the client understands, and do not be embarrassed by the client's terminology. The client may perceive the interview as less threatening if the discussion begins with more general questions and then progresses to questions specific to the reproductive system. For example, first ask a female client about menstrual and childbirth histories before asking questions about sexually transmitted diseases. Interview questions are also less threatening if they are asked in a way that gives the client permission to report behaviors and manifestations. For example, rather than asking a man if he has difficulty achieving or maintaining an erection, ask him to describe any changes he has noticed in having an erection.

## Health Assessment Interview for Men

The health assessment for the male reproductive system is often a part of the assessment of the urinary system (see Chapter 25). ⊕ Before asking questions about sexual history, explain that this information is part of a general health assessment. If a health problem is identified, collect information specific to its onset, characteristics, duration, frequency, precipitating or relieving factors, treatment and/or self-care, and outcome. For example, ask the client:

- When did you first notice that you were having difficulty urinating?
- Did you use a different brand of condoms before you noticed the rash on your penis?
- Describe the changes that occurred in your ability to have an erection after you started taking medicine for high blood pressure.

In questioning the client about past medical history, ask about chronic illnesses such as diabetes, chronic renal failure, cardiovascular disease, multiple sclerosis, spinal cord tumors or trauma, or thyroid disease. The effects of these illnesses as well as the treatment of the illnesses may cause **impotence** (inability to achieve or maintain an erection). The following drugs may cause sexual function problems: antihypertensives, antidepressants, antispasmodics, tranquilizers, sedatives, and histamine$_2$-receptor antagonists. Psychosocial stressors also may contribute to impotence.

If the man was born to a woman treated during pregnancy with diethylstilbestrol (DES), a drug used in the 1940s and 1950s to prevent miscarriage, he may have congenital deformities of the urinary tract as well as decreased semen levels. If the man had mumps as a child, sterility is possible. The risk for testicular cancer is greatest in men who have a history of an undescended testicle, an inguinal hernia, testicular swelling with mumps, a history of maternal use of DES or oral contraceptives, and a family history of testicular cancer.

Explore the lifestyle and social history of the man; the use of alcohol, cigarettes, or street drugs may affect sexual function. Frequent sexual intercourse, especially if unprotected, increases the potential for sexually transmitted diseases including HIV infection. Sexual intercourse with same-sex partners further increases the risk for HIV infection. Other questions about sexuality may include number of sexual partners; history of premature ejaculation, impotence, or other sexual problems; any history of sexual trauma; use of condoms or other contraceptives; and current level of sexual satisfaction.

Specific questions and leading statements, categorized by functional health patterns, can be found on the Companion Website.

## Health Assessment Interview for Women

The focused interview for the female reproductive system is usually extensive. However, the questions may in many instances be tailored to the specific health problem of the client. As with the assessment of other body systems, analyze and document the onset of the problem, its duration, frequency, precipitating and relieving factors, any associated symptoms, treatment, self-care, and outcome. For example, ask the client:

- Did you notice that you had increased vaginal bleeding after intercourse?
- Does the over-the-counter medication relieve the vaginal itching and discharge?
- Have you had any fever or abdominal pain with this vaginal infection?

Ask about menstrual history, obstetric history, use of contraceptives, sexual history, use of medications, and reproductive system examinations. Also assess the use of condoms during intercourse; unprotected sexual intercourse increases the risk of sexually transmitted diseases, including HIV infection. Also ask about smoking; a history of smoking increases the risk of circulatory problems in the woman taking oral contraceptives. Smoking also increases the risk for cancer of the cervix.

Chronic illnesses may affect the function of the female reproductive system. Diabetes increases the risk of vaginal infections and vaginal dryness, both of which interfere with sexual pleasure. Chronic heavy menstrual flow may result in anemia. Thyroid and adrenal disorders may affect secondary sex characteristics, the menstrual cycle, and the ability to become pregnant.

Obtaining any family history of cancer is important. The risk for endometrial cancer is higher in women with a family history of endometrial, breast, or colon cancer; the risk for ovarian cancer is higher in women with a family history of ovarian or breast cancer; and the risk for breast cancer is higher in women with a family history of breast cancer. Exposure to diethylstilbestrol (DES) in utero increases the risk of cancer of the cervix and vagina. Exposure to asbestos poses a risk of cancer of the ovary. The risk for breast cancer is also greater if the client has a history of fibrocystic disease.

Carefully explore any history of vaginal bleeding and vaginal discharge. Ask about the onset of vaginal bleeding, any related factors, the color (pink, red, dark red, brown), the character (thin, watery, presence of mucus, size and number of clots), the amount (spotting, how many pads or tampons in a specific amount of time) and relationship to menstrual cycle. Regarding vaginal discharge, ask about the onset, color (white, green, gray), character (thin, curdlike, infected), odor, itching, and rash.

Questions about sexuality may include number of sexual partners; history of **anorgasmia** (absence of orgasm), **dyspareunia** (painful intercourse), or other problems; history of sexual trauma; use of condoms or other contraceptives, and current level of sexual satisfaction.

Specific questions and leading statements, categorized by functional health patterns, can be found on the Companion Website.

## Physical Assessment

Physical assessment of the reproductive system usually is conducted as part of a scheduled screening (e.g., for an annual Papanicolaou smear) or for a specific reproductive health problem. If conducted as part of a total physical assessment, this is usually the final system to be assessed. The nurse must feel comfortable with the examination of clients of the opposite gender; if either the nurse or the client is not comfortable, a nurse of the same gender should be asked to conduct this part of the assessment.

The reproductive system is assessed by inspection and palpation. Ask the client to void before having the examination. Prior to the examination, collect all necessary equipment and explain the techniques to the client to decrease anxiety. Put on disposable gloves before beginning the examination and wear them throughout the examination.

### The Male Reproductive System

The equipment necessary for assessing the male reproductive system includes disposable gloves, lubricant, and a flashlight. If a culture is to be taken of any drainage or discharge, sterile cotton swabs and culture media should be available. Explain the procedures for the examination thoroughly; if the man is unfamiliar with his internal genitalia, charts may be used to demonstrate the parts that will be examined.

Ask the client to remove his clothing and put on a gown. The assessment may be done with the client sitting or standing. Ensure that the examining room is warm and private.

### Breast and Lymph Node Assessment with Abnormal Findings (✓)

(Note: Assessment of male breasts is less complicated than assessment of female breasts but should not be overlooked.)

- Inspect and palpate both breasts, including areola and nipple.
  - ✓ A smooth, firm, mobile, tender disc of breast tissue behind the areola indicates *gynecomastia,* abnormal enlargement of the breast(s) in men. Gynecomastia requires additional investigation to determine cause.
  - ✓ A hard, irregular nodule in the nipple area suggests carcinoma.
- Palpate the axillary lymph nodes.
  - ✓ Enlarged axillary nodes are common with infections of the hand or arm but may be caused by cancer.
  - ✓ Enlarged supraclavicular nodes may indicate metastasis.

### External Assessment with Abnormal Findings (✓)

- Inspect and palpate the inguinal and femoral area for bulges. Ask the client to bear down or cough as you palpate (Figure 46–6 ■).
  - ✓ A bulge that increases with straining suggests a hernia.
- Inspect the penis. If the client is uncircumcised, retract the foreskin or ask the client to do so.
  - ✓ **Phimosis** (tightness of prepuce that prevents retraction of foreskin) may be congenital or due to recurrent *balanoposthitis* (generalized infection of glans penis and prepuce).

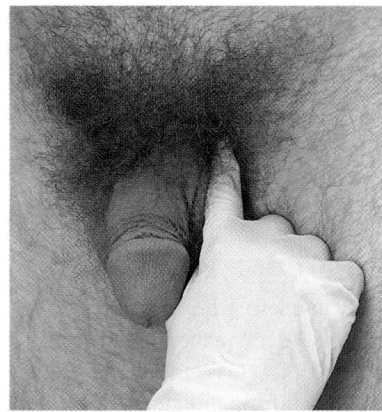

**Figure 46–6** ■ Palpating the male inguinal area for bulges.

- ✓ Narrow or inflamed foreskin can cause paraphimosis, retraction of the foreskin that causes painful swelling of the glans.
- ✓ **Balanitis** (inflammation of the glands) is associated with bacterial or fungal infections.
- ✓ Ulcers, vesicles, or warts suggest sexually transmitted infection.
- ✓ Nodules or sores seen in uncircumcised men may be cancer.
- Inspect the external urinary meatus. Press the glans between the thumb and forefinger (Figure 46–7 ■). Replace the foreskin if appropriate.
  - ✓ Erythema or discharge indicates inflammatory disease. Further assessment is required.
- Inspect the skin around the base of the penis.
  - ✓ Excoriation or inflammation suggests lice or scabies.
- Palpate the shaft of the penis.
  - ✓ Induration with tenderness along with ventral surface suggests urethral stricture with inflammation.
- Inspect the scrotum. Further assess any swelling in the scrotum using transillumination: Darken the room and place a lighted flashlight against the skin of the scrotum. The normal scrotum and epididymis appear as dark masses with regular borders.

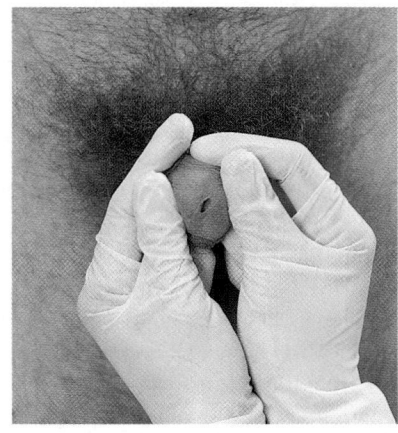

**Figure 46–7** ■ Inspecting the external urinary meatus of the male.

✓A unilateral or bilateral poorly developed scrotum suggests **cryptorchidism** (failure of one or both testes to descend into the scrotum).

✓Swelling of the scrotum may indicate indirect inguinal hernia, **hydrocele** (accumulation of fluid in the scrotum), or scrotal edema. Swellings containing serous fluid will transilluminate. Swellings containing blood or tissue will not transilluminate.

- Palpate each testis and epididymis.

✓Tender, painful scrotal swelling occurs in acute epididymitis, acute orchitis, torsion of the spermatic cord, and strangulated hernia.

✓A painless nodule in the testis is associated with testicular cancer.

### Prostate Assessment with Abnormal Findings (✓)

(Note: The prostate gland is assessed by digital rectal examination. See Chapter 23 ⊖⊃ for technique for palpation of the rectal wall.)

- Palpate the posterior surface of the prostate gland. With a gloved index finger, palpate the anterior rectal wall for the rounded, two-lobed structure of the posterior prostate.

✓Enlargement (1-cm protrusion into the rectum) with obliteration of the median sulcus suggests benign prostatic hypertrophy.

✓Enlargement with asymmetry and tenderness suggests prostatitis.

✓A hard irregular nodule is seen in carcinoma.

## The Female Reproductive System

The equipment necessary for assessing the female reproductive system includes disposable latex gloves, a good light source, sterile cotton swabs, a spatula, water-soluble lubricant, slides, cytologic fixative, and specula of various sizes. If cultures are to be taken, culture media is necessary. Carefully explain the procedure for the examination, and show the speculum to the woman. If the woman is unfamiliar with her genitalia, charts may be used to demonstrate the parts that will be examined.

Ask the client to remove her clothing and put on a gown. Ensure that the examining room is private and warm.

The examination usually begins with examination of the breasts with the client in the sitting and supine positions. The nurse then helps the client move to the lithotomy position on the examining table, with the feet in the stirrups and the buttocks even with the foot of the table. Older or frail clients may not be able to tolerate this position. In this case, the client is examined in the supine position. Use draping throughout the examination so that only the part of the body being examined is exposed. Although the entire examination is described here, the internal examination is conducted only by a nurse with advanced practice in the procedure.

### Breast Assessment with Abnormal Findings (✓)

- Inspect both breasts simultaneously with the client seated in the following positions: arms at sides, arms overhead, hands pressed on hips, leaning forward. Inspect breast size, symmetry, contour, skin color, texture, venous patterns, and lesions. Lift the breasts, and inspect the lower and lateral aspects.

✓Retractions, dimpling, and abnormal contours suggest benign lesions, but may also suggest malignancy.

✓Thickened, dimpled skin with enlarged pores (called peau d'orange, orange peel, or pig skin) and unilateral venous patterns are also associated with malignancy.

✓Redness may be seen with infection or carcinoma.

- Inspect the areolae and nipples.

✓Peau d'orange may be noted first in the areola.

✓Recent unilateral inversion of the nipple or asymmetry in the directions in which the nipples point suggests cancer.

- Palpate both breasts, axillae, and supraclavicular areas. Figure 46–8 ■ illustrates a possible pattern for breast palpation. Various palpation patterns may be used as long as every part of each breast is palpated, including the axillary tail (also called tail of Spence), which is the breast tissue that extends from the upper outer quadrant toward and into the axillae. Ask the client to assume a supine position with a small pillow under the shoulder and the arm over the head, and repeat the systematic palpation sequence. Findings of nonpathologic breast enlargement, nodularity, and tenderness are more common the week preceding and during menstrual flow. Describe identified masses by location, size, shape, consistency, tenderness, mobility, and delineation of borders.

✓Tenderness may be related to premenstrual fullness, fibrocystic disease, or inflammation. Tenderness may also indicate cancer.

✓Nodules in the tail of the breast may be enlarged lymph nodes.

✓Hard, irregular, fixed unilateral masses that are poorly delineated suggest carcinoma.

✓Bilateral, single or multiple, round, mobile, well-delineated masses are consistent with fibrocystic breast disease or fibroadenoma.

✓Swelling, tenderness, erythema, and heat may be seen with mastitis.

- Palpate the nipple then compress it between the thumb and index finger. Note the color of any discharge.

✓Loss of nipple elasticity is seen in cancer.

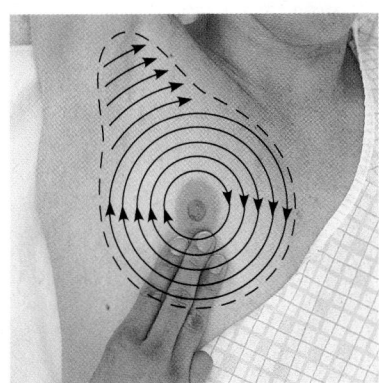

**Figure 46–8** ■ Possible pattern for palpation of the breast.

✓ Bloody or serous discharge is associated with intraductal papilloma.

✓ Milky discharge not due to prior pregnancy and found on both sides suggests **galactorrhea** (lactation not associated with pregnancy or nursing), which is sometimes associated with a pituitary tumor.

✓ Unilateral discharge from one or two ducts can be seen in fibrocystic breast disease, intraductal papilloma, or carcinoma.

### Axillary Assessment with Abnormal Findings (✓)

• Inspect the skin of the axillae.

✓ Rash may be due to allergy or other causes.

✓ Signs of inflammation and infection may be due to infection of the sweat glands.

✓ Palpate all sections of both axillae for palpable nodes (Figure 46–9 ■).

✓ Enlarged axillary nodes are most often due to infection of the hand or arm but can be caused by malignancy.

✓ Enlarged supraclavicular nodes are associated with lymphatic metastases from abdominal or thoracic carcinoma.

### External Assessment with Abnormal Findings (✓)

Help the client to the lithotomy position with the knees flexed and separated.

• Inspect and palpate the labia majora.

✓ Excoriation, rashes, or lesions suggest inflammatory or infective processes.

✓ Bulging of the labia that increases with straining suggests a hernia.

✓ Varicosities may be present on the labia.

• Inspect the labia minora. Use a gloved hand to separate the labia majora for better visualization.

✓ Inflammation, irritation, excoriation, or caking of discharge in tissue folds suggests vaginal infection or poor hygiene.

✓ Ulcers or vesicles may be symptoms of sexually transmitted infection.

• Palpate the inside of the labia minora between gloved thumb and forefinger.

✓ Small, firm, round cystic nodules in labia suggest sebaceous cysts.

✓ Wartlike lesions suggest condylomata acuminata (genital warts).

✓ Firm, painless ulcers suggest chancre of primary syphilis.

✓ Shallow, painful ulcers suggest herpes infection.

✓ Ulcerated or red raised lesions in older women suggest vulvar carcinoma.

• Inspect the clitoris.

✓ Enlargement may be a symptom of a masculinizing condition.

• Inspect the vaginal opening.

✓ Swelling or discoloration may be caused by trauma.

✓ Discharge or lesions may be symptoms of infection.

✓ Fissures or fistulas may be related to injury, infection, spreading of a malignancy, or trauma.

• Palpate Skene's glands. Using the index finger, "milk" Skene's glands on both sides and over the urethra and inspect for possible discharge (Figure 46–10 ■).

✓ Discharge from Skene's glands and/or tenderness suggests infection.

• Palpate Bartholin's glands. Palpate Bartholin's glands at the posterior labia majora (Figure 46–11 ■).

✓ A nontender mass in the posterolateral portion of the labia majora is indicative of a Bartholin's cyst.

✓ Swelling, redness, or tenderness, especially if unilateral, may indicate abscess of Bartholin's glands.

• Inspect the vaginal orifice for bulging and urinary incontinence. Ask the client to strain or "bear down."

✓ Bulging of the anterior vaginal wall and urinary incontinence suggest a cystocele.

✓ Bulging of the posterior wall suggests a rectocele.

✓ Protrusion of the cervix or uterus into the vagina indicates uterine prolapse.

• Inspect and palpate the perineum.

✓ Episiotomy scarring may be apparent.

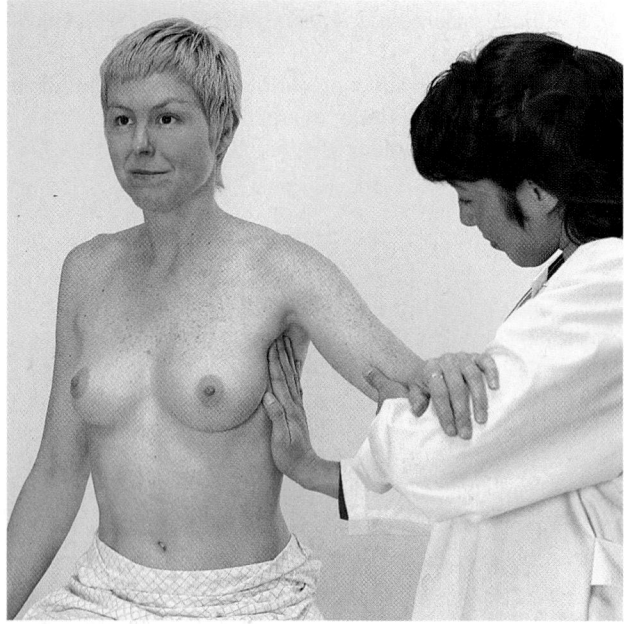

**Figure 46–9** ■ Palpating the axillary lymph nodes.

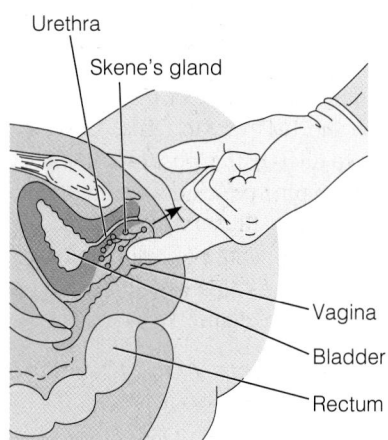

Urethra
Skene's gland
Vagina
Bladder
Rectum

**Figure 46–10** ■ Palpating Skene's glands.

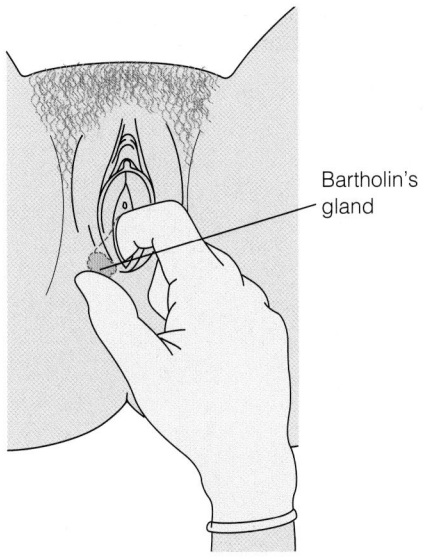

**Figure 46–11 ■** Palpating Bartholin's glands.

✓ Inflammation, lesions, and growths may be seen in infections or cancer.

✓ Fistulas may be the result of injury, trauma, infection, or spreading of a malignancy.

## Vaginal and Cervical Assessment with Abnormal Findings (✓)

• Use a vaginal speculum to inspect the vaginal walls and cervix. See the guidelines in Box 46–1.

✓ Bluish color of the cervix and vaginal mucosa may be a sign of pregnancy.

✓ A pale cervix is associated with anemia.

✓ A cervix to the right or left of the midline may indicate a pelvic mass, uterine adhesions, or pregnancy.

✓ Projection of the cervix more than 3 cm into the vaginal canal may indicate a pelvic or uterine mass.

✓ Transverse or star-shaped cervical lacerations reflect trauma causing tearing of the cervix.

✓ An enlarged cervix is associated with infection.

---

## BOX 46–1 ■ Guidelines for Intravaginal Assessment and Use of the Vaginal Speculum

The size of the speculum that is used for an internal examination of the female reproductive system depends on the age of the woman and size of the vagina. Two types of specula are available. The Graves speculum, used most often for examinations of adult women, is available in lengths of 3½ to 5 inches and widths of ¾ to 1½ inches. The Pederson speculum, which is narrower, may be used to examine adolescents or adult women who are virgins, who have never had a baby, or who are postmenopausal with vaginal atrophy. The speculum should be warm: A heating pad is used in many institutions. If cultures or smears are to be obtained, neither water nor gel should be used either to warm or to lubricate the speculum.

If cells are to be taken for cytologic studies, the client should not douche, use vaginal medications, or take a tub bath for 24 hours before the examination. Finally, the examination is usually deferred if the client is menstruating or has a vaginal infection.

The general procedure is as follows:

1. Place the index and middle finger of one hand into the vagina, just inside the introitus, and press the fingers toward the rectum. Hold the speculum in the other hand.
2. Ask the client to bear down, and insert the closed blades of the speculum into the vagina at an oblique angle until the ends of the blades reach the fingertips (see the accompanying figure). Withdraw the fingers and rotate the speculum to a transverse position.
3. Continue to insert the speculum until it reaches the end of the vagina. Depress the lever of the speculum to open the blades. If the cervix is not in full view, try closing the blades, withdrawing the speculum about halfway, and inserting it again at a more downward angle. When the cervix is in full view, fix the depressed lever to an open position.
4. Inspect the cervix. The normal cervix is pink and midline. Assess color, position, size, projection into the vagina, surface and shape, and any discharge.

If a Papanicolaou (Pap) smear to collect cervical cells for cytologic studies is done, the following procedure may be used:

1. To collect cells from the vaginal pool, roll a sterile cotton-tipped applicator on the vaginal wall below the cervix. Paint the smear on the slide, and spray the slide with fixative.
2. To collect endocervical cells, place the groove of the spatula snugly against the cervical os, and rotate it 360 degrees. In a single stroke, spread the material from both sides of the spatula on a slide, and immediately spray with fixative.

If cultures are to be done, take a specimen from the vagina and/or cervix with a sterile, cotton-tipped applicator, and then either spread the specimen on a culture plate or place it in a culture container. Follow institutional protocols for preparing specimens for vaginal infections from suspected organisms.

At the end of the examination, loosen the lever control and slowly withdraw the speculum, closing the blades slowly and rotating the speculum while observing all areas of the vaginal wall. Assess the color of the mucosa and the color and appearance of any discharge.

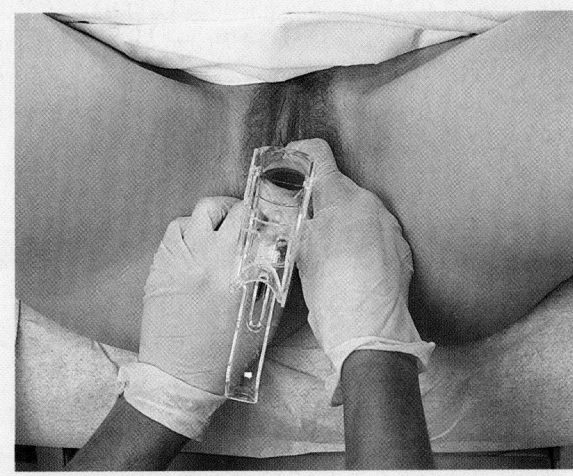

Inserting the vaginal speculum.

## BOX 46–2 ■ Guidelines for Bimanual Pelvic Examination

The bimanual pelvic examination is done to palpate the cervix, uterus, and ovaries. The examiner's hand that will be used intravaginally is held with the index and middle fingers extended, the thumb abducted, and the fourth and fifth fingers folded on the palm of the hand. The extended fingers are lubricated.

The general procedure is as follows:

1. Spread the labia with the thumb and finger of the opposite hand and insert the lubricated fingers into the vagina with the palm upward.
2. Place the opposite hand on the abdomen; it is used to press on the abdomen and gently move the internal genitals toward the intravaginal fingers (see the accompanying figure).
3. Ask the client to take deep breaths to relax the abdominal wall.
4. Palpate the cervix, assessing size, contour, position, surface, consistency, tenderness, and mobility. The cervix should be freely movable and non-tender.
5. Palpate the uterus by pressing downward on the abdomen while placing the intravaginal fingers in the anterior fornix and gently lifting against the abdominal hand. Assess the size, shape, surface; consistency, position, mobility, and tenderness of the uterus. The normal uterus is freely movable and nontender.
6. Palpate the adnexal areas, which surround the uterus and contain the fallopian tubes and ovaries. Because these struc-

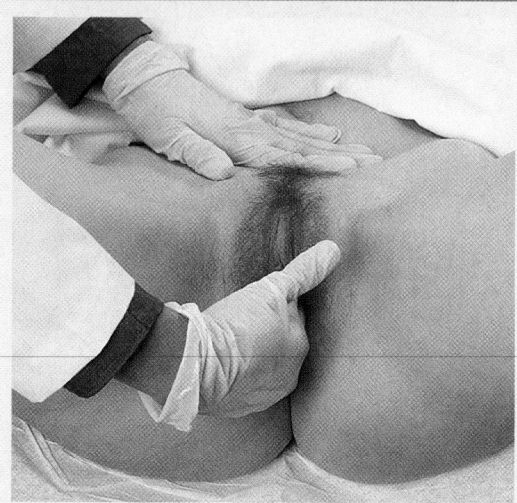

Bimanual pelvic examination.

tures are small, palpation may not be possible. If the ovaries are palpable, they should be smooth and firm. The normal ovary is sensitive to touch, firm, and highly movable.

7. Withdraw the fingers. Provide tissues for the client's use in wiping the genital area.

---

✓ An ectropion (eversion of columnar epithelium lining the cervical canal) appears plush red around the central cervical os and may bleed easily.

✓ Nabothian cysts (small, white, or yellow raised, round areas on the cervix) are considered normal but may become infected.

✓ Cervical polyps may be cervical or endometrial in origin.

• Palpate the cervix, uterus, and ovaries. See the guidelines in Box 46–2.

✓ The uterus may be retroverted (tilted backward) or retroflexed (angled backward).

✓ Pain on movement of the cervix during manual examination suggests pelvic inflammatory disease (PID).

✓ Softening of the uterine isthmus (Hegar's sign), softening of the cervix (Goodell's sign), and uterine enlargement may be objective signs of pregnancy.

✓ Firm, irregular nodules that vary greatly with size and are continuous with the uterine surface are likely to be myomas (fibroids).

✓ Unilateral or bilateral smooth, compressible adnexal masses are found in ovarian tumors.

✓ Profuse menstrual bleeding is seen with endometrial polyps, dysfunctional uterine bleeding (DUB), and use of an intrauterine device.

✓ Irregular bleeding may be associated with endometrial polyps, DUB, uterine or cervical carcinoma, or oral contraceptives.

✓ Postmenopausal bleeding is seen with endometrial hyperplasia, estrogen therapy, and endometrial cancer.

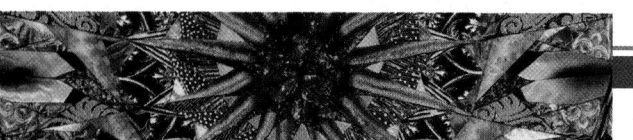

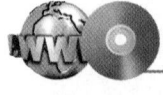

## EXPLORE MediaLink

# TEST YOURSELF

1. In the male, sperm and testosterone are produced by the:
   a. Epididymis
   b. Seminal vesicles
   c. Testes
   d. Cowper's glands

2. In the female, what structure is analogous to the penis in the male?
   a. Ovaries
   b. Labia majora
   c. Labia minora
   d. Clitoris

3. Suspected abnormalities of the scrotum may be further assessed through:
   a. Transillumination
   b. Auscultation
   c. Palpation
   d. Percussion

4. What assessment technique is **primarily** used to determine abnormalities of the breast?
   a. Inspection
   b. Auscultation
   c. Palpation
   d. Percussion

5. At what anatomic location would you palpate Bartholin's glands?
   a. Above the clitoris
   b. Posterior labia majora
   c. Inferior to the urinary meatus
   d. Internal vaginal wall

See Test Yourself answers in Appendix C.

# BIBLIOGRAPHY

Andresen, G. (1998). Assessing the older patient. *RN, 61*(3), 46–56.

Billington, A. (1997). Running a nurse-led prostate assessment clinic. *Community Nurse, 3*(7), 26.

Blackwell, J., & Blackwell, D. (1997). Menopause: Life event or medical disease? *Clinical Nurse Specialist, 11*(1), 7–11.

Dumesic, D. (1996). Pelvic examinations: What to focus on in menopausal women. *Consultant, 36*(1), 39–46.

Frizzell, J. (1998). The PSA test. *American Journal of Nursing, 98*(4), 14–15.

Heath, H., & White, I. (2001). Sexuality and older people: An introduction to nursing assessment. *Nursing Older People, 13*(4), 29–31.

Klingman, L. (1999). Assessing the female reproductive system: A guide through the gynecologic exam. *American Journal of Nursing, 99*(8), 37–43.

Padbury, V. (1997). Women's health check. *Practice Nurse, 13*(9), 547–549.

Parker, S. (1997). Well-women clinics: Breast and pelvic examinations. *Practice Nurse, 14*(9), 582.

Weber, J., & Kelley, J. (2002). *Health assessment in nursing* (2nd ed.). Philadelphia: Lippincott-Raven.

Wilson, S., & Giddens, J. (2001). *Health assessment for nursing practice.* St. Louis: Mosby.

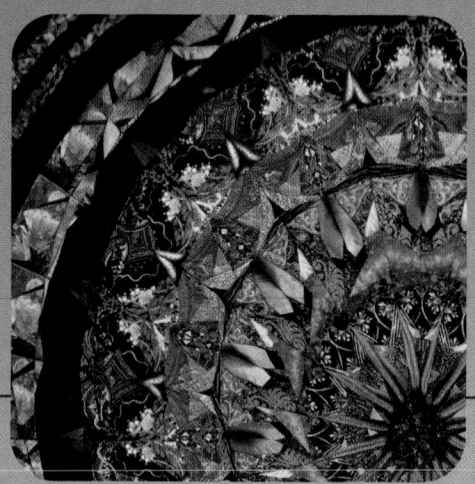

# CHAPTER 47

# Nursing Care of Men with Reproductive System Disorders

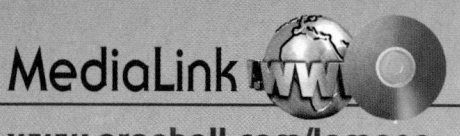

## MediaLink

### www.prenhall.com/lemone

Additional resources for this chapter can be found on the Student CD-ROM accompanying this textbook, and on the Companion Website at www. prenhall.com/lemone. Click on Chapter 47 to select the activities for this chapter.

**CD-ROM**
- Audio Glossary
- NCLEX Review

**Companion Website**
- More NCLEX Review
- Case Study
  Benign Prostatic Hyperplasia (BPH)
- Care Plan Activity
  Radical Prostatectomy
- MediaLink Application
  Prostate Cancer Prevention

## LEARNING OUTCOMES

After completing this chapter, you will be able to:

- Apply knowledge of normal male anatomy, physiology, and assessments when providing care for men with reproductive system disorders (see Chapter 46).

- Explain the pathophysiology of disorders of the male reproductive system.

- Discuss risk factors for cancers of the male reproductive system.

- Discuss the collaborative care, with related nursing implications, for men with disorders of the reproductive system.

- Provide appropriate nursing care for the man having prostate surgery.

- Use the nursing process as a framework for providing individualized care to men with disorders of the reproductive system.

Men are subject to disorders of the penis, scrotum and testes, prostate gland, and breast. These disorders may be inflammatory, structural, benign, or malignant. Young men are at increased risk for testicular cancer. As men age, both benign and malignant problems with the prostate gland become common. Many of the disorders pose significant risk to the man's fertility and sexual and urinary function, and some are life threatening. This chapter discusses disorders of the male reproductive system, including disorders of sexual expression and the male breast. As many of the treatments and disorders of the male reproductive system have the potential to affect erection and ejaculation, these problems are discussed first.

## DISORDERS OF SEXUAL EXPRESSION

### THE MAN WITH ERECTILE DYSFUNCTION

**Erectile dysfunction** is the inability of the male to attain and maintain an erection sufficient to permit satisfactory sexual intercourse. **Impotence,** a term often used synonymously with erectile dysfunction, may involve a total inability to achieve erection, an inconsistent ability to achieve erection, or the ability to sustain only brief erections. Erectile dysfunction has many possible causes (Table 47–1). Erectile dysfunction may or may not be associated with a loss of **libido** (sexual desire).

The incidence of erectile dysfunction is difficult to estimate because many affected men may not report the disorder. An estimated 10 million men in the United States have erectile dysfunction, and most are older than 65. A prevalence of 5% is noted at age 40, increasing to approximately 25% at age 65 or older (Tierney et al., 2001). Most problems with erection have an organic cause. Because this is a problem primarily of aging men, the discussion of pathophysiology focuses on this age group.

### PATHOPHYSIOLOGY

Age-related changes in sexual function involve cellular and tissue changes in the penis, decreased sensory activity, hypogonadism, and the effects of chronic illness. In the penis, a change from elastic collagen to a more rigid collagen results in decreased distensibility (a less rigid erection). This, in turn, interferes with the veno-occlusive mechanism, which prevents blood from "leaking" out of the penis into the general vasculature

### TABLE 47–1  Causes of Erectile Dysfunction

| Major Pathologic Causes | | Major Iatrogenic Causes | |
|---|---|---|---|
| | | **Medications** | **Procedures and Infections** |
| *Neurogenic*<br>Spinal cord injury<br>Cerebrovascular accident<br>Parkinson's disease<br>Multiple sclerosis<br><br>*Endocrinologic*<br>Diabetes mellitus<br>Hypogonadism<br>Hypothyroidism<br><br>*Inflammatory*<br>Prostatitis<br>Cystitis<br><br>*Activity Intolerance*<br>Pulmonary problems<br>Anemias<br>Myocardial infarction<br>Congestive heart failure<br>Hepatic diseases<br>Renal failure<br><br>*Substance Dependency*<br>Alcohol<br>Marijuana<br>Narcotics<br>Sedatives<br>Tobacco | *Arterial*<br>Atherosclerosis<br>Hypertension<br>Aortic aneurysm<br>Sickle cell anemia<br><br>*Mechanical*<br>Decreased penile<br>distensibility<br>Congenital disorders<br>Morbid obesity<br>Hydrocele<br>Hip or pelvic fractures<br><br>*Psychogenic*<br>Depression<br>Stress<br>Fatigue<br>Fear of failure<br><br>*Compulsive Food Disorders*<br>Compulsive overeating<br>Anorexia nervosa<br>Bulimia | *Antihypertensives*<br>Hydrochlorothiazide<br>Spironolactone<br>Methyldopa<br>Clonidine<br>Prazosin<br>Propranolol<br>Reserpine<br><br>*Psychotropic Agents*<br>Phenothiazines<br>Butyrophenones<br>Tricyclic antidepressants<br>MAO inhibitors<br>Diazepam<br>Chlorodiazepoxide<br><br>*Endocrinologic Agents*<br>LHRH agonists<br>Estrogen compounds<br>Progesterone<br><br>*Other*<br>Antiparkinsonian agents<br>Anticholinergic agents<br>Immunosuppressive agents<br>Antihistamines | *Surgery*<br>Coronary artery bypass<br>Pelvic lymphadenectomy<br>Radical prostatectomy<br>Radical cystectomy<br>Abdominal perineal resection<br>Sympathectomy<br>Aortic aneurysm repair<br>Transplant surgeries<br><br>*Other*<br>Severe nosocomial infection<br>Radiation therapy to pelvis |

prematurely. Problems with this mechanism result in incomplete erections. Vibrotactile sensation over the skin of the penis declines with age. This decline may explain why some older men require longer stimulation to achieve an erection. Hypogonadism, common in aging men, results in decreased testosterone levels. There may be a relationship between lower androgen levels and erectile function.

Many illnesses affect erectile function. Damage to arteries, smooth muscles, and fibrous tissues are the most common causes of impotence. Diseases such as diabetes, kidney disease, chronic alcoholism, atherosclerosis, and vascular disease are responsible for about 70% of erectile dysfunction. Innervation and blood flow to the penis may be damaged during surgery, prostate surgery in particular. Given the effects of aging on erectile function, the increased incidence of chronic illness, and the multiple treatments required to manage those illnesses, it is not surprising that many older men have difficulty with erectile function.

## COLLABORATIVE CARE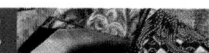

The management of men with erectile dysfunction is growing in importance and scale, because the population as a whole is aging, so the incidence is increasing proportionately. Another factor is the gradual change in the willingness of men and their partners to be forthcoming about sexual concerns. Although sexuality is still a very sensitive and private area for most people, the knowledge that help is available is causing men to seek answers. Many older men are coming to believe that loss of erectile function is not an inevitable part of aging.

## Diagnostic Tests

The following diagnostic tests may be ordered.

- *Blood profiles,* including chemistry and testosterone, prolactin, thyroxin, and PSA levels, are performed to identify metabolic and endocrine problems that may be causing the dysfunction.
- *Nocturnal penile tumescence and rigidity (NPTR) monitoring* helps differentiate between psychogenic and organic causes. These tests can be performed in a sleep laboratory, although home testing with portable devices is an alternative. The number and quality of erections occurring during REM sleep can be determined.
- *Cavernosometry* and *cavernosography* of the corpora are used to evaluate arterial inflow and venous outflow of the penis.

## Medications

Erectile dysfunction can be treated with oral medications, self-administered intracavernous injections, or by topical agents.

- *Oral medications:* Sildenafil citrate (Viagra) interferes with the breakdown of a biochemical involved in the smooth muscle relaxation of the corpus cavernosum necessary to produce an erection. While sildenafil citrate has no direct effect on the corpus cavernosum, it enhances the effect of nitric oxide (NO) released during sexual stimulation. At recommended doses, no effect occurs in the absence of sexual stimulation. See the box below for nursing implications of this drug.

## Medications Administration

### Sildenafil (Viagra)

#### Sildenafil citrate (Viagra)

Sildenafil citrate is an oral medication used to treat erectile dysfunction in men. In the presence of nitric oxide released during sexual stimulation, sildenafil citrate increases smooth muscle relaxation in the corpus cavernosum, increasing the ability to achieve and maintain an erection. It may be taken once per day, approximately 1 hour before sexual activity.

#### Nursing Responsibilities

- Assess the client's health and medication history for use of nitrates. Sildenafil citrate is contraindicated for men who are currently taking nitrates such as nitroglycerine in short- or long-acting forms (including oral, sublingual transdermal, and other forms such as nitrolingual spray). Combining these drugs may cause significant hypotension.
- Inquire about the use of recreational nitrates such as amyl nitrate or nitrite ("poppers") or butyl nitrate. Use of these substances also contraindicates the use of sildenafil citrate.
- Clients who are at risk for priapism, including men with sickle cell disease, multiple myeloma, or leukemia, or who have an anatomic abnormality of the penis should not take sildenafil citrate.
- Drugs such as ketoconazole, erythromycin, and cimetidine reduce the clearance of sildenafil citrate; concurrent administration may necessitate a reduced dosage.
- This drug is approved only for use in adult males; it is not approved for children or women.

#### Client and Family Teaching

- Take this drug as needed, approximately 1 hour before sexual activity. It can be taken within 30 minutes to 4 hours of sexual activity, although the response may be diminished after 2 hours.
- Do not take this drug more than once a day.
- Taking the drug after a high-fat meal may delay the onset of effects.
- Do not combine with other treatments for erectile dysfunction.
- If you experience chest pain or shortness of breath while using this drug, contact your physician.

- *Injectable medications:* Papaverine and prostaglandin E injections may be used. When injected directly into the penis, papaverine relaxes the arterioles and smooth muscles of the cavernosum, thus inducing tumescence (swelling). An erection usually develops that lasts from 30 minutes to 4 hours. Prostaglandin E functions much as papaverine does, but has fewer side effects. One problem with this treatment is its mode of delivery. There is a high attrition rate, and clients report dissatisfaction with lack of spontaneity, loss of interest in sex, physical limitations, cost, and occasionally, pain. Alprostadil (Caverject) is another injectable medication that may be used to treat erectile dysfunction. It may be injected into the penis or placed in the urethra as a minisuppository.
- *Hormone replacement therapy:* Testosterone injections (200 mg IM every 3 weeks) or topical patches may be used for men with documented androgen deficiency and who do not have prostate cancer.
- *Transdermal medications:* Transdermal nitroglycerin paste has restored erectile function to a few men when applied directly to the penis. The mechanism of action is probably arteriolar dilation.

## Mechanical Devices

The most frequently prescribed mechanical device for erectile dysfunction is the vacuum constriction device (VCD). The VCD draws blood into the penis with a vacuum, trapping it there with a constricting band at the base of the penis. After the device is removed for intercourse, a single small band, often called an O-ring, is left at the base of the penis to maintain the erection. If the man can attain an erection but cannot maintain it, then an O-ring alone can be used.

## Surgery

Surgical treatment for erectile dysfunction involves either revascularization procedures or implantation of prosthetic devices. Venous or arterial procedures are generally not successful. The result is often temporary, because the underlying cause of the vascular insufficiency is usually not corrected. Implantation of penile prostheses is now common (Figure 47–1 ■). Men are generally satisfied with their prostheses, and they rank the inflatable type highest. Partners are also more likely to report satisfaction with the penile implant, although not to the same degree as clients. Some partners report that the implanted penis is harder than a normal erect penis and therefore causes pain. Also, the man can have intercourse for a prolonged period of time, and some partners do not find prolonged penetration enjoyable. Client and partner teaching is mandatory. Counseling by a sex therapist may be needed to facilitate adaptation to the implant.

## NURSING CARE

Nurses in almost any health care setting may encounter men with erectile dysfunction, either through routine examinations or through careful assessment of clients' conditions and treatments that may incidentally cause erectile dysfunction. Nurses employed in clinics, operating rooms, and surgical units with urological services commonly encounter men being treated for erectile dysfunction. Nurses in a variety of settings, including long-term care, encounter men who have had surgical interventions, such as penile implants.

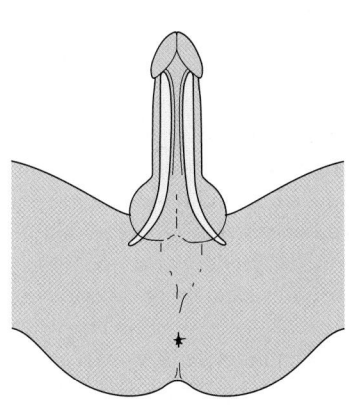

**A** Semirigid

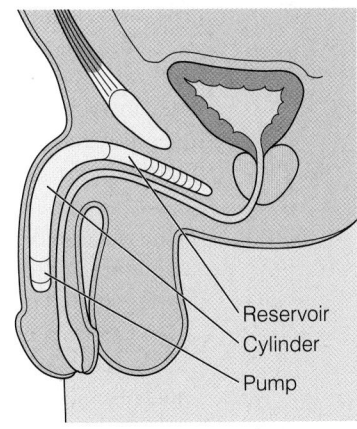

**B** Self-contained

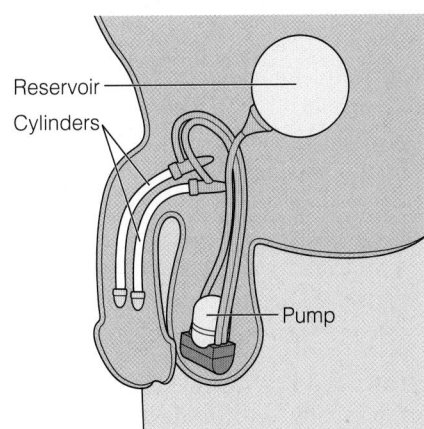

Reservoir
Cylinders
Pump

**C** Inflatable

**Figure 47–1** ■ Types of penile implants. *A,* With semirigid rods implanted in the corpora cavernosa, the penis is always in a state of semi-erection, which may not be acceptable to the man. *B,* With a self-contained penile implant, the penis remains flaccid until the man compresses a pump at the head of the penis, which transfers fluid from a reservoir to a cylinder within the penis to achieve an erection. The man presses a release valve to return the fluid to the reservoir. *C,* With an inflatable penile implant, the penis remains flaccid until the man compresses a pump in the scrotum, which transfers fluid from an abdominal reservoir to cylinders in the corpora cavernosa to achieve an erection. Pressing a release valve returns the fluid to the reservoir.

## Nursing Diagnoses and Interventions

Because nurses are usually accessible, they are most likely to discover problems of erectile dysfunction. Once a problem is known, nurses are involved in giving information, providing emotional support, and referring clients to physicians or counselors. Although there are many possible nursing diagnoses, this section focuses on nursing care related to sexual dysfunction and self-esteem.

### Sexual Dysfunction

Many men who lose erectile function are not aware of the cause. Often the man blames the loss on unrelated factors, such as age, a medication for an illness, a dangerous illness, or his sexual partner. Not knowing causes anxiety, which may disrupt the relationship with his partner or lead him to discontinue an important medication.

- Assess for risk factors for erectile dysfunction. Be especially alert to men who have recently begun medications or had recent surgeries that could cause erectile dysfunction. *Awareness of risk factors helps the nurse to prioritize care, although nurses must remember that almost all aging clients have at least one risk factor.*
- Assess for sexual dysfunction. Men have shown increasing willingness to discuss sexual concerns and expect nurses to be aware of the physiologic effects of their disease and side effects of treatment on all aspects of their health. *If a problem exists, information obtained in a sexual assessment guides the nurse in deciding if the next step should be client teaching, referral, or both.*

> **PRACTICE ALERT** *Many men will not volunteer information about sexual function unless asked, but then are open about concerns and appreciate being asked.* ■

- Perform a detailed assessment of current sexual practices. *It is essential for health care providers to understand the client and partner's sexual pattern in order to provide appropriate, individualized care.*
- Discuss previous methods of coping with erectile dysfunction. *Awareness of coping strategies can provide insight for the nurse and guide teaching.*
- Provide information about treatment options. *The man needs to know the details of the intervention, the chances for success, and the possible complications.*

### Situational Low Self-Esteem

The man with erectile dysfunction often believes himself to be "less than a man." In addition, the insertion of a penile implant with a semirigid prosthesis may result in disturbances in body image related to changes in sexual activity as well as the appearance and embarrassment of a permanent semierection.

- Collect data during the health history, in a nonjudgmental manner, about physiologic function, other chronic illnesses, and feelings about sexual inadequacy. *This infor-*

*mation is necessary to establish the database for individualized interventions.*

- If the man has had a penile implant, teach him and his partner how to use the pump, including how to inflate and deflate the device. Suggest he practice inflation and deflation during the postoperative period. Suggest wearing snug-fitting underwear with the penis placed in an upright position on the abdomen and loose trousers. Provide information about length of healing, and that sexual activity may resume within 6 to 8 weeks following surgery. *Practice using the pump will maintain the pump position and promote tissue growth around the implant. The type of clothing worn can improve the ability to conceal the semi-rigid prosthesis and decrease embarrassment. Recovery from surgery is necessary before resuming sexual activity.*

### Home Care

Many nurses find that men with erectile dysfunction and their partners have lived in isolation with the problem for many years. The partner may even be unaware of the problem. The partner may believe that the man is seeing someone else or that the man has lost his attraction to the partner. The man may have kept his problem a secret because an intense feeling of shame makes him unable to admit that he cannot perform sexually. Many men greet the information about the high incidence of erectile dysfunction with a sense of relief that they are not alone in having this problem. All men and their partners also need to be aware of support services available to them.

# THE MAN WITH EJACULATORY DYSFUNCTION

There are many types of ejaculatory dysfunction. *Premature ejaculation* is usually psychogenic in origin, although diabetes can cause the problem as well. *Delayed ejaculation* can be related to aging changes, such as decreased vibrotactile sensation over the penis or decreased libido secondary to hypogonadism. Delayed ejaculation and inability to ejaculate at all may be caused by certain medications, such as antihypertensives, antidepressants, anxiolytics, and narcotics. *Retrograde ejaculation* (seminal fluid discharged into the bladder) may develop in aging men but is usually related to treatment of prostatic conditions or testicular cancer.

Among these problems, premature ejaculation has proved most responsive to medical management. The man can experiment with ways (such as wearing condoms) to decrease sensitivity. Using relaxation and guided imagery can delay sexual excitement. Mechanical devices, such as constrictive rings around the base of the penis, can help the man delay ejaculation and sustain an erection.

Nursing care focuses on assessment of the problem and teaching. The man's partner can be taught how to avoid excessive stimulation until ejaculation. If the problem persists, the man should be referred to a specialist.

# DISORDERS OF THE PENIS

## THE MAN WITH PHIMOSIS OR PRIAPISM

Two less common disorders of the penis are phimosis and priapism. Although uncommon, these disorders can cause problems with urination and sexual activity. In some cases, they are considered a medical emergency, as decreased blood flow to the penis may result in tissue ischemia and necrosis.

**Phimosis** is constriction of the foreskin so that it cannot be retracted over the glans penis. Phimosis may be congenital, or it may be related to chronic infections under the foreskin, which lead to adhesions. The major problem with this condition is that it prevents adequate hygiene, which may lead to malignant changes of the penis. It also may interfere with urinary elimination and intercourse. In a related disorder, called *paraphimosis,* the foreskin is tight and constricted, and is not able to cover the glans penis. The glans becomes engorged and edematous, and is painful. Paraphimosis may result from long-term retraction of the foreskin, such as occurs in placement of an indwelling catheter in the uncircumcised male (Porth, 2002). The tight foreskin can result in ischemia of the glans.

**Priapism** is an involuntary, sustained, painful erection that is not associated with sexual arousal. The prolonged erection may result in ischemia and fibrosis of the erectile tissue with high risk of subsequent impotence (Porth, 2002). The disorder, classified as either primary or secondary, is caused by impaired blood flow in the corpora cavernosa. Primary priapism results from conditions such as tumors, infection, or trauma. Secondary priapism is caused by blood disorders (e.g., leukemia, sickle cell anemia, and thrombocytopenia), neurologic disorders (e.g., spinal cord injury or stroke), renal failure, and some medications (see Box 47-1). Men who use intracavernous injection therapy for erectile dysfunction are at risk for priapism.

## COLLABORATIVE CARE

Severe phimosis or paraphimosis may require surgical circumcision. If infection is present, the appropriate antibiotic is administered.

| BOX 47-1 | ■ Factors Implicated in the Etiology of Priapism |
| --- | --- |

**Illnesses/Conditions**
- Sickle cell disease
- Leukemia
- Metastatic cancer
- Spinal cord trauma

**Drugs**
- Papaverine
- Psychotropic drugs
- Alcohol
- Marijuana

Conservative treatment of priapism includes iced saline enemas, intravenous ketamine (Ketalar) administration to induce anesthesia, and spinal anesthesia. Blood may be aspirated from the corpus through the dorsal glans, followed by catheterization and pressure dressings to maintain decompression. If necessary, more aggressive surgery to create vascular shunts to maintain blood flow is performed. When priapism is prolonged, up to 50% of men have subsequent erectile dysfunction.

## NURSING CARE

Nursing care for priapism focuses on assessing the penis, monitoring urinary output, and providing pain control. Assessment of the penis includes inspection for degree of erection and changes in color due to ischemia, and palpation of the penis for firmness and degree of rigidity. Monitor urine output, assessing for oliguria or signs of acute urinary retention. Pain is treated with analgesics.

The man usually has moderate to severe anxiety related to pain, the treatment, and the threat to his sexual function. The treatment may sound bizarre and painful, especially since the area is already extremely sensitive. The man may be acutely embarrassed by the erection and needs reassurance that the nurse understands that the erection is not within his control.

## THE MAN WITH CANCER OF THE PENIS

Cancer of the penis is a rare cancer in North America, occurring in approximately 1200 men per year (American Cancer Society [ACS], 2002). It most commonly affects men between the ages of 45 and 60. The cause is unknown. Penile cancer is rare in Jewish and Muslim men, populations in which routine circumcision is practiced, although the correlation between circumcision and this cancer is unclear. Phimosis is a risk factor, as are viral HPV and HIV infections. Ultraviolet light exposure (such as that used to treat psoriasis) also may play a role (Porth, 2002).

### PATHOPHYSIOLOGY AND MANIFESTATIONS

Squamous cell carcinoma accounts for 95% of all penile cancers. The tumor usually develops as a nodular or wartlike growth or a red velvety lesion on the glans or foreskin. The tumors tend to grow slowly. Penile cancer spreads to the superficial or deep inguinal nodes, and very late in the disease may spread to the bone, liver, or lungs. If the lesion is treated before inguinal node involvement, chances for a cure are good. Most of these lesions are painless but there may be significant ulceration and bleeding. Purulent, foul-smelling discharge may be evident under the foreskin. Occasionally, men with penile cancer may present with enlarged inguinal lymph nodes.

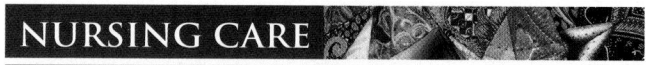

## COLLABORATIVE CARE

Cancer of the penis is diagnosed by a biopsy of the lesion, including any suspicious inguinal lymph nodes. The cancer is staged according to the size of the tumor, extent of invasion, status of inguinal lymph nodes, and presence or absence of distant metastasis. Small, localized lesions may be treated with fluorouracil cream, external-beam radiation, laser therapy, or surgical excision. Larger lesions with superficial or deep infiltration of penile structures require partial or total amputation of the penis. Chemotherapy may be administered to men with distant metastasis.

## NURSING CARE

Education can help prevent this disease or provide early detection. Teach men about the risks of unprotected sex and encourage condom use. Also encourage men to shield their genitals when having ultraviolet light therapy or using tanning salons. Discuss the importance of seeking prompt treatment for any lesion or abnormal drainage noted on the penis.

If the man has a penile amputation, nurses help cope with the problems of a shortened or absent penis, including the potentially devastating effect on body image and self-concept. If a total penectomy is performed, the surgeon creates a perineal urethrostomy, preserving urinary continence. However, the man must void in the sitting position, reinforcing the feeling of loss. Dribbling of urine after voiding may be a problem for a few weeks. The man should be taught to perform careful perineal hygiene following surgery, using mild soap and water. Sitz baths may be helpful to relieve pain and to promote healing. If an inguinal lymph node dissection is performed, the man may experience persistent lymphedema of the lower extremities.

# DISORDERS OF THE TESTIS AND SCROTUM

## THE MAN WITH A BENIGN SCROTAL MASS

Most scrotal masses are benign and can be managed in a manner that is satisfactory to the client. The most common are hydroceles, spermatoceles, and varicoceles (Figure 47–2 ■).

- A **hydrocele,** the most common cause of scrotal swelling, is a collection of fluid within the tunica vaginalis. The swelling ranges from slightly larger than the testicle to larger than a grapefruit. The cause of chronic hydrocele in men over the age of 40 years is an imbalance between production and reabsorption of fluid within the layers of the scrotum. Hydroceles also may occur secondary to trauma, infection, or a tumor. A hydrocele may be differentiated from a solid mass by transillumination or ultrasound of the scrotum. If the hydrocele becomes large enough to cause embarrassment or sig-nificant pain, the fluid is aspirated and an agent is injected into the scrotal sac to sclerose the tunica vaginalis. Hydroceles are not associated with infertility.

- A **spermatocele** is a mobile, usually painless mass that forms when efferent ducts in the epididymis dilate and form a cyst. It is thought to result from leakage of sperm due to trauma or infection. Treatment is usually not necessary. Spermatoceles are not associated with infertility.

- A **varicocele** is an abnormal dilation of a vein within the spermatic cord. It is caused by incompetent or congenitally missing valves that allow blood to pool in the spermatic cord veins. The dilated vein forms a soft mass that may be painful. Most varicoceles occur after puberty on the left side. A major concern with this condition is that it can decrease blood flow through the testis, interfere with spermatogenesis, and cause infertility. Varicoceles can be felt by scrotal palpation. Sonography is also frequently used for diagnosis. If infertil-

**Figure 47–2 ■** Common disorders of the scrotum. Hydroceles and spermatoceles do not usually require treatment unless they become large and cause pain. Varicoceles are usually treated to prevent infertility.

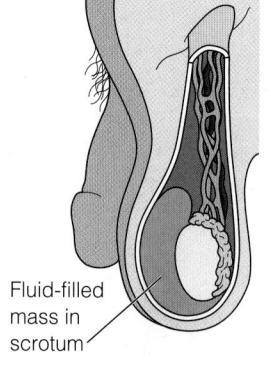

Fluid-filled mass in scrotum

**Hydrocele**

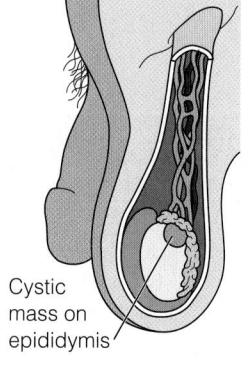

Cystic mass on epididymis

**Spermatocele**

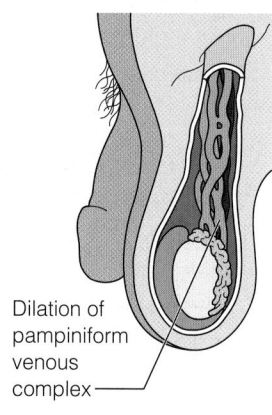

Dilation of pampiniform venous complex

**Varicocele**

ity is a concern, the spermatic vein may be ligated or occluded with a sclerosing agent or balloon catheter. If the varicocele is small and infertility is not a concern, a scrotal support is recommended.

## NURSING CARE

Nursing care focuses on reducing anxiety and teaching about comfort measures. Almost all men are aware of the possible pain associated with scrotal manipulation. They need information and reassurance about pain management if surgical treatment is necessary. External bleeding is minimal after surgery; however, some men do develop scrotal hematomas, manifested by scrotal edema and a purple discoloration.

## THE MAN WITH EPIDIDYMITIS

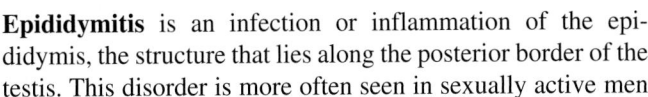

**Epididymitis** is an infection or inflammation of the epididymis, the structure that lies along the posterior border of the testis. This disorder is more often seen in sexually active men who are less than 35 years of age.

Sexually transmitted urethritis caused by *C. trachomatis* or *N. gonorrhoeae* is the usual precipitating factor for epididymitis in younger men. Men who practice unprotected anal intercourse may acquire sexually transmitted epididymitis from *E. coli, H. influenzae, Cryptococcus,* or tuberculosis (McCance & Huether, 2002). In men older than 35, epididymitis usually is associated with a urinary tract infection or prostatitis. Chemical epididymitis is associated with an inflammatory response to the reflux of urine into the ejaculatory ducts from urethral strictures, congenital structural anomalies, or increased abdominal pressure from excessive heavy lifting. This type is usually self-limiting and does not require treatment.

## PATHOPHYSIOLOGY AND MANIFESTATIONS

Infectious epididymis spreads by ascending the vas deferens from an already infected urethra or bladder. Early manifestations include pain and local edema, which can progress to erythema and edema of the entire scrotum, especially on the side of the involved epididymis. Complications of the disorder include abscess formation, infarction of the testis, and infertility.

## COLLABORATIVE CARE

The infection is diagnosed with a specimen culture from a urethral swab or epididymial aspiration. Severe epididymitis may be treated with intravenous antibiotics and hospitalization. Less acute forms of the disease are treated with outpatient antibiotic therapy. The man's sexual partner should be treated with antibiotics if the causative organism is sexually transmitted.

## NURSING CARE

Nursing care involves symptomatic relief. Ice packs and a scrotal support may be applied to the scrotum to relieve pain. Ensure the man knows that complete resolution of the infection may take weeks to months, and that treatment should continue until the infection is gone. Provide information about the possibility of infertility, as the man may wish to seek evaluation for this problem at a later date.

## THE MAN WITH ORCHITIS

**Orchitis** is an acute inflammation or infection of the testes. It most commonly occurs as a complication of a systemic illness or as an extension of epididymitis. Infection may reach the testes through the vas deferens and the lymphatic and vascular channels. Trauma, including vasectomy and other scrotal surgeries, may cause inflammation of the testes.

## PATHOPHYSIOLOGY AND MANIFESTATIONS

The most common infectious cause of orchitis in postpubertal men is mumps. The manifestations have a sudden onset, usually within 3 to 4 days after the swelling of the parotid glands. Manifestations include a high fever, increased WBCs, and unilateral or bilateral scrotal redness, swelling, and pain. In about 30% of cases, atrophy of the testes with irreversible damage to spermatogenesis occurs (McCance & Huether, 2002). Although androgen production is not affected, permanent sterility may result.

## COLLABORATIVE CARE

Treatment is supportive and symptomatic, including antibiotic therapy if urine cultures are positive. Bed rest, scrotal support and elevation, hot or cold compresses, and analgesics for pain are prescribed. If a hydrocele occurs, it is aspirated. Nursing care is similar to that of the client with epididymitis and other scrotal disorders.

## THE MAN WITH TESTICULAR TORSION

**Testicular torsion,** twisting of the spermatic cord with scrotal swelling and pain, is a potential medical emergency. The condition occurs most often between birth and age 20, but can occur at any age. Testicular torsion may occur spontaneously, or it may follow trauma or physical exertion. The torsion of the arteries and veins decreases or stops testicular circulation with resultant vascular engorgement and ischemia.

Testicular torsion is usually diagnosed by history and physical examination. Testicular scanning may be used to determine if blood flow to the testicle is reduced. Treatment, which involves detorsion of the testicle and fixation to the scrotum, must begin as quickly as possible. If the testicle is necrotic or has sustained significant damage, an *orchiectomy* (surgical removal of a testes) is performed.

## THE MAN WITH TESTICULAR CANCER

Testicular cancer accounts for only 1% of all cancers in men; however, it is the most common cancer in men between the ages of 15 and 35. Annually, an estimated 7500 young men in the United States are diagnosed with this cancer (ACS, 2002). Survival from testicular cancer has improved dramatically as a result of treatment with effective combination chemotherapy.

The cause of testicular cancer is unknown, but both congenital and acquired factors have been associated with tumor development. About 5% develop in a man with a history of undescended testicle (**cryptorchidism**). Testicular cancer is more common on the right side, which parallels the incidence of cryptorchidism (Tierney et al., 2001).

## PATHOPHYSIOLOGY AND MANIFESTATIONS

Approximately 95% of testicular malignancies are germ cell tumors (Porth, 2002). Germ cell tumors are classified, depending on their origin and ability to differentiate, as seminomas and nonseminomas. Seminomas are the most common type, and are believed to arise from the seminiferous epithelium of the testes. Nonseminomas contain more than one cell type; they include embryonal carcinoma, teratoma, choriocarcinoma, and yolk cell carcinoma. The most common type in men age 20 to 30 is embryonal carcinomas. Testicular cancer may also arise from specialized cells of the gonadal stroma. These tumors are named for the cells from which they originate: Leydig cell, Sertoli cell, granulosa cell, and theca cell tumors.

Local spread of the cancer to the epididymis or spermatic cord is inhibited by the outer covering of the testicles, the tunica albuginea. Therefore, spread by lymphatic and vascular channels to other organs often causes distant disease before large masses develop in the scrotum. Lymphatic dissemination usually leads to disease in retroperitoneal lymph nodes, whereas vascular dissemination can lead to metastasis in the lungs, bone, or liver. Bilateral presentation of testicular cancer is unusual. The classic presenting manifestation of testicular cancer is a painless hard nodule. Other manifestations are summarized in the box on this page. Manifestations of metastasis include lower extremity edema, back pain, cough, hemoptysis, or dizziness. HCG-producing tumors may cause breast enlargement (*gynecomastia*).

### Risk Factors

Risk factors for testicular cancer include the following:

- Cryptorchidism
- Genetic predisposition, especially in identical twins and brothers
- Disorders of testicular development (such as Klinefelter's syndrome)
- Maternal estrogen administration during pregnancy

## Manifestations of Testicular Cancer

**Common**
- Painless swelling on one testicle
- Painless nodule on one testicle

**Occasional**
- Dull ache in pelvis or scrotum

**Uncommon (10%)**
- Acute pain in scrotum

**Metastatic symptoms**
- Neck mass
- Respiratory symptoms
- Gastrointestinal disturbance
- Lumbar back pain

**Rare (5%)**
- Infertility
- Gynecomastia

## COLLABORATIVE CARE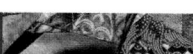

Care focuses on diagnosis, elimination of the cancer, and prevention or treatment of metastasis. Once testicular cancer is suspected, the man undergoes a number of screening tests to help determine the likelihood of the disease and its stage. If the disease is confined to the testicle, it is classified as stage I. Stage II disease is limited to the testicle and regional lymph nodes. Stage III disease involves metastasis above the diaphragm or extensive visceral involvement. Often, the man does not undergo biopsy before the beginning of treatment, but instead receives a definitive diagnosis after orchiectomy. Most men treated for testicular cancer will live a normal life span.

### Diagnostic Tests

The following diagnostic tests may be ordered.

- *Serum studies* for tumor markers. Germ cell tumors, which account for 95% of testicular cancers, produce biochemical markers such as human chorionic gonadotropin (hCG) and alpha-fetoprotein (AFP) that can be measured using radioimmunoassay techniques. Elevated levels provide strong evidence of testicular cancer. These markers are also measured after surgery to help determine the presence of residual disease that remains undetected by other means. Persistent elevation may indicate the need for further therapy.
- *Serum lactic acid dehydrogenase (LDH) levels* are elevated in testicular cancer, and may be significantly elevated when metastatic disease is present. The LDH is a less specific indicator of testicular cancer than the hCG and AFP.
- *Liver function tests, X-ray,* and *CT scans* of the chest and abdomen may be performed to evaluate the possibility of metastasis.

### Medications

Progress in chemotherapy to treat testicular cancer is one of the chief reasons why most men survive the disease. The client with advanced disease receives platinum-based combination chemotherapy. Two frequently used combinations are (1) cisplatin, bleomycin, and etoposide (BEP), and (2) etoposide plus cisplatin (EP). Toxicity from the BEP regimen can be significant, with nausea, vomiting, hair loss, bone marrow suppression, nephrotoxicity, ototoxicity, and peripheral neuropathy. Decreasing BEP cycles to 3 (rather than 4) or using the EP regimen reduces both the mortality and morbidity associated with chemotherapy. Chemotherapy is discussed in Chapter 10. ⊖⊙

## Surgery

*Radical orchiectomy* is the treatment used in all forms and stages of testicular cancer. A modified retroperitoneal lymph node dissection that preserves the nerves necessary for ejaculation often is performed at the same time.

## Radiation Therapy

Radiation therapy is used for stage I seminoma to treat cancer in the retroperitoneal lymph nodes, the most frequent site for distant metastasis. The man may experience temporary diarrhea, nausea, or a decline in bone marrow function, such as thrombocytopenia or leukopenia. These problems are usually mild and respond well to symptomatic treatment or time. Damage to the contralateral testicle is minimized by careful shielding. Pretreatment and posttreatment analysis of sperm number and function is necessary. The most common long-term complication is dyspepsia or ulcer disease. Radiation therapy is discussed in Chapter 10. ⊖⊙

## NURSING CARE

## Health Promotion

Unfortunately, even when risk factors are considered, most men who develop testicular cancer have none. Therefore, beginning at the age of 15, all men should perform monthly testicular self-examination, as described in Box 47–2.

## Nursing Diagnoses and Interventions

Nursing care of the man with testicular cancer is complex. The nurse must consider the reactions to the diagnosis, the change in body image accompanying treatment, and sexual and reproductive issues. Although chances of a cure are excellent, the long-term effect on quality of life may be extensive, requiring a change in life goals.

## Deficient Knowledge

The nurse often initiates and reinforces teaching about what to expect after radical orchiectomy. The man's knowledge about surgery is assessed, and postoperative routines such as early ambulation are explained (see Chapter 7). ⊖⊙

- Explain pain control methods. In addition to the usual analgesics used to control postoperative incisional pain, ice bags may be applied to the scrotum. A scrotal support provides relief, especially when the client ambulates. *Surgery results in incisional pain, and the scrotum is tender and slightly swollen.*
- Teach the signs and symptoms of complications. The incision is closed with Steri-Strips or staples, and, although rare, wound dehiscence is possible. If the incision gapes open, or

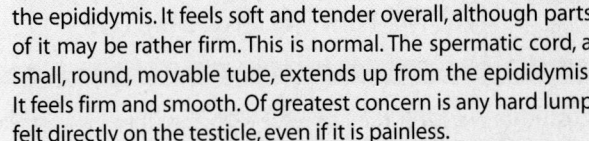

**BOX 47–2  ■  Testicular Self-Examination**

- Examine your testicles when you are taking a warm shower or bath, or just after if you prefer to use a mirror to compare size.
- The scrotum, testicles, and hands should be soapy to allow easy manipulation of the tissue.
- Gently roll each testicle between the thumb and fingers of each hand. If one testicle is substantially larger than the other, or if you feel any hard lumps, consult your physician immediately.
- Normal scrotal contents may be confusing. Just above and behind the testicle is the epididymis. It feels soft and tender overall, although parts of it may be rather firm. This is normal. The spermatic cord, a small, round, movable tube, extends up from the epididymis. It feels firm and smooth. Of greatest concern is any hard lump felt directly on the testicle, even if it is painless.
- Choose a day out of each month on which to examine yourself. Most men choose an easy day to remember, such as the first or last day of the month. Star this day on your calendar to help you remember.

if there is bleeding beyond slight oozing after 24 hours, the man should call the surgeon. Another rare complication is a hematoma in the scrotum caused by bleeding from the spermatic cord stump. Rapid onset of scrotal edema is a sign of this problem. *Because the man is usually discharged early, complications may not become apparent until he is at home.*
- Reinforce knowledge concerning the effect of surgery on sexuality. *If treatment involves only a unilateral orchiectomy, there should be no lasting effects on the client's sexual or reproductive function.*

## Ineffective Sexuality Patterns

The effect of testicular cancer and its treatment on sexual and reproductive function is varied. If the man has a retroperitoneal lymph node dissection, severing of the sympathetic plexus may result in retrograde ejaculation or failure to ejaculate. Infertility may be caused by ejaculation disorders, surgery, chemotherapy, or radiation therapy.

- Assess the man's prediagnosis sexual function. To assess this area, the nurse must establish an atmosphere of openness and permission to discuss sexual concerns. After the initial shock of the diagnosis, men report intense concern about sexual and reproductive issues, which can be relieved only by information. *Knowledge of the man's usual sexual function can guide teaching.*
- Discuss the possibility of preserving sperm in a bank prior to treatment. *This option may help relieve the man's fears about his ability to father children in the future, but must be completed prior to initiating treatment with surgery, chemotherapy, or radiation therapy.*

- Help coping with feelings about altered sexual function and appearance. Explain that testicular implants can be inserted to preserve appearance. *Many clients, regardless if they are in a significant relationship, deeply grieve the loss of the ability to father children. It is important to maintain body image despite disfiguring surgery.*

## Home Care

Families need to be included in teaching for a variety of reasons. If the man is of reproductive age, his partner will have significant anxiety and will require information. For the teenager, parents need information about the effect on sexual function and are often very involved in postoperative care. The man needs the support of the people he loves, and knowledgeable loved ones can give more effective support.

Provide teaching and reinforcement of the need for follow-up, especially if the retroperitoneal lymph nodes were not surgically explored. For men with a risk for recurrence, surveillance with periodic physical examinations, chest X-ray films, tumor markers, and CT scans of the retroperitoneal nodes could continue for a minimum of 5 years and possibly 10 years after orchiectomy.

# DISORDERS OF THE PROSTATE GLAND

## THE MAN WITH PROSTATITIS

**Prostatitis** is a term used to refer to different types of inflammatory disorders of the prostate gland. **Prostatodynia** is a condition in which the client experiences the symptoms of prostatitis but shows no evidence of inflammation or infection. Manifestations of prostatitis and prostatodynia are summarized in the box below.

## PATHOPHYSIOLOGY AND MANIFESTATIONS

The National Institutes of Health have defined four types of prostatitis: acute bacterial prostatitis, chronic bacterial prostatitis, chronic prostatitis/pelvic pain syndrome, and asymptomatic inflammatory prostatitis. Men with asymptomatic inflammatory prostatitis have no subjective symptoms, but are diagnosed when a biopsy or prostatic fluid examination is conducted.

## Acute Bacterial Prostatitis

Acute bacterial prostatitis is most often caused by an ascending infection from the urethra or reflux of infected urine into the ducts of the prostate gland. The organism most often responsible for the infection is *E. coli;* other causative organisms include *Pseudomonas, Klebsiella,* and *Chlamydia.*

Manifestations of acute bacterial prostatitis include increased temperature, malaise, muscle and joint pain, urinary frequency and urgency, dysuria, and urethral discharge. The man often experiences dull, aching pain in the perineum, rectum, or lower back. On rectal examination, the prostate is enlarged and painful.

## Chronic Bacterial Prostatitis

Men with chronic bacterial prostatitis often present with a history of recurrent urinary tract infections. The causative organisms are most often *E. coli, Proteus,* or *Klebsiella.* Calculi may form in the prostate and contribute to the chronicity of the problem.

The manifestations of chronic bacterial prostatitis include urinary frequency and urgency, dysuria, low back pain, and perineal discomfort. Epididymitis may be associated with the prostatitis.

## Chronic Prostatitis/Chronic Pelvic Pain Syndrome

This type of prostatitis is both the most common and the least understood of the syndromes (Porth, 2002). The two types (inflammatory and noninflammatory) are based on the presence of white blood cells in the prostatic fluid.

- *Inflammatory prostatitis* is believed to be an autoimmune disorder, but the actual cause is unknown. Men with this type of prostatitis have low back pain; urinary manifestations; pain in the penis, testicles, scrotum, lower back, and rectum; decreased libido, and painful ejaculations. They do not have bacteria in their urine, but do have abnormal inflammatory cells in prostatic secretions.

---

### Manifestations of Prostatitis and Prostatodynia

**Acute Bacterial Prostatitis**
- Onset (may be abrupt): obstruction, irritation, or pain upon voiding; frequency; and urgency
- Positive cultures of infectious organism
- Nonurinary symptoms: chills, fever, low back and pelvic floor pain

**Chronic Bacterial Prostatitis**
- Urinary symptoms sometimes similar to those of the acute form, except less sudden, less dramatic, or even absent
- Positive cultures of causative organism not always obtainable

**Chronic Prostatitis**
- Perineal, suprapubic, low back, or genital pain
- Irritation upon voiding
- Postejaculatory pain
- Negative cultures of organisms

**Prostatodynia**
- Pelvic, low back, or perineal pain
- Irritation or obstruction upon voiding
- No evidence of inflammation in the prostate
- No urinary tract infections
- Normal prostatic secretions

• *Noninflammatory prostatitis* (prostatodynia) has manifestations similar to those of inflammatory prostatitis, but no evidence of urinary or prostatic infection or inflammation can be found. The cause is not known, but is believed to be the result of a problem outside the prostate gland, such as obstruction of the bladder neck.

## COLLABORATIVE CARE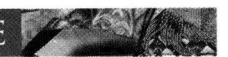

### Diagnostic Tests

It is often difficult to diagnose prostatitis. Urine and prostatic secretion examination and cultures are obtained to determine the presence and type of blood cells and bacteria. X-ray studies and ultrasound to visualize pelvic structures also may be useful.

### Medications

Bacterial prostatitis is treated with appropriate antibiotics. Men with the chronic form must take antibiotics for a much longer period, often up to 4 months, and may still relapse as soon as the antibiotic is discontinued. Nonbacterial prostatitis does not usually respond satisfactorily to drug therapy, although relief from symptoms is possible. Nonsteroidal anti-inflammatory drugs are useful for pain, and anticholinergics may reduce voiding symptoms. Prostatodynia is treated symptomatically to relieve muscle tension, usually with alpha-adrenergic blocking agents or muscle relaxants.

## NURSING CARE

Teaching for the man with prostatitis focuses on symptom management. Men with acute and chronic bacterial prostatitis should be taught to increase fluid intake to around 3 L daily and to void often. These measures help decrease irritation when voiding. Regular bowel movements helps ease pain associated with defecation. Local heat, such as sitz baths, may be helpful to relieve pain and irritation. It is important to teach the man to finish the course of antibiotic therapy. Men with chronic prostatitis/chronic pelvic pain syndrome need to know that the condition is not contagious and does not cause cancer (Porth, 2002).

## THE MAN WITH BENIGN PROSTATIC HYPERPLASIA (BPH)

**Benign prostatic hyperplasia (BPH),** an age-related, nonmalignant enlargement of the prostate gland, is a common disorder of the aging male. The prostate, very small at birth, grows at puberty, and reaches adult size around age 20. Benign hyperplasia (increased number of cells) begins at 40 to 45 years of age, and continues slowly through the rest of life. It is estimated that one-fourth of men over age 55 and one-half of men over 75 have manifestations of BPH (Porth, 2002). The problem that brings men to a health care provider is the associated urinary dysfunction.

## PATHOPHYSIOLOGY AND MANIFESTATIONS

The cause of BPH is unknown, but risk factors include age, family history, race, ethnicity, and hormonal factors. The incidence, which increases with age, is highest in African Americans and lowest in native Japanese. Higher rates have been associated with a family history of BPH.

The two necessary preconditions for BPH are age of 50 or greater and the presence of testes. Men who are castrated before puberty do not develop BPH. The androgen that mediates prostatic growth at all ages is dihydrotestosterone (DHT), which is formed in the prostate from testosterone. Although androgen levels decrease in aging men, the aging prostate appears to become more sensitive to available DHT. Estrogen, produced in small amounts in men, appears to sensitize the prostate gland to the effects of DHT. Increasing estrogen levels associated with aging or a relative increase in estrogen related to testosterone levels may contribute to prostatic hyperplasia.

BPH begins as small nodules in the periurethral glands, which are the inner layers of the prostate. The prostate enlarges through formation and growth of nodules (hyperplasia) and enlargement of glandular cells (hypertrophy). These changes occur over a long period of time. The pathophysiologic effects result from a combination of factors, including urethral resistance to the effects of BPH, intravesical pressure during voiding, detrusor muscle strength, neurologic functioning, and general physical health (McCance & Huether, 2002).

The expanding prostatic tissue compresses the urethra (Figure 47–3 ■) and causes partial or complete obstruction of the outflow of urine from the urinary bladder. The detrusor muscles hypertrophy to compensate for increased resistance to urinary flow; however, eventually decreased bladder compliance and bladder instability result. As a result, the man with BPH has manifestations from obstruction (weak urinary stream, increased time to void, hesitancy, incomplete bladder emptying, and postvoid dribbling) and irritation (frequency, urgency, incontinence, nocturia, dysuria, and bladder pain). Urinary retention may become chronic, resulting in overflow incontinence with any increase in intraabdominal pressure. There is little correlation between the size of the prostate gland and the urinary manifestations.

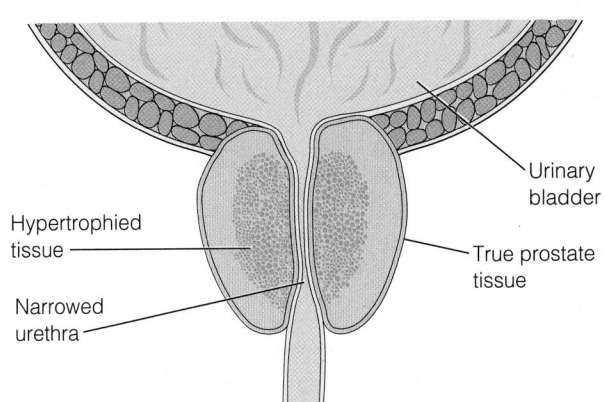

**Figure 47–3** ■ Benign prostatic hyperplasia.

*Labels:* Urinary bladder · True prostate tissue · Hypertrophied tissue · Narrowed urethra

## Manifestations of Benign Prostatic Hyperplasia

- Diminished force of urinary stream
- Hesitancy in initiating voiding
- Postvoid dribbling
- Sensation of incomplete emptying
- Urinary retention

- Nocturia
- Frequency
- Urgency
- Urge incontinence
- Dysuria
- Hematuria

Manifestations of BPH are summarized in the box above.

Unless the enlarging mass is reduced, multiple complications may occur. As urine is retained in the bladder, increasing bladder distention occurs. Diverticula (outpouchings) on the bladder wall result from the distention. The distention may also obstruct the ureters. Infection, more common in retained urine and in diverticula, may ascend from the bladder to the kidneys. Hydroureter, hydronephrosis, and renal insufficiency are possible complications.

## COLLABORATIVE CARE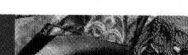

Care of men with BPH focuses on diagnosing the disorder, correcting or minimizing the urinary obstruction, and preventing or treating complications. There is no way to reverse BPH. Treatment is often determined by the severity of the manifestations and the presence of complications. Mild cases are often monitored over time, and may remain stable or improve.

### Diagnostic Tests

The following diagnostic tests may be ordered, and include those outlined in the clinical guidelines published by the Agency for Health Care Policy and Research (1994).

- *Urinalysis* detects bacteria, WBCs, or microscopic RBCs.
- *Serum creatinine levels* are determined to estimate renal function.
- *Prostate-specific antigen (PSA) levels* are obtained to rule out prostate cancer. PSA is a glycoprotein produced only in the cytoplasm of benign and malignant prostate cells; the serum level corresponds with the volume of both benign and malignant prostate tissue.
- *DRE* examines the external surface of the prostate gland. In BPH, the prostate is asymmetrical and enlarged.
- *Residual urine* (amount of urine remaining in the bladder after voiding) may be measured with ultrasonography or postvoiding catheterization (more than 100 mL is considered high).
- *Uroflowmetry* measures urine flow rate; normal is greater than 14 mL/second. A finding of less than 10 mL/second indicates obstruction.

In addition, the man's own subjective experiences with BPH are included in the diagnosis and treatment. For example, the International Prostate Symptom Score uses a scale of 0 (not at all) to 5 (almost always) to collect data about areas such as feeling as though the bladder did not empty with urinating, need to urinate within 2 hours after urinating, starting and stopping the stream several times while urinating, and straining to urinate. This questionnaire also asks how many times during the night the man gets up to urinate and how the man feels about having the disorder (Lepor, 2000).

### Medications

Treatment with medications is based on two considerations: The hyperplastic tissue is androgen dependent, and smooth muscle contraction within the prostate can exacerbate urinary obstruction. The first consideration is usually addressed by treatment for mild prostate enlargement with finasteride (Proscar), an antiandrogen agent that inhibits the conversion of testosterone to DHT and causes the enlarged prostate to shrink in size. Finasteride does cause impotence, decreased libido, and decreased volume of ejaculate. Client and family education includes the information that crushed tablets should not be handled by pregnant women, as the drug may be absorbed through the skin and be harmful to a male fetus.

Excessive smooth muscle contraction in BPH may be blocked with the alpha-adrenergic antagonists such as terazosin (Hytrin), doxazosin (Cardura), and tamsulosin (Flomax). These medications relieve obstruction and increase the flow of urine. They may cause orthostatic hypotension. Client and family teaching includes advice about making position changes slowly to avoid dizziness and accidental falls, how to take and record blood pressure, and to check with the health care provider before taking any medication for coughs, colds, or allergies (as these OTC medications may contain an adrenergic agent).

### Surgery

Men who have urinary retention, recurrent urinary tract infection, hematuria, bladder stones, or renal insufficiency secondary to BPH are candidates for surgical intervention. *Transurethral resection of the prostate (TURP), transurethral incision of the prostate (TUIP),* and open *prostatectomy* are the most common procedures.

A TURP is the surgical procedure used most often. Obstructing prostate tissue is removed using the wire loop of a resectoscope and electrocautery, inserted through the urethra (Figure 47–4 ■). This surgery has potential risks, however, including postoperative hemorrhage or clot retention, inability to void, and urinary tract infection. Other possible complications are incontinence, impotence, and retrograde ejaculation.

In the TUIP procedure, a YAG laser is used to make small incisions in the smooth muscle where the prostate is attached to the bladder. The gland is split to reduce pressure on the urethra. No tissue is removed, so this procedure is most appropriate for men with smaller prostate glands. TUIP can be done on an outpatient basis, and has the additional advantage of less risk of postoperative retrograde ejaculation than is associated with TURP or other prostatectomy procedures.

When the prostate gland is very large, an open prostatectomy may be used. These procedures are discussed in the section on prostate cancer that follows. Nursing care for the client having prostate surgery is outlined on pages 1539–1540.

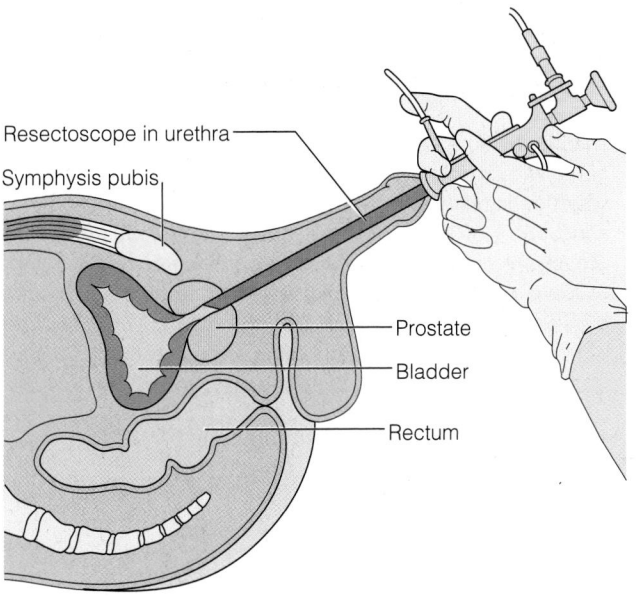

**A**  Transurethral resection of the prostate

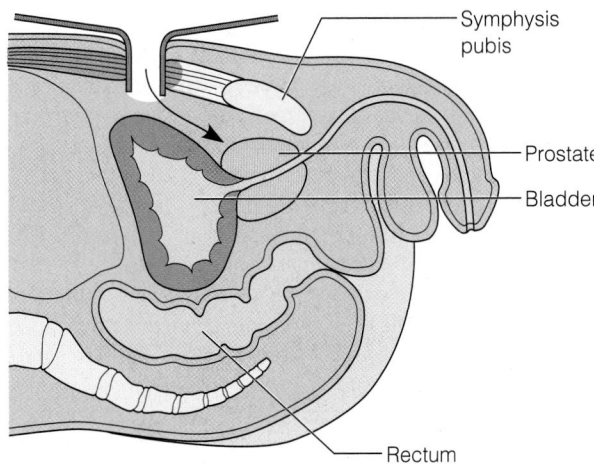

**B**  Retropubic prostatectomy

**Figure 47–4** ■ *A,* In a transurethral resection of the prostate (TURP), a resectoscope inserted through the urethra is used to remove excess prostate tissue. *B,* In a retropubic prostatectomy, prostate tissue is removed through an abdominal incision.

## NURSING CARE OF THE MAN UNDERGOING PROSTATECTOMY

### PREOPERATIVE NURSING CARE

- Assess the man's and family's knowledge about the surgery. *Some men are confused about the surgical approach, because there are several, quite different, methods.*
- Inform the man that he will have a urinary catheter when he returns from surgery, and he may have a drain(s) in his incision. He also will be wearing sequential pneumatic compression stockings. *This knowledge can reduce anxiety postoperatively and increase cooperation with postoperative care.*
- Ensure that a signed consent form is in the chart and that all other preoperative tasks outlined in Chapter 7 are done. ⬡
- Bowel preparation with a 2% neomycin enema may be ordered. *This cleanses the bowel if a perineal approach will be used.*
- Communicate willingness to address any concerns or anxiety. *Men may be anxious about the outcome of their surgery and potential long-term effects of the surgery on their sexuality. When a prostatectomy is performed for prostate cancer, additional fears include the extent of the cancer and surgery, chances for cure, and possible end-of-life issues.*

### POSTOPERATIVE CARE

- Maintain the usual postoperative assessments (see Chapter 7) and follow aseptic techniques in urinary drainage and irrigation care. Monitor vital signs closely for the first 24 hours and regularly thereafter. *The man who has had prostate surgery is at risk*

for hemorrhage and other postoperative complications. Vital sign changes may be early manifestations.
- Maintain accurate intake and output records, including amounts of irrigating solution used. Frequently assess patency of any catheters and drains. Monitor color and character of urine. *Catheters may become occluded by blood clots or kinks, interfering with urinary drainage and increasing the risk of hemorrhage.*
- Assess and manage the man's pain. *The man may have at least three types of pain: incisional pain, bladder spasm, and abdominal cramps due to intestinal gas. Analgesics and nonsteroidal anti-inflammatory drugs (NSAIDs) are administered on a routine and prn basis to control incisional pain. Bladder spasms may be accompanied by strong urges to void and urine leakage around the catheter. Belladona and opium (B & O) suppositories may be used to relieve bladder spasms.*
- Maintain antiembolic stockings and pneumatic compression devices as ordered. Assist with leg exercises and ambulation as ordered, usually the first postoperative day. *The man who has had prostate surgery is at risk for developing thromboemboli; these are important preventive measures.*
- Encourage the man to maintain a liberal fluid intake of 2 to 3 L a day. *Increased fluids reduce burning on urination after catheter removal and the risk of urinary tract infection.*

*(continued on page 1540)*

# NURSING CARE OF THE MAN UNDERGOING PROSTATECTOMY (continued)

## The Man with a Transurethral Resection of the Prostate (TURP)

- For the first 24 to 48 hours, monitor for hemorrhage, evidenced by frankly bloody urinary output, presence of large blood clots, decreased urinary output, increasing bladder spasms, decreased hemoglobin and hematocrit, tachycardia, and hypotension. Notify the physician if any of these manifestations occur. *Postoperative hemorrhage may be either arterial or venous, and may be precipitated by movement, bladder spasms, or an obstructed urinary drainage system.*

- Instruct the man with a three-way indwelling catheter with traction to keep the leg straight while the traction is applied. *A No. 18 to 22 Fr three-way catheter with a 30 to 45 mL balloon usually is inserted following a TURP. The inflated balloon is pulled down into the prostatic fossa and the catheter tubing is pulled down and taped to the man's leg to apply pressure against the operative site, preventing bleeding.*

- Explain that the presence of a urinary catheter will cause the sensation of needing to void, but it is important not to strain to try to void around the catheter or when having a bowel movement. Explain that bladder spasms, experienced as lower abdominal pressure or pain and a desire to urinate, may occur. Ensure that the man understands that this is an expected sensation, and that medications can help alleviate this discomfort. *Pressure on the urethra by the large catheter and on the internal sphincter by the catheter's balloon stimulate the micturition reflex. Straining to void or to have a bowel movement may stimulate bladder spasms and increase pain; it also may increase the risk for bleeding. Administer pain medications at regular intervals.*

- If the man has a continuous bladder irrigation (CBI), assess the catheter and the drainage tubing at regular intervals. Maintain the rate of flow of irrigating fluid to keep the output light pink or colorless. Assess the urinary output every 1 to 2 hours for color, consistency, amount, and presence of blood clots; assess for bladder spasms. *CBI is used to prevent the formation of blood clots, which could obstruct urinary output. Bladder distention resulting from output obstruction increases the risk of bleeding. Irrigating fluids are continuously infused and drained at a rate to keep urine light pink or colorless. Urine that is frankly bloody, contains many blood clots, or is decreased in amount, as well as bladder spasms, are indicators of obstruction and bleeding.*

- Assess for fluid volume excess and hyponatremia, called TURP syndrome, which is manifested by hyponatremia, decreased hematocrit, hypertension, bradycardia, nausea, and confusion. If these manifestations occur, notify the physician. *TURP syndrome results from the absorption of irrigating fluids during and after surgery. Untreated, it may result in dysrhythmias, seizures, or both.*

- If the man does not have CBI, follow agency procedure and physician orders for irrigating the indwelling catheter (usually when the urine is frankly bloody or has numerous larger blood clots, or when bladder spasms increase). In most in-

stances, using sterile technique, the catheter is gently irrigated with 50 mL of irrigating solution at a time, until the obstruction is relieved or the urine is clear. Ensure equal input and output of irrigating fluid. *Intermittent irrigation may be used to prevent obstruction of urinary drainage.*

- Following catheter removal, assess the amount, color, and consistency of urine. Explain that the man may experience burning on urination, that dribbling after urination is a common experience, and that the urine may contain small blood clots after catheter removal. *The CBI and catheter usually are removed in the 24 to 48 hours following surgery. Urinary control may be improved by teaching the man to start and stop the urine stream several times during each voiding and by practicing Kegel exercises. Regaining full control may take up to 1 year.*

## The Man with a Retropubic Prostatectomy

- Assess the abdominal incision for the presence of urine. *As the bladder is not entered during a retropubic prostatectomy, no urine should be found on the dressing.*

- Assess the abdominal incision for increased or purulent drainage, and the man for an increased temperature and pain. *These manifestations indicate the presence of infection.*

## The Man with a Suprapubic Prostatectomy

- Assess urinary output from both the suprapubic and the urethral catheters. *The man with a suprapubic prostatectomy often has two separate closed drainage systems: one from the suprapubic incision and one from a urethral catheter.*

- Assess the abdominal dressing for urinary drainage, and change saturated dressings frequently. Consult with a skin care specialist if necessary. *Urine is highly irritating to the skin.*

- Following removal of the urethral catheter (usually 2 to 4 days after surgery) and based on physician orders, clamp the suprapubic catheter and encourage the man to void. Assess residual urine by unclamping the suprapubic catheter and measuring urinary output after voiding. *If residual urine is 75 mL or less with several voidings, the suprapubic catheter is removed.*

## The Man with a Perineal Prostatectomy

- Assess perineal incision for drainage and manifestations of infection. *Location of the incision in the perineum increases the risk of infection.*

- Do not take rectal temperatures or administer enemas. *Insertion of a thermometer or enema tubing into the rectum may precipitate bleeding.*

- Use a T-binder or padded scrotal support to hold the dressing in place. Following removal of the dressing and perineal sutures, heat lamps or sitz baths may be used. *The location of the dressing makes application difficult: Heat lamps or sitz baths provide heat and promote healing.*

- Teach the man to perform perineal irrigations with sterile normal saline as ordered and after each bowel movement. *Because of the proximity of the incision to the anus, special wound care is necessary to prevent infection.*

Newer treatments for BPH include minimally invasive procedures such as balloon urethroplasty, destruction of excess prostate tissue using laser energy, microwave hyperthermia, and placement of intraurethral stents to maintain patency of the urethra. Balloon urethroplasty is a simple procedure in which a balloon-tipped catheter is inserted into the narrowed portion of the urethra. Inflation of the balloon widens the urethra, relieving obstruction. Obstructing prostate tissue can be destroyed using laser energy or desiccated by microwave hyperthermia. These procedures can be done as outpatient surgery.

## Phytotherapy

Phytotherapy is the use of plants or plant extracts for medical treatment. Several plant extracts have been used for years in Europe to treat BPH and are being used more often in the United States. The phytotherapy used include saw palmetto berry, the bark of *Pygeum africanum,* the roots of *Echinacea, purpurea,* and *Hypoxis rooperi,* and the leaves of the trembling poplar. The mechanisms of action of these extracts is unknown, but men report they are effective in relieving manifestations (Tierney, et al., 2001).

## NURSING CARE

Most men are unsure of the function of the prostate gland and even the prostate's exact location, though its relationship to sexual and urinary function is at least generally known. This lack of knowledge, coupled with the growing number of treatment options, is confusing to many men. There are many similarities between the nursing care of men with BPH and that of men with prostate cancer (see the section that follows). Nursing approaches to problems of urinary incontinence, sexual dysfunction, and pain are discussed there. This section provides interventions related to deficient knowledge, urinary retention, and risk of infection.

## Nursing Diagnoses and Interventions

### Deficient Knowledge

- Explain the anatomy and physiology of the prostate gland, as well as normal changes that occur with aging. *Men must know about their bodies in order to make accurate decisions about treatment.*
- Discuss treatment options, including information about effects on erectile function, ejaculation, and fertility. Counsel the man to discuss specific concerns with his urologist. *There are many different treatment options available; the choice should be a mutual decision between the man, his partner, and the urologist.*
- Discuss effects of TURP, including urinary retention and urinary incontinence. *These common transient postoperative effects are related to the surgical procedure and the postoperative indwelling catheter.*

- Explain to the man having a TURP that a catheter will be placed into the bladder, with the tubing taped to his inner thigh, and that irrigation fluid will be infusing into and out of the catheter for the first 36 to 72 hours following surgery. *The catheter and irrigation are necessary to remove blood clots from the bladder and allow drainage of urine. Gentle traction is applied to the catheter to apply pressure to the operative site (prostatic fossa) and prevent excessive bleeding.*
- Explain that, following removal of the catheter, he will most likely have urinary frequency and urgency. He may also experience dribbling of urine after voiding. Stress the importance of increasing oral fluid intake and regular Kegel exercises. *Urinary manifestations are related to the surgical procedure and the indwelling catheter. Increased fluid intake helps decrease dysuria. Kegel exercises strengthen periurethral muscles and decrease postvoiding urine leakage.*

### Urinary Retention

- Teach the manifestations of acute urinary retention: dysuria, overflow incontinence, bladder pain and distention, no urine output. *Acute urinary retention is a potential complication of BPH, requiring immediate medical attention.*
- Teach that the risk of developing urinary retention increases when the man with BPH takes over-the-counter diet or decongestant medications, or prescription medications such as antidepressants, anticholinergics, calcium channel blockers, antipsychotics, and medications to treat Parkinson's disease. *Over-the-counter decongestants and diet pills may contain alpha-adrenergic agonists that increase smooth muscle tone of the prostate, bladder neck, and proximal urethra. The prescribed medications may relax detrusor muscle contractions. Both actions may increase the risk of urinary retention (Gray & Brown, 2002).*
- Suggest avoiding intake of large volumes of liquid at any one time. *A single intake of a large volume of liquid results in rapid bladder filling and increases the risk of urinary retention.*

**PRACTICE ALERT**  *In addition to avoiding a large amount of fluids at one time, it is also important to teach the man to limit liquids that stimulate voiding, such as coffee and alcoholic beverages.* ■

- Teach how to use double-voiding technique: Urinate, then sit on the toilet for 3 to 5 minutes, then urinate again. *This technique may relieve mild to moderate urinary retention.*

### Risk for Infection

- Monitor WBC and vital signs. *Infection is indicated by an increase in WBCs, body temperature, and pulse rate.*
- Maintain sterile procedures when changing irrigation fluids and emptying Foley catheter draining bag. *Sterile procedures are necessary to prevent infection.*

## Risk for Imbalanced Fluid Volume

A prostatectomy brings increased risk of imbalanced fluid volume as a result of excessive bleeding from the operative site (prostatic fossa) as well as absorption of irrigating fluid.

- Monitor pulse and blood pressure. *Manifestations of hypovolemic shock include an increasing pulse and a decreasing blood pressure.*
- Monitor color of drainage in urinary drainage bag (Table 47–2). *The appearance of urine and irrigation fluid in the urinary drainage bag is an excellent indicator of bleeding after a prostatectomy.*

| TABLE 47–2 | Significance of Character of Urine After Prostatectomy and Related Nursing Care |
|---|---|
| **Urine Color** | **Nursing Implications** |
| Light red to red | Normal day of surgery and first postoperative day |
| Very dark red | May indicate increased venous bleeding or inadequate dilution. Catheter at risk for occlusion. Increase flow rate of irrigant. If urine does not clear, notify physician. |
| Bright red | May indicate arterial bleeding. Increase flow rate of irrigant, monitor vital signs, and notify physician. |
| Contains blood clots | Occasional blood clot normal. If clots are frequent, catheter may become obstructed. Increase flow rate of irrigant. |
| Clear to light pink | Normal throughout hospitalization. |

- Monitor for manifestations of transurethral resection (TURP) syndrome: nausea and vomiting, confusion, hypertension, bradycardia, and visual disturbances. *The absorption of isotonic bladder irrigating fluids during and after surgery may cause this hypervolemic, hyponatremic state. Treatment includes diuresis and, in severe cases, hypertonic saline administration (Tierney et al., 2001).*

## Home Care

Depending on the man's choice of treatment, the procedure may be performed on an outpatient basis. If there are no complications, the man having a TURP may be discharged within 2 days after surgery. Discharge instructions after prostate surgery are given in the box below. Home care often involves care of an indwelling urinary catheter. Teaching includes the following information.

- Change from the daytime leg drainage bag to a larger night drainage bag. A larger bag suspended from the bed frame at night permits gravity drainage of urine and prevents reflux of urine back into the bladder.
- Avoid strapping the leg bag on too tightly, which can decrease venous return and increase risk for thrombophlebitis and embolic complications such as pulmonary emboli.
- Place a soft cloth between the leg bag and thigh to decrease friction and absorb dampness under the bag, reducing the risk of skin irritation.
- Empty the leg bag every 3 to 4 hours to prevent overfilling.
- Promptly report any unexpected changes in urine color, consistency, or odor; hematuria, evidence of frank bleeding, or large blood clots, as well as a lack of or significant decrease in urine output to the urologist.

## Meeting Individualized Needs

### DISCHARGE INSTRUCTIONS FOR MEN AFTER PROSTATE SURGERY

#### ACTIVITY

The healing period lasts from 4 to 8 weeks. Avoid strenuous activity and heavy lifting. Do not drive for 2 weeks, except for short rides. Do take long walks, but take stairs slowly and carefully. Continue dorsiflexion exercises that you did in the hospital to prevent blood clots in the legs. You can take showers, but avoid tub baths while the catheter is in place.

#### BLEEDING

Bleeding can occur any time after surgery. It is fairly common after a bowel movement, coughing, or increased exercise. If you notice blood in the urine, increase fluids and rest until the urine is clear. If heavy bleeding plugs the channel, call the care provider immediately. Avoid aspirin and NSAIDS for at least 2 weeks.

#### BOWEL MOVEMENTS

Keep bowel movements regular and soft to avoid pressure on the prostate area. Drink fruit juices and take mild laxatives or stool softeners as ordered.

#### DIET

Resume your normal diet. Increase fluids to ten glasses (8 oz) daily. Avoid alcohol unless otherwise advised by your physician.

#### SEXUAL INTERCOURSE

Do not have sex for 6 weeks after surgery to avoid bleeding. You may still have erections even with the catheter in place. When you resume sex, ejaculate flows back into the bladder, so you will express little or no semen.

#### URINATION

After your catheter is removed, you may experience some burning, stinging, or leakage for several weeks, and you may pass small blood clots occasionally. These symptoms will disappear as the area heals. It is best to use pads to control leakage.

#### WORK

If work is not strenuous, you may return in 4 weeks; otherwise, wait 6 to 8 weeks.

#### PLEASE CALL IMMEDIATELY IF:

- You are unable to urinate.
- Bleeding is not controlled by fluids and rest, or is excessive.
- You have chills and fever or severe abdominal pain.
- Your scrotum becomes swollen and tender.
- You have pain in one calf, chest pain, or difficulty breathing.

## THE MAN WITH PROSTATIC CANCER

Cancer of the prostate is the most common type of cancer and the second leading cause of death in North America (ACS, 2002). It is primarily a disease of older men, increasing in incidence with age, with the majority of cases diagnosed in men older than 65 years. It is estimated that each year, approximately 189,000 men will be diagnosed with prostate cancer, and 30,000 will die of it. Prostate cancer is a major health problem for older men, but the death rate is decreasing due to advances in diagnosis and treatment.

When diagnosed early, prostate cancer is curable. When the cancer is confined to the prostate at diagnosis, the 5-year survival rate is 100%. Even when the cancer has spread regionally, approximately 95% of clients are alive after 5 years. More than 75% of prostate cancer diagnoses are made at one of these stages (ACS, 2002). Many men are found to have prostate cancer on autopsy; usually the cancer has produced no manifestations or complications.

## PATHOPHYSIOLOGY AND MANIFESTATIONS

The prostate gland consists primarily of glandular epithelial cells. The exact etiology of prostate cancer is unknown, although androgens are believed to have a role in its development. Almost all primary prostate cancers are adenoncarcinomas, and develop in the peripheral zones of the prostate gland. This location increases the risk of local spread to the prostatic capsule. Despite its proximity to the rectum, metastasis to the bowel is uncommon because a tough sheet of tissue, Denonvilliers' fascia, acts as an effective physical barrier.

As the tumor enlarges, it may compress the urethra, obstructing urinary flow. The tumor may metastasize and involve the seminal vesicles or bladder by direct extension. Metastasis by lymph and venous channels is common.

Men with early-state prostate cancer are often asymptomatic. Pain from metastasis to bones is often the initial manifestation noted. Urinary manifestations depend on the size and location of the tumor and the stage of the malignancy. They are often much like manifestations of BPH: urgency, frequency, hesitancy, dysuria, and nocturia. The man may also notice hematuria or blood in the ejaculate (Porth, 2002). Manifestations are summarized in the box on this page.

Death usually occurs secondary to debility caused by multiple sites of skeletal metastasis, especially to the vertebrae. Compression fractures of the spine are common, resulting in the possible loss of mobility and bowel and bladder function. Tumors may eventually involve bone marrow, resulting in severe anemias and impaired immune function.

### Risk Factors

In addition to age, race is a significant risk factor for prostate cancer (see the Focus on Diversity box on this page). Other risk factors are as follows:

- Genetic and hereditary factors, with risk increased in men who have a family history of the disease

## Manifestations of Prostate Cancer

**Genitourinary**
- Dysuria
- Frequency of urination
- Reduction in urinary stream
- Nocturia

- Nocturia
- Hematuria
- Abnormal prostate on digital rectal examination

**Musculoskeletal**
- Bone or joint pain
- Migratory bone pain

- Back pain

**Neurologic**
- Nerve pain
- Bilateral lower extremity weakness

- Bowel or bladder dysfunction
- Muscle spasms

**Systemic**
- Weight loss

- Fatigue

## Focus on Diversity

### RISK AND INCIDENCE OF PROSTATE CANCER

- African Americans have the highest incidence of prostate cancer in the United States and the world, with rates more than twice as high as whites.
- African Americans also are more likely to be diagnosed later and to die of prostate cancer, with a mortality rate more than double that of other racial and ethnic groups.
- Asians and Native Americans have the lowest incidence of prostate cancer.

- Having a vasectomy, believed to increase the levels of circulating free testosterone
- Dietary factors, including a diet high in fat and red meats, low in vitamin A, vitamin D, lycopene, and selenium (McCance & Huether, 2002)
- Low exposure to sunlight

## COLLABORATIVE CARE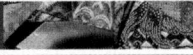

Care of the man with prostate cancer focuses on diagnosis, elimination or containment of the cancer, and prevention or treatment of complications. There are currently no proven clinical strategies to prevent the development of prostate cancer. Therefore, strategies for early detection remain the major emphasis for control of this disease.

### Diagnostic Tests

Although an increasing number of clients are now diagnosed with asymptomatic prostate cancer, many clients with prostate cancer have either locally advanced cancer or distant metastasis at the time of diagnosis. The definitive diagnosis can be made only by biopsy; however, other tests may suggest the presence of prostate cancer.

- *DRE*, with the prostate gland being nodular and fixed in prostate cancer.

• *Prostate-specific antigen (PSA) levels* are used to diagnose and stage prostate cancer, and to monitor response to treatment (normal levels are <4 ng/mL). Although men with BPH also have elevated PSA levels, almost two-thirds of those with a PSA greater than 10 ng/mL have prostate cancer (Tierney et al., 2001).

• *Transrectal ultrasonography (TRUS)* is used when the DRE is abnormal or if the PSA is elevated.

• *Prostatic biopsy* must be performed and interpreted before the diagnosis of prostate cancer can be established.

Either needle biopsy or a TRUS-guided biopsy is performed. Implications for nursing care are presented in the box below.

• *Grade* and *stage* help to determine prognosis and guide treatment decisions. Grade (cancer cell differentiation) is determined by the pathologist. Prostate cancer is staged with a variety of tests. Table 47–3 outlines treatment options according to the stage of the cancer.

• *Bone scan, MRI, or CT scans* may be performed to determine the presence of tumor metastasis.

## Nursing Implications for Diagnostic Tests

### Prostate Biopsy

#### Preparation

• Assess the man's understanding of the procedure. The procedure is becoming common, and many men will have heard about it from friends or family and may have significant anxiety. Especially if the man has experienced uncomfortable or perhaps painful rectal examinations in the past, the prospect of a needle advanced through the rectum into the gland can be frightening. Be sure to describe the procedure fully, and explain what the man will feel. Inform the man that he will be awake and lying on his side. (The examination can also be performed in the sitting, supine, or lithotomy position.) A local anesthetic (2% lidocaine jelly) will be applied to the rectum to minimize pain caused by stretching of the rectal wall. Because the pain receptors in the rectum respond only to stretch, the man will feel no pain as the needle penetrates the rectal wall. The ultrasound probe is inserted in the rectum approximately 10 cm, and then a balloon covering the probe is inflated with water to visualize the prostate. The man will feel a sensation of rectal fullness and possibly pain. Many men describe it as very uncomfortable. The biopsy instrument is inserted next to the probe. Men may feel a sharp pain (a "pinch") as the biopsy is obtained. Reassure the man that the nurse will be with him throughout the procedure to provide support.

• A signed consent should be in the man's chart, as this procedure is invasive.

• Some urologists require a preoperative bleeding profile and complete blood count. The man is often advised to avoid aspirin products and nonsteroidal anti-inflammatory agents for a week before the biopsy.

• An enema is usually administered prior to the examination to ensure a clean rectum.

#### Teaching

• You will be monitored for approximately 1 hour after the examination to ensure that your vital signs are stable and that you can urinate without difficulty.

• Avoid any strenuous activity for the rest of the day.

• Hematuria (blood in the urine) and some bloody streaks in the stool are expected for 24 to 48 hours after the procedure. You can also expect hematospermia (blood in the ejaculate) for a few days to 2 weeks afterward, depending on how often you ejaculate.

• Report any signs of unusual bleeding, such as blood clots in your urine or bloody stools, or infection, such as rectal pain, dysuria, and urgency.

### TABLE 47–3  Prostate Cancer Staging and Treatment

| Stage | Description | Treatment |
|-------|-------------|-----------|
| I | Confined to prostate, nonpalpable, focal involvement; well differentiated | Observation and follow-up<br>Interstitial or external-beam radiation therapy<br>Radical prostatectomy |
| II | Confined to prostate, palpable, involves one or both lobes; poorly differentiated | Careful observation in selected clients<br>Radical prostatectomy<br>Interstitial or external-beam radiation therapy<br>Ultrasound-guided percutaneous cryosurgery |
| III | Extension of the tumor outside the prostate capsule, possible seminal vesicle involvement | External-beam radiation therapy<br>Interstitial radiation<br>Radical prostatectomy<br>Adjunctive hormone therapy<br>Palliative surgery (TURP) |
| IV | Extension of the tumor into surrounding tissues; lymph node involvement or distant metastasis | Hormone therapy<br>External-beam radiation therapy<br>Palliative treatment with radiation therapy and/or TURP<br>Radical prostatectomy with orchiectomy<br>Chemotherapy |

## Treatments

The treatment of prostate cancer is complex and depends on the grade and stage of the cancer as well as the age, general health, and preference of the client. In some cases, for example, when the client with a slow-growing tumor is elderly or has a limited life expectancy, watchful waiting is the treatment of choice. Treatments for prostate cancer include surgery, radiation therapy, and hormone manipulation.

### Surgery

Surgery for prostate cancer includes several types of prostatectomies. For very early disease in older men, cure may be achieved with a simple prostatectomy (TURP).

- *Radical prostatectomy* involves removal of the prostate, prostatic capsule, seminal vesicles, and a portion of the bladder neck. Many clients experience varying degrees of urinary incontinence and erectile dysfunction. Refer to the box on pages 1539–1540 for nursing care of men having a prostatectomy.
- *Retropubic prostatectomy* is most often performed because it allows adequate control of bleeding, visualization of the prostate bed and bladder neck, and access to pelvic lymph nodes.
- *Perineal prostatectomy* is often preferred for older men or those who are poor surgical risks. This approach requires less time, and involves less bleeding.
- *Suprapubic prostatectomy* is rarely used, usually when problems with the bladder are expected. Control of bleeding is more difficult because the surgical approach is through the bladder.

For clients with stage III, locally advanced (beyond the prostatic capsule) cancer, surgery is controversial because of the likelihood of hidden lymph node metastasis and relapse. TURP is not performed as curative therapy but may be used to relieve urinary obstruction for men with advanced disease (stage III or IV).

Surgical intervention is now available for men with urinary sphincter insufficiency, which is the major cause of incontinence after prostatectomy. An artificial urinary sphincter is surgically implanted (Figure 47–5 ■). To be eligible, the man must be able to manipulate the pump placed in the scrotum and have adequate cognitive function to know when a problem with the appliance occurs.

### Radiation Therapy

Radiation therapy may be used as a primary treatment for prostate cancer. Long-term problems of impotence and urinary incontinence may be avoided, and survival rates often are comparable. Radiation may be delivered either by external beam or interstitial implants of radioactive seeds of iodine, gold, palladium, or iridium (*brachytherapy*). Interstitial radiation has a lower risk of impotence and rectal damage than external-beam radiation. See Chapter 10 ⬡⬡ for nursing care of the client receiving radiation therapy. Table 47–4 compares the possible complications of radiation therapy with those of surgery.

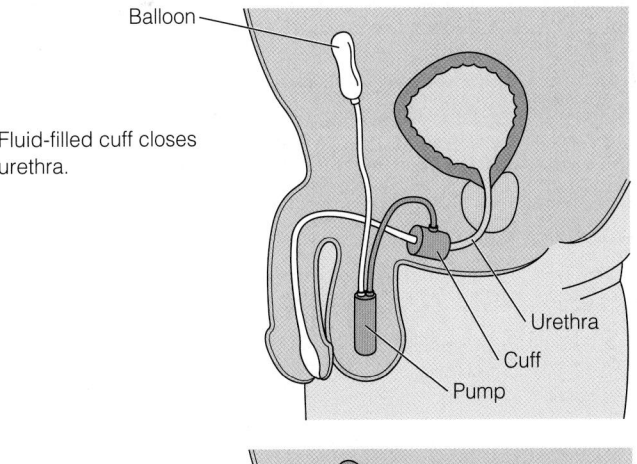

Fluid-filled cuff closes urethra.

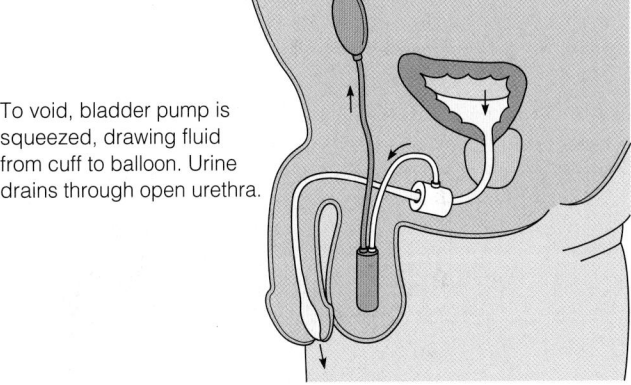

To void, bladder pump is squeezed, drawing fluid from cuff to balloon. Urine drains through open urethra.

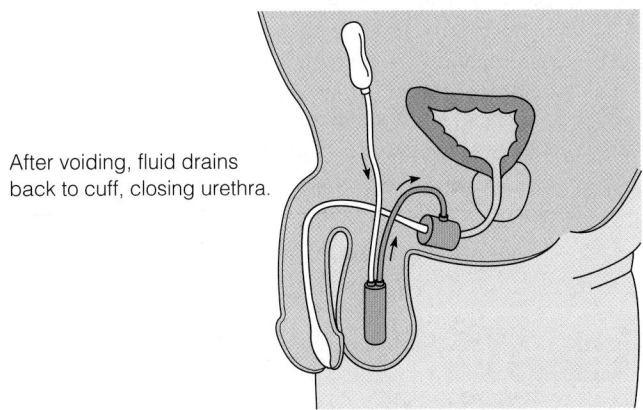

After voiding, fluid drains back to cuff, closing urethra.

**Figure 47–5 ■** Method of operation of an artificial urinary sphincter.

Radiation therapy has a palliative role for clients with metastatic prostate cancer, reducing the size of bone metastasis, controlling pain, and restoring function, such as continence or the ability to ambulate for clients with spinal cord compression.

### Hormonal Manipulation

Androgen deprivation therapy is used to treat advanced prostate cancer. Many cells in the growing tumor are androgen dependent and either cease to grow or die if deprived of androgens. Unfortunately, other cancer cells thrive without androgen and are unaffected by therapy to reduce circulating androgens. Therefore, the effects of hormone manipulations vary from complete but temporary regression of the tumor to no response

| TABLE 47-4 | Potential Complications Related to Radical Prostatectomy and Radiation Therapy |
| --- | --- |

| Radical Prostatectomy | Radiation Therapy |
| --- | --- |
| Erectile dysfunction | Erectile dysfunction* |
| Urethral stricture | Urethral stricture |
| Fistula/rectal injury | Rectal/anal stricture* |
| Urinary incontinence | Cystitis |
| Surgical/anesthetic risk | Diarrhea |
|  | Proctitis |
|  | Rectal ulcer |
|  | Bowel obstruction* |
|  | Urinary incontinence |

*Delayed complications; may appear months or years after completion of therapy.

at all. Strategies to induce androgen deprivation vary from orchiectomy to oral administration of hormonal agents. Table 47–5 lists hormone therapies and the advantages and disadvantages of each.

## NURSING CARE

### Health Promotion

Nurses are in a unique position to increase public awareness about detecting early prostate cancer. Every encounter with men and their families—in clinics, hospital units, or in the home—is an opportunity to provide information about early detection and identify needs. Several studies have shown a positive correlation between increased awareness of and participation in prostate cancer screening procedures. The American Cancer Society has free pamphlets about early detection of prostate cancer, which are useful in educating the public.

All men should be given information about the limitations and benefits of testing for early detection and treatment so they can make an informed decision. The American Cancer Society (2002) recommends that the PSA and DRE should be offered each year, beginning at age 50, to all men with a life expectancy of at least 10 years. Men at high risk (men of African descent and those with a first-degree relative diagnosed at a younger age) should begin testing at age 45. In addition, men with an even higher risk, due to multiple first-degree relatives diagnosed at an early age, could begin testing at age 40, with the following criteria:

PSA <1.0 ng/mL, no additional testing needed until age 45
PSA >1.0 ng/mL but <2.5 ng/mL, have annual testing
PSA >2.5 ng/mL, further evaluation with a biopsy

### Assessment

Collect the following data through the health history and physical examination (see Chapter 46). Note that a rectal examination is an advanced nursing assessment.

- Health history: risk factors, urinary elimination patterns and manifestations, hematuria, pain
- Physical assessment: DRE to assess prostate size, symmetry, firmness, and nodules

### Nursing Diagnoses and Interventions

The nursing care of men with prostate cancer must be holistic, sensitive, and individualized. The nursing diagnoses discussed for the man with BPH may also be appropriate. This section focuses on problems with urinary incontinence, sexual function, and pain.

### Urinary Incontinence (Reflex, Stress, Total)

Urinary incontinence is a disturbing complication following treatment for prostate cancer. Both radical prostatectomy and external-beam radiation therapy can cause incontinence, rang-

| TABLE 47-5 | Surgical and Hormone* Therapy in the Management of Advanced Prostate Cancer | | |
| --- | --- | --- | --- |
| **Treatment** | **Advantages** | | **Disadvantages** |
| Orchiectomy | Inexpensive Immediate effect; i.e., men report diminished pain from metastasis in the recovery room | | Body image problems due to loss of testicles |
| Estrogen compounds (diethylstilbestrol) | Inexpensive Effects reversible | | Increased risk of cardiovascular problems More likely to cause gynecomastia, hypertrophy of breast tissue |
| Luteinizing hormone-releasing hormone agonist (LHRH) (leuprolide) | Effects reversible No cardiovascular risk Monthly administration | | Very expensive Subcutaneous injection route Slow onset: up to 4 weeks |
| Steroidal antiandrogens (megestrol [Megace]) | Effects reversible No cardiovascular risk Inexpensive | | May not drop testosterone levels sufficiently Weight gain |
| Nonsteroidal antiandrogens (flutamide; often used in conjunction with LHRH) | Does not alter circulating androgens Blocks some side effects of LHRH May be effective if other methods fail | | Very expensive |

*All hormonal manipulations have the potential disadvantage of loss of libido, erectile dysfunction, hot flashes, and gynecomastia.

ing from a drop or two when the client lifts a heavy object (**stress incontinence**) to no control at all. Older men may experience **urge incontinence,** the involuntary passage of urine soon after a strong sense of urgency to void. Total and unpredictable loss of urine is classified as total incontinence. The man's reaction to incontinence may be severe even if the incontinence is not great. Many men have significant anxiety at the prospect of an incontinent episode in public, because they feel shame and often guilt about the loss of control.

- Assess the degree of incontinence and its effects on lifestyle. *The nurse needs to determine the client's previous urinary patterns and the type of incontinence currently being experienced to plan appropriate interventions.*
- Teach Kegel exercises to help restore continence. *Pelvic muscle or Kegel exercises can often either eliminate or improve stress incontinence.*
- Teach methods to control dampness and odor from stress incontinence.
  - Do not attempt to prevent accidental voiding by restricting fluids. *Not only will the client continue to have incontinent episodes, but also his urine will become concentrated, exacerbating the problem with odor.*
  - Manage occasional episodes (one to three small volume accidents per day) with absorbent pads worn inside the underwear and changed as needed. Most pads are made with a polymer gel that controls odor. *Appropriate measures help promote good hygiene, decrease anxiety, and increase comfort.*
- Refer to physical therapy or a continence specialist for additional measures to promote continence. *Special exercises, restricting some types of fluids, and other measures such as bladder training can help the client deal with incontinence.*

- Explore options such as an external collection device (external catheter or Texas catheter) for the man with total incontinence. *This device may improve the client's self-esteem and allow resumption of social activities.*
- Encourage verbalizing feelings about the impact of incontinence on his quality of life. *The degree of incontinence does not necessarily correlate to the client's perceived level of suffering. Listening to these concerns with sensitivity can help the client work through these feelings and may allow him to move toward a healthy adaptation to his disability.*

## Sexual Dysfunction

Surgical treatment for prostate cancer may cause erectile dysfunction and changes in ejaculatory function. Hormone therapy for advanced prostate cancer lowers libido and may also cause erectile dysfunction. The diagnosis of cancer and body image changes caused by hormone therapy may lower self-esteem, which in turn can diminish sexual desire and willingness to interact sexually with a partner. Most older men are active sexually and fully capable of sustaining an erection. They are likely to fear the effect of treatment on their sexual health. They may allow this concern to guide their decision about the treatment course, or they may refuse all therapy because of this fear. Client reactions vary greatly, and the nurse must maintain a nonjudgmental approach to education and support.

- Assess the man's pretreatment sexual function. *Knowledge of previous sexual function is necessary to plan appropriate interventions.*
- Teach the man about the actual or potential effects of therapy on sexual function (see the box below). *The incidence of erectile dysfunction varies with different therapies for prostate cancer.*

---

## Nursing Research

### Evidence-Based Practice to Identify Sexual Needs in Men with BPH and Prostate Cancer

The consequences of treatment for prostatic hyperplasia and prostate cancer often include postoperative physical effects such as erectile dysfunction, retrograde ejaculation, and loss of sexual desire. This study (Jakobsson, 2001) compared sexual problems in men with prostate cancer in comparison to men with prostatic hyperplasia and men in the general population. The men with hyperplasia and cancer, in comparison to men in the general population, reported more problems with sexual pleasure and attraction, erectile function and sexual satisfaction, and sexual performance (including a lower intercourse frequency). Despite these problems, neither the men nor their partners used medications, masturbation, or artificial aids to achieve erection. The disease and the treatment of prostatic hyperplasia and prostate cancer were found to interfere with sexual intimacy between men and their partners.

#### IMPLICATIONS FOR NURSING

Men with prostate disease need information about the effects of treatment on their sexual functioning. It is important to assess the man's knowledge about his body, a past history of sexual function and satisfaction, and current dysfunction and concerns. When used as part of the total assessment, questions about sexual function

legitimize sexual concerns, establish an understanding of terminology, determine understanding of the disease and treatment options, and determine understanding of the side effects of treatments and medications and their effects on body image and sexuality.

If time is limited for assessment or if the nurse is not comfortable discussing this area of human functioning, a questionnaire may be used. In addition to information about the potential effects of treatment, men and their partners also need education about options available to achieve erection and sexual intimacy.

#### Critical Thinking in Client Care

1. You are caring for a 75-year-old man who has a TURP for BPH. His wife tells you that they have always had an active sex life and she hopes this will not ruin that. What would you say to her?
2. Consider the implications for sexual dysfunction in the man diagnosed with prostate cancer. Do you believe the diagnosis of cancer, when combined with the effects of treatment, might affect sexual function even more? Why or why not?
3. Health care providers sometimes view the older adult as asexual. How does this view affect assessments and teaching? What can be done to change this situation?

- Provide an opportunity for the man and his partner to discuss implications of and concerns about the diagnosis and treatment on sexual function. *The treatments for prostate cancer often affect the physiology of erection. The man and his partner need support and counseling during the period of adjustment.*
- Discuss medical and surgical treatments for erectile dysfunction (see first section of this chapter). *Many men are as devastated by the loss of erectile function as they are by the diagnosis of cancer. Information about achieving erection and maintaining sexual intimacy is essential to quality of life.*

**PRACTICE ALERT** *A therapeutic approach to assessing how the man feels is to use an opening statement such as, "Some men are very concerned about effects of (type of treatment) on their ability to have an erection. Tell me how you feel about it."* ■

- Refer for sexual counseling as appropriate. *The man and his partner may require therapy beyond that provided by nurses.*

## Acute/Chronic Pain

The causes of pain in clients with advanced prostate cancer are many. It is not unusual for a client to have three or four distinct pains simultaneously, all from different sources. The most common cause of pain is metastasis to the spinal column, usually the thoracic spine. Other sources of pain include fractures, lymphedema of the lower extremities, gynecomastia, and mus-cle spasms. Because most clients are over the age of 65, many also have pain associated with preexisting conditions, such as osteoarthritis, unrelated to the cancer.

- Assess the intensity, location, and quality of the client's pain. *A cardinal rule of successful pain management is the importance of reducing or eliminating the cause of pain. Appropriate interventions are based on a careful assessment of the client's pain.*
- Provide optimal pain relief with prescribed analgesics. *It is important that the man and his family understand that pain medications should be used on a regular basis to maintain comfort and should not be delayed until pain is severe.*
- Teach the client and family noninvasive methods of pain control. *Various modalities can be successful in alleviating pain or reducing its perception, thus enhancing the comfort of the client (see Chapter 4).* ⊘

## Using NANDA, NIC, and NOC

Chart 47–1 shows links between NANDA nursing diagnoses, NIC, and NOC when caring for the man with surgical treatment for prostate cancer.

## Home Care

Depending on the type of treatment, the following topics should be addressed in preparing the man and his family for home care.

---

### CHART 47–1 NANDA, NIC, AND NOC LINKAGES

#### The Client with Surgical Treatment of Prostate Cancer

| NURSING DIAGNOSES | NURSING INTERVENTIONS | NURSING OUTCOMES |
|---|---|---|
| • Acute Pain | • Analgesia Administration<br>• Anxiety Reduction<br>• Pain Management | • Pain Level<br>• Symptom Severity |
| • Risk for Infection | • Infection Control<br>• Nutrition Management<br>• Skin Surveillance<br>• Wound Care | • Risk Control<br>• Nutritional Status<br>• Tissue Integrity: Skin |
| • Impaired Urinary Elimination | • Urinary Elimination Management<br>• Bladder Irrigation<br>• Fluid Management<br>• Tube Care: Urinary<br>• Pain Management | • Urinary Elimination |
| • Disturbed Body Image | • Active Listening<br>• Coping Enhancement<br>• Teaching: Sexuality<br>• Support Group | • Acceptance: Health Status<br>• Grief Resolution |

*Note. Data from* Nursing Outcomes Classification (NOC) *by M. Johnson & M. Maas (Eds.), 1997, St. Louis: Mosby;* Nursing Diagnoses: Definitions & Classification 2001–2002 *by North American Nursing Diagnosis Association, 2001, Philadelphia: NANDA;* Nursing Interventions Classification (NIC) *by J.C. McCloskey & G. M. Bulechek (Eds.), 2000, St. Louis: Mosby. Reprinted by permission.*

- For the man having a surgical procedure: manifestations of infection and excessive bleeding, catheter care, wound care pain management
- For the man having radiation therapy (Greifzu, 2000):
  - Danger of radiation damage to others (sleep in a room alone for a week, avoid close contact with pregnant women, infants, and children)
  - Condom use during sexual contact (ejaculate may be discolored, distressing sexual partner)

- The importance of keeping appointments with health care providers and having yearly PSA and rectal examinations
- If appropriate, community services, such as support groups, home health nurses, and hospice
- Helpful resources:
  - American Cancer Society
  - American Urological Association
  - National Cancer Institute

## Nursing Care Plan
## A Man with Prostate Cancer

William Turner, a 71-year-old African American, lives with his wife in a small retirement community in Florida. His wife had a stroke 2 years ago, and Mr. Turner does all the cooking and housework. He has been in good health for most of his life, having only "a small touch" of osteoarthritis in his knees and hands. He has noticed a gradual onset of urinary urgency and frequency over the past 2 years, but has never had incontinence. During a routine checkup, the nurse practitioner at the local health clinic performs a digital rectal examination and palpates a hard nodule on the surface of Mr. Turner's prostate. After his PSA is found to be elevated, he is referred to a urologist, who diagnoses prostate cancer. Mr. Turner chooses to have surgery, and a radical retropubic prostatectomy and lymph node dissection are performed. The lymph nodes are negative for metastasis. Following surgery, his recovery is uncomplicated. However, the nurse caring for Mr. Turner is concerned about his ability to care for his indwelling catheter because of his arthritis and his wife's physical disabilities from the stroke. The nurse makes a referral to a home health agency to ensure Mr. Turner can manage his care at home. An initial home health assessment is scheduled for the day after Mr. Turner is discharged from the hospital.

### ASSESSMENT

The home health nurse notes that the house is clean and neat. Mr. Turner is dressing, but still wearing his night urinary drainage bag, even though it is 1300. Mr. Turner tells the nurse that his main problem is going to get groceries, because he is embarrassed to be seen with the drainage bag. He says he has not been able to remove the drainage bag and attach the leg bag because of his arthritis. Physical assessment findings include the pelvic incision to be healing without signs of infection. There is no tenderness in his calves, chest pain, or shortness of breath. The urine is yellow, without odor. Mr. Turner does state that he sees no need for the pelvic exercises since he is no longer in the hospital. He also expresses the belief that he is cured of cancer and questions the need for follow-up care.

### DIAGNOSES

- *Risk for stress urinary incontinence* related to surgical procedure
- *Ineffective health maintenance* related to inability to care for the urinary drainage system, not understanding need for postoperative exercises, and questions about follow-up care

### EXPECTED OUTCOMES

- Regain urinary continence after catheter removal.
- Change the urinary drainage bag with the appropriate assistance.
- Verbalize the rationale for performing postoperative exercise.
- Verbalize the need for continued follow-up care.

### PLANNING AND IMPLEMENTATION

- Discuss the possibility of stress incontinence after the catheter is removed.
- Reinforce the need for Kegel exercises while the catheter is still in place.
- Explore Mr. Turner's support system to identify people who could assist him with catheter care and arrange a teaching session with them.
- Teach Mr. Turner the importance of follow-up care, relating the care to the history of the disease.

### EVALUATION

Good friends from Mr. Turner's church have assisted him with care of his drainage bag, and have reminded him to do his Kegel exercises several times a day while the catheter is in place. When the catheter is removed, Mr. Turner has only a small amount of leaking of urine after voiding. He understands that it may take several weeks for this to resolve. Efforts to help him understand the need for continued medical care are less successful. Mr. Turner continues to state that he is cured, his wife needs him, and he sees no need to go back to the doctor.

### Critical Thinking in the Nursing Process

1. Outline a teaching plan for Mr. Turner for the risk for altered skin integrity related to urinary incontinence.
2. As a result of Mr. Turner's refusal to have ongoing medical care, he might be labeled as noncompliant. Would you make this nursing diagnosis? Why or why not?
3. If you were the home health nurse making a home visit and found that Mr. Turner had no urinary drainage for 16 hours, what assessments would you make? How would you handle this problem?

See Evaluating Your Response in Appendix C.

# MALE BREAST DISORDERS

## THE MAN WITH GYNECOMASTIA

**Gynecomastia,** the abnormal enlargement of the male breast, is thought to result from a high ratio of estradiol to testosterone. It is common during puberty, affecting as many as 50% of adolescent males, but usually resolves within 1 to 2 years. Any condition that increases estrogen activity or decreases testosterone production can contribute to gynecomastia. Conditions that increase estrogen activity include obesity, testicular tumors, liver disease, and adrenal carcinoma; conditions that decrease testosterone production include chronic illness such as tuberculosis or Hodgkin's disease, injury, and orchitis. Drugs such as digitalis, opiates, and chemotherapeutic agents are also associated with gynecomastia. Gynecomastia is usually bilateral. If it is unilateral, biopsy may be necessary to rule out breast cancer.

No treatment is necessary for the transient gynecomastia of puberty. If the condition becomes chronic, however, creating psychologic discomfort, surgery may be necessary to remove the subcutaneous breast tissue. When related to an underlying disorder such as tuberculosis, treatment of that disorder is required. In severe cases, tamoxifen is given to decrease estrogen activity.

Nursing care for the client with gynecomastia includes education about the cause and treatment of the condition, and emotional support for the psychosocial implications of this feminizing condition.

## THE MAN WITH BREAST CANCER

Although male breast cancer is rare, accounting for about 1% of all breast cancer cases, it is as serious to the men who have it as it is to the women. About 1500 men in the United States are estimated to be diagnosed with breast cancer each year, accounting for 400 deaths (ACS, 2002). The etiology of male breast cancer is unclear; hormonal, genetic, and perhaps environmental factors appear to be important.

Male breast cancer is clinically and histologically similar to female breast cancer, although lobular cancer is rare in males. Most tumors are estrogen-receptor positive. Because many men believe that breast cancer is only a woman's disease, they often delay seeking medical attention for symptoms and thus may present with advanced disease.

Treatment of male breast cancer is much like the treatment of female breast cancer, beginning with modified radical mastectomy, node dissection, and staging to determine the therapeutic options. Radiation, chemotherapy, or hormonal therapy (usually tamoxifen), are the conventional adjuncts to surgery. Castration is the most successful palliative measure in men with advanced breast cancer, resulting in tumor regression and prolonging life.

Nursing care for the man with breast cancer is essentially the same as for the woman with breast cancer (see Chapter 48). The nurse has an opportunity to help the man and his family cope with the psychosocial effects of having breast cancer. He may feel embarrassment or shame about his condition as well as fear about the life-threatening nature of the disease. His family may share those feelings. By listening with understanding and empathy, the nurse can help the client and family resolve their feelings and move toward healing.

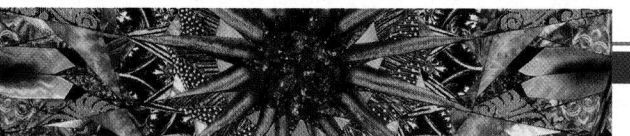

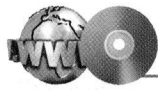

## EXPLORE MediaLink

NCLEX review questions, case studies, care plan activities, MediaLink applications, and other interactive resources for this chapter can be found on the Companion Website at www.prenhall.com/lemone.

Click on Chapter 47 to select the activities for this chapter. For animations, video clips, more NCLEX review questions, and an audio glossary, access the Student CD-ROM accompanying this textbook.

# TEST YOURSELF

1. When conducting a health assessment, which of the following statements would most likely elicit information about sexual concerns?

    a. "Following your prostate surgery, did you first notice you had problems with sexual intercourse?"
    b. "Why do you think you should be sexually active at your age?"
    c. "Do you miss having sex?"
    d. "Tell me about your experience with sexual function since you developed prostate enlargement."

2. You are conducting a health teaching session for young men. What topic would be appropriate to reduce the risk of cancer of the penis?

    a. Wearing a condom during sexual intercourse
    b. Retracting the foreskin of the penis when showering
    c. Avoiding tight pants and very hot showers
    d. Maintaining a regular testicular self-examination schedule

3. Which of the following interventions would be appropriate for the man with prostatitis?

    a. Wear a scrotal support during the day
    b. Increase fluid intake and void often

    c. Know the manifestations of testicular torsion
    d. Surgical intervention may be necessary

4. The enlarging prostate in BPH typically is manifested by assessment of problems with:

    a. Bowel elimination
    b. Urinary elimination
    c. Peripheral vascular function
    d. Skin integrity

5. You are caring for a man who has returned to the unit following recovery from a TURP. His urinary drainage bag is filled with dark red fluid with obvious clots. He is having painful bladder spasms. What would you do first?

    a. Assess his intake and output since surgery
    b. Administer pain medication in the form of a B & O suppository
    c. Report your assessments to his urologist
    d. Nothing, as these manifestations are expected following a TURP

See Test Yourself answers in Appendix C.

# BIBLIOGRAPHY

Agency of Health Care Policy and Research. (1994). *Clinical practice guidelines for benign prostatic hyperplasia.* AHCPR Pub. no. a94-0582. Rockville, MD: U.S. Department of Health and Human Services.

American Cancer Society. (2002). *Cancer facts and figures 2002.* Atlanta: Author.

Angelucci, P. A. (1997). Caring for patients with benign prostatic hyperplasia. *Nursing, 27*(11), 54–55.

Center for Disease Control. (2001). Prostate cancer. Available www.cdc.gov/cancer/prostate/prostate.htm

Chan, E. (2001). Promoting informed decision-making about prostate cancer screening. *Comprehensive Therapy, 27*(3), 195–201, 265–266.

Germino, B. B., Mohler, J., Ware, A., Harris, L., Belyea, M., & Mishel, M. H. (1998). Uncertainty in prostate cancer. Ethnic and family patterns. *Cancer Practitioner, 6*(2), 107–113.

Gray, M., & Brown, K. (2002). Genitourinary system. In J. Thompson, G. McFarland, J. Hirsch, & S. Tucker, *Mosby's clinical nursing* (5th ed.) (pp. 917–999). St. Louis: Mosby.

Greifzu, S. (2000). Prostate cancer. *RN, 63*(6), 27–32.

Hellerstedt, B., & Pienta, K. (2002). The current state of hormonal therapy for prostate cancer. *CA: A Cancer Journal for Clinicans, 52*(3), 154–179.

Jakobsson, L. (2001). Sexual problems in men with prostate cancer in comparison with men with benign prostatic hyperplasia and men from the general population. *Journal of Clinical Nursing, 10*(4), 573–582.

Jakobsson, L., Hallberg, I., & Loven, L. (2000). Experiences of micturition problems, indwelling catheter treatment and sexual life consequences in men with prostate cancer. *Journal of Advanced Nursing, 31*(1), 59–67.

Johnson, M., Maas, M., & Moorhead, S. (Eds.). (2000). *Nursing outcomes classification (NOC)* (2nd ed.). St. Louis: Mosby.

Kee, J. (1998). *Handbook of laboratory and diagnostic tests with nursing implications* (4th ed.). Upper Saddle River, NJ: Prentice Hall.

Lepor, H. (Ed.). (2000). *Prostatic diseases.* Philadelphia: Saunders.

McCance, K., & Huether, S. (2002). *Pathophysiology: The biologic basis for disease in adults & children.* St. Louis: Mosby.

McCloskey, J. C. & Bulecheck, G. M. (Eds.). (2000). *Nursing interventions classification (NIC)* (3rd ed.). St. Louis: Mosby.

North American Nursing Diagnosis Association. (2001). *Nursing diagnoses: Definitions and classification, 2001–2002.* Philadelphia: NANDA.

Ord-Lawson, S., & Fitch, M. (1997). The relationship between perceived social support and mood of testicular cancer patients. *Canadian Oncology Nursing Journal, 7*(2), 90–95.

Porth, C. M. (2002). *Pathophysiology: Concepts of altered health states* (6th ed.). Philadelphia: Lippincott.

Shannon, M., Wilson, B., & Stang, C. (2002). *Health professional's drug guide 2002.* Upper Saddle River, NJ: Prentice Hall.

Shuster, J. (1998). Megestrol and impotence—teaching patients about this dose-related adverse effect. *Nursing, 28*(3), 25.

Therapies for the treatment of benign prostatic hyperplasia (BPH). Available http://cpmcnet.columbia.edu/dept/urology/bphtherapy.html

Tierney, L. M., McPhee, S. J., & Papadakis, M. A. (Eds.). (2001). *Current medical diagnosis & treatment* (40th ed.). Stamford, CT: Appleton & Lange.

Weinrich, S. P., Atkinson, C., Boyd, M. D., & Weinrich, M. C. (1998). The impact of prostate cancer knowledge on cancer screening. *Oncology Nursing Forum, 25*(3), 527–534.

Weinrich, S. P., Weinrich, M., Frank-Stromborg, M., Johnson, A., Cover, K., Creanga, D., Boyde, M., & Holdford, D. (1998). Prostate cancer education in African American churches. *Public Health Nursing, 15*(3), 188–195.

Yarbro, C., & Ferrans, C. (1998). Quality of life of patients with prostate cancer treated with surgery or radiation therapy. *Oncology Nursing Forum, 25*(4), 685–693.

Yarbo, C., Frogge, M., Goodman, M., & Groenwald, S. (Eds.). (2001). *Cancer nursing: Principles and practice* (5th ed.). Sudbury, MA: Jones & Bartlett.

Zaccagnini, M. (1999). Clinical snapshot: Prostate cancer. *American Journal of Nursing, 99*(4), 34–35.

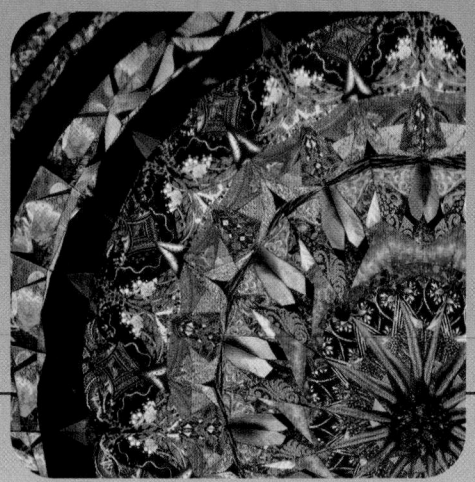

# CHAPTER 48

# Nursing Care of Women with Reproductive System Disorders

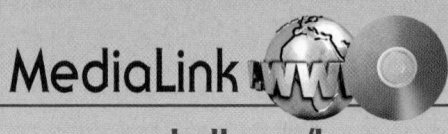

## MediaLink

**www.prenhall.com/lemone**

Additional resources for this chapter can be found on the Student CD-ROM accompanying this textbook, and on the Companion Website at www. prenhall.com/lemone. Click on Chapter 48 to select the activities for this chapter.

**CD-ROM**
• Audio Glossary
• NCLEX Review

**Companion Website**
• More NCLEX Review
• Case Study
   Breast Cancer
• Care Plan Activity
   Postoperative Hysterectomy Care
• MediaLink Application
   Premenstrual Syndrome

## LEARNING OUTCOMES

After completing this chapter, you will be able to:

▪ Apply knowledge of normal female anatomy, physiology, and assessments when providing nursing care for women with reproductive system disorders (see Chapter 46).

▪ Explain the pathophysiology of disorders of the female reproductive system.

▪ Describe the physiologic process of menopause.

▪ Discuss risk factors for cancers of the female reproductive system.

▪ Discuss the collaborative care, with related nursing implications, for women with disorders of the reproductive system.

▪ Provide appropriate nursing care for women having diagnostic tests and gynecologic surgery.

▪ Provide accurate information to women about health-promoting behaviors that prevent disorders of the female reproductive system or facilitate their early diagnosis.

▪ Use the nursing process as a framework for providing individualized care to women with disorders of the reproductive system.

Disorders of the female reproductive system range from the minor discomfort of menstrual cramps to life-threatening diseases such as cancer. Many of these disorders can occur at any point in a woman's adult life. They may affect her ability to bear children, her sexuality, and her sense of well-being as a woman.

Women who experience reproductive system changes and disorders require a holistic approach to meet their physical, emotional, and educational needs. Because the ability to reproduce affects self-esteem, feelings of femininity, and general health, both sensitivity and understanding of caregivers are essential. Providing personal medical and family history and undergoing diagnostic tests often require women to disclose personal, intimate information, which they may find embarrassing and uncomfortable. When planning and implementing care, nurses must consider the woman within the context of her culture, socioeconomic and educational level, and lifestyle. It is also important that the nurse not make assumptions or judgments about sexual orientation.

This chapter discusses the physiologic process of menopause, menstrual disorders, structural disorders of the female reproductive system, and disorders of female reproductive tissue, including the breast. Disorders of female sexual expression are summarized. Sexually transmitted diseases, including vaginal infections and pelvic inflammatory disease, are discussed in Chapter 49. Many of the disorders result in actual or potential health problems requiring nursing care based on similar nursing diagnoses. To avoid repeating those diagnoses and interventions for each disorder, they have been divided among the nursing care discussions as appropriate. Treatment of cancer with chemotherapy and radiation is discussed in Chapter 10. ∞

## THE PERIMENOPAUSAL WOMAN

**Menopause** is the permanent cessation of menses. The *climacteric*, or *perimenopausal*, period denotes the time during which reproductive function gradually ceases. For most women, the perimenopausal period lasts several years. It begins with a decline in the production of the hormone estrogen, includes the permanent cessation of menstruation due to loss of ovarian function, and extends for 1 year after the final menstrual period, at which time a woman is said to be *postmenopausal*. The average woman will live one-third of her life after menopause.

Menopause is neither a disease nor a disorder, but a normal physiologic process. However, the hormonal changes that occur can be accompanied by unpleasant side effects. There is wide variation in how individual women experience these side effects. In the United States, most women stop menstruating between 48 and 55 years of age. A woman who had not menstruated for 1 full year or has a follicular-stimulating hormone (FSH) level of more than 30 mIU/mL is considered menopausal (Porth, 2002). Certain health risks increase after menopause, including heart disease, osteoporosis, and breast cancer.

## THE PHYSIOLOGY OF MENOPAUSE

The menopausal period marks the natural biologic end of reproductive ability. *Surgical menopause* occurs when the ovaries are removed in premenopausal women, dramatically reducing the production of estrogen and progestins. *Chemical menopause* often occurs during cancer chemotherapy, when cytotoxic drugs arrest ovarian function.

As ovarian function decreases, the production of estradiol ($E_2$), the most biologically active estrogen, decreases and is ultimately replaced by estrone as the major ovarian estrogen. Estrone is produced in small amounts and has only about one-tenth the biologic activity of estradiol. With decreased ovarian function, the second ovarian hormone, progesterone, which is produced during the luteal phase of the menstrual cycle, also is markedly reduced.

## MANIFESTATIONS

As estrogen decreases, various tissues are affected. The breast tissue, body hair, skin elasticity, and subcutaneous fat decreases. The ovaries and uterus become smaller, and the cervix and vagina also decrease in size and become pale in color. These changes may result in problems with vaginal dryness, dyspareunia, urinary stress incontinence, urinary tract infections, and vaginitis. Vasomotor instability often results in hot flashes, palpitations, dizziness, and headaches. Other problems resulting from vasomotor instability include insomnia, frequent awakening, and perspiration (night sweats). The woman may experience irritability, anxiety, and depression as a result of these events.

Long-term estrogen deprivation results in an imbalance in bone remodeling and osteoporosis, leading to fractures and kyphosis. The risk for cardiovascular diseases increases. Manifestations of the perimenopausal period are listed in the box below. These manifestations vary widely. Some women experience severe symptoms, others experience moderate symptoms, and some women experience few or no symptoms.

### Manifestations of the Perimenopausal Period

- Menstrual cycles become erratic. Menstrual flow varies widely in amount and duration and eventually ceases.
- Vaginal, vulval, and urethral tissues begin to atrophy.
- Vaginal pH rises, predisposing the woman to bacterial infections.
- Vaginal lubrication decreases, and vaginal rugae decrease in number. This may result in dyspareunia (pain during sexual intercourse), injury, and fungal infections.
- Vasomotor instability due to a decrease in estrogen may result in hot flashes and night sweats. A hot flash starts in the chest and moves upward toward the face and may last from seconds to several minutes.
- Psychologic symptoms may include moodiness, nervousness, insomnia, headaches, irritability, anxiety, inability to concentrate, and depression.

## COLLABORATIVE CARE

Care of the woman experiencing menopausal symptoms focuses on relieving symptoms and minimizing postmenopausal health risks.

### Diagnostic Tests

As estrogen secretion diminishes, levels of FSH and LH rise and remain elevated.

### Medications

Hormone replacement therapy (HRT) may be prescribed to alleviate the unpleasant manifestations of menopause. HRT may include estrogen alone for women who have had a hysterectomy, or a combination of estrogen and progestin. The addition of progestin stimulates monthly shedding of the interuterine lining, decreasing the risk of uterine cancer. HRT relieves hot flashes and night sweats and decreases problems of vaginal dryness and urogenital tissue atrophy, which can lead to painful intercourse and urinary incontinence.

Long-term benefits of HRT were once believed to be a reduced risk of coronary heart disease, osteoporosis, and Alzheimer's disease; however, research has demonstrated that estrogen plus progestin does not reduce the overall rate of coronary artery disease in postmenopausal women with established coronary disease but does increase the rate of thromboembolic events (blood clots) in the same women (Grady et al., 2000; Hulley et al., 1998). In addition, Hulley et al. (1999) and Torgerson and Bell-Syer (2001) found little evidence of the benefits of HRT in preventing fractures. In 2002, a major study of HRT was stopped, as government scientists reported that long-term use of estrogen and progestin significantly increased women's risk of breast cancer, strokes, and heart attacks. Although HRT did decrease the risk of colon cancer and hip fractures, there are other means of preventing these illnesses. Further studies are planned to evaluate using lower dose HRT, other methods of administrations (such as the patch), and estrogen alone for women who have had a hysterectomy.

Nausea, vomiting, weight gain, breast tenderness and engorgement, and vaginal bleeding are common side effects of HRT. Fluid retention may develop, worsening existing problems such as asthma, epilepsy, migraine headache, and heart and kidney diseases.

Contraindications for HRT include:

- Current diagnosis of endometrial cancer; current or past history of estrogen-dependent breast, ovarian, or cervical cancer.
- Hypertriglyceridemia.
- Active thrombotic disorders or inherited clotting disorders.
- Acute or chronic liver disease or kidney failure.
- Unexplained vaginal bleeding.
- Pregnancy.

Selective estrogen receptor modulators (SERMs) such as raloxifene (Evista) provide an alternative to HRT for preventing osteoporosis. SERMs act like estrogen in some tissues but

not in others, and appear to significantly reduce the risk of breast cancer in menopausal women. Although they do not prevent manifestations of menopause, they provide an alternative for women who cannot take HRT.

### Complementary Therapies

The following complementary therapies are examples of those used by menopausal women to reduce associated discomforts (Fontaine, 2000):

- Aromatherapy: geranium, rose, fennel in bathwater or lotions
- Herbs: black cohosh, vitex, agnue castii, rehmannia, ginseng, Chinese tonic of He Shou Wu, dong quai
- Supplements: vitamin E, soy protein
- Meditation

## NURSING CARE

Nursing care during and after the menopausal period focuses on minimizing the symptoms associated with hormonal changes, reducing the risk of cardiovascular disease and osteoporosis, and educating the woman about lifestyle changes important to health and well-being.

### Health Promotion

The American Cancer Society (2002) recommends a cancer-related checkup every year after the age of 40. This checkup includes examination for cancers of the thyroid, ovaries, lymph nodes, oral cavity, and skin. Other important checkups include screening for cervical, breast, and colorectal cancer. Health counseling should also include information about alcohol and tobacco use, sun exposure, diet and nutrition, exercise, risk factors, sexual practices, and environmental and occupational exposures. It is important to discuss the benefits of rest and exercise, as well as a diet that includes fruits, vegetables, and fiber. Other health-promotion teaching is discussed later.

### Assessment

Collect the following data through the health history and physical examination (see Chapter 46). When assessing the older woman, be aware of normal changes with aging, as outlined in the box below.

## Nursing Care of the Older Adult

### VARIATIONS IN ASSESSMENT FINDING

- Menstrual irregularities during the perimenopausal period, hot flashes, night sweats
- Decreased size of vulva, loss of vaginal lubrication and flattened vaginal rugae
- Decreased size of clitoris, vagina, cervix, and ovaries
- Reduced size of breasts
- Loss of skin elasticity and turgor
- Loss of pubic and axillary hair, growth of facial hair, loss of hair pigment

- Health history: problems with urinary frequency, urgency, or incontinence; menstrual history; sexual history; dyspareunia; use of alcohol, nicotine, and drugs; medications, sleep patterns, hot flashes, night sweats, changes in emotional responses
- Physical assessment: height and weight, posture, vital signs, breast examination, pelvic examination, abdominal assessment

## Nursing Diagnoses and Interventions

Although each nursing care plan must be individualized, interventions often focus on problems with lack of information, sexuality, and self-esteem.

### Deficient Knowledge

Because menopausal manifestations vary widely, it is difficult to predict their effect on an individual woman. However, the well-informed woman is better prepared to deal with whatever symptoms she experiences.

- Discuss physiologic manifestations, such as hot flashes and night sweats. *The underlying cause of hot flashes is not known (Porth, 2002). Many physiologic effects of menopause are amenable to nonpharmacologic methods of relief, such as lifestyle changes.*

**PRACTICE ALERT**  *When hot flashes occur at night and are accompanied by perspiration, they are called night sweats. Night sweats often interfere with normal sleep patterns, leading to increased fatigue and irritability.* ■

- Provide information about dietary recommendations. The recommended daily intake of calcium for women over 50 is 1200 mg. *Some women need to use calcium supplements or calcium-containing antacid tablets to meet this requirement.*
- Emphasize the importance of weight-bearing exercise. *Weight-bearing exercise reduces the rate of bone loss, helps maintain optimum weight, and reduces cardiovascular risk.*
- Provide information about the benefits and risks of HRT. Not every woman will need or want it. *Every woman needs to understand both the risks and the benefits before deciding whether to undergo HRT.*
- Encourage the woman to obtain yearly mammograms, clinical breast examinations, and Pap tests, and to perform monthly breast self-examination at the same day each month. *The increased risk for cancer of the breast and pelvic reproductive organs makes self-examination and health care provider screening during and after menopause even more important.*
- Suggest the following resources
  - National Institute on Aging
  - North American Menopause Society
  - The Hormone Foundation
  - Women's Health Initiative
  - National Women's Health Information Center

### Ineffective Sexuality Patterns

Vaginal dryness and atrophy, together with the emotional effect of menopause, can interfere with sexual expression and satisfaction. Suggesting measures to help the woman and her partner cope with these changes can enable them to continue or resume a mutually satisfying sexual relationship.

- Encourage expression of feelings and concerns about how menopause is changing her sex life. *Midlife and older women may not be comfortable in discussing their intimate sexual behavior.*
- Suggest ways to increase vaginal lubrication, such as spending more time in foreplay and/or using water-soluble gels (e.g., Replens) for vaginal lubrication. *A more leisurely approach to sexual activity can be mutually gratifying for both the woman and her partner. Use of water-soluble gels can prevent vaginal pain and irritation and improve the quality of the sexual experience.*

**PRACTICE ALERT**  *Plant estrogens, found in food such as brown rice, corn, green beans, lemon and orange peels, and tofu, are mildly estrogenic and may improve vaginal dryness.* ■

- Explain that as women age, it may take longer for vaginal lubrication and orgasm to occur. *This information is important to prevent the woman from believing something is wrong with her, or her partner believing he or she is no longer interesting or sexually exciting.*

### Situational Low Self-Esteem

Each woman responds to the aging process in her own way, and most women have coping skills that adequately equip them to deal with the gradual changes associated with aging. Among the factors that may provoke a self-esteem disturbance are the loss of youth, a sense of emptiness as children leave home, and the need to redefine one's self-concept and roles as parenting becomes less important. Women who place a high value on their physical attractiveness may experience a painful psychologic response to the physical changes of menopause.

- Encourage expression of fears and concerns related to changes in interpersonal and family functions. *Many women associate aging with "uselessness" and unattractiveness.*
- Suggest volunteer activities or employment for the woman who has extra time. *This enables the woman to feel that she is still a contributing member of society. Volunteering for activities involving young people can help reduce anxiety about the loss of reproductive ability or any late regrets about not having had children.*
- Discuss the importance of a healthy lifestyle in maintaining physical attractiveness. Identify risk factors and high-risk behaviors. *Lifestyle habits and behaviors affect many body systems and physical appearance. For example, cigarette smoking and overexposure to the sun make the skin age faster, contributing to wrinkles. Active women who exercise and eat a well-balanced diet look and feel better.*

## Disturbed Body Image

As women progress through the perimenopausal period, changes in appearance and the loss of childbearing ability may combine to make the woman feel "old, ugly, and useless." Although this is far from the truth, with women living at least one-third of their lives after menopause in productive careers and activities, it nevertheless is the perception of women as well as society. The physical changes the woman often experiences include growth of facial hair, excessive perspiration and flushing of the face, and weight gain.

- Encourage the woman to describe her perceptions of her own body. *This information is necessary to obtain data to establish an individualized plan of care.*

- Encourage verbalization of feelings of concern, anger, anxiety, loss, and fear over body changes. *Expressing these emotions can facilitate the grieving process and acceptance of change.*
- Stress that certain physical characteristics of a person cannot be changed; emphasize the importance of learning to recognize and appreciate one's own special strengths. *These help the woman gain acceptance and a realistic appraisal of self.*
- Refer, as appropriate, for dietary management, exercise, stress management and cosmetic assistance (e.g., for aggravating facial hair). *These actions increase wellness and a positive sense of self.*

# MENSTRUAL DISORDERS

Monthly menstruation normally involves some minor discomfort, including breast tenderness, a feeling of heaviness and congestion in the pelvic area, uterine cramping, and lower backache. Many women, however, experience more serious effects, both physiologic and psychologic. This section discusses premenstrual syndrome, dysmenorrhea, and abnormal uterine bleeding. (The menstrual cycle is discussed in Chapter 46).

## THE WOMAN WITH PREMENSTRUAL SYNDROME

**Premenstrual syndrome (PMS)** is a complex of manifestations (e.g., mood swings, breast tenderness, fatigue, irritability, food cravings, and depression) that are limited to 3 to 14 days before menstruation and relieved by the onset of menses. It is estimated that 25% to 40% of all adult women experience mild to moderate symptoms and 1% to 8% have severe symptoms (Porth, 2002). For about 7% of women, PMS is so disabling that it is called *premenstrual dysphoric disorder (PMDD)*. The syndrome is seen less frequently during the teens and 20s, reaching a peak in women in their mid-30s. Major life stressors, age greater than 30, and depression are risk factors associated with PMS. Premenstrual syndrome can be a factor in absenteeism at school or work, decreased productivity, interpersonal relationship difficulties, and lifestyle disruption.

## PATHOPHYSIOLOGY AND MANIFESTATIONS

Although the pathophysiology of PMS is not clearly understood, it is believed that hormonal changes such as altered estrogen–progesterone ratios, increased prolactin levels, and rising aldosterone levels during the luteal phase of the menstrual cycle contribute to the problem. Increased production of aldosterone results in sodium retention and edema. Decreased

levels of monamine oxidase in the brain are associated with depression, and reduced levels of serotonin can lead to mood swings.

Manifestations of PMS occur during the luteal phase of the menstrual cycle (7 to 10 days prior to the onset of the menstrual flow), abating when the menstrual flow begins. The *Multisystem Effects of PMS* are shown on page 1557. Although PMS may produce a variety of physiologic and psychologic manifestations, the exact nature of these manifestations and their intensity are individualized for each woman with this disorder (see the Nursing Research box on page 1558). The manifestations may even differ from month to month in the same woman.

## COLLABORATIVE CARE

If no organic cause can be identified, the goals of care are to relieve manifestations and to help develop self-care patterns that will help the woman anticipate and cope more effectively with future episodes of PMS. There are no definitive diagnostic tests for PMS. The regular recurrence of manifestations preceding the onset of menses for at least 3 months leads to a diagnosis of PMS. The treatment of PMS integrates this self-monitored record of manifestations, regular exercise, avoiding caffeine, and a diet low in simple sugars and high in lean proteins (Porth, 2002).

### Medications

If the manifestations of PMS are severe or incapacitating, ovulation may be suppressed by the use of gonadotropin-releasing hormone (GnRH) agonists, oral contraceptives, or danazol. Progesterone and antiprostaglandin agents such as NSAIDs may help relieve cramping. Diuretics may be prescribed to relieve bloating. Selective serotonin reuptake inhibitors such as fluoxetine (Prozac), sertraline (Zoloft), and paroxetine (Paxil) may be used to manage mood and some physical manifestations of PMS.

# Multisystem Effects of Premenstrual Syndrome

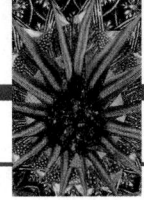

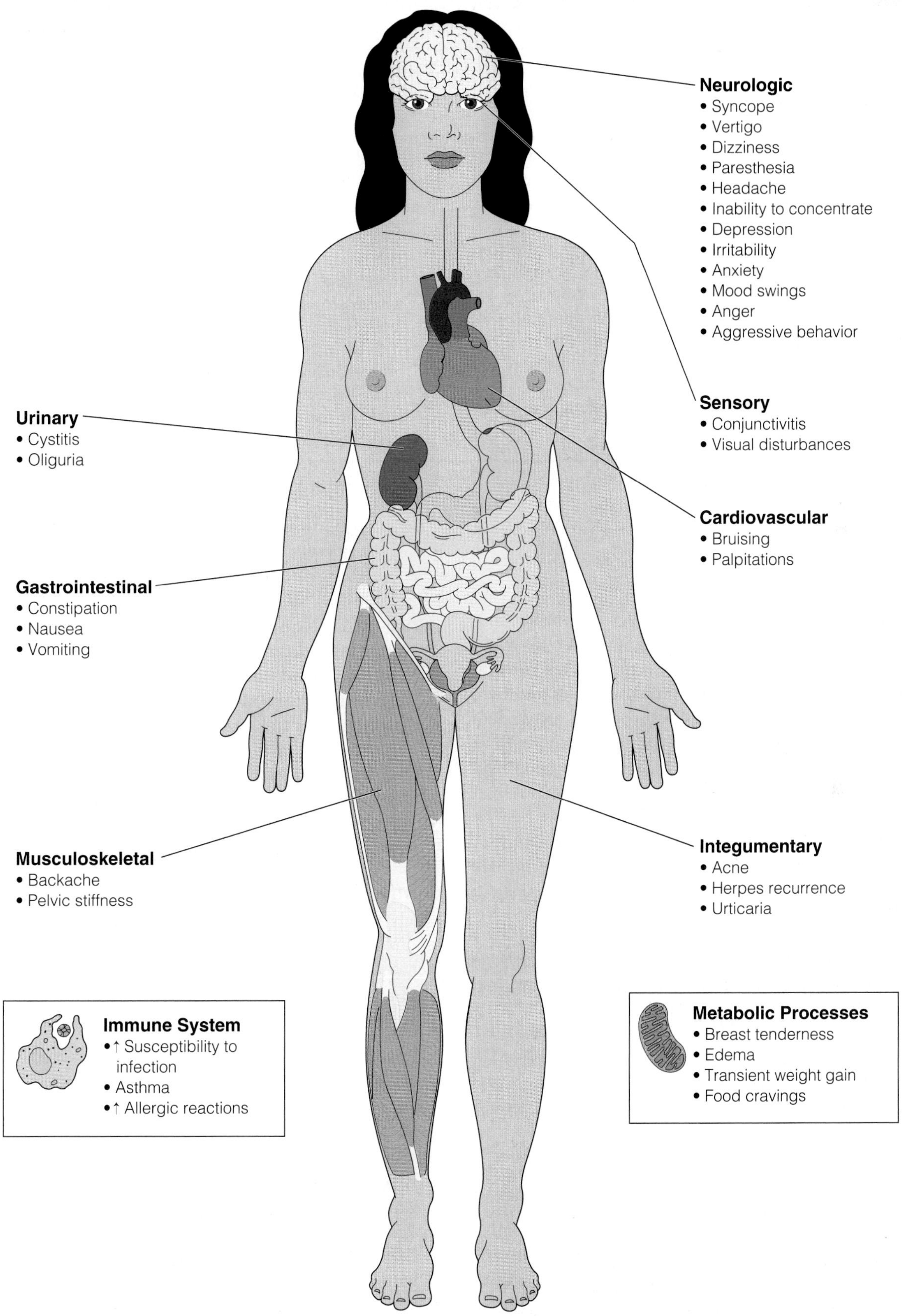
Neurologic
• Syncope
• Vertigo
• Dizziness
• Paresthesia
• Headache
• Inability to concentrate
• Depression
• Irritability
• Anxiety
• Mood swings
• Anger
• Aggressive behavior
Sensory
• Conjunctivitis
• Visual disturbances
Urinary
• Cystitis
• Oliguria
Cardiovascular
• Bruising
• Palpitations
Gastrointestinal
• Constipation
• Nausea
• Vomiting
Musculoskeletal
• Backache
• Pelvic stiffness
Integumentary
• Acne
• Herpes recurrence
• Urticaria
Immune System
• ↑ Susceptibility to infection
• Asthma
• ↑ Allergic reactions
Metabolic Processes
• Breast tenderness
• Edema
• Transient weight gain
• Food cravings

## Nursing Research

### Evidence-Based Practice for PMS

Many women experience varying degrees of premenstrual symptoms. Despite its prevalence, the behavioral and physiologic causes of PMS are poorly understood. This lack of understanding contributes to ineffective treatment based on symptoms rather than etiology of the disorder. Evidence suggests that stress contributes to the occurrence of premenstrual symptoms and that changes in stress hormone regulation may alter mood and affect.

In this study (Cahill, 1998), the researcher monitored symptom and cortisol secretion patterns for three menstrual cycles in three distinct groups of women: those with few premenstrual symptoms, those experiencing PMS patterns, and women with premenstrual symptoms. During the luteal phase, women in the PMS group had lower cortisol levels than did women in either of the other groups. Findings suggest that transient changes in stress hormone regulation may contribute to mood alterations associated with PMS.

### IMPLICATIONS FOR NURSING

Further study of the biochemical, physiologic, and psychologic factors that are involved in PMS is needed. With better understanding of its causes, more effective interventions for PMS can be developed. This study suggests that nursing interventions designed to limit stress effects in treating women with turmoil-type premenstrual symptoms may be appropriate.

### Critical Thinking in Client Care

1. This study looked at the effects of the menstrual cycle on mood and affect. What other manifestations of PMS do women commonly experience? What biochemical, physiologic, and psychologic factors might contribute to symptoms such as gastrointestinal, musculoskeletal, genitourinary, and other manifestations of PMS?
2. What effects might PMS have on a woman's family, social, and work interactions? What self-care measures would you suggest to the woman?

## Complementary Therapies

Complementary therapies for the woman with PMS focus on diet, exercise, relaxation, and stress management.

- A diet high in complex carbohydrates with limited simple sugars and alcohol is recommended to minimize reactive hypoglycemia, which can contribute to the manifestations of PMS.
- Reduced sodium intake helps minimize fluid retention. Increased intake of calcium (1200 mg per day), magnesium (200 mg per day), and vitamin E (400 IU per day) may be helpful (Mayo Foundation for Medical Education and Research, 2002).
- Caffeine is restricted to reduce irritability.
- Exercise is beneficial, but adequate rest also is necessary.
- Techniques for relaxation and stress management include deep abdominal breathing, meditation, muscle relaxation, and guided imagery.

## NURSING CARE

### Nursing Diagnoses and Interventions

Nursing care for the woman with PMS focuses on relieving manifestations. Most women experiencing PMS require interventions to manage pain and enhance coping.

### Acute Pain

The woman with PMS may have pain from headache (including migraine), cramps, excessive fluid retention, breast swelling, joint and muscle pain, and backache.

- Teach effective pharmacologic and nonpharmacologic self-care measures to relieve pain: application of heat, relaxation techniques (such as breathing exercises, imagery techniques, or meditation), and exercise. *Heat relieves muscle spasms and causes blood vessels to dilate, increasing blood supply to the pelvis and uterine muscles. Relaxation and exercise aid the release of naturally produced pain relievers called endorphins.*
- Review daily activities and suggest ways to balance rest periods and activity. *During rest periods, energy and oxygen requirements decrease, increasing the amount of energy and oxygen available to muscles.*
- Review manifestations and, if possible, correlate these with dietary patterns and activity levels. Encourage the woman to keep a diary of PMS manifestations. *Maintaining a diary of PMS manifestations, activity, and foods eaten can provide data to identify modifiable causes of discomfort.*
- Suggest sexual activity as a way to lessen cramps. *Orgasm may help relieve dysmenorrhea.*

### Ineffective Coping

Many women experience wide mood swings during episodes of PMS, sometimes exhibiting self-destructive or aggressive behaviors toward others. These mood swings can interfere with a woman's ability to manage her responsibilities at home or at work.

- Encourage the woman to keep a journal of her menstrual cycle and to document her mood changes in the 7 to 10 days prior to menstruation. *Recognizing the signs and timing of PMS is the first step in developing methods to cope with the problem.*
- Explore possible ways to rearrange or reschedule activities when experiencing PMS. *Planning ahead enables the woman to assume more control and promotes coping methods.*
- Explore what, if any, self-care measures have helped cope with mood alterations in the past. *Encourage healthful coping mechanisms, such as relaxation techniques and exercise. Some women may rely on alcohol or other drugs during PMS, which only exacerbate the manifestations.*

## Home Care

Teach the woman and family that PMS is not caused by a pathologic process but is a physiologic response to hormonal changes of the menstrual cycle. With an understanding of the condition, the woman is better able to manage anxiety and to become actively involved in techniques to reduce the manifestations. Teaching should also include dietary measures, relaxation techniques and exercise, stress reduction techniques, and support systems.

# THE WOMAN WITH DYSMENORRHEA

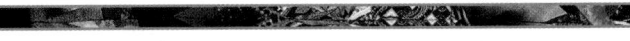

**Dysmenorrhea,** pain or discomfort associated with menstruation, is experienced by a significant number of menstruating women. *Primary dysmenorrhea* occurs without specific pelvic pathology, whereas *secondary dysmenorrhea* is related to identified pelvic disease, such as endometriosis or pelvic inflammatory disease.

## PATHOPHYSIOLOGY AND MANIFESTATIONS

In primary dysmenorrhea, excessive production of prostaglandins stimulates uterine muscle fibers to contract. As the muscles contract, uterine circulation is compromised, resulting in uterine ischemia and pain. These contractions can range from mild cramping to severe muscle spasms. Psychologic factors, such as anxiety and tension, may contribute to dysmenorrhea. Childbirth tends to decrease the incidence and severity of manifestations, possibly because of dilation of the internal cervical os. Manifestations of primary dysmenorrhea (see the box below) may be severe enough to disrupt activities of daily living, sexual function, and even fertility.

Secondary dysmenorrhea is related to underlying organic conditions that involve scarring or injury to the reproductive tract. Endometriosis, fibroid tumors, pelvic inflammatory disease, or ovarian cancer may result in painful menses.

# COLLABORATIVE CARE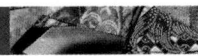

Care of the woman with menstrual pain focuses on identifying the underlying cause, reestablishing functional capacity, and managing pain.

## Manifestations of Primary Dysmenorrhea

- Abdominal pain beginning with onset of menses and lasting 12 to 48 hours
- Pain radiating to lower back and thighs
- Headache
- Nausea
- Vomiting
- Diarrhea
- Fatigue
- Breast tenderness

A careful history and physical are performed to rule out any underlying organic cause of dysmenorrhea. If no organic cause can be found, the diagnosis is primary dysmenorrhea. In addition, attitudes and expectations about menstruation and lifestyle disruption are identified and explored.

## Diagnostic Tests

Various diagnostic tests are performed to identify structural abnormalities, hormonal imbalances, and pathologic conditions that could cause menstrual pain.

- *Pelvic examination,* including a Papanicolaou (PAP) smear and cervical and vaginal cultures, is performed to detect structural abnormalities, malignancy, or infections.
- *Follicle-stimulating hormone (FSH) and luteinizing hormone (LH) levels* are measured to assess the function of the pituitary gland. The results are correlated with the time of the menstrual cycle.
- *Progesterone* and *estradiol levels* are measured to assess ovarian function.
- *Thyroid function tests* ($T_3$ and $T_4$) are performed to assess thyroid function.
- *Vaginal or pelvic ultrasonography* is used to detect the presence of space-occupying lesions, including fibroid tumors, cysts, abscesses, and neoplasms (see the box below).
- *CT scan* or *MRI* can be used to detect pelvic tumors.
- *Laparoscopy* is used to diagnose structural defects and blockages caused by scarring, endometriosis, tumors, and cysts (Figure 48–1 ■). See the box on page 1560 for nursing care for the woman having a laparoscopy.
- *Dilation and curettage (D&C)* of the uterus is performed to obtain tissue for evaluation or to relieve dysmenorrhea and heavy bleeding. (This procedure is presented later in this chapter in the discussion on surgery.)

## Nursing Implications for Diagnostic Tests

### Ultrasound Examination

- If indicated, ensure that the woman's bladder is full by forcing fluids and instructing her not to void. If she is NPO, a Foley catheter may be inserted into the bladder and sterile water instilled. The catheter is then clamped to prevent the water from leaving the bladder. The full bladder lifts the pelvic organs higher into the abdomen and improves visualization.
- Explain to the woman that she will be allowed to empty her bladder as soon as possible.
- Coat the abdomen with ultrasonic transducing gel. The gel provides a better image when the scanner is applied to the abdomen. For vaginal ultrasound, a transducer is covered with a condom or vinyl glove, coated with transducing gel, and introduced into the vagina.
- Explain the procedure to the woman, indicating that she can watch the procedure and ask questions about the images on the screen. If appropriate, point out landmarks on the screen.

If it is determined that a woman has secondary dysmenorrhea due to an underlying organic cause, therapeutic measures are directed at the specific condition.

## Medications

Dysmenorrhea may be treated with analgesics, prostaglandin inhibitors such as NSAIDs, or oral contraceptives (see the Medication Administration box on this page).

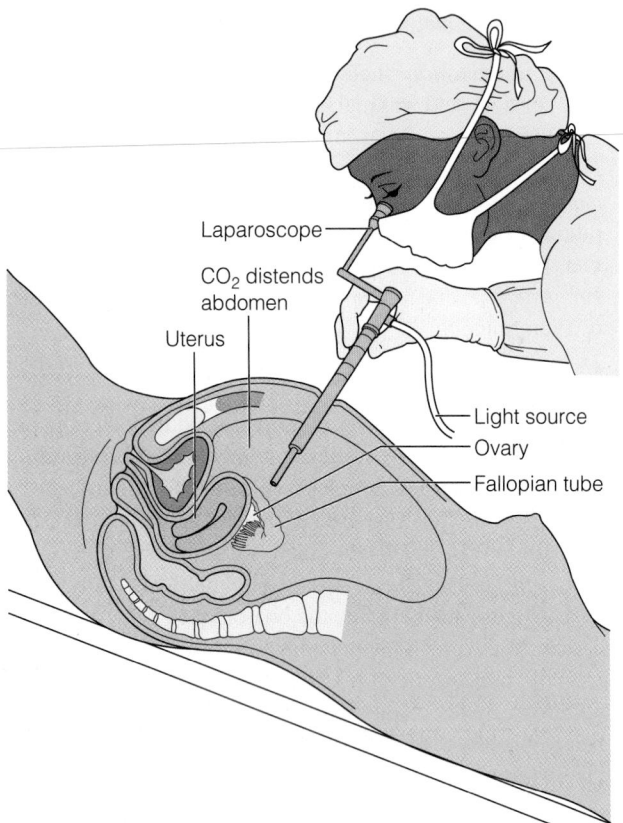

Laparoscope

$CO_2$ distends abdomen

Uterus

Light source
Ovary
Fallopian tube

**Figure 48–1** ■ Laparoscopy. In this surgical procedure, a flexible, lighted instrument (laparoscope) is inserted through a periumbilical incision. Laparoscopy allows visualization of the pelvic cavity.

## Complementary Therapies

The complementary therapies listed for the woman with PMS may also be useful for the woman with dysmenorrhea. Using a heating pad on the abdomen also helps reduce pain.

## Medication Administration

### The Woman with Dysmenorrhea

#### ORAL CONTRACEPTIVES

Norethindrone and ethinyl estradiol (Brevicon, Norinyl)
Norgestrel and ethinyl estradiol (Ovral)

Oral contraceptives inhibit ovulation and help reduce cramping and bleeding. Side effects of oral contraceptives include breast tenderness, weight gain, nausea, midcycle bleeding, mood swings, depression, chloasma (skin discoloration) on the face and chest, hypertension, vascular complications, vaginal candidiasis, migraines, and glucose intolerance. Oral contraceptives are contraindicated in women with personal or family history of breast cancer in first-degree relatives, hypertension, history of stroke or transient ischemic attack (TIA), smoking, history of estrogen-dependent cancer, pregnancy, liver disease, or thrombophlebitis.

#### Nursing Responsibilities
- Assess the client for potential contraindications to drug therapy.

#### Client and Family Teaching
- Take the drug as prescribed until the physician indicates otherwise or until side effects prevent you from continuing to take them.
- If you are taking oral contraceptives, be sure to take them at the same time every day.
- Report to the physician suspected pregnancy and any side effects such as nausea, rash, drowsiness, stomach pain, ringing in the ears, tenderness in the calf of the leg, and shortness of breath.
- Do not smoke while taking oral contraceptives.

## NURSING CARE OF THE WOMAN UNDERGOING LAPAROSCOPY

### PREOPERATIVE CARE
- Instruct the woman to empty the bladder prior to the surgical procedure.
- Explain to the woman that referred shoulder pain or expulsion of gas through the vagina may occur postoperatively. *During the procedure, the woman's abdomen is insufflated with carbon dioxide gas to distend the abdomen and facilitate visualization of the pelvic organs. The surgical table is then tilted so that the intestines will fall away from the pelvic organs. Some carbon dioxide gas may remain in the abdomen after the procedure.*

- Explain that pain should be minimal. Instruct the woman to report excessive pain to the nurse or physician at once. *Excessive pain signals infection or other postoperative complication.*

### POSTOPERATIVE CARE
- Apply a perineal pad. Teach the woman proper perineal hygiene, emphasizing the need to change pads at least every 4 hours. Keep a pad count. *Proper perineal hygiene reduces the risk of postoperative infection. Pad count is an indication of blood loss.*
- Assess for excessive vaginal bleeding. *Minor bleeding is normal; excessive bleeding may indicate hemorrhage.*

## NURSING CARE

Nursing care for the woman with primary dysmenorrhea focuses on controlling manifestations and providing education about the normal physiology of the menstrual cycle and self-care measures. Care of the woman with secondary dysmenorrhea varies according to the underlying cause and is discussed within sections on specific disorders. Nursing interventions for the woman with PMS are also appropriate for the woman with dysmenorrhea.

## THE WOMAN WITH DYSFUNCTIONAL UTERINE BLEEDING

**Dysfunctional uterine bleeding (DUB)** refers to vaginal bleeding that is usually painless but abnormal in amount, duration, or time of occurrence. The types of DUB include primary and secondary amenorrhea, oligomenorrhea, menorrhagia, metrorrhagia, and postmenopausal bleeding.

- **Amenorrhea** is the absence of menstruation. *Primary amenorrhea,* absence of menarche by age 16, or by age 14 if secondary sex characteristics fail to develop, may be caused by structural abnormalities, hormonal imbalances, polycystic ovary disease, or an imperforate hymen. Because a certain percentage of body fat is required for menstruation to occur, anorexia nervosa, bulimia, or excessive athletic training can also cause primary amenorrhea. *Secondary amenorrhea,* absence of menses for at least 6 months in a previously menstruating female, may also be caused by anorexia nervosa, excessive athletic activity or training, or a large weight loss. Other causes include hormonal imbalances and ovarian tumors. Normal, or physiologic, secondary amenorrhea occurs during pregnancy, breastfeeding, and menopause.
- **Oligomenorrhea,** scant menses, usually is related to hormonal imbalances.
- **Menorrhagia,** excessive or prolonged menstruation, may result from thyroid disorders, endometriosis, pelvic inflammatory disease, functional ovarian cysts, or uterine fibroids or polyps. Clotting disorders and anticoagulant medications also can cause menorrhagia. A single heavy or long cycle is not in itself a cause for concern; however, repetitive long or heavy cycles can lead to excessive blood loss, fatigue, anemia, hemorrhage, and sexual dysfunction.
- **Metrorrhagia,** bleeding between menstrual periods, may be caused by hormonal imbalances, pelvic inflammatory disease, cervical or uterine polyps, uterine fibroids, or cervical or uterine cancer. Because cancer is a possible cause of metrorrhagia, early evaluation and treatment are extremely important. *Mittleschmerz* (midcycle spotting associated with ovulation) occurs in many women and is not considered metrorrhagia.
- **Postmenopausal bleeding** may be caused by endometrial polyps, endometrial hyperplasia, or uterine cancer. The possibility of cancer makes early evaluation and treatment essential.

A number of factors may predispose a woman to DUB. These factors include stress, extreme weight changes, use of oral contraceptive agents or intrauterine devices (IUDs), and postmenopausal status. Dysfunctional uterine bleeding is usually related to hormonal imbalances or pelvic neoplasms, either benign or malignant.

## PATHOPHYSIOLOGY

Hormonal imbalances, especially progesterone deficiency with relative estrogen excess, results in endometrial hyperplasia. Estrogen stimulates endometrial proliferation. However, without the support provided by progesterone, sloughing occurs, resulting in vaginal bleeding that may be irregular, prolonged, or profuse. Defects in the follicular phase shorten the proliferative phase of the menstrual cycle, resulting in spotting and breakthrough bleeding. Defects during the luteal phase result in excessive amount or duration of flow due to persistence of the corpus luteum. This leads to a deficiency of progesterone, resulting in vaginal bleeding. *Anovulation,* absence of ovulation, is associated with both estrogen and progesterone deficiencies. Emotional upsets or stress can cause hormonal imbalances and thus affect menstruation. Pelvic neoplasms, discussed later, also cause abnormal bleeding.

## COLLABORATIVE CARE

The care of the woman with DUB focuses on identifying and treating the underlying disease. A careful history and physical examination are performed. Abdominal and pelvic examinations are performed to rule out abdominal masses. The woman may need to keep a menstrual history and basal body temperature chart for several months to determine whether ovulation is occurring.

### Diagnostic Tests

Diagnostic tests that may be ordered include the following:

- *CBC* is performed to rule out systemic disease as a contributing factor to DUB and to evaluate its effects.
- *Thyroid function studies,* including measurement of triiodothyronine ($T_3$), thyroxine ($T_4$), and thyroid-stimulating hormone (TSH) levels, are performed to rule out hyper- or hypothyroidism as a cause of DUB.
- *Endocrine studies* are done to evaluate pituitary and adrenal function. Pituitary dysfunction may first be manifested by menstrual irregularities.
- *Serum progesterone levels* are measured to determine the level of progesterone deficiency.
- *Pap smear* rules out or identifies cervical carcinoma.
- *Pelvic ultrasound* identifies luteal cysts.
- *Hysteroscopy* detects abnormalities of the uterine cavity.
- *Endometrial biopsy* is performed to obtain endometrial tissue for histologic examination.

### Medications

For many women, hormonal agents can correct menstrual irregularities. For anovulatory DUB, oral contraceptives may be prescribed for 3 to 6 months. Progesterone or medroxyprogesterone also may be prescribed to regulate uterine bleeding.

Ovulatory DUB may be treated with progestins during the luteal phase. Oral iron supplements may be prescribed to replace iron lost through menstrual bleeding.

## Surgery

Surgical intervention emphasizes the least invasive method that proves effective relief, beginning with a therapeutic dilation and curettage (D&C), then endometrial ablation, and, finally, hysterectomy.

### Therapeutic D&C

In a therapeutic D&C, the cervical canal is dilated and the uterine wall is scraped. D&C, the most frequently performed minor gynecologic surgical procedure, is used to diagnose and treat DUB and other disorders of the female reproductive system. It may be performed to correct excessive or prolonged bleeding. D&C is contraindicated in any woman who has been taking anticoagulant drugs or whose condition precludes the use of regional or general anesthesia. Nursing care of the woman having a D&C is described in the box below.

### Endometrial Ablation

In an endometrial ablation, the endometrial layer of the uterus is permanently destroyed using laser surgery or electrosurgical resection. It is performed in women who do not respond to pharmacologic management or D&C. The woman needs to understand that this procedure ends menstruation and reproduction.

### Hysterectomy

Hysterectomy, or removal of the uterus, may be performed when medical management of bleeding disorders is unsuccessful or malignancy is present, particularly if the woman no longer wishes to bear children. In premenopausal women, the ovaries are usually left in place; in postmenopausal women, a total hysterectomy, or panhysterectomy, may be performed; this procedure involves removal of the uterus, fallopian tubes, and ovaries.

Hysterectomy may involve either an abdominal or a vaginal approach. The choice depends on the underlying disorder, the need to explore the abdominal cavity, and the preference of the surgeon and woman. Nursing care of the woman undergoing a hysterectomy is described in the box on page 1563.

*Abdominal hysterectomy* is performed when a preexisting abdominal scar is present, when adhesions are thought to be present, or when a large operating field is necessary. For example, the woman with endometriosis is more likely to have an abdominal hysterectomy because endometrial tissue implants that may be present on other abdominal organs need to be removed. The surgical incision may be either longitudinal, made in the midline from umbilicus to pubis, or a *pfannenstiel incision,* also known as the bikini cut.

*Vaginal hysterectomy,* removal of the uterus through the vagina, is desirable when the uterus has descended into the vagina or if the urinary bladder or rectum have prolapsed into the vagina. Vaginal hysterectomy leaves no visible abdominal scar.

## NURSING CARE

### Nursing Diagnoses and Interventions

DUB usually causes the woman anxiety. Her self-image, sexuality, or reproductive capacity may be threatened, and she may fear the possibility of cancer. She may be embarrassed to discuss her menstrual history and hygiene practices. Interventions for the woman with DUB commonly address problems with anxiety and sexual function.

### Anxiety

The anxiety associated with abnormal uterine bleeding can be intense. Until the cause of the bleeding is identified and has been addressed, the woman may fear cancer or other life-threatening conditions.

- Discuss the results of tests and examinations with the woman. *This allows for open exchange of information.*
- Provide information about the causes, treatments, risks, long-term effects of treatments, and prognosis. *This allows the woman to assume responsibility for her own health and become involved in her own treatment plan.*

## NURSING CARE | OF THE WOMAN UNDERGOING DILATION AND CURETTAGE (D&C)

### PREOPERATIVE CARE

- If ordered, ask the woman to come in 24 hours before surgery for insertion of a laminaria tent. *This device absorbs cervical secretions and slowly dilates the cervix.*
- Ensure that the woman remains NPO after midnight on the day of surgery.

### POSTOPERATIVE CARE

- Monitor circulation and sensation in the legs, and avoid compression of the popliteal area. *The lithotomy position requires the woman's legs to be elevated in stirrups, which can impair circulation.*

- Instruct the woman to use perineal pads and avoid tampons for 2 weeks. *This reduces the risk of infection and allows tissues to heal.*
- Explain that the onset of the next menstrual period may be delayed.
- Explain that intercourse should be avoided until after the postoperative checkup and after vaginal discharge has ceased. *This precaution reduces the risk of infection.*
- Instruct the woman to rest for several days after surgery, avoid heavy lifting, and report any bleeding that is bright red or exceeds that of a normal menstrual period. *Vigorous activity, lifting, or straining interferes with healing and may cause hemorrhage.*

## NURSING CARE OF THE WOMAN UNDERGOING A HYSTERECTOMY

### PREOPERATIVE CARE

- Assess the woman's understanding of the procedure. Provide explanation, clarification, and emotional support as needed. Reassure that the anesthesia will eliminate any pain during surgery and that medication will be administered postoperatively to minimize discomfort. *The woman who understands about the procedure to be performed and what to expect after surgery will be less anxious.*
- Cleanse the abdominal and perineal area, and, if ordered, shave the perineal area.
- If ordered, administer a small cleansing enema and ask the woman to empty her bladder. *This precaution helps prevent contamination from the bowel or bladder during surgery.*
- Administer preoperative medications as ordered.
- Check the chart to ensure that the consent form has been signed.

### POSTOPERATIVE CARE

- Assess for signs of hemorrhage. *Hemorrhage is more common after vaginal hysterectomy than after abdominal hysterectomy.*
- Monitor vital signs every 4 hours, auscultate lungs every shift and measure intake and output. *These data are important indicators of hemodynamic status and complications.*
- Once the catheter has been removed, measure the amount of urine voided.
- Assess for complications, including infection, ileus, shock or hemorrhage, thrombophlebitis, and pulmonary embolus.
- Assess vaginal discharge; instruct the woman in perineal care.
- Assess incision and bowel sounds every shift.
- Encourage turning, coughing, deep breathing, and early ambulation.
- Encourage fluid intake.

- Teach to splint the abdomen and cough deeply. Teach the use of the incentive spirometer.
- Instruct to restrict physical activity for 4 to 6 weeks. Heavy lifting, stair climbing, douching, tampons, and sexual intercourse should be avoided. The woman should shower, avoiding tub baths, until bleeding has ceased. *Infection and hemorrhage are the greatest postoperative risks; restricting activities and preventing the introduction of any foreign material into the vagina helps reduce these risks.*
- Explain to the woman that she may feel tired for several days after surgery and needs to rest periodically.
- Explain that appetite may be depressed and bowel elimination may be sluggish. *These are after effects of general anesthesia, handling of the bowel during surgery, and loss of muscle tone in the bowel while empty.*
- Teach the woman to recognize signs of complications that should be reported to the physician or nurse:
  a. Temperature greater than 100°F (37.7°C)
  b. Vaginal bleeding that is greater than a typical menstrual period or is bright red
  c. Urinary incontinence, urgency, burning, or frequency
  d. Severe pain
- Encourage the woman to express feelings that may signal a negative self-concept. Correct any misconceptions. *Some women believe that hysterectomy means weight gain, the end of sexual activity, and the growth of facial hair.*
- Provide information on risks and benefits of hormone replacement therapy, if indicated. *If the ovaries have also been removed, the woman is immediately thrust into menopause and may want or need hormone replacement therapy.*
- Reinforce the need to obtain gynecologic examinations regularly even after hysterectomy.

---

- Evaluate coping strategies and psychosocial support systems. Teach coping strategies if indicated. *The possibility of surgery or cancer represents a crisis for the woman and her support system. Support groups can provide assistance for the woman through crisis intervention.*

### Sexual Dysfunction

The woman with DUB may be unwilling to express herself sexually, particularly if bleeding is frequent or heavy. Additionally, fatigue may prevent her from participating in sexual activity.

- Offer information about engaging in sexual activity during menstruation. Explain that conception is possible during this time and that orgasm may help relieve symptoms. *Some women mistakenly believe that birth control measures are unnecessary during menstruation. Orgasm causes a release of tension and vascular congestion and frequently provides at least temporary relief of symptoms.*
- Provide an opportunity for the expression of concerns related to alterations in lifestyle and sexual functioning. *Some women have had a prolonged period of sexual abstinence related to DUB. Allowing women to verbalize concerns can assist them*

*in working collaboratively with the health care provider to minimize the impact of illness and optimize function.*
- Encourage frequent rest periods. *This conserves energy and may allow sexual activities to resume.*
- Provide information about alternative methods of sexual expression. *Methods of sexual expression other than vaginal intercourse may satisfy the needs of both partners.*

**PRACTICE ALERT** *If the nurse is not comfortable with frank discussions about sexual activities, referral is indicated.* ■

### Home Care

Provide support, appropriate reassurance, and information to help the woman and her family better understand her disorder and the therapeutic interventions indicated. Teaching also includes self-care measures that help minimize the effects of DUB on the daily functioning of the woman. The following topics should be included.

- Administration and side effects of prescribed medications, including iron

- The need to maintain a balanced diet, increasing iron-rich foods such as eggs, beans, liver, beef, and shrimp (Inform the woman that while orange juice may improve the absorption of iron, foods high in calcium and oxalic acid, such as spinach, may reduce its absorption.)

- Importance of maintaining a fluid intake of 2000 to 3000 mL a day
- The need to immediately report recurring episodes of DUB, particularly in postmenopausal women, to the health care provider

## STRUCTURAL DISORDERS

Structural disorders of the female reproductive system include displacement disorders and fistulas.

### THE WOMAN WITH A UTERINE DISPLACEMENT

The uterus may be displaced within the pelvic cavity or may descend into the vaginal canal. Displacement of the uterus within the pelvic cavity is classified according to the direction of the displacement (Figure 48–2 ■):

- **Retroversion** of the uterus is a backward tilting of the uterus toward the rectum.
- **Retroflexion** involves a flexing or bending of the uterine corpus in a backward manner toward the rectum.
- **Anteversion** is an exaggerated forward tilting of the uterus.
- **Anteflexion** is a flexing or folding of the uterine corpus upon itself.

**Prolapse** of the uterus into the vaginal canal can vary from mild to complete prolapse outside of the body. First-degree, or mild, prolapse involves a descent of less than half the uterine

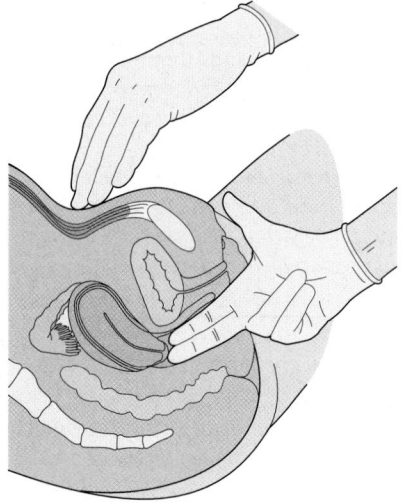

**A** Retroversion

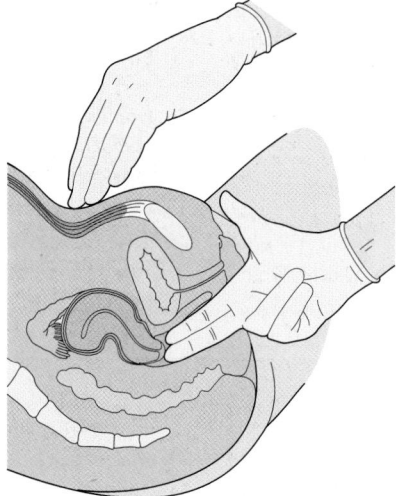

**B** Retroflexion

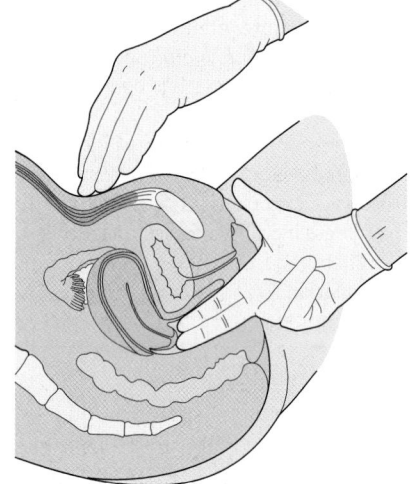

**C** Anteversion

**Figure 48–2** ■ Displacements of the uterus within the uterine cavity. *A*, Retroversion is a backward tilting. *B*, Retroflexion is a backward bending. *C*, Anteversion is a forward tilting. *D*, Anteflexion is a forward bending.

**D** Anteflexion

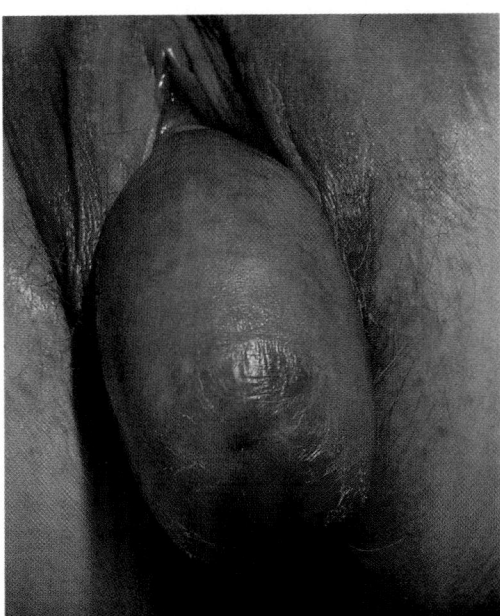

**Figure 48–3** ■ Prolapse of the uterus can vary from mild to complete. In third-degree uterine prolapse, or procidentia, the uterus prolapses completely outside the body, with inversion of the vagina.

*Source: M. English/Custom Medical Stock Photo.*

corpus into the vagina. Second-degree, or marked, prolapse involves the descent of the entire uterus into the vaginal canal, so that the cervix is at the introitus to the vagina. Third-degree prolapse, or *procidentia,* is complete prolapse of the uterus outside the body, with inversion of the vaginal canal (Figure 48–3 ■). Prolapse of the uterus is often accompanied by **cystocele** (herniation of the bladder into the vagina) or **rectocele** (herniation of the rectum into the vagina).

## PATHOPHYSIOLOGY AND MANIFESTATIONS

Displacement or prolapse of the uterus, bladder, or rectum can be a congenital or acquired condition. Congenital tilting or flexion of the uterus is rare. More commonly, tilting or flexion disorders in which the uterus remains within the pelvic cavity are related to scarring and inflammation of pelvic inflammatory disease, endometriosis, pregnancy, and tumors.

Downward displacement of the pelvic organs into the vagina results from weakened pelvic musculature, usually attributable to stretching of the supporting ligaments and muscles during pregnancy and childbirth. Unrepaired lacerations from childbirth, rapid deliveries, multiple pregnancies, congenital weakness, or loss of elasticity and muscle tone with aging may contribute to these disorders. The manifestations of displacement disorders are listed in the box on this page.

## COLLABORATIVE CARE

Collaborative care focuses on identifying the cause of the structural disorder, correcting or minimizing the condition, relieving pain, preventing or treating infection, and supporting and educating the woman.

### Manifestations of Displacement Disorders

**Uterine Displacement within the Pelvic Cavity**
- Dysmenorrhea
- Dyspareunia
- Backache
- Infertility

**Uterine Prolapse**
- Backache
- Bearing-down sensation
- Constipation
- Urinary incontinence
- Hemorrhoids
- Dyspareunia

**Cystocele/Rectocele**
- Bearing-down sensation
- Constipation
- Fecal incontinence
- Hemorrhoids
- Urinary incontinence

A careful history and physical examination are performed. Diagnosis of uterine displacement is made after physical examination. If herniation of the rectum or bladder is suspected, the woman is asked to bear down or cough during the examination so the prolapse can be palpated and any leakage of urine or feces visualized. A history of infections, multiple pregnancies in rapid succession, and rapid labors support this diagnosis.

Treatment may include Kegel exercises to strengthen weakened pelvic muscles. Kegel exercises can be useful in the early stages of downward displacement. These exercises are discussed in Chapter 26. ⌘

### Surgery

Several surgical procedures are used to repair structural disorders. For women presenting with a cystocele, anterior *colporrhaphy* (repair of the cystocele) is the most common procedure. The anterior repair shortens the pelvic muscles, providing tighter support for the bladder. The *Marshall-Marchetti-Krantz procedure* involves resuspension of the urinary bladder in correct anatomic position. A rectocele is repaired with a posterior colporrhaphy, which shortens the pelvic muscles, providing a tighter support for the rectum.

A prolapsed uterus may be surgically repositioned and the supporting muscles shortened to provide greater support. In postmenopausal women or women with procidentia, hysterectomy is the preferred treatment.

### Pessary

When surgery is contraindicated, a *pessary* (a removable device) may be inserted into the vagina to provide temporary support for the uterus or bladder. At regular intervals, the pessary is removed, cleaned, and reinserted.

## NURSING CARE

### Nursing Diagnoses and Interventions

Nursing care focuses on education about the disorder, proposed treatments, and self-care measures for relief of symptoms.

Nursing interventions for the woman with a displacement disorder address problems with urinary incontinence and anxiety.

### Stress Incontinence

Relaxation of the pelvic floor can lead to stress incontinence. This can prove both troublesome and embarrassing and can increase the incidence of urinary tract infection.

- Teach Kegel exercises. *These exercises strengthen perineal muscle tone, minimize urinary leakage, and minimize descent of the bladder and rectum into the vagina. In post-menopausal women, estrogen supplements also can improve muscle tone in the perineal area.*
- Suggest the use of perineal pads (ranging from thin pantiliners to full-thickness incontinence pads) or special underwear (such as Depends) to absorb urine leakage. *Using pads or undergarments often allows the woman to once again take part in her usual social activities.*
- Explain perineal care and proper use of perineal pads. *Cleansing the perineum from front to back, and applying and removing perineal pads the same way minimizes cross infection from the anus to the vaginal and urethral openings. Incontinence pads need to be changed frequently to minimize surface bacterial counts.*
- Suggest reducing or eliminating caffeine intake. *Reducing caffeine intake can reduce urinary frequency and urgency.*
- Stress the importance of cleaning the perineal area. *Urine is very irritating to the skin.*

### Anxiety

Anxiety is common among women with a displacement disorder. Many women have only a cursory understanding of their reproductive anatomy. This lack of knowledge often compounds the anxiety. The nurse can use drawings and models to explain structural disorders and treatment options available.

- Encourage questions from the woman and her partner. *This helps assess the level of understanding so that teaching can be more effective.*
- Explain that the relief from discomfort and fatigue may positively influence sexual expression, and reassure the woman that the capacity for orgasm will not be affected. *Many women and their partners have major concerns about the effects of the disorder and its treatment on their sex life and capacity for sexual pleasure.*
- Explore coping mechanisms that have been previously successful. *This can help relieve anxiety and boost self-esteem.*

## Home Care

If surgery is the treatment of choice, teaching centers on what to expect in the preoperative and postoperative periods. If medical treatment is used initially, teaching focuses on measures to relieve the manifestations, such as Kegel exercises, use of incontinence pads, or the use, care, and insertion of a pessary.

Because obesity is a risk factor associated with relaxation of the pelvic and abdominal muscles, dietary counseling may be indicated. Preoperatively, a diet high in fiber may alleviate constipation, a particular concern during the postoperative period.

# THE WOMAN WITH A VAGINAL FISTULA

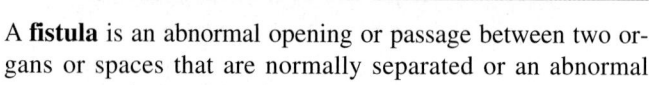

A **fistula** is an abnormal opening or passage between two organs or spaces that are normally separated or an abnormal passage to the outside of the body. The two types of vaginal fistulas are as follows:

- *Vesicovaginal fistula* is an abnormal opening between the urinary bladder and the vagina, leading to incontinent leakage of urine through the vagina.
- *Rectovaginal fistula* (less common) is an abnormal opening between the rectum and vagina, causing incontinent leakage of stool or flatus through the vagina.

Fistulas between the bladder and the vagina or between the rectum and the vagina may develop as a complication of childbirth, gynecologic or urologic surgery, or radiation therapy for gynecologic cancer. Cancer of the bladder is sometimes involved. The woman with a vaginal fistula often presents with a complaint of involuntary leakage of urine or flatus and symptoms of infection.

## COLLABORATIVE CARE

Fistulas are diagnosed by pelvic examination. Diagnosis of vesicovaginal fistula can be made by instilling dye into the urinary bladder through a catheter and observing the vagina for leakage. If no leakage is detected, a tampon or vaginal pack is inserted into the vagina, and the woman is asked to ambulate. If an abnormal opening is present, the tampon will absorb the dye. Dye may also be injected intravenously because it is excreted by the kidneys. Urine and vaginal cultures may be performed to rule out infections. Antibiotics are administered if infection is present.

A small vaginal fistula may resolve spontaneously. Otherwise, surgery is performed after inflammation has subsided, often a period of several months. Rarely, in the presence of a large, highly inflamed rectovaginal fistula, a temporary colostomy is performed, allowing inflammation and irritation to subside (see Chapter 24). ∞

## NURSING CARE

Nursing care for the woman with repair of a vaginal fistula is similar to that for the woman with a displacement disorder. Teaching is an important component of nursing care. Stress the importance of careful perineal cleansing to reduce irritation and prevent further tissue breakdown. Suggest perineal irrigation or sitz baths for cleansing. Perineal pads or special underwear may be used to absorb urine or fecal drainage. For the woman with a rectovaginal fistula, provide information about avoiding gas-forming foods to minimize embarrassment from odor.

# DISORDERS OF FEMALE REPRODUCTIVE TISSUE

Both benign and malignant tissue disorders affect the female reproductive system. Benign tumors and cysts include Bartholin's gland cysts, cervical polyps, endometrial cysts and polyps, ovarian cysts, and uterine leiomyomas (fibroids). **Endometriosis** is a condition in which endometrial tissue implants outside the uterus in various locations in the pelvic cavity. Malignant tumors of reproductive tissue include cervical cancer, endometrial cancer, ovarian cancer, and vulvar cancer.

## THE WOMAN WITH CYSTS OR POLYPS

A **cyst** is a fluid-filled sac. A **polyp** is a highly vascular solid tumor attached by a pedicle, or stem. Cysts or polyps of the female reproductive system can occur in the vulva, cervix, endometrium, or ovaries.

## PATHOPHYSIOLOGY AND MANIFESTATIONS

Following are different types of female reproductive tissue cysts and polyps.

- *Bartholin's gland cysts* are the most common cystic disorder of the vulva. These cysts are caused by the infection or obstruction of Bartholin's gland.
- *Cervical polyps* are the most common benign cervical lesion in women of reproductive age. These polyps tend to occur in women over age 40 who have borne several children and have a history of using oral contraceptives. It is possible that cervical polyps develop from endocervical hyperplasia. The polyp develops at the vaginal end of the cervix, has a stem, and is highly vascular.
- *Endometrial cysts and polyps* are caused by endometrial overgrowth and are often filled with old blood (the dark color leads to the label "chocolate cysts"). Endometrial cysts are the result of endometrial implants on the ovary and are associated with endometriosis. Endometrial polyps, in contrast, are intrauterine overgrowths, similar to cervical polyps, and usually have a stalk.

- *Ovarian cysts* are classified as follicular cysts and corpus luteum cysts. Follicular cysts develop as a result of failure of the mature follicle to rupture or failure of an immature follicle to reabsorb fluid after ovulation. Corpus luteum cysts develop as a result of increased hormone secretion by the corpus luteum after ovulation. Most functional cysts regress spontaneously within two or three menstrual cycles.
- *Polycystic ovary syndrome (POS)* is an endocrine disorder characterized by numerous follicular cysts; anovulation; elevated serum estrogen, androgen, and LH levels; amenorrhea or irregular menses; hirsutism; obesity; and infertility. Women with POS often have insulin resistance and are at increased risk for early-onset type II diabetes, as well as breast and endometrial cancer.

The causes and manifestations of benign cysts and polyps of the female reproductive system are presented in Table 48–1. Complications associated with these disorders include infection, rupture, infertility, hemorrhage, and recurrence.

## COLLABORATIVE CARE

Care focuses on identifying and correcting the disorder and preventing its recurrence. A careful history and physical examination are performed, including inspection and visualization. Examination of the reproductive tract reveals the presence of most cysts and polyps. The menstrual history may reveal menstrual irregularities.

### Diagnostic Tests

The following diagnostic tests may be used to diagnose cysts and polyps of the female reproductive system.

- *Luteinizing hormone (LH) level* and *serum testosterone* are elevated and *FSH/LH ratio* is reversed in POS. *Glucose tolerance tests* also may be performed.
- *Pregnancy test* is performed to rule out early pregnancy when luteal cysts are suspected.
- *Laparoscopy* is performed to visualize ovarian cysts.
- *Ultrasonography* or *X-ray examination* is used to differentiate cysts from solid tumors.

TABLE 48–1  Benign Cysts and Polyps of the Female Reproductive System

| Site | Type | Etiologic Origin | Manifestations |
|------|------|------------------|----------------|
| Ovary | Functional cysts | Ovulation—include follicular cysts and corpus luteum cysts | May resolve spontaneously; can cause pain, menstrual irregularity, or amenorrhea |
| | Polycystic ovarian syndrome | Unknown; possible hypothalamic-pituitary dysfunction | Hirsutism, obesity; amenorrhea or irregular menses; hyperinsulinemia; infertility |
| Vulva | Bartholin cysts | Obstruction or infection of Bartholin's gland | Pain, redness, perineal mass, dyspareunia |
| Endometrium | Chocolate cysts | Endometrial overgrowth; filled with old blood | |
| | Endometrial polyps | Unknown | Bleeding between periods |
| Cervix | Cervical polyps | Unknown | Bleeding after intercourse or between periods |

## Medications

Pharmacologic intervention includes antibiotic treatment of any infection or abscess and, for functional ovarian cysts, regulation of ovarian hormones through administration of oral contraceptives to achieve regression of the cyst. Clomiphene (Clomid, Serophene) may be prescribed to stimulate ovulation in the woman with POS who wishes to become pregnant. Dexamethasone (Decadron) suppresses ACTH and adrenal androgens, and may be added to increase the likelihood of ovulation.

## Surgery

Cervical polyps are readily visible through a vaginal speculum and usually are removed with a clamp, using a twisting motion. To remove endometrial cysts or polyps, a transcervical approach is used. The specimen is sent to the laboratory for evaluation, and chemical or electrical cauterization is applied after cyst removal. For Bartholin's gland cysts and any abscesses, the lesion is incised and drained, and a drainage device is left in place. Follicular cysts may be punctured through laser surgery, or a wedge resection of the ovary may be performed to restore ovulation. Rarely, oophorectomy (removal of the ovary) is performed if the cysts are very large.

## NURSING CARE

Nursing care focuses on relieving pain, implementing measures to correct the disorder, and preventing recurrence and complications. Address the following topics for self-care at home.

- The condition, its treatment, and measures to relieve pain
- The importance of keeping follow-up appointments
- Manifestations of infection (for postsurgical care) and the need to notify the physician should they occur
- If cervical polypectomy is performed, the use of external pads for 1 week (The woman must be able to state the signs of excessive bleeding and recognize that saturating more than one pad in an hour indicates the need for immediate follow-up.)
- The importance of long-term follow-up care for the woman with POS

## THE WOMAN WITH LEIOMYOMA

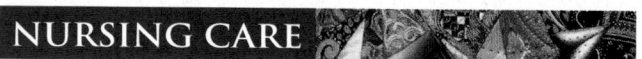

**Leiomyomata (fibroid tumors)** are benign tumors that originate from smooth muscle of the uterus. They are the most common form of pelvic tumor, believed to occur in 1 of every 4 or 5 women older than 35 years of age (Porth, 2002). Fibroids are seen more often and grow more rapidly in African Americans.

Fibroid tumors usually develop in the uterine corpus, and may be intramural, subserous, or submucous (Figure 48–4 ■).

- Intramural fibroid tumors (the most common type) are embedded in the myometrium. They usually present as an enlargement of the uterus.

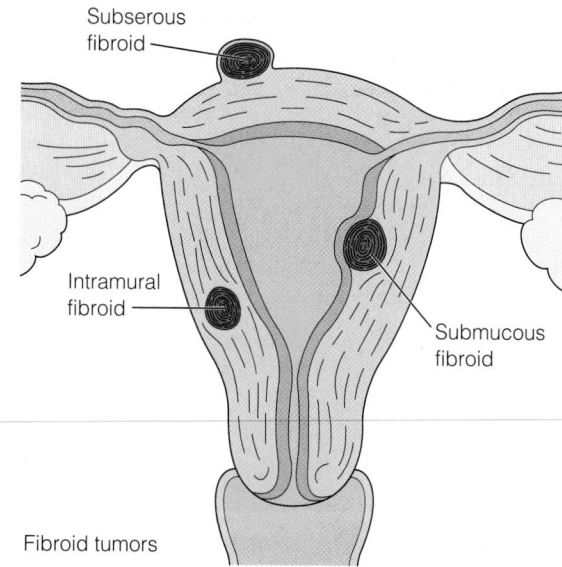

**Figure 48–4 ■** Types of uterine fibroid tumors (leiomyomata). Intramural fibroid tumors lie within the uterine wall. Subserous fibroid tumors lie beneath the serous lining of the uterus and project into the peritoneum. Submucous fibroid tumors lie beneath the endometrial lining of the uterus.

- Subserous fibroid tumors lie beneath the serous lining of the uterus and project into the peritoneal cavity. They may become pedunculated (on a stem) and displace or compress other tissues, such as the ureter or bladder.
- Submucous fibroid tumors lie beneath the endometrial lining of the uterus. They displace endometrial tissue and are more likely to cause bleeding, infection, and necrosis than the other types.

The actual cause of fibroid tumors is not clearly understood, but the association with estrogen stimulation is strong. Small tumors may be asymptomatic. The rate of growth varies, but they may increase in size during pregnancy or with use of oral contraceptives or HRT. Large fibroid tumors can crowd other organs, leading to pelvic pressure, pain, dysmenorrhea, menorrhagia, and fatigue. Depending on the location of the tumor, constipation and urinary urgency and frequency may occur. Most fibroid tumors shrink with menopause.

## COLLABORATIVE CARE

Treatment of the woman with uterine fibroids depends on the size and location of the tumors, the severity of the manifestations, and her age and childbearing status. Tests used to diagnose uterine fibroids may include an ultrasound to differentiate leiomyomata from endometriosis and a laparoscopy to visualize subserosal leiomyomata.

In asymptomatic women who wish to bear children, the fibroid tumors are monitored. Follow-up two to three times per year to monitor growth and the woman's response is recommended.

## Medications

Leuprolide acetate (Lupron) is used to decrease the size of the tumor if surgery is contraindicated or not desired. Gonadotropin-releasing hormone (GnRH) agonists are also administered.

## Surgery

*Myomectomy,* removal of the tumor without removing the entire uterus, is the surgical procedure of choice for young women who wish to retain reproductive capability. Laparoscopic laser technique is used for many women. A hysterectomy is performed if tumors are large, and if bleeding or other problems continue in perimenopausal women. A hysterectomy usually requires a hospital stay of 3 to 4 days, and a 6-week recovery time. A new method of treatment is with a *uterine fibroid embolization.* In this procedure, a catheter is guided through the femoral artery to the uterus, where tiny particles are injected into the artery supplying the fibroid to cut off the fibroid's blood supply. This procedure requires only an overnight hospital stay with a return to normal activities in 1 week.

If surgery is deferred, teaching emphasizes the importance of regular follow-up assessments to monitor tumor growth. If a hysterectomy is performed, teaching emphasizes appropriate preoperative and postoperative care. Dietary modifications to increase iron intake, prevent constipation, and promote healing are important.

## THE WOMAN WITH ENDOMETRIOSIS

**Endometriosis** is a condition in which multiple, small, usually benign implantations of endometrial tissue develop throughout the pelvic cavity. Endometriosis affects from 10% to 15% of women of childbearing age and is more common in women who postpone childbearing. Risk factors for endometriosis include early menarche, regular periods with a cycle of less than 27 days, menses lasting more than 7 days, heavier flow, increased menstrual pain, and a history of the condition in first-degree female relatives (Porth, 2002).

## PATHOPHYSIOLOGY AND MANIFESTATIONS

The cause of endometriosis is unclear, but several theories have been proposed. The metaplasia theory asserts that endometrial tissue develops from embryonic epithelial cells as a result of hormonal or inflammatory changes. The theory of retrograde menstruation suggests that menstrual tissue backs up through the fallopian tubes during menses, implants on various pelvic structures, and survives. The transplantation theory asserts that endometrial implants spread via lymphatic or vascular routes.

The abnormally located endometrial tissue responds to cyclic ovarian hormone stimulation, and bleeding occurs at the sites of implantation. Scarring, inflammation, and adhesions may develop. Endometriosis is a slowly progressive disease, responsive to ovarian hormone stimulation. Thus, the implants regress during pregnancy and atrophy at menopause unless the

### Manifestations of Endometriosis

- Heavy, throbbing pain of the lower abdomen and pelvis, radiating down the thighs and around the back. (The degree of pain, however, is not indicative of the severity of the disease.)
- Feeling of rectal pressure and discomfort when having a bowel movement
- Dyspareunia
- Dysfunctional uterine bleeding
- Infertility

woman is receiving HRT. Because progressive scarring may interfere with ability to conceive, women with significant endometriosis are encouraged to have children early if they wish to do so. Manifestations of endometriosis, which usually present during the luteal phase of the menstrual cycle, are summarized in the box above.

### COLLABORATIVE CARE

Endometriosis may be difficult to diagnose, but a history of dysmenorrhea, dyspareunia, and infertility strongly suggests this diagnosis. Interventions depend on the severity of symptoms, the extent of the disease, and the woman's age and desire for childbearing. Treatment goals focus on pain management and restoring fertility.

## Diagnostic Tests

Diagnostic tests are ordered to rule out other medical conditions and identify the endometrial implants.

- *Pelvic ultrasonography* may be performed to rule out other causes for pain and discomfort, including space-occupying masses
- *CBC with differential* is used to rule out pelvic abscesses and infectious processes. A low hemoglobin and hematocrit may be noted if menorrhagia accompanies endometriosis or tissue implants bleed significantly during the menses.
- *Laparoscopy* is used to visualize implants, and is the only method for definitive diagnosis.

## Medications

Medications include analgesics to control pain and prostaglandin synthesis inhibitors such as NSAIDs. Hormone therapy may include oral contraceptives or progesterone to induce pseudopregnancy, or danazol (Danocrine) to induce amenorrhea and involution of both endometrial tissue. Prolonged use of danazol, however, may result in masculinizing effects. GnRH is used to elevate levels of estrogen and progesterone and minimize bleeding.

## Surgery

Surgical interventions include laparoscopy with laser ablation (excision or removal) of endometrial implants. Refractory endometriosis may be treated with total hysterectomy.

# NURSING CARE

## Nursing Diagnoses and Interventions

Nursing care includes providing pain relief, providing education about the condition and the treatment options, and helping the woman cope with treatment outcomes. The severity of the disease and its manifestations are not necessarily related. Advanced disease may exhibit few manifestations, whereas early disease may be quite painful. Interventions for pain, discussed previously, are also appropriate for the woman with endometriosis. A priority diagnosis for the young woman with this disorder is anxiety related to loss of reproductive function.

### Anxiety

Anxiety about the unsure prognosis related to infertility is a particular problem for young women who plan to have a family in the near or distant future.

- Encourage expression of fears and anxiety about infertility, and answer questions honestly. *Knowledge helps relieve anxiety and fear.*
- Provide information on fertility awareness methods, including measurement of basal body temperature and other techniques for recognizing ovulation. *Understanding these techniques helps the woman and her partner optimize the conditions for conception.*

## Using NANDA, NIC, and NOC

Chart 48–1 shows links between NANDA nursing diagnoses, NIC, and NOC when caring for the woman with endometriosis.

## Home Care

Explain the cause of the disorder and the various treatment options, including their side effects. Discuss fertility awareness methods and the risks and benefits of long-term use of oral contraceptives. Stress the importance of exercise, smoking cessation, and weight control. If surgical treatment is chosen, provide preoperative and postoperative teaching.

# THE WOMAN WITH CERVICAL CANCER

The American Cancer Society (2002) estimates that 13,000 cases of cervical cancer will be diagnosed, with approximately 4100 deaths attributed to the disease, annually. The incidence is greater in blacks than whites. Effective screening with the Papanicolaou smear (Pap test) has reduced the death rate by 55% over the last 30 years, although the death rates for blacks continues to be more than 2 times that of whites. The age of diagnosis is between 50 and 55 years; however, it begins to appear in women in their 20s.

## PATHOPHYSIOLOGY AND MANIFESTATIONS

Most cervical cancers (90%) are squamous cell carcinomas that begin as neoplasia in the cervical epithelium. *Precancerous dysplasia (cervical intraepithelial neoplasia [CIN], cervical carcinoma in situ)* is estimated to occur in 1 of 8 women before the age of 20, often associated with human papillomavirus (HPV) infection. Studies have also found a strong association with reproductive infections with *Chlamydia trachomatis.* (These infections are discussed in Chapter 49). The precursor lesions may spontaneously regress (60%), persist (30%), or progress and undergo malignant change (10%). Only about 1% become invasive (Porth, 2002). The CIN system of grading dysplastic changes is based on the extent of involvement of the epithelial thickness of the cervix. Carcinoma in situ is localized; invasive cancer spreads to deeper layers.

Cancer in situ most often develops in the transformation zone where the columnar epithelium of the cervical lining meets the squamous epithelium of the outer cervix and vagina. Squamous cell cancers spread by direct invasion of accessory structures, including the vaginal wall, pelvic wall, bladder, and rectum. Although metastasis is most frequently confined to the pelvic area, distant metastasis may occur through the lymphatic system. Clinical staging is based on the International Federation of Gynecology and Obstetrics (FIGO) system (Table 48–2).

---

**CHART 48–1 NANDA, NIC, AND NOC LINKAGES**

### The Client with Endometriosis

| NURSING DIAGNOSES | NURSING INTERVENTIONS | NURSING OUTCOMES |
|---|---|---|
| • Fatigue | • Energy Management | • Energy Conservation |
| • Deficient Knowledge | • Teaching: Disease Process | • Knowledge: Disease Process |
| | • Teaching: Sexuality | |
| | • Preconception Counseling | |
| • Powerlessness | • Emotional Support | • Social Support |
| | • Self-Esteem Enhancement | • Health Beliefs: Perceived Control |

*Note. Data from Nursing Outcomes Classification (NOC) by M. Johnson & M. Maas (Eds.), 1997, St. Louis: Mosby; Nursing Diagnoses: Definitions & Classification 2001–2002 by North American Nursing Diagnosis Association, 2001, Philadelphia: NANDA; Nursing Interventions Classification (NIC) by J.C. McCloskey & G. M. Bulechek (Eds.), 2000, St. Louis: Mosby. Reprinted by permission.*

## Nursing Care Plan
## A Woman with Endometriosis

Angela Hall is a 31-year-old married accountant, who relates a history of severe dysmenorrhea and menorrhagia, a feeling of pelvic heaviness and pain that radiates down her thighs. Because of her discomfort, her husband has complained about the quality of their sex life and has expressed concerns about their plans for having children. Mrs. Hall reports being so tired she doesn't care whether she has sex or not, and, in fact, would really prefer not to: "Sex hurts so much, I just can't stand it." Endometriosis is suspected, and a diagnostic laparoscopy has been scheduled.

### ASSESSMENT

Christine Brigham, RN, NP, interviews Mrs. Hall and makes the following assessments: BP 110/70, P 68, R 18, T 98.2°F (36.7°C). Mrs. Hall's weight is 130 lb (59 kg) and within normal limits for her height. Review of laboratory findings indicate a hemoglobin level of 9.8 g/dL (normal range: 12 to 16 g/dL) and a hematocrit of 33.1% (normal range: 35% to 45%). Physical examination reveals pelvic tenderness on manipulation of the cervix, and small masses that are palpable on abdominal/pelvic examination.

### DIAGNOSIS

- *Chronic pain* related to endometrial pelvic implants
- *Anxiety* related to effect of endometriosis on fertility
- *Deficient knowledge* related to diagnosis and treatment options
- *Ineffective sexuality patterns* related to the manifestations of endometriosis

### EXPECTED OUTCOMES

- Develop effective self-care measures to deal with the pain and discomfort.
- Verbalize decreased anxiety.
- Demonstrate understanding of the disease and treatment options.
- Verbalize an improvement in sexual functioning and a decrease in interpersonal stress between herself and her husband.

### PLANNING AND IMPLEMENTATION

- Identify the location, type, duration, and history of the pain.
- Recommend analgesics and heat therapy.
- Provide information on biofeedback, relaxation, and imagery to lessen pain.
- Discuss with Mr. and Mrs. Hall the causes of endometriosis and its manifestations.
- Encourage the Halls to discuss their feelings about the effect of the disease on their sex life, lifestyle, and fertility.
- Refer the couple to the local mental health center if appropriate.

### EVALUATION

Two years after the initiation of treatment, Mr. and Mrs. Hall have become parents of a baby girl. Mrs. Hall states that the discomfort and other manifestations of endometriosis have eased. Relaxation and imagery have effectively minimized her pain and brought about improvement in her function as wife, mother, and sexual partner. Counseling has improved the interpersonal and sexual relations between the Halls. Dietary management has improved her anemia, although the menorrhagia persists. The Halls are trying to have a second child, understanding the advantages of rapid succession of pregnancies. They will be followed in the nursing clinic and referred to an infertility clinic if conception does not occur within 1 year.

### Critical Thinking in the Nursing Process

1. Explain the pathophysiologic basis for Mrs. Hall's anemia.
2. How would you handle the situation if Mr. and Mrs. Hall were extremely uncomfortable and embarrassed about discussing their sexual problems?
3. Develop a plan of care for Mrs. Hall for the nursing diagnosis, *Situational low self*-esteem, related to the manifestations of endometriosis.

See Evaluating your Response in Appendix C.

| TABLE 48-2 | FIGO Staging Classification for Cervical Cancer |
|---|---|
| **Stage** | **Description** |
| 0 | Carcinoma in situ, intraepithelial carcinoma |
| I | Carcinoma that is strictly confined to the cervix |
| II | Involvement of the vagina, limited to the upper two-thirds of the vagina, or infiltration of the parametria (connective tissue surrounding the uterus) but not the side wall of the pelvis |
| III | Involvement of the lower third of the vagina or extension to the pelvic side wall |
| IV | Extension outside the reproductive tract |

Preinvasive cancer is limited to the cervix and rarely causes symptoms. Invasive cancer produces vaginal bleeding after intercourse or between menstrual periods, and vaginal discharge that increases as the cancer progresses. These changes are subtle, and may be more readily noticed by the postmenopausal woman. Manifestations of advanced disease include referred pain in the back or thighs, hematuria, bloody stools, anemia, and weight loss.

### Risk Factors

As described by the American Cancer Society (2001), risk factors for cervical cancer include infection of the external genitalia and anus with HPV, first intercourse before 16 years of age, multiple sex partners or male partners with multiple sex partners, a history of sexually transmitted infections, and infection with HIV. The most important risk factor is infection by the HPV. Other risk factors include smoking and poor nutritional status, family history of cervical cancer, and exposure to DES (diethylstilbestrol) in utero.

## COLLABORATIVE CARE

The goals of treatment are to eradicate the cancer and minimize complications and metastasis. The type of treatment depends on the degree of malignant change, the size and location of the lesion, and the extent of metastasis.

## Diagnostic Tests

Diagnostic tests used to diagnose cervical cancer include the following:

- *Pap smear* is the primary screening tool for cervical carcinoma (see the box below). If the results show atypical cells, the test is repeated. Pap test results may be reported in descriptive terms with abnormal cells described as benign, which may include infectious, inflammatory, atrophic, or other cell changes, or as epithelial cell abnormalities, including atypical squamous cells to squamous cell carcinoma, and atypical glandular cells to adenocarcinoma.

## Nursing Implications for Diagnostic Tests

### Papanicolaou (Pap) Test

The Papanicolaou smear (Pap test) is used to screen for cervical intraepithelial neoplasia (CIN) and cervical cancer. It can also be used to assess hormonal status and identify the presence of sexually transmitted diseases, such as human papilloma virus (HPV) infection.

With the woman in the lithotomy position, a speculum is inserted to visualize the cervix. A plastic or wooden spatula is used to scrape the cervical os and any suspicious-looking areas, and the material is transferred to a slide for histologic analysis. A cotton-tipped applicator or cytobrush is used to obtain a specimen from the endocervix; this specimen is then transferred to a second slide.

### Client Preparation
- Instruct the woman to empty her bladder.
- Explain that the test should be painless and quick, although slight cramping may be experienced when the endocervical specimen is obtained.

### Client and Family Teaching
- Teach the woman about recommended frequency of screening, every 3 years until age 65 after two successive negative results a year apart or more frequently if the woman has specific risk factors for cervical cancer.
- Teach the woman to schedule the Pap test for a time when she is not menstruating. Blood interferes with interpretation of the smear.
- Teach the woman to avoid intercourse, douching, or placing of any medication in the vagina for 36 hours prior to the test.

## Nursing Implications for Diagnostic Tests

### Cervical Biopsy

Cervical biopsy is performed for women whose Pap smear findings indicate possible cervical cancer or cervical intraepithelial neoplasia (CIN). The biopsy is also used to screen women at high risk for vaginal and cervical cancers due to intrauterine DES exposure. With the woman in the lithotomy position, the cervix is cleaned with 3% acetic acid, and tissue samples are taken for biopsy. Afterward, the area is cleaned and a perineal pad applied.

### Client Preparation
- Explain the procedure, indicating that the test usually involves minimal discomfort although a cramping sensation may be experienced as the cervix is dilated to obtain the specimen.
- Have the woman empty her bladder prior to the procedure.

### Client and Family Teaching
- Explain that minor bleeding and vaginal discharge are expected following this procedure. Perineal pads should be used and tampons avoided for at least one week.
- Caution to avoid sexual intercourse until discharge has stopped.
- Instruct to notify the physician if heavy bleeding or manifestations of infection (pain, foul smelling discharge, fever, malaise) occur.

- *Colposcopy* and *cervical biopsy* of the suspicious area may be performed if the second Pap test yields abnormal findings (see the box above).
- *Loop diathermy technique* (loop electrosurgical excision procedure [LEEP]) allows simultaneous diagnosis and treatment of dysplastic lesions found on colposcopy. This procedure is performed in the office, using a wire for both cutting and coagulation during excision of the dysplastic region of the cervix.
- *MRI* or *CT* of the pelvis, abdomen, or bones may be performed to detect the spread of the tumor.

## Medications

Chemotherapy is used for tumors not responsive to other therapy, tumors that cannot be removed, or as adjunct therapy if metastasis has occurred (see Chapter 10). ∞

## Treatments

The treatment for cervical cancer may include surgery and radiation therapy.

### Surgery

When combined with colposcopy, laser surgery is a viable treatment method provided that the cancer is limited to the cervical epithelium. Cryosurgery, which involves the use of a probe to freeze tissue, causing necrosis and sloughing, is also used for noninvasive lesions. Conization (Figure 48–5 ■) is performed to treat microinvasive carcinoma when colposcopy cannot define the limits of the invasion. For invasive lesions,

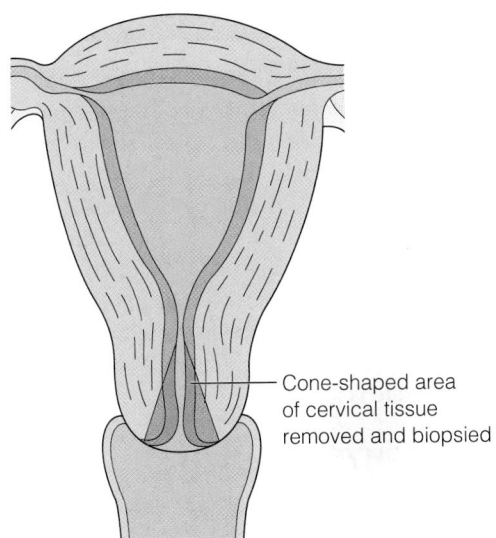

**Figure 48–5** ■ Conization, the surgical removal of a cone-shaped section of the cervix, is used to treat microinvasive carcinoma of the cervix.

Cone-shaped area of cervical tissue removed and biopsied

hysterectomy or radical hysterectomy (removal of the uterus, fallopian tubes, lymph nodes, and ovaries) is performed.

A **pelvic exenteration,** the removal of all pelvic contents, including the bowel, vagina, and bladder, is performed if the cancer recurs without involvement of the lymphatic system. An anterior exenteration is the removal of the uterus, ovaries, fallopian tubes, vagina, bladder, urethra, and lymphatic vessels and nodes. An ileal conduit is created for excretion of urine (see Chapter 26). A posterior exenteration is the removal of the uterus, ovaries, uterine tubes, bowel, and rectum. A colostomy is created for excretion of feces (see Chapter 24). ⊂⊃

### Radiation Therapy

Radiation therapy is used to treat invasive cervical cancer. External radiation beam therapy and intracavity cesium irradiation can be used.

## NURSING CARE

Nursing care involves helping the woman deal with the physical and psychologic effects of a potentially life-threatening illness, providing information needed to make informed decisions, and minimizing the adverse effects of therapy. Pain relief measures are important, as is grief work on the part of the woman and family. The woman should be encouraged to perform self-care activities and resume normal everyday activities and sexual functioning to the extent possible.

### Health Promotion

The American Cancer Society (2002) recommends that women should begin annual screening for cervical cancer with the Pap test at the age of 18, or after beginning sexual activity, whichever comes first. After three consecutive negative Pap tests, screening can be performed less frequently, at the discretion of the health care provider.

It is vital that nurses educate women of all ages about controlling risk factors for cervical cancer and about the importance of screening for this cancer throughout the life span. Teach young women about the relationship between early sexual activity, multiple partners, and risk for sexually transmitted diseases and cervical cancer. Discuss safer sex alternatives and using condoms for protection. Emphasize the importance of continued screening exams for the older woman who may not see a gynecologic specialist on a regular basis.

### Assessment

Collect the following data through a health history and physical examination (see Chapter 46).

- Health history: history of sexually transmitted infections, sexual history, family history of cervical cancer, vaginal bleeding or discharge, smoking history, maternal treatment with DES
- Physical assessment: pelvic examination, abdomen, lymph glands

### Nursing Diagnoses and Interventions

This section discusses nursing interventions for the woman who has been diagnosed with cervical cancer and requires surgical and/or radiation treatment. Other nursing diagnoses and interventions that may be appropriate for the woman with cervical cancer are discussed in the sections discussing other female reproductive system cancers.

### Fear

Many people believe that cancer equals death; however, this is no longer true in many cases, especially with early diagnosis. For cervical cancer that is diagnosed at an early stage, the 5-year survival rate is 92%. If the disease is in situ, the rate is nearly 100%.

- Explain that 70% of all women with cervical cancer survive for 5 years or more and that the earlier the cancer is detected, the better the prognosis. *This gives the woman hope, an essential ingredient in recovery.*
- Allow adequate time for the woman and her partner to express their concerns and to ask questions. *Unexpressed feelings and fears and lack of understanding may cause the woman to view the situation as worse than it is.*
- Refer to cancer counselor or support groups for additional information. *Cancer survivors who visit clients in the hospital provide proof that people can survive the diagnosis and treatment of cancer and lead normal, productive lives.*

### Impaired Tissue Integrity

Surgery interrupts the integrity of the skin surface, providing a potential portal of invasion for bacteria. Radiation therapy causes an inflammatory response in the skin and mucous membranes within the field of radiation, creating further risk of tissue reaction and breakdown.

- Teach wound and skin care, particularly if pelvic exenteration is performed. Irrigations with saline or solutions of saline and hydrogen peroxide are performed at intervals, with dry heat applied thereafter to dry the area. *Open and damaged tissue increases the risk for infection. Meticulous skin and wound care is necessary to prevent infection and further tissue destruction.*

- If appropriate, teach stoma care, and care for the skin surrounding the stoma. (These procedures are discussed in Chapters 24 and 26.) 🔗 *Urine and stool are irritating to the skin. Without proper care, the skin surrounding the stoma can become excoriated.*
- Apply non-oil-based lotions to skin surface. This may minimize itching and help maintain integrity. *Oil-based lotions are not recommended for tissue undergoing radiation.*
- Instruct the woman not to remove the markings used to localize the radiation beam to the target area. *Markings are used in future radiation treatments.*
- Monitor for evidence of fistula formation, and teach the woman to do the same. *Fistula formation is a potential complication of radiation to the pelvic or abdominal cavities. Vaginal fistulas may form between the vagina and the bladder or rectum. Fistulas may also develop between the bladder and rectum, resulting in the expulsion of stool in the urine or loss of urine through the anus.*

## Using NANDA, NIC, and NOC

Chart 48–2 shows links between NANDA nursing diagnoses, NIC, and NOC when caring for the woman with cervical cancer.

## Home Care

Teaching varies according to the stage of the cancer and the treatment selected. Provide information concerning radiation, chemotherapy, or surgery, as indicated. Preoperative teaching focuses on postoperative expectations, including management of urinary or fecal diversion, if indicated (see Chapters 24 and 26). Help the woman and family recognize signs of infection and understand the importance of follow-up care. In addition, suggest the following resources:

- American Cancer Society
- National Cancer Institute
- Women's Cancer Network

# THE WOMAN WITH ENDOMETRIAL CANCER

Endometrial carcinoma is the most frequently diagnosed pelvic cancer in the United States. The American Cancer Society (2002) estimates that each year approximately 39,000 women are diagnosed with endometrial cancer, and 6600 die from this disease. The incidence is higher in whites than blacks, but the mortality rate is nearly twice as high in blacks. Most endometrial cancer is diagnosed in postmenopausal women, with the peak incidence in the late 50s and early 60s. When diagnosed and treated early in the disease, the 5-year survival rate is about 90%.

## PATHOPHYSIOLOGY AND MANIFESTATIONS

Most endometrial malignancies are adenocarcinomas that are slow to grow and metastasize. These cancers develop in the glandular cells or endometrial lining of the uterus (the same tissue that is shed each month during a normal menstrual period). Endometrial hyperplasia (excessive growth) is a precursor of endometrial cancer. These tumors tend to grow slowly in the early stages.

Tumor growth usually begins in the fundus, invades the vascular myometrium, and spreads throughout the female reproductive tract. Metastasis occurs by means of the lymphatic system, through the fallopian tubes to the peritoneal cavity, and to the rest of the body via the bloodstream. Target areas for metastasis include the lungs, liver, and bone. The FIGO classification of endometrial cancer is presented in Table 48–3.

The major manifestation of endometrial hyperplasia or overt endometrial cancer is abnormal, painless vaginal bleeding. In menstruating women, this bleeding is manifested as menorrhagia or metrorrhagia. In postmenopausal women, any bleeding is abnormal. Later manifestations include pelvic cramping, bleeding after intercourse, and lower abdominal pressure. In advanced disease, lymph node enlargement, pleural effusion, abdominal masses, and ascites may be present.

## CHART 48-2 NANDA, NIC, AND NOC LINKAGES

### The Client with Cervical Cancer

| NURSING DIAGNOSES | NURSING INTERVENTIONS | NURSING OUTCOMES |
|---|---|---|
| • Deficient Knowledge | • Teaching: Safe Sex<br><br>• Teaching: Disease Process | • Knowledge: Infection Control<br>• Risk Control: STD<br>• Knowledge: Disease Process<br>• Knowledge: Health Behaviors |
| • Anticipatory Grieving | • Active Listening<br>• Emotional Support | • Coping<br>• Grief Resolution |
| • Ineffective Protection | • Risk Identification<br>• Chemotherapy Management<br>• Surgical Precautions | • Infection Status |

*Note. Data from Nursing Outcomes Classification (NOC) by M. Johnson & M. Maas (Eds.), 1997, St. Louis: Mosby; Nursing Diagnoses: Definitions & Classification 2001–2002 by North American Nursing Diagnosis Association, 2001, Philadelphia: NANDA; Nursing Interventions Classification (NIC) by J.C. McCloskey & G. M. Bulechek (Eds.), 2000, St. Louis: Mosby. Reprinted by permission.*

## Nursing Care Plan
## A Woman with Cervical Cancer

Anna Eliza Gillam is a 45-year-old divorced mother of four children ranging in age from 16 to 23. She was married at age 18 and had several sexual partners prior to her marriage. She has had three sexual partners since her marriage ended. Last year she was treated with cryosurgery for venereal warts. The Pap smear taken 2 weeks ago showed atypical cells, and she has come in for a repeat test.

### ASSESSMENT

Judy Davis, RN, the admitting nurse, interviews Mrs. Gillam and records the following assessment findings: BP 130/80, P 72, R 18, T 99.2°F (37.3°C). Ms. Gillam weighs 142 lb (64.5 kg), approximately 15% over her ideal body weight. Examination of the cervix reveals a large necrotic lesion at the 7 o'clock position. She has reduced her smoking to less than 10 cigarettes per day, and she does not drink alcohol.

Ms. Gillam is extremely fearful and anxious and has told no one about her abnormal Pap smear. She reveals that she has had back pain radiating down her thighs for several months and a foul vaginal discharge that increases after intercourse. Until 2 weeks ago, she had not had a Pap smear for 5 years. Ms. Davis performs the repeat Pap smear, which is positive for squamous cell carcinoma of the cervix. A CT scan and lymphangiography are scheduled. Laparoscopy shows the disease to be widespread in the pelvic cavity.

### DIAGNOSES

- *Decisional conflict* related to treatment options
- *Chronic and acute pain* related to metastasis and surgery
- *Risk for impaired skin integrity* related to radiation
- *Fear* related to diagnosis of cervical cancer
- *Anticipatory grieving* related to potential loss of life

### EXPECTED OUTCOMES

- Gain knowledge to make informed decisions about treatment options.
- Develop strategies for pain control.
- Maintain skin and tissue integrity during radiation treatment.
- Express her feelings about the fear of cancer and death.

- Develop effective coping strategies for dealing with life-threatening illness and pain.

### PLANNING AND IMPLEMENTATION

- Discuss treatment alternatives, including the prognosis with each option.
- Administer pain medications as prescribed.
- Inspect skin surfaces daily before and after radiation therapy.
- Provide information on biofeedback training and relaxation techniques for control of moderate pain.
- Refer to a local cancer support group so that she can interact with cancer survivors.
- Refer Mrs. Gillam to a social worker in preparation for her altered level of functioning.

### EVALUATION

Mrs. Gillam has begun radiation therapy following pelvic extenteration. She controls her pain with relaxation and imagery techniques, requiring only occasional analgesics. She uses a water-based lotion to soothe the skin surface and is careful not to remove the skin markings. She seems optimistic and has quit smoking. She and her family have continued to attend the cancer support group meetings. Mrs. Gillam is planning for the future and has talked with her family about what it means to live with cancer.

### Critical Thinking in the Nursing Process

1. Compare and contrast your teaching plan for health promotion interventions to decrease the risks of cervical cancer for a young woman of 17 and an older woman of 70. Would they differ, and if so, how?
2. Develop a teaching plan to help Mrs. Gillam cope with the effects of radiation.
3. During a home visit, Mrs. Gillam tells the nurse that she has been so tired since beginning radiation treatments that all she can do is sit in her chair. Design a plan of care for the nursing diagnosis, *Fatigue*.

See Evaluating Your Response in Appendix C.

---

| TABLE 48–3 | FIGO Staging Classification for Endometrial Cancer |
| --- | --- |
| **Stage** | **Description** |
| I | Tumor limited to endometrium or myometrium |
| II | Endocervical glandular involvement or invasion of cervical stroma |
| III | Metastasis or invasion of serosa, adnexae, vagina, and pelvic or para-aortic lymph nodes |
| IV | Tumor invasion of bladder or bowel mucosa; distant metastases |

## Risk Factors

A significant risk factor for endometrial cancer is prolonged estrogen stimulation with hyperplasia. Other factors that increase the risk are obesity, anovulatory menstrual cycles, decreasing ovarian function (as with menopause), estrogen-secreting tumors, and unopposed estrogen (e.g., estrogen therapy without progesterone). Medical conditions that may alter estrogen metabolism and increase the risk of endometrial cancer are diabetes mellitus, hypertension, and polycystic ovary syndrome (Porth, 2002). Tamoxifen, a drug that blocks estrogen receptor sites and is used to treat breast cancer, has a weak estrogenic effect on the endometrium, and is also a risk factor.

## COLLABORATIVE CARE

The goals of care for the woman with endometrial cancer are to eradicate the cancer and minimize complications and metastasis.

### Diagnostic Tests

Tests used to diagnose cancer of the endometrium include the following:

- *Vaginal ultrasonography* is sometimes used to determine endometrial thickening, which may indicate hypertrophy or malignant changes.
- *Endometrial biopsy* (see the box below) or dilation and curettage (D&C) provides definitive diagnosis.
- *Transvaginal ultrasound* is used to measure endometrial thickness.
- *Laparoscopy* may be performed to determine the stage of the cancer.
- Other tests to determine the extent of the disease include *chest X-ray, intravenous urography, cystoscopy, barium enema, sigmoidoscopy, MRI,* and *bone scans.*

### Medications

Although the treatment of choice for primary endometrial carcinoma is surgery, progesterone therapy may be used for recurrent disease. About one-third of women respond favorably, primarily those with well-differentiated tumors. Chemotherapy is less effective than other forms of therapy, although cisplatin or combination chemotherapy may be used for women with disseminated disease.

### Surgery

After the diagnosis is confirmed, a total abdominal hysterectomy and bilateral salpingo-oophorectomy is performed. A radical hysterectomy with node dissection is performed if the disease is stage II or beyond.

### Radiation Therapy

Treatment with external and internal radiation may be performed as a preoperative measure or as adjuvant treatment in advanced cases.

## NURSING CARE

### Health Promotion

All perimenopausal and postmenopausal women need annual pelvic examinations. Those in high-risk groups are advised to have endometrial biopsies every 2 years. Any vaginal bleeding in postmenopausal women should be reported at once to the physician. In addition, control of diseases such as diabetes mellitus and hypertension decreases the risk of endometrial hyperplasia.

### Assessment

Collect the following data through a health history and physical examination (see Chapter 46).

- Health history: abnormal vaginal bleeding, menstrual history, use of estrogen (without progesterone) to treat menopausal symptoms, breast cancer treated with tamoxifen, childbearing status, presence of chronic illnesses
- Physical assessment: height and weight, pelvic examination, abdomen, lymph glands

### Nursing Diagnoses and Interventions

Nursing care involves helping the woman deal with the physical and psychologic effects of a potentially life-threatening illness, make informed decisions, and minimize the adverse effects of therapy. Pain relief is a key component of care, as is grief work on the part of the woman and family. Encourage the woman to perform self-care and resume normal activities of daily living.

#### Acute Pain

Total abdominal hysterectomy can involve severe and prolonged pain, not only from the surgical incision but also from the manipulation of internal organs during surgery. Abdominal viscera are highly vascular and easily bruised by handling.

- Administer analgesics as ordered. *Analgesics provide pain relief and promote early ambulation.*
- Encourage ambulation. *Ambulation facilitates the expulsion of flatus, which can cause distention as well as discomfort.*

## Nursing Implications for Diagnostic Tests

### Endometrial Biopsy

Endometrial biopsy is performed to detect endometrial cancer or hyperplasia. With the woman in the lithotomy position, the cervix is cleaned with iodine solution and the biopsy specimen is taken from the endometrial lining, using a transcervical approach and either curettage or vacuum aspiration.

#### Client Preparation

- Explain that this procedure is uncomfortable but that postprocedure pain medication can offer relief.
- Explain that the procedure causes vaginal bleeding, and instruct the woman to use perineal pads rather than tampons.

- When the physician has informed the woman about the results of the biopsy, encourage her to ask questions and express her feelings and concerns.

#### Client and Family Teaching

- Instruct to avoid intercourse until advised by the physician.
- Provide information about treatment options or health maintenance activities related to regular examinations and health screening.

- Apply heat to the abdomen, and recommend that the woman use a heating pad at home. *Heat dilates blood vessels, increasing blood supply to the pelvis.*

### Disturbed Body Image

For many women, the side effects of cancer treatment can be almost as difficult and painful as the disease itself. Although side effects of the different therapies vary among individuals, the woman's body image and quality of life are always affected. Such side effects as alopecia (hair loss), nausea, vomiting, fatigue, diarrhea, stomatitis, and surgical scarring disturb body image.

- Review the side effects of the treatment regimen proposed, and assist the woman to develop a plan to deal with these effects. *This promotes a sense of control.*
- Remind the woman and family that side effects are usually manageable and may be temporary. *Over-the-counter agents can be used to alleviate stomatitis. Frequent rest periods can relieve fatigue. Medications can be prescribed for nausea, vomiting, and diarrhea.*

### Ineffective Sexuality Patterns

Altered sexuality may result from a feeling of unattractiveness, fatigue, or pain and discomfort. The woman's partner may fear that sexual activity will be harmful.

- Encourage expression of feelings about the effect of cancer on their lives and sexual relationship. *Verbalizing feelings helps relieves stress and maximizes relaxation.*
- Suggest that the couple explore alternative sexual positions and coordinate sexual activity with rest periods and periods that are relatively free from pain. *This creates a more favorable environment for satisfying sexual activity.*

## Home Care

Provide information about the specific treatment and prognosis for the cancer. Explain the expected side effects of radiation implant therapy (see Chapter 10). ⊂⊃ Pain control measures are also an essential part of the teaching plan (see Chapter 4). ⊂⊃ The resources listed for the woman with cervical cancer are also appropriate for the woman with endometrial cancer.

## THE WOMAN WITH OVARIAN CANCER

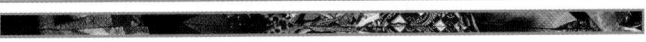

Ovarian cancer is the second most common gynecologic cancer. It is the most lethal, killing an estimated 14,000 women in the United States each year. Approximately 23,000 women in the United States were diagnosed with ovarian cancer in 2002 (ACS, 2002). The incidence increases with age, peaking in women between the ages of 40 and 80 years; half of all cases are in women over 65 years of age. Ovarian cancer is more common in whites than blacks, and mortality rate is highest in whites.

| Stage | Description |
|-------|-------------|
| I | Growth limited to the ovaries |
| II | Growth involving one or both ovaries with pelvic extension |
| III | Tumor involving one or both ovaries, with peritoneal implants outside the pelvis or positive retroperitoneal or inguinal nodes |
| IV | Growth involving one or both ovaries with distant metastasis |

TABLE 48-4 FIGO Staging Classification for Ovarian Cancer

## PATHOPHYSIOLOGY AND MANIFESTATIONS

There are several types of ovarian cancers: epithelial tumors, germ cell tumors, and gonadal stromal tumors. Most ovarian cancers are epithelial tumors, originating from the surface epithelium of the ovary. Ovarian cancer usually spreads by local shedding of cancer cells into the peritoneal cavity and by direct invasion of the bowel and bladder. Cancer cells in peritoneal fluid can implant in the intestines, bladder, and mesentary. Tumor cells also spread through the lymph and blood to such organs as the liver, and across the diaphragm to involve the lungs. Both pelvic and para-aortic lymph nodes may be involved and tumor cells can block lymphatic drainage from the abdomen, resulting in ascites. Staging for ovarian cancer is based on surgical and histologic evaluation (Table 48–4).

In early stages, ovarian cancer generally causes no warning signs or manifestations. When manifestations do develop, they are often vague and mild, such as indigestion, urinary frequency, abdominal bloating, and constipation. Abnormal vaginal bleeding may occur if the endometrium is stimulated by a hormone-secreting tumor or if the tumor erodes the vaginal wall. Pelvic pain sometimes occurs. An enlarged abdomen with ascites signals later-stage disease.

## Risk Factors

Family history is a significant risk factor, with a 50% risk of developing the disease if two or more first- or second-degree relatives have site-specific ovarian cancer. Other types of inherited risk are *breast-ovarian cancer syndrome* (first- and second-degree relatives have both breast and ovarian cancer) and *family cancer syndrome* (Lynch syndrome II), in which male or female relatives have a history of colorectal, endometrial, ovarian, pancreatic, or other types of cancer (Porth, 2002). The breast cancer susceptibility genes BRAC1 and BRAC2 are implicated in 5% to 10% of hereditary ovarian cancers.

Risk factors also include a high-fat diet and use of powders containing talc in the genital area. Other factors associated with increased risk are prior use of fertility drugs or HRT, and a diet low in fruits and vegetables (ACS, 2001a).

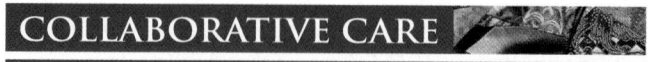

As with other malignancies, care of the woman with ovarian cancer is focused on surgery to determine the stage of the tumor and to remove as much of the tumor as possible. Unfortunately, because there are no early manifestations, the disease is often well advanced prior to diagnosis.

## Diagnostic Tests

Tests used in the diagnosis of ovarian cancer may include the following:

- *Blood test* in which patterns of proteins in blood serum can reflect the presence of disease. This preliminary test was able to accurately identify 100% of a small sample of patients with stage I ovarian cancer (National Cancer Institute, 2002).
- *Laparoscopy* is performed to determine definitive diagnosis and organ involvement.
- *Pap smears* are abnormal in up to 30% of women with ovarian cancer.
- *CA125 antigen level* can be useful in detecting ovarian cancer. CA125 is a tumor marker that is highly specific to epithelial ovarian cancer. Transvaginal or transabdominal ultrasonography is used to measure ovarian size and detect small masses. These tests, however, are not appropriate screening measures because they cannot differentiate between cystic or benign ovarian masses and malignancy.
- *CT scans* and *X-ray films* can reveal areas of metastasis.

## Medications

While surgery is the treatment of choice for ovarian cancer, chemotherapy may be used to achieve remission of the disease. Chemotherapy is not curative for ovarian cancer. Combination chemotherapy regimens using cyclophosphamide and cisplatin or other agents may be employed. Chemotherapy with paclitaxel (Taxol) may prolong survival. Close monitoring of bone marrow and renal function is vital while the woman is on chemotherapy because these drugs have significant toxic effects.

## Surgery

In young women with stage I disease who wish to bear children, treatment may be limited to removal of one ovary. Usually, however, total hysterectomy with bilateral salpingo-oophorectomy (removal of the ovaries and fallopian tubes) and removal of the omentum are performed.

## Radiation Therapy

Radiation therapy using external-beam or intracavitary implants is performed for palliative purposes only and is directed at shrinking the tumor at selected sites.

Nursing care for the woman with ovarian cancer is similar to the nursing care for women with other gynecologic cancers.

The side effects of treatment and generally poor prognosis diminish the woman's quality of life and involve major psychosocial implications (see Chapter 10). ⮌

## Home Care

Address the following topics in preparing the woman and her family for home care.

- If a positive family history of the disease or previous breast cancer exists, stress the importance of obtaining regular pelvic examinations. Inform women in this risk group that annual screening with transvaginal ultrasound and CA125 measurements may be recommended.
- Long-term use of oral contraceptives may reduce the risk of developing ovarian cancer.
- It is crucial not to ignore symptoms such as indigestion, nausea, or urinary frequency, as these seemingly unrelated manifestations may be early signs of ovarian tumors. Emphasize, however, that ovarian cancer usually is asymptomatic in early stages.
- Discuss treatment options and their side effects and provide information on ways to minimize or manage side effects.
- Refer to hospice services when appropriate. The resources suggested for the woman with cervical cancer are also appropriate for the woman with ovarian cancer.

# THE WOMAN WITH CANCER OF THE VULVA

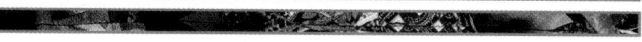

Cancer of the vulva occurs most often in women between the ages of 60 and 70. The prognosis of vulvar carcinoma depends on the degree of invasion, general health status of the woman, presence of chronic diseases, and ability to withstand treatment. The 5-year survival rate for early vulvar carcinoma without lymphatic involvement is 85% to 90% (McCance & Huether, 2002).

## PATHOPHYSIOLOGY AND MANIFESTATIONS

The cause of vulvar cancer is unknown, but there is evidence to associate it with sexually transmitted diseases, particularly human papilloma virus (HPV). Nearly 85% of malignant and premalignant cervical and vulvar lesions have been found to contain HPV DNA, HPV structural antigens, or both. Herpes simplex type 2 (HSV2) infection has also been associated with vulvar cancer. Other risk factors include advanced age, diabetes, and a history of leukoplakia.

Most vulvar cancers are epidermoid or squamous cell carcinomas. The primary site is usually the labia majora, but vulvar cancer is also found on the labia minora, clitoris, vestibule, and occasionally in multiple locations. Metastasis occurs by direct extension into the vagina, perineal skin, anus, and urethra. The cancer also spreads through the lymphatic system via the superficial and deep inguinal and femoral nodes, and to the pelvic lymph nodes.

The woman with vulvar cancer is often asymptomatic, and lesions are discovered on routine examination or self-examination. Discoloration can vary from white macular patches to red painless sores. Lesions may be *exophytic* (proliferating outwardly), *endophytic* (proliferating inwardly), ulcerative, or *verrucous* (resembling a wart).

Pruritus is the most common manifestation, and the woman often has had a history of prolonged vulvar irritation. Perineal pain and bleeding indicate large tumors and advanced disease. In very advanced disease, dysuria related to urethral involvement may be the presenting symptom.

## COLLABORATIVE CARE

The report of itching, burning, or a sore on the vulva merits careful investigation and biopsy of any lesions found. Inguinal lymph nodes may be enlarged. The goal of care is to eradicate the lesion and reduce the risk of recurrence. Surgical resection is the preferred treatment. If lymph nodes are involved, radiation therapy is used postoperatively. Chemotherapy is reserved for distant metastases.

Diagnosis is based on the results of an excisional biopsy of the lesion. Metastasis, if suspected, can be evaluated by chest X-ray examination, barium enema, intravenous pyelogram, cystoscopy, CT and MRI scans, and proctoscopy. Lymphangiography can also be used.

Surgery is the most common treatment for vulvar cancer. The specific procedure depends on the stage of the cancer. Early, noninvasive lesions may be treated with laser surgery, cryosurgery, or electrocautery. For more advanced disease, vulvectomy may be performed (Figure 48–6 ■). A simple vulvectomy involves the removal of the vulva, labia majora and minora, clitoris, and prepuce. A radical vulvectomy is performed if invasion is suspected. This procedure involves removal of all the tissue in a simple vulvectomy, as well as the subcutaneous tissue and regional lymph nodes.

## NURSING CARE

### Nursing Diagnoses and Interventions

Nursing care is similar to that for the woman with endometrial cancer. The woman fears death as the ultimate outcome as well as the possible pain and suffering that surgery and other treatments may cause. Many older women are still sexually active, and radical surgery represents a great loss to them. Disruption of perineal tissues is a priority nursing problem for these women.

### Impaired Tissue Integrity

The woman who has undergone a vulvectomy is at high risk for infection and impaired healing because of proximity of the surgical site to urinary and anal orifices. In addition, the women are often older and may have age-related changes in healing and immune function.

- Teach the woman and/or her partner or other family member the procedure for irrigation of the vulvectomy. If neither is able to perform this procedure, arrange for home health nursing. *Irrigation helps prevent skin breakdown and infection.*
- After irrigation, apply dry heat using a heat lamp positioned about 18 inches from the area; emphasize safety precautions, including use of a low-wattage bulb (40 to 60 watts). *Dry heat helps promote healing and comfort.*
- Provide information on maintaining a diet high in protein, iron, and vitamin C. *These nutrients promote collagen formation and wound healing.*

### Home Care

Explain the association between sexually transmitted diseases such as human papilloma virus (genital warts) and cancer of the vulva. Provide information about safer sex practices such as abstinence, limiting the number of sexual partners, and using condoms (male or female). Explain that early diagnosis and treatment of STIs and other irritative conditions of the external genitalia may reduce the risk of developing vulvar cancer. Teaching for the woman undergoing a vulvectomy should emphasize the potential for skin breakdown, particularly with radiation therapy. Explain that removal of lymph nodes leads to lymphedema and that recurrent cellulitis and sexual dysfunction are common complications of vulvar cancer.

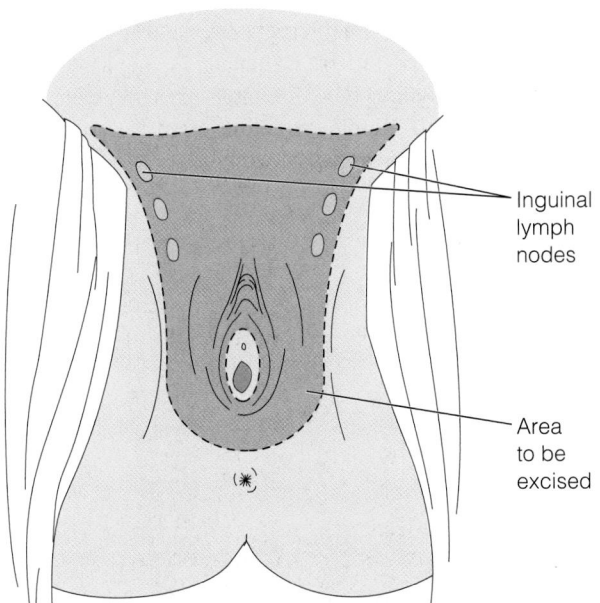

**Figure 48–6** ■ Vulvectomy for vulvar carcinoma. A radical vulvectomy involves removal of the vulva, labia majora, labia minora, clitoris, prepuce, subcutaneous tissue, and regional lymph nodes.

Inguinal lymph nodes

Area to be excised

# DISORDERS OF THE FEMALE BREAST

Breast disorders are common conditions that primarily affect women (disorders of the male breast are discussed in Chapter 24). 🔗 When a woman discovers a breast lump, her first response is often fear: of breast cancer, of losing her breast, and perhaps of losing her life. Because American society views the breast as a significant component of feminine beauty, any problem that threatens the breast often strikes at the core of a woman's self-image.

Nurses play a critical role in the care of women experiencing breast disorders by providing education, support, and advocacy. Part of the nurse's role is educating women about normal breast tissue, common benign breast disorders, available screening techniques and risk factors for breast cancers, and breast self-examination.

## THE WOMAN WITH A BENIGN BREAST DISORDER

Benign breast disorders occur frequently in women and may be a source of anxiety. Changes in a woman's breast tissue often correspond to hormonal changes of the menstrual cycle. Most women notice increased tenderness and lumpiness prior to menses. (For this reason, it is best to perform BSE after the menstrual period.) Breast tissue changes in response to hormonal, nutritional, physical, and environmental stimuli. More than half of all women who menstruate regularly will find a lump in the breast; 80% of these lumps are benign. Benign breast disorders include fibrocystic breast changes, fibroadenomas, intraductal papillomas, duct ectasia, fat necrosis, and mastitis (Table 48–5).

## PATHOPHYSIOLOGY AND MANIFESTATIONS
### Fibrocystic Changes

**Fibrocystic changes (FCC)** (*fibrocystic breast disease*) is the physiologic nodularity and breast tenderness which increases and decreases with the menstrual cycle. An estimated 50% to 80% of all women experience some of these changes, which include fibrosis, epithelial proliferation, and cyst formation. FCC is most common in women 30 to 50 years of age, and is rare in postmenopausal women who are not taking hormone replacement (Porth, 2002).

FCC includes many different lesions and breast changes. The more common nonproliferative form does not increase the risk for breast cancer. The proliferative form, accompanied by giant cysts and proliferative epithelial lesions, does increase the risk for breast cancer.

Nonproliferative changes may be cystic or fibrous. Cystic change refers to the dilation of ducts in the subareolar, lobular, or lobe areas. Cysts often go unnoticed unless there is pain and tenderness associated with menses. Fibrous changes are infrequent but can occur during the menstrual years. A firm, palpable mass, 2 to 3 cm in size, is typically located in the upper outer breast quadrant following an inflammatory response to ductal irritation.

Women with fibrocystic changes experience bilateral or unilateral pain or tenderness in the upper, outer quadrants of their breasts, and report that their breasts feel particularly thick and lumpy the week prior to menses. Nipple discharge may be present. Pain is due to edema of the connective tissue of the breast, dilation of the ducts, and some inflammatory response; some women report an increase in breast size. Multiple, mobile cysts may form, usually in both breasts (Figure 48–7 ■). Fluid aspirated from these cysts ranges in color from milky white to yellow, brown, or green. If the fluid is tinged with blood, there is reason to suspect malignancy.

### Intraductal Disorders

An **intraductal papilloma** is a tiny, wartlike growth on the inside of the peripheral mammary duct that causes discharge from the nipple. The discharge may be clear and sticky or bloody. When more than one of these growths is present, the condition is called *intraductal papillomatosis*. This condition is most common in women in their 30s and 40s. The lesion must be investigated to rule out malignancy.

**Mammary duct ectasia** (*plasma cell mastitis*) is a palpable lumpiness found beneath the areola. Duct ectasia involves periductal inflammation, dilation of the ductal system, and accumulation of fluid and dead cells that block the involved ducts. The condition usually occurs in perimenopausal women and is difficult to differentiate from cancer.

Manifestations of mammary duct ectasia include sticky, thick nipple discharge with burning and itching around the nipple, and inflammation. The discharge may be green, greenish brown, or bloody. Nipple retraction often is associated with duct ectasia in postmenopausal women.

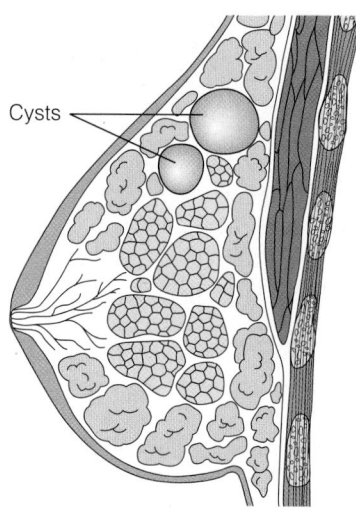

Cysts

**Figure 48–7** ■ Fibrocystic breast changes.

### TABLE 48-5   Summary of Common Breast Disorders

| Condition | Age | Pain | Nipple Discharge | Location | Consistency and Mobility | Diagnosis and Treatment |
|---|---|---|---|---|---|---|
| Duct ectasia | 35 to 55 years; median age 40 | Burning around nipple | Sticky, multicolored; usually bilateral | No specific location | Retroareolar mass with advanced disease | Open biopsy; local excision of diseased portion of breast |
| Fibroadenoma | 15 to 39 years; median age 20 | No | No | No specific location | Mobile, firm, smooth, well delineated mass | Mammography, surgical or needle biopsy; excision of the tumor |
| Fibrocystic breast disease | 20 to 49 years; median age 30 (may subside with menopause) | Yes | No | Upper outer quadrant | Bilateral multiple lumps influenced by the menstrual cycle | Needle aspiration; observation; biopsy if there is an unresolved mass or mammographic changes |
| Intraductal papilloma | 35 to 55 years; median age 40 | Yes | Serous or sanguineous; usually unilateral from one duct | No specific location | Usually soft, poorly delineated mass | Pap smear of nipple discharge; biopsy; wedge resection |
| Mastitis, acute | Childbearing years | Tenderness, pain | No | No specific location | Generalized redness of overlying skin | Antibiotic therapy; incision and drainage if mastitis progresses to an abscess |
| Mastitis, chronic | Any age | Tenderness, pain; headache; high fever | No | No specific location | Generalized redness and swelling | Antibiotics, usually penicillin |
| Fat necrosis | Any age | Tenderness | No | No specific location | Firm, irregular, palpable | Surgical biopsy to rule out cancer |

## COLLABORATIVE CARE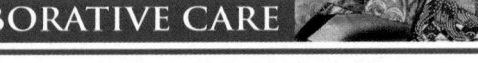

Diagnosis of fibrocystic breast changes is based on complete history, physical examination, and imaging studies. A biopsy may be required for diagnosis.

Analysis of nipple discharge, mammography, and possibly ductography may be used to diagnose ductal disorders. The affected duct is excised in an open biopsy procedure. Nursing care for the woman is similar to that for any client with an open biopsy. It also is important to reassure the woman that these disorders are not breast cancer.

The treatment is usually symptomatic. Cyst aspiration may relieve pain, and also allows examination of fluid to confirm the cystic nature of the disease. A well-fitting brassiere that provides good support worn day and night helps relieve discomfort. Some women report that eliminating xanthines (found in coffee, tea, cola and chocolate) from the diet decreases symptoms. Aspirin, mild analgesics, local heat or cold, and vitamin E may help relieve breast pain. Hormone therapy is controversial because of the benign nature of the disease and potential adverse effects of therapy. Danazol, a synthetic androgen, may be prescribed for women with severe pain.

## NURSING CARE

When a woman presents with a breast mass, nursing responsibilities include taking a careful history and facilitating follow-up care. If a palpable mass is present, it is important to ask how long the lesion has been present and whether the woman has noticed any pain associated with the mass, any change in its size, and any changes in association with the menstrual cycle.

In many cases, definitive diagnosis of the breast disorder requires surgical biopsy to rule out cancer. During the diagnostic process, the nurse can provide emotional support and education about diagnostic and therapeutic procedures, self-care and comfort measures, and resources to help the woman cope with the experience.

## THE WOMAN WITH BREAST CANCER

**Breast cancer** is the unregulated growth of abnormal cells in breast tissue. Breast cancer is the most commonly occurring cancer in women and the second leading cause of death in women in the United States. The American Cancer Society (2002a) estimates that more than 200,000 women will be diagnosed with breast cancer each year, and approximately 40,000 women will die from it annually. There are racial differences in the incidence and mortality of breast cancer (see the Focus on Diversity box below).

Possible causes of breast cancer include environmental, hormonal, reproductive, and hereditary factors. Two breast cancer susceptibility genes have been identified: BRCA1 on chromosome 17 and BRCA2 on chromosome 13. These genes may be responsible for the approximately 8% of women with hereditary breast cancer. A woman with identified mutations in BRCA1 (known to be involved in tumor suppression) has a lifetime risk of 56% to 85% for breast cancer and also has an increased risk for ovarian cancer (Porth, 2002). Mutations of a tumor suppressor gene, are also linked to increased risk for breast cancer

### PATHOPHYSIOLOGY

Cancer of the breast begins as a single transformed cell and is hormone dependent. Cancers of the breast are classified as noninvasive (in situ) or invasive, depending on the penetration of the tumor into surrounding tissue. Breast cancer may remain a noninvasive disease, or an invasive disease without metastasis, for long periods of time. Two atypical types of breast cancer are inflammatory carcinoma and Paget's disease.

Breast cancer may be categorized as carcinoma of the mammary ducts, carcinoma of mammary lobules, or sarcoma of the breast. Most breast cancers are adenocarcinomas and

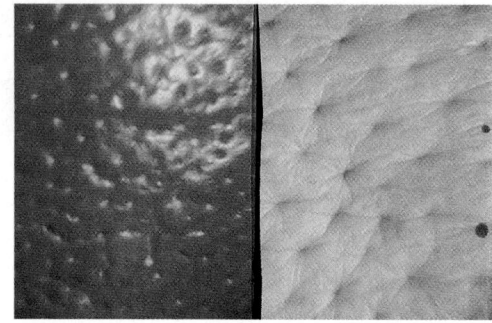

**Figure 48–8** ■ *Left,* Orange peel; *Right,* Peau d'orange sign.

*Source: CNRI/Phototake, Inc.*

appear to arise in the terminal section of the breast ductal tissue. There are many histologic types of breast cancer, and only examples are described here. The most common type is *infiltrating ductal carcinoma,* accounting for approximately 70% of cases (McCance & Huether, 2002). Inflammatory carcinoma of the breast, a systemic disease, is the most malignant form of breast cancer. Edema of the skin (*peau d'orange*) is usually present (Figure 48–8 ■). *Paget's disease* is a rare type of breast cancer involving infiltration of the nipple epithelium (Figure 48–9 ■).

Breast cancer can metastasize to other sites through the bloodstream or lymphatic system. The common sites of metastasis of breast cancer are bone, brain, lung, liver, skin, and lymph nodes. Staging is a system of classifying cancer according to the size of the tumor, involvement of lymph nodes, and metastasis to distant sites, and the presence/absence of distant metastasis (Table 48–6). The staging of the breast cancer provides important information for making decisions about treatment options and is also used as a basis for prognosis.

### MANIFESTATIONS

The manifestations of breast cancer may include a nontender lump in the breast (most often in the upper outer quadrant, the area with the most glandular tissue), abnormal nipple discharge, a rash around the nipple area, nipple retraction, dim-

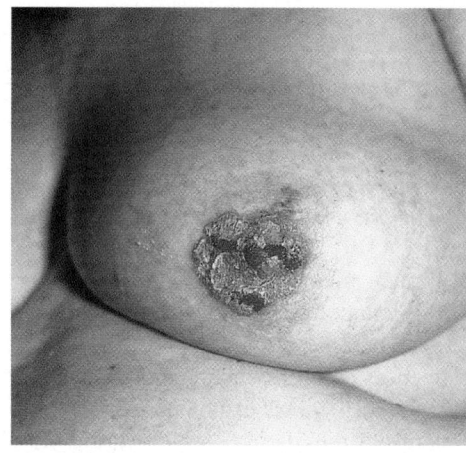

**Figure 48–9** ■ Paget's disease of the nipple.

*Source: Carroll H. Weiss/Camera M.D. Studios.*

## Focus on Diversity

### INCIDENCE AND MORTALITY FOR BREAST CANCER IN WOMEN

- Breast cancer is more prevalent in African American women up to the age of 40 years.
- Breast cancer is more prevalent in Caucasian women over the age of 40 years.
- Asian, Hispanic, and American Indian women have a lower risk of developing breast cancer.
- African American women are more likely to die from the cancer because they are often diagnosed at an advanced stage.

| Stage | Tumor | Node | Metastasis |
|---|---|---|---|
| 0 | Tis–Carcinoma in situ or Paget's disease of the nipple | N0–No regional lymph node metastasis | M0–No evidence of distant metastasis |
| I | T1–Tumor no larger than 2 cm | N0 | M0 |
| IIA | T0–No evidence of primary tumor | N1–Metastasis to movable ipsilateral axillary nodes | M0 |
|  | T1 |  |  |
|  | T2–Tumor no larger than 5 cm | N0 | M0 |
| IIB | T2 | N1 | M0 |
|  | T3–Tumor larger than 5 cm | N0 | M0 |
| IIIA | T0 | N2–Metastasis to ipsilateral fixed axillary nodes | M0 |
|  | T1 |  |  |
|  | T2 |  |  |
|  | T3 | N1 | M0 |
|  |  | N2 | M0 |
| IIIB | T4–Tumor of any size with direct extension to chest wall or skin | Any N | M0 |
|  | Any T | N3–Metastasis to ipsilateral internal mammary lymph nodes | M0 |
| IV | Any T | N0 and N1 | M1–Distant metastasis |

TABLE 48–6  Staging of Breast Cancer

## Manifestations of Breast Cancer

- Breast mass or thickening
- Unusual lump in the underarm or above the collarbone
- Persistent skin rash near the nipple area
- Flaking or eruption near the nipple
- Dimpling, pulling, or retraction in an area of the breast
- Nipple discharge
- Change in nipple position
- Burning, stinging, or pricking sensation

pling of the skin, or a change in the position of the nipple (see the box above). Breast cancer is usually painless, but some women report a burning or stinging sensation. Many women with breast cancer have no symptoms, and their tumors are detected by mammography. However, most breast cancers are found by the women themselves (during breast self-examination or a shower) or by their partners during sexual activity.

## Risk Factors

Of the various kinds of risk factors for breast cancer, some can be changed and some cannot. Those that cannot be changed are:

- Being an aging woman (see the box below). Women are 100 times more likely to have breast cancer than are men, with the risk increasing with age. About 77% of women with breast cancer are over the age of 50 when diagnosed (ACS, 2001).
- Genetic risk factors (as previously described).

## Nursing Care of the Older Adult

### OLDER WOMEN WITH BREAST CANCER

- Although the incidence of breast cancer is increasing among premenopausal women, it is still primarily a disease of older women. However, the needs of older women with breast cancer have been inadequately addressed in the professional literature and in the popular media.
- Women between the ages of 50 and 65 are the group most likely to benefit from annual screening mammography, yet many women in this age group have never had a mammogram. Failure of physicians to refer older women for mammography is the reason most frequently cited for this statistic; nurse practitioners and female physicians are more likely to refer women for mammography. Promotional campaigns for mammography send a confusing message by showing images of women in their 20s and 30s for whom mammography is largely ineffective, rather than women in older age groups who are more likely to benefit from mammography.

- For too long, mastectomy was perceived as the only treatment option open to most older women with breast cancer, even those with early-stage disease. Slowly that perception is changing as breast-conservation treatment gains greater acceptance. The choice of surgical treatment, particularly for older women, is highly individual. Many older women wish to preserve their breasts.
- Although older women with breast cancer may experience coexisting chronic illnesses and impaired physical function, research suggests that they show lower levels of emotional distress than younger women. Obviously the need for services such as personal care, shopping, housekeeping, and transportation increases as the ages of the woman and the caregiver increase.

- Family history of breast cancer. Relatives from either the maternal or paternal side of the family. Having a first-degree relative (mother, sister, or daughter) with breast cancer approximately doubles the risk, and having two first-degree relatives increases it fivefold. Having a male family member with breast cancer also poses an increased risk.
- Personal history of breast cancer. A woman with cancer in one breast has a three to fivefold increase in risk for developing a new cancer in the other breast or in a different part of the same breast.
- Previous breast biopsy. If earlier breast biopsies were diagnosed as proliferative, then breast disease without atypical hyperplasia increases risk by 1.5 to 2 times. A previous biopsy of atypical hyperplasia increases risk by 4 to 5 times.
- Previous breast irradiation. Radiation of the chest as a child or young woman for other cancer (such as Hodgkin's disease) significantly increases the risk.
- Menstrual history. Women who begin menstruating before the age of 12 or who have menopause after the age of 50 are at a slightly higher risk.

Lifestyle related factors and breast cancer risk include using oral contraceptives, not having children or having them after the age of 30, using HRT for more than 5 years, not breast feeding, drinking alcohol (especially two to five drinks daily), obesity, high-fat diets, physical inactivity, and (possibly) environmental pollution. Risk factors that have been postulated, but have not been proven, include using antiperspirants, wearing underwire bras, smoking, induced abortion, and breast implants.

## COLLABORATIVE CARE

Diagnosis of breast cancer begins with detection, either detection of asymptomatic lesions discovered through screening or symptomatic lesions discovered by the woman. Any palpable mass requires evaluation. Once the diagnosis is made, a number of treatment options are available. The choice of treatment depends on several factors, such as the stage of the cancer, the age of the woman, and the woman's preferences.

### Diagnostic Tests

The following diagnostic tests may be ordered to diagnoses breast cancer.

- *Clinical breast examination (CBE)* is the inspection and palpation of the breasts and axillae performed by a trained health professional. The physical examination includes inspection, palpation, and a check for nipple discharge (see Chapter 46).
- *Mammogram* is a low-dose X-ray study of the breast used to detect breast lesions. Although mammography can detect breast tumors 2 years before they reach palpable size, most of these tumors have been present for 8 to 10 years. Although controversy exists about the ability of screening mammography to improve mortality rates for women under 50, the American Cancer Society (2002) recommends annual screening beginning at age 40.

- *Percutaneous needle biopsy* defines cystic masses or fibrocystic changes and provides specimens for cytologic examination. In aspiration biopsy or fine-needle aspiration biopsy, a fine needle is used to remove cells or fluid from the breast lesion (Figure 48–10A ■). In many facilities, fine-needle aspiration biopsies are performed using a stereotactic biopsy device; mammography and a computer are used to guide the needle.
- *Stereotactic needle biopsy* obtains cells for histologic evaluation.
- *Excisional biopsy* removes the entire lump (Figure 48–10B). See the box on page 1585 for nursing implications for a breast biopsy.
- *Ductal lavage and nipple aspiration* withdraw fluid to analyze for abnormal cells.

### Medications

Adjuvant (additional) systemic therapy following primary treatment for early-stage breast cancer refers to the administration of chemotherapy or hormonal therapy. This type of therapy has been widely studied; its use reduces the rates of recurrence and death from breast cancer.

Tamoxifen citrate (Nolvadex) is an oral medication that interferes with estrogen activity. It is used to treat advanced breast

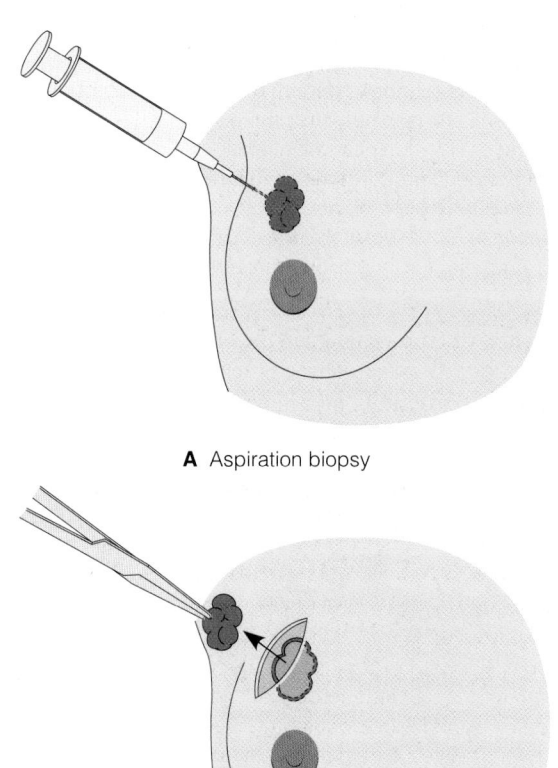

**A** Aspiration biopsy

**B** Excisional biopsy

**Figure 48–10** ■ Types of breast biopsy. *A,* In an aspiration biopsy, a needle is used to aspirate fluid or tissue from the breast. *B,* In an excisional biopsy, tissue from the breast lesion is removed surgically.

## Nursing Implications for Diagnostic Tests

### Breast Biopsy

#### PREPARATION OF THE WOMAN

##### All Biopsies
- Ensure that the consent form is signed.
- Acknowledge that preoperative anxiety is normal. It is important to remember that 80% of all breast lesions are benign.

#### WOMAN AND FAMILY TEACHING

##### Aspiration Biopsy (Fine-Needle Aspiration Biopsy)
- A needle will be used to remove tissue and/or fluid from the breast lesion. This procedure may be done in the surgeon's office and takes only a few minutes.
- Aspirated tissue is sent for histologic examination to determine whether it is cancerous. Results are sent to the surgeon within a few days.
- Mild analgesics are usually sufficient to relieve postbiopsy pain.

##### Stereotactic Core Biopsy (Tru-Cut Biopsy)
- The woman lies face down on a special stereotactic biopsy table with a hole through which her breast protrudes. The breast is anesthetized, the lesion located by mammography, and a computer-guided hollow-core needle enters the breast at high speed and withdraws a core of tissue.
- The tissue is sent for histologic examination to determine whether it is cancerous. Results are available within 36 hours.
- Mild analgesics are usually sufficient to relieve postbiopsy pain.

##### Incisional or Excisional Biopsy
- The needle-wire localization procedure provides a guide for the surgeon to follow. This procedure involves a mammogram followed by insertion of a hollow needle and one or more wires into the lesion. Dye may be injected through the hollow needle; the dye may cause a stinging sensation. The woman is then taken to the operating room with the wires in place for the biopsy.
- The biopsy is generally performed in an ambulatory surgery center using local anesthesia. If the woman has large breasts or is at high risk for complications, the surgeon may prefer to use the standard operating room.
- In an incisional biopsy, a section of tissue is removed from the breast lesion and sent for histologic examination.
- In an excisional biopsy, the entire lesion is removed along with a surrounding margin of normal-looking tissue. The specimen is then sent for mammographic and histologic analysis, to be sure that the entire lesion has been removed and to determine whether it is cancerous.
- A screen shields the operative area from view. A nurse stands within view of the woman to explain what's happening, answer questions, and offer emotional support.
- If there is any painful sensation, the woman needs to ask for additional anesthesia.
- The surgeon closes the internal incision with absorbable sutures and secures the skin with sutures or tape. A gauze dressing is applied to protect the area.
- Postoperative pain, bruising, or scarring varies according to the surgeon's technique and the woman's tissue. It is helpful to wear a bra and to apply ice packs periodically. Mild analgesics are generally sufficient to control pain.
- Results of the biopsy are usually available within a few days.

## Medication Administration

### Tamoxifen

**Tamoxifen (Nolvadex)**

Tamoxifen is the most widely prescribed breast cancer drug, commonly given to prevent recurrence of estrogen-positive breast cancer in postmenopausal women. It inhibits tumor growth by blocking the estrogen receptor sites of cancer cells. Tamoxifen increases a woman's risk of developing endomerial cancer, deep vein thrombosis (DVT), and pulmonary embolism.

#### Nursing Responsibilities
- Assess for potential contraindications to therapy.
- Assess liver function tests; tamoxifen may interfere with liver function.

#### Client and Family Teaching
- If in childbearing years, use a nonhormonal, barrier form of contraception; tamoxifen has adverse effects on the developing fetus.
- Take the drug as prescribed until the physician indicates otherwise.
- Side effects such as hot flashes, vaginal dryness, irregular periods, and weight gain are commonly experienced by women taking tamoxifen.
- Do not smoke while taking tamoxifen; smoking further increases the risk of DVT.
- Promptly report any abnormal vaginal bleeding (nonmenstrual bleeding, bleeding after menopause) to your primary care provider.

cancer, as an adjuvant for early-stage breast cancer, and as a preventive treatment for women at high risk of developing breast cancer. Nursing implications for tamoxifen are presented in the Medication Administration box above.

Chemotherapy has become the standard of care for the majority of breast cancer cases with axillary node involvement. In late metastatic disease, chemotherapy becomes the primary treatment to prolong the woman's life. Chemotherapy is discussed in Chapter 10. ⊘⊘

Immunotherapy, using trastuzumab (Herceptin), is used to stop the growth of breast tumors that express the HER2/neu receptor (which binds an epidermal growth factor that contributes to cancer cell growth) on their cell surface. This drug is a recombinant DNA-derived monoclonal antibody that binds to the receptor, inhibiting tumor cell proliferation.

## Treatments

The choice of systemic treatment depends on the woman's age, stage of cancer, and other individual factors. Breast cancer tends to be more aggressive in premenopausal women, probably because of hormonal factors. Thus, treatment regimens for premenopausal women are also more aggressive.

### Surgery

Until recently, the treatment of choice for breast cancer was a radical mastectomy. The trend now is toward more conservative surgery combined with chemotherapy, hormone therapy, or radiation, depending on the stage of the tumor and the age of the woman.

**MASTECTOMY.** There are various types of mastectomy for breast cancer. *Radical mastectomy* is the removal of the entire affected breast, the underlying chest muscles, and the lymph nodes under the arms. *Simple mastectomy* is the removal of the complete breast only. *Segmental mastectomy* or *lumpectomy* (Figure 48–11A ■) is the removal of the tumor and the surrounding margin of breast tissues. *Modified radical mastectomy* is the removal of the breast tissue and lymph nodes under the arm (axillary node dissection), leaving the chest wall muscles intact (Figure 48–11B). See the box on page 1587 for the nursing care of a woman having a mastectomy.

Axillary node dissection is generally performed with all invasive breast carcinoma to stage the tumor. Because this surgery can cause **lymphedema** (accumulation of fluid in the soft tissues of the arm caused by removal of lymph channels), nerve damage, and adhesions, and because of the role of the lymph nodes in immune system function, nonsurgical methods of detecting lymph node involvement are being used. *Sentinel node biopsy* is conducted by injecting a radioactive substance or dye into the region of the tumor. The dye is carried to the first (sentinel) lymph node to receive lymph from the tumor and would therefore be the node most likely to contain cancer cells if the cancer had metastasized. If the sentinel node is positive, more nodes are removed. If it is negative, further node evaluation is usually not indicated.

Breast conservation surgery (*lumpectomy*) may be defined as excision of the primary tumor and adjacent breast tissue followed by radiation therapy. Many women are candidates for this procedure; however, women who have multicentric breast neoplasms and those who have large tumors in relation to their breast size are examples of unsuitable candidates. Selection of women for this procedure is guided by the need for local control of the lesion, cosmetic results, and personal preference.

**BREAST RECONSTRUCTION.** After a mastectomy, some women may choose to have their breast reconstructed. They report that surgical reconstruction of the breast simplifies their lives and restores a sense of body integrity. Other women choose to use a removable breast prosthesis, and some women are comfortable without reconstruction or a prosthesis.

Breast reconstruction may be performed at the time of the mastectomy or at any time thereafter, depending on the woman's preference. A number of procedures may be used for the breast reconstruction (Figure 48–12 ■). These include placement of a submuscular implant, the use of a tissue expander followed by an implant, the transposition of muscle and blood supply from the abdomen or back, or using (most often) the transverse rectus abdominis myocutaneous (TRAM) free tissue flap. Nursing implications for the care of women undergoing breast reconstruction surgery are summarized in the box on page 1588.

### Radiation Therapy

Radiation therapy is typically used following breast cancer surgery to destroy any remaining cancer cells that could cause

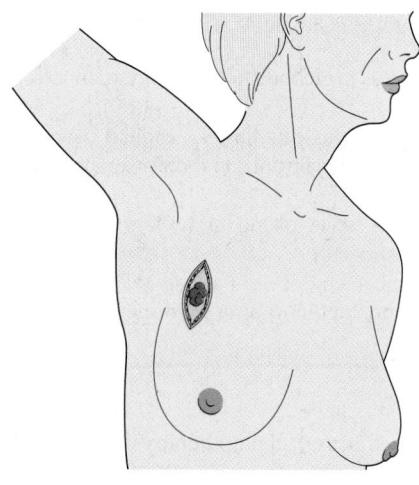
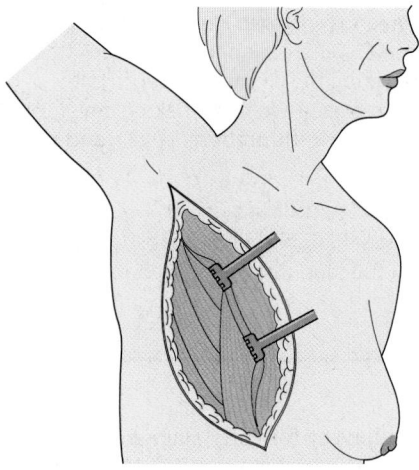

**A** Lumpectomy          **B** Modified radical mastectomy

**Figure 48–11 ■** Types of mastectomy. *A,* In a lumpectomy, only the tumor and a small margin of surrounding tissue are removed. *B,* In a modified radical mastectomy, all breast tissue and the underarm lymph nodes are removed, but the underlying muscles remain.

## NURSING CARE OF THE WOMAN HAVING A MASTECTOMY

### NURSING RESPONSIBILITIES

- Ensure that the woman or family member signs informed consent form.
- See Chapter 7 ⊂⊃ for preoperative preparation.

### Client and Family Teaching

- Deep-breathing exercises are important because after general anesthesia, it is difficult for air to reach the lungs, particularly with the restrictive surgical dressing that decreases chest expansion.
- A suction apparatus will be placed in the wound to allow drainage of excess body fluids that accumulate when the lymph nodes are removed. This device is usually removed 3 to 5 days after surgery.
- An IV line may be in place for fluid replacement and antibiotics to reduce the risk of postoperative infection.
- Control pain by using the patient-controlled analgesia device or requesting analgesics before pain becomes severe. Take analgesics as needed before performing recommended exercises to facilitate full movement.
- Note any signs of bleeding on the dressing or on the bedding.
- Numbness or feelings of "pins and needles" in the axillary area are common.

- Lying on one's back or on the side not operated on helps fluid drain from the site.
- Moving the arm on the operated side helps regain mobility; specific exercises will be prescribed for increasing mobility after the incisions have healed.
- If fluid builds up after the drains have been removed, it can be aspirated by the surgeon.
- Use caution about lifting heavy objects with the arm on the operated side.
- Be careful about injury and infection on the affected side; wear rubber gloves when washing dishes, garden gloves when working outside. Request that caregivers not perform blood pressures or venipunctures on the operative side to reduce the risk of injury and infection.
- Feelings of anxiety, sadness, and fear of looking at the incision are normal; mastectomy means abrupt change in body image. It is normal to mourn the loss of a breast and to fear the loss of one's life after a cancer diagnosis.
- Sexual intimacy can be affected by mastectomy; it often helps to be able to discuss potential sexual problems with one's partner, with a counselor, or with a breast cancer support group.

---

recurrence or metastasis. If a tumor is unusually large, radiation may be used to shrink the tumor prior to surgery. Radiation therapy is most commonly used in combination with lumpectomy for early stage (I or II) breast cancer. Palliative radiation therapy is also used to treat chest wall recurrences and some bone metastases to help control pain and prevent fractures. Radiation therapy is administered by means of an external-beam or tissue implants (see Chapter 10). ⊂⊃

A new experimental radiation treatment (*intraoperative radiotherapy*) is provided by a single, concentrated dose of radiation. During surgery, a probe is inserted into the cavity created by the lumpectomy and radiation equivalent to 6 weeks of doses is emitted for about 25 minutes. If this proves successful, the treatment could make lumpectomy available to more women and prevent the woman from having 6 weeks of daily radiation treatments following surgery.

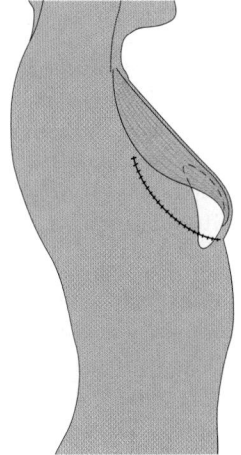 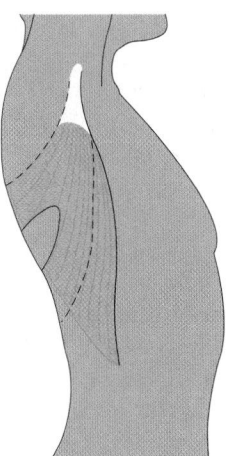 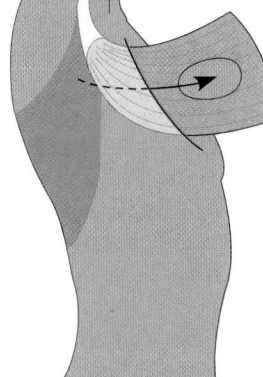

**A** Implant          **B** Latissimus dorsi musculocutaneous flap

**Figure 48–12** ■ Types of breast reconstruction surgeries. *A,* A breast implant is inserted under the pectoris muscle. *B,* Autogenous procedures transfer a flap of skin, muscle, and fat from the donor site on the woman's body to the mastectomy site. The most frequently used donor muscle sites are the latissimus dorsi and the rectus abdominis (the TRAM-flap or transrectus abdominis muscle flap).

## NURSING CARE OF THE WOMAN HAVING BREAST RECONSTRUCTION

### CLIENT AND FAMILY TEACHING

- Controversy exists about the health effects of silicone. While there is no conclusive evidence that silicone implants induce cancer or autoimmune disease, they are associated with hardening and pain due to contracture of the capsule around the implant. The implant may rupture, releasing silicone gel, or infection may occur. Saline-filled breast implants may be an alternative.
- Reconstruction can be done immediately after a mastectomy, or at any time later on. Some surgeons believe that delayed reconstruction offers better cosmetic results.
- Reconstructive surgery can create a natural looking breast that makes clothes fit better. Since it has no nerve endings, however, the reconstructed breast has no feeling or sensations.
- If a simple mastectomy is done, an implant approximately the same size as the other breast is placed under the pectoral muscle on the operative side. This creates a breast mound that closely resembles the natural breast in shape and softness. If the implant is placed over the pectoral muscle, a high degree of firmness may occur.

- With a simple mastectomy or modified radical mastectomy, a tissue expander may be used to replace the breast. The tissue expander is placed under the pectoral muscle and gradually expanded with saline injections every 2 to 3 weeks to stretch the overlying skin and create a pocket. After a period of time, usually 1 to 2 months, the tissue expander is exchanged for a saline implant.
- With more extensive surgery such as radical mastectomy, a flap of skin, fat, or muscle is transferred from a donor site to the operative area. A new nipple may be created by using tissue from the opposite nipple or from the inner thigh.
- Reconstructive surgery may require multiple surgeries, including all the risks associated with anesthesia. As the complexity of the procedures increases, so does the risk of complications such as infection.
- To decrease the risk of a fibrous capsule forming around the implant, it is important to perform breast massage as instructed.

## NURSING CARE

Breast cancer is not one disease entity, but many, depending on the affected breast tissue, the tissue's estrogen dependency, and the age of the person at onset. The psychosocial impact of breast cancer extends beyond the fear and threat of death. The diagnosis may transform the woman's sense of self and lead to reintegration or negotiation of family relationships.

### Health Promotion

The American Cancer Society (2002a) recommends that all women conduct a monthly breast self-examination (BSE) beginning at age 20, have a clinical breast examination every 3 years from ages 20 to 39 years, and have a clinical breast examination and mammogram each year starting at age 40 years.

All women should be taught to perform BSE monthly (Figure 48–13 ■). Premenopausal women should perform BSE after their menstrual period, because hormonal changes increase breast tenderness and lumpiness prior to menses.

Educational messages about breast cancer screening need to be culturally sensitive to the intended audience. Media campaigns promoting mammography often show young white women, an approach that has proved ineffective among women of color (see the Nursing Research box on page 1590). By working with women of different races and cultures, nurses can help make breast cancer education more meaningful to women in these groups.

### Assessment

Collect the following data through the health history and physical examination (see Chapter 46). Further focused assessments are described with nursing interventions following.

- Health history: family history of breast cancer, breast changes, nipple discharge, use of HRT, personal history of breast cancer, previous diagnostic tests and treatment for cancer, menstrual history, pregnancies, alcohol intake, physical activity, dietary history
- Physical assessment: height and weight, breast, lymph glands

## Nursing Diagnoses and Interventions

Although each woman has individual needs, nursing diagnoses prior to surgery are concerned with anxiety, decisional conflict, knowledge deficit, and grief over the loss of a breast. Because the typical hospital stay is short, usually 2 to 3 days, preoperative teaching is done on an outpatient basis.

### Anxiety

The woman with breast cancer is often anxious about the diagnoses, the surgery, the outcome of surgery if nodal involvement is found, and the possible changes in sexual and family relationships. Studies show that young women with breast cancer, a growing population, are particularly vulnerable for anxiety and other psychosocial effects, as are their spouses and their children.

- Provide opportunities to express thoughts and feelings. In this process, the woman can name her fears. *Once the fears are named, the nurse may simply listen, educate, or dispel fears that stem from lack of understanding.*
- Discuss with the woman her knowledge of breast cancer. *Assessing the woman's knowledge of breast cancer helps the nurse plan more effective teaching.*
- Encourage discussion relating to immediate concerns about resuming her life at home and the changes she must make. *Anticipatory guidance can help plan for and cope with changes in her life and relationships.*

**Figure 48–13** ■ Teaching Breast Self-Examination (BSE)

**Step 1** Teach the woman to observe her breasts in front of a mirror and in good lighting. Tell her to observe her breasts in four positions:

- With her arms relaxed and at her sides
- With her arms lifted over her head
- With her hands pressed against her hips
- With her hands pressed together at her waist, leaning forward

Instruct her to look at each breast individually, and then to compare them. She should observe for any visible abnormalities, such as lumps, dimpling, deviation, recent nipple retraction, irregular shape, edema, discharge, or asymmetry.

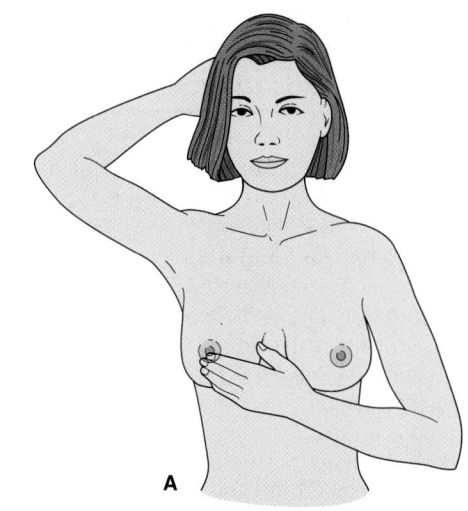

A

**Step 2** Teach the woman to palpate both breasts while standing or sitting, with one hand behind her head (Figure *A*). Tell her that many women palpate their breasts in the shower because water and soap make the skin slippery and easier to palpate. Show the woman how to use the pads of her fingers to palpate all areas of her breast, using the concentric circles technique (Figure B). Tell her to press the breast tissue gently against the chest wall, and to be sure to palpate the axillary tail.

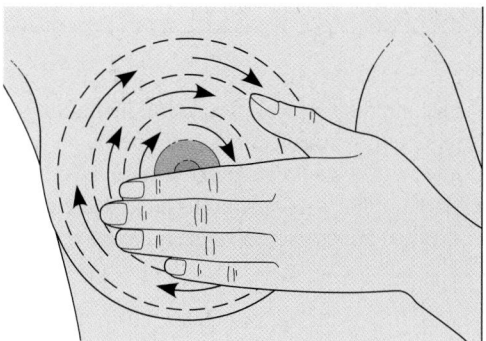

B

**Step 3** Instruct the client to palpate her breasts again while lying down, as described in step 2. Suggest that she place a folded towel under the shoulder and back on the side to be palpated. The arm on the examining side should be over the head, with the hand under the head (Figure C).

**Step 4** Teach the woman to palpate the areola and nipples next. Show her how to compress the nipple to check for discharge (Figure D).

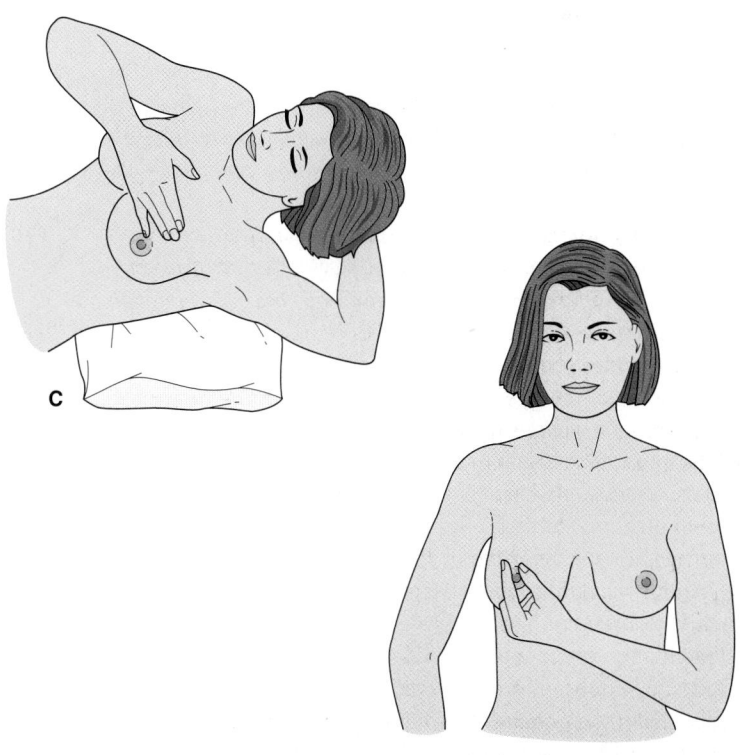

C

**Step 5** Remind the woman to use a calendar to keep a record of when she performs BSE. Teach her to perform BSE at the same time each month, usually 5 days after the onset of menses, when there is less hormonal influence on tissues.

D

1589

## Nursing Research

### Evidence-Based Practice for Cancer Screening for African American Women

African American women have a higher mortality from breast cancer than do European American women, despite a lower incidence. This difference may be due to the later stage of diagnosis for African American women when compared with European American women. This study (Champion & Scott, 1997) describes the development of culturally sensitive scales to measure beliefs related to mammography and breast self-examination screening. The researchers found that barriers to mammography such as understanding the procedure, scheduling, child care, and transportation are more relevant to low-income African American than to the predominantly European American, middle-class population with whom previous screening scales were developed. It is important to note that many of the identified barriers related to socioeconomic status rather than race; tools used for screening purposes may translate better among socioeconomic groups than ethnic groups.

### IMPLICATIONS FOR NURSING

Further study is needed to identify the barriers to breast cancer screening among different populations of women. Increasing breast self-examination practices and mammography can eventually help decrease the mortality from breast cancer among African American women.

### Critical Thinking in Client Care

1. What other barriers to breast cancer screening would you identify in women in lower socioeconomic groups? Why are these barriers specific to this group of women?
2. Are there barriers to breast cancer screening that are unique to African American women? To Hispanic women? To Asian American women? How could your teaching and interventions to increase breast cancer screening be tailored to women of different cultural groups?

---

- Explain the surgical procedure, including information about preoperative medications, anesthesia, and recovery. *Knowing what to expect helps to decrease anxiety.*
- Explain that it is normal to have decreased sensation in the surgical area. *Severed or damaged nerves reduce sensation.*

### Decisional Conflict

The woman with breast cancer must make life-changing decisions about treatment within a relatively brief and highly stressful time. Her age, menopausal status, and stage of cancer are only some of the factors that affect her decisions. Culture, values, lifestyle, socioeconomic status, and self-esteem also are considered.

- Provide an opportunity for the woman to ask questions; answer questions as simply and directly as possible. Make eye contact and pay attention to body language. *During this time, the woman can process information and make informed decisions.*
- Focus on immediate concerns, and provide up-to-date written material for the woman to review. *Written material provides easy reference to information not processed immediately because of anxiety and stress.*
- Listen to the woman in a nonjudgmental manner during her decision-making process. *Nonjudgmental, empathic listening helps the woman process information and make informed decisions. Only she knows the context of her life.*
- If the woman wishes, provide opportunities for her to meet with other women who have had breast cancer surgery. *Not all women are ready to meet others in their situation, but opening the door to this resource is appropriate. The woman may choose to talk with these women after the surgery.*
- Facilitate a team approach with the surgeon, anesthesiologist, oncologist, plastic surgeon, and other health professionals. *Being the woman's advocate during this time of anxiety and decision making reduces the stress of coordinating multiple health care provider schedules.*

### Anticipatory Grieving

Breast surgery, even lumpectomy, alters the appearance of the breast. This loss is expressed through grief.

- Listen attentively to expressions of grief and watch for nonverbal cues (failure to make eye contact, crying, silence). *Not all women will express grief clearly; sometimes unspoken grief is the most painful. Grief is relieved only when expressed in a nonthreatening environment.*
- Allow time to interact and do not rush interactions. *Taking time to be with the woman communicates caring.*
- Explain that it is normal to have periods of depression, anger, and denial after breast surgery. *All these feelings are appropriate expressions of grief.*
- If the woman wishes to do so, involve the partner in helping the woman cope with her grief. *Remember that the partner may also be grieving. Not all women want to share their grief, and not all partners are interested and supportive.*

### Risk for Infection

Like any surgical client, the woman who has breast surgery is at risk for infection. Removal of lymph nodes and the presence of a draining wound increase the risk.

- Assess the surgical dressings for bleeding, drainage, color, and odor every 4 hours for 24 hours and document your findings. Circle any visible bleeding and drainage on the dressing as a baseline for subsequent assessment. *Excessive bleeding or drainage signals postoperative complications that may require emergency attention.*
- Observe the incision and IV sites for pain, redness, swelling, and drainage. Assess the drainage system for patency and adequate suction; note the color and amount of drainage. *Careful observation for any signs of infection is essential because the woman's immune system is compromised. IV catheters should be placed on the uninvolved side only.*
- Change dressings and IV tubing using aseptic technique. *Moist dressings and intravenous tubing provide sites for bac-*

*terial growth. Routine dressing and IV tubing changes using aseptic technique reduce the risk for infection.*

- Encourage a protein-rich diet. Discuss the woman's nutritional status with the dietitian and request a consultation for the woman. *Adequate nutrition promotes healing and boosts the immune system.*
- Teach the woman how to care for the drainage system, if present (clean the site, empty the device, and record the amount, color, and type of drainage). *The woman is often discharged prior to removal of the drainage system and dressings and needs teaching to provide self-care.*
- At discharge, teach the woman to watch for and report to her health care provider the manifestations of infection: fever, redness or hardness at the surgical site, or purulent drainage. *Any of these manifestations should be reported to the physician/surgeon. Knowing the signs and symptoms of infection prepares the woman to seek prompt treatment if infection occurs.*
- Explain that she may experience scaling, flaking, dryness, itching, rash, or dry desquamation of the skin, particularly after radiation therapy. *Impaired skin integrity increases the risk of infection.*
- Tell the woman to avoid deodorants and talcum powder on the affected side until the incision is completely healed. *These substances may irritate the skin and impede healing.*

### Risk for Injury
Removal of the lymph nodes puts the woman at risk for injury and long-term complications such as lymphedema and infection.

- When obtaining blood pressure and starting IVs, use the nonsurgical side. *Compression of the arm on the surgical side may cause lymphedema.*
- Elevate the affected arm on a pillow higher than shoulder, but do not abduct it; the hand should be higher than the elbow. *Elevating the arm permits drainage, prevents swelling, and promotes circulation.*
- Encourage range-of-motion exercises in the affected arm. *Exercise helps develop collateral drainage.*
- Explain that lymphedema massage and an elastic compression bandage may help control the swelling after she has recovered from surgery. *It is important that women know about the resources available after recovery.*

### Body Image Disturbance
Breast surgery can change the woman's body image. The surgical changes may be compounded by weight gain and other side effects of chemotherapy or hormone therapy. Self-esteem also affects adjustment to a changed body image.

- Assess how the woman views her body. Discuss with the woman what image of herself she had prior to surgery. *Self-image is related to self-esteem. Discuss whether her self-image has changed.*
- Explain that redness and swelling in the scar will fade with time. *The knowledge that the scar will fade may give the woman a more realistic view of the changes.*

- Include the partner and family if possible when discussing the plan of care and ADLs. Request consultation with a psychologist or other professional if the woman is interested. *Discussion with the partner and family can facilitate the woman's emotional healing process.*
- Offer pamphlets and suggest books and videos that might increase knowledge about what lies ahead. *Knowing what to expect can help the woman cope.*

**PRACTICE ALERT** *Offer referral to support groups with women experiencing similar problems. Some women may prefer one-on-one counseling.* ■

- Encourage the woman to look at her incision when she feels ready; often the reality is not as frightening as the woman had imagined. Explain that it is normal to be afraid to look. *Reassurance that her behavior is normal decreases anxiety.*
- If the woman is interested in breast reconstruction, provide written material and encourage her to talk with a plastic surgeon and with women who have had reconstruction. *It is important that the woman is fully informed about available options to make an informed decision.*

## Using NANDA, NIC, and NOC
Chart 48–3 shows links between NANDA nursing diagnoses, NIC, and NOC when caring for the woman with breast cancer.

## Home Care
The woman with breast cancer and her family have much to learn to provide self-care at home. Address the following topics in preparation for home care.

- Manifestations of infection and the need to report any that occur to her health care provider
- The importance of ADLs, such as eating, combing her hair, and washing her face
- Postmastectomy exercises (Figure 48–14 ■) as discussed with physicians and physical therapists
- The need for adequate rest and emotional support
- Participation in a breast cancer support group and on-line information services and bulletin boards for sources of education and support
- Prosthesis management, if this option is chosen (A temporary lightweight prosthesis may be worn immediately after the drains and sutures have been removed from the surgical site. Because prostheses are expensive, a permanent one should not be purchased until the wound has completely healed. Prostheses are available at medical stores and many larger department stores. Most private and government insurance policies pay for the first prosthesis.)
- Helpful resources:
  - Reach to Recovery
  - American Cancer Society
  - National Breast Cancer Coalition
  - National Lymphedema Network

## CHART 48–3 NANDA, NIC, AND NOC LINKAGES

### The Client with Breast Cancer/Mastectomy

| NURSING DIAGNOSES | NURSING INTERVENTIONS | NURSING OUTCOMES |
|---|---|---|
| • Acute Pain | • Analgesia Administration<br>• Anxiety Reduction<br>• Pain Management | • Pain Level<br>• Symptom Severity |
| • Risk for Infection | • Infection Control<br>• Nutrition Management<br>• Skin Surveillance<br>• Wound Care | • Risk Control<br>• Nutritional Status<br>• Tissue Integrity: Skin |
| • Risk for Injury<br>• Impaired Physical Mobility | • Postanesthesia Care<br>• Exercise Promotion: Stretching<br>• Teaching: Prescribed Activity/Exercises | • Safety Status<br>• Mobility Level |
| • Fear | • Anxiety Reduction<br>• Progressive Muscle Relaxation<br>• Spiritual Support<br>• Support Group | • Fear Control |

*Note. Data from* Nursing Outcomes Classification (NOC) *by M. Johnson & M. Maas (Eds.), 1997, St. Louis: Mosby;* Nursing Diagnoses: Definitions & Classification 2001–2002 *by North American Nursing Diagnosis Association, 2001, Philadelphia: NANDA;* Nursing Interventions Classification (NIC) *by J.C. McCloskey & G. M. Bulechek (Eds.), 2000, St. Louis: Mosby. Reprinted by permission.*

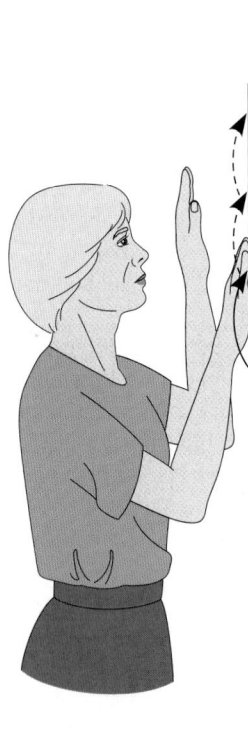

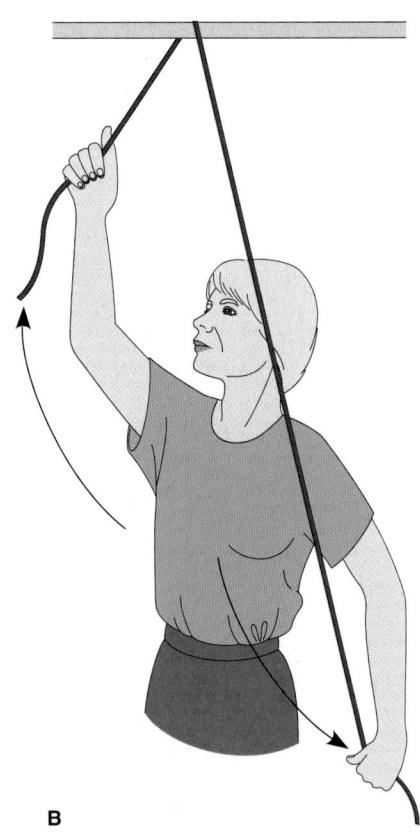

**A**          **B**

**Figure 48–14** ■ Postmastectomy exercises. *A,* Wall climbing: Stand facing wall with toes 6 to 12 inches from wall. Bend elbows and place palms against wall at shoulder level. Gradually move both hands up the wall parallel to each other until incisional pulling or pain occurs. (Mark that spot on wall to measure progress.) Work hands down to shoulder level. Move closer to wall as height of reach improves. *B,* Overhead pulley: Using operated arm, toss 6-foot rope over shower curtain rod (or over top of a door that has a nail in the top to hold the rope in place for the exercise). Grasp one end of rope in each hand. Slowly raise operated arm as far as comfortable by pulling down on the rope on opposite side. Keep raised arm close to your head. Reverse to raise unoperated arm by lowering the operated arm. Repeat.

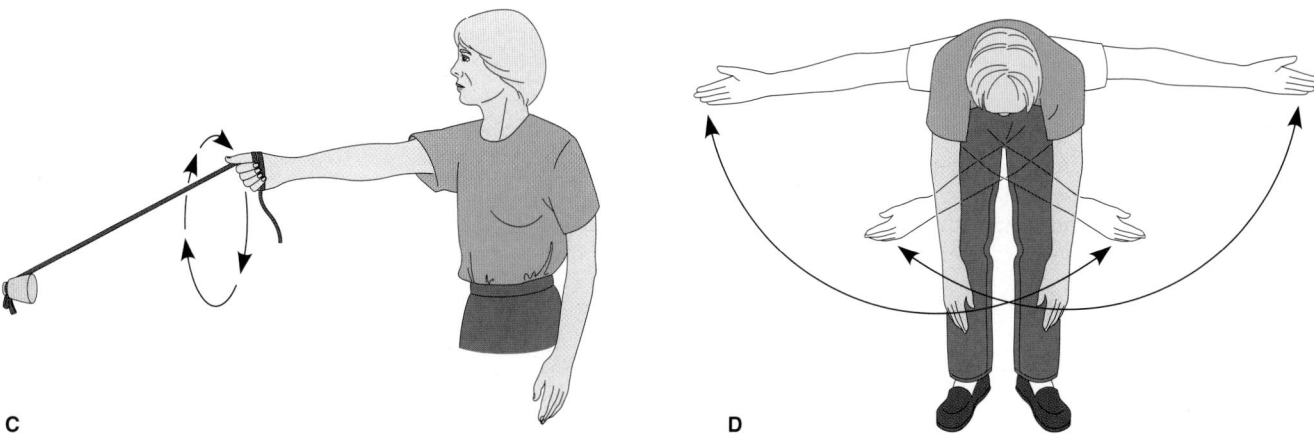

**Figure 48–14** ■ (*Continued*) *C,* Rope turning: Tie rope to door handle. Hold rope in hand of operated side. Back away from door until arm is extended away from body, parallel to floor. Swing rope in as wide a circle as possible. Increase size of circle as mobility returns. *D,* Arm swings: Stand with feet 8 inches apart. Bend forward from waist, allowing arms to hang toward floor. Swing both arms up to sides to reach shoulder level. Swing back to center, then cross arms at center. Do not bend elbows. If possible, do this and other exercises in front of mirror to ensure even posture and correct motion.

## Nursing Care Plan
### A Woman with Breast Cancer

Rachel Clemments is a 42-year-old mother of two, Sarah, age 12, and Jennifer, age 18. Because of a family history of breast cancer, she has been closely monitored (annual mammograms and clinical breast examination, monthly BSE, a needle aspiration biopsy with negative findings) for 4 years prior to her diagnosis. Mrs. Clemments discovers a lump in her left breast during her monthly BSE. An incisional biopsy reveals invasive lobular carcinoma in the left breast. Mrs. Clemments is debating whether to have reconstructive breast surgery. Her oncologist has recommended a 6-month course of adjuvant chemotherapy, and she is concerned about side effects. One of her greatest concerns is how her illness will affect her ability to support and care for her daughters. She is afraid that recovering from the mastectomy and completing the chemotherapy regimen will limit her ability to keep her part-time job, complete her academic work, and continue to meet the needs of her daughters. Also, this breast cancer diagnosis seems part of the family legacy. She wonders, "When will it happen to Jennifer? To Sarah?"

### ASSESSMENT
During the history, Laura Nelson, RN, the nurse admitting Mrs. Clemments, learns that her mother, two of her aunts, and one sister had been diagnosed with breast cancer. Her mother and one of the aunts died before age 45. Physical assessment findings include T 98.5°F (37.0°C), BP 110/62, P 65, R 14. Her weight is 120 lb (54 kg); she is 66 inches (168 cm) tall. Modified radical mastectomy is performed; histologic examination shows a 3 cm tumor; axillary node dissection shows that 4 of 16 lymph nodes are positive.

### DIAGNOSES
- *Risk for infection* related to surgical incision
- *Ineffective tissue perfusion* related to edema
- *Acute pain* related to surgery
- *Disturbed body image* related to loss of breast

- *Decisional conflict* about treatment, related to concerns about risks and benefits
- *Interrupted family processes* related to effect of surgery and therapy on family roles and relationships
- *Fear* related to disease process/prognosis

### EXPECTED OUTCOMES
- Remain free of infection.
- Maintain adequate tissue perfusion.
- Experience minimal pain or discomfort during her recovery.
- Maintain a positive body image, regardless of her decision about reconstruction.
- Evaluate the treatment options in relation to personal values and decide on a course of action.
- Together with her daughters, acknowledge the need for a change in family roles during her illness and identify new coping patterns.
- Identify the sources of her fear and demonstrate behaviors that may reduce fears.

### PLANNING AND IMPLEMENTATION
- Teach her about handwashing and wound care.
- Discuss the postoperative drainage device and its management after she goes home.
- Assess her pain tolerance and administer analgesics as prescribed.
- Teach her to use caution when moving the arm on the operated side, to avoid lifting heavy objects, and to wear gloves when gardening.
- Encourage her to discuss her thoughts and feelings about her body changes.
- Suggest that she talk with a Reach to Recovery volunteer about her thoughts and feelings.

(continued on page 1594)

## Nursing Care Plan
### A Woman with Breast Cancer *(continued)*

- Assess her interest in spiritual/religious support and refer if appropriate.
- Discuss medication and dietary changes that will minimize the effects of chemotherapy; request a consultation with the dietitian.
- Provide a list of educational resources about chemotherapy and breast reconstruction.
- Discuss the use of a temporary prosthesis and later the fitting of a permanent prosthesis (6 to 8 weeks after surgery), the need to be fitted by an experienced person, and insurance reimbursement for the prosthesis.
- Discuss the possibility of attending a breast cancer support group where she can draw on the experiences of other women who have undergone mastectomy, chemotherapy, or radiation.
- Refer her and her daughters to social services for a consultation about the changed family roles during her recovery and treatment.
- Encourage her to verbalize her fears about her own prognosis and about her daughters' future risk of breast cancer; assess the need/interest for referral to psychologic counseling.
- Teach her about dietary and lifestyle changes that can help reduce the risk of breast cancer for her daughters (low-fat, high-fiber diet; regular exercise; avoidance of obesity, alcohol, and oral contraceptives).

### EVALUATION

At discharge, Mrs. Clemments has no signs of physical complications and is looking forward to being at home with her daughters as temporary caregivers. Together they decide to try a vegetarian diet and buy a new vegetarian cookbook. Mrs. Clemments met with a Reach to Recovery volunteer, who brought her a temporary prosthesis and booklets about postmastectomy exercises, chemotherapy, and breast reconstruction. The volunteer also referred her to a local breast cancer support group. Mrs. Clemments has talked about her concerns related to breast reconstruction, which center on the possible health risks of silicone. "I want to wait and talk with women who have had reconstruction before I decide," she said. "I want to avoid anything that would increase the risk of complications. The possibility of recurrence and my fear for my daughters' future health are more than enough to worry about."

### Critical Thinking in the Nursing Process

1. What role could genetic counseling play in helping Mrs. Clemments and her daughters better understand the daughters' risk of breast cancer?
2. Describe the types of mastectomies and their implications for nursing care.
3. What medications might help minimize the side effects of chemotherapy?
4. Develop a plan of care for Mrs. Clemments for the nursing diagnosis, *Sleep pattern disturbance.*

See Evaluating Your Response in Appendix C.

# DISORDERS OF SEXUAL EXPRESSION

The normal female sexual drive can persist well into the eighth and ninth decade. The body maintains the capacity for sexual activity and orgasm long after menopause (see the Meeting Individualized Needs box on page 1595). In a typical sexual event, two physiologic sexual responses occur: vasocongestion and myotonia. Sexual stimulation results in vasocongestion of the blood vessels surrounding the vagina, causing engorgement, increased lubrication, and genital swelling and enlargement. Arousal, or myotonia, increases muscular tension, resulting in voluntary and involuntary muscle contraction.

The sexual response cycle has four phases: excitement, plateau, orgasm, and resolution. These phases always occur in the same sequence; however, the duration of each phase may vary. Sexual arousal typically ends in orgasm, or climax, but sometimes fails to do so. The refractory period, or period in which the sexual organs are incapable of responding to stimulus, does not occur in the female. Multiple orgasms are physically possible in all women.

Although nurses may not do sexual counseling, they should be able to obtain a sexual history without embarrassment, discuss sexual concerns with women, and make appropriate referrals.

## PATHOPHYSIOLOGY

Disorders of sexual expression may include dyspareunia, inhibited sexual desire, and orgasmic dysfunction.

### Dyspareunia

The woman with **dyspareunia** (pain during intercourse) may find it difficult to express her feelings to her partner. This condition is more likely to manifest itself as decreased desire or inhibited orgasm. The causes of dyspareunia range from organic to psychogenic.

Physical conditions, such as imperforate hymen, vaginal scarring, or vaginismus, may cause dyspareunia. *Vaginismus* is a rare condition in which the vaginal muscles at the introitus contract so tightly that an erect penis cannot be inserted. An

## Meeting Individualized Needs

### SEXUAL FUNCTION IN THE AGING WOMAN

Myths, taboos, and stereotypes held by society may foster the belief that older women are no longer interested in expressing their sexuality. Two commonly held myths are that menopause is the death of a woman's sexuality and that hysterectomy results in the inability to function sexually. Loss of sexual function is not an inevitable result of aging, although physical changes related to aging do affect the female sexual response. These physical changes, along with chronic conditions common in aging women, may alter a woman's sexual function. In addition, some medications used to treat the chronic conditions associated with aging can also alter the sexual response. It is the role of the nurse to educate women about the myths and misinformation about changes in sexual functioning and to provide information about ways to achieve optimal sexual health.

#### Physiologic Changes

Changes in aging women's sexual function begin in the perimenopausal period as estrogen levels decrease. Estrogen-sensitive cells are found throughout the central nervous system and the cardiovascular system. These cells are involved in the female sexual response. With menopause comes a decrease in the levels of estradiol, which affects nerve transmission and the response in the peripheral vascular system. As a result, the timing and degree of vasocongestion during the sexual response are affected.

Specific changes in the female sexual response occur in all phases. During the plateau phase, the capacity for vasocongestion decreases, as does muscle tension. In the orgasmic phase, the contractions are fewer and less intense. During the resolution phase, vasocongestion subsides more quickly.

#### Nursing Care

The nurse's role in assisting aging women to reach optimal sexual functioning centers on teaching them about the physiologic and psychologic changes associated with menopause. In addition, the nurse should instruct the woman in how the effects of chronic illness and the medications used to treat these illnesses affect sexual functioning. The woman should be taught the importance of maintaining a healthy lifestyle, which includes a balanced diet, weight-bearing and aerobic exercises, stress management, and routine health examinations.

For problems related to vaginal dryness and dyspareunia, the nurse can recommend water-soluble vaginal lubricants or vaginal gels before intercourse. Intercourse on a regular basis and estrogen replacement therapy can also be recommended for these problems. Women who experience joint pain or other musculoskeletal pain due to conditions such as arthritis can benefit from instruction in how to adapt positions for intercourse.

---

early traumatic event, such as sexual abuse, fear of men, rape, or ignorance of sexual functioning contribute to this disorder. However, it is estimated that 90% of dyspareunia is psychogenic in origin. The woman develops an anxiety-fear-guilt cycle in which negative thoughts become associated with the act of vaginal penetration, initiating a conditioned involuntary reflex. Other sexual activity may be quite pleasurable.

## Inhibited Sexual Desire

Inhibited sexual desire may be a result of pathophysiologic processes or may be psychogenic in origin. Often, inhibited sexual desire is rooted deeply in childhood teaching or experiences that may be too painful to recall. Cultural and religious values can also affect the processing of sexual stimuli. Fear of pregnancy or sexually transmitted diseases and depression also contribute to decreased libido.

## Orgasmic Dysfunction

Inhibited female orgasm (**anorgasmia**) is the most prevalent sexual problem among women. However, fewer than 20% of cases are physiologic in origin. It is estimated that from 8% to 15% of women have never experienced an orgasm in the waking state. Psychogenically induced anorgasmia may result from unresolved conflicts about sexual activity. Organic causes of anorgasmia include the presence of disease that re-

sults in general debilitation or that affects the sexual response cycle, and the use of drugs that depress the central nervous system.

Primary anorgasmia exists when a woman has never experienced an orgasm during the waking state, either through self-stimulation or intercourse. Secondary anorgasmia exists when a woman who previously experienced orgasms is no longer able to do so.

## NURSING CARE

Nursing care focuses on identifying the type of disorder of sexual expression through a thorough history, including the onset, duration, frequency, and context or situation in which the problem occurs. The woman's partner should be included in discussions when possible.

Teach the woman and her partner about varied normal and acceptable sexual responses. The goal is to increase self-awareness and understanding of communication and their relationship to sexual desire. Explain the differences in the behaviors that men and women consider sexually stimulating. Sex therapists may provide training in autostimulation techniques (masturbation) after inhibitions against this practice are discussed. Group therapy may be encouraged to help the woman discuss her problem and to decrease the sense of isolation it gives her.

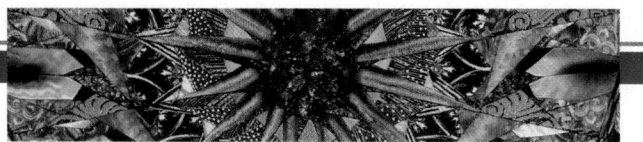

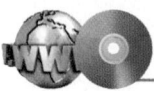 EXPLORE MediaLink

NCLEX review questions, case studies, care plan activities, MediaLink applications, and other interactive resources for this chapter can be found on the Companion Website at www.prenhall.com/lemone.

Click on Chapter 48 to select the activities for this chapter. For animations, video clips, more NCLEX review questions, and an audio glossary, access the Student CD-ROM accompanying this textbook.

## TEST YOURSELF

1. Your aunt tells you that her health care provider has asked her to begin short-term HRT. She asks you to tell her what good it would do her. Your reply is based on the knowledge that HRT:

   a. Prevents breast cancer
   b. Relieves perimenopausal discomforts, such as hot flashes and vaginal dryness
   c. Increases the risk of bone loss
   d. Has little effect on the physiologic effects of menopause

2. An intervention for the woman with a uterine displacement disorder is to teach Kegel exercises. These exercises may help reduce:

   a. Stress incontinence
   b. Menorrhagia
   c. Vaginal discharge
   d. Retroversion

3. Which of the following topics would you include in a health-promotion seminar to reduce the risk of cervical cancer?

   a. Weight loss
   b. Safe sex methods
   c. Yearly mammograms
   d. A diet high in iron

4. Of the following women, which one would be most at risk for breast cancer?

   a. Age 23, two children
   b. Age 33, never pregnant
   c. Age 45, very thin
   d. Age 64, positive family history

5. You are caring for a woman who is scheduled to have a lumpectomy later in the day. She is crying. What would be an appropriate nursing diagnosis?

   a. *Disturbed body image*
   b. *Fatigue*
   c. *Anticipatory grieving*
   d. *Risk for injury*

See Test Yourself answers in Appendix C.

## BIBLIOGRAPHY

American Cancer Society. (2002a). *Cancer facts & figures 2002.* Atlanta: Author.

_____ . (2002b). *New test may spot women at high risk for breast cancer.* Available wysiwyg://19?http://www.cancer.org/epris. . . pot_women_at_high_risk_for_breast_cancer

_____ . (2001a). *What are the risk factors for breast cancer?* Available wysiwyg://13/http:/www.cancer.org/epris. . . factors_for_breast_cancer

_____ . (2001b) *What are the risk factors for ovarian cancer?* Available http://www.c. . . /CRI_2_4_2X_What_are_the_risk_factors_for_ovarian_cancer

_____ . (2001c) *What are the risk factors for cervical cancer?* Available http://What_are_the_risk_factors_for_cervical_cancer

Andrews, G. (2000). Alleviating the misery of premenstrual syndrome. *Community Nurse, 5*(12), 23–24.

Cadman, L. (1998). Lifelong protection from cervical cancer. *Community Nurse, 3*(12), 12–13.

Cahill, C. (1998). Differences in cortisol, a stress hormone, in women with turmoil-type premenstrual symptoms. *Nursing Research, 47*(5), 278–284.

Champion, V. L., & Scott, C. (1997). Reliability and validity of breast cancer screening belief scales in African American women. *Nursing Research, 46*(6), 331–337.

Eliopoulos, C. (2001). *Gerontological nursing* (5th ed.). Philadelphia: Lippincott.

Fentiman, I., & Hamed, H. (2001). Assessment of breast problems. *International Journal of Clinical Practice, 55*(7), 458–460.

Fontaine, K. (2000). *Healing practices: alternative therapies for nursing.* Upper Saddle River, NJ: Prentice Hall.

Foxall, M. J., Barron, C. R., & Houfek, J. (1998). Ethnic differences in breast self-examination practice and health beliefs. *Journal of Advanced Nursing, 27*(2), 419–428.

Grady, D., Wenger, N., Herrington, D., Khan, S., Furberg, C., Hunninghake, D., Vittinghoff, E., & Hulley, S. (2000). Hormone replacement therapy and blood clots. *Annals of Internal Medicine,* May 2. Available www.coloradohealthsite.org/CHNReports/hrtandclots.html

Hoskins, C., & Haber, J. (2000). Adjusting to breast cancer. *American Journal of Nursing, 100*(4), 26–32.

Hulley, S., Grady, D., Bush, T., Furberg, C., Herrinton, D., Riggs, B., & Vittinghoff, E. (1999). Randomized trial of estrogen plus progestin for secondary prevention of coronary heart disease in postmenopausal women. *Journal of the American Medical Association,* August 19, p. 605. Available www.coloradohealthsite.org/women/women_estrogen.html

Institute of Medicine. (2002). Hormone replacement therapy: Project summary. Available www4/matopma;academies.org/IO

Irvine, D. M., Vincent, L., Graydon, J. E., & Bubela, N. (1998). Fatigue in women with breast cancer receiving radiation therapy. *Cancer Nursing, 21*(2), 127–135.

Jemal, A., Thomas, A., Murray, T., & Thun, M. (2002). Cancer statistics, 2002. *CA: A Cancer Journal for Clinicians, 52*(1), 45.

Johnson, M., & Maas, M. (Eds.). (1997). *Nursing outcomes classification.* St. Louis: Mosby.

Kee, J. (1998). *Handbook of laboratory and diagnostic tests with nursing implications* (4th ed.). Upper Saddle River, NJ: Prentice Hall.

Machia, J. (2001). Breast cancer: Risk, prevention, and tamoxifen. *American Journal of Nursing, 101*(4), 26–36.

Mayo Foundation for Medical Education and Research. (2002). Premenstrual syndrome. Available www.mayoclinic.com/diseases & conditions A-Z.>P> Premenstrual syndrome

Mazmanian, C. (1999). Hysterectomy: Holistic care is key. *RN, 62*(6), 32–35.

McCance, K., & Huether, S. (2002). *Pathophysiology: The biologic basis for disease in adults & children* (4th ed.). St. Louis: Mosby.

McCloskey, J. C., & Bulecheck, G. M. (Eds.). (2000). *Nursing interventions classification (NIC)* (3rd ed.). St. Louis: Mosby.

Murray, R., & Zentner, J. (2001). *Health promotion strategies through the life span* (7th ed.). Upper Saddle River, NJ: Prentice Hall.

National Cancer Institute. (February 7, 2002). Protein patterns may identify ovarian cancer. Available wysiwyg://23/http://newscenter. cancer.gov/pressreleases/proteomics07feb02. html

North American Nursing Diagnosis Association. (2001). *Nursing diagnoses: Definitions and classification, 2001–2001.* Philadelphia: NANDA.

Peters, S. (1997). The puzzle of premenstrual syndrome: Putting the pieces together. *Advance for Nurse Practitioners, 5*(10), 41–42, 44, 79.

Peters, S. (1998). Menopause: A new era. *Advance for Nurse Practitioners, 6*(7), 61–64.

Porth, C. M. (2002). *Pathophysiology: Concepts of altered health states* (6th ed.). Philadelphia: Lippincott.

Resnick, B., & Belcher, A. (2002). Breast reconstruction. *American Journal of Nursing, 102*(4), 26–34.

Shannon, M., Wilson, B., & Stang, C. (2002). *Health professional's drug guide 2002.* Upper Saddle River, NJ: Prentice Hall.

Smith, A., & Hughes, P. L. (1998). The estrogen dilemma. *American Journal of Nursing, 98*(4), 17–20.

Smith, R. et al. (2002). American Cancer Society guidelines for the early detection of cancer. *CA A Cancer Journal for Clinicians, 52*(1), 8–22.

Tiedemann, D. (2000). Ovarian cancer. *RN, 63*(10), 36–42.

Tierney, L. M., McPhee, S. J., & Papadakis, M. A. (Eds.). (2001). *Current medical diagnosis & treatment* (40th ed.). Stamford, CT: Appleton & Lange.

Torgerson, D., & Bell-Syer, S. (2001). Hormone replacement therapy and prevention of nonvertebral trials: A meta-analysis of randomized trials. *Journal of the American Medical Association,* June 13. Available www. coloradohealthsite.org/CHNReports/HRT_ fractures.html.

U.S. National Library of Medicine. (2002). Caution on hormone replacement therapy. Available www.nlm.nih.gov/medlilneplus/ news/fullstory_8434.html

Wolf, L. (1999). Dysmenorrhea. *Journal of the American Academy of Nurse Practitioners, 11*(3), 125–133.

Yarbo, C., Frogge, M., Goodman, M., & Groenwald, S. (Eds.). (2001). *Cancer nursing: Principles and practice* (5th ed.). Sudbury, MA: Jones & Bartlett.

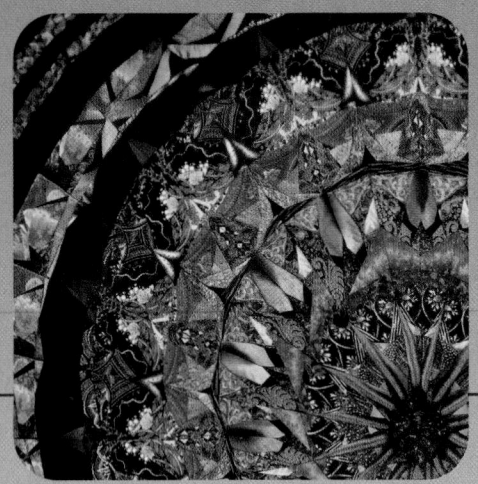

# CHAPTER 49

# Nursing Care of Clients with Sexually Transmitted Infections

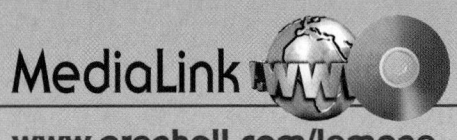

## MediaLink

**www.prenhall.com/lemone**

Additional resources for this chapter can be found on the Student CD-ROM accompanying this textbook, and on the Companion Website at www. prenhall.com/lemone. Click on Chapter 49 to select the activities for this chapter.

**CD-ROM**
• Audio Glossary
• NCLEX Review

**Companion Website**
• More NCLEX Review
• Case Study
   Syphilis
• Care Plan Activity
   Gonorrhea

## LEARNING OUTCOMES

After completing this chapter, you will be able to:

■ Apply knowledge of normal anatomy, physiology, and assessments when providing nursing care for the client with a sexually transmitted infection (STI) (see Chapter 46).

■ Explain the pathophysiology and manifestations of the most common STIs.

■ Identify diagnostic tests and collaborative care used to diagnose and treat STIs.

■ Describe teaching to prevent and control STIs.

■ Use the nursing process as a framework for providing individualized care to clients with STIs.

Any infection transmitted by sexual contact, including vaginal, oral, and anal intercourse, is referred to as a **sexually transmitted infection (STI)**. Infections transmitted by sexual intercourse are also labeled as **sexually transmitted diseases (STDs)** or venereal diseases. STIs are transmitted by intimate and sexual contact, and include systemic diseases (such as tuberculosis and hepatitis) that can be transmitted from an infected person to a partner. This chapter discusses STIs that involve the urogenital system and are sexually transmitted. Every sexually active person is at risk for STIs, and some of these diseases can be life threatening, particularly for women and infants.

This chapter provides an overview of the most common STIs with related collaborative and nursing care. Vaginal infections and pelvic inflammatory disease are included in this chapter as they are often transmitted by intimate contact.

## OVERVIEW OF STIs

### Incidence and Prevalence

STIs have reached epidemic proportions in the United States and continue to increase worldwide. They are the most frequent infections encountered by professionals in the field of reproductive health. According to the Centers for Disease Control and Prevention (CDC) (2000a, b), an estimated 15 million people contract an STI from an infected person each year in the United States and more than two-thirds of those infected are younger than age 25. In addition, viral STIs (considered incurable) affect more than 56 million people: 1 million with HIV, 20 million with genital warts, and 45 million with genital herpes. Some authorities believe that at least half of all Americans have been infected by an STI by age 35.

Women and infants are disproportionately affected by STIs. Many STIs are more easily transmitted from a man to a woman than from a woman to a man. Women often experience few early manifestations of the infection, delaying diagnosis and treatment. Furthermore, women are at greater risk for complications of STIs such as PID and genital cancers.

Several factors help explain the escalating incidence of STIs. The so-called sexual revolution of the 1960s and 1970s, fueled by "the pill" and the freedom from unplanned pregnancy, led to a more permissive attitude about sexuality and increases in sexual activity and the number of sexual partners. In addition, since oral contraceptives were introduced to American women in 1961, they have replaced the condom as a birth control method for many couples. However, oral contraceptives do not protect against STIs, a fact of increasing importance in the age of HIV/AIDS. Indeed, by making the vaginal environment less acidic, oral contraceptives predispose women to infection.

Finally, the emergence of HIV/AIDS has created a kind of "epidemiologic synergy" among all STIs. Other STIs, such as syphilis, HSV, and chancroid, facilitate the transmission of HIV/AIDS, and the immune suppression caused by HIV potentiates the infectious process of other STIs. In fact, individuals who are infected with STIs are 2 to 5 times more likely than uninfected individuals to acquire HIV if they are exposed to the virus. This is the result of several factors: Genital ulcers create a portal of entry for HIV, nonulcerative STIs increase the concentration of cells in genital secretions that can be targets for HIV, and infection with both an STI and HIV results in an increased likelihood of having HIV in genital secretions and semen.

The incidence of STIs is highest in populations with multiple sexual partners and among people of color in urban populations of lower socioeconomic status. People in these groups generally have little information about prevention of STIs and limited access to medical care, two factors that often delay diagnosis and treatment and sometimes limit compliance. Drug abuse, unprotected sexual activity, and sexual activity with multiple partners also are associated with increased incidence of STIs.

All states require reporting of syphilis, gonorrhea, and AIDS to state and federal agencies. Chlamydia is reportable in most states; however, requirements for reporting other STIs vary by state. This uneven reporting of cases means that the exact incidence of many STIs is unknown.

### Characteristics of STIs

Although sexually transmitted diseases are caused by various organisms, they have several common characteristics.

- Most can be prevented by the use of latex condoms.
- They can be transmitted during both heterosexual and homosexual activities.
- For treatment to be effective, sexual partners of the infected person must also be treated.
- Two or more STIs frequently coexist in the same client.

The complications of STIs include pelvic inflammatory disease (PID), ectopic pregnancy, infertility, chronic pelvic pain, neonatal illness and death, and genital cancer. Some STIs can be cured through appropriate early treatment with antibiotics. Others, such as genital herpes and genital warts, are chronic conditions that can be managed but not cured. The most serious STI is AIDS, which at this time is incurable. HIV/AIDS is discussed in Chapter 9. 🔗 Treatment guidelines for STIs are updated regularly and are available from the Centers for Disease Control and Prevention. Nurses have a critical role in the prevention of STIs by teaching clients about these diseases, their prevention, treatment, and potential complications. Table 49–1 summarizes the most common STIs.

### Prevention and Control

The prevention and control of STIs is based on the principles of education, detection, effective diagnosis, and treatment of infected persons; and evaluation, treatment, and counseling of sex partners of people who are infected. The ability of the health care provider to obtain an accurate sexual history is essential to prevention and control efforts.

The most effective way to prevent sexual transmission of HIV and other STIs is to avoid sexual intercourse with an

## TABLE 49–1 Selected Sexually Transmitted Infections*

| Condition/Organism | Signs & Symptoms | Medical Treatment[†] | Complications |
|---|---|---|---|
| Syphilis[‡]<br>*Treponema pallidum* | **Primary:** Painless chancre at site of exposure; regional lymphadenopathy<br>**Secondary:** Skin rash; oral mucous patches; generalized lymphadenopathy; condyloma lata; fever; malaise; patchy alopecia<br>**Tertiary (late):** Infiltrating tumors of skin, bone, liver; *cardiovascular changes:* aortitis, aneurysms; *central nervous system degeneration:* paresthesias, shooting pains, abnormal reflexes, dementia, psychoses | Benzathine penicillin G IM in a single injection *or* doxycycline PO for 14 days<br>Syphilis of indeterminate length or more than 1 year's duration: benzathine penicillin G IM weekly for 3 weeks *or* doxycycline PO for 28 days | Disease progression and transmission<br><br>Disease progression and transmission<br><br><br>Disease progression and transmission<br>Heart failure, blindness, paralysis, skin ulcers, liver failure, mental illness |
| Gonorrhea[‡]<br>*Neisseria gonorrhoeae* | **In females:** Often asymptomatic, but can include abnormal vaginal discharge, abnormal menses, dysuria<br>**In males:** Dysuria, increased urinary frequency, purulent urethral discharge | Cefixime PO *or* ciprofloxacin PO *or* ceftriaxone IM in a single injection *plus* azithromycin PO in a single dose *or* doxycycline PO for 7 days to treat possible coexisting chlamydia | **In females:** Pelvic inflammatory disease (PID), sterility, ectopic pregnancy, abdominal adhesions<br>**In males:** Prostatitis, urethritis, nephritis, epididymitis, sterility |
| Chancroid[‡] (rare in U.S.)<br>*Haemophilus ducreyi* | **In females:** Frequently asymptomatic<br>**In males:** Painful penile ulcers and lymphadenopathy | Azithromycin PO once *or* ceftriaxone IM once *or* ciprofloxacin PO for 3 days *or* erythromycin PO for 7 days | Secondary infection of lesions, fistulas, chronic ulcers |
| Granuloma inguinale[‡] (donovanosis)<br>(rare in U.S.)<br>*Calymmatobacterium granulomatis* | Single or multiple subcutaneous nodules that erode to form painless, bleeding, enlarging ulcers | Trimethoprim-sulfamethoxazole PO for 21 days *or* doxycycline PO for 21 days | Secondary infection of lesions, keloid formations on genitals, tissue necrosis, fever, malaise, secondary anemia, cachexia, and death |
| Lymphogranuloma venereum[‡] (LGV) (rare in U.S.)<br>*Chlamydia trachomatis* (immunotypes L1, L2, or L3) | Painless vesicle or nonindurated ulcer, followed by regional lymphadenopathy, inguinal abscess | Doxycycline PO for 21 days *or* erythromycin PO for 21 days | Ruptured inguinal or perianal abscesses producing draining sinuses or fistulas, nephropathy, hepatomegaly, or phlebitis |
| Chlamydial infections<br>*Chlamydia trachomatis* | **In females:** Asymptomatic but can include dysuria, mucopurulent vaginal or cervical discharge, vaginal bleeding or pelvic pain<br>**In males:** Sometimes asymptomatic but can include dysuria, white or clear urethral discharge, testicular pain (epididymitis) | Doxycycline PO for 7 days *or* azithromycin PO once | **In females:** Pelvic inflammatory disease (PID), infertility, pelvic abscesses, spontaneous abortion, still-birth, postpartum endometritis<br>**In neonates:** Ophthalmia neonatorum or pneumonia<br>**In males:** Nongonococcal urethritis, epididymitis, prostatitis, disease transmission |

\* This table does not include the following STIs discussed in other chapters: AIDS/HIV, viral hepatitis, sexually transmitted enteritis and proctitis, and ectoparasitic infections.
† Treatment recommendations are based on 1998 treatment guidelines by the Centers for Disease Control and Prevention.
‡ Reporting to state and federal agencies required by law.

## TABLE 49–1  Selected Sexually Transmitted Infections* (continued)

| Condition/Organism | Signs & Symptoms | Medical Treatment† | Complications |
|---|---|---|---|
| Genital herpes<br>Herpes simplex virus, usually type 2 but rarely type 1 | Single or multiple vesicles, on the genitals with associated pruritus, followed by painful ulcers | No cure; acyclovir PO or famcyclovir PO or valacyclovir PO for 7–10 days or until symptoms resolve | **In females:** Potentially fatal infection of fetus or neonate; possible cervical cancer<br>**In neonates:** Neonatal herpes affecting eye, skin, mucous membranes, and possibly central nervous system<br>**In males:** Neuralgia, meningitis, ascending myelitis, urethral strictures, lymphatic suppuration<br>**In both males and females:** Herpes keratitis, a severe eye infection, caused by autoinoculation |
| Genital warts<br>(Condyloma acuminatum) Human papillomavirus (HPV) | Single or multiple painless warts on genitals or perianal area | No cure, recurrence in 80% of cases; cryotherapy with liquid nitrogen or cryoprobe, or podophyllin 10%–25% in tincture of benzoin compound applied to wart, or client-applied podofilox topical solution or gel or imiquimod cream | **In females:** Enlargement during pregnancy and obstruction of the birth canal; transmission to fetus or neonate; increased risk of cancer of the cervix, vagina, vulva, and anus<br>**In neonates:** Respiratory papillomatosis, a chronic condition requiring multiple surgeries<br>**In males and females:** Urinary obstruction and bleeding |
| Bacterial vaginosis<br>Gardnerella vaginalis, Mycoplasma hominis | Excessive or foul-smelling vaginal discharge; erythema, edema, and pruritus of the external genitals | Metronidazole PO or clindamycin cream 2% or metronidazole gel intravaginally for 7 days | Recurrent infections; increased risk of PID |
| Mucopurulent cervicitis<br>Chlamydia trachomatis, Neisseria gonorrhoeae | Mucopurulent cervical discharge | Depends on causative organism; Chlamydia involved in 50% of cases | **In females:** Pelvic inflammatory disease (PID), infertility, pelvic abscesses, spontaneous abortion, stillbirth, postpartum endometritis<br>**In neonates:** Opthalmia neonatorum or pneumonia |
| Nongonococcal urethritis (NGU)<br>Chlamydia trachomatis, Urea plasma urealyticum, Trichomonas vaginalis, herpes simplex | Dysuria, urinary frequency, mucoid to purulent urethral discharge; some men asymptomatic | Depends on causative organism; azithromycin PO in a single dose or doxycycline PO for 7 days | Urethral strictures or epididymitis; if transmitted to female partners, may result in mucopurulent cervicitis and PID; if female is pregnant, can cause neonatal ophthalmia or pneumonia |
| Pelvic inflammatory disease (PID)<br>Chlamydia trachomatis, Neisseria gonorrhoeae, Mycoplasma hominis, and others | Asymptomatic or can include pain and tenderness in lower abdomen, uterus and adnexa, possibly with fever, chills, and elevated white blood count and erythrocyte sedimentation rate | Combined drug therapy such as cefotetan IV plus doxycycline IV or PO or clindamycin IV plus gentamicin IV or IM; may require hospitalization | Ectopic pregnancy, pelvic abscess; infertility, recurrent or chronic PID, chronic abdominal pain, pelvic adhesions, depression |
| Trichomoniasis<br>Trichomonas vaginalis | **In females:** Asymptomatic or can include frothy, excessive vaginal discharge, erythema, edema and pruritus<br>**In males:** Usually asymptomatic but can include urethritis, penile lesions, or inflammation | Metronidazole PO in a single dose or for 7 days | **In females:** Recurrent infections, salpingitis, low birth weight infants, prematurity |

## Meeting Individualized Needs

### HEALTH PROMOTION IN CLIENTS WITH STIs

| Barrier Protection | Teaching Topics |
| --- | --- |
| • Male condoms | ✓ Use a new condom with each act of sexual intercourse.<br>✓ Handle carefully to avoid damaging the condom.<br>✓ Be sure no air is trapped in the end of the condom.<br>✓ Put the condom on when the penis is erect and before genital contact with partner.<br>✓ Ensure adequate lubrication exists during intercourse, using only water-based lubricants (e.g., K-Y® Jelly, Astroglide®, AquaLube, and glycerine) and latex condoms. Oil-based lubricants, such as petroleum jelly, massage oil, mineral oil, or body lotions can weaken latex.<br>✓ Withdraw while the penis is erect and hold the condom firmly against the base of the penis during withdrawal. |
| • Female condoms | ✓ The female condom (Reality®) is a lubricated polyurethane sheath with a ring on each end that is inserted into the vagina. It is an effective mechanical barrier to viruses. |
| • Vaginal spermicides, sponges, diaphragms | ✓ Vaginal spermicides used alone without condoms reduce the risk for cervical gonorrhea and chlamydia. They do not reduce the risk of HIV infection.<br>✓ The vaginal sponge has the same benefit as spermicides.<br>✓ The diaphragm protects against cervical gonorrhea, chlamydia, and trichomoniasis, but not HIV. |

infected partner. It is recommended that both partners be tested for STIs, including HIV, before beginning to have sexual intercourse. If a person chooses to have intercourse with an infected partner or one whose infection status is unknown, a new condom should be used for each act of intercourse (CDC, 1998). See the box above for recommended STI barrier guidelines (CDC, 1998).

Prevention teaching for the person who is an injecting-drug user includes:

- Enroll or continue in a drug treatment program.
- Do not use injection equipment that has been used by another person. If equipment is shared, first clean the syringe and needle with bleach and water (to reduce the rate of HIV transmission).
- If needles can legally be obtained in the community, obtain and use clean needles.

Eliminating further transmission and reinfection of STIs is critical to control. For treatable STIs, this means that referral of sex partners for diagnosis, treatment, and counseling is essential. Gonorrhea, syphilis, and AIDS are reportable diseases in every state, and chlamydial infections are reportable in most states. When a health care professional refers infected clients to a local or state department of health, every effort is made to identify and contact sex partners. Reports of STI and HIV infections are maintained in strictest confidence, and are protected by law from subpoena. Suggested resources for people with STIs are listed in Box 49–1.

### BOX 49–1 ■ Resources for Clients with STIs

- CDC National STD Hotline
- CDC National Prevention Information Network
- National Center for HIV, STD, and TB Prevention
- National HPV and Cervical Cancer Resource Center and Hotline
- National Herpes Hotline
- American Social Health Association

## THE CLIENT WITH A VAGINAL INFECTION

The vagina may be infected by yeasts, protozoa, or bacteria. These infections can be sexually transmitted, but the male partner does not usually have manifestations of the infection. Risk factors include the use of oral contraceptives or broad-spectrum antibiotics, obesity, diabetes, pregnancy, unprotected sexual activity, multiple sexual partners, and poor personal hygiene. Manifestations of vaginal infections are outlined in Table 49–2.

Preventive measures include educating women about personal hygiene practices and safer sex. Women need to avoid frequent douching and wearing nylon underwear and/or tight pants. Unprotected sexual activity, particularly with multiple partners, increases the risk of vaginal infections.

TABLE 49-2   Vaginal Infections

| Infection | Type of Discharge | Typical Manifestations | Treatment | Nursing Care |
|---|---|---|---|---|
| Candidiasis (*Monilia*, yeast) | Thick white patches adhering to cervix and vaginal wall, resembling cottage cheese; little odor | Itching of vulva and vaginal area, redness, painful intercourse | Miconazole, clotrimazole, or terconazole creams or suppositories; povidone-iodine (Betadine) or vinegar douches | Teach perineal hygiene and proper use of vaginal applicators. Instruct the client to complete the entire treatment. |
| Simple vaginalis (bacterial vaginosis, *Gardnerella* vaginosis) | Thin, white, "milklike," or gray with fishy odor, especially when mixed with potassium hydroxide | None to mild itching or burning in vulvar area; clue cells on microscopic examination | Oral metronidazole for client; topical metronidazole or clindamycin for client's sexual partner | Teach proper perineal hygiene. Instruct client to complete treatment. Teach client relationship of infection to PID. |
| Trichomoniasis | Frothy, yellow or white, foul odor | Burning and itching of vulva | Oral metronidazole for client and sexual partner | Teach perineal hygiene |
| Atrophic vaginitis (Senile vaginitis) | Thin, opaque discharge, occasionally blood-tinged, odorless; pale, smooth, thin, dry vaginal walls | Painful intercourse, itching, vaginal dryness | Use of topical estrogen cream; use of water-soluble lubricant for intercourse. Evaluate need for HRT and antibiotic therapy | Counsel client on symptoms of menopause and sexual techniques to minimize trauma |

## PATHOPHYSIOLOGY

Alterations in pH, changes in the normal flora, and low estrogen levels are conducive to the development of vaginal infections. When conditions are favorable, microorganisms invade the vulva and vagina.

## Bacterial Vaginosis

**Bacterial vaginosis** (nonspecific vaginitis) is the most common cause of vaginal infection in women of reproductive age. *Gardnerella vaginalis* is one of the causative organisms, but others are also implicated. The relationship of sexual activity to this infection is not clear, and is believed to be the catalyst instead of the cause. The primary manifestation is a vaginal discharge that is thin and grayish-white, and has a foul, fishy odor. Complications include pelvic inflammatory disease, preterm labor, premature rupture of the membranes, and postpartum endometritis.

## Candidiasis

**Candidiasis** (moniliasis or yeast infection) is caused by the organism *Candida albicans,* which has several strains of different virulence. Candida organisms are part of the normal vaginal environment, causing problems only when they multiply rapidly. When increased estrogen levels, antibiotics, diabetes mellitus, fecal contamination, or other factors alter the normal vaginal flora, the organism proliferates, resulting in a yeast infection. The manifestations include an odorless, thick, cheesy vaginal discharge. This is often accompanied by itching and irritation of the vulva, dysuria, and dyspareunia.

## Trichomoniasis

**Trichomoniasis** is caused by *Trichomonas vaginalis,* a protozoan parasite. Symptoms usually appear in 5 to 28 days of exposure. It most commonly infects the vagina in women and the urethra in men. Most men are asymptomatic. Women have a frothy, green-yellow vaginal discharge with a strong odor, often accompanied by itching and irritation of the genitalia. Trichomoniasis during pregnancy may cause premature rupture of the membranes and preterm delivery. A woman with HIV who becomes infected has an increased risk of transmitting HIV to her sex partner.

## COLLABORATIVE CARE

Collaborative care focuses on identifying and eliminating the infection and preventing recurrence.

## Diagnostic Tests

Diagnostic tests vary with the suspected organism. The following tests may be ordered.

- *Culture of vaginal secretions* is performed and discharge is examined microscopically for the presence of "clue cells" if bacterial vaginitis is suspected.
- If candidiasis is suspected, the discharge is examined microscopically to detect hyphae (filaments or threads) and spores.
- *Normal saline wet prep* is used to detect the presence of protozoa if trichomoniasis is suspected
- *Glucose tolerance tests* or *HIV screening* are performed at the time of the initial assessment, if indicated.

## Medications

The pharmacologic treatment varies with the organism, as shown in Table 49–2. The sexual partner must also be treated to prevent reinfection. Some antifungal agents are available without prescription, which can lead to self-medication with the incorrect agent or allow repeated infections to go unreported.

## NURSING CARE

### Nursing Diagnoses and Interventions

Nursing care focuses on teaching the client and, if necessary, her sexual partner to comply with the treatment regimen, use safer sex practices, and prevent future transmission of the infection. Careful history taking may also reveal high-risk sexual practices that require intervention, particularly if the client has had repeated yeast infections. The initial presenting symptom for many HIV-positive women is vaginal candidiasis, which may be refractory to over-the-counter treatments. Treatment with some antibiotics destroys normal vaginal flora, resulting in superinfection with yeast. Although each nursing care plan must be individualized, nursing diagnoses that often apply to clients with vaginal infections are presented below.

### Deficient Knowledge

Many women are unaware of the causes of vaginal infections and the self-care measures to prevent and treat these infections. If possible, both the woman and her sexual partner should be taught the following information.

- Explain the transmission of the infection. Many infections are transmitted most easily during certain times of the menstrual cycle; some can also be transmitted by towels or other inanimate objects, or by certain types of sexual activity. *A frank discussion of disease transmission and prevention with the woman and her partner can reduce the risk of reinfection.*
- The need to complete the course of treatment. *Many infections are asymptomatic in one partner. Incomplete treatment allows for recurrence of the infection and reinfection of the partner.*

---

**BOX 49–2 ■ Self-Care Comfort Measures**

- Do not wear pantyhose; wear loose fitting pants or skirts.
- Double-rinse underwear; do not use fabric softener on underwear.
- Do not use bubble bath, perfumed soaps, or feminine hygiene products.
- Use 100% cotton menstrual pads and tampons.
- Use white, unscented toilet paper.
- Use a water-soluble lubricant for intercourse.
- Apply ice or a frozen blue gel pack wrapped in a towel to the vulva after intercourse to relieve burning.
- Rinse vulva with cool water after voiding and intercourse.

---

### Acute Pain

The symptoms of vaginitis can lead to dysuria, painful excoriation or ulceration of tissue, and painful intercourse (**dyspareunia**). Often these symptoms can be relieved by relatively simple self-care measures. See Box 49–2 for additional comfort measures.

- Suggest the use of cool compresses and vinegar or povidone-iodine douches (if approved by the primary health care provider). *Cool compresses relieve itching. Vinegar and iodine are fungicidal and bactericidal in effect.*
- Recommend sitz baths to alleviate discomfort. *Sitz baths cleanse the perineal area and the warmth is soothing to inflamed, irritated skin and membranes.*
- Wear cotton underwear. *Cotton absorbs moisture and allows better air circulation than other types of material.*
- Avoid sexual contact until treatment is completed. *Treatment of the infected woman and her sex partner as well as sexual abstinence are necessary to prevent reinfection.*

### Home Care

Teaching focuses on eradicating the infection, preventing further disease transmission, and relieving discomfort associated with the condition. Educating the client and her partner(s) about safer sex and improved genital hygiene practices can reduce the incidence of recurrence. Unless contraindicated, encourage the client with repeated mild candidiasis infections to consume 8 oz of yogurt containing live active cultures daily to help restore normal vaginal flora.

## INFECTIONS OF THE EXTERNAL GENITALIA

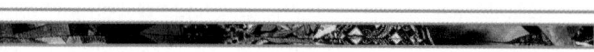

### THE CLIENT WITH GENITAL HERPES

**Genital herpes** (*herpes simplex genitalis*) is the most common infectious genital ulceration in the United States, and is considered epidemic. Although not a reportable disease, it is estimated to affect 1 million individuals each year. Recurrent infections affect an estimated 45 million people annually. The incidence is highest in teens and young adults, and in nonwhite lower socioeconomic populations (McCance & Huether, 2002). Genital herpes is chronic and, in many people, largely asymptomatic. Currently, it is incurable.

While the majority of infected people are asymptomatic, others experience frequent, painful recurrences. Other than recurrences, however, men are not likely to experience serious physical complications of genital herpes. Women, however, face concerns about childbearing (and infection of the newborn during delivery, resulting in death for 6 of 10 infants) and possible cervical cancer, although the risk of malignancy is not clearly established.

## PATHOPHYSIOLOGY AND MANIFESTATIONS

Genital herpes is transmitted by vaginal, anal, or oral-genital contact. Although it may be caused by either the herpes simplex viruses HSV-type 1 (HSV-1) or HSV-type 2 (HSV-2), 80% of initial infections and 95% of recurrent infections are caused by HSV-2. The incubation period is 3 to 7 days. Within 1 week after exposure to genital herpes, painful red papules appear in the genital area. In men, the lesions generally occur on the glans or shaft of the penis. In women, the lesions commonly occur on the labia, vagina, and cervix. Anal intercourse may result in lesions in and around the anus.

Soon after the papules appear, they form small painful blisters filled with clear fluid containing virus particles (Figure 49–1 ■). The blisters break, shedding the highly infectious virus and creating patches of painful ulcers that last 6 weeks (or longer if they become infected). Touching these blisters and then rubbing or scratching in another place can spread the infection to other areas of the body (*autoinoculation*).

The first outbreak of herpes lesions is called *first episode infection,* with an average duration of 12 days. Subsequent occurrences, usually less severe, are termed *recurrent infections* (average duration of 4 to 5 days). The period between episodes is called *latency,* during which time the person remains infectious even though no symptoms are present. During latency, the virus withdraws into the nerve fibers that lead from the infected site to the lower spine, remaining dormant until recurrence, at which time it retraces its path to the genital area.

The manifestations of genital herpes are presented in the box on this page. Prodromal symptoms of recurrent outbreaks of genital herpes can include burning, itching, tingling, or throbbing at the sites where lesions commonly appear. These sensations may be accompanied by pain in the legs, groin, or buttocks. Some authorities believe that prodromal symptoms signal increased levels of infectiousness, during which sexual contact should be avoided.

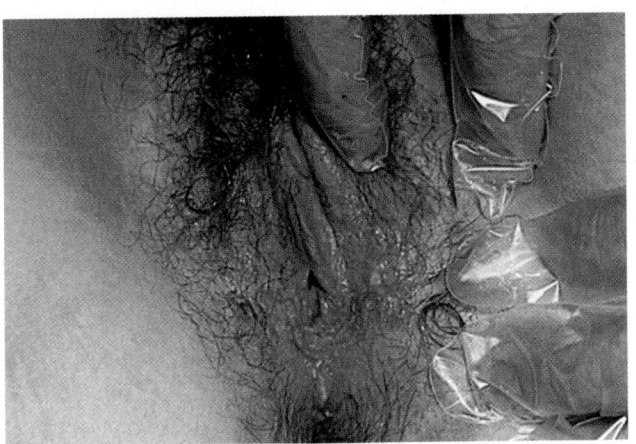

**Figure 49–1** ■ Genital herpes blisters as they appear on the labia.

*Source: Biophoto Associates/Photo Researchers, Inc.*

### Manifestations of Genital Herpes

- Herpetic lesions
- Regional lymphadenopathy
- Headache
- Fever
- General malaise
- Dysuria
- Urinary retention
- Vaginal discharge
- Urethral discharge (men)

In rare cases, the herpes virus spreads to the brain, causing herpes encephalitis, a life-threatening disorder. Prompt treatment with acyclovir (Zovirax) can cure the encephalitis, but more than 60% of survivors have permanent neurologic damage.

## COLLABORATIVE CARE

Because there is no cure for genital herpes, treatment focuses on relieving symptoms and preventing spread of the infection. Client education is essential to prevent further transmission of the disease and to help clients integrate management of a chronic disease into their lifestyles.

Presumptive diagnosis of genital herpes is based on history and physical examination of the client, including lesions and patterns of recurrence. Definitive diagnosis requires isolation of the virus in tissue culture. Ideally, tissue specimens should be obtained within 48 hours of the appearance of the blisters.

### Medications

Acyclovir (Zovirax) helps reduce the length and severity of the first episode and is the treatment of choice for genital herpes. The oral form is considered most effective for first episode as well as recurrences and is given for 7 to 10 days or until lesions heal. It may also be administered intravenously. Evidence shows that some strains of HSV are becoming resistant to acyclovir, particularly in HIV-positive people. In those cases, foscarnet (Foscavir) is used. Other antivirals used for treatment and prevention are valacyclovir (Valtrex), penciclovir (Denavir), and famcyclovir (Famvir).

## NURSING CARE

### Nursing Diagnoses and Interventions

In planning and implementing holistic nursing care for the client with genital herpes, the nurse needs to consider both short-term and long-term implications. Although the immediate priority is symptom relief and prevention of further transmission, the client needs assistance to deal with the life-changing diagnosis of a chronic disease (see the Nursing Research box on page 1606). Nursing diagnoses discussed in this section focus on pain, sexual dysfunction, and anxiety regarding childbearing and possible malignancy.

## Nursing Research

### Evidence-Based Practice for the Client with Genital Herpes

Researchers studied 70 young adults to determine the physical and psychosocial effects of living with genital herpes (Swanson et al., 1995). Stress was found to be the major cause of recurrence, headaches the major stress symptom, and acyclovir the major treatment. Findings indicated that young adults with genital herpes had lower self-concept, more psychopathology, greater frequency of daily hassles, and less intense emotional uplifts than non-patient control subjects. The researchers found no differences between the two groups in scores on depression.

#### IMPLICATIONS FOR NURSING

Clients with genital herpes need psychosocial support and counseling as well as education in self-care measures to deal with physical effects of the disease. Teaching stress-management techniques and suggesting alternatives to sexual intercourse, such as masturbation, may be useful. Allowing clients to express feelings and perceptions about how genital herpes has affected their lives can be an important part of counseling. Teaching safer sex practices and communication skills to use with a partner needs to be part of the care of all clients with STIs.

#### Critical Thinking in Client Care

1. Do you believe that the threat of contracting genital herpes or another chronic STI will change established sexual behavior patterns among high school and college students? Why or why not?
2. Do people with genital herpes who take appropriate precautions have the right to enter into sexual relationships without revealing that they are infected? Why or why not?
3. Why would the presence of genital herpes increase the likelihood of contracting other STIs?

### Acute Pain

Herpetic lesions are very painful and can become infected. Because the virus resides in the nerve ganglia, pain may also occur in the legs, thighs, groin, or buttocks. Although acyclovir diminishes the pain of herpes and accelerates the healing process, additional measures can relieve the discomfort further.

- Teach how to keep herpes blisters clean and dry. A solution of warm water, soap, and hydrogen peroxide can be used to cleanse the lesions two or three times daily. Burrow's solution can also be used. Lesions should be dried using a hair dryer turned to a cool setting. It is important to wear loose cotton clothing that will not trap moisture; panty hose and tight jeans are to be avoided. *Keeping the lesions clean and dry reduces the possibility of secondary infection and speeds the healing process.*
- For dysuria, suggest pouring water over the genitals while urinating. Drinking additional fluids also helps dilute the acidity of the urine; however, fluids that increase acidity, such as cranberry juice, should be avoided. *These measures dilute the acid content of urine and thereby reduce the burning sensation.*

### Sexual Dysfunction

Clients who learn that they are infected with an incurable STI may believe they can no longer have a normal sex life. Fortunately, many people have learned to live with and manage genital herpes without infecting their partners or their children.

- Provide a supportive, nonjudgmental environment for the client to discuss feelings and ask questions about what this diagnosis means to future sexual relationships. *Feelings of guilt, shame, and anger are natural responses to such a diagnosis and can lead to a total avoidance of sexual intimacy.*

- Offer information about support groups and other resources for people with herpes such as the National Herpes Information Hotline. *Information about how others cope with this disease can offset feelings of shame and hopelessness.*

### Anxiety

The woman with genital herpes faces two serious potential complications: elevated risk of cervical cancer and infection of her neonate during delivery. Some evidence suggests that the risk of cervical cancer is higher among women with genital herpes, although a direct causal link has not been identified. There is no question about the risk of neonatal infection from a mother with herpes, however, and such infection can range from asymptomatic to widely disseminated fatal disease. Transmission occurs during passage through the birth canal. The risk is highest during the first episode of infection.

- Advise the client about need for regular Papanicolaou (Pap) smears; some authorities suggest Pap smears every 6 months for women with genital herpes. *Careful monitoring will detect cervical dysplasia at a time when treatment is most likely to be effective.*
- Discuss with women of childbearing age that cesarean delivery can prevent transmission of infection to the neonate. In women without signs or symptoms of recurrence, vaginal delivery is possible. *Understanding that infection of the neonate can be prevented helps relieve anxiety.*

### Home Care

Health teaching for clients with genital herpes involves helping them manage this chronic disease with the least possible disruption in lifestyle and relationships. Understanding the disease process and factors that affect it helps the client regain a sense of control and see the potential for future sexual intimacy without transmission of infection. The following topics should be addressed.

- How to recognize prodromal symptoms of recurrence and factors that seem to trigger recurrences (such as emotional stress, acidic food, sun exposure)
- The need for abstinence from sexual contact from the time prodromal symptoms appear until 10 days after all lesions have healed
- If lesions become infected, use of topical acyclovir. (Painful lesions can be protected with sterile vaseline or aloe vera gel.)
- Use of latex condoms due to viral shedding at any time and careful hygiene practices (such as not sharing towels or other personal items) even during latency periods

## THE CLIENT WITH GENITAL WARTS

**Genital warts,** also known as *condyloma acuminatum* or *venereal warts,* are caused by human papilloma virus (HPV) and are transmitted by all types of sexual contact. The incubation period for genital warts ranges from 6 weeks to 8 months, with an average of 3 months. The four specific types of warts are as follows:

- *Condyloma acuminata:* cauliflower-shaped lesions that appear on moist skin surfaces such as the vagina or anus
- *Kerototic warts:* thick, hard lesions that develop on dry keratinized skin such as the labia major, penis, or scrotum
- *Papular warts:* smooth lesions that also develop on keratinized skin
- *Flat warts:* slightly raised lesions, often invisible to the naked eye, also develop on kertinized skin

HPV is not a reportable disease, so its exact incidence is unknown, but it is believed to be one of the most common STIs in the United States. Most HPV infections are asymptomatic or unrecognized. An estimated 20 million Americans are infected with the virus, and up to 1 million new cases are diagnosed annually. Like most STIs, genital warts are most commonly found in young, sexually active adults and are associated with early onset of sexual activity and multiple sexual partners.

Several subtypes of HPV are strongly associated with cervical dysplasia. More than 90% of cervical cancers contain DNA of oncogenic (cancer-promoting) HPV subtypes. HPV also is associated with a higher risk of vaginal, vulvar, penile, and anal cancers.

## PATHOPHYSIOLOGY AND MANIFESTATIONS

Although most people carry HPV without symptoms, others exhibit characteristic manifestations: single or multiple painless, cauliflowerlike growths on the vulvovaginal area, perineum, penis, urethra, or anus (Figure 49–2 ■). In women, the growths may appear in the vagina or on the cervix and be apparent only during a pelvic examination.

Potential complications of genital warts include obstruction of the urethra, causing bleeding, and transmission of the virus to the fetus during pregnancy or delivery. Infants infected with HPV can develop respiratory papillomatosis, a respiratory condition causing chronic distress and requiring multiple surgeries. There is also a relationship between HPV and the development of genital malignancies, with the risk believed to be increased by smoking, immunosuppression, and using oral contraceptives.

## COLLABORATIVE CARE

Treatment is directed at removal of the warts, relief of symptoms, and health teaching to reduce the risk of recurrence and future transmission. The HPV is considered chronic, however, with recurrence experienced in 80% of those infected.

### Diagnostic Tests

Genital and anal warts are diagnosed primarily by clinical appearance or by examination of Pap smear specimens. However, therapy is not determined until a VDRL test for syphilis and a gonorrheal culture have been done. Because HPV infection has been associated with various genital and anal cancers, biopsy is performed if lesions bleed.

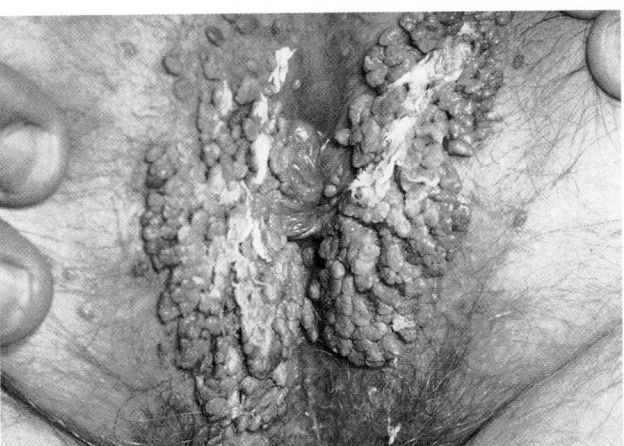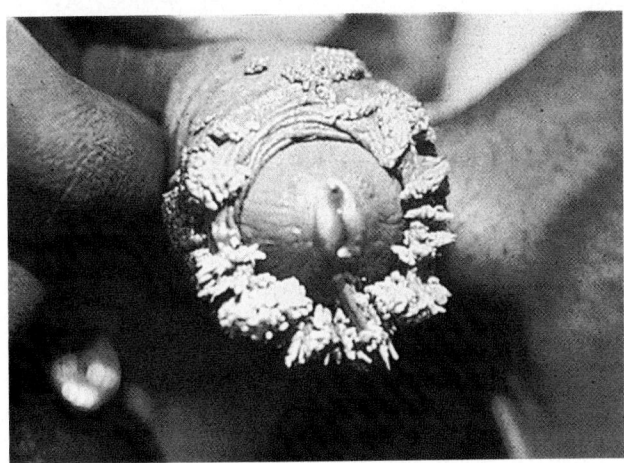

**Figure 49–2** ■ Genital warts (condyloma acuminatum) on the vulva and penis.

*Source: Kenneth Greer/Visuals Unlimited; National AV Center.*

## Medication Administration

### The Client with Genital Warts

#### TOPICAL APPLICATIONS

Podophyllin resin (Pod-Ben-25, podofilox 0.5% solution)
Trichloroacetic acid

Although cryotherapy using liquid nitrogen or a cryoprobe is more commonly used to treat genital warts, podophyllum preparations or trichloroacetic acid are sometimes used. Podophyllin resin, 25% in compound tincture of benzoin, is applied topically to the warts by the physician once weekly for 3 to 5 weeks.

Podophyllin resin is contraindicated during pregnancy; the alternative is cryotherapy or topical treatment with trichloroacetic acid. Podophyllin resin is also contraindicated in cervical, urethral, oral, or anorectal warts. It is important to avoid contact of podophyllin resin with the eyes.

Adverse effects of podophyllin resin include local irritation, severe ulceration of surrounding tissue, nausea, diarrhea, lethargy, paralysis, and coma.

#### Nursing Responsibilities

- Establish baseline data, including mental status, vital signs, and weight.
- Document and report any existing lesions (genital, anal, or oral).
- Cover the tissue surrounding the warts with petrolatum or a paste of baking soda and water to protect the tissue from the caustic treatment solution.

#### Client and Family Teaching

- Wash off the treated area thoroughly within 1 to 4 hours after the first application; gradually increase this period to 6 to 8 hours after the second and subsequent applications.
- Return for regular treatment until warts are gone.
- Refer partners for examination and any necessary treatment.
- Report any adverse effects (nausea, diarrhea, local irritation, lethargy, numbness)
- Avoid sexual activity until you and your partners have been free of disease for 1 month.
- Use condoms to prevent future infections.
- Return for an annual Pap smear.

## Medications

Topical agents used to treat genital warts include podofilox or podophyllin. Podophyllin (Condylox, Podofin) is contraindicated during pregnancy and can have serious side effects in any client, ranging from nausea, diarrhea, and lethargy to paralysis and coma (see the box above).

## Other Treatments

Genital warts may also be removed by cryotherapy, electrocautery, or surgical excision. Carbon dioxide laser surgery is becoming increasingly common for removal of extensive warts (see Chapter 14 ⊂⊃ for a discussion of these procedures).

## NURSING CARE

### Nursing Diagnoses and Interventions

Nursing care for the client with genital warts includes pretreatment teaching, treatment of the lesions, health teaching for self-care, and health promotion.

### Deficient Knowledge

HPV is spread by contact with infectious lesions or secretions, with up to 70% of genital warts spread by people who do not know they have the infection. Although there is no known cure, it is essential to prevent secondary infections.

- Discuss the need for prompt treatment and the necessity for sexual abstinence until lesions have healed. *This reduces the risk of reinfection and further transmission of the disease.*

- Discuss the increased risk of cervical cancer and the importance of an annual Pap smear. *Understanding the risk, the client will be more motivated to seek annual screening.*
- Stress the importance of thorough handwashing. *Handwashing is essential to prevent hand-to-eye spread of HPV, which is the most frequent cause of corneal damage and subsequent blindness in the United States (Porth, 2002).*

### Fear

Surgery engenders some degree of fear in most clients: fear of the procedure itself, of pain and possible complications. Surgery or cryotherapy in the genital area involves all these fears plus fear of possible impaired sexual function.

- Allow the client to express specific fears and feelings about the procedure. Explain the procedure, approximate recovery time, possible complications and ways to avoid them, and ways to cope with complications that do occur. *Knowing what to expect reduces the client's fear and helps the client feel a greater sense of control.*
- Explain that the procedure is performed with a local anesthesia. *Being awake during surgery gives the client a greater sense of participation in the treatment process.*

### Home Care

Health teaching emphasizes the need for the client and infected partners to return for regular treatment until lesions have resolved, and to use condoms to prevent reinfection. Because of the increased risk of cervical cancer, annual Pap smears are essential for female clients.

# UROGENITAL INFECTIONS

## THE CLIENT WITH CHLAMYDIA

**Chlamydia** are a group of syndromes, all caused by *Chlamydia trachomatis,* a bacterium that behaves like a virus, reproducing only within the host cell. The bacterium is spread by any sexual contact and to the neonate by passage through the birth canal of an infected mother. The syndromes include acute urethral syndrome, nongonococcal urethritis, mucopurulent cervicitis, and pelvic inflammatory disease (PID); all are commonly called chlamydia.

Chlamydia is the most commonly reported bacterial STI in the United States, affecting an estimated 3 million people each year. Of that number, three of every four reported cases occurred in people under age 25. Chlamydia is so common in young women, that by age 30, 50% of sexually active women have evidence that they have had chlamydia at some time during their lives (CDC, 2001). Risk factors for chlamydia are listed in Box 49–3.

Because chlamydia is asymptomatic in most women until they have invaded the uterus and uterine tubes, treatment is delayed, resulting in devastating long-term complications. Nearly a third of men with urethral chlamydia are also asymptomatic. Chlamydia is a leading cause of preventable blindness, particularly in the newborn.

## PATHOPHYSIOLOGY AND MANIFESTATIONS

The incubation period is from 1 to 3 weeks; however, chlamydia may be present for months or years without producing noticeable symptoms in women. Chlamydia typically invades the same target organs as gonorrhea (cervix and male urethra) and result in similar manifestations (dysuria, urinary frequency, and discharge). Clients may be asymptomatic; however, they are still potentially infectious.

If chlamydial infections in women are not treated, they ascend into the upper reproductive tract, causing such complications as PID, which includes endometritis, salpingitis, and chronic pelvic pain. These infections are a major cause of infertility and ectopic pregnancy, a potentially life-threatening disorder in women. Complications of chlamydial infections in men include epididymitis, prostatitis, sterility, and Reiter's syndrome.

| BOX 49–3 | ■ Risk Factors for Chlamydial Infection |
| --- | --- |

- Personal or partner history of STD
- Pregnancy
- Adolescent sexual activity
- Oral contraceptive use
- Unprotected sexual activity
- Multiple sexual partners

## COLLABORATIVE CARE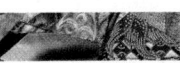

*C. trachomatis* is treated with medications to eradicate the infection. Its prevalence, particularly in younger populations, makes widespread screening necessary if the disease is to be controlled. Because chlamydia is often asymptomatic, treatment is often begun on a presumptive basis. The CDC recommends screening asymptomatic women who are at high risk for chlamydial infection.

### Diagnostic Tests

The following diagnostic tests may be ordered.

- *Cultures of tissue* from the female endocervix and urethra, or from the male urethra
- *Tests for antibodies* to chlamydia such as direct fluorescent antibody (DFA) test and an enzyme-linked immunosorbent assay (ELISA)
- *Polymerase chain reaction (PCR)* or *ligase chain reaction (LCR) tests,* highly sensitive and specific tests, on urine and vaginal swab specimens (Porth, 2002)

### Medications

The drug of choice for chlamydial infections in men and nonpregnant women is oral azithromycin (Zithromax) or doxycycline (Vibramycin, Vivox) given as prescribed for 7 days. For pregnant women, erythromycin (E.E.S., Wyamycin E) is the alternative therapy. Ofloxacin (Floxin, Ocuflox) given twice daily for 7 days is another alternative treatment.

## NURSING CARE

Nursing care of the client with chlamydia focuses on eradication of the infection, prevention of future infections, and management of any chronic complications. Nursing diagnoses for the client with chlamydia are the same as for clients with any STI. Interventions are similar to those previously discussed for gonorrhea and genital herpes.

### Home Care

Health teaching for the client with chlamydia centers on the need to comply with the treatment regimen, refer partners for examination and necessary treatment, and the use of condoms to avoid reinfection. If the infection has progressed to pelvic inflammatory disease (discussed later), the client needs additional information on self-care and health promotion. The CDC recommends annual screening for chlamydia for clients who are young, sexually active, and do not use condoms correctly with every act of sexual intercourse. All pregnant women should be screened for chlamydia.

## THE CLIENT WITH GONORRHEA

**Gonorrhea,** also known as **GC** or **clap,** is caused by *Neisseria gonorrhoeae,* a gram-negative diplococcus. The incubation period is 2 to 8 days after exposure. Gonorrhea is transmitted by direct sexual contact and during delivery as the neonate passes through the birth canal. Gonorrhea is the most common reportable communicable disease in the United States. The CDC estimates that approximately 300,000 new cases occur annually, with the rate of reported gonorrhea increasing. Women age 15 to 19 have the highest rate, along with men age 20 to 24 (CDC, 2000).

Gonorrhea rates for African Americans are 30% higher than for non-Hispanic whites. Other risk factors include residence in large urban areas, transients, early onset of sexual activity, multiple serial or consecutive sex partners, drug use, prostitution, and previous gonorrheal or concurrent STI infection (McCance & Huether, 2002).

## PATHOPHYSIOLOGY AND MANIFESTATIONS

The organism initially targets the female cervix and the male urethra. Without treatment, the disease ultimately disseminates to other organs. In men, gonorrhea can cause acute, painful inflammation of the prostate, epididymis, and periurethral glands and can lead to sterility. In women, it can cause pelvic inflammatory disease (PID), endometritis, salpingitis, and pelvic peritonitis. In the neonate, gonorrhea can cause ophthalmia neonatorum, rhinitis, or anorectal infection.

Manifestations of gonorrhea in men include dysuria and serous, milky, or purulent discharge. Some men also experience regional lymphadenopathy. About 20% of men and 80% of women remain asymptomatic until the disease is advanced. Those women with symptoms experience dysuria, urinary frequency, abnormal menses (increased flow or dysmenorrhea), increased vaginal discharge, and dyspareunia (pain with intercourse).

Anal and rectal gonorrhea occurs in 30% to 50% of women diagnosed with gonorrhea. In women it is often asymptomatic and may not be connected with anal intercourse. Anorectal gonorrhea is seen most often in homosexual men. The manifestations include pruritus, mucopurulent rectal discharge, rectal bleeding and pain, and constipation. Gonococcal pharyngitis occurs primarily in homosexual or bisexual men or heterosexual women after oral sexual contact (fellatio) with an infected partner. The manifestations include fever, sore throat, and enlarged lymph glands.

### Complications

The complications of untreated gonorrhea in both men and women may be permanent and serious. They include:

- Pelvic inflammatory disease (PID) in women, leading to internal abscesses, chronic pain, ectopic pregnancy, and infertility.
- Blindness, infection of joints, and potentially lethal infections of the blood in the newborn, contracted during delivery.
- Epididymitis and prostatitis in men, resulting in infertility and dysuria.
- Spread of the infection to the blood and joints.
- Increased susceptibility to and transmission of HIV

## COLLABORATIVE CARE

The goals of treatment for the client with gonorrhea include eradication of the organism and any coexisting disease, and prevention of reinfection or transmission. It is important to emphasize the importance of taking all medications as prescribed and abstaining from sexual contact until the infection is cured in both client and partners. Condom use to prevent future infections is essential, particularly for pregnant women whose partners may be infected.

### Diagnostic Tests

Diagnosis of gonorrhea is based on the following diagnostic tests.

- *Fluid analysis* from the infected mucous membranes (cervix, urethra, rectum, or throat)
- *Urinalysis* from an infected person
- *Gram stain,* allowing visualization of the bacteria under the microscope

### Medications

Because of the many penicillin-resistant strains of *N. gonorrhoeae,* an alternative antibiotic, such as oral cefixime (Suprax), ciproflaxacin (Cipro), or ofloxacin (Floxin); or intramuscular ceftriaxone (Rocephin), is used to treat gonorrhea. A single dose of oral azithromycin (Zithromax) or a 7-day course of oral doxycycline (Vibramycin, Vivox) usually is added to treat any coexisting chlamydial infection. Infected sexual partners also need to be treated.

## NURSING CARE

### Nursing Diagnoses and Interventions

In planning and implementing care for the client with gonorrhea, the nurse considers the possible coexistence of other STIs such as syphilis and HIV, the impact of the disease and its treatment on the client's lifestyle, and the likelihood of noncompliance. Nursing diagnoses discussed in this section focus on noncompliance and impaired social interaction.

#### Noncompliance

Although one-time treatment with the recommended antibiotic is highly effective in curing gonorrhea, noncompliance with the doxycycline regimen may leave any coexisting chlamydial infection unresolved. Noncompliance with recommendations for abstinence, follow-up, or condom use fosters a high rate of reinfection. Failure to refer partners for examination and treatment also leads to reinfection.

- Reinforce the need for taking all medications as directed and keeping follow-up appointments to be sure no reinfection has occurred. Discuss the prevalence of gonorrhea and the potential complications if it is not cured. *The client who understands the complications of incomplete or failed treatment is more likely to comply with the medication regimen.*

- Discuss the importance of sexual abstinence until the infection is cured, referral of partners, and condom use to prevent reinfection. *Understanding that cure is possible and reinfection is avoidable helps the client cope with the disease and its treatment and is likely to increase compliance.*

### Impaired Social Interaction

Diagnosis of any STI can make clients feel "dirty," ashamed, and guilty about their sexual behaviors, and unworthy to be with others.

- Provide privacy, confidentiality, and a safe, nonjudgmental environment for expression of concerns. Help the client un-

derstand that gonorrhea is a consequence of sexual behavior, not a punishment, and that it can be avoided in the future. *Being treated with respect and privacy helps the client realize that the disease does not change an individual's worth as a person. This knowledge enhances the client's ability to relate to others.*

## Home Care

Health teaching focuses on helping clients understand the importance of (1) taking any and all prescribed medication, (2) referring sexual partners for evaluation and treatment, (3) abstaining from all sexual contact until the client and partners are cured, and (4) using a condom to avoid transmitting or contracting infections in the future. Clients also need to understand the need for a follow-up visit 4 to 7 days after treatment is completed.

## Nursing Care Plan
## A Client with Gonorrhea

Janet Cirit, a 33-year-old legal secretary, lives in a suburban midwestern community. She is unmarried but dating a man named Jim Adkins, who lives in an adjacent suburb. Ms. Cirit visits her gynecologist because her periods have become irregular and she is experiencing pelvic pain and an abnormal amount of vaginal discharge. Recently she has developed a sore throat. The pelvic pain has begun to disrupt her sleeping pattern, and she is concerned that she might have cancer because her mother recently died of ovarian cancer.

### ASSESSMENT

When Ms. Cirit arrives for her appointment at the gynecologist's office, Marsha Davidson, the nurse practitioner, interviews her. Ms. Davidson completes a thorough medical and sexual history, including questions about her menstrual periods, pain associated with urination or sexual intercourse, urinary frequency, most recent Pap smear, birth control method, history of STI and drug use, and types of sexual activity. Ms. Cirit reports her symptoms and her concern about ovarian cancer. She also indicates that she is taking oral contraceptives and therefore sees no need for her boyfriend to use a condom because she believes their relationship is monogamous.

Physical examination reveals both pharyngeal and cervical inflammation, and lower abdominal tenderness. Her temperature is 98.5°F (37.0°C). There are no signs or symptoms of pregnancy.

The gynecologist orders a Pap smear and cultures of the cervix, urethra, and pharynx to evaluate for gonorrhea and chlamydial infection. Blood is drawn for WBC. Test results are positive for gonorrhea and negative for chlamydia. The WBC is slightly elevated, indicating possible salpingitis. Because Mr. Adkins has been Ms. Cirit's only sexual partner, it is clear that he is the source of infection and needs to be treated as well.

### DIAGNOSIS

- *Pain* related to the infectious process
- *Anxiety* related to fear about possible cancer
- *Situational low self-esteem* related to shame and guilt because of having an STI

- *Ineffective sexuality patterns* related to the impaired relationship and fear of reinfection

### EXPECTED OUTCOMES

- Experience relief of pain, indicating that the infection had been eradicated.
- Express relief that the Pap smear showed no abnormal cells.
- Verbalize that she has nothing to be ashamed of and that she has been wise to seek treatment as soon as symptoms occurred.
- Verbalize that she will insist her partner use condoms during future sexual activity.

### PLANNING AND IMPLEMENTATION

- Administer ceftriaxone IM as ordered.
- Emphasize the need for regular Pap smears and pelvic examinations because of the family history of ovarian cancer.
- Discuss feelings and concerns about the diagnosis of gonorrhea. Stress that such a diagnosis does not reflect on one's self-worth as a person.
- Teach how to talk with a future sexual partner about condom use.

### EVALUATION

A week later during her follow-up visit, Ms. Cirit states that she is feeling much better and sleeping well at night since the pain has ended. She has terminated her relationship with Mr. Adkins and is considering joining a health club in the hope of increasing her level of fitness and perhaps meeting someone new.

### Critical Thinking in the Nursing Process

1. How are Ms. Cirit's manifestations related to the infectious process of gonorrhea?
2. Should the nurse have suggested that Ms. Cirit also be tested for HIV? Why or why not?
3. Develop a care plan for Ms. Cirit for the nursing diagnosis, *Impaired social interaction*.

See Evaluating Your Response in Appendix C.

## THE CLIENT WITH SYPHILIS

**Syphilis** is a complex systemic STI caused by a spirochete, *Treponema pallidum,* which may infect almost any body tissue or organ. It is transmitted from open lesions during any sexual contact (genital, oral-genital, or anal-genital). The organism is highly susceptible to heat and drying, but can survive for days in fluids; thus, it may also be transmitted by infected blood or other body fluid such as saliva. The incubation period ranges from 10 to 90 days, averaging 21 days. If not treated appropriately, syphilis can lead to blindness, paralysis, mental illness, cardiovascular damage, and death. Syphilis often occurs with one or more other STIs, such as HIV/AIDS or chlamydial infection. Pregnant women with syphilis can also infect the fetus, causing eye damage, dental and bone deformities, blindness, brain damage, and death.

With the advent of penicillin in the 1940s and 1950s, the incidence of syphilis plummeted. While in 1996 the rate of syphilis infection reached its lowest level in many years, it remains a significant problem in certain geographic regions, and among specific populations such as African Americans. Rates also remain high in many urban centers, with higher infection rates found in drug users, transients, and the homeless. The rate of syphilis infection is declining among most racial and ethnic groups, with the exception of American Indians and Alaska Natives (CDC, 2001).

## PATHOPHYSIOLOGY AND MANIFESTATIONS

Any break in the skin or mucous membrane is vulnerable to invasion by the spirochete. Once it has entered the system, the spirochete is spread through the blood and lymphatic system. Congenital syphilis is transferred to the fetus through the placental circulation. Syphilis is generally characterized by three clinical stages: primary, secondary, and tertiary. Each stage has characteristic manifestations (see the box below). The client with syphilis also may experience a latency period when no signs of the disease are evident.

### Primary Syphilis

The primary stage of syphilis is characterized by the appearance of a **chancre** (Figure 49–3 ■) and by regional enlargement of lymph nodes; little or no pain accompanies these warning signs. The chancre appears at the site of inoculation (genitals, anus, mouth, breast, finger) 3 to 4 weeks after the infectious contact. In women, a genital chancre may go unnoticed, disappearing within 4 to 6 weeks. In both primary and secondary stages, syphilis remains highly infectious, even if no symptoms are evident.

### Secondary Syphilis

Manifestations of secondary syphilis may appear any time from 2 weeks to 6 months after the initial chancre disappears. These symptoms can include a skin rash, especially on the

## Manifestations of Syphilis

**REPRODUCTIVE**

Primary
- Genital chancre (may be internal in female)

Secondary
- Condyloma lata

**INTEGUMENTARY SYSTEM**

Secondary
- Rash on palms and soles

Tertiary
- Granulomatous lesions involving mucous membranes and skin

**GASTROINTESTINAL SYSTEM**

Secondary
- Anorexia
- Oral mucous patches

**NEUROLOGIC SYSTEM**

Secondary
- Asymptomatic
- Headache
- Meningitis
- Cranial neuropathies

Tertiary
- Asymptomatic
- Neurosyphilis
- Tabes dorsalis
- Seizures, hemiparesis, hemiplegia
- Personality changes, hyperactive reflexes, Argyll Robertson pupil, decreased memory, slurred speech, optic atrophy

**MUSCULOSKELETAL SYSTEM**

Secondary
- Arthralgia
- Bone and joint arthritis
- Myalgia
- Periostitis

Tertiary
- Gummas

**CARDIOVASCULAR SYSTEM**

Tertiary
- Aortic insufficiency
- Aortic aneurysm
- Stenosis of openings to coronary arteries

**RENAL SYSTEM**

Secondary
- Glomerulonephritis
- Nephrotic syndrome

**OTHER**

Primary
- Regional lymphadenopathy

Secondary
- Generalized lymphadenopathy
- Fever
- Malaise
- Hepatitis
- Alopecia

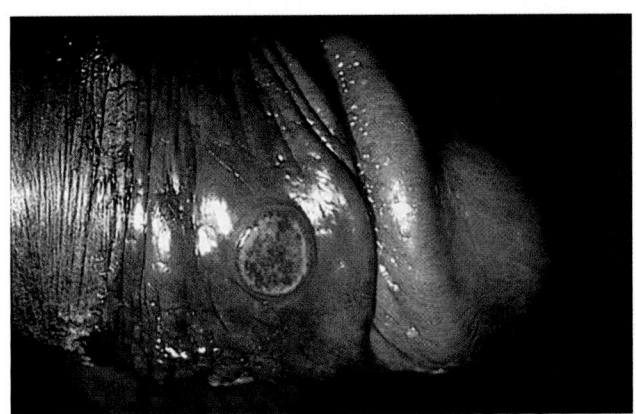

**Figure 49–3** ■ Chancre of primary syphilis on the penis.

*Source: Biophoto Associates/Photo Researchers, Inc.*

palms of the hands (Figure 49–4 ■) or soles of the feet, mucous patches in the oral cavity; sore throat; generalized lymphadenopathy; condyloma lata (flat, broad-based papules, unlike the pedunculated structure of genital warts) on the labia, anus or corner of the mouth; flulike symptoms; and alopecia. These manifestations generally disappear within 2 to 6 weeks, and an asymptomatic latency period begins.

## Latent and Tertiary Syphilis

The latent stage of syphilis begins 2 or more years after the initial infection and can last up to 50 years. During this stage, no symptoms of syphilis are apparent, and the disease is not transmissible by sexual contact. It can be transmitted by infected blood, however; thus, all prospective blood donors must be screened for syphilis. In two-thirds of all cases, the latent stage persists without further complications. Unless treated, the remaining one-third of infected people progress to late-stage or tertiary syphilis. In the presence of HIV infection, disease progression seems to be more rapid.

Two types of late-stage syphilis occur. Benign late syphilis, of rapid onset, is characterized by localized devel-

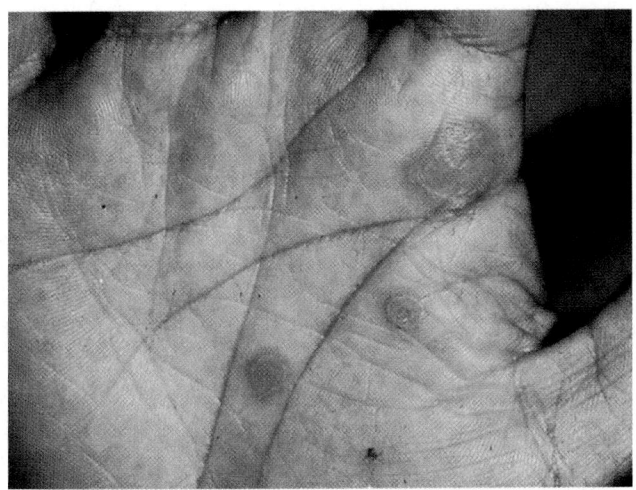

**Figure 49–4** ■ Palmar rash of secondary syphilis.

*Source: Dr. Carroll Weiss, Camera MD Studios.*

opment of infiltrating tumors (*gummas*) in skin, bones, and liver, generally responding promptly to treatment. Of more insidious onset is a diffuse inflammatory response that involves the central nervous system and the cardiovascular system. Though the disease can still be treated at this stage, much of the cardiovascular and central nervous system damage is irreversible.

## COLLABORATIVE CARE

The goals of treatment are to inactivate the spirochete and educate the client about how to prevent reinfection or further transmission. Treatment includes antibiotic therapy and identification and referral of partners for testing and treatment if necessary, follow-up testing, and education about condom use to prevent reinfection of self and transmission of disease to partners. In addition, clients should be screened for chlamydial infection and advised to have an HIV test.

### Diagnostic Tests

Diagnosis of syphilis is complex because it mimics many other diseases. A careful history and physical examination are obtained, as well as laboratory evaluations of lesions and blood. The following tests are widely used.

- The *VDRL (Venereal Disease Research Laboratory)* and *RPR (rapid plasma reagin) blood tests* measure antibody production. People with syphilis become positive about 4 to 6 weeks after infection. However, these tests are not specific for syphilis, and other diseases may also cause positive results. Additional tests are required for definitive diagnosis.
- *FTA-ABS (fluorescent treponemal antibody absorption) test* is specific for *T. pallidum* and can be used to confirm VDRL and RPR findings. It may be used for clients whose clinical picture indicates syphilis but who have negative VDRL results.
- *Immunofluorescent staining* during which a specimen obtained from early lesions or aspiration of lymph nodes is specially treated and examined microscopically for the presence of *T. pallidum.*
- *Darkfield microscopy* involves examining a specimen from the chancre for the presence of *T. pallidum* using a darkfield microscope.

### Medications

The treatment of choice for primary and secondary syphilis is benzathine penicillin G, given intramuscularly (IM) in a single dose. For syphilis of indeterminate length or more than 1 year's duration, the total dosage is increased and given in three weekly injections. Clients allergic to penicillin are given oral doxycycline. The length of therapy depends on the estimated duration of infection. If the client cannot tolerate doxycycline, oral erythromycin is substituted.

Treatment of syphilis in pregnant women may result in a severe reaction called the *Jarisch-Herxheimer reaction*, involving fever, musculoskeletal pain, tachycardia, and sometimes hypotension. This is not a reaction to the penicillin itself, but to

MediaLink | SYPHILIS CASE STUDY

the sudden and massive destruction of spirochetes by the penicillin and the resulting release of toxins into the bloodstream. The Jarisch-Herxheimer reaction generally begins within 24 hours of treatment and subsides in another 24 hours. Treatment should not be discontinued unless symptoms become life threatening.

## NURSING CARE

### Nursing Diagnoses and Interventions

In planning and implementing nursing care for the client with syphilis, the nurse needs to consider the client's age, lifestyle, access to health care, and educational level. Although each client has individualized needs, nursing diagnoses for the client with syphilis would be the same as for any client with an STI. Nursing diagnoses discussed in this section focus on high risk for injury, anxiety, and self-esteem.

### Risk for Injury

If syphilis is not diagnosed and treated promptly and effectively, it can have devastating effects on all body systems, particularly the neurologic and cardiovascular systems, eventually leading to a painful death.

- Teach the importance of taking any prescribed oral medication. *Completion of the prescribed course of antibiotic is important to ensure eradication of the infecting organism.*
- Encourage referral of any sexual partners for evaluation and any necessary treatment. *Without treatment of both partners, reinfection can occur or the disease may be transmitted to other people through sexual activity.*
- Teach abstinence from sexual contact until client and partners are cured and to use condoms to prevent future infections. *Abstinence until the organism is eradicated prevents reinfection. Condoms provide barrier protection, reducing the risk of infection during sexual activity.*
- Emphasize the importance of returning for follow-up testing at 3- and 6-month intervals for early syphilis, and 6- and 12-month intervals for late latent syphilis. *Follow-up testing is performed to assure eradication of the disease.*
- Provide information about signs and symptoms of reinfection. *Successful treatment of the disease does not prevent possible subsequent infections.*

### Anxiety

The diagnosis of syphilis understandably causes the client anxiety, not only about personal well-being but about the well-being of partners and, in the expectant woman, her fetus.

- Emphasize that syphilis can be effectively treated, preventing the serious complications of late-stage disease. *This information provides a sense of control and helps decrease anxiety.*
- Teach the pregnant client that taking medications as directed and returning each month for follow-up testing will help ensure the well-being of her baby. *Knowing that treatment can reduce the risk to her baby relieves anxiety and possibly increases compliance.*

### Low Self-Esteem

Living with any chronic disease can be damaging to a person's self-esteem. However, the client with syphilis or any STI needs additional support to cope with the stigma of this kind of infection. Unfortunately, the populations most affected by STIs often lack family and other social support networks.

- Create an environment where the client feels respected and safe to discuss questions and concerns about the disease and its effect on the client's life. *Being treated with respect helps enhance self-esteem.*
- Provide privacy and confidentiality. *Clients are often embarrassed to discuss the intimate details of their sex lives.*
- Let clients know that the nurse and other health care providers care about them and the successful treatment of their disease. *Feeling valued enhances self-esteem.*

### Home Care

Education is an essential part of nursing care for the client with any STI, and syphilis is no exception. The nurse emphasizes that syphilis is a chronic disease that can be spread to others even though no symptoms are evident. Address the following topics.

- Taking any and all prescribed medication
- Referring sexual partners for evaluation and treatment
- Abstaining from all sexual contact for a minimum of 1 month after treatment
- Using a condom to avoid transmitting or contracting infections in the future
- The need for follow-up testing (at 3 and 6 months for clients with primary or secondary syphilis, and at 6 and 12 months for those with late-stage disease). If clients are HIV-positive, follow-up visits are recommended 1, 2, 3, 6, 9, and 12 months after treatment

## THE CLIENT WITH PELVIC INFLAMMATORY DISEASE

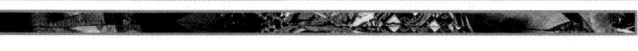

**Pelvic inflammatory disease (PID)** is a term used to describe infection of the pelvic organs, including the fallopian tubes (**salpingitis**), ovaries (**oophoritis**), cervix (**cervicitis**), endometrium (**endometritis**), pelvic peritoneum, and the pelvic vascular system. PID can be caused by one or more infectious agents, including *Neisseria gonorrhoeae, Chlamydia trachomatis, Escherichia coli,* and *Mycoplasma hominis. N. gonorrhoeae* and *C. trachomatis* are responsible for as much as 80% of PID; dual infection with both agents is common.

PID is not a reportable disease in the United States; however, it is estimated that about 1 million women experience PID each year. As a result of the infection, more than 100,000 women become infertile and a large proportion of the ectopic pregnancies occurring each year are the result of PID. The disease may also cause pelvic abscesses and chronic abdominal pain.

Sexually active women ages 16 to 24 years are most at risk. Risk factors include a history of sexually transmitted disease (especially gonorrhea and chlamydia), bacterial vaginosis,

## Nursing Care Plan
## A Client with Syphilis

Eddie Kratz, age 22, works as a bellman at a large hotel. For the past year, he has shared a small apartment with Marla Jones, who is 5 months pregnant with his child. Although he intends to marry Ms. Jones before the baby is born, he has continued a previous relationship with a woman named Justine Simpson. His sexual activities with Ms. Simpson have increased in frequency as Ms. Jones's pregnancy has advanced. Recently Mr. Kratz has noticed a swelling in his groin and a sore on his penis.

### ASSESSMENT

When Mr. Kratz comes to the community clinic, he is interviewed by the nurse practitioner, Sally Morovitz. She takes a thorough medical and sexual history, including questions about drug use, allergies, difficulty with urination, urinary frequency, itching or discharge from the penis, recent sexual activities, precautions taken against infection, history of STIs, and sexual function. She determines that Mr. Kratz has been having unprotected sex with both Ms. Jones and Ms. Simpson. He believes that Ms. Jones is not having sex with anyone except him, but he is not sure.

Physical assessment reveals a classic syphilitic chancre on the shaft of the penis and regional lymphadenopathy. A specimen of exudate from the chancre is sent for darkfield examination. Ms. Morovitz discusses with Mr. Kratz the likelihood that he has syphilis and the need to tell both Ms. Jones and Ms. Simpson so that they can be tested and, if necessary, treated. Ms. Morovitz also suggests that Mr. Kratz be tested for HIV since he has been having unprotected sex with two women, at least one of whom may be sexually active with other partners. He agrees, and blood is drawn for an ELISA test. Darkfield analysis of the chancre exudate confirms the diagnosis of syphilis; the ELISA results are negative for HIV.

### DIAGNOSES

- *Risk for injury* to the client, his partners, and the infant, related to the disease process
- *Ineffective health maintenance* related to a lack of knowledge about the disease process, its transmission, and the need for treatment
- *Interrupted family processes* related to the effects of the diagnosis of syphilis on the couple's relationship
- *Anxiety* related to the effects of the infection on the unborn child

### EXPECTED OUTCOMES

- Prompt treatment will cure the syphilis.

- Will verbalize understanding for the need to abstain from sexual contact during treatment, complete all medications, return for follow-up visits, and use condoms to prevent reinfection.
- Will verbalize ability to cope with the effect of diagnosis and treatment on the relationship.
- Will verbalize decreased anxiety following education and treatment.

### PLANNING AND IMPLEMENTATION

- Administer IM injection of benzathine penicillin G as ordered, and document.
- Discuss the importance of abstaining from sexual activity until he and his partners are cured, and of using condoms to prevent reinfection.
- Explain the need to return for follow-up testing in 3 months and again at 6 months. Provide a copy of the STI prevention checklist, and document that reminders need to be sent at 3- and 6-month intervals.
- Notify sexual partners that they need to come to the clinic for testing.
- Refer to a social worker for counseling about the impact of the disease on their relationship.
- Teach the couple about the importance of treatment to the health of their infant.

### EVALUATION

At the 3-month follow-up visit, the chancre on Mr. Kratz's penis has healed, and he reports that he is using a condom any time he has sex. Ms. Jones has also tested positive for syphilis and negative for HIV, so she, too, is given benzathine penicillin G, and verbal and written follow-up instructions, including follow-up until the infant is born. The couple is meeting every other week with the social worker and say that their relationship is improving. Ms. Simpson has received similar test results and is given a prescription for doxycycline because she is allergic to penicillin.

### Critical Thinking in the Nursing Process

1. What signs and symptoms might a client with early syphilis experience?
2. List some appropriate questions for taking a sexual history when you suspect the presence of one or more STIs.
3. How might you counsel Mr. Kratz to help him break the news of the diagnosis to Ms. Jones?

See Evaluating Your Response in Appendix C.

---

multiple sexual partners, douching, and previous PID. Oral contraceptives and barrier contraceptive devices such as condoms reduce the risk of PID.

The prognosis depends on the number of episodes, promptness of treatment, and modification of risk-taking behaviors. Prevention includes educating women, especially young women, regarding the causes and transmission of infection and methods of self-protection, such as appropriate personal hygiene and avoiding unprotected sexual activity.

## PATHOPHYSIOLOGY AND MANIFESTATIONS

Pelvic inflammatory disease is usually polymicrobial (caused by more than one microbe) in origin. Pathogenic microorganisms enter the vagina and travel to the uterus during intercourse or other sexual activity. They can also gain direct access to the uterus during childbirth, abortion, or surgery of the reproductive tract. The organisms ascend to the endocervical canal to the fallopian tubes and ovaries. Abscess formation is common.

Manifestations of PID include fever, purulent vaginal discharge, severe lower abdominal pain, and a painful cervical movement. However, the manifestations may be so mild that the infection is not recognized. Complications include pelvic abscess, infertility, ectopic pregnancy, chronic pelvic pain, pelvic adhesions, dyspareunia, and chronic pelvic pain.

## COLLABORATIVE CARE

The goals of treatment are to eliminate the infection and prevent complications and recurrence. The physical examination may reveal abdominal, adnexal, and cervical pain.

### Diagnostic Tests

Tests used in the diagnosis of PID may include the following:

- *CBC* with differential reveals a markedly elevated WBC.
- *Sedimentation rate* increases with infection.
- *Laparoscopy* or *laparotomy* may reveal inflammation, edema, or hyperemia of the fallopian tubes, or tubal discharge and, possibly, generalized pelvic involvement, abscesses, and scarring.

### Medications

Combination antibiotic therapy with at least two broad-spectrum antibiotics administered IV or orally is the typical treatment for PID. If PID is not acute, outpatient antibiotic therapy is prescribed. In acute cases, however, the client may be hospitalized. Analgesics are given, and antibiotics and fluids are administered intravenously. Commonly prescribed antibiotics include doxycycline (Vibramycin), cefoxitin (Mefoxin), clindamycin (Cleocin), gentamicin (Garamycin), ofloxacin (Floxin), and ceftriaxone (Rocephin). The antiprotozoal agent, metronidazole (Flagyl) may also be administered. Nursing implications for these drugs are discussed in Chapter 8. ⊙⊘

### Surgery

The surgeon may insert a drain into an abscess, if present, and remove any adhesions. If the client does not respond to conservative therapy, surgical removal of the uterus, uterine tubes, and ovaries may be necessary.

## NURSING CARE

### Nursing Diagnoses and Interventions

The goals of nursing care are to treat the infection and to prevent complications, such as scarring and infertility. The client who is hospitalized maintains bed rest in the semi-Fowler's position to promote drainage and to localize the infectious process in the pelvic cavity. Nursing diagnoses that often apply to the client with PID are described below.

### Risk for Injury

PID can have severe, even life-threatening, complications. Scarring of fallopian tubes can lead to ectopic pregnancy or pelvic abscess. Infertility is a common complication, as are re-

current or chronic PID, chronic abdominal pain, pelvic adhesions, premature hysterectomy, and depression.

- Administer antibiotic therapy as ordered, and monitor closely for adverse effects. *Antibiotics used in acute PID are potent agents; some can have life-threatening side effects.*
- Practice thorough handwashing and strict adherence to universal precautions when handling perineal pads and linens. Appropriate disinfection of bedpans, toilet seats, linens, and utensils is also important. *These practices help avoid disseminating the infection to others.*

### Deficient Knowledge

PID is most common in young women, many of whom have limited understanding of their own anatomy and physiology, and of sexually transmitted disease. Diagnosis and treatment of PID offer an opportunity to increase that understanding, thereby preventing complications and recurrent infection.

- Explain how infection is spread and what measures to take to prevent future infection. *Understanding can improve compliance with treatment regimens and perhaps change high-risk behavior.*
- Explain the need to complete the treatment regimen and the importance of follow-up visits. If the client or partner fails to take all of the medication as prescribed, the infection may not be completely cured. *Noncompliance and recurrence are common, particularly if follow-up appointments are not kept.*
- Teach proper perineal care, especially wiping from front to back. *This reduces transmission of fecal organisms to reproductive tissues and reduces the incidence of urinary tract infections.*
- Caution the client about using tampons, particularly if they previously have caused problems. Instruct the client to change tampons or pads at least every 4 hours. *Menstrual flow and other discharges provide a favorable environment for microorganisms to multiply.*
- Provide information about safer sex practices and family planning. Instruct the client to remove diaphragms within 6 hours after use. IUDs are contraindicated. Latex condoms offer the most effective protection against infection. *These measures help prevent recurrence of infection.*
- Teach the client to report any unusual vaginal discharge or odor to the health care provider. *Treatment is most effective early in the disease process.*

### Home Care

Teach measures to eradicate the infection and prevent recurrence, and help the client deal with the physical and psychosocial implications of treatment, including possible infertility. Provide general information related to sexually transmitted diseases. Inform the client that the patency of the fallopian tubes can be evaluated after several menstrual cycles; this delay allows for complete resolution of the inflammatory process.

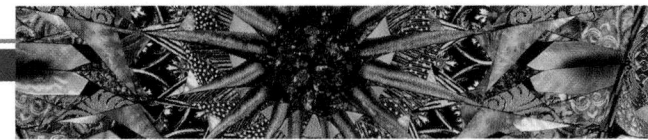

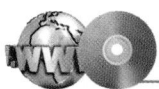

## EXPLORE MediaLink

NCLEX review questions, case studies, care plan activities, MediaLink applications, and other interactive resources for this chapter can be found on the Companion Website at www.prenhall.com/lemone.

Click on Chapter 49 to select the activities for this chapter. For animations, video clips, more NCLEX review questions, and an audio glossary, access the Student CD-ROM accompanying this textbook.

## TEST YOURSELF

1. Which population is most often affected by STIs?
   a. Men
   b. Women and infants
   c. Adolescent males
   d. Older adults

2. Which of the following statements would indicate a client understands teaching to treat an STI?
   a. "My sex partner and I must both take medications."
   b. "I know I can never have sex again."
   c. "I will douche after every sexual encounter with my partner."
   d. "My sex partner does not have an infection, so won't need medications."

3. You are assessing a young male. He has both blisters and ulcerations on the shaft of his penis. What is his most likely medical diagnosis?
   a. Chlamydia
   b. Gonorrhea

   c. Genital warts
   d. Genital herpes

4. The infective organism responsible for gonorrhea *initially* targets what body parts?
   a. Male urethra and female cervix
   b. Female vulva and vagina
   c. Male prostate
   d. Male and female external genitalia

5. Which of the following is true about syphilis?
   a. Syphilis is caused by a virus
   b. Syphilis is transmitted only through intimate genital contact
   c. Syphilis is spread through the blood and lymphatic system
   d. Syphilis has no effect on the developing fetus

See Test Yourself answers in Appendix C.

## BIBLIOGRAPHY

Centers for Disease Control and Prevention. (1998). Guidelines for treatment of sexually transmitted diseases. *MMWR, 47* (No. RR-1).

Centers for Disease Control and Prevention. (2001a). *Division of sexually transmitted diseases; facts.* Available www.cdc.gov/nchstp/dstd/Fact_Sheets

_____. (2001b). National Center for Health Statistics. *Fastats A to Z: Sexually transmitted disease* Available www.cdc.gov/nchswww/fastats/stds.htm

_____. (2000). *STD surveillance 2000.* Available www.cdc.gov/std/stats/2000NatOverview.htm

Champion, J., Piper, J., Shain, R., Perdue, S., & Newton, E. (2001). Minority women with sexually transmitted diseases: Sexual abuse and risk for pelvic inflammatory disease. *Research in Nursing & Health, 24*(1), 38–43.

Currie, S. (2001). Sexually transmitted infections and older people. *Elderly Care, 12*(1), 15–19.

Hutchinson, M., Sosa, D., & Thompson, A. (2001). Sexual protective strategies of late adolescent females: More than just condoms. *JOGHN-*

*Journal of Obstetric, Gynecologic, & Neonatal Nursing, 30*(4), 429–438.

McCance, K., & Huether, S. (2002). *Pathophysiology: The biologic basis for disease in adults & children* (4th ed.). St. Louis: Mosby.

McEwan, A., & Pittam, D. (2001). Clinical update: Sexually transmissible infections. *Australian Nursing Journal, 9*(2) (insert 1-4), 23–26.

Miller, K., & Graves, J. (2000). Update on the prevention and treatment of sexually transmitted diseases. *American Family Physician, 61*(2), 379–386.

Nicholas, H. (1998). Sexually transmitted diseases. Gonorrhoea: Symptoms and treatment. *Nursing Times, 94*(8), 52–54.

North American Nursing Diagnosis Association. (2001). *Nursing diagnoses: Definitions and classification 2001–2002.* Philadelphia: NANDA.

Porth, C. M. (2002). *Pathophysiology: Concepts of altered health states* (6th ed.). Philadelphia: Lippincott.

Ricchini, W. (1997). Break the silence: Talking to your patients about STDs. *Advance for Nurse Practitioners, 5*(6), 55–56, 83.

Shannon, M., Wilson, B., & Stang, C. (2002). *Health professional's drug guide 2002.* Upper Saddle River, NJ: Prentice Hall.

Slade, C. S. (1998). HPV and cervical cancer: Breaking the deadly link. *Advance for Nurse Practitioners, 6*(3), 39–40, 42, 54.

Swanson, J., Dibble, S., & Chenitz, W. (1995). Clinical features and psychosocial factors in young adults with genital herpes. *Image: Journal of Nursing Scholarship, 27*(1), 16–22.

Thomas, D. (2001). Sexually transmitted viral infections: Epidemiology and treatment. *Journal of Obstetric, Gynecologic, & Neonatal Nursing, 30*(3), 316–323.

Tierney, L. M., McPhee, S. J., & Papadakis, M. A. (Eds.). (2001). *Current medical diagnosis & treatment* (40th ed.). Stamford, CT: Appleton & Lange.

Weston, A. (1998). Striking back at syphilis. *Nursing Times, 94*(3), 30–32.

_____. (1998). Warts and all. *Nursing Times, 94*(3), 26–28.

Wright, T. (1998). Genital warts: Their etiology and treatment. *Nursing Times, 94*(7), 52–54.

# APPENDIX A

## Standard Precautions

Standard precautions are designed to reduce the risk of transmission of microorganisms from both recognized and unrecognized sources of infection. They are the primary strategies for preventing nosocomial infections within institutions, and are important to protect health care workers as well. Standard precautions apply to (1) blood; (2) all body fluids, secretions, and excretions except sweat, regardless of whether or not they contain visible blood; (3) nonintact skin; and (4) mucous membranes. Standard precautions are applied to all clients receiving care in hospitals, regardless of their diagnosis or presumed infection status. These precautions are specifically designed for hospitals; however, they also may be implemented in extended and long-term care facilities, and to a more limited extent in providing home care or in other community-based care settings.

### HANDWASHING

- Wash your hands (a) after touching blood, body fluids, secretions, excretions, and contaminated items, whether or not gloves are worn; (b) immediately after removing gloves, even if gloves appear to be intact; (c) between contacts with clients; and (d) when otherwise indicated to prevent transfer of organisms to other clients. You may need to wash your hands between tasks and procedures on the same client to prevent cross-contaminating different body sites.

- Use soap and warm water for handwashing when hands are visibly dirty or contaminated with blood or other body fluids.

- If hands are not visibly soiled, use an alcohol-based hand rub for routinely decontaminating hands in all other situations.

### GLOVES

- Wear clean, nonsterile gloves when touching blood, body fluids, secretions, excretions, and contaminated items.

- Put on clean gloves just before touching mucous membranes and nonintact skin.

- Change your gloves between tasks and procedures on the same client after contacting material that may contain a high concentration of microorganisms.

- Wear gloves for all invasive procedures such as performing venipuncture or other vascular or surgical procedures.

- Wear gloves if you have cuts, scratches, or other breaks in the skin.

- Remove gloves promptly after use, before touching noncontaminated items and surfaces, and before going to another client; wash hands immediately after removing gloves.

### MASK, EYE PROTECTION, FACE SHIELD

Wear a mask and eye protection or a face shield to protect mucous membranes of your eyes, nose, and mouth during procedures and client care activities that are likely to generate splashes or sprays of blood, body fluids, secretions, or excretions.

### GOWN

Wear a gown (clean, disposable) to protect your skin and prevent soiling of clothing during procedures and client care activities that are likely to generate splashes or sprays of blood, body fluids, secretions, or excretions. Remove soiled gowns promptly, washing your hands immediately after gown removal.

### EQUIPMENT

Handle used client care equipment that is soiled with blood, body fluids, secretions, and excretions in a way that prevents exposing your skin and mucous membranes, contaminating your clothing, and transferring microorganisms to other clients or environments. Ensure that reusable equipment is cleaned and appropriately reprocessed before using for the care of another client.

### ENVIRONMENTAL CONTROL

Follow hospital procedures for routine care, cleaning, and disinfecting environmental surfaces, beds, bed rails, bedside equipment, and other frequently touched surfaces.

### LINEN

Handle and transport linens soiled with blood, body fluids, secretions, and excretions in a manner that prevents exposing your skin and mucous membranes, contaminating your clothing, and transferring microorganisms to other clients and environments. Place soiled linen in leakage-resistant bags at the location where it is used.

### OCCUPATIONAL HEALTH AND BLOODBORNE PATHOGENS

- Take care to prevent injuries when using needles, scalpels, and other sharps; when handling sharp instruments after

*Sources.* Centers for Disease Control and Prevention (2002). Guidelines for hand hygiene in health-care settings: Recommendations of the Healthcare Infection Control Practices Advisory Committee and the HICPAC/SHEA/ APIC/IDSA Hand Hygiene Taskforce. *MMWR, 51*(RR-16), 1–56; Hospital Infection Control Practices Advisory Committee (1997). Part II. Recommendations for isolation precautions in hospitals. Atlanta: Public Health Service, U.S. Department of Health and Human Services, Centers for Disease Control and Prevention.

procedures; when cleaning used instruments; and when disposing of used needles.

- Never recap used needles, manipulate them using both hands, or handle them in a manner that directs the point of a needle toward any part of your body. If it is necessary to protect the needle prior to disposal, use a one-handed "scoop" technique or mechanical device to hold the needle sheath.

- Do not remove used needles from disposable syringes by hand; do not bend, break, or otherwise manipulate used needles by hand.

- Place used disposable syringes and needles, scalpel blades, and other sharp items in appropriate puncture-resistant containers located as close as practical to the area in which the items were used.

- Place reusable syringes and needles in a puncture-resistant container for transport to the reprocessing area.

- Use mouthpieces, resuscitation bags, or other ventilation devices as an alternative to mouth-to-mouth resuscitation methods whenever possible.

## CLIENT PLACEMENT

Place clients who contaminate the environment or who do not (or are not expected to) assist in maintaining appropriate hygiene or environmental control (e.g., an ambulatory, confused client with fecal incontinence) in a private room.

# 2003–2004 NANDA-Approved Nursing Diagnoses

Activity Intolerance
Activity Intolerance, Risk for
Adaptive Capacity: Intracranial, Decreased
Adjustment, Impaired
Airway Clearance, Ineffective
Anxiety
Anxiety, Death
Aspiration, Risk for
Attachment, Parent/Infant/Child, Risk for Impaired
Body Image, Disturbed
Body Temperature: Imbalanced, Risk for
Bowel Incontinence
Breastfeeding, Effective
Breastfeeding, Ineffective
Breastfeeding, Interrupted
Breathing Pattern, Ineffective
Cardiac Output, Decreased
Caregiver Role Strain
Caregiver Role Strain, Risk for
Communication, Readiness for Enhanced
Communication: Verbal, Impaired
Confusion, Acute
Confusion, Chronic
Constipation
Constipation, Perceived
Constipation, Risk for
Coping: Community, Ineffective
Coping: Community, Readiness for Enhanced
Coping, Defensive
Coping: Family, Compromised
Coping: Family, Disabled
Coping: Family, Readiness for Enhanced
Coping (Individual), Readiness for Enhanced
Coping, Ineffective
Decisional Conflict (Specify)
Denial, Ineffective
Dentition, Impaired
Development: Delayed, Risk for
Diarrhea
Disuse Syndrome, Risk for
Diversional Activity, Deficient
Dysreflexia, Autonomic
Dysreflexia, Autonomic, Risk for
Energy Field, Disturbed
Environmental Interpretation Syndrome, Impaired
Failure to Thrive, Adult
Falls, Risk for
Family Processes, Dysfunctional: Alcoholism
Family Processes, Interrupted
Family Processes, Readiness for Enhanced
Fatigue
Fear
Fluid Balance, Readiness for Enhanced
Fluid Volume, Deficient
Fluid Volume, Deficient, Risk for
Fluid Volume, Excess
Fluid Volume, Imbalanced, Risk for
Gas Exchange, Impaired
Grieving, Anticipatory
Grieving, Dysfunctional
Growth, Disproportionate, Risk for
Growth and Development, Delayed

Health Maintenance, Ineffective
Health-Seeking Behaviors (Specify)
Home Maintenance, Impaired
Hopelessness
Hyperthermia
Hypothermia
Identity: Personal, Disturbed
Infant Behavior, Disorganized
Infant Behavior: Disorganized, Risk for
Infant Behavior: Organized, Readiness for Enhanced
Infant Feeding Pattern, Ineffective
Infection, Risk for
Injury, Risk for
Knowledge, Deficient (Specify)
Knowledge (Specify), Readiness for Enhanced
Latex Allergy Response
Latex Allergy Response, Risk for
Loneliness, Risk for
Memory, Impaired
Mobility: Bed, Impaired
Mobility: Physical, Impaired
Mobility: Wheelchair, Impaired
Nausea
Neurovascular Dysfunction: Peripheral, Risk for
Noncompliance (Specify)
Nutrition, Imbalanced: Less than Body Requirements
Nutrition, Imbalanced: More than Body Requirements
Nutrition, Imbalanced: More than Body Requirements, Risk for
Nutrition, Readiness for Enhanced
Oral Mucous Membrane, Impaired
Pain, Acute
Pain, Chronic
Parenting, Impaired
Parenting, Readiness for Enhanced
Parenting, Risk for Impaired
Perioperative Positioning Injury, Risk for
Poisoning, Risk for
Posttrauma Syndrome
Posttrauma Syndrome, Risk for
Powerlessness
Powerlessness, Risk for
Protection, Ineffective
Rape-Trauma Syndrome
Rape-Trauma Syndrome: Compound Reaction
Rape-Trauma Syndrome: Silent Reaction
Relocation Stress Syndrome
Relocation Stress Syndrome, Risk for
Role Conflict, Parental
Role Performance, Ineffective
Self-Care Deficit: Bathing/Hygiene
Self-Care Deficit: Dressing/Grooming
Self-Care Deficit: Feeding
Self-Care Deficit: Toileting
Self-Concept, Readiness for Enhanced
Self-Esteem, Chronic Low
Self-Esteem, Situational Low
Self-Esteem, Risk for Situational Low
Self-Mutilation

Self-Mutilation, Risk for
Sensory Perception, Disturbed (Specify: Visual, Auditory, Kinesthetic, Gustatory, Tactile, Olfactory)
Sexual Dysfunction
Sexuality Patterns, Ineffective
Skin Integrity, Impaired
Skin Integrity, Risk for Impaired
Sleep Deprivation
Sleep Pattern Disturbed
Sleep, Readiness for Enhanced
Social Interaction, Impaired
Social Isolation
Sorrow, Chronic
Spiritual Distress
Spiritual Distress, Risk for
Spiritual Well-Being, Readiness for Enhanced
Spontaneous Ventilation, Impaired
Sudden Infant Death Syndrome, Risk for
Suffocation, Risk for
Suicide, Risk for
Surgical Recovery, Delayed
Swallowing, Impaired
Therapeutic Regimen Management: Community, Ineffective
Therapeutic Regimen Management, Effective
Therapeutic Regimen Management: Family, Ineffective
Therapeutic Regimen Management, Ineffective
Therapeutic Regimen Management, Readiness for Enhanced
Thermoregulation, Ineffective
Thought Processes, Disturbed
Tissue Integrity, Impaired
Tissue Perfusion, Ineffective (Specify: Renal, Cerebral, Cardiopulmonary, Gastrointestinal, Peripheral)
Transfer Ability, Impaired
Trauma, Risk for
Unilateral Neglect
Urinary Elimination, Impaired
Urinary Elimination, Readiness for Enhanced
Urinary Incontinence, Functional
Urinary Incontinence, Reflex
Urinary Incontinence, Stress
Urinary Incontinence, Total
Urinary Incontinence, Urge
Urinary Incontinence, Risk for Urge
Urinary Retention
Ventilatory Weaning Response, Dysfunctional
Violence: Other-Directed, Risk for
Violence: Self-Directed, Risk for
Walking, Impaired
Wandering

*Source. NANDA Nursing Diagnoses: Definitions and Classification, 2003–2004.* Philadelphia: North American Nursing Diagnosis Association. Used with permission.

# APPENDIX C

## Evaluate Your Response and Test Yourself Answers

### Answers to Test Yourself

Chapter 1: The Medical-Surgical Nurse
1. D 2. A 3. B 4. C 5. C

Chapter 2: The Adult Client in Health and Illness 1. D 2. A 3. B 4. B 5. B

Chapter 3: Community-Based and Home Care of the Adult Client 1. B 2. D 3. C 4. A 5. B

Chapter 4: Nursing Care of Clients in Pain 1. B 2. A 3. B 4. D 5. C

Chapter 5: Nursing Care of Clients with Altered Fluid, Electrolyte, or Acid-Base Balance 1. A 2. D 3. B 4. D 5. A

Chapter 6: Nursing Care of Clients Experiencing Trauma and Shock 1. D 2. A 3. B 4. C 5. B

Chapter 7: Nursing Care of Clients Having Surgery 1. B 2. D 3. C 4. B 5. D

Chapter 8: Nursing Care of Clients with Infection 1. C 2. B 3. D 4. A 5. B

Chapter 9: Nursing Care of Clients with Altered Immunity 1. D 2. A 3. C 4. D 5. B

Chapter 10: Nursing Care of Clients with Cancer 1. C 2. A 3. C 4. B 5. C

Chapter 11: Nursing Care of Clients Experiencing Loss, Grief, and Death 1. C 2. D 3. B 4. A 5. C

Chapter 12: Nursing Care of Clients with Problems of Substance Abuse 1. B 2. A 3. D 4. C 5. B

Chapter 13: Assessing Clients with Integumentary Disorders 1. B 2. C 3. A 4. D 5. D

Chapter 14: Nursing Care of Clients with Integumentary Disorders 1. C 2. B 3. D 4. A 5. B

Chapter 15: Nursing Care of Clients with Burns 1. A 2. C 3. D 4. B 5. C

Chapter 16: Assessing Clients with Endocrine Disorders 1. D 2. A 3. C 4. B 5. B

Chapter 17: Nursing Care of Clients with Endocrine Disorders 1. A 2. C 3. C 4. D 5. B

Chapter 18: Nursing Care of Clients with Diabetes Mellitus 1. A 2. C 3. D 4. C 5. C

Chapter 19: Assessing Clients with Nutritional and Gastrointestinal Disorders 1. A 2. C 3. D 4. A 5. D

Chapter 20: Nursing Care of Clients with Nutritional Disorders 1. C 2. B 3. A 4. C 5. D

Chapter 21: Nursing Care of Clients with Upper Gastrointestinal Disorders 1. D 2. B 3. A 4. D 5. C

Chapter 22: Nursing Care of Clients with Gallbladder, Liver, and Pancreatic Disorders 1. A 2. C 3. D 4. B 5. C

Chapter 23: Assessing Clients with Bowel Elimination Disorders 1. D 2. A 3. D 4. D 5. C

Chapter 24: Nursing Care of Clients with Bowel Disorders 1. B 2. C 3. A 4. D 5. B

Chapter 25: Assessing Clients with Urinary System Disorders 1. D 2. C 3. B 4. C 5. A

Chapter 26: Nursing Care of Clients with Urinary Tract Disorders 1. B 2. D 3. A 4. C 5. C

Chapter 27: Nursing Care of Clients with Kidney Disorders 1. B 2. D 3. A 4. C 5. B

Chapter 28: Assessing Clients with Cardiac Disorders 1. C 2. D 3. C 4. A 5. B

Chapter 29: Nursing Care of Clients with Coronary Heart Disease 1. C 2. B 3. D 4. A 5. B

Chapter 30: Nursing Care of Clients with Cardiac Disorders 1. A 2. C 3. B 4. D 5. C

Chapter 31: Assessing Clients with Hematologic, Peripheral Vascular, and Lymphatic Disorders 1. D 2. A 3. B 4. C 5. A

Chapter 32: Nursing Care of Clients with Hematologic Disorders 1. C 2. D 3. A 4. B 5. A

Chapter 33: Nursing Care of Clients with Peripheral Vascular and Lymphatic Disorders 1. C 2. A 3. D 4. B 5. A

Chapter 34: Assessing Clients with Respiratory Disorders 1. D 2. C 3. B 4. D 5. C

Chapter 35: Nursing Care of Clients with Upper Respiratory Disorders 1. B 2. D 3. C 4. A 5. C

Chapter 36: Nursing Care of Clients with Lower Respiratory Disorders 1. D 2. B 3. A 4. C 5. D

Chapter 37: Assessing Clients with Musculo-skeletal Disorders 1. C 2. A 3. B 4. D 5. A

Chapter 38: Nursing Care of Clients with Musculoskeletal Trauma 1. B 2. C 3. C 4. A 5. D

Chapter 39: Nursing Care of Clients with Musculoskeletal Disorders 1. B 2. D 3. D 4. A 5. C

Chapter 40: Assessing Clients with Neurologic Disorders 1. D 2. C 3. B 4. A 5. B

Chapter 41: Nursing Care of Clients with Cerebrovascular and Spinal Cord Disorders 1. B 2. D 3. C 4. A 5. B

Chapter 42: Nursing Care of Clients with Intracranial Disorders 1. D 2. B 3. B 4. A 5. C

Chapter 43: Nursing Care of Clients with Neurologic Disorders 1. C 2. A 3. B 4. D 5. B

Chapter 44: Assessing Clients with Eye or Ear Disorders 1. B 2. C 3. A 4. D 5. C

Chapter 45: Nursing Care of Clients with Eye and Ear Disorders 1. B 2. D 3. C 4. A 5. D

Chapter 46: Assessing Clients with Reproductive System Disorders 1. C 2. D 3. A 4. C 5. B

Chapter 47: Nursing Care of Men with Reproductive System Disorders 1. D 2. A 3. B 4. B 5. C

Chapter 48: Nursing Care of Women with Reproductive System Disorders 1. B 2. A 3. B 4. D 5. C

Chapter 49: Nursing Care of Clients with Sexually Transmitted Infections 1. B 2. A 3. D 4. A 5. C

### Evaluate Your Response: Cues for Critical Thinking Questions

Chapter 4: Nursing Care of Clients in Pain

A Client with Chronic Pain

1. Review the factors that affect an individual's response to pain. What have you observed in your own family and friends, as well as clients for whom you have cared?

2. Reflect on the benefits and disadvantages of each alternative. Make your decision based on knowledge about pain and about medications for pain.

3. What factors in Ms. Akers's illness and treatment increase her risk for constipation? What would you include in the plan specific to fluid intake and diet?

## Chapter 5: Nursing Care of Clients with Altered Fluid, Electrolyte, or Acid-Base Balance

### A Client with Fluid Volume Excess

1. Review the homeostatic mechanisms that control fluid balance and cardiac output. Which mechanisms are employed in this situation?

2. Review the anatomy and physiology of the respiratory system, including cardiopulmonary blood flow. Think about the effects of the upper abdominal organs on respiratory function as well.

3. Use therapeutic communication techniques: What is behind the client's statement? How can you facilitate Mrs. Rainwater's involvement in care decisions?

4. Review the actions and precautions for diuretic therapy. Think about what the client needs to know in terms of timing, possible adverse effects, and other information about diuretic therapy.

### A Client with Hypokalemia

1. Review the physiologic effects of potassium, especially its intracellular and neuromuscular effects.

2. Review the potential sites and causes of excess potassium loss.

3. Think about the effects of diuretics on potassium balance and the effects of hypokalemia on digitalis therapy. What is the primary indication for digitalis therapy and how does this contribute to the interaction of these three factors?

4. Review the section in Chapter 24 on constipation and its management. 

### A Client with Hyperkalemia

1. Review the causes and manifestations of hyperkalemia.

2. What are the potential effects of hyperkalemia on cardiac conduction? At what level of hyperkalemia are these likely to be seen?

3. Review collaborative treatment measures to rapidly reduce potassium levels. Why would these be used with a K+ of 8.5?

4. Think about the effects of anxiety on learning as you develop a plan to provide teaching to avoid future episodes of hyperkalemia. As you develop your plan, remember the potential long-term effects of chronic renal failure.

### A Client with Acute Respiratory Acidosis

1. Review normal gas exchange across the alveolar-capillary membrane and the processes that drive this exchange. Then review the role that carbon dioxide plays as a potential acid.

2. Describe the effect of acidosis on mental function.

3. Consider risk factors for choking: alcohol consumption, taking large bites of food, inadequate chewing, and so forth.

## Chapter 6: Nursing Care of Clients Experiencing Trauma and Shock

### A Client with Multiple Injuries

1. The definition of *Deficient fluid volume* is decreased intravascular, interstitial, and/or intracellular fluid. Which of Mrs. Souza's vital signs would support this definition? What other assessments could you make that would further support this diagnosis?

2. Consider the physiology of cellular metabolism. How long do brain cells live without oxygen? What happens if circulation is improved but the airway is blocked?

3. What can cause restlessness? Consider comfort, elimination, oxygenation, emotional status, and immobility.

4. List the multiple possibilities for entry of pathogens into the human body. Would age and physical condition increase the risk? What about transmission from health care personnel?

### A Client with Septic Shock

1. Review the pharmacologic effects of vasopressors. Consider the pathologic basis for septic shock and how these medications may be effective.

2. Review the content on respiratory acidosis in Chapter 5.  What do these findings tell you? What is present in Ms. Huang's physical status that would cause these manifestations?

3. Review the content about colloidal intravenous solutions in the chapter. What would you expect them to do when they are administered? How does this correlate to cardiac output? How do you assess increased circulatory volume?

## Chapter 7: Nursing Care of Clients Having Surgery

### A Client Having Surgery

1. Safety concerns include ambulating and not tripping over scatter rugs or clutter. See information in Chapter 3 on safety in the home. 

2. Medications used to prevent an occurrence such as infection are called prophylactic medications. Her risks for infection are from the surgical wound and microvascular circulation in bone. Teach her to take the complete course of antibiotics prescribed and the possible side effects of the antibiotic. Encourage her to notify the physician if side effects or adverse events occur.

3. When blood stops flowing, it clots. Her immobility is a concern and puts her at risk for thrombosis and emboli. She has a risk for bleeding secondary to the anticoagulant and should inform any health care providers such as dentists that she is taking the anticoagulant.

4. Consider the risk for osteoporosis in addition to the degenerative changes Mrs. Overbeck experienced. She will need calcium sources and vitamin D.

## Chapter 8: Nursing Care of Clients with Infection

### A Client with Acquired Immunity

1. Review the adult immunizations listed in Table 8–8.  Consider the geographical area in which the client lives. For example, clients living in areas at risk for Lyme disease should check with their physician about the new Lyme disease vaccine.

2. Review the concept of acquired immunity and the discussion of immunization in this chapter. What affect could nonimmunized persons have on their family and community?

3. Identify possible systemic and local reactions associated with immunizations. List manifestations that the client should report to the primary caregiver.

### Chapter 9: Nursing Care of Clients with Altered Immunity

#### A Client with HIV Infection

1. Considering Ms. Lu's age, how effective is her immune system? How could lifestyle factors affect immune status?

2. At this stage of Ms. Lu's diagnosis, would you expect the physician to order a viral load test? Why or why not?

3. You have been asked to discuss AIDS and safe sex practices to a group of high school freshmen. What information would you present to them?

4. What resources could you provide to Ms. Lu and her fiancé regarding their desire to have a child?

### Chapter 10: Nursing Care of Clients with Cancer

1. Review content on altered nutrition in Chapter 20 and the content in this chapter on the nursing diagnosis Altered Nutrition: Less than Body Requirements. Make a list of diagnostic tests for malnutrition with normal values.

2. Consider the type of cancers Mr. Casey has been diagnosed as having. Where in the body do these malignancies commonly metastasize? What would cause the pain?

3. Review a pharmacology book for medications that increase appetite and make a list of those appropriate to Mr. Casey.

4. Sepsis is discussed in Chapter 6. ⊖⊕ Review the content in that chapter on septic shock and outline manifestations. Develop a plan of care for Mr. Casey that is structured by priority of nursing diagnoses.

### Chapter 11: Nursing Care of Clients Experiencing Loss, Grief, and Death

#### A Client Experiencing Loss and Grief

1. Review the physical manifestations of grief described in the chapter and compare and contrast those with the ones verbalized by Mrs. Rogers.

2. Consider the benefits of including Mrs. Rogers's daughter in a meeting of the staff. What type of questions would be most useful in making the daughter feel a part of the plan of care? Why would a statement such as, "Why don't you do more for your mother," be inappropriate?

3. Consider the losses Mrs. Rogers has experienced. Review the material in the chapter on responses to loss. Think about the reasons you would not say, "Oh, you have a lot to live for." Think of two or three questions or statements that would help you assess the reason why Mrs. Rogers said this to you.

### Chapter 12: Nursing Care of Clients with Problems of Substance Abuse

1. Consider the interactions of prescribed or over-the-counter medications with alcohol. What if the client has not taken prescribed medications because of chronic alcoholism?

2. Review the effects of Anatbuse. Make a list of possible interactions and side effects.

3. *Imbalanced nutrition: Less than body requirements* is an appropriate nursing diagnosis when a client does not have sufficient nutritional intake to meet metabolic needs. What in Mr. Russell's history and physical assessment supports this diagnosis? What nutritional information should you provide?

### Chapter 14: Nursing Care of Clients with Integumentary Disorders

#### A Client with Herpes Zoster

1. Consider environmental, economic, and language barriers. What agencies in your own city or state exist to provide help? What can you do other than make referrals? If you do make a referral, to whom would it be?

2. Review skin assessment guidelines in Chapter 13. ⊖⊕ How would you determine that the lesions had not improved? What manifestations would indicate secondary infection of the lesions? What would you do next if the lesions are still very painful and have not improved?

3. *Ineffective role performance* is defined as patterns of behavior and self-expression that do not match the environmental context, norms, and expectations. Related factors include inadequate or inappropriate linkage with the health care system and poverty. Based on this information, what interventions would you use? How would you evaluate the effectiveness of your interventions?

#### A Client with Malignant Melanoma

1. List reasons why people do not seek health care. Do you believe nurses can effect change? If so, what community activities would be most effective?

2. Consider attitudes toward the possibility of future illnesses. How would this affect your plan? What do you believe would be most effective in teaching this age group?

3. Think about what you know about taking prescribed antibiotics as well as the side effects of antibiotic therapy. What would you suggest that Mr. Sanders do?

4. *Powerlessness* is the perception that one's own actions will not significantly affect an outcome. Is this a common response to the diagnosis of cancer? Consider types of communications and interventions that would allow greater decision making for Mr. Sanders.

### Chapter 15: Nursing Care of Clients with Burns

#### A Client with a Major Burn

1. Review the effects of the major burn wound on the renal and gastrointestinal systems. What assessments would indicate effective fluid resuscitation?

2. What type of burns did Mr. Howard have on his arms? Consider the effect of compression on the peripheral vascular system. What assessments would you make to identify this complication?

3. Consider the type of pain the client has. What do you think might happen if the narcotics were given by other routes, such as oral or intramuscularly?

4. Review the effects of a major burn. Consider the damage to cell wall integrity and capillary beds. What effect does the shift of proteins and sodium have on intravascular volume?

## Chapter 17: Nursing Care of Clients with Endocrine Disorders

### A Client with Graves' Disease

1. What effect does increased TH have on metabolism and cardiac rate and stroke volume? How does this effect compare to that of sympathetic stimulation?

2. Consider the effect of elevating any body part, such as elevating your leg above heart level for a sprained ankle. How does this affect venous return?

3. You will need to consider Mrs. Manuel from both a medical and a surgical perspective. How would you teach her to care for her incision? With removal of most of the thyroid gland, what symptoms would you be sure she knew about? What should she do if these occur?

### A Client with Hypothyroidism

1. Make a list of changes in body systems with aging and with decreased TH levels. How would you determine what assessment findings were abnormal?

2. Consider the effects of the following factors: weakness, fatigue, problems with memory. What would you recommend she do in her home to increase her safety?

3. Prepare a list of manifestations of hyperthyroidism. Be sure they are in terms a client would understand.

### A Client with Cushing's Syndrome

1. Review Ms. Domico's lab results and compare them to normal results. What altered the findings in her case?

2. How many ways can you think of to assess fluid balance? Consider weight, I&O, and skin. What other assessments provide information?

3. Review Box 17–3. ⚭ How does fatigue differ from "just being tired"? Would increasing hours of sleep be an intervention you would include? Why or why not?

### A Client with Addison's Disease

1. Review the functions of the hormones of the adrenal cortex in Chapter 16. ⚭ Consider the effects of stress, and formulate your response with rationale.

2. Review content on fluid imbalance in Chapter 5. ⚭ Make a list of assessments you might make that would indicate severe dehydration. What is the pathophysiology of fluid loss in the client with Addison's disease?

3. Review content on sodium and potassium in Chapter 5 ⚭ and make a list of foods you would suggest Mr. Sardoff eat.

## Chapter 18: Nursing Care of Clients with Diabetes Mellitus

### A Client with Type 1 Diabetes

1. How do the increased urinary output and increased osmolarity of the blood plasma affect the fluid status of the body? What is the response of the body to decreased intravascular volume?

2. Consider the effects of nicotine on blood vessels. How would these effects, when combined with the pathologic effects of long-standing hyperglycemia, affect blood vessel walls?

3. Review the information about chronic illness in Chapter 2. ⚭ *Powerlessness* is a perceived lack of control over a situation and/or one's ability to significantly affect an outcome. What types of statements by a client would help you make this nursing diagnosis?

4. Compare and contrast the developmental needs and tasks of the young adult and the older adult (see Chapter 2 ⚭ ). Consider the teaching materials that might have to be adapted to physical changes in the older adult.

## Chapter 20: Nursing Care of Clients with Nutritional Disorders

### A Client with Obesity

1. Review the physiology of cholesterol formation in the body and the factors that affect this process.

2. Consider developmental stages and teaching strategies for adult learners.

3. Think about individual factors, family and support group influences, and cultural factors that may affect recommended weight loss and exercise strategies.

### A Client with Malnutrition

1. Review the physiology of albumin and cholesterol formation in the body.

2. Review Mrs. Chow's diet and compare it to the food pyramid or recommendations for food intake to formulate your response.

3. Consider cultural influences and the client's preferred foods as you plan a diet that is high in calories and protein.

## Chapter 21: Nursing Care of Clients with Upper Gastrointestinal Disorders

### A Client with Oral Cancer

1. Review the major risk factors for oral cancer and identify the populations most likely to have these risk factors.

2. Work with your classmates to plan (and implement) an education program, considering the developmental/teaching needs of this group of young people.

3. Think about the possible causes for Mr. Chavez's refusal to talk (remember that assessment is the first step of the nursing process). How will you identify factors contributing to his behavior?

### A Client with Peptic Ulcer Disease

1. Review the physiology of the gastric mucosal barrier and the pathogenesis of peptic ulcer disease, and the effect of *H. pylori* infection on these processes.

2. Review physiologic responses to stress in your physiology or nursing fundamentals text; compare and apply this information with the physiology of the gastric mucosal barrier and the pathophysiology of ulcer development.

3. Consider Mr. O'Donnell's occupation and schedule, as well as the prescribed medications and when each should be taken.

4. Using journal and text resources as well as your classmates, identify as many stress reduction techniques as possible. Then sort your list into those which could be used while working, and identify ways to effectively teach each technique.

### A Client with Gastric Cancer

1. Review the healing process and the normal physiology of the stomach as you formulate your answer to this question.

2. Consider the surgery, immediate postoperative care, and what the client and family should expect in developing your teaching plan.

3. Review Chapter 10 ⬤ and nursing care related to chemotherapy.

4. Again, review Chapter 10 ⬤ for nursing care measures for clients with cancer; also review Chapter 20 ⬤ for strategies to prevent and manage malnutrition.

### Chapter 22: Nursing Care of Clients with Gallbladder, Liver, and Pancreatic Disorders

### A Client with Cholelithiasis

1. Review the composition of gallstones, as well as the physiology of gallbladder function and bile. Research and discuss dietary practices of the Chickasaw tribe (or of Native Americans).

2. Review Chapter 7 ⬤ for care related to a laparotomy (incision into the abdomen).

3. As you develop your plan, consider Mrs. Red Wing's culture, job, and family obligations.

### A Client with Hepatitis A

1. In your plan, consider the transmission and pathophysiology of hepatitis A. Review developmental considerations when teaching clients to adapt your teaching to Mr. Johns's level.

2. Review Table 22–2, ⬤ as well as the pathophysiology of hepatitis.

3. Review Tables 22–2 and 22–3, ⬤ as well as standard precautions.

4. In your plan, consider the living situation (group home), the developmental level of the residents, and the resident care managers (largely

unskilled). Work with your study or clinical group to develop this plan.

### A Client with Alcoholic Cirrhosis

1. Review the anatomy and physiology of the liver and its circulation, as well as the pathophysiology of cirrhosis and its complications.

2. Consult your nutrition textbook as needed for foods that are high in calories but low in protein and sodium. When planning for limited protein intake, be sure to include high-quality proteins and limit intake of lower-quality proteins such as legumes.

3. Review the pathophysiology of hepatic encephalopathy and the medication box on page 591 ⬤ to develop your responses to this question.

4. Review therapeutic communication skills; consult your nursing diagnosis and care planning text book as you develop this care plan.

### A Client with Acute Pancreatitis

1. Review Chapter 12 ⬤ for assessment data indicative of alcohol withdrawal.

2. Review both the pathophysiology of acute pancreatitis and the acute inflammatory process.

3. Consult your nutrition textbook or the American Dietetic Association web site: www.eatright.org

4. Consult your nursing care planning textbook to develop this care plan.

### Chapter 24: Nursing Care of Clients with Bowel Disorders

### A Client with Acute Appendicitis

1. Review the acute inflammatory response to an infectious process and the role WBCs play in the immune response.

2. Review Chapter 7. ⬤ Consider factors such as incision size, abdominal muscle disruption, and manipulation of the bowel in developing your response.

3. Consider points such as pain management, resumption of activities, incision care, and potential complications in developing your teaching plan. Consider the client's education and developmental stage as well.

4. Review the effects of anxiety on recovery and learning. Identify nursing measures to reduce situational anxiety.

### A Client with Ulcerative Colitis

1. Review normal functions of the small and large intestine. Review the usual location of an ileostomy. Review fluid volume deficit in Chapter 5 ⬤ for manifestations and assessment data.

2. Think about the effect of chronic blood loss and review the effect of malnutrition on the hemoglobin and hematocrit.

3. Review the home care section of inflammatory bowel disease for teaching points to include.

4. Review nursing care for the client with diarrhea, as well as the procedure for ileostomy care.

### A Client with Colorectal Cancer

1. Review peripheral innervation and impulse transmission in your anatomy and physiology textbook; think about how nerves in the rectal region are disrupted in an abdominoperineal resection. Also review the phantom pain phenomenon in Chapter 4. ⬤

2. Compare elimination through a colostomy with "normal" bowel elimination through the anus. How do they differ in terms of the passage of flatus?

3. Review Procedure 24–1 ⬤ and the nursing care box on page 672. ⬤ Also review the procedure for administering an enema in your fundamentals or skills textbook.

4. Review this nursing diagnosis in your nursing diagnosis or nursing care planning handbook; be sure to individualize your plan to Mr. Cunningham's situation and needs.

### A Client with Diverticulitis

1. Review Mrs. Ukoha's presenting symptoms and laboratory data. Then review the collaborative care section related to diverticulitis.

2. Consider how long Mrs. Ukoha may have been on bowel rest (NPO) prior to having a bowel movement, and the manifestations of diverticular disease.

3. Review the risk factors for and pathophysiology of diverticular disease and diverticulitis.

4. Consult your nutrition textbook and see Table 24–13 ⊜ to develop your teaching plan.

## Chapter 26: Nursing Care of Clients with Urinary Tract Disorders

### A Client with Cystitis

1. Consider risk factors for UTI as well as factors affecting Mrs. Waisanen's immune function.

2. Consider the indications for short-course antibiotic therapy and the indications for conventional therapy. Think about factors such as cost, compliance, and the risk for adverse effects, as well as how antibiotics work to eradicate bacteria.

3. Identify why *Ineffective health maintenance* may be an appropriate nursing diagnosis for Mrs. Waisanen and the individual factors contributing to this diagnosis as you plan care.

### A Client with Urinary Calculi

1. Review the risk factors for urinary lithiasis.

2/3. Using the medications section of collaborative care for the client with urinary calculi in Chapter 26 ⊜ as well as Chapter 4, ⊜ and your pharmacology textbook or drug handbook, review analgesia for the client with renal colic and the intended and adverse effects of the drugs given to Mr. Leton.

### A Client with a Bladder Tumor

1. Review the physiology of the bladder and the risk factors for urinary tract tumors.

2. Review Mr. Hussain's health history for possible contributing factors.

3. See Chapter 12 ⊜ for nursing care of clients with problems of substance abuse.

4. Use your nursing care planning and nursing diagnoses textbooks to identify possible outcomes and interventions for *Sexual dysfunction*.

### A Client with Urinary Incontinence

1. Review the desired and adverse effects of the prescribed medications.

2. Review the effects of menopause and estrogen deficiency on perineal tissues.

3. Review Mrs. Giovanni's physical examination findings and risk factors for UTI.

4. Identify factors that may contribute to *Situational low self-esteem* in Mrs. Giovanni and nursing measures to address this diagnosis.

## Chapter 27: Nursing Care of Clients with Kidney Disorders

### A Client with Acute Glomerulonephritis

1. Review Chapter 8 ⊜ and the use of antibiotics to treat infection.

2. Review Mr. Chang's history and the risk factors for acute glomerulonephritis.

3. Review the diagnostic tests used to differentiate different forms of glomerulonephritis on page 750. ⊜

### A Client with Acute Renal Failure

1. Review common causes and the pathophysiology of acute renal failure.

2. Review the sections on peptic ulcer disease and stress gastritis in Chapter 21. ⊜

3. Consider the position requirements to maintain body and bone alignment in skeletal traction (Chapter 38). ⊜

### A Client with End-Stage Renal Disease

1. Review the usual onset, pathophysiology, and long-term effects of type 1 and type 2 diabetes (Chapter 18). ⊜

2. Consider the effects of urea and ammonia (both neurologic toxins) on brain function.

3. Review the manifestations of uremia.

4. Consider the composition of the dialysate and its possible effect on blood glucose control.

## Chapter 29: Nursing Care of Clients with Coronary Heart Disease

### A Client with Coronary Artery Bypass Surgery

1. Identify Mr. Clements's modifiable risk factors as you develop your plan. What barriers might need to be overcome to implement strategies to reduce his risk factors?

2. What strategies can you use to overcome denial without creating hostility or impairing the client-nurse relationship?

3. Consider traditional family roles as well as those roles that are unique to these individuals. Identify measures you can use to enlist the spouse's support.

4. Think about therapeutic communications as you formulate your response. Will your age or gender potentially affect your ability to respond effectively to these concerns? Would referral to another health care provider be appropriate?

### A Client with Acute Myocardial Infarction

1. Review immediate treatment measures for MI. Are other means available for reestablishing coronary artery perfusion? If you are in a rural area without immediate access to a cardiac catheterization lab, how will this affect your response?

2. Review the section of this chapter on dysrhythmias and their treatment. Research protocols for treating frequent PVCs in the post-MI client at your clinical facility.

3. Review the goals of cardiac rehabilitation and Mrs. Williams's individual risk factors as you develop your teaching plan.

4. Consider the value of using a therapeutic response to Mrs. Williams's statement concerning smoking. Also consider the risks associated with cigarette smoke. How can you respond without supporting Mrs. Williams's desire to smoke and without precipitating anger or resistance? Review Chapter 12. ⊜

### A Client with Supraventricular Tachycardia

1. Review the effects of sympathetic and parasympathetic nervous system stimulation on cardiac function.

2. Review the section on supraventricular tachycardias, as well as the antidysrhythmic medications for other treatment options.

3. Use your pharmacology textbook as you develop your teaching plan.

## Chapter 30: Nursing Care of Clients with Cardiac Disorders

### A Client with Heart Failure

1. Review the prescribed medications and their interactions. Do not forget to consider Mr. Jackson's age in assessing his risk for toxicity and interactions.

2. Review therapeutic communications skills and the use of open-ended statements to evaluate the underlying message of Mr. Jackson's statement.

3. Review exercise recommendations for the client with heart failure (page 885) ⌸ as well as cardiac rehabilitation principles (Chapter 29). ⌸

4. Review the rationale for aspirin therapy in the client with CHD and its effects on platelets and clotting as you formulate your response.

5. Review Chapter 41 ⌸ for causes of CVA and the section of Chapter 29 ⌸ on atrial fibrillation.

### A Client with Mitral Valve Prolapse

1. Review the pathophysiology and manifestations of MVP, as well as the general treatment measures for valve disorders.

2. Think about the effects of progressive conditioning on cardiac function.

3. Consider the anxiety associated with heart conditions and with a potentially progressive disorder that could affect childbearing and other life activities, as well as ultimately necessitate surgery.

4. Review the manifestations of MVP and of mitral regurgitation.

## Chapter 32: Nursing Care of Clients with Hematologic Disorders

### A Client with Anemia

1. Consider the effects of Mrs. Matthews's rapid weight loss on fluid balance, as well as the effects of tissue hypoxia on cardiac output.

2. Refer to Box 32–6 ⌸ and your nutrition text. Be sure to consider Mrs. Matthews's age in designing your menu.

3. Consider factors such as Mrs. Matthews's recent dietary history, the folic acid content of foods, and

other pertinent factors in the history and physical assessment

4. In addition to general factors to consider for the older adult (don't forget transportation among other factors), also consider the possible effect of Mrs. Matthews's recent loss and the grieving process.

### A Client with Hemophilia

1. Review the pathophysiology of hemophilia and its effect on the clotting process.

2. Consider both the ABCs and Maslow's hierarchy of needs as you respond to this question.

3. Think about the genetic transmission of hemophilia. How might Mr. Cruise's hemophila affect any children that he has? Grandchildren?

4. Review your nursing fundamentals book, nursing skills book, and intravenous therapy text to develop your teaching plan. Also consider previous learning and developmental levels.

5. Consult your nursing care planning text. Consider why this might be an appropriate nursing diagnosis for Mr. Cruise.

### A Client with Leukemia

1. Review the physiology of white blood cells, and the immune and inflammatory responses.

2. Think about the risks created by hospitalization in terms of exposure to infection and invasive procedures.

3. Think about the effect of inability to perform self care on self-esteem, self-confidence, and perception of power and control.

4. Use information provided in the nursing care and home care sections of this chapter as well as in Chapter 8. ⌸

5. Use your nursing care planning and fundamentals texts to develop your care plan.

### A Client with Hodgkin's disease

1. Review Chapter 10 ⌸ and the effects of chemotherapy and radiation on cancerous cells. Think about the advantages of combining these two therapies in terms of short and long-term desired and adverse effects.

2. Consider the primary and potential risks for infection in community settings as you design your teaching plan. What teaching strategies will you use for a young adult with Mr. Quito's education and experience?

3. Review theories of development and the developmental tasks for the young adult.

4. Use your nursing fundamentals and nursing care planning texts for reference in developing your care plan.

## Chapter 33: Nursing Care of Clients with Peripheral Vascular and Lymphatic Disorders

### A Client with Hypertension

1. Review Mrs. Spezia's assessment data and the risk factors for primary hypertension.

2. Review the pathophysiology of primary hypertension and of obesity (Chapter 20), ⌸ as well as the relationship between hypertension and coronary heart disease.

3. Think about resources that are available in your community for homeless people. Talk to community health and social service agencies to identify additional resources.

4. Again, review Mrs. Spezia's assessment data, the pathophysiology of hypertension, and the long-term effects of stress.

5. Use your nursing care planning and nursing diagnosis textbooks to help develop your care plan.

### A Client with Peripheral Atherosclerosis

1. Review treatments for peripheral atherosclerosis, as well as lifestyle measures for preventing and treating atherosclerosis and coronary heart disease (Chapter 29). ⌸

2. Compare the pathophysiology of peripheral atherosclerosis, intermittent claudication, and coronary heart disease (Chapter 29 ⌸) to identify similarities and differences.

3. Review the actions of beta blockers and their role in angina prophylaxis.

4. Use your nursing care planning and nutrition textbooks to help develop your care plan.

**A Client with Deep Vein Thrombosis**

1. Review the pathophysiologic processes of venous thrombosis and inflammation as you develop your answer.

2. Think about questions you could ask for further information as well as potential resources for Mrs. Hipps.

3. Consider assessment data to evaluate Mrs. Hipps's limitations and resources, as well as community resources to help meet her needs.

4. Use your nursing diagnosis and care planning textbooks to develop your plan of care.

## Chapter 35: Nursing Care of Clients with Upper Respiratory Disorders

**A Client with Peritonsillar Abscess**

1/2. Review the manifestations of upper respiratory infections and management of these disorders.

3. Think about the primary uses of the nose, mouth, and pharynx as you consider nursing diagnoses related to upper respiratory disorders.

**A Client with Nasal Fracture**

1. Consider other measures to restore the client's sense of control over the situation. Consider the potentially traumatic effects of suction on the mucous membranes as well as possible infection control risks.

2. Review the implications and potential dangers of CSF leakage to help you develop your care plan.

3. Think about the benefits and drawbacks of immediate and delayed rhinoplasty.

**A Client with Total Laryngectomy**

1. Review the options for speech rehabilitation. If available, practice using a speech generator. Practice esophageal speech.

2. Use your nursing care planning and nursing diagnoses handbook to develop your care plan. Consider Mr. Tom's age, occupation, and marital status in your plan of care.

3. Review Chapter 7 ⊜ for surgical nursing care interventions, as well as your nursing fundamentals textbook for wound care strategies.

4. Consider measures to promote airway clearance and ventilation of all lung fields.

## Chapter 36: Nursing Care of Clients with Lower Respiratory Disorders

**A Client with Pneumonia**

1. Review Mrs. O'Neal's assessment data and compare her history with identified risk factors for pneumonia.

2. Review normal immune and inflammatory responses and the role of white blood cells in these processes.

3. Review Chapter 9 ⊜ and altered immune responses for the physiology and effects of anaphylactic shock.

4. Use your nursing care planning and nursing diagnosis textbooks to help develop your care plan.

**A Client with Tuberculosis**

1. Consider available resources for mentally ill clients, as well as community and public health resources. Consider measures to ensure compliance with the prescribed treatment.

2. Contact your local public health department, the discharge planner for your unit, or the social services department in your clinical facility to help identify available resources.

3. Use your nursing fundamentals text, the nursing care section under Pneumonia, and your nursing diagnosis or care planning handbook as you develop your care plan.

**A Client with COPD**

1. Review the processes by which cigarette smoke inflicts damage on lung tissue. Use your pediatric and pathophysiology texts for additional information.

2. Review the physiology of the respiratory drive, as well as the effects of chronic elevated carbon dioxide levels in the blood.

3. Review the manifestations of COPD and its complications as well as the section of this chapter on respiratory failure.

4. Use your nursing diagnosis handbook to help identify appropriate goals and interventions for this nursing diagnosis.

**A Client with Lung Cancer**

1. Review Chapter 10 ⊜ and use your pharmacology text to research the effects of these drugs and the rationale for combination chemotherapy.

2. Use Chapter 10 ⊜ and your pharmacology text to identify probable side effects of this treatment regimen. Then use your nursing care planning book to identify appropriate nursing diagnoses and interventions.

3. Review the pathophysiology and collaborative care sections for lung cancer to develop your response to this question.

**A Client with ARDS**

1. As you respond to this question, consider additional treatment measures for ARDS and respiratory failure. Also consider the potential long-term consequences and complications of intubation and mechanical ventilation. Discuss strategies for communicating with Ms. Adamson's family and supporting coping and decision-making by Ms. Adamson and her family in an instance such as this.

2. Think about the precipitating factors for ARDS and the factors that may precipitate respiratory failure in a client with COPD. Consider the probable overall respiratory and general health status of the individual affected by each of these conditions.

3. Review the precipitating factors for ARDS and discuss strategies to prevent them.

4. Use your nursing care planning book to identify appropriate goals and nursing interventions for this nursing diagnosis.

## Chapter 38: Nursing Care of Clients with Musculoskeletal Trauma

**A Client with a Hip Fracture**

1. Consider Mrs. Carbolito's age and the fact that she is postmenopausal. What effect does estrogen have on bone health? What might have increased her risk for falls?

2. Review the principles of traction application. What purpose does it

serve prior to surgery? What words could you use that she would understand? Think about the effects of trauma, pain, and suddenly finding oneself in a strange environment on listening and understanding verbal communications.

3. List how each of these manifestations would affect skin integrity, food intake, and bone healing.

### A Client with a Below-the-Knee Amputation

1. Design a sequential plan for Mr. Rocke's self-care of the stump. Consider his readiness to learn and the complexity of the care. Is there a risk in letting him assume total responsibility from the beginning? Why or why not?

2. List the factors used to describe Mr. Rocke. How do these affect his ability or willingness to follow up with medical care? What community agencies are available where you live or go to school that would be good sources of assistance and support for Mr. Rocke?

3. Review the information about exercise. How would Mr. Rocke's choice not to do exercises affect his ability to use a prosthesis to walk?

### Chapter 39: Nursing Care of Clients with Musculoskeletal Disorders

### A Client with Osteoporosis

1. Review the effects of nicotine and caffeine on blood circulation to bones. What effect does alcohol play in bone loss?

2. Review foods that increase blood cholesterol levels. What is considered a normal cholesterol level? You may need to read content in Chapter 29. ᏀᎠ Knowing the client needs calcium, what type of dairy products would you recommend?

3. List activities for the client who is not able to be ambulatory. How many of the activities on your list would help prevent osteoporosis?

4. *Risk for trauma* is defined as an increased risk for accidental tissue injury, such as a fracture. What

interventions would you teach Mrs. Bauer to reduce this risk?

### A Client with Osteoarthritis

1. Review information about serum creatinine and BUN in a laboratory studies textbook or on the web. What medications is Mr. Cerulli taking that may be affecting these findings? Consider what teaching is necessary related to these findings.

2. What assessments are significant for confusion? If necessary, review content related to confusion. Review Mr. Cerulli's history in the case study and determine factors that may have contributed to his risk for confusion before, during, and after surgery.

3. *Acute confusion* is defined as an abrupt onset of a cluster of global, transient changes and disturbances in attention, cognition, psychomotor activity, level of consciousness, and/or sleep/wake cycle. What assessments could you make to support this diagnosis for Mr. Cerulli? What interventions might you design for this diagnosis?

### A Client with Rheumatoid Arthritis

1. Think about the role differences in a 42-year-old woman and a 72-year-old woman. On the other hand, consider the effects of a chronic illness that may have been present for 30 years. Would your plan differ? Why or why not?

2. List the possible disabilities that may be caused by rheumatoid arthritis. How do you believe these would affect Mrs. James? What agencies in your community are available for support of people with this type of illness? Where would you go for literature to give Mrs. James?

3. *Ineffective role performance* is defined as behaviors and expressions that do not match norms or expectations. Do you believe this is an appropriate nursing diagnosis for Mrs. James? Why or why not? What interventions could be implemented for this diagnosis?

### Chapter 41: Nursing Care of Clients with Cerebrovascular and Spinal Cord Disorders

### A Client with a Stroke

1. What subjective manifestations does the client with hypertension have? (Review content in Chapter 33.) ᏀᎠ

2. How does increased blood pressure affect the walls of blood vessels in the cerebral circulation?

3. Consider referral to community resources as a volunteer tutor for adult literacy, gardening, and/or woodworking. Tutoring college students is another option.

4. Use statements that will encourage Mr. Boren to talk about his arm and how he feels about being unable to use it.

### A Client with a SCI

1. What are the developmental tasks of a 19-year-old? How does the inability to meet these tasks affect emotional responses?

2. Think about questions that explore Mr. Valdez's fears in relation to sexuality. Practice questions and statements with friends until you are not embarrassed to ask them.

3. Consider how your own values and beliefs may differ from those of a client.

4. What baseline assessments and information are necessary before developing a plan for urinary elimination needs? Why would self-catheterization be an option? What are the risks of long-term Foley catheterization?

### A Client with an Intervertebral Disk

1. What emergency management of any possible spinal cord injury is necessary, and why?

2. Consider social and economic needs. What types of community and health care resources are available for a young single mother?

3. What type of clothing would be most useful for Mrs. Ivans? In what sequence should she dress? What about shoes?

## Chapter 42: Nursing Care of Clients with Intracranial Disorders

### A Client with a Migraine Headache

1. Review the content in the chapter on migraine headaches. List questions that you would ask specific to onset, length, manifestations, stages, pain, diet, and factors associated with the headache onset.

2. Consider foods that are high in sodium. What would you suggest if Ms. Friedman eats fast foods at least five times a week? Review the food pyramid in Chapter 2 ⬤ and outline a weekly meal plan for Ms. Friedman.

3. Discuss with members of your class those factors that interfere with their normal sleep patterns. What suggestions might you give Ms. Friedman to help her improve her sleep? Why is this important?

### A Client with a Seizure Disorder

1. List the teaching topics you would include for Ms. Carlson. Consider how her needs (e.g., for safety) would differ if she lived alone.

2. Describe statements you could use to help Ms. Carlson understand not only the dangers but also the legal issues involved. What if Ms. Carlson does not recognize these concerns?

3. What type of questions could you ask Ms. Carlson to determine why she feels this way? Would you personally find it embarrassing? How can you facilitate Ms. Carlson's understanding for this recommendation?

### A Client with Subdural Hematoma

1. Review the manifestations of the types of intracranial hematomas. What assessments are specific to a subdural hematoma? Why is it important to know this?

2. What are some other interventions that might be used? How could family help? What if no family members are available?

3. Acute confusion is a sudden onset of changes in attention, cognition, psychomotor activity, level of consciousness, and/or sleep/wake cycle. What would you determine as priority nursing diagnoses and interventions for Mr. Lee?

### A Client with Bacterial Meningitis

1. List the environmental stimuli in the hospital setting. How could these be decreased? What effect do these stimuli have on cognition and behavior that is altered by an intracranial infection?

2. Think about how you would feel if Mr. Cook tried to hit you. How would you respond to him? To whom would you report this?

3. Why would Mr. Cook have pain? How would pain be manifested during the initial treatment period for Mr. Cook? Is it important to consider the respiratory effects of narcotics for him? Defend your answer.

### A Client with a Brain Tumor

1. Review content in the chapter on increased intracranial pressure and intracranial surgery. List collaborative and nursing interventions to decrease increased intracranial pressure.

2. What do these manifestations indicate? What would be your priority assessment? Who would you notify?

3. Practice the use of therapeutic communications and what response you would make.

4. Consider the reasons Ms. Lange feels powerless. What nursing interventions might decrease this feeling?

## Chapter 43: Nursing Care of Clients with Neurologic Disorders

### A Client with AD

1. Think about what information you would need and how you would collect it. Consider such factors as the age of family members, educational level of family members, and stage of the client's AD. What else would you need to know?

2. Review the suggested activities in this section of the chapter. What others can you think of or have you seen used successfully? Osteoarthritis often results in joint stiffness and pain as well as problems with mobility. Would this affect your interventions? If so, how could they be adapted?

3. Consider the type of foods that might be prepared, the timing of meals, and interventions that might be used to decrease agitation before or during meals.

### A Client with MS

1. Outline a typical day's activities for Mr. McMurphy that would provide a balance between activity and rest. What assessments would you make to evaluate the effectiveness of this plan?

2. Consider how respiratory infections are spread. Why is Mr. McMurphy at increased risk?

3. The definition of *Risk for injury* is that one is at risk as a result of environmental conditions interacting with the person's adaptive and defensive resources. What factors in this client's history and physical status would support this diagnosis? What interventions would you include in the care plan and why?

### A Client with Parkinson's Disease

1. Consider the adaptations that might be made to clothing and shoes. What adaptive devices might be useful?

2. What information would you need to know before you develop your interventions? Include that from Mr. Avneil and what might be available in the community and the long-term care facility.

3. *Chronic sorrow* is a recurring pattern of sadness in response to continual loss. Consider the type of communications you would need to use with Mr. Avneil to identify his degree of sorrow. What other assessment might provide cues to support this diagnosis (think about eating and sleeping)? How might an activity such as reminiscence help?

### A Client with Myasthenia Gravis

1. Review the pathophysiology of myasthenia gravis. What is the action of Tensilon?

2. Consider teaching topics for Mrs. Avis that would assist her in conserving energy while preparing meals. List suggestions to conserve energy while eating.

3. *Ineffective role performance* is the state in which behaviors and self-expression do not match such factors as norms and expectations. What changes occur as a result of this illness? What do you think Mrs. Avis expects of herself? What are some interventions you could implement to facilitate acceptance of the change she is experiencing?

### Chapter 45: Nursing Care of Clients with Eye and Ear Disorders

#### A Client with Glaucoma and Cataracts

1. What is the pathophysiology of glaucoma? How does a cataract affect glaucoma?

2. Consider the effects of corticosteroids on glaucoma. If Mrs. Rainey is to administer several medications at home, identify specific teaching guidelines for her.

3. Consider referral for home health visits. Think about the effect of transferring her for a brief admission to an assisted-living facility.

### Chapter 47: Nursing Care of Men with Reproductive System Disorders

#### A Man with Prostate Cancer

1. Why would Mr. Turner be at risk for altered skin integrity? Outline the interventions you would include on his teaching plan that would promote skin integrity as he cares for himself at home.

2. *Noncompliance* is defined as behaviors that do not coincide with the therapeutic plan agreed upon by the person and the health care professional. Do you think Mr. Turner fully understood his treatment and agreed with his follow-up care? What could be done in the preoperative phase of Mr. Turner's care to better ensure his understanding and desire to have continued medical care?

3. What assessments indicate that Mr. Turner does or does not have bladder distention? Would you report this? If so, to whom?

### Chapter 48: Nursing Care of Women with Reproductive System Disorders

#### A Woman with Endometriosis

1. What is the relationship between Mrs. Hall's manifestations and a decreased RBC count? Review the information in Chapter 32 ⊂⊃ and list assessments you would make to identify anemia.

2. List nonthreatening questions you would use to begin the discussion. How might it help to ask these questions at the beginning of the interview? Then list questions that you might use to collect data about the couple's sexual history. Would you be embarrassed to ask them? If so, how might this in turn affect their responses?

3. *Situational low self-esteem* is the state in which a person develops a negative perception of self-worth in response to a current situation. What information in Mrs. Hall's history might provide data to support this nursing diagnosis?

#### A Woman with Cervical Cancer

1. Review the risk factors for cervical cancer. Consider what might differ for a young woman and an older woman.

2. Review the information in Chapter 10 ⊂⊃ on radiation as a treatment for cancer. What interventions would be appropriate for Ms. Gillam?

3. Based on your review of the information on radiation, explain how radiation might cause fatigue. How does fatigue differ from being tired? What interventions would you include in a plan of care for this nursing diagnosis?

#### A Woman with Breast Cancer

1. Review the information in the chapter on the genetic factors that pose a risk for developing breast cancer. How could you explain this in terms understandable by Mrs. Clemments and her daughters?

2. List the different types of mastectomies. Consider the implications of the differences, and how this would affect your nursing care.

3. Review the information on chemotherapy in Chapter 10. ⊂⊃ List the types of chemotherapy and its common side effects. Consider the classifications of medications that are used to treat these side effects.

4. What factors in the treatment of Mrs. Clemments treatment might disrupt the amount and quality of her sleep? What interventions might be used to improve her sleep pattern?

### Chapter 49: Nursing Care of Clients with Sexually Transmitted Infections

#### A Client with Gonorrhea

1. What manifestations does Ms. Cirit have that are typical of the disease? Would you make other assessments? If so, what are they?

2. Review the discussion of HIV in Chapter 9. ⊂⊃ Do you believe it is true that infection with gonorrhea may increase the risk of HIV? If so, how would you explain this to Ms. Cirit?

3. *Impaired social interaction* is a state of aloneness or rejection experienced by an individual that is perceived as negative. What assessments of Ms. Cirit might support this diagnosis? What interventions and expected outcomes would you develop?

#### A Client with Syphilis

1. Describe the assessments you would expect to find in a man with early syphilis.

2. Consider topics such as number of sex partners, patterns of sexual activity, and use of safe sex practices. What other topics should be explored? How can you ask these questions without being embarrassed or embarrassing the client?

3. List possible statements you might make. Do you believe this is a nursing responsibility? If you do not feel comfortable with this topic, what could you do?

# CREDITS

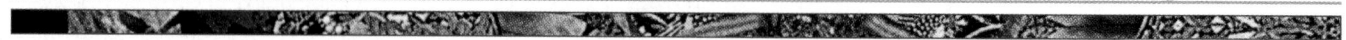

All photographs/illustrations not credited on page, under or adjacent to the piece, or not credited below, were photographed/rendered on assignment and are property of Pearson Education/Prentice Hall Health.

**Illustrations:**

| | |
|---|---|
| Figure 28–3 | Todd A. Buck |
| Figure 28–7 | Todd A. Buck |
| Figure 34–1 | Todd A. Buck |
| Figure 19–1 | Todd A. Buck |
| Figure 12–2 | Todd A. Buck |
| Figure 44–1 | Todd A. Buck |
| Figure 37–1 | Todd A. Buck |
| Figure 37–4 | Todd A. Buck |
| Figure 44–11 | Todd A. Buck |

# INDEX

## M

# SINGLE PC LICENSE AGREEMENT AND LIMITED WARRANTY

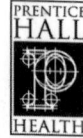
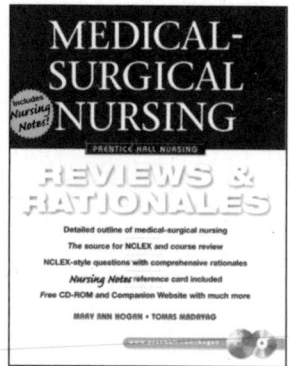
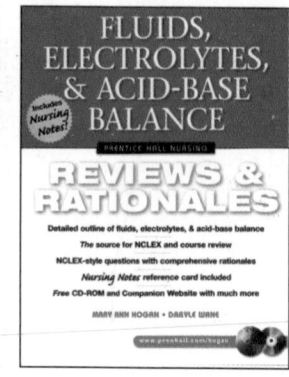
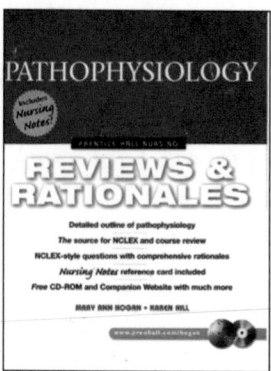
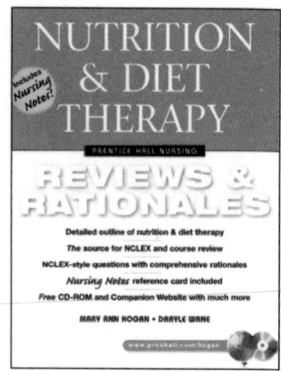
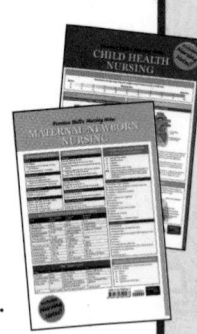